W9-DDK-570

MATERNAL-FETAL MEDICINE

MATERNAL-FETAL MEDICINE

Fifth Edition

EDITORS

ROBERT K. CREASY, MD

Professor Emeritus
Department of Obstetrics, Gynecology, and Reproductive Sciences
University of Texas Medical School at Houston
Houston, Texas
Corte Madera, California

ROBERT RESNIK, MD

Professor of Reproductive Medicine
University of California, San Diego,
School of Medicine
La Jolla, California

ASSOCIATE EDITOR

JAY D. IAMS, MD

Professor and Frederick P. Zuspan Endowed Chair in Obstetrics and Gynecology
Division of Maternal-Fetal Medicine
The Ohio State University College of Medicine and Public Health
Columbus, Ohio

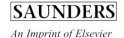

SAUNDERS

An Imprint of Elsevier

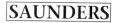

An Imprint of Elsevier

The Curtis Center
Independence Square West
Philadelphia, Pennsylvania 19106-3399

MATERNAL-FETAL MEDICINE   ISBN 0-7216-0004-2
FIFTH EDITION
Copyright © 2004, 1999, 1994, 1989, 1984, Elsevier Inc. (USA). All rights reserved.

NOTICE

Medicine in an ever-changing field. Standard safety precautions must be followed, but as new research and clinical experience broaden our knowledge, changes in treatment and drug therapy may become necessary or appropriate. Readers are advised to check the most current product information provided by the manufacturer of each drug to be administered to verify the recommended dose, the method and duration of administration, and contraindications. It is the responsibility of the treating physician, relying on experience and knowledge of the patient, to determine dosages and the best treatment for each individual patient. Neither the Publisher nor the editors assume any liability for any injury and/or damage to persons or property arising from this publication.

The Publisher

Library of Congress Cataloging-in-Publication Data

Maternal-fetal medicine / [edited by] Robert K. Creasy, Robert Resnik, Jay D. Iams.—5th ed.
    p. ; cm.
  Includes bibliographical references and index.
  ISBN 0-7216-0004-2
   1. Obstetrics. 2. Perinatology. I. Creasy, Robert K. II. Resnik, Robert. III. Iams, Jay D.
  [DNLM: 1. Fetal Diseases. 2. Pregnancy Complications. 3. Prenatal Diagnosis. WQ 211
M425 2004]
RG526.M34 2004
618.2—dc21

                              2003041522

Acquisitions Editor: Stephanie Smith Donley
Developmental Editor: Melissa Dudlick

Printed in the United States of America

Last digit is the print number: 9 8 7 6 5 4 3 2

For
Judy, Lauren, and Pat
with love and gratitude—for everything

CONTRIBUTORS

Barbara Abrams, DrPH
Professor, School of Public Health, University of California, Berkeley, California.
Maternal Nutrition

Emad Abu-Hamda, MD
Gastroenterology Fellow, University of Texas Health Science Center, Houston, Texas.
Gastrointestinal Disease in Pregnancy

Michael J. Aminoff, MD, DSc, FRCP
Professor of Neurology, University of California, San Francisco, School of Medicine; Attending Physician, University of California, San Francisco, Medical Center, San Francisco, California.
Neurologic Disorders

Robert L. Andres, MD
Associate Professor, Department of Obstetrics and Gynecology, University of Utah School of Medicine, Salt Lake City, Utah; Attending Physician and Medical Director, Labor and Delivery, McKay-Dee Hospital Center, Ogden, Utah.
Effects of Therapeutic, Diagnostic, and Environmental Agents and Exposure to Social and Illicit Drugs

Kurt Benirschke, MD
Professor Emeritus, University of California, San Diego, La Jolla, California.
Normal Early Development; Multiple Gestation: The Biology of Twinning

Michael L. Berman, MD
Professor of Obstetrics and Gynecology, University of California, Irvine, Medical Center; Director, Fellowship Training Program in Gynecologic Oncology, Chac Family Comprehensive Care Center, University of California, Irvine, Medical Center, Orange, California.
Pelvic Malignancies, Gestational Trophoblastic Neoplasia, and Nonpelvic Malignancies

Daniel G. Blanchard, MD, FACC
Professor of Clinical Medicine, Division of Cardiology, Department of Internal Medicine, University of California, San Diego, School of Medicine; Director, Cardiac Noninvasive Laboratories, University of California, San Diego, Medical Center, San Diego, California.
Cardiac Diseases

Watson A. Bowes Jr., MD
Professor of Obstetrics and Gynecology, Emeritus, University of North Carolina, Chapel Hill, North Carolina.
Clinical Aspects of Normal and Abnormal Labor

Robert A. Brace, PhD
Professor Emeritus, Department of Reproductive Medicine, University of California, San Diego, La Jolla, California.
Amniotic Fluid Dynamics

D. Ware Branch, MD
Professor, University of Utah School of Medicine, Department of Obstetrics-Gynecology, Salt Lake City, Utah.
The Immunology of Pregnancy

John R. G. Challis, DSc, FRSC
Vice President, Research, and Associate Provost, University of Toronto; Professor, Departments of Physiology, Obstetrics and Gynecology, and Medicine, University of Toronto, Toronto, Ontario, Canada.
Characteristics of Parturition

Steven L. Clark, MD
Professor of Obstetrics and Gynecology, University of Utah School of Medicine; LDS Hospital, Salt Lake City, Utah.
Placenta Previa and Abruptio Placentae

Ronald Clyman, MD
Professor of Pediatrics, Senior Staff, Cardiovascular Research Institute, University of California at San Francisco, San Francisco, California.
Fetal Cardiovascular Physiology

Joshua A. Copel, MD
Professor, Obstetrics/Gynecology and Pediatrics, and Director, Maternal-Fetal Medicine, Yale University School of Medicine, New Haven, Connecticut.
Fetal Cardiac Arrhythmias: Diagnosis and Therapy

Robert K. Creasy, MD
Professor Emeritus, Department of Obstetrics, Gynecology, and Reproductive Sciences, University of Texas Medical School at Houston, Houston, Texas; Corte Madera, California.
Preterm Labor and Delivery; Intrauterine Growth Restriction

Mary E. D'Alton, MD
Professor and Chair, Obstetrics and Gynecology, Columbia University College of Physicians and Surgeons; Chair, Department of Obstetrics and Gynecology, Columbia Presbyterian Medical Center, New York, New York.
Multiple Gestation: Clinical Characteristics and Management

John M. Davison, MD
Professor of Obstetric Medicine, Department of Obstetrics and Gynaecology, University of Newcastle upon Tyne Medical School; Consultant Obstetrician and Gynaecologist, Directorate of Women's Services, Royal Victoria Infirmary, Newcastle upon Tyne, United Kingdom.
Renal Disorders

Philip J. Di Saia, MD
Professor and Director, Division of Gynecologic Oncology, The Dorothy Marsh Chair in Reproductive Biology, University of California, Irvine, Medical Center, Orange, California.
Pelvic Malignancies, Gestational Trophoblastic Neoplasia, and Nonpelvic Malignancies

Mitchell P. Dombrowski, MD
Professor with Tenure, Wayne State University; Chief, Department of Obstetrics and Gynecology, St. John Hospital, Detroit, Michigan.
Respiratory Diseases in Pregnancy

W. Patrick Duff, MD
Professor, Department of Obstetrics and Gynecology, University of Florida College of Medicine, Gainesville, Florida.
Maternal and Fetal Infectious Disorders

Jeffrey R. Fineman, MD
Professor of Pediatrics, University of California at San Francisco, San Francisco, California.
Fetal Cardiovascular Physiology

Avroy A. Fanaroff, MB, BCh(RAND), FRCP(E), FRCPCN
Professor of Pediatrics and Reproductive Biology, Case Western Reserve University School of Medicine; Eliza Henry Barnes Professor in Neonatology, Rainbow Babies and Children's Hospital, Cleveland, Ohio.
Identification and Management of Problems in the High-Risk Neonate

Alan W. Flake, MD
Professor of Surgery and Obstetrics and Gynecology, University of Pennsylvania, Children's Hospital of Philadelphia; Director, Children's Institute for Surgical Science, University of Pennsylvania, Children's Hospital of Philadelphia, Philadelphia, Pennsylvania.
Fetal Therapy: Medical and Surgical Approaches

Michael Raymond Foley, MD
Clinical Professor, Department of Obstetrics and Gynecology, University of Arizona Medical School at the Arizona Health Sciences Center, Tucson, Arizona; Director, Obstetric Intensive Care Unit, Good Samaritan Regional Medical, Phoenix, Arizona; Medical Director, Phoenix Perinatal Associates, Phoenix, Arizona.
Intensive Care Monitoring of the Critically Ill Pregnant Patient

Robert Gagnon, MD, FRCS(C)
Professor, Departments of Obstetrics and Gynecology and Physiology, University of Western Ontario Faculty of Medicine; Active Teaching Staff, St. Joseph's Health Centre of London, London, Ontario, Canada.
Fetal Breathing and Body Movements

Thomas J. Garite, MD
The E. J. Quilligan Professor and Chair, Obstetrics and Gynecology, University of California at Irvine, Orange, California.
Premature Rupture of the Membranes

Ronald S. Gibbs, MD
Professor and Chair, E. Stewart Taylor Chair in Obstetrics and Gynecology, Department of Obstetrics and Gynecology, University of Colorado Health Sciences Center, Denver, Colorado.
Maternal and Fetal Infectious Disorders

Larry C. Gilstrap III, MD
Emma Sue Hightower Professor and Chairman, Department of Obstetrics, Gynecology, and Reproductive Sciences, University of Texas Medical School at Houston, Houston, Texas.
Fetal Acid-Base Balance

J. Christopher Glantz, MD, MPH
Associate Professor of Obstetrics and Gynecology, Division of Maternal-Fetal Medicine, University of Rochester School of Medicine and Dentistry, Rochester, New York.
Significance of Amniotic Fluid Meconium

Robert L. Goldenberg, MD
Charles E. Flowers Professor of Obstetrics and Gynecology, University of Alabama, Birmingham, Alabama.
Cerebral Palsy

Bernard Gonik, MD
Professor and Fann Srere Chair of Perinatal Medicine, Department of Obstetrics and Gynecology, Wayne State University School of Medicine, Detroit, Michigan.
Intensive Care Monitoring of the Critically Ill Pregnant Patient

Bruce A. Hamilton, PhD
Departments of Medicine and Cellular and Molecular Medicine, University of California, San Diego, School of Medicine, La Jolla, California.
Basic Genetics and Patterns of Inheritance

Gary D. V. Hankins, MD
Professor and Vice Chairman, Department of Obstetrics and Gynecology, and Chief, Division of Maternal-Fetal Medicine, The University of Texas Medical Branch, Galveston, Texas.
Rheumatologic and Connective Tissue Disorders

Christopher R. Harman, MD
Professor, Vice Chair, and Head, Division of Maternal and Fetal Medicine, Department of Obstetrics, Gynecology, and Reproductive Sciences, University of Maryland, Baltimore, School of Medicine; Director, Center for Advanced Fetal Care, University of Maryland Medical System, Baltimore, Maryland.
Assessment of Fetal Health

Michael A. Heymann, MD
Professor of Pediatrics, Emeritus, and Senior Investigator, Emeritus, Cardiovascular Research Institute, University of California at San Francisco, San Francisco, California.
Fetal Cardiovascular Physiology

Joseph A. Hill, MD
Associate Professor, Department of Obstetrics and Gynecology, Harvard Medical School, Boston, Massachusetts; Reproductive Endocrinologist, Fertility Center of New England, Reading, Massachusetts.
Recurrent Pregnancy Loss

Jay D. Iams, MD
Professor and Frederick P. Zuspan Endowed Chair in Obstetrics and Gynecology, Division of Maternal-Fetal Medicine, The Ohio State University College of Medicine and Public Health, Columbus, Ohio.
Abnormal Cervical Competence; Preterm Labor and Delivery

Thomas M. Jenkins, MD
Assistant Professor, University of Wisconsin Medical School, Madison, Wisconsin.
Prenatal Diagnosis of Congenital Disorders

Alan H. Jobe, MD, PhD
Professor of Pediatrics, University of Cincinnati School of Medicine; Professor of Pediatrics, Cincinnati Children's Hospital, Cincinnati, Ohio.
Fetal Lung Development

Sarah J. Kilpatrick, MD, PhD
Professor and Interim Head, Department of Obstetrics and Gynecology, University of Illinois, Chicago, Illinois.
Maternal Hematologic Disorders

Charles S. Kleinman, MD
Professor of Clinical Pediatrics in Obstetrics and Gynecology, Columbia University College of Physicians and Surgeons and Medical College of Cornell University, New York, New York; Professor of Pediatric Cardiac Imaging and Fetal Cardiology, New York–Presbyterian Hospital, New York, New York.
Fetal Cardiac Arrhythmias: Diagnosis and Therapy

Krzysztof M. Kuczkowski, MD
Assistant Clinical Professor of Anesthesiology and Reproductive Medicine and Codirector of Obstetric Anesthesia, Departments of Anesthesiology and Reproductive Medicine, University of California at San Diego, San Diego, California.
Anesthetic Considerations for Complicated Pregnancies

Mark B. Landon, MD
Professor and Vice Chairman, Department of Obstetrics and Gynecology, The Ohio State University College of Medicine and Public Health; Director of Maternal-Fetal Medicine and Clinical Chief of Obstetrics, The Ohio State University Hospitals, Columbus, Ohio.
Diseases of the Liver, Biliary System, and Pancreas

Russell K. Laros Jr., MD, MSc
Professor of Obstetrics and Gynecology, University of California at San Francisco, San Francisco, California.
Thromboembolic Disease; Maternal Hematologic Disorders

Robert M. Lawrence, MD
Clinical Associate Professor, Pediatric Immunology and Infectious Diseases, Department of Pediatric Immunology and Infectious Diseases, University of Florida, College of Medicine, Gainesville, Florida.
The Breast and the Physiology of Lactation

Ruth A. Lawrence, MD
Professor of Pediatrics, Obstetrics, and Gynecology, University of Rochester, School of Medicine and Dentistry, Rochester, New York.
The Breast and the Physiology of Lactation

Marshall D. Lindheimer, MD
Professor of Medicine, Obstetrics and Gynecology, and Clinical Pharmacology, Emeritus, University of Chicago, Division of Biological Sciences, Pritzker School of Medicine, Chicago, Illinois.
Renal Disorders

James H. Liu, MD
Professor and Chair, Department of Reproductive Biology, Case Western Reserve University; Professor and Chair, Department of Obstetrics and Gynecology, University Hospitals of Cleveland, Cleveland, Ohio.
　Endocrinology of Pregnancy

Charles J. Lockwood, MD
Professor and Chairman, Obstetrics and Gynecology, Yale University School of Medicine; Chief, Obstetrics and Gynecology, Yale–New Haven Hospital, New Haven, Connecticut.
　Thrombophilias in Pregnancy

Stephen J. Lye, PhD
Professor of Obstetrics and Gynaecology, Physiology, and Medicine, University of Toronto; Vice President, Research, Mount Sinai Hospital; Associate Director, Samuel Lunenfeld Research Institute of Mount Sinai Hospital, Toronto, Ontario, Canada.
　Characteristics of Parturition

George A. Macones, MD, MSCE
Associate Professor, Director of Maternal-Fetal Medicine, Director of Obstetrics, University of Pennsylvania, School of Medicine, Philadelphia, Pennsylvania.
　Evidence-Based Practice in Perinatal Medicine

Fergal D. Malone, MD
Associate Professor, Obstetrics and Gynecology, Columbia University College of Physicians and Surgeons; Director, Division of Maternal-Fetal Medicine, Columbia Presbyterian Medical Center, New York, New York.
　Multiple Gestation: Clinical Characteristics and Management

Frank A. Manning, MD, MSc(OXON), FRCS
Professor, New York University School of Medicine; Professor and Chair, Department of Obstetrics and Gynecology; New York University–Downtown Hospital, New York, New York.
　General Principles and Applications of Ultrasonography

Richard J. Martin, MBBS, FRACP
Professor of Pediatrics, Reproductive Biology, and Physiology and Biophysics, Case Western Reserve University School of Medicine; Director, Division of Neonatology, Rainbow Babies and Children's Hospital, Cleveland, Ohio.
　Identification and Management of Problems in the High-Risk Neonate

Brian M. Mercer, MD
Professor, Reproductive Biology, Case Western Reserve University; Vice Chair and Director of Maternal-Fetal Medicine, Department of Obstetrics and Gynecology, MetroHealth Medical Center, Cleveland, Ohio.
　Assessment and Induction of Fetal Pulmonary Maturity

Giacomo Meschia, MD
Professor of Physiology, Emeritus, University of Colorado, School of Medicine, Denver, Colorado.
　Placental Respiratory Gas Exchange and Fetal Oxygenation

Dzovag Minassian, MPH
Research Assistant, School of Public Health, University of California at Berkeley, Berkeley, California.
　Maternal Nutrition

Howard L. Minkoff, MD
Distinguished Professor of Obstetrics and Gynecology, State University of New York Health Science Center at Down State Medical Center; Chairman, Department of Obstetrics and Gynecology, Maimonides Medical Center, Brooklyn, New York.
　Human Immunodeficiency Virus

Kenneth J. Moise Jr., MD
UpJohn Distinguished Professor of Obstetrics and Gynecology and Director, Division of Maternal-Fetal Medicine, University of North Carolina at Chapel Hill, Chapel Hill, North Carolina.
　Hemolytic Disease of the Fetus and Newborn

Manju Monga, MD
Associate Professor and Program Director, Department of Obstetrics, Gynecology, and Reproductive Sciences, University of Texas, Houston, Medical School, Houston, Texas.
　Biology and Physiology of the Reproductive Tract and Control of Myometrial Contraction; Maternal Cardiovascular and Renal Adaptation to Pregnancy

Thomas R. Moore, MD
Professor and Chairman, Department of Reproductive Medicine, University of California, San Diego, School of Medicine; Director, Division of Perinatal Medicine, University of California, San Diego, Medical Center, San Diego, California.
　Diabetes in Pregnancy

Shahla Nader, MD
Professor, Department of Obstetrics and Gynecology and Department of Internal Medicine (Endocrinology), University of Texas Medical School at Houston; Teaching Staff, Hermann Hospital, Houston, Texas.
　Thyroid Disease and Pregnancy; Other Endocrine Disorders of Pregnancy

Michael P. Nageotte, MD
Professor, Department of Obstetrics and Gynecology, University of California at Irvine, Orange, California; Executive Careline Director, Obstetrics/Gynecology/Newborn, Long Beach Memorial Medical Center, Long Beach, California.
　Intrapartum Fetal Surveillance

Rodrigo Nehgme, MD
Cardiologist-Electrophysiologist, Nemours Cardiac Center, A. I. duPont Hospital for Children, Wilmington, Delaware.
Fetal Cardiac Arrhythmias: Diagnosis and Therapy

Julian T. Parer, MD, PhD
Professor, Department of Obstetrics, Gynecology, and Reproductive Sciences, University of California at San Francisco, San Francisco, California.
Intrapartum Fetal Surveillance

Barbara L. Parry, MD
Professor of Psychiatry, University of California at San Diego, La Jolla, California; Associate Director, Medical Student Clerkship, University of California at San Diego, La Jolla, California; Codirector, Primary Care Clinic, Veterans Administration Hospital, La Jolla, California.
Management of Depression and Psychoses during Pregnancy and the Puerperium

Morgan R. Peltier, PhD
Reproductive Sciences Laboratory, Division of Maternal-Fetal Medicine, Department of Obstetrics and Gynecology, University of Utah School of Medicine, Salt Lake City, Utah.
The Immunology of Pregnancy

Kate E. Pickett, PhD
Assistant Professor, Department of Health Studies and Department of Obstetrics and Gynecology, University of Chicago, Chicago, Illinois.
Maternal Nutrition

Ronald P. Rapini, MD
Professor and Chairman, Department of Dermatology, University of Texas Medical School and M. D. Anderson Cancer Center, Houston Texas.
The Skin and Pregnancy

Laurence S. Reisner, MD
Professor Emeritus, Anesthesiology and Reproductive Medicine, University of California, San Diego; Director of Obstetric Anesthesia, University of California, San Diego, Medical Center, San Diego, California.
Anesthetic Considerations for Complicated Pregnancies

Jamie L. Resnik, MD
Assistant Adjunct Professor, Department of Reproductive Medicine, University of California at San Diego, San Diego and La Jolla, California.
Post-term Pregnancy

Robert Resnik, MD
Professor of Reproductive Medicine, University of California, San Diego, School of Medicine, La Jolla, California.
The Puerperium; Intrauterine Growth Restriction; Post-term Pregnancy

Bryan S. Richardson, MD, FRCS(C)
Professor, Department of Obstetrics and Gynecology and Department of Physiology and Pediatrics, University of Western Ontario Faculty of Medicine; Chair, Division of Fetal and Neonatal Health, The Lawson Health Research Institute, London, Ontario, Canada.
Fetal Breathing and Body Movements

James M. Roberts, MD
Professor and Vice Chair (Research), Department of Obstetrics, Gynecology, and Reproductive Sciences, and Professor of Epidemiology, University of Pittsburgh; Elsie Hilliard Hillman Chair of Women's and Infants' Health Research and Director, Magee-Women's Research Institute; Vice President, Research, Magee-Women's Hospital, Pittsburgh, Pennsylvania.
Pregnancy-Related Hypertension

Ricardo J. Rodriguez, MD, FAAP
Assistant Professor of Pediatrics, Case Western Reserve University; Attending Neonatologist, Department of Pediatrics, Division of Neonatology, Rainbow Babies and Children's Hospital, Cleveland, Ohio.
Identification and Management of Problems in the High-Risk Neonate

Barbara M. Sanborn, PhD
Professor, Department of Biochemistry and Molecular Biology, University of Texas Medical School at Houston, Houston, Texas.
Biology and Physiology of the Reproductive Tract and Control of Myometrial Contraction

Larry D. Scott, MD, MA
Professor of Medicine, Division of Gastroenterology, University of Texas Medical School, Houston, Texas.
Gastrointestinal Disease in Pregnancy

Ralph Shabetai, MD
Professor of Medicine, Emeritus, University of California at San Diego, San Diego, California; Cardiologist, VA Health Care System, La Jolla, California, and University of California, San Diego, Medical Center, San Diego, California.
Cardiac Diseases

Robert M. Silver, MD
Associate Professor, University of Utah, Salt Lake City, Utah.
The Immunology of Pregnancy; Thrombophilias in Pregnancy

Victor R. Suarez, MD
Maternal-Fetal Medicine Fellow, The University of Texas Medical Branch, Galveston, Texas.
   Rheumatologic and Connective Tissue Disorders

Richard L. Sweet, MD
Professor, University of California, Davis; Director, Women's Center for Health, University of California, Davis, Health System, Sacramento, California.
   Maternal and Fetal Infectious Disorders

Krishnansu S. Tewari, MD
Assistant Clinical Professor, University of California, Irvine, Medical Center, Orange, California; Division of Gynecologic Oncology—Tricentral Service Area, Department of Obstetrics and Gynecology, The Southern California Permanente Medical Group, Kaiser Foundation Hospitals of Baldwin Park, Bellflower, and Harbor City, California.
   Pelvic Malignancies, Gestational Trophoblastic Neoplasia, and Nonpelvic Malignancies

John M. Thorp Jr., MD
McAllister Distinguished Professor of Obstetrics and Gynecology, University of North Carolina School of Medicine; Adjunct Professor of Epidemiology, University of North Carolina School of Public Health, Chapel Hill, North Carolina.
   Clinical Aspects of Normal and Abnormal Labor

Ronald J. Wapner, MD
Professor, Drexel University College of Medicine, Philadelphia, Pennsylvania.
   Prenatal Diagnosis of Congenital Disorders

Janice E. Whitty, MD
Associate Professor, Wayne State University School of Medicine; Director, Maternal Special Care Unit, Wayne State University/Hutzel Women's Hospital, Detroit, Michigan.
   Respiratory Diseases in Pregnancy

Isabelle Wilkins, MD
Associate Professor and Director, Division of Maternal-Fetal Medicine, Baylor College of Medicine, Houston, Texas.
   Nonimmune Hydrops

James R. Woods Jr., MD
Professor and Chair, Department of Obstetrics and Gynecology, University of Rochester School of Medicine and Dentistry, Rochester, New York.
   Significance of Amniotic Fluid Meconium

Anthony Wynshaw-Boris, MD, PhD
Associate Professor, University of California, San Diego, School of Medicine, La Jolla, California.
   Basic Genetics and Patterns of Inheritance

PREFACE

Although it has been a challenging task to put together what is now the fifth edition of *Maternal-Fetal Medicine*, it has also been a rewarding and extraordinarily stimulating endeavor. We have had the opportunity to continue collaboration with many repeat contributors and to call upon the expertise and knowledge of several new authors. Their scholarly efforts have combined to contribute a unique vitality and to ensure that the basic scientific and clinical material presented reflects the most contemporary information available in order that we may provide a solid foundation for the modern management of pregnancy complications.

In addition to a revised and updated version of each chapter, the fifth edition includes a newly rewritten section on genetics and prenatal diagnostic screening and new chapters that address the congenital and acquired thrombophylic disorders, diagnosis and management of the depressive/mood disorders and more common psychoses, and statistical considerations in perinatal medicine.

We express our deep gratitude to the practitioners, residents, and medical students who continually challenge us and who have made both teaching and the production of this book such a rewarding experience. We are also indebted to Mary Murrell for her many hours of hard work in the preparation of materials for the text. Finally, we extend appreciation to our editor, Stephanie Donley; to our senior development editor, Melissa Dudlick; and to Deborah Thorp and Kim Davis, all at Elsevier, for capably guiding the fifth edition to fruition.

Robert K. Creasy
Robert Resnik
Jay D. Iams

CONTENTS

Part IV
THE NEONATE

Part I
SCIENTIFIC BASIS
OF PERINATAL BIOLOGY

Chapter 1

BASIC GENETICS AND PATTERNS OF INHERITANCE

Bruce A. Hamilton, PhD, and Anthony Wynshaw-Boris, MD, PhD

IMPACT OF GENETICS AND THE HUMAN GENOME PROJECT ON MEDICINE IN THE 21ST CENTURY

For most of the 20th century, geneticists were seen as working outside the everyday clinical practice of medicine. The exceptions were those medical geneticists who studied rare chromosomal abnormalities and rare causes of birth defects and metabolic disorders. As recently as 20 years ago, genetics was generally not taught as part of the medical school curriculum, and most physicians' understanding of genetics was derived from undergraduate studies. How things have changed in the 21st century! Genetics is now recognized to be a contributing factor to virtually all human illnesses. In addition, the widespread reporting of genetic discoveries in the lay press and the plethora of genetic information available via the Internet has led to a great increase in the sophistication of patients and their families as medical consumers regarding genetics.

The importance of genetics in medical practice has grown as a consequence of the immense progress made in genetics and molecular biology during the 20th century. In the early years of the century, Mendel's laws were rediscovered and applied to many fields, including human disease. Fifty years ago, Watson and Crick published the structure of DNA and ushered in the era of molecular biology. At nearly the same time, the era of cytogenetics began with the determination of the correct number of human chromosomes (46). Twenty-five years ago, Sanger and Gilbert independently published techniques for determining the sequence of DNA. These findings led scientists, most prominently Renato Dulbecco and James Watson, to propose and initiate the Human Genome Project in the 1980s, with the goal of obtaining the complete human DNA sequence. At the time, it was hard to imagine that this goal could be achieved, but in the first year of the 21st century, a draft of the human genome was published simultaneously by the publicly funded Human Genome Project and a private company, Celera. In 2003 the complete human sequence should be available from the Human Genome Project, and a number of public consortia and private companies are determining the variations in DNA sequences over populations by cataloging single nucleotide polymorphisms (SNPs). The concepts, tools, and techniques of modern genetics and molecular biology available today have already had a profound impact on biomedical research and will clearly revolutionize our approach to diagnosis and treatment of human disease over the next decade and beyond.

Genetics plays an important role in day-to-day practice of obstetrics and gynecology, perhaps more so than any other specialty of medicine with the possible exception of pediatrics. In obstetric practice, genetic issues often arise before, during, and after pregnancy. Amniocentesis or chorionic villus sampling may detect potential chromosomal defects in the fetus. Fetuses examined during pregnancy by ultrasound may have possible birth defects. Specific prenatal diagnostic tests for genetic diseases may be requested by couples attempting to conceive who have a family history of that disorder. Infertile couples often require a workup for genetic causes of their infertility. In gynecology, genetics is particularly important in disorders of sexual development and gynecologic malignancies.

WHAT IS A GENE?

Genes are the fundamental unit of heredity. As a concise description, a gene includes all the structural and regulatory information required to produce its encoded RNA or protein products. In this section we outline the chemical nature of genes, the biochemistry of gene function, and the classes and consequences of genetic mutations.

Chemical Nature of Genes

Human genes are composed of deoxyribonucleic acid (DNA, Fig. 1-1). DNA is a negatively charged polymer of *nucleotides*. Each nucleotide is composed of a "base" attached to a 5-carbon deoxyribose sugar. Four bases are used in cellular DNA: two purines, adenine (A) and guanine (G), and two pyrimidines, cytosine (C) and thymine (T). The polymer is formed through phosphodiester bonds that connect the 5′ carbon atom of one sugar to the 3′ carbon of the next, which imparts directionality to the polymer.

Cellular DNA is a double-stranded helix. The two strands run antiparallel; that is, the 5′ to 3′ orientation of one strand runs in the opposite direction along the helix from its *complementary* strand. The bases in the two strands are paired: A with T and G with C. Hydrogen bonds between the base pairs hold the strands together: two hydrogen bonds for A:T pairs and three for G:C pairs. Each base thus has a complementary base, and the sequence of bases on one strand implies the

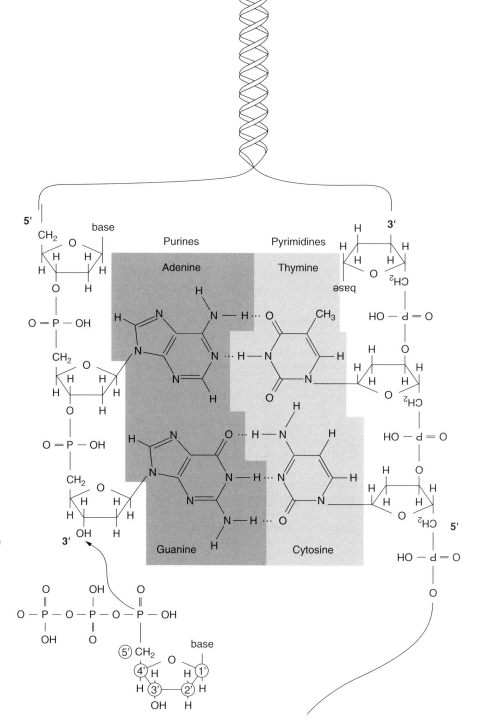

FIGURE 1-1 ■ Schematic diagram of DNA structure. Each strand of the double helix is a polymer of deoxyribonucleotides. Hydrogen bonds between base pairs (shown here as dots [···]) hold the strands together. Each base pair includes one purine base (adenine or guanine) and its complementary pyrimidine base (thymine or cytosine). Two hydrogen bonds form between A:T pairs and three between G:C pairs. The two polymer strands run antiparallel to each other according to the polarity of their sugar backbone. As shown at the bottom, DNA synthesis proceeds in the direction 5′ to 3′ by addition of new nucleoside triphosphates. Energy stored in the triphosphate bond is used for the polymerization reaction. The numbering system for carbon atoms in the deoxyribose sugar is indicated.

complementary sequence of the opposite strand. DNA is replicated in the 5′ to 3′ direction using the sequence of the complementary strand as a template. Nucleotide precursors used in DNA synthesis have 5′ triphosphate groups. Polymerase enzymes use the energy of this triphosphate to catalyze formation of a phosphoester bond with the hydroxyl group attached to the 3′ carbon of the extending strand.

The chemical attributes of DNA are the basis for clinical and forensic molecular diagnostic tests. Because nucleic acids form double-stranded duplexes, synthetic DNA and RNA molecules can be used to probe the integrity and composition of specific genes from patient samples.

Biochemistry of Gene Function

Information Transfer

DNA is an information molecule. The central dogma of molecular biology is that information in DNA is *transcribed* to make RNA and information in messenger RNA (mRNA) is

Second letter

First letter	U	C	A	G	Third letter
U	UUU UUC } phe UUA UUG } leu	UCU UCC UCA UCG } ser	UAU UAC } tyr UAA UAG } ter*	UGU UGC } cys UGA ter* UGG trp	U C A G
C	CUU CUC CUA CUG } leu	CCU CCC CCA CCG } pro	CAU CAC } his CAA CAG } gln	CGU CGC CGA CGG } arg	U C A G
A	AUU AUC AUA } ile AUG met	ACU ACC ACA ACG } thr	AAU AAC } asn AAA AAG } lys	AGU AGC } ser AGA AGG } arg	U C A G
G	GUU GUC GUA GUG } val	GCU GCC GCA GCG } ala	GAU GAC } asp GAA GAG } glu_	GGU GGC GGA GGG } gly	U C A G

FIGURE 1-2 ■ The genetic code. The letters U, C, A, and G correspond to the nucleotide bases in DNA. In this diagram, U (uracil) is substituted for T (thymidine) to reflect the genetic code as it appears in messenger RNA. Three distinct triplets (codons)—UAA, UAG, and UGA—are "nonsense" codons and result in termination of messenger RNA translation into a polypeptide chain. All amino acids except methionine and tryptophan have more than one codon; thus the genetic code is degenerate. This is the primary reason why so many single base-change mutations are "silent." For example, changing the terminal U in a UUU codon to a terminal C (UUC) still codes for phenylalanine. In contrast, an A to T(U) change (GAG to GUG) in the β-globin gene results in substitution of valine for glutamic acid at position 6 in the β-globin amino acid sequence, thus yielding "sickle cell" globin.

translated to make protein. DNA is also the template for its own replication. In some instances, such as in retroviruses, RNA is reverse transcribed into DNA. Although proteins are used to catalyze the synthesis of DNA, RNA, and proteins, proteins do not confer information back to genes. The sequence of RNA nucleotides (A, C, G, and uracil [U] bases coupled to ribose) is the same as the *coding* or *sense strand* of DNA from which it is transcribed (except that U replaces T). The sequence of amino acids in a protein is determined by a three-letter code of nucleotides in its mRNA (Fig. 1-2). The phase of the reading frame for these three-letter codons is set from the first codon, usually an AUG, encoding the initial methionine.

Quality Control in Gene Expression

Several mechanisms protect the specificity and fidelity of gene expression in cells. *Promoter* and *enhancer* sequences are binding sites on DNA for proteins that direct transcription of RNA. Promoter sequences are typically adjacent and 5′ to the start of mRNA encoding sequences (although some promoter elements are also found downstream of the start site, particularly in introns), whereas enhancers may act at considerable distance from either the 5′ or 3′ direction. The combinations of binding sites present determine under what conditions the gene is transcribed.

Newly transcribed RNA is generally processed before it is used by a cell. Pre-mRNAs generally receive a 5′ "cap" structure and a polyadenylated 3′ tail. Protein coding genes typically contain *exons* that remain in the processed RNA and one or more *introns* that must be removed by *splicing* (Fig. 1-3). Nucleotide sequences in the RNA that are recognized by protein and RNA splicing factors determine where splicing occurs. Many RNAs can be spliced in more than one way to encode a related series of products. Some splicing factors remain associated with the RNA and act as a "mark." For most genes, only spliced RNA is exported from the nucleus. Spliced RNAs that retain premature stop codons are rapidly degraded. Mutations in genes involved in these quality control steps appear in the clinic as early and severe genetic disorders, including spinal muscular atrophy (caused by mutations in *SMN1*, which encodes a splicing accessory factor) and fragile

X syndrome (mutations in *FMR1*, an RNA-binding protein). Protein synthesis is also highly regulated. Translation, folding, modification, transport, and sometimes cleavage to create an active form of the protein are all regulated steps in the expression of protein coding genes.

Mutations

Changes in the nucleotide sequence of a gene may occur through environmental damage to DNA, through errors in DNA replication, or through unequal partitioning during meiosis. Ultraviolet light, ionizing radiation, and chemicals that intercalate, bind to, or covalently modify DNA are examples of mutation-causing agents. Replication errors often involve changes in the number of a repeated sequence; for example, changes in the number of (CAG)n repeats encoding polyglutamine in the *Huntintin* gene can result in alleles prone to Huntington disease. Replication also plays a crucial role in other mutations. Cells generally respond to high levels of DNA damage by blocking DNA replication and inducing a variety of DNA repair pathways. However, for any one site of DNA damage, replication may occur before repair. A frequent source of human mutation is spontaneous deamination of cytosine (Fig. 1-4). The modified base can be interpreted as a thymine if replication occurs before repair of

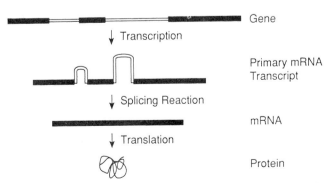

FIGURE 1-3 ■ Transcription of DNA to RNA and translation of RNA to protein. Introns (□) are spliced out of the primary messenger RNA (mRNA) transcript and exons (■) are joined together to form mature mRNA.

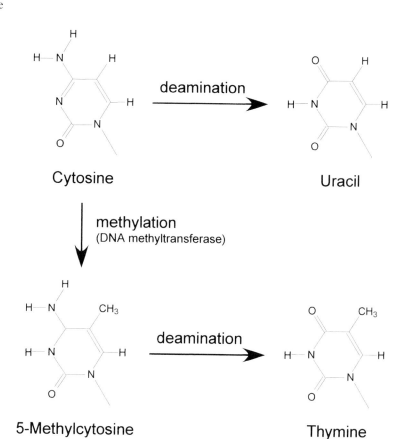

FIGURE 1-4 ■ Deamination of cytosine or its 5-methyl derivative produces a pyrimidine capable of pairing with adenine rather than guanine. Repair enzymes may remove the mispaired base before replication, but replication before repair (or repair of the wrong strand) results in the change becoming permanent. Spontaneous deamination of cytosine is a major mechanism of mutation in humans. Deamination of cytosine is also accelerated by some mutagenic chemicals, such as hydrazine.

the G:T mismatch pair. Ultraviolet light causes photochemical dimerization of adjacent thymine residues that may then be altered during repair or replication; in humans this is more relevant to somatic mutations in exposed skin cells than to germline mutations. Ionizing radiation, by contrast, penetrates tissues and can cause both base changes and double-strand breaks in DNA. Errors in repair of double-strand breaks result in deletion, inversion, or translocation of large regions of DNA. Many chemicals, including alkylating agents and epoxides, can form chemical adducts with the bases of DNA. If the adduct is not recognized during the next round of DNA replication, the wrong base may be incorporated into the opposite strand. In addition, the human genome includes hundreds of thousands of endogenous retroviruses, retrotransposons, and other potentially mobile DNA elements. Movement of such elements or recombination between them is a source of spontaneous insertions and deletions, respectively.

Changes in the DNA sequence of a gene create distinct alleles of that gene. Alleles can be classified based on how they affect the function of that gene. An *amorphic* allele is a complete loss of function, *hypomorphic* is a partial loss of function, *hypermorphic* is a gain of normal function, *neomorphic* is a gain of novel function not encoded by the normal gene, and an *antimorphic* or dominant negative allele antagonizes normal function. A practical impact of allele classes is that distinct clinical syndromes may be caused by different alleles of the same gene. For example, different allelic mutations in the androgen receptor gene have been tied to partial or complete androgen insensitivity (Brown et al., 1988) (including hypospadias and Reifenstein syndrome), prostate cancer sus-

ceptibility, and spinal and bulbar muscular atrophy (La Spada et al., 1991). Similarly, mutations in the *CFTR* chloride channel cause cystic fibrosis, but some alleles are associated with pancreatitis or other less severe symptoms; mutations in the *DTDST* sulfate transporter cause diastrophic dysplasia, atelosteogenesis, or achondrogenesis depending on the type of mutation present.

A small fraction of changes in genomic DNA affect gene function. Approximately 2% to 5% of the human genome encodes protein or confers regulatory specificity. Even within the protein coding sequences, many base changes do not alter the encoded amino acid, and these are called *silent substitutions*. Changes in DNA sequence that occurred long ago and do not alter gene function or whose impact is uncertain are often referred to as *polymorphisms*, whereas *mutation* is reserved for newly created changes and changes that have significant impacts on gene function, such as in disease-causing alleles of disease-associated genes. Mutations that do affect gene function may occur in coding sequences or in sequences required for transcription, processing, or stability of the RNA. The rate of spontaneous mutation in humans can vary tremendously depending on the size and structural constraints of the gene involved, but estimates range from 10^{-4} per generation for large genes such as *NF1* down to 10^{-6} or 10^{-7} for smaller genes. Given current estimates of 30,000 to 40,000 human genes (Lander et al., 2001; Venter et al., 2001) and given that more than 6 billion humans inhabit the earth, one may be sure that each human is mutant for some gene and each gene is mutated in some humans. Several public databases that curate information about human genes and mutations are now available online (Table 1-1).

TABLE 1-1. ONLINE RESOURCES FOR HUMAN GENETICS

Information on individual genes:	
Online Mendelian Inheritance in Man (OMIM),	*http://www.ncbi.nlm.nih.gov/entrez/ query.fcgi?db=OMIM*
GeneCards,	*http://bioinfo.weizmann.ac.il/cards/index.html*
GenBank,	*http://www.ncbi.nlm.nih.gov/GenBank*
Genome browsers:	
European Molecular Biology Organization/EBI,	*http://www.ensembl.org/*
NCBI,	*http://www.ncbi.nlm.nih.gov/*
University of California, Santa Cruz,	*http://genome.ucsc.edu/*
GeneLynx,	*http://www.genelynx.org/*

CHROMOSOMES IN HUMANS

Most of the 30,000 to 40,000 or more coding genes reside in the nucleus and are packaged on the *chromosomes*. In the human, there are 46 chromosomes in a normal cell: 23 pairs of autosomes, and the X and Y sex chromosomes (see later). The autosomes are numbered from the largest (1) to the smallest (21 and 22). Each chromosome contains a *centromere*, a constricted region that forms the attachments to the mitotic spindle and govern chromosome movements during mitosis. The *chromosomal arms* radiate on each side of the centromere, terminating in the *telomere*, or end of each arm. Each chromosome contains a distinct set of genetic information. Each pair of autosomes is homologous and has an identical set of genes. Normal females have two X chromosomes, whereas normal males have one X and one Y chromosome. In addition to the nuclear chromosomes, the mitochondrial genome contains approximately 37 genes on a single chromosome that resides in this organelle.

Each chromosome is a continuous DNA double helical strand, packaged into *chromatin*, which consists of protein and DNA. The protein moiety consists of basic *histone* and acidic *nonhistone* proteins. Five major groups of histones are important for proper packing of chromatin, whereas the heterogeneous nonhistone proteins are required for normal gene expression and higher order chromosome packaging. Two each of the four core histones (H2A, H2B, H3, and H4) form a histone octamer nucleosome core that binds with DNA in a fashion that permits tight supercoiling and packaging of DNA in the chromosome-like thread on a spool. The fifth histone, H1, binds to DNA at the edge of each nucleosome in the spacer region. A single nucleosome core and spacer consists of about 200 base pairs of DNA. The nucleosome "beads" are further condensed into higher order structures called solenoids, which can be packed into loops of chromatin that are attached to nonhistone matrix proteins. The orderly packaging of DNA into chromatin performs several functions, not the least of which is the packing of an enormous amount of DNA into the small volume of the nucleus. This orderly packing allows each chromosome to be faithfully wound and unwound during replication and cell division. Additionally, chromatin organization plays an important role in the control of gene expression.

Cell Cycle, Mitosis, and Meiosis

Cell Cycle

In replicating somatic cells, the complete diploid set of chromosomes is duplicated and the cell divides into two identical "daughter" cells, each with chromosomes and genes identical to those of the parent cell. The process of cell division is called *mitosis*, and the period between divisions is called *interphase*. Interphase can be divided into G_1, S, and G_2 *phases*, and a typical cell cycle is depicted in Figure 1-5. During the G_1 phase, synthesis of RNA and proteins occurs. In addition, the cell prepares for DNA replication. *S phase* ushers in the period of DNA replication. Not all chromosomes are replicated at the same time, and within a chromosome DNA is not synchronously replicated. Rather, DNA synthesis is initiated at thousands of origins of replication scattered along each chromosome. Between replication and division, called the G_2 *phase*, chromosome regions may be repaired and the cell is made ready for mitosis. In the G_1 phase, DNA of every chromosome of the diploid set (2n) is present once. Between the S and G_2 phases, every chromosome doubles to become two identical polynucleotides, referred to as *sister chromatids*. Thus, all DNA is now present twice ($2 \times 2n = 4n$).

Mitosis

The process of mitosis ensures that each daughter cell contains an identical and complete set of genetic information from the parent cell; this process is diagrammed in Figure 1-6. Mitosis is a continuous process that can be artificially divided into four stages based on the morphology of the chromosomes and mitotic apparatus. The beginning of mitosis is characterized by swelling of chromatin, which becomes visible under the light microscope by the end of *prophase*. Only 2 of the 46 chromosomes are shown in Figure 1-6. In prophase, the two sister chromatids (chromosomes) lie closely adjacent. The

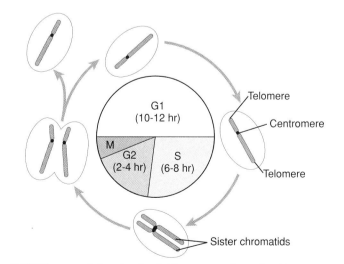

FIGURE 1-5 ■ Cell cycle of a dividing mammalian cell, with approximate times in each phase of the cycle. In the G_1 phase, the diploid chromosome set (2n) is present once. After DNA synthesis (S phase), the diploid chromosome set is present in duplicate (4n). After mitosis (M), the DNA content returns to 2n. The telomeres, centromere, and sister chromatids are indicated. (From Nussbaum RL, McInnes RR, Willard HF: Thompson and Thompson Genetics in Medicine, 6th ed. Philadelphia, WB Saunders, 2001.)

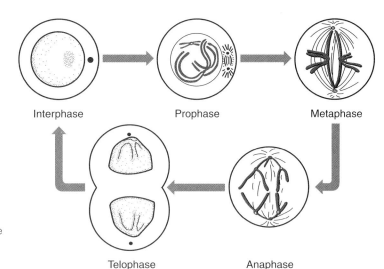

FIGURE 1-6 ■ Schematic representation of mitosis. Only 2 of the 46 chromosomes are present. (From Vogel F, Motulsky AG: Human Genetics: Problems and Approaches. New York, Springer-Verlag, 1979.)

nuclear membrane disappears, the nucleolus vanishes, and the spindle fibers begin to form from the microtubule organizing centers, or *centrosomes*, that take positions perpendicular to the eventual plane of cleavage of the cell. A protein called *tubulin* forms the microtubules of the spindle and connects with the centromeric region of each chromosome. The chromosomes condense and move to the middle of the spindle at the eventual point of cleavage.

After prophase, the cell is in *metaphase*, when the chromosomes are maximally condensed. The chromosomes line up with the centromeres located on an equatorial plane between the spindle poles. In addition, this is the important phase for cytogenetic technology. In metaphase, virtually all clinical methods of examining chromosomes cause arrest of further steps in mitosis. Thus, we see all sister chromatids (4n) in a standard clinical karyotype.

Anaphase begins as the two chromatids of each chromosome separate, connected at first only at the centromere region (early *anaphase*). Once the centromeres separate, the sister chromosomes of each chromosome are drawn to the opposite poles by the spindle fibers. During *telophase*, chromosomes lose their visibility under the microscope, spindle fibers are degraded, tubulin is stored away for the next division, and a new nucleolus and nuclear membrane develop. The cytoplasm also divides along the same plane as the equatorial plate in a process called *cytokinesis*. Cytokinesis occurs once the segregating chromosomes approach the spindle poles. Thus, the elaborate process of mitosis and cytokinesis of a single cell results in the segregation of an equal complete set of chromosomes and genetic material in each of the resulting daughter cells.

Meiosis and the Meiotic Cell Cycle

In mitotic cell division, the number of chromosomes remains constant for each daughter cell. In contrast, a property of meiotic cell division is the reduction in the number of chromosomes from the diploid number in the germline to the haploid number in gametes (from 46 to 23 in humans). To accomplish this reduction, two successive rounds of meiotic division occur. The first division is a reduction division where the chromosome number is reduced by one half and is accomplished by pairing to homologous chromosomes. The second meiotic division is similar to most mitotic divisions, except the total number of chromosomes is haploid rather than diploid. The haploid number is found only in the germline; thus, after fertilization the diploid chromosome number is restored. The selection of chromosomes from each homologous pair in the haploid cell is completely random, thereby ensuring genetic variability in each germ cell. In addition, recombination occurs during the initial stages of chromosome pairing during the first phase of meiosis, providing an additional layer of genetic diversity in each of the gametes.

STAGES OF MEIOSIS

Figure 1-7 depicts the stages of meiosis. DNA synthesis has already occurred before the first meiotic division and does not again occur during the two stages of meiotic division. A major feature of *meiotic division I* is the pairing of homologous chromosomes at homologous regions during prophase I, a complex stage were many tasks are accomplished that can be subdivided into substages based on morphology of meiotic chromosomes. These stages are termed *leptonema, zygonema, pachynema, diplonema,* and *diakinesis.* Condensation and pairing occur during leptonema and zygonema (Fig. 1-7C and *D*). The paired homologous chromosome regions are connected at a double-structured region, the synaptonemal complex during pachynema. In diplonema, four chromatids of each kind are seen in close approximation side by side (see Fig. 1-7D). Nonsister chromatids become separated, whereas the sister chromatids remain paired; the chromatid crossings (chiasmata) between nonsister chromatids can be seen (see Fig. 1-7D). The chiasmata are believed to be sites of recombination. The chromosomes separate at diakinesis (see Fig. 1-7). The chromosomes now enter meiotic metaphase I and telophase I (Fig. 1-7E and *F*).

Meiotic division II is essentially a mitotic division of a fully copied set of haploid chromosomes. From each meiotic metaphase II, two daughter cells are formed (Fig. 1-7H_1 and H_2), and a random assortment of DNA along the chromosome is accomplished at division (Fig. 1-7I). After meiosis II, the genetic material is distributed to four cells as haploid chromosomes (23 in each cell). In addition to random crossing over, there also is random distribution of nonhomologous chromo-

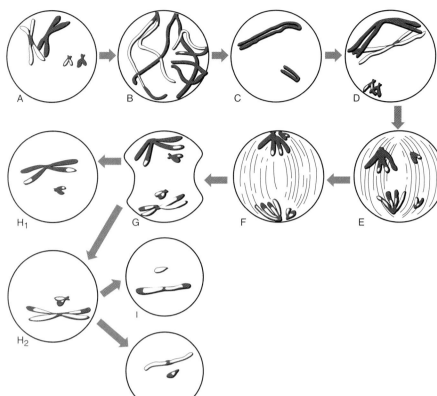

FIGURE 1-7 ■ The stages of meiosis. Paternal chromosomes are black; maternal chromosomes are white. **A**, Condensed chromosomes in mitosis. **B**, Leptotene. **C**, Zygotene. **D**, Diplotene with crossing over. **E**, Diakinesis–anaphase I. **F**, Anaphase I. **G**, Telophase I. **H₁** and **H₂**, Metaphase II. **I**, Telophase II. (From Vogel F, Motulsky AG: Human Genetics: Problems and Approaches. New York, Springer-Verlag, 1979.)

somes to each of the final four haploid daughter cells. For these 23 chromosomes, the number of possible combinations in a single germ cell is 2^{23}, or 8,388,608. Thus $2^{23} \times 2^{23}$ equals the number of possible genotypes in the children of any particular combination of parents. This impressive number of variable genotypes is further enhanced by crossing over during prophase I of meiosis. Chiasma formation occurs during pairing and may be essential to this process, because there appears to be at least one chiasma per chromosome arm. A chiasma appears to be a point of crossover between two nonsister chromatids that occurs through breakage and reunion of nonsister chromatids at homologous points (Fig. 1-8).

GENDER DIFFERENCES IN MEIOSIS

There are crucial distinctions between the two sexes in meiosis.

MALES. In the male, meiosis is continuous in spermatocytes from puberty through adult life. After meiosis II, sperm cells acquire the ability to move effectively. The primordial fetal germ cells that produce oogonia in the female give rise to gonocytes at the same time in the male fetus. In these gonocytes, the tubules produce Ad (dark) spermatogonia (Fig. 1-9). During the middle of the second decade of life in males, spermatogenesis is fully established. At this point, the number of Ad spermatogonia is approximately 4.3×10^8 to 6.4×10^8 per testis. Ad spermatogonia undergo continuous divisions. During a given division, one cell may produce two Ad cells, whereas another produces two Ap (pale) cells. These Ap cells develop into B spermatogonia and hence into spermatocytes that undergo meiosis (see Fig. 1-9). Primary spermatocytes are in meiosis I, whereas secondary spermatocytes are in meiosis II. Vogel and Rathenberg (1975) calculated approximations of

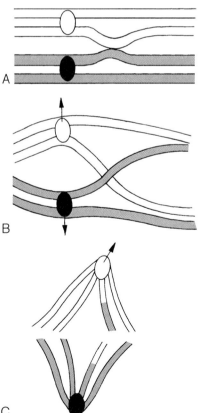

FIGURE 1-8 ■ Crossing over and chiasma formation. **A**, Homologous chromatids are attached to each other. **B**, Crossing over with chiasma occurs. **C**, Chromatid separation occurs. (From Vogel F, Motulsky AG: Human Genetics: Problems and Approaches. New York, Springer-Verlag, 1979.)

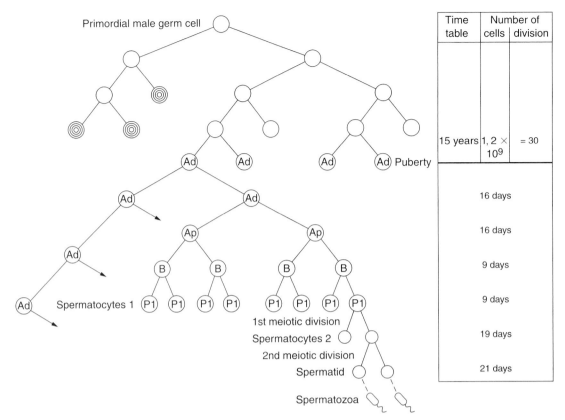

FIGURE 1-9 ■ Cell divisions during spermatogenesis. The overall number of cell divisions is much higher than in oogenesis. It increases with advancing age. Ad, dark spermatogonia; Ap, pale spermatogonia; B, spermatogonia; P1, spermatocytes. *Concentric circles* indicate cell atrophy. (From Vogel F, Motulsky AG: Human Genetics: Problems and Approaches. New York, Springer-Verlag, 1979.)

the number of cell divisions according to age. On the basis of these approximations, it can be estimated further that from embryonic age to 28 years, the number of cell divisions of human sperm is approximately 15 times greater than the number of cell divisions in the life history of an oocyte.

FEMALES. In the primitive gonad destined to become female, the number of ovarian stem cells increases rapidly by mitotic cell division. Between the 2nd and 3rd months of fetal life, oocytes begin to enter meiosis (Fig. 1-10). By the time of birth, mitosis in the female germ cells is finished and only the two meiotic divisions remain to be fulfilled. After birth, all oogonia are either transformed into oocytes or degenerate. Fetal germ cells increase from 6×10^5 at 2 months' gestation to 6.8×10^6 during the 5th month. Decline begins at this time, to about 2×10^6 at birth. Meiosis remains arrested in the viable oocytes until puberty. At puberty, some oocytes start the division process again. An individual follicle matures at the time of ovulation. At the completion of meiosis I, one of the cells becomes the secondary oocyte, accumulating most of the cytoplasm and organelles, whereas the other cell becomes the first *polar body*. The maturing secondary oocyte completes meiotic metaphase II at the time of ovulation. If fertilization occurs, meiosis II in the oocyte is completed, with the formation of the second polar body. Only about 400 oocytes eventually mature during the reproductive lifetime of a woman, whereas the rest degenerate. In the female, only one of the four meiotic prod-

ucts develops into a mature oocyte; the other three become polar bodies that usually are not fertilized.

There are, then, three basic differences in meiosis between males and females:

1. In females, one division product becomes a mature germ cell and three become polar bodies. In the male, all four meiotic products become mature germ cells.
2. In females, a low number of embryonic mitotic cell divisions occurs very early, followed by early embryonic meiotic cell division that continues to occur up to around the 9th month of gestation; division is then arrested for many years, commences again at puberty, and is completed only after fertilization. In the male, there is a much longer period of mitotic cell division, followed immediately by meiosis at puberty; meiosis is completed when spermatids develop into mature sperm.
3. In females, very few gametes are produced one at a time, whereas in males, a large number of gametes are produced virtually continuously.

FERTILIZATION

The chromosomes of the egg and sperm are segregated after fertilization into the pronuclei, and each is surrounded by a nuclear membrane. The DNA of the diploid zygote replicates soon after fertilization and after division two diploid daughter cells are formed, initiating embryonic development.

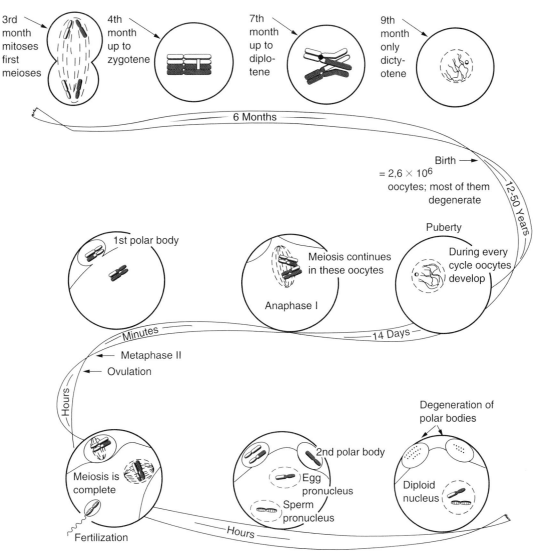

FIGURE 1-10 ■ Meiosis in the human female. Meiosis starts after 3 months of development. During childhood, the cytoplasm of oocytes increases in volume, but the nucleus remains unchanged. About 90% of all oocytes degenerate at the onset of puberty. During the first half of every month, the luteinizing hormone of the pituitary stimulates meiosis, which is now almost completed (end of the prophase that began during embryonic stage; metaphase I, anaphase I, telophase I, and—within a few minutes—prophase II and metaphase II). Then meiosis stops again. A few hours after metaphase I is reached, ovulation is induced by luteinizing hormone. Fertilization occurs in the fallopian tube, and then the second meiotic division is complete. Nuclear membranes are formed around the maternal and paternal chromosomes. After some hours, the two "pronuclei" fuse and the first cleavage division begins. (From Bresch C, Haussmann R: Klassiche und Moleculare Genetik, 3rd ed. Berlin, Springer-Verlag, 1972.)

CLINICAL SIGNIFICANCE OF MITOSIS AND MEIOSIS

The proper segregation of chromosomes during meiosis and mitosis ensures that the progeny cells contain the appropriate genetic instructions. When errors occur in either process, the result is that an individual or cell lineage contains an abnormal number of chromosomes and an unbalanced genetic complement. *Meiotic nondisjunction*, occurring primarily during oogenesis, is responsible for chromosomally abnormal fetuses in several percent of recognized pregnancies. *Mitotic nondisjunction* can occur during tumor formation. In addition, if it occurs early after fertilization, it may result in chromosomally unbalanced embryos or *mosaicism* that may result in birth defects and mental retardation.

Analysis of Human Chromosomes

The era of clinical human cytogenetics began just a little more than 35 years ago with the discovery that somatic cells in humans contain 46 chromosomes. The utilization of a simple procedure—hypotonic treatment for spreading the chromosomes of individual cells—enabled medical scientists and physicians to microscopically examine and study chromosomes in single cells rather than tissue sections. Between 1956 and 1959, it was recognized that visible changes in the number or structure of chromosomes could result in a number of birth defects, such as Down syndrome, Turner syndrome, Klinefelter syndrome, Patau syndrome, and cri du chat syndrome. Chromosome disorders represent a large proportion of fetal loss, congenital defects, and mental retardation, and there are a number of clinical indications for chromosome analysis. Regarding the practice of obstetrics and gynecology, these include abnormal phenotype in a newborn infant, unexplained first-trimester spontaneous abortion with no fetal karyotype, pregnancy resulting in stillborn or neonatal death, fertility problems, and pregnancy in women of advanced ages.

Preparation of Human Metaphase Chromosomes

Metaphase chromosomes can be prepared from any cell undergoing mitosis. During the day-to-day activity of almost any clinical or research cytogenetic laboratory, chromosome analysis will be obtained in cells derived from peripheral blood, bone marrow, amniotic fluid, skin, or other tissues *in situ* and in tissue cultures. For clinical cytogenetic diagnosis in living non-leukemic individuals, metaphase cells from peripheral blood samples are the easiest to obtain. To obtain adequate numbers of metaphase cells from peripheral blood, mitosis must be induced artificially, and in most procedures, *phytohemagglutinin*, a mitogen, is used for this purpose.

Specifically, T-cell lymphocytes are induced to undergo mitosis; thus, almost all chromosome analyses of human peripheral blood samples produce karyotypes of T lymphocytes. In general descriptive terms, a suspension of peripheral blood cells is incubated at 37°C in tissue culture media with mitogen for 72 hours to produce an actively dividing population of cells. The cells are then incubated for 1 to 3 hours in a dilute solution of a mitotic spindle poison such as colchicine to stop the cells in metaphase when chromosomes are condensed. Next, the nuclei containing the chromosomes are made fragile by swelling in a short treatment (10 to 30 minutes) in a hypotonic salt solution. The chromosomes are fixed in a mixture of alcohol and acetic acid and then gently spread on a glass slide for drying and staining.

Most cytogenetic laboratories use one or more of the staining procedures that stain each chromosome with variable intensity at specific regions, thereby providing "bands" along the chromosome; hence, the term *banding patterns* is used to identify chromosomes. All procedures are effective and provide different types of morphologic information about individual chromosomes. For convenience in descriptive terminology, various banding patterns have been named for the methods by which they were revealed. Some of the more commonly used methods are as follows:

1. G *bands* are revealed by Giemsa staining in association with various other secondary steps. This is probably the most widely used banding technique.
2. Quinacrine mustard and similar fluorochromes provide fluorescent staining for Q *bands*. The banding patterns are identical to those in G bands, but a fluorescence microscope is required. Q banding is particularly useful for identifying the Y chromosomes in both metaphase and interphase cells.
3. R *bands* are the result of "reverse" banding. They are produced by controlled denaturation, usually with heat. The pattern in R banding is opposite to that in G and Q banding; light bands produced on G and Q banding are dark on R banding, and dark bands on G and Q banding are light on R banding.

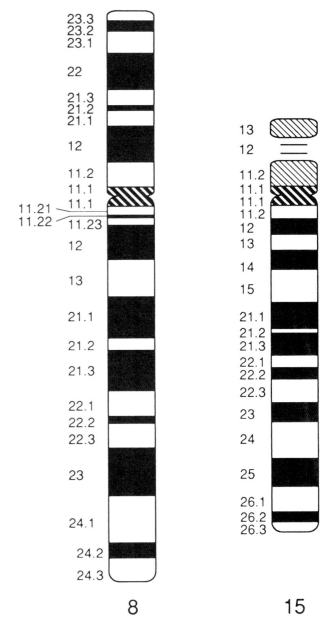

FIGURE 1-11 ■ An ideogram of two representative chromosomes. Chromosome 8 and chromosome 15 represent arbitrary examples of schematic high-resolution mid-metaphase Giemsa banding. At the level of resolution demonstrated in this figure, a haploid set of 23 chromosomes has a combined total of approximately 550 bands. Broad cross-hatched areas represent the centromere, and the narrow cross-hatched areas represent regions of variable size and staining intensity. A detailed ideogram of the entire human haploid set of chromosomes was published by the Standing Committee on Human Cytogenetic Nomenclature. (ISCN: Report of the Standing Committee on Human Cytogenetic Nomenclature. Basel, Karger, 1995.)

4. T *bands* produce specific staining of the telomeric regions of the chromosome.
5. C *bands* reflect constitutive heterochromatin and are located primarily on the pericentric regions of the chromosome.

Modifications and new procedures of band staining are constantly being developed. For example, a silver stain can be used to identify specifically the nucleolus organizer regions that were functionally active during the previous interphase. Other techniques enhance underlying chromosome instability and are useful in identifying certain aberrations associated with malignancies. Recent modifications of the basic culture-staining procedures have resulted in more elongated chromosomes, prophase-like in appearance, with more readily identifiable banding patterns.

Figure 1-11 depicts an ideogram of G banding of two normal chromosomes. Starting from the centromeric region, each chromosome is organized into two regions: the P region (*short arm*) and the q region (*long arm*). Within each region, the area is further subdivided numerically. These numerical band designations greatly facilitate the descriptive identification of specific chromosomes. A complete male karyogram is depicted in Figure 1-12. A female karyogram would have two X chromosomes.

Molecular Cytogenetics: Fluorescence *in Situ* Hybridization and Multicolor Karyotyping

Besides routine karyotyping methods, more specific and sophisticated techniques have been developed that make use of fluorescence techniques and specific DNA sequences isolated by molecular biological techniques. These techniques allow the evaluation of a chromosomal preparation for gain or loss of specific genes or chromosome regions and for the presence of translocations. In *fluorescence in situ hybridization* (FISH), DNA probes representing specific genes, chromosomal regions, and even whole chromosomes can be labeled with fluorescently tagged nucleotides. After hybridization to metaphase and/or interphase preparations of chromosomes, these probes will specifically bind to the gene, region, or chromosome of interest (Fig. 1-13, Color Plate 1). This technique facilitates the detection of fine details of chromosome structure. For example, any single copy gene will normally be present in two copies in a diploid cell, one copy on each homologous chromosome. If one of the genes is missing in certain disease states, then only one copy will be detected by FISH with a probe specific for that gene. If the gene is present in numerous copies, as often occurs to certain oncogenes in tumors, multiple copies will be detected.

Similarly, entire chromosomes can be isolated by flow cytometry and probes prepared by labeling the entire chromosomal DNA complement (called a *chromosome paint probe*). When hybridized under appropriate conditions to metaphase and/or interphase preparations of chromosomes, these probes will specifically detect the chromosome of interest. A translocation that occurs between two chromosomes can be easily detected with a chromosomal paint probe to one of the translocation partners. Normally, this probe would identify two diploid chromosomes, and the entire length of each chromosome will be fluorescent. In contrast, the paint probe will identify a normal completely labeled chromosome and two new

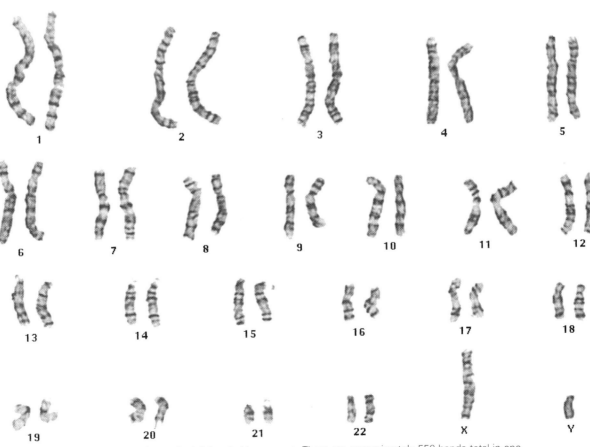

FIGURE 1-12 ■ A standard G-banded karyogram. There are approximately 550 bands total in one haploid set of chromosome in this karyogram. The sex karyotype is XY (male). A female karyogram would show two X chromosomes.

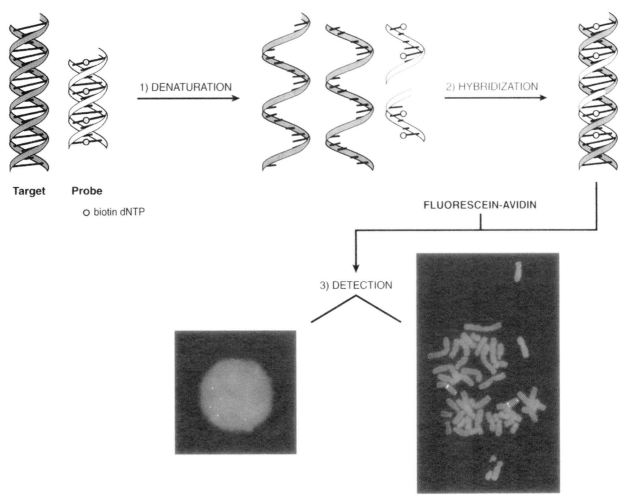

FIGURE 1–13 ■ A schematic representation of fluorescence *in situ* hybridization. The DNA target (chromosome) and a short DNA fragment "probe" containing nucleotides labeled with biotin (dNTP) are denatured. The probe is specific for a chromosomal region containing the gene or genes of interest. During renaturation, some of the DNA molecules containing the region of interest hybridize with complementary nucleotide sequences in the probe, and with subsequent binding to a fluorochrome marker (fluorescein-avidin) a signal (yellow-green) is produced. The two lower panels demonstrate a metaphase cell and an interphase cell. The probe used is specific for chromosome 7. A control probe for band q36 on the long arm establishes the presence of two number 7 chromosomes. The second probe is specific for the Williams syndrome region at band 7q11.23. This signal is more intense and demonstrates no deletion at region 7q11.23 and essentially excludes the diagnosis of Williams syndrome. The signals are easily visible in both the metaphase and interphase cells. See also Color Plate 1.

incompletely labeled chromosomes, representing the translocated fragments.

Recently, an extension of this methodology has been developed that is useful for the fluorescent detection and analysis of all chromosomes simultaneously. One such method is called *spectral karyotyping* (Fig. 1-14; Color Plate 2). A large number of fluorescent tags are available that can be used individually or in combination to prepare labeled chromosomes. It is possible to individually label each chromosome with unique combinations of these tags so that each one will emit a unique fluorescent signal upon hybridization to chromosomal preparations. If all uniquely labeled chromosomal paint probes are mixed and hybridized to metaphase preparations simultaneously, each chromosome will emit a unique wavelength of light. These different wavelengths can be detected by a microscopically mounted spectrophotometer linked to a high-resolution camera. Sophisticated image analysis programs can then

distinguish individual chromosomes, and a metaphase spread will appear as a multicolored array (see Fig. 1-14). With knowledge of the expected emission from each chromosome, the signal from each chromosome can be specifically identified, and the entire metaphase can be displayed as a karyogram. This method is particularly useful for the identification of translocations between chromosomes.

Characteristics of the More Common Chromosome Aberrations in Humans

Abnormalities in Chromosome Number

Alteration of the number of chromosomes is called *heteroploidy*. A heteroploid individual is *euploid* if the number of chromosomes is a multiple of the haploid number of 23 and *aneuploid* if there is any other number of chromosomes.

PLATE 1

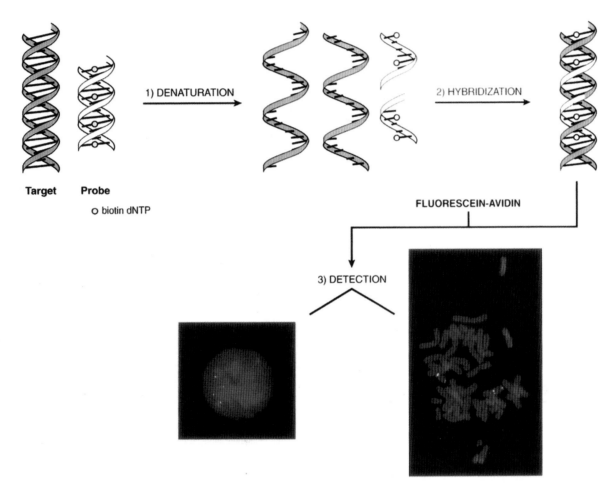

FIGURE 1–13 ■ A schematic representation of fluorescence *in situ* hybridization. The DNA target (chromosome) and a short DNA fragment "probe" containing nucleotides labeled with biotin (dNTP) are denatured. The probe is specific for a chromosomal region containing the gene or genes of interest. During renaturation, some of the DNA molecules containing the region of interest hybridize with complementary nucleotide sequences in the probe, and with subsequent binding to a fluorochrome marker (fluorescein-avidin) a signal (yellow-green) is produced. The two lower panels demonstrate a metaphase cell and an interphase cell. The probe used is specific for chromosome 7. A control probe for band q36 on the long arm establishes the presence of two number 7 chromosomes. The second probe is specific for the Williams syndrome region at band 7q11.23. This signal is more intense and demonstrates no deletion at region 7q11.23 and essentially excludes the diagnosis of Williams syndrome. The signals are easily visible in both the metaphase and interphase cells.

PLATE 2

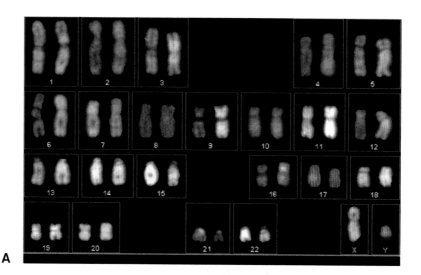

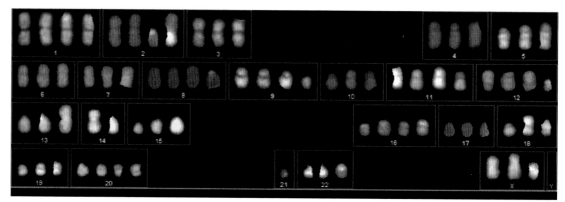

FIGURE 1-14 ■ Spectral karyotyping (SKY). **A**, A normal human karyotype after SKY analysis, showing the presence of two copies of each chromosome, each pair with a different color. In addition, the X and Y chromosomes are different colors. **B**, SKY analysis of a tumor cell line, displaying extra copies of nearly all chromosomes, as well as translocations. These can be appreciated as chromosomes consisting of two colors. (Photos courtesy of Dr. Karen Arden, Ludwig Cancer Institute, UCSD School of Medicine.)

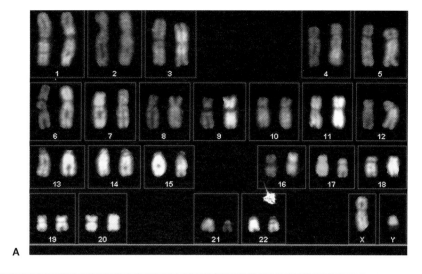

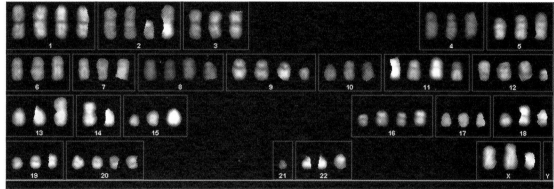

FIGURE 1-14 ■ Spectral karyotyping (SKY). **A**, A normal human karyotype after SKY analysis, showing the presence of two copies of each chromosome, each pair with a different color. In addition, the X and Y chromosomes are different colors. **B**, SKY analysis of a tumor cell line, displaying extra copies of nearly all chromosomes, as well as translocations. These can be appreciated as chromosomes consisting of two colors. See also Color Plate 2. (Photos courtesy of Dr. Karen Arden, Ludwig Cancer Institute, UCSD School of Medicine.)

Abnormalities of single chromosomes are usually due to nondisjunction or anaphase lag, whereas whole genome abnormalities are referred to as *polyploidization*.

Aneuploidy

Aneuploidy is the most frequently seen chromosome abnormality in clinical cytogenetics, occurring in 3% to 4% of clinically recognized pregnancies. Aneuploidy occurs during both meiosis and mitosis. The most significant cause of aneuploidy is *nondisjunction*. Nondisjunction may occur in both mitosis and meiosis but is observed more frequently in meiosis. One pair of chromosomes fails to separate (disjoin) and is transferred in anaphase to one pole. Meiotic nondisjunction can occur in meiosis I or II. The result is that one product will have both members of the pair and one will have neither of that pair (Fig. 1-15). After fertilization, the embryo will contain either an extra third chromosome (trisomy) or will have only one of the normal chromosome pair (monosomy).

Anaphase lag is another event that can lead to abnormalities in chromosome number. In this process, one chromosome of a pair does not move as rapidly during the anaphase process as its sister chromosome and is lost. Often this loss leads to a mosaic cell population, one euploid and one monosomic (e.g., 45,XO/46,XX mosaicism).

Polyploidy

In affected fetuses that are polyploid, the whole genome is present more than once in every cell. When the increase is by a factor of one for each cell, the result is *triploidy*, with 69 chromosomes per cell. Triploidy is most often caused by fertilization of a single egg with two sperm, but it may rarely result from the duplication of chromosomes during meiosis without division.

Alterations of Chromosome Structure

Structural alterations in chromosomes constitute the other major group of cytogenetic abnormalities. Such defects are seen less frequently in newborns than numerical defects and occur in about 0.0025% of newborns. However, chromosome rearrangements are a common occurrence in malignancies. Structural rearrangements are balanced if there is no net loss or gain of chromosomal material or unbalanced if there is an abnormal genetic complement.

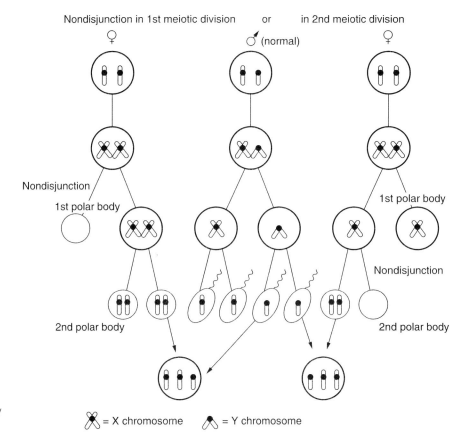

FIGURE 1-15 ■ Nondisjunction of the X chromosome in the first and second meiotic divisions in a female. Fertilization is by a Y-bearing sperm. An XXY genotype/phenotype can result from both first and second meiotic division nondisjunction. (From Vogel F, Motulsky AG: Human Genetics: Problems and Approaches. New York, Springer-Verlag, 1979.)

DELETIONS AND DUPLICATIONS

Deletions refer to the loss of a chromosome segment. Deletions may occur on the terminal segment of the short or long arm. Alternatively, an interstitial deletion may occur anywhere on the chromosome. Deletions can result from chromosomal breakage and when loss of the deleted fragment lacks a centromere (Fig. 1-16) or from unequal crossover between homologous chromosomes. One of the chromosomes carries a deletion, whereas the other reciprocal event is a duplication. A *ring chromosome* results from terminal deletions on both the short and long arms of the same chromosome (Fig. 1-17).

INSERTIONS

In the process of insertion, an interstitial deleted segment is inserted into a nonhomologous chromosome (Fig. 1-18).

INVERSIONS

Inversions more often involve the centromere (*pericentric*) rather than noncentromeric areas (*paracentric*). Figure 1-19 is a diagrammatic representation of a pericentric inversion. Inversions reduce pairing between homologous chromosomes. Thus, crossing over may be suppressed within inverted heterozygote chromosomes. For homologous chromosomes to pair, one must form a loop in the region of the inversion (Fig. 1-20). If the inversion is pericentric, the centromere lies within the loop. When crossing over occurs, each of the two chromatids within the crossover has both a duplication and a deletion. If gametes are formed with the abnormal chromosomes, the fetus will be monosomic for one portion of the chromosome and trisomic for another portion. One result of abnormal chromosome recombinants might be increased fetal demise from duplication or deficiency of a chromosomal region.

When pericentric inversion occurs as a new mutation, usually the result is a phenotypically normal individual. However, when a carrier of a pericentric inversion reproduces, the pairing events just described may occur. If fertilization involves the abnormal gametes, there is a risk for abnormal progeny. When pericentric inversion is observed in a phenotypically abnormal child, parental karyotyping is indicated.

An exception to this rule involves a pericentric inversion in chromosome 9, the most common inversion noted in humans. An approximate 5% frequency of this inversion has been observed in nearly 14,000 amniotic fluid cultures. In the 30 or so instances in which parental karyotyping was performed, invariably one or the other parent carried a pericentric inversion on one number 9 chromosome. One explanation for the apparently benign status of pericentric inversion in this chromosome is that the pericentric region on chromosome 9 contains many highly repetitive or genetically silent regions in the nucleotide sequence, so that inversion in this region is of no clinical consequence. Alternatively, inversions involving relatively short DNA sequences may not be involved in crossing over.

TRANSLOCATIONS

A translocation is the most common form of chromosome structural rearrangement in humans. There are two types: *reciprocal* (Fig. 1-21) and *Robertsonian* (Fig. 1-22).

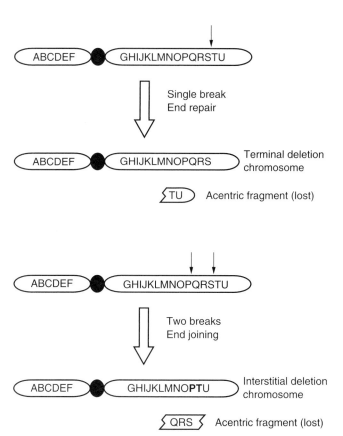

FIGURE 1-16 ■ Schematic representation of two kinds of deletion events. A single double-strand break (*arrow*) may produce a terminal deletion if the end is repaired to retain telomere function. The telomeric fragment lacks a centromere (indicated by the *filled oval* in the intact chromosome) and will generally be lost in the next cell division. A chromosome with two double-strand breaks may suffer an interstitial deletion if the break is repaired by end joining of the centromeric and telomeric fragments.

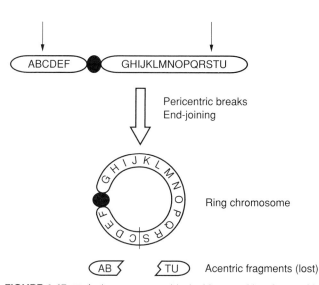

FIGURE 1-17 ■ A chromosome with double-strand breaks on either side of its centromere (*filled oval*) can result in terminal deletions (see Fig. 1-16), pericentric inversion, or formation of a *ring chromosome* by joining the two centromeric ends from the breaks. In the case of ring chromosome formation, the acentric fragments would be lost in the next cell division.

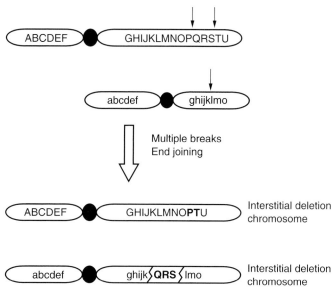

FIGURE 1-18 ■ Interstitial translocations can result from repair by end joining of fragments from nonhomologous chromosomes. In the example illustrated, a fragment QRS is liberated from one chromosome and inserted at a break between k and l in the recipient chromosome.

RECIPROCAL TRANSLOCATION. If a reciprocal translocation is balanced, phenotypic abnormalities are uncommon. Unbalanced translocations result in miscarriage, stillbirth, or live birth with multiple malformations, developmental delay, and mental retardation. Reciprocal translocations nearly always involve nonhomologous chromosomes among any of the 23 chromosome pairs, including chromosomes X and Y.

Gametogenesis in heterozygous carriers of translocations is especially significant because of the increased risk for chromosome segregation that produces gametes with unbalanced chromosomes in the diploid set (see Fig. 1-21). In a reciprocal translocation, there will be four chromosomes with segments in common (see Fig. 1-21). During meiosis, homologous segments must match for crossing over so that in a translocation set of four a *quadrivalent* is formed. During meiosis I, the four chromosomes may segregate randomly in two daughter cells with several results.

In 2:2 alternate segregation (see Fig. 1-21), one centromere segregates to one daughter cell and the next centromere segregates to the other daughter cell. This is the only mode that leads to a normal or balanced normal karyotype. Adjacent segregation and 3:1 nondisjunction segregation all produce unbalanced gametes.

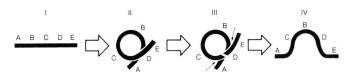

FIGURE 1-19 ■ An illustrative example of a possible mechanism for development of a pericentric inversion. **I,** Normal sequence of coded information on the chromosome. **II,** Formation of a loop involving a chromosome region. **III,** Breakage and reunion at the arrows, where the chromosome loop intersects itself. **IV,** Formation of the inverted information sequence after reunion.

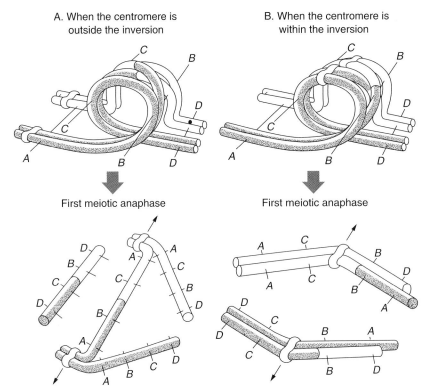

A. When the centromere is
outside the inversion

B. When the centromere is
within the inversion

First meiotic anaphase

First meiotic anaphase

FIGURE 1-20 ■ Crossing over within the inversion loop of an inversion heterozygote results in aberrant chromatids with duplications or deficiencies. (From Srb AM, Owen RD, Edgar RS: General Genetics, 2nd ed. San Francisco, WH Freeman, 1965.)

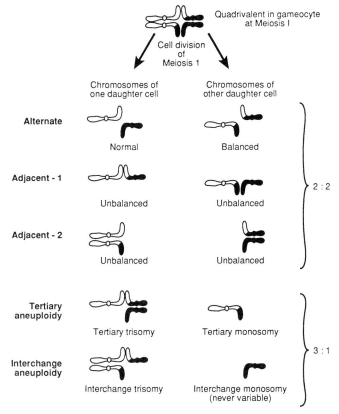

FIGURE 1-21 ■ Chromosome segregation during meiosis in a reciprocal translocation heterozygote. (Modified from Gardner RJM, Sutherland GR: Chromosome Abnormalities and Genetic Counseling. New York, Oxford University Press, 1989.)

If a gamete is chromosomally unbalanced, the odds are increased for spontaneous abortion. In familial translocations, the risk of unbalanced progeny seems to depend on the method of ascertainment. For example, if a familial reciprocal translocation is ascertained by a chromosomally unbalanced live birth or stillbirth, the risk for subsequent chromosomally unbalanced children is approximately 15% and the risk for spontaneous abortion or stillbirth is approximately 25%. In contrast, if the ascertainment is unbiased, risk for chromosomally unbalanced live birth is 1% to 2% but the risk for miscarriage or stillbirth remains at 25%.

There appears to be a parental sex influence on the risk for chromosomally unbalanced progeny associated with certain types of segregants. In general, the risk for unbalanced progeny is higher if the female parent carries the translocation than it is with the paternal carrier. In addition, a viable conceptus is influenced by type of configuration produced during meiosis by the translocated chromosomes. In general, larger translocated fragments and more asymmetrical pairing are associated with a greater likelihood for abnormal outcome of pregnancy.

ROBERTSONIAN TRANSLOCATION. Robertsonian translocations involve only *acrocentric* chromosome pairs 13, 14, 15, 21, and 22. They are joined end to end at the centromere and may be homologous (i.e., t21;21) or nonhomologous (i.e., t13;14). Robertsonian translocation is named for an insect cytogeneticist, W. R. B. Robertson, who in 1916 was the first to describe a translocation involving two acrocentric chromosomes. The Robertsonian translocation is unique because the fusion of two acrocentric chromosomes usually

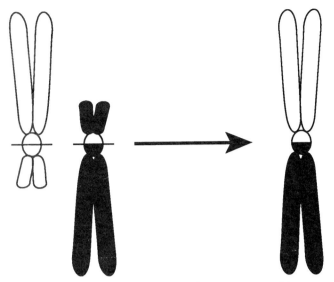

FIGURE 1-22 ■ Formation of a centric fusion (monocentric) Robertsonian translocation. Robertsonian translocations involve only the acrocentric chromosomes.

involves the centromere (see Fig. 1-22) or regions close to the centromere. However, reciprocal translocations may also include acrocentric chromosomes.

Robertsonian translocations are nearly always nonhomologous. Most homologous Robertsonian translocations produce nonviable conceptuses. For example, translocation 14;14 would result in either trisomy 14 or monosomy 14, and both are nonviable.

The most common nonhomologous Robertsonian translocation in humans is 13;14. Approximately 80% of all nonhomologous Robertsonian translocations involve chromosomes 13, 14, and 15. The next most common are translocations involving one chromosome from pairs 13, 14, and 15 and one chromosome from pairs 21 and 22.

Figure 1-23 illustrates gametogenesis in a nonhomologous 14;21 Robertsonian translocation carrier and also represents the model for segregation during gametogenesis with any Robertsonian translocation. Translocation carriers theoretically produce six types of gametes in equal proportions. Monosomic gametes are generally nonviable as are many trisomies (e.g., trisomy 14 or 15). As illustrated, three gametes may result in viable conceptuses and one (B_1) may produce a liveborn abnormal infant.

Robertsonian translocation 14;21 is the most medically significant in terms of incidence and genetic risk. In contrast, the most frequent Robertsonian translocation, 13;14, rarely produces chromosomally unbalanced progeny. Nonetheless, genetic counseling and at least consideration of prenatal diagnosis is recommended for all families with a chromosome Robertsonian or reciprocal translocation.

ISOCHROMOSOMES

An isochromosome is a structural rearrangement in which one arm of a chromosome is lost and the other arm is duplicated. The resulting chromosome is a mirror image of itself. Isochromosomes often involve the long arm of the X chromosome.

Autosomal Deletion and Duplication Syndromes

Autosomal deletions and duplications are often associated with clinically evident birth defects or milder dysmorphisms. Often the chromosomal defect is unique to that individual, and it is difficult to provide prognostic information to the family. In a few cases, a number of patients with similar phenotypic abnormalities were found to display similar cytogenetic defects. Some of these are cytogenetically detectable, whereas others are smaller and require molecular cytogenetic techniques. These are termed "microdeletion" and microduplication syndromes and merely reflect the size of the deletion or duplication. Table 1-2 summarizes some of the deletion and duplication syndromes that have been described and for which commercial FISH probes are available.

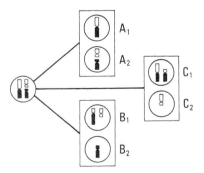

FIGURE 1-23 ■ Gametogenesis for Robertsonian translocation. A_1 is balanced with 22 chromosomes, including t (14q21q). A_2 is normal with 22 chromosomes. B_1 is abnormal with 23 chromosomes, including t(14q21q) and 21. This gamete would produce an infant with Down syndrome. B_2 is abnormal with 22 chromosomes and monosomy for chromosome 21. C_1 is abnormal with 23 chromosomes, including t(14q21q) and 14. C_2 is abnormal with 22 chromosomes and no chromosome 14.

TABLE 1-2. DIAGNOSIS OF MICRODELETION SYNDROMES

Syndrome	Chromosome Band	Chromosome Defect
Alagille	20p12.1–p11.23	Deletion
Angelman	15q11–q13	Deletion (maternal genes)
Cri du chat	5p15.2–p15.3	Deletion
DiGeorge*	22q11.21–q11.23	Deletion
Miller-Diecker	17p13.3	Deletion
Prader-Willi	15q11–q13	Deletion (paternal genes)
Rubenstein-Taybi	16p13.3	Deletion
Smith-Magenis	17p11.2	Deletion
WAGR	11p13	Deletion
Williams	7q11.23	Deletion
Wolf-Hirschhorn	4p16.3	Deletion

* Patients with velocardiofacial and *Schprinzen* (Catch 22) syndromes also have deletions at 22q11.21–q11.23.

WAGR, Wilms tumor, aniridia, genital anomalies, growth retardation.

Clinical and Biological Considerations of the Sex Chromosomes

The X and Y chromosomes merit separate discussion. They have distinct patterns of inheritance and are structurally different. However, they pair in male meiosis because of the presence of the pseudoautosomal region at the ends of the short arms of the X and Y chromosomes. The pseudoautosomal region is the only region of homology between the X and Y chromosomes, and pairing as well as recombination occur in this region.

The primitive gonad is undifferentiated, and phenotypic sex in human beings is determined by the presence or absence of the Y chromosome. This is the case for two reasons. First, in the absence of the Y chromosome, the primitive gonad will differentiate into an ovary, and female genitalia will form. Thus, the female sex is the default sex. Second, the *SRY* gene, present on the Y chromosome, is necessary and sufficient for testis formation, as well as male external genitalia.

The X chromosome is present in two copies in females but only in one copy in males. To equalize dosage differences in critical genes on the X chromosomes between the two sexes, one of the X chromosomes is randomly inactivated in somatic cells of the female (Lyon, 1961). In addition, in cells with more than two X chromosomes, all but one of them are inactivated. This ensures that in any diploid cell, regardless of sex, only a single active X chromosome is present. X inactivation results in the complete inactivation of about 90% of the genes on the X chromosome. This is noteworthy because 10% of genes on the X chromosome escape X *inactivation*. Many of these are clustered on the short arm of X, so aneuploidies involving this region may have greater clinical significance than those on the long arm. X chromosome inactivation occurs because of the presence of an X inactivation center on Xq13 that contains a gene called *XIST* that is expressed on the allele of the inactive X chromosome. At the moment, the mechanism of action of *XIST* in X chromosome inactivation is unclear.

Although X inactivation is random in normal somatic cells, structural abnormalities of the X chromosome often result in nonrandom X inactivation. In general, when a structural abnormality involves only one X chromosome (i.e., deletion, isochromosome, ring chromosome), the abnormal X chromosome always appears to be the one inactivated. If the structural abnormality is a translocation between part of one X chromosome and an autosome, the "normal" X seems to be the one genetically inactive. Although this pattern is not proven, it is assumed that if the X chromosome translocated to an autosome is genetically inactivated, part or all of that autosome might also become inactive, rendering that cell functionally monosomic for the autosome and thus nonviable. This phenomenon helps to explain why some females heterozygous for X-linked recessive biochemical disorders, such as Duchenne muscular dystrophy, have phenotypic expression of that disorder. In this instance, if the mutant X chromosome is the one involved in the X autosome translocation and the normal allele is inactive by virtue of being on the normal inactive X chromosome, it is likely that the female will express the disease.

Abnormalities of the sex chromosomes or genes on the sex chromosomes may affect any of the stages of sexual and reproductive development. Although an increased number of either the X or the Y chromosome enhances the likelihood of mental retardation and other anatomic anomalies, irrespective of the sex phenotype, aneuploidy of the sex chromosome does not alter prenatal fetal development nearly as much as aneuploidy of an autosome. Of note, a high frequency of mutations or deletions of the X chromosome do result in X-linked mental retardation. Numeric and structural sex chromosome aneuploidies are summarized in Table 1-3, and we briefly describe only a few of the more common sex chromosome aberrations.

Turner Syndrome

Although Turner syndrome occurs in approximately 1 per 10,000 liveborn females, it is one of the chromosome abnormalities most commonly observed in studies of spontaneous abortuses. It is unknown why the same chromosomal defect usually results in spontaneous fetal loss but is also compatible with survival. It is often detected prenatally through ascertainment of a cystic hygroma by fetal ultrasound examination during the second trimester. Although there is wide variability in the phenotypic expression of Turner syndrome, it represents

 TABLE 1-3. NUMERIC AND STRUCTURAL X CHROMOSOMAL ANEUPLOIDIES IN HUMANS

Karyotype	Phenotype	Approximate Frequency
XXY	Klinefelter syndrome	1 per 700 males
XXXY	Klinefelter variant	~1 per 2500 males
XXXXY	Low-grade mental deficiency; severe sexual underdevelopment; radioulnar synostosis	Rare
XXX	Sometimes mild oligophrenia; occasionally disturbances of gonadal function	1 per 1000 females
XXXX XXXXX	Physically normal; severe mental retardation	Rare
XXY/XY and XXY/XX mosaics	Klinefelter-like, sometimes milder in symptomatology	~5–25% of all "Klinefelter-like" patients
XXX/XX mosaics	Like XXX	Rare
XO	Turner syndrome	~1 per 2500 females at birth
XO/XX and XO/XXX mosaics	(Turner); very different degree of manifestation	Not uncommon
Various structural anomalies of X chromosomes		Not uncommon
XYY	Increased stature; occasional behavioral abnormalities	1 per 800 males
XXYY	Increased stature; otherwise resembling Klinefelter syndrome	Rare

From Vogel F, Motulsky AG: Human Genetics: Problems and Approaches. New York, Springer-Verlag, 1979.

one sex chromosome abnormality that should be identifiable by physical examination of the newborn.

Turner syndrome is associated with a 45,XO genotype. Sex chromosome mosaics (such as 46,XX/45,XO) and structurally abnormal genotypes (such as 46,X/delX and 46,X/isoX) are all phenotypic females like those with 45,XO Turner syndrome, but they have fewer of the typical manifestations associated with the 45,XO phenotype. The paternally derived X chromosome is more often missing in the 45,XO genotype.

Some of the common features of the 45,XO phenotype and the frequency with which they are seen are listed in Table 1-4. Mental retardation is not normally seen in this syndrome unless a small ring X chromosome is present. Although there is inadequate information at present to permit assessment of longevity and cause of death in adult life, the general health prognosis is good for childhood and young adult life with this phenotype. Renal anomalies, when present, rarely cause significant health problems, and when congenital heart disease is part of the phenotype, surgery is generally effective. The congenital lymphedema usually disappears during infancy, and when webbing of the neck poses a cosmetic problem, it may be corrected by plastic surgery. Short stature is a persistent problem. If a diagnosis is achieved early, height increase and external sexual development may be achieved, with the collaboration of a knowledgeable endocrinologist. In particular, growth hormone therapy is standard and results in significant increases in adult height. Affected patients are nearly always sterile, and the emotional adjustment to this issue should be part of any medical management of gonadal dysgenesis.

When the diagnosis of 45,XO genotype or a variant is missed during infancy or childhood, a complaint of persisting short stature or amenorrhea finally brings the patient to the physician. Often this delay precludes any specific therapy for the short stature. In rare variants of Turner syndrome, some cells may carry a Y chromosome, suggesting that such an individual was initially an X,Y male but the Y chromosome was lost. Occasionally, the Y chromosome line is found only in the germ cells, and the clinical manifestation in the individual may be virilization during adolescence or an unexplained growth spurt. In these cases, it is imperative to perform a gonadal biopsy for histologic and chromosome analysis. If a Y chromosome cell line is demonstrated in gonadal tissue, extirpation is indicated to prevent subsequent malignant transformation in gonadal cells.

Klinefelter Syndrome

Klinefelter syndrome, which occurs in approximately 1 per 700 to 1000 liveborn males, is associated with a 47,XXY genotype. Major physical features of Klinefelter syndrome are as follows:

1. Relatively tall and slim body type, with relatively long limbs (especially the legs) is seen beginning in childhood.
2. Hypogonadism is seen at puberty, with small, soft testes and usually a small penis. Infertility is the rule. Gynecomastia is frequent, and cryptorchidism or hypospadias may be seen. Lack of virilization at puberty is common; indeed, it is often the reason for the patient to seek medical attention.
3. There is a tendency toward lower verbal comprehension and poorer performance on intelligence quotient tests, with learning disabilities a common feature. There is a higher incidence of behavioral and social problems often requiring professional help.

There are several karyotypic variants of Klinefelter syndrome with more than two X chromosomes (such as the genotype 48,XXXY). As the number of X chromosomes increases, there is a corresponding increase in the severity of the phenotype, with a greater incidence of mental retardation and with more physical abnormalities than those typical of Klinefelter syndrome. Approximately 15% of individuals with some of the Klinefelter phenotype will be 47,XXY/46,XY mosaic. Such mosaic individuals have more variable phenotypes and have a somewhat better prognosis for testicular function. In general, chromosome aneuploidies that include the Y chromosome are less likely to be diagnosed clinically during infancy or childhood. In fact, individuals are often first diagnosed during evaluation for infertility.

Prevalence of Chromosome Disorders in Humans

Identifiable abnormalities in the human karyotype occur more frequently than mutations, leading to mendelian hereditary disease. Table 1-5 summarizes studies on incidence of sex chromosome and autosomal chromosomal abnormalities (Hsu, 1998).

The most common autosomal numerical disorders in liveborn humans are trisomy 21, trisomy 18, and trisomy 13. Numerous studies have shown that trisomy 21 is the most common aneuploidy among liveborn humans. On the other hand, balanced reciprocal translocations occur almost as frequently. Trisomy 13 occurs at a much lower frequency than trisomy 18 or trisomy 21, possibly because of increased fetal demise with this mutation. Among sex chromosomes, aneuploidies 45,X, 47,XYY, and 47,XXY are seen in liveborn babies.

It is noteworthy that the incidence of common chromosome abnormalities such as trisomy 21 is nearly 10 times greater than the incidence of genetic diseases such as achondroplasia, hemophilia A, and Duchenne muscular dystrophy.

TABLE 1-4. 45,XO PHENOTYPE: MAJOR FEATURES AND THEIR INCIDENCE

Feature	Incidence (%)
Small stature, often noted at birth	100
Ovarian dysgenesis with variable degree of hypoplasia of germinal elements	90+
Transient congenital lymphedema, especially notable over the dorsum of the hands and feet	80+
Shield-like, broad chest with widely spaced, inverted, and/or hypoplastic nipples	80+
Prominent auricles	80+
Low posterior hairline, giving the appearance of a short neck	80+
Webbing of posterior neck	50
Anomalies of elbow, including cubitus valgus	70
Short metacarpal and/or metatarsal	50
Narrow, hyperconvex, and/or deepset nails	70
Renal anomalies	60+
Cardiac anomalies (coarctation of the aorta in 70% of cases)	20+
Perceptive hearing loss	50

TABLE 1-5. INCIDENCE OF CHROMOSOMAL ABNORMALITIES IN NEWBORN SURVEYS

Type of Abnormality	Number	Approximate Incidence
Sex chromosome aneuploidy		
Males (43,612 newborns)		
47,XXY	45	1/1000
47,XYY	45	1/1000
Other X or Y aneuploidy	32	1/1350
Total	**122**	**1/360 male births**
Females (24,547 newborns)		
45,X	6	1/4000
47,XXX	27	1/900
Other X aneuploidy	9	1/2700
Total	**42**	**1/580 female births**
Autosomal aneuploidy (68,159 newborns)		
Trisomy 21	82	1/830
Trisomy 18	9	1/7500
Trisomy 13	3	1/22,700
Other aneuploidy	2	1/34,000
Total	**96**	**1/700 live births**
Structural abnormalities (68,159 newborns) (Sex chromosomes and autosomes)		
Balanced rearrangements		
Robertsonian	62	1/1100
Other	77	1/885
Unbalanced rearrangements		
Robertsonian	5	1/13,600
Other	38	1/1800
Total	**182**	**1/375 live births**
All chromosome abnormalities	**442**	**1/154 live births**

From Hsu LYF: Prenatal diagnosis of chromosomal abnormalities through amniocentesis. *In* Milunsky A (ed): Genetic Disorders and the Fetus, 4th ed. Baltimore, Johns Hopkins University Press, 1998, p. 179.

The cumulative data on chromosome abnormalities reveal an unanticipated finding. Chromosome analysis in newborns from several worldwide population samples shows the overall incidence of chromosome abnormalities to be 0.5% to 0.6%. In a large study series of nearly 55,000 infants, more than two thirds had no significant physical abnormality in association with these chromosomal defects, and of the one third with significant phenotype abnormalities, nearly 66% had trisomy 21.

Chromosome Abnormalities in Abortuses and Stillbirths

About 15% of pregnancies terminate in spontaneous abortions, and at least 80% of those do so in the first trimester. The incidence of chromosome abnormalities in spontaneous abortuses during the first trimester has been reported to be as high as 61.5% (Boueá et al., 1975). Table 1-6 summarizes the genotype incidence in chromosomally abnormal abortuses (Hsu, 1998). For comparison, note the incidence of chromosome abnormalities in liveborn babies (see Table 1-5). At an incidence of 19%, 45,XO is the most common chromosome abnormality found in first trimester spontaneous abortions. Comparison with the relatively low incidence of 45,XO in liveborn babies suggests that most conceptuses with this genotype are aborted spontaneously. Trisomic embryos are seen for all autosomes except chromosomes 1, 5, 11, 12, 17, and 19.

TABLE 1-6. FREQUENCY OF CHROMOSOME ABNORMALITIES IN SPONTANEOUS ABORTIONS WITH ABNORMAL KARYOTYPES

Type	Approximate Proportion of Abnormal Karyotypes
Aneuploidy	
Autosomal trisomy	0.52
Autosomal monosomy	<0.01
45,X	0.19
Triploidy	0.16
Tetraploidy	0.06
Other	0.07

Based on analysis of 8841 unselected spontaneous abortions, as summarized by Hsu LYF: Prenatal diagnosis of chromosomal abnormalities through amniocentesis. *In* Milunsky A (ed): Genetic Disorders and the Fetus, 4th ed. Baltimore, Johns Hopkins University Press, 1998, p. 179.

The studies of Creasy and colleagues (1976) and Nussbaum and colleagues (2001) offer a comparison between karyotypic abnormalities in live births and in spontaneous abortions (Table 1-7). Triploidy/tetraploidy and trisomy 16 are the most common autosomal abnormalities in spontaneous abortuses but are never seen in live births. Comparison of the overall incidence of about 1 per 830 live births for trisomy 21 with the incidence in abortuses suggests that approximately 78% of trisomy 21 conceptuses are aborted spontaneously.

Summary of Maternal-Fetal Indications for Chromosome Analysis

Among all genetic aspects of maternal-fetal medicine, chromosome mutations and clinical syndromes associated with a dysmorphic phenotype constitute the category that most often requires the physician's attention. It is worthwhile, therefore, to review indications for at least the consideration of chromo-

TABLE 1-7. OUTCOME OF 10,000 CONCEPTIONS

Outcome	Conceptions	Spontaneous Abortions No.	Spontaneous Abortions Percent	Live Births
Total	10,000	1500	15	8500
Normal chromosomes	9200	750	8	8450
Abnormal chromosomes				
Total	800	750	94	50
Triploid/tetraploid	170	170	100	—
45,X	140	139	99	1
Trisomy 16	112	112	100	—
Trisomy 18	20	19	95	1
Trisomy 21	45	35	78	10
Trisomy, other	209	208	99.5	1
47,XXY, 47,XXX, 47,XYY	19	4	21	15
Unbalanced rearrangements	27	23	85	4
Balanced rearrangements	19	3	16	16
Other	39	37	95	2

some analysis as part of the evaluation of fetus, infant, or parents. The following situations would justify chromosome analysis.

Abnormal Phenotype in a Newborn Infant

Most abnormal phenotypes in the newborn due to chromosome abnormalities reflect abnormal autosomes. The important findings that should prompt karyotyping include (1) low birth weight and/or early evidence of failure to thrive; (2) any indication of developmental delay, in particular mental retardation; (3) abnormal (dysmorphic) features of the head and face, such as microcephaly, micrognathia, and abnormalities of eyes, ears, and mouth; (4) abnormalities of the hands and feet; and (5) congenital defects of various internal organs.

A single isolated malformation or mental retardation without an associated physical malformation significantly reduces the likelihood of a chromosome abnormality. Disorders of the sex chromosomes are more likely to be associated with phenotypic ambiguity of the external genitalia and perhaps slight abnormality in growth pattern. Certainly, any newborn manifesting sexual ambiguity should undergo a chromosome analysis. In addition to helping to exclude the possibility of a life-threatening genetic disorder (e.g., adrenogenital syndrome), the identification of sex genotype by chromosome analysis will assist attending physicians in their decisions about therapy and counseling for the parents. For the infant suspected of having autosome abnormalities, in whom the chromosomal genotype is urgently needed for making decisions about the infant's care, rapid chromosome analysis can be obtained by culture of bone marrow aspirate. When a familial chromosome mutation, such as unbalanced translocation, is detected in the infant, karyotyping of other kindred is indicated.

Unexplained First-Trimester Spontaneous Abortion with No Fetal Karyotype

Usually, couples seek medical help because of recurrent first-trimester abortions, and there is no previous karyotype for aborted tissue. Many genetic centers now recommend parental karyotyping after several (usually two or three) spontaneous abortions have occurred. The likelihood of a parental genome mutation is probably greatest if the couple has already produced a child with birth defects. When a parental chromosome structural abnormality is identified, genetic counseling and prenatal fetal monitoring in all subsequent pregnancies are advised.

Stillbirth or Neonatal Death

Unless an explanation is obvious, any evaluation of a stillborn infant or a child dying in the neonatal period should include chromosome analysis. There is an approximately 10% incidence of chromosomal abnormalities in such individuals, compared with less than 1% for liveborn infants surviving the neonatal period. The likelihood of finding a chromosome mutation is increased significantly if intrauterine growth retardation or phenotypic birth defects are present.

Fertility Problems

In women presenting with amenorrhea and couples presenting with a history of infertility or spontaneous abortion, the incidence of chromosomal defects is between 3% and 6%.

Neoplasia

All cancers present with some element of genomic instability, and specific chromosomal defects are often pathopneumonic of certain specific cancers, especially hematologic malignancies.

Pregnancy in a Woman of Advanced Age

There is an increased risk of chromosomal abnormalities in fetuses conceived in women older than 30 to 35 years. A karyotypic analysis of the fetus is part of routine care in such pregnancies.

■ PATTERNS OF INHERITANCE

Single-gene traits are those inherited from a single locus. They segregate based on two fundamental laws of genetics in diploid organisms established by Gregor Mendel using garden peas in 1857. These two laws are *segregation* (Fig. 1-24A) and *independent assortment* (Fig. 1-24B). In medical genetics, *mendelian disorders* refer to single-gene phenotypes that segregate distinctly within families and generally occur in the proportions noted by Mendel in his experiments. Specific phenotypic or genotypic traits are inherited in distinct fashions, depending on whether the responsible gene is on the X chromosome or an autosome and whether one or two copies of a gene are necessary for a phenotype. A phenotype is *dominant* if it is expressed when present on only one chromosome of a pair, whereas *recessive* traits are expressed only when present on both chromosomes. A purely dominant trait has the same

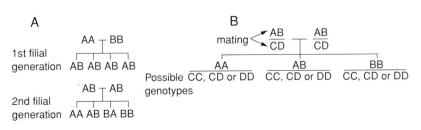

FIGURE 1-24 ■ Mendel's first and second laws. **A**, With A and B representing alleles at the same locus, a mating of homozygous A and homozygous B individuals results in heterozygotes for A and B in each offspring. Mating of heterozygotes A,B results in the 1-2-1 segregation ratio in offspring. **B**, The segregation of genotypes for A and B at locus 1 is independent of the segregation of alleles C and D at locus 2. (From Kelly TE: Clinical Genetics and Genetic Counseling. Chicago, Year Book Medical Publishers, 1980.)

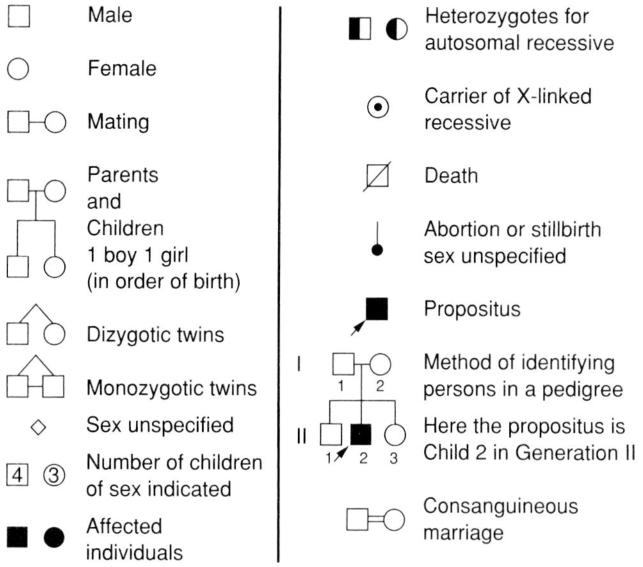

Male

Female

Mating

Parents and Children 1 boy 1 girl (in order of birth)

Dizygotic twins

Monozygotic twins

◇ Sex unspecified

Number of children of sex indicated

Affected individuals

Heterozygotes for autosomal recessive

Carrier of X-linked recessive

Death

Abortion or stillbirth sex unspecified

Propositus

Method of identifying persons in a pedigree

Here the propositus is Child 2 in Generation II

Consanguineous marriage

FIGURE 1-25 ■ Symbols commonly used in pedigree charts. (From Thompson MW: Thompson and Thompson's Genetics in Medicine, 4th ed. Philadelphia, WB Saunders, 1986.)

phenotype when present on either one or two chromosome pairs. However, if a phenotype is expressed when present as a single copy but is expressed more strongly when present on two chromosomes, the trait is *codominant*. Victor McKusick's catalog of single-gene phenotypes and mendelian disorders (McKusick, 1998) is now available online (OMIM, see Table 1-1) and is an indispensable reference for human genetic traits and disorders.

Virtually any aspect of genetic evaluation requires development of a pedigree: a graphic representation of family history data. Figure 1-25 illustrates some of the symbols useful in this process. This aspect of data gathering serves several functions:

1. It assists the determination of transmission for the gene expression in question (recessive, dominant, sex-linked, or autosomal).
2. There is a greater likelihood that all possible genetic issues will be included in the data gathering when a formal pedigree chart is assembled.
3. When consanguinity is present, the pedigree chart helps to relate the consanguinity to individuals in subsequent generations who are expressing the phenotype of a particular inheritable disorder.

Autosomal Dominant Mode of Inheritance

In autosomal dominant inheritance, the disease is expressed in the heterozygote and the probability of transmitting the gene to progeny is 50% with each pregnancy.

The pedigree in Figure 1-26 demonstrates the features of inheritance of an autosomal dominant disease: gene expression in each generation, approximately half of the offspring affected (both males and females), and father-to-son transmission.

Criteria for Autosomal Dominant Inheritance

The criteria for autosomal dominant inheritance may be summarized as follows:

1. Expression of the gene rarely skips a generation.
2. Affected individuals, if reproductively fit, transmit the gene expression to progeny with a probability of 50%.
3. The sexes are affected equally, and there is father-to-son transmission.
4. A person in the kindred at risk who is not affected will not transmit the gene to progeny.

Other Characteristics

Other characteristics, although not exclusive properties of autosomal dominant disease, seem to be associated with this group of diseases more frequently.

VARIABLE EXPRESSIVITY

Variable expressivity refers to the degree of severity of expression of a trait and is commonly seen in kindreds with autosomal dominant traits. In neurofibromatosis, for example, a kindred may have a range of phenotypic expression in affected individuals, from some cafe au lait spots with a few tumors to extensive cafe au lait spots with massive neurofibromata.

PENETRANCE

Penetrance refers to whether or not there is any recognition of phenotypic expression of a particular mutant allele. If a gene is fully penetrant, it is always expressed as part of the genome of that individual. On the other hand, if a gene displays incomplete penetrance, not all individuals with that gene display any recognizable phenotype. For example, in the autosomal dominant form of retinoblastoma, the mutant gene is only 80% penetrant. This means that a person who receives the gene for retinoblastoma from a parent has a 20% chance that the gene will not be expressed by the usual identifiable means.

Penetrance may also be influenced by the means available to detect expression of the gene. For example, in autosomal dominant hypercholesterolemia, a myocardial infarct (a manifestation of gene expression and penetrance) may not appear until well into adult life. In this disorder, there is a laboratory test for gene expression, namely the serum cholesterol level, which becomes elevated quite early in life, well before the first chest pain of angina pectoris.

FIGURE 1-26 ■ Stereotype pedigree of autosomal dominant inheritance. Half the offspring of affected persons (7 of 14) are affected. The condition is transmitted only by affected family members, never by unaffected ones. Equal numbers of males and females are affected. Male-to-male transmission is seen. (From Thompson MW: Thompson and Thompson's Genetics in Medicine, 4th ed. Philadelphia, WB Saunders, 1986.)

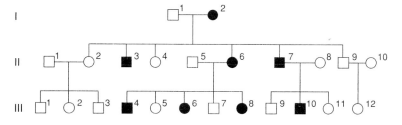

NEW MUTATIONS

It is not uncommon for an autosomal dominant disorder to become manifest for the first time in a kindred as a new mutation. New mutations are also seen with sex-linked recessive disorders. For example, in a form of autosomal dominant dwarfism called achondroplasia, nearly 80% of individuals represent new mutations. When this phenomenon can be identified with certainty, parents may be reassured that the recurrence risk is probably no greater than that for the general population. The recurrence risk for offspring of the affected "new mutant" is 50%. New mutations for autosomal dominant diseases appear to be related to paternal age.

Autosomal Recessive Mode of Inheritance

For autosomal recessive diseases, mutant genes are expressed only in homozygous individuals. Consanguinity often is a clue for autosomal inheritance when the specific gene mutation has not been identified. A pedigree consistent with autosomal recessive inheritance is shown in Figure 1-27. Primary features consistent with autosomal recessive inheritance may be summarized as follows:

1. Both males and females are affected.
2. Unless consanguinity or random selection of heterozygous matings in each generation occurs, mutant gene expression may appear to skip generations, in contrast to autosomal dominant inheritance, which rarely skips generations.
3. Parents are usually unaffected, but unaffected sibs of affected homozygotes may be heterozygous carriers. Affected individuals rarely have affected children.
4. Subsequent to identification of a propositus, the recurrence risk for homozygous affected progeny in each subsequent pregnancy is one chance in four.
5. If the incidence of the disorder is rare, consanguineous parentage is often seen.

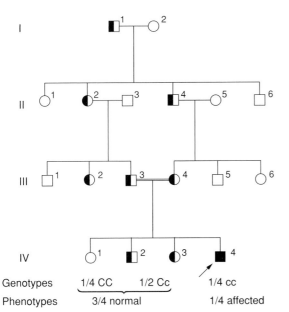

Genotypes   1/4 CC   1/2 Cc   1/4 cc
             └── 3/4 normal ──┘   1/4 affected
Phenotypes

FIGURE 1-27 ■ Stereotype pedigree of autosomal recessive inheritance, including a cousin marriage. A gene from a common ancestor I-1 has been transmitted down two lines of descent to "meet itself" in IV-4. (From Thompson MW: Thompson and Thompson's Genetics in Medicine, 4th ed. Philadelphia, WB Saunders, 1986.)

Sex-Linked Mode of Inheritance

In this instance, *sex-linked* refers to inheritance from the X chromosome. For this group of genetic diseases, the male is considered to be hemizygous in relation to X-linked genes, whereas females are almost always heterozygous. However, because of patterns of X inactivation, females of some X-linked disorders may be more mildly affected than males with the same disorder.

Hemophilia A is among the best-known X-linked recessive diseases. For illustrative purposes, we shall use the symbol Xh to represent the recessive allele for hemophilia A on the X chromosome and XH to represent the normal or dominant allele. The diagrams in Figure 1-28 demonstrate progeny genotypes in matings between affected males and normal females as well as matings between normal males and heterozygous phenotypically normal females. When the father is affected, all sons will be normal and all daughters will be heterozygous carriers and phenotypically normal (Fig. 1-28A). In the other mating cross, each daughter will have a 50% chance of being normal and a 50% chance of being a heterozygous carrier that is phenotypically normal (Fig. 1-28B). Each son will have a 50% chance of being normal and a 50% chance of being affected.

Characteristics of X-linked recessive inheritance may be summarized as follows:

1. A higher incidence of the disorder is noted in males than in females.
2. The mutant gene expression is never transmitted directly from father to son.
3. The mutant gene is transmitted from an affected male to all his daughters.
4. The trait is transmitted through a series of carrier females, and affected males in a kindred are related to one another through the females.
5. For sporadic cases, there is an increase in the age of the maternal grandfather at which he fathered the mother of an affected child—similar to the increase in paternal age for certain new dominant mutations.

In contrast to X-linked recessive inheritance, X-linked dominant disorders are nearly twice as common in females as in males (Fig. 1-29). For example, none of the sons of a male affected with vitamin D–resistant rickets is affected, but all his daughters receive the mutant gene from him, and because the mutant is dominant, they all have the disease. A female with one X-linked mutant dominant allele will have the disease, and the transmission to her progeny, assuming a hemizygous normal mate, will be indistinguishable from that seen in autosomal dominant inheritance. As a group, the X-linked dominant disorders are relatively uncommon. Vitamin D–resistant rickets (hypophosphatemia) is one, and the X-linked blood group X is another.

The distinguishing features of X-linked dominant inheritance are summarized as follows:

1. All daughters of affected males have the disorder, but no sons are affected.
2. Heterozygous affected females transmit the mutant allele at a rate of 50% to progeny of both sexes. If the affected female is homozygous, all her children will be affected.
3. The incidence of X-linked dominant disease may be twice as common in females as in males.

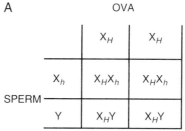

A   OVA

	X_H	X_H
X_h	$X_H X_h$	$X_H X_h$
Y	$X_H Y$	$X_H Y$

SPERM

Daughters: 100 percent heterozygotes
Sons: 100 percent normal

B   OVA

	X_H	X_h
X_H	$X_H X_H$	$X_H X_h$
Y	$X_H Y$	$X_h Y$

SPERM

Daughters: 50 percent normal, 50 percent carriers
Sons: 50 percent normal, 50 percent affected

FIGURE 1-28 ■ Sex-linked recessive inheritance patterns. See text. (From Thompson MW: Thompson and Thompson's Genetics in Medicine, 4th ed. Philadelphia, WB Saunders, 1986.)

Some rare disorders that are exclusively or nearly exclusively seen in females, such as Rett syndrome and incontinentia pigmenti type 2, appear to be X-linked dominant conditions in which affected males die before birth.

Multifactorial Inheritance

In this age of genes and genomes, we should remember that not everything that runs in families is genetic and not everything that is genetic runs in families. Environmental and sociologic factors such as diet, age at first pregnancy, socioeconomic level, access to health care, and other environmental conditions often segregate in families along with the genes. An excellent example is the occurrence in families of cholera or tuberculosis. Although susceptibility to infectious diseases may be under some form of genetic control, the susceptibility of a family to these diseases is likely the result of unsanitary conditions (cholera) or chromic exposure (tuberculosis). On the other hand, some genetic disorders are sufficiently devastating that they are rarely if ever transmitted between generations, and most cases occur as *de novo* mutations. Examples of genetic disorders for which many patients have no family history include chromosomal abnormalities such as Down syndrome;

contiguous gene syndromes such as Prader-Willi, Angelman, or Smith-Magenis syndromes; and single-gene disorders for which one copy of the gene is not enough (called *haploinsufficiency*) such as neurofibromatosis type I. On the other hand, many common disorders have both genetic and nongenetic components to their etiology. A clinician who might encounter either familial clusters or rare genetic disorders should be familiar with the concepts used to distinguish genetic from nongenetic transmission.

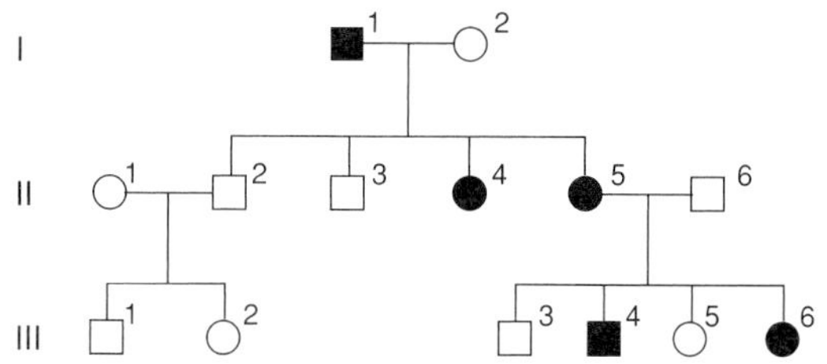

Heritability

A measure of the genetic contribution to disease is *heritability*, which is the amount of phenotypic variation explained by genes relative to the total amount of variation. A more detailed treatment of statistical estimates of heritability can be found in texts devoted to genetic analysis (Hartl and Clark, 1997; Ott, 1999). High heritability does not imply the action of a single gene. Monogenic, oligogenic, and polygenic disorders are distinguished. A disease with high heritability may also be inherited in different families through different genes. A disease caused by any of several mutations in the same gene is said to show allelic heterogeneity. A disease caused by changes in any of several different genes is said to show locus heterogeneity. Disease caused by environmental factors that mimic a genetic disorder is said to phenocopy that disorder.

Recurrence Risk

One common statistical measure used to estimate heritability is the *recurrence risk* to family members of an index case or proband. This is often expressed as the ratio of risk to a first-degree relative divided by the risk in the general population. Recurrence risk to full siblings is a common measure, but depending on the structure of available patient populations first cousin, grandparent/grandchild, and other comparisons have been used.

FIGURE 1-29 ■ Stereotype pedigree of X-linked dominant inheritance. Affected males have no sons and no normal daughters. (From Thompson MW: Thompson and Thompson's Genetics in Medicine, 4th ed. Philadelphia, WB Saunders, 1986.)

Twin Studies

Twin studies are often extremely valuable in distinguishing effects of shared genes from effects of shared environment, particularly for diseases with complex etiology. A genetic component to a trait or disease can be seen as a difference in recurrence risk or concordance rate between monozygotic twins (derived from a single fertilization event and therefore genetically identical) and dizygotic twins (derived by independent fertilization of two eggs released in the same cycle and therefore sharing half of their genes). All twins generally share both prenatal and postnatal environments. Monozygotic twins also share all their genetic complement, but dizygotic twins share only half of theirs. Any substantial difference in concordance rate (or recurrence risk) between monozygotic and dizygotic twins as a group is taken as evidence of a genetic component.

Complex Inheritance

Many common disorders show complex inheritance. Allergy, asthma, autism, cleft lip and palate, diabetes, dizygotic twinning, handedness, hypertension, multiple sclerosis, neural tube defects, and schizophrenia are all examples of such complex traits with population frequencies above 1%. Some complex disorders have rare single-gene (monogenic) forms, but most cases have more complex etiology. Complex disorders will include examples of polygenic inheritance, in which several genes contribute to the disease in the absence of environmental effects, and multifactorial inheritance, in which genes and environment interact to produce disease. In practice, a complex trait may have monogenic, polygenic, and multifactorial forms. Although such etiologic heterogeneity makes identification of the underlying genes (and environmental risk factors) more difficult, several characteristic features help to identify disorders with complex inheritance.

Complex inheritance may involve either *quantitative traits* or *qualitative traits*. In a quantitative trait, each causal gene or nongenetic factor contributes incrementally to a measurable outcome, such as height, body mass index, or age at onset of disease. A qualitative trait has alternative outcomes that are either nonquantitative in nature or very imprecisely quantified in practice; each causal gene contributes to meeting a threshold for expression of the trait or to the probability of expressing the trait, such as susceptibility to disease. Note that these modes are not completely distinct: Susceptibility genes may act quantitatively on the probability of disease for each individual, but clinical outcome may be qualitative as the presence or absence of disease. Disease genes may also act additively to reach a qualitative threshold for disease and beyond threshold contribute to increased severity of disease. Stratifying patients by subphenotypes or risk factors may simplify the inheritance patterns of some complex traits.

Genes that underlie complex traits have been extremely difficult to identify. However, the recent availability of new methods of linkage analysis and high-throughput genotyping, public availability of a nearly complete human genome sequence, and the prospect of genome-wide association studies, together with improved repositories of clinical and family data and samples, are fueling renewed interest and optimism in disorders. We should expect to see much progress in identifying such genes over the next several years. This places additional importance on the ability of practicing doctors to identify clinical presentations and families that fit particular inheritance patterns.

CHARACTERISTIC FEATURES OF COMPLEX TRAITS

REGRESSION TO THE MEAN. Because complex traits involve the inheritance (or environmental presence) of many factors, offspring from extreme individuals tend to be less extreme than the parents or regress to the mean of the population. Independent assortment in meiosis results in different combinations of genes being passed to offspring and changing environments result in different factors being experienced by the offspring. Using a familiar example of a nondisease trait, very tall parents will have taller than average children, but in general children of the tallest parents will not inherit all of the "tall factors" that the parents have.

HERITABILITY. Complex traits have heritability estimates over a wide range. They are by definition less heritable than fully penetrant monogenic traits but more heritable than would be expected by chance alone. The range of heritability reflects the varying degree to which genes determine the outcome of each trait. The higher the ratio of recurrence risk to a family member to risk in the general population (or the higher the ratio of monozygotic twin concordance to dizygotic twin concordance), the more genetically tractable the disease will likely be.

THRESHOLD TRAITS. The rate of development can determine outcome in a *threshold trait*. The idea of a threshold trait is that if a developmental event does not happen by a specified time in development (a developmental threshold), then a malformation or other phenotype will occur. Developmental rates are generally determined by a combination of genetic and environmental factors.

PENETRANCE, PROBABILITY, AND SEVERITY. The likelihood of having the disorder or trait, given the right genotype, is called the *penetrance*. For simple mendelian disorders penetrance may be at or near 100%. For traits with environmental cofactors or developmental threshold effects, the penetrance can be much lower. For some disorders, the penetrance (in terms of either likelihood or severity of the disorder) is part of the pattern of inheritance within a family. Affected relatives of a severely affected proband are likely to be more severely affected than the average case. This is the other side of regression to the mean: Returning to our nondisease example, the children of very tall parents may not be as tall as their parents but will likely be taller than average. Taking a disease example, if a liveborn infant has unilateral cleft lip, the recurrence risk to future siblings is 2.5%, but for a liveborn infant with bilateral cleft lip and palate, the recurrence risk is 6%.

INCREASED RISK ACROSS DIAGNOSTIC CATEGORIES. Another frequent feature of complex inheritance is that relatives of the proband may be at increased risk for related diagnostic categories. This has been suggested for categories of psychiatric illness, for some autoimmune disorders, and for some malformation syndromes. The implication of this is that overlapping sets of genes and environmental factors can lead to dysfunctions that present as related clinical entities.

RARER FORMS SHOW INCREASED RELATIVE RISK. Forms of multifactorial disease that are less frequent in the general population tend to have higher recurrence risk ratios for families of an affected proband. For example, pyloric stenosis is five times more common in males than females in the general population. As Table 1-8 shows, male relatives of any proband face

TABLE 1-8. RECURRENCE RISK OF PYLORIC STENOSIS FOR FIRST-DEGREE RELATIVES

	Risk (%)	General Population Risk
Male relatives of male patients	4.6	×10
Female relatives of male patients	2.6	×25
Male relatives of female patients	18.2	×35
Female relatives of female patients	8.1	×80

From Kelly TE: Clinical Genetics and Genetic Counseling. Copyright © 1980 by Year Book Medical Publishers, Chicago. Reproduced with permission.

a higher risk than their sisters, but relatives of female probands face much higher risk than relatives of male probands.

Common Disorders with Multifactorial Inheritance

CLEFT LIP AND CLEFT PALATE

The malformation of cleft lip may occur with or without cleft palate (orofacial cleft) but is etiologically distinct from cleft palate alone (Fraser, 1970). These common malformations occur in more than 200 described human syndromes (McKusick, 2002), including several single-gene disorders, chromosomal abnormalities, and syndromes of teratogen exposure (including thalidomide). Developmentally, cleft lip with or without cleft palate results from a failure in the fusion of the frontal prominence with the maxillary process at about 7 weeks of fetal development. Incidence is two- to fourfold higher in males than females and varies among ethnogeographic groups: 0.4 per 1000 births in African Americans, 1 per 1000 births in whites, and 1.7 per 1000 births in Japanese. However, the recurrence risk to first-degree relatives is lower in Japan than in Europe, suggesting a higher environmental influence in Japan (Koguchi, 1975). Within a population, the recurrence risk varies with the severity of defect in the proband, as noted previously. Examples are shown in Table 1-9.

CLEFT PALATE

In cleft palate without cleft lip, the secondary palate fails to fuse. The general incidence is approximately 1 in 2500 and is more common in females than males. Little ethnic variation is noted, and the recurrence risk is approximately 2%.

NEURAL TUBE DEFECTS

This group of malformations is of special importance because of the possibility of mid-trimester prenatal diagnosis and current considerations for prenatal screening of these disorders in all pregnancies. Expression of neural tube defects can be highly variable among individuals, ranging from anencephaly at one extreme to lumbar meningocele with little or no neurologic impairment at the other. The spectrum includes encephalocele, iniencephaly, meningomyelocele (usually involving the lower thoracic and lumbar spine and often called spina bifida cystica), and spina bifida. Defects arise through failure of the embryonic neural tube to close within 28 days from conception. The incidence in European-derived populations can vary substantially. For example, the overall incidence in the British Isles is 4.5 to 5.0 per 1000 births but has been as high as 7.8 per 1000 in Ireland, Scotland, and Wales. The

overall U.S. incidence is 1.5 to 2.0 per 1000 but is lower for individuals of African or Asian ancestry. Recurrence risks for anencephaly and spina bifida probands are shown in Table 1-9. Epidemiologic and experimental animal studies have suggested that neural tube defects have characteristics of threshold traits as well as substantial environmental factors. Among environmental influences on neural tube defects, recent attention has been paid to the importance of dietary folate in preventing neural tube defects, and preliminary work has suggested inositol as another potential factor (Copp, 1998; Beemster et al., 2002; Cavalli and Copp 2002).

PYLORIC STENOSIS

Pyloric stenosis is the most common disorder requiring corrective surgery in infants, with an incidence of 1 to 5 per 1000 live births. Heritability is inferred from the high recurrence risk to relatives. Males are at higher risk than females, irrespective of family history, but the ratio of recurrence risk to general risk is higher in females (see Table 1-8). Mitchell and Risch (1993) concluded that family studies were inconsistent with a single major locus causing pyloric stenosis and set model-based limits for the effect of any single locus at no more than a fivefold increase in recurrence risk. Evidence from patient material (Subramaniam et al., 2001) and targeted mutations in mice (Huang et al., 1993; Gyurko et al., 2002) suggest that neuronal nitric oxide synthase may be one genetic locus for some instances of pyloric stenosis.

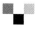

TABLE 1-9. EXAMPLES OF RECURRENCE RISKS FOR CLEFT LIP WITH OR WITHOUT CLEFT PALATE AND NEURAL TUBE MALFORMATIONS

Family History	Risk for Cleft Lip ± Cleft Palate (%)	Risk for Anencephaly and Spina Bifida (%)
No sibs affected		
Neither parent affected	0.1	0.3
One parent affected	3.0	4.5
Both parents affected	34.0	30.0
One sib affected		
Neither parent affected	3.0	4.0
One parent affected	11.0	12.0
Both parents affected	40.0	38.0
Two sibs affected		
Neither parent affected	9.0	10.0
One parent affected	19.0	20.0
Both parents affected	45.0	43.0
One sib and one second-degree relative affected		
Neither parent affected	6.0	7.0
One parent affected	16.0	18.0
Both parents affected	43.0	42.0
One sib and one third-degree relative affected		
Neither parent affected	4.0	5.5
One parent affected	14.0	16.0
Both parents affected	44.0	42.0

Adapted from Thompson MW: Thompson and Thompson's Genetics in Medicine, 4th ed. Philadelphia, WB Saunders, 1986: Based on data from Bonaiti-Pellié C: Risk tables for genetic counselling in some common congenital malformations. J Med Gene **11:**374, 1974.

CELIAC DISEASE

Autoimmune reaction in celiac disease causes inflammatory injury to the mucosa of the small intestine, resulting in malabsorption. Once thought uncommon, celiac disease (or gluten-sensitive enteropathy) is now thought to affect as many as 1 in 120 to 1 in 300 people in Europe and North America. Several factors point to multifactorial inheritance. Recurrence risk to siblings is 10% or higher. Concordance rates for monozygotic twins is more than fourfold higher than for dizygotic twins (Greco et al., 2002). Exposure to wheat gluten (or other grains, such as rye and barley) are environmental factors. Genetic linkage to human leukocyte antigen and non–human leukocyte antigen genetic effects have been reported, although studies in different populations suggest linkage to different genetic loci in addition to human leukocyte antigen (Zhong et al., 1996; Greco et al., 2001; Liu et al., 2002).

INFLAMMATORY BOWEL DISEASE (CROHN DISEASE)

Genetic components of autoimmune disease directed against the gastrointestinal tract have also been mapped for findings of Crohn disease and ulcerative colitis. Together these somewhat overlapping diagnoses occur in 2 to 3 people per 1000 in the United States. Genetic effects of at least eight distinct "*IBD*" loci have been identified in this complex trait, including linkage to the human leukocyte antigen region of chromosome 6p. As an interesting example of molecular analysis in a complex trait, Rioux and coworkers (2001) mapped one locus on chromosome 5q, *IBD5*, to a cluster of inflammatory cytokine genes; several of the genes in this interval were polymorphic between patients and population control subjects, but causality for any one gene could not be determined because of strong linkage disequilibrium across the implicated region.

HIRSCHSPRUNG DISEASE

Congenital megacolon caused by lack of enteric ganglia along the intestine is a relatively well-studied complex genetic trait. Both dominant and recessive forms are known, and penetrance is variable. Several single-gene mutations associated with varying penetrance for Hirschsprung disease have been identified that illuminate biochemical pathways with unique importance for the establishment of enteric ganglia. Aganglionic megacolon also occurs within more complicated disorders, including cartilage-hair hypoplasia, Smith-Lemli-Opitz syndrome type II, and primary central hypoventilation syndrome. Variations in the *RET* oncogene are a major finding in human Hirschsprung patients, and mutations in endothelin 3, endothelin receptor B, glial-derived neurotrophic factor, and the transcriptional regulator *SOX10* have been identified in both human and animal studies. Most recently, an exhaustive search for genetic linkage implicated two additional loci (whose molecular nature is not yet known) that act as oligogenic determinants of the expression of mild *RET* alleles (Gabriel et al., 2002).

CONGENITAL HEART DEFECTS

The overall incidence of congenital heart disease is 5 to 7 live births per 1000 and is the leading cause of death from birth defects (Hoess et al., 2002). These defects are heterogeneous and caused by single-gene defects, chromosomal abnormalities (trisomy 21), and teratogens such as rubella and maternal diabetes. Table 1-10, abstracted from Nora (1968), summarizes the empiric recurrence risk for six common con-

TABLE 1-10. FREQUENCY OF SIX COMMON CONGENITAL HEART DEFECTS IN SIBS OF PROBANDS

Anomaly	Frequency in Sibs (%)*	Expected Frequency (%)†
Ventricular septal defect	4.3	4.2
Patent ductus arteriosus	3.2	2.9
Tetralogy of Fallot	2.2	2.6
Atrial septal defect	3.2	2.6
Pulmonary stenosis	2.9	2.6
Aortic stenosis	2.6	2.1

* Data from Nora JJ: Multifactorial inheritance hypothesis for the etiology of congenital heart disease: The genetic-environmental interaction. Circulation **38**:604, 1968.
†$\sqrt{p}$, where p is the population frequency of the specific defect.

From Thompson MW: Thompson and Thompson's Genetics in Medicine, 4th ed. Philadelphia, WB Saunders, 1986.

genital heart defects. Heart malformations associated with chromosomal abnormalities often show different presentations for the same cytologic findings; allelic heterogeneity at some single-gene loci may also account for some diversity in clinical findings.

Mitochondrial Inheritance

Mutations in mitochondria produce unique patterns of inheritance. All mitochondria inherited at conception come from the mother, termed *matrilineal* inheritance. Mitochondria are the only organelles in animal cells that carry their own DNA (mitochondrial DNA [mtDNA]). Human mitochondria contain a circular genome of 16,571 base pairs that encodes just 37 genes (GenBank reference sequence NC_001807). In contrast to nuclear genes, which are present in two copies per diploid cell, the mitochondrial genome is present once per mitochondrion and therefore in a variable number of copies per cell. mtDNA is subject to a relatively high rate of mutation, perhaps because of the generation of free radicals during energy production. Mutations in mtDNA create a mixture of normal and mutant mitochondria, called *heteroplasmy*. At cell division, mitochondria segregate randomly to the two daughter cells. This *replicative segregation* can ultimately result in a cell lineage inheriting only mutant mtDNA (*homoplasmy*). Segregation of either inherited or *de novo* mtDNA mutations among cell lineages can also result in a mosaic pattern across tissues of a single individual.

Phenotypic expression of mitochondrial mutations depends on the extent of heteroplasmy, the cell type involved, and the fraction of the cell type affected. Organ systems most frequently affected by mitochondrial mutations are those with high energy requirements, particularly muscle and brain. Mutations that reduce energy production by mitochondria may produce disease whenever energy production capacity falls below a threshold level. This may be episodic if the energy threshold is only crossed during exertion or other stressors. Leiber optic atrophy is perhaps the best-known example of inherited disease caused by mutations in mtDNA. Mitochondrial myopathy (a complex including neurodegeneration, pigmentary retinopathy, and Leigh syndrome), MERRF disease (myoclonic epilepsy with ragged red fibers), MELAS (mitochondrial encephalomyopathy, lactic acidosis, and stroke-like episodes), and hypertrophic cardiomyopathy are also attributable to mutations in mtDNA. Most of these are not identifiable at birth but become evident with age as later onset maternally inherited disorders.

DYNAMIC MUTATIONS AND TRINUCLEOTIDE REPEATS

Repetitive DNA sequences can give rise to mutations through a variety of mechanisms. Repeats of two, three, or four nucleotides are prone to changes in repeat length. The mutation rate depends on repeat length of the starting allele, genomic context, and other factors. Small changes in repeat length alleles have been attributed to "slippage" of the DNA polymerase (or more probably the DNA fragment) during replication. Much larger changes in repeat length are more likely due to unequal crossing over during meiosis (Warren, 1997). Alleles that can change within a pedigree are said to be dynamic. Dynamic mutations can show other unusual features of inheritance. "Premutation alleles" are those that are expanded sufficiently to be highly dynamic but are not disease causing. Disease alleles are themselves dynamic and if transmitted may give rise to alleles with more severe phenotypes and earlier onset. This is called *anticipation*. Most dynamic mutations seen in humans thus far are caused by instability of *trinucleotide repeats*, specifically CAG repeats encoding polyglutamine in the protein and other trinucleotides in noncoding sequences that alter expression of the encoded products.

Expanded polyglutamine repeats cause neurodegenerative disorders that have several features in common. These disorders show dominant inheritance, mature onset, and neurologic symptoms that include motor signs. Examples include Huntington disease (HD), several forms of spinocerebellar ataxia, dentatorubropallidoluysian atrophy, and spinobulbar muscular atrophy. Although these disorders typically have mature onset, age at onset varies inversely with the length of repeat, and extremely rare childhood Huntington disease patients have been reported as young as 2 years of age. Expanded polyglutamine-containing proteins have been shown to be cytotoxic in several experimental contexts. The interpretation of these disorders is that expanded polyglutamine destabilizes protein structure and that the misfolded protein, often found in insoluble aggregates, impairs cell function and ultimately leads to cell death. For a given repeat length, toxicity increases with solubility (Watase et al., 2002), which favors a surface area model for toxicity (Floyd and Hamilton, 1999).

Amplification of other amino acid homopolymers can also be associated with disease, including some evident at birth. An amplified GCG repeat encoding polyalanine in the poly(A)-binding protein gene (*PABPN1*) is associated with autosomal dominant oculopharyngeal muscular dystrophy, also apparently through a toxic gain-of-function mechanism (Brais et al., 1998). Nondynamic amplification of polyalanine (including each of the alanine codons) in the homeobox gene *HOXD13* causes synpolydactyly, and the severity of phenotypes correlates with the extent of amplification (Muragaki et al., 1996; Goodman et al., 1997). Expanded polyalanine in another homeobox gene, *ARX*, results in an X-linked infantile spasm syndrome equivalent to that seen by inactivating mutations of the same gene and recessive in female carriers, suggesting that in at least one example polyalanine expansions may act by inactivating the protein rather than through gain of toxicity. Interestingly, all six polyalanine expansions associated with human disease to date have been nucleic acid–binding proteins.

Trinucleotide repeat expansions in noncoding sequences can also cause disease by altering gene expression. One example is Friedreich ataxia, an autosomal recessive neurologic disorder with juvenile onset. The most common form is caused by loss-of-function alleles of the *FRDA* (*frataxin*) gene. The most frequent class of *FRDA* allele in patients is expansion of a GAA repeat in an intron of the gene, accounting for 98% of mutant alleles (Delatycki et al., 1999). Extremely long repeats induce an epigenetic loss of expression of that copy of the gene. GAA expansion alleles and rare protein-inactivating alleles have roughly the same effect on gene function. Another example of mutation caused a noncoding repeat expansion is fragile X syndrome (which includes mental retardation, macroorchidism, and facial dysmorphology). The most frequent cause of fragile X syndrome is expansion of a CGG repeat in the 5' untranslated region of the *FMR1* gene. CpG dinucleotides are targets for methylation (Bird, 1992), and DNA of the expanded allele is hypermethylated compared with both normal and premutation (stable intermediate length repeat) alleles. Hypermethylation in or near transcriptional control elements results in loss of *FMR1* expression of the expanded allele in affected males. Expanded CGG alleles are equivalent to isolated cases hemizygous for missense and splice site mutations, confirming that this repeat expansion acts as a loss-of-function allele. Autosomal dominant myotonic dystrophy (MD1) is a third example. Expansion of a CTG trinucleotide repeat in the 3' untranslated region of the *DMPK* protein kinase gene is strongly correlated with the disease and shows anticipation in families; however, the pathogenic mechanism remains unclear.

Imprinting

Besides the modes of inheritance already discussed, several atypical patterns of inheritance have been described. We discuss one of these patterns, called *imprinting*. Although most genes seem to have equivalent expression from alleles inherited from the father and the mother, it is now known that the expression of several genes differs from the parental alleles. This phenomenon has been termed genomic imprinting, because it appears that the two parental alleles are distinguished by some sort of mark. It appears that this mark is a reversible form of chromatin modification, perhaps methylation of one of the parental alleles, that occurs during gametogenesis and before fertilization. The mark then suppresses expression of this allele after conception. This mark is reversible in the germline, so that the parent of origin mark can be placed anew during gametogenesis (Tilghman, 1999).

Prader-Willi and Angelman syndromes are good examples of the phenotypic effects of imprinting. Prader-Willi syndrome is characterized by neonatal hypotonia, childhood obesity with excessive eating, small hands and feet, hypogonadism, and mild mental retardation. Angelman syndrome is characterized by severe mental retardation, seizures, a characteristic spastic movement disorder, and an abnormal facial appearance. Although it is now known that these syndromes are caused by different genes, both syndromes can result from deletions of the same region of chromosome 15q11-q13. In about 70% of the time, Prader-Willi syndrome results from the deletion of this region inherited from the father, so they have only the maternal copy of this region. Strikingly, in about 70% of cases of Angelman syndrome, the same region is deleted and inherited from the mother, so they have only the paternal copy of this region.

Several rare disorders have now been attributed to imprinting effects. At this point, it is unclear if imprinting is an important factor in more common disorders, but it is likely that imprinting is involved in several human genetic disorders.

GENETIC TESTING AND DNA DIAGNOSTICS

The realization in the 1980s that DNA variations, or polymorphisms, between individuals occur fairly frequently led to the development of both DNA forensics and molecular diagnostics for genetic disorders and risk factors (Botstein et al., 1980). DNA diagnostics in medicine can use either *direct* assays for a specific mutation or *linkage analysis* with polymorphisms linked to a disease locus. Direct assays for specific mutations are most useful when a relatively small number of distinct mutations account for most patients with a particular form of disease. As analysis methods become faster, cheaper, and more highly automated, performing direct tests on each nucleotide of a disease gene without knowing will become increasingly practical, particularly for genes in which a high proportion of patients have *de novo* mutations. Indirect assays by linkage analysis (Fig. 1-30) have traditionally been most useful for risk assessment when a disease gene has been mapped in pedigrees but not yet identified at the molecular level. Linkage analysis requires cooperation of other family members, usually including at least one affected member, to identify markers alleles on the disease-associated chromosome in that particular pedigree. Recombination between the marker and the disease gene is a potential caveat if a single marker is used; use of markers on each side of the disease gene at least makes this evident, and the likelihood of recombination can be built into the risk assessment. In practice, linkage assays for identified disease gene becomes a smaller clinical need as a higher proportion of

significant disease genes can be assayed directly. However, linkage analysis and family studies remain crucial to the successful identification of disease and disease susceptibility genes.

The initial molecular diagnostics to come out of the recombinant DNA revolution were based on restriction fragment length polymorphisms (RFLPs, see Fig. 1-30). RFLPs are typically assayed by Southern blotting (Southern, 1975), which requires substantial amounts of DNA, and are relatively labor intensive and difficult to automate, making them relatively expensive. This approach is still used to identify large repeat expansions for genes known to be subject to dynamic mutations. Development of the polymerase chain reaction (PCR) by Mullis and coworkers in the mid-1980s allowed selective amplification of any desired sequence of DNA and radically changed the power of DNA diagnostics in terms of sample requirements and in terms of the kinds of assays one could perform (Mullis and Faloona, 1987). Linkage markers in current use include simple sequence repeat length polymorphisms (SSLPs, or microsatellites) and, increasingly, biallelic SNPs. SNPs in particular have the advantage of being assayable in multiplex formats, such that many distinct polymorphic sites may be interrogated in a single biochemical reaction. Several different technologies for SNP detection have been and continue to be developed to allow simultaneous detection of larger numbers of loci at smaller marginal cost.

Methods Used in Genetic Testing

Hybridization-Based Methods

Nucleic acid hybridization is a simple physical chemical process with well-described parameters (Wetmur and Davidson, 1968; Wetmur, 1976) and forms the basis for a wide variety of molecular genetic tests. The rate and stability of nucleic acid duplexes depend on the concentration of each strand, temperature, ionic strength of the solution, and the presence of hydrogen bond competitors like urea and formamide. Tests based on whole-genome Southern blots were among the first available for mutations with no cytologic correlate. As discussed earlier, hybridization of fluorescently labeled probes to fixed chromosomal spreads (FISH, spectral karyotyping) allow the identification of microdeletions, microduplications, translocations, and other cytologic abnormalities that would be difficult to detect without molecular probes. Other methods include hybridization of patient DNA to allele-specific oligonucleotides to discriminate single base changes. An example of detection by allele-specific oligonucleotides is given in the reverse dot-blot analysis shown in Figure 1-31. In a reverse dot-blot analysis, the probe sequence is bound to the support matrix while the amplified patient sample is labeled and hybridized to the oligonucleotides; using this approach, a patient sample can be tested for several mutations in a single assay.

Southern blotting is used to detect variations in size or amount of a defined DNA fragment (Fig. 1-32). To produce the defined fragments from whole genomic DNA, *restriction endonuclease* enzymes are used to cut intact DNA at specific sites. Restriction enzymes occur in bacteria where they form part of the host defense against bacterial viruses. Different bacterial species produce enzymes that recognize and cleave DNA at different sites. Each restriction enzyme cuts DNA at a defined sequence, usually a palindrome 4 to 8 base pairs

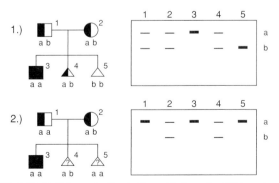

FIGURE 1-30 ■ Schematic illustration of linkage by DNA probe analysis of restriction fragment length polymorphisms (RFLPs). *Left,* Pedigree for two families. The darkened symbols represent heterozygosity or homozygosity for the disease gene. Members tested are listed numerically. *Open triangles* represent fetuses in putative pregnancies. (a) and (b) represent DNA restriction fragment lengths. *Right,* Gel electrophoresis patterns for RFLPs. (Modified from Emery AEH: An Introduction to Recombinant DNA. New York, John Wiley & Sons, 1980.)

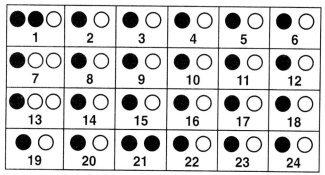

FIGURE 1-31 ■ Reverse dot-blot analysis for cystic fibrosis (CF) mutations. Twenty-seven CF mutations were analyzed in this study. The complete panel in this figure represents a single filter, subdivided into 24 sections. Each section is numbered for specific mutation analysis. Sections 1, 7, and 13 analyze two separate mutations. Circles on the left in each numbered section contain normal oligonucleotide sequences from the CF gene region on chromosome 7. The sequences in each section represent different regions on the gene where a mutation has been identified. Thus, complementary normal sequences, amplified by polymerase chain reaction (PCR), hybridize as indicated by the *dark circles*. The *open circles* represent effort at hybridization between mutant sequences fixed to the filter and DNA sequences obtained from the patient and amplified by PCR. If the patient does not have a CF mutation among the group of 27 in this analysis, there is no hybridization and the circle remains open. In this analysis, sections 1 and 21 demonstrate that this patient has two CF mutations and would be designated a compound heterozygote. This individual most likely would have clinical manifestations of CF.

in length. For example, *Eco*RI cuts the palindromic site 5'-GAATTC-3' between the G and the A:

$$5'\text{-GAATTC-}3' \rightarrow 5'\text{-G} \qquad \text{AATTC-}3'$$
$$3'\text{-CTTAAG-}5' \qquad 3'\text{-CTTAA} \qquad \text{G-}5'$$

After digestion with restriction enzymes, DNA is size fractionated by gel electrophoresis (moving through a gel matrix that retards larger fragments more than smaller fragments as they move in response to an electric field). DNA is then denatured into single strands by hydroxide and then transferred (blotted) from the gel to a membrane capable of binding the DNA, usually nitrocellulose or derivitized nylon. Single-stranded DNA on the membrane is then available for hybridization by base pairing with a "probe" sequence. The probe is labeled with either a radionuclide (usually ^{32}P) or chemical (biotin, digoxigenin, or fluorescein) tag for detection. After hybridization and removal of excess probe, the hybrid fragments are detected by film autoradiography for ^{32}P probes or antibody conjugate-based methods (chemiluminescence or chromatogenic reactions). By quantifying the radiologic signal from a Southern blot, it is also possible to assess the *copy number* of the DNA fragment in the genome relative to known standards. Southern blots have been used to detect insertions and deletions that change the length of the restriction fragment, sequence changes that affect a specific restriction site, and duplications and deficiencies that change the copy number of the fragment.

Polymerase Chain Reaction

Amplification of DNA segments through PCR revolutionized DNA diagnostics for both medicine and forensics beginning in the mid-1980s (Saiki et al., 1985, 1986, 1988;

Mullis et al., 1986). Synthetic oligonucleotides are used to prime DNA synthesis such that synthesis directed from each primer includes the sequence complementary to the other primer (Fig. 1-33). Multiple cycles of DNA denaturation, primer annealing, and elongation of DNA synthesis create an exponential amplification of the DNA sequence between the two primers. The phases of this cycle are controlled by temperature. Using PCR to amplify specific DNA fragments, multiple diagnostic tests can be performed on minimal amounts of starting material.

Variations in length, such as occur in dynamic mutations, can be assayed directly by PCR amplification followed by gel electrophoresis to determine the size of the PCR product. For example, diagnostic tests for expanded alleles are available for dentatorubropallidoluysian atrophy, Huntington disease, and

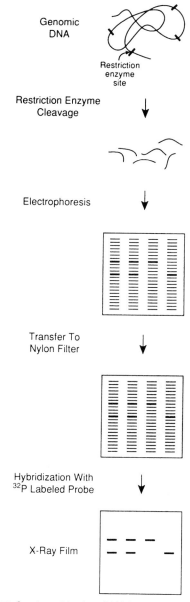

Genomic DNA

Restriction enzyme site

Restriction Enzyme Cleavage

Electrophoresis

Transfer To Nylon Filter

Hybridization With ^{32}P **Labeled Probe**

X-Ray Film

FIGURE 1-32 ■ Southern blotting. DNA is cleaved by a restriction enzyme, separated according to size by agarose gel electrophoresis, and transferred to a filter. After hybridization of the DNA to a labeled probe and exposure of the filter to x-ray film, complementary sequences can be identified.

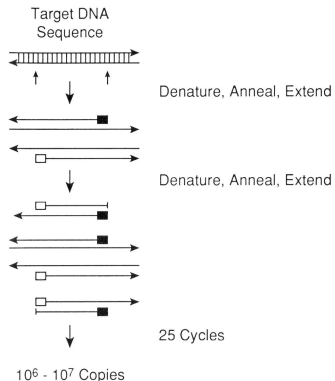

Target DNA
Sequence

Denature, Anneal, Extend

Denature, Anneal, Extend

25 Cycles

10^6 - 10^7 Copies
of Target Sequence

FIGURE 1-33 ■ Polymerase chain reaction (PCR). Repeated synthesis of a specific target DNA sequence (*upper arrows*) results in exponential amplification. The reaction proceeds from the primers (□, ■) in the 3′ direction on each strand. The first two cycles of the PCR are shown.

fragile X syndrome that are based on determining the size of the allele by amplification of patient DNA using oligonucleotide primers that flank the site of expansion.

Anonymous marker loci, such as SSLPs, can be assayed in the same way for gene mapping and forensic studies. More recently, SNPs are amplified singly or in a multiplex combination of loci and detected by electrophoretic, hybridization, or spectroscopic methods. SNP-based assays are expected to have increasing clinical impact in coming years because they allow highly parallel analysis. *Multiplex* PCR amplifications can allow parallel analysis of many genetic loci simultaneously.

Common mutations can also be assayed by PCR using primers specific for each allele or by allele-specific oligonucleotide hybridization. For genes in which no single mutation is common among patients, such as the hereditary hearing loss gene *JGB2*, novel sequence variations can be identified by direct DNA sequencing of PCR products from that gene.

DNA Sequencing

Modern genetics, and clinical diagnostics in particular, rely heavily on knowing the exact sequence of nucleotides in genes. Methods to identify sequences of small RNA molecules first began to appear in the late 1960s. However, the appearance of two methods for DNA sequencing of longer fragments in 1977 was a major breakthrough. The *chemical cleavage method* (Maxam and Gilbert, 1977) uses base-specific chemistries to cleave a

specified base from its sugar, followed by a second reaction to cleave the phosphodiester bond adjacent to the resulting abasic site. The *chain termination method* (Sanger et al., 1977) uses enzymatic synthesis of DNA in the presence of dideoxynucleotides; dideoxynucleotides prevent further synthesis beyond their site of incorporation because they lack the 3′ hydroxyl group (see Fig. 1-1). The chain termination method is by far the most widely used today. It has been further developed to include fluorescent labels for automated detection and thermostable polymerase enzymes to allow multiple cycles of DNA synthesis for each template molecule. An important extension of this approach for diagnostics is the use of single nucleotide extension products (termed *mini-sequencing*) to determine alleles based on a single nucleotide change without the added labor and expense of a gel or capillary electrophoresis. For example, tests for hereditary hemochromatosis use a version of mini-sequencing called *pyrosequencing* to detect the C282Y mutation and the H63D and S65C alleles of the *HFE* gene.

Other Considerations

Current technology is quite powerful and still developing. Vanishingly small specimens can now be used to query ever expanding numbers of known genes and anonymous DNA markers. Future developments seem likely to continue this trend toward making molecular genetic tests faster, less expensive, and more reliable. This technologic facility and the link between diagnostics and forensics raises numerous ethical, legal, and social issues (often referred to as ELSI). In current practice, one needs to pay particular attention to informed consent, restrictions on use of clinical material in research, and what has been termed genetic privacy. These issues are beyond the scope of this chapter but are as vital to the practitioner who requests genetic testing as they are to the practitioner in the diagnostic laboratory.

Linkage Analysis

Linkage analysis uses DNA polymorphisms as markers to follow the inheritance of a gene within a family. This approach is used to identify unknown genes that contribute to disease and to follow disease-associated chromosomal segments in affected families before pinpointing the causal mutation. Linkage analysis takes advantage of meiotic recombination by counting how frequently two loci are inherited together. By comparing the inheritance of a disease with inheritance of alleles at several known DNA polymorphisms (*marker* loci), it is possible to map the positions of disease genes. Theoretically, any single-gene disorder should be amenable to carrier identification and prenatal diagnosis by linkage analysis once the gene is mapped.

DNA polymorphisms are codominantly inherited, meaning each allele carried by an individual should be detected in a well-designed assay. Several kinds of DNA polymorphisms are frequent in the human genome and have been used in linkage studies.

RFLPs arise through insertions (often of mobile repetitive elements, such as Alu), deletions, and base changes at restriction sites (particularly through deamination of C residues in CG dinucleotides). Assays for RFLP markers by Southern blotting are described previously. RFLPs that have diagnostic importance are usually either converted to a PCR-based assay for the underlying sequence change or replaced for diagnostic use by a linked polymorphism that is more easily assayed.

Insertions and deletions occur frequently in the human genome. These range from one to thousands of base pairs and arise by multiple mechanisms. Small insertion/deletion polymorphisms most likely occur through errors in DNA replication and repair, and the rate of new mutation is probably sensitive to environmental exposures. Larger insertions and deletions arise through several mechanisms, including retrotransposition (such as for Alu repeat sequences) and illegitimate recombination at sites of sequence homology (a frequent finding in microdeletion syndromes). Insertions and deletions were initially detected as RFLPs by Southern blotting. Now *indel* polymorphisms are usually detected using PCR-based methods designed to be compatible with detecting either simple sequence length repeats of SNPs.

Variable number tandem repeats are more polymorphic than RFLPs and can occur in several alleles, varying by the number of repeat copies present at the locus. Variable number tandem repeats can be detected by Southern blot more sensitively than RFLPs because multiple copies are present. Some variable number tandem repeats are small enough to be assayed by PCR and can be used along with other PCR-based markers.

SSLPs (also called short tandem repeats, simple sequence repeats, or microsatellites) are simple repeats of two, three, or four nucleotides (such as CACACACACA). Like variable number tandem repeats, SSLPs can have several possible alleles. The spontaneous mutation rate to a new allele size ranges from 10^{-3} to 10^{-6}. This high mutation rate makes microsatellites useful as markers for genetic mapping: They mutate frequently enough to be highly polymorphic in a population but are stable enough to be transmitted reliably in a pedigree. Simple sequence repeats (microsatellites) occur approximately every 30 kilobases in the human genome (depending on the repeat length threshold one sets), and a high proportion are polymorphic to some extent across human populations. These markers are easily assayed on a moderate scale but still must be resolved by electrophoresis. Although this is practicable for a modest scale, such as diagnostics for linkage to a mapped but still unknown disease mutation segregating within a family, and has been used for genome-wide scans for genetic linkage, identifying the correct size of each allele is the most significant bottleneck for applications requiring very high throughput with many markers.

SNPs are by far the most frequent class of polymorphism in the human genome. On average, any two copies of the human genome will have a polymorphism approximately every 1000 base pairs. Millions of SNPs have been cataloged across the human genome (Sachidanandam et al., 2001). On a small scale, these polymorphisms can be detected using the direct analysis methods described for detecting specific mutations. However, for large linkage studies, the number of single genotypes that must be generated is quite large, and higher throughput methods have been and continue to be developed. Competing methods for large-scale genotyping include variations on allele-specific PCR that allow detection by hybridization, highly parallel allele-specific oligonucleotides hybridization on high-density oligonucleotide arrays produced by photolithography (Wang et al., 1998), and mini-sequencing detected by mass spectroscopy (Tang et al., 1999). These recently developed methods will impact DNA diagnostics in both the discovery of new genes involved in disease and in parallel testing for multiple disorders.

Identifying New Disease Genes

Linkage data to identify new disease genes are analyzed by computer algorithms to assess their statistical significance. Although many linkage analysis packages are available, a recurrent question arises with respect to the statistical threshold for declaring linkage. As pointed out by Lander and Kruglyak (1995), each genome scan is really a series of discreet hypotheses. Statistical thresholds must be set to account for the number of hypotheses tested. Lander and Kruglyak argue that in the current era, the number of hypotheses that must be accounted for in linkage studies is a function of genome size, as one could (and does) continue testing markers until the genome is covered. They suggested using statistical thresholds based on the likelihood of false-positive findings in a complete genome linkage scan (genome-wide significance) rather than in a discrete test of any one specific locus (point-wise significance). Computer simulations in the absence of linkage and permutation testing of real linkage data support the idea that genome-wide significance levels are needed to minimize reporting of false-positive findings.

Association and Linkage Disequilibrium

A related concept to linkage analysis is genetic association. In this study design, case and control samples are compared for alleles at each locus to ask whether one or more alleles is significantly overrepresented (disease-associated alleles) or underrepresented (protective alleles) in disease cases. One of the best studied examples of genetic association is the increased risk of late-onset Alzheimer's disease for individuals with certain alleles of the apolipoprotein E gene (Corder et al., 1993; Roses, 1996). The amino acid variants encoded by the E4 allele of *APOE* are thought to be directly responsible for the increased risk. However, a strong association of a polymorphism with disease does not necessarily mean that the polymorphism causes the disease, although it does provide immediate diagnostic value. Associations that are not causal occur by *linkage disequilibrium*. Linkage disequilibrium essentially means that specific alleles at two loci are inherited together throughout a population. This occurs when the genetic distance between the loci is small compared with the number of generations in which the two alleles could have separated by recombination in that population. Association studies that take best advantage of population-based linkage disequilibrium may provide the next opportunity to discover genes that act in multifactorial and genetically heterogeneous diseases. Current efforts in this area include both maps of human DNA polymorphisms (Sachidanandam et al., 2001) and maps of regions co-inherited by linkage disequilibrium in the general population (Gabriel et al., 2002).

IMPACT OF THE HUMAN GENOME PROJECT AND GENOMICS

In 2001, a draft of the human genome was published simultaneously by the publicly funded Human Genome Project (Lander et al., 2001) and a private company, Celera (Venter et al., 2001). Both groups had covered approximately 90% of the genome, and, as discussed previously, estimates of the number of genes had ranged from 30,000 to 40,000 human genes in these first published studies (Lander et al., 2001; Venter et al., 2001) to substantially higher estimates (Liang et al., 2000; Hogenesch et al., 2001). As we have noted, in 2003 the complete human sequence should be available from the Human Genome Project, and a number of public consortia and private companies are determining the variations in DNA sequences over populations by cataloging SNPs. As discussed in the introduction to this chapter, these tremendous advances have already had a profound impact on biomedical research. It is the consensus that this research will revolutionize our approach to diagnosis and treatment of human disease over the next decade and beyond, especially with respect to the identification of genetic risk factors for some of the most common disorders today, including cancer, hypertension, coronary artery disease, diabetes, susceptibility to infectious diseases, and obesity. Certainly, diagnostic testing by methods outlined in this chapter will be improved with this information. It is difficult to estimate when these advances will make their way into clinical practice, although others have ventured to gaze into the future (Collins and McKusick, 2001).

CONCLUSION

As noted in the beginning of this chapter, genetics plays an important role in the day-to-day practice of obstetrics and gynecology. We have summarized the basic concepts of genetics as they apply to the understanding and treatment of human diseases and have emphasized those areas most pertinent to the practice of obstetrics and gynecology. Increasingly, clinical genetics will become one of the disciplines physicians will be expected to use for the care of their patients. The expanding knowledge gained through research in molecular biology and molecular genetics, along with the use of genetic information provided by the Human Genome Project and genomics, will provide new information necessary for physicians to formulating new clinical approaches to medical diagnostics and therapeutics.

■ A C K N O W L E D G M E N T S

We acknowledge the contributions of the authors of the previous edition of this book, O. W. Jones and T. C. Cahill, for the organization and many of the figures and tables used in the present chapter. We also thank Dr. Karen Arden for providing the spectral karyotyping image (see Fig. 1-14).

R E F E R E N C E S

Beemster P, Groenen P, Steegers-Theunissen R: Involvement of inositol in reproduction. Nutr Rev **60**:80, 2002.

Bird A: The essentials of DNA methylation. Cell **70**:5, 1992.

Botstein D, White RL, Skolnick EM, et al: Construction of a genetic linkage map in man using restriction fragment length polymorphisms. Am J Hum Genet **32**:314, 1980.

Boueá J, Boueá A, Lazar P: Retrospective and prospective epidemiological studies of 1500 karyotyped spontaneous human abortions. Teratology **12**:11, 1975.

Brais B, Bouchard JP, Xie YG, et al: Short GCG expansions in the PABP2 gene cause oculopharyngeal muscular dystrophy. Nat Genet **18**:164, 1998.

Bresch C, Hausmann R: Klassiche und Moleculare Genetik, 3rd ed. Berlin, Springer-Verlag, 1972.

Brown TR, Lubahn DB, Wilson EM, et al: Deletion of the steroid-binding domain of the human androgen receptor gene in one family with complete androgen insensitivity syndrome: evidence for further genetic heterogeneity in this syndrome. Proc Natl Acad Sci USA **85**:8151, 1988.

Cavalli P, Copp AJ: Inositol and folate resistant neural tube defects. J Med Genet **39**:E5, 2002.

Collins FS, McKusick VA: Implications of the Human Genome Project for medical science. JAMA **285**:540, 2001.

Copp AJ: Prevention of neural tube defects: vitamins, enzymes and genes. Curr Opin Neurol **11**:97, 1998.

Corder EH, Saunders AM, Strittmatter WJ, et al: Gene dose of apolipoprotein E type 4 allele and the risk of Alzheimer's disease in late onset families. Science **261**:921, 1993.

Creasy MR, Crolla JA, Alberman ED: A cytogenetic study of human spontaneous abortions using banding techniques. Hum Genet **31**:177, 1976.

Delatycki MB, Knight M, Koenig M, et al.: G130V, a common FRDA point mutation, appears to have arisen from a common founder. Hum Genet **105**:343, 1999.

Floyd JA, Hamilton BA: Intranuclear inclusions and the ubiquitin-proteasome pathway: digestion of a red herring? Neuron **24**:765, 1999.

Fraser FC: The genetics of cleft lip and cleft palate. Am J Hum Genet **22**:336, 1970.

Gabriel SB, Salomon R, Pelet A, et al: Segregation at three loci explains familial and population risk in Hirschsprung disease. Nat Genet **31**:89, 2002.

Gabriel SB, Schaffner SF, Nguyen H, et al: The structure of haplotype blocks in the human genome. Science **23**:23, 2002.

Goodman FR, Mundlos S, Muragaki Y, et al: Synpolydactyly phenotypes correlate with size of expansions in HOXD13 polyalanine tract. Proc Natl Acad Sci USA **94**:7458, 1997.

Greco L, Babron MC, Corazza GR, et al: Existence of a genetic risk factor on chromosome 5q in Italian coeliac disease families. Ann Hum Genet **65**:35, 2001.

Greco L, Romino R, Coto I, et al: The first large population based twin study of coeliac disease. Gut **50**:624, 2002.

Gyurko R, Leupen S, Huang PL: Deletion of exon 6 of the neuronal nitric oxide synthase gene in mice results in hypogonadism and infertility. Endocrinology **143**:2767, 2002.

Hartl DL, Clark AG: Principles of Population Genetics. Sunderland, MA, Sinauer Associates, 1997, p. 542.

Hassold TJ: A cytogenetic study of repeated spontaneous abortions. Am J Hum Genet **32**:723, 1980.

Hoess K, Goldmuntz E, Pyeritz RE: Genetic counseling for congenital heart disease: New approaches for a new decade. Curr Cardiol Rep **4**:68, 2002.

Hogenesch JB, Ching KA, Batalov S, et al: A comparison of the Celera and Ensembl predicted gene sets reveals little overlap in novel genes. Cell **106**:413, 2001.

Hsu LYF: Prenatal diagnosis of chromosomal abnormalities through amniocentesis. *In* Milunsky A (ed): Genetic Disorders in the Fetus, 4th ed. Baltimore, Johns Hopkins University Press, 1998, p. 179.

Huang PL, Dawson TM, Bredt DS, et al: Targeted disruption of the neuronal nitric oxide synthase gene. Cell **75**:1273, 1993.

ISCN: Report of the Standing Committee of Human Cytogenetic Nomenclature. Basel, Karger, 1995.

Koguchi H: Recurrence rate in offspring and siblings of patients with cleft lip and/or cleft palate. Jinrui Idengaku Zasshi **20**:207, 1975.

Lamson SH, Hook EB: A simple function for maternal-age-specific rates of Down syndrome in the 20- to 49-year age range and its biological implications. Am J Hum Genet **32**:743, 1980.

Lander E, Kruglyak L: Genetic dissection of complex traits: guidelines for interpreting and reporting linkage results. Nat Genet **11**:241, 1995.

Lander ES, Linton LM, Birren B, et al: Initial sequencing and analysis of the human genome. Nature **409**:860, 2001.

La Spada AR, Wilson EM, Lubahn DB, et al: Androgen receptor gene mutations in X-linked spinal and bulbar muscular atrophy. Nature **352**:77, 1991.

Liang F, Holt I, Pertea G, et al: Gene index analysis of the human genome estimates approximately 120,000 genes. Nat Genet **25**:239, 2000.

Liu J, Juo SH, Holopainen P, et al: Genomewide linkage analysis of celiac disease in Finnish families. Am J Hum Genet **70**:51, 2002.

Lyon MF: Gene action in the X-chromosome of the mouse (*Mus musculus* L). Nature **190**:372, 1961.

Maxam AM, Gilbert W: A new method of sequencing DNA. Proc Natl Acad Sci USA **74**:560, 1977.

McKusick VA: Mendelian Inheritance in Man, 12th ed. Baltimore, Johns Hopkins University Press, 1998.

McKusick VA: Online. Mendelian Inheritance in Man (National Center for Biotechnology Information). Available at *http://www.ncbi.nlm.nih.gov/entrez/query.fcgi?db=OMIM*. Accessed 2002.

Mitchell LE, Risch N: The genetics of infantile hypertrophic pyloric stenosis. A reanalysis. Am J Dis Child **147:**1203, 1993.

Mullis KB, Faloona F: Specific synthesis of DNA in vitro via a polymerase-catalyzed chain reaction. Methods Enzymol **155:**335, 1987.

Mullis K, Faloona F, Scharf S, et al: Specific enzymatic amplification of DNA in vitro: the polymerase chain reaction. Cold Spring Harb Symp Quant Biol **51:**263, 1986.

Muragaki Y, Mundlos S, Upton J, et al: Altered growth and branching patterns in synpolydactyly caused by mutations in HOXD13. Science **272:**548, 1996.

Nora JJ: Multifactorial inheritance hypothesis for the etiology of congenital heart diseases: The genetic-environmental interaction. Circulation **38:**604, 1968.

Nussbaum RL, McInnes RR, Willard HF: Thompson and Thompson Genetics in Medicine, 6th ed. Philadelphia, WB Saunders, 2001.

Ott J: Analysis of Human Genetic Linkage, 3rd ed. Baltimore, Johns Hopkins University Press, 1999.

Rioux JD, Daly MJ, Silverberg MS, et al: Genetic variation in the 5q31 cytokine gene cluster confers susceptibility to Crohn disease. Nat Genet **29:**223, 2001.

Roses AD: Apolipoprotein E alleles as risk factors in Alzheimer's disease. Annu Rev Med **47:**387, 1996.

Sachidanandam R, Weissman D, Schmidt SC, et al: A map of human genome sequence variation containing 1.42 million single nucleotide polymorphisms. Nature **409:**928, 2001.

Saiki RK, Bugawan TL, Horn GT, et al: Analysis of enzymatically amplified β-globin and HLA-DQα DNA with allele-specific oligonucleotide probes. Nature **324:**163, 1986.

Saiki RK, Gelfand DH, Stoffel S, et al: Primer-directed enzymatic amplification of DNA with a thermostable DNA polymerase. Science **239:**487, 1988.

Saiki RK, Scharf S, Faloona F, et al: Enzymatic amplification of β-globin genomic sequences and restriction site analysis for diagnosis of sickle cell anemia. Science **230:**1350, 1985.

Sanger F, Nicklen S, Coulson AR: DNA sequencing with chain-terminating inhibitors. Proc Natl Acad Sci USA **74:**5463, 1977.

Southern EM: Detection of specific sequences among DNA fragments separated by gel electrophoresis. J Mol Biol **98:**503, 1975.

Subramaniam R, Doig CM, Moore L: Nitric oxide synthase is absent in only a subset of cases of pyloric stenosis. J Pediatr Surg **36:**616, 2001.

Tang K, Fu DJ, Julien D, et al: Chip-based genotyping by mass spectrometry. Proc Natl Acad Sci USA **96:**10016, 1999.

Tilghman SM: The sins of the fathers and mothers: Genomic imprinting in mammalian development. Cell **96(2):**185, 1999.

Venter JC, Adams MD, Myers EW, et al: The sequence of the human genome. Science **291:**1304, 2001.

Vogel F, Motulsky AG: Human Genetics: Problems and Approaches. New York, Springer-Verlag, 1979.

Vogel F, Rathenberg R: Spontaneous mutation in man. Adv Hum Genet **5:**223, 1975.

Wang DG, Fan JB, Siao CJ, et al.: Large-scale identification, mapping, and genotyping of single-nucleotide polymorphisms in the human genome. Science **280:**1077, 1998.

Warren ST: Polyalanine expansion in synpolydactyly might result from unequal crossing-over of HOXD13. Science **275:**408, 1997.

Watase K, Weeber EJ, Xu B, et al: A long CAG repeat in the mouse Sca1 locus replicates SCA1 features and reveals the impact of protein solubility on selective neurodegeneration. Neuron **34:**905, 2002.

Wetmur JG: Hybridization and renaturation kinetics of nucleic acids. Annu Rev Biophys Bioeng **5:**337, 1976.

Wetmur JG, Davidson N: Kinetics of renaturation of DNA. J Mol Biol **31:**349, 1968.

Zhong F, McCombs CC, Olson JM, et al: An autosomal screen for genes that predispose to celiac disease in the western counties of Ireland. Nat Genet **14:**329, 1996.

Chapter 2
NORMAL EARLY DEVELOPMENT

Kurt Benirschke, MD

The developing fertilized ovum enters the uterine cavity on about the 4th day after fertilization. The first differentiation of a human ovum into embryonic and future placental cells occurred in a 58-cell morula described by Hertig (1968). The specimen was 6 days old and had five embryonic cells (the "inner cell mass," or "stem cells"), and 53 trophoblastic cells constituted the wall of this uterine blastocyst. The polar bodies and an apparently degenerating zona pellucida were still present in the specimen, features destined to be lost shortly before implantation.

Proliferation of the trophoblastic shell after this stage of development is rapid, and a segmentation cavity develops, with the more slowly reproducing embryonic cells assuming a marginal "polar" position. The adjacent trophoblastic cells enlarge and secure implantation, which is assumed to take place on the 6th day after fertilization, although such a human specimen has not yet been described. With the very rapid enlargement occurring in the anchoring trophoblastic cells, the endometrial cells are dissociated by mechanisms discussed in this chapter. The entire blastocyst thus assumes an "interstitial" position (i.e., it sinks entirely into the endometrium at the site of attachment). The process may well be aided by the collapse of the blastocyst cavity that occurs at this time. Through this invasive activity, the blastocyst collapses, and through the deposition of fibrin or occasionally a coagulum at the site of penetration, the implanted trophoblastic shell comes to be surrounded by endometrium (decidua) on all sides. Perhaps some endometrial proliferation at the edges seals the defect.

The portion of decidua lying between blastocyst and myometrium is the *decidua basalis*; the portion covering the defect is the *decidua capsularis*. Eventually, the latter comes to lie on the outside of the placental membranes. The decidua of the opposite side of the uterus is the *decidua vera*. At the time of implantation (day 6), the 0.1-mm blastocyst can be detected only by a dissecting microscope. Within a few days, however, it will constitute a polypoid protrusion that can be detected readily by careful inspection of the endometrium. Thus, the approximately 14-day-old ovum (Figs. 2-1 and 2-2) appeared to be a polyp.

Occasionally, a small blood clot is attached to its surface, the *Schlusskoagulum*, whose presence may be detected clinically by spotting (Hartman sign) and may lead to misinterpretation of the length of gestation. Decidual hemorrhages and small areas of necrosis at the site of trophoblastic penetration are common at this time and later.

MACROSCOPIC DEVELOPMENT

In most recorded sites of early implantation, the ovum was found in the upper portion of the fundus. More recently, it has been possible to follow the development of the placenta by ultrasonographic techniques. Thus, Rizos and colleagues (1979) found the 16-week placenta to be attached anteriorly in 37% of patients, posteriorly in 24%, in a fundal position in 34%, and both anteriorly and posteriorly in 4%. Others have used sonography to measure placenta size and volume prenatally and have correlated their findings with fetal outcome (Hoogland et al., 1980). Of interest in this context is the finding from sonographic study that low implantation of the placenta in the uterus occurs frequently, with the formation of an apparent placenta previa. Moreover, a low implantation may change through differential growth of the placenta and uterus and apparent marginal placental atrophy, so that at term the situation does not clinically resemble placenta previa (King, 1973). In the report of Rizos and colleagues, only 5 of 47 patients in whom placenta previa was diagnosed with ultrasound between 16 and 18 weeks actually had this condition when delivery occurred at term. These findings are important in the interpretation of the shape of the placenta at term and necessitate revision of former impressions.

Most commonly, the placenta develops at the uterine fundus. Through rapid expansion of the extraembryonic cavity (the exocoelom) and proliferation of the trophoblastic shell, the ovum bulges into the endometrial cavity at the time of the first missed menstrual period. The surface is flecked by tiny hemorrhages and necrotic decidua. With continued expansion of the embryonic cavity, the surface bulges into the endometrial cavity and becomes attenuated. The peripheral villi atrophy and the future placental "membranes" form. They consist of decidua capsularis on the outside, hyalinized villi and trophoblast in the middle, and the membranous chorion laeve (and amnion) on the inside.

The relationship of these membranes to the remainder of the uterus was sequentially traced in numerous pregnant uteri in a series collected by Boyd and coworkers (1970). Their observations suggested that the membranes truly fuse with the decidua vera of the side opposite to implantation in the 4th month of pregnancy, thereby obliterating the endometrial cavity. The decidua capsularis appeared to degenerate in their specimens before this time, and what is present on the outside of the term-delivered placenta was construed to be decidua vera attached to chorion. With the atrophy of peripheral villi

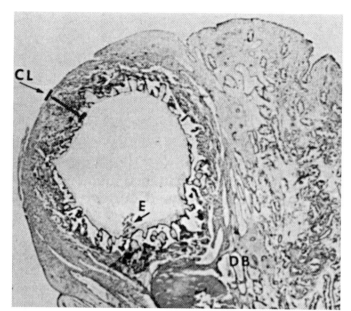

FIGURE 2-1. ■ Implanted human embryo of approximately 14 days' gestational age. The implantation site projects into the endometrial cavity. Villi are just beginning to form. The secretory endometrium is undergoing decidualization. CL, chorion laeve; DB, decidua basalis; E, embryo. H&E, ×16.

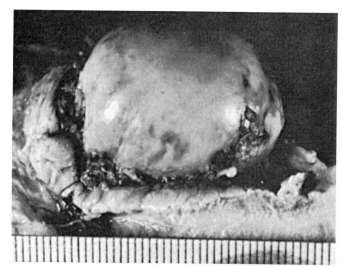

FIGURE 2-3. ■ Endometrium with 7-week pregnancy. Note protuberance of flattened membrane projecting into endometrial cavity. (Courtesy of Dr. Jirasek, Prague.)

and attachment of the membranes to the opposite side of the uterus, the macroscopic delineation of the placenta is essentially completed. Next, the formation of amnion, yolk sac, and body stalk is described.

Figures 2-3 to 2-5 demonstrate the developing placenta and embryo at 7 weeks with an embryonic crown–rump length of 15 mm; the width of the entire specimen is approximately 25 mm. Through the "herniation" of the chorion laeve into the endometrial cavity, its surface has been smoothed and stretched. At the edge, the decidua is thrown into a fold and

minute coagula are present (see Fig. 2-3). When a tangential section is removed, the extension of the villous tissue for some distance onto the abembryonic pole of the cavity can be seen. The villi have already completely atrophied at the apex. The embryo is contained within the amniotic sac, which does not completely fill the chorionic cavity (see Fig. 2-4). It is suspended within the cavity by a gel (the *magma reticulare*) that liquefies on touching. When the sac is opened, the embryo and umbilical cord emerge (see Fig. 2-5).

An understanding of the morphogenesis of these structures is essential and can be gained from a study of Figure 2-2. In this histologic section, the embryo is sectioned longitudinally. The ectoderm appears as a dark streak and is contiguous with the amniotic sac epithelium that lies below. On the other side of the embryo lie the endoderm and yolk sac. The mesoderm is seen to "flow" from the left caudal pole of the embryo onto the

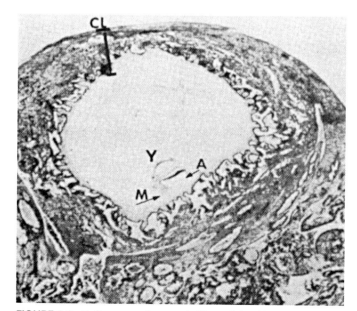

FIGURE 2-2. ■ Same specimen as in Figure 2-1, with embryo sectioned longitudinally. A, amnion; CL, chorion laeve (future membranes); M, mesoderm (developing cord); Y, yolk sac (endoderm).

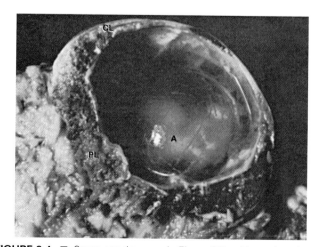

FIGURE 2-4. ■ Same specimen as in Figure 2-3, with portion of chorion laeve (CL) removed to show partial atrophy of membranous villi, formation of definitive placenta (PL), and amniotic sac (A), which only partially fills chorionic cavity at this age. (Courtesy of Dr. Jirasek, Prague.)

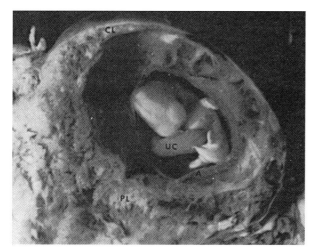

FIGURE 2-5. ■ Same specimen as in Figure 2-3, with amnion (A) opened to disclose the 15-mm embryo and its umbilical cord (UC). CL, chorion laeve; PL, placenta. (Courtesy of Dr. Jirasek, Prague.)

inner surface of the trophoblastic shell. This streak of mesoderm ultimately becomes the substance of the umbilical cord. As the embryo grows and folds in such a manner as to enclose the endoderm, the amnion enlarges and the embryo may be construed to herniate into this amniotic sac. A portion of the primitive yolk sac will be enclosed by the embryo to become its gut; another portion will be exteriorized (lying outside the amniotic sac) and will be connected by the omphalomesenteric (vitelline) vessels and duct. Most often, these yolk structures disappear completely in later development; only in occasional term placentas can the calcified atrophic remnant of yolk sac be found at the periphery as a tiny (3-mm), yellow, extra-amniotic disk.

Once the amniotic sac has enclosed the entire embryo, it reflects on the umbilical cord, whose entire length it will eventually cover. At 8 weeks, the amnion is a thin translucent membrane (Fig. 2-6). It does not fully expand to cover the inside of the entire sac until about 12 weeks. It never completely grows together with the chorion, however, so that in most term placentas the amnion may be dislodged from the chorion and the placental surface. The amnion does not have any blood vessels but is composed of a single layer of ectodermal epithelium, peripheral to which is a layer of delicate connective tissue with some macrophages (Bourne, 1962). Sophisticated studies have now shown that amnion and chorion also possess sheets of delicate elastic membranes (Hieber et al., 1997). It is presumed that these aid in the elasticity of the membranes and help prevent premature rupture. Betraying the ectodermal origin of the amnion are small plaques of squamous metaplasia near the insertion of the term placenta's umbilical cord that must not be mistaken for amnion nodosum.

When the embryonic cells differentiate into mesoderm, endoderm, and ectoderm, the mesoderm is first clearly seen at the caudal pole of the embryonic disk (see Fig. 2-2). The mesodermal cells rapidly proliferate and send a column of cells streaming toward the inner surface of the trophoblastic cavity, which they then come to line. This column is ultimately destined to become the umbilical cord, and blood vessels and a rudimentary allantoic sac grow into this body stalk from the primitive yolk sac—hence the term *chorioallantoic vessels*. It is commonly thought that the *inner cell mass*, the future embryo, lies centrally in the early stages of implantation and that for

this reason the umbilical cord comes to be attached to the center of the placenta.

Aberrant attachment, such as at the margin or to the membranes (velamentous insertion), may be explained by one of two contradictory hypotheses. According to one hypothesis, the embryo had a less than perfect central position at the time of implantation and was perhaps even on the opposite side; thus, when the mesoderm proliferated the location of the cord was established on the surface of the endometrium, the area destined to become membranes. The second hypothesis suggests that normal central implantation occurred but the area of implantation was less than optimal for placental development. Subsequently, the expansion of the placenta occurred to one side rather than in a uniform centrifugal manner. The already established location of the cord therefore changed from a central to a lateral position, a process called *trophotropism*.

This second hypothesis is supported by the much more common marginal or velamentous position of cords in multiple pregnancy, in which one can imagine there is competition for space by and collision of expanding placentas. In term placentas, moreover, marginal placental atrophy is often found, and the finding of succenturiate (accessory) lobes can best be explained by this mechanism. Also, the ultrasonographic finding of a "wandering" placenta favors this assumption, as does the fact that most of the few early embryos studied had a relatively central implantation. The first hypothesis is supported by the finding of a much higher frequency of velamentous insertion of the cord in aborted specimens than in term placentas (Monie, 1965).

The umbilical cord measures approximately 55 cm in length at term, but extreme variations occur for largely unknown reasons. Because a normal cord weighs as much as 100 g and the segments of cord supplied with the placenta vary so much, the cord and membranes should be removed before the placental weight is ascertained. More often than not, the cord is spiraled, most commonly in a sinistral manner. Numerous theories have been presented to explain this helical arrangement, but the cause remains largely unknown. Because such twists do not exist in species with longitudinal orientation in bicornuate uteri and because of the observed mobility of the primate fetus

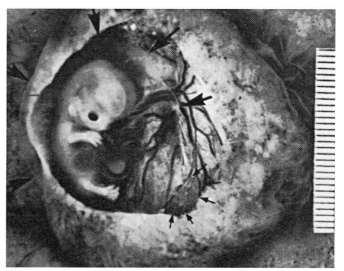

FIGURE 2-6. ■ Pregnancy at 8 weeks with 20-mm embryo. The top portion of chorion laeve has been removed, thus disclosing amnion (*large arrows*) and extra-amniotic yolk sac (*small arrows*).

in its uterus simplex, it is most likely that fetal movements are the cause of the cord twisting (Benirschke, 1981; Lacro et al., 1987). Further support for this explanation comes from the entwinement of cords in monoamniotic twins.

The cord contains two umbilical arteries and one vein. A second rudimentary vein, the omphalomesenteric (vitelline) vessels, and the allantoic duct of early embryonic stages atrophy, and only on rare occasions are remnants of these structures found in the term cord. The two umbilical arteries anastomose through a variably constructed vessel within 2 cm of the insertion of the cord in almost all normal placentas, the so-called Hyrtl anastomosis. There are no nerves in the cord. True knots occur in a few umbilical cords, particularly in very long ones, but much more common are so-called *false knots*. They represent redundancies (varicosities) of umbilical vessels that may protrude on the cord surface and have no clinical significance (Fig. 2-7).

The surface vessels of the placenta represent ramifications of the umbilical vessels and pursue a predictable course on the chorionic surface. In general, one arterial branch is accompanied by one branch of the vein, and each terminal pair of vessels supplies one fetal cotyledon. The arteries may be recognized by their superficial location (i.e., they cross over the veins). Anastomoses between superficial vessels do not occur; for that matter, no such connections ever develop between villous vessels. Each district is isolated and distinct from the others (see Fig. 2-7).

Two types of surface vascular arrangements have been observed, a very coarse and sparse vasculature and finely dispersed vessels. No significantly different fetal outcomes correlate with these features, however, and mixtures of the two types exist in single placentas. The number of terminal perforating vessels determines the number of fetal–placental cotyledons or districts. In most placentas this number is about 20, somewhat more than the number of lobules that can be seen from the maternal side of mature placentas. In general, there is correspondence of fetal lobules with maternal septal subdivisions when injection studies are performed of both circulations (Wigglesworth, 1967).

Authors who have performed such dual injections envisage that the intervillous circulation is achieved by the injection of blood from a decidual artery into the center of a fetal cotyledon, which there disperses from a central cavity in the villous tissue to the periphery of the cotyledon and to the undersurface of the chorion, from where it is drained by veins in the septa and decidual base (Ramsey, 1969). The loose central structure of cotyledons can be well demonstrated when a placenta is horizontally sectioned. This more conventional model of cotyledonary arrangement of villous structure and intervillous circulation has been challenged by Gruenwald (1975). He envisaged a different lobular architecture, with arterial openings occurring at the periphery of cotyledons, a concept that has not yet been unequivocally refuted. The former notion that all intervillous blood flows laterally to the *marginal sinus*, however, is no longer acceptable.

The normal term placenta from which membranes and cord have been trimmed weighs between 400 and 500 g. There is enormous variability in placental size and shape, as there is in fetal weight. Some variations can be explained by racial differences, altitude, pathologic circumstances of implantation, diseases, or maternal habits such as smoking. In many cases, however, the deviations from "normal" are as difficult to explain as the factors that ultimately determine fetal and placental growth in general. Systematic studies of placental structure have given some insight into the complexities; they have been summarized in the careful analysis by Teasdale (1980). Absolute growth, as determined by DNA, RNA, and protein content, occurs in the placenta to the 36th week of gestation. Thereafter, proliferation of cells does not normally occur, and the placenta undergoes only further maturational changes. Previous studies have suggested an expansion of villous surface to between 11 and 13 m^2 at term, whereas Teasdale's careful measurements suggest that the maximum is reached with 10.6 m^2 at 36 weeks, decreasing to 9.4 m^2 at term. The fetal-to-placental ratio is estimated to change from 5:1 in the third trimester to 7:1 at term, most rapidly increasing during the last month of gestation. Reasons for discrepancies of these measurements reported in the literature are partly explained by inconsistent handling of the organ at delivery. Thus, a variable amount of blood may be trapped, depending on the time of cord clamping. It is widely accepted now that the delivered placenta has a smaller volume, in particular is less thick, than before delivery, as ascertained by sonography (Bleker et al., 1977). Therefore, for quantitative assessment a histometric analysis must accompany such correlative study. Apparently, the slight increase in placental volume occurring in the last month of pregnancy results from an expansion of the "nonparenchymal" space (i.e., villous capillary size, decidua, septa, and fibrin). Thus, during the last month of gestation, fetal growth occurs without a commensurate increase in placental volume, indicating that changes must occur in perfusion or transport function of the placenta to ensure enhanced delivery of metabolic substrates to the fetus.

Macroscopically, a delivered normal term placenta can be described as a disk-shaped, round, or ovoid structure measuring 18 × 20 cm in diameter and approximately 2 cm thick. The cord is normally inserted near the center of the disk (marginal in 7% and on the membranes in 1%); it measures 40 to 60 cm in length and 1.5 cm in thickness. It has two arteries, one vein, and a number of helical spirals. The membranes are attached at the periphery and have some degenerated yellow decidua on their outer surface and a smooth glistening inner amniotic

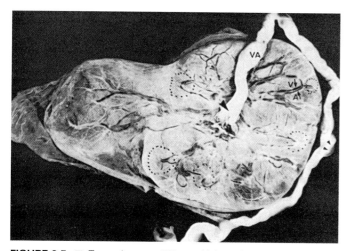

FIGURE 2-7. ■ Term placenta, 530 g, with lateral accessory (succenturiate) lobe to the left. The centrally inserted cord has a varicosity (VA) and a false knot (*small arrowheads*). At the base of the cord (*large arrowhead*) is the anastomosis between the two umbilical arteries. A surface artery (A) and vein (V) are labeled at top right, and several fetal cotyledons are indicated by *dotted circles*.

surface. The amnion is only slightly adherent to the chorionic face of the placenta, from which it can be stripped by forceps, but it is firmly attached to the cord, upon which it reflects.

The fetal surface of the placenta is blue because of the fetal villous blood content seen through the membranes. Irregular whitish plaques of subchorionic fibrin slightly project between fetal vessels and produce what has been referred to as a "bosselated" surface; it is indicative of a mature organ.

The maternal surface usually has a film of loosely attached blood clot, which when removed discloses the thin, grayish layer of decidua basalis and fibrin that come away with delivery. In the fibrin, yellow granules and streaks of calcification characterize maturity. They are extremely variable in amount. The maternal surface is usually broken up into irregular lobules (cotyledons) by crevices that continue into partial or complete septa between fetal cotyledons. These septa are constructed of decidual cells and cellular trophoblast. On sectioning, the dark red villous tissue reflects the content of fetal blood. Loosely structured areas represent intervillous lakes, the presumed sites of first blood injections ("spurts") from decidual arteries.

■ MICROSCOPIC DEVELOPMENT

It is likely that some adhesion molecules are essential for blastocyst attachment to the endometrium (Enders, 2001). Once the trophoblastic shell has attached, marked changes occur on its surface and invasion is accomplished by dissociation and ingestion of endometrial cells. Completely interstitial implantation of the blastocyst is accomplished on the ninth day of gestation. The trophoblastic shell has proliferated appreciably, particularly at its basal portions, and most trophoblastic cells possess disproportionately large nuclei and form a syncytium. Within this mass of trophoblastic cells develop clefts (*lacunae*) that coalesce to form the most primitive type of the future intervillous space.

At about this time or on the next day, the somewhat congested decidual vessels are tapped by the trophoblast. The first maternal leukocytes have been observed on day 11 in this primitive intervillous space, later to be followed by blood, thus establishing the primitive intervillous circulation (Hertig, 1968). At the same time, the trophoblastic cells can be seen to differentiate into a central cellular type (*cytotrophoblast*, the future Langhans layer) and peripheral syncytiotrophoblast (Fig. 2-8). The syncytium never shows mitoses and grows by incorporation of cytotrophoblastic nuclei and cytoplasm, only the latter cells being capable of mitosis (Richart, 1961; Galton, 1962). Recent studies indicate that the formation of the syncytium from cytotrophoblast is a very complex one and requires a protein ("syncytin") derived from a genetic contribution of a retroviral envelope gene (Mi et al., 2000; Pötgens et al., 2002).

On day 13, the first connective tissue may be observed in the central portion of the future villi. It will rapidly expand peripherally into the cell columns of trophoblast. Evidence suggests that this connective tissue core derives from the mesoderm of the extraembryonic space and perhaps the body stalk (see Fig. 2-2) and not by central "delamination" from trophoblast. By the 30th day, a truly villous ovum is formed, and the basic future development of the villous structure is delineated. Villi are found around the entire circumference at first, only to atrophy over the pole later. Commencing almost simultaneously, on the 14th day and subsequently, is the development of villous capillaries.

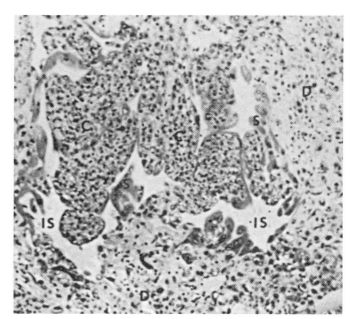

FIGURE 2-8. ■ Trophoblastic shell of a 13-day-old human ovum. Cell columns composed of solid cytotrophoblast (C) are covered by syncytiotrophoblast (S) lining the entire intervillous space (IS), which is still devoid of maternal blood. D, decidua. H&E, ×300.

Although Hertig (1968) discussed in great detail how such a process also derives from delaminated trophoblastic cells by the internal detachment of angioblastic cells, more likely their origin is from fetal mesoderm or endoderm. These are not idle problems of the embryologist but pertain directly to an understanding of the genesis of hydatidiform moles. If villous connective tissue and vessels are definitely derived from the embryo (rather than the trophoblast), hydatidiform moles must at one time have had an embryo. Occasional complete hydatidiform moles have been shown to contain degenerated embryos, but in most complete hydatidiform moles the embryo and its vessels have disappeared (Benirschke and Kaufmann, 1995; Baergen et al., 1996). Villous vessels coalesce and connect to the omphalomesenteric and later allantoic vessels of the embryonic body stalk, and a true fetal circulation is active by 21 days (Moore and Persaud, 1993). The initial fetal blood cells come from yolk sac, and only after the 2nd month do they issue from fetal hematopoietic islands. With an established circulation, the villi are now called *tertiary* villi (Enders, 2001).

The villous structure changes appreciably during further development, and gestational age can be crudely estimated from the histologic appearance of the villi. In young placentas, the mesenchymal core of villi is extremely loosely structured, appearing almost edematous (Fig. 2-9). Capillaries are filled with nucleated cells and lie very close to the villous surface. This surface is uniformly covered by an inner cellular cytotrophoblast, which contains numerous mitoses and in turn is covered by a thick layer of syncytium that contains abundant organelles in its metabolically active cytoplasm. The syncytium is functionally the most important part of the placenta. With advancing age the villi elongate, lose their central edema, branch successively, and decrease in diameter. At term they contain little mesenchyma and are filled with distended capillaries. Cytotrophoblastic mitoses are rare after 36 weeks in normal placentas. The syncytium tends to form buds and "knots," some of which break loose and are swept into the intervillous circulation, where they reach the maternal lung. Fibrin

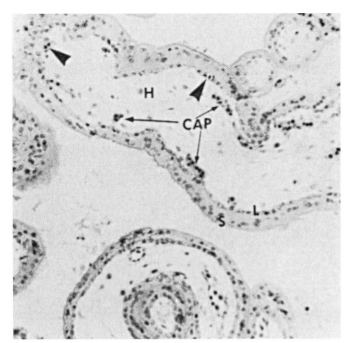

FIGURE 2-9. ■ Villi of 30-day-old placenta. Note the very loosely structured mesenchymal core containing isolated macrophages, thin-walled fetal capillaries (CAP) filled with nucleated red blood cells, and the double-layered trophoblastic surface. H, Hofbauer cells; L, Langhans cells with mitoses at *heavy arrows* (cytotrophoblast); S, syncytium. H&E, ×160.

although flow was of low resistance and pulsatility from day 20 on. The population of Hofbauer cells derives from circulating fetal blood and increases in the first 36 weeks and falls thereafter (Teasdale, 1980). Although their precise function is not well understood, immunohistochemical studies show that this large population of cells represents fully differentiated phagocytes (Wood, 1980). After hemolysis, they are seen to produce hemosiderin; in the chorionic surface, they actively transport meconium after its discharge, and it is speculated that they remove antifetal antibodies.

At the site of implantation, trophoblastic cells intermingle extensively with decidua basalis; indeed, they penetrate into the superficial portions of myometrium. These areas are often characterized by scattered lymphocyte infiltration and decidual necrosis (Pijnenborg et al., 1980). Cytotrophoblastic cells enter the opened mouths of maternal arterioles and penetrate deeply along their endothelial linings. Some trophoblastic cells infiltrate the decidua and myometrium, often fusing to form *placental giant cells* (Fig. 2-11); others invade the spiral arterioles from the outside. They cause considerable local change, including fibrin deposition, and alter the normally contractile vessels to presumably rigid uteroplacental arteries. Thrombosis is not found normally but is a common finding when hypertensive changes are superimposed.

Electron microscopic study of placental villi in general supports the findings made by light microscopy, but it adds significant new details. The arborization of villi and their complexity are best appreciated in scanning electron micrographs

and fibrinoid, also eosinophilic but composed of a variety of novel protein compounds, are normally accumulated in ever-increasing quantities on the surface of villi, in the subchorionic area, and along the floor of the placenta, where Rohr and Nitabuch's fibrin layers mingle with decidua basalis. Fibrinoid of the placenta is a complex admixture of true fibrin and a variety of proteins such as laminins and collagens (Kaufmann et al., 1996). Near term, some of these fibrin deposits become calcified as a normal process that may become excessive in the postmature placenta. The amount of calcium varies greatly but has no deleterious influence on placental function. The placental septa, composed of cellular extravillous trophoblast ("X cells" or intermediate trophoblast) and decidua, often undergo cystic change as a sign of maturity (Fig. 2-10).

The X cell has recently been the focus of attention. It is a separate lineage of trophoblast that is intimately related to fibrinoid deposition, the production of the *major basic protein* and placental lactogen. Most so-called placental site giant cells are X cells and are often confused with decidual stromal elements (Wasmoen et al, 1987; Benirschke and Kaufmann, 1995). From these basal trophoblastic elements come a variety of enzymes, especially stromelysin-3, to prepare the invasion of the decidual floor and blood vessels (Maquoi et al., 1997). These cells also infiltrate into the orifices of basal decidual spiral arterioles.

Hustin and Schaaps (1987) and their colleagues (1988) offered evidence that these extravillous trophoblastic cells completely occlude these vessels in early pregnancy, thus allowing only a filtrate of maternal blood to enter the intervillous space. This hypothesis was challenged with studies using Doppler flow in rhesus monkeys (Simpson et al., 1997). These investigations showed an early vascular connection of the maternal arterial circulation with the intervillous space,

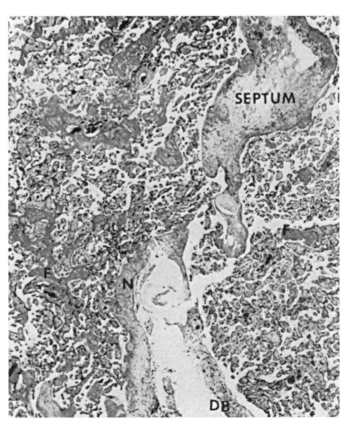

FIGURE 2-10. ■ Term placenta; basal portion with septum constructed of decidua and trophoblast, forming small cysts. Villi are finely branched, and grayish masses of fibrin (F) are found throughout. At the bottom of the figure is the decidua basalis (DB), the only maternal tissue in a delivered placenta. Nitabuch's fibrin layer (N) is discontinuous. H&E, ×64.

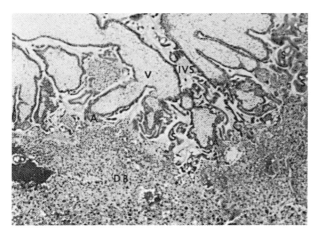

FIGURE 2-11. ■ Implantation site of first trimester placenta.
A, anchoring villi composed of cytotrophoblast; DB, decidua basalis
with maternal vessels and diffusely infiltrated placental giant cells;
IVS, intervillous space; S, syncytial buds; V, villi. H&E, ×40. (From
Benirschke K, Kaufmann P: The Pathology of the Human Placenta,
3rd ed. New York, Springer-Verlag, 1995.)

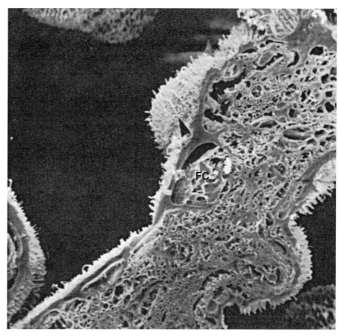

FIGURE 2-13. ■ Freeze-fracture scanning electron microphotograph
of term placental villus to show microvillous surface, often in rows
(*arrowhead*), grayish trophoblast cytoplasm, and proximity of the fetal
capillary (FC) to the black intervillous space (×250). (From Sandstedt B:
The placenta and low birth weight. Curr Top Pathol **66**:1, 1979.)

(Fig. 2-12). In the more peripheral areas of cotyledons, the villi
appear histologically more mature (i.e., they are smaller and
have more branches and less stroma). The syncytial surface is
covered by numerous minute microvilli, and syncytial bridges
are occasionally seen. In the central portion of the cotyledon,
the villi are plump and less branched. Freeze-fracture scanning
electron microscopy discloses the proximity of fetal vessels to
the basement membrane and the profusely microvillous surface
of the syncytium (Fig. 2-13). With advancing maturity, the
Langhans cytotrophoblastic layer not only becomes less prominent but also is interrupted in many more places. Here, then,
the fetal capillaries abut a thin layer of syncytium, presumably
the most efficient site of transfer.

These electron micrographic features of maturity are also
found more frequently in the periphery of cotyledons than
in their more immature-appearing centers, but qualitative
differences do not exist (Schuhmann and Wynn, 1980). The
slightly different electron micrographic features of villi in
part relate to the state of contraction of fetal capillaries
(Fig. 2-14), and they may in part be the result of oxygen supply.

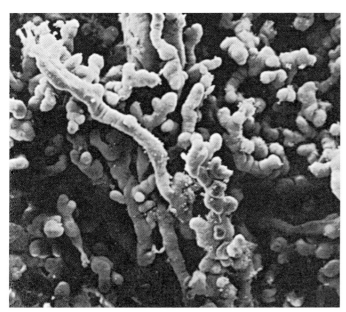

FIGURE 2-12. ■ Scanning electron micrograph of mature villi at the
periphery of the cotyledon. Note the fine uniform structure, rare
adherence, and microvillous velvety surface of the terminal villi (×100).
(From Sandstedt B: The placenta and low birth weight. Curr Top
Pathol **66**:1, 1979.)

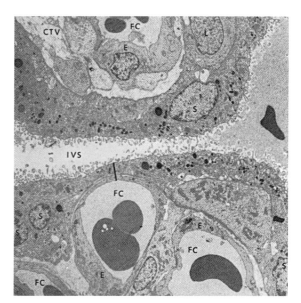

FIGURE 2-14. ■ Transmission electron micrograph of two placental
villi at 30 weeks' gestation. *Top*, The fetal capillary (FC) is contracted;
bottom, several capillaries are dilated. Note microvilli and shortest
maternal–fetal exchange distance (indicated by *bar*). CTV, connective
tissue of villus (×5000); E, fetal capillary endothelium; IVS, intervillous
space; L, Langhans cell nucleus; S, syncytial nuclei. (Courtesy of
Dr. R. M. Wynn., Department of Obstetrics, Gynecology, and
Pathology, SUNY Health Sciences Center, Brooklyn, NY.)

Desmosomes have been identified by scanning and transmission electron microscopy in trophoblast (Reale et al., 1980). They interlock syncytium with cytotrophoblast, and when found with free membranes in the cytoplasm of the syncytium, they presumably represent the remnants of the fusion-incorporation process of cytotrophoblast into syncytium. The structure of the syncytiotrophoblastic cytoplasm is extremely complex. It is filled with minute vacuoles, ribosomes, mitochondria, and the other usual cytoplasmic components. Conversely, the cytotrophoblastic cytoplasm is relatively simple, reflecting its presumed primary function as precursor cells for syncytium.

REFERENCES

Baergen RN, Kelly T, McGinnis MJ, et al: Complete hydatidiform mole with coexisting embryo. Hum Pathol 27:731, 1996.

Benirschke K: Anatomy. In Berger GS, Brenner WE, Keith LG (eds): Second Trimester Abortion. Boston, John Wright, 1981, p 39.

Benirschke K, Kaufmann P: The Pathology of the Human Placenta, 3rd ed. New York, Springer-Verlag, 1995.

Bleker OP, Kloosterman GJ, Breur W, et al: The volumetric growth of the human placenta: A longitudinal ultrasonic study. Am J Obstet Gynecol 127:657, 1977.

Bourne GL: The Human Amnion and Chorion. London, Lloyd-Luke, 1962.

Boyd JD, Hamilton WJ: The Human Placenta. Cambridge, Heffer and Sons, 1970.

Enders AC: Perspectives on human implantation. Infertil Reprod Med Clin North Am 12:251, 2001.

Galton M: DNA content of placental nuclei. J Cell Biol 13:183, 1962.

Gruenwald P: Lobular architecture of primate placentas. In Gruenwald P (ed): The Placenta and Its Maternal Supply Line. Baltimore, University Park Press, 1975.

Hertig AT: Human Trophoblast. Springfield, IL, Charles C Thomas, 1968.

Hieber AD, Corcino D, Motosue J, et al: Detection of elastin in the human fetal membranes: Proposed molecular basis for elasticity. Placenta 18:301, 1997.

Hoogland HJ, deHaan J, Martin CB: Placental size during early pregnancy and fetal outcome: A preliminary report of a sequential ultrasonographic study. Obstet Gynecol 138:441, 1980.

Hustin J, Schaaps JP: Echocardiographic and anatomic studies of the maternotrophoblastic border during the first trimester of pregnancy. Am J Obstet Gynecol 157:162, 1987.

Hustin J, Schaaps JP, Lambotte R: Anatomical studies of the utero-placental vascularization in the first trimester of pregnancy. Trophoblast Res 3:49, 1988.

Kaufmann P, Huppertz B, Frank H-G: The fibrinoids of the human placenta: origin, composition and functional relevance. Ann Anat 178:485, 1996.

King DL: Placental migration demonstrated by ultrasonography. Radiology 109:167, 1973.

Lacro RV, Jones KL, Benirschke K: The umbilical cord twist: Origin, direction, and relevance. Am J Obstet Gynecol 157:833, 1987.

Maquoi E, Polette M, Nawrocki B, et al: Expression of stromelysin-3 in the human placenta and placental bed. Placenta 18:277, 1997.

Mi S, Lee X, Veldman GM, et al: Syncytin is a captive retroviral envelope protein involved in human placental morphogenesis. Nature 403:785, 2000.

Monie IW: Velamentous insertion of the cord in early pregnancy. Am J Obstet Gynecol 93:276, 1965.

Moore KL, Persaud TVN: The Developing Human: Clinically Oriented Embryology, 3rd ed. Philadelphia, WB Saunders, 1993.

Pijnenborg R, Dixon G, Robertson WB, et al: Trophoblastic invasion of human decidua from 8 to 18 weeks by pregnancy. Placenta 1:3, 1980.

Pötgens AJG, Schmitz U, Bose P, et al: Mechanism of syncytial fusion: A review. Placenta 23 (Suppl A):S107, 2002.

Ramsey EM: New appraisal of an old organ: The placenta. Proc Am Philos Soc 113:296, 1969.

Reale E, Wang T, Zaccheo D, et al: Junctions on the maternal blood surface of the human placental syncytium. Placenta 1:245, 1980.

Richart R: Studies of placental morphogenesis. I. Radioautographic studies of human placenta utilizing tritiated thymidine. Proc Soc Exp Biol 106:829, 1961.

Rizos N, Doran TA, Miskin M, et al: Natural history of placenta previa ascertained by diagnostic ultrasound. Obstet Gynecol 133:287, 1979.

Sandstedt B: The placenta and low birth weight. Curr Top Pathol 66:1, 1979.

Schuhmann RA, Wynn RM: Regional ultrastructural differences in placental villi in cotyledons of a mature human placenta. Placenta 1:345, 1980.

Simpson NAB, Nimrod C, De Vermette R, et al: Determination of intervillous flow in early pregnancy. Placenta 18:287, 1997.

Teasdale F: Gestational changes in the functional structure of the human placenta in relation to fetal growth: A morphometric study. Am J Obstet Gynecol 137:560, 1980.

Wasmoen TL, Benirschke K, Gleich GJ: Demonstration of immunoreactive eosinophil granule major basic protein in the plasma and placentae of nonhuman primates. Placenta 8:283, 1987.

Wigglesworth JS: Vascular organization of the human placenta. Nature 216:1120, 1967.

Wood GW: Mononuclear phagocytes in the human placenta. Placenta 1:113, 1980.

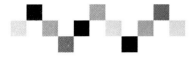

Chapter 3
AMNIOTIC FLUID DYNAMICS

Robert A. Brace, PhD

This chapter supplies quantitative information about amniotic fluid volume (AFV) and describes the current evidence regarding its formation and regulation.

GESTATIONAL CHANGES

Intrauterine water content increases progressively throughout normal human gestation. At term, total water accumulation is approximately 3500 mL, with 2400 mL in the fetus, 400 mL in the placenta, and 700 mL in the amniotic fluid. Volumes of amniotic fluid at various gestational ages have been studied by use of direct volumetric methods, indicator dilution techniques, and, more recently, quantitative ultrasonographic methods. In normal pregnancies, a wide range of volumes occurs, particularly during the latter half of gestation. Figure 3-1 illustrates the progressive increase in AFV from 30 mL at 10 weeks to 190 mL at 16 weeks and to a mean of 780 mL at 32 to 35 weeks' gestation, after which a decrease occurs. Figure 3-1 also provides a statistical definition of polyhydramnios and oligohydramnios as a function of gestational age. For example, 500 mL at 14 weeks is far in excess of normal, whereas 2000 mL at 33 weeks is not outside the 95% confidence interval for normal pregnancies.

The gestational pattern of volume changes can vary considerably in individual women in that AFV may increase progressively until delivery or may begin to decrease as early as 24 weeks' gestation. As seen in Figure 3-1, a decrease in mean volume begins to occur after 36 weeks and becomes progressive, especially in post-term pregnancies. The rate of change in AFV is a strong function of gestational age. Figure 3-2 shows that AFV increases at a rate of 10 mL/wk at the beginning of the fetal period. This increases to 50 to 60 mL/wk at 19 to 25 weeks' gestation before undergoing a gradual decrease until the rate of change equals zero (i.e., AFV is a maximum) at 34 weeks. Thereafter, AFV falls, with the decrease averaging 60 to 70 mL/wk at 40 weeks. The decrease in post-term pregnancies has been found to be as high as 150 mL/wk from 38 to 43 weeks' gestation (Elliott and Inman, 1961). Although the basic mechanisms that produce these alterations in AFV throughout gestation are unclear, it is important to note that, when expressed as a percentage (see Fig. 3-2), the rate of change decreases monotonically throughout the fetal period. Thus, the late decrease in amniotic volume represents a natural progression rather than an aberration.

The volume of amniotic fluid is important clinically because volumes in excess of 1.5 to 2 liters (polyhydramnios) or less than 0.5 liters (oligohydramnios) between 32 and 36 weeks' gestation are often associated with fetal abnormalities and/or poor perinatal outcome (Chamberlain et al., 1984a,b). Polyhydramnios (also termed hydramnios) occurring during the second trimester spontaneously resolves in 40% to 50% of cases; the resolution is associated with a normal perinatal outcome (Zamah et al., 1982). Conversely, oligohydramnios in mid-pregnancy frequently is associated with poor outcome (Mercer et al., 1984; Bastide et al., 1986). These conditions are discussed in more detail in the context of pregnancy disorders elsewhere in the text.

BASIC MECHANISMS OF WATER TRANSPORT

An understanding of the mechanisms that regulate amniotic fluid dynamics requires knowledge of the biology of water transport. For a review of these principles as they apply to amniotic fluid accumulation, see the comprehensive review by Seeds (1980).

Briefly, the active transport of water has not been demonstrated in biological tissues. Thus, net water accumulation across body membranes, including the placenta, occurs only by passive mechanisms in response to hydrostatic and/or osmotic pressure gradients. If no such gradients exist, no net transfer of volume takes place. Seeds (1980) reported that careful investigations to demonstrate the existence of transplacental chemical gradients that would be responsible for the net water transfer over the 9 months of gestation have been unsuccessful. However, because only exceedingly small chemical gradients would be necessary to explain the small daily net water transfer, it is entirely possible that current experimental techniques are not sufficiently sensitive to demonstrate their presence. Net transplacental water transfer also depends on differences in placental permeability characteristics for each solute, and these only have been explored using mathematical modeling (Wilbur et al., 1978).

A second difficulty in understanding the factors involved in regulating water accumulation is that confusion has occurred over interpretation of studies that explored the movement of isotopically labeled water. As Seeds (1980) discussed in detail, data describing the diffusional movement of water molecules do not provide any information relevant to net volume changes, whereas only net volume changes affect AFV. This is illustrated by the fact that as blood passes through a single capillary, each water molecule in the blood diffuses back and forth

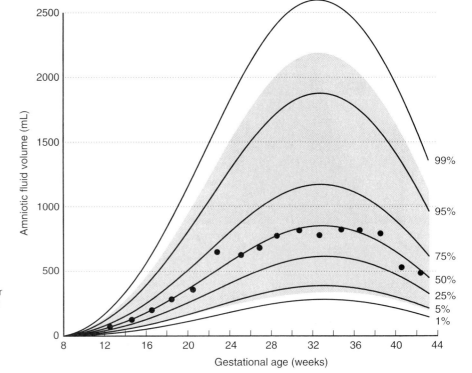

FIGURE 3-1 ■ Amniotic fluid as a function of gestational age. Closed circles (●) are means for 2-week intervals from 705 women. Shaded area is 95% confidence interval. Percentiles are calculated from polynomial regression. (From Brace RA, Wolf EJ: Normal amniotic fluid volume changes throughout pregnancy. Am J Obstet Gynecol **161**:382, 1989.)

across the capillary wall 100 times, in contrast to a net volume movement across the capillary membrane of less than 1% (Landis and Pappenheimer, 1963). Because present techniques for measurement of the diffusional movement of water do not have a resolution anywhere near this ratio of 1 part in 10,000, they cannot be used to study the factors that affect the net changes in AFV. Thus, for the regulatory mechanisms to be explored, net volume changes must be measured and related to the conditions being studied.

PATHWAYS FOR FLUID MOVEMENT

AFV is the integrated sum of the inflows and outflows of the amniotic space. Thus, a knowledge of the pathways for fluid movement is a prerequisite for understanding the volume regulatory mechanisms. In early gestation, significant amounts of amniotic fluid are present before the establishment of fetal micturition or deglutition. Although the formation of amniotic fluid at this early stage is virtually unexplored, the most

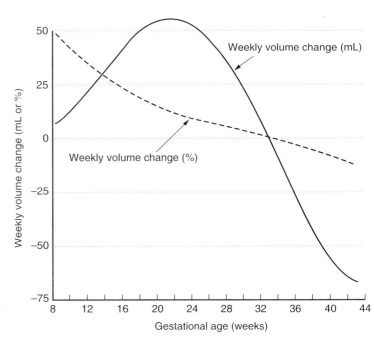

FIGURE 3-2 ■ Weekly changes in mean amniotic volume. (From Brace RA, Wolf EJ: Normal amniotic fluid volume changes throughout pregnancy. Am J Obstet Gynecol **161**:382, 1989.)

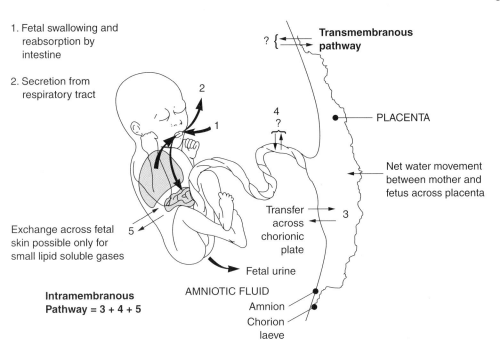

1. Fetal swallowing and reabsorption by intestine

2. Secretion from respiratory tract

Exchange across fetal skin possible only for small lipid soluble gases

Transmembranous pathway

PLACENTA

Net water movement between mother and fetus across placenta

Transfer across chorionic plate

Fetal urine

AMNIOTIC FLUID

Amnion

Chorion laeve

Intramembranous Pathway = 3 + 4 + 5

FIGURE 3-3 ■ Summary of the significant pathways of water and solute exchange between the amniotic fluid and fetus. (Modified from Seeds AE: Current concepts of amniotic fluid dynamics. Am J Obstet Gynecol **138**:575, 1980.)

likely mechanism is an active transport of solute (probably sodium or chloride) by the amnion into the amniotic space, with water moving passively down the chemical potential gradient. Much more is known about the pathways involved in the regulation of AFV during the second half of gestation after the fetal skin keratinizes. Figure 3-3 summarizes these pathways; it is important to note that a total of six potential pathways may allow fluid to enter and/or leave the amniotic space in late gestation, with four of these being major pathways and two minor pathways. The excretion of fetal urine and the swallowing of amniotic fluid by the fetus are the major pathways for the formation and clearance, respectively, of amniotic fluid (see Fig. 3-3). The secretion of large volumes of fluid each day by the fetal lungs is now well established, so the fetal lungs are the second major source of amniotic fluid during the second half of gestation.

The most significant advance in our understanding of amniotic volume regulatory mechanisms over the past two decades is quantitative documentation that both water and solutes rapidly move between amniotic fluid and fetal blood within the placenta and membranes (Gilbert and Brace, 1989; Brace, 1995; Ross et al., 2001). The latter pathway is referred to as the *intramembranous pathway*, which is the fourth of four major pathways. Movement of water and solutes between amniotic fluid and maternal blood within the wall of the uterus is exchanged through the *transmembranous pathway*. This is a minor pathway often ignored because of very low or nonexistent fluxes. Finally, fluid secreted by the fetal oral–nasal cavities most likely contributes to AFV, and this is the second minor pathway. The integration of flows through these six potential pathways leads to the regulation of AFV. These pathways and their respective flows are described later.

The amniotic fluid was once considered to be a stagnant pool. However, this view is far from accurate because, relative to AFV, large amounts of fluid enter and leave the amniotic space each day. Gitlin and colleagues (1972) injected several different high molecular weight proteins into the amniotic

fluid of pregnant women and found that they were all cleared at essentially the same rate, averaging a 63% per day decrease in amniotic concentrations. Because of the exponential nature of clearances, this corresponds to a net volume turnover in excess of 95% AFV per day. Thus, amniotic fluid circulates with a turnover time of approximately 1 day in late gestation. This turnover rate of 1 volume per day is only a small fraction of that determined with isotopically labeled water (Liley, 1972; Lotgering and Wallenburg, 1986). As already discussed, however, the latter represents the diffusional exchange of water molecules rather than net volume movements and does not depict amniotic fluid movements.

Fetal Urine

Fetal urine is a major, and most likely *the* major, source of amniotic fluid during the latter half of pregnancy. Urine first enters the amniotic space at 8 to 11 weeks' gestation (Abramovich and Page, 1973). Early studies using real-time ultrasonographic techniques found that the urine production rate rose steadily throughout the latter half of gestation (Fig. 3-4). Urine production per kilogram of body weight increased from approximately 110 mL/kg in 24 hours at 25 weeks to approximately 190 mL/kg in 24 hours at 39 weeks (Lotgering and Wallenburg, 1986). At term, fetal urine flow rate was 500 to 600 mL/day. Subsequent studies (Rabinowitz et al., 1989) found human fetal urine flow rates equal to twice those shown in Figure 3-4 when bladder volume measurements were made at 2- to 5-minute intervals rather than the 15- to 30-minute intervals used in earlier studies, suggesting that term fetal urinary output in humans may be 1000 to 1200 mL/day. This difference is attributed to the fact that fetal micturition occurs at 20- to 25-minute intervals. In near-term fetal sheep, with direct methods used for measuring urine production rates, similar high values have been found (Gresham et al., 1972; Wlodek et al., 1988; Brace and Moore, 1991). Other studies (Hedriana, 1997), however, suggest that

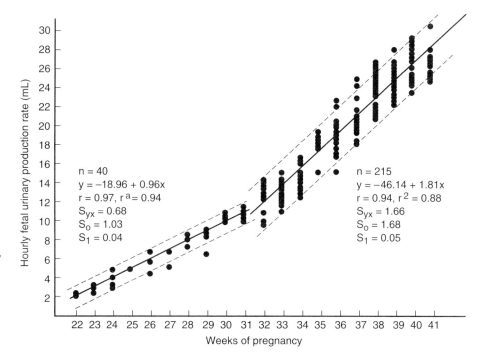

FIGURE 3-4 ■ Increase in hourly fetal urinary production rates as determined by ultrasonographic techniques during human pregnancy. (From Kurjak A, Kirkinen P, Latin V, et al: Ultrasonic assessment of fetal kidney function in normal and complicated pregnancies. Am J Obstet Gynecol **141**:266, 1981.)

ultrasonographic studies with measurements at 2- to 5-minute intervals overestimate urine production rates by roughly 35% because the human fetal urinary bladder is nonellipsoidal. Thus, the current best estimate of near-term urine flow in the human fetus averages 700 to 900 mL/day. As seen in Figure 3-4, there is a tendency for the urine flow rate to decrease after 40 weeks' gestation, but this may be better characterized as a failure to increase with advancing gestational age rather than as a decrease. Others found a clear reduction in human fetal urinary output in post-term pregnancies, particularly if oligohydramnios is present (Trimmer et al., 1990).

Any condition that prevents either the formation of urine or the entry of urine into the amniotic sac almost invariably results in oligohydramnios in the second half of gestation. Bain and Scott (1960) reviewed 50 cases of fetal urinary tract malformations, including 28 of renal agenesis, 17 of severe cystic dysplasia, and 5 of urethral atresia. In all but one case, oligohydramnios was observed. More recent reports fully support the concept that anuria or oliguria is a frequent cause of oligohydramnios (Chamberlain et al., 1984a). Even under less severe conditions, there is an association between a reduced fetal urine production rate and amniotic volume. In growth-restricted fetuses, AFV is low, as is urine flow rate (VanOtterlo et al., 1977), although this is not found in all cases (Creasy, 1984). In addition, it has long been observed that fetal pulmonary hypoplasia is associated with reduced AFV in an entity known as *Potter's syndrome*. The oligohydramnios-associated pulmonary hypoplasia appears to be due to compression of the fetal chest and body by the uterine wall (Nakayama et al., 1983). Excess fluid loss from the lungs because of this compression also contributes (Harding et al., 1990).

In contrast to the relationship between oligohydramnios and low urine flow rates, there may not be a consistent association between excess fetal urine production and hydramnios. Abramovich and coworkers (1979) reported that urine production in normal fetuses was not different from that in those with hydramnios. In diabetic pregnancy, it might be expected that fetal hyperglycemia would result in an increased solute load and urinary production rate. However, only 16 of 42 diabetic patients (32%) and only 1 of 10 hydramniotic patients had fetal urinary production rates greater than the 95th percentile (Kurjak et al., 1981). Furthermore, VanOtterlo and associates (1977) found no increase in urinary output in diabetic pregnancies with hydramnios. In contrast, Yasuhi and colleagues (1994), using more frequent ultrasound measurements, found fetal urine production to be elevated in fasting diabetics. Further, an acute glucose load given to pregnant sheep elevated fetal glomerular filtration rate and urinary output (Smith and Lumbers, 1989), again suggesting that alterations in fetal renal function may contribute to the association between polyhydramnios and diabetes. The positive relationship between high fetal urine production and elevated AFV has led to therapeutic treatment with indomethacin, a prostaglandin synthesis inhibitor. At moderate concentrations, this reduces fetal urine production and AFV through a combination of mechanisms (Walker et al., 1994).

Fetal Swallowing

The human fetus begins swallowing at roughly the same age at which urine first enters the amniotic space (i.e., 8 to 11 weeks' gestation). Earlier studies suggested that the volume of amniotic fluid swallowed in late gestation averages 210 to 760 mL/day (Pritchard, 1965). Volumes in excess of 1000 mL/day have been measured in near-term fetal sheep when more detailed methods were used (Tomoda et al., 1985). Relative to ovine fetal weight, swallowed volume increased from 100 mL/kg/day at the beginning of the third trimester to 500 mL/kg/day at term (Tomoda et al., 1985). These daily volumes do not include the amount of tracheal fluid from the lungs (see later) that is swallowed before it enters the amniotic space, so the total swallowed volume may be higher than these figures indicate. Studies have shown that the fetus swallows usually during episodes of breathing activity (Harding et al., 1984) and that fetal breathing is suppressed or absent before the onset of labor (Carmichael et al., 1984). This suggests that the above estimates of the amount of amniotic fluid swallowed by the normal human fetus at or near term may have been underestimated if breathing activity was concomitantly reduced.

Fetal swallowing plays an important role in determining AFV during the last half of gestation. In a review of 169 cases of hydramnios, Scott and Wilson (1957) were able to attribute the excess AFV to a disturbance in the fetal swallowing mechanism in 54 patients (32%). Furthermore, all cases of esophageal atresia are associated with hydramnios unless there is a communication with the trachea that provides a route for swallowing. A large review of 1745 cases of hydramnios revealed esophageal abnormalities in 27% and other conditions that interfered with fetal swallowing in 18% (Moya et al., 1960). These suggestions that a lack of swallowing mediates the hydramnios are supported by the observation that in fetal monkeys, esophageal ligation during the last trimester elevated AFV (Minei and Suzuki, 1976); however, AFV returned to or was below normal with esophageal ligation before delivery. This demonstrates amniotic fluid clearance in primates by a pathway(s) in addition to swallowing, most likely reflecting an increased intramembranous absorption. Studies in fetal sheep have found consistent increases in intramembranous absorption when fetal swallowing of amniotic fluid is prevented (Matsumoto et al., 2000).

The role of taste in regulating fetal swallowing has been little studied. In the human fetus, swallowing is reduced after intra-amniotic injection of an oil that tastes "vile," but injection of saccharin produced inconsistent results (Liley, 1972). Animal studies have shown that neither the frequency nor the extent of swallowing depends on outflow from the trachea or the volume of the gastric compartment. Further, fetal hypoxia suppresses fetal swallowing activity, whereas fetal hypertonicity and angiotensin II may enhance swallowing (Ross and Nijland, 1997; Ross et al., 1989).

Fetal Respiratory Tract

For many years there had been widespread acceptance of the idea that amniotic fluid entered the fetal lungs by way of the trachea and was absorbed by the capillaries lining the alveoli. Starting in the 1960s, considerable evidence began to accumulate suggesting that an outflow of lung fluid occurred through the trachea rather than an inflow of amniotic fluid. In 1972, Liley reviewed the topic and reported that after intra-amniotic injection of contrast medium in more than 800 patients, "in only four instances, all highly pathological pregnancies, was any contrast medium detectable radiologically or histologically in the fetal or neonatal lung." This is supported by the observation that although meconium staining of amniotic fluid is common, meconium aspiration is rare and usually occurs only under conditions of severe fetal asphyxia. Studies in near-term fetal sheep showed a normal outflow from the lungs of 200 to 400 mL/day (Adamson et al., 1973) and that this flow of 10% of body weight a day is mediated by an active transport of chloride ions across the epithelial lining of the developing lung. In addition, tracheal ligation in different mammalian species always leads to an abnormal distention of

the fetal lungs. Thus, ample data support the concept that there is a relatively large volume of liquid flowing out of the lungs of the human fetus during normal pregnancy, although this has yet to be quantified.

Even though it is clear that an outflow of fetal lung fluid occurs, the relative contribution of lung liquid to amniotic fluid is not clear. Early studies in anesthetized animals suggested that the lung fluid exiting the trachea was usually swallowed before it entered the amniotic space. In a study in which flows and compositions were measured in chronically catheterized fetal sheep, it was found that an average of 50% of the fluid secreted by the fetal lungs entered the amniotic sac and the remainder was swallowed as it exited the trachea (Brace et al., 1994). In humans, the phospholipids (either the lecithin-to-sphingomyelin ratio or the relative amounts of phosphatidylglycerol and phosphatidylinositol) measured in amniotic fluid as tests of fetal lung maturity are of pulmonary origin and are not passed in significant quantities through the urine. Thus, a significant fraction of the secreted lung liquid in the human fetus appears to enter the amniotic fluid.

Fetal Skin

It is possible that amniotic fluid may be derived from water transport across the highly permeable skin of the fetus during the first half of gestation. At 22 to 25 weeks, keratinization of the skin occurs; it is generally accepted that significant amounts of water and solute are not transferred across this membrane after keratinization except for small lipid-soluble molecules, such as carbon dioxide. As has been reviewed (Brace, 1986), however, there is ample evidence that the rate of water metabolism and transepidermal water loss is greater in premature newborns (32 to 37 weeks) than in full-term infants, and in very preterm infants (28 to 30 weeks) a further increase occurs.

Fetal Membranes

The amnion and chorion provide a large surface area for the potential transfer of both water and solute and hence may play an important role in the regulation of amniotic fluid balance. Until recently, little was known about either net volume or solute movement across the membranes except for a few isolated pieces of information in combination with speculation. As noted earlier, an inward transfer of solute across the amnion with water following passively is believed to be the source of amniotic fluid very early in gestation. In the latter half of gestation, Liley (1972) and others have suggested that the net water transfer across the amnion is outward, whereas the net electrolyte transfer is inward. Rodeck and Nicolini (1988) noted that water and solutes readily cross the fetal surface of the placenta between amniotic fluid and fetal blood. It is also known that AFV usually decreases after fetal death. The latter should be interpreted cautiously because the membranes are undoubtedly changed with fetal death. Thus, the membranes and fetal surface of the placenta allow water and solute movement.

By summing best estimates of inflows and outflows in the near-term fetus (Fig. 3-5), one can estimate that 200 to 500 mL/day leaves the amniotic space across the fetal membranes during late gestation. Measurements in late gestation fetal sheep (Gilbert and Brace, 1989; Jang and Brace, 1992;

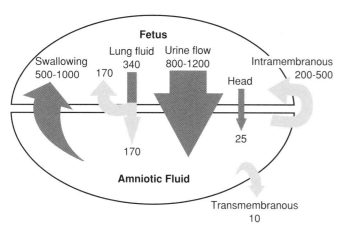

FIGURE 3-5 ■ Estimates of inflows to and outflows from amniotic fluid in the near-term fetus. (Modified from Gilbert WM, Moore TR, Brace RA: Amniotic fluid dynamics. Fetal Med Rev **3**:89, 1991.)

Brace, 1995) support the concept that 200 to 500 mL/day of ovine amniotic fluid are absorbed by the fetal blood that perfuses the fetal surface of the placenta and the membranes (the amnion and chorion are vascularized in sheep but not in humans). This is *intramembranous* flow (Gilbert and Brace, 1989), and similar volumes may be absorbed across the fetal surface of the placenta in humans (Gilbert et al., 1991, 1997; Mann et al., 1996; Curran et al., 1998). Gitlin and colleagues (1972) noted that the clearance of high molecular weight proteins from the amniotic fluid is elevated in laboring women. Because labor is associated with suppressed fetal swallowing, intramembranous absorption appears responsible for the elevated protein clearance. This is consistent with recent animal studies that demonstrated rapid intramembranous albumin clearance (Mann et al., 2001; Faber and Anderson, 2002).

In contrast to an increasing role of intramembranous flow in the regulation of AFV as suggested by recent data, there is little support for transmembranous flow contributing to AFV regulation in the latter half of gestation. Highly diffusible solutes such as urea and carbon dioxide have nondetectable transmembranous fluxes. Quantitative estimates suggest that only 10 mL/day may cross the *transmembranous route* and be absorbed by the uterus in late gestation sheep when amniotic osmolality is normal (Anderson et al., 1988). However, the decrease in AFV after fetal death shows that our knowledge of transmembranous fluxes is far from complete. More study is needed.

Experimental studies indicate that the fetal membranes may be abnormal when AFV falls outside its normal range. The amniotic epithelial cell layer is one-half normal thickness in pregnancies complicated by oligohydramnios, whereas thicknesses greater than normal frequently occur with hydramnios (Hebertson et al., 1986). In addition, a chorionic lactogen receptor deficiency occurs in various forms of chronic hydramnios (Healy et al., 1985). Whether these produce or are caused by the aberrations in AFV has yet to be established. However, the observation that fetal prolactin levels are low in diabetic pregnancies (Saltzman et al., 1986) supports the possibility that altered membrane transport may play a role in the etiology of polyhydramnios and oligohydramnios.

A major driving force for both intramembranous and transmembranous fluid movements is present because amniotic fluid normally has a lower osmolality than either fetal or maternal blood after the fetal skin keratinizes. Experimental studies demonstrated that intramembranous absorption varies with the amniotic-to-fetal blood osmotic gradient when amniotic osmolality is varied over a large range (Faber and Anderson, 2002). However, with a normal osmotic gradient, only 35% of the intramembranous flux depended on the osmotic gradient, so other nonpassive mechanisms contribute to intramembranous absorption. This is consistent with the observation that radiolabeled albumin rapidly crosses from amniotic fluid to fetal blood in pregnant sheep, whereas no flux of radiolabeled albumin occurs in the opposite direction from fetal blood to amniotic fluid (Faber and Anderson, 2002).

Because of the large surface area of the chorioamnion, it has often been suggested that large amounts of water and solutes move across the membranes. Thus, it is not surprising that membrane permeability frequently has been proposed to be an important regulator of AFV (Lingwood and Wintour, 1984). Although membrane permeability is critically important, little is known about the filtration and permeability characteristics of the membranes *in vivo* as they relate to amniotic fluid dynamics because of a sparsity of studies and sometimes conflicting interpretations. For example, the increase in amniotic fluid osmolality after the intravenous injection of hypertonic fluids into pregnant sheep was interpreted to be due to a net transmembranous movement of water (Ross et al., 1983). However, this was shown to be due to an increase in fetal urine osmolality (Woods, 1986). A great deal more information about intramembranous and transmembranous movements is needed to put in perspective the role of the membranes and fetal surface of the placenta in determining AFV.

Other Sources

It has been suggested that significant volumes of water are transferred between the amniotic fluid and the fetal vessels in the umbilical cord (Plentl, 1961). However, with the small surface area and a thickness that is thousands of times that of most membranes across which transfer occurs, it is unlikely that any significant volume exchange occurs across this surface. A more likely site of water and solute exchange is the fetal surface of the placenta, in that the chorionic plate has a larger surface area and a rich supply of fetal blood just beneath its surface. Another relevant observation is that the density of sweat glands in the fetus is higher than in later life (Liley, 1972), but it is unknown whether the fetus sweats *in utero*.

Finally, secretions from the nasal and buccal mucosa should be considered. The large amounts of saliva produced by the newborn suggest a similar production by the fetus, and experimental studies in late-gestation sheep found that approximately 25 mL/day of fluid was secreted from the fetal head (Brace, 1986). Because this flow is small compared with the other main flows, it is not considered to be a main source of amniotic fluid.

■ COMPOSITION OF AMNIOTIC FLUID

During the first third of gestation, amniotic fluid has an electrolyte composition and osmolality that are essentially the same as those of fetal and maternal blood (Fig. 3-6). When

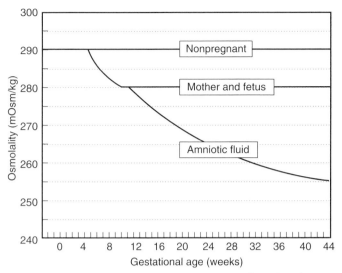

FIGURE 3-6 ■ Gestational changes in osmolality of amniotic fluid and fetal and maternal blood. (From Gilbert WM, Moore TR, Brace RA: Amniotic fluid dynamics. Fetal Med Rev **3**:89, 1991.)

fetal urine begins to enter the amniotic sac, amniotic osmolality decreases slightly compared with fetal blood. As keratinization of the fetal skin occurs, amniotic fluid osmolality continues to decrease with advancing gestational age, reaching values of 250 to 260 mOsm/kg water near term compared with blood osmolality of 280 mOsm/kg (see Fig. 3-6). The amniotic fluid concentration of major solutes, such as sodium and chloride ions, parallels the changes in osmolality, and disease states involving major alterations in amniotic fluid electrolyte concentrations are virtually unknown. The low amniotic fluid osmolality is produced by the inflow of markedly hypotonic fetal urine (60 to 140 mOsm/kg water) in combination with a lesser volume of isotonic lung liquid. Modeling studies also suggest that the passive diffusional entry of small molecular weight solutes through the intramembranous pathway have a major impact on amniotic fluid composition (Curran et al., 1998).

In fetal monkeys, partial exchange of amniotic fluid with distilled water was followed by a restoration of solute concentrations within 24 hours while volume was reduced (Schruefer et al., 1972). In fetal sheep, infusion of 1 liter of an artificial amniotic saline was followed by a return to normal volume within 24 hours, whereas infusion of 1 liter of isotonic mannitol reduced sodium concentration and elevated volume for more than 24 hours (Tomoda et al., 1987). These data show that both amniotic osmolality and amniotic composition play an important role in determining AFV. This occurs primarily by altering the intramembranous movement of solutes and water, although transmembranous flow, if such occurs, may change as well. From theory, the extent of intramembranous and transmembranous water and solute movements depends on the filtration and permeability characteristics of the fetal membranes, but these have yet to be determined *in vivo* in humans. In sheep, the filtration coefficient of the intramembranous pathway averages 5% that of the placenta (Gilbert and Brace, 1990), whereas that of the transmembranous pathway is about 10-fold lower (Anderson et al., 1988).

REGULATION OF AMNIOTIC FLUID VOLUME

Although many theories have been advanced to explain the accumulation of amniotic fluid, little is known about the determinants of AFV in most circumstances. It is safe to state that if AFV is regulated, one or more of the inflows or outflows must be adjusted so as to maintain AFV close to normal; however, it is not known whether AFV is, in fact, regulated. It has often been argued that AFV must be regulated because most of the time volume late in gestation falls within the range of 0.5 to 2 liters. This concept is supported by animal studies in which AFV returned toward normal after experimental increases or decreases in volume (Tomoda et al., 1987), but these observations do not prove that volume regulation exists and do not provide insight as to mechanisms.

One approach to understanding the regulation of AFV is to examine the individual flows that enter and leave the amniotic space. A considerable amount is known about the regulation of fetal urine flow and composition. These are modulated by arginine vasopressin, aldosterone, angiotensin II, and atrial natriuretic peptide in ways that are qualitatively similar to regulation in the adult. The rate of fluid production by the fetal lungs is affected by several hormones circulating in fetal blood, including arginine vasopressin and epinephrine (Brace, 1986), and the progressive decrease in lung liquid production that begins 3 days before delivery correlates inversely with plasma cortisol concentrations (Kitterman et al., 1979). Fetal swallowing varies with fetal osmolality and angiotensin II concentrations and is suppressed by hypoxia. Thus, of the four major flows to and from the amniotic sac, all except intramembranous are regulated to meet the needs of the fetus, not to maintain AFV. This conclusion is the basis of the current concept that if AFV is regulated, this occurs through regulation of intramembranous absorption (Ross et al., 2001).

Recent studies support this concept in that under a variety of experiment conditions, intramembranous absorption increases greatly and thereby prevents polyhydramnios (Faber and Anderson, 1999, 2002; Matsumoto et al., 2000, Matsumoto, Cheung, et al., 2001). Further, increased intramembranous absorption appears to be responsible for the oligohydramnios that occurs with severe placental insufficiency (Gagnon et al., 2002). The increased absorption may be mediated by vascular endothelial growth factor, because vascular endothelial growth factor mRNA levels within the membranes and placenta are elevated under all conditions studied thus far when intramembranous flow is increased (Matsumoto, Bogic, et al., 2001, 2002). The currently emerging concept is that vascular endothelial growth factor modulates intramembranous absorption by promoting vesicular transport across the amnion and into the fetal blood perfusing the fetal surface of the placenta.

Finally, the mother's fluid status may affect AFV. Because fluid moves with relative ease between fetal and maternal blood across the placenta, the maternal effects on fetal hydration could be a major determinant of AFV under certain circumstances. Ample data show that acute changes in maternal osmolality alter fetal hydration. In a study yet to be confirmed, Goodlin and coworkers (1983) reported that if fetal anomalies and diabetes are excluded, there is a strong relationship between maternal plasma volume expansion during pregnancy and AFV, so that subnormal plasma volume expansion is associated with oligohydramnios and elevated plasma volume with hydramnios. In addition, when the maternal plasma volume deficit was corrected with intravenous fluids, the oligohydramnios frequently was resolved. Animal studies of maternal water deprivation similarly have found reduced AFV. In contrast, studies in pregnant sheep have shown that severe sodium depletion over 6 days caused a large decrease in maternal plasma volume and sodium ion concentration with an increase in AFV (Phillips and Sundaram, 1966). Thus, the maternal effects on amniotic fluid have yet to be clearly delineated. Nonetheless, important studies are beginning to characterize the maternal effects on AFV in humans. For example, ingestion of 2 liters of water in women with a low amniotic fluid index resulted in a significant increase in the amniotic fluid index (Kilpatrick et al., 1991; Hofmeyr and Gulmezoglu, 2002).

■ SUMMARY

There is a wide range of AFVs during normal human pregnancy. When fetal anomalies are excluded, there are three major determinants of AFV: movements of water and solutes within and across the membranes; physiologic regulation by the fetus of three major flow rates, including urine production, swallowing, and intramembranous absorption; and maternal effects on transplacental fluid movement. Active regulation of AFV appears to occur through modulation of the rate of intramembranous absorption that, in turn, may be regulated by vascular endothelial growth factor.

REFERENCES

Abramovich DR, Garden A, Landial J, et al: Fetal swallowing and voiding in relation to hydramnios. Obstet Gynecol **54**:15, 1979.

Abramovich DR, Page KP: Pathways of water transfer between liquor amnii and the feto-placental unit at term. Eur J Obstet Gynaecol **3**:155, 1973.

Adamson TM, Brodecky V, Lambert TF, et al: The production and composition of lung liquid in the in-utero foetal lamb. *In* Comline RS, Cross KW, Dawes GS, et al (eds): Foetal and Neonatal Physiology. Cambridge, Cambridge University Press, 1973.

Anderson DF, Faber JJ, Parks CM: Extraplacental transfer of water in the sheep. J Physiol **406**:75, 1988.

Bain AD, Scott JS: Renal agenesis and severe urinary tract dysplasia: A review of 50 cases with particular reference to the associated anomalies. Br Med J **1**:841, 1960.

Bastide A, Manning F, Harmon C, et al: Ultrasound evaluation of amniotic fluid: Outcome of pregnancies with severe oligohydramnios. Am J Obstet Gynecol **154**:895, 1986.

Brace RA: Amniotic fluid volume and its relationship to fetal fluid balance: Review of experimental data. Semin Perinatol **10**:103, 1986.

Brace RA: Progress toward understanding the regulation of amniotic fluid volume: Water and solute fluxes in and through the fetal membranes. Placenta **16**:1, 1995.

Brace RA, Moore TR: Diurnal rhythms in fetal urine flow, vascular pressures, and heart rate in sheep. Am J Physiol **261**:R1015, 1991.

Brace RA, Wlodek ME, Cock ML, et al: Swallowing of lung liquid and amniotic fluid by the ovine fetus under normoxic and hypoxic conditions. Am J Obstet Gynecol **171**:764, 1994.

Brace RA, Wolf EJ: Normal amniotic fluid volume changes throughout pregnancy. Am J Obstet Gynecol **161**:382, 1989.

Carmichael L, Campbell K, Patrick J: Fetal breathing, gross fetal body movements, and maternal and fetal heart rates before spontaneous labor at term. Am J Obstet Gynecol **148**:675, 1984.

Chamberlain PF, Manning FA, Morrison I, et al: Ultrasound evaluation of amniotic fluid volume. I. The relationship of marginal and decreased amniotic fluid volumes to perinatal outcome. Am J Obstet Gynecol **150**:245, 1984a.

Chamberlain PF, Manning FA, Morrison I, et al: Ultrasound evaluation of amniotic fluid volume. II. The relationship of increased amniotic fluid volumes to perinatal outcome. Am J Obstet Gynecol **150**:250, 1984b.

Creasy RK: Biophysical aspects of management of the growth retarded fetus. Semin Perinatol **8**:56, 1984.

Curran MA, Nijland MJ, Mann SE, et al: Human amniotic fluid mathematical model: Determination and effect of intramembranous sodium flux. Am J Obstet Gynecol **178**:484, 1998.

Elliott PM, Inman WHW: Volume of liquor amnii in normal and abnormal pregnancy. Lancet **2**:836, 1961.

Faber JJ, Anderson DF: Regulatory response of intramembranous absorption of amniotic fluid to infusion of exogenous fluid in sheep. Am J Physiol **277**:R236, 1999.

Faber JJ, Anderson DF: Absorption of amniotic fluid by amniochorion in sheep. Am J Physiol **282**:H850, 2002.

Gagnon R, Harding R, Brace RA: Amniotic fluid and fetal urinary responses to severe placental insufficiency in sheep. Am J Obstet Gynecol **186**:1076, 2002.

Gilbert WM, Brace RA: The missing link in amniotic fluid volume regulation: Intramembranous absorption. Obstet Gynecol **74**:748, 1989.

Gilbert WM, Brace RA: Novel determination of filtration coefficient of ovine placenta and intramembranous pathway. Am J Physiol **259**:R1281, 1990.

Gilbert WM, Eby-Wilkens E, Tarantal AF: The missing link in rhesus monkey amniotic fluid volume regulation: Intramembranous absorption. Obstet Gynecol **89**:462, 1997.

Gilbert WM, Moore TR, Brace RA: Amniotic fluid dynamics. Fetal Med Rev **3**:89, 1991.

Gitlin D, Dumate J, Morales C, et al: The turnover of amniotic fluid protein in the human conceptus. Am J Obstet Gynecol **113**:632, 1972.

Goodlin RC, Anderson JC, Gallagher TF: Relationship between amniotic fluid volume and maternal plasma volume expansion. Am J Obstet Gynecol **146**:505, 1983.

Gresham EL, Rankin JH, Makowski EL, et al: An evaluation of fetal renal function in a chronic sheep preparation. J Clin Invest **51**:149, 1972.

Harding R, Bocking AD, Sigger JN, et al: Composition and volume of fluid swallowed by fetal sheep. Q J Exp Physiol **69**:487, 1984.

Harding R, Hooper SB, Dickson KA: A mechanism leading to reduced lung expansion and lung hypoplasia in fetal sheep during oligohydramnios. Am J Obstet Gynecol **163**:1904, 1990.

Healy DL, Herington AC, O'Herlihy C: Chronic polyhydramnios is a syndrome with a lactogen receptor defect in the chorion laeve. Br J Obstet Gynaecol **92**:461, 1985.

Hebertson RM, Hammond ME, Bryson MJ: Amniotic epithelial ultrastructure in normal, polyhydramnic, and oligohydramnic pregnancies. Obstet Gynecol **68**:74, 1986.

Hedriana HL: Ultrasound measurement of fetal urine flow. Clin Obstet Gynecol **40**:337, 1997.

Hofmeyr GJ, Gulmezoglu AM: Maternal hydration for increasing amniotic fluid volume in oligohydramnios and normal amniotic fluid volume. Cochrane Database Syst Rev **1**:CD000134, 2002.

Jang PR, Brace RA: Amniotic fluid composition changes during urine drainage and tracheo-esophageal occlusion in fetal sheep. Am J Obstet Gynecol **167**:1732, 1992.

Kilpatrick SJ, Safford KL, Pomeroy T, et al: Maternal hydration increases amniotic fluid index. Obstet Gynecol **78**:1098, 1991.

Kitterman JA, Ballard PL, Clements JA, et al: Tracheal fluid in fetal lambs: Spontaneous decrease prior to birth. J Appl Physiol **47**:985, 1979.

Kurjak A, Kirkinen P, Latin V, et al: Ultrasonic assessment of fetal kidney function in normal and complicated pregnancies. Am J Obstet Gynecol **141**:266, 1981.

Landis EM, Pappenheimer JR: Exchange of substances through capillary walls. *In* Hamilton WF, Dow P (eds): Handbook of Physiology, Circulation, vol. 2, section 2. Bethesda, Md, American Physiological Society, 1963.

Liley AW: Disorders of amniotic fluid. *In* Assali NS (ed): Pathophysiology of Gestation. New York, Academic Press, 1972.

Lingwood BE, Wintour EM: Amniotic fluid volume and in vivo permeability of ovine fetal membranes. Obstet Gynecol **64**:368, 1984.

Lotgering FK, Wallenburg HCS: Mechanisms of production and clearance of amniotic fluid. Semin Perinatol **10**:94, 1986.

Mann SE, Lee JJ, Ross MG: Ovine intramembranous pathway permeability: Use of solute clearance to determine membrane porosity. J Matern Fetal Med **10**:335, 2001.

Mann SE, Nijland MJ, Ross MG: Mathematic modeling of human amniotic fluid dynamics. Am J Obstet Gynecol **175**:937, 1996.

Matsumoto LC, Bogic L, Brace RA, et al: Fetal esophageal ligation induces VEGF mRNA expression in fetal membranes. Am J Obstet Gynecol **184**:175, 2001.

Matsumoto LC, Bogic L, Brace RA, et al: Prolonged hypoxia upregulates vascular endothelial growth factor messenger RNA expression in ovine fetal membranes and placenta. Am J Obstet Gynecol **186:**303, 2002.

Matsumoto LC, Cheung CY, Brace RA: Effect of esophageal ligation on amniotic fluid volume and urinary flow rate in fetal sheep. Am J Obstet Gynecol **182:**699, 2000.

Matsumoto LC, Cheung CY, Brace RA: Increased urinary flow without development of polyhydramnios in response to prolonged hypoxia in the ovine fetus. Am J Obstet Gynecol **184:**1008, 2001.

Mercer LJ, Brown LG, Petres RE, et al: A survey of pregnancies complicated by decreased amniotic fluid. Am J Obstet Gynecol **149:**355, 1984.

Minei LJ, Suzuki K: Role of fetal deglutition and micturition in the production and turnover of amniotic fluid in the monkey. Obstet Gynecol **48:**177, 1976.

Moya F, Apgar V, St. James L, et al: Hydramnios and congenital anomalies. JAMA **173:**1552, 1960.

Nakayama PD, Glick PL, Harrison MR, et al: Experimental pulmonary hypoplasia due to oligohydramnios and its reversal by relieving thoracic compression. J Pediatr Surg **18:**347, 1983.

Phillips GD, Sundaram SK: Sodium depletion of pregnant ewes and its effects on foetuses and foetal fluids. J Physiol **184:**889, 1966.

Plentl AA: Transfer of water across perfused umbilical cord. Proc Soc Exp Biol Med **107:**622, 1961.

Pritchard JA: Deglutition by normal and anencephalic fetuses. Obstet Gynecol **25:**289, 1965.

Rabinowitz R, Peters MT, Vyas S, et al: Measurement of fetal urine production in normal pregnancy by real-time ultrasonography. Am J Obstet Gynecol **161:**1264, 1989.

Rodeck CH, Nicolini U: Physiology of the mid-trimester fetus. Br Med Bull **44:**826, 1988.

Ross MG, Brace RA, NIH Workshop Participants: National Institute of Child Health and Human Development Conference Summary: Amniotic fluid biology—basic and clinical aspects. J Matern Fetal Med **10:**2, 2001.

Ross MG, Ervin MG, Leake RD, et al: Bulk flow of amniotic water in response to maternal osmotic challenge. Am J Obstet Gynecol **147:**697, 1983.

Ross MG, Nijland MJ: Fetal swallowing: Relation to amniotic fluid regulation. Clin Obstet Gynecol **40:**352, 1997.

Ross MG, Sherman DJ, Ervin MG, et al: Stimuli for fetal swallowing: Systemic factors. Am J Obstet Gynecol **161:**1559, 1989.

Saltzman DH, Barbieri RL, Frigoletto FD: Decreased fetal cord prolactin concentration in diabetic pregnancies. Am J Obstet Gynecol **154:**1035, 1986.

Schruefer JJ, Seeds AE, Behrman RE, et al: Changes in amniotic fluid volume and total solute concentration in the rhesus monkey following replacement with distilled water. Am J Obstet Gynecol **112:**807, 1972.

Scott JS, Wilson LK: Hydramnios as an early sign of oesophageal atresia. Lancet **2:**569, 1957.

Seeds AE: Current concepts of amniotic fluid dynamics. Am J Obstet Gynecol **138:**575, 1980.

Smith FG, Lumbers E: Effects of maternal hyperglycemia on fetal renal function in sheep. Am J Physiol **255:**F11, 1989.

Tomoda S, Brace RA, Longo LD: Amniotic fluid volume and fetal swallowing rate in sheep. Am J Physiol **249:**R133, 1985.

Tomoda S, Brace RA, Longo LD: Amniotic fluid volume regulation: Basal values and responses to fluid infusion and withdrawal in sheep. Am J Physiol **252:**R380, 1987.

Trimmer KJ, Leveno KJ, Peters MT, et al: Observations on the cause of oligohydramnios in prolonged pregnancy. Am J Obstet Gynecol **163:**1900, 1990.

VanOtterlo LC, Wladimiroff JW, Wallenburg HCS: Relationship between fetal urine production and amniotic fluid volume in normal pregnancy and pregnancy complicated by diabetes. Br J Obstet Gynaecol **84:**205, 1977.

Walker MPR, Moore TR, Brace RA: Indomethacin and arginine vasopressin interaction in the fetal kidney: A mechanism of oliguria. Am J Obstet Gynecol **171:**1234, 1994.

Wilbur WJ, Power GG, Longo LD: Water exchange in the placenta a mathematical model. Am J Physiol **235:**R181, 1978.

Wlodek ME, Challis JRG, Patrick J: Urethral and urachal urine output to the amniotic and allantoic sacs in fetal sheep. J Dev Physiol **10:**309, 1988.

Woods LL: Fetal renal contribution to amniotic fluid osmolality during maternal hypertonicity. Am J Physiol **250:**R235, 1986.

Yasuhi I, Ishimaru T, Hirai M, et al: Hourly fetal urine production rates in the fasting and the postprandial state of normal and diabetic pregnant women. Obstet Gynecol l **84:**64, 1994.

Zamah NM, Gillieson MS, Walters JH, et al: Sonographic detection of polyhydramnios: A five-year experience. Am J Obstet Gynecol **143:**523, 1982.

Chapter 4
MULTIPLE GESTATION
The Biology of Twinning

Kurt Benirschke, MD

INCIDENCE OF TWINNING

The incidence of twinning is surely underestimated. Figures usually given derive from national or regional birth statistics and rely on the reporting by physicians or other personnel attending births. They do not accurately reflect the occurrence of twins at conception because the much higher prenatal mortality of twins (as abortion or fetus papyraceus) is not taken into account. Moreover, the widespread practice of assisted reproductive technology has led to a much enhanced frequency in developed countries, accompanied at times with significant problems (Gleicher et al., 2000).

Guttmacher (1953) suggested that 1.05% to 1.35% of pregnancies were twins, the reason for such wide variation of incidence being that the frequency of the twinning process varies widely in different populations. Data collated from various countries reveal that the variability relates largely to the ethnic stock of the population under consideration. Moreover, although the dizygotic (DZ) twinning rate varies widely under different circumstances, the monozygotic (MZ) twinning rate is "remarkably constant," usually between 3.5 and 4 per 1000 (Bulmer, 1970), although Murphy and Hey (1997) found the rate to have slightly increased in recent years.

When the twinning rate of a population is known, one can roughly calculate the frequencies of triplets, quadruplets, and so on by using *Hellin's hypothesis*. This hypothesis states that when the frequency of twinning is n, that of triplets is n^2, of quadruplets n^3, and so on. The highest number recorded so far is nine offspring (Benirschke and Kim, 1973). Since 1973, there has been a steady rise in the incidence of twins and triplets, so that currently 1 in 43 births is a twin and 1 in 1341 pregnancies results in triplets (Luke, 1994). In part, this increase was attributed to delayed childbearing, but the use of ovulation-enhancing drugs has also been implicated. Although acknowledging the increased DZ twinning frequency attributed to clomiphene, Tong and coworkers (1997) found that the DZ-to-MZ ratio has significantly declined from 1.12 (1960) to 0.05 (1978) and suggested adverse environmental factors as a possible cause.

TYPES OF TWINS

Twins who possess characteristics that make them virtually indistinguishable are referred to as "identical," whereas other twins who are unlike are considered "fraternal." Identical twins always have the same gender, but fraternal twins may be of different genders. The terms identical and fraternal, although popular, are scientifically less useful and are best replaced by the terms *monozygotic* and *dizygotic*, respectively, to indicate the mechanism of origin of the two types of twins. An important reason for this preference is that MZ twins with discordant phenotypes (e.g., cleft lip) would be misclassified as fraternal.

To assess the frequency of MZ and DZ twins, investigators have commonly used *Weinberg's differential method*. This method suggests that the frequency of MZ twins can be deduced from a twin sample when the sex of the twin pairs is known. Thus, if male and female conceptuses were approximately equal and all twins were fraternal (DZ), there would be 50 male–female pairs, 25 male–male pairs, and 25 female–female pairs in every 100 pairs of twins. Any excess of like-sex twins is assumed to be the population of MZ twins. This number then can be calculated by using the following formula:

$$\text{MZ twins} = \text{like-sex pairs} - \text{unlike-sex pairs/number of pregnancies.}$$

When this formula is applied to national birth statistics, approximately one third of twins in the United States are MZ. Moreover, the very high twinning rate of the Yoruba tribe in Nigeria results from a higher frequency of double ovulation, whereas the low twinning rate in Japan is the result of a lower frequency of double ovulation. This formula also supports the notion that MZ twinning occurs with a relatively uniform incidence in different populations and rises only slightly with advancing maternal age (Bulmer, 1970). In contrast, the rate of DZ twinning increases with maternal age to about 35 years and then falls abruptly. The rate also increases with parity, is higher in conceptions that occur in the first 3 months of marriage, and decreases in periods of malnutrition, such as during World War II. James (1981) deduced that DZ twinning also increases with coital frequency, and numerous studies indicate that DZ twins occur in certain families, presumably because of the presence of genetic factors leading to double ovulation. These factors are expressed in the mother but may be transmitted through males. Only a few pedigrees suggest that MZ twinning is inherited, and most authorities conclude that it is a random event. There is also evidence that assisted reproductive technology has increased the frequency of MZ twin births as well, perhaps because of damage to the blastocyst (Sills et al., 2000; Platt et al., 2001).

Much has been written about the possible occurrence of "third twins" or twins that may arise from possibly irregular ovulation events, such as polar body fertilization. Bulmer (1970) concluded that such an event is unlikely to have been described. Bieber and colleagues (1981), however, suggested that the development of an *acardiac* triploid twin (a malformed MZ twin without a heart) represents such an example. As explained later, the topic is important because the evidence that DZ twins come from two ovulations does not rest on very firm knowledge. Goldgar and Kimberling (1981) developed a genetic model to discriminate between DZ and polar body twins. They found that only near-centromeric genetic loci can confidently be used to make such a crucial distinction.

Twins may also originate from fertilization by sperm of two fathers, and the suggestion by James (1981) that DZ twinning is influenced by coital rates relates to this phenomenon of superfecundation. Few cases have been verified. In the ninth reported case, one white twin male and one African-American twin male were presumably conceived by two documented events 1 week apart (Harris, 1982).

CAUSES OF TWINNING

The causes of both MZ and DZ twinning are poorly understood. It is commonly assumed that DZ twinning occurs because of double ovulation, and occasional cases support this assumption. Meyer and Meyer (1981) described two 14-day implantation sites with two corpora lutea of similar age in contralateral ovaries. Moreover, multiple pregnancy can be induced by induction of ovulation, and the polyovulation can be followed via ultrasonography (Schenker et al., 1981; Martin et al., 1991). Serum gonadotropin levels in twin-prone Nigerian women are higher than in control subjects (Nylander, 1981), and lower levels are found in Japanese women, who are less likely to produce fraternal twins (Soma et al., 1975). For these and other reasons, we assume that DZ twinning is the result of somewhat elevated serum gonadotropin levels, leading to double ovulation. Moreover, it is assumed that gonadotropin levels are influenced by maternal age, nutrition, parity, and, among other factors, maternal genotype. It has now been found that DZ twinning correlates with a mutation on chromosome 3 that codes for a receptor gene (Busjahn et al., 2000), whereas Healey and colleagues (1997) questioned a relation to the fragile X syndrome.

Although these assumptions may be correct, they are not proven, and the existence of two corpora lutea is rarely ascertained. It is of interest to learn that the use of ovulation-enhancing agents has also led to an increase in MZ twins but is most easily identified in triplets (Derom et al., 1987). We observed the same phenomenon in placental examination of triplets and quadruplets. This finding seems at first contradictory, but accidents in preservation of the zona pellucida have been witnessed in assisted reproduction of domestic animals, and these accidents are presumably also the basis for these unexpected events. In addition, the occurrence of two ova in one follicle is well documented, as are many abnormal fertilization events.

More important questions about the validity of this concept of DZ twinning are statistical, however, and as yet unanswered. Non–right-handedness is found not only in MZ and DZ twins but also in their close relatives at a higher rate than would be expected in the general population (Boklage, 1981). The same observations have been made with respect to certain forms of schizophrenia, suggesting that the traditional MZ and DZ divisions may be incorrect, a full spectrum may exist between the two classes, and the MZ twinning process relates to a factor interfering with the brain symmetry development of the embryo.

The mechanism leading to MZ twinning is even more obscure. That such twins exist can be verified not only by their physical similarity but also by their identity in genetic characters. Exhaustive blood group analysis, finding no differences in the face of different parental markers, was formerly used to verify identity. Chromosomal markers have been used for the diagnosis of MZ twins with apparently greater assurance (McCracken et al., 1978; Morton et al., 1981), but most recently direct comparison of DNA variations is being used for zygosity diagnosis. The determination of restriction fragment length polymorphism compares fragments of DNA and is decisive. Moreover, this technique can use a variety of tissues, including blood and placenta (Derom et al., 1985; Hill and Jeffreys, 1985). This methodology has now been greatly simplified and automated so that zygosity diagnosis can be achieved quickly, reliably, and inexpensively (Becker et al., 1997). The facts that MZ twins occur slightly more frequently with advancing maternal age (Bulmer, 1970), that malformations often occur, that *conjoined twins* develop, and that MZ twinning can be induced by teratogens (Kaufman and O'Shea, 1978) have led to the hypothesis that MZ twins result from a teratologic event. Boklage (1981) suggested a disturbance in the process of symmetry development in the embryo. It has been possible to produce MZ twins by the separation of early blastomeres in several animal species (*Triturus* sp., *Ovis* sp., *Bos* sp., *Mus* sp., and others), but such physical events do not occur in early embryonic stages.

Because of these uncertainties, it has been convenient to speak of the "twinning impetus," an external and perhaps teratogenic agency, that is randomly distributed and that may lead to twins only up to a certain stage before the embryonic axis is established. Experiments in mice with vincristine support this hypothesis (Kaufman and O'Shea, 1978). If teratogens had their effect later, twins would not be seen but anomalies in the singleton would develop. It is further assumed that this twinning impetus may lead to separation of embryonic cells but that it will not lead to a splitting of already formed cavities. Therefore, when the embryonic events are plotted against embryonic age, one may deduce from the placental configuration the approximate timing of the twinning process (Fig. 4-1).

PLACENTATION IN TWINNING

There are two principally different placental types, *monochorionic* and *dichorionic* (Fig. 4-2), and it is essential that they are so identified at birth. Indeed, it is also desirable to differentiate these placentas prenatally by ascertaining the thickness of the "dividing membranes" sonographically. Winn and associates (1989) established criteria for this measurement and suggested, with an 82% accuracy, that a maximal thickness of 2 mm is diagnostic of monochorionicity. More recent studies showed the reliability of this methodology, especially in the mid-trimester. Oligohydramnios is its most serious limitation (Stagiannis et al., 1995; Vayssiere et al., 1996). Numerous

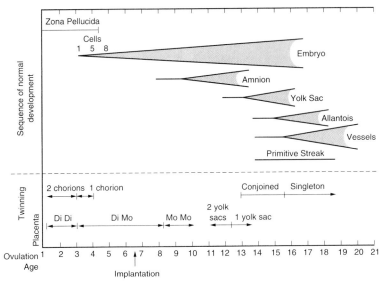

FIGURE 4-1 ■ Schematic representation of monozygotic twinning event superimposed on temporal events of embryogenesis. The embryonic events in the upper portion are sketched according to the publications of early human embryos by Hertig (1968). The twinning event is depicted in the lower portion with resulting placental types indicated. Di Di, diamniotic dichorionic; Di Mo, diamniotic monochorionic; Mo Mo, monoamniotic monochorionic. (From Benirschke K, Kim CK: Multiple pregnancy. N Engl J Med **288**:1276, 1973. Reprinted by permission from The New England Journal of Medicine.)

surveys of placental types of twins have shown that heterosexual (assuredly DZ) twins virtually always have a dichorionic placenta and that monochorionic twins have always been of the same sex. These basic facts led us to assume that all monochorionic twins are MZ. Only very rare exceptions have been identified.

Some MZ twins may be endowed with dichorionic placentas (i.e., twins that separated in the first 2 days after fertilization) (see Fig. 4-1). Most MZ twins, however, have a placenta with diamniotic and monochorionic membranes. Monoamniotic twins, which are by necessity also monochorionic, occur least commonly (incidence, ~1%). Conjoined twins are monoamniotic and are less common still, because it becomes increasingly difficult for a rapidly growing embryo to submit to the twinning impetus.

DZ twins always have dichorionic placentation. Their placentas may be separated or intimately fused (Fig. 4-3). If the placentas are fused, a ridge develops in the central fusion plane that allows easy distinction from the monochorionic placenta. With rare exceptions (King et al., 1995; Molnar-Nadasdy and Altshuler, 1996), blood vessels never cross from one side to the other, and when the dividing membranes (that portion separating the two sacs) are carefully dissected, four separate layers can be identified: one amnion on either side and two chorions in the middle. Between the two chorions one finds degenerated trophoblast and atrophied villi, features that render the dividing membranes of a diamniotic dichorionic twin pair

opaque. Differential expansion of the fetal sacs often causes the membranes of one placenta to push away those of the other (Fig. 4-4), a feature that must not be confused with monochorionic placentation. Very few verified DZ twins with monochorionic placenta have occurred, even with occasional anastomoses and consequent blood chimerism. They are so rare that most have not been reported.

Although 20% to 30% of MZ twins have a dichorionic placentation, most often their placentas are monochorionic. The latter type is invariably fused, and the dividing membranes consist of two translucent amnions only. When these amnions are separated from each other, the single chorion on the placental surface is evident. The chorion carries the fetal blood vessels and various types of interfetal vascular communications that occur regularly in monochorionic twins.

The two principal types of membrane relationships are shown in Figures 4-5 and 4-6. Monoamniotic twins are least common and carry a mortality rate of approximately 50% to 60% because frequent encircling of the cords and knotting lead to cessation of umbilical blood flow. Fetal demise usually occurs in the first part of pregnancy; after 32 weeks' gestation, no further mortality can be expected from entangling (Carr et al., 1990; Tessen and Zlatnik, 1991). The possibility exists, however, that formerly diamniotic membranes become disrupted during gestation with increased fetal mortality ensuing (Gilbert et al., 1991). The perinatal mortality rate of diamniotic monochorionic twins is next highest (~25%), because of the high frequency of the *interfetal*

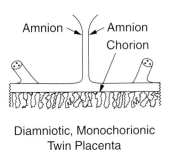

Diamniotic, Monochorionic
Twin Placenta

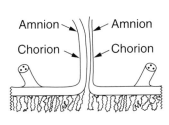

Diamniotic, Dichorionic
Twin Placenta

FIGURE 4-2 ■ The two principal types of twin placentation. *Left,* Diamniotic monochorionic placenta, always monozygotic. *Right,* Diamniotic dichorionic placenta, which may or may not be fused.

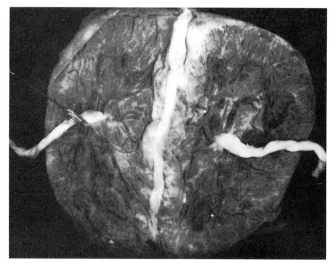

FIGURE 4-3 ■ Diamniotic dichorionic twin placenta, fused. The umbilical cord on the left had a single umbilical artery. Note the close approximation of two placental disks with ridge formed by membranes in center.

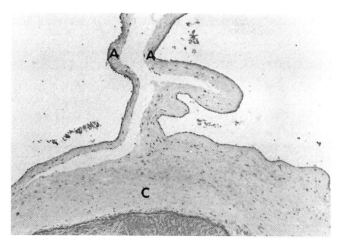

FIGURE 4-5 ■ T section at the point of dividing membranes in diamniotic (A) monochorionic (C) twin placenta.

transfusion syndrome. The mortality rate is lowest for dichorionic twins (8.9%). This has been verified by a large study of twins in Belgium (Loos et al., 1998).

The relationship of placentas among triplets, quadruplets, and higher orders of multiple births generally follows the same principles, except that monochorionic and dichorionic placentations may coexist (Fig. 4-7). With these higher numbers, there is more frequent association of placental anomalies, particularly marginal and *velamentous insertions* of the umbilical cord (Fig. 4-8; see Fig. 4-7) and single umbilical artery (see Fig. 4-3). The etiology of these anomalies may be related to the crowding of placentas and competition for space or to primary disturbances of nidation of the blastocysts.

Velamentous Insertion of Umbilical Cord and Vasa Previa

With the six to nine times higher incidence of velamentous umbilical cord insertion in twin placentas and an even higher incidence in higher order multiple births, the presence of vasa

previa in multiple pregnancy must be anticipated. It is a serious complication and is often lethal because of exsanguination during delivery. Membranous vessels originating from a cord with velamentous insertion radiate toward the placental surface and are not protected by Wharton jelly. Therefore, they may thrombose or may be compressed during labor. Sinusoidal fetal heart patterns may indicate this complication (Antoine et al., 1982). When the membranes are ruptured during delivery and these vessels accidentally have a transcervical position (vasa previa), the rupture may lead to exsanguinating hemorrhage. Not only may the first twin exsanguinate but, as has been described, the second twin may exsanguinate through interfetal placental anastomoses if the placentation is monochorionic. Vasa previa may exist not only over the cervical os but also over the dividing membrane when the second twin's cord has a velamentous insertion on the dividing membranes. Fetal hemorrhage leading to death within 3 minutes has been observed when the diamniotic dichorionic membranes of the second twin were ruptured (Benirschke and Kaufmann, 2000). In nine cases collected by Antoine and colleagues (1982), no

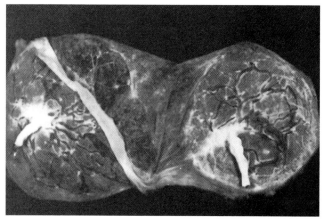

FIGURE 4-4 ■ Diamniotic dichorionic (separate) twin placenta in which the membranous sac of the right twin has pushed away the left membranes so that fusion of dividing membranes occurs over the left placenta ("irregular chorionic fusion").

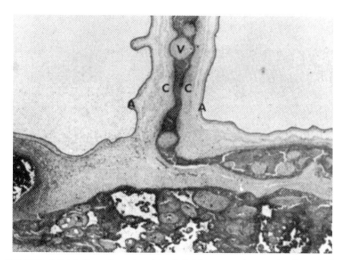

FIGURE 4-6 ■ T section at point of dividing membranes in diamniotic (A) dichorionic (C) fused twin placenta showing degenerated villi (V) and trophoblast (*dark area*) between the membranes. Inflammation of the chorial vessel is present (*left*).

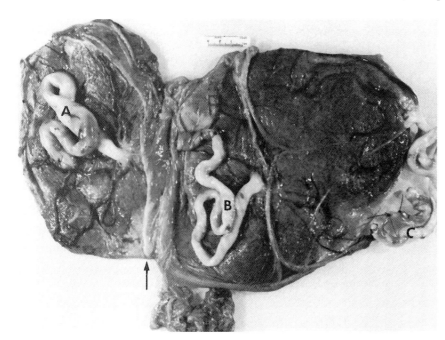

FIGURE 4-7 ■ Placenta of male triplets at 36 weeks. Triplet A has a separate chorion (ridge indicated by *arrow*) from diamniotic monochorionic pair B and C (*right*). Note marginal cord insertion of C. Anastomoses existed between B and C, but A was isolated.

first twin survived and 62.5% of the second twins eventually succumbed as the result of this hemorrhage. In addition, marginal and velamentous insertions of the cord are significantly correlated with smaller fetal weight (Redline et al., 2001).

The gloom with which this entity has formerly been discussed is no longer warranted (Vandriede and Kammeraad, 1981). When vaginal bleeding is not judged with certainty to be the result of a placenta previa, the use of 1-hour hemoglobin electrophoresis is helpful for the detection of fetal blood, as is the Kleihauer-Betke technique, particularly because it can be done more quickly and in the delivery suite at any time.

However, massive external hemorrhage may not always occur to alert the obstetrician to the presence of vasa previa (Fig. 4-9). Anticipation of the possible existence of vasa previa in multiple births is therefore necessary.

Monoamniotic Twins

Monoamniotic twins are all MZ, because all must also have a single chorion. Monoamniotic twins are the least common. Their occurrence is variably recorded as from 1 in 33 to 1 in 661 twin births. In the series reported by Benirschke and

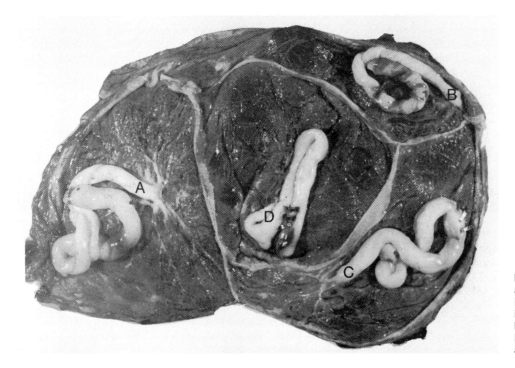

FIGURE 4-8 ■ Placenta of quadruplets at 28.5 weeks. A, C, and D are female; B is male. Placenta is tetrachorionic and intimately fused. Birth order is indicated by letters. Cord B is marginally inserted. Despite intimate fusion, there are no anastomoses.

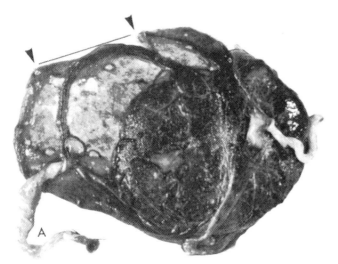

FIGURE 4-9 ■ Fatal vasa previa in twin A of an intimately fused diamniotic dichorionic twin placenta. The disrupted vessel is indicated by *arrowheads*. The mother was admitted 4 hours after rupture of membranes with no history of significant bleeding. Twin A had an Apgar score of 1 and could not be resuscitated. Twin B lived. The left half of the placenta had marked pallor (on maternal surface) because of fetal hemorrhage.

Kaufmann (2000), 3 of 250 pairs had this type of placenta, and three of the six fetuses died from various complications.

The most common complication is encircling and knotting of cords with cessation of umbilical blood flow. Indeed, double survival of monoamniotic twins is so uncommon that such cases were deemed worthy of report (Colburn and Pasquale, 1982). The extent of the knotting of cords is at times astonishing and testimony to the degree of fetal movements. Care must be exercised when the cord of the first-delivered twin is clamped because the cord of the second twin may be inadvertently severed before its birth (McLeod and McCoy, 1981).

Locking is another less common complication associated with monoamniotic twins. Most monochorionic twins have interfetal placental anastomoses, but such vessel communications are not invariably found. It was formerly believed that blood was exchanged between the twins through these anastomoses and that if one twin succumbed before birth, thromboplastin, possibly originating in the macerating fetus, might lead to disseminated intravascular coagulation in the surviving twin. This phenomenon is restricted to monochorionic placentation and occurs in triplets as well (Thomas, 1974). An alternative view for demise of the second twin has now assumed greater likelihood: that severe and acute hypotension develops through exsanguination into an already dead twin via large anastomoses (Yoshioka et al., 1979; Yoshida and Soma, 1986; Benirschke, 1993).

Because of the high mortality rate—the survival rate is only 40% (Colburn and Pasquale, 1982)—antenatal diagnosis is desirable. This has been achieved by amniography and, more recently, by ultrasonography (see Chapters 20 and 29). With such a diagnosis, however, a clear course of action awaited accumulation of adequate statistics that delineate exactly when in the course of pregnancy one or both twins are likely to succumb from cord encircling. Rodis and colleagues (1997) provided some of these data; they showed a 90% survival when adequate antenatal care was provided.

The umbilical cords of monoamniotic twins usually arise near each other on the placenta, and in rare circumstances they are partially fused. Less often, they are velamentous (McLeod and McCoy, 1981). The fusion of cords, of course, represents a gradual transition to the invariably monoamniotic conjoined twins that are thought to form only slightly later, at the end of the twinning spectrum shown in Figure 4-1. Conjoined twins may have two cords with three vessels each, forked cords, anomalous vessels, or, at the other end of the spectrum, one cord with only one artery and one vein. Congenital anomalies, although more common among twins in general, are particularly common in monoamniotic and conjoined twins. The more frequent occurrence of *sirenomelia*—100 to 150 times more common in twins than in singletons (Wright and Christopher, 1982)—has led to insight into the relationship of this anomaly with pulmonary hypoplasia, a regular finding in sirens due to a deficient urinary tract. When one monoamniotic twin is a siren and the other is normal, the amniotic fluid produced by the second twin apparently protects the siren from experiencing pulmonary hypoplasia. When the placenta is diamniotic, this protection does not occur (Wright and Christopher, 1982).

Diamniotic Monochorionic Twins

Diamniotic monochorionic twins are MZ, the placenta is fused, and the umbilical cords often have a marginal or velamentous insertion. The diagnosis is readily apparent from the absence of a ridge at the base of the dividing membranes (see Figs. 4-3, 4-7, and 4-9) and the translucency of the dividing membranes. When the membranes are dissected, one amnion can be readily stripped from the other, leaving a single (placental) chorionic plate that carries the fetal blood vessels. The amnions do not necessarily meet at the vascular equator of the two placental beds but may shift irregularly from one side to the other, presumably because of fetal movements and the relative fluid contents of the two sacs. The diamniotic monochorionic placenta is the most common type seen in MZ twins; approximately 70% have this conformation (see Fig. 4-1).

The diamniotic monochorionic placenta and, less commonly, the monoamniotic twin placenta nearly always possess interfetal blood vessel communications. The anastomosis is more often an artery-to-artery (arterioarterial) than a vein-to-vein communication, and sometimes both types are present and multiple. These vessels allow blood to shift readily from one side to the other, equalizing volumes and pressures. They are most readily demonstrated, after the amnion has been removed, by careful inspection, by stroking blood from one side to the other, or by injection. It is generally impractical to inject the entire placenta from the cord, because rather large volumes are needed and the blood must not be clotted. One can verify the existence of anastomoses more readily by first cutting off the cords and then injecting water or milk into those vessels that are thought to be anastomotic.

The large anastomoses have important practical clinical implications. Through these communications, the second twin may exsanguinate if vasa previa of the first twin are ruptured or, of course, if the cord of the first twin is not clamped. Indeed, because twins are sometimes not detected before delivery, the occasional practice of permitting placental transfusion to occur should be done only when it is confirmed that twins do not exist. Otherwise, the second twin may rapidly exsanguinate through these commonly large-caliber vessels.

It must also be realized that the interfetal anastomoses of larger caliber may lead to significant shifts of blood between fetuses. This is particularly important when one fetus dies. The vascular bed of the dead twin relaxes, and a substantial amount of blood from the survivor may enter the dead twin, causing anemia in the survivor, possibly with destructive consequences. It now appears likely that the appreciable frequency of cerebral palsy of a surviving monochorionic twin results from acute hypotension after one twin dies because of major blood shifts between the twins through placental anastomoses (Yoshioka et al., 1979; Liu et al., 1992). This feature is then grossly similar to the appearance of the twins shown in Figure 4-12, who died from the transfusion syndrome, here with an arteriovenous anastomosis. One twin has much more blood than the other, and when this is due to large blood vessel anastomoses rather than the arteriovenous shunt to be described next, such twins have been erroneously said to have the classic *transfusion syndrome*. Twins with such marked differences in blood content near term are never the result of the twin–twin transfusion syndrome.

The most important anastomosis, the *arteriovenous shunt*, is also the most difficult to diagnose. It is not a direct communication; instead, it occurs when one cotyledon is fed by an artery from one twin and is drained by a vein into the other twin. The arteriovenous shunt is diagrammatically shown in Figure 4-10; the common vascular relationships at a twin vascular equator are seen in Figure 4-11. To recognize such a shared cotyledon, one must follow all terminal arterial branches (arteries cross over veins) and ascertain whether a vein is returning to the same twin, as is normal (see Fig. 4-11, *left*) or whether the cotyledon is drained to the other twin (see Fig. 4-11, *right*). To verify the existence of a common or shared cotyledon, one may inject the artery with water; the shared cotyledon rises and blanches and the water then drains from the vein of the other twin. This arrangement has been referred to as the "third circulation." It is incorrect, however to assume that there are other "deep" anastomoses, as are often discussed. Villi are never connected deep in the placenta, and they can exchange blood only through common shared cotyledons.

Arteriovenous shunts may exist singly or may be multiple, and they may be in opposing directions. When they are not accompanied by artery-to-artery or vein-to-vein anastomoses,

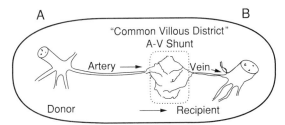

FIGURE 4-10 ■ A and **B**, Monochorionic placenta with shared cotyledon, the basis for the twin transfusion syndrome.

one fetus continuously donates blood into the recipient (see Fig. 4-10), which is the basis of the *twin transfusion syndrome*. This syndrome leads to plethora and hypervolemia (hypertension) of the recipient and anemia (hypotension) of the donor. Cardiac compensation (hypertrophy in the recipient) ensues first, followed by a wide spectrum of bodily growth differences (Figs. 4-12 and 4-13). A common symptom is rapid uterine growth due to hydramnios of the recipient; it is thought to be secondary to excessive fetal urination. The hydramnios usually manifests between 20 and 30 weeks of pregnancy, may reach enormous quantities, and is frequently the cause of premature delivery. The amniotic sac of the donor may be dry, and amnion nodosum may develop. The severity and time of noted growth discrepancy probably depend on the size and the number as well as the direction of arteriovenous shunts. On occasion the syndrome first becomes symptomatic when a formerly balanced blood exchange becomes unstable because of spontaneous thrombosis of a placental vein (Nikkels et al., 2002).

At times, one twin dies *in utero*, the hydramnios disappears, and the pregnancy goes to term with one twin normal and the other a fetus papyraceus (Benirschke and Kaufmann, 2000). When the twins are born, usually prematurely, they may differ remarkably in size; indeed, they may be so discordant that they seem to be DZ twins. Catch-up growth occurs postnatally but often is incomplete, and the twins remain discordant even though they are MZ. This is one more reason not to use the term "identical" twins.

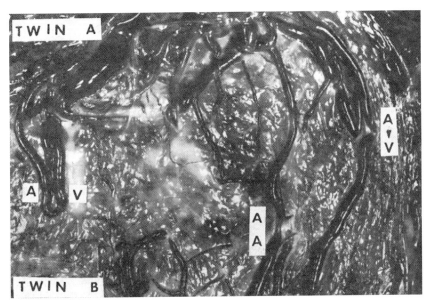

FIGURE 4-11 ■ Diamniotic monochorionic placenta showing a portion of the "vascular equator." The amnions have been stripped off; only the chorionic surface is seen. *Left*, Twin A has a normal cotyledonary supply, with an artery (above veins) feeding a cotyledon that is drained back into twin A. *Middle*, An interfetal arterioarterial anastomosis is seen. *Right*, An arteriovenous shunt (A to B) is demonstrated. These twins came to term because the arterioarterial anastomosis immediately compensated for any inequality of blood volume arising from the arteriovenous shunt. A, artery; V, vein.

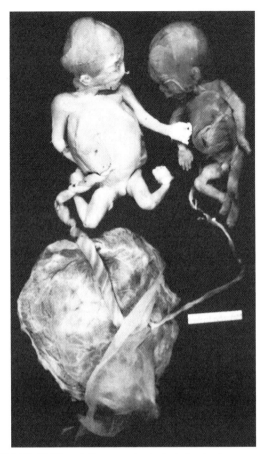

FIGURE 4-12 ■ Diamniotic monochorionic twin abortus secondary to the twin transfusion syndrome. The "donor" (*right*) appears plethoric because he died *in utero* (maceration) and blood returned to him through the arteriovenous shunt. Note discrepancy in size, thick cord of recipient, and hydramneic (large) sac.

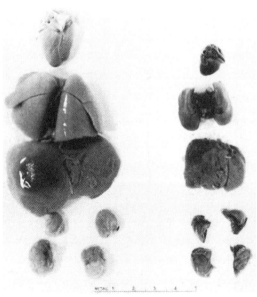

FIGURE 4-13 ■ Hearts, lungs, livers, adrenals, and kidneys of monozygotic twins with transfusion syndrome shown in Figure 4-12. Most marked discrepancies of size exist in hearts, lungs, and livers.

The prenatal diagnosis of the transfusion syndrome can usually be made when mid-trimester hydramnios complicates a twin pregnancy. Wittmann and coworkers (1981) differentiated the condition from other discrepancies of twin growth by the use of ultrasonography. The recipient is more active, and the hydramnios can be associated with the larger twin, whereas the smaller donor twin is the "stuck twin," constrained by oligohydramnios in its amnion. These authors advocate the use of tocolytic agents and report that amniocentesis is rapidly followed by reaccumulation of hydramnios. We believe that the most accurate diagnosis is made by the ascertainment of the relative sizes of the twins' hearts rather than by neonatal blood studies. There is much blood exchanged acutely during delivery in monochorionic twins that make the diagnosis more haphazard.

Digoxin therapy and other means of prenatal treatment have been attempted, generally with mediocre success (De Lia et al., 1985). More incisive is the obliteration of interfetal placental anastomoses at the height of hydramnios by laser fetoscopy (De Lia et al., 1993, 1995). Recent improvements in this technique now make it possible even when the placenta has a posterior location; it is definitive and has greatly prolonged pregnancies that were formerly doomed (see also Chapter 29).

■ ABNORMALITIES OF TWIN GESTATION

Fetus Papyraceus

When one of the fetuses in a multiple gestation dies before birth and the pregnancy continues, the fluid of the dead twin's tissues is gradually absorbed, the amniotic fluid disappears, and the fetus is compressed and becomes incorporated into the membranes. Hence, it is called a *fetus compressus, fetus papyraceus,* or *membranous twin.* The condition occurs in both DZ and MZ twins and is a regular finding when multiple gestations are surgically reduced.

The existence of the fetus papyraceus has important practical and theoretical implications. First, a birth with such an association is not usually entered into statistics as a twin gestation; hence, the frequency of twinning is underestimated. Further, fetus papyraceus is often not recognized at birth. Figure 4-14 shows a twin placenta from what was thought to be an abruptio placentae of a singleton birth. One placenta was normal and the other was a shriveled, diminutive, and separate organ of a DZ fetus papyraceus. The small embryo must have died early, but the preservation of the cord is remarkable. It is possible that this fetus papyraceus was a chromosomally abnormal conceptus that would ordinarily have been aborted had it not been for the normal twin. This would support one hypothesis for the rapid fall in the rate of twin gestations in women over age 35 years. Another less well-understood hypothesis purports ovarian failure in older women to be the cause of the decline (Bulmer, 1970).

Fetus papyraceus in diamniotic monochorionic twins is also often overlooked. The example illustrated in Figure 4-15 was so small and compressed that its formerly presumably normal structure could be deduced only from radiographs (Fig. 4-16) for it to be differentiated from an acardiac twin. This fetus papyraceus is particularly interesting because it was associated with aplasia cutis of the surviving twin. The diffuse form of this

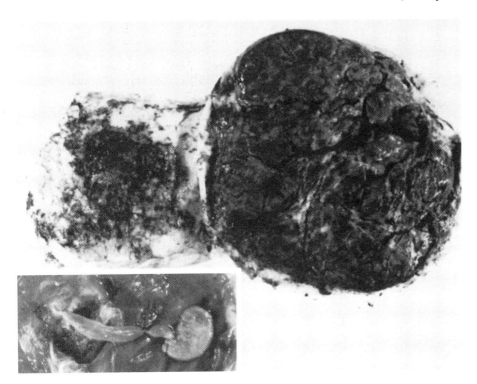

FIGURE 4-14 ■ Placenta of a 35-year-old woman thought to have abruptio placentae. Diamniotic dichorionic separate twin placentas, maternal surface. Normal twin placenta (*right*). Degenerated twin placenta (*left*). *Inset*, Fetus papyraceus, attached to cord. Embryo was golden-yellow, about 1 cm.

unusual skin condition has always been associated with MZ twins, one a fetus papyraceus, in cases in which the placenta has been examined (Mannino et al., 1977). The inference is that diffuse patchy aplasia cutis (in contrast to that in scalp midline) is the result of a prenatal insult associated with the death of one MZ twin.

Another insight into prenatal life afforded by the fetus papyraceus relates to the mechanism that leads to amnion nodosum. When one twin dies, so does the amnion of its sac. This occurs earliest on the diamniotic dividing membranes (Fig. 4-17). Because the amnion does not possess blood vessels, its growth and maintenance must be supported by nutrients and oxygen from adjacent tissues. The large area of dividing

membranes, which are in contact only with amniotic fluid, must be maintained by this fluid. The amnion dies because of the disappearance of fluid or deficiency of its oxygen content. Amnion nodosum, or impaction of vernix, occurs secondarily after epithelial death.

Acardiac Twin

The most bizarre malformation recorded, acardiac twin, occurs only in one twin of a pair of MZ twins. The normal twin maintains the acardiac twin by perfusion through two anastomoses, one artery to artery and one vein to vein. The circulation of the acardiac twin is therefore reversed, and most

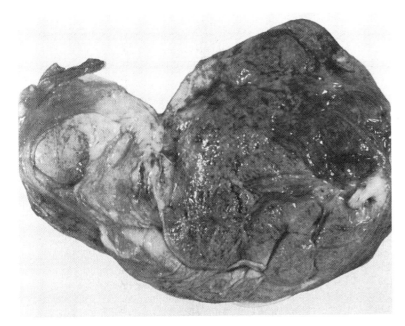

FIGURE 4-15 ■ Diamniotic monochorionic twin placenta with small round fetus papyraceus (see Fig. 4-16) compressed in the thickened membranes at left. Surviving twin associated with right had aplasia cutis.

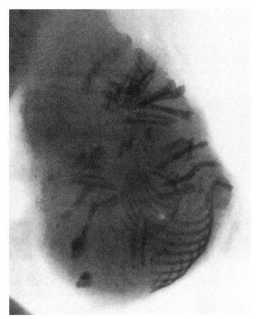

FIGURE 4-16 ■ Radiograph of fetus papyraceus shown in Figure 4-15. The complete presence of skeleton, including skull (*top left*) of fetus, rules out an acardiac twin.

authors have assumed that this reversal of circulation may also be the cause of the malformation (Benirschke and Harper, 1977). This concept is challenged by the occasional observation of an acardiac twin with different chromosomal constitution from that of the always diploid normal twin. Two trisomic acardiac fetuses and one triploid acardiac have been described, findings that suggest major errors in fertilization (Bieber et al., 1981; Moore et al., 1990). Genetic study in the case of Bieber and colleagues indicated the likelihood of origin by fertilization of a polar body for the triploid embryo. It is then remarkable that for every acardiac twin for which adequate placental examination has been made, a monochorionic (usually monoamniotic) placenta has been found, thought to be diagnostic of monozygosity.

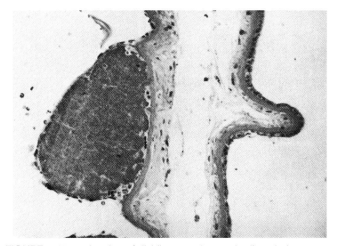

FIGURE 4-17 ■ Amnion of dividing membranes in diamniotic monochorionic twin placenta. The twin and amnion at right were living. The twin at left had died, and a nodule of impacted vernix is present on degenerated amniotic surface.

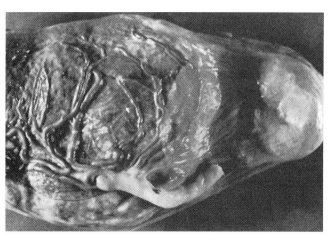

FIGURE 4-18 ■ Diamniotic monochorionic twin placenta with acardiac fetus papyraceus in a separate amnion at right. Diagnosis of acardiac nature was accomplished only by roentgenography.

Occasionally, an acardiac fetus is also a fetus papyraceus (Fig. 4-18), and only radiographs disclose its identity. Acardiac fetuses usually have no heart, as the name implies. Occasionally, however, a misshapen heart is found, commonly two chambered. The wide range of sizes and shapes among acardiac twins has led to a complex taxonomy. Most often, acardiac twins possess legs but lack arms and often have no head or have a head that is markedly abnormal. An acardiac fetus may look like an inside-out teratomatous mass (Fig. 4-19), although the fetus can be distinguished from a teratoma by the presence of an umbilical cord. The cord is invariably short, betraying the immobility of the acardiac fetus, and usually it possesses only one artery. Of course, acardiac fetuses do not survive and have occasionally been removed before term (Robie et al., 1989).

Acardiac fetuses are often referred to as representing the *twin reversed arterial perfusion syndrome*; they can now be detected prenatally sonographically by the absence of cardiac activity and reversal of flow by Doppler (Zucchini et al., 1993). Because the normal twin perfuses this acardiac fetus in a reversed fashion, cardiac hypertrophy and failure may develop in the donor. Healey (1994) identified a 35% mortality rate for the so-called pump twin, and prenatal removal, cord ligation, and other therapy have been advocated.

Other Anomalies

It has long been known that malformations occur more commonly in twins than in singletons; this increase is due to the higher incidence of structural defects in MZ twins (Schinzel et al., 1979). These anomalies may be concordant, but more frequently they are discordant, even in MZ twins. The reasons for the genesis of some anomalies are more readily comprehended than for others, such as the discordant development of conjoined twins and perhaps acardiac anomaly and aplasia cutis. Perhaps some other disruptions, such as porencephaly, occur as a result of interfetal vascular embolization or coagulation, and deformations caused by crowding are explicable. In a large number of structural defects, however, the pathogenesis appears to be linked in some way to the twinning process itself. Thus, anencephaly and sirenomelia occur inexplicably commonly as discordant

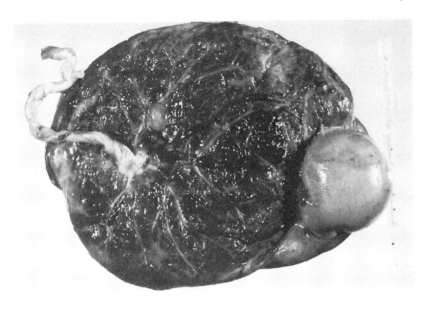

FIGURE 4-19 ■ Diamniotic monochorionic term twin placenta with acardiac twin (amorphus) at right. It was a skin-covered ball of fat with few bones. The umbilical cord was very short. (Courtesy of the late N. Eastman, Johns Hopkins School of Medicine, Baltimore Md.)

anomalies in MZ twins. These and other considerations, detailed by Schinzel and colleagues (1979), suggest that further studies may provide significant insight into not only the poorly understood twinning process but also the pathogenesis of many congenital anomalies (Benirschke and Masliah, 2001).

Perhaps the most perplexing discordance occurs in the so-called *heterokaryotic* MZ twins (i.e., MZ twins with different karyotypes and phenotypes). On first impression, the idea of MZ twins with different karyotypes appears to be contradictory. If chromosomal nondisjunction of cells occurs just before or at the time of twinning, however, the process that causes mosaicism in a singleton may lead to MZ twins with different chromosome sets. Most often this has been described for the sex chromosomes, and XO/XXX, XO/XX, and even XO/XY twins have been reported with appropriate divergence of phenotypes. Sixteen such cases of divergence in gonadal dysgenesis were described by Pedersen and colleagues (1980), to which cases of discordance for trisomy 21 and some cases of acardiac twin must be added. These are the exceptional events, but they indicate the complexities of the twinning process.

"Disappearance" of a Twin

A word may be said about the apparent frequency of twins detected in early pregnancy by ultrasonography and their "disappearance" in later development. Figure 4-14 clearly indicates that even early embryonic death can be recognized in term placentas. I have critically examined a number of term placentas from pregnancies in which a diagnosis of twins had been confirmed by ultrasonography in early stages but no fetus papyraceus or other structure resembling a twin was found. Spontaneous reduction of twin pregnancies observed sonographically were found in 36%, of triplets in 53%, and of quadruplets in 65% (Dickey et al., 2002).

Another reason for a vanishing twin, of course, is the selective fetal reduction of multifetal pregnancies. These multiple pregnancies are often hormonally induced, and selective reduction from triplets to twins improves the outcome of pregnancy (Smith-Levitin et al., 1996). The "reduced" twin may

be detected in the placental membranes, but more often it is represented merely by a small amount of necrotic tissue. The many complications of selective reduction have been summarized by Berkovitz and associates (1996).

Chimeras

On rare occasions, blood grouping or lymphocyte karyotype examination of *fraternal twins* has shown the coexistence of two genetically dissimilar cell types. This state is referred to as *blood chimerism* because the solid tissues do not participate in the admixture. Blood chimerism is best explained by the existence of transplacental anastomoses in fraternal twins that allow migration of the bone marrow-like blood cell precursors circulating in one embryo to settle in the other twin. Because blood chimerism happens so early in embryonic life, this graft is tolerated as "self" and settles permanently without any ill effect. Although blood chimerism occurs with regularity in marmosets and frequently in twin cattle, it must be very uncommon in humans, in whom such anastomoses between the presumably dichorionic twins have been identified only rarely (Lage et al., 1989). The very tight junction between intimately fused placentas in DZ twins and tetrachorionic quadruplets has never been associated with such chimerism.

■ IDENTIFICATION OF TWIN ZYGOSITY

The zygosity of twins is of interest to the twins, their parents, physicians who may treat the children in the future, and scientists. An attempt should be made to establish the zygosity at birth and to register the objective findings in the chart. This time is particularly valuable because of the availability of the placenta, examination of which can aid materially in the process. A good example for this need was provided by St. Clair and colleagues (1998), who treated presumed DZ twins for renal transplantation. DNA tests established "identity" only 15 years later when the transplant had been successful; immunosuppressive therapy was discontinued only then.

The most efficient way to identify zygosity is as follows. Gender examination allows the classification of male–female pairs as fraternal or DZ. The twins should also have a dichorionic placenta that may be separated or fused. Next, the placenta is studied in detail, and twins with a monochorionic placenta (monoamniotic or diamniotic) can be set aside as being of MZ ("identical") origin, whether or not they have dissimilar phenotypes. If doubt exists on gross examination of the dividing membranes, a transverse section (see Figs. 4-5 and 4-6) should be studied histologically. There then remain the like-sex twins with dichorionic placental membranes whose zygosity cannot instantly be known. They must be studied genetically, and several means of discriminating study exist.

One may study a variety of enzyme markers (complex) or, more conventionally, the blood groups. If parents have dissimilar blood groups, DZ twins will, more likely, have dissimilar blood groups. The larger the dissimilarity of parents, the more likely will DZ twins differ in one marker or another. The difficulty occurs when parents have very similar antigenic distribution and also when the blood bank undertaking these studies does not possess all antibodies needed to completely type the blood. Moreover, it is impossible to ensure monozygosity with this method, although one can approach very high probabilities. For these reasons, chromosome markers have been used; they are considered by some to be more discriminating and easier to use (McCracken et al., 1978; Morton et al., 1981). MZ twins always have an identical pattern, and DZ twins do not. The only reservation about this method is that the twin pairs who have been studied for chromosomal polymorphism were not newborns and their chorionic status was unknown; most of them must have been monochorionic (see Fig. 4-1). In each case, the placental anastomoses of the monochorionic placenta, by necessity, would have led to admixtures of would-be different cells. It is therefore mandatory to conduct such studies only in dichorionic twins in the future. The study of DNA polymorphism is currently the best way to approach these difficult problems (Derom et al., 1985; Hill and Jeffreys, 1985; Becker et al., 1997).

Cameron (1968) examined gender, placentas, and genotypes of 668 consecutive twin pairs in Birmingham, England, and found the following distribution:

- 35% DZ, because they were male and female
- 20% MZ, because they were monochorionic (and had the same gender)
- 45% of the same gender but with dichorionic membranes; when these last were genotyped, 36% were DZ because of genetic differences
- 8% MZ, because of genetic identity

REFERENCES

Antoine C, Young BK, Silverman F, et al: Sinusoidal fetal heart rate pattern with vasa previa in twin pregnancy. Obstet Gynecol **27**:295, 1982.

Becker A, Busjahn A, Faulhaber HD, et al: Twin zygosity diagnosis: Automated determination with microsatellites. J Reprod Med **42**:260, 1997.

Benirschke K: Intrauterine death of a twin: Mechanisms, implications for surviving twin, and placental pathology. Semin Diagn Pathol **10**:222, 1993.

Benirschke K, Harper V: The acardiac anomaly. Teratology **15**:311, 1977.

Benirschke K, Kaufman P: The Pathology of the Human Placenta. New York, Springer-Verlag, 2000.

Benirschke K, Kim CK: Multiple pregnancy. N Engl J Med **288**:1276, 1973.

Benirschke K, Masliah E: The placenta in multiple pregnancy: outstanding issues. Reprod Fertil Dev **13**:6, 2001.

Berkovitz RL, Lynch L, Stone J, et al: The current status of multifetal pregnancy reduction. Am J Obstet Gynecol **174**:1265, 1996.

Bieber FR, Nance WE, Morton CC, et al: Genetic studies of an acardiac monster: Evidence of polar body twinning in man. Science **213**:775, 1981.

Boklage CE: On the distribution of nonrighthandedness among twins and their families. Acta Genet Med Gemellol (Roma) **30**:775, 1981.

Bulmer MG: The Biology of Twinning in Man. Oxford, Clarendon Press, 1970.

Busjahn A, Knoblauch H, Faulhaber H-D, et al: A region on chromosome 3 is linked to dizygotic twinning. Nat Genet **4**:398, 2000.

Cameron AH: The Birmingham twin survey. Proc Soc Med **61**:229, 1968.

Carr SR, Aronson MP, Coustan DR: Survival rates of monoamniotic twins do not decrease after 30 weeks' gestation. Am J Obstet Gynecol **163**:719, 1990.

Colburn DW, Pasquale SA: Monoamniotic twin pregnancy. J Reprod Med **27**:165, 1982.

De Lia JE, Emery MG, Sheafor SA, et al: Twin transfusion syndrome: Successful in utero treatment with digoxin. Int J Gynaecol Obstet **23**:197, 1985.

De Lia JE, Kuhlmann RS, Cruikshank DP, et al: Current topic: Placental surgery–a new frontier. Placenta **14**:477, 1993.

De Lia JE, Kuhlmann RS, Harstad TW, et al: Fetoscopic laser ablation of placental vessels in severe previable twin-twin transfusion syndrome. Am J Obstet Gynecol **172**:1202, 1995.

Derom C, Bakker E, Vlietinck R, et al: Zygosity determination in newborn twins using DNA variants. J Med Genet **22**:279, 1985.

Derom C, Vlietinck R, Derom R, et al: Increased monozygotic twinning rate after ovulation induction. Lancet **1**:1236, 1987.

Dickey R, Taylor SN, Lu PY, et al: Spontaneous reduction of multiple pregnancy: Incidence and effect on outcome. Am J Obstet Gynecol **186**:77, 2002.

Gilbert WM, Davis SE, Kaplan C, et al: Morbidity associated with prenatal disruption of the dividing membrane in twin gestations. Obstet Gynecol **78**:623, 1991.

Gleicher N, Oleske DM, Tur-Kaspa I, et al: Reducing the risk of high order multiple pregnancy after ovarian stimulation with gonadotropins. N Engl J Med **343**:57, 2000.

Goldgar DE, Kimberling WJ: Genetic expectations of polar body twinning. Acta Genet Med Gemellol (Roma) **30**:257, 1981.

Guttmacher AF: The incidence of multiple births in man and some other uniparae. Obstet Gynecol **2**:22, 1953.

Harris DW: Letter to the editor. J Reprod Med **27**:39, 1982.

Healey MG: Acardia: Predictive risk factors for the co-twin survival. Teratology **50**:205, 1994.

Healey SC, Duffy DL, Martin NG, et al: Is fragile X syndrome a risk factor for dizygotic twinning? Am J Med Genet **72**:245, 1997.

Hertig AT: Human Trophoblast. Springfield, IL, Charles C Thomas, 1968.

Hill AVS, Jeffreys AJ: Use of minisatellite DNA probes for determination of twin zygosity at birth. Lancet **2**:1394, 1985.

James WH: Dizygotic twinning, marital stage and status and coital rates. Ann Hum Biol **8**:371, 1981.

Kaufman MH, O'Shea KS: Induction of monozygotic twinning in the mouse. Nature **276**:707, 1978.

King AD, Soothill PW, Montemagno R, et al: Twin-to-twin blood transfusion in a dichorionic pregnancy without the oligohydramnious-polyhydramnious sequence. Br J Obstet Gynaecol **102**:334, 1995.

Lage JM, Vanmarter LJ, Mikhail E: Vascular anastomoses in fused, dichorionic twin placentas resulting in twin transfusion syndrome. Placenta **10**:55, 1989.

Liu S, Benirschke K, Scioscia AL, et al: Intrauterine death in multiple gestation. Acta Genet Med Gemellol (Roma) **41**:5, 1992.

Loos R, Derom C, Vlietinck R, et al: The East Flanders prospective twin survey (Belgium): a population-based register. Twin Res **1**:167, 1998.

Luke B: The changing pattern of multiple births in the United States: Maternal and infant characteristics, 1973–1990. Obstet Gynecol **84**:101, 1994.

Mannino FL, Jones KL, Benirschke K: Congenital skin defects and fetus papyraceus. J Pediatr **91**:559, 1977.

Martin NG, Shanley S, Butt K, et al: Excessive follicular recruitment and growth in mothers of spontaneous dizygotic twins. Acta Genet Med Gemellol (Roma) **40**:291, 1991.

McCracken AA, Daly PA, Zolnick MR, et al: Twins and Q-banded chromosome polymorphisms. Hum Genet **45**:253, 1978.

McLeod FN, McCoy DR: Monoamniotic twins with an unusual cord complication: Case report. Br J Obstet Gynaecol 88:774, 1981.

Meyer WR, Meyer WW: Report on a very young dizygotic human twin pregnancy. Arch Gynecol 231:51, 1981.

Molnar-Nadasdy G, Altshuler G: Perinatal pathology casebook. J Perinatol 16:507, 1996.

Moore TR, Gale S, Benirschke K: Perinatal outcome of forty-nine pregnancies complicated by acardiac twinning. Am J Obstet Gynecol 163:907, 1990.

Morton CC, Covey LA, Nance WE, et al: Quinacrine mustard and nucleolar organizer region heteromorphisms in twins. Acta Genet Med Gemellol (Roma) 30:39, 1981.

Murphy M, Hey K: Twinning rates. Lancet 349:1349, 1997.

Nikkels PJ, van Gemert MJC, Sollie-Szarynska KM, et al: Rapid onset of severe twin-twin transfusion syndrome caused by placental venous thrombosis. Pediatr Devel Pathol 5:310, 2002.

Nylander PPS: The factors that influence twinning rates. Acta Genet Med Gemellol (Roma) 30:189, 1981.

Pedersen IK, Philip J, Sele V, et al: Monozygotic twins with dissimilar phenotypes and chromosome complements. Acta Obstet Gynecol Scand 59:459, 1980.

Platt MJ, Marshall A, Pharoah POD: The effects of assisted reproduction on the trends and zygosity of multiple births in England and Wales 1974–1999. Twin Res 4:417, 2001.

Redline RW, Shah D, Sakar H, et al: Placental lesions associated with abnormal growth in twins. Pediatr Devel Pathol 4:473, 2001.

Robie GF, Payne GG, Morgan MA: Selective delivery of an acardiac, acephalic twin. N Engl J Med 320:512, 1989.

Rodis JF, McIlveen P, Egan JFX, et al: Monoamniotic twins: Improved perinatal survival with accurate prenatal diagnosis and antenatal fetal surveillance. Am J Obstet Gynecol 177:1046, 1997.

Schenker JG, Yarkoni S, Granat M: Multiple pregnancies following induction of ovulation. Fertil Steril 35:105, 1981.

Schinzel AAGL, Smith DW, Miller JR: Monozygotic twinning and structural defects. J Pediatr 95:921, 1979.

Sills ES, Tucker MJ, Palermo GD: Assisted reproductive technologies and monozygous twins: Implications for future study and clinical practice. Twin Res 3:217, 2000.

Smith-Levitin M, Kowalik A, Birnholz J, et al: Selective reduction of multifetal pregnancies to twins improves outcome over nonreduced triplet gestations. Am J Obstet Gynecol 175:878, 1996.

Soma H, Takayama M, Kiyokawa T, et al: Serum gonadotropin levels in Japanese women. Obstet Gynecol 46:311, 1975.

Stagiannis KD, Sepulveda W, Southwell D, et al: Ultrasonographic measurement of the dividing membrane in twin pregnancy during the second and third trimesters: A reproducibility study. Am J Obstet Gynecol 173:1546, 1995.

St. Clair DM, St. Clair JB, Swainson CP, et al: Twin zygosity testing for medical purposes. Am J Med Genet 77:412, 1998.

Tessen JA, Zlatnik FJ: Monoamniotic twins: A retrospective controlled study. Obstet Gynecol 77:832, 1991.

Thomas DB: Intrauterine intraventricular haemorrhage and disseminated intravascular coagulation in a triplet pregnancy. Aust Paediatr J 10:25, 1974.

Tong S, Caddy D, Short RV: Use of dizygotic to monozygotic twinning ratio as a measure of fertility. Lancet 349:843, 1997.

Vandriede DM, Kammeraad LA: Vasa previa: Case report, review and presentation of a new diagnostic method. J Reprod Med 26:577, 1981.

Vayssiere CF, Heim N, Camus EP, et al: Determination of chorionicity in twin gestations by high-frequency abdominal ultrasonography: Counting the layers of the dividing membrane. Am J Obstet Gynecol 175:1529, 1996.

Winn HN, Gabrielli S, Reece EA, et al: Ultrasonographic criteria for the prenatal diagnosis of placental chorionicity in twin gestations. Am J Obstet Gynecol 161:1540, 1989.

Wittmann BK, Baldwin VJ, Nichol B: Antenatal diagnosis of twin transfusion syndrome by ultrasound. Obstet Gynecol 58:123, 1981.

Wright JCY, Christopher CR: Sirenomelia, Potter's syndrome and their relationship to monozygotic twinning: A case report and discussion. J Reprod Med 27:291, 1982.

Yoshida K, Soma H: Outcome of the surviving cotwin of a fetus papyraceus or a dead fetus. Acta Genet Med Gemellol (Roma) 35:91, 1986.

Yoshioka H, Kadomoto Y, Mino M, et al: Multicystic encephalomalacia in liveborn twin with a stillborn macerated co-twin. J Pediatr 95:798, 1979.

Zucchini S, Borghesani F, Soffriti G, et al: Transvaginal ultrasound diagnosis of twin reversed arterial perfusion syndrome at 9 weeks' gestation. Ultrasound Obstet Gynecol 3:209, 1993.

Chapter 5

BIOLOGY AND PHYSIOLOGY OF THE REPRODUCTIVE TRACT AND CONTROL OF MYOMETRIAL CONTRACTION

Manju Monga, MD, and Barbara M. Sanborn, PhD

Knowledge of the normal changes that occur in the reproductive tract during pregnancy, the processes that give rise to uterine contraction/relaxation, and the mechanisms controlling these processes is critical to an understanding of myometrial activity and to the rational use of agents to control that activity. Underlying the actions of uterine contractants and relaxants are a number of electrical and biochemical pathways that operate in a time-dependent and pregnancy stage-dependent manner.

MORPHOLOGIC CHANGES IN THE REPRODUCTIVE TRACT DURING PREGNANCY

The Uterus

The uterus undergoes a dramatic increase in size, weight, and capacity during pregnancy. The nonpregnant uterus weighs 40 to 70 g and has a capacity of 10 mL. The uterus at term weighs 1100 to 1200 g and has an average capacity of 5 liters. Early in pregnancy, there is an increase in the number of myometrial cells (hyperplasia); however, mitoses in myometrial cells are rarely seen after the initial period of pregnancy that is followed by an almost exclusive increase in cell size (hypertrophy) (Sanborn, 1987). Hypertrophy occurs early in pregnancy because of the hormonal influence of progesterone and particularly estrogen, with an increase in cellular protein synthesis documented shortly after estrogen exposure (Katzenellenbogen et al., 1979; Sanborn, 1987). Mechanical distension results in stretch-induced hypertrophy as the size of the conceptus increases later in pregnancy. Stretch-induced hypertrophy is associated with increased edema and enlargement of small blood vessels. Myometrial cell size increases from 50 to 500 μm in length and 5 to 15 μm in width. As myometrial cell size increases, there is an increase in oxytocin receptor protein per cell and an increase in the number of smooth muscle cells expressing oxytocin receptors, suggesting an increase in cellular differentiation and an increase in cell size (Ivell et al., 2001).

The increase in myometrial cell size is accompanied by an increase in fibrous and connective tissue that surrounds the myometrial cells. There is hypertrophy of fibrous and elastic tissue throughout the uterus, associated with an increase in the size and number of blood vessels and lymphatics. In addition, trophoblastic invasion of the uterus occurs early in pregnancy, with colonization of the subendometrial myometrium by extravillous interstitial and endovascular trophoblast (Uduwela et al., 2000). This facilitates successful hemochorial placentation and access of fetal cells to nutrients from maternal circulation through the placenta.

Uterine shape changes from predominantly pear shaped to a globular–spherical shape by 12 to 16 weeks' gestation. As pregnancy enters the late second trimester, the uterus becomes more ovoid in shape as length increases out of proportion to width, and this is associated with gradual thinning of the uterine wall. The isthmus, or lowest part of the uterus, fails to undergo hypertrophy and becomes quite distensible, decreasing in cellular content and becoming thin (Danforth, 1947; Sanborn, 1987).

Uterine Blood Flow

Associated with the increase in uterine size is a 10-fold increase in uterine blood flow. Studies in ovine pregnancy indicate blood flow of 800 to 1200 mL/min at term (Rosenfeld, 1977) as compared with measurements obtained by indirect means in humans of 450 to 650 mL/min (Metcalfe et al., 1955; Assali et al., 1960; Rekonen et al., 1976; Edman et al., 1981). This increase in uterine blood flow represents a shift from 2% of cardiac output in the nonpregnant state to 17% at term (see Chapter 8). Studies in sheep have demonstrated that the increase in uterine blood flow is associated with redistribution of flow within the uterus. In the nonpregnant state, uterine blood flow is equally divided between myometrium and endometrium. As pregnancy progresses, blood flow to the placenta accounts for 80% to 90% of uterine blood flow, with the remainder distributed between the endometrium and myometrium (Makowski et al., 1968, Rosenfeld et al., 1974).

The mechanism by which uteroplacental blood flow increases so dramatically is incompletely understood. However, the increase in flow parallels an increase in number and size and concomitant decrease in resistance (vasodilatation) of placental vessels (Teasdale, 1976). Studies in sheep have shown that vasodilatation and uterine blood flow, and specifically flow to placental tissues, increase in response to estradiol (Resnik et al., 1974), by 25% to 43% at term (Rosenfeld et al., 1976), suggesting that sensitivity of uterine vasculature to estrogen may play a role. In addition, expression of vascular endothelial growth factor increases in response to estrogen and may be associated with new vessel growth (Cullinan-Bove and Koos, 1993). There is exaggerated blunting of uterine vascular resistance to angiotensin II as compared with systemic vascular resistance, and this may also result in increased distribution of cardiac output to the uterus (Rosenfeld, 1984).

Recent attention has focused on the role of nitric oxide as a mediator of increased uterine blood flow in pregnancy. Magness and coworkers showed that uterine, but not systemic, artery endothelial nitric oxide synthase protein and mRNA expression and activity are elevated in ovine pregnancy (Magness et al., 1996, 1997, 2001), and this increase is associated with an increase in agonist-stimulated production of prostacyclin and nitric oxide at a cellular level (Bird et al., 2000). The increase in prostacyclin production is accompanied by specific upregulation of cyclooxygenase-1 expression in uterine artery, but not in systemic artery, endothelium (Habermehl et al., 2000). Increased levels of prostacyclin and nitric oxide (and cyclic guanosine monophosphate, the physiologic messenger of nitric oxide) in pregnancy are associated with vasodilatation of the maternal systemic circulation and increased uteroplacental flow (Sladek et al., 1997). In addition, nitric oxide levels have been shown to increase in response to chronic hypoxia, possibly providing a protective regulation of uterine vasomotor tone (Xiao et al., 2001).

Cervix

In contrast to the uterus, which is primarily composed of smooth muscle, the cervix is dominated by fibrous connective tissue composed of extracellular matrix (collagen, elastin, and proteoglycans) and a cellular portion (smooth muscle, fibroblasts, epithelium, and blood vessels). There is extensive remodeling of the cervix during pregnancy, with decrease in collagen content associated with an increase in a low molecular weight dermatan sulfate proteoglycan, decorin. As decorin, which coats collagen fibrils, increases, there is dispersion and disorganization of collagen fibrils (Rechberger and Woessner, 1993). Enzymatic degradation of the cervical extracellular matrix occurs with increased activity of matrix metalloproteinases and elastases. The activity of these enzymes is enhanced by cytokines, including interleukin-1β and interleukin-8, and may contribute to cervical changes associated with infection-precipitated preterm labor (Watari et al., 1999). Hyaluronic acid production is also stimulated by cytokines, and increased levels are found with advancing gestational age and the onset of labor. Increased hyaluronic acid is associated with increased water content and loosening and dispersal of collagen fibers in the cervi (Winkler and Rath, 1999). Finally, the hormonal influence of estrogen, progesterone, and relaxin may result in increased collagenase activity and increased glycosaminoglycan content (Leppert, 1995; Hwang et al., 1996). These changes that result in progressive softening and shortening (ripening and effacement) of the cervix were recently summarized by Ludmir and Sehdev (2000).

The cervix is lined with columnar epithelium. The endocervical glands increase in size and produce mucus throughout pregnancy that forms the *mucous plug*. These proliferating endocervical mucosal glands commonly spread onto the portio

vaginalis of the uterus, resulting in eversion of the squamocolumnar junction that often appears red and velvety in appearance during pregnancy.

Vagina

There is an increase in vascularity of the vagina, with thickening of the vaginal mucosa and enlargement of the papillae. The vagina appears violet-blue in color because of the increase in vascularity, a change that is termed *Chadwick's sign*. There is loosening of collagen and hypertrophy of smooth muscle tissue of the vagina and an increase in cervical and vaginal secretions.

Adnexa

The uterine tubes (fallopian tubes) show little anatomic change during pregnancy, although marked increase in vascularity of the tubes and ovaries is noted. The ovaries cease ovulation during pregnancy, and a single corpus luteum persists, producing progesterone maximally for the first 7 weeks of pregnancy (first 5 weeks after conception). Thereafter, corpus luteal function is of minimal importance, because it is surpassed by placental production of progesterone. The corpus luteum also produces relaxin. Relaxin production continues to increase for the duration of pregnancy; however, its role in human pregnancy has not been well defined (Eddie et al., 1986). Exaggerated luteinization of the ovary may result in a pregnancy luteoma (solid) or theca lutein cysts (multicystic), causing maternal virilization and less commonly virilization of the female fetus (Cohen et al., 1982). Theca lutein cysts are often associated with high maternal human chorionic gonadotropin levels and are commonly seen in molar pregnancies. A decidual reaction on the surface of the ovaries is commonly observed as friable elevated patches of tissue that bleed easily when handled.

CONTROL OF MYOMETRIAL CONTRACTION

Relation of Electrical Activity of Myometrial Contraction

Changes in electrical activity underlie uterine contraction/relaxation. The plasma membrane of cells constitutes a permeability barrier to many biological molecules. The potential difference across the plasma membrane (*membrane potential*) derives from an unequal distribution of ions inside relative to outside the cell (Marshall, 1990; Parkington and Coleman, 1990; Sanborn, 1995). This is attributable to the presence of large negatively charged intracellular biomolecules that cannot exit and of selective plasma membrane channels that regulate the entry and efflux of ions such as sodium (Na^+), potassium (K^+), calcium (Ca^{2+}), and chloride (Cl^-). The permeability of these ion channels is regulated by a variety of signals. Ions move through these channels in a direction that is determined both by the concentration of the ion on each side of the barrier and by the membrane potential.

The resting membrane potential is determined primarily by the permeabilities and relative concentrations of Na^+, K^+, and Cl^-. The concentrations of Na^+, Ca^{2+}, and Cl^- are higher outside the cell, whereas the concentration of K^+ is higher inside the cell. The resting membrane potential in myometrium is generally approximately –40 to –50 mV (Sanborn, 1995; Parkington et al., 1999). It becomes more negative (approximately –60 mV) during pregnancy and increases to approximately –45 mV near term.

The myometrium exhibits rhythmic alterations in membrane potential, termed slow waves (Marshall, 1990; Parkington and Coleman, 1990; Sanborn, 1995). At the *threshold potential*, there is a fast depolarization that generates an *action potential* on top of the slow wave. The action potential is attributed to entry of Ca^{2+} through voltage-sensitive Ca^{2+} channels and, possibly at the end of pregnancy, also through fast Na^+ channels (Sperelakis et al., 1992; Sanborn, 1995). During pregnancy, the pattern of electrical activity in the myometrium changes from irregular spikes to regular activity. Near term, the action potentials generated on top of slow waves correlate with contractions (Fig. 5-1). Frequency of contraction is correlated with the frequency of action potentials, force of contraction with the number of spikes in the action potential and the number of cells activated together, and duration of contraction with the duration of the train of action potentials (Marshall, 1990). As labor progresses, electrical activity becomes more organized and increases in amplitude and duration.

Intercellular Communication Via Gap Junctions

The coordination of contractions is critically dependent on the formation of gap junctions. *Gap junctions* are intercellular channels that when open facilitate electrical and metabolic communication between myometrial cells (Garfield et al., 1990, 1995; Garfield, 1994). Gap junctions consist of pores composed of proteins known as *connexins*, which connect the interior of two cells and which allow current and molecules, up to 1000 Da, to pass between cells. The 42-kDa protein, connexin 43, is the major component of myometrial gap junctions. Each gap junction may consist of a few to thousands of channels, and each channel is constructed from a group of six connexin proteins symmetrically aligned with six connexins in an adjacent cell.

Gap junction function is regulated by the number of gap junctions (structural coupling), their permeability (functional coupling), and their degradation (Garfield et al., 1995). The onset and progression of labor, term or preterm, is preceded by a rapid and dramatic increase in the number and size of gap junctions in lower mammals (Garfield et al., 1990, 1995; Garfield, 1994). In human myometrium, gap junctions are increased in number in women in spontaneous labor compared with nonpregnant women or pregnant women not in labor (Kilarski et al., 1994; Ciray et al., 1995). It is not clear, however, whether gap junctions increase during late pregnancy (Chow and Lye, 1994) or during the active phase of labor (Roomans et al., 1993).

In many species, progesterone appears to *suppress* the number and permeability of gap junctions, whereas estrogen is associated with an *increased* number and permeability of gap junctions (Garfield, 1994). Gap junction channels rapidly transform between the open and closed state; this functional regulation has been correlated with phosphorylation of connexin proteins. Although studies in other cells indicate that cyclic adenosine monophosphate (cAMP)–dependent protein

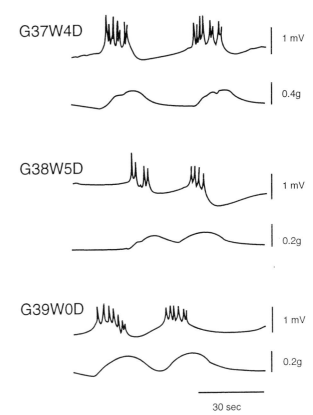

FIGURE 5-1 ■ Simultaneous recordings of electrical (*top recording*) and mechanical (*bottom recording*) activity in uteri of pregnant women at three different gestations (G) of 37 to 39 weeks (W) and of 4, 5, and 0 days (D). (From Kawarabayashi T, Ikeda M, Sugimori H, et al: Spontaneous electrical activity and effects of noradrenaline on pregnant human myometrium recorded by the single sucrose gap method. Acta Physiol Hung **67**:71, 1986.)

kinases regulate phosphorylation of connexin proteins and result in closure of gap junctions (Garfield, 1994), Burghardt and coworkers (1996) demonstrated that cAMP increased gap junction expression and intercellular communication in an immortalized myometrial cell line derived from a pregnant human at term.

Gap junctions rapidly disappear after delivery as a result of internalization, endocytosis, and digestion; this is accompanied by decreased excitability and contractile function of myometrial smooth muscle (Garfield et al., 1990). The mechanisms responsible for this degradation process remain to be delineated.

Link of Ca^{2+} to Contraction and Contractile Proteins

A rise in intracellular calcium (Ca_i^{2+}) triggers muscle contraction. The structural basis for contraction is the relative movement of thick and thin filaments in the contractile apparatus. Although this movement is similar in all muscles, several structural and regulatory features are specific to smooth muscles, including myometrium (Jiang and Stephens, 1994; Somlyo and Somlyo, 1994). In smooth muscle, the extensive sarcomere arrangement of thick and thin filaments seen in striated muscle is present on a much smaller scale. Intermediate filaments contribute to the cytoskeletal network that is thought

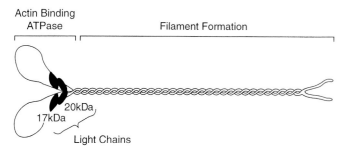

FIGURE 5-2 ■ Schematic representation of smooth muscle myosin showing the globular head region of each 200-kDa heavy chain, with associated 17- and 20-kDa light chain subunits, and the filamentous tail region that interacts with similar regions of other myosin molecules to form the thick filament. (Modified from Adelstein RS, Sellers JR: Myosin structure and function. *In* Barany MS [ed]: Biochemistry of Smooth Muscle Contraction. San Diego, Academic Press, 1996, p. 3.)

to maintain the structural integrity of "mini-sarcomeres." The thin filaments insert into dense bands that are linked by the cytoskeletal network, allowing generation of force in any direction in the cell. Smooth muscles generally maintain high force with relatively little energy expenditure, and they exhibit greater shortening than striated muscles.

Myosin makes up the thick filaments of the contractile apparatus. Smooth muscle myosin is a hexamer consisting of two heavy chain subunits (~200 kDa) and two pairs each of 20- and 17-kDa light chains (Fig. 5-2). Each heavy chain has a globular head that contains actin binding sites and adenosine triphosphate (ATP) hydrolysis (ATPase) activity. A neck region connects the globular head to the remainder of each myosin molecule, which consists of a long α-helical tail that interacts with the tail of the other heavy chain subunit. Multiple myosin molecules interact via the α-helical tail in a coiled coil rod, forming the thick filament from which the globular heads pro-

trude. Thin filaments are composed of actin and polymerized into a double-helical strand and associated proteins. When the myosin head interacts with actin, the ATPase activity in the myosin head is activated. The energy generated as a result of the hydrolysis of ATP is conserved as conformational energy that allows the myosin head to move in the neck region, changing the relative position of the thick and thin filaments. The myosin head then detaches and can reattach at another site on the actin filament when reactivated.

The actin–myosin interaction is regulated by Ca_i^{2+}. In the myometrium, as in other smooth muscle, the effect of Ca_i^{2+} is mediated through the Ca^{2+} binding protein calmodulin (CaM) (Fig. 5-3) (Word, 1995; Gallagher et al., 1997; Sanborn, 2001). The Ca^{2+} CaM complex binds to and increases the activity of myosin light chain kinase (MLCK) by a mechanism that decreases the influence of an autoinhibitory region of the kinase (Gallagher et al., 1997). MLCK phosphorylates the myosin 20-kDa light chain on a specific serine residue near the N-terminus. Phosphorylation of myosin correlates with an increase in actomyosin ATPase activity and is proposed to facilitate the actin–myosin interaction by increasing the flexibility of the head–neck junction (Jiang and Stephens, 1994).

A number of other proteins may be involved in regulation at the level of the thin filament. Associated with the actin filament are tropomyosin, caldesmon, and calponin. Both tropomyosin and caldesmon increase the binding of actin to myosin and both proteins bind Ca^{2+} CaM. Interaction with Ca^{2+} CaM diminishes the effect of caldesmon on actin–myosin interaction. Both caldesmon and calponin inhibit actomyosin ATPase activity; this inhibition is reversed by the Ca^{2+} CaM complex or by phosphorylation by a Ca^{2+} sensitive kinase. Thus, these proteins provide a means for regulation of actin–myosin interaction and associated ATPase activity and are implicated in the regulation of cross-bridge cycling.

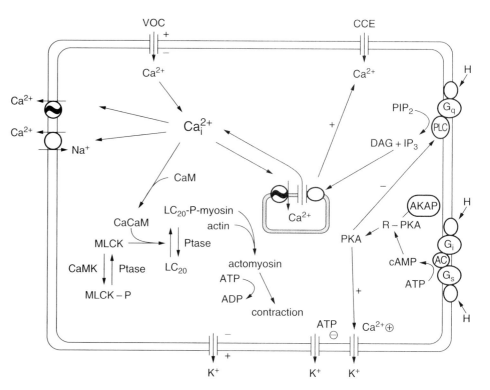

FIGURE 5-3 ■ Pathways leading to control of $Ca^{2+?}$ in smooth muscle. AC, adenylyl cyclase; ADP, adenosine diphosphate; AKAP, adenosine kinase associated protein; ATP, adenosine triphosphate; Ca_i^{2+}, intercellular calcium; CaM, calmodulin; CaMK, Ca^{2+} calmodulin-dependent protein kinase; cAMP, cyclic adenosine monophosphate; Ca^{2+} transport ATPases, Na^+/Ca^{2+} exchanger, Ca^{2+}-activated K^+ channel, ATP-sensitive K^+ channel; CCE, capacitative calcium entry; DAG, diacylglycerol; G, GTP-binding protein; IP_3, inositol-1,4,5-triphosphate; LC_{20}, myosin light chain; MLCK, myosin light chain kinase; PIP_2, phosphatidyl inositol biphosphate; PKA, protein kinase A; PLC, phospholipase C; Ptase, phosphatase; VOC, voltage-operated Ca^{2+} channel. (Modified from Sanborn BM, Yue C, Wang W, Dodge KL: G protein signaling pathways in myometrium: Affecting the balance between contraction and relaxation. Rev Reprod **3**:196–205, 1998.)

In human myometrium, an increase in tension is associated with an increase in Ca_i^{2+} and in myosin light chain phosphorylation (Word, 1995; Savineau and Marthan, 1997). Increases in Ca_i^{2+} precede myosin light chain phosphorylation, and maximal phosphorylation occurs before maximal force is achieved. For the same amount of force generated, less phosphorylation occurs in myometrium from late pregnant than from nonpregnant women (Word et al., 1993). The stress-to-light chain phosphorylation ratio is 2.2-fold greater in tissue from pregnant women. At present, the physiologic basis for this apparent increased efficiency is not understood. Although the amounts of actin and myosin increase per cell in pregnancy, there is no increase per gram of tissue or per milligram of protein and no difference in the specific activity of the MLCK or the phosphatase that removes the phosphate group (Word, 1995). Interestingly, pregnant sheep myometrium also develops greater force per stimulus without differences in myosin light chain phosphorylation than nonpregnant tissue, but in this case the contents of myosin and actin per gram wet weight are increased (Ipson et al., 1996).

Although regulation of myosin phosphorylation by Ca^{2+} has a major effect on smooth muscle contraction, other mechanisms also pertain. For example, tension increases in myometrium, and other smooth muscle can occur in response to external signals in the absence of a change in membrane potential or Ca_i^{2+} (Jiang and Stephens, 1994; Somlyo and Somlyo, 1994). Ca^{2+} sensitization, exemplified by an increase in force-to-Ca_i^{2+} ratio in response to contractants, may involve the participation of additional intracellular signaling pathways (Sanborn, 2001).

Multiple mechanisms contribute to relaxation and include reduction in Ca_i^{2+}, inhibition of MLCK, activation of phosphatases, and alteration in membrane potential (Sanborn, 1995, 2001; Word, 1995; Somlyo and Somlyo, 2000). In human myometrium, spontaneous contraction/relaxation cycles are associated with phosphorylation/dephosphorylation of myosin light chain and alterations in MLCK activity (Fig. 5-4) (Word et al., 1994). During stretch-induced contraction of human myometrium, both force and light chain phosphorylation decline, whereas Ca_i^{2+} is still significantly elevated (Word et al., 1994).

The increase in Ca_i^{2+} results in an activation of Ca^{2+} CaM-dependent kinase II. This enzyme phosphorylates MLCK, resulting in a decrease in MLCK activity as a consequence of a decreased affinity for Ca^{2+} CaM (Gallagher et al., 1997). Thus, phosphorylation of MLCK decreases the Ca^{2+} sensitivity (desensitization) of myosin light chain phosphorylation. The decrease in MLCK activity in human myometrium correlates with a decreased rate of myosin phosphorylation (Word et al., 1994).

Phosphatases play an important role in determining the sensitivity of the contractile apparatus to stimuli and changes in Ca_i^{2+} (Savineau and Marthan, 1997; Hartshorne et al., 1998; Somlyo and Somlyo, 2000). Phosphatases can be regulated by direct effects on the catalytic subunits or effects on targeting of regulatory subunits (Pato et al., 1994; Hartshorne, 1998). Myosin light chain phosphatase removes phosphates from myosin light chains; phosphatases also remove phosphate from and relieve the inhibitory actions of the thin filament associated regulatory proteins calponin and caldesmon (Pato et al., 1994; Savineau and Marthan, 1997). Some data suggest

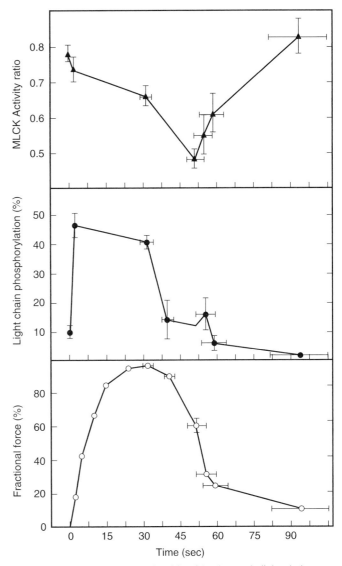

FIGURE 5-4 ■ Temporal relationship of (*top*) myosin light chain kinase (MLCK) activity, (*middle*) myosin light chain phosphorylation, and (*bottom*) force in longitudinal muscle strips from nonpregnant human myometrium undergoing spontaneous contractions. (From Word RA, Tang DC, Kamm KE: Activation properties of myosin light chain kinase during contraction/relaxation cycles of tonic and phasic smooth muscles. J Biol Chem **269**:21596, 1994.)

that calcium sensitization may play an important role as pregnancy progresses (Szal et al., 1994; Savineau and Marthan, 1997; McKillen et al., 1999).

Control of Intracellular Ca^{2+} in Myometrium

Extracellular Ca^{2+} concentrations are in the millimolar range, whereas resting Ca_i^{2+} in myometrium is 100 to 140 nM and can rise to 300 to 800 nM with stimulation (Sanborn, 1995). A variety of ion channels controls Ca^{2+} entry into the myometrium. L-type voltage-operated Ca^{2+} channels (L-VOCs) have been described in human myometrium and are active at physiologic membrane potentials. Studies in lower mammals indicate that L-VOC density increases during gestation. These channels are sensitive to the action of dihydropyridines and are currently the target of tocolytic therapy with agents such as nifedipine and ritodrine (Monga and Creasy, 1995). The depolarization that accompanies an action potential is attributed, in large part, to Ca^{2+} entry through these channels. Depolarization, in turn, stimulates L-VOCs, although Ca^{2+} inactivates them. There is ample evidence that sustained spontaneous and stimulated myometrial contractions require the presence of functioning L-VOCs. However, data conflict concerning the ability of contractants, such as oxytocin, to stimulate L-VOC current (Sanborn et al., 1998). The activity of L-VOCs can be reduced by membrane hyperpolarization (Sanborn, 1995). Ca^{2+}-activated K^+ channels, activated in response to the increase in Ca_i^{2+} or stimulated by relaxants (see later), can perform this role. Stimulation of other types of K^+ channels would have similar effects.

Ca^{2+} can also enter cells through channels that are opened in response to a signal generated by the release of Ca^{2+} from intracellular stores (Montell et al., 2002; Putney et al., 2001). Evidence for intracellular Ca^{2+} release-activated or capacitative calcium entry has been obtained in human myometrial cells (Monga et al., 1999; Young et al., 2001; Yang et al., 2002). The presence of multiple Trp proteins, postulated to constitute these channels, was recently documented in human myometrium (Yang et al., 2002). The relative importance of these channels versus L-VOC in myometrium has yet to be determined; it may be possible to target them for inhibition in the control of inappropriate myometrial contractions. Other types of Ca^{2+} channels, including T (transient)-type Ca^{2+} channels and nonselective ATP-activated cation channels, have been reported in myometrium (Sanborn, 1995). The relative importance of these channels with respect to increasing Ca_i^{2+} or altering membrane potential is not clear.

Calcium release from intracellular stores is another major mechanism by which Ca_i^{2+} is increased (see Fig. 5-3) (Sanborn, 2001). Many stimulatory agents act to increase Ca_i^{2+} via their specific receptors. These receptors activate phospholipase C (PLC) either directly or indirectly. PLC hydrolyzes phosphatidylinositol biphosphate to generate inositol-1,4,5-triphosphate and diacylglycerol (see Fig. 5-3). Inositol triphosphate stimulates the release of Ca^{2+} from intracellular stores and diacylglycerol activates protein kinase C. There are several forms of PLC, each of which appears to stimulate distinct signal transduction pathways. PLC-γ is activated by receptors that possess tyrosine kinase activity and is responsible for the action of agonists such as epidermal growth factor in myometrium (Anwer et al., 1996), whereas PLC-β isoforms are activated by agonists such as oxytocin that stimulate heterotrimeric guanosine triphosphate binding proteins of the $G\alpha_{q/11}$ family (Ku et al., 1995). PLC-β can also be stimulated by the βγ subunits released from the heterotrimeric G proteins.

The regulation of myometrial phosphoinositide turnover appears to be species, agonist, and hormonal state specific (Sanborn, 2001). Phosphoinositide turnover is inhibited by adenyl cyclase activity, cAMP generation, and protein kinase A activation (see Fig. 5-3) (Yue et al., 1998; Dodge et al., 1999a). This mechanism is stimulated by the guanosine triphosphate binding protein $G\alpha_s$ and inhibited by $G\alpha_i$ (Fuchs, 1995). Protein kinase A inhibition of phosphoinositide turnover involves phosphorylation of PLC-β3 (Yue et al., 1998). This effect requires anchoring of protein kinase A to the plasma membrane via an A kinase–associated protein (Dodge et al., 1999a). During pregnancy, the expression of $G\alpha_s$

is increased in the myometrium and functional coupling of $G\alpha_s$ to adenyl cyclase is increased, perhaps contributing to uterine quiescence during pregnancy; however, its influence may decline at the end of pregnancy (Europe-Finner et al., 1994). Furthermore, in the rat the association of protein kinase A with the A kinase–associated protein is altered during late gestation (Dodge et al., 1999b), and this may diminish sensitivity to the cAMP system.

Energy-dependent systems transport Ca^{2+} against its concentration gradient and contribute to myometrial cell relaxation (see Fig. 5-3) (Kosterin et al., 1994). A plasma membrane ATP driven Ca^{2+} pump is inhibited by oxytocin; in contrast, relaxants stimulate Ca^{2+} efflux (Kosterin et al., 1994; Sanborn et al., 1994). An Na^+-Ca^{2+} exchanger is also present in the plasma membrane. It has a much lower affinity for Ca^{2+} and therefore may play a smaller role in regulating Ca_i^{2+} concentration. Ca^{2+} pumps are also located in the endoplasmic reticulum and mitochondria of uterine smooth muscle cells and may play a role in refilling inositol triphosphate sensitive intracellular Ca^{2+} stores and preventing Ca^{2+} overload, respectively (Kosterin et al., 1994).

HORMONAL REGULATION OF MYOMETRIAL CONTRACTION

Uterine Contractants

Oxytocin receptors are present in the myometrium and a number of other reproductive tissues (Fuchs, 1995). Uterine responsiveness to oxytocin is dependent on receptor concentration (Fuchs, 1995; Zeeman et al., 1997). Myometrial concentrations of oxytocin receptors increase 50- to 100-fold in the first trimester of pregnancy compared with the nonpregnant state, and they increase 300-fold by parturition in human myometrium (Fuchs, 1995; Zeeman et al., 1997). Oxytocin receptor concentration in myometrial cells is increased by estrogen and suppressed by progesterone (Zeeman et al., 1997). Myometrial oxytocin receptor activation results in interaction with the guanosine triphosphate binding proteins of the $G\alpha_{q/11}$ subfamily that stimulate PLC activity and subsequently increase production of inositol triphosphate (see Fig. 5-3) (Ku et al., 1995; Sanborn, 2001). Oxytocin also stimulates influx of Ca^{2+} across the plasma membrane, in part by activation of capacitative calcium entry (Yang et al., 2002).

Prostaglandin levels increase in maternal plasma, urine, and amniotic fluid with labor, and prostaglandins stimulate uterine contractility both *in vivo* and *in vitro* (Olson et al., 1995). Pregnant and nonpregnant human myometrium contains all receptors and subtypes of the naturally occurring prostanoids (prostaglandins E_2, $F_{2\alpha}$, D_2, I_2, and thromboxane) (Fuchs, 1995). Myometrial contractions appear to be mediated by prostaglandin $F_{2\alpha}$, thromboxane, and prostaglandin E_1 and E_3, whereas inhibition of contractions is mediated by prostaglandins D, E_2, and I_2 (Fuchs, 1995). At the cellular level, prostaglandins raise Ca_i^{2+} levels by increasing Ca^{2+} influx across the cell membrane, stimulating calcium release from intracellular stores and enhancing myometrial gap junction formation (Hertelendy and Molnar, 1990; Phaneuf et al., 1993; Garfield, 1994).

Endothelin receptors have been isolated in amnion, chorion, endometrium, and myometrium (Yallampalli, 1994;

Fuchs, 1995). Endothelin receptors increase in myometrium during delivery and may contribute to the enhanced contractile response to endothelin at term (Yallampalli, 1994; Honore et al., 2000). At the cellular level, endothelin increases Ca_i^{2+} by receptor–PLC coupling and by calcium influx via nifedipine-sensitive channels (Fuchs, 1995; Kaya et al., 1999). In addition, endothelin may act in a paracrine manner, stimulating prostaglandin production by the endometrium and fetal membranes (Yallampalli, 1994).

Epidermal growth factor receptors are present in endometrium and myometrium plasma membrane and appear to be induced by estrogen (Fuchs, 1995). Epidermal growth factor stimulates mobilization of arachidonic acid via both lipoxygenase and cyclooxygenase-catalyzed pathways (Yallampalli, 1994). In human myometrial cells, the effect of epidermal growth factor appears to be independent of arachidonic acid mobilization and involves stimulation of the tyrosine kinase PLC-γ pathway with resultant increase in Ca_i^{2+} (Anwer et al., 1996).

Uterine Relaxants

β_2-Adrenergic receptors are prevalent in the smooth muscle of the uterus. Agents such as ritodrine, salbutamol, terbutaline, and fenoterol display selectivity for membrane-bound β_2-adrenergic receptors in the myometrium, which results in activation of the adenylate cyclase enzyme via stimulation of the $G\alpha_s$ protein. These agonists increase intracellular cAMP concentration, resulting in activation of cAMP-dependent protein kinase A. Protein kinase A inhibits myosin light chain phosphorylation (Wen et al., 1992) (see Fig. 5-3). In addition, protein kinase A activity is associated with decreased Ca^{2+} entry, increased Ca^{2+} efflux from myometrial cells, and increased K^+ conductance (see Fig. 5-3) (Sanborn, 1995, 2001). The net result of these effects is myometrial relaxation.

Synthetic oxytocin receptor antagonists such as atosiban (mixed vasopressin/oxytocin receptor specificity) and L-371,257 (specific oxytocin antagonist) inhibit both *in vitro* and *in vivo* contractile activity of the uterus (Goodwin et al., 1996; Buscher et al., 2001; Wilson et al., 2001) as a result of competitive inhibition of oxytocin binding. The clinical use of specific oxytocin receptor antagonists is potentially attractive because the lack of appreciable receptor sites in tissues other than myometrium and fetal membranes may minimize side effects. In several clinical trials, atosiban exhibited fewer cardiovascular effects but similar efficacy as β-adrenergic agents in arresting preterm labor, although in one trial it was no more effective than placebo in preventing delivery in women who presented at less than 28 weeks' gestation (Valenzuela et al., 2000; European Atosiban Study Group, 2001; French/Australian Atosiban Investigators Group 2001; Thornton et al., 2001; Worldwide Atosiban versus Beth-agonists Study Group, 2001).

Relaxin is secreted by the corpus luteum, placenta, and myometrium, and relaxin binding sites have been localized in myometrial cells (Hollingsworth et al., 1994). Relaxin increases intracellular cAMP levels and inhibits agonist-stimulated increases in Ca_i^{2+} via protein kinase A but also inhibits myometrial contractile activity by stimulation of Ca^{2+}-activated K^+ channels and possibly ATP-sensitive K^+ channels (Hollingsworth et al., 1994; Sanborn, 1995). Relaxin also inhibits agonist-stimulated inositol triphosphate generation, increases Ca^{2+} efflux and inhibits myosin light chain phospho-

rylation. Despite its selective properties as a myometrial relaxing agent *in vitro*, its use has been limited clinically as a tocolytic, and there has been a lack of consistent inhibition of uterine contractile activity in response to relaxin administration *in vivo* (Kelly et al., 2001). The role of corticotropin-releasing hormone in myometrial quiescence is complicated by the presence of pregnancy-related alternative splice forms and a diminished role in cAMP generation near the end of pregnancy (Grammatopoulos et al., 1999; Grammatopoulos and Hillhouse, 1999).

L-Arginine, the substrate of nitric oxide, and nitric acid have been shown to effect relaxation of myometrial contractile activity *in vitro*, in an effect that is reversed by L-nitro-arginine methyl ester (a nitric oxide synthase inhibitor) (Garfield et al., 1995). Nitric oxide donors activate guanylate cyclase and generate cyclic guanosine monophosphate, which decreases Ca^{2+} sensitivity of myosin light chain phosphorylation and increases myosin light chain phosphatase activity (Wu et al., 1996; Van Riper et al., 1997). These results suggest that nitric oxide donors such as sodium nitroprusside might be used to suppress uterine contractility, although effectiveness may diminish near term (Garfield et al., 1995; Barber et al., 1999; Ekerhovd et al., 1999; Longo et al., 1999). Nonetheless, the role of cyclic guanosine monophosphate in maintaining human uterine quiescence has been questioned (Cornwell et al., 2001).

High extracellular magnesium concentrations (10 mM) gradually increase intracellular magnesium levels, inhibit Ca^{2+} entry into myometrial cells via L-type and T-type VOCs, and enhance Ca^{2+} sensitivity of K^+ channels favoring hyperpolarization (Monga and Creasy, 1995; Sanborn, 1995). Because myometrial cell contraction is dependent on cell membrane depolarization and an increase in Ca_i^{2+} levels with subsequent activation of MLCK activity, hyperpolarization and inhibition of calcium influx across the plasma membrane contribute to myometrial cell relaxation. Also, magnesium competes with Ca^{2+} and decreases the CaM binding affinity for MLCK, further favoring myometrial cell relaxation (Ohki et al., 1997).

Calcium channel blockers such as nifedipine, nitrendipine, diltiazem, and verapamil function primarily by inhibiting the entry of Ca^{2+} via voltage-dependent L-type Ca^{2+} channels (Hollingsworth et al., 1994; Monga and Creasy, 1995). The dihydropyridines (nifedipine and nitrendipine) are more often used clinically as uterine relaxants because they have less effect on the atrioventricular conduction pathway in the heart than verapamil or diltiazem.

Finally, inhibition of prostaglandin production is a potential target for tocolysis. Prostaglandin synthesis inhibitors inactivate the cyclooxygenase enzyme responsible for the conversion of arachidonic acid to the intermediate endoperoxide prostaglandin G_2, which is subsequently converted to prostaglandins E_2 and $F_{2\alpha}$ (Monga and Creasy, 1995). Aspirin causes irreversible acetylation of the cyclooxygenase enzyme, whereas indomethacin is a competitive inhibitor.

■ REGULATION OF GENE TRANSCRIPTION WITH PREGNANCY AND LABOR

Molecular approaches are providing new insights into regulation of myometrial activity in the pregnant state and during labor. A functional progesterone withdrawal has been suggested as a result of changes in progesterone receptor A and B isoform ratios (Mesiano et al., 2002). This could affect expression and/or intracellular localization of key signaling components. Suppression subtractive hybridization and microarray technology are emerging as important tools to identify candidates involved in maintaining pregnancy and/or labor, and quantitative polymerase chain reaction has improved documentation of gene regulation. Upregulation of genes during labor that are involved in immune, inflammatory, and contractile responses; down-regulation of genes related to the relaxation response; and identification of genes involved with a variety of cellular responses or of unknown function have been reported (Aguan et al., 2000; Chan et al., 2002). These data present the challenge to distinguish causality and consequence in these types of studies.

■ S U M M A R Y

The female reproductive tract undergoes dramatic changes during pregnancy and labor. These changes are crucial for retention of pregnancy, prevention of preterm labor, and the timely initiation of labor at term. An understanding of the morphologic changes in the reproductive tract and the biochemical mechanisms that control uterine contraction and relaxation outlined above may improve our understanding of the physiologic basis of uterine contractile activity. This in turn may facilitate further development of pharmacologic agents for use in clinical situations that require the use of uterine stimulants or tocolytics.

R E F E R E N C E S

Adelstein RS, Sellers JR: Myosin structure and function. *In* Barany MS (ed): Biochemistry of Smooth Muscle Contraction. San Diego, Academic Press, 1996.

Aguan K, Carvajal JA, Thompson LP, et al: Application of a functional genomics approach to identify differentially expressed genes in human myometrium during pregnancy and labour. Mol Hum Reprod **6**:1141, 2000.

Anwer K, Monga M, Sanborn BM: Epidermal growth factor increases phosphoinositide turnover and intracellular free calcium in an immortalized human myometrial cell line independent of the arachidonic acid metabolic pathway. Am J Obstet Gynecol **174**:676, 1996.

Assali NS, Rauramo I, Peltonen T: Measurement of uterine blood low and uterine metabolism. Am J Obstet Gynecol **79**:86, 1960.

Barber A, Robson SC, Lyall E. Hemoxygenase and nitric oxide synthase do not maintain human uterine quiescence during pregnancy. Am J Pathol **155**:831, 1999.

Bird IM, Sullivan JA, Di T, et al: Pregnancy-dependent changes in cell signaling underlie changes in differential control of vasodilator production in uterine artery endothelial cells. Endocrinology **141**:1107, 2000.

Burghardt RC, Barhoumi R, Stickney M, et al: Correlation between connexin-43 expression, cell-cell communication, and oxytocin-induced calcium responses in an immortalized human myometrial cell line. Biol Reprod **55**:433, 1996.

Buscher U, Chen FC, Riesenkampff E, et al: Effects of oxytocin receptor antagonist atosiban on pregnant myometrium in vitro. Obstet Gynecol **98**:117, 2001.

Chan EC, Fraser S, Yin S, et al: Human myometrial genes are differentially expressed in labor: A suppression subtractive hybridization study. J Clin Endocrinol Metab **87**:2435, 2002.

Chow L, Lye SJ: Expression of the gap junction protein connexin 43 is increased in the human myometrium toward term and with the onset of labor. Am J Obstet Gynecol **170**:788, 1994.

Ciray HN, Guner H, Hakansson H, et al: Morphometric analysis of gap junctions in nonpregnant and term pregnant human myometrium. Acta Obstet Gynaecol Scand **74**:497, 1995.

Cohen DA, Daughaday WH, Weldon VV: Fetal and maternal virilization associated with pregnancy. Am J Dis Child **136**:353, 1982.

Cornwell TL, Li J, Sellak H, et al: Reorganization of myofilament proteins and decreased cGMP-dependent protein kinase in the human uterus during pregnancy. J Clin Endocrinol Metab **86**:3981, 2001.

Cullinan-Bove K, Koos RD: Vascular endothelial growth factor/vascular permeability factor expression in the rat uterus. Rapid stimulation by estrogen correlates with estrogen induced increases in uterine capillary permeability and growth. Endocrinology **133**:829, 1993.

Danforth DN: The fibrous nature of the human cervix and its relation to the isthmic segment in the gravid and non-gravid uteri. Am J Obstet Gynecol **53**:541, 1947.

Dodge KL, Carr DW, Sanborn BM: PKA anchoring to the myometrial plasma membrane is required for cAMP regulation of phosphatidylinositide turnover. Endocrinology **140**:5165, 1999a.

Dodge KL, Carr DW, Yue C, et al: A role for AKAP scaffolding in the loss of a cAMP inhibitory response in late pregnant rat myometrium. Mol Endocrinol **13**:1977, 1999b.

Eddie LW, Bell RJ, Lester Aet al: Radioimmunoassay of relaxin in pregnancy with an analogue of human relaxin. Lancet. **1**:1344, 1986.

Edman CD, Toofanian A, MacDonald PC, et al: Placental clearance rate of maternal plasma androstenedione through placental estradiol formation: An indirect method of assessing uteroplacental blood flow. Am J Obstet Gynecol **131**:1029, 1981.

Ekerhovd E, Weidegard B, Brannstrom M, et al: Nitric oxide-mediated effects on myometrial contractility at term during prelabor and labor. Obstet Gynecol **93**:987, 1999.

Europe-Finner GN, Phaneuf S, Tolkovsky JM, et al: Downregulation of Gαs in human myometrium in term and preterm labor: A mechanism for parturition. J Clin Endocrinol Metab **79**:1835, 1994.

European Atosiban Study Group: The oxytocin antagonist atosiban versus the beta-agonist terbutaline in the treatment of preterm labor. A randomized, double-blind, controlled study. Acta Obstet Gynaecol Scand **80**:413, 2001.

French/Australian Atosiban Investigators Group: Treatment of preterm labor with the oxytocin antagonist atosiban: A double-blind, randomized, controlled comparison with salbutamol. J Obstet Gynecol Reprod Biol **98**:177, 2001.

Fuchs AR: Plasma membrane receptors regulating myometrial contractility and their hormonal modulation. Semin Perinatol **19**:15, 1995.

Gallagher PJ, Herring BP, Stull JT: Myosin light chain kinases. J Muscle Res Cell Motil **18**:1, 1997.

Garfield RE: Role of cell to cell coupling in control of myometrial contractility and labor. *In* Garfield RE, Tabb TN (eds): Control of Uterine Contractility. Boca Raton, FL, CRC Press, 1994, p. 39.

Garfield RE, Ali M, Yallampalli C, et al: Role of gap junctions and nitric oxide in control of myometrial contractility. Semin Perinatol **19**:41, 1995.

Garfield RE, Tabb T, Thilander G: Intercellular coupling and modulation of uterine contractility. *In* Garfield RE (ed): Uterine Contractility. Norwell, Serono Symposia, 1990, p. 21.

Goodwin TM, Valenzuela G, Silver H, et al: Dose ranging study of the oxytocin antagonist atosiban in the treatment of preterm labor. Obstet Gynecol **88**:331, 1996.

Grammatopoulos DK, Dai Y, Randeva HS, et al: A novel spliced variant of the type 1 corticotropin-releasing hormone receptor with a deletion in the seventh transmembrane domain present in the human pregnant term myometrium and fetal membranes. Mol Endocrinol **13**:2189, 1999.

Grammatopoulos DK, Hillhouse EW: Role of corticotropin-releasing hormone in onset of labour. Lancet **354**:1546, 1999.

Habermehl DA, Hanowiak MA, Vagnoni KE, et al: Endothelial vasodilator production by uterine and systemic arteries. IV. Cyclooxygenase isoform expression during the ovarian cycle and pregnancy in sheep. Biol Reprod **62**:781, 2000.

Hartshorne DJ: Myosin phosphatase: Subunits and interactions. Acta Physiol Scand **164**:483, 1998.

Hartshorne DJ, Ito M, Erdodi F: Myosin light chain phosphatase: Subunit composition, interactions and regulation. J Muscle Res Cell Motil **19**:325, 1998.

Hertelendy F, Molnar M: Mode of action of prostaglandins in myometrial cells. *In* Garfield RE (ed): Uterine Contractility. Norwell, Serono Symposia, 1990, p. 221.

Hollingsworth M, Downing SJ, Cheuk JMS, et al: Pharmacological strategies for uterine relaxation. *In* Garfield RE, Tabb TN (eds): Control of Uterine Contractility. Boca Raton, FL, CRC Press, 1994, p. 401.

Honore JC, Robert B, Vacher-Lavenu MC, et al: Expression of endothelin receptors in human myometrium during pregnancy and in uterine leiomyomas. J Cardiovasc Pharmacol **36**(5 Suppl 1):S386, 2000.

Hwang JJ, Macinga D, Rorke EA: Relaxin modulates human cervical stromal activity. J Clin Endocrinol Metab **81**:3379, 1996.

Ipson MA, Rosenfeld CR, Magness RR, et al: Alterations in myometrial stress during ovine pregnancy and the puerperium. Am J Physiol **217**:R446, 1996.

Ivell R, Kimura T, Muller D, et al: The structure and regulation of the oxytocin receptor. Exp Physiol **86:**289, 2001.

Jiang H, Stephens NL: Calcium and smooth muscle contraction. Mol Cell Biochem. **135:**1, 1994.

Katzenellenbogen BS, Bhakoo HS, Ferguson ER, et al: Estrogen and anti-estrogen action in reproductive tissues and tumors. Rec Prog Horm Res **35:**259, 1979.

Kawarabayashi T, Ikeda M, Sugimori H, et al: Spontaneous electrical activity and effects of noradrenaline on pregnant human myometrium recorded by the single sucrose gap method. Acta Physiol Hung **67:**71, 1986.

Kaya T, Cetin A, Cetin M, et al: Effects of endothelin-1 and calcium channel blockers on contractions in human myometrium. A study on myometrial strips from normal and diabetic pregnant women. J Reprod Med **44:**115, 1999

Kelly AJ, Kavanagh J, Thomas J. Relaxin for cervical ripening and induction of labour. Cochrane Database Syst Rev **2:**CD03103, 2001.

Kilarski WM, Rezapour M, Backstrom T, et al: Morphometric analysis of gap junction density in human myometrium at term. Acta Obstet Gynaecol Scand **73:**377, 1994.

Kosterin SA, Burdyga TV, Fomin VP, et al: Mechanisms of calcium transport in myometrium. *In* Garfield RE, Tabb TN (eds): Control of Uterine Contractility. Boca Raton, FL, CRC Press, 1994, p. 129.

Ku CY, Qian A, Wen Y, et al: Oxytocin stimulates myometrial GTPase and phospholipase C activities via coupling to Gαq/11. Endocrinology **136:**1509, 1995.

Leppert PC: Anatomy and physiology of cervical ripening. Clin Obstet Gynecol **38:**267, 1995.

Longo M, Jain V, Vedernikov YP, et al: Effect of nitric oxide and carbon monoxide on uterine contractility during human and rat pregnancy. Am J Obstet Gynecol **181:**981, 1999.

Ludmir J, Sehdev HM: Anatomy and physiology of the uterine cervix. Clin Obstet Gynecol **43:**433, 2000.

Magness RR, Rosenfeld CR, Hassan A, et al: Endothelial vasodilator production by uterine and systemic arteries. I. Effects of ANG II on PGI2 and NO in pregnancy. Am J Physiol **270:**H1914, 1996.

Magness RR, Shaw CE, Phernetton TM, et al: Endothelial vasodilator production by uterine and systemic arteries. II. Pregnancy effects on NO synthase expression. Am J Physiol **272:**J1730, 1997.

Magness RR, Sullivan JA, Li Y, et al: Endothelial vasodilator production by uterine and systemic arteries. VI. Ovarian and pregnancy effects on eNOS and NOx. Am J Physiol **280:**H1692, 2001.

Makowski EL, Meschia G, Droegemueller W, et al: Distribution of uterine blood flow in the pregnant sheep. Am J Obstet Gynecol **101:**409, 1968.

Marshall JM: Relation between membrane potential and spontaneous contraction of the uterus. *In* Garfield RE (ed): Uterine Contractility. Norwell, Serono Symposia, 1990, pp. 3–8.

McKillen K, Thornton S, Taylor CW: Oxytocin increases the [Ca2+]i sensitivity of human myometrium during the falling phase of phasic contractions. Am J Physiol **276:**E345, 1999.

Mesiano S, Chan EC, Fitter JT, et al: Progesterone withdrawal and estrogen activation in human parturition are coordinated by progesterone receptor a expression in the myometrium. J Clin Endocrinol Metab **87:**2924, 2002.

Metcalfe J, Romney SL, Ramsey LH, et al: Estimation of uterine blood flow in normal human pregnancy at term. J Clin Invest **34:**1632, 1955.

Monga M, Campbell DF, Sanborn BM: Oxytocin-stimulated capacitative calcium entry in human myometrial cells. Am Obstet Gynecol **181:**424, 1999.

Monga M, Creasy RK: Pharmacologic management of preterm labor. Semin Perinatol **19:**84, 1995.

Montell C, Birnbaumer L, Flockerzi V: The TRP channels, a remarkably functional family. Cell **108:**595, 2002.

Ohki S, Ikura M, Zhang M: Identification of magnesium binding sites and the role of magnesium on target recognition by calmodulin. Biochemistry **36:**4309, 1997.

Olson DM, Mijovic JE, Sadowsky DW: Control of human parturition. Semin Perinatol **19:**52, 1995.

Parkington HC, Coleman HA: The role of membrane potential in the control of uterine motility. *In* Carsten ME, Miller JD (eds): Uterine Function: Molecular and Cellular Aspects. New York, Plenum Press, 1990.

Parkington HC, Tonta MA, Brennecke SP, et al: Contractile activity, membrane potential, and cytoplasmic calcium in human uterine smooth muscle in the third trimester of pregnancy and during labor. Am J Obstet Gynecol **181:**1445, 1999.

Pato MD, Tulloch AG, Walsh MP, et al: Smooth muscle phosphatases: Structure, regulation, and function. Can J Physiol Pharmacol **72:**1427, 1994.

Phaneuf S, Europe-Finner GN, Varney M, et al: Oxytocin-stimulated phosphoinositide hydrolysis in human myometrial cells: Involvement of pertussis toxin-sensitive and insensitive G-proteins. J Endocrinol **136:**497, 1993.

Putney JW Jr, Broad LM, Braun FJ, et al: Mechanisms of capacitative calcium entry. J Cell Sci **114:**2223, 2001.

Rechberger T, Woessner JF Jr. Collagenase, its inhibitors and decorin in the lower uterine segment in pregnant women. Am J Obstet Gynecol **168:**1598, 1993.

Rekonen A, Lutola H, Pitkanene M, et al: Measurement of intervillous and myometrial blood flow by an intravenous 133Xe method. Br J Obstet Gynaecol **83:**723, 1976.

Resnik R, Killam AP, Battaglia FC, et al: The stimulation of uterine blood flow by various estrogens. Endocrinology **94:**1192, 1974.

Roomans GM, Kilarski WM, Ciray N, et al: Structural and functional studies of gap junction in human myometrium. Eur J Morphol **31:**55, 1993.

Rosenfeld CR: Distribution of cardiac output in ovine pregnancy. Am J Physiol **232:**H231, 1977.

Rosenfeld CR: Consideration of the uteroplacental circulation in intrauterine growth. Semin Perinatol **8:**42, 1984.

Rosenfeld CR, Morriss FH JR, Battaglia FC, et al: Effect of estradiol-17 on blood flow to reproductive and nonreproductive tissues in pregnant ewes. Am J Obstet Gynecol **124:**618, 1976.

Rosenfeld CR, Morriss FH Jr, Makowski EL, et al: Circulatory changes in the reproductive tissue of ewes during pregnancy. Gynecol Invest **5:**127, 1974.

Sanborn BM: Hypertrophy of uterine smooth muscle. *In* Seidel CL, Weisbrodt NW (eds): Hypertrophic Response in Smooth Muscle. Boca Raton, FL, CRC Press, 1987, p. 85.

Sanborn BM: Ion channels and the control of myometrial electrical activity. Semin Perinatol **19:**31, 1995.

Sanborn BM: Hormones and calcium: Mechanisms controlling uterine smooth muscle contractile activity. Exp Physiol **86:**223, 2001.

Sanborn BM, Anwer K, Wen Y, et al: Modification of calcium regulatory systems. *In* Garfield RE, Tabb TN (eds): Control of Uterine Contractility. Boca Raton, FL, CRC Press, 1994, p. 105.

Sanborn BM, Dodge K, Monga M, et al: Molecular mechanisms regulating the effects of oxytocin on myometrial intracellular calcium. Adv Exp Med Biol **449:**277, 1998.

Savineau JP, Marthan R: Modulation of the calcium sensitivity of the smooth muscle contractile apparatus: Molecular mechanisms, pharmacological and pathophysiological implications. Fund Clin Pharmacol **11:**289, 1997.

Sladek SM, Magness RR, Conrad KP: Nitric oxide in pregnancy. Am J Physiol **272:**R441, 1997.

Somlyo AP, Somlyo AV: Signal transduction and regulation of smooth muscle. Nature **372:**231, 1994.

Somlyo AP, Somlyo AV: Signal transduction by G-proteins, rho-kinase and protein phosphatase to smooth muscle and non-muscle myosin II. J Physiol (Lond) **522:**177, 2000.

Sperelakis N, Inoue Y, Ohya Y: Fast Na+ and slow Ca2+ current in smooth muscle from pregnant rat uterus. Mol Cell Biochem **114:**78, 1992.

Szal SE, Repke JT, Seely EW, et al: [Ca2+]i signaling in pregnant human myometrium. Am J Physiol **267:**E77, 1994.

Teasdale F: Numerical density of nuclei in the sheep placenta. Anat Rec **185:**186, 1976.

Thornton S, Vatish M, Slater D: Oxytocin antagonists: Clinical and scientific considerations. Exp Physiol **86:**825, 2001.

Uduwela AS, Perera MAK, Aigin L, et al: Endometrial-myometrial interface: Relationship to adenomyosis and changes in pregnancy. Obstet Gynecol Surv **55:**390, 2000.

Valenzuela GJ, Sanchez-Ramos L, Romero R, et al: Maintenance treatment of preterm labor with the oxytocin antagonist atosiban. The Atosiban PTL-098 Study Group. Am J Obstet Gynecol **182:**1184, 2000.

Van Riper DA, McDaniel NL, Rembold CM: Myosin light chain kinase phosphorylation in nitrovasodilator-induced swine carotid artery relaxation. Biochim Biophys Acta **1355:**323, 1997.

Watari M, Watari H, DiSanto ME, et al: Pro-inflammatory cytokines induce expression of matrix-metabolizing enzymes in human cervical smooth muscle cells. Am J Pathol **154L:**1755, 1999.

Wen Y, Anwer K, Singh SP, et al: Protein kinase A inhibits phospholipase C activity and alters protein phosphorylation in rat myometrial plasma membranes. Endocrinology **131:**1377, 1992.

Wilson RJ, Allen MJ, Nandi M, et al: Spontaneous contractions of myometrium from humans, non-human primate and rodents are sensitive to selective oxytocin receptor antagonism in vitro. Br J Obstet Gynaecol **108:**960, 2001.

Winkler M, Rath W: Changes in the cervical extracellular matrix during pregnancy and parturition. J Perinat Med **27:**45, 1999.

Word RA: Myosin phosphorylation and the control of myometrial contraction/relaxation. Semin Perinatol **19:**3, 1995.

Word RA, Stull JT, Casey ML, et al: Contractile elements and myosin light chain phosphorylation in myometrial tissue from nonpregnant and pregnant women. J Clin Invest **92:**29, 1993.

Word RA, Tang DC, Kamm KE: Activation properties of myosin light chain kinase during contraction/relaxation cycles of tonic and phasic smooth muscles. J Biol Chem **269:**21596, 1994.

Worldwide Atosiban versus Beta-agonists Study Group. Effectiveness and safety of the oxytocin antagonist atosiban versus beta-adrenergic agonists in the treatment of preterm labour. The Worldwide Atosiban versus. Beta-agonists Study Group. Br J Obstet Gynaecol **108:**133, 2001.

Wu X, Somlyo AV, Somlyo AP: Cyclic GMP-dependent stimulation reverses G-protein–coupled inhibition of smooth muscle myosin-light chain phosphatase. Biochem Biophys Res Commun **220:**658, 1996.

Xiao D, Bird IM, Magness RR, et al: Upregulation of eNOS in pregnant ovine uterine arteries by chronic hypoxia. Am J Physiol **280:**H812, 2001.

Yallampalli C: Role of growth factors and cytokines in the control of uterine contractility. *In* Garfield RE, Tabb TN (eds): Control of Uterine Contractility. Boca Raton, FL, CRC Press, 1994, p. 285.

Yang M, Gupta A, Shlykov SG, et al: Expression of Trp proteins implicated in regulated calcium entry in human myometrium and a human myometrial cell line. Biol Reprod **67:**988, 2002.

Young RC, Schumann R, Zhang P: Nifedipine block of capacitative calcium entry in cultured human uterine smooth-muscle cells. J Soc Gynecol Invest **8:**210, 2001.

Yue C, Dodge KL, Weber G, et al: Phosphorylation of serine 1105 by protein kinase A inhibits phospholipase Cβ3 stimulation by Gαq. J Biol Chem **273:**18023, 1998.

Zeeman GG, Khan-Dawood FS, Dawood MY: Oxytocin and its receptor in pregnancy and parturition: Current concepts and clinical implications. Obstet Gynecol **89:**874, 1997.

Chapter 6

CHARACTERISTICS OF PARTURITION

John R.G. Challis, DSc, FRSC, and Stephen J. Lye, PhD

Parturition results from a complex interplay and interaction between maternal, placental, and fetal factors. The process requires that the uterus, maintained in a state of relative quiescence during pregnancy, develops coordinated contractility and that the cervix dilates to allow passage of the fetus through the birth canal. To be fully successful, parturition requires that maturation of the fetal organ systems necessary for extrauterine life has occurred and that the mother has undergone changes necessary for lactation in the postpartum period. Preterm birth, where there is asynchrony between these processes, occurs in 8% to 10% of all human pregnancies (Meis et al., 1998) (see Chapter 34). Its incidence has changed little over the past 40 years. A variety of factors, such as socioeconomic status, maternal age, and work-related stress, is known to increase predisposition to preterm birth, although the mechanisms underlying these effects are poorly understood at the present time. In some centers the recent tendency to increased preterm labor rates is associated with multiple gestations, in part as a result of assisted reproductive treatments.

Causes of preterm birth fall into three general categories: indicated, in which a demonstrable complication of pregnancy such as preeclampsia or fetal distress requires obstetric intervention; premature rupture of membranes with or without infection; and idiopathic preterm birth. Generally, approximately 30% to 40% of preterm births are associated with an underlying infective process, whereas 40% to 50% are idiopathic and may be potentially preventable.

In this chapter we refer to experimental studies in sheep, the species of choice for many investigators examining the birth process. In this species there is coordinated activation of the hypothalamic-pituitary-adrenal (HPA) axis in the fetus, resulting in increased fetal cortisol output in late gestation. This increased output provides a key signal resulting in altered placental and maternal hormone production. In the human, the role of the fetus is less well defined. However, in idiopathic preterm birth, it is clear that a similar pathway to that described in sheep may well be implicated. In both species, increased output of prostaglandins appears to represent a final stimulatory pathway to the myometrium, and the production of these compounds is examined in some more detail.

PATTERNS OF UTERINE ACTIVITY

Myometrial activity during pregnancy is characterized by poorly coordinated contractures or Braxton Hicks contractions of human gestation. The development of coordinated uterine contractions at term results in a myometrium that is excitable and generating high-frequency, high-amplitude activity. It is spontaneously active and responds to exogenous uterotonins. We term the transition of the myometrium from a quiescent to an active state as an "activation" process. When this has occurred, the myometrium can then undergo "stimulation" in response to endogenous and/or exogenous agonists (Lye et al., 1998).

The uterine phenotype can then be examined as different phases of the parturition process. For much of pregnancy the uterus is relatively quiescent, representing phase 0 of parturition. Activation corresponds to phase 1 and is effected through mechanical and uterotropic inputs. Stimulation corresponds to phase 2 when endogenous uterotonins act on the activated myometrium. Phase 3 corresponds to postpartum involution of the uterus. In this sequence, the "initiation" of parturition corresponds to the transition from phase 0 to phase 1.

Myometrial contractility depends on conformational changes in the actin and myosin filaments of the myometrium that allow them to slide over each other, ultimately leading to shortening of the myocyte (see Chapter 5). These changes require adenosine triphosphate, which is generated by myosin after phosphorylation of the 20-kDa light chains by the enzyme myosin light chain kinase. Myosin light chain kinase is activated through interaction with the calcium-binding protein calmodulin, which in turn requires four Ca^{2+} ions for its own activation. The regulation of myosin light chain kinase was reviewed elsewhere (MacKenzie et al., 1990). Activity of the enzyme is altered by intracellular pathways that regulate levels of calcium and of cyclic adenosine monophosphate (cAMP). Uterotonins are effective by increasing intracellular calcium levels or by increasing the flux of calcium through receptor-operated channels or calcium release from sarcoplasmic reticulum. Inhibitors of myometrial activity may work by increasing levels of intracellular cAMP, which block calcium release.

Coordinated myometrial contractility at term requires cell-to-cell coupling, effected through the formation of intercellular gap junctions. The proteins forming gap junctions are termed connexins, and their alignment to form an interconnecting pore allows low resistance electrical or ionic coupling between adjacent cells. Regulation of connexins occurs at both the transcription and translation level and can be influenced by steroids and by mechanical stretch. The pioneering studies of Garfield (1988) established a massive increase in the numbers of gap junctions with the onset of labor, and this appears to be a consistent finding across species. In the rat, highest levels of connexin-43 (CX-43) messenger RNA (mRNA) and protein were found in myometrium during the process of delivery and continued synthesis of gap junctions would be required to maintain labor (Chow and Lye, 1994). Inhibition or reversal of gap junction formation clearly offers an important therapeutic target for preventing preterm uterine contractility.

■ MYOMETRIAL ACTIVATION

It is generally clear that regulation of myometrial quiescence during pregnancy and increased contractile activity at labor are influenced by the integration of mechanical and endocrine signals. These signals have their origin within the fetal genome (Fig. 6-1). Hormonal signals emanating from the fetal HPA axis are programmed to regulate, in most species, relative levels of estrogen, progesterone, and prostaglandins during pregnancy and labor. Mechanical signals also originate within the fetal genome in that it is the growth of the fetus itself that imparts mechanical stimulation to the uterus. Myometrial activation results from coordinated expression of a cassette of proteins termed contraction-associated proteins (CAPs). These include increased expression of CX-43 and the oxytocin receptor and prostaglandin F (PGF) receptor. Expression of CAPs is regulated positively by estrogen and negatively by progesterone. CAP expression is increased in preterm labor but does not increase when labor is blocked by progesterone (Chow and Lye, 1994).

Regulation of CAP gene expression by steroids probably occurs indirectly through synthesis of mediating transcription factors. Thus, although estrogen increases transcription of the CX-43 and oxytocin receptor genes, these lack the consensus palindromic sequence typically found in the 5′ promoter region of estrogen-responsive genes. Further, inhibition of *de novo* protein synthesis blocks estrogen-induced increases in CX-43 expression. It is likely that members of the *fos* family of transcription factors mediate estrogen-induced increases in CAP gene expression. Thus, estrogen increases levels of mRNA encoding the AP-1 protein *c-fos* in the myometrium and the onset of term and preterm labor in the rat is associated with increased expression of *c-fos* and the *fos* family members,

Fra-1 and Fra-2. Progesterone attenuates the expression of these transcription factors as well as CX-43 (Lye et al., 2001).

Uterine stretch is also a major regulator of smooth muscle contractility (Lye et al., 2001). Stretch of the uterus induces increased CAP gene expression and myometrial activation, but the development of myometrial tension is attenuated during pregnancy due to increased myometrial growth. Progesterone appears to block stretch-induced gene expression in the myometrium. Thus, withdrawal or reversal of progesterone action at term allows activation at that time. Moreover, preterm labor in multifetal pregnancies may arise because the stretch-attenuating pathways are overwhelmed by the greatly increased myometrial tensile stress, shifting the balance for regulating myometrial contractility toward activation.

In unilaterally pregnant rats, CAP gene expression is increased in the gravid horn at the time of labor (Lye et al., 2001). This effect was reproduced by placing a small tube into one horn of bilaterally ovariectomized nonpregnant animals. Administration of progesterone blocked stretch-induced increases in CX-43 expression. In unilaterally pregnant animals, upregulation of CAP gene expression occurred in the nonpregnant horn implanted with a small 3-mm Silastic tube (mechanical stretch) as it did in the contralateral pregnant horn at the time of labor. CX-43 transcripts were not upregulated in the nonpregnant control horn. When tissues were examined from animals on day 20 of pregnancy 3 days earlier, when circulating progesterone levels are still high, there was no effect of mechanical stretch on CX-43 transcripts. These data suggest that stretch can upregulate CAPs, but the ability to do so depends on the prevailing maternal endocrine environment. During pregnancy, stretch is inadequate to induce CX-43 because circulating progesterone concentrations are high. At term, when systemic progesterone levels have decreased, stretch itself is adequate to produce the same level of CX-43 expression as in a pregnant horn containing the fetus. The mechanisms by which stretch regulates CX-43 expression in the myometrium are unknown. Stretch increases *c-fos* within 15 minutes in *in vitro* systems, and this effect depends on activation of mitogen activated protein kinase signaling. Stretch of uterine myocytes in culture induces rapid and intensity-dependent activation of the mitogen activated protein kinases extracellular signal-regulated kinase 1/2, P38, and c-Jun NH$_2$-terminal kinase. Moreover, activation of extracellular signal-regulated kinase 1/2 and P38 is required for the induction of *c-fos* expression. These *in vitro* data are supported by *in vivo* data that found increased expression of extracellular signal-regulated kinase 1/2 and P38 in the gravid (but not nongravid) uterine horns of unilaterally pregnant rats during labor. These data suggest that *c-fos*, and possible other AP-1 family members, might mediate actions of both endocrine signals and tensile stress in regulating CAP gene expression and myometrial activity.

Lye and coworkers (2001) suggested that growth factors such as insulin-like growth factor I and epidermal growth factor mediate hormone (estrogen)-induced myocyte proliferation during early pregnancy. As pregnancy progresses, fetal growth induces uterine stretch, which in the presence of elevated progesterone leads to a switch from proliferation to myocyte hypertrophy. This stretch-induced uterine growth attenuates development of tension in the myometrium and hence inhibits the activation of CAP genes. The ability of the myometrium to undergo hypertrophy is supported by elevated focal adhesion kinase activity, which requires elevated progesterone. With the fall (functional or actual) of proges-

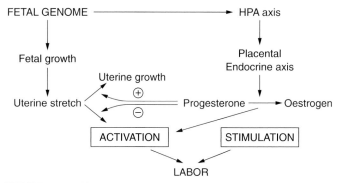

FIGURE 6-1 ■ The onset of labor is dictated by the fetal genome proceeding through either a fetal growth pathway with increases in uterine stretch or a fetal endocrine pathway involving activation of the fetal hypothalamic-pituitary-adrenal (HPA) axis. These two arms are not independent because changes in progesterone and estrogen modulate the ability of uterine stretch to increase expressions of genes associated with myometrial activation.

terone at term, focal adhesion kinase activity is reduced, leading to formation of stable focal adhesion sites anchoring the myocytes to their extracellular matrix. This curtails myometrial hypertrophy while fetal growth is continuing, thereby causing an increase in tension within the myometrium. This in turn increases expression of CAP genes affecting myometrial activation. Elevated levels of stimulatory uterotonins then act on the activated myometrium to induce labor contractions.

MYOMETRIAL ACTIVATION

Fetal Hypothalamic-Pituitary-Adrenal Axis

The pioneering studies of Professor Sir Graham (Mont) Liggins and Geoffrey Thorburn, working in the sheep and goat, showed conclusively in those species that the fetus *in utero* provided the trigger for the onset of parturition and did so through activation of the fetal HPA axis (Liggins and Thorburn, 1994). It is now clear that in virtually every species studied, including the human, there are increases in the concentration of the major adrenal glucocorticoid product (cortisol in the sheep and human; corticosterone in the rat and mouse) in the fetal circulation in late gestation. This cortisol helps ensure that fetal maturation occurs synchronously with processes leading to birth. In the sheep fetus, plasma adrenocorticotropin (ACTH) and cortisol concentrations rise progressively over the last 15 to 20 days of pregnancy (Matthews and Challis, 1996). These hormone changes are associated with upregulation of key genes at different levels of the HPA axis: corticotropin-releasing hormone (CRH) in the fetal hypothalamus, proopiomelanocortin in the fetal pituitary, and ACTH receptor and steroidogenic enzymes in the fetal adrenal gland. Importantly, an adverse intrauterine environment, for example in association with hypoxemia, results in precocious activation of the fetal HPA axis. Fetal sheep exposed to acute hypoxemia generate increases in circulating ACTH and cortisol concentrations. The rises in cortisol tend to be greater in later gestation consistent with progressive fetal adrenal maturation. Within 6 hours of provoking hypoxemia, there is increased

expression of mRNA encoding CRH in the fetal hypothalamus and of proopiomelanocortin in the fetal pituitary gland (Matthews and Challis, 1996). With sustained hypoxemia, proopiomelanocortin mRNA in the *pars distalis* was still elevated, although levels of proopiomelanocortin in the *pars intermedia* of the fetal pituitary had declined. Recent studies have reported that periconceptual undernutrition of the mother leads, in later gestation, to altered feedback set points in the fetal HPA axis, and in a high proportion of animals there is a premature rise in fetal plasma ACTH and cortisol and premature birth (Bloomfield et al., 2003).

Coincident with prepartum increases of cortisol, there is an increase in the concentration of PGE_2 in the circulation of the fetal sheep (Challis et al., 2000). Fetal PGE_2 appears to be derived in large part from the placenta. $PGF_{2\alpha}$ increases in the maternal circulation, but only during the last 24 to 48 hours before birth. In sheep, the difference in time course and profile of PGE_2 in the fetus and $PGF_{2\alpha}$ in the mother has suggested that these different prostaglandins might be derived from different intrauterine tissues. Recent studies have provided evidence that in sheep there is a progression in PG output in late gestation from fetal tissues (trophoblast) to maternal tissues (endometrium, myometrium). It is likely that in human gestation there is a similar progressive change from trophoblast-derived cells in the fetal membranes (amnion and chorion) through to maternal decidua and myometrium (see later). In sheep, evidence is now accumulating to suggest that earlier descriptions of the sequence of events occurring prepartum were incorrect and require revision (Whittle et al., 2001(11)) (Fig. 6-2). More recent studies support the increase in fetal HPA axis function during late gestation leading directly to fetal cortisol upregulating prostaglandin H_2 synthase type 2 (PGHS-2) in the placenta and increasing placental PGE_2 output. Because, in turn, PGE_2 increases activity of the fetal HPA axis, this results in the establishment of a feed-forward endocrine loop. We suggested that increased placental PGE_2 then mediates through autocrine/paracrine mechanisms, an increase in trophoblast $P450_{C17}$ expression and activity. This allows, in the term placenta, metabolism of C-21 steroids to C-19 steroids, which are then aromatized to estrogen, accounting in part for the coincident decline in maternal

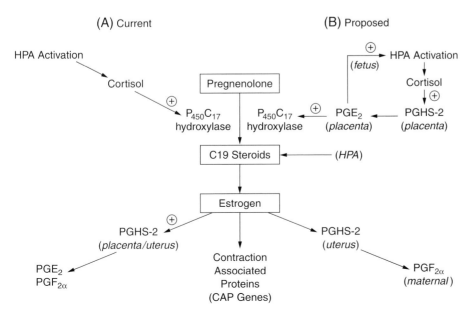

(A) Current   (B) Proposed

FIGURE 6-2 ■ Endocrine pathways leading to the onset of parturition in sheep. **A**, Current model. **B**, Proposed sequence of hormone events. In the current model, activation of the fetal hypothalamic-pituitary-adrenal (HPA) axis leads to increased cortisol thought to upregulate expression of $P450_{C17}$ in the placenta. In the new proposed hypothesis, increased fetal adrenal output of cortisol results in upregulation of prostaglandin H_2 synthase type 2 (PGHS-2) gene expression in the placenta with increased production of prostaglandin (PG)E_2. PGE_2 feeds back to further upregulate fetal HPA function but is itself responsible for upregulation of $P450_{C17}$ gene expression in the placenta. Increased placental estrogen is required for upregulation of PGHS-2 in maternal tissues but not in fetal tissues. Thus, with the onset of parturition there is progression from fetal trophoblast within the placenta to the maternal uterine tissues. CAP, contraction-associated protein.

plasma progesterone concentrations and sharp prepartum increase in placental estrogen output. The late gestation increase in estrogen upregulates expression of maternal endometrial PGHS, resulting in $PGF_{2\alpha}$ being secreted into the maternal circulation and also acting locally within the uterine tissues to effect myometrial contractility (see Fig. 6-2). Thus, in sheep there is separation between regulation of PGHS in fetal tissues from maternal tissues, different PGs produced in trophoblast and in endometrium, and coordinated signaling by which the stimulus to myometrial contractility follows the endocrine and tensile changes that have provoked myometrial activation.

Maturation of HPA axis function occurs in the primate fetus in a manner generally analogous to that discussed in the sheep. A pituitary stimulus is required for adrenal maturation; adrenal development is impaired in anencephaly, and pituitary proopiomelanocortin mRNA, fetal adrenal ACTH receptor, and 3β-hydroxysteroid dehydrogenase (3β-HSD) mRNA are suppressed by betamethasone administration to the baboon fetus (Pepe and Albrecht, 1995). The primate fetal adrenal is divided into an outer definitive zone that produces predominantly aldosterone, the fetal zone that produces dehydroepiandrosterone sulfate, and the transitional zone that produces predominantly cortisol. Thus, $P450_{Scc}$ is expressed throughout the primate fetal adrenal, whereas $P450_{C17}$ is not expressed in the definitive zone but is expressed in the transitional and fetal zones. ACTH stimulates steroidogenesis in the transitional and fetal zones; the major products in late pregnancy are cortisol from the former and dehydroepiandrosterone sulfate from the latter. Interestingly, more recent studies have indicated that CRH, potentially of placental origin, can also stimulate the fetal zone to produce dehydroepiandrosterone sulfate.

Therefore, in primates, late gestation is associated with increased capacity for cortisol and C-19 steroid production from the fetal adrenal gland. When androstenedione was infused into pregnant rhesus monkeys at about three fourths of the way through gestation, there was an increase in maternal plasma estrogen concentrations and premature birth (Mecenas et al., 1996). This activity was blocked by the coinfusion of the aromatase inhibitor 4-hydroxyandrostenedione, which prevented the maternal endocrine changes and blocked the nocturnal increases in uterine myometrial contractility. However, elevations of maternal systemic estrogen concentrations by direct infusion increased myometrial activity but did not produce premature delivery, suggesting the need for estrogen to be generated locally, near to its autocrine/paracrine site of action.

The differences in fetal adrenal–placental relationships and estrogen production between the primate and sheep in late gestation are more of detail than substance (Challis et al., 2000). In both species the fetal adrenal produces increasing amounts of cortisol in late pregnancy. In both sheep and primate the fetoplacental unit produces increased amounts of estrogen. In the primate, estrogen results from placental aromatization of precursors generated within the fetal adrenal gland and there is no induction of $P450_{C17}$ in the placenta. In sheep it is likely that a similar fetoplacental unit is responsible for the progressive increase of estrogen output during the course of gestation. Superimposed on that background at term, an adrenal steroid (cortisol) triggers changes in placental steroidogenesis so that C-19 steroid for estrogen production is generated within trophoblast. We submit that for most of pregnancy fetal–placental interaction is responsible for estrogen production by aromatization of fetal adrenal C-19 steroids in both species. Because placental estrogen output in human gestation is so high and systemic levels are already at their K_d for the receptor, there would be no need for an additional mechanism to boost estrogen output at term, as occurs in the ovine species.

Withdrawal of the Progesterone Block

A fall in plasma progesterone concentration is a common endocrine event associated with parturition across species except primates (Challis et al., 2000). Administration of exogenous progesterone at term blocks the expression of CAP genes and the onset of labor. Even in the human, administration of the progesterone receptor antagonist RU 486 leads to increased uterine activity and induction of labor.

It is clear now that by analogy with information obtained from animal models, there is in the human functional, rather than systemic, withdrawal of progesterone action on the myometrium in late pregnancy. Progesterone action in large part is mediated through a nuclear ligand-inducible transcription factor, the PR. It is obvious that antagonism of progesterone action at the level of the PR or PR interaction with transcriptional machinery could affect progesterone withdrawal. Mechanisms might include a decrease in PR expression, a switch in PR isoform, a change in expression of receptor accessory proteins, or increased expression of endogenous antagonists of progesterone or PR (such as cortisol, transforming growth factor β, or phospholipids). There are three isoforms of the PR: a full-length PR-B and truncated isoforms PR-A and PR-C. PR-B functions predominantly as an activator of progesterone-responsive genes, whereas PR-A acts as a modulator or repressor of PR-B function, possibly because it lacks one of the three activation function domains (AF3) contained within PR-B. There is now clear evidence from several groups that PR-A inhibits PR-B–mediated progesterone action. Recent studies showing differentially increased expression of PR-A mRNA in human myometrium during late pregnancy (Mesiano, 2001), potentially in response to increased output of estrogen, provide a clear mechanism by which functional progesterone withdrawal could be effected in primate species.

It is possible, however, that even this story will require further refinement. A regionalization of myometrial function in the human is well established. Some years ago, Wikland and colleagues (1984) found that although $PGF_{2\alpha}$ had little effect on fundal myometrium taken before labor, it was stimulatory in lower segment specimens. However, $PGF_{2\alpha}$ and PGE_2 always stimulated fundal myometrium collected during spontaneous labor. In lower segment samples collected at that time, PGE_2 induced inhibition, whereas $PGF_{2\alpha}$ had no effect. We and others have suggested that in the myometrium, functional withdrawal of progesterone in the fundus induces CAP gene expression and myometrial activation (Challis et al., 2000). In contrast, there are no significant changes in expression of CX-43 or oxytocin receptor in lower segment myometrium, but there is upregulation of CX-26 and CRH-R1, which would be expected to promote myometrial relaxation. Progesterone signaling may be required in the lower uterine segment to promote expression of genes that induce relaxation, facilitating passage of the fetus.

MYOMETRIAL STIMULATION: PHASE 2 OF PARTURITION

Uterine stimulation follows activation. Although many agonists have been described to stimulate myometrial contractility, the most convincing information is available for PGs and oxytocin. The physiologic role of other putative agonists such as CRH is uncertain, as discussed later.

Overwhelming evidence supports a role for PGs in the labor process, at term, and at preterm (Challis et al., 2000). PGs contribute to the transition from phase 1 to phase 2, although as seen above through their endocrine effects in the fetus, they may have additional activity in the transition from phase 0 to phase 1. Delayed labor onset occurs in knockout mice lacking $PGF_{2\alpha}$ receptor, cytosolic phospholipase A_2, and prostaglandin H_2 synthase type 1 (PGHS-1) enzymes (Muglia, 2000). Lack of $PGF_{2\alpha}$ receptor prevents luteolysis at the end of gestation, plasma progesterone levels are maintained, and oxytocin receptor gene expression in the uterus is suppressed. In human pregnancy there is increased PG output before the appearance of labor-like myometrial contractions, and drugs that block PG synthesis prolong gestational length.

Regulation of PG synthesis may occur at several different levels of the arachidonic acid cascade. PGs are formed from membrane phospholipids through the initial activity of phospholipase A_2 or C isozymes, forming unesterified arachidonic acid. Expression of phospholipase A_2 increases gradually in human fetal membranes during gestation but does not appear to show further increase at the time of labor. In turn, arachidonic acid is metabolized to the intermediate PGH_2 by PGHS enzymes, which have both cyclooxygenase and peroxidase activities. There are two forms of PGHS. Both are heme proteins, with 60% to 65% homology at the cDNA level, although they are products of distinct genes. The constitutive form (PGHS-1) has similar properties to other housekeeping genes. The inducible form (PGHS-2) is characteristically upregulated by growth factors and cytokines. The activities of PGHS isozymes can be inhibited by various nonsteroidal anti-inflammatory drugs. The current search is for compounds specific for PGHS-2 because this enzyme appears to be most involved in the increased output of PG that occurs at the time of labor.

PGH_2 is converted to specific PGs through different PG synthase enzymes. Recent studies have shown two forms of prostaglandin E_2 synthase, a cytosolic form and a membrane-bound form. In human intrauterine tissues, membrane-bound prostaglandin E_2 synthase expression is upregulated by cytokines and may be coordinately regulated with PGHS-2. However, neither we nor others have been able to detect dramatic changes in membrane-bound prostaglandin E_2 synthase expression at the time of labor that would be indicative of a critical role in the increased output of PG that occurs at this time.

Metabolism of primary PG is another point of regulation. The major pathway in the breakdown of PGE_2 and $PGF_{2\alpha}$ involves the action of a type 1 NAD^+-dependent 15-hydroxyprostaglandin dehydrogenase (PGDH) that catalyzes oxidation of 15-hydroxy groups, resulting in formation of 15-keto and 13,14-dihydro-15-keto compounds with reduced biological activity. PGDH is abundantly expressed in human chorion and regulated by a variety of factors, including cytokines and steroid hormones.

PG action is effected through specific receptors, including PGF for $PGF_{2\alpha}$ and four major subtypes for PGE_2 (EP-1, EP-2, EP-3, and EP-4). EP-1 and EP-3 receptors are coupled through intracellular signaling pathways that lead to increased free calcium and decreased cAMP and thus promote contractility. EP-2 and EP-4 receptors are coupled through pathways that increase cAMP formation, leading to relaxation of smooth muscle.

Compartmentalization of Prostaglandin Synthesis and Metabolism

PG synthesizing and metabolizing enzymes are discretely compartmentalized within human fetal membranes (Challis et al., 2000). Amnion is a major site of PG synthesis, in which PGHS activity and PGHS-2 mRNA expression is increased at term and preterm. Chorion expresses both PGHS and PGDH enzymes, although the latter predominates. Thus, there is very little transfer of biologically active PG from amnion, and presumably chorion, through pregnancy to underlying decidua and myometrium. We have argued that increased output of PG by amnion and chorion at the time of labor represents an initial step in the fetal to maternal progression of PG synthesis. However, biologically the major role of PG generated within the membranes may be to effect increased expression and biologic activity of a variety of matrix metalloproteinase enzymes with collagenolytic activity responsible for membrane breakdown. In addition, they may participate in a newly described feed-forward loop that determines the local biologically active level of glucocorticoid by affecting the enzyme 11β-HSD (see later). Thus, chorion has been described as a protective barrier preventing the free transfer of primary PGs generated within amnion and chorion from reaching underlying decidua and/or myometrium (Sangha et al., 1994). Decidua contains both PGHS and some PGDH activity, but there are minimal changes in decidual PGHS-2 expression at the time of labor. In myometrium, different reports have stated that PGHS activity either increases, decreases, or remains about the same. Presumably, this reflects in large part the difficulty of obtaining representative samples of human myometrium and the likelihood of regional regulation of myometrial PGHS expression. Studies from our own laboratory have failed to detect changes in PGHS-2 protein with labor at term in human myometrium, although PGDH protein was lower in samples collected from women at term in labor, providing an alternate mechanism to increased primary PG output.

Regulation of Prostaglandin Synthesis and Metabolism

Regulation of PGHS-2 expression is clearly multifactorial. There are two nuclear factor (NF)-κB binding elements within the proximal promoter region of PGHS-2 (Wang et al., 1993). p50 and p65, key members of the NF-κB *rel* family of proteins, are present in trophoblasts and likely serve as mediators of cytokine-induced upregulation of PGHS-2 expression. The PGHS-2 promoter also includes response elements resembling NF-IL6, CRE, GRE, and AP2 sites (Wang et al., 1993). *In vitro* studies indicate that PGHS-2 mRNA, protein, and activity may be increased several-fold in response to various cytokines and growth factors, raising the possibility that where these compounds are present or elevated, they may be important regulators of PG biosynthesis. Although glucocorticoids inhibit PG output in many cell types, in trophoblast-derived cells, including amnion and chorion, glucocorticoids increase PGE_2 output and increase levels of PGHS-2 mRNA and PGHS protein (Zakar et al., 1995). It seems likely that cytokine mediation of PG synthesis is a major pathway associated with infection-driven preterm labor. The effects of glucocorticoids on PGHS may be important in circumstances of idiopathic preterm labor. The relative importance of these two pathways, or of others, involving growth factors in mechanisms leading to parturition at full term remains, unfortunately, little more than speculation at the current time.

Cytokine-driven uterine stimulation is an established mechanism leading to preterm parturition. Recent reports indicating increased levels of cytokines in patients at term suggest that this pathway could be of more general importance. The amniotic fluid of preterm labor patients contains high concentrations of a variety of cytokines, including interleukin (IL)-1α, IL-6, IL-8, IL-10, and tumor necrosis factor (Kniss and Iams, 1998). It is thought that bacterial organisms secrete endotoxins such as lipopolysaccharide, which provoke cytokine output from macrophages in amnion or chorion. Cytokines in turn elevate PG production and decrease PG metabolism, provoking a feed-forward cascade. Administration of cytokines such as IL-1 or of bacterial endotoxin to pregnant mice provokes premature parturition. Cytokines might also promote release of other uterotonins, including oxytocin and perhaps CRH in decidua, myometrium, and/or placenta. Pro-inflammatory cytokines such as IL-1β upregulate PGE_2 synthesis in cultures of cells from human fetal membranes or myometrium (see Challis et al., 2000). IL-1β increases levels of both phospholipase A_2 and PGHS-2 mRNA in WISH cells and amnion, without change in PGHS-1. Recently it has been postulated (Kniss, 2002, unpublished data) that there is both positive and negative regulation of the PGHS-2 gene. It is clear from several studies that NF-κB is involved in upregulation of PGHS-2 gene expression in response to pro-inflammatory cytokines such as IL-1β or tumor necrosis factor α. It is suggested that during the majority of pregnancy (phase 0 of parturition) the nuclear hormone receptor, PPARγ, inhibits PGHS-2 expression. Thus, the balance of PPARγ and NF-κB expression determines the level of PGHS-2 regulation. Overexpression of PPARγ would result in downregulation in levels of PGHS-2 mRNA by preventing NF-κB activation, and term contractility may require diminution of the effect of PPARγ so that NF-κB activation of PGHS-2 gene expression can occur.

It is also clear that the effects of pro-inflammatory cytokines such as IL-1β can be blocked or reversed *in vitro* by coculture with the anti-inflammatory cytokines such as IL-10 (Pomini et al., 1999). Importantly, IL-10 alone produces a modest stimulation of PGE_2 output and PGHS-2 mRNA levels in explants of human chorion. Clearly, integration of IL-1β and IL-10 effects, with changes in PPARγ and NF-κB, may be crucial to understanding the molecular basis of PGHS-2 gene regulation and expression. It is also clear (see later) that cytokines have multiple sites of action, including effects on phospholipases, PG synthases, and PGDH, all of which contribute to the net stimulation of PG output.

Prostaglandin Inactivation

The net output of bioactive PGs may be determined not only by rates of synthesis but also by rates of metabolism. Thus, the predominant localization of PGDH in chorion trophoblast cells appears to effect a metabolic barrier to the transfer of primary prostaglandins from amnion and chorion to underlying decidua and myometrium (Sangha et al., 1994), and *in vitro* studies have estimated the transfer of unmetabolized PG in the order of 2% to 3%. We did not find changes in PGDH expression or activation in association with labor at term but did find significant decreases in chorionic PGDH in association with preterm labor after infection (Van Meir et al., 1997). In that circumstance, the chorion trophoblast cells are destroyed, thereby eliminating the site of the metabolizing enzyme. PGDH mRNA, protein, and activity were also reduced overall in patients with idiopathic preterm labor and, in a subset of these patients, were reduced by 85% compared with levels in patients presenting at term in the absence of infection. Thus, relative PGDH deficiency may represent a cause of preterm labor in a subset of women. Importantly, at the time of labor, PGDH activity in chorion collected from the region over the internal os of the cervix was reduced compared with tissue from nonlaboring term patients. This was not associated with loss of trophoblast cells, suggesting hormonal regulation of PGDH expression, perhaps through diminished tonic upregulation by progesterone in this site as a normal event of term labor.

The changes in PGDH mRNA indicate that regulation of this enzyme may take place at a transcriptional level. Regulation of PGDH is clearly multifactorial, and both cytokines and steroids appear to play key roles. The 1.6 kb promoter region of PGDH has been sequenced and contains several potential regulatory elements, including AP1, AP2, NF-IL6, ATF-CRE, and GRE sites (Patel and Challis, 2002). IL-1β and tumor necrosis factor α decrease PGDH mRNA and activity in placental and chorion trophoblasts potentially acting through the NF-IL6 element in the promoter region. Anti-inflammatory cytokines such as IL-10 reverse the pro-inflammatory cytokine effects. Steroid hormones also affect PGDH gene expression. Treatment of patients with RU 486 decreased PGDH activity in early pregnancy endometrium. Recently, we found that human chorion or placental trophoblast cells expressed reduced amount of PGDH after treatment with RU 486 or onapristone (progestin antagonists) or trilostane (3β-hydroxysteroid dehydrogenase inhibitor) *in vitro*, whereas administration of exogenous progesterone to these treated cells restored PGDH activity to basal values (Patel and Challis, 2002). This suggests that endogenous progesterone, sequestered from the systemic circulation or generated locally through the 3β-HSD activity of chorion trophoblast cells, could sustain PGDH activity in an autocrine/paracrine manner. This action could be regarded as contributing to the progesterone-derived block on the myometrium during pregnancy.

In early studies we found that chorion and placental trophoblast cells in culture exhibited a dose-dependent decrease in PGDH activity and a significant decrease in levels of PGDH mRNA when treated in a dose-dependent manner with synthetic glucocorticoids, betamethasone or dexamethasone, and cortisol (Patel et al., 1999). The effects of glucocorticoids are presumably exerted through the glucocorticoid receptor, localized by *in situ* hybridization and by immunohistochemistry in human fetal membranes. We have seen previously the presence of several glucocorticoid response elements within the PGDH promoter region. Interestingly, progesterone attenuated cortisol-induced inhibition of PGDH activity and expression.

Conversely, the ability of exogenous progesterone to restore PGDH in chorion trophoblast cells pretreated with the 3β-HSD inhibitor, trilostane, was blocked by coincubation with a specific glucocorticoid receptor antagonist. Thus, regulation of PGDH appears to be influenced, at least in part, by opposing activities of cortisol and progesterone. We have suggested that progesterone maintains tonically the activity of this enzyme in a local fashion through the course of gestation (Challis et al., 2000). The action of progesterone may be exerted through the progesterone receptor, through other activator proteins, or through binding to the glucocorticoid receptor. At term, increased levels of endogenous glucocorticoid displace progesterone from the glucocorticoid receptor, thereby diminishing PGDH expression and activity, allowing increased output of biologically active prostaglandin and providing an additional mechanism to effect PG withdrawal.

Corticotropin-Releasing Hormone

A surprising observation made over a decade ago was that CRH was easily detectable in maternal plasma during the course of human gestation and increased dramatically toward term (Petraglia et al., 1996). Several studies showed that CRH concentrations were elevated in patients destined to give birth preterm and were lower in patients who went on to deliver post-term. CRH in the peripheral circulation is derived from the placenta and fetal membranes, and the increased concentrations reflect increased expression of CRH mRNA. In these sites, control of CRH production is multifactorial. Expression is inhibited by progesterone and nitric oxide and stimulated by a variety of agents, including cytokines, neuropeptides, and glucocorticoids (Petraglia et al., 1996). *In vivo* studies have extended these *in vitro* observations, and in separate sets of patients we showed that prenatal betamethasone administration to women presenting in preterm labor resulted in significant increases in maternal plasma CRH concentrations, whereas there were 60% to 80% decreases in maternal plasma ACTH and cortisol concentrations. These observations led us and others to propose a mechanism by which altered production of placental CRH might mediate the fetal placental response to an adverse intrauterine environment, resulting in idiopathic preterm birth (Challis et al., 2000). Fetal stress, for example in response to hypoxemia and/or reduced uteroplacental perfusion, results in activation of the fetal HPA axis with increased output of cortisol from the fetal adrenal gland. Fetal cortisol stimulates placental CRH gene expression, apparently through a mechanism that might require generation of cAMP. We suggested that CRH might act initially as a vasodilator within the placenta to increase uteroplacental blood flow in an attempt to enhance placental oxygen transfer to the fetus. In the event that this correction fails, HPA axis activation is sustained, placental CRH output enhanced further, and a threshold reached by which placental CRH stimulates PG production within the fetal membranes. In addition, CRH stimulates directly from the fetal zone of the fetal adrenal gland an increased output of C-19 steroids, which are aromatized to estrogen in the placenta, thereby facilitating uterine activation. Enhanced production of PG is then able to effect stimulation of the myometrium and premature delivery. Evidence in support of this hypothesis includes the observations that maternal plasma CRH concentrations are significantly higher in the plasma of women at 28 to 32 weeks' gestation who present with the diagnosis of preterm labor and who deliver within 12 to 24 hours, compared with patients with the same diagnosis but in whom delivery did not occur and in whom circulating CRH concentrations were the same as those of a control group of patients who continued to term (Korebrits et al., 1998). This observation suggests the possibility of using measurements of maternal plasma CRH as one of a battery of markers to discriminate among patients with an initial diagnosis of preterm labor and those who would proceed to preterm delivery and in whom tocolytic management might be introduced.

It is clear that placental CRH output may be increased not only in response to fetal stress, but also in response to elevations of maternal glucocorticoids. Hobel and colleagues (1999) reported that maternal peripheral plasma CRH concentrations are increased in patients with increased scores in anxiety tests and that elevations in maternal CRH values in the second trimester may be predictive of preterm labor.

The mechanism by which CRH might influence myometrial function has been delineated in an elegant series of studies from Hillhouse and Grammatopoulos (2001), who pointed out that in early pregnancy, placentally derived CRH is inactive because it binds in the peripheral circulation to the CRH-binding protein. CRH-binding protein concentrations decrease prepartum, thereby increasing free CRH concentrations at that time. There are multiple forms of CRH receptor in myometrium placenta and fetal membranes. During pregnancy, CRH effects on myometrium include inhibition of PGE_2, increases in intracellular cAMP, and upregulation of nitric oxide synthase with relaxation of myometrial function. At term, with increased expression of oxytocin receptors the CRH receptor reverts to a low affinity state, reducing intracellular cAMP generation and allowing an increase in myometrial excitability. These data suggest that during pregnancy CRH plays a protective role for the myometrium by preventing uterine contractions, whereas at term CRH enhances the myometrial contractile responses to $PGF_{2\alpha}$, PGE_2, and oxytocin. Recent observations showing that CRH increases expression of PGDH in chorion trophoblast cells is consistent with this protective role (McKeown and Challis, 2003). In this event, it may be that the elevated levels of CRH in maternal plasma during gestation with impending preterm labor are not causal to stimulating myometrial contractility but reflect a response of the fetal–placental unit to compromise with feedback-increased production of substances that might inhibit uterine contractility. Conversely, in patients proceeding post-term, there would be less generation of CRH required as myometrial inhibitor.

Regulation of Intrauterine Glucocorticoid Concentrations

We have seen that expression of PGHS-2, PGDH, and CRH within human intrauterine tissues is regulated by glucocorticoids (Fig. 6-3). Those glucocorticoids may be derived from the systemic circulation, the fetus, or from amniotic fluid. In addition, levels of bioactive glucocorticoid within the placenta and fetal membranes may be regulated locally through the activity of the 11β-HSD isoforms, 11β-HSD-1 and 11β-HSD-2. Expression of 11β-HSD-2 predominates in the placenta in the syncytiotrophoblast layer. 11β-HSD-2 acts

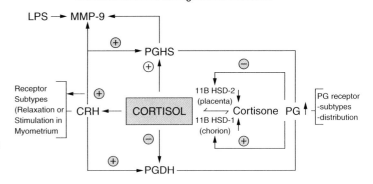

FIGURE 6-3 ■ Interrelationship between cortisol, prostaglandin H₂ synthase type 2 (PGHS-2), 15-hydroxyprostaglandin dehydrogenase (PGDH), and corticotropin-releasing hormone (CRH). In chorion, cortisone can be converted to cortisol through the activity of 11β-hydroxysteroid dehydrogenase-1 (11β-HSD-1), and the activity of this enzyme is increased locally by prostaglandins (PGs). LPS, lipopolysaccharide; MMP-9, matrix metalloproteinase-9.

predominantly as a dehydrogenase, converting maternal cortisol to inactive cortisone and thereby preventing excess passage of maternal cortisol down the concentration gradient into the fetal compartment. Importantly, levels of placental 11β-HSD-2 are decreased in association with conditions such as preeclampsia (Alfaidy et al., 2002). Thus, in this circumstance, there would be diminished placental inactivation of cortisol through the 11β-HSD-2 pathway. More maternally derived glucocorticoid would cross the placenta into the fetal compartment, potentially contributing to growth inhibition. In addition, one would expect levels of cortisol to be higher in the placental environment itself, and this may contribute to increased rates of apoptosis in the placentas of preeclamptic pregnancies. It is clear that the level of activity of 11β-HSD-2 should also regulate the availability of cortisol to influence stimulation of placental CRH output. Studies are obviously required to correlate changes in placental CRH expression with altered placental 11β-HSD-2 in different pathophysiologic states. The recent observation that placental 11β-HSD-2 increases dramatically around the 10th week of gestation in association with increased placental vascularity suggests that its expression might be responsive to changes in oxygen tension. The finding that first and third trimester placental tissue, incubated in 3% oxygen, expressed lower levels of 11β-HSD-2 protein and activity compared with tissue maintained at 20% oxygen is consistent with this observation (Alfaidy et al., 2002). We have proposed that hypoxemia either lowers placental 11β-HSD-2 expression or prevents the normal gestation-induced increase in 11β-HSD-2, resulting in less maternal cortisol metabolism and higher local cortisol concentration.

Recently, Alfaidy and colleagues (2001) demonstrated that chorion trophoblast cells have the potential to generate cortisol locally. These cells express a variety of steroidogenic enzymes but in particular 11β-HSD-1, which acts predominantly as a reductase enzyme. The expression and activity of 11β-HSD-1 to form cortisol from cortisone increases progressively in chorion trophoblast cells during the course of gestation. Importantly, these investigators have shown short-term regulation of 11β-HSD-1 in chorion trophoblasts in response to prostaglandins. PGF₂α and the synthetic PGF receptor agonist, fluprostenol, stimulated 11β-HSD-1 reductase activity in a dose-dependent fashion. This response increases the potential for local cortisol generation from circulating cortisone, thereby creating a positive feed-forward loop by which increased cortisol contributes to increased PG production,

which increases cortisol by activating 11β-HSD-1. We have demonstrated by immunostaining the presence of PGF receptors in chorion trophoblasts *in vivo* and *in vitro* and have shown increased expression of chorion trophoblast PGF receptor in tissue collected from patients at term in labor, compared with those in the absence of labor. Thus, the sensitivity of these cells to respond to exogenous PG should increase at that time.

Application to Clinical Preterm Labor

The rates of preterm labor have remained relatively unchanged in North America over the last 30 to 40 years; if anything, increases have occurred as a result of increased multiple gestations. There is a clear need to recognize first those preterm labors in which prevention is undesirable because it constitutes a greater compromise to fetal health than delivery. There is also a need to develop diagnostic indicators specific for particular windows of gestation to determine the patient in true preterm labor. Methods of tocolysis might then be related on a patient-specific basis to the underlying cause of preterm labor in that individual. Hence, diagnosis of preterm labor should encompass a multiple test approach.

The development of specific PGHS-2 inhibitors offers great promise for tocolysis, because increased expression of PGHS-2 within intrauterine tissues clearly defines a final common pathway in birth mechanisms among species. The potential to develop specific antagonists to PGF or EP receptors linked to enhanced contractility is also of clear therapeutic potential. The ability to modulate CRH effects on the myometrium will require a proper understanding of its physiologic effects. The emerging picture of regionalization of myometrial contractility will require understanding of differential regulation of agonists to receptors in different parts of the uterus. It is possible also that development of agonists to EP-2 or EP-4 receptors would promote relaxation of myometrial function.

A more fundamental approach involves recognition and regulation of candidate genes leading to phase 1 myometrial activation. Animal studies have suggested that an inhibition of PGHS-2 might also suppress CAP gene expression, but the applicability of this information to primates and the potential for reversal remains untested. It is abundantly clear that our improved understanding of fundamental labor mechanisms has not yet been translated into better diagnoses of preterm labor either in the general population or in high-risk patients. For reasons discussed, it is unlikely that a single test will meet that objective. Recent advances in gene chip technology, however, do suggest that alterations of particular gene clusters may occur in relation to preterm labor, and its seems inevitable that this line of investigation must be an important focus of activity in the immediate future.

REFERENCES

Alfaidy N, Gupta S, DeMarko C, et al: Oxygen regulation of placental 11-beta-hydroxysteroid dehydrogenase-2: Physiological and pathological implications. J Clin Endocrinol Metab **87**:4797, 2002.

Alfaidy N, Xiong ZG, Myatt L, et al: Prostaglandin F2alpha potentiates cortisol production by stimulating 11beta-hydroxysteroid dehydrogenase 1: A novel feedback loop that may contribute to human labor. J Clin Endocrinol Metab **86**:5585, 2001.

Bloomfield FH, Oliver MH, Hawkins P, et al: A peri-conceptual nutritional origin for non-infectious preterm birth. Science (in press), 2003.

Challis JRG, Matthews SG, Gibb W, et al: Endocrine and paracrine regulation of birth at term and preterm. Endocr Rev **21**:514, 2000.

Chow L, Lye SJ: Expression of the gap junction protein, connexin-43, is increased in the human myometrium towards term and with the onset of labour. Am J Obstet Gynecol **170**:788, 1994.

Garfield RE: Structural and functional studies of the control of myometrial contractility and labour. *In* McNellis D, Challis JRG, MacDonald PC, et al. (eds): The Onset of Labour: Cellular and Integrative Mechanisms. Perinatology Press, Ithaca, NY, 1988, p. 55.

Hillhouse EW, Grammatopoulos DK: Control of intracellular signalling by corticotropin-releasing hormone in human myometrium. *In* Smith R (ed): The Endocrinology of Parturition: Basic Science and Clinical Application. Karger, Basel, Switzerland, 2001, p. 66.

Hobel CJ, Dunkel-Schetter C, Roesch SC, et al: Maternal plasma corticotropin-releasing hormone associated with stress at 20 weeks' gestation in pregnancies ending in preterm delivery. Am J Obstet Gynecol **180**:257, 1999.

Kniss DA, Iams JD: Regulation of parturition update: Endocrine and paracrine effectors of term and preterm labor. Clin Perinatol **25**:819, 1998.

Korebrits C, Ramirez MM, Watson L, et al: Maternal corticotropin-releasing hormone is increased with impending preterm birth. J Clin Endocrinol Metab **83**:1585, 1998.

Liggins GC, Thorburn GD: Initiation of parturition. *In* Lamming GE (ed): Marshall's Physiology of Reproduction. Chapman and Hall, London, UK, 1994, p. 863.

Lye SJ, Mitchell J, Nashman N, et al: Role of mechanical signals in the onset of term and preterm labor. *In* Smith R (ed): The Endocrinology of Parturition: Basic Science and Clinical Application. Karger, Basel, Switzerland, 2001, p. 165.

Lye SJ, Ou CW, Teoh TG, et al: The molecular basis of labour and tocolysis. Fetal Matern Med Rev **10**:121, 1998.

MacKenzie LW, Word RA, Casey ML, et al: Myosin light chain phosphorylation in human myometrial smooth muscle cells. Am J Physiol **258**:92, 1990.

Matthews SG, Challis JRG: Regulation of the hypothalamo-pituitary-adrenocortical axis in fetal sheep. Trends Endocrinol Metab **7**:239, 1996.

McKeown KJ, Challis JRG: Regulation of expression of 15-hydroxyprostaglandin dehydrogenase (PGDH) by corticotrophin-releasing hormone (CRH) through a calcium-dependent pathway in human chorion trophoblast cells. J Clin Endocrinol Metab (in press), 2003.

Mecenas CA, Giussani DA, Owiny J, et al: Production of premature delivery in pregnant rhesus monkeys by androstenedione infusion. Nat Med **2**:443, 1996.

Meis PJ, Goldenberg RL, Mercer JE, et al: The preterm prediction study: Risk factors for indicated preterm births. Maternal-Fetal Medicine Units Network of the National Institute of Child Health and Human Development. Am J Obstet Gynecol **178**:562, 1998.

Mesiano S: Roles of estrogen and progesterone in human parturition. *In* Smith R (ed): The Endocrinology of Parturition: Basic Science and Clinical Application. Karger, Basel, Switzerland, 2001, p. 86.

Muglia LJ: Genetic analysis of fetal development and parturition control in the mouse. Pediatr Res **47**:437, 2000.

Patel FA, Challis JRG: Cortisol progesterone antagonism in the regulation of 15-hydroxy prostaglandin dehydrogenase activity and mRNA levels in human chorion and placental trophoblast cells at term. J Clin Endocrinol Metab **87**:700, 2002.

Patel FA, Clifton VL, Chwalisz K, et al: Steroid regulation of prostaglandin dehydrogenase activity and expression in human term placenta and chorio-decidua in relation to labor. J Clin Endocrinol Metab **84**:291, 1999.

Pepe GJ, Albrecht ED: Actions of placental and fetal adrenal steroid hormones in primate pregnancy. Endocr Rev **16**:608, 1995.

Petraglia F, Florio P, Nappi C, et al: Peptide signaling in human placenta and membranes: Autocrine, paracrine and endocrine mechanisms. Endocr Rev **17**:156, 1996.

Pomini F, Caruso A, Challis JR: Interleukin-10 modifies the effects of interleukin-1beta and tumor necrosis factor-alpha on the activity and expression of prostaglandin H synthase-2 and the NAD+-dependent 15-hydroxyprostaglandin dehydrogenase in cultured term human villous trophoblast and chorion trophoblast cells. J Clin Endocrinol Metab **84**:4645, 1999.

Sangha RK, Walton JC, Ensor CM, et al: Immunohistochemical localization, messenger ribonucleic acid abundance, and activity of 15-hydroxyprostaglandin dehydrogenase in placenta and fetal membranes during term and preterm labor. J Clin Endocrinol Metab **78**:982, 1994.

Van Meir CA, Matthews SG, Keirse MJ, et al: 15-Hydroxyprostaglandin dehydrogenase: Implications in preterm labor with and without ascending infection. J Clin Endocrinol Metab **82**:969, 1997.

Wang LH, Hajibeigi A, Xu XM, et al: Characterization of the promoter of human prostaglandin H synthase-1 gene. Biophys Res Commun **190**:406, 1993.

Whittle WL, Patel FA, Alfaidy N, et al: Glucocorticoid regulation of human and ovine parturition: The relationship between fetal hypothalamic-pituitary-adrenal axis activation and intrauterine prostaglandin production. Biol Reprod **64**:1019, 2001.

Wikland M, Lingwood BE, Wiqvist N: Myometrial response to prostaglandins during labour. Gynecol Obstet Invest **17**:131, 1984.

Zakar T, Hirst JJ, Mijovic JE, et al: Dexamethasone stimulates arachidonic acid conversion to prostaglandin E2 in human amnion cells. Endocrinology **136**:1610, 1995.

Chapter 7

THE IMMUNOLOGY OF PREGNANCY

Robert M. Silver, MD, Morgan R. Peltier, PhD, and D. Ware Branch, MD

Two unique and fascinating immunologic stories unfold during pregnancy. First, a fetus living in an isolated sterile environment develops the essential framework of the immune system so it can mount a respectable, albeit somewhat immature, immunologic response. Second, at the maternal-fetal interface a combination of fetal and maternal immunologic factors conspires to allow, and perhaps encourage, the growth of the semi-allogeneic conceptus.

To fully understand how these two stories evolve would be to completely understand immunology itself; as yet, only part of either story is revealed. In this chapter we review the ontogeny of the fetal immune response and the immunologic relationship between the mother and conceptus. A basic understanding of these issues is of more than academic interest; many disorders of the fetus or mother are due to aberrations in the normal immunology of pregnancy. Most clinicians recognize the immunologic pathophysiology of red blood cell and platelet alloimmunization, neonatal systemic lupus erythematosus, idiopathic thrombocytopenic purpura, myasthenia gravis, and heritable congenital immunodeficiencies. In addition, common obstetric conditions, such as spontaneous abortion, fetal death, preeclampsia, fetal growth retardation, placental insufficiency, and preterm labor, are known or suspected to be at least in part immunologically mediated.

OVERVIEW OF THE IMMUNE RESPONSE

The immune system is often described as two interactive and often complementary defense systems or responses: *innate* (Fig. 7-1) and *adaptive* (Fig. 7-2). The innate immune response is a *nonspecific reaction to foreign antigens*. Specific antigens are not required to elicit innate immunity nor does the response improve after reexposure to a specific antigen. In contrast, *adaptive immunity occurs in response to specific antigens*. Adaptive immune responses are altered when an organism has been previously exposed to a foreign antigen, a concept termed *immunologic memory*.

Both innate and adaptive immune responses are primarily *mediated* by specialized cellular constituents and soluble factors. Many of these soluble factors are cytokines, small proteins secreted by cells that nonenzymatically regulate cellular function (Nathan and Sporn, 1991). Cytokines were originally characterized in lymphoid tissues. It is now clear, however, that cytokines are produced by, and exert effects on, a wide variety of other cells, including gestational tissues. Detailed reviews of the complex regulation and multiple functions of cytokines are published elsewhere (Nathan and Sporn, 1991; Lanzavecchia and Sallusto, 2000).

Briefly, cytokines can be loosely divided into inflammatory cytokines, T-cell–derived lymphokines, hematopoietic growth factors, peptide growth factors, and chemokines (Table 7-1). Other soluble components of the immune system include immunoglobulins (Igs), complement, fibronectin, C-reactive protein, prostaglandins, and hormones.

INNATE IMMUNE RESPONSE

Innate immunity includes physical and biochemical barriers to the entry of foreign material. These barriers include skin, mucous membranes, ciliated epithelial linings, endothelial cells, and active components of secretions, such as lysozymes. *In utero* the fetus is protected by several layers of maternal and fetal tissues. Some layers, such as amniotic fluid, have additional bacteriostatic properties.

The primary effector cells of innate immunity are granulocytes (neutrophils), macrophages and monocytes, and natural killer (NK) cells, all of which are derived from bone marrow stem cells. Neutrophils and macrophages protect against invading organisms by engulfing and destroying them in a process termed phagocytosis. These cells are located throughout the body in areas where they are likely to encounter organisms.

Consider, for example, the strategic location of alveolar macrophages and the tissue macrophages of the spleen and liver. These cells are capable of chemotaxis, "honing" to areas of infection or inflammation. NK cells are a heterogeneous nonphagocytic population of cells that resemble T lymphocytes. In contrast to most lymphocytes, NK cells do not require specialized antigen presentation for the recognition of foreign antigen. They are particularly adept at recognizing the surface markers on virus-infected or tumor cells and are responsible for mediating spontaneous cell-mediated cytotoxicity.

A new class of membrane-bound molecules, termed toll-like receptors, has recently been identified. These cell surface receptors are present on phagocytes and other cell types and play a critical role in the innate immune response to pathogenic organisms. Humans have at least 10 toll-like receptors that all have intracellular domains that are highly homologous to the interleukin (IL)-1 receptor. The extracellular domains are less homologous and recognize conserved molecules on various classes of pathogens. For example, toll-like receptor-2 recognizes peptidoglycans and

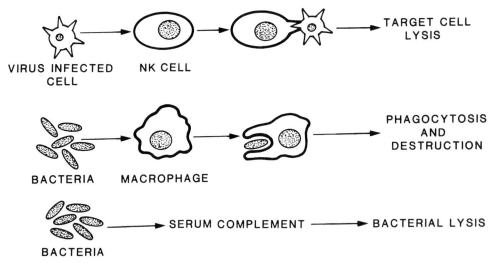

FIGURE 7-1 ■ Summary of innate immunity. Surface antigens of viruses, bacteria, and tumors induce innate immune function. In this system, natural killer (NK) cells and phagocytes, such as macrophages, can recognize certain antigens in a nonspecific fashion and either lyse the offending infected cells or ingest and destroy the offending organisms. Only the foreign nature of the antigen is required; antigen processing and major histocompatibility antigen participation are not necessary.

common bacterial lipoproteins from spirochetes and mycoplasmas, whereas toll-like receptor-4 recognizes the lipid A portion of lipopolysaccharide and lipoteichoic acid (Medzhitov, 2001). Several other cell surface receptors recognize specific microbial products and are integral to innate immunity. These include mannan-binding lectin, mannose receptors, and the macrophage scavenger receptor (Medzhitov and Janeway, 2000).

Endothelial cells are also an important component to innate immunity. Endothelial cells respond directly to lipopolysaccharide and other bacterial components through an extracellular complex that includes toll-like receptor-4 and soluble CD14. Activation of signal transduction pathways by these receptors causes increased expression of adhesion molecules capable of recruiting leukocytes, pro-inflammatory cytokine secretion, and upregulation of tissue factor expression that may activate the coagulation pathway (Henneke and Golenbock, 2002; Levi et al., 2002).

Circulating factors, such as *complement* and the *acute phase proteins*, are also part of the innate immune system. The complement system is composed of multiple proteins and can be activated through either a classic or alternative pathway. Each pathway converges onto a final common cascade of reactions, leading to the destruction of microbial pathogens. Components of the complement cascade can bind to foreign organisms, lyse bacteria, facilitate phagocytosis, and attract circulating phagocytes.

Acute phase proteins, such as C-reactive protein, are induced by the cytokine IL-6 and can bind to the surface of certain types of bacteria, promoting phagocytosis. Many other soluble factors, including cytokines, are integral to innate immunity. One of the most important groups is interferons (IFNs), which are produced by virus-infected cells. IFNs activate NK cells and can induce resistance to viral infections in neighboring host cells. IL-12, a cytokine produced by macrophages, is also a powerful activator of NK cells.

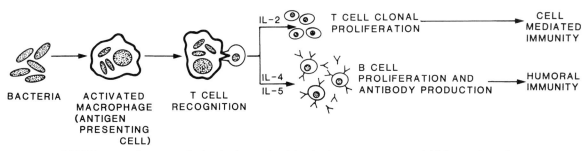

FIGURE 7-2 ■ Summary of adaptive immunity. Adaptive immune responses initially require antigen processing and subsequent presentation to T cells. A T cell with a receptor specific for an inciting antigen will be activated and undergo clonal proliferation. In part, the type of cytokine produced by the activated T cell dictates the nature of the subsequent response. Interleukin-2 (IL-2) is the primary growth factor required for clonal proliferation of T cells and stimulates the proliferation of cytotoxic and memory T cells. IL-4 and IL-5 stimulate B-cell proliferation, differentiation, and antibody production.

TABLE 7-1. CELLULAR SOURCES, TARGET CELLS, AND PRINCIPAL ACTIVITIES OF CYTOKINES RELEVANT TO REPRODUCTIVE IMMUNOLOGY

Cytokine	Cellular Sources	Target Cells	Principle Activities
Inflammatory Cytokines			
Interleukin-1α	Macrophages	T and B cells	Lymphocyte activation, prostaglandin production
Interleukin-1β	Monocytes, B cells, endothelial cells	Macrophages, endothelial cells, fibroblasts	Macrophage stimulation, prexia, enhanced leukocyte-endothelial interaction, tissue regeneration, enhances MHC expression
Tumor necrosis factor-α	Macrophages, cytotoxic T cells, NK cells	Macrophages, neutrophils, fibroblasts	Cachexia, enhanced leukocyte endothelial interaction, macrophage activation, enhanced cytotoxicity
Interleukin-6	Macrophages, fibroblasts, activated CD4+ T cells	Macrophages, endothelial cells, hepatocytes, B cells	Acute phase response, T-cell activation, prostaglandin production, B-cell differentiation into plasma cells and antibody production
Interleukin-12	Mononuclear phagocytes, dendritic cells	NK cells, T cells	Activates NK cells, stimulates production of a pro-inflammatory phenotype in T cells
Interleukin-15	Mononuclear phagocytes	NK cells	Stimulates proliferation of NK cells
Anti-inflammatory Cytokines			
Interleukin L-10	T cells, macrophages	Macrophages	Potent inhibitor of macrophages
Interleukin L-13	Activated T cells	B cells	Stimulates B-cell development
Chemokines			
Interleukin-8	Macrophages, monocytes, endothelial cells, keratinocytes, fibroblasts	Neutrophils, T cells, basophils	Neutrophil activations and degranulation, chemotactic for neutrophils and T cells
T-cell–derived Lymphokines			
Interleukin-2	Activated CD4+ T cells, NK cells	CD4+ and CD8+ T cells	T-cell growth and proliferation
Interleukin-3	Activated CD4+ T cells	Hematopoietic precursors, stem cells	Promotes growth and differentiation of myeloid progenitor cells
Interleukin-4	Activated CD4+ T cells	B cells, eosinophils	B-cell growth and differentiation, IgE production, eosinophilia
Interleukin-5	Activated CD4+ T cells	B cells	B-cell differentiation, antibody isotype switching
Interferon-γ	Activated CD4+ T cells, NK cells	CD4+ and CD8+ T cells, macrophages	Enhances MHC class II expression, macrophage activation, enhances endothelial-leukocyte interaction
Interferon-α	Mononuclear phagocytes	Virus-infected cells, NK cells	Inhibits viral replication, inhibits cell proliferation, increases MHC expression, activates NK cells
Colony-Stimulating Factors (CSFs)			
Granulocytc CSF	Mononuclear phagocytes, endothelial cells, fibroblasts	Granulocyte progenitors	Maturation of progenitors into granulocytes
Granulocyte-macrophage CSF	T cells, mononuclear phagocytes, endothelial cells, fibroblasts	Granulocyte and macrophage progenitors	Maturation of progenitors into granulocytes and macrophages
Macrophage CSF	Mononuclear phagocytes, endothelial cells, fibroblasts	Macrophage progenitors	Maturation of progenitors into macrophages
Peptide Growth Factors			
Transforming growth factor-β	T cells, mononuclear phagocytes	T cells, mononuclear phagocytes, other cells	Inhibits the activation of mononuclear phagocytes, inhibits activation and proliferation of T cells

Ig, immunoglobulin; MHC, major histocompatibility complex; NK, natural killer.

ADAPTIVE IMMUNE RESPONSE

The adaptive immune response consists of two types of antigen-specific responses: *cellular* and *humoral*. These responses are mediated by T and B lymphocytes, the cellular constituents of the adaptive immune system, and ultimately result in the clearance of pathogens via antibody binding, cytolysis, and phagocytosis. For many adaptive responses, the phagocytic cells described earlier, as part of the innate immune system, must first process ingested antigen and present it for recognition by mature lymphocytes. Presented antigens are then recognized by specific receptors on the surface of T and B cells. The specificity of T and B cells is derived from a complex and elegant process termed *gene rearrangement*, which generates myriad possible antigen recognition sites and accounts for the diversity and specificity of the adaptive immune response. The primary function of B lymphocytes is the production of Igs, also termed *antibodies*, that recognize specific foreign antigens. There are five primary Ig isotypes: IgG, IgM, IgD, IgA, and IgE.

B cells mature in two stages. The first stage is *antigen independent* and involves the differentiation of stem cells into pre-B cells, characterized by cell-surface Ig molecules that function as receptors. The second stage is *antigen dependent* and occurs when a specific antigen binds to the cell's specific Ig receptor. This induces the pre-B cell to undergo clonal proliferation and differentiate into plasma cells, the mature antibody-secreting descendant of B lymphocytes. The secreted antibodies have the same binding specificity as the original pre-B-cell receptor. Antibodies facilitate the immune destruction of organisms or infected cells to which they are bound by promoting phagocytosis and membrane lysis.

Ig proteins are composed of two identical heavy and two identical light chains of amino acids (Fig. 7-3). The heavy and light chains are encoded by separate genes, and regions within

each chain are encoded by corresponding gene segments. The antigen-binding portion of the molecule is composed of a combination of highly variable regions within the heavy and light chains. An astonishingly wide diversity of Ig molecules can be generated by rearrangement of the gene segments responsible for the molecule in the developing B cell.

Although a detailed description is beyond the scope of this review, the process of gene rearrangement allows a large number of different Ig molecules to be made from a relatively small number of genes. Rearranged genes are present in pre-B cells and B cells, and each cell makes only one Ig, which is expressed on the cell surface as an antigen receptor. When an antigen is recognized by a B-cell surface Ig, the B cell is stimulated to proliferate (clonal proliferation). Cells expressing antibody that binds the antigen more avidly are most strongly stimulated to proliferate. In this fashion, specific antibody-secreting cells are selected by antigen exposure.

T cells also undergo a maturation process, beginning with the differentiation of pluripotent stem cells into T-cell precursors. As these cells mature, they express a variety of cell-surface adhesion molecules. One of these molecules is the *T-cell receptor* (TcR), an antigen recognition molecule. Like Ig, it uses gene rearrangement to generate specificity. The TcR is a disulfide-linked heterodimer composed of either αβ or γδ subunits. The structure of the TcR is similar to that of Ig and is thought to be derived from the same superfamily of genes (Royer and Reinherz, 1987). Although TcRs capable of recognizing "self" antigens are generated, such T cells are deleted before maturation during a complex differentiation process in the thymus.

Another important T-cell surface molecule is the CD3 protein complex. When CD3 becomes linked to the αβ TcR, the T cell becomes activated, differentiates, and generates clones with identical antigen specificity. This TcR-CD3 complex recognizes foreign antigen only when it is presented by a phagocytic antigen processing cell in the context of other self-antigens, termed major histocompatibility complex (MHC) antigens in the human (Fig. 7-4). This absolute requirement for MHC antigen is known as "MHC restriction."

Two types or classes of *classic* MHC molecules have been described (Hansen and Sachs, 1989). Class I MHC molecules, encoded by the human leukocyte antigen (HLA) locus, include HLA-A, -B, and -C and are found on most cells. The HLA-D locus encodes class II MHC molecules, which are expressed on antigen-presenting cells and B cells. Both class I and II classic MHC molecules are highly polymorphic and, to a large degree, are the molecules recognized as foreign that lead to allograft rejection. *Nonclassic* MHC molecules also exist, known as HLA-E, -F, and -G; they are class I-like and are nonpolymorphic or oligomorphic.

Mature T cells usually express one of two additional surface molecules, CD4 or CD8. CD4-positive T cells recognize antigens presented in association with class II MHC molecules, whereas T cells expressing CD8 bind to antigens presented with class I MHC molecules. CD4-positive T cells are often referred to as *helper T cells* and can facilitate immune responses.

Two distinct types of helper T cells have been described (Mosmann et al., 1986). The first type of cell, termed *Th1*, secretes IL-2, IFN-γ, and lymphotoxin, cytokines important to T-cell cytotoxicity and delayed hypersensitivity reactions. In contrast, *Th2* cells secrete IL-4, IL-5, IL-6, and IL-10, all cytokines that foster antibody production and allergic reac-

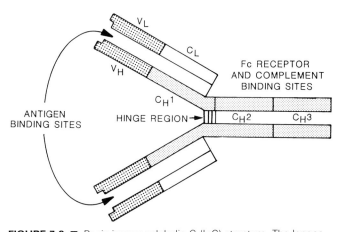

FIGURE 7-3 ■ Basic immunoglobulin G (IgG) structure. The longer, inside chain is the "heavy" chain. It is structurally distinct for each class or subclass of antibody. The outside, shorter chain is the "light" chain. There is sequence variability at the amino-terminal end of both the heavy and light chains (V_H and V_L regions, respectively). The antigen-binding sites are at the amino-terminal ends of these variable regions. The rest of the molecule has a relatively constant (C) structure, with three distinct domains (C_H1, C_H2, and C_H3, respectively). The hinge region between the C_H1 and C_H2 domains allows each binding site of the antibody to operate independently.

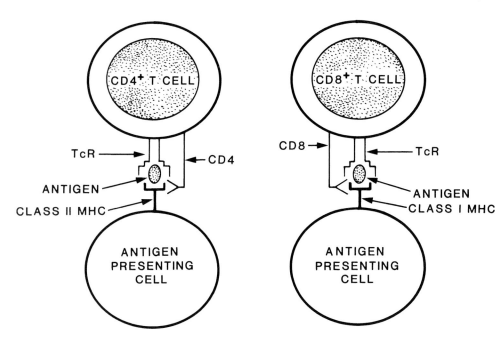

FIGURE 7-4 ■ T-cell receptor (TcR) and antigen recognition. T cells recognize foreign antigen in the context of self major histocompatibility antigen (MHC) when it is presented in this context by antigen-presenting cells (e.g., macrophages). Antigen presented with class II MHC molecules (*left*) is recognized by T cells bearing the CD4 adhesion molecule. Such cells usually act as T "helper" cells. Antigen presented with class 1 MHC molecules (*right*) is recognized by T cells bearing the CD8 adhesion molecule. Such T cells usually act as cytotoxic T cells or T "suppressor" cells.

tions. T cells expressing CD8 often have either cytotoxic activity or specifically suppress the activity of macrophages, B cells, and helper T cells. These are sometimes referred to as *cytotoxic* and *suppressor* T cells, respectively.

In general, viruses and parasites stimulate primarily T-cell–mediated adaptive immune responses, whereas bacteria elicit both an innate phagocytic response and a humoral (antibody-mediated) adaptive response. Of course, there is a large degree of overlap and interplay among the various components of the immune system. Through modulation and regulation by cytokines, the final adaptive immune response is an impressive and changing array that can respond to virtually any foreign antigen.

FETAL AND NEONATAL IMMUNITY

Although the structural framework of the normal immune system is built *in utero*, immune development continues during the neonatal period, infancy, and childhood. Next, we present the development of the fetal immune response and important differences between the developing fetal and adult immune responses.

Development of Innate Immunity

The skin of fetuses and preterm infants is poorly developed compared with that in term newborns and adults. Preterm infants (<30 weeks' gestation) are at increased risk of infection as a result of the inability of the epidermis to adequately block the invasion of microbial pathogens. Regardless of gestational age, the skin completes functional development in 2 to 3 weeks after birth (Holbrook, 1992).

The immune effector cells of the innate immune system arise from hematopoietic progenitor cells first noted in the blood islands of the embryonic yolk sac. By 8 weeks' gestation, the yolk sac is replaced by the fetal liver as the source of these cells. By 20 weeks' gestation, almost all hematopoietic progenitor cells are derived from fetal bone marrow. These pluripotent hematopoietic cells respond to a variety of stimuli by differentiation and proliferation (Fauser and Messner, 1978, 1979; Messner and Fauser, 1980; Messner et al., 1981), giving rise to granulocytes and macrophages.

Macrophage-like cells are found as early as 4 weeks of human gestation, appearing at the yolk sac stage of embryonic development (Keleman and Janossa, 1980; Beelen et al., 1990). Circulating monocytes, which differentiate into macrophages in tissues, are present in the fetus by 16 weeks' gestation (Stiehm, 1975). The number of circulating monocytes in term neonates is similar to that in adults, but there are fewer tissue macrophages. This appears to be due to diminished monocyte infiltration into sites of inflammation in the neonate (Klein et al., 1977). The number of tissue macrophages does not reach adult levels until ages 6 to 10 years. Although the phagocytic and antigen-processing capacities of neonatal and adult macrophages are similar, neonatal cells have a relatively decreased capacity to produce and respond to several cytokines (Li et al., 1996).

Granulocytes appear in the fetal spleen and liver at 8 weeks' gestation and in the fetal circulation by 12 to 14 weeks' gestation. In contrast to adults, no more than 10% of the leukocytes in the fetal circulation are granulocytes, and a substantial number of these are functionally immature granulocyte precursors (Forestier et al., 1986). After delivery, the number of granulocytes increases dramatically, reaching or exceeding adult levels by 48 to 72 hours. Compared with adults, however, neonates have poor ability to increase neutrophil production, a deficit that may contribute to the relatively high rate of neutropenia seen in severe neonatal infection. Neonatal granulocytes are inferior to adult cells in many functional capacities, including the ability to migrate to sites of inflammation, adhere to endothelial surfaces, and kill bacteria (Shigeoka et al., 1979; Anderson et al., 1981, 1985).

Although NK cells are of uncertain lineage, they may be detected in the fetal liver between 8 and 13 weeks' gestation (Uksila et al., 1983). The number of NK cells increases during gestation but remains lower than in adults, even at term (Berry et al., 1992). The cytolytic activity of NK cells, as measured by lysis of virally infected target cells, improves during gestation, the newborn period, and early childhood. At birth, neonatal NK cells have 15% to 65% of adult cytolytic activity (Lubens et al., 1982; Harrison and Waner, 1985). Adult levels are reached at approximately 5 years of age.

Many circulating components of the innate immune system are present by the middle of the second trimester. The fetal liver makes C2 and C4 as early as 8 weeks' gestation (Colten, 1976; Colten and Goldberger, 1979). Other complement proteins, including C1, C3, C5, C7, and C9, are detectable in fetal serum by 18 weeks' gestation, but the concentrations remain relatively low. It does not appear that maternal complement is transferred across the placenta. Serum levels of complement proteins increase during the third trimester, reaching approximately 50% of adult levels by term (Ballow et al., 1974). Complement levels gradually increase after birth, approaching adult levels by about 1 year of age. Complement activity is also decreased in neonates. At term, the hemolytic activity of complement is about 40% of adult levels for the classic pathway and 55% of adult levels for the alternative pathway (Johnston et al., 1979; Notarangelo et al., 1984).

Development of Adaptive Immunity

Cells destined to become B cells differentiate from hematopoietic precursors in the fetal liver by 8 weeks' gestation and the fetal bone marrow by 12 weeks' gestation. Mature plasma cells expressing IgM appear at 15 weeks' gestation, whereas those secreting IgG and IgA are present by 20 to 30 weeks' gestation. In the normal fetus, IgM is undetectable until the third trimester, when production is increased. In fact, only minimal levels of IgM and IgA are present at term, reaching 10% and 1% of adult levels, respectively (Stiehm and Fudenberg, 1966; Ballow et al., 1986). Neonatal levels of IgM can be increased in infants with intrauterine infections, indicating that the fetus is capable of an antibody response. Total cord IgM concentrations above 20 mg/dL suggest an intrauterine infection, and organism-specific IgM may be found. However, the ability of a neonate—and, presumably, of the fetus—to respond to antigens is limited. For example, the neonatal antibody response to bacterial polysaccharides is decreased, accounting in part for the neonate's susceptibility to certain bacterial infections (Baker et al., 1981).

In contrast to IgM or IgA, late third-trimester fetal and neonatal concentrations of IgG approach adult levels. This is primarily due to the transplacental passage of maternal IgG, the only isotype to cross the placenta. Maternal IgG can be detected in the fetus as early as 8 weeks' gestation, but the efficiency of transport is poor (Morell et al., 1986). Although active transport of maternal IgG increases throughout gestation, it is limited before the third trimester. For this reason, premature infants are not well protected by maternal antibodies and are at increased risk for infection during the first year of life. Even at term fetal–neonatal IgG production is limited, and IgG levels drop after birth. IgG levels do not reach adult titers until late childhood or early puberty. Some maternal infections (e.g., gram-negative pathogens, including *Escherichia coli* and *Salmonella*) initiate primarily an IgM antibody response. Because these antibodies do not cross the placenta, the fetus is not protected by maternal Ig.

The maturation of B lymphocytes into antibody-secreting plasma cells is regulated by the type of antigen, local factors, and other immune effector cells. For example, the production of Ig in response to many protein antigens requires antigen processing by macrophages, antigen recognition by helper T cells, and the stimulation of B cells by cytokines secreted from T cells. Antibodies can also be generated independently of T cells in response to other antigens, particularly large compounds, such as polysaccharides and lipopolysaccharides. This T-cell–independent B-cell response is the last to appear in the human neonate, in part accounting for the poor neonatal antibody response to certain bacterial antigens, such as the capsule of group B streptococci (Baker et al., 1981). The neonatal response to antigens requiring a T-cell response appears to be normal (Van Tol et al., 1983).

The unfortunate consequences of poor antibody production are seen in X-linked hypogammaglobulinemia, a disease of males characterized by the absence of B cells in the peripheral circulation, markedly low levels of IgG, and the absence of IgM and other classes of antibodies. Affected infants usually become ill with chronic bacterial infections as maternally acquired IgG declines below significant levels starting at 4 to 6 months of age.

T cells are also derived from the pluripotent hematopoietic cells first seen in the yolk sac. To differentiate into T cells, these cells must first migrate to the thymus, an organ whose sole function appears to be T-cell maturation and development. The fetal thymus is colonized with T-cell precursors by 8 weeks' gestation.

As T cells mature, they express several different adhesion molecules on their surface. The most immature intrathymic T cells are termed *stage I* thymocytes. They account for 10% of intrathymic cells and do not express the surface proteins CD3, CD4, or CD8. They are sometimes called "triple negative" cells (Haynes et al., 1989). *Stage II* thymocytes express both CD4 and CD8 but do not express the TcR-CD3 complex. These cells constitute 50% of the thymocyte population and can distinguish between self and foreign antigens. Most stage II thymocytes recognize self-antigens and are eliminated within the thymus (Schwartz, 1989). After maturation is completed, stage III thymocytes express either the CD4 or CD8 molecule as well as the TcR-CD3 complex. *Stage III* thymocytes make up the remaining 40% of the thymocyte population. By 12 to 16 weeks' gestation, the fetal thymus contains similar proportions of T cells in each stage of development as the adult (Lobach et al., 1985). In contrast to that in adults, the mass of the thymus relative to body weight is relatively large in late fetal life, infancy, and childhood, suggesting that the immune system is somehow triggered to greatly expand the T-cell pool over this period. The gland begins to involute around the onset of puberty.

T cells bearing the γδ TcR are the first to appear in the fetus, but their functional significance is unknown. They represent a very small proportion of all T cells in postnatal life. Most mature circulating T cells express the αβ heterodimer, which requires cross-linkage to the CD3 protein to be functional. Some circulating T cells in the neonate do not express CD3 and are probably immature T cells. The proportion of these immature cells is greater in premature infants, possibly contributing to their relative lack of T-cell immunity.

In the newborn, the total number of circulating T cells, as well as the proportions of CD4 and CD8 cells, is similar to those found in the adult (Griffiths-Chu et al., 1984; Solinger, 1985; Harris et al., 1992), and T helper cell function appears intact. Several aspects of neonatal T cells, however, are seemingly immature. For example, neonatal T cells make little IFN-γ in response to mitogen or antigen (Wilson et al., 1986). Furthermore, neonatal T cells have only about 50% of the cytotoxic activity of adult cells after sensitization (Granberg and Hirvonen, 1980). Studies of perinatally acquired neonatal viral infections show that the specific T-cell response is delayed compared with that of adults (Sullender et al., 1987), becoming normal after 2 months of age.

Interestingly, neonatal T suppressor cells can suppress the proliferative response of adult T cells (e.g., maternal T-cell proliferation) but not neonatal T-cell proliferation (Olding et al., 1977; Oldstone et al., 1977). This paradoxical characteristic of fetal suppressor T cells is present by 8 weeks' gestation (Unander and Olding, 1981) and may represent one way in which the conceptus is protected from a potentially harmful maternal immune response. Stimulated neonatal T cells also suppress adult B-cell Ig production (Oldstone et al., 1977).

The crucial role of the thymus to the development of a normal cellular immune system is evident in infants born with *DiGeorge syndrome*, a condition associated with aplasia or hypoplasia of the thymus. The embryologic lesion involves a failure of normal development of the thymus from the pharyngeal pouch. The condition is also associated with a failure of parathyroid gland development, also a pharyngeal pouch derivative, with temporally related developmental abnormalities of the philtrum of the lip, ears, and aortic arch. Immunologically, the infants have moderate to severe T-cell deficiency, resulting in lymphopenia, susceptibility to viruses, and a propensity to graft-versus-host reactions after blood transfusions. The most severe of the congenital immunodeficiency syndromes is known as *severe combined immunodeficiency* syndrome. This disease occurs as an X-linked recessive, an autosomal recessive, or a sporadic form and is characterized by an absence of B-cell and T-cell immunity. The etiologic mechanism is probably a failure of the differentiation of hematopoietic stem cells. Patients are susceptible to virtually any infection, viral or bacterial, and rarely live beyond the age of 1 year.

In summary, aspects of both the innate and adaptive immune responses of the normal neonate are more limited than in the adult. In the adaptive system, both T-cell and antibody responses are diminished. Neonatal protection by passively acquired maternal IgG is likely substantial but is imperfect. As a consequence of these limitations, the neonate, and particularly the premature neonate, is relatively susceptible to systemic bacterial and viral infections.

MATERNAL-FETAL IMMUNOLOGY

Many reproductive immunologists consider the conceptus to be a *semi-allograft*, because it bears antigens of both paternal and maternal origin. Much of what is known about maternal-fetal immunology comes from investigations designed to explain how the fetal and placental semi-allograft avoids immunologic attack by the mother. Such an approach is not surprising, given medicine's tendency to focus on immunology as it pertains to transplantation. As a result, reproductive immunologists have spent more than two decades trying to make maternal-fetal immunology fit the immunologic concepts and assumptions derived from studies of allograft acceptance and rejection.

A growing body of evidence, however, suggests that the immunologic relationship between the mother and conceptus does not easily fit into the allograft paradigm. Rather than being primarily destructive and thus requiring abrogation, the normal immunologic interactions between mother and fetal tissues may serve to promote the growth and development of the conceptus, a precept that makes far better teleologic sense. It seems unlikely that nature would engineer a complex alloimmune system primarily so that it would have to be overcome for the sake of reproduction (or manipulated when we learned to transplant tissues from the body of one individual into the body of another). Yet, pathologic alloimmune interactions between mother and conceptus may occur, and at least part of maternal-fetal immunology involves avoiding these potentially harmful events.

We next review the constituents of the immune system at the maternal-fetal interface, grouped as trophoblast antigens, cellular components, and soluble factors. Potential roles for these constituents in normal pregnancy and several adverse reproductive outcomes are discussed. Finally, we describe changes in the maternal immune system that occur during pregnancy.

Trophoblast Antigens

The primary fetal tissue in contact with the maternal immune system is the placenta (Fig. 7-5), prompting reproductive immunologists to search for alloantigens expressed on trophoblast. In humans, the placental villus is composed mainly of syncytiotrophoblast cells, with an underlying layer of villous cytotrophoblast and a mesenchymal core. The villi are bathed in circulating maternal blood and its constituent immune cells. Thus, syncytiotrophoblast represents the majority of conceptus tissue in contact with the maternal immune system. Extravillous cytotrophoblasts form columns of cells that invade into the maternal decidua. These cells usually replace the endothelium of spiral arteries in the decidua and myometrium during the first 18 weeks of gestation, forming another interface between fetal tissues and maternal immune cells.

Classic MHC antigens are highly polymorphic and, to a large degree, account for the "foreignness" of an allograft. As such, MHC expression in the placenta has been the focus of much investigation. Syncytiotrophoblast lacks both class I and class II antigens (Faulk and Temple, 1976; Sunderland et al., 1981; Bulmer and Johnson, 1985a; Hunt et al., 1988). Hence, most trophoblast in contact with maternal tissues lacks the determinants required for maternal T-cell activation or for destruction by cytotoxic T cells.

Extravillous cytotrophoblast also does not express class II MHC antigens (Bulmer and Johnson, 1985a). In contrast to syncytiotrophoblast, however, some populations of extravillous cytotrophoblast express common framework determinants of class I MHC antigens. These cells include cytotrophoblast of the anchoring columns, interstitial cytotrophoblast in the decidua and walls of the spiral arteries (Sunderland et al., 1981), and the cytotrophoblast of the chorion laeve (Redman et al., 1984). Although this cytotrophoblast is recognized by antibodies directed at monomorphic determinants of class I

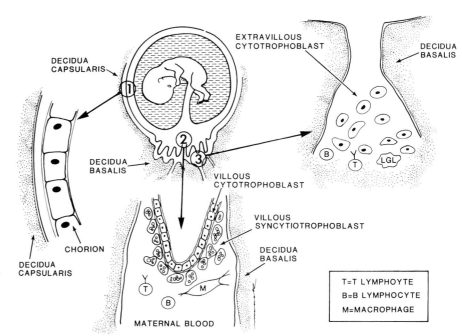

FIGURE 7-5 ■ Maternal-fetal interface in the hemochorial placenta. There are three interfaces, including syncytiotrophoblast-maternal blood, extravillous cytotrophoblast-maternal decidua, and chorion leave-decidua capsularis, where potential maternal-fetal immune interactions may occur. LGL, large granular lymphocyte. (From Heyborne KD, Silver RM: Immunology of postimplantation pregnancy. *In* Bronson RA, Alexander NJ, Anderson OJ, et al [eds]: Reproductive Immunology. Cambridge, Mass, Blackwell Scientific Publications, 1996, p. 383.)

MHC antigens, the cells are not reactive with antibodies directed against MHC class I polymorphic determinants (Hsi et al, 1984; Redman et al., 1984; Hunt et al., 1989). These findings indicate that the MHC antigens expressed by extravillous cytotrophoblast are partial or muted in some way (Redman et al., 1984; Ellis et al., 1986) and are qualitatively different from those expressed by other tissues. Elegant studies have determined that this molecule is HLA-G, a nonclassic class I (or class Ib) MHC antigen (Ellis et al., 1990; Kovats et al., 1990). The weight of HLA-G is about 39 kDa; the weight of classic MHC class I molecules is 45 kDa (Ellis et al., 1990). Like classic class I molecules, HLA-G is associated with β_2-microglobulin. It is expressed in few tissues, including the placenta and possibly the eye, liver, and lymphocytes (Shukla et al., 1990; Houlihan et al., 1992; Kirszenbaum et al., 1994). HLA-G polymorphism is uncommon, perhaps allowing cytotrophoblast cells to express MHC genes without engendering an immunologic response from the mother.

HLA-G expression is both temporally and spatially regulated. First-trimester extravillous cytotrophoblast has both HLA-G messenger RNA and protein (Hunt, Fishback et al., 1990; Yelavarthi et al., 1991); first-trimester syncytiotrophoblast and villous cytotrophoblast are positive for HLA-G messenger RNA but negative for HLA-G protein on an immunohistologic basis (Sunderland et al., 1981; Hunt, Fishback et al., 1990; Yelavarthi et al., 1991; Lata et al., 1992). In the term placenta, the expression of HLA-G in extravillous cytotrophoblast increases, whereas the presence of HLA-G messenger RNA in syncytiotrophoblast substantially decreases (Hunt et al., 1988; Yelavarthi et al., 1991). These data indicate that the expression of HLA-G (and other MHC molecules) is regulated at the transcriptional and immediate post-transcriptional and the translational levels. MHC gene regulation is complex and may involve *imprinting*, a phenomenon wherein maternal and paternal genes are differentially regulated.

It is possible that classic MHC class I molecules may be expressed in trophoblast under certain conditions. For example, MHC class I expression is upregulated in many tissues in the setting of inflammatory cytokines, such as IFN-γ and tumor necrosis factor (TNF)-α (Rosa et al., 1985; Collins et al., 1986). Indeed, class I molecules can be somewhat upregulated by IFN in dispersed cell cultures of cytotrophoblasts and some trophoblast cell lines (Zuckerman and Head, 1986; Feinman et al., 1987; Hunt, Atherton et al., 1990). However, class I antigens are generally not expressed in response to IFN-γ in explant cultures of placental villi and in murine *in vivo* studies (Hunt et al., 1987; Mattsson et al., 1989; Peyman and Hammond, 1992). These data suggest that cell–cell interactions may be important in resisting the induction of class I antigens by IFN-γ in trophoblast.

Given the strict temporal and tissue-specific regulation of class Ib MHC expression in trophoblast, it is likely that HLA-G has an important role in normal reproduction. One possibility is that HLA-G is involved in antigen presentation. Sanders and colleagues (1991) showed that CD8 receptors can bind HLA-G in a fashion similar to that in which CD8 receptors bind to classic MHC class I antigens. Also, HLA-G may actually interact with CD4 cells by forming a class II-like structure (Ishitani and Geraghty, 1992). Thus, HLA-G may serve to present foreign intracellular antigens to T cells.

HLA-G expression may also serve a protective role for trophoblast. HLA-G inhibits proliferation of $CD4^+$ T lymphocytes (Bainbridge et al., 2000) and decreases decidual cell production of TNF-α and IFN-γ (Kanai et al., 2001b). Addition of HLA-G, purified from the placenta, to mixed lymphocyte cultures causes a shift from a Th1 to Th2 phenotype by increasing production of IL-10 and decreasing production of TNF-α and IFN-γ (Kapsi et al., 2000). Cytotoxic activities of peripheral blood NK and cytotoxic T lymphocyte (CTL) cells and decidual large granular lymphocytes are also inhibited when the target cells express HLA-G (Sanders et al., 1991; Riteau et al., 2001; Rieger et al., 2002). HLA-G may interact with a variety of inhibitory receptors on decidual leukocytes to suppress NK-cell activity, including killer cell Ig-like receptors, Ig-like transcripts, and a heterodimer of CD94 and NKG2 (King et al., 2000b).

Six isoforms of HLA-G arise from differential splicing of the HLA-G gene, including two that are soluble. Soluble HLA-G is the product of a messenger RNA species with a premature stop codon that is secreted by trophoblasts and is present in amniotic fluid. Peripheral blood levels of soluble HLA-G are significantly higher in women during pregnancy than in nonpregnant control subjects (Hunt et al., 2000). Soluble HLA-G also inhibits alloproliferative responses in mixed lymphocyte cultures (Lila et al., 2001). In contrast to membrane-bound HLA-G, soluble HLA-G stimulates release of TNF-α and IFN-γ. This increase in Th1 cytokines is accompanied, however, by an increase in IL-10 (Kanai et al., 2001a) that may suppress the abortogenic effects of TNF-α and IFN-γ.

In addition to HLA-G, two other nonclassic MHC-I molecules, HLA-C and HLA-E, are expressed on placental cells. HLA-C is present on extravillous trophoblast of first-trimester placentas, upregulated by IFN-γ, and binds to killer inhibitory receptors present on some classes of NK cells (King et al., 2000a). HLA-E is also present on first trimester trophoblast (King, Allan et al., 2000) and interacts with CD94/NKG2 receptors on decidual NK cells to inhibit their cytotoxic activity (King, Allen et al., 2000; King et al., 2000b). Taken together, these observations suggest that nonclassic MHC class I molecules may play a role in suppressing T- and NK-cell activity against the placenta. Other proposed functions of trophoblast MHC antigens include binding of peptide hormones important to placental growth and development (Due et al., 1986) and regulation of trophoblast invasion (Loke et al., 1991).

Although these potential functions are intriguing, they must be considered in light of the successful reproduction of mice lacking functional MHC class I molecules secondary to gene targeting (Grusby et al., 1993). The lack of classic MHC class I and class II antigens may well be a primary mechanism by which the conceptus maintains immunologic inertness. A broader question is whether there are any alloantigens on the trophoblast, MHC or otherwise, that might be recognized by the mother and induce an alloimmune response. Several investigators have attempted to study trophoblast antigenicity by inducing antibody formation in animals after immunization with membrane preparations of human trophoblast. Although numerous monoclonal and polyclonal antibodies to human trophoblast surface antigens have been generated (Bulmer and Johnson, 1985a), none of the antibodies thus identified appears to be entirely trophoblast specific.

One antigen system identified in this fashion is the so-called trophoblast lymphocyte cross-reactive antigen system (McIntyre and Faulk, 1982; McIntyre et al., 1983). Trophoblast lymphocyte cross-reactive antibodies react with trophoblast as well as several other cells, and heterozygosity in trophoblast lymphocyte cross-reactive antigens had been proposed as a requirement for normal pregnancy (McIntyre et al., 1983). The trophoblast lymphocyte cross-reactive antigen is now known to be CD46, or membrane cofactor protein, a membrane-bound complement receptor (Purcell et al., 1990). This receptor binds C3b and C4b, allowing them to be inactivated by factor I. Thus, CD46 may prevent complement-mediated damage to trophoblast. The molecule is polymorphic but is expressed on numerous cell types and does not represent a specific trophoblast antigen.

Several other cell-surface proteins are expressed by trophoblast, some of which are polymorphic. In theory, these can lead to maternal immune recognition, although no data currently exist. Such proteins include placental alkaline phosphatase (Purcell et al., 1990), the transferrin receptor (Galbraith et al., 1980), and the Fc receptor used to transport IgG (Johnson and Brown, 1981). On the whole, trophoblast is remarkable for its lack of expression of antigens that might result in a harmful immune response.

Other cell-surface proteins present in trophoblast may play active roles in suppressing maternal immunity to the fetus. Fas ligand (also called Fas L or CD95L) is a protein belonging to the TNF family that induces apoptosis of T cells expressing the membrane receptor Fas (CD95). Interactions of these two surface proteins are important in the process of removing autoreactive T cells in the thymus. Fas L is expressed in murine placentas, especially in labyrinthine trophoblast and giant cells (Hunt et al., 1997). Placentas from mice that lack Fas L (the *gld* strain) have extensive leukocytic infiltrates and necrosis in the decidual–placental interface (Hunt et al., 1997). Fas L is also expressed on the surface of the placenta in human pregnancy (Runic et al., 1996; Bamberger et al., 1997), immunolocalizing to cytotrophoblast and syncytiotrophoblast of first-trimester and term placentas (Runic et al., 1996). Staining for Fas L is especially strong in the invasive interstitial trophoblast cells of first-trimester pregnancies (Hammer et al., 1999) and is colocalized with CD45+ cells (leukocytes) in the maternal decidua (Hammer et al., 1999; Kauma et al., 1999). There is evidence that Fas L induces apoptosis in these CD45+ cells in human placentas. Apoptosis is increased in activated lymphocytes cultured with human trophoblast. The apoptosis is partially abrogated when monoclonal antibody to Fas L is added to the culture (Kauma et al., 1999).

Cytotoxic T lymphocyte-associated antigen-4 (CTLA-4) is another cell-surface molecule that may prevent T-cell–mediated harm to gestational tissues. This molecule binds to CD80 and CD86 on activated antigen-presenting cells and functions to inactivate previously activated lymphocytes, thus controlling T-cell proliferation. Administration of a soluble form of CTLA-4, CTLA-Ig, enables long-term survival of xenografts (Lenschow et al., 1992) and has been actively investigated as a pharmaceutical to improve transplantation success. Placentas at all stages (trimesters) of gestation have significant staining for this molecule in the villous mesenchyme but not in trophoblast or endothelial cells (Kaufmann et al., 1999). The functional significance of this molecule in the placenta is uncertain, however, because CTLA –/– mouse embryos survive through pregnancy (Chambers et al., 1997).

Cellular Constituents

Four maternal immune effector cell populations are present in the luteal phase of the endometrium and decidua: (1) a unique population of cells, known as *large granular lymphocytes* (LGLs), (2) macrophages, (3) T lymphocytes, and (4) granulocytes.

Large Granular Lymphocytes

LGLs are characterized by abundant cytoplasm, eccentric nuclei, and large azurophilic granules (Bulmer et al., 1987). The numbers of LGL increase during the luteal phase, and by early pregnancy they constitute the largest population of immune cells in the decidua (Bulmer and Johnson, 1985b; Bulmer et al., 1987; Starkey et al., 1988). They are especially abundant in the decidua basalis and parietalis and around spiral arteries and invading trophoblasts (Zheng et al., 1991) and are quite proliferative (Kammerer et al., 1999). The cell-surface antigen phenotype of LGLs suggests a relationship to NK cells (Bulmer et al., 1987). LGLs typically express asialo-GM_1, CD45, and CD56 (NKH-1) antigens but do not have T-cell markers, such as CD3, CD4, and CD8. During early pregnancy the cells seem to take on an activated phenotype, as indicated by their high expression of CD69 and CD45RO (Kodama et al., 1998). A very small number of similar cells are present in the peripheral circulation. Numbers of decidual LGLs decrease during midpregnancy, and few are present in term gestational tissues.

The similarities of LGLs to NK cells has prompted speculation that LGLs might have cytotoxic activity, perhaps functioning to limit trophoblast invasion or to destroy infected or damaged cells. Indeed, decidual LGLs kill standard NK cell targets (e.g., tumor cells) (King et al., 1989), and their cytotoxic activity is enhanced by IL-2 (Redman et al., 1991). However, LGLs do not consistently lyse trophoblast *in vitro* (King et al., 1989). LGLs are capable of secreting immune mediators, such as IL-1, IL-2, TNF-α, and colony-stimulating factors (CSFs). In turn, these cytokines may influence the regulation of trophoblast growth and invasion.

Evidence from animal models suggests that the LGLs may facilitate placental development. Mice that are genetically deficient for uterine NK cells (Tgε26 strain), the murine equivalent of human decidual LGLs, have lower litter sizes and birth weights compared with wild-type mice; this effect can be reversed by grafting the Tgε26 mice with bone marrow from severe combined immunodeficient mice (Guimond et al., 1997, 1998, 1999). Placentas associated with fetal deaths in this strain of mice are very small and are characterized by arteriosclerosis that resembles what is observed in preeclampsia in humans (Guimond et al., 1997). It is likely that the uterine NK cells contribute to the growth of the placenta through their secretion of IFN-γ because mouse strains that lack IFN-γ or the α chain of the IFN-γ receptor have similar pregnancy outcomes as Tgε26 mice (Ashkar and Croy, 1999). Similarly, bone marrow grafts into uterine NK–cell–deficient mice are only able to restore the physiologic changes in placental vascularity when the donor cells are from IFN-γ competent mice (Ashkar et al., 2000).

Macrophages

Abundant macrophages are present in the luteal phase endometrium, but their numbers decline in the late secretory phase. During pregnancy, macrophages are widely distributed in the decidua and are concentrated in the portion of decidua underlying the point of trophoblastic invasion (Bulmer and Johnson, 1984). They are the predominant leukocyte in close proximity to cytotrophoblast.

Unlike LGLs, decidual macrophages persist as pregnancy advances. The function of decidual macrophages is unknown but might include antigen presentation to resident T cells or phagocytosis of bacteria or immune complexes. The ability of decidual macrophages to migrate, become activated, and kill bacteria is impaired in a murine model of *Listeria monocytogenes* infection (Redline and Lu, 1987). Decidual macrophage func-

tion appears to be inhibited by the substratum formed by decidual cells as opposed to an intrinsic quality of the macrophages (Redline et al., 1990). At term, some of the macrophages at the basal plate of the placenta are fetal in origin (Hofbauer cells). Their function is also uncertain, but they may act as phagocytic cells to remove debris at the maternal-fetal interface (Bulmer and Johnson, 1984). The antigen-processing capacity of these fetal macrophages is reduced compared with that of systemic monocytes (Chang et al., 1993).

The placenta is a rich source of Hofbauer cells that may play an important role in pregnancy maintenance and the survival of the fetal allograft. These cells are mitotic and contain many intracytoplasmic granules. They are present as early as day 18 post-conception and persist until term, accounting for 15% to 40% of villous cells (Goldstein et al., 1988; Yagel et al., 1990; Castellucci and Kaufmann, 2000).

Mice homozygous for the osteoporotic mutation lack the CSF gene and are macrophage deficient. Homozygotic females (op/op) are infertile when bred with op/op males but not when bred with +/op males (Pollard et al., 1991). The proliferation of placental macrophages depends on CSF production by villous stroma that binds to CSF receptors on placental macrophages (Boocock et al., 1992; Kanzaki et al., 1992; Jokhi et al., 1993). It has been shown that placental macrophage-conditioned medium stimulated the growth of cytotrophoblasts and their differentiation into syncytiotrophoblasts and regulate their secretion of human chorionic gonadotropin and human placental lactogen (Cervar et al., 1999; Khan et al., 2000). Placental macrophages do not produce human chorionic gonadotropin or human placental lactogen themselves. However, they produce IL-1, which increases human chorionic gonadotropin production by first-trimester trophoblasts (Yagel et al., 1989). The effects of macrophages on trophoblast proliferation and differentiation may be regulated by vasoendothelial growth factor and macrophage CSF, which stimulate cytotrophoblast cell proliferation and syncytiotrophoblast formation (Saito et al., 1993; Athanassiades et al., 1998). Both of these hormones are produced and secreted by placental macrophages *ex vivo* (Ahmed et al., 1995; Khan et al., 2000). Also, placental macrophages may have immunosuppressive effects in the placenta. They can suppress mixed lymphocyte reactions or mitogen-stimulated lymphocyte proliferation in a dose-dependent manner through the secretion of prostaglandin E_2 (Yagel et al., 1988). Other molecules produced by placental macrophages with immunosuppressive properties include Fas L (Zorzi et al., 1998), which can interact with Fas on activated T cells to induce apoptosis, and secretory HLA-G (Chu et al., 1998), which can inhibit T-cell proliferation and NK-cell activity.

T Lymphocytes

T lymphocytes with both αβ and γδ receptors are present in the decidua throughout pregnancy. αβ T cells, which can be divided into CD4+ and CD8+ subsets, may interact with class Ib antigens or with other antigen-presenting cells in the decidua to fight infection. There appears to be a greater number of CD8+ T cells than CD4+ T cells, especially in association with endometrial glands. These CD8+ cells have immunosuppressive activity (Nagarkatti and Clark, 1983; Thomas and Erickson, 1986).

Although data are conflicting, most carefully done studies suggest that the percentage of γδ T cells is enriched in early

(Mincherva-Nilsson et al., 1992) and late human (Ditzian-Kadanoff et al., 1993) and murine decidua (Heyborne et al., 1992). These cells are also present in the placental villi after 12 weeks of pregnancy but are absent by term (Bonney et al., 2000). Unlike αβ T cells, γδ T cells do not always require MHC restriction for cytotoxicity and may serve an antimicrobial function. They are typically enriched at mucosal sites and may play important roles in innate immunity through their NK-like activities.

The γδ T cells in the reproductive tract are phenotypically distinct in that they typically express the Vγ1 chain as opposed to the Vγ9 chain (Christmas et al., 1993; Hayakawa et al., 1996) normally expressed in γδ T cells in peripheral blood. In contrast, the proportion of Vγ9/δ2-positive T cells (relative to the Vγ1-positive cells) was increased in one population of women with recurrent spontaneous abortion compared with those with normal pregnancy outcomes (Barakonyi et al., 1999). A subpopulation of murine decidual γδ T cells has been shown to recognize a conserved mammalian trophoblast antigen (Heyborne et al., 1994). Thus, recognition of trophoblast by Vγ1-positive γδ T cells may be important for normal pregnancy outcome.

Granulocytes

B cells are not routinely found in gestational tissues. Although granulocytes are present in the decidua, little is known about their function.

Soluble Factors

Many of the complex immunologic cellular interactions that occur at the maternal-fetal interface are mediated by soluble factors. Most of these are cytokines, but prostaglandins, hormones, and Igs are other important soluble constituents of the immune system. In addition to immune effector cells, these molecules are produced by gestational tissues, such as decidua, trophoblast, and chorion.

Several considerations make it difficult to delineate the specific role of individual soluble factors. These molecules can exhibit autocrine, paracrine, and endocrine activity, affecting cells in adjacent and distant tissues. In addition, *in vivo* relationships are difficult to discern from *in vitro* studies, and the regulation of these factors is complex and intertwined. Also, many factors have numerous, diverse, and sometimes apparently opposite activities. Finally, many soluble factors have redundant effects, ensuring the function of the immune system but impairing our ability to dissect out the role of each individual molecule.

Despite these problems, advances in molecular biology have enhanced our ability to study these factors. For a detailed review of cytokine production in gestational tissues, the reader is referred to a review (Heyborne and Silver, 1996) and to Table 7-2. We now focus on the potential favorable and adverse effects of cytokines and other soluble factors during pregnancy (Fig. 7-6).

Immunodystrophism

Focus on the enigma of how the fetal "semi-allograft" avoids immunologic attack by the mother led investigators to assume that a maternal response to fetal antigens would be

TABLE 7-2. CYTOKINES AT THE MATERNAL–FETAL INTERFACE IN HUMAN PREGNANCY

Cytokine	Tissue	Possible Function
Interleukin-1	Placenta (macrophages)	Immunodystrophism
	Decidua (macrophages)	
	Amniotic fluid (third trimester)	
Tumor necrosis factor-α	Placenta	Immunodystrophism
	Uterus (decidual macrophages)	
	Amniotic fluid	
Interleukin-6	Placenta	Immunotrophism
	Decidua	Immunodystrophism
	Chorion	
	Amniotic fluid	
Interleukin-8	Decidua	Immunodystrophism
	Chorion	
	Amnion	
	Amniotic fluid	
Interleukin-10	Placenta	Immunosuppression
	Decidua	
	Amnion	
	Amniotic fluid	
Interleukin-12	Placenta	Immunotrophism
	Decidua	
Interleukin-13	Endometrium	Immunosuppression
	Placenta	
Interleukin-15	Endometrium	Immunotrophism
	Placenta	
	Decidua	
	Membranes	
Interleukin-2	Trophoblast	Immunodystrophism
	Amnio	
Interferon-γ	Placenta	Immunodystrophism
	Decidual glands	
Interferon-α	Placenta	Immunodystrophism
	Decidua (macrophages)	
Granulocyte CSF	Placenta	Immunotrophism
	Decidua (macrophages)	
Granulocyte-macrophage CSF	Placenta	Immunotrophism
Macrophage-CSF	Placenta	Immunotrophism
	Decidua	
	Amniotic fluid	
Transforming growth factor-β₁	Placenta	Immunosuppression
	Decidua	
	Fetal membranes	
Transforming growth factor-β₂	Decidua (CD3 leukocytes)	Immunosuppression

CSF, colony-stimulating factor.

harmful to the conceptus. This paradigm is known as immunodystrophism (Anderson et al., 1991). Recent data from mice with a disruption in the TATA binding protein gene support this concept (Hobbs et al., 2002). Over 90% of these mice die in mid-gestation from a placental defect. However, survival is increased if a wild-type placenta is supplied, the mice are reared in immunocompromised mothers,

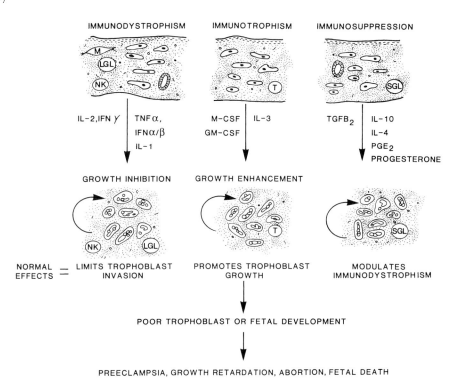

FIGURE 7-6 ■ Immunodystrophism, immunotrophism, and immunosuppression at the maternal-fetal interface. Soluble factors are produced by decidua and trophoblast, which affect trophoblast growth and development in a paracrine and autocrine fashion. GM-CSF, granulocyte-macrophage colony-stimulating factor; IL, interleukin; IFN, interferon; M-CSF, macrophage colony-stimulating factor; PGE, prostaglandin E; TGF, transforming growth factor; TNF, tumor necrosis factor. (From Heyborne KD, Silver RM: Immunology of postimplantation pregnancy. *In* Bronson RA, Alexander NJ, Anderson OJ, et al [eds]: Reproductive Immunology. Cambridge, Mass, Blackwell Scientific Publications, 1996, p. 383.)

or fetal/placental β_2-microglobulin was disrupted. These findings suggest that the TATA binding protein regulates a placental $\beta_2$microglobulin–dependent process that helps the placenta evade rejection by the maternal immune system (Hobbs et al., 2002).

Inhibitory effects of the immune system do not need to be deleterious to the fetus, however. For example, they may serve to limit the extent of trophoblast invasion during normal pregnancy. Histologic evaluation of ectopic pregnancies (Paterson and Grant, 1975; Steven and Morris, 1975) in which trophoblast is dramatically more invasive and destructive suggests that local factors in the decidua and/or endometrium inhibit trophoblast invasiveness. Too much inhibition may lead to poor trophoblast growth and development, resulting in pregnancy loss, fetal growth impairment, or preeclampsia.

TNF-α, IFN-γ, and IFN-α/β can inhibit *in vitro* rodent trophoblast cultures (Hunt, Atherton et al., 1990), and similar cytokines, including CSF, can restrict the growth of the human choriocarcinoma cell line, JEG-3 (Berkowitz et al., 1988). This restriction may be due to an inhibition of trophoblast cell DNA synthesis by the cytokines (Hunt et al., 1989). It is uncertain whether cytokines have direct toxicity against trophoblasts. Although one group demonstrated that trophoblast monolayers can be disrupted by TNF-α or IFN-γ (Yui et al., 1993), another found that TNF-α did not kill trophoblast cells *in vitro* (Drake and Head, 1990). Cytokines can also inhibit the proliferation of human endometrial cells (Tabizadeh et al., 1988) and can disrupt the embryonic development of preimplantation embryos (Hill et al., 1987). Hill and coworkers (1992) showed that supernatants taken from mononuclear cells from women with recurrent pregnancy loss and then cultured with either sperm or trophoblast antigens are toxic to both murine embryo development and

trophoblast growth. The exact nature of the embryotoxic factors is unknown, but it may be IFN-γ or TNF-α (Hill et al., 1995).

The systemic administration of IL-1 (Silen et al., 1989; Romero et al., 1991; Silver, 1996), IL-2 (Tezabwala et al., 1989; Chaouat et al., 1990; Lala et al., 1990), TNF-α (Silen et al., 1989; Chaouat et al., 1990; Silver et al., 1994), and IFN-γ (Chaouat et al., 1990) can all cause pregnancy loss in rodents. Although "physiologic levels" of these cytokines are present during normal pregnancy, harmful levels may be produced in certain pathologic conditions. For example, cytokine production increases in the setting of infection (Bone, 1991) and hypoxia (Benyo et al., 1997).

Potential *in vivo* sources for the production of these immunodystrophic cytokines include NK cells, T cells, and macrophages. NK cells produce IL-2 and IFN-γ, and increased numbers of decidual NK cells expressing the cell-surface marker asialo-GM$_1$ have been reported in a murine model of recurrent abortion (Gendron and Baines, 1988). Moreover, activation of NK cells can increase the rate of abortion in this model, whereas depleting NK cells decreases the rate of pregnancy loss (de Fougerolles and Baines, 1987). Although decidual NK cells and LGLs have cytotoxic activity against conventional NK-cell targets (Ferry et al., 1990), it is unclear whether these cells are capable of lysing trophoblast. Naive and IFN-activated NK cells do not have cytotoxic activity against trophoblast (Zuckerman and Head, 1988; Ferry et al., 1991), whereas studies of IL-2–activated NK cells yield mixed results (Johnson, 1989; King and Loke, 1990; Ferry et al., 1991).

Trophoblast appears to be resistant to cellular immune destruction by cytotoxic T lymphocytes (Zuckerman and Head, 1985, 1987; Clark and Chaouat, 1986) except under special conditions (Drake and Head, 1989). Macrophages can also produce immunodystrophic cytokines. Like NK cells and T cells, macrophages appear to be incapable of lysing trophoblast (Lu et al., 1989). No single immune effector cell population has been clearly shown to be responsible for immunodystrophism.

Immunosuppression

Several investigators have theorized that cytokines with immunosuppressive activity prevent the maternal immune system from destroying the implanting conceptus. Clark and McDermott (1978) reported the presence of suppressor cells in murine decidua that act to prevent the generation of cytotoxic T lymphocytes *in vitro*. The most important cells appear to be a decidual population of small granulated lymphocytes that lack T-cell– and NK-cell–surface markers (Clark et al., 1983). Similar cells have been found in human decidua (Daya et al., 1987). These cells release a soluble factor that can suppress the generation of cytotoxic T cells and the activation of NK cells by blocking the action of IL-2 (Clark et al., 1985, 1988; Daya et al., 1987). A deficiency of these cells has been associated with pregnancy loss in both mice and humans (Clark et al., 1990, 1991). This suppressive factor has many similarities to transforming growth factor (TGF)-β_2 and is considered to be a TGF-β_2–like molecule (Clark et al., 1990, 1991). The TGF-β family has well-known immunosuppressive properties (Rook et al., 1986; Tsunawaki et al., 1988).

An immunosuppressive factor is also elaborated by trophoblast. This factor can inhibit the proliferation of cytotoxic T cells and the lytic activity of NK cells (Chaouat and Kolb, 1984; Kolb et al., 1984; Menu et al., 1989). Supernatants from cultures of several human choriocarcinoma cell lines have similar activity, suppressing IL-2–dependent T-cell proliferation (Chaouat et al., 1991). This trophoblast product is inhibited by antibodies neutralizing TGF-β_2 and therefore may be a TGF-β_2–like molecule similar to the one described by Clark and colleagues. Similarly, a powerful immunosuppressive factor in amniotic fluid also has properties similar to those of TGF-β_2 (Altman et al., 1990). Interestingly, this TGF-β_2–like molecule can bind α-fetoprotein in amniotic fluid; perhaps this explains the immunosuppressive activity that has been attributed to α-fetoprotein (Tomasi, 1978; Van Oers et al., 1989).

Another cytokine with potent immunosuppressive activity is IL-10 (Moore et al., 1990, 1993). IL-10 is present in gestational tissues (Lin et al., 1993) and is capable of inhibiting the production of the potentially harmful cytokines IL-1, IFN-γ, and TNF-α (Mosmann and Moore, 1991). Thus, IL-10 may have an important immunosuppressive role at the maternal-fetal interface. IL-4 also has the potential to inhibit immune responses via the suppression of IL-2–induced lymphokine-activated killer cell formation (Swisher et al., 1990) and the inhibition of TNF-α and IFN-γ production by monocytes (Martinez et al., 1990).

In addition to cytokines, several other types of molecules appear to have immunosuppressive activity in gestational tissues. Prostaglandin E_2 is abundantly produced by gestational tissues and has a variety of immunosuppressive activities (Goodwin and Ceuppens, 1983). Decidual prostaglandin E_2 has been reported to inhibit the activity of murine decidual NK cells (Scodras et al., 1990) by downregulating IL-2 receptor expression and inhibiting IL-2 production by T cells (Lala

et al., 1988; Parhar et al., 1989). Data from *in vivo* experiments support an immunosuppressive role for prostaglandin E_2 in normal pregnancy. Pregnant mice treated early in gestation with indomethacin, an inhibitor of prostaglandin production, have an increased rate of pregnancy loss associated with elevated NK cell activity (Lala et al., 1990). In this model, inhibition of NK cells prevents fetal loss. Although these data are intriguing, successful pregnancies occur in most women who inadvertently take cyclooxygenase inhibitors during early pregnancy. Thus, it is uncertain that immunosuppression by prostaglandins is crucial to normal gestation.

Indoleamine 2,3-dioxygenase (IDO) is another soluble factor with immunosuppressive properties. IDO is produced by macrophages and other cells in response to IFN-γ and prevents the proliferation of local T-cell populations by catabolizing tryptophan, an essential amino acid for lymphocyte proliferation. Inhibition of this enzyme in mice with 1-methyl-tryptophan results in T-cell rejection and pregnancy loss in allogeneic, but not syngeneic, matings (Munn et al., 1998). These pregnancy losses are associated with a dense influx of mononuclear cells into the decidua and embryo. Allogeneic pregnancies of RAG –/– mice that lack mature T cells do not experience any pregnancy losses in response to IDO inhibition (Munn et al., 1998), confirming that the effect is mediated by lymphocytes. IDO is present in the decidua basalis of first trimester and villous endothelial cells of term placentas in humans (Sedlmayr et al., 2002). Thus, IDO may play a role in the maintenance of human allogeneic pregnancies. Indeed, one report noted decreased IDO in the placentas of pregnancies complicated by preeclampsia compared with those from normotensive control subjects (Santoso et al., 2002). The role of IDO in human recurrent pregnancy loss, however, has not been studied.

Steroid hormones may also play a role in immunosuppression at the maternal-fetal interface. Their role in the regulation of the immune system in general is complex and currently the subject of intense investigation. Progesterone has immunosuppressive effects on both cell- and humoral-mediated immunity (Stites and Siiteri, 1983; Ansar and Talal, 1990). Maternal T cells bear progesterone receptors, and T cells incubated with progesterone release an immunosuppressive factor (Szekeres-Bartho et al., 1985, 1986). This factor blocks some NK-cell activity (Chaouat et al., 1991). Many immunosuppressive effects of progesterone occur only at levels that are much higher than are present in maternal serum. However, such concentrations are found in gestational tissues (Stites and Siiteri, 1983), providing an attractive potential mechanism for immunotolerance of the fetus while maintaining systemic immunity.

Estrogen suppresses T-cell proliferation and delayed-type hypersensitivity (Ansar and Talal, 1990), although some investigators believe that it enhances antibody responses (Sthoeger et al., 1988). Free cortisol levels are slightly elevated in pregnancy, and glucocorticoids have a variety of well-known immunosuppressive effects. The steroid hormone 1,25-dihydroxyvitamin D, abundant in the placenta and decidua, also has immunosuppressive activities. This hormone can inhibit the T-cell production of IL-2, IFN-γ, and granulocyte-macrophage CSF (GM-CSF) (Tsoukas et al., 1984; Reichel et al., 1987; Tobler et al., 1988). Another hormone with immunosuppressive activity is human chorionic gonadotropin, which can inhibit the proliferation of cultured lymphocytes in response to mitogen (Ricketts and Jones, 1985).

Finally, there may be an immunologic role for the numerous pregnancy-specific proteins produced by the endometrium and early gestational tissues. Placental protein 14, also known as endometrial α_2-globulin, is believed to exert an important local immunosuppressive effect (Van Cong et al., 1991). Its expression is under the influence of progesterone, again implicating this steroid hormone in an immunologic role.

Pregnancy-specific glycoproteins are a major syncytiotrophoblast product with purported immunosuppressive function. Pregnancy-specific glycoproteins can inhibit cytokine production and mitogen-induced lymphocyte proliferation (Johannsen et al., 1976; Cerni et al., 1977). These molecules are members of the Ig supergene family and share extensive structural homology with known cell-adhesion molecules, thus suggesting a role in cell adhesion (Chou and Zilberstein, 1990).

Immunotrophism

Contrary to the tenets of immunodystrophism and immunosuppression, some studies suggest that a maternal immune response to fetal antigens may be beneficial to the conceptus and necessary for fetal survival. Instead of being harmful molecules that need to be suppressed, cytokines derived from maternal T cells may act as placental growth factors, leading to improved placental function and, ultimately, fetal survival. This concept has been named placental immunotrophism by Wegmann (1984).

Cytokines of the CSF family most likely relevant to immunotrophism include GM-CSF, macrophage CSF (also called CSF-1), and IL-3. These cytokines can stimulate the growth and phagocytic capacity of murine placental cells *in vitro* (Athanassakis et al., 1987; Armstrong and Chaouat, 1989). Although the exact cell population stimulated by these cytokines is uncertain, GM-CSF has its greatest effect on murine ectoplacental cone trophoblast early in gestation (Armstrong and Chaouat, 1989). This effect progressively lessens on placental cells taken from later in pregnancy. GM-CSF also has a trophic effect on preimplantation murine embryos (Robertson et al., 1991).

Macrophage CSF is particularly compelling because it is abundant in murine gestational tissues but is minimal in nonpregnant endometrium (Bartocci et al., 1986; Pollard et al., 1987; Arceci et al., 1989). In fact, the macrophage CSF concentration increases 1000-fold during pregnancy in the murine uterus. Intrauterine macrophage CSF is upregulated by estrogen and progesterone through synergistic action on uterine glandular epithelial cells (Pollard et al., 1987).

In vivo studies also support the immunotrophism hypothesis. Systemically administered CSFs have been shown to reduce pregnancy loss in murine models of spontaneous abortion. Abortion rates were reduced and placental and fetal weights increased after the administration of either GM-CSF or IL-3 in the CBA/J_DBA/2 model (Wegmann et al., 1989; Chaouat et al., 1990). Similarly, pregnancy outcome was improved after IL-3 administration in a murine model of antiphospholipid syndrome (Fishman et al., 1993).

The depletion of these cytokines can also have adverse effects on murine pregnancy. In some matings, the depletion of maternal T cells results in increased abortion rates and decreased fetal and placental weights (Chaouat et al., 1989;

Athanassakis et al., 1990). This may be due to a reduction of GM-CSF and IL-3, because T cells are the primary source of these cytokines.

These observations support a role for immunotrophism in normal pregnancy, and the concept is attractive. Most immunodeficient mice, however, either from naturally occurring mutations (e.g., mice with severe combined immunodeficiency) (Schultz and Sidman, 1987) or gene targeting (e.g., MHC "knockout" mice) (Grusby et al., 1993) normally can reproduce. Successful pregnancy in these mice does not exclude a beneficial effect of cytokines during normal pregnancy, but it raises the question about the relevance of any single experiment or observation and underscores the complexity of pregnancy immunology. Redundancy in the immune system makes it unlikely that any one cell type or single molecule is entirely responsible for successful reproduction.

Also, cytokines thought to be immunodystrophic may also have immunotrophic qualities. For example, IFN-γ, IL-1β, and TNF-α increase vasoendothelial growth factor expression (a vascular growth factor) in a first-trimester trophoblast cell line (Choi et al., 2002). This further illustrates the complexity of the system. Indeed, low levels of some soluble factors may be required for normal pregnancy, whereas elevated levels of the same factors may be harmful.

A maternal humoral response to fetal antigens has also been proposed as being helpful to the conceptus (Beer et al., 1981). In the most popular hypothesis, antifetal ("blocking") antibodies were thought to prevent a maternal antifetal cell-mediated immune response. In turn, the absence of blocking would result in spontaneous abortion (Beer et al., 1981). This concept formed the basis for the mixed lymphocyte reaction and the use of paternal leukocyte immunization in the evaluation and treatment of recurrent abortion.

Most data do not, however, support the clinical relevance of blocking antibodies for the following reasons:

1. Many women with normal pregnancies do not have blocking antibodies (Rocklin et al., 1982), whereas many women with unexplained recurrent abortion do (Sargent et al., 1988).
2. Mixed lymphocyte reaction inhibition appears to be nonspecific and may be due to factors other than antibodies (Duc et al., 1985).
3. Mice completely lacking Igs are able to successfully reproduce (Rodger, 1985).

Maternal humoral recognition of fetal antigens does occur in a substantial proportion of normal pregnancies. Antipaternal (antifetal) leukocytotoxic antibodies are found in 35% to 65% of multiparas and nearly 25% of primiparas (Berke and Johansen, 1974; Beard et al., 1983). These antibodies are primarily of the IgG isotype and are directed against paternal MHC antigens. Although once thought to be potentially harmful to the fetus, these antibodies cannot actually damage trophoblast (Billington and Davies, 1987), and they are present in many normal women (Berke and Johansen, 1974). Thus, most investigators do not believe that blocking, cytotoxic, or other alloantibodies are helpful, harmful, or necessary for human pregnancy (Coulam, 1992; Cowchock and Smith, 1992).

Another potentially beneficial effect of immune mediators is the temporal and spatial regulation of trophoblast growth. Cell–cell or cell–extracellular matrix interactions (Cunningham, 1991) are regulated by morphoregulatory molecules, known as cell-adhesion molecules; substrate adhesion; and cell junctional molecules. Morphoregulatory molecules, such as E-cadherin (Coutifaris et al., 1991), integrins (Damsky et al., 1992), and oncofetal fibronectin (Feinberg et al., 1991), are all important to normal placental growth and development. Cell adhesion is also crucial to many aspects of immune function (Dustin and Springer, 1991), and several morphoregulatory molecules participate in both immunologic and developmental processes (Hynes, 1987). Strong integrin expression has been demonstrated on LGLs (Burrows et al., 1993), but there are few other data regarding the interplay between morphoregulatory molecules and immune effector cells in the placenta.

The precise and unique regulation of cell–cell interactions in the placenta are reminiscent of cancer biology. In fact, the regulatory controls of cell–cell contact inhibition are temporarily inhibited during trophoblast invasion, prompting some authors to consider placental development a "pseudomalignant process" (Ohlsson et al., 1993). These investigators emphasize the role of growth factors and proto-oncogenes in placental growth and maturation. A variety of soluble factors and cell-surface molecules, including immune mediators, is now recognized as relevant to placental development.

Th1- and Th2-Type Cytokines

Mosmann and colleagues (1986) first described two mutually inhibitory types of murine T helper cells. T helper type 1 (Th1) cells secrete IL-2, IFN-γ, and lymphotoxin, whereas T helper type 2 (Th2) cells produce IL-4, IL-5, IL-6, and IL-10 (Mosmann and Moore, 1991). Th1 cytokines facilitate cell-mediated immunity and delayed-type hypersensitivity reactions. In contrast, cytokines produced by Th2 cells promote antibody-mediated responses and allergic reactions.

In general, Th1 cytokines are immunodystrophic and considered harmful to pregnancy. Because IL-10, a Th2 cytokine, can downregulate the production of Th1 cytokines, Wegmann and coworkers (1993) proposed that normal pregnancy is balanced in favor of Th2 cells. Indeed, cultures of murine placental and decidual cells constitutively produce Th2 cytokines (Lin et al., 1993). Moreover, the ratio of Th2 to Th1 cytokines is much greater in supernatants from cultured decidual cells compared with spleen cells. The notion of a Th2 bias during pregnancy is also consistent with clinical observations in humans. Disorders associated with autoantibodies may worsen during pregnancy, whereas cell-mediated autoimmune conditions (e.g., rheumatoid arthritis) often improve (Varner, 1991).

Recent evidence, however, suggests that this model may be overly simplistic. Knockout mice for IL-10 (Kuhn et al., 1993) and double knockout mice for IL-10 and IL-4 have normal pregnancies (Svensson et al., 2001). Additional Th1 and Th2 cytokines have been discovered since this model was first built. Studies on the expression of these more recently discovered cytokines at the maternal-fetal interface did not conform to a clear Th1 or Th2 pattern (Chaouat et al., 2002). Furthermore, the pro-inflammatory Th1 cytokine, IFN-γ, from uterine NK cells is important to placental development in mice and may be required to stimulate IDO production (see previous).

In summary, the immunologic relationship between mother and fetus is complex; much of it remains cloaked in mystery. Nonetheless, newer investigations and advances in molecular biology have dramatically enhanced our knowledge of the immunobiology of the maternal-fetal interface. The fetus likely benefits from mechanisms to protect the conceptus from attack by the maternal immune system. No doubt these mechanisms are multiple and complementary, including the complex regulation of MHC gene regulation in the placenta, HLA-G expression on extravillous cytotrophoblast, and the elaboration of soluble immunosuppressive factors, such as TGF-α. In pathologic conditions, such as infection, hypoxia, or perhaps some cases of recurrent miscarriage, immunodystrophic Th1 cytokines, such as IFN-γ and TNF-α, may harm the pregnancy. However, there is much more to maternal-fetal immunology than immunotolerance of the fetal allograft. Indeed, immunologic interactions between mother and fetus appear to be helpful and possibly necessary for fetal survival. Maternally produced cytokines may serve as placental growth factors, limit trophoblast invasion, and mediate tissue remodeling. Instead of conforming to traditional paradigms, it is now apparent that the maternal-fetal interface has evolved novel immune mechanisms that allow for the coexistence of host defense mechanisms and reproduction.

MATERNAL IMMUNE RESPONSE

Clinicians have long perceived that the maternal immune response is suppressed or altered during pregnancy. This belief is rooted in a need to explain maternal tolerance of the fetal allograft as well as in anecdotal clinical observations. Indeed, numerous reports indicate that pregnant women have increased susceptibility to a variety of infections. Impaired maternal immune responses have been reported after infection with hepatitis, influenza, varicella, variola, cytomegalovirus, polio, listerial and streptococcal organisms, gonorrhea, salmonella, leprosy, malaria, and coccidioidomycosis (Heyborne and Silver, 1996). In general, there appears to be a trend toward increased susceptibility to viral infections, consistent with suppressed cell-mediated immunity and a relative decrease in Th1 responses during pregnancy. However, most of these reports are uncontrolled case series. More recent carefully analyzed data do not indicate that maternal immunity is substantially impaired, and most pregnant women are able to adequately respond to most infectious diseases.

Although systemic immunity remains largely intact, local immunity appears to be altered in utero. Studies in both mice (Dudley et al., 1990) and humans (Fuchs et al., 1977) indicate differences between peripheral leukocytes and leukocytes associated with gestational tissues. In these studies, leukocytes in gestational tissues were less responsive than their systemic counterparts. Data from a murine model of infection with L. monocytogenes, a cause of serious in utero infections in humans, are consistent with these observations. L. monocytogenes is not cleared from the placenta despite a normal immune response against Listeria in the liver and spleen (Redline and Lu, 1987). Susceptibility to listerial infection in gestational tissues appears to be due to a local impairment of macrophage function (Redline et al., 1990).

TABLE 7-3. ALTERATIONS IN MATERNAL CELLULAR AND HUMORAL IMMUNITY DURING PREGNANCY

Immune System Component	Alteration with Pregnancy	Reference
B-cell numbers	No change	Sridama et al., 1982
		Dodson et al., 1977
T-cell numbers and subsets	No change	Siegel and Gleicher, 1981
		Moore et al., 1983
		Bardequez et al., 1991
		Coulam et al., 1983
		Lucivero et al., 1983
		Tallon et al., 1984
T-cell function	No change	Gill and Repetti, 1979
		Beer, 1988
	Decreased	Gehrz et al., 1981
		Petrucco et al., 1976
NK-cell function	Decreased	Vaquer et al., 1987
		Toder et al., 1984
IgG, IgM, IgA	No change	Margoulis et al., 1971
ADCC	No change	Gonik et al., 1987
Complement	No change	Kovar and Riches, 1988
		Johnson and Gustavii, 1987

ADCC, antibody-dependent cell-mediated cytotoxicity; Ig, immunoglobulin; NK; natural killer.

Many investigators have attempted to characterize the maternal immune response by determining immune-cell subsets, immune cell function, and circulating levels of soluble factors during pregnancy. In general, immune function is similar in pregnant and nonpregnant women (Table 7-3). Some, but not all, studies suggest that both T-cell and NK-cell function may be decreased during pregnancy. However, the maternal response to vaccines and the delayed-type hypersensitivity response remain intact (Murray et al., 1979; Jones et al., 1983). Also, pregnancy does not diminish transplantation rejection in animal models. Taken together, there is no clear trend toward either the suppression or enhancement of systemic immune function during pregnancy.

REFERENCES

Ahmed A, Li XF, Dunk C, et al: Colocalization of vascular endothelial growth factor and its FLT-1 receptor in human placenta. Growth Factors 12:235, 1995.

Altman DJ, Schneider SS, Thompson DA, et al: A transforming growth factor β2 (TGF-β2)-like immunosuppressive factor in amniotic fluid and localization of TGF-β2 mRNA in the pregnant uterus. J Exp Med 172:1391, 1990.

Anderson DC, Freeman KB, Hughes BJ, et al: Secretory determinants of impaired adherence and motility of neonatal PMNs. Pediatr Res 19:257A, 1985.

Anderson DC, Hughes BJ, Smith CW: Abnormal mobility of neonatal polymorphonuclear leukocytes. J Clin Invest 68:863, 1981.

Anderson DJ, Hill JA, Haimovici F, et al: Adverse effects of immune cell products in pregnancy. In Wegmann TF, Gill TJ, Nisbet-Brown E (eds): Molecular and Cellular Immunobiology of the Maternal-Fetal Interface. New York, Oxford University Press, 1991, p. 207.

Ansar AS, Talal N: Sex hormones and the immune system. Part 2. Animal data. Ballieres Clin Rheumatol 4:13, 1990.

Arceci RJ, Shanahan F, Stanley ER, et al: Temporal expression and location of colony stimulating factor-1 (CSF-1) and its receptor in the female reproductive tract are consistent with CSF-1 regulated placental development. Proc Natl Acad Sci USA 86:8818, 1989.

Armstrong DT, Chaouat G: Effects of lymphokines and immune complexes on murine placental cell growth in vitro. Biol Reprod 40:466, 1989.

Ashkar AA, Croy BA: Interferon-γ contributes to the normalcy of murine pregnancy. Biol Reprod 61:493, 1999.

Ashkar AA, Di Santo JP, Croy BA: Interferon gamma contributes to initiation of uterine vasculature modification, decidual integrity and uterine natural killer cell maturation during normal murine pregnancy. J Exp Med 192:259, 2000.

Athanassakis I, Bleackley PC, Paetkau V, et al: The immunostimulatory effect of T cells and T cell lymphokines on murine fetally derived placental cells. J Immunol 138:37, 1987.

Athanassakis I, Chaouat G, Wegmann TG: The effects of anti-CD4 and anti-CD8 antibody treatment on placental growth and function in allogeneic and syngeneic murine pregnancy. Cell Immunol 129:13, 1990.

Athanassiades A, Hamilton GS, Lala PK: Vascular endothelial growth factor stimulates proliferation but not migration or invasiveness in human extravillous trophoblast. Biol Reprod 59:643, 1998.

Bainbridge DRJ, Ellis SA, Sargent IL: HLA-G suppresses proliferation of CD4+ T-lymphocytes. J Reprod Immunol 48:17, 2000.

Baker CJ, Edwards MS, Kasper DL: Role of antibody to native type III polysaccharide group B streptococcus in infant infection. Pediatrics 68:544, 1981.

Ballow M, Cates KL, Rowe JC, et al: Development of the immune system in very low birth weight (less than 1500 g) premature infants: Concentrations of plasma immunoglobulins and patterns of infections. Pediatr Res 20:899, 1986.

Ballow M, Fung F, Good RA, et al: Developmental aspects of complement components in the newborn. Clin Exp Immunol 18:257, 1974.

Bamberger AM, Schulte HM, Thuneke I, et al: Expression of the apoptosis inducing Fas ligand (FasL) in human first and third trimester placenta and choriocarcinoma cells. J Clin Endocrinol Metab 82:3173, 1997.

Barakonyi A, Polgar B, Szekeres-Bartho J: The role of gamma/delta T-cell receptor-positive cells in pregnancy. Part II. Am J Reprod Immunol 42:83, 1999.

Bardequez AD, McNerney R, Frieri M, et al: Cellular immunity in preeclampsia: Alterations in T-lymphocyte subpopulations during early pregnancy. Obstet Gynecol 77:859, 1991.

Bartocci A, Pollard JW, Stanley ER: Regulation of colony stimulating factor-1 during pregnancy. J Exp Med 164:956, 1986.

Beard RW, Braude P, Mowbray JF, et al: Protective antibodies and spontaneous abortion. Lancet 2:1990, 1983.

Beelen RHJ, van Rees EP, Bos HJ, et al: Ontogeny of antigen-presenting cells. In Chaouat G (ed): The Immunology of the Fetus. Boca Raton, FL, CRC Press, 1990.

Beer A: Immunology of reproduction. In Samter M, Talmage DW, Frank MM, et al (eds): Immunological Diseases. Boston, Little, Brown & Co, 1988, p. 329.

Beer AE, Quebbeman JF, Ayers JWI, et al: Major histocompatibility complex antigens, maternal and fetal immune responses and chronic habitual abortion in humans. Am J Obstet Gynecol 141:987, 1981.

Benyo DF, Miles TM, Conrad KP: Hypoxia stimulates cytokine production by villous explants from the human placenta. J Clin Endocrinol Metab 82:1582, 1997.

Berke J, Johansen K: The formation of HLA antibodies in pregnancy: The antigenicity of aborted and term fetuses. J Obstet Gynaecol Br Commonw 81:222, 1974.

Berkowitz RS, Hill JA, Kurtz CB, et al: Effects of products of activated leukocytes (lymphokines and monokines) on the growth of malignant trophoblast cell in vitro. Am J Obstet Gynecol 158:199, 1988.

Berry SM, Fine N, Bichalski JA, et al: Circulating lymphocyte subsets in second and third trimester fetuses: Comparison with newborns and adults. Am J Obstet Gynecol 167:895, 1992.

Billington WD, Davies M: Maternal antibody to placental syncytiotrophoblast during pregnancy. In Wegmann TG, Gill TJ (eds): Immunology of Reproduction. New York, Oxford University Press, 1987.

Bone R: The pathogenesis of sepsis. Ann Intern Med 115:457, 1991.

Bonney EA, Pudney J, Anderson DJ, et al: Gamma-delta T cells in midgestation human placental villi. Gynecol Obstet Invest 50:153, 2000.

Boocock CA, Hayes M, Chang MY, et al: Isolation and characterization of four CSF-1-dependent placental macrophage cell lines. J Leukoc Biol 51:532, 1992.

Bulmer JN, Johnson PM: Macrophage populations in the human placenta and amniochorion. Clin Exp Immunol 57:393, 1984.

Bulmer JN, Johnson PM: Antigen expression by trophoblast populations in the human placenta and their possible immunobiological relevance. Placenta 6:127, 1985a.

Bulmer JN, Johnson PM: Immunohistological characterisation of the decidual leukocytic infiltrate related to endometrial gland epithelium in early human pregnancy. J Reprod Immunol **7**:364, 1985b.

Bulmer JN, Johnson PM, Bulmer D: Leukocyte populations in human decidua and endometrium. *In* Gill TJ, Wegmann TG, Nisbet-Brown E (eds): Immunoregulation and Fetal Survival. New York, Oxford University Press, 1987.

Burrows TD, King A, Loke YW: Expression of adhesion molecules by human decidual large granular lymphocytes. Cell Immunol **147**:81, 1993.

Castellucci M, Kaufmann P: Basic structure of the villous trees. *In* Benirschke K, Kaufmann P (eds): Pathology of the Human Placenta. Springer, New York, 2000.

Cerni C, Tatra G, Bohn H: Immunosuppression by human placental lactogen (HPL) and the pregnancy specific B_1-glycoprotein (SP_1). Arch Gynecol **223**:1, 1977.

Cervar M, Blaschitz A, Dohr G, et al: Paracrine regulation of distinct trophoblast functions in vitro by placental macrophages. Cell Tissue Res **295**:297, 1999.

Chambers CA, Cado D, Truong T, et al: Thymocyte development is normal in CTLA-4 deficient mice. Proc Natl Acad Sci USA **94**:9296, 1997.

Chang MY, Pollard JW, Khalili H, et al: Mouse placental macrophages have a decreased ability to present antigen. Proc Natl Acad Sci USA **90**:462, 1993.

Chaouat G, Kolb JP: Immunoactive products of murine placenta. II. Afferent suppression of maternal cell mediated immunity by supernatants from short term enriched cultures of murine trophoblast enriched maternal cell populations. Ann Immunol (Institut Pasteur) **135C**:205, 1984.

Chaouat G, Menu E, Athanassakis I, et al: Maternal T cells regulate placental size and fetal survival. Reg Immunol **1**:143, 1989.

Chaouat G, Menu E, Clark DA, et al: Control of fetal survival in CBA_DBA/2 mice by lymphokine therapy. J Reprod Fertil **89**:447, 1990.

Chaouat G, Menu E, Szekeres-Bartho J, et al: Immunological and endocrinological factors that contribute to successful pregnancy. *In* Wegmann TG, Gill TJ, Nisbet-Brown E (eds): Molecular and Cellular Immunobiology of the Maternal-Fetal Interface. New York, Oxford University Press, 1991, p. 277.

Chaouat G, Zourbas S, Ostojic S, et al: A brief review of recent data on some cytokine expressions at the materno-foetal interface which might challenge the classical Th1/Th2 dichotomy. J Reprod Immunol **53**:241, 2002.

Choi SJ, Park JY, Lee YK, et al: Effects of cytokines on VEGF expression and secretion by human first trimester trophoblast cell line. Am J Reprod Immunol **48**:70, 2002.

Chou JY, Zilberstein M: Expression of the pregnancy specific β1 glycoprotein gene in cultured human trophoblasts. Endocrinology **127**:2127, 1990.

Christmas SE, Brew R, Deniz G, et al: T-cell receptor heterogeneity of γδ T-cell clones from human female reproductive tissues. Immunology **78**:436, 1993.

Chu W, Fant ME, Geraghty DE, et al: Soluble HLA-G in human placentas: Synthesis in trophoblasts and interferon-gamma-activated macrophages but not placental fibroblasts. Hum Immunol **59**:435, 1998.

Clark DA, Chaouat G: Characterization of the cellular basis for the inhibition of cytotoxic effector cells by the murine placenta. Cell Immunol **102**:43, 1986.

Clark DA, Chaput A, Walker C, et al: Active suppression of host-vs-graft reaction in pregnant mice. VI. Soluble suppressor activity obtained from decidua blocks the response to IL-2. J Immunol **134**:1659, 1985.

Clark DA, Falbo M, Rowley RB, et al: Active suppression of host-vs-graft reaction in pregnant mice. IX. Soluble suppressor activity obtained from allopregnant mouse decidua that blocks the response to interleukin 2 is related to TGF-α. J Immunol **141**:3833, 1988.

Clark DA, Flanders KC, Banwatt D, et al: Murine pregnancy decidua produces a unique immunosuppressive molecule related to transforming growth factor β2. J Immunol **144**:3008, 1990.

Clark DA, Lea RG, Rowley B, et al: Transforming growth factor-β related suppressor factor in mammalian pregnancy decidua: Homologies between the mouse and human in successful pregnancy and recurrent spontaneous abortion. *In* Chaouat G (ed): Maternofetal Relationship: Molecular and Cellular Biology. Proceedings INSERM Colloque, John Libbey Eurotext, Paris, **212**:171, 1991.

Clark DA, McDermott MR: Active suppression of host-vs-graft reaction in pregnant mice. I. Suppression of cytotoxic T cell generation in lymph nodes draining the uterus. J Immunol **121**:1389, 1978.

Clark DA, Slapsys RM, Croy BA, et al: Suppressor cell activity in uterine decidua correlates with success or failure of murine pregnancies. J Immunol **131**:540, 1983.

Collins T, LaPierre LA, Fiers W, et al: Recombinant human tumor necrosis factor increases mRNA levels and surface expression of HLA-A, B antigens in vascular endothelial cells and dermal fibroblasts in vitro. Proc Natl Acad Sci USA **83**:446, 1986.

Colten HR: Biosynthesis of complement. Adv Immunol **22**:67, 1976.

Colten HR, Goldberger G: Ontogeny of serum complement proteins. Pediatrics **64**:775, 1979.

Coulam C, Silverfield J, Kazmar RE, et al: T lymphocyte subsets during pregnancy and the menstrual cycle. Am J Reprod Immunol **4**:88, 1983.

Coulam CB: Immunologic tests in the evaluation of reproductive disorders: A critical review. Am J Obstet Gynecol **167**:1844, 1992.

Coutifaris C, Kao L, Sehdev HM, et al: E-cadherin expression during the differentiation of human trophoblasts. Development **113**:767, 1991.

Cowchock FS, Smith JB: Predictors for live birth after unexplained spontaneous abortions: Correlations between immunologic test results, obstetric histories, and outcome of next pregnancy without treatment. Am J Obstet Gynecol **167**:1208, 1992.

Cunningham BA: Cell adhesion molecules and the regulation of development. Am J Obstet Gynecol **164**:939, 1991.

Damsky CH, Fitzgerald ML, Fisher SJ: Distribution patterns of extracellular matrix components and adhesion receptors are intricately modulated during first trimester cytotrophoblast differentiation along the invasive pathway, in vivo. J Clin Invest **89**:210, 1992.

Daya S, Rosenthal KL, Clark DA: Immunosuppressor factor(s) produced by decidua-associated suppresor cells: A proposed mechanism for fetal allograft survival. Am J Obstet Gynecol **156**:344, 1987.

de Fougerolles AR, Baines MG: Modulation of the natural killer cell activity in pregnant mice alters the spontaneous abortion rate. J Reprod Immunol **11**:147, 1987.

Ditzian-Kadanoff R, Garon J, Verp MS, et al: γδ T cells in human decidua. Am J Obstet Gynecol **168**:831, 1993.

Dodson MG, Kerman RH, Lange CF, et al: T and B cells in pregnancy. Obstet Gynecol **49**:299, 1977.

Drake BL, Head JR: Murine trophoblast can be killed by allospecific cytotoxic T lymphocytes generated in GIBCO Opti-MEM medium. J Reprod Immunol **15**:71, 1989.

Drake BL, Head JR: Murine trophoblast cells are not killed by tumor necrosis factor-α. J Reprod Immunol **17**:93, 1990.

Duc HT, Masse A, Bobe P, et al: Deviation of humoral and cellular alloimmune reactions by placental extracts. J Reprod Immunol **7**:27, 1985.

Dudley DJ, Mitchell MD, Creighton K, et al: Lymphokine production during term human pregnancy: Differences between peripheral leukocytes and decidual cells. Am J Obstet Gynecol **163**:1890, 1990.

Due C, Simonsen M, Olsen L: The major histocompatibility complex class I heavy chain as a structural subunit of the human cell membrane insulin receptor: Implications for a range of biological functions of histocompatibility antigens. Proc Natl Acad Sci USA **83**:6007, 1986.

Dustin ML, Springer TA: Role of lymphocyte adhesion receptors in transient interactions and cell locomotion. Annu Rev Immunol **9**:27, 1991.

Ellis SA, Palmer MS, McMichael AJ: Human trophoblast and the choriocarcinoma cell line BeWo express a truncated HLA class I molecule. J Immunol **144**:731, 1990.

Ellis SA, Sargent IL, Redman CWG, et al: Evidence for a novel HLA antigen on human extravillous cytotrophoblast and a choriocarcinoma cell line. Immunology **59**:595, 1986.

Faulk WP, Temple A: Distribution and beta-2 microglobulin and HLA in chorionic villi of human placenta. Nature (London) **262**:799, 1976.

Fauser AA, Messner HA: Granuloerythropoietic colonies in human bone marrow, peripheral blood and cord blood. Blood **52**:1243, 1978.

Fauser AA, Messner HA: Identification of megakaryocytes, macrophages and eosinophils in colonies of human bone marrow containing neutrophilic granulocytes and erythroblasts. Blood **53**:1023, 1979.

Feinberg RF, Kliman HJ, Lockwood CJ: Is oncofetal fibronectin a trophoblast glue for human implantation? Am J Pathol **138**:537, 1991.

Feinman MA, Kliman HJ, Main EK: HLA antigen expression and induction by γ-interferon in cultured human trophoblasts. Am J Obstet Gynecol **157**:1429, 1987.

Ferry BL, Sargent IL, Starkey PM, et al: Cytotoxic activity, against trophoblast and choriocarcinoma cells, of large granular lymphocytes from human early pregnancy decidua. Cell Immunol **132**:140, 1991.

Ferry BL, Starkey PM, Sargent IL, et al: Cell populations in the human early pregnancy decidua: Natural killer cell activity and response to interleukin-2 of CD56-positive large granular lymphocytes. Immunology **70**:446, 1990.

Fishman P, Falach-Vaknine E, Zigelman R, et al: Prevention of fetal loss in experimental antiphospholipid syndrome by in vivo administration of recombinant interleukin-3. J Clin Invest **91**:1834, 1993.

Forestier F, Daffos F, Galacteros F, et al: Hematological values of 163 normal fetuses between 18 and 30 weeks of gestation. Pediatr Res **20**:342, 1986.

Fuchs T, Hammarstrom L, Smith E, et al: *In vivo* suppression of uterine lymphocytes during early pregnancy. Acta Obstet Gynaecol Scand **56**:151, 1977.

Galbraith GMP, Galbraith RM, Faulk WP: Immunological studies of transferrin and transferrin receptors on human placental trophoblast. Placenta **1**:33, 1980.

Gehrz RC, Christianson WR, Linner KM: A longitudinal analysis of lymphocyte proliferative responses to mitogens and antigens during human pregnancy. Am J Obstet Gynecol **140**:665, 1981.

Gendron RL, Baines MG: Infiltrating decidual natural killer cells are associated with spontaneous abortion in mice. Cell Immunol **113**:261, 1988.

Gill TJ III, Repetti CF: Immunological and genetic factors influencing reproduction. Am J Pathol **95**:463, 1979.

Goldstein J, Braverman M, Salafia C, et al: The phenotype of human placental macrophages and its variation with gestational age. Am J Pathol **133**:648, 1988.

Gonik B, Loo LS, West S, et al: Natural killer cytotoxicity and antibody-dependent cellular cytotoxicity to herpes simplex virus-infected cells in human pregnancy. Am J Reprod Immunol Microbiol **13**:23, 1987.

Goodwin J, Ceuppens J: Special article: Regulation of the immune response by prostaglandins. J Clin Immunol **3**:295, 1983.

Granberg C, Hirvonen T: Cell-mediated lympholysis by fetal and neonatal lymphocytes in sheep and man. Cell Immunol **51**:13, 1980.

Griffiths-Chu S, Patterson JAK, Berger CL, et al: Characterization of immature T cell subpopulations in neonatal blood. Blood **64**:296, 1984.

Grusby MJ, Auchincloss H, Lee R, et al: Mice lacking major histocompatibility complex class I and class II molecules. Proc Natl Acad Sci USA **90**:3913, 1993.

Guimond M, Wang B, Croy BA: Immune competence involving the natural killer cell lineage promotes placental growth. Placenta **20**:441, 1999.

Guimond MJ, Luross JA, Wang B, et al: Absence of natural killer cells during murine pregnancy is associated with reproductive compromise in Tgε26 mice. Biol Reprod **56**:169, 1997.

Guimond MJ, Wang B, Croy BA: Engraftment of bone marrow from severe combined immunodeficient (SCID) mice reverses the reproductive deficits in natural killer cell–deficient tgε26 mice. J Exp Med **187**:217, 1998.

Hammer A, Blaschitz A, Daxbock C, et al: Fas and Fas-ligand are expressed in the uteroplacental unit of first-trimester pregnancy. Am J Reprod Immunol **41**:41, 1999.

Hansen TH, Sachs DH: The major histocompatibility complex. *In* Paul WE (ed): Fundamental Immunology. New York, Raven Press, 1989, p. 445.

Harris DT, Schumacher MJ, Locasio J, et al: Phenotypic and functional immaturity of human umbilical cord blood T lymphocytes. Proc Natl Acad Sci USA **89**:10,006, 1992.

Harrison CJ, Waner JL: Natural killer cell activity in infants and children excreting cytomegalovirus. J Infect Dis **151**:301, 1985.

Hayakawa S, Shiraishi H, Saitoh S, et al: Decidua as a site of extrathymic Vg1 T-cell differentiation. Am J Reprod Immunol **35**:233, 1996.

Haynes BF, Denning SM, Singer KH, et al: Ontogeny of T cell precursors: A model for the initial stages of human T-cell development. Immunol Today **10**:87, 1989.

Henneke P, Golenbock DT: Innate immune recognition of lipopolysaccharide by endothelial cells. Crit Care Med **30**:S207, 2002.

Heyborne KD, Cranfill RL, Carding SR, et al: Characterization of γδ T lymphocytes at the maternal-fetal interface. J Immunol **149**:2872, 1992.

Heyborne KD, Fu YX, Nelson A, et al: Recognition of trophoblasts by γδ T cells. J Immunol **153**:2918, 1994.

Heyborne KD, Silver RM: Immunology of postimplantation pregnancy. *In* Bronson RA, Alexander NJ, Anderson OJ, et al (eds): Reproductive Immunology. Cambridge, MA, Blackwell Scientific Publications, 1996, p. 383.

Hill JA, Haimovici F, Anderson DJ: Products of activated lymphocytes and macrophages inhibit mouse embryo development in vitro. J Immunol **139**:2250, 1987.

Hill JA, Polgar K, Anderson DJ: T-helper 1-type immunity to trophoblast in women with recurrent spontaneous abortion. JAMA **273**:1933, 1995.

Hill JA, Polgar K, Harlow BL, et al: Evidence of embryo and trophoblast toxic cellular immune response(s) in women with recurrent spontaneous abortion. Am J Obstet Gynecol **166**:1044, 1992.

Hobbs NK, Bondavera AA, Barnett S, et al: Removing the vertebrate-specific TBP N terminus disrupts placental β2m-dependent interactions with the maternal immune system. Cell **110**:43, 2002.

Holbrook KA: Structural and biochemical organogenesis of skin and cutaneous appendages in the fetus and neonate. *In* Polin RA, Fox WW (eds): Fetal and Neonatal Physiology. Philadelphia, WB Saunders, 1992, p. 527.

Houlihan JM, Biro PA, Fergar-Payne A, et al: Evidence for the expression of non-HLA-A, -B, -C class I genes in the human fetal liver. J Immunol **149**:668, 1992.

Hsi BL, Yeh CJG, Faulk WP: Class I antigens of the major histocompatibility complex on cytotrophoblasts of human chorion laeve. Immunology **52**:621, 1984.

Hunt JS, Andrews GK, Wood GW: Normal trophoblasts resist induction of class I HLA. J Immunol **138**:2481, 1987.

Hunt JS, Atherton RA, Pace JL: Differential responses of rat trophoblast cells and embryonic fibroblasts to cytokines that regulate proliferation and class I MHC antigen expression. J Immunol **145**:184, 1990.

Hunt JS, Fishback JL, Andrews GK, et al: Expression of class I HLA genes by trophoblast cells: Analysis by in situ hybridization. J Immunol **140**:1293, 1988.

Hunt JS, Fishback JL, Chumbley G, et al: Identification of class I MHC mRNA in human first trimester trophoblast cells by in situ hybridization. J Immunol **144**:4420, 1990.

Hunt JS, Jadhav L, Chu W, et al: Soluble HLA-G circulates in maternal blood during pregnancy. Am J Obstet Gynecol **183**:682, 2000.

Hunt JS, Lessin D, King CR: Ontogeny and distribution of cells expressing HLA-B locus-specific determinants in the placenta and extraplacental membranes. J Reprod Immunol **15**:21, 1989.

Hunt JS, Vassmer D, Ferguson TA, et al: Fas ligand is positioned in mouse uterus and placenta to prevent trafficking of activated leukocytes between the mother and the conceptus. J Immunol **158**:4122, 1997.

Hynes RO: Integrins: A family of cell surface receptors. Cell **48**:549, 1987.

Ishitani A, Geraghty DE: Alternative splicing of HLA-G transcripts yields proteins with primary structures resembling both class I and class II antigens. Proc Natl Acad Sci USA **89**:3947, 1992.

Johannsen R, Haupt H, Bohn H, et al: Inhibition of the mixed leukocyte culture (MLC) by proteins: Mechanism and specificity of the reaction. Z Immun Forsch Exp Ther **152**:280, 1976.

Johnson PM: Immunological intercourse at the feto-maternal interface. Immunol Today **10**:215, 1989.

Johnson PM, Brown PJ: Fcγ receptors in the human placenta. Placenta **2**:355, 1981.

Johnson U, Gustavii B: Complement components in normal pregnancy. Acta Pathol Microbiol Immunol Scand **95**:97, 1987.

Johnston RB, Altenburger KM, Atkinson AW, et al: Complement in the newborn infant. Pediatrics **645**:781, 1979.

Jokhi PP, Chumbley G, King A, et al: Expression of the colony stimulating factor-1 receptor (c-fms product) by cells at the human uteroplacental interface. Lab Invest **68**:308, 1993.

Jones WR, Hawes CS, Kemp AS: Studies on cell-mediated immunity in human pregnancy. *In* Wegmann TG, Gill TJ (eds): Immunology of Reproduction. New York, Oxford University Press, 1983, p. 363.

Kammerer U, Marzusch K, Krober S, et al: A subset of CD56+ large granular lymphocytes in first-trimester human deciduas are proliferating cells. Fertil Steril **71**:74, 1999.

Kanai T, Fujii T, Kozuma S, et al: Soluble HLA-G influences the release of cytokines from allogeneic peripheral blood mononuclear cells in culture. Mol Hum Reprod **7**:195, 2001a.

Kanai T, Fujii T, Unno N, et al: Human leukocyte antigen-G-expressing cells differently modulate the release of cytokines from mononuclear cells present in the deciduas versus peripheral blood. Am J Reprod Immunol **45**:94, 2001b.

Kanzaki H, Yui J, Iwai M, et al: The expression and localization of mRNA for colony-stimulating factor (CSF)-1 in human term placenta. Hum Reprod **7**:563, 1992.

Kapsi K, Albert SE, Yie S-M, et al: HLA-G has a concentration-dependent effect on the generation of an allo-CTL response. Immunology **101**:191, 2000.

Kaufman KA, Bowen JA, Tsai AF, et al: The CLTA-4 gene is expressed in placental fibroblasts. Mol Hum Reprod **5**:84, 1999.

Kauma SW, Huff TF, Hayes N, et al: Placental Fas ligand expression is a mechanism for maternal immune tolerance to the fetus. J Clin Endocrinol Metab **84**:2188, 1999.

Keleman E, Janossa M: Macrophages are the first differentiated blood cells formed in human embryonic liver. Exp Hematol **8**:996, 1980.

Khan S, Katabuchi H, Araki M, et al: Human villous macrophage-conditioned media enhance human trophoblast growth and differentiation *in vitro*. Biol Reprod **62**:1075, 2000.

King A, Allan DSJ, Bowen M, et al: HLA-E is expressed on trophoblast and interacts with CD94/NKG2 receptors on decidual NK cells. Eur J Immunol **30**:1623, 2000.

King A, Birkby C, Loke TW: Early human decidual cells exhibit NK activity against K562 cell line but not against first trimester trophoblast. Cell Immunol **118**:337, 1989.

King A, Burrows TD, Hilby SE, et al: Surface expression of HLA-C antigen by human extravillous trophoblast. Placenta **21**:376, 2000a.

King A, Hilby SE, Gardner L, et al: Recognition of trophoblast HLA class I molecules by decidual NK cell receptors—a review. Placenta **14**:S81, 2000b.

King A, Loke YW: Human trophoblast and JEG choriocarcinoma cells are sensitive to lysis by IL-2 stimulated decidual NK cells. Cell Immunol **129**:435, 1990.

Kirszenbaum M, Moreau P, Gluckman E, et al: An alternatively spliced form of HLA-G mRNA in human trophoblasts and evidence for the presence of HLA-G transcript in adult lymphocytes. Proc Natl Acad Sci USA **91**:4209, 1994.

Klein RB, Fischer TJ, Gard SE, et al: Decreased mononuclear and polymorphonuclear chemotaxis in human newborns, infants and young children. Pediatrics **60**:467, 1977.

Kodama T, Hara T, Oamoto E, et al: Characteristic changes of large granular lymphocytes that strongly express CD56 in endometrium during the menstrual cycle and early pregnancy. Hum Reprod **13**:1036, 1998.

Kolb JP, Chaouat G, Chassoux DJ: Immunoactive products of placenta. III. Suppression of natural killing activity. J Immunol **132**:2305, 1984.

Kovar IZ, Riches PG: C3 and C4 complement proteins in late pregnancy and parturition. J Clin Pathol **41**:650, 1988.

Kovats S, Main EK, Librach C, et al: A class I antigen, HLA-G, expressed in human trophoblasts. Science **248**:220, 1990.

Kuhn R, Lohler J, Rennick D, et al: Interleukin-10-deficient mice develop chronic enterocolitis. Cell **75**:263, 1993.

Lala PK, Kennedy TG, Parhar RS: Suppression of lymphocyte alloreactivity by early gestational human decidua. Cell Immunol **116**:411, 1988.

Lala PK, Scodras JM, Graham CH, et al: Activation of maternal killer cells in the pregnant uterus with chronic indomethacin therapy, IL-2 therapy, or a combination therapy is associated with embryonic demise. Cell Immunol **127**:368, 1990.

Lanzavecchia A, Sallusto F: Dynamics of T lymphocyte responses: intermediates, effectors, and memory cells. Science **290**:92, 2000.

Lata JA, Tuan RS, Shepley KJ: Localization of major histocompatibility complex class I and II mRNA in human first trimester chorionic villi by in situ hybridization. J Exp Med **175**:1027, 1992.

Lenschow DJ, Zeng Y, Thistlethwaite JR, et al: Long-term survival of xenogeneic pancreatic islet grafts induced by CTLA4 Ig. Science **257**:789, 1992.

Levi M, ten Cate H, van der Poll T: Endothelium: interface between coagulation and inflammation. Crit Care Med **30**:S220, 2002.

Li Y, Ohls RK, Christensen RD: Effects of recombinant granulocyte-macrophage colony stimulating factor on the capacity of mononuclear cells from preterm infants to generate interleukin-6 and granulocyte colony-stimulating factor. Int J Pediatr Hematol Oncol **3**:63, 1996.

Lila N, Rouass-Freiss N, Dausset J, et al: Soluble HLA-G protein secreted by allo-specific CD4+ T cells suppresses the allo-proliferative response: A CD4+ T cell regulatory mechanism. Proc Natl Acad Sci USA **98**:12150, 2001.

Lin H, Mossmann TR, Guilbert L, et al: Synthesis of T helper 2-type cytokines at the maternal fetal interface. J Immunol **151**:4562, 1993.

Lobach DF, Hensley LL, Ho W, et al: Human T cell antigen expression during the early stages of fetal thymic maturation. J Immunol **135**:1752, 1985.

Loke YW, Grabowska A, King A: Human trophoblast-decidua interaction in vitro. In Wegmann TG, Gill TJ, Nisbet-Brown E (eds): Molecular and Cellular Immunobiology of the Maternal-Fetal Interface. New York, Oxford University Press, 1991, p. 99.

Lu CY, Redline R, Shea CM: Pregnancy as a model of allograft tolerance: Interactions between adherent macrophages and trophoblast populations. Transplantation **48**:848, 1989.

Lubens RG, Gard SE, Soderberg-Warner M, et al: Lectin-dependent T-lymphocyte and natural killer cytotoxic deficiencies in human newborns. Cell Immunol **74**:40, 1982.

Lucivero G, Selvaggi A, Dell'osso A, et al: Mononuclear cell subpopulations during normal pregnancy. I. Analysis of cell surface markers using conventional techniques and monoclonal antibodies. Am J Reprod Immunol **4**:142, 1983.

Margoulis GV, Buckley RH, Younger JB: Serum immunoglobulin concentrations during normal pregnancy. Am J Obstet Gynecol **109**:971, 1971.

Martinez OM, Gibbons RS, Garovoy MR, et al: IL-4 inhibits IL-2 receptor expression and IL-2 dependent proliferation of human T cells. J Immunol **144**:2211, 1990.

Mattsson R, Holmdahl R, Shcenynius A, et al: Allopregnancy in mice treated with recombinant rat interferon-gamma (abstr). J Reprod Immunol (Suppl)**16**:151, 1989.

McIntyre JA, Faulk WP: Allotypic trophoblast-lymphocyte cross-reactive (TLX) cell surface antigen. Hum Immunol **4**:27, 1982.

McIntyre JA, Faulk WP, Verhulst SJ, et al: Human trophoblast lymphocyte cross-reactive (TLX) antigens define a new alloantigen system. Science **222**:1135, 1983.

Medzhitov R: Toll-like receptors and innate immunity. Nat Rev Immunol **1**:135, 2001.

Medzhitov R, Janeway C Jr: Innate immunity. N Engl J Med **343**:338, 2000.

Menu E, Kaplan L, Andreu G, et al: Immunoactive products of human placenta. I. An immunoregulatory factor obtained from explant cultures of human placenta inhibit CTL generation and cytotoxic effector cell generation. Cell Immunol **119**:341, 1989.

Messner HA, Fauser AA: Culture studies of human pluripotent hematopoietic progenitors. Blut **41**:327, 1980.

Messner HA, Izaquirre CA, Jamal N: Identification of T lymphocytes in human mixed hematopoietic colonies. Blood **58**:402, 1981.

Mincherva-Nilsson L, Hammarstrom S, Hammarstrom ML: Human decidual leukocytes from early pregnancy contain high numbers of γδ T cells and show selective downregulation of alloreactivity. J Immunol **149**:2203, 1992.

Moore KW, O'Garra A, de Waal Malefyt R, et al: Interleukin-10. Annu Rev Immunol **11**:165, 1993.

Moore KW, Vieira P, Fiorentino DF, et al: Homology of cytokine synthesis inhibitory factor (IL-10) to the Epstein-Barr virus gene BCRF1. Science **248**:1230, 1990.

Moore MP, Carter NP, Redman CW: Lymphocyte subsets in normal and pre-eclamptic pregnancies. Br J Obstet Gynaecol **90**:326, 1983.

Morell A, Sidiropoulos D, Herrmann U, et al: IgG subclasses and antibodies to group B streptococci, pneumococci, and tetanus toxoid in preterm neonates after intravenous infusion of immunoglobulin to the mothers. Pediatr Res **20**:933, 1986.

Mosmann TR, Cherwinski H, Bond MW, et al: Two types of murine helper T cell clone. I. Definition according to profiles of lymphokine activities and secreted proteins. J Immunol **136**:2348, 1986.

Mosmann TR, Moore KW: The role of IL-10 in cross-regulation of TH1 and TH2 responses. Immunol Today **12**:A49, 1991.

Munn DH, Zhou M, Attwood JT, et al: Prevention of allogeneic fetal rejection by tryptophan catabolism. Science **281**:1191, 1998.

Murray DL, Imagawa DT, Okada DM, et al: Antibody response to monovalent A/New Jersey/8/76 influenza vaccine in pregnant women. J Clin Microbiol **10**:184, 1979.

Nagarkatti PS, Clark DA: In vitro activity and in vivo correlates of alloantigen-specific murine suppressor T cells induced by allogeneic pregnancy. J Immunol **131**:638, 1983.

Nathan C, Sporn M: Cytokines in context. J Cell Biol **113**:981, 1991.

Notarangelo LD, Chirico G, Chiara A, et al: Activity of classical and alternative pathways of complement in preterm and small for gestational age infants. Pediatr Res **18**:281, 1984.

Ohlsson R, Glaser A, Holmgren L, et al: The molecular biology of placental development. In Redman CWG, Sargent IL, Starkey PM (eds): The Human Placenta. Oxford, Blackwell Scientific Publications, 1993, p. 33.

Olding LB, Murgita RA, Wigzell H: Mitogen-stimulated lymphoid cells from human newborns suppress the proliferation of maternal lymphocytes across a cell-impermeable membrane. J Immunol **119**:1109, 1977.

Oldstone MBA, Tishon A, Moretta L: Active thymus derived suppressor lymphocytes in human cord blood. Nature **269**:333, 1977.

Parhar RS, Yagel S, Lala PK: PGE₂-mediated immunosuppression by first trimester human decidual cells blocks activation of maternal leukocytes in the decidua with potential anti-trophoblast activity. Cell Immunol **120**:61, 1989.

Paterson WG, Grant KA: Advanced intraligamentous pregnancy: Report of a case, review of the literature and a discussion of the biological implications. Obstet Gynecol Surv **30**:715, 1975.

Petrucco O, Seamark RF, Holmes K, et al: Changes in lymphocyte function during pregnancy. Br J Obstet Gynaecol **83**:245, 1976.

Peyman JA, Hammond GL: Localization of IFN-γ receptor in first trimester placenta to trophoblasts but lack of stimulation of HLA-DRA, -DRB, or invariant chain mRNA expression by IFN-γ. J Immunol **149**:2675, 1992.

Pollard JW, Bartocci A, Arceci R, et al: Apparent role of the macrophage growth factor, CSF-1, in placental development. Nature **330**:484, 1987.

Pollard JW, Hunt JS, Wiktor-Jedvzejczak W, et al: A pregnancy defect in the osteoporetic (op/op) mouse demonstrates the requirement for CSF-1 in female fertility. Dev Biol **148**:273, 1991.

Purcell DFJ, McKenzie IFC, Lublin DM, et al: The human cell-surface glyco-proteins Huly-m5, membrane cofactor protein (MCP) of the complement system, and trophoblast-leukocyte common (TLX) antigen are CD46. Immunology **70**:155, 1990.

Redline RW, Lu CY: Role of local immunosuppression in murine fetoplacental listeriosis. J Clin Invest **79**:1234, 1987.

Redline RW, McKay DB, Vasquez MA, et al: Macrophage functions are regulated by the substratum of murine decidual stromal cells. J Clin Invest **85**:1951, 1990.

Redman CWG, Ferry BL, Jackson MC, et al: Immune cell populations in human early pregnancy decidua. *In* Wegmann TF, Gill TJ, Nisbet-Brown E (eds): Molecular and Cellular Immunobiology of the Maternal-Fetal Interface. New York, Oxford University Press, 1991, p. 110.

Redman CWG, McMichael AJ, Stirrat GM, et al: Class I MHC antigens on extravillus trophoblast. Immunology **52**:457, 1984.

Reichel H, Koeffler HP, Tobler A, et al: 1-Alpha,25-dihydroxyvitamin D$_3$ inhibits gamma-interferon synthesis by normal human peripheral blood lymphocytes. Proc Natl Acad Sci USA **84**:3385, 1987.

Ricketts RM, Jones DB: Differential effect of human chorionic gonadotrophin on lymphocyte proliferation induced by mitogens. J Reprod Immunol **7**:225, 1985.

Rieger L, Hofmeister V, Probe C, et al: Th1- and Th2-like cytokine production by first trimester decidual large granular lymphocytes is influenced by HLA-G and HLA-E. Mol Hum Reprod **8**:255, 2002.

Riteau B, Rouas-Freiss N, Menier C, et al: HLA-G2, -G3, and -G4 isoforms expressed as nonmature cell surface glycoproteins inhibit NK and antigen-specific CTL cytolysis. J Immunol **166**:5018, 2001.

Robertson SA, Lavranos T, Seamark RF: In vitro models of the maternal-fetal interface. *In* Wegmann TF, Gill TJ, Nisbet-Brown E (eds): Molecular and Cellular Immunobiology of the Maternal-Fetal Interface. New York, Oxford University Press, 1991, p. 191.

Rocklin RE, Kitzmiller JL, Garvey MR: Maternal-fetal relation: Further characterization of an immunologic blocking factor that develops during pregnancy. Clin Immunol Immunopathol **22**:305, 1982.

Rodger JC: Lack of a requirement for a maternal humoral immune response to establish and maintain successful allogeneic pregnancy. Transplantation **40**:372, 1985.

Romero R, Mazor M, Tartakovsky B: Systemic administration of interleukin-1 induces preterm parturition in mice. Am J Obstet Gynecol **165**:969, 1991.

Rook AH, Rehrl JH, Wakefield LM, et al: Effects of transforming growth factor-β on the functions of natural killer cells: Depressed cytolytic activity and blunting of interferon-responsiveness. J Immunol **136**:3916, 1986.

Rosa F, Hatat D, Abdadie A, et al: Regulation of histocompatibility antigens by interferon. Ann Immunol **136**:103, 1985.

Royer HD, Reinherz EL: T lymphocytes: Ontogeny, function and relevance to clinical disorders. N Engl J Med **317**:1136, 1987.

Runic R, Lockwood CJ, Ma Y, et al: Expression of Fas ligand by human cytotrophoblasts: Implications in placentation and fetal survival. J Clin Endocrinol Metab **81**:3119, 1996.

Saito S, Motoyoshi K, Saito M, et al: Localization and production of human macrophage colony-stimulating factor (hM-CSF) in human placental and decidual tissues. Lymphok Cytok Res **12**:101, 1993.

Sanders SK, Giblin PA, Kavathas P: Cell-cell adhesion mediated by CD8 and human histocompatibility complex class 1 molecule on cytotrophoblasts. J Exp Med **174**:737, 1991

Santoso DI, Rogers P, Wallace EM, et al: Localization of indoleamine 2,3-dioxygenase and 4-hydroynoneal in normal and pre-eclamptic placentae. Placenta **23**:373, 2002.

Sargent IL, Wilkins T, Redman CWG: Maternal immune responses to the fetus in early pregnancy and recurrent miscarriage. Lancet **2**:1099, 1988.

Schultz LD, Sidman CL: Genetically determined models of immunodeficiency. Annu Rev Immunol **5**:367, 1987.

Schwartz RH: Acquisition of immunologic self-tolerance. Cell **57**:1073, 1989.

Scodras JM, Parhar RS, Kennedy TG, et al: Prostaglandin-mediated inactivation of natural killer cells in the murine decidua. Cell Immunol **127**:352, 1990.

Sedlmayr P, Blaschitz A, Wintersteiger R, et al: Localization of indoleamine 2,3-dioxygenase in human female reproductive organs and the placenta. Mol Hum Reprod **84**:385, 2002.

Shigeoka AO, Santos JI, Hill HR: Functional analysis of neutrophil granulocytes from healthy, infected, and stressed neonates. J Pediatr **95**:454, 1979.

Shukla H, Swaroop A, Srivastava R, et al: The mRNA of a human class I gene HLA G/HLA 6.0 exhibits a restricted pattern of expression. Nucleic Acids Res **18**:2189, 1990.

Siegel I, Gleicher N: Changes in peripheral mononuclear cells in pregnancy. Am J Reprod Immunol **1**:154, 1981.

Silen ML, Firpo A, Morgello S, et al: Interleukin-1α and tumor necrosis factor α cause placental injury in the rat. Am J Pathol **135**:239, 1989.

Silver RM: Bacterial lipopolysaccharide-mediated murine fetal death: The role of interleukin-1. Am J Obstet Gynecol **176**:544, 1996.

Silver RM, Lohner SL, Daynes RA, et al: Lipopolysaccharide-induced fetal death: The role of tumor necrosis factor alpha. Biol Reprod **50**:1108, 1994.

Solinger AM: Immature T lymphocytes in human neonatal blood. Cell Immunol **92**:115, 1985.

Sridama V, Pacini F, Yang S-L, et al: Decreased levels of T helper cells: A possible cause of immunodeficiency in pregnancy. N Engl J Med **307**:352, 1982.

Starkey PM, Sargent IL, Redman CWG: Cell populations in human early pregnancy decidua: Characterisation and isolation of large granular lymphocytes by flow cytometry. Immunology **65**:129, 1988.

Steven DH, Morris G: Development of the fetal membranes. *In* Steven DH (ed): Comparative Placentation: Essays in Structure and Function. New York, Academic Press, 1975, p. 58.

Sthoeger ZM, Chiorazzi N, Lahita RG: Regulation of the immune response by sex hormones. I. In vitro effects of estradiol and testosterone on Pokeweed mitogen-induced human B cell differentiation. J Immunol **141**:91, 1988.

Stiehm ER: Fetal defense mechanisms. Am J Dis Child **129**:438, 1975.

Stiehm ER, Fudenberg HH: Serum levels of immune globulins in health and disease: A survey. Pediatrics **37**:715, 1966.

Stites DP, Siiteri PK: Steroids as immunosuppressants in pregnancy. Immunol Rev **75**:117, 1983.

Sullender WM, Miller JL, Yasukawa LL, et al: Humoral and cell-mediated immunity in neonates with herpes simplex virus infection. J Infect Dis **155**:28, 1987.

Sunderland CA, Redman CWG, Stirrat GM: HLA-A,B,C antigens are expressed on nonvillous trophoblasts of the early human placenta. J Immunol **127**:2614, 1981.

Svensson L, Arvola M, Sallstrom MA, et al: The Th2 cytokines IL-4 and IL-10 are not crucial for the completion of allogeneic pregnancy in mice. J Reprod Immunol **51**:3, 2001.

Swisher SG, Economou JS, Holmes EC, et al: TNF-α and IFN-γ reverse IL-4 inhibition of lymphokine activated killer cell function. Cell Immunol **128**:450, 1990.

Szekeres-Bartho J, Hadnagy J, Pacsa AS: The suppressive effect of progesterone during pregnancy: Unique sensitivity of pregnancy lymphocytes. J Reprod Immunol **7**:121, 1986.

Szekeres-Bartho J, Kilar F, Falkay G, et al: Progesterone-treated lymphocytes release a substance inhibiting cytotoxicity and prostaglandin synthesis. Am J Reprod Immunol **9**:15, 1985.

Tabibzadeh SS, Satyaswaroop PG, Rao PN: Antiproliferative effect of interferon-γ in human endometrial epithelial cells in vitro: Potential local growth modulatory role in endometrium. J Clin Endocrinol Metab **67**:131, 1988.

Tallon DF, Corcoran DJD, O'Dwyer EM, et al: Circulating lymphocyte sub-populations in pregnancy: A longitudinal study. J Immunol **132**:1784, 1984.

Tezabwala BU, Johnson PM, Rees RC: Inhibition of pregnancy viability in mice following IL-2 administration. Immunology **67**:115, 1989.

Thomas IK, Erickson KL: Gestational immunosuppression is mediated by specific Ly2 T cells. Immunology **57**:201, 1986.

Tobler A, Miller CW, Norman AW, et al: 1,25-Dihydroxyvitamin D$_3$ modulates the expression of a lymphokine (granulocyte-macrophage colony stimulating factor) posttranscriptionally. J Clin Invest **81**:1819, 1988.

Toder V, Nebel L, Gleicher N: Studies of natural killer cells in pregnancy. I. Analysis at the single cell level. J Clin Lab Immunol **14**:123, 1984.

Tomasi TB: Suppressive factors in amniotic fluid and newborn serum: Is α-fetoprotein involved? Cell Immunol **37**:459, 1978.

Tsoukas CD, Provvedini DM, Manolagas SC: 1,25-Dihydroxyvitamin D$_3$: A novel immunoregulatory hormone. Science **224**:1438, 1984.

Tsunawaki S, Sporn M, Ding A, et al: Deactivation of macrophages by transforming growth factor-β. Nature **334**:260, 1988.

Uksila J, Lassila O, Hirveonen T, et al: Development of natural killer cell function in the human fetus. J Immunol **130**:154, 1983.

Unander AM, Olding LB: Ontogeny and postnatal persistence of a strong suppressor activity in man. J Immunol **127**:1182, 1981.

Van Cong N, Vaisse C, Gross M-S, et al: The human placental protein 14 (PP14) gene is localized on chromosome 9q34. Hum Genet **86**:515, 1991.

Van Oers NSC, Cohen BL, Murgita RA: Isolation and characterization of a distinct immunoregulatory isoform of ?-fetoprotein produced by the normal fetus. J Exp Med **170**:811, 1989.

Van Tol MJD, Zijlstra J, Heijnen CJ, et al: Antigen-specific plaque-forming cell response of human cord blood lymphocytes after in vitro stimulation by T cell-dependent antigens. Eur J Immunol **13**:390, 1983.

Vaquer S, de la Hera A, Jorda J, et al: Diminished natural killer activity in pregnancy: Modulation by interleukin 2 and interferon gamma. Scand J Immunol **26**:691, 1987.

Varner MW: Autoimmune disorders and pregnancy. Semin Perinatol **15**:238, 1991.

Wegmann TG: Fetal protection against abortion: Is it immunosuppression or immunostimulation? Ann Immunol **135D**:309, 1984.

Wegmann TG, Athanassakis I, Guilbert L, et al: The role of M-CSF and GM-CSF in fostering placental growth, fetal growth, and fetal survival. Transplant Proc **21**:566, 1989.

Wegmann TG, Lin H, Guilbert L, et al: Bidirectional cytokine interactions in the maternal-fetal relationship: Is successful pregnancy a Th2 phenomenon? Immunol Today **15**:353, 1993.

Wilson CB, Westall J, Johnston L, et al: Decreased production of interferon-gamma by human neonatal cells. J Clin Invest **77**:860, 1986.

Yagel S, Lala PK, Powell WA, et al: Interleukin-1 stimulates human chorionic gonadotrophin secretion by first trimester human trophoblast. J Clin Endocrinol Metab **68**:992,1989.

Yagel S, Livni N, Zacut D, et al: Characterization and localization of human placental mononuclear phagocytes by monoclonal antibodies and other cell markers. Isr J Med Sci **26**:243, 1990.

Yagel S, Palti Z, Gallily R: Prostaglandin E_2-mediated suppression of human maternal lymphocyte alloreactivity by first-trimester fetal macrophages. Obstet Gynecol **72**:648, 1988.

Yelavarthi KK, Fishback JL, Hunt JS: Analysis of HLA-G mRNA in human placental and extraplacental membrane cells by in situ hybridization. J Immunol **146**:2847, 1991.

Yui J, Garcia-Lloret MI, Wegmann TG, et al: Disruption of trophoblast monolayers by TNF-α and IFN-γ and antagonism by GM-CSF. Boston, Serono Symposia, 1993.

Zheng LM, Ojcius DM, Young JD: Role of granulated metrial gland cells in the immunology of pregnancy. Am J Reprod Immunol **25**:72, 1991.

Zorzi W, Thellin O, Coumans B, et al: Demonstration of the expression of CD95 ligand transcript and protein in human placenta. Placenta **19**:269 1998.

Zuckerman F, Head JR: Susceptibility of mouse trophoblast to antibody and complement-mediated damage. Transplant Proc **17**:925, 1985.

Zuckerman F, Head JR: Possible mechanism of nonrejection of the feto-placental allograft: Trophoblast resistance to lysis by cellular immune effectors. Transplant Proc **19**:554, 1987.

Zuckerman FA, Head JR: Expression of MHC antigens on murine trophoblast and their modulation by interferon. J Immunol **137**:846, 1986.

Zuckerman FA, Head JR: Murine trophoblast resists cell-mediated lysis. II. Resistance to natural cell-mediated cytotoxicity. Cell Immunol **116**:274, 1988.

Chapter 8

MATERNAL CARDIOVASCULAR AND RENAL ADAPTATION TO PREGNANCY

Manju Monga, MD

There are profound changes in the cardiovascular and renal systems during pregnancy. These remarkable adaptations begin early after conception and continue as gestation advances, yet most are almost totally reversible within weeks to months after delivery.

Physiologic adaptations of the cardiovascular system, which include changes in anatomy, blood volume, cardiac output, and systemic vascular resistance, result in cardiac enlargement, sinus tachycardia, cardiac murmurs, and peripheral edema. Although these adaptations are normal in pregnancy, they are signs of cardiovascular dysfunction in the nonpregnant patient. Similarly, normal anatomic and functional changes in the renal system during pregnancy, such as dilatation of the collecting systems, may lead one to a misdiagnosis of urinary tract disease. These physiologic adaptations are usually well tolerated by the pregnant patient, but they must be understood so that normal may be distinguished from abnormal.

CARDIOVASCULAR SYSTEM

Blood Volume

Plasma volume increases progressively from 6 to 8 weeks' gestation and reaches a maximal volume of 4700 to 5200 mL at 32 weeks, an increase of 45% (1200 to 1600 mL) above nonpregnant values (Pritchard, 1965a; Lund and Donovan, 1967). This increment is greater in multiple gestations and is also correlated with fetal weight (Rovinsky and Jaffin, 1965; Duffus et al., 1971; Duvekot et al., 1995). The mechanism of this plasma volume expansion is unclear but may be related to nitric oxide-mediated vasodilatation that subsequently induces the renin-angiotensin-aldosterone system and stimulates sodium and water retention (Carbillon et al., 2000). Because maternal hypervolemia is present in cases of hydatidiform mole, it is unlikely that the presence of a fetus per se is necessary for this to occur (Pritchard, 1965b).

Red blood cell mass increases by 250 to 450 mL by term, an increment of 20% to 30% from prepregnancy values. This rise, which is even greater in women receiving exogenous iron supplementation, reflects increased production of red blood cells rather than prolongation of red blood cell life (Pritchard, 1965a). Placental chorionic somatomammotropin, progesterone, and perhaps prolactin are responsible for this increase in erythropoiesis (Jepson, 1968), which consequently increases the maternal demand for iron by 500 mg during pregnancy.

This is in addition to 300 mg of iron transferred from maternal stores to the fetus and 200 mg of iron required to compensate for normal daily losses over the course of pregnancy. Erythrocyte 2,3-diphosphoglycerate concentration increases in pregnancy, thus lowering the affinity of maternal hemoglobin for oxygen. This facilitates the dissociation of oxygen from hemoglobin, which enhances oxygen transfer to the fetus (Bille-Brahe and Rorth, 1979).

The changes mentioned above result in a 45% increase in circulating blood volume. This may protect the pregnant woman from hemodynamic instability after blood loss. Because plasma volume increases disproportionately to red blood cell mass, physiologic hemodilution occurs, resulting in a mild decrease in maternal hematocrit, which is maximal in the middle of the third trimester. This may have a protective function by decreasing blood viscosity to counter the predisposition to thromboembolic events in pregnancy (Koller, 1982) and may be beneficial for intervillous perfusion (Pieters et al., 1987). See Chapter 47 for changes in other blood constituents during pregnancy.

Anatomic Changes

Histologic and echocardiographic studies indicate that ventricular wall muscle mass and end-diastolic volume increase in pregnancy without an associated increase in end-systolic volume or end-diastolic pressures (Rubler et al., 1977; Lard-Meeter et al., 1979). Ventricular mass increases in the first trimester (Thompson et al., 1986), in contrast to the increment in end-diastolic volume that occurs in the second and early third trimesters (Rubler et al., 1977). This increases cardiac compliance (resulting in a physiologically dilated heart) without a concomitant reduction in ejection fraction, implying that myocardial contractility must also increase. This is supported by studies of systolic time intervals in pregnancy (Rubler et al., 1972; Burg et al., 1974) and echocardiographic demonstration of a decreased ratio of load-independent wall stress to velocity of circumferential fiber shortening (Gilson et al., 1997). Left atrial diameter increases parallel to the rise in blood volume, starting early in pregnancy and plateauing by 30 weeks (Vered et al., 1991).

Finally, a general softening of collagen occurs in the entire vascular system, associated with hypertrophy of the smooth muscle components (Marazita, 1946). This results in increased compliance of capacitive (predominantly elastic

111

wall) and conductive (predominantly muscular wall) arteries and veins that is evident as early as 5 weeks of amenorrhea (Spaanderman et al., 2000).

Cardiac Output

Cardiac output, the product of heart rate and stroke volume, is a measure of the functional capacity of the heart. Cardiac output may be calculated by invasive heart catheterization with dye dilution or thermodilution or by noninvasive methods, such as impedance cardiography and echocardiography. Limited data have been obtained from normal pregnant women by means of invasive methods (Bader et al., 1955; Walters et al., 1966; Clark et al., 1989). M-mode echocardiography (Mashini et al., 1987) and Doppler studies (Ihlen et al., 1984; Easterling et al., 1987, 1990b) have also been used to determine cardiac output during pregnancy and have demonstrated good correlation with thermodilution methods. These validation studies have not been performed in healthy pregnant women, and reports are limited to critically ill patients. Yet to be determined is the most appropriate echocardiographic technique (pulsed-wave or continuous Doppler) and the most reproducible site through which to measure blood flow (Duvekot and Pieters, 1994). In contrast, thoracic electrical bioimpedance, which is influenced by intrathoracic fluid volume, hemoglobin, and chest configuration (all of which change in pregnancy), has had poor correlation with thermodilution techniques in pregnancy, with large underestimation of cardiac output (Milsom et al., 1983; Easterling et al., 1989; Masaki et al., 1989).

Cardiac output increases by 30% to 50% during pregnancy (Bader et al., 1955; Walters et al., 1966; Clark et al., 1989; Robson et al., 1989; Easterling et al., 1990a; Gilson et al., 1997), with 50% of this increase occurring by 8 weeks' gestation (Capeless and Clapp, 1989). A slower rate of increase occurs until the third trimester of pregnancy. There is a small decline in cardiac output at term due to a fall in stroke volume (Ueland et al., 1969; Rubler et al., 1977; McLennan et al., 1987; Easterling et al., 1990a).

Increased maternal cardiac output is due to an increase in both stroke volume and heart rate. Stroke volume is primarily responsible for the early increase in cardiac output (Capeless and Clapp, 1989; Robson et al., 1989), probably reflecting the increase in ventricular muscle mass and end-diastolic volume. Stroke volume declines toward term (Ueland et al., 1969). In contrast, maternal heart rate, which rises from 5 weeks' gestation to a maximal increment of 15 to 20 beats/min by 32 weeks' gestation, is maintained (Ueland et al., 1969; Robson et al., 1989, Stein et al., 1999) (Fig. 8-1). Therefore, in the late third trimester, the relatively mild maternal tachycardia is primarily responsible for maintaining cardiac output.

Maternal posture significantly affects cardiac output. Turning from the left lateral recumbent to the supine position at term can result in a drop in cardiac output by as much as 25% to 30% (Ueland et al., 1969). This is due to caval compression by the gravid uterus, which diminishes venous return from the lower extremities, decreasing stroke volume and cardiac output. Although most women do not become hypotensive with this maneuver, up to 8% of women will demonstrate the supine hypotensive syndrome, which is manifest by a sudden drop in blood pressure, bradycardia, and

syncope (Holmes, 1960). This may be due to inadequacy of the paravertebral collateral blood supply in these women.

There is selective regional distribution of this physiologic increase in cardiac output. Uterine blood flow increases 10-fold to between 500 and 800 mL/min (Gant and Worley, 1989). This represents a shift from 2% of total cardiac output in the nonpregnant state to 17% at term. Renal blood flow increases significantly (by 50%) during pregnancy (Chesley and Sloan, 1964), as does perfusion of the breasts and skin (Katz and Sokal, 1980; Frederiksen, 2001). There does not appear to be any major alteration in blood flow to the brain or liver.

Blood Pressure

Arterial blood pressure decreases in pregnancy beginning as early as the 7th week (Capeless and Clapp, 1989). This early drop probably represents incomplete compensation for the fall in peripheral vascular resistance by the increase in cardiac output. When measured in the sitting or standing positions, systolic blood pressure remains relatively stable throughout pregnancy, whereas diastolic blood pressure decreases by a maximum of 10 mm at 28 weeks and then increases toward nonpregnant levels by term (Wilson et al., 1980). In contrast, when measured in the left lateral recumbent position, both systolic and diastolic blood pressures decrease to a level 5 to 10 mm Hg and 10 to 15 mm Hg, respectively, below nonpregnant values. This nadir occurs at 24 to 32 weeks' gestation and is followed by a rise toward nonpregnant values at term (Wilson et al., 1980) (Fig. 8-2). Because diastolic pressures fall to a greater extent than systolic pressures, there is a slight increase in pulse pressure in the early third trimester. Because arterial blood pressures are approximately 10 mm Hg higher in the standing or sitting positions than in the lateral or supine positions, consistency in position during successive blood pressure measurements is essential for the accurate documentation of a trend during pregnancy.

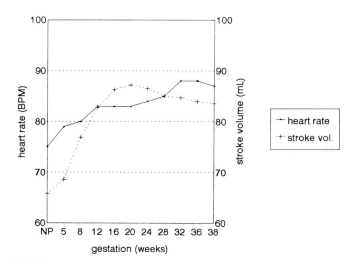

FIGURE 8-1 ■ Alteration in stroke volume and heart rate during pregnancy. Stroke volume increases maximally during the first half of gestation. There is a slight decrease in stroke volume toward term. The mild increase in heart rate begins early in gestation and continues until term. (Adapted from Robson SC, Hunter S, Boys RJ, et al: Serial study of factors influencing changes in cardiac output during human pregnancy. Am J Physiol **256**:H1060, 1989.)

Confusion has arisen with regard to the definition of diastolic blood pressure in pregnancy. Measurement of *Korotkoff phase 4* (the point of muffling) results in mean diastolic pressures 13 mm Hg higher than measurement of *Korotkoff phase 5* (the point of disappearance) (Wickman et al., 1984). Use of Korotkoff phase 4 may be less reproducible (Johenning and Barron, 1992). Intra-arterial measurements of diastolic pressures may be 15 mm Hg lower than manual determinations (Koller, 1982), whereas they may be significantly higher than automated cuff diastolic measurements (Kirshon et al., 1987). For these reasons, one should be consistent in the method by which blood pressure is recorded throughout pregnancy and ascertain the definition of diastolic blood pressure when reviewing studies of arterial blood pressure in pregnant women.

The use of ambulatory blood pressure monitoring has been validated in pregnancy (Clark et al., 1991; Shennan et al., 1993). Twenty-four–hour monitoring has shown measurements that are either significantly lower (Halligan et al., 1993) or higher (Churchill and Beevers, 1996) than office measurements. These differences cannot be explained by activity level, although work and job-related stress has been shown to increase blood pressure in late pregnancy (Churchill and Beevers, 1996; Walker et al., 2001). This suggests that ambulatory blood pressure measurements should not be considered directly comparable with office blood pressure readings in pregnancy and that further study is needed before obstetric outcome can be predicted on the basis of ambulatory recordings (Churchill and Beevers, 1996). Ambulatory blood pressure monitoring has shown marked circadian variation in blood pressure during pregnancy, with nadir of systolic and diastolic blood pressures in the early morning hours and peak in late afternoon and evening (Hermida et al., 2000).

Systemic Vascular Resistance

Systemic vascular resistance is calculated by the following equation:

$$[\text{mean arterial pressure} - \text{central venous pressure}] \times 80 \text{ dynes-seconds cm}^{-5}/\text{cardiac output}$$

Systemic vascular resistance decreases from as early as 5 weeks of pregnancy as a result of the vasodilatory effect of progesterone and prostaglandins and perhaps the arteriovenous fistula–like function of the low-resistance uteroplacental circulation (Greiss and Anderson, 1970; Gerber et al., 1981; Duvekot et al., 1993; Gilson et al., 1997). Alternatively, it has been proposed that increased production of endothelium-derived relaxant factors, such as nitric oxide, initiates vasodilation and a drop in systemic vascular resistance (Duvekot and Pieters, 1994; Carbillon et al., 2000). This decrease in systemic vascular tone may be the primary trigger for increasing heart rate, stroke volume, and cardiac output in the first few weeks of pregnancy (Duvekot et al., 1993; Carbillon et al., 2000). The fall in systemic vascular resistance is paralleled by an increase in vascular compliance, which reaches a nadir at 14 to 24 weeks' gestation and then rises progressively toward term (Bader et al., 1955; Spaanderman et al., 2000).

Venous Vascular Bed

Venous compliance increases progressively during pregnancy; this results in a decrease in flow velocity and subsequent stasis (Fawer et al., 1978). This increase in venous capacitance may be due to the relaxant effect of progesterone or endothelium-derived relaxant factors on the smooth muscle of the blood vessels or to altered elastic properties of the venous wall. As a result of this decrease in venous vascular resistance, pregnant women are more sensitive to autonomic blockade, which results in further venous pooling, decreased venous return, and a fall in cardiac output manifested as a sudden drop in arterial blood pressure. This may be seen in response to conduction anesthesia and ganglionic blockade. Forearm venous pressure increases throughout normal pregnancy by 40% to 50% above nonpregnant values. Calf venous pressures are always higher than those of the forearm, and this difference becomes more exaggerated as gestation advances, due in part to the enlarging uterus (Barwin and Roddie, 1976).

Antepartum Hemodynamics

Clark and colleagues (1989) studied the effect of pregnancy on central hemodynamics by placing Swan-Ganz catheters and arterial lines in 10 normal primiparous women at 35 to 38 weeks' gestation and again at 11 to 13 weeks' postpartum (Table 8-1). Late pregnancy was characterized by significant elevations in heart rate, stroke volume, and cardiac output in concert with significant decreases in systemic and pulmonary vascular resistance and serum colloid osmotic pressure. There was no significant alteration in pulmonary capillary wedge pressure, central venous pressure, or mean arterial blood pressure. Clark and colleagues (1989) suggested that pulmonary

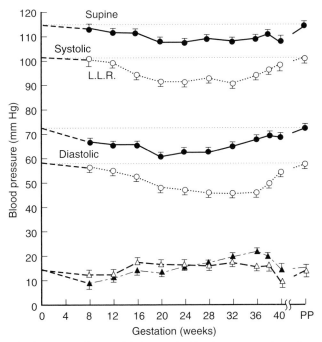

FIGURE 8-2 ■ Sequential changes in blood pressures throughout pregnancy with subjects in supine (*closed circles*) and left lateral recumbent (L.L.R.; *open circles*) positions. The change in systolic (*open triangles*) and diastolic (*closed triangles*) blood pressures produced by movement from the left lateral recumbent to the supine position is illustrated in the bottom part of figure. (From Wilson M, Morganti AA, Zervoudakis I, et al: Blood pressure, the renin-aldosterone system and sex steroids throughout normal pregnancy. Am J Med **68**:97, 1980.)

TABLE 8-1. HEMODYNAMIC PROFILES FOR NONPREGNANT AND PREGNANT PATIENTS IN THE THIRD TRIMESTER

	Nonpregnant	Pregnant	Change
Cardiac output (liters/min)	4.3 ± 0.9	6.2 ± 1.0	+43%
Heart rate (beats/min)	71 ± 10	83 ± 10	+17%
SVR (dyne-sec-cm^{-5})	1530 ± 520	1210 ± 266	−21%
PVR (dyne-sec-cm^{-5})	119 ± 47	78 ± 22	−34%
CVP (mm Hg)	3.7 ± 2.6	3.6 ± 2.5	NS
COP (mm Hg)	20.8 ± 1.0	18.0 ± 1.5	−14%
PCWP (mm Hg)	6.3 ± 2.1	7.5 ± 1.8	NS
COP-PCWP (mm Hg)	14.5 ± 2.5	10.5 ± 2.7	−28%

COP, colloid osmotic pressure; COP-PCWP, gradient between COP and PCWP; CVP, central venous pressure; nonpregnant, 11–13 weeks' postpartum; PCWP, pulmonary capillary wedge pressure; pregnant, 36–38 weeks' gestation; PVR, pulmonary vascular resistance; SVR, systemic vascular resistance.

Adapted with permission from Clark SL, Cotton DB, Lee W, et al: Central hemodynamic assessment of normal term pregnancy. Am J Obstet Gynecol **161:**1439, 1989.

capillary wedge pressure does not increase, despite significant increases in blood volume and stroke volume, because of ventricular dilatation and the fall in pulmonary vascular resistance. They noted, however, that pregnant women were still at higher risk for pulmonary edema because of the significantly decreased gradient between colloid osmotic pressure and pulmonary capillary wedge pressure (gradient of 10.5 ± 2.7 mm Hg) compared with the nonpregnant state (gradient of 14.5 ± 2.5 mm Hg).

Circulation time demonstrates a slight but progressive decline during pregnancy, reaching a minimal value of 10.2 seconds in the third trimester (Manchester and Loube, 1946). These findings have been interpreted to mean that blood flow velocity increases slightly in pregnancy.

Autonomic cardiovascular control in pregnancy has been investigated (Ekholm and Erkkola, 1996; Stein et al., 1999). These studies have indicated a blunted heart rate and blood pressure response to the Valsalva maneuver, possibly resulting from adaptation to increased blood volume, and decreased heart rate variability, possibly because of decreased vagal control of the heart. Heart rate and blood pressure increase with standing in early pregnancy, and this implies increased sympathetic outflow to the heart. In contrast, pregnancy near term is characterized by increased hemodynamic stability in response to orthostatic stress.

Arterial Blood Gases

Maternal tidal volume increases by 40% in pregnancy (see also Chapter 46), and this increase results in maternal hyperventilation and hypocapnia (Awe et al., 1979). There is a decrease in partial pressure of carbon dioxide from a normal pregnancy level of 39 mm Hg to approximately 28 to 31 mm Hg. This is partially compensated by increased renal secretion of hydrogen ions, with a resultant serum bicarbonate level of 18 to 22 mEq/liter. A mild respiratory alkalosis is therefore normal in pregnancy, with an arterial pH of 7.44 compared with 7.40 in the nonpregnant state. There is also a narrowing of the difference between arterial and central venous oxygen saturation in pregnancy (Guzman and Caplan, 1970). This implies that the increase in cardiac output is more than adequate to compensate for the increased metabolic demands of pregnancy.

Symptoms and Signs of Normal Pregnancy

Pregnant women report dyspnea with increased frequency as gestation advances (15% in the first trimester compared with 75% by the third) (Milne et al., 1978). The mechanism for this is unclear but may relate to the exaggerated ventilatory response (perhaps progesterone mediated) in response to increased metabolic demand. Easy fatigability and decreased exercise tolerance are also commonly reported, although mild to moderate exercise is well tolerated under normal circumstances (Kulpa et al., 1987; Wolfe et al., 1989). Increased lower extremity venous pressure, caused by compression by the gravid uterus and lower colloid osmotic pressure, is commonly manifest as dependent edema—most often found in the distal lower extremities at term. Thigh-high support stockings significantly increase systemic vascular resistance by preventing venous pooling in the lower extremities and may be effective in decreasing peripheral edema in pregnancy (Hobel et al., 1996).

Cutforth and MacDonald (1966) clearly documented the alterations in heart sounds in pregnancy by phonocardiographic study of 50 normal primigravid women. Briefly, the first heart sound increased in loudness and was more widely split in approximately 90% of women (30 to 45 msec compared with 15 msec in the nonpregnant state). This is due to early closure of the mitral valve as demonstrated by the shortened interval between the Q wave of the electrocardiogram and the first heart sound. There was no significant change in the second heart sound until 30 weeks' gestation, when there may be persistent splitting that does not vary with respiration. A loud third heart sound was heard in up to 90% of pregnant women, whereas less than 5% had an audible fourth heart sound.

Systolic murmurs develop in more than 95% of pregnant women. These are heard best along the left sternal border and are most often either aortic or pulmonary in origin. Doppler echocardiography demonstrated an increased incidence of functional tricuspid regurgitation during pregnancy that may also lead to a systolic precordial murmur (Limacher et al., 1985). Although most of these changes in heart sounds are first audible between 12 and 20 weeks' gestation and regress by 1 week postpartum, nearly 20% have a persistent systolic murmur beyond the 4th week after delivery (Cutforth and MacDonald, 1966). Systolic murmurs louder than grade 2/4 and diastolic murmurs of any intensity are considered abnormal during pregnancy. However, 14% of women may have a continuous murmur of mammary vessel origin, which is heard maximally in the second intercostal space (Cutforth and MacDonald, 1966).

Uterine growth results in upward displacement of the diaphragm, which is associated with superior, lateral, and anterior displacement of the heart within the thorax. This leads to lateral displacement of the point of maximal impulse and may suggest cardiomegaly on chest radiographs. This appearance is further enhanced by straightening of the left heart border and prominence of the pulmonary outflow tracts; however, the cardiothoracic ratio is only slightly increased, if at all, in normal pregnancy (Turner, 1975).

Intrapartum Hemodynamic Changes

Labor results in significant alterations in the cardiovascular measurements, as discussed previously. The first stage of labor is associated with a 12% to 31% rise in cardiac output, primarily because of a 22% increase in stroke volume (Ueland and Hansen, 1969; Robson, Dunlop et al., 1987). The second stage of labor is associated with an even greater increase in cardiac output (49%). Laboring in the left lateral decubitus position or analgesia decreases the magnitude of this increment. The increase in cardiac output is not completely abolished by relief of pain, however, because contractions result in the transfer of 300 to 500 mL of blood from the uterus to the general circulation (Adams and Alexander, 1958; Hendricks and Quilligan 1958). Systolic blood and diastolic blood pressures transiently increase by 35 and 25 mm Hg, respectively, during labor (Robson, Dunlop et al., 1987). For these reasons, women who have cardiovascular compromise may experience decompensation with labor, especially during the second stage.

Postpartum Hemodynamic Changes

Pregnant women with cardiac disease are perhaps at greatest risk for pulmonary edema in the immediate postpartum period. The immediate puerperium is associated with an 80% increase in cardiac output within 10 to 15 minutes after vaginal delivery with local anesthesia compared with 60% with caudal anesthesia (Ueland and Metcalfe, 1975; Robson, Hunter et al., 1987). This immediate increase in cardiac output is due to release of venocaval obstruction by the gravid uterus, autotransfusion of uteroplacental blood, and rapid mobilization of extravascular fluid. All these changes result in increased venous return to the heart and increased stroke volume. Cardiac output returns to prelabor values 1 hour after delivery (Robson, Hunter et al., 1987). Cesarean section does not cause as dramatic a shift in hemodynamics, although there is still a 25% increase in cardiac output using the most controlled form of analgesia (epidural anesthesia without epinephrine) (Ueland et al., 1968; James et al., 1989).

Vaginal delivery is associated with a blood loss of approximately 500 mL, whereas cesarean section may cause a loss of 1000 mL (Ueland, 1976). The pregnant woman is protected from postpartum blood loss in part by the expansion of blood volume associated with pregnancy. In fact, there may be a slight rise in hematocrit values several days after an uncomplicated vaginal delivery because of the normal postpartum diuresis (Ueland, 1976).

M-mode echocardiographic studies have shown that left atrial dimensions increase 1 to 3 days postpartum, perhaps because of mobilization of excessive body fluids and increased venous return (Robson, Hunter et al., 1987). Atrial natriuretic levels also increase in the immediate postpartum period, which may stimulate diuresis and natriuresis in the early puerperium (Pouta et al., 1996).

Whereas left atrial dimensions and heart rate normalize within the first 10 days postpartum, left ventricular dimensions decrease gradually for 4 to 6 months. Cardiovascular measurements, such as stroke volume, cardiac output, and systemic vascular resistance, as measured by M-mode echocardiography, do not completely return to prepregnancy values by 12 weeks' postpartum and may continue to decrease for 24 weeks before stabilizing (Robson, Hunter et al., 1987; Capeless and Clapp, 1991). Therefore, the early postpartum period may not accurately reflect the nonpregnant state in studies of pregnancy-related hemodynamic changes.

KIDNEYS AND LOWER URINARY TRACT

The marked hemodynamic and hormonal changes of normal pregnancy are associated with striking alterations in renal physiology involving structure, dynamics, tubular function, and volume homeostasis.

Structure and Dynamics

Renal size and weight increase during pregnancy due to an increase in renal vascular and interstitial volume. Kidney length increases by approximately 1 cm (Bailey and Rolleston, 1971), and renal volume, as determined by computed nephrosonography, increases by approximately 30% (Christensen et al., 1989).

More dramatic, however, is dilatation of the urinary collecting system, which occurs in more than 80% of gravidas by mid-gestation (Rasmussen and Nielse, 1988). Caliceal and ureteral dilatation are more common on the right side than the left (Schulman and Herlinger, 1975; Hertzberg et al., 1993), and the degree of caliceal dilatation is more pronounced on the right than on the left (15 versus 5 mm) (Fried et al., 1983). The prominence of these changes on the right side may be due to dextrorotation of the pregnant uterus, the location of the right ovarian vein that crosses the ureter, and/or the protective "cushion" effect of the sigmoid colon on the left side. Ureteral dilatation is rarely present below the level of the pelvic brim, and sonographic visualization demonstrates tapering of the ureters as they cross the common iliac artery (MacNeily et al., 1991). Therefore, it has been suggested that obstruction or compression of the ureters by the enlarging uterus and ovarian vein plexus is the primary etiology for the physiologic hydronephrosis and hydroureter of pregnancy. Although obstruction plays a role in the physiologic pyelectasis of pregnancy, there has been no consistently documented associated increase in renal arterial resistance (Hertzberg et al., 1993). One reason for this may be the poor reproducibility of pulsed Doppler measurements in the maternal renal circulation due to high inter- and intraobserver variability (Nakai et al., 2002). Progesterone may play a concomitant role in ureteral smooth muscle relaxation, but there is no consensus on the influence of hormones on these anatomic alterations (Marchant, 1972).

The dilatation of the urinary collecting system has several important clinical consequences, including an increase in ascending urinary tract infection, perhaps related to urinary stasis; difficulty in interpreting radiologic examinations of the urinary tract; and interference with evaluation of glomerular and tubular function, because these tests require high urine flow rates. Renal volume returns to normal within the first week of delivery (Christensen et al., 1989), but hydronephrosis and hydroureter may persist for 3 to 4 months postpartum (Fried et al., 1983). This fact should be considered when radiologic or renal function studies on postpartum women are being interpreted.

Ureteral peristalsis does not change in pregnancy. However, ureteral tone progressively increases, possibly as a result of mechanical obstruction, and then returns to normal shortly after delivery (Sala and Rubi, 1967). Controversy exists with regard to changes in urinary bladder pressures and capacity. In one study, urinary bladder pressure doubled between the first and third trimesters of pregnancy, implying a decrease in bladder capacity (Iosif et al., 1980). Previous studies demonstrated a relatively hypotonic bladder, with decreased pressure and increased capacity near term (Youssef, 1956). Urethral length and intraurethral closure pressure in pregnancy have also been determined by urodynamic studies and have been found to increase by 20% (Iosif et al., 1980). The latter may counter the increase in bladder pressure in an attempt to reduce stress incontinence, which is more common in pregnancy occurring in 29% to 41% at term (Kristiansson et al., 2001).

Renal Function

Renal plasma flow, as estimated by para-aminohippurate clearance, increases by 60% to 80% over nonpregnant values by the middle of the second trimester and then falls to 50% above prepregnancy values in the third trimester (Dunlop, 1981). Renal plasma flow, like cardiac output, is significantly higher when the patient is in the left lateral recumbent position than when she is sitting, standing, or supine. This reflects maximal venous return in the left lateral position (Equimokhai et al., 1981; Davison and Dunlop, 1984).

Glomerular filtration rate (GFR) is estimated by determination of inulin, iohexol, or creatinine clearance. Creatinine clearance, although most commonly used, is the least precise of the determinations because creatinine is secreted by the tubules in addition to being cleared by the glomeruli. One can calculate creatinine clearance by dividing the total amount of urinary creatinine (in mg) by the duration of collection (in minutes). This value is then divided by the creatinine concentration in serum (in mg/mL). This yields a creatinine clearance in mL/min.

GFR begins to increase by as early as 6 weeks' gestation, with a peak of 50% over nonpregnant values by the end of the first trimester (Davison and Dunlop, 1984). Although there are few data on the measurement of GFR after 36 weeks' gestation, GFR does not appear to decrease at term. Creatinine clearance is thus moderately increased in pregnancy (110 to 150 mL/min). This rate has a circadian variation of 80% to 125%, with maximal creatinine excretion between 2 PM and 10 PM and lowest excretion rates between 2 AM and 10 AM (Kalousek et al., 1969).

The mechanisms behind the changes in renal hemodynamics are unclear, although study of pregnant rats would suggest that GFR rises secondary to vasodilatation of preglomerular and postglomerular resistance vessels without any alteration in glomerular capillary pressure (Baylis, 1987). This is further supported by the lack of continued increase in GFR after the first trimester of pregnancy despite decreasing serum albumin, implying independence from changes in oncotic pressure (Duvekot et al., 1993).

Because the increase in renal plasma flow is initially greater than the rise in GFR, the filtration fraction (GFR/renal plasma flow) decreases until the third trimester of pregnancy, when a fall in renal plasma flow results in the return of the filtration fraction to prepregnancy values of 1/5 (Davison and Dunlop, 1984). This alteration in filtration fraction parallels the change in mean arterial pressure described previously and may be related to circulating progesterone levels (Davison and Dunlop, 1980; Dunlop, 1981).

Filtration capacity, which is estimated by the maximal GFR in response to a vasodilator stimulus, appears to be intact in pregnancy, as documented by studies of amino acid administration in rats (Baylis, 1987) and protein loading in pregnant women (Ronco et al., 1988). As the resting GFR rises during pregnancy, the functional renal reserve (the difference between the filtration capacity and the resting GFR) decreases. One can therefore accurately assess renal function in pregnant patients with early renal disease by determining filtration capacity but not by functional renal reserve (Ronco et al., 1988).

The pregnancy-associated rise in GFR (which occurs without any concomitant increase in production of urea or creatinine) results in decreased serum creatinine and urea concentrations in pregnancy (Davison and Dunlop, 1980). Serum creatinine falls from prepregnancy values of 0.83 mg/dL to 0.73, 0.58, and 0.5 mg/dL in successive trimesters. Blood urea nitrogen decreases from 12 mg/dL in the nonpregnant state to 11, 9, and 10 mg/dL in the first, second, and third trimesters, respectively.

Renal Tubular Function

Sodium

Several factors promote sodium excretion in pregnancy. There is an increase in the filtered load of sodium from approximately 20,000 mEq/day to 30,000 mEq/day as a result of the 50% rise in GFR. Hormones that favor sodium excretion include the following:

1. Progesterone, a competitive inhibitor of aldosterone (Barron and Lindheimer, 1984)
2. Vasodilatory prostaglandins (Davison and Dunlop, 1984)
3. Atrial natriuretic factor (although increased pregnancy-related production of atrial natriuretic factor has not been universally demonstrated) (Bond et al., 1989; Marlettini et al., 1991)

Despite these forces, there is a cumulative *retention* of approximately 950 mg of sodium during pregnancy. This is distributed between the maternal intravascular and interstitial compartments, the fetus, and the placenta (Hytten and Leitch, 1971). The net reabsorption of sodium is one of the most remarkable adaptations of renal tubular function to pregnancy.

Factors that promote this sodium *reabsorption* include the increased production and secretion of aldosterone, deoxycorti-

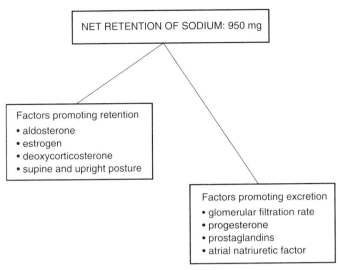

FIGURE 8-3 ■ Factors influencing the regulation of sodium excretion in pregnancy.

costerone, and estrogen (Barron and Lindheimer, 1984) (Fig. 8-3). These hormones may be regulated, in part, by the rise in plasma progesterone and vasodilatory prostaglandins, but they are also mediated by stimulation of the renin-angiotensin system. All components of the renin-angiotensin-aldosterone system increase in the first trimester of pregnancy and peak at 30 to 32 weeks' gestation (Carbillon et al., 2000). Hepatic renin substrate is stimulated by estrogens and results in elevated renal production of renin. Renin stimulates increased conversion of angiotensinogen to angiotensins I and II. Sodium retention is also favored by postural changes in pregnancy; the supine and upright positions are associated with a marked decrease in sodium excretion (Chesley and Sloan, 1964).

Potassium

Although the pregnancy-associated increase in plasma aldosterone would favor potassium excretion, a net *retention* of 300 to 350 mEq of potassium actually occurs. Increased kaliuresis may be prevented by the influence of progesterone on renal potassium excretion (Lindheimer et al., 1987). Because potassium reabsorption from the distal tubule and Henle's loop decreases with pregnancy, it has been deduced that a significant increase in proximal tubular reabsorption occurs (Garland and Green, 1982).

Calcium

Urinary calcium excretion increases as a result of increased calcium clearance (Roelofsen et al., 1988). This is balanced by increased absorption of calcium from the small intestine, and therefore serum ionic (unbound) calcium levels remain stable. Total calcium levels fall in pregnancy from 4.75 mEq/liter in the first trimester to 4.3 mEq/liter at term because of a decrease in plasma albumin (Pitkin et al., 1979). There is a rise in calcitriol in early pregnancy, paralleled by suppression of the parathyroid hormone and increase in renal tubular phosphorus reabsorption (Weiss et al., 1998). This increase in calcitriol promotes reabsorption of calcium and phosphorus from the intestine and may facilitate bone mineralization in the fetus.

Glucose

Glucose excretion increases in pregnant women 10-fold to 100-fold over nonpregnant values of 100 mg/day (Davison and Hytten, 1975). This glycosuria, which occurs despite increased plasma insulin and decreased plasma glucose levels, is due to impaired collecting tubule and Henle's loop reabsorption of the 5% of the filtered glucose that normally escapes proximal convoluted tubular reabsorption (Bishop and Green, 1981). The clinical significance of this is that glycosuria cannot be accurately used to monitor pregnant women with diabetes mellitus. In addition, increased glycosuria may predispose these patients to urinary tract infections.

Uric Acid

Plasma uric acid levels decrease by 25% as early as 8 weeks' gestation, reaching a nadir of 2 to 3 mg/dL at 24 weeks' gestation, and then increase toward nonpregnant levels at term (Lind et al., 1984). This may be due to an alteration in the fractional clearance of uric acid (uric acid clearance/GFR), with a net decrease in renal tubular uric acid reabsorption (Dunlop and Davison, 1977). Conditions that lead to volume contraction, such as preeclampsia, may be associated with decreased uric acid clearance and increased plasma levels.

Amino Acids

The fractional excretion of alanine, glycine, histidine, serine, and threonine increases in pregnancy (Hytten and Cheyne, 1972). Cystine, leucine, lysine, phenylalanine, taurine, and tyrosine excretion increases early in pregnancy but then decreases in the second half of gestation. The excretion of arginine, asparagine, glutamic acid, isoleucine, methionine, and ornithine does not change. The mechanism of this selective amino aciduria is unknown. It is unclear whether renal excretion of albumin decreases (Misiani et al., 1991) or remains stable (Wright et al., 1987) in normal pregnancy. Urinary protein excretion does not normally exceed 300 mg/ 24 hours.

Volume Homeostasis

Body weight increases by an average of 30 to 35 pounds in pregnancy (Abrams and Laros, 1986). Two thirds of this gain may be accounted for by an increase in total body water, with 6 to 7 liters gained in the extracellular space and approximately 2 liters gained in the intracellular space. Plasma volume expansion, as outlined previously, accounts for 25% of the increase in extracellular water, with the rest of the increment appearing as interstitial fluid (Hytten, 1981).

As water is retained, plasma sodium and urea levels fall slightly, from 140.3 ± 1.7 to 136.6 ± 1.5 mM/liter and from 4.9 ± 0.9 to 2.9 ± 0.5 mM/liter, respectively (Davison et al., 1981). By 4 weeks after conception, plasma osmolality has decreased by 10 mOsm/kg, from 289 to 280.9. Because water deprivation in pregnant women leads to an appropriate increase in vasopressin and urine osmolality and water loading results in a proportional decrease, it appears that the osmoregulation system is functioning normally but is "reset" at a lower threshold (Davison et al., 1984, 1988). Further evidence to support this conclusion is that the osmotic threshold for thirst is decreased by 10 mOsm/kg in pregnancy (Lindheimer et al., 1989). The mechanism for this readjustment of the osmoregulatory system is unclear but may involve placental secretion of human chorionic gonadotropin (Davison et al., 1988).

REFERENCES

Abrams BF, Laros RK Jr: Prepregnancy weight, weight gain, and birth weight. Am J Obstet Gynecol **154:**503, 1986.

Adams JQ, Alexander AM: Alterations in cardiovascular physiology during labor. Obstet Gynecol **12:**542, 1958.

Awe RJ, Nicotra MB, Newsom TD, et al: Arterial oxygenation and alveolar-arterial gradients in term pregnancy. Obstet Gynecol **53:**182, 1979.

Bader RA, Bader MG, Rose DJ, et al: Hemodynamics at rest and during exercise in normal pregnancy as studied by cardiac catheterization. J Clin Invest **34:**1524, 1955.

Bailey RR, Rolleston GLI: Kidney length and ureteric dilatation in the puerperium. J Obstet Gynaecol Br Commonw **78:**55, 1971.

Barron WM, Lindheimer MD: Renal sodium and water handling in pregnancy. Obstet Gynecol Annu **13:**35, 1984.

Barwin BN, Roddie IC: Venous distensibility during pregnancy determined by graded venous congestion. Am J Obstet Gynecol **125:**921, 1976.

Baylis C: The determinants of renal hemodynamics in pregnancy. Am J Kidney Dis **9:**260, 1987.

Bille-Brahe NE, Rorth M: Red cell 2,3,-diphosphoglycerate in pregnancy. Acta Obstet Gynaecol Scand **58:**19, 1979.

Bishop JHV, Green R: Effects of pregnancy on glucose reabsorption by the proximal convoluted tubule in the rat. J Physiol (Lond) **319:**271, 1981.

Bond AL, August P, Druzin ML, et al: Atrial natriuretic factor in normal and hypertensive pregnancy. Am J Obstet Gynecol **160:**1112, 1989.

Burg J, Dodek A, Kloster F, et al: Alterations of systolic time intervals during pregnancy. Circulation **49:**560, 1974.

Capeless EL, Clapp JF: Cardiovascular changes in early phase of pregnancy. Am J Obstet Gynecol **161:**1449, 1989.

Capeless EL, Clapp JF: When do cardiovascular parameters return to their preconception values? Am J Obstet Gynecol **165:**883, 1991.

Carbillon L, Uzasn M, Uzan S: Pregnancy, vascular tone, and maternal hemodynamics: A crucial adaptation. Obstet Gynecol Surv **55:**574, 2000.

Chesley LC, Sloan DM: The effect of posture on renal function in late pregnancy. Am J Obstet Gynecol **89:**754, 1964.

Christensen T, Klebe JG, Bertelsen V, et al: Changes in renal volume during normal pregnancy. Acta Obstet Gynaecol Scand **68:**541, 1989.

Churchill D, Beevers DG: Differences between office and 24-hour ambulatory blood pressure measurement during pregnancy. Obstet Gynecol **88:**455, 1996.

Clark S, Hofemyr JG, Coats AJ, et al: Ambulatory blood pressure monitoring in pregnancy: Validation of the TM-420 monitor. Obstet Gynecol **77:**152, 1991.

Clark SL, Cotton DB, Lee W, et al: Central hemodynamic assessment of normal term pregnancy. Am J Obstet Gynecol **161:**1439, 1989.

Cutforth R, MacDonald CB: Heart sounds during normal pregnancy. Am Heart J **71:**741, 1966.

Davison JM, Dunlop W: Renal hemodynamics and tubular function in normal human pregnancy. Kidney Int **18:**152, 1980.

Davison JM, Dunlop W: Changes in renal hemodynamics and tubular function induced by normal human pregnancy. Semin Nephrol **4:**198, 1984.

Davison JM, Gilmore EA, Durr J, et al: Altered osmotic thresholds for vasopressin secretion and thirst in human pregnancy. Am J Physiol **246:**F105, 1984.

Davison JM, Hytten FE: The effect of pregnancy on the renal handling of glucose. J Obstet Gynaecol Br Commonw **82:**374, 1975.

Davison JM, Shiells EA, Philips PR, et al: Serial evaluation of vasopressin and thirst in human pregnancy: Role of human chorionic gonadotropin on the osmoregulatory changes of gestation. J Clin Invest **81:**798, 1988.

Davison JM, Vallotton MB, Lindheimer MD: Plasma osmolality and urinary concentration and dilution during and after pregnancy. Br J Obstet Gynaecol **88:**472, 1981.

Duffus GM, MacGillivaray I, Dennis KJ: The relationship between baby weight and changes in maternal weight, total body water, plasma volume, electrolytes, and proteins and urinary oestriol excretion. J Obstet Gynaecol Br Commonw **78:**97, 1971.

Duvekot JJ, Cheriex EC, Pieters FAA, et al: Early pregnancy changes in hemodynamics and volume homeostasis are consecutive adjustments triggered by a primary fall in systemic vascular tone. Am J Obstet Gynecol **169:**1382, 1993.

Duvekot JJ, Cheriex EC, Pieters FAA, et al: Maternal volume homeostasis in early pregnancy in relation to fetal growth restriction. Obstet Gynecol **85:**361, 1995.

Duvekot JJ, Pieters LLH: Maternal cardiovascular hemodynamic adaptation to pregnancy. Obstet Gynecol Surv **49:**S1, 1994.

Dunlop W: Serial changes in renal hemodynamics during normal human pregnancy. Br J Obstet Gynaecol **88:**1, 1981.

Dunlop W, Davison JM: The effect of normal pregnancy upon the renal handling of uric acid. Br J Obstet Gynaecol **84:**13, 1977.

Easterling TR, Benedetti TJ, Carlson KL, et al: Measurement of cardiac output in pregnancy by thermodilution and impedance techniques. Br J Obstet Gynaecol **96:**67, 1989.

Easterling TR, Benedetti TJ, Schmucker BC, et al: Maternal hemodynamics in normal and preeclamptic pregnancies: A longitudinal study. Obstet Gynecol **76:**1061, 1990a.

Easterling TR, Carlson KL, Schmucker BC, et al: Measurement of cardiac output in pregnancy by Doppler technique. Am J Perinatol **7:**220, 1990b.

Easterling TR, Watts H, Schmucker BC, et al: Measurement of cardiac output during pregnancy: Validation of Doppler technique and clinical observations in preeclampsia. Obstet Gynecol **69:**845, 1987.

Ekholm EMK, Erkkola RU: Autonomic cardiovascular control in pregnancy. Eur J Obstet Gynecol Reprod Biol **64:**29, 1996.

Equimokhai M, Davison JM, Philips PR, et al: Non-postural serial changes in renal function during the third trimester of normal human pregnancy. Br J Obstet Gynaecol **88:**465, 1981.

Fawer R, Dettling A, Weihs D, et al: Effect of the menstrual cycle, oral contraception and pregnancy on forearm blood flow, venous distensibility and clotting factors. Eur J Clin Pharmacol **13:**251, 1978.

Frederiksen MC: Physiologic changes in pregnancy and their effect on drug disposition. Semin Perinatol **25:**120, 2001.

Fried A, Woodring JH, Thompson TJ: Hydronephrosis of pregnancy. J Ultrasound Med **2:**255, 1983.

Gant NF, Worley RJ: Measurement of uteroplacental blood flow in the human. *In* Rosenfeld CR (ed): The Uterine Circulation. Ithaca, Perinatology Press, 1989, p. 53.

Garland HO, Green R: Micropuncture study of changes in glomerular filtration and ion and water handling in the rat kidney during pregnancy. J Physiol (Lond) **329:**389, 1982.

Gerber JG, Payne HA, Murphy RC, et al: Prostacyclin produced by the pregnant uterus in the dog may act as a circulating vasodepressor substance. J Clin Invest **67:**632, 1981.

Gilson GJ, Samaan S, Crawford MH, et al: Changes in hemodynamics, ventricular remodeling, and ventricular contractility during normal pregnancy: A longitudinal study. Obstet Gynecol **89:**957, 1997.

Greiss FC, Anderson SG: Effect of ovarian hormones on the uterine vascular bed. Am J Obstet Gynecol **107:**829, 1970.

Guzman C, Caplan R: Cardiorespiratory response to exercise during pregnancy. Am J Obstet Gynecol **108:**600, 1970.

Halligan A, O'Brien E, O'Malley K, et al: Twenty four hour ambulatory blood pressure measurement in a primigravid population. J Hypertens **11:**869, 1993.

Hendricks CH, Quilligan EJ: Cardiac output during labor. Am J Obstet Gynecol **76:**969, 1958.

Hermida RC, Auala DE, Mojon A, et al: Blood pressure patterns in normal pregnancy, gestational hypertension, and preeclampsia. Hypertension **36:**149, 2000.

Hertzberg BS, Carroll BA, Bowie JD, et al: Doppler USS assessment of maternal kidneys: Analysis of intrarenal resistivity indexes in normal pregnancy and physiologic pelvocaliectasis. Radiology **186:**689, 1993.

Hobel CJ, Castro L, Rosen D, et al: The effect of thigh-length support stockings on the hemodynamic response to ambulation in pregnancy. Am J Obstet Gynecol **174:**1734, 1996.

Holmes F: Incidence of the supine hypotensive syndrome in late pregnancy. J Obstet Gynaecol Br Emp **67:**254, 1960.

Hytten FE: Weight gain in pregnancy. *In* Hytten F, Chamberlain G (eds): Clinical Physiology in Obstetrics. Oxford, Blackwell Scientific Publications, 1981.

Hytten FE, Cheyne GA: The aminoaciduria of pregnancy. J Obstet Gynaecol Br Commonw **79:**424, 1972.

Hytten FE, Leitch I: The Physiology of Human Pregnancy, 2nd ed. Oxford, Blackwell Scientific Publications, 1971.

Ihlen H, Amlie JP, Dale J, et al: Determination of cardiac output by Doppler echocardiography. Br Heart J **54**:51, 1984.

Iosif S, Ingermarsson I, Ulmsten U: Urodynamics studies in normal pregnancy and in puerperium. Am J Obstet Gynecol **137**:696, 1980.

James CF, Banner T, Caton D: Cardiac output in women undergoing cesarean section with epidural or general anesthesia. Am J Obstet Gynecol **160**:1178, 1989.

Jepson JH: Endocrine control of maternal and fetal erythropoiesis. Can Med Assoc J **98**:884, 1968.

Johenning AR, Barron WM: Indirect blood pressure measurement in pregnancy: Korotkoff phase 4 versus phase 5. Am J Obstet Gynecol **167**:577, 1992.

Kalousek G, Hlavecek C, Nedoss B, et al: Circadian rhythms of creatinine and electrolyte excretion in healthy pregnant women. Am J Obstet Gynecol **103**:856, 1969.

Katz M, Sokal MM: Skin perfusion in pregnancy. Am J Obstet Gynecol **137**:30, 1980.

Kirshon B, Lee W, Cotton DB, et al: Indirect blood pressure monitoring in the obstetric patient. Obstet Gynecol **70**:799, 1987.

Koller O: The clinical significance of hemodilution during pregnancy. Obstet Gynecol Surv **37**:649, 1982.

Kristiansson P, Samuelsson E, Von Schoultz B, et al: Reproductive hormones and stress urinary incontinence in pregnancy. Act Obstet Gynaecol Scand **80**:1125, 2001.

Kulpa PJ, White BM, Visscher R: Aerobic exercise in pregnancy. Am J Obstet Gynecol **156**:1395, 1987.

Lard-Meeter K, van de Ley G, Bom T, et al: Cardiocirculatory adjustments during pregnancy: An echocardiographic study. Clin Cardiol **49**:560, 1979.

Limacher MC, Ware JA, O'Meara ME, et al: Tricuspid regurgitation during pregnancy: Two-dimensional and pulsed Doppler echocardiographic observations. Am J Cardiol **55**:1059, 1985.

Lind T, Godfrey KA, Otun H: Changes in serum uric acid concentration during normal pregnancy. Br J Obstet Gynaecol **91**:128, 1984.

Lindheimer MD, Barron WM, Davison JM: Osmoregulation of thirst and vasopressin release in pregnancy. Am J Physiol **257**:F59, 1989.

Lindheimer MD, Richardson DA, Ehrlich EN, et al: Potassium homeostasis in pregnancy. J Reprod Med **32**:517, 1987.

Lund CJ, Donovan JC: Blood volume during pregnancy. Am J Obstet Gynecol **98**:393, 1967.

MacNeily AE, Goldenberg SL, Allen GJJ, et al: Sonographic visualization of the ureter in pregnancy. J Urol **146**:298, 1991.

Manchester B, Loube SD: The velocity of blood flow in normal pregnant women. Am Heart J **32**:215, 1946.

Marazita AJD: The action of hormones on varicose veins in pregnancy. Med Rec **159**:422, 1946.

Marchant DJ: Effects of pregnancy and progestational agents on the urinary tract. Am J Obstet Gynecol **112**:487, 1972.

Marlettini MG, Cassani A, Boschi S, et al: Plasma concentrations of atrial natriuretic factor in normal pregnancy and early puerperium. Clin Exp Hypertens A **13**:1305, 1991.

Masaki DI, Greenspoon JS, Ouzounizn JG: Measurement of cardiac output by thoracic electrical bioimpedance and thermodilution. Am J Obstet Gynecol **161**:680, 1989.

Mashini IS, Albazzaz SJ, Fadel HE, et al: Serial noninvasive evaluation of cardiovascular hemodynamics during pregnancy. Am J Obstet Gynecol **156**:1208, 1987.

McLennan FM, Haites NE, Rawles JM: Stroke and minute distance in pregnancy: A longitudinal study using Doppler ultrasound. Br J Obstet Gynaecol **94**:499, 1987.

Milne JA, Howie AD, Pack AL: Dyspnoea during normal pregnancy. Br J Obstet Gynaecol **85**:260, 1978.

Milsom I, Forssman L, Sivertsson R, et al: Measurement of cardiac stroke volume by impedance cardiography in the last trimester of pregnancy. Acta Obstet Gynaecol Scand **62**:473, 1983.

Misiani R, Marchesi D, Tiraboschi G, et al: Urinary albumin excretion in normal pregnancy and pregnancy-induced hypertension. Nephron **59**:416, 1991.

Nakai A, Miyake H, Oya A, et al: Reproducibility of pulsed Doppler measurements of the maternal renal circulation in normal pregnancies and those with pregnancy-induced hypertension. Ultrasound Obstet Gynecol **19**:598, 2002.

Pieters LLH, Verkeste CM, Saxena PR, et al: Relationship between maternal hemodynamics and hematocrit and hemodynamic effects of isovolemic hemodilution and hemoconcentration in the awake late-pregnant guinea pig. Pediatr Res **21**:584, 1987.

Pitkin RM, Reynolds WA, Williams GA, et al: Calcium metabolism in pregnancy: A longitudinal study. Am J Obstet Gynecol **133**:781, 1979.

Pouta AM, Raasanen JP, Airaksinen KEJ, et al: Changes in maternal heart dimensions and plasma atrial natriuretic peptide levels in the early puerperium of normal and pre-eclamptic pregnancies. Br J Obstet Gynaecol **103**:988, 1996.

Pritchard JA: Changes in the blood volume during pregnancy and delivery. Anesthesiology **26**:393, 1965a.

Pritchard JA: Blood volume changes in pregnancy and the puerperiums. IV. Anemia associated with hydatidiform mole. Am J Obstet Gynecol **91**:621, 1965b.

Rasmussen PE, Nielse FR: Hydronephrosis during pregnancy: A literature survey. Eur J Obstet Gynaecol Reprod Biol **27**:249, 1988.

Robson SC, Dunlop W, Boys RJ, et al: Cardiac output during labor. Br Med J **295**:1169, 1987.

Robson SC, Hunter S, Boys RJ, et al: Serial study of factors influencing changes in cardiac output during human pregnancy. Am J Physiol **256**:H1060, 1989.

Robson SC, Hunter S, Moore M, et al: Haemodynamic changes during the puerperium: A Doppler and M-mode echocardiographic study. Br J Obstet Gynaecol **94**:1028, 1987.

Roelofsen JMT, Berkel GM, Uttendorfsky OT, et al: Urinary excretion rates of calcium and magnesium in normal and complicated pregnancies. Eur J Obstet Gynaecol Reprod Biol **27**:227, 1988.

Ronco C, Brendolan A, Bragantini L, et al: Renal functional reserve in pregnancy. Nephrol Dial Transplant **2**:157, 1988.

Rovinsky JJ, Jaffin H: Cardiovascular hemodynamics in pregnancy. I. Blood and plasma volumes in multiple pregnancy. Am J Obstet Gynecol **93**:1, 1965.

Rubler S, Damani P, Pinto E: Cardiac size and performance during pregnancy estimated with echocardiography. Am J Cardiol **49**:534, 1977.

Rubler S, Hammer N, Schneebaum R: Systolic time intervals in pregnancy and the postpartum period. Am Heart J **86**:182, 1972.

Sala NL, Rubi RA: Ureteral function in pregnant women. II. Ureteral contractility during normal pregnancy. Am J Obstet Gynecol **99**:228, 1967.

Schulman A, Herlinger H: Urinary tract dilatation in pregnancy. Br J Radiol **48**:638, 1975.

Shennan AH, Kissane J, de Sweit M: Validation of the Spacelabs 90207 ambulatory blood pressure monitor for use in pregnancy. Br J Obstet Gynaecol **100**:904, 1993.

Spaanderman MEA, Willekes C, Hoeks APG, et al: The effect of pregnancy on the compliance of large arteries and veins in healthy parous control subjects and women with a history of preeclampsia. Am J Obstet Gynecol **183**:1278, 2000.

Stein PK, Hagley MT, Cole PL, et al: Changes in 24-hour heart rate variability during normal pregnancy. Am J Obstet Gynecol **180**:978, 1999.

Thompson JA, Hayes PM, Sagar KB, et al: Echocardiographic left ventricular mass to differentiate chronic hypertension from preeclampsia during pregnancy. Am J Obstet Gynecol **155**:994, 1986.

Turner AF: The chest radiograph during pregnancy. Clin Obstet Gynecol **18**:65, 1975.

Ueland K: Maternal cardiovascular dynamics. VII. Intrapartum blood volume changes. Am J Obstet Gynecol **126**:671, 1976.

Ueland K, Akamatsu TJ, Eng M, et al: Maternal cardiovascular hemodynamics. I. Cesarean section under subarachnoid block anesthesia. Am J Obstet Gynecol **100**:42, 1968.

Ueland K, Hansen JM: Maternal cardiovascular hemodynamics. III. Labor and delivery under local and caudal anesthesia. Am J Obstet Gynecol **103**:8, 1969.

Ueland K, Metcalfe J: Circulatory changes in pregnancy. Clin Obstet Gynecol **18**:41, 1975.

Ueland K, Novy M, Peterson E, et al: Maternal cardiovascular dynamics. IV. The influence of gestational age on the maternal cardiovascular response to posture and exercise. Am J Obstet Gynecol **104**:856, 1969.

Vered Z, Poler SM, Gibson P, et al: Noninvasive detection of the morphologic and hemodynamic changes during normal pregnancy. Clin Cardiol **14**:327, 1991.

Walker SP, Permezel M, Brennecke SP, et al: Blood pressure in late pregnancy and work outside the home. Obstet Gynecol **97**:361, 2001.

Walters WAW, MacGregor WG, Hills M: Cardiac output at rest during pregnancy and the puerperium. Clin Sci (Colch) **30**:1, 1966.

Weiss M, Eisenstein Z, Ramot Y, et al: Renal reabsorption of inorganic phosphorus in pregnancy in relation to the calciotropic hormones. Br J Obstet Gynaecol **105**:195, 1998.

Wickman K, Ryden G, Wickman G: The influence of different positions and Korotkoff sounds on the blood pressure measurements in pregnancy. Acta Obstet Gynaecol Scand **118** (Suppl):25, 1984.

Wilson M, Morganti AA, Zervoudakis I, et al: Blood pressure, the renin-aldosterone system and sex steroids throughout normal pregnancy. Am J Med **68:**97, 1980.

Wolfe LA, Hall P, Webb KA: Prescription of aerobic exercise during pregnancy. Sports Med **8:**273, 1989.

Wright A, Steeke P, Bennet JR, et al: The urinary excretion of albumin in normal pregnancy. Br J Obstet Gynaecol **94:**408, 1987.

Youssef AF: Cystometric studies in gynecology and obstetrics. Obstet Gynecol **8:**181, 1956.

Chapter 9
ENDOCRINOLOGY OF PREGNANCY

James H. Liu, MD

The concept of the fetus, the placenta, and the mother as a functional unit originated in the 1950s. More recent is the recognition that the placenta itself is an endocrine organ capable of synthesizing virtually every hormone, growth factor, and cytokine thus far identified. The premise that the placenta, composed chiefly of two cell types—syncytiotrophoblast and cytotrophoblast—can synthesize and secrete a vast array of active substances could not even be contemplated until it was recognized in the 1970s that a single cell can, in fact, synthesize more than a single product. This concept is even more remarkable because the placenta has no neural connections to either the mother or the fetus and is discarded after childbirth. Yet the placenta, an integral part of the fetal–placental–maternal unit, can be viewed as the most amazing endocrine organ of all. In this chapter we detail the hormonal interactions of the fetal–placental–maternal unit and the neuroendocrine and metabolic changes that occur in the mother and in the fetus during pregnancy and at parturition.

IMPLANTATION

The process of embryo implantation takes place between 6 and 7 days after ovulation (Hertig et al., 1956; O'Rahilly, 1973). More contemporary studies suggest that in most successful human pregnancies, the embryo implants 8 to 10 days after ovulation (Wilcox et al., 1999). This event involves a series of complex steps: (1) orientation of the blastocyst with respect to the endometrial surface; (2) initial adhesion of the blastocyst to endometrium; (3) meeting of the microvilli on the surface of trophoblast with pinopodes, microprotrusions from the apical end of the uterine epithelium; (4) trophoblastic migration through the endometrial surface epithelium; (5) embryonic invasion with localized disruption of the endometrial capillary beds; and (6) remodeling of the capillary bed and formation of trophoblastic lacunae (Edelman and Crossin, 1991, Norwitz et al., 2001). By day 10, the blastocyst is completely encased within the uterine stromal tissue. Although recent work with *in vitro* fertilization (IVF)–related techniques such as embryo donation and frozen embryo transfer has contributed significantly to our understanding of this process, much of our present physiologic information is derived from other mammalian species because human tissue experiments are limited by ethical constraints. This implantation process has been reviewed recently by Norwitz et al. (2001).

Results from assisted reproductive technologies suggest a window for implantation in which the endometrium is "receptive" to embryo implantation. In this concept, synchronization between embryonic and uterine receptivity is required for successful nidation. IVF-generated data suggest that implantation is successful usually after embryo transfer between days 15 and 19 of the menstrual cycle (Bergh and Navot, 1992). If the embryo arrives outside this window or is in a different location, embryo demise or the likelihood of ectopic pregnancy increases. Although the process of embryo implantation requires a receptive endometrium, the process is not exclusive to the endometrium because advanced ectopic (e.g., abdominal) pregnancies have been reported with a viable fetus.

During a typical IVF cycle, embryos are transferred to the uterus on day 3 or day 5 after oocyte retrieval and fertilization. By day 3 of embryo culture, embryo development is at the six- to eight-cell stage. Embryos placed back into the uterus at this stage remain unattached to the endometrium and continue developing to the blastocyst stage, "hatch" or escape from the zona pellucida, and implant by day 7. In IVF programs that transfer on day 3, the chance of each embryo implanting is approximately 12% to 25%. Thus, to achieve a reasonable chance of overall pregnancy, most women undergoing IVF will have three to four good quality embryos placed back into the uterus to achieve clinical pregnancy rates of 35% to 45% per IVF cycle. Because the implantation potential for each embryo cannot be determined by embryo morphology alone, this procedure can result in higher order multiple pregnancies such as twins, triplets, or occasionally quadruplets. In 1997, the use of assisted reproductive technologies accounted for more than 40% of all triplets born in the United States (MMWR, 2000).

Some IVF programs have the capability to culture embryos up to 5 days. Embryos at this stage are at the blastocyst or morula stage. The overall implantation rate for each good quality embryo at this stage is between 30% and 50% per embryo. Thus, to achieve a reasonable chance of pregnancy, most women will have only two good quality blastocyst-staged embryos transferred to the uterus, reducing the changes of higher order multiple pregnancies. A recent study from population-based control data indicate that the use of assisted reproductive technology accounts for a disproportionate number of low-birth-weight and very-low-birth-weight infants because of multiple pregnancies and in part because of higher rates of low birth weight among singleton infants conceived with assisted reproductive technologies (Schieve et al., 2002).

The cellular differentiation and remodeling of the endometrium induced by sequential exposure to estradiol and progesterone may play a major role in endometrial receptivity. The beginning of endometrial receptivity coincides with the downregulation of progesterone and estrogen receptors induced by the corpus luteum production of progesterone. It was thought that this process required tight regulation such that the morphologic development of microvilli (pinopodes) in glandular epithelium (Rogers et al., 1989) and increased angiogenesis were required for successful embryo nidation. Experience with IVF techniques, however, suggests marked differences in endometrial morphology in women at the same time of the cycle or between the same women from cycle to cycle (Rogers, 1993). Nevertheless, the current concept is that developmental expression of factors by the blastocyst and the endometrium allows cell-to-cell communications so that successful nidation can take place.

Reviews of embryo implantation have identified an increasing number of factors such as integrins, mucins, cytokines, proteinases, and glycoproteins localized to either the embryo or the endometrium during the window of implantation (Lindhard et al., 2002). Much of the information is derived from animal studies, and its application to human implantation is primarily circumstantial. Table 9-1 lists several of the factors believed to mediate embryo implantation.

Ultrasound studies of early human gestation show that most implantation sites are localized to the upper two thirds of the uterus and are closer to the side of the corpus luteum (Kawakami et al., 1993). A growing body of literature suggests that the *integrins*, a class of adhesion molecules, are involved in implantation. Integrins are also essential components of the extracellular matrix and function as receptors that anchor extracellular adhesion proteins to cytoskeletal components (Hynes, 1992).

Integrins are heterodimers composed of different α subunits and a common β subunit. At present, the integrin receptor family is composed of at least 14 distinct α subunits and more than 9 β subunits (Sueoka et al., 1997), making up to 20 integrin heterodimers (Lessey, 1998). Integrins are cell-surface receptors for fibrinogen, fibronectin, collagen, and laminin. These receptors recognize a common amino acid tripeptide, Arg-Gly-Asp (RGD), present in extracellular matrix proteins, such as fibronectin. Integrins have been localized to sperm, oocyte, blastocyst, and endometrium.

One particular integrin, $\alpha_v\beta_3$, is expressed on endometrial cells after day 19 of the menstrual cycle. This integrin appears to be a marker for the implantation window. $\alpha_v\beta_3$ is also localized to trophoblast cells, suggesting that this integrin may participate in cell-to-cell interactions between the trophoblast

and endometrium acting through a common bridging ligand. It is postulated that after hatching, the blastocyst, through its trophoblastic integrin receptors, attaches to the endometrial surface. Mouse primary trophoblast cells appear to interact with the fibronectin exclusively through the RGD recognition site (Armant et al., 1986). The appearance of the β_3 integrin subunit is dependent on the downregulation of progesterone and estrogen receptors in the endometrial glands (Lessey et al., 1996). Subsequent changes in trophoblast adhesive and migratory behavior appear to stem from alterations in the expression of various integrin receptors. Antibodies to α_v or β-integrins inhibit the attachment activity of intact blastocysts (Schultz and Armant, 1995).

The role of integrins in trophoblast migration is not clear, but the expression of β_1-integrins appears to promote this latter phenomenon (Ruoslahti and Pierschbacher, 1987). Work in the rhesus monkey suggests that the trophoblast migrates into the endometrium directly beneath the implantation site, invading small arterioles but not veins (Enders and King, 1991).

Controlled invasion of the maternal vascular system by the trophoblast is necessary for the establishment of the hemochorial placenta. Studies with human placental villous explants suggest that chorionic villous cytotrophoblasts can differentiate along two distinct pathways: by fusing to form the syncytiotrophoblast layer or as extravillous trophoblasts that have the potential to invade the inner basalis layer of endometrium and the myometrium to reach the spiral arteries. Once trophoblasts have breached the endometrial blood vessels, decidualized stromal cells are believed to promote endometrial hemostasis by release of tissue factor and thrombin generation (Lockwood et al., 1997).

Three growth factors have been implicated in the regulation of this process. Epidermal growth factor (EGF) (Bass et al., 1994) and interleukin-1β (Librach et al., 1994) stimulate invasion by the extravillous trophoblast, whereas transforming growth factor-β appears to inhibit the differentiation toward the invasive phenotype and serves to limit the invasiveness of extravillous trophoblast and to induce syncytium formation (Graham et al., 1992). The process of invasion appears to peak by 12 weeks' gestation (Aplin, 1991). These trophoblasts proceed to form the chorionic villi, the functional units of the placenta, consisting of a central core of loose connective tissue and abundant capillaries connecting it with the fetal circulation. Around this core are the outer syncytiotrophoblast layer

TABLE 9-1. GROWTH FACTORS AND PROTEINS THAT PLAY A SIGNIFICANT ROLE DURING EMBRYO IMPLANTATION

Factors	Putative Role	Reference
Leukemia inhibitory factor	Cytokine involved in implantation	Cullinan et al., 1996
Integrins	Cell-to-cell interactions	Sueoka et al., 1997
Transforming growth factor-β	Inhibits trophoblast invasion, stimulates syncytium formation	Graham et al., 1992
Epidermal growth factor	Mediates trophoblast invasion	Bass et al., 1994
Interleukin-1β	Mediates trophoblast invasion	Librach et al., 1994
Interleukin-10	Mediates implantation	Stewart et al., 1997
Matrix metalloproteinases	Mediates implantation	Stewart et al., 1997
Vascular endothelial growth factor	Mediates implantation	Stewart et al., 1997

and the inner layer of cytotrophoblast. In general, both cytotrophoblast and syncytiotrophoblast produce peptide hormones, whereas the syncytiotrophoblast produces all of the steroid hormones.

HUMAN CHORIONIC GONADOTROPIN PRODUCTION

Human chorionic gonadotropin (hCG) is one of the earliest products of the cells forming the embryo and should be viewed as one of the first embryonic signals elaborated by the embryo even before implantation (Hay and Lopata, 1988). This glycoprotein is a heterodimer (36 to 40 kDa). It is composed of a 92-amino acid α subunit that is homologous to thyroid-stimulating hormone, luteinizing hormone (LH), and follicle-stimulating hormone and a 145-amino acid β subunit that is similar to LH. The α subunit gene for hCG has been localized to chromosome 6; the β subunit gene is located on chromosome 19, fairly close to the LH-β gene. In contrast to LH, the presence of sialic acid residues on hCG-β accounts for its prolonged half-life in the circulation. After implantation, hCG is produced principally by the syncytiotrophoblast layer of the chorionic villus and is secreted into the intervillous space. Cytotrophoblasts also seem able to produce hCG.

On a clinical basis, hCG can be detected in either the serum or urine 7 to 8 days before expected menses and is the earliest biochemical marker for pregnancy (Fig. 9-1). In studies during IVF cycles in which embryos were transferred 2 days after fertilization, β-hCG messenger RNA was detected as early as the eight-cell stage, whereas intact hCG was not detectable until 8 days after egg retrieval. The increase in hCG levels between days 5 and 9 after ovum collection is principally due to free β-hCG production, whereas by day 22 most of the circulating hCG is in the dimer form.

These observations correspond to *in vitro* studies that indicate a two-phase control of dimer hCG synthesis mediated principally through a supply of subunits. In contrast to LH secretion in the pituitary gland, hCG is secreted constitutively as subunits are available and is not stored in secretory granules (Muyan and Boime, 1997). Initially, immature syncytiotrophoblast produces free β-hCG subunits, whereas the ability to produce the α subunit by cytotrophoblast appears to lag by several days (Hay, 1985). As the trophoblast matures, the ratio of α subunit to β subunit reaches a 1:1 ratio and reaches a peak of approximately 100,000 mU/mL by the 9th or 10th week of gestation (Fig. 9-2). By 22 weeks' gestation, the placenta produces more α subunit than β-hCG. At term gestation, the ratio of α subunit to hCG release is approximately 10:1 (Takemori et al., 1981).

The exponential rise of hCG after implantation is characterized by a doubling time of 30.9 ± 3.7 hours (Lenton and Woodward, 1988). The hCG doubling time has been used as a characteristic marker by clinicians to differentiate normal from abnormal gestations (i.e., ectopic pregnancy). The inability to detect an intrauterine pregnancy by endovaginal ultrasound when serum hCG levels reach 1100 to 1500 mU/mL strongly suggests an abnormal gestation or ectopic pregnancy. Higher than normal hCG levels may indicate a molar pregnancy or multiple-gestational pregnancies. Levels of hCG in combination with maternal α-fetoprotein and unconjugated estriol

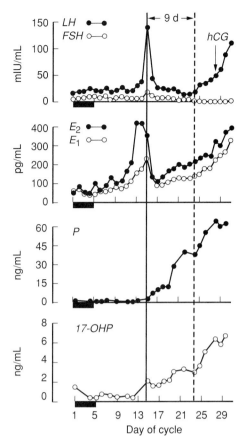

FIGURE 9-1 ■ Hormonal patterns of human chorionic gonadotropin (hCG), luteinizing hormone (LH), follicle-stimulating hormone (FSH), estradiol (E$_2$), estrone (E$_1$), progesterone (P), and 17α-hydroxyprogesterone (17-OHP) during a conception cycle. Note the rise in hCG, which is detectable on cycle days 26 and 27. (Adapted with permission from S.S.C. Yen, MD, DSc, University of California, San Diego.)

have been used as a screening test for detection of fetal anomalies (see Chapter 18).

MAINTENANCE OF EARLY PREGNANCY: HUMAN CHORIONIC GONADOTROPIN AND CORPUS LUTEUM OF PREGNANCY

The major biological role of hCG during early pregnancy is to "rescue" corpus luteum from its premature demise while maintaining progesterone production. Although the secretory pattern of hCG is not well characterized, hCG is required for rescue and maintenance of the corpus luteum until the luteal–placental shift in progesterone synthesis occurs. This concept is supported by observations that immunoneutralization of hCG results in early pregnancy loss (Stevens, 1975; Csapo and Pulkkiven, 1978).

Studies in early pregnancy show that secretion of hCG and progesterone from the corpus luteum appears to be irregularly episodic with varying frequencies and peaks (Owens et al., 1981; Nakajima et al., 1990). In first-trimester explant experiments, intermittent gonadotropin-releasing hormone administration enhances the pulse-like secretion of hCG from these explants, indirectly implicating placental

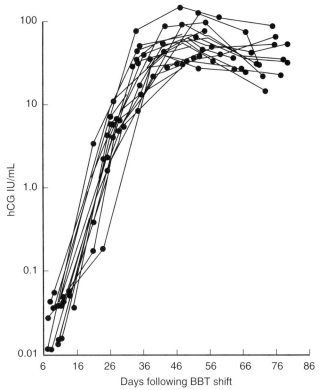

FIGURE 9-2 ■ Exponential rise of circulating human chorionic gonadotropin (hCG) after implantation during the first trimester of pregnancy, with a subsequent plateau between the 11th to 12th week of gestation. BBT, basal body temperature. (From Braunstein GD, Kamdar V, Rasor J, et al: A chorionic gonadotropin-like substance in normal human tissues. J Clin Endocrinol Metab **49**:917, 1979. Copyright © by the Endocrine Society.)

gonadotropin-releasing hormone as a paracrine regulator of hCG secretion (Barnea et al., 1991). During nonconception cycles, the corpus luteum is preprogrammed to undergo luteolysis, a process that is not well understood. Acting through the LH receptor, hCG is also able to stimulate parallel production of estradiol, 17-hydroxyprogesterone, and other peptides, such as relaxin and inhibin, from the corpus luteum.

TIMING OF THE LUTEAL–PLACENTAL SHIFT

Ovarian progesterone production is essential for maintenance of early pregnancy. If progesterone action is blocked by a competitive progesterone antagonist, such as mifepristone, pregnancy termination results. During later gestation, placental production of progesterone is sufficient to maintain pregnancy. To uncover the timing of this luteal placental shift, Csapo and colleagues performed luteectomy experiments. They demonstrated that removal of the corpus luteum before, but not after, the 7th week of gestation usually resulted in subsequent abortion (Csapo et al., 1973; Csapo and Pulkkinen, 1978). Removal of the corpus luteum after the 9th week appears to have little or no influence on gestation (Fig. 9-3). Thus, progesterone supplementation is required if corpus luteum function is compromised before 9 to 10 weeks of gestation.

FETOPLACENTAL UNIT AS AN ENDOCRINE ORGAN

The fetus and placenta must function together in an integrated fashion to control the growth and development of the unit and subsequent expulsion of the fetus from the uterus. Contributing to fetal and placental activity are the changes occurring in the maternal endocrine milieu. Estrogens, androgens, and progestins are involved in pregnancy from before implantation to parturition. They are synthesized and metabolized in complex pathways involving the fetus, the placenta, and the mother.

The fetal ovary is not active and does not secrete estrogens until puberty. In contrast, the Leydig cells of the fetal testes are capable of production of large amounts of testosterone such that the circulating testosterone concentrations in the first-trimester male fetus is similar to the adult man (Tapanainen et al., 1981). Initial stimulus of the testes is by hCG. Fetal testosterone is required for promoting differentiation and masculinization of the male external and internal genitalia. In addition, local conversion of testosterone to dihydrotestosterone by 5α-reductase in the genital target tissues ensures final maturation of the external male genital structures. The maternal environment is protected from the testosterone produced by the male fetus because of excess placental aromatase enzyme that can convert testosterone to estradiol.

Progesterone

During most of pregnancy, the major source of progesterone is the placenta; for the first 6 to 10 weeks, however, the major source of progesterone is the corpus luteum. Exogenous progesterone must be administered only during the first trimester to oocyte recipients who have no ovarian function (Rebar and Cedars, 1992).

Progesterone is synthesized within the placenta mainly from circulating maternal cholesterol (Simpson and MacDonald, 1981). By the end of pregnancy, the placental production of progesterone approximates 250 mg/day, with circulating levels in the mother of about 130 to 150 mg/mL. In comparison, in the follicular phase, production of progesterone approximates 2.5 mg/day; in the luteal phase, it is about 25 mg/day. About 90% of the progesterone synthesized by the placenta enters the

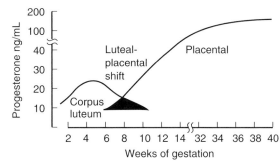

FIGURE 9-3 ■ Diagrammatic representation of the shift in progesterone production from the corpus luteum to the placenta between the 7th and 9th weeks of gestation. (Adapted with permission from S.S.C. Yen, MD, DSc, University of California, San Diego.)

maternal compartment. Most of the progesterone in the maternal circulation is metabolized to pregnanediol and is excreted in the urine as a glucuronide.

17α-Hydroxyprogesterone is also elevated in the maternal circulation during the first 6 weeks of pregnancy, paralleling the levels of progesterone (Tulchinsky and Hobel, 1973). After 6 weeks of gestation, 17α-hydroxyprogesterone levels decrease progressively, becoming undetectable during the middle third of pregnancy, whereas progesterone levels fall transiently between 8 and 10 weeks of gestation and then increase thereafter. The decrease in 17α-hydroxyprogesterone and the dip in progesterone levels reflect the transition of progesterone secretion from the corpus luteum to the placenta. The secretion of 17α-hydroxyprogesterone during the last third of pregnancy is derived largely from the fetoplacental unit.

Estrogens

The major estrogen formed in pregnancy is estriol. Estriol is not secreted by the ovary of nonpregnant women, but it makes up more than 90% of the known estrogen in the urine of pregnant women and is excreted as sulfate and glucuronide conjugates. Maternal serum levels of estriol increase to between 12 and 20 ng/mL by term (Fig. 9-4). Generally, circulating levels of estradiol are even higher than those of estriol. This is true because circulating estriol, in contrast to estrone and estradiol, has a very low affinity for sex hormone–binding globulin and is cleared much more rapidly

from the circulation. During pregnancy a woman produces more estrogen than a normal ovulatory woman could produce in more than 150 years (Tulchinsky and Hobel, 1973).

The biosynthesis of estrogens demonstrates the interdependence of the fetus, the placenta, and the mother. To form estrogens, the placenta, which has active aromatizing capacity, uses circulating androgens, primarily from the fetal adrenal glands. The major androgenic precursor to placental estrogen formation is dehydroepiandrosterone sulfate (DHEAS), which is the major androgen produced by the fetal adrenal cortex. DHEAS transported to the placenta is cleaved by sulfatase, which the placenta has in abundance, to form free unconjugated dehydroepiandrosterone and is then aromatized by placental aromatase to estrone and estradiol. Very little estrone and estradiol are converted to estriol by the placenta. Near term, about 60% of the estradiol-17β and estrone is formed from fetal androgen precursors and about 40% is formed from maternal DHEAS (Siiteri and MacDonald, 1963).

The major portion of fetal DHEAS undergoes 16α-hydroxylation, primarily in the fetal liver but also in the fetal adrenal gland (Fig. 9-5). Fetal adrenal DHEAS in the circulation is taken up by syncytiotrophoblast cells where steroid sulfatase, a microsomal enzyme, converts it back to DHEA that is then aromatized to estriol (Salido et al., 1990). Estriol is then secreted into the maternal circulation and conjugated in the maternal liver to form estriol sulfate, estriol glucosiduronate, and mixed conjugates and is excreted via the maternal urine.

Estetrol is an estrogen unique to pregnancy; it is the 15α-hydroxy derivative of estriol and is derived exclusively from fetal precursors. Although the measurement of estetrol in pregnancy had been proposed as an aid in monitoring a fetus at risk for intrauterine death, it has not proved to be any better than measurement of urinary estriol (Tulchinsky et al., 1975). Neither is used in a clinical setting.

Hydroxylation at the C_2 position of the phenolic A ring results in the formation of so-called catecholestrogens (2-hydroxyestrone, 2-hydroxyestradiol, and 2-hydroxyestriol) and is a major process in estrogen metabolism. 2-Hydroxyestrone is excreted in maternal urine in the largest amounts during pregnancy with marked individual variation (100 to 2500 mg/24 hours). Apparently, 2-hydroxyestrone levels increase during the first and second trimesters and decrease in the third trimester (Gelbke et al., 1975). The physiologic significance of the catecholestrogens is unclear, particularly because they are rapidly cleared from the circulation; however, they do have the capacity to alter catecholamine synthesis and metabolism during pregnancy (inhibiting catecholamine inactivation via competition for carboxyl-o-methyl transferase and reducing catecholamine synthesis via inhibition of tyrosine hydroxylase). Catecholestrogens also function as antiestrogens, competing with estrogens for their receptors. Thus, catecholestrogens, present in large quantities, may have significant effects in pregnancy. About 90% of the estradiol-17β and estriol secreted by the placenta enters the maternal compartment. Estrone is preferentially secreted into the fetal compartment (Gelbke et al., 1975).

In the past, maternal estriol measurements were often used as an index of fetoplacental function. The numerous problems that have been documented in interpreting low estradiol levels have limited the usage of estriol. The normal range of urinary estradiol concentrations at any given stage of gestation is quite large (typically ±1 standard deviation). A single

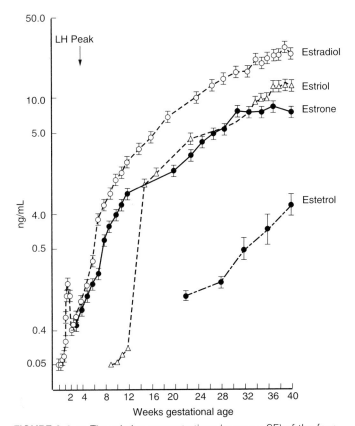

FIGURE 9-4 ■ The relative concentrations (means ± SE) of the four major estrogens plotted on log scale during the course of pregnancy. LH, luteinizing hormone. (Courtesy of John Marshall, University of Virginia.)

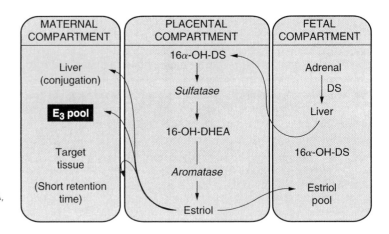

FIGURE 9-5 ■ Diagram of the roles of each compartment in the formation of estriol (E₃) from the fetal precursor 16α-hydroxydehydroepiandrosterone sulfate (16α-OH-DS). DHEA, dehydroepiandrosterone. (Adapted with permission from S.S.C. Yen, MD, DSc, University of California, San Diego.)

plasma measurement is meaningless because of moment-to-moment fluctuations. Body position (i.e., bed rest and ambulation) affect blood flow to the uterus and kidney and, therefore, estriol levels. Moreover, numerous drugs, including glucocorticoids and ampicillin, affect estriol levels.

Two genetic diseases document that placental estrogen synthesis, at least at high levels, is apparently not required for maintenance of pregnancy. Human gestation proceeds to term when the fetus and placenta lack sulfatase (Bradshaw and Carr, 1986). In this disorder, the gene has been localized to the distal short arm of the X chromosome and the resulting male offspring manifest ichthyosis during the first few months of life. Pregnancies also reach term accompanied by severe fetal and placental aromatase deficiency (Harada, 1993). Although pregnancy is maintained in both cases in the face of low placental estrogen synthesis, the changes in the reproductive tract that normally precede parturition, particularly ripening of the cervix, do not occur, revealing a significant role for placental estrogens in preparation for labor and birth. In addition, in the case of aromatase deficiency, both the fetus and the mother are virilized as a consequence of diminished aromatization of androgens.

Low levels of estrogens also occur after fetal demise and in most anencephalic pregnancies in which fetal signals from the fetal hypothalamic–pituitary unit are diminished and do not stimulate synthesis of fetal adrenal androgens. In the absence of a fetus, as occurs in molar pregnancy and in pseudocyesis, estrogen levels are low as well.

Roles of Estrogens and Progestins during Pregnancy

Estrogens and progestins appear to play several important roles in pregnancy. They clearly induce the secretory endometrium, required for implantation. Progesterone appears to be important in maintaining uterine quiescence during pregnancy by actions on uterine smooth muscle (Roberts et al., 1984). Progesterone apparently suppresses uterine contraction by action through cell surface gama-aminobutyric acid-a receptors that may be similar to its action on human brain neurons (Strauss et al., 1995). Progesterone also inhibits uterine prostaglandin production (Cane and Villee, 1975), presumably promoting uterine quiescence and delaying cervical ripening. Progesterone may also help to maintain pregnancy by inhibiting T-lymphocyte–mediated processes that play a role in tissue rejection (Siiteri et al., 1977). Thus, the high local concentrations of progesterone appear to contribute to the immunologically privileged status of the pregnant uterus. Progesterone is important in creating a barrier to penetration of pathogens into the uterus.

Estrogens are important for parturition at the appropriate time. The stimulatory effects of estrogen on phospholipid synthesis and turnover, prostaglandin production, and increased formation of lysosomes in the uterine endometrium, as well as estrogen modulation of adrenergic mechanisms in uterine myometrium, may be means by which estrogens act to time the onset of labor (Casey et al., 1983). Estrogens also increase uterine blood flow (Resnik et al., 1974), which ensures an adequate supply of oxygen and nutrients to the fetus. In this regard, it appears that estriol, an extremely weak estrogen, is just as effective as other estrogens in increasing uteroplacental blood flow (Resnik et al., 1974).

Estrogens are important in preparing the breast for lactation (Martin and Oakey, 1982). They also affect other endocrine systems during pregnancy, such as the renin–angiotensin system (Carr and Gant, 1983), and stimulate production of hormone-binding globulins in the liver. Estrogens may play a role in fetal development and organ maturation, including increasing fetal lung surfactant production (Parker et al., 1987).

Placenta and Growth Factors

The functional roles for growth factors in the placenta can be divided into three areas:

1. Regulation of cell growth and differentiation
2. Local regulation of hormone release
3. Regulation of uterine contractility

Growth factors that are elaborated by the placenta are responsible for the following:

1. Regulation of amino acid transport
2. Increased glucose uptake
3. DNA synthesis and cell replication
4. RNA and protein synthesis

These processes may be regulated in an autocrine or paracrine manner within the placenta.

Although much of the research has been conducted in other mammalian systems and may not be directly applicable to

■ TABLE 9-2. GROWTH FACTORS, NEUROPEPTIDES, AND PROTEINS IDENTIFIED IN PLACENTAL TISSUES

Protein/Peptide Hormone	Neurohormone/ Neuropeptides	Growth Factors	Binding Proteins	Cytokines
Human chorionic gonadotropin	Gonadotropin-releasing hormone	Activin	Corticotropin-releasing hormone-binding protein (CRH-BP)	Interleukin-I (IL-1)
Human placental lactogen	Thyroid-releasing hormone	Follistatin	Insulin-like growth factor binding protein (IGFBP-1)	IL-2
Growth hormone variant	Growth hormone-releasing hormone	Inhibin	IGFBP-2	IL-6
Adrenocorticotropic hormone	Somatostatin	Transforming growth factor-β and -α	IGFBP-3	IL-8
	Corticotropin-releasing hormone	Epidermal growth factor	IGFBP-4	Interferon-α
	Oxytocin	Insulin-like growth factor-I (IGF-I)	IGFBP-5	Interferon-β
	Neuropeptide Y	IGF-II	IGFBP-6	Interferon-γ
	β-Endorphin	Fibroblastic growth factor		Tumor necrosis factor-α
	Met-enkephalin	Platelet-derived growth factor		
	Dynorphin			

humans, major similarities probably exist in the way growth factors operate to ensure continuing growth and development of the fetus. In the human, most of our knowledge has been limited to descriptive studies demonstrating localization of many growth factor systems. Unfortunately, our understanding of their functional roles has only begun. Table 9-2 is a partial listing of growth factors that have been identified in the placenta. A detailed description of their respective roles is beyond the scope of this chapter. Only major growth factor systems are discussed.

Insulin-Like Growth Factor, Epidermal Growth Factor, and Transforming Growth Factor-α

In preimplantation embryos, the insulin-like growth factor (IGF), the transforming growth factor-α, and the EGF systems have been studied extensively. In general, IGF-II/IGF-I receptors are primarily responsible for regulation of cell proliferation, whereas cell differentiation is regulated by the transforming growth factor-α and EGF-receptor systems.

IGF-I appears to be an important modulator of fetal growth. IGF-I is normally produced in response to pituitary growth hormone (GH) by the liver (Fig. 9-6). In pregnancy, the levels of IGF-I may be regulated in part by placental GH, a variant of pituitary GH. Fetal cord plasma IGF-I levels are positively correlated to birth weight and length of the fetus (Caufriez et al., 1993; Kniss et al., 1994).

EGF and *transforming growth factor-α* in the placenta both interact with the EGF receptor. Both growth factors are present in cytotrophoblast and syncytiotrophoblast. In these latter cells, EGF stimulates secretion of hCG and human placental lactogen (Maruo et al., 1992). The proliferative activities induced by a number of growth factors appear to overlap. These factors include IGF, platelet-derived growth factors, EGF, and fibroblastic growth factors.

Human Chorionic Somatomammotropin

Human chorionic somatomammotropin (hCS), initially named human placental lactogen when it was isolated from the human placenta in the 1960s (Josimovich and MacLaren, 1962), has structural, biological, and immunologic similarities to both pituitary human growth hormone (hGH) and prolactin. hCS is now known to be a single-chain polypeptide (~22 kDa) containing 191 amino acids and two disulfide bonds. It shares up to 96% homology with GH and about 67% homology with prolactin (Bewley et al., 1972; Cooke et al., 1981). The hCS/hGH gene cluster has been localized to the long arm of chromosome 17 and consists of five genes, two coding for hGH and three for hCS (Owerbach et al., 1980). Two of the three hCS genes are expressed at approximately equivalent rates in term placenta and synthesize identical proteins, and the third gene appears to be a pseudogene (Barrera-Saldana et al., 1983).

hCS is produced only by syncytiotrophoblast and appears to be transcribed at a constant rate throughout gestation (McWilliams and Boime, 1980; Hoshina et al., 1982). As a consequence, serum levels of hCS correlate very well with placental mass as the placenta increases in size during pregnancy. At term, placental production approximates 1 to 4 g/day and maternal serum levels of hCS range from 5 to 15 μg/mL (Fig. 9-7), making it the most abundant secretory product of the placenta.

Despite the huge quantities produced during pregnancy, the function of hCS remains poorly understood. It has been suggested that hCS must exert its major metabolic effects on the mother to ensure that the nutritional demands of the fetus are met, functioning as the "growth hormone" of pregnancy (Grumbach et al., 1966). During pregnancy, maternal plasma glucose levels are decreased, plasma free fatty acids are increased, and insulin secretion is increased with resistance to endogenous insulin as a consequence of the GH-like and contrainsulin effects of hCS (Fig. 9-8). Peripheral glucose uptake is inhibited in the mother but crosses the placenta freely. Amino acids are actively transported to the fetus against a concentration gradient, and transplacental passage of free fatty acids is slow. As a consequence, when the mother is in the unfed or starved state, glucose should be reserved largely for the fetus and free fatty acids would be used preferentially by the mother. The placenta is impermeable to insulin and other protein hormones.

Despite these presumptions, the regulation of hCS is poorly understood. Factors that regulate pituitary GH secretion are largely ineffective in altering concentrations of hCS. In addition, despite its structural homology to GH and prolactin, hCS has very little (although definite) growth-promoting and lactogenic activity in humans (Grumbach et al., 1966). Moreover, normal pregnancies resulting in delivery of healthy infants have been reported in individuals with very low to absent production of hCS (Nielsen et al., 1979; Parks et al., 1985). Thus, it is possible that hCS is not essential for pregnancy but may serve as an evolutionary redundancy for pituitary GH and prolactin. Whether pregnancies with diminished hCS production would have good outcomes in the presence of nutritional deprivation, however, remains unknown.

Human Placental Growth Hormone

Only in the last several years has the existence of a placental GH been documented. The two forms of human placental GH present include a 22-kDa form and a glycosylated 25-kDa

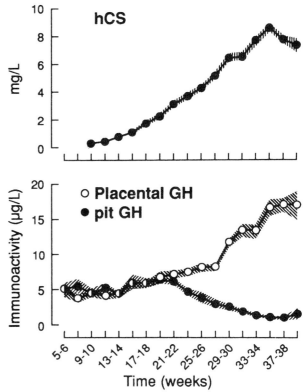

FIGURE 9-7 ■ The time course of human chorionic somatomammotropin (hCS), placental growth hormone (GH), and pituitary growth hormone (pit GH) during human pregnancy. (Modified from Frankenne F, Closset J, Gomez F, et al: The physiology of growth hormones (GHs) in pregnant women and partial characterization of the placental GH variant. J Clin Endocrinol Metab **6**:1171, 1988. Copyright © by the Endocrine Society.)

form. Both are encoded by the hGH-V gene in the hCS/hGH gene cluster on chromosome 17 (DeNoto et al., 1981; Seeburg, 1982). Pituitary hCG is encoded by the hGH-N gene in the same gene cluster (Igout et al., 1988).

During the first trimester, pituitary GH is measurable in maternal serum and is secreted in a pulsatile fashion (Eriksson et al., 1989). Human placental GH levels begin to rise thereafter as pituitary GH levels decrease; human placental GH is secreted in a relatively constant (in contrast to a pulsatile) manner (Eriksson et al., 1989). It appears as if human placental GH stimulates IGF-I production, which in turn suppresses

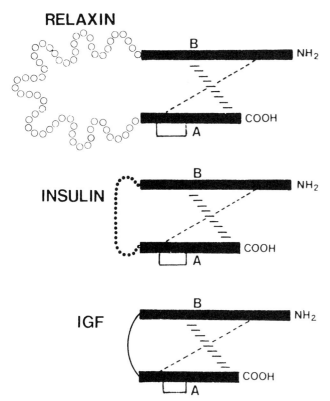

FIGURE 9-6 ■ Comparison of the structural similarities for relaxin, insulin, and insulin-like growth factor (IGF). (Adapted with permission from S.S.C. Yen, MD, DSc, University of California, San Diego.)

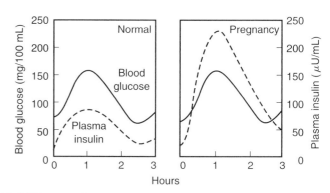

FIGURE 9-8 ■ Comparison of the plasma insulin response to an oral glucose load (100 g) in women during late pregnancy and in nonpregnant (normal) women. (Adapted with permission from S.S.C. Yen, MD, DSc, University of California, San Diego.)

pituitary GH secretion in the second half of pregnancy (Frankenne, 1988).

ENDOCRINE–METABOLIC CHANGES IN PREGNANCY

Pregnancy is accompanied by a series of metabolic changes, including hyperinsulinemia, insulin resistance, relative fasting hypoglycemia, increased circulating plasma lipids, and hypoaminoacidemia. All these changes seem intended to ensure an uninterrupted supply of metabolic fuels to the growing fetus. It is also now clear that these changes are directed by hormones elaborated by the fetoplacental unit.

The insulin resistance associated with pregnancy has been recognized for many years and is known to be accompanied by maternal islet cell hyperplasia (Fig. 9-9). The mechanism responsible for increasing insulin resistance throughout pregnancy is not entirely clear. It appears that hCS and human placental GH in particular reduce insulin receptor sites and glucose transport in insulin-sensitive tissues in the mother (Ciaraldi et al., 1992) (Fig. 9-10). There is no evidence that glucagon plays a significant role as a diabetogenic factor. The rapid return to normal glucose metabolism after delivery in women with gestational diabetes has been regarded as the best evidence that fetoplacental hormones are largely diabetogenic in the mother (Yen et al., 1971).

Total plasma lipids increase significantly and progressively after 24 weeks of gestation, with the increases in triglycerides, cholesterol, and free fatty acids being most marked (Freinkel et al., 1973) (Table 9-3). Pre-β-lipoprotein, a very-low-density lipoprotein that normally represents a very small percentage of total lipoprotein, is increased in pregnancy. High-density-lipoprotein cholesterol levels increase in early pregnancy, whereas low-density-lipoprotein cholesterol levels increase later in pregnancy (Potter and Nestel, 1979).

Plasma triglyceride levels increase more in response to an oral glucose load in late pregnancy than in the nonpregnant state (Freinkel et al., 1973). Because the placenta is poorly permeable to fat but readily permeable to glucose and amino acids, this mechanism helps to ensure an adequate supply of glucose for the fetus.

Prolonged fasting in pregnancy is accompanied by exaggerated hypoglycemia, hypoinsulinism, and hyperketonemia (Felig et al., 1972). Gluconeogenesis, however, is not increased, as would be expected. Thus, even though the demands of the fetus during maternal fasting are met in part by accelerated muscle breakdown, it is at the expense of the mother, in whom homeostatic mechanisms do not include sufficient gluconeogenesis to prevent maternal hypoglycemia. It is not clear whether normal muscle catabolism simply cannot keep up with the loss of glucose and amino acids to the fetus during fasting or whether there are additional restraints on muscle breakdown during pregnancy.

Although cortisol is a potent diabetogenic hormone, inhibiting peripheral glucose uptake and promoting insulin secretion, and serum free cortisol levels clearly increase in late pregnancy (Cousins et al., 1983; Abou-Samra et al., 1984), it is unclear just how great a role cortisol plays in the diabetogenic nature of pregnancy. The increased circulating concentrations of estrogen and progesterone in pregnancy may also be important in the altered glucose-insulin homeostasis present during pregnancy.

Inhibin-Related Proteins

The human placenta has the capacity to synthesize inhibin, activin, and follistatin (Petraglia et al., 1996). *Inhibin* is a dimeric protein composed of an α subunit (18 kDa) and a β subunit (14 kDa), originally shown to have an inhibitory effect on pituitary follicle-stimulating hormone release. Two different β subunits have been characterized and have been designated as β_A and β_B. Each different β subunit can thus give rise to two different inhibins (inhibin A, β_A, and inhibin B, β_B). Activin is a closely related protein that was discovered soon after inhibin and was named because of its ability to stimulate pituitary follicle-stimulating hormone release.

Activin is composed of two β subunits. All three possible configurations of activin have been identified—$\beta_A\beta_A$, $\beta_A\beta_B$, and $\beta_B\beta_B$. *Follistatin* is a single-chain glycoprotein that can functionally inhibit pituitary follicle-stimulating hormone release by binding of activin. Besides the human trophoblast, the maternal decidua, amnion, and chorion have been demonstrated to express messenger RNAs and immunoreactive proteins for inhibin, activin, and follistatin.

High levels of inhibin-like proteins have been reported in patients with fetal Down syndrome (Van Lith et al., 1992) and in patients with hydatidiform mole (Yohkaichiya et al., 1989); low levels have been observed in women with abnormal gestations, such as ectopic pregnancies (Yohkaichiya et al., 1993) and pregnancies that end in abortion (Norman et al., 1993). High levels of maternal activin A have been observed in pregnancies complicated by preeclampsia, diabetes, and preterm labor (Petraglia et al., 1996).

At this point, there are no *in vivo* models to study the functional roles of inhibin-related proteins on placental hormone secretion and thus the biological roles of this system have been derived from *in vitro* cell cultures. In cultured placental cells, activin appears to increase the release of hCG and progesterone (Steele et al., 1993), whereas inhibins decrease hCG and progesterone levels. Follistatin has been reported to reverse the activin-induced release of hCG and progesterone. These regulatory events appear to be parallel to that of the

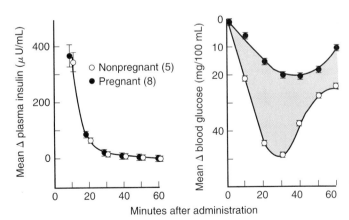

FIGURE 9-9 ■ *Left,* Almost identical disappearance curves of circulating insulin after a bolus intravenous insulin injection (0.1 U/kg) in pregnant and nonpregnant women. *Right,* A marked decline in blood glucose in response to exogenous insulin levels in nonpregnant versus pregnant women suggesting increased insulin resistance in the latter group. (From Burt RL, Davidson WF: Insulin half-life and utilization in normal pregnancy. Obstet Gynecol **4:**161, 1974. Reprinted with permission from the American College of Obstetricians and Gynecologists.)

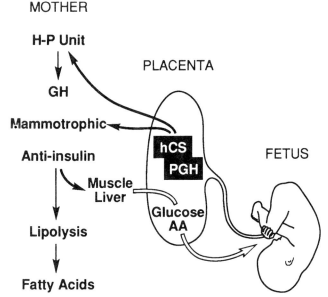

FIGURE 9-10 ■ The proposed functional role of human chorionic somatomammotropin (hCS) and placental growth hormone (PGH) in the readjustment of maternal metabolic homeostasis with preferential transfer of amino acid (AA) and glucose to the fetus. GH, pituitary growth hormone; H-P Unit, hypothalamic-pituitary unit. (Adapted with permission from S.S.C. Yen, MD, DSc, University of California, San Diego.)

pituitary gland, where activin increases follicle-stimulating hormone release, whereas follistatin and inhibin oppose this effect.

Corticotropin-Releasing Hormone and Corticotropin-Releasing Hormone Binding Protein System

The placenta, chorion, amnion, and decidua are all capable of synthesizing corticotropin-releasing hormone (CRH). This 41-amino acid peptide was first isolated from the hypothalamus and is responsible for stimulation of adrenocorticotropic hormone and pro-opiomelanocortin

peptides from the pituitary. CRH is detectable by 7 to 8 weeks' gestation (Frim et al., 1988), and maternal plasma levels of CRH rise progressively throughout gestation (Goland et al., 1988). Maternal CRH levels increase significantly with labor, reaching a peak at delivery; levels remain stable in the absence of labor with cesarean section (Petraglia et al., 1990). In the term placenta, CRH has been localized to both cytotrophoblast and syncytiotrophoblast (Warren and Silverman, 1995). The addition of CRH to human placental cells or amnion stimulates release of prostaglandin E and prostaglandin $F_{2\alpha}$, suggesting that locally elaborated CRH plays a major role in the initiation of myometrial contractility and labor (Jones and Challis, 1989).

CRH-binding protein has also been identified in the placenta and appears to be produced by syncytiotrophoblast (Berkowitz et al., 1996), decidua, and fetal membranes (Challis et al., 1995). This protein conceptually functions as a CRH receptor in the circulation, reduces the biological activity of CRH, and thus may serve a modulatory role for localized CRH action.

Oxytocin

Oxytocin, a nonapeptide produced by the supraoptic and paraventricular nuclei of the hypothalamus, has now also been localized to the syncytiotrophoblast. In placental cell cultures, increased concentrations of estradiol are associated with increased levels of oxytocin mRNA. The content of immunoreactive oxytocin increases throughout gestation and is parallel to maternal blood levels. The placental oxytocin content is estimated to be fivefold greater than in the posterior pituitary lobe, suggesting that the placenta may be the main source of oxytocin during pregnancy (Nakazawa et al., 1984).

The role of maternal oxytocin in pregnancy and in parturition remains unclear. Circulating levels of oxytocin are low throughout pregnancy and increase markedly only during the second stage of labor (Leake et al., 1981). Oxytocin receptors are present in myometrium and increase dramatically in number only shortly before the onset of labor (Fuchs et al., 1984). The sensitivity of the myometrium, therefore, changes more dramatically in preparation for labor than do the circulating levels of the hormone. Oxytocin also can stimulate the production of prostaglandins by human decidua (Fuchs et al., 1982). These data do not document any role for oxytocin in parturition and imply that it is unlikely to be the initiator of human parturition.

Relaxin

Relaxin, a peptide hormone of approximately 6 kDa, belongs to the insulin family. It is composed of two disulfide-linked chains, A and B (see Fig. 9-6). Relaxin is produced in a number of sites, including the corpus luteum in pregnant and nonpregnant women, the decidua, the placenta, the prostate, and the atria of the heart.

Relaxin first appears in the serum of pregnant women at the same time as hCG does. Levels during pregnancy approximate 1 ng/mL. Relaxin concentrations are highest during the first trimester and peak at about 1.2 ng/mL between the 8th and 12th weeks of pregnancy and then gradually decrease to 1 ng/mL for the duration of pregnancy (Bell et al., 1987). There is no evidence of any circadian rhythm, and no significant changes have been noted during labor.

TABLE 9-3. BASAL VALUES FOR INSULIN, GLUCAGON, AND PLASMA METABOLIC FUELS IN YOUNG WOMEN AFTER OVERNIGHT FAST

Measurements	Nongravid	Late Pregnancy
Glucose (mg/dL)	79 ± 2.4	68 ± 1.5*
Insulin (µU/mL)	9.8 ± 1.1	16.2 ± 2.0*
Glucagon (pg/mL)	126 ± 6.1	130 ± 5.2 (NS)
Amino acids (µmol/liter)	3.82 ± 0.13	3.18 ± 0.11*
Alanine (µmol/liter)	286 ± 15	225 ± 9*
FFA (µmol/liter)	626 ± 42	725 ± 21*
(mg/dL)	76.2 ± 7.0	181 ± 10*
Cholesterol (mg/dL)	163 ± 8.7	205 ± 5.7*

* Significant difference between nongravid and late pregnancy values.
NS, not significant; FFA, free fatty acid.

Data from Freinkel N, Metzger BE, Nitzan M, et al: Facilitated anabolism in late pregnancy: Some novel maternal compensations for accelerated starvation. *In* Malaisse WJ, Pirart J (eds): Diabetes. International Series No. 312. Amsterdam, Excerpta Medica, 1973, p. 474.

The available evidence suggests that all relaxin circulating in the mother during pregnancy is of luteal origin. The relaxin concentration is highest in the blood draining the corpus luteum (Weiss et al., 1976). By immunohistochemistry profiles, relaxin can be detected only within the corpus luteum in the ovary. Luteectomy at term results in a prompt fall in circulating relaxin with a half-life of less than 1 hour. In the absence of luteectomy, relaxin levels fall to undetectable levels over the first 3 days after delivery, consistent with the time frame for postpartum luteolysis. Perhaps most convincing is the observation that relaxin is undetectable in the serum of women pregnant by IVF and egg donation who have no corpora lutea (Eddie et al., 1990; Emmi et al., 1991).

Relaxin appears to have a broad range of biological activities. These include collagen remodeling and softening of the cervix and lower reproductive tract and inhibition of uterine contractility (Bani, 1997). However, circulating relaxin does not seem to be necessary for pregnancy maintenance or normal delivery in women. Women who become pregnant by egg donation go into labor at term and are capable of delivery vaginally (Eddie et al., 1990). It is possible, however, that the placenta and decidua may provide sufficient relaxin for normal parturition under such circumstances.

Two conditions associated with an increase in circulating relaxin levels are multiple gestation and ovarian stimulation with the use of ovulation-inducing agents. Relaxin concentrations are higher in patients who become pregnant from IVF and exogenous gonadotropin treatment than in untreated pregnant control subjects. In both circumstances there are multiple corpora lutea, and multiple gestations independently produce a significant increase in serum relaxin concentrations. Multiple gestations are associated with a higher risk of premature delivery, according to one group who suggested that first-trimester hyperrelaxinemia can predict the risk of preterm delivery (Weiss et al., 1993). This observation, potentially important, warrants further investigation.

Prolactin

During the first trimester of pregnancy, maternal serum prolactin levels rise progressively to achieve levels of approximately 125 to 180 ng/mL (Riggs et al., 1977) (Fig. 9-11).

The dramatic 10-fold increase in prolactin levels is believed to be a reflection of the estrogen-stimulated increase in size of the pituitary lactotropes, which contributes to a 2- to 3-fold enlargement of pituitary volume. Despite the increased magnitude of prolactin concentrations during pregnancy, the normal sleep-associated increase in prolactin remains preserved (Boyar et al., 1975). At delivery, the higher level of prolactin is responsible for priming the breast tissue in preparation for lactation.

After delivery, prolactin levels remain elevated at 200 to 250 ng/mL and fall gradually toward the normal range (<25 ng/mL) during a 3- to 4-week interval in non–breast-feeding mothers (Liu and Park, 1988). In women who are breast-feeding, prolactin levels remain elevated and increase with each nursing episode. This constant hyperprolactinemic state may be partly responsible for the delay in return of ovulatory function in the breast-feeding woman.

The decidua is the major source of amniotic fluid prolactin. Decidual cells are capable of secretion of prolactin after day 23 of the menstrual cycle. Decidual prolactin is immunologically identical to the 23-kDa prolactin produced by the pituitary gland and the complementary DNA from decidua appears virtually identical to pituitary prolactin (Bigazzi, 1983; Tyson and McCoshen, 1983). Unlike the pituitary gland, decidua prolactin is not regulated by dopamine or thyrotropin-releasing hormone. The decidual prolactin synthesis is coupled to progesterone-induced decidualization. Once cells are stimulated to decidualize, prolactin production continues in culture even in the absence of progesterone. Because abnormal levels of amniotic fluid prolactin levels have been found in pregnancies complicated by polyhydramnios or oligohydramnios, it is believed that the biological role of locally produced prolactin is to regulate solute and water transport in the amniotic compartment (Handwerger and Brar, 1992).

Prostaglandins

Although concentrations of prostaglandin precursors are high in the endometrial compartment during pregnancy, there is a marked decrease in the production of prostaglandins by the endometria decidua. Levels of cyclooxygenase 1, the constitutive expressed cyclooxygenase enzyme, fall precipitously during

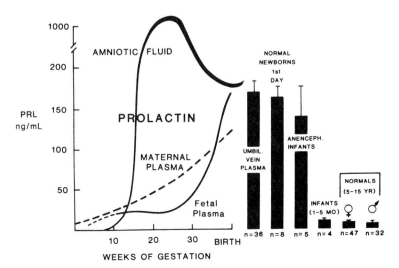

FIGURE 9-11 ■ Approximate levels of prolactin (PRL) in amniotic fluid, maternal plasma, and fetal plasma during the time course of pregnancy. Plasma levels of normal and anencephalic newborns are compared with normal infants and adults. (Modified from Aubert ML, Grumbach MM, Kaplan SL: The ontogenesis of human fetal hormones. III. Prolactin. J Clin Endocrinol Metab **56**:155, 1975. Copyright © by the Endocrine Society.)

the mid-luteal phase of the menstrual cycle at the time of implantation. Under the influence of progesterone, the endometria decidua produces secretory component, an endogenous inhibitor of prostaglandin synthesis (Norwitz and Wilson, 2000). The exogenous administration of prostaglandins is capable of inducing abortion or labor in all species, including humans. Taken together, these observations suggest multiple mechanism(s) that inhibit prostaglandin production during pregnancy. Progesterone may be one factor that suppresses synthesis of prostaglandins.

REFERENCES

Abou-Samra AB, Pugeat M, Dechaud H, et al: Increased concentration of N-terminal lipotrophin and unbound cortisol during pregnancy. Clin Endocrinol 20:221, 1984.

Aplin JD: Implantation, trophoblast differentiation and haemochorial placentation: Mechanistic evidence in vivo and in vitro. J Cell Sci 99:681, 1991.

Armant DR, Kaplan HA, Mover H, et al: The effect of hexapeptides on attachment and outgrowth of mouse blastocysts cultured in vitro: Evidence for the involvement of the cell recognition tripeptide Arg-Gly-Asp. Proc Natl Acad Sci USA 83:6751, 1986.

Aubert ML, Grumbach MM, Kaplan SL: The ontogenesis of human fetal hormones. III. Prolactin. J Clin Endocrinol Metab 56:155, 1975.

Bani D: Relaxin: A pleiotropic hormone. Gen Pharmol 28:13, 1997.

Barnea ER, Kaplan M, Naor Z: Comparative stimulatory effect of gonadotropin releasing hormone (GnRH) and GnRH agonist upon pulsatile human chorionic gonadotropin secretion in superfused placental explants: Reversible inhibition by a GnRH antagonist. Hum Reprod 6:1063, 1991.

Barrera-Saldana HA, Seeburg PH, Saunders GF: Two structurally different genes produce the same secreted human placental lactogen hormone. Bio Chem 258:3787, 1983.

Bass KE, Morrish D, Roth I, et al: Human cytotrophoblast invasion is upregulated by epidermal growth factor: Evidence that paracrine factors modify this process. Dev Biol 164:550, 1994.

Bell RJ, Eddie LW, Lester AR: Relaxin in human pregnancy serum measured with an homologous radioimmunoassay. Obstet Gynecol 69:585, 1987.

Bergh PA, Navot D: Oocyte donation—extending a woman's reproductive life span. Reprod Rev 2:126, 1992.

Berkowitz GS, Lapinski RH, Lockwood CJ, et al: Corticotropin-releasing factor and its binding protein: Maternal serum levels in term and preterm deliveries. Am J Obstet Gynecol 174:1477, 1996.

Bewley TA, Dixon JS, Li CH: Sequence comparison of human pituitary growth hormone, human chorionic somatomammotropin, and ovine pituitary growth and lactogenic hormones. Int J Pept Protein Res 4:281, 1972.

Bigazzi M: Specific endocrine function of human decidua. Semin Reprod Endocrinol 1:343, 1983.

Boyar RM, Finkelstein JW, Kapen S, et al: Twenty-four hour prolactin (PRL) secretory patterns during pregnancy. J Clin Endocrinol Metab 40:1117, 1975.

Bradshaw KD, Carr BR: Placental sulfatase deficiency: maternal and fetal expressions of steroid sulfatase deficiency and X-linked ichthyosis. Obstet Gynecol Surv 68:505, 1986.

Burt RL, Davidson WF: Insulin half-life and utilization in normal pregnancy. Obstet Gynecol 43:161, 1974.

Cane EM, Villee CA: The synthesis of prostaglandin F by human endometrium in organ culture. Prostaglandins 9:281, 1975.

Carr BR, Gant NF: The endocrinology of pregnancy-induced hypertension. Clin Perinatol 10:737, 1983.

Casey ML, Winkel CA, Porter JC, et al: Endocrine regulation of the initiation and maintenance of parturition. Clin Perinatol 10:709, 1983.

Caufriez A, Frankenne F, Hennen G, et al: Regulation of maternal IGF-I by placental GH in normal and abnormal human pregnancies. Am J Physiol 265:E572, 1993.

Challis JRG, Matthews SG, Van Meir C, et al: Current topic: The placental corticotropin-releasing hormone-adrenocorticotrophin axis. Placenta 16:481, 1995.

Ciaraldi TP, Kettel LM, El-Roeiy A, et al: Mechanisms of cellular insulin resistance in human pregnancy. J Clin Endocrinol Metab 75:577, 1992.

Cooke NE, Coit D, Shine J: Human prolactin cDNA structural analysis and evolutionary comparisons. J Biol Chem 256:4007, 1981.

Cousins L, Rigg L, Hollinsworth D, et al: Qualitative and quantitative assessment of the circadian rhythm of cortisol in pregnancy. Am J Obstet Gynecol 145:411, 1983.

Csapo AI, Pulkkinen M: Indispensability of the human corpus luteum in the maintenance of early pregnancy: Luteectomy evidence. Obstet Gynecol Surv 33:69, 1978.

Csapo AI, Pulkkinen MO, Wiest WG: Effect of luteectomy and progesterone replacement therapy in early pregnant patients. Am J Obstet Gynecol 115:756, 1973.

Cullinan EB, Abbondanzo SJ, Anderson PS, et al: Leukemia inhibitory factor (LIF) and LIF receptor expression in human endometrium suggests a potential autocrine/paracrine function in regulating embryo implantation. Proc Natl Acad Sci USA 93:3115, 1996.

DeNoto FM, Moore DD, Goodman HM: Human growth hormone DNA sequence and mRNA structures: Possible alternative splicing. Nucleic Acids Res 9:719, 1981.

Eddie LW, Cameron IT, Leeton JF: Ovarian relaxin is not essential for dilatation of cervix. Lancet 336:243, 1990.

Edelman GM, Crossin KL: Cell adhesion molecules: Implications for molecular histology. Annu Rev Biochem 60:155, 1991.

Emmi AM, Skurnick J, Goldsmith LT: Ovarian control of pituitary hormone secretion in early human pregnancy. J Clin Endocrinol Metab 72:1359, 1991.

Enders AC, King BF: Early stages of trophoblastic invasion of the maternal vascular system during implantation in the macaque and baboon. Am J Anat 192:329, 1991.

Eriksson L, Frankenne F, Eden S, et al: Growth hormone 24-hour serum profiles during pregnancy: Lack of pulsatility for the secretion of the placental variant. Br J Obstet Gynaecol 96:949, 1989.

Felig P, Kim YJ, Lynch V, et al: Amino acid metabolism during starvation in human pregnancy. J Clin Invest 51:1195, 1972.

Frankenne F, Closset J, Gomez F, et al: The physiology of growth hormones (GHs) in pregnant women and partial characterization of the placental GH variant. J Clin Endocrinol Metab 66:1171, 1988.

Freinkel N, Metzger BE, Nitzan M, et al: Facilitated anabolism in late pregnancy: Some novel maternal compensations for accelerated starvation. In Malaisse WJ, Pirart J (eds): Diabetes. International Series No. 312. Amsterdam, Excerpta Medica, 1973, p. 474.

Frim DM, Emanuel RL, Robinson BG, et al: Characterization and gestational regulation of corticotropin-releasing hormone messenger RNA in human placenta. J Clin Invest 82:287, 1988.

Fuchs A-R, Fuchs R, Husslein P: Oxytocin receptors and human parturition: A dual role for oxytocin in the initiation of labor. Science 214:1396, 1982.

Fuchs A-R, Fuchs F, Husslein P, et al: Oxytocin receptors in the human uterus during pregnancy and parturition. Am J Obstet Gynecol 150:734, 1984.

Gelbke HP, Bottger M, Knuppen R: Excretion of 2-hydroxyestrone in urine throughout human pregnancies. J Clin Endocrinol Metab 41:744, 1975.

Goland RS, Wardlaw SL, Blum M, et al: Biologically active corticotropin-releasing hormone in maternal and fetal plasma during pregnancy. Am J Obstet Gynecol 159:884, 1988.

Graham CH, Lysiak JJ, McCrae KR, et al: Localization of transforming growth factor-beta at the human fetal-maternal interface: Role in trophoblast growth and differentiation. Biol Reprod 46:561, 1992.

Grumbach MM, Kaplan SL, Abrams CL, et al: Plasma free fatty acid response to the administration of chorionic "growth hormone-prolactain." J Clin Endocrinol Metab 26:476, 1966.

Handwerger S, Brar A: Placental lactogen, placental growth hormone, and decidual prolactin. Semin Reprod Endocrinol 10:106, 1992.

Harada N: Genetic analysis of human aromatase deficiency. J Steroid Biochem Mol Biol 44:331, 1993.

Hay DL: Discordant and variable production of human chorionic gonadotropin and its free alpha- and beta-subunits in early pregnancy. J Clin Endocrinol Metab 61:1195, 1985.

Hay DL, Lopata A: Chorionic gonadotropin secretion by human embryos in vitro. J Clin Endocrinol Metab 67:1322, 1988.

Hertig AT, Rock J, Adams EC: A description of 34 human ova within the first 17 days of development. Am J Anat 98:435, 1956.

Hoshina M, Boothby M, Boime I: Cytological localization of chorionic gonadotropin α and placental lactogen mRNAs during development of the human placenta. J Cell Biol 93:190, 1982.

Hynes RO: Integrins: Versatility, modulation, and signaling in cell adhesion. Cell 69:11, 1992.

Igout A, Scippo ML, Frankenne F, et al: Cloning and nucleotide sequence of placental hGH-V cDNA. Arch Int Physiol Biochim 96:63, 1988.

Jones SA, Challis JRG: Local stimulation of prostaglandin production by corticotropin-releasing hormone in human fetal membranes and placenta. Biochem Biophys Res Commun 159:192, 1989.

Josimovich JB, MacLaren JA: Presence in the human placenta and term serum of a highly lactogenic substance immunologically related to pituitary growth hormone. Endocrinology 71:209, 1962.

Kawakami Y, Andoh K, Mizunuma H, et al: Assessment of the implantation site by transvaginal ultrasound. Fertil Steril 59:1003, 1993.

Kniss DA, Shubert PJ, Zimmerman PD, et al: Insulin like growth factors: Their regulation of glucose and amino acid transport in placental trophoblasts isolated from first trimester chorionic villi. J Reprod Med 39:249, 1994.

Leake RD, Weitzman RE, Glatz TH, et al: Plasma oxytocin concentrations in man, nonpregnant women and pregnant women before and during spontaneous labor. J Clin Endocrinol Metab 53:730, 1981.

Lenton EA, Woodward AJ: The endocrinology of conception cycles and implantation in women. J Reprod Fertil 36 (Suppl):1, 1988.

Lessey BA: Endometrial integrins and the establishment of uterine receptivity. Hum Reprod 13:347, 1998.

Lessey BA, Yeh I, Castelbaum AJ, et al: Endometrial progesterone receptors and markers of uterine receptivity in the window of implantation. Fertil Steril 65:477, 1996.

Librach CL, Feigenbaum SL, Bass KE, et al: Interleukin-1 β-regulates human cytotrophoblast metalloproteinase activity and invasion in vitro. J Biol Chem 269:17125, 1994.

Lindhard A, Bentin-Ley U, Ravn V, et al: Biochemical evaluation of function at the time of implantation. Fertil Steril 78:221, 2002.

Liu JH, Park KH: Gonadotropin and prolactin secretion increases during sleep during the puerperium in nonlactating women. J Clin Endocrinol Metab 66:839, 1988.

Lockwood CJ, Krikun G, Hausknecht V, et al: Decidual cell regulation of hemostasis during implantation and menstruation. Ann N Y Acad Sci 828:188, 1997.

Martin RH, Oakey RE: The role of antenatal oestrogen in postpartum human lactogenesis: Evidence from oestrogen-deficient pregnancies. Clin Endocrinol 17:403, 1982.

Maruo T, Matsuo H, Murata K, et al: Gestational age-dependent dual action of epidermal growth factor on human placenta early in gestation. Endocrinology 75:1366, 1992.

McWilliams D, Boime I: Cytological localization of placental lactogen messenger ribonucleic acid in syncytiotrophoblast layers of human placenta. Endocrinology 107:761, 1980.

MMWR. Contribution of assisted reproductive technology and ovulation-induction drugs to triplet and higher-order multiple births—United States, 1980–1997. Morb Mortal Wkly Rep 49:535, 2000.

Muyan M, Boime I: Secretion of chorionic gonadotropin from human trophoblasts. Placenta 18:237, 1997.

Nakajima ST, McAuliffe T, Gibson M: The 24-hour pattern of the levels of serum progesterone and immunoreactive human chorionic gonadotropin in normal early pregnancy. J Clin Endocrinol Metab 71:345, 1990.

Nakazawa K, Makino T, Iizuka R, et al: Immunohistochemical study on oxytocin-like substance in the human placenta. Endocrinol Jpn 31:763, 1984.

Nielsen PV, Pedersen H, Kampmann EM: Absence of human placental lactogen in an otherwise uneventful pregnancy. Am J Obstet Gynecol 135:322, 1979.

Norman RJ, McLoughlin JW, Borthwick GM, et al: Inhibin and relaxin concentrations in early singleton, multiple, and failing pregnancy: Relationship to gonadotropin and steroid profiles. Fertil Steril 59:130, 1993.

Norwitz ER, Schust DJ, Fisher SJ: Implantation and the survival of early pregnancy. N Engl J Med 345:1400, 2001.

Norwitz ER, Wilson T: Secretory component: A potential regulator of endometrial-decidual prostaglandin production in early human pregnancy. Am J Obstet Gynecol 183:108, 2000.

O'Rahilly R: Developmental Stages in Human Embryos. Part A. Embryos of the First 3 Weeks (Stages 1 to 9). Publication No. 631. Washington, DC, Carnegie Institution, 1973.

Owens OM, Ryan KJ, Tulchinsky D: Episodic secretion of human chorionic gonadotropin in early pregnancy. J Clin Endocrinol Metab 53:1307, 1981.

Owerbach D, Rutter WJ, Martial JA: Genes for growth hormone chorionic somatomammotropin and growth hormone–like gene on chromosomes 17 in humans. Science 209:289, 1980.

Parker CR Jr, Hankins GD, Guzick DS: Ontogeny of unconjugated estriol in fetal blood and the relation of estriol levels at birth to the development of respiratory distress syndrome. Pediatr Res 21:386, 1987.

Parks JS, Nielsen PV, Sexton LA, et al: An effect of gene dosage on production of human chorionic somatomammotropin. J Clin Endocrinol Metab 60:994, 1985.

Petraglia F, Florio P, Carmine N, et al: Peptide signaling in human placenta and membranes: Autocrine, paracrine, and endocrine mechanisms. Endocrinol Rev 17:156, 1996.

Petraglia F, Giardino L, Coukos G, et al: Corticotrophin-releasing factor at parturition: Plasma and amniotic fluid levels and placental binding. Obstet Gynecol 75:784, 1990.

Potter JM, Nestel PJ: The hyperlipidemia of pregnancy in normal and complicated pregnancies. Am J Obstet Gynecol 133:165, 1979.

Rebar RW, Cedars MI: Hypergonadotropic forms of amenorrhea in young women. Pediatr Clin North Am 21:173, 1992.

Resnik R, Killam AP, Battaglia FC, et al: Stimulation of uterine blood flow by various estrogens. Endocrinology 94:1192, 1974.

Riggs LA, Lein A, Yen SSC: The pattern of increase in circulating prolactin levels during human gestation. Am J Obstet Gynecol 129:454, 1977.

Roberts JM, Lewis VL, Riemer RK: Hormonal control of uterine adrenergic response. In Bottari J, Thomas P, Vokser A, et al (eds): Uterine Contractility. New York, Masson, 1984, p. 161.

Rogers PAW: Uterine receptivity. In Gardner D, Trounson AO (eds): Handbook of In Vitro Fertilization. Boca Raton, FL, CRC Press, 1993, p. 263.

Rogers PAW, Murphy CR, Leeton J, et al: An ultrastructural study of human uterine epithelium from a patient with a confirmed pregnancy. Acta Anat 135:176, 1989.

Ruoslahti E, Pierschbacher MD: New perspective in cell adhesion: RGD and integrins. Science 238:491, 1987.

Salido EC, Yen PH, Barajas L, et al: Steroid sulfatase expression in human placenta: Immunocytochemistry and in situ hybridization study. J Clin Endocrinol Metab 70:1564, 1990.

Schieve LA, Meikle SF, Ferre C, et al: Low and very low birth weight in infants with use of assisted reproductive technology. N Engl J Med 346:731, 2002.

Schultz JF, Armant DR: Beta$_1$- and beta$_3$-class integrins mediate fibronectin binding activity at the surface of developing mouse peri-implantation blastocysts. J Biol Chem 270:11522, 1995.

Seeburg PH: The human growth hormone gene family: Nucleotide sequences show recent divergence and predict a new polypeptide hormone. DNA 1:239, 1982.

Siiteri PK, Febres F, Clemens LE, et al: Progesterone and maintenance of pregnancy: Is progesterone nature's immunosuppressant? Ann N Y Acad Sci 286:384, 1977.

Siiteri PK, MacDonald PC: The utilization of circulating dehydroisoandrosterone sulfate for estrogen synthesis during human pregnancy. Steroids 2:713, 1963.

Simpson ER, MacDonald PC: Endocrine physiology of the placenta. Annu Rev Physiol 43:163, 1981.

Steele GL, Currie WD, Yuen BH, et al: Acute stimulation of human chorionic gonadotropin secretion by recombinant human activin-A in first trimester human trophoblast. Endocrinology 133:297, 1993.

Stevens VC: Antifertility effects from immunisation with intact subunits and fragments of hCG. In Edwards RG, Johnson MG (eds): Physiological Effects of Immunity Against Reproductive Hormones. London, Cambridge University Press, 1975, p. 249.

Stewart CL, Cullinan EB: Preimplantation development of mammalian embryo and its regulation by growth factors. Dev Genet 21:91, 1997.

Strauss JF III, Gfvels ME, King BE: Placental hormones. In Degroot (ed): Endocrinology. WB Saunders, Philadelphia, 1995, p. 2171.

Sueoka K, Shiokawa S, Miyazaki T, et al: Integrins and reproductive physiology: Expression and modulation in fertilization, embryogenesis, and implantation. Fertil Steril 67:799, 1997.

Takemori M, Nishimura R, Ashitaka Y, et al: Release of human chorionic gonadotropin (hCG) and its alpha-subunit (hCGa) from perifused human placenta. Endocrinol Jpn 28:757, 1981.

Tapanainen J, Kellokumpu-Lehtinen P, Pelliniem L, et al: Age-related changes in endogenous steroids of human testis during early and mid-pregnancy. J Clin Endocrinol Metab 52:98, 1981.

Tulchinsky D, Frigoletto F, Ryan KJ, et al: Plasma estetrol as an index of fetal well-being. J Clin Endocrinol Metab 40:560, 1975.

Tulchinsky D, Hobel CJ: Plasma human chorionic gonadotropin, estrone, estradiol, estriol, progesterone and 17α-hydroxyprogesterone in human pregnancy. III. Early normal pregnancy. Am J Obstet Gynecol 117:884, 1973.

Tyson JE, McCoshen JA: Decidual prolactin: An enigmatic cyber in human reproduction. Semin Reprod Endocrinol 1:197, 1983.

Van Lith JM, Pratt JJ, Beekhuis JR, et al: Second trimester maternal serum immunoreactive inhibin as a marker for fetal Down's syndrome. Prenat Diagn **12:**801, 1992.

Warren WB, Silverman AJ: Cellular localization of corticotrophin releasing hormone in the placenta, fetal membranes, and decidua. Placenta **9:**16, 1995.

Weiss G, Goldsmith LT, Sachdev R: Elevated first-trimester serum relaxin concentrations in pregnant women following ovarian stimulation predict prematurity risk and preterm delivery. Obstet Gynecol **82:**821, 1993.

Weiss G, O'Byrne EM, Steinetz BTG: Relaxin: A product of the human corpus luteum of pregnancy. Science **194:**948, 1976.

Wilcox A, Baird DD, Weinberg C: Time of implantation of the conceptus and loss of pregnancy. N Engl J Med **340:**1796, 1999.

Yen SSC, Tsai CC, Vela P: Gestational diabetogenesis: Quantitative analyses of glucose-insulin interrelationship between normal pregnancy and pregnancy with gestational diabetes. Am J Obstet Gynecol **11:**792, 1971.

Yohkaichiya T, Fudaya T, Hoshiai H, et al: Inhibin, a new circulating marker in hydatidiform mole. Br Med J **298:**1684, 1989.

Yohkaichiya T, Polson DW, Hughes EG, et al: Serum immunoreactive inhibin levels in early pregnancy after in vitro fertilization and embryo transfer. Fertil Steril **59:**1081, 1993.

Chapter 10

THE BREAST AND THE PHYSIOLOGY OF LACTATION

Robert M. Lawrence, MD, and Ruth A. Lawrence, MD

Universal breast-feeding is recommended by the American College of Obstetrics and Gynecology, the World Health Organization, United Nations International Children's Emergency Fund, the American Academy of Pediatrics (AAP), and the Women, Infants and Children's Nutrition Program, but recommendations alone are not sufficient to promote breast-feeding. It is the responsibility of every physician to recommend and support breast-feeding enthusiastically. This is especially true in obstetrics where a physician's advice can immediately influence a woman's informed decision concerning breast-feeding and create or decrease barriers to successful breast-feeding. It is essential that a discussion of the benefits of breast-feeding to infants, mothers, and families (fathers included) is presented alongside any potential risks or contraindications. In contrast to the tremendous benefits of breast-feeding, the risks and contraindications are few. Summarized here are the conditions in which the risks of breast-feeding outweigh its benefits (Lawrence, 1997). Women who fit any of the following criteria should not breast-feed:

- Women who take street drugs or do not control their alcohol
- A woman who has an infant with galactosemia because both human and cow's milk exacerbate the condition (a lactose-free formula is required)
- Women who are infected with the human immunodeficiency virus (HIV; see later)
- Women who have active untreated tuberculosis—because of the increased risk of airborne transmission associated with close contact—until after appropriate treatment has been initiated
- Women who are known or suspected to be infected with Ebola or Marburg virus or Lassa fever (see later)
- Women who take certain medications (see later)
- Women who are undergoing treatment for breast cancer

Medical situations that indicate a potential risk from breast-feeding must be considered along with the benefits of breast-feeding in each maternal-infant dyad's unique situation.

BENEFITS OF BREAST-FEEDING

Breast-feeding provides benefits for both the mother and infant. Breast milk is species specific, made uniquely for the human infant (Lawrence and Lawrence, 1999). Protein in breast milk is readily digested and is present in appropriate amounts to be handled by the developing kidney. Various minerals (iron) and nutrients exist in a form and in conjunction with other components that make them easily absorbed to meet infants' needs during the periods of rapid growth (Dewey, 2001; Lawrence and Lawrence, 1999). Cholesterol and docosahexaenoic acid have been shown to play a role in central nervous system development and may contribute to the enhanced intelligence quotient measurements reported in breast-fed infants (SanGiovanni et al., 2000a; Horwood et al., 2001).

Protection against infections, including otitis media, croup, pneumonia, and gastrointestinal infections, is mediated by the over 50 immunologically active components found in breast milk. (AAP, 1997; Lawrence and Lawrence, 1999) These immunologically active components include viable functioning cells (T and B lymphocytes, macrophages), T-cell–secreted products, immunoglobulins (especially secretory IgA), carrier proteins like lactoferrin and transferrin, enzymes (lysozyme and lipoprotein lipase), and nonspecific factors such as complement, bifidus factor, gangliosides, and nucleotides. Other immune factors in breast milk include hormones, hormone-like factors, and growth factors that contribute to the normal maturation of the mucosal barrier of the respiratory and gastrointestinal tracts as well as the developing infant's immune system. Breast milk is a very dynamic fluid, varying with the maternal-infant dyads' environment and needs, especially in the face of infection and/or stress (e.g., nucleotides, secretory IgA, interleukin, interferon, and cytokines) (Butte et al., 1984; Quan et al., 1990; Srivastava et al., 1996; Pickering et al., 1998). There is also evidence that breast-feeding provides protection against some noninfectious illnesses like wheezing/asthma and eczema, childhood lymphoma, insulin-dependent childhood-onset diabetes, and obesity (AAP, 1997; von Kries et al., 1999; Lawrence and Lawrence, 1999) in children who are exclusively breast-fed for the first 4 to 6 months of life.

Cognitive and psychological benefits for breast-fed infants have been suggested, including developmental performance (Lucas et al., 1992), visual acuity (Neuringer, 2000; Jorgensen 1996; SanGiovanni et al., 2000b), school performance (Horwood and Fergusson, 1998), and performance on standardized (Horwood and Fergusson, 1998) and intelligence quotient (Horwood et al., 2001) tests. More recent articles continue the debate over the relative contributions of nutrition, genetics, and environment to the intellectual development of infants and the possible influence on the child's or adult's future cognitive abilities as measured by intelligence quotient testing (Lucas et al., 1998; Jacobson et al., 1999). The psychological benefits are more difficult to measure but are readily described by most mothers who successfully breast-fed their infants.

Potential benefits to the mother include improved postpartum recovery, a lower incidence of subsequent obesity (Subcommittee on Nutrition During Lactation, 1991), a decreased risk of osteoporosis, and reduced incidence of both breast and ovarian cancers (Labbok, 2001). Calcium and phosphorous concentrations are higher in lactating women, and the risk of osteoporosis is measurably less for women who have breast-fed their infants (Kalkwarf and Specker, 1995; Kalkwarf et al., 1996). Increasing number of pregnancies, longer oral contraceptive use, and increasing duration of lactation are all protective against ovarian cancer (Whitemore, 1994; John et al., 1993; Rosenblatt and Thomas, 1993). The incidence of breast cancer is lower among women who have nursed (Newcomb et al., 1994).

ROLE OF OBSTETRICIANS IN PROMOTING BREAST-FEEDING

Obstetricians have many responsibilities for breast-feeding, including the following:

1. Enthusiastic promotion and support for breast-feeding, based on the published literature of its benefits
2. Clinical knowledge about the physiology of lactogenesis (Neville et al., 2001) and lactation and in the prenatal, intrapartum, and postpartum support of the lactating mother
3. Development and support of hospital policies to facilitate breast-feeding and remove barriers to breast-feeding
4. Community efforts to provide women with adequate information to make an informed decision about breast-feeding including links to community breast-feeding resources
5. Fostering acceptance of breast-feeding among the general public by promoting a normative portrayal of breast-feeding in the media and supporting sufficient time and facilities in the workplace
6. Performing breast examinations in the prenatal, intrapartum, and postpartum periods and emphasizing lactation as the primary function of the breast
7. Participation in breast-feeding education in medical and other health profession schools (AAP, 1997)

The mother's plan for infant feeding should be addressed early in prenatal care, including counseling, a medical history focused on breast health and breast-feeding, and a physical examination of the breast. Counseling can be modeled after "The Best Start Three Step Breastfeeding Counseling Strategy" (Beststart@mindspring.com; Lazarov and Evans, 2000), a publication that advises beginning with open-ended questions about breast-feeding. An acknowledgment that feelings of doubt about the ability to breast-feed successfully are normal is a good place to begin. Education about breast-feeding then continues with discussion of how others have dealt with these concerns. This conversation will elucidate much about the woman's knowledge of breast-feeding, her previous experiences with breast-feeding, and her own attitudes and those of the infant's father, the extended family, and other potentially supportive persons in the mother's life.

To support breast-feeding adequately throughout the first 6 months of an infant's life, the concerns of family and friends must be answered positively to foster support for breast-feeding on many levels. Misconceptions and potential barriers must be identified and reasonable solutions developed in partnership with the woman. These often include feelings of responsibility for every unexplained problem the infant displays; conflicts among a woman's several roles as mother, sexual partner, and worker outside the home; and, most commonly, a greater time commitment and fatigue than was expected. It is important to address these and other questions repeatedly throughout pregnancy and not just in the immediate postpartum period.

EXAMINATION OF THE BREAST

The medical history related to the breasts should include their development, previous experience with breast-feeding, systemic illnesses, infections, breast surgery or trauma, medications, allergies, self–breast examinations and findings, and any anatomic/physical concerns the mother has about her breasts.

The breast examination at prenatal and postpartum visits should include careful inspection and palpation. Inspection of the breasts is most effective in the sitting position, first with the arms overhead and then with hands on the hips. Skin changes, distortions in shape or contour, and the form and size of the areola and nipple should be noted. Palpation can begin in the sitting position, looking for axillary and supraclavicular adenopathy. Palpation in the supine position is easier for the complete examination of the breast and surrounding anterolateral chest wall. Size, shape, consistency, masses, scars, tenderness, and any abnormalities can be noted in both descriptive and picture form for future comparison. Serial examinations should document maturational changes of pregnancy (size, shape, fullness, enlargement of areola) and nipple position (inversion/eversion). With the increased frequency of cosmetic breast surgery, it is important to be aware of the nature of any surgery and to examine carefully for the location of the surgical scars. Many women successfully breast-feed after surgery for benign breast disease, breast augmentation, or breast reduction. However, a periareolar incision or "nipple translocation technique" for breast reduction can damage nerves and/or ducts, making this more difficult. Nipple piercing is another increasingly common procedure after which breast-feeding can be successful with the jewelry removed. Such surgeries do not preclude successful breast-feeding but rather remind us that additional early support should be provided to these mothers from physicians, nurses, lactation consultants, and peer support groups.

Perinatal Period

The obstetrician can make important contributions to successful breast-feeding through the conduct of the labor, delivery, and puerperium. A stressful or exhausting labor and delivery has been shown to affect lactation adversely (Neville et al., 1988). A safe delivery for both the mother and infant is the most important. Selection of medications during the delivery and postpartum that are compatible with breast-feeding and do not interfere with the bonding and first feeding is another important way to facilitate breast-feeding. Immediate skin-to-skin contact with the mother and a first feeding within 1 hour of delivery are probably the most important intrapartum steps to increase the likelihood of successful breast-feeding. Having the infant room with the mother, feeding on demand, and early breast-feeding support and assessment of appropriate techniques within the first 24 to 36 hours can also help. Supplementation should be avoided unless medically indicated.

Medication choices with breast-feeding in mind is very important (see Table 10-6D). Most women and many health professionals assume that no medication can be safely administered to a lactating woman, when in fact the number of drugs that are contraindicated is actually quite small. Rather than assume a medication is unsafe, it is better to consult one of several readily available texts or a drug information website before offering any opinion about a particular medication.

Early follow-up (2 to 4 days) after discharge with the infant's doctor should be arranged for all breast-feeding mothers. Continued support of breast-feeding should occur through the 6-week postpartum visit for the mother. Inquiry about breast-feeding should include discussion of techniques to ensure complete emptying of the breast, nipple soreness or trauma, plugged duct (in the form of a small lump), mastitis, breast abscess, breast masses, or bloody nipple discharge. All the above can usually be treated without stopping breast-feeding.

Lactogenesis

Lactation is the physiologic completion of the reproductive cycle. The human infant is the most immature and dependent of all mammals except for marsupials, and thus the breast provides the most physiologic nutrients required by the human infant at birth. Throughout pregnancy, the breast develops and prepares to take over the role of fully nourishing the infant when the placenta is expelled. The breast is prepared for full lactation after 16 weeks' gestation. The physiologic adaptation of the mammary gland to its role in infant survival is a complex system, only the outline of which is discussed here. There are a number of complete reviews of the newer scientific studies on the physiology of lactation (Neville, 1997; Neville et al., 2001). The hormonal control of lactation can be described in relation to the five major changes in the development of the mammary gland: embryogenesis, mammogenesis or mammary growth, lactogenesis or initiation of milk secretion, lactation or full milk secretion, and involution (Table 10-1). Detailed explanation of mammary growth is beyond the scope of this discussion. The two most important hormones involved in lactation itself are prolactin and oxytocin, and these are described with relationship to their impact on lactogenesis.

■ THE BREAST

To fully understand the process of lactation, one needs to understand the anatomy and physiology of the breast as it applies to this important function of the breast. The human mammary gland is the only organ that does not contain all the rudimentary tissues at birth. It experiences dramatic changes in size, shape, and function from birth through menarche, pregnancy, and lactation and ultimately during involution. There are three major phases of growth and development before pregnancy and lactation: *in utero*, during the first 2 years of life, and at puberty (Fig. 10-1).

Embryonic Development

The milk streak appears in the 4th week of gestation when the embryo is approximately 2.5 mm long. It becomes the milk line or milk ridge during the 5th week of gestation (2.5 to

TABLE 10-1. STAGES OF MAMMARY DEVELOPMENT

Developmental Stage	Hormonal Regulation	Local Factors	Description
Embryogenesis	?	Fat pad necessary for ductal extension	Epithelial bud develops in 18- to 19-week-old fetus, extending short distance into mammary fat pad with blind ducts that become canalized; some milk secretion may be present at birth
Mammogenesis			Anatomic development
Puberty			
Before onset of menses	Estrogen, GH	IGF-I, hGF, TGF-β, ? others	Ductal extension into mammary fat pad; branching morphogenesis
After onset of menses	Estrogen, progesterone, ? PRL		Lobular development with formation of terminal duct lobular unit
Pregnancy	Progesterone, PRL, hPL	HER, ? others	Alveolus formation; partial cellular differentiation
Lactogenesis	Progesterone withdrawal, PRL, glucocorticoid	Not known	Onset of milk secretion Stage I: midpregnancy Stage II: parturition
Lactation	PRL, oxytocin	FIL	Ongoing milk secretion
Involution	PRL withdrawal	Milk stasis, ? FIL	Alveolar epithelium undergoes apoptosis and remodeling; gland reverts to prepregnant state

FIL, feedback inhibition of lactation; GH, growth hormone; HER, herregulin; hGF, human growth factor; hPL, human placental lactogen; IGF-I, insulin-like growth factor I; PRL, prolactin; TGF, transforming growth factor.

Modified from Neville MC: Mammary gland biology and lactation: A short course. Presented at the biannual meeting of the International Society for Research on Human Milk and Lactation, Plymouth, Mass., October 1997.

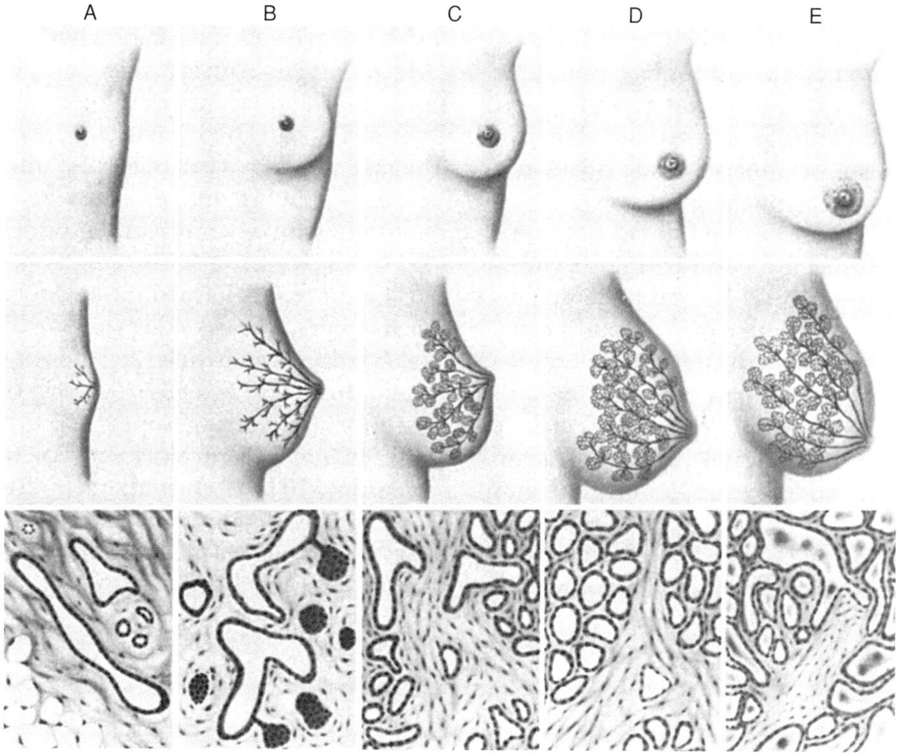

FIGURE 10-1 ■ Female breast from infancy to lactation with corresponding cross-section and duct structure. **A**, **B**, and **C**, Gradual development of well-differentiated ductular and peripheral lobular–alveolar system. **D**, Ductular sprouting and intensified peripheral lobular–alveolar development in pregnancy. Glandular luminal cells begin actively synthesizing milk fat and proteins near term; only small amounts are released into lumen. **E**, With postpartum withdrawal of luteal and placental sex steroids and placental lactogen, prolactin is able to induce full secretory activity of alveolar cells and release of milk into alveoli and smaller ducts. (From Lawrence RA, Lawrence RM: Breastfeeding: A Guide for the Medical Profession, 5th ed. St. Louis, Mosby, 1999, p. 38, Fig. 2-3.)

5.5 mm). The mammary gland itself begins to develop at 6 weeks of embryonic life with the continuation of the proliferation of the milk ducts throughout embryonic growth. The process of forming the nipple in the human embryo begins with a thickened raised area of ectoderm in the region of the future gland by the 4th week of pregnancy. This thickened ectoderm becomes depressed into the underlying mesoderm, and thus the surface of the mammary area soon becomes flat and finally sinks below the level of the surrounding epidermis. The mesoderm that is in contact with the ingrowth of the ectoderm is compressed, and its elements become arranged in concentric layers that at a later stage give rise to the gland's stroma. The ingrowing mass of ectodermal cells by dividing and branching gives rise to the future lobes and lobules and much later to the alveoli.

By 16 weeks' gestation in the fetus, the branching stage has produced 15 to 25 epithelial strips that represent the future secretory alveoli. By 28 weeks' gestation, placental sex hormones enter the fetal circulation and induce canalization. The lactiferous ducts and their branches are developed from outgrowth in the lumen. They open into a shallow epidermal depression known as the mammary pit. The pit becomes elevated as a result of mesenchymal proliferation, forming the nipple and areola. An inverted nipple is the failure of this pit to elevate (Bland and Romnell, 1991). At 32 weeks' gestation, the lumen has formed in the branching system, and by term there are 15 to 25 mammary ducts that form the fetal mammary gland (Fig. 10-2).

The nipple, areola, and breast bud have become important landmarks for the determination of gestational age in the newborn. At 40 weeks, the nipple and areola are clearly seen and the breast bud is up to 1.0 cm in diameter. In the first weeks after delivery, the breast bud is visible and palpable; however, the gland then regresses to a quiescent stage as maternal hormones in the infant are diminished and grows only in proportion to the rest of the body until puberty.

Pubertal Development

With the onset of puberty in the female, further growth of the breast occurs and the areolae enlarge and become more pigmented. The further development of the breast involves two distinct processes: organogenesis and milk production. The ductal and lobular growth is organogenesis, and this is initiated before and throughout puberty, resulting in the growth of breast parenchyma with its surrounding fat pad. The formation of alveolar buds begins within 1 to 2 years of the onset of menses and continues for several years, producing alveolar lobes. This menarchial stimulus begins with the extension of the ductal tree and the generation of its branching pattern. The existing ducts elongate, dichotomously branching the growing ductal tips. The ducts can develop bulbous terminal end buds that are the forerunners of alveoli. The formation of the alveolar bud begins within 1 to 2 years of the onset of menses. During this ductal growth, the alveoli enlarge and the nipple and areola become more pigmented. This growth involves an increase in connective tissue, adipose tissue, and vascular channels and is stimulated by estrogen and progesterone released by the ovary (Osbourne, 1996).

During the menstrual cycle, there continues to be cyclic microscopic proliferation and regression of ductal breast tissue. The breast continues to enlarge slightly with further division of the ductal system until about the age of 28, unless pregnancy intervenes.

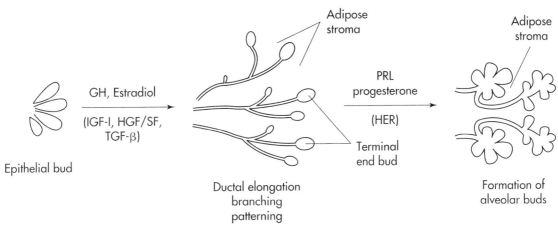

FIGURE 10-2 ■ Scheme for regulation of mammary development in the mouse. GH, growth hormone; HER, herregulin; HGF/SF, human growth factor/secretory factor; IGF-I, insulin-like growth factor I; PRL, prolactin; TGF-β, transforming growth factor-β. (From Neville MC: Mammary gland biology and lactation: A short course. Presented at the annual meeting of the International Society for Research on Human Milk and Lactation. Plymouth, Mass, October 1997.)

The Mature Breast

The mature breast is located in the superficial fascia between the second and sixth intercostal cartilages and is superficial to the pectoralis muscle. It measures 10 to 12 cm in diameter. It is located horizontally from the parasternal to the mid-axillary line. The central thickness of the gland is 5 to 7 cm. In the nonpregnant state, the breast weighs about 200 g. During pregnancy, however, the size and weight increase to about 400 to 600 g and to 600 to 800 g during lactation. A projection of mammary tissue into the axilla is known as the tail of Spence and is connected to the central duct system. The breast is usually dome shaped or conic, becoming more hemispheric in the adult and pendulous in the older parous female.

Abnormalities

In some women, mammary tissue develops at other sites in the galactic band. This is referred to as hypermastia, which is the presence of accessory mammary glands that are phylogenic remnants. These remnants may include accessory nipples or accessory gland tissue located anywhere along the milk line. From 2% to 6% of women have hypermastia. These remnants remain quiet until pregnancy when they may respond to the hormonal milieu by enlarging and even secreting milk during lactation. If left unstimulated, they will regress postpartum. Major glandular tissue in the axilla may pose a cosmetic or management problem if the tissue enlarges significantly during pregnancy and lactation, secreting milk. It is distinct from the tail of Spence.

Other abnormalities may include amastia, absence of the breast and/or nipple, amazia, hyperadenia, hypoplasia, polythelia, and symmastia (Table 10-2). Abnormalities of the kidneys have been associated with polythelia. Other variations include hyperplasia or hypoplasia in various combinations, as outlined in Table 10-3. Gigantomastia is the excessive enlargement of the breasts in pregnancy and lactation, sometimes to life-threatening proportions. This enlargement may occur with the first or any pregnancy and may or may not recur. The enlarge-ment recedes but rarely back to original size (Lawrence and Lawrence, 1999). Breast-feeding has been successful in some cases of gigantomastia with appropriate professional support.

Mothers with congenital abnormalities of the breast may wish to breast-feed. Not all abnormalities or variations preclude breast-feeding, and the question should be considered on a case-by-case basis.

Nipple and Areola

The skin of the breast includes the nipple and areola and the thin flexible elastic skin that covers the body of the breast. The nipple is a conic elevation in the center of the areola at the level of about the fourth intercostal space, just below the midline of the breast. The nipple contains smooth muscle fibers and is richly innervated with sensory and pain fibers. It has a verrucous surface and has sebaceous and apocrine sweat glands, but not hair.

The areola surrounds the nipple and is also slightly pigmented and becomes deeply pigmented during pregnancy and lactation. The average diameter is 15 to 16 mm, but the range may exceed 5 cm during pregnancy. The sensory innervation is less than that of the nipple. The nipple and areola are very elastic and elongate into a teat when drawn into the mouth by the suckling infant.

 TABLE 10-2. BREAST ABNORMALITIES

Accessory breast: Any tissue outside the two major glands
Amastia: Congenital absence of breast and nipple
Amazia: Nipple without breast tissue
Hyperadenia: Mammary tissue without nipple
Hypoplasia: Underdevelopment of breast
Polythelia: Supernumerary nipple(s) (also *hyperthelia*)
Symmastia: Webbing between breasts

From Lawrence RA, Lawrence RM: Breastfeeding: A Guide for the Medical Profession, 5th ed. St. Louis, Mosby, 1999, p. 41, Box 2-1.

TABLE 10-3. TYPES OF BREAST HYPOPLASIA, HYPERPLASIA, AND ACQUIRED ABNORMALITIES

Unilateral hypoplasia, contralateral breast normal
Bilateral hypoplasia with asymmetry
Unilateral hyperplasia, contralateral breast normal
Bilateral hyperplasia with asymmetry
Unilateral hypoplasia, contralateral breast hyperplasia
Unilateral hypoplasia of breast, thorax, and pectoral muscles (Poland syndrome)
Acquired abnormalities caused by trauma, burns, radiation treatment for hemangioma or intrathoracic disease, chest tube insertion in infancy, and preadolescent biopsy

From Lawrence RA, Lawrence RM: Breastfeeding: A Guide for the Medical Profession, 5th ed. St. Louis, Mosby, 1999, p. 41, Box 2-2.

The surface of the areola contains Montgomery glands, which hypertrophy in pregnancy and lactation and resemble vesicles. They secrete a sebaceous material to lubricate the nipple and areola and protect the tissue while suckling during lactation. These glands atrophy after weaning and are not visible to the naked eye except during pregnancy or lactation.

Each nipple contains 15 to 25 lactiferous ducts surrounded by fibromuscular tissue. These ducts end as small orifices at the tip of the nipple from which the milk flows. The ducts tract in the areola and have a dilation at the nipple base, forming a milk sinus, called lactiferous sinus, that functions as a temporary collecting area during suckling.

The corpus mammae is an orderly conglomeration of a number of independent glands known as lobes. The morphology of the gland includes parenchyma that contains the ductular-lobular-alveolar structures. It also includes the stroma, which is the connective tissue, fat tissue, blood vessels, nerves, and lymphatics.

The mass of breast tissue consists of the tubuloalveolar glands embedded in the adipose tissue, which gives the gland its smooth rounded contour. The mammary fat pad is essential for the proliferation and differentiation of the ductal arborization. Each lobe forms a gland separated by connective tissue and opens into a duct that opens into the nipple. The extension of ducts is orderly and protected by an inhibitory zone into which other ducts cannot penetrate (Fig. 10-3).

Blood is supplied to the breast from branches of the intercostal arteries and perforating branches of the internal thoracic artery. The main blood supply comes from the internal mammary artery and the lateral thoracic artery. The venous supply parallels the arterial supply.

Lymphatic drainage has been thoroughly studied by researchers of breast cancer. The main drainage is to axillary nodes and the parasternal nodes along the thoracic artery within the thorax. The lymphatics of the breast originate in lymph capillaries of the mammary connective tissue and drain through the deep substance of the breast.

The breast is innervated from the branches of the fourth, fifth, and sixth intercostal nerves. The sensory innervation of the nipple and areola is extensive and includes both autonomic and sensory nerves. The innervation of the corpus mammae is meager by comparison and is predominantly autonomic. Neither parasympathetic nor cholinergic fibers supply any part of the breast. The efferent nerves are sympathetic adrenergic. Most of the mammary nerves follow the arteries. A few fibers course along the walls of the ducts. They may be sensory fibers that sense milk pressure. No innervation has been identified to supply the myoepithelial cells. Thus, the conclusion is that secretory activities of the acinar epithelium of the ducts depend on hormonal stimulation, such as oxytocin.

When sensory fibers are stimulated, the release of adenohypophyseal prolactin and neurohypophyseal oxytocin occurs. The areola is most sensitive to the stimulus of suckling, the nipple the least, and the skin of the breast intermediate. The large number of dermal nerve endings results in high responsiveness to suckling. Pain fibers are more numerous in the

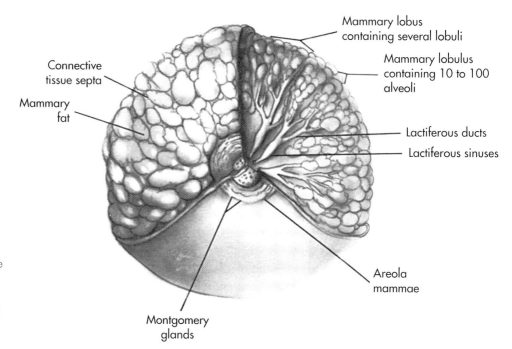

FIGURE 10-3 ■ Morphology of mature breast with dissection to reveal mammary fat and duct system. (From Lawrence RA, Lawrence RM: Breastfeeding: A Guide for the Medical Profession, 5th ed. St. Louis, Mosby, 1999, p 43, Fig. 2-7.)

nipple, with few in the areola. All cutaneous nerves run radially toward the nipple. Breast nerves can influence the mammary blood supply and therefore also influence the transport of oxytocin and prolactin to the myoepithelial cells and the lacteal cells, respectively.

MAMMARY GLAND IN PREGNANCY

During the first trimester, there is rapid growth and branching from the terminal duct system into the adipose tissue stimulated by the changing levels of circulating hormones. As epithelial structures proliferate, adipose tissue decreases. There is increased infiltration of the interstitial tissue with lymphatics, plasma cells, and eosinophils. By the third trimester, parenchymal cell growth slows and alveoli become distended with early colostrum. Alveolar proliferation is extensive.

The lactating mammary gland has a large number of alveoli that are made up of cuboidal, epithelial, and myoepithelial cells. Little connective tissue separates the alveoli. Lipid droplets are visible in the cells. By complex interplay of the nervous system and endocrine factors (progesterone, estrogen, thyroid, insulin, and growth factors), the mammary gland begins to function (lactogenesis stage I) and other hormones establish the milk secretion and maintain it (lactogenesis stage II).

Human prolactin has a significant role in both pregnancy and lactation. The levels are high during pregnancy, but the influence of prolactin on the breast itself is inhibited by a hormone produced by the placenta, originally referred to as prolactin-inhibiting hormone but believed to be progesterone.

PHYSIOLOGY OF LACTATION

Lactogenesis is the initiation of milk secretion, beginning with the changes in the mammary epithelium in early pregnancy to full lactation. Stage I lactogenesis occurs during pregnancy and is achieved when the gland is sufficiently differentiated to secrete milk. It is prevented from doing so by high circulating plasma concentrations of progesterone (Kuhn, 1977). Stage II is the onset of copious milk secretion associated with delivery of infant and the placenta. The progesterone level decreases sharply, by 10-fold in the first 4 days (Neville, 2001). This is accompanied by the programmed transformation of the mammary epithelium (Chen et al., 1998). By day 5, 500 to 750 mL of milk is available to the infant (Fig. 10-4). The changes in milk composition that occurs in the first 10 days postpartum should be viewed as part of a continuum where the first 4 days see rapid changes followed by slower changes of various components of milk throughout lactation (Neville et al., 2001). This is due to the change in permeability of the paracellular pathways, resulting in a shift from high concentrations of sodium, chloride, and the protective immunoglobulins and lactoferrin, little lactose, and no casein in colostrum to increasing amounts of all milk components (Morton, 1994).

Lactogenesis stage II results in an increase of milk of 100 mL in the first 24 hours to large volumes (500 to 750 mL/day) by day 4 or 5, gradually leveling off by day 8 (Neville et al., 1988). These volume changes are associated with a decrease in sodium and chloride concentration and an increase in lactose concentration. The production of lactose drives the production of milk. The early changes in sodium and chloride are a function of the closure of the tight junctions that block the paracellular pathway (Kulski et al., 1978; Aperia et al., 1979). Secretory IgA and lactoferrin represent 10% by weight of the milk produced in the first 48 hours, and although their volumes continue, the increase in volume of milk produced decreases their concentration. At 8 days secretory IgA and lactoferrin are 1% by weight and 2 to 3 g/day (Neville, 1995b).

At 36 hours postpartum in multiparas and up to 72 hours in primiparas, milk production increases 10-fold (from 50 to 500 mL/day). This is described by women as their milk coming in. This reflects a massive increase in synthesis and secretion of the components of mature milk, including lactose, protein, and lipid (Neville et al., 1991).

During pregnancy, hormones have two essential roles: to maintain the pregnancy and to produce mammary tissue that is prepared to produce milk but does not do so. Progesterone, prolactin, and possibly placental lactogen are credited with the development of the alveoli. Progesterone has been identified as

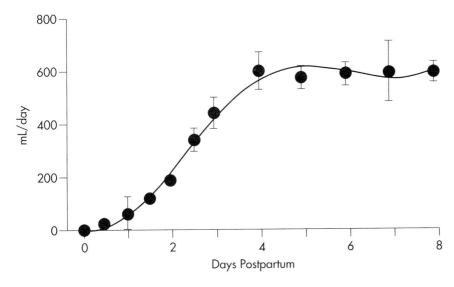

FIGURE 10-4 ■ Milk volumes during 1st week postpartum. Mean values from 12 multiparous white women who test weighed their infants before and after every feeding for first 7 days postpartum. (Redrawn from Neville MC: Determinants of milk volume and composition. *In* Jensen RG (ed): Handbook of Milk Composition. San Diego, Academic Press, 1995, p. 1375.)

the major inhibitor of milk production during pregnancy (Kuhn, 1983). Prolactin levels in pregnancy are over 200 ng/mL. It is apparently the continued high level of prolactin and a decrease in progesterone that are necessary for stage II lactogenesis after parturition (Kuhn, 1983). The placenta is the main source of progesterone in pregnancy. It is further established that progesterone receptors are lost in the human breast postpartum. Estrogen levels drop precipitously postpartum.

In addition to prolactin, insulin and corticoids are essential to milk synthesis (Neubauer et al., 1993). Delayed lactogenesis is seen in retained placenta, cesarean section, diabetes, and stress during delivery (Neifert et al., 1981; Neville et al., 1988; Sozmen, 1992; Neubauer et al., 1993). Stressful labors were first noted by Jackson (1950) to influence the early breastfeeding experience in the rooming-in unit in the 1940s. Except for retained placenta, stress may be the trigger for delayed lactogenesis in the other conditions. The significance of high milk sodium syndrome requires further study (Morton, 1994). It has been observed that high sodium levels in early milk samples are seen in pregnancy, mastitis, involution (weaning), premature birth, and inhibition of prolactin secretion (bromocriptine). These observations suggest that junctional closure depends on adequate suckling and/or effective milk removal in the first 3 days postpartum.

If milk removal does not begin by 72 hours, the changes in milk composition associated with lactogenesis are reversed and the probability that lactation will be successful decreases. Thus, the clinical efforts that facilitate early suckling by the newborn do enhance the probability of lactation success. Further early stimulation of the breast by pumping before 72 hours postpartum is essential when the infant is unable to nurse directly.

■ LET-DOWN (EJECTION) REFLEX

An effective let-down reflex is key to successful lactation. This reflex, also known as the ejection reflex, was first described in humans by Peterson and Ludwick in 1942 but was later demonstrated clinically by Newton and Newton (1948) to be due to the release of oxytocin by the pituitary.

Since that time, many refinements in the understanding of the process have been published but the fundamental principles are unchanged (Fig. 10-5).

A mother may produce milk, but if it is not excreted, further production is eventually suppressed. The reflex is a complex function that depends on hormones, nerves, and glandular response and can be inhibited most easily by psychological influences.

Oxytocin is the hormone responsible for the stimulus of the myoepithelial cells to contract and eject the milk from the ductal system. The ducts begin at the alveoli, which are surrounded by a basket-like structure of myoepithelial cells that also surround the ducts all the way to the nipple. When the infant stimulates the breast by suckling, impulses sent to the central nervous system and to the posterior pituitary release oxytocin, which in turn is carried by the bloodstream to the myoepithelial cells. This is a neuroendocrine reflex. Oxytocin release can also be stimulated by other pathways of sight, sound, and smell that represent the infant. Oxytocin also stimulates the myoepithelial cells in the uterus, which are very sensitive to oxytocin during parturition and for a week or so postpartum. This causes the uterus to contract, decreases blood loss, and hastens postpartum involution. The uterus of a mother who breast-feeds returns to a prepregnant state more rapidly. The uterine cramping experienced while breastfeeding is a result of this stimulus (see Fig. 10-5).

Newton and Newton (1948) demonstrated that pain and stress interfered with the let-down reflex because it interfered with oxytocin release. In their experimental model, they used pain, loud noises, or pressure to solve mathematical problems to stimulate stress. In other species, oxytocin release has been shown to stimulate mothering behaviors (Pedersen et al., 1994). Levels of adrenocorticotropin and plasma cortisol are decreased in lactating women compared with nonlactating women in response to stress.

Prolactin is central to the production of milk and regulates the rate of synthesis. Its release depends on the suckling of the infant or the stimulation of the nipple by mechanical pumping or manual expression. Prolactin is also released through a neuroendocrine reflex. Its influence is modified, however, by the actual release of milk from the alveoli. Local factors in the

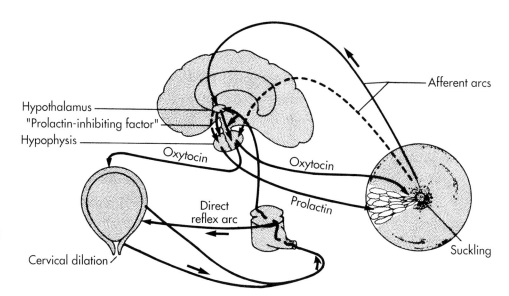

FIGURE 10-5 ■ Neuroendocrine control of milk ejection. (Modified from Vorherr H: The Breast: Morphology, Physiology and Lactation. New York, Academic Press, 1974.)

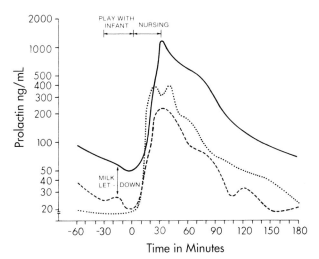

FIGURE 10-6 ■ Plasma prolactin measured by radioimmunoassay before, during, and after period of nursing in three mothers, 22 to 26 days postpartum. Prolactin levels rose with suckling and not with infant contact. (Modified from Josimovich JB, Reynolds M, Cobo E: Lactogenic hormones, fetal nutrition, and lactation. *In* Josimovich JB, Reynolds M, Cobo E (eds): Problems of Human Reproduction, vol. 2. New York, John Wiley & Sons, 1974. p. 1.)

ductal system or in the accumulated milk can inhibit milk release and thus inhibit further milk production. Prolactin is not released as a result of sound, sight, or smell of the infant, as is the case with oxytocin, only suckling (Fig. 10-6).

INITIATION OF LACTATION

Although breast-feeding is a natural process in postpartum women, it is a learned skill, not a reflex. Because the incidence of breast-feeding in developed countries dropped to about 10% in the 1950s and 1960s, there are few experienced role models available for new mothers to support, encourage, and assist them to feed their infants at the breast. In the late 1940s, Edith Jackson at Yale in cooperation with Herbert Thoms established the first rooming-in unit in the United States, introduced "child birth without fear," and reestablished breast-feeding as the norm for mothers and infants at the Yale New Haven Hospital (Jackson et al., 1948). Obstetric and pediatric residents were well schooled in the practical aspects of breast-feeding and human lactation. Jackson and her pediatric colleagues published the classic article on the management of breast-feeding (Barnes et al., 1953) upon which decades of publications for both the public and the professional were based.

The obstetrician and pediatrician have become more involved in the decision to breast-feed and the practical management of the mother–baby dyad. Medical schools are adding breast-feeding and lactation to their curriculum gradually. Although it is not the physician's role to put the infant to the breast, it is important to understand the process, to recognize problems, and to know how to solve them. Breast-feeding support is a team event where the physician works with many health care professionals, including nurses, midwives, doulas, and dietitians, to provide complete care to the perinatal patient. There are now lactation specialists who may be nurses, dietitians, or nonmedical individuals with special training or

physicians with specialty designation. The physician should be sure the consultant is licensed and board certified by the International Board of Lactation Consultant Examiners or, if another physician, is recognized as a fellow of the Academy of Breastfeeding Medicine.

Except in extreme cases, breast size does not influence milk production. Augmentation mammoplasty does not interfere with lactation unless a periareolar incision was made and nerves were interrupted. If augmentation was done for cosmetic enhancement, the tissue should function well, but if there was little or no palpable breast tissue before surgery, lactation may be improbable.

Reduction mammoplasty is more invasive surgery, and results depend on the technique used. If many ducts were severed and the nipple and areolar transplanted, it will interfere with lactation. If, however, the nipple and areolar remained intact on a pedicle of ducts, lactation could be successful. Other incisions for lump removal should be discussed but usually do not interfere with lactation.

During pregnancy, the obstetrician should document the changes in the breasts in response to pregnancy when the nipple and areola should become more pigmented and enlarged and the breast should enlarge several cup sizes. Lack of breast changes should also be communicated to the pediatrician. This failure of breast changes is a risk for early failure to thrive because of insufficient milk supply. A breast examination should be conducted late in the pregnancy to check for any new findings of masses, lumps, discharge, or pain. Berens (2001) described the role of the obstetrician throughout pregnancy in detail.

INITIATING BREAST-FEEDING

The ideal time to initiate breast-feeding is immediately after birth (the Baby Friendly Initiative recommends within a half hour of birth). When left on the mother's abdomen to explore, the unmedicated newborn will move toward the breast and latch on and begin suckling. This usually takes 20 to 30 minutes if left unassisted (Righard and Alade, 1990). The infant is ready to feed and has been sucking *in utero* since about 14 weeks, consuming amniotic fluid daily (about 1 g protein/kg of fetal weight is received daily from amniotic fluid). The infant at 28 weeks' gestation already has a rooting, sucking, and coordinated swallow while breast-feeding. The ability to coordinate suck and swallow while bottle feeding does not occur until 34 weeks.

Shortly after delivery, the mother should be offered the opportunity to breast-feed and should be assisted to assume a comfortable position, usually lying on her side. The infant can be placed beside her, tummy to tummy facing the breast. The mother should support her breast with her hand, keeping her fingers behind the areolar so the infant can latch on. The mother should stroke the center of the lower lip with the breast. The infant should open the mouth wide, extend the tongue, and draw the nipple and areolar into the mouth to form a teat. This teat is compressed against the palate by the tongue, and the gums and lips form a seal with the breast. It is the peristaltic motion of the tongue that stimulates the let-down reflex and milks the lactiferous sinuses that eject the milk. The continued peristaltic motion to the posterior tongue, the pharynx, and down the esophagus is one coordinated motion so that swallowing is automatically coordinated with suckling when breast-feeding. Sucking an artificial nipple is a very different tongue motion that is not coordinated with swallow. A newborn should not be given a bottle to test feeding ability before breast-feeding. It is wise to avoid all artificial nipples (bottles or pacifiers) in the early weeks of breast-feeding. If, for a medical necessity, the infant requires artificial formula, it can be given by medicine cup (cup feeding) (Fredeen, 1948; Malhotra, et al., 1999)

The initial contact may be limited to the exploration of the breast by the infant, with licking and nuzzling of the nipple, or the infant may latch on and suck for minutes. Timing is not necessary because the infant will interrupt him- or herself. The first hour after birth, the full-term unmedicated infant will be quietly alert. It is an opportunity for the mother, father, and infant to get acquainted before each slips into a deep refreshing sleep that may last several hours.

Ideally, mother and infant recover in the same room together. The infant is fed when he or she wakens, and the mother learns the early signs of hunger. Crying is a very late sign. She also learns about caring for her infant. There should be no schedules and no intervention unless an infant does not feed for over 6 hours. The nursing staff and lactation consultants ensure that the infant latches on well and the mother's questions are answered. Breast-feeding should not hurt; when it does the process should be observed and adjusted. The pediatrician should observe a feeding as part of the infant's discharge examination. The mother should be aware of the milk letting down by tingling in the breast or dripping from the opposite breast. The infant should be noted to swallow (Fig. 10-7).

The weight is measured daily and again just before discharge. A weight loss of over 5% in the first 48 hours should be assessed by checking the feeding process and reviewing voidings and stoolings. Maximum weight loss should not exceed 7% in a breast-fed infant by 72 hours. The weight should plateau after 72 hours. Birth weight should be regained by 7 days or, at the latest, 10 days. A healthy infant voids at least once and stools at least once in the first 24 hours, at least twice in the second 24 hours, and at least three times in the third 24 hours. From then on voidings should occur at least six times daily. An infant should stool at least once (and preferably three times) every day in the first month of life. At 3 to 4 months of age, a perfectly healthy breast-fed infant may go a week without stooling and then pass a soft yellow stool, but this should not occur under 1 month of age.

Early discharge from the hospital has increased the need for newborn care visits within a few days after discharge and as required thereafter at 2- to 4-week intervals for assessment of weight and hydration. The AAP recommends a visit at 3 to 5 days of age for infants discharged at 48 hours or less (AAP, 1997).

ISSUES IN THE POSTPARTUM PERIOD

Breast Engorgement and Nipple Tenderness

A little engorgement of the breast in the first 24 hours is physiologic as the vascular supply shifts from the once-gravid uterus to the breasts. Absence of any engorgement, like absence of breast growth during pregnancy, is of concern. Excess engorgement is not only painful but the increased vascular pressure compresses the alveoli and ducts and interferes with milk production and release (Humerick et al., 1994). Prevention of excessive engorgement is the best treatment and involves the following: (1) wearing a well-fitting nursing brassiere even before the breasts are engorged and around the clock; (2) frequent feedings for the infant, being sure to balance the use of both breasts; (3) gentle massage and softening of the areola before offering the breast to the infant so that proper latch-on can be accomplished; (4) if necessary, applying cold packs or cold compresses after a feeding; and (5) taking acetaminophen or ibuprofen, which may be safely used by the mother for discomfort.

Peak engorgement usually occurs between 72 and 96 hours postpartum. At the peak of discomfort, standing in a warm shower to let milk drip or warm compresses before pumping to relieve the pressure will provide relief before the phenomenon subsides.

Sore nipples are a common complaint when early lactation has gone unassisted. It should not hurt to breast-feed. When it does hurt, the infant should be taken off the breast by breaking the suction with a finger and reattaching the infant, following the steps previously described carefully. The major cause of sore nipples is inadequate latch-on and not breast-feeding too long or too frequently. A newborn usually feeds about every 2 hours in the first few weeks of life. Persistent sore nipples, cracks, or oozing may require the assistance of a

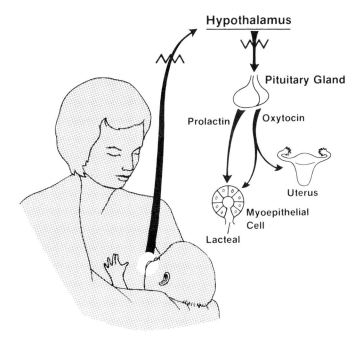

FIGURE 10-7 ■ Diagram of ejection reflex arc. When infant suckles breast, mechanoreceptors in nipple and areola are stimulated, which sends a stimulus along nerve pathways to hypothalamus, which stimulates posterior pituitary gland to release oxytocin. Oxytocin is carried via the bloodstream to breast and uterus. Oxytocin stimulates myoepithelial cells in breast to contract and eject milk from alveolus. Prolactin is responsible for milk production in alveolus. Prolactin is secreted by anterior pituitary gland in response to suckling. Stress such as pain and anxiety can inhibit let-down reflex. Sight or cry of infant can stimulate release of oxytocin but not prolactin. (From Lawrence RA, Lawrence RM: Breastfeeding: A Guide for the Medical Profession, 5th ed. St. Louis, Mosby, 1999, p. 266, Fig. 8-17.)

licensed certified lactation consultant who can take the time to work with the mother to identify the cause, determine effective treatment, and assist the dyad in maintaining pain-free breast-feeding.

Faltering Milk Supply

Many misconceptions lead to the impression that failing milk supply is a common occurrence. Many women discontinue breast-feeding before 3 months postpartum, believing their milk is diminishing because their breasts are no longer engorged. Once supply and demand have been equilibrated and the breast makes what the infant needs, the breasts are soft and do not constantly drip. The emptying time of the stomach of the infant with human milk is 90 minutes, with formula it is 3 to 4 hours, and with cow's milk it is 6 hours. Continuing to feed every 3 hours is a testimony to its digestibility, not its inadequacy. Weight gain in the infant is the better barometer of success. The American College of Obstetrics and Gynecology supports the AAP statement that exclusive breast-feeding should continue for 6 months, with continued breast-feeding while adding weaning foods for the next 6 months, and then as long thereafter as mutually desired by mother and child (Lau, 2001).

Genuine failure to produce enough milk may be due to infant causes, such as increased need, increased fluid losses, or lack of adequate suckling, or to maternal causes, such as failure to let down or failure of production. Each case should be carefully reviewed because most situations are remediable. Ideally, the pediatrician is experienced in lactation management or has a staff member who is. Working together with a licensed certified lactation specialist, the issues can be resolved and breast-feeding can continue successfully.

BREAST-FEEDING AFTER PREMATURE OR MULTIPLE BIRTHS

Human milk is beneficial in the management of the premature infant according to the Policy Statement of the AAP. The benefits include infection protection qualities; improvement in gastrointestinal function, digestion, and absorption of nutrients; and neurodevelopmental outcomes. The psychological well-being of the mother is enhanced by providing her milk for her compromised infant (Schanler, 2001). Meeting the intrauterine rates of growth and nutrient accretion requires attention. Although human milk satisfies these needs for larger premature infants, it can be carefully supplemented for smaller infants and still preserve the benefits of human milk.

Twins and triplets present problems of time management for the mother (Gromada and Spangler, 1998). The mother will make enough milk, as supply will meet demand. Twins learn quickly to nurse simultaneously and will continue to do so for months or years. Breast-feeding ensures a mother's interaction with her infants. Helpful friends and relatives can perform the other household duties. The mother can also provide enough milk for triplets. Some mothers prefer to nurse two at a feeding, giving the third a bottle but rotating the three feeding by feeding. Any breast milk is valuable in this situation. Mothers of multiples need help. It may be necessary for the physician to prescribe help and careful attention to proper rest. Mothers have also breast-fed quadruplets and higher. Usually, they will nurse several at each feeding and rotate bottle feeding.

CONTRACEPTION

Lactation suppresses ovulation and thus helps prevent pregnancy for the first several months after delivery but should not be relied on as a sole method of contraception. Many couples resume coitus before the first postpartum visit and should be educated about the effects of breast-feeding on sexual function and fertility. Interest in sex may be reduced, not only by the endocrine environment of lactation but also by maternal fatigue, reduced vaginal lubrication during lactation, and the altered roles of wife and mother. Contraceptive choices are consequently affected by lactation.

Nonhormonal choices are preferred until ovulation resumes. The American College of Obstetricians and Gynecologists recommends prelubricated condoms or other lubricated barrier methods such as a diaphragm. Intrauterine devices are appropriate once uterine involution has occurred. Supplemental lubrication may be required.

Use of hormonal contraceptives in breast-feeding women raises questions about maternal–fetal transfer of hormones, but the principal concerns relate to the effect on milk production and risk to the mother. Progestin-only contraceptives, such as the mini-pill tablet, depo-injection of medroxyprogesterone acetate, and levonorgestrel implants, are the hormonal methods of choice when nonhormonal methods are not acceptable. Unlike combined estrogen–progestin pills, the progestin-only methods have no effect on the quantity or quality of milk. The package inserts for progestin-only methods recommend initiation of use at 6 weeks postpartum for women who are breast-feeding exclusively and at 3 weeks for those who supplement formula along with breast milk. The injectable medroxyprogesterone acetate is recommended only after 6 weeks following delivery. The reasons for the delayed use of the progestin-only methods are primarily theoretical, related to concerns about an immediate effect on the onset of milk production if used within 3 days of birth and on the uncertain ability of the newborn to metabolize progesterone. However, concern about the impact of early initiation of progestin-only pills has been ameliorated by a recent report that found no adverse effects on continuation rates, exclusive breast-feeding, or use of supplements (Halderman and Nelson, 2002)

Combined estrogen–progestin contraceptive tablets are not ideal during lactation because they reduce both the quantity and quality of milk and may increase the risk of maternal thromboembolism in the already hypercoagulable postpartum period. If used at all, they should not be started until at least 6 weeks postpartum and after lactation is well established.

MATERNAL INFECTIONS DURING BREAST-FEEDING

There is a tremendous amount of concern and worry about the risk to a breast-feeding infant when the mother has an infectious illness. Maternal infection is not a contraindication to breast-feeding in most infectious illnesses and in most situations despite the amount of worry. Proscribing breast-feeding out of fear of infection deprives the infant of the significant immunologic, nutritional, and emotional benefits of breast-feeding when they are most needed (Lawrence and Lawrence, 1999).

Decision-making about breast-feeding in the face of infection should include consideration of the usual route of transmission, reasonable infection control precautions, potential severity of infection in the infant/child, medications to treat the mother that are compatible with breast-feeding, the utility of prophylaxis for the infant, the protective effect of breast milk, and the acceptability of using expressed breast milk temporarily. The decision to continue breast-feeding should be made in discussion with the mother/parents, weighing the known and potential risks of the infection against the known benefits of breast-feeding (Lawrence and Lawrence, 2001).

For example, diphtheria or active pulmonary tuberculosis in the mother is commonly transmitted via the respiratory route, such that infant contact with the mother should be proscribed regardless of whether the infant is breast-feeding or formula-fed. As long as there are no lesions on the breast, cutaneous diphtheria, or tuberculosis mastitis, expressed breast milk can be given to the infant during the initial treatment of the mother (probable infectious period is 5 days for diphtheria and 14 days or until the sputum is negative for tuberculosis per acid-fast bacillus smear). Diphtheria and tuberculosis are not transmitted in the milk. Prophylactic antibiotics for the infant are appropriate in each case, penicillin or erythromycin for diphtheria and isoniazid for tuberculosis (Snider and Powell, 1984; Lawrence and Lawrence, 1999; AAP, 2000).

In certain highly infectious and serious infections, such as the hemorrhagic fevers—specifically with Ebola or Marburg viruses and Lassa fever—the risk of transmission from any contact with the infected mother is high, and the potential severity of the illness in mother or infant necessitates separation of infant (breast-fed or formula-fed) from the mother and proscription of breast-feeding as well as expressed breast milk. For Dengue virus or Hantavirus, standard precautions are appropriate along with temporary use of expressed breast milk and subsequent breast-feeding in the recovering mother (Lawrence and Lawrence, 1999). In the case of infections at specific sites, the management may vary with the specific etiologic organism. For example, mastitis due to *Staphylococcus* or group A *Streptococcus* requires contact precautions, delaying breast-feeding for 24 hours after beginning therapy in the mother and discarding the expressed breast milk for the first 24 hours. For endometritis due to group B *Streptococcus*, standard precautions, breast-feeding after the initial 24 hours of therapy in the mother, and the use of expressed breast milk in the interim are appropriate. An example of the probable protective effect of breast-feeding is botulism (Arnon, 1980, 1986; Arnon et al., 1982) Candida mastitis is a situation in which breast-feeding should continue while the mother and infant are treated simultaneously for at least 2 weeks to prevent reinfection of the breast from contact with the infant's oral candidiasis.

In mothers with hepatitis, identification of the etiologic agent is required before the appropriate management can be determined. Before the etiologic agent is identified, care must include precautions for all potential organisms. Suspension of breast-feeding (pumping and discarding breast milk) until the etiology is determined may be required. Consultation with an infectious disease specialist is often appropriate. For hepatitis A virus, infection in the newborn or young infant is uncommon and not associated with severe illness. Breast-feeding can continue, and if the diagnosis is made within 2 to 3 weeks of the infant's initial exposure to the infected mother, then immune serum globulin and hepatitis A virus vaccine simultaneously can decrease infection in the infant. With hepatitis B virus, the risk of chronic hepatitis B virus infection and its serious complications is high (up to 90%) when infection occurs perinatally or in early infancy. The hepatitis B immune globulin and the hepatitis B virus vaccine given simultaneously will prevent hepatitis B virus transmission in over 95% of cases, irrespective of infant feeding practices (breast-feeding or formula-feeding). Therefore, it is very appropriate to continue breast-feeding as soon as effective immune therapy is given (AAP, 2000).

No clear data indicate hepatitis C virus transmission via breast milk in HIV-negative mothers (L. S. Barden, personal communication, 2000) However, given the multiple issues involved (e.g., low risk of hepatitis C virus transmission via breast milk, increased risk of transmission in association with HIV infection and high levels of hepatitis C virus-RNA in maternal serum, lack of effective preventive treatments [vaccines or immune serum globulin] and the risk of chronic hepatitis C virus infection, and serious liver disease), it is essential to educate the parents about the possible risks of continued breast-feeding. If the mother is symptomatic, breast-feeding may not be indicated. If mother is not symptomatic, breast-feeding is usually appropriate.

Maternal retroviral infection and breast-feeding is a highly controversial issue that continues to be evaluated and debated. HIV-1 is transmissible via breast-feeding and can significantly increase the risk of HIV infection in infants born to HIV-positive mothers. One meta-analysis of five studies of infants born to HIV-infected mothers reported the risk of HIV transmission to infants strictly from breast-feeding as 14% (confidence intervals, 7% to 22%) (Dunn et al., 1992). Among the many concerns about HIV and breast-feeding are the risk of transmission related to the duration of breast-feeding, the relative risks of exclusive versus nonexclusive breast-feeding, the risk of mortality and morbidity resulting from other infections and malnutrition associated with not breast-feeding, the significance of HIV viral loads and CD4 counts in the mother relative to transmission from breast milk, the potential protective effects of breast milk against HIV infection, and the degree to which antiretroviral therapy for the mother and/or infant will be protective against HIV infection. Social issues involved in this debate include the right of the mother to make choices for herself and her infant, the social stigma of not breast-feeding in certain cultures and communities, and the possibility that breast-feeding rates in HIV-negative mothers will be adversely affected by the advice given to HIV-positive mothers. In many countries neither choice is optimal: Breast-feeding risks HIV infection in the infant, but not breast-feeding increases the risks of other infections and malnutrition. The lack of adequate data from controlled trials about the various factors contributing to infection adds to the difficulty of making straightforward recommendations applicable to diverse situations around the world. In the United States, it is appropriate to advise no breast-feeding for infants of HIV-infected mothers to decrease the risk of HIV transmission to the infant (Lawrence, 1997).

There are limited reports concerning the risk of HIV-2 transmission via breast-feeding. Studies suggest that HIV-2 transmission via breast milk is less common than with HIV-1 (Ekpini et al., 1997). However, until adequate information is available, it is appropriate to use the same guidelines as for HIV-1.

Human T-cell leukemia virus type I infection is associated with breast-feeding, although short-term breast-feeding (<6 months) may pose no greater risk than for formula-fed infants (Hino, 1989, 1993; Takezaki et al., 1997). In Japan, where high rates of human T-cell leukemia virus type I infection occur, proscription of breast-feeding is common. In the United States, it is appropriate in the face of documented maternal human T-cell leukemia virus type I infection to discuss the options and risks and benefits of breast-feeding in this situation and to consider short-term breast-feeding. There are many uncertainties concerning human T-cell leukemia virus type II infection related to the diseases associated with infection and the actual transmission via breast milk. Here again, a discussion of the available data and including an infectious disease consultant in the discussion are appropriate (Lawrence and Lawrence, 1999).

Numerous reviews (DeCock et al., 2000; Weinberg, 2000; WHO Collaborative Study, 2000; Andiman, 2002) and studies (Mbori-Ngacha et al., 2001; Wolf et al., 2001) attempt to address the numerous issues of breast-feeding by HIV-positive mothers. The two most helpful resources related to breast-feeding and infection are the AAP's report of the Committee on Infectious Diseases (2000) and a guide for medical professionals by Lawrence and Lawrence (1999) that contains a chapter and an appendix dedicated to the issue. See also Table 10-4.

COMPLICATIONS OF THE BREAST

Plugged Ducts

Tender lumps in the breast in a mother who is otherwise well are probably caused by plugging of a collecting duct. The best treatment is to continue nursing while manually massaging the area to initiate and ensure complete drainage. Holding the infant in a different position and/or hot packs before a feeding may encourage flow. If repeated plugging occurs, a check should be made for possible obstruction from a brassiere strap or other external forces. Some women can actually see small plugs ejected when they massage. For some, reducing polyunsaturated fats in the diet and adding lecithin (Lawrence and Lawrence, 1999) provides relief.

Galactocele

Milk retention cysts are uncommon and are usually associated with lactation. The swelling is smooth and rounded and nontender. The cyst may be aspirated to confirm the diagnosis and to avoid surgery, but it will fill up again. The cyst can be moved with local anesthesia without interrupting breast-feeding. The diagnosis can also be confirmed by ultrasound: A cyst and milk look similar and tumor will be distinguishable (Lawrence and Lawrence, 1999).

Mastitis

Mastitis is an infectious process in the breast producing localized tenderness, redness, and heat, together with systemic symptoms of a flu-like illness with fever and malaise. It is dis-

tinguished from engorgement and plugged duct (Table 10-5). There is usually a red, tender, hot, swollen, wedge-shaped area of the breast corresponding to a lobe that is visible (Fig. 10-8). The common organisms are *Staphylococcus aureus*, *Escherichia coli*, and, rarely, streptococcus.

The major points of management are as follows:

1. Breast-feeding should continue on both breasts.
2. Antibiotics appropriate to probable cause and local sensitivities should be prescribed.
3. Antibiotics should be given for no less than 10 days, and preferably 14. The antibiotic should be safe for the infant.
4. Bed rest is necessary, and the mother should bring the infant to bed to nurse. She will need assistance for the rest of the household responsibilities.

The most common cause of recurrent mastitis is delayed or inadequate treatment of the initial disease. On recurrence, cultures of a midstream flow of milk should be sent and antibiotics chosen accordingly.

Candidiasis of Nipple and Breast

Candidiasis of the breast is frequently overdiagnosed because there are several causes for stabbing burning pain in the breast that is described by mothers as feeling like "a stab with a hot poker." On examination, there may be little to see except a pinkish hue to the nipple and central areola. Rarely are white plaques seen on the nipple. If the mother has a history of vaginal candidiasis, the infant's mouth may have become colonized with consequent inoculation of the nipples. The infant should also be examined for both thrush and diaper rash and treated simultaneously with the mother for a full 2 weeks. Nystatin ointment is applied after each feeding to nipples and areolae. The infant receives nystatin drops orally to the oral mucous membranes after each feeding. A recurrent episode can be treated with 200 mg oral fluconazole systemically once daily for 3 days for the mother. The infant can be given 6 mg/kg on day 1 and then 3 mg/kg per dose 24 hours orally; pacifiers and bottle nipples that are put in the mouth should be discarded.

MEDICATIONS WHILE BREAST-FEEDING

Questions about medication are the most commonly asked regarding breast-feeding. The transfer of maternal drugs to the infant during lactation is different from transfer to the fetus during pregnancy. Although it is almost always better to breast-feed, the physician must weigh the benefit and risk of a medication against the substantial benefit of being breast-fed for the infant. The risk-to-benefit ratio differs for each drug and clinical setting. Both scientific information and experienced clinical judgment are required to assess the risks and benefits and determine the therapeutic choice.

The AAP Committee on Drugs has published a list of commonly used drugs and chemicals that may transfer into human milk (AAP, 2001). The list is not all-inclusive and is revised intermittently. Absence of a drug from the list merely indicates the committee did not study it in reference to lactation. The categories are as follows:

TABLE 10-4. PRECAUTIONS AND BREAST-FEEDING RECOMMENDATIONS FOR SELECTED MATERNAL INFECTIONS

Organism, Syndrome, or Condition*	Breast-Feeding Acceptable†	Compatibility of Medications with Breast-Feeding‡
Candidiasis		
Mucocutaneous infection, vulvovaginitis	Yes (therapy for the infant simultaneous with mother's therapy)§	Topical agents, fluconazole, ketoconazole, itraconazole, amphotericin B, flucytosine
Candida albicans		
Candida krusei		
Candida tropicalis invasive infections		
Chlamydia		
Chlamydia trachomatis	Yes (consider treating the infant)	Erythromycin, azithromycin, clarithromycin, doxycycline, tetracycline, sulfisoxazole
Urethritis, vaginitis, endometritis salpingitis, lymphogranuloma venereum, conjunctivitis, pneumonia		
Cytomegalovirus		
Asymptomatic infection	Yes (for full-term infants)	
Infectious mononucleosis	No (for premature or immunodeficient infants; do not give expressed breast milk)	
Endometritis, pelvic inflammatory disease		
Anaerobic organisms	Yes	Clindamycin, metronidazole, cefoxitin, cefmetazole
Chlamydia trachomatis	Yes	Erythromycin, azithromycin, tetracycline
Enterobacteriaceae	Yes	Ampicillin, aminoglycosides, cephalosporins
Group B streptococci	Yes (after 24 hr of therapy, breast milk is okay; observation	Penicillin, cephalosporin, macrolides
Mycoplasma hominis	Yes	Clindamycin, tetracycline
Neisseria gonorrhoeae	Yes#	Ceftriaxone, spectinomycin, doxycycline, azithromycin
Ureaplasma urealyticum	Yes	Erythromycin, azithromycin, clarithromycin, tetracycline
Gonorrhea		
Genital, pharyngeal, conjunctival, or disseminated infection		
Neisseria gonorhoeae	Yes#	Ceftriaxone, ciprofloxacin, spectinomycin, azithromycin, doxycycline
Hepatitis§		
A—Acute only	Yes (after immune serum globulin and vaccine)	
B—Chronic hepatitis, cirrhosis, hepatocellular carcinona	Yes (after HBIG and vaccine)	
C—Chronic hepatitis, cirrhosis, hepatocellular carcinoma	Yes	
D—Associated with hepatitis B	Yes (after HBIG and vaccine)	
E—Severe disease in pregnant women	Yes	
G	Inadequate data	
Herpes simplex		
Type 1,2 (HSV$_{1,2}$)		
Mucocutaneous	Yes (in the absence of breast lesions)	Acyclovir, valacyclovir, famcyclovir
Neonatal		
Encephalitis		
Human immunodeficiency viruses§		
Type 1	No/yes**	Little or no available information on antiretrovirals in breast milk
Type 2	No/yes**	
Human T-cell leukemia viruses		
Type I		
T-cell leukemia/lymphoma, myelopathy, dermatitis, adenitis, Sjögren syndrome	No§	
Type II		
Myelopathy, arthritis, glomerulonephritis	No§	
Lyme disease		
Borrelia burgdorferi		
Multistaged illness of skin, joint, and peripheral or central nervous system	Yes, with informed discussion	Ceftriaxone, ampicillin, doxycycline

TABLE 10-4. PRECAUTIONS AND BREAST-FEEDING RECOMMENDATIONS FOR SELECTED MATERNAL INFECTIONS—cont'd

Organism, Syndrome, or Condition*	Breast-Feeding Acceptable†	Compatibility of Medications with Breast-Feeding‡
Mastitis		
Candida albicans	Yes, with simultaneous treatment of the infant	Nystatin, ketoconazole
Enterobacteriaceae	Yes	Fluconazole
Staphylococcus aureus Group A streptococcus	Yes (after 24 hr of therapy, during which milk must be discarded)	First-generation cephalosporin, dicloxacillin, oxacillin, erythromycin
Mycobacterium tuberculosis§	No§ breast milk or breast-feeding for 2 weeks of maternal therapy, consider prophylactic INH for the infant	Isoniazid, rifampin, ethambutol, pyrazinamide ethionamide
Mycobacterium tuberculosis§ Pulmonary, extrapulmonary	Yes, expressed breast milk can be used during initial 2 weeks of maternal therapy, then breast-feeding can continue	Antituberculous medications are acceptable during breast-feeding
Trichomonas vaginalis Vaginitis, urethritis, or asymptomatic infections	Yes	Metronidazole
Adenoviruses Conjunctivitis Upper/lower respiratory infections Gastroenteritis	Yes‖	

* Patients with the syndromes or conditions listed may present with atypical signs and symptoms (e.g., pertussis in neonates and adults may not have paroxysmal or severe cough). The clinician's index of suspicion should be guided by the prevalence of specific conditions in the community and clinical judgment. The organisms listed are not intended to represent the complete or even most likely diagnoses but rather possible etiologic agents.
† Yes means that if in a hospitalized mother and infant the proposed precautions are followed, breast-feeding is acceptable and may be beneficial to the infant. Any infant breast-feeding during a maternal infection should be observed closely for signs or symptoms of illness.
‡ To ensure that appropriate empiric precautions are always implemented, hospitals must have systems in place to routinely evaluate patients according to these criteria as part of their preadmission and admission care.
§ See text for more explanation.
‖ Adenovirus types 4 and 7 have been known to cause severe respiratory disease in premature infants or individuals with immunodeficiency or underlying respiratory disease. In certain situations, feeding of expressed breast milk to the infant may not be advisable.
Breast-feed immediately if mother receives ceftriaxone intramuscularly or intravenously. Breast-feed after 24-hr antibiotic therapy for other treatment regimens, with feeding expressed breast milk for the first 24 hr.
** No, in the United States and many other countries. Yes, when no safe alternative to breast milk is available.
HBIG, hepatitis B immunoglobulin; HSV, herpes simplex virus; INH, isoniazid.
Modified from Lawrence RA, Lawrence RM: Breastfeeding: A Guide for the Medical Profession, 5th ed. St. Louis, Mosby, 1999.

1. Cytotoxic drugs that may interfere with cellular metabolism of the nursing infant (Table 10-6A)
2. Drugs of abuse for which adverse effects on the infant during breast-feeding have been reported (Table 10-6B)
3. Radioactive compounds that require temporary cessation of breast-feeding (Table 10-6C)
4. Drugs for which the effect on nursing infants is unknown but which may be of concern, for example, bromocriptine, ergotamine compounds, and lithium (AAP and American College of Obstetricians and Gynecologists, 1997)
5. Drugs that have been associated with significant effects on some nursing infants and should be given to nursing mothers with caution
6. Maternal medication usually compatible with breast-feeding (Table 10-6D)
7. Food and environmental agents that might have an effect on the breast-feeding infant

TABLE 10-5. COMPARISON OF FINDINGS OF ENGORGEMENT, PLUGGED DUCT, AND MASTITIS

Characteristics	Engorgement	Plugged Duct	Mastitis
Onset	Gradual, immediately postpartum	Gradual, after feedings	Sudden, after 10 days
Site	Bilateral	Unilateral	Usually unilateral
Swelling and heat	Generalized	May shift; little or no heat	Localized, red, hot, swollen
Pain	Generalized	Mild but localized	Intense but localized
Body temperature	<38.4°C (101°F)	<38.4°C	>38.4°C
Systemic symptoms	Feels well	Feels well	Flu-like symptoms

From Lawrence RA, Lawrence RM: Breastfeeding: A Guide for the Medical Profession, 5th ed. St. Louis, Mosby, 1999, p. 279, Table 8-5.

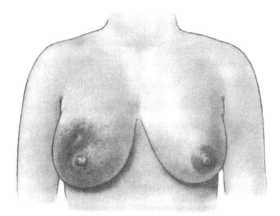

FIGURE 10-8 ■ Mastitis of right breast, upper outer quadrant. (From Lawrence RA, Lawrence RM: Breastfeeding: A Guide for the Medical Profession, 5th ed. St. Louis, Mosby, 1999, p. 279, Fig. 8-24.)

 TABLE 10-6. DRUG GROUPS 1, 2, 3, AND 6

A. Group 1: Cytotoxic Drugs That May Interfere with Cellular Metabolism of the Nursing Infant
Possible immune suppression; unknown effect on growth or association with carcinogenesis; neutropenia
    Cyclophosphamide
    Cyclosporine
    Doxorubicin*
    Methotrexate

B. Group 2: Drugs of Abuse for Which Adverse Effects on the Infant during Breast-Feeding Have Been Reported†
Amphetamine*
Cocaine
Heroin
Marijuana
Phencyclidine

C. Group 3: Radioactive Compounds That Require Temporary Cessation of Breast-Feeding
Copper 64 (^{64}Cu)
Gallium 67 (^{67}Ga)
Indium 111 (^{111}In)
Iodine 123 (^{123}I)
Iodine 125 (^{125}I)
Iodine 131 (^{131}I)
Radioactive sodium
Technetium 99m (^{99m}Tc)
Macroaggregates, ^{99m}Tc O$_4$

D. Group 6: Partial List of Selected Maternal Medications Usually Compatible with Breast-Feeding
Analgesics
    Acetaminophen
    Ibuprofen
    Codeine
    Antacids

D. Group 6—cont'd
Antibiotics that can also be given to infants
    Acyclovir
    Amoxicillin
    Cephalosporins
    Erythromycin
    Fluconazole
    Gentamicin
    Kanamycin
    Miconazole
    Penicillins
    Spironolactone
    Streptomycin
    Vancomycin
Cardiovascular/antihypertensive
    Captopril
    Digoxin
    Enalapril
    Hydralazine
    Labetalol
    Metoprolol
    Nifedipine
    Nitrofurantoin
    Quinidine
    Quinine
    Sotalol
    Timolol
Miscellaneous compounds
    Lidocaine
    Progesterone-only contraceptive pill
    Magnesium sulfate
    Prednisolone
    Prednisone
    Propylthiouracil
    Scopolamine
    Warfarin
    Laxatives (bulk forming and stool softening)
    Vaccines

* Drug is concentrated in human milk.
† The Committee on Drugs strongly believes that nursing mothers should not ingest drugs of abuse, because they are hazardous to the nursing infant and to the health of the mother.

From American Academy of Pediatrics, Committee on Drugs: The transfer of drugs and other chemicals into human milk. Pediatrics **108**:776, 2001.

TABLE 10-7. STEPS IN THE PASSAGE OF DRUGS INTO BREAST MILK

1. Mammary alveolar epithelium represents a lipid barrier with water-filled pores and is most permeable for drugs during colostral phase of milk secretion (1st week postpartum).
2. Drug excretion into milk depends on the drug's degree of ionization, molecular weight, solubility in fat and water, and relation of pH of plasma (7.4) to pH of milk (7.0).
3. Drugs enter mammary cells basally in the non-ionized non–protein-bound form by diffusion or active transport.
4. Water-soluble drugs of molecular weight below 200 pass through water-filled membranous pores.
5. Drugs leave mammary alveolar cells by diffusion or active transport.
6. Drugs may enter milk via spaces between mammary alveolar cells.
7. Most ingested drugs appear in milk; drug amounts in milk usually do not exceed 1% of ingested dosage, and levels in the milk are independent of milk volume.
8. Drugs are bound much less to milk proteins than to plasma proteins.
9. Drug-metabolizing capacity of mammary epithelium is not understood.

Modified from Lawrence RA, Lawrence RM: Breastfeeding: A Guide for the Medical Profession, 5th ed. St. Louis, Mosby, 1999.

A lack of information does not necessarily require cessation of breast-feeding. Understanding the pharmacology of the drugs, dosing schedule, and the stage of growth and development of the infant may permit a decision about the possibility that the active drug would affect the infant. Characteristics of the drug that influence its passage into milk include the size of the molecule, its solubility in lipid or water, whether it binds to protein, the pH, and the diffusion rates (Table 10-7). The routes of administration will influence the blood levels and therefore the milk levels. Passive diffusion is the principal transport mechanism. The metabolism of the drug influences the presence in the milk of the active form or an inactive metabolite (Fig. 10-9).

The infant's ability to absorb, digest, metabolize, store, or excrete a drug must be considered when choosing a medication for a nursing mother. A drug that is not orally bioavailable will not be absorbed from the milk by the infant. The ability to absorb and metabolize a drug depends on the infant's developmental age and the chronologic age. An 18 month old who nurses briefly about four times a day for comfort will get little medication, has substantial other diet, and can metabolize and excrete more efficiently than a newborn. In the first weeks of life, the maturation or gestational age should be considered in determining the safety of a medication because the less mature the infant, the less mature the liver and kidneys.

Milk-to-Plasma Ratio

The milk-to-plasma ratio is a common term applied to drugs in lactation that by definition is the level in the milk compared with the level in the plasma at a given time. One must know the dose of the drug, time, and route of dosing to interpret the ratio. If there is a very low level in the plasma and the same very low level in the milk, the ratio is 1. In this case, a ratio of 1 would imply the level is of concern, but actually the level in milk is low. Most drugs have a milk-to-plasma ratio of less than 1. It is also important to know peak plasma and peak milk levels and peak plasma and milk times to make appropriate recommendations to avoid feeding the infant when transfer would be greatest.

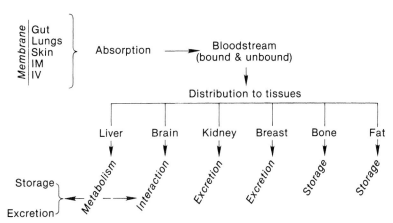

FIGURE 10-9 ■ Distribution pathways for drugs, during lactation. IM, intramuscular; IV, intravenous. (Modified from Rivera-Calimlim L: Distribution pathways for drugs, once absorbed during lactation. Clin Perinatol **14**:51, 1976.)

REFERENCES

American Academy of Pediatrics: Red Book 2000: Report of the Committee on Infectious Diseases, 25th ed. Elk Grove Village, IL, American Academy of Pediatrics, 2000.

American Academy of Pediatrics, American College of Obstetricians and Gynecologists: Guidelines for Perinatal Care, 4th ed. Elk Grove Village, IL, American Academy of Pediatrics; Washington, DC, American College of Obstetricians and Gynecologists, 1997.

American Academy of Pediatrics, Committee on Drugs: The transfer of drugs and other chemicals into human milk. Pediatrics **108**:776, 2001.

American Academy of Pediatrics, Work Group on Breastfeeding: Breastfeeding and the use of human milk. Pediatrics **100**:1035, 1997.

Andiman W: Transmission of HIV-1 from mother to infant. Curr Opin Pediatr **14**:78, 2002.

Aperia A, Broberger O, Herin P, et al: Salt content in human breast milk during the first three weeks after delivery. Acta Paediatr Scand **68**:441, 1979.

Arnon SS: Infant botulism. Annu Rev Med **31**:541, 1980.

Arnon SS: Infant botulism: Anticipating the second decade. J Infect Dis **154**:201, 1986.

Arnon SS, Damus K, Thompson B, et al: Protective role of human milk against sudden death from infant botulism. J Pediatr **100**:568, 1982.

Barnes GR, Lethin AN, Jackson EB, et al: Management of breastfeeding. JAMA **151**:192, 1953.

Berens PD: Prenatal, intrapartum, and postpartum support of the lactating mother. Pediatr Clin North Am **48**:365, 2001.

Bland KJ, Romnell LJ: Congenital and acquired disturbances of breast development and growth. In Bland KI, Copeland EM III (eds): The Breast: Comprehensive Management of Benign and Malignant Diseases. Philadelphia, WB Saunders, 1991, p. 69.

Butte NF, Goldblum RM, Fehl LM, et al: Daily ingestion of immunologic components in human milk during the first four months of life. Acta Paediatr Scand **73**:206, 1984.

Chen DC, Nommsen-Rivers L, Dewey KG, et al: Stress during labor and delivery and early lactation performance. Am J Clin Nutr **68**:335, 1998.

DeCock K, Fowler M, Mercier E, et al: Prevention of mother-to-child HIV transmission in resource-poor countries. JAMA **283**:1175, 2000.

Dewey KG: Nutrition, growth, and complementary feeding of the breastfed infant. Pediatr Clin North Am **48**:87, 2001.

Dunn DT, Newell ML, Ades AE, et al: Risk of human immunodeficiency virus type 1 transmission through breastfeeding. Lancet **340**:585, 1992.

Ekpini ER, Wiktor SZ, Satten GA, et al: Late postnatal mother-to-child transmission of HIV-1 in Abidjan, Cote D'Ivoire. Lancet **349**:1054, 1997.

Fredeen R: Cup feeding of newborn infants. Pediatrics **2**:544, 1948.

Gromada KK, Spangler AK: Breastfeeding twins and higher-order multiples. J Obstet Gynecol Neonatal Nurs **27**:441, 1998.

Halderman LD, Nelson AL: Impact of early postpartum administration of progestin-only hormonal contraceptives compared with nonhormonal contraceptives on short-term breast-feeding patterns. Am J Obstet Gynecol **186**:1250, 2002.

Hino S: Milk-borne transmission of HTLV-I as a major route in the endemic cycle. Acta Pediatr Jpn **31**:428, 1989.

Hino S, Katamine S, Kawase K, et al: Intervention of maternal transmission of HTLV-I in Nagasaki, Japan. Leukemia **94**:S68, 1993.

Horwood LJ, Darlow BA, Mogridge N: Breast milk feeding and cognitive ability at 7–8 years. Arch Dis Child Fetal Neonatal Ed **84**:F23, 2001.

Horwood LJ, Fergusson DM: Breastfeeding and later cognitive and academic outcomes. Pediatrics **101**:91, 1998.

Humerick SS, Hill PD, Anderson MA: Breast engorgement: Patterns and selected outcomes. J Hum Lactat **10**:87, 1994.

Jackson EB: Pediatric and psychiatric aspects of the Yale room-in project. Conn State Med J **14**:616, 1950.

Jackson EB, Olmsted RW, Foord A, et al: A hospital rooming-in unit for four newborn infants and their mothers. Pediatrics **1**:28, 1948.

Jacobson SW, Chiodo LM, Jacobson JL: Breastfeeding effects on intelligence in 4- and 11-year old children. Pediatrics **103**:71, 1999.

John EM, Whitemore AS, Harris R, et al: Characteristics relating to ovarian cancer risk: Collaborative analysis of seven US case-control studies—epithelial ovarian cancer in black women. Collaborative Ovarian Cancer Group. J Natl Cancer Inst **85**:142, 1993.

Jorgensen MH, Hernell O, Lund P, et al: Visual acuity and erythrocyte docosahexaenoic acid-status in breast-fed and formula-fed term infants during first four months of life. Lipids **31**:99, 1996.

Josimovich JB, Reynolds M, Cobo E: Lactogenic hormones, fetal nutrition, and lactation. In Josimovich JB, Reynolds M, Cobo E (eds): Problems of Human Reproduction, vol. 2. New York, John Wiley & Sons, 1974, p. 1.

Kalkwarf HJ, Specker BL: Bone mineral loss during lactation and recovery after weaning. Obstet Gynecol **86**:26, 1995.

Kalkwarf HJ, Specker BL, Heubi JE, et al: Intestinal calcium absorption of women during lactation and after weaning. Am J Clin Nutr **63**:526, 1996.

Kuhn NJ: Lactogenesis: The search for trigger mechanisms in different species. In Peaker M (ed): Comparative Aspects of Lactation. London, Academic Press, 1977, p. 165.

Kuhn NJ: The biochemistry of lactogenesis. In Mepham TB (ed): Biochemistry of Lactation. Amsterdam, Elsevier, 1983, p. 351.

Kulski JK, Hartmann PE, Martin JD, et al: Effects of bromocriptine mesylate on the composition of the mammary section in non-breastfeeding women. Obstet Gynecol **52**:38, 1978.

Labbok MH: Effects of breastfeeding on the mother. Pediatr Clin North Am **48**:143, 2001.

Lau C: Effect of stress on lactation. Pediatr Clin North Am **48**:221, 2001.

Lawrence RA: A Review of the Medical Benefits and Contraindications to Breastfeeding in the United States. Maternal and Child Health Technical Information Bulletin. Arlington, VA, National Center for Education in Maternal and Child Health, 1997.

Lawrence RA, Lawrence RM: Breastfeeding: A Guide for the Medical Profession, 5th ed. St. Louis, Mosby, 1999.

Lawrence RA, Lawrence RM: Given the benefits of breastfeeding, what contraindications exist? Pediatr Clin North Am **48**:235, 2001.

Lazarov M, Evans A: Encouraging the best for low-income women. Zero to three. Aug/Sept 2000, p. 15. Electronic journal available at *http://www.zerotothree.org (professional.htmp)*.

Lucas A, Morley R, Cole TJ, et al: Breast milk and subsequent intelligence quotient in children born preterm. Lancet **339**:261, 1992.

Lucas A, Morley R, Cole TJ, et al: Randomized trial of early diet in preterm babies and later intelligence quotient. BMJ **317**:1481, 1998.

Malhotra N, Vishwambaran L, Sundaram KR, et al.: A controlled trial of alternative methods of oral feeding in neonates. Early Hum Dev **54**:29, 1999.

Mbori-Ngacha D, Nduati R, John G, et al: Morbidity and mortality in breast-fed and formula-fed infants of HIV-1 infected women: A randomized clinical trial. JAMA **286**:2413, 2001.

Morton JA: The clinical usefulness of breast milk sodium in the assessment of lactogenesis. Pediatrics **93**:802, 1994.

Neifert MR, McDonough SL, Neville MC: Failure of lactogenesis associated with placental retention. Am J Obstet Gynecol **140**:477, 1981.

Neubauer SH, Ferris AM, Chase CG, et al: Delayed lactogenesis in women with insulin-dependent diabetes mellitus. Am J Clin Nutr **58**:54, 1993.

Neuringer M: Infant vision and retinal function in studies of dietary long-chain polyunsaturated fatty acids: Methods, results, and implications. Am J Clin Nutr **71** (Suppl):256, 2000.

Neville MC: Determinants of milk volume and composition. In Jensen RG (ed): Handbook of Milk Composition. San Diego, Academic Press, 1995a, p. 87.

Neville MC: Lactogenesis in women: A cascade of events revealed by milk composition. In Jensen RD (ed): The Composition of Milks. San Diego, Academic Press, 1995b, p. 87.

Neville MC: Mammary gland biology and lactation: A short course. Presented at biannual meeting of the International Society for Research on Human Milk and Lactation, Plymouth, MA, October 1997.

Neville MC: Anatomy and physiology of lactation. Pediatr Clin North Am **48**:13, 2001.

Neville MC, Allen JC, Archer P, et al: Studies in human lactation: Milk volume and nutrient composition during weaning and lactogenesis. Am J Clin Nutr **54**:81, 1991.

Neville MC, Keller RP, Seacat J, et al: Studies in human lactation: Milk volumes in lactating women during the onset of lactation and full lactation. Am J Clin Nutr **48**:1375, 1988.

Neville MC, Morton J, Umemura S: Lactogenesis: Transition from pregnancy to lactation. Pediatr Clin North Am **48**:35, 2001.

Newcomb PA, Storer BE, Longnecker MP, et al: Lactation and a reduced risk of premenopausal breast cancer. N Engl J Med **330**:81, 1994.

Newton M, Newton NR: The let-down reflex in human lactation. J Pediatr **33**:698, 1948.

Osbourne MP: Breast development and anatomy. In Harris JR, Lippman ME, Morrow M, et al (eds): Diseases of the Breast. Philadelphia, Lippincott-Raven, 1996.

Pedersen CA, Caldwell JD, Walker C: Oxytocin activates the postpartum onset of rat maternal behavior in the ventral tegmental and medial preoptic areas. Behav Neurosci **108**:1163, 1994.

Peterson WE, Ludwick TM: Humoral nature of the factor causing let down of milk. Federation Proceeding **1**:66, 1942.

Pickering LK, Granoff DM, Erickson JD, et al: Modulation of the immune system by human milk and infant formula containing nucleotides. Pediatrics **101**:242, 1998.

Quan R, Barness LA, Uawy R: Do infants need nucleotide supplemented formula for optimal nutrition? J Pediatr Gastroenterol Nutr **11**:429, 1990.

Righard L, Alade MO: Effect of delivery room routine on success of first breast-feed. Lancet **336**:1105, 1990.

Rosenblatt KA, Thomas DB: WHO collaborative study of neoplasia and steroid contraceptives: Lactation and the risk of epithelial ovarian cancer. Int J Epidemiol **22**:192, 1993.

SanGiovanni JP, Berkey CS, Dwyer JT, et al: Dietary essential fatty acids, long-chain polyunsaturated fatty acids, and visual resolution acuity in healthy fullterm infants: A systematic review. Early Hum Dev **57**:165, 2000a.

SanGiovanni JP, Parra-Cabrera S, Colditz GA, et al: Meta-analysis of dietary essential fatty acids and long-chain polyunsaturated fatty acids as they relate to visual resolution acuity in healthy preterm infants. Pediatrics **105**:1292, 2000.

Schanler RJ: The use of human milk for premature infants. Pediatr Clin North Am **48**:207, 2001.

Snider DE Jr, Powell KE: Should women taking antituberculous drugs breast-feed? Arch Intern Med **144**:589, 1984.

Sozmen M: Effects of early suckling of cesarean-born babies on lactation. Biol Neonate **62**:67, 1992.

Srivastava MD, Srivastava A, Brouhard B, et al: Cytokines in human milk. Res Common Mol Pathol Pharmacol **93**:263, 1996.

Subcommittee on Nutrition during Lactation, Institute of Medicine: Nutrition during lactation. National Academy of Sciences, National Academy Press, Washington, DC, 1991.

Takezaki T, Tajima K, Ito M, et al: Short-term breastfeeding may reduce the risk of vertical transmission of HTLV-I. Leukemia **11** (Suppl 3):60, 1997.

von Kries R, Koletzko B, Sauerwald, et al: Breastfeeding and obesity: Cross sectional study. Br Med J **319**:147, 1999.

Vorherr H: The Breast: Morphology, Physiology and Lactation. New York, Academic Press, 1974.

Weinberg GA: The dilemma of postnatal mother-to-child transmission of HIV: To breastfeed or not? Birth **27**:199, 2000.

Whitemore AS: Characteristics relating to ovarian cancer risk: Implications for prevention and detection. Gynecol Oncol **55** (3 pt 2):515, 1994.

WHO Collaborative Study Team on the Role of Breastfeeding on the Prevention of Infant Mortality: Effect of breastfeeding on infant and child mortality due to infectious diseases in less developed countries: A pooled analysis. Lancet **355**:451, 2000.

Wolf LE, Lo B, Beckerman KP, et al: When parents reject interventions to reduce postnatal human immunodeficiency virus transmission. Arch Pediatr Adolesc Med **155**:927, 2001.

SUGGESTED READINGS

Briggs GG, Freeman RK, Yaffe SJ: Drugs in Pregnancy and Lactation, 6th ed. Philadelphia, Lippincott Williams & Wilkins, 2002.

Hale T: Medications and Mother's Milk, 12th ed. Amarillo, Pharmasoft Publishing, 2002.

Lawrence RA, Lawrence RM: Breastfeeding: A Guide for the Medical Profession, 5th ed. St. Louis, Mosby, 1999.

Telephone Consultation Service for Physicians at the Breastfeeding and Human Lactation Study Center at the University of Rochester School of Medicine, (585) 275-0088. Available weekdays.

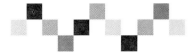

Chapter 11
MATERNAL NUTRITION

Barbara Abrams, DrPH, Dzovag Minassian, MPH, and Kate E. Pickett, PhD

BACKGROUND

Healthy maternal nutrition during pregnancy increases the likelihood of a full-term well-developed infant, uncomplicated pregnancy and childbirth, low risk of maternal postpartum obesity, and sufficient nutrient and energy stores to support lactation and long-term maternal health, including preparation for a subsequent pregnancy. The most recent guidelines for prenatal nutrition are found in the 1990 Institute of Medicine (IOM) report, *Nutrition during Pregnancy*, which reviews the scientific evidence regarding weight gain, dietary intake, and nutrient supplementation (IOM, 1990).

Nutrition and reproduction do not operate within a vacuum. Genetic, social, cultural, economic, and personal factors interrelate and make it extremely difficult to identify the independent influence of maternal nutritional status. It is rarely possible to directly study the effect of poor nutrition on pregnancy outcome. Instead, we must piece together evidence from clinical observations, epidemiology, metabolic and laboratory investigations, and experimental trials of food supplementation or other nutrition interventions. Difficulties in obtaining accurate measures of nutritional status and reliable definitions of outcomes complicate the interpretation of research. The effect of a nutritional insult may depend on its timing during gestation, its severity, or both. Furthermore, major changes in maternal metabolism may conserve nutrients to provide for fetal needs, but some women do not manifest these protective changes, and the mechanisms underlying these adaptations are not well understood (King, 2000b). Nonetheless, there is now more scientific evidence of the importance of maternal nutrition than ever before.

The "fetal origins hypothesis," first proposed by Barker in the early 1990s, suggests that fetal nutrition has lifelong effects on metabolism, with a far-reaching impact on risk of chronic disease in adulthood (Barker, 1998). Over the past decade, a large body of epidemiologic evidence has accumulated linking birth weight to hypertension, glucose intolerance, type II diabetes, and coronary heart disease and mortality (Frankel et al., 1996; Rich-Edwards et al., 1997; Huxley et al., 2000; Law et al., 2001). Much of the early work in this area, involving painstaking construction of study cohorts based on rare collections of birth-weight records from early 20th century England, was criticized for failing to account for selection bias or important confounding factors, such as socioeconomic status (Paneth and Susser, 1995; Gillman and Rich-Edwards, 2000). More recent work has overcome many of these limitations. However, it is still not clear how much fetal growth matters, in comparison with postnatal growth, or whether particular periods of gestation are more important than others (Gillman, 2002). A pattern of fetal growth restriction, followed by fast postnatal growth and later obesity, seems to confer the highest risk of adult chronic disease. Further research is needed to sort out the roles of genetic and environmental factors and the respective contributions of maternal nutrition, maternal physiology, placental factors, and fetal metabolism to the "birthweight effect" (Hattersley and Tooke, 1999; Harding, 2001). In the meantime, the potential importance of fetal health for long-term adult health is an additional reason to emphasize the importance of health promotion and maintenance for all women of reproductive age.

NUTRITIONAL INFLUENCES ON PREGNANCY OUTCOME

Maternal Body Size and Weight Gain during Pregnancy

Women who begin pregnancy underweight and those with low pregnancy weight gains are at higher risk for delivering a low-birth-weight infant (<2500 g); low-birth-weight rates are highest when both factors are present. Women who are overweight before pregnancy and those with a large gestational gain are more likely to deliver macrosomic babies. Figure 11-1 illustrates these relationships and also shows that maternal weight gain has less effect on birth weight as prepregnancy weight for height increases (IOM, 1990).

Based on these findings, the IOM made new recommendations (Table 11-1) in the form of specific ranges of gestational weight gain based on maternal prepregnancy weight for height or body mass index. Although the IOM proposed modified weight gain goals for groups of women at high risk for either low birth weight (teenagers, African-American women) or cesarean delivery (short women), to date, there is little evidence to establish the validity of these modifications (data not presented).

The IOM guidelines have been widely adopted, but critics argue that the higher amount of gain recommended for underweight and normal weight women is unlikely to improve perinatal outcomes and might increase negative consequences for mother or infant. Published data to date suggest otherwise. A recent systematic review of studies examined the association between the IOM weight gain ranges and maternal and fetal outcomes (low birth weight, macrosomia, spontaneous preterm

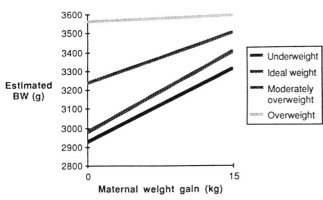

FIGURE 11-1 ■ Birth weight (BW) of liveborn infants at term by prepregnancy body mass and weight gain adjusted for maternal age, race, parity, socioeconomic status, cigarette consumption, and gestational age (*n* = 2964). (From Abrams BF, Laros RK: Prepregnancy weight, weight gain, and birth weight. Am J Obstet Gynecol **154**:503, 1986.)

TABLE 11-1. RECOMMENDED TOTAL WEIGHT GAIN RANGES FOR PREGNANT WOMEN BY PREPREGNANCY BODY MASS INDEX (BMI)*

Weight for Height	BMI	Recommended Total Gain	
		kg	lb
Underweight	<19.8	12.5–18	28–40
Normal weight	19.8–26.0	11.5–16	25–35
Overweight†	>26.0–29.0	7–11.5	15–25

* BMI is calculated using metric units.
† The recommended target weight gain for obese women (BMI > 29.0) is at least 6.0 kg (15 pounds).

Reprinted with permission from Institute of Medicine: Nutrition during Pregnancy, Weight Gain and Nutrient Supplements. Report of the Subcommittee on Nutritional Status and Weight Gain during Pregnancy, Subcommittee on Dietary Intake and Nutrient Supplements during Pregnancy, Committee on Nutritional Status during Pregnancy and Lactation, Food and Nutrition Board. Washington, DC, National Academy Press, 1990. Copyright © 1990 by the National Academy of Sciences. Published by National Academy Press, Washington, DC.

delivery, cesarean delivery, and maternal postpartum obesity); women who gained within the recommended ranges experienced the healthiest pregnancy outcomes compared with those who gained above or below the recommended amount (Abrams et al., 2000). However, in a diverse array of study populations, only about 30% to 40% of women gained within the recommended ranges.

In actual practice, clinicians must assess the rate and pattern of weight gain during pregnancy because total maternal weight gain is unknown until delivery. Maternal gain during the second trimester may be more strongly associated with fetal growth than gain in the first or third, and a lower rate of weight gain than recommended by the IOM during the last trimester of pregnancy is associated with increased risk of spontaneous preterm delivery (Abrams et al., 2000). Though it is not yet understood whether low maternal weight gain causes

these outcomes or simply marks them, avoiding low weight gain during pregnancy, if possible, seems prudent.

Plotting a woman's weight at each prenatal visit against the recommended pattern as shown in Figure 11-2 provides a visual assessment of the weight gain pattern. This graph is based on the recommended total target gain in Table 11-1 as the end points and reflects the recommended rate of gain of 0.5 kg/wk for underweight women, 0.4 kg/wk for normal weight-for-height women, and 0.3 kg/wk for overweight women. The IOM suggests that the target for obese women should be determined individually, but some clinicians apply the recommended ranges for overweight women (6.8 to 11 kg). Low gestational weight gain is defined as less than 0.5 kg/mo for obese women and less than 1 kg/mo for nonobese women. Gains of greater than 3 kg/mo are defined as potentially excessive (IOM, 1990).

FIGURE 11-2 ■ Prenatal weight gain chart, *Dotted line* represents prepregnancy body mass index (BMI) < 19.8; *small-dashed line* represents prepregnancy BMI 19.8–26.0; *large-dashed line* represents BMI > 26.0. (Reprinted from Institute of Medicine: Nutrition during Pregnancy and Lactation: An Implementation Guide. Subcommittee for a Clinical Application Guide, Committee on Nutritional Status during Pregnancy and Lactation, Food and Nutrition Board. Washington, DC, National Academy Press, 1992. Copyright © 1992 by the National Academy of Sciences. Published by National Academy Press, Washington, DC.)

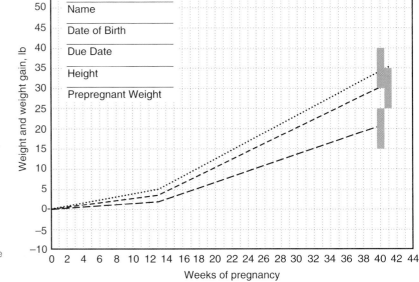

The process of interpreting weight gain during pregnancy is complicated because the actual range of weight gain associated with good pregnancy outcome in populations of women is far wider than the ranges recommended by the IOM (Carmichael et al., 1997). Though weight gain alone is not a sensitive or specific diagnostic tool for poor pregnancy outcome, the IOM recommends that clinicians set a weight gain target with each mother at her first prenatal visit based on her prepregnancy body mass index and provide education on nutrition and physical activity. As the pregnancy progresses, if maternal weight gain deviates from expected, an individualized assessment of the quantity and quality of dietary intake, activity patterns, and other risk factors can either identify areas for change or reassure the clinician and mother that her prenatal weight gain is appropriate. Although delivery of such care is a challenge in our current medical care delivery system, the "obesity toxic" environment in the United States places pregnant and postpartum women in great need of these services. Several resources describe in detail how to deliver this standard of care (Abrams and Parker, 1990; IOM, 1992a,b; Abrams, 1994; Cogswell et al., 2001). Ideally, a nutritionist or registered dietitian skilled in counseling perinatal patients should perform such an assessment.

Additional research is urgently needed to understand how to best support healthy prenatal weight gains and postpartum weight loss in all women. Given the growing epidemic of obesity among women of childbearing age in the United States, more research is also needed to better understand how to manage the pregnancies of obese women and how to prevent or treat postpartum obesity (Gunderson and Abrams, 2000; Lu et al., 2001).

Diet

Periconceptional Issues

We now know that a mother's nutrition at the time of conception influences the health of her infant. It is well established that periconceptional supplementation with folic acid can reduce the incidence of neural tube defects by approximately one half, and the U.S. Centers for Disease Control and Prevention recommends that all women of childbearing age who are capable of becoming pregnant consume 0.4 mg/day of folic acid from diet or supplements (Centers for Disease Control, 1992). Women with a history of pregnancy affected by neural tube defects should supplement their diets with 4 mg of folic acid from 1 month before they plan to become pregnant and throughout the first trimester. Since 1998, the food supply in the United States has been fortified with folate, but some argue that both the level of fortification and recommended preconceptional supplemental dose may be too low to prevent all neural tube defects (Wald et al., 2001). More research is needed to determine if additional vitamins are involved and whether preconceptional vitamin supplementation can reduce the risk of other birth defects or childhood cancers (Moyers and Bailey, 2001).

Although periconceptional vitamin supplementation appears to have benefits, women should be advised to avoid doses above the Recommended Dietary Allowance for pregnancy and drugs that contain high amounts of nutrients (e.g., retinoid therapies). In a study of 20,000 pregnant women, intakes of more than 15,000 IU/day of preformed vitamin A were significantly associated with an increased risk of birth defects (Rothman et al., 1995). Intensive periconceptional management of blood glucose (including dietary counseling) for women with diabetes and of serum phenylalanine for women with phenylketonuria is essential, because these groups of women, as well as those with other metabolic disorders, are at high risk for poor pregnancy outcome (Jovanovic, 2000; Hellekson, 2001).

Postconception

After conception, the mother's diet must provide adequate nutrients to support the development of new maternal and fetal tissues, to meet maternal maintenance costs, and to provide for maternal activity. Additionally, fat deposits are laid down as energy reserves for lactation. Requirements vary by nutrient, stage of gestation, and number of fetuses and may be further influenced by maternal body size and lifestyle factors (e.g., cigarette smoking). Increased requirements are met both through increased dietary intake and through physiologic adjustments in nutrient absorption, excretion, and metabolism.

Energy

Total caloric intake appears to be the most important nutritional influence on birth weight. It has been estimated that a typical pregnancy costs 80,000 additional kcal over prepregnancy requirements or about 300 extra kcal/day, which theoretically produces a maternal weight gain of 10 to 12 kg at term (National Research Council, 1989). However, it has been suggested that the actual requirements for energy vary highly and may range from zero to more than 120,000 calories over the course of a pregnancy (King et al., 1994). Generally, thin or undernourished women require higher energy intakes than other women, but actual predictors of energy requirements are poorly understood. The only practical approach available to clinicians is to use gestational weight gain as a barometer of energy intake. If weight gain is adequate, energy intake is sufficient; if weight gain is low or excessive, an individual assessment is warranted.

Although energy intake and maternal weight gain are important parameters of nutritional status, overall nutrition is more important than caloric intake alone. *Nutrient density*, defined as the quantity of protein, vitamins, and minerals per 100 kcal of food, is an important concept, given the widespread use of processed foods with low nutrient density. The current recommended addition of 300 kcal/day represents a 17% increase over prepregnancy requirements; for vitamins and minerals the pregnancy-related increase ranges from 20% to 100%. For example, a 300-kcal increase can be achieved by choosing one of several snacks: a pint of low-fat milk, a peanut butter sandwich on whole-grain bread, six small cookies, or a 12-ounce can of soda and 10 potato chips. The milk or sandwich has a superior nutrient-density profile, providing excellent amounts of additional nutrients besides calories; the cookies or soda and chips are nutritionally empty. A recent study of more than 2200 pregnant American women concluded that low nutrient-dense foods were major sources of energy, fat, and carbohydrates and fortified foods the major contributors of iron, folate, and vitamin C (Siega-Riz et al., 2002). Another study linked high sugar intake with increased risk of low birth weight among low-income adolescents in several racial and ethnic groups and increased preterm delivery among adolescents of Puerto Rican ethnicity (Lenders et al., 1994, 1997). Because the prepregnancy diets of many American women are less than optimal in nutrient density, eating "to appetite" without additional education and guidance may result in dietary intake well below standards in vital nutrients but excessive in calories, fat, and sodium.

Protein

Eating patterns in the United States tend toward diets that are adequate or even excessive in protein-rich foods. The estimated daily requirement for protein in pregnancy is 60 g, about 15 g over nonpregnant requirements (National Research Council, 1989). It is likely that a woman's prepregnancy intake of protein already includes the recommended increase that is essential for fetal growth and development. Protein-containing foods can be excellent sources of vitamins and minerals such as iron, vitamin B_6, and zinc. However, animal proteins, such as red meats and whole-fat dairy products, can provide excessive (and calorie-dense) fat if used in abundance. Consumption of lean animal foods (such as chicken and fish), low-fat or nonfat dairy products, and vegetable proteins (such as legumes) should be encouraged, especially in women with normal or high body mass indices.

Despite claims that pregnancy-induced hypertension can be prevented or treated with a high-protein diet, there is no evidence that high-protein intake during pregnancy is beneficial, and there is some evidence that "excessive amounts" of protein may be harmful (Zlatnick and Burmeister, 1983; Rush, 1989).

Fatty Acids

In the last decade, new attention has been focused on the role of the essential fatty acids linoleic and α-linolenic acid (one of the omega-3 fatty acids) during pregnancy. Omega-3 fatty acids contribute to neural and visual function development of the fetus. Good sources of these fatty acids include vegetable oils like canola and soybean (α-linolenic) and fatty fish (omega-3) (Hornstra, 2000; Olsen and Secher, 2002). However, a high seafood diet offers the potential for exposure to contaminants such as methylmercury and polychlorinated biphenyls), which are implicated in congenital poisoning, neurologic abnormalities, and neurobehavioral delays in infants (Steuerwald et al., 2000). The U.S. Environmental Protection Agency posts guidelines for safe levels of seafood consumption during pregnancy (www.epa.gov/waterscience/fishadvice).

Trans-fatty acids are created when vegetable oils are hydrogenated to produce margarine, shortening, and other fats commonly used to process foods, particularly commercial baked goods. These isomeric fatty acids inhibit normal fatty acid metabolism and may increase heart disease in adults and reduce fetal birth weight and head circumference (Ascherio and Willett, 1997; Craig-Schmidt, 2001).

Future research is required to fully understand the best type and amount of fat for pregnancy, whether fish oil supplementation is safe and effective, and the health impacts of *trans*-fatty acid consumption during pregnancy. In the meantime, women can be encouraged to consume their fat from unhydrogenated vegetable sources, to eat a moderate amount of seafood, and to emphasize unprocessed foods.

Sodium

In the past, salt was forbidden to pregnant women, and diuretics were used at the first sign of edema. Because diuretics are now known to potentially cause electrolyte imbalance, hyperglycemia, hyperuricemia, a decrease in blood volume, and other problems during pregnancy, they are rarely prescribed. A randomized trial of a low-sodium diet in pregnancy showed that sodium restriction was associated with a significant decrease in overall diet quality. Although this intervention showed no significant effects on birth or placental weight, it also had no impact on maternal blood pressure (van der Maten et al., 1997).

Although sodium should not be restricted during pregnancy, excessive use should not be condoned. A diet of primarily natural foods can be safely salted "to taste." Processed foods are already high in sodium and should be consumed in moderation.

Iron

Hemodilution during pregnancy decreases hemoglobin concentration. Increasing iron intake through diet or supplements can limit the decrease. The average pregnant woman requires approximately 1000 mg of iron during the last two trimesters of pregnancy to increase maternal red blood cell volume and for fetal erythropoiesis (IOM, 1990). Evidence suggests that without supplemental iron, women can exhaust their serum ferritin (iron stores) markedly between the 12th and 25th week of gestation, probably to increase maternal red blood cell mass (Allen, 2001). Large epidemiologic studies have reported that both low (suggesting anemia) and high (suggesting hypovolemia) hematocrit levels before the third trimester are associated with low birth weight, preterm birth, and fetal death (Scholl and Reilly, 2000; Bodnar et al., 2001). Maternal anemia during pregnancy appears to reduce fetal iron stores, and this deficit persists well into the 1st year of the baby's life. Iron-deficiency anemia has adverse consequences on infant development; therefore, maternal anemia should be prevented and treated (Allen, 2000).

To avoid iron-deficiency anemia during pregnancy, the IOM recommends daily supplementation of 30 mg of elemental iron during the second and third trimesters for all pregnant women (IOM, 1990). Therapeutic iron is prescribed in doses of 60 to 120 mg/day for women with diagnosed iron-deficiency anemia. This is defined by a hemoglobin concentration of less than 11 g/100 mL (hematocrit of less than 33%) during the first and third trimesters and a hemoglobin concentration of less than 10.5 g/100 mL (hematocrit of less than 32%) during the second trimester. Adjustments to these criteria accounting for altitude and maternal smoking are available (IOM, 1992a). Women taking therapeutic doses of iron should also supplement their diets with 15 mg of zinc and 2 mg of copper, because high doses of iron may interfere with the absorption and utilization of these nutrients. Additional guidelines for the diagnosis and management of anemia have been published (IOM, 1992a).

To improve iron nutrition through diet, women should be aware of the best food sources of iron: meats, chicken, fish, legumes, leafy vegetables, and whole-grain or enriched breads and cereals. Animal protein, which provides heme iron, enhances iron absorption from the gut as does ascorbic acid, and their effects are additive. Food cooked in cast-iron pans contains significant amounts of iron. Tea and coffee can bind iron in the gut and should be avoided at meals at which good sources of iron are eaten. Large doses of calcium or magnesium salts also decrease iron absorption. Because erythropoiesis depends on protein, vitamin B_{12}, and folate, dietary assessment and improvement of intake for those nutrients can be therapeutic in the treatment of anemia.

Calcium

Data on the effectiveness of calcium in preventing or treating pregnancy-induced or gestational hypertension are contradictory (Ritchie and King, 2000). For example, a 1997 meta-analysis concluded that calcium supplementation during pregnancy leads to a reduction in blood pressure and preeclampsia, but calcium supplementation did not reduce the incidence of preeclampsia, other hypertensive disorders, or poor fetal outcome in a randomized trial of more than 4500 women that was published later (Bucher et al., 1996; Levine et al., 1997).

Whatever its effect on maternal blood pressure, the current recommendation for calcium intake is 1000 mg/day for women 19 to 50 years old and 1300 mg/day for women less than 18 years old (IOM, 1998). This reflects newer knowledge of calcium metabolism during pregnancy and is equivalent to the requirement for nonpregnant women (Allen, 1998). Three servings of calcium-rich foods, such as low-fat milk, cheese, yogurt, or calcium-fortified orange juice, for adults and four servings for adolescents will provide the recommended amount.

Lactase deficiency is common among certain ethnic groups, including persons of Asian, African, and Middle Eastern descent. Although symptoms of lactose intolerance include abdominal cramping, bloating, flatulence, and diarrhea, there is some evidence that lactose intolerance improves during pregnancy, and some of these women may tolerate dairy products well (Szilagyi et al., 1996). Women who do not use milk because of personal preference or lactose intolerance benefit from counseling about culturally acceptable alternative food sources. Lower lactose foods include cheese, yogurt, and special lactose-reduced milk. Calcium-fortified orange juice or soy milk, tofu (soybean curd) made with calcium sulfate, canned fish with bones (such as salmon and sardines), ground sesame seeds, and leafy green vegetables also provide calcium.

Low calcium intake has been defined as less than 600 mg/day (equivalent to a diet containing only one serving of a calcium-rich food in addition to nondairy foods). Women who are unable to increase their intake of calcium foods to achieve the Recommended Dietary Allowance should be given a calcium supplement of 600 mg/day, especially if they are younger than age 25 years and thus still increasing their own bone density (IOM, 1990).

Folate

Maternal folate nutrition is not only important during the periconceptional period. Folate plays an essential role in nucleic acid synthesis and is required to increase red blood cell mass and growth of the uterus, placenta, and fetus. Poor maternal folate status can result from low dietary intake, maternal genetic factors that are, as yet, poorly understood, or an inter-

action of the two. Populations with high rates of adverse pregnancy outcomes often also consume diets low in micronutrients, including folate. Cigarette smoking, alcohol abuse, and previous use of oral contraceptives are associated with poor maternal folate status. Low serum folate has been linked epidemiologically with increased risk of preterm delivery and fetal growth restriction. Elevated maternal homocysteine levels, which result from folate inadequacy and may reflect a maternal chromosomal abnormality, have been associated with higher rates of habitual spontaneous abortions, placental abruptions, and preeclampsia (Scholl and Johnson, 2000).

The recommended intake for folate during pregnancy is 600 µg/day, which is higher than the amount usually consumed through food. Therefore, most pregnant women will require a vitamin supplement in addition to a well-balanced diet that includes fortified grains and cereals and foods naturally high in folate, such as strawberries, leafy vegetables, and broccoli (Bailey, 2000).

Zinc

The trace mineral zinc is involved in several important biochemical reactions, and adequate zinc status is required for human growth. Some studies have suggested that low maternal zinc status is associated with adverse pregnancy outcome, but results are inconsistent, possibly because the lack of a reliable biochemical marker of zinc status hinders research. Zinc absorption is reduced among women who have cereal-based diets high in phytate, who take large amounts of supplemental iron, and who have gastrointestinal disease. In addition, those who smoke, abuse alcohol, or undergo acute stress may experience further compromised plasma zinc concentrations and transport to the fetus and may therefore benefit from a supplement (King, 2000a).

Fluoride

A randomized controlled trial of prenatal fluoride supplementation showed no effect on caries prevention in the 5-year-old offspring of the study mothers. Thus, the benefits of fluoride supplementation during pregnancy remain controversial (Leverett et al., 1997).

Supplementation

Because there is little scientific evidence that supplementation improves pregnancy outcome, the routine use of prenatal vitamin–mineral supplements has traditionally been a controversial topic among nutritionists (Hemminki, 1982; Keen and Zidenberg-Cherr, 1994). However, a study of low-income teenagers found that prenatal multivitamin–mineral supplements were associated with significant reductions in preterm delivery and low birth weight (Scholl et al., 1997).

After examining all the available evidence regarding the safety issues and justification for vitamin and mineral supplementation during pregnancy, the IOM concluded that routine supplementation of any nutrient, except iron, is unnecessary. They recommended an assessment of the dietary practices of each pregnant woman and prescription of a supplement at the beginning of the second trimester for those who are unlikely to consume an adequate diet and who are in high-risk categories (Table 11-2) (IOM, 1990). In a survey of pregnant women in

TABLE 11-2. NUTRITIONAL RISK FACTORS IN PREGNANCY

Significant deviation of pregravid weight from ideal weight
Inadequate or excessive weight gain
Adolescence, particularly age within 2 years of menarche
Psychological, social, cultural, religious, or economic factors that limit or affect adequacy of nutrition
History of obstetric problems, including previous low-birth-weight infant
Chronic illness, such as diabetes, thyroid, phenylketonuria, or sickle cell disease
Multiple gestation
Abnormal laboratory values, such as low hemoglobin level, glycosuria, abnormal blood glucose level, albuminuria, and ketonuria
Substance abuse
Eating disorders
Pica
Food allergies or intolerances
Bed rest

North Carolina, food alone provided recommended amounts of iron in only about 30% and folate in only 60% of those studied (Siega-Riz et al., 2002). This supports previous findings that American women, including those with high incomes, do not meet dietary requirements through food alone (Block and Abrams, 1993) and suggests that a substantial proportion of pregnant women may benefit from supplementation.

Table 11-3 gives the recommended composition of this supplement and additional guidelines for complete vegetarians and women with low calcium intake. However, because pills contain only a small number of the essential nutrients and other substances found in foods, supplementation should be viewed as an adjunct to a healthy diet, not a replacement. Furthermore, data from the 1988 U.S. National Maternal and Infant Health Survey suggest that about one third of African-American mothers did not consume their prescribed supplements. Multivariate analysis suggested that women with the characteristics of low education, young age, unmarried, non-smokers, or participants in the Women, Infants, and Children program were less likely to use their prescribed prenatal supplements (Yu et al., 1996). Thus, even when prescribed, supplements may not improve maternal nutrition, even in groups of women who might most benefit from them.

Currently, about 20% of pregnant women in the United States participate in the Special Supplemental Food Program for Women, Infants, and Children, which provides food, education, and referrals to low-income pregnant women at nutritional risk. Prenatal Women, Infants, and Children program participation is associated with a reduction in the incidence of low birth weight and preterm delivery (Abrams, 1993). Furthermore, the program is cost effective. A General Accounting Office meta-analysis (Avruch and Cackley, 1995) suggested that for every federal dollar invested in the Women, Infants, and Children program, $2.89 was saved during the infant's first year of life.

Dietary Guidance

Pregnancy creates a special demand for high-quality nutrients and is an excellent impetus for changing poor food habits. Nutritional counseling can improve both weight gain

during pregnancy and birth weight (IOM, 1992b). Although pregnancy is considered a "teachable moment," dietary guidance becomes effective only if the patient sees merit in the suggestions made and can apply the information to her own life.

Guidelines have been developed to translate nutritional recommendations into actual foods. Table 11-4 is a food guide for the reproductive years that can provide adequate amounts of nutrients, except for iron and perhaps calories. As stated earlier, energy needs are highly individual; therefore, the need to add additional foods is influenced by many maternal characteristics, including the following:

- Prepregnancy weight for height
- Weight gain pattern during pregnancy
- Metabolic differences
- Number of fetuses
- Maternal activity
- Appetite
- Maternal age

A North Carolina study found that low nutrient-dense foods were the major source of calories during the second trimester of pregnancy. Intake of saturated fat and refined carbohydrates such as soft drinks and refined baked goods was prevalent, and more than one half of the women consumed a low-fiber diet (Siega-Riz et al., 2002). This is quite different from the ideal prenatal diet that includes small frequent meals of nutrient-dense vegetables, fruits, lean protein sources, dairy products, and unrefined grains or complex carbohydrates that are high in dietary fiber and yield healthier glucose metabolism.

Nutrition education to improve maternal diet should be available to all women before or early in pregnancy, whether in a group or individually. Essential topics should include hazardous substances, including cigarettes and alcohol; weight

TABLE 11-3. RECOMMENDED LEVELS OF VITAMIN AND MINERAL SUPPLEMENTATION

Multivitamin–mineral preparation for women with poor diets or in high-risk categories

Iron	30 mg	Vitamin B_6	2 mg
Zinc	15 mg	Folate	300 µg
Copper	2 mg	Vitamin C	50 mg
Calcium	250 mg	Vitamin D	5 µg

Supplementation for women in special circumstances
Complete vegetarians (consume no animal products whatsoever)
10 µg (400 IU) vitamin D
2 µg vitamin B_{12}
Women under age 25 whose daily intake of calcium is less than 600 mg
600 mg calcium
Women with low intake of vitamin D–fortified milk, especially those who have minimal exposure to sunlight
10 µg (400 IU) vitamin D

gain recommendations and goals; adequate exercise; and a description of how to achieve a healthy prenatal diet.

Information on infant feeding options, including encouragement and support for breast-feeding, is also part of the nutritional care plan. Individualized assessment of all patients includes a review of prepregnancy weight for height, gestational weight gain, use of drugs, laboratory values (hemoglobin, hematocrit), medical and social problems, and dietary habits. Research is needed to determine the most effective ways of delivering nutrition services in prenatal care. A pragmatic approach is to elicit an estimate of "usual" diet or intake during the previous 24 hours and compare it with a recommended diet guide. The presence of particular factors may indicate that a woman is at high risk for nutritional problems and needs in-depth nutritional assessment, counseling, and follow-up (see Table 11-2).

Basic nutritional assessment and guidance should be provided by the woman's primary health care provider before, during, and after pregnancy. If problems are identified, intensive nutritional assessment and counseling are best performed by an experienced dietitian who understands the physiologic needs of pregnancy and the cultural food habits of the patients served and who also is an effective communicator and counselor. Because nutrition is only one aspect of prenatal care, nutritional recommendations should support and complement the care given by other members of the medical team. A practical guide to the delivery of perinatal nutrition care is available (IOM, 1992a) and is summarized in Table 11-5.

TABLE 11-5. GENERAL GUIDELINES FOR MATERNAL NUTRITION CARE

Preconceptional
1. Assess weight status, hemoglobin or hematocrit, dietary intake, exercise habits, eating disorders, and other parameters of nutritional status.
2. Offer basic guidance regarding healthful diet, exercise, and avoidance of harmful substances.
3. Provide individualized care to address risk factors such as obesity, anemia, phenylketonuria, or previous birth of infant with neural tube defect.

During pregnancy
1. Assess dietary intake; encourage a varied diet with good nutrient density.
2. Recommend and monitor weight gain based on prepregnancy weight for height.
3. Encourage moderate exercise as appropriate.
4. Counsel to avoid exposure to drugs and chemicals.
5. Supplement with prophylactic (30 mg elemental) iron; other nutrients based on assessments.
6. Provide education to all women on diet, weight gain, management of common pregnancy discomforts, and benefits of and preparation for breast-feeding.
7. Provide individual assessment and counseling by a perinatal nutritionist for women at risk for nutritional problems.

Postpartum period
1. Assist with initiation and maintenance of breast-feeding, including recommendations for nutritional needs of lactation.
2. Encourage varied diet with good nutrient density for all women.
3. Provide realistic health-promoting advice regarding weight loss.
4. Counsel to avoid exposure to drugs and other harmful substances.

TABLE 11-4. DAILY FOOD GUIDE FOR WOMEN OF CHILDBEARING AGE

	No. of Daily Servings	
Food Category	**Nonpregnant**	**Pregnant/ lactating**
Protein-rich foods (meat, poultry, fish, eggs, legumes, nuts; servings equivalent to 1 oz meat)	5	7
Dairy products or other calcium-rich foods, such as tofu (servings equivalent to 1 cup milk)	3*	3*
Grain products (emphasize whole-grain breads and cereals; serving size: 1 slice bread: 1 oz dry cereal; 1/2 cup cooked pasta, hot cereal, or rice)	6+	6+
Fruits and vegetables (serving size: approx. 1/2 cup cooked; 1/2–1 cup raw: 6 oz juice):		
Vitamin C sources	2+	2+
Leafy green vegetables	1+	1+
Other fruits and vegetables	2+	2+

* Women aged 11–24 years should consume one extra serving of dairy products daily.

Modified from California Department of Health Services, Maternal and Child Health Branch and WIC Supplemental Food Branch: Nutrition during Pregnancy and the Postpartum Period: A Manual for Health Care Professionals. Sacramento, Calif., Department of Health Services, 1990.

CLINICAL ISSUES

Clinicians are likely to encounter a number of nutrition problems in day-to-day prenatal care. Some of the issues frequently encountered are summarized.

Adolescent Pregnancy

Girls under 17 years of age are at higher risk for short gestation, perinatal mortality, and low-birth-weight babies. Sociocultural and psychological factors heavily influence the outcome of these pregnancies. Physiologically, the pregnant adolescent within 2 years of menarche is at highest risk, presumably because of the growth demands of her own body and of the fetus, although studies have suggested that older adolescents are also still growing (Scholl et al., 1994; Hediger et al., 1997). Diets chosen by female adolescents are notoriously variable. Ingestion of vitamin supplements is erratic, and abuse of drugs, tobacco, and alcohol may be a problem. In addition, adolescent concerns about body image may lead to dieting during pregnancy, resulting in inadequate energy and nutrient intake (Lenders et al., 2000).

Bed Rest

Some women require bed rest during pregnancy because of hypertensive disorders, preterm labor, and other problems. Nutritional counseling is important in these cases to help achieve (or control) weight gain, to alleviate symptoms such as poor appetite or constipation secondary to medication or inactivity, and to assist the woman in creating a plan that allows access to foods that are both easy to prepare and nutritious (Herron and Dulock, 1987; IOM, 1992a).

Constipation

Constipation can be treated by increasing dietary fiber, fluid intake, and exercise. Good sources of dietary fiber include whole grains, bran, legumes, and fresh fruits and vegetables.

Diabetes

The diabetic pregnancy is discussed in Chapter 49.

Eating Disorders

The prevalence of anorexia nervosa, bulimia nervosa, pica (eating of nonfoods), and other eating disorders is not known, but these conditions can lead to poor pregnancy outcome and require specialized nutritional management using a team approach (IOM, 1992a,b).

Eating and Drinking during Labor

Restrictions on eating and drinking during labor were instituted in the 1940s to reduce the risk of aspiration pneumonia among parturient women who received general anesthesia. Since that time, general anesthesia has become much less common in obstetrics, and modern anesthetic techniques have reduced the risk of aspiration under general anesthesia. There is also no evidence in the medical literature of benefits from restricting oral fluids during labor or of risks associated with drinking clear fluids (Elkington, 1991). As a consequence, many clinical practices have relaxed restrictions and allow various clear fluids by mouth (Ludka and Roberts, 1993). In Europe, policies permitting food and drink are often much more relaxed, with no accompanying increase in aspiration-related mortality or morbidity (Broach and Newton, 1988; Michael et al., 1991; Scheepers et al., 2001). The nutritional requirements of laboring women have not been well studied, although evidence from one clinical trial showed that women assigned to a light diet during labor were less likely to develop ketosis than those restricted to water (Scrutton et al., 1999). The increased energy needs of all persons involved in physiologically demanding or vigorous activity suggests the benefits of careful attention to energy and fluid intake.

Heartburn and Acid Indigestion

Heartburn and acid indigestion are common complaints during pregnancy. Eating small, frequent, dry meals separately from fluid intake; avoiding greasy foods; and wearing loose-fitting clothing can provide some relief. Because antacids taken for symptomatic relief may bind iron in the gastrointestinal tract, excessive use should be discouraged, especially if iron-deficiency anemia is a problem. If antacids are used, those containing calcium are preferred.

Multiple Gestation

The incidence of multiple gestation is increasing, and women carrying two or more fetuses have higher nutritional requirements. A recent review supported the IOM recommendation that women gain from 16 to 20.5 kg when carrying twins and suggested that a gain of 22.7 kg was consistent with good outcome for women carrying triplets (Brown and Carlson, 2000). Pattern of gain has been shown to affect birth weight in multifetal pregnancy; thus gains during the second and third trimester of 1.5 kg per week for twins and 1.5 kg per week throughout pregnancy for triplets are advised. Underweight women might benefit from a higher rate of gain, and overweight women might benefit from less.

Women carrying multiple fetuses require the nutrient supplementation described in Table 11-3. They also may benefit from the increased energy intake of high-quality foods. Physical discomfort is common during late pregnancy and may interfere with adequate intake. Small frequent meals of high-quality foods and additional healthy snacks, such as milkshakes, may enhance energy and nutrient intake.

Nausea and Vomiting

Nausea and vomiting, which usually occurs during the first trimester but can persist throughout pregnancy, is a common medical condition. It most likely results from the presence of human chorionic gonadotropin or estrogens. Though it is a medical condition, nausea and vomiting can be exacerbated by psychological factors. It can cause discomfort and anxiety as well as weight loss, ketosis, and dehydration in more severe cases. Management includes sympathetic reassurance that nausea is common, is not harmful to the fetus, and will resolve. Eating small frequent meals consisting of dry starchy foods and avoidance of strong odors and flavors also can help. Results of clinical trials indicate that vitamin B_6 supplementation (25 mg three times a day) may help in the relief of vomiting and severe nausea during pregnancy (Sahakian et al., 1991). In severe cases, if other gastrointestinal illnesses are ruled out, psychological counseling and hospitalization may be necessary (Goodwin and Romero, 2002) (see also Chapter 52).

Vegetarian Diets

Since the 1970s, diets that exclude some or all animal products have become relatively popular. Such diets can provide adequate nutrition during pregnancy if they are correctly balanced. Plans that include dairy products provide a good balance of nutrients for pregnancy. Vegetarian diets that exclude all animal products (vegan) can also be used successfully during pregnancy, but they demand closer assessment, counseling, and surveillance to ensure nutritional adequacy. Avoidance of all animal products can result in vitamin B_{12} deficiency. The vegan diet also is often extremely low in fat and high in fiber; it is sometimes difficult for a woman to eat enough to satisfy caloric requirements during pregnancy. Calcium, riboflavin, and vitamin D intake may be marginal if dairy products are not used, and iron and zinc intake may be low as well.

Dietary assessment and counseling can dramatically upgrade the quality of the diet while the vegetarian pattern is maintained. Supplements may be indicated (see Table 11-3).

Food-Borne Infections and Environmental Hazards

Intracellular food-borne pathogens that are controlled by cellular immunity can be particularly deleterious to pregnancy because progesterone production during pregnancy may lead to a suppression of cell-mediated immune function. Pregnant women are more susceptible to certain food-borne infections from the hepatitis E virus, *Coxiella burnetii*, and, most concerning, *Toxoplasma gondii* and *Listeria monocytogenes* (Smith, 1999). The *Listeria* bacterium, found in luncheon meats, unpasteurized soft cheeses, and refrigerated smoked seafood, can cause miscarriage, fetal death, and severe illness of the newborn. Pregnant women should be advised to wash hands frequently, cook and refrigerate food properly, and avoid cross-contamination of raw foods. More detailed advice to pregnant women concerning food-borne illness precautions can be found at the U.S. Environmental Protection Agency website (www.epa.gov).

Toxic heavy metals such as lead (found in food and water and lead-based products such as paint and utensils), cadmium (found in contaminated soil affecting food crops and animal feed), and organic mercury (found in contaminated water and fish products) have the most severe cumulative health effects on the pregnant woman and fetuses (March of Dimes, 2002).

REFERENCES

Abrams B: Preventing low birth weight: Does WIC work? A review of evaluations of the Special Supplemental Food Program for Women, Infants and Children. Ann N Y Acad Sci **678**:306, 1993.

Abrams B: Weight gain and energy intake during pregnancy. Clin Obstet Gynecol **37**:515, 1994.

Abrams B, Altman S, Pickett K: Pregnancy weight gain: still controversial. Am J Clin Nutr **71** (Suppl):1233S, 2000.

Abrams B, Parker J: Maternal weight gain in women with good pregnancy outcome. Obstet Gynecol **76**:1, 1990.

Allen LH: Women's dietary calcium requirements are not increased by pregnancy or lactation. Am J Clin Nutr **67**:591, 1998.

Allen LH: Anemia and iron deficiency: Effects on pregnancy outcome. Am J Clin Nutr **71**(5 Suppl):1280S, 2000.

Allen LH: Anemia and iron deficiency: effects on pregnancy outcome. Am J Clin Nutr **71** (Suppl):1280S, 2001.

Ascherio A, Willett WC: Health effects of trans fatty acids. Am J Clin Nutr **66** (Suppl):1006S, 1997.

Avruch S, Cackley AP: Savings achieved by giving WIC benefits to women prenatally. Public Health Rep **110**:27, 1995.

Bailey LB: New standard for dietary folate intake in pregnant women. Am J Clin Nutr **71** (Suppl):1304S, 2000.

Barker DJP: Mothers, Babies and Disease in Later Life, 2nd ed. London, Harcourt Brace, 1998.

Block G, Abrams B: Vitamin and mineral status of women of childbearing potential. Ann N Y Acad Sci **678**:244, 1993.

Bodnar LM, Scanlon KS, Freedman DS, et al: High prevalence of postpartum anemia among low-income women in the United States. Am J Obstet Gynecol **185**:438, 2001.

Broach J, Newton N: Food and beverages in labor. Part I. Cross-cultural and historical practices. Birth **15**:81, 1988.

Brown JE, Carlson M: Nutrition and multifetal pregnancy. J Am Diet Assoc **100**:343, 2000.

Bucher HC, Guyatt GH, Cook RJ, et al: Effect of calcium supplementation on pregnancy-induced hypertension and preeclampsia: A meta-analysis of randomized controlled trials. JAMA **275**:1113, 1996.

Carmichael S, Abrams B, Selvin S: Am J Public Health **87**:1984, 1997.

Centers for Disease Control: Recommendations for the use of folic acid to reduce the number of cases of spina bifida and other neural tube defects. MMWR Morb Mortal Wkly Rep **41** (RR14):1, 1992.

Cogswell ME, Perry GS, Shieve LA, et al: Obesity in women of childbearing age: Risks, prevention and treatment. Prim Care Update Obstet Gynecol **8**:89, 2001.

Craig-Schmidt MC: Isomeric fatty acids: evaluation status and implications for maternal and child health. Lipids **36**:997, 2001.

Elkington KW: At the water's edge: where obstetrics and anesthesia meet. Obstet Gynecol **77**:304, 1991.

Frankel S, Elwood P, Sweetnam P, et al: Birthweight, body-mass index in middle age and incident coronary heart disease. Lancet **348**:1478, 1996.

Gillman MW: Epidemiological challenges in studying the fetal origins of adult chronic disease. Int J Epidemiol **31**:294, 2002.

Gillman MW, Rich-Edwards J: The fetal origins of adult disease: from skeptic to convert. Pediatr Perinatal Epidemiol **14**:192, 2000.

Goodwin TM, Romero R: Understanding and treating nausea and vomiting of pregnancy. Am J Obstet Gynecol **186**:181S, 2002.

Gunderson EP, Abrams B: Epidemiology of gestational weight gain and body weight changes after pregnancy. Epidemiol Rev **22**:261, 2000.

Harding JE: The nutritional basis of the fetal origins of adult disease. Int J Epidemiol **30**:15, 2001.

Hattersley AT, Tooke JE: The fetal insulin hypothesis: an alternative explanation of the association of low birthweight with diabetes and vascular disease. Lancet **353**:789, 1999.

Hediger M, Scholl TO, Schall JI, et al: Implications of the Camden Study of adolescent pregnancy: Interactions among maternal growth, nutritional status, and body composition. Ann N Y Acad Sci **817**:281, 1997.

Hellekson KL: NIH consensus statement on phenylketonuria. Am Fam Physician **63**:1430, 2001.

Hemminki E: Effects of routine haematinic and vitamin administration in pregnancy. *In* Enkin E, Chalmers I (eds): Effectiveness and Satisfaction in Antenatal Care. Philadelphia, Lippincott, 1982, Chapter 7.

Herron M, Dulock H: Preterm Labor. White Plains, NY, March of Dimes Foundation, 1987.

Hornstra G: Essential fatty acids in mothers and their neonates. Am J Clin Nutr **71** (Suppl):1262S, 2000.

Huxley RR, Shiell AW, Law CM: The role of size at birth and postnatal catch-up growth in determining systolic blood pressure: a systematic review of the literature. J Hypertens **18**:815, 2000.

Institute of Medicine: Nutrition during Pregnancy, Weight Gain and Nutrient Supplements. Report of the Subcommittee on Nutritional Status and Weight Gain during Pregnancy, Subcommittee on Dietary Intake and Nutrient Supplements during Pregnancy, Committee on Nutritional Status during Pregnancy and Lactation, Food and Nutrition Board. Washington, DC, National Academy Press, 1990.

Institute of Medicine: Nutrition during Pregnancy and Lactation: An Implementation Guide. Subcommittee for a Clinical Application Guide, Committee on Nutritional Status during Pregnancy and Lactation, Food and Nutrition Board. Washington, DC, National Academy Press, 1992a.

Institute of Medicine: Nutrition Services in Perinatal Care, Report of the Committee on Nutritional Status during Pregnancy and Lactation, Food and Nutrition Board. Washington, DC, National Academy Press, 1992b.

Institute of Medicine: Dietary Reference Intakes: Calcium, Phosphorus, Magnesium, Vitamin D, and Fluoride. Washington, DC, National Academy Press, 1998.

Jovanovic L: Medical nutritional therapy in pregnant women with pregestational diabetes mellitus. J Matern Fetal Med **9**:21, 2000.

Keen C, Zidenberg-Cherr S: Should vitamin-mineral supplements be recommended for all women with child-bearing potential? Am J Clin Nutr **59**(2 Suppl):532S, 1994.

King J: Determinants of maternal zinc status during pregnancy. Am J Clin Nutr **71** (Suppl):1334S, 2000a.

King JC: Physiology of pregnancy and human metabolism. Am J Clin Nutr **71** (Suppl):1218S, 2000b.

King JC, Butte NF, Bronstein MN, et al: Energy metabolism during pregnancy: Influence of maternal energy status. Am J Clin Nutr **59**:439S, 1994.

Law CM, Fall CHD, Newsome CA, et al: Is birthweight related to glucose and insulin metabolism? A systematic review. Pediatr Res **50**:60A, 2001.

Lenders CM, Hediger ML, Scholl TO, et al: Effect of high-sugar intake by low-income pregnant adolescents on infant birth weight. J Adolesc Health **15**:596, 1994.

Lenders CM, Hediger ML, Scholl TO, et al: Gestational age and infant size at birth are associated with dietary sugar intake among pregnant adolescents. J Nutr **127**:1113, 1997.

Lenders CM, McElrath TF, Scholl TO: Nutrition in adolescent pregnancy. Curr Opin Pediatr **12**:291, 2000.

Leverett DH, Adair SM, Vaughan BW, et al: Randomized clinical trial of the effect of prenatal fluoride supplements in preventing dental caries. Caries Res **31**:174, 1997.

Levine RJ, Hauth JC, Curet LB, et al: Trial of calcium to prevent preeclampsia. N Engl J Med **337**:69, 1997.

Lu GC, Rouse DJ, DuBard M, et al: The effect of increasing prevalence of maternal obesity on perinatal morbidity. Am J Obstet Gynecol **185**:845, 2001.

Ludka LM, Roberts CC: Eating and drinking in labor. A literature review. J Nurs Midw **38**:199, 1993.

March of Dimes: Nutrition Today Matters Tomorrow: A Report from the March of Dimes Task Force on Nutrition and Optimal Human Development, Wilkes-Barre, Pa, March of Dimes Education Services, 2002.

Michael S, Reilly CS, Caunt JA: Policies for oral intake during labour. A survey of maternity units in England and Wales. Anaesthesia **46**:1071, 1991.

Moyers S, Bailey LB: Fetal malformations and folate metabolism: review of recent evidence. Nutr Rev **59**:215, 2001.

National Research Council: Recommended Dietary Allowances. Washington, DC, National Academy Press, 1989.

Olsen SF, Secher NJ: Low consumption of seafood in early pregnancy as a risk factor for preterm delivery: Prospective cohort study. BMJ **324**:1, 2002.

Paneth N, Susser M: Early origin of coronary heart disease (the "Barker hypothesis"). BMJ **310**:411, 1995.

Rich-Edwards JW, Stampfer MJ, Manson JE, et al: Birthweight and the risk of cardiovascular disease in adult women. Br Med J **315**:396, 1997.

Ritchie LD, King JC: Dietary calcium and pregnancy-induced hypertension: Is there a relation? Am J Clin Nutr **71** (Suppl):1371S, 2000.

Rothman KJ, Moore LL, Singer MR, et al: Teratogenicity of high vitamin A intake. N Engl J Med **333**:1369, 1995.

Rush D: Effects of changes in protein and calorie intake during pregnancy on the growth of the human fetus. *In* Enken M, Chalmers I (eds): Effective Care in Pregnancy and Childbirth. Vol. 1. Oxford, Oxford University Press, 1989, p. 255.

Sahakian V, Rouse D, Sipes S, et al: Vitamin B$_6$ is effective therapy for nausea and vomiting of pregnancy: A randomized, double-blind placebo-controlled study. Obstet Gynecol **78**:33, 1991.

Scheepers HC, Thans MC, de Jong PA, et al: Eating and drinking in labor: The influence of caregiver advice on women's behavior. Birth **28**:119, 2001.

Scholl TO, Hediger ML, Schall JI, et al: Maternal growth during pregnancy and the competition for nutrients. Am J Clin Nutr **60**:183, 1994.

Scholl TO, Hediger ML, Bendich A, et al: Use of multivitamin/mineral prenatal supplements: Influence on the outcome of pregnancy. Am J Epidemiol **146**:134, 1997.

Scholl TO, Johnson WG: Folic acid: Influence on the outcome of pregnancy. Am J Clin Nutr **71** (Suppl):1295S, 2000.

Scholl TO, Reilly T: Anemia, iron, and pregnancy outcome. J Nutr **130** (2 Suppl):443S, 2000.

Scrutton MJ, Metcalfe GA, Lowy C, et al: Eating in labour. A randomised controlled trial assessing the risks and benefits. Anaesthesia **54**:329, 1999.

Siega-Riz AM, Bodnar LM, Savitz DA: What are pregnant women eating? Nutrient and food group differences by race. Am J Obstet Gynecol **186**:480, 2002.

Smith JL: Foodborne infections during pregnancy. J Food Prot **62**:818, 1999.

Steuerwald U, Weihe P, Jorgensen PJ, et al: Maternal seafood diet, methylmercury exposure, and neonatal neurologic function. J Pediatr **136**:599, 2000.

Szilagyi A, Salomon R, Martin M, et al: Lactose handling by women with lactose malabsorption is improved during pregnancy. Clin Invest Med **19**:416, 1996.

van der Maten GD, van Raaij JM, Visman L, et al: Low-sodium diet in pregnancy: Effects on blood pressure and maternal nutritional status. Br J Nutr **77**:703, 1997.

Wald NJ, Law MR, Morris JK, et al: Quantifying the effect of folic acid. Lancet **358**:2069, 2001.

Yu SM, Keppel KG, Singh GK, et al: Preconceptional and prenatal multivitamin-mineral supplement use in the 1988 National Maternal and Infant Health Survey. Am J Public Health **86**:240, 1996.

Zlatnick F, Burmeister L: Dietary protein and preeclampsia. Am J Obstet Gynecol **147**:345, 1983.

Chapter 12
THE PUERPERIUM

Robert Resnik, MD

REPRODUCTIVE ORGANS

Uterus

The puerperium begins immediately after delivery of the placenta. Frequent strong myometrial contractions rapidly induce a decrease in size, and within 24 hours the uterus becomes a globular hard mass approximately the size it was at 20 weeks' gestation. Uterine blood flow alterations take place quite rapidly. Within 2 days of delivery, abdominal Doppler ultrasonography reveals a sharp increase in uterine vascular resistance (Tekay and Jouppila, 1993). The figure-of-eight interlaced muscle bundle of the middle uterine layer compresses blood vessels supplying the placental site, preventing hemorrhage. Within 1 week postpartum, the uterus has decreased in size by 50%, to 500 g. After 2 weeks, normal involution is such that the uterus cannot be felt by abdominal examination. By 6 weeks, it has returned almost to its nonpregnant dimensions. Recently, Mulic-Lutvica and colleagues (2001) conducted a detailed ultrasonic evaluation of the uterus and cavity from postpartum days 1 through 56. This study of 42 women after a normal vaginal delivery demonstrated that the maximum anteroposterior diameter of the uterus decreased from 92 mm on day 1 to 39 mm 8 weeks postpartum. (The latter measurement was made with transvaginal examination.) Measurements of the uterine cavity diminished from 16 mm on day 1 to 4.0 mm at 8 weeks.

Appropriate involution of the placental site is of great importance. After the placenta separates, only the basal portion of the decidua remains. Within 72 hours postpartum, two layers become apparent. The first layer is superficial and is sloughed with the lochia. The underlying layer contains residual endometrial glands and is a source of the new endometrium. By day 7, the surface epithelium and stroma begin to assume a nonpregnant appearance. By the 16th day, proliferative endometrium has been completely restored. At this point, the endometrium is identical to that of the nonpregnant uterus in the proliferative phase of the cycle, except that remnants of hyalinized decidua remain and leukocytic infiltrates may be observed in the stroma (Sharman, 1953). The appearance of blood vessels underlying the placental site is shown in Figure 12-1.

The placental site itself takes longer to regenerate. Immediately after delivery, marked constriction of arterioles supplying the placental site occurs and a fibrinoid endarteritis develops in a matter of hours. The area then undergoes hyalinization. Venous sites also become thrombotic and hyalinized (Anderson and Davis, 1968). The area then heals either by decidual sloughing produced by endometrial growth from areas adjacent to the placental site or by a process similar to that by which any denuded epithelial area regenerates. If this process does not proceed properly, *subinvolution* is said to occur, which may result in significant late postpartum hemorrhage. The normal histologic appearance of the placental site 6 weeks postpartum is shown in Figure 12-2.

Cervix

After delivery of the placenta, the cervix has little tone and bears little resemblance to its nonpregnant state. Within 2 to 3 days, it resumes its customary appearance but is still dilated to 2 or 3 cm. At 1 week postpartum, the gross appearance of the cervix is very much like that in the nonpregnant state, although histologic examination shows regression of the endocervical hypertrophy (Glass and Rosenthal, 1950). As late as 6 weeks postpartum, involution is still occurring, with evidence of stromal edema and round cell infiltration, the latter persisting up to 3 or 4 months (McLaren, 1952). Thus, any evaluation of the cervix relative to repetitive mid-trimester loss should be delayed until at least 3 months after termination of pregnancy.

Vagina

Immediately after delivery, the prominent vaginal rugae are not visible and the vagina appears smooth and swollen. Within 3 weeks, the vascularity and edema regress and rugae reappear. Histologically, the vaginal epithelium returns to its normal nonpregnant appearance in 6 to 10 weeks. At 6 weeks, the vagina has completed involution, although varying degrees of mucosal and fascial relaxation may remain, manifested by a persistent cystocele and/or rectocele (Kistner, 1978).

RETURN OF OVULATION AND MENSTRUATION

Hormone patterns in the postpartum period are characterized by low levels of gonadotropins and sex steroids and by elevated concentrations of prolactin. Consequently, it is not surprising that the return to ovulation and menstruation largely depends on whether and for how long lactation and nursing occur (Campbell and Gray, 1993).

Early studies demonstrated that the initial ovulation after delivery in nonlactating women occurred at a mean of

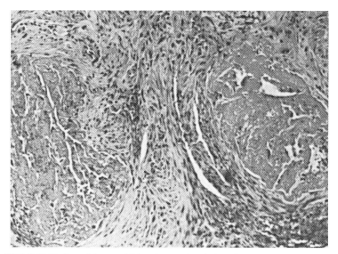

FIGURE 12-1 ■ Maternal blood vessels of the placental site 2 weeks postpartum. Both vessels are filled with contracted thrombotic material, and early fibrocytic ingrowth is beginning at the periphery. Magnification ×160.

10 weeks and for nursing women, 17 weeks (Lyon and Stamm, 1946). With use of sequential endometrial biopsies, a secretory pattern may be observed as early as day 44 (Sharman, 1951a). Other studies have corroborated these earlier findings but show that women who breast-feed for less than 28 days will ovulate at approximately the same time as women who do not breast-feed. Furthermore, ovulation can take place as early as 27 days after delivery (Cronin, 1968), although the appearance of vaginal bleeding in breast-feeding women in the first 8 weeks postpartum does not represent a return to ovulatory function (Visness et al., 1997).

Return of menstruation in nonlactating women increases linearly up to 12 weeks postpartum, and 70% will have menstruated by that time (Sharman, 1951b). The mean time to first menses is 7 to 9 weeks; in lactating women, the longer the period of lactation, the longer the mean time to the first menstrual period. It is generally agreed that any menstrual period in the first 6 weeks is anovulatory, but once menstruation ensues, the percentage of subsequent menses that are ovulatory rises rapidly. The role of prolactin, as well as other polypeptide and steroid hormones, in ovarian function during the puerperium has been studied in detail (Rolland et al., 1975).

The physiologic basis for postpartum amenorrhea is not entirely clear, although it is known that gonadotropin activity is minimal for 2 to 3 weeks after delivery. It has been postulated that this may be due to a transient pituitary insensitivity to luteinizing hormone–releasing factor, and earlier data suggest that normal postpartum women have a deficiency in endogenous luteinizing hormone–releasing factor secretion (Sheehan and Yen, 1979; Liu and Park, 1988). It has been shown that fully breast-feeding women treated with exogenous gonadotropin-releasing hormone develop a hormone profile consistent with return to ovulation and follicular development confirmed by transvaginal sonography (Zinaman et al., 1995). These data clearly demonstrate that the pituitary is sensitive to gonadotropin-releasing hormone and that the low ovarian function observed in breast-feeding women is due, at least in part, to suckling-induced alterations in hypothalamic gonadotropin-releasing hormone production and release. Chapter 10 addresses the physiology of lactation in detail.

Lactation is well known to predispose to increased bone turnover and loss of bone density. This loss is not prevented by calcium supplementation (Kalkwarf and Specker, 1995; Sowers et al., 1995; Kalkwarf et al., 1997). At 3 months postpartum in breast-feeding women, bone densitometry performed on 47 nursing mothers revealed a decrease in bone mineral content of 4% in the spine and 2.4% in the femoral neck. This decrease was not observed in formula-feeding women or nonpregnant control subjects (Laskey et al., 1998). The improvement in bone density after weaning is thought to be due to restoration of normal menstrual function and to an increase in intestinal calcium absorption (Kalkwarf et al., 1996).

Disappearance of Chorionic Gonadotropin

After normal term vaginal delivery, the disappearance of human chorionic gonadotropin-β from the maternal circulation follows a biexponential curve. The initial rapid half-life component averages 4.75 hours, and the slow component averages 32.2 hours. Total elimination from the circulation occurs at a median time of 14 days (Reyes et al., 1985). This is in contrast to that observed after first-trimester therapeutic abortions, after which the total elimination time is 37 days. Among pregnant women undergoing hysterectomy, human chorionic gonadotropin-β disappears from the maternal circulation in 12 days, similar to that observed after term delivery. These differences are presumably due to more definitive placental separation in term deliveries compared with therapeutic abortions (Marrs et al., 1975).

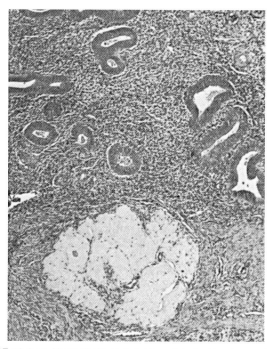

FIGURE 12-2 ■ Normally involuted placental site blood vessels 6 weeks postpartum. Endometrium shows some inflammatory cell infiltration, irregular glandular lumen, and hemosiderin. Formerly thrombosed uteroplacental vessel is now completely "organized," and hyaline tissue has replaced thrombus. This vessel will now gradually become recanalized by new vascular growth. Magnification ×64.

SYSTEMIC CHANGES

The changes that occur in other organ systems during the puerperium are of interest from a physiologic perspective and because the clinician often must distinguish between a normal postpartum finding and a pathophysiologic change. It is frequently stated that return to nonpregnant anatomy and function requires 6 to 8 weeks, implying a linear return to baseline values. Because this is not always the case, it is worthwhile to examine some of these changes in greater depth.

Cardiovascular System

Most of the major circulatory changes that occur during pregnancy return to basal nonpregnant levels early in the puerperium. The changes of greatest hemodynamic significance observed in response to pregnancy include a dramatic augmentation of cardiac output and blood volume and a decrease in peripheral vascular resistance (see Chapters 8 and 41). Although these alterations do return to baseline levels within 6 weeks after delivery, less is known about the rate of return, which appears to be variable.

Data obtained in postpartum sheep demonstrate that much of the return to baseline nonpregnant physiology actually occurs within 2 weeks. In animals studied from days 8 to 14 postpartum, cardiac output falls from 100 mL/kg/min in late pregnancy to 82 mL/kg/min during the 2nd week. Nonpregnant values average 65 mL/kg/min, and it is therefore apparent that 50% of the return to nonpregnant cardiac output is accomplished in the first 2 weeks. The same is true of systemic vascular resistance (Dilts et al., 1969).

Studies in humans using a combination of Doppler ultrasonography and echocardiography reveal that cardiac output remains increased for at least 48 hours postpartum as a result of an increase in stroke volume, despite a decrease in heart rate. This is presumably a consequence of increased venous return secondary to the rapid decrease in uterine blood flow and of mobilization of interstitial fluids. By 2 weeks postpartum, cardiac output had decreased by almost 30% from the early puerperium, probably as a result of decreased blood volume. Myocardial contractility is also enhanced during pregnancy, and this temporary remodeling of the myocardium returns to the nonpregnant state by 6 weeks postpartum (Robson et al., 1987; Gilson et al., 1997).

More recent data obtained by M-mode electrocardiography suggest that stroke volume, cardiac output, end-diastolic volume, and systemic vascular resistance remain strikingly elevated over the nonpregnant state as long as 12 weeks postpartum (Capeless and Clapp, 1991) and that left ventricular volume and cardiac output are significantly elevated compared with nulliparas at 1 year postpartum (Clapp and Capeless, 1997). These authors pointed out that the contribution of stroke volume to the total change in cardiac output has been underestimated in the past, and their data are summarized in Table 12-1.

Blood volume alterations also take place rapidly. A normal vaginal delivery is associated with a blood loss of approximately 500 mL, and losses may reach 1000 mL or more with cesarean section (Pritchard, 1965). By the 3rd postpartum day, the blood volume increase observed during pregnancy has declined by 16% of the predelivery peak (Ueland, 1976).

There is additional evidence that other parameters, such as heart rate, blood pressure, oxygen consumption, and total body water, return to nonpregnant levels within a few days postpartum. Consequently, it appears that the rate of return of cardiovascular parameters to nonpregnant values is quite variable, with some functions returning in a matter of days and others still elevated 12 weeks postpartum. It is no longer accurate to assume a linear return to the nonpregnant state in 6 weeks.

Urinary Tract

The functional changes that occur in the renal system during pregnancy appear to return to their nonpregnant baseline levels promptly postpartum. Renal plasma flow increases by about 200 to 250 mL/min in late pregnancy, concomitant with inulin (glomerular filtration rate) and creatinine clearance. Studies of women throughout pregnancy and the postpartum period demonstrate that renal plasma flow, glomerular filtration rate, and serum creatinine clearance have returned to nonpregnant levels by 6 weeks (Sims and Krantz, 1958). Little information exists regarding very early changes, although renal plasma flow decreases substantially in the first 5 days.

In contrast to the physiologic dynamics, renal morphologic changes secondary to pregnancy may persist for several months. The classic changes in pregnancy include dilation of the calyces, renal pelvis, and ureters. By 5 days postpartum, intravenous pyelogram studies reveal the mean kidney length to be 1.5 cm greater than in nonpregnant women (Bailey and Rolleston, 1971). It has also been noted that 80% of postpartum women demonstrate significant nonobstructive dilation of the lumbar aspect of at least one ureter, usually the right. Bladder function is altered, and 20% of postpartum women experience incomplete emptying, as demonstrated by residual contrast medium in the bladder after micturition. This generalized dilation may last 3 months or longer, and as many as 10% of women have long-term persistent changes in urinary tract anatomy (Spino and Fry, 1970).

Liver

During pregnancy, many of the alterations observed in protein synthesis and serum levels are induced by increasing circulatory estrogen levels. These include α and β globulins as well as fibrinogen and other clotting factors of liver origin,

TABLE 12-1. CARDIOVASCULAR MEASUREMENTS OBTAINED BEFORE PREGNANCY AND AT 6 AND 12 WEEKS POSTPARTUM

	Before Pregnancy	6 Weeks Postpartum	12 Weeks Postpartum
Cardiac output (L/min)	4.3 ± 0.2	4.6 ± 2	4.9 ± 0.2*
Stroke volume (mL)	68 ± 3	81 ± 4*	79 ± 3*
End-diastolic volume (mL)	107 ± 6	124 ± 7*	119 ± 5*
Systemic vascular resistance	349 ± 83	1277 ± 65	1154 ± 70*

*Statistically significant difference compared with prepregnancy values at $P = 0.025$ or less.

From Capeless EL, Clapp JF: When do cardiovascular parameters return to their preconception values? Am J Obstet Gynecol **165**:55, 1991.

ceruloplasmin, and sex steroid–binding, corticosteroid-binding, and thyroid-binding globulins. The return to normal levels usually occurs within 3 weeks postpartum. Serum albumin concentrations decrease in pregnancy because of plasma volume increases and an accelerated catabolic degradation. Levels of free fatty acids, cholesterol, triglycerides, and lipoproteins are in the normal nonpregnant range by 10 days, with a significant decrease noted within 24 hours (Fabian et al., 1968; Potter and Nestel, 1979).

It is important to emphasize that the transaminase enzymes are not altered by pregnancy, and their elevation in the pregnancy should be considered to represent a pathologic alteration. However, recent data suggest that liver enzymes, including the aspartate, alanine, and gamma glutamyl transferases, may rise significantly postpartum in the normal pregnancy for up to 10 days, particularly after cesarean delivery (David et al., 2000). During pregnancy, alkaline phosphatase is derived from the placenta and from liver and bone. The total serum alkaline phosphatase level, usually the only measurement made because most laboratories do not routinely measure and report the heat-labile and heat-stable fractions separately, does not return to the nonpregnant baseline level until 20 days postpartum (Zuckerman et al., 1965).

REFERENCES

Anderson WR, Davis J: Placental site involution. Am J Obstet Gynecol **102**:23, 1968.

Bailey RR, Rolleston GL: Kidney length and ureteral dilatation in the puerperium. J Obstet Gynaecol Br Commonw **78**:55, 1971.

Campbell OM, Gray RH: Characteristics and determinants of postpartum ovarian function in women in the United States. Am J Obstet Gynecol **169**:55, 1993.

Capeless EL, Clapp JF: When do cardiovascular parameters return to their preconception values? Am J Obstet Gynecol **165**:883, 1991.

Clapp JF, Capeless EL: Cardiovascular function before, during, and after the first and subsequent pregnancies. Am J Cardiol **80**:1469, 1997.

Cronin TJ: Influence of lactation upon ovulation. Lancet **2**:422, 1968.

David AL, Kolecha M, Girling JC: Factors influencing postnatal liver function tests. B J Obstet Gynaecol **107**:1421, 2000.

Dilts PV Jr, Brinkman CR III, Kirschbaum TH, et al: Uterine and systemic hemodynamic interrelationships and their response to hypoxia. Am J Obstet Gynecol **103**:138, 1969.

Fabian E, Stark A, Kucerova L, et al: Plasma levels of free fatty acids, lipoprotein lipase, and post-heparin esterase in pregnancy. Am J Obstet Gynecol **100**:904, 1968.

Gilson GJ, Samaan S, Crawford MH, et al: Changes in hemodynamics, ventricular remodeling, and ventricular contractility during normal pregnancy: A longitudinal study. Obstet Gynecol **89**:957, 1997.

Glass M, Rosenthal AH: Cervical changes in pregnancy, labor and the puerperium. Am J Obstet Gynecol **60**:353, 1950.

Kalkwarf HJ, Specker BL: Bone mineral loss during lactation and recovery after weaning. Obstet Gynecol **86**:26, 1995.

Kalkwarf HJ, Specker BL, Bianchi DC, et al: The effect of calcium supplementation on bone density during lactation and after weaning. N Engl J Med **337**:523, 1997.

Kalkwarf HJ, Specker BL, Heubi JE, et al: Intestinal calcium absorption of women during lactation and after weaning. Am J Clin Nutr **63**:526, 1996.

Kistner RW: Physiology of the vagina. *In* Havez ESE, Evans TN (eds): The Human Vagina. Amsterdam, North Holland, 1978.

Laskey MA, Prentice A, Hanratty LA, et al: Bone changes after 3 months of lactation: Influence of calcium intake, breast-milk output, and vitamin D-receptor genotype. Am J Clin Nutr **67**:685, 1998.

Liu JH, Park KH: Gonadotropin and prolactin secretion increases during sleep during the puerperium in nonlactating women. J Clin Endocrinol Metab **66**:839, 1988.

Lyon RA, Stamm MJ: The onset of ovulation during the puerperium. Cal Med **65**:99, 1946.

Marrs RP, Kletzky OA, Howard WF, et al: Disappearance of human chorionic gonadotropin and resumption of ovulation following abortion. Am J Obstet Gynecol **135**:731, 1975.

McLaren HC: The involution of the cervix. Br Med J **1**:347, 1952.

Mulic-Lutvica A, Bekuretnion M, Bakes O, et al: Ultrasonic evaluation of the uterus and uterine cavity after normal, vaginal delivery. Ultrasound Obstet Gynecol **18**:491, 2001.

Potter JM, Nestel PJ: The hyperlipidemia of pregnancy in normal and complicated pregnancies. Am J Obstet Gynecol **133**:165, 1979.

Pritchard JA: Changes in blood volume during pregnancy and delivery. Anesthesiology **26**:393, 1965.

Reyes FI, Winter JSD, Faiman C: Postpartum disappearance of chorionic gonadotropin from the maternal and neonatal circulations. Am J Obstet Gynecol **153**:486, 1985.

Robson SC, Dunlop W, Hunter S: Haemodynamic changes during the early puerperium. Br Med J **294**:106, 1987.

Rolland R, Leguin RM, Schellekens LA, et al: The role of prolactin in the restoration of ovarian function during the early postpartum period in the human female. I. A study during physiological lactation. Clin Endocrinol **4**:15, 1975.

Sharman A: Ovulation after pregnancy. Fertil Steril **2**:371, 1951a.

Sharman A: Menstruation after childbirth. J Obstet Gynaecol Br Commonw **58**:440, 1951b.

Sharman A: Postpartum regeneration of the human endometrium. J Anat **87**:1, 1953.

Sheehan KL, Yen SSC: Activation of pituitary gonadotropic function by an agonist of luteinizing hormone–releasing factor in the puerperium. Am J Obstet Gynecol **135**:755, 1979.

Sims EAH, Krantz KE: Serial studies of renal function during pregnancy and the puerperium in normal women. J Clin Invest **37**:1764, 1958.

Sowers M, Eyre D, Hollis BW, et al: Biochemical markers of bone turnover in lactating and nonlactating postpartum women. J Clin Endocrinol Metab **80**:2210, 1995.

Spino FI, Fry IA: Ureteral dilatation in nonpregnant women. Proc R Soc Med **63**:462, 1970.

Tekay A, Jouppila P: A longitudinal Doppler ultrasonographic assessment of the alterations in peripheral vascular resistance of uterine arteries and ultrasonographic findings of the involuting uterus during the puerperium. Am J Obstet Gynecol **168**:190, 1993.

Ueland K: Maternal cardiovascular dynamics. VII. Intrapartum blood volume changes. Am J Obstet Gynecol **126**:671, 1976.

Visness CM, Kennedy KI, Gross BA, et al: Fertility of fully breast feeding women in the early postpartum period. Obstet Gynecol **89**:164, 1997.

Zinaman MG, Cartledge T, Tomai T, et al: Pulsatile GnRH stimulates normal cyclic ovarian function in amenorrheic lactating postpartum women. J Clin Endocrinol Metab **80**:2088, 1995.

Zuckerman H, Sadovsky E, Kallner B: Serum alkaline phosphatase in pregnancy and puerperium. Obstet Gynecol **25**:819, 1965.

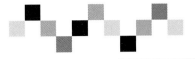

Chapter 13
FETAL CARDIOVASCULAR PHYSIOLOGY

Jeffrey R. Fineman, MD, Ronald Clyman, MD, and Michael A. Heymann, MD

BLOOD FLOW PATTERNS AND OXYGEN DELIVERY

In the mammalian adult oxygenation occurs in the lungs, and oxygenated blood returns via the pulmonary veins to the left side of the heart to be ejected by the left ventricle into the systemic circulation. In the fetus gas exchange occurs in the placenta, and the fetal lungs are nonfunctional as far as the transfer of oxygen and carbon dioxide is concerned. For oxygenated blood derived from the placenta to reach the systemic circulation, the fetal circulation is so arranged that several sites of intercommunication (shunts) are present. In addition, preferential flow and streaming occur to limit the disadvantages of intermixing of the oxygenated and deoxygenated blood returning to the heart. The patterns of blood flow to and from the fetal heart are shown diagrammatically in Figure 13-1. With fetal stress, these preferential streaming patterns may be modified even more to mitigate the adverse effects of disorders such as reduced umbilical blood flow and fetal hypoxemia. Little quantitative information regarding primate fetal circulation is available; the data presented here were obtained mainly from fetal lambs.

Venous Return to the Heart

About 40% (~200 mL/kg fetal weight/min) of total fetal cardiac output is distributed to the placental circulation; a similar amount will return to the heart via the umbilical venous system. Because umbilical venous blood is the most highly saturated blood in the fetal circulation (Fig. 13-2), distribution of umbilical venous return is most important in determining oxygen delivery to fetal tissues. After entering the intra-abdominal portion of the umbilical vein, a portion of umbilical venous blood flow supplies the liver; the remainder passes through the ductus venosus, which directly connects the umbilical vein–portal sinus confluence to the inferior vena cava (see Figs. 13-1 and 13-2). Unlike the umbilical and portal veins, the ductus venosus has no direct branches to the liver. Umbilical venous blood can enter the ductus venosus directly. Portal venous return, however, can reach the ductus venosus only through the portal sinus (see Fig. 13-2) (Bristow et al., 1981). Approximately 50% of umbilical blood flow passes through the ductus venosus; the remainder enters the hepatic–portal venous system and passes through the hepatic vasculature (Edelstone et al., 1978).

The fetal liver receives its blood supply not only from the umbilical vein but also from the portal vein and hepatic artery.

In normal fetal lambs *in utero*, umbilical venous blood flow contributes approximately 75% to 80% of total blood supply of the liver (Edelstone et al., 1978, 1980; Bristow et al., 1983). Portal venous blood flow accounts for about 15%, and hepatic arterial blood flow from the aorta represents only 4% to 5%. The distribution of blood flow from these sources to various parts of the liver is quite different. Hepatic arterial blood flow to the liver is equally distributed to the right and left lobes, but the left lobe is supplied almost exclusively by umbilical venous blood (>95%). In contrast, the right lobe receives both umbilical venous blood (~60%) and portal venous blood (~30%). Because umbilical venous blood supplies a major portion of flow to the right liver lobe by traversing the portal sinus, little if any portal venous blood reaches the ductus venosus. The blood in the ductus venosus, therefore, has pH, blood gas values, and hemoglobin oxygen saturation similar to those of umbilical venous blood. The portion of umbilical venous blood flow that passes via the ductus venosus directly into the inferior vena cava meets the systemic venous drainage from the lower body.

Blood flow through the thoracic inferior vena cava represents approximately 65% to 70% of venous return to the heart; flow from the ductus venosus accounts for about one third of this (Rudolph and Heymann, 1970; Edelstone et al., 1978). The two streams (one from the abdominal inferior vena cava and one from the ductus venosus) do not mix, and they demonstrate definite streaming within the thoracic inferior vena cava; the well-oxygenated blood derived from the ductus venosus occupies the dorsal and leftward portion of the inferior vena cava (Edelstone and Rudolph, 1979). This separation of the more highly saturated umbilical venous stream and the desaturated inferior vena caval stream returning from the lower body produces preferential flow of umbilical venous return into the left atrium and then the left ventricle and ascending aorta (Behrman et al., 1970; Edelstone and Rudolph, 1979; Reuss et al., 1981). Of particular importance is preferential streaming of umbilical venous blood to the brain and myocardium.

The preferential streaming of umbilical venous return to the left lobe of the liver and portal venous return to the right lobe also affects the distribution of oxygenated blood to the fetal body. The left hepatic lobe is perfused with umbilical venous blood, which has an oxygen saturation of 80% to 85%; the right lobe is perfused by a mixture of umbilical and portal venous blood, which has a much lower oxygen saturation (~35%) (see Fig. 13-2). The oxygen saturation of blood in the hepatic veins reflects this difference in perfusion saturation

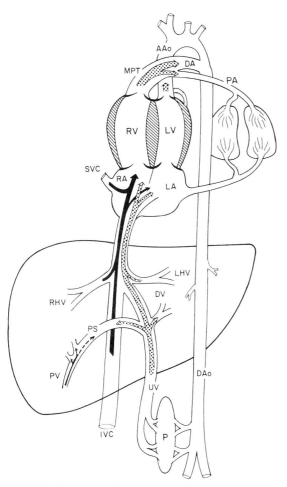

FIGURE 13-1 ■ Diagrammatic representation of the normal fetal circulation and major fetal flow patterns. AAo, ascending aorta; DA, ductus arteriosus; DAo, descending aorta; DV, ductus venosus; IVC, inferior vena cava; LA, left atrium; LHV, left hepatic vein; LV, left ventricle; MPT, main pulmonary trunk; P, placenta; PA, main branch pulmonary arteries; PS, portal sinus; PV, portal vein; RA, right atrium; RHV, right hepatic vein; RV, right ventricle; SVC, superior vena cava; UV, umbilical vein.

heart (Bristow et al., 1983). Similarly, right hepatic blood flow follows the distribution pattern of abdominal inferior vena caval blood flow.

The inferior vena caval blood then enters the right atrium, and because of the position of the foramen ovale, more preferential streaming occurs. The foramen ovale is situated low in the interatrial septum, close to the inferior vena cava. The cephalad margin of the foramen, formed by the lower margin of the septum secundum, lies on the right side of the atrial septum; it is called the *crista dividens* and is positioned so that it overrides the orifice of the inferior vena cava. The crista dividens therefore splits the inferior vena caval bloodstream into an anterior and rightward stream that enters the right atrium and a posterior and leftward stream that passes through the foramen ovale into the left atrium. It is this latter stream that has the more highly saturated blood returning from the umbilical circulation through the ductus venosus and left hepatic lobe. Despite this anatomic arrangement and the preferential streaming within the inferior vena cava, some mixing of blood does occur; a portion of the more highly saturated umbilical venous blood passes directly into the right atrium, and some desaturated abdominal inferior vena caval blood passes into the left atrium. The net result, however, is still a significantly higher saturation in the left atrium than in the right (Fig. 13-3).

Blood returning to the heart via the superior vena cava also streams preferentially once it reaches the right atrium. The crista interveniens, situated in the posterolateral aspect of the right atrial wall, effectively directs superior vena caval blood toward the tricuspid valve. The coronary sinus, which drains blood from the left ventricular myocardium, enters the right atrium between the crista dividens and the tricuspid valve; the very desaturated coronary venous return (saturation ~20%) therefore is also preferentially directed toward the tricuspid valve. This preferential streaming of superior vena caval and coronary sinus venous return to the right ventricle is also advantageous in the fetal circulation, because this very desaturated blood is preferentially directed toward the placenta for

(Bristow et al., 1981, 1983). The oxygen saturation in left hepatic venous blood is about 10% lower than that in umbilical venous blood but about 10% higher than that in right hepatic venous blood, in which the saturation more closely approximates that in the descending aorta.

In fetal lambs, the ductus venosus and left hepatic vein drain into the inferior vena cava, essentially at a common point; partial valves are seen over the entrance of the hepatic vein and ductus venosus into the inferior vena cava (Bristow et al., 1981). Similarly, the entrance of the right hepatic vein into the inferior vena cava has a valve-like membrane overlying the ostium. This arrangement probably allows left hepatic venous blood to be distributed in a manner similar to that of ductus venosus blood, whereas right hepatic venous blood is distributed similarly to the abdominal inferior vena caval stream. This is particularly important because about half of umbilical venous return passes through the liver, thereby accounting for about 20% of total venous return to the heart. In fetal lambs, left hepatic venous blood flow follows the same pattern as ductus venosus flow, with preferential streaming to the brain and

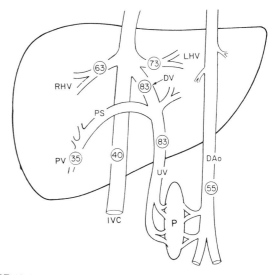

FIGURE 13-2 ■ Representative normal hemoglobin oxygen saturation data (numbers indicate percent saturation) in the umbilical, inferior vena caval, and hepatic venous drainage in fetal lambs. See Figure 13-1 for abbreviations.

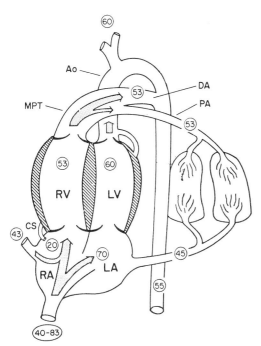

FIGURE 13-3 ■ Representative normal hemoglobin oxygen saturation data (numbers indicate percent saturation) in the heart and major vascular channels in fetal lambs. Ao, aorta; CS, coronary sinus. See Figure 13-1 for abbreviations.

reoxygenation. Pulmonary venous return to the heart enters the left atrium, where it mixes with the portion of inferior vena caval blood that has crossed the foramen ovale to enter the left atrium.

Approximately 65% of total cardiac output reaches the lower body and placenta and returns via the thoracic inferior vena cava to the heart (Fig. 13-4). Of this inferior vena caval return, approximately 40% crosses the foramen ovale to the left atrium; the remaining 60% enters the right ventricle across the tricuspid valve. The amount of inferior vena caval return crossing the foramen ovale therefore represents about 27% of total fetal cardiac output. This blood then combines with pulmonary venous return (~8% of total fetal cardiac output) and represents the output of the left ventricle, or approximately

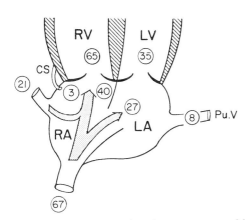

FIGURE 13-4 ■ Representative values for percentages of fetal cardiac output (combined ventricular output) returning to the heart in fetal lambs. CS, coronary sinus; Pu.V, pulmonary vein. See Figure 13-1 for abbreviations.

35% of total fetal cardiac output. The venous return from the superior vena cava, the coronary sinus, and the remainder of the inferior vena caval return (~40% of total fetal cardiac output) enters the right ventricle and represents the portion of total fetal cardiac output ejected by the right ventricle (~65% of total fetal cardiac output).

Cardiac Output and Its Distribution

In the fetus, because of the blood flow across the ductus arteriosus into the descending aorta, lower body organs are perfused by both the right and left ventricles (across the aortic isthmus). For this reason and because of intracardiac shunting, it is customary to consider fetal cardiac output the total output of the heart, or combined ventricular output. In fetal lambs, this is about 450 mL/kg/min. Unlike the adult, and because of the various sites of intracardiac and extracardiac shunting, the left and right ventricles in the fetus do not eject in series and therefore do not need to have the same stroke volume. In fact, as shown in Figure 13-5, the right ventricle ejects approximately two thirds of total fetal cardiac output (~300 mL/kg/min), whereas the left ventricle ejects only a little more than one third (~150 mL/kg/min) (Heymann et al., 1973).

Echocardiographic studies in human pregnancy have suggested that the right ventricle also dominates the left (Sahn et al., 1980; Reed et al., 1986; DeSmedt et al., 1987; Rasanen et al., 1996; Harada et al., 1997). Of the 65% of cardiac output ejected by the right ventricle, only a small amount (8%) flows through the pulmonary arteries to the lungs. The remainder (57%) crosses the ductus arteriosus and enters the descending aorta. Because right ventricular output contains all superior vena caval and coronary sinus return, it allows this unoxygenated venous blood to be preferentially returned to the placenta. Left ventricular output (~35% of cardiac output) enters the ascending aorta; in the fetal lamb, approximately 21% reaches the brain, head, upper limbs, and upper thorax. About 10% of cardiac output traverses the aortic isthmus and joins the blood flowing across the ductus arteriosus to perfuse the descending aorta.

As shown in Figure 13-3, the level of hemoglobin oxygen saturation in the ventricles and great arteries is determined by the streaming patterns into, through, and out of the fetal heart. The highly saturated umbilical venous return streams preferentially across the foramen ovale into the left atrium, where it mixes with the relatively small amount of desaturated blood returning from the pulmonary veins. The net result is that blood ejected by the left ventricle to the ascending aorta is relatively well oxygenated (saturation about 60%). On the other hand, the extremely desaturated coronary sinus venous return and the desaturated blood returning from the brain and upper body flow almost exclusively across the tricuspid valve into the right ventricle. This blood mixes with the inferior vena caval stream, which is primarily composed of desaturated blood returning from the lower body, but also contains some umbilical venous return. The net result is that the oxygen saturation of blood in the right ventricle is lower than that in the left. This blood perfuses the fetal lungs and traverses the ductus arteriosus to the descending aorta, from which it perfuses lower body organs and reaches the placenta for reoxygenation.

Blood gas and pH values in the fetus also reflect the preferential streaming patterns (Table 13-1). The data shown represent values usually found in healthy, catheterized, fetal

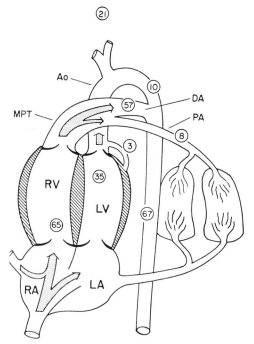

FIGURE 13-5 ■ Representative normal values for percentages of total cardiac output (combined ventricular output) ejected by the heart and passing through the major arteries leaving the heart in fetal lambs. Ao, aorta. See Figure 13-1 for abbreviations.

TABLE 13-1. NORMAL FETAL pH AND BLOOD GAS DATA

	Umbilical Vein	Descending Aorta	Ascending Aorta
pH	7.40–7.43	7.36–7.39	7.37–7.40
Po$_2$ (torr)	28–32	20–23	21–25
Pco$_2$ (torr)	38–42	43–48	41–45

Pco$_2$, partial pressure of carbon dioxide; Po$_2$, partial pressure of oxygen.

combined output of both ventricles (i.e., the combined ventricular output). Typical values are shown in Figure 13-6 (Rudolph and Heymann, 1970; Peeters et al., 1979). These values remain fairly constant throughout the latter third of gestation, the period in which such measurements have been made. There is, however, a slight increase in the percentage of combined ventricular output distributed to the heart, brain, and gastrointestinal tract in the 10 days before parturition. The flow distributed to the lungs increases from approximately 4% to 8% of combined ventricular output between 125 and 130 days (0.85) of gestation. Organ blood flows are shown in Table 13-2. Umbilical placental blood flow is usually not considered in relation to placental weight, which is quite variable, but rather is expressed in relation to fetal weight, like combined ventricular output. Placental blood flow is approximately 200 mL/kg/min.

Intracardiac and Vascular Pressures

Vascular pressure in the fetus reflects the preferential streaming patterns described previously. Although the ductus venosus is a fairly large widely dilated structure, there is a high flow returning from the placenta through the umbilical veins, and therefore this structure offers some resistance to flow. Umbilical venous pressure is generally 3 to 5 mm Hg higher than that in the inferior vena cava (Fig. 13-7). Right atrial pressure is also higher than left atrial pressure because

animals. Both inter-animal and daily variability are seen. During a normal uterine contraction, arterial blood has a lower partial pressure of oxygen than under truly resting conditions. In addition, during the last 7 to 10 days of gestation, partial pressure of oxygen declines slightly and partial pressure of carbon dioxide increases commensurately.

The distribution of blood flow to individual organs is shown in Figure 13-6. Because arterial blood supply to lower body organs is derived from both the left and right ventricles, it is customary to express organ flow as a percentage of the

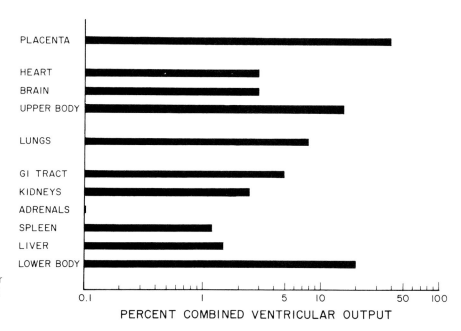

FIGURE 13-6 ■ Representative normal values for the percentages of total cardiac output (combined ventricular output) distributed to different organs or parts in fetal lambs. GI, gastrointestinal.

TABLE 13-2. ORGAN BLOOD FLOWS IN NORMAL FETAL LAMBS CLOSE TO TERM

Organ	Blood Flow (mL/100 g organ weight/min)
Heart	180
Brain	125
Upper body	25
Lungs	100
Gastrointestinal tract	70
Kidneys	150
Adrenals	200
Spleen	200
Liver (hepatic arterial)	20
Lower body	25

of the greater volume of flow through the right atrium. Although the ductus arteriosus is widely patent, it too offers a small resistance to flow. Therefore, systolic pressures in the main pulmonary trunk and the right ventricle are slightly higher (1 to 2 mm Hg) than those in the aorta and left ventricle.

The representative pressure data shown in Figure 13-7 would be expected in a fetus close to term. Arterial pressures increase slowly and progressively over the last third of gestation, reaching these values shortly before parturition. Measurement of intravascular pressures in the fetus reflects the additional amniotic pressure not found after birth. Because intra-amniotic pressure is used as the zero reference point, the values presented exclude this additional pressure and are therefore true vascular pressures.

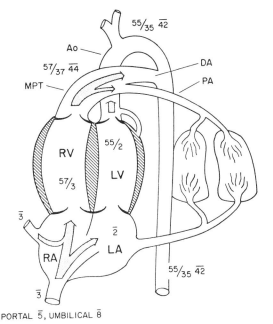

FIGURE 13-7 ■ Representative normal pressures in millimeters of mercury (mm Hg) in various vessels and cardiac chambers in fetal lambs. Ao, aorta. See Figure 13-1 for abbreviations.

MYOCARDIAL FUNCTION

Cardiac output is determined by the interrelationships of preload, afterload, myocardial contractility, and heart rate. *Preload* (ventricular filling pressure) reflects the initial muscle length, which by the Frank-Starling principle influences the development of myocardial force. *Afterload* (the impedance to ejection from the ventricles) is reflected basically by arterial pressure. *Contractility* reflects the intrinsic inotropic capability of the myocardium.

Studies of fetal myocardium show immaturity of structure, function, and sympathetic innervation relative to the adult (Friedman, 1973; Heymann and Rudolph, 1973; Kirkpatrick et al., 1976; Gilbert, 1980, 1982). At all muscle lengths along the length–tension curve, the active tension generated by fetal myocardium is lower compared with adult myocardium (Friedman, 1973). In addition, resting, or passive, tension is higher in fetuses than in adults, suggesting lower compliance of fetal myocardium.

Studies in chronically instrumented intact fetal lambs showed that after volume loading by the infusion of blood or saline, the right ventricle is unable to increase stroke work or output to the same extent as in the adult (Heymann and Rudolph, 1973). This is particularly true in less mature fetuses, in whom right ventricular end-diastolic pressure is markedly elevated without any obvious change in right ventricular stroke work (Fig. 13-8). Similar results are found for both the left and right ventricles but with some ability to increase output or work at lower pressures, between 2 and 5 mm Hg (Kirkpatrick et al., 1976; Gilbert, 1980, 1982). Limitations in stroke work increase with increasing filling pressure have been shown to be afterload dependent and, for the left ventricle, are probably affected by right ventricular mechanical constraint (Hawkins et al., 1989; Teitel et al., 1991).

Fetal and adult sarcomeres have equivalent lengths (Sheldon et al., 1976), but there are major ultrastructural differences between fetal myocardium and adult myocardium. The diameter of the fetal cells is smaller and, perhaps more importantly, the proportion of noncontractile mass (i.e., of nuclei, mitochondria, and surface membranes) to the number of myofibrils is significantly greater than in the adult. In the fetal myocardium, only about 30% of the muscle mass consists of contractile elements; in the adult, the proportion is about 60%. These ultrastructural differences are probably responsible for the age-dependent differences in performance (Friedman, 1973).

In newborn lambs, stroke volume is decreased at afterload levels considered low for adult animals (Downing et al., 1965). Gilbert (1982) showed that in fetal animals an increase in arterial pressure of about 15 mm Hg, produced by methoxamine infusion, depresses the cardiac function curve so that cardiac output averages 25% to 30% less than normal. The extent of shortening is less in the fetus at any level of tension than in the adult, a potential explanation for the effects of afterload on stroke volume (Friedman, 1973).

In chronically instrumented fetal lambs, there is a close relationship between cardiac output and heart rate. Spontaneous and induced changes in heart rate are associated with corresponding changes in left or right ventricular output. Increasing heart rate from the resting level of about 180 up to

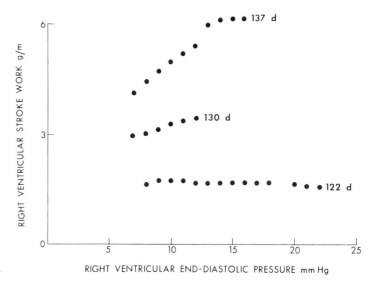

FIGURE 13-8 ■ Right ventricular function curves in three fetal lambs of different gestational ages (term is about 145 days). d, days.

250 to 300 beats/min increases cardiac output 15% to 20%. Likewise, decreasing heart rate below the resting level significantly decreases ventricular output.

The fetal heart normally appears to operate near the top of its cardiac function curve. An increase in heart rate results in only a modest increase in output; however, bradycardia can reduce output significantly. Above an atrial filling pressure of approximately 8 mm Hg, there is little or no increase in output because the length–tension relationship has reached a plateau. In addition, the fetal heart is sensitive to changes in afterload.

Sympathetic and Parasympathetic Innervation

Isolated fetal cardiac tissue has a lower threshold of response to the inotropic effects of norepinephrine than adult cardiac tissue and is more sensitive to norepinephrine throughout dose–response curves (Friedman, 1973). Because isoproterenol, a direct β-adrenergic agonist that is not taken up and stored in sympathetic nerves, has similar effects on fetal and adult myocardium, the supersensitivity of fetal myocardium to norepinephrine is probably due to incomplete development of sympathetic innervation in fetal myocardium. Myocardial concentrations of norepinephrine in the fetus within several weeks of term are significantly lower than in newborn animals, and activity of tyrosine hydroxylase, the intraneuronal enzyme responsible for the first transformation in catecholamine biosynthesis, is also reduced (Friedman, 1973). In contrast, adrenal gland tyrosine hydroxylase activity at the same gestational age is not suppressed, possibly because the decrease in myocardial activity is related to delayed sympathetic innervation rather than to a generalized immaturity.

Monoamine oxidase, the enzyme responsible for oxidative deamination of norepinephrine, is also present in lower concentrations in the fetal heart than in the adult. Histochemical evaluation of the development of sympathetic innervation using the monoamine fluorescence technique has further substantiated the delayed development of sympathetic innervation of the fetal myocardium. At term, sympathetic innervation is incomplete. Patterns of staining indicate a progression of innervation, starting at the area of the sinoatrial node and progressing toward the left ventricular apex (Friedman et al., 1968; Lebowitz et al., 1972).

Although sympathetic nervous innervation appears to begin developing in the fetal heart by about 0.55 of gestation, β-adrenergic receptors seem to be present much earlier and can be stimulated by appropriate agonists before 0.4 of gestation (Barrett et al., 1972). Before about 0.55 of gestation (80 days of gestation in the lamb), fetal myocardium may be affected by circulating catecholamines, but local reflex activity through the sympathetic nervous system is not likely to play a major role in circulatory regulation.

Vagal stimulation at about 0.85 of gestation produces bradycardia. Administering atropine at 0.55 of gestation produces a modest increase in fetal heart rate (Vapaavouri et al., 1973), indicating that vagal innervation is present by this stage of development. Histochemical staining for acetylcholinesterase in close-to-term fetuses has shown that the concentrations of this enzyme, which is responsible for metabolism of acetylcholine, are similar to those found in adults.

Energy Metabolism

In the normal unstressed fetus, myocardial blood flow is about 180 mL/min/100 g tissue, approximately 80% more than in the adult. Fetal myocardial oxygen consumption, as measured in the left ventricular free wall, is about 400 mM/100 g/min, similar to that in the adult. In adult sheep, free fatty acids provide the major source of energy for the myocardium, and carbohydrate accounts for only about 40% of myocardial oxygen consumption (Fisher et al., 1980). In fetal sheep under normal conditions, however, free fatty acid concentrations are extremely low, and almost all the oxygen consumed can be accounted for by carbohydrate metabolism—glucose for 33%, pyruvate for 6%, and lactate for 58% of the oxygen consumed by the left ventricular free wall.

ATPase activity in fetal myocardium is equal to that in adult myocardium, suggesting that energy utilization by the contractile apparatus is similar in fetal and adult myocardium (Friedman, 1973). Mitochondria from fetal myocardium demonstrate higher oxidative phosphorylation than those from adult myocardium. The higher oxygen consumption in fetal mitochondria uncoupled by deoxyribonucleoprotein suggests that the augmented respiratory rate in mitochondria is a reflection of increased electron transport (Friedman, 1973). This is consistent with the greater cytochrome oxidase activity in fetal mitochondria.

CONTROL OF THE CARDIOVASCULAR SYSTEM

Maintenance of normal cardiovascular function, blood pressure, heart rate, and distribution of blood flow represents a complex interrelationship between local vascular and reflex effects. These effects are initiated by the stimulation of various receptors and are mediated through the autonomic nervous system as well as through hormonal influences. Although some information is available about how these mechanisms affect the circulation after stress, little is known about their role in normal fetal cardiovascular homeostasis. To complicate the situation, other factors, such as sleep state, electrocortical activity, and uterine activity, transiently affect the circulation. As a result, this area of fetal physiology is difficult to study and the data are difficult to interpret.

Local Regulation

As the oxygen content of blood perfusing the fetus falls, blood flow to the brain, myocardium, and adrenal gland increases; conversely, pulmonary blood flow falls as oxygen content decreases. Local effects of changes in oxygen environment are less clearly established for other organs.

Many adult organs exhibit *autoregulation*, the ability to maintain constant blood flow over a fairly wide range of perfusion pressures. In the fetus, the umbilical–placental circulation does not exhibit autoregulation and blood flow changes in relation to changes in arterial perfusion pressure (Berman et al., 1976). On the other hand, the cerebral circulation in fetal lambs does show autoregulatory capability (Papile et al., 1985).

Baroreflex Regulation

In chronically instrumented fetal lambs, the fetal heart rate slows after an acute increase in systemic arterial pressure (Shinebourne et al., 1972; Maloney et al., 1977). This baroreflex response, although present by 0.55 (80 days) of gestation, is poorly developed early on, but the sensitivity of the reflex to induced changes in pressure increases with advancing gestation. Carotid denervation partially inhibits the response, and combined carotid and aortic denervation abolishes it. Parasympathetic blockade with atropine also abolishes the reflex. Although the existence of the arterial baroreflex is established, Dawes and associates (1980) suggested that the threshold for fetal baroreflex activity is above the range of the normal fetal arterial blood pressure and that this reflex is not important in controlling cardiovascular function *in utero.*

Carotid sinus and vagus nerve activity are synchronous with the arterial pulse, suggesting continuous baroreceptor activity (Biscoe et al., 1969; Ponte and Purves, 1973). Marked fluctuations in the arterial blood pressure and heart rate are observed after sinoaortic denervation, although the average arterial blood pressure and heart rate are not different from control (Itskovitz et al., 1983).

The baroreflex in fetal animals requires fairly marked changes in pressures to produce relatively minor responses. Sinoaortic denervation increases heart rate and blood pressure variability, however. Under normal circumstances, therefore, baroreceptor function acts to stabilize the heart rate and blood pressure. In the fetus, as in the adult, baroreflex control is also influenced by hormonal systems (Segar, 1997).

Chemoreflex Regulation

In general, chemoreceptor stimulation by sodium cyanide injection induces hypertension and bradycardia (Dawes et al., 1969; Goodlin and Rudolph, 1972). Central or carotid chemoreceptor stimulation causes hypertension and mild tachycardia with increased respiratory activity, whereas aortic chemoreceptor stimulation produces bradycardia with modest increases in arterial blood pressure. Because the carotid chemoreceptors are less sensitive than the aortic chemoreceptors, hypertension and bradycardia usually result. In chronically instrumented fetal lambs, sodium cyanide produces bradycardia with variable blood pressure changes, responses abolished by sinoaortic denervation (Itskovitz and Rudolph, 1982). Fetal hypoxia produces bradycardia and hypertension that are abolished by carotid sinus denervation (Bartelds et al., 1993).

Autonomic Nervous System and Adrenal Medulla

As described earlier, sympathetic innervation of the heart is not complete until term or, in some species, until after delivery. In contrast, cholinergic innervation, as measured by the presence of acetylcholinesterase, appears to be fully developed during fetal life. The innervation of other vascular beds also appears to proceed at different rates during gestation (Zink and Van Petten, 1981).

Adrenergic receptors are present in the fetus and have been demonstrated in myocardium (Cheng et al., 1980, 1981; Whitsett et al., 1982). Receptor populations that have been studied in the fetus exhibit characteristics similar to those in adults (Nuwayhid et al., 1975; Harris and Van Petten, 1979). The fetus possesses mature adrenergic receptors fairly early in gestation, but the concentration of receptors is different from that in adult organs (Cheng et al., 1980). The fetal concentration of receptors can be altered by administering thyroid hormone or isoxsuprine to the mother.

Injecting cholinergic or adrenergic agonists into fetal sheep produces responses as early as 0.4 (60 days) of gestation (Barrett et al., 1972; Assali et al., 1977). α-Adrenergic stimulation with methoxamine produces an increase in arterial blood pressure, a small decrease in cardiac output, an increase in blood flow to the lungs, and a marked decrease in kidney and peripheral blood flow as early as 0.5 of gestation. β-Adrenergic stimulation by isoproterenol causes a response earlier in gestation and an increase in heart rate with little or no change in arterial blood pressure and cardiac output. Blood flow to both the myocardium and the lungs is increased. Administration of acetylcholine decreases blood pressure and heart rate and increases pulmonary blood flow markedly, particularly in fetuses close to term.

Although receptor affinity is well developed during fetal life, the response to a specific agonist is blunted relative to the adult. The maximal constrictor response to norepinephrine or nerve stimulation increases throughout the latter part of gestation and even more after birth (Wyse et al., 1977). The increase might result from gestational differences in neurotransmitter release in the fetus. During the last trimester of gestation, there is a progressive increase in maximal pressor response to ephedrine, which exerts its effect indirectly through neurotransmitter release; phenylephrine has a direct pressor effect (Harris and Van Petten, 1978). In addition, neurotransmitter reuptake in sympathetic nerve terminals is not fully mature in the fetus (Harris and Van Petten, 1979). Similarly, the differences between fetal and adult myocardium with respect to threshold and sensitivity to norepinephrine indicate an immature reuptake mechanism for norepinephrine in the fetus (Friedman, 1973).

As gestation progresses, these variable rates of maturation of different components of the autonomic nervous system modify control mechanisms relating to the autonomic nervous system. The role of β-adrenergic stimulation in resting circulatory regulation has been evaluated by pharmacologic blockade of β-adrenergic receptors with propranolol. This component of the sympathetic nervous system exerts a positive influence over fetal heart rate that first appears at about 0.6 (80 to 90 days) of gestation (Vapaavouri et al., 1973), but this influence is relatively small (Walker et al., 1978). During stress such as hypoxia or hemorrhage, however, β-adrenergic activity appears to be increased because propranolol produces much greater changes in heart rate.

α-Adrenergic control of the circulation has a somewhat clearer developmental pattern. α-Adrenergic blockade with phentolamine or phenoxybenzamine reduces arterial blood pressure very little, if at all, before 0.75 (100 to 110 days) of gestation; thereafter, there is a progressive increase in response, indicating a progressive increase in resting vascular tone attributed to α-adrenergic nervous activity. The parasympathetic nervous system exerts an inhibitory influence over fetal heart rate that is present by 0.55 (80 days) of gestation (Vapaavouri et al., 1973; Walker et al., 1978). Parasympathetic blockade with atropine produces small changes at this age, with a progressive increase in parasympathetic control as gestation advances. After approximately 0.85 (120 to 130 days) of gestation, no further increase is evident.

Hypoxemia or asphyxia increases circulating plasma catecholamine concentrations in fetal sheep (Comline et al., 1965; Jones and Robinson, 1975; Lewis et al., 1982). In fetuses younger than about 120 days' gestation, when the adrenal gland becomes innervated, extremely low fetal blood oxygen concentrations are required to stimulate the adrenal gland; thereafter, catecholamine secretion can be induced by more moderate hypoxemia (Comline et al., 1965). Infusing catecholamines to reach plasma concentrations that mimic those observed during hypoxemia produces circulatory changes similar to those seen during hypoxemia (Lorijn and Longo, 1980). Adrenal medullary responses to stress appear to play a role in circulatory adjustments; whether catecholamine secretion exerts a continuous regulatory function is not clear.

Hormonal Regulation of the Circulation

Renin-Angiotensin System

The renin-angiotensin system is important in regulating the normal fetal circulation and its response to hemorrhage. The juxtaglomerular apparatus in the kidneys is well developed in

fetuses and is present by 0.6 (90 days) of gestation (Smith et al., 1974). Plasma renin activity, as well as circulating angiotensin II, is present in fetal plasma as early as about 0.6 (90 days) of gestation (Broughton-Pipkin et al., 1974; Iwamoto and Rudolph, 1979; Iwamoto et al., 1979). The effects of fetal stress such as hemorrhage and hypoxia on the renin-angiotensin system are not absolutely clear. Small amounts of hemorrhage increase plasma renin activity (Broughton-Pipkin et al., 1974; Smith et al., 1974); other studies, however, have shown little effect (Robillard and Weitzman, 1980). Similarly, the effects of hypoxemia on the renin-angiotensin system in the fetus are controversial, but most likely hypoxemia is of little consequence.

When angiotensin II is infused to achieve plasma concentrations similar to those that occur after a moderate (15% to 20%) hemorrhage, there are broad cardiovascular effects (Iwamoto and Rudolph, 1982). Arterial blood pressure increases markedly, and after an initial abrupt bradycardia, heart rate increases. Combined ventricular output increases, as does blood flow to the lungs and myocardium. Renal blood flow decreases, but umbilical placental flow is unchanged; this latter phenomenon indicates vascular constriction in the umbilical–placental circulation because arterial blood pressure increases but flow does not. The increase in myocardial blood flow is probably caused by an increase in stroke work, and the large increase in pulmonary blood flow probably reflects the release of some other local pulmonary vasodilating substance, such as one of the prostaglandins (Gryglewski, 1980).

Inhibiting the action of angiotensin II by specific inhibitors, such as saralasin, has somewhat variable effects. In unstressed fetal animals, however, generally a fall in mean arterial pressure and a slight decrease in heart rate occur (Iwamoto and Rudolph, 1979). Combined ventricular output is unaltered, but umbilical–placental blood flow falls, probably in association with the fall in systemic arterial pressure. Blood flow to the peripheral tissues, adrenal glands, and myocardium increases. During hemorrhage, the effects of saralasin are markedly accentuated and result in profound hypotension and bradycardia.

Under normal resting conditions, endogenous angiotensin II appears to exert a tonic vasoconstriction on the peripheral vascular bed, thereby maintaining systemic arterial blood pressure and umbilical–placental blood flow. In response to hemorrhage, angiotensin II is released and produces more vasoconstriction in the periphery, as well as other cardiovascular effects, thereby maintaining systemic arterial blood pressure and umbilical blood flow.

Vasopressin

Arginine vasopressin (antidiuretic hormone) has been detected as early as 0.4 (60 days) of gestation in fetal lambs (Drummond et al., 1980). Although hypoxia and hemorrhage, as well as many other stimuli such as hypotension and hypernatremia, induced a marked increase in plasma vasopressin concentrations (Rurak, 1978; Drummond et al., 1980), it is unlikely that vasopressin plays a major role in normal circulatory regulation. Maximal antidiuresis in adults occurs with vasopressin concentrations that have no discernible effects on systemic blood pressure. Fetal vasopressin concentrations are below this level.

Infusing vasopressin into fetal sheep to produce concentrations similar to those observed during fetal hypoxemia produces hypertension and bradycardia (Iwamoto et al., 1979). Combined ventricular output decreases slightly, but the proportion distributed to the gastrointestinal tract and peripheral circulations falls, whereas that to the umbilical–placental, myocardial, and cerebral circulations increases. These findings indicate that vasopressin probably participates in fetal circulatory responses to stress not only directly but also by enhancing pressor responses to other vasoactive substances. Under resting conditions, however, vasopressin apparently has little regulatory function.

Atrial Natriuretic Factor

Atrial natriuretic factor, a potent volume-regulating family of peptides released from the atria and ventricles as well as other sites in response to stretch, also has vasoregulatory functions. It is present in fetal plasma, and concentrations are highest in blood leaving the right ventricle, indicating production in the right side of the heart (Hargrave et al., 1990). In the fetus, when infused to produce concentrations equivalent to those induced by stress, such as hypoxemia or volume loading, it produces pulmonary vasodilatation, suggesting a possible role in modulating right ventricular afterload.

Arachidonic Acid Metabolites

Although prostaglandins generally are locally active substances that do not normally circulate in adult blood, relatively high concentrations do normally circulate in the fetus (Mitchell et al., 1978; Challis and Patrick, 1980). It is likely that these prostaglandins are derived from the placenta. The fetal vasculature is also capable of producing prostaglandins, and the umbilical vessels, ductus arteriosus, and aorta produce significant amounts of prostaglandin E and prostacyclin (PGI_2).

Prostaglandins administered to the fetus have diverse and extensive cardiovascular effects. Prostaglandin E_1 (PGE_1) and prostaglandin E_2 (PGE_2) constrict the umbilical–placental circulation (Novy et al., 1974; Berman et al., 1978). Prostaglandin $F_{2\alpha}$ and thromboxane also cause constriction, whereas PGI_2 dilates the umbilical–placental circulation. PGE_1, PGE_2, PGI_2, and prostaglandin D_2 produce pulmonary vasodilatation in the fetus, whereas prostaglandin $F_{2\alpha}$ produces constriction (Cassin, 1987). Infusing PGE_1 into fetal sheep has no effect on cardiac output or systemic pressure, but in addition to a reduction in umbilical–placental blood flow, there are increases in flow to the myocardium, adrenals, gastrointestinal tract, and peripheral tissues (Tripp et al., 1978).

Of great interest is the role of prostaglandins in maintaining patency of the ductus arteriosus in the fetus. Circulating prostaglandins, as well as PGE_2 and PGI_2 produced locally in the ductus arteriosus, play a major role in maintaining the ductus arteriosus in a dilated state in utero (Olley et al., 1975; Clyman, 1980, 1987). For details of the overall physiological regulation of the ductus arteriosus, see later.

The role of endogenous prostaglandin production in regulating other fetal vascular beds has been elucidated by administering inhibitors of prostaglandin synthesis to the fetus. Although PGE_2 produces umbilical–placental vasoconstriction, inhibition of prostaglandin synthesis has little effect on umbilical–placental vascular resistance, suggesting that prostaglandins do not normally regulate the umbilical–placental circulation. When prostaglandin synthesis is inhibited, the proportion of blood flow to the gastrointestinal tract, kidneys, and peripheral circulation decreases, indicating an increase in vascular resistance in these tissues. Vascular resistances to other tissues are essentially unchanged.

Although prostaglandins do not appear to be central to regulation of the resting fetal pulmonary circulation, PGI_2 may act to modulate tone and thereby maintain pulmonary vascular resistance relatively constant. However, leukotrienes, also metabolites of arachidonic acid and potent smooth muscle constrictors, may play an active role in maintenance of the normally high fetal pulmonary vascular resistance. In newborns (Schreiber et al., 1985), leukotriene inhibition attenuates hypoxic pulmonary vasoconstriction. In fetal lambs, leukotriene receptor blockade (Soifer et al., 1985) or synthesis inhibition (LeBidois et al., 1987) increases pulmonary blood flow about eightfold, suggesting a role for leukotrienes in maintenance of the normally high fetal pulmonary vascular resistance; the presence of leukotrienes in fetal tracheal fluid further supports this (Velvis et al., 1990).

Endothelial-Derived Factors and Endothelin

In addition to PGI_2, vascular endothelial cells can be stimulated to produce other important vasoactive factors, including potent vasoconstrictors, such as endothelin, and potent vasodilators, such as endothelium-derived relaxing factor. Endothelium-derived relaxing factor is now known to be nitric oxide (NO) and generally is called endothelium-derived nitric oxide (EDNO) (Ignarro, 1989). EDNO is produced by most endothelial cells in response to varied stimuli, generally involving specific receptors or changes in shear stress; smooth muscle relaxation is produced through several messenger systems, such as guanylyl cyclase/cyclic guanosine monophosphate, K channels, or PGI_2/cyclic adenosine monophosphate. In the fetus, EDNO is produced by umbilical vascular endothelium (Van de Voorde et al., 1987; Chaudhuri et al., 1991); nitroso-compounds reduce umbilical vascular resistance in vitro (Myatt et al., 1991), and EDNO modulates resting umbilical vascular tone in fetal sheep in utero (Chang et al., 1992). Disturbances in normal EDNO production may also be involved in the genesis of preeclampsia (Pinto et al., 1991).

EDNO clearly is involved in regulation of vascular tone in the fetal pulmonary circulation, although it plays a far more important role in postnatal transition to air breathing (Fineman et al., 1995). Superfused fetal sheep pulmonary arteries release endothelium-derived relaxing factor when stimulated with bradykinin (Glasgow et al., 1990). In fetal lambs, the vasodilating effects of bradykinin are attenuated by methylene blue and resting tone increases with $N\omega$-nitro-L-arginine, an inhibitor of NO synthesis by NO synthase from precursor L-arginine (Moore et al., 1992), suggesting that a cyclic guanosine monophosphate–dependent mechanism, such as EDNO production, continuously modulates or offsets the increased tone of the resting fetal pulmonary circulation. Inhibition of EDNO synthesis also blocks the pulmonary vasodilatation with oxygenation of fetal lungs in utero and markedly attenuates the increase in pulmonary blood flow with ventilation at birth (Moore et al., 1992; Fineman et al., 1994).

Endothelin-1 (ET-1), a 21 amino acid polypeptide, also produced by vascular endothelial cells, has potent vasoactive properties (Yanagisawa et al., 1988). The hemodynamic effects of ET-1 are mediated by at least two distinct receptor populations, ET_A and ET_B, the densities of which are different depending on the vascular bed studied. The ET_A receptors are located on vascular smooth muscle cells and mediate vasoconstriction, whereas the predominant subpopulation of ET_B receptors is located on endothelial cells and mediates vasodilation (Arai et al., 1990; Sakurai et al., 1990; Wong et al., 1995). However, a second subpopulation of ET_B receptors is located on smooth muscle cells and mediates vasoconstriction (Shetty et al., 1993). The vasodilating effects of ET-1 are associated with the release of NO and potassium channel activation (Cassin et al., 1991; Ivy et al., 1994; Wong et al., 1993; Wong, Fineman et al., 1994; Wong, Vanderford et al., 1994). The vasoconstricting effects of ET-1 are associated with phospholipase activation, the hydrolysis of phosphoinositol to inositol-1,4,5-triphosphate and diacylglycerol, and the subsequent release of Ca^{2+} (La and Reid, 1995). In addition to its vasoactive properties, ET-1 has mitogenic activity on vascular smooth muscle cells and may participate in vascular remodeling (Hassoun et al., 1992).

The predominant effect of exogenous ET-1 in the fetal and newborn sheep pulmonary circulation is vasodilation, mediated via ET_B receptor activation and NO release. However, the predominant effect in the juvenile and adult pulmonary circulations is vasoconstriction, mediated via ET_A receptor activation. In fetal lambs, selective ET_A receptor blockade produces small decreases in resting fetal pulmonary vascular resistance. This suggests a potential minor role for basal ET-1–induced vasoconstriction in maintaining the high fetal pulmonary vascular resistance (Ivy et al., 1994; Wong, Fineman et al., 1994). Although plasma and urinary concentrations of ET-1 are increased at birth (Malamitsi-Puchner et al., 1995; Sulyok et al., 1993), in vivo studies suggest that basal ET-1 activity does not play an important role in mediating the transitional pulmonary circulation (Winters et al., 1996). ET-1 causes fetal renal vasodilation (Bogaert et al, 1996) and thus may be involved in the regulation of fetal renal blood flow.

Other factors, such as calcitonin gene-related peptide and a related substance, adrenomedullin, have vasodilatory effects on the fetal pulmonary circulation and too may play a role in the regulation of pulmonary vascular tone in the fetus (DeVroomen et al., 1997, 1998). The effects of these substances probably also are mediated by NO release (Takahashi et al., 2000a).

DUCTUS ARTERIOSUS

Patency of the fetal ductus arteriosus is regulated by both dilating and contracting factors. The factors that promote ductus arteriosus constriction in the fetus have yet to be fully identified. The ductus arteriosus maintains a tonic degree of constriction in utero that appears to be both dependent and independent of extracellular calcium (Kajino et al., 2001). ET-1 also appears to play a role in producing the basal tone of the ductus arteriosus (Coceani et al., 1999).

The factors that oppose ductus arteriosus constriction in utero are better understood. The vascular pressure within the ductus arteriosus lumen opposes ductus arteriosus constriction (Clyman et al., 1989). Vasodilator prostaglandins appear to be the most important factors opposing ductus arteriosus constriction in the latter part of gestation (Momma and Toyono, 1999; Kajino et al., 2001). Inhibitors of prostaglandin synthesis (e.g., indomethacin) constrict the fetal ductus arteriosus both in vitro and in vivo (Sharpe et al., 1975; Heymann and Rudolph, 1976; Clyman, 1980). Both the cyclooxygenase-1 and cyclooxygen-

ase-2 isoforms of cyclooxygenase are present within the fetal ductus arteriosus and are responsible for synthesizing the prostaglandins that maintain ductus arteriosus patency (Takahashi et al., 2000b). Inhibitors of both cyclooxygenase-1 and cyclooxygenase-2 will individually produce fetal ductus arteriosus constriction in vivo (Takahashi et al., 2000b). Conversely, PGE_2 will dilate the constricted ductus arteriosus both in vitro and in vivo. PGE_2 produces ductus arteriosus relaxation by interacting with several of the PGE receptors (EP2, EP3, and EP4) (Bouayad et al., 2001). The EP4 receptor appears to play a prominent role in ductus arteriosus vasodilation (Smith et al., 1994; Nguyen et al., 1997). NO also is made by the fetal ductus arteriosus and appears to play an important role in maintaining ductus arteriosus patency in rodent fetuses (Momma and Toyono, 1999). Although NO is also made in the ductus arteriosus of larger species, its importance in maintaining ductus arteriosus patency under normal conditions has not been conclusively demonstrated (Fox et al., 1996) (see next paragraph for the role in fetuses exposed to indomethacin tocolysis).

Although pharmacologic inhibition of prostaglandin synthesis produces ductus arteriosus constriction in utero, genetic interruptions of either prostaglandin synthesis (i.e., homozygous combined cyclooxygenase-1 and cyclooxygenase-2 "knockout" mice [Loftin et al., 2001]) or signaling (i.e., homozygous EP4 receptor "knockout" mice [Nguyen et al., 1997]) do not lead to ductus arteriosus constriction in utero. Contrary to expectations, both genetic interruptions produce newborn mice in which the ductus arteriosus fails to close after birth. The mechanisms through which the absence of prostaglandins early in gestation alter the normal balance of other vasoactive factors in the ductus arteriosus have yet to be elucidated. It is interesting to note that pharmacologic inhibition of prostaglandin synthesis in human pregnancy also is associated with an increased incidence of patent ductus arteriosus after birth (Norton et al., 1993). When the fetus is exposed to indomethacin in utero, the ductus arteriosus constricts. Ductus arteriosus constriction in utero produces ischemic hypoxia, increased NO production, and smooth muscle cell death within the ductus arteriosus wall. These factors prevent the ductus arteriosus from constricting normally after birth and make it resistant to the constrictive effects of indomethacin administered postnatally (Clyman et al., 2001; Goldbarg et al., 2002).

REFERENCES

Arai H, Hori S, Aramori I, et al: Cloning and expression of a cDNA encoding an endothelin receptor. Nature **348:**730, 1990.

Assali NS, Brinkman CR III, Woods JR Jr, et al: Development of neurohumoral control of fetal, neonatal, and adult cardiovascular functions. Am J Obstet Gynecol **129:**748, 1977.

Barrett CT, Heymann MA, Rudolph AM: Alpha and beta adrenergic function in fetal sheep. Am J Obstet Gynecol **112:**1114, 1972.

Bartelds B, van Bel F, Teitel DF, et al: Carotid, not aortic, chemoreceptors mediate the fetal cardiovascular response to acute hypoxemia in lambs. Pediatr Res **34:**51, 1993.

Behrman RE, Lees MH, Peterson EN, et al: Distribution of the circulation in the normal and asphyxiated fetal primate. Am J Obstet Gynecol **108:**956, 1970.

Berman W Jr, Goodlin RC, Heymann MA, et al: Pressure-flow relationships in the umbilical and uterine circulations of the sheep. Circ Res **38:**262, 1976.

Berman W Jr, Goodlin RC, Heymann MA, et al: Effects of pharmacologic agents on umbilical blood flow in fetal lambs in utero. Biol Neonate **33:**225, 1978.

Biscoe TJ, Purves MJ, Sampson SR: Types of nervous activity which may be recorded from the carotid sinus nerve in the sheep foetus. J Physiol (Lond) **202**:1, 1969.

Bogaert GA, Kogan BA, Mevorach RA, et al: Exogenous endothelin-1 causes renal vasodilation in the fetal lamb. J Urol **156**:847, 1996.

Bouayad A, Kajino H, Waleh N, et al: Characterization of PGE_2 receptors in fetal and newborn lamb ductus arteriosus. Am J Physiol **280**:H2342, 2001.

Bristow J, Rudolph AM, Itskovitz J: A preparation for studying liver blood flow, oxygen consumption, and metabolism in the fetal lamb in utero. J Dev Physiol **3**:255, 1981.

Bristow J, Rudolph AM, Itskovitz J, et al: Hepatic oxygen and glucose metabolism in the fetal lamb. J Clin Invest **71**:1, 1983.

Broughton-Pipkin F, Lumbers ER, Mott JC: Factors influencing plasma renin and angiotensin II in the conscious pregnant ewe and its foetus. J Physiol (Lond) **243**:619, 1974.

Cassin S: Role of prostaglandins, thromboxanes, and leukotrienes in the control of the pulmonary circulation in the fetus and newborn. Semin Perinatol **11**:53, 1987.

Cassin S, Kristova V, Davis T, et al: Tone-dependent responses to endothelin in isolated perfused fetal sheep pulmonary circulation in situ. J Appl Physiol **70**:1228, 1991.

Challis JRG, Patrick JE: The production of prostaglandins and thromboxanes in the feto-placental unit and their effects on the developing fetus. Semin Perinatol **4**:23, 1980.

Chang J-K, Roman C, Heymann MA: Effect of endothelium-derived relaxing factor inhibition on the umbilical-placental circulation in fetal lambs in utero. Am J Obstet Gynecol **166**:727, 1992.

Chaudhuri G, Buga GM, Gold ME, et al: Characterization and actions of human umbilical endothelium derived relaxing factor. Br J Pharmacol **102**:331, 1991.

Cheng JB, Cornett LE, Goldfien A, et al: Decreased concentration of myocardial alpha-adrenoceptors with increasing age in foetal lambs. Br J Pharmacol **70**:515, 1980.

Cheng JB, Goldfien A, Cornett LE, et al: Identification of beta-adrenergic receptors using (3H)dihydroalprenolol in fetal sheep heart: Direct evidence of qualitative similarity to the receptors in adult sheep heart. Pediatr Res **15**:1083, 1981.

Clyman RI: Ontogeny of the ductus arteriosus response to prostaglandins and inhibitors of their synthesis. Semin Perinatol **4**:115, 1980.

Clyman RI: Ductus arteriosus: Current theories of prenatal and postnatal regulation. Semin Perinatol **11**:64, 1987.

Clyman RI, Chen YQ, Chemtob S, et al: In utero remodeling of the fetal lamb ductus arteriosus: The role of antenatal indomethacin and avascular zone thickness on vasa vasorum proliferation, neointima formation, and cell death. Circulation **103**:1806, 2001.

Clyman RI, Mauray F, Heymann MA, et al: Influence of increased pulmonary vascular pressures on the closure of the ductus arteriosus in newborn lambs. Pediatr Res **25**:136, 1989.

Coceani F, Liu Y, Seidlitz E, et al: Endothelin A receptor is necessary for O_2 constriction but not closure of ductus arteriosus. Am J Physiol **277**:H1521, 1999.

Comline RS, Silver IA, Silver M: Factors responsible for the stimulation of the adrenal medulla during asphyxia in the foetal lamb. J Physiol (Lond) **178**:211, 1965.

Dawes GS, Duncan LB, Lewis BV, et al: Cyanide stimulation of the systemic arterial chemoreceptors in foetal lambs. J Physiol (Lond) **201**:117, 1969.

Dawes GS, Johnston BM, Walker DW: Relationship of arterial pressure and heart rate in fetal, newborn, and adult sheep. J Physiol (Lond) **309**:405, 1980.

DeSmedt MCH, Visser GHA, Meijboom EJ: Fetal cardiac output estimated by Doppler echocardiography during mid and late gestation. Am J Cardiol **60**:338, 1987.

DeVroomen M, Takahashi Y, Gournay V, et al: Adrenomedullin increases pulmonary blood flow in fetal sheep. Pediatr Res **41**:493, 1997,

DeVroomen M, Takahashi Y, Roman C, et al: Calcitonin gene-related peptide increases pulmonary blood flow in fetal sheep. Am J Physiol **274**:H277, 1998.

Downing SE, Talner NS, Gardner TM: Ventricular function in the newborn lamb. Am J Physiol **208**:931, 1965.

Drummond WH, Rudolph AM, Keil LC, et al: Arginine vasopressin and prolactin after hemorrhage in the fetal lamb. Am J Physiol **238**:E214, 1980.

Edelstone DI, Rudolph AM: Preferential streaming of ductus venosus blood to the brain and heart in fetal lambs. Am J Physiol **237**:H724, 1979.

Edelstone DI, Rudolph AM, Heymann MA: Liver and ductus venosus blood flows in fetal lambs in utero. Circ Res **42**:426, 1978.

Edelstone DI, Rudolph AM, Heymann MA: Effects of hypoxemia and decreasing umbilical flow on liver and ductus venosus blood flows in fetal lambs. Am J Physiol **238**:H656, 1980.

Fineman JR, Soifer SJ, Heymann MA: Regulation of pulmonary vascular tone in the perinatal period. Annu Rev Physiol **57**:115, 1995

Fineman JR, Wong J, Morin FC, et al: Chronic nitric oxide inhibition in utero produces persistent pulmonary hypertension in newborn lambs. J Clin Invest **93**:2675, 1994.

Fisher DJ, Heymann MA, Rudolph AM: Myocardial oxygen and carbohydrate consumption in fetal lambs in utero and in adult sheep. Am J Physiol **238**:H399, 1980.

Fox JJ, Ziegler JW, Dunbar DI, et al: Role of nitric oxide and cGMP system in regulation of ductus arteriosus tone in ovine fetus. Am J Physiol **271**:H2638, 1996.

Friedman WF: The intrinsic physiologic properties of the developing heart. In Friedman WF, Lesch M, Sonnenblick EH (eds): Neonatal Heart Disease. New York, Grune & Stratton, 1973.

Friedman WF, Pool PE, Jacobowitz D, et al: Sympathetic innervation of the developing rabbit heart. Circ Res **23**:25, 1968.

Gilbert RD: Control of fetal cardiac output during changes in blood volume. Am J Physiol **238**:H80, 1980.

Gilbert RD: Effects of afterload and baroreceptors on cardiac function in fetal sheep. J Dev Physiol **4**:299, 1982.

Glasgow RE, Heymann MA: Endothelium-derived relaxing factor as a mediator of bradykinin-induced perinatal pulmonary vasodilatation. Clin Res **38**:211A, 1990.

Goldbarg SH, Takahashi Y, Cruz C, et al: In utero indomethacin alters O_2 delivery to the fetal ductus arteriosus: Implications for postnatal patency. Am J Physiol **282**:R184, 2002.

Goodlin RC, Rudolph AM: Factors associated with initiation of breathing. In Hodari AA, Mariona FG (eds): Proceedings of the International Symposium on Physiological Biochemistry of the Fetus. Springfield, Ill, Charles C Thomas, 1972.

Gryglewski RJ: The lung as a generator of prostacyclin. Ciba Found Symp **78**:147, 1980.

Harada K, Rice MJ, Shiota T, et al: Gestational age- and growth-related alterations in fetal right and left ventricular diastolic filling patterns. Am J Cardiol **79**:173, 1997.

Hargrave B, Roman C, Morville P, et al: Pulmonary vascular effects of exogenous atrial natriuretic peptide in sheep fetuses. Pediatr Res **27**:140, 1990.

Harris WH, Van Petten GR: Development of cardiovascular responses to sympathomimetic amines and autonomic blockade in the unanesthetised fetus. Can J Physiol Pharmacol **56**:400, 1978.

Harris WH, Van Petten GR: Development of cardiovascular responses to noradrenaline, normetanephrine and metanephrine in the unanesthetised fetus. Can J Physiol Pharmacol **57**:242, 1979.

Hassoun PM, Thappa V, Landman MJ, et al: Endothelin 1: Mitogenic activity on pulmonary artery smooth muscle cells and release from hypoxic endothelial cells. Proc Exp Bio Med **199**:165, 1992.

Hawkins J, Van Hare GF, Schmidt KG, et al: Effects of increasing afterload on left ventricular output in fetal lambs. Circ Res **65**:127, 1989.

Heymann MA, Creasy RK, Rudolph AM: Quantitation of blood flow patterns in the fetal lamb in utero. In Comline RS, Cross KW, Dawes GS, et al (eds): Proceedings of the Sir Joseph Barcroft Centenary Symposium: Foetal and Neonatal Physiology. Cambridge, Cambridge University Press, 1973.

Heymann MA, Rudolph AM: Effects of increasing preload on right ventricular output in fetal lambs in utero [abstract]. Circulation **48**:IV-37, 1973.

Heymann MA, Rudolph AM: Effects of acetylsalicylic acid on the ductus arteriosus and circulation in fetal lambs in utero. Circ Res **38**:418, 1976.

Ignarro LJ: Biological actions and properties of endothelium-derived nitric oxide formed and released from artery and vein. Circ Res **65**:1, 1989.

Itskovitz J, LaGamma EF, Rudolph AM: Baroreflex control of the circulation of chronically instrumented fetal lambs. Circ Res **52**:589, 1983.

Itskovitz J, Rudolph AM: Denervation of arterial chemoreceptors and baroreceptors in fetal lambs in utero. Am J Physiol **242**:H916, 1982.

Ivy DD, Kinsella JP, Abman SH: Physiologic characterization of endothelin A and B receptor activity in the ovine fetal pulmonary circulation. J Clin Invest **93**:2141, 1994.

Iwamoto HS, Rudolph AM: Effects of endogenous angiotensin II on the fetal circulation. J Dev Physiol **1**:283, 1979.

Iwamoto HS, Rudolph AM: Effects of angiotensin II on the blood flow and its distribution in fetal lambs. Circ Res **48**:183, 1982.

Iwamoto HS, Rudolph AM, Keil LC, et al: Hemodynamic responses of the sheep fetus to vasopressin infusion. Circ Res **44**:430, 1979.

Jones CT, Robinson RD: Plasma catecholamines in fetal and adult sheep. J Physiol (Lond) **248**:15, 1975.

Kajino H, Chen YQ, Seidner SR, et al: Factors that increase the contractile tone of the ductus arteriosus also regulate its anatomic remodeling. Am J Physiol 281:R291, 2001.

Kirkpatrick SE, Pitlick PT, Naliboff JB, et al: Frank-Starling relationship as an important determinant of fetal cardiac output. Am J Physiol **231**:495, 1976.

La M, Reid JJ: Endothelin-1 and the regulation of vascular tone. Clin Exp Pharmacol Physiol **22**:315, 1995.

LeBidois J, Soifer SJ, Clyman RI, et al: Piriprost: A putative leukotriene synthesis inhibitor increases pulmonary blood flow in fetal lambs. Pediatr Res **22**:350, 1987.

Lebowitz EA, Novick JS, Rudolph AM: Development of myocardial sympathetic innervation in the fetal lamb. Pediatr Res **6**:887, 1972.

Lewis AB, Evans WN, Sischo W: Plasma catecholamine responses to hypoxemia in fetal lambs. Biol Neonate **41**:115, 1982.

Loftin CD, Trivedi DB, Tiano HF, et al: Failure of ductus arteriosus closure and remodeling in neonatal mice deficient in cyclooxygenase-1 and cyclooxygenase-2. Proc Natl Acad Sci USA **98**:1059, 2001.

Lorijn RWH, Longo LD: Norepinephrine elevation in the fetal lamb: Oxygen consumption and cardiac output. Am J Physiol **239**:R115, 1980.

Malamitsi-Puchner A, Economou E, Efstathopoulos T, et al: Endothelin 1-21 plasma concentrations on days 1 and 4 of life in healthy and ill preterm neonates. Biol Neonate **67**:317, 1995.

Maloney JE, Cannata JP, Dowling MH, et al: Baroreflex activity in conscious fetal and newborn lambs. Biol Neonate **31**:340, 1977.

Mitchell MD, Flint AP, Bibby J, et al: Plasma concentrations of prostaglandins during late human pregnancy: Influence of normal and preterm labor. J Clin Endocrinol Metab **46**:947, 1978.

Momma K, Toyono M: The role of nitric oxide in dilating the fetal ductus arteriosus in rats. Pediatr Res **46**:311, 1999.

Moore P, Velvis H, Fineman JR, et al: Endothelium derived relaxing factor inhibition attenuates the increase in pulmonary blood flow due to oxygen ventilation in fetal lambs. J Appl Physiol **73**:2151, 1992.

Myatt L, Brewer A, Brockman D: The action of nitric oxide in the perfused human fetal-placental circulation. Am J Obstet Gynecol **164**:687, 1991.

Nguyen M, Camenisch T, Snouwaert JN, et al: The prostaglandin receptor EP4 triggers remodelling of the cardiovascular system at birth. Nature **390**:78, 1997.

Norton ME, Merrill J, Cooper BAB, et al: Neonatal complications after the administration of indomethacin for preterm labor. N Engl J Med **329**:1602, 1993.

Novy MJ, Piasecki G, Jackson BT: Effect of prostaglandins E2 and F2-alpha on umbilical blood flow and fetal hemodynamics. Prostaglandins **5**:543, 1974.

Nuwayhid B, Brinkman CR III, Su C, et al: Systemic and pulmonary hemodynamic responses to adrenergic and cholinergic agonists during fetal development. Biol Neonate **26**:301, 1975.

Olley PM, Bodach E, Heaton J, et al: Further evidence implicating E-type prostaglandins in the patency of the lamb ductus arteriosus. Eur J Pharmacol **34**:247, 1975.

Papile L, Rudolph AM, Heymann MA: Autoregulation of cerebral blood flow in the preterm fetal lamb. Pediatr Res **19**:159, 1985.

Peeters LLH, Sheldon RE, Jones MD Jr, et al: Blood flow to fetal organs as a function of arterial oxygen content. Am J Obstet Gynecol **135**:637, 1979.

Pinto A, Sorrentino R, Sorrentino P, et al: Endothelial-derived relaxing factor released by endothelial cells of human umbilical vessels and its impairment in pregnancy-induced hypertension. Am J Obstet Gynecol **164**:507, 1991.

Ponte J, Purves MJ: Types of afferent nervous activity which may be measured in the vagus nerve of the sheep foetus. J Physiol (Lond) **229**:51, 1973.

Rasanen J, Wood DC, Weiner S, et al: Role of the pulmonary circulation in the distribution of human fetal cardiac output during the second half of pregnancy. Circulation **94**:1068, 1996.

Reed KL, Meijboom EJ, Sahn DJ, et al: Cardiac Doppler flow velocities in human fetuses. Circulation **73**:41, 1986.

Reuss ML, Rudolph AM, Heymann MA: Selective distribution of microspheres injected into the umbilical veins and inferior venae cavae of fetal sheep. Am J Obstet Gynecol **141**:427, 1981.

Robillard JE, Weitzman RE: Developmental aspects of the fetal renal response to exogenous arginine vasopressin. Am J Physiol **238**:F407, 1980.

Rudolph AM, Heymann MA: Circulatory changes during growth in the fetal lamb. Circ Res **26**:289, 1970.

Rurak DW: Plasma vasopressin levels during hypoxaemia and the cardiovascular effects of exogenous vasopressin in foetal and adult sheep. J Physiol (Lond) **277**:341, 1978.

Sahn DJ, Lange LW, Allen HD, et al: Quantitative real-time cross-sectional echocardiography in the developing normal human fetus and newborn. Circulation **62**:588, 1980.

Sakurai T, Yanagisawa M, Takuwa Y, et al: Cloning of a cDNA encoding a non-isopeptide-selective subtype of the endothelin receptor. Nature **348**:732, 1990.

Schreiber MD, Heymann MA, Soifer SJ: Leukotriene inhibition prevents and reverses hypoxic pulmonary vasoconstriction in newborn lambs. Pediatr Res **19**:437, 1985.

Segar JL: Ontogeny of the arterial and cardiopulmonary baroreflex during fetal and postnatal life. Am J Physiol **273**:R457, 1997.

Sharpe GL, Larsson KS, Thalme B: Studies on closure of the ductus arteriosus. XII. In utero effects of indomethacin and sodium salicylate in rats and rabbits. Prostaglandins **9**:585, 1975.

Sheldon CA, Friedman WF, Sybers HD: Scanning electron microscopy of fetal and neonatal lamb cardiac cells. J Mol Cell Cardiol **8**:853, 1976.

Shetty SS, Toshikazu O, Webb RL, et al: Functionally distinct endothelin b receptors in vascular endothelium and smooth muscle. Biochem Biophys Res Commun **191**:459, 1993.

Shinebourne EA, Vapaavouri EK, Williams RL, et al: Development of baroreflex activity in unanesthetized fetal and neonatal lambs. Circ Res **31**:710, 1972.

Smith FG Jr, Lupu AN, Barajas L, et al: The renin-angiotensin system in the fetal lamb. Pediatr Res **8**:611, 1974.

Smith GCS, Coleman RA, McGrath JC: Characterization of dilator prostanoid receptors in the fetal rabbit ductus arteriosus. J Pharmacol Exp Ther **271**:390, 1994.

Soifer SJ, Loitz RD, Roman C, et al: Leukotriene end-organ antagonists increase pulmonary blood flow in fetal lambs. Am J Physiol **249**:H570, 1985.

Sulyok E, Ertl T, Adamovits K, et al: Urinary endothelin excretion in the neonate: Influence of maturity and perinatal pathology. Pediatr Nephrol **7**:881, 1993.

Takahashi Y, de Vrooman M, Roman C, et al: Mechanisms of calcitonin gene related peptide (CGRP)-induced increases of pulmonary blood flow in fetal sheep. Am J Physiol **279**:H1654, 2000a.

Takahashi Y, Roman C, Chemtob S, et al: Cyclooxygenase-2 inhibitors constrict the fetal lamb ductus arteriosus both in vitro and in vivo. Am J Physiol **278**:R1496, 2000b.

Teitel DF, Dalinghaus M, Cassidy SC, et al: In utero ventilation augments the left ventricular response to isoproterenol and volume loading in fetal sheep. Pediatr Res **29**:466, 1991.

Tripp ME, Heymann MA, Rudolph AM: Hemodynamic effects of prostaglandin E₁ on lambs in utero. In Coceani F, Olley PM (eds): Prostaglandins and Perinatal Medicine. Advances in Prostaglandin and Thromboxane Research, vol 4. New York, Raven Press, 1978.

Van de Voorde J, Vanderstichele H, Leusen I: Release of endothelium-derived relaxing factor from human umbilical vessels. Circ Res **60**:517, 1987.

Vapaavouri EK, Shinebourne EA, Williams RL, et al: Development of cardiovascular responses to autonomic blockade in intact fetal and neonatal lambs. Biol Neonate **22**:177, 1973.

Velvis H, Krusell J, Roman C, et al: Leukotrienes C₄, D₄, and E₄ in fetal lamb tracheal fluid. J Dev Physiol **14**:13, 1990.

Walker AM, Cannata J, Dowling MH, et al: Sympathetic and parasympathetic control of heart rate in unanesthetised fetal and newborn lambs. Biol Neonate **33**:135, 1978.

Whitsett JA, Pollinger J, Matz S: β-Adrenergic receptors and catecholamine-sensitive adenylate cyclase in developing rat ventricular myocardium: Effect of thyroid status. Pediatr Res **16**:463, 1982.

Winters J, Wong J, Van Dyke D, et al: Endothelin receptor blockade does not alter the increase in pulmonary blood flow due to oxygen ventilation in fetal lambs. Pediatr Res **40**:152, 1996.

Wong J, Fineman JR, Heymann MA: The role of endothelin and endothelin receptor subtypes in regulation of fetal pulmonary vascular tone. Pediatr Res **35**:664, 1994.

Wong J, Vanderford PA, Fineman JR, et al: Endothelin-1 produces pulmonary vasodilation in the intact newborn lamb. Am J Physiol **265**:H1318, 1993.

Wong J, Vanderford PA, Fineman JR, et al: Developmental effects of endothelin-1 on the pulmonary circulation in sheep. Pediatr Res **36**:394, 1994.

Wong J, Vanderford PA, Winters J, et al: Endothelin b receptor agonists produce pulmonary vasodilation in the intact newborn lamb with pulmonary hypertension. J Cardiovasc Pharm **25**:207, 1995.

Wyse DG, Van Petten GR, Harris WH: Responses to electrical stimulation, noradrenaline, serotonin, and vasopressin in the isolated ear artery of the developing lamb and ewe. Can J Physiol Pharmacol **55**:1001, 1977.

Yanagisawa M, Kurihara H, Kimura S, et al: A novel potent vasoconstrictor peptide produced by vascular endothelial cells. Nature **332**:411, 1988.

Zink J, Van Petten GR: Noradrenergic control of blood vessels in the premature lamb fetus. Biol Neonate **39**:61, 1981.

Chapter 14

FETAL BREATHING AND BODY MOVEMENTS

Bryan S. Richardson, MD, FRCS(C), and Robert Gagnon, MD, FRCS(C)

During the last several years, fetal activity has been extensively studied with systematic investigation in animals, primarily the catheterized ovine fetus. In addition, the widespread use of real-time ultrasonic sector scanners has allowed for direct measurement of fetal movement in humans. It has become evident that fetal breathing and body movements are important functions in utero and are necessary for the normal growth and development of organ systems. These activities also serve to characterize the healthy fetus and become altered when oxygenation is compromised, providing a basis for the use of activity parameters in the biophysical assessment of fetal health. The study of activity patterns in utero has also firmly established the existence of fetal behavioral states, with similarities to postnatal sleep states. Moreover, a developmental process has become apparent that may have functional importance for the growth and development of the brain and provide a means for neurobehavioral assessment. However, physiologic and pathologic factors have been shown to affect fetal breathing and body movements, and an understanding of these is fundamental to the interpretation of fetal movement activity in the high-risk pregnant patient.

FETAL BREATHING MOVEMENTS

Animal Studies

Physiology and Biological Patterns

Fetal breathing movements were initially reported in the ovine fetus some 30 years ago by Dawes and coworkers (1972), who used measurements from chronically implanted tracheal pressure catheters. Two types of breathing movements were distinguished. The first occurred infrequently and consisted of single, brief, relatively deep inspiratory efforts recurring irregularly at a slow rate. The second, described as rapid irregular breathing, consisted of bursts of activity of much higher frequency (1 to 2 Hz) lasting from a few seconds to an hour; the inspiratory movements were irregular in both rate and depth. Diaphragmatic electromyographic (EMG) recordings demonstrate that after initiation of electrical activity in the diaphragm, tracheal pressure falls and tracheal flow begins and moves inward in the direction of the lungs at the rate of approximately 0.5 mL per breath (Maloney et al., 1975). On completion of each fetal diaphragmatic EMG burst, tracheal pressure returns to

normal; lung liquid flow is directed out of the lung and returns to zero between diaphragmatic EMG bursts. These observations confirm that the negative tracheal pressure measurements represent periods during which the fetal diaphragm descends into the abdomen, creating negative pressure in the chest and positive pressure in the fetal abdomen.

Although there is no evidence of a causal relationship between changes in arterial blood gas tension or pH and the onset of spontaneous fetal breathing movements, induced hypercapnia (Boddy et al., 1974) and metabolic acidosis (Hohimer and Bissonnette, 1981) have been found to affect the incidence and amplitude of respiratory movements in the ovine fetus, indicating the existence of functional chemoreceptors in the fetus. Further studies in the sheep fetus indicate that both central (Hohimer et al., 1983) and peripheral (Murai et al., 1985) chemoreceptor structures are active and capable of modulating the incidence of these movements.

Episodes of rapid irregular fetal breathing movements occur up to 40% of the time in chronically instrumented fetal sheep during the last third of pregnancy. As in postnatal life, these respiratory movements are affected by behavioral or sleep states and for the ovine fetus occur only during times of low-voltage electrocortical activity and electroocular activity characteristic of rapid eye movement (REM) sleep (Fig. 14-1) (Dawes et al., 1972). Although the to and fro movement of tracheal fluid is small for individual respiratory movements (<1 mL), there is an overall flow of fluid away from the lungs that is approximately fivefold greater during episodes of breathing movements than during apnea (Harding et al., 1984). A circadian rhythm in breathing activity has also been observed and is characterized by a twofold increase in the incidence of rapid irregular breathing movements during the late evening over that measured during early morning hours (Boddy et al., 1973). Fetal breathing movements in primates also are episodic, with an incidence in the chronic rhesus monkey preparation noted to be approximately 50% of the time near term (Martin et al., 1974). Studies in the baboon fetus report a similar overall incidence for breathing movements, which for this species are evident during times of electrocortical activity characteristic of both non-REM and REM sleep, albeit at an increased incidence and respiratory rate for the latter (Stark and Myers, 1992).

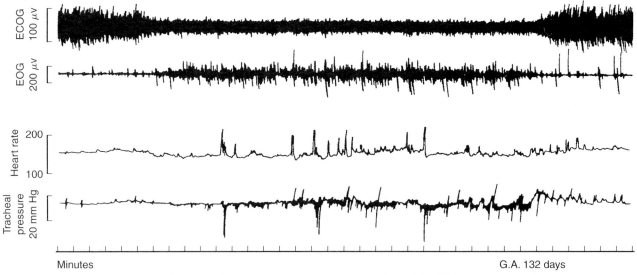

FIGURE 14-1 ■ Chart recording demonstrating that electro-ocular activity (EOG) and fetal breathing movements normally occur during times of low-voltage electrocortical activity (ECOG).

Developmental Changes

Developmental changes in fetal breathing activity are noted for the ovine species and are clearly dependent on the means by which this activity is measured. Whereas the incidence of fetal breathing movements as measured from tracheal pressure changes is lower in the younger gestational aged fetus (~20% of the time at 90 days' gestation; term 147 days), diaphragmatic EMG activity is almost continuous, with increasing apneic modulation as gestation advances (Ioffe et al., 1987; Matsuda et al., 1992). However, the diaphragmatic EMG activity of the fetus of younger gestational age is primarily tonic in nature, with a prolonged burst duration. With advancing gestation, phasic diaphragmatic activity becomes more pronounced in keeping with the increased incidence of fetal breathing movements as measured by tracheal pressure change in animals near term. A developmental change in the pattern of breathing is also noted and appears to be related to the development of episodic variations in electrocortical activity characteristic of sleep states (Clewlow et al., 1983). Before 105 days' gestation and with electrocortical activity still undifferentiated, breathing movements are nonepisodic and occur over short durations at frequent intervals. Thereafter, breathing movements become distinctly episodic and are associated with REM as the electrocorticogram begins to differentiate into high-voltage and low-voltage patterns.

Parturition

The incidence of fetal lamb breathing movements decreases 2 or 3 days before the onset of labor and remains reduced until delivery despite fetal blood gas and glucose concentrations within the normal range (Berger et al., 1986; Patrick et al., 1987b). The mechanism for this decrease in fetal breathing activity may relate to increasing concentrations of prostaglandin E_2, which is thought to play an important role in the onset of labor in sheep and is known to diminish fetal breathing activity (Kitterman et al., 1983). Such a mechanism is further supported by the findings of Patrick and colleagues (1987b), during the last 12 hours before the onset of adrenocorticotropic hormone–induced labor in sheep, of a significant negative relationship between fetal arterial prostaglandin E_2 concentrations and the incidence of fetal breathing movements, which fell to approximately 15% of the time during early labor.

Hypoxia and Asphyxia

Neuromuscular blockade in the ovine fetus results in an approximate 20% decrease in oxygen (O_2) consumption, presumably in part because of a decrease in breathing activity and other movements (Rurak and Gruber, 1983b). Conversely, fetal O_2 consumption is increased to a similar extent during periods of fetal breathing movements when compared with apneic periods (Rurak and Gruber, 1983a). As such, a decrease in fetal movements when oxygenation becomes compromised may serve as a protective mechanism, whereby energy expenditure and thus O_2 requirements are also decreased.

In the near-term ovine fetus, moderate hypoxemia of short-term duration (reduction of arterial partial pressure of oxygen [P_{O_2}] from approximately 24 to 14 mm Hg for 1 to 2 hours) results in a decrease in fetal breathing movements to less than 10% of the time (Bocking and Harding, 1986). Similar responses to fetal hypoxemia are observed in chronic rhesus monkey preparations (Martin et al., 1974). However, if this degree of hypoxemia is maintained in the absence of incipient metabolic acidemia, breathing activity returns toward normal after several hours, indicating an adaptive process (Bocking et al., 1988; Koos et al., 1988).

With sustained hypoxemia of a moderate to severe degree and leading to metabolic acidosis, fetal breathing movements are again markedly decreased and more so than for other biophysical activities (Matsuda et al., 1994) (Fig. 14-2). As such, fetal breathing movements would appear to be a more sensitive biophysical indicator for worsening hypoxemia. However, with the removal of the asphyxial insult, there is a rapid normalization of biophysical activity, including that of breathing move-

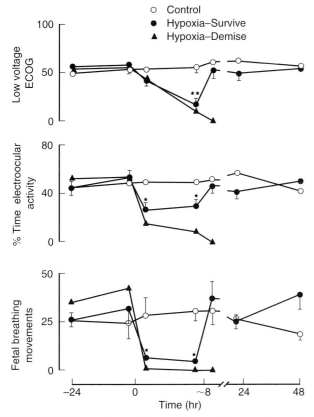

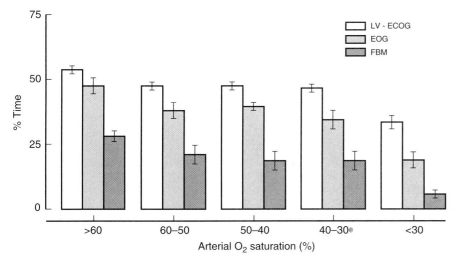

FIGURE 14-2 ■ Percentage of time with low-voltage electrocortical activity (ECOG), electro-ocular activity, and fetal breathing movements plotted for 2-hour time intervals before, during, and after experimental period (0 to approximately 8 hours). Values are means ± SE. *Asterisk, P* < .05; *two asterisks, P* < .01 versus control group values. Statistical analysis was not performed for hypoxia–demise group. (From Matsuda Y, Patrick J, Carmichael L, et al. Recovery of the ovine fetus from sustained hypoxia: Effects on endocrine, cardiovascular and biophysical activity. Am J Obstet Gynecol **170**:1433, 1994.)

ments for those animals surviving (Matsuda et al., 1994). With prolonged and graded reductions in fetal oxygenation over several days, a marked decrease in fetal movement activity is only seen as the degree of hypoxemia approaches the level at which acidemia becomes apparent (Richardson et al., 1992) (Fig. 14-3). Fetal breathing assessment should thus be seen as a potential marker of moderate to severe hypoxemic changes, with heightened surveillance required for the extremely high-risk pregnancy, because the time course for alteration before fetal demise may be relatively short. A maturational process is also apparent for the biophysical response of the ovine fetus to hypoxic insults, with the preterm fetus showing less reduction in breathing activity at 0.7 to 0.8 of gestation (Clewlow et al., 1983; Bocking and Harding, 1986) and no reduction in breathing activity at 0.6 of gestation (Matsuda et al., 1992). This may then affect survival and the success of antenatal assessment protocols.

Intrauterine Growth Restriction

Growth is known to account for a consequential fraction of the substrate consumption of fetal sheep near term (Battaglia and Meschia, 1978). With both prolonged reduction in fetal O_2 delivery over several days (Anderson et al., 1986) and induced intrauterine growth restriction (IUGR) (Clapp et al., 1981), total O_2 consumption by the fetus is reduced approximately 20%. This decrease in oxidative metabolism represents the energy "savings" from decreased tissue growth but also reflects, in part, changes in movement activity and associated energy requirements. The ovine fetus thus demonstrates a rapid adaptation to a limitation in substrate delivery with a decrease in growth rate and movement activity and thereby substrate needs, resulting in metabolic normality with a variable degree of hypoxemia and usually little evidence of metabolic acidosis or anaerobic metabolism (Clapp et al., 1981; Worthington et al., 1981). Of note, if decreased fetal growth is sufficient, the fall-off in O_2 consumption may balance that for O_2 delivery such that fetal oxygen levels are in fact normalized (Mostello et al., 1991). As such, movement activity in some IUGR fetuses may be little affected.

Worthington and colleagues (1981) studied the effects of reduction of placental size in sheep with resultant asymmetrical IUGR and chronic hypoxia without acidemia. The incidence

FIGURE 14-3 ■ Percentage of time with low-voltage electrocortical activity (LV-ECOG), electro-ocular activity (EOG), and fetal breathing movement (FBM) during graded reductions in fetal arterial oxygen saturation over 5 days of study. (From Richardson B: Metabolism of the fetal brain: Biological and pathological development. *In* Hanson M: The Fetal and Neonatal Brain Stem. Cambridge, Cambridge University Press, 1991, p. 87.)

of fetal breathing movements was marginally decreased, occurring approximately 20% of the time. This finding was statistically significant but involved 24-hour periods of observation, which would limit the effects of other influencing factors, including the diurnal and periodic nature of breathing activity.

Other Factors Affecting Breathing Movements

See Table 14-1 for other factors that alter breathing activity in chronic fetal animal preparations.

Human Studies

Physiology and Biological Patterns

In the mid-1970s it became possible to quantify fetal breathing and body movements by means of linear-array real-time imaging techniques, with most investigators documenting visual interpretations of movement by means of an event marker from echoes displayed on a video screen (Patrick et al., 1978). Human fetal breathing movements are most readily visualized on longitudinal scanning, thus permitting visualization of both anterior fetal chest and abdominal wall echoes. During each fetal breathing movement, the anterior chest wall echoes move inward 0.5 to 5 mm and the anterior abdominal wall echoes move outward in the opposite direction about 3 to 8 mm. As in the ovine fetus, the amplitude of chest and abdominal wall movements during episodes of fetal breathing is variable. Similarly, the fetal diaphragm appears to be the primary muscular force generating these movements, because echoes that represent this structure descend into the fetal abdomen during and return after each fetal breath.

The incidence of human fetal breathing movements has been shown to correlate with induced changes in maternal end-tidal partial pressure of carbon dioxide, increasing with maternal breathing of 2% and 4% carbon dioxide and decreasing with maternal hyperventilation (Connors et al., 1988a). This again suggests the existence of functional fetal chemoreceptors, as previously noted for the ovine fetus. Increasing maternal arterial P_{O_2} with high concentrations (50%) of inspired oxygen has no effect on fetal respiratory activity in normal fetuses (Devoe et al., 1984).

Breathing movements made by healthy human fetuses are episodic and separated by periods of apnea. Measurement of breath-to-breath intervals during the last 10 weeks of pregnancy reveals that only 3% of these intervals are 6 seconds or longer (Patrick et al., 1980a). Therefore, in the absence of gross fetal body movements, it is reasonable to define fetal apnea as a period of 6 seconds or longer in humans. Human fetal breathing movements are seen to occur approximately 30% of the observed time during the last 10 weeks of pregnancy (Patrick et al., 1978, 1980b). Near term there is a clustering of fetal breathing and gross body movements into episodes lasting 20 to 60 minutes and recurring every 60 to 90 minutes, suggesting a relationship to behavioral state activity, as previously noted for animal studies (Patrick et al., 1978, 1980b). This behavioral state relationship has been quantified by Junge and Walter (1980), with breathing movements reported to be present approximately 30% of the time during fetal "active" periods (analogous to the REM state) as determined by coincident recording of heart rate and body movements. Although breathing movements are decreased, they are still present approximately 14% of the time during fetal "quiet" periods (analogous to the non-REM state). The character of fetal breathing is also affected by

TABLE 14-1. FACTORS AFFECTING FETAL BREATHING MOVEMENTS (FBMs) IN SHEEP

Glucose concentration	
Hypoglycemia	Decreased FBM (Boddy and Dawes, 1975)
Glucose infusions	Increased FBM in fetuses with low blood glucose; no effect in normoglycemic fetuses (Richardson et al., 1982)
Temperature	
Increased core temperature	Increased FBM for 2–3 hr (Walker, 1988)
Barbiturates	
Phenobarbitone	Decreased FBM in mature fetuses (Boddy et al., 1976)
Caffeine	Increased FBM for 10–15 min (Piercy et al., 1977; Jansen et al., 1983)
Catecholamines	Increased FBM (Boddy and Dawes, 1975)
Cocaine	Increased FBM during labor (Derks et al., 1993)
Diazepam	Decreased FBM (Piercy et al., 1977)
Doxapram	Increased FBM (Hogg et al., 1977; Jansen et al., 1983)
Ethanol	Variable effect on FBM depending on acute or chronic exposure (Patrick et al., 1985; Smith et al., 1989)
Fluoxetine	Variable effect on FBM depending on acute or chronic exposure (Morrison et al., 2001)
Narcotics	
Methadone	Initial decrease followed by an increase in FBM with acute exposure
Morphine	(Szeto, 1983; Bennet et al., 1986; Hasan et al., 1988)
Prostaglandin E_2	Arrest of FBM (Kitterman et al., 1979)
Prostaglandin inhibitors	
Indomethacin	Increased FBM for 12–18 hr (Kitterman et al., 1979; Patrick et al., 1987a)
Meclofenamate	
Theophylline	Increased FBM (Bissonnette et al., 1990)

sleep states, as Nijhuis and colleagues (1983) reported fetal breathing rhythm to be more regular during quiet periods than during active periods.

As a result of the episodic nature of human fetal breathing movements, the percentage of time spent breathing can be substantially altered by the length of recording time. It is thus necessary to record for a long enough period to be certain that the recording interval does not entirely consist of a normal period of fetal apnea. Patrick and colleagues (1978, 1980a,b) studied healthy patients over 24-hour observation intervals through the last 10 weeks of pregnancy. Analysis of successive 5-minute intervals in each patient was performed to determine the percentage of intervals of 5 minutes and multiples of 5 minutes during which no fetal breathing movements were observed. This study demonstrated that approximately 25% of 5-minute intervals, 15% of 15-minute intervals, and 8% of 30-minute intervals contained no fetal breathing movements (Fig. 14-4). It was also evident from this study that episodes of fetal apnea of up to 2 hours can occasionally occur in healthy human fetuses when recordings are made without attention to time of day.

Throughout the last 10 weeks of pregnancy, the percentage of time a fetus spends breathing is increased significantly during the 2nd and 3rd hours after maternal meals, with the increase appearing to follow the normal postprandial increase in maternal blood glucose concentration (Patrick et al., 1978,

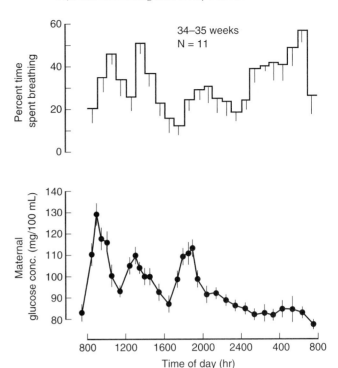

FIGURE 14-5 ■ Percentage of time spent breathing by 11 fetuses at 34 to 35 weeks each hour of the day. Mothers were given meals at 8 A.M., 12 noon, and 5:00 P.M. Fetuses made breathing movements a greater percentage of the time during the 2nd and 3rd hours after breakfast, lunch, and dinner. There was a prolonged significant increase in the percentage of time spent breathing between 1 A.M. and 7 A.M. Peak glucose concentrations occurred at 9 A.M., 1 P.M. and 6 P.M. (From Patrick J, Natale R, Richardson B: Patterns of human fetal breathing activity at 34 to 35 weeks' gestational age. Am J Obstet Gynecol **132**:507, 1978.)

1980b) (Fig. 14-5). A prolonged significant increase in fetal breathing movements is also observed overnight while mothers are asleep (Patrick et al., 1978, 1980b; Natale et al., 1988) (see Fig. 14-5). This may represent a circadian rhythm in fetal breathing activity, as previously described for the ovine fetus. There is also a circadian rhythm in the maternal plasma estriol concentration, which is inversely related to the circadian rhythm in the cortisol level at 30 to 35 weeks of pregnancy (Patrick, Challis et al., 1980). This finding is consistent with the hypothesis that maternal cortisol or placental metabolites of cortisol might cross to the fetus and influence fetal hypothalamic pituitary and adrenal function. It is notable that the overnight increase in the maternal cortisol level coincides with the overnight increase in fetal breathing movements.

Developmental Changes

Rhythmic breathing movements can be observed from 10 weeks of gestation onward, with a trend toward an increase in incidence thereafter, although they are still only evident 6% of the recording time by 19 weeks of gestation (de Vries et al., 1985). Continuous 24-hour recordings of fetal breathing activity at 24 to 28 weeks of gestation were reported by Natale et al. (1988), with the mean incidence found to be 14%. Fetal breathing activity was now distinctly episodic and clustered with other behavioral variables, but the longest period of apnea was only 14 minutes, which is significantly less than that

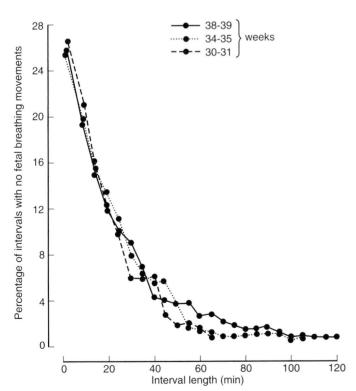

FIGURE 14-4 ■ Composite plot of the percentage of intervals with no fetal breathing movements in nine fetuses at 30 to 31 weeks, 11 at 34 to 35 weeks, and 11 at 38 to 39 weeks, demonstrating a similar distribution at these different gestational ages. The longest apneic interval was 65 minutes at 30 to 31 weeks, 105 minutes at 34 to 35 weeks, and 120 minutes at 38 to 39 weeks. (From Patrick J, Campbell K, Carmichael L, et al: A definition of human fetal apnea and the distribution of fetal apneic intervals during the last ten weeks of pregnancy. Am J Obstet Gynecol **136**:471, 1980.)

seen during the last 10 weeks of pregnancy. This suggests that different normal values need to be used in the evaluation of fetal health at earlier gestations.

Although the overall percentage of time the fetus spends breathing changes little between 30 and 40 weeks of gestation, differences in patterns of breathing activity and in distributions of breath-to-breath intervals are evident (Patrick et al., 1980a). The mean rate of fetal breathing movements at 30 to 31 weeks is 58 breaths/min and at 38 to 39 weeks falls to 41 breaths/min. The distribution of breath-to-breath intervals is much broader at 30 to 31 weeks than at 38 to 39 weeks, when breath-to-breath intervals are more regular. These changes in respiratory rate and variability over this period suggest a maturation in the control of fetal breathing movements, which probably reflects the emergence of behavioral state influences.

Parturition

A number of reports suggest that patterns of human fetal breathing movements are changed in relation to human labor at term. In healthy patients with either spontaneous or induced labor and subsequently shown to have normal outcomes, fetal breathing movements are decreased to less than 10% of the time on average during the latent phase of labor and are further decreased during the active phase of labor (Richardson et al., 1979; Wittman et al., 1979). In 24-hour studies of fetal activity at term, a decrease in fetal breathing movements is also noted in patients subsequently entering spontaneous labor within 3 days when compared with patients delivering more than 7 days after study (Carmichael et al., 1984). These data additionally indicate that a significant decrease in breathing activity normally occurs in the days immediately preceding the onset of labor at term.

Assessment of Preterm Labor

Because fetal breathing activity is known to decrease during labor, its incidence has been proposed as a means of predicting fetuses at risk of preterm delivery in women who present with signs of premature labor. Several studies have shown that fetal apnea of 20 to 60 minutes' duration is a reliable indicator of true premature labor, with subsequent premature delivery within 48 to 72 hours in almost all these patients (Castle and Turnbull, 1985; Besinger et al., 1987; Devoe et al., 1994). However, these patients also have a lower success rate with tocolytic therapy (Castle and Turnbull, 1985; Devoe et al., 1994), suggesting more advanced premature labor. This suggestion is further supported by our study result for electively induced labor at term, when prolonged fetal apnea was only evident during active labor (Richardson et al., 1979). In those same clinical studies of prematurely laboring patients, the presence of fetal breathing movements did not appear to be as reliable in predicting false premature labor, with a number of patients still delivering within the subsequent 48 to 72 hours. Given the wide range in the incidence of fetal breathing movements when monitored over short time intervals and the finding that fetal apnea is only consistently seen in advanced labor, the observation of a decrease in this activity is unlikely to be clinically useful in the management of women with preterm labor.

Premature Rupture of the Membranes and Chorioamnionitis

Rupture of the membranes per se, whether prematurely or at term, would not appear to affect either fetal breathing movements or body movements, as measured from an incidence standpoint or component parts of biophysical profile (BPP) scoring (Richardson et al., 1979; Vintzileos et al., 1985). With associated increases in uterine contractility and those endocrine events leading to the onset of labor, there is a decrease in fetal breathing movements and, to a lesser extent, in body movements (Castle and Turnbull, 1985; Devoe et al., 1994), as discussed in relation to parturition.

Clinical studies of patients with preterm rupture of the membranes have also noted a decrease in fetal breathing movements and body movements or in BPP scores (especially absent fetal breathing and nonreactive non-stress testing) in those patients with subsequent positive amniotic fluid testing for infection, clinical chorioamnionitis, or neonatal sepsis (Vintzileos et al., 1985; Vintzileos, Campbell, et al., 1986; Goldstein et al., 1988, Gauthier et al., 1992; Carroll et al., 1995; Rosemond et al., 1995). This may relate to the fetal response to bacterial products, whereby "inflammatory" cytokines are released in turn, affecting fetal behavioral activity. As such, BPP monitoring of fetal activity has been proposed for patients with preterm rupture of the membranes as a screen for whether amniotic fluid testing for infection is required (Vintzileos, Campbell, et al., 1986; Goldstein et al., 1988) and as an indicator of an onsetting infective process and thus the need for delivery (Vintzileos et al., 1985; Vintzileos, Campbell, et al., 1986; Goldstein et al., 1988). However, studies to date have reported varying sensitivities in the prediction of intrauterine infection, which probably relate to the severity of the infective process, the degree of any fetal inflammatory response, and the proximity of activity testing to the time of delivery. Additionally, some of these patients show a decrease in fetal breathing and movement activity in relation to impending labor and without subsequent evidence of infection, contributing to a lowered specificity for such testing as also reported in a number of these studies. A recent study by Ghidini and coworkers (2000) with BPP assessment within 24 hours of delivery in patients with preterm rupture of the membranes found no predictive value of such testing for subsequent histopathologic evidence of acute placental inflammation. The monitoring of fetal activity is thus unlikely to be useful in the management of women with preterm rupture of the membranes as a measure of impending infection.

Intrauterine Growth Restriction

The human fetus also undergoes IUGR in response to limitations in substrate availability, including that of oxygen. Cordocentesis data indicate variable degrees of hypoxemia (Soothill et al., 1987; Cox et al., 1988), although in many instances blood gas values are within the normal range, suggesting a degree of normalization with the fall-off in growth. In patients with IUGR, the incidence of fetal breathing movements is reported to be variably decreased and appears to depend on the severity of IUGR and the conditions and duration of study (van Vliet et al., 1985; Ruedrich et al., 1989; Gagnon et al., 1990; Bekedam et al., 1991). Although of probable biological importance with an associated decrease in energy expenditure, there is considerable overlap with population norms, which limits the usefulness of this parameter, at least as used clinically, as a marker of IUGR.

Maternal hyperoxia increases the incidence of breathing movements in the IUGR fetus, with no such increases noted for the well-grown fetus (Ruedrich et al., 1989; Gagnon et al., 1990; Bekedam et al., 1991). Although fetal hypoxemia is thus implicated as the basis for the reduced incidence of breathing movements in the IUGR fetus, the induced increase in such activity is to a level similar to that of the well-grown fetus and, given the inherent periodicity of fetal breathing activity, is again unlikely to serve as a useful clinical marker.

Assessment of Fetal Health

The present use of fetal breathing and body movements in the assessment of fetal health is largely confined to their component parts in BPP scoring (see Chapter 21). As used in the BPP, fetal movement activity has been scored in an "all or none" manner and related to a number of outcomes, including subsequent intrauterine demise, fetal distress in labor requiring operative intervention, abnormal 5-minute Apgar score, abnormal umbilical cord gases or pH, and IUGR. Although these end points differ somewhat, the physiologic basis for the use of fetal activity in the biophysical assessment of fetal health is the same; that is, with a compromise in oxygenation leading to hypoxemia with or without associated acidosis, fetal movement activity will decrease as an adaptive response whereby energy expenditure is also decreased.

As currently scored within the BPP, fetal breathing movements are more likely to be falsely abnormal at 26 to 33 weeks' gestation when compared with 34 to 41 weeks (Baskett, 1988). This is not surprising, given the lower incidence of breathing activity in younger fetuses, and emphasizes the need to estab-lish population norms reflecting the biological patterns and known factors affecting this activity. Likewise, non-stress testing is more likely to be falsely nonreactive before 32 weeks' gestation (Vintzileos, Feinstein, et al., 1986), again reflecting well-described maturational changes whereby the amplitude in fetal heart rate (FHR) acceleration in association with body movements is normally less prior to this gestational age (Natale et al., 1985).

The negative predictive value for a normal perinatal outcome is high and similar among the three dynamic biophysical variables—fetal breathing movements, gross body movements, and non-stress heart rate testing—and in the order of 95% with little improvement when test results are combined (Manning et al., 1980; Baskett et al., 1984). However, the positive predictive value for an abnormal perinatal outcome is improved when test results are combined. For the dynamic fetal variables, the monitoring of body movements appears to improve the positive predictive value of the BPP more than the monitoring of breathing movements or non-stress testing (Platt et al., 1983; Vintzileos et al., 1983). As noted by Devoe and colleagues (1988), however, such comparisons are without statistical relationship to physiologic incidence data, because the unweighted and somewhat arbitrary scoring system currently used does not provide for the quantification of the dynamic fetal variables and their normal population standards.

In the 24-hour observation studies by Patrick and coworkers (1980a, 1982) on healthy patients through the last 10 weeks of pregnancy, the percentage of 30-minute intervals with no fetal breathing movements was close to 8% on average, whereas that for no gross fetal body movements was only 4% on average (Figs. 14-4 and 14-6). Moreover, sequential rather than concurrent monitoring of these fetal activities, as used in BPP scoring, does not respect the interdependence of these

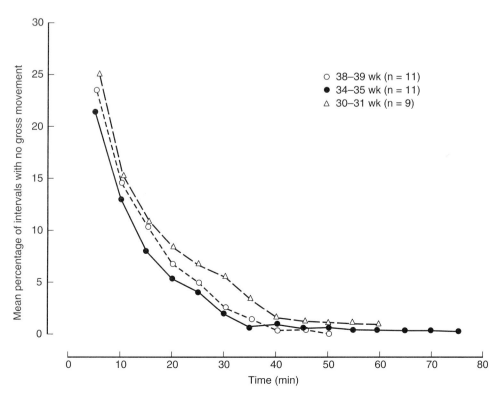

FIGURE 14-6 ■ Composite plot of the percentage of intervals with no gross fetal body movements in nine fetuses at 30 to 31 weeks, 11 at 34 to 35 weeks, and 11 at 38 to 39 weeks. A similar distribution was demonstrated at these different gestational ages. The longest period of fetal quiescence was 60 minutes at 30 to 31 weeks, 75 minutes at 34 to 35 weeks, and 50 minutes at 38 to 39 weeks. (From Patrick J, Campbell K, Carmichael L, et al: Patterns of gross fetal body movements over a 24-hour observation interval during the last 10 weeks of pregnancy. Am J Obstet Gynecol **142**:363, 1982.)

variables with behavioral state organization. Given the cyclic nature of fetal behavioral activity, 70 minutes of observational testing with BPP scoring should be more predictive of a poor fetal outcome than either 30 minutes of ultrasound scanning or 40 minutes of non-stress testing alone. It has yet to be determined whether prolongation of the monitoring interval for any of the dynamic variables, as previously suggested for non-stress testing (Brown and Patrick, 1981), would be equally successful in improving the positive predictive value for poor perinatal outcome. Despite such concerns, a study by Devoe et al. (1992) in high-risk pregnant patients, with concurrent biophysical testing and using established population norms, again found the monitoring of body movements to have a better positive predictive value for adverse perinatal outcome than the other dynamic variables.

Fetal movement activity in the high-risk obstetric patient has also been related to umbilical cord gases and pH obtained at the time of subsequent delivery by elective cesarean section (Vintzileos et al., 1987, 1991; Ribbert, Nicolaides et al., 1993) or by cordocentesis (Ribbert et al., 1990; Manning et al., 1993). From these studies, it appears that decreased FHR reactivity and the absence of breathing movements are earlier manifestations of fetal hypoxemia with onsetting acidemia. This implies a hierarchy within the fetal brain for the control of these activities in response to onsetting hypoxemia or acidemia. Although this may be true, as suggested by studies in the ovine fetus (Richardson et al., 1992), the clinical evidence to date shows considerable overlap of blood gas and pH values among test groupings and is again largely based on arbitrary standards without relation to population norms.

In a longitudinal study of IUGR fetuses, Ribbert, Visser and associates (1993) observed that heart rate reactivity was reduced with the onset of hypoxemia and was followed by a gradual decrease in fetal body movement. The percent time of fetal breathing was little changed with chronic hypoxemia alone but fell to zero with the onset of associated acidemia. Thus, as fetal oxygenation becomes compromised, body movements may be decreased before breathing movements; however, body movements continue to be evident longer because the decrease in body movements is gradual, whereas that for breathing movements is more abrupt. Nonetheless, as clinically used in BPP scoring, the increased sensitivity of non-reactive non-stress testing and absent fetal body movements for predicting adverse perinatal outcome (Vintzileos et al., 1983) is in keeping with their earlier occurrence as fetal oxygenation worsens.

Although the negative predictive value for a normal perinatal outcome is high with BPP scoring, there continues to be a small number of patients with adverse perinatal outcome that is not predicted on the basis of dynamic fetal monitoring (Manning et al., 1987). This serves to emphasize that the monitoring of fetal breathing movements, as well as the other dynamic fetal variables, allows the assessment of fetal health only at the time of testing, from which a probability of continued health may be formulated. An improvement in negative predictive value might occur with more frequent testing, but the time course over which these fetal variables become abnormal before fetal death is not known and may well change with the assorted disease processes and their severity. Anecdotal clinical reports indicate that in some instances deterioration in scoring profiles may occur over as short a time interval as 2 to 3 days (Baskett et al., 1984; Manning et al., 1987). The

TABLE 14-2. FACTORS AFFECTING FETAL BREATHING MOVEMENTS (FBMs) IN HUMANS

Glucose concentration	
Glucose infusions	Increased FBM in patients who have fasted (Natale et al., 1978)
Cigarette smoking	Increased frequency of FBM although incidence unchanged (Fox et al., 1977; Thaler et al., 1980)
Caffeine	Increased FBM with chronic exposure; no effect with acute exposure (McGowan et al., 1987)
Ethanol	Dramatic decrease in FBM (Fox et al., 1978; McLeod et al., 1984)
Methadone	Decreased FBM with chronic exposure (Richardson et al., 1984)
Tocolytics	Dramatic increase in FBM (Hallak et al., 1992)
Other drugs	Small-series reports have appeared on the effects of amylobarbital, diazepam, meperidine, methyldopa, salbutamol, and terbutaline (Lewis and Boylan, 1979)

marked decrease in fetal movement activity required for an abnormal BPP score with the "all or none" criteria appears to be a marker for moderate to severe hypoxemic change with onsetting acidemia as determined by related changes in umbilical cord gases and pH. This is similar to the study of movement activity in the ovine fetus with prolonged reductions in oxygenation (Richardson et al., 1992) and again suggests the need for heightened surveillance in the extremely high-risk pregnancy, perhaps with daily monitoring, because metabolic deterioration may occur rapidly as acidemia worsens.

Other Factors Affecting Breathing Movements

Table 14-2 lists other factors that alter breathing activity in human fetuses.

FETAL BODY MOVEMENTS

Animal Studies

Physiology and Biological Patterns

Study of fetal body movements using fetal animal preparations has been limited; again, most information has been obtained from the ovine fetus. Dawes and colleagues (1972) provided one of the first descriptions in sheep near term delivered into a warm saline bath with intact umbilical cords. Three types of movement activity were observed. In the first, the lamb appeared awake, moved its limbs, raised its head, and opened its eyes. The second type involved slow gentle extension of the limbs and seemed to correspond to non-REM sleep. The third type appeared to correspond to REM sleep and entailed movements of the eyes and twitching of ears, lips, and limbs. Fetal movement activity has subsequently been characterized by the use of EMG leads or transit time ultrasonography on different skeletal muscles, including forelimb, neck (postural muscle activity), and trunk (Ruckebusch et al., 1977; Natale et al., 1981; Szeto and

Hinman, 1985). Simple fetal movements, such as extension of the head and flexion or extension of the limbs, have been identified, as have complex movements characterized by two to three repetitive elements involving combined movements of the neck, limb, and trunk.

Ovine fetal movement activity is also affected by the behavioral state, although the relationship is much less clear than that reported for breathing movements. Simple fetal movements, although episodic in nature, are seen during both high-voltage and low-voltage electrocortical activity characteristic of non-REM and REM sleep, respectively (Ruckebusch et al., 1977; Natale et al., 1981). Complex movements likewise usually occur in clusters and are particularly prevalent during the transition between electrocortical states, although this can also occur both in high-voltage and, to a lesser extent, low-voltage electrocortical activity. Near term, the ovine fetus also demonstrates short periods of wakefulness characterized by low-voltage electrocortical activity and nuchal muscle tone and a marked increase in gross movement activity (Ruckebusch et al., 1977; Szeto and Hinman, 1985). A circadian rhythm in body movements has also been observed characterized by an increase in gross movement activity overnight, which becomes more pronounced near term with the establishment of the awake state (Ruckebusch et al., 1977).

Developmental Changes

A developmental change in the pattern of nuchal muscle activity is evident and appears to be related to behavioral state development (Clewlow et al., 1983). Before 105 days of gestation and with electrocortical activity still undifferentiated, nuchal muscle activity is almost continuous and without obvious pattern or relationship to the other biophysical variables. Thereafter, nuchal muscle activity becomes episodic and, with the distinct differentiation of electrocortical activity after 120 days of gestation, is clearly related to the high-voltage state. Gross body movement activity is also increased in the last few days before birth and probably relates to the appearance at this time of fetal wakefulness (Ruckebusch et al., 1977; Szeto and Hinman, 1985).

Parturition

In the ovine fetus, forelimb movements, although decreased by approximately 50%, continue to be evident throughout labor and are linked to behavioral state activity (Natale et al., 1981). As labor becomes well established, movements are often associated with uterine contractions.

Hypoxia and Asphyxia

In the unanesthetized sheep fetus, moderate hypoxemia of short-term duration (reduction of arterial Po_2 from ~22 to 14 mm Hg for 1 to 2 hours) results in a decrease in fetal forelimb and nuchal muscle activity to less than 30% of control values. (Natale et al., 1981; Bocking and Harding, 1986). This degree of hypoxemia is sufficient to result in metabolic acidemia. With mild hypoxemia (reduction of arterial Po_2 to ~16 mm Hg), nuchal muscle activity is decreased by only 10% to 15% from control values (Woudstra et al., 1990). Although of probable biological significance and representing a protective adaptive mechanism, this small fall in fetal movement activity would be of little clinical use as an indicator of mild fetal hypoxemia. Fetal body movements should also be seen as a potential marker for moderate to severe hypoxemic change and, when markedly decreased, probably reflect a degree of hypoxemia close to that required for the onset of metabolic acidemia.

Human Studies

Physiology and Biological Patterns

Human fetal body movements have been systematically studied over the last half of pregnancy by the use of linear-array real-time imaging techniques, as previously described for the study of human fetal breathing movements. These studies of fetal activity in healthy pregnancies have relied on longitudinal scanning of the fetus, thus permitting the simultaneous measurement of fetal breathing activity. Although these techniques provide accurate measurement of fetal rolling and stretching movements, isolated movements of the fetal limbs are not as well visualized.

Human fetal gross body movements occur approximately 10% of the time over the last 10 weeks of pregnancy, with an average of 31 movements per hour over a 24-hour period (Patrick et al., 1982). As previously noted, near term there is a clustering of fetal breathing and gross body movements, suggesting a relationship to behavioral state activity (Patrick et al., 1978, 1980b). Studies by Nijhuis and coworkers (1982) identified an inextricable linkage of gross body movement activity to other behavioral parameters, thus firmly establishing the existence of fetal behavioral states. Fetal body movements are frequent during *state 2F* (active periods analogous to the REM state) but much reduced or absent during *state 1F* (quiet periods analogous to the non-REM state). This gives rise to an "activity–quiescent" cycle with a duration of approximately 60 minutes by term, although with considerable variability. An additional active fetal period, called *state 4F*, is characterized by frequent and vigorous gross body movements and, by inference from human neonatal studies, appears to represent periods of fetal wakefulness. These are usually seen no more than 10% of the time and are of relatively short duration (5 to 10 minutes).

As a result of the episodic nature of human fetal gross body movements, it is again important to record for a long enough period to be certain that the recording interval does not entirely consist of a normal period of fetal quiescence. From 24-hour observation studies on healthy pregnant patients through the last 10 weeks of pregnancy, it was determined that approximately 25% of 5-minute intervals, 10% of 15-minute intervals, and 5% of 30-minute intervals contained no gross body movement activity (see Fig. 14-6) (Patrick et al., 1982). It was also evident that episodes of fetal quiescence of up to 75 minutes can occasionally occur in healthy human fetuses when recordings are made without attention to time of day.

Near term there is an increase in the incidence and number of gross fetal body movements in the late evening, and this increase may correspond to increased periods of wakefulness (Fig. 14-7) (Patrick et al., 1982). In contrast to fetal breathing movements, gross body movements are not influenced by maternal plasma glucose concentrations or maternal meals during the day (see Fig. 14-7).

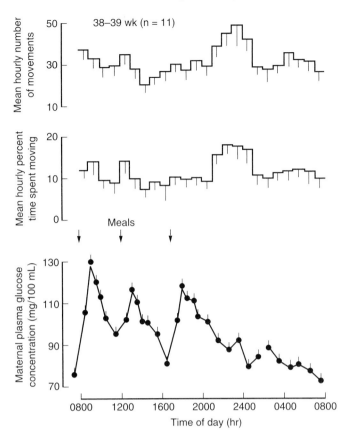

FIGURE 14-7 ■ Maternal glucose concentrations, average number of movements, and percentage of time spent moving by fetuses plotted each hour of the day (± SEM) in 11 fetuses at 38 to 39 weeks' gestational age. There was a peak in activity between 9 PM and 1 AM (From Patrick J, Campbell K, Carmichael L, et al: Patterns of gross fetal body movements over a 24-hour observation interval during the last 10 weeks of pregnancy. Am J Obstet Gynecol **142**:363, 1982.)

Relationship of Body Movements to Heart Rate Accelerations

The relationship of fetal body movements to heart rate accelerations provides the basis for non-stress heart rate testing. Timor-Tritsch and associates (1978), using strain gauges placed on the maternal abdomen wall, reported that 99.8% of all fetal movements of greater than 3 seconds' duration are associated with FHR accelerations (>10 beats/min). Patrick and coworkers (1984), using real-time ultrasound and abdominal electrocardiographic methods, reported that near term 92% of all evident gross body movements were associated with FHR accelerations (≥10 beats/min and lasting ≥10 seconds), whereas 85% of all accelerations occurred in association with body movements. Thus, quantitative observations of fetal movements appear to be interchangeable with FHR accelerations over the last few weeks of pregnancy. However, it remains to be determined whether the compromised fetus with a nonreactive nonstress test has a loss of FHR accelerations with body movements or becomes inactive and stops moving.

Developmental Changes

Longitudinal study of fetal movement activity over the first half of pregnancy reveals that movements even of the young fetus appear to be specific and with recognizable patterning (de

Vries et al., 1985). Fetal movements can be observed from 8 weeks of gestation onward, with a developmental trend in the various movements evident, including a gradual increase in incidence (e.g., breathing movements and swallowing), an increase in incidence until a plateau is reached (e.g., general movements), or an increase in incidence followed by a decrease (e.g., startles). Most of these movements, however, seem to occur at no regular interval, with fetal quiescence usually no longer than 5 to 10 minutes (de Vries et al., 1985).

Recordings of gross fetal body movements at 24 to 28 weeks of gestation have been reported by Nasello-Paterson and coworkers (1988), who found the mean incidence to be approximately 13%, which is similar to the incidence reported over the last 10 weeks of pregnancy (Patrick et al., 1982). However, the total number of movements per hour shows a maturational decrease, suggesting that fetuses between 24 and 28 weeks of gestation move significantly more often but with a shorter duration of movement than do fetuses between 30 and 39 weeks of gestation. Although fetal movement activity is now becoming episodic and clustered with other behavioral variables, the longest period of quiescence was only 24 minutes, which is significantly less than that observed during the last 10 weeks of pregnancy, again suggesting that different norms need to be used in the evaluation of fetal health at earlier gestations. This group also noted a maturational change in the relationship of body movements to heart rate accelerations, whereby the proportion of larger amplitude accelerations (i.e., ≥15 beats/min) increased with gestational age and the proportion of total heart rate accelerations associated with fetal body movements shifted from low amplitude types of accelerations (i.e., <15 beats/min) to accelerations of higher amplitude (i.e., ≥15 beats/min) as fetuses reached 32 weeks of gestation (Natale et al., 1985). These maturational changes have obvious implications for nonstress test scoring in the fetus of younger gestational age.

Although the incidence of fetal body movements changes little over the last half of pregnancy, the emergence of behavioral states has a marked effect on the patterns of movement activity. As periods of coincidence of behavioral parameters give rise to clearly defined behavioral states, a maturational change in the duration of the so-called activity–quiescent cycle is seen, with a progressive increase from approximately 20 minutes' duration at 28 weeks of gestation to approximately 60 minutes by term, which is similar in length to the sleep state cycling of the newborn infant (Nijhuis et al., 1982; Drogtrop et al., 1990).

Parturition

Gross fetal body movements, although somewhat reduced, continue to be evident throughout labor, with a periodicity suggestive of activity–quiescent cycling (Richardson et al., 1979). Unlike fetal breathing movements, the incidence of gross body movements remains unchanged during the last 3 days before spontaneous labor at term (Carmichael et al., 1984).

Intrauterine Growth Restriction

The incidence and number of gross body movements are also variably decreased in patients with IUGR (Bekedam et al., 1985; Gagnon et al., 1988a, 1990; Ruedrich et al., 1989). Although of probable biological significance, with a decrease in energy expenditure and thus oxygen requirements anticipated, considerable overlap with population norms is again evident, as previously discussed for fetal breathing movements. Whether maternal hyperoxia increases the incidence of these movements to a level similar to that of the well-grown fetus is controversial (Ruedrich et al., 1989; Gagnon et al., 1990). Given the inherent periodicity of fetal movement activity, this again is unlikely to serve as a useful clinical marker for IUGR.

Assessment of Fetal Health

The potential usefulness of maternally perceived fetal movement activity as a measure of fetal health has long been recognized (Sadovsky and Polishuk, 1977). Recording of movement by the mother is simple, inexpensive, and readily available and does not require sophisticated equipment. However, maternal perception of fetal activity can be misleading, because some movements go undetected and others are wrongly recorded, instead possibly representing Braxton Hicks contractions or maternal aortic pulsation and respiration. This contributes to the large intrapatient and interpatient variation in the monitoring of fetal movements and the difficulty in establishing population norms.

Connors and colleagues (1988b) studied maternal perception of fetal activity from 24 weeks of gestation until term. Although large interpatient variation in movement counts per hour was evident, only 2% (28 to 40 weeks) to 4% (24 to 27 weeks) of 1-hour observation periods were without perceived movement. When the observation period was extended to 2 consecutive hours, only five observations in one patient contained no movement. These findings correlate closely with the objective ultrasonography data reported by Patrick et al. (1982) and suggest that 2 hours is a sufficient period of time to allow for the normal periodicity of fetal movement activity. Although the ideal number of movements to be counted has not been defined, perception of 10 distinct movements in a period of up to 2 hours is considered reassuring (Moore and Piacquadio, 1989). In the absence of a reassuring count, a biophysical means of fetal assessment with either non-stress testing or ultrasound scanning for fetal movements should be used.

The present use of fetal body movements in the assessment of fetal health also depends on its component part in BPP scoring (see Chapter 21). Thus, much of the discussion on the predictive value of fetal breathing movements in the assessment of fetal health also applies to that for fetal gross body movements.

FETAL GROWTH AND DEVELOPMENT

The abundance of *in utero* movement activity in the healthy fetus and the poor outcome associated with its restriction in animal experimentation and in the human fetus support an important role for movement activity in fetal growth and development.

Breathing Movements

Evidence from animal experimentation and from observations of human fetuses has indicated that fetal breathing movements are important for the normal development of the fetal lungs. Studies in fetal rabbits (Wigglesworth and Desai, 1979) and sheep (Harding et al., 1993) have shown that, following section of the upper cervical spinal cord and elimination of phasic respiratory movements of the diaphragm, the DNA content of the lungs was reduced. Circumstantial evidence from anomalous development of human fetuses also supports the conclusion that loss of fetal breathing movements plays a role in abnormal lung growth with pulmonary hypoplasia, although loss of thoracic volume may be just as important (Liggins, 1984). By opposing lung recoil, breathing movements help to maintain the high level of lung expansion that is now known to be essential for normal growth and structural maturation of the fetal lungs (Harding, 1997). The prolonged absence or impairment of fetal breathing is likely to result in a reduced level of lung expansion, which can then lead to hypoplasia of the lungs.

Body Movements

The neural activity of fetal motility and its motor effects may contribute to the development of muscles, joints, and even the fine structure of the central nervous system itself (Prechtl, 1987). However, there has been little study, either experimentally or of a clinical nature, in this area to date.

FETAL ACTIVITY AND VIBROACOUSTIC STIMULATION

Fetal Response to Stimulation

It is clinically important that periods of fetal quiescence combined with absence of heart rate accelerations may normally occur in human fetuses for up to 75 minutes, as described previously. As a result, there is some difficulty in separating healthy fetuses at rest from sick fetuses who are not moving because of hypoxemia or asphyxia. Neither external physical manipulation of human fetuses (Richardson et al., 1981) nor administration of glucose to women (Bocking et al., 1982) changes the overall pattern of gross fetal body movements. External vibroacoustic stimulation (VAS) is the only stimulus that can reproducibly alter FHR and fetal movement patterns during the third trimester of human pregnancy (Gagnon et al., 1987b). This has led to substantial investigation into the safety and efficacy of the use of external VAS in assessing fetal health.

Structural Development of Fetal Sensory Receptors

The embryonic ear forms from an ectodermal thickening of the auditory placode, which is present in the 23-day-old human embryo (Altmann, 1950). As the placode invaginates into surrounding mesenchyma, a pit develops that assumes a vesicular shape and is termed the otocyst. In the 4- to 5-week-old embryo, the otocyst divides into two lobes; one lobe becomes the cochlea and the other the labyrinth (Ormerod, 1960). At 6 months, both the organ of Corti and the tunnel of Corti are present in all turns of the cochlea. Peripheral vibration-sensitive endings, including Meissner and pacinian corpuscles, which transmit vibrotactile stimuli, have been described in the hands of human fetuses at 24 weeks of gestation. Therefore, by about the 24th week of intrauterine life, the cochlea and peripheral sensory end-organs have reached their normal development.

Functional Development of Fetal Sensory Receptors

In the adult, the ear responds to sound frequencies between approximately 20 and 20,000 Hz. Optimal response occurs at 2000 Hz (Schmidt, 1986). The nature of this frequency response is determined in large measure by the physical characteristics of the receiving organ, the nature of the external auditory canal, the tympanic membrane, and the ossicles that link the tympanic membrane through the middle ear to the fluids in the inner ear. The ear is an impedance-matching device designed to receive sounds transmitted in air. *In utero*, the middle ear and external canals are filled with fluid, which tends to dampen the frequency response of the tympanic membrane and ossicles and may prevent the middle ear from impedance matching. Therefore, fetuses probably require very high sound pressure levels (SPLs) to be able to detect sound.

Some evidence that human fetal auditory receptors are functional comes from records of evoked responses made from scalp electrodes during labor (Scibetta et al., 1971). Newborns exposed to sound stimuli have auditory brain responses that are neuroelectric signals recorded from electroencephalogram electrodes placed on the scalp. Auditory brain responses are now considered valuable in evaluation of newborn hearing function (Despland and Galambos, 1980). Auditory brain responses first appear between 26 and 28 weeks' gestation in preterm human infants, and no auditory brain responses can be detected before 26 weeks. The minimum stimulus intensity required to elicit evoked responses is 65-dB SPL at 25 weeks (Starr et al., 1977); it decreases to 50 dB at 30 to 32 weeks (Uziel et al., 1980) and is adult-like at 35 weeks' gestation (Uziel et al., 1980). The observation of auditory brain responses and maturational changes has been confirmed in catheterized fetal lambs (Woods et al., 1984).

Fetal Sound Environment during Vibroacoustic Stimulation

In contrast to the neonate, the human fetus is surrounded by the fluid-filled amniotic cavity. Until recently, it was not technically feasible to measure the fetal sound environment during the application of VAS on the surface of the maternal abdomen using an electronic artificial larynx. Estimations of intrauterine SPLs during VAS have varied from 90 to 111 dB (Smith et al., 1990) and up to 139 dB (Gerhardt et al., 1988).

We measured the intrauterine background noise in 10 women in active labor using a miniaturized hydrophone placed at the level of the fetal neck under ultrasonographic guidance (Benzaquen et al., 1990). In eight women no cardiovascular sound was audible, and the background intrauterine noise consisted predominantly of low-frequency (<100 Hz) noise with maximum intensity of 85 dB at 12.5 Hz, which is the resonance frequency of the human body (Wasserman, 1990). Intermittent maternal bowel sounds and maternal vocalization featured well above the intrauterine background noise. During VAS, as used in clinical practice during active labor, the intrauterine SPL increased to an average of 95 dB at frequencies between 87 and 20,000 Hz (Gagnon et al., 1992) (Fig. 14-8), which was similar to the overall SPL reported by Smith and associates (1990). In addition, our data indicated that a minimum threshold of 94 dB intrauterine SPL was necessary to elicit a reproducible FHR response (Gagnon et al., 1992).

Gross Fetal Body Movements and Vibroacoustic Stimulation

The presence of a fetal "startle reflex" has been demonstrated during VAS (Leader et al., 1982). This reflex was defined as an immediate marked fetal response involving either trunk or limb movement that occurs during VAS and for about 2.5 seconds afterward.

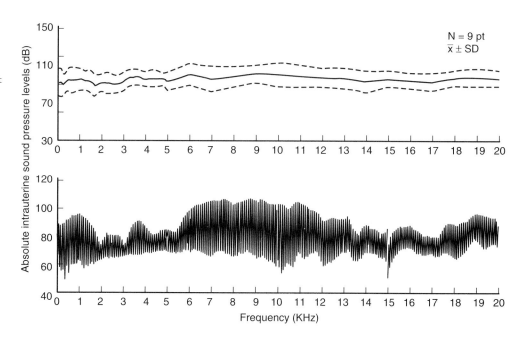

FIGURE 14-8 ■ The mean (95 dB) ± 1 SD (15 dB) intrauterine sound pressure levels (re: 2 × 10^{-3} newtons/m²) during vibroacoustic stimulation at 0 cm from the surface of the maternal abdomen were plotted for frequencies between 87 and 20,000 (Hz) (*top*). A typical example of intrauterine sound pressure levels recorded for frequencies between 87 and 20,000 Hz during vibroacoustic stimulation at 0 cm (*bottom*). (From Gagnon R, Benzaquen S, Hunse C: The fetal sound environment during vibroacoustic stimulation in labor: Effect on fetal heart rate response. Obstet Gynecol **79**:950–955, 1992. Reprinted by permission from the American College of Obstetricians and Gynecologists.)

Gelman and associates (1982) reported a significant increase in the number of fetal movements after a 2000-Hz 110-dB stimulus applied on the maternal abdomen for 1 minute, but not after a 500-Hz stimulus. This increase in fetal activity persisted for 30 minutes after the stimulus. However, Schmidt and associates (1985), using sound stimulation without touching the maternal abdomen, were not able to observe any change in patterns of fetal activity or heart rate.

A prolonged increase in the incidence of fetal body movements has been reported after VAS with an electronic artificial larynx (Gagnon et al., 1986, 1987b; Yao et al., 1990). There was a significant but delayed increase in both the number and incidence of gross fetal body movements between 10 and 30 minutes after a 5-second vibroacoustic stimulus. This delayed increase in body movements occurred in human fetuses only after 33 weeks' gestation (Gagnon et al., 1986, 1987b). In fetuses between 26 and 32 weeks' gestation, gross fetal body movements are not altered after VAS, which demonstrates a maturational change in the fetal responses to VAS possibly related to the development of fetal behavioral states.

Fetal Breathing Movements and Vibroacoustic Stimulation

A significant decrease in fetal breathing movements has been reported only in term (>36 weeks) fetuses after VAS (Gagnon et al., 1987b). Analysis of the mean percentage of total breath-to-breath intervals in successive 0.5-second increments in 10 healthy term fetuses during the hour after control ($n = 5$) or VAS ($n = 5$) demonstrated a skewed distribution of breath-to-breath intervals with a peak of 1.0 to 1.5 seconds after control, but during the hour after stimulus there was a broad distribution of breath-to-breath intervals at 1 to 2.5 seconds without a well-defined peak. This suggested that fetuses were breathing not only less frequently but also more irregularly after stimulation, as is typical of a state of wakefulness (Nijhuis et al., 1982, 1983).

Fetal Heart Rate Response to Vibroacoustic Stimulation

In an attempt to detect deafness during the antenatal period, Johansson and associates (1964) found a significant increase in FHR for 5 seconds after application of a 3000-Hz stimulus at an SPL of 110 dB for 1 second on the surface of the maternal abdomen. This effect on FHR has been noted by many authors (Grimwade et al., 1971; Davey et al., 1984; Jensen, 1984; Serafini et al., 1984) using different frequencies (range of 500 to 3000 Hz) and SPLs (range of 70 to 130 dB). External stimulation with the electronic artificial larynx has produced the most reliable FHR response and is now widely used in clinical practice.

With the use of computerized FHR analysis, responses to VAS in healthy human fetuses have been shown to be altered by gestational age (Gagnon et al., 1987b). There is an immediate FHR response after stimulation characterized by an increase in duration of accelerations in fetuses from 26 weeks to term and an increase in basal FHR after 30 weeks' gestation. There is also a delayed FHR response after 33 weeks' gestation, which consists of an increase in the number of accelerations between 10 and 20 minutes after stimulus (Fig. 14-9) (Gagnon et al.,

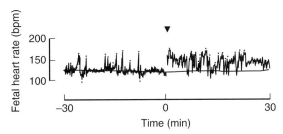

FIGURE 14-9 ■ A typical example of an increase in basal fetal heart rate (FHR) and FHR accelerations after the application of a 5-second vibratory acoustic stimulus with an electronic artificial larynx. (From Gagnon R, Benzaquen S, Hunse C: The fetal sound environment during vibroacoustic stimulation near term: Fetal heart rate and heart rate variability responses. Am J Obstet Gynecol **156:**323, 1987.)

1987a,b), and on occasion a persistent fetal tachycardia can last up to 1.5 hours after stimulation (Gagnon et al., 1987a,b; Visser et al., 1989). The FHR response to VAS is believed to be due to a switch in fetal behavioral states from state 1F to state 4F or to a disruption of normal behavioral states. Numerous factors besides gestational age and unrelated to fetal hypoxemia or acidosis can alter FHR response to VAS (Table 14-3).

Clinical Significance

It is well documented that the presence of fetal body movements and FHR accelerations in response to VAS is associated with minimal risk (<1%) of intrauterine death within a week (Smith et al., 1986). Although FHR accelerations induced by VAS may have the same predictive value for fetal outcome compared with currently used tests of antepartum fetal assessment, no randomized clinical trials have shown that VAS can definitely replace BPP testing (Richards, 1990).

VAS decreases testing time during antepartum FHR testing (Smith et al., 1986) and, in combination with assessment of amniotic fluid volume, may reduce the incidence of unexpected intrauterine fetal deaths (Clark et al., 1989). Goodwin

TABLE 14-3. FACTORS AFFECTING FETAL HEART RATE (FHR) RESPONSE TO VIBROACOUSTIC STIMULATION

Prestimulatory basal FHR	Inversely correlated with amplitude of first FHR acceleration (Gagnon et al., 1988b)
Prestimulus fetal behavioral state	FHR response more consistent during quiet (1F) sleep state (Devoe et al., 1990)
Intrauterine growth retardation	
≥32 weeks	Smaller amplitude and shorter duration of FHR response than normally grown fetus (Gagnon et al., 1988a)
<32 weeks	Rare FHR response (Gagnon et al., 1989)
Rupture of membranes	Decreased occurrence of FHR response (Richards et al., 1988)
Cervical dilatation	Inversely correlated with FHR response (Richards et al., 1988)
Intrauterine sound pressure level reached during stimulus	Positively correlated with duration of first FHR acceleration (Gagnon et al., 1992)

and associates (1994) reported that the use of intrapartum VAS virtually eliminated the use of fetal scalp blood sampling on a large clinical service without increasing the cesarean section rate or the incidence of perinatal asphyxia defined by low Apgar score (<3) at 5 minutes of life.

Under certain conditions, the FHR response to VAS may be difficult to interpret. The fetus may receive a subthreshold stimulus (Gagnon et al., 1992), may have a high prestimulation baseline FHR (Gagnon et al., 1988b), or may be immature (Gagnon et al., 1987b)—all factors that can lead to a falsely nonreactive test. Of more concern is the potentially reactive fetus after VAS in the presence of significant metabolic acidosis (Ingemarrsson et al., 1989; Irion et al., 1996), indicating that VAS may occasionally be a stimulus too strong to differentiate the healthy from the acidotic fetus. This is exemplified in the recent meta-analysis on the use of intrapartum fetal stimulation tests to predict fetal metabolic acidosis (Skupski et al., 2002). It has been demonstrated that the likelihood of fetal metabolic acidosis after a negative VAS test (presence of FHR acceleration in response to the stimulus) was 2.41%. Similarly, the likelihood of fetal metabolic acidosis after a positive test (absence of FHR acceleration in response to the stimulus) following intrapartum VAS was 38.5%. This important information on intrapartum VAS test performance of a false-negative rate of approximately 2.5% and a false-positive rate of approximately 60% should be taken into account for subsequent clinical management decisions during labor. Therefore, if VAS is used to complement non-stress testing or intrapartum FHR monitoring, one should take these limitations into account when interpreting test results.

■ SUMMARY

The abundance of in utero movement activity and/or the resultant outcome from its limitation in either animal experimentation or human case reports supports an important role for such activity in fetal growth and development. With impairments in fetal oxygenation, a decrease in fetal neuromuscular activity may provide an adaptive mechanism whereby energy expenditure and thus oxygen requirements are decreased. Thus, a lack of fetal activity, including both breathing and gross body movements, may serve as a marker for fetal hypoxemia or acidemia. However, a number of biological factors also affect these activities, the most important being the developmental aspects of the fetal behavioral state, which gives rise to the periodic nature of these movements. Gestational age, time of day, relationship to maternal meals, and maternal drug ingestion are also important considerations in interpreting fetal activity measurements. Additionally, it appears that hypoxemia of a chronic nature must approach the level at which acidemia becomes apparent before a marked change in fetal behavioral activity is noted. Fetal biophysical assessment should be seen as a marker for moderate to severe hypoxemic change, with heightened surveillance required for the extremely high-risk pregnancy, because the time course for biophysical alteration before fetal demise may be relatively short.

REFERENCES

Altmann E: Normal development of the ear and its mechanics. Arch Otolaryngol 52:725, 1950.

Anderson DF, Parks CM, Faber JJ: Fetal O$_2$ consumption in sheep during controlled long-term reductions in umbilical blood flow. Am J Physiol 250:H1037, 1986.

Baskett TF: Gestational age and fetal biophysical assessment. Am J Obstet Gynecol 158:332, 1988.

Baskett TF, Gray JH, Prewett SJ, et al: Antepartum fetal assessment using a fetal biophysical profile score. Am J Obstet Gynecol 148:630, 1984.

Battaglia FC, Meschia G: Principal substrates of fetal metabolism. Physiol Rev 58:499, 1978.

Bekedam DJ, Mulder EJH, Snijders RJM, et al: The effects of maternal hyperoxia on fetal breathing movements, body movements and heart rate variation in growth retarded fetuses. Early Hum Dev 27:223, 1991.

Bekedam DJ, Visser GHA, de Vries JJ, et al: Motor behavior in the growth retarded fetus. Early Hum Dev 12:155, 1985.

Bennet L, Johnston BM, Gluckman PD: The central effects of morphine on fetal breathing movements in the fetal sheep. J Dev Physiol 8:297, 1986.

Benzaquen S, Gagnon R, Hunse C, et al: The intrauterine sound environment of the human fetus during labor. Am J Obstet Gynecol 163:484, 1990.

Berger PJ, Walker AM, Horne R, et al: Phasic respiratory activity in the fetal lamb during late gestation and labour. Respir Physiol 65:55, 1986.

Besinger RE, Compton AA, Hayashi RH: The presence or absence of fetal breathing movements as a predictor of outcome in preterm labor. Am J Obstet Gynecol 157:753, 1987.

Bissonnette JM, Hohimer AR, Conrad R, et al: Theophylline stimulates fetal breathing movements during hypoxia. Pediatr Res 28:83, 1990.

Bocking A, Adamson L, Cousin A, et al: Effects of intravenous glucose injections on human fetal breathing movements and gross fetal body movements at 38 to 40 weeks' gestational age. Am J Obstet Gynecol 142:606, 1982.

Bocking AD, Gagnon R, Milne KM, et al: Behavioral activity during prolonged hypoxemia in fetal sheep. J Appl Physiol 65:2420, 1988.

Bocking AD, Harding R: Effects of reduced uterine blood flow on electrocortical activity breathing and skeletal muscle activity in fetal sheep. Am J Obstet Gynecol 154:655, 1986.

Boddy K, Dawes GS: Fetal breathing. Br Med Bull 32:1, 1975.

Boddy K, Dawes GS, Fisher R, et al: Foetal respiratory movements, electrocortical and cardiovascular responses to hypoxaemia and hypercapnia in sheep. J Physiol (Lond) 243:500, 1974.

Boddy K, Dawes GS, Fisher RL, et al: The effects of pentobarbitone and pethidine on foetal breathing movements in sheep. Br J Pharmacol 57:311, 1976.

Boddy K, Dawes GS, Robinson JS: A 24-hour rhythm in the fetus. In Comline RS, Cross KW, Dawes GS, et al (eds): Foetal and Neonatal Physiology. Proceedings of the Sir Joseph Barcroft Centenary Symposium. London, Cambridge University Press, 1973.

Brown R, Patrick J: The nonstress test: How long is enough? Am J Obstet Gynecol 141:646, 1981.

Carmichael L, Campbell K, Patrick J: Fetal breathing, gross fetal body movements and maternal and fetal heart rates before spontaneous labor at term. Am J Obstet Gynecol 148:675, 1984.

Carroll SG, Papaioannou S, Nicolaides KH: Assessment of fetal activity and amniotic fluid volume in the prediction of intrauterine infection in preterm prelabor amniorrhexis. Am J Obstet Gynecol 172:1427, 1995.

Castle BM, Turnbull AC: The significance of preterm breathing. In Beard RW, Sharp F (eds): Preterm Labor and its Consequences. London, The Royal College of Obstetricians and Gynaecologists, 1985.

Clapp JF, Szeto HH, Larrow R, et al: Fetal metabolic response to experimental placental vascular damage. Am J Obstet Gynecol 140:446, 1981.

Clark SL, Sobey P, Jolley K: Nonstress testing with acoustic stimulation and amniotic fluid volume measurement: 5973 tests without unexpected fetal death. Am J Obstet Gynecol 160:694, 1989.

Clewlow F, Dawes GS, Johnston BM, et al: Changes in breathing electrocortical and muscle activity in unanaesthetized fetal lambs with age. J Physiol 341:463, 1983.

Connors G, Hunse C, Carmichael L, et al: The role of carbon dioxide in the generation of human fetal breathing movements. Am J Obstet Gynecol 158:322, 1988a.

Connors G, Natale R, Nasello-Paterson C: Maternally perceived fetal activity from twenty-four weeks' gestation to term in normal and at-risk pregnancies. Am J Obstet Gynecol 158:294, 1988b.

Cox WL, Daffos F, Forestier F, et al: Physiology and management of intrauterine growth retardation: A biologic approach with fetal blood sampling. Am J Obstet Gynecol 159:36, 1988.

Davey DA, Dommisse J, Macnab M, et al: The value of an auditory stimulatory test in antenatal fetal cardiotocography. Eur J Obstet Gynaecol Reprod Biol 18:273, 1984.

Dawes GS, Fox HE, Leduc BM, et al: Respiratory movements and rapid eye movement sleep in the foetal lamb. J Physiol (Lond) 220:119, 1972.

de Vries JIP, Visser GHA, Prechtl HFR: The emergence of fetal behaviour. II. Quantitative aspects. Early Hum Dev **12**:99, 1985.

Derks JB, Owiny J, Sadowski D, et al: Effects of repeated administration of cocaine to the fetal sheep in the last days of pregnancy. Am J Obstet Gynecol **168**:719, 1993.

Despland PA, Galambos R: The auditory brain stem response: A useful diagnostic tool in the intensive care nursery. Pediatr Res **14**:154, 1980.

Devoe LD, Abduljabbar H, Carmichael L, et al: The effects of maternal hyperoxia on fetal breathing movements in third-trimester pregnancies. Am J Obstet Gynecol **148**:790, 1984.

Devoe LD, Castillo RA, Searle N, et al: Prognostic components of computerized fetal biophysical testing. Am J Obstet Gynecol **158**:1144, 1988.

Devoe LD, Murray C, Faircloth D, et al: Vibroacoustic stimulation and fetal behavioural state in normal term human pregnancy. Am J Obstet Gynecol **163**:1156, 1990.

Devoe LD, Youssef AA, Croom CS, et al: Can fetal biophysical observations anticipate outcome in preterm labor or preterm rupture of membranes? Obstet Gynecol **84**:432, 1994.

Devoe LD, Youssef AA, Gardner P, et al: Refining the biophysical profile with a risk-related evaluation of test performance. Am J Obstet Gynecol **167**:346, 352, 1992.

Drogtrop AP, Ubels R, Nijhuis JG: The association between fetal body movements, eye movements, and heart rate patterns in pregnancies between 25 and 30 weeks of gestation. Early Hum Dev **23**:67, 1990.

Fox HE, Hohler CW: Fetal evaluation by real-time imaging. Clin Obstet Gynecol **20**:339, 1977.

Fox HE, Steinbrecher M, Pessel D, et al: Maternal ethanol ingestion and the occurrence of human fetal breathing movements. Am J Obstet Gynecol **132**:354, 1978.

Gagnon R, Benzaquen S, Hunse C: The fetal sound environment during vibroacoustic stimulation in labor: Effect on fetal heart rate response. Obstet Gynecol **79**:950, 1992.

Gagnon R, Hunse C, Carmichael L, et al: Effects of vibratory acoustic stimulation on human fetal breathing and gross fetal body movements near term. Am J Obstet Gynecol **155**:1227, 1986.

Gagnon R, Hunse C, Carmichael L, et al: External vibroacoustic stimulation near term: Fetal heart rate and heart rate variability responses. Am J Obstet Gynecol **156**:323, 1987a.

Gagnon R, Hunse C, Carmichael L, et al: Human fetal responses to vibratory acoustic stimulation from twenty-six weeks to term. Am J Obstet Gynecol **157**:1375, 1987b.

Gagnon R, Hunse C, Carmichael L, et al: Vibratory acoustic stimulation in the 26- to 32-week small-for-gestational-age fetus. Am J Obstet Gynecol **160**:160, 1989.

Gagnon R, Hunse C, Fellows F, et al: Fetal heart rate and activity patterns in growth-retarded fetuses: Changes after vibratory acoustic stimulation. Am J Obstet Gynecol **158**:265, 1988a.

Gagnon R, Hunse C, Patrick J: Fetal responses to vibratory acoustic stimulation: Influence of basal heart rate. Am J Obstet Gynecol **159**:835, 1988b.

Gagnon R, Hunse C, Vijan S: The effect of maternal hyperoxia on behavioral activity in growth-retarded human fetuses. Am J Obstet Gynecol **163**:1894, 1990.

Gauthier DW, Meyer WJ, Bieniarz A: Biophysical profile as a predictor of amniotic fluid culture results. Obstet Gynecol **80**:102, 1992.

Gelman SR, Wood S, Spellacy WN, et al: Fetal movements in response to sound stimulation. Am J Obstet Gynecol **143**:484, 1982.

Gerhardt KJ, Abrams RM, Kovaz B, et al: Intrauterine noise levels in pregnant ewes produced by sound applied to the abdomen. Am J Obstet Gynecol **159**:228, 1988.

Ghidini A, Salafia CM, Kirn V, et al: Biophysical profile in predicting acute ascending infection in preterm rupture of membranes before 32 weeks. Am J Obstet Gynecol **96**:201, 2000.

Goldstein I, Romero R, Merrill S, et al: Fetal body and breathing movements as predictors of intraamniotic infection in preterm premature rupture of membranes. Am J Obstet Gynecol **159**:363, 1988.

Goodwin TM, Milner-Masterson L, Paul RH: Elimination of fetal scalp blood sampling on a large clinical service. Obstet Gynecol **83**:971, 1994.

Grimwade JG, Walker DW, Bartlett M, et al: Human fetal heart rate change and movement in response to sound and vibration. Am J Obstet Gynecol **109**:86, 1971.

Hallak M, Moise KJ, Lira N, et al: The effect of tocolytic agents (indomethacin and terbutaline) on fetal breathing and body movements: A prospective, randomized, double-blind, placebo-controlled clinical trial. Am J Obstet Gynecol **167**:1059, 1992.

Harding R: Fetal pulmonary development: the role of respiratory movements. Equine Vet J **24** (Suppl):32, 1997.

Harding R, Hooper SB, Han VKM: Abolition of fetal breathing movements by spinal cord transection leads to reductions in fetal lung liquid volume, lung growth and IGF-II gene expression. Pediatr Res **34**:148, 1993.

Harding R, Sigger JN, Wickham PJD, et al: The regulation of flow of pulmonary fluid in fetal sheep. Respir Physiol **57**:47, 1984.

Hasan SU, Lee DS, Gibson DA, et al: Effect of morphine on breathing and behavior in fetal sheep. J Appl Physiol **64**:2058, 1988.

Hogg MIJ, Golding RH, Rosen M: The effect of doxapram on fetal breathing in the sheep. Br J Obstet Gynaecol **84**:48, 1977.

Hohimer AR, Bissonnette JM: Effect of metabolic acidosis on fetal breathing movements in utero. Respir Physiol **43**:99, 1981.

Hohimer AR, Bissonnette JM, Richardson BS, et al: Central chemical regulation of breathing movements in fetal lambs. Respir Physiol **51**:99, 1983.

Ingemarsson I, Alulkumaran S: Reactive fetal heart rate response to vibroacoustic stimulation in fetuses with low scalp blood pH. Br J Obstet Gynaecol **96**:562, 1989.

Ioffe S, Jansen AH, Chernick V: Maturation of spontaneous fetal diaphragmatic activity and fetal response to hypercapnia and hypoxemia. J Appl Physiol **63**:609, 1987.

Irion O, Stuckelberger P, Moutquin JM, et al: Is intrapartum vibratory acoustic stimulation a valid alternative to fetal pH determination? Br J Obstet Gynaecol **103**:642, 1996.

Jansen AH, Ioffe S, Chernick V: Drug-induced changes in fetal breathing activity and sleep state. Can J Physiol Pharmacol **61**:315, 1983.

Jensen OH: Fetal heart rate response to a controlled sound stimulus as a measure of fetal well-being. Acta Obstet Gynaecol Scand **63**:97, 1984.

Johansson B, Wedenberg E, Westen B: Measurement of tone response by the human fetus: A preliminary report. Acta Otolaryngol **57**:188, 1964.

Junge HD, Walter H: Behavioral states and breathing activity in the fetus near term. J Perinat Med **8**:150, 1980.

Kitterman JA, Liggins GC, Clements JA, et al: Stimulation of breathing movements in fetal sheep by inhibitors of prostaglandin synthesis. J Dev Physiol **1**:453, 1979.

Kitterman JA, Liggins GC, Fewell JE, et al: Inhibition of breathing movements in fetal sheep by prostaglandins. J Appl Physiol **54**:687, 1983.

Koos BJ, Kitanaka T, Matsuda Y, et al: Fetal breathing adaptation to prolonged hypoxaemia in sheep. J Dev Physiol **10**:161, 1988.

Leader LR, Baillie P, Martin B, et al: The assessment and significance of habituation to a repeated stimulus by human fetus. Early Hum Dev **7**:211, 1982.

Lewis P, Boylan P: Fetal breathing: A review. Am J Obstet Gynecol **134**:587, 1979.

Liggins GC: Growth of the fetal lung. J Dev Physiol **6**:237–248, 1984.

Maloney JE, Adamson TM, Brodecky V, et al: Diaphragmatic activity and lung liquid flow in unanesthetized fetal sheep. J Appl Physiol **39**:587, 1975b.

Manning FA, Morrison I, Harman CR, et al: Fetal assessment based on fetal biophysical profile scoring: Experience in 19,221 referred high-risk pregnancies. Am J Obstet Gynecol **157**:880, 1987.

Manning FA, Platt LD, Sipos L: Antepartum fetal evaluation: Development of a fetal biophysical profile. Am J Obstet Gynecol **136**:787, 1980.

Manning FA, Snijders R, Harman CR, et al: Fetal biophysical profile score. VI. Correlation with antepartum umbilical venous fetal pH. Am J Obstet Gynecol **169**:755, 1993.

Martin CB, Murata Y, Petrie RH, et al: Respiratory movements in fetal rhesus monkeys. Am J Obstet Gynecol **119**:939, 1974.

Matsuda Y, Patrick J, Carmichael L, et al: Effects of sustained hypoxemia on the sheep fetus at mid-gestation: Endocrine cardiovascular and biophysical responses. Am J Obstet Gynecol **167**:531, 1992.

Matsuda Y, Patrick J, Carmichael L, et al: Recovery of the ovine fetus from sustained hypoxia: Effect on endocrine, cardiovascular, and biophysical activity. Am J Obstet Gynecol **170**:1433, 1994.

McGowan J, Devoe LD, Searle N, et al: The effects of long- and short-term maternal caffeine ingestion on human fetal breathing and body movements in term gestations. Am J Obstet Gynecol **157**:726, 1987.

McLeod W, Brien J, Carmichael L, et al: Maternal glucose injections do not alter the suppression of fetal breathing following maternal ethanol ingestion. Am J Obstet Gynecol **148**:634, 1984.

Moore TR, Piacquadio K: A prospective evaluation of fetal movement screening to reduce the incidence of antepartum fetal death. Am J Obstet Gynecol **160**:1075, 1989.

Morrison JM, Chien C, Gruber N, et al: Fetal behavioural state changes following maternal fluoxetine infusion in sheep. Dev Brain Res **131**:47, 2001.

Mostello D, Chalk C, Khoury J, et al: Chronic anemia in pregnant ewes: Maternal and fetal effects. Am J Physiol **261**:R1075, 1991.

Murai DT, Lee C-CH, Wallen LD, et al: Denervation of peripheral chemoreceptors decreases breathing movements in fetal sheep. J Appl Physiol **59:**575, 1985.

Nasello-Paterson C, Natale R, Connors G: Ultrasonic evaluation of fetal body movements over twenty-four hours in the human fetus at 24 to 28 weeks' gestation. Am J Obstet Gynecol **158:**312, 1988.

Natale R, Clewlow F, Dawes GS: Measurement of fetal forelimb movements in lambs in utero. Am J Obstet Gynecol **158:**545, 1981.

Natale R, Nasello-Paterson C, Connors G: Patterns of fetal breathing activity in the human fetus at 24 to 28 weeks' gestation. Am J Obstet Gynecol **158:**317, 1988.

Natale R, Nasello-Peterson C, Turliuk R: Longitudinal measurements of fetal breathing body movements, heart rate and heart rate accelerations and decelerations at 24 to 32 weeks of gestation. Am J Obstet Gynecol **151:**256, 1985.

Natale R, Patrick J, Richardson B: Effects of maternal venous plasma glucose concentrations on fetal breathing movements. Am J Obstet Gynecol **132:**36, 1978.

Nijhuis JG, Martin CB, Gommers S, et al: The rhythmicity of fetal breathing varies with behavioural state in the human fetus. Early Hum Dev **9:**1, 1983.

Nijhuis JG, Prechtl HFR, Martin CB, et al: Are there behavioural states in the human fetus? Early Hum Dev **6:**177, 1982.

Ormerod FC: The pathology of congenital deafness in the child. *In* Ewing A (ed): The Modern Educational Treatment of Deafness. Manchester, Manchester University Press, 1960, p. 811.

Patrick J, Campbell K, Carmichael L, et al: A definition of human fetal apnea and the distribution of fetal apneic intervals during the last 10 weeks of pregnancy. Am J Obstet Gynecol **136:**471, 1980a.

Patrick J, Campbell K, Carmichael L, et al: Patterns of human fetal breathing during the last 10 weeks of pregnancy. Obstet Gynecol **56:**24, 1980b.

Patrick J, Campbell K, Carmichael L, et al: Patterns of gross fetal body movements over a 24-hour observation interval during the last 10 weeks of pregnancy. Am J Obstet Gynecol **142:**363, 1982.

Patrick J, Carmichael L, Chess L, et al: Accelerations of the human fetal heart rate at 38 to 40 weeks gestational age. Am J Obstet Gynecol **148:**35, 1984.

Patrick J, Challis J, Campbell K, et al: Circadian rhythms in maternal plasma cortisol and estriol concentrations at 30 to 31, 34 to 35, and 38 to 39 weeks' gestational age. Am J Obstet Gynecol **136:**325, 1980.

Patrick J, Challis JRG, Cross J: Effects of maternal indomethacin administration on fetal breathing movements in sheep. J Dev Physiol **9:**295, 1987a.

Patrick J, Challis JRG, Cross J, et al: The relationship between fetal breathing movements and prostaglandin E$_2$ during ACTH-induced labour in sheep. J Dev Physiol **9:**287, 1987b.

Patrick J, Natale R, Richardson B: Patterns of human fetal breathing activity at 34 to 35 weeks' gestational age. Am J Obstet Gynecol **132:**507, 1978.

Patrick J, Richardson B, Hasen G, et al: Effects of maternal ethanol infusion on fetal cardiovascular and brain activity in lambs. Am J Obstet Gynecol **151:**859, 1985.

Piercy WN, Day MA, Neims AH, et al: Alteration of ovine fetal respiratory-like activity by diazepam, caffeine and doxapram. Am J Obstet Gynecol **127:**43, 1977.

Platt LD, Eglinton GS, Sipos L, et al: Further experience with the biophysical profile. Obstet Gynecol **61:**480, 1983.

Prechtl HFR: Perinatal development of postnatal behaviour. *In* Rauh H, Steinhausen H (eds): Psychobiology and Early Development. North-Holland, Elsevier, 1987, p. 231.

Ribbert LS, Nicolaides KH, Visser GHA: Prediction of fetal acidaemia in intrauterine growth retardation: Comparison of quantified fetal activity with biophysical profile score. Br J Obstet Gynaecol **100:**653, 1993.

Ribbert LSM, Snijders RJM, Nicolaides KH, et al: Relationship of fetal biophysical profile and blood gas values at cordocentesis in severely growth-retarded fetuses. Am J Obstet Gynecol **163:**569, 1990.

Ribbert LSM, Visser GHA, Mulder EJH, et al: Changes with time in fetal heart rate variation, movement incidences and haemodynamics in intrauterine growth-retarded fetuses: A longitudinal approach to the assessment of fetal well-being. Early Hum Dev **31:**195, 1993.

Richards DS: The fetal vibroacoustic stimulation test: An update. Semin Perinatol **14:**305, 1990.

Richards DS, Cefalo RC, Thorpe JM, et al: Determinants of fetal heart rate response to vibroacoustic stimulation in labor. Obstet Gynecol **71:**535, 1988.

Richardson B, Campbell K, Carmichael L, et al: Effects of external physical stimulation on fetuses near term. Am J Obstet Gynecol **139:**344, 1981.

Richardson B, Hohimer AR, Mueggler P, et al: Effects of glucose concentration on fetal breathing movements and electrocortical activity in fetal lambs. Am J Obstet Gynecol **142:**678, 1982.

Richardson B, Natale R, Patrick J: Human fetal breathing activity during induced labor at term. Am J Obstet Gynecol **133:**147, 1979.

Richardson B, O'Grady JP, Olsen GD: Fetal breathing movements and the response to carbon dioxide in patients on methadone maintenance. Am J Obstet Gynecol **150:**400, 1984.

Richardson BS, Carmichael L, Homan J, et al: Electrocortical activity, electroocular activity and breathing movements in fetal sheep with prolonged and graded hypoxemia. Am J Obstet Gynecol **167:**553, 1992.

Rosemond RI, Glass CA, Wingo CE: Daily fetal movement and breathing assessments in the management of preterm membrane rupture. J Matern Fetal Invest **5:**236, 1995.

Ruckebusch Y, Gaujoux M, Eghbali B: Sleep cycles and kinesis in the foetal lamb. Electroencephalogr Clin Neurophysiol **42:**226, 1977.

Ruedrich DA, Devoe LD, Searle N: Effects of maternal hyperoxia on the biophysical assessment of fetuses with suspected intrauterine growth retardation. Am J Obstet Gynecol **161:**188, 1989.

Rurak DW, Gruber NC: Increased oxygen consumption associated with breathing activity in fetal lambs. J Appl Physiol **54:**701, 1983a.

Rurak DW, Gruber NC: The effect of neuromuscular blockade on oxygen consumption and blood gases in the fetal lamb. Am J Obstet Gynecol **145:**258, 1983b.

Sadovsky E, Polishuk WZ: Fetal movement in utero: Nature assessment, prognostic value, timing of delivery. Obstet Gynecol **50:**49, 1977.

Schmidt RF: Fundamentals of Sensory Physiology, 3rd ed. Berlin, Springer-Verlag, 1986.

Schmidt W, Boos R, Gnirs LA, et al: Fetal behavioural states and controlled sound stimulation. Early Hum Dev **12:**145, 1985.

Scibetta JJ, Rosen MG, Hochburg CI, et al: Human fetal brain response to sound during labor. Am J Obstet Gynecol **109:**82, 1971.

Serafini P, Lindsay MJB, Nages DA, et al: Antepartum fetal heart rate response to sound stimulation: The acoustic stimulation test. Am J Obstet Gynecol **148:**41, 1984.

Skupski DW, Rosenberg CR, Eglinton GS: Intrapartum fetal stimulation tests: A meta-analysis. Obstet Gynecol **99:**129, 2002.

Smith CV, Phelan JP, Platt LD: Fetal acoustic stimulation testing (the Fas test). II. A randomized clinical comparison with the non-stress test. Am J Obstet Gynecol **155:**131, 1986.

Smith CV, Satt B, Phelan JP, et al: Intrauterine sound levels: Intrapartum assessment with an intrauterine microphone. Am J Perinatol **7:**312, 1990.

Smith GN, Brien JF, Carmichael L, et al: Development of tolerance to ethanol-induced suppression of breathing movements and brain activity in the near-term fetal sheep during short-term maternal administration of ethanol. J Dev Physiol **11:**189, 1989.

Soothill PW, Nicolaides KH, Campbell S: Prenatal asphyxia hyperlacticaemia, hypoglycaemia, and erythroblastosis in growth retarded fetuses. Br Med J **294:**1051, 1987.

Stark RI, Myers MM: Effect of electroencephalographic state on fetal breathing activity in the baboon. Abstract presented at the Proceedings of the 39th Annual Meeting of the Society for Gynecologic Investigation, March 18–21, 1992, San Antonio, Texas.

Starr A, Amlie RN, Martin WH, et al: Development of auditory function in newborn infants revealed by auditory brainstem potentials. Pediatrics **60:**831, 1977.

Szeto HH: Effects of narcotic drugs on fetal behavioral activity: Acute methadone exposure. Am J Obstet Gynecol **146:**211, 1983.

Szeto HH, Hinman DJ: Prenatal development of sleep-wake patterns in sheep. Sleep **8:**347, 1985.

Thaler JS, Goodman JDS, Dawes GS: The effect of maternal smoking on fetal breathing rate and activity patterns. Am J Obstet Gynecol **138:**282, 1980.

Timor-Tritsch IE, Dierker LJ, Zador I, et al: Fetal movements associated with fetal heart rate accelerations and decelerations. Am J Obstet Gynecol **131:**276, 1978.

Uziel A, Marot M, Germain M: Les potentiels eávoqueá du nerf auditif et du tronc ceáreábral chez le nouveau-neá et l'enfant. Rev Laryngol Otol Rhinol **101:**55, 1980.

van Vliet MAT, Martin CB, Nijhuis JG, et al: The relationship between fetal activity and behavioral states and fetal breathing movements in normal and growth-retarded fetuses. Am J Obstet Gynecol **153:**582, 1985.

Vintzileos AM, Campbell WA, Ingardia CJ, et al: The fetal biophysical profile and its predictive value. Obstet Gynecol **62:**271, 1983.

Vintzileos AM, Campbell WA, Nochimson DJ, et al: The fetal biophysical profile in patients with premature rupture of the membranes: An early predictor of fetal infection. Am J Obstet Gynecol **152:**510, 1985.

Vintzileos AM, Campbell WA, Nochimson DJ, et al: Fetal biophysical profile versus amniocentesis in predicting infection in preterm premature rupture of the membranes. Obstet Gynecol **68:**488, 1986.

Vintzileos AM, Feinstein SJ, Lodeiro JG, et al: Fetal biophysical profile and the effect of premature rupture of the membranes. Obstet Gynecol **67:**818, 1986.

Vintzileos AM, Fleming AD, Scorza WE, et al: Relationship between fetal biophysical activities and umbilical cord blood gas values. Am J Obstet Gynecol **165:**707, 1991.

Vintzileos AM, Gaffney SE, Salinger LM, et al: The relationship among the fetal biophysical profile, umbilical cord pH, and Apgar scores. Am J Obstet Gynecol **157:**627, 1987.

Visser GHA, Mulder HH, Wit HP, et al: Vibro-acoustic stimulation of the human fetus: Effects on behavioral state organization. Early Hum Dev **19:**285, 1989.

Walker DW: Effects of increased core temperature on breathing movements and electrocortical activity in fetal sheep. J Dev Physiol **10:**513, 1988.

Wasserman DE: Vibration: Principles, measurements and health standards. Semin Perinatol **14:**311, 1990.

Wigglesworth JD, Desai R: Effects on lung growth of cervical cord section in the rabbit fetus. Early Human Dev **3:**51, 1979.

Wittman BK, Davison BM, Lyons E, et al: Real-time ultrasound observation of fetal activity in labor. Am J Obstet Gynecol **86:**178, 1979.

Woods JR, Plessinger M, Mack C: The fetal auditory brainstem response. Pediatr Res **18:**83, 1984.

Worthington D, Piercy WN, Smith BT: Effects of reduction of placental size in sheep. Obstet Gynecol **58:**215, 1981.

Woudstra BR, Aarnoudse JG, de Wolf THM, et al: Nuchal muscle activity at different levels of hypoxemia in fetal sheep. Am J Obstet Gynecol **162:**559, 1990.

Yao QW, Jakobsson J, Nymon M, et al: Fetal responses to different intensity levels of vibroacoustic stimulation. Obstet Gynecol **75:**206, 1990.

Chapter 15

PLACENTAL RESPIRATORY GAS EXCHANGE AND FETAL OXYGENATION

Giacomo Meschia, MD

Knowledge of respiratory gas exchange across the human placenta depends on the integrating of observations in pregnant patients with experimental findings in laboratory animals. This integration is necessary because data on the physiology of the human fetus are scant and cannot be interpreted correctly in the absence of experimental evidence. The evidence in laboratory animals consists of a fairly comprehensive set of data in sheep with chronically implanted vascular catheters in the maternal and fetal circulation and a more limited but important set of data in nonhuman primates and other mammals.

TRANSPORT OF ATMOSPHERIC OXYGEN TO THE GRAVID UTERUS

The transport of oxygen (O_2) from the atmosphere to fetal tissues can be visualized as a sequence of six steps that alternate bulk transport with transport by diffusion (Fig. 15-1). The first three steps of this process are part of general physiologic knowledge and therefore are presented here briefly.

In *step 1*, transport from the atmosphere to the alveoli is by action of the respiratory muscles, which move air in and out of the lungs. This action maintains the partial pressure of oxygen (P_{O_2}) in the alveoli at a level that is regulated by several physiologic mechanisms, some of which are driven by sensors of the P_{O_2}, partial pressure of carbon dioxide (P_{CO_2}), and pH of maternal blood. During pregnancy, the maternal organism is set to regulate arterial P_{CO_2} at a lower level than in the nonpregnant state.

In *step 2*, oxygen diffuses from the alveoli into the maternal red blood cells that circulate through the lungs. In the normal organism at sea level, the diffusion rate is so rapid that the P_{O_2} at the venous end of the pulmonary capillaries becomes virtually equal to the P_{O_2} in the adjacent alveoli. Nevertheless, the P_{O_2} of maternal arterial blood is somewhat less than the P_{O_2} in a sample of alveolar air, in part because some deoxygenated blood bypasses the lungs and in part because ventilation and perfusion of the alveoli are not matched evenly throughout the lungs. Under pathologic conditions that prevent the equilibration of P_{O_2} between alveoli and blood, increase the degree of uneven ventilation-perfusion, or shunt more deoxygenated blood directly into the arterial system, the P_{O_2} difference between alveolar air and arterial blood becomes larger.

In *step 3*, maternal blood, propelled by action of the maternal heart, transports oxygen from the lungs to the gravid uterus via the pulmonary veins, left atrium, left ventricle, aorta, uterine arteries, and branches of the ovarian and vaginal arteries. Oxygen is transported by blood in two forms, free and bound to hemoglobin. In any blood samples, these two forms are in reversible equilibrium. The special nomenclature for the components of this equilibrium is summarized in Table 15-1.

OXYGEN UPTAKE BY THE UTERUS AND FETUS

The oxygen uptake by the uterus and the fetus can be calculated by measuring simultaneously uterine and umbilical blood flows and the oxygen content of blood samples drawn from four blood vessels: maternal artery, uterine vein, umbilical vein, and umbilical artery. A numerical example of these calculations is presented in Figure 15-2.

The rationale, commonly known as the *Fick principle*, is as follows. Each milliliter of maternal blood in passing through the pregnant uterus gives up a certain amount of oxygen, which one can calculate by measuring the difference in oxygen content between maternal arterial blood and uterine venous blood. The quantity of oxygen lost by each milliliter of blood is then multiplied by the milliliters of blood flowing through the pregnant uterus to obtain the uterine oxygen uptake. To calculate the rate at which the fetus takes up oxygen from the placenta, one would apply exactly the same reasoning to the umbilical blood data. Note that the oxygen uptake by the gravid uterus is greater than the oxygen uptake by the fetus. This is so because the placenta is metabolically active and consumes a relatively large fraction of the oxygen that the uterine circulation delivers to the gravid uterus.

Fetal growth is accompanied by an increase in fetal oxygen uptake. However, oxygen uptake and fetal weight do not grow proportionally. A 200-g mid-gestation fetal lamb has an average oxygen uptake of 0.460 μmol/min/g, whereas a 3000-g near-term fetus has an average uptake of 0.340 μmol/min/g (Bell et al., 1986). The differences in uptake are much larger if the uptake is related to fetal dry weight because fetal growth is accompanied by a decrease in fetal water content. Oxygen uptake expressed per unit fetal dry weight is about 2.5 times higher at mid-gestation.

Given this complexity and the lack of comparable information for the human fetus, it is important to ask whether fetal oxygen uptake measurements in experimental animals can be

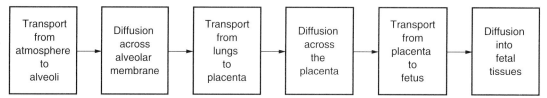

FIGURE 15-1 ■ Transport of oxygen from the atmosphere to the fetal tissues in a sequence of steps that alternate bulk and diffusional transport. (From Meschia G: Supply of oxygen to the fetus. J Reprod Med **23**:160, 1979.)

used to estimate human fetal oxygen uptake. If the aim is an accurate estimate, the answer must be no because several interspecies differences are likely to affect oxygen demand. For example, in comparing near-term ovine and human fetuses of equal body weight, one must note that the human fetus has a much larger brain mass, has more adipose tissue, lives at a lower body temperature, and grows more slowly. It would be surprising if all these differences did not add up to a significant difference in oxygen uptake. However, attempts to measure near-term fetal oxygen consumption rates in different species (i.e., horse, cattle, rhesus monkey, guinea pig) have yielded values of oxygen uptake per gram wet weight that are within ±20% of the fetal lamb value despite very large differences in body size, rate of growth, and body composition (Battaglia and Meschia, 1986). Therefore, one may assume that data in experimental animals provide an approximate estimate of human fetal oxygen demand.

Oxygen Pressures in Uterine and Umbilical Circulations

In chronic sheep preparations, the P_{O_2} of umbilical venous blood, which is the most oxygenated blood of the fetal organism, is low in comparison with maternal arterial P_{O_2} (Table 15-2).

The major reason for this large P_{O_2} difference is that the ovine placenta functions as a venous equilibration system. To understand how such a system works, one must consider its prototype, the concurrent exchanger presented in Figure 15-3.

Two channels are separated by a semipermeable membrane. Maternal blood is pumped through one channel and fetal blood is pumped through the other channel in such a way that both streams run in the same direction. The mother's arterial blood enters the exchanger with a P_{O_2} higher than that of fetal arterial blood. This establishes at the arterial end of the system a maternal–fetal P_{O_2} gradient that moves oxygen across the membrane.

As the two bloodstreams proceed toward the venous end, there is a progressive decrease of P_{O_2} in the maternal blood and a progressive increase of P_{O_2} in the fetal blood. If the streams flow sufficiently slowly or if the membrane is sufficiently permeable to oxygen, maternal and fetal blood can exit the exchanger with identical P_{O_2} values. Note the important boundary condition that under no circumstances can the recipient stream exit with a venous P_{O_2} higher than the venous P_{O_2} of the donor stream.

The structure of the ovine placenta is more complex than that of a concurrent exchanger. Nevertheless, it shares with the concurrent model a basic property, namely that the venous P_{O_2} of the umbilical circulation depends on and cannot be higher than the venous P_{O_2} of the uterine circulation (Rankin et al., 1971). An experimental demonstration of this fact is presented in Figure 15-4. In every instance, the umbilical venous P_{O_2} is less than the uterine venous P_{O_2}. This means

TABLE 15-1. BLOOD OXYGEN TRANSPORT: NOMENCLATURE, SYMBOLS, UNITS, METHODS OF MEASUREMENT, AND INTERRELATIONSHIPS

Nomenclature	Symbol	Units	Methods of Measurement
Free O_2	$[O_2]$	mM*	
O_2 bound to hemoglobin	$[HbO_2]$	mM*	
O_2 content	$[O_2\,Tot]$	mM*	e.g., Van Slyke apparatus
O_2 pressure	P_{O_2}	mm Hg†	P_{O_2} electrode
Hemoglobin	$[Hb]$	mM*	Spectrophotometer
O_2 capacity	$[O_2\,CAP]$	mM*	
O_2 saturation	S	—	Spectrophotometer
O_2 saturation × 100	% S	—	

$[O_2\,Tot] = [HbO_2] + [O_2]$
$[O_2\,CAP] = 4\,[Hb]$‡
$S = [HbO_2] \div [O_2\,CAP]$
$[O_2] = \alpha_{O_2}\,P_{O_2}$ (where α_{O_2} = O_2 solubility coefficient)

* Another unit used often in reporting quantities of O_2 is mL_{STP} (1 millimol = 22.4 mL_{STP}).
† The unit millimeters of mercury (mm Hg) is also called the torr.
‡ Each hemoglobin molecule can combine with four molecules of oxygen.

Measured Quantities

Maternal arterial O_2 content (A): 0.143 ml_{STP}/ml of blood
Uterine venous O_2 content (V): 0.109 ml_{STP}/ml of blood
Umbilical arterial O_2 content (a): 0.078 ml_{STP}/ml of blood
Umbilical venous O_2 content (v): 0.115 ml_{STP}/ml of blood
Uterine blood flow (F): 1412 ml/min
Umbilical blood flow (f): 716 ml/min
Fetal body weight (BW): 4.0 kg
Uteroplacental unit weight (UPW): 1.0 kg

Calculations

O_2 uptake by the gravid uterus:	$(A - V) \times F = 48.0\ ml_{STP}$/min
O_2 uptake by the fetus:	$(v - a) \times f = 26.5\ ml_{STP}$/min
O_2 uptake per kg by fetus:	$(v - a) \times f \div BW =$ 6.6 ml_{STP}/min/kg
O_2 uptake per kg by fetus and uteroplacental unit:	$(A - V) \times F \div (BW + UPW)$ = 9.6 ml_{STP}/min/kg

FIGURE 15-2 ■ Numerical example of the application of the Fick principle to a calculation of the oxygen uptake by the pregnant uterus and the fetus. Representative data from experiments in chronic sheep preparations during the last 2 weeks of pregnancy.

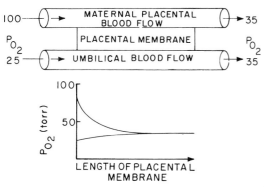

FIGURE 15-3 ■ Concurrent model of transplacental oxygen diffusion. P_{O_2}, partial pressure of oxygen.

TABLE 15-2. REPRESENTATIVE P_{O_2} VALUES IN UTERINE AND UMBILICAL CIRCULATIONS OF SHEEP

Location	P_{O_2} (mm Hg)
Uterine artery	72
Uterine vein	42
Umbilical vein	28
Umbilical artery	19

that the transfer of oxygen from the uterine to the umbilical circulation does not attain the maximum level of performance of a venous equilibrator. To explain this inefficiency, the following factors must be considered:

1. *Shunts.* Part of the uterine blood flow is shunted away from the area of exchange and perfuses the myometrium and the endometrial gland. A fraction of umbilical blood flow does not perfuse the placental cotyledons. In addition to anatomic shunts are diffusional shunts within the maternal and fetal placental microcirculations (Fig. 15-5).
2. *Uneven perfusion.* Both within and among the placental cotyledons there is a certain degree of uneven perfusion (i.e., the maternal-to-fetal blood flow ratio can be high in some parts of the placenta and low in others). This unevenness is a source of inefficiency. The greater the unevenness of perfusion ratios, the greater the P_{O_2} difference between the major placental veins of the mother and the fetus.
3. *Oxygen-diffusing capacity.* Placental oxygen-diffusing capacity is the rate of oxygen transport from placenta to fetus divided by the *mean* P_{O_2} difference between maternal and

fetal red blood cells. Its value is a function of the surface and thickness of the placental barrier (the larger the surface and smaller the thickness, the higher the diffusing capacity) and of the reaction rates of oxygen with hemoglobin (Longo et al., 1972). Placental oxygen-diffusing capacity has not been measured directly but has been estimated from measurements of the diffusing capacity of the placenta for carbon monoxide (Bissonnette et al., 1979). In simple terms, we may consider oxygen-diffusing capacity to be the *permeability* of the placental barrier to oxygen. Similarly, the reciprocal of oxygen-diffusing capacity is the *resistance* of the placental barrier to the diffusion of oxygen.

In the obstetrical literature, the statement is often made that "placental oxygen transport is blood flow limited." This statement depends on theoretical models that are not realistic. It implies that placental oxygen-diffusing capacity is a negligible hindrance to placental oxygen transport. To the contrary, experimental evidence in sheep indicates that most of the P_{O_2} difference between uterine and umbilical venous blood is due to a low oxygen-diffusing capacity that prevents the equilibration of maternal and fetal P_{O_2} across the placental barrier (Wilkening and Meschia, 1992). The concept that placental oxygen-diffusing capacity limits placental O_2 transport is important for understanding pathologic

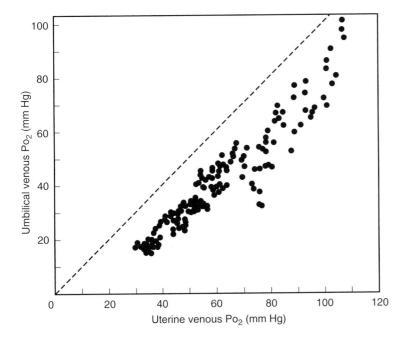

FIGURE 15-4 ■ Relationship of umbilical venous partial pressure of oxygen (P_{O_2}) to uterine venous P_{O_2} in sheep. The *dashed line* is the line of identity. Uterine venous P_{O_2} was varied by administration of different gas mixtures to the mother and by displacing the oxyhemoglobin dissociation curve of maternal blood through changes of maternal blood pH. Note that each point is below the identity line. (From Rankin JHG, Meschia G, Makowski EL, et al: Relationship between uterine and umbilical P_{O_2} in sheep. Am J Physiol **220**:1688, 1971.)

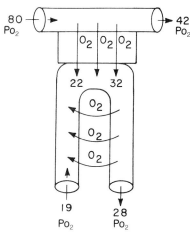

FIGURE 15-5 ■ Example of a diffusional shunt. Fetal blood exiting the area of exchange decreases its partial pressure of oxygen (P_{O_2}) by donating oxygen to the incoming fetal arterial blood.

conditions. In the ovine fetus, severe intrauterine growth restriction is associated with an abnormally low umbilical venous P_{O_2} (Bell et al., 1987). This low P_{O_2} is due to a very small placental oxygen-diffusing capacity that requires the fetus to maintain a large transplacental P_{O_2} gradient to draw oxygen from the mother across the placenta. In the human fetus, intrauterine growth restriction is also associated with a uterine–umbilical venous P_{O_2} difference that is greater than normal (Fig. 15-6), thus indicating that the hypoxia of the human intrauterine growth restriction fetus is due also to an abnormally low placental oxygen-diffusing capacity. In human populations living at high altitude, there is a significant increase in the capillary volume fraction of the placental terminal villi. This increase is responsible for an increase of placental oxygen-diffusing capacity, which compensates, in part, for the low P_{O_2} of maternal blood (Reshetnikova et al., 1994).

Is the Human Placenta a Venous Equilibrator?

In several species (e.g., guinea pig, rabbit), the placenta forms a countercurrent exchanger, which is more effective in transporting oxygen than a venous equilibrator. The effectiveness of the human placenta has been difficult to establish. One of the major problems has been variability in placental venous drainage. Experiments in the rhesus monkey, which has a placenta similar to the human placenta, demonstrated that maternal placental venous drainage of fetally infused tritiated water was via either the left or right ovarian vein or via both (Wallenburg and vanKreel, 1977). Furthermore, in some cases drainage shifted from one vein to the other during the course of the experiment, showing that the position of the placenta in the uterus is not a reliable indicator of which vein draws the placenta preferentially (Battaglia et al., 1970).

Thus, attempts to demonstrate the relation between maternal and fetal placental venous P_{O_2} in primates require a multiple venous sampling approach on the maternal side. With this approach, a study of human placental venous drainage at elective cesarean section (Pardi et al., 1992) has found umbilical venous P_{O_2} to be lower than the P_{O_2} in the least oxygenated of the maternal veins (see Fig. 15-6). This result agrees with previous findings in the rhesus monkey (Parer and Behrman, 1967) and favors the concept that the human placenta, like the ovine placenta, is a venous equilibrator.

Factors That Determine Uterine Venous P_{O_2}

The evidence in sheep, rhesus monkeys, and humans focuses attention on uterine venous P_{O_2} as the primary determinant of the upper limit of umbilical venous blood P_{O_2} in these species. The factors that determine uterine venous P_{O_2} are shown in Figure 15-7. The immediately causative factors that determine uterine venous P_{O_2} are the oxygen saturation and the oxyhemoglobin dissociation curve of venous blood. The position of the oxyhemoglobin dissociation curve is shifted by pH, so that at any given saturation the P_{O_2} is inversely related to pH (*Bohr effect*). Because of the Bohr effect, maternal alkalosis can be detrimental to fetal oxygenation via its effect on uterine venous P_{O_2} (Fig. 15-8).

The oxygen saturation of uterine venous blood, S_V, is a function of four variables:

1. Oxygen saturation of maternal arterial blood (S_A)
2. Oxygen capacity of maternal blood (O_2 CAP)

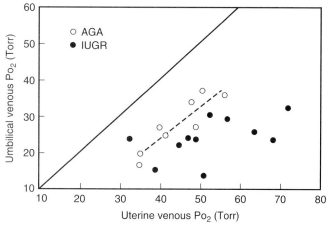

FIGURE 15-6 ■ Relationship between uterine venous and umbilical venous partial pressure of oxygen (P_{O_2}) in normal (○) and intrauterine growth restriction (IUGR) (●) human pregnancies. AGA, appropriate for gestational age. (From Pardi G, Cetin I, Marconi AM, et al: Venous drainage of the human uterus: Respiratory gas studies in normal and fetal growth-retarded pregnancies. Am J Obstet Gynecol **166**:699, 1992).

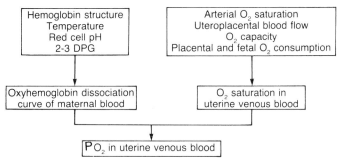

FIGURE 15-7 ■ Factors that determine uterine venous partial pressure of oxygen (P_{O_2}). 2-3 DPG, 2,3-diphosphoglycerate.

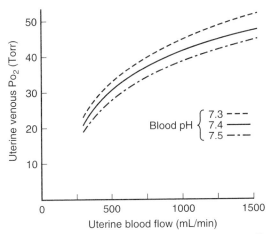

FIGURE 15-8 ■ Uterine venous partial pressure of oxygen (Po₂) as a function of uterine blood flow in a pregnant patient close to term. The figure was constructed on the assumption that the following values were constant: maternal arterial Po₂, 80 torr; maternal oxygen capacity, 17.4 volumes percent; oxygen consumption rate of the gravid uterus, 30 mL_STP/min.

3. Uterine blood flow (F)
4. Oxygen consumption rate of the gravid uterus ($\dot{V}O_2$):

$$S_V = S_A - \dot{V}O_2/F\,[O_2\,CAP]$$

This equation is an application of the Fick principle.* It is an approximation that neglects the small contribution of free oxygen to the oxygen content of blood. Implicit in the equation are the three main types of hypoxia listed in textbooks of physiology:

1. Low saturation of arterial blood (hypoxic hypoxia)
2. Reduced oxygen capacity (anemic hypoxia)
3. Reduction in blood flow (circulatory hypoxia)

These types of hypoxia, alone or in combination, decrease uterine venous saturation. A decrease in uterine venous oxygen saturation implies a decrease of uterine venous Po₂ and impairment of fetal oxygenation.

An important consequence of the inefficiency of a placenta, which is a venous equilibrator and has a low oxygen-diffusing capacity, is that it requires a relatively high uterine blood flow to provide a normal level of fetal oxygenation. For example, if we consider as valid the evidence that under normal physiologic conditions the umbilical venous Po₂ of a 35-week-old human

---

* Derivation of equation for oxygen saturation of venous blood. Let $\dot{V}O_2$ = uterine oxygen consumption (mmol/min), F = uterine blood flow (mL/min), A = arterial oxygen content (mmol/mL), V = uterine venous oxygen content (mmol/mL), [O₂ CAP] = oxygen capacity (mmol/mL), S_A = oxygen saturation of arterial blood, and S_V = oxygen saturation of uterine venous blood. According to the Fick principle,

$$\dot{V}O_2 = F(A - V)$$

Divide both sides of the equation by oxygen capacity:

$$\dot{V}O_2/[O_2\,CAP] = F\,A/[O_2\,CAP] - V/[O_2\,CAP]$$

If we neglect the contribution of free oxygen to A and V,

$$A/[O_2\,CAP] = S_A \text{ and } V/[O_2\,CAP] = S_V$$

Therefore, $\dot{V}O_2/[O_2\,CAP] =$

$$F\,(S_A - S_V) \text{ and } S_V = S_A - \dot{V}O_2/F\,[O_2\,CAP]$$

fetus is about 30 torr (Bozzetti et al., 1987) and that uterine venous Po₂ must be at least 10 mm Hg higher than umbilical venous Po₂ (Pardi et al., 1992), according to Figure 15-8 the uterine blood flow in late human pregnancy should be normally about 1 liter. Early estimates based on Doppler technology were considerably lower (Thaler et al., 1990). However, using improved Doppler imaging, Konje and colleagues (2001) reported the mean blood flow carried by the two uterine arteries to be 942 mL/min at 36 weeks. Note that knowledge about the normal value of uterine blood flow is of crucial importance in constructing a correct model of fetal oxygenation.

TRANSPORT OF OXYGEN TO FETAL TISSUE

In recent years, there has been considerable progress in the exploration of human fetal physiology by means of techniques for blood flow measurement and umbilical venous blood sampling *in utero*. The results of this effort, together with comparative data in sheep, allow us to construct a tentative picture of normal human fetal oxygenation and blood oxygen transport (Table 15-3).

In both the human and ovine fetus, arterial Po₂ is about one fourth the maternal arterial Po₂ at sea level. This is a consequence partly of the structural and functional characteristics of the placenta, which require that the oxygenation of fetal blood take place at a low Po₂, and partly of the anatomy of the fetal circulation, which forms arterial blood by mixing the blood that returns from the placenta with deoxygenated blood returning from the fetal tissues.

Despite the very low Po₂ of its blood, the fetus is capable of transporting large amounts of oxygen from the placenta to the sites of oxygen consumption within the fetal body. Three major adaptations make this possible:

1. The hemoglobin of fetal red blood cells has a high affinity for oxygen (i.e., it binds oxygen at low Po₂ values). This property enables the fetal red blood cells that circulate through the placenta to become highly saturated with oxygen.
2. The fetus has a very high cardiac output relative to its body size and metabolic rate.

TABLE 15-3. REPRESENTATIVE DATA FOR BLOOD OXYGEN TRANSPORT IN A 35-WEEK HUMAN FETUS AND A SHEEP FETUS AT A COMPARABLE DEVELOPMENTAL STAGE

	Human Fetus (35-week)	Sheep Fetus (19-week)
Blood O₂ capacity (mM)	9.4	6.7
Umbilical venous O₂ saturation (%)	70.0	81.0
Umbilical venous O₂ content (mM)	6.6	5.4
Umbilical venous Po₂ (torr)	28.0	28.0
Umbilical arterial O₂ saturation (%)	40.0	56.0
Umbilical arterial O₂ content (mM)	3.8	3.8
Umbilical arterial Po₂ (torr)	19.0	19.0
Cardiac output (mL/min/kg)	500.0	500.0
Umbilical blood flow (mL/min /kg)	120.0	216.0
Umbilical flow/cardiac output	0.24	0.43

3. The distribution of cardiac output between placenta and fetus and within the fetus creates a well-balanced oxygen uptake and delivery system.

Available data for the human fetus indicate that this adaptive strategy has some intriguing quantitative differences from the ovine model. At mid-gestation, the oxygen capacity of human fetal blood is approximately 6.5 mM; umbilical venous oxygen saturation and P_{O_2} are about 90% and 50 torr, respectively (Bozzetti et al., 1987). The high P_{O_2} suggests that maternal placental blood flow is very high with respect to oxygen demand. By comparison, the mid-gestation ovine fetus has a somewhat lower oxygen capacity (5.7 ± 0.3 mM) and equally high umbilical venous oxygen saturation (89% ± 1%). Note that a 90% oxygen saturation is close to the highest value that one can reasonably expect for the oxygenation of blood by any respiratory organ.

As gestation progresses toward term, umbilical venous oxygen saturation and P_{O_2} decline concomitantly with an increase in oxygen capacity. These changes occur in both species, but those described in humans are larger (Soothill et al., 1986; Bozzetti et al., 1987), so that in late gestation the human fetus has blood with substantially greater oxygen capacity and about 10% lower umbilical venous oxygen saturation than the ovine fetus.

Despite the difference in oxygen saturation, the two species have comparable umbilical venous P_{O_2} values because human fetal blood has slightly lower oxygen affinity than ovine fetal blood. Although the oxygen affinity of human fetal blood is not as high as in sheep, it still represents an important adaptation to the low P_{O_2} at which the human placenta oxygenates the fetus. Figure 15-9 compares the oxyhemoglobin dissociation curves of human adult and fetal blood. At a P_{O_2} of 30 torr and blood pH 7.4, fetal blood is 73% saturated with oxygen; adult blood is only 60% saturated.

In addition to umbilical venous P_{O_2} and oxygen saturation, we must consider oxygen content, which is the product of oxygen saturation and capacity. In this regard, the late-gestation human fetus has umbilical venous blood with higher oxygen content compared with the sheep fetus because the

higher oxygen capacity more than compensates for the lower saturation.

The next two important factors to be considered are umbilical blood flow and fetal cardiac output. The human umbilical blood flow is approximately 120 mL/min/kg fetus (Gill et al., 1984), which is about 40% lower than umbilical blood flow measured in sheep (Battaglia and Meschia, 1986). Initial attempts to measure human fetal cardiac output suggested that it is also relatively small, but further investigations indicate that cardiac output is as high in the human as in the sheep fetus and approximately equal to 500 mL/min/kg fetus (Kenny et al., 1986; DeSmedt et al., 1987; Rizzo and Arduini, 1991). Therefore, there seems to be a major difference between the two species in the distribution of fetal cardiac output. In fetal sheep, umbilical blood flow represents approximately 40% of cardiac output; in the late-gestation human fetus, umbilical blood flow is less than 30% of cardiac output (see Table 15-3). This large difference may result, in part, from errors of measurement. It seems clear, however, that in comparison with the ovine fetus, a high blood oxygen capacity (i.e., high hemoglobin content and hematocrit) and a low umbilical blood flow-to-cardiac output ratio are distinctive normal characteristics of the human fetus. Umbilical blood flow and oxygen capacity are interrelated. In anemic human fetuses, umbilical blood flow becomes greater than 120 mL/min/kg fetus and can be as high as in the sheep fetus (Jouppila and Kirkinen, 1984).

The function of the fetal circulation as an oxygen delivery system depends on an appropriate balance between umbilical blood flow and fetal somatic blood flow. It is intuitive that directing too much cardiac output into the somatic circulation would impair the umbilical uptake of oxygen and that directing too much cardiac output into the umbilical circulation would impair the supply of oxygen to fetal organs. It may seem that, theoretically, the optimal balance is to split the distribution of cardiac output evenly between the umbilical and somatic circulations; in fact, however, the experimental evidence shows a balance tilted toward the somatic circulation. The enormous growth of the human fetal brain is probably the major factor that creates the demand for a smaller umbilical flow in the human than in the ovine fetus. At term, the human fetus and the ovine fetus weigh about the same, but the mass of the fetal human brain is about eight times greater. A larger cerebral mass implies greater oxygen demand and requires a greater percentage of cardiac output directed to the fetal upper body at the expense of the fetal lower body and the umbilical circulation. The high O_2 capacity of human fetal blood can be viewed as a compensatory mechanism that allows the human fetus to maintain a relatively low umbilical blood flow without compromising umbilical O_2 uptake.

Because of its low blood P_{O_2}, the fetus is more hypoxic than the neonate. Normally, however, the fetus has access to all the oxygen that it needs and does not use anaerobic glycolysis as a terminal source of energy (Battaglia and Meschia, 1978). Furthermore, the low level of P_{O_2} in fetal arterial blood is physiologically useful because it is an essential component of the mechanisms that keep the ductus arteriosus open and the pulmonary vascular bed constricted. To counteract the pathologic connotation of the word "hypoxia," it is advisable to use the expression "physiologic hypoxia" to refer to the normal state of fetal oxygenation.

In the ordinary usage of the term, *fetal hypoxia* means any decrease below normal in the level of fetal oxygenation. Such a

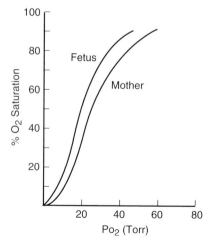

FIGURE 15-9 ■ The oxyhemoglobin dissociation curves of maternal and fetal human blood at pH 7.4 and 37°C. P_{O_2}, partial pressure of oxygen. (Adapted from Hellegers AE, Schruefer JJ: Nomograms and empirical equations relating oxygen tension, percentage saturation, and pH in maternal and fetal blood. Am J Obstet Gynecol **81**:377, 1961.)

decrease may come about in different ways, most commonly as a reduction in the P_{O_2} of umbilical venous blood, which in turn determines a decrease of fetal arterial P_{O_2}, in the oxygen capacity of fetal blood (anemic hypoxia, elevated levels of carbon monoxide), or in the perfusion rate of the umbilical circulation.

The circulation of a nonanesthetized otherwise healthy fetus reacts to an acute decrease in umbilical venous and arterial P_{O_2} in a predictable manner (Sheldon et al., 1979). As the P_{O_2} falls, blood flow is increased to the central nervous system (CNS) and the heart, although cardiac output and placental blood flow tend to remain constant. As a consequence, acute fetal hypoxia is characterized by a redistribution of cardiac output favoring CNS and heart at the expense of other parts of the fetal body.

The fraction of cardiac output directed to CNS and heart increases hyperbolically as the arterial oxygen content decreases (Fig. 15-10). The functional meaning of this relationship is that to mount a successful defense against hypoxia, the fetus must keep constant (or nearly so) the flow of oxygen to the CNS and heart (i.e., the product of blood flow times the oxygen content per milliliter of arterial blood). The limit of a successful circulatory defense against acute hypoxia is reached when the perfusion rate of the CNS and the heart has reached its maximum. In the fetal lamb, this limit is attained when the oxygen content in the supraductal arteries is approximately 1 mM. At this level, the flow of blood per gram of tissue is extremely high in the brain (~4 mL/min/g) and in the heart (~7 mL/min/g). Furthermore, the combined CNS and heart flow has become 26% of fetal cardiac output (see Fig. 15-10). The circulations of the human and ovine fetus react similarly to acute hypoxia. Under normal physiologic conditions, however, the large oxygen demand of the human fetal brain requires a larger contribution of cardiac output to cerebral perfusion than in the fetal lamb. As a consequence, in response to acute hypoxia the human fetus may not be able to produce a percentage increase in cerebral blood flow as dramatic as in a species with a small brain.

Between the region of oxygenation that defines physiologic hypoxia and the limit below which there is an insufficient oxygen supply to the CNS and heart, there is a broad region (approximately between 2.5 and 1 mM arterial oxygen content in the fetal lamb) in which the supply of oxygen to some parts of the fetal body other than the CNS and heart (e.g., skeletal muscle) cannot sustain a normal level of O_2 consumption. In this region of oxygenation, fetal blood accumulates lactic acid.

OXYGEN THERAPY

The inhalation of oxygen by a pregnant patient can increase dramatically the P_{O_2} of maternal arterial blood but causes only a small increase in fetal arterial P_{O_2} (Table 15-4). This observation seems to contradict the empirical knowledge that oxygen therapy can be an effective measure for the improvement of fetal oxygenation. Indeed, some investigators have claimed that maternal oxygen inhalation cannot ameliorate fetal hypoxia because its effect on fetal P_{O_2} is "negligible." Others have claimed that the discrepancy of P_{O_2} changes in mother and fetus is the consequence of severe placental vasoconstriction in response to the high P_{O_2} of maternal blood. To dispel these misconceptions, it is necessary first to understand why fetal arterial P_{O_2} increases much less than maternal arterial P_{O_2} and then to focus attention on the effect that oxygen therapy has on the oxygen content of fetal blood.

The venous equilibration model of placental exchange and the characteristics of the maternal and fetal oxyhemoglobin dissociation curves readily explain the "small" effect of oxygen therapy on fetal P_{O_2}. In the example shown in Figure 15-11, the oxygen contents of maternal and fetal blood are plotted against P_{O_2}:

- The inhalation of 100% oxygen by the mother causes the P_{O_2} of maternal arterial blood to increase from 90 to 500 torr (*step a*).
- This increase in P_{O_2} causes an increase of maternal arterial oxygen content equal to 1 mM (*step b*). These changes in arterial P_{O_2} and oxygen content do not cause any appreciable change in the uterine blood flow.
- If we assume they do not increase the uterine oxygen consumption rate—a correct assumption if fetal oxygen

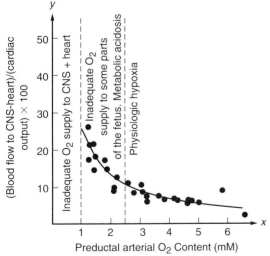

FIGURE 15-10 ■ Hyperbolic relationship between the oxygen content in the preductal arteries of a fetal lamb and the percentage of cardiac output directed to the heart and the central nervous system (CNS). The curve was drawn according to the equation $y \bullet x = 0.26$. (Data from Peeters LLH, Sheldon RE, Jones MD Jr, et al: Blood flow to fetal organs as a function of arterial oxygen content. Am J Obstet Gynecol **135**:1071, 1979.)

TABLE 15-4. P_{O_2} OF MATERNAL AND UMBILICAL BLOOD AT DIFFERENT LEVELS OF MATERNAL OXYGENATION

Location	P_{O_2} (mm Hg)			
	Rhesus Monkey*		Human†	
Maternal artery	108	257	91	583
Uterine vein	37	44	—	—
Umbilical vein	22	30	32	40
Umbilical artery	15	21	11	16

* Data from Behrman RE, Peterson EN, Delannoy CW: The supply of O_2 to the primate fetus with two different O_2 tensions and anesthetics. Respir Physiol 6:271, 1969.
† Data from Wulf KH, Künzel W, Lehmann V: Clinical aspects of placental gas exchange. In Longo LD, Bartels H (eds): Respiratory Gas Exchange and Blood Flow in the Placenta. Washington, DC, DHEW Publication (National Institutes of Health), 1972.

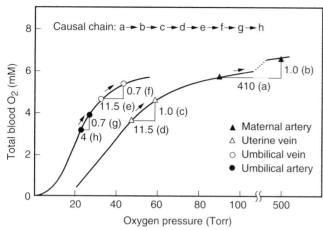

FIGURE 15-11 ■ Example of the relationship between oxygen content and partial pressure of oxygen in maternal and fetal blood before and after maternal inhalation of 100% oxygen. (From Meschia G: Transfer of oxygen across the placenta. *In* Gluck L (ed): Intrauterine Asphyxia and the Developing Fetal Brain. Chicago, Year Book Medical Publishers, 1977.)

moglobin dissociation curve and by the position of the umbilical venous point on that curve.

■ In this example, the oxygen content of umbilical venous blood increases 0.7 mM. If we assume no appreciable change in umbilical blood flow or oxygen uptake, it follows (again by application of the law of conservation of matter) that the oxygen content in the umbilical artery must increase also 0.7 mM (*step g*).

■ Because the arterial point is positioned on the steep part of the fetal oxyhemoglobin dissociation curve, an increase of 0.7 mM in oxygen content is associated with a Po_2 increase of only 4 torr (*step h*).

The end result of this chain of events is that a Po_2 change of 410 torr in maternal arterial blood results in a Po_2 change of 4 torr in umbilical arterial blood.

If we focus our attention on fetal Po_2 changes by excluding other considerations, we might be tempted to conclude that maternal oxygen therapy has no appreciable effect on fetal oxygenation. To the contrary, it should be noted that oxygen therapy can cause similar increments in the *oxygen content* of maternal and fetal blood. In the example, an increase of 1 mM in maternal blood was associated with an increase of 0.7 mM in fetal blood. Under somewhat different circumstances, the oxygen content of fetal blood can actually increase more than the oxygen content of maternal blood (Fig. 15-12).

Oxygen therapy is commonly used in the treatment of acute fetal hypoxia. It may be valuable also in the treatment of chronic fetal hypoxia. In two studies, 55% oxygen was administered for several days to pregnant patients with intrauterine growth restriction (Nicolaides et al., 1989; Battaglia et al., 1992). There were significant increases in umbilical venous Po_2 and oxygen saturation, a significant improvement in Doppler flow patterns, and preliminary evidence of decreased perinatal mortality. There was no evidence of increased fetal growth rate in response to the increased level of fetal oxygenation. This negative result agrees with the hypothesis that the placenta of a growth-retarded fetus has a reduced transport capacity for all metabolic substrates. Maternal hyperoxia improves the transport of oxygen but may not have any effect on the placental transport capacity of nutrients, and therefore it may not remove the hindrance to fetal growth.

Finally, it is important to consider the issue of oxygen toxicity. Breathing oxygen at high concentrations can be harmful to the lungs of the mother. Because of this concern, breathing

supply was already adequate before oxygen therapy—the law of conservation of matter requires that uterine venous oxygen content increase also 1 mM (*step c*).

■ The increase in uterine venous oxygen content causes the uterine venous Po_2 to increase 11.5 torr (*step d*). Note that the "S" shape of the maternal oxyhemoglobin dissociation curve and the different positions of the arterial and venous points on this curve determine that an equal change of oxygen content is associated with a markedly smaller change of Po_2 in the uterine vein than in the maternal arteries. Note also that the assumption of a constant oxygen consumption rate maximizes the increase in venous Po_2. If the oxygen consumption of the gravid uterus were to increase in response to oxygen therapy, the increase of venous Po_2 would be less than indicated.

■ Given an increase of 11.5 torr in the uterine venous Po_2, the umbilical venous Po_2 will increase by an approximately equal value (*step e*) (see experimental data in Fig. 15-4).

■ The increase in umbilical venous Po_2 is associated with an increase in umbilical venous oxygen content (*step f*), whose magnitude is dictated by the slope of the oxyhe-

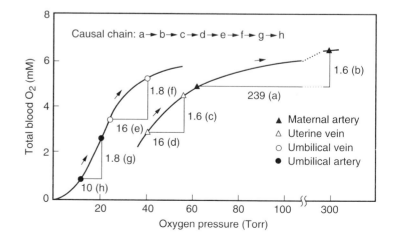

FIGURE 15-12 ■ Example of the pronounced effect of oxygen therapy on fetal oxygen content in a case of fetal hypoxia secondary to maternal hypoxia. (From Meschia G: Transfer of oxygen across the placenta. *In* Gluck L (ed): Intrauterine Asphyxia and the Developing Fetal Brain. Chicago, Year Book Medical Publishers, 1977.)

100% oxygen at atmospheric pressure must be limited to a few hours only. Breathing 50% oxygen at atmospheric pressure is considered safe. However, the question whether pregnancy alters the tolerance of the mother to hyperoxia has not been addressed. In general, there is no concern that maternal hyperoxia would increase fetal P_{O_2} to toxic levels, as long as the oxygen is administered at atmospheric pressure and for the purpose of treating fetal hypoxia.

PLACENTAL CARBON DIOXIDE TRANSFER

Carbon dioxide is an end product of fetal metabolism. In the fetal lamb, the respiratory quotient (i.e., the moles of CO_2 produced per mole of oxygen consumed) is approximately 0.94.

The CO_2 produced by the fetus diffuses from the umbilical circulation into the placenta and from the placenta into the maternal blood, which brings it to the lungs for excretion. The diffusional transfer of CO_2 from fetus to mother requires the P_{CO_2} of fetal blood to be higher than the P_{CO_2} of maternal blood. In chronic sheep preparations, umbilical venous P_{CO_2} is approximately 5 torr higher than uterine venous P_{CO_2}. The factors responsible for determining the magnitude of the P_{CO_2} gradient between fetal and maternal blood have not been analyzed in detail. A consequence of the high diffusibility of CO_2 across the placenta is that respiratory disturbances of acid-base balance in the mother cause—with a delay of a few minutes only—analogous disturbances in the fetus, as long as the two organisms are in communication via a well-perfused placenta. An abnormally low fetal P_{CO_2} (fetal respiratory alkalosis) is always secondary to a low maternal P_{CO_2}. To the contrary, an abnormally high fetal P_{CO_2} (fetal respiratory acidosis) can be due to a high maternal arterial P_{CO_2}, inadequate gas exchange across the placenta, or a combination of these two conditions.

There are probably substantial differences among mammals in the permeability of the placental barrier to bicarbonate ions. The epitheliochorial placenta of sheep has a very low permeability to bicarbonate and to other small anions, such as chloride ions and ketoacids. If maternal metabolic acidosis or alkalosis develops, the bicarbonate concentration of fetal blood remains normal for several days; however, the hemochorial placenta of the rabbit or rhesus monkey is much more permeable to chloride ions than an epitheliochorial placenta. This suggests that the hemochorial placenta is permeable to bicarbonate and other ions, in which case metabolic disturbances of acid-base balance in the mother would cause analogous disturbances in the fetus. Unfortunately, there is no exact information, in the human or any other species with a hemochorial placenta, about the rate at which a metabolic disturbance of acid-base balance in the maternal compartment is transmitted to the fetal compartment.

REFERENCES

Battaglia C, Artini PG, B'Ambrogio G, et al: Maternal hyperoxygenation in the treatment of intrauterine growth retardation. Am J Obstet Gynecol **167**:430, 1992.

Battaglia FC, Makowski EL, Meschia G: Physiologic study of the uterine venous drainage of the pregnant rhesus monkey. Yale J Biol Med **42**:218, 1970.

Battaglia FC, Meschia G: Principal substrates of fetal metabolism. Physiol Rev **58**:499, 1978.

Battaglia FC, Meschia G: An Introduction to Fetal Physiology. New York, Academic Press, 1986.

Behrman RE, Peterson EN, Delannoy CW: The supply of O_2 to the primate fetus with two different O_2 tensions and anesthetics. Respir Physiol **6**:271, 1969.

Bell AW, Kennaugh JM, Battaglia FC, et al: Metabolic and circulatory studies of fetal lamb at midgestation. Am J Physiol **250**:E538, 1986.

Bell AW, Wilkening RB, Meschia G: Some aspects of placental function in chronically heat-stressed ewes. J Dev Physiol **9**:17, 1987.

Bissonnette JM, Longo LD, Nevy MJ, et al: Placental diffusing capacity and its relation to fetal growth. J Dev Physiol **1**:351, 1979.

Bozzetti P, Buscaglia M, Cetin I, et al: Respiratory gases, acid-base balance and lactate concentrations of the midterm human fetus. Biol Neonate **51**:188, 1987.

DeSmedt MCH, Visser GHA, Meijboom EJ: Fetal cardiac output estimated by Doppler echocardiography during mid and late gestation. Am J Cardiol **60**:338, 1987.

Gill RW, Kossoff G, Warren PS, et al: Umbilical venous flow in normal and complicated pregnancy. Ultrasound Med Biol **10**:349, 1984.

Hellegers AE, Schruefer JJ: Nomograms and empirical equations relating oxygen tension, percentage saturation and pH in maternal and fetal blood. Am J Obstet Gynecol **81**:377, 1961.

Jouppila P, Kirkinen P: Umbilical vein blood flow in the human fetus in cases of maternal and fetal anemia and uterine bleeding. Ultrasound Med Biol **10**:365, 1984.

Kenny JF, Plappert T, Doubilet P, et al: Changes in intracardiac blood flow velocities and right and left ventricular stroke volumes in the gestational age in the normal human fetus: A prospective Doppler echocardiographic study. Circulation **74**:1208, 1986.

Konje J, Kaufmann P, Bell SC et al: A longitudinal study of quantitative uterine blood flow with the use of color power angiography in appropriate for gestational age pregnancies. Am J Obstet Gynecol **185**:608, 2001.

Longo LD, Hill EP, Power GG: Theoretical analysis of factors affecting placental O_2 transfer. Am J Physiol **222**:730, 1972.

Meschia G: Transfer of oxygen across the placenta. *In* Gluck L (ed): Intrauterine Asphyxia and the Developing Fetal Brain. Chicago, Year Book Medical Publishers, 1977.

Meschia G: Supply of oxygen to the fetus. J Reprod Med **23**:160, 1979.

Nicolaides KH, Econimides DL, Soothill PW: Blood gases, pH and lactate in appropriate-and-small-for-gestational-age fetuses. Am J Obstet Gynecol **161**:996, 1989.

Pardi G, Cetin I, Marconi AM, et al: Venous drainage of the human uterus: Respiratory gas studies in normal and fetal growth retarded pregnancies. Am J Obstet Gynecol **166**:699, 1992.

Parer GT, Behrman RE: The oxygen consumption of the pregnant uterus and fetus of *Macaca mulatta*. Respir Physiol **3**:288, 1967.

Peeters LLH, Sheldon RE, Jones MD Jr, et al: Blood flow to fetal organs as a function of arterial oxygen content. Am J Obstet Gynecol **135**:637, 1979.

Rankin JHG, Meschia G, Makowski EL, et al: Relationship between uterine and umbilical venous P_{O_2} in sheep. Am J Physiol **220**:1688, 1971.

Reshetnikova OS, Burton GJ, Milovanov AP: Effects of hypobaric hypoxia on the fetoplacental unit: The morphometric diffusing capacity of the villous membrane at high altitude. Am J Obstet Gynecol **171**:1560, 1994.

Rizzo G, Arduini D: Fetal cardiac function in intrauterine growth retardation. Am J Obstet Gynecol **165**:876, 1991.

Sheldon RE, Peeters LLH, Jones MD Jr, et al: Redistribution of cardiac output and oxygen delivery in the hypoxemic fetal lamb. Am J Obstet Gynecol **135**:1071, 1979.

Soothill P, Nicolaides KH, Rodeck CH, et al: Effect of gestational age on fetal and intervillous blood gas and acid base values in human pregnancy. Fetal Ther **1**:168, 1986.

Thaler I, Manor D, Itskovitz G, et al: Changes in uterine blood flow during human pregnancy. Am J Obstet Gynecol **162**:121, 1990.

Wallenburg HCS, vanKreel BK: Placental and nonplacental drainage of the uterus in the pregnant rhesus monkey. Eur J Obstet Gynaecol Reprod Biol **7**:79, 1977.

Wilkening RB, Meschia G: Comparative physiology of placental oxygen transport. Placenta **13**:1, 1992.

Wulf KH, Künzel W, Lehmann V: Clinical aspects of placental gas exchange. *In* Longo LD, Bartels H (eds): Respiratory Gas Exchange and Blood Flow in the Placenta. Washington, DC, DHEW Publications (National Institutes of Health), 1972.

Chapter 16
FETAL LUNG DEVELOPMENT

Alan H. Jobe, MD, PhD

In the recent past, lung immaturity in the preterm newborn uniformly resulted in rapid death. With intensive clinical management, lung function no longer limits survival of the preterm newborn in many cases. That management includes attempts to delay delivery, the use of corticosteroids to mature the fetal lung, improvements in neonatal ventilatory techniques, and surfactant treatments. Lung maturation involves considerations of anatomy, physiology, and cell biology, all of which must be appreciated for a balanced understanding of lung functional development and maturation. Although the anatomy and physiology of lung development in the human and in experimental animals have been characterized, cell biology and genetics are just beginning to reveal the mechanisms underlying the developmental program.

Hyaline membranes were described in association with respiratory deaths early in this century. However, there was no substantial increase in the understanding of lung immaturity until Avery and Mead (1959) correlated respiratory failure with decreased surfactant levels in saline extracts of the lungs of infants with respiratory distress syndrome (RDS). Once the association between atelectasis with hyaline membranes and surfactant levels was appreciated, a large research effort was focused on the surfactant system. The first direct clinical benefit was the development by Gluck and colleagues (1971) of the lecithin-to-sphingomyelin ratio using amniotic fluid to predict the risk of RDS in preterm infants. The utility of phosphatidylglycerol measurements for lung maturity testing then was recognized (Hallman et al., 1976). The maturational effects of corticosteroids on developing systems were apparent by the late 1960s, and in 1972 Liggins and Howie demonstrated a decreased incidence in RDS with maternal corticosteroid treatments. The development of surfactant treatment for RDS and other neonatal lung diseases has had a major beneficial impact on outcomes (Jobe, 1993a). Further progress in the pulmonary outcomes of infants will result from new information about how antenatal and postnatal abnormalities contribute to lung development, injury, and repair.

LUNG STRUCTURAL DEVELOPMENT

Embryonic Development

Lung development is divided into three periods: embryonic, fetal, and postnatal (Boyden, 1977). The lung first appears as a ventral bud off the esophagus just caudal to the laryngotra-

cheal sulcus. The grooves between the lung bud and the esophagus deepen, and the bud elongates within the surrounding mesenchyme and divides to form the future main stem bronchi (Fig. 16-1). Using transgenic mouse models, several factors that determine lung bud formation have been identified as homologs of developmental regulatory genes in *Drosophila* (Perl and Whitsett, 1999). Deletion of fibroblast growth factor-10 (FGF-10) or a compound deletion of the zinc finger DNA binding proteins Gli2 and Gli3 prevent lung development by disrupting tracheal development. Subsequent dichotomous branching of the trachea gives rise to the conducting airways and lobar structures of the lungs. Branching is controlled by the underlying mesoderm because removal of the mesenchyme stops branching, and transplantation of the mesenchyme from a branching airway to a more proximal airway or the trachea induces budding in the new location. Lobar airways are formed by about 37 days with progression to segmental airways by 42 days and subsegmental bronchi by 48 days in the human (Burri, 1985).

Some of the diffusable factors responsible for airway branching have been identified (Cardoso and Williams, 2001). Several members of the large family of fibroblast growth factors acting through a specific fibroblast growth factor receptor modulate airway branching and parenchymal development. For example, overexpression of fibroblast growth factor-7 (also known as keratinocyte growth factor) results in lung tumors similar to cystic adenomatoid malformations. Deletion of thyroid transcription factor-1, a number of the Nkx2 transcription factor family, results in a cystic lung beyond the first-order bronchus. Several factors are associated with the development of tracheal–esophageal fistula in transgenic mice. These and other genes have very precise spacial and temporal expression patterns that choreograph lung structural development. Newly developed techniques to turn on or turn off specific genes in mouse models will result in a more complete understanding of early lung development.

Fetal Lung Development

Fetal lung development is divided into the pseudoglandular, canalicular, and saccular/alveolar stages based on the histologic appearance of the lung and the development of airways and vasculature. The alveolarization of the lung is a postnatal event in rodents, but the saccular stage merges with alveolarization at about 32 weeks' gestation in the human (Zeltner and Burri, 1987) (Fig. 16-2).

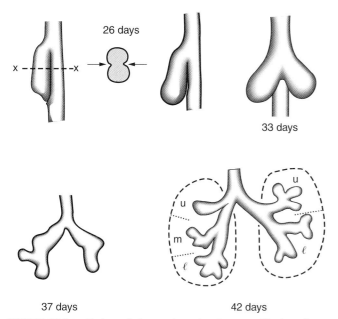

26 days

33 days

u

u

m

ℓ

ℓ

37 days   42 days

FIGURE 16-1 ■ Embryonic human lung development. The lung first appears as a protrusion of the foregut at 26 days. The lung bud becomes more prominent with deepening of the laryngotracheal grooves. The lung bud has branched by 33 days, and the prospective main bronchi are penetrating the mesenchyme by 37 days. By 42 days, lobar and initial segmental bronchi have formed. (Modified from Burri PW: Development and growth of the human lung. *In* Fishman AP, Fisher AB (eds): Handbook of Physiology: The Respiratory System. Bethesda, Md., American Physiological Society, 1985, p. 1.)

Pseudoglandular Stage

The pseudoglandular period, from about the 7th to 17th week of human gestation, is characterized by progressive division to generate 15 to 20 generations of airways depending on airway segment length and lobar position (Zeltner and Burri, 1987). The developing airways are lined with simple cuboidal cells that contain large amounts of glycogen. Epithelial differentiation is centrifugal in that the most distal tubules are lined with undifferentiated cells with progressive differentiation in the more proximal airways (Burri, 1985). Upper lobar development occurs earlier than lower lobe development in animals, and a similar pattern of development probably occurs in humans. Pulmonary arteries grow in conjunction with the airways, and the principal arterial pathways are present by 14 weeks. The pulmonary microvasculature develops in the mesenchyme around the developing airways by the processes of angiogenesis by remodeling and sprouting of new vessels from preexisting vessels and by vasculogenesis, which is the formation of primitive vascular plexuses that then fuse and connect with vessels. Pulmonary venous development occurs in parallel by both angiogeneses and vasculogeneses but with a different pattern that demarcates lung segments and subsegments. By the end of the pseudoglandular stage, airways, arteries, and veins have developed in the pattern corresponding to that found in the adult.

Canalicular Stage

The canalicular stage, between about 16 and 25 weeks' gestation, represents the transformation of the previable lung to the potentially viable lung that can exchange gas. The three major events during this stage are the "birth" of the acinus, epithelial differentiation with the development of the potential air–blood barrier, and the start of surfactant synthesis within recognizable type II cells (Burri, 1985). The acinus is the tuft of airways and alveoli originating from a terminal bronchiole. Its initial development is the critical first step for the development of the future gas exchange surface of the lung. The initially poorly vascularized mesenchyme surrounding the airways becomes more vascular and more closely aligned with the airway epithelial cells. The capillaries initially form a double capillary network between future air spaces. These capillaries subsequently fuse to form a single capillary between the future gas exchange surfaces with close apposition to the saccular walls to form a structure by about 19 weeks similar to the thin air–blood barrier in the adult lung. If the double capillary network does not fuse, the infant will have severe hypoxemia and the histopathologic findings of alveolar-capillary dysplasia. The total surface area occupied by the air–blood barrier increases exponentially through the canalicular stage with a resultant fall in the mean wall thickness and with an increased potential for gas exchange.

Epithelial differentiation is characterized by proximal-to-distal thinning of the epithelium by transformation of cuboidal cells into thin cells that line wide tubes. The tubes grow both in length and in width with attenuation of the mesenchyme, which is simultaneously becoming vascularized. After about 20 weeks' gestation in the human fetus, these cuboidal cells rich in glycogen begin to have more lamellar bodies in their cytoplasm, indicating the initiation of surfactant production.

Saccular and Alveolar Stages

The saccular stage initiates the period of lung development from the potentially viable stages of prematurity from about 24 weeks to term. The saccule is the terminal airway structural element of the fetal lung. Alveolarization is initiated at about 32 weeks from the terminal saccules by the appearance of septa comprised of capillaries, elastin fibers, and collagen fibers (Burri, 1985). Langston and coworkers (1984) estimated that the term human lung contains about 50 million alveoli, and Hislop and associates (1986) found about 150 million alveoli in term human lungs. These variable estimates result from somewhat different definitions for the morphometric identification of developing alveoli. For comparison, the adult human lung contains about 300 million alveoli. From about 25 weeks' gestation to term, there is a progressive increase in potential lung gas volume and epithelial surface area. The increase in alveoli, lung volume, and surface area establishes the anatomic potential for gas exchange and thus the potential for fetal viability.

Alveolarization and the associated vascularization are the critical terminal stages of lung development that are influenced by common obstetric interventions. The important concept is that alveolar development is a late fetal event that is at its maximal rate during the stages of fetal development when preterm labor and delivery are frequent (Fig. 16-3). Once alveoli are formed, the lung subsequently looses alveoli with age, although under some circumstances the adult lung may be able to develop new alveoli (Massaro and Massaro, 2002). However, if alveolarization is disrupted during the period of rapid accumulation between about 32 weeks' gestation and term, then there may be adverse short-term and long-term effects on lung function in the newborn.

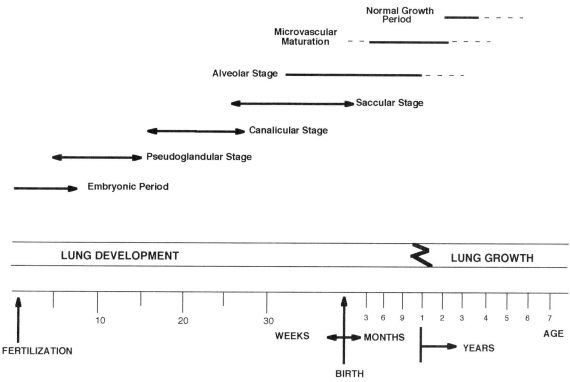

FIGURE 16-2 ■ Timetable for lung development. The period of lung development continues to 1 to 2 years of age, and subsequently lung growth occurs. The timing of the saccular and alveolar stages and the period of microvascular maturation overlap with indeterminate initiation and end points. (Modified from Zeltner TB, Burri PH: The postnatal development and growth of the human lung. II. Morphology. Respir Physiol **67**:269, 1987.)

The factors that modulate normal alveolarization are not known. However, a number of clinical interventions and agents are known to disrupt normal alveolarization in developing animals (Table 16-1). Hyperoxia, hypoxia, and mechanical ventilation all can interfere with alveolarization (Massaro and Massaro, 2002). The preterm infant that is mechanically ventilated will be exposed to these factors as well as nutritional deficits. Recent human pathology from very-low-birth-weight infants who have died of bronchopulmonary dysplasia (BPD) demonstrates an arrest of alveolar development with lungs that contain fewer and larger alveoli (Thibeault et al., 2000). These lungs also demonstrate less airway injury, inflammation, and fibrosis than the lungs of infants who died from bronchopulmonary dysplasia in earlier eras.

New concepts about inflammatory mediators are being developed that link the clinical observations that chorioamnionitis can be associated with the subsequent development of bronchopulmonary dysplasia (Jobe, 1999). In transgenic mouse models, the overexpression of pro-inflammatory cytokines during the period of postnatal alveolarization disrupts alveolar formation. These same cytokines are elevated in amniotic fluid, cord blood, and tracheal aspirate samples of infants exposed to

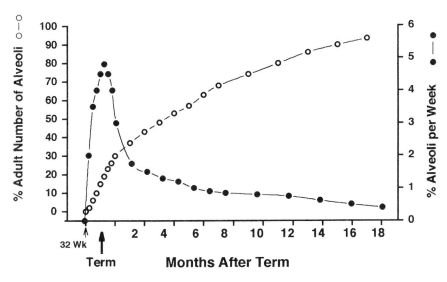

FIGURE 16-3 ■ Alveolar number increases from about 32 weeks' gestation to achieve the average number of alveoli in the adult lung of 300 million. The period of most rapid increase in alveolar number expressed as percent appearing per week is between about 32 weeks and term. Curves are based on the morphologic measurements of Langston and coworkers (1984) and Hislop and coworkers (1986) assuming 30% of the alveoli have formed by term.

TABLE 16-1. MODULATORS OF ALVEOLARIZATION

Factors that delay or interfere with alveolarization
  Mechanical ventilation of the preterm infant
  Glucocorticoids
  Pro-inflammatory cytokines (TNF-α, TGF-α, IL-11, IL-6)
  Chorioamnionitis
  Hyperoxia or hypoxia
  Poor nutrition
  Nicotine
Factors that stimulate alveolarization
  Vitamin A (retinoic acid)
  Thyroxine

IL, interleukin; TGF-α, transforming growth factor-α; TNF-α, tumor necrosis factor-α.

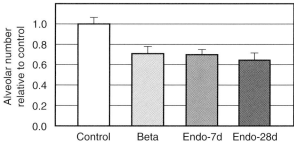

FIGURE 16-4 ■ Effect of maternal betamethasone (Beta) and intra-amniotic endotoxin (Endo) on alveolar number in preterm lambs. The betamethasone treatment (0.5 mg/kg) was given 7 days before preterm delivery at 125 days' gestation. Endotoxin (*Escherichia coli* 055:B5) (20 mg) was given by intra-amniotic injection 6 days before preterm delivery at 125 days or continuously from day 80 to day 108 at a rate of 0.6 mg/day into the amniotic fluid using an Alzet pump. The interventions decreased alveolarization of the fetal lung. (Data from Willet KE, Jobe AH, Ikegami M, et al: Antenatal endotoxin and glucocorticoid effects on lung morphometry in preterm lambs. Pediatr Res **48**:782, 2000; and Moss TJM, Newnham JP, Willet KE, et al: Early gestational intra-amniotic endotoxin: Lung function, surfactant and morphometry. Am J Respir Crit Care Med **165**:805, 2002.)

chorioamnionitis before preterm delivery. In an experimental model of chorioamnionitis caused by an intra-amniotic injection of endotoxin in sheep, a single dose of endotoxin given 7 days before preterm delivery or a continuous 28 day intra-amniotic infusion of endotoxin decreased alveolar numbers after preterm delivery (Willet et al., 2000) (Fig. 16-4).

Another clinically relevant observation is that glucocorticoids can cause a profound arrest in alveolarization in rodents and other animals. Postnatal glucocorticoids can cause permanent abnormalities in alveolar and vascular development in mice and rats (Massaro and Massaro, 2002). In the monkey, maternal glucocorticoids given at the saccular stage of lung development decrease the mesenchyme and make the lung appear more mature, but at term the lung has a lower gas volume and fewer alveoli (Johnson et al., 1981). A high dose of glucocorticoids given to monkeys for 3 days during the pseudoglandular stage of lung development results in fewer alveoli at term (Bunton and Plopper, 1984). In sheep, single or repetitive weekly maternal glucocorticoid treatments cause a decrease in alveolar number and an increase in alveolar size after preterm birth (see Fig. 16-4). However, in the sheep the alveolar numbers were normal at term despite three weekly betamethasone treatments (Willet et al., 2001a). This result demonstrates that recovery from an inhibition of alveolar development is possible. A concern is that many very-low-birth-weight infants are exposed to antenatal and postnatal glucocorticoid therapy and that both may interfere with lung development.

Pulmonary Hypoplasia

Although embryonic developmental anomalies occasionally result in unilateral pulmonary atresias and abnormal lung segmentation syndromes, pulmonary hypoplasia syndromes are much more common. Pulmonary hypoplasia diagnosed by low lung weight was found in 15% to 20% of unselected autopsy series (Wigglesworth and Desai, 1982). The diagnosis of pulmonary hypoplasia by the anatomic criteria of decreased airway numbers and radial alveolar counts is time-consuming and not routine. Measurements of lung DNA content relative to body weight also separate infants with pulmonary hypoplasia from infants with normal lung development. However, generally the diagnosis is made clinically based on the severity of respiratory failure and the clinical associations. The fetus must maintain the appropriate volume of fetal lung fluid in the airways and have the normal frequency and amplitude of fetal breathing movements for the lung to grow normally (Liggins, 1984). Fetal lung fluid volume can be decreased either by external chest compression (e.g., oligohydramnios) or by space occupation in the chest cavity (e.g., diaphragmatic hernia). Classifications of conditions associated with pulmonary hypoplasia are listed in Table 16-2. Thoracic compression syndromes are most destructive to lung growth during the canalicular period of human lung development from 16 to 24 weeks' gestation. Oligohydramnios not associated with renal anomalies does not invariably result in pulmonary hypoplasia; however, the earlier in gestation, the more severe and the longer the oligohydramnios lasts, the more likely severe pulmonary hypoplasia will occur (Thibeault et al., 1985). Infants delivered after many weeks of oligohydramnios secondary to premature preterm rupture of membranes can have good lung function (Lindner et al., 2002). Pulmonary hypoplasia, despite

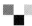

TABLE 16-2. CLINICAL ASSOCIATIONS WITH PULMONARY HYPOPLASIA

Thoracic compression
  Renal agenesis (Potter syndrome)
  Urinary tract outflow obstruction
  Oligohydramnios before 28 weeks' gestational age
  Extra-amniotic fetal development
Decreased intrathoracic space
  Diaphragmatic hernia
  Pleural effusions
  Abdominal distention sufficient to limit chest volume
  Thoracic dystrophies
Decreased fetal breathing
  Intrauterine central nervous system damage
  Fetal Werdnig-Hoffmann syndrome
  Other neuropathies and myopathies
Other associations
  Primary pulmonary hypoplasia
  Trisomy 21
  Multiple congenital anomalies
  Erythroblastosis fetalis

maintenance of apparently normal fetal lung fluid and amniotic fluid volumes, can occur in infants with severe central nervous system damage from infectious or developmental neuropathies and myopathies.

Diaphragmatic hernia is the most common cause of pulmonary hypoplasia caused by lung compression. The lung on the side of the diaphragmatic hernia is often severely hypoplastic, but the contralateral lung also is hypoplastic, although less so. Studies in animal models indicate that maturation of the surfactant system is delayed in the lungs, and surfactant components are decreased in amniotic fluid from infants with diaphragmatic hernia (Wilcox et al., 1997). Attempts to surgically correct the diaphragmatic hernia in utero have seldom succeeded. Obstruction of the trachea to stimulate lung growth by distention with fetal lung fluid is being evaluated. The tracheal obstruction causes the fetal lung to overdistend with fetal lung fluid secreted by the lung. Although the lung grows larger, the constant stretch results in decreased type II cell numbers and decreased surfactant (Kay et al., 2001). The fetal lung will develop abnormally if it collapses because of loss of fetal lung fluid or if it is overstretched.

Infants with diaphragmatic hernia and with less severe degrees of pulmonary hypoplasia can be supported with mechanical ventilation. The attempt to achieve normal gas exchange and oxygenation with excessive mechanical ventilation will result in severe lung injury (Muratore and Wilson, 2000). Gentle approaches to mechanical ventilation together with the selective use of extracorporeal membrane oxygenation and delayed surgical correction of diaphragmatic hernias is resulting in survivals of 80% or better. Infants with trisomy 21 or other syndromes may have anomalous lung development or may have abnormal fetal breathing patterns that may result in pulmonary hypoplasia.

Fetal Lung Fluid

The fetal airways are filled with fluid until delivery and the initiation of ventilation. Quantitative information about fetal lung fluid is from the fetal lamb, with sonographic and pathologic correlates available for the human. The fetal lung close to term contains enough fluid to maintain the airway volume approximately at the same volume as the functional residual capacity once air breathing is established. This volume is about 25 mL/kg body weight in the fetal lamb. The composition of fetal lung fluid is unique relative to other fetal fluids (O'Brodovich, 2001). The chloride content is high, and the bicarbonate and protein contents are low. The fetal epithelium is essentially impermeable to protein. The fetal lung fluid is in equilibrium with fetal partial pressure of carbon dioxide values of about 45 mm Hg, which results in a low pH in fetal lung fluid. This electrolyte composition is maintained by transepithelial Cl^- secretion with bicarbonate reabsorption. However, there are species differences in fetal lung fluid, and bicarbonate and pH are higher in the primate. Active chloride transport by epithelial cells results in passive water movement into the fetal air spaces with a net production rate for fetal lung fluid of 4 to 5 mL/kg/hour (Bland and Chapman, 1994). The production of fetal lung fluid will be about 400 mL/day for a 4-kg fetus. In humans, some of this fluid is swallowed and some mixes with the amniotic fluid. The pressure in the fetal trachea exceeds that in the amniotic fluid by about 2 mm Hg, generating an outflow resistance that maintains the fetal lung fluid volume in the fetal lung. The secretion of fetal lung fluid is primarily an intrinsic metabolic function of the developing alveolar and airway epithelium because changes in vascular hydrostatic pressures, tracheal pressures, and fetal breathing movements do not greatly affect fetal lung fluid production.

Although the presence of fetal lung fluid is essential for normal lung development, its clearance is equally essential for normal neonatal respiratory adaptation. Fetal lung fluid production can be completely stopped and fluid adsorption initiated in near-term fetal sheep by vascular infusions of epinephrine at concentrations that approximate the levels of epinephrine present during labor (Brown et al., 1983). The epinephrine-responsive change in the air space epithelium from fluid secretion to absorption is absent in preterm fetal sheep and can be induced by short-term cortisol and triiodothyronine infusions (Barker et al., 1990). In term guinea pigs, the Na^+ channel blocker amiloride mixed with fetal lung fluid delays fluid clearance and causes respiratory distress, demonstrating that Na^+K^+ adenosine triphosphatase function is essential for the clearance of airway fluid after birth (O'Brodovich, 2001).

Fetal lung fluid production may decrease in the days just before labor. Fetal lung fluid volume decreases in fetal sheep to about 65% of the maximal volumes present during fetal life (Bland and Chapman, 1994). During active labor and delivery, another 30% of the fluid is cleared from the airways and alveoli, leaving only about 35% of the fetal lung fluid to be adsorbed and cleared from the lungs with breathing. Most of the fluid moves rapidly into the interstitial spaces and subsequently directly into the pulmonary vasculature, with less than 20% of the fluid being cleared by pulmonary lymphatics. Clearance of the fluid from the interstitial spaces occurs over many hours. Alveolar fluid volume in the normal lung is only about 0.3 mL/kg. The sequence of prelabor, labor, and delivery is an important regulator of the fetal lung fluid volume present at the initiation of air breathing.

Cesarean delivery of fetuses who have not experienced labor can result in decreased lung compliance, early respiratory distress, and transient tachypnea of the newborn (Faxelius et al., 1982). The magnitude of the potential problem can be appreciated by the following estimates. Assume the apneic term newborn born without labor has a fetal lung fluid volume of 25 mL/kg, a normal blood volume of 80 mL/kg, and hematocrit of 50%. The fetal lung fluid, which contains essentially no protein, would be equivalent to 62% of the plasma volume. Cesarean delivery, intubation, and ventilation could result in a crystalloid volume challenge of 25 mL/kg, which could destabilize cardiopulmonary function. Although this scenario is the extreme, many subtle abnormalities and a few severe difficulties of neonatal adaptation are likely to result from the presence of large amounts of alveolar and interstitial fluid in the lungs of infants.

■ SURFACTANT

Lipids

Surfactant from lungs of all mammalian species contains 70% to 80% phospholipids, about 8% protein, and about 8% neutral lipids, primarily cholesterol (Fig. 16-5). The phosphatidylcholine species of the phospholipids contribute about 70% by weight to surfactant and are about 80% of the

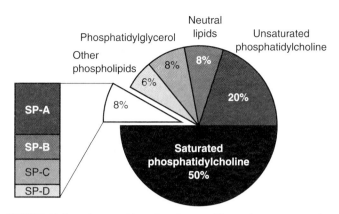

FIGURE 16-5 ■ Composition of surfactant. The major component is saturated phosphatidylcholine. The surfactant proteins contribute about 8% to the mass of surfactant.

phospholipids (Veldhuizen et al., 1998). The composition of the phospholipids in surfactant is unique relative to the lipid composition of the lung or other organs. About 50% of the phosphatidylcholine species are saturated in that both fatty acids esterified to the glycerol-phosphorylcholine backbone are predominantly the 16-carbon saturated fatty acid, palmitic acid. The other major phosphatidylcholine species of surfactant has a fatty acid with one double bond in the 2-acyl position of the molecule.

Saturated phosphatidylcholine is the principal surface-active component of surfactant. The acidic phospholipid, phosphatidylglycerol, is 4% to 15% of the phospholipids in surfactant from different species. The composition of the phospholipids in the surfactant lipoprotein complex changes during late gestation. Surfactant phospholipids from the immature fetus or newborn contain relatively large amounts of phosphatidylinositol, which then decrease as phosphatidylglycerol appears with lung maturity (Kulovich et al., 1979). Although phosphatidylglycerol is a convenient marker for lung maturity, its presence is not necessary for normal surfactant function.

Proteins

Much of the protein isolated with surfactant from alveolar lavages is serum protein that is not specific to surfactant. However, four surfactant-specific proteins have been characterized and their functions in part elucidated (Weaver and Conkright, 2001). Two of the proteins (SP-A and SP-D) have related structures and are classified as collectins because they bind carbohydrate lectins in a calcium-dependent manner.

The 26-kDa monomer of SP-A is heavily glycosylated and assembled as a six tetramer complex of about 650 kDa (Crouch and Wright, 2001). The protein has a collagen-like domain that facilitates tetramer formation and a carbohydrate recognition domain. In the late gestation and mature lung, SP-A is expressed predominantly in type II cells and Clara cells. SP-A appears in fetal lung fluid and amniotic fluid in parallel with the surfactant phospholipids during late gestation. It is secreted constitutively and separately from the surfactant complex contained in the lamellar bodies. Once in the air space, SP-A associates with surfactant and is required for tubular myelin formation. SP-A may contribute to the biophysical function of surfactant primarily by making surfactant less sensitive to inactivation by edema fluid and inflammatory

products in the injured lung. Mice that lack SP-A have essentially normal surfactant function and metabolism unless the lung is injured.

SP-A functions primarily as an innate host defense protein in the alveolus and airways (Crouch and Wright, 2001). The ability of SP-A to bind carbohydrates and to interact with immune cells in the lungs contributes to host defense. It binds endotoxin avidly, and it also binds a wide range of gram-positive and gram-negative organisms, fungi (such as *Aspergillus fumigatus*), and other organisms such as mycobacteria and *Pneumocystis carinii*. Macrophages have receptors for SP-A, and SP-A promotes phagocytosis and killing of microorganisms by alveolar macrophages. SP-A also acts as an opsonin for the phagocytosis of viruses, such as herpes simplex, influenza A, and respiratory syncytial virus. Mice that lack SP-A have less effective clearance and killing of bacteria and viruses, and the infections are more likely to become systemic (LeVine et al., 1999). The defect in host defenses can be corrected by treating SP-A–deficient mice with SP-A.

Another component to the host defense role of SP-A is modulation of the inflammatory response to infection. Nitric oxide production by macrophages is increased by SP-A to promote pathogen killing. SP-A also downregulates the general inflammatory response of the lung that generates tumor necrosis factor-α and other pro-inflammatory cytokines.

Two closely related genes express SP-A in humans, and no genetically based deficiency state has been identified. However, genetic polymorphisms in SP-A have been linked to an increased risk of RDS (Ramet et al., 2000). Infants born with low SP-A to surfactant phospholipid ratios are at increased risk of death and bronchopulmonary dysplasia (Hallman et al., 1991). SP-A levels also are low in preterm baboon models of BPD, in infants with respiratory syncytial virus pneumonia, and in the acute RDS.

SP-D has similarities in structure and function to SP-A, but distinct differences also are apparent (Crouch and Wright, 2001). The 43-kDa monomer of SP-D forms tetramers by collagen domains and then associates into a 560-kDa multimer. The carbohydrate recognition domain of SP-D binds endotoxin, gram-negative organisms, and a variety of other lung pathogens with a specificity that overlaps with SP-A. SP-D is minimally associated with surfactant lipids. The protein is present in alveolar lavage fluid at 10% to 33% of the level of SP-A. SP-D is expressed in the lung in type II cells, Clara cells, and other airway cells and glands. Expression of SP-D in the lung increases from late gestation to achieve adult levels after term, and glucocorticoids increase SP-D expression.

SP-D has the characteristics of an innate host defense protein. It binds bacteria and fungi, aggregates viruses, and promotes opsonization and phagocytosis by macrophages. It also may modulate the pro-inflammatory responses of leukocytes in the lung. In contrast to SP-A, SP-D increases with acute lung injury. Mice that lack SP-D have increased tissue and alveolar pools of surfactant lipids, although surfactant function is normal (Wert et al., 2000). These mice develop emphysema after several months of age, probably because of increased metalloproteinase activity. Mice that are SP-D deficient have a greater inflammatory response when given respiratory syncytial virus (LeVine et al., 2001). No SP-D deficiency has been identified in humans, and its contribution to the pathogenesis of BPD and lung infections in newborns has not been defined.

SP-B is a small 79 amino acid homodimer of about 18 kDa that comprises about 2% of surfactant by weight (Weaver and Conkright, 2001). The essential function of SP-B is its absolute requirement for normal packaging of the surfactant phospholipids into lamellar bodies for secretion. In the absence of SP-B in transgenic mice or term infants, type II cells have no lamellar bodies and SP-C is incompletely processed. Therefore, functionally SP-B deficiency also results in SP-C deficiency. Mice and humans that lack SP-B die soon after birth with a severe RDS-like syndrome (Cole et al., 2000). Surfactant treatment is not effective, presumably because there are no pathways for reprocessing of the surfactant components.

Deficiency of SP-B most frequently occurs because of a frame shift mutation, although multiple compound mutations have been described. The gene frequency of this frame shift maturation is 1 per 1000 to 3000 individuals (Cole et al., 2000). Deficiency of SP-B from all mutations accounts for about 30% of term infants that die of severe RDS at birth as a result of possible genetic causes for the respiratory failure. An antenatal diagnosis of SP-B deficiency can be made using amniotic fluid. Some mutations result in low expression that may increase with glucocorticoid treatment. Infants with low expression may have a chronic progressive lung disease indistinguishable from bronchopulmonary dysplasia. Acute lung injury and inflammation resulting in tumor necrosis factor-α release in the lungs will depress SP-B levels.

SP-C is a 35 amino acid monomer of 4.5 kDa that is about 2% of surfactant by weight (Weaver and Conkright, 2001). This extremely hydrophobic protein promotes surfactant film adsorption. The SP-C sequence is highly conserved across species, and messenger RNA is expressed in the developing tips of the branching airways during early lung development. During late gestation, SP-C is expressed, processed, and secreted with SP-B and the surfactant lipids in lamellar bodies only by type II cells. A deficiency of SP-C in mice results in no lung developmental abnormalities or striking abnormalities in surfactant function (Glasser et al., 2001). However, the mice get a progressive interstitial lung disease as they age. SP-C deficiency in humans also can cause a progressive interstitial lung disease that can present in infancy and may make the individual susceptible to developing acute RDS (Nogee et al., 2002). The clinical spectrum of genetically based SP-C abnormalities in humans has not been well defined yet. Acute lung injury will decrease the expression of SP-C, but how this may affect lung function is not known.

Surfactant Metabolism

Type II cells and macrophages are the cells responsible for the major pathways involved in surfactant metabolism (Fig. 16-6). The synthesis and secretion pathways are a complex sequence of biochemical events involving lipids,

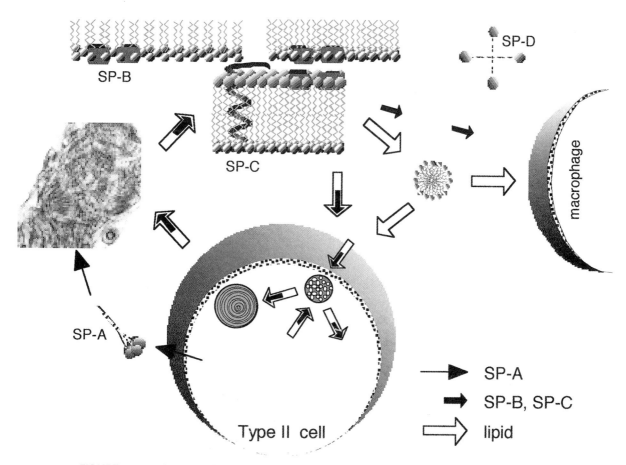

FIGURE 16-6 ■ Drawing of surfactant metabolism. The lipid-associated surfactant proteins B (SP-B) and SP-C (*solid arrows*) track with the lipid from synthesis to secretion and surface film formation. The small vesicular forms of surfactant do not contain SP-B or SP-C.

SP-B, and SP-C that result in the release of the lamellar bodies to the alveolus via exocytosis. Specific enzymes within the endoplasmic reticulum use glucose, phosphate, and fatty acids as substrates for phospholipid synthesis. The uniqueness of a phospholipid is determined by the fatty acid side chains esterified to the glycerol carbon backbone and by the head group (e.g., choline, glycerol, inositol) linked to the phosphate. The interrelated pathways for the synthesis of lung phospholipids are outlined in Figure 16-7, and the enzymes discussed in the next paragraph are identified by roman numerals on that figure.

The 3-carbon backbone of each phospholipid enters the pathway as glycerol-3-phosphate. The *de novo* synthetic pathway then proceeds through two sequential acyltransferase reactions. A saturated fatty acyl-coenzyme A (usually palmitic acid) is esterified to the 1-acyl position of glycerol-3-phosphate by glycerol-phosphate acyltransferase (I). Then the 1-acyl-glycerol-phosphate phosphotransferase (II) esterifies either an unsaturated or saturated fatty acid to the 2-acyl position, generating diacylglycerophosphate (phosphatidic acid), which is the common precursor of the phospholipids. Phosphatidic acid is then either dephosphorylated to diacylglycerol by phosphatidic acid phosphatase (III) or converted to cytidine-5'-diphospho-diacylglycerol by phosphatidate cytidyltransferase (VIII). Cytidine-5'-diphospho-diacylglycerol is the common precursor of phosphatidylglycerol and phospha-

tidylinositol. Phosphatidylglycerol is synthesized by a two-step pathway involving the enzymes glycerol-phosphate phosphatidyltransferase (IX) and phosphatidylglycerolphosphatase (X). The diacylglycerol is the direct precursor of both phosphatidylethanolamine and phosphatidylcholine after the transfer of ethanolamine or choline from the cytidine-5'-diphospho-ethanolamine or cytidine-5'-diphospho-choline to the diacylglycerol by the appropriate phosphotransferase (IV, XII). However, the resulting phosphatidylcholines are largely 1-acyl saturated, 2-acyl unsaturated.

A remolding of some of the 2-acyl-unsaturated phosphatidylcholines resulting from this *de novo* synthetic pathway occurs within the type II cell before packaging of the resulting saturated phosphatidylcholine into lamellar bodies for secretion. Two pathways for the synthesis of saturated phosphatidylcholine from unsaturated phosphatidylcholine have been identified. The direct reacylation of lysophosphatidylcholine with palmitoyl-coenzyme A (enzyme VI) is the important pathway for saturated phosphatidylcholine synthesis in type II cells (Van Golde et al., 1988).

Although the overall synthetic pathways are known, the details of how the components of surfactant condense to form the surfactant lipoprotein complex containing the phospholipids SP-B and SP-C within lamellar bodies remain obscure. The hydrophobic surfactant proteins are essential to lamellar body formation because the lamellar bodies are absent from

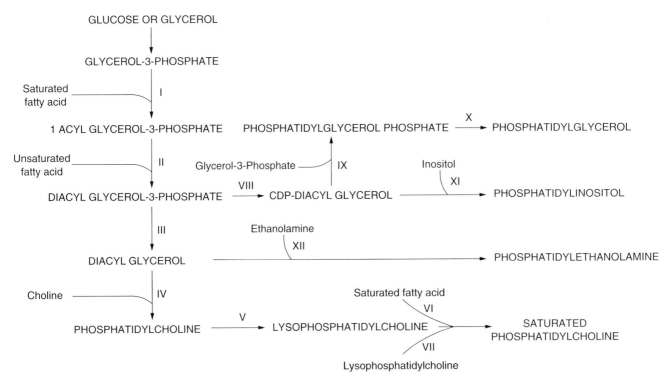

FIGURE 16-7 ■ Biosynthesis of lung phospholipids. The major pathways and precursors for the synthesis of saturated phosphatidylcholine, phosphatidylethanolamine, phosphatidylinositol, and phosphatidylglycerol are outlined. The enzymes specific for each step are indicated by roman numerals: I, glycerophosphate acyltransferase; II, 1-acyl-glycerol-phosphate phosphotransferase; III, phosphatidic acid phosphatase; IV, cytidine-5'-diphospho (CDP)-choline diacylglycerol phosphotransferase; V, phospholipase A_2; VI, lysophosphatidylcholine acyl transferase; VII, lysophosphatidylcholine-lysophosphatidylcholine acyl transferase; VIII, phosphatidate cytidyltransferase; IX, glycerophosphate phosphatidyltransferase; X, phosphatidylglycerol phosphatase; XI, CDP-ethanolamine diacylglycerol phosphotransferase.

type II cells that lack SP-B. The development and maturation of the ability of the immature lung to process surfactant lipids from synthesis to secretion are essential if the fetus is to ventilate successfully after birth.

Once the type II cell has matured sufficiently to have surfactant stores, secretion can be stimulated by a number of mechanisms (Mason and Voelker, 1998). Type II cells have β receptors and respond to β agonists by increased surfactant secretion. Purines, such as adenosine triphosphate, are more potent stimulators of surfactant secretion than β agonists and may be important for surfactant secretion at birth. Surfactant secretion also occurs with mechanical stimuli, such as lung distention and hyperventilation. The surfactant secretion that occurs with the initiation of ventilation after birth probably results from multiple stimuli, such as the combined effects of elevated catecholamines and lung expansion.

After Avery and Mead (1959) observed that saline extracts of the lungs of infants with RDS had high minimum surface tensions, decreased alveolar and tissue surfactant pools were documented in developing animals. In general, increasing surfactant pool sizes correlate with improving compliance during development, although other factors, such as structural maturation of the lung, also influence compliance measurements. Infants with RDS have surfactant pool sizes on the order of 2 to 10 mg/kg of body weight (Hallman et al., 1986). The quantity is similar to the amount of surfactant found in the alveoli of healthy adult animals and humans but much less than the amount of surfactant recovered from healthy term animals, which have surfactant pool sizes of 100 mg/kg of body weight.

The rate of increase in the pool size of alveolar surfactant after preterm birth has been measured in ventilated preterm monkeys recovering from RDS (Jackson et al., 1986). The surfactant pool size increases from about 5 mg/kg toward the 100 mg/kg value measured in term monkeys within 3 to 4 days. Although there are no comparable pool size measurement for humans, the concentration of saturated phosphatidylcholine in airway samples from infants recovering from RDS increased over a 4- to 5-day period to become comparable with values for normal or surfactant-treated infants (Hallman et al., 1991). This slow increase in pool size explains why the uncomplicated clinical course of RDS lasts from 3 to 5 days. The explanation for why surfactant pool sizes increase slowly after preterm birth is apparent from measurements of the kinetics of surfactant secretion and clearance in the newborn (Ikegami et al., 1989). After the intravascular injection of radiolabeled precursors of surfactant phosphatidylcholine, incorporation into lung phosphatidylcholine is rapid. However, there are long time delays between synthesis and the movement of surfactant components from the endoplasmic reticulum through the Golgi to lamellar bodies for eventual secretion. The time lag from surfactant phospholipid synthesis to peak secretion of labeled surfactant is about 40 hours in term newborn lambs. Ventilated preterm baboons with RDS that are developing BPD have small alveolar pool sizes of surfactant, a low percent secretion of de novo synthesized lipids, and decreased surfactant function (Seidner et al., 1998). Using stable isotope, the peak time for secretion of surfactant lipids labeled with ^{13}C-glucose infused over the first 24 hours of life in infants with RDS was about 70 hours (Bunt et al., 2000) (Fig. 16-8).

The slow increase in the alveolar surfactant pool from de novo synthesis is balanced in the term and preterm lung by slow catabolism and clearance (Jobe, 1993b). Radiolabeled surfactant phospholipids given into the air spaces of term lambs are cleared from the lung with a half-life on the order of 6 days. This slow lung clearance is in striking contrast with the more rapid catabolism characteristic of the adult lung with half-life values on the order of 12 hours. Preterm ventilated baboons that are developing BPD degrade a treatment dose of surfactant with a half-life of about 2 days (Seidner et al., 1998). Using ^{13}C-dipalmitoylphosphatidylcholine, the biological half-life of surfactant lipids in infants with RDS was about 35 hours (Torresin et al., 2000) (see Fig. 16-8). Although the measurements of surfactant metabolism in preterm infants are limited, the consistency of the values between infants with RDS and the preterm animal models clearly indicate that the preterm lung requires a number of days to achieve normal surfactant function and metabolism.

Surfactant does not remain static in the air spaces. The surfactant phospholipids move from the air spaces back to type II cells, where they are taken up by an endocytotic process into multivesicular bodies (see Fig. 16-6). In the term and preterm lung, about 90% of the phospholipids are recycled back to lamellar bodies and resecreted to the air space. In the adult lung, this process is about 25% efficient. The phospholipids are recycled as intact molecules without degradation and resynthesis. In the adult lung, about 50% of the catabolism of surfactant is by uptake by macrophages. There are few macrophages in the preterm lung at birth, but their numbers increase with inflammation and injury.

An understanding of the dynamics of surfactant metabolism is further complicated by form transitions within the alveolar space (Jobe, 1993b). The surfactant phosphatidylcholine moves from secretion as lamellar bodies to a tubular myelin pool that is the reservoir in the hypophase from which the surface film is maintained. SP-A is essential for this transition. Area compression of the surface film is then thought to concentrate saturated phosphatidylcholine by squeezing out other lipids and surfactant proteins. New surfactant facilitated by SP-B and SP-C adsorbs into the surface film and "used" surfactant leaves in the form of small vesicles, which then are cleared from the air spaces. The major compositional difference between the large surface active aggregates of surfactant and the small vesicular forms is that the small forms contain little of the surfactant-specific proteins SP-A, SP-B, or SP-C. Lamellar bodies are secreted at birth to form an alveolar pool of primarily large aggregate forms. As the newborn goes through neonatal transition, surfactant begins to function and the percentage of large aggregate forms falls and the small forms increase. The distribution of aggregate forms within a few hours of birth approximates that found in the adult animal. The ratio of small to large aggregate forms increases with lung injury.

Physiologic Effects of Surfactant on the Preterm Lung

The effect of surfactant on the preterm surfactant-deficient lung can be demonstrated by the pressure–volume relationships during quasi-static inflation and deflation (Jobe, 1993a). Preterm surfactant-deficient rabbit lungs do not accumulate much gas on inflation until pressures exceed 25 cm H_2O (Fig. 16-9). The pressure needed to open a lung unit is related to the radius of curvature and surface tension of the meniscus of fluid in the airway to each uninflated lung unit. The uninflated lung contains many different units with different radii. The units with

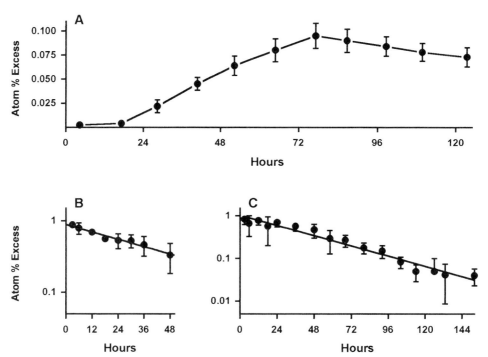

FIGURE 16-8 ■ Measurements of surfactant metabolism in preterm infants with respiratory distress syndrome using stable isotopes. **A**, Mean ± standard error curve for the ^{13}C labeling of palmitate in phosphatidylcholine recovered from airway aspirates of 11 preterm infants that received ^{13}C-glucose infusion for the first 24 hours of life. The time to maximum enrichment expressed as atom percent excess ^{13}C was 77 ± 8 hours. The half-life after peak enrichment was about 100 hours. (Data from Bunt JE, Carnielli VP, Darcos Wattimena JL, et al: The effect in premature infants of prenatal corticosteroids on endogenous surfactant synthesis as measured with stable isotopes. Am J Respir Crit Care Med **162**:844, 2000.) Loss of ^{13}C-dipalmitoylphosphatidylcholine from treatment doses of surfactant given to eight preterm infants at a mean age of 4.6 hours (**B**) and for a second dose of surfactant given at a mean age of 37 hours (**C**). The half-life of the label in the airway aspirates was about 34 hours. (Data from Torresin M, Zimmermann LJ, Cogo PE, et al: Exogenous surfactant kinetics in infant respiratory distress syndrome: A novel method with stable isotopes. Am J Respir Crit Care Med **161**:1584, 2000.)

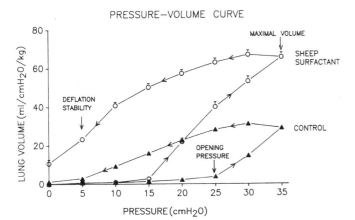

FIGURE 16-9 ■ Pressure–volume relationships for the inflation and deflation of surfactant-deficient and surfactant-treated preterm rabbit lungs. The *arrowheads* on the curves indicate the direction of the inflation–deflation sequence. The control lungs are from 27-day preterm rabbits. Surfactant deficiency is indicated by the high opening pressure, the low maximal volume at a distending pressure of 35 cm H_2O, and the lack of deflation stability at low pressures on deflation. In contrast, treatment of 27-day preterm rabbits with a natural surfactant strikingly alters the pressure–volume relationships.

larger radii and lower surface tensions "pop" open first, because with partial expansion the radius increases and the forces needed to finish opening the unit fall.

Surfactant treatment results in a striking decrease in the opening pressure to about 15 cm H_2O. Because the treatment does not alter the radii of the airways, the decreased opening pressure results from adsorption of the surfactant to the menisci. Inflation is more uniform because more units are opening at lower pressures so that there is less overdistention of the units that do open, as occurs in the surfactant-deficient lung.

An important effect of surfactant on the surfactant-deficient lung is the increase in maximal volume at maximal pressure. In Figure 16-9, maximal volume at 35 cm H_2O increased 2.5 times with surfactant treatment to a volume that is similar to that achieved in a term newborn rabbit lung. Increased pressures above 35 cm H_2O in control lungs result in lung rupture with little further volume accumulation. This volume difference, which can be achieved only with the surfactant treatment, is lung volume that will provide better gas exchange. The opening pressures of many distal lung units in the surfactant-deficient lung exceed 35 cm H_2O and exceed the rupture pressure of the preterm lung. Surfactant also stabilizes the lung on deflation. The surfactant-deficient lung collapses completely at low transpulmonary pressures, but the surfactant-treated lung retains about 40% of the lung volume on deflation to 5 cm H_2O.

SURFACTANT FOR RESPIRATORY DISTRESS SYNDROME

Fujiwara and associates (1980) first reported improved oxygenation in infants with severe RDS treated with surfactant. Surfactant for RDS became generally available with the licensure of surfactant in 1990 after extensive clinical trials (Soll and Morley, 2001). Three surfactants prepared from pig or cow lungs are currently in use in the United States. These surfactants are not equivalent to natural surfactant in composition or function because they have altered surfactant protein and/or phospholipid compositions and somewhat different biophysical characteristics. However, the metabolic characteristics of surfactant in the preterm are favorable for surfactant treatment (Jobe, 1993b). Alveolar and tissue pool sizes are small, and the alveolar pool increases slowly after birth. Treatment acutely increases both the alveolar and tissue pools because the exogenously administered surfactant is taken up into type II cells and processed for resecretion. Although the surfactants used clinically are not equivalent in function to native surfactant, the surfactant recovered by alveolar wash has improved function within hours after surfactant treatment of preterm animals (Ikegami et al., 1993). The preterm lung, if uninjured, can rapidly improve the function of the surfactant used for treatment. Also of benefit is the slow catabolic rate of surfactant. The surfactant used for treatment remains in the lungs and is not rapidly degraded (see Fig. 16-8). Treatment doses of surfactant do not feed-back inhibit the endogenous synthesis of saturated phosphatidylcholine or the surfactant proteins. No adverse metabolic consequences of surfactant treatment on the endogenous metabolism of surfactant or other lung functions have been identified. There are no clinically important differences between the surfactants used clinically to treat RDS.

Surfactants have been evaluated for two indications: the treatment of tiny preterm infants at risk for RDS immediately after birth and the treatment of infants with established RDS (Soll and Morley, 2001). Either treatment strategy is effective in decreasing the severity of respiratory symptoms and infant mortality. The choice of treatment strategy probably does not influence complications or outcomes for larger infants with RDS, but early treatment may benefit the very immature infant weighing less than 1 kg at birth (Kendig et al., 1998).

In the initial trials, delivery room treatment was compared with treatment many hours after birth. In clinical practice, the two treatment strategies now are less distinct because treatment is given as soon after birth as is practical and when some respiratory distress is apparent. A surfactant treatment should not interfere with neonatal resuscitation and initial stabilization. Clinical treatment strategies also include the use of continuous positive end-expiratory pressure with surfactant treatments to avoid mechanical ventilation (Verder et al., 1999).

The clinical trials consistently showed that mortality from RDS and overall infant mortality rates decreased with surfactant treatment (Soll and Morley, 2001) (Fig. 16-10). Surfactant treatments also decrease the incidence of pneumothorax, oxygen requirements, and ventilatory requirements over the first several days of life. A disappointment has been the lack of a consistent decrease in the incidence of BPD in surfactant-treated survivors of RDS. Presumably, infants whose lives are saved by surfactant treatment are those most likely to develop BPD, thus in part explaining the lack of decrease of this chronic lung disease. Fortunately, the severity of BPD has decreased despite the survival of more immature infants. Although isolated trials report either increases or decreases in the occurrences of common neonatal problems, such as patent ductus arteriosus and intraventricular hemorrhage, surfactant treatments do not seem to affect the nonpulmonary complications of prematurity.

Although surfactant treatments are effective, infants still die of RDS and other complications of prematurity. The only

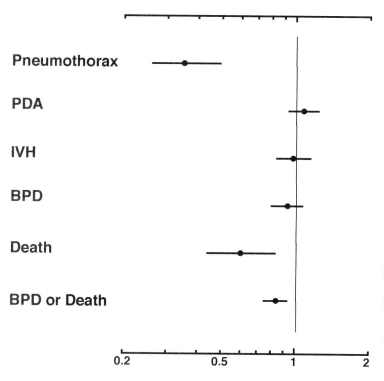

FIGURE 16-10 ■ Meta-analysis of eight randomized controlled trials of surfactant from animal lungs used for the treatment of respiratory distress syndrome. Results are given as odds ratios and 95% confidence intervals for the 988 randomized patients. BDP, bronchopulmonary dysplasia; IVH, intraventricular hemorrhage; PDA, patent ductus arteriosis. (Data from Soll RF, Morley C: Prophylactic versus Selective Use of Surfactant for Preventing Morbidity and Mortality in Preterm Infants. The Cochrane Library, Issue 2. Oxford, Update Software, 2001.)

way to prevent RDS is to prevent preterm delivery. If preterm delivery is inevitable, attempts to "mature the fetus" are reasonable. Infants exposed to antenatal corticosteroids respond better to surfactant compared with untreated infants (Jobe et al., 1993). This clinical observation is supported by animal models demonstrating that augmented surfactant treatment responses follow fetal exposure to corticosteroids. The availability of surfactant to treat RDS is not a reason to withhold maternal glucocorticoids because of the better response to surfactant and a decreased incidence of intraventricular hemorrhage and other complications of prematurity.

INDUCED LUNG MATURATION

Normally lung maturation does not occur until after 36 or 37 weeks' gestation in an infant destined to deliver at term. However, the incidence of RDS is only about 30% at 30 weeks' gestation, and infants as early as 25 weeks' gestation occasionally do not have RDS. Therefore, spontaneous "early maturation" is frequent and is thought to result from fetal stress inducing endogenous fetal cortisol and other hormones that result in early lung maturation response. Clinical experience and recent results in transgenic mouse models suggest that endogenous cortisol is not as absolutely required for normal lung development as previously thought (Jobe and Ikegami, 2000). Explants of fetal human lung from midgestation will differentiate and develop mature type II cells and surfactant in the absence of glucocorticoids. Infants born at term without hypothalamic-pituitary function generally have normal lungs. The simplest interpretation of these two observations is that the fetal human lung can develop without cortisol. However, some maternal cortisol crosses the placenta to the fetus, and transgenic mouse experiments clarify these observations. Disruption of the corticotropin-releasing hormone (CRH) gene (CRH-/-) result in adult mice with very low plasma corticosterone levels that require corticosterone supplementation to reproduce (Muglia et al., 1999). CRH-/- fetuses from the CRH-/- mice die after birth with respiratory failure. The lungs are cellular and appear to have an arrest in thinning of the saccules, although the surfactant system matures relatively normally in the CRH-/- mice. Corticosterone supplementation in the water of the CRH-/- dam prevents the delayed lung development in CRH-/- fetuses, because glucocorticoids leak from dam to fetus. The lungs of CRH-/- fetuses developed normally in CRH+ dams because corticosterone is transferred to the fetus during the circadian peak in maternal glucocorticoid secretion (Venihaki et al., 2000). Very low levels of fetal glucocorticoid exposure are sufficient to support normal lung maturation, and there may be no requirement for the normal glucocorticoids for development of the surfactant system.

The clinical issues regarding diagnosis and induction of fetal lung maturation are detailed in Chapter 25. However, a few additional issues pertaining to basic mechanisms are pertinent at this juncture. Pharmacologic induction of early lung maturation is the rationale for the clinical use of antenatal glucocorticoids in women at risk of preterm delivery. Numerous animal models and the clinical trials demonstrate that glucocorticoids can induce lung and other organ maturation. However, the fetal stress presumed to accompany fetal growth restriction, preeclampsia, or premature rupture of membranes

is not consistently associated with a decrease in the incidence of RDS in the clinical literature (Tyson et al., 1995). No good clinical data on fetal cortisol levels directly correlate with clinical stress and lung maturation.

A provocative clinical observation is that histologic chorioamnionitis is associated with decreased RDS and death in very-low-birth-weight infants (Costeloe et al., 2000). This observation has been explored in fetal sheep using an intra-amniotic injection of endotoxin as an inflammatory stimulus. The endotoxin induces chorioamnionitis and lung inflammation followed by a change in lung structure comparable with the maternal betamethasone effect and stimulation of the surfactant system (Jobe et al., 2000) (Fig. 16-11). Fetal plasma cortisol is not increased by the endotoxin stimulus, demonstrating that the lung maturational effect is not mediated by cortisol. Similar induced lung maturation also can be achieved with an intra-amniotic injection of the pro-inflammatory interleukin-1 (Willet et al., 2001a). In fetal sheep, maternal betamethasone causes fetal growth restriction and thymic involution, and both adverse effects are prevented if the fetus also is exposed to intra-amniotic endotoxin (Newnham et al., 2001). These results with endotoxin and the clinical observations indicate that unidentified mediators are contributing to the early lung maturation that frequently accompanies preterm birth.

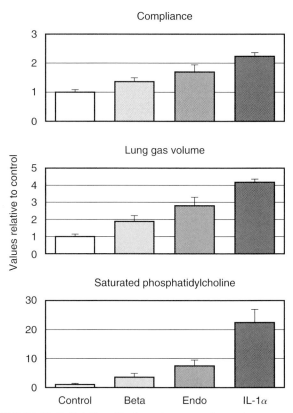

FIGURE 16-11 ■ Relative effects on lung compliance, lung gas volume measured at 40 cm H_2O pressure, and the amount of saturated phosphatidylcholine in alveolar washes 7 days after fetal exposure to 0.5 mg/kg maternal betamethasone (Beta), 10 mg intra-amniotic endotoxin (Endo), or 150 μg recombinant ovine interleukin-1α (IL-1α). The pro-inflammatory endotoxin or IL-1α stimulus improved lung function and increased surfactant. (Data from Jobe AH, Newnham JP, Willet KE, et al: Endotoxin induced lung maturation in preterm lambs is not mediated by cortisol. Am J Respir Crit Care Med **162**:1656, 2000; and Willet K, Kramer BW, Kallapur SG, et al: Intra-amniotic injection of IL-1 induces inflammation and maturation in fetal sheep lung. Am J Physiol 282:L411, 2001.)

TABLE 16-3. EFFECTOR SUBSTANCES THAT ALTER LUNG MATURATION IN *IN VITRO* SYSTEMS

Accelerate maturation
    Corticosteroids
    Thyrotropin-releasing hormone
    Triiodothyronine
    β Agonists
    Prolactin
    Epidermal growth factor
    Transforming growth factor-α
    Estrogen
    Bombesin
Delay maturation
    Insulin
    Androgens
    Transforming growth factor-α

Although multiple hormones influence lung maturation (Table 16-3), the only lung maturational agent other than corticosteroids that has been systematically evaluated in the human is thyrotropin-releasing hormone (TRH). The rationale for the use of TRH is that thyroid hormones induce lung maturation when given to the fetus, and the combined use of thyroid hormones and corticosteroids stimulate surfactant synthesis *in vitro* in human lung explants and lung tissues from other animals more rapidly and to a greater extent than either agent alone (Gross, 1990). Thyroid hormones are not a good choice for maternal treatment because high and toxic maternal doses would be required to achieve placental transfer. TRH does cross the placenta, and maternal TRH elevates fetal triiodothyronine, thyroxine, and prolactin levels.

A meta-analysis of small trials demonstrated that the combination of prenatal TRH and corticosteroids decreased RDS compared with prenatal corticosteroids alone (Moya and Gross, 1993). The provocative result from the individual trials was that TRH decreased the incidence of BPD. However, three large trials have not confirmed a beneficial effect of maternal TRH, and one trial suggested some acute risks and concerns about longer term outcomes for infants that received TRH (ACTOBAT, 1995). At this time, the use of TRH cannot be recommended to induce early lung maturation.

REFERENCES

ACTOBAT: Australian collaborative trial of antenatal thyrotropin-releasing hormone (ACTOBAT) for prevention of neonatal respiratory disease. Lancet **345**:877, 1995.

Avery ME, Mead J: Surface properties in relation to atelectasis and hyaline membrane disease. Am J Dis Child **97**:517, 1959.

Barker PM, Markiewicz M, Parker KA, et al: Synergistic action of triiodothyronine and hydrocortisone on epinephrine induced readsorption of fetal lung fluid. Pediatr Res **27**:588, 1990.

Bland RD, Chapman DL: Adsorption of liquid from the lungs at birth. *In* Effros RM (ed): Fluid and Solute Transport in the Airspaces of the Lungs. New York, Marcel Dekker, 1994, p. 303.

Boyden EA: Development and growth of the airways. *In* Hodson WA (ed): Development of the Lung. New York, Marcel Dekker, 1977, p. 3.

Brown MJ, Oliver RE, Ramoden CA, et al: Effects of adrenaline and of spontaneous labor on the secretion and adsorption of lung liquid in the fetal lamb. J Physiol (Lond) **344**:137, 1983.

Bunt JE, Carnielli VP, Darcos Wattimena JL, et al: The effect in premature infants of prenatal corticosteroids on endogenous surfactant synthesis as measured with stable isotopes. Am J Respir Crit Care Med **162**:844, 2000.

Bunton TE, Plopper CG: Triamcinolone-induced structural alterations in the development of the lung of the fetal rhesus macaque. Am J Obstet Gynecol **148**:203, 1984.

Burri PW: Developmental and growth of the human lung. *In* Fishman AP, Fisher AB (eds): Handbook of Physiology: The Respiratory System. Bethesda, Md, American Physiologic Society, 1985, p. 1.

Cardoso WV, Williams MC: Basic mechanisms of lung development: Eighth Woods Hole Conference on Lung Cell Biology 2000. Am J Respir Cell Mol Biol **25**:137, 2001.

Cole FS, Hamvas A, Rubinstein P, et al: Population-based estimates of surfactant protein B deficiency. Pediatrics **105**:538, 2000.

Costeloe K, Hennessy E, Gibson AT, et al: The EPICure study: Outcomes to discharge from hospital for infants born at the threshold of viability [In Process Citation]. Pediatrics **106**:659, 2000.

Crouch E, Wright JR: Surfactant proteins a and d and pulmonary host defense. Annu Rev Physiol **63**:521, 2001.

Faxelius G, Bremme K, Lagercrantz H: An old problem revisited—hyaline membrane disease and caesarean section. Eur J Pediatr **139**:121, 1982.

Fujiwara T, Chida S, Watabe Y, et al: Artificial surfactant therapy in hyaline-membrane disease. Lancet **1**:55, 1980.

Glasser SW, Burhans MS, Korfhagen TR, et al: Altered stability of pulmonary surfactant in SP-C-deficient mice. Proc Natl Acad Sci USA **98**:6366, 2001.

Gluck L, Kulovich M, Borer RC, et al: Diagnosis of the respiratory distress syndrome by amniocentesis. Am J Obstet Gyncol **109**:440, 1971.

Gross I. Regulation of fetal lung maturation. Am J Physiol **259**:L337, 1990.

Hallman M, Kulovich M, Kirkpatrick E, et al: Phosphatidylinositol and phosphatidylglycerol in amniotic fluid: indices of lung maturity. Am J Obstet Gynecol **125**:613, 1976.

Hallman M, Merritt TA, Akino T, et al: Surfactant protein-A, phosphatidylcholine, and surfactant inhibitors in epithelial lining fluid—correlation with surface activity, severity of respiratory distress syndrome, and outcome in small premature infants. Am Rev Respir Dis **144**:1376, 1991.

Hallman M, Merritt TA, Pohjavuori M, et al: Effect of surfactant substitution on lung effluent phospholipids in respiratory distress syndrome: Evaluation of surfactant phospholipid turnover, pool size, and the relationship to severity of respiratory failure. Pediatr Res **20**:1228, 1986.

Hislop AA, Wigglesworth JS, Desai R: Alveolar development in the human fetus and infant. Early Hum Dev **13**:1, 1986.

Ikegami M, Jobe A, Yamada T, et al: Surfactant metabolism in surfactant-treated preterm ventilated lambs. J Appl Physiol **67**:429, 1989.

Ikegami M, Ueda T, Absolom D, et al: Changes in exogenous surfactant in ventilated preterm lamb lungs. Am Rev Respir Dis **148**:837, 1993.

Jackson JC, Palmer S, Truog WE, et al: Surfactant quantity and composition during recovery from hyaline membrane disease. Pediatr Res **20**:1243, 1986.

Jobe AH: Pulmonary surfactant therapy. N Engl J Med **328**:861, 1993a.

Jobe AH: Surfactant metabolism. Clin Perinatol **20**:683, 1993b.

Jobe AH: The new BPD: An arrest of lung development. Pediatr Res **46**:641, 1999.

Jobe AH, Ikegami M: Fetal responses to glucocorticoids. *In* Mendelson CR (ed): Endocrinology of the Lung. Totowa, NJ, Humana Press, 2000, p. 45.

Jobe AH, Mitchell BR, Gunkel JH: Beneficial effects of the combined use of prenatal corticosteroids and postnatal surfactant on preterm infants. Am J Obstet Gynecol **168**:508, 1993.

Jobe AH, Newnham JP, Willet KE, et al: Endotoxin induced lung maturation in preterm lambs is not mediated by cortisol. Am J Respir Crit Care Med **162**:1656, 2000.

Johnson JWC, Mitzner W, Beck JC, et al: Long-term effects of betamethasone on fetal development. Am J Obstet Gynecol **141**:1053, 1981.

Kay S, Laberge JM, Flageole H, et al: Use of antenatal steroids to counteract the negative effects of tracheal occlusion in the fetal lamb model. Pediatr Res **50**:495, 2001.

Kendig JW, Ryan RM, Sinkin RA, et al: Comparison of two strategies for surfactant prophylaxis in very premature infants: A multicenter randomized trial. Pediatrics **101**:1006, 1998.

Kulovich MV, Hallman M, Gluck L: The lung profile: Normal pregnancy. Am J Obstet Gynecol **135**:57, 1979.

Langston C, Kida D, Reed M, et al: Human lung growth in late gestation and in the neonate. Am Rev Respir Dis **129**:607, 1984.

LeVine AM, Kurak KE, Wright JR, et al: Surfactant protein-A (SP-A) binds group B streptococcus enhancing phagocytosis and clearance from lungs of surfactant protein-A deficient mice. Am J Respir Mol Cell Biol **20**:279, 1999.

LeVine AM, Whitsett JA, Hartshorn KL, et al: Surfactant protein D enhances clearance of influenza A virus from the lung in vivo. J Immunol **167**:5868, 2001.

Liggins GC: Growth of the fetal lung. J Dev Physiol **6**:237, 1984.

Liggins GC, Howie RN: A controlled trial of antepartium glucocorticoid treatment for prevention of RDS in premature infants. Pediatrics **50**:515, 1972.

Lindner W, Pohlandt F, Grab D, et al: Acute respiratory failure and short-term outcome after premature rupture of the membranes and oligohydramnios before 20 weeks of gestation. J Pediatr **140**:177, 2002.

Mason RJ, Voelker DR: Regulatory mechanisms of surfactant secretion. Biochim Biophys Acta **1408**:226, 1998.

Massaro D, Massaro GD: Pulmonary alveoli: Formation, the "call for oxygen," and other regulators [invited review]. Am J Physiol Lung Cell Mol Physiol **282**:L345, 2002.

Moya FR, Gross I: Combined hormonal therapy for the prevention of respiratory distress syndrome and its consequences. Semin Perinatol **17**:267, 1993.

Muglia LJ, Bae DS, Brown TT, et al: Proliferation and differentiation defects during lung development in corticotropin-releasing hormone-deficient mice. Am J Respir Cell Mol Biol **20**:181, 1999.

Muratore CS, Wilson JM: Congenital diaphragmatic hernia: Where are we and where do we go from here? Semin Perinatol **24**:418, 2000.

Newnham JP, Moss TJ, Padbury JF, et al: The interactive effects of endotoxin with prenatal glucocorticoids on short-term lung function in sheep. Am J Obstet Gynecol **185**:190, 2001.

Nogee LM, Dunbar AE 3rd, Wert S, et al: Mutations in the surfactant protein C gene associated with interstitial lung disease. Chest **121**:20S, 2002.

O'Brodovich H: Fetal lung liquid secretion: Insights using the tools of inhibitors and genetic knock-out experiments. Am J Respir Cell Mol Biol **25**:8, 2001.

Perl AK, Whitsett JA: Molecular mechanisms controlling lung morphogenesis. Clin Genet **56**:14, 1999.

Ramet M, Haataja R, Marttila R, et al: Association between the surfactant protein A (SP-A) gene locus and respiratory-distress syndrome in the Finnish population. Am J Hum Genet **66**:1569, 2000.

Seidner SR, Jobe AH, Coalson JJ, et al: Abnormal surfactant metabolism and function in preterm ventilated baboons. Am J Respir Crit Care Med **158**:1982, 1998.

Soll RF, Morley C: Prophylactic Versus Selective Use of Surfactant for Preventing Morbidity and Mortality in Preterm Infants. The Cochrane Library, Issue 2. Oxford, Update Software, 2001.

Thibeault DW, Beatty EC Jr, Hall RT, et al: Neonatal pulmonary hypoplasia with premature rupture of fetal membranes and oligohydramnios. J Pediatr **107**:273, 1985.

Thibeault DW, Mabry SM, Ekekezie I, et al: Lung elastic tissue maturation and perturbations during the evolution of chronic lung disease. Pediatrics **106**:1452, 2000.

Torresin M, Zimmermann LJ, Cogo PE, et al: Exogenous surfactant kinetics in infant respiratory distress syndrome: A novel method with stable isotopes. Am J Respir Crit Care Med **161**:1584, 2000.

Tyson JE, Kennedy K, Broyles S, et al: The small for gestational age infant: Accelerated or delayed pulmonary maturation? Increased or decreased survival? Pediatrics **95**:534, 1995.

Van Golde LM, Batenburg JJ, Robertson B: The pulmonary surfactant system: biochemical aspects and functional significance. Physiol Rev **68**:374, 1988.

Veldhuizen R, Nag K, Orgeig S, et al: The role of lipids in pulmonary surfactant. Biochim Biophys Acta **1408**:90, 1998.

Venihaki M, Carrigan A, Dikkes P, et al: Circadian rise in maternal glucocorticoid prevents pulmonary dysplasia in fetal mice with adrenal insufficiency. Proc Natl Acad Sci USA **97**:7336, 2000.

Verder H, Albertsen P, Ebbesen F, et al: Nasal continuous positive airway pressure and early surfactant therapy for respiratory distress syndrome in newborns of less than 30 weeks' gestation. Pediatrics **103**:E24, 1999.

Weaver TE, Conkright JJ: Function of surfactant proteins B and C. Annu Rev Physiol **63**:555, 2001.

Wert SE, Yoshida M, LeVine AM, et al: Increased metalloproteinase activity, oxidant production, and emphysema in surfactant protein D gene-inactivated mice. Proc Natl Acad Sci USA **97**:5972, 2000.

Wigglesworth JS, Desai R. Is fetal respiratory function a major determinant of perinatal survival? Lancet **1**:264, 1982.

Wilcox DT, Glick PL, Karamanoukian HL, et al: Contributions by individual lungs to the surfactant status in congenital diaphragmatic hernia. Pediatr Res **41**:686, 1997.

Willet K, Jobe A, Ikegami M, et al: Antenatal endotoxin and glucocorticoid effects on lung morphometry in preterm lambs. Pediatr Res **48**:782, 2000.

Willet K, Kramer BW, Kallapur SG, et al: Intra-amniotic injection of IL-1 induces inflammation and maturation in fetal sheep lung. Am J Physiol **282**:L411, 2001a.

Willet KE, Jobe AH, Ikegami M, et al: Lung morphometry after repetitive antenatal glucocorticoid treatment in preterm sheep. Am J Respir Crit Care Med **163**:1437, 2001b.

Zeltner TB, Burri PH: The postnatal development and growth of the human lung. II. Morphology. Respir Physiol **67**:269, 1987.

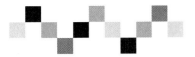

Chapter 17

EVIDENCE-BASED PRACTICE IN PERINATAL MEDICINE

George A. Macones, MD, MSCE

All those who drink of this remedy recover in a short time, except those whom it does not help, who die. Therefore, it is obvious that it fails only in incurable cases.

—Galen (circa 100 AD)

EVIDENCE-BASED MEDICINE IN PERSPECTIVE

Great strides have been made in the past 25 years in the care of women. Many of these improvements have come about as a result of carefully designed studies of interventions aimed at improving health. Before this time, physicians relied on anecdote and personal experience to guide patient care.

Evidence-based medicine is a style of practice best described as "... integrating individual clinical expertise with the best-available external clinical evidence from systematic research" (Centre for Evidence-Based Medicine, Oxford University). Thus, contrary to what many believe, evidence-based medicine combines an understanding of the literature *and* individual expertise. It is this blend of evidence and clinical intuition that makes evidence-based medicine so attractive and essential to the practice of modern medicine.

Why is the practice of evidence-based medicine so important in maternal-fetal medicine? First, the practice of evidence-based medicine will allow for the best care of our patients. We can look to the history of obstetrics for examples of where an incomplete or improper assessment of the evidence has led to problems with care today. The classic example is the emergence of electronic fetal heart rate monitoring (see Chapter 22). This device was quite novel when it was introduced. It was generally assumed that implementation of this new device would obviously lead to improved perinatal outcomes. Unfortunately, electronic fetal monitoring was widely implemented before such evidence existed, and now it is rooted in the practice of obstetrics in the United States and in many other countries. As has been well documented, it is uncertain whether continuous electronic fetal monitoring confers any benefit above intermittent auscultation in low-risk patients. In fact, electronic fetal monitoring has been blamed as a major contributing factor in the rise in the rate of cesarean section.

Second, clinical research is growing exponentially, as evidenced by the number of medical journals, research publications, and scientific societies. Some have estimated that 1000 articles are added to MEDLINE per day. In addition, clinical research has gained in importance, with programs at the National Institutes of Health and other funding agencies focused on clinical research. With the volume and rapid access to such information (for both physicians and patients), it is essential for practicing clinicians to be able to assess the medical literature to determine a best course of action for an individual patient.

Finally, today in perinatal medicine we are faced with a number of important yet unanswered questions:

- Does the fetal pulse oximeter reduce the rate of cesarean section and improve neonatal outcome?
- Does *in utero* fetal surgery improve function in infants with neural tube defects compared with standard management?
- Should we screen women with a history of poor pregnancy outcome for inherited thrombophilias? If so, how should we treat those who are positive?

How do we, as physicians and researchers, reach sound decisions for such questions? We reach them by being able to assess the medical evidence. In the sections that follow, we review the principles that serve as a basis for learning to interpret clinical research, including clinical research study designs, measures of effect, sources of error in clinical research (systematic and random), and screening and diagnosis. This will provide the reader with the information that will advance the journey toward becoming an evidence-based medicine practitioner.

TYPES OF CLINICAL RESEARCH STUDIES

A number of study designs are reported in the medical literature.

Descriptive Studies

Case reports and case series are simple descriptions of either a single case or number of cases and are termed a *descriptive* study (Peipert and Phipps, 1998). Often they focus on an unusual disease, unusual presentation of a disease, or unusual treatment for a disease. In case reports and case series, there is no control group. Because of this, drawing any inference on causality is impossible. Such studies are useful mainly for hypothesis *generation*, rather than hypothesis *testing*. That said, case reports and case series can be very valuable in the scientific process, because many important observations were initially made by a single case or series of cases. An excellent example of the importance of case reports or series occurred in the early 1980s, where physicians in California noted an unusual respiratory illness that was occurring in homosexual young men. The observation of these astute physicians led to the early discovery of the acquired immunodeficiency syndrome epidemic in the United States.

Observational Studies

The two main types of *observational* studies are case-control studies and cohort studies (Hennekens and Buring, 1987; Kelsey et al., 1996; Peipert and Phipps, 1998). Both of these study designs attempt to assess the relationship between an exposure and an outcome (Table 17-1).

In case-control studies, subjects are identified on the basis of disease rather than on exposure. Groups of subjects with and without disease are identified, and then exposures of interest are retrospectively sought. Comparisons of the distribution of exposures are then made between cases and controls. Case-control studies are useful for the study of rare conditions. Advantages of case-control studies include the following: They can assess the impact of multiple exposures, they can be done quickly, and they are inexpensive. Disadvantages include the following: they cannot be used to calculate an incidence of disease given a particular exposure and there is potential for confounding and bias.

Cohort studies identify subjects based on exposure and then assess the relationship between the exposure and the clinical outcome of interest. Cohort studies can be either retrospective or prospective. In a retrospective cohort study, the exposed population is identified after the event of interest has occurred. In a prospective cohort study, exposed and unexposed subjects are followed over time to see if the outcome of interest occurs. Cohort studies are useful in the study of rare exposures. The advantages of cohort studies are that the incidence of disease in exposed and unexposed individuals can be assessed and there is less potential for bias (especially if prospective). The main disadvantage of prospective cohort studies is that they can be time-consuming and expensive and can take years to complete (if prospective).

A clinical example may help to distinguish these designs. Suppose one is interested in the relationship between anticonvulsant use in pregnancy and the occurrence of neural tube defects. Such a question could be assessed with either a case-control or cohort study. For the case-control study, one would identify a group of cases of fetuses/neonates with neural tube defects and a group of controls (i.e., children without a neural

tube defect). One could then review the maternal record to see if exposure to anticonvulsants has occurred. The cohort version of this study would be to identify a population of women taking anticonvulsants in pregnancy and a group not taking anticonvulsants. Both groups would then be followed during pregnancy to see if the fetus/neonate had a neural tube defect.

Interventional Studies

The randomized clinical trial is the gold standard of clinical research design (Meinert, 1986). In a clinical trial, eligible consenting participants are randomly allocated to receive different therapies. Differences in clinical outcomes can then be compared based on treatment assignment. The reason that clinical trials are so powerful is that the likelihood of confounding and bias influencing the results is minimized. However, there are some drawbacks with clinical trials. Clinical trials are logistically difficult, expensive, and can take years to complete. There are also concerns about whether the results of clinical trials can be "generalized," that is, applied to clinical practice with the expectation that the same results will occur. Specifically, it has been documented that those who consent to be part of a trial are "different" from those who do not consent. In addition, well-done clinical trials often have strict inclusion and exclusion criteria, with strict follow-up procedures. In real-life clinical situations, such rigor in follow-up rarely occurs. Standards for reporting prospective randomized trials have been developed. These have been published as the CONSORT statement (Moher et al., 2001).

Despite these concerns, clinical trials provide the best evidence upon which to base our practice. An excellent example of a practice-guiding clinical trial was the screening and treatment study of bacterial vaginosis in pregnancy performed by the Maternal-Fetal Medicine Units Network (Carey et al., 2000). A variety of studies from around the world suggested that symptomatic and asymptomatic bacterial vaginosis was associated with spontaneous preterm birth (Kurki et al., 1992; Riduan et al., 1993; Hillier et al., 1995). In addition, small clinical trials in high-risk women suggested that screening and treating bacterial vaginosis in pregnancy could reduce the occurrence of spontaneous preterm delivery (Hauth et al., 1995). Many assumed that screening and treating all pregnant women could, on a population level, reduce the incidence of preterm birth. To answer this question, the MFMU Network performed a placebo-controlled clinical trial comparing metronidazole with placebo for women who screened positive for bacterial vaginosis in pregnancy (Carey et al., 2000). This study demonstrated that treating asymptomatic bacterial vaginosis in pregnancy did not reduce the occurrence of preterm birth.

Other Study Designs

Two other study designs deserve mention: meta-analysis and decision analysis. Both are valuable tools for the evidence-based medicine practitioner.

Meta-Analysis

Meta-analysis is a methodology in which the results of a series of randomized clinical trials (or observational studies) can be statistically combined to obtain a "summary estimate"

TABLE 17-1. ADVANTAGES AND DISADVANTAGES OF CASE-CONTROL STUDIES VERSUS COHORT STUDIES

Case-Control Study	Cohort Study
Good for rare disease	Good for common disease
Study multiple exposures	Study multiple outcomes
Done quickly	Long follow-up
Inexpensive	Expensive (prospective)
No incidence data	Can directly calculate incidence
Prone to bias	Less prone to bias

for the effect of a given treatment (Peipert and Bracken, 1997). The strength of a meta-analysis comes from the combined analysis of results from multiple small clinical trials, thereby increasing the "power" to detect differences in treatment. Numerous meta-analyses have been performed for topics in obstetrics (Sanchez-Ramos et al., 1999; Tsatsaris et al. 2001), including many performed within the Cochrane Database of Systemic Reviews (2002). Two such analyses are shown in Figures 17-1 and 17-2, taken from the Cochrane Library meta-analysis of the effect on neonatal outcome of antibiotics given antenatally to women with preterm prematurely ruptured amniotic membranes (Kenyon et al., 2002). In Figure 17-1, a comparison of neonatal infectious complications between those who received antibiotics and those who did not are made and pooled for all available studies. Each of 11 randomized trials that met inclusion criteria in this analysis is listed, with the number of subjects and the frequency of the outcome in the treatment and control groups noted. The relative risk and 95% confidence interval for each study (see under Assessing Random Error) weighted for their sample size are shown. The total number of subjects with the outcome of interest is summed and the combined relative risk and 95% confidence interval calculated. In this example, a number of small trials show a nonsignificant trend in favor of antibiotic treatment. The "pooled" (i.e., statistically combined) relative risk was 0.67, with a 95% confidence interval from 0.52 to 0.85. The point estimate suggests the "best guess" is that antibiotics reduce the risk of neonatal infection by 33%. The confidence interval suggests that the data are consistent with as much as a 48% reduction in risk (1 − 0.52) or as little as a 15% (1 − 0.85) reduction in risk. But still, even the upper bound of the confidence interval suggests a protective effect of antibiotics on neonatal infection.

Compare this summary graph with that for the effect of antibiotics on perinatal death in women with preterm prema-ture rupture of membranes (Fig. 17-2). Here the pooled estimate yields a point estimate relative risk of 0.89 with a 95% confidence interval from 0.67 to 1.18. The point estimate suggests the best estimate is that antibiotics reduce the occurrence of perinatal death by 11%. The confidence interval suggests that the data are also consistent with as much as a 33% reduction in perinatal death or an 18% *increase* in perinatal death with antibiotics. Because the confidence interval crosses a relative risk of 1.0, the data are consistent with "no difference" between the groups.

A notable negative of meta-analysis is that among clinical trials on the same general topic, seldom are the populations exactly the same and seldom are the treatments the same in each trial. Thus, at times, meta-analysis can seem like "mixing apples with oranges" (Cook and Guyatt, 1994; LeLorier et al., 1997; Peipert and Bracken, 1997; Villar et al., 1997). It is incumbent on the reader to make such a determination. Guidelines for publication of quality meta-analyses have been promulgated by the QUOROM statement proposed by a consortium of journal editors (Moher et al., 1999) and, like the CONSORT statement, are subscribed to by *The American Journal of Obstetrics and Gynecology*, *Obstetrics and Gynecology*, and general medical journals such as *Lancet*, *The New England Journal of Medicine*, and JAMA.

Decision Analysis

Decision analysis is a methodology in which the component parts of a complex decision are broken down and analyzed in a theoretical model. Decision models often compare different therapeutic strategies for a clinical dilemma, using the existing literature. The ultimate goal of any decision analysis is to reach a clinical decision. Importantly, decision models are often the foundation for formal economic analysis, such as cost-effectiveness analysis (Macones et al., 1999). Decision and

Study	Treatment	Control	Relative Risk (Fixed) 95% CI	Weight %	Relative Risk (Fixed) 95% CI
Cox 1995	0 / 31	1 / 31		1.1	0.33 [0.01, 7.88]
Ernest 1994	0 / 77	2 / 67		2.0	0.17 [0.01, 3.57]
Garcia 1995	4 / 30	5 / 30		3.8	0.80 [0.24, 2.69]
Johnston 1990	3 / 40	11 / 45		7.9	0.31 [0.09, 1.02]
Kurki 1992	0 / 57	1 / 58		1.1	0.34 [0.01, 8.15]
Lockwood 1993	2 / 37	4 / 35		3.1	0.47 [0.09, 2.42]
McGregor 1991	1 / 24	1 / 27		0.7	1.13 [0.07, 17.02]
Mercer 1992	14 / 109	19 / 114		14.1	0.77 [0.41, 1.46]
Mercer 1997	46 / 299	67 / 312		49.9	0.72 [0.51, 1.01]
Ovalle Salas 1997	7 / 42	7 / 43		5.3	1.02 [0.39, 2.67]
Svare 1997	7 / 30	16 / 37		10.9	0.54 [0.26, 1.14]
Total (95% CI)	84 / 776	134 / 799		100.0	0.67 [0.52, 0.85]

Review: Antibiotics for preterm premature rupture of membranes
Comparison: 01 Any antibiotic versus placebo
Outcome: 16 Neonatal infection including pneumonia

Test for heterogeneity chi-square = 4.56 df = 10 p = 0.9186
Test for overall effect Z = 3.21 p = 0.00

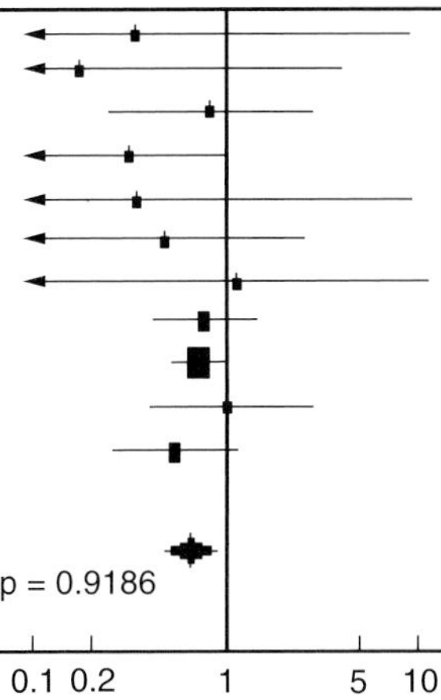

0.1 0.2   1   5 10

FIGURE 17-1 ■ Meta-analysis summary graph of the effect of maternal antibiotic administration on the occurrence of neonatal infection in women with preterm premature rupture of membranes. 95% CI, 95% confidence interval. (From Kenyon S, Boulvain M, Neilson J: Antibiotics for preterm premature rupture of membranes (Cochrane Review). *The Cochrane Library*, issue 4. Oxford, Update Software, 2002.)

Review: Antibiotics for preterm premature rupture of membranes
Comparison: 03 Macrolide antibiotics versus placebo
Outcome: 28 Perinatal death/death before discharge

Study	Treatment	Control	Relative Risk (Fixed) 95% CI	Weight %	Relative Risk (Fixed) 95% CI
Garcia 1995	2 / 30	5 / 30		5.2	0.40 [0.08, 1.90]
Kenyon 2001	70 / 1190	82 / 1225		84.2	0.88 [0.65, 1.20]
McGregor 1991	6 / 28	0 / 27		0.5	12.55 [0.74, 212.53]
Mercer 1992	6 / 106	10 / 114		10.0	0.65 [0.24, 1.71]
Total (95% CI)	84 / 1354	97 / 1396		100.0	0.89 [0.67, 1.18]

Test for heterogeneity chi-square = 4.80 df = 3 p = 0.1868
Test for overall effect Z = 0.79 p = 0.40

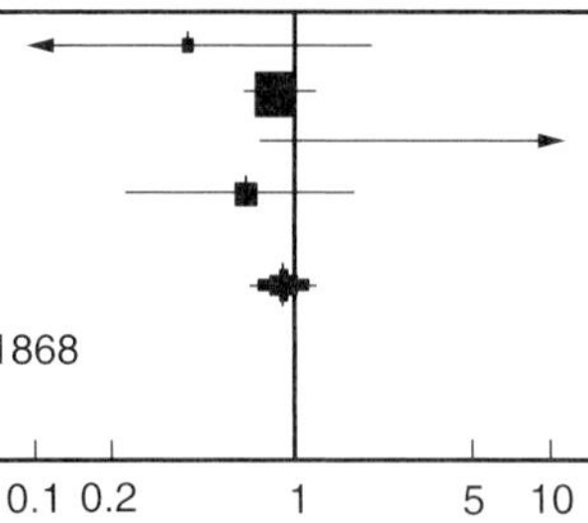

0.1 0.2   1   5   10

FIGURE 17-2 ■ Meta-analysis summary graph of the effect of maternal antibiotic administration on the occurrence of perinatal death/death before discharge in women with preterm premature rupture of membranes. 95% CI, 95% confidence interval. (From Kenyon S, Boulvain M, Neilson J: Antibiotics for preterm premature rupture of membranes (Cochrane Review). *The Cochrane Library*, issue 4. Oxford, Update Software, 2002.)

economic analyses are fairly common in the obstetric literature. Such analyses have been published on GBS screening (Rouse et al., 1994), indomethacin use for preterm labor (Macones and Robinson, 1997), and tocolysis at advanced gestational ages (Macones et al., 1998). Although a detailed discussion of this powerful methodology is outside the scope of this chapter, interested readers should consider reading review articles on this subject (Macones et al., 1999).

SOURCES OF ERROR IN CLINICAL RESEARCH

Broadly speaking, two types of error can occur in clinical research studies: systematic error and random error (Hennekens and Buring, 1987; Kelsey et al., 1996). Systematic error is generally introduced by the investigator through an issue with study design. Sources of systematic error include confounding and bias (Datta, 1993; Sitthi-amorn and Poshyachinda, 1993; Grimes and Schulz, 2002). Random error is assessed using various methods for hypothesis testing, as described below. As readers of clinical research, our goals are to understand and to try to interpret the role of these errors in the studies we read.

Confounding

Confounding is a type of systematic error that can be present in observational research studies (Datta, 1993; Leon, 1993; Grimes and Schulz, 2002). Confounding can be described as occurring when two factors are associated with each other and the effect of one factor on a given outcome is distorted by the effect of the other factor. Importantly, randomized clinical trials generally cannot be confounded, because randomization itself should lead to an equal distribution of confounding factors between various treatment groups (Meinert, 1986).

An example of a case that illustrates possible confounding comes from observational studies of indomethacin for tocolysis. Norton and colleagues (1993) performed a matched retrospective cohort study of infants delivered at less than 30 weeks.

These authors identified 57 infants whose mothers were exposed to indomethacin delivered at or below 30 weeks' gestation and 57 infants whose mothers did not receive indomethacin. The results of this study suggested that the antepartum administration of indomethacin was an independent risk factor for necrotizing enterocolitis and grades II to IV intraventricular hemorrhage. This observational study suggested a positive association between antenatal indomethacin exposure and adverse neonatal outcomes, as did others (Itskovitz et al., 1980; Major et al., 1994; Iannucci et al., 1996). However, to properly interpret observational studies as an evidence-based practitioner, it is important to assess sources of systematic error that may explain the observed results, such as confounding and bias. In this example, it is possible that confounding may explain the association between indomethacin and neonatal morbidity observed in this observational study (Macones et al., 2001).

Specifically, in the observational studies of indomethacin and neonatal morbidity, it is likely that indomethacin was used mainly in subjects who failed first-line tocolysis, because indomethacin is generally not a first-line tocolytic in practice. If "failing" first-line tocolysis is itself a risk factor for adverse neonatal outcome, then the association between indomethacin and adverse neonatal outcome can be confounded. Thus, a principal question in the interpretation of these studies is whether patients who are failing first-line tocolysis are themselves at higher risk for adverse neonatal outcomes (whether exposed to indomethacin or not) than those who respond to first-line tocolysis. Existing data suggest that women whose labor does not stop after first-line tocolysis have an increased risk of adverse neonatal consequences because of the well-established relationship between tocolytic failure and subclinical and intra-amniotic infection, both of which themselves are associated with adverse neonatal outcome.

Because of the relationships between refractory preterm labor and subclinical infection and between subclinical infection and major neonatal morbidity (Romero et al., 1989, 1998; Yoon et al., 1997), it is uncertain whether the association between indomethacin and adverse neonatal outcome in these retrospective observational studies is a "true" or a spurious association resulting from confounding. We hypothesize that in the observational studies, exposure to indomethacin may be nothing more than a sign of more severe preterm labor, which itself is associated with major neonatal complications (Macones et al., 2001).

Bias

Bias is defined as a "process at any stage of inference tending to produce results that depart systematically from true results" (Last, 1995). Bias is usually something that enters at the study design stage (Sitthi-amorn and Poshyachinda, 1993; Grimes and Schulz, 2002). There are two main types of bias to consider when reading clinical research. *Selection bias* occurs when an error is made in the selection of a study population. *Information bias* occurs when a systematic error takes place in the measurement of information on exposure or outcome.

An example of bias may be helpful. Recall bias is a type of information bias that occurs when subjects differentially recall past events based on either an exposure status or disease outcome. A classic example of recall bias can occur in observational studies of teratogenesis. Consider a case-control study to assess whether exposure to medications is associated with cleft lip (Czeizel and Rockenbauer, 1998). In this example, cases of cleft lip were ascertained after delivery occurred; the controls were women who delivered children without a birth defect. Mothers of cases and controls were queried regarding medication use during the pregnancy. The question when reading such a study is whether women who have delivered a child with a birth defect are more likely to recall medication use than a woman who has delivered a normal child. To the extent that there is differential recall, there may be significant recall bias that would lead to an inflated estimate of the relationship between medications and cleft lip.

Assessing the Role of Systematic Error in Clinical Research

It is essential for clinicians to be able to assess the role of systematic error in clinical research. Although a detailed discussion is beyond the scope of this chapter, there are several useful maxims for reading clinical research:

1. Systematic error is more of a concern for observational studies than for clinical trials. Because of randomization, confounding seldom occurs in clinical trials (Schulz and Grimes, 2002).
2. Retrospective observational studies are often more likely to be biased than prospective studies (though bias still can occur in prospective observational studies).
3. In any observational study, one should always carefully read the methods section and consider whether there is the potential for bias.
4. Even if one believes a study to have a serious bias, it should not automatically be discarded. It is important to consider not just the *presence* of bias but also the *direction* of the bias (Grimes and Schulz, 2002). Consider again the example of the case-control study of medications and cleft palate described above. Now assume that the results of the study suggested no association between medications and cleft palate. Concern about recall bias given the study design is appropriate, but in this case the recall bias would have led to an *overestimate* of the association between medications

and cleft lip. Given that the study showed no association, it is unlikely that the recall bias would lead to a change in the overall interpretation of the results of the study.

5. Likewise, confounding should always be considered as an explanation of observed results. Readers should consider whether relevant confounding factors were measured and, if unmeasured, the direction of the possible confounding. There are statistical techniques to "adjust" for measured confounding factors, such as multivariate analysis and logistic regression (Hosmer and Lemeshow, 1989). In modern observational clinical research, *it is unacceptable to report only unadjusted associations when measured confounders can be adjusted for using appropriate statistical techniques.*

Assessing Random Error: Hypothesis Testing and Measures of Effect in Clinical Research

In clinical research, one is often interested in whether an exposure is significantly associated with an outcome or whether an intervention can improve a given outcome. Commonly, interpretation of the results of clinical research is focused on the assessment of a "significance test," such as a probability value. This type of testing provides information on the role of chance (i.e., random error) to explain the observed results in a given study. Although assessing the role of *random* error is important when reading medical literature, it is equally important to assess the role of *systematic* error (i.e., bias and confounding) in clinical research.

Let us consider the randomized clinical trial cited previously of a program to screen and treat bacterial vaginosis during pregnancy (Carey et al., 2000). The goal of the study was to see whether treating asymptomatic bacterial vaginosis in pregnancy could reduce the risk of spontaneous preterm birth. To answer this question, a large-scale, multicenter, randomized, clinical trial was undertaken. Low-risk and high-risk women were screened for bacterial vaginosis with a Gram stain of a vaginal smear. Enrolled women who were found to have bacterial vaginosis were then randomized to receive either oral metronidazole or placebo. The primary outcome was the occurrence of delivery at less than 35 weeks' gestation. The primary results of the study are summarized in Table 17-2.

The association between treatment with metronidazole and preterm birth can be expressed in several ways: by probability value; by relative risk with 95% confidence intervals; and by several other measures of effect, including odds ratio and risk difference.

TABLE 17-2. METRONIDAZOLE VERSUS PLACEBO TO PREVENT PRETERM BIRTH

| | Delivery < 37 Weeks | | |
	Yes	No	Total
Metronidazole	116	837	953
Placebo	121	845	966
Total	237	1682	1919

Data from Carey JC, Klebanoff MA, Hauth JC, et al, for the National Institute of Child Health and Human Development Network of Maternal-Fetal Medicine Units: Metronidazole to prevent preterm delivery in pregnant women with asymptomatic bacterial vaginosis. N Engl J Med **342**:534, 2000.

Probability Value

A *probability value* is defined as the probability of obtaining the observed differences in the sample if there is no true difference in the population. For example, a probability value of 0.05 means that there is a 5% probability of achieving the observed difference, if in fact the null hypothesis of no true difference is true. Thus, the smaller the probability value, the smaller the possibility of chance as the explanation of an observed difference. In the above example, the probability value is 0.95, indicating a high likelihood that chance explains the small difference in the rate of preterm birth between the groups.

Traditionally, a probability value of less than 0.05 has been termed "significant," whereas a probability value of more than 0.05 is "not significant." In fact, many journals still allow probability values to be reported in this way. However, with the above definition of a probability value in mind, readers should wonder whether a probability value of 0.049 is different from a probability value of 0.051? Clearly, there is more to the interpretation of a probability value than the absolute number itself.

Relative Risk with 95% Confidence Intervals

A relative risk is defined as the incidence of the outcome in the exposed group divided by the incidence of disease in the unexposed (untreated) group. Thus, using Table 17-2, the relative risk is as follows:

$$\text{Relative risk} = \frac{116/953}{121/966} = \frac{0.122}{0.125} = 0.98$$

A relative risk of 1.0 means that the incidence of the outcome is identical in the exposed and unexposed subjects. A relative risk of less than 1.0 means that the incidence of the outcome is less in the exposed group, whereas a relative risk of more than 1.0 means that the incidence is greater in the exposed group.

The *point estimate* is the best estimate of the association between an exposure and outcome but does not give information about the stability or statistical precision of the estimate. Obviously, the precision of such an estimate is related to the power of the study. The precision of a relative risk or other measure of effect is often described as a 95% confidence interval (Shakespeare et al., 2001). A 95% confidence interval is interpreted as follows: If a study is without bias, there is a 95% chance that the true point estimate lies within the bounds of the confidence interval. The narrower the confidence interval, the greater precision in the estimate. The wider the confidence interval, the less certainty there is in the estimate.

Confidence intervals also provide information about statistical significance. In general, if a relative risk of 1.0 falls within the bounds of the 95% confidence interval for a given association, then the corresponding probability value will be more than 0.05. Likewise, if a relative risk of 1.0 is not included in the bounds of a 95% confidence interval, then the corresponding probability value will likely be less than 0.05.

Other Measures of Effect

An *odds ratio* is another popular measure of effect that can be calculated from either observational studies or clinical trials (Victora, 1993). Odds ratios are good approximations of relative risks in cases where the disease of interest is rare. Odds ratios are most commonly calculated for case-control studies where the calculation of a relative risk is impossible. Odds ratios are also the output for most statistical packages when multivariable logistic regressions are performed. In general, relative risks are preferred over odds ratios when data are available to calculate a relative risk, such as in cohort studies or clinical trials.

Using the example from the MFMU Network trial of a protocol to screen and treat bacterial vaginosis to prevent preterm birth (see Table 17-2), the odds ratio for the association between treatment and preterm birth is as follows:

$$\text{Odds ratio} = \frac{116 \times 845}{121 \times 837} = 0.97$$

An odds ratio is interpreted in exactly the same manner as a relative risk. Thus, an odds ratio of 2.0 would be interpreted as a twofold increase in risk, whereas an odds ratio of 0.5 would mean a 50% reduction in risk. Ninety-five percent confidence intervals are also interpreted in the same fashion as those for relative risks. Remember that the preferred measure of effect to calculate in clinical trials and cohort studies is a relative risk (or risk difference). Odds ratios can be used as surrogates for relative risks in cases where the disease under question is rare.

The *risk difference* is the simple arithmetic difference in incidence between groups and can be calculated from clinical trial data or from cohort studies (but not from case-control studies). In the case of the preterm birth data from the MFMU Network study above, the risk difference is 0.122 − 0.125 = −0.003.

A risk difference is interpreted differently from a relative risk or odds ratio. A risk difference of zero means that there is no difference in the incidence of disease between groups. A positive risk difference means that the incidence of the outcome is greater in the experimental group, whereas a negative risk difference means that the incidence of the outcome is greater in the control group. In the above example, the risk difference means that there is a 0.3% reduction in the risk of preterm birth in those exposed to metronidazole. If the 95% confidence interval includes zero, this signifies that the data are consistent with there being no difference in the incidence between groups (and corresponds to a probability value of more than 0.05).

Which measure of effect is appropriate is largely determined by the aims of the study and the study design (Victora, 1993).

ASSESSING RESEARCH ON SCREENING AND DIAGNOSIS

Screening and diagnostic tests are an integral part of our everyday lives in clinical medicine. For example, when we are seeing a routine obstetric patient in the office, we often will check the fundal height. This, in essence, is a screening test for fetal growth disturbances and amniotic fluid abnormalities. If the fundal height measures significantly less than anticipated, we will perform a "diagnostic" test, in this case an ultrasound examination. The same sequence of screening followed by diagnostic testing occurs commonly in obstetric practice, for example, a family history (screening test) that leads to a "targeted ultrasound" (that may be diagnostic for some disorders or a screening test for others) and eventually to amniocentesis (diagnostic test). Because such testing dominates our clinical lives, it is essential that physicians understand the principles of screening and diagnostic tests (Boardman and Peipert, 1998). It is through this understanding that physicians will make rational decisions about whether the next new test should be used in clinical practice.

Screening versus Diagnosis

Screening has been defined as "the presumptive identification of an unrecognized disease or defect by the application of tests, examination or other procedures which can be applied rapidly. . . . A screening test is not meant to be diagnostic. Persons with positive or suspicious findings must be referred to their physicians for diagnosis and treatment" (Last, 1995). Thus, screening tests are those that are widely applied to a population and require follow-up with a "diagnostic test" (if an individual screens positive). In general, a successful screening program must meet the following criteria:

- The condition screened for must have a significant burden.
- There must be effective early treatment for those who screen positive.
- The test must be sufficiently sensitive and specific (see later).
- The screening test must be inexpensive and easy to perform.
- The screening test must be safe and acceptable to patients.

Cervical cytology screening for premalignant lesions of the cervix is an example of a successful screening program that fulfills all the above criteria. In contrast, although cytomegalovirus infection of the fetus and neonate creates a significant burden of disease, a screening program for this virus has no value because there is no successful intervention. Similarly, although cervicovaginal fetal fibronectin screening can identify as many as 60% of women destined for preterm birth before 28 weeks (Goldenberg et al., 1996), there is currently no effective intervention that could be applied to screen-positive women to reduce the risk of preterm delivery (Andrews et al., 2003).

Sensitivity, Specificity, and Predictive Values

For any test, whether screening or diagnostic, it is critical to understand its test characteristics. Sensitivity and specificity are characteristics inherent in the test and are independent of the prevalence of the disease (Clarke, 1990; Boardman and Peipert, 1998). *Sensitivity* is the probability, expressed as a percentage, that if the disease is present, the test is positive. The numerator is the number of subjects with the disease who have a positive test, and the denominator is the total number of diseased subjects. *Specificity* is the probability, expressed as a percentage, that if the disease is absent, the test is negative. The numerator is the number of subjects without disease who have a negative test, and the denominator is the total number of nondiseased subjects. Although the sensitivity and specificity of a test are important considerations when deciding whether or not to order a test, we become more interested in the *predictive values* when the test results have returned. As opposed to sensitivity and specificity, predictive values are dependent on the prevalence of the outcome.

A *positive predictive value* (PPV) is the probability that if the test is positive, the subject has the disease. The numerator is the number of subjects with the disease who have a positive test, and the denominator is the total number of those with positive tests. A *negative predictive value* (NPV) is the probability that if the test is negative, the subject does not have the disease. The numerator is the number of subjects without disease who have a negative test, and the denominator is the total number of those with negative tests. Given the same sensitivity and specificity, as the prevalence rises, the PPV will increase and the NPV will decrease. Likewise, as the prevalence decreases, the PPV decreases and the NPV increases.

These abstract concepts are best demonstrated with a clinical example. Peaceman and colleagues (1997) performed a prospective cohort study at multiple centers to assess whether cervicovaginal fetal fibronectin could be used as a *diagnostic* test in women with symptoms of preterm labor; fetal fibronectin has also been assessed in other studies as a *screening* test (Goldenberg et al., 1996). In the Peaceman study, women with symptoms of early preterm labor were enrolled, and cervicovaginal swabs for fibronectin testing were obtained. Both treating physicians and patients were blinded to the results of the fibronectin test, a strength of the study. The outcomes assessed were the occurrence of delivery within 7 days, within 2 weeks, and before 37 weeks' gestation. The results of the analysis of delivery within 7 days (Table 17-3) may be used as an example to illustrate sensitivity, specificity, and PPV and NPV.

Some would look at these results and the high NPV and suggest that fetal fibronectin is a useful tool in this setting to "rule out" an imminent delivery. Another way of looking at these same data would be to look closely at the low prevalence of delivery within 7 days (3%). After reading this article, the following questions emerge: Is it appropriate to use a diagnostic test in such a low prevalence group? And more importantly, what would be the impact of testing a higher prevalence population (i.e., a greater chance of preterm birth within 7 days)?

Physicians may look at these results differently. Some may argue that the treatment for preterm labor has risk, is of questionable efficacy, and is overused. Thus, a test that could avoid overtreatment with tocolytics might be helpful. Others could argue that the very high NPV with fetal fibronectin was

TABLE 17-3. FETAL FIBRONECTIN (FFN) TO PREDICT DELIVERY WITHIN 7 DAYS OF TESTING

	Delivery < 7 Days		
	Yes	**No**	**Total**
FFN +	20	130	150
FFN −	3	610	613
Total	23	740	763

Prevalence $= \frac{23}{763} = 3\%$

Sensitivity $= \frac{20}{23} = 87\%$ Specificity $= \frac{610}{740} = 82\%$

PPV $= \frac{20}{150} = 13\%$ NPV $= \frac{610}{613} = 99.5\%$

NPV, negative predictive value; PPV, positive predictive value.

Data from Peaceman AM, Andrews WW, Thorp JM, et al: Fetal fibronectin as a predictor of preterm birth in patients with symptoms: A multicenter trial. Am J Obstet Gynecol **177**:13, 1997.

obtained only when testing patients with a very low prevalence of preterm delivery and that no "diagnostic" test is needed in such a low prevalence population. Furthermore, when this test is used in a higher prevalence group, the NPV will decrease, making it much less useful. The value of a test with these characteristics clearly is population dependent, according to the prevalence of preterm birth and the prevailing pattern of clinical care regarding tocolytic drugs for women with minimal symptoms.

For example, assuming the population tested could be selected by additional clinical data to define a group with a higher prevalence of delivery within 7 days, Table 17-4 illustrates the effect of the increased prevalence on PPV and NPV. Remember that the same sensitivity and specificity stay constant regardless of the disease prevalence. As expected, the PPV increases somewhat, and the NPV is decreased to 97%. Another way of looking at the NPV is that 3% of those with a negative test will go on to deliver within 7 days. Is this rate of false-negative testing acceptable for a patient who presents at 24 weeks with symptoms of preterm labor? Once again, the answer is determined by clinical factors regarding both patients and physicians that are unique to the clinical setting.

Likelihood Ratios

Likelihood ratios are another method of describing test performance and can be used to calculate post-test probabilities, just like predictive values. In literature from the United States, predictive values are commonly reported, whereas in many European and South American journals, likelihood ratios are preferred. A likelihood ratio is defined as the probability of the test result in the presence of outcome divided by the probability of the result in those without the outcome. Separate likelihood ratios are calculated for positive tests and negative tests. Simply put, likelihood ratios express how many times more (or less) likely a test result is to be found in those with the outcome compared with those without the outcome.

As an example, the positive likelihood ratios from the data on delivery within 7 days in the Peaceman study used previously can be calculated as shown here, by dividing the proportion of women with a positive test who did deliver within 7 days by the proportion of women with a positive test who did not deliver within 7 days (Peaceman et al., 1997):

$$\text{Positive likelihood ratio} = \frac{20/23}{130/740} = \frac{0.87}{0.18} = 4.8$$

Likelihood ratios can also be used to calculate a post-test probability (PPVs), which is what we use in clinical practice. To do this, however, the pretest probability (prevalence) must be converted to pretest odds using the formula

Odds = probability of event/1 − probability of event
Probability = odds/1 + odds

Using the Peaceman data for a positive test, the prevalence of delivery within 7 days is 3%. In odds, this translates to 0.031. Then, we can calculate the post-test odds using the formula

Pretest odds × likelihood ratio = Post-test odds

In this case, the post-test odds is 0.031 × 4.8 = 0.1488. When the post-test odds are converted to a post-test probability (i.e., a PPV), the result is 0.1488/1.1488 = 13.0%, the same as the PPV calculation above in Table 17-3.

TABLE 17-4. FETAL FIBRONECTIN (FFN) TO PREDICT DELIVERY WITHIN 7 DAYS OF TESTING: HYPOTHETICAL ANALYSIS OF A HIGH PREVALENCE GROUP

| | Delivery < 7 Days | | |
	Yes	No	Total
FFN +	99	117	216
FFN −	15	532	547
Total	114	649	763

Prevalence $= \frac{114}{763} = 15\%$

Sensitivity $= \frac{99}{114} = 87\%$ Specificity $= \frac{532}{649} = 82\%$

PPV $= \frac{99}{216} = 45\%$ NPV $= \frac{532}{547} = 97\%$

NPV, negative predictive value; PPV, positive predictive value.

Thus, likelihood ratios are another method to assess the utility of a test (by looking at the positive and negative likelihood ratio) and to convert pretest probabilities to post-test probabilities. For the latter issue, this can be somewhat cumbersome, and many individuals prefer simply using a 2 × 2 table to calculate predictive values.

Receiver Operating Characteristic Curves

Although test results may be categorical (i.e., positive or negative), they are more often expressed in clinical medicine as a point on a continuum. As clinicians, we evaluate test results and try to discriminate "normal" from "abnormal." Although it would be ideal to have tests that are simultaneously very sensitive and specific, this is seldom the case. Thus, we are faced with selecting thresholds that trade off degrees of sensitivity versus specificity. A graphic method that makes these trade-offs explicit and aids in the selection of cut points is the receiver operating characteristic (ROC) curve. The sensitivity is placed on the y axis versus 1 minus the specificity (false-positive rate) on the x axis for the entire range of cut points. Tests that discriminate well tend to generate a curve that occupies the upper left corner of the graph. Poorly discriminating tests will generate a curve that falls along the diagonal that follows from the lower left corner to the upper right corner. A 45-degree line along this diagonal describes a nondiscriminating test, which is one that has no threshold value.

ROC curves have three primary uses: to select a cut point for an individual test, to assess the overall accuracy of the individual test, and to compare the overall accuracy of two tests for the same condition. The last is most often done by calculating and comparing the area under the ROC curve.

A recent example of the clinical use of ROC curves in selecting an appropriate cut point was published by Owen and colleagues (2000) and focused on mid-trimester transvaginal cervical length measurements to predict preterm birth before 35 weeks' gestation in high-risk women. To assess this question, the authors performed a multicenter prospective study of transvaginal ultrasound cervical measurements every 2 weeks in 183 women with a prior birth at less than 32 weeks. Figure 17-3 depicts a comparison of ROC

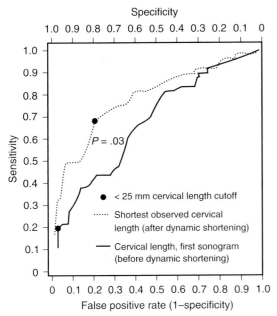

FIGURE 17-3 ■ Receiver operating characteristic curves of cervical length cutoffs for the prediction of spontaneous preterm birth before 35 weeks' gestation. (From Owen J, Yost N, Berghella V, et al: Mid-trimester endovaginal sonography in women at high risk for spontaneous preterm birth. JAMA **286**:1340, 2000.)

curves for shortest observed cervical length to the cervical length at the first examination for the prediction of spontaneous preterm birth before 35 weeks' gestation. Figure 17-3 suggests the following:

1. The shortest observed cervical length is a better discriminator than the initial cervical length for the prediction of spontaneous preterm birth less than 35 weeks.
2. Although the shortest observed cervical length is better than the initial examination, neither test is particularly dis-

criminating (as evidenced by the fact that neither curve is very close to the left upper corner of the graph).

3. The optimal cut point for the shortest observed cervical length is 25 mm. At this level, however, the sensitivity is only approximately 70%, with a false-positive rate of approximately 20%.

Iams and colleagues (2002) reported a study of several tests to predict preterm birth in pregnant women. Cervical examinations by digital examination (expressed as a Bishop score) and by ultrasound (expressed as the length of the cervical canal) were compared with monitored uterine contraction frequency and fetal fibronectin in cervicovaginal secretions using ROC curves. The performance of each test was displayed on a common graph of their ROC curves (Fig. 17-4). Cervical length by ultrasound, though far from an ideal test, had the "best" performance as the uppermost line of the curves displayed.

■ S U M M A R Y

This overview of study design and methods to analyze and report data in perinatal medicine may serve as a starting point to integrate research data appropriately into clinical care. As with any skill, it is mastered by frequent repetition and especially by analyzing and presenting one's own data with one of the methods described.

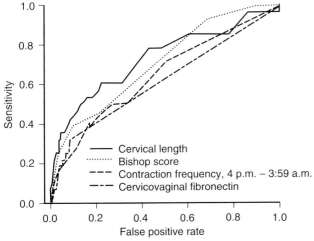

FIGURE 17-4 ■ Receiver operating characteristic curves for cervical length, Bishop score, frequency of contractions, and presence or absence of fetal fibronectin in cervicovaginal secretions at 27 to 28 weeks in the prediction of spontaneous preterm delivery (less than 35 weeks). (From Iams JD, Newman RB, Thom EA, et al, for the National Institute of Child Health and Human Development Network of Maternal-Fetal Medicine Units: Frequency of uterine contractions and the risk of spontaneous preterm delivery. N Engl J Med **346**:250, 2002.)

R E F E R E N C E S

Andrews WW, for the National Institute of Child Health and Human Development: Maternal-Fetal Medicine Units Network. Randomized Clinical Trial of Metronidazole Plus Erythromycin to Prevent Spontaneous Preterm Delivery in Fetal Fibronectin Positive Women. Obstet Gynecol, 2003.

Boardman LA, Peipert JF: Screening and diagnostic testing. Clin Obstet Gynecol **41**:267, 1998.

Carey JC, Klebanoff MA, Hauth JC, et al, for the National Institute of Child Health and Human Development Network of Maternal-Fetal Medicine Units: Metronidazole to prevent preterm delivery in pregnant women with asymptomatic bacterial vaginosis. N Engl J Med **342**:534, 2000.

Clarke J: A scientific approach to surgical reasoning. I. Diagnostic accuracy. Theoret Surg **5**:206, 1990.

Cochrane Database of Systematic Reviews: The Cochrane Library, issue 4. Oxford, 2002. Update software; available online at www.cochrane.org. Look for the Cochrane Pregnancy and Childbirth Group. Abstracts of Cochrane Reviews.

Cook D, Guyatt G: The professional meta-analyst: An evolutionary advantage. J Clin Epidemiol **47**:1327, 1994.

Czeizel AE, Rockenbauer M: A population based case-control teratologic study of oral metronidazole treatment during pregnancy. Br J Obstet Gynaecol **105**:322, 1998.

Datta M: You cannot exclude the explanation you have not considered. Lancet **342**:345, 1993.

Goldenberg RL, Mercer BM, Meis PJ, et al: The preterm prediction study: Fetal fibronectin testing and spontaneous preterm birth. NICHD Maternal Fetal Medicine Units Network. Obstet Gynecol **87**:643, 1996.

Grimes DA, Schulz KF: Bias and causal associations in observational research. Lancet **359**:248, 2002.

Hauth JC, Goldenberg RL, Andrews WW, et al: Reduced incidence of preterm delivery with metronidazole and erythromycin in women with bacterial vaginosis. N Engl J Med **333**:1732, 1995.

Hennekens CH, Buring JE: Epidemiology in Medicine. Boston, Little, Brown, 1987.

Hillier SL, Nugent RP, Eschenbach DA, et al: Association between bacterial vaginosis and preterm delivery of a low-birth-weight infant. The Vaginal Infections and Prematurity Study Group. N Engl J Med **333**:1737, 1995.

Hosmer D, Lemeshow D: Applied Logistic Regression. New York, Wiley, 1989.

Iams JD, Newman RB, Thom EA, et al, for The National Institute of Child Health and Human Development Network of Maternal-Fetal Medicine Units: Frequency of uterine contractions and the risk of spontaneous preterm delivery. N Engl J Med **346**:250, 2002.

Iannucci T, Besinger R, Fisher S, et al: Effect of dual tocolysis on the incidence of severe intraventricular hemorrhage among extremely low-birth-weight infants. Am J Obstet Gynecol **175**:1043, 1996.

Itskovitz J, Abramovici H, Brandes J: Oligohydramnion, meconium and perinatal death concurrent with indomethacin treatment in human pregnancy. J Reprod Med **24**:137, 1980.

Kelsey JL, Whittemore AS, Evans AE, et al: Methods in Observational Epidemiology. New York, Oxford University Press, 1996.

Kenyon S, Boulvain M, Neilson J: Antibiotics for preterm premature rupture of membranes (Cochrane Review). *The Cochrane Library*, issue 4. Oxford, Update Software, 2002.

Kurki T, Sivonen A, Renkonen O, et al: Bacterial vaginosis in early pregnancy and pregnancy outcome. Obstet Gynecol **80**:173, 1992.

Last JL: A Dictionary of Epidemiology. New York, Oxford University Press, 1995.

LeLorier J, Gregoire G, Benhaddad A, et al: Discrepancies between meta-analyses and subsequent large randomized, controlled trials. N Engl J Med **337**:536, 1997.

Leon D: Failed or misleading adjustment for confounding. Lancet **342**:479, 1993.

Macones G, Goldie S, Peipert J: Economic analyses in obstetrics and gynecology: A guide for clinicians and researchers. Obstet Gynecol Surv **54**:663, 1999.

Macones G, Marder S, Clothier B, et al: The controversy surrounding indomethacin for tocolysis. Am J Obstet Gynecol **184**:264, 2001.

Macones G, Robinson C: Is there justification for using indomethacin in preterm labor? An analysis of risks and benefits. Am J Obstet Gynecol **177**:819, 1997.

Macones GM, Bader TJ, Asch DA: Optimising maternal-fetal outcomes in preterm labour: A decision analysis. Br J Obstet Gynaecol **105**:541, 1998.

Major C, Lewis D, Harding J, et al: Tocolysis with indomethacin increases the incidence of necrotizing enterocolitis in the low birth weight neonate. Am J Obstet Gynecol **170**:102, 1994.

Meinert CL: Clinical Trials: Design, Conduct, and Analysis. New York, Oxford University Press, 1986.

Moher D, Cook DJ, Eastwood S, et al: Improving the quality of reports of meta-analyses of randomised controlled trials: the QUOROM statement. Quality of Reporting of Meta-analyses. Lancet **354**:1896, 1999.

Moher D, Schulz KF, Altman D: The CONSORT statement: Revised recommendations for improving the quality of reports of parallel-group randomized trials. JAMA **285**:1987, 2001.

Norton ME, Merrill J, Cooper BA, et al: Neonatal complications after the administration of indomethacin for preterm labor. N Engl J Med **329**:1602, 1993.

Owen J, Yost N, Berghella V, et al: Mid-trimester endovaginal sonography in women at high risk for spontaneous preterm birth. JAMA **286**:1340, 2000.

Peaceman AM, Andrews WW, Thorp JM, et al: Fetal fibronectin as a predictor of preterm birth in patients with symptoms: a multicenter trial. Am J Obstet Gynecol **177**:13, 1997.

Peipert JF, Bracken MB: Systematic reviews of medical evidence: The use of meta-analysis in obstetrics and gynecology. Obstet Gynecol **89**:628, 1997.

Peipert JF, Phipps MG: Observational studies. Clin Obstet Gynecol **41**:235, 1998.

Riduan JM, Hillier SL, Utomo B, et al: Bacterial vaginosis and prematurity in Indonesia: Association in early and late pregnancy. Am J Obstet Gynecol **169**:175, 1993.

Romero R, Gomez R, Ghezzi F, et al: A fetal systemic inflammatory response is followed by the spontaneous onset of preterm parturition. Am J Obstet Gynecol **179**:186, 1998.

Romero R, Sirtori M, Oyarzun E: Infection and labor. V. Prevalence, microbiology, and clinical significance of intraamniotic infection in women with preterm labor and intact membranes. Am J Obstet Gynecol **161**:817, 1989.

Rouse D, Goldenberg R, Cliver S, et al: Strategies for the prevention of early-onset neonatal group B streptococcal sepsis: A decision analysis. Obstet Gynecol **83**:483, 1994.

Sanchez-Ramos L, Kaunitz AM, Gaudier FL, et al: Efficacy of maintenance therapy after acute tocolysis: A meta-analysis. Am J Obstet Gynecol **181**:484, 1999.

Schulz KF, Grimes DA: Generation of allocation sequences in randomised trials: Chance not choice. Lancet **359**:515, 2002.

Shakespeare TP, Gebski VJ, Veness MJ, et al: Improving interpretation of clinical studies by use of confidence levels, clinical significance curves, and risk-benefit contours. Lancet **357**:1349, 2001.

Sitthi-amorn C, Poshyachinda V: Bias. Lancet **342**:286, 1993.

Tsatsaris V, Papatsonis D, Goffinet F, et al: Tocolysis with nifedipine or beta-adrenergic agonists: A meta-analysis. Obstet Gynecol **97**:840, 2001.

Victora C: What's the denominator? Lancet **342**:97, 1993.

Villar J, Paggio G, Carroli G, et al: Factors affecting the comparability of meta-analyses and largest trials results in perinatology. J Clin Epidemiol **50**:997, 1997.

Yoon B, Kim C, Romero R, et al: Experimentally induced intrauterine infection causes fetal brain white matter lesions in rabbits. Am J Obstet Gynecol **177**:797, 1997.

Part II
FETAL DISORDERS: DIAGNOSIS AND THERAPY

Chapter 18

PRENATAL DIAGNOSIS OF CONGENITAL DISORDERS

Thomas M. Jenkins, MD, and Ronald J. Wapner, MD

Prenatal diagnosis, a term once seen as synonymous with invasive fetal testing and karyotype evaluation, now encompasses pedigree analysis, population screening, fetal risk assessment, genetic counseling, and fetal diagnostic testing. Although prenatal evaluation of the fetus for genetic disorders can have a huge impact on individual families, most screening and testing is done for events that occur in less than 1% of pregnancies. In this chapter we describe different modalities available for *in utero* fetal diagnosis of congenital disorders, the approach to screening ongoing pregnancies for genetic disease, and the requisite counseling requirement for each.

SCREENING FOR FETAL GENETIC DISORDERS

Detecting or defining risk for disease in an asymptomatic low-risk population is the goal of screening. As opposed to diagnostic testing, intended to identify or confirm an affected individual, screening is intended to identify populations having an increased risk for a specific disorder and for whom diagnostic testing may be warranted. An ideal perinatal genetic screening test should fulfill the following criteria:

- Identify common or important fetal disorders
- Be cost effective and easy to perform
- Have a high detection rate and a low false-positive rate
- Be reliable and reproducible
- Test for disorders for which a diagnostic test exists
- Be positive early enough in gestation to permit safe and legal options for pregnancy termination if desired

Sensitivity and specificity are two key concepts in screening test performance (see Chapter 17). Sensitivity is the percent of affected pregnancies that are screen positive. Specificity is the percent of individuals with unaffected pregnancies who screen negative. The reciprocal of specificity is the false-positive rate. Sensitivity and specificity are independent of disease frequency and describe the anticipated performance of a screening test in the population. Alternatively, positive and negative predictive values are dependent on disease prevalence and are vital in the interpretation of the test result for an individual patient. These latter two values represent, respectively, the likelihood that a person with a positive or negative test does or does not have an

affected pregnancy. The impact of the prevalence of the disease on the positive and negative predictive values is described in Chapter 17 and is shown in Tables 17-3 and 17-4. In the example of screening for Down syndrome based on age, a 29-year-old woman has an expected prevalence of 0.1%, whereas a 44-year-old woman has a prevalence of 4%.

Use of screening tests requires that cutoff values for "positive" tests be set. Performance of the test is dependent on this cutoff; for example, increased detection rate can be obtained by lowering the cutoff threshold but with a concomitant lowered specificity resulting in more false-positive results. Table 18-1 shows the performance of second-trimester maternal serum screening for Down syndrome based on various cutoffs (Huang et al., 1997). A receiver operating curve can be used as a statistical method to find the "best" balance between sensitivity and specificity. A line diagram is plotted with sensitivity on the vertical axis and the false-positive rate plotted horizontally (Fig. 18-1). The further the plot is toward the upper left corner, the better the test's performance, with increasing sensitivity and a reduced false-positive rate. When screening for Down syndrome, these cutoff values are important for the clinicians and laboratories that provide the testing. When viewed from the patient's perspective, reporting tests as positive or negative can be confusing. Receipt of a "positive" result of 1 in 250 may lead to a choice of a diagnostic test that carries a risk of complications, whereas a "negative" result of 1 in 290 may provide greater reassurance than intended, when in fact the actual risk of Down syndrome is similar for both patients. Ideally, a prescreen explanation of the significance of a positive or negative result will assist patients in understanding their results. Many centers report the absolute risk to the patient to further help in interpretation. Regardless of the counseling approach, understanding the concept of screening is difficult for many patients. From the perspective of the laboratory or clinician, selection of a cutoff that is too high or too low will lead to over- or underutilization of diagnostic tests and their consequent risks of procedure-related pregnancy loss or false reassurance, respectively.

Likelihood Ratios

The impact of a positive screening test is dependent on the pretest (*a priori*) risk of an affected pregnancy. Likelihood ratios are statistical means to modify an individual's risk based on

TABLE 18-1. DOWN SYNDROME DETECTION AND FALSE-POSITIVE RATES (FPR) USING DIFFERENT CUTOFF VALUES

Triple Screen	Detection Rate	FPR	Quadruple Screen	Detection Rate	FPR
1:200	57	4.3	1:200	60	3.5
1:250	61	5.6	1:250	64	4.5
1:300	64	6.8	1:300	67	5.5
1:350	67	8.1	1:350	69	6.5
1:400	69	9.3	1:400	72	7.6

Data from Huang T, Watt H, Wald N: The effect of differences in the distribution of maternal age in England and Wales on the performance of prenatal screening for Down's syndrome. Prenat Diagn **17**:615, 1997.

TABLE 18-2. ADJUSTING THE RISK FOR DOWN SYNDROME USING LIKELIHOOD RATIOS FOR BINARY ULTRASOUND MARKERS

A priori risk of Down syndrome (age or triple screen)	1:1000
Positive ultrasound marker for Down syndrome	
Rate in Down syndrome population (sensitivity of marker)	10%
Rate in general population (FPR of marker)	1.0%
Likelihood ratio (sens/FPR)	10.0
Adjusted risk for Down syndrome	
(*A priori* risk × likelihood ratio) = $\frac{1}{1000} \times 10$	1:100

FPR, false-positive rate.

known data for a population. For binary risk factors that are either present or absent, likelihood ratios are determined by comparing the frequency of positive tests in affected pregnancies to the frequency in normal pregnancies. This is calculated as the sensitivity of the test divided by its false-positive rate (likelihood ratio = sensitivity/false-positive rate). For tests that use continuous variables (such as serum marker measurements), likelihood ratios are calculated from the log gaussian distributions of normal and affected pregnancies. Once a likelihood ratio is determined, it can be used to modify the *a priori* risk (Table 18-2). If more than one likelihood ratio is available and is independent of other parameters, it also can be used to modify risk. In this way, multiple factors (such as maternal age, serum analytes, and ultrasound findings) can be simultaneously used to modify risk.

ANTENATAL SCREENING FOR DOWN SYNDROME

There is presently a general consensus in the United States that invasive testing for Down syndrome be offered to those with a second-trimester risk of 1:270 or higher (liveborn risk of 1:380). The cutoff level and subsequent public policy was determined over 25 years ago and was based on a maternal age risk of 35 years at delivery. The factors considered in determining this value included the prevalence of disease, a perceived significant increase in the trisomy 21 risk after this age, the risk of invasive testing, the availability of resources, and a cost-to-benefit analysis. Since that time, a number of additional screening tests for Down syndrome have become available that challenge the validity of maternal age as a single indication for invasive testing.

Maternal Age as a Screening Test

The association of Down syndrome with advancing maternal age was first reported in 1909 (Shuttleworth, 1909). Fifty years later, karyotype analysis was developed and correlated the Down syndrome phenotype with an extra G chromosome (Lejeune, 1959). This subsequently led to the development of genetic amniocentesis through which the prenatal diagnosis of Down syndrome became feasible. To standardize the use of this emerging technology, a consensus report from the National Institutes of Health in 1979 suggested that amniocentesis be routinely offered to women aged 35 years or older at delivery. At that time, maternal age risks of Down syndrome were only available in 5-year groupings. Using these data, the age of 35 seemed a natural cutoff, because women in the 30- to 34-year grouping had a risk of 1:880, and the risk for women aged 35 to 40 was almost fourfold higher. This cutoff was based on a number of factors, including the availability of experienced operators and cytogenetics laboratories, the cost-to-benefit ratio, and the balance between procedure-related losses and the possibility of a positive finding. This cutoff continues to be used, and the second-trimester risk of 1:270 or liveborn risk of 1:380 remains the standard value for offering women invasive testing. The risk for Down syndrome is now recognized to be continuous, which emphasizes the arbitrary nature of an absolute age threshold of 35. In addition to maternal age, the risk of trisomy 21 is dependent on the gestational age at which testing is performed, because only 69% of first-trimester and 76% of second-trimester Down syndrome pregnancies are

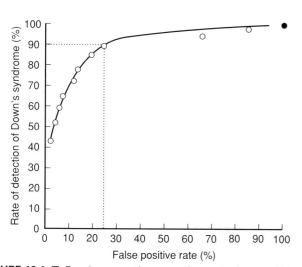

FIGURE 18-1 ■ Receiver operating curve demonstrating sensitivity for Down syndrome detection versus false-positive rate. Cutoff points for sensitivity versus false-positive rate are determined by these curves. (From Haddow JE, Palomaki GE, Knight GJ, et al: Reducing the need for amniocentesis in women 35 years of age or older with serum markers for screening. N Engl J Med **330**:1114, 1994.)

viable (Morris et al., 1999) (Table 18-3). Currently, more than 80% of diagnostic procedures to determine fetal karyotype performed in the United States are performed solely for "advanced maternal age," yet 70% of affected pregnancies are born to women outside this group. With many women delaying childbirth until later in life, more than 7.5% of pregnant women in the United States are being offered testing based on age alone. In Switzerland and the United Kingdom, almost 15% of births now occur in women over 35.

Second-Trimester Serum Analyte Screening

Serum analyte screening may be used to identify the 70% of Down syndrome pregnancies in women less than 35 years of age. This approach is derived from a 1984 report of lower maternal serum α-fetoprotein (MSAFP) levels in women carrying a Down syndrome fetus. Women with Down syndrome pregnancies had a median MSAFP value of 0.75 multiples of the unaffected median (MoM) (Merkatz et al., 1984; Haddow and Palomaki, 1993). Using this deviation to calculate a likelihood ratio, the age-related risk for Down syndrome could be adjusted. When the standard 1:270 cutoff was used, approximately 25% of Down syndrome pregnancies among women less than 35 years of age were screen positive (Cuckle et al., 1984; DiMaio et al., 1987; New England Regional Genetics Group Prenatal Collaborative Study of Down Syndrome Screening, 1989).

Elevated human chorionic gonadotropin (hCG) (mean, 2.3 MoM) and reduced levels of unconjugated estriol (mean, 0.7 MoM) were subsequently linked to an increased risk of trisomy 21 (Bogart et al., 1987; Canick et al., 1988; Haddow and Palomaki, 1993). hCG or reduced levels of unconjugated estriol used alone to modify the maternal age risk has a Down syndrome detection rate of only 20% to 30%. However, because they are independent variables, they can be analyzed simultaneously with maternal age to form a composite risk calculation (frequently called a triple screen).

The sensitivity of the triple screen for Down syndrome detection in women under age 35 years ranges between 57% and 67% if the false-positive rate is held constant at 5% (Wald et al., 1988; Heyl et al., 1990; MacDonald et al., 1991; Phillips et al., 1996). Overall, the odds of having an affected pregnancy with a positive screen is approximately 1 in 33 to 1 in 62, depending on the age range of the population studied (Burton, Prins, et al., 1993; Haddow et al., 1992), an improvement over the 1:100 odds when maternal age is the sole screening parameter. Because of the impact of maternal age on the risk analysis, screening women who will be 35 years of age or more increases the sensitivity of the same cutoffs to approximately 87% but with a false-positive rate of nearly 25% (Heyl et al., 1990; Haddow et al., 1994).

Other analytes or combinations of analytes have been tested to further increase sensitivity. The most commonly added is inhibin A, an analyte produced initially by the corpus luteum and later by the placenta. Inhibin A levels are elevated in Down syndrome pregnancies (1.3 to 2.5 MoM) and do not vary with gestational age in the second trimester. There is, however, a small correlation with hCG levels, making the added sensitivity for Down syndrome detection less robust (Renier et al., 1998). Detection rates when a "quad screen" of α-fetoprotein (AFP), hCG, unconjugated estriol, and inhibin A are used are about 70% in the population under age 35 years.

Hyperglycosylated hCG excreted in maternal urine has been tested as a marker for Down syndrome. One study of nearly 1500 women (1448 control subjects and 39 Down syndrome pregnancies) reported a sensitivity of 96% of affected pregnancies with a 5% false-positive rate and 71% detection with a 1% false-positive rate when a combination of hyperglycosylated hCG, urine β-core hCG fragment, MSAFP, and maternal age was used (Cole et al., 1999). This detection rate, however, has not been duplicated by others.

With the addition of extra markers, the potential benefit versus the cost must be balanced. With each additional marker, costs to society can balloon into the millions secondary to the numbers of pregnancies tested each year. The relative cost and value of raising the sensitivity or lowering the false-positive rate a few percentage points is an ongoing debate.

Abnormal Maternal Serum Markers in Pregnancies with a Normal Karyotype

Unexplained Elevated Maternal Serum α-Fetoprotein

When an elevated MSAFP is reported in pregnancies in which the gestational age is correctly assigned, the fetus is structurally normal, and the amniotic fluid AFP (AFAFP) is normal, the biological explanation is almost always a breach in the maternal-fetal interface. This leads to higher AFP levels in the maternal circulation. Not surprisingly, women with this combination of findings have been found to have an increased risk of numerous obstetric complications, including fetal growth restriction, fetal death, prematurity, oligohydramnios, abruptio placenta, and preeclampsia. The data in Table 18-4 summarize the numerous reports. The higher the MSAFP level, the greater the risk. Crandall and colleagues (1991) studied 1002 women with MSAFP values greater than 2.5 MoM and stratified them by the degree of elevation. In those with a normal ultrasound and amniocentesis, the risk of

TABLE 18-3. RISK FOR DOWN SYNDROME BASED ON MATERNAL AND GESTATIONAL AGE

Maternal Age (Yr)	Gestational Age			
	12 Wk	**16 Wk**	**20 Wk**	**Liveborn**
20	1/1068	1/1200	1/1295	1/1527
25	1/946	1/1062	1/1147	1/1352
30	1/626	1/703	1/759	1/895
31	1/543	1/610	1/658	1/776
32	1/461	1/518	1/559	1/659
33	1/383	1/430	1/464	1/547
34	1/312	1/350	1/378	1/446
35	1/249	1/280	1/302	1/356
36	1/196	1/220	1/238	1/280
37	1/152	1/171	1/185	1/218
38	1/117	1/131	1/142	1/167
39	1/89	1/100	1/108	1/128
40	1/68	1/76	1/82	1/97
42	1/38	1/43	1/46	1/55
44	1/21	1/24	1/26	1/30
45	1/16	1/18	1/19	1/23

Data from Hook EB: Rates of chromosome abnormalities at different maternal ages. Obstet Gynecol **58**:282, 1981.

TABLE 18-4. STUDIES EVALUATING THE RELATION OF UNEXPLAINED ELEVATIONS OF MSAFP AND POOR PREGNANCY OUTCOME

Source	Location (Year)	Pregnancies Screened	MoM Cutoff	LBW Risk	IUGR Risk	Premature Delivery Risk	Abruption Risk	IUFD Risk	Perinatal Death
Brock et al.	Scotland (1977, 1979)	15,481	2.3	2.5×				+	+
Wald et al.	England (1977, 1980)	3,194 4,198	3.0	4.7×		5.8×			3.5×
Macri	New York (1978)	6,031	2.0	2.0×					
Gordon et al.	England (1978)	1,055	2.0			3.5×			4.5×
Smith	England (1980)	1,500	2.0	+	+	+			+
Evans and Stokes	Wales (1984)	2,913	2.0	3.0×			+		8.0×
Burton et al.	North Carolina (1983, 1988)	42,037	2.5	2.0×				8.0×	10.0×
Persson et al.	Sweden (1983)	10,147	2.3	2.8×		2.0×	10.0×		3.0×
Haddow et al.	Maine (1983)	3,636	2.0	3.6×		2.0×			
Purdie et al.	Scotland (1983)	7,223	2.5	2.5×			20.0×		
Fuhrmann and Weitzel	West Germany (1985)	50,000	2.5	3.5×				8.6×	
Williamson et al.	Iowa (1986)	1,161		Poor outcomes					
Robinson et al.	California (1989)	35,787	2.0	3.5×					
Ghosh et al.	Hong Kong (1986)	9,838	2.0	+					
Schnittger and Kjessler	Sweden (1984)	18,037	2.0	+			+		
Hamilton et al.	Scotland (1985)	10,885	2.5	10.0×	2×	>10.0×	3.0×		8.0×
Doran et al.	Ontario (1987)	8,140	2.0	6.0×				+	
Milunsky et al.	Massachusetts (1989)	13,486	2.0	4.0×			3.0×	8.0×	+

IUFD, intrauterine fetal demise; IUGR, intrauterine growth retardation; LBW, low birth weight; MoM, multiple of the median; MSAFP; maternal serum α-fetoprotein; +, increased risk but unquantified.

Data from Milunsky A (ed): Genetic disorders and the fetus: Diagnosis, prevention, and treatment. 3rd ed. Baltimore, Md, Johns Hopkins University Press, 1992, p. 656.

adverse outcome was 27% overall but varied with the degree of elevation. Adverse outcome occurred in 16% when the MSAFP was 2.5 to 2.9 MoM, 29% when it was 3.0 to 5.0 MoM, and 70% when it was over 5.0 MoM. Waller and coworkers investigated 51,008 women screened with MSAFP in California to evaluate the predictive value of high MSAFP compared with low levels. The risk of delivery before 28 weeks was 0.4% with low values (<0.81 MoM) and 3.2% for those with high values (>2.5 MoM), an eightfold difference (Waller et al., 1991, 1993, 1996). The rates for delivery before 37 weeks were 2.6% for the low MSAFP group and 24.3% for the high MSAFP group. Notably, women with MSAFP values over 2.5 MoM had a 10.5-fold increase in preeclampsia and a 10-fold increased risk of placental complications, suggesting that an elevated value in the absence of an anomaly may derive from a fetal–maternal hemorrhage of sufficient volume to have clinical significance. This observation may explain the elevation in MSAFP, but to date no management protocol has been demonstrated to improve outcome in these cases.

Unexplained Elevated Human Chorionic Gonadotropin Levels

The risk for adverse pregnancy outcome with elevated hCG levels appears to be independent of those associated with elevated AFP. Studies have shown that unexplained elevated hCG is associated with an increased risk of preeclamp-

sia, preterm birth, low birth weight, fetal demise, and possibly hypertension (Yaron et al., 1999). It appears that the higher the hCG, the greater the risk.

Elevated Human Chorionic Gonadotropin and Maternal Serum α-Fetoprotein

The combination of an elevated MSAFP and hCG occurs rarely but may have an overall pregnancy complication rate exceeding 50%. A study of 66 singleton and 33 multiple pregnancies with an MSAFP more than 2 MoM and an hCG more than 3.0 MoM found that 60% of singletons and 81% of twins had at least one obstetric complication, including preeclampsia, preterm birth, growth restriction, placental abnormalities, or fetal death (Kuller et al., 1995). Confined placental mosaicism for chromosome 16 has been reported to be associated with extremely high levels of both analytes as well as with similar poor outcomes (Morssink et al., 1995; Benn, 1998).

Low Second-Trimester Maternal Serum Estriol Levels

Low maternal serum unconjugated estriol levels have been linked to adverse pregnancy outcomes (Santolaya-Forgas et al., 1996; Kowalczyk et al., 1998). Very low or absent estriol levels of 0.0 to 0.15 MoM suggest biochemical abnormalities of the fetus or placenta, including placental steroid sulfatase deficiency, Smith-Lemli-Opitz syndrome, congenital adrenal hypoplasia, adrenocorticotropin deficiency, hypothalamic corticotropin deficiency, and anencephaly.

Smith-Lemli-Opitz syndrome is an autosomal recessive disorder secondary to a defect in 3β-hydroxysteroid-δ7-reductase, altering cholesterol synthesis and resulting in low cholesterol levels and the accumulation of the cholesterol precursor 7-dehydrocholesterol in blood and amniotic fluid. Because cholesterol is a precursor of estriol, the defect results in reduced or undetectable levels of estriol in maternal serum and amniotic fluid. Smith-Lemli-Opitz syndrome is characterized by low birth weight, failure to thrive, and moderate to severe mental retardation. It is associated with multiple structural anomalies, including syndactyly of the second and third toes, microcephaly, ptosis, and a typical-appearing facies (Bitzer et al., 1994; Canick et al., 1997; Tint et al., 1998)

Bradley and colleagues (1999) summarized findings in 33 women who delivered infants with Smith-Lemli-Opitz syndrome. Twenty-four of 26 women who had second-trimester estriol values obtained had levels less than the 5th percentile (<0.5 MoM). The median level in this group was 0.23 MoM (below the first percentile). A risk assessment based on low maternal serum unconjugated estriol levels has been suggested but is not presently available (Palomaki et al., 2002). Reliable and inexpensive prenatal testing for Smith-Lemli-Opitz syndrome is available based on amniotic fluid cholesterol or 7-dehydrocholesterol levels (Kratz et al., 1999).

Placental steroid sulfatase deficiency is an X-linked recessive disorder resulting from deletion of Xp22.3. This enzyme deficiency prevents removal of the sulfate molecule from fetal estrogen precursors, preventing conversion to estriol. The fetal phenotype depends on the extent of the deletion with over 90% of cases presenting as X-linked ichthyosis that can be treated with topical keratolytic agents. However, in about 5% of cases, there can be a deletion of contiguous genes causing mental retardation. The deletion can, on occasion, extend to cause Kallman syndrome or chondrodysplasia punctata. The lack of estrogen biosynthesis may result in delayed onset of labor, prolonged labor, or stillbirth.

Prenatal diagnosis for the deletion leading to placental sulfatase deficiency and congenital ichthyosis can be performed by identifying the gene deletion by karyotype or fluorescent *in situ* hybridization (Zalel et al., 1996; Bradley et al., 1997; Santolaya-Forgas et al., 1997). Although very low estriol levels, usually below the level of detection, can detect males at risk for this disorder, testing in these cases is not routinely offered because the phenotype is usually mild. However, the rarer more serious cases of extensive deletions will be missed (Schleifer et al., 1995).

Second-Trimester Ultrasound Markers for Down Syndrome

The clinical diagnosis of Down syndrome is suggested when an infant is found to have a compilation of specific physical findings that can also occur in normal individuals. These include a simian crease, a short femur, clinodactyly, and excessive nuchal skin. Similarly, the *in utero* diagnosis of Down syndrome can be suspected when anomalies or physical features that occur more frequently in Down syndrome than in the general population are noted on an ultrasound examination. Certain of these congenital anomalies, such as atrioventricular canal or duodenal atresia, strongly suggest the possibility of

Down syndrome and are independent indications to offer invasive testing. Although when present there is a high risk of trisomy 21, these anomalies have low sensitivity and thus are not useful in screening. For example, when duodenal atresia is identified, there is an approximate 40% risk of Down syndrome, yet it is seen in only 8% of affected fetuses. Physical characteristics that are not themselves anomalies but that occur more commonly in fetuses with Down syndrome are called *markers*. By comparing the prevalence of markers in Down syndrome fetuses to their prevalence in the normal population, a likelihood ratio can be calculated that can be used to modify the *a priori* age or triple screen risk. This is the basis for ultrasound screening for Down syndrome.

For a marker to be useful for Down syndrome screening, it should be sensitive (i.e., present in a high proportion of Down syndrome pregnancies), specific (i.e., rarely seen in normal fetuses), easily imaged in standard sonographic examination, and present early enough in the second trimester that subsequent diagnostic testing by amniocentesis can be performed so that results are available when pregnancy termination remains an option. A list of presently available markers and their likelihood ratios are seen in Tables 18-5 and 18-6, respectively.

Before considering each marker individually, it is important to remember that the predictive value of any test (e.g., a marker) is dependent on the prevalence in the population of the condition being tested for. In the case of sonographic markers for trisomy 21, the clinical importance of a marker, therefore, varies according to the *a priori* risk as determined by maternal age, the results of multiple serum markers, and the presence of any other sonographic markers detected at the same examination. It is wise, therefore, to defer discussion of the impact of markers until the ultrasound examination has been completed and the results of serum screening have been reported. Markers commonly sought to assess the risk of Down syndrome include the following:

- An *increased nuchal fold* in the second trimester is the most distinctive marker. The fetal head is imaged in a transverse plane similar to that for measuring the biparietal diameter. The thalami and the upper portion of the cerebellum should be in the plane of the image. The distance between the external surface of the occipital bone and the external surface of the skin is then measured. About 35% of Down syndrome fetuses but only 0.7% of normal fetuses will have a nuchal skin fold measurement greater than 5 mm. This ratio yields a likelihood ratio of 50 but includes fetuses with more than one marker. When an increased nuchal fold is an isolated finding, the likelihood ratio is still strong at 20-fold. This high likelihood ratio is obtained because

TABLE 18-5. SECOND-TRIMESTER ULTRASOUND MARKERS ASSOCIATED WITH DOWN SYNDROME

Brachycephaly	Hypoplasia of the mid-phalynx of the fifth digit
Increased nuchal thickness	Echogenic intracardiac focus
Congenital heart defects	"Sandal gap" of the foot
Hyperechoic bowel	Widened ischial spine angle
Shortened femur	Foot length
Shortened humerus	Short or absent nasal bone
Renal pyelectasis	
Duodenal atresia	

TABLE 18-6. LIKELIHOOD RATIOS AND 95% CONFIDENCE LIMITS FOR ISOLATED MARKERS IN THREE STUDIES: AAURA, Nyberg et al. 1998 (*n* = 1042), Nyberg et al. 2001 (*n* = 8830); and Smith-Bindman et al. 2001 (*n* = Meta-analysis of >131,000)

Sonographic Marker	AAURA LR*	Nyberg et al. LR (95% CI)†	Smith-Bindman et al. LR (95% CI)‡
Nuchal thickening	18.6	11.0 (5.2–22)	17.0 (8.0–38)
Hyperechoic bowel	5.5	6.7 (2.7–16.8)	6.1 (3.0–12.6)
Short humerus	2.5	5.1 (1.6–16.5)	7.5 (4.7–12)
Short femur	2.2	1.5 (0.8–2.8)	2.7 (1.2–6)
EIF	2.0	1.8 (1.0–3)	2.8 (1.5–5.5)
Pyelectasis	1.5	1.5 (0.6–3.6)	1.9 (0.7–5.1)

* LR assumed by the original AAURA model, Nyberg DA, Luthy DA, Resta RG, et al: Age-adjusted ultrasound risk assessment for fetal Down's syndrome during the second trimester: Description of the method and analysis of 142 cases. Ultrasound Obstet Gynecol **12**:8, 1998.
† Nyberg DA, Souter VL, El-Bastawissi A, et al: Isolated sonographic markers for detection of fetal Down syndrome in the second trimester of pregnancy. J Ultrasound Med **20**:1053, 2001.
‡LR of meta-analysis by Smith-Bindman R, Hosmer W, Feldstein VA, et al: Second-trimester ultrasound to detect fetuses with Down syndrome: A meta-analysis, JAMA **285**:1044, 2001.

AAURA, age adjusted ultrasound risk adjustment; CI, confidence interval; EIF, echogenic intracardiac focus; LR, likelihood ratio.

of the rarity of an increased nuchal fold in an unaffected population (i.e., high sensitivity). For women with an *a priori* risk of less than 1:1600 (age-related risk for a 20 year old), a 20-fold increase results in a risk estimate of at least 1:270. Thus, the presence of an increased nuchal fold alone is an indication to offer invasive testing. (Benacerraf et al., 1987; Perella et al., 1988; Nyberg et al., 1990; Crane and Gray, 1991; Donnenfeld, 1992; Borrell et al., 1996).

- Down syndrome fetuses in the second trimester may have *short proximal extremities* relative to the length expected from their biparietal diameter. This can be used to identify at-risk pregnancies by calculating a ratio of observed to expected femur length based on the fetus's biparietal diameter. An observed-to-expected ratio of less than 0.91 or a biparietal diameter-to-femur ratio of more than 1.5 has a reported likelihood ratio of 1.5 to 2.7 when present as an isolated finding. A short humerus is more strongly related to Down syndrome, with reported likelihood ratios ranging from 2.5 to 7.5. Bahado-Singh and coworkers (1998) combined humerus length with nuchal skin fold to estimate Down syndrome risk and calculated the likelihood ratios for various measurements to adjust estimated Down syndrome risk for each patient.
- *Echogenic intracardiac foci* occur in up to 5% of normal pregnancies and in approximately 13% to 18% of Down syndrome gestations (Bromley et al., 1998). The likelihood ratio for Down syndrome when an echogenic focus is present as an isolated marker has ranged from 1.8 to 2.8. The risk does not seem to vary if the focus is in the right or left ventricle or if it is unilateral or bilateral.
- *Increased echogenicity of the fetal bowel,* when brighter than the surrounding bone, has a Down syndrome likelihood ratio of 5.5 to 6.7 (Nyberg, Resta, Mahony,

et al., 1993; MacGregor et al., 1995; Corteville et al., 1996). This finding can also be seen with fetal cystic fibrosis (CF), congenital cytomegalovirus infection, swallowed bloody amniotic fluid, and severe intrauterine growth restriction. Therefore, if amniocentesis is performed for this finding, testing for the other potential etiologies should be considered.

- *Mild fetal pyelectasis* (a renal anterior posterior diameter greater than 4 mm) has been suggested as a potential marker for Down syndrome. As an isolated marker, the likelihood ratio has ranged from 1.5 to 1.9 (see Table 18-6). This has been found by Snijders and coworkers (1995) not to be significantly more frequent in Down syndrome pregnancies than in normal pregnancies (low specificity).
- Other markers described include a hypoplastic fifth middle phalanx of the hand (Benacerraf et al., 1988), short ears, a sandal gap between the first and second toes (Drugan et al., 2000; Shipp and Benacerraf, 2002), an abnormal iliac wing angle (Paladini et al., 2000), an altered foot-to-femur ratio (Johnson, Barr, et al., 1993), and a short or absent nasal bone (Cicero et al., 2001). These markers are inconsistently used because of the time and expertise required to obtain them.

Use of Ultrasound to Estimate the Risk of Down Syndrome

As with other screening modalities, second-trimester ultrasound can be used to alter the *a priori* risk in either direction. A benign second-trimester scan having none of the known markers and no anomalies has been suggested to have a likelihood ratio of 0.4, assuming the image quality is satisfactory. Nyberg and coworkers (1998) used this approach to calculate an age-adjusted ultrasound risk assessment for Down syndrome in 8914 pregnancies (186 fetuses with Down syndrome, 8728 control subjects). Some type of sonographic finding (major abnormality, minor marker, or both) was observed in 68.8% of fetuses with trisomy 21 compared with 13.6% of control fetuses (*P* < .001). The observation that about one third of fetuses with Down syndrome have neither a marker nor an anomaly has been used to adjust the estimated risk of Down syndrome downward by approximately 60% to 65% (likelihood ratio, 0.4) when the "genetic ultrasound" is normal. This sensitivity was observed in a single experienced center. It is doubtful that the same sensitivity can be achieved in every center (Crane et al., 1994).

A positive likelihood ratio can be used to estimate an increase in risk. The magnitude of the increase depends on the marker(s) or anomalies seen. Nyberg and colleagues reviewed their own data (1998, 2001) and the data of others (Smith-Bindman et al., 2001) to estimate a likelihood ratio for each marker as an isolated finding (see Table 18-6). An isolated minor or "soft" marker was the only sonographic finding in 42 (22.6%) of 186 fetuses with trisomy 21 compared with 987 (11.3%) of 8728 control fetuses (*P* < .001). Nuchal thickening and hyperechoic bowel showed the strongest association with trisomy 21 as isolated markers, followed by shortened humerus, echogenic intracardiac focus, shortened femur, and pyelectasis. Echogenic intracardiac focus was the single most common isolated marker in both affected fetuses (7.1%) and control fetuses (3.9%) but carried a low risk.

Combined Ultrasound and Multiple Marker Risk Assessment in the Second Trimester

Ultrasound markers can also be combined with serum markers if they are independent. Souter and coworkers (2002) demonstrated a relatively small correlation that needs to be taken into consideration if a quantitative approach is used. Bahado-Singh and colleagues (2002) combined ultrasound markers with maternal analytes, including urinary hyperglycosylated hCG and urinary β-core fragment of hCG. In a sample of 585 pregnancies, the sensitivity was 93.7%, with a false-positive rate of 5%.

Ultrasound Screening for Other Chromosomal Abnormalities

Fetal aneuploidy other than Down syndrome can be suspected based on ultrasound findings (Table 18-7). Choroid plexus cysts occur in 1% of fetuses between 16 and 24 weeks' gestation and have been associated with trisomy 18. Thirty percent to 35% of fetuses with trisomy 18 will have choroid plexus cysts. Among fetuses with a choroid plexus cyst, about 3% will have trisomy 18, most (65% to 90%) of whom will have other ultrasound findings (Table 18-8). Although an iso-

lated choroid plexus cyst was estimated to yield a probability of trisomy 18 in 1 of 150 in one review, many of the series reviewed contained a high proportion of older women, which would overstate the risk. Snijders and coworkers (1994) calculated that an isolated choroid plexus cyst has a likelihood ratio for trisomy 18 of 1.5 and can be used to calculate an individual's risk for trisomy 18. The size, location, or persistence of the cyst does not alter this risk (Shunagshoti et al., 1966; Nadel et al., 1992; Riebel et al., 1992; Porto et al., 1993; Nava et al, 1994).

Table 18-7 displays the magnitude of the associations between various ultrasound findings and aneuploid conditions as estimated from a referral population. The rates noted may overestimate the strength of the association when such findings are noted on a screening examination.

First-Trimester Screening for Aneuploidy

Nuchal Translucency

In his initial description of the syndrome that bears his name, Langdon Down described skin so deficient in elasticity that it appeared to be too large for the body. This was particularly noticeable in the neck area. The skin in the fetal neck can now be seen with ultrasound as early as 10 to 12 weeks of

TABLE 18-7. ASSOCIATION OF ULTRASOUND MARKERS WITH ANEUPLOIDY

U.S. Finding	Isolated (%)	Multiple (%)	Trisomy 13	Trisomy 18	Trisomy 21	Other	45X
Holoprosencephaly n = 132	4	39	30	7	—	7	—
Choroid plexus cysts n = 1806	1	46	11	121	18	11	—
Facial cleft n = 118	0	51	25	16	—	6	—
Cystic hygroma n = 276	52	71	—	13	26	11	163
Nuchal skin fold	19	45	—	9	85	19	10
Diaphragmatic hernia n = 173	2	34	—	18	—	14	—
Ventriculomegaly n = 690	2	17	10	23	13	14	—
Posterior fossa cyst n = 101	0	52	10	22	—	8	—
Major heart defects n = 829	16	66	30	82	68	31	30
Duodenal atresia n = 44	38	64	—	—	21	2	—
Hyperechoic bowel n = 196	7	42	—	—	22	17	—
Omphalocoele n = 475	13	46	28	108	—	31	—
Renal anomalies n = 1825	3	24	40	52	48	62	—
Mild hydronephrosis n = 631	2	33	8	6	27	9	—
IUGR (early) n = 621	4	38	11	47	—	18	36 (triploidy)
Talipes n = 127	0	33	—	—	—	—	—

Isolated, isolated finding; multiple, multiple findings on ultrasound. Renal anomalies defined as mild hydro, moderate, severe hydro, multicystic kidney, obstruction, or renal agenesis.

IUGR, intrauterine growth restriction; US, ultrasound.

Adapted from Snijders RJM, Nicolaides KH: ULtrasound Markers for Fetal Chromosomal Defects. New York, Parthenon Publishing Group, 1996.

TABLE 18-8. ULTRASOUND FINDINGS ASSOCIATED WITH TRISOMY 18

Finding	Percentage
Growth restriction	46
Hand or feet abnormalities	39
Rocker bottom feet	
Overlapping fingers	
Cardiac abnormality	31
CNS abnormality	29
Diaphragmatic hernia	13
Ventral wall defect	10
Facial abnormality	7
At least one abnormality	90

CNS, central nervous system.

From Gupta JK, Cave M, Lilford RJ, et al: Clinical significance of fetal choroid plexus cysts. Lancet **346**:724, 1995.

gestation and is known as a nuchal translucency (NT). The quantification of this additional "skin behind the neck" can be used for first-trimester Down syndrome screening (Nicolaides et al., 1999).

The NT is a fluid-filled space in the posterior fetal nuchal area. NT is defined as a collection of fluid under the skin behind the neck in fetuses between 11 and 14 weeks' gestation. This can be successfully measured by transabdominal ultrasound examination in approximately 95% of cases.

Studies conducted in women with increased risk of aneuploidy demonstrated an association between increased NT and chromosomal defects (Cullen et al., 1990; Szabo and Gellen, 1990; Nicolaides et al., 1992; Schulte-Vallentin and Schindler, 1992; Shulman et al., 1992; Suchet et al., 1992; van Zalen-Sprock et al., 1992; Ville et al., 1992; Wilson et al., 1992; Hewitt, 1993; Johnson, Johnson, et al., 1993; Nadel et al., 1993; Savoldelli et al., 1993; Trauffer et al., 1994; Brambati et al., 1995; Comas et al., 1995; Pandya, Kondylios, et al., 1995; Szabo et al., 1995). Subsequent studies demonstrated that a NT thickness above the 95th percentile was present in approximately 80% of trisomy 21 fetuses (Pandya, Kondylios, et al., 1994). As for other serum and ultrasound markers, the significance of the NT thickness is dependent on the *a priori* risk for a chromosomal abnormality. NT thickness increases with gestational age or crown-rump length. Figure 18-2 illustrates the NT between 11 and 14 weeks' gestation. These observations suggested that NT could be used as a screening test for Down syndrome by converting the deviation from the expected mean to a likelihood ratio.

NT combined with the maternal and gestational age to assess the risk for Down syndrome was studied in more than 100,000 pregnancies (Snijders et al., 1998). NT was greater than the 95th percentile in more than 70% of fetuses with trisomy 21. The risk of Down syndrome was calculated by the maternal age and gestational age prevalence multiplied by the likelihood ratio. A cutoff of 1:300 was used. The studied sample included 326 fetuses with trisomy 21. Eighty-two percent of trisomy 21 fetuses were identified, with a false-positive rate of 8.3% (Snijders et al., 1998). When a screen-positive rate of 5% was selected, the sensitivity was 77% (95% confidence interval, 72% to 82%). Subsequent studies have

demonstrated similar Down syndrome detection rates between 70% and 75% (Table 18-9).

The screening paradigm using an ultrasound measurement to determine a likelihood ratio is reliable only if NT is measured in a standard fashion. Standards for NT measurements include the following:

1. The minimum crown length should be 45 mm and the maximum 84 mm. The success rate for accomplishing a measurement for gestational age is between 98% and 100%. The success rate falls to 90% at 14 weeks and onward (Whitlow and Economides, 1998).
2. Either transabdominal or transvaginal scanning can be used, with about 95% of cases able to be imaged by the transabdominal route (Braithwaite and Economides, 1995).
3. A true sagittal section of the fetus as for measuring the fetal crown-rump length must be obtained.
4. The magnification must be such that the fetus occupies at least three fourths of the image. The magnification should be increased so that each increment in the distance between calipers should only be 0.1 mm. Studies have demonstrated that ultrasound measurements can be accurate to the nearest 0.1 to 0.2 mm (Braithwaite et al., 1996).
5. Care must be taken to clearly distinguish between the fetal skin and the amnion. At this gestation, both structures appear as thin membranes. This can be accomplished by either waiting for spontaneous fetal movement away from the amniotic membrane or by bouncing the fetus off the amnion by asking the mother to cough or tap on her abdomen (Figure 18-3).
6. The maximum thickness of this subcutaneous translucency between the skin and the soft tissue overlying the cervical spine should be measured by placing the calipers on the lines as illustrated in Figure 18-4.
7. During the scan, the measurement should be taken and the maximum one recorded and used for Down syndrome risk calculation.
8. The NT should be measured with the fetus in the neutral position. When the fetal neck is hyperextended, the measurement can be increased by 0.6 mm, and when the neck is

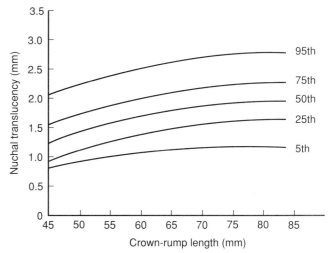

FIGURE 18-2 ■ Normative curves for nuchal translucency measurement between 11 and 14 weeks' gestation. (From Nicolaides KH, Sebire NJ, Snijders RJM: The 11–14 Week Scan. New York, Parthenon, 1999.)

TABLE 18-9. STUDIES EXAMINING THE IMPLEMENTATION OF FETAL NUCHAL TRANSLUCENCY (NT) SCREENING

Source	Gestation (Wk)	n	Successful Measurement	NT cutoff (mm)	FPR	DR Trisomy 21
Pandya et al., 1995	10–14	1,763	100%	>2.5	3.6%	3 of 4 (75%)
Szabo et al., 1995	9–12	3,380	100%	>3.0	1.6%	28 of 31 (90%)
Bewley et al., 1995	8–13	1,704	66%	>3.0	6.0%	1 of 3 (33%)
Bower et al., 1995	8–14	1,481	97%	>3.0	6.3%	4 of 8 (50%)
Kornman et al.,1996	8–13	923	58%	>3.0	6.3%	2 of 4 (50%)
Zimmerman et al., 1996	10–13	1,131	100%	>3.0	1.9%	2 of 3 (67%)
Taipale et al., 1997	10–16	10,010	99%	>3.0	0.8%	7 of 13 (54%)
Hafner et al., 1998	10–14	4,371	100%	>2.5	1.7%	4 of 7 (57%)
Pajkrt et al., 1998	10–14	1,547	96%	>3.0	2.2%	6 of 9 (67%)

DR, detection rate; FPR, false-positive rate.

Adapted from Nicolaides KH, Sebire NJ, Snijders RJM: The 11–14 Week Scan. New York, Parthenon, 1999.

flexed, the measurement can be decreased by 0.4 mm (Whitlow et al., 1998).

9. The umbilical cord may be found around the fetal neck in approximately 5% to 10% of cases, which may produce a falsely increased NT adding about 0.8 mm to the measurement (Schaefer et al., 1998). In such cases, the measurement of NT above and below the cord will be different, and the smallest measurement is the most appropriate.

Even with these criteria, debate about the feasibility of standardized NT measurements remains. Certification courses are available with continuous quality assessment to maintain proper technique. The ability to achieve a reliable measurement has been linked to the motivation of the sonographer. A study comparing the results obtained from hospitals where NT was clinically used compared with those where they were merely measured but were not acted on reported that, in the interventional groups, successful measurement was achieved in 100% of cases, whereas the noninterventional centers were successful in only 85% (Roberts et al., 1995). In a recent prospective study (Pandya, Altman, et al., 1995), the NT was measured by two to four operators in 200 pregnant women, demonstrating that after an initial measurement, a second one made by the same operator or another operator varied from the initial measurement by less than 0.5 and 0.6 mm, respectively, in 95% of cases. It is suggested that a large part of the variation between operators can be accounted for by placement of the calipers rather than generation of the appropriate image. Subsequent studies (Herman et al., 1999; Pajkrt et al., 2000; Snijders et al., 2002) have continued to report small interoperator differences.

First-Trimester Biochemical Screening

Two serum analytes are useful for first-trimester screening. Pregnancy-associated plasma protein A has been demonstrated to have a mean value of 0.4 MoM in trisomy 21 pregnancies. The free β subunit of hCG is elevated in Down syndrome pregnancies, with a mean value of 1.8 MoM. Screening using pregnancy-associated plasma protein A alone will identify about 40% to 45% of trisomy 21 pregnancies, and free β-hCG will identify about 23%, both with a false-positive rate of 5%

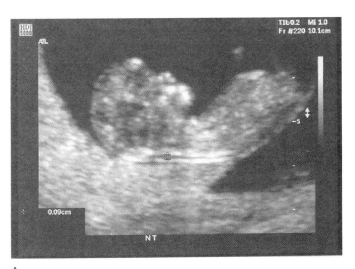

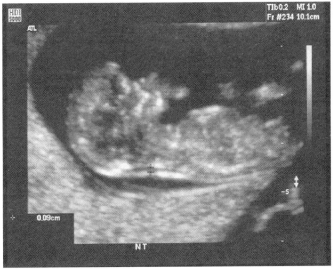

A   B

FIGURE 18-3 ■ First-trimester nuchal translucency (NT) measurement. Clear distinction of the amnion versus the skin edge is made by waiting for fetal movement. More accurate measurement with fetal movement is demonstrated.

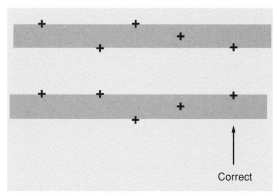

FIGURE 18-4 ■ Proper placement of the calipers for measuring the nuchal translucency. (From Nicolaides KH, Sebire NJ, Snijders RJM: The 11–14 Week Scan. New York, Parthenon, 1999.)

(Macri et al., 1994; Berry et al., 1995; Cuckle and van Lith, 1999). Combining both free β-hCG and pregnancy-associated plasma protein A can identify 60% to 65% of trisomy 21 pregnancies, for a similar 5% false-positive rate (Krantz et al., 1996). This is a serum analyte detection rate similar to that seen with triple screening in the second trimester.

Combined Nuchal Translucency and Biochemical First-Trimester Screening

Combining NT with serum analytes will improve the first-trimester Down syndrome detection rate. Krantz and colleagues (2000) showed a 90% detection rate for a 5% false-positive rate in 5718 pregnancies screened in the first trimester. Wapner and coworkers (2001) showed a 79% detection rate for a 5% false-positive rate. Wapner (2002) and Crossley and coworkers (2002) found an 82% detection rate. In women over age 35, 90% of trisomy 21 pregnancies were identified with a 16% false-positive rate (Wapner, 2002). First-trimester screening can also identify trisomy 18 pregnancies. Over 90% of such pregnancies will be screen positive when combined biochemical and NT screening is used (Wapner, 2002).

A potential disadvantage of earlier screening is that chromosomally abnormal pregnancies that are destined to miscarry will be identified. The impact of this can be evaluated because 69% of trisomy 21 fetuses living in the first trimester and 76% of those alive in the second trimester will be born alive (Morris et al., 1999). Using this information, Dunston and Nix (1998) calculated that a detection rate of 80% in the first trimester is approximately equivalent to a second-trimester sensitivity of 75%, suggesting that when early spontaneous losses of trisomy 21 pregnancies are considered, first-trimester screening is superior to that presently available in the second trimester.

First-trimester screening would be less desirable if screen-positive pregnancies or those with enlarged NTs were preferentially lost. In a study of 108 fetuses with trisomy 21 diagnosed in the first trimester because of increased NT, Nicolaides and colleagues found that six patients elected to continue the pregnancy (Hyett et al., 1996). In five of the six fetuses the translucency resolved, and at the second-trimester scan the nuchal fold thickness was normal. All six of these trisomy 21 fetuses were born alive. Wapner (2002) calculated that over 80% of screen-positive trisomy 21 pregnancies would be born alive.

Integrated Screening: Combining Both First- and Second-Trimester Tests

Wald and colleagues (1999) described a protocol for screening for Down syndrome based on tests performed during both the first (NT and pregnancy-associated plasma protein A) and second trimester (AFP and hCG). They calculated that 85% of affected pregnancies would be detected with a false-positive rate of only 0.9%. These results, although quite impressive, are based solely on previous studies, some rather small. This protocol has not been performed prospectively. Although this screening approach may be quite sensitive and specific, delaying the diagnosis until late in the second trimester is not an acceptable approach for many women (Jenkins and Wapner, 1999).

Can Maternal Age Be Eliminated as an Indication for Invasive Prenatal Diagnosis?

Maternal age of 35 or older has been a standard indication for invasive testing for over 35 years, despite a sensitivity of only 30% for a 7.5% rate of amniocentesis (number of births to women over 35 in the United States). As serum screening has emerged, the importance of maternal age as a single indication for testing is being reevaluated.

In women aged 35 years and older, 87% of Down syndrome pregnancies and 25% of unaffected pregnancies will be screen positive at a cutoff of 1:250 (Haddow et al., 1994). The incidence of Down syndrome in this age group is approximately 1:100. Table 18-10 demonstrates that performing an amniocentesis on screen-negative (risk < 1:270) women aged 35 years or older would lead to the loss of three normal pregnancies from procedure-induced complications for every Down syndrome pregnancy identified. If first-trimester screening becomes commonplace and is confirmed to have a 90% sensitivity for a 15% false-positive rate in women aged 35 years or older (Wapner, 2002), the benefits of screening as opposed to offering an invasive test are even greater.

Screening the entire population of pregnant women regardless of age provides the most effective use of resources. Presently, 7.5% of women over age 35 are offered invasive testing, as are about 5% of women under age 35 who are screen positive, making 12.1% of pregnant women eligible for testing. If second-trimester screening were used and only screen-positive patients were offered invasive testing, the number of procedures would be reduced to only 6.4% of the pregnant population. If first-trimester screening is used, the number of eligible patients is only 3.8%.

Age-related autosomal and sex chromosome trisomies other than trisomy 21 would potentially be missed if invasive testing for age were abandoned. Presently, both second- and first-trimester screening for trisomy 18 are available and efficient. Wapner (2002) showed a 100% detection rate using first-trimester combined screening in women aged 35 years and older. About 50% of the sex chromosome abnormalities will be screen positive in the second trimester in women aged 35 years and older (Rose et al., 1994). Presently, many centers offer women aged 35 years and older the option of screening before invasive testing. This approach has to be preceded by explicit patient counseling to explain the risks of both options.

TABLE 18-10. COMPARISON OF SCREENING APPROACHES FOR WOMEN AGED 35 YEARS AND OLDER*

	Based on population of 10,000 pregnant women ≥35 years old		
	Invasive Procedures for All Women ≥35 Years (*n* = 10,000)	First-Trimester Screening for All Women ≥35 Years (*n* = 10,000)	Second-Trimester Screening for All Women ≥35 Years (*n* = 10,000)
Down syndrome pregnancies	100	100.0	100
Down syndrome detected	100	90.0	87
Down syndrome missed	0	10.0	13
Invasive procedures performed	10,000	1500.0	2500
Pregnancies lost due to procedure	50	7.5	13
Pregnancies lost to diagnosis	N/A	4.3	3
1 trisomy 21 pregnancy in screen-negative women			

*Assumes one procedure-related loss for every 200 invasive procedures performed. First-trimester screening: sens 90%, FPR 16%. Second-trimester screening: sens 87%, FPR 25%.

FPR, false-positive rate; sens, sensitivity.

MATERNAL SERUM α-FETOPROTEIN SCREENING FOR NEURAL TUBE AND OTHER STRUCTURAL DEFECTS

Maternal serum screening for neural tube defects was the initial foray into pregnancy screening for congenital anomalies. Because 95% of neural tube defects occurred in families without a history of a previously affected offspring, prenatal detection of these defects was largely fortuitous before 1980. Screening is based on elevated levels of MSAFP, which occurs in anencephaly and spina bifida.

AFP is a fetal-specific globin similar to albumin in molecular weight and charge but with a different primary structure and distinct antigenic properties. The gene for AFP is located on chromosome 4q. It is synthesized early in gestation by the yolk sac and subsequently by the gastrointestinal tract and fetal liver. The kidneys and placenta also produce trace amounts of AFP. The level of fetal plasma AFP peaks between 10 and 13 weeks of gestation and declines exponentially from 14 to 32 weeks and then more sharply until term. The exponential fall in fetal plasma AFP is most likely due to the dilution effect of increasing fetal blood volume, as well as a decline in the amounts synthesized by the fetus.

AFP enters the fetal urine and is excreted into the amniotic fluid. Peak levels of AFAFP are reached between 12 and 14 weeks' gestation, decline between 10% and 15% per week during the second trimester, and are almost nondetectable at term. The concentration gradient between fetal plasma and AFAFP is about 150 to 200:1. The concentration differential between fetal and maternal serum is about 50,000:1. Hence, the presence of a small volume of fetal blood or serum within the amniotic fluid can raise the AFP level significantly.

AFP levels in maternal plasma or serum rise above nonpregnant levels as early as the 7th week of gestation. Maternal serum levels are significantly lower than amniotic fluid levels and actually increase during gestation until 28 and 32 weeks, when they peak. This apparent paradoxical rise in MSAFP when amniotic fluid and serum levels are decreasing is believed to be accounted for by increasing placental permeability to fetal plasma proteins. In normal pregnancies, transport of AFAFP contributes little to the MSAFP compartment. The

significant difference in fetal serum AFP compared with that in the amniotic fluid and maternal serum serves as the basis of using this fetal protein to screen for fetal lesions such as neural tube defects, which potentially will leak high levels of AFP into the amniotic fluid and, hence, the maternal serum.

MSAFP screening for neural tube defects is ideally performed between 16 and 18 weeks of pregnancy. Cutoffs between 2.0 and 2.5 MoM as upper limits will yield detection rates of almost 100% for anencephaly and 85% to 92% for open spina bifida, with a false-positive rate between 2% and 5%. As with all screening modalities, the positive predictive value for an individual patient is dependent on the population risk. Table 18-11 demonstrates the odds of an individual woman having a child with a neural tube defect based on the degree of elevation of her serum AFP, and her *a priori* risk of having a child with a neural tube defect. Because MSAFP values rise between 16% and 18% per week during the second trimester, use of MoM at a gestational week for comparison between laboratories is recommended. The median is preferred to the mean because it is less influenced by occasional outliers.

TABLE 18-11. THE ODDS OF INDIVIDUAL WOMEN WITH PARTICULAR SERUM α-FETOPROTEIN (AFP) LEVELS AT 16–18 WEEKS' GESTATION OF HAVING A FETUS WITH OPEN SPINA BIFIDA

	A Priori Birth Incidence*	
Serum AFP (MoM)	1 per 1000	2 per 1000
2.0	1:800	1:400
2.5	1:290	1:140
3.0	1:120	1:59
3.5	1:53	1:27
4.0	1:26	1:13
4.5	1:14	1:7
5.0	1:7	1:4

* In the absence of antenatal diagnosis. Multiple pregnancies excluded by ultrasonography.

MoM, multiple of the median.

From Milunsky A (ed): Genetic Disorders and the Fetus: Diagnosis, Prevention, and Treatment. 3rd ed. Baltimore, Md, Johns Hopkins University Press, 1992, p. 656.

MSAFP is performed using an enzyme immunoassay. All laboratories performing this test should have their own normal ranges and a mechanism for continuous quality control assessment. The College of American Pathologists operates a nationwide external proficiency test in the United States, which is an essential element in population-based screening programs. Most laboratories presently use an upper limit cutoff of 2.0 MoM. Some laboratories use a somewhat higher cutoff up to 2.5 MoM. The choice of a specific cutoff is a balance between the anticipated detection rate and the false-positive rate. Because ultrasound screening for the evaluation of elevated neural tube defects has replaced the need for amniocentesis in many cases, a trend toward choosing a lower AFP threshold to gain a higher detection rate with slightly more false positives has occurred.

Because of interlaboratory variation and interassay variation, many clinics will repeat an MSAFP that initially falls between 2 and 3 MoM. If the repeat value is normal, no further evaluation is required. However, the variance of MSAFP by gestational week related to assay precision or individual fluctuation yields no practical value in performing a repeat MSAFP on either the same or a second sample taken up to 1 month later. Most centers thus choose to obtain an ultrasound after any elevated MSAFP.

A number of factors can influence the interpretation of an MSAFP value. The most important factor for efficient MSAFP screening is the accuracy of the gestational age determination. Because there is an exponential rise in MSAFP over the recommended screening period of 15 to 20 weeks, a variation of 2 weeks between the actual gestational age and that used for MSAFP interpretation can be misleading. A potential confounding factor is that fetuses with spina bifida may have biparietal diameters that are reduced by approximately 2 weeks. Consequently, femur length and biparietal diameter should be measured to confirm gestational age for AFP screening. A first-trimester ultrasound is the preferable means of documenting gestational age; results of this ultrasound can be submitted to the laboratory in place of the last menstrual period.

Maternal weight affects the MSAFP concentration. The heavier the woman, the lower the MSAFP value as a result of dilution in the larger blood volume. Adjusting MSAFP values for maternal weight will increase the detection rate for open spina bifida. Dividing the observed MoM by the expected MoM for a given weight enables adjustment for differences in weight. Correction for weights over 250 pounds significantly increases the rate of elevated MSAFP results, suggesting overcorrection. Therefore, some laboratories recommend linear correction of MSAFP only up to a weight of 200 pounds. Presently, weight correction of MSAFP reports is routinely performed.

Maternal ethnicity may also alter the interpretation of an MSAFP level, because black women have a 10% to 15% higher MSAFP than non-blacks (O'Brien et al., 1997). This is important because the incidence of neural tube defects in blacks is lower. Other ethnic groups also have slightly different MSAFP levels but do not vary sufficiently to warrant corrections. Pregnant women with insulin-dependent diabetes mellitus have MSAFP values that are significantly lower than nondiabetic women in the second trimester (Wald et al., 1979; Crossley et al., 1996), which requires adjustments in the interpretation. This is critical because there is up to a 10-fold higher frequency of neural tube defects in the offspring of these patients. MSAFP also must be altered in multiple gestations, and this adjustment is discussed later.

There may be a genetic component to raised MSAFP. Women with an elevated MSAFP in one pregnancy appear to have an increased risk of elevated values in subsequent gestations. False-positive AFP has been seen in multiple members of some families (Crandall and Matsumoto, 1986; Heinonen et al., 1996).

Once an elevated MSAFP has been detected, the initial step is ultrasound evaluation to confirm the gestational age, rule out twin gestations, identify other causes of elevated MSAFP such as fetal demise and oligohydramnios, and identify other structural defects that can cause elevated MSAFP, such as omphaloceles, gastroschisis, and duodenal atresia (Table 18-12). The most important aspect of this initial ultrasound is confirmation of gestational age. In up to 50% of cases, incorrect dating will be identified, and adjustment of the initial value resolves the issue. If the elevated MSAFP remains unexplained, further testing by either amniocentesis or targeted ultrasound is required.

Until recently, the standard diagnostic test for an elevated MSAFP had been amniocentesis with evaluation of amniotic fluid AFP and acetylcholinesterase (AChE) levels. AFAFP determination has nearly a 100% detection rate for anencephaly and a 96% to 99% detection rate for open spina bifida, with a false-positive rate of 0.7% to 1.0% (Crandall and Matsumoto, 1986). The accuracy of amniotic fluid determination is enhanced by the addition of AChE. As opposed to AFP, which is a fetal serum analyte, AChE is predominately neuronally derived, giving it additional specificity for nervous system lesions. The most common assay for AChE is a polychromic gel electrophoresis in which AChE can be distinguished from nonspecific cholinesterases on the basis of mobility. A combined use of AFP and AChE together appears to be the most sensitive and specific in determining neural tube defects.

As with AFP, there are a number of potential confounders with AChE. When fetal blood is present in the amniotic fluid, interpretation of AChE might be complicated and inaccurate. In addition, false-positive AChE results have been clearly documented in normal pregnancies before 15 weeks' gestation and may be seen in up to one third of cases under 12 weeks' gestation.

 TABLE 18-12. FETAL ANOMALIES ASSOCIATED WITH AN ELEVATED AMNIOTIC FLUID α-FETOPROTEIN

Positive AChE	Negative AChE
Anencephaly	Aneuploidy
Open spina bifida	IUFD
Encephalocele	Obstructive uropathy
Omphalocele	Cleft lip/palate
Gastroschisis	Omphalocele
Esophageal atresia	Gastroschisis
Teratoma	Fetal hydrops
IUFD	IUGR
Cystic hygroma	Congenital nephrosis
Acardiac twin	Normal gestation
Cloacal extrophy	
Epidermolysis bullosa	
Aplasia cutis congenital	
Normal gestation	

AChE, acetylcholinesterase; IUFD, intrauterine fetal demise; IUGR, intrauterine growth restriction.

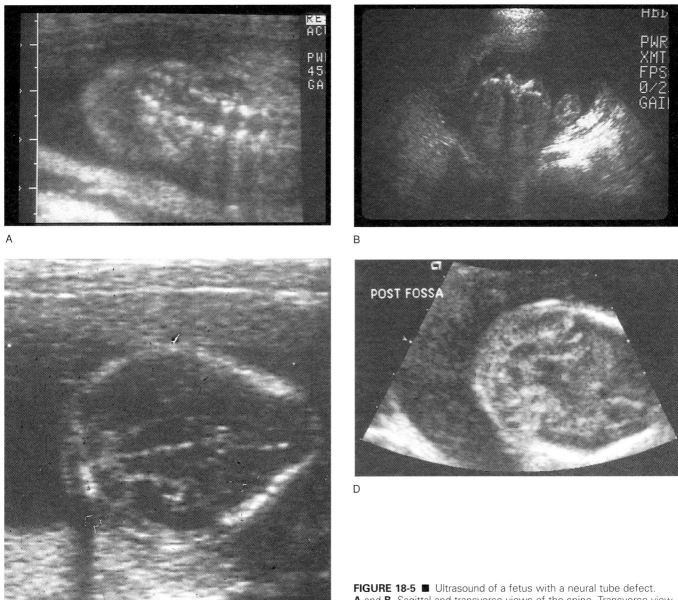

FIGURE 18-5 ■ Ultrasound of a fetus with a neural tube defect. **A** and **B**, Sagittal and transverse views of the spine. Transverse view of the skull with (**C**) scalloping of the frontal bones, the "lemon sign," and (**D**) the herniation of the cerebellum, the "banana sign."

In experienced hands, targeted ultrasound for elevated MSAFP has been found to be as sensitive and specific as amniotic fluid AFP and AChE levels (Lennon and Gray, 1999; Boyd et al., 2000). Although ultrasound as a primary screening tool for spina bifida may only identify 60% to 80% of neural tube defects, targeted sonographic evaluation in high-risk cases is remarkably accurate. Sensitivity has been reported between 97% and 100%, with 100% specificity.

Ultrasound diagnosis of meningomyelocele is frequently based on the finding of a cystic mass protruding from the dorsal vertebral bodies without skin covering. This is ideally seen in the transverse plane as a wide separation of the lateral processes of the lamina. In the coronal plane, widening of the parallel lines of the normal spine can be seen. It should be cautioned that occasionally coronal and sagittal views can be misleading, and the present standard for spina bifida screening by ultrasound is an image of transverse planes of individual vertebrae. Some cases of meningomyelocele will not have a cystic structure and will only be identified by subtle widening of the posterior processes.

Indirect sonographic signs of meningomyelocele have been found to be as important as visualization of the spinal lesion and are somewhat easier to image. These include ventriculomegaly, microcephaly, frontal bone scalloping (lemon sign), and obliteration of the cisterna magna with either an "absent" cerebellum or abnormal anterior curvature of the cerebellar hemispheres (banana sign) (Nicolaides et al., 1986) (Fig. 18-5). These findings are seen in over 95% of cases of neural tube defects imaged in the middle of the second trimester. The banana sign and lemon sign may not be present after 22 to 24 weeks' gestation. Anencephaly should routinely be identified by ultrasound as early as 11 or 12 weeks' gestation but should be reconfirmed by a scan at around 13 weeks because ossification of the skull in some cases may not be completed until that time.

Presently, the best approach to evaluate an elevated MSAFP uses a combination of ultrasound imaging and amniocentesis. In cases in which ultrasound expertise is available and optimal images can be obtained of both the spine and the central nervous system, amniocentesis can be avoided. If ultrasound expertise or high-resolution equipment is not available or fetal position or maternal body habitus prevents optimal fetal visualization, further evaluation by amniocentesis should be offered.

Other Fetal Causes of Elevated Maternal Serum α-Fetoprotein and Amniotic Fluid α-Fetoprotein

The greater the elevation in both MSAFP and AFAFP, the greater the risk of fetal abnormalities. Crandall and Chen (1997) analyzed 1086 amniotic fluid samples with elevated AFP levels and found abnormalities associated with AFAFP elevations of 2.0 to 4.9, 5.0 to 9.9, and more than 10.0 MoM in 25%, 88.1%, and 97.7% of pregnancies, respectively.

In addition to neural tube defects, other lesions leaking fetal serum into the amniotic fluid can cause elevations of both MSAFP and AFAFP. These include fetal abdominal wall defects such as omphalocele, gastroschisis, or extrophy of the bladder; weeping skin lesions such as epidermolysis bullosa or aplasia cutis; and some cases of sacrococcygeal teratoma and fetal urinary tract obstruction. Table 18-12 lists other fetal conditions associated with elevated MSAFP with and without elevations of AChE.

Because AFP is made in the gastrointestinal tract and in the fetal liver, reduced intestinal AFP clearance with regurgitation of intestinal contents has been associated with elevated MSAFP and AFAFP. Reflux of lung fluid can also cause elevated levels. This occurs with duodenal atresia, annular pancreas, intestinal atresia, pharyngeal teratoma, and congenital cystic adenomatoid malformation of the lung.

Exceedingly high MSAFP and AFAFP is seen in congenital nephrosis (Seppala and Ruoslahti, 1972; Seppala et al., 1972, 1976; Kjessler et al., 1975). The elevated AFP is a result of altered or defective filtering capabilities of the fetal glomeruli. Congenital nephrosis is an autosomal recessive disorder with the most common mutations mapping to chromosome 19q, the nephrin gene (*NPHS1*). In the Finnish population, 36 mutations have been located within the gene, with two, Fin_{major} and Fin_{minor}, accounting for 94% of cases (Kestila et al., 1998). Lenkkeri and colleagues (1999) reported that 20% (7 of 35) of non-Finnish cases have no detectable mutation along the nephrin gene sequence. Therefore, non-Finnish cases may have mutations in other sequences or on other chromosomes (Kestila et al., 1998; Lenkkeri et al., 1999).

The condition is lethal in infancy if untreated, with an average lifespan of 7 months (Hallman and Hjelt, 1959). More aggressive treatments have been attempted, including dialysis and bilateral nephrectomy with subsequent renal transplant, resulting in some survivors. Unfortunately, a transplant cannot be performed until 2 years of age on average (Holmberg et al., 1991).

In Finland, where the disorder occurs in 1 of 2600 to 8000 pregnancies, screening programs using mid-trimester MSAFP have been used successfully to identify this condition (Ryynanen et al., 1983; Heinonen et al., 1996). In other areas of the world, when markedly elevated AFP levels are found without ultrasound associated anomalies, congenital nephrosis must be considered.

The finding of an elevated MSAFP (usually over 5 to 6 MoM) followed by an extremely elevated (frequently more than 10 MoM) level in the amniotic fluid is the primary means of antenatal detection. Although one case of congenital nephrosis with a low AFP level (<2.5) has been described (Heinonen et al., 1996), this is extremely unusual and probably was related to too early testing because the degree of elevation of AFAFP increases with gestational age, proportionate to the contribution that fetal urine makes to the amniotic fluid. Consistent with this is a case report in which serial amniocentesis showed a rapid increase in AFP levels between 14 and 18 weeks (Crow et al., 1997). Other amniotic fluid markers of congenital proteinuria such as transferrin and albumin have been examined to help make a more definitive diagnosis, but the sensitivity of these substances is not sufficient (Suren et al., 1993; Ghidini et al., 1994).

The difficulty in confirming congenital nephrosis *in utero* is the lack of ultrasound findings. Although echogenic and slightly enlarged kidneys have been described, in most the kidneys appear normal, the amount of amniotic fluid is normal, and placentomegaly, which may occur, does not appear until late in gestation. If no ultrasound anomalies are seen, the karyotype is normal, and elevated AFAFP is confirmed, congenital nephrosis must be suspected, but a normal gestation (false positive) is possible (Heinonen et al., 1996). In these cases, *in utero* fetal kidney biopsy provides a means to examine the renal cortex, glomerular basement membrane structure, and podocyte morphology (Wapner et al., 2001) because the pathologic characteristics are present in the second trimester (Rapola, 1981). Electron microscopic evaluation of the biopsy sample is required to visualize altered podocyte morphology diagnostic of this condition.

ULTRASOUND SCREENING FOR FETAL CONGENITAL ANOMALIES

The value of routine second-trimester ultrasound as a screening test is unknown. The Routine Antenatal Diagnostic Imaging Ultrasound Study (Crane et al., 1994) was a randomized controlled trial to test whether routine ultrasound during pregnancy would reduce perinatal morbidity and mortality. This study concluded that routine ultrasound did not alter perinatal outcomes and therefore should not be routinely performed on all women. Limitations to this study are numerous; for example, nearly 70% of the control group received an ultrasound examination at some point in their pregnancy, more congenital anomalies were detected in the screened group, but the overall rate of detected anomalies was only 35%, and experienced referral centers demonstrated a 23% higher detection (35 versus 13%) compared with nontertiary centers.

At present, the American College of Obstetricians and Gynecologists does not recommend ultrasound as a routine part of prenatal care (American College of Obstetricians and Gynecologists Committee on Technical Bulletins, 1993), but some authors argue that denial of access to universal ultrasound with its current abilities may be unethical (Chasen and Chervenak, 1998). Whether routine or targeted, anatomic screening should be done by experienced centers to increase detection of anomalies and limit false-positive results (Filly and Crane, 2002).

Increased Nuchal Translucency and Normal Karyotype

An increased NT has been described with certain nonchromosomal fetal disorders (van Zalen-Sprock et al., 1992; Ville et al., 1992; Hewitt, 1993; Johnson, Johnson, et al., 1993; Nadel et al., 1993; Shulman et al., 1994; Trauffer et al., 1994; Salvesen et al., 1995; Hewitt et al., 1996; Moselhi and Thilaganathan, 1996; Fukada et al., 1997; Hernadi and Torocsik, 1997; Reynders et al., 1997; Thilaganathan et al., 1997; Hafner et al., 1998; Bilardo et al., 1998; Pajkrt et al., 1998; Van Vugt et al., 1998; Adekunle et al., 1999). In some cases, this may be coincidental. However, in others, such as cardiac defects, diaphragmatic hernias, and fetal skeletal and neurologic abnormalities, a true relationship appears likely. Additionally, an association between increased NT and poor perinatal outcomes, including miscarriage and perinatal death, exists (Souka et al., 1998). This information is important in counseling patients who have an elevated NT and a normal karyotype.

In approximately 90% of cases in which the NT is greater than the 99th percentile but below 4.5 mm, a healthy infant can be expected. With NTs between 4.5 and 6.4 mm, about 80% of births will result in a healthy newborn. Measurements over 6.5 mm have only a 45% incidence of normal results (Souka et al., 1998).

The association of increased NT with fetal cardiac and great vessel defects is significant (Bronshtein et al., 1990; Gembruch et al., 1990, 1993; Achiron et al., 1994; Hyett et al., 1995a–d; Hyett, Moscoso, et al., 1997; Hyett, Perdu, et al., 1997) (Table 18-13). A large series from the Fetal Medicine Foundation Project showed that the prevalence of major cardiovascular abnormalities increase with increasing NT (Souka et al., 1998). With an NT measurement between the 95th percentile and 3.4 mm, the frequency of heart and great vessel anomalies was 4 per 1000. When the NT was between 3.5 and 4.5 mm, the incidence increased to 27 per 1000, and when the NT was greater than 6.5 mm, the frequency was 170 per 1000. In a similar, but retrospective, study of approximately 30,000 chromosomally normal singleton pregnancies, the prevalence of cardiac defects increased from 0.8 per 1000 in individuals with an NT below the 95th percentile to almost 64 per 1000 when the NT was above the 99th percentile (Hyett et al., 1999). Alternatively, approximately 40% of all fetuses with cardiac defects will have an NT above the 99th percentile, and 66% will be above the 95th percentile (Hyett et al., 1999). This information strongly suggests that the presence of an NT above the 99th percentile, and perhaps above the 95th, should be followed with a fetal echocardiogram. In this group of individuals, the frequency of major cardiac defects would be anticipated to be about 2%, which is higher than the threshold risk for pregnancies presently receiving echocardiograms, such as those with a mother affected with diabetes mellitus or a family history of an affected offspring. If a cutoff at the 95th percentile is used and 5% of all pregnancies would be offered testing, there may be insufficient resources to accomplish this. However, if a 99th percentile NT measurement is used, only about 1% of patients would require echocardiograms, with an incidence of positive findings of approximately 6%. Recent improvements in the resolution of ultrasound and increasing experience with first-trimester cardiac scanning suggest that major cardiac defects could be identified by the end of the first trimester (Dolkart and Reimers, 1991; Gembruch et al., 1993; Carvalho et al., 1998; Sharland, 1998; Zosmer et al., 1999). This means that patients identified with an enlarged NT who presently have their echocardiograms performed at 20 weeks may not need to delay testing.

Fetal anomalies occur frequently enough after an elevated NT that follow-up scans in the second trimester are recommended. These anomalies include diaphragmatic hernias, severe skeletal defects, and omphaloceles (Souka et al., 1998). Table 18-14 lists the anomalies with a possible relationship with an increased NT.

The most difficult counseling issue involves patients with an elevated NT, a normal karyotype, and a normal second-trimester ultrasound. In a certain percentage of these cases, genetic syndromes not identifiable by ultrasound may be present, including Noonan syndrome, as well as others listed in Table 18-14. Recently, there has also been some speculation of an increased frequency of unexplained developmental delay in some of these infants (E. Pergament, personal communication, 2002). Presently, there is insufficient information to counsel patients specifically; however, in most cases, patients can be reassured that this frequency appears to be less than 10% (Pergament, 2000).

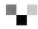

SCREENING FOR GENE MUTATIONS LEADING TO FETAL DISEASE

Certain populations have an increased frequency of specific identifiable disease causing gene mutations. This may occur because the population has remained relatively isolated, many individuals in the population are descended from a few common relatives having a specific mutation (founder effect),

TABLE 18-13. PREVALENCE OF MAJOR DEFECTS OF THE HEART AND GREAT ARTERIES IN CHROMOSOMALLY NORMAL FETUSES BY NUCHAL TRANSLUCENCY THICKNESS

Nuchal Translucency (mm)	n	Major Cardiac Defects	Prevalence (per 1000)
<95th centile	27,332	22	0.8
≥95th centile-3.4	1,507	8	5.3
3.5–4.4	208	6	28.9
4.5–5.4	66	6	90.0
≥5.5	41	8	195.1
Total	29,154	50	1.7

From Hyett J, Perdu M, Sharland G, et al. Using fetal nuchal translucency to screen for major congenital cardiac defects at 10–14 weeks of gestation: Population based cohort study. Br Med J **318**:81, 1999.

TABLE 18-14. FETAL ABNORMALITIES AND GENETIC SYNDROMES ASSOCIATED WITH INCREASED NUCHAL TRANSLUCENCY

Diaphragmatic hernia	Joubert syndrome
Cardiac defects	Jarcho-Levin syndrome
Exomphalos	Meckel-Gruber syndrome
Achondrogenesis type II	Nance-Sweeny syndrome
Achondroplasia	Noonan syndrome
Asphyxiating thoracic dystrophy	Osteogenesis imperfecta type II
Beckwith-Wiedemann syndrome	Perlman syndrome
Blomstrand osteochondrodysplasia	Roberts syndrome
Body stalk anomaly	Short-rib polydactyly syndrome
Campomelic dysplasia	Smith-Lemli-Opitz syndrome
EEC syndrome	Spinal muscular atrophy type 1
Fetal akinesia deformation sequence	Thanatophoric dysplasia
Fryn syndrome	Trigonocephaly "C" syndrome
GM$_1$ gangliosidosis	VACTERL association
Hydrolethalus syndrome	Zellweger syndrome

EEC syndrome, ectrodactyly-ectodermal dysplasia-cleft palate syndrome; VACTERL association, vertebral abnormality, anal atresia, cardiac defect, tracheoesophageal fistula, renal and radial limb abnormality.

of a comprehensive screening program. Components of this program should include patient education, counseling, and a relationship with medical facilities capable of performing invasive diagnostic testing when needed. To be responsive to patient needs, information related to genetics, in general and specific to their individual risks, should be given. This should include basic inheritance patterns, variable nature of disease expression, risk of occurrence, and the diagnostic and therapeutic options available. Educating a couple can be accomplished by using direct counseling, printed materials, or interactive online systems.

Before carrier testing is performed, informed consent should be obtained. This should demonstrate that the individual has fully understood the multiple options that ensue from testing. It is equally important to ensure that those who decline testing do so knowledgeably, and this should be documented. Any testing performed must be voluntary, and patients must be assured that every effort will be made to ensure confidentiality. As molecular diagnostics has become more available, the complexity of gene-based diagnosis and screening has also become obvious. The vast number of mutations with their varying phenotypic consequences will frequently require sophisticated laboratory capabilities and subsequent counseling by individuals explicitly trained in this area.

Cystic Fibrosis Screening

CF is a multisystem genetic disorder in which defective chloride transport across membranes causes dehydrated secretions, leading to tenacious mucus in the lungs, mucous plugs in the pancreas, and high sweat chloride levels. CF is an autosomal recessive disorder with the responsible gene on chromosome 7 coding for the CF transmembrane conductance regulator. CF can have a highly variable presentation and course ranging from severe pulmonary and gastrointestinal

or the carrier state may have a beneficial effect on survival in a particular environment (sickle cell carrier state protection from malaria). It has become a part of routine obstetric care to identify these at-risk individuals. Presently, candidates for screening are identified because of their race or heritage. Table 18-15 lists the standard screening tests that should be offered to appropriate pregnant patients based on their ethnicity.

The goal of testing is to provide individuals with information that will permit them to make informed reproductive decisions. Such testing is of maximum benefit when it is part

TABLE 18-15. COMMON AUTOSOMAL RECESSIVE DISORDERS IN VARIOUS ETHNIC GROUPS FOR WHICH CARRIER SCREENING IS RECOMMENDED

Ethnic Group	Genetic Disorder	Carrier Frequency in Ethnic Group	Frequency of Carrier Couples	Screening Test Available?	Detection Rate (%)
African ancestry	Sickle cell disease (HbS and C)	1:10—HbS	1:130	Hb electrophoresis	100
	Sickle cell S/β-thalassemia	1:20—HbC		MCV, Hb electrophoresis	
	α-Thalassemia			MCV, DNA	
Ashkenazi Jews (and Jews of unknown descent)	Tay Sachs disease	1:30	1:150	Hexosaminidase A level	98
	Canavan disease	1:40	1:1600	DNA mutation	
Chinese	α-Thalassemia		1:625	MCV	
French Canadian Cajun	Tay Sachs disease			Hexosaminidase A level	
Mediterranean (Italian/Greek/ Turks/Spaniards)	β-Thalassemia		1:900	MCV	
All patients seeking preconceptional counseling (especially whites of European origin)	Cystic fibrosis	1:25–29	1:625	DNA mutation	80*

* Depends on ethnic group: 70% for southern European descent, 90% for northern European descent.
Hb, hemoglobin; MCV, mean corpuscular volume.

TABLE 18-16. CARRIER FREQUENCY DISTRIBUTION OF COMMON CYSTIC FIBROSIS ALLELES IN VARIOUS ETHNIC GROUPS

Group	Incidence	Carrier Frequency	Delta F508 (%)	Common White Alleles (%)	Group-Specific Alleles (%)	Approximate Mutation Dectection Rate (%)
Whites in North America	1/3,300	1/29	70	14	—	80–85
Hispanics	1/8,9000	1/46	46	11	—	57
Ashkenazi Jews		1/29	30	67	—	97
Native Americans	1/3,970, 1/1,500		0	25	69	94
African Americans	1/15,300	1/60–65	48	4	23	75
Asian Americans	1/32,100	1/90	30			30

From Cutting GR. Genetic epidemiology and genotype/phenotype correlations. Presented at the NIH Consensus Development Conference on Genetic Testing for Cystic Fibrosis, Washington, DC, April 14–16, 1997.

disease in infancy to relatively mild disease with initial presentation during young adulthood. Mutations of the CF gene can lead to otherwise normal males with congenital absence of the vas deferens or women with chronic sinusitis or bronchitis as their only morbidity.

CF is one of the most common genetic diseases in whites, with an incidence of about 1:3300 individuals. The gene is also relatively common in Ashkenazi Jews and has a fairly high incidence among Hispanics (1:9550). The disease is rare in native Africans and Asians (<1:50,000) but somewhat higher in American populations of these ethnic groups (1:15,300 and 1:32,100, respectively). Table 18-16 demonstrates the incidence of CF and the carrier frequency in various ethnic groups.

The gene causing CF was first cloned in 1989 and provided the initial ability to screen individuals with no family history. More than 600 mutations and DNA sequence variations have since been identified. The Δ F508 mutation is the most common and is a frame shift mutation caused by a 3-base pair deletion in exon 10 of the CF transmembrane conductance regulator that codes for phenylalanine at the 508th amino acid. Although present in almost all populations, its relative frequency varies among different geographies and ethnic groups. The highest frequency is observed in the white population, where it accounts for approximately 70% of CF mutations. Some 15 to 20 other "common" mutations account for

2% to 15% of CF alleles, depending on the ethnic composition of the patient group.

The sensitivity of CF screening using DNA mutation analysis is dependent on the frequency of common identifiable mutations in the screened population. Although over 90% carrier detection is presently possible in a number of ethnic groups, a standard panel of mutations has been developed to maximize overall screening efficiency that provides the greatest pan-ethnic detection and can be practically performed (Table 18-17). This panel is composed of 25 mutations and contains all CF-causing mutations with an allele frequency of at least 0.1% in the general U.S. population. An understanding of the distribution of mutations in the CF transmembrane conductance regulator is continually advancing, and it is likely that this panel will continue to evolve.

There has been much discussion and debate over which ethnic and racial groups should be offered CF carrier testing. Some maintain that screening should be limited to the highest risk populations, such as non-Jewish whites of European ancestry and Ashkenazi Jews, in which both the carrier frequency (1:25 to 1:30) and the mutation detection rate (25 mutations detect more than 80% of CF alleles) are sufficiently high to justify cost-effective screening. This would exclude African Americans with a detection rate of only about 75%. Hispanics would also be excluded, despite their relatively high incidence of the disease, because detectable alleles account for only 57%

TABLE 18-17. RECOMMENDED CORE MUTATION PANEL FOR GENERAL POPULATION CYSTIC FIBROSIS CARRIER SCREENING

Standard mutation panel

ΔF508	ΔI507	G542X	G551D	W1282X	N1_
R553X →	621+1G T	R117H	1717-G1 A	A455E	R5_
R1162X →	G85E	R334W	R347P	711+1G T	189
2184delA → →	1078delT	3849+10kbC T	2789+5G A	3659delC	114
3120+1G → A					

Reflex tests

1506V,* 1507V,* F508C[†]

5T/7T/9T[†]

* Benign variants. This test distinguishes between a cystic fibrosis mutation and these benign variants. 1506V, 1507V, and F508C are performed tests for unexpected homozygosity for ΔF508 and/or Δ1507.
[†] 5T in *cis* can modify R117H phenotype or alone can contribute to congenital bilateral absence of vas deferens (CBA VD); 5T analysis.

of their CF mutations. Screening would be even less effective in Asian Americans, who would have only 30% sensitivity. Others argue that the admixture of populations in the United States makes it difficult to exclude patients based on specific ethnic group and that even attempting to make such a determination in a busy clinical setting may place an undue burden on primary care physicians.

To resolve this debate, the National Institutes of Health issued a consensus statement in 1997. This concluded that CF testing should be offered to adults with a positive family history of CF, to partners of people with CF, to all couples planning a pregnancy, and to couples seeking prenatal testing, particularly those in high-risk populations. It was believed that genetic testing should be offered in the prenatal setting to enhance the ability to make reproductive choices and to engage individuals when their interest and use of the information was maximal.

A second National Institutes of Health-sponsored conference focusing on implementation of the consensus recommendations was held in 1998. Shortly thereafter, the American Colleges of Medical Genetics and Obstetrics and Gynecology, in conjunction with the National Human Genome Research Institute, issued a joint opinion entitled "Preconception and Prenatal Carrier Screening for Cystic Fibrosis." This document recommended narrowing the population screened to non-Jewish whites and Ashkenazi Jews. Information about screening should be made available to other ethnic and racial groups through educational brochures and/or other efficient methods. These lower risk groups should be informed of the availability of testing but should also be advised of the limitations encountered for their particular situation. For example, Asian Americans, African Americans, and Native Americans without significant white mixture should be informed of the rarity of the disease and the low yield of the test in their respective populations (Mennuti et al., 1999; Grody et al., 2001). Preconception testing should be encouraged, but for practical purposes, most testing should continue to occur in the prenatal setting.

In appropriate populations, there are two possible approaches to screening. In *sequential* screening, one member of the couple (usually the woman) is tested first, and only if a positive result is obtained is the partner tested. Alternatively, *couple-based* screening analyzes specimens from both partners, with each informed of their specific results. Present recommendations are that either is appropriate, with the method depending on the target population, the nature of the clinical setting, and the judgment of the practitioner. Couple-based testing is recommended for white couples with Northern European and Ashkenazi Jewish decent, particularly when concurrently testing for other common genetic disorders. Sequential screening is believed to be more useful for groups in which the carrier frequency is lower and for situations where obtaining a simultaneous sample from the partner is impractical. In general, the individual provider or center should choose whichever method they believe is most practical for their setting.

All patients with negative screen results should be reminded that carrier screening is not 100% sensitive. This is particularly pertinent in couples in which one partner is found to carry a mutation. The residual risk after a negative CF carrier test is dependent on the ethnic and racial group of the patient (Table 18-18). In Northern and Eastern European pop-

ulations in which CF mutation screening detects up to 90% of mutant alleles and in which the carrier frequency is 1:25, a negative screen reduces the risk of being a carrier to 1 in 241. Screen-negative couples will then reduce their risk of having an affected child from 1 in 2500 ($1/4 \times 1/25 \times 1/25$) to 1 in 232,324 ($1/4 \times 1/241 \times 1/241$). If one parent has a mutation and the other is negative, the risk of an affected child is 1 in 964 ($1/4 \times 1 \times 1/241$). In cases in which both parents are found to have identifiable mutations, the risk of an affected child is 1 in 4. Prenatal diagnosis by either chorionic villus sampling (CVS) or amniocentesis, along with genetic counseling, would be recommended.

In most cases, interpretation of the screening results is straightforward, but complicated situations may occur and frequently involve finding the 5T variant polymorphism. This is one of three poly(T) alleles (5T, 7T, and 9T) in intron 8 of the CF transmembrane conductance regulator gene. Both the 5T and the 7T mutation along with the R117H mutation can cause congenital bilateral absence of the vas deferens. This occurs when the 7T mutation is on the same allele (in *cis*) with the R117H mutation or when the 5T allele is in *trans* with a common CF allele. Accordingly, testing for the R117H mutation and the poly(T) intron 8 polymorphisms in a screening panel will produce complicated counseling issues, because it expands the risk ascertainment beyond classic CF. Unfortunately, this cannot be avoided by not screening for the poly(T) alleles, because the relatively common R117H mutation can also cause classic CF when in *cis* with a 5T allele. It is presently recommended that the R117H mutation be included in the routine screening panel, while recognizing that this will potentially screen for male infertility. Thus, to distinguish the genotypes of R117H associated with CF from those associated with congenital bilateral absence of the vas deferens, reflex testing for the 5T/7T/9T variant is recommended only when the R117H mutation is positive. If also positive for 5T, the laboratory will request specimens from appropriate family members to determine if the 5T is in *cis* or *trans* with the R117H allele to provide definitive genetic counseling. In this way, the initial screening is for classic CF rather than fertility

TABLE 18-18. IMPACT OF A NEGATIVE CF SCREENING PANEL (25 MUTATIONS) ON THE CARRIER RISK*

Ethnic Group	Detection Rate (%)	Estimated Carrier Risk	
		Before Test	After Negative Test
Ashkenazi Jewish	97	1/29	Approx. 1 in 930
European white	80	1/29	Approx. 1 in 140
African American	69	1/65	Approx. 1 in 207
Hispanic American†	57	1/46	Approx. 1 in 105
European white with positive family history	80		
Sibling with CF		2/3	Approx. 1 in 3.5
Carrier parent		1/2	Approx. 1 in 6
Carrier grandparent		¼	Approx. 1 in 14

* Residual carrier risk after a negative test is modified by the presence of a positive family history.
† This is a pooled set of data and requires additional information to accurately predict risk for specific Hispanic populations.
CF, cystic fibrosis.

of the fetus, because about 5% of the population will have the 5T polymorphism.

Jewish Disease Testing

A number of recessive disorders occur more frequently in the Ashkenazi Jewish population. Carrier testing for two of these, Tay-Sachs disease and Canavan disease, is now considered standard of care (American College of Obstetricians and Gynecologists Committee on Obstetricians Screening for Tay-Sachs Disease, 1995).

Tay-Sachs disease is an autosomal recessive lysosomal storage disorder caused by deficiency of the enzyme hexosaminidase A. This results in a group of neurodegenerative disorders caused by intralysosomal storage of the specific glycosphingolipid G_{M2} ganglioside. Classic Tay-Sachs disease is characterized by loss of motor skills beginning between 3 and 6 months of age, with progressive neurodegeneration, including seizures, blindness, and eventual total incapacitation and death usually before the age of 4. There are juvenile, chronic, and adult onset variants of hexosaminidase A deficiency having a later onset, slower progression, and more variable neurologic findings.

The incidence of the Tay-Sachs carrier state is between 1:27 and 1:30 in the Ashkenazi Jewish population (i.e., from Central and Eastern Europe), resulting in a birth prevalence of 1:3600 infants. Among Sephardic Jews and all non-Jews, the disease frequency is approximately 100 times less, corresponding to a 10-fold lower carrier frequency (1:250 to 1:300). As the result of extensive genetic counseling of carriers and prenatal diagnosis, the incidence of Tay-Sachs disease in Ashkenazi Jews in North America has already been reduced by greater than 90% (Kaback et al., 1993; Kaback, 2000)

In addition to Ashkenazi Jews, Tay-Sachs disease can occur in children of any ethnic, racial, or religious group, but certain populations that are relatively isolated genetically, such as French Canadians of the Eastern St. Lawrence River valley area of Quebec, Cajuns from Louisiana, and the Amish in Pennsylvania, have been found to carry hexosaminidase A mutations with frequencies comparable with, or even greater than, those observed in Ashkenazi Jews.

Population screening for the carrier state of Tay-Sachs disease uses serum or leukocyte determination of hexosaminidase A enzyme activity using synthetic substrate. Carriers will have significantly reduced levels compared with noncarriers. Serum samples are used for testing all males and for nonpregnant women not on oral contraceptives. Pregnant women, those on oral contraceptives, and women who have a tissue destructive disorder such as diabetes mellitus, hepatitis, or rheumatoid arthritis should have white blood cell determination of enzyme activity, because these conditions artificially lower the serum hexosaminidase level, leading to a false diagnosis of the carrier state. When the enzymatic testing is abnormal or inconclusive, DNA analysis of the hexosaminidase A gene is performed to confirm the diagnosis, identify the specific mutation, and rule out the presence of a pseudodeficiency allele that is present in approximately 2% of the Ashkenazi Jewish population and approximately 35% of the non-Jewish population (Akerman et al., 1997).

Two pseudodeficiency alleles exist and can be tested for. Individuals heterozygous for the pseudodeficiency allele have an apparent deficiency of hexosaminidase A enzymatic activity with the synthetic substrate but not with the natural substrate, G_{M2} ganglioside. Their levels are similar to those of Tay-Sachs carriers, leading to a potential incorrect determination of a carrier. Homozygous pseudodeficient individuals have extremely low or absent hexosaminidase A levels similar to individuals affected with Tay-Sachs disease. Neither compound heterozygotes having one Tay-Sachs allele and one pseudodeficient allele nor homozygotes for the pseudodeficient allele have any neurologic abnormality.

There are over 90 disease-causing mutations in the hexosaminidase A gene, but routine mutation analysis tests for only the six most common mutations (Gravel et al., 2001). Molecular analysis of the six mutation hexosaminidase panel will identify between 92% and 98% of Jewish carriers but only between 23% and 46% of non-Jewish carriers (Table 18-19).

TABLE 18-19. MOLECULAR GENETIC TESTING USED IN HEXOSAMINIDASE A DEFICIENCY

		% of Heterozygotes			
		Obligate*		Screening[†]	
Allele	Allele Status	Jewish	Non-Jewish	Jewish	Non-Jewish
+TAC1278	Null	81	32	80	8.0
+1 IVS 12	Null	15	0	9	0.0
+1 IVS 9	Null	0	14	0	10.3[‡]
G269S	Adult onset	2	0	3	5.0
R247W	Pseudodeficiency	0	0	2	32.0
R249W	Pseudodeficiency	0	0	0	4.0
% of disease-causing alleles detected using the 6-mutation *HEX A* panel		98	46	92	23.0

* Obligate heterozygotes (i.e., parents of a child with hexosaminidase A deficiency).
† Individuals identified in screening programs as having levels of hexosaminidase A enzymatic activity in the heterozygous range.
‡ Primarily persons of Celtic, French, Cajun, Pennsylvania Dutch background.

From Kaback M, Lim-Steele J, Dabholkar D, et al. Tay-Sachs disease—carrier screening, prenatal diagnosis, and the molecular era. An international perspective, 1970 to 1993. The International TSD Data Collection Network. JAMA **270**:2307, 1993.

It is not uncommon for a couple in which one partner is Jewish and the other is not to inquire about testing. It is presently recommended that such couples be offered carrier analysis by enzymatic testing, because DNA analysis with the routine six mutation panel would fail to detect a significant proportion of the non-Jewish carriers. Also, individuals who have French Canadian, Cajun, and Amish ancestry should be offered carrier testing. Individuals who are pursuing reproductive technologies that involve gamete donation and who are at increased risk of being heterozygous for hexosaminidase A because of their ethnic background should also be screened.

Prenatal diagnosis for Tay-Sachs disease is available by enzymatic analysis of either amniocytes or chorionic villi. Hexosaminidase A deficiency can be identified on chorionic villus samples within 30 minutes of retrieval or from uncultured amniotic fluid (Grebner and Jackson, 1979; Grebner et al., 1982, 1985). Alternatively, if the disease-causing mutation has been identified in both parents, prenatal testing can be performed by mutation analysis. Prenatal testing is predominantly performed when both parents are known but may also be recommended when one parent is a known heterozygote and the other has inconclusive enzymatic activity without a disease-causing mutation found on DNA analysis. It also may be recommended when the mother is a known heterozygote and the father is either unknown or unavailable for testing. Both of these latter scenarios require intensive genetic counseling.

Screening of Ashkenazi Jewish patients or couples for Canavan disease is recommended (American College of Medical Genetics position statement on carrier testing for Canavan disease, 1998; American College of Obstetricians and Gynecologists position statement on screening for Canavan Disease, 1998; New England Regional Genetics Group Position Statement on Carrier Testing for Canavan Disease, 2/2000). This disorder is caused by a deficiency in aspartoacylase and is characterized by developmental delay by the age of 3 to 5 months with severe hypotonia and failure to achieve independent sitting, ambulation, or speech (Elpeleg et al., 1994). Hypotonia eventually changes to spasticity,

requiring assistance with feeding. Life expectancy is usually into the teens (Matalon et al., 1995). Because about 99% of disease-causing mutations in persons of Ashkenazi Jewish heritage is identified by only three alleles, carrier testing is done by DNA mutation analysis (Kaul, Gao, Aloya, et al., 1994; Kaul, Gao, Balamurugan, et al., 1994b). Testing by biochemical analysis is not routinely available because it relies on a complex enzyme assay and cultured skin fibroblasts (Matalon and Michals-Matalon, 1998). Fifty-five percent of disease-causing alleles in non-Jewish individuals are identified by analysis of these three alleles as well (Kaul et al., 1996). Prenatal testing for pregnancies that are at 25% risk can be performed either by amniocentesis or CVS using mutation analysis. For the unusual couple where one partner is known to be a carrier and a mutation or the carrier status of the other is uncertain or unknown, prenatal testing can be performed by measuring the level of N-acetyl aspartic acid in amniotic fluid at 16 to 18 weeks (Bennett et al., 1993; Kelley, 1993).

A number of other disorders have been found to occur more frequently among the Ashkenazi Jewish population (Sugarman and Allitto, 2001) (Table 18-20). The gene frequency for these disorders varies as compared with those for Tay-Sachs or Canavan disease (Kronn et al., 1995). In some of these disorders, such as Gaucher disease type I, the phenotype in some individuals is relatively benign or treatable. Although this autosomal recessive lysosomal storage disease has a carrier frequency of 1 in 18 in Ashkenazi Jewish individuals, the clinical course is heterogeneous, ranging from early onset of severe disease with major disability or death in childhood to a mild disease compatible with a normal productive life. The phenotype in this disorder is well correlated with the genotype. Of the more than 200 mutations in the affected acid β-glucosidase gene, four mutations (N370S, 84GG, L444P, and IVS2) account for 95% of those in Ashkenazi Jews. Although an affected individual who carries two copies of any combination of the 84GG, L444P, or IVS2 mutations will have severe neurodegenerative disease, individuals homozygous for the most common N370S mutation have a non-neurologic disorder

TABLE 18-20. POTENTIAL SCREENING AVAILABLE FOR AUTOSOMAL RECESSIVE DISORDERS IN THE ASHKENAZI JEWISH POPULATION

Disease	Status	Genetic Defect	Carrier Frequency in Ashkenazi Jews	Comments
Tay-Sachs	S	Hexosaminidase A deficiency	1:30	Screening done by enzyme analysis. Carrier screening during pregnancy, while on oral contraceptives, or with debilitating illness requires leukocyte analysis. Pseudodeficient allele exists.
Canavan	S	Aspartoacylase (ASPA) deficiency	1:40	Three common mutations account for 99% of disease-causing alleles.
Niemann-Pick type A	A	Acid sphingomyelinase deficiency	1:90	
Gaucher type I	A	Glucocerebrosidase deficiency	1:14	The type I Gaucher disease seen in this population is the mild variant with no CNS involvement.
Fanconi anemia	A	Chromosome breakage	1:29	
Bloom syndrome	A	Chromosome breakage	1:100	
Congenital deafness	A	Connexin 26 mutation	1:21	Wide variability in severity of disease.
Familial dysautonomia	A	IKBKAP gene mutation	1:30	

A, available for screening at-risk families (could be used for population screening); CNS, central nervous system; S, standard of care.

with an average age at onset of 30. Some individuals may never come to medical attention. Individuals having the N370S mutation with one of the other three common mutations will also have non-neurologic disease but of a somewhat more severe phenotype than in N370S homozygotes. This predominance of relatively mild non-neurologic disease in the Ashkenazi Jewish population has led some to question whether screening in this population is appropriate. In addition, effective treatment of type I Gaucher disease with enzyme replacement exists.

Presently, in some centers the availability of these carrier tests is discussed with Jewish couples so they can make individualized decisions on their utilization. Overall, if these nine diseases are screened for, one in six Ashkenazi Jews will be determined to be a carrier for at least one disorder. To avoid the anxiety that such a high carrier rate may engender, it is recommended that both members of a couple be screened simultaneously, so that genetic counseling only needs to be provided to carrier couples (Eng and Desnick, 2001).

Hemoglobinopathies

Sickle Cell Syndromes

Sickle cell diseases are a common group of inherited hemoglobin disorders characterized by chronic hemolytic anemia, heightened susceptibility to infection, end-organ damage, and intermittent attacks of vascular occlusion causing both acute and chronic pain. Approximately 70,000 Americans of different ethnic backgrounds have sickle cell disease. In the United States, sickle cell syndromes are most frequently present in African Americans and occur at a frequency of 1:400. The disease is also found in high frequency in individuals from certain areas of the Mediterranean basin, the Middle East, and India (Stein et al., 1984).

Sickle cell syndromes include sickle cell anemia, hemoglobin SC disease, and hemoglobin S β-thalassemia. Normal hemoglobin consists of hemoglobin A (α, β), hemoglobin F (α, γ), and hemoglobin A_2 (α, δ). The protein sequences are coded on chromosome 11 for the β, δ, and γ chains, and the β variants such as hemoglobin S, hemoglobin C, and hemoglobin D all occur from a mutation of this gene. Sickle cell anemia is the most common variant and results when an individual inherits a substitution of valine for the normal glutamic acid in the sixth amino acid position of the β globin chain. This substitution alters the hemoglobin molecule so that it crystallizes and alters the red cell into a sickle shape once the hemoglobin loses oxygen. Hemoglobin C is caused by a substitution of lysine in the same location.

β-Thalassemias are caused by mutations that reduce or abolish the production of the β globin subunits of hemoglobin. Compound heterozygotes of β-thalassemia and hemoglobin S have very significant clinical problems. In hemoglobin S β^0-thalassemia, no normal hemoglobin A is made so that a hemoglobin electrophoresis will show only hemoglobin S, increased hemoglobin A_2, and increased hemoglobin F. In hemoglobin S β^+-thalassemia, hemoglobin A is reduced so hemoglobin electrophoresis will show hemoglobin A (5% to 25%), hemoglobin F, hemoglobin S, and increased hemoglobin A_2. The severity of the clinical manifestations with sickle thalassemia can vary greatly between patients. Most individuals with the hemoglobin S β^+-thalassemia will have preserva-

tion of spleen function with fewer problems with infections, fewer pain episodes, and less organ damage than sickle cell disease. Individuals with hemoglobin S β^0-thalassemia may have very severe disease identical to homozygotes sickle cell anemia.

Screening for sickle cell disease should be offered to individuals of African and African American descent and those from the Mediterranean basin, the Middle East, and India. The definitive test to determine the carrier state of sickle cell disease is a hemoglobin electrophoresis, which is based on the altered electrical charge of abnormal hemoglobins caused by the amino acid substitutions. A simple sickle cell prep/Sickledex will fail to identify individuals carrying β-thalassemia or certain sickle cell variants (hemoglobins C, D, and E) and is no longer acceptable for screening. In addition, routine cellulose acetate gel hemoglobin electrophoresis cannot delineate all hemoglobin variants. If this routine electrophoresis is abnormal, further testing by high-performance liquid chromatography may be necessary.

Hemoglobin C occurs in higher frequency in individuals with heritage from West Africa, Italy, Greece, Turkey, and the Middle East. Individuals who are hemoglobin C homozygotes have a mild hemolytic anemia, microcytosis, and target cell formation. They may very occasionally have episodes of joint and abdominal pain. Splenomegaly is common, and aplastic crisis and gallstones may occur. Compound heterozygotes with hemoglobin S and C have a sickle syndrome that is very similar to sickle cell anemia. Hemoglobin C carriers have no anemia but will usually have target cells on blood smear and may have a slightly low mean corpuscular volume (MCV) with no other clinical problems. Individuals who are compound heterozygotes for hemoglobin C and β-thalassemia who inherit a β^0 mutation have a moderately severe anemia, splenomegaly, and may have bone changes. Individuals who inherit a β^+ mutation with hemoglobin C only have a mild anemia, low MCV, and target cells.

On occasion, hemoglobin E will be seen on an electrophoresis. This is a structurally abnormal hemoglobin caused by a substitution of lysine for glutamic acid at the 26th position of the β globin chain, which causes abnormal processing of pre-messenger RNA to functional messenger RNA, resulting in decreased synthesis of hemoglobin E. The hemoglobin E gene is very common in areas of Southeast Asia, India, and China. Heterozygotes for hemoglobin E and hemoglobin A have no anemia, a low MCV, and target cells on blood smear. Hemoglobin electrophoresis will show approximately 75% hemoglobin A and 25% hemoglobin E. Homozygotes for hemoglobin E may have normal hemoglobin levels or only a slight anemia. The MCV will be low, and many target cells will be present. There will be a single band in the hemoglobin C/A position on cellulose acetate electrophoresis and increased hemoglobin F (10% to 15%). There will be no clinically significant problems. Individuals who are compound heterozygotes for hemoglobin E and β^0-thalassemia can have a severe disease with profound anemia, microcytosis, splenomegaly, jaundice, and expansion of marrow space. Hemoglobin electrophoresis in these individuals will show hemoglobin E and a significant increase in hemoglobin F (30% to 60%). Individuals who are compound heterozygote for hemoglobin E and β^+-thalassemia have a moderate disease with anemia, microcytosis, splenomegaly, and jaundice. Hemoglobin electrophoresis will show hemoglobin E at

TABLE 18-21. MOLECULAR GENETIC TESTING USED IN β-THALASSEMIA

Population	Patients with % Results Positive	Most Common HB Mutations in At-Risk Populations
Mediterranean	91–95	-87 C→G, IVS1-1 G→A, IVS1-6 T→C, IVS1-110 G→A, cd 39 C-
Middle East	91–95	cd 8 -AA, cd 8/9 + G, IVS1-5 G→C, cd 39 C→T, cd 44-C, IVS2-1 G→A
Indian	91–95	-619 bp deletion, cd 8/9 + G, IVS1-1 G→T, IVS1-5 G→C, 41/42 - TTCT
Thai	91–95	-28 A→G, 17 A→T, 19 A→G, IVS1-5 G→C, 41/42 - TTCT, IVS2-654 C→T
Chinese	91–95	-28 A→G, 17 A→T, 41/42 - TTCT, IVS2-654 C→T
African/ African American	75–80	-88 C→T, -29 A→AG, IVS1-5 G→T, cd 24 T→A, IVS11-949 A→G, A→C

Hb; hemoglobin.

approximately 40%, hemoglobin A at 1% to 30%, and a significant increase in hemoglobin F (at approximately 30% to 50%).

Sickle cell anemias are inherited as autosomal recessive disorders. Therefore, couples in which both parents carry the hemoglobin S gene have a 1:4 risk of having an affected child. Prenatal diagnosis using molecular DNA detection of the mutation is routine. Individuals in which one parent has a hemoglobin S mutation and the other is a carrier of β-thalassemia have a 25% risk of a child having sickle thalassemia. If the specific parental mutation responsible for thalassemia is known, the gene can be detected by molecular analysis of villi or amniocytes and an effected child identified. If the thalassemia mutation is not identifiable, fetal blood sampling for globin chain synthesis may be required.

β-Thalassemia

β-Thalassemia is characterized by reduced hemoglobin β chain production and results in microcytic, hypochromic anemia, and an abnormal peripheral blood smear with nucleated red cells. There is reduced (β+) to absent (β0) amounts of hemoglobin A on hemoglobin electrophoresis (Cao et al.,

1997). Patients homozygous for a β-thalassemia mutation have thalassemia major with severe anemia and hepatosplenomegaly. They usually come to medical attention within the first 2 years of life, and without treatment affected children will have severe failure to thrive and a shortened life expectancy. Treatment requires a program of regular transfusions and chelation therapy, which can result in normal growth and development.

β-Thalassemia is inherited in an autosomal recessive manner, with two carrier parents having a 25% chance of an affected child. Heterozygotes are clinically asymptomatic and may only have slight anemia. Carriers are referred to as having thalassemia minor (Flint et al., 1998). The β-thalassemias result from more than 200 different hemoglobin β chain mutations (Huisman et al., 1997). Despite this marked molecular heterogeneity, the prevalent molecular defects are limited in each at risk population, that is, each racial or ethnic population will have only 4 to 10 mutations that account for the large majority of their disease-causing alleles (Table 18-21). For instance, in individuals of Mediterranean, Middle Eastern, Indian, Tai, and Chinese extraction, a limited number of population-specific mutations account for between 90% and 95% of the disease genes. In Africans and African Americans, common mutations account for approximately 75% to 80%. This phenomenon has significantly facilitated molecular genetic testing.

Screening for thalassemia should be offered to all individuals of Mediterranean, Middle Eastern, Transcaucasus, Central Asian, Indian, and Far Eastern groups. It is also common in individuals of African heritage, and carrier testing should be offered to all African Americans. As with sickle cell disease, the distribution is probably related to selective pressure from malaria, because the disease distribution is similar to that of endemic *Plasmodium falciparum* malaria (Flint et al., 1998). However, because of population migration and, in a limited part, the slave trade, β-thalassemia is now also commonly seen in northern Europe, North and South America, the Caribbean, and Australia.

Carriers are identified by evaluation of the red blood cell indices, quantitative hemoglobin analysis, and hemoglobin β chain mutation studies. Carriers are initially identified by their red blood cell indices that show microcytosis (low MCV < 80) and a reduced content of hemoglobin per cell (low mean corpuscular hemoglobin). This is followed up by a hemoglobin electrophoresis that will display a hemoglobin A_2 of more than 3.5% (Table 18-22). It should be noted that, on rare occasions, carrier identification using MCV can be misleading. For example, if there is co-inheritance of an α-thalassemia gene, this may normalize red blood cell indices. Also, co-inheritance

TABLE 18-22. RED BLOOD CELL INDICES IN β-THALASSEMIA

Red Blood Cell Index	Normal		Affected	Carrier
	Male	Female	β-Thalassemia Major	β-Thalassemia Minor
Mean corpuscular volume, fL	80.0–100.0	80.0–100.0	50–70	<80
Mean corpuscular hemoglobin, pg	27.5–33.2	27.5–33.2	12–20	18–22
Hemoglobin, g/dL	14–18	12–16	<7	11–14

From Hann IM, Gibson BES, Letsky EA: Fetal and Neonatal Haematology. Philadelphia, WB Saunders, 1991.

of the δ-thalassemia gene can reduce the normal increased hemoglobin A_2 levels typical of β-thalassemia. Likewise, screening using only a routine hemoglobin electrophoresis as the primary test is insufficient, because thalassemia carriers can be easily missed because hemoglobin levels may be normal and the electrophoresis may only show subtle increases in hemoglobin A_2 and F, which can be overlooked. Therefore, a complete blood count with MCV and red cell count should be obtained and a quantitative hemoglobin electrophoresis performed, because the MCV is almost always low in β-thalassemia and the red cell count is elevated. Quantitative hemoglobin electrophoresis for hemoglobin A_2 and F is diagnostic (Cao et al., 1997).

When the initial hematologic analysis is abnormal and the couple is at risk for having a child with either homozygous β-thalassemia or thalassemia sickle cell disease syndrome, DNA analysis of the hemoglobin β chain is indicated to identify the disease-causing mutation. This will help identify carriers of mild and silent mutations of β-thalassemia resulting in attenuated forms of the disease. Knowledge of the specific mutations will also be required if subsequent prenatal diagnosis is performed. However, the sensitivity of molecular testing remains less than 100%, so there will be individuals in whom a specific mutation cannot be identified.

Prenatal diagnosis is offered to couples when both members are carriers of β-thalassemia and their gene mutations have been identified. In these cases, mutation analysis can be performed by DNA extracted from either CVS or amniocentesis. Prenatal testing is occasionally offered to families in which one parent is a definitive heterozygote and the other parent has a β-thalassemia–like hematologic picture but no mutation can be identified by sequence analysis. Very occasionally, the father of a pregnancy with a known heterozygote mother is unavailable for testing. If this father belongs to a population at risk, prenatal diagnosis can be offered. In the latter two situations, if the known mutation is identified by CVS or amniocentesis, globin chain synthesis analysis is available for definitive diagnosis.

α-Thalassemia

α-Thalassemia is a hemoglobinopathy caused by the deficiency or absence of α globin chain synthesis. The α globin gene cluster is located on chromosome 16 and includes two adult genes (α1 and α2) so that normal individuals have four α globin genes (α1α2/α1α2). α-Thalassemia can be divided into two forms based on the number of functioning genes. A severe form called $α^0$-thalassemia results in a typical thalassemic blood picture in heterozygotes and a severe perinatal lethal form in homozgotes. $α^0$-Thalassemia results from 1 of 17 gene deletions, all of which delete both α globin genes on each chromosome. Alternatively, $α^+$-thalassemia is milder and is almost completely silent in heterozygotes. This form is commonly caused by one of six deletions that remove one of the two α globin genes on chromosome 16.

The homozygous state of $α^0$-thalassemia resulting from deletions of all four α globin genes (--/--) causes severe hydrops fetalis and the predominance of hemoglobin Barts ($γ_4$) and a small amount of hemoglobin Portland ($ζ_2γ2$) in the fetus. This is routinely lethal *in utero* or in the early neonatal period if untreated. Although cases of *in utero* transfusions with fetal survival have been described, this must be followed by repeti-

tive transfusions of the infant and subsequent bone marrow transplant. This approach is not routinely recommended. Maternal risks of hemoglobin Barts hydrops fetalis syndrome include preeclampsia and postpartum hemorrhage.

Hemoglobin H disease results from the compound heterozygous state for $α^0$ and $α^+$-(--/-α)thalassemia, leading to the deletion of three of the four α chain genes. These individuals have a moderately severe hypochromic microcytic anemia and produce large amounts of hemoglobin H ($β_4$) because of the excessive quantities of β chains in their reticulocytes. In the most common form, these individuals lead a relatively normal life but may have fatigue, general discomfort, and splenomegaly. They rarely require hospitalization. There is a rare more severe form of hemoglobin H disease arising from a compound heterozygous state of $α^0$-thalassemia and nondeletion $α^+$-thalassemia involving the more dominant α2 gene.

$α^0$-Thalassemia gene deletions are found in high frequency in individuals from Southeast Asia, South China, the Philippine Islands, Thailand, and a few Mediterranean countries, such as Greece and Cyprus. Because these populations are at risk for the homozygous state leading to hemoglobin Barts disease, they should be screened for the presence of the gene. Alternatively, $α^+$-thalassemia genes are frequent in Africa, the Mediterranean area, the Middle East, the Indian subcontinent, Melanesia, Southeast Asia, and the Pacific area. Because this leads to a mild form of thalassemia, routine screening for α-thalassemia in these populations is not recommended.

The carrier state for $α^0$-thalassemia is identified by performing a complete blood count with indices. Carriers (--/αα) will have a decreased MCV (<80 fL) and mean corpuscular hemoglobin (<27 pg) as with β-thalassemia but are differentiated by having a normal hemoglobin A_2 (<3.5%) level. The diagnosis is confirmed by DNA testing, which can identify the specific deletion. Prenatal diagnosis is available by CVS or amniocentesis and is based on the molecular determination of the gene status.

Fragile X Syndrome

Fragile X syndrome is characterized by relatively typical phenotypic characteristics and moderate mental retardation in affected males. Affected females have somewhat milder mental retardation (Curry et al., 1997). Classic features become more prevalent with age, including long face, large ears, prominent jaw, and macrotestes. There is delayed attainment of motor milestones and speech. Abnormal temperament is frequently associated with hyperactivity, hand flapping, hand biting, and, very occasionally, autism. Behaviors in postpubertal males include tactile defensiveness, poor eye contact, and preservative speech. Physical and behavioral features can be seen in female heterozygotes, both with a lower frequency and milder involvement.

Prevalence estimates of the fragile X syndrome have been revised downward since the isolation of the gene in 1991. Despite this, the original estimates are still occasionally quoted in the fragile X literature. Most recent studies using molecular genetic testing have estimated a prevalence of 16 to 25:100,000 males. The prevalence of affected females is presumed to be approximately one half of the male prevalence.

Fragile X syndrome is inherited in X-linked dominant fashion. The molecular mutations leading to this syndrome result from expansion of a trinucleotide repeat (CGG) causing aberrant methylation of the gene. This results in decreased or complete absence of the protein gene product termed "fragile X mental retardation 1 protein" (FMR-1). This protein is found in the cytoplasm of many cells but is most abundant in neurons (Devys et al., 1993). The function of the protein remains unknown, but its absence leads to developmental abnormalities.

The size of the trinucleotide repeat and the sex of the individual determine the clinical manifestation. Unaffected individuals have between 6 and 54 CGG repeats. Those having between 55 and 230 repeats are considered to be premutation carriers. Affected individuals have more than 230 repeats. The phenotype of males is entirely dependent on the size of the mutation. The phenotype of females, although also dependent on the size of the mutation, can be modified by random inactivation of either the normal or mutated X chromosome in the brain (Franke et al., 1996). Males with more than 230 CGG repeats are said to have a full fragile X mutation and will have moderate to severe mental retardation with the typical fragile X phenotype. Approximately 50% of females who have a full fragile X mutation will be mentally retarded but are usually less severely affected than males with the full mutation (Riddle et al., 1998). Importantly, about 50% of females who are heterozygotes for the full mutation will be intellectually normal (Turner et al., 1996).

The probability of a carrier of a premutation having a child with a full mutation is dependent on both the size of the pre-mutation and the sex of the carrier. When premutations are transmitted by the father, only small increases in the trinucleotide repeat number may occur and will not result in full mutations. All daughters of "transmitting males" will be unaffected premutation carriers, with the potential of subsequent expansion in their offspring.

Females who are premutation carriers have a 50% risk of transmitting the abnormal chromosome in each pregnancy (Nolin et al., 1996). Their risk of having an offspring with a full mutation is based on their premutation size. Table 18-23 demonstrates the likelihood of expansion to a full mutation

based on the maternal premutation size. Although the likelihood for repeat instability increases with the increasing number of CGG trinucleotide repeats (Fu et al., 1991), the percentages should be viewed only as approximations, because they are derived from a relatively small number of patients. In these cases, prenatal diagnosis should be offered.

The presence of normal transmitting males and the variable likelihood of full expansion by females carrying a premutation will lead to pedigrees with skipped generations or the seemingly spontaneous occurrence of the fragile X syndrome (Toledano-Alhadef et al., 2001). Therefore, carrier testing should be offered to all individuals seeking reproductive counseling who have either a family history of fragile X syndrome or undiagnosed mental retardation in individuals of either sex (Curry et al., 1997).

Some centers offer all women seeking prenatal diagnosis the opportunity to have fragile X testing performed as part of routine screening. This approach is based on evidence that the frequency of the premutation is relatively high in the general population. One study of a French Canadian population found that 1:259 women had a premutation in the FMR-1 gene (Rousseau et al., 1995). The benefits of such a screening strategy have not been demonstrated.

Methodologies for molecular testing vary from laboratory to laboratory. Most screen patient DNA samples by the polymerase chain reaction (PCR) specific for the trinucleotide repeat region of the FMR-1 gene (Oostra and Willemsen, 2001). This technique has high sensitivity for FMR-1 repeats in the normal and lower premutation range but may rarely fail to detect FMR-1 alleles in the upper premutation range. It also can fail to detect full mutations with a high repeat number (especially when used for prenatal testing). Because of these limitations, many laboratories also perform Southern blot analysis, which will detect the presence of full mutations and large premutations. When PCR reveals a normal or premutation allele size in male patients or two alleles within the normal or premutation range in female patients, further testing by Southern blot is not necessary (Tarleton and Saul, 1993; Maddalena et al., 2001).

Prenatal testing for fetuses at increased risk for FMR-1 full mutations is performed using DNA extracted from either amniocytes or chorionic villi. The Southern blot patterns for DNA expansions derived from amniocytes are identical to those found in adult tissues. However, unreliable methylation patterns can occur in DNA from cells obtained by CVS because methylation of villus tissue may occur at varying gestational ages (Sutcliffe et al., 1992). Because the methylation pattern is predictive of gene function, it is occasionally used to make the distinction between a large premutation and a small full mutation. As a result, on occasion, follow-up amniocentesis or testing using PCR to determine the size of the FMR-1 alleles may be required. Chromosome analysis for fragile X status using modified culture techniques to induce the fragile sites seen in the effected X chromosomes is no longer used for diagnosis due to low sensitivity and increased cost when compared with DNA testing. Because of the complexity of FMR-1 trinucleotide repeat expansion detection and the accompanying methylation issues, a laboratory with known competence for FMR-1 prenatal molecular testing is strongly suggested (Hagerman, 1996; Maddalena et al., 2001; Oostra and Willemsen, 2001).

TABLE 18-23. FRAGILE X SYNDROME: RISK THAT A MOTHER WITH A PREMUTATION WILL HAVE AN AFFECTED CHILD WITH A FULL MUTATION

Number of Maternal CGG Repeats	Approximate Risk of Having an Affected Son	Approximate Risk of Having an Affected Daughter*
56–59	7%	3.5%
60–69	10%	5.0%
70–79	29%	15.0%
80–89	36%	18.0%
90–99	47%	24.0%
>100	50%	25.0%

* Unlike classic X-linked dominant disorders where all females with a mutation are affected, only about 50% of females with a full mutation are mentally retarded. This variability in phenotype is likely to be related to variability in X chromosome inactivation, a phenomenon independent of FMR-1 mutations.

Adapted from Nolin SL, Lewis FA, 3rd, Ye LL, et al. Familial transmission of the FMR1 CGG repeat. Am J Hum Genet **59**: 1252, 1996.

DIAGNOSTIC TESTS

Indications for Invasive Testing

Indications for diagnostic testing are dominated by advanced maternal age (>35 years) and positive screening tests and are discussed previously in detail. A prior history of a fetus with a chromosomal abnormality is the next most frequent indication for cytogenetic testing. The recurrence risk after the birth of one child with trisomy 21 varies in the literature, with most studies quoting an empiric risk of approximately 1% to 1.5% for any trisomy (Gardner and Sutherland, 1996). Closer scrutiny suggests that the risk is dependent on the age of the mother at the birth of the initial trisomic child. Warburton and colleagues (1991) demonstrated that if the initial trisomic child is born when a mother is less than 30 years old, a future pregnancy born while the mother is still under 30 years old has an eightfold increased risk over maternal age risk. This usually results in a risk of just under 1%. If the initial trisomy 21 birth occurred when the mother was over 30, the risk of another trisomic child is not statistically greater than her age-related risk at the time of the next pregnancy.

The risk of a liveborn trisomic child after a trisomy 21 conception that was either spontaneously or electively terminated is uncertain. The work of Warburton and colleagues (1987) suggests that the karyotype of a miscarried pregnancy may predict the karyotype of subsequent miscarriages, but the relevance of this to live births is uncertain. Presently, most authorities recommend the conservative approach of offering the same risks as for a liveborn conception so that prenatal diagnosis in subsequent pregnancies is recommended.

After the birth of two or more trisomy 21 pregnancies, the possibility that one of the parents is either a somatic or germ cell mosaic for Down syndrome must be considered, and peripheral blood chromosomes on the parents should be offered. Uchida and Freeman (1986) reported parental mosaicism in 2.7% to 4.3% of peripheral karyotypes in such parents. Mothers appeared to have a higher risk than fathers. The risk of recurrence in these families may be as high as 10% to 20%, and prenatal testing is indicated.

About 3% to 5% of Down syndrome cases are secondary to either a *de novo* or inherited Robertsonian translocation. If the translocation is *de novo*, risk of another affected child is minimal, although gonadal mosaicism leading to a recurrence has been suspected in some families. Prenatal diagnosis may be offered in these cases. If the balanced translocation is present in the mother, the overall risk of an unbalanced liveborn Down syndrome child is 10% to 15% but varies according to the specific translocation (Table 18-24). If the translocation is paternal, the risk of an unbalanced offspring is approximately 0.5%, but also depends on the nature of the translocation. In all cases of parental translocation, prenatal diagnosis is indicated.

Some offspring with inherited balanced Robertsonian translocations have been found to have uniparental disomy (UPD). This can have phenotypic consequences if chromosomes 14 or 15 are involved. In pregnancies in which a balanced Robertsonian translocation involving one of these acrocentric chromosomes is present, additional testing for UPD is indicated (Berend et al., 2000).

The recurrence risk after the birth of a child with a trisomy other than 21 is poorly quantified. In a recent collaborative

TABLE 18-24. PARENTAL CARRIER OF ROBERTSONIAN TRANSLOCATION: EMPIRIC RISK OF DOWN SYNDROME LIVE BIRTHS

Carrier	Risk of Down Syndrome Live Births
Mother: 13/21, 14/21, 15/21 translocation	10.0–15%
Mother: 21/22 translocation	4.0–15%
Father: 13/21, 14/21, 15/21 translocation	0.5–5%
Father: 21/22 translocation	0.5–2%
Either parent: 21/21	100%

study of 1076 Japanese women with a history of a previous trisomy in whom second-trimester amniocentesis was performed, none of the 170 women with previous trisomy 18 offspring and none of the 46 women with a previous trisomy 13 offspring had another such fetus (Uehara et al., 1999). In general, an empiric risk of about 1% is appropriate, and prenatal diagnosis should be offered.

A previous 45X pregnancy does not significantly increase the risk of a recurrence, but cases of maternal 45X,46XX mosaicism leading to a second affected child have been described (Kher et al., 1994). The recurrence after a triploid pregnancy is exceedingly low but has been reported to recur (Pergament, 2000).

Other cytogenetic indications for invasive testing include a parental reciprocal translocation or inversion, a parent or previous child with a mosaic karyotype or marker chromosome, or a sex chromosome/autosome translocation. The risk of an unbalanced offspring in these cases is dependent on the mode of ascertainment and the specific rearrangement, and genetic counseling is recommended.

Prenatal invasive testing is also indicated to obtain material for biochemical or DNA studies. The molecular abnormalities responsible for many disorders are being identified at a rapid rate, and any listing of these is soon outdated. A list of the more common genetic conditions for which DNA-based prenatal diagnosis is available is given in Table 18-25. A more detailed list, and a list of the centers performing each test, can be found at www.genetests.org. Many of these conditions are rare and their diagnosis complex, so that consultation with a genetics unit is encouraged before performing an invasive test.

Ultrasound identification of fetal structural anomalies is increasing in frequency as an indication for invasive testing. In addition to major structural defects that have long been known to be associated with fetal aneuploidy, more subtle markers have been demonstrated to increase the risk (Nyberg, Resta, Luthy, et al., 1993; Rotmensch et al., 1997). In addition, ultrasound markers for fetal infection, anemia, or other disorders frequently may require evaluation by amniocentesis.

Amniocentesis

Historical Perspective

Amniocentesis was first performed in the 1880s for decompression of polyhydramnios (Lambl, 1881; Schatz, 1992). It was during the 1950s that amniocentesis became a significant diagnostic tool when measurement of amniotic fluid bilirubin

TABLE 18-25. LIST OF COMMON CONDITIONS IN WHICH MOLECULAR PRENATAL DIAGNOSIS IS AVAILABLE

Disorder	Mode of Inheritance	Prenatal Diagnosis
α_1-Antitrypsin deficiency	AR	Determine PiZZ allele. Not all homozygotes have liver involvement, pre-procedure genetic counseling critical
α-Thalassemia	AR	α Hemoglobin gene mutation (see text).
Adult polycystic kidney	AD	PKD1 and PKD2 gene mutations. In large families linkage is possible in >90%. Gene mutation identifiable in ~50% of PKD1 and 75% of PKD2.
β-Thalassemia	AR	β Hemoglobin gene mutation (see text).
Congenital adrenal hyperplasia	AR	CYP21A2 gene mutations/deletions. Nine common mutations/deletions detect 90–95% of carriers. Sequencing available.
Cystic fibrosis	A	CFTR gene mutation (see text).
Duchenne/Becker muscular dystrophy	XLR	Dystrophin gene mutation.
Fragile X syndrome	XLR	CGG repeat number (see text).
Hemoglobinopathy (SS, SC)	AR	β-Chain gene mutation (see text).
Hemophilia A	XLR	Factor VIII gene inversion 45%, other gene mutations 45% (not available in all labs), linkage analysis in appropriate families.
Huntington disease	AD	CAG repeat length (PGD and non-informing PND possible to avoid disclosing presymtomatic parents disease status).
Marfan syndrome	AD	Fibrilin (FBN-1) gene mutation. Linkage in large families. Approx 70% have mutation identified (not always clinically available).
Myotonic dystrophy	AD	CTG expansion in the DMPK gene.
Neurofibromatosis type 1	AD	NF1 gene mutation identifiable in >95% of cases but requires sequencing. Linkage in appropriate families.
Phenylketonuria	AR	4 to 15 common mutations 40–50% detection. Further mutation analysis >99%.
Spinal muscular atrophy	AR/AD	
Tay-Sachs disease	AR	Enzyme absence; gene mutation (see text).

AD, autosomal dominant; AR, autosomal recessive; PGD, preimplantation genetic diagnosis; PND, prenatal diagnosis; XLR, X-linked recessive.

concentration began to be used in the monitoring of Rh isoimmunization (Bevis, 1950; Walker, 1957). In that same decade, amniocentesis for fetal chromosome analysis was initiated as laboratory techniques for cell culture and karyotype were developed. The first reported applications were limited to fetal sex determination by Barr body analysis (Fuchs and Riis, 1956). The feasibility of culturing and karyotyping amniotic fluid cells was demonstrated in 1966 (Steele and Breg, 1966), and the first prenatal diagnosis of an abnormal karyotype, a balanced translocation, was reported in 1967 (Jacobson and Barter, 1967).

Technique of Amniocentesis

Mid-trimester amniocentesis for genetic evaluation is most commonly performed between 15 and 18 weeks' gestation. At this age, the amount of fluid is adequate (approximately 150 mL), and the ratio of viable to nonviable cells is greatest. Before the procedure, an ultrasound scan is performed to determine the number of fetuses, confirm gestational age, ensure fetal viability, document anatomy, and locate the placenta and cord insertion. After an appropriate sampling path has been chosen, the maternal abdomen is washed with antiseptic solution. Continuously guided by ultrasound, a 20- to 22-gauge needle is introduced into a pocket of amniotic fluid free of fetal parts and umbilical cord (Fig. 18-6). The pocket should be large enough to allow advancement of the needle tip through the free-floating amniotic membrane that may occasionally obstruct the flow of fluid. The first 2 mL of aspirated amniotic fluid is discarded to prevent maternal cell contamination of the tissue culture, and then 20 to 30 mL of amniotic

fluid is withdrawn. Fetal heart rate and activity are documented immediately after the procedure.

Transplacental passage of the needle should be avoided when possible, but if unavoidable, attempts should be made to traverse the thinnest portion, away from the placental edge (Lenke, Ashwood, et al., 1985). If the placenta must be traversed, color Doppler is helpful in avoiding any large fetal vessels at the sampling site. The area close to the placental cord insertion should be avoided, because it contains the largest vessels. Using this approach, transplacental amniocentesis does not increase fetal loss rates in the hands of experienced operators (Bombard et al., 1995; Marthin et al., 1997).

Amniocentesis should be performed using continuous ultrasound guidance. Guidance should be maintained throughout the procedure to avoid inadvertent puncture of the fetus and to identify uterine contractions that occasionally retract the needle tip back into the myometrium. Romero and colleagues (1985) showed that continuous guidance decreases the number of insertions as well as dry and bloody taps.

The procedure may be performed either free-hand or with a needle guide (Lenke, Cyr, et al., 1985b; Jeanty et al., 1990). The free-hand technique allows easier manipulation of the needle if the position of the target is abruptly altered by a uterine contraction or fetal movement. Alternatively, a needle guide allows more certain ascertainment of the needle entry point and a more precise preentry determination of the sampling path. The guide may allow easier sampling in certain situations, such as oligohydramnios or morbidly obese patients. A needle guide is especially helpful for relatively inexperienced operators or sonographers. Most guides now allow easy intra-

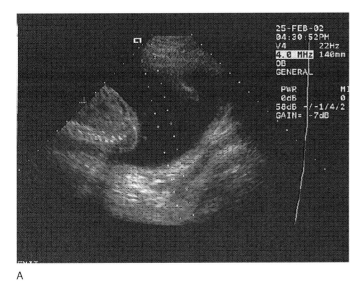
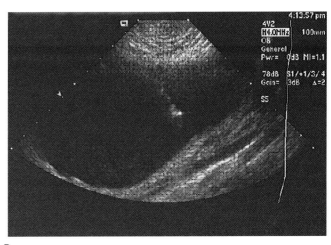

A   B

FIGURE 18-6 ■ Ultrasound of amniocentesis with a needle guide (**A**) or free-hand technique
(**B**). Both techniques can be used and are usually chosen by practitioner preference. Needle guides can be
helpful when one member of the team (operator or sonographer) is less experienced or when dealing with
oligohydramnios or morbid obesity.

operative removal of the needle from the guide and quick
adaptation to free-hand guidance once the uterus has been
entered (Sonek et al., 1989).

If the initial attempt to obtain fluid is unsuccessful, a second
attempt in another location should be performed after reevaluation of the fetal and placental positions. Amniotic membrane tenting and the development of needle-induced uterine
wall contractions are most frequently the cause of initial
failure. No more than two attempts should be made at any
single session. If unsuccessful after two attempts, the patient
may be rescheduled in several days. Studies have demonstrated
that fetal loss rate increases with the number of insertions.
Marthin and coworkers (1997) reported a postamniocentesis
loss rate of 3.8% after three insertions compared with 1.2%
after a single pass. Loss rates do not increase with the number
of separate procedures. In experienced centers, return visits are
rarely required, occurring in less than 1% of cases (Johnson
et al., 1999).

Laboratory Considerations for Amniocentesis

The cells within the amniotic fluid arise from the fetal skin,
respiratory tract, urinary tract, gastrointestinal tract, and placenta. After retrieval, the cells are put into tissue culture,
either in flasks or more often on coverslips. After 3 to 7 days of
growth, sufficient mitoses are present for staining and karyotype analysis. Cells grown in flasks are harvested and analyzed
together, whereas those grown on coverslips are analyzed *in situ*
as individual colonies. Amniocyte culture is quite reliable,
with failure occurring in less than 1% of cases.

MOSAIC RESULTS

Chromosomal mosaicism is the presence of two or more cell
lines with different karyotypes in a single sample and occurs in
approximately 0.1% to 0.3% of amniocentesis cases. This most
frequently results from postzygotic nondisjunction (Hsu and
Perlis, 1984) but can also occur from meiotic errors with tri-

somic rescue (see Laboratory Aspects of Chorionic Villus
Sampling, later). The most common etiology is pseudomosaicism (Hsu and Perlis, 1984), where the abnormality is
evident in only one of several flasks or confined to a single
colony on a coverslip. In this case, the abnormal cells have
arisen *in vitro*, are not present in the fetus, and are not clinically important. Even the observation of multiple cell lines on
more than one coverslip or in more than one flask in a sample
does not necessarily mean that the fetus is mosaic, because the
results are confirmed in only 70% of cases (Bui et al., 1984).
Some mosaic results (e.g., trisomy 20) occur in the amniotic
fluid relatively frequently but are rarely confirmed in the fetus
(Johnson and Wapner, 1997).

Alternatively, true fetal mosaicism is rare, occurring in
0.25% of amniocenteses but can be clinically important,
leading to phenotypic or developmental abnormalities (Hsu
and Perlis, 1984). In many cases the question of whether amniotic fluid mosaicism involves the fetus may be resolved by karyotyping fetal lymphocytes obtained by percutaneous umbilical
blood sampling (PUBS) (Gosden et al., 1988). However, this
approach may not be valid in all cases, because the mosaic cell
line may involve fetal tissues but may be excluded from the
fetal hematopoietic compartment and therefore not present in
a fetal blood sample (Johnson and Wapner, 1997). Certain
chromosomes, such as 22, are notorious for exclusion from fetal
blood and may require testing of additional fetal tissues such as
the skin (Berghella et al., 1998). Evaluation of mosaic results
should also include detailed ultrasound assessment to assess
fetal growth and exclude structural anomalies. If both ultrasound and fetal sampling are normal, the parents can be reassured that, in most cases, the fetus is unaffected (Gosden et al.,
1988). However, a small chance of fetal involvement still
exists because the presence of an undetectable but clinically
significant abnormal cell line can never be absolutely
excluded. Because of the complexity of interpreting mosaic
amniotic fluid results, consultation with a cytogenetics laboratory and a clinical geneticist is recommended.

Use of Fluorescence *In Situ* Hybridization

Fluorescence *in situ* hybridization (FISH) probes are relatively short fluorescently labeled DNA sequences that are hybridized to a known location on a specific chromosome and allow for determination of the number and location of specific DNA sequences. Interphase cells are evaluated by counting the number of discrete fluorescent signals from each probe. A normal diploid cell queried with a probe for the centromere of chromosome 18 would have two signals, whereas a trisomy 18 cell would have three.

Prenatal interphase evaluation of uncultured amniotic fluid can detect aneuploidies caused by monosomies, free trisomies, trisomies associated with Robertsonian translocations, triploidy, and other numerical chromosomal abnormalities. In standard practice, probes involving chromosomes 13, 18, 21, X, and Y are used. This technology will not routinely detect cytogenetic abnormalities such as mosaics, translocations, or rare aneuploidies (Klinger et al., 1992; Ward et al., 1993).

Since 1993 the position of the American College of Medical Genetics has been that prenatal FISH is investigational. In 1997, the U.S. Food and Drug Administration cleared the specific FISH probes to enumerate chromosomes 13, 18, 21, X, and Y for prenatal diagnosis. Subsequent studies demonstrate an extremely high concordance rate between FISH and standard cytogenetics (99.8%) for specific abnormalities that the assay is designed to detect (Cheong Leung et al., 2001; Sawa et al., 2001; Tepperberg et al., 2001; Weremowicz et al., 2001). These performance characteristics support the utilization of FISH for prenatal testing when a diagnosis of aneuploidy of chromosome 13, 18, 21, X, or Y is highly suspected by virtue of maternal age, positive maternal serum biochemical screening, or abnormal ultrasound findings (Technical and clinical assessment of fluorescence *in situ* hybridization: An ACMG/ASHG position statement, 2000).

Presently, it is suggested that FISH analysis not be used as a primary screening test on all genetic amniocenteses because of its inability to detect structural rearrangements, mosaicism, markers, and uncommon trisomies. Evans and coworkers (1999) surveyed the results of almost 73,000 prenatal cases from seven centers and reported that only 67% of abnormalities would have been detected by routine FISH. This interpretation may be misleading in that some of the missed abnormalities would not have had an impact on fetal development. Because all abnormalities would be detectable by tissue culture, FISH analysis is not cost effective. Presently, most laboratories use FISH to offer quick reassurance to patients with an unusually high degree of anxiety or to test fetuses at the highest risk, such as those with ultrasound anomalies. It is also beneficial in cases where rapid results are crucial to subsequent management, such as advanced gestational age.

FISH on metaphase chromosomes using probes for unique sequences has greatly expanded the "resolution" of conventional chromosome analysis. This has been demonstrated in countless case reports by the diagnosis of structural changes at the submicroscopic level (e.g., microdeletion syndromes) or by the determination of the origin of marker chromosomes and complex structural changes (Pergament, 2000).

Complications of Amniocentesis

A common finding after amniocentesis is cramping lasting for 1 to 2 hours. Lower abdominal discomfort may occur for up to 48 hours after the procedure but is usually not severe. Fortunately, serious maternal complications such as septic shock are rare. Amnionitis occurs in 0.1% of cases (Turnbull and MacKenzie, 1983) and can occur from contamination of the amniotic fluid with skin flora or from inadvertent puncture of the maternal bowel. It may also follow procedure-induced amnion rupture. Postamniocentesis chorioamnionitis can have an insidious onset and frequently presents with flu-like symptoms with few early localizing signs. This can evolve into a systemic infection with marked maternal morbidity unless early aggressive treatment is undertaken. Therefore, a high index of suspicion is necessary.

The development of rhesus isoimmunization will occur in approximately 1% of Rh-negative women undergoing amniocentesis (Golbus et al., 1979; Hill et al., 1980; Tabor, Jerne et al., 1986) but can be avoided by prophylactic administration of anti-D immunoglobulin after the procedure.

Amniotic fluid leakage or vaginal bleeding is noted by 2% to 3% of patients after amniocentesis. Unlike spontaneous second-trimester amnion rupture, which has a dismal prognosis, fluid leakage after amniocentesis will usually resolve after a few days of bed rest. Successful pregnancy outcome after such an event is common (Kishida et al., 1994). Occasionally, leakage of amniotic fluid will persist throughout pregnancy (NICHD Amniocentesis Registry, 1976; Simpson et al., 1981), but if the amniotic fluid volume remains adequate, a good outcome may be anticipated.

Pregnancy Loss after Mid-Trimester Amniocentesis

The safety of mid-trimester amniocentesis was documented in the mid-1970s by three collaborative studies performed in the United Kingdom, United States, and Canada (Medical Research Council, 1977; NICHD Amniocentesis Registry, 1978; Working Party on Amniocentesis, 1978). These studies were not randomized but rather included unsampled matched control groups. The U.S. and Canadian studies showed similar loss rates (spontaneous abortions, stillbirths, and neonatal deaths) between the two groups. A greater risk of loss occurred with needles of 19 gauge or larger and with more than two needle insertions per procedure. Both studies reported total post-procedure loss rates of 3% to 4%.

In contrast to these studies, the British Collaborative Study found an excess of fetal loss (1% to 1.5%) in the amniocentesis group compared with control subjects. This study has been criticized for a number of concerns, including a significant proportion of sampled patients with elevated MSAFP levels, an unusually low complication rate in the control group, and a change in the matching criteria during the study.

The only prospective, randomized, controlled trial evaluating the safety of second-trimester amniocentesis is a Danish study, which reported on 4606 low-risk healthy women, 25 to 34 years old, who were randomly allocated to either amniocentesis or to ultrasound examination (Tabor, Philip, et al., 1986). The total fetal loss rate in the amniocentesis group was 1.7% and in the control subjects, 0.7% ($P < .01$). The observed difference of 1% (95% confidence interval, 0.3, 1.5) gave a relative risk of 2.3. The conclusions of this study were initially criticized because the original report stated that an 18-gauge needle (which is associated with higher risks than smaller needles) was used. Tabor and colleagues (1988) subsequently reported that they had in fact used a 20-gauge needle for most of the procedures. Most contemporary studies using ultrasound guidance report total post-procedure loss rates to 28 weeks between 1% and 2% (Anonymous, 1998). These studies are consistent with a procedure-induced loss rate of approximately 1 in 200, which is the most commonly quoted in pre-procedure counseling.

Both the U.K. and Danish studies (Working Party on Amniocentesis, 1978; Tabor, Philip, et al., 1986) found an increase in respiratory distress syndrome and pneumonia in neonates from the amniocentesis groups. Other studies have not found this association. The U.K. study also showed an increased incidence of talipes and dislocation of the hip in the amniocentesis group (Working Party on Amniocentesis, 1978). This finding has not been confirmed.

In early experience with amniocentesis, needle puncture of the fetus was reported in 0.1% to 3.0% of cases (Karp and Hayden, 1977; NICHD Amniocentesis Registry, 1978) and was associated with fetal exsanguination (Young et al., 1977), intestinal atresia (Swift et al., 1979; Therkelsen and Rehder, 1981), ileocutaneous fistula (Rickwood, 1977), gangrene of a fetal limb (Lamb, 1975), uniocular blindness (Merin and Beyth, 1980), porencephalic cysts (Youroukos et al., 1980), patellar tendon disruption (Epley et al., 1979), skin dimples (Broome et al., 1976), and peripheral nerve damage (Karp and Hayden, 1977). Continuous use of ultrasound to guide the needle minimizes needle puncture of the fetus and, in experienced centers, is an exceedingly rare complication.

No long-term adverse effects have been demonstrated in children undergoing amniocentesis. Baird and colleagues (1994) compared 1296 liveborn children whose mothers had a mid-trimester amniocentesis to unsampled control subjects. With the exception of hemolytic disease due to isoimmunization, the offspring of women who had amniocentesis were no more likely than control subjects to have a disability during childhood and adolescence. Finegan and colleagues (1990) reported an increased incidence of middle-ear abnormalities in children whose mothers had amniocentesis.

Amniocentesis Performed before 15 Weeks' Gestation (Early Amniocentesis)

The desire for a first-trimester diagnosis stimulated interest in the feasibility of performing amniocentesis under 15 weeks' gestation. The technique at this gestational age varies from conventional amniocentesis in that less fluid is available and incomplete fusion of the amnion and chorion frequently cause tenting of the membranes, resulting in failed procedures in 2% to 3% of cases (Anonymous, 1998; Johnson et al., 1999).

Although initial experience with early amniocentesis were reassuring (Penso et al., 1990; Assel et al., 1992; Hanson et al., 1992; Henry and Miller, 1992), subsequent studies have raised serious concerns about its safety. In 1994, Nicolaides and coworkers (1994) reported on over 1300 women undergoing first-trimester diagnoses. In this study, significantly higher rates of fetal loss (5.3% versus 2.3%) were seen in the early amniocentesis group. This finding was echoed by Vandenbussche and coworkers (1994), who reported a 6.7% higher occurrence of pregnancy loss for early amniocentesis versus CVS. Sundberg and colleagues (1997), in a prospective randomized comparison of CVS to early amniocentesis, also found a higher loss rate with early amniocentesis but had to terminate the study early because of an unanticipated increase in talipes equinovarus in the early amniocentesis group. Higher loss rates have also been found when comparing early amniocentesis to second-trimester amniocentesis. The Canadian Early and Mid-trimester Amniocentesis trial reported a 1.7% higher incidence of fetal loss in the early amniocentesis group compared with second-trimester sampling when taking all fetal losses into account (7.6% versus 5.9%) (Anonymous, 1998).

There is also an increased frequency of culture failure and ruptured membranes compared with later procedures (Nicolaides et al., 1994; Sundberg et al., 1997; Anonymous, 1998). Of most concern, however, is that fetal talipes equinovarus (club feet) occurred in 1% to 2% of cases sampled by early amniocentesis. This rate is 10-fold higher than the 1 per 1000 births seen in the U.S. population. The club foot deformities are believed to occur secondary to procedure-induced fluid leakage, because they occurred in 1% of cases in which no leakage occurred and in 15% of cases when leakage occurred (Anonymous, 1998). For these reasons, amniocentesis should rarely, if ever, be performed before the 13th week of gestation. The safety of amniocentesis in weeks 13 and 14 is uncertain. Until its safety can be ensured, it is best to delay routine sampling until week 15 or 16 of pregnancy.

Chorionic Villus Sampling

The major drawbacks of conventional second-trimester genetic amniocentesis are the delayed availability of the karyotype and the increased medical risks of a pregnancy termination late in pregnancy. Furthermore, delaying the procedure until after fetal movement is believed to inflict a severe emotional burden on the patient. Secondary to these concerns, attempts have been made to move prenatal diagnosis into the first trimester. CVS, which samples the developing placenta rather than penetrating the amniotic membrane, has been the most successful approach to date at accomplishing this.

History of Chorionic Villus Sampling

The ability to sample and analyze villus tissue was demonstrated over 25 years ago by the Chinese, who, in an attempt to develop a technique for fetal sex determination, inserted a thin catheter into the uterus guided only by tactile sensation (Department of Obstetrics and Gynecology, Tietung Hospital, 1975). When resistance from the gestational sac was felt, suction was applied and small pieces of villi were aspirated. Although this approach seems relatively crude by today's standards of ultrasonically guided invasive procedures, their diagnostic accuracy and low miscarriage rate demonstrated the feasibility of first-trimester sampling.

Initial experiences in other parts of the world were not as promising. In 1968, Hahnemann and Mohr attempted blind transcervical trophoblast biopsy in 12 patients using a 6-mm diameter instrument. Although successful tissue culture was possible, half of these subjects subsequently aborted. In 1973, Kullander and Sandahl used a 5-mm diameter fiberoptic endocervoscope with biopsy forceps to perform transcervical CVS in patients requesting pregnancy termination. Although tissue culture was successful in approximately half of the cases, two subjects subsequently became septic.

In 1974, Hahnemann described further experience with first-trimester prenatal diagnosis using a 2.5-mm hysteroscope and a cylindrical biopsy knife. Once again, significant complications, including inadvertent rupture of the amniotic sac, were encountered. By this time, the safety of mid-trimester genetic amniocentesis had become well established, and further attempts at first-trimester prenatal diagnosis were temporarily abandoned in the Western Hemisphere.

Two technological advances occurred in the early 1980s that allowed reintroduction of CVS. The first of these was the development of real-time sonography, making continuous guidance possible. At the same time, sampling instruments were miniaturized and refined. In 1982, Kazy and associates reported the first transcervical CVS performed with real-time sonographic guidance. That same year, Old and colleagues (1982) reported the first-trimester diagnosis of β-thalassemia major using DNA from chorionic villi obtained by sonographically guided transcervical aspiration with a 1.5-mm diameter polyethylene catheter. Using a similar sampling technique, Brambati and Simoni (1983) diagnosed trisomy 21 at 11 weeks' gestation.

After these preliminary reports, several CVS programs were established both in Europe and the United States, with the outcomes informally reported to a World Health Organization (WHO)-sponsored registry maintained at Jefferson Medical College in Philadelphia. This registry, along with single center reports, was used to estimate the safety of CVS until 1989, when two prospective multicentered studies, one from Canada (Canadian Collaborative CVS/Amniocentesis Clinical Trial Group, 1989) and one from the United States (Rhoads et al., 1989), were published and confirmed the safety of the procedure.

Technique of Transcervical Chorionic Villus Sampling

Ultrasound examination immediately before the procedure confirms fetal heart activity, appropriate size, and placental location. The position of the uterus and cervix is determined, and a catheter path is mapped. If the uterus is anteverted, addi-

tional filling of the bladder can be used to straighten the uterine position. Although most procedures require a moderately filled bladder, an overfilled bladder is discouraged, because it lifts the uterus out of the pelvis, lengthening the sampling path, which can diminish the flexibility required for catheter manipulation. Occasionally, a uterine contraction may interfere with passage of the catheter. Delaying the procedure until the contraction dissipates is suggested (Fig. 18-7).

When the uterine condition and location are favorable, the patient is placed in the lithotomy position, and the vulva and vagina are aseptically prepared with povidone-iodine solution. A speculum is inserted, and the cervix is similarly prepared. The distal 3 to 5 cm of the sampling catheter is molded into a slightly curved shape and the catheter gently passed under ultrasound guidance through the cervix until a loss of resistance is felt at the endocervix. The operator then waits until the sonographer visualizes the catheter tip. The catheter is then advanced parallel to the chorionic membranes to the distal edge of the placenta. The stylet is then removed and a 20-mL syringe containing nutrient medium is attached. Negative pressure is applied by means of the syringe and the catheter removed slowly.

The syringe is then visually inspected for villi. These can frequently be seen with the naked eye as white branching structures floating in the media. On occasion, however, viewing the samples under a low-power dissecting microscope is necessary to confirm the presence of sufficient villi. Maternal decidua is frequently retrieved with the sample but is usually easily recognized by its amorphous appearance. If sufficient villi are not retrieved with the initial pass, a second insertion can be made with minimal impact on pregnancy loss rate.

Technique of Transabdominal Chorionic Villus Sampling

Continuous ultrasound is used to direct a 19- or 20-gauge spinal needle into the long axis of the placenta (Fig. 18-8). After removal of the stylet, villi are aspirated into a 20-mL

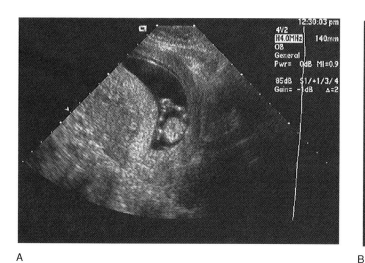

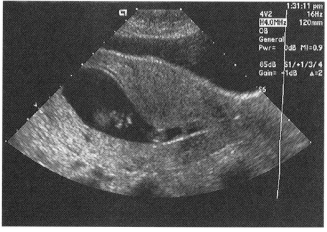

A

B

FIGURE 18-7 ■ Ultrasound photos of a transcervical chorionic villus sampling. **A,** Typical uterine focal contraction characteristic of this gestational age involving the posterior wall of the uterus. **B,** The same patient 60 minutes later is pictured. The contraction has dissipated, the bladder has filled, and the operator is now able to pass the catheter into the posterior chorionic frondosum.

More chorionic tissue is obtained by the transcervical method, but the proportion of cases in which less than 10 mg is obtained is similar in both groups. There are no differences in birth weight, gestational age at delivery, or congenital malformations with either method.

Laboratory Aspects of Chorionic Villus Sampling

Chorionic villi have three major components: an outer layer of hormonally active and invasive syncytiotrophoblast, a middle layer of cytotrophoblast from which syncytiotrophoblast cells are derived, and an inner mesodermal core containing blood capillaries.

The average sample from a transcervical aspiration contains 15 to 30 mg of villous material. The villi identified in the syringe are carefully and aseptically transferred for inspection and dissection under a microscope. The villi are cleaned of adherent decidua and then exposed to trypsin to digest and separate the cytotrophoblast from the underlying mesodermal core. The cytotrophoblast has a high mitotic index, with many spontaneous mitoses available for immediate chromosome analysis. The liquid suspension containing the cytotrophoblast is either dropped immediately onto a slide for analysis or may undergo a short incubation (Gregson and Seabright, 1983; Simoni et al., 1983). This "direct" chromosome preparation can give preliminary results within 2 to 3 hours. However, most laboratories now use an overnight incubation to improve karyotype quality and thus report results within 2 to 4 days. The remaining villus core is placed in tissue culture and is typically ready for harvest and chromosome analysis within 1 week (Chang et al., 1982). The direct method has the advantage of providing a rapid result and minimizing the decidual contamination, whereas tissue culture is better for interpreting discrepancies between the cytotrophoblast and the actual fetal state. Ideally, both the direct and culture methods should be used, because they each evaluate slightly different tissue sources. Although the direct preparation is less likely to be representative of the fetus, its use will minimize the likelihood of maternal cell contamination, and, if culture fails, a nonmosaic normal direct preparation result can be considered conclusive, although rare cases of false-negative rates for trisomy 21 and 18 have been reported (Martin, Simpson, et al., 1986; Bartels et al., 1989). Abnormalities in either may have clinical implications.

Most biochemical diagnoses that can be made from amniotic fluid or cultured amniocytes can usually be made from chorionic villi (Poenaru, 1987). In many cases, the results are available more rapidly and efficiently when villi are used because sufficient enzyme is present to allow direct analysis rather than the products of tissue culture being required. However, for certain rare biochemical diagnosis, villi will not be an appropriate or reliable diagnostic source (Gray et al., 1995). To ensure that appropriate testing is possible, the laboratory should be consulted before sampling.

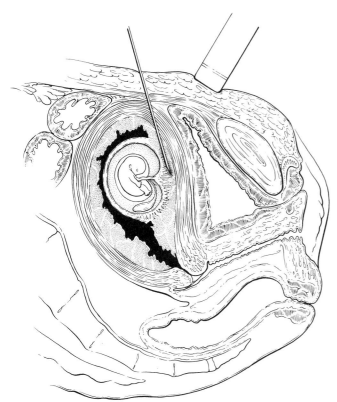

FIGURE 18-8 ■ Transabdominal chorionic villus sampling. Continuous ultrasound guidance is used to allow guidance of the needle into the chorionic frondosum, remaining parallel to the plate. The sample is then obtained by "back and forth" movement of the needle while maintaining negative pressure. The needle tip is kept in sight through ultrasound continuously. (From Scioscia AL: Reproductive genetics. In Moore TR, Reiter RC, Rebar RW, et al (eds): Obstetrics and Gynecology: A Longitudinal Approach. New York, Churchill Livingstone, 1993, p. 72.)

syringe containing tissue culture media. Because the needle is somewhat smaller than the cervical sampling catheter, three or four to-and-fro passes of the needle tip through the body of the placenta are required to retrieve the villi. Unlike transcervical CVS, which is best performed before 14 weeks' gestation, the transabdominal procedure can be performed throughout pregnancy and therefore constitutes an alternative to amniocentesis or PUBS when a karyotype is needed. If oligohydramnios is present, transabdominal CVS may be the only approach available.

Comparison of Transcervical and Transabdominal Chorionic Villus Sampling

The transabdominal and transcervical approaches to villus sampling have been shown to be equally safe (Brambati, Terzian, et al., 1991; Jackson et al., 1992). In most cases, operator or patient choice will determine the sampling route; however, in about 3% to 5% of cases, one approach is clearly preferred so operators must be skilled in both. For example, a posterior placenta is sampled most easily by the transcervical route, whereas a fundal placenta is more simply approached transabdominally. Bowel in the sampling path may preclude transabdominal CVS in some cases, whereas necrotic cervical polyps or an active herpetic lesion should lead to transabdominal sampling.

Accuracy of Chorionic Villus Sampling Cytogenetic Results

CVS is now considered a reliable method of prenatal diagnosis, but early in its development incorrect results were reported (Simoni et al., 1983; Martin, Elias, et al., 1986;

Cheung et al., 1987). The major sources of these errors included maternal cell contamination and misinterpretation of mosaicism confined to the placenta. Today, genetic evaluation of chorionic villi provides a high degree of success and accuracy, particularly in regard to the diagnosis of common trisomies (Mikkelsen and Ayme, 1987; Ledbetter et al., 1990). The U.S. collaborative study revealed a 99.7% rate of successful cytogenetic diagnosis, with only 1.1% of the patients requiring a second diagnostic test such as amniocentesis or fetal blood analysis to further interpret the results (Ledbetter et al., 1990). In most cases, the additional testing was required to delineate the clinical significance of mosaic or other ambiguous results (76%), whereas laboratory failure (21%) and maternal cell contamination (3%) also required follow-up testing.

MATERNAL CELL CONTAMINATION

Chorionic villus samples typically contain a mixture of placental villi and maternally derived decidua. Although specimens are thoroughly washed and inspected under a microscope after collection, some maternal cells may remain and grow in the culture. As a result, two cell lines, one fetal and the other maternal, may be identified. In other cases, the maternal cell line may completely overgrow the culture, thereby leading to diagnostic errors, including incorrect sex determination (Williams et al., 1987; Ledbetter et al., 1992; Boehm et al., 1993) and potentially to false-negative diagnoses, although there are no published reports of the latter. Direct preparations of chorionic villi are generally thought to prevent maternal cell contamination (Gregson and Seabright, 1983; Williams et al., 1987), whereas long-term culture has a rate varying from 1.8% to 4% (Ledbetter et al., 1992). Because, in contrast to cytotrophoblast, maternal decidua has a low mitotic index, it is highly desirable for laboratories to offer a direct chromosome preparation as well as a long-term culture on all samples of chorionic villus. Even in culture, the contaminating cells are easily identified as maternal and should not lead to clinical errors. Interestingly, for reasons still uncertain, maternal cell contamination occurs more frequently in specimens retrieved by the transcervical route (Ledbetter et al., 1992).

Contamination of samples with significant amounts of maternal decidual tissue is almost always due to small sample size, making selection of appropriate tissue difficult. In experienced centers in which adequate quantities of villi are available, this problem has disappeared. Choosing only whole clearly typical villus material and discarding any atypical fragments, small pieces, or fragments with adherent decidua will avoid confusion (Elles et al., 1983). Therefore, if the initial aspiration is small, a second pass should be performed rather than risk inaccurate results. When proper care is taken and good cooperation and communication exist between the sampler and the laboratory, absence of even small amounts of contaminating maternal tissue can be accomplished.

CONFINED PLACENTAL MOSAICISM

The second major source of potential diagnostic error associated with CVS is mosaicism confined to the placenta. Although the fetus and placenta have a common ancestry, chorionic villus tissue will not always reflect fetal genotype (Karkut et al., 1985; Ledbetter et al., 1990). Although initially there was concern that this might invalidate CVS as a prenatal diagnostic tool, subsequent investigations have led to a clearer understanding of villus biology, so that accurate clinical interpretation is now possible. This understanding has also revealed new information about the etiology of pregnancy loss, discovered a new cause of intrauterine growth retardation, and clarified the basic mechanism of UPD.

Discrepancies between the cytogenetics of the placenta and fetus occur because the cells contributing to the chorionic villi become separate and distinct from those forming the embryo in early development. Specifically, at approximately the 32- to 64-cell stage, only 3 to 4 become compartmentalized into the inner cell mass to form the embryo, whereas the remainder become precursors of the extra embryonic tissues (Wolstenholme, 1996). Mosaicism can then occur through two possible mechanisms (Wolstenholme, 1996). An initial meiotic error in one of the gametes can lead to a trisomic conceptus that normally would spontaneously abort. However, if during subsequent mitotic divisions one or more of the early aneuploid cells loses one of the trisomic chromosomes through anaphase lag, the embryo can be "rescued" by reduction of a portion of its cells to disomy. This will result in a mosaic morula with the percentage of normal cells dependent on the cell division at which rescue occurred. More abnormal cells will be present when correction is delayed to the second or a subsequent cell division. Because most cells in the morula proceed to the trophoblast cell lineage (processed by the direct preparation), it is highly probable that that lineage will continue to contain a significant number of trisomic cells. Alternatively, because only a small proportion of cells are incorporated into the inner cell mass, involvement of the fetus will depend on the random distribution of the aneuploid progenitor cells. Involvement of the mesenchymal core of the villus, which also evolves from the inner cell mass, is similarly dependent on this random cell distribution. Noninvolvement of the fetal cell lineage will produce "confined placental mosaicism," in which the trophoblast and perhaps the extra embryonic mesoderm will have aneuploid cells but the fetus will be euploid.

In the second mechanism, mitotic postzygotic errors produce mosaicism with the distribution and percent of aneuploid cells in the morula or blastocyst dependent on the timing of nondisjunction. If mitotic errors occur early in the development of the morula, they may segregate to the inner cell mass and have the same potential to produce an affected fetus as do meiotic errors. Mitotic errors occurring after primary cell differentiation and compartmentalization has been completed led to cytogenetic abnormalities in only one lineage.

Meiotic rescue can lead to UPD. This occurs because the original trisomic cell contained two chromosomes from one parent and one from the other. After rescue, there is a theoretical one in three chance that the resulting pair of chromosomes came from the same parent, which is called UPD. UPD may have clinical consequences if the chromosomes involved carry imprinted genes in which expression is based on the parent of origin. For example, Prader-Willi syndrome may result from uniparental maternal disomy for chromosome 15. Therefore, a CVS diagnosis of confined placental mosaicism for trisomy 15 may be the initial clue that UPD could be present and lead to an affected child (Cassidy et al., 1992; Purvis-Smith et al., 1992). Because of this, all cases in which trisomy 15 (either complete or mosaic) is confined to the placenta should be evaluated for UPD by amniotic fluid analysis.

In addition to chromosome 15, chromosomes 7, 11, 14, and 22 are believed to be imprinted and require similar follow-up (Ledbetter and Engel, 1995).

Confined placental mosaicism (unassociated with UPD) can alter placental function and lead to fetal growth failure or perinatal death (Worton and Stern, 1984; Kalousek et al., 1987, 1991; Goldberg et al., 1990; Johnson et al., 1990; Wapner et al., 1992; Wolstenholme, 1996). The exact mechanism by which abnormal cells within the placenta alter function is unknown, but the effect is limited to specific chromosomes. For example, confined placental mosaicism for chromosome 16 leads to severe intrauterine growth restriction, prematurity, or perinatal death, with less than 30% of pregnancies resulting in normal, appropriate-for-gestational-age, full-term infants (Breed et al., 1991; Post and Nijhuis, 1992; Kalousek et al., 1993; Phillips et al., 1996; Benn, 1998).

Mosaicism occurs in about 1% of all CVS samples (Mikkelsen and Ayme, 1987; Vejerslev and Mikkelsen, 1989; Breed et al., 1991; Ledbetter et al., 1992) but is confirmed in the fetus in only 10% to 40% of these cases. In most cases, if the mosaic results are confined to the placenta, fetal development will be normal. If the mosaic cell line involves the fetus, significant phenotypic consequences are possible. The probability of fetal involvement appears to be related to the tissue source in which the aneuploid cells were detected with culture results more likely than direct preparation, reflecting a true fetal mosaicism.

The specific chromosome involved also predicts the likelihood of fetal involvement (Ledbetter and Engel, 1995). Phillips and coworkers (1996) demonstrated that autosomal mosaicism involving common trisomies (i.e., 21, 18, and 13) was confirmed in the fetus in 19% of cases, whereas uncommon trisomies involved the fetus in only 3%. When sex chromosome mosaicism was found in the placenta, the abnormal cell line was confirmed in the fetus in 16% of cases.

When placental mosaicism is discovered, amniocentesis can be performed to elucidate the extent of fetal involvement. When mosaicism is limited to the direct preparation, amniocentesis correlates perfectly with fetal genotype (Phillips et al., 1996). When a mosaicism is observed in tissue culture, amniocentesis will predict the true fetal karyotype in approximately 94% of cases, with both false-positive and false-negative results seen (Phillips et al., 1996). Three cases were reported of

mosaic trisomy 21 on villus culture, a normal amniotic fluid analysis, followed by a fetus or newborn with mosaic aneuploidy (Ledbetter et al., 1990).

The following clinical recommendations may be used to assist in evaluation of CVS mosaicism. Analysis of CVS samples should, if possible, include both direct preparation and tissue culture. If mosaicism is found, follow-up amniocentesis should be offered. Under no circumstances should a decision to terminate a pregnancy be based entirely on a CVS mosaic result. For CVS mosaicism involving sex chromosome abnormalities, polyploidy, marker chromosomes, structural rearrangements, and uncommon trisomies, the patient can be reassured if amniocentesis results are euploid and detailed ultrasonographic examination is normal. However, no guarantees should be made, and, as described previously, in certain cases testing for UPD will be indicated. If common trisomies 21, 18, and 13 are involved, amniocentesis should be offered, but the patient must be advised of the possibilities of a false-negative result. Follow-up may include detailed ultrasonography, fetal blood sampling, or fetal skin biopsy. At present, the predictive accuracy of these additional tests is uncertain.

Pregnancy Loss after Chorionic Villus Sampling

Data evaluating the safety of CVS comes primarily from three collaborative reports (Table 18-26). In 1989, the Canadian Collaborative CVS/Amniocentesis Clinical Trial Group reported a prospective randomized trial comparing CVS to amniocentesis performed at 15 to 20 weeks' gestation. To account for potential differences in the background loss rates in the two different sampling windows, all patients were enrolled in the first trimester and the frequency of all subsequent spontaneous abortions, induced abortions, and later losses occurring before 28 weeks were compared. The results demonstrated equivalent safety of the two procedures. There was a 7.6% loss rate in the CVS group and a 7.0% loss rate in the amniocentesis group. The excess loss rate of 0.6% for CVS over amniocentesis was not statistically significant. No significant differences were noted in the incidence of preterm birth, low birth weight, or rate of maternal complication.

A multicenter U.S. study involved a prospective, though nonrandomized, trial of 2235 women who were enrolled in the first trimester and chose either transcervical CVS or second-

TABLE 18-26. TOTAL PREGNANCY LOSS RATES OF CHORIONIC VILLUS SAMPLING (CVS) AND AMNIOCENTESIS (AC) IN THREE COLLABORATIVE TRIALS

Study	Eligible or Attempted (n)		Total Loss Rate (%)		CVS Excess Loss Rate (%)
	CVS	AC	CVS	AC	
Canadian Collaborative CVS/Amniocentesis Clinical Trial Group	1191	1200	7.6	7.0	0.6
Rhoads and associates	2235	651	7.2	5.7	0.8*
Medical Research Council	1609	1592	13.6	9.0	4.6

* Corrected for difference in maternal age and gestational age.

trimester amniocentesis (Rhoads et al., 1989). An excess pregnancy loss rate of 0.8% in the CVS group over the amniocentesis group was calculated, which was not statistically significant. Repeated catheter insertions were significantly associated with pregnancy loss, with cases requiring three or more passes having a 10.8% spontaneous abortion rate, compared with 2.9% in cases that required only one pass.

A prospective, randomized, collaborative comparison of more than 3200 pregnancies, sponsored by the European Medical Research Council, reported CVS having a 4.6% greater pregnancy loss rate than amniocentesis (95% confidence interval, 1.6% to 7.5%) (MRC Working Party on the Evaluation of Chorion Villus Sampling, 1991). This difference reflected more spontaneous deaths before 28 weeks' gestation (2.9%), more terminations of pregnancy for chromosomal anomalies (1.0%), and more neonatal deaths (0.3%). Villus sampling was performed by both the transcervical and transabdominal routes. Repeat procedures were significantly higher in the CVS group compared with the amniocentesis group.

Most likely, operator inexperience in the European centers accounts for this discrepancy. The U.S. trial consisted of seven experienced centers and the Canadian trial 11, whereas the Medical Research Council trial used 31 centers, some relatively inexperienced, contributing various numbers of cases and using different sampling and cytogenetic procedures. There were, on average, 325 cases per center in the U.S. study, 106 in the Canadian study, and 52 in the European trial. These results demonstrate a relatively prolonged learning curve for CVS before safety is maximized. Saura and colleagues (1994) showed that over 400 cases may be required.

Other Complications of Chorionic Villus Sampling

Postprocedure bleeding is the most common complaint after CVS. Most centers report postprocedure bleeding in 7% to 10% of patients sampled transcervically, whereas bleeding or spotting is relatively uncommon after transabdominal sampling, occurring in 1% or less of cases (Rhoads et al., 1989). Minimal spotting may occur in up to one third of women sampled by the transcervical route (Rhoads et al., 1989). On occasion, a small subchorionic hematoma may be seen after sampling (Brambati, Oldrini, et al., 1987). This usually resolves spontaneously within a few weeks and is rarely associated with adverse outcome. Hematomas occur when the catheter is passed too deeply into the underlying vascular decidua basalis. Because passage into the decidua gives a "gritty" sensation, careful attention to the feel of the catheter can minimize this complication. Operators should also avoid sampling near or within large placental "lakes," which will also lead to bleeding (Liu et al., 1991).

Since the initial development of transcervical CVS, there has been concern that transvaginal passage of an instrument would introduce vaginal flora into the uterus. Although cultures of catheter tips have isolated bacteria in 30% of transcervical CVS cases (Brambati and Varotto, 1985; McFadyen et al., 1985; Wass and Bennett, 1985; Brambati, Matarelli, et al., 1987), the incidence of chorioamnionitis is extremely low and occurs equally infrequently after either the transcervical or transabdominal procedure. In the U.S. collaborative trial, infection was suspected as a possible etiology of pregnancy loss in only 0.3% of cases (Rhoads et al., 1989).

Early in the development of transcervical CVS, two life-threatening pelvic infections were reported (Blakemore et al., 1985; Barela et al., 1986). The practice of using a new sterile catheter for each insertion has subsequently been universally adopted, and there have been no additional reports of serious infections. Infection after transabdominal CVS has been demonstrated and may result from inadvertent bowel puncture by the sampling needle (Brambati, Terzian, et al., 1991).

Acute rupture of membranes is exceedingly rare in experienced centers (Rhoads et al., 1989). Fluid leakage with oligohydramnios has been reported days to weeks after the procedure (Hogge et al., 1986; Cheng et al., 1991). In most cases, this is unrelated to the procedure but occasionally may be secondary to a procedure-induced hematoma.

An acute rise in MSAFP after CVS has consistently been reported, implying a detectable degree of fetomaternal bleeding (Blakemore et al., 1986; Brambati et al., 1986; Shulman and Elias, 1990). The MSAFP elevation is not related to the technique used to retrieve villi but seems to depend on the quantity of tissue aspirated (Shulman and Elias, 1990). Levels return to normal ranges by 16 to 18 weeks of gestation, thus allowing MSAFP serum screening to proceed according to usual prenatal protocols. All Rh-negative nonsensitized women undergoing CVS should receive Rh-D immune globulin subsequent to the procedure. Exacerbation of preexisting Rh immunization after CVS has been described. Existing Rh sensitization, therefore, represents a contraindication to the procedure (Moise and Carpenter, 1990).

Risk of Fetal Abnormality after Chorionic Villus Sampling

Firth and colleagues (1991) reported five occurrences of severe limb abnormalities out of 289 pregnancies sampled by CVS between 56 and 66 days. Four of these cases had the unusual but severe oromandibular-limb hypogenesis syndrome, which occurs in the general population at a rate of 1 per 175,000 births (Firth et al., 1991). Burton, Schulz, and coworkers (1993) then reported on 14 more post-CVS cases of limb reduction defects (LRD) ranging from mild to severe, only two of which occurred when sampling was performed beyond 9.5 weeks. After these two early reports, the WHO gathered additional data from its CVS registry, published reports (Firth et al., 1991; Burton, Schulz, et al., 1993), and case-controlled studies (Mastroiacovo et al., 1992; Olney et al., 1994) and concluded that "far greater data supporting CVS not being associated with LRD were available in various collaborative studies, in individual centers having the greatest experience, and in the WHO-initiated registry comprising 138,996 procedures" (WHO/PAHO, 1999). They further concluded that CVS was not associated with LRD when performed after 8 completed weeks of pregnancy (Froster and Jackson, 1996). This infrequent occurrence of LRD after CVS was echoed by the American College of Obstetricians and Gynecologists, who stated that a risk for LRD of 1 in 3000 would be a prudent upper limit for counseling patients. Data on 216,381 procedures are now in the WHO CVS registry and have been reported (WHO/PAHO, 1999). This report analyzed the frequency of limb anomalies, their pattern, and their associated gestational age at sampling and found no overall increased risk of LRD or any difference in the pattern of defects compared with the general population. To analyze a possible temporal relationship between CVS and LRD, a subset of 106,383 cases was stratified by the week at which the procedure was performed. The incidence of LRD was 11.7, 4.9, 3.8, 3.4, and 2.3 per 10,000 CVS procedures in weeks 8, 9, 10, 11, and more than 12, respectively. Only the rate at week 8 exceeded the background risk of 6.0 per 10,000 births. If cases from the cluster seen in the original report of Firth and coworkers (1991) are removed, the rate for week 8 procedures also falls below baseline. Brambati and colleagues (1992), in a small series of early CVS cases, had an LRD incidence of 1.6% for procedures performed in weeks 6 and 7, 0.1% in week 8, and (population frequency) 0.059% in week 9.

Present data confirm that performing CVS in the standard gestational window of 10 to 13 weeks does not increase the risk of LRD. Sampling before 10 weeks is not recommended, except in very unusual circumstances, such as when a patient's religious beliefs may preclude a pregnancy termination beyond a specific gestational age (Wapner et al., 2002). These patients, however, must be informed that the incidence of severe LRD could be as high as 1% to 2%.

PRENATAL DIAGNOSIS AND MULTIPLE GESTATION

Risk of Fetal Aneuploidy in Multiple Gestations

The overall probability that a given multiple gestation contains an aneuploid fetus is dependent on its zygosity. Because monozygotic twins originate from the same gamete, both fetuses possess the same karyotype, and the overall risk of aneuploidy is that of a singleton. Although this construct ignores the very small possibility of mitotic nondisjunction, such a possibility is such a rare occurrence that it should not change the overall risk calculation. In dizygotic twins, on the other hand, either one or both fetuses may be affected, with the chance for aneuploidy in either fetus being independent. The risk of both dizygotic twins fetuses being affected is low (the singleton risk squared), whereas the risk of at least one affected fetus is approximately twice the singleton risk (Rodis et al., 1990). These risks can be used to counsel patients if the zygosity is known.

If zygosity is unknown, the risk of at least one fetus being aneuploid can be approximated as 5:3 the risk of a singleton gestation. This approximation is based on the assumption that one third of all twin gestations are monozygotic twins. Despite the slight inaccuracy of this approach secondary to varying rates of monozygotic twins and dizygotic twins twinning with maternal age and ethnicity, this approximation is quite satisfactory for patient counseling. A more accurate determination taking these variations into account has been published by Myers and colleagues (1997). Based on these calculations, a 32-year-old woman with twins has nearly the risk of at least one aneuploid fetus as that of a 35-year-old woman with a singleton. Present recommendations are that invasive prenatal diagnosis be offered at this cutoff. Table 18-27 demonstrates the risk of fetal aneuploidy at different maternal ages in twin gestations using these calculations.

Higher-order multiple gestations resulting from assisted reproductive techniques have a greater preponderance for polyzygosity than naturally occurring multiples. The risk of at

TABLE 18-27. CALCULATED RISK AT TERM OF DOWN SYNDROME IN AT LEAST ONE FETUS FOR TWIN GESTATIONS

Maternal Age (yr)	Singleton Risk	Twin Risk	Equivalent Age (Yr)
25	1/1,250	1/679	32.5
30	1/952	1/508	33.8
32	1/769	1/409	34.7
35	1/378	1/199	37.5
40	1/106	1/56	42.5

From Meyers C, Adam R, Dungan J, et al. Aneuploidy in twin gestations: When is maternal age advanced? Obstet Gynecol **89**:248, 1997.

least one aneuploid fetus can be approximated as the singleton risk multiplied by the number of fetuses. Despite the fact that recent studies have shown that monozygotic twin pregnancies occur more frequently than anticipated after the use of assisted reproductive techniques (Hook, 1981; Wenstrom et al., 1993), their frequency still remains low enough so that the above estimation remains appropriate.

An even steeper increase in the risk of transmission for pregnancies at risk for mendelian disorders occurs with multiple gestations. For example, for a twin gestation at risk for an autosomal recessive disorder, there is a three in eight chance of at least one fetus being affected and a one in eight chance that both will inherit the affected genes.

Biochemical Screening

For singleton pregnancies, second-trimester biochemical screening is a routine practice. For twins, however, the value and accuracy of serum screening is much less certain because the contribution of an abnormal fetus will, on average, be brought closer to the normal mean by an unaffected cotwin. This tends to decrease the overall screening sensitivity. Screening, however, can still be useful despite this lower sensitivity.

The mean and median values of MSAFP, unconjugated estriol, and hCG in twins have been studied and are presented in Table 18-28. Dividing the measured result by the twin median can be used to estimate a twin MoM for each analyte. These MoM values can then be used in singleton algorithms to estimate a risk of aneuploidy. Neveux and coworkers (1996) evaluated this approach and, based on a calculated model, predicted that 73% of monozygotic twin and 43% of dizygotic twin cases with a Down syndrome fetus would be detected with

TABLE 18-28. AFP, hCG, AND UNCONJUGATED ESTRIOL VALUES IN TWIN GESTATIONS

Source	n	AFP	hCG	Unconjugated Estriol
Wald et al., 1991	200	2.13	1.84	1.67
Canick et al., 1990	35	2.30	1.90	1.70
Alpert et al., 1990	51	1.60	1.70	1.50
Foundation for Blood Research	58	2.00	2.30	1.70
All	344	2.04	1.90	1.60

AFP, α-fetoprotein; hCG, human chorionic gonadotropin.

a 5% false-positive rate. In their clinical sample of 274 twin pregnancies, 5.5% screened positive. They had no cases of Down syndrome, making evaluation of the sensitivity difficult. Presently, the use of biochemical markers for aneuploidy screening in multiple gestations is extremely limited and is not recommended for general practice.

For the detection of neural tube defects, the levels of maternal AFP are again affected by the presence of a cofetus. The mean MSAFP level in twin pregnancies ranges from 2.0 to 2.5 MoM. This is not surprising, considering double production. In singleton gestations, an MSAFP upper cutoff of 2.5 MoM will identify 75% of fetuses with a neural tube defect and have a false-positive rate between 2% and 3.3%. A similar cutoff in twin gestations would identify 99% of anencephalic fetuses and 89% of open neural tube defects (Cuckle et al., 1990), but this would be associated with an unacceptably high false-positive rate of 30%. A twin false-positive rate similar to that for singletons can be calculated by doubling the singleton cutoff level; for example, choosing an MSAFP cutoff value of 5.0 MoM for twins would have the same false-positive rate as a 2.5 MoM cutoff in singletons. The detection rate will be lower, however, because, when only one fetus has a neural tube defect, the normal coexisting fetus will contribute an AFP level near the singleton median. Maintaining the 75% sensitivity accomplished with singleton screening would require an MSAFP elevation of approximately 3.5 MoM, which would have a false-positive rate of 15%.

Presently, there is no standard agreement on the MSAFP elevation that warrants further evaluation in twins. Some centers use a cutoff of 4.0 MoM, which would identify approximately 60% of open spina bifida fetuses but has approximately an 8% incidence of false-positive results. Other centers use a cutoff of 4.5 MoM, which has a sensitivity of approximately 50%.

Amniocentesis in Multifetal Gestations

Amniocentesis in multifetal pregnancy involves puncture of the first sac, withdrawal of amniotic fluid, injection of dye to "mark the sampled sac," and then a new needle insertion to puncture the second sac (Elias et al., 1980). If the fluid aspirated after the second puncture is clear, this is confirmation that the first sac was not resampled. If blue-tinged fluid is retrieved, the needle should be removed and another attempt at sampling the second sac should be made.

History has shown the possible toxic effects of dye instillation. Methylene blue is associated with small bowel atresia

(Nicolini and Monni, 1990; Van der Pol et al., 1992) and an increased risk of fetal death (Kidd et al., 1996). Its use is now contraindicated. Use of indigo carmine (the dye of choice) has been reviewed in large series by both Cragan and coworkers (1993) and Pruggmayer and coworkers (1992), and no increased risk for small bowel atresia or any other congenital anomaly has been found. However, because of the theoretical risk of intra-amniotic dye, instillation-free techniques have evolved (Jeanty et al., 1990; Sebire et al., 1996).

A single-puncture method has been described in which the site of needle insertion is determined by the position of the dividing membrane (Jeanty et al., 1990). After entry into the first sac and aspiration of amniotic fluid, the needle is advanced through the dividing membrane into the second sac. To avoid contamination of the second sample with fluid from the first, the first 1 mL of fluid from the second sample is discarded. This method may cause iatrogenic rupture of the dividing membrane, with creation of a monoamniotic sac and its attendant risk of cord entanglement (Megory et al., 1991). This appears to occur almost exclusively in monochorionic gestations.

Bahado-Singh and colleagues (1992) described a technique of twin amniocentesis that entails identifying the separating membranes with a curvilinear or linear transducer. The first needle is inserted, fluid retrieved, and the needle left in place while a second needle is inserted into the coexisting sac. Visualization of the two needle tips on alternate sides of the membrane confirms sampling of both fetuses. Patient tolerance of this technique may be a problem, as well as the potential requirement of two operators when sampling.

Complications of Amniocentesis in Multiple Gestation

A comparison of the relative safety of any invasive procedure in multiple gestations must take into consideration that, at any gestational age, loss rates for multiples are significantly higher than for singletons. Evaluation of the safety of invasive procedures, therefore, needs to be kept in context. Most series report postprocedure loss rates between 2% and 5% (Table 18-29). Literature evaluating the risk of pregnancy loss before 28 weeks in unsampled twins with a normal second-trimester ultrasound demonstrates rates of 4.5% (Prompelan et al., 1989), 5.8% (Coleman et al., 1987), and 7.2% (Pretorious et al., 1993), which helps to put the increase in postprocedure rates into perspective. However, the ideal way to evaluate procedure-induced loss rates is to

TABLE 18-29. PREGNANCY OUTCOMES AFTER TWIN AMNIOCENTESIS

Source	Years of Procedures	Continuous Guidance	n	Success Rate	Loss to 20 Wk	Loss to 28 Wk
Pijpers, 1988	1980–1985	N	83	93%	1.2%	4.8%
Anderson, 1991	1969–1990	N	330	99%	—	3.6%
Antsaklis, 1991	1978–1988	N	53	100%	0.0%	1.9%
Pruggmayer, 1991	1982–1989	Y	98	100%	6.1%	8.1%
Pruggmayer, 1992	1981–1990	Y	529	100%	2.3%	3.7%
Wapner, 1993	1984–1990	Y	73	100%	1.4%	2.9%
Ghidini, 1993	1987–1992	Y	101	100%	0.0%	3.0%
Ko, 1998	1986–1997	Y	128	100%	4.5%	—
Yukobowich, 2001	1990–1997	Y	476	100%	2.7%*	—

* Loss within 4 weeks of procedure.

compare similar cohorts of sampled and unsampled twins. Ghidini and colleagues (1993) evaluated the risk of amniocentesis in twins by comparing 101 sampled pregnancies with an unsampled control group scanned at a matching gestational age. No significant difference in total loss rate was detected. A recent report attributed a 2% higher loss rate with amniocentesis (2.7% versus 0.6%) as compared with singletons or nonsampled twin gestations, with 13 losses in 476 pregnancies (95% confidence interval, 1.5, 4.6) (Yukobowich et al., 2001). The make-up of the sampled group was 47% maternal age of at least 35 years, 21% abnormal MSAFP, and 11% abnormal ultrasound, which could have affected loss rates. No study in the literature currently has the power to definitively quantify the procedure-induced loss rate in twins. Empirically, the procedure-related loss rate is 1% to 1.5%.

Patients with twins must also be counseled about the risk of finding a karyotypically abnormal child, which, because of the presence of two fetuses, is approximately twice that after a singleton procedure (Rodis et al., 1990). Amniocentesis in twins does raise some very painful questions. Families need to consider the possibility of a test showing that one of the twins is normal and the other has an abnormality. Selective termination of the affected fetus is now a routine procedure and can be accomplished in 100% of cases with a postprocedure loss rate of 5% to 10% in experienced centers (Evans et al., 1999). However, this approach is also associated with an increased risk of preterm birth, especially when performed after 20 weeks' gestation or if the lower fetus is terminated (Lynch et al., 1996).

Chorionic Villus Sampling in Multiple Gestations

Twin, as well as higher-order multiple, gestations have been sampled successfully using CVS (Brambati, Tului, et al., 1991; Pergament et al., 1992; Wapner et al., 1993; De Catte et al., 2000). Each distinct placental site must be identified and sampled individually. Because no dye marker is available to ensure retrieval from a gestation, if there is any suspicion that two separate samples have not been obtained, a back-up amniocentesis should be offered if the fetal genders are concordant (Brambati, Tului, et al., 1991). However, this is rarely required if meticulous intraoperative ultrasound placement of the needle or catheter is performed. Another difficulty is the possible cross-contamination of samples when both placentas are on the same uterine wall (i.e., both anterior or both posterior). In these cases, sampling the lower sac transcervically and the upper transabdominally minimizes the chance of contamination. When a biochemical diagnosis is required, the potential for misinterpretation is even greater because a small amount of normal tissue could significantly alter the test result. These cases should only be sampled in experienced centers.

Complications of Chorionic Villus Sampling in Multiple Gestations

Studies assessing procedure-related loss rates after CVS sampling of twins are shown in Table 18-30. In experienced centers, no increased procedure-related loss risks are seen compared with second-trimester amniocentesis.

TABLE 18-30. SAFETY OF CHORIONIC VILLUS SAMPLING WITH TWINS

Source	n	Success Rate	Pregnancy Loss Rate to 28 wk
Wapner, 1993	161	100.0%	2.8%
Pergament, 1992	128	99.2%	2.4%
Brambati, 1991	66	100.0%	1.6%
DeCatte, 2000	262	99.0%	3.1%*

* Loss before 22 weeks.

Which Procedure to Perform?

Whether to perform a first- or second-trimester procedure depends on a number of factors, including local availability of the procedures described. If both CVS and amniocentesis are available, the relative risks and the advantages of an earlier diagnosis need to be considered. Second-trimester amniocentesis is more readily available and technically easier to perform; however, CVS provides the information more than 1 month sooner, thus providing earlier reassurance. When discordant results are encountered, if selective termination is chosen, its complications and loss rates are markedly decreased if performed at less than 16 weeks' gestation (Evans et al., 1999).

Only one study to date has analyzed outcomes for twins after CVS compared with second-trimester amniocentesis (Wapner et al., 1993). In this work, 81 women had amniocentesis and 161 had CVS. Loss of the entire pregnancy before the 28th week followed amniocentesis in 2.9% of the cases and CVS in 3.2%. The fetal loss rate, which included loss of one fetus, was 9.3% for amniocentesis and 4.9% for CVS.

PERCUTANEOUS UMBILICAL BLOOD SAMPLING

In 1983, Daffos and coworkers described a method of obtaining fetal blood using ultrasound guidance of a 20- to 22-gauge spinal needle through the maternal abdomen into the umbilical cord. This technique (variously called PUBS, fetal blood sampling, cordocentesis, or funipuncture) offered considerable advantage in both efficacy and safety over the fetoscopic methods previously used to obtain fetal blood.

Until recently, a common reason for PUBS was the need for rapid karyotype. With the advent of rapid and safer cytogenetic diagnosis by either FISH of amniocytes or the rapid analysis of chorionic villi obtained by placental biopsy, the diagnostic indications for PUBS has changed. Currently, the primary genetic indication is evaluation of mosaic results found on amniocentesis or CVS. Most fetal mendelian disorders that previously required fetal blood for diagnosis are now made using molecular DNA analysis of amniocytes or chorionic villi. PUBS is only necessary for the rare cases in which the specific mutation is not known. The most frequent nongenetic indications are assessment for fetal anemia, infection, and thrombocytopenia. These indications are described in detail in Chapters 27, 30, 31, and 39.

The main complication of PUBS is fetal loss, which is estimated to be approximately 2% higher than background risk

(Daffos et al., 1985; Shulman and Elias, 1990). This exact risk is difficult to quantify because many of the fetuses studied had severe congenital malformations.

Best estimates for procedure-related risk are from the North American PUBS registry, which collected data from 16 centers in the United States and Canada. Information on 7462 diagnostic procedures performed on 6023 patients is available (Ludomirsky, 1993). Fetal loss is defined as intrauterine fetal death within 14 days of the procedure. The fetal loss rate in these cases is calculated to be 1.1% per procedure and 1.3% per patient.

The major causes for fetal loss were chorioamnionitis, rupture of membranes, puncture site bleeding, severe bradycardia, and thrombosis. The range of losses for participating centers varied from 1% to 6.7%, which reflects operator experience and differences in patient selection. These figures are subjective, relying on the operator's impression that a pregnancy loss was directly related to the procedure and not to the underlying fetal condition.

Technique of Percutaneous Umbilical Blood Sampling

Fetal vessels can be accessed within either the cord or the fetus itself. The cord is most reliably entered at the placental insertion site where it is anchored. Color Doppler imaging enhances visualization of the insertion site and is especially useful when oligohydramnios is present. Entering the cord near the umbilical insertion site or into a free loop is possible but can be more difficult. The hepatic vein is the most accessible and safe intrafetal location (Nicolini et al., 1990).

It is essential to verify that the blood sample is fetal in origin. The most definitive way to establish this is to compare the MCV of the retrieved red cells with a sample of maternal blood. This comparison is easily performed on small aliquots of blood by a standard channeling instrument. Fetal red blood cells are considerably larger than those of an adult, but the value is gestational age dependent. The mean MCV decreases from 145 fL at 16 weeks to 113 fL at 36 weeks of gestation (Alter et al., 1988). Alternatively, one can visually confirm appropriate location of the needle by injecting a small amount of sterile saline. If the needle is in the umbilical vein, microbubbles will be seen moving toward the fetus.

Forestier and colleagues (1988) recommended performing biochemical studies on the aspirated blood that include a complete blood count with differential analysis and determination of anti-I and anti-i cold agglutinin, β-hCG, factors IX and VIIIC, and AFP levels. It is not general practice to perform all these studies.

OTHER INVASIVE DIAGNOSTIC PROCEDURES

On infrequent occasions, analysis of other fetal tissues may be required. Fetal skin biopsies are performed to diagnosis fetal genetic skin disorders when molecular testing is not available. It can also be helpful in the workup of fetal mosaicism for chromosomes (such as 22) known not to be manifest in fetal blood (Berghella et al., 1998). Fetal muscle biopsy for dystrophin analysis is used to diagnose muscular dystrophy in a male fetus if DNA testing is not informative (Evans et al., 1995). Fetal

kidney biopsy has diagnosed congenital nephrosis in utero (Wapner et al., 2001), and aspiration and analysis of fetal urine is imperative in the preshunt evaluation of fetal renal function (Johnson et al., 1994). Each of these procedures is performed under ultrasound guidance. Because they are only rarely required, their use is usually confined to only a few regional referral centers in hopes of limiting procedural risk.

PREIMPLANTATION GENETIC DIAGNOSIS

Over the last two decades, methods of in vitro fertilization and embryo culture and transfer have developed into routine clinical practice. Simultaneously, advances in our knowledge of genomics and the introduction of increasingly sophisticated genetic diagnostic procedures now allow prenatal diagnoses to be performed even before pregnancy by testing one or two cells of a developing preimplantation embryo. This technique was developed initially to benefit patients at high risk for a fetal genetic disorder and for whom termination of an affected fetus was not an option. Most of these diagnoses were for relatively rare mendelian disorders. However, as the technology has progressed and the ability to perform cytogenetic analysis by FISH on single cells has improved, preimplantation genetic diagnosis (PGD) offers improved outcomes for in vitro fertilization patients, patients with repetitive miscarriages, and women of advanced maternal age.

The techniques available to retrieve preimplantation cells for diagnosis include polar body biopsy of prefertilized oocytes, biopsy of one or two cells (called blastomeres) from the 6- to 8-cell early cleavage stage embryo on day 3, or removal of 5 to 12 cells from the trophectoderm of the 5- to 7-day blastocyst (Harper and Delhanty, 2000). In all cases, removal of the cells is well tolerated, with continued development of the embryo and no increased risk of congenital anomalies (Hardy et al., 1990).

At present, the number of cycles performed worldwide exceeds 2500, yielding approximately 600 clinical pregnancies. The most common indication is chromosomal evaluation for aneuploidy, including evaluation for both structural rearrangements and numerical abnormalities. Reciprocal translocations are the most common structural anomaly for which PGD is used. Analysis of chromosome number using FISH for chromosomes 21, 13, 18, X, and Y is performed for maternal age, a previous child with aneuploidy, repeated in vitro fertilization failures, recurrent spontaneous abortions, or a combination of these.

As techniques have improved, cytogenetic results can be obtained in almost 90% of cases (Munne et al., 1995; Geraedts et al., 1999). However, clinical interpretive errors have occurred, probably because early-stage embryos are frequently mosaic, with mosaicism rates of 42% to 50% (Munne et al., 1995; Laverge et al., 1998). Abnormal-appearing zygotes have the highest rates of mosaicism (Munne et al., 1995; Kligman et al., 1996), but those appearing "normal" still carry a risk of approximately 20% (Munne et al., 1995). Rates of mosaicism within the inner cell mass are similar to those in trophoblast precursors (Evsikov and Verlinsky, 1998), showing that there is not a selection bias against aneuploid cells from integrating into the fetal precursor cells. Accordingly, the rate of misdiagnosis with one biopsied blastomere is at least 5.4%. In contrast to blastomere biopsy, no misdiagnosis of aneuploidy has been reported with polar body biopsy to date. However, secondary to the potential for error, invasive prenatal diagnosis by CVS or amniocentesis is still performed for appropriate indications even when PGD has been performed.

Aneuploid screening and preselection of normal embryos is now used to improve *in vitro* fertilization implantation and pregnancy rates even if no genetic indication for testing is present. When this is performed, about 40% of embryos are suitable for transfer. The success of this approach has led to its extended use to other indications, such as repetitive aborters with normal parental karyotypes and multiple *in vitro* fertilization failures.

PGD for monogenetic disorders requires the ability to evaluate the DNA of a single cell. To accomplish this, the DNA content of a single blastomere is amplified by PCR and then analyzed. The most common monogenetic disorders evaluated by PGD are CF, thalassemia, and spinal muscular atrophy among the autosomal recessive disorders; myotonic dystrophy, Huntington disease, and Charcot-Marie-Tooth disease among the dominant disorders; and fragile X, Duchenne/Becker muscular dystrophy, and hemophilia among the X-linked disorders. PGD is especially valuable for adult-onset autosomal disorders such as Huntington disease where the parents want to avoid the birth of an affected child but do not wish to have their own diagnosis confirmed. Using PGD, only unaffected zygotes can be implanted without informing the parents of whether the gene was present. However, to maintain parental nondisclosure, this approach must be performed on all subsequent pregnancies, even if no evidence of the gene is seen in prior cycles.

Although the molecular diagnosis is considered to be quite accurate, errors have occurred. For example, the PCR may fail or an error may occur as a result of a failure of a primer to anneal to the relevant sequence, a phenomenon called "allele dropout." This may lead to an incorrect diagnosis, especially when there is a compound heterozygote. Recent improvements in this technology have made these errors exceedingly uncommon, with some centers now reporting 100% accuracy. Despite this, invasive prenatal diagnosis should still be performed.

FETAL CELLS AND DNA WITHIN THE MATERNAL CIRCULATION

Cytogenetic evaluation of fetal cells retrieved from the maternal peripheral circulation for analysis has demonstrated potential to become a noninvasive diagnostic test (Bianchi, 2000). The most promising results have been with the retrieval of fetal nucleated red blood cells. This cell line appears to be the most appropriate target, because they have specific antigens that can be used to enhance isolation (Adinolfi, 1995) and contaminating maternal nucleated red cells are rare. Over the years, laboratory techniques such as diffusion gradients, fluorescent cell sorting, and magnetic cell separation have been used to improve the yield and concentration of the fetal cells. The staggeringly small number of fetal cells (0 to 20 cells within 20 mL of maternal blood) and their low concentration (one fetal cell per 100,000 to 10 million maternal cells) have hampered consistent retrieval. Despite this, there have been a number of reports of successful retrieval of aneuploid cells from the maternal circulation of women carrying affected pregnancies (Bianchi et al., 1994, 1997, 1999; de la Cruz et al., 1998).

Although fetal cell retrieval remains an intriguing option for noninvasive prenatal diagnosis, it is likely that routine feasibility will require the development of newer technologies. Work is underway on a number of possibilities. In one approach, computer scanning technology is being used that can rapidly survey the large number of cells on a slide and selectively identify those that are fetal. This technique requires the development of markers that are uniquely fetal, such as stains for early embryonic fetal hemoglobin. Once these rare cells are identified, there still remains the task of analyzing their genetic content. Although FISH for specific chromosomes has been used, fetal cell isolation and detection techniques cause cell injury, making FISH interpretation difficult and at times unreliable. The development of techniques to remove single cells from a slide and individually evaluate them using molecular technology is underway. Single-cell PCR may also allow the diagnosis of single-gene disorders (Hahn et al., 2000).

Free fetal DNA has also been detected within maternal plasma and has been explored as a potential approach to fetal diagnosis. This has certain technical advantages. It is less labor intensive because the amount of free fetal DNA is relatively greater than the number of fetal cells and may account for over 3% of the total DNA in a maternal sample (Lo et al., 1998). The free fetal DNA is suspected to be of placental (trophoblast) origin and is released into the maternal serum throughout pregnancy (Houfflin-Debarge et al., 1999). After delivery and removal of the placenta, the DNA disappears rapidly, with most women having complete clearance within 2 hours (Lo et al., 1999).

Prenatal diagnostic techniques using free fetal DNA are limited because the sequence of interest must be distinguishable from those of the mother; that is, mutations in the maternal DNA of a carrier mother cannot be differentiated from those of the fetus. This would prevent fetal diagnosis of an autosomal recessive disorder if the father carried the same mutation. However, if the father carries a mutation different from that of the mother, lack of detection of the paternal mutation in the maternal circulation would preclude the need for invasive testing. To diagnose an autosomal dominant disorder, the mutation would have to be of paternal origin.

An interesting and practical use of evaluating fetal DNA in the maternal circulation is the determination of fetal Rh-D status if the mother is Rh negative. This is possible because individuals who are Rh negative lack the D gene sequence. Therefore, detection of this sequence in a pregnant woman would identify an Rh-positive fetus and its absence an Rh-negative pregnancy. Presently, determination of fetal blood type in Rh-negative women can be performed with almost complete accuracy (Lo et al., 1998, 1999; Zhang et al., 2000).

REFERENCES

Achiron R, Rotstein Z, Lipitz S, et al: First-trimester diagnosis of fetal congenital heart disease by transvaginal ultrasonography. Obstet Gynecol **84**:69, 1994.

Adekunle O, Gopee A, el-Sayed M, et al: Increased first trimester nuchal translucency: Pregnancy and infant outcomes after routine screening for Down's syndrome in an unselected antenatal population. Br J Radiol **72**:457, 1999.

Adinolfi M: Non- or minimally invasive prenatal diagnostic tests on maternal blood samples or transcervical cells. Prenat Diagn **15**:889, 1995.

Akerman BR, Natowicz MR, Kaback MM, et al: Novel mutations and DNA-based screening in non-Jewish carriers of Tay-Sachs disease. Am J Hum Genet **60**:1099, 1997.

Alter BP, Goldberg JD, Berkowitz RL: Red cell size heterogeneity during ontogeny. Am J Pediatr Hemat Oncol 10:279, 1988.

American College of Medical Genetics position statement on carrier testing for Canavan disease. 1998.

American College of Obstetricians and Gynecologists Committee on Obstetrics Screening for Tay-Sachs Disease. Number 162. Washington, DC, American College of Obstetricians and Gynecologists, 1995.

American College of Obstetricians and Gynecologists Committee on Technical Bulletins. Ultrasonography in Pregnancy. Technical Bulletin Number 187. Washington, DC, American College of Obstetricians and Gynecologists, 1993.

American College of Obstetricians and Gynecologists position statement on screening for Canavan disease. 1998.

Anonymous: Randomized trial to assess safety and fetal outcome of early and midtrimester amniocentesis. The Canadian Early and Mid-Trimester Amniocentesis Trial (CEMAT) Group. Lancet 351:242, 1998.

Assel BG, Lewis SM, Dickerman LH, et al: Single-operator comparison of early and mid-second-trimester amniocentesis. Obstet Gynecol 79:940, 1992.

Bahado-Singh R, Deren O, Oz U, et al: An alternative for women initially declining genetic amniocentesis: Individual Down syndrome odds on the basis of maternal age and multiple ultrasonographic markers. Am J Obstet Gynecol 179:514, 1998.

Bahado-Singh R, Schmitt R, Hobbins J: New technique for genetic amniocentesis in twins. Obstet Gynecol 70:304, 1992.

Bahado-Singh R, Shahabi S, Karaca M, et al: The comprehensive midtrimester test: High-sensitivity Down syndrome test. Am J Obstet Gynecol 186:803, 2002.

Baird PA, Yee IM, Sadovnick AD: Population-based study of long-term outcomes after amniocentesis. Lancet 344:1134, 1994.

Barela AI, Kleinman GE, Golditch IM, et al: Septic shock with renal failure after chorionic villus sampling. Am J Obstet Gynecol 154:1100, 1986.

Bartels I, Hansmann I, Holland U, et al: Down syndrome at birth not detected by first-trimester chorionic villus sampling. Am J Med Genet 34:606, 1989.

Benacerraf BR, Gelman R, Frigoletto FD Jr: Sonographic identification of second-trimester fetuses with Down's syndrome. N Engl J Med 317:1371, 1987.

Benacerraf BR, Osathanondh R, Frigoletto FD: Sonographic demonstration of hypoplasia of the middle phalanx of the fifth digit: A finding associated with Down syndrome. Am J Obstet Gynecol 159:181, 1988.

Benn P: Trisomy 16 and trisomy 16 mosaicism: A review. Am J Med Genet 79:121, 1998.

Bennett MJ, Gibson KM, Sherwood WG, et al: Reliable prenatal diagnosis of Canavan disease (aspartoacylase deficiency): comparison of enzymatic and metabolite analysis. J Inherit Metab Dis 16:831, 1993.

Berend SA, Horwitz J, McCaskill C, et al: Identification of uniparental disomy following prenatal detection of Robertsonian translocations and isochromosomes. Am J Hum Genet 66:1787, 2000.

Berghella V, Wapner RJ, Yang-Feng T, et al: Prenatal confirmation of true fetal trisomy 22 mosaicism by fetal skin biopsy following normal fetal blood sampling. Prenat Diagn 18:384, 1998.

Berry E, Aitken DA, Crossley JA, et al: Analysis of maternal serum alpha-fetoprotein and free beta human chorionic gonadotrophin in the first trimester: implications for Down's syndrome screening. Prenat Diagn 15:555, 1995.

Bevis D: Composition of liquor amnii in haemolytic disease of the newborn. Lancet 2:443, 1950.

Bianchi DW: Fetal cells in the mother: from genetic diagnosis to diseases associated with fetal cell microchimerism. Eur J Obstet Gynaecol Reprod Biol 92:103, 2000.

Bianchi DW, Shuber AP, DeMaria MA, et al: Fetal cells in maternal blood: Determination of purity and yield by quantitative polymerase chain reaction. Am J Obstet Gynecol 171:922, 1994.

Bianchi DW, Simpson JL, Jackson LG, et al: Fetal cells in maternal blood: NIFTY clinical trial interim analysis. DM-STAT. NICHD fetal cell study (NIFTY) group. Prenat Diagn 19:994, 1999.

Bianchi DW, Williams JM, Sullivan LM, et al: PCR quantitation of fetal cells in maternal blood in normal and aneuploid pregnancies. Am J Hum Genet 61:822, 1997.

Bilardo CM, Pajkrt E, de Graaf I, et al: Outcome of fetuses with enlarged nuchal translucency and normal karyotype. Ultrasound Obstet Gynecol 11:401, 1998.

Bitzer MG, Kelley RI, Schwartz MF: Abnormal maternal serum marker pattern associated with Smith-Lemli-Opitz (SLO) syndrome. Am J Hum Genet 55:A277, 1994.

Blakemore KJ, Baumgarten A, Schoenfeld-Dimaio M, et al: Rise in maternal serum alpha-fetoprotein concentration after chorionic villus sampling and the possibility of isoimmunization. Am J Obstet Gynecol 155:988, 1986.

Blakemore K, Mahoney J, Hobbins J: Infection and chorionic villus sampling. Lancet 2:339, 1985.

Boehm FH, Salyer SL, Dev VG, et al: Chorionic villus sampling: quality control—A continuous improvement model. Am J Obstet Gynecol 168:1766, 1993.

Bogart MH, Pandian MR, Jones OW: Abnormal maternal serum chorionic gonadotropin levels in pregnancies with fetal chromosome abnormalities. Prenat Diagn 7:623, 1987.

Bombard AT, Powers JF, Carter S, et al: Procedure-related fetal losses in transplacental versus nontransplacental genetic amniocentesis. Am J Obstet Gynecol 172:868, 1995.

Borrell A, Costa D, Martinez JM, et al: Early midtrimester fetal nuchal thickness: Effectiveness as a marker of Down syndrome. Am J Obstet Gynecol 175:45, 1996.

Boyd PA, Wellesley DG, De Walle HE, et al: Evaluation of the prenatal diagnosis of neural tube defects by fetal ultrasonographic examination in different centres across Europe. J of Med Screen 7:169, 2000.

Bradley LA, Canick JA, Palomaki GE, et al: Undetectable maternal serum unconjugated estriol levels in the second trimester: Risk of perinatal complications associated with placental sulfatase deficiency. Am J Obstet Gynecol 176:531, 1997.

Bradley LA, Palomaki GE, Knight GJ, et al: Levels of unconjugated estriol and other maternal serum markers in pregnancies with Smith-Lemli-Opitz (RSH) syndrome fetuses. Am J Med Genet 82:355, 1999.

Braithwaite JM, Economides DL: The measurement of nuchal translucency with transabdominal and transvaginal sonography—Success rates, repeatability and levels of agreement. Br J Radiol 68:720, 1995.

Braithwaite JM, Morris RW, Economides DL: Nuchal translucency measurements: Frequency distribution and changes with gestation in a general population. Br J Obstet Gynaecol 103:1201, 1996.

Brambati B, Cislaghi C, Tului L, et al: First-trimester Down's syndrome screening using nuchal translucency: A prospective study in patients undergoing chorionic villus sampling. Ultrasound Obstet Gynecol 5:9, 1995.

Brambati B, Guercilena S, Bonacchi I, et al: Feto-maternal transfusion after chorionic villus sampling: Clinical implications. Hum Reprod 1:37, 1986.

Brambati B, Matarrelli M, Varotto F: Septic complications after chorionic villus sampling. Lancet 1:1212, 1987.

Brambati B, Oldrini A, Ferrazzi E, et al: Chorionic villus sampling: an analysis of the obstetric experience of 1,000 cases. Prenat Diagn 7:157, 1987.

Brambati B, Simoni G: Diagnosis of fetal trisomy 21 in first trimester. Lancet 1:586, 1983.

Brambati B, Simoni G, Travi M, et al: Genetic diagnosis by chorionic villus sampling before 8 gestational weeks: Efficiency, reliability, and risks on 317 completed pregnancies. Prenat Diagn 12:789, 1992.

Brambati B, Terzian E, Tognoni G: Randomized clinical trial of transabdominal versus transcervical chorionic villus sampling methods. Prenat Diagn 11:285, 1991.

Brambati B, Tului L, Lanzani A, et al: First-trimester genetic diagnosis in multiple pregnancy: Principles and potential pitfalls. Prenat Diagn 11:767, 1991.

Brambati B, Varotto F: Infection and chorionic villus sampling. Lancet 2:609, 1985.

Breed AS, Mantingh A, Vosters R, et al: Follow-up and pregnancy outcome after a diagnosis of mosaicism in CVS. Prenat Diagn 11:577, 1991.

Bromley B, Lieberman E, Shipp TD, et al: Significance of an echogenic intracardiac focus in fetuses at high and low risk for aneuploidy. J Ultrasound Med 17:127, 1998.

Bronshtein M, Siegler E, Yoffe N, et al: Prenatal diagnosis of ventricular septal defect and overriding aorta at 14 weeks' gestation, using transvaginal sonography. Prenat Diagn 10:697, 1990.

Broome DL, Wilson MG, Weiss B, et al: Needle puncture of fetus: a complication of second-trimester amniocentesis. Am J Obstet Gynecol 126:247, 1976.

Bui TH, Iselius L, Lindsten J: European collaborative study on prenatal diagnosis: Mosaicism, pseudomosaicism and single abnormal cells in amniotic fluid cell cultures. Prenat Diagn 4:145, 1984.

Burton BK, Prins GS, Verp MS: A prospective trial of prenatal screening for Down syndrome by means of maternal serum alpha-fetoprotein, human chorionic gonadotropin, and unconjugated estriol. Am J Obstet Gynecol 169:526, 1993.

Burton BK, Schulz CJ, Burd LI: Spectrum of limb disruption defects associated with chorionic villus sampling. Pediatrics 91:989, 1993.

Canadian Collaborative CVS/Amniocentesis Clinical Trial Group: Multicentre randomized clinical trial of chorionic villus sampling and amniocentesis. Lancet **1**:1, 1989.

Canick JA, Abuelo DN, Bradley LA, et al: Maternal serum marker levels in two pregnancies affected with Smith-Lemli-Opitz syndrome. Prenat Diagn **17**:187, 1997.

Canick JA, Knight GJ, Palomaki GE, et al: Low second trimester maternal serum unconjugated oestriol in pregnancies with Down's syndrome. Br J Obstet Gynaecol **95**:330, 1988.

Cao A, Saba L, Galanello R, et al: Molecular diagnosis and carrier screening for beta thalassemia. JAMA **278**:1273, 1997.

Carvalho JS, Moscoso G, Ville Y: First-trimester transabdominal fetal echocardiography. Lancet **351**:1023, 1998.

Cassidy SB, Lai LW, Erickson RP, et al: Trisomy 15 with loss of the paternal 15 as a cause of Prader-Willi syndrome due to maternal disomy. Am J Hum Genet **51**:701, 1992.

Chang HC, Jones OW, Masui H: Human amniotic fluid cells grown in a hormone-supplemented medium: Suitability for prenatal diagnosis. Proc Natl Acad Sci USA **79**:4795, 1982.

Chasen ST, Chervenak FA: What is the relationship between the universal use of ultrasound, the rate of detection of twins, and outcome differences? Clin Obstet Gynecol **41**:66, 1998.

Cheng EY, Luthy DA, Hickok DE, et al: Transcervical chorionic villus sampling and midtrimester oligohydramnios. Am J Obstet Gynecol **165**:1063, 1991.

Cheong Leung W, Chitayat D, Seaward G, et al: Role of amniotic fluid interphase fluorescence in situ hybridization (FISH) analysis in patient management. Prenat Diagn **21**:327, 2001.

Cheung SW, Crane JP, Beaver HA, et al: Chromosome mosaicism and maternal cell contamination in chorionic villi. Prenat Diagn **7**:535, 1987.

Cicero S, Curcio P, Papageorghiou A, et al: Absence of nasal bone in fetuses with trisomy 21 at 11–14 weeks of gestation: an observational study. Lancet **358**:1665, 2001.

Cole LA, Shahabi S, Oz UA, et al: Hyperglycosylated human chorionic gonadotropin (invasive trophoblast antigen) immunoassay: A new basis for gestational Down syndrome screening. Clin Chem **45**:2109, 1999.

Coleman B, Grumback K, Arger P, et al: Twin gestations: monitoring of complications and anomalies with ultrasound. Radiology **165**:449, 1987.

Comas C, Martinez JM, Ojuel J, et al: First-trimester nuchal edema as a marker of aneuploidy. Ultrasound Obstet Gynecol **5**:26, 1995.

Corteville JE, Gray DL, Langer JC: Bowel abnormalities in the fetus—Correlation of prenatal ultrasonographic findings with outcome. Am J Obstet Gynecol **175**:724, 1996.

Cragan JD, Martin ML, Khoury MJ, et al: Dye use during amniocentesis and birth defects. Lancet **341**:1352, 1993.

Crandall BF, Chua C: Risks for fetal abnormalities after very and moderately elevated AF-AFPs. Prenat Diagn **17**:837, 1997.

Crandall BF, Matsumoto M: Routine amniotic fluid alphafetoprotein assay: Experience with 40,000 pregnancies. Am J Med Genet **24**:143, 1986.

Crandall BF, Robinson L, Grau P: Risks associated with an elevated maternal serum alpha-fetoprotein level. Am J Obstet Gynecol **165**:581, 1991.

Crane JP, Gray DL: Sonographically measured nuchal skinfold thickness as a screening tool for Down syndrome: Results of a prospective clinical trial. Obstet Gynecol **77**:533, 1991.

Crane JP, LeFevre ML, Winborn RC, et al: A randomized trial of prenatal ultrasonographic screening: Impact on the detection, management, and outcome of anomalous fetuses. The RADIUS Study Group. Am J Obstet Gynecol **171**:392, 1994.

Crossley JA, Aitken DA, Cameron AD, et al: Combined ultrasound and biochemical screening for Down's syndrome in the first trimester: A Scottish multicentre study. BJOG **109**:667, 2002.

Crossley JA, Berry E, Aitken DA et al: Insulin-dependent diabetes mellitus and prenatal screening results: Current experience from a regional screening programme. Prenat Diagn **16**:1039, 1996.

Crow YJ, Tolmie JL, Crossley JA, et al: Maternal serum alpha-fetoprotein levels in congenital nephrosis. Prenat Diagn **17**:1089, 1997.

Cuckle H, Wald N, Stevenson JD, et al: Maternal serum alpha-fetoprotein screening for open neural tube defects in twin pregnancies. Prenat Diagn **10**:71, 1990.

Cuckle HS, van Lith JM: Appropriate biochemical parameters in first-trimester screening for Down syndrome. Prenat Diagn **19**:505, 1999.

Cuckle HS, Wald NJ, Lindenbaum RH: Maternal serum alpha-fetoprotein measurement: A screening test for Down syndrome. Lancet **1**:926, 1984.

Cullen MT, Gabrielli S, Green JJ, et al: Diagnosis and significance of cystic hygroma in the first trimester. Prenat Diagn **10**:643, 1990.

Curry CJ, Stevenson RE, Aughton D, et al: Evaluation of mental retardation: Recommendations of a Consensus Conference: American College of Medical Genetics. Am J Med Genet **72**:468, 1997.

Daffos F, Capella-Pavlovsky M, Forestier F: Fetal blood sampling via the umbilical cord using a needle guided by ultrasound. Report of 66 cases. Prenat Diagn **3**:271, 1983.

Daffos F, Capella-Pavlovsky M, Forestier F: Fetal blood sampling during pregnancy with use of a needle guided by ultrasound: a study of 606 consecutive cases. Am J Obstet Gynecol **153**:655, 1985.

De Catte L, Liebaers I, Foulon W: Outcome of twin gestations after first trimester chorionic villus sampling. Obstet Gynecol **96**:714, 2000.

de la Cruz F, Shifrin H, Elias S, et al: Low false-positive rate of aneuploidy detection using fetal cells isolated from maternal blood. Fetal Diagn Ther **13**:380, 1998.

Department of Obstetrics and Gynecology, Tietung Hospital of Anshan Iron and Steel Co., Anshan, China: Fetal sex prediction by sex chromatin of chorionic villi cells during early pregnancy. Chin Med J (Engl) **1**:117, 1975.

Devys D, Lutz Y, Rouyer N, et al: The FMR-1 protein is cytoplasmic, most abundant in neurons and appears normal in carriers of a fragile X premutation. Nat Genet **4**:335, 1993.

DiMaio MS, Baumgarten A, Greenstein RM, et al: Screening for fetal Down's syndrome in pregnancy by measuring maternal serum alpha-fetoprotein levels. N Engl J Med **317**:342, 1987.

Dolkart LA, Reimers FT: Transvaginal fetal echocardiography in early pregnancy: Normative data. Am J Obstet Gynecol **165**:688, 1991.

Donnenfeld AE: Sonographic screening for Down syndrome. Genet Teratol **1**:1, 1992.

Drugan A, Johnson MP, Evans MI: Ultrasound screening for fetal chromosome anomalies. Am J Med Genet **90**:98, 2000.

Dunstan FDJ, Nox ABJ: Screening for Down's syndrome: The effect of test date on the diction rate. Am Clin Biochem **35**:57, 1998.

Elias S, Gerbie A, Simpson J, et al: Genetic amniocentesis in twin gestations. Am J Obstet Gynecol **138**:169, 1980.

Elles RG, Williamson R, Niazi M, et al: Absence of maternal contamination of chorionic villi used for fetal-gene analysis. N Engl J Med **308**:1433, 1983.

Elpeleg ON, Shaag A, Anikster Y, et al: Prenatal detection of Canavan disease (aspartoacylase deficiency) by DNA analysis. J Inherit Metab Dis **17**:664, 1994.

Eng CM, Desnick RJ: Experiences in molecular-based prenatal screening for Ashkenazi Jewish genetic diseases. Adv Genet **44**:275, 2001.

Epley SL, Hanson JW, Cruikshank DP: Fetal injury with midtrimester diagnostic amniocentesis. Obstet Gynecol **53**:77, 1979.

Evans MI, Goldberg JD, Horenstein J, et al: Selective termination for structural, chromosomal, and mendelian anomalies: International experience. Am J Obstet Gynecol **181**:893, 1999.

Evans MI, Krivchenia EL, Johnson MP, et al: In utero fetal muscle biopsy alters diagnosis and carrier risks in Duchenne and Becker muscular dystrophy. Fetal Diagn Ther **10**:71, 1995.

Evsikov S, Verlinsky Y: Mosaicism in the inner cell mass of human blastocysts. Hum Reprod **13**:3151, 1998.

Filly RA, Crane JP: Routine obstetric sonography. J Ultrasound Med **21**:713, 2002.

Finegan JA, Quarrington BJ, Hughes HE, et al: Child outcome following midtrimester amniocentesis: Development, behaviour, and physical status at age 4 years. Br J Obstet Gynaecol **97**:32, 1990.

Firth HV, Boyd PA, Chamberlain P, et al: Severe limb abnormalities after chorion villus sampling at 56–66 days' gestation. Lancet **337**:762, 1991.

Flint J, Harding RM, Boyce AJ, et al: The population genetics of the haemoglobinopathies. Baillieres Clin Haematol **11**:1, 1998.

Forestier F, Cox WL, Daffos F, et al: The assessment of fetal blood samples. Am J Obstet Gynecol **158**:1184, 1988.

Franke P, Maier W, Hautzinger M, et al: Fragile-X carrier females: evidence for a distinct psychopathological phenotype? Am J Med Genet **64**:334, 1996.

Froster UG, Jackson L: Limb defects and chorionic villus sampling: results from an international registry, 1992–94. Lancet **347**:489, 1996.

Fu YH, Kuhl DP, Pizzuti A, et al: Variation of the CGG repeat at the fragile X site results in genetic instability: Resolution of the Sherman paradox. Cell **67**:1047, 1991.

Fuchs F, Riis P: Antenatal sex determination. Nature **177**:330, 1956.

Fukada Y, Yasumizu T, Takizawa M, et al: The prognosis of fetuses with transient nuchal translucency in the first and early second trimester. Acta Obstet Gynaecol Scand **76**:913, 1997.

Gardner RJM, Sutherland GR: Chromosome Abnormalities and Genetic Counseling. New York, Oxford University Press, 1996, p. 243.

Gembruch U, Knopfle G, Bald R, et al: Early diagnosis of fetal congenital heart disease by transvaginal echocardiography. Ultrasound Obstet Gynecol 3:310, 1993.

Gembruch U, Knopfle G, Chatterjee M, et al: First-trimester diagnosis of fetal congenital heart disease by transvaginal two-dimensional and Doppler echocardiography. Obstet Gynecol 75:496, 1990.

Geraedts J, Handyside A, Harper J, et al: ESHRE Preimplantation Genetic Diagnosis (PGD) Consortium: Preliminary assessment of data from January 1997 to September 1998. ESHRE PGD Consortium Steering Committee. Hum Reprod 14:3138, 1999.

Ghidini A, Alvarez M, Silverberg G, et al: Congenital nephrosis in low-risk pregnancies. Prenat Diagn 14:599, 1994.

Ghidini A, Lynch L, Hicks C, et al: The risk of second-trimester amniocentesis in twin gestations: A case-control study. Am J Obstet Gynecol 169:1013, 1993.

Golbus MS, Loughman WD, Epstein CJ, et al: Prenatal genetic diagnosis in 3000 amniocenteses. N Engl J Med 300:157, 1979.

Goldberg JD, Porter AE, Golbus MS: Current assessment of fetal losses as a direct consequence of chorionic villus sampling. Am J Med Genet 35:174, 1990.

Gosden C, Nicolaides KH, Rodeck CH: Fetal blood sampling in investigation of chromosome mosaicism in amniotic fluid cell culture. Lancet 1:613, 1988.

Gravel RA, Kaback MM, Proia RL, et al: The GM2 gangliosidoses. In Scriver CR, Beaudet AL, Sly WS, et al (eds): The Metabolic and Molecular Bases of Inherited Diseases, vol 3, 8th ed. New York, McGraw-Hill, 2001, p. 3827.

Gray RG, Green A, Cole T, et al: A misdiagnosis of X-linked adrenoleukodystrophy in cultured chorionic villus cells by the measurement of very long chain fatty acids. Prenat Diagn 15:486, 1995.

Grebner EE, Jackson LG: Prenatal diagnosis of Tay-Sachs disease: Studies on the reliability of hexosaminidase levels in amniotic fluid. Am J Obstet Gynecol 134:547, 1979.

Grebner EE, Jackson LG: Prenatal diagnosis of neurolipidoses. Ann Clin Lab Sci 12:381, 1982.

Grebner EE, Jackson LG: Prenatal diagnosis for Tay-Sachs disease using chorionic villus sampling. Prenat Diagn 5:313, 1985.

Gregson N, Seabright N: Handling of chorionic villi for direct chromosome studies. Lancet 2:1491, 1983.

Grody WW, Cutting GR, Klinger KW, et al: Laboratory standards and guidelines for population-based cystic fibrosis carrier screening. Genet Med 3:149, 2001.

Haddow J, Palomaki G: Prenatal screening for Down syndrome. In Simpson J, Elias S (eds): Essentials of Prenatal Diagnosis. New York, Churchill Livingstone, 1993, p. 185.

Haddow JE, Palomaki GE, Knight GJ, et al: Prenatal screening for Down's syndrome with use of maternal serum markers. N Engl J Med 327:588, 1992.

Haddow JE, Palomaki GE, Knight GJ, et al: Reducing the need for amniocentesis in women 35 years of age or older with serum markers for screening. N Engl J Med 330:1114, 1994.

Hafner E, Schuchter K, Liebhart E, et al: Results of routine fetal nuchal translucency measurement at weeks 10–13 in 4233 unselected pregnant women. Prenat Diagn 18:29, 1998.

Hagerman RJ: Medical follow-up and pharmacotherapy. In Hagerman RJ, Cronister A (eds): Fragile X Syndrome: Diagnosis, Treatment and Research, 2nd ed. Baltimore, The Johns Hopkins University Press, 1996, p. 283.

Hahn S, Zhong XY, Troeger C, et al: Current applications of single-cell PCR. Cell Mol Life Sci 57:96, 2000.

Hahnemann N: Early prenatal diagnosis; a study of biopsy techniques and cell culturing from extraembryonic membranes. Clin Genet 6:294, 1974.

Hahnemann N, Mohr J: Genetic diagnosis in the embryo by means of biopsy from extraembryonic membranes. Bull Eur Soc Hum Genet 2:23, 1968.

Hallman N, Hjelt L: Congenital nephrotic syndrome. J Pediatr 55:152, 1959.

Hanson F, Tennant F, Hune S, et al: Early amniocentesis: outcome, risks, and technical problems at less than or equal to 12.8 weeks. Am J Obstet Gynecol 166:1707, 1992.

Hardy K, Martin KL, Leese HJ, et al: Human preimplantation development in vitro is not adversely affected by biopsy at the 8-cell stage. Hum Reprod 5:708, 1990.

Harper JC, Delhanty JD: Preimplantation genetic diagnosis. Curr Opin Obstet Gynecol 12:67, 2000.

Heinonen S, Ryynanen M, Kirkinen P, et al: Prenatal screening for congenital nephrosis in east Finland: Results and impact on the birth prevalence of the disease. Prenat Diagn 16:207, 1996.

Henry GP, Miller WA: Early amniocentesis. J Reprod Med 37:396, 1992.

Herman A, Maymon R, Dreazen E, et al: Utilization of the nuchal translucency image-scoring method during training of new examiners. Fetal Diagn Ther 14:234, 1999.

Hernadi L, Torocsik M: Screening for fetal anomalies in the 12th week of pregnancy by transvaginal sonography in an unselected population. Prenat Diagn 17:753, 1997.

Hewitt B: Nuchal translucency in the first trimester. Aust N Z J Obstet Gynaecol 33:389, 1993.

Hewitt BG, de Crespigny L, Sampson AJ, et al: Correlation between nuchal thickness and abnormal karyotype in first trimester fetuses. Med J Aust 165:365, 1996.

Heyl PS, Miller W, Canick JA: Maternal serum screening for aneuploid pregnancy by alpha-fetoprotein, hCG, and unconjugated estriol. Obstet Gynecol 76:1025, 1990.

Hill LM, Platt LD, Kellogg B: Rh sensitization after genetic amniocentesis. Obstet Gynecol 56:459, 1980.

Hogge WA, Schonberg SA, Golbus MS: Chorionic villus sampling: experience of the first 1000 cases. Am J Obstet Gynecol 154:1249, 1986.

Holmberg C, Jalanko H, Koskimies O, et al: Renal transplantation in small children with congenital nephrotic syndrome of the Finnish type. Transplant Proc 23:1378, 1991.

Hook EB: Rates of chromosome abnormalities at different maternal ages. Obstet Gynecol 58:282, 1981.

Houfflin-Debarge V, O'Donnell H, Overton T, et al: High sensitivity of fetal DNA in plasma compared to serum and nucleated cells using unnested PCR in maternal blood. Fetal Diagn Ther 15:102, 1999.

Hsu LY, Perlis TE: United States survey on chromosome mosaicism and pseudomosaicism in prenatal diagnosis. Prenat Diagn 4:97, 1984.

Huang T, Watt H, Wald N: The effect of differences in the distribution of maternal age in England and Wales on the performance of prenatal screening for Down's syndrome. Prenat Diagn 17:615, 1997.

Huisman THJ, Carver MFH, Baysal E: A Syllabus of Thalassemia Mutations. Augusta, Ga, The Sickle Cell Anemia Foundation, 1997.

Hyett J, Moscoso G, Nicolaides K: Increased nuchal translucency in trisomy 21 fetuses: Relationship to narrowing of the aortic isthmus. Hum Reprod 10:3049, 1995a.

Hyett J, Moscoso G, Nicolaides K: Morphometric analysis of the great vessels in early fetal life. Hum Reprod 10:3045, 1995b.

Hyett J, Moscoso G, Nicolaides KH: Cardiac defects in 1st-trimester fetuses with trisomy 18. Fetal Diagn Ther 10:381, 1995c.

Hyett J, Moscoso G, Nicolaides KH: First-trimester nuchal translucency and cardiac septal defects in fetuses with trisomy 21. Am J Obstet Gynecol 172:1411, 1995d.

Hyett J, Moscoso G, Nicolaides K: Abnormalities of the heart and great arteries in first trimester chromosomally abnormal fetuses. Am J Med Genet 69:207, 1997.

Hyett J, Perdu M, Sharland GK, et al: Increased nuchal translucency at 10–14 weeks of gestation as a marker for major cardiac defects. Ultrasound Obstet Gynecol 10:242, 1997.

Hyett J, Perdu M, Sharland G, et al: Using fetal nuchal translucency to screen for major congenital cardiac defects at 10–14 weeks of gestation: Population based cohort study. Br Med J 318:81, 1999.

Hyett JA, Sebire NJ, Snijders RJ, et al: Intrauterine lethality of trisomy 21 fetuses with increased nuchal translucency thickness. Ultrasound Obstet Gynecol 7:101, 1996.

Jackson LG, Zachary JM, Fowler SE, et al: A randomized comparison of transcervical and transabdominal chorionic-villus sampling. The U.S. National Institute of Child Health and Human Development Chorionic-Villus Sampling and Amniocentesis Study Group. N Engl J Med 327:594, 1992.

Jacobson C, Barter R: Intrauterine diagnosis and management of genetic defects. Am J Obstet Gynecol 99:795, 1967.

Jeanty P, Shah D, Roussis P: Single-needle insertion in twin amniocentesis. J Ultrasound Med 9:511, 1990.

Jenkins TM, Wapner RJ: Integrated screening for Down's syndrome. N Engl J Med 341:1935, 1999.

Johnson A, Wapner RJ: Mosaicism: implications for postnatal outcome. Curr Opin Obstet Gynecol 9:126, 1997.

Johnson A, Wapner RJ, Davis GH, et al: Mosaicism in chorionic villus sampling: An association with poor perinatal outcome. Obstet Gynecol 75:573, 1990.

Johnson JM, Wilson RD, Singer J, et al: Technical factors in early amniocentesis predict adverse outcome. Results of the Canadian Early (EA) versus Mid-trimester (MA) Amniocentesis Trial. Prenat Diagn 19:732, 1999.

Johnson M, Bukowdki T, Reitleman C, et al: In utero surgical treatment of fetal obstructive uropathy: A new comprehensive approach to identify appropriate candidates for vesicoamniotic shunt therapy. Am J Obstet Gynecol 170:1770, 1994.

Johnson MP, Barr M Jr, Treadwell MC, et al: Fetal leg and femur/foot length ratio: A marker for trisomy 21. Am J Obstet Gynecol **169**:557, 1993.

Johnson MP, Johnson A, Holzgreve W, et al: First-trimester simple hygroma: Cause and outcome. Am J Obstet Gynecol **168**:156, 1993.

Kaback M, Lim-Steele J, Dabholkar D, et al: Tay-Sachs disease—Carrier screening, prenatal diagnosis, and the molecular era. An international perspective, 1970 to 1993. The International TSD Data Collection Network. JAMA **270**:2307, 1993.

Kaback MM: Population-based genetic screening for reproductive counseling: The Tay-Sachs disease model. Eur J Pediatr **159** (Suppl 3):S192, 2000.

Kalousek DK, Dill FJ, Pantzar T, et al: Confined chorionic mosaicism in prenatal diagnosis. Hum Genet **77**:163, 1987.

Kalousek DK, Howard-Peebles PN, Olson SB, et al: Confirmation of CVS mosaicism in term placentae and high frequency of intrauterine growth retardation association with confined placental mosaicism. Prenat Diagn **11**:743, 1991.

Kalousek DK, Langlois S, Barrett I, et al: Uniparental disomy for chromosome 16 in humans. Am J Hum Genet **52**:8, 1993.

Karkut I, Zakrzewski S, Sperling K: Mixed karyotypes obtained by chorionic villi analysis: Mosaicism and maternal contamination. *In* Fraccaro M, et al. (ed): First Trimester Fetal Diagnosis. Heidelberg, Springer-Verlag, 1985.

Karp LE, Hayden PW: Fetal puncture during midtrimester amniocentesis. Obstet Gynecol **49**:115, 1977.

Kaul R, Gao GP, Aloya M, et al: Canavan disease: mutations among Jewish and non-Jewish patients. Am J Hum Genet **55**:34, 1994.

Kaul R, Gao GP, Balamurugan K, et al: Spectrum of Canavan mutations among Jewish and non-Jewish patients. Am J Hum Genet **55**:A212, 1994.

Kaul R, Gao GP, Matalon R, et al: Identification and expression of eight novel mutations among non-Jewish patients with Canavan disease. Am J Hum Genet **59**:95, 1996.

Kazy Z, Rozovdky I, Bakhaev V: Chorion biopsy in early pregnancy: a method of early prenatal diagnosis for inherited disorders. Prenat Diagn **2**:39, 1982.

Kelley RI: Prenatal detection of Canavan disease by measurement of N-acetyl-L-aspartate in amniotic fluid. J Inherit Metab Dis **16**:918, 1993.

Kestila M, Lenkkeri U, Mannikko M, et al: Positionally cloned gene for a novel glomerular protein–nephrin is mutated in congenital nephrotic syndrome. Mol Cell **1**:575, 1998.

Kher AS, Chattopadhyay A, Datta S, et al: Familial mosaic Turner syndrome. Clin Genet **46**:382, 1994.

Kidd S, Lancaster P, Anderson J, et al: Fetal death after exposure to methylene blue dye during mid-trimester amniocentesis in twin pregnancy. Prenat Diagn **16**:39, 1996.

Kishida T, Yamada H, Sagawa T, et al: Spontaneous reseal of high-leak PROM following genetic amniocentesis. Int J Gynaecol Obstet **47**:55, 1994.

Kjessler B, Johansson SG, Sherman M, et al: Alpha-fetoprotein in antenatal diagnosis of congenital nephrosis. Lancet **1**:432, 1975.

Kligman I, Benadiva C, Alikani M, et al: The presence of multinucleated blastomeres in human embryos is correlated with chromosomal abnormalities. Hum Reprod **11**:1492, 1996.

Klinger K, Landes G, Shook D, et al: Rapid detection of chromosome aneuploidies in uncultured amniocytes by using fluorescence in situ hybridization (FISH). Am J Hum Genet **51**:55, 1992.

Kowalczyk TD, Cabaniss ML, Cusmano L: Association of low unconjugated estriol in the second trimester and adverse pregnancy outcome. Obstet Gynecol **91**:396, 1998.

Krantz DA, Hallahan TW, Orlandi F, et al: First-trimester Down syndrome screening using dried blood biochemistry and nuchal translucency. Obstet Gynecol **96**:207, 2000.

Krantz DA, Larsen JW, Buchanan PD, et al: First-trimester Down syndrome screening: Free beta-human chorionic gonadotropin and pregnancy-associated plasma protein A. Am J Obstet Gynecol **174**:612, 1996.

Kratz LE, Kelley RI: Prenatal diagnosis of the RSH/Smith-Lemli-Opitz syndrome. Am J Med Genet **82**:376, 1999.

Kronn D, Oddoux C, Phillips J, et al: Prevalence of Canavan disease heterozygotes in the New York metropolitan Ashkenazi Jewish population. Am J Hum Genet **57**:1250, 1995.

Kullander S, Sandahl B: Fetal chromosome analysis after transcervical placental biopsies during early pregnancy. Acta Obstet Gynecol Scand **52**:355, 1973.

Kuller JA, Sellati LE, Chescheir NC, et al: Outcome of pregnancies with elevation of both maternal serum alpha-fetoprotein and human chorionic gonadotropin. Am J Perinatol **12**:93, 1995.

Lamb MP: Gangrene of a fetal limb due to amniocentesis. Br J Obstet Gynaecol **82**:829, 1975.

Lambl D: Ein seltener Fall von Hydramnios. Zentrabl Gynaskol **5**:329, 1881.

Laverge H, Van der Elst J, De Sutter P, et al: Fluorescent in-situ hybridization on human embryos showing cleavage arrest after freezing and thawing. Hum Reprod **13**:425, 1998.

Ledbetter DH, Engel E: Uniparental disomy in humans: development of an imprinting map and its implications for prenatal diagnosis. Hum Mol Genet **4**:1757, 1995.

Ledbetter DH, Martin AO, Verlinsky Y, et al: Cytogenetic results of chorionic villus sampling: High success rate and diagnostic accuracy in the United States collaborative study. Am J Obstet Gynecol **162**:495, 1990.

Ledbetter DH, Zachary JM, Simpson JL, et al: Cytogenetic results from the U.S. Collaborative Study on CVS. Prenat Diagn **12**:317, 1992.

Lejeune J: Les chromosomes humains en culture de tissues. C R Acad Sci **248**:602, 1959.

Lenke RR, Ashwood ER, Cyr DR, et al: Genetic amniocentesis: Significance of intraamniotic bleeding and placental location. Obstet Gynecol **65**:798, 1985.

Lenke RR, Cyr DR, Mack LA: Midtrimester genetic amniocentesis with simultaneous ultrasound guidance. J Clin Ultrasound **13**:371, 1985.

Lenkkeri U, Mannikko M, McCready P, et al: Structure of the gene for congenital nephrotic syndrome of the Finnish type (NPHS1) and characterization of mutations. Am J Hum Genet **64**:51, 1999.

Lennon CA, Gray DL: Sensitivity and specificity of ultrasound for the detection of neural tube and ventral wall defects in a high-risk population. Obstet Gynecol **94**:562, 1999.

Liu D, Agbaje R, Preston C, et al: Intraplacental sonolucent spaces: incidences and relevance to chorionic villus sampling. Prenat Diagn **11**:805, 1991.

Lo Y, Zhang J, Leung T, et al: Rapid clearance of fetal DNA from maternal plasma. Am J Hum Genet **64**:218, 1999.

Lo YM, Tein MS, Lau TK, et al: Quantitative analysis of fetal DNA in maternal plasma and serum: Implications for noninvasive prenatal diagnosis. Am J Hum Genet **62**:768, 1998.

Ludomirsky A: Intrauterine fetal blood sampling—A multicenter registry. Evaluation of 7462 procedures between 1987–1991 (abstr). Am J Obstet Gynecol **168**:318, 1993.

Lynch L, Berkowitz RL, Stone J, et al: Preterm delivery after selective termination in twin pregnancies. Obstet Gynecol **87**:366, 1996.

MacDonald ML, Wagner RM, Slotnick RN: Sensitivity and specificity of screening for Down syndrome with alpha-fetoprotein, hCG, unconjugated estriol, and maternal age. Obstet Gynecol **77**:63, 1991.

MacGregor SN, Tamura R, Sabbagha R, et al: Isolated hyperechoic fetal bowel: Significance and implications for management. Am J Obstet Gynecol **173**:1254, 1995.

Macri JN, Spencer K, Garver K, et al: Maternal serum free beta hCG screening: results of studies including 480 cases of Down syndrome. Prenat Diagn **14**:97, 1994.

Maddalena A, Richards CS, McGinniss MJ, et al: Technical standards and guidelines for fragile X: The first of a series of disease-specific supplements to the Standards and Guidelines for Clinical Genetics Laboratories of the American College of Medical Genetics. Quality Assurance Subcommittee of the Laboratory Practice Committee. Genet Med **3**:200, 2001.

Marthin T, Liedgren S, Hammar M: Transplacental needle passage and other risk-factors associated with second trimester amniocentesis. Acta Obstet Gynaecol Scand **76**:728, 1997.

Martin A, Elias S, Rosinsky B, et al: False-negative findings on chorionic villus sampling. Lancet **2**:391, 1986.

Martin AO, Simpson JL, Rosinsky BJ, et al: Chorionic villus sampling in continuing pregnancies. II. Cytogenetic reliability. Am J Obstet Gynecol **154**:1353, 1986.

Mastroiacovo P, Botto LD, Cavalcanti DP, et al: Limb anomalies following chorionic villus sampling: A registry based case-control study. Am J Med Genet **44**:856, 1992.

Matalon R, Michals K, Kaul R: Canavan disease: From spongy degeneration to molecular analysis. J Pediatr **127**:511, 1995.

Matalon R, Michals-Matalon K: Molecular basis of Canavan disease. Eur J Paediatr Neurol **2**:69, 1998.

McFadyen I, Taylor-Robinson D, Furr P, et al: Infections and chorionic villus sampling. Lancet **2**:610, 1985.

Medical Research Council: Diagnosis of Genetic Disease by Amniocentesis during the Second Trimester of Pregnancy. Ottawa, Canada, MRC, 1977.

Megory E, Weiner E, Shalev E, et al: Pseudomonoamniotic twins with cord entanglement following genetic funipuncture. Obstet Gynecol **78**:915, 1991.

Mennuti MT, Thomson E, Press N: Screening for cystic fibrosis carrier state. Obstet Gynecol **93**:456, 1999.

Merin M, Beyth Y: Uniocular congenital blindness as a complication of midtrimester amniocentesis. Am J Ophthalmol **89**:299, 1980.

Merkatz IR, Nitowsky HM, Macri JN, et al: An association between low maternal serum alpha-fetoprotein and fetal chromosomal abnormalities. Am J Obstet Gynecol **148**:886, 1984.

Meyers C, Adam R, Dungan J, et al: Aneuploidy in twin gestations: When is maternal age advanced? Obstet Gynecol **89**:248, 1997.

Mikkelsen M, Ayme S: Chromosomal findings in chorionic villi. *In* Vogel F, Sperling K (ed): Human Genetics. Heidelberg, Springer-Verlag, 1987.

Moise KJ Jr, Carpenter RJ Jr: Increased severity of fetal hemolytic disease with known rhesus alloimmunization after first-trimester transcervical chorionic villus biopsy. Fetal Diagn Ther **5**:76, 1990.

Morris JK, Wald NJ, Watt HC: Fetal loss in Down syndrome pregnancies. Prenat Diagn **19**:142, 1999.

Morssink LP, Kornman LH, Beekhuis JR, et al: Abnormal levels of maternal serum human chorionic gonadotropin and alpha-fetoprotein in the second trimester: Relation to fetal weight and preterm delivery. Prenat Diagn **15**:1041, 1995.

Moselhi M, Thilaganathan B: Nuchal translucency: A marker for the antenatal diagnosis of aortic coarctation. Br J Obstet Gynaecol **103**:1044, 1996.

MRC Working Party on the Evaluation of Chorion Villus Sampling: Medical Research Council European trial of chorion villus sampling. Lancet **337**:1491, 1991.

Munne S, Sultan KM, Weier HU, et al: Assessment of numeric abnormalities of X, Y, 18, and 16 chromosomes in preimplantation human embryos before transfer. Am J Obstet Gynecol **172**:1191, 1995.

Nadel A, Bromley B, Benacerraf BR: Nuchal thickening or cystic hygromas in first- and early second-trimester fetuses: Prognosis and outcome. Obstet Gynecol **82**:43, 1993.

Nadel AS, Bromley BS, Frigoletto FD Jr, et al: Isolated choroid plexus cysts in the second-trimester fetus: Is amniocentesis really indicated? Radiology **185**:545, 1992.

Nava S, Godmilow L, Reeser S, et al: Significance of sonographically detected second-trimester choroid plexus cysts: A series of 211 cases and a review of the literature. Ultrasound Obstet Gynecol **4**:448, 1994

Neveux LM, Palomaki GE, Knight GJ, et al: Multiple marker screening for Down syndrome in twin pregnancies. Prenat Diagn **16**:29, 1996.

New England Regional Genetics Group position statement on carrier testing for Canavan disease. 2/2000.

New England Regional Genetics Group Prenatal Collaborative Study of Down Syndrome Screening: Combining maternal serum alpha-fetoprotein, human chorionic gonadotropin, and unconjugated estriol. Am J Obstet Gynecol **169**:526, 1989.

NICHD Amniocentesis Registry: Midtrimester amniocentesis for prenatal diagnosis: Safety and accuracy. JAMA **236**:1471, 1976.

NICHD Amniocentesis Registry: The Safety and Accuracy of Mid-Trimester Amniocentesis. DHEW Publication No. (NIH) 78-190. Washington, DC, Department of Health, Education and Welfare, 1978.

Nicolaides K, Brizot Mde L, Patel F, et al: Comparison of chorionic villus sampling and amniocentesis for fetal karyotyping at 10–13 weeks' gestation. Lancet **344**:435, 1994.

Nicolaides KH, Azar G, Byrne D, et al: Fetal nuchal translucency: ultrasound screening for chromosomal defects in first trimester of pregnancy. BMJ **304**:867, 1992.

Nicolaides KH, Campbell S, Gabbe SG, et al: Ultrasound screening for spina bifida: Cranial and cerebellar signs. Lancet **2**:72, 1986.

Nicolaides KH, Sebire NJ, Snijders RJM: The 11–14 Week Scan. New York, Parthenon, 1999.

Nicolini U, Monni G: Intestinal obstruction in babies exposed in utero to methylene blue. Lancet **336**:1258, 1990.

Nicolini U, Nicolaidis P, Fisk NM, et al: Fetal blood sampling from the intrahepatic vein: Analysis of safety and clinical experience with 214 procedures. Obstet Gynecol **76**:47, 1990.

Nolin SL, Lewis FA 3rd, Ye LL, et al: Familial transmission of the FMR1 CGG repeat. Am J Hum Genet **59**:1252, 1996.

Nyberg DA, Luthy DA, Resta RG, et al: Age-adjusted ultrasound risk assessment for fetal Down's syndrome during the second trimester: Description of the method and analysis of 142 cases. Ultrasound Obstet Gynecol **12**:8, 1998.

Nyberg DA, Resta RG, Hickok DE, et al: Femur length shortening in the detection of Down syndrome: Is prenatal screening feasible? Am J Obstet Gynecol **162**:1247, 1990.

Nyberg DA, Resta RG, Luthy DA, et al: Humerus and femur length shortening in the detection of Down's syndrome. Am J Obstet Gynecol **168**:534, 1993.

Nyberg DA, Resta RG, Mahony T, et al: Fetal hyperechogenic bowel and Down's syndrome. Ultrasound Obstet Gynecol **3**:330, 1993.

Nyberg DA, Souter VL, El-Bastawissi A, et al: Isolated sonographic markers for detection of fetal Down syndrome in the second trimester of pregnancy. J Ultrasound Med **20**:1053, 2001.

O'Brien JE, Dvorin E, Drugan A, et al: Race-ethnicity-specific variation in multiple-marker biochemical screening: Alpha-fetoprotein, hCG, and estriol. Obstet Gynecol **89**:355 1997.

Old JM, Ward RH, Petrou M, et al: First-trimester fetal diagnosis for haemoglobinopathies: Three cases. Lancet **2**:1413, 1982.

Olney RS, Khoury MJ, Botto LD, et al: Limb defects and gestational age at chorionic villus sampling. Lancet **344**:476, 1994.

Oostra BA, Willemsen R: Diagnostic tests for fragile X syndrome. Expert Rev Mol Diagn **1**:226, 2001.

Pajkrt E, Mol BW, Boer K, et al: Intra- and interoperator repeatability of the nuchal translucency measurement. Ultrasound Obstet Gynecol **15**:297, 2000.

Pajkrt E, van Lith JM, Mol BW, et al: Screening for Down's syndrome by fetal nuchal translucency measurement in a general obstetric population. Ultrasound Obstet Gynecol **12**:163, 1998.

Paladini D, Tartaglione A, Agangi A, et al: The association between congenital heart disease and Down syndrome in prenatal life. Ultrasound Obstet Gynecol **15**:104, 2000.

Palomaki GE, Bradley LA, Knight GJ, et al: Assigning risk for Smith-Lemli-Opitz syndrome as part of 2nd trimester screening for Down's syndrome. J Med Screen **9**:43, 2002.

Pandya PP, Altman DG, Brizot ML, et al: Repeatability of measurement of fetal nuchal translucency thickness. Ultrasound Obstet Gynecol **5**:334, 1995.

Pandya PP, Brizot ML, Kuhn P, et al: First-trimester fetal nuchal translucency thickness and risk for trisomies. Obstet Gynecol **84**:420, 1994.

Pandya PP, Kondylios A, Hilbert L, et al: Chromosomal defects and outcome in 1015 fetuses with increased nuchal translucency. Ultrasound Obstet Gynecol **5**:15, 1995.

Penso CA, Sandstrom MM, Garber MF, et al: Early amniocentesis: Report of 407 cases with neonatal follow-up. Obstet Gynecol **76**:1032, 1990.

Perella R, Duerinckx AJ, Grant EG, et al: Second-trimester sonographic diagnosis of Down syndrome: Role of femur-length shortening and nuchal-fold thickening. AJR Am J Roentgenol **151**:981, 1988.

Pergament E: The application of fluorescence in-situ hybridization to prenatal diagnosis. Curr Opin Obstet Gynecol **12**:73, 2000.

Pergament E, Schulman JD, Copeland K, et al: The risk and efficacy of chorionic villus sampling in multiple gestations. Prenat Diagn **12**:377, 1992.

Phillips O, Tharapel A, Lerner J, et al: Risk of fetal mosaicism when placental mosaicism is diagnosed by chorionic villus sampling. Am J Obstet Gynecol **174**:850, 1996.

Poenaru L: First trimester prenatal diagnosis of metabolic diseases: a survey in countries from the European community. Prenat Diagn **7**:333, 1987.

Porto M, Murata Y, Warneke LA, et al: Fetal choroid plexus cysts: an independent risk factor for chromosomal anomalies. J Clin Ultrasound **21**:103, 1993.

Post JG, Nijhuis JG: Trisomy 16 confined to the placenta. Prenat Diagn **12**:1001, 1992.

Pretorious D, Budorick N, Scioscia A, et al: Twin pregnancies in the second trimester in an α-fetoprotein screening program: Sonographic evaluation and outcome. AJR Am J Roentgenol **161**:1001, 1993.

Prompelan H, Madiam H, Schillinger H: Prognose von sonographisch früh diagnostizierter awillingsschwangerschafter. Geburtsh Frauv **49**:715, 1989.

Pruggmayer M, Johoda M, Van der Pol J: Genetic amniocentesis in twin pregnancies: Results of a multicenter study of 529 cases. Ultrasound Obstet Gynecol **2**:6, 1992.

Purvis-Smith SG, Saville T, Manass S, et al: Uniparental disomy 15 resulting from "correction" of an initial trisomy 15. Am J Hum Genet **50**:1348, 1992.

Rapola J: Renal pathology of fetal congenital nephrosis. Acta Pathol Microbiol Scand [A] **89**:63, 1981.

Renier MA, Vereecken A, Van Herck E, et al: Second trimester maternal dimeric inhibin-A in the multiple-marker screening test for Down's syndrome. Hum Reprod **13**:744, 1998.

Reynders CS, Pauker SP, Benacerraf BR: First trimester isolated fetal nuchal lucency: Significance and outcome. J Ultrasound Med **16**:101, 1997.

Rhoads GG, Jackson LG, Schlesselman SE, et al: The safety and efficacy of chorionic villus sampling for early prenatal diagnosis of cytogenetic abnormalities. N Engl J Med **320**:609, 1989.

Rickwood AM: A case of ileal atresia and ileocutaneous fistula caused by amniocentesis. J Pediatr **91**:312, 1977.

Riddle JE, Cheema A, Sobesky WE, et al: Phenotypic involvement in females with the FMR1 gene mutation. Am J Ment Retard **102**:590, 1998.

Riebel T, Nasir R, Weber K: Choroid plexus cysts: a normal finding on ultrasound. Pediatr Radiol **22**:410, 1992.

Roberts LJ, Bewley S, Mackinson AM, et al: First trimester fetal nuchal translucency: Problems with screening the general population. 1. Br J Obstet Gynaecol **102**:381, 1995.

Rodis JF, Egan JF, Craffey A, et al: Calculated risk of chromosomal abnormalities in twin gestations. Obstet Gynecol **76**:1037, 1990.

Romero R, Jeanty P, Reece EA, et al: Sonographically monitored amniocentesis to decrease intraoperative complications. Obstet Gynecol **65**:426, 1985.

Rose NC, Palomaki GE, Haddow JE, et al: Maternal serum alpha-fetoprotein screening for chromosomal abnormalities: A prospective study in women aged 35 and older. Am J Obstet Gynecol **170**:1073, 1994.

Rotmensch S, Liberati M, Bronshtein M, et al: Prenatal sonographic findings in 187 fetuses with Down syndrome. Prenat Diagn **17**:1001, 1997.

Rousseau F, Rouillard P, Morel ML, et al: Prevalence of carriers of premutation-size alleles of the FMRI gene—And implications for the population genetics of the fragile X syndrome. Am J Hum Genet **57**:1006, 1995.

Ryynanen M, Seppala M, Kuusela P, et al: Antenatal screening for congenital nephrosis in Finland by maternal serum alpha-fetoprotein. Br J Obstet Gynaecol **90**:437, 1983.

Salvesen DR, Goble O: Early amniocentesis and fetal nuchal translucency in women requesting karyotyping for advanced maternal age. Prenat Diagn **15**:971, 1995.

Santolaya-Forgas J, Cohen L, Vengalil S, et al: Prenatal diagnosis of X-linked ichthyosis using molecular cytogenetics. Fetal Diagn Ther **12**:36, 1997.

Santolaya-Forgas J, Jessup J, Burd LI, et al: Pregnancy outcome in women with low midtrimester maternal serum unconjugated estriol. J Reprod Med **41**:87, 1996.

Saura R, Gauthier B, Taine L, et al: Operator experience and fetal loss rate in transabdominal CVS. Prenat Diagn **14**:70, 1994.

Savoldelli G, Binkert F, Achermann J, et al: Ultrasound screening for chromosomal anomalies in the first trimester of pregnancy. Prenat Diagn **13**:513, 1993.

Sawa R, Hayashi Z, Tanaka T, et al: Rapid detection of chromosome aneuploidies by prenatal interphase FISH (fluorescence in situ hybridization) and its clinical utility in Japan. J Obstet Gynaecol Res **27**:41, 2001.

Schaefer M, Laurichesse-Delmas H, Ville Y: The effect of nuchal cord on nuchal translucency measurement at 10–14 weeks. Ultrasound Obstet Gynecol **11**:271, 1998.

Schatz F: Eine besondere Art von ein seitiger Oligohydramnie bei Zwillingen. Arch Gynecol **65**:329, 1992.

Schleifer RA, Bradley LA, Richards DS, et al: Pregnancy outcome for women with very low levels of maternal serum unconjugated estriol on second-trimester screening. Am J Obstet Gynecol **173**:1152, 1995.

Schulte-Vallentin M, Schindler H: Non-echogenic nuchal oedema as a marker in trisomy 21 screening. Lancet **339**:1053, 1992.

Sebire NJ, Noble PL, Odibo A, et al: Single uterine entry for genetic amniocentesis in twin pregnancies. Ultrasound Obstet Gynecol **7**:26, 1996.

Seppala M, Rapola J, Huttunen NP, et al: Congenital nephrotic syndrome: prenatal diagnosis and genetic counselling by estimation of amniotic-fluid and maternal serum alpha-fetoprotein. Lancet **2**:123, 1976.

Seppala M, Ruoslahti E: Alpha fetoprotein in amniotic fluid: An index of gestational age. Am J Obstet Gynecol **114**:595, 1972.

Sharland G: First-trimester transabdominal fetal echocardiography. Lancet **351**:1662, 1998.

Shipp TD, Benacerraf BR: Second trimester ultrasound screening for chromosomal abnormalities. Prenat Diagn **22**:296, 2002.

Shulman LP, Elias S: Percutaneous umbilical blood sampling, fetal skin sampling, and fetal liver biopsy. Semin Perinatol **14**:456, 1990.

Shulman LP, Emerson DS, Felker RE, et al: High frequency of cytogenetic abnormalities in fetuses with cystic hygroma diagnosed in the first trimester. Obstet Gynecol **80**:80, 1992.

Shulman LP, Emerson DS, Grevengood C, et al: Clinical course and outcome of fetuses with isolated cystic nuchal lesions and normal karyotypes detected in the first trimester. Am J Obstet Gynecol **171**:1278, 1994.

Shunagshoti S, Netsky MG: Neuroepithelial (colloid) cysts of the nervous system. Further observation of pathogenesis, location, incidence and histochemistry. Neurology **16**:887, 1966.

Shuttleworth G: Mongolian imbecility. Br Med J **2**:661, 1909.

Simoni G, Brambati B, Danesino C, et al: Efficient direct chromosome analyses and enzyme determinations from chorionic villi samples in the first trimester of pregnancy. Hum Genet **63**:349, 1983.

Simpson JL, Socol ML, Aladjem S, et al: Normal fetal growth despite persistent amniotic fluid leakage after genetic amniocentesis. Prenat Diagn **1**:277, 1981.

Smith-Bindman R, Hosmer W, Feldstein VA, et al: Second-trimester ultrasound to detect fetuses with Down syndrome: A meta-analysis. JAMA **285**:1044, 2001.

Snijders RJ, Noble P, Sebire N, et al: UK multicentre project on assessment of risk of trisomy 21 by maternal age and fetal nuchal-translucency thickness at 10–14 weeks of gestation. Fetal Medicine Foundation First Trimester Screening Group. Lancet **352**:343, 1998.

Snijders RJ, Sebire NJ, Faria M, et al: Fetal mild hydronephrosis and chromosomal defects: Relation to maternal age and gestation. Fetal Diagn Ther **10**:349, 1995.

Snijders RJ, Shawa L, Nicolaides KH: Fetal choroid plexus cysts and trisomy 18: Assessment of risk based on ultrasound findings and maternal age. Prenat Diagn **14**:1119, 1994.

Snijders RJ, Thom EA, Zachary JM, et al: First-trimester trisomy screening: Nuchal translucency measurement training and quality assurance to correct and unify technique. Ultrasound Obstet Gynecol **19**:353, 2002.

Sonek J, Nicolaides K, Sadowsky G, et al: Articulated needle guide: report on the first 30 cases. Obstet Gynecol **74**:821, 1989.

Souka AP, Snijders RJ, Novakov A, et al: Defects and syndromes in chromosomally normal fetuses with increased nuchal translucency thickness at 10–14 weeks of gestation. Ultrasound Obstet Gynecol **11**:391, 1998.

Souter VL, Nyberg DA, El-Bastawissi A, et al: Correlation of ultrasound findings and biochemical markers in the second trimester of pregnancy in fetuses with trisomy 21. Prenat Diagn **22**:175, 2002.

Steele M, Breg W Jr: Chromosome analysis of human amniotic-fluid cells. Lancet **1**:383, 1966.

Stein J, Berg C, Jones JA, et al: A screening protocol for a prenatal population at risk for inherited hemoglobin disorders: Results of its application to a group of Southeast Asians and blacks. Am J Obstet Gynecol **150**:333, 1984.

Suchet IB, van der Westhuizen NG, Labatte MF: Fetal cystic hygromas: further insights into their natural history. Can Assoc Radiol J **43**:420, 1992.

Sugarman EA, Allitto BA: Carrier testing for seven diseases common in the Ashkenazi Jewish population: Implications for counseling and testing. Obstet Gynecol **97**:S38, 2001.

Sundberg K, Bang J, Smidt-Jensen S, et al: Randomised study of risk of fetal loss related to early amniocentesis versus chorionic villus sampling. Lancet **350**:697, 1997.

Suren A, Grone HJ, Kallerhoff M, et al: Prenatal diagnosis of congenital nephrosis of the Finnish type (CNF) in the second trimester. Int J Gynaecol Obstet **41**:165, 1993.

Sutcliffe JS, Nelson DL, Zhang F, et al: DNA methylation represses FMR-1 transcription in fragile X syndrome. Hum Mol Genet **1**:397, 1992.

Swift PG, Driscoll IB, Vowles KD: Neonatal small-bowel obstruction associated with amniocentesis. Br Med J **1**:720, 1979.

Szabo J, Gellen J: Nuchal fluid accumulation in trisomy-21 detected by vaginosonography in first trimester. Lancet **336**:1133, 1990.

Szabo J, Gellen J, Szemere G: First-trimester ultrasound screening for fetal aneuploidies in women over 35 and under 35 years of age. Ultrasound Obstet Gynecol **5**:161, 1995.

Tabor A, Jerne D, Bock JE: Incidence of rhesus immunisation after genetic amniocentesis. Br Med J (Clin Res Ed) **293**:533, 1986.

Tabor A, Philip J, Bang J, et al: Needle size and risk of miscarriage after amniocentesis. Lancet **1**:183, 1988.

Tabor A, Philip J, Madsen M, et al: Randomised controlled trial of genetic amniocentesis in 4606 low-risk women. Lancet **1**:1287, 1986.

Tarleton JC, Saul RA: Molecular genetic advances in fragile X syndrome. J Pediatr **122**:169, 1993.

Technical and clinical assessment of fluorescence in situ hybridization: An ACMG/ASHG position statement. I. Technical considerations. Test and Technology Transfer Committee. Genet Med **2**:356, 2000.

Tepperberg J, Pettenati MJ, Rao PN, et al: Prenatal diagnosis using interphase fluorescence in situ hybridization (FISH): 2-year multi-center retrospective study and review of the literature. Prenat Diagn **21**:293, 2001.

Therkelsen AJ, Rehder H: Intestinal atresia caused by second trimester amniocentesis. Case report. Br J Obstet Gynaecol **88**:559, 1981.

Thilaganathan B, Slack A, Wathen NC: Effect of first-trimester nuchal translucency on second-trimester maternal serum biochemical screening for Down's syndrome. Ultrasound Obstet Gynecol **10**:261, 1997.

Tint GS, Abuelo D, Till M, et al: Fetal Smith-Lemli-Opitz syndrome can be detected accurately and reliably by measuring amniotic fluid dehydrocholesterols. Prenat Diagn **18**:651, 1998.

Toledano-Alhadef H, Basel-Vanagaite L, Magal N, et al: Fragile-X carrier screening and the prevalence of premutation and full-mutation carriers in Israel. Am J Hum Genet **69**:351, 2001.

Trauffer PM, Anderson CE, Johnson A, et al: The natural history of euploid pregnancies with first-trimester cystic hygromas. Am J Obstet Gynecol **170**:1279, 1994.

Turnbull AC, MacKenzie IZ: Second-trimester amniocentesis and termination of pregnancy. Br Med Bull **39**:315, 1983.

Turner G, Webb T, Wake S, et al: Prevalence of fragile X syndrome. Am J Med Genet **64**:196, 1996.

Uchida IA, Freeman VCP: Trisomy 21 Down syndrome. II. Structural chromosome rearrangements in the parents. Hum Genet **72**:118, 1986.

Uehara S, Yaegashi N, Maeda T, et al: Risk of recurrence of fetal chromosomal aberrations: Analysis of trisomy 21, trisomy 18, trisomy 13, and 45,X in 1,076 Japanese mothers. J Obstet Gynaecol Res **25**:373, 1999.

Van der Pol J, Volf H, Boer K, et al: Jejunal atresia related to the use of methylene blue in genetic amniocentesis in twins. Br J Obstet Gynaecol **99**:141, 1992.

Van Vugt JM, Tinnemans BW, Van Zalen-Sprock RM: Outcome and early childhood follow-up of chromosomally normal fetuses with increased nuchal translucency at 10–14 weeks' gestation. Ultrasound Obstet Gynecol **11**:407, 1998.

van Zalen-Sprock MM, van Vugt JMG, van Geijn HP: First-trimester diagnosis of cystic hygroma—Course and outcome. Am J Obstet Gynecol **167**:94, 1992.

Vandenbussche FP, Kanhai HH, Keirse MJ: Safety of early amniocentesis. Lancet **344**:1032, 1994.

Vejerslev LO, Mikkelsen M: The European collaborative study on mosaicism in chorionic villus sampling: Data from 1986 to 1987. Prenat Diagn **9**:575, 1989.

Ville Y, Lalondrelle C, Doumerc S, et al: First-trimester diagnosis of nuchal anomalies: Significance and fetal outcomes. Ultrasound Obstet Gynecol **2**:314, 1992.

Wald NJ, Cuckle H, Boreham J, et al: Maternal serum alpha-fetoprotein and diabetes mellitus. Br J Obstet Gynaecol **86**:101, 1979.

Wald NJ, Cuckle HS, Densem JW, et al: Maternal serum screening for Down's syndrome in early pregnancy. Br Med J **297**:883, 1988.

Wald NJ, Watt HC, Hackshaw AK: Integrated screening for Down's syndrome on the basis of tests performed during the first and second trimesters. N Engl J Med **341**:461, 1999.

Walker A: Liquor amnii studies in the prediction of haemolytic disease of the newborn. Br Med J **2**:376, 1957.

Waller DK, Lustig LS, Cunningham GC, et al: Second-trimester maternal serum alpha-fetoprotein levels and the risk of subsequent fetal death. N Engl J Med **325**:6, 1991.

Waller DK, Lustig LS, Cunningham GC, et al: The association between maternal serum alpha-fetoprotein and preterm birth, small for gestational age infants, preeclampsia, and placental complications. Obstet Gynecol **88**:816, 1996.

Waller DK, Lustig LS, Smith AH, et al: Alpha-fetoprotein: A biomarker for pregnancy outcome. Epidemiology **4**:471, 1993.

Wapner R: First trimester aneuploid screening: results of the NICHD multicenter study. Am J Obstet Gynecol **185**:S70, 2002.

Wapner RJ, Evans MI, Davis G, et al: Procedural risks versus theology: chorionic villus sampling for Orthodox Jews at less than 8 weeks' gestation. Am J Obstet Gynecol **186**:1133, 2002.

Wapner RJ, Jenkins TM, Silverman N, et al: Prenatal diagnosis of congenital nephrosis by in utero kidney biopsy. Prenat Diagn **21**:256, 2001.

Wapner RJ, Johnson A, Davis G, et al: Prenatal diagnosis in twin gestations: A comparison between second-trimester amniocentesis and first-trimester chorionic villus sampling. Obstet Gynecol **82**:49, 1993.

Wapner RJ, Simpson JL, Golbus MS, et al: Chorionic mosaicism: association with fetal loss but not with adverse perinatal outcome. Prenat Diagn **12**:347, 1992.

Warburton D, Byrne J, Canki N: Chromosome Anomalies and Prenatal Development: An Atlas. Oxford Monographs on Medical Genetics No. 20. New York, Oxford University Press, 1991.

Warburton D, Kline J, Stein Z, et al: Does the karyotype of a spontaneous abortion predict the karyotype of a subsequent abortion?—Evidence from 273 women with two karyotyped spontaneous abortions. Am J Hum Genet **41**:465, 1987.

Ward BE, Gersen SL, Carelli MP, et al: Rapid prenatal diagnosis of chromosomal aneuploidies by fluorescence in situ hybridization: Clinical experience with 4,500 specimens. Am J Hum Genet **52**:854, 1993.

Wass D, Bennett M: Infection and chorionic villus sampling. Lancet **2**:338, 1985.

Wenstrom KD, Syrop CH, Hammitt DG, et al: Increased risk of monochorionic twinning associated with assisted reproduction. Fertil Steril **60**:510, 1993.

Weremowicz S, Sandstrom DJ, Morton CC, et al: Fluorescence in situ hybridization (FISH) for rapid detection of aneuploidy: experience in 911 prenatal cases. Prenat Diagn **21**:262, 2001.

Whitlow BJ, Chatzipapas IK, Economides DL: The effect of fetal neck position on nuchal translucency measurement. Br J Obstet Gynaecol **105**:872, 1998.

Whitlow BJ, Economides DL: The optimal gestational age to examine fetal anatomy and measure nuchal translucency in the first trimester. Ultrasound Obstet Gynecol **11**:258, 1998.

WHO/PAHO: Consultation on CVS: evaluation of chorionic villus sampling safety. Prenat Diagn **19**:97, 1999.

Williams J, Madearis A, Chun W, et al: Maternal cell contamination in cultured chorionic villi: Comparison of chromosome Q-polymorphisms derived from villi, fetal skin, and maternal lymphocytes. Prenat Diagn **7**:315, 1987.

Wilson RD, Venir N, Farquharson DF: Fetal nuchal fluid—Physiological or pathological?—In pregnancies less than 17 menstrual weeks. Prenat Diagn **12**:755, 1992.

Wolstenholme J: Confined placental mosaicism for trisomies 2, 3, 7, 8, 9, 16, and 22: Their incidence, likely origins, and mechanisms for cell lineage compartmentalization. Prenat Diagn **16**:511, 1996.

Working Party on Amniocentesis: An assessment of hazards of amniocentesis. Br J Obstet Gynaecol **85**:1, 1978.

Worton RG, Stern R: A Canadian collaborative study of mosaicism in amniotic fluid cell cultures. Prenat Diagn **4**:131, 1984.

Yaron Y, Cherry M, Kramer RL, et al: Second-trimester maternal serum marker screening: Maternal serum alpha-fetoprotein, beta-human chorionic gonadotropin, estriol, and their various combination as predictors of pregnancy outcome. Am J Obstet Gynecol **181**:968, 1999.

Young PE, Matson MR, Jones OW: Fetal exsanguination and other vascular injuries from midtrimester genetic amniocentesis. Am J Obstet Gynecol **129**:21, 1977.

Youroukos S, Papadelis F, Matsaniotis N: Porencephalic cysts after amniocentesis. Arch Dis Child **55**:814, 1980.

Yukobowich E, Anteby EY, Cohen SM, et al: Risk of fetal loss in twin pregnancies undergoing second trimester amniocentesis (1). Obstet Gynecol **98**:231, 2001.

Zalel Y, Kedar I, Tepper R, et al: Differential diagnosis and management of very low second trimester maternal serum unconjugated estriol levels, with special emphasis on the diagnosis of X-linked ichthyosis. Obstet Gynecol Surv **51**:200, 1996.

Zhang J, Fidler C, Murphy M, et al: Determination of fetal RhD status by maternal plasma DNA analysis. Ann N Y Acad Sci **906**:153, 2000.

Zosmer N, Souter VL, Chan CS, et al: Early diagnosis of major cardiac defects in chromosomally normal fetuses with increased nuchal translucency. Br J Obstet Gynaecol **106**:829, 1999.

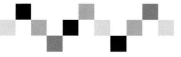

Chapter 19

EFFECTS OF THERAPEUTIC, DIAGNOSTIC, AND ENVIRONMENTAL AGENTS AND EXPOSURE TO SOCIAL AND ILLICIT DRUGS

Robert L. Andres, MD

THERAPEUTIC, DIAGNOSTIC, AND ENVIRONMENTAL AGENTS

A common issue encountered by those caring for pregnant women is whether or not a drug is thought to cause birth defects, or its teratogenic potential. The word teratogen is derived from the Greek *teratos* or monster. Sheppard (1998) defined a teratogen as any agent that acts during embryonic or fetal development to produce a permanent alteration of form or function. The drugs most commonly described as established teratogens are listed in Table 19-1.

The baseline risk of major malformations is often quoted at 2% to 4%. Although teratogens make up only 3% of these malformations (Nelson and Holmes, 1989), they represent, for the most part, the only preventable cause (Table 19-2).

Several factors may influence the teratogenic potential of a given drug exposure: the degree to which the drug crosses the placenta, the gestational age at which the exposure occurs, the genetic sensitivity (predisposition) of a given fetus (e.g., epoxide metabolism in the hydantoin syndrome), and concurrent environmental factors (inadequate folic acid intake in patients exposed to valproic acid). The U.S. Food and Drug Administration (FDA, 1980a) published a classification system that addresses the relative safety of medications during pregnancy. These classifications are detailed in Table 19-3.

Therapeutic Agents

Analgesics

ASPIRIN

The use of salicylic acid is reported by nearly half of all pregnant women. Concerns over the drug's potential teratogenicity were raised by the description of an increase in the incidence of both oral clefts and fetal deaths (Cote et al., 1974) among infants born to women who used aspirin while pregnant. A possible association with truncus arteriosus was later reported by Zierler and Rothman (1985). Other investigators failed to show an association between the use of aspirin and congenital cardiac disease (Werler et al., 1984). The

Collaborative Perinatal Project included over 5000 infants who were exposed to aspirin with no apparent increase in the incidence of congenital anomalies (Scone et al., 1976).

INDOMETHACIN

Indomethacin is a nonsteroidal anti-inflammatory drug that is used as an analgesic and as a tocolytic agent. Although the drug is not considered to be teratogenic, data support its association with reversible constriction of the fetal ductus arteriosus. This narrowing has been shown to be dose related and to occur most commonly when the drug is administered after 32 weeks' gestation (Van den Veyver et al., 1993). Persistent pulmonary hypertension in the neonate has also been reported after *in utero* exposure (Csaba et al., 1978). Additional adverse effects of the drug include decreased fetal urine output, oligohydramnios (Goldenberg et al., 1989), and neonatal renal insufficiency (Kirshon et al., 1988a).

Antibiotics and Anti-infectious Agents

TETRACYCLINE

There is no evidence that first-trimester exposure to tetracycline is associated with an increased risk of congenital anomalies (Aselton et al., 1985; Czeizel and Rockenbauer, 1997). The use of tetracycline beyond the first trimester is associated with brownish discoloration of the deciduous teeth, hypoplasia of the enamel, and inhibition of bone growth (Cohlan et al., 1963; Kutscher et al., 1966).

SULFONAMIDES

There is no evidence that sulfonamides pose a teratogenic risk to the human fetus. Given the drug's competition with free bilirubin for binding sites, use of the drug near delivery of a preterm infant has been associated with hyperbilirubinemia (Landers et al., 1983). Theoretic concerns of neonatal kernicterus have not been documented (Baskin et al., 1980).

SULFAMETHOXAZOLE AND TRIMETHOPRIM

The available information on the teratogenic potential of this combination is controversial. The concern over the use of trimethoprim is based on the drug's mechanism of action as a

TABLE 19-1. ESTABLISHED TERATOGENS

Drug	Potential Defect	Comments
ACE inhibitors	Renal dysgenesis, oligohydramnios, IUGR, and skull ossifications defects. Neonatal renal failure.	Risk increases with use in 2nd and 3rd trimester.
Alcohol	Prenatal and postnatal growth restriction, CNS abnormalities (microcephaly and mental retardation), and craniofacial dysmorphology (fetal alcohol syndrome). Renal, cardiac, and other major malformations.	Risk not limited to 1st trimester. Late pregnancy use associated with IUGR and developmental delay. Incidence of defects > 30% among "heavy drinkers."
Aminopterin and methotrexate	SAB, craniofacial dysmorphology, limb defects, NTDs, craniosynostosis, and IUGR.	Folic acid antagonists. Anomalies in 30% of liveborn fetuses.
Androgens and norprogesterones	Masculinization of external female genitalia.	Labioscrotal fusion can occur with exposure < 9 weeks. Clitiromegaly possible at any gestational age.
Carbamazepine	NTDs, craniofacial abnormalities, nail hypoplasia, IUGR, and developmental delay.	Risk of NTDs 1–2%
Diethylstilbestrol	Clear cell adenocarcinoma of the vagina, vaginal adenosis, abnormalities of the cervix and uterus, testicular abnormalities, and male/female infertility.	Risk of carcinoma rare. Exposure in 1st trimester = 50% vaginal adenosis.
Isotretinoin	CNS defects, abnormal ears, thymic abnormalities, cardiac defects, and fetal death.	As many as 50% of exposed are affected.
Lithium	Cardiac defects (Ebstein anomaly).	Greatest risk (1%) in first trimester.
Penicillamine	Cutis laxa.	Seen with chronic use.
Phenytoin	Craniofacial dysmorphology, IUGR, nail hypoplasia, microcephaly, and developmental delay.	Full syndrome in 10%. As many as 30% exhibit some manifestations.
Streptomycin	Hearing loss, eighth nerve damage.	
Tetracycline	Discoloration of deciduous teeth and enamel hypoplasia	Risk only in 2nd and 3rd trimester.
Thalidomide	Limb reduction defects, ear and cardiac abnormalities.	Critical period 38–50 days postconception. 20% of exposed are affected.
Trimethadione	Developmental delay, V-shaped eyebrows, oral clefts, and craniofacial abnormalities.	80% rate of abnormalities associated with 1st-trimester exposure.
Valproic acid	NTDs, minor facial defects.	Risk of NTDs 1%.
Warfarin	Nasal hypoplasia, stippled epiphyses, and CNS abnormalities.	Greatest risk from 6–9 weeks; 15–25% affected.

ACE, angiotensin-converting enzyme; CNS, central nervous system; IUGR, intrauterine growth restriction; NTD, neural tube defect; SAB, spontaneous abortion.

Modified from Martinez L: Pregnancy Risk Line. Utah State Department of Health and American College of Obstetricians and Gynecologists Educational Bulletin, Number 236, Salt Lake City, State of Utah Department of Health, 1997.

folate antagonist and on the observation that large doses of the drug have been shown to cause structural defects in various animal models. Data from a cohort of over 2000 Michigan Medicaid recipients suggested an increased risk of cardiovascular anomalies (Briggs et al., 1998). Although a number of clinical investigations reported no increase in the incidence of birth defects (Williams et al., 1969; Ochoa, 1971; Brumfitt and Pursell, 1972), more recent data suggest an increase in the risk of anomalies. Hernandez-Diaz and coworkers (2000) published a case-control study of patients with neural tube defects, congenital heart disease, or oral clefts. Their comparison of 1242 infants with neural tube defects to a control group demonstrated that trimethoprim use was five times more common in the study group (odds ratio [OR], 4.8; 95th confidence interval [CI], 1.5 to 16.1). In patients with congenital heart disease (n = 3870) the odds ratio for trimethoprim use was 3.4 (95th CI, 1.8 to 6.4), and in patients with oral clefts (n = 1962) the odds ratio was 2.6 (95th CI, 1.6 to 6.1).

AMNIOGLYCOSIDES

In utero exposure to aminoglycosides (especially streptomycin and kanamycin) has been associated with a 1% to 2% risk of neonatal ototoxicity (Conway and Birt, 1965). No known teratogenic effect other than congenital deafness has been associated with the use of aminoglycosides.

QUINOLONES

There is little information about the potential teratogenic potential for this relatively new class of antibiotics (e.g., ciprofloxacin, norfloxacin). Berkovitch and colleagues (1994) evaluated 38 infants who were exposed to quinolones during the first trimester of fetal life and did not find any malformations. Two hundred women who used quinolones during their pregnancy were evaluated prospectively (Loebstein et al., 1998). The incidence of major congenital malformations did not vary between those exposed to quinolones (2.2%) and the control (nonexposed) group (2.6%) (relative risk, 0.85; 95th CI, 0.98 to 20.57). Despite these data, the manufacturer recommends that the drugs should not be used during pregnancy.

ETHAMBUTOL, RIFAMPIN, AND ISONIAZID

With the exception of streptomycin, there is no evidence that the drugs commonly used to treat tuberculosis are associated with an increase in the risk of anomalies among exposed fetuses (Warkany, 1979; Snider et al., 1980).

TABLE 19-2. CAUSES OF MALFORMATIONS AMONG AFFECTED INFANTS

Causes	Number	Percent
Chromosome abnormalities	157	10.1
Single mutant genes	48	3.1
Familial	225	14.5
Multifactorial inheritance	356	23.0
Teratogens	49	3.2
Uterine factors	39	2.5
Twinning	6	0.4
Unknown cause	669	43.2

Modified from Nelson K, Holmes LB: Malformations due to spontaneous mutations on newborn infants. N Engl J Med **320**:19, 1989.

METRONIDAZOLE

Although case reports have described malformations in infants exposed to metronidazole (Cantu and Garcia-Cruz, 1982; Greenberg, 1985), significant evidence shows the drug is not teratogenic in humans. Two meta-analyses (Burtin et al., 1995; Caro-Paton et al., 1997) have been published in the past decade, both of which concluded no increased risk of malformations associated with first-trimester exposure to metronidazole. A prospective, controlled, cohort study involving 228 women with exposure to metronidazole during pregnancy (Diav-Citrin et al., 2001b) found major congenital malformations in 1.6% of exposed newborns and in 1.4% of the control group.

ACYCLOVIR

The Acyclovir in Pregnancy Registry was established in 1984, and the initial report documented nine cases of malformations (3.8%) among 312 exposed infants, an incidence similar to the general population (Andrews et al., 1992). An update from the registry (739 cases) reported no demonstrable increase in the incidence of malformations and no identifiable pattern of anomalies among exposed offspring (Acyclovir Pregnancy Registry, 1998) (see Chapter 40).

ANTIRETROVIRAL AGENTS

Antiretroviral drugs have become a mainstay in the management of pregnant women infected with the human immunodeficiency virus. Their general mechanism of action (interference with intracellular viral replication) has generated appropriate concern over the potential teratogenicity of these medications. The nucleoside reverse transcriptase inhibitors (e.g., zidovudine, lamivudine, didanosine, etc.) are the most widely studied in terms of the possible association with congenital malformations. The Antiretroviral Pregnancy Registry, established in 1989, reported on over 400 women who were exposed to either zidovudine or lamivudine during the first trimester of pregnancy. There has been no overt increase in the rate of congenital malformations in the infants born to this cohort of women (Interim Report, 2001). There is significantly less information available about the teratogenic potential of both nonnucleoside reverse transcriptase inhibitors and protease inhibitors (Watts, 2002).

Anticoagulants

HEPARIN

Neither unfractionated nor low-molecular-weight heparin cross the placenta and as such are not associated with congenital anomalies or other adverse fetal effects.

WARFARIN

The suggestion that warfarin may be a human teratogen is frequently credited to Kerber and associates (1968). The specific pattern of anomalies observed in newborns exposed to warfarin was described by Barr and Burdi (1976) and include prenatal growth deficiency, mental deficiency, seizures, nasal hypoplasia, and epiphyseal stippling. The critical period for exposure appears to be the later half of the first trimester, with exposure during the second and third trimester linked to abnormalities of the central nervous system (CNS) (e.g., Dandy-Walker malformation, agenesis of the corpus callosum, etc.), possibly as a result of fetal hemorrhage (Pettiflor and Benson, 1975; Hall et al., 1980). The incidence of anomalies among exposed pregnancies has

TABLE 19-3. FOOD AND DRUG ADMINISTRATION CATEGORIES FOR DRUGS AND MEDICATIONS

Category A	Controlled studies in women fail to demonstrate a risk to the fetus in the first trimester (and there is no evidence of a risk in later trimesters), and the possibility of fetal harm appears to be remote.
Category B	Either animal-reproduction studies have not demonstrated a fetal risk but there are no controlled studies in pregnant women or animal-reproduction studies have shown an adverse effect (other than a risk in fertility) that was not confirmed in controlled studies in women in the first trimester (and there is no evidence of a risk in the later trimesters).
Category C	Either studies in animals have revealed adverse effects on the fetus (teratogenic or embryocidal or other) and there are no controlled studies in women or studies in women and animals are not available. Drugs should be given only if the potential benefit justifies the potential risk to the fetus.
Category D	There is positive evidence of human fetal risk, but the benefits from use in pregnant women may be acceptable despite the risk (e.g., if the drug is needed in a life-threatening situation for a serious disease for which safer drugs cannot be used or are ineffective).
Category X	Studies in animals or human beings have demonstrated fetal abnormalities or there is evidence of fetal risk based on human experience or both, and the risk of the drug in pregnant women clearly outweighs any possible benefit. The drug is contraindicated in women who are or may become pregnant.

From Food and Drug Administration: Drug Bulletin. Fed Reg **44**:37434, 1980.

been reported to be in the range of 10% to 15% (Hall et al., 1980; Ginsberg and Hirsh, 1989) (also see Chapters 41, 42, and 48).

Antiepileptic Drugs

As a group, drugs used to treat seizure disorders are associated with an increase in the risk of congenital malformations (Gilmore et al., 1998; Canger et al., 1999) (see Chapter 55). Each of the commonly used antiepileptic drugs (AEDs) has been implicated as a teratogen. Studies have reported the risk of congenital malformations among women exposed to AEDs to be approximately 70 in 1000 compared with 18 to 30 in 1000 for nonexposed pregnancies (Annegers et al., 1974; Kelly, 1984). The structural defects observed most commonly include congenital heart disease, neural tube defects, and cleft lip and palate. Minor defects reported include hypoplasia of the digits and nails, hypertelorism, broad nasal bridge, epicanthal folds, abnormal ears, and a short upturned nose. Recent studies (Canger et al., 1999; Holmes et al., 2001) challenged the long-held belief that the risk of malformations is increased with epileptics in general, regardless of the use of AEDs (Yerby, 1993). The use of multiple anticonvulsant medications (polytherapy) is associated with a significantly greater risk of structural defects (Kaneko et al., 1988; Koch et al., 1992; Holmes et al., 2001) than is observed among newborns exposed to a single agent.

TRIMETHADIONE

This agent is an established teratogen, and its use is contraindicated during pregnancy. A characteristic pattern of malformations has been described (Zackai et al., 1975) that includes intrauterine growth restriction (IUGR), mental deficiency, cardiac septal defects, and craniofacial abnormalities (e.g., short upturned nose with a low nasal bridge, prominent forehead, upslanted eyebrows, and an abnormal helix of the external ear). Although the exact risk is unknown, estimates range from 50% to 80% (Delgado-Escueta and Janz, 1992).

DIPHENYLHYDANTOIN

Hanson and Smith (1975) are credited with the description of a pattern of anomalies associated with *in utero* exposure to hydantoin. The findings included IUGR, microcephaly, mental deficiency, hypoplasia of the digits and nails, and craniofacial abnormalities (e.g., short nose with low nasal bridge, ocular hypertelorism, abnormal ears, and a wide mouth with a prominent upper lip). Further studies suggested that approximately 10% of exposed fetuses exhibit findings consistent with the fetal hydantoin syndrome, whereas as many as one third will have one or more of the more minor abnormalities (Hanson et al., 1976; Kelly, 1984). The susceptibility of a given fetus to the teratogenic effect of hydantoin (as well as carbamazepine and phenobarbital) is thought to be related to the activity of epoxide hydroxylase. This enzyme is responsible for the metabolism of the epoxide intermediate (metabolic by product of hydantoin), which is thought to be the agent responsible for the teratogenic effects, rather than the drug itself (Beuhler et al., 1990).

Scolnik and coworkers (1994) found the mean intelligence quotient score for 34 infants exposed to hydantoin to be 10.6 points lower than that observed in their control group.

This finding of impaired cognitive functioning remains unsettled, with studies both supporting (Hanson, 1986) and refuting (Adams et al., 2000) long-term developmental sequelae associated with *in utero* exposure to hydantoin.

VALPROIC ACID

The possibility of an association between *in utero* exposure to valproic acid and spina bifida was reported approximately 20 years ago (Robert and Guiband, 1982). Since that initial report, numerous studies reinforced the risk of spina bifida (primarily lumbosacral defects) among fetuses exposed to valproic acid, with the specific risk ranging from 1% to 5% (Lammer, 1987; Omtzigt et al., 1992).

Valproic acid use during pregnancy has been associated with a pattern of minor anomalies and developmental delay, termed the "fetal valproate syndrome" (DiLiberti et al., 1984). The minor anomalies included epicanthal folds, a flat nasal bridge, small upturned nose, a long upper lip with a relatively shallow philtrum, a thin upper vermillion border, and downturned angles of the mouth (Fig. 19-1). This pattern of minor facial anomalies has been reported by other investigators (Clayton-Smith and Donnai, 1995).

The risk of an increase in other anomalies is less clear. Data support an increase in anomalies affecting the musculoskeletal, cardiovascular, pulmonary, and genital systems (Kozma, 2000) as well as specific concerns over limb reduction defects (Rodriguez-Pinella et al., 2000) and craniosynostosis (Lajeunie et al., 1998). Reports demonstrated an increase in the risk of multiple congenital anomalies associated with prenatal exposure to valproic acid (Samren et al., 1997; Kaneko et al., 1999). Kaneko and coworkers (1999) reported on 983 women who used various AEDs during pregnancy and found multiple congenital anomalies in 11.1% of those who used valproic acid as monotherapy. The risk of anomalies was correlated with both the total daily dose and the serum level of valproic acid. Samren and colleagues (1997) also noted a significant increase

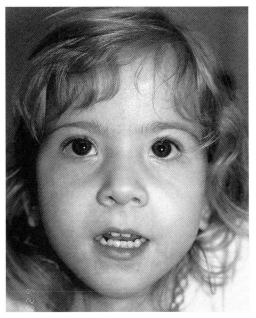

FIGURE 19-1 ■ Six-year-old girl with the characteristic findings associated with *in utero* exposure to valproic acid.

in the risk of congenital anomalies among women who took greater than 1000 mg of valproic acid daily when compared with those fetuses exposed to less than 600 mg daily (relative risk, 6.8; 95th CI, 1.4 to 32.7).

Relatively few reports address the potential for an association between in utero exposure to valproic acid and cognitive deficits and/or developmental abnormalities. A recent review of the literature (Kozma, 2000) suggested that development deficits were reported in approximately 20% and mental retardation observed in 10% of infants exposed to valproic acid before birth.

CARBAMAZEPINE

Jones and colleagues (1989) followed a cohort of 35 infants exposed to carbamazepine, noting a pattern of malformations similar to that observed with in utero exposure to hydantoin and valproic acid. The specific findings included craniofacial abnormalities (microcephaly, upslanting palpebral fissures, and a long philtrum), nail hypoplasia, and developmental delay. Since that report several publications reinforced the association of prenatal carbamazepine use and abnormalities in fetal growth, developmental delay, and craniofacial anomalies (Nulman et al., 1997; Moore et al., 2000; Wide et al., 2000).

Carbamazepine has also been associated with an increased risk of spina bifida (Rosa, 1992; Kaneko et al., 1993; Hernandez-Diaz et al., 2001). The reported risk ranges from 0.5% to 1.7% (Sheppard et al., 2002). Hernandez-Diaz and coworkers (2001) showed that dietary supplementation with folic acid (4 to 5 mg daily) was associated with a reduction in the risk of neural tube defects in fetuses exposed to carbamazepine. The American College of Obstetricians and Gynecologists (1997) suggested that all pregnant women taking folic acid antagonists supplement their diet with 4 mg daily of folic acid.

Several investigators suggested that carbamazepine is associated with an increased risk of major congenital anomalies (Pearse et al., 1992; Nulman et al., 1997; Diav-Citrin et al., 2001a). A prospective study of 210 patients (Diav-Citrin et al., 2001a) who took carbamazepine during the first trimester of pregnancy demonstrated a twofold increase in the incidence of congenital anomalies among those exposed infants. The relative risk of major congenital anomalies in the carbamazepine-exposed infants was 2.24 (95th CI, 1.1 to 4.56).

BARBITURATES

These agents (e.g., phenobarbital and primidone) have been used extensively in the treatment of epilepsy. Although the data are limited, there appears to be an increased risk of anomalies similar to those observed with other AEDs (hydantoin, valproic acid, and carbamazepine) (Myhree and Williams, 1981; Krauss et al., 1984; Jones et al., 1992). Data from the International Database on Malformations and Drug Exposure supported a threefold increase in the risk of cleft lip and palate with the use of phenobarbital (Arpino et al., 2000). There is disagreement about whether the anomalies associated with barbiturate use are seen with monotherapy or are the result of exposure to other AEDs used along with barbiturates in patients who require polytherapy.

MISCELLANEOUS ANTIEPILEPTIC DRUGS

A number of newer agents have been introduced into practice over the past several years, including lamotrigine, gabapentin, felbamate, and tiagabine. Limited data are available on the use of lamotrigine, which suggests that the risk of congenital anomalies among infants born to women using this drug while pregnant is not increased over the baseline risk (Reiff-Eldridge et al., 2000). The safety of these drugs should be considered unproven until more data are made available.

Antihypertensive Agents

No data support a teratogenic effect of the vast majority of drugs used in the modern treatment of hypertension (Rosenthal and Oparil, 2002). This includes methyldopa, hydralazine, beta-blockers, calcium channel blockers, and clonidine.

ANGIOTENSIN-CONVERTING ENZYME INHIBITORS

The use of angiotensin-converting enzyme inhibitors (enalapril, captopril, and lisinopril) in the second and third trimesters has been associated with oligohydramnios, IUGR, neonatal anuria, skull hypoplasia, pulmonary hypoplasia, and neonatal death (Brent and Beckman, 1991; Hanssens et al., 1991). These abnormalities are thought to result from prolonged fetal hypotension and hypoperfusion of the fetal kidneys, leading to renal ischemia and tubular dysgenesis (Pryde et al., 1993). The resultant oligohydramnios is associated with pulmonary hypoplasia and an increase in perinatal morbidity and mortality.

Antithyroid Drugs

METHIMAZOLE (TAPAZOLE)

Although both propylthiouracil and methimazole are known to cross the placenta, only methimazole has been associated with an increased risk of congenital anomalies. Milham and Elledge (1972) described characteristic scalp defects in 11 newborns, 2 of which had been exposed to methimazole for the treatment of maternal hyperthyroidism. A number of additional cases have been reported since that initial observation (Mujtaba and Burrow, 1975; Milham, 1985). Although the risk of this abnormality among exposed newborns is unknown, it is likely to be extremely rare. The use of methimazole during pregnancy has been linked to other congenital anomalies, including esophageal atresia, tracheoesophageal fistula, choanal atresia, and ectodermal anomalies (Ramirez et al., 1992; Martin-Denavit et al., 2000). Clementi and coworkers (1999) suggested the term "methimazole syndrome," which includes scalp defects, choanal atresia, and tracheoesophageal fistula. The association with multiple congenital anomalies was recently reviewed by Ornoy and Diav-Citrin (2002).

[131]I THERAPY

The fetal thyroid begins to concentrate iodide at approximately 10 weeks' gestation. Exposure to ablative doses of ^{131}I beyond that gestational age is associated with significant risk to the fetal thyroid. Although the exact risk is unknown, there is a potential for fetal hypothyroidism secondary to destruction of the gland. Stoffer and Hamber (1976) reviewed the outcome of pregnancies complicated by first- or second-trimester exposure to ablative doses of ^{131}I, noting 6 cases of neonatal hypothyroidism among 178 live births.

Chemotherapeutic and Immunosuppresive Agents

CYCLOPHOSPHAMIDE

It is generally accepted that cyclophosphamide and other alkylating agents are best avoided during the first trimester of pregnancy. Numerous case reports have described anomalies in infants born to women who ingested cyclophosphamide during the first trimester of pregnancy. The reported anomalies included hypoplastic fingers and toes, oral clefts, single coronary artery, imperforate anus, IUGR, and microcephaly (Manson et al., 1982; Kirshon et al., 1988b). The interpretation of data related to the teratogenic potential of cyclophosphamide (as is true with many of the chemotherapeutic agents) is often complicated by the concurrent use of other drugs and/or radiation therapy. The FDA classified cyclophosphamide as a category D agent (Briggs et al., 1998).

METHOTREXATE AND AMINOPTERIN

These drugs are classified as folic acid antagonists and are thought to cause either embryonic death or anomalies based on their inhibition of dihydrofolate reductase, leading to cellular death. The pattern of anomalies associated with first-trimester exposure includes microcephaly, cleft palate, neural tube defects, delayed fetal growth, abnormal cranial ossification, ocular hypertelorism, small low-set ears, severe micrognathia, and limb abnormalities (Milunsky et al., 1968). A review of 41 cases of prenatal exposure to aminopterin and 20 cases of methotrexate reinforced the risks of these folic acid antagonists (Feldkamp and Carey, 1993). These investigators found that all the infants exposed to aminopterin were anomalous, and 3 of 17 liveborn infants exposed to methotrexate had birth defects consistent with the aminopterin syndrome. Based on this literature review, the authors suggested that the methotrexate dose required to produce the described pattern of anomalies was approximately 10 mg/wk. Nguyen and associates (2002) described a newborn with multiple anomalies (gastrointestinal, cardiopulmonary, craniofacial, and skeletal) that was exposed to a significantly lower dose of methotrexate before 6 weeks' gestation.

AZATHIOPRINE

Azathioprine is a derivative of 6-mercaptopurine that decreases the production of antibodies and the proliferation of T cells. Several reports suggested that the use of azathioprine during the first trimester of pregnancy is not associated with an increase in the risk of congenital anomalies. The drug, however, has been shown to significantly increase the risk of IUGR (Scott, 1977; Pirson et al., 1985; Haugen et al., 1994). Armenti and coworkers (1994) described a cohort of 146 renal transplant patients who were treated with azathioprine and corticosteroids. There were no anomalies noted among the newborns, although greater than 50% were classified as small for gestational age.

CYCLOSPORINE

The available data do not support an increased risk of anomalies associated with the use of cyclosporine (Armenti et al., 1994).

Hormones

PROGESTATIONAL AGENTS AND ESTROGEN–PROGESTOGEN COMBINATIONS

Given the frequent use of progestational agents in various clinical settings (contraception, medical management of dysfunctional bleeding, early medical abortion, and recurrent pregnancy loss), it is not surprising that they are inadvertently administered to patients who are unaware of an early pregnancy. The teratogenic potential of these drugs has been questioned since the late 1960s. Studies from the late 1960s and early 1970s suggested that the use of progestational drugs were associated with an increased risk of both cardiovascular abnormalities and limb reduction defects (Gal et al., 1967; Gal, 1972; Janerich et al., 1974, 1977). Heinonen and coworkers (1977a) analyzed data from the Collaborative Perinatal Project and found an increased risk of cardiac anomalies associated with first-trimester exposure to oral contraceptives and female hormones. These data were later re-evaluated by Wiseman and associates (1984), who noted that a significant number of newborns with cardiac malformations had been exposed outside the time period (gestational age) that would impact cardiac development. These authors also excluded a number of newborns diagnosed with Down syndrome. Their analysis of the data from the Collaborative Perinatal Project suggested no increase in the risk of cardiac malformations associated with *in utero* exposure to these agents.

A number of other studies failed to support an association between progestational drugs and congenital malformations (Ferencz et al., 1980; Wilson and Brent, 1981; Katz et al., 1985; Ressequie et al., 1985; Rock et al., 1985; Check et al., 1986; Yovich et al., 1988; Brent, 1989). The FDA concluded that the available evidence does not support an increased risk of limb reduction defects, congenital heart disease, or neural tube defects after exposure to either progestins or oral contraceptives (Brent, 1989).

The potential for masculinization of the female fetus exists with exposure to certain testosterone-derived progestins during weeks 7 through 12. These preparations include ethinyl testosterone, 19-norethinyl testosterone, norgestrel, and norethynodrel (Schardein, 1980).

DIETHYLSTILBESTROL

Herbst and associates (1971) published a landmark study describing eight women diagnosed with vaginal adenocarcinoma in young adulthood whose mothers had taken diethylstilbestrol while pregnant. It is estimated that the absolute risk of diethylstilbestrol-related clear cell adenocarcinoma of the vagina or cervix is 1 per 1000 exposures (Melnick et al., 1987). Structural abnormalities of the reproductive tract (male and female) were also observed after exposure to the drug within the first 20 weeks of pregnancy. Abnormalities of the cervix and/or vagina (cervical collars, hoods, and septa) have been reported in 25% (Robboy et al., 1984), and abnormalities of the uterus (T-shaped cavity) are seen in as many as two thirds (Kaufman et al., 1980) of exposed females.

ADRENAL CORTICOSTEROIDS

As early as the 1960s, glucocorticoid use was associated with cleft lip and palate (Bongiovanno and McPadden, 1960). More recent evidence supports this association (Rodriguez-Pinella and Martinez-Frias, 1998; Carmichael and Shaw, 1999;

Park-Wyllie et al., 2000). A meta-analysis published by Park-Wyllie and coworkers (2000) concluded that the use of corticosteroids during pregnancy was associated with a 3.5-fold increase in the risk of oral clefts. The authors pointed out that this represents an extremely small increase (1 to 2 per 1000) in cases of cleft lip and palate among treated women. As always, the potential benefits of a medication must be balanced against the risks.

Psychoactive Medications

BENZODIAZEPINES

This group of drugs (all category D) includes lorazepam, alprazolam, chlordiazepoxide, and diazepam. Diazepam is the most widely studied among these drugs, and studies published in the 1970s suggested an association between the drug and cleft lip and palate (Aarskog, 1975; Safra and Oakley, 1975; Saxen, 1975). Several follow-up studies failed to show a significant increase in oral clefts among patients with first-trimester exposure to benzodiazepines (Rosenberg et al., 1983; Shiono and Mills, 1984; Czeizel, 1988). Rosenberg and associates (1983) conducted a case-control study of over 600 patients with cleft lip and palate and approximately 2500 control subjects who had other congenital abnormalities. The relative risk of oral clefts among patients with exposure to benzodiazepines during the first 4 months of pregnancy was 0.8 (95th CI, 0.4 to 1.7). Early reports linking the use of diazepam to congenital cardiac defects (Rothman et al., 1979; Bracken and Holford, 1981) have also not been duplicated. Investigations by both Bracken (1986) and Zierler and Rothman (1985) failed to show any significant increase in the risk of congenital heart disease related to maternal use of diazepam.

Although most data regarding the teratogenic potential of benzodiazepines is specific to diazepam, there are limited data on other agents used in the treatment of anxiety disorders. An increase in the risk of major malformations has been reported with both chlordiazepoxide (Kullander and Kallen, 1976; Heinonen et al., 1977b) and meprobamate (Milkovich and van den Berg, 1974; Saxen, 1975). Most published studies, however, suggest no increase in the risk of congenital anomalies among fetuses exposed to either chlordiazepoxide (Hartz et al., 1975; Czeizel, 1988) or meprobamate (Belafsky et al., 1969; Hartz et al., 1975).

In general, the published data do not support an overt increase in the risk of congenital malformations among fetuses exposed to benzodiazepines. Observed neonatal complications include a neonatal withdrawal syndrome (Rementeria and Bhatt, 1977) and the "floppy infant syndrome" (Gillberg 1977), described as hypotonia, feeding difficulties, and lethargy.

TRICYCLIC ANTIDEPRESSANTS

Early reports raised the possibility of cardiovascular (Briggs et al., 1998) and limb reduction abnormalities (McBride, 1972) among children exposed to either imipramine or amitriptyline. However, numerous reports show that these drugs are not associated with an increase in the risk of birth defects (Rachelefsky et al., 1972; Sim, 1972; Briggs et al., 1998). The Michigan Medicaid study analyzed data from 467 newborns exposed to amitriptyline (Briggs et al., 1998) and failed to find a significant difference in the number of birth defects. Nulman and associates (1997) reported on 80 infants

with in utero exposure to tricyclics, concluding no demonstrable impact of the exposure on language, intelligence quotient, or behavior.

LITHIUM

The initial report of lithium-associated congenital malformations is credited to Lewis and Suris (1970). The defects described included heart and great vessel abnormalities, Ebstein anomaly (misplaced tricuspid valve within right ventricle), neural tube defects, talipes, microtia, and thyroid abnormalities (Warkany, 1988). An international registry was established to better define the risk of these defects. Early reports from the registry (Weinstein and Goldfield, 1975) included information on 143 infants exposed to lithium in utero. Of the 13 noted to have malformations, 9 were cardiac abnormalities; 4 of the cardiac abnormalities were diagnosed with Ebstein anomaly. This finding of several newborns with Ebstein anomaly is dramatic when compared with the background risk in the general population (1 per 20,000). The methodologic shortcomings of these early reports led to a prospective study analyzing the outcome of 148 women who were identified through the Teratogen Information Services in North America. In this cohort of women, there was only one case of Ebstein anomaly discovered with no other cardiac malformations noted (Jacobson et al., 1992). A case-control study published by Zalzstein et al. (1990) found no increase in the use of lithium among 59 patients with Ebstein anomaly.

The available data suggest that the use of lithium is associated with an extremely small increase in the risk of cardiac abnormalities. It seems reasonable to include a fetal echocardiographic examination in the management of these pregnancies. If there is consideration given to discontinuation of the drug, this should be done slowly, over a 10- to 14-day period given the high risk of relapse among these patients (Cohen et al., 1994).

SELECTIVE SEROTONIN REUPTAKE INHIBITORS

Drugs within this class of antidepressants (fluoxetine, paroxetine, sertraline, etc.) are among the most widely prescribed medications among reproductive-aged women. In short, there is no apparent increase in the risk of congenital malformations among newborns born to women using these medications during pregnancy (category B). Fluoxetine is the most widely studied of these agents, with several investigations concluding that the risk of major malformations was not increased among women taking the drug during pregnancy (Pastuszak et al., 1993; Chambers et al., 1996; Goldstein et al., 1997). In addition, Nulman and coworkers (1997) evaluated over 200 children with an average age of 3 years who were exposed to fluoxetine in utero. No significant increase in neurobehavioral sequelae was noted in these infants. Although less data are available with regard to other serotonin reuptake inhibitors used in the treatment of depression, the available data (Kulin et al., 1998; Einarson et al., 2001) suggest that these newer agents are not associated with an increase in birth defects. A prospective, controlled, multicenter study conducted by Kulin and associates (1998) analyzed the pregnancy outcome of 267 women who used various selective serotonin reuptake inhibitors (fluvoxamine, paroxetine, and sertraline) during pregnancy. The incidence of major malformations among the study group (4.1%) was not significantly different from the control group (3.8%) (relative risk, 1.06; 95th CI, 0.43 to 2.62).

Vitamin A and Its Synthetic Derivatives

VITAMIN A

The teratogenic potential of excessive doses of vitamin A is well described in a number of animal models (Geelen, 1979; Rosa et al., 1986). There are also reports detailing congenital anomalies in humans associated with the consumption of excessive amounts (up to 500,000 IU) of vitamin A (Bernhardt and Dorsey, 1974; Von Lennep and El Khazen, 1985). A prospective study of over 22,000 pregnancies resulted in the identification of 339 newborns with congenital abnormalities. Among this cohort, there were 121 newborns with anomalies thought to originate in the cranial neural crest (the defects commonly associated with excessive vitamin A intake). The relative risk for these defects was 3.5 (95th CI, 1.7 to 7.3) among women ingesting more than 15,000 IU/day from diet and supplements combined and 4.8 (95th CI, 2.2 to 10.5) for women taking more than 10,000 IU/day from supplements alone (Rothman et al., 1995). The current recommendation for the intake of vitamin A by pregnant women states that supplementation, if necessary, should be limited to 5,000 IU daily.

ISOTRETINOIN

Various animal models demonstrated the teratogenicity of isotretinoin (Monga, 1997). Given these animal data, isotretinoin was classified as a category X drug by the FDA upon its release in the early 1980s (FDA, 1983). Shortly after it became available for the treatment of acne, observations of congenital anomalies among exposed newborns were reported (Rosa, 1983; Hill, 1984). A pattern of anomalies emerged that included cardiovascular defects (transposition and ventricular septal defect), dysmorphic ears, CNS abnormalities (hydrocephalus), thymic abnormalities, cleft palate, and abnormalities of the retinal or optic nerve. Lammer and colleagues (1985) detailed the outcome of 154 pregnancies complicated by first-trimester exposure to isotretinoin. Among the 59 patients that elected to continue their pregnancy (95 elective abortions) there were 12 spontaneous abortions and 21 live births with major congenital malformations. The reported risk of major malformations among fetuses exposed to isotretinoin ranged from 23% to 33% (Lammer, 1987; Dai et al., 1992). There does not appear to be a risk of malformations when the drug is discontinued at least 2 months before conception (Dai et al., 1989). A specialized program was established in 1988 aimed at clinicians prescribing the drug to reproductive-aged women. This program reinforced the need for both the documentation of a negative pregnancy test before prescribing isotretinoin and strict adherence to the use of two forms of contraception for the duration of drug use. Despite these efforts, isotretinoin-exposed pregnancies continue to occur. The Boston University Accutane Survey enrolled almost 500,000 reproductive-aged women during the years 1989 to 1999, and close follow-up documented 900 Accutane-exposed pregnancies (Centers for Disease Control and Prevention, 2000).

ETRETINATE

This drug is a synthetic retinoid used in the treatment of psoriasis. It is classified as a category X drug, associated with a pattern of anomalies similar to that seen with the use of isotretinoin (Geiger et al., 1994; Rothman et al., 1995).

Unlike isotretinoin, etretinate has a long half-life (120 days) and has been detected in the serum years after its discontinuation. Congenital malformations were reported in a patient who conceived approximately 1 year after stopping the drug (Lammer, 1988). It has been suggested that pregnancy should be delayed for at least 2 years after the discontinuation of etretinate (Geiger et al., 1994).

Miscellaneous

PENICILLAMINE

Most pregnancies in which penicillamine is used (primarily for Wilson disease) result in normal newborns. However, a connective tissue defect similar to generalized cutis laxa has been reported after the use of this drug (Mjolnerod et al., 1971; Rosa, 1986). The defects appear to be limited to the offspring of patients who are treated for a prolonged period of time, as in the case of chronic treatment for a pregnant woman with Wilson disease.

THALIDOMIDE

The association of thalidomide and congenital anomalies was first reported by Lenz and Knapp (1962). Exposure to this drug during a critical period (22 to 36 days after conception) is associated primarily with limb reduction defects, although other abnormalities have been reported. These anomalies include facial hemangiomas, intestinal atresias, deafness, and defects of both the renal and the cardiovascular systems (Knapp et al., 1962; Brent and Holmes, 1988; Lenz, 1988). The incidence of malformations among exposed fetuses has been estimated at 20% to 30% (Koren et al., 1998). The exact mechanism of thalidomide-induced embryopathy is controversial. The proposed mechanisms were reviewed by Stephens (1988). The recent reintroduction of thalidomide for the treatment of erythema nodosum leprosum has raised concern over the potential for inadvertent administration to a patient with an unrecognized pregnancy (Marwick, 1997; Ances, 2002).

MISOPROSTOL

The use of misoprostol has been associated with both Mobius syndrome (congenital facial paralysis) and limb reduction defects (Gonzalez et al., 1998; Pastuszak et al., 1998). Data from the Latin American Collaborative Study of Congenital Malformations suggested an increase in various malformations (transverse limb defects, arthrogryposis, hydrocephalus, holoprosencephaly, and exstrophy of the bladder) among newborns exposed to misoprostol. However, interpretation of the results from these studies is complicated by the concurrent use of other medications (e.g., methotrexate) that may also be teratogenic.

Diagnostic Agents

Ionizing Radiation

As early as the 1920s, the potential adverse effects of high-dose radiation on the fetus were recognized. In general, the effects noted to occur with greater frequency among infants exposed to high-dose radiation (e.g., 25 to 20 rads and greater) include microcephaly, growth restriction, and mental retardation (Hall, 1991). Data from the survivors of the atomic bomb in Nagasaki and Hiroshima showed an increasing risk of mental retardation and microcephaly associated with an increase in the fetal exposure to radiation. The risk appears to be the greatest when exposure occurred between 8 and 15 weeks' gestation. Higher doses were required to produce the same results as gestational age advanced (Yamazaki and Schull, 1990). The available data do not support an increase in the risk of mental retardation associated with radiation exposure beyond 25 weeks' or before 8 weeks' gestation. It has been suggested that the minimum dose associated with an increased risk of mental retardation is in the range of 20 to 40 rads (Committee on Biological Effects, 1990).

The clinical use of diagnostic imaging studies during pregnancy is rarely, if ever, associated with adverse fetal effects. This is a function of the relative low level of radiation to the fetus as a result of these procedures (Table 19-4). The American College of Radiologists (Hall, 1991) maintained "no single diagnostic procedure results in a radiation dose significant enough to threaten the well-being of the developing embryo and fetus." In summary, there is no evidence that supports an increase in pregnancy loss, congenital malformation, or growth restriction at cumulative doses less than 5 rad (Brent, 1989).

Magnetic Resonance Imaging

There is a growing list of obstetric indications for which magnetic resonance imaging is being used. These include the clarification of suspected fetal malformations, the characterization of maternal pelvic masses, suspected placenta accreta, and the evaluation of suspected tumors in the maternal abdomen and retroperitoneal space. The available data suggest no reported harmful human effects (including mutagenic) from the use of magnetic resonance imaging (Wagner et al., 1997; American College of Radiology, 1998).

Ultrasound

The safety of diagnostic ultrasonography has been studied extensively. There have been no fetal risks associated with the use of real-time imaging of the fetus (Miller et al., 1998).

TABLE 19-4. ESTIMATED FETAL EXPOSURE ASSOCIATED WITH VARIOUS DIAGNOSTIC IMAGING PROCEDURES

Procedure	Level of Exposure
Chest radiograph (posteroanterior and lateral)	0.02–0.07 mrad
Abdominal film (single view)	100 mrad
Intravenous pyelography	1 rad or greater
Hip film (single view)	200 mrad
Mammography	7–20 mrad
Barium enema or small bowel series	2–4 rad
CT of head or chest	<1 rad
CT of abdomen and lumbar spine	3.5 rad
CT pelvimetry	230 mrad

CT, computed tomography.

Modified from American College of Obstetricians and Gynecologists: Guidelines for Diagnostic Imaging during Pregnancy. Committee Opinion No. 158. Washington, DC, American College of Obstetricians and Gynecologists, 1995.

Nuclear Medicine Studies

The potential fetal complications associated with the use of radioactive iodine were discussed previously in this chapter. The other common use of nuclear medicine imaging techniques during pregnancy is that of the ventilation-perfusion scan. This procedure, which typically involves the use of technetium-labeled albumin (99^mTc) and inhaled xenon gas (^{127}Xe or ^{133}Xe), is safe. The dose of radiation delivered to the fetus has been estimated to be no greater than 50 mrad (Ginsberg et al., 1989).

Environmental Agents

Organic Solvents

Several publications reviewed the complex subject of occupational exposure and offered suggestions for counseling these women about the potential for teratogenicity (Bentur and Koren, 1991; Giacoia, 1992). McMartin and associates (1998) published a meta-analysis of epidemiologic investigations in which they showed an increased risk of major malformations associated with first-trimester exposure to occupational organic solvents. An analysis of five studies (n = 7036 patients) suggested a significant increase in the risk of malformations among the offspring of women with reported occupational exposures (OR, 1.64; 95th CI, 1.16 to 2.30). There was also a trend toward an increase in the risk of spontaneous abortion (OR, 1.25; 95th CI, 0.99 to 1.58).

A prospective, observational, controlled study of 125 pregnant women with first-trimester exposure to occupational organic solvents was conducted through the Motherisk Program at the University of Toronto (Khattak et al., 1999). The incidence of major malformations in the study patients was compared with a control group of pregnant women exposed to a nonteratogenic agent. The relative risk for anomalies in the study group was 13 (95th CI, 1.8 to 99.5). Among the 13 anomalous fetuses, 12 were delivered to women who reported being symptomatic as a result of their exposure.

Pesticides

Despite hundreds of studies, available data are insufficient to allow conclusions regarding a possible association between exposure to pesticides and congenital anomalies. Interested readers are referred to detailed discussions outlining the investigations in this field (Nurminen, 1995; Garcia, 1998).

Mercury

Exposure to significant amounts of methylmercury, primarily by the consumption of contaminated seafood, has been associated with neurodevelopmental deficits since the Japanese epidemics of 1956 (Minamata) and 1965 (Niigata). The reported effects included cerebral palsy and mental retardation (Minamata disease) (Matsumoto et al., 1965). A recent study (Kondo, 2000; Steuerwald et al., 2000) reinforced the concern over the fetal effects of maternal ingestion of seafood contaminated with methylmercury. One hundred eighty-two singleton term births from the Faeroe Islands in the North Atlantic were analyzed. Numerous fetal and maternal tissue samples were obtained and evaluated for contaminants, including methylmercury and polychlorinated biphenyls. The authors

TABLE 19-5. SOURCES OF CURRENT
TERATOGEN INFORMATION

Massachusetts Teratogen Information Service
Boston, Massachusetts
(617) 466-8474

Texas Teratogen Information Services
(800) 733-4727

Pregnancy Riskline
Salt Lake City, Utah
(801) 328-2229

Reproductive Toxicology Center
REPROTOX
Columbia Hospital for Women Medical Center
Washington, DC
(202) 293-5137

Organization of Teratogen Information Services
http://orphues.ucsd.edu/ctis

Motherisk Program, Toronto
(416) 813-6780
www.motherisk.org

concluded that higher levels of cord-blood mercury levels were associated with an increased risk of the association of both mercury and lead and with neurodevelopmental deficits (Mendola et al., 2002).

Lead

In utero exposure to high levels of lead has been associated with an increase in pregnancy loss and with mental retardation (ACOG, 1997b). Interested readers are referred to a recent review of the association of both mercury and lead with neurodevelopmental abnormalities in the offspring (Mendola et al., 2002).

In summary, it is important to provide the pregnant woman and her family with accurate information regarding exposure to therapeutic, diagnostic, and environmental agents. This crucial responsibility can be extremely challenging, and the ramifications of relaying inaccurate information are far reaching. The reader should be aware of the various teratogen information services and computer databases that are available to assist in obtaining the most appropriate information (Table 19-5).

SOCIAL AND ILLICIT DRUG USE

The use of illicit drugs during pregnancy has received significant attention over the past 15 years. Although a great deal has been learned regarding the implications of perinatal drug use, many important issues remain unsettled. In addition, far too little attention is given to the consequences of the use of social drugs (i.e., alcohol and tobacco), which are by far the most commonly used substances during pregnancy and contribute significantly to adverse perinatal outcome. Fetal alcohol syndrome (FAS), for example, is the most common nongenetic cause of mental retardation in the Western world (Abel and Sokol, 1987), and tobacco use is the most common

preventable cause of low birth weight, with an attributable risk of approximately 15% (Ventura et al., 1995).

Numerous issues complicate the interpretation of data generated from clinical investigations that deal with pregnancies among women who use alcohol, tobacco, or illicit drugs:

1. Concurrent use of multiple drugs
2. Timing of exposure (trimester)
3. Degree of exposure (amount and purity of drug)
4. Social support and environmental effects (e.g., availability of prenatal care, nutrition, parenting skills)
5. Selection of an appropriate control group

Ongoing research in the area of perinatal substance use is focusing on an explanation for the broad spectrum of effects observed among pregnancies. The potential for variation in genetic susceptibility of the fetus to a given drug may explain to some degree the variability in perinatal outcome. Studies are also being designed to address the importance of timing, frequency, and degree of exposure as well as the contribution of confounding environmental factors (nutrition, adequacy of prenatal care, etc.).

Prevalence and Drug Screening

The most recent data available are included in the results from the National Household Survey on Drug Abuse, conducted by the National Institute on Drug Abuse (Substance Abuse and Mental Health Services Administration, 2000) (Table 19-6). This report details findings from a cohort of over 50,000 women (45,875 nonpregnant and 2387 pregnant) who were asked about their use of alcohol, tobacco, or illicit drugs within the preceding month. Among pregnant females, 64% were white, 15% African American, 14% Hispanic, 3% Asian, and less than 1% were Native Americans or Alaskans. Among pregnant women, 3.3% (80,000) reported having used an illicit drug within the preceding month, the most common drug being marijuana (2.5%). This compares with the prevalence among nonpregnant women (any illicit drug 7.7%, marijuana 5.7%). Cocaine use was reported by 0.1% of pregnant and 0.8% of nonpregnant women. Among pregnant women, illicit drug use is reportedly more common by younger women (aged 15 to 17 years) and by African American women. As expected, tobacco and alcohol use are reported significantly more commonly than illicit drugs. Tobacco use was reported by 17% (416,000) of pregnant women interviewed (31.6% of nonpregnant women) and was more common among younger women and white women. Thirteen percent of pregnant women (316,000) admitted to the use of alcohol within the past month, with 3% (80,000) of pregnant women admitting to "binge" drinking (five or more drinks at one sitting). Heavy drinking (five or more drinks on the same occasion on each of 5 or more days during the past month) was reported by 0.7% of pregnant women. The use of alcohol was more common among women between the ages of 26 and 44, whereas heavy and binge drinking was common in the 15- to 17-year-old subset. Alcohol use was reported more commonly among white women, with both binge drinking and heavy drinking more common among Native Americans and Alaskans.

Given the well-documented discrepancies between self-reporting of drug use and toxicology results, many investigators have relied on toxicology studies (urine and/or meconium) to estimate the prevalence of drug use among

TABLE 19-6. PREVALENCE OF SOCIAL AND ILLICIT DRUG USE DURING PREGNANCY

	Alcohol (%)	Tobacco (%)	Cocaine (%)	Amphetamines (%)	Marijuana (%)	Opiates (%)
National Pregnancy and Health Survey, 1995* (n = 2163)	18.8	20.4	1.1	—	2.9	—
Vega et al., 1993† (n = 29,494)	6.5	8.9	1.1	0.7	1.9	1.5
Ostrea et al., 1992‡ (n = 3010)	—	—	30.7	—	11.9	20.5
Chasnoff et al., 1990 (n = 715)	—	—	3.4	—	11.9	0.3
CDC, Rhode Island, 1990 (n = 465)	—	—	2.6	0.2	3.0	1.7
Gillogley et al., 1990 (n = 1643)	—	—	8.5	6.5	—	1.2
Lester et al., 2001 (n = 8527)‡	—	—	9.5	—	7.2	2.3
National Household Survey on Drug Abuse, 2000 (n = 2387)	13	17	0.1	—	3.3	—

*Screening by self-report (patient history).
†Screening on maternal urine and by self-report (tobacco).
‡Screening on neonatal meconium samples.
CDC, Centers for Disease Control and Prevention.

pregnant women. Numerous studies reinforce the poor correlation between maternal self-report and urine toxicology (Zuckerman et al., 1989; Gillogley et al., 1990; Markovic et al., 2000; Ostrea et al., 2001). Among the patients with positive urine drug screens in the intrapartum screening done by Gillogley and coworkers (1990), 48% denied drug use on hospital admission.

A large population-based epidemiologic study in California surveyed more than 200 hospitals and nearly 30,000 women (Vega et al., 1993). The most frequently identified drug (urine toxicology) was alcohol (6.5%), followed by cannabinoid (1.9%), opiates (1.5%), cocaine (1.15%), and amphetamines (0.7%). The use of meconium samples has generally yielded a higher rate of perinatal drug exposure. A prospective study of more than 3000 neonates found that 44% of the meconium samples collected were positive for cocaine, marijuana, or opiates. Among the women admitting to illicit drug use (11%), urine toxicology was positive in 52%, whereas meconium testing identified 88% as positive (Ostrea et al., 1992). Lester and coworkers (2001) analyzed the meconium of 8527 newborns as a part of the multicenter Maternal Lifestyle Study. Cocaine metabolites were identified in 9.5%, opiates in 2.3%, and marijuana metabolites in 7.2%.

Although meconium and hair are more sensitive methods in the detection of drug use, testing of maternal urine remains the most frequently used tool for screening. Even though the analysis of meconium and hair (Chiarotti et al., 1996; Kline et al., 1997) are significantly more sensitive than urine toxicology, false-positive results (thought to be a result of passive exposure) are encountered with the use of hair samples (Ostrea et al., 2001), whereas meconium testing is not widely available and is significantly more expensive (Kwong and Ryan, 1997). The major disadvantage of urine drug screening is that it detects only relatively recent drug use. The metabolites of alcohol are detectable for 8 hours, whereas cocaine, amphetamine, and opiate metabolites can be found for 24 to 72 hours after use. Only the metabolites of marijuana and benzodiazepines persist for a period of weeks (Hawks and Chiang, 1986). Selective drug screening (most commonly urine) is thought by many to be a necessary adjunct to history taking in the detection of illicit drug use.

Numerous drug-screening criteria have been suggested, and a proposed set of indications is listed in Table 19-7. The design and implementation of any drug-screening program should

include input from legal counsel and social services staff to address specific liability issues and local reporting laws.

Alcohol

The effects of alcohol on the fetus and newborn have been recognized for centuries. Aristotle said "foolish, drunk, or hare brained women for the most part bring forth children like unto themselves, difficult and listless" (Rosett and Weiner, 1984).

TABLE 19-7. CRITERIA FOR URINE DRUG SCREENING

Physical appearance and demeanor
  Altered mental status
  Pupils extremely dilated or constricted
  Track marks or abscesses in extremities
  Inflamed or indurated nasal mucosa
Obstetric (past or present)
  Preterm labor or preterm delivery
  Low-birth-weight infant
  Intrauterine growth restriction
  Preterm premature rupture of membranes
  Placental abruption
  Fetal death
  Unexplained congenital anomalies
  Suspected neonatal withdrawal symptoms
  Absent or erratic prenatal care
Medical
  Human immunodeficiency virus/acquired immunodeficiency
    syndrome
  Cellulitis
  Cirrhosis
  Endocarditis
  Hepatitis
  Pancreatitis
  Pneumonia
  Sexually transmitted diseases
Social
  Illicit drug use by partner
  Incarceration
  Prostitution
  Domestic violence

Modified from Chasnoff IJ: Perinatal effects of cocaine. Contemp Obstet Gynecol **29:**163, 1987.

In 1973, a pattern of anomalies was described in infants born to alcoholic women (Jones et al., 1973). In the years that followed, numerous studies reinforced the adverse fetal effects of maternal alcohol use (Ouellette et al., 1977; Clarren and Smith, 1978; Hanson et al., 1978; Olegard et al., 1979; Sokol et al., 1980). These data led to a report from the U.S. Surgeon General, who recommended that without an identifiable threshold, the safest course was abstinence (FDA, 1981).

Despite this recommendation and a report suggesting that FAS is the most common nongenetic cause of mental retardation (Abel and Sokol, 1986), women have continued to drink alcohol while pregnant. The Centers for Disease Control and Prevention (2002a) reported the results from the Behavioral Risk Factor Surveillance System completed in 1999. This self-report telephone survey conducted throughout all 50 states demonstrated that alcohol consumption among pregnant women increased from 12.4% in 1991 to a high of 16.3% in 1995 with a small decrease in 1999 to 12.8%. Frequent drinking, defined as at least seven drinks in a week or at least five drinks on at least one occasion, increased from 0.8% in 1991 to 3.5% in 1995 ($P < .01$) and 3.3% in 1999. Binge drinking, defined as at least five drinks at one sitting, was less than 1.0% in 1991, 2.9% in 1995, and 2.7% in 1995.

Gladstone and coworkers (1997) reported binge drinking (mean drinks daily, 7.2) among 3.1% of pregnant women interviewed. These women were more likely to be single, to smoke cigarettes, and to report the use of illicit drugs than the control group. The prevalence of heavy or problem drinkers varies from 6% to 11%, depending on methodology and terminology (Sokol et al., 1981; Abel and Sokol, 1989). These pregnancies are thought to be the most consistently and severely affected (Rosett et al., 1983).

Ethanol is metabolized to acetaldehyde by nicotinamide adenine dinucleotide–dependent alcohol dehydrogenase. Both ethanol and acetaldehyde are toxic to the fetus. The pharmacokinetics of ethanol in the maternal–fetal unit have been studied extensively, with data demonstrating an unimpeded and bidirectional movement of alcohol between the maternal and fetal compartments. Studies in human subjects (Idanpann-Heikkila et al., 1972), sheep (Brien et al., 1985, 1987; Clarke et al., 1988), guinea pigs (Clarke et al., 1986), and mice (Blakeley and Scott, 1984) demonstrate that maternal and fetal concentrations of alcohol (serum) are equivalent. Investigations in the human (Brien et al., 1983) and in the pregnant ewe (Brien et al., 1987; Clarke et al., 1988) suggest that amniotic fluid levels rise more slowly than fetal blood levels but remain detectable after the disappearance of ethanol from the fetal circulation. The activity of alcohol dehydrogenase in fetal liver is less than 10% of that observed in the adult liver (Pikkarainen and Raiha, 1967; Cumming et al., 1985; Clarke et al., 1989). Therefore, the fetus is reliant on maternal hepatic transformation of ingested ethanol and may be exposed to prolonged levels of ethanol in the amniotic fluid.

The mechanisms by which ethanol exerts its effects on the developing fetus are complex and not completely understood. Various animal models have suggested that ethanol exposure interferes with protein synthesis (Henderson et al., 1980; Dresoti et al., 1981; Inselman et al., 1985) and with the placental transfer of amino acids and glucose (Fisher et al., 1981; Marquis et al., 1984; Gordon et al., 1985; Snyder et al., 1986). Fetal hypoglycemia, hypoinsulinemia, and a decrease in fetal thyroid hormones and liver glycogen stores were also demon-

strated (Rose et al., 1981; Singh et al., 1984, 1986) and may contribute to abnormalities of fetal growth. Alterations in urinary metabolites of prostacyclin and thromboxane have been reported in neonates born to alcoholic women (Ylikorkala et al., 1988), suggesting that an alteration in the prostacyclin-to-thromboxane ratio and resultant vasoconstriction may contribute to the various fetal effects. Halmesmaki and coworkers (1990) hypothesized that ethanol-exposed fetuses are subjected to chronic hypoxemia, reflected by elevated levels of erythropoietin in umbilical cord blood samples. Interested readers are referred to a recent review discussing the mechanisms surrounding free oxygen radicals, growth regulatory factors, acetaldehyde formation, and retinoic acid (Chaudhuri, 2000).

FAS (Sokol and Clarren, 1989) is a specific recognizable pattern of malformations (Figs. 19-2 and 19-3) generally defined as follows:

1. Prenatal and postnatal growth deficiency
2. CNS abnormalities
3. Craniofacial abnormalities

These criteria, along with an expanded list (Table 19-8), comprise the clinical spectrum of neonates/infants with FAS. It is interesting to note that most clinical findings are supported by research using various animal models (Randall et al., 1977; Ellis and Pick, 1980; Clarren and Bowden, 1982). Nwaogu and Ihemelandu (1999) showed a decrease in muscle mass among neonatal rats treated with ethanol *in utero* corresponding to the consistent pattern of growth delay seen in FAS. Others showed abnormalities in the ultrastructure of neurons in both the motor and sensory cortex in rats treated with ethanol (Ashwell and Zhang, 1996). Daft and colleagues (1986) found an increase in several complex cardiac defects in ethanol-treated mice.

The reported incidence of FAS varies from 1 in 50 to 1 in 2500 live births (Clarren and Smith, 1978; Obe and Majewski,

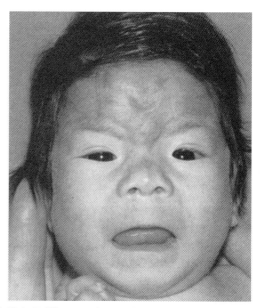

FIGURE 19-2 ■ Nine-month-old infant with fetal alcohol syndrome. (From Streissguth AP, Aase JM, Clarren SK, et al: Fetal alcohol syndrome in adolescents and adults. JAMA **265**:1961, 1991. Copyright 1991, American Medical Association.)

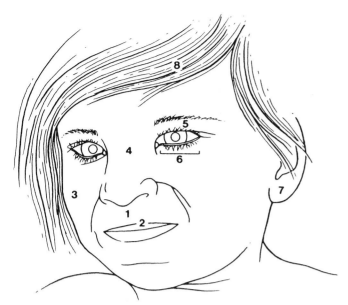

FIGURE 19-3 ■ Facial features associated with fetal alcohol syndrome. *1,* Absent philtrum; *2,* thinned upper vermilion; *3,* hypoplastic midface; *4,* low nasal bridge; *5,* epicanthal fold; *6,* shortened palpebral fissure; *7,* low-set ears; *8,* microcephaly. (From Coles CD: Impact of prenatal alcohol exposure on the newborn and the child. Clin Obstet Gynecol **36:**255, 1993.)

1978; Olegard et al., 1979; Sokol et al., 1980; Abel, 1995). A review of the data concluded that the overall rate of FAS in the Western world is 0.33 per 1000 live births (Abel and Sokol, 1991). The incidence of FAS among parents who are heavy drinkers is significantly greater, possibly as high as 8% (Abel, 1988). Data from the Birth Defects Monitoring Program from the Centers for Disease Control and Prevention (1995) suggested a fourfold increase in the incidence of FAS over the years 1979 to 1993. The most recent data available from the Centers for Disease Control and Prevention (2002b) and the Fetal Alcohol Syndrome Surveillance Network reported a relatively stable incidence of FAS. Data collected from four states showed the incidence of FAS to be 0.3 to 0.4 per 1000 live births.

Although a few reports have not shown a significant effect of alcohol on birth weight (Tennes and Blackard, 1980; Marbury et al., 1983; Coles et al., 1985), most studies support this association (Little, 1977; Ouellette et al., 1977; Hanson et al., 1978; Kaminski et al., 1978; Rosett et al., 1983; Halmesmaki, 1988; Day et al., 1989). Studies conducted in both cultured rat embryos (Brown et al., 1979) and CH3 mice (Lochry et al., 1982) showed a dose-dependent reduction in growth associated with ethanol exposure. Similarly, a decrease in mean fetal weight has been documented in the ovine fetus after a chronic infusion of intravenous ethanol (Rose et al., 1981) and in beagles after chronic gastric lavage with ethanol (Ellis and Pick, 1980).

Mills and coworkers (1984) prospectively followed more than 30,000 pregnancies, noting a decrease in mean birth weight of 165 g in women reporting the consumption of three to five drinks per day. Sokol and coinvestigators (1980) observed a similar effect on birth weight (190 g) when they compared nondrinkers with those admitting to alcohol use during their pregnancy. Data from the National Natality Survey conducted by the National Center for Health Statistics

demonstrated a significant difference in mean birth weight among those patients with moderate (0 to 13 drinks a week) alcohol use (3181 g) and heavy (more than two drinks a day) alcohol use (2808 g) compared with patients who were abstinent during pregnancy (3301 g). Both Virji (1991) and Mills and coworkers (1984) demonstrated a dose-dependent increase in the likelihood of delivering a low-birth-weight infant. Among heavy drinkers, 33% (11 of 33) delivered an infant weighing less than 2500 g (Virji, 1991). These differences were independent of tobacco use, maternal weight gain, parity, and level of education.

The impact of ethanol on growth extends into infancy. In a follow-up study of more than 400 inner city infants whose mothers used social or illicit drugs, infants exposed to alcohol late in pregnancy had a slower rate of growth over the first 6 months of life than infants exposed to cocaine, tobacco, or opiates (Jacobson et al., 1994). The evidence also supports a decrease in mean birth length and in mean head circumference among infants with *in utero* exposure to ethanol (Ouellette et al., 1977; Smith et al., 1986; Day et al., 1989).

Data from both animal models (Clarren and Astley, 1992) and human subjects (Harlap and Shiono, 1980; Kline et al., 1980; Kaminski et al., 1981) suggested that the use of alcohol is associated with an increased risk of spontaneous abortion. Several of the clinical studies supporting this association (Kline et al., 1980; Russell and Skinner, 1988; Armstrong et al., 1992) demonstrated a "dose-dependent" effect of alcohol, with odds ratios ranging from 1.02 to 2.62. In contrast, several investigations were unable to duplicate this finding (Parazzini et al., 1990; Cavallo et al., 1995). Abel (1997) published a thorough review of this subject .

There is evidence that abnormalities in fetal growth (i.e., decreased head circumference and low birth weight) and, possibly, the entire FAS can be significantly lowered by a reduced alcohol intake during pregnancy (Rosett et al., 1983; Halmesmaki, 1988). Given this possibility, it is clear that identifying the pregnant alcohol user is of great importance.

TABLE 19-8. CLINICAL FEATURES OF FETAL ALCOHOL SYNDROME

A. Common presentations
 1. Prenatal and/or postnatal growth retardation*
 2. Mental retardation*
 3. Facial dysmorphogenesis*
 4. Cardiac septal defects
 5. Minor joint abnormalities
B. Less common presentations
 1. Ocular abnormalities
 2. Retinal abnormalities
 3. Hearing and vestibular disturbances
 4. Urinary abnormalities
 5. Hepatic anomalies
 6. Cardiac defects (heart rate pattern abnormalities)
 7. Immune system impairment
 8. Skeletal system abnormalities
 9. Cutaneous abnormalities
 10. Nail dysplasia

* Included in the original description of fetal alcohol syndrome.

From Chaudhuri JD: Alcohol and the developing fetus. Med Sci Monit **6:**1031, 2000.

However, Sokol and Miller (1980) found that three of every four pregnant patients with alcohol abuse went undetected by the clinician.

Several approaches to detecting alcohol use by way of patient interview were studied (Pokorny et al., 1972; Ewing, 1984). Sokol and colleagues (1989) described the T-ACE questionnaire (Table 19-9), an instrument consisting of four questions used to identify the at-risk (heavy) drinker. The probability of risk drinking increased from 1.5% in those responding negatively to all four questions to 63% for those answering positively to all four items. This brief screening tool for alcohol abuse should be included in every initial prenatal visit.

Although it is generally agreed that heavy alcohol use places the patient at a significant risk for delivery of a low-birth-weight infant or an infant with FAS, a "safe" level of alcohol consumption has not been determined. FAS has been described with the consumption of as little as 2 ounces of alcohol daily, and partial expression of FAS (i.e., fetal alcohol effects) has been reported in women using only 1 ounce per day (Abel, 1988; Little et al., 1992). *At present, there is no clear minimum threshold for the effects of alcohol on the fetus, and pregnant women should be counseled to abstain from its use.*

Smoking

The deleterious effects of cigarette smoking on pregnancy outcome have been recognized for decades. The original report associating cigarette smoking to prematurity (defined as birth weight less than 2500 g) was published in the late 1950s (Simpson, 1957). Since that time, the published evidence implicating cigarette smoking as a major cause of perinatal morbidity and mortality has been overwhelming. Tobacco use during pregnancy is recognized to be responsible for 15% to 25% of all low-birth-weight infants (Institute of Medicine, 1985; Ventura, 1995), 10% to 15% of all preterm births (Shiono, Klebanoff, Rhoads, 1986), and 5% of all perinatal deaths (Prager et al., 1984).

Many studies support the link between the use of tobacco and an increase in overall perinatal mortality (Meyer and Tonascia, 1977; Schramm, 1997; Kleinman et al., 1988). The Ontario Perinatal Mortality Study concluded that the relative risk of perinatal mortality among smokers was 1.27, which translates to an attributable risk of 10.5% (Meyer et al., 1976). Data from the State of Missouri vital statistics (360,000 births, 2500 fetal deaths, and 3800 infant deaths) reinforced the association between smoking and an increase in perinatal

TABLE 19-10. PERINATAL COMPLICATIONS ASSOCIATED WITH TOBACCO USE

Spontaneous abortion
Premature rupture of membranes
Preterm delivery
Low birth weight
Intrauterine growth restriction
Placenta previa
Placental abruption
Sudden infant death syndrome

mortality (Kleinman et al., 1988). Among primigravidas smoking at least one pack per day, the odds ratio for fetal death was 1.62 (95th CI, 1.34 to 1.97) and 1.42 (95th CI, 1.16 to 1.74) for neonatal death. The odds ratio for both fetal and neonatal death among multiparous women was 1.30. This increase in adverse perinatal outcome may be secondary to the association of smoking with low birth weight, preterm birth, placenta previa, placental abruption, premature rupture of the membranes (PROM), and spontaneous abortion (Andres et al., 1996) (Table 19-10).

The physiologic mechanisms responsible for the adverse consequences of cigarette smoking during pregnancy center on carbon monoxide and nicotine. Carbon monoxide crosses the placenta (Longo and Ching, 1977) and binds to hemoglobin, forming carboxyhemoglobin, which reduces the oxygen-carrying capacity of blood (Astrup, 1972). Similarly, carbon dioxide increases the affinity of hemoglobin for oxygen, which in turn interferes with oxygen delivery to the tissues (Longo, 1977). Studies in the pregnant ewe (Longo and Hill, 1977) and in the human (Bureau et al., 1982) show that fetal carboxyhemoglobin levels exceed maternal carboxyhemoglobin levels, leading to a relatively prolonged fetal exposure to the effects of carboxyhemoglobin (Fig. 19-4).

Nicotine crosses the placenta (Manning and Feyerabend, 1976) and is detectable in the fetal circulation. The concentration of nicotine in fetal serum exceeds maternal serum

TABLE 19-9. T-ACE QUESTIONS FOUND TO BE SIGNIFICANT IDENTIFIERS OF RISK DRINKING*

T   How many drinks does it take to make you feel high (**T**OLERANCE)?
A   Have people **A**NNOYED you by criticizing your drinking?
C   Have you felt you ought to **C**UT DOWN on your drinking?
E   Have you ever had a drink first thing in the morning to steady your nerves or to get rid of a hangover (**E**YE-OPENER)?

* Alcohol intake sufficient to cause potential damage to embryo or fetus.

From Sokol RJ, Martier SS, Ager JW: The T-ACE questions: Practical prenatal detection of risk-drinking. Am J Obstet Gynecol **160**:863, 1989.

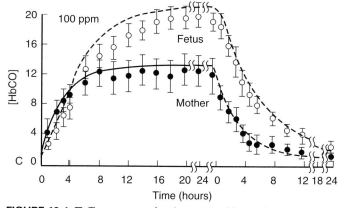

FIGURE 19-4 ■ Time course of carbon monoxide uptake in maternal and fetal sheep exposed to carbon monoxide. The experimental results for the ewe (●) and fetal lamb (○) are the mean values (± SEM). The theoretical predictions of the changes in maternal and fetal carboxyhemoglobin (HbCO) levels for the ewe and lamb are shown by the solid and interrupted lines, respectively. (From Longo LD: The biological effects of carbon monoxide on the pregnant woman, fetus, and newborn infant. Am J Obstet Gynecol **129**:69, 1977.)

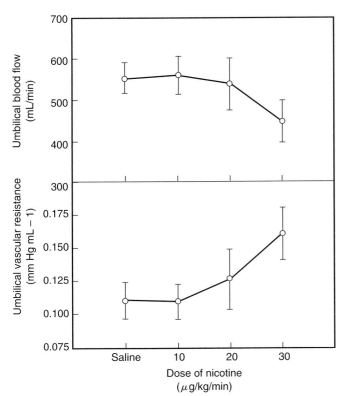

FIGURE 19-5 ■ Umbilical blood flow and umbilical vascular resistance response to maternally administered nicotine. Maternal administration produced a decrease in umbilical blood flow from a baseline of 554 ± 37 to 449 ± 52 mL/min, which was significant only at the 30-µg/kg/min dose (P < .05). Umbilical vascular resistance increased from a baseline of 0.110 ± 0.013 to 0.161 ± .020 mm Hg/mL, which was significant only at the 30-µg/kg/min dose (P < .05). For the 20-µg/kg/min dose, n = 6. For saline solution and all other doses, n = 8. (From Clark KE, Irion GL: Fetal hemodynamic response to maternal intravenous nicotine administration. Am J Obstet Gynecol **167**:1624, 1992.)

maturity) among women who smoked, the risk increasing with the number of cigarettes smoked daily (Fig. 19-6). Since that time, a dose-response effect of smoking on the incidence of low birth weight has been noted in several investigations (Meyer et al., 1976; Miller and Jekel, 1987; McDonald et al., 1992a).

Data from the Ontario Perinatal Mortality Study demonstrated that women smoking more than one pack of cigarettes daily had a 130% increased risk for delivering an infant weighing under 2500 g; women who smoked less than one pack per day increased their risk by only 53% (Meyer et al., 1976). The association with low birth weight is thought to be primarily due to IUGR and is observed across gestational ages (Davies et al., 1976; Hoff et al., 1986; Horta et al., 1997). A study by McDonald and colleagues (1992a) concluded that the odds ratio for the delivery of a small-for-gestational age infant (birth weight less than the 5th percentile) among those women smoking more than 20 cigarettes a day was 3.19 (95th CI, 2.82 to 3.60).

Studies show that the average difference in birth weight between smokers and nonsmokers ranges from 127 to 274 g (Jeanty et al., 1987; Kline et al., 1987; Hebel et al., 1988; Pulkkinen, 1990). Perkins and coworkers (1997) demonstrated a significant negative correlation (r = –0.19) between maternal serum cotinine levels (metabolic product of nicotine) and mean birth weight. There was a 100-g decrease in mean birth weight for each 1 µg/L increase in serum cotinine (Perkins et al., 1997). As is true with the incidence of low birth weight, the effect of smoking on the difference in mean birth weight is thought to be dose dependent (Hoff et al., 1986; Beaulac-Baillargeon and Desrosiers, 1987; Haddow et al., 1987; Hebel et al., 1988).

Smoking has also been reported to be an independent risk factor for preterm labor and delivery. Several studies suggested an increase in the relative risk (range, 1.4 to 1.8) of preterm delivery among smokers compared with women who do not

levels in the pregnant ewe (Monheit et al., 1983), the rhesus monkey (Suzuki et al., 1974), and, more recently, the human (Luck et al., 1985). Suzuki and colleagues (1980) showed that uterine blood flow is reduced by as much as 38% after the intravascular infusion of nicotine to the pregnant rhesus monkey. Similar alterations in uterine blood flow (Monheit et al., 1983; Clark and Irion, 1992) and umbilical blood flow (Clark and Irion, 1992) (Fig. 19-5) were reported by investigators who used the pregnant ewe. The effect of nicotine on fetal oxygenation and acid-base balance is controversial, with some studies noting significant hypoxemia and acidemia (Manning et al., 1978; Suzuki et al., 1980) and others failing to demonstrate significant changes in either arterial partial pressure of oxygen or pH (Clark and Irion, 1992; Monheit et al., 1983). The uterine artery vasoconstriction may be explained by the increase in circulating catecholamines.

Resnik and coworkers (1979) demonstrated a significant increase in both epinephrine (60.4%) and norepinephrine (70.1%) levels over control values after an infusion of nicotine to the pregnant ewe. In the human, amniotic fluid catecholamine levels are significantly higher in smokers than in nonsmokers (Divers et al., 1981). Simpson (1957) is credited with reporting the relationship between cigarette smoking and an increase in the incidence of low birth weight. She observed a twofold increase in the incidence of low birth weight (pre-

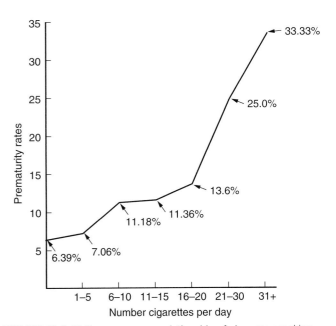

FIGURE 19-6 ■ Dose–response relationship of cigarette smoking and prematurity. (From Simpson WJ: A preliminary report on cigarette smoking and the incidence of prematurity. Am J Obstet Gynecol **73**:808, 1957.)

smoke during pregnancy (Meyer et al., 1976; Guzick et al., 1984; Virji and Cottington, 1991; Heffner et al., 1993; Kolas et al., 2000; Ohmi et al., 2002).

A recent prospective study from the National Institute of Child Health and Development showed that preterm birth (less than 37 weeks' gestation) occurred in 6.8% of nonsmokers compared with 8.1% of women smoking more than one pack of cigarettes daily. The adjusted odds ratio for preterm birth among the smokers was 1.2 (95th CI, 1.1 to 1.4) with an attributable risk due to smoking of 4% (Shiono, Klebanoff, Rhoads, 1986). Among a large (n = 40,445) cohort of singleton pregnancies, the relative risk of preterm birth among those smoking at least 10 cigarettes daily was 1.43 (95th CI, 1.27 to 1.60) (McDonald et al., 1992a). Kyrklund-Blomberg and Cnattingius (1998) analyzed over 300,000 singleton births over a 2-year period in Sweden. In this cohort, smoking was associated with an increase in the risk (OR, 1.7) of spontaneous preterm birth and preterm birth at less than 32 weeks' gestational age. This increased risk persisted after controlling for smoking-associated complications, leading to elective preterm delivery.

Several authors noted an increase in the risk of both placenta previa (Kramer et al., 1989; Williams et al., 1991; Monica and Lilja, 1995; Ananth et al., 1996; Andres, 1996; Chemlow et al., 1996; Mortensen et al., 2001) and placental abruption (Meyer and Tonascia, 1977; Naeye, 1980; Eriksen et al., 1991; Spinillo et al., 1994; Ananth et al., 1996; Mortensen et al., 2001) among smokers. A case-control study of 32 cases of placenta previa and 96 matched control subjects showed a relative risk for placenta previa of 3.0 (95th CI, 1.3 to 9.9), which persisted after controlling for parity, age, previous cesarean birth, and previous spontaneous abortion (Chemlow et al., 1996). A large epidemiologic study (87,184 pregnancies) analyzed data from 17 hospitals in Nova Scotia, where the incidence of smoking among pregnant women was 33%. Placenta previa was diagnosed in 3.6 per 1000 pregnancies, with smokers having a relative risk of 1.36 (95th CI, 1.04 to 1.79) (Ananth et al., 1996). It has been suggested that the placental hypertrophy observed in women who smoke increases the risk of implantation in the lower uterine segment.

A population-based cohort study (Mortensen et al., 2001) of nearly 50,000 singleton births demonstrated that smoking was also associated with a twofold risk of placental abruption (OR, 1.88; 95th CI, 1.72 to 2.30). Spinillo and coworkers (1994) noted the same 2.5-fold increased risk by their analysis of preterm deliveries complicated by placental abruption. Multivariate analysis confirmed that the use of tobacco was an independent risk factor for abruption among preterm deliveries (adjusted OR, 2.36; 95th CI, 1.29 to 4.33). The proposed mechanisms for placental abruption among smokers include decidual necrosis at the periphery of the placenta, microinfarcts, and atheromatous and fibrinoid changes in the placenta (Naeye, 1979). Hypovascular and atrophic villi have also been observed with greater frequency among smokers (Mochizuki et al., 1984).

Limited data link cigarette smoking to PROM. Neither the Perinatal Collaborative Project nor the Ontario Perinatal Mortality Study was able to offer firm conclusions regarding PROM. Two case-control studies (Hadley et al., 1990; Shubert et al., 1992) demonstrated a significant increase in the risk of preterm PROM among smokers.

The risk of spontaneous abortion appears to be increased among smokers, with studies demonstrating a relative risk ranging from 1.1 to 1.8 (Kline et al., 1977; Himmelberger et al., 1978; Armstrong et al., 1992). A case-control study of women presenting to an inner city emergency department with spontaneous abortion showed an independent association of cotinine in the maternal urine with spontaneous abortion (OR, 1.8; 95th CI, 1.3 to 2.6) (Ness et al., 1999). Despite published reports demonstrating an increase in the incidence of cleft lip and palate among the offspring of smokers (Lieff et al., 1999; Lorente et al., 2000), there does not appear to be consistent support for an association between smoking and congenital anomalies (Evans et al., 1979; Hemminki et al., 1983; Shiono, Klebanoff, Berendes, 1986; McDonald et al., 1992b).

Reducing the number of cigarettes smoked per day appears to lower the incidence of placental abruption (Naeye, 1980), low birth weight (Sexton and Hebel, 1984; Dolan-Mullen et al., 1994), and preterm birth (Mainous and Hueston, 1994). Several studies showed that the discontinuation of smoking by the end of the second trimester reduces the patient's risk of delivering a low-birth-weight infant to the level of the nonsmoker (MacArthur and Knox, 1988; McDonald et al., 1992a; Lindley et al., 2000). Several authors suggested that with even a modest rate of successful smoking cessation, as many as 2000 low-birth-weight deliveries would be prevented annually, with a reduction in health care costs of $20 to $50 million (O'Campo et al., 1995; Lightwood et al., 1999).

These findings have led to a growing interest in the development and implementation of smoking cessation programs (Dolan-Mullen et al., 1994; Mullen, 1999; Klesges et al., 2001). Given the documented effectiveness of even a brief counseling session (5 to 15 minutes) and the distribution of pregnancy-specific educational materials (Mullen, 1999; Melvin et al., 2000; Klesges et al., 2001), clinicians caring for pregnant women are capable of effecting significant improvements in perinatal outcome by offering these interventions. Although various methods of pharmacotherapy (i.e., nicotine gum, nicotine patches, or bupropion) have been used in pregnant women (Wright et al., 1997; Ogburn et al., 1999; Benowitz et al., 2000), very little data are available on their efficacy. It is likely that the use of these therapies, as an adjunct to behavioral interventions, will be the focus of numerous investigations and will eventually become a readily accepted part of a smoking cessation program.

Passive smoke exposure (second-hand smoking) has been linked to a small decrease (20 to 70 g) in mean birth weight (Martin and Bracken, 1986; Rubin et al., 1986; Windham et al., 1999; Dejmek et al., 2002). However, the association between passive smoke exposure and both low birth weight and IUGR is controversial (Chen and Pettiti, 1995; Windham et al., 1999; Dejmek et al., 2002).

Maternal smoking has also been associated with numerous postnatal complications. The increase in the risk of sudden infant death syndrome (Blair et al., 1996; MacDorman et al., 1997; Wisborg et al., 2000) is well supported by published data. It has been suggested that maternal tobacco use may be responsible for 20% to 30% of all deaths from sudden infant death syndrome (Taylor and Sanderson, 1995; Pollack, 2001). An evaluation of the lungs of infants undergoing autopsy showed a significantly greater concentration of nicotine in those whose cause of death was listed as sudden infant death syndrome compared with control subjects (McMartin et al., 2002)

Maternal smoking during pregnancy is associated with various behavioral problems, hypertension, and respiratory disorders in childhood (Higgins, 2002).

Caffeine

Caffeine-containing beverages, including coffee, are widely consumed by pregnant women. There is rapid transplacental passage of caffeine (1,3,7-trimethylxanthine), with fetal plasma levels reaching equilibrium with maternal levels (Aldridge et al., 1981). Concerns over the ingestion of caffeine during pregnancy extend back to a report linking caffeine with skeletal malformations in mice (Nishimura and Nakai, 1960). Since then, several other animal models have reinforced the potential for an association between caffeine use and birth defects (Nolen, 1988). These data led to a report from the FDA (1980b) recommending a limitation on caffeine intake during pregnancy. Later in the decade (1988), the FDA reported that there was "insufficient evidence to conclude that caffeine adversely affects reproductive function in the human."

Although two studies reported an association between caffeine consumption and ectrodactyly and cleft palate (Borlee et al., 1978; Furuhashi et al., 1985), numerous clinical investigations refute any causal link between caffeine and congenital anomalies. In fact, several authors (Linn et al., 1982; Rosenberg et al., 1982; Kurpa et al., 1983; McDonald et al., 1992b) showed no increase in the risk of skeletal malformations, orofacial clefts, neural tube defects, or cardiac defects among coffee drinkers. A thorough review of the published literature addressing the potential teratogenicity of caffeine (Christian and Brent, 2001) concluded that this chemical is a potential teratogen only at very large amounts or with the concurrent use of alcohol or tobacco.

Numerous studies showed no overt association between caffeine use and preterm delivery (Linn et al., 1982; McDonald et al., 1992a; Fortier et al., 1993). However, the association between spontaneous abortion and caffeine use is unsettled. Several authors reported an increased risk of miscarriage (Furuhashi et al., 1985; Srispuphan and Bracken, 1986; Wilcox et al., 1990; Cnattingius et al., 2000), whereas others were unable to demonstrate any significant effect of caffeine on early pregnancy loss (Linn et al., 1982; Watkinson and Fried, 1985; Mills et al., 1993; Klebanoff et al., 1999). A meta-analysis of six investigations (over 40,000 pregnancies) concluded that the overall risk ratio for spontaneous abortion among "moderate to heavy" (more than 150 mg/day) caffeine users was 1.36 (95th CI, 1.29 to 1.45) (Fernandes et al., 1998).

Whereas data from animal models (Gilbert and Pistey, 1973; Dunlop and Court, 1981) support the association between caffeine and alterations in fetal growth, the results from published clinical investigations are less conclusive. Martin and Bracken (1987) prospectively studied 3891 patients, of whom 77% consumed caffeine during pregnancy. Women ingesting caffeine-containing products were divided into low (1 to 150 mg/day), moderate (151 to 300 mg/day), and heavy (more than 301 mg/day) users. The relative risk of delivering a low-birth-weight infant was 1.4, 2.3, and 4.6, respectively. A population-based study of more than 7000 women investigated the effect of caffeine use on fetal growth (Fortier et al., 1993). Although caffeine intake was not related to low birth weight or preterm delivery, there was a dose-dependent increase in the risk of IUGR, defined as birth weight less than the 10th percentile for gestational age. Among those women consuming more than 300 mg/day of caffeine, the adjusted odds ratio for delivering a newborn with IUGR was 1.57 (95% CI, 1.05 to 2.33). More recently, a prospective study of 873 women delivering singleton infants in Sweden failed to show an effect of caffeine consumption on fetal growth. This investigation controlled for the impact of smoking using maternal cotinine levels as a measure of tobacco use (Clausson et al., 2002). Similarly, Klebanoff and cohorts (2002) used data from the Collaborative Perinatal Project (1959 to 1966) to compare the serum concentration of paraxanthine (major metabolite of caffeine) as a marker of caffeine exposure with the risk of delivering a small-for-gestational age infant. These authors concluded that there was an association between paraxanthine levels and fetal growth restriction only among women who smoked cigarettes.

In balance, most published studies suggest an increased risk of fetal growth delay among women ingesting more than 300 mg/day of caffeine (three to four cups of coffee). The previously referenced meta-analysis (Fernandes et al., 1998) concluded that among women with "moderate to heavy" caffeine consumption, the overall risk ratio for delivering a low-birth-weight infant was 1.51 (95th CI, 1.39 to 1.63). Given the available information, it seems prudent to recommend that pregnant women who choose to consume coffee or other caffeine-containing substances limit their intake to less than 300 mg/day.

Cocaine

Cocaine is derived from the leaves of the *Erythroxylon coca* plant. It exerts its effect by interfering with the reuptake of neurotransmitters, such as dopamine and norepinephrine, at the presynaptic nerve terminals. This results in vasoconstriction, tachycardia, hypertension, and an increase in circulating catecholamines (Ritchie and Greene, 1985). The drug can be administered intravenously or by "snorting" (intranasal route) the powder form. Alkaloidal cocaine, often referred to as "crack," is a heat-stable preparation that can be smoked as a cigarette, with absorption through the alveolar membranes (Crack, 1986). The drug is metabolized by the action of plasma and hepatic cholinesterases (Stewart et al., 1979).

Plasma cholinesterase activity may be diminished in pregnant women and in the fetus, leading to an accumulation of cocaine and an increase in the potential for toxicity (Telsey et al., 1988; Hadeed and Siegel, 1989). In addition, there is increasing evidence that placental metabolism of cocaine may play an important part in determining the degree of fetal exposure (Roe et al., 1990; Simone et al., 1994). The medical complications of cocaine use in adults are well described (Cregler and Marx, 1986). The cardiovascular effects of cocaine appear to be more pronounced during pregnancy (Plessinger and Woods, 1990). This may be due to the effect of progesterone, which increases the metabolism of cocaine to norcocaine (a biologically active metabolite), or to the increasing sensitivity of α-adrenergic receptors associated with pregnancy (Woods and Plessinger, 1990).

The association between cocaine use and congenital anomalies remains controversial. In general, the anomalies reported to occur more frequently among cocaine-exposed fetuses involve the genitourinary system, cardiovascular system, and CNS as well as the extremities. The proposed mechanism centers on the deformation or destruction of normally formed embryonic structures secondary to an interruption of blood supply. Several authors (Fantel et al., 1992; Zimmerman et al., 1994) proposed that cocaine-mediated vasoconstriction and hypoperfusion result in the production of reactive oxygen molecules.

Basic science investigation offers support for cocaine as a teratogen. Webster and Brown-Woodman (1990), treating Sprague-Dawley rats with cocaine, noted that the offspring had hemorrhages involving the head, limbs, tail, and genital tubercle. They hypothesized that an interruption of blood flow led to necrosis and to disruption of both developing and normally formed structures. Other investigators reported an increase in anomalies related to *in utero* exposure to cocaine (Mahalik et al., 1982; Finnell et al., 1990). Finnell and coworkers (1990) concluded that intraperitoneal injections of cocaine resulted in dose-dependent genitourinary and cardiovascular defects in their mouse model. Although studies reporting negative findings have been published (Fantel and McPhail, 1982; Church et al., 1987), the specific anomalies observed in animal models closely resemble the pattern of abnormalities described clinically.

Chasnoff and coworkers (1985) reported two cases of genitourinary tract anomalies among a cohort of 23 neonates whose mothers used cocaine during pregnancy. This observation was followed by a number of retrospective studies published in the late 1980s and early 1990s that reinforced the association between cocaine use and congenital anomalies. In two case-control studies (Chavez et al., 1989; Ferris et al., 1992), a significant increase in genitourinary tract abnormalities was observed among cocaine-exposed infants compared with nonexposed subjects. Analysis of the data from the Atlanta Birth Defects Case-Control Study (Chavez et al., 1989) demonstrated a greater incidence of *in utero* cocaine exposure among the 276 infants with genitourinary tract anomalies (1.4%) than in the 2837 control subjects (0.5%) (OR, 4.39; 95th CI, 1.12 to 17.24). Cardiac abnormalities were more common (relative risk, 3.9; 95th CI, 1.4 to 9.4) among a cohort of 214 cocaine-exposed infants than in a control group of 340 drug-free neonates (Lipschultz et al., 1991).

Prospective studies evaluating the teratogenicity of cocaine have been inconclusive. Bingol and associates (1987) reported an increase in the incidence of congenital anomalies (primarily cardiac and CNS) among 50 cocaine-exposed newborns (10%) compared with 110 polydrug noncocaine (4.5%) and 340 drug-free newborns (2%). Numerous clinical investigations failed to show a significant increase in the risk of anomalies among cocaine users (Madden et al., 1986; Cherukuri et al., 1988; Hadeed and Siegel, 1989; Gillogley et al., 1990). Investigators from the University of Florida (Behnke et al., 2001) conducted a prospective, longitudinal, cohort study that included 272 offspring of identified cocaine users and 154 control subjects. Experienced examiners (blinded to maternal drug history) completed a neonatal assessment that included a detailed standardized checklist of physical features designed to identify both minor and major anomalies. Although the birth weight and head circumference of the cocaine-exposed infants were significantly smaller than the control subjects, there was no significant difference noted in congenital anomalies.

Although the association between cocaine and congenital anomalies remains unsettled, a recent meta-analysis deserves mention (Addis et al., 2001). In this meta-analysis, 13 studies comparing cocaine-only users to drug-free control subjects (polydrug users were analyzed separately) were included in their review. Their weighted analysis resulted in a relative risk of 1.70 (95th CI, 1.11 to 2.60) for major congenital malformations among infants exposed only to cocaine.

The impact of cocaine use on fetal growth has been studied extensively. A decrease in mean fetal weight has been demonstrated after the administration of cocaine HCl to pregnant rats (Fantel and McPhail, 1982; Church et al., 1987). This decrease developed independently of maternal weight changes, suggesting a direct effect of cocaine on fetal growth rather than simply the effect of maternal malnutrition.

The impairment of fetal growth may be explained by the drug's vasoconstrictive effect on the uteroplacental circulation. Studies in both the pregnant ewe (Moore et al., 1986; Woods et al., 1987) and the pregnant baboon (Morgan et al., 1991) demonstrated a decrease in uterine blood flow after the intravenous administration of cocaine (Fig. 19-7). Significant changes in hemodynamics and oxygenation have been demonstrated in both acute and chronic models of cocaine administration in the pregnant ewe (Idia et al., 1994; Arbeille et al., 1997). Arbeille and associates (1997) also documented significant alterations in both umbilical and cerebral blood flow and a 15% to 20% decrease in fetal weight when compared with a control (placebo) group. Chronic fetal hypoxemia (Soothill et al., 1986) and diminished uteroplacental blood flow (Creasy et al., 1972; Clapp et al., 1980) have been associ-

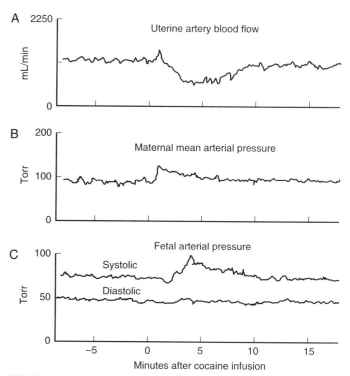

FIGURE 19-7 ■ Maternal and fetal cardiovascular responses to cocaine infusion. **A**, Maternal uterine artery blood flow after infusion of 0.5 mg/kg of cocaine during 1 minute. **B**, Maternal mean arterial blood pressure response to cocaine infusion. **C**, Fetal arterial (systolic/diastolic) pressure response to infusion of 0.5 mg/kg of cocaine. (From Moore TR, Sorg J, Miller L, et al: Hemodynamic effects of intravenous cocaine on the pregnant ewe and fetus. Am J Obstet Gynecol **155**:883, 1986.)

ated with suboptimal fetal growth. The drug's effect on fetal growth may also be explained by impairment in transplacental transport of amino acids (Dicke et al., 1994) or by alterations in protein synthesis by the placenta (Salhab et al., 1994).

Clinically, cocaine use has been associated with a decrease in mean birth weight and an increase in the incidence of both low-birth-weight infants and of IUGR (Bingol et al., 1987; Oro and Dixon, 1987; Ryan et al., 1987; Cherukuri et al., 1988; Chouteau et al., 1988; Zuckerman et al., 1989; Chasnoff et al., 1989; Dixon and Bejar, 1989; Fulroth et al., 1989; Hadeed and Siegel, 1989; Kaye et al., 1989; MacGregor et al., 1989; Gillogley et al., 1990; McCalla et al., 1991; Spence et al., 1991; Bateman et al., 1993; Eyler et al., 1994; Wehbeh et al., 1995; Sprauve et al., 1997; Bandstra et al., 2001). Only a few studies failed to duplicate the finding of delayed fetal growth (Kliegman et al., 1994; Miller et al., 1995; Shiono et al., 1995).

The difference in mean birth weight ranges from approximately 300 to 500 g (McCalla et al., 1991; Spence et al., 1991; Bateman et al., 1993; Eyler et al., 1994; Wehbeh et al., 1995; Sprauve et al., 1997). In a study of 361 cocaine-exposed infants born at an inner city hospital, the difference in mean birth weight (compared with 387 drug-free control subjects) was 401 g. Multivariate analysis, controlling for race, tobacco use, alcohol, gestational age, and prenatal care, demonstrated a difference in mean birth weight of 154 g (95th CI, 68 to 240 g; $P < .01$).

Low-birth-weight infants are more common among the offspring of women whose pregnancy is complicated by cocaine use. Two studies (Bateman et al., 1993; Sprauve et al., 1997) that controlled for confounding variables (e.g., alcohol, prenatal care, race, body weight, gestational age) demonstrated a statistically significant increase in the incidence of low birth weight. Sprauve and coinvestigators (1997), in a retrospective cohort study of 483 cocaine users and 3158 cocaine-free patients, reported an adjusted odds ratio of 1.59 (95th CI, 1.03 to 2.43) for low birth weight ($P < .05$). Bateman and coworkers (1993), reporting on a cohort of 168 cocaine-exposed neonates, demonstrated that the risk of low birth weight was essentially doubled, with an adjusted odds ratio of 2.10 (95th CI, 1.23 to 3.67).

The diagnosis of IUGR is frequently difficult in this population, given the erratic nature of their prenatal care and the uncertainty of the gestational age. Several studies suggested an increased risk of IUGR in this subset of women (Keith et al., 1989; MacGregor et al., 1989; Sprauve et al., 1997), but others noted only a trend (statistically insignificant) toward an increased incidence of IUGR (Ryan et al., 1987; Mastrogiannis et al., 1990; Miller et al., 1995). In the study of 483 cocaine users by Sprauve and associates (1997), the risk of delivering an infant with IUGR (less than the 10th percentile for gestational age) was almost tripled (crude OR, 2.74). Following multiple logistic regression analysis, the use of cocaine was found to be an independent risk factor for IUGR (adjusted OR, 1.70; 95th CI, 1.24 to 2.32).

Mirochnick and coauthors (1995) supported the cause-and-effect relationship of cocaine and delayed fetal growth. In a study of 95 cocaine-exposed infants delivered at term, benzoyl-ecgonine was measured in meconium samples. The level of benzoylecgonine was compared with the neonate's birth weight, birth length, and head circumference (Fig. 19-8). In each measure of fetal growth, there was a significant negative correlation with the level of benzoyl ecgonine in the neonatal meconium: birth weight ($r = -0.22$), birth length ($r = -0.28$), and head circumference ($r = -0.20$). Other studies duplicated the finding of a dose-dependent effect of cocaine on fetal growth (Chiriboga et al., 1999; Katikaneni et al., 2002).

Several studies suggested that cocaine exposure has a significant impact on head circumference (Bingol et al., 1987; Oro and Dixon, 1987; Ryan et al., 1987; Cherukuri et al., 1988; Chasnoff et al., 1989; Fulroth et al., 1989; Hadeed and Siegel, 1989; Little et al., 1989; Gillogley et al., 1990; Little and Snell, 1991; Chiriboga et al., 1999). Studies showed a negative correlation between head circumference and cocaine metabolites (benzoylecgonine) in both maternal (Bateman and Chiriboga, 2000) and neonatal hair (Sallee et al., 1995). A study comparing 28 neonates exposed to cocaine *in utero* with 33 drug-free control subjects demonstrated a smaller head circumference (31.3 versus 33.1 cm) and head circumference percentiles (55th versus 33rd percentile for gestational age) in the exposed group. In addition, the level of benzoylecgonine in neonatal hair was negatively correlated ($r = -0.36$) with head circumference ($P = .06$) (Sallee et al., 1995). As stated previously, Mirochnick and coworkers (1995) reported a similar negative correlation between benzoylecgonine levels in neonatal meconium and head circumference ($r = -0.20$; $P = .04$).

Abnormalities of the CNS have been noted among infants exposed to cocaine. These include cerebral infarction (Chasnoff et al., 1986; Heier et al., 1991) (Fig. 19-9), electroencephalographic changes, and seizure activity (Doberczak et al., 1988; Kramer et al., 1990). Studies both support (Dixon and Bejar, 1989; Singer et al., 1994) and refute (Heier et al., 1991; Dusick et al., 1993) an increase in the incidence of intraventricular and periventricular hemorrhages in these infants. Dusick and coworkers (1993) prospectively enrolled 323 very-low-birth-weight infants (86 cocaine-exposed) who underwent cranial sonographic examinations. The incidence of intraventricular hemorrhage was 36% in both groups, and the incidence of grades III and IV lesions was the same (14%) in both groups. Recent work has heightened the suspicion that cocaine may be associated with congenital anomalies of the CNS (Dominguez et al., 1991; Heier et al., 1991; Dogra et al., 1994). A prospective investigation of 43 cocaine-exposed neonates and 63 drug-free control subjects, with ultrasound, magnetic

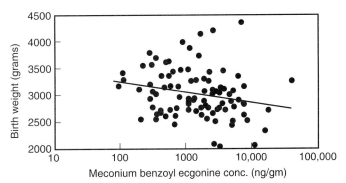

FIGURE 19-8 ■ Relationship between meconium benzoylecgonine concentration and birth weight. (From Mirochnick M, Frank DA, Cabral H, et al: Relation between meconium concentration of the cocaine metabolite benzoylecgonine and fetal growth. J Pediatr **125**:636, 1995.)

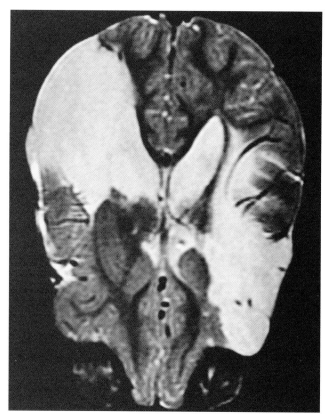

FIGURE 19-9 ■ Magnetic resonance image of bihemispheric cerebral infarction in a neonate with *in utero* exposure to cocaine. (Courtesy of J. Slopis, MD, University of Texas, Houston, Health Sciences Center.)

resonance imaging, and computed tomography of the intracranial anatomy, demonstrated a 12% incidence of anomalies in the cocaine group with no such anomalies noted in the control patients (Heier et al., 1991).

Studies involving the pregnant rat (Daniel, 1964; Nakahara et al., 1996), baboon (Morgan et al., 1994), and human (Monga et al., 1993) suggested that cocaine may have a stimulatory effect on myometrial contractility. In contrast, the administration of cocaine to the near-term pregnant ewe did not result in a significant increase in myometrial electromyographic activity or maternal plasma oxytocin concentrations (Owiny et al., 1992). An increase in plasma oxytocin levels was demonstrated in the pregnant baboon after the administration of cocaine (Morgan et al., 1996).

Several mechanisms for the increase in myometrial activity have been proposed. Studies in the pregnant ewe suggested that repeated hypoxemic episodes increase the likelihood of myometrial contractile activity (Braaksma et al., 1995). Increased levels of circulating catecholamines may lead to an increase in the stimulation of α-adrenergic receptors (Hurd et al., 1991a,b). Both Hurd and coworkers (1993) and other investigators (Hertelendy and Molnar, 1992; Smith et al., 1995; Wang et al., 1996) showed that cocaine use is associated with a decrease in β-adrenergic receptor activity. Cocaine-induced alterations in placental prostanoid production (Monga et al., 1994) may offer yet another mechanism for the increased uterine activity observed clinically in this subset of patients. Other investigators, using human myometrial cell culture, showed that cocaine has an inhibitory effect

on adenylate cyclase and leads to the intracellular mobilization of calcium (Hertelendy and Molnar, 1992; Molnar et al., 1992).

Most data from clinical investigations published during the 1980s supported an increased incidence of preterm delivery among women using cocaine (MacGregor et al., 1987; Oro and Dixon, 1987; Cherukuri et al., 1988; Chasnoff et al., 1989; Hadeed and Siegel, 1989; Keith et al., 1989; Little et al., 1989; Neerhof et al., 1989; Gillogley et al., 1990) (Table 19-11). Eyler and coworkers (1994) analyzed the pregnancy outcome among 168 cocaine users, 168 matched control subjects, and 6914 additional patients delivering during the study period. Preterm delivery (less than 37 weeks) was noted in 43.4% of the cocaine users, 31.5% of the matched control subjects, and 22.9% of the remaining sample. After evaluating their data by multivariate analysis, both Kliegman and coworkers (1994) and Bateman and coworkers (1993) demonstrated that cocaine use was an independent risk factor for preterm birth. Kliegman and associates found the preterm birth rate among cocaine users (*n* = 65) to be 19.3% compared with 3.2% in the control group (relative risk, 13.4; 95th CI, 1.2 to 145.0). Other published investigations do not show an increase in preterm delivery among cocaine users (Sprauve et al., 1997; Little et al., 1999; Miller and Boudreaux, 1999). Sprauve and associates (1997) noted that although the incidence of preterm delivery was increased in the 483 cocaine-dependent women (28.2%), in comparison with the control group (17.1%), this difference did not persist after controlling for tobacco use, prenatal care, abruption, or hypertension (adjusted OR, 1.9; 95th CI, 0.63 to 1.22). Miller and Boudreaux (1999) found an increase in the incidence of preterm delivery among cocaine users delivering at their institution (28 of 135) compared with a drug-free control group (12 of 137). However, analysis of these data using logistic regression demonstrated that the use of cocaine was not an independent risk factor for prematurity (OR, 0.6; 95th CI, 0.2 to 1.9).

Even in studies where there is a significant increase in the risk of preterm delivery, the mean gestational age at delivery among cocaine users tends to be within 2 weeks of the control group (Eyler et al., 1998; Addis et al., 2001). This observation

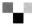

TABLE 19-11. PRETERM DELIVERY AMONG COCAINE USERS: SELECTED STUDIES CONTROLLING FOR RACE, PRENATAL CARE, SMOKING, AND ALCOHOL USE

Reference	Sample Size (Cocaine Users)	Sample Size (Controls)	Odds Ratio (95th CI)
MacGregor et al., 1987	70	70	10.9(2.3–71.6)
Oro and Dixon, 1987	46	45	4.0(1.1–6.4)
Ryan et al., 1987	50	50	2.7(0.4–21.6)
Bateman et al., 1993	361	387	1.94(1.21–3.11)
Kliegman et al., 1994	20	405	13.40(1.23–145.0)
Shiono et al., 1995	93	7377	1.3(0.9–2.0)
Sprauve et al., 1997	483	3158	0.88(0.57–2.30)
Miller et al., 1999	135	137	0.6(0.2–1.9)

CI, confidence interval.

suggests that most preterm births in the cocaine group occur in the 34- to 37-week age group and that deliveries at earlier gestational ages are less common.

Although limited data support the association between cocaine use and PROM (Keith et al., 1989; Cherukuri et al., 1988; Mastrogiannis et al., 1990; McCalla et al., 1991), these studies are limited by both the sample size and the failure to control for potential confounding variables, especially tobacco use. Miller and coworkers (1995) observed an increase in the incidence of PROM in their cocaine-dependent patients (37 of 138) relative to the control group (42 of 276) (OR, 2.04; 95th CI, 1.24 to 3.36) but noted that both tobacco use and inadequate prenatal care were significantly more common in the cocaine users. A twofold increase in the incidence of preterm PROM (OR, 2.1; 95th CI, 1.1 to 4.8) was reported by Little and coinvestigators (1999). Among 538 patients with preterm PROM delivering at Hutzel Hospital in Detroit, 16.1% (85) had a positive urine screen for cocaine metabolites (Refuerzo et al., 2002). Their hypothesis was that among patients with preterm PROM, the use of cocaine would be associated with an increase in perinatal morbidity and mortality. Interestingly, the patients in the cocaine-positive group had a more favorable neonatal outcome (less pneumonia and sepsis) even though there was no difference in gestational age at the time of ruptured membranes, gestational age at delivery, or length of latent period. It is uncertain whether there is a difference in the length of the latent period in cocaine users, with some investigations demonstrating a shorter latent phase (Myles et al., 1998) and others noting a longer latent phase (Delaney et al., 1997).

It has been suggested that the production of reactive oxygen species after cocaine-mediated ischemia and reperfusion may impact the integrity of the membranes, leading to rupture. Interested readers are referred to a detailed discussion of reactive oxygen species and its role in adverse perinatal outcome associated with substance abuse (Woods et al., 1998).

In 1983, Acker and colleagues reported two cases of placental abruption occurring in women admitting to cocaine use. After this report, Chasnoff and coworkers (1985) published their experience with a small group of cocaine-using women receiving prenatal care at their institution. Placental abruption was noted in 4 of 23 cocaine-using women in contrast to 15 opiate-dependent women and 15 drug-free control subjects in whom there were no cases of abruption. Most investigations published since that time have been limited by a relatively small sample size, a lack of uniformity in diagnostic criteria for abruption, and inconsistent pathologic examinations of the placentas. Most studies support an increase in the relative risk of abruption among cocaine users, with several authors demonstrating a statistically significant increase in incidence (Bingol et al., 1987; Chasnoff et al., 1987, 1989; MacGregor et al., 1987; Oro and Dixon, 1987; Hadeed and Siegel, 1989; Neerhof et al., 1989; Kistin et al., 1996; Little et al., 1999). Data from the Maternal Lifestyle Study (Bauer et al., 2002) showed abruptio placenta to be twice as common among cocaine users (relative risk, 2.1; 95th CI, 1.1 to 4.0).

One investigation retrospectively reviewed the records of 592 cocaine users and 4687 drug-free control patients. Placental abruption was diagnosed more frequently among the cocaine users (11 of 592; 1.9%) than the control subjects (45 of 4677; 1.0%) (P < .05) (Dombrowski et al., 1991). However, Sprauve and colleagues (1997), controlling for both tobacco use and hypertension, observed that the incidence of placental abruption (adjusted OR, 1.41; 95th CI, 0.64 to 3.10) was not significantly greater in the women using cocaine.

Placenta previa has also been reported to occur with greater frequency among women using cocaine (Handler et al., 1994; Macones et al., 1997). Handler and coworkers (1994) studied 304 patients with placenta previa and over 2000 control subjects. Women using cocaine were 1.4 times more likely to have the diagnosis of placenta previa (95th CI, 0.8 to 2.4) than were control subjects. This risk persisted after controlling for other known risk factors for previa, including the use of tobacco.

Available data offer little support for an increase in depressed Apgar scores (MacGregor et al., 1987; Oro and Dixon, 1987; Kaye et al., 1989; Keith et al., 1989) or abnormal umbilical artery pH and blood gas values (Andres and Day, 2000) among the infants of cocaine-using women. Although precipitate delivery has been reported more commonly in cocaine users (Chasnoff et al., 1987), two studies suggested that cocaine has no consistent effect on the duration of labor (Dombrowski et al., 1991; Wehbeh et al., 1995).

Sudden infant death syndrome has been reported to occur with greater frequency among cocaine-exposed infants. A meta-analysis of 10 studies calculated an odds ratio of 4.10 (95th CI, 3.17 to 5.30) for cocaine-exposed infants relative to drug-free control subjects (Fares et al., 1997).

There is disagreement regarding the long-term consequences of *in utero* cocaine exposure. Overall, the mortality rate in the first 2 years of life does not appear to be increased (Ostrea et al., 1997) except for the cocaine-exposed infants weighing under 2500 g. Among low-birth-weight infants, those exposed to either cocaine or opiates had a higher mortality rate than the drug-free infants (OR, 5.9; 95th CI, 1.4 to 24.0). Early reports suggested that these infants had a higher incidence of neurobehavioral abnormalities (e.g., abnormal sleeping patterns, feeding problems, hypertonia, tremors, and learning disabilities) (Chasnoff et al., 1989). Since those initial reports in the later half of the 1980s, most investigations have suggested that the developmental outcome of these infants is not significantly different than "well-matched," drug-free, control infants. Reviews of this complex subject have been published by Landry and Whitney (1996) and more recently by Frank and associates (2001).

Opiates

Opiates refer to naturally occurring substances including morphine and codeine recovered from the *Papaver somniferum* poppy. The term *opioid* refers to synthetic narcotics, such as heroin, meperidine, fentanyl, propoxyphene, and methadone. Most available data regarding the effect of opiates on pregnancy outcome are drawn from patients using intravenous heroin and, since its introduction in 1965 to treat opiate dependence (Dole and Nyswander, 1965), the oral administration of methadone.

The most common perinatal complications associated with the use of heroin, methadone, or other opioids are fetal growth restriction (Blinick et al., 1969; Stone et al., 1971; Naeye et al., 1973b; Zelson et al., 1973; Pellosi et al., 1975; Kandall et al., 1976, 1977; Ostrea et al., 1976; Fricker and Segal, 1978; Chasnoff et al., 1982; Doberczak et al., 1987; Little et al., 1990) and the neonatal abstinence syndrome (Stone et al., 1971; Wilson et al., 1973; Levy and Spino, 1993). Several other perinatal complications have been reported to occur with greater frequency in opiate-dependent women. These include preterm delivery (Stone et al., 1971; Pellosi et al., 1975; Fricker and Segal, 1978; Little et al., 1990), fetal death (Rementeria and Nunag, 1973; Zuspan et al., 1975; Fricker and Segal, 1978), decreased head circumference (Chasnoff et al., 1982; Doberczak et al., 1987), depressed Apgar scores (Ostrea et al., 1976), meconium staining of the amniotic fluid (Blinick et al., 1969; Ostrea et al., 1976; Little et al., 1990), PROM (Ostrea et al., 1976), multiple gestations (Ostrea et al., 1976), and chorioamnionitis (Naeye et al., 1973b).

It is important to emphasize that many of these reports include primarily heroin-dependent women, where neither the dose nor the frequency of drug use is known. The concurrent use of alcohol and tobacco as well as the coexistence of medical complications (e.g., gonorrhea, hepatitis, human immunodeficiency virus, etc.) are extremely common in opiate-dependent pregnant women (Kaltenbach et al., 1998; Bauer et al., 2002). Most clinical investigations have not adequately controlled for these confounding variables.

The association of maternal opiate use with altered fetal growth is supported by work in animal models. Investigations in the pregnant rabbit (Roloff and Howalt, 1973; Taeusch et al., 1973; Raye et al., 1975) and in the pregnant mouse (Naeye et al., 1973a) demonstrated delayed growth in the opiate-exposed offspring. Postmortem examination of 59 heroin-exposed newborns demonstrated a decrease in cell number in all organs studied (Naeye et al., 1973b). Other proposed mechanisms for altered fetal growth include decreased fetal growth hormone concentration (Cushman, 1972) and chronic fetal hypoxemia from cyclic opiate withdrawal (Cohen et al., 1980).

Clinical reports offer support for an association between opiate use and IUGR. A study of heroin-dependent pregnant women ($n = 24$) delivering at Parkland Hospital in Dallas found the mean birth weight (2870 ± 500 g) to be significantly less than observed among 100 unexposed control subjects (3296 ± 433 g) ($P < .05$) (Little et al., 1990). A recent meta-analysis (Hulse et al., 1997) compared the mean birth weight and the incidence of low birth weight among infants born to women using heroin, methadone, or a combination of the two with a control group of opiate-free women. The reduction in mean birth weight was 489 g (95th CI, 284 to 693) among heroin users, 279 g (95th CI, 229 to 328) among methadone users, and 557 g (95th CI, 403 to 710) among women using both drugs concurrently. The relative risk of low birth weight was 4.61 (95th CI, 2.78 to 7.65) for women using only heroin, 1.36 (95th CI, 0.83 to 2.22) among methadone-exposed infants, and 3.28 (95th CI, 2.47 to 4.39) for patients using both heroin and methadone. Although this meta-analysis suggested that the use of either heroin or methadone is associated with delayed fetal growth, the authors pointed out that the studies analyzed did not control for the use of tobacco, an overt confounding variable. One of the few studies that controlled for the use of tobacco among opiate-dependent pregnant women concluded that differences in birth weight among heroin users was not observed after adjustments for various confounding variables (e.g., tobacco use, prenatal care, nutrition) (Lifschitz et al., 1983).

Although several studies suggested an increased rate of preterm delivery (Stone et al., 1971; Pellosi et al., 1975; Ostrea et al., 1976), others failed to demonstrate such an association (Lifschitz et al., 1983; Doberczak et al., 1987). In balance, there is little support for an increase in the risk of preterm delivery among opiate-dependent women.

The use of methadone maintenance for opiate-dependent pregnant women is thought to improve perinatal outcome and, more specifically, to reduce the incidence of fetal growth restriction. Several authors observed improved birth weight (Zelson et al., 1973; Kandall et al., 1976, 1977; Doberczak et al., 1987; Finnegan, 1991), whereas others did not demonstrate a significant impact on fetal growth (Rajegowda et al., 1972; Edelin et al., 1988).

Regardless of the issue of fetal growth, the use of methadone in the opiate-dependent pregnant woman has several important advantages:

1. The avoidance of intravenous drug use decreases the patient's risk of human immunodeficiency virus, hepatitis, and subacute bacterial endocarditis.
2. The scheduled administration of methadone circumvents the pattern of recurrent withdrawal, which results in significant fetal effects. The risks include fetal hypoxemia, hypertension, bradycardia, and intrauterine demise (Rementeria and Nunag, 1973; Zuspan et al., 1975; Cohen et al., 1980; Umans and Szeto, 1985).
3. "Drug-seeking" behaviors, including prostitution, and the accompanying increased risk of sexually transmitted diseases may also be minimized by the scheduled administration of methadone.

Several issues specific to the antepartum and intrapartum management of the pregnant opiate user deserve mention. Testing for sexually transmitted diseases (e.g., human immunodeficiency virus, syphilis, gonorrhea, and chlamydia) and acute and chronic hepatitis is essential. The clinician should be able to recognize the signs and symptoms of both opiate withdrawal and intoxication (Table 19-12) (Hoegerman and Schnoll, 1991). The heroin-dependent patient should, when possible, be counseled regarding the reported benefits of methadone maintenance. The patient should be started on a low dose of methadone (10 to 20 mg) in an inpatient setting, with gradual adjustment of the dose based on the signs and symptoms of withdrawal (Table 19-13). Given the risk of fetal compromise, the withdrawal of a patient from methadone maintenance, when appropriate, must be approached gradually by clinicians experienced in caring for opiate-dependent pregnant women.

No clear association has been established between opiate exposure and structural defects in the offspring. There is, however, a well-defined picture of neonatal withdrawal referred to as the *neonatal abstinence syndrome*. This disorder occurs in 50% to 95% of exposed infants (Stone et al., 1971; Wilson et al., 1973; Levy and Spino, 1993). It is more common in methadone-exposed neonates than in heroin-exposed neonates (Rajegowda et al., 1972). The clinical syndrome is generally clinically apparent within 3 days, although its onset has been described as late as 2 weeks of life. Clinical findings associated with neonatal abstinence syndrome are listed in Table 19-14 (Stimmel and Jerez, 1985). The most common finding is CNS irritability, observed in approximately 70% of neonates (Cooper et al., 1983).

Treatment consists of supportive therapy (a calm, warm, quiet environment) or various drugs (phenobarbital, paregoric, diazepam, chlorpromazine) (Levy and Spino, 1993). Although controversial, published data support a positive correlation

TABLE 19-12. SIGNS OF OPIOID INTOXICATION AND WITHDRAWAL IN THE ADULT

Intoxication
  Clouded mentation
  Drowsiness
  Analgesia
  Euphoria
  Decreased respirations
  Diminished peristalsis with resultant constipation
  Diminished drug seeking
  Miosis
Withdrawal
  Drug craving
  Lacrimation
  Rhinorrhea
  Yawning
  Sweating
  Restless sleep
  Mydriasis
  Anorexia
  Vomiting
  Diarrhea
  Abdominal cramping
  Chills
  Flushing
  Muscle spasms and aches
  Tremors and irritability
  Hypertension
  Hyperventilation
  Tachycardia
  Piloerection

From Hoegerman G, Schnoll S: Narcotic use in pregnancy. Clin Perinatol **18**:58, 1991.

TABLE 19-13. METHADONE MAINTENANCE FOR OPIATE-DEPENDENT PREGNANT WOMEN

Initiation of methadone treatment
  Starting dose (day 1)
    10–20 mg (depending on severity of initial symptoms)
  Additional dose based on medical evaluations at 6-hour intervals
    5–10 mg for persistent signs and symptoms of opiate withdrawal (see Table 19-7)
  Dose for day 2
    Total methadone in first 24 hr (10–60 mg); may be given as single dose or split dose (every 12 hr)
Methadone withdrawal during pregnancy
  Inpatient
    2-mg/day decrease in daily dose
  Outpatient
    5- to 10-mg/wk decrease in dose

Osterloh and Lee, 1989), as is the use of tobacco and alcohol. Women who use marijuana tend to be younger, unmarried, less well educated, and in a lower socioeconomic group than nonusers (Fried et al., 1980).

Available data linking marijuana use to congenital anomalies are weak. Early case reports linking its use to limb reduction defects (Hecht et al., 1968; Carakushansky et al., 1969) are difficult to interpret because of the concurrent exposure to

TABLE 19-14. NEONATAL WITHDRAWAL SYNDROME

Central nervous system symptoms
  Disturbance in sleep patterns
  Hyperactivity
  Hyperreflexia
  Tremors
  Increased muscle tone
  Myoclonic jerks
  Shrill cry
  Convulsions
Metabolic symptoms
  Fever
  Hypoglycemia
  Mottling
  Sweating
  Yawning
  Vasomotor instability
Respiratory symptoms
  Nasal flaring
  Nasal stuffiness
  Sneezing
  Tachypnea
  Yawning
  Hiccups
Gastrointestinal symptoms
  Excessive sucking
  Poor feeding
  Vomiting
  Diarrhea

From Stimmel B, Jerez E: Alcohol and substance abuse during pregnancy. In Cherry SH, Berkowitz RL, Kase NG (eds): Medical, Surgical, and Gynecologic Complications of Pregnancy. Baltimore, Williams & Wilkins, copyright © 1985.

between both the daily methadone dose at delivery and the cumulative intake for the 3 months before delivery and the severity of the neonatal withdrawal (Harper et al., 1974; Doberczak et al., 1993; Malpas et al., 1995). In the Doberczak and colleagues cohort of 21 patients enrolled in a methadone maintenance program, the severity of neonatal abstinence syndrome (using a standardized scoring system) was correlated with the daily methadone dose in the third trimester (range, 20 to 80 mg), maternal plasma levels at delivery, cord blood levels, and the rate of decline of neonatal plasma methadone levels. The authors found a significant correlation between drug levels and severity of neonatal symptoms. Other investigators have not demonstrated any association between methadone dose and severity of withdrawal (Mack et al., 1991). Long-term developmental sequelae have been reported in infants exposed to opiates and include an increased risk of behavioral and school-related problems (Wilson, 1989).

Marijuana

The active ingredient in marijuana, tetrahydrocannabinol, causes a mild tachycardia, a slight increase in arterial pressure, and a generalized euphoria. The effects generally are evident within 30 to 60 minutes and persist for as long as 3 to 5 hours. Estimates of marijuana use during pregnancy range from 3% (self-report) to 35% (maternal urine). Concurrent use of other illicit drugs is common (Gibson et al., 1983; Linn et al., 1983;

other illicit drugs. Numerous authors failed to observe an increase in the incidence of congenital anomalies in neonates exposed to marijuana in utero (Linn et al., 1983; O'Connell and Fried, 1984; Tennes et al., 1985; Zuckerman et al., 1989). Reports of an increase in FAS-type features in exposed newborns (Hingson et al., 1982; Qazi et al., 1985) merit scrutiny and additional investigation.

Several studies suggested an association between marijuana use and a decrease in birth weight and birth length (Hingson et al., 1982; Zuckerman et al., 1989). Many of the studies suggesting an impairment of fetal growth did not adequately control for confounding variables, such as the use of other illicit drugs, alcohol, or tobacco (Gibson et al., 1983; Hatch and Bracken, 1986). Both the Avon Longitudinal Study of Pregnancy (Fergusson et al., 2002) and the Vaginal Infections in Prematurity study (Shiono et al., 1995) examined the impact of marijuana use on fetal growth, controlling for confounding variables such as tobacco use. The Avon Longitudinal Study of Pregnancy concluded that the difference in mean birth weight among the women who smoked marijuana at least weekly was not statistically significant. The Vaginal Infections in Prematurity study showed no increased risk of delivering a low-birth-weight infant.

There is little support for marijuana use as an independent risk factor for preterm delivery. One study reported a mean estimated gestational age at delivery of 39.7 weeks among nonusers, 40.2 weeks among irregular and moderate users, and 38.8 weeks among heavy users (Fried and O'Connell, 1987). Several other reports failed to show an increased incidence of preterm delivery in patients using marijuana (Linn et al., 1983; Tennes et al., 1985; Shiono et al., 1995).

Although newborns exposed prenatally to marijuana demonstrated changes in performance on the Brazelton Neonatal Behavioral Assessment Score (i.e., increased tremors and startles) (Fried and Makin, 1987), other investigators showed no alterations in neonatal behavior (Tennes et al., 1985; Dreher et al., 1994). There appears to be no effect of in utero exposure on neurodevelopmental testing or on postnatal growth (Tennes et al., 1985; Fried and Watkinson, 1988).

Amphetamine and Methamphetamine

Amphetamine and methamphetamine belong to the general group of sympathomimetic amines. Their stimulatory effect on the sympathetic nervous system is mediated by an increase in the release of neurotransmitters from the presynaptic terminal. These drugs can be used orally or intravenously. The appearance of crystal methamphetamine ("ice"), a smokable form of the drug, has renewed concerns over the perinatal complications of amphetamine-like drugs (Cho, 1990). Methamphetamine, when administered to the pregnant ewe, results in a decrease in uterine blood flow and fetal hypoxemia (Burchfield et al., 1991; Andres et al., 1992; Stek et al., 1995). Other authors, using the same model, observed fetal hyperglycemia, hyperinsulinemia, lactic acidemia, and an increase in circulating catecholamines (Dickinson et al., 1994).

Methamphetamine and amphetamine have been associated with a significant decrease in both birth weight and birth length (Naeye, 1983; Oro and Dixon, 1987; Little et al., 1988; Gillogley et al., 1990). Data collected from the University of California, Davis (Gillogley et al., 1990), showed that the

mean birth weight among neonates of 106 amphetamine users (2947 g) was significantly lower than neonates born to drug-free control subjects (3165 g). However, the incidence of alcohol use in the amphetamine users was significantly greater than in the control group.

There is no clear association between amphetamine or methamphetamine use and preterm delivery. Although Oro and Dixon (1987) found a significant increase in the incidence of preterm delivery among patients using cocaine and/or methamphetamine, other investigators showed no difference in either the incidence of preterm birth or the estimated gestational age at delivery (Little et al., 1988; Gillogley et al., 1990).

Studies in both animal models and humans suggested that amphetamine use may be associated with significant CNS effects. Rumbaugh and associates (1971) demonstrated areas of cerebral ischemia and infarction in rhesus monkeys given intravenous methamphetamine. Similarly, cerebral hemorrhage and ischemic stroke have been reported in adults using amphetamines (Delaney and Estes, 1980; Rothrock et al., 1988). Sonographic examination of term neonates exposed to methamphetamine suggests an increase in the incidence of intraventricular hemorrhage, to the level of that seen among preterm neonates at risk for hypoxemic encephalopathy (Dixon and Bejar, 1989). This difference was not noted in opiate-exposed neonates with similar demographic and lifestyle variables.

Although early investigations suggested an increased risk for congenital anomalies in amphetamine-exposed fetuses (Nora et al., 1970; Nelson and Forfar, 1971), most available data do not support the association of amphetamine and methamphetamine and congenital anomalies (Heinonen et al., 1977b; Milkovich and van den Berg, 1977).

Recommendations

Various methods for screening the obstetric population for the use of alcohol, tobacco, and illicit drug use are available. Because women who use tobacco and/or alcohol tend to diminish their use when pregnant, even before their initial prenatal visit, a distinct window of opportunity exists for the physician to intervene and to influence not only the pregnancy but also the overall health of these women. In addition, cessation programs are often successful, not only in reducing drug use but also in improving overall perinatal outcome. The task of identifying women who use illicit drugs and enrolling them in formal prenatal care programs is further complicated not only by the illegality of the substances but also by the complex social and economic circumstances common in this population. These women often fear legal consequences when participating in organized medical clinics and therefore participate erratically or avoid care completely. Nevertheless, the overall perinatal outcome among illicit drug users appears to be improved by regular prenatal care (MacGregor et al., 1989; Racine et al., 1993). Obstetric care of the drug-dependent woman, as with all patients, must be individualized. Table 19-15 outlines a number of major components in patient care.

In general, a nonjudgmental and factual approach, with attention to promoting compliance, offers the best outcome for these frequently complex pregnancies.

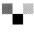

TABLE 19-15. KEY ISSUES IN CARING FOR THE PREGNANT WOMAN USING SOCIAL OR ILLICIT DRUGS

1. Referral to multispecialty clinic if available
2. Referral to drug counseling program
3. Screening for domestic violence
4. Screening for sexually transmitted diseases
5. Frequent urine toxicology to monitor drug use
6. Targeted ultrasound examination to rule out congenital abnormalities
7. Serial ultrasound studies to evaluate fetal growth
8. Patient education
   a. Effects of specific drugs on pregnancy outcome
   b. Signs and symptoms of preterm labor
   c. Parenting classes
9. Antepartum testing
10. Pediatric referral
11. Close postpartum follow-up

REFERENCES

Aarskog D: Association between maternal intake of diazepam and oral clefts. Lancet 2:921, 1975.

Abel E: Fetal Alcohol Exposure and Effects: A Comprehensive Bibliography. Westport, Conn, Greenwood Press, 1988.

Abel E, Sokol, R: Incidence of fetal alcohol syndrome and economic impact of FAS-related mental retardation. Drug Alcohol Depend 19:51, 1987.

Abel EL: An update on the incidence of FAS: FAS is not an equal opportunity birth defect. Neurotoxicol Teratol 17:437, 1995.

Abel EL: Maternal alcohol consumption and spontaneous abortion. Alcohol 32:211, 1997.

Abel EL, Sokol RJ: Fetal alcohol syndrome is now the leading cause of mental retardation. Lancet 1:222, 1986.

Abel EL, Sokol RJ: Fetal diagnosis and therapy. Alcohol 2:140, 1989.

Abel EL, Sokol RJ: A revised conservative estimate of the incidence of FAS and its economic impact. Alcohol Clin Exp Res 15:514, 1991.

Acker D, Sachs BP, Tracey KJ, et al: Abruptio placentae associated with cocaine use. Am J Obstet Gynecol 146:220, 1983.

Acyclovir Pregnancy Registry: Interim Report. Project Office. Research Triangle Park, NC, Glaxo Wellcome, July 31, 1998.

Adams J, Harvey EA, Holmes LB: Cognitive deficits following gestational monotherapy with phenobarbital and carbamazepine. Neurotoxicol Teratol 22:466, 2000.

Addis A, Moretti ME, Syed FA, et al: Fetal effects of cocaine: An updated meta-analysis. Reprod Toxicol 15:341;2001.

Aldridge A, Bailey J, Neims AH: The disposition of caffeine during and after pregnancy. Semin Perinatol 5:310, 1981.

American College of Obstetricians and Gynecologists: Guidelines for Diagnostic Imaging during Pregnancy. Committee Opinion No. 158, Washington, DC, American College of Obstetricians and Gynecologists, 1995.

American College of Obstetricians and Gynecologists: Teratology. Educational Bulletin, Number 236, Washington, DC, American College of Obstetricians and Gynecologists, 1997.

American College of Radiology: MR safety and sedation. In 1998 American College of Radiology Standards. Philadelphia, Pa, American College of Radiology, 1998, p. 457.

Ananth CV, Savitz DA, Luther ER: Maternal cigarette smoking as a risk factor for placental abruption, placenta previa and uterine bleeding in pregnancy. Am J Epidemiol 144:881, 1996.

Ances BM: New concerns about thalidomide. Obstet Gynecol 99:125, 2002.

Andres RL: The association of cigarette smoking with placenta previa and abruptio placentae. Semin Perinatol 20:154, 1996.

Andres RL, Day MC: Recent cocaine use is not associated with fetal acidemia or other manifestations of intrapartum fetal distress. Am J Perinatol 17:63, 2000.

Andres RL, Day MC, Larrabee KD: The perinatal consequences of smoking and alcohol use. Curr Probl Obstet Gynecol Fertil 19:171, 1996.

Andres RL, Dickinson JE, Deaver JE, et al: Ovine maternal and fetal vascular responses to acute methamphetamine administration. Abstract presented at the 39th Annual Meeting of the Society for Gynecologic Investigation, 1992, San Antonio, Texas.

Andrews EB, Yankaskas BC, Cordero JF, et al: Acyclovir in pregnancy registry: Six years experience. Obstet Gynecol 79:7, 1992.

Annegers JF, Elveback LR, Hauser WA, et al: Do anticonvulsants have a teratogenic effect? Arch Neurol 31:364, 1974.

Arbeille P, Maulik D, Salihagic A, et al: Effect of long-term cocaine administration to pregnant ewes on fetal hemodynamics, oxygenation and growth. Obstet Gynecol 90:795, 1997.

Armenti V, Ahlswede K, Ahlswede B, et al: National transplantation pregnancy registry: Outcome of 154 pregnancies in cyclophosphamide-treated female kidney transplant recipients. Transplantation 57:502, 1994.

Armstrong BG, McDonald AD, Sloan M: Cigarette, alcohol and coffee consumption and spontaneous abortion. Am J Public Health 82:85, 1992.

Arpino C, Brescianini S, Robert E, et al: Teratogenic effects of antiepileptic drugs: Use of an International Database on Malformations and Drug Exposure (MADRE). Epilepsia 41:1436, 2000.

Aselton P, Jick H, Mulnsky A, et al: First-trimester drug use and congenital disorders. Obstet Gynecol 89:524, 1985.

Ashwell KW, Zhang LL: Forebrain hypoplasia following acute prenatal ethanol exposure: Quantitative analysis of effects on specific forebrain nuclei. Pathology 28:161, 1996.

Astrup P: Some physiological and pathological effects of moderate carbon monoxide exposure. Br Med J 4:447, 1972.

Bandstra ES, Morrow CE, Anthony JC, et al: Intrauterine growth of full-term infants: Impact of prenatal cocaine exposure. Pediatrics 108:1309, 2001.

Barr M, Burdi AR: Warfarin-associated embryopathy in a 17-week abortus. Teratology 14:129, 1976.

Baskin C, La S, Wenger NK: Sulfadiazine rheumatic fever prophylaxis during pregnancy: Does it increase the risk of kernicterus in the newborn? Cardiology 65:222, 1980.

Bateman DA, Chiriboga CA: Dose-response effect of cocaine on newborn head circumference. Pediatrics 106:33, 2000.

Bateman DA, Ngm SKC, Hansen CA, et al: The effects of intrauterine cocaine exposure in newborns. Am J Public Health 83:190, 1993.

Bauer CR, Shankaran S, Bada HS, et al: The maternal lifestyle study: Drug exposure during pregnancy and short-term maternal outcomes. Am J Obstet Gynecol 186:487, 2002.

Beaulac-Baillargeon L, Desrosiers C: Caffeine-cigarette interaction on fetal growth. Am J Obstet Gynecol 157:1236, 1987.

Behnke M, Eyler FD, Garvan CW, et al: The search for congenital malformations in newborns with fetal cocaine exposure. Pediatrics 107:74, 2001.

Belafsky HA, Breslow S, Hirsch LM, et al: Meprobamate during pregnancy. Obstet Gynecol 34:378, 1969.

Benowitz NL, Dempsey DA, Goldenberg RL, et al: The use of pharmacotherapies for smoking cessation during pregnancy. Tobacco Control 9 (Suppl 3):91, 2000.

Bentur Y, Koren G: The three most common occupation exposures reported by pregnant women. Am J Obstet Gynecol 165:429, 1991.

Berkovitch M, Pastuszak A, Gazarian M, et al: Safety of the new quinolones in pregnancy. Obstet Gynecol 84:535, 1994.

Bernhardt IB, Dorsey DJ: Hypervitaminosis A and congenital renal abnormalities in a human infant. Obstet Gynecol 43:750, 1974.

Beuhler BA, Delimont D, VanWase M, et al: Prenatal prediction of risk of the fetal hydantoin syndrome. N Engl J Med 322:1657, 1990.

Bingol N, Fuchs M, Diaz V, et al: Teratogenicity of cocaine in humans. J Pediatr 110:93, 1987.

Blair PS, Fleming PJ, Bensley D, et al: Smoking and sudden infant death syndrome: Results from 1993–5 case control study for confidential inquiry into stillbirths and deaths in infancy. BMJ 313:195, 1996.

Blakeley PM, Scott WJ: Determination of the proximate teratogen of the mouse F.A.S. 2. Pharmacokinetics of the placental transfer of ethanol and acetaldehyde. Toxicol Appl Pharmacol 72:364, 1984.

Blinick G, Wallach RC, Jerez E: Pregnancy in narcotic addicts treated by medical withdrawal. Am J Obstet Gynecol 105:997, 1969.

Bongiovanni AM, McPadden AL: Steroids during pregnancy and possible fetal consequences. Fertil Steril 11:181, 1960.

Borlee I, Lechat MF, Bouckaert P, et al: Le cafe à facteur de risque pendant la grossesse? Louvain Med 97:279, 1978.

Braaksma M, Woudstra B, Sikkema M, et al: Hypoxia increases the duration of spontaneous uterine contracture in the near-term pregnant ewe.

Abstract presented at the 42nd Annual Meeting of the Society for Gynecologic Investigation, 1995, Chicago, Illinois.

Bracken MB: Drug use in pregnancy and congenital heart disease in offspring. N Engl J Med **314**:1120, 1986.

Bracken MB, Holford TR: Exposure to prescribed drugs in pregnancy and association with congenital malformations. Obstet Gynecol **58**:336, 1981.

Brent RL: Kudos to the Food and Drug Administration: reversal of the package insert warning for birth defects for oral contraceptives [editorial comment]. Teratology **39**:93, 1989.

Brent RL, Beckman DA: Angiotensin converting enzyme inhibitors, an embryopathic class of drugs with unique properties: Information for clinical teratology counselors. Teratology **43**:543, 1991.

Brent RL, Holmes LB: Clinical and basic science lessons from the thalidomide tragedy: What have we learned about the causes of limb defects? Teratology **38**:241, 1988.

Brien J, Clark D, Smith G, et al: Disposition of acute, multiple dose ethanol in the near-term pregnant ewe. Am J Obstet Gynecol **157**:204, 1987.

Brien JF, Clarke DW, Richardson B, et al: Disposition of ethanol in maternal blood, fetal blood and amniotic fluid of third-trimester pregnant ewes. Am J Obstet Gynecol **152**:583, 1985.

Brien JF, Loomis CW, Tranmer J, et al: Disposition of ethanol in human maternal venous blood and amniotic fluid. Am J Obstet Gynecol **146**:181, 1983.

Briggs GC, Freeman RK, Yaffe SJ: Drugs in pregnancy and lactation, 5th ed. Baltimore, Williams & Wilkins, 1998.

Brown NA, Goulding EH, Fabro S: Ethanol embryotoxicity: Direct effects on mammalian embryos in vitro. Science **206**:573, 1979.

Brumfitt W, Pursell R: Double-blind trial to compare ampicillin, cephalexin, co-trimoxazole, and trimethoprim in treatment of urinary tract infection. Br Med J **2**:673, 1972.

Burchfield DJ, Lucas VW, Abrams RM, et al: Disposition and pharmacodynamics of methamphetamine in pregnant sheep. JAMA **254**:1968, 1991.

Bureau MA, Monette J, Shapcott D, et al. Carboxyhemoglobin concentration in fetal cord blood and in blood of mothers who smoked in labor. Pediatrics **69**:371, 1982.

Burtin P, Taddio A, Ariburnu O, et al: Safety of metronidazole in pregnancy: A meta-analysis. Am J Obstet Gynecol **172**:525, 1995.

Canger R, Battino D, Canevini MP, et al: Malformations in offspring of women with epilepsy: A prospective study. Epilepsia **40**:1231, 1999.

Cantu JM, Garcia-Cruz D: Midline facial defect as a teratogenic effect of metronidazole. Birth Defects **18**:85, 1982.

Carakushansky G, Neu RL, Gardner LI: Lysergide and cannabis as possible teratogens in man. Lancet **1**:150, 1969.

Carmichael SL, Shaw GM: Maternal corticosteroid use and the risk for selected anomalies. Am J Med Genet **86**:242, 1999.

Caro-Paton T, Carvajal A, Martin di Diego I, et al: Is metronidazole teratogenic? A meta-analysis. Br J Clin Pharmacol **44**:179, 1997.

Cavallo F, Russo R, Zotti C, et al: Moderate alcohol consumption and spontaneous abortion. Alcohol **30**:195, 1995.

Centers for Disease Control: Current trends: Statewide prevalence of illicit drug use by pregnant women—Rhode Island. MMWR Morb Mortal Wkly Rep **39**:225, 1990.

Centers for Disease Control and Prevention: Update: Trends in fetal alcohol syndrome—United States, 1979–1993. MMWR Morb Mortal Wkly Rep **44**:249, 1995.

Center for Disease Control and Prevention: Accutane-exposed pregnancies. MMWR Morb Mortal Wkly Rep **49**:28, 2000.

Centers for Disease Control and Prevention: Alcohol use among women of childbearing age—United States, 1991–1999. MMWR Morb Mortal Wkly Rep **51**:273, 2002a.

Centers for Disease Control and Prevention: Fetal alcohol syndrome—Alaska, Arizona, Colorado and New York. MMWR Morb Mortal Wkly Rep **51**:433, 2002b.

Chambers CD, Johnson KA, Dick LM, et al: Birth outcomes in pregnant women taking fluoxetine. N Engl J Med **335**:1010, 1996.

Chasnoff I, Griffith D, MacGregor S, et al: Temporal patterns of cocaine use in pregnancy. JAMA **261**:1741, 1989.

Chasnoff IJ: Perinatal effects of cocaine. Contemp Obstet Gynecol **29**:163, 1987.

Chasnoff IJ, Burns K, Burns W: Cocaine use in pregnancy: Perinatal morbidity and mortality. Neurotoxicol Teratol **9**:291, 1987.

Chasnoff IJ, Burns WJ, Schnoll SH, et al: Cocaine use in pregnancy. N Engl J Med **313**:666, 1985.

Chasnoff IJ, Bussey M, Savich R, et al: Perinatal cerebral infarction and maternal cocaine use. J Pediatr **108**:456, 1986.

Chasnoff IJ, Hatcher R, Burns WJ: Polydrug and methadone-addicted newborns: A continuum of impairment? Pediatrics **70**:210, 1982.

Chasnoff IJ, Landress HJ, Barrett ME: The prevalence of illicit drug or alcohol use during pregnancy and discrepancies in mandatory reporting in Pinellas County, Florida. N Engl J Med **322**:1202, 1990.

Chaudhuri JD: Alcohol and the developing fetus—A review. Med Sci Monit **6**:1031, 2000.

Chavez GF, Mulinare J, Cordero JF: Maternal cocaine use during early pregnancy as a risk factor for congenital anomalies. JAMA **262**:795, 1989.

Check JH, Rankin A, Teichman M: The risk of fetal anomalies as a result of progesterone therapy during pregnancy. Fertil Steril **45**:575, 1986.

Chemlow D, Andrew E, Baker ER: Maternal cigarette smoking and placenta previa. Obstet Gynecol **87**:703, 1996.

Chen L, Pettiti DP: Case-control study of passive smoking and the risk of small-for-gestational-age at term. Am J Epidemiol **142**:158, 1995.

Cherukuri R, Minkoff H, Hansen RL, et al: A cohort study of alkaloidal cocaine ("crack") in pregnancy. Obstet Gynecol **72**:147, 1988.

Chiarotti M, Satrano-Rossi S, Offidani C, et al: Evaluation of cocaine use during pregnancy through toxicological analysis of hair. J Anal Toxicol **20**:555, 1996.

Chiriboga CA, Brust JCM, Bateman D, et al: Dose-response effect of fetal cocaine exposure of newborn neurologic functioning. Pediatrics **103**:79, 1999.

Cho AK: Ice: A new dosage form of an old drug. Science **249**:631, 1990.

Chouteau M, Namerow PB, Leppert P: The effect of cocaine abuse on birthweight and gestational age. Obstet Gynecol **72**:351, 1988.

Christian MS, Brent RL. Teratogen update: Evaluation of the reproductive and developmental risks of caffeine. Teratology **64**:51, 2001.

Church MW, Dintcheff BA, Gessner PK: Dose-dependent consequences of cocaine on pregnancy outcome in the Long-Evans rat. Neurotoxicol Teratol **10**:51, 1987.

Clapp JF, Szeto HH, Larro R, et al: Umbilical blood flow response to embolization of the uterine circulation. Am J Obstet Gynecol **138**:60, 1980.

Clark KE, Irion GL: Fetal hemodynamic response to maternal intravenous nicotine administration. Am J Obstet Gynecol **167**:1624, 1992.

Clarke DW, Smith GN, Patrick J, et al: Disposition of ethanol and its proximate metabolite, acetaldehyde, in the near-term pregnant ewe for short-term maternal administration of moderate-dose ethanol. Drug Metab Dispos **16**:464, 1988.

Clarke DW, Smith GN, Patrick J, et al: Activity of alcohol dehydrogenase and aldehyde dehydrogenase in maternal liver, fetal liver and placenta of the near-term pregnant ewe. Dev Pharmacol Ther **12**:35, 1989.

Clarke DW, Steenhart NA, Brien JF: Disposition of ethanol and activity of hepatic and placental ADH and ALDH in the third-trimester pregnant guinea pig for single and short-term oral ethanol administration. Alcohol Clin Exp Res **10**:330, 1986.

Clarren SK, Astley SJ: Pregnancy outcome after weekly oral administration of ethanol during gestation in the pig-tailed macaque: Comparing early gestational exposure to full gestational exposure. Teratology **45**:1, 1992.

Clarren SK, Bowden DM: The fetal alcohol syndrome: A new primate mode for binge drinking and its relevance to human ethanol teratogenesis. J Pediatr **101**:819, 1982.

Clarren SK, Smith DW: The fetal alcohol syndrome. N Engl J Med **298**:1063, 1978.

Clausson B, Granath F, Ekborn A, et al. Effect of caffeine exposure during pregnancy on birth weight and gestational age. Am J Epidemiol **155**:429, 2002.

Clayton-Smith J, Donnai D: Fetal valproate syndrome. J Med Genet **32**:724, 1995.

Clementi M, Di Gianatonio E, Pelo E, et al: Methimazole embryopathy. Delineation of the phenotype. Am J Med Genet **83**:43, 1999.

Cnattingius S, Signorello LB, Anneren G, et al: Caffeine intake and the risk of first-trimester spontaneous abortion. N Engl J Med **343**:1839, 2000.

Cohen LS, Friedman MJ, Jefferson JW: A reevaluation of risk of in utero exposure to lithium. JAMA **271**:146, 1994.

Cohen MS, Rudolph AM, Melmon KL: Antagonism of morphine by naloxone in pregnant ewes and fetal lambs. Dev Pharmacol Ther **1**:58, 1980.

Cohlan SQU, Bevelander G, Tiamsic T: Growth inhibition of premature receiving tetracycline. Am J Dis Child **105**:453, 1963.

Coles CD: Impact of prenatal alcohol exposure on the newborn and the child. Clin Obstet Gynecol **36**:255, 1993.

Coles CD, Smith I, Fernhoff PM, et al: Neonatal neurobehavioral characteristics as correlates of maternal alcohol use during gestation. Alcohol Clin Exp Res 9:454, 1985.

Committee on Biological Effects of Ionizing Radiation, National Research Council: Other somatic and fetal effects. In Bier V (ed): Effects of Exposure to Low Levels of Ionizing Radiation. Washington, DC, National Academy Press, 1990, p. 352.

Conway N, Birt DN: Streptomycin in pregnancy: Effect on the fetal ear. BMJ 2:260, 1965.

Cooper JR, Altman F, Brown BS, et al: Research on the Treatment of Narcotic Addiction—State of the Art. Treatment Research Monograph Series NIDA. Rockville, Md, U.S. Department of Health and Human Services, 1983.

Cote C, Menwissen H, Bickering R: Effects on the neonate of prednisone and azathioprine administered to the mother during pregnancy. J Pediatr 85:324, 1974. Crack. Med Lett Drugs Ther 28:69, 1986.

Creasy RK, Barrett CT, de Sweit M, et al: Experimental intrauterine growth retardation in the sheep. Am J Obstet Gynecol 112:566, 1972.

Cregler L, Marx H: Medical complications of cocaine abuse. N Engl J Med 315:1495, 1986.

Csaba I, Sulyok FE, Ertl T: Relationship of maternal treatment with indomethacin to persistence of fetal circulation syndrome. J Pediatr 92:484, 1978.

Cumming ME, Ong BY, Wade JG, et al: Ethanol disposition in newborn lambs and comparison of alcohol dehydrogenase activity in placenta and maternal sheep, fetal and neonatal lamb liver. Dev Pharmacol Ther 8:338, 1985.

Cushman P: Growth hormone in narcotic addiction. J Clin Endocrinol Metab 35:352, 1972.

Czeizel A: Lack of evidence of teratogenicity of benzodiazepine drugs in Hungary . Reprod Toxicol 1:183, 1988.

Czeizel AE, Rockenbauer M: Teratogenic study of doxycycline. Obstet Gynecol 89:524, 1997.

Daft PA, Johnston MC, Sulik KK: Abnormal heart and great vessel development following acute ethanol exposure in mice. Teratology 33:93, 1986.

Dai WS, Hsu MA, Itri LM: Safety of pregnancy after discontinuation of isotretinoin. Arch Dermatol 125:362, 1989.

Dai WS, LaBraico JM, Stern RS; Epidemiology of isotretinoin exposure during pregnancy. J Am Acad Dermatol 26:599, 1992.

Daniel EE: Effects of cocaine and adrenaline on contracture and downhill ion movements induced by inhibitors of membrane ATPase in rat uteri. Can J Physiol Pharmacol 42:497, 1964.

Davies DP, Gray OP, Elwood PC, et al: Cigarette smoking in pregnancy: Associations with maternal weight gain and fetal growth. Lancet 1:385, 1976.

Day NL, Jasperse D, Richardson G, et al: Prenatal exposure to alcohol: Effect on infant growth and morphologic characteristics. Pediatrics 84:536, 1989.

Dejmek J, Solansky I, Podrazilova K, et al: The exposure of nonsmoking and smoking mothers to environmental tobacco smoke during different gestational ages and fetal growth. Environ Health Perspect 110:601, 2002.

Delaney DB, Larrabee KD, Monga M: Preterm premature rupture of the membranes associated with recent cocaine use. Am J Perinatol 14:285, 1997.

Delaney P, Estes M: Intracranial hemorrhage associated with amphetamine abuse. Neurology 30:1125, 1980.

Delgado-Escueta A, Janz D: Consensus guidelines: Preconception counseling, management, and care of the pregnant woman with epilepsy. Neurology 42 (Suppl 5):149, 1992.

Diav-Citrin O, Shechtman S, Arnon J, et al: Is carbamazepine teratogenic? A prospective controlled study of 210 pregnancies. Neurology 57:321, 2001a.

Diav-Citrin O, Shechtman S, Gotteiner T, et al: Pregnancy outcome after exposure to metronidazole: A prospective controlled cohort study. Teratology 63:186, 2001b.

Dicke JM, Verges CK, Polakoski KL: The effects of cocaine in neutral amino acid uptake by human placental basal membrane vesicles. Am J Obstet Gynecol 171:485, 1994.

Dickinson JE, Andres RL, Parisi VM: The ovine sympathoadrenal response to the maternal administration of methamphetamine. Am J Obstet Gynecol 170:1452, 1994.

DiLiberti J, Farndon PA, Dennis NR, et al: The fetal valproate syndrome. Am J Med Genet 19:473, 1984.

Divers WA, Wilkes MM, Babakina A, et al: Maternal smoking and elevation of catecholamines and metabolites in the amniotic fluid. Am J Obstet Gynecol 141:265, 1981.

Dixon SD, Bejar R: Echoencephalographic findings in neonates associated with maternal cocaine and methamphetamine use: Incidence and clinical correlates. J Pediatr 115:770, 1989.

Doberczak TM, Kandall SR, Friedmann P: Relationships between maternal methadone dosage, maternal-neonatal methadone levels and neonatal withdrawal. Obstet Gynecol 81:936, 1993.

Doberczak TM, Shanzer S, Senie RT, et al: Neonatal neurologic and electroencephalographic effects of intrauterine cocaine exposure. J Pediatr 113:354, 1988.

Doberczak TM, Thorton JC, Berstein J, et al: Impact of maternal drug dependency on birthweight and head circumference of offspring. Am J Dis Child 141:1163, 1987.

Dogra VS, Shyken JM, Menon PA, et al: Neurosonographic abnormalities associated with maternal history of cocaine use in neonates of appropriate size for their gestational age. Am J Neuroradiol 15:697, 1994.

Dolan-Mullen P, Ramirez G, Groff JY: A meta-analysis of randomized trials of prenatal smoking cessation interventions. Am J Obstet Gynecol 171:1328, 1994.

Dole VP, Nyswander ME: A medical treatment for diacetylmorphine (heroin) addiction: A clinical trial with methadone hydrochloride. JAMA 193:646, 1965.

Dombrowski MP, Wolfe HM, Welch RA, et al: Cocaine abuse is associated with abruptio placentae and decreased birthweight, but not shorter labor. Obstet Gynecol 77:139, 1991.

Dominguez R, Vila-Coro AA, Slopis JM, et al: Brain and ocular abnormalities in infants with in utero exposure to cocaine and other street drugs. Am J Dis Child 145:688, 1991.

Dreher MC, Nugent K, Hudgins R: Prenatal marijuana exposure and neonatal outcomes in Jamaica: An ethnographic study. Pediatrics 93:254, 1994.

Dresoti IE, Ballard J, Belling B, et al: The effects of ethanol and acetaldehyde on DNA synthesis in growing cells and on fetal development in the rat. Alcohol Clin Exp Res 5:357, 1981.

Dunlop M, Court JM. Effects of maternal caffeine ingestion on neonatal growth rats. Biol Neonate 39:178, 1981.

Dusick AM, Covert RF, Screiber MD, et al: Risk of intraventricular hemorrhage and other adverse outcomes after cocaine exposure in a cohort of very low birth weight infants. J Pediatr 122:438, 1993.

Edelin KC, Gurganious L, Golar K, et al: Methadone maintenance in pregnancy: Consequences to care and outcome. Obstet Gynecol 71:399, 1988.

Einarson A, Fatoye B, Sarkar M, et al: Pregnancy outcome following gestational exposure to venlafaxine: A multicenter prospective controlled study. Am J Psychiatry 158:1728, 2001.

Ellis FW, Pick JR: An animal model for the fetal alcohol syndrome in beagles. Clin Exp Res 4:123, 1980.

Eriksen G, Wohlert M, Ersbak V, et al: Placental abruption: A case control investigation. Br J Obstet Gynaecol 98:448, 1991.

Evans DR, Newcombe RG, Campbell H: Maternal smoking habits and congenital malformations: A population study. Br Med J 2:171, 1979.

Ewing JA: Detecting alcoholism: The CAGE questionnaire. JAMA 252:1905, 1984.

Eyler FD, Behnke M, Conlon M, et al: Prenatal cocaine use: A comparison of neonates matched on maternal risk factors. Neurotoxicol Teratol 16:81, 1994.

Eyler FD, Behnke M, Conlon M, et al: Birth outcome from a prospective, matched study of prenatal crack/cocaine use. I. Interactive and dose effects on health and growth. Pediatrics 101:229, 1998.

Fantel AG, McPhail BJ: The teratogenicity of cocaine. Teratology 26:17, 1982.

Fantel AG, Barber CV, Mackler B: Ischemia/reperfusion: A new hypothesis for the developmental toxicity of cocaine. Teratology 46:285, 1992.

Fares I, McCulloch KM, Raju TNK: Intrauterine cocaine exposure and the risk of sudden infant death syndrome: A meta-analysis. J Perinatol 17:179, 1997.

Feldkamp M, Carey JC: Clinical teratology counseling and consultation case report: Low dose methotrexate exposure in the early weeks of pregnancy. Teratology 47:533, 1993.

Ferencz C, Matanoski GM, Wilson PD, et al: Maternal hormone therapy and congenital heart disease. Teratology 21:225, 1980.

Fergusson DM, Horwood LJ, Northstone K. ALSPAC Study Team: Maternal use of cannabis and pregnancy outcome. Br J Obstet Gynaecol 109:21, 2002.

Fernandes O, Sabharwal M, Smiley T, et al: Moderate to heavy caffeine consumption during pregnancy and relationship to spontaneous abortion and abnormal fetal growth: A meta-analysis. Reprod Toxicol 12:435, 1998.

Ferris EF, Mendoza SA, Griswold WR, et al: Prenatal risk factors for urinary tract abnormalities. Pediatr Res 31:92A, 1992.

Finnegan LP: Treatment issues for opioid-dependent pregnant women during the perinatal period. J Psychoactive Drugs **23**:191, 1991.

Finnell RH, Toloyan S, VanWaes M, et al: Preliminary evidence for a cocaine-induced embryopathy in mice. Toxicol Appl Pharmacol **103**:228, 1990.

Fisher SE, Atkinson M, Holzman I, et al: Effect of ethanol upon placental uptake of amino acids. Prog Biochem Pharmacol **18**:216, 1981.

Food and Drug Administration: Drug Bulletin. Fed Reg **44**:37434, 1980a.

Food and Drug Administration: Report on Caffeine. Washington, DC, U.S. Government Printing Office, 1980b.

Food and Drug Administration: Surgeon General's advisory on alcohol and pregnancy. FDA Drug Bull **11**:9, 1981.

Food and Drug Administration: Drug bulletin. Adverse effects with isotretinoin. FDA Drug Bull **13**:21, 1983.

Food and Drug Administration: Consumer. Washington, DC, U.S. Government Printing Office, December 1987 to January 1988, p. 22.

Fortier I, Marcoux S, Beaulac-Baillargeon L: Relation of caffeine intake during pregnancy to intrauterine growth retardation and preterm birth. Am J Epidemiol **137**:931, 1993.

Frank DA, Augustyn M, Knight WG, et al: Growth, development and behavior in early childhood following prenatal cocaine exposure. A systematic review. JAMA **285**:1613, 2001.

Fricker HS, Segal S: Narcotic addiction, pregnancy and the newborn. Am J Dis Child **132**:360, 1978.

Fried PA, Makin JE: Neonatal behavioral correlates of prenatal exposure to marijuana in a low risk population. Neurotoxicol Teratol **9**:1, 1987.

Fried PA, O'Connell CM: A comparison of the effects of prenatal exposure to tobacco, alcohol, cannabis and caffeine on birth size and subsequent growth. Neurotoxicol Teratol **9**:79, 1987.

Fried PA, Watkinson B: Twelve and twenty-four month neurobehavioral follow-up of children prenatally exposed to marijuana cigarettes and alcohol. Neurobehav Toxicol Teratol **10**:305, 1988.

Fried PA, Watkinson B, Grant A, et al: Changing patterns of soft drug use prior to and during pregnancy: A prospective study. Drug Alcohol Depend **6**:323, 1980.

Fulroth R, Phillips B, Durand DJ: Perinatal outcome of infants exposed to cocaine and/or heroin in utero. Am J Dis Child **143**:905, 1989.

Furuhashi N, Sato S, Suzuki M, et al: Effects of caffeine ingestion during pregnancy. Gynecol Obstet Invest **19**:187, 1985.

Gal I: Risks and benefits of the use of hormonal pregnancy test tablets. Nature **240**:241, 1972.

Gal I, Kirman B, Stern J: Hormonal pregnancy tests and congenital malformations. Nature **216**;83, 1967.

Garcia AM: Occupational exposure to pesticides and congenital malformations: A review of mechanisms, methods and results. Am J Ind Med **33**:232, 1998.

Geelen JAG: Hypervitaminosis A induced teratogenesis. Crit Rev Toxicol **16**:351, 1979.

Geiger JM, Baudin M, Saurat JH: Teratogenic resin with etretinate and acitretin treatment. Dermatology **189**:109, 1994.

Giacoia GP: Reproductive hazards in the workplace. Obstet Gynecol Surv **47**:679, 1992.

Gibson GT, Baghurst PA, Colley DP: Maternal alcohol, tobacco and cannabis consumption and the outcome of pregnancy. Aust N Z J Obstet Gynaecol **23**:15, 1983.

Gilbert EF, Pistey WR: Effect on the offspring of repeated caffeine administration to pregnant rats. J Reprod Fertil **34**:495, 1973.

Gillberg C: "Floppy-infant syndrome" and maternal diazepam. Lancet **2**:244, 1977.

Gillogley KM, Evans AT, Hansen RL, et al: The perinatal impact of cocaine, amphetamine and opiate use detected by universal intrapartum screening. Am J Obstet Gynecol **163**:1535, 1990.

Gilmore J, Pennell PB, Stern BJ: Medication use during pregnancy and for neurologic conditions. Neurol Clin **16**:189, 1998.

Ginsberg JS, Hirsh J: Anticoagulants during pregnancy. Annu Rev Med **40**:79, 1989.

Ginsberg JS, Hirsh J, Rainbow AJ, et al: Risks to the fetus of radiologic procedures used in the diagnosis of maternal venous thromboembolic disease. Thromb Haemost **61**:189, 1989.

Gladstone J, Levy M, Nulman I, et al: Characteristics of pregnant women who engage in binge alcohol consumption. Can Med Assoc J **156**:789, 1997.

Goldenberg R, Davis R, Baker R: Indomethacin induced oligohydramnios. Am J Obstet Gynecol **160**:1196, 1989.

Golding J: Reproduction and caffeine consumption: A literature review. Early Hum Dev **43**:1, 1995.

Goldstein DJ, Corbin LA, Sundell KL: Effects of first trimester fluoxetine on the newborn. Obstet Gynecol **89**:713, 1997.

Gonzalez CH, Marques-Dias MJ, Kim CA, et al: Congenital abnormalities in Brazilian children associated with misoprostol misuse in the first trimester of pregnancy. Lancet **351**:1624, 1998.

Gordon BHJ, Streeter ML, Rosso P, et al: Prenatal alcohol exposure: Abnormalities in placental growth and fetal amino acid uptake in the rat. Biol Neonate **47**:113, 1985.

Greenberg F: Possible metronidazole teratogenicity and clefting [letter]. Am J Med Genet **22**:825, 1985.

Guzick DS, Daikoku NH, Kaltreider DF: Predictability of pregnancy outcome in preterm delivery. Obstet Gynecol **63**:645, 1984.

Haddow JE, Knight GJ, Palomaki GE, et al: Cigarette consumption and serum cotinine in relation to birthweight. Br J Obstet Gynaecol **94**:678, 1987.

Hadeed AJ, Siegel SR: Maternal cocaine use during pregnancy: Effect on the newborn infant. Pediatrics **84**:205, 1989.

Hadley C, Main D, Gabbe S: Risk factors for preterm premature rupture of the fetal membranes. Am J Perinatol **7**:374, 1990.

Hall EJ: Scientific view of low-level radiation risks. Radiographics **11**:509, 1991.

Hall JG, Pauli RM, Wilson RM: Maternal and fetal sequelae of anti-coagulation during pregnancy. Am J Med **68**:12, 1980.

Halmesmaki E: Alcohol counselling of 85 pregnant problem drinkers: Effect on drinking and fetal outcome. Br J Obstet Gynaecol **95**:243, 1988.

Halmesmaki E, Teramo AK, Widness AJ, et al: Maternal alcohol abuse is associated with elevated fetal erythropoietin levels. Obstet Gynecol **76**:219, 1990.

Handler AS, Mason ED, Rosenberg DL, et al: The relationship between exposure during pregnancy to cigarette smoking and cocaine use and placenta previa. Am J Obstet Gynecol **170**:884, 1994.

Hanson JW: Teratogen update: Fetal hydantoin effects. Teratology **33**:349, 1986.

Hanson JW, Myrianthopolous NC, Harvey MAS, et al: Risks to the offspring of women treated with hydantoin anticonvulsants, with emphasis on the fetal hydantoin syndrome. J Pediatr **89**:662, 1976.

Hanson JW, Smith DW: The fetal hydantoin syndrome. J Pediatr **87**:285, 1975.

Hanson JW, Streissguth AP, Smith DW: The effect of moderate alcohol consumption on fetal growth and morphogenesis. J Pediatr **92**:947, 1978.

Hanssens M, Kierse MJNC, Vankelecom F, et al: Fetal and neonatal effects of treatment with angiotensin converting enzyme inhibitors in pregnancy. Obstet Gynecol **78**:128, 1991.

Harlap S, Shiono PH: Alcohol, smoking and the incidence of spontaneous abortions in the first and second trimester. Lancet **1**:173, 1980.

Harper RG, Solish GI, Feingold E, et al: Maternal ingested methadone, body fluid methadone and the neonatal withdrawal syndrome. Am J Obstet Gynecol **129**:417, 1974.

Hartz SC, Heinonen OP, Shapiro S, et al: Antenatal exposure to meprobamate and chlordiazepoxide in relation to malformations, mental development and childhood mortality. N Engl J Med **292**:726, 1975.

Hatch EE, Bracken MB: Effect of marijuana use in pregnancy on fetal growth. Am J Epidemiol **124**:986, 1986.

Haugen G, Fauchald P, Sodal G, et al: Pregnancy outcome in renal allograft recipients in Norway: The importance of immunosuppressive drug regimen and health status before pregnancy. Acta Obstet Gynaecol Scand **73**:541, 1994.

Hawks RL, Chiang CN (eds): Urine Testing for Drugs of Abuse. NIDA Research Monograph 73, Rockville, Md, DHHS, 1986.

Hebel JR, Fox NL, Sexton M: Dose-response of birth weight to various measures of maternal smoking during pregnancy. J Clin Epidemiol **41**:483, 1988.

Hecht F, Beals R, Lees MH, et al: Lysergic-acid-diethylamide and cannabis as possible teratogens in man. Lancet **2**:1087, 1968.

Heffner LJ, Sherman CB, Speizer FE, et al: Clinical and environmental predictors of preterm delivery. Obstet Gynecol **81**:750, 1993.

Heier LA, Carpanzaon CR, Mast J, et al: Maternal cocaine abuse: The spectrum of radiologic abnormalities in the neonatal CNS. Am J Neuroradiol **12**:951, 1991.

Heinonen OP, Slone D, Monson RR, et al: Cardiovascular birth defects and antenatal exposure to female sex hormones. N Engl J Med **296**:67, 1977a.

Heinonen OP, Slone D, Shapiro S: Birth Defects and Drugs in Pregnancy. Littleton, Mass, Publishing Sciences Group, 1977b.

Hemminki K, Mutanen P, Saloniemi I: Smoking and the occurrence of congenital malformations and spontaneous abortions: Multivariate analysis. Am J Obstet Gynecol **145**:61, 1983.

Henderson GI, Hoyumpa AM, Rothschild MA, et al: Effect of ethanol and ethanol-induced hypothermia on protein synthesis in pregnant and fetal rats. Alcohol Clin Exp Res **4:**165, 1980.

Herbst AL, Ulfelder H, Poskanzer DC: Adenocarcinoma of the vagina. Association of maternal stilbestrol therapy. N Engl J Med **284:**878, 1971.

Hernandez-Diaz S, Werler MM, Walker AM: Folic acid antagonists during pregnancy and the risk of birth defects. N Engl J Med **343:**1608, 2000.

Hernandez-Diaz S, Werler MM, Walker AM, et al: Neural tube defects in relation to use of folic acid antagonists during pregnancy. Am J Epidemiol **153:**961, 2001.

Hertelendy F, Molnar M: Cocaine directly affects signal transduction on human myometrial cells [abstract no. 44]. Am J Obstet Gynecol **166:**292, 1992.

Higgins S: Smoking in pregnancy. Curr Opin Obstet Gynecol **14:**145, 2002.

Hill RM: Isotretinoin teratogenicity. Lancet **2:**1465, 1984.

Himmelberger DU, Brown BW, Cohen EN: Cigarette smoking during pregnancy and the occurrence of spontaneous abortion and congenital anomaly. Am J Epidemiol **108:**470, 1978.

Hingson R, Alpert JJ, Day N, et al: Effects of maternal drinking and marijuana use on fetal growth and development. Pediatrics **70:**539, 1982.

Hoegerman G, Schnoll S: Narcotic use in pregnancy. Clin Perinatol **18:**58, 1991.

Hoff C, Wetelecki W, Blackburn WR, et al: Trend associations of smoking with maternal, fetal, and neonatal morbidity. Obstet Gynecol **68:**317, 1986.

Holmes LB, Harvey EA, Coull BA, et al: The teratogenicity of anticonvulsant agents. N Engl J Med **344:**1132, 2001.

Horta BL, Victora CG, Menezes AM, et al: Low birthweight, preterm births and intrauterine growth retardation in relation to maternal smoking. Paediatr Perinatal Epidemiol **11:**140, 1997.

Hulse GK, Milne E, English DR, et al: The relationship between maternal use of heroin and methadone and infant birth weight. Addiction **92:**1571, 1997.

Hurd WW, Cavin JM, Dombrowski MP, et al: Cocaine selectively inhibits the beta-adrenergic receptor binding in pregnant human myometrium. Am J Obstet Gynecol **169:**644, 1993.

Hurd WW, Robertson PA, Riemer RK, et al: Cocaine directly augments the alpha-adrenergic contractile response of the pregnant rabbit uterus. Am J Obstet Gynecol **164:**182, 1991a.

Hurd WW, Smith AJ, Gauvin JM, et al: Cocaine blocks extraneuronal reuptake of norepinephrine by the pregnant human uterus. Obstet Gynecol **78:**249, 1991b.

Idanpann-Heikkila J, Jouppila P, Akerblom HK, et al: Elimination and metabolic effects of ethanol in mother, fetus and newborn infant. Am J Obstet Gynecol **112:**387, 1972.

Idia H, Gleason CA, O'Brien TP, et al: Fetal response to acute fetal cocaine injection in sheep. Am J Physiol **267:**H1968 , 1994.

Inselman LS, Fisher SE, Spencer H, et al: Effects of intrauterine ethanol exposure on fetal lung growth. Pediatr Res **19:**12, 1985.

Institute of Medicine: Preventing Low Birthweight. Washington, DC, National Academy Press, 1985.

Interim Report: 1/1/89–1/31/01. Wilmington, NC, Antiretroviral Pregnancy Registry, May 2001.

Jacobson J, Jacobson S, Sokol R: Effects of prenatal exposure to alcohol, smoking and illicit drugs on postpartum somatic growth. Alcohol Clin Exp Res **18:**317, 1994.

Jacobson SJ, Jones K, Johnson K, et al: Prospective multicenter study of pregnancy outcome after lithium exposure during the first trimester. Lancet **339:**530, 1992.

Janerich DT, Dugan JM, Standfast SJ, et al: Congenital heart disease and prenatal exposure to exogenous sex hormones. BMJ **1:**1058, 1977.

Janerich DT, Piper JM, Glebatis DM: Oral contraceptives and congenital limb reductions defects. N Engl J Med **291:**697, 1974.

Jeanty P, Cousaert E, deMaertalaer V, et al: Sonographic detection of smoking-related decreased fetal growth. J Ultrasound Med **6:**13, 1987.

Jones KL, Lacro RV, Johnson KA, et al: Pattern of malformations in the children of women treated with carbamazepine during pregnancy. N Engl J Med **320:**1661, 1989.

Jones KL, Smith DW, Ulleland CN, et al: Patterns of malformations in offspring of chronic alcoholic mothers. Lancet **1:**1267, 1973.

Jones LL, Johnson KA, Chambers CC: Pregnancy outcome in women treated with phenobarbital monotherapy. Teratology **45:**452, 1992.

Kaltenbach K, Berghella V, Finnegan L: Opioid dependence during pregnancy. Obstet Gynecol Clin North Am **25:**139, 1998.

Kaminski M, Franc M, Lebouiver M, et al: Moderate alcohol use and pregnancy outcome. Neurobehav Toxicol Teratol **3:**173, 1981.

Kaminski M, Ruimeau-Roquette C, Schwartz D: Alcohol consumption in pregnant women and the outcome of pregnancy. Alcohol Clin Exp Res **1:**155, 1978.

Kandall SR, Albin S, Gart LM, et al: The narcotic-dependent mother: Fetal and neonatal consequences. Early Hum Dev **1:**161, 1977.

Kandall SR, Albin S, Lowinson J, et al: Differential effects of maternal heroin and methadone use on birthweight. Pediatrics **58:**681, 1976.

Kaneko S, Battino D, Andermann E, et al: Congenital malformation due to antiepileptic drugs. Epilepsy **33:**145, 1999.

Kaneko S, Otani K, Fukushima Y, et al: Teratogenicity of antiepileptic drugs: Analysis of possible risk factors. Epilepsia **29:**459, 1988.

Kaneko S, Otani K, Kondo T, et al: Teratogenicity of antiepileptic drugs and drug specific malformations. Jpn J Psychiatry Neurol **47:**306, 1993.

Katikaneni LD, Salle FR, Hulsey TC: Neonatal hair analysis for benzoylecgonine: A sensitive and semiquantitative biological marker for chronic gestational cocaine exposure. Biol Neonate **81:**29, 2002.

Katz Z, Lancet M, Skomik J, et al: Teratogenicity of progestogens given during the first trimester of pregnancy. Obstet Gynecol **65:**775, 1985.

Kaufman RH, Adam E, Binder GI, et al: Upper genital tract changes and pregnancy outcome in offspring exposed in utero to diethylstilbestrol. Am J Obstet Gynecol **137:**299, 1980.

Kaye K, Eklind L, Goldberg D, et al: Birth outcomes for infants of drug abusing mothers. N Y State J Med **89:**256, 1989.

Keith L, MacGregor S, Friedell S, et al: Substance abuse in pregnant women: Recent experience at the Perinatal Center for Chemical Dependence of Northwestern Memorial Hospital. Obstet Gynecol **73:**15, 1989.

Kelly TE: Teratogenicity of anticonvulsant drugs. 1. Review of the literature. Am J Med Gen **19:**413, 1984.

Kerber IJ, Warr OS, Richardson C: Pregnancy in a patient with a prosthetic mitral valve. JAMA **203:**223, 1968.

Khattak S, K-Moghtader G, McMartin K, et al: Pregnancy outcome following gestational exposure to organic solvents: A prospective controlled study. JAMA **281:**1106, 1999.

Kirshon B, Moise K, Wasserstrum M: Influence of short term indomethacin therapy on fetal urine output. Obstet Gynecol **72:**51, 1988a.

Kirshon B, Wasserstrum N, Willis R, et al: Teratogenic effects of first trimester cyclophosphamide therapy. Obstet Gynecol **72:**462, 1988b.

Kistin N, Handler A, Davis F, et al: Cocaine and cigarettes: a comparison of risks. Paediatr Perinat Epidemiol **10:**269, 1996.

Klebanoff MA, Levine RJ, Clemens JD, et al: Maternal serum caffeine metabolites and small-for-gestational age birth. Am J Epidemiiol **155:**32, 2002.

Klebanoff MA, Levine RJ, DerSimonian R, et al: Maternal serum paraxanthine, a caffeine metabolite, and the risk of spontaneous abortion. N Engl J Med **341:**1639, 1999.

Kleinman JC, Pierre MB, Madans JH, et al: Effects of maternal smoking on fetal and infant mortality. Am J Epidemiol **127:**274, 1988.

Klesges LM, Johnson KC, Ward KD, et al: Smoking cessation in pregnant women. Obstet Gynecol Clin North Am **28:**269, 2001.

Kliegman RM, Madura D, Eisenberg I, et al: Relation of maternal cocaine use to the risks of prematurity and low birth weight. J Pediatr **124:**751, 1994.

Kline J, Ng SK, Schittini M, et al: Cocaine use during pregnancy: Sensitive detection by hair assay. Am J Public Health **87:**352, 1997.

Kline J, Shrout P, Stein Z, et al: Drinking during pregnancy and spontaneous abortion. Lancet **2:**176, 1980.

Kline J, Stein Z, Hutzler M: Cigarettes, alcohol and marijuana: Varying associations with birth weight. Int J Epidemiol **16:**44, 1987.

Kline J, Stein ZA, Susser M, et al: Smoking: A risk factor for spontaneous abortion. N Engl J Med **297:**793, 1977.

Knapp K, Lenz W, Nowack E: Multiple congenital anomalies. Lancet **2:**725, 1962.

Koch S, Losche G, Jager-Roman E, et al: Major birth malformations and antiepileptic drugs. Neurology **42** (Suppl 5):83, 1992.

Kolas T, Nakling J, Salvesen KA: Smoking during pregnancy increases the risk of preterm births among parous women. Acta Obstet Gynaecol Scand **79:**644, 2000.

Kondo K: Congenital Minamata disease: warning from Japan's experience. J Child Neurol **15:**458, 2000.

Koren G, Pastuszak A, Ito S: Drugs in pregnancy. N Engl J Med **338:**1128, 1998.

Kozma C: Valproic acid embryopathy: report of two siblings with further expansion of the phenotypic abnormalities and a review of the literature. Am J Med Genet **98:**165, 2000.

Kramer LD, Locke GE, Ogunyemi A, et al: Neonatal cocaine related seizures. J Child Neurol **5:**60, 1990.

Kramer MD, Taylor V, Hickok DE, et al: Smoking and placenta previa. Am J Epidemiol **130:**804, 1989.

Krauss CM, Holmes LB, Van Lang QN, et al: Four siblings with similar malformations after exposure to phenytoin and primidone. J Pediatr **105**:750, 1984.

Kulin NA, Pastuszak A, Sage SR, et al: Pregnancy outcome following maternal use of the new selective serotonin reuptake inhibitors. A prospective controlled multicenter study. JAMA **279**:609, 1998.

Kullander S, Kallen B: A prospective study of drugs and pregnancy. Acta Obstet Gynaecol Scand **55**:25, 1976.

Kurpa K, Holmberg PC, Kuosma E, et al: Coffee consumption during pregnancy and selected congenital malformations: A nationwide case-control study. Am J Public Health **73**:1397, 1983.

Kutscher AH, Zegarelli EV, Tovell HM, et al: Discoloration of deciduous teeth induced by administration of tetracycline antepartum. Am J Obstet Gynecol **96**:291, 1966.

Kwong TC, Ryan RM: Detection of intrauterine illicit drug exposure by newborn drug testing. Clin Chem **43**:235, 1997.

Kyrklund-Blomberg NB, Cnattingius S: Preterm birth and maternal smoking: Risks related to gestational age and onset of delivery. Am J Obstet Gynecol **179**:1051, 1998.

Lajeunie E, Le Merrer M, Marchac D, et al: Syndromal and non-syndromal primary trigonocephaly: Analysis of 237 patients. Am J Med Genet **75**:211, 1998.

Lammer EJ: Teratogen update: Valproic acid. Teratology **35**:465, 1987.

Lammer EJ: Embryopathy in an infant conceived one year after termination of maternal etretinate. Lancet **2**:1080, 1988.

Lammer EJ, Chen DT, Hoar RM, et al: Retinoic acid embryopathy. N Engl J Med **313**:837, 1985.

Landers DV, Green JR, Sweet RL: Antibiotic use during pregnancy and the postpartum period. Clin Obstet Gynecol **26**:391, 1983.

Landry SH, Whitney JA: The impact of prenatal cocaine exposure: Studies of the developing infant. Semin Perinatol **20**:99, 1996.

Lenz W: A short history of thalidomide embryopathy. Teratology **38**:203, 1988.

Lenz W, Knapp K: Thalidomide embryopathy. Arch Environ Health **5**:100, 1962.

Lester BM, El Sohly M, Wright LL, et al: The maternal lifestyle study: Drug use by meconium toxicology and maternal self-report. Pediatrics **107**:309, 2001.

Levy M, Spino M: Neonatal withdrawal syndrome: Associated drugs and pharmacologic management. Pharmacotherapy **13**:202, 1993.

Lewis WH, Suris OR: Treatment with lithium carbonate: Results in 35 cases. Tex Med **66**:58, 1970.

Lieff S, Olshan AF, Werler M, et al: Maternal cigarette smoking during pregnancy and risk of oral clefts in newborns. Am J Epidemiol **150**:683, 1999.

Lifschitz MH, Wilson GS, Smith E, et al: Fetal and postnatal growth of children born to narcotic-dependent women. J Pediatr **102**:686, 1983.

Lightwood JM, Phibbs CS, Glantz SA: Short-term health and economic benefits of smoking cessation: Low birthweight. Pediatrics **104**:1312, 1999.

Lindley AA, Becker S, Gray RH, et al: Effect of continuing or stopping smoking during pregnancy on infant birth weight, crown-heel length, head circumference, ponderal index, and brain:body weight ratio. Am J Epidemiol **152**:219, 2000.

Linn S, Schoenbaum S, Monson R, et al: The association of marijuana use with outcome of pregnancy. Am J Public Health **73**:1161, 1983.

Linn SC, Shoenbaum RR, Monson B, et al: No association between coffee consumption and adverse outcomes of pregnancy. N Engl J Med **306**:141, 1982.

Lipschultz SE, Frassica JJ, Orav EJ: Cardiovascular abnormalities in infants prenatally exposed to cocaine. J Pediatr **118**:44, 1991.

Little BB, Snell LM: Brain growth among fetuses exposed to cocaine in utero. Obstet Gynecol **77**:361, 1991.

Little BB, Snell LM, Gilstrap LC: Methamphetamine abuse during pregnancy: Outcome and fetal effects. Obstet Gynecol **72**:541, 1988.

Little BB, Snell LM, Gilstrap LC: Alcohol use during pregnancy and maternal alcoholism. In Gilstrap LC, Little BB (eds): Drugs and Pregnancy. New York, Elsevier, 1992, p. 367.

Little BB, Snell LM, Klein VR, et al: Cocaine abuse during pregnancy: Maternal and fetal implications. Obstet Gynecol **73**:157, 1989.

Little BB, Snell LM, Klein VR, et al: Maternal and fetal effects of heroin addiction during pregnancy. J Reprod Med **35**:159, 1990.

Little BB, Snell LM, Trimmer KJ, et al: Peripartum cocaine use and adverse pregnancy outcome. Am J Hum Biol **11**:598, 1999.

Little RE: Moderate alcohol use during pregnancy and decreased infant birth weight. Am J Public Health **67**:1154, 1977.

Lochry EA, Randall CL, Goldsmith AA, et al: Effects of acute alcohol exposure during selected days of gestation in CH3 mice. Neurobehav Toxicol Teratol **4**:15, 1982.

Loebstein R, Addis A, Ho E, et al: Pregnancy outcome following gestational exposure to fluoroquinolones: a multicenter prospective controlled study. Antimicrob Agents Chemother **42**:1336, 1998.

Longo LD: The biological effects of carbon monoxide on the pregnant woman, fetus, and newborn infant. Am J Obstet Gynecol **129**:69, 1977.

Longo LD, Ching KS: Placental diffusing capacity for carbon monoxide and oxygen in unanesthetized sheep. J Appl Physiol **43**:885, 1977.

Longo LD, Hill ED: Carbon monoxide uptake and elimination in fetal and maternal sheep. Am J Obstet Gynecol **232**:324, 1977.

Lorente C, Cordier S, Goujard J, et al: Tobacco and alcohol use during pregnancy and risk of oral clefts. Occupational Exposure and Congenital Malformation Working Group. Am J Public Health **90**:415, 2000.

Luck W, Ngu H, Hansen R, et al: Extent of nicotine and cotinine transfer to the human fetus, placenta and amniotic fluid of smoking mothers. Dev Pharmacol Ther **8**:384, 1985.

MacArthur C, Knox EG: Smoking and pregnancy: Effects of stopping at different stages. Br J Obstet Gynaecol **95**:551, 1988.

MacDorman MF, Cnattingius S, Hoffman HJ, et al: Sudden infant death syndrome and smoking in the United States and Sweden. Am J Epidemiol **146**:249, 1997.

MacGregor S, Keith L, Bachicha J, et al: Cocaine abuse during pregnancy: Correlation between prenatal care and perinatal outcome. Obstet Gynecol **74**:882, 1989.

MacGregor S, Keith L, Chasnoff I, et al: Cocaine use during pregnancy: Adverse perinatal outcome. Am J Obstet Gynecol **157**:686, 1987.

Mack G, Thomas D, Giles W, et al: Methadone levels and neonatal withdrawal. J Pediatr Child Health **27**:96, 1991.

Macones GA, Sehdev HM, Parry S, et al: The association between maternal cocaine use and placenta previa. Am J Obstet Gynecol **177**:1097, 1997.

Madden JD, Payne TE, Miller S: Maternal cocaine abuse and effect on the newborn. Pediatrics **77**:209, 1986.

Mahalik MP, Gautieri RF, Mann DE: Teratogenic potential of cocaine hydrochloride in CF-a mice. J Pharm Sci **69**:703, 1982.

Mainous A, Hueston W: The effect of smoking cessation during pregnancy on preterm delivery and low birthweight. J Fam Pract **38**:262, 1994.

Malpas TJ, Darlow BA, Lennox R, et al: Maternal methadone dosage and neonatal withdrawal. Aust N Z J Obstet Gynaecol **35**:175, 1995.

Manning F, Walker D, Feyerabend C: The effect of nicotine on fetal breathing movements in conscious pregnant ewes. Obstet Gynecol **52**:563, 1978.

Manning FA, Feyerabend C: Cigarette smoking and fetal breathing movements. Br J Obstet Gynaecol **83**:262, 1976.

Manson JM, Papa L, Miller ML, et al: Studies of DNA damage and cell death in embryonic limb buds induced by teratogenic exposure to cyclophosphamide. Teratog Carcinog Mutagen **2**:47, 1982.

Marbury MC, Linn S, Monson R, et al: The association of alcohol consumption with outcome of pregnancy. Am J Public Health **73**:1165, 1983.

Markovic N, Ness RB, Cefilli D, et al: Substance abuse measures among women in early pregnancy. Am J Obstet Gynecol **183**:627, 2000.

Marquis S, Leichter J, Lee M: Plasma amino acids and glucose levels in the rat fetus and dam after chronic maternal alcohol consumption. Biol Neonate **46**:36, 1984.

Martin TR, Bracken MB: Association of low birth weight with passive smoke exposure in pregnancy. Am J Epidemiol **124**:633, 1986.

Martin TR, Bracken MB: The association between low birth weight and caffeine consumption during pregnancy. Am J Epidemiol **126**:813, 1987.

Martin-Denavit T, Edery P, Planchu H, et al: Ectodermal abnormalities associated with methimazole intrauterine exposure. Am J Med Genet **94**:337, 2000.

Marwick C: Thalidomide back—Under strict control. JAMA **278**:1135, 1997.

Mastrogiannis D, Decavalas G, Verma U, et al: Perinatal outcome after recent cocaine usage. Obstet Gynecol **75**:8, 1990.

Matsumoto H, Koyo G, Takeuchi T: Fetal miramata disease. A neuropathological study of two cases of intrauterine intoxication by a methylmercury compound. J Neuropathol Exp Neurol **24**:563, 1965.

McBride WG: Limb deformities associated with iminodibenzyl hydrochloride. Med J Aust **1**:492, 1972.

McCalla S, Minkoff HL, Feldman J, et al: The biologic and social consequences of perinatal cocaine use in an inner-city population: Results of an anonymous cross-sectional study. Am J Obstet Gynecol **164**:625, 1991.

McDonald AD, Armstrong BG, Sloan M: Cigarette, alcohol, and coffee consumption and prematurity. Am J Public Health **82**:87, 1992a.

McDonald AD, Armstrong BG, Sloan M: Cigarette, alcohol, and coffee consumption and congenital defects. Am J Public Health **82**:91, 1992b.

McMartin KI, Chu M, Kopecky E, et al: Pregnancy outcome following maternal organic solvent exposure: A meta-analysis of epidemiologic studies. Am J Ind Med **34**:288, 1998.

McMartin KL, Platt MS, Hackman R, et al: Lung tissue concentrations of nicotine in sudden infant death syndrome (SIDS). J Pediatr **140**:205, 2002.

Melnick S, Cole P, Anderson D, et al: Rates and risks of diethystilbestrol-related clear cell adenocarcinoma of the vagina and cervix. N Engl J Med **316**:514, 1987.

Melvin C, Dolan Mullen P, Windsor RA, et al: Recommended cessation counseling for pregnant women who smoke: a review of the evidence. Tobacco Control **9** (Suppl 3):80, 2000.

Mendola P, Selevan SG, Gutter S, et al: Environmental factors associated with a spectrum of neurodevelopmental deficits. Ment Retard Disabil Res Rev **8**:188, 2002.

Meyer MB, Jonas BS, Tonascia JA: Perinatal events associated with maternal smoking during pregnancy. Am J Epidemiol **103**:464, 1976.

Meyer MB, Tonascia JA: Maternal smoking, pregnancy complications and perinatal mortality. Am J Obstet Gynecol **55**:701, 1977.

Milham S: Scalp defects in infants of mothers treated for hyperthyroidism with methimazole or carbimazole during pregnancy. Teratology **32**:321, 1985.

Milham S, Elledge W: Maternal methimazole and congenital defects in children [letter]. Teratology **5**:125, 1972.

Milkovich L, van den Berg BJ: Effects of prenatal meprobamate and chlordiazepoxide hydrochloride on human embryonic and fetal development. N Engl J Med **291**:1268, 1971.

Milkovich L, van den Berg BJ: Effects of antenatal exposure to anorectic drugs. Am J Obstet Gynecol **129**:637, 1974.

Miller HC, Jekel JF: Incidence of low birthweight infants born to mothers with multiple risk factors. Yale J Biol Med **60**:397, 1987.

Miller JM, Boudreaux MC: A study of antenatal cocaine use—chaos in action. Am J Obstet Gynecol **180**:1427, 1999.

Miller JM, Boudreaux MC, Regan FA: A case-control study of cocaine use in pregnancy. Am J Obstet Gynecol **172**:180, 1995.

Miller MW, Brayman AA, Abramowicz JS: Obstetrical ultrasonography: A biophysical consideration of patient safety—The "rules" have changed. Am J Obstet Gynecol **179**:241, 1998.

Mills J, Graubard B: Is moderate drinking during pregnancy associated with an increase in the risk for malformations? Pediatrics **80**:309, 1987.

Mills J, Graubard BI, Harley EE, et al: Maternal alcohol consumption and birth weight: How much drinking during pregnancy is safe? JAMA **252**:1875, 1984.

Mills JL, Holmes LB, Aarons JH, et al: Moderate caffeine use and the risk of spontaneous abortion and intrauterine growth retardation. JAMA **269**:593, 1993.

Milunsky A, Graef JW, Gaynor MF: Methotrexate-induced congenital malformations with a review of the literature. J Pediatr **72**:790, 1968.

Mirochnick M, Frank DA, Cabral H, et al: Relation between meconium concentration of the cocaine metabolite benzoylecgonine and fetal growth. J Pediatr **125**:636, 1995.

Mjolnerod OK, Rasmussen K, Dommerud SA, et al: Congenital connective tissue defect probably due to D-penicillamine treatment in pregnancy. Lancet **1**:673, 1971.

Mochizuki M, Mauro T, Masuko K, et al: Effects of smoking on fetoplacental-maternal system during pregnancy. Am J Obstet Gynecol **149**:313, 1984.

Molnar M, Winn H, Hertelendy F: Cocaine activates the inositol cycle and potentiates the action of oxytocin in human myometrial cells. Abstract presented at the meeting of the Society for Gynecologic Investigation, March 1992, San Antonio, Texas, p. 224.

Monga M: Vitamin A and its congeners. Semin Perinatol **21**:135, 1997.

Monga M, Chimielowiec S, Andres RL, et al: Cocaine alters placental production of thromboxane and prostacyclin. Am J Obstet Gynecol **171**:965, 1994.

Monga M, Weisbrodt NW, Andres RL, et al: The acute effect of cocaine exposure on pregnant human myometrial activity. Am J Obstet Gynecol **169**:782, 1993.

Monheit AG, van Vunakis H, Key TC, et al: Maternal and fetal cardiovascular effects of nicotine infusion in pregnant sheep. Am J Obstet Gynecol **145**:290, 1983.

Monica G, Lilja C: Placenta previa, maternal smoking and recurrence risk. Acta Obstet Gynaecol Scand **74**:341, 1995.

Moore SJ, Turnpenny P, Quinn A, et al: A clinical study of 57 children with fetal anticonvulsive syndromes. J Med Genet **37**:489, 2000.

Moore TR, Sorg J, Miller L, et al: Hemodynamic effects of intravenous cocaine on the pregnant ewe and fetus. Am J Obstet Gynecol **155**:883, 1986.

Morgan MA, Honnebier M, Mecenas C, et al: Cocaine's effect on plasma oxytocin concentrations in the baboon during late pregnancy. Am J Obstet Gynecol **174**:1026, 1996.

Morgan MA, Silavin SL, Randolph M, et al: Effect of intravenous cocaine on uterine blood flow in the gravid baboon. Am J Obstet Gynecol **164**:1021, 1991.

Morgan MA, Wentworth RA, Silavin SL, et al: Intravenous administration of cocaine stimulates gravid baboon myometrium in the last third of gestation. Am J Obstet Gynecol **170**:416, 1994.

Mortensen JT, Thulstrup AM, Larsen H, et al: Smoking, sex of the offspring, and risk of placental abruption, placenta previa and preeclampsia: a population-based cohort study. Acta Obstet Gynaecol Scand **80**:894, 2001.

Mujtaba Q, Burrow GN: Treatment of hyperthyroidism in pregnancy with propylthiouracil and methimazole. Obstet Gynecol **46**:282, 1975.

Mullen P: Maternal smoking during pregnancy and evidence-based intervention to promote cessation. Prim Care **26**:578, 1999.

Myhree SA, Williams R: Teratogenic effects associated with maternal primidone therapy. J Pediatr **99**:160, 1981.

Myles TD, Espinoza R, Meyer W, et al: Effects of smoking, alcohol, and drugs of abuse on the outcome of "expectantly" managed cases of preterm premature rupture of the membranes. J Matern Fetal Med **7**:157, 1998.

Naeye R: The duration of maternal cigarette smoking, fetal and placental disorders. Early Hum Dev **3**:229, 1979.

Naeye RL: Abruptio placentae and placenta previa: Frequency, perinatal mortality and cigarette smoking. Obstet Gynecol **55**:701, 1980.

Naeye RL: Maternal use of dextroamphetamine and growth of the fetus. Pharmacology **26**:117, 1983.

Naeye RL, Blanc W, Leblanc W: Heroin and the fetus. Pediatr Res **7**:321, 1973a.

Naeye RL, Blanc W, Leblanc W, et al: Fetal complications of maternal heroin addiction: Abnormal growth, infections and episodes of stress. J Pediatr **83**:1055, 1973b.

Nakahara K, Iso A, Chao CR, et al: Pregnancy enhances cocaine-enhanced stimulation of uterine contractions in the chronically instrumented rat. Am J Obstet Gynecol **175**:188, 1996.

Neerhof MG, MacGregor SN, Retzky SS, et al: Cocaine abuse during pregnancy: Peripartum prevalence and perinatal outcome. Am J Obstet Gynecol **161**:633, 1989.

Nelson K, Holmes LB: Malformations due to spontaneous mutations in newborn infants. N Engl J Med **320**:19, 1989.

Nelson MM, Forfar JO: Associations between drugs administered during pregnancy and congenital abnormalities of the fetus. Br Med J **1**:523, 1971.

Ness RB, Grisso JA, Hirschinger MA, et al: Cocaine and tobacco use and the risk of spontaneous abortion. N Engl J Med **340**:333, 1999.

Nguyen C, Duhl AJ, Escallon CS, et al: Multiple anomalies in a fetus exposed to low-dose methotrexate in the first trimester. Obstet Gynecol **99**:599, 2002.

Nishimura H, Nakai K: Congenital malformations in offspring of mice treated with caffeine. Proc Soc Exp Biol Med **104**:140, 1960.

Nolen GA: The developmental toxicology of caffeine. Issues Rev Teratol **4**:305, 1988.

Nora JL, Vargo TA, Nora AH, et al: Dexamphetamine: A possible environmental trigger in cardiovascular malformations. Lancet **1**:1290, 1970.

Nulman I, Scolnik D, Chitayat D, et al: Findings in children exposed in utero to phenytoin and carbamazepine monotherapy: independent effects of epilepsy and medications. Am J Med Genet **68**:18, 1997.

Nurminen T: Maternal pesticide exposure and pregnancy outcome. J Occup Environ Med **37**:935, 1995.

Nwaogu IC, Ihemelandu EC: Effects of maternal alcohol consumption on the allometric growth of muscles in fetal and neonatal rats. Cell Tiss Organ **164**:167, 1999.

Obe G, Majewski F: No elevation of exchange type aberrations in lymphocytes of children with an alcohol embryopathy. Hum Genet **43**:31, 1978.

O'Campo P, Davis M, Gielen A: Smoking cessation intervention programs for pregnant women: Review and future directions. Semin Perinatol **19**:279, 1995.

Ochoa AG: Trimethoprim and sulfamethoxazole in pregnancy. JAMA **217**:1244, 1971.

O'Connell CM, Fried PA: An investigation of prenatal cannabis exposure and minor physical anomalies in a low risk population. Neurobehav Toxicol Teratol **6**:345, 1984.

Ogburn PL, Hurt RD, Crighan IT, et al: Nicotine patch use in pregnant smokers: Nicotine and cotinine levels and fetal effects. Am J Obstet Gynecol **181**:736, 1999.

Ohmi H, Hirooka K, Mochizuki Y: Fetal growth and the timing of exposure to maternal smoking. Periatr Int **44**:55, 2002.

Olegard R, Sabel KG, Aronsson M, et al: Effects on the child of alcohol abuse during pregnancy: Retrospective and prospective studies. Acta Paediatr Scand **275**:112, 1979.

Omtzigt JGC, Los FJ, Grobee DE, et al: The risk of spina bifida aperta after first trimester exposure to valproate in a prenatal cohort. Neurology **42** (Suppl 5):119, 1992.

Ornoy A, Diav-Citrin O: Teratogen update: antithyroid drugs. Methimazole and propylthiouracil. Teratology **65**:38, 2002.

Oro AS, Dixon SD: Perinatal cocaine and methamphetamine exposure: Maternal and neonatal correlates. J Pediatr **111**:571, 1987.

Osterloh JD, Lee BL: Urine drug screening in mothers and newborns. Am J Dis Child **143**:791, 1989.

Ostrea EM, Brady M, Gauge S, et al: Drug screening of newborns by meconium analysis: A large-scale, prospective, epidemiologic study. Pediatrics **89**:107, 1992.

Ostrea EM, Chavez CJ, Strauss ME: A study of factors that influence the severity of neonatal narcotic withdrawal. J Pediatr **88**:642, 1976.

Ostrea EM, Knapp DK, Tannenbaum L, et al: Estimates of illicit drug use during pregnancy by maternal interview, hair analysis and meconium analysis. J Pediatr **138**:344, 2001.

Ostrea EM, Ostrea AR, Simpson PM: Mortality within the first 2 years in infants exposed to cocaine, opiate or cannabinoid during gestation. Pediatrics **100**:79, 1997.

Ouellette EM, Rosett HL, Rosman NP, et al: Adverse effects on offspring of maternal alcohol abuse during pregnancy. N Engl J Med **297**:528, 1977.

Owiny JR, Myers T, Massmann GA, et al: Lack of effect of maternal cocaine administration on myometrial electromyogram and maternal plasma oxytocin concentrations in pregnant sheep at 124–126 days' gestational age. Obstet Gynecol **79**:82, 1992.

Parazzini F, Bocciolone L, La Vecchia C, et al: Maternal and paternal moderate alcohol consumption and unexplained miscarriages. Br J Obstet Gynaecol **97**:618, 1990.

Park-Wyllie L, Mazzotta P, Pastuszak A, et al: Birth defects after maternal exposure to corticosteroids: Prospective cohort study and meta-analysis of epidemiologic studies. Teratology **62**:385, 2000.

Pastuszak A, Schick-Boschetto B, Zuber C, et al: Pregnancy outcome following first trimester exposure to fluoxetine. JAMA **269**:2446, 1993.

Pastuszak SL, Schuler L, Speck-Martin CE, et al: Use of misoprostol during pregnancy and Mobuis' syndrome in infants. N Engl J Med **338**:1881, 1998.

Pearse SB, Rodriguez LAG, Hartwell C, et al: A pregnancy register of patients receiving carbamazepine in the U.K. Drug Safety **1**:321, 1992.

Pellosi MA, Fratarola M, Apuzzio J, et al: Pregnancy complicated by heroin addiction. Obstet Gynecol **45**:512, 1975.

Perkins SL, Belcher JM, Livesey JF: A Canadian tertiary care center study of maternal and umbilical cord cotinine levels as markers of smoking during pregnancy: Relationship to neonatal effects. Can J Public Health **88**:232, 1997.

Pettiflor JM, Benson R: Congenital malformations associated with the administration of oral anticoagulants during pregnancy. J Pediatr **86**:459, 1975.

Pikkarainen PH, Raiha NC: Development of alcohol dehydrogenase activity in the human liver. Pediatr Res **1**:165, 1967.

Pirson Y, van Lierden M, Ghysen J, et al: Retardation of fetal growth in patients receiving immunosuppressive therapy. N Engl J Med **313**:328, 1985.

Plessinger MA, Woods JR: Progesterone increases cardiovascular toxicity to cocaine in nonpregnant ewes. Am J Obstet Gynecol **163**:1659, 1990.

Pokorny AD, Miller BA, Kaplan HB: The MAST: A shortened version of the Michigan Alcoholism Screening Test. Am J Psychiatry **129**:118, 1972.

Pollack HA: Sudden infant death syndrome, maternal smoking during pregnancy and the cost-effectiveness of smoking cessation intervention. Am J Public Health **91**:432, 2001.

Prager K, Malin H, Spiegler D, et al: Smoking and drinking behavior before and during pregnancy of married mothers of liveborn infants and stillborn infants. Public Health Reports **99**:117, 1984.

Pryde PG, Sedman AB, Nugent CE, et al: Angiotensin converting enzyme inhibitor fetopathy. J Am Soc Nephrol **3**:1575, 1993.

Pulkkinen P: Smoking in pregnancy, with special reference to fetal growth and certain trace element distribution between mother, placenta and fetus. Acta Obstet Gynaecol Scand **69**:543, 1990.

Qazi QH, Mariano E, Milman DH, et al: Abnormalities in offspring associated with prenatal marijuana exposure. Dev Pharmacol Ther **8**:141, 1985.

Rachelefsky GS, Flynt JW, Ebbin AJ, et al: Possible teratogenicity of tricyclic antidepressants. Lancet **1**:838, 1972.

Racine A, Joyce T, Anderson R: The association between prenatal care and birth weight among women exposed to cocaine in New York City. JAMA **270**:1581, 1993.

Rajegowda BK, Glass L, Evans HE, et al: Methadone withdrawal in newborn infants. J Pediatr **81**:532, 1972.

Ramirez A, de los Monteros E, Parra A, et al: Esophageal atresia and tracheoesophageal atresia fistula in two infants born to hyperthyroid women receiving methimazole (Tapazole) during pregnancy. Am J Med Genet **44**:200, 1992.

Randall CL, Taylor WJ, Walker DW: Ethanol-induced malformations in mice. Alcohol Clin Exp Res **1**:219, 1977.

Raye JR, Dubin JW, Blechner JN: Fetal growth restriction following maternal narcotic administration: Nutritional or drug effect. Pediatr Res **9**:279, 1975.

Refuerzo JS, Sokol RJ, Blackwell SC, et al: Cocaine use and preterm premature rupture of the membranes: Improvement in neonatal outcome. Am J Obstet Gynecol **186**:1150, 2002.

Reiff-Eldridge R, Heffner CR, Ephross SA, et al: Monitoring pregnancy outcomes after prenatal drug exposure through prospective pregnancy registries: A pharmaceutical company commitment. Am J Obstet Gynecol **182**:159, 2000.

Rementeria JL, Bhatt K: Withdrawl symptoms in neonates from intrauterine exposure to diazepam. J Pediatr **90**:123, 1977.

Rementeria JL, Nunag NN: Narcotic withdrawal in pregnancy: Stillbirth incidence with a case report. Am J Obstet Gynecol **116**:1152, 1973.

Resnik R, Brink GW, Wilkes M: Catecholamine-mediated reduction in uterine blood flow after nicotine infusion in the pregnant ewe. J Clin Invest **63**:1133, 1979.

Ressequie LK, Hick JF, Bruen JA, et al: Congenital malformations among offspring exposed in utero to progestins: Olmstead County, Minnesota, 1936–1974. Fertil Steril **43**:514, 1985.

Ritchie J, Greene N: Local anesthetics. In Goodman A, Gillman L, Rall T, et al (eds): The Pharmacological Basis of Therapeutics, 7th ed. New York, Macmillan, 1985, p. 309.

Robboy SJ, Noller KL, O'Brien P, et al: Increased incidence of cervical and vaginal dysplasia in 3,980 diethystilbestrol-exposed young women. Experience of the National Collaborative Diethystilbestrol Adenosis Project. JAMA **252**:2979, 1984.

Robert E, Guiband P: Maternal valproic acid and congenital neural tube defects. Lancet **2**:934, 1982.

Robert E, Vollset SE, Botto L, et al: Malformation surveillance and maternal drug exposure: The Madre project. Risk Safety Med **6**:78, 1984.

Rock JA, Wentz AC, Cole KA, et al: Fetal malformations following progesterone therapy during pregnancy: A preliminary report. Fertil Steril **44**:17, 1985.

Rodriguez-Pinella E, Arroyo I, Fondevilla J, et al: Prenatal exposure to valproic acid during pregnancy and limb deficiencies: A case-control study. Am J Med Genet **90**:376, 2000.

Rodriguez-Pinella E, Martinez-Frias ML: Corticosteroids during pregnancy and oral clefts: a case-control study. Teratology **58**:2, 1998.

Roe DA, Little BB, Bawdon RE, et al: Metabolism of cocaine by human placentas: Implications for fetal exposure. Am J Obstet Gynecol **163**:715, 1990.

Roloff DW, Howalt WF: The effect of chronic maternal morphine administration on lung development and growth of fetal rabbits. Pediatr Res **7**:321, 1973.

Rosa FW: Teratogenicity of isotretinoin. Lancet **2**(8348):513, 1983.

Rosa FW: Teratogenic update: Penicillamine. Teratology **33**:127, 1986.

Rosa FW: Spina bifida in infants of women treated with carbamazepine during pregnancy. N Engl J Med **324**:672, 1992.

Rosa FW, Wilk AL, Kelsey FO: Teratogen update: Vitamin A congeners. Teratology **33**:355, 1986.

Rose J, Strandhoy JW, Meis PJ: Acute and chronic effects of maternal ethanol administration on the ovine maternal-fetal unit. Prog Biochem Pharmacol **18**:1, 1981.

Rosenberg L, Mitchell AA, Parsells JL, et al: Lack of relation of oral clefts to diazepam use in pregnancy. N Engl J Med **309**:1282, 1983.

Rosenberg L, Mitchell AA, Shapiro S, et al: Selected birth defects in relation to caffeine-containing beverages. JAMA **247**:1249, 1982.

Rosenthal T, Oparil S: The effect of antihypertensive drugs on the fetus. J Hum Hyperten **16**:293, 2002.

Rosett HL, Weiner L: Alcohol and the Fetus. New York, Oxford University Press, 1984.

Rosett HL, Weiner L, Lee A, et al: Patterns of alcohol consumption and fetal development. Obstet Gynecol **61**:539, 1983.

Rothman JK, Fyler DC, Goldblatt A, et al: Exogenous hormones and other drug exposures of children with congenital heart disease. Am J Epidemiol **109**:433, 1979.

Rothman KJ, Moore LL, Singer MR, et al: Teratogenicity of high vitamin A intake. N Engl J Med **333**:1369, 1995.

Rothrock JF, Rubenstein R, Lyden P: Ischemic stroke associated with methamphetamine inhalation. Neurology **38**:589, 1988.

Rubin D, Krasilnikoff P, Leventhal J, et al: Effect of passive smoking on birthweight. Lancet **2**:1415, 1986.

Rumbaugh CL, Bergeron RT, Scanlan RL, et al: Cerebral vascular changes secondary to amphetamine abuse in the experimental animal. Radiology **101**:345, 1971.

Russell M, Skinner JB: Early measures of maternal alcohol misuse as predictors of adverse pregnancy outcomes. Alcohol Clin Exp Res **12**:824, 1988.

Ryan L, Ehrlich S, Finnegan L: Cocaine abuse in pregnancy: Effects on the fetus and newborn. Neurotoxicol Teratol **9**:295–9, 1987.

Safra MJ, Oakley GP Jr: Association between cleft lip with or without cleft palate and prenatal exposure to diazepam. Lancet **2**:478, 1975.

Salhab AS, DeVane CL, Medrano T, et al: Fetoplacental growth and placental protein synthesis in rats after chronic maternal cocaine administration. J Pharmacol Exp Ther **270**:392, 1994.

Sallee FR, Katikaneni LP, McArthur PD, et al: Head growth in cocaine-exposed infants: Relationship to neonate hair level. J Dev Behav Pediatr **16**:77, 1995.

Samren EB, von Duijin CM, Koch S, et al: Maternal use of anti-epileptic drugs and the risk of major congenital malformations: A joint European prospective study of human teratogenesis associated with maternal epilepsy. Epilepsia **38**:981, 1997.

Saxen I: Association between oral clefts and drugs taken during pregnancy. Int J Epidemiol **4**:37, 1975.

Schardein JL: Congenital abnormalities and hormones during pregnancy: A clinical review. Teratology **22**:251, 1980.

Schramm WF: Smoking during pregnancy: Missouri longitudinal study. Paediatr Perinat Epidemiol **11** (Suppl 1):73, 1997.

Scolnik D, Nulman I, Rovet J, et al: Neurodevelopment of children exposed in utero to phenytoin and carbamazepine monotherapy. JAMA **271**:767, 1994.

Scone D, Heinonen O, Kaufman D, et al: Aspirin and congenital malformations. Lancet **1**:1373, 1976.

Scott JR: Fetal growth retardation associated with maternal administration of immunosuppressive drugs. Am J Obstet Gynecol **128**:668, 1977.

Sexton M, Hebel JR: A clinical trial of change in maternal smoking and its effect on birth weight. JAMA **251**:911, 1984.

Sheppard TH: The Catalog of Teratogenic Agents, 9th ed. Baltimore, Johns Hopkins University Press, 1998.

Sheppard TH, Brent RL, Jones KL, et al: Update on new developments in the study of human teratogens. Teratology **65**:153, 2002.

Shiono PH, Klebanoff MA, Berendes HW: Congenital malformations and maternal smoking during pregnancy. Teratology **34**:65, 1986.

Shiono PH, Klebanoff MA, Nugent RP, et al: The impact of cocaine and marijuana use on low birthweight and preterm birth: A multicenter study. Am J Obstet Gynecol **172**:19, 1995.

Shiono PH, Klebanoff MA, Rhoads GG: Smoking and drinking during pregnancy: Their effects on preterm birth. JAMA **255**:82, 1986.

Shiono PH, Mills JL: Oral clefts and diazepam use during pregnancy. N Engl J Med **311**:919, 1984.

Shubert PJ, Diss E, Iams L: Etiology of preterm premature rupture of the membranes. Obstet Gynecol Clin North Am **19**:251, 1992.

Sim M: Imipramine and pregnancy. Br Med J **2**:45, 1972.

Simone C, Derewlany LO, Oskamp M, et al: Acetylcholinesterase and butyrylcholinesterase activity in the human term placenta: Implications for fetal cocaine exposure. J Lab Clin Med **123**:400, 1994.

Simpson WJ: A preliminary report on cigarette smoking and the incidence of prematurity. Am J Obstet Gynecol **73**:808, 1957.

Singer LT, Yamashita TS, Hawkins S, et al: Increased incidence of intraventricular hemorrhage and developmental delay in cocaine-exposed very low birth weight infants. J Pediatr **124**:765, 1994.

Singh SP, Snyder AK, Pullen GL: Fetal alcohol syndrome: Glucose and liver metabolism in term rat fetus and neonate. Alcohol Clin Exp Res **10**:54, 1986.

Singh SP, Snyder AK, Singh SK: Effects of ethanol ingestion on maternal and fetal glucose homeostasis. J Lab Clin Med **104**:176, 1984.

Smith IE, Coles CD, Lancaster J, et al: The effect of volume and duration of prenatal ethanol exposure on neonatal physical and behavioral development. Neurobehav Toxicol Teratol **8**:375, 1986.

Smith YR, Dombrowski MP, Leach KC, et al: Decrease in myometrial beta-adrenergic receptors with prenatal cocaine use. Obstet Gynecol **85**:357, 1995.

Snider DE, Layde PM, Johnson MW, et al: Treatment of tuberculosis during pregnancy. Am Rev Respir Dis **122**:65, 1980.

Snyder AK, Singh SP, Pullen GL: Ethanol-induced intrauterine growth retardation: Correlation with placental glucose transfer. Alcohol Clin Exp Res **10**:176, 1986.

Sokol RJ, Clarren SK: Guidelines for use of terminology describing the impact of prenatal alcohol on the offspring. Alcoholism **13**:597, 1989.

Sokol RJ, Martier SS, Ager JW: The T-ACE questions: Practical prenatal detection of risk-drinking. Am J Obstet Gynecol **160**:863, 1989.

Sokol RJ, Miller SI: Identifying the alcohol-abusing obstetric/gynecologic patient: A practical approach. Alcohol Health Res World **4**:36, 1980.

Sokol RJ, Miller SI, Debanne S, et al: The Cleveland/NIAA prospective alcohol-in-pregnancy study: The first year. Neurobehav Toxicol Teratol **3**:203, 1981.

Sokol RJ, Miller SI, Reed G: Alcohol abuse during pregnancy: An epidemiologic study. Alcohol Clin Exp Res **4**:135, 1980.

Soothill PW, Nicolaides KH, Bilardo K, et al: Uteroplacental blood velocity index and umbilical venous PO_2, PCO_2, pH, lactate and erythroblast count in growth retarded fetuses. Fetal Ther **1**:174, 1986.

Spence MR, Williams R, DiGregorio GJ, et al: The relationship between recent cocaine use and pregnancy outcome. Obstet Gynecol **78**:326, 1991.

Spinillo A, Capuzzo E, Colonna C, et al: Factors associated with abruptio placentae in preterm deliveries. Acta Obstet Gynaecol Scand **73**:307, 1994.

Sprauve ME, Lindsay MK, Herbert S, et al: Adverse perinatal outcome in parturients who use crack cocaine. Obstet Gynecol **89**:674, 1997.

Srispuphan W, Bracken MB: Caffeine consumption during pregnancy and association with late spontaneous abortion. Am J Obstet Gynecol **154**:14, 1986.

Stek AM, Baker RS, Fisher BK, et al: Fetal responses to maternal and fetal methamphetamine administration in sheep. Am J Obstet Gynecol **173**:1592, 1995.

Stephens TD: Proposed mechanisms of action of thalidomide embryopathy. Teratology **38**:229, 1988.

Steuerwold U, Weilie P, Jorgensen PJ, et al: Maternal seafood diet, methylmercury exposure, and neonatal neurologic function. J. Pediatr **136**:599, 2000.

Stewart DJ, Inaba T, Lucassen M, et al: Cocaine metabolism: Cocaine and norcocaine hydrolysis by liver and serum esterases. Clin Pharmacol Ther **252**:464, 1979.

Stimmel B, Jerez E: Alcohol and substance abuse during pregnancy. In Cherry SH, Berkowitz RL, Kase NG (eds): Medical, Surgical, and Gynecologic Complications of Pregnancy. Baltimore, Williams & Wilkins, 1985, p. 566.

Stoffer SS, Hamber JI: Inadvertent ^{131}I therapy for hyperthyroidism in the first trimester of pregnancy. J Nucl Med **17**:146, 1976.

Stone ML, Salerno LJ, Green M, et al: Narcotic addiction in pregnancy. Am J Obstet Gynecol **109**:717, 1971.

Substance Abuse and Mental Health Services Administration: Summary of Findings from the National Household Survey on Drug Abuse. NHSDA Series: H-13, DHHS, Publication No. SMA 01-3549. Rockville, Md, DHHS, 2000.

Suzuki K, Horiguchi T, Comas-Urrutia CA, et al: Placental transfer and distribution of nicotine in the pregnant Rhesus monkey. Am J Obstet Gynecol **119**:253, 1974.

Suzuki K, Minei LJ, Johnson EE: Effect of nicotine upon uterine blood flow in the pregnant rhesus monkey. Am J Obstet Gynecol **136**:1009, 1980.

Taeusch HW, Carson SH, Wang NS, et al: Heroin induction of lung maturation and growth retardation in fetal rabbits. J Pediatr **82**:5, 1973.

Taylor JA, Sanderson M: A reexamination of the risk factors for sudden infant death syndrome. J Pediatr **126**:887, 1995.

Telsey A, Merrit A, Dixon S: Cocaine exposure in a term neonate: Necrotizing enterocolitis as a complication. Clin Pediatr **27**:547, 1988.

Tennes K, Avitable N, Blackard C, et al: Marijuana: Prenatal and postnatal exposure in the human. NIDA Res Monogr **59**:48, 1985.

Tennes K, Blackard C: Maternal alcohol consumption, birthweight and minor physical anomalies. Am J Obstet Gynecol **138**:774, 1980.

Umans JG, Szeto HH: Precipitated opiate abstinence in utero. Am J Obstet Gynecol **151**:441, 1985.

U.S. Department of Health and Human Services (DHHS): National Pregnancy and Health Survey, Substance Abuse and Mental Health Service Administration, National Institute on Drug Abuse, 1995.

U.S. Department of Health and Human Services: National Household Survey on Drug Abuse. Substance Abuse and Mental Health Service Administration. National Institute on Drug Abuse, 2000.

Van den Veyver IB, Moise KJ Jr, Ou CN, et al: The effect of gestational age and fetal indomethacin levels on the incidence of constriction of the fetal ductus arteriosus. Obstet Gynecol **82**:500, 1993.

Vega WA, Kolody B, Hwang J, et al: Prevalence and magnitude of perinatal substance exposures in California. N Engl J Med **329**:850, 1993.

Ventura S, Martin J, Taffel S, et al: Advanced report of final natality statistics, 1993. Month Vital Stat Rep. **44:**1,1995.

Virji SK: The relationship between alcohol consumption during pregnancy and infant birthweight. Acta Obstet Gynaecol Scand 70:303, 1991.

Virji SK, Cottington E: Risk factors associated with preterm deliveries among racial groups in a national sample of married mothers. Am J Perinatol **8:**347, 1991.

Von Lennep E, El Khazen: A case of partial sirenomelia and possible vitamin A teratogenesis. Prenat Diagn **5:**30, 1985.

Wagner LK, Lester RG, Saldana LR: Exposure of the Pregnant Patient to Diagnostic Radiation. Philadelphia, Medical Physics Publishing, 1997, p. 26.

Wang FL, Dombrowski MP, Hurd WW: Cocaine and beta-adrenergic receptor function in pregnant myometrium. Am J Obstet Gynecol 175:1651, 1996.

Warkany J: Antituberculosis drugs. Teratology **20:**133, 1979.

Warkany J: Teratogen update: Lithium. Teratology 38:593, 1988.

Watkinson B, Fried PA: Maternal caffeine use before, during and after pregnancy and effects upon offspring. Neurobehav Toxicol Teratol 7:9, 1985.

Watts DH: Management of the human immunodeficiency virus infection in pregnancy. N Engl J Med 346:1879, 2002.

Webster WS, Brown-Woodman PDC: Cocaine as a cause of congenital malformation of vascular origin: Experimental evidence in the rat. Teratology **41:**689, 1990.

Wehbeh H, Matthews RP, McCalla S, et al: The effect of recent cocaine use on the progress of labor. Am J Obstet Gynecol 172:1014, 1995.

Weinstein MR, Goldfield M: Cardiovascular malformations with lithium use during pregnancy. Am J Psychiatry **132:**529, 1975.

Werler M, Mitchell A, Shapiro S: The relation of aspirin use during the first trimester of pregnancy to congenital cardiac defects. N Engl J Med **321:**1169, 1984.

Wide K, Winbladh B, Tomson T, et al: Psychomotor development and minor anomalies in children exposed to antiepileptic drugs in utero: a population-based study. Dev Med Child Neurol 42:87, 2000.

Wilcox AJ, Weinberg CR, Baird DD: Risk factors for early pregnancy loss. Epidemiology 1:382, 1990.

Williams JD, Condie AP, Brumfitt W, et al: The treatment of bacteriuria in pregnant women with sulphamethoxazole and trimethoprim. Postgrad Med J **45:**71, 1969.

Williams MA, Mittendorf R, Lieberman E, et al: Cigarette smoking during pregnancy in relation to placenta previa. Am J Obstet Gynecol **165:**28, 1991.

Wilson G: Clinical studies of infants and children exposed prenatally to heroin. Ann N Y Acad Sci **562:**183–194, 1989.

Wilson GS, Desmond MM, Verniaud WM: Early development of infants of heroin-addicted mothers. Am J Dis Child **126:**457, 1973.

Wilson JG, Brent RL: Are female sex hormones teratogenic? Am J Obstet Gynecol **114:**567, 1981.

Windham GC, Eaton A, Hopkins B: Evidence for an association between environmental tobacco smoke exposure and birthweight: a meta-analysis and new data. Paediatr Perinat Epidemiol 13:35, 1999.

Wisborg K, Kesmodel U, Henriksen TB, et al: A prospective study of smoking during pregnancy and SIDS. Arch Dis Child **83:**203, 2000.

Wiseman RA, Dodds-Smith IC: Cardiovascular birth defects and antenatal exposure to female sex hormones: A reevaluation of some base data. Teratology 30:359, 1984.

Woods JR, Plessinger MA: Pregnancy increases cardiovascular toxicity to cocaine. Am J Obstet Gynecol **162:**529, 1990.

Woods JR, Plessinger MA, Clark KE: Effect of cocaine on uterine blood flow and fetal oxygenation. JAMA **257:**957, 1987.

Woods JR, Plessinger MA, Fantel A: An introduction to reactive oxygen species and their possible roles in substance abuse. Obstet Gynecol Clin North Am 25:219, 1998.

Wright LN, Thorp JM, Juller JA, et al: Transdermal nicotine replacement in pregnancy: pharmacokinetics and fetal effects. Am J Obstet Gynecol **176:**1090, 1997.

Yamazaki JN, Schull WJ: Perinatal loss and neurological abnormalities among children of the atomic bomb: Nagasaki and Hiroshima revisited, 1949 to 1989. JAMA **264:**605, 1990.

Yerby MS: Epilespy and pregnancy. New issues for an old disorder. Neurol Clin 1:777, 1993.

Ylikorkala O, Halmesmaki E, Viinikka L: Urinary prostacyclin and thromboxane metabolites in drinking pregnant women and in their infants: Relations to the fetal alcohol effects. Obstet Gynecol 71:61, 1988.

Yovich JL, Turner SR, Draper R: Medroxyprogesterone acetate therapy in early pregnancy has no apparent fetal effects. Teratology 38:135, 1988.

Zackai EH, Mellman WJ, Neiderer B, et al: The fetal trimethadone syndrome. J Pediatr 87:280, 1975.

Zalzstein E, Koren G, Einarson T, et al: A case-control study on the association between first trimester exposure to lithium and Ebstein's anomaly. Am J Cardiol 65:817, 1990.

Zelson C, Lee SJ, Casalino M: Neonatal narcotic addiction: Comparative effects of maternal intake of heroin and methadone. N Engl J Med **289:**1216, 1973.

Zierler S, Rothman KJ: Congenital heart disease in relation to maternal use of bendectin and other drugs in early pregnancy. N Engl J Med **313:**347, 1985.

Zimmerman EF, Potturi RB, Resnick E, et al: Role of oxygen free radicals in cocaine induced vascular disruption in mice. Teratology 49:192, 1994.

Zuckerman B, Frank DA, Hingson R, et al: Effects of maternal marijuana and cocaine use on fetal growth. N Engl J Med **320:**762, 1989.

Zuspan FP, Gumpel JA, Mejia-Zelaya A, et al: Fetal stress from methadone withdrawal. Am J Obstet Gynecol **122:**43, 1975.

Chapter 20

GENERAL PRINCIPLES AND APPLICATIONS OF ULTRASONOGRAPHY

Frank A. Manning, MD, MSc(OXON), FRCS

Diagnostic ultrasound imaging, now ubiquitous in nearly all fields of medicine, began as an obstetric tool. Toward the end of the 1950s, the late Scottish obstetrician Sir Ian Donald modified the sonar technology developed as a submarine detection method to provide images of the fetus *in utero* (Donald et al., 1958). Since its introduction, the method has undergone remarkable modifications and improvements. The contemporary method uses synthetic crystals (zirconate) to generate low-energy (less than 100 mW/cm^2) high-frequency (3.5 to 9 MHz) sound waves. As applied to tissues, the reflected sound waves are detected by the emitting transducer and displayed on a cathode ray tube according to the intensity of the echo (brightness) as a range of 128 intensity shades (gray scale) and the time lag of the returning echo (distance). Electronic switching (sector transducer) or sequential firing of multiple crystals (curvilinear transducer) can be used to emit and receive the ultrasound waves fast enough (more than 40 frames/sec) to detect motion of the target structure (real-time, or dynamic, ultrasonography). The original transducers were designed for *transabdominal* access.

More recently, end-fire transducers have become available, permitting a *transvaginal* approach to uterine and fetal imaging. The selective use of either a transabdominal or transvaginal approach allows one to obtain images of remarkable quality and detail in virtually all cases, regardless of maternal obesity and other limiting factors. The selection of transducer and imaging route varies according to clinical indications, physician experience, and patient preference, but clearly there is a trend toward greater use of the transvaginal approach, especially in earlier pregnancy evaluation and even in later gestation.

The improvements in technology are ongoing. Most new equipment now includes a system for detecting the Doppler shift and power spectral analysis of reflected echoes as may be produced by blood flow within major arteries and veins and within the heart, movement of the intracardiac structures, and fluid flow in the trachea and upper airways. The Doppler signal may be displayed as either a waveform (Doppler ultrasound) or colors assigned according to frequency and direction of flow (color Doppler). Virtually all ultrasound equipment now incorporates electronic calipers to measure linear, area, and circumference parameters and has built-in software to correlate observed measurements (e.g., fetal head circumference) with standard nomograms. Newer innovations include three-dimensional ultrasound derived by off-line, rapid, computer-driven reconstruction of the data lines and, most recently,

four-dimensional ultrasound (three-dimensional ultrasound displayed in real time are now coming on stream in clinical practice) (Fig. 20-1). The added diagnostic value of three-dimensional imaging remains to be established (Platt et al., 1998). The images produced by these new techniques can be spectacular in clarity and detail, but high-resolution images are not easily obtained in many patients, especially those who are moderately obese. It may not be possible to obtain any more information with the three-dimensional technique than available with the standard two-dimensional method. In contrast, the four-dimensional imaging method appears to be a diagnostic breakthrough, on par with the significance of the introduction of ultrasound. The four-dimensional technique allows for integration of fetal anatomy and function, approaching the clarity of the naked eye. It seems likely that this new technology will open new vistas to the understanding of the fetus in health and disease. However, like all new technologies, proof of the clinical value of four-dimensional ultrasound is pending. Concurrent with the improved image quality has been a dramatic fall in energy level of the ultrasound signals. The safety of ultrasonography in obstetrics has been studied extensively (Lyons et al., 1988). Because no reproducible study has described any adverse fetal or maternal effects at the intensity and frequency used in obstetrics, it seems reasonable to conclude that ultrasonography is safe. Furthermore, because the method has now been used safely in up to three generations of pregnant patients who themselves were exposed to diagnostic ultrasonography *in utero*, it seems reasonable to conclude that the imaging energies cause no adverse long-term effects.

With its continued and dramatic improvement in image quality, dynamic range, and clinical applications, ultrasonography has profoundly affected the very nature of obstetric care in general and of high-risk obstetrics in particular. The ability to "see" the fetus, its activities, its contiguous structures, and its environment has led to the concept of fetus as patient. Clinical perinatal medicine is now largely directed at the integration of the fetal information, derived almost exclusively by dynamic ultrasound imaging, with maternal risk factors and obstetric variables. Today, virtually all invasive uterine and fetal procedures are performed under real-time ultrasound guidance. Hence, dynamic ultrasound imaging has become common in general obstetric care and essential in the evaluation and care of the high-risk pregnancy. About 80% of all pregnant women in the United States undergo at least one ultrasound examination.

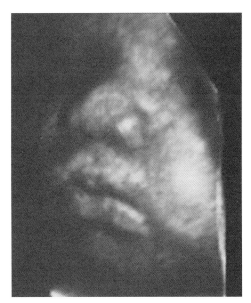

FIGURE 20-1 ■ The frontal view of the face of a near-term fetus produced by three-dimensional ultrasound imaging. Note the striking clarity of detail of the lips, philtrum, and nose. (Courtesy of Professor Delores Pretoius, Department of Radiology, University of California, San Diego.)

ROUTINE ULTRASONOGRAPHY IN PREGNANCY

The Controversy

The clinical value of diagnostic ultrasonography in the evaluation and management of the high-risk pregnancy is accepted. The value of applying the technology to either low-risk pregnancy or all pregnancies (routine ultrasonography) is controversial and remains a topic of active research and debate. Given the value of the technology in the high-risk pregnancy, one might assume that ultrasonography can improve the outcome of the pregnancy without clinical risk factors, albeit less commonly. Early nonrandomized studies of relatively few patients appeared to confirm this assumption (Youngblood, 1989; Ewigman et al., 1991).

Controlled clinical trials of routine ultrasonography have yielded conflicting results. In Finland, a randomized clinical trial of a systematic single ultrasound examination in pregnancy yielded positive results (Saari-Kemppainen et al., 1990). In this study, the perinatal mortality rate was 4.6 per 1000 live births, a rate more than 50% lower than the perinatal mortality rate of 9 per 1000 in the untested control patients (P < .05). The lowered mortality rate in the tested patients was primarily due to detection of lethal anomalies that resulted in pregnancy termination. In the United States, the Routine Antenatal Diagnostic Imaging with Ultrasound (RADIUS) trial examined the value of routine ultrasonography in low-risk pregnancies (Ewigman et al., 1993). This prospective randomized study determined perinatal outcome among 15,530 low-risk patients recruited from 109 practice sites and assigned either to routine ultrasonography at 18 to 20 weeks and again at 30 to 33 weeks (7812 tested patients) or to ultrasonography only as indicated by clinical risk factors (7718 control patients). The tested population and the control population showed little difference in terms of the incidence of adverse perinatal outcome (4.9% and

5%, respectively), the incidence of delivery before 37 weeks (5.5% and 5.9%, respectively), or mean birth weight (3433 ± 544 and 3429 ± 544 g, respectively). The authors of this study concluded that "the adoption of routine ultrasound screening in the United States would add considerably to the cost of care in pregnancy (estimate $500 million per annum), with no improvement in perinatal outcome."

The value of routine ultrasound screening for the detection of the anomalous fetus is still debated, although the preponderance of newer data appears to support routine screening. In the RADIUS trial, although the detection of anomalies was more than twofold higher in the group subjected to routine ultrasound as compared with control subjects, the sensitivity for the tested group (16.6%) was surprisingly low (Crane et al., 1994). These results led the authors of this randomized study to conclude that, given the projected cost of the routine use of ultrasound to screen for fetal anomalies among all pregnant women in the United States (estimate $500,000.00 per annum), the cost-to-benefit ratio could not support routine screening. In contrast, in a study of 2031 patients routinely screened between 15 and 22 weeks' gestation, Van Dorsten and colleagues (1998) reported a 75% sensitivity and a 99.9% specificity for anomaly detection in the presence of a 3% prevalence of anomaly. The importance of resolving the value of routine ultrasound screening for fetal anomaly has become even more important, because in many areas routine screening has been incorporated into standard practice.

Safety of Ultrasound Imaging

Because ultrasound information is created by spectral analysis of echoes produced when the target tissue is bombarded with sound energy, ultrasound imaging must be considered an invasive procedure carrying theoretical risks of tissue damage. Ultrasound energy is absorbed by tissues and transformed into other energy forms. Most sound energy is converted to heat, and the proportion of conversion increases directly with the emitting frequency. With low-level frequencies, a proportion of the energy is converted to movements within the target tissue, producing mechanical motion (vibration) called *resonance*. Low-frequency ultrasonography can be used to create tissue disruption. This principle is applied therapeutically in physiotherapy.

With diagnostic ultrasonography, resonance does not occur and most of the ultrasound energy is dissipated as heat. The amount of heat released per gram of tissue per unit of time varies directly with the intensity of the signal and inversely with the square of the distance from the emitting source. By convention, ultrasound energies are measured at the source and recorded as power per area or watts per square centimeter. It is important to recognize that energy delivered to tissue varies inversely with the square of the distance. Thus, for example, if a target is 8 cm from an emitting source of 100 W/cm², the target receives only $\frac{1}{64}$, or 0.156%, of the originally emitted energy. In special circumstances, high-energy low-frequency ultrasonography causes tissue disruption by cavitation, but that effect does not occur with diagnostic ultrasonography.

For practical purposes, a safe level of tissue ultrasound exposure has been arbitrarily defined as less than or equal to 100 mW/cm². Most commercial ultrasonography instruments operate at ranges far lower than the maximal safe standard and produce energies of 10 to 20 mW/cm². Thus, a fetal target 8 cm from the course receives on average 0.01 to 0.03 mW/cm², or 0.01% to 0.03% of the maximal safe levels. The total tissue energy is a function of exposure time. Diagnostic units use pulsed ultrasound with a usual duty cycle of $\frac{1}{1000}$, which produces only 86 seconds of ultrasound exposure during 24 hours of continuous scanning. Thus, ultrasound energy delivered to tissues varies with the following:

- Frequency
- Intensity (power)
- Exposure time
- Distance from the emitting source

At present, there are no known examples of damage to target tissue from use of conventional diagnostic ultrasound imaging. Prospective studies of the biological effects of *in utero* exposure to ultrasound energies in the diagnostic range have failed to yield any differences between exposed offspring and nonexposed sibling control subjects (Lyons et al., 1988). Long-term follow-up studies of infants exposed to at least one ultrasound examination *in utero* failed to demonstrate any effect of ultrasound on cognitive development, although a significant variation in left-hand preference has been observed (Salversen et al., 1993). This latter finding is more likely an effect of the randomness of statistical significance than a physiologic effect. There is no doubt that high-energy (more than 100 mW/cm²) continuous ultrasound in frequencies within the range used for diagnostic ultrasonography can produce tissue damage (Edmonds, 1972). The relevance of this observation to current use of ultrasonography in clinical obstetrics is questionable. It seems reasonable to state that diagnostic ultrasonography in indicated circumstances carries no recognized inherent risk per se to the mother or fetus and that it provides information that can produce major benefits in pregnancy outcome.

CLINICAL APPLICATIONS OF OBSTETRIC ULTRASONOGRAPHY

Overview

The accepted and potential applications of ultrasonography in pregnancy are broad and continue to increase. In general, applications can be segregated according to the information sought. Information about the fetus is the most common and important indication for ultrasound examination in pregnancy. The basic and minimum information to be acquired about the fetus can be summarized according to a series of specific queries. If the fetus were amenable to providing a history, the questions to be asked and that are answered by ultrasound examination might be as follows:

1. *How old are you?* (gestational age determination based on fetal morphometrics)
2. *Are you alone?* (identification of multiple pregnancy by type and number)
3. *Are you intact?* (fetal anomaly screening by systematic anatomic and functional review)
4. *Are you receiving adequate nourishment?* (determination of fetal weight percentile from combined morphometric measures and subjective assessment of physical characteristics of intrauterine growth restriction [IUGR] or macrosomia)

5. *Is your environment safe?* (assessment of amniotic fluid volume, placental site and architecture, cord anatomy and position, umbilical artery blood flow velocity waveform, and possibly the characteristics of the internal os and the length of the cervix)
6. *Are you safer inside or outside the uterus?* (determination of fetal well-being by fetal biophysical profile score)

This ultrasonography-derived fetal data should be determined at each fetal ultrasound examination and always interpreted within the context of maternal health and well-being and obstetric factors. Thus, obstetric ultrasonography becomes a means of integrating fetal, maternal, and obstetric variables into a rational management scheme tailored to the needs of the individual patient.

Guidelines for Obstetric Ultrasonography: Standard Criteria

In many countries, including Canada, the United Kingdom, Germany, Norway, and Sweden (all countries with a socialized universal health care system), systematic "routine" ultrasonography is recommended in pregnancy. In the United States, routine ultrasonography has not been sanctioned, and a National Institutes of Health consensus meeting developed and published guidelines for indicated ultrasonography (U.S. Department of Health and Human Services, 1984). Twenty-eight indications are described. As reflected by the RADIUS trial, at least 60% of all pregnant patients meet one or more of these criteria.

Guidelines for General Application: The Minimal Examination

Ultrasound imaging methods are used widely in perinatal medicine, and their use continues to expand in both frequency and utility of application. Although this tool has been responsible for major advances in the practice of the specialty, there is no uniform agreement regarding its routine use. The minimal criteria for conduct of an ultrasound examination in pregnancy have been developed and published by the Section of Obstetrics and Gynecology of the American Institute for Ultrasound in Medicine–Standards for Ob/Gyn Ultrasound Practice 1995 and are listed in Table 20-1. These criteria apply to the general examination and do not replace those for more detailed and specialized examinations in selected high-risk pregnancies (Table 20-2). The guidelines assume that the operator is trained in the use of ultrasound equipment, has at least a minimal understanding of fetal anatomy and physiology, and is familiar with the pregnancy risk factors as they relate to the expected ultrasound findings. Only dynamic (real-time) ultrasonography equipment should be used; fetal examination with the older static ultrasound scanners is considered inappropriate and unsatisfactory. The transducer is selected according to the indication for the procedure, gestational age, and maternal body habitus. Up to the middle of the second trimester (20 weeks) and in the obese patient, a transvaginal probe usually yields the best image quality. In selected cases, such as the evaluation of cervical length and shape (Iams et al., 1994; Timor-Trisch et al., 1996) and in the confirmation of a diagnosis of placenta previa, the transvaginal route is best. Adequate documentation of the results is considered essential

TABLE 20-1. AMERICAN INSTITUTE OF ULTRASOUND IN MEDICINE GUIDELINES (MINIMAL) FOR OBSTETRIC ULTRASOUND EXAMINATION

First trimester
  1. The location of the gestational sac should be documented; the embryo should be identified and the crown-rump length recorded.
  2. Presence or absence of fetal life should be reported.
  3. Fetal number should be documented.
  4. Evaluation of the uterus (including cervix) and adnexal structures should be performed.

Second and third trimesters
  1. Fetal life, number, and presentation should be documented.
  2. An estimate of the amount of amniotic fluid (increased, decreased, normal) should be reported.
  3. The placental location should be recorded and its relationship to the internal cervical os determined.
  4. Assessment of gestational age should be accomplished by using a combination of biparietal diameter (or head circumference) and femur length. Fetal growth assessment (as opposed to age) requires the addition of abdominal circumference. If previous studies have been performed, an estimate of the appropriateness of interval change should be given.
  5. Evaluation of the uterus and adnexal structures should be performed.
  6. The study should include, but not necessarily be limited to, the following fetal anatomy: cerebral ventricles, spine, stomach, urinary bladder, umbilical cord insertion site on the anterior abdominal wall, and renal region.

for high-quality patient care. The American Institute for Ultrasound in Medicine recommendation is to maintain permanent records of the ultrasound images, appropriately labeled to identify the patient, the date of examination, and the scan orientation. High-quality thermal imaging devices are readily available, are inexpensive to purchase, are compatible with all modern ultrasound machines, and are cheap and easy to operate. The photographs obtained by this method are generally of good quality and provide excellent hard-copy records. Videotape records of the dynamic portion of the scan are not considered a requirement. The permanent record should also include a written interpretation of the observations, and the examination should be described in the patient's medical record.

First-Trimester Obstetric Ultrasound Examination

In the first trimester, the focus of the examination is directed primarily toward determination of fetal age, number, and viability and toward detection of disease of contiguous structures. In the early first trimester (6 to 10 weeks' gestation), the fetal crown-rump length measurement is the recommended method for determining gestational age. In the late first trimester, crown-rump length measurements may be less reliable because of active extension of the fetal head and trunk. After 10 weeks' gestation, fetal age generally is best determined by head measurements (biparietal diameter [BPD] and head circumference). More recently, detailed assessment of fetal anatomy in the first-trimester scan has been emphasized; the transvaginal approach allows detailed assessment of fetal anatomy in the late first trimester in more than 80% of patients, and the combined transvaginal/transabdominal approach permits such assessment in 95% (Braithwaite et al., 1996). The high-quality imaging made possible by the transvaginal approach permits early detection of some anomalies, including anencephaly (Rottem et al., 1989), and assessment of the cervix, and consequently in most centers the transvaginal scan has become the primary and preferred method for first-trimester screening. Pandya and associates (1995) described an association between chromosomal abnormalities,

especially aneuploidies, and increased nuchal thickness and translucency. First-trimester nuchal lucency screening has been reported to be an effective means of increasing detection of the fetus with aneuploidy in an American population (Wapner for the BUN group, 2001), and comparative trials are ongoing (D'Alton, personal communication, 2002).

Second- and Third-Trimester Obstetric Ultrasound Examination

In the second and third trimesters, the guidelines are more extensive and include assessment of the following:

- Fetal presentation
- Placental position (with particular reference to the relationship of the lower margin of the placenta to the lower uterine segment and the cervix)
- Amniotic fluid volume
- Fetal anatomy (a general survey to include evaluation of the cerebral ventricles, spine, stomach, urinary bladder, kidney, and region of insertion of the umbilical vessels into the fetal abdomen)

Fetal measurements that should be documented by hard copy are as follows:

- An estimate of head size, either by BPD or by head circumference, and usually both
- Femur length
- Abdominal circumference in a plane at or near the intrahepatic junction of the umbilical vein and the portal sinus

When possible, current measurement should be compared with previous measurements and reported. Assessment of placental position relative to the internal os is much improved by the transvaginal route of scanning. The incidence of placenta previa as diagnosed by transvaginal ultrasonography at 15 to 20 weeks' gestation is 1.1%, with only 14% of cases persisting to term. The method identifies patients at risk for placenta previa at delivery, with a sensitivity of 100% and a specificity of 85% (Lauria et al., 1996).

■ **TABLE 20-2.** ULTRASOUND ASSESSMENT OF THE HIGH-RISK FETUS: EXTENDED CRITERIA

Criterion	Standard Method/Procedures	Ancillary Methods/Procedures	Examples of Clinical Application
Fetal age determination	Parameter of head size (BPD, head circumference); femur length, abdominal circumference	Other long bone length (humerus, tibia, etc.); facial structures (mandible length, intraorbital diameter, pinna size); foot length	Differentiation of mistaken dates and IUGR; determination of risk to neonatal viability in threatened preterm labor
Fetal mass determination	Abdominal circumference alone; head circumference; femur length	Calculated fetal volume methods; total intrauterine volume	Detection of IUGR/macrosomia; determination of volume of blood for fetal transfusion
Determination of fetal number	General uterine survey; estimate of zygosity; assessment of membranes; determination of type of placentation; determination of fetal positions	US-guided invasive diagnostic/therapeutic procedures (decompressing amniocentesis, selective fetal reduction)	Identification of twin–twin transfusion syndrome and identification and management of twin disparity growth syndrome
Fetal structural/functional integrity	Anatomic survey notation and assessment of dynamic physiologic variables	US-guided invasive diagnostic procedures (PUBS, CVS, amniocentesis, fetal biopsy)	Site selection for delivery of a fetus with treatable anomaly; avoidance of intervention for a lethal anomaly; specific intrauterine therapy
Environmental assessment	Assessment of position and morphology of the placenta and cord; amniotic fluid volume and its reflective characteristics; evaluation for the presence of abnormal structures within the uterine cavity (e.g., amniotic bands), uterine wall (fibroids); determination of fetal position	Doppler assessment of umbilical artery blood flow velocity waveform	Identification of placenta previa; identification of cord presentation; detection of intraplacental and intra-amniotic bleeding
Evaluation of immediate fetal risk	Amniotic fluid volume; fetal movement, breathing, and tone (modified biophysical profile score)	US-guided cordocentesis for fetal blood gas determination; blood flow velocity waveform assessment of intrafetal vessels	Balancing the risk of fetal vs. neonatal morbidity and mortality

BPD, biparietal diameter; CVS, chorionic villus sampling; IUGR, intrauterine growth retardation; PUBS, percutaneous fetal blood sampling; US, ultrasound.

Guidelines for Ultrasound Assessment of the Fetus at Risk: The Extended Examination

The guidelines of the American Institute for Ultrasound in Medicine need to be viewed in perspective; they describe the bare minimum of ultrasound information that should be obtained without reference to the expertise of the examiner or to the presence of specific pregnancy risk factors. The principles of ultrasound fetal assessment for the perinatologist are different and may be summarized as follows.

Criteria for assessment of the fetus at risk exceed the minimal criteria described for the general examination. In the specialized practice of maternal-fetal medicine, it is usual and recommended practice to collect considerably more information regarding the status of the fetus and its environment. The standard fetal ultrasound information regarding estimates of age, growth, structural integrity, and amniotic fluid volume should be supplemented with the following:

■ Evaluation of fetal morphometric proportions
■ Notation of the presence and character of dynamic fetal biophysical activities as an indicator of fetal well-being (biophysical profile score)
■ Umbilical cord structure and position
■ Placental morphology

In selected cases (e.g., IUGR), umbilical artery and intrafetal (middle cerebral artery, inferior vena cava) blood-flow velocity waveforms are usually recorded. Routine umbilical artery velocity waveform analysis has not been of value as a screening method for IUGR or other fetal manifestations of chronic uteroplacental insufficiency and is neither required nor recommended as a routine measure (Low, 1990).

Criteria for the assessment of the fetus at risk may be expected to vary by maternal and fetal risk factors. The focus of ultrasound assessment may also be expected to vary according to the associated maternal risk factors and by the results of the current or preceding ultrasound examination. This concept, called *disease-specific assessment*, has become a critical and necessary aspect of the complete ultrasound examination. As with most aspects of ultrasound assessment, disease-specific assessment is merely an intrauterine extension of a traditional and time-honored principle of extrauterine medicine: The search for the signs of a disease process varies according to the understanding of the pathophysiology of the condition. Fetal medicine is replete with examples of application of this principle:

1. Detection of a variance in fetal weight below the normal range for gestational age should trigger a detailed search for the underlying etiologic mechanism.
2. In the diabetic pregnancy, the ultrasound examination is focused toward detection of macrosomia and the

complication of shoulder dystocia (Cohen et al., 1996) and of such anomalies as caudal regression syndrome and cardiac defects, which are common in this condition.

3. In alloimmune syndromes, fetal liver size and morphology, the presence of early ascites, and an abnormal fetal biophysical profile score provide insight as to the severity and progression of fetal anemia and help guide the timing and appropriateness of repeated intravascular transfusion.

4. In multiple gestation, the ultrasound examination is extended so as to obtain information on the type of twinning and the presence or absence of complications specific to the condition.

When the principle of disease-specific assessment is considered in terms of the range and complexities of fetal disease, it is clear that annotation of appropriate universal criteria for ultrasound examination is neither simple nor direct; rather, it must include both the basics and the focused examination.

In the fetus at risk, dynamic ultrasound assessment is used as both a diagnostic and a management tool. The impact of this principle on the practice of fetal medicine is best viewed historically. At its inception, ultrasound imaging in pregnancy was seen as a way to estimate fetal viability, age, and number. As a diagnostic tool, it was confined to the domain of imaging specialists, usually radiologists, who were somewhat removed from direct clinical care and whose function was to provide a diagnosis but not a management plan. The concepts of monitoring the pathophysiology of a given condition and of integrating a wide spectrum of critical information into a rational management plan have become integral aspects of ultrasound fetal assessment. The fetus is now viewed as a separate patient in whom the detection of a disease process, usually by ultrasound assessment, is the beginning step in formulating management. In this contemporary age, the managing perinatologist collects the needed uterine and fetal ultrasound information, which includes the following:

- Determining the presence or absence of a given fetal risk condition
- Monitoring the progression of such a condition
- Estimating the probability that a given condition, associated complication, or both will cause serious or even lethal fetal or neonatal sequelae
- Balancing the relative risks and benefits of continued intrauterine existence versus delivery and neonatal care
- Considering the applicability and efficacy of the various forms of disease-specific intrauterine fetal therapy
- Weighing the potential value of ultrasound-guided invasive diagnostic procedures
- Integrating these data within the context of the maternal condition and the usual obstetric considerations

The relationship between the diagnostic and management aspects of ultrasound fetal assessment is both intimate and dynamic. Once a diagnosis of a potentially serious fetal disorder has been established, the focus of ultrasound assessment is turned toward the balancing of fetal versus neonatal risks. In some clinical instances, the diagnosis per se dictates management. The ultrasound diagnosis of a lethal fetal anomaly, such as anencephaly, precludes the need for any further fetal assessment, and fetal considerations give way to management directed solely at avoiding maternal morbidity. Similarly, in the mature fetus, the diagnosis of severe dysmature IUGR obviates further assessment and intervention is directed toward fetal indications. Usually, however, an ultrasound diagnosis is only the first (albeit critical) aspect of ultrasound assessment, and subsequent evaluation is directed toward monitoring the progression of the fetal disease and balancing relative fetal and neonatal risks.

The ability to exclude fetal disease despite the presence of historical or maternal risk factors is an important aspect of ultrasound assessment. In the pre-ultrasound era, management protocols were empirical, based on the probability of existing fetal complications as derived from general experience. For example, for patients with diabetes, hypertension, suspected IUGR, and pregnancies that extended beyond 42 completed weeks, management by delivery at a predescribed fetal age was commonly recommended. In contemporary perinatal medicine, it has become possible to modify management of these high-risk circumstances according to the presence or absence of signs of fetal compromise as determined by direct ultrasound fetal assessment. The approach does not entirely obviate an aggressive obstetric approach to the management of many high-risk circumstances, but it does permit many of these pregnancies to continue longer with more appropriate delivery timing and without undue fetal risk. Ultrasound-guided selective conservative management of the high-risk pregnancy can reduce the incidence of neonatal complications associated with immaturity and can be expected to reduce the incidence of induction and operative delivery in the mother, thereby reducing her risk of associated complications. A summary of the ultrasound evaluation of the high-risk fetus is shown in Table 20-2.

Ultrasound data in the high-risk fetus must be interpreted within the overall clinical context. The highly reliable ultrasound information regarding the presence, progression, and risk associated with a fetal disease state cannot be interpreted in isolation but instead needs to be considered in the light of maternal and obstetric factors. Integration of the maternal, fetal, and obstetric factors determines the need for, the frequency of, and the management plan that flows from any ultrasound examination. The fetal aspects of this equation were discussed previously. The maternal aspects are of equal importance, and clearly fetal management decisions must be made in light of the maternal condition.

Serious or progressive pregnancy-related maternal disease is considered an indication for intervention and overrides fetal considerations. Thus, for example, serial antepartum fetal assessment by ultrasound methods in the presence of severe progressive maternal hypertension is not warranted. Similarly, a diagnosis of a lethal fetal anomaly may not influence the mode of delivery in a patient with a history of a previous classic cesarean section.

Assessment of the maternal condition also influences the frequency of fetal ultrasound assessment. In the diabetic patient under poor control or in the patient with a medical condition associated with increased fetal risk (e.g., systemic lupus erythematosus), assessment of the fetus may be frequent. Interpretation of the fetal ultrasound findings also is influenced by obstetric factors. The favorableness of the cervix for induction, the fetal position, and a history of previous cesarean section can be expected to influence management decisions that arise as a result of ultrasound fetal assessment.

SPECIFIC APPLICATION OF ULTRASONOGRAPHY IN PERINATAL MEDICINE

Determination of Fetal Age by Ultrasonography

Determination of gestational age and its correlate, the *estimated date of confinement*, is standard obstetric practice. Virtually all obstetric management decisions depend on an accurate assessment of fetal age. These measurements also form the critical base from which pathologic deviations from the normal are recognized. The accuracy of the age estimate is not only critical in the planning of appropriate management, but also may profoundly alter the actual incidence of suspected high-risk factors in a population. For example, regarding the incidence of IUGR in a given population, the incidence of suspected disease is as high as 20% when gestational age is based on menstrual history and as low as 5% when based on ultrasound-derived dates. Similarly, the incidence of prolonged or post-term pregnancy (more than 294 completed days) is 9% when menstrual dates are used but only 3% when ultrasound dates are used (Grennert et al., 1978).

Mongelli and coworkers (1996) evaluated the predictive accuracy of gestational age determination by composite ultrasound-derived fetal morphometric measures in 34,249 pregnancies with certain menstrual dating. Delivery occurred within ±7 days of the estimated date of confinement in 49.5% of cases as determined by menstrual dates compared with 55.2% according to the ultrasound-determined estimated date of confinement. These differences were significant. These authors suggested that even if menstrual dates are considered to be "certain," there is no advantage to using them to determine the estimated date of confinement if data from a dating ultrasound before 24 weeks' gestation are available. In this study, the incidence of postdate pregnancy (at least 42 completed weeks) was 0.8%.

The importance of accurate gestational age estimates is now becoming more apparent earlier in pregnancy. For example, an accurate estimate of fetal age is essential in plotting distribution of maternal serum α-fetoprotein and triple screen values (see Chapter 18). Selection of the appropriate temporal window for chorionic villus sampling depends on such accurate estimates. In the future, new therapies, such as stem cell transfusion and gene therapy, will likely depend on accurate dates.

Estimation of gestational age by ultrasound study is based on the known relationship between fetal age and fetal size, in part and in whole. Because contemporary ultrasound methods allow accurate measurement of a wide range of fetal physical parameters, it becomes possible to construct distribution plots (*nomograms*) of given measurements against gestational age. From such nomograms, one can calculate mean fetal age and range of estimate. Interestingly, virtually all such nomograms yield an accuracy at least comparable with that of data based on the last normal menstrual period (LNMP) and usually even better.

The ultrasound method of fetal age determination has several other inherent advantages, including providing the following opportunities:

- Selecting the most accurate variable for a given fetal age range (e.g., crown-rump length instead of BPD)
- Combining variables to refine predictive accuracy (e.g., BPD and femur length)
- Measuring variables sequentially

The selection of the optimal method and the interpretation of predictive accuracy depend on several basic principles.

Accuracy of the ultrasound estimate of fetal age is inversely related to fetal age. The rate at which a fetus grows is not constant but rather shows a progressive and sustained transition from the exponential rate evident at conception toward the linear rate evident in late pregnancy. The more rapid the growth rate, the more pronounced the incremental change in a given physical parameter per unit of time. Further fetal growth is the net result of the interaction between intrinsic growth potential and environmental factors that may enhance or inhibit growth. The influence of environmental factors become progressively more apparent as gestational age advances. Hence, the distribution of physical measurements for a population of fetuses of the same age broadens as age advances (Fig. 20-2). Accordingly, the accuracy of a physical measurement parameter in predicting gestational age is inversely proportional to gestational age. This important clinical phenomenon has been observed for virtually every physical determinant of fetal age that can be measured by ultrasound.

The optimal method for ultrasound determination of fetal age varies with gestational age. A gestational sac, signaling intrauterine pregnancy, has been identified from as early as the 25th day after the first day of the LNMP (conceptual age, 11 days). The developing embryo has been visualized as early as the 34th day after LNMP (conceptual age, 20 days) and fetal heart motion as early as the 38th day after LNMP (conceptual age, 24 days). Although gestational sac volume can be used to estimate gestational age from as early as 4 weeks from LNMP, crown-rump length determination is the most practical early measure used. Crown-rump length can be determined from as early as 5 to 12 weeks' gestation and remains one of the most accurate methods of fetal age determination (Fig. 20-3). The range of error of estimate with crown-rump length is approximately 3 days (Robinson, 1973)—substantially more accurate than estimates based on menstrual history.

From about the 10th week onward, crown-rump length determination becomes more difficult because of deflexion and variable position of the developing fetal head and flexion of the fetal trunk. At about the 10th week, the fetal head may be well visualized by either transvaginal or transabdominal sonography and intracranial anatomic landmarks identified. The BPD can be measured from about 10 weeks onward; such measurements between the 16th and 20th weeks yield an estimate error of less than 7 days (Hadlock et al., 1982a). Although fetal long bone structures (humerus and femur) can be seen as early as 10 weeks' gestation, accurate measurement of length is difficult before about 14 weeks' gestation. Fetal long bone measurements are technically possible from about 14 to 16 weeks' gestation onward.

The technical error of measurement is relatively constant. The axial resolution of a given ultrasound line is high, yielding discrimination up to 0.2 mm, and this axial resolution does not vary with absolute target size. Therefore, if it is assumed that the target insonation angle is appropriate and the guiding landmarks are visible, the error of estimate due to axial resolution is constant and minimal. However, because ultrasound resolution has increased, selection of the start and end points

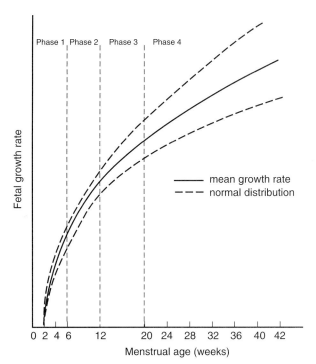

FIGURE 20-2 ■ Theoretical plot of fetal growth rate against menstrual age. Phase 1: 0–6 weeks. Conceptual growth is exponential at the onset with initial transition toward linear growth. Individual variability is minimal at this stage. Gestational sac volume can be measured by 4 weeks. The embryo is seen as early as 4.5 weeks (20 days conceptual age), and fetal heart activity is seen from as early as 5 weeks (24 days conceptual age). Phase 2: 6–12 weeks. Growth rate is slowing, but individual variability still remains sharply restricted. Crown-rump measurement can be made from as early as 6 weeks and yields an estimated error of ±3 days. At about 10 weeks, the biparietal diameter (BPD) can be measured. Phase 3: 12–20 weeks. Growth rate continues to slow and individual variability becomes more apparent. BPD can be measured from as early as 10 weeks; femur length and abdominal circumference are measured from as early as 14 weeks. Composite age estimates yield an error of estimate of about 1 week. Phase 4: 20 weeks onward. Growth rate is slowing and individual variability becomes progressively more apparent as age advances. Composite age estimates yield an error of at least ±1.5 weeks. Serial estimates of the growth rate derived from composite variables become the method of choice for age estimation. In late phase 4 (more than 32 weeks) the range of error of estimate (more than ±2.5 weeks) precludes accurate estimate of fetal age. Alternate clinical methods must be used.

for a given measurement has become more difficult. For example, BPD measurement by the older bistable B-mode methods was relatively simple because only the bony table of the calvarium produced a recognizable signal. Modern equipment reveals not only the bone of the calvarium but also hair, skin, and subcutaneous tissue. Therefore, one must assume that the beginning point of measurement is set at the calvarium surface and not the scalp surface.

Accuracy of gestational age estimates by ultrasonography increases as more variables are measured. There is a clear relationship between a growing fetal physical parameter and gestational age. In the early days of ultrasound determination of fetal age, the dimensions of the fetal head were the only fetal landmarks that could be measured in a reproducible and certain manner. Hence, these dimensions, particularly the BPD, became the mainstay of fetal age estimates. Now, contemporary high-resolution ultrasound methods allow simple

and accurate measurement of a large spectrum of fetal physical parameters. To date, all such parameters have been shown to be subject to the vicissitudes of the inherent population variability characteristic of later pregnancy, and no single variable shows an appreciable advantage in predictive accuracy.

The inherent variability in a fetal population of equal age is not constant across physical variables but instead varies for each parameter. This principle has considerable clinical importance because it means that the error of estimate for the mean of composite variables is always less than the error for any single variable. Thus, for example, Hadlock and colleagues (1983a), using a composite estimate of BPD, abdominal circumference, head circumference, and femur length, improved predictive accuracy by 8% in early pregnancy (12 to 18 weeks) and by up to 28% in late pregnancy (36 to 42 weeks). It thus seems reasonable to conclude that all ultrasound estimates of fetal age beyond the crown-rump measurement stage should be based on a range of variables. This principle is now easy to apply because all ultrasound machines have built-in software that contains a wide choice of nomograms and have the capability of calculating estimated fetal age from the composite measurement obtained.

Although gestational age nomograms can use many fetal morphometric variables, most clinicians use a composite estimate of gestational age based on measurements of the BPD, head circumference, femur length, and abdominal circumference. Estimates of fetal age based on a single variable such as BPD should and will disappear from clinical practice. With contemporary ultrasound equipment, one can measure at least two variables (abdominal circumference plus either head circumference or femur length) in virtually every fetus and the head, abdomen, and femur in most fetuses (more than 95%).

In later gestation, the accuracy of fetal age determination is enhanced by serial measurements. For reasons cited previously, determination of fetal age in later pregnancy (more than

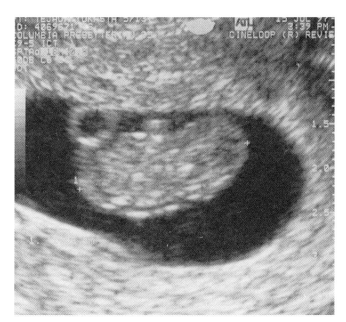

FIGURE 20-3 ■ Crown-rump measurement (2.08 cm) in a 9-week fetus. The fetal head at this age is very large relative to the thorax and abdomen. The fetal yolk sac is still present at this gestational age. Determination of fetal age by crown-rump measurement is the most accurate method available, yielding an estimate error of about 3 days.

20 weeks), as based on a single ultrasound examination, can be fraught with considerable error, the magnitude of which increases as gestational age advances (see Fig. 20-2). This clinical dilemma is common and usually occurs in the patient with an unknown or uncertain menstrual history who, for whatever reason, begins prenatal care at an advanced gestation. Because it is rare for dates to be underestimated by whatever menstrual data may be available, such patients are frequently considered to have possible IUGR. The method of choice for evaluating such patients is determination of the rate of fetal growth by serial estimates of fetal physical parameters spaced widely enough to account for the inherent measurement error (usually more than 2 weeks). The concept is based on the curvilinear characteristics of the mean growth curve of the normal fetus (see Fig. 20-2) and requires a composite estimate rather than any single variable.

An alternative method that depends on the same principle involves serial composite measurements, usually two and, preferably, three such measurements, spaced at least 2 weeks apart and plotted against standard fetal growth curves. The method, when applied between 24 and 32 weeks' gestation, yields an estimate error of ± 10 days. Fetal age estimates beyond 32 weeks' gestation are subject to major error and are not of real clinical value. In such cases, management is best based on assessment of fetal well-being and detection of ancillary signs of either excessive or reduced fetal growth.

Specific Fetal Measurements

Fetal Head Measurements

By convention, the physical dimensions of the fetal head are measured in the plane of the BPD. This transverse plane transcribes the fetal head at an angle approximately 30 degrees to a line connecting the orbits and occiput and is just above the internal auditory meatus (Fig. 20-4). Within the plane lie the anterior falx, the cavum septum pellucidum, the anterior horn and lateral walls of the lateral ventricles, the choroid plexus, and the midbrain nucleus, the thalamus. Portions of the middle cerebral arteries and the vessels of the circle of Willis are usually visible in this plane. The definition of structure improves with advancing gestation, but accurate measurement depends on recognition of most of these landmarks. Attention to detail is critical to measurement accuracy. Measurements at a plane above the true BPD underestimate the true dimension, and tangential or oblique angulation may overestimate the true dimension.

Three fetal head dimensions are commonly measured:

1. The BPD is measured as the distance from the outer surface of the proximal calvarium (outer skull table) to the inner surface of the distal calvarium (inner skull table) at the maximal width of the head in the previously described BPD plane.
2. The long axis of the fetal head is measured from the outer surface of the front of the skull to the outer surface at the back of the skull.
3. The head circumference is measured along the outer surface of the fetal skull in the plane of the BPD.

With all modern equipment, electronic planimetric calipers are used to obtain the measurements simultaneously. For the most part, BPD and head circumference may be used

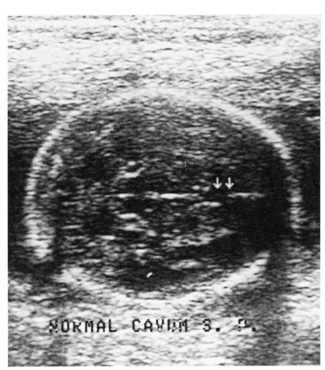

FIGURE 20-4 ■ The fetal head in the plane of the biparietal diameter. Note the ovoid shape. The midline structure (the septum cavum pellucidum) is well visualized, as are the lateral walls of the lateral ventricle, the anterior horn, and the choroid plexus. Portions of the middle cerebral artery in the sylvian gyrus and branches of the circle of Willis are seen with dynamic mode imaging.

interchangeably to estimate fetal age, with BPD being the most commonly used variable. The accuracy of estimate for either varies with gestational age, yielding an estimate error of ±8 days before 20 weeks' gestation, ±12 days between 18 and 24 weeks, and ±15 days after 24 weeks (Hadlock, 1985).

Because variation in fetal head shape is not uncommon and because BPD may vary with head shape, using head circumference yields no theoretical advantages. One must consider variation in head shape and in interpreting BPD measurements. *Dolichocephaly*, a fetal head shape in which the longitudinal axis is exaggerated and the transverse axis (BPD) is foreshortened, is common with breech presentation and with severe oligohydramnios. A BPD determination in the dolichocephalic head underestimates fetal age. In contrast, *brachycephaly*, in which the longitudinal axis is foreshortened and the transverse axis (BPD) is exaggerated, although uncommon, may be observed. A BPD determination performed in the brachycephalic head overestimates fetal age. The observation of inward collapse and pointing of the anterior calvarium, yielding a "lemon-shaped" appearance, is an almost uniform finding among fetuses with a neural tube defect; this observation should always prompt a detailed scan of the fetal spine (Nicolaides et al., 1986).

The *cephalic index* is designed to avoid the potential errors that variation in head shape can introduce to the measurement of the BPD (Hohler, 1982). The predictive accuracy of the BPD is maintained, provided the cephalic index, defined as the longitudinal length divided by BPD × 100, is 78% ± 8%. When the cephalic index falls outside this normal range, the use of head circumference rather than BPD is recommended.

The estimate of fetal age is determined from published nomograms. Many such nomograms are derived from study populations that vary by ethnical and geographic factors. The selection of the appropriate nomogram varies with the individual population characteristics.

Fetal Long Bone and Limb Measurements

Fetal limb anatomy, including the bony structures, may now be assessed easily by means of conventional high-resolution ultrasound equipment. The growth of the long bones (femur, tibia, fibula, humerus, radius, and ulna), all of which may be measured, is directly related to fetal age (Jeanty, Kirkpatrick et al., 1981). By convention, femur length is the long bone measurement conventionally used as a fetal age determinant (O'Brien and Queenan, 1981). This measurement is made from the outer surface of the proximal end of the femur (greater trochanter) along the shaft of the femur to the distal end, not including the distal femoral epiphysis (Fig. 20-5). Such measurements become technically possible from about 14 weeks' gestation onward. The range of estimate error of fetal age by femur length varies with gestational age, ranging from as low as ±7 days when measured before 20 weeks of gestation to as high as ±16 days when measured beyond 36 weeks of gestation (Hadlock, 1985).

The value of long bone assessment extends beyond determination of fetal age. Abnormalities of limb growth (e.g., short limb dystrophy) are detected by such assessment. Furthermore, long bone growth, particularly femur growth, bears a direct relationship to linear growth of the fetus. By this association, fetal length may be determined according to the following formula (Fazekas and Kosa, 1978):

$$\text{Fetal length} = (\text{femur length [cm]} \times 6.44) + 4.51$$

This method yields an estimate of fetal length to within 1 cm when performed after 36 weeks' gestation (Manning

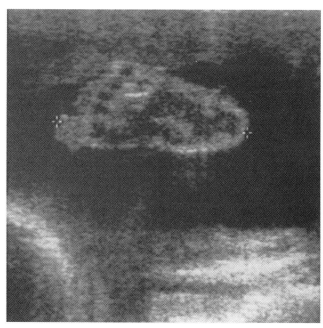

FIGURE 20-6 ■ Fetal foot. Foot length is measured from the tip of the great toe to the heel. In this fetus, the foot measures 5.8 cm, consistent with a gestational age of 27.5 weeks. Fetal foot measurements are usually obtained without difficulty and are used in calculation of composite ultrasound fetal age estimates.

et al., 1983a). Fetal length determination is a critical component of fetal mass-to-length ratios (ponderal index) and may be used for recognition of abnormalities of fetal growth.

Another promising ancillary method for determination of fetal age and condition is assessment of anatomy and length of the fetal foot (Fig. 20-6). The measurement is made from the outer surface of the heel to the distal end of the great toe. Fetal foot length yields an estimate of error comparable with that of femur length and BPD (Mercer et al., 1987). Fetal foot position may be used to detect contraction deformities; soft tissue defects may be seen with a variety of chromosomal abnormalities (Fig. 20-7).

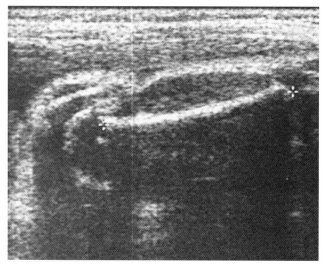

FIGURE 20-5 ■ Ultrasound image of the femur in a fetus at term. The calipers are placed proximally on the greater trochanter and distally at the edge of the femur shaft. The slight curvature of the femur shaft is a usual and normal observation. The ossified distal femoral epiphysis appears as an echogenic structure at the distal end of the femur. Bone shadowing is observed, and this is also a normal finding.

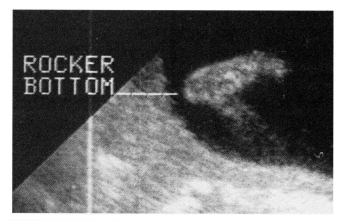

FIGURE 20-7 ■ Fetal foot at 17 weeks of gestation in a fetus with trisomy 13. The foot exhibits edema with loss of normal contour. This finding is not diagnostic of underlying karyotype abnormality; rather, it is only an indication for further investigation.

Fetal Abdominal Circumference Determination

Fetal abdominal circumference, measured at a plane just slightly superior to the umbilicus, may be used to assess both fetal age and fetal mass (Campbell, 1977). Abdominal circumference is measured in the maximal transverse plane of the upper abdomen. Included within this plane are fetal liver, stomach, spleen, and a portion of the umbilical vein within the hepatic structure (Fig. 20-8). The abdominal circumference may be measured directly by planimetric methods or calculated from the mean of two perpendicular diameters. Because the fetal abdomen is ovoid in the midline sagittal plane, the accuracy of abdominal circumference measurement depends critically on selection of the largest transverse plane. All fetal biometric parameters introduce estimate error into composite calculations, and unavoidable measurement inaccuracies may compound age/weight estimate error (Dudley and Chapman, 2002). Fetal abdominal circumference determination yields an estimate error of ±12 days when measured before 20 weeks' gestation and ±21 days when measured after 36 weeks (Hadlock et al., 1982b).

Ancillary Ultrasound Measures of Fetal Age

As stated previously, virtually any physical parameter of the growing developing fetus may be expected to bear a direct relationship to fetal age. If one uses contemporary high-resolution dynamic ultrasound imaging, one can measure a wide range of such fetal physical variables. Accordingly, the literature now contains many reports relating new parameters to fetal age.

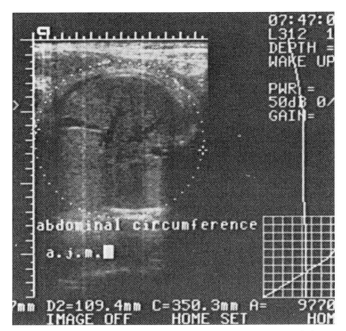

FIGURE 20-8 ■ Transverse scan of the abdomen in a 36-week fetus. The fetal spine is at 3 o'clock. The echolucent intrahepatic portion of the umbilical vein is seen at 9 o'clock. Note the relatively homogeneous fetal liver and the echolucent branching of the hepatic vein. The inferior vena cava is seen as an echolucent circle just anterior and inferior to the fetal spine. This is the correct view from which to measure the fetal abdominal circumference. In this fetus, electronic calipers are used to record an abdominal circumference of 35.0 cm.

These variables include distal femoral epiphyseal size (Chinn et al., 1983), intraorbital diameter (Mayden et al., 1982), renal diameter (Jeanty et al., 1982), and gut structural characteristics (Goldstein et al., 1987). Even such variables as the morphology of the fetal external ear may be used to assess fetal age (Birnholz, 1983). With the dynamic mode, it has been possible to assess developmental movement patterns (Nijhuis et al., 1982) and gut peristalsis as markers of fetal age. What remains unclear is whether such ancillary measures, when considered alone or in combination, will be of any measurable value in refining the predictive accuracy of fetal age estimates compared with estimates based on a composite assessment of head, long bone, and abdominal circumference measurements.

Estimation of Fetal Weight (Mass)

Fetal weight estimates, like fetal age estimates, commonly play a pivotal role in perinatal management decisions. Because perinatal weight correlates with neonatal survival, fetal weight estimates may strongly influence decisions regarding the appropriateness of intervention, observation, and management in the high-risk premature fetus. As the field of fetal therapy continues to unfold, accurate fetal weight estimates have become even more important in calculating drug dosage and blood transfusion volumes (Harman et al., 1990). Most importantly, however, fetal weight estimates, when considered against age estimates, provide the basis for recognition of abnormal fetal growth patterns; the increased risk of perinatal death at the extremes of the normal growth curve has been well described (Lubchenco et al., 1972; Morrison and Olsen, 1985).

Because the recognition of fetal weight and age discrepancies is of such clinical importance, there is a great need for accurate methods to detect these aberrations of growth. Examination of the relationship between fetal physical dimension, as measured by ultrasound, and fetal mass presents an alternative and more direct method of calculating fetal weight. Such relationships have been explored extensively and a variety of formulas reported. Ultrasound estimates of fetal weight are subject to at least two critical sources of error (see Chapters 28 and 49).

First, these measures assume a uniform relationship between linear measures of fetal structure and fetal volume. Although such relationships clearly exist, some variability is to be expected. Second, these estimates assume that in a given normal fetal population the relationship between volume and mass (density) is constant. Studies in normal neonates and in stillbirths indicate that perinatal density is not constant (Thompson et al., 1983). The average perinatal density is slightly less than water (mean, 0.919 ± 0.7 g/mL) but may range from 0.833 to 1.012 g/mL. Thus, even in a population of normal fetuses in which volume is known with certainty, the average error of weight estimate is about 8% and may be as high as 21%.

Among fetuses with abnormal growth patterns, subcutaneous fat may be either reduced (as in IUGR) or increased (as in diabetic macrosomia); therefore, variation in fetal density may be even greater than in the normal population. Furthermore, within the individual fetus, the density of various structures differs; the mean density of the head is 0.571 g/mL and of the body is 1.118 g/mL. Therefore, variation in relative contribution to total mass, as may occur with asymmetrical ("head-sparing") IUGR, may be expected to further compound the estimate error.

Because the fetus does not exhibit uniform density, estimates based on the physical dimension of any given structure may vary in accuracy. Estimates of fetal weight based on head dimension alone, in which the fetal head contributes to only 20% of total mass, are so variable as to be of no clinical value. In contrast, estimates derived from body dimension (e.g., abdominal circumference) are considerably more accurate because the fetal body accounts for 80% of total mass and the density of the trunk more closely approximates mean density. Following a principle that appears ingrained in all aspects of perinatal ultrasonography, fetal weight estimates based on a combination of fetal physical variables are substantially more accurate than most single variables.

As would be predicted, the least error in estimate is achieved when true volume is known with certainty; true volume as measured by water displacement yields an estimate error of about 7.6% (±2 standard deviations [SD]) (Thompson et al., 1983). Neonatal volume derived from direct measurement of physical dimensions yields an estimate error of about 8.2%; the slight increase in estimate error is assumed to be due to the introduction of measurement error. The most exact estimate of fetal volume is based on multiple serial ultrasound planes; it is time-consuming and cumbersome but yields an estimate error comparable with that of direct displacement methods (approximately 6.5%; ±2 SD) (McCallum and Brinkley, 1979).

Composite measurement of head, abdominal, and femur dimensions yields an estimate error of about 15% (Hadlock, 1985). Fetal weight estimates based on the summed volumes of fetal head, trunk, and limbs, as reported by Thompson and associates (1983), yielded an estimate error of ±16.2%. Warsof and coworkers (1977) and Shepard and colleagues (1982) used head measurements (BPD) and trunk measurements (abdominal circumference) to estimate fetal weight; despite the method's ease of use, it remains one of the least accurate, yielding a range of error of about 21.2% (±2 SD). Interestingly and inexplicably, estimates of fetal weight based on abdominal circumference alone are reported to yield a range of estimate error of not greater than about 15% (2 SD) (Campbell and Wilkin, 1975). The various ultrasonic methods for determining fetal weight are summarized in Table 20-3. Because the error of estimate appears relatively constant for each method and because the normal fetus exhibits sustained growth, serial estimates made at intervals wide enough (usually more than 2 weeks) to account for estimate error permit detection of deviation from the expected normal growth rate. This method, then, is important in detecting growth rate abnormalities (Divon et al., 1986).

Although the accuracy of fetal weight estimate by ultrasound in a population is good, the assumption that in the individual fetus the ultrasound estimated weight must therefore fall within a ±15% estimate can be very misleading. The actual ultrasound derived estimate will vary by the morphometric parameters used in the calculation, and this variation can be considerable at term. For example, in a term infant with average (50th percentile) individual morphometrics, the calculated weight difference between the Hadlock and Shepard method may be as great as 300 g. The impact of relative proportions on fetal weight estimates is also evident in comparison with the weight estimates among macrosomic fetuses in diabetic and nondiabetic mothers (Wong et al., 2001). Fetal weight estimates by ultrasound were more than four times as likely to underestimate weight in diabetic fetuses, and this estimate error increased as actual weight increased.

Evaluation of Fetal Growth

From conception to delivery and beyond, the developing infant exhibits circumferential and linear growth at a progressively slowing rate, resulting in continuous incremental increases in volume and mass (see Fig. 20-2). Fetal growth may be viewed as the net integration of stimulatory and inhibitory influences arising intrinsically and environmentally. Accordingly, and not surprisingly, fetal growth provides clear insight into a wide range of pathologic perinatal conditions.

The complexities of fetal growth result in a wide spectrum of responses to abnormal growth-regulating factors. Consequently, there are no simple algorithms for ultrasound detection of growth abnormalities, which instead depend on a consideration and evaluation of a number of morphologic and

TABLE 20-3. ESTIMATION OF FETAL WEIGHT BY ULTRASOUND METHODS

Method	Variables Measured	Range of Estimate Error ± 2 SD (%)
Neonatal volume (Thompson et al., 1983)	Total volume by water displacement	7.6
Neonatal volume	Head, trunk, limb volume	8.2
Composite fetal volume (McCallum and Brinkley, 1979)	Serial ultrasound planes	6.5
Composite fetal volume (Hadlock, 1985)	Head circumference, abdominal circumference, femur	15
Composite fetal volume (Thompson et al., 1983)	Head, trunk, limb volume	16.2
Head/trunk volume (Shepard et al., 1982)	Biparietal diameter and abdominal circumference	21.2
Trunk volume only (Campbell and Wilkin, 1975)	Abdominal circumference	15

SD, standard deviation.

functional variables. One may achieve maximal discrimination of abnormal from normal fetal growth only by considering such a wide range of variables. Diagnosis of abnormality based on assessment of any single set of variables, such as fetal morphometrics, is less accurate. This point merits added emphasis because it remains common practice for some ultrasound laboratories to report only fetal morphometrics (e.g., BPD, femur length, abdominal circumference) in cases of suspected growth abnormality.

Reduced Fetal Growth

The ultrasound diagnosis of impaired or retarded fetal growth is of crucial interest to perinatologists because this problem is among the most frequent complications associated with fetal and neonatal death (Morrison and Olsen, 1985) and because ultrasound-based diagnosis, etiologic determination, and management can significantly reduce perinatal morbidity and mortality. In a population of 10,135 infants with birth weights less than the 10th percentile for gestational age and sex, the mortality rate in the ultrasound-screened and managed group was reduced by 60% compared with the unscreened group (8.4 per 1000 versus 21.3 per 1000, respectively) (Manning, 1995b) (Table 20-4). Chapter 28 covers the pathophysiology of fetal growth restriction, but some additional comments are warranted here to underscore the importance of ultrasonography in the diagnosis and management of this condition.

The population of fetuses with growth failure is heterogeneous by etiology and prognosis. Growth failure, or IUGR, is defined by a birth weight at or below the 10th percentile for gestational age and sex. There is a direct exponential relationship between the birth weight percentile and both perinatal mortality and morbidity (Manning, 1995b) (Fig. 20-9). Assuming a normal (gaussian) distribution, 10% of the fetal population is classified as having IUGR by this definition; in practice, the observed incidence of IUGR by this definition is 5%. This population of small fetuses is heterogeneous by etiology and perinatal prog-

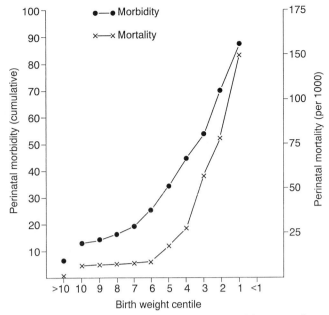

FIGURE 20-9 ■ The relationship between birth weight percentile as determined at birth and the risk of perinatal mortality or morbidity. Observations were made in 1560 perinates with a birth weight at or below the 10th percentile for gestational age and sex. No increase in abnormal perinatal outcome was observed until the birth-weight percentile fell to the 5th percentile or less. Note the exponential increase in adverse perinatal outcome as the rank fell below the 5th percentile. (From Manning FA: Fetal Medicine: Principles and Practice. Norwalk, Conn, Appleton & Lange, 1995.)

nosis. Most IUGR fetuses (80% to 85%) are categorized as "constitutionally small"; they are not at increased perinatal risk and do not require aggressive intervention. They account for only a small proportion of the perinatal deaths associated with IUGR, and the fetal mortality rate of this group of IUGR fetuses is comparable with that of the appropriate-for-gestational-age nonanomalous fetuses (stillbirth rate, 1.9 per 1000).

True growth failure secondary to extrinsic factors, commonly called *uteroplacental failure*, occurs in 10% to 15% of IUGR fetuses. These fetuses, described as having asymmetrical IUGR, are at extreme perinatal risk and usually require early intervention to avoid mortality and major morbidity. The remaining 5% to 10% of fetuses with IUGR exhibit intrinsic growth failure secondary to one or more organ system anomalies (e.g., renal agenesis, short limb dystrophy), to chromosomal anomaly (e.g., trisomy 18), or to chronic intrauterine viral infection (e.g., cytomegalic inclusion disease virus, rubella).

The prognosis for fetuses with intrinsic growth failure varies but is usually grim. Forewarning of the presence of lethal anomalies can prevent operative delivery and the attendant maternal risks. Assessment of fetal morphometric, morphologic, and functional data improves diagnostic accuracy and the development of rational management strategies.

Ultrasound methods for detection of significant fetal growth failure are undergoing constant revision. Fetal morphometrics have been very useful in identifying the population of fetuses with IUGR. Diagnostic accuracy by ultrasound methods now exceeds 85% compared with about 40% detection by clinical means alone, and the clinical problem of "overdiagnosis" (false-positive diagnosis) is also sharply reduced.

TABLE 20-4. CORRECTED PERINATAL MORTALITY (PNM) RATIOS (EXCLUDE LETHAL ANOMALY) AMONG LOW-RISK AND HIGH-RISK (SCREENED/UNSCREENED) PREGNANCIES AND AMONG SMALL-FOR-GESTATIONAL AGE (SGA) FETUSES (SCREENED/UNSCREENED), MANITOBA EXPERIENCE

Category	No. of Cases	Corrected PNM (per 1000 Live Births)
All cases	144,786	5.6
All low risk	101,350	3.8
All high risk	43,436	9.8
Screened high risk	31,740	2.2
All SGA (7% total population)	10,135	17.8
Unscreened SGA	7,460	21.3
Screened SGA*	2,675	8.4

* Serial fetal assessment management.

From Manning FA: Intrauterine growth retardation: Etiology, pathophysiology, diagnosis and treatment. *In* Fetal Medicine: Principles and Practice. Norwalk, Conn, Appleton & Lange, 1995, p. 313 ff.

Two major problems result from basing diagnosis and management of IUGR solely on fetal morphometrics. The primary purpose of fetal morphometric evaluation is to identify the subset having a fetal weight below the limits for the normal range. The lower limit of normal weight per given gestation may vary among centers. Most centers use the 10th percentile for gestational age as a lower cutoff to define the group at risk for pathologic fetal growth restriction. Thus, one should first recognize that morphometrics alone do not define the etiology or pathophysiology of the disease process. Second, the concept of growth failure "in evolution" must be considered. The ultimate disposition of extrinsic fetal growth failure depends on fetal age at onset, rate of progression, and the interval between disease onset and initial diagnostic observation.

Consider, for example, the fetus with growth potential that falls in the 90th percentile of the normal population with late-onset extrinsic growth failure. Such a fetus may exhibit severe compromise and even die before the reduced growth rate propels it to less than the 10th percentile. In practice, this scenario is rare and is usually not an indication for either extended antepartum testing or early intervention. Consideration of the wide spectrum of fetal information provided by dynamic ultrasound scanning can overcome these limitations. The additional information should include assessment of factors such as amniotic fluid volume. Recognition of a major organ or chromosomal anomaly excludes most fetuses with IUGR because of intrinsic growth failure. Distinguishing the otherwise normal small fetus from the asymmetrical IUGR fetus, although more difficult, is essential because the management strategies are distinctly disparate. The asymmetrical IUGR fetus often exhibits morphologic changes. Body proportion changes are characterized by a lesser effect on head growth and a more pronounced effect on trunk and limb growth (Hadlock et al., 1983b). A significant alteration in the ratio of head circumference to abdominal circumference (more than ±2 SD above the mean) yields a true-positive diagnostic rate of 85% (Campbell, 1977). An abnormal fetal ponderal index yields a true-positive rate of 46.6% (Hadlock et al., 1983b). Loss of subcutaneous fat, best measured in the region of the mid-thigh or paraspinal area, strongly suggests asymmetrical IUGR. Evaluation of the functional sequelae of growth failure provides insight to both the etiology and the severity of disease.

The volume of amniotic fluid can be assessed either subjectively or more objectively by measurement of the largest pocket of fluid, or amniotic fluid index. The observation of oligohydramnios in fetuses known to have an intact genitourinary system and intact membranes is a powerful predictor of impending fetal jeopardy (Chamberlain et al., 1984b). Oligohydramnios in a fetus with morphometric evidence of IUGR virtually always indicates asymmetrical severe (dysmature) IUGR, and some authors consider it an immediate indication for delivery (Bastide et al., 1986). The presence of normal amniotic fluid volume does not differentiate the normal small fetus from the fetus with less severe dysmature IUGR (Manning et al., 1983b; Hoddick et al., 1984).

Abnormalities in Doppler flow velocity waveform in the umbilical artery and in select intrafetal vessels (middle cerebral artery, thoracic aorta) may be useful in defining the presumed etiology of IUGR and are discussed in greater detail in Chapter 28. An absence of diastolic flow in the fetus with an estimated weight below the 10th percentile strongly suggests

evidence of uteroplacental dysfunction and a pathologic type of growth failure (Arduini et al., 1987; Beattie and Dornan, 1989) (see also Chapter 21). When Doppler flow and the biophysical profiles are normal, it becomes reasonable and safe to extend the interval between observations, thereby permitting assessment of fetal growth rate.

Both diagnostic accuracy and management criteria vary with the certainty of fetal age estimates. Virtually all ultrasound-derived fetal morphometric measures used to assess the adequacy of fetal growth and its pathologic deviation depend on accuracy of the gestational age estimate. As described previously, estimates of fetal age from menstrual history carry considerable potential for error; as estimate error increases, the accuracy in ranking the growth parameter percentile decreases. The important clinical corollary is that when fetal age is overestimated, the frequency of diagnosis of IUGR increases.

Campbell (1974) similarly reported a high incidence of overdiagnosis of IUGR. When dates are known with certainty, as with known LNMP, early ultrasound measurements, or both, the diagnosis of IUGR is easily achieved by confirmation of a major deviation of growth parameters below the lower distribution limit of the expected mean. When dates are certain, IUGR can usually be confirmed from a single ultrasound examination. When dates are uncertain—a common clinical situation—the diagnosis becomes more difficult, and serial assessment is required. By plotting the incremental change over time, one can determine the rate of growth. The interval between serial examinations varies directly with gestational age (see Fig. 20-1) and is usually at least 2 weeks. For each individual variable (BPD, head circumference, abdominal circumference, femur, fetal weight estimate), the growth rate may be plotted against the normal curve. Assessment of fetal well-being is used adjunctively for each visit and offers considerable assurance that continued observation until the next scheduled visit is a safe and reasonable approach. A fetus exhibiting sustained growth in all variables may be safely categorized either as a normal small fetus or as of mistaken gestational age. Sharp differentiation of these two categories is inconsequential because obstetric intervention is unwarranted. Absence of or severe delay in fetal growth over serial examinations strongly suggests IUGR, and early intervention is warranted. The management of the IUGR fetus is discussed in detail in Chapter 28.

Fetal Macrosomia

The fetus with enhanced general growth or macrosomia is defined by a birth weight equal to or greater than the 90th percentile for gestational age and sex. The condition can usually be ascribed to one of three general causes. The most common reason is enhanced intrinsic growth potential, and the normal large fetus accounts for about 50% to 60% of macrosomia cases. The condition is characterized by exaggerated, but proportional, linear and circumferential growth. Such fetuses are not at risk for fetal asphyxia but are at risk for birth trauma. Abnormal maternal glucose homeostasis accounts for about 35% to 40% of macrosomic fetuses (see Chapter 49). Although such fetuses may exhibit some enhancement of both linear and circumferential growth, they invariably exhibit abnormal fat deposition most evident in the malar cheek pad and the paraspinal area (Fig. 20-10). Fetuses with macrosomia caused by maternal glucose intolerance are at increased risk for intrauterine death and birth trauma. Underestimation of fetal

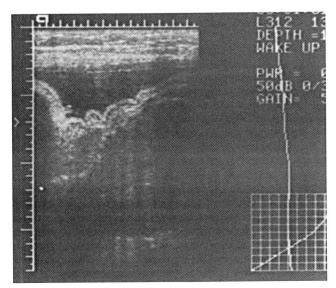

FIGURE 20-10 ■ An ultrasound view of the occiput and posterior cervical region of a macrosomic fetus. The undulations of the skin are a typical feature in the fetus with increased subcutaneous fat.

age is an unusual clinical error, accounting for only about 5% of perinatal macrosomia. Fetuses described as macrosomic on this basis are not at risk for fetal death or birth trauma.

Accurate detection of macrosomia beyond 36 weeks' gestation would be of great value in avoiding the risk of birth trauma. Unfortunately, there is no reliable way to identify the fetus weighing more than 4000 g, a weight beyond which the risk of birth trauma rises sharply (Benedetti and Gabbe, 1978). Fetal weight estimates at this range yield significant error; the standard formulas for estimation of fetal weight based on a composite of fetal measures (head circumference, abdominal circumference, femur length) yield a range of error of up to 22% in 95% of cases. For detection of fetuses with an actual weight of 4000 g or greater, these formulas have a maximal sensitivity and specificity of about 75% (Delepa and Mueller-Heubach, 1991). Because ultrasonography tends to result in overestimates of weight as weight increases, the false-positive rate for estimation of macrosomia is relatively high, reaching 35% in some studies (Levine et al., 1992; Sandmire, 1993).

Chest circumference or biacromial diameter as a predictor of shoulder dystocia has been studied (Elliott et al., 1982). The method, except in extreme cases, is relatively poor in predicting subsequent shoulder dystocia. Furthermore, whether induction of labor at term is of any clinical benefit for macrosomia suspected on the basis of ultrasonography alone or combined with clinical estimation of fetal weight remains unproven. In a prospective randomized trial of 284 near-term pregnancies complicated by clinical/ultrasound-confirmed macrosomia (between 4000 and 4500 g), induction of labor for suspected macrosomia decreased neither the rate of cesarean section (20% overall) nor the incidence of shoulder dystocia (5.1%) or neonatal injury (9.2%) (Ofer et al., 1997).

Fetal weight estimates derived from three-dimensional ultrasound data (fractional limb volume and abdominal circumference) have been reported to be ±7.8% of true weight (Lee et al., 2001). This approach holds promise as a means of improving weight estimates but awaits rigorous clinical testing.

Detection of Fetal Development Anomalies

When discovery at delivery is used as the temporal reference, the frequency of overt congenital anomalies is about 3% (Marden et al., 1964). The rate of anomalies at birth appears to be relatively constant across different populations and time periods. The reported incidence of congenital anomaly at delivery must underestimate true incidence because lethal embryonic and early fetal anomalies are excluded, as are anomalies not manifested until later life. Although congenital anomalies have always been a major prenatal problem and their rate of occurrence is constant, their relative clinical significance has increased dramatically since the introduction of dynamic ultrasound imaging. Among the unscreened population, anomalies account for about 25% of all perinatal mortality, whereas in the screened population in whom asphyxial death is reduced, anomalies now account for more than 80% of all perinatal deaths. A continuing fall in overall perinatal mortality, with a continuing rise in the proportion ascribed to anomaly, is the expected benefit of antenatal ultrasound fetal assessment.

In a study of 159,990 pregnancies, the perinatal mortality rate attributable to anomalies was 3.12 per 1000, accounting for 33% of the total mortality rate (Manning, 1995a). Among 55,612 high-risk patients subjected to repeated ultrasound examination for assessment of fetal well-being, the mortality rate secondary to anomalies was 5.85 per 1000, accounting for 83% of all causes of death (Manning, 1995a).

The very definition of *anomaly* is under constant revision. On the basis of high-resolution dynamic ultrasound imaging methods, a spectrum of fetal anomalies is recognized ranging from primary *functional* defects (e.g., myotonic dystrophies and cardiac dysrhythmias without overt anatomic defect) to primary *structural defects* without overt functional fetal components (e.g., cleft palate) to the most common condition of *mixed functional and structural defects* (e.g., obstructive uropathy with renal dysgenesis and pulmonary hypoplasia). Anatomic derangements with functional defects may be primary (e.g., bradyarrhythmias with atrioventricular canal defects) or secondary (ascites with tachyarrhythmia), and they may be remote from the defective organ system (e.g., hydramnios with duodenal atresia, oligohydramnios with obstructive uropathy). In some conditions, such as esophageal atresia and tracheoesophageal fistula, alteration of amniotic fluid volume, a functional sequela, may be the only manifestation of the structural lesion. The high mortality rate associated with these conditions is largely the result of hydramnios-induced prematurity.

Prenatal detection of congenital anomalies, although of obvious clinical importance, is only the first step in unraveling this difficult and common clinical dilemma. The subsequent development of rational management strategies for the anomalous fetus must take into consideration both the fetus and the mother. Management depends on consideration of such variables as the following:

- Expected prognosis for a fetus with the lesion
- Demonstration of progressive pathophysiology
- Availability of treatment modalities (if any)
- Fetal age at the time of diagnosis

Consideration of these variables presents a wide range of management options. When fetal prognosis is hopeless, all efforts are directed toward minimizing maternal risk. When a structural lesion is identified and exhibits no progressive pathophysiology on serial evaluation (e.g., arrested hydrocephalus), conservative management may be indicated. In the mature fetus, the presence of an anomaly amenable to neonatal therapy (e.g., omphalocele) should prompt appropriate referral and planning for postdelivery surgical repair. In highly selected cases, *in utero* therapy may be indicated for a progressive potentially lethal anomaly discovered in the grossly immature fetus. Such therapy may be either medical (e.g., chronotropic agents for fetal tachyarrhythmia with heart failure) or surgical (e.g., chronic diversion therapy for obstructive uropathy). A proposed clinical classification of fetal anomalies is presented in Table 20-5. Medical and surgical approaches to specific fetal disorders are discussed in Chapter 27.

The accuracy of fetal anomaly detection by ultrasonography is as difficult to define as the actual incidence of anomalies, is subject to the same compounding factors, and remains highly variable. The detection rate depends on the age of the fetus at examination. In general, the more mature the anomalous fetus at ultrasound examination, the higher the diagnostic rate. The ultrasound sensitivity for detection of major anomalies among patients routinely screened before 24 weeks' gestation has been reported to be as low as 17% (Ewigman et al., 1993) to as high as 75% (Van Dorsten et al., 1998). The detection rate of major (life-threatening) anomalies in the screened group was 79.7% (59 of 74 cases).

Beyond 36 weeks of gestation, more than 85% of all major anomalies can be detected by ultrasound assessment (Manning et al., 1983b). Chromosomal anomalies without overt structural or functional markers are not identified by ultrasound methods. The detection rate falls dramatically in earlier gestation because the anomalous condition may not yet be expressed (e.g., ureteropelvic obstruction) or the lesion may be too small to be visualized (e.g., small myelomeningocele). As a rule, the earlier in gestation a lesion is detected, the less the prognostic significance. Furthermore, an anomaly in one system should alert the clinician to the possibility of associated anomalies, not all of which may be detected by ultrasonography. For example, the presence of obstructive uropathy is associated with karyotypic anomalies in about 8% of cases (Manning et al., 1986).

Almost all reports of anomaly detection by ultrasonography emphasize the positive diagnostic accuracy, but few reports detail the negative predictive accuracy. Accordingly, the predictive accuracy parameters of ultrasound screening for anomalies, when applied to the population at large, remain essentially unexplored. The diagnostic acuity of ultrasonography depends directly on the intensity of examination. Although there are probably few, if any, structural abnormalities visible to the naked eye that cannot be detected by ultrasound imaging, the practicalities of the time constraints of examination introduce unavoidable error. A detection rate of 100%, although a theoretic possibility, has not been achieved in the practical clinical setting. In general, the probability of detection of a lesion is directly related to the index of suspicion. This factor accounts for the difficulties in achieving comparable diagnostic accuracy between the general population and that population referred with historical or other indicators of an increased risk of underlying anomaly.

Anomalies of the Head, Neck, and Face

The ultrasound assessment of the fetal head and face may be divided into general assessment of shape and proportion and specific assessment of facial and intracranial architecture. The examiner uses sequential views, rotating through the sagittal, parasagittal, coronal, and transverse planes. In general assessment, the presence and shape of the calvarium are noted. Absence of the bony calvarium is the characteristic feature of the severe neural tube defect anencephaly (Fig. 20-11). This uniformly lethal anomaly may be detected from as early as 10 weeks' gestation (menstrual age) and always is overt by 16 weeks' gestation. The lesion is associated with absence, to varying degrees, of cerebral tissue and gross distortion of intracranial architecture.

Herniation of meninges or cerebral tissue through a defect in the calvarium is the hallmark of encephalocele (Fig. 20-12). A variant of neural tube defect, it is a midline lesion and is usually posterior. The prognosis of a *posterior encephalocele* is guarded. The overall reported survival rate ranges from 40% to 75% (Mealy et al., 1970; Simpson et al., 1984). Ultrasound findings that portend a poor to hopeless prognosis include a large defect with herniation of the brain, collapse of the anterior calvarium, ventriculomegaly, and associated malformations of other organ systems. The prognosis for survival is much better with small posterior defects, especially when there is no

TABLE 20-5. A CLINICAL CLASSIFICATION OF FETAL ANOMALIES

Type	Prognosis	Progression*	Pulmonary Maturity	Management	Examples[†]
I	Good	Nonprogressive	NA	Conservative	Intermittent fetal arrhythmia, unilateral multicystic renal disease, cystic hygroma, arrested hydrocephalus
II	Good	Progressive	Present	Delivery; give neonatal treatment	Chylothorax, ureteropelvic obstruction, arrhythmia with congestive heart failure
III	Good	Progressive	Absent	Intrauterine therapy or early delivery	Obstructive uropathy, arrhythmia with congestive heart failure, obstructive hydrocephalus
IV	Hopeless	NA		Conservative	Anencephaly, renal agenesis, holoprosencephaly, hypoplastic left ventricle

* As determined by serial ultrasound fetal assessment.
† For illustrative purposes only.
NA, not applicable.

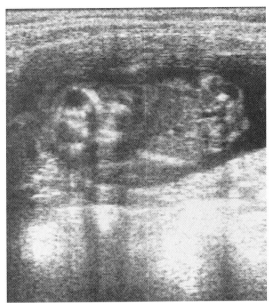

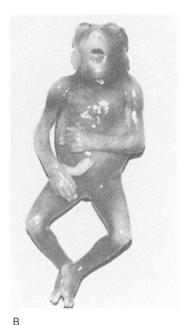

FIGURE 20-11 ■ **A,** An ultrasound view in the longitudinal coronal plane of an anencephalic fetus. The fetal calvarium is totally absent, and the fetal orbits appear relatively large and prominent. **B,** Same anencephalic fetus as in **A.** Note the prominence of the eyes and the complete absence of the calvarium.

A

B

herniation of the brain. Up to 25% of surviving infants with posterior encephalocele exhibit severe long-term neurologic disabilities (Brown and Sheridan-Periera, 1992). *Iniencephaly,* a condition associated with a neural tube defect in the high cervical spine, is a variant of posterior encephalocele; the prognosis is extremely poor. *Anterior encephalocele* is exceedingly rare and usually only occurs in patients of Asian extraction. The prognosis is generally better than that for the posterior variety, but it remains guarded (Brown and Sheridan-Periera, 1992). Surviving infants with an anterior encephalocele often have major distortion of the face, and effective cosmetic repair is usually difficult (Lipschitz et al., 1969).

Distortion and enlargement of the calvarium without herniation may occur with thanatophoric dwarfism, the various cleidocranial dysplasias, and achondrospondylodysplasias. Marked cranial asymmetry may occur with primary synostosis and with autosomal dominant conditions such as Apert, Crouzon, Pheiffer, and Jackson-Weiss syndromes and the autosomal recessive conditions such as Christian and Summitt syndromes. Chromosomal abnormalities (5p+, 7p–, 13q–) have been associated with craniosynostosis as has the teratogen, aminopterin.

Symmetrical reduction in head size, called *microcephaly,* is among the most difficult of fetal anomalies to classify. There is no clear relationship, except in the extreme, between head and brain size and the presence of normal brain function. Primary microcephaly may be due to either a nonpathologic normal distribution phenomenon or an arrest of cerebral growth with resultant diminished head growth. Both conditions may be associated with reduced head dimensions, decrease in the ratio of head circumference to abdominal circumference, and reduced growth rate evident on serial measurement.

Differentiation of normal from pathologic microcephaly can be extremely difficult. Such differentiation is of major importance because the subsequent management strategies are widely divergent. Unequivocal diagnosis of pathologic microcephaly carries a grim prognosis and should be reserved for cases exhibiting extreme microcephaly (head circumference more than 4 SD below the mean for gestational age), absence or marked reduction in cerebral hemisphere volume, or extreme variance in the ratio of head circumference to abdominal circumference (less than 4 SD of the mean), or when environmental etiologic factors (e.g., high-dose radiation exposure, proven fetal cytomegalovirus infection) have been identified. Pathologic microcephaly has been associated with aneuploidy (trisomy 21, 13, 18, 22), chromosome defects (deletions of 4p, 5p, 18p, 18q), and single gene disorders such as Smith-Lemil-Opitz, Roberts, Angelman, and Bloom syndromes.

Soft tissue abnormalities of the fetal head and neck may be cystic or solid and often indicate underlying fetal functional or karyotypic abnormality. Generalized scalp edema is a characteristic feature of immune and nonimmune hydrops and of

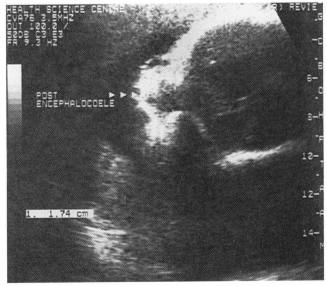

FIGURE 20-12 ■ A transverse scan of the head in a fetus with a posterior encephalocele. Note the defect in the posterior skull (1.74 cm) and the protrusion of cerebral meninges through the defect.

fetal congestive heart failure. *Cystic hygroma* is manifested as multiple discrete cystic masses of varying size, primarily of the paraspinal cervical region but occasionally involving the anterior neck or axilla (Fig. 20-13). Cystic hygroma frequently is associated with the XO karyotype and variants (70% of cases) and with trisomy 21 (20% of cases), but it also may be associated with a normal fetal karyotype (Phillips and McGahan, 1981). It is most commonly observed in the second trimester and usually decreases in size with advancing gestation. Based on extensive first-trimester screening data, it would appear that cystic hygroma is a much more common fetal anomaly than previously known and that the lethality of the anomaly is high (Malone et al., 2002). At least one third of fetuses with cystic hygroma will have other anomalies (usually cardiac). The neck webbing typical of Turner syndrome is presumed to be a residual effect of cystic hygroma in early fetal life. The complication of hydrops in fetuses with cystic hygroma, most commonly observed in the third trimester, carries an extremely poor prognosis (Chervenak, 1983). Cystic hygroma must be differentiated from cavernous hemangioma. With Doppler flow ultrasonography, this differentiation is simple because cystic hygroma never exhibits flow within the cystic mass, whereas venous flow is characteristic of cavernous hemangioma. Detection of cystic hygromas is an indication for fetal karyotype determination.

When observed before 20 weeks' gestation, localized nonedematous thickening or lucency (more than 5 mm) of the posterior nuchal subcutaneous tissue has been reported as a sonographic sign of trisomy 21 (Benacerraf and Frigoletto, 1985). In the initial reports, however, this finding was present in only 4 of 11 fetuses with Down syndrome (36%) and in 1 fetus with a normal karyotype. Furthermore, determination of subcutaneous thickness is angle dependent, and false-positive results are reported (Toi et al., 1987). Nonetheless, this finding should be considered an indication for further karyotypic evaluation. The use of increased nuchal lucency for diagnosis of chromosomal disorders in the first trimester is discussed in Chapter 18.

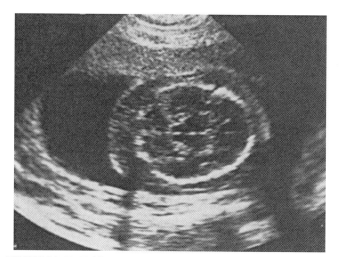

FIGURE 20-13 ■ Ultrasound scan of the fetal head in the plane of the biparietal diameter demonstrating massive scalp edema secondary to immune (Rh) hydrops fetalis. The subcutaneous tissues of the scalp are grossly distended as a result of fluid accumulation. Scalp edema of this degree usually portends an ominous prognosis.

Evaluation of fetal facial structure, now possible with some considerable clarity, may offer insight on the presence of genetic and associated structural anomalies. The fetal face is visualized in the sagittal (profile), serial coronal (frontal), and serial transverse views (Fig. 20-14). Facial dimensions are assessed in the profile view. Mandibular shortening and jaw retraction suggest Pierre Robin and Treacher Collins syndromes and may occur with trisomy 13 and trisomy 18. The prognosis of fetuses with micrognathia is very poor. Among 56 affected fetuses, Nicolaides and colleagues (1993) noted that 37 had trisomy (most commonly trisomy 18). Among the 19 fetuses with micrognathia and a normal karyotype, most had major anomalies, and only 1 of these fetuses survived. A nomogram for mandible length has been published (Chitty et al., 1993). Facial clefts ranging from cleft lip and palate to major facial cleft (bifid face) are best identified in the frontal and transverse scan planes (Fig. 20-15A). The fetal lips and hard palate may be seen in great detail, and the diagnosis of cleft lip, palate, or both are possible. However, the specificity and sensitivity of ultrasound diagnosis of these conditions remain undetermined. Observation of facial cleft should alert the clinician to the possibility of underlying karyotypic abnormality, especially trisomy 13 and trisomy 18.

Dynamic ultrasound imaging may permit visualization of the fetal tongue. Macroglossia may occur in Beckwith syndrome, with fetal hypothyroidism, and with some forms of gangliosidosis. Approximately 9% of fetuses with overt macroglossia will have trisomy 21. The fetal eye and orbits are well visualized, and nomograms for interorbital diameters have been published (Mayden et al., 1982). Both hypotelorism and hypertelorism may be identified and are suggestive but not diagnostic of associated anomalies. The exception is extreme hypotelorism, which is highly suggestive of holoprosencephaly. Examination of the fetal ear, although possible by ultrasonography, has yet to be shown to be of diagnostic value. Diminished pinna length is characteristic of trisomy 21, but a nomogram for fetal pinna length has not been reported. Determination of relative ear position is possible and may shed light on the presence of associated anomalies. In the normal fetus, a line extended from the mid-orbit transects the pinna just above the external auditory meatus (Fig. 20-16). In the fetus with low-set ears, the superior edge of the pinna falls below the extended mid-orbital line. Low-set ears occur in a variety of conditions, including Turner syndrome, Potter syndrome, trisomy 13, and trisomy 18. The clinical usefulness of ultrasound determination of ear level remains to be determined by prospective study.

Abnormalities of intracranial architecture are among the most common and most significant developmental anomalies. By means of contemporary high-resolution ultrasound methods, especially the transvaginal transducer, the fetal brain may be examined in remarkable detail (Timor-Trisch et al., 1996).

Anomalies of the fetal brain can generally be assigned to two general categories: primary ventriculomegaly and primary brain tissue lesions. *Ventriculomegaly* is defined as bilateral enlargement of the ventricular system beyond the upper limit (± 2 SD) of distribution for the normal population of equal age; in practice, the ventricle-to-hemisphere ratio is used to determine ventriculomegaly (Jeanty, Dramaix-Wilmet et al., 1981). In clinical practice, the terms ventriculomegaly and *hydrocephalus* are used synonymously, although strictly speaking such interchange of terms is incorrect. Ventriculomegaly is of

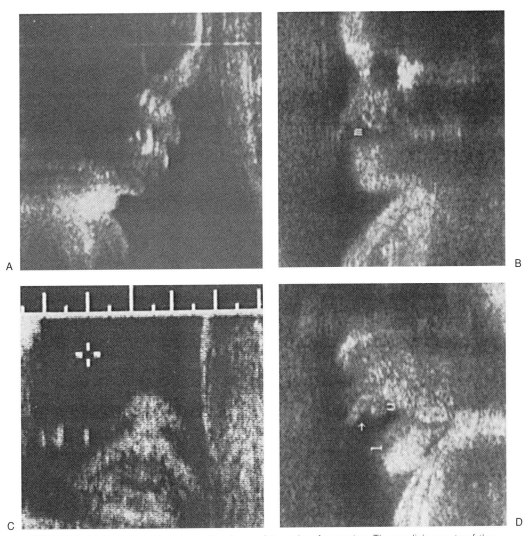

FIGURE 20-14 ■ **A,** Fetal face in profile view at 24 weeks of gestation. The medial aspects of the orbit, the nose, and the mouth are well visualized. **B,** A slightly rotated profile view of a 26-week fetus with a major cleft of the lip (m). **C,** A view of the fetal mouth and nose from an inferior angle. The lips are well seen and are normal. The mouth is slightly open, permitting a view of the anterior gingiva. **D,** A slightly rotated inferior angle view of the mouth in a fetus with major clefting of the upper lip (*arrow*). l, lower lip; u, upper lip.

greatest clinical significance when shown to be progressive or associated with recognized underlying abnormalities, although long-term morbidity may be associated with mild nonprogressive fetal ventriculomegaly (Bloom et al., 1997). Pathologic ventriculomegaly is usually associated with one of four underlying conditions (holoprosencephaly, aqueductal stenosis, major neural tube defect, or unilateral or occasionally bilateral cystic cerebellar degeneration), and the prognosis varies substantially with these associations.

1. *Holoprosencephaly* results from disordered forebrain development and is characterized by the presence of a single ventricle (usually enlarged), absence of the corpus callosum, major forebrain dysgenesis, and facial abnormalities almost always involving the fetal eyes. In its most advanced and most common form, alobar holoprosencephaly involves a markedly detailed single ventricle, absent forebrain, and cyclopia. The diagnosis can be confirmed by transvaginal sonography as early as 14 weeks (Bronshtein and Weiner, 1991). The prognosis is extremely poor, perinatal death is common, and severe mental retardation is uniform (Laurence and Coates, 1962; Chervenak et al., 1985). Accordingly, when the diagnosis is made, heroic efforts for the fetus in the antepartum period (e.g., ventriculoamniotic shunt), intrapartum period (operative delivery for fetal indication), or neonatal period should be actively discouraged.

2. Ventriculomegaly due to *aqueductal stenosis* presents a major management dilemma. The condition is characterized by progressive dilatation of the lateral ventricle beginning initially in the anterior horn and then involving the entire lateral ventricle, with lateral displacement of the choroid plexus and of the middle cerebral artery and compression of the cerebral cortex (Fig. 20-17). Although proximal dilatation of the third ventricle may occur, this sign is not uniform. The diagnosis of ventriculomegaly due to aqueduct stenosis is one of exclusion—that is, by ruling out posterior fossa lesion (e.g., Dandy-Walker cyst) and associated neural tube defects. Characteristically, the fetal calvarium is normal in shape and not enlarged with early disease; symmetrical enlargement is observed with advanced

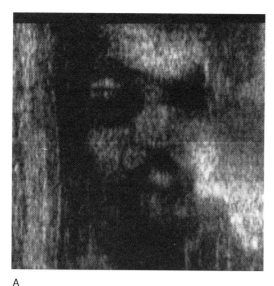
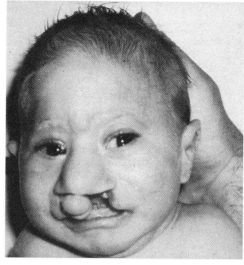
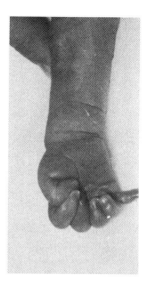

A   B

FIGURE 20-15 ■ A, A sonogram of the face from the frontal coronal perspective in a fetus with trisomy 18. Note the large facial cleft. **B,** Face of the child at delivery. Trisomy 18 was confirmed.

disease. The appropriate management is difficult to determine(Vintzileos et al., 1987). Except in the extreme case, neither the extent of ventriculomegaly nor the degree of cortical tissue compression is a reliable prognostic indicator of adverse neurologic or intellectual sequelae. Perinatal outcome with ventriculomegaly due to aqueductal stenosis is usually, but not invariably, poor (Laurence and Coates, 1962; McCullough

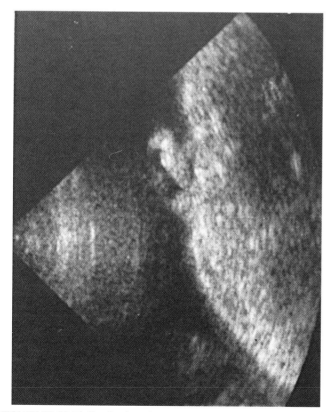

FIGURE 20-16 ■ The fetal ear in the coronal view. In this normal fetus note the midorbital plane transects the external auditory meatus.

and Balzer-Martin, 1982). Spontaneous arrest of ventriculomegaly is reported (Laurence and Coates, 1967). Chronic ventricular decompression in the neonate is associated with high survival (more than 85%) and may be associated with normal neurologic development and intellectual function in most cases (65%). However, it is invariably associated with major associated morbidity (infection, shunt revision, growth failure) (McCullough and Balzer-Martin, 1982). The value, if any, of fetal ventricular decompression remains unknown, although the procedure is technically possible and may be associated with intact outcome (Manning et al., 1986). Although clear prognostic indicators are not available, the earlier the fetal age at diagnosis and the more progressive the ventriculomegaly, the worse the prognosis seems to be. Instability of the falx, called the *wavering midline*, indicates severe disease associated with a particularly poor outcome (Nelson et al., 1984). No reliable clinical evidence suggests that neurologic outcome, including cognition, is improved by early delivery of infants with ventriculomegaly secondary to aqueduct stenosis.

3. Ventriculomegaly due to *major neural tube defect* is usually associated with definitive ultrasound signs and can be recognized with some certainty. The concordance of spinal neural tube defects and the Arnold-Chiari malformation is high, approaching 100%. The Arnold-Chiari malformation, characterized by herniation of the cerebellar tonsils and midbrain structures into the foramen magnum, causes ventriculomegaly due to compression of the fourth and occasionally the third ventricle. Downward traction of the brain causes a reduction in the anterior calvarium, in turn producing a triangular head in the plane of the BPD, known as the "lemon sign." Compression of the cerebellar hemisphere creates the "banana sign" (Fig. 20-18). When these two signs are observed, the probability of a spinal defect approaches 100%. Conversely, their absence conveys a high probability of a normal intact spinal canal.

4. Unilateral or occasionally bilateral *cystic cerebellar degeneration* (Dandy-Walker cysts) can cause ventriculomegaly due to compression of either the fourth or the third ventricle

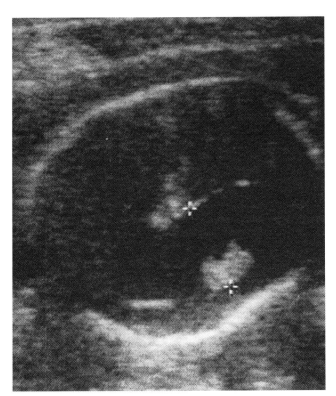

FIGURE 20-17 ■ Fetal ventriculomegaly at 21 weeks' gestation secondary to aqueductal stenosis. The fetal head is normal in shape and size. The key diagnostic features are the increase in ventricle size, as evidenced by an abnormal ventricle-to-hemisphere ratio (0.8125 in this case) and a prominent lateral shift of the choroid plexus. The midline structures were stable, and the cortical mantle was seen. Disease was rapidly progressive; the fetus was delivered at 24 weeks and died.

(Fig. 20-19). The salient ultrasound characteristics of Dandy-Walker syndrome are agenesis of the cerebellar vermis, splaying of the cerebellar hemispheres, and dilation of the fourth ventricle. In the normal fetus the cerebellar vermis do not fuse before about 18 weeks' gestation (Bromley et al., 1994), and accordingly the diagnosis of Dandy-Walker syndrome should not be considered before 18 completed weeks of gestation. The prognosis of Dandy-Walker syndrome, although variable, is generally poor (Vintzileos et al., 1987), and 75% of infants with this condition will have evidence of significant hydrocephalus by 3 months of age.

Agenesis of the corpus callosum is a relatively rare brain anomaly. The salient ultrasound findings are "tear-shaped" lateral ventricles with wide separation of the anterior horn and dilatation of the occipital horn, elevation and dilation of the third ventricle, and inability to visualize the fibers of the corpus callosum (Pilu et al., 1993). Agenesis of the corpus callosum is usually an isolated finding but can be associated with trisomy 18, 13, and 8 and with craniofacial defects as may be seen in Apert syndrome. The prognosis varies according to the extent of the agenesis and the presence of associated abnormalities (Taylor and David, 1998). Partial agenesis of the corpus callosum may be exceedingly difficult to recognize and may be associated with craniofacial abnormalities, including facial clefting.

Cysts of the choroids plexus are a common finding and may be seen in upward of 15% of all early pregnancies. A weak association between choroid plexus cysts and trisomy 18 is

reported. In the absence of ultrasound signs of trisomy 18 (ventricular septal defect, overlapping fingers, IUGR), the presence of choroid plexus cysts(s) does not connote an ominous outcome and is not an indication for amniocentesis or chorionic villus sampling (Nadel et al., 1992). Rarely, isolated saccular herniation of the ventricular wall, usually the posterior horn of the lateral ventricle, causes extrinsic compression of the cerebrospinal fluid circulation (porencephalic cyst).

Abnormalities of the Neural Tube

Abnormal closure of the neural tube is a relatively common lesion (approximately 1 per 1000 births) that produces a spectrum of anomalies ranging from absence of the dorsal laminae of the vertebral bodies (spina bifida), herniation of meninges

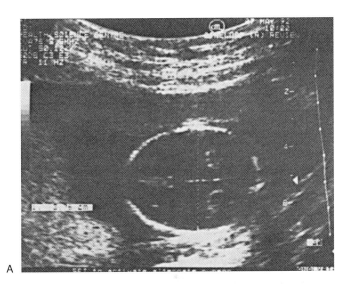

A

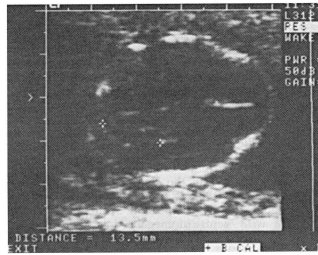

B

FIGURE 20-18 ■ **A,** Normal fetal calvarium at 17 weeks of gestation. This ultrasound image, in the biparietal diameter plane, demonstrates the normal symmetrical shape of the calvarium and the normal cerebellar hemispheres (seen as faint circular echogenic structures in the posterior region of the image). **B,** The fetal calvarium at 18 weeks in a fetus with proven lumbosacral myelomeningocele. Note the collapse of the anterior calvarium disrupting the normal oval shape of the skull (lemon sign). The fetal cerebellar hemisphere (marked on the inferior side by the calipers) is elongated and flattened (banana sign). These are the typical cranial ultrasound signs of the Arnold-Chiari malformation seen in most fetuses with neural tube defect.

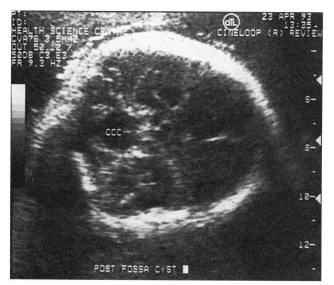

FIGURE 20-19 ■ Dandy-Walker syndrome. Note the centrally located echolucent cyst in the posterior fossa with splaying of the cerebellar hemispheres. This fetus exhibited mild associated ventriculomegaly (not shown).

(myelocele), and herniation of meninges and neural elements (myelomeningocele) to absence of development of the forebrain and midbrain elements (anencephaly). The spinal lesion (excluding encephalocele and anencephaly) is most commonly located in the lumbar spine (approximately 70%) or the sacral spine (approximately 20%) and less commonly involves the thoracic or cervical spine. The prognosis varies with the location of the defect, being best with a low sacral lesion, and with the extent and nature of the defect. The smaller lesion without neural elements carries the most favorable prognosis. The lesion may involve single or multiple vertebral bodies (Fig. 20-20).

Prenatal diagnosis of neural tube defects has improved dramatically in recent years because of the use of maternal serum α-fetoprotein screening, amniotic fluid α-fetoprotein and N-acetylcholinesterase determination, and high-resolution dynamic ultrasound imaging (see Chapter 18). Accuracy parameters of the ultrasound diagnosis or exclusion of neural tube defects is now of major importance because subsequent clinical management depends on the certainty of diagnosis. There is little doubt that the positive predictive accuracy of the ultrasound diagnosis of neural tube defect is high; collapse of the anterior calvarium (lemon sign) and compressive distortion of the cerebellar hemispheres (banana sign) is a near certain indicator of a neural tube defect.

In contrast, a normal head shape and normal cerebellar shape are extremely reliable indicators of the absence of a neural tube defect. In a study of more than 7500 patients with elevated maternal serum α-fetoprotein (more than 2.5 multiples of the median) at 16 to 18 weeks referred for ultrasound assessment in the middle of the second trimester, the false-negative rate of a normal head shape and cerebellum was 0%. This high reliability of a negative scan should eliminate the use of amniocentesis for evaluation of elevated α-fetoprotein (Kyle et al., 1994).

In utero surgical repair of neural tube defect has been reported (Bruner et al., 2001). The benefits of fetal repair of neural tube lesions are not established to date. Initial reports

suggesting some improvement in spinal function have not been substantiated (Tulipan et al., 2003). The severity of hindbrain herniation (Arnold-Chiari defect) appears lessened in fetuses who have had an *in utero* repair of myelomeningocele, but whether this observed effect will result in a reduced incidence of postnatal ventricle shunts and long-term brain development is not established. The benefit, if any, of fetal surgical repair of neural tube defect is being addressed in a randomized multicenter trial (effective start date September 2002).

Abnormalities of the Fetal Thorax

In the normal fetus, the thoracic cavity is bell-shaped, with the inferior margin delineated by the markedly concave diaphragmatic leaves, which appear sonolucent (Fig. 20-21). Gross reduction in thoracic volume or distortion of shape is typical of a variety of disorders, including severe pulmonary hypoplasia associated with renal agenesis, asphyxiating thoracic dystrophy typical of thanatophoric dwarfism, and osteogenesis imperfecta and other skeletal dysplasias.

Diaphragmatic hernia is characterized by herniation of abdominal contents into the thoracic cavity (Fig. 20-22). The hernia, which may contain stomach, liver, spleen, and small bowel, causes displacement of the heart, usually anteriorly and to the right. The defect in the diaphragm is usually not visible. Lethal pulmonary hypoplasia may occur in association with diaphragmatic hernia presumed secondary to lung compression.

The mortality rate for diaphragmatic hernia varies directly with the fetal age at diagnosis and with the presence or absence of hydramnios; the slope of the mortality curve reflects both the extent of the fetal lesion and the natural selection process occurring at the time of transition to pulmonary dependence. Untreated diaphragmatic hernia confers a high

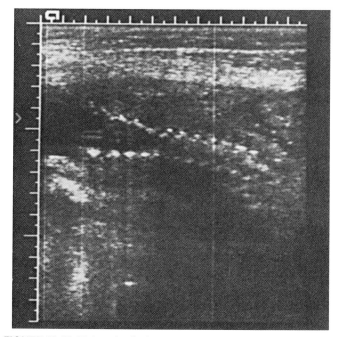

FIGURE 20-20 ■ Longitudinal coronal scan of the fetal spine in a fetus with a large lumbosacral myelomeningocele. The splaying of the spinal process is a typical and diagnostic finding in this condition. The two echogenic parallel lines at the end of the splayed spine are a portion of the herniated spinal cord.

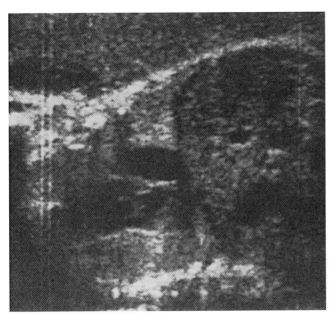

FIGURE 20-21 ■ Coronal view (linear array) of fetal thorax and abdomen at 35 weeks of gestation. Lung tissue and liver tissue vary in echodensity. The sonolucent diaphragm is well visualized bilaterally. The central echolucent structure in the thorax is the fetal heart.

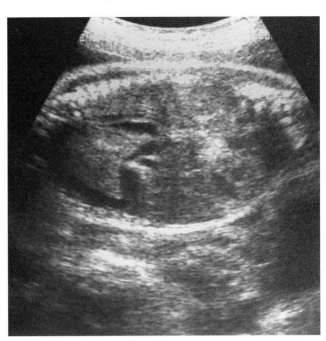

FIGURE 20-23 ■ Sagittal scan of the thorax in a 31-week fetus with bilateral pleural effusions. The effusion is greater in the right hemithorax, and there is no associated ascites or skin edema. In this fetus, the discovery of pleural effusion was incidental. The pleural effusion was the result of chylothorax. It is likely that this observation was critical in the survival of this perinate.

probability of mortality (85% to 90%), and when the lesion is associated with hydramnios, survival is unusual (Benacerraf and Adzick, 1987). The prognosis has improved dramatically in recent years, primarily because of advances in immediate neonatal ventilation and delaying corrective neonatal surgery to allow for the natural diminution in pulmonary vascular resistance. A randomized clinical trial failed to demonstrate any benefit to *in utero* repair of diaphragmatic hernia, and the procedure has been abandoned (Harrison et al., 1997). At the

present time, neonatal survival rates of infants with an antenatal diagnosis of diaphragmatic hernia now exceed 80% (Wenstrom et al., 1991). This advance has further reduced the value of prenatal (fetal) surgical repair of the lesion.

Pleural effusions are readily identified (Fig. 20-23) and may be secondary to anomalies of the thoracic duct (chylothorax), to generalized hypoproteinemia as occurs with nonimmune hydrops, or to acquired immune hydrops. Forewarning of pleural effusion can be lifesaving for the newborn, although whether decompression should occur at or before delivery remains controversial (Lange and Manning, 1981; Benacerraf and Frigoletto, 1985). Clinical experience with chronic pleuroamniotic shunt placement has been encouraging (Rodeck et al., 1988).

Lung tissue is well visualized, and specific malformations such as *cystic adenomatoid malformation* (CAM) and bronchial inclusion cysts may be identified (Fig. 20-24). CAM is classified as type I (few large cysts), type II (multiple small cysts visible by ultrasound), and type III (microcystic mass appearing as solid mass by ultrasound). Perinatal prognosis varies by CAM type (Adzick et al., 1998). The prognosis with type I is good, and survival is expected. In some instances type I CAM may resolve spontaneously *in utero*. Type II CAM may be associated with abnormalities. Type III CAM has a variable prognosis, but when associated with fetal hydrops, the outcome with type III CAM is exceedingly poor.

The prenatal diagnosis of pulmonary hypoplasia by ultrasonography has been reported, although the specificity and sensitivity of current techniques are not yet satisfactory (Nimrod et al., 1988; Sherer et al., 1990). Equating prenatal estimates of thoracic volume and lung volume to postnatal lung function falls outside the existing discrimination of contemporary ultrasound methods. Tracheoesophageal fistula may

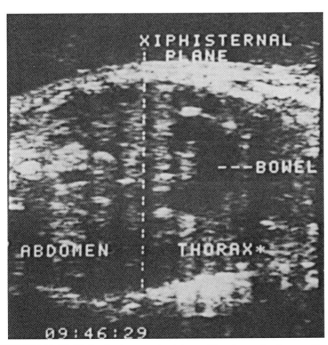

FIGURE 20-22 ■ Sagittal scan of a fetus with a large diaphragmatic hernia. The echolucent mass in the fetal chest is a dilated loop of small bowel.

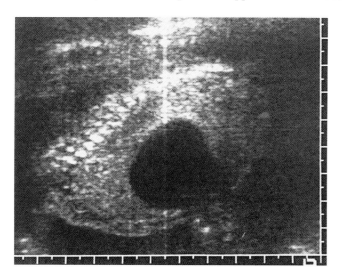

FIGURE 20-24 ■ Sagittal view of the fetal thorax in a fetus with a huge unilateral bronchial cyst. The cyst was aspirated (38 mL of fluid) and did not recur.

be suspected by ultrasound detection of hydramnios and failure to visualize the fetal stomach on repeated examination. At present, however, definitive ultrasound diagnosis of tracheo-esophageal fistula is not yet possible.

Abnormalities of the Fetal Heart

Structural abnormalities of the fetal heart are among the most common fetal anomalies, affecting anywhere from 0.4% to 1% of all pregnancies (Hoffman and Christianson, 1978). Cardiac anomalies occur rarely in isolation and are usually associated with other defects in the heart, other organ systems, or in association with single gene defects, syndromes, or chromosomal abnormalities, including deletions and aneuploidies. About 25% of all fetuses with a detected fetal heart anomaly will have an associated chromosomal defect (Allan, 1998). Conversely, nearly all fetuses (99%) with trisomy 18 will have a cardiac defect, more than 90% of fetuses with trisomy 13 will have a defect, and about half (50%) of fetuses with trisomy 21 will have a defect. Further about 50% of fetuses with chromosome deletions or partial trisomies will have a cardiac defect, as will about 40% of fetuses with XO. Because of the peculiarities of the fetal circulation, most fetal cardiac defects are not associated with functional deficits in fetal life and are for the most part silent in their pathologic expression. The true pathophysiology of most fetal cardiac defects is not evident until the conversion to adult circulation. Accordingly, the recognition of significant fetal cardiac structural defects usually depends on detection of the anatomic defect without the leading clues of a functional sequelae. Thus, the antenatal detection of fetal cardiac anomalies is very dependent on a detailed and systematic evaluation of fetal cardiac structures. Given the size of the fetal heart and the fact that all structures within are moving continuously and rapidly, recognition of fetal cardiac defects is among the most challenging of all aspects of fetal ultrasound. It should be acknowledged that not all fetal cardiac defects will be recognized even when the scan is done by an experienced observer. Conversely, it should be noted that the more inexperienced the observer, the more likely a cardiac defect will be missed. The sensitivity of ultra-

sound diagnosis of fetal cardiac abnormalities has been reported to range from 70% to 85% (Davis et al., 1990; Achiron et al., 1992; Bromley et al., 1992). The sensitivity of ultrasound detection of cardiac defects varies according to three factors: the index of suspicion, the gestational age at examination, and the magnitude and character of the defect.

1. *The index of suspicion* (Table 20-6): Risk factors that should enhance the index of suspicion include a family history of cardiac defects (the risk of recurrence with one previously affected infant is 5% and with two previously affected infants is 10%) (Allan et al., 1986), an increased risk of aneuploidy (as may be indicated by nuchal lucency measurements, abnormal maternal serum screening), maternal age, diabetes, autoimmune collagen diseases, exposure to drugs (such as lithium, aminopterin, and alcohol), and various viral infections, including rubella and mumps.

2. *The gestational age at examination:* As a general principle, the older the fetus at the time of ultrasound evaluation, the higher the detection rate of structural cardiac defects. A four-chamber view of the fetal heart (the minimal diagnostic view) can be obtained as early as 10 to 12 weeks' gestation using high-resolution transvaginal ultrasound (Bronshtein et al., 1991), but for all practical purposes the sensitivity curve for detection remains close to zero until about the middle of the second trimester and then accelerates thereafter. The detection rate is improved not only because with advancing age the heart structures are larger and more echo defined, but

TABLE 20-6. INDICATIONS FOR DETAILED FETAL ECHOCARDIOGRAPHIC EXAMINATION

Fetal Risk Factors

    Extracardiac anomalies
        Chromosomal
        Anatomic
    Fetal cardiac dysrhythmia
        Irregular rhythm
        Tachycardia (+200 beats/min)
        Bradycardia (nonperiodic)
    Nonimmune hydrops fetalis
    Suspected cardiac anomaly on level I scan
    Abnormal fetal situs

Maternal Risk Factors

    Congenital heart disease
    Cardiac teratogen exposure
        Lithium carbonate
        Alcohol
        Anticonvulsants
            Phenytoin
            Trimethadione
        Isoretinoin
    Maternal metabolic disorders
        Diabetes mellitus
        Phenylketonuria

Familial Risk Factors

    Congenital heart disease
        Previous sibling
        Paternal
    Syndromes
        Marfan
        Noonan
        Tuberous sclerosis

also because some cardiac anomalies evolve and in so doing become more evident. Hypoplastic ventricle syndrome is the classic example of an evolving anomaly. In early gestation (before 16 weeks) the hypoplastic ventricle may appear completely normal or even slightly larger than normal. As the hyperplasia evolves, the ventricle shrinks in size, becomes echo dense, and ultimately appears as a nonfunctional slit-like cavity with an echo-dense intimal lining (endocardial fibroelastosis).

3. *The magnitude and character of the defect:* The detection of a cardiac defect will vary according to the defect. The more severe defects, including hypoplastic ventricle, univentricular heart, severe outflow tract obstructions, and major endocardial cushion, are among the most easily recognized and most commonly diagnosed. In contrast, relatively common defects such as ventricular septal defects (both membranous and muscular), atrial septal defects, coarctation, supravalvular stenosis (usually aortic stenosis), and tetralogy of Fallot are very frequently missed, even with a high-quality scan done by an experienced operator. The detection of ventricular septal defect may be particularly difficult. In a series of over 7000 fetuses examined routinely at 18 weeks' gestation, Tegander and coworkers (1995) reported that the detection rate of ventricular septal defect (53 cases in total) was 0%. In contrast, in a focused study of cardiac defects among 1022 fetuses from 18 weeks to term, Copel and coworkers (1987) identified 71 of 74 fetuses (96%) with a major structural defect.

ULTRASOUND EXAMINATION OF THE FETAL HEART: TECHNICAL CONSIDERATIONS

The ultrasound examination of the fetal heart may be divided in two separate aspects. The fetal heart is first identified and a general evaluation done noting the size of the heart relative to the thoracic cavity, the position of the apex of the heart, the general symmetry of the four chambers, the rate, the subjective contractility of the ventricles, the appearance of any echogenic foci or distorting structures within the chambers, the presence of fluid within the pericardium, and the presence of other effusions and skin edema (suggestive of cardiac failure). The specific and detailed examination of the fetal heart is based on rotation of the ultrasound images around the long axis, the coronal axis, and the transverse axis of the heart and a longitudinal (sagittal) view of the ascending aorta and aortic arch. The specific views required to achieve maximal discrimination are the four-chamber view (coronal view; Fig. 20-25), the long axis (sagittal) view of the left and subsequently the right ventricle (Fig. 20-26), and the aortic outflow tract (Fig. 20-27). These views can be obtained in most fetuses, although occasionally a fetus may remain in a spine-up position, straddling the maternal spine and obscuring the four-chamber view. In such instances it is usually necessary to bring the patient back at a later time to evaluate the fetal heart. Maternal abdominal wall obesity can obscure the fetal cardiac anatomy. Intracardiac Doppler flow velocity measurement, color Doppler flow mapping, and power Doppler analysis, although of considerable value in evaluating the postnatal heart and circulation, have been of minimal value in assessing the fetal heart. There is no convincing evidence to date that the addition of these Doppler-based parameters have enhanced the sensitivity of ultrasound for detection of structural cardiac defects. Similarly the use of M-mode ultrasound is of limited value in the evaluation of the fetal heart structure and function.

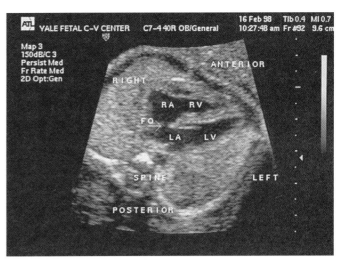

FIGURE 20-25 ■ Four-chamber view of the fetal heart at 24 weeks of gestation. The fetal left atrium (LA) is the structure that is closest to the fetal spine. The right atrium (RA) is anterior to it, and the foramen ovale (FO) is visible in the atrial septum. The two fetal ventricles (LV, RV) are relatively equal in size, although the interventricular septum appears to bow slightly to the left, suggesting volume overload of the fetal right ventricle. In this view the inflow portion of the interventricular septum is visualized, and the integrity of the atrioventricular septum can be examined. The two atrioventricular valves are well seen. The septal leaflet of the tricuspid valve is inserted slightly farther toward the cardiac apex than is the anterior leaflet of the mitral valve. The pulmonary veins can be seen entering the left atrium, giving it an irregular shape. The apical aspect of the right ventricle appears foreshortened as a result of the moderator band. The coarse trabeculation of the right ventricular septum and the apical insertion of the tricuspid valve identify the right ventricle.

SPECIFIC CARDIAC ANOMALIES

Atrial septal and *ventricular septal defects* are among the most common cardiac defects. Ostium primum atrial defects are the most common form of atrial septal defect (Allan, 1998). These defects occur close to the endocardial cushion. Large ostium premium atrial septal defects are also known as endocardial cushion defects or atrioventricular canal defects. These defects have a strong association with chromosomal abnormalities. It is estimated that 50% of fetuses with an endocardial cushion defect will have a chromosomal abnormality of which the most common are trisomy 21 (60%) and trisomy 18 (25%) (Machado et al., 1988). The prognosis for perinates with endocardial cushion defects is generally poor even among those with normal karyotype (Machado et al., 1988). Ostium secundum atrial defects occur in the region of the foramen ovale. These lesions are usually isolated and are generally insignificant in fetal and early neonatal life but may be a cause of pulmonary hypertension in adult life. Ventricular septal defects may affect either the muscular or membranous portion of the septum (or both). These defects are notoriously hard to detect *in utero*. They have no functional significance and are only important to recognize as markers of other fetal anomalies. At least 25% of ventricular septal defects will close spontaneously, often *in utero*.

Ventricular hypoplasia accounts for approximately 10% of all fetal cardiac defects. The left ventricle is most commonly affected, possibly as a consequence of critical aortic stenosis. Left ventricular hypoplasia evolves *in utero*: Ventricle size is initially normal or even slightly dilated, progressing to a

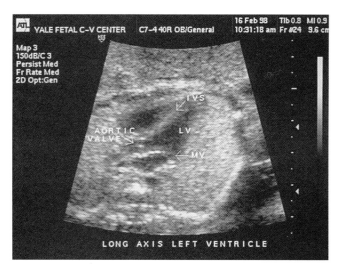

FIGURE 20-26 ■ Normal long-axis (sagittal) view of the left ventricular outflow tract in a 24-week fetus. In this view the interventricular septum (IVS) is in continuity with the anterior wall of the aorta. This view provides appreciation of the integrity of the anterior aspect of the interventricular septum. The aorta is completely committed to the left ventricle (LV). In addition, the mitral valve (MV) is seen separating the left atrium from the left ventricle.

thickened ventricular wall with obliteration of the ventricular cavity. In end-stage disease the ventricle is small and non-motile. The perinatal prognosis of hypoplastic left ventricle is exceedingly poor. In a study of 11 fetuses diagnosed and followed, 4 died *in utero* and 5 died within the 1st week of neonatal life (Blake et al., 1991). Staged surgical repair of hypoplastic left ventricle (Norwood procedure) is possible in the relatively few newborns who survive the critical transition from fetal to adult circulation: The 5-year survival in these infants is reported to be about 60% (Kern et al., 1997). *In utero* correction of the critical aortic stenosis has been attempted as a corrective measure to halt the progression of fetal disease (Allan et al., 1995), but the results have been poor and the procedure abandoned.

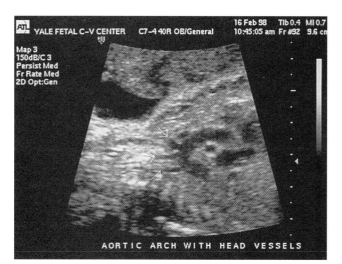

FIGURE 20-27 ■ Normal aortic arch view in a 24-week fetus. The three head vessels (*arrows*) are indicated. The fetal head is to the left, and the legs are to the right in this image.

Tetralogy of Fallot accounts for about 10% of all fetal cardiac defects. This lesion is not easily or reliably recognized by ultrasound. The salient features are the relatively large right ventricle, the large ventricular septal defect, and the large aortic orifice. Recognition of an overriding of the aorta in the fetus is not always possible. The prognosis of tetralogy of Fallot is generally good but will vary according to associated anomalies. Tetralogy of Fallot is associated with trisomy 13, 18, and 21; with microdeletion of chromosome 22q; and with DiGeorge syndrome, CHARGE, and the complex of vertebral defects, anal atresia, tracheoesophageal fistula with esophageal atresia, and radial and renal anomalies.

Transposition of the great vessels accounts for about 10% of all fetal cardiac defects. In the complete (noncorrected) version of this defect, the aorta arises from the right ventricle and the pulmonary artery arises from the left ventricle. The salient ultrasound feature is seen in the outflow tracts where the normal association of the pulmonary artery and the aorta is not seen, cross-over does not occur, and the two outflow tracts run parallel. Postnatal surgical repair of transposition of the great vessels is possible, and the prognosis is generally good.

Coarctation of the aorta accounts for about 8% of cases of congenital heart disease. Coarctation commonly presents and evolves as a postnatal event but can occur in fetal life (Allan et al., 1988). The salient ultrasound features in the fetus are an enlarged right ventricle, enlarged pulmonary outflow tract, and a visible narrowing of the aorta. Other cardiac defects are commonly associated with aortic coarctation (90%), and other organ system anomalies occur in about 15% of perinates with coarctation. The association between coarctation and Turner syndrome (XO) is well recognized. About 10% of all perinates with Turner syndrome will have coarctation of the aorta.

Ebstein anomaly is a relatively rare fetal cardiac anomaly characterized by a large right ventricle, downward migration of the tricuspid valve, a large ventricular septal defect, and often visible tricuspid regurgitation. The fetal prognosis with Ebstein anomaly is poor and about one third of all affected fetuses will die *in utero*. Long-term postnatal survival with Ebstein anomaly is rare (Celermajer et al., 1994).

Rare cardiac anomalies include *double-outlet right ventricle* (an anomaly associated with maternal lithium exposure), cardiac tumors such as *rhabdomyoma* (associated with tuberous sclerosis), and *pulmonary stenosis* and *anomalous venous return* (prenatal diagnosis not possible).

Abnormalities of the Gastrointestinal Tract

The fetal stomach, small and large bowel, liver, pancreas, and spleen are usually easily visualized. Because the fetal gastrointestinal tract normally contains fluid (swallowed amniotic fluid and local secretion), obstructive disorders are characterized by proximal dilatation creating echolucent masses. Persistent absence of stomach fluid, particularly when associated with hydramnios, strongly suggests esophageal atresia. Occlusion of the pylorus of the stomach, which is rarely observed *in utero*, results in a distended stomach and associated hydramnios. Duodenal atresia is the most common congenital gastrointestinal obstruction and results in the dilatation of the proximal duodenum and the antrum of the fetal stomach (prepyloric region); these areas of dilatation result in the classic "double-bubble" sign of duodenal atresia (Fig. 20-28).

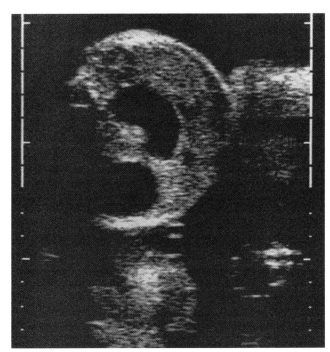

FIGURE 20-28 ■ Transverse view of the fetal abdomen exhibiting the classic "double-bubble" sign of proximal gut (duodenal) atresia. The two echolucent masses represent the dilated fluid-filled stomach and the dilated fluid-filled duodenum proximal to the atretic obstruction. Note the associated hydramnios, an almost uniform finding. Trisomy 21 is commonly associated with duodenal atresia.

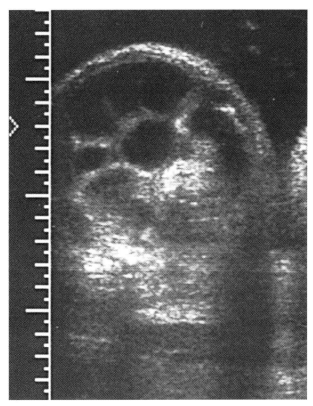

FIGURE 20-29 ■ Transverse view of the fetal abdomen in a fetus with distal ileal atresia. Note the multiple loops of dilated small bowel. During real-time ultrasound scanning hyperperistaltic activity in most of the dilated bowel loops was observed.

Because duodenal atresia is frequently associated with trisomy 21 (30% of cases), fetal karyotype determination is indicated when this lesion is detected. Jejunal or ileal atresia produces proximal dilatation, which appears as multiple echolucent areas (Fig. 20-29). Using dynamic ultrasound imaging, one can observe marked preobstruction peristalsis. Large-bowel obstruction rarely produces proximal dilatation, although this occasionally occurs with anal atresia. Large-bowel rupture due to meconium ileus is reported, producing complex echolucent abdominal mass with multiple scattered echogenic lesions (calcified meconium) (Brugman et al., 1979). Increased second-trimester bowel echogenicity has been associated with a significant risk of aneuploidy; the differential diagnosis should also include cystic fibrosis (Scioscia et al., 1992) (Fig. 20-30).

Anterior abdominal wall defects generally fall into one of two diagnostic categories. *Omphalocele* is an exaggerated umbilical hernia in which fetal liver and frequently fetal bowel extrude (Fig. 20-31). The omphalocele sac (peritoneum) is usually visible. Associated defects are common, and about 30% of cases involve an abnormal karyotype, usually trisomy 13. Hence, fetal karyotype determination is indicated. The diagnosis of omphalocele may be confirmed from as early as 12 weeks' gestation by transvaginal scan (Fig. 20-32).

Pentalogy of Cantrell is characterized by a midline high (epigastric) omphalocele, defect in the lower sternum, absence of the anterior portion of the diaphragm, absent diaphragmatic pericardium, and major cardia defects, usually large ventricular septal defect. The prognosis with this syndrome is exceedingly poor.

Gastroschisis is a rupture of the upper anterior abdominal wall, invariably on the right side, with extrusion of intestines but rarely fetal liver. Because the defect is not covered with peritoneum, the fetal intestine floats freely and may be scattered within the amniotic cavity (Fig. 20-33). Gastroschisis is not associated with an increased risk of karyotype anomaly.

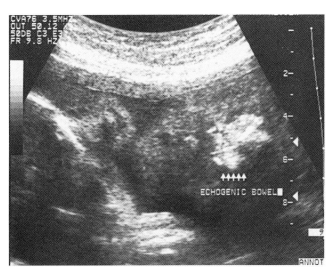

FIGURE 20-30 ■ A transverse scan of the abdomen in a 19-week fetus demonstrating intense echogenicity of the small bowel. The bowel echogenicity is comparable with that of bone.

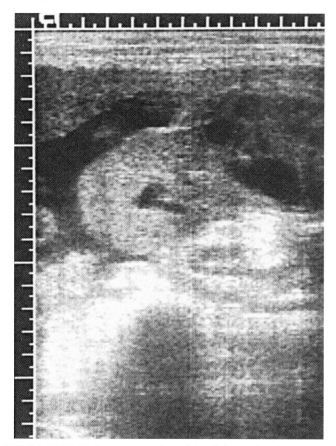

FIGURE 20-31 ■ A transverse view of the abdomen in a 28-week fetus with omphalocele. Note the protrusion of the fetal liver through the hernial sac. The karyotype of this fetus was normal.

Nonimmune hydrops is characterized by ascites, pleural and pericardial effusion, and generalized and often massive subcutaneous edema. The fetal prognosis varies with the underlying cause (Romero et al., 1986; Warsof et al., 1986). Nonimmune hydrops is always a diagnosis of exclusion and is considered after an immune etiology has been ruled out. Ultrasound-guided cordocentesis (percutaneous fetal blood sampling) is indicated in most cases of nonimmune hydrops for both diag-

nostic and therapeutic purposes. Fetal parvovirus type B viral infection is a relatively common cause of nonimmune hydrops (18% of cases) and can often be successfully treated by fetal intravascular transfusion.

Abnormalities of the Genitourinary Tract

The genitourinary tract, including the fetal kidney, ureter, and bladder (Fig. 20-34), is readily assessed by conventional ultrasound examination. Abnormalities of the genitourinary tract may be broadly classified as *primary renal dysgenesis* of variable type and severity and as *obstructive disorders*. Ultrasound diagnosis of fetal renal disease is subject to error (Avni et al., 1985).

Renal dysgenesis presents as a spectrum of disorders that may affect one or both kidneys. The most severe variant of dysgenesis, it is usually bilateral, characterized by absence of recognizable renal tissue, absent fetal bladder, extreme oligohydramnios, and lethal pulmonary hypoplasia. Oligohydramnios is invariably present after 16 weeks' gestation.

The diagnosis of renal dysgenesis is usually problematic because oligohydramnios makes visualization of the renal fossa difficult and adrenal tissue may be confused with renal tissue. Serial evaluation over a 4- to 6-hour period to confirm absence of urine production, as evidenced by failure to visualize the fetal bladder, may be extremely useful in establishing the certainty of the diagnosis. Because fetal urine production is subject to diurnal variation, observation for less than 3 hours may produce false-positive results (Chamberlain et al., 1984a).

In late gestation, the differential diagnosis of severe oligohydramnios and reduced fetal size is either severe IUGR or renal agenesis. Because the perinatal prognosis and appropriate management are radically different, establishing the correct diagnosis with certainty requires considerable effort. Such determination may include ultrasound assessment by different examiners on different occasions. Less severe renal dysgenesis may present as unilateral (common) or bilateral (uncommon) *multicystic dysplasia* (Fig. 20-35). Such lesions are characterized by increase in renal volume, distortion of renal architecture, multiple irregularly sized echolucent renal cysts, and areas of increased echogenicity and calcification. Bilateral disease may

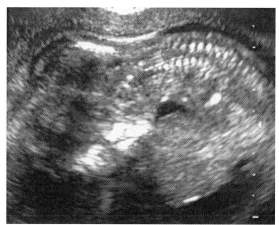
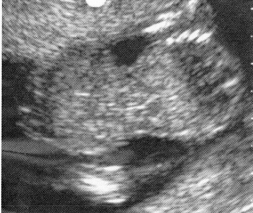

FIGURE 20-32 ■ Fetal omphalocele, diagnosed by transvaginal sonography at 13 weeks of gestation. Note the protrusion of the fetal liver through the hernial sac. (Courtesy of Dr. Timor, Columbia Presbyterian Hospital, New York.)

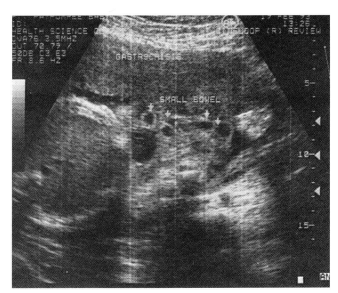

FIGURE 20-33 ■ Gastroschisis in a third-trimester fetus. Multiple loops of dilated small bowel float freely in the amniotic fluid. The fetal liver is within the fetal abdomen. By real-time image, bowel peristalsis appeared diminished in this fetus.

be associated with oligohydramnios and is invariably fatal. Unilateral disease is associated with normal amniotic fluid volume, evidence of contralateral renal function (bladder filling), and a favorable prognosis. Multicystic dysplastic disease must be differentiated from simple obstructive disorders. "Finnish" renal dysgenesis (infantile polycystic kidneys) is characterized by massive enlargement of both kidneys and a general increase in echogenicity (Fig. 20-36) (Hobbins et al., 1979; Romero et al., 1984). Oligohydramnios is commonly but not invariably present. The condition is uniformly fatal.

Congenital urinary tract obstruction may occur at several sites. The most common site of obstruction is the ureteropelvic junction, producing renal pelvis dilatation (pyelectasis) in milder cases and renal calyceal dilatation (hydronephrosis)

with more severe obstruction (Fig. 20-37). The lesion is usually but not invariably bilateral and is associated with normal fetal urine production and normal amniotic fluid volume. Most often, the disease is slowly progressive, and early delivery usually is not indicated. A pediatric urologist should assess the newborn. Minor bilateral dilatation of the renal pelvis has been associated with trisomy 21, although the association is weak and as an isolated finding is not an indication for amniocentesis to determine fetal karyotype.

Outlet tract obstruction may be caused by posterior urethral valve syndrome (male fetus), urethral atresia, or persistent cloacal syndrome. Outlet production produces megalocystis, hydroureter, and hydronephrosis. Oligohydramnios is common but not invariable. Pulmonary hypoplasia is a common associated finding. Posterior urethral valve syndrome may be recognized by observing dilatation of the proximal urethra (Fig. 20-38). Persistent outlet obstruction, particularly when caused by posterior urethral valve syndrome, may be an indication for *in utero* diversion therapy (Manning et al., 1986). *In utero* vesicoamniotic shunts should be reserved for those patients with isolated bladder outlet obstruction and normal renal function as manifest in a fresh fetal urine sample by a sodium of less than 100 mEq/liter ("salt saving"), an osmolality of less than 240 mOsm ("ability to concentrate"), and a β_2-microglobulin of less than 2 mg/liter (absence of tubular damage).

Anomalies of the Musculoskeletal System

As with all organ system anomalies, those of the musculoskeletal system are manifested as functional, structural, or combined lesions. Accordingly, a skeletal survey should include assessment of long bones, extremities, and digits and determination of normal functional activities. Abnormalities of the calvarium, face, spine, and thoracic cage frequently occur in conjunction with limb abnormalities.

Individual long bones are assessed for presence, length, proportion, shape, calcification, and epiphyseal and metaphyseal structure. As with most anomalies, the detail of examination is

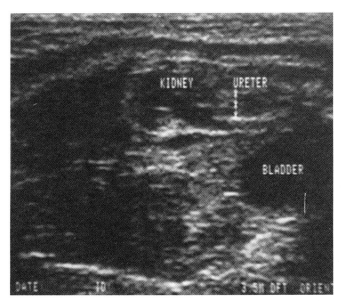

FIGURE 20-34 ■ Coronal view of the fetal abdomen demonstrating a normal left kidney and ureter and a normal bladder.

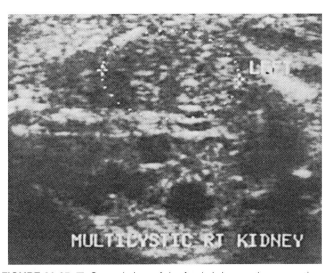

FIGURE 20-35 ■ Coronal view of the fetal abdomen demonstrating a normal left kidney and a markedly enlarged multicystic right kidney. Note the very irregular outline of the right kidney and the presence of coarse cysts and areas of increased echogenicity. At surgery (neonatal), the multicystic dysplastic right kidney was removed.

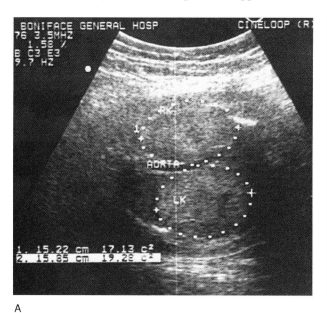

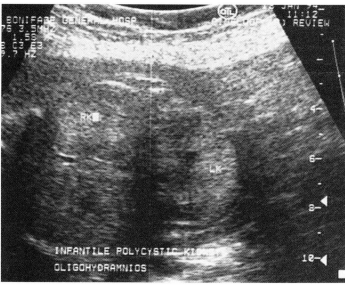

A   B

FIGURE 20-36 ■ **A,** Coronal view of the abdomen in a fetus with infantile polycystic kidneys. The massively enlarged echolucent kidneys appear to fill up most of the abdominal cavity. **B,** Transverse scan of the abdomen in the same fetus. Again, note kidney size and increased echogenicity. RK, right kidney; LK, left kidney.

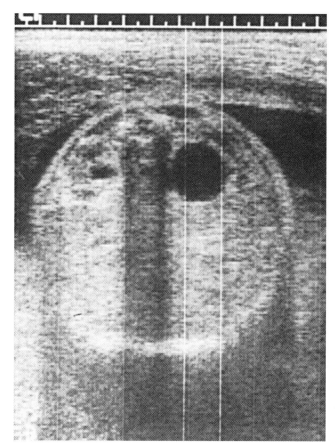

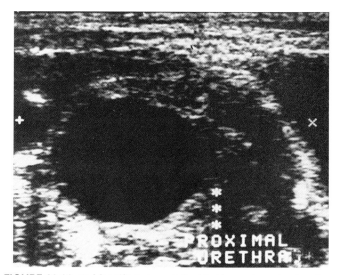

a function of the index of suspicion (as when there has been a previously affected child).

The *skeletal dysplasias*, also called *short-limb dystrophies*, are a complex group of anomalies with varying morphometric characteristics and prognosis. The diagnosis of skeletal dysplasia is based on objective morphometric data pertaining to limb length and growth and subjective assessment of shape, density, and proportion. Nomograms for individual bone length and growth have been published (Jeanty, Kirkpatrick, et al., 1981).

Thanatophoric dysplasia presents as extreme shortening of limbs, thoracic cage deformity (with associated pulmonary hypoplasia), and relative cephalomegaly (Hobbins and Mahoney, 1985; McGuire et al., 1987). Although the mortal-

FIGURE 20-37 ■ Severe bilateral ureteropelvic obstruction at 31 weeks of gestation. Note the asymmetrical dilatation of renal pelvis (greatest on the left) and the less pronounced dilatation of calyces. Amniotic fluid volume is normal.

FIGURE 20-38 ■ Magnified view of the bladder and proximal urethra in a fetus with posterior urethral valves. Note the dilatation of the proximal urethra and the absence of visualization of the distal urethra. The bladder wall is thickened and relatively echogenic.

ity associated with this condition is high, long-term survival with normal intelligence with this condition is possible. Associated anomalies include micrognathia and cleft palate.

Camptomelic dysplasia is characterized by limb reduction and extreme bowing of the long bones. Although the prognosis varies, perinatal death is usual. *Diastrophic dysplasia*, an autosomal recessive condition, involves severe limb shortening and frequently radical displacement of the thumbs (Hobbins and Mahoney, 1985).

Osteogenesis imperfecta is a spectrum of disease, ranging from mild camptomelia (bowing) to extreme demineralization, fracture, and short limbs (Chervenak et al., 1982). Spontaneous intrauterine fracture, indicated by displacement of bone elements and seen most often in the ribs, is diagnostic of a severe form of the disease. Long bone growth may be normal in early pregnancy, and abnormalities may not be evident until the mid to late second trimester.

Achondroplasia presents as short limbs with marked flaring and enlargement of the metaphyses. *Chondroectodermal dysplasia* (Ellis-van Creveld syndrome) is part of an anomalad including cranial anomalies, limb shortening, chest deformity, and frequently polydactyly.

Hypophosphatasia is characterized by short-limb dystrophy and often extreme demineralization of the long bones. Absence of long bones occurs with the *TAR syndrome* (thrombocytopenia and absent radius) and with forms of syringomyelia and phocomelia.

The fetal extremities may be visualized with some clarity; such evaluation offers insight into the presence of both localized and generalized anomalies. Abnormal fixed flexor position of the fetal fingers is a near-universal finding in fetuses with trisomy 18 (Fig. 20-39). Malrotation and malflexion of the feet (equinovalgus or equinovarus) may be diagnosed *in utero*. With subtle deformity, prolonged or repeated observation is necessary to avoid the false-positive result. Soft tissue edema of the feet may be recognized and is associated with a variety of chromosomal abnormalities, including trisomy 13 and trisomy 18, and with Turner syndrome and its variants. Multiple extreme flexion deformities typical of arthrogryposis multiplex congenita may be visible. In such cases, complete absence of normal flexion and extension motion of the limb is typical.

Functional abnormalities characterized by either excessive abnormal limb motion or absence of motion may be visible. Fetal tonic-clonic seizure disorders have been observed, associated with severe degenerative central nervous system disease, with spontaneous fetal intracerebral hemorrhage, and with opiate withdrawal. Hypomotility and hypotonia or paresis may be observed with primary anterior horn cell diseases, such as Werdnig-Hoffmann syndrome, and with severe myotonic dystrophy. Recognition of abnormal muscle group wasting or hypertrophy, both of which are typical of some muscular dystrophies and muscle glycogen storage disease, may theoretically be of clinical value.

Ultrasound Assessment of the Fetal Environment

Evaluation of the fetal environment (including amniotic fluid volume, umbilical cord structure, blood flow, fetal position, and placental morphology and site) is an integral part of ultrasound fetal assessment, shedding light on the presence of, or potential for, fetal disease.

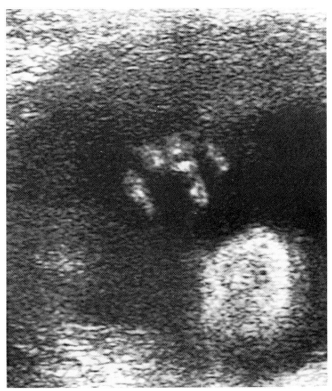
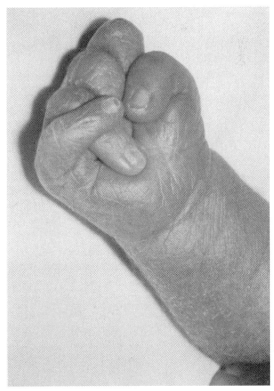

A   B

FIGURE 20-39 ■ A, An abnormal fetal hand (*right*). Flexion of the fourth finger was sustained throughout this and subsequent scans. **B,** Hand of the perinate at delivery. Again, note the abnormal flexion of the fourth finger. A diagnosis of trisomy 18 was confirmed in this child.

TABLE 20-7. CAUSES OF POLYHYDRAMNIOS IN 102 PREGNANCIES

Diagnosis	No.	%
Idiopathic	68	67
Anomalies	13	13
Gestational and insulin-dependent diabetes	15	15
Twins	5	5

Adapted from Hill LM, Breckle R, Thomas ML, et al: Polyhydramnios: Ultrasonically detected prevalence and neonatal outcome. Obstet Gynecol **69**:21, 1987. Reprinted with permission from the American College of Obstetricians and Gynecologists.

Amniotic Fluid Volume

Clinicians have long recognized that abnormalities of amniotic fluid volume, either excessive or diminished, are associated with impending fetal disorders (Chamberlain et al., 1984c) (Tables 20-7 and 20-8). The amniotic fluid is readily displayed with ultrasound, and it is therefore possible to assess adequacy of volume. The volume of amniotic fluid may be judged by either subjective or objective methods; in experienced hands, both methods yield comparable rates of predictive accuracy. By definition, the criteria for subjective assessment are difficult to categorize but include, in the case of oligohydramnios, the absence of fluid pockets throughout the uterine cavity, the impression of crowding of fetal small parts, and in severe cases the overlapping of the fetal ribs (Fig. 20-40). In the case of hydramnios, the criteria include multiple large pockets greater than 12 cm in vertical axis, the impression of the floating fetus, and free movement of the fetal limbs (Fig. 20-41). Objective determination of amniotic fluid volume is based on identification of the largest pocket of fluid and measurement of the vertical diameter. The objective method is subject to error owing to variation in pocket size created by fetal movement. Accordingly, it is of real value only in detecting the extremes of fluid volume distribution and variation within the normal range.

Two methods are reported for determination of amniotic fluid volume. The first is a measurement of the single largest pocket on a general scan of the uterus. It is initially performed to identify the presence and distribution of amniotic fluid; then the largest pocket is identified and the vertical depth is measured. Amniotic fluid is described as "decreased" if the largest single pocket is less than 2 cm.

The alternative method is the amniotic fluid index. The uterus is divided arbitrarily into four equal quadrants, and the vertical depth of the largest pocket in each quadrant is measured; these results are summed and expressed in millimeters (Rutherford et al., 1987). The normal limits for the amniotic fluid index per week of gestational age have been published (Table 20-9). In this method, amniotic fluid volume is described as normal if the summed value is greater than 80 mm and less than 180 mm. The single-pocket method and the amniotic fluid index are largely comparable in terms of predictive accuracy, and the method used in any given center is a matter of personal preference (Fig. 20-42).

In using the objective method to determine oligohydramnios, one must avoid confusing approximated loops of cord with fluid pockets. Occasionally, amniotic fluid of extreme turbidity can suggest oligohydramnios (Fig. 20-43); one can avoid this error by noting the characteristics of the umbilical cord and vessels. In day-to-day practice, subjective and objective methods of assessment of fluid volume may be used interchangeably. For reporting purposes, the objective method is preferred because it is less subject to interobserver variability.

The risk of adverse perinatal outcome is increased in pregnancies associated with hydramnios (Hill et al., 1987a) and oligohydramnios (see Table 20-8). Perinatal mortality shows a bimodal distribution, with values for the largest pocket of fluid increasing when the fluid pocket is greater than 8 cm or is 2 cm or less (Fig. 20-44). The selection of the end point for intervention for oligohydramnios in the structurally normal fetus should probably be set at less than 2 cm.

Oligohydramnios (fluid pocket less than 2 cm; amniotic fluid index less than 80 mm) is in general related to one of three conditions: rupture of membranes, congenital absence of functioning renal tissue or obstructive uropathy, or diminished renal perfusion with a resultant chronic reduction in fetal urine production, a consequence of hypoxemia-induced redistribution of fetal cardiac output. The presence of oligohydramnios in the fetus with intact membranes and a functional genitourinary tract usually signals significant fetal compromise and, in the fetus capable of extrauterine survival, an indication for prompt delivery. Aggressive management of oligohydramnios has been associated with a sharp fall in the corrected perinatal mortality rate (Bastide et al., 1986). The most common high-risk factors associated with oligohydramnios are post-term gestation and IUGR (Manning et al., 1981; Chamberlain et al., 1984b). The management and outcome of post-term gestation are sharply altered by amniotic fluid volume monitoring (Johnson et al., 1986). The relationship between oligohydramnios and IUGR is less

TABLE 20-8. THE RELATIONSHIP OF AMNIOTIC FLUID POCKET TO PERINATAL OUTCOME

Largest Pocket of Amniotic Fluid	No. of Patients	% Total	Gross PNM	Corrected PNM	% Major Anomaly	% IUGR (<10th)	% Macrosomia (>90th)
>8 cm	243	3.2	32.9	4.12	4.3	3.8	33.3
2–8 cm	7096	93.8	4.65	1.97	0.54	4.9	8.7
1–2 cm	159	2.1	56.6	37.8	2.52	20.0	—
<1 cm	64	0.85	187.7	109.4	9.37	38.6	—

IUGR, intrauterine growth restriction: PNM, perinatal mortality.

From Chamberlain PF, Manning FA, Morrison I, et al: Ultrasound evaluation of amniotic fluid volume. I. The relationship of marginal and decreased amniotic fluid volumes to perinatal outcome. Am J Obstet Gynecol **150**:245, 1984.

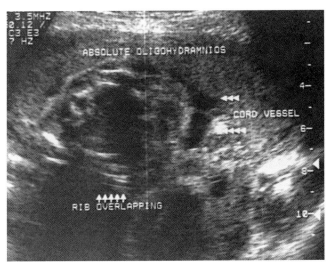

FIGURE 20-40 ■ Sonogram of a fetus with near absolute oligohydramnios. In this fetus, no cord-free pockets of amniotic fluid could be identified, and the only echolucent spaces within the amniotic cavity were created by bunched-up loops of cord. Note the overlapping of the fetal ribs. On real-time scanning, the fetal limbs were observed to move. Extension of the arms and legs was not seen.

clear. However, the presence of oligohydramnios in a fetus with suspected growth failure is a powerful indicator of underlying asymmetrical IUGR.

The quality of amniotic fluid may be assessed by ultrasound. Turbidity created by vernix, debris, meconium, and intrauterine bleeding may be visible, and occasionally the fluid appears opaque (see Fig. 20-43). Meconium cannot be reliably identified by ultrasound assessment. In one study, amniotic fluid turbidity (free-floating particles) was noted to indicate a mature lecithin-to-sphingomyelin (L/S) ratio (Gross et al., 1985). This association cannot be reliable because debris may be visible as early as 14 weeks' gestation. Prospective studies have also been unable to confirm this association (Helewa et al., 1989). Chapter 3 provides more details on amniotic fluid physiology.

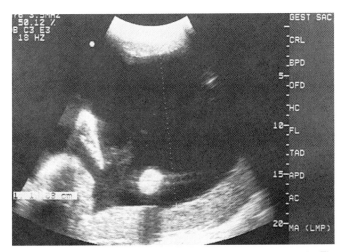

FIGURE 20-41 ■ Hydramnios in a fetus with esophageal atresia. The largest pocket of amniotic fluid, as measured in this image, was 19.88 cm. The hydramnios in this case was treated by serial reduction amniocentesis. The child was delivered at 35 weeks and survived.

TABLE 20-9. AMNIOTIC FLUID INDEX PERCENTILE VALUES (mm)

| Week | \multicolumn{5}{c}{Percentile} | N |
	2.5	5	50	95	97.5	
16	73	79	121	185	201	32
17	77	83	127	194	211	26
18	80	87	133	202	220	17
19	83	90	137	207	225	14
20	86	93	141	212	230	25
21	88	95	143	214	233	14
22	89	97	145	216	235	14
23	90	98	146	218	237	14
24	90	98	147	219	238	23
25	89	97	147	221	240	12
26	89	97	147	223	242	11
27	85	95	156	226	245	17
28	86	94	146	228	249	25
29	84	92	145	231	254	12
30	82	90	145	234	258	17
31	79	88	144	238	263	26
32	77	86	144	242	269	25
33	74	83	143	245	274	30
34	72	81	142	248	278	31
35	70	79	140	249	279	27
36	68	77	138	249	279	39
37	66	75	135	244	275	36
38	65	73	132	239	269	27
39	64	72	127	226	255	12
40	63	71	123	214	240	64
41	63	70	116	194	216	162
42	63	69	110	175	192	30

From Moore TR, Cayle JE: The amniotic fluid index in normal pregnancy. Am J Obstet Gynecol **162**:1168, 1990.

Assessment of the Umbilical Cord

The umbilical cord may be assessed in its entirety. The number of vessels may be determined (Fig. 20-45), the presence of cord knotting (Fig. 20-46), or entwining in monoamniotic twins (Fig. 20-47) noted, and cystic and degenerative lesions identified (Hill et al., 1987b). The absence of normal cord twisting has been reported to be associated with increased perinatal morbidity and mortality. Recognition of cord presentation is now possible, making prevention of cord prolapse possible in select cases (Lange and Manning, 1985).

Evaluation of the Placenta

The placenta can first be clearly recognized on ultrasonography between 14 and 16 weeks' gestation. Before this time, it is usually possible to identify the site of placental implantation, which is characterized by a thickened portion of the intrauterine cavity. However, clear discrimination of the placental edge from adjacent thickened decidua is difficult.

Normally, the implantation site is in the region of the fundus, with an approximately equal anteroposterior distribution. In early gestation (less than 16 weeks), a low implantation site is associated with increased early fetal loss, although the association is by no means absolute. With

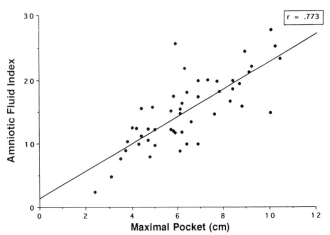

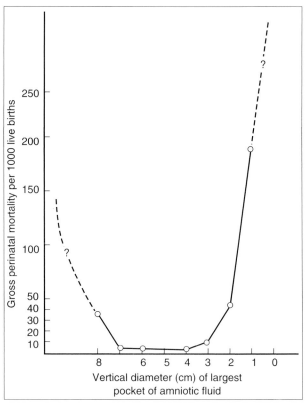

FIGURE 20-42 ■ Correlation between the amniotic fluid index and the largest pocket method for determination of adequacy of amniotic fluid volume. Either method may be used clinically. (From Croom CS, Barias BB, Ramos-Santos E, et al: Do semi-quantitative amniotic fluid indexes reflect actual outcome? Am J Obstet Gynecol **167**:995, 1992.)

advancing gestation, it becomes progressively easier to define the limits of the placenta and to evaluate its structural characteristics.

Definition of the lower edge of the placenta in relation to the internal os is important in establishing the diagnosis of placenta previa. The use of transvaginal scanning has greatly improved the diagnosis of placental previa, and this is now the imaging method of choice. The procedure is safe, provided the

FIGURE 20-44 ■ Relationship between perinatal mortality rate and the largest pocket of amniotic fluid as measured before delivery in 9760 high-risk patients.

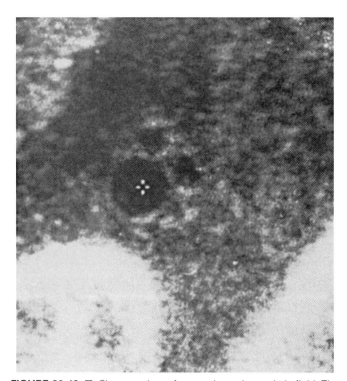

FIGURE 20-43 ■ Close-up view of very echogenic amniotic fluid. The fetal umbilical cord and vessels (echolucent) are outlined. It is possible to confuse very echogenic amniotic fluid with oligohydramnios. With serial scan, the echogenic amniotic fluid may suddenly become echolucent. The explanation for this phenomenon is unknown, but it may be caused by precipitation of amniotic fluid debris or blood.

transducer is introduced slowly into the vagina and is not inserted deep enough to contact the cervix directly. Evaluation of placental position and structural characteristics provides useful information in the management of the high-risk patient. The umbilical vein at its placental origin may be easily recognized by ultrasonography (Fig. 20-48); this is the usual target site for cordocentesis (percutaneous fetal blood sampling).

Placenta accreta is a dangerous obstetric condition in which placental villi invade beyond the decidua basalis. The depth of the invasion may be superficial (accreta), may penetrate deep into the myometrium (increta), or may penetrate through the uterus to involve the serosa and contiguous structures (bladder, small bowel, omentum). The risk factors, diagnosis, and management of this abnormal placentation are discussed in detail in Chapter 37.

DEVELOPMENTAL ANOMALIES OF THE PLACENTA

In about 35% of all mature placentas, cystic spaces called *placental cavities* occur (Fig. 20-49) (Fujikura and Sho, 1997). These cystic spaces, which are usually multiple, are characterized by the absence of blood flow within as determined by Doppler ultrasound evaluation. Placental cavities are not known to be associated with an increase in perinatal morbidity or mortality.

Chorioangiomas develop within the placenta. They may be multiple or single and may become very large. As a rule, this degenerative disorder is of no clinical significance. Large vascular channels are common within the normal placenta and may be confused with placental cysts. The vascular channel

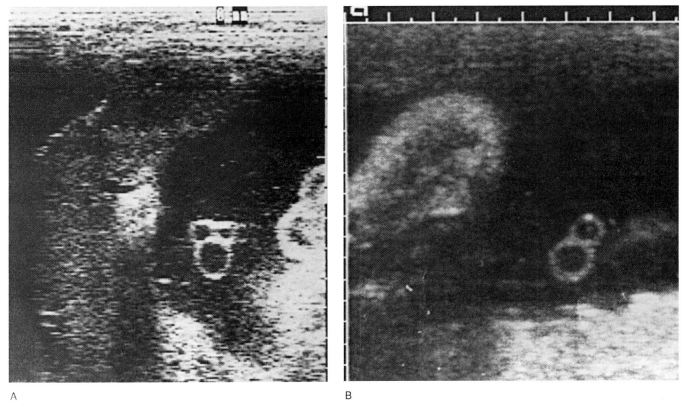

A   B

FIGURE 20-45 ■ **A,** Transverse scan of a normal umbilical cord demonstrating three vessels. The single umbilical vein has a diameter of nearly twice that of each artery. **B,** Transverse scan of the umbilical cord demonstrating a single umbilical artery. The single artery is larger in diameter than that observed within the two-artery cord.

usually represents large fetal veins coursing over the fetal surface of the placenta, and Doppler scanning usually reveals a flow pattern within this vessel. Longitudinal scanning of the area confirms that the cystic areas represent vascular channels. Amniotic bands may also be identified.

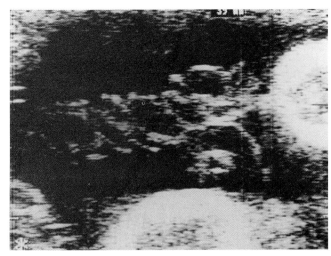

FIGURE 20-46 ■ Sonogram of a true cord knot. The umbilical arteries and vein at the level of the knot create a widening of the cord. The finding of a cord knot was an incidental discovery in this fetus and was confirmed at delivery. This perinate was delivered by elective cesarean section.

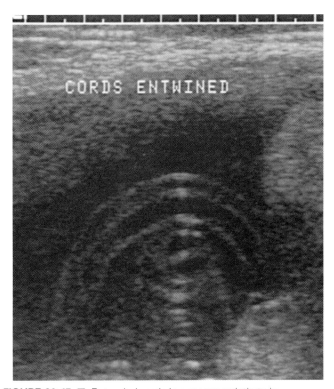

FIGURE 20-47 ■ Entangled cords in a monoamniotic twin pregnancy. The umbilical cord of one twin wraps around the cord of the other twin. At delivery (by cesarean section), the cords were completely entangled and four loose cord knots were present.

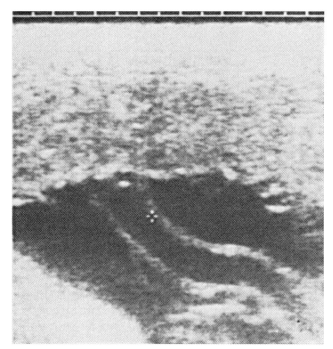

FIGURE 20-48 ■ The fetal umbilical vein at its placental insertion. This is the usual and preferred site for ultrasound-guided fetal blood sampling and for intravascular transfusion.

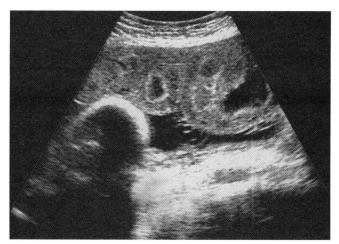

FIGURE 20-49 ■ Sonogram of the placenta demonstrating multiple echolucent cavities. Increased echogenicity is present around each cavity. Placental lucencies are relatively common and do not appear to be associated with increased fetal risk.

failure to observe fetal heart motion with adequate thoracic visualization indicates fetal demise. As gestation advances, the fetal cardiac motion becomes easier to detect. Dynamic ultrasound scanning is the primary method for establishing the diagnosis of fetal death, and ancillary methods (e.g., radiography for *Spalding sign* and intravascular gas) are of less

GRADING OF PLACENTAL MATURITY

Grannum and colleagues (1979) reported a method of categorizing ultrasonographic characteristics of the maturing placenta. This method was based primarily on the identification and distribution of calcium deposits within the fetal component of placenta (Fig. 20-50). In their preliminary report, these authors noted a relationship between advancing placental grade and fetal pulmonary maturity, so that in the 23 patients with placental maturity grade III, the incidence of a mature L/S ratio (more than 2.0) was 100%. In 28 patients with grade II placental maturity, the incidence of a mature L/S ratio was 87.5%, and in 21 patients with grade I maturity, the incidence of a mature L/S ratio was 67.7%. The authors postulated that the observation of grade III placenta could lead to fewer amniocenteses and hence could reduce infant risk.

In an expanded series of 314 patients, Harman and associates (1982) noted similar relationships but also observed that 3 of 84 patients (3.4%) with grade III placenta had immature phospholipid profiles (L/S ratio less than 2, phosphatidyl glycerol absent). In these patients, addition of BPD was not useful in reducing false-positive results. These data suggest that placental grading alone may not be accurate enough to predict pulmonary maturity and eliminate the need for amniocentesis. Because of its limited clinical value, placental grading is rarely performed and reported in contemporary obstetric ultrasonography.

Confirmation of Fetal Death

Dynamic ultrasound imaging methods can provide an absolute diagnosis of death *in utero*. Fetal heart motion can be identified routinely from 8 weeks' gestation onward, and

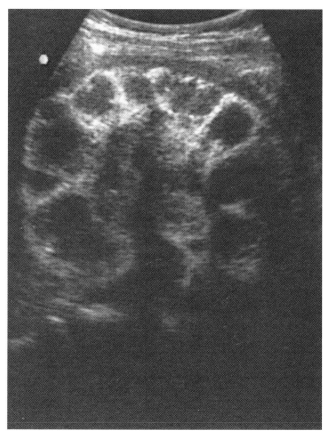

FIGURE 20-50 ■ A grade III placenta at term (Grannum criteria). Calcium accumulation at the periphery of individual cotyledons produces a ring-like structure.

value. When the fetus has been dead for 2 or more days, fetal scalp edema (maceration) and overlap of cranial bones become visible. The inexperienced observer should be cautious, however, because transmitted maternal pulsation can produce fetal heart structure motion, leading to an incorrect diagnosis of fetal bradycardia.

Determination of Fetal Lie, Position, and Attitude

Ultrasound imaging of the fetus allows the physician to determine fetal lie with certainty and to evaluate fetal position and attitude. Breech presentation is easily recognized, and one can identify the type of breech presentation with detailed scanning.

Use of Ultrasound Scanning in Multiple Gestation

Multiple fetuses occur in up to 1% of all pregnancies and are associated with a disproportionately high rate of perinatal morbidity. Ultrasound scanning is an extremely reliable method for detection of multiple pregnancies and should result in a false-negative rate approaching zero.

Although recognition of the presence of a multiple gestation is the first and key diagnostic step, it is also essential to attempt to define the type of multiple gestation. Whereas the risk of fetal and maternal complications is increased with all types of twinning, the fetal risks are greatest for monozygous twins. One can estimate the type of multiple gestation by assessing placental number, fetal gender, and the presence or absence of a separating membrane as well as its thickness. The diagnosis of dizygotic twins can be confirmed with almost complete certainty when the fetuses are of different sex. Only ultrasonography can confirm a diagnosis of monoamniotic twins, the typical findings being the inability to demonstrate a membrane on repeated scans and the observation of cord entanglement. Aggressive management of monoamniotic twins is strongly recommended, because the mortality rate for this condition exceeds 50%. Successful outcome with monoamniotic twinning diagnosed by antenatal ultrasound examination has been reported (Sutter et al., 1986).

Twin gestation may be detected by ultrasonography as early as 6 to 8 weeks' gestation and with reliability by 8 to 12 weeks. Detection is based on identification of two or more separate gestational sacs or fetuses. Interestingly, early detection of twins leads to a false-positive diagnostic rate of 60% to 70%. In our experience, only one third of patients in whom a diagnosis of multiple fetuses is made before 20 weeks' gestation subsequently deliver more than one infant. This observation confirms the very high fetal wastage associated with multiple gestation. In early gestation (before 20 weeks), death of one twin is associated with gradual resorption of both twin and gestation sac. These changes can be monitored by ultrasonography. Death of a twin fetus in late gestation is characterized by gradual decrease in fetal size and increasing echodensity; the latter phenomenon is likely a result of loss of tissue fluid and to fetal compression.

From approximately 16 weeks onward, the fused amnions in diamniotic twins are clearly visible, particularly with a dynamic ultrasound method. Differentiation of the placentas in dichorionic twins is difficult except in late gestation. Early

indices of gestational age (gestational sac volume, crown-rump length) are as accurate in multiple gestation as in singleton pregnancy. Similarly, in nondiscordant twins, BPD and abdominal circumference measurements are reliable indices of gestational age and weight. The BPD becomes less reliable after 28 to 30 weeks' gestation in twin pregnancies.

Ultrasound monitoring of fetal growth and well-being is an important part of management of the twin gestation. Discordance of growth complicates up to 30% of all twin gestations and is a major cause of fetal death and neonatal morbidity and mortality. Detection of discordant twins is relatively simple by ultrasound methods. At each visit, fetal weight is calculated from abdominal circumference measurements, head growth is determined by BPD measurement, and qualitative amniotic fluid volume is determined for each twin. In addition, biophysical profile scoring is performed for each twin. When discordance is defined as a birth-weight difference of at least 30%, this approach detects in excess of 95% of all cases. When discordance is detected, amniocentesis of the larger twin is indicated and delivery may be considered if pulmonary maturity has been reached. See Chapters 4 and 29 for a detailed discussion of multiple gestation.

Fetal Sex Determination

In the active fetus, one can visualize the perineum and external genitalia and therefore assign fetal phenotypic sex. External genitalia may be differentiated from as early as 16 weeks' gestation and reliably from about 22 weeks onward. The diagnosis of the male fetus is direct, by notation of the penis and scrotum (Fig. 20-51). The characteristic undulating movement of the scrotum with fetal limb motion makes confusion with a loop of umbilical cord highly unlikely. The diagnosis of female sex may be confirmed either directly or by

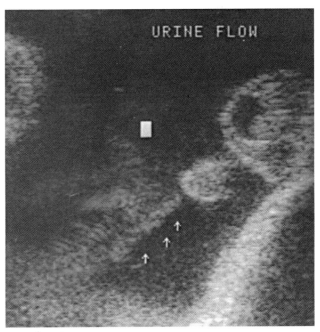

FIGURE 20-51 ■ Penis and scrotum in a normal male fetus. This sonogram was taken during fetal micturition, and a stream of fetal urine can be seen. The echolucency within the fetal scrotum is a small hydrocele, a normal finding in the fetus.

exclusion (i.e., failure to identify the male genitalia). The latter method may lead to error if the male genitalia are flattened between the buttocks. Because an error in the assignment of fetal sex may result in considerable consternation, the diagnosis should be withheld unless certain.

Ultrasound Assessment of the Cervix

The cervix may be visualized by either transabdominal or transvaginal scanning techniques, the latter being the method of choice. An ultrasound assessment of the cervix provides an objective method for determining cervical length (Fig. 20-52) and the shape of the internal os during and after uterine contractions. The relationship between cervical length and the risk of premature delivery has been a subject of active ongoing research.

In their landmark study, Iams and associates (1996) confirmed that the risk of preterm delivery was directly proportional to the measured cervical length (Fig. 20-53). Ultrasound cervical length measurement is at least equal to and probably superior to clinical assessment of cervical length and consistency (see Chapter 34).

The value of ultrasound measurement of cervical length in the prevention of preterm birth has not been established, almost certainly because of the lack of effective long-term tocolytic agents. Combining cervical length measurement with biochemical markers of impending preterm labor, such as assay of fetal fibronectin in vaginal secretions (Pearceman et al., 1997), holds promise as a highly precise method to stratify individual patient risk for preterm delivery. However, random-

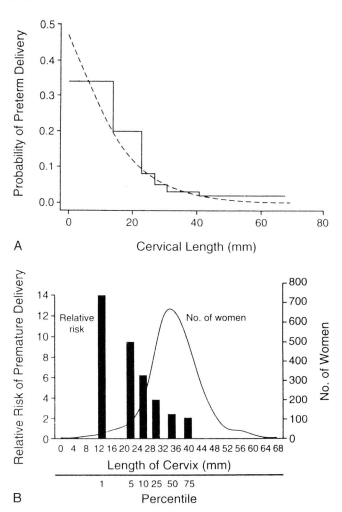

A, The observed probability (rate) of preterm delivery (less than 35 weeks of gestation) according to cervical length measured by transvaginal ultrasound at 24 weeks. **B,** The relation of distribution of cervical length measurement and relative risk of preterm delivery. (From Iams JD, Goldenberg RL, Meis PJ, et al: The length of the cervix and the risk of spontaneous premature delivery. Reprinted from N Engl J Med **34**:567, 1996.)

ized clinical trials of the efficacy of cervical cerclage based on selection by ultrasound evidence of cervical shortening or dilation have not shown any evidence of prolonged gestations or improved perinatal survival (Rust et al., 2000).

REFERENCES

Achiron R, Galseer J, Gelnernter I, et al: Extended fetal echocardiography examination for detecting cardiac malformations in low risk pregnancies. Br Med J **304**:671, 1992.

Adzick NS, Harrison MR, Crombleholme TM, et al: Fetal lung lesions: Management and outcome. Am J Obstet Gynecol **179**:884, 1998.

Allan LD: Fetal echocardiography. Clin Obstet Gynecol **31**:61, 1998.

Allan LD, Chita SK, Anderson RH, et al: Coarctation of the aorta in prenatal life: An echocardiography, anatomy and functional study. Br Heart J **59**:539, 1988.

Allan LD, Crawford DC, Chita SK, et al: Familial recurrence of congenital heart disease in a prospective series of mothers referred for echocardiography. Am J Cardiol **58**:334, 1986.

Allan LD, Maxwell DJ, Carminiti M, et al: Survival after fetal balloon valvoplasty. Ultrasound Obstet Gynecol **5**:90, 1995.

Arduini D, Rizzo G, Romanini C, et al: Fetal blood flow velocity waveforms as predictors of growth retardation. Obstet Gynecol **70**:7, 1987.

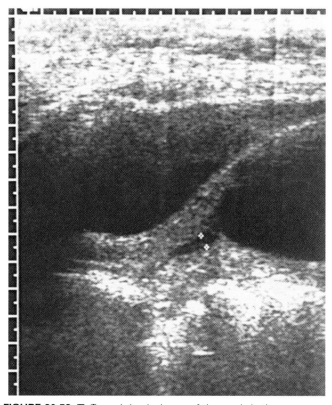

FIGURE 20-52 ■ Transabdominal scan of the cervix in the longitudinal plane. The internal os is dilated 4.8 mm; cervical length is 35 mm.

Avni EF, Rodesch F, Schulman CC: Fetal uropathies: Diagnostic pitfalls and management. J Urol **134**:921, 1985.

Bastide A, Manning FA, Harman CR, et al: Ultrasound evaluation of amniotic fluid: Outcome of pregnancies with severe oligohydramnios. Am J Obstet Gynecol **154**:895, 1986.

Beattie RB, Dornan JC: Antenatal screening for fetal growth retardation with umbilical artery Doppler ultrasonography. Br Med J **298**:631, 1989.

Benacerraf BR, Adzick NS: Fetal diaphragmatic hernia: Ultrasound diagnosis and clinical outcome in 19 cases. Am J Obstet Gynecol **156**:573, 1987.

Benacerraf BR, Frigoletto FD: Mid-trimester fetal thoracentesis. J Clin Ultrasound **13**:202, 1985.

Benedetti TJ, Gabbe SG: Shoulder dystocia: A complication of fetal macrosomia and prolonged second stage of labour with midpelvic delivery. Obstet Gynecol **52**:526, 1978.

Birnholz JC: The fetal external ear. Radiology **1417**:819, 1983.

Blake DM, Copel JA, Kleinman CS: Hypoplastic left ventricle syndrome: Prenatal diagnosis, clinical profile and management. Am J Obstet Gynecol **165**:529, 1991.

Bloom SL, Bloom DD, Dellanebbia C, et al: The development outcome of children with mild isolated ventriculomegaly. Obstet Gynecol **90**:93, 1997.

Braithwaite JM, Armstrong MA, Economides DL: Assessment of fetal anatomy at 12–13 weeks' gestation by transabdominal and transvaginal sonography. Br J Obstet Gynaecol **103**:82, 1996.

Bromley B, Estroff JA, Sanders SP, et al: Fetal echocardiography: accuracy and limitations in a population at high-risk and low-risk for heart defects. Am J Obstet Gynecol **166**:1473, 1992.

Bromley B, Nadel AS, Pauker S, et al: Closure of the cerebellar vermis: Evaluation in the second trimester. Radiology **153**:761, 1994.

Bronshtein M, Weiner Z: Early sonographic diagnosis of alobar holoprosencephaly. Prenat Diagn **11**:459, 1991.

Bronshtein M, Zimmer EZ, Milo S, et al: Fetal cardiac abnormalities detected by transvaginal sonography at 12–16 weeks' gestation. Obstet Gynecol **78**:374, 1991.

Brown MS, Sheridan-Periera M: Outlook for a child with a cephalocoele. Pediatrics **90**:914, 1992.

Brugman SM, Jjelland JJ, Thomasson JE, et al: Sonographic findings with radiologic correlation in meconium peritonitis. J Clin Ultrasound **7**:306, 1979.

Bruner J, Tulipan N, Reed G, et al: Intrauterine repair of spina bifida: Preoperative predictors of shunt dependent hydrocephalus. Am J Obstet Gynecol **185** (Suppl):S28, 2001.

Campbell S: The assessment of fetal growth by diagnostic ultrasound. Clin Perinatol **1**:507, 1974.

Campbell S: Ultrasound measurement of the fetal head to abdomen circumference ratio in assessment of growth retardation. Br J Obstet Gynaecol **84**:165, 1977.

Campbell S, Wilkin P: Ultrasonic measurement of fetal abdominal circumference in the estimation of fetal weight. Br J Obstet Gynaecol **82**:689, 1975.

Celermajer DS, Bull C, Till JA, et al: Ebstein's anomaly: Presentation and outcome from fetus to adult. J Am Coll Cardiol **23**:170, 1994.

Chamberlain PF, Manning FA, Morrison I, et al: Circadian rhythm in bladder volumes in the term human fetus. Obstet Gynecol **64**:657, 1984a.

Chamberlain PF, Manning FA, Morrison I, et al: Ultrasound evaluation of amniotic fluid volume. I. The relationship of marginal and decreased amniotic fluid volumes to perinatal outcome. Am J Obstet Gynecol **150**:245, 1984b.

Chamberlain PF, Manning FA, Morrison I, et al: Ultrasound evaluation of amniotic fluid volume. II. The relationship of increased amniotic fluid volume to perinatal outcome. Am J Obstet Gynecol **150**:250, 1984c.

Chervenak FA: Fetal cystic hygroma: Etiology and natural history. N Engl J Med **309**:822, 1983.

Chervenak FA, Berkowitz RL, Tontora M, et al: The management of fetal hydrocephalus. Am J Obstet Gynecol **155**:933, 1985.

Chervenak FA, Romero RR, Berkowitz RL, et al: Antenatal sonographic findings of osteogenesis imperfecta. Am J Obstet Gynecol **143**:228, 1982.

Chinn DH, Bolding DB, Callen PW, et al: Ultrasonographic identification of fetal lower extremity epiphyseal ossification centers. Radiology **147**:815, 1983.

Chitty S, Campbell S, Altman DG: Measurement of the fetal mandible—feasibility and construction of a centile chart. Prenat Diagn **13**:749, 1993.

Cohen B, Penning S, Major C, et al: Sonographic prediction of shoulder dystocia in infants of diabetic mothers. Obstet Gynecol **88**:10, 1996.

Copel JA, Pilu G, Green J, et al: Fetal echocardiography screening for congenital heart disease. The importance of the four-chamber view. Am J Obstet Gynecol **158**:409, 1987.

Crane JP, LeFevre ML, Winborn RC, et al: A randomized trial of prenatal ultrasonographic screening: Impact on the detection, management, and outcome of anomalous fetuses. Am J Obstet Gynecol **171**:392, 1994.

Davis GK, Farquhar CM, Allan LD, et al: Structural cardiac abnormalities in the fetus: Reliability of prenatal diagnosis and outcome. Br J Obstet Gynaecol **97**:27, 1990.

Delepa EH, Mueller-Heubach E: Pregnancy outcome following ultrasound diagnosis of macrosomia. Obstet Gynecol **78**:340, 1991.

Divon MY, Chamberlain PF, Sipos L, et al: Identification of the small for gestational age fetus with the use of gestational age-independent indices of fetal growth. Am J Obstet Gynecol **155**:1197, 1986.

Donald I, Mac Vicar J, Brown TG: Investigation of abdominal masses by abdominal ultrasound. Lancet **1**:1188, 1958.

Dudley NJ, Chapman E: The importance of quality management in fetal measurement. Ultrasound Obstet Gynecol **19**:190, 2002.

Edmonds PD: Interactions of Ultrasound and Biological Tissues. U.S. Department of Health, Education, and Welfare (DHEW) Publications (FDA) 73-8008. Washington, DC, U.S. Food and Drug Administration, 1972.

Elliott JP, Garite TJ, Freeman RJ, et al: Ultrasound prediction of fetal macrosomia in diabetic pregnancies. Obstet Gynecol **60**:159, 1982.

Ewigman B, Corneilson S, Horman D, et al: Use of routine prenatal ultrasound by private practice obstetricians in Iowa. J Ultrasound Med **10**:427, 1991.

Ewigman B, Crane JP, Frigoletto FD, et al: Effect of prenatal ultrasound screening on perinatal outcome. N Engl J Med **329**:821, 1993.

Fazekas IG, Kosa F: Forensic Fetal Osteology. Budapest, Akademia Kiado, 1978, p. 256.

Fujikura T, Sho S: Placental cavities. Obstet Gynecol **90**:112, 1997.

Goldstein I, Lockwood C, Hobbins JC: Ultrasound assessment of fetal intestinal development in the evaluation of gestational age. Presented at the Proceedings of the Society of Perinatologists and Obstetricians, 1987, Tampa, Florida.

Grannum PAT, Berkowitz RL, Hobbins JC: The ultrasonic changes in the maturing placenta and their relationship to fetal pulmonic maturity. Am J Obstet Gynecol **133**:915, 1979.

Grennert L, Persson P, Gerrser G, et al: Benefits of ultrasound screening of a pregnant population. Acta Obstet Gynaecol Scand **78** (Suppl):5, 1978.

Gross TL, Wolfson RN, Kuhnerol PM: Sonographically detected free floating particles in amniotic fluid predict a mature lecithin-sphingomyelin ratio. J Clin Ultrasound **13**:405, 1985.

Hadlock FP: Determination of fetal age. *In* Athey PA, Hadlock FP (eds): Ultrasound in Obstetrics and Gynecology. St. Louis, Mosby, 1985.

Hadlock FP, Deter RL, Harrist RB, et al: Fetal abdominal circumference: Relation to menstrual age. Am J Radiol **139**:367, 1982a.

Hadlock FP, Deter RL, Harrist RB, et al: Fetal biparietal diameter: A critical re-evaluation of the relation to menstrual age by means of real-time ultrasound. J Ultrasound Med **1**:97, 1982b.

Hadlock FP, Deter RL, Harrist RB, et al: A date-independent predictor of intrauterine growth retardation: Femur length/abdominal circumference ratio. Am J Radiol **141**:979, 1983a.

Hadlock FP, Deter RL, Harrist RB, et al: Computer assisted analysis of fetal age in the third trimester using multiple fetal growth parameters. J Clin Ultrasound **11**:313, 1983b.

Harman CR, Bowman JM, Manning FA, et al: Intrauterine transfusion—intraperitoneal versus intravascular approach: A case-control comparison. Am J Obstet Gynecol **162**:1053, 1990.

Harman CR, Manning FA, Stearns E, et al: The correlation of ultrasonic placental grading and fetal pulmonic maturation in 563 pregnancies. Am J Obstet Gynecol **143**:941, 1982.

Harrison MR, Adzick NS, Bullard K, et al: Correction of congenital diaphragmatic hernia in utero. VII. A prospective trial. J Pediatr Surg **31**:1637, 1997.

Helewa M, Manning FA, Harman CR, et al: Sonographic amniotic fluid free floating particles: Any relationship to fetal lung maturity. Obstet Gynecol **74**:893, 1989.

Hill LM, Breckle R, Thomas ML, et al: Polyhydramnios: Ultrasonically detected prevalence and neonatal outcome. Obstet Gynecol **69**:21, 1987a.

Hill LM, Kislak S, Runco P: An ultrasonic view of the umbilical cord. Obstet Gynecol Surv **42**:82, 1987b.

Hobbins JC, Grannum PAT, Berkowitz RL, et al: Ultrasound in the diagnosis of congenital anomalies. Am J Obstet Gynecol **134**:331, 1979.

Hobbins JC, Mahoney MJ: Skeletal dysplasias. *In* Sarden RC, James AM (eds): The Principles and Practice of Ultrasonography in Obstetrics and Gynecology. Norwalk, Conn, Appleton-Century-Crofts, 1985, p. 267.

Hoddick WK, Callen PW, Filly RA, et al: Ultrasonographic determination of qualitative amniotic fluid volume in intrauterine growth retardation: Reassessment of the 1 cm rule. Am J Obstet Gynecol 149:758, 1984.

Hoffman JIE, Christianson R: Congenital heart disease in a cohort of 19502 births with long-term follow-up. Am J Cardiol 42:641, 1978.

Hohler CW: Cross-checking pregnancy landmarks by ultrasound. Contemp Obstet Gynecol 20:169, 1982.

Iams JD, Goldenberg RL, Meis PJ, et al: The length of the cervix and the risk of spontaneous premature delivery. N Engl J Med 334:567, 1996.

Iams JD, Paraskos J, Landon MB, et al: Cervical sonography in preterm labor. Obstet Gynecol 84:40, 1994.

Jeanty P, Dramaix-Wilmet M, Delbeke D, et al: Ultrasonic evaluation of fetal ventricular growth. Neuroradiology 21:127, 1981.

Jeanty P, Dramaix-Wilmet M, Elkhazen N, et al: Measurement of fetal kidney growth on ultrasound. Radiology 144:159, 1982.

Jeanty P, Kirkpatrick C, Dramaix-Wilmet M, et al: Ultrasound evaluation of fetal limb growth. Radiology 140:165, 1981.

Johnson JM, Harman CR, Lange IR, et al: Biophysical profile scoring in the management of the post-term pregnancy: An analysis of 307 patients. Am J Obstet Gynecol 154:269, 1986.

Kern JH, Hayes CJ, Michler RC, et al: Survival and risk factors for analysis of the Norwood procedure for hypoplastic left ventricle syndrome. Am J Cardiol 80:170, 1997.

Kyle PM, Harman CR, Evans JA, et al: Life without amniocentesis: Elevated maternal serum alpha-fetoprotein (MSAFP) in the Manitoba program 1986–1991. J Ultrasound Obstet Gynecol 4:1,1994.

Lange IR, Manning FA: Antenatal diagnosis of congenital pleural effusions. Am J Obstet Gynecol 140:839, 1981.

Lange IR, Manning FA: Cord prolapse: Is antenatal diagnosis possible? Am J Obstet Gynecol 151:1083, 1985.

Laurence KM, Coates JS: The natural history of hydrocephalus: Detailed analysis of 182 unoperated cases. Arch Dis Child 37:345, 1962.

Laurence KM, Coates JS: Spontaneously arrested hydrocephalus: Results of the re-examination of 82 survivors from a series of 182 unoperated cases. Dev Med Child Neurol 13 (Suppl):4, 1967.

Lauria MR, Smith RS, Treadwell MC, et al: The use of second-trimester transvaginal sonography to predict placenta previa. Ultrasound Obstet Gynecol 8:337, 1996.

Lee W, Deter RL, Ebersole JD, et al: Birth weight prediction by three-dimensional ultrasonography: Fractional limb volume. J Ultrasound Med 20:1283, 2001.

Levine AB, Lockwood CJ, Brown B, et al: Sonographic diagnosis of the large for gestational age fetus at term: Does it make a difference? Obstet Gynecol 79:55, 1992.

Lipschitz R, Beck JM, Froman C: An assessment of the treatment of encephalomeningocoeles. East Afr Med J 43:609, 1969.

Low JA: The current status of maternal and fetal blood flow velocimetry. Trans Am Gynecol Obstet Soc 9:139, 1990.

Lubchenco LO, Searle DT, Brazie JV: Neonatal mortality rate: Relationship to birth weight of gestational age. J Pediatr 81:814, 1972.

Lyons EA, Dyke C, Cheang M: In utero exposure to diagnostic ultrasound: A six year follow-up. Radiology 166:687, 1988.

Machado MV, Crawford DC, Anderson RH, et al: Atrioventricular septal defect in prenatal life. Br Heart J 59:352, 1988.

Malone F, Ball RH, Nyberg DA, et al: First trimester cystic hygroma—a population based screening study (the Faster trial). Am J Obstet Gynecol 185 (Suppl):S99, 2002.

Manning FA: Aspects of fetal life. In Fetal Medicine: Principles and Practice. Norwalk, Conn, Appleton & Lange, 1995a, p 3.

Manning FA: Intrauterine growth retardation: Etiology, pathophysiology, diagnosis and treatment. In Fetal Medicine: Principles and Practice. Norwalk, Conn, Appleton & Lange, 1995b, p. 313.

Manning FA, Harrison MR, Rodick C: Catheter shunts for fetal hydronephrosis and hydrocephalus: Report of the International Fetal Surgery Registry. N Engl J Med 315:336, 1986.

Manning FA, Hill LM, Platt LD: Qualitative amniotic fluid volume determination by ultrasound: Antepartum detection of intrauterine growth retardation. Am J Obstet Gynecol 139:254, 1981.

Manning FA, Lange IR, Morrison I, et al: Calculation of fetal length in utero: An ultrasound method. Abstract presented at the Proceedings of the Society of Obstetricians and Gynecologists, June 1983a, Vancouver, British Columbia, Canada.

Manning FA, Lange IR, Morrison I, et al: Determination of fetal health: Methods for antepartum and intrapartum fetal assessment. Curr Probl Obstet Gynecol 7:1, 1983b.

Marden PM, Smith DW, McDonald MJ: Congenital anomalies in the newborn infant, including minor variations. J Pediatr 64:357, 1964.

Mayden KL, Tortora M, Berkowitz RL: Orbital diameters: A new parameter for prenatal diagnosis and dating. Am J Obstet Gynecol 144:289, 1982.

McCallum WD, Brinkley TF: Estimation of fetal weight from ultrasound measurement. Am J Obstet Gynecol 133:195, 1979.

McCullough DC, Balzer-Martin LA: Current prognosis in overt neonatal hydrocephalus. J Neurosurg 57:378, 1982.

McGuire J, Manning FA, Lange IR, et al: Antenatal diagnosis of skeletal dysplasia using ultrasound. Birth Defects 23:367, 1987.

Mealy J, Dzenitis AJ, Hockey AA: The prognosis of encephalocoeles. J Neurosurg 32:209, 1970.

Mercer BM, Sklar S, Shariatnadar A, et al: Fetal foot length as a predictor of gestational age. Am J Obstet Gynecol 156:350, 1987.

Mongelli M, Wilcox M, Gardosi J: Estimating the date of confinement: Ultrasonographic biometry versus certain menstrual dates. Am J Obstet Gynecol 174:278, 1996.

Morrison I, Olsen J: Weight specific stillbirth and associated causes of death: An analysis of 765 stillbirths. Am J Obstet Gynecol 152:975, 1985.

Nadel A, Bromberg B, Frigoletto F, et al: Isolated choroids plexus cyst in the second trimester—is amniocentesis really indicated? Radiology 185:545, 1992.

Nelson LH, Anderson SG, Perry MF: The wavering midline: A diagnostic sign of fetal hydrocephalus. Am J Obstet Gynecol 149:662, 1984.

Nicolaides KH, Gabbe SG, Guidetti R: Ultrasound screening for spina bifida: Cranial and cerebellar signs. Lancet 1:71, 1986.

Nicolaides KH, Salversen DR, Snijders RJM, et al: Fetal facial defects: associated malformations and chromosomal abnormalities. Fetal Diagn Ther 8:1, 1993.

Nijhuis JG, Prechtl HFR, Martin CB Jr, et al: Are there behavioural states in the human fetus? Early Hum Dev 6:177, 1982.

Nimrod C, Nicholson S, Davies D, et al: Pulmonary hypoplasia testing in clinical obstetrics. Am J Obstet Gynecol 158:277, 1988.

O'Brien GD, Queenan JT: Growth of the ultrasound fetal femur during normal pregnancy. Am J Obstet Gynecol 141:833, 1981.

Ofer G, Rosen DJD, Dolfin Z, et al: Induction of labor versus expectant, management: A randomized study. Obstet Gynecol 89:913, 1997.

Pandya PP, Snijders RJM, Johnson SP, et al: Screening for fetal trisomies by maternal age and fetal nuchal translucency thickness at 10 to 14 weeks' gestation. Br J Obstet Gynaecol 102:957, 1995.

Pearceman AM, Andrews WA, Thorp JM, et al: Fetal fibronectin as a predictor of preterm birth in patients with symptoms: A multicenter trial. Am J Obstet Gynecol 177:13, 1997.

Phillips HE, McGahan PP: Intrauterine fetal cystic hygromas: Sonographic detection. Am J Radiol 136:799, 1981.

Pilu G, Sandri F, Perolo A, et al: Sonography of agenesis of the corpus callosum: A survey of 35 cases. Ultrasound Obstet Gynecol 3:318, 1993.

Platt LD, Santulli T Jr, Carlson DE, et al: Three-dimensional ultrasound ultrasonography in obstetrics and gynecology: Preliminary experience. Am J Obstet Gynecol 178:119, 1998.

Robinson HP: Sonar measurement of fetal crown-rump length as a means of assessing maturity in the first trimester of pregnancy. Br Med J 4:28, 1973.

Rodeck CH, Fisk NM, Fraser DI, et al: Long term in utero drainage of fetal hydrothorax. N Engl J Med 319:1135, 1988.

Romero R, Copel J, Jeanty P, et al: Causes, diagnosis and management of non-immune hydrops. Clin Diagn Ultrasound, 19:31, 1986.

Romero R, Cullen M, Jeanty P: The diagnosis of congenital renal anomalies with ultrasound. II. Infantile polycystic kidney disease. Am J Obstet Gynecol 150:219, 1984.

Rottem S, Bronshtein M, Thaler I: First trimester transvaginal sonographic diagnosis of fetal anomalies. Lancet 1:444, 1989.

Rust O, Atlas R, Jones K, et al: A randomized trial of cerclage vs. no cerclage in patients with sonographically detected 2nd trimester premature dilatation of the internal os. Am J Obstet Gynecol 182:S13, 2000.

Rutherford SE, Phelan JP, Smith CV, et al: The four-quadrant assessment of amniotic fluid volume: An adjunct to antepartum fetal heart rate testing. Obstet Gynecol 70:353, 1987.

Saari-Kemppainen A, Karjalainen O, Ylostalo P, et al: Ultrasound screening and perinatal mortality: Controlled trial of systematic one-stage screening in pregnancy. Lancet 336:278, 1990.

Salversen KA, Vatter LJ, Eik-Ness SH, et al: Routine sonography in utero and subsequent handness and neurological development. BMJ 307:159, 1993.

Sandmire HF: Whither ultrasound prediction of macrosomia? Obstet Gynecol 82:860, 1993.

Scioscia AL, Pretorius DH, Budorick NE: Second trimester echogenic bowel and chromosomal abnormalities. Am J Obstet Gynecol **167:**889, 1992.

Shepard MJ, Richards VA, Berkowitz RL, et al: An evaluation of two equations for predicting fetal weight by ultrasound. Am J Obstet Gynecol **152:**47, 1982.

Sherer DM, Davis JM, Woods JR Jr: Hypoplasia: A review. Obstet Gynecol Surv **45:**792, 1990.

Simpson DA, David DJ, White J: Cephalocoeles: Treatment, outcome and antenatal diagnosis. Neurosurgery **15:**14, 1984.

Sutter JA, Arab H, Manning FA: Monoamniotic twins: Antenatal diagnosis and management. Am J Obstet Gynecol **155:**836, 1986.

Taylor M, David AS: Agenesis of the corpus callosum: a UK series of 56 cases. J Neurol Neurosurg Psychiatry **64:**131, 1998.

Tegander E, Eik-Nes SH, Johansen OJ, et al: Prenatal detection of heart defects at the routine fetal examination at 18 weeks in a non-selected population. Ultrasound Obstet Gynecol **5:**372, 1995.

Thompson TE, Manning FA, Morrison I: Determination of fetal volume *in utero* by an ultrasound method correlation with neonatal birth weight. J Ultrasound Med **2:**113, 1983.

Timor-Trisch IE, Boozajomehri F, Masakowski Y, et al: Can a "snapshot" sagittal view of the cervix by transvaginal ultrasonography predict active preterm labor? Am J Obstet Gynecol **174:**990, 1996.

Toi A, Simpson GF, Filly RA: Ultrasonically evident fetal nuchal skin thickening: Is it specific for Down's syndrome? Am J Obstet Gynecol **156:**150, 1987.

Tulipan N, Sutton LN, Bruner JP, et al: The effect of intrauterine myelomeningocele repair on the incidence of rhunt-dependent hydrocephalus. Pediat Neurosurg **38:**27, 2003.

U.S. Department of Health and Human Services: Diagnostic Ultrasound in Pregnancy. National Institutes of Health (NIH) Publication No. 84-667. Washington, DC, NIH, 1984.

Van Dorsten JP, Hulsey TC, Newman RB, et al: Fetal anomaly detection by second trimester ultrasonography in a tertiary center. Am J Obstet Gynecol **178:**742, 1998.

Vintzileos AM, Campbell WA, Weinbaum PJ, et al: Perinatal management and outcome of fetal ventriculomegaly. Obstet Gynecol **69:**5, 1987.

Wapner R for the BUN Group: First trimester aneuploid screening: Results of the NICHD Multicenter Study. Amer J Obstet Gynecol **185:**S70, 2001.

Warsof SL, Gohari P, Berkowitz RL, et al: The estimation of fetal weight by computer assisted analysis. Am J Obstet Gynecol **128:**881, 1977.

Warsof SL, Nicholades KH, Rodeck C: Immune and non-immune hydrops. Clin Obstet Gynecol **29:**533, 1986.

Wenstrom KD, Weiner CP, Hanson TW: A five-year statewide experience with congenital diaphragmatic hernia. Am J Obstet Gynecol **165:**838, 1991

Wong SF, Chan FY, Cincotta RB, et al: Sonographic estimation of fetal weight in macrosomic fetuses: Diabetic versus non-diabetic pregnancies. Aust N Z Obstet Gynecol **41:**429, 2001.

Youngblood JP: Should ultrasound be used routinely in pregnancy? J Fam Pract **29:**657, 1989.

Chapter 21

ASSESSMENT OF FETAL HEALTH

Christopher R. Harman, MD

Fetal status is the fulcrum for many perinatal decisions. If fetal evaluation is satisfactory and imminent critical change is unlikely, management may be confidently conservative, seeking further maturation. If fetal status is uncertain, management will depend on gestational age. Near term, delivery may be the best option; before then, enhanced surveillance and preparation for delivery is indicated; and remote from term, intrauterine therapy might be attempted. When serious fetal compromise is certain, the balance shifts to delivery and neonatal management—down to the frontiers of viability. Thus, what we do is determined by what we believe of fetal status.

Just as management pivots on fetal status, the monitoring process must vary with fetal and maternal condition. Because the fetal environment determines the acuity of our monitoring, risk assignment is a process of constant revision. Historical factors are important, but give way as more specific information becomes available from first- and second-trimester screening and the individual behavior of the subject fetus. Maternal conditions change as well, with advancing gestation, worsening disease, the impacts of maternal treatment, superimposed on changes in placental function and fetal demands, and monitoring must cope with these many complexities.

As the interlocutor between maternal-fetal status and clinical action, assessment of fetal well-being must meet many demands. These requirements, and the complex situations in which they must apply, dictate the prime directive of all fetal assessment: No single parameter can suffice. The aim of this chapter is to describe the integration of multiple components in a comprehensive approach to fetal assessment.

FETAL CONTEXT

The broad range of fetal activity provides many avenues for the evaluation of fetal status. We reliably equate the presence of normal behavior with normal healthy status. Beginning with pioneering work focused on fetal breathing (Dawes et al., 1970, 1972), it became clear that the absence of specific fetal behaviors could mean serious hypoxemia and/or acidosis (Boddy et al., 1974; Nijhuis et al., 1982; Bocking, Gagnon, White, et al., 1988). The number of parameters has multiplied, and their application has extended to progressively lower gestational ages. In a few cases, specific abnormal behavior is directly linked to abnormal fetal status (e.g., intrauterine fetal seizures), but the general pattern has endured for most variables: present = normal and absent = abnormal.

Normal Fetal Behavior

There are many changing patterns of normal human fetal behavior. These overlap and in some cases are influenced by maternal and placental factors, with the result that most fetal behaviors are episodic and irregular. A number of fetal behavioral characteristics must be understood to recognize the fetal context of monitoring.

Basic Functions

Even the most primary functions are subject to marked variability that conditions monitoring techniques and interpretation. Fetal heart rate (FHR) comes under increasing parasympathetic dominance as pregnancy progresses, resulting in a gradual decrease in heart rate, increase in variability, increasing responsiveness (accelerations and decelerations), and the emergence of complex relationships with other behaviors (Pillai and James, 1990b) Variability in basic functions is not restricted to neurologic interactions; as placental and fetal vascular systems mature, so do resistance characteristics, regionalization of blood flow, and cardiovascular reflexes (Van Eyck et al., 1985). In short, the interpretation of fetal vital functions requires detailed understanding of the fetal environment.

Individual Behaviors

Coordinated activity such as thumb-sucking, respiratory movements, and apparently deliberate changes in position begin very early. A large repertoire of fetal activities is already established by 10 to 12 weeks. These individual behaviors change throughout pregnancy, and their distribution may alter dramatically. For example, fetal hiccups are the most dominant form of early diaphragmatic activity, and these give way to sustained patterns of rhythmic fetal breathing movements (Pillai and James, 1990a). Fetal breathing movements, in turn, become much more responsive to maternal glucose levels, the emergence of behavioral states, and circadian rhythms and may even show patterns of carbon dioxide responsiveness identical to newborn infants as pregnancy progresses (Baier et al., 1990, 1992). Fetal movement demonstrates increasing sophistication with advancing gestation. The wriggling activity seen at 8 to 10 weeks gives way to the total body jumping activity that gradually diminishes as the second trimester begins. By that time, defined kicking, delicate hand movements, fetal breathing, and virtually all the individual behaviors of the term fetus can be demonstrated. The distribution of individual behaviors changes markedly over the remainder of pregnancy, including the often dramatic reduction in fetal kicking at 34 to 38 weeks with the onset of small-amplitude highly coordinated movements typical of infants. Chapter 14 addresses fetal breathing and body movements in greater detail.

Patterned Behavior

As individual behaviors change, so do their relationships with one another. In the first trimester, individual behaviors appear, to the virtual exclusion of others (e.g., the fetus almost never hiccups while moving). By 18 to 20 weeks, there are periods of high and low activity, during which many behaviors may appear simultaneously. Beginning at this time, diurnal patterns are evident in fetal urine production, adrenal steroid production, heart rate, Doppler arterial velocities, and virtually all complex behaviors (Patrick et al., 1980; Chamberlain et al., 1984a; Arduini et al., 1986).

Fetal Behavioral States

By the beginning of the third trimester, behavioral states 1F–4F can be defined (Pillai and James, 1990a; Martin, 1981; Nijhuis et al., 1982), which are directly analogous to the neonatal behavioral states originally described by Prechtl (1974). Two patterns dominate—quiet sleep and active sleep. In quiet sleep, state 1F, rapid eye movements and repetitive mouthing movements are present, but almost all other movements are absent. As term approaches, this level of inactivity extends, from a mean of about 220 seconds in midtrimester, to as long as 110 minutes by 40 weeks (Pillai and James, 1990a; de Vries et al., 1987). Clustering of movements during state 2F, active sleep, provides excellent opportunity for monitoring, because multiple activities overlap. In state 4F (active awake), the "jogging fetus" illustrates a high level of voluntary activity, and sustained high heart rate where return to baseline may be interpreted as decelerations. As with its neonatal equivalent, state 3F (quiet awake) is unusual and short and is seldom present before term. Clearly, fetal assessment using any or all of these variables must account for their complex presentation.

Coupled Behaviors

Several behavioral characteristics provide advantages for monitoring because they are coupled. The classic association of FHR accelerations with fetal movement, the basis of the non-stress test (NST), is so reliable that an acceleration of significant amplitude can be inferred to prove fetal activity (Lee et al., 1975). Fetal breathing movements and maternal glucose levels are reliably connected, so that fetal assessment units operate most efficiently in the 2 to 3 hours after each mealtime (Harman et al., 1999). Of course, fetal breathing movements produce effects in many other individual parameters (Fig. 21-1; Color Plates 3 and 4). Over the longer term,

the pairing of sleep and wake cycles may be the most reliable evidence available of normal fetal oxygen status (Arduini and Rizzo, 1990).

Fetal/Neonatal Transition

Evidence of true "infant" behavior in term fetuses is seen in many systems. Sometimes this responsiveness is problematic; even earlier than term, the fetal ductus arteriosus may begin to close with indomethacin exposure (de Vries et al., 1988). During behavioral state 4F, in addition to unusually vigorous activity, the "jogging fetus" coordinates combined facial and chest movements that can be seen clearly as "crying." During these short periods, at term it appears the fetus is actually awake. Finally, the fetus exposed to high concentrations of oxygen will initiate carbon dioxide–dependent breathing activity that includes deep inhalation/expiration movements, moving much more pulmonary fluid than in normal fetal breathing movement activity (Baier et al., 1992). This "true breathing" includes a series of cardiovascular changes similar to those of infancy, all of which may be reversed by allowing fetal oxygen levels to decline back to normal. These levels of responsiveness, including Doppler evaluation of flow changes, may provide detailed information about fetal maturity (de Vries et al., 1988).

Fetal Responses to Hypoxemia

Every tool for fetal evaluation relies on an association between altered fetal homeostasis and altered fetal behavior. Because fetal partial pressure of oxygen normally declines throughout gestation, many of these responses constitute normal adaptation. When abnormally decreased placental respiratory function occurs (typically illustrated by hypoxemia), these responses may be invoked permanently or temporarily in response to acute changes, chronic changes, or superimposed acute-on-chronic insults (Richardson, 1989). Thus, for each individual fetus, the circumstances of decline and the timing and proportion of compensation will be highly individualized (Rudolph, 1984; Bocking, Gagnon, Milne, et al., 1988). For the purposes of discussion, the phases of fetal compensation can be grouped conveniently into three categories: increase oxygen supply, control oxygen distribution, and reduce oxygen consumption.

1. *Increase oxygen supply.* Several temporary responses will increase oxygen availability. Although these produce the marginal increments necessary to respond to most incidental issues, they are unlikely to suffice in the case of placental insufficiency or marginal fetal status subject to the onset of labor. These include increase in baseline heart rate, increase in hemoglobin concentration, improved cardiac contractility/efficiency, and increased oxygen extraction (Richardson, 1989; Rurak et al., 1990). These steps are limited in capacity: Whereas mild intrauterine growth restriction (IUGR) features increased nucleated red cell liberation and a tendency toward polycythemia, more severe IUGR features even higher liberation of premature red cell forms but worsening anemia (Baschat et al., 1999). On the other hand, during "normal" situations of decreased oxygen (e.g., during contractions in term labor), increased oxygen extraction may contribute up to 14% additional oxygen on a virtually instantaneous basis (Rurak et al., 1987).

2. *Control oxygen distribution.* The distribution of blood flow results in preservation of oxygenation in vital centers of the brain, heart, adrenals, and placenta, with corresponding reduction to mesenteric, renal, and distal aortic outflow tracts (Sheldon et al., 1979; Baschat, Gembruch, Reiss, et al., 2000). The resulting differences in perfusion will lead to differential growth rates and asymmetrical IUGR and will have long-term implications far beyond fetal and neonatal health. Many of these hemodynamic adaptations can be depicted on serial Doppler evaluation of placental and fetal systemic circulations (see later), which occur before acute changes in other fetal

behaviors. Thus, "brain-sparing" depiction of increased brain flow in the face of rising placental vascular resistance may signal shunting of blood away from somatic arterial beds (Baschat et al., 2001). "Heart-sparing" dilatation of the fetal coronary arteries appears to be a much later hemodynamic change, associated with marked placental insufficiency (Baschat, Gembruch, Gortner, et al., 2000). The onset of these hemodynamic responses may be very subtle, including minor shifts in the cortical proportion of renal blood flow or slight reductions in gut perfusion. Progressive redistribution, up until cardiac decompensation, is an effective means of rationing the limited/declin-

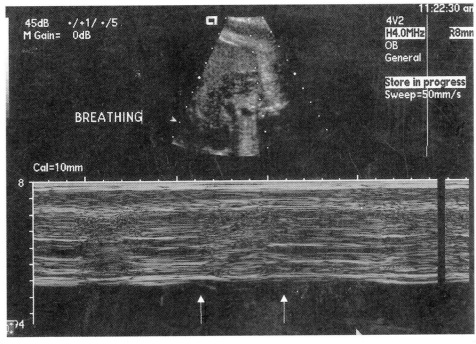

A

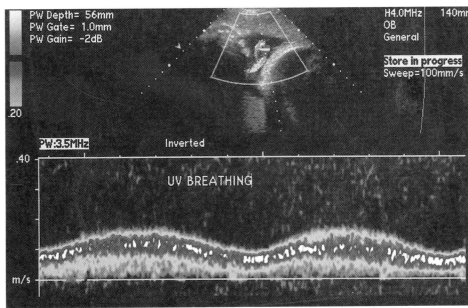

B

FIGURE 21-1 ■ Depictions of fetal breathing movement. **A,** Diaphragmatic movement on M-mode ultrasound; note broad (3 to 4 second) excursions typical of deep breathing, one of many normal patterns. **B,** Umbilical venous fluctuations. See also Color Plate 3.

Continued

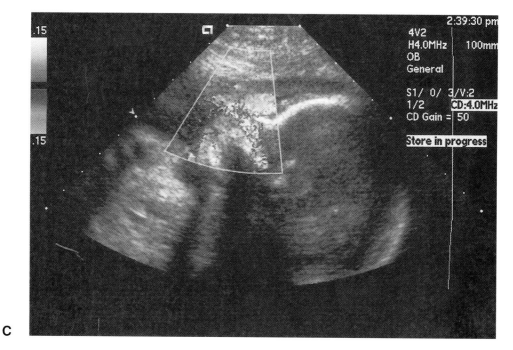

C

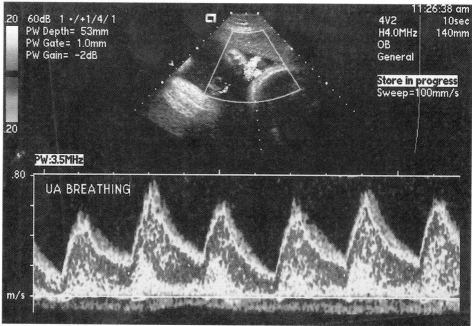

D

FIGURE 21-1, cont'd ■ **C,** Nasal flaring of expelled lung fluid during fetal breathing movement. **D,** Fetal heart rate variability; "respiratory arrhythmia" is depicted in umbilical artery. See also Color Plate 4.

ing oxygen supply (Nijhuis et al., 1982). Most fetuses experiencing chronic limitations in oxygen can maintain normal pH, neurologic function, and cardiac efficiency through a very low range of umbilical venous partial pressure of oxygen (Bocking, Gagnon, Milne, et al., 1988; Pillai and James, 1991a).

3. Reduce oxygen consumption. This sophisticated mechanism of fetal adaptation to oxygen limits should not be confused with the obtundation induced by severe absolute cerebral hypoxemia. Most fetal responses that decrease oxygen consumption are voluntary and can be rapidly turned on and off (Anderson et al., 1986). These are initiated with minor increases in time between activity cycles and may extend all

the way to complete abolition of fetal activity, rapidly reversible bare minutes after delivery. Fetal oxygen consumption may fall more than 15% during inactivity, and when this is coupled with redistribution and extraction, there may even be significant increases in oxygen supply to critical organs (Rurak and Gruber, 1983). Different elements of fetal behavior may illustrate different sensitivities to declining oxygen levels. Heart rate reactivity tends to disappear before fetal breathing movements, which are almost always absent before fetal movements disappear (Fig. 21-2) (Harman, 1999).

These pathways of response are sequential, overlapping, and potentially reversible (Koos et al., 1988). The IUGR fetus, for

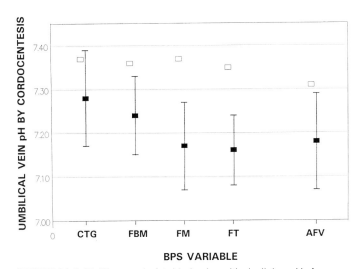

FIGURE 21-2 ■ Changes in fetal behavior with declining pH. As umbilical venous pH falls, various behaviors become less frequent and eventually disappear. The graph summarizes cordocentesis data relating antepartum pH to individual biophysical profile score (BPS) variables. □, mean pH when variable present (normal); ■ ± 1 standard deviation, mean pH of fetuses where variable absent (abnormal). Data suggest sequential loss of individual variables.

example, may deal effectively with increasing placental insufficiency with a combination of increasing oxygen extraction, increased hemoglobin concentration, and diversion of flow, such that temporary reduction in fetal activity may be restored and amniotic fluid volume maintained (Kitanaka et al., 1989). The extent to which these changes are reversible *in utero* will vary but include increased fetal activity with maternal supplemental oxygen and improved Doppler resistance patterns when oligohydramnios is restored by amnioinfusion.

Absent Fetal Behavior: How Long Is Too Long?

With the establishment of behavioral state cycles, state 1F categorizes the phase of "quiet sleep." Electroencephalographic features low-frequency, high-voltage patterns, occasional twitches but few voluntary movements, individual breathing movements without sustained episodes, marked diminution in heart rate variability, odd "mouthing" movements, and absence of acceleration/movement coupling (Pillai and James, 1991b).

Near term, such profound inactivity, illustrated by the nonreactive NST (Fig. 21-3), is readily confused with fetal compromise. This confusion led to many inappropriate interventions during the initial development of FHR monitoring. Although state 1F and the unreactive NST seldom persist longer than 40 minutes, intervals approaching 2 hours are still most likely normal (Brown and Patrick, 1981). The definition of these abnormal periods will depend very much on the modality of testing. Multitransducer real-time observation of fetal activity often discloses frequent small movements of hands, mouth, and trunk when less rigorous assessment describes complete inactivity. Clearly, any fetal testing modality must address the critical distinction: nearly dead or just napping.

■ PRINCIPLES OF MONITORING

Accounting for all these potential variables, the ideal monitoring system would gather a wide range of information, with versatility for all maternal and fetal conditions and flexibility for all gestational ages, allowing for varying degrees of onset, severity, and duration of intrauterine challenges (Harman, 1999). In meeting these objectives, an ideal antenatal monitoring system would do the following:

1. Detect fetal peril with specificity, sensitivity, and timeliness to allow preventive intervention. These qualities imply
   a. Correlation with measurable standards of fetal compromise (antepartum pH, postdelivery outcome such as blood gases, Apgar scores, and neonatal performance)
   b. Proportionality between test results and outcome (the worst score = highest risk of permanent handicap or perinatal mortality)
   c. A low false alarm rate, especially as prematurity deepens
   d. Application to all ranges of perinatal morbidity and basic perinatal mortality
   e. A reliable relationship to compromise that yields intervention early enough to prevent permanent damage but late enough to be certain of the need for intervention and to minimize the risks of prematurity
2. Reliably exclude stillbirth or permanent injury over a significant period of time. However, allowing for the possibility of acute change such as placental abruption, a

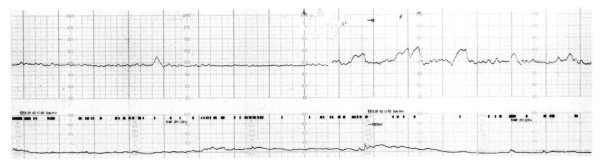

FIGURE 21-3 ■ Eighteen-minute sleep–wake cycle in term fetus. Virtually no activity (one kick, one acceleration) in first 9 minutes, with low variability fetal heart rate, behavioral state 1F. Next 9 minutes 60 discreet fetal movements on real-time ultrasound, multiple accelerations, increased variation between accelerations (2F).

normal test must exclude abnormal outcomes for a clinically important length of time, most commonly 7 days.

3. Exclude lethal congenital anomalies. This mandates at least one high-resolution comprehensive fetal examination but does not dictate that this must be repeated at every testing opportunity.
4. Incorporate multiple variables. This principle reflects the only way in which a monitoring system can address the interwoven cycles of behaviors and the many ways in which the normal fetus can manifest that normality.
5. Apply to fetal compromise from a variety of basic sources, including asphyxia, poisoning, metabolic abnormalities, anemia, and chance obstetric factors such as cord accident to address the many origins of adverse outcome. These should be applicable in outpatient settings, with readily available equipment, accessible technicality, and high reproducibility.
6. Have measurable benefits to high-risk populations, in reduction of perinatal mortality and perinatal morbidity, at least in part by safely extending intrauterine time. Meeting these objectives simultaneously will, by definition, be cost effective.

No single variable or measurement could possibly meet these objectives in the context of the great variability in normal behavior, the complex cascades of responsiveness to abnormal conditions, in the complicated balance between stillbirth from intrauterine decompensation and neonatal death from prematurity. *It appears that the time-worn lesson of fetal assessment is that only through a broad combination of variables can fetal status, normal or abnormal, be depicted with accuracy.* Nevertheless, the search goes on for the "silver bullet," the single parameter that will tell all. Our recent perinatal literature is full of such examples, including the use of the biparietal diameter as the unequivocal measurement for definition of IUGR (Duff and Evans, 1981), non-stress testing as the single parameter to determine obstetric management (Devoe, 1990), or a series of Doppler parameters (absent diastolic velocities, cerebralization of blood flow, umbilical-venous pulsations, in that historical order) where knee-jerk responses, in the form of delivery as soon as the observation was made, have resulted in a litany of iatrogenic problems (Woo et al., 1987).

The most recent trial of single-parameter intervention analyzed the potential benefits of early delivery as soon as umbilical artery Dopplers reached a critical level of abnormality (GRIT, 2003). This study demonstrated two fundamental pitfalls that have recurred throughout the history of fetal monitoring: (1) single parameter monitoring causes unnecessary iatrogenic injury and demise from prematurity and (2) ensuring fetal safety while reaching for more maturation time is even more demanding than simple delivery. *Only by integration of information from multiple physiologic sources, with multiple time periods, can the assessment of fetal health reach these goals.*

TESTS OF FETAL HEALTH

Fetal testing focuses on the detection of chronic and intermediate term compromise to prevent stillbirth, decrease neonatal mortality, and minimize long-term morbidity. No system of fetal monitoring has been devised to detect acute antenatal compromise, chance events such as placental abrup-

tion or cord accident, or the unmonitored onset of labor. Most reported testing schemes feature a core system of multiple variables, with a number of ancillary tests applied in specific unusual circumstances. The discussion that follows focuses on the application of biophysical profile scoring, with additional important inputs from other modalities. There are many appropriate variations on this theme. However, the fundamental principle of multiple variables giving the most reliable evidence of fetal status remains.

Monitoring Tools

Biophysical Profile Scoring

The biophysical profile score (BPS) presumes that multiple parameters of well-being are better predictors of outcome than single parameters (Manning et al., 1980). Figure 21-4 shows one example of the detailed evaluation of outcome variables performed during the development of biophysical profile scoring (Platt et al., 1978; Manning, Platt, et al., 1979). The five variables illustrated are those of traditional biophysical profile scoring, but many variations have been included. Vintzileos and colleagues (1983) added placental grading, for a total possible score of 12. Several authors proposed a "modified" biophysical profile that usually includes heart rate monitoring and amniotic fluid evaluation (Nageotte et al., 1994; Miller et al., 1996). The following discussion does not deal with potential differences in these approaches but focuses on the value of multivariable fetal assessment.

BIOPHYSICAL PROFILE SCORE VARIABLES

Table 21-1 lists the BPS variables. Important interpretive points are expanded upon here.

AMNIOTIC FLUID VOLUME. Amniotic fluid volume less than 2 cm or greater than 8 cm is not normal, and a detailed evaluation of the fetus must be carried out to exclude anatomic and anomalous explanations (Chamberlain et al., 1984b; Harman, 1989). In normal fetuses, moderate hydramnios

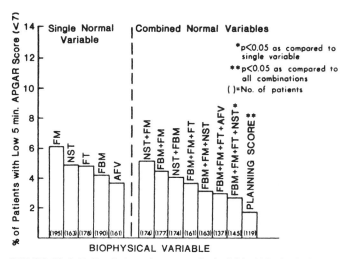

FIGURE 21-4 ■ Prediction of outcome by individual biophysical profile score variables (*left*) or combinations of variables (*right*). In this example, a 5-minute Apgar score less than 7 was best predicted by a combination of all five variables. (The "Planning Score," named for Platt and Manning, was the first full biophysical profile score.) AFV, amniotic fluid volume; FBM, fetal breathing movement; FM, fetal movement; FT, fetal tone; NST, non-stress test.

TABLE 21-1. INTERPRETATION OF BPS VARIABLES

Fetal Variable	Normal Behavior (Score = 2)	Abnormal Behavior (Score = 0)
Fetal breathing movements	Intermittent multiple episodes of more than 30-sec duration, within 30-min BPS time frame. Hiccups count. Continuous FBM for 30 min = exclude fetal acidosis.	Continuous breathing without cessation. Completely absent breathing or no sustained episodes.
Body or limb movements	At least four discrete body movements in 30 min. Continuous active movement episodes = single movement. Includes fine motor movements, rolling movements, and so on, but not REM or mouthing movements.	Three or fewer body/limb movements in a 30-min observation period.
Fetal tone/posture	Demonstration of active extension with rapid return to flexion of fetal limbs and brisk repositioning/trunk rotation. Opening and closing of hand, mouth, kicking, and so on.	Low-velocity movement only. Incomplete flexion, flaccid extremity positions, abnormal fetal posture. Must score = 0 when FM completely absent.
Cardiotocogram	Normal mean variation (computerized FHR interpretation), accelerations associated with maternal palpation FM (accelerations graded for gestation), 20-min CTG.	Fetal movement and accelerations not coupled. Insufficient accelerations, absent accelerations, or decelerative trace. Mean variation < 20 on numerical analysis of CTG.
Amniotic fluid evaluation	At least one pocket > 3 cm with no umbilical cord. See text regarding subjectively decreased fluid.	No cord-free pocket > 2 cm or elements of subjectively reduced amniotic fluid volume definite.

BPS, biophysical profile score; CTG, cardiotocogram; FBM, fetal breathing movements; FHR, fetal heart rate; FM, fetal movement; REM; rapid age movement.

(amniotic fluid largest pocket depth, 8 to 12 cm), anatomic issues, idiopathic hydramnios, and fetal macrosomia due to maternal diabetes are the most common explanations, and fetal testing will likely reflect fetal neurologic status accurately (Chamberlain et al., 1984c). For pockets greater than 12 cm in depth in singleton pregnancies, neurologic issues, and structural defects associated with aneuploidy are much more likely, in which case biophysical profile scoring may be invalid (Manning, Baskett, et al., 1981). Thus, one variable may lead to suspicion about the validity of testing and call for additional evaluation. Amniotic fluid pockets are identified in real time, and clear fluid is proven because the fetus readily moves through it. When there is doubt, a cord-free pocket is confirmed by pulsed Doppler. There is evidence that application of continuous color imaging may lead to the false impression of oligohydramnios (Magann et al., 2001) (Fig. 21-5; Color Plate 5).

SUBJECTIVELY REDUCED AMNIOTIC FLUID. This suggests fluid that is significantly less than average, although it does meet minimum criteria of 2-cm pocket depth. Although subjective, most of these are readily quantified, including restricted extension of movements that have normal tone, the uterus and/or placenta molding to the contours of the fetus, FHR decelerations with transducer pressure, spontaneous decelerations associated with fetal movement, maternal reports of decreased fetal movement, no cord-free pocket greater than 3 cm in depth, or a sharp drop in the maximum pocket depth between serial visits (Harman, 1998).

SINGLE POCKET DEPTH VERSUS AMNIOTIC FLUID INDEX. Classic biophysical profile scoring uses single pocket depth. The maximum vertical pocket measurable with the transducer in a normal vertical attitude to the maternal abdomen is recorded. The transducer is then rotated 90 degrees, in the same vertical axis, to confirm that the measured pocket has true biplanar dimensions. The phrase "2 × 2 pocket" applied to this standard is misleading, because it suggests that a pocket 2 cm deep and 2 cm wide is required, which is not the case.

This standard for oligohydramnios has good reliability as a test for potential fetal compromise, as a correlate of IUGR, and as a correlate of repetitive decelerations in labor leading to a decision for cesarean section delivery. This measurement does not correlate perfectly with absolute amniotic fluid volume measured by dye infusion or with other ultrasound methods of amniotic fluid estimate (Croom et al., 1992). Of course, the vertical pocket method was intended as a reflection of the relative amount of amniotic fluid, with a cutoff value producing high sensitivity and reasonable specificity for outcome, and not meant as an absolute physiologic parameter (Manning, Hill, et al., 1981). We continue to use maximum single pocket depth in all biophysical profile scoring (Bastide et al., 1986).

The amniotic fluid index (AFI) is another ultrasound method of estimating amniotic fluid volume, which measures vertical pocket depth in four quadrants and then sums them (Phelan et al., 1987). This total can be evaluated by simple cutoff values (AFI less than 5 by some authors, less than 6 by others, defining oligohydramnios; AFI of 24 or more defining hydramnios) or by gestational age-related tables (Moore and Cayle, 1990). Reference to such tables, which illustrate average AFI across mid and third trimester, shows only a modest change in AFI across gestation. For the average fetus, an AFI greater than 10 is maintained (Moore and Cayle, 1990). Thus, because several standards exist in the literature, direct comparison of results between groups of observers or between methods of ultrasound evaluation of amniotic fluid volume is not precise. The weight of evidence, correlating amniotic fluid assessment with outcome, favors the single pocket method, because it has been applied longer, and outcomes have been studied in more detail (Manning, Hill, et al., 1981; Manning, 1995a; Johnson et al., 1986). Several studies of single pocket depth versus AFI have been concluded in large populations, with no clear determinant between the two (Moore, 1990; Magann et al., 2000). In dye-dilution studies, it would appear that AFI predicts actual volume of amniotic fluid better within the normal range, but the single pocket method

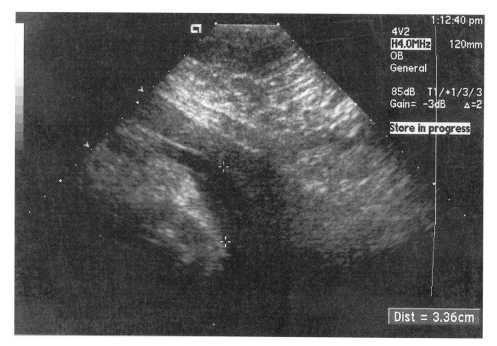

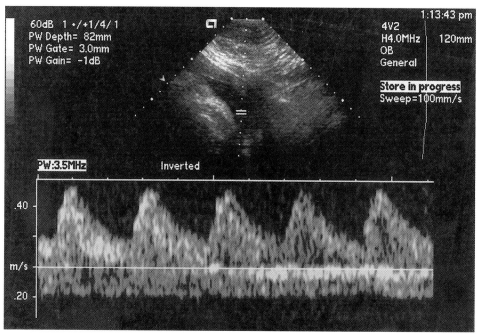

FIGURE 21-5 ■ Fluid pocket verification. **A,** Amniotic fluid apparently meets biophysical profile score vertical pocket criteria. **B,** Pulsed Doppler demonstrates this is actually a vertical pocket of umbilical cord, with no measurable amniotic fluid. See also Color Plate 5.

predicts with higher accuracy the amniotic fluid volumes at the lower limits of normal and in the oligohydramnios range (Croom et al., 1992; Manning, 1995a). Although the differences are rather modest, these factors, as well as improved interobserver error with the simpler method, favor retention of single pocket depth measurement for BPS. The critical principle, fetal oliguria, is illustrated well by the single pocket method. The concept that reduced urine output was a direct consequence of hypoxemia (Nicolaides et al., 1990) has given way to more complicated mechanisms involving redistribution of blood flow and segmental renal hemodynamics (Groome et al., 1991).

FETAL BREATHING MOVEMENTS. The presence of rhythmic fetal diaphragm contractions and/or hiccups lasting more than 30 seconds constitutes a normal score. Isolated individual breaths and/or hiccups do not. Fetal "gasping" is a rare phenomenon, probably related to serious acidosis in the near-term fetus. This must be verified by observations of the fetal face and neck, which show the facial equivalent of gasping, not the vigorous diaphragmatic movement of the hyperglycemic fetus of a diabetic mother. Further, gasping motions do not occur in the presence of normal fetal activity patterns and/or normally reactive non-stress testing. Because the amplitude of fetal breathing depends on gestational age, maternal glucose, exposure to increased oxygen concentrations, and many medications (e.g., xanthines), careful evaluation of all parameters is necessary before intervention is precipitated (Manning, Martin, et al., 1979).

Their defined episodic nature means fetal breathing movements are the most frequently absent parameter during normal testing (Manning, Morrison, et al., 1990). Although this can be averted in some populations by scheduling BPS within 2 to 3 hours of mealtime or can be promoted in given fetuses by glucose-rich drinks such as orange juice (Natale et al., 1981), this is the most common reason for performing cardiotocography in the normal fetus monitored with BPS. The use of fetal breathing movements in separate testing schemes for infection in preterm premature rupture of membranes (Vintzileos et al., 1986; Roussis et al., 1991), differentiating true from false preterm labor (Castle and Turnbull, 1983; Boylan et al., 1985), in pulmonary hypoplasia (Broth et al., 2002), and in indicating the likelihood of labor in patients with ruptured membranes (Vintzileos et al., 1986) has limited statistical validity. Our experience in hundreds of thousands of patients suggests that the large number of exceptions to each of these theories mean that formatted application is unlikely to be completely successful. The unusual presence of continuous monotonous fetal breathing, with complete absence of all other behavior for an extended period, may indicate acidosis, especially in the diabetic fetus (Molteni et al., 1980; Hohimer and Bissonnette, 1981; Manning, Heaman, et al., 1981).

FETAL MOVEMENT AND TONE. One of the interpretive pitfalls of biophysical profile scoring is that at least some movements must be necessary to evaluate tone (Harman, 1999). It is emphasized that tone is not simply the flexed posture of a normal fetus. (Our experience is that all but the most obtunded fetus, or those paralyzed with pancuronium for intrauterine procedures, will have normal curved posture.) Although the evaluation of tone is indeed subjective, there must be at least some movements to assess it.

The original description of movement called for large amplitude movements of the fetal body and/or limbs, because ultrasound was so primitive at that time it was sometimes difficult to tell if the fetus was moving at all (Manning,

1995c). Current application using high-resolution machines allows virtually any movement of the fetus, including fine motor movement of the face, hands, purposeful movement such as swallowing, facial expressions, sucking, yawning, large kicks, small kicks, rolling motions, and so on. In a fetus who does not move over 30 minutes, extended testing is required (Manning et al., 1990a), and completion of heart rate testing is also performed to extend the time of continuous observation, but also to allow the near-term sleeping fetus to "wake up." Causing state changes by acoustic stimulation, shaking the fetus, intravenous glucose boluses, and so on have not been studied in trial situations where gold standard ultrasound observation of fetal status can be documented. In practice, the frequency of fetal movement is referenced to previous BPS experience with this fetus, maternal reports, and gestational age. The markedly preterm fetus moves virtually all the time, and a movement frequency of only five to eight movements per hour would be considered markedly reduced movement and calls for an increased frequency of testing, even though minimum criteria are met.

CARDIOTOCOGRAM. Systematic recording of the FHR with simultaneous documentation of uterine activity constitutes cardiotocography (Fig. 21-6) (Martin, 1978). When spontaneous contractions occur and are sufficiently well-defined to document their timing, a spontaneous contraction stress test (CST) is denoted. The same pattern elicited by intravenous infusion of oxytocin is called an oxytocin challenge test (OCT). These tests are discussed later. When criteria relating fetal movement to standardized interpretation of FHR accelerations are applied, an NST is defined (Lavery, 1982). Finally, these data can be digitally acquired by a computerized system that interprets not only accelerations and decelerations, but also numerically analyzes FHR variability within gestational age-normalized paradigms (Dawes et al., 1991b; Guzman et al., 1996).

An experienced observer can derive much information from the cardiotocogram (CTG). Contraction patterns may suggest uterine irritability as in preterm labor, uterine infection, or impending abruptio placentae. The minimal deceleration pattern illustrated in Figure 21-7 is highly suggestive

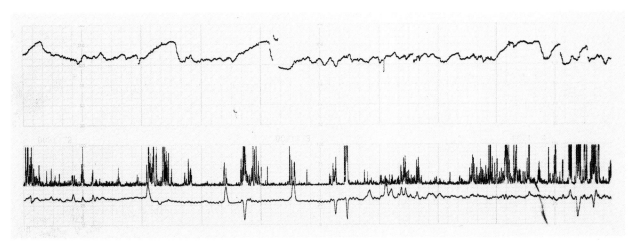

FIGURE 21-6 ■ Reactive non-stress test. Prominent fetal heart rate accelerations associated with palpated fetal movements (also documented by this type of monitor, second tracing from bottom). Between large accelerations, normal variability, classified as moderate by the National Institute of Child Health and Human Development criteria. No detectable uterine contractions (*bottom tracing*).

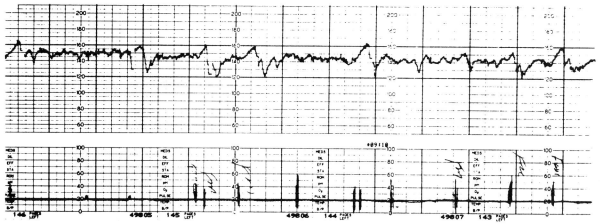

FIGURE 21-7 ■ "Minimal variable" fetal heart rate pattern. Numerous fetal movements, marked FM on *lower tracing*, were associated with small decelerations due to cord compression. Biophysical profile score was 6/10, with equivocal non-stress test and no amniotic fluid pocket more than 2.0 cm. Fetus failed induction because of repetitive decelerations despite amnioinfusion in labor.

of oligohydramnios. Fetal breathing will often produce characteristic deflections of the tocodynamometer as well as irregularities in FHR (Fig. 21-8) (Fouron et al., 1975). Normal variability with a monotonous repetitive pattern (saw tooth), especially 40 minutes in duration, may be an indication of fetal anemia, whereas overt sinusoidal heart rate is indicative of more severe concerns of the fetus that may include anemia to the point of hydrops, drug intoxica-

tion (e.g., narcotics), or abnormalities of the central nervous system with decorticate behavior (Nijhuis et al., 1990; Yaffe et al., 1989).

The abiding principle of the use of CTG in biophysical profile scoring is that it is never used alone (Manning et al., 1984; Manning, Morrison, Lange, et al., 1987). Any of the above patterns would immediately call for performance of all ultrasound parameters in the BPS. The CTG must be inter-

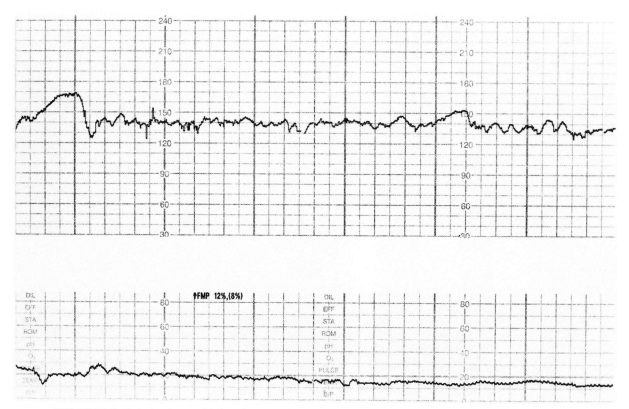

FIGURE 21-8 ■ Active fetus with "respiratory arrhythmia." Simultaneous real-time ultrasound shows episodic fetal breathing for most of this tracing after the first large acceleration. *Upper tracing* shows increased short-term variability; *lower tracing* shows maternal abdomen moving in small amplitude waves 20 to 30/min and fetal chest movements.

■ **TABLE 21-2.** SYSTEMATIC APPLICATION OF BIOPHYSICAL PROFILE SCORING

Biophysical Profile Score	Interpretation	Predicted PNM/1000*	Recommended Management
10/10 8/8 8/10 (AFV normal)	No evidence of fetal asphyxia present.	Less than 1/1000	No acute intervention on fetal basis. Serial testing indicated by disorder-specific protocols.
8/10-OLIGO	Chronic fetal compromise likely.	89/1000	For absolute oligohydramnios, prove normal urinary tract, disprove asymptomatic rupture of membranes, then deliver at any viable gestation.
6/10 (AFV normal)	Equivocal test, fetal asphyxia is not excluded.	Depends on progression (61/1000 on average)	Repeat testing immediately, before assigning final value. If score is 6/10, then 10/10, in two continuous 30-min periods, manage as 10/10. For persistent 6/10, deliver the mature fetus, repeat within 24 hr in the immature fetus, then deliver if less than 6/10.
4/10	Acute fetal asphyxia likely. If AFV-OLIGO, acute on chronic asphyxia very likely.	91/1000	Deliver by obstetrically appropriate method, with continuous monitoring.
2/10	Acute fetal asphyxia, most likely with chronic decompensation.	125/1000	Deliver for fetal indications (usually cesarean section).
0/10	Severe acute asphyxia virtually certain.	600/1000	Deliver immediately by cesarean section.

* Per 1000 live births, within 1 week of the test result shown, if no intervention. For scores of 0, 2, or 4, intervention should commence virtually immediately, provided the fetus is viable.

AFV, amniotic fluid volume; PNM, perinatal mortality.

preted within the gestational age context (Castillo et al., 1989). Modification of the interpretation of the NST is shown in Table 21-1 and reflects the potential benefits of computerized CTG in the preterm fetus (Baskett, 1988; Ribbert et al., 1991).

PERFORMANCE OF BIOPHYSICAL PROFILE SCORING

Interpretation of the BPS is meant to dictate action according to the systematic application in Table 21-2. More detailed instructions on the application of biophysical profile scoring are available elsewhere (Manning, 1995c; Harman, 1998, 1999), but several technical points deserve emphasis.

SCORE OUT OF 10. A score of "6/8" is not a BPS. When the four ultrasound variables are performed first, if any of these is absent, the CTG *must* be performed before the BPS is complete, and the score will be x/10. The only score that is allowed to stand after the ultrasound variables have been evaluated is 8/8. In that case, the CTG does not need to be performed. In units that conform to this original design of BPS (which was based on the performance of a randomized controlled trial), FHR monitoring is used in only about 10% of cases (Manning, Morrison, Lange, et al., 1987; Harman, 1999). Exceptions to this application include high-risk fetuses with vascular abnormalities; multiple medical disorders (especially the combination of hypertension and diabetes); unstable situations such as chronic abruption, fetal infection, and fetal arrhythmias; or other high-risk maternal situations. Of critical importance, always requiring all five variables to be performed ("score out of 10"), are fetuses with Doppler-defined placental abnormalities, especially those with reversed end-diastolic velocities (REDV) or absent end-diastolic velocities (AEDV) and/or umbilical venous pulsations.

8/10–OLIGO. Above the lower limits of viability, after documentation of severe oligohydramnios, with no visible vertical pocket measuring more than 2 cm, delivery is a primary consideration (Bastide et al., 1986). Although the application of

the AFI and its more flexible definition of oligohydramnios have caused confusion on this point (the above definition means the AFI will almost always be less than 6), adherence to the single pocket rule will avoid undue interference. Especially if the fetus has otherwise normal behavior, normal measurements, and normal Dopplers, a high index of suspicion would suggest amnioinfusion to exclude rupture of membranes (Fisk et al., 1991). In a few cases, invasive fetal testing to confirm normal oxygen and pH levels may also prove important. In anhydramnios, if delivery is to be delayed for administration of steroids or other temporizing, either continuous monitoring or biophysical profile scoring up to several times daily is needed. It should be emphasized that oligohydramnios does not require immediate cesarean delivery, especially when all other parameters of fetal behavior are within normal limits, but induction of labor under these circumstances carries a risk of cesarean delivery of about 45%.

EQUIVOCAL OR ABNORMAL SCORES. The correlation between abnormal scores and high risk of poor outcome has been demonstrated in large population studies and produces a characteristically shaped outcome curve (Manning et al., 1985) (Fig. 21-9). Before acting, however, one must consider the differential diagnosis of this abnormal behavior. Because so many factors may influence biophysical profile scoring (Table 21-3), prolonged testing, retesting after a brief interval, or adding ancillary tests (discussed later) are important steps before the action illustrated in the systematic response for equivocal scores. When the score is 0 to 4/10, especially in the fetus with reduced fluid, IUGR, and in whom serial observations have previously been normal, undue delay in delivery for these ancillary tests would not be reasonable. Thus, confirmatory tests are applied if diagnosis is uncertain but not as a complicated formula of responses in the biophysical profile scoring system.

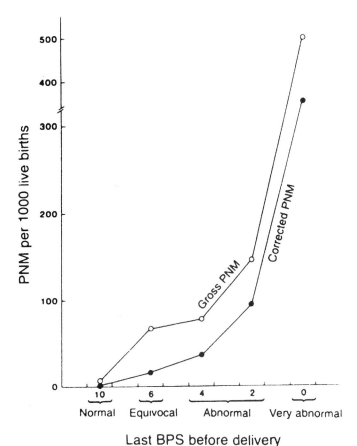

FIGURE 21-9 ■ Perinatal mortality (PNM) varies exponentially with declining biophysical profile score (BPS). The important contribution of lethal fetal anomalies accounts for the difference in the two curves.

INTERACTIVE FETAL MONITORING

Rigid application of rote versions of biophysical profile scoring protocols may ignore valuable information (Yoon et al., 1993). When the operator is astute, listens to information volunteered by the mother, pays attention to uterine contractility during the examination, and adapts the testing parameters to the individual clinical situation, the methodology will usually succeed. It is emphasized that the motivated obstetrically inclined ultrasonographer may gather information on a variety of levels, stimulating further investigation, excluding preterm labor and incipient abruption, recognizing maternal input about fetal status, and so on (Manning, Morrison, Harman, et al., 1987). That the situation in Figure 21-10 (Color Plate 6) featured normal biophysical profile scoring is overshadowed by the lifesaving intervention of immediate admission to the labor floor (Lange et al., 1985). Many facets of real-time observation can be obtained in the short time required to perform a normal BPS. BPS is based on the principle of accepting information from all possible sources: the five classic parameters; all routine ultrasound observations of uterus, placenta, and membranes; fetal growth parameters; comprehensive Doppler survey; maternal reports; maternal abdominal palpation; and even information volunteered by the family during the scan.

There is no doubt that the team applying this methodology is critical to the success of biophysical profile scoring. This emphasizes the importance of integration of testing into an overall program of fetal evaluation, common sense, and good judgment while highlighting the flexibility of BPS.

Fetal Heart Rate Monitoring

Much of this topic has been reviewed previously under cardiotocography. The isolated use of FHR testing, whether by classic NST or by the introduction of contraction challenges, is not considered standard of care for high-risk fetuses. There may be economic or logistic reasons why ultrasound is not

TABLE 21-3. MANY FACTORS INFLUENCE BPS PERFORMANCE

Agent	Fetal Effect
Drugs	
Sedatives/sedative side effects (e.g., Aldomet)	Diminished activity of all varieties; abolition of none
Excitatory (e.g., theophylline)	Continuous "picket fence" FBM
Street drugs (e.g., crack cocaine)	Rachitic, rigid, furious, bizarre FM
Indomethacin	Oligohydramnios
Maternal cigarette smoking	Various observations:
	FBM abolished or attenuated but some report no change
	FM reduced
Maternal Hyperglycemia (Iatrogenic or Unregulated)	Sustained FBM/acidosis, diminution or abolition of FM/FT/CTG-reactivity
Maternal Hypoglycemia (e.g., Poor Nutrition, Insulin Excess)	Abnormal paucity of all behaviors, normal AFV
Single Parameter Removed by Perinatal Condition	
Persistent fetal arrhythmia	Uninterpretable CTG
Spontaneous premature rupture of membranes	Obligatory oligohydramnios
Periodic decelerations (e.g., in proteinuric preeclampsia)	CTG defined as nonreactive
Acute Disasters (Eclampsia, Abruptio Placentae, Ketoacidosis)	Invalidates BPS predictive accuracy

AFV, amniotic fluid volume; BPS, biophysical profile score; CTG, cardiotocogram; FBM, fetal breathing movements; FM, fetal movement; FT, fetal tone.

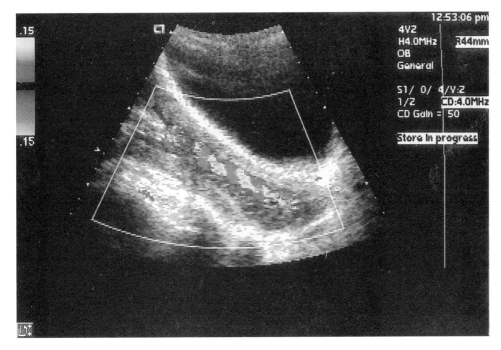

FIGURE 21-10 ■ Color Doppler shows umbilical cord trapped in prolapsed membranes filling entire endocervical canal. As the patient was transferred from the stretcher to the operating room table, the membranes ruptured and the cord prolapsed. The 32-week fetus survived intact after immediate cesarean section. See also Color Plate 6.

available to women undergoing routine prenatal care with no identifiable risks, but even in that population there are substantial problems with using the NST as the only method of surveillance (Table 21-4). A valuable component of virtually all multivariable systems, the NST recognizes the unique coupling of fetal neurologic status to cardiovascular reflex responses (Baser et al., 1992). It is one of the factors that tends to disappear earliest during progressive fetal compromise (Vintzileos et al., 1991; Harman, 1998), and many studies have shown it to be the most sensitive of the four shorter term variables to worsening hypoxemia and/or acidosis (Manning et al., 1993; Morrison et al., 1994). In modified BPS systems, a fully reactive NST may be used to infer fetal movement. Any abnormality in such testing, including the nonreactive NST, occasional decelerations, decreased variability, and persistent minor decelerations, calls for detailed ultrasound evaluation.

THE NON-STRESS TEST

Lee and colleagues (1975, 1976) described the original method, and there have been many minor variations. In fact, whereas the presence of coupled acceleration–palpable movement pairs has been evaluated under many circumstances, no absolute value for amplitude or duration of accelerations has been determined to be significant in predicting fetal status (Devoe, 1990). The classic accepted criteria for a reactive NST are at least two FHR accelerations lasting at least 15 seconds and rising at least 15 beats/min above the established baseline heart rate (Druzin, 1989). Most term fetuses have many of these accelerations in each 20- to 30-minute period of active sleep (behavioral state 2F), and the term fetus will seldom go more than 60 minutes, and not more than 100 minutes, without meeting these criteria (Brown and Patrick, 1981). On the other hand, preterm fetuses, IUGR fetuses at similar gestations, or fetuses with maternal medication such as sedatives or magnesium sulfate will frequently have paired accelerations–movements that do not meet these criteria (Castillo et al., 1989). Modification of these criteria in biophysical profile scoring (e.g., including accelerations of 10 beats/min lasting 10 seconds on a back-

ground of normal FHR variability) accepts the principle that earlier fetuses have smaller accelerations but that they should always demonstrate some degree of FHR acceleration with palpated fetal movements.

NST reactivity may be inferred in a number of ways. Experienced nurses listening from a distance to the audible output of a heart rate monitor can detect accelerations and properly classify reactive NSTs without looking at the paper record (Baskett et al., 1981). Real-time ultrasound observation of concurrent FHR accelerations and movements also correlates perfectly with reactive NST.

False reassuring NSTs do exist, at a rate of 4 to 5 per 1000 in the largest studies (Druzin et al., 1980; Freeman et al., 1982; Devoe, 1990). These are most problematic in fetuses with asymmetrical IUGR, oligohydramnios, and metabolic problems associated with severe macrosomia. In other words, NST

TABLE 21-4. PROBLEMS WITH NON-STRESS TEST ALONE

Method Fails to Detect

Oligohydramnios
Lethal anomalies
Cord presentation, abnormalities
Placental abnormalities
Growth disorders
Twin demise
Anomalies requiring intervention
Overall sensitivity 50% (all outcomes)

Nonreactive Test

Poor specificity for compromise
Poor specificity for fetal death

Reactive Test

False-reassuring rate 6/1000
Unreliable as backup test*

* False reassuring rate for post-dates pregnancy 20/1000, false reassuring rate for decreased fetal movement 24/1000.

has significant liabilities among the highest risk groups. It should not be used in isolation in determining antenatal status of such fetuses.

The nonreactive NST is defined by an FHR monitoring interval that does not meet the above criteria. However, a large variation in the total duration allowed for this is documented, ranging from a minimum of 10 minutes of monitoring to 40 minutes or even 60 minutes according to some authors (Nochimson et al., 1978; Schifrin et al., 1979). In the context of biophysical profile scoring, 30 minutes are allowed for the NST to reach reactivity. About 10% to 12% of fetuses in the third trimester will not meet these criteria at 30 minutes, whereas this number falls below 6% by 40 minutes (Brown and Patrick, 1981). Clearly then, the choice of time end point will be the most critical issue in determining the false-alarm rate of non-stress testing, its major clinical drawback. In fact, because most normal fetuses will demonstrate normal ultrasound variables in biophysical profile scoring (i.e., reach a score of 8/8) within 15 minutes, the additional time to perform non-stress testing is optional and unnecessary in a large number of monitored fetuses (see previously). It is economical, therefore, to start antenatal testing with the ultrasound biophysical variables, proceeding to NST if not all of these are normal. By far the most common explanation for the nonreactive NST is the presence of a longer-than-average sleep cycle in a normal fetus (Pillai and James, 1990b). A nonreactive NST, especially if variability remains present and there are no decelerations, should not be assumed to indicate fetal compromise. There should be a clear protocol of responses and follow-up evaluation for any system using non-stress testing as the primary means of ensuring fetal well-being.

Although such protocols have in the past used CSTs (see previously) or other manipulations of FHR as the backup test for a nonreactive NST, the standard of care now indicates that ultrasound evaluation (some form of fetal BPS) must be carried out, virtually immediately. As well, although fetal non-stress testing in isolation was frequently the reference test for post-term pregnancies, decreased fetal movement on maternal movement counting programs, and other published protocols for first-line monitoring, the standard of care now indicates a much more comprehensive evaluation (American College of Obstetricians and Gynecologists, 2001).

COMPUTERIZED INTERPRETATION OF FETAL HEART RATE MONITORING

A number of systems are available with computerized storage and interpretation of FHR records obtained with conventional monitors. The principle behind such applications is that visual interpretation of FHR variability, and perhaps the arguments about the technical definition of actual accelerations, can be resolved by objective interpretation using digitized analysis of heart rate patterns (Borgatta et al., 1988; Dawes et al., 1991a). This is essentially a computerized extension of the classification of heart rate variability, as is proposed by the National Institutes of Health workshop on electronic heart rate monitoring (National Institute of Child Health & Human Development, 1997). That system categorizes heart rate variability as undetectable, minimal, moderate, marked, and sinusoidal. Computerized analysis can depict variability as a continuous output variable, analyzing beat-to-beat variability (short-term variation, which has a mean of 3 to 8 msec), or as overall variation, depicted as mean minute variability from the

established baseline (Dawes and Redman, 1981). Normal mean minute variation is correlated with gestational age, and an example is shown in Figure 21-11. The interpretation algorithm is very complex and includes correlation of gestational age for the definitions of accelerations, variability, baseline heart rate, movement frequency, and the depiction of fetal state (Dawes et al., 1991b). Although the subtleties of states 3F and 4F are not depicted, states 1F (low variability, fetal movements) and 2F (high variability and significantly increased movement frequency) are correctly classified (Pillai and James, 1990c). Finally, variations within periods of high episodes and low episodes are also analyzed and compared with gestational age-corrected means. Data are stored on a hard disk and therefore available for serial comparison, analysis for gestational age trends, and research involving various factors such as drugs, maternal oxygen, and so on, in examining effects on central nervous system regulation of FHR.

This technology really represents a more exacting analysis of information currently available from standard heart rate monitors. Quality control information such as percentage signal loss and a more objective definition of baseline heart rate, may also be advantageous. The precise depiction of beat-to-beat variability, the objective analysis of multiple variables within the FHR record, the nonarbitrary definition of accelerations, baseline, and variability with gestational age norms all have scientific appeal in reducing the arguments about interpretation of non-stress testing. However, this methodology has not gained large practical acceptance. The explanation would appear to be fairly simple: There are not many fetuses for whom such precision is required. Most fetuses with equivocal testing on heart rate evaluation will simply be referred to ultrasound-based backup testing schemes. As the limits of viability are extended progressively downward, however, this system may find its true role. The immature heart rate regulation seen in fetuses before 28 weeks in all cases and before 32 weeks in many fetuses may preclude normal NST interpretation but may still be interpretable by computer-based models (Snijders et al., 1997). Further, the delayed maturation of heart rate regulation seen in IUGR fetuses is not an absolute impediment to computerized interpretation (Van Vliet et al., 1985; Weiner et al., 1996). Finally, because the analysis generates continuous variables rather than arbitrary cutoff ranges, excellent correlation between abnormal FHR variability and abnormal perinatal outcome, including mortality, short-term morbidity, and abnormal cord blood gases and pH, are readily analyzed. Thus, in specialized circumstances, computerized interpretation of the FHR record has distinct advantages over the "eyeball" methods.

ABNORMALITIES ON NON-STRESS TESTING

PERSISTENT NONREACTIVE TRACING. As discussed previously, the patient is referred immediately for detailed evaluation using biophysical profile scoring. In a fetus who has normal ultrasound variables and repetitive nonreactive tracings despite extended periods of heart rate observation, central nervous system abnormalities, drug ingestion, or prior fetal central nervous system injury should be considered.

REPETITIVE FETAL HEART RATE DECELERATIONS (NO DETECTABLE UTERINE CONTRACTIONS). Classic patterns of late deceleration and variable decelerations may occur in the context of NST monitoring, with no deflection of the uterine pressure monitor. It is probable that uterine activity is respon-

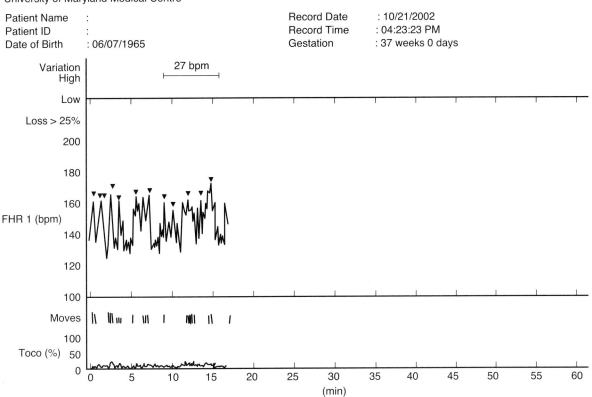

Oxford Instruments Medical Ltd
University of Maryland Medical Centre

Sonicaid FetalCare v.1.1

Patient Name   :
Patient ID   :
Date of Birth   : 06/07/1965

Record Date   : 10/21/2002
Record Time   : 04:23:23 PM
Gestation   : 37 weeks 0 days

ADVICE ONLY. THIS IS NOT INTENDED AS A DIAGNOSIS.

Dawes / Redman criteria for FHR1 met at 16 mins.

Results for FHR1:

Signal loss (%)	0
Contraction peaks	1
Fetal movements (per hour)	40
per min in high	1.10
Basal Heart Rate (bpm)	136
Accelerations > 10 bpm & 15 sec	12
Accelerations > 15 bpm & 15 sec	9
Decelerations > 20 lost beats	0
High episodes (min)	7 (26.75 bpm)
at 37 weeks gestation 87.4% of normal fetuses have less variation	
Low episodes (min)	0
Short term variation (ms)	11.9 (4.26 bpm)

FIGURE 21-11 ■ Output from Oxford Sonicaid System 8002 computerized cardiotocogram interpretation algorithm. bpm, beats per minute; FHR, fetal heart rate.

sible, but the situation (placental insufficiency in the case of late decelerations, umbilical cord compression in the case of variable decelerations) is so susceptible that even minor changes in uterine tone may provoke them. Either pattern should call for immediate evaluation by real-time ultrasound to exclude IUGR, direct fetal compromise, oligohydramnios, or more acute events such as placental abruption. This should be done immediately—the explanation may be imminent cord prolapse or evolving placental separation without significant maternal findings. Ultrasound can also demonstrate cord entanglement, multiple loops of nuchal cord, or the normal fetus grasping its cord and applying repetitive pressure.

Significant variable decelerations lasting up to 2 minutes may occur as the term fetus squeezes the cord with its hand (Petrikovsky and Kaplan, 1993). In the context of modern fetal evaluation, all these issues suggest that FHR monitoring should be done in a unit capable of immediate ultrasound evaluation.

Doppler Ultrasound Evaluation

This is extensively discussed in Chapter 28 regarding IUGR. In the overall context of fetal evaluation, Doppler provides a critical role. Doppler velocimetry defines the placental status and therefore the relative risk of sudden deterioration

(Baschat et al., 2001; Baschat and Harman, 2001). Doppler categories of risk may be used to dictate frequency of immediate fetal monitoring by biophysical profile scoring (Table 21-5) (Harman, 1998). Although Doppler should not be taken out of context or used in isolation, extreme abnormalities may indicate a need for very prompt intervention, and detailed evaluation of fetal status using all available tools should be instituted. It is emphasized, therefore, that the following discussion takes place within the context of multivariable testing and evaluation of the fetus: Waveform analysis by itself, no matter how complex, is not sufficient.

Fetal Doppler Velocimetry

Fetal Doppler studies have evolved from simple evaluation of the umbilical outflow to assess the placenta (Snijders and Hyett, 1997) to comprehensive multivessel evaluation of fetal circulatory status (Baschat and Harman, 2001). Although most literature is focused on umbilical artery velocimetry by itself, this does not meet current standards of practice. Integration of both placental (primarily umbilical artery) and fetal systemic (at least middle cerebral artery [MCA] and precordial veins) are required to adequately assess the compromised fetus (Harman and Baschat, 2003).

UMBILICAL ARTERY

HEMODYNAMICS. The umbilical arteries arise from the common iliac arteries and represent the dominant outflow of distal aortic circulation. Because there are no somatic branches after the umbilical arteries curve around the fetal bladder and rise to the level of the umbilicus where they join the umbilical vein, the umbilical arteries purely reflect placental circulation.

TABLE 21-5. DOPPLER ABNORMALITY DICTATES BPS FREQUENCY*

Abnormality[†]	BPS Frequency[‡]	Decision to Deliver (Fetal)[§]
Elevated indices Only	Weekly	Abnormal BPS[¶] or term or >36 weeks with no fetal growth
AEDV	Twice weekly	Abnormal BPS[¶] or >34 weeks proven maturity, or conversion to REDV
REDV	Daily	Any BPS <10/10** or >32 weeks, antenatal steroids given
REDV-UVP	Three times daily	Any BPS <10/10** or >28 weeks, antenatal steroids given

* BPS determines management. Must be viable to enter: >25 weeks' gestation, >500 g, normal anatomy, normal karyotype.
† Umbilical artery and complete venous-tree Doppler. Cerebralization of blood flow confirms umbilical artery abnormality as serious, does not directly alter management.
‡ *Minimum* frequency, increased on basis of severity: maternal condition(s), degree of IUGR, gestation.
§ Neonatal consultation, maternal condition/instability, direct fetal parameter by cordocentesis, all will impact this family—perinatology decision.
¶ Any BPS ≤ 4/10, or 8/10—Oligo, or repeated 6/10.
** BPS 8/10 cyclic absence of FBM is the only exception—in that case, repeat BPS < 6 h.

A or REDV, absent or reversed end-diastolic velocity; BPS, biophysical profile score; FBM, fetal breathing movement; IUGR, intrauterine growth restriction; UVP, umbilical venous pulsations.

Normal umbilical artery resistance falls progressively through pregnancy, reflecting increased numbers of tertiary stem, villous, small vessels (Fig. 21-12; Color Plate 7) (Stuart et al., 1980). Umbilical artery resistance may be increased in a number of pathologic conditions and may change dramatically to reflect acute changes such as sublethal infarction, partial abruption of the placenta, placental scarring from intervillous thrombosis, and damage from villitis, viral or bacterial. In classic IUGR, increased resistance in the umbilical arteries represents placental injury with loss of cross-sectional arterial outflow (Giles et al., 1985). In the sheep model, infarcting multiple small vessels by infusing microspheres can be titrated to induce precise rises in umbilical artery resistance (Trudinger et al., 1987; Morrow et al., 1989). As umbilical artery resistance rises (Fig. 21-13; Color Plate 8), diastolic velocities fall, and ultimately these are absent (AEDV) (Trudinger et al., 1987). As resistance rises even further, an elastic component is added, which will induce REDV, as the insufficient, rigid, placental circulation recoils after being distended by pulse pressure (Arabin et al., 1988). This latter condition is terminal and can only exist for a short period of time; our longest recorded healthy survivor had 13 days of REDV, contrasted to our longest survivor with AEDV of more than 14 weeks (Harman, 1998).

MEASUREMENT TECHNIQUES. As with all Doppler evaluations, the Doppler gate is enlarged to encompass the entire vessel, and transducer position is adjusted to eliminate aliasing, to minimize the Doppler angle, and to sample a single umbilical artery (Eik-Nes et al., 1984). In the initial Doppler evaluation of any compromised fetus, both umbilical arteries should be sampled, and information from the best umbilical artery should be used in clinical decisions (Maulik et al., 1982). There is no established standard as to where along the course of the umbilical artery the definitive evaluation should be made. Especially for the compromised IUGR fetus, the length of the cord may represent substantial resistance in itself. Figure 21-14 (Color Plate 9) demonstrates reversed, absent, and present end-diastolic velocities in the umbilical cord in a severely growth restricted fetus. Although all these waveforms are abnormal, the midcord waveform may be most representative of the challenges faced by the fetal circulation in perfusing the placenta. Work is underway to quantify these relationships across all gestations with IUGR fetuses.

CLINICAL SIGNIFICANCE. Elevated umbilical artery indices suggest placental liability but correlate with IUGR in less than 60% of cases (Pollack and Divon, 1995). Although indicating a need for ongoing monitoring of fetal growth, proportions, amniotic fluid volume, and well-being, *elevated umbilical artery indices alone represent statistical markers for fetal surveillance rather than indicators for intervention in themselves.* In fetuses thought not to be at risk for placental insufficiency, markedly elevated umbilical artery resistance indices should suggest previously undiagnosed placental injury and increased fetal surveillance. Elevated umbilical artery indices mandate performance of multivessel systemic Doppler assessment and BPS (Divon et al., 1989; Hecher, Campbell, et al., 1995).

AEDV may exist in equilibrium for an extended period of time. Further, because standardization varies widely between studies, it is difficult to be certain what AEDV means over large populations. In many fetuses, AEDV is not stable and will progress to REDV over time. Many fetuses with AEDV also have altered brain blood flow, with increased diastolic veloci-

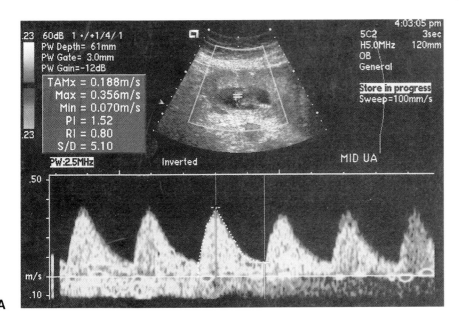

A

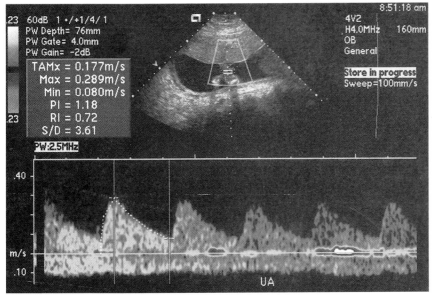

B

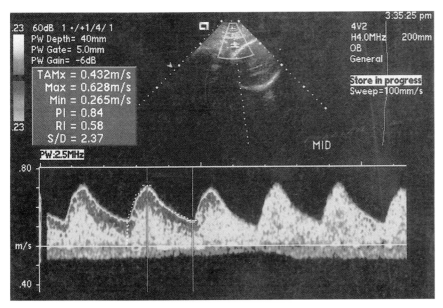

C

FIGURE 21-12 ■ Evolution of normal umbilical artery resistance, measured in midcord. Although there is an increase in diastolic velocities and corresponding gradual decline in S/D ratio from first trimester to third (**A** to **C**), note there is already well-developed diastolic flow in the earlier waveform. See also Color Plate 7.

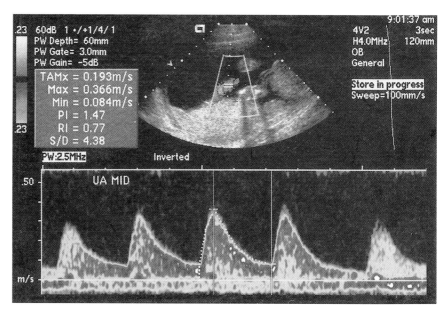

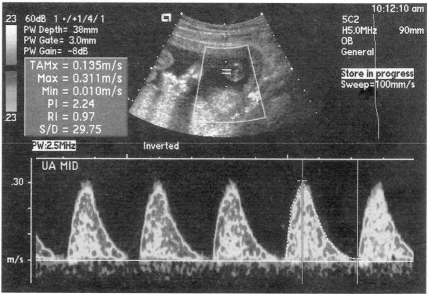

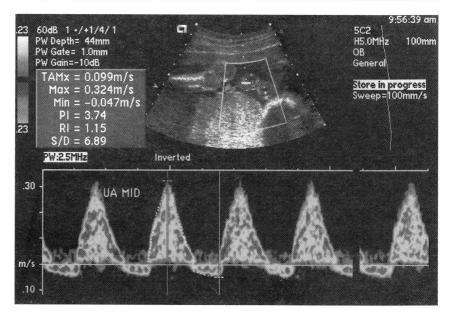

FIGURE 21-13 ■ Progressive abnormality of umbilical artery resistance. Initially nearly normal at 18 weeks (P.I. 147 [**A**]), by 24 weeks (**B**) the umbilical artery shows absent end-diastolic velocities that progressed to reversal of flow for 25% of the cardiac cycle (**C**). The infant had an umbilical venous pH of 7.18 after nonlabored cesarean section. All measurements in midcord. See also Color Plate 8.

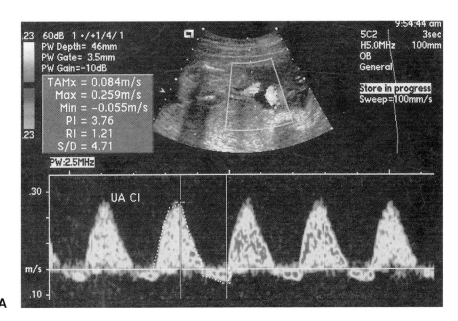

A

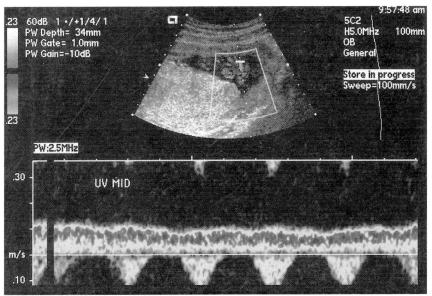

B

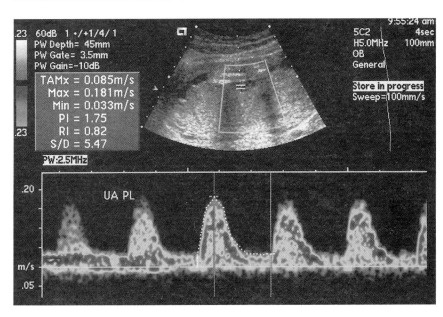

C

FIGURE 21-14 ■ Umbilical artery resistance may vary extremely from one point on cord to another. **A,** Abdominal cord insertion shows reversed end-diastolic velocities. **B,** Midcord shows absent end-diastolic velocities (waveforms inverted in this image). **C,** Placental cord insertion has elevated resistance but does demonstrate positive diastolic flow. During the 3-minute period shown in the three panels, there were no uterine contractions. See also Color Plate 9.

ties, the "brain-sparing" phenomenon (Baschat, Gembruch, Reiss, et al., 2000). Most fetuses with AEDV will have estimated fetal weight below the 10th percentile, thus qualifying as placenta-based IUGR (Farine et al., 1995). As well, at least half the mothers of such fetuses will have chronic hypertension and/or proteinuric preeclampsia. Although AEDV beyond 10 weeks' gestation is not a normal finding, not all fetuses with this degree of placental resistance have functional evidence of placental insufficiency in the form of acidosis or hypoxemia. AEDV is not usually compatible with term pregnancy, and so it is not surprising that the majority (80% to 100%) of such fetuses are delivered by cesarean section, often electively, or provoked by fetal distress in labor. Clearly, the combination of prematurity, IUGR, and potential placental respiratory insufficiency suggests that tertiary delivery is indicated for most of these fetuses.

AEDV is an indication for preparation for delivery, including appropriate referral, administration of antenatal steroids, and detailed maternal evaluation to exclude undiagnosed hypertension, renal disorders, connective tissue disorders, or thrombophilias. Further, because up to 20% of such fetuses will have malformations or overt aneuploidy, a diligent review of fetal anatomy, and in some cases invasive fetal testing for fetal karyotype, is indicated (Hsieh et al., 1988). Although the latter may seem unduly invasive considering the short intrauterine time remaining, avoidance of maternal morbidity (about 35% of those requiring cesarean delivery undergo *classic* cesarean sections) and exclusion of fetal karyotypic abnormality are important. It is noted that even in fetuses with no visible anomalies, the combination of IUGR, including fetal disproportion, and abnormal placental Dopplers may be associated with 5% to 8% aneuploidy (Farine et al., 1995).

Finding AEDV calls for immediate evaluation of fetal behavior, amniotic fluid volume, and FHR variability (BPS, scored out of 10). Subsequent interval monitoring with biophysical profile scoring remains our standard. Monitoring these fetuses with non-stress testing alone is not adequate, because most of these fetuses will have reduced variability and small accelerations in any case. Relying on composite scoring of the BPS means a lower rate of false-positive tests but does require the observer to become attuned to the movement pattern of the individual fetus. In this precarious situation, subjectively reduced amniotic fluid volume, overall reductions in total fetal activity, long intervals between periods of fetal breathing, and spontaneous FHR decelerations observed on real-time ultrasound may lie above the baseline threshold for BPS variables but indicate progressive deterioration in fetal status. This level of awareness required of the ultrasound observer may explain some authors' dissatisfaction in withholding delivery in these fetuses (Yoon et al., 1992; Battaglia et al., 1993). Infants who had AEDV as fetuses are at risk for many neonatal complications because of placental insufficiency, asphyxial events surrounding delivery, and the significant impacts of prematurity (Table 21-6) (Trudinger et al., 1991; Kelly et al., 1993; Zelop et al., 1996). The aim of pregnancy monitoring is to extend the pregnancy as far as possible, under safe fetal conditions, to reduce as much as possible the impact of prematurity.

REDV magnifies the dangers and risks noted above. In almost every fetal situation, this is a very unstable, often rapidly changing fetal-placental process. In many cases, overt abruption, intraplacental bleeding, or fetal maternal hemor-

rhage is the end point of observation. Thus, many authors continue to recommend delivery as soon as possible (Farine et al., 1995, Pollack and Divon, 1995; Pattinson et al., 1995). Because many cases of REDV are discovered on the first evaluation (e.g., on referral for evaluation of clinical IUGR), the progression for an individual fetus is difficult to determine. In our experience, if the BPS is normal *and* amniotic fluid is adequate *and* there are no decelerations on the CTG *and* mean minute variation is greater than 3 msec, time can be taken to administer antenatal steroids *and* to evaluate maternal condition before delivery. Because REDV is always associated with very significant abnormalities of cerebral perfusion (marked centralization) and often with abnormal venous circulation (abnormal ductus venosus and/or pulsatile umbilical vein), REDV is associated with the highest frequency of fetal compromise, neonatal complications, perinatal mortality, and perinatal morbidity. Despite this, measures to reduce the superimposed impacts of prematurity in such infants may be effective in achieving the highest rate of intact survival (Divon et al., 1989; Baschat and Harman, 2001).

MIDDLE CEREBRAL ARTERY

HEMODYNAMICS. Two features about the anatomy of the MCA are important. First, it represents a readily accessible fetal vessel depicting brain blood flow. Although this vessel has been used in adults to infer downstream (brain parenchymal) small-vessel resistance (Aaslid et al., 1982, 1984), in the fetus such resistance is uniformly high, and the primary relationship studied is the flow in the vessel itself. The MCA is short, straight, and uniformly positioned relative to the fetal skull and other intracranial landmarks (Fig. 21-15; Color Plate 10). Thus, Doppler measurements taken from this vessel are more reproducible than other vascular beds and have few collateral circulatory influences, while representing a critical component of the fetal circulation, which is usually readily accessible throughout gestation (Van den Wijngaard et al., 1989).

MCA peak velocities in systole generally reflect measured peak velocities in other vascular beds. Because the Doppler

TABLE 21-6. ABNORMAL UMBILICAL ARTERY DOPPLER INDICATES NEONATAL COMPROMISE*

Cesarean section for fetal distress
Acidosis
Hypoxemia
Low Apgar-5
Ventilator required
Long-term oxygen
BPD
Anemia
Increased NRBC
Thrombocytopenia
Prolonged NRBC release
Neutropenia
Transfusions required
IVH
NEC
Perinatal mortality

* For all these outcomes, their frequency rises exponentially from abnormal indices to absent end-diastolic velocities to reversed end-diastolic velocities.
BPD, bronchopulmonary dysplasia; IVH, intraventricular hemorrhage; NEC, necrotizing enterocolitis; NRBC, nucleated red blood cells.

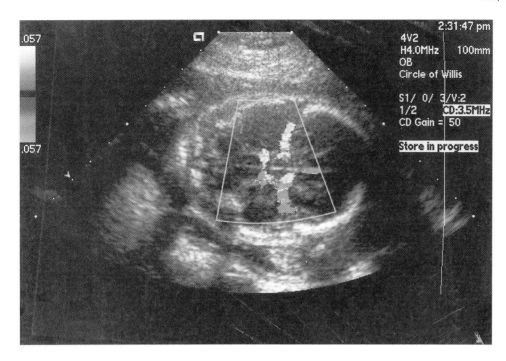

FIGURE 21-15 ■ Doppler color flow mapping illustrates the fetal Circle of Willis (vertical vessel, middle cerebral artery). See also Color Plate 10.

angle can be minimized reproducibly, this feature allows direct interpretation of the peak velocity rather than inference from vascular indices. One of the roles of MCA Doppler, therefore, is to evaluate the absolute speed of blood flow, which has direct application in fetal anemia (Harman, 1996; Mari et al., 2000). As the blood becomes thinner, cardiac ejection fraction increases, transaortic velocities increase, and the MCA offers an ideal location for direct interpretation of this increase in velocity as a decline in fetal hematocrit (Fig. 21-16) (Copel et al., 1988).

Although the many complications of placental insufficiency may also include anemia and elevation of the peak velocity, the key MCA abnormality expressed by the compromised fetus is centralization (Fig. 21-17; Color Plate 11) (Chandran et al., 1993; Hecher, Ville, et al., 1995). This is an increase in diastolic velocities, representative of increased brain blood flow. A significant question is whether such changes are compensatory (parenchymal vasodilatation by active mechanisms) or involuntary (increased shunting of blood away from somatic circulations, under the force of hypertension dictated by accelerating placental vascular resistance). That a positive mechanism is in place (the first explanation) is suggested by maintenance of normal fetal activities, continued brain growth, and normal pH, even as centralization is taking place (Baschat et al., 2001). Cerebral blood flow as depicted by the MCA may be responsive to a number of stimuli, including maternal administration of oxygen (increased resistance) (Arduini et al., 1989), carbon dioxide (decreased resistance) (Potts et al., 1992), or nicotine (increased resistance, and lack of responsiveness) (Arbeille et al., 1992). These changes may occur gradually, indicated by subtle changes in the "cerebroplacental ratio" (Arbeille et al., 1987). The cerebroplacental ratio reflects the calculated ratio of resistance indices in the MCA and umbilical artery and may change subtly in response to shifts in circulation representing the earliest stages of brain sparing (Wladimiroff et al., 1987; Arbeille et al., 1988). The cerebroplacental ratio may therefore provide an early warning system to initiate more detailed fetal surveillance.

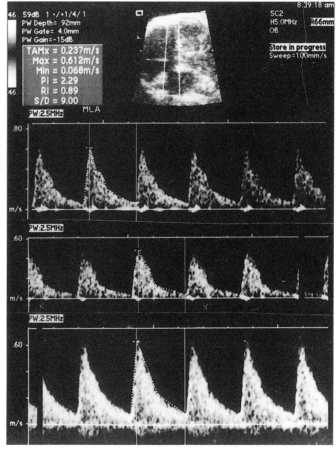

FIGURE 21-16 ■ The peak systolic velocity in the middle cerebral artery (MCA) reflects fetal hematocrit accurately. This fetus had serious anti-D isoimmune anemia. *Top,* Pretransfusion, the MCA peak of 60 cm/sec correctly predicted anemia, hematocrit 19.0. After intrauterine transfusion, the MCA peak fell to 41 cm/sec as hematocrit rose to 44.0. Before the next transfusion (*bottom*) middle cerebral artery rose to 62 cm/sec and hematocrit had fallen to 20.0.

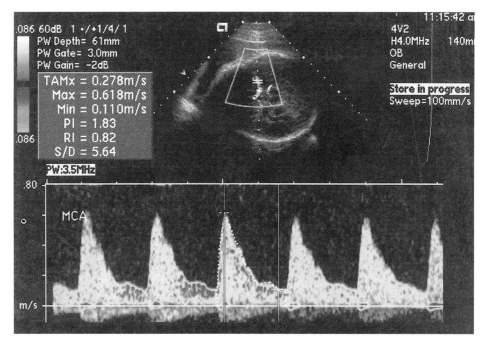

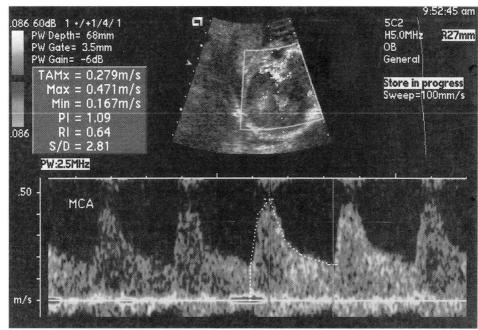

FIGURE 21-17 ■ Centralization of blood flow. Normal middle cerebral artery shows high resistance, low diastolic velocities (**A**). As placental resistance rises, brain blood flow increases with falling resistance and increased diastolic velocities in the middle cerebral artery (**B**). See also Color Plate 11.

MEASUREMENT TECHNIQUES. As demonstrated in Figures 21-15 to 21-17, the MCA is readily identified, and its short straight course provides little technical challenge. The gate is opened to encompass the vessel, and short periods of insonation are used to minimize the amount of direct multiformat ultrasound delivered to the fetal brain. For this reason, most authorities recommend fetal MCA velocimetry should not be studied in the first trimester.

CLINICAL SIGNIFICANCE. As IUGR worsens and compensatory mechanisms take place, MCA diastolic velocities rise. This centralization continues to increase in most fetuses with AEDV, and many with REDV (Karsdorp et al., 1994). At the point when REDV and fetal hypoxemia result in cardiac decompensation, MCA diastolic velocities may fall, returning to an apparently high-resistance pattern because cardiac output is no longer sufficient to force blood into the fetal circulation (fetal cerebrovascular tone and fetal brain edema are thought to contribute here). This reversion resulting from heart failure has been called "normalization" and is an ominous sign meriting consideration for delivery (Jensen et al., 1999). Other than this infrequent extreme, the MCA *indicates need for further testing rather than dictating clinical management by itself.* Shifts in the cerebroplacental ratio or overt centralization of the MCA indicates a need for comprehensive fetal examination, testing using multivessel Doppler, and biophysical profile scoring, scored out of 10, on a frequent basis (Baschat and Harman, 2001). An exception to this rule occurs close to term, where MCA centralization without abnormal umbilical arteries or precordial veins has been associated with acidosis and hypoxemia and poor perinatal outcome (Hershkovitz et al., 2000). The frequency of this finding in completely normal fetuses is unknown but definite. At present, as further clinical investigation into this phenomenon is carried out, we institute comprehensive monitoring including biophysical profile scoring and fetal growth surveillance, but we do not automatically move to delivery with this finding. Many centers now use the MCA as an indication for invasive fetal testing in situations where fetal anemia may exist (e.g., viral infection, transplacental hemorrhage, alloimmunization, and hereditary red cell abnormalities) (Harman, 1996).

Fetal Venous Dopplers

DUCTUS VENOSUS

This vessel reflects volume management by the right atrium and is responsive to fetal oxygenation, dilating as hypoxemia worsens. Many authorities use this as a direct reflection of overall fetal cardiac function. Although various indices have been applied, none seems to have superiority, and simple waveform shape—the reversed A wave (generated by atrial contraction)—has high sensitivity for fetal cardiac failure, decompensation due to severe afterload increase as seen in placental insufficiency, or heart failure associated with fetal hydrops, as in end-stage anemia, viral infection, or nonimmune causes (Huisman, 2001). In twin-to-twin transfusion syndrome, this pattern in the recipient twin indicates myocardial failure due to volume overload (which may occur as a result of intrauterine fetal myocardial infarction), whereas in the donor twin it indicates myocardial dysfunction due to preterminal placental failure and hypoxemia (Hecher et al., 1995). Severe abnormalities of ductus venosus flow may be temporarily responsive to maternal oxygenation, amnioinfusion to relieve fetal cord compression (Harman, Baschat, Muench, in press), or other maneuvers to assist the compromised fetal heart, but in general this finding is another reason to consider preparation for delivery in the short term (Fig. 21-18; Color Plate 12). A notable exception occurs in the first trimester, where severe decreases in forward flow through the ductus venosus during the A wave do not indicate structural or functional heart failure but indicate increases in backward fluid volume, compatible with congenital heart disease or aneuploidy, as depicted by increased nuchal translucency (Matias et al., 1998).

UMBILICAL VEIN

Venous pulsations represent the only reproducible abnormality of diagnostic significance of this vessel. "Double pulsation" is most frequently seen in association with increased afterload, as in abnormal umbilical resistance, and is thought to indicate excessive volume in the precordial venous system, with a constricted ductus venosus and normal heart mechanics (Falkensammer et al., 2001). Triple pulsations, on the other hand, may be due to a partially or completely dilated ductus venosus, volume failure, and hypoxemic myocardial dysfunction. (Fig. 21-19; Color Plate 13) (Baschat and Gembruch, 1996; Hofstaetter et al., 2001). Although several groups have demonstrated that umbilical venous pulsations are an ominous finding and frequently lead to intrauterine demise or serious neonatal compromise, definitions are not well standardized (Harman, Baschat, Gembruch, et al., in press). It is a frequent finding, for example, that umbilical venous pulsations occur when the umbilical cord is mildly compressed or at the end of large-volume fetal transfusions when the circulation is full (but in the complete absence of cardiac failure) (Oepkes et al., 1993; Baz et al., 1999). Isolated umbilical venous pulsations (in the absence of IUGR, abnormal umbilical arteries, and without centralization of MCA flow) have uncertain significance. Thus, umbilical venous pulsations represent the best example of the dictum: Doppler investigations are not to be taken in isolation, out of context with other fetal observations (Kiserud, 2001).

Maternal Dopplers

UTERINE ARTERY

The maternal uterine artery normally demonstrates progressive reduction in resistance and increased diastolic velocities throughout gestation (Fig. 21-20) (Trudinger et al., 1985a). This depends on absence of maternal hypertension and presence of normal placental invasion (Rotmensch et al., 1995). Abnormal placentation results in maintenance of the prepregnancy high impedance characteristics of uterine artery circulation (Schulman et al., 1986). High resistance, persistence of diastolic notching, and even absent end-systolic forward flow can persist throughout pregnancy if placentation is inadequate. Different components of uterine artery abnormality have different sensitivities and specificity for placental malfunction, maternal hypertensive disorders, or their combination. Uterine artery "lateralization" has the highest positive predictive accuracy (Chan et al., 1995). In this situation, indices remain elevated and notching (reflective of the elastic component of unmodified maternal uterine artery muscle) and a marked difference between the side where the placenta is (which is usually much better than the contralateral side) demonstrate inadequate placentation. In more than 50% of women, this is associated with hypertensive disorders and overt preeclampsia, with or without IUGR (Bewley et al., 1991). In patients with thrombophilias, history of prior severe preeclampsia/eclampsia, and/or severe IUGR, persistence of placental lateralization may be an indication for heparin therapy in mid-trimester (Fig. 21-21). These findings will differ from the woman with persistent arterial muscle hypertrophy due to long-standing chronic hypertension. In that case, although notching will persist bilaterally and resistance indices will be higher than normal, the gestational age increase in diastolic velocities will occur. Although this may represent a less-severe form of inadequate placental effect, superimposed preeclampsia and late IUGR may occur.

MATERNAL CEREBRAL DOPPLERS

Initial interest in maternal MCA Doppler in the monitoring and pharmacologic management of serious preeclampsia has not become standard of practice (Williams and McLean, 1993; Williams and Wilson, 1994). The maternal MCA can be visualized through the temporal "window" of thin bone just anterior to the temporal artery, allowing depiction of the normal MCA waveform. The characteristics of this waveform in normal and

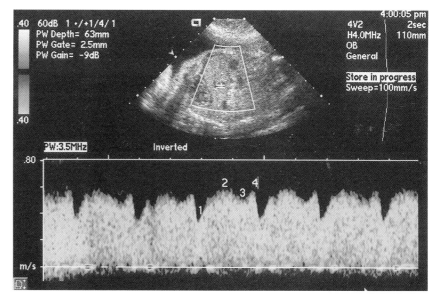

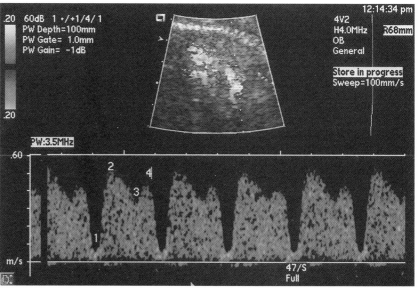

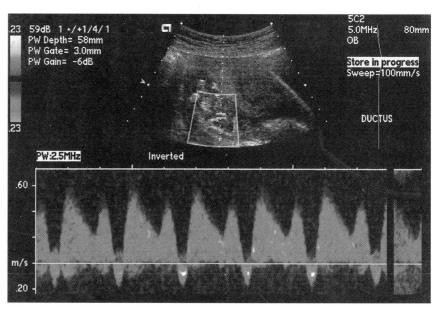

FIGURE 21-18 ■ Ductus venosus waveforms. **A,** Normal four-phase waveform (1, atrial contraction; 2, ventricular systole; 3, ascent of annulus; 4, diastole) with a wave showing only modest normal reduction in forward flow. **B,** Markedly increased afterload (from placental resistance) is reflected through the heart as markedly abnormal forward cardiac function, with nearly retrograde a wave. **C,** Preterminal cardiac failure. Note severe retrograde a wave as well as distorted cardiac function producing distortion of y-descent. See also Color Plate 12.

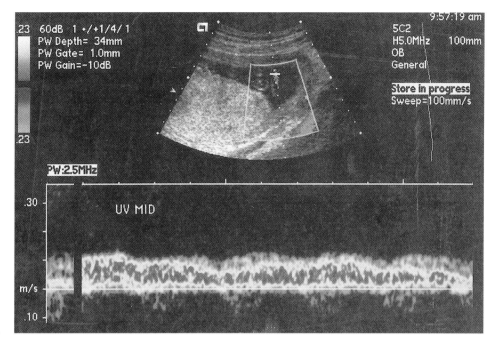

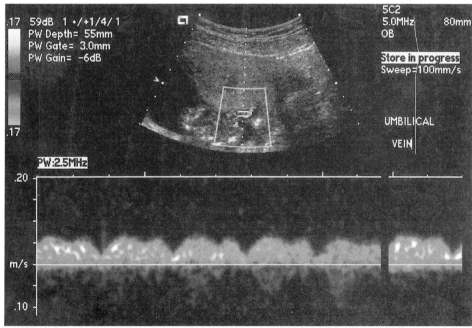

FIGURE 21-19 ■ Umbilical venous pulsations. **A,** Moderate pulsatility, increased placental resistance in intrauterine growth restriction. **B,** Cardiac failure with tricuspid regurgitation reflected as retrograde flow all the way back to midcord. Note timing relationship to arterial pulsations (below line). See also Color Plate 13.

hypertensive pregnancies are shown in Figure 21-22 (Color Plate 14). In units with practice at this technically exacting method, monitoring of maternal cerebral circulation, especially in posteclampsia women being managed with multiple antihypertensive drugs including acute vasodilators such as nitroprusside, there may be a role for serial monitoring of these vessels (Kyle et al., 1993). In general, however, the research demonstrating the powerful and almost immediate effect of magnesium sulfate in producing dilatation of the cerebrovasculature, releasing arterial spasm, means that clinical application of these Doppler techniques is seldom mandatory (Belfort and Moise, 1992).

Patterns of Deterioration

In general, placental abnormalities may persist for months before other Doppler parameters deteriorate. As placental resistance increases (probably as more and more placental infarcts occur), brain sparing is invoked, with progressive abnormalities in umbilical artery circulation (AEDV, progressing to REDV) being associated with higher and higher diastolic velocities in the MCA. By this time subjective elements of behavior, such as increasing intervals of quiet sleep (state 1F), decreased velocity of fetal movements (often per-

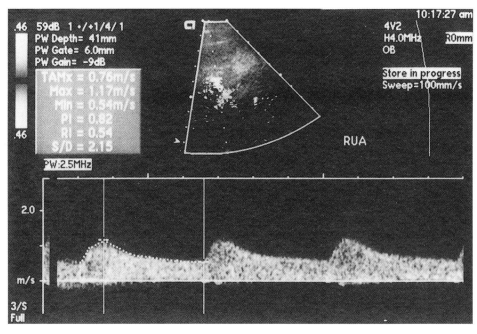

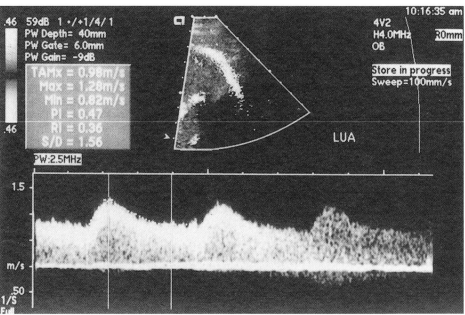

FIGURE 21-20 ■ Normal maternal Dopplers from right (RUA) and left (LUA) uterine arteries. Low-resistance high-diastolic flow, little difference from one side to the other, characterize normal placentation.

ceived by the mother as "weaker" movements), and elements of subjectively decreased amniotic fluid, may begin to appear (Hecher et al., 2001). With onset of AEDV, progressive changes in the cerebroplacental ratio, and overt centralization, oligohydramnios becomes more common. The NST often becomes flatter, with overt nonreactivity at or just before deterioration of precordial veins, including retrograde ductus venosus A wave. About this time, reversal of end-diastolic velocities in the umbilical artery may occur (although this progression is completed in only 20% of severe IUGR), with progressive loss of fetal breathing movements, followed by fetal tone, and then abolition of all movements, as the BPS becomes overtly abnormal (Fig. 21-23) (Baschat et al., 2001).

Integration of Doppler Results and Other Tests

Although the stereotypical deterioration depicted above is not always followed and does not always progress at a regular rate, the onset of these changes calls for many management steps. As investigations with Dopplers and correlation with other aspects of placental monitoring become better understood, the timing of onset of these placental markers of insufficiency moves progressively earlier in gestation. Although AEDV may be considered normal in early gestation, by 12 to 14 weeks they occur in only 10% of patients (Gurel et al., in press, 2003). Among these 10% are fetuses who subsequently develop IUGR. Although the false-positive rate of

PLATE 3

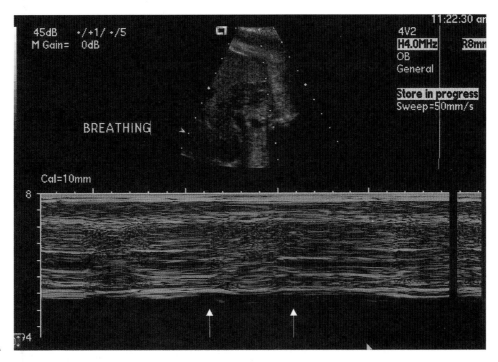

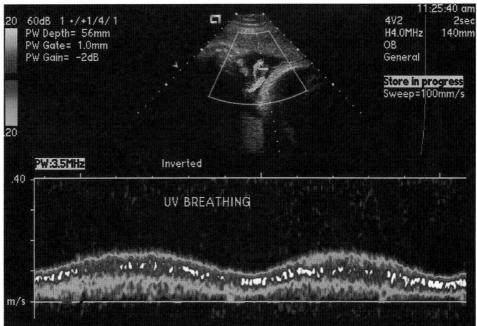

FIGURE 21-1 ■ Depictions of fetal breathing movement. **A,** Diaphragmatic movement on M-mode ultrasound; note broad (3 to 4 second) excursions typical of deep breathing, one of many normal patterns. **B,** Umbilical venous fluctuations.

Continued

PLATE 4

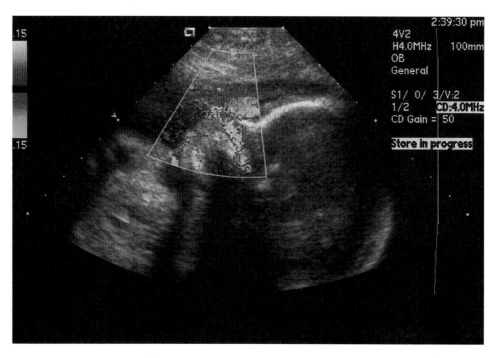

C

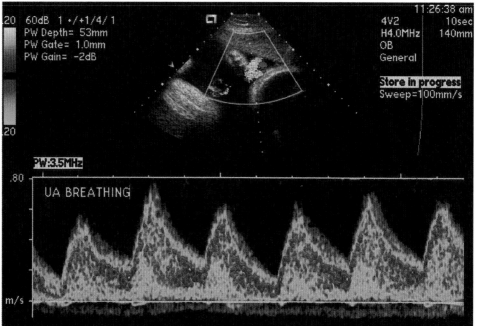

D

FIGURE 21-1, cont'd ■ **C,** Nasal flaring of expelled lung fluid during fetal breathing movement. **D,** Fetal heart rate variability; "respiratory arrhythmia" is depicted in umbilical artery.

PLATE 5

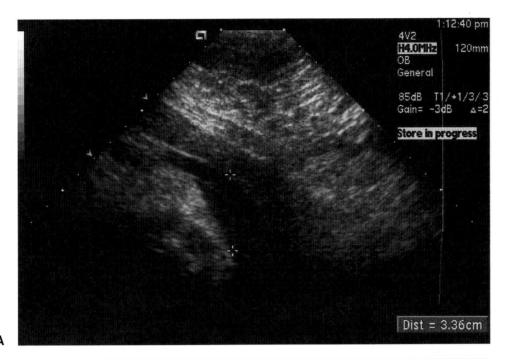

A

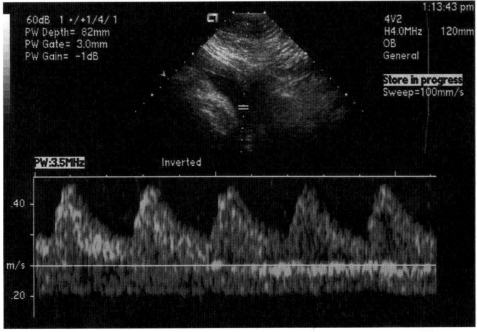

B

FIGURE 21-5 ■ Fluid pocket verification. **A,** Amniotic fluid apparently meets biophysical profile score vertical pocket criteria. **B,** Pulsed Doppler demonstrates this is actually a vertical pocket of umbilical cord, with no measurable amniotic fluid.

PLATE 6

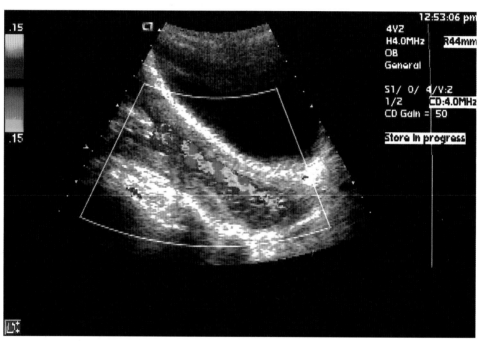

FIGURE 21-10 ■ Color Doppler shows umbilical cord trapped in prolapsed membranes filling entire endocervical canal. As the patient was transferred from the stretcher to the operating room table, the membranes ruptured and the cord prolapsed. The 32-week fetus survived intact after immediate cesarean section.

PLATE 7

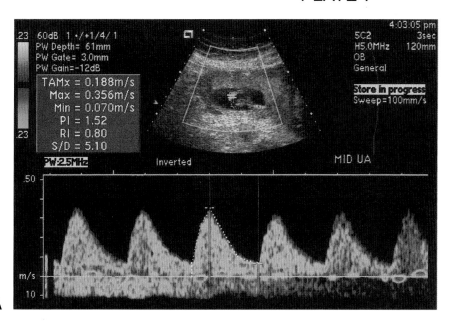

A

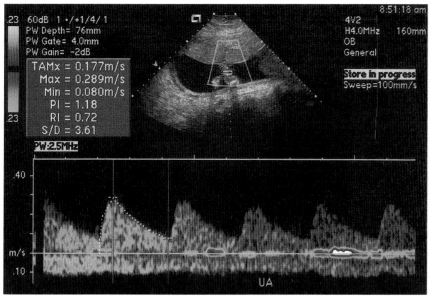

B

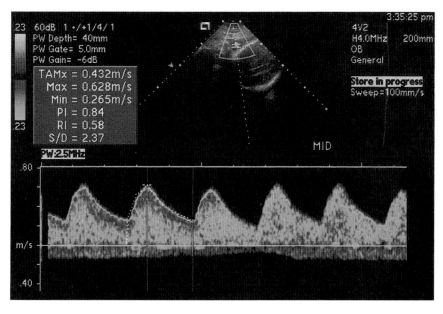

C

FIGURE 21-12 ■ Evolution of normal umbilical artery resistance, measured in midcord. Although there is an increase in diastolic velocities and corresponding gradual decline in S/D ratio from first trimester to third (**A** to **C**), note there is already well-developed diastolic flow in the earlier waveform.

PLATE 8

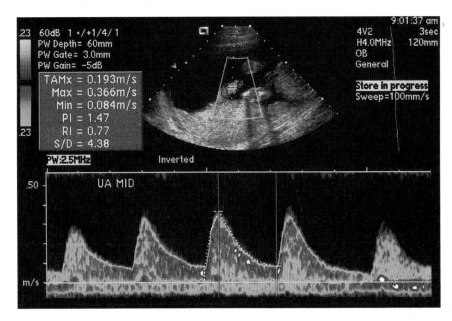

A

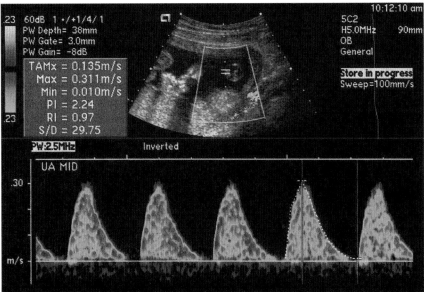

B

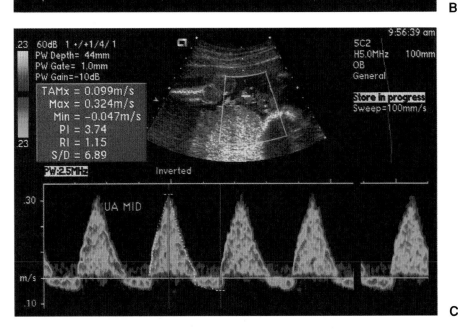

C

FIGURE 21-13 ■ Progressive abnormality of umbilical artery resistance. Initially nearly normal at 18 weeks (P.I. 147 [**A**]), by 24 weeks (**B**) the umbilical artery shows absent end-diastolic velocities that progressed to reversal of flow for 25% of the cardiac cycle (**C**). The infant had an umbilical venous pH of 7.18 after nonlabored cesarean section. All measurements in midcord.

PLATE 9

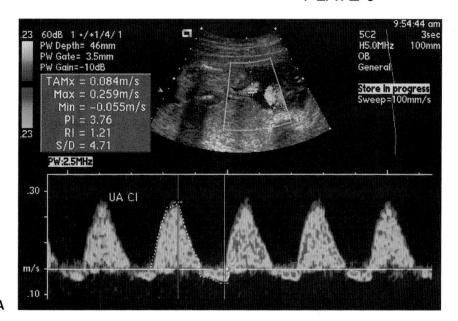

A

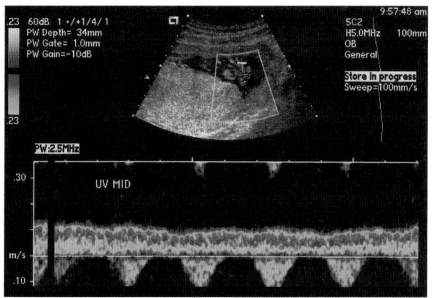

B

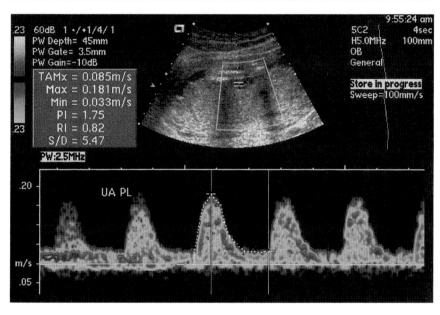

C

FIGURE 21-14 ■ Umbilical artery resistance may vary extremely from one point on cord to another. **A,** Abdominal cord insertion shows reversed end-diastolic velocities. **B,** Midcord shows absent end-diastolic velocities (waveforms inverted in this image). **C,** Placental cord insertion has elevated resistance but does demonstrate positive diastolic flow. During the 3-minute period shown in the three panels, there were no uterine contractions.

PLATE 10

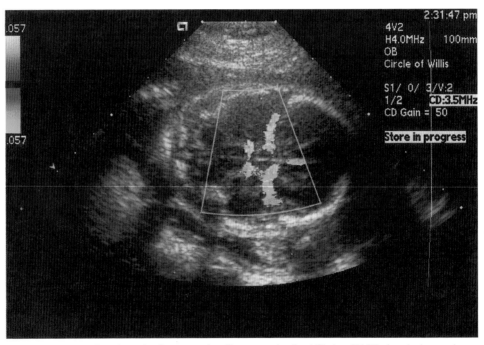

FIGURE 21-15 ■ Doppler color flow mapping illustrates the fetal Circle of Willis (vertical vessel, middle cerebral artery).

PLATE 11

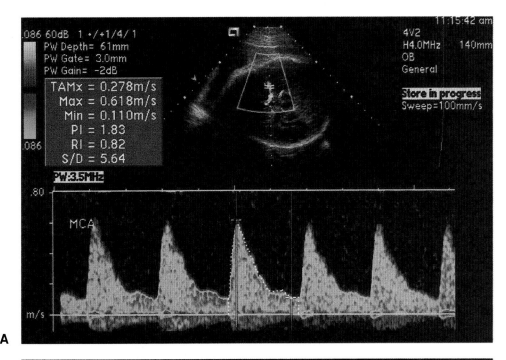

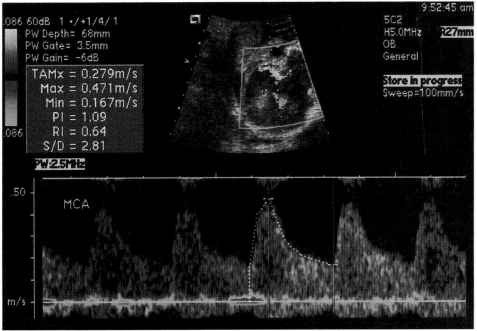

FIGURE 21-17 ■ Centralization of blood flow. Normal middle cerebral artery shows high resistance, low diastolic velocities (**A**). As placental resistance rises, brain blood flow increases with falling resistance and increased diastolic velocities in the middle cerebral artery (**B**).

PLATE 12

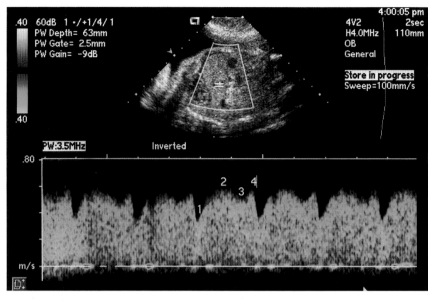

A

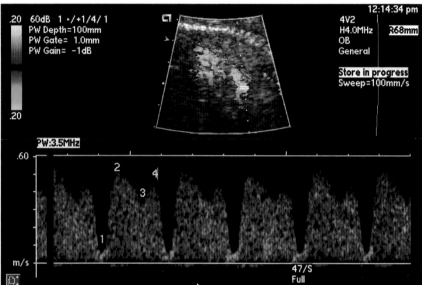

B

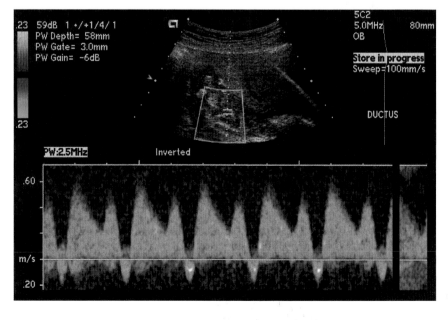

C

FIGURE 21-18 ■ Ductus venosus waveforms. **A,** Normal four-phase waveform (1, atrial contraction; 2, ventricular systole; 3, ascent of annulus; 4, diastole) with a wave showing only modest normal reduction in forward flow. **B,** Markedly increased afterload (from placental resistance) is reflected through the heart as markedly abnormal forward cardiac function, with nearly retrograde a wave. **C,** Preterminal cardiac failure. Note severe retrograde a wave as well as distorted cardiac function producing distortion of y-descent.

PLATE 13

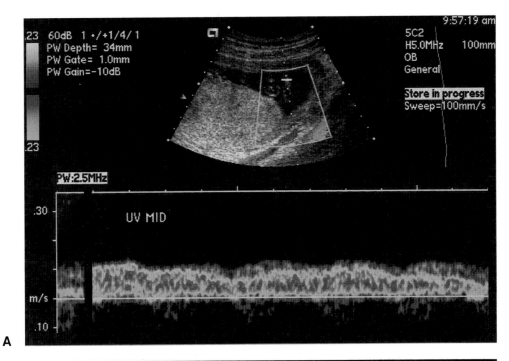

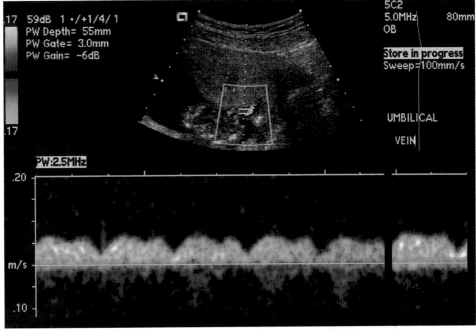

FIGURE 21-19 ■ Umbilical venous pulsations. **A,** Moderate pulsatility, increased placental resistance in intrauterine growth restriction. **B,** Cardiac failure with tricuspid regurgitation reflected as retrograde flow all the way back to midcord. Note timing relationship to arterial pulsations (below line).

PLATE 14

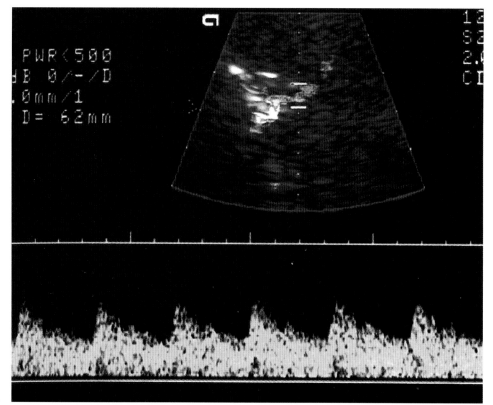

A

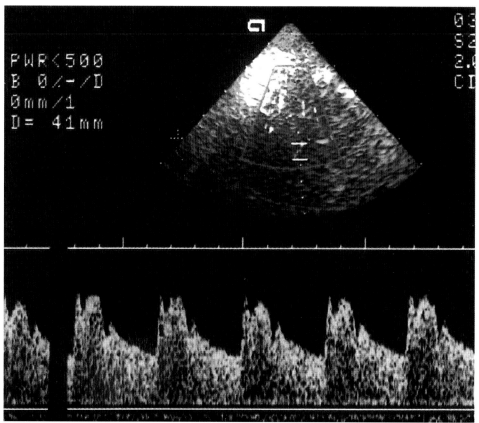

B

FIGURE 21-22 ■ Maternal intracranial Doppler examination. **A,** Normal middle cerebral artery Doppler waveform has modest systolic peak less than 60 cm/sec, diastolic peak less than 30 cm/sec, and slight notching. **B,** Abnormal maternal middle cerebral artery in preeclamptic woman at 26 weeks has higher velocities (102 and 50 cm/sec, respectively), with systolic and diastolic notching.

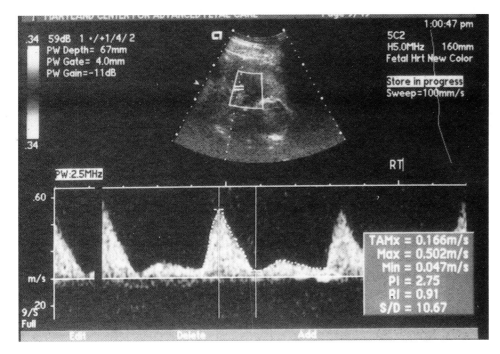

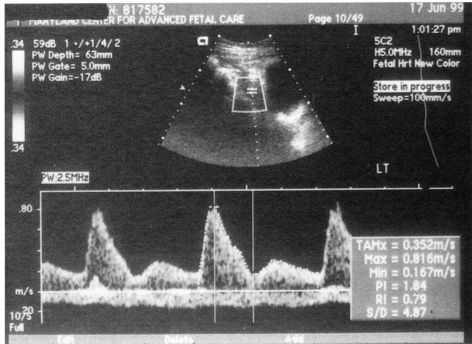

FIGURE 21-21 ■ Markedly abnormal uterine arteries in a mother with lupus, hypertension, superimposed preeclampsia, and intrauterine growth restriction at same gestation as the woman in Figure 21-20. Note: Increased resistance, persistent diastolic notching, significant difference between right (RT) and left (LT).

such screening is high, it does focus early attention on the role of primary placentation on determining IUGR (Dixon and Robertson, 1958; Robertson et al., 1975). Such patients frequently manifest placental injury by elevated maternal serum α-fetoprotein tests, an indication in our monitoring regimen for the institution of low-dose aspirin therapy. This constellation of placental markers calls for early, and frequent, serial evaluation of fetal growth, amniotic fluid volume maintenance, markers of IUGR such as lagging abdominal circumference, or isolated lagging skeletal growth parameters, as well as head-to-abdomen disproportion early in gestation. Detailed evaluation for cofactors, including placental anomalies, single umbilical artery, markers for fetal aneuploidy, and markers for other syndromes associated with fetal growth restriction, all should be carried out. Maternal laboratory investigations will establish risks for superimposed preeclampsia or maternal disorders such as thrombophilia and antiphospholipid antibody syndrome that would mandate the addition of heparin to the established low-dose aspirin therapy. In such patients, biophysical profile scoring, including computerized interpretation of FHR variability, is begun as early as 25 weeks' gestation. Acute events such as placental abruption, cardiac decompensation, and superimposed maternal preeclampsia will make the situation volatile. *The 7-day interval of routine biophysical profile scoring is inappropriate here.*

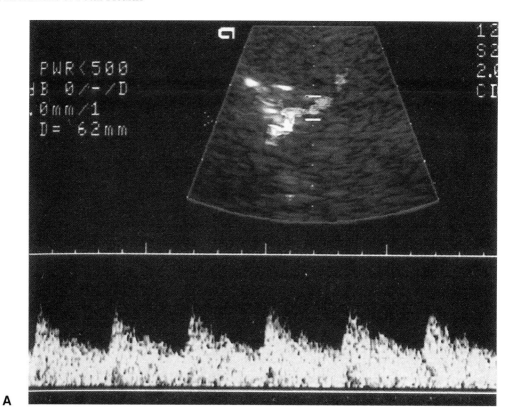

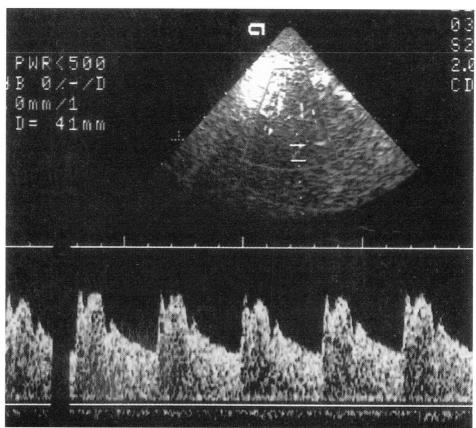

FIGURE 21-22 ■ Maternal intracranial Doppler examination. **A,** Normal middle cerebral artery Doppler waveform has modest systolic peak less than 60 cm/sec, diastolic peak less than 30 cm/sec, and slight notching. **B,** Abnormal maternal middle cerebral artery in preeclamptic woman at 26 weeks has higher velocities (102 and 50 cm/sec, respectively), with systolic and diastolic notching. See also Color Plate 14.

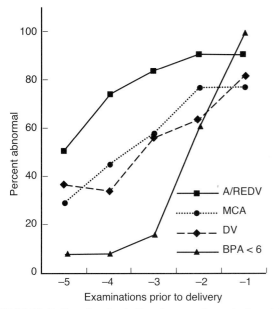

FIGURE 21-23 ■ Deterioration in Doppler waveforms before delivery for abnormal biophysical profile score (BPS). All fetuses had prospective Dopplers, and management decisions were made according to biophysical profile score. A/REDV, absent or reversed diastolic velocity; DV, ductus venosus; MCA, middle cerebral artery.

ANCILLARY TESTS

Fetal Patient

As with any patient, detailed evaluation of the fetus's history and physical examination may be highly revealing. As such, family history, further pregnancy screening (including nuchal translucency and maternal serum analytes), detailed review of fetal anatomy, serial evaluation of growth, amniotic fluid volume, and Doppler patterns all set the stage for the detailed monitoring protocols described here. The careful analysis of maternal risk factors, such as cigarette smoking, hypertension, antiphospholipid antibody syndromes, thrombophilia, vascular effects of diabetes, cocaine and other toxic substance abuse, and other sources of placental impairment, have a primary role in directing fetuses to surveillance. Overlapping risk factors mean modifying surveillance protocols to focus on vascular issues, reduce interval between testing based on severity, and apply ancillary testing (e.g., score out of 10 in all diabetics with vascular disease). These sources of information are not static—sonographers interact with patients at every visit and, in addition to routine inquiries, should have immediate access to a perinatologist to pursue any clinically indicated line of inquiry. This receptiveness to all channels of information about maternal and fetal well-being is a statistically important supplement to any monitoring technique.

Contraction Stress Test
Oxytocin Challenge Test

The CST and the OCT are two forms of testing that use FHR responses to uterine activity in evaluating fetal health. The CST uses spontaneously occurring contractions, or contractions induced by maternal nipple stimulation (Lenke and Nemes, 1984), whereas OCT uses intravenously administered oxytocin to cause repetitive uterine activity (Ray et al., 1972) (Fig. 21-24). In either case, interpretation includes observation of standard non-stress testing parameters (accelerations, FHR baseline, and category of variability) and the response of the heart rate once a contraction pattern has been established.

Technique is similar to the NST, except the mother may not be monitored sitting or supine. In either case postural artifact and restriction of fetal movement in response to contractions may generate falsely alarming tests. Once a contraction pattern is established, with at least three contractions in 10 minutes, evaluation is possible. *Negative OCT* has no decelerations or other unclassifiable changes from baseline with contractions (Ray et al., 1972). There may be isolated decelerations or times when the FHR is not adequately monitored, so the interpretive criteria suggested by Schifrin (1979) is that any monitored segment where three consecutive contractions are not associated with significant deflections in FHR baseline is considered negative (normal).

There are also interpretive arguments about designation of a *positive* (abnormal) CST/OCT. The classic standard for OCT interpretation is that FHR decelerations must accompany at least three consecutive contractions (Schifrin, 1979). Another interpretation scheme categorizes the CST as positive if at least 50% of the contractions cause late decelerations (when there are at least three contractions in 10 minutes) or in situations where all the contractions are associated with late decelerations but there are fewer than three in 10 minutes (Huddlestone et al., 1984). An *equivocal* CST/OCT demonstrates repetitive decelerations not late in timing and pattern, usually classified as variable decelerations. Because this is a marker for oligohydramnios or cord entrapment, further assessment is required for this category of tests as well (Collea and Holls, 1982; Merrill et al., 1995).

When contractions are not occurring spontaneously, intravenous oxytocin is given, as for induction of labor, initiating infusion at 0.5 mU/min, titrating upward in 1-mU increments until the contraction pattern has been established. Clearly, such manipulation of the intrauterine environment is done in a hospital setting to enable the emergency response that may be necessary in cases of hyperstimulation, unrelenting contractions despite discontinuing the oxytocin, tetanic contractions, and fixed fetal bradycardia. Although the more dangerous consequences of these events are rare, hyperstimulation occurs in more than 10% of tests (Freeman and Lagnew, 1990).

Clinical application of these tests is infrequent in modern fetal assessment units. Even those clinical groups who established, tested, and validated clinical implementation of the CST/OCT now report fetal evaluation based on modifications of biophysical profile scoring in the nonstressed uterine environment (Nageotte et al., 1995; Merrill et al., 1995). Several factors are responsible for the marginalization of this previously popular technique. First, the method may have significant complications. Second, even for normal testing, the method is time consuming and expensive, usually taking up to 40 minutes to provoke contractions and ensure normality, and much longer if the test is equivocal or abnormal. Third, although these tests are very good indicators of fetal well-being when negative (negative predictive values exceeding 99.8%), a positive test is not accurate enough to form the basis for clinical action. Positive predictive values for perinatal mortality of 8.7% to 14.9% and for morbidity up to 70% for low 5-minute Apgar scores, fetal distress, and cesarean

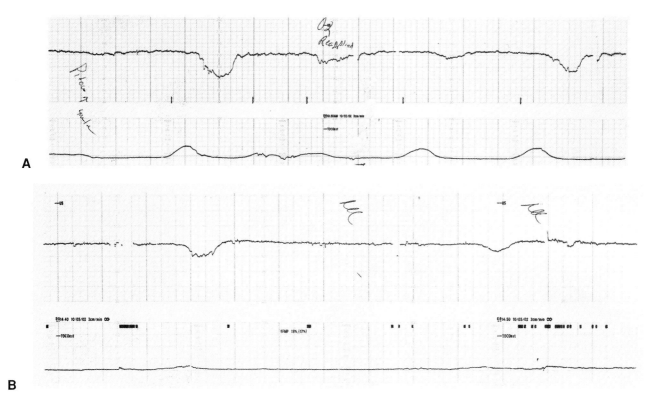

FIGURE 21-24 ■ **A,** Oxytocin challenge test. Once contractions were established, repetitive late decelerations occurred with each contraction (positive oxytocin challenge test). Delivery was by cesarean section because of fetal distress as induction of labor was attempted. Note that different strengths of contractions produced different depths of deceleration, all late in timing. **B,** Contraction stress test. Even trivial uterine activity caused late decelerations in this fetus, severe intrauterine growth restriction with abnormal Dopplers. Biophysical profile score 4/10 at 25 weeks (positive contraction stress test).

delivery for abnormal FHR in labor show correlations but do not justify emergency delivery. When biophysical profile scoring is the backup test for a positive CST/OCT, at least 50% of pregnancies may be safely allowed to continue 1 week or more and the remainder demonstrate outcomes that correlate better with the biophysical profile variables than with elements of the CST/OCT (Nageotte et al., 1994). Few centers use either of these tests as a first-line method for high-risk pregnancy fetal monitoring.

In our center, where biophysical profile scoring is the primary method for fetal surveillance, two roles remain for uterine stimulation as a fetal challenge. In the compromised IUGR fetus with oligohydramnios, it is likely, but not certain, that cesarean delivery is required. If the OCT is negative and there is no change in fetal baseline heart rate, induction of labor will be successful for vaginal delivery in about 45% of cases. If the OCT is positive, safe vaginal delivery is rare. Although much of this outcome is predetermined by our responses to a positive OCT, it does demonstrate that reassurance from negative OCT may avoid maternal morbidity. Currently, this approach is applied only to fetuses greater than 32 weeks' gestation and weighing more than 1500 g, presenting by the vertex, with at least some residual amniotic fluid present.

Before delivery we use the CST/OCT to monitor some fetuses with unique presentations. In the fetus with normal amniotic fluid and normal biophysical profile scoring who has markedly abnormal Doppler velocimetry in multiple vessels, highly suggestive of placental insufficiency, the combination of stressed testing and fetal blood sampling for pH and cord blood gases may be used to allow for continuation of the pregnancy. Although our information is restricted to a relatively small number of fetuses, it would appear that when both of these ancillary tests are normal, the BPS is validated as a method for delaying delivery up to 10 weeks, in the face of markedly abnormal Doppler patterns.

Vibroacoustic Stimulation

Where NST or other forms of FHR monitoring are the primary means of evaluating fetal health, the nonreactive test due to fetal quiet sleep (state 1F) is a major source of false-alarming tests and consumes an inordinate amount of time waiting for state change. Because time (usually nursing time) is an expensive commodity, many efforts have focused on shortening this mandatory waiting time by rapidly provoking a state change to generate a reactive tracing. How the OCT and BPS address these issues was discussed previously. Another method of addressing the nonreactive NST is vibroacoustic stimulation (VAS). Stimulating the fetus with a noxious vibration/noise is effective in producing state change, fetal startle movements, and increased FHR variability and shortening the time it takes to demonstrate fetal well-being (Ohel et al., 1986; Gagnon et al., 1986).

Mechanism of Action

It is not clear whether vibration alone is sufficient to provoke these responses or whether the combination of vibration and audible noise is necessary. Although vibration sense is fully developed throughout the body by 22 to 24 weeks (Patrick and Gagnon, 1990), auditory responses are functional about a month later (Woods et al., 1984). It is clear that from this time on, the fetal sound environment is significant.

Under normal circumstances, the fetus is exposed to low-frequency sound energy from a variety of sources. Direct human data are scarce, but detailed evaluation of hearing in the fetal sheep and other models appears to be analogous (Vince and Armitage, 1980; Lecanuet et al., 1998). High-frequency sound is attenuated significantly, whereas low-frequency sound, such as thunder, airport noise, or the rhythm section of music, produces measurable evoked potentials in the cerebrum and appropriate deformation within the fetal ear (Bauer et al., 1997). High-decibel impact may even produce damage in the appropriate low-frequency areas (Abrams et al., 1997). This discrimination probably extends to differentiation of vowels (low frequency, easily heard) from consonants (higher frequency, probably heard poorly) and produces apparent learning behavior (Gerhardt and Abrams, 2000). The latter includes recognition/favoring the maternal voice over other voices, apparent recognition of music played in fetal life (whether it is the actual music and its multiple tones or simply the rhythm is unclear), and perceived responsiveness to intrauterine music (Poreba et al., 2000). Again, it is unclear whether it is the actual music or merely its pattern that the fetus favors; apparently low-amplitude music with a slow rhythm is soothing, whereas high-amplitude, high-frequency, high-rate rhythmic music produces significant accelerations (Groome et al., 1999) and perhaps even a state change to hyperactive 4F (Gingras and O'Donnell, 1998).

Given these observations about fetal hearing and the exquisite sense of vibration that is developed even earlier, it is not surprising the fetus can be "stimulated" by electromechanical devices that induce a very broad band of atonal "white" noise from 0.1 to 10 kHz (Abrams et al., 1995). Depending on the instrument used, this may deliver sound pressure exceeding 130 decibels (enough to produce permanent damage) and at almost all points in the entire range in excess of 70 decibels (comfortable hearing) (Gerhardt et al., 1988). Placement of the emitter makes an important difference on delivery of sound amplitude. If the instrument is held a few inches above the maternal abdomen, direct conduction is not facilitated, and the maximum amplitude delivered is probably less than 100 decibels. If, as in some sheep experiments, the transmitter is pressed directly against the fetal skull, sound as well as vibration is transmitted at an extremely high sound pressure, with combined effects easily capable of producing injury (Abrams et al., 1997). A commercially produced vibroacoustic stimulator is available, and many units continue to use the electronic artificial larynx originally adapted to this purpose. A number of different instruments, including ordinary alarm clocks, tin cans, electric toothbrushes, clapping hands, and electric door buzzers, have been used to provoke the classic fetal response.

VAS induces reproducible state changes in fetuses (Gingras and O'Donnell, 1998). When the fetus is in quiet sleep (1F), even short bursts of VAS provoke the movement patterns, type of movements, fetal posture, FHR, and FHR variability typical of state 2F. If the fetus is already in state 2F (moving actively), the VAS may generate conversion to 4F (hyperactive "jogging" fetus) and almost always results in increased frequency of movements, amplitude of movements, rise in heart rate, and exaggerated FHR variability. On occasion, fetal bradycardia has been incited (Sherer et al., 1988). The high frequency of state change in the human fetus, especially close to term, means that VAS achieves its purpose of shortening the monitoring time, converting a nonreactive NST to a reactive one and avoiding prolonged testing times (Newnham et al., 1990). Some authors proposed that this approach does not need to be limited to a nonreactive NST, but that a modified BPS can be constructed by measuring amniotic fluid volume and then FHR responses on M-mode ultrasound after VAS (Kamel et al., 1999). A trial was conducted comparing three testing schemes: full BPS, NST alone, and the modified biophysical profile of AFI plus VAS. AFI plus VAS was better than NST and equalled BPS in sensitivity and negative predictive value. The significantly high false-positive rate (67%) called for backup testing using the full BPS. One might consider whether the investigators demonstrated the superiority of their proposed technique, because ultrasound was used to determine the AFI and was standing by to perform the full BPS within minutes, rather than performing a biophysical profile at the outset.

Problems with the Methodology

A large number of studies demonstrated similar high false-positive rates (Gagnon, 1989). Of more concern is the potential for false-reassuring rates. Because the frequency of true fetal compromise, manifest as asphyxia before labor, intrapartum fetal distress, low Apgar scores, and abnormal pH, is very low in most of these populations, very large numbers of patients must be studied to evaluate the liability of failed detection. It is notable that in trials of VAS, where prevalence of adverse outcome was reasonably high, the false-negative rate was unacceptable. For example, Serafini and colleagues (1984) documented a 55% false-reassuring rate in the detection of intrapartum fetal distress (prevalence 20%), and Kuhlman and colleagues (1988) showed a 53% false-reassuring rate for pH less than 7.20 (prevalence 16%). It is clear that this methodology may shorten testing time in all subjects by provoking state changes that are not limited by the presence of fetal compromise. Further, because most trials excluded patients with oligohydramnios, known IUGR, and were conducted only on term fetuses, much of the available literature does not apply to those patients most in need of highly accurate antenatal testing.

Among the higher risk target groups, there are further drawbacks to this methodology. Although safety improves with advancing gestational age, preterm infants may require more sound to elicit significant responses, raising the odds of hearing injury when VAS is applied before 33 weeks' gestation (Bartnicki et al., 1998; Kisilevsky et al., 2000). Responsiveness is decreased in abnormal fetuses (Vindla et al., 1999), fetuses of mothers with hypertension (Warner et al., 2002), fetuses exposed to cocaine in fetal life (Gingras and O'Donnell, 1998), fetuses whose mothers have depression (Allister et al., 2001), and fetuses with severe IUGR (Gagnon et al., 1989) treated with magnesium, antenatal steroids, or β-mimetics for preterm labor (Rotmensch et al., 1999; Sherer, 1994). Thus, the greatest liability for inaccuracies with VAS are compounded in those fetuses at greatest need for monitoring.

A fundamental issue with this testing modality is not addressed by any of the studies. There are anecdotal reports of permanent arrhythmias, sudden decelerations, numerous examples of hearing deficit, and the unavoidable conclusion of those using these techniques that this is a truly noxious, perhaps even harmful, stimulus. State change alterations produce significant changes in brain neurotransmitter levels, psychic organization, and even gross motor function in adult subjects (Devoe et al., 1990). That VAS is useful in persuading a breech-presenting fetus to turn spontaneously into the transverse position with one or two applications (Johnson and Elliott, 1995) is seen by some as a useful or even essential adjunct to external cephalic version (Hofmeyr, 2002) but by others as undue punishment for malpresentation (Kiuchi et al., 2000). Given the array of antenatal tests available to discriminate periods of fetal quiescence from true compromise, especially considering the combination of BPS scored out of 10 with Doppler velocimetry of multiple fetal vessels, all completed in under 30 minutes in 96% of subjects, a major role of VAS in many modern surveillance programs is questionable.

Fetal Movement Counting

Maternal awareness of fetal activity in the unprovoked setting has been documented for many generations. Systematic application of this awareness has demonstrated incomplete efficacy. Multiple factors may impact on the reliability of maternal movement counting as a method of fetal surveillance (Table 21-7). Sudden absolute cessation of fetal movements is a cause for alarm. However, this may be a premortem event rather than one with any realistic warning period. Second, simple NST has been proven ineffective in monitoring the fetus with sudden decreased fetal movement, including the largest randomized trial of fetal movement counting conducted in England (Grant et al., 1982). That study, which used the "count to 10" method, produced several interesting effects. First, the control group experienced a very significant drop in

perinatal mortality compared with patients not enrolled in the study at all—a clear example of the so-called Hawthorne effect, where the presence of a trial within the community produces responses even in those not undergoing the experimental maneuver. Second, the compliance for immediate reporting of decreased fetal movement was low, relative to many other studies of fetal movement counting. It is critical, of course, that women report the decrease on the day it happens and not at their next prenatal visit. Finally, the rescue methodology was simple FHR monitoring, resulting in a large proportion of fetuses who ultimately died, being monitored and discharged without ultrasound evaluation. Thus, although the authors concluded that "routine daily counting . . . seems to offer no advantage over informal inquiry about movements during standard antenatal care," it may well be that the information about fetal activity, especially focusing on significant changes in routine rather than absolute loss of movement, may be effective, especially in the context of multisystem monitoring.

 ## INVASIVE FETAL TESTING

Fetal Blood Sampling

The ability to sample the fetal circulation, as early as 17 to 18 weeks and conveniently by 22 weeks, led to a wealth of experience in determining fetal metabolic, respiratory, hematologic, and genetic correlates with altered fetal status. As experience was gained, it became clear that virtually any test possible in the newborn or infant could be obtained and evaluated with reliability in the fetus. Although the risks of these techniques were measurable, experienced teams were able to perform ultrasound-guided fetal blood sampling in normal-appearing fetuses (e.g., for rapid karyotype of women who attended genetic counseling late) with fetal loss rates much less than 1%, and in several series only modestly more than amniocentesis (Weiner, 1988; Nicolini et al., 1990).

Fetal blood sampling has specific applications:

- For fetal abnormalities (for investigating fetal karyotype, evidence of viral infection, evidence of asphyxial injury)
- Where history, maternal titers, or MCA Dopplers indicate a risk of anemia

 TABLE 21-7. PROBLEMS WITH FETAL MOVEMENT COUNTING

Factors	Effect
Highly variable methodology	Confusion and inconsistent instructions.
Efficacy	Physician noncompliance.
Fetal/maternal variation	
Different activity between fetuses	These factors require flexible, individualized FMC methodology.
Changing activity in the same fetus	
Different perceptions between mothers	
Different perceptions by same mother	
Public misinformation (e.g. infant stops moving before labor, it's okay)	Failure to follow protocol directions in unusual circumstances.
Poor maternal compliance	Up to 20% of women do not count but may falsify records.
Faulty clinical response	Despite proper maternal performance, no definitive testing/ intervention is undertaken or too much reliance is placed on CTG alone. Biophysical profile scoring is the only acceptable response to bona fide decreased fetal movement.

CTG, cardiotocogram; FMC, fetal movement counting.

- For specific metabolic, hematologic, or gene disorders testable only by fetal blood sampling
- Infrequent confirmation of ambiguous testing from amniocentesis or chorionic villus sampling
- Even more rarely, for documentation of fetal respiratory status

This list is shorter than a decade ago, because the experience gained through fetal blood sampling has led to its elimination as an essential test. In other words, the noninvasive correlates, proven through the experience of fetal blood sampling, have rendered the actual blood test less important. Key examples are the use of MCA Doppler peak velocity to assess the degree of fetal anemia, which has markedly reduced the need for initial blood samples and delayed the timing of those samples in other cases (see Chapter 30). The clear correlation between biophysical profile scoring and fetal pH on cordocentesis (Figs. 21-2 and 21-25) mean that the BPS can be safely relied on to indicate fetal pH without the blood test (Manning et al., 1993). Further, the application of sensitive polymerase chain reaction techniques for gene amplification and the emergence of many new genetic markers have replaced essential blood tests with tests of improved accuracy from fetal cells obtained by simple amniocentesis. Table 21-8 lists the change in the indication for cordocentesis, noting that the modern distribution of the procedure also reflects a 70% to 80% reduction in application of cordocentesis.

Cordocentesis Procedure

The umbilical vein is the target of choice of many teams (Daffos et al., 1983; Manning, 1995b), and it may be approached at virtually any point in its course. At the placental insertion it is stable and usually easily entered, but this is also true of free loops of cord that may be pinned against the

TABLE 21-8. CHANGES IN INDICATIONS FOR CORDOCENTESIS 1991–2003

	Then	Now
Rapid karyotype	28%	5%
Investigate other abnormal tests	10%	10%
Red blood cell alloimmunization	23%	18%
Infection	10%	15%
Nonimmune hydrops	7%	20%
Blood gases and pH	5%	5%
Twin–twin transfusion	5%	8%
Neonatal alloimmune thrombocytopenia	5%	10%
Immune thrombocytopenia	2%	—
Immune deficiency	2%	1%
Coagulopathy	1%	—
Hemoglobinopathy	1%	—
Paralysis for fetal MRI	—	4%
Late fetocide (anomalies)	—	4%

MRI, magnetic resonance imaging.

posterior wall of the uterus, the umbilical vein at the abdominal skin insertion, or within the intrahepatic portion of the vessel. As much time as necessary is spent identifying the ideal approach to the most clear imaged target. Once this is done, the procedure itself has been greatly simplified and can usually be accomplished in a few minutes. Several adjuncts previously advocated in regard to fetal blood sampling have been discarded by most groups. These include maternal sedation, narcotic analgesia, prophylactic antibiotics, tocolysis, and admission to the hospital. Except in unusual circumstances, the mother is not prepared for emergency surgery and does not have an intravenous catheter, standby services such as obstetric anesthesia, or a reserved operating room. Suggested prerequisites for this procedure are shown in Table 21-9.

EQUIPMENT

A 22-gauge spinal needle of appropriate length usually suffices. Echo-tip needles and larger-bore introducers are no longer used.

NEEDLE GUIDE

Various designs exist for needle guides. These guides are fixed to the ultrasound transducer (Fig. 21-26). This limits excursion and angulation of the needle shaft, and the path of the needle is illustrated by software additions to standard ultrasound machines. Whereas debate has been vigorous in the last decade about measurable differences in outcome related to the use of the needle guide (Weiner and Okamura, 1996), it now appears to be truly a matter of personal preference. Most senior authors reporting large series do not use needle guides.

ULTRASOUND GUIDANCE

The maternal skin is marked for the approximate point of needle insertion before preparation with an operative wash. Sterile drapes are placed on the abdomen, primarily to allow operator and ultrasonographer to maintain a sterile field while making appropriate adjustments to fetal movement, necessary changes in maternal position, and so on. The needle is inserted into the skin, and then the ultrasound transducer in a sterile sheath is placed on the maternal abdomen. (This avoids any

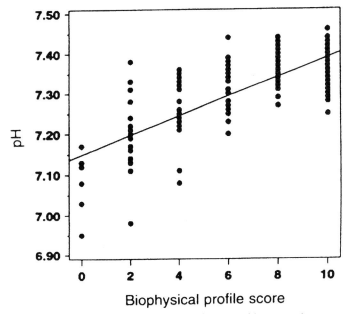

FIGURE 21-25 ■ Cordocentesis in 493 fetuses with concomitant biophysical profile score shows correlation of score with unlabored fetal umbilical venous pH. Biophysical profile score 10/10, pH greater than 7.20 in 100%. Biophysical profile score 0/10, pH always less than 7.20. Note wide variation in pH for scores of 2 to 4/10.

TABLE 21-9. PREREQUISITES FOR CORDOCENTESIS

Experienced Team

Comprehensive follow-up
Complete database
Multidisciplinary approach
Technical expertise

Facility (Tertiary Center)

Neonatal intensive care unit
Full laboratory capability
Postprocedure monitoring facility

Equipment

Bedside testing: optional (e.g., potassium hydroxide for alkaline
 precipitation test, Coulter counter)
Needle guide: optional
High-resolution ultrasonography
Pulsed-wave and color-flow Doppler
Image storage

Preparation

Skin preparation and drapes
Neonatal resuscitation tray
Syringes, sample containers, heparin
Injectable normal saline, pancuronium 2 mg/mL

Detailed Maternal Procedural Orientation

Written Informed Consent

accidental contact with the tip of the needle and ensures a sterile field.) The aim is to image the needle tip continuously, using small side-to-side excursions of the transducer with a small bobbing motion of the needle to assist in resolution. As the needle approaches the target vessel, the magnified field feature of the ultrasound machine is used, and the last few millimeters are completed to allow the needle tip to rest against the vessel wall. This is followed by a sharp 3- to 5-mm "pop" to overcome the resistance of the tissue around the vessel and the vessel wall itself. Once the needle is seen within the lumen of the vessel, the stylette is removed and backflow is observed, which will usually gently fill the needle hub. In many circumstances, however, surface tension must be overcome by a small amount of suction on the needle to demonstrate free flow. The sample is obtained by directed flow rather than vigorous suction, the latter which will pull the vessel wall up against the needle and stop flow altogether. If free blood flow is not obtained, the needle is withdrawn in very small increments, with continuous gentle suction and rotation of the needle through a few degrees. The stylette is not replaced unnecessarily, because each stylette insertion introduces an echogenic microbubble into the ultrasound field directly above the target.

VESSEL CONFIRMATION

Vessel identity is confirmed by infusion of a small bolus (0.2 to 0.3 mL) of normal saline. Turbulence in the vein is usually unmistakable (Fig. 21-27), whereas arterial turbulence may be more difficult to see. If uterine activity, the small caliber of very early vessels, fetal interference, or maternal intolerance shorten the procedure, the samples obtained are prioritized to address the most critical elements. Samples that may have been contaminated by amniotic fluid should not be discarded because they are as reliable as pure fetal blood for

polymerase chain reaction techniques or other genetic testing. On the other hand, metabolic measurements, fetal blood gasses and pH, and especially hematologic measurements require absolutely pure fetal blood obtained under free-flowing conditions without heparin in the syringe delivered immediately into the appropriate tubes for testing (Moniz et al., 1985; Forestier et al., 1986; Weiner, 1995; Nava et al., 1996).

FETAL PARALYSIS

Paralyzing the fetus with intravenous pancuronium, 0.2 to 0.3 mg/kg of estimated fetal weight, was done in virtually all procedures by many teams. Its use remains very common in transamniotic intrauterine fetal transfusion procedures and may indeed provide some physiologic benefit (Weiner and Anderson, 1989). For routine blood sampling, however, the needle is actually in the vessel for a very short time (usually less than 2 minutes) and fetal movement is not perilous. Pancuronium is rarely used (Harman, 1995), and the prior difficulty differentiating pancuronium effect from postprocedure fetal distress is now avoided (Pielet et al., 1988).

NEEDLE REMOVAL

The needle is withdrawn gently but firmly, without changing the angle used to insert it. Bleeding from the needle puncture site will be visible with all transamniotic punctures, but because this is variable, it is always monitored to cessation. Later in gestation, when a free loop is used, Wharton jelly within the cord is usually completely hemostatic, and only one or two drops will escape. If vessel puncture through an anterior placenta has been completely extra-amniotic, bleeding may exist but will be invisible, so post-procedure monitoring would

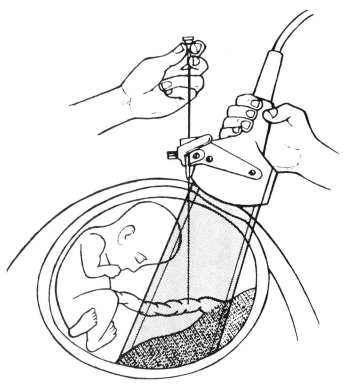

FIGURE 21-26 ■ A needle guide is attached to the transducer, and the shaft of the needle is visualized in the ultrasound plane for this style of cordocentesis.

POSTPROCEDURAL MONITORING

When the immediate procedural monitoring is completed, the fetus should be moving and should have a stable heart beat with no active bleeding. The uterus should relax completely between any contractions that may have been provoked by the procedure, and the absence of a prelabor contraction pattern is confirmed by a brief (30 minutes or less) period of cardiotocography. Sample validation and verification of normal maternal and fetal status after the procedure allow discharge from the hospital, usually within 1 hour.

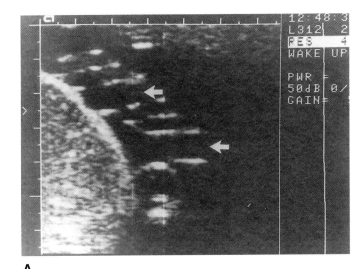

A

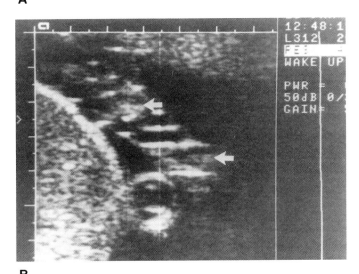

B

FIGURE 21-27 ■ **A,** The umbilical cord in longitudinal section, adjacent to the fetal abdomen. The needle produced excellent return of fetal blood. No infusion. **B,** Infusion of 250 μL of normal saline demonstrates bright turbulence, identifying the umbilical vein (*arrows*).

be hemodynamic rather than visible. Ten minutes of direct Doppler-assisted ultrasound monitoring will account for that small possibility. In the Rh-negative woman, anti-D immunoglobulin is given at the end of the procedure.

SAMPLE VALIDATION

Typical turbulence and a free-flowing blood sample provide assurance the needle was properly placed. Laboratory confirmation should be obtained that the sample is pure fetal blood without maternal contamination, which can be ensured by a variety of tests. At term, there may be a broad distribution of fetal cell sizes as adult hemoglobin concentration rises, so the final confirmation of pure fetal origin is not by Coulter counter (Fig. 21-28) but by the Kleihauer-Betke test (Kleihauer et al., 1967). This test takes 45 to 70 minutes to complete and is thus not suitable for bedside use; only after it is reported to show 100% fetal cells should a final interpretation of results be made.

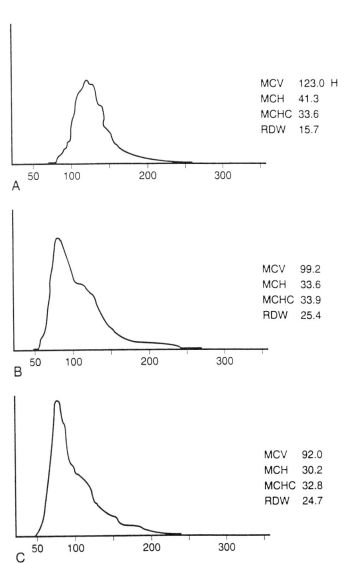

FIGURE 21-28 ■ **A,** Coulter counter histogram of mean corpuscular volume (MCV) on a pure fetal sample at the time of fetal intrauterine transfusion. MCV = 123 fL, hemoglobin 8.6 g/dL, 100% fetal red blood cells. **B,** Part way through the first intravascular fetal transfusion, the hemoglobin is 12.9 g/dL, 65% fetal, 35% donor-adult red blood cells. The histogram shows two peaks, representing these two red blood cell populations. MCV = 99.2 fL. **C,** With completion of the transfusion, the total hemoglobin is 15.9 g/dL, 50% fetal, 50% donor red blood cells. The higher peak of smaller more uniform donor-adult red blood cells is obvious on the left. MCV = 92 fL. MCH, mean corpuscular hemoglobin; MCHC, mean corpuscular hemoglobin concentration; RDW, red blood cell distribution width.

COMPLICATIONS

Overall pregnancy loss rate depends largely on the fetal condition for which the cordocentesis is done (Duchatel et al., 1993; Manning, 1995a) (Table 21-10). The rate of pregnancy loss is worse in cases of fetal hydrops, multiple anomalies, and abnormal karyotype (Wilson et al., 1994).

IMMEDIATE COMPLICATIONS. *Fetal bradycardia* has been reported in as many as 52% of procedures and is the most common complication of cordocentesis. It is almost always of short duration, self-limited, and usually with no long-term consequences. First, the maternal left tilt is used to eliminate the possibility of maternal supine hypotension. Uterine contractile status is evaluated, and on rare occasions terbutaline is administered to promote uterine relaxation. (In this case, bradycardia may be due to contraction of the uterus directly at the cord insertion or to pinning the fetus against the umbilical cord by the contraction; the fetus may be moved away from the area of contraction). More serious bradycardia may occur as often as 3% of the time and may indicate umbilical artery spasm. Maternal oxygen administration may relieve this spasm, and frequently it relents after a few minutes, without untoward fetal effect (Baier et al., 1992).

In about 1 in 300 cordocentesis procedures, profound or prolonged bradycardia occurs. Undetected cord hematoma, transplacental hemorrhage, uterine activity, or combinations of these may lead to fetal death on these rare occasions (Harman, 1995; Paidas et al., 1995). Reinsertion of the needle to try to aspirate a hematoma is usually unsuccessful and may cause further intrafunic bleeding.

Fetal bleeding is common and includes 50% to 60% of simple vein punctures bleeding for 15 to 60 seconds. Bleeding over 300 seconds or massive hemorrhage requiring resuscitation occurs less than once per 200 cordocentesis procedures (Harman, 1995). When this does occur, frequently the result of severe fetal thrombocytopenia, the time to act is short (Harman et al., 1988). The approach is dictated by the gestational age. *This plan must be made before starting the procedure.* A viable fetus should be delivered by emergency cesarean delivery.

Most often, *cord hematoma* is not specifically detected but noted incidentally after delivery or as a result of the emergency intervention for intractable bradycardia. The overall incidence may be very high if one includes the small bruise that almost always occurs when Wharton jelly is perforated with intraamniotic cordocentesis (Fig. 21-29). The incidence of sympto-

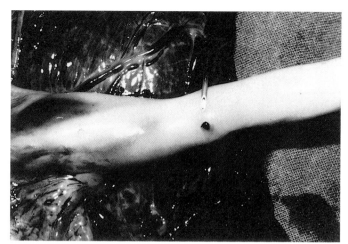

FIGURE 21-29 ■ Normal small bruise when transamniotic needle insertion is through Wharton jelly. Cordocentesis produced no visible bleeding when needle was withdrawn.

matic cord hematoma causing significant fetal bradycardia is very low (Jauniaux et al., 1990). This is more commonly the result of difficult procedures with multiple attempts, including infusion of saline to try to identify the needle tip, infusion of pancuronium to paralyze a very active fetus (Seeds et al., 1989), or by deliberate infusion of platelets or blood (Doyle et al., 1993), with malposition of the needle tip (Harman, 1995). The occurrence of an intrafunic hematoma requiring delivery seldom occurs at previable gestations; the cord is probably not thick enough to retain the hematoma but may require emergency delivery later in gestation.

Acute maternal complications are also seen. Cordocentesis takes longer than amniocentesis, and the mother will likely have more discomfort. The test is less uncomfortable than transabdominal chorion villus sampling, so for most women pain, contractions, and anxiety are not dominant complaints. Acute rupture of membranes is rare, usually associated with gross hydramnios or prolonged difficult procedures. Preterm labor is very rare.

DELAYED COMPLICATIONS. Evidence for transmission of viral *infection* to the fetus from contaminated amniotic fluid or transplacentally from mothers with active diseases is not convincing. Amniocentesis does not increase hepatitis B transmission (Ko et al., 1994), so it has been argued that cordocentesis for human immunodeficiency virus testing may also be safe (Viscarello et al., 1992). However, the possibility of vertical transmission exists (Mandelbrot et al., 1994). Therefore the application of fetal blood sampling in mothers with human immunodeficiency virus may be of very limited value. Chorioamnionitis after cordocentesis in previously uninfected women is unusual but may be severe on rare occasions (Wilkins et al., 1989). Infectious agents are skin *Staphylococcus* species and enteric organisms.

In the case of *maternal alloimmunization,* fetal transfusion with donor blood may cause new red cell antibody development in up to 20% of women. For simple cordocentesis, however, serologic data are much less pronounced. Between 15% and 26% of women do show significant volumes of transplacental bleeding, as judged by maternal Kleihauer-Betke test, or up to 40% as judged by elevation of maternal serum α-fetoprotein after the test (Nicolini et al., 1988). This is associated with transplacental insertion, and infrequently

TABLE 21-10. FETAL CONDITION AND CORDOCENTESIS LOSS

Condition	Average (%)	Range (%)
Nonimmune hydrops	35.00	3–80
Hydramnios	20.00	5–33
IUGR/oligohydramnios	9.30	1–14
Single anomaly*	5.80	1–13
Multiple anomalies*	4.80	1–12
Rh, platelets	3.40	0–17
Risk of infection	0.60	1–1.3
Normal, DS risk only	0.48	0–1.3

* Statistically not different.

DS, Down syndrome; IUGR, intrauterine growth restriction.

TABLE 21-11. FETAL BLOOD GASES AND pH

Parameter (Mean Value)	22 Weeks	28 Weeks	34 Weeks	40 Weeks
UV (pH)	7.416	7.407	3.398	7.388
UV (Po_2)	47.600	42.000	36.300	30.600
UV (Pco_2)	33.600	34.900	36.200	37.500
UV (Hco_3)	22.300	23.000	23.700	24.300
UA (pH)	7.390	7.379	7.368	7.357
UA (Po_2)	28.300	26.300	24.300	22.300
UV pressure (mm Hg)	3.800	5.200	6.500	–

UA, umbilical artery; UV, umbilical vein.

Data from Soothill PW, Nicolaides KH, Rodeck CH, et al: Effect of gestational age on fetal and intervillous blood gas and acid-base values in human pregnancy. Fetal Ther **1**:168, 1986; Nicolaides KH, Economides DL, Soothill PW: Blood gases, pH, and lactate in inappropriate- and small-for-gestational-age fetuses. Am J Obstet Gynecol **161**:996, 1989; and Weiner CP, Sipes SL, Wenstrom K: The effect of fetal age upon normal fetal laboratory values and venous pressure. Obstet Gynecol **79**:713, 1992.

(7 of 90 women) it results in elevation of already present red cell antibody levels (Bowman et al., 1994). No cases of clinically significant new alloimmunization developed as a consequence of cordocentesis within a 17-year surveillance window (Harman, 1995). This experience includes the following:

- Knowing maternal Rh before all procedures
- Administration of Rh immune globulin at the end of the procedure
- Maternal Kleihauer test after all procedures
- Follow-up additional Rh immune globulin for any case of transplacental hemorrhage of more than 10 mL of fetal red blood cells
- Avoiding the placenta if at all possible in women with known fetal–maternal incompatibility

FETAL RESPIRATORY STATUS BY CORDOCENTESIS

Table 21-11 presents normative data for fetal blood gases and pH and demonstrates the progression of changes in these values with advancing gestation (Soothill et al., 1986; Nicolaides et al., 1989; Weiner et al., 1992). Of course, on the rare occasions where fetal blood sampling is performed to evaluate indices of infection, acidosis in the macrosomic diabetic fetus, hematologic indices in cases of hydrops, intracranial hemorrhage, or other presentation with abnormal fetal testing, specific knowledge of the individual variables, within the gestational age limitations, is essential.

PRACTICAL FETAL TESTING

Biophysical Profile Scoring Performance

Performance characteristics and distribution of test results are shown in Table 21-12. The false-negative rate of 0.54 per 1000 tests describes the number of fetuses who have died within 7 days of the last BPS, which was a normal score (Dayal et al., 2000; Manning, Morrison, Harman, et al., 1987). Excluded are fetuses with lethal congenital anomalies and cases where fetuses died remote from testing. This false-negative rate does not apply to non-normal scores; incremental morbidity and mortality is seen with decreasing scores despite intervention or where intervention was precluded by previable gestation or fetal size.

Disorder-Specific Testing

Benefits of testing in specific maternal and/or fetal conditions will be amplified by the addition of different variables, different testing intervals, or prioritizing subsets of observation variables. For example, in chronic placental insufficiency with asymmetrical IUGR, the combination of Doppler velocimetry, fetal growth parameters, and delayed maturation of variability of FHR will provide important modification of BPS interpretation (Baschat and Harman, 2001). On the other hand, where fetal metabolic risks dominate, well-being is ensured by biophysical profile scoring, with specific invasive testing (e.g., fetal lung maturity amniocentesis and maternal glucose) providing essential prognostic detail.

Modification of the BPS protocol and the use of additional tests also reflects severity of disease. This would include fetuses with decelerative heart rate tracings, abnormal Dopplers,

TABLE 21-12. BPS PERFORMANCE STATISTICS

Normal score 8/8	Completion mean 11 min	
Abnormal score	Requires 30-min scan to meet definition of abnormal	
Test score distribution		
Normal score	10/10 8/8	97.84%
Equivocal score	6/10	1.00%
Abnormal scores	4/10	0.56
	2/10	0.19
	0/10	0.07
Negative predictive value (BPS normal, 7-day duration)		99.946%

Positive predictive values (Change with test score, endpoint)

Examples:

BPS	End Point	PPV
0/10	Perinatal mortality	100% (no intervention)
0/10	Neonatal mortality	43% (despite intervention)
0/10	Perinatal morbidity	100%
4/10	Perinatal morbidity	63%
6/10	Perinatal morbidity	35%

BPS, biophysical profile score; PPV, positive predictive value.

equivocal biophysical profile scoring, and those at the margin of viability for whom even a few further days of intrauterine life may be critical. In such vulnerable situations, monitoring frequency is increased, up to two or three times a day. Each center should develop protocols for the management of typical referral concerns, reflecting local needs and practices. A typical scheme for monitoring the post-term pregnancy (Johnson et al., 1986) is shown in Figure 21-30. Approaches to testing of the IUGR fetus are discussed in Chapter 28.

Clinical Impact of Fetal Monitoring

This area of discussion is in flux. Outcome studies of children monitored and managed according to Doppler protocols are just now becoming available. A significant amount of data is available from large populations studied with biophysical profile scoring alone, and much of this is discussed later. However, the principles of integrated fetal testing, using both biophysical and Doppler data to determine intervention in high-risk fetuses (IUGR, preterm, and preterm IUGR), have been in place for a limited time and in relatively limited populations. Thus, the following discussion is more likely representative of the potential benefit of comprehensive monitoring.

Perinatal Mortality

The application of comprehensive fetal testing, with biophysical profile scoring at the core, is associated with significant declines in perinatal mortality (Table 21-13)

TABLE 21-13. PERINATAL MORTALITY CHANGES WITH BPS APPLICATION

Program	n	PNM Tested	PNM Not Tested
Ireland*	3,200	4.1	10.7
Nova Scotia†	5,000	3.1	6.6
Manitoba‡	56,000	1.9	7.7
California§	15,000	1.3	8.8

* Chamberlain, 1991.
† Baskett et al., 1987.
‡ Manning, 1995b.
§ Miller et al., 1996.
BPS, biophysical profile score; *n*, number tested; PNM, perinatal mortality/1000.

(Baskett et al., 1987; Chamberlain, 1991; Manning, 1995b; Miller et al., 1996). These data reflect practical application of biophysical profile scoring and its management scheme, not merely statistical associations with outcome. Because such management schemes are now considered standard of practice, it becomes difficult to further evaluate the relationship between abnormal findings and outcome, that is, "natural history" can no longer be observed. Although many factors in addition to the actual testing scheme may be important in generating these markedly improved perinatal mortality rates, it is clear that an ultrasound-based system of fetal assessment can produce important benefits. The power of these studies is in the large number of subjects, giving these data effective strength similar to a smaller randomized trial.

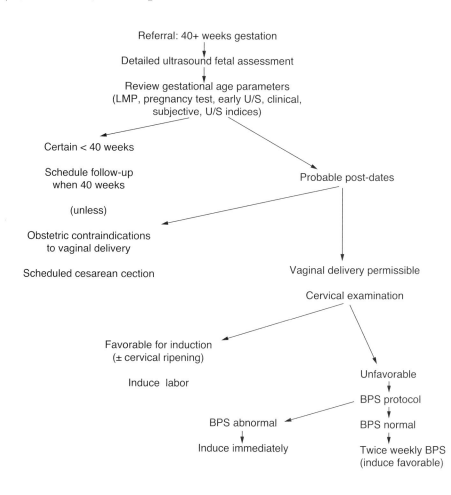

FIGURE 21-30 ■ Schematic diagram of management of the post-term pregnancy, using biophysical profile scoring and induction of labor when the cervix is favorable. BPS, biophysical profile score; LMP, last menstrual period; U/S, ultrasound.

Impact on Perinatal Morbidity

The relationship of fetal condition illustrated by BPS with neonatal consequences is well documented (Fig. 21-31) (Baskett et al., 1984; Vintzileos et al., 1987; Manning et al., 1990b). The data relating Doppler abnormalities to neonatal consequences, as illustrated in Table 21-6, provide even more specific detail (Baschat et al., 1999, 2001, 2002; Baschat, Gembruch, Reiss, et al., 2000). Clearly the studies currently underway relating antenatal findings and patterned perinatal measures responsive to these issues will be instructive. Perhaps as important as these shorter-term measures are the impacts on long-term development.

Neurologic Development in Children Managed by the Biophysical Profile Scoring Protocol

Table 21-14 illustrates the beneficial effect of biophysical profile scoring used to manage high-risk populations on the occurrence of a number of permanent handicaps (Manning, 1995c; Manning et al., 1998, 2000a, b). In the samples shown in Table 21-14, the population referred for BPS had higher

TABLE 21-14. CHILDHOOD NEUROLOGIC SEQUELLAE IN BPS-TESTED AND NONTESTED POPULATIONS*

Variable	Tested	Nontested	*P*
Deliveries followed	26,288	58,659	
Mean birth weight	2.09 ± 0.99 kg	2.28 ± 0.32 kg	NS
<1.0 kg	14%	6.7%	NS
Mean gestational age	33.4 ± 5.6 wk	34.4 ± 2.1 wk	NS
<32 wk	40.5%	37.8%	NS
<28 wk	13.5%	10.9%	NS
Cerebral palsy rate	1.33	4.74	<.001
Cortical blindness	0.66	1.04	<.01
Cortical deafness	0.90	2.2	<.005
Mental retardation	0.80	3.1	<.001
ADHD	4.7	28.1	<.001
EDOC	1.2	1.0	NS

*All rates expressed per 1000 liveborn.
ADHD, attention deficit hyperactivity disorder; BPS, biophysical profile score; EDOC, emotional disorders of childhood (control variable); NS; not significant.

risks, earlier birth gestations, and lighter birth weights but better outcomes. The untested population, screened by routine antenatal care at the same rate as the referred population, determined to have no identifiable risk factors before delivery, and having statistically identical maternal characteristics, with the same frequency of genetic/congenital abnormalities, provides a baseline rate of these disorders, which is higher than the monitored population. A further definitive control is seen in the diagnostic grouping for emotional disorders for childhood, which was not different between groups, eliminating the theory of ascertainment bias (Manning et al., 2000c). The critical outcome of cerebral palsy diagnosed at 3 years of age deserves a more detailed discussion.

Biophysical Profile Score and Cerebral Palsy

With an abnormal BPS, the likelihood of cerebral palsy becomes increasingly more likely (Fig. 21-32) (Manning et al., 1997). Most of these cases have identifiable antenatal causes (Table 21-15) (Harman, 1998). The normal BPS is highly reassuring (cerebral palsy rate less than 0.85 per 1000 liveborn). An abnormal score, frequently the trigger for intervention, was associated with a higher rate of cerebral palsy compared with normal tested subjects (Manning et al., 1998). However, most fetuses experiencing cerebral palsy with a low BPS had low scores on their one and only fetal evaluation—they were then promptly delivered. Review of the origins of cerebral palsy demonstrates meaningful reduction in intrapartum causes (6% in the tested group, 9% in the untested group) and neonatal time period (28% versus 33%, respectively).

■ SUMMARY

Fetal monitoring is a progressive process of risk assignment. A combination of family, historical, and maternal data are assembled to indicate relative risks at the beginning of the pregnancy. Fetal data are gathered through ultrasound examination, screening modalities, and initial observations of fetal performance to further refine that evaluation and initiate the process of detailed fetal assessment.

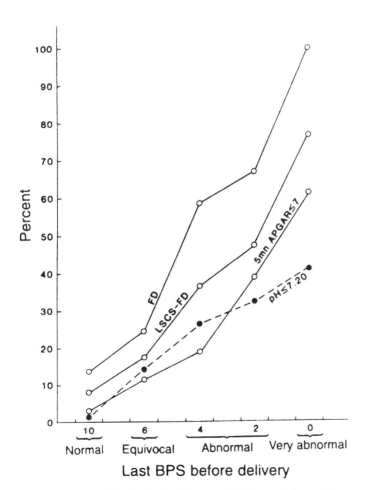

FIGURE 21-31 ■ Biophysical profile score (BPS) accurately predicts perinatal morbidity. Declining scores strongly predict increasing frequency of fetal distress (FD), cesarean section for fetal distress (LSCS-FD), low 5-minute Apgar score, and umbilical vein pH less than 7.20.

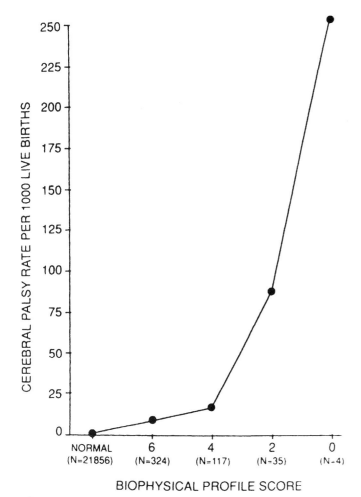

FIGURE 21-32 ■ Cerebral palsy rate is exponentially related to worsening biophysical profile score.

Multivariable evaluation, with biophysical profile scoring at the core, and the liberal addition of Doppler velocimetry of placental and fetal circulations can achieve optimal extension of the pregnancy in the safest fashion and delivery of the healthiest neonate. The process is always one of balancing the risks of neonatal injury against the dangers of adverse intrauterine events. That balance will continue to shift as antenatal interventions, better screening tools, and the success of our neonatal colleagues change. The principles of multivariable testing, flexible regimes responsive to maternal and fetal conditions, and continuous validation by reliable outcome measures endure.

 TABLE 21-15. PRIMARY ETIOLOGY OF CEREBRAL PALSY IN BPS-MANAGED POPULATIONS

	RR
Antenatal causes	.38*
Intrapartum causes	.195*
Neonatal causes	.245*
Postnatal causes	.25*
All cerebral palsy	.280*

* Confidence limits do not cross 1.0, i.e., statistically significant.

BPS, biophysical profile score; RR, relative risk compared with low-risk population managed without BPS.

REFERENCES

Aaslid R, Huber P, Nornes H: Evaluation of cerebrovascular spasm with transcranial Doppler ultrasound. J Neurosurg **60**:37, 1984.

Aaslid R, Markwalder T-M, Nornes H: Noninvasive transcranial Doppler ultrasound recording of flow velocity in basal cerebral arteries. J Neurosurg **57**:769, 1982.

Abrams RM, Gerhardt KJ, Rosa C, et al: Fetal acoustic stimulation test: stimulus features of three artificial larynges recorded in sheep. Am J Obstet Gynecol **173**:1372, 1995.

Abrams RM, Peters AJ, Gerhardt KJ: Effect of abdominal vibroacoustic stimulation on sound and acceleration levels at the head of the fetal sheep. Obstet Gynecol **90**:216, 1997.

Allister L, Lester BP, Carr S, et al: The effects of maternal depression on fetal heart rate response to vibroacoustic stimulation. Dev Neuropsychol **20**:639, 2001.

American College of Obstetricians and Gynecologists: ACOG Practice Bulletin. Antepartum Fetal Surveillance. *In* Compendium 2001. Washington, DC, ACOG, 2001, p. 119.

Anderson DF, Parks CM, Faber JJ: Fetal O₂ consumption in sheep during controlled long-term reductions in umbilical blood flow. Am J Physiol **250**:H1037, 1986.

Arabin B, Siebert M, Jimenez R, et al: Obstetrical characteristics of a loss of end diastolic velocities in the fetal aorta and/or umbilical artery using Doppler ultrasound. Gynecol Obstet Invest **25**:173, 1988.

Arbeille P, Body G, Saliba E, et al: Fetal cerebral circulation assessment by Doppler ultrasound in normal and pathological pregnancies. Eur J Obstet Gynecol Reprod Biol **29**:261, 1988.

Arbeille P, Bosc M, Vaillant MC, et al: Nicotine-induced changes in the cerebral circulation in ovine fetuses. Am J Perinatol **9**:270, 1992.

Arbeille P, Roncin A, Berson M, et al: Exploration of the fetal cerebral blood flow by duplex Doppler–linear array system in normal and pathological pregnancies. Ultrasound Med Biol **13**:329, 1987.

Arduini D, Rizzo G: Fetal behavioural states. *In* Dawes GS, Burruto F, Zacutti A, et al (eds): Fetal Autonomy and Adaptation. Chichester, Wiley, 1990, p. 55.

Arduini D, Rizzo G, Parlati E, et al: Modifications of ultradian and circadian rhythms of fetal heart rate after fetal-maternal adrenal gland suppression: A double blind study. Prenat Diagn **6**:409, 1986.

Arduini D, Rizzo G, Romanini C, et al: Hemodynamic changes in growth retarded fetuses during maternal oxygen administration as predictors of fetal outcome. J Ultrasound Med **8**:193, 1989.

Baier RJ, Hasan SU, Cates DB, et al: Effects of various concentrations of O₂ and umbilical cord occlusion on fetal breathing and behavior. J Appl Physiol **68**:1597, 1990.

Baier RJ, Hasan SU, Cates DB, et al: Hyperoxemia profoundly alters breathing pattern and arouses the fetal sheep. J Dev Physiol **18**:143, 1992.

Bartnicki J, Dimer JA, Hertqig K, et al: Computerized cardiotocography following vibroacoustic stimulation of premature fetuses. Gynecol Obstet Invest **45**:73, 1998.

Baschat AA, Gembruch U: Triphasic umbilical venous blood flow with prolonged survival in severe intrauterine growth retardation: A case report. Ultrasound Obstet Gynecol **8**:201, 1996.

Baschat AA, Gembruch U, Gortner L, et al: Coronary artery blood flow visualization signifies hemodynamic deterioration in growth-restricted fetuses. Ultrasound Obstet Gynecol **16**:425, 2000.

Baschat AA, Gembruch U, Harman CR: The sequence of changes in Doppler and biophysical parameters as severe fetal growth restriction worsens. Ultrasound Obstet Gynecol **18**:571, 2001.

Baschat AA, Gembruch U, Reiss I, et al: Neonatal nucleated red blood cell counts in growth-restricted fetuses: Relationship to arterial and venous Doppler studies. Am J Obstet Gynecol **181**:190, 1999.

Baschat AA, Gembruch U, Reiss I, et al: Relationship between arterial and venous Doppler and perinatal outcome in fetal growth restriction. Ultrasound Obstet Gynecol **16**:407, 2000.

Baschat AA, Gembruch U, Viscardi RM, et al: Antenatal prediction of intraventricular hemorrhage in fetal growth restriction: What is the role of Doppler? Ultrasound Obstet Gynecol **19**:334, 2002.

Baschat AA, Harman CR: Antenatal assessment of the growth restricted fetus. Curr Opin Obstet Gynecol **13**:161, 2001.

Baser I, Johnson TRB, Paine LL: Coupling of fetal movement and fetal heart rate accelerations as an indicator of fetal health. Obstet Gynecol **80**:62, 1992.

Baskett TF: Gestational age and fetal biophysical assessment. Am J Obstet Gynecol **158**:332, 1988.

Baskett TF, Allen AC, Gray JH, et al: Fetal biophysical profile and perinatal death. Obstet Gynecol **70**:357, 1987.

Baskett TF, Boyce CD, Lohre MA, et al: Simplified antepartum fetal heart assessment. Br J Obstet Gynaecol **88**:395, 1981.

Baskett TF, Gray JH, Prewett SJ, et al: Antepartum fetal assessment using a fetal biophysical profile score. Am J Obstet Gynecol **148**:630, 1984.

Bastide A, Manning F, Harman CR, et al: Ultrasound evaluation of amniotic fluid: Outcome of pregnancies with severe oligohydramnios. Am J Obstet Gynecol **154**:895, 1986.

Battaglia C, Artini PG, Galli PA, et al: Absent or reversed end-diastolic flow in umbilical artery and severe intrauterine growth retardation. An ominous association. Acta Obstet Gynecol Scand **72**:167, 1993.

Bauer R, Schwab M, Abrams RM, et al: Electrocortical and heart rate response during vibroacoustic stimulation in fetal sheep. Am J Obstet Gynecol **177**:66, 1997.

Baz E, Zikulnig L, Hackeloer BJ, et al: Abnormal ductus venosus blood flow: a clue to umbilical cord complication. Ultrasound Obstet Gynecol **13**:204, 1999.

Belfort MA, Moise KJ: Effect of magnesium sulfate on maternal brain blood flow in preeclampsia: A randomized, placebo-controlled study. Am J Obstet Gynecol **167**:661, 1992.

Bewley S, Cooper D, Campbell S: Doppler investigation of uteroplacental blood flow resistance in the second trimester: A screening study for pre-eclampsia and intrauterine growth retardation. Br J Obstet Gynaecol **98**:871, 1991.

Bocking AD, Gagnon R, Milne KM, et al: Behavioral activity during prolonged hypoxemia in fetal sheep. J Appl Physiol **65**:2420, 1988.

Bocking AD, Gagnon R, White SE, et al: Circulatory responses to prolonged hypoxemia in fetal sheep. Am J Obstet Gynecol **159**:1418, 1988.

Boddy K, Dawes GS, Fisher R, et al: Foetal respiratory movements, electrocortical and cardiovascular responses to hypoxaemia and hypercapnia in sheep. J Physiol (Lond) **243**:599, 1974.

Borgatta A, Shrout L, Divon MY: Reliability and reproducibility of nonstress test readings. Am J Obstet Gynecol **159**:554, 1988.

Bowman JM, Pollock JM, Peterson LE, et al: Fetomaternal hemorrhage following funipuncture: Increase in severity of maternal red cell alloimmunization. Obstet Gynecol **84**:839, 1994.

Boylan P, O'Donovan P, Owens OJ: Fetal breathing movements and the diagnosis of labor: A prospective analysis of 100 cases. Obstet Gynecol **66**:517, 1985.

Broth RE, Wood DC, Rasanen J, et al: Prenatal prediction of lethal pulmonary hypoplasia: The hyperoxygenation test for pulmonary artery reactivity. Am J Obstet Gynecol **187**:940, 2002.

Brown R, Patrick J: The nonstress test: How long is enough. Am J Obstet Gynecol **151**:646, 1981.

Castillo RA, Devoe LD, Arthur M, et al: The preterm nonstress test: effects of gestational age and length of study. Am J Obstet Gynecol **160**:172, 1989.

Castle BM, Turnbull AC: The presence or absence of fetal breathing movements predicts the outcome of preterm labour. Lancet **2**:471, 1983.

Chamberlain PF: Later fetal death—Has ultrasound a role to play in its prevention? Irish J Med Sci **160**:251, 1991.

Chamberlain PF, Manning FA, Morrison I, et al: Circadian rhythm in bladder volumes in the term human fetus. Obstet Gynecol **64**:657, 1984a.

Chamberlain PF, Manning FA, Morrison I, et al: Ultrasound evaluation of amniotic fluid volume. I. The relationship of marginal and decreased amniotic fluid volumes to perinatal outcome. Am J Obstet Gynecol **150**:245, 1984b.

Chamberlain PF, Manning FA, Morrison I, et al: Ultrasound evaluation of amniotic fluid volume. II. The relationship of increased amniotic fluid volume to perinatal outcome. Am J Obstet Gynecol **150**:250, 1984c.

Chan FY, Pun TC, Lam C, et al: Pregnancy screening by uterine artery Doppler velocimetry—Which criterion performs best? Obstet Gynecol **85**:596, 1995.

Chandran R, Serra-Serra V, Sellers SM, et al: Fetal cerebral Doppler in the recognition of fetal compromise. Br J Obstet Gynaecol **100**:139, 1993.

Collea JV, Holls WM: The contraction stress test. Clin Obstet Gynecol **4**:707, 1982.

Copel JA, Grannum PA, Belanger K, et al: Pulsed Doppler flow-velocity waveforms before and after intrauterine intravascular transfusion for severe erythroblastosis fetalis. Am J Obstet Gynecol **158**:768, 1988.

Croom CS, Barias BB, Ramos-Santos E, et al: Do semiquantitative amniotic fluid indexes reflect actual outcome? Am J Obstet Gynecol **167**:986, 1992.

Daffos F, Capella-Pavlovsky M, Forestier F: Fetal blood sampling via the umbilical cord using a needle guided by ultrasound: Report of 66 cases. Prenat Diagn **3**:271, 1983.

Dawes GS, Fox HE, Leduc BM, et al: Respiratory movements and paradoxical sleep in the foetal lamb. J Physiol (Lond) **210**:47, 1970.

Dawes GS, Fox HE, Leduc BM, et al: Respiratory movements and rapid eye movement sleep in the foetal lamb. J Physiol (Lond) **220**:119, 1972.

Dawes GS, Moulden M, Redman CWG: The advantages of computerized fetal heart rate analysis. J Perinat Med **19**:39, 1991a.

Dawes GS, Moulden M, Redman CWG: System 8000: Computerized antenatal FHR analysis. J Perinat Med **19**:47, 1991b.

Dawes GS, Redman CWG: Numerical analysis of the normal human antenatal fetal heart rate. Br J Obstet Gynaecol **88**:792, 1981.

Dayal AK, Manning FA, Berck DJ, et al: Fetal death after normal biophysical profile score: An eighteen-year experience. Am J Obstet Gynecol **183**:783, 2000.

Devoe LD: The non-stress test. In Eden RD, Boehm FH (eds): Assessment and Care of the Fetus: Physiological, Clinical and Medicolegal Principles. Norwalk, Conn, Appleton & Lange, 1990, 265 ff.

Devoe LD, Murray C, Faircloth R, et al: Vibroacoustic stimulation and fetal behavioral state in normal term human pregnancy. Am J Obstet Gynecol **163**:1156, 1990.

de Vries JIP, Visser GHA, Mulder EJH, et al: Diurnal and other variations in fetal movement and heart rate patterns at 20 to 22 weeks. Early Human Dev **15**:333, 1987.

de Vries JIP, Visser GHA, Prechtl HFR: The emergence of fetal behaviour. III. Individual differences and consistencies. Early Human Dev **16**:85, 1988.

Divon MY, Girz BA, Lieblish R, et al: Clinical management of the fetus with markedly diminished umbilical artery end-diastolic flow. Am J Obstet Gynecol **161**:1523, 1989.

Dixon HG, Robertson WB: A study of the vessels of the placental bed in normotensive and hypertensive women. J Obstet Gynaecol Br Emp **65**:803, 1958.

Doyle LW, de Crespigny L, Kelly EA: Haematoma complicating fetal intravascular transfusions. Aust N Z J Obstet Gynaecol **33**:208, 1993.

Druzin ML: Antepartum fetal heart rate monitoring—State of the art. Clin Perinatol **16**:627, 1989.

Druzin ML, Gratacos J, Paul RH: Antepartum fetal heart rate testing. VI. Predictive reliability of "normal" tests in the prevention of antepartum deaths. Am J Obstet Gynecol **137**:745, 1980.

Duchatel F, Oury JF, Mennesson B, et al: Complications of diagnostic ultrasound-guided percutaneous umbilical blood sampling: Analysis of a series of 341 cases and review of the literature. Eur J Obstet Gynaecol Reprod Biol **52**:95, 1993.

Duff GB, Evans LJ: Measurement of the fetal biparietal diameter by ultrasound is not an accurate method of detecting fetal growth retardation. N Z Med J **94**:312, 1981.

Eik-Nes SH, Marshal K, Kristoffersen K: Methodology and basic problems related to blood flow studies in the human fetus. Ultrasound Med Biol **10**:329, 1984.

Falkensammer CB, Paul J, Huhta JC: Fetal congestive heart failure: Correlation of Tei index and cardiovascular score. J Perinat Med **29**:390, 2001.

Farine D, Kelly EN, Ryan G, et al: Absent and Reversed Umbilical Artery End-Diastolic Velocity. In Copel JA, Reed KL (eds): Doppler Ultrasound in Obstetrics and Gynecology. New York, Raven Press, 1995, p. 187.

Fisk NM, Ronderos-Dumit D, Soliani A, et al: Diagnostic and therapeutic transabdominal amnioinfusion in oligohydramnios. Obstet Gynecol **78**:270, 1991.

Forestier F, Daffos F, Galacteros F, et al: Hematological values of 163 normal fetuses between 18 and 30 weeks of gestation. Pediatr Res **20**:342, 1986.

Fouron J-C, Korcaz Y, Leduc B: Cardiovascular changes associated with fetal breathing. Am J Obstet Gynecol **123**:868, 1975.

Freeman RK, Anderson G, Dorchester W: A prospective multi-institutional study of antepartum fetal heart rate monitoring. I. Risk of perinatal mortality and morbidity according to antepartum fetal heart rate results. Am J Obstet Gynecol **143**:771, 1982.

Freeman RK, Lagnew DC Jr: The contraction stress test. In Eden RD, Boehm FM (eds): Assessment and Care of the Fetus: Physiological, Clinical and Medicolegal Principles. Norwalk, Conn, Appleton & Lange, 1990, 351 ff.

Gagnon R: Acoustic stimulation: effect on heart rate and other biophysical variables. Clin Perinatol **16**:643, 1989.

Gagnon R, Hunse C, Carmichael L, et al: Effects of vibratory acoustic stimulation on human fetal breathing and gross body movements near term. Am J Obstet Gynecol **155**:1227, 1986.

Gagnon R, Hunse C, Carmichael L, et al: Vibratory acoustic stimulation in 26- to 32-week, small-for-gestational-age fetus. Am J Obstet Gynecol **160**:160, 1989.

Gerhardt KJ, Abrams RM: Fetal exposures to sound and vibroacoustic stimulation. J Perinatol **30**:S21, 2000.

Gerhardt KJ, Abrams RM, Kovatz BM, et al: Intrauterine noise levels produced in pregnant ewes by sound applied to the abdomen. Am J Obstet Gynecol **159**:228, 1988.

Giles WB, Trudinger BJ, Baird PJ: Fetal umbilical artery flow velocity waveforms and placental resistance: Pathological correlations. Br J Obstet Gynaecol **92**:31, 1985.

Gingras JL, O'Donnell KJ: State control in the substance-exposed fetus. I. The fetal neurobehavioral profile: An assessment of fetal state, arousal, and regulation competency. Ann N Y Acad Sci **846**:262, 1998.

Grant A, Elbourne D, Valentin L, et al: Routine formal fetal movement counting and risk of antepartum late death in normally formed singletons. Lancet **2**:345, 1982.

GRIT Study Group: A randomized trial of timed delivery for the compromised pre-term fetus: Short-term outcomes and Bayesian interpretation. Br J Obstet Gynaecol **110**:27, 2003.

Groome LJ, Mooney DM, Holland SB, et al: Behavioral state affects heart rate response to low-intensity sound in human fetuses. Early Hum Dev **54**:39, 1999.

Groome LJ, Owen J, Neely CL: Oligohydramnios: Antepartum fetal urine production and intrapartum fetal distress. Am J Obstet Gynecol **165**:1077, 1991.

Gurel A, Baschat AA, Harman CR: Umbilical, uterine and precordial venous Doppler characteristics in the first trimester: Relation to perinatal outcome. Ultrasound Obstet Gynecol (in press, 2003).

Guzman ER, Vintzileos AM, Martins M, et al: The efficacy of individual computer heart rate indices in detecting acidemia at birth in growth-restricted fetuses. Obstet Gynecol **87**:969, 1996.

Harman CR: Comprehensive examination of the human fetus. Fetal Med **1**:125, 1989.

Harman CR: Invasive techniques in the management of alloimmune anemia. In Harman CR (ed): Invasive Fetal Testing and Treatment. Cambridge, Blackwell, 1995, p. 109.

Harman CR: Ultrasound in the management of the alloimmunized pregnancy. In Fleisher AC, Manning FA, Jeanty P, et al (eds): Sonography in Obstetrics and Gynecology, 5th ed. Norwalk, Conn, Appleton & Lange, 1996, p. 683.

Harman CR: Fetal biophysical variables and fetal status. In Maulik D (ed): Asphyxia and Brain Damage. New York, Wiley-Liss, 1998, p. 279.

Harman CR, Baschat AA: Comprehensive assessment of fetal wellbeing: Which Doppler tests should be performed? Curr Opin Obstet Gynecol **15**:147, 2003.

Harman CR, Baschat AA, Gembruch U, et al: Fetal venous Doppler in IUGR: Which vessel? Which parameter? Am J Obstet Gynecol (in press).

Harman CR, Baschat AA, Muench M: Acute cardiovascular responses to amnioinfusion in severe IUGR. Am J Obstet Gynecol (in press).

Harman CR, Bowman JM, Menticoglou SM, et al: Profound fetal thrombocytopenia in Rhesus disease: Serious hazard at intravascular transfusion. Lancet **2**:741, 1988.

Harman CR, Menticoglou SM: Fetal surveillance in diabetic pregnancy. Curr Opin Obstet Gynecol **9**:83, 1997.

Harman CR, Menticoglou S, Manning FA: Assessing fetal health. In James DK, Steer PJ, Weiner CP, et al (eds): High Risk Pregnancy Management Options. New York, WB Saunders, 1999, p. 249.

Hecher K, Bilardo CM, Stigter RH, et al: Monitoring of fetuses with intrauterine growth restriction: A longitudinal study. Ultrasound Obstet Gynecol **18**:564, 2001.

Hecher K, Campbell S, Doyle P, et al: Assessment of fetal compromise by Doppler ultrasound investigation of the fetal circulation. Circulation **91**:129, 1995.

Hecher K, Ville Y, Snijders R, et al: Doppler studies of the fetal circulation in twin-twin transfusion syndrome. Ultrasound Obstet Gynecol **5**:318, 1995.

Hershkovitz R, Kingdom JC, Geary M, et al: Fetal cerebral blood flow redistribution in late gestation: Identification of compromise in small fetuses with normal umbilical artery Doppler. Ultrasound Obstet Gynecol **15**:209, 2000.

Hofmeyr GJ: Interventions to help external cephalic version for breech presentation at term. Cochrane Database Syst Rev **2**:CD000184, 2002.

Hofstaetter C, Dubiel M, Gudmundsson S: Two types of umbilical venous pulsations and outcome of high-risk pregnancy. Early Hum Dev **61**:111, 2001.

Hohimer AR, Bissonnette JM: Effect of metabolic acidosis on fetal breathing movements in utero. Respir Physiol **43**:99, 1981.

Hsieh FJ, Chang FM, Ko TM, et al: Umbilical artery flow velocity waveforms in fetuses dying with congenital abnormalities. Br J Obstet Gynecol **95**:478, 1988.

Huddlestone JF, Sutliff G, Robinson D: Contraction stress test by intermittent nipple stimulation. Obstet Gynecol **63**:660, 1984.

Huisman TW: Doppler assessment of the fetal venous system. Semin Perinatol **25**:21, 2001.

Jauniaux E, Nicolaides KH, Campbell S, et al: Hematoma of the umbilical cord secondary to cordocentesis for intrauterine fetal transfusion. Prenat Diagn **10**:477, 1990.

Jensen A, Garnier Y, Berger R: Dynamics of fetal circulatory responses to hypoxia and asphyxia. Eur J Obstet Gynaecol Reprod Biol **84**:155, 1999.

Johnson JM, Harman CR, Lange IR, et al: Biophysical profile scoring in the management of the post term pregnancy: An analysis of 307 patients. Am J Obstet Gynecol **154**:269, 1986.

Johnson RL, Elliott JP: Fetal acoustic stimulation, an adjunct to external cephalic version: A blinded, randomized crossover study. Am J Obstet Gynecol **173**:1369, 1995.

Kamel HS, Makhlouf AM, Youssef AA: Simplified biophysical profile: An antepartum fetal screening test. Gynecol Obstet Invest **47**:223, 1999.

Karsdorp VH, van Vugt JM, van Geijn HP, et al: Clinical significance of absent or reversed end diastolic velocity waveforms in umbilical artery. Lancet **344**:1664, 1994.

Kelly E, Ryan G, Farine D, et al: Absent end diastolic umbilical artery velocity (AEVD): Short and long-term outcome. J Mat-Fet Invest, **3**:203, 1993.

Kiserud T: The ductus venosus. Semin Perinatol **25**:11, 2001.

Kisilevsky BS, Pang L, Hains SM: Maturation of human fetal responses to airborne sound in low- and high-risk fetuses. Early Hum Dev **58**:179, 2000.

Kitanaka T, Alonso JG, Gilbert RD, et al: Fetal responses to long-term hypoxaemia in sheep. Am J Physiol **256**:R1340, 1989.

Kiuchi M, Nagata N, Ikeno S, et al: The relationship between the response to external light stimulation and behavioral states in the human fetus: how it differs from vibroacoustic stimulation. Early Hum Dev **58**:153, 2000.

Kleihauer E, Stein G, Schmidt G: Demonstration of fetal hemoglobin in blood stains dependent upon their age. Z Gesamte Exp Med **144**:105, 1967.

Ko TM, Tseng LH, Chang MH, et al: Amniocentesis in mothers who are hepatitis B virus carriers does not expose the infant to an increased risk of hepatitis B virus infection. Arch Gynecol Obstet **255**:25, 1994.

Koos B, Kitanaka T, Matsuda K, et al: Fetal breathing adaptation to prolonged hypoxaemia in sheep. J Dev Physiol **10**:161, 1988.

Kuhlman KA, Kayreen AB, Depp R, et al: Ultrasonic imaging of normal fetal response to external vibratory acoustic stimulation. Am J Obstet Gynecol **158**:47, 1988.

Kyle PM, Buckley D, Redman CWG: Noninvasive assessment of the maternal cerebral circulation by transcranial Doppler ultrasound during angiotensin II infusion. Br J Obstet Gynaecol **100**:85, 1993.

Lange IR, Manning FA, Morrison I, et al: Cord prolapse: Is antenatal diagnosis possible? Am J Obstet Gynecol **151**:1083, 1985.

Lavery JP: Nonstress fetal heart rate testing. Clin Obstet Gynecol **25**:689, 1982.

Lecanuet JP, Gautheron B, Locatelli A, et al: What sounds reach fetuses: Biological and nonbiological modeling of the transmission of pure tones. Dev Psychobiol **33**:203, 1998.

Lee CY, DiLoreto PC, O'Lane JM: A study of fetal heart rate acceleration patterns. Obstet Gynecol **45**:142, 1975.

Lee CY, DiLoreto PC, Longrand B: Fetal activity acceleration determination for the evaluation of fetal reserve. Obstet Gynecol **48**:19, 1976.

Lenke RR, Nemes JML: Use of nipple stimulation to obtain contraction stress test. Obstet Gynecol **63**:345, 1984.

Magann EF, Chauhan SP, Barrilleaux PS, et al: Amniotic fluid index and single deepest pocket: Weak indicators of abnormal amniotic volumes. Obstet Gynecol **96**:737, 2000.

Magann EF, Chauhan SP, Barrilleaux PS, et al: Ultrasound estimate of amniotic fluid volume: Color Doppler overdiagnosis of oligohydramnios. Obstet Gynecol **98**:71, 2001.

Mandelbrot L, Schlienger I, Bongain A, et al: Thrombocytopenia in pregnant women infected with human immunodeficiency virus: Maternal and neonatal outcome. Am J Obstet Gynecol **171**:252, 1994.

Manning FA: Amniotic fluid volume. In Fetal Medicine Principles and Practice. Norwalk, Conn, Appleton & Lange, 1995a, p. 173.

Manning FA: Cordocentesis: Clinical considerations. In Harman CR (ed): Invasive Fetal Testing and Treatment. Cambridge, Blackwell, 1995b, p. 49.

Manning FA: Fetal biophysical profile scoring: Theoretical considerations and clinical application. In Fetal Medicine Principles and Practice, vol 6. Norwalk, Conn, Appleton & Lange, 1995c, p. 221.

Manning FA, Baskett TF, Morrison I, et al: Fetal biophysical profile scoring: A prospective study in 1184 high-risk patients. Am J Obstet Gynecol **140**:289, 1981.

Manning FA, Bondagji N, Harman CR, et al: Fetal assessment based on the fetal biophysical profile score. VII. Relationship of last BPS result to subsequent cerebral palsy. J Gynecol Obstet Biol Reprod **26**:720, 1997.

Manning FA, Bondagji N, Harman CR, et al: Fetal assessment based on biophysical profile scoring. VIII. The incidence of cerebral palsy in tested and non-tested perinates. Am J Obstet Gynecol **178**:696, 1998.

Manning FA, Harman CR, Menticoglou S, et al: Attention deficit disorder: Relationship to fetal biophysical profile. Am J Obstet Gynecol **182**:S72, 2000a.

Manning FA, Harman CR, Menticoglou S, et al: Mental retardation: Prevalence and etiologic factors in a large obstetric population. Am J Obstet Gynecol **182**:S110, 2000b.

Manning FA, Harman CR, Menticoglou S, et al: The prevalence of non-specific emotional disorder of childhood is unrelated to adverse perinatal factors. Am J Obstet Gynecol **182**:S110, 2000c.

Manning FA, Harman CR, Morrison I, et al: Fetal assessment based on fetal biophysical profile scoring. III. Positive predictive accuracy of the very abnormal test (biophysical profile score = 0). Am J Obstet Gynecol **162**:398, 1990a.

Manning FA, Harman CR, Morrison I, et al: Fetal assessment based on fetal biophysical profile scoring. IV. An analysis of perinatal morbidity and mortality. Am J Obstet Gynecol **162**:703, 1990b.

Manning FA, Heaman M, Boyce D, et al: Intrauterine fetal tachypnea. Obstet Gynecol **58**:398, 1981.

Manning FA, Hill LM, Platt LD: Qualitative amniotic fluid volume determination by ultrasound: Antepartum detection of intrauterine growth retardation. Am J Obstet Gynecol **139**:254, 1981.

Manning FA, Lange IR, Morrison I, et al: Fetal biophysical profile score and the nonstress test: A comparative trial. Obstet Gynecol **64**:326, 1984.

Manning FA, Martin CB Jr, Murata Y, et al: Breathing movements before death in the primate fetus. Am J Obstet Gynecol **135**:71, 1979.

Manning FA, Morrison I, Harman CR, et al: Fetal assessment based on fetal biophysical profile scoring: Experience in 19,221 referred high-risk pregnancies. II. An analysis of false-negative fetal deaths. Am J Obstet Gynecol **157**:880, 1987.

Manning FA, Morrison I, Harman CR, et al: The abnormal fetal biophysical profile score. V. Predictive accuracy according to score composition. Am J Obstet Gynecol **162**:918, 1990.

Manning FA, Morrison I, Lange IR, et al: Fetal assessment based on fetal biophysical profile scoring: Experience in 12,620 referred high-risk pregnancies. I. Perinatal mortality by frequency and etiology. Am J Obstet Gynecol **151**:343, 1985.

Manning FA, Morrison I, Lange IR, et al: Fetal biophysical profile scoring: Selective use of the nonstress test. Am J Obstet Gynecol **156**:709, 1987.

Manning FA, Platt LD, Sipos L, et al: Fetal breathing movements and the nonstress test in high-risk pregnancies. Am J Obstet Gynecol **135**:511, 1979.

Manning FA, Platt LD, Sipos L: Antepartum fetal evaluation: Development of a fetal biophysical profile score. Am J Obstet Gynecol **136**:787, 1980.

Manning FA, Snijders R, Harman CR, et al: Fetal biophysical profile scoring. VI. Correlations with antepartum umbilical venous pH. Am J Obstet Gynecol **169**:755, 1993.

Mari G, Deter RL, Carpenter RL, et al: Noninvasive diagnosis by Doppler ultrasonography of fetal anemia due to maternal red-cell alloimmunization. N Engl J Med **342**:9, 2000.

Martin CB Jr: Regulation of the fetal heart rate and genesis of FHR patterns. Semin Perinat **2**:131, 1978.

Martin CB Jr: Behavioural states in the human fetus. J Reprod Med **26**:425, 1981.

Matias A, Gomes C, Flack N, et al: Screening for chromosomal abnormalities at 10–14 weeks: The role of ductus venosus blood flow. Ultrasound Obstet Gynecol **12**:380, 1998.

Maulik D, Saini VD, Nanda NC, et al: Doppler evaluation of fetal hemodynamics. Ultrasound Med Biol **8**:705, 1982.

Merrill PA, Porto M, Lovett SM, et al: Evaluation of the nonreactive positive contraction stress test prior to 32 weeks: The role of the biophysical profile. Am J Perinatol **12**:229, 1995.

Miller DA, Rabello YA, Paul RH: The modified biophysical profile: Antepartum testing in the 1990s. Am J Obstet Gynecol **174**:812, 1996.

Molteni RA, Melmed MH, Sheldon RE, et al: Induction of fetal breathing by metabolic acidemia and its effect on blood flow to the respiratory muscles. Am J Obstet Gynecol **36**:609, 1980.

Moniz CF, Nicolaides KH, Bamforth FJ, et al: Normal reference ranges for biochemical substances relating to renal, hepatic, and bone function in fetal and maternal plasma throughout pregnancy. J Clin Pathol **38**:468, 1985.

Moore TR: Superiority of the four-quadrant sum over the single-deepest-pocket technique in ultrasonographic identification of abnormal amniotic fluid volumes. Am J Obstet Gynecol **163**:762, 1990.

Moore TR, Cayle JE: The amniotic fluid index in normal pregnancy. Am J Obstet Gynecol **162**:1168, 1990.

Morrison I, Menticoglou S, Manning FA, et al: Comparison of antepartum test results to perinatal outcome. J Matern Fetal Med **3**:75, 1994.

Morrow RJ, Adamson SL, Bull SB, et al: Effect of placental embolization on the umbilical arterial waveform in fetal sheep. Am J Obstet Gynecol **161**:1055, 1989.

Nageotte MP, Towers CV, Asrat T, et al: The value of a negative antepartum test: Contraction stress test and modified biophysical profile. Obstet Gynecol **84**:231, 1994.

Nageotte MP, Towers CV, Asrat T, et al: Perinatal outcome with the modified biophysical profile. Am J Obstet Gynecol **172**:1329, 1995.

Natale R, Clewlow F, Dawes GS: Measurement of fetal forelimb movements in the lamb in utero. Am J Obstet Gynecol **140**:545, 1981.

National Institute of Child Health & Human Development Research Planning Workshop: Electronic fetal heart rate monitoring: Research guidelines for interpretation. J Obstet Gynecol Neonat Nurs **26**:635, 1997.

Nava S, Bocconi L, Zuliani G, et al: Aspects of fetal physiology from 18 to 37 weeks' gestation as assessed by blood sampling. Obstet Gynecol **87**:975, 1996.

Newnham JP, Burns SE, Roberman BD: Effect of vibratory acoustic stimulation on the duration of fetal heart rate monitoring tests. Am J Perinatol **7**:232, 1990.

Nicolaides KH, Economides DL, Soothill PW: Blood gases, PH, and lactate in appropriate- and small-for-gestational-age fetuses. Am J Obstet Gynecol **161**:996, 1989.

Nicolaides KH, Peters MT, Vyas S, et al: Relation of rate of urine production to oxygen tensions in small-for-gestational-age fetuses. Am J Obstet Gynecol **162**:387, 1990.

Nicolini U, Nicolaidis P, Fisk NM, et al: Fetal blood sampling from the intrahepatic vein: Analysis of safety and clinical experience with 214 procedures. Obstet Gynecol **76**:47, 1990.

Nicolini U, Santolaya I, Ojo OE, et al: The fetal intrahepatic umbilical vein as an alternative to cord needling for prenatal diagnosis and therapy. Prenat Diagn **8**:665, 1988.

Nijhuis JG, Crevels AJ, van Dongen PWJ: Fetal brain death: The definition of a fetal heart rate pattern and its clinical consequences. Obstet Gynecol Surv **45**:229, 1990.

Nijhuis JG, Prechtl HFR, Martin CB Jr, et al: Are there behavioural states in the human fetus? Early Hum Dev **6**:177, 1982.

Nochimson DJ, Turbeville JS, Terry JE, et al: The non-stress test. Obstet Gynecol **51**:419, 1978.

Oepkes D, Vandenbussche FP, Van Bel F, et al: Fetal ductus venosus blood flow velocities before and after transfusion in red-cell alloimmunized pregnancies. Obstet Gynecol **82**:237, 1993.

Ohel G, Birkenfield A, Rabinowitz R, et al: Fetal response to vibratory acoustic stimulation in periods of low heart rate reactivity and low activity. Am J Obstet Gynecol **154**:619, 1986.

Paidas MI, Berkowitz RL, Lynch L, et al: Alloimmune thrombocytopenia: Fetal and neonatal losses related to cordocentesis. Am J Obstet Gynecol **172**:475, 1995.

Patrick J, Campbell K, Carmichael L, et al: Patterns of human fetal breathing movements during the last 10 weeks of pregnancy. Obstet Gynecol **56**:24, 1980.

Patrick JE, Gagnon R: Adaptation to vibroacoustic stimulation. *In* Dawes GS, Zacutti A, Borruto F, et al (eds): Fetal Autonomy and Adaptation. Chichester, England, Wiley, 1990, p. 39.

Pattinson RC, Norman K, Kirsten G, et al: Relationship between the fetal heart rate pattern and perinatal mortality in fetuses with absent end-diastolic velocities of the umbilical artery: A case-controlled study. Am J Perinatol **12**:286, 1995.

Petrikovsky BM, Kaplan GP: Fetal grasping of the umbilical cord causing variable fetal heart rate decelerations. J Clin Ultrasound **21**:642, 1993.

Phelan JP, Ahn MO, Smith CV, et al: Amniotic fluid index measurements during pregnancy. J Reprod Med **32**:601, 1987.

Pielet BW, Socol ML, MacGregor SN, et al: Fetal heart rote changes after fetal intravascular treatment with pancuronium bromide. Am J Obstet Gynecol **159**:640, 1988.

Pillai M, James D: Development of human fetal behaviour: A review. Fetal Diagn Ther **5**:15, 1990a.

Pillai M, James D: The development of fetal heart rate patterns during normal pregnancy. Obstet Gynecol **76**:812, 1990b.

Pillai M, James D: The importance of the behavioural state in biophysical assessment of the term human fetus. Br J Obstet Gynaecol **97**:1130, 1990c.

Pillai M, James D: Continuation of normal neurobehavioural development in fetuses with absent umbilical arterial end diastolic velocities. Br J Obstet Gynaecol **98**:277, 1991a.

Pillai M, James D: Human fetal mouthing movements: A potential biophysical variable for distinguishing state 1F from abnormal fetal behaviour. Report of four cases. Eur J Obstet Gynaecol Reprod Biol **38**:151, 1991b.

Platt LD, Manning FA, LeMay M, et al: Human fetal breathing: relationships to fetal condition. Am J Obstet Gynecol **132**:514, 1978.

Pollack RN, Divon MY: Intrauterine Growth Retardation: Diagnosis. *In* Copel JA, Reed KL (eds): Doppler Ultrasound in Obstetrics and Gynecology. New York, Raven Press, 1995, p. 171.

Poreba A, Dudkieqicz D, Drygalski M: The influence of the sounds of music on chosen cardiotocographic parameters in mature pregnancies. Ginekol Pol **71**:915, 2000.

Potts P, Connors G, Gillis S, et al: The effect of carbon dioxide on Doppler flow velocity waveforms in the human fetus. J Dev Physiol **17**:119, 1992.

Prechtl HFR: The behavioural states of the newborn infant [review]. Brain Res **76**:185, 1974.

Ray M, Freeman RK, Pine S: Clinical experience with the oxytocin challenge test. Am J Obstet Gynecol **114**:1, 1972.

Ribbert LSM, Fidler V, Visser GHA: Computer-assisted analysis of normal second trimester fetal heart rate patterns. J Perinat Med **19**:53, 1991.

Richardson BS: Fetal adaptive responses to asphyxia. Clin Perinat **16**:595, 1989.

Robertson WB, Brosen I, Dixon G: Uteroplacental vascular pathology. Eur J Obstet Gynaecol Reprod **5**:47, 1975.

Rotmensch S, Celentano C, Liberati M, et al: The effect of antenatal steroid administration on the fetal response to vibroacoustic stimulation. Acta Obstet Gynaecol Scand **78**:847, 1999.

Rotmensch S, Liberati M, Santolaya-Forgas J, et al: Uteroplacental and intraplacental circulation. *In* Copel JA, Reed KL (eds): Doppler Ultrasound in Obstetrics and Gynecology, vol 11. New York, Raven, 1995, p. 115.

Roussis P, Rosemond RL, Glass C, et al: Preterm premature rupture of membranes: Detection of infection. Am J Obstet Gynecol **165**:1099, 1991.

Rudolph AM: The fetal circulation and its response to stress. J Dev Physiol **16**:595, 1984.

Rurak DW, Gruber NC: Effect of neuromuscular blockade on oxygen consumption and blood gases. Am J Obstet Gynecol **145**:258, 1983.

Rurak DW, Richardson BS, Patrick JE, et al: Oxygen consumption in the fetal lamb during sustained hypoxemia with progressive acidemia. Am J Physiol **258**:1108, 1990.

Rurak DW, Selke P, Fisher M, et al: Fetal oxygen extraction: comparison of the human and sheep. Am J Obstet Gynecol **156**:360, 1987.

Schifrin BS: The rationale for antepartum fetal heart rate monitoring. J Reprod Med **23**:213, 1979.

Schifrin BS, Foye G, Amato J, et al: Routine fetal heart rate monitoring in the antepartum period. Obstet Gynecol **54**:21, 1979.

Schulman H, Fleischer A, Fannakides G, et al: Development of uterine artery compliance in pregnancy as detected by Doppler ultrasound. Am J Obstet Gynecol **155**:1031, 1986.

Seeds JW, Chescheir NC, Bowes WA Jr, et al: Fetal death as a complication of intrauterine intravascular transfusion. Obstet Gynecol **74**:461, 1989.

Serafini P, Lindsay MBJ, Nagy DA, et al: Antepartum fetal heart rate response to sound stimulation: The acoustic stimulation test. Am J Obstet Gynecol **148**:41, 1984.

Sheldon RE, Peeters LLH, Jones MD, et al: Redistribution of cardiac output and oxygen delivery in the hypoxemic fetal lamb. Am J Obstet Gynecol **135**:1071, 1979.

Sherer DM: Blunted fetal response to vibroacoustic stimulation associated with maternal intravenous magnesium sulfate therapy. Am J Perinatol **11**:401, 1994.

Sherer DM, Menashe M, Sadovsky E: Severe fetal bradycardia caused by external vibratory acoustic stimulation. Am J Obstet Gynecol **159**:334, 1988.

Snijders R, Hyett J: Fetal testing in intra-uterine growth retardation. Curr Opin Obstet Gynecol **9**:91, 1997.

Snijders RJM, McLaren R, Nicolaides KH: Computer-assisted analysis of fetal heart rate patterns at 20–41 weeks' gestation. Fetal Diagn Ther **5**:79, 1997.

Soothill PW, Nicolaides KH, Rodeck CH, et al: Effect of gestational age on fetal and intervillous blood gas and acid-base values in human pregnancy. Fetal Ther **1**:168, 1986.

Soothill PW, Sherer DM: Blunted fetal response to vibroacoustic stimulation associated with maternal intravenous magnesium sulfate therapy. Am J Perinatol **11**:401, 1994.

Stuart B, Drumm J, Fitzgerald DE, et al: Fetal blood velocity waveforms in normal pregnancy. Br J Obstet Gynaecol **87**:780, 1980.

Trudinger BJ, Cook CM, Giles WB, et al: Fetal umbilical artery velocity waveforms and subsequent neonatal outcome. Br J Obstet Gynecol **98**:378, 1991.

Trudinger BJ, Giles WB, Cook CM: Uteroplacental blood flow velocity-time waveforms in normal and complicated pregnancy. Br J Obstet Gynaecol **92**:39, 1985a.

Trudinger BJ, Giles WB, Cook CM, et al: Fetal umbilical artery flow velocity waveforms and placental resistance: Clinical significance. Br J Obstet Gynaecol **92**:23, 1985b.

Trudinger BJ, Stevens D, Connelly A, et al: Umbilical artery flow velocity waveforms and placental resistance. The effects of embolization of the umbilical circulation. Am J Obstet Gynecol **157**:1443, 1987.

Van den Wijngaard JAGW, Groenenberg IAL, Wladimiroff JW, et al: Cerebral Doppler ultrasound of the human fetus. Br J Obstet Gynaecol **96**:845, 1989.

Van Eyck J, Wladimiroff JW, Noordam MJ, et al: The blood flow velocity waveform in the fetal descending aorta: Its relationship to fetal behaviour state in normal pregnancy at 37–38 weeks. Early Hum Dev **12**:137, 1985.

Van Vliet MAT, Martin CB Jr, Nijhuis JG, et al: Behavioural states in growth retarded human fetuses. Early Hum Dev **12**:183, 1985.

Vince MA, Armitage SE: Sound stimulation available to the sheep fetus. Reprod Nutr Dev **20**:801, 1980.

Vindla S, James D, Sahota D: Comparison of unstimulated and stimulated behaviour in human fetuses with congenital abnormalities. Fetal Diagn Ther **14**:156, 1999.

Vintzileos AM, Campbell WA, Ingardia CJ, et al: The fetal biophysical profile and its predictive value. Obstet Gynecol **62**:271, 1983.

Vintzileos AM, Campbell WA, Nochimson DL, et al: Fetal biophysical profile versus amniocentesis in predicting infection in premature rupture of the membranes. Obstet Gynecol **68**:488, 1986.

Vintzileos AM, Flemming AD, Scorza WE, et al: Relationship between fetal biophysical activities and umbilical cord blood gas values. Am J Obstet Gynecol **165**:707, 1991.

Vintzileos AM, Gaffney SE, Salinger LM, et al: The relationship among the fetal biophysical profile, umbilical cord pH, and Apgar scores. Am J Obstet Gynecol **157**:627, 1987.

Viscarello RR, Cullen MT, DeGennaro NJ, et al: Fetal blood sampling in human immunodeficiency virus-seropositive women before elective midtrimester termination of pregnancy. Am J Obstet Gynecol **167**:1075, 1992.

Warner J, Hains SM, Kisilevsky BS: An exploratory study of fetal behavior at 33 and 36 weeks gestational age in hypertensive women. Dev Psychobiol **41**:156, 2002.

Weiner CP: The role of cordocentesis in fetal diagnosis. Clin Obstet Gynecol **31**:285, 1988.

Weiner CP: The biochemical assessment of the human fetus: Norms and applications. *In* Harman CR (ed): Invasive Fetal Testing and Treatment. Cambridge, Blackwell, 1995, p. 93.

Weiner CP, Anderson TL: The acute effect of cordocentesis with or without fetal curarization and of intravascular transfusion upon umbilical artery waveform indices. Obstet Gynecol **73**:219, 1989.

Weiner CP, Gonick B (eds): High Risk Pregnancy Management Options. New York, Saunders, 1999, p. 249.

Weiner CP, Okamura K: Diagnostic fetal blood sampling technique-related losses. Fetal Diagn Ther **11**:169, 1996.

Weiner CP, Sipes SL, Wenstrom K: The effect of fetal age upon normal fetal laboratory values and venous pressure. Obstet Gynecol **79**:713, 1992.

Weiner Z, Farmakides G, Schulman H, et al: Surveillance of growth-retarded fetuses with computerized fetal heart rate monitoring combined with Doppler velocimetry of the umbilical and uterine arteries. J Reprod Med **41**:112, 1996.

Wilkins I, Mezrow G, Lynch L, et al: Amnionitis and life-threatening respiratory distress after percutaneous umbilical blood sampling. Am J Obstet Gynecol **160**:427, 1989.

Williams K, McLean C: Maternal cerebral vasospasm in eclampsia assessed by transcranial Doppler. Am J Perinatol **10**:243, 1993.

Williams K, Wilson S: Maternal middle cerebral artery blood flow velocity variation with gestational age. Obstet Gynecol **84**:445, 1994.

Wilson RD, Farquharson DF, Wittmann BK, et al: Cordocentesis: Overall pregnancy loss rate as important as procedure loss rate. Fetal Diagn Ther **9**:142, 1994.

Wladimiroff JW, van den Wijngaard JA, Degani S, et al: Cerebral and umbilical arterial blood flow velocity waveforms in normal and growth-retarded pregnancies. Obstet Gynecol **69**:705, 1987.

Woo JSK, Liang ST, Lo RLS: Significance of an absent or reversed end diastolic flow in Doppler umbilical artery waveforms. J Ultrasound Med **6**:291, 1987.

Woods JR, Plessinger M, Mack C: The fetal auditory brainstem response. Pediatr Res **18**:83, 1984.

Yaffe H, Kreisberg GA, Gale R: Sinusoidal heart rate pattern and normal bio-physical profile in a severely compromised fetus. Acta Obstet Gynaecol Scand **68**:561, 1989.

Yoon BH, Romero R, Roh CR, et al: Relationship between the fetal biophys-ical profile score, umbilical artery Doppler velocimetry, and fetal blood acid-base status determined by cordocentesis. Am J Obstet Gynecol **169**:1586, 1993.

Yoon BH, Syn HC, Kim SW: The efficacy of Doppler umbilical artery velocimetry in identifying fetal acidosis. A comparison with fetal biophys-ical profile. J Ultrasound Med **11**:1, 1992.

Zelop CM, Richardson DK, Heffner LJ: Outcomes of severely abnormal umbil-ical artery Doppler velocimetry in structurally normal singleton fetuses. Obstet Gynecol **87**:434, 1996.

Chapter 22
INTRAPARTUM FETAL SURVEILLANCE

Julian T. Parer, MD, PhD, and Michael P. Nageotte, MD

FACTORS CONTROLLING FETAL HEART RATE

Fetal heart rate (FHR) analysis is the prime means by which a fetus is evaluated for adequacy of oxygenation. Knowledge of its rate and regulation are thus of great importance to the obstetrician. The average heart rate in the normal term fetus before labor is 140 beats/min. Earlier in pregnancy it is higher but not substantially so. At 20 weeks, the average FHR is 155 beats/min; at 30 weeks, it is 144 beats/min. Variations of 20 beats/min above or below these values are seen in normal fetuses.

The fetal heart is similar to the adult heart in that it has its own intrinsic pacemaker activity that results in rhythmic contractions. The sinoatrial node, found in one wall of the right atrium, has the fastest rate of contraction and sets the rate in the normal heart. The next fastest pacemaker rate is found in the atrium. Finally, the ventricle has a slower rate of beating than either the sinoatrial node or the atrium. In cases of complete or partial heart block in the fetus, variations in rate below normal can be seen. The rate in a fetus with a complete heart block is about 50 to 60 beats/min.

Variability of the FHR from beat to beat and longer term trends in heart rate over periods of less than 1 minute are important properties. Variability has prognostic importance clinically; valuable empiric interpretations can be made from its presence, its decrease, or its absence. The mean FHR is the result of many physiologic factors that modulate the intrinsic rate of the heart, the most obvious being signals from the autonomic nervous system.

Parasympathetic Nervous System

The parasympathetic nervous system consists primarily of the vagus nerve (10th cranial nerve), which originates in the medulla oblongata. Fibers from this nerve supply the sinoatrial and the atrioventricular nodes, the neuronal bridge between atrium and ventricle. Stimulation of the vagus nerve or injection of acetylcholine, the substance secreted at the nerve endings, results in a decrease in heart rate in the normal fetus owing to vagal influence on the sinoatrial node that decreases its rate of firing and the rate of transmission of impulses from atrium to ventricle. In a similar fashion, blocking of this nerve in a normal fetus by injecting a substance that blocks the effect of acetylcholine (e.g., atropine) causes an increase in the FHR of approximately 20 beats/min at term (Mendez-Bauer et al., 1963). This finding demonstrates a normally constant vagal influence on the heart rate, tending to decrease it from its normal intrinsic rate.

The vagus nerve also has another very important function: It is responsible for transmission of impulses causing beat-to-beat variability of FHR. Blocking the vagus nerve with atropine results in a disappearance of this variability. Hence, there are two possible vagal influences on the heart: a tonic influence tending to decrease its rate and an oscillatory influence that results in FHR variability (DeHaan et al., 1973). The vagal tone is not necessarily constant. Its influence increases with gestational age (Schifferli and Caldeyro-Barcia, 1973). In fetal sheep, vagal activity increases as much as fourfold during acute hypoxia (Parer, 1997) or experimentally produced fetal growth restriction (Llanos et al., 1980).

Sympathetic Nervous System

Sympathetic nerves are widely distributed in the muscle of the heart at term. Stimulation of the sympathetic nerves releases norepinephrine and causes increases in the FHR and the vigor of cardiac contractions, resulting in higher cardiac output. The sympathetic nerves are a reserve mechanism to improve the pumping activity of the heart during intermittent stressful situations. There is normally a tonic sympathetic influence on the heart. Propranolol, which blocks the action of these sympathetic nerves, causes a decrease in FHR of approximately 10 beats/min when administered to the normal sheep fetus. As with the vagal tone, tonic influence increases as much as twofold during fetal hypoxia.

FHR variability decreases only slightly after blocking of the sympathetic nerves in primates. There is a commonly held theory that FHR variability is a result of the two neuronal inputs to the fetal heart (*vagal* and *β-adrenergic*), each with a different time constant. However, because atropine almost abolishes FHR variability and propranolol decreases it only a little, it is unlikely that this theory is correct for the primate (Parer et al., 1981). There appear to be important species differences in the transmission of FHR variability impulses. Both vagal and β-adrenergic influences are probably important in the sheep (Dalton et al., 1983). One must keep this in mind, because sheep are frequently used in fetal physiology studies.

Alpha-adrenergic activity is also important in altering the distribution of blood flow to specific organs during stress. During hypoxia, therefore, vasoconstriction of certain vascular beds (e.g., gut, liver, lung) allows preferential flow of blood with the available oxygen to vital organs (e.g., brain, heart, and adrenals), and blood flow to the placenta is maintained (see Chapter 15). Factors that influence the activity of the parasympathetic and sympathetic nervous systems are discussed next.

Chemoreceptors

Chemoreceptors are found in both the peripheral nervous system and the central nervous system. They have their most dramatic effects on the regulation of respiration but are also important in the control of the circulation. The peripheral chemoreceptors are in the carotid and aortic bodies, located in the arch of the aorta and the area of the carotid sinus. The central chemoreceptors in the medulla oblongata respond to changes in the oxygen and carbon dioxide tensions in blood or cerebrospinal fluid perfusing this area.

In the adult, when oxygen is decreased or the carbon dioxide content is increased in the arterial blood perfusing the central chemoreceptors, a reflex tachycardia occurs. There is also a substantial increase in arterial blood pressure, particularly when carbon dioxide concentration is increased. Both effects are thought to be protective, in an attempt to circulate more blood through the affected areas to bring about a decrease in carbon dioxide tension or an increase in oxygen tension. Selective hypoxia or hypercapnia of the peripheral chemoreceptors alone in the adult produces a bradycardia, in contrast to the tachycardia and hypertension seen with central hypoxia or hypercapnia.

The interaction of the central and peripheral chemoreceptors in the fetus is poorly understood. It is known that the net result of hypoxia or hypercapnia in the unanesthetized fetus is bradycardia with hypertension. During basal conditions, the chemoreceptors contribute to the stabilization of the heart rate and blood pressure (Hanson, 1988).

Baroreceptors

In the arch of the aorta and in the carotid sinus at the junction of the internal and external carotid arteries are small stretch receptors in the vessel walls that are sensitive to increases in blood pressure. When pressure rises, impulses are sent from these receptors via the vagus or glossopharyngeal nerve to the mid-brain, resulting in further impulses via the vagus nerve to the heart, tending to slow it. This is an extremely rapid response, being seen with almost the first systolic rise of blood pressure. It is a protective, stabilizing attempt by the body to lower blood pressure by decreasing heart rate and cardiac output when blood pressure is increasing.

Central Nervous System

In the adult, the higher centers of the brain influence heart rate. Heart rate is increased by emotional stimuli such as fear and sexual arousal. In fetal lambs and monkeys, the electroencephalogram or electro-oculogram shows increased activity at times in association with variability of the heart rate and body movements. At other times, apparently when the fetus is sleeping, body movement slows and the FHR variability decreases, suggesting an association between these two factors and central nervous system activity (Nijhuis et al., 1982).

The hypothalamus is the area of dispatch of nerve impulses produced by physical expressions of emotion, including acceleration of the heart rate and elevation of the blood pressure. In the fetal lamb, stimulating an electrode in the hypothalamus causes the FHR to increase, at least initially, followed by a decrease, probably because of the protective baroreflex mentioned earlier. The increases in blood pressure and heart rate are mediated by the sympathetic nerves.

The medulla oblongata contains the vasomotor centers, integrative centers where the net result of all the inputs is either acceleration or deceleration of the heart rate. It is probably in these centers that the net result of numerous central and peripheral inputs is processed to generate irregular oscillatory vagal impulses, giving rise to FHR variability.

Hormonal Regulation

Adrenal Medulla

The fetal adrenal medulla produces epinephrine and norepinephrine in response to stress. Both substances act on the heart and cardiovascular system in a way similar to sympathetic stimulation to produce a faster heart rate, greater force of contraction of the heart, and higher arterial blood pressure. It is not clear, however, whether catecholamines exert a regulatory function in the resting fetus, at least in sheep.

Renin-Angiotensin System

Angiotensin II may play a role in fetal circulatory regulation at rest, but its main activity is observed during hemorrhagic stress on a fetus.

Arginine Vasopressin

Vasopressin affects the distribution of blood flow in fetal sheep. However, this is probably operative only during hypoxia and possibly other stressful situations. A possible influence of arginine vasopressin in producing the sinusoidal FHR pattern is discussed later.

Prostaglandins

Arachidonic acid metabolites are found in high concentrations in the fetal circulation and in many tissues. Their main roles seem to be regulating umbilical blood flow and maintaining the patency of the ductus arteriosus during fetal life.

Other Hormones

Other hormones, such as nitric oxide, α-melanocyte–stimulating hormone, atrial natriuretic hormone, neuropeptide Y, thyrotropin-releasing hormone, cortisol, and metabolites such as adenosine are also present in the fetus and participate in the circulatory function regulation. However, their relative quantitative importance is still not determined.

Blood Volume Control

Capillary Fluid Shift

In the adult, when the blood pressure of the body is elevated by excessive blood volume, some fluid moves out of the capillaries into interstitial spaces, thereby decreasing the blood volume toward normal. Conversely, if the adult loses blood through hemorrhage, some fluid shifts out of the interstitial spaces into the circulation, thereby increasing the blood volume toward normal. There is normally a delicate balance between the pressures inside and outside the capillaries. This mechanism of regulating blood pressure is slower than the almost-instantaneous regulation found with the reflex mechanisms discussed previously. Its role in the fetus is imperfectly understood, although imbalances may be responsible for the hydrops seen in some cases of red cell alloimmunization and the high output failure sometimes seen with extreme fetal tachycardia. In addition, studies performed in sheep show that blood volume is kept closer to normal in a fetus than in an adult after reductions or expansions of volume (Brace, 1995).

Intraplacental Pressures

Fluid moves down hydrostatic pressure gradients and also in response to osmotic pressure gradients. The actual value of these factors within the human placenta, where fetal and maternal blood closely approximate, is controversial. It seems likely, however, that some delicate balancing mechanisms within the placenta prevent rapid fluid shifts between mother and fetus. The arterial blood pressure of the mother is much higher (approximately 100 mm Hg) than that of the fetus (approximately 55 mm Hg), and osmotic pressures are not substantially different. Hence, some compensatory mechanism must be present to equalize the effective pressures at the exchange points.

Frank-Starling Mechanism

The amount of blood pumped by the heart is determined by the amount of blood returning to the heart; that is, the heart pumps all the blood that flows into it without excessive damming of blood in the veins. When the cardiac muscle is stretched before contraction by an increased inflow of blood, it contracts with a greater force than before and is able to pump out more blood. This mechanism has been studied in the unanesthetized fetal lamb, where it is seen to be less well developed than in the adult sheep (Rudolph and Heymann, 1973), probably because the fetal heart muscle is not as well developed. The same is likely true of the human fetus, which is generally more immature at birth than the lamb. As a consequence, increases in the filling pressure or preload produce minor if any changes in combined ventricular output, suggesting that the fetal heart normally operates near the top of its function curve.

The output of the fetal heart is also related to the heart rate. Some researchers have shown that spontaneous variations of heart rate relate directly to cardiac output (i.e., as rate increases, output increases). However, different responses have been observed during right or left atrial pacing studies. No changes were observed in left ventricular output when the right atrium was paced, whereas the output decreased during left atrial pacing (Anderson et al., 1986). Similarly, right ventricular output was unchanged with left atrial pacing and reduced with right atrial pacing (Anderson et al., 1987). Clearly, additional factors are required to explain such differences. In addition to heart rate and preload, cardiac output depends on afterload and intrinsic contractility (Anderson et al., 1986, 1987). This relationship between FHR and cardiac output has not been confirmed in human fetuses under physiologic conditions because the spontaneous increase in heart rate has been found to be associated with a decrease in stroke volume, maintaining the cardiac output unchanged (Kenny et al., 1987).

The fetal heart appears to be highly sensitive to changes in the afterload, represented by the fetal arterial blood pressure.

In this way, increases in afterload dramatically reduce the stroke volume or cardiac output. As already stated, the fetal heart, in contrast to the adult heart, is incompletely developed. Many ultrastructural differences between the fetal and adult heart account for a lower intrinsic capacity of the fetal heart to contract. None of these four determinants of cardiac output works separately; instead, each interacts dynamically to modulate the fetal cardiac output during physiologic conditions. Cardiac output responses during hypoxic bradycardia are described later.

In clinical practice, it is reasonable to assume that at modest variations of heart rate from the normal range, there are relatively small effects on the cardiac output. However, at extremes (e.g., tachycardia above 240 beats/min or a bradycardia below 60 beats/min), cardiac output and umbilical blood flow are likely to be substantially decreased.

UMBILICAL BLOOD FLOW

Umbilical blood flow measured by ultrasonography is about 360 mL/min or 120 mL/min/kg in an undisturbed fetus at term (Gill et al., 1981). This figure is considerably less than that in a sheep (approximately 200 mL/min/kg). The differences may be explained by the somewhat higher metabolic rate (body temperature 39°C) and lower hemoglobin concentration (10 g/dL) in the fetal sheep. Once again, this species difference is important because most information on fetal circulatory physiology has come from fetal sheep. The umbilical blood flow is approximately 40% of the combined ventricular output, and about 20% of this blood flow is shunted (it does not exchange with maternal blood in sheep). Either it is carried through actual vascular shunts within the fetal side of the placenta, or it does not approach maternal blood closely enough to exchange with it.

Umbilical blood flow is unaffected by acute moderate hypoxia but is decreased by severe hypoxia. There is no innervation of the umbilical cord, but umbilical blood flow decreases with the administration of catecholamines. Flow is also decreased by acute cord occlusion. There are no known means of increasing umbilical flow when it is thought to be decreased chronically. However, variable decelerations in the FHR occur with transient umbilical cord compression during labor. Manipulation of maternal position either to the lateral or Trendelenburg position or replenishing amniotic fluid volume can sometimes abolish these patterns; the implication is that cord compression has been relieved.

HYPOXIA/ACIDEMIA

Fetal Responses

Studies of chronically prepared animals have shown that a number of responses occur during acute hypoxia or acidemia in the previously normoxemic fetus. Little or no change in combined cardiac output and umbilical (placental) blood flow occurs, but there is a redistribution of blood flow favoring certain vital organs—namely, heart, brain, and adrenal gland—and a decrease in the blood flow to the gut, spleen, kidneys, and carcass (Cohn et al., 1974). This initial response is presumed to be advantageous to a fetus in the same way as the diving reflex is in an adult seal, in that the blood containing the available oxygen and other nutrients is supplied preferentially to vital organs.

Fetal oxygen consumption decreased to values as low as 60% of control (from approximately 8 to 5 mL/min/kg) during fetal hypoxia in the chronically instrumented fetus with arterial oxygen tension of 10 mm Hg (Parer, 1980). This decrease is rapidly instituted, stable for periods up to 45 minutes, proportional to the degree of hypoxia, and rapidly reversible on cessation of maternal hypoxia. It is accompanied by a fetal bradycardia of about 30 beats/min below control (approximately 170 beats/min control to 140 beats/min hypoxia in fetal sheep) and an increase in fetal arterial blood pressure (approximately 54 mm Hg control to 61 mm Hg hypoxia mean pressure). There is also progressive fetal acidosis during fetal isocapnic hypoxia (fetal arterial pH 7.38 control to 7.33 after 25 minutes of hypoxia). This is a metabolic acidosis due to lactic acid accumulation as a result of anaerobic metabolism primarily in those partially vasoconstricted beds where oxygenation is inadequate for normal basic needs (Mann, 1970). During fetal acidemia, the increase in carbon dioxide tension superimposes a respiratory component on the acidosis.

The series of responses just described (redistribution of blood flow favoring vital organs, decreased total oxygen consumption, and anaerobic glycolysis) may be thought of as temporary compensatory mechanisms that enable a fetus to survive moderately long periods (e.g., up to 30 minutes) of limited oxygen supply without decompensation of vital organs, particularly the brain and heart. The close matching of blood flow to oxygen availability to achieve a constancy of oxygen consumption has been demonstrated in the fetal cerebral circulation (Jones et al., 1977) and in the fetal myocardium (Fisher et al., 1982). In studies on hypoxic lamb fetuses, cerebral oxygen consumption was constant over a wide range of arterial oxygen contents because the decrease in arteriovenous oxygen content accompanying hypoxia was compensated for by an increase in cerebral blood flow. However, during more severe acidemia or sustained hypoxemia, these responses are no longer maintained, and a decrease in the cardiac output, arterial blood pressure, and blood flow to the brain and heart has been described (Yaffe et al., 1987). These changes may be considered to be a stage of decompensation, after which tissue damage and even fetal death may follow (Myers, 1972).

Metabolic Effects

The fetus depends partially on anaerobic metabolism for its energy needs during oxygen insufficiency (Mann, 1970; Low et al., 1975). It has also been shown in experimental animals that a newborn's ability to tolerate hypoxia depends on cardiac carbohydrate reserves; whether this also applies to a human fetus is unknown, but clinical observations support the view that carbohydrate-depleted fetuses succumb more readily than those with normal reserves. A nutritionally growth-restricted fetus also is more susceptible to intrauterine hypoxia and depression than a normal fetus (Mann et al., 1974).

The prime aim of compensatory responses in hypoxia is maintenance of the circulation, and maintenance of the integrity of cardiac function is paramount in this regard. Carbohydrate availability is critical in supplying substrates for glycolysis at more severe degrees of hypoxia.

Mechanisms of Responses

The cardiovascular responses to hypoxia are instituted rapidly and are mediated by neural and hormonal mechanisms (Parer, 1997). The tonic influence of the autonomic nervous system on heart rate, blood pressure, and umbilical circulation in a normoxemic fetus is quantitatively minor. This is in marked contrast to autonomic activity during hypoxia.

In studies using total pharmacologic blockade, parasympathetic activity is augmented three- to fivefold, and β-adrenergic activity doubled when measured by heart rate response. The net result of these changes is a decrease in FHR during hypoxia. Augmented β-adrenergic activity also may be important in maintaining cardiac output and umbilical blood flow during hypoxia, probably by increased inotropic effect on the heart.

Alpha-adrenergic activity is important in determining regional distribution of blood flow in hypoxic fetal sheep by selective vasoconstriction. Blood flow to the brain, heart, and adrenals is preserved, with decreased supply to the carcass, lungs, kidneys, and gut. Alpha-adrenergic blockade reverses the hypertension and increases the peripheral resistance observed during fetal hypoxia. These changes are due to a decrease in the resistance in the gut, spleen, lungs, and probably carcass, indicating a participation of the α-adrenergic system in their vasoconstriction (Reuss et al., 1982).

Plasma concentrations of catecholamines, arginine vasopressin, β-endorphin, and atrial natriuretic factor increase during hypoxia in the fetus. The contributions of catecholamines to the circulatory responses to hypoxia were described earlier. Vasopressin contributes to the increase in blood pressure observed during hypoxia by decreasing umbilical and gut blood flows. β-Endorphin and other endogenous opioids also participate in the response to hypoxia. The blockade of its receptors with naloxone further increases the hypertensive response by increasing the vasoconstriction in the kidneys and carcass. During hypoxia, a decrease in the fetal blood volume has been described. Atrial natriuretic factor may play a role in this response. In addition, nitric oxide, prostaglandins, and adenosine have all been implicated in regulation of the fetal circulation during hypoxia.

Most of these results have been obtained from the chronically catheterized fetal sheep model. The relative contributions of these and other mediators to the cardiovascular response to hypoxia in a human fetus continue to be explored, because it is clear that the redistribution of blood flow is a powerful mechanism for protection of fetal organs from damage during periods of oxygen insufficiency.

■ FETAL HEART RATE MONITOR

The FHR monitor is a device with two components: One recognizes and processes heart rate, and the other recognizes uterine contractions (Hon, 1968). To recognize FHR, the device uses the R wave of the fetal electrocardiogram complex or a signal generated by the movement of a cardiovascular structure using ultrasound and the Doppler principle. Uterine contractions are detected either by a catheter inserted transcervically into the amniotic cavity, which contains or is attached to a pressure transducer, or by an external device called a *tocodynamometer*, or tocometer, which is placed on the maternal abdomen and recognizes the tightening of the maternal abdomen during a contraction. Monitoring with devices attached directly to the fetus or placed within the uterine cavity is called "direct," "internal," or "invasive." Devices that do not require direct connection with the fetus are called "noninvasive" or "external."

A critical component of the fetal monitor is the cardiotachometer. An understanding of its mode of action is essential for appreciating FHR variability. Within the monitor is a device for recognizing the cardiac event. Another device measures the interval between the events, and a third device rapidly divides the interval in seconds into 60 to give a rate for each interval between beats. These individual rates are then traced on a strip chart recorder moving at a specific speed. When the paper moves slowly, the recording appears as a jiggly line, representing the variability. If the intervals between heart beats are identical, the line is straight, representing absence of variability or a flat or silent baseline.

Fetal Heart Rate Detection

Fetal Electrode

The internal means of detecting FHR consists of a small stainless steel spiral electrode attached to the fetal scalp. A second contact is bathed by the vaginal fluids. The wires traverse the vaginal canal and are connected to the machine. This mode gives the most accurate FHR tracing because of the discreteness of the signal, so that it accurately depicts beat-to-beat variability.

Doppler Ultrasound Transducer

The Doppler ultrasound transducer consists of a device affixed to the maternal abdominal wall that transmits a high-frequency sound of approximately 2.5 MHz. The signal is reflected from a moving structure (e.g., the ventricle wall), and the reflected beam is changed in frequency, depending on whether the wall moves away from or toward the source. The change in frequency with each systole is recognized as the cardiac event and is processed by the machine.

Although this device is simple to apply and can be used before rupture of membranes, it is sometimes unreliable during labor because of maternal and fetal movements. A greater disadvantage is that it may not give a valid indication of beat-to-beat variability, because the Doppler signal is broad and slurred and the machine is not always able to accurately and consistently select a point on this slurred curve representing the exact time of a cardiac event. Hence, an artificial short-term variability can be portrayed by this device. Long-term variability, however, is usually displayed reasonably accurately.

Improvements in construction and logic have made the Doppler devices more accurate and easier to use. In particular, the technique of autocorrelation can be used to define the timing of the cardiac contraction more accurately by taking a number of points on the "curve" depicting the Doppler frequency shift. Earlier systems selected a threshold or peak of the curve, thereby making small errors in the timing of the contraction, which resulted in the artifactual "variability" noted above.

Sources of Artifact and Error

There are a number of opportunities for misinterpretation of FHR records (Klapholz et al., 1974). These can be due to electrical or signal defects, limitations of the machinery, or errors in interpretation of the records. These errors and their solutions are shown in Table 22-1.

Uterine Activity Detection

Intra-amniotic Catheter

The internal invasive means of detecting uterine activity uses a soft plastic, open-ended, or balloon- or transducer-tipped catheter placed transcervically into the amniotic cavity (Parer, 1997). The catheters transmit pressure changes caused by contractions to a transducer. The pressure changes are translated to an electrical signal displayed and calibrated directly in millimeters of mercury of pressure.

Tocodynamometer

The tocodynamometer, an external device, is strapped to the maternal abdominal wall, generally over the uterine fundus. The tightening of the fundus with each contraction is

TABLE 22-1. TYPES OF ERRORS IN FETAL HEART RATE (FHR) MONITORING AND THEIR SOLUTIONS

Type of Error	Solution
Electrical or Signal Errors	
Faulty electrode material, leg plate, or monitor	Replace defective parts
Intrinsic fetal ECG voltage too low	Use Doppler method Ground the machine
Interference by maternal signal (e.g., movement)	Recognize
Limitations of Machinery	
Halving or doubling (very slow rates may be doubled and very fast rates [>240 beats/min] may be halved by machine)	Auscultation or ultrasound imaging
Short-term variability in Doppler signal resulting from indistinct FHR signal	Realize that short-term variability cannot always be reliably determined with a Doppler method
Interpretive Errors	
Maternal signal being picked up instead of fetal signal	Compare FHR pattern with maternal rate (use maternal pulse oximeter)
Scaling error (using two speeds on some machines, which are capable of 1 and 3 cm/min)	Recognize that FHR pattern changes with recording rate and use one rate all the time, preferably 3 cm/min
Nonrecognition of artifact (e.g., noisy signal)	Recognize
Arrhythmias (tend to be regular) confused with artifact (tend to be irregular)	Record fetal ECG directly

ECG, electrocardiogram.

detected by pressure on a small button in the center of the transducer, and uterine activity is displayed on the recorder. In a sense, it acts just like the hand placed on the abdomen to detect uterine activity. This simple device detects frequency and duration of uterine contractions, but it cannot be calibrated for intensity as in direct pressure measurements. A modification of this device uses a circumferential ring that allows its attachment with a standard tension. This device can be at least partially calibrated.

A potential disadvantage is that the tocodynamometer works best with the mother in the supine position and moving as little as possible. This requirement may not be compatible with maternal comfort, fetal well-being, or progression of labor.

CHARACTERISTICS OF FETAL HEART RATE PATTERNS

Basic Patterns

The characteristics of the FHR pattern are classified as *baseline* or *periodic/episodic* (Hon and Quilligan, 1967; National Institute of Child Health and Human Development [NICHD], 1997). The baseline features—heart rate and variability—are those recorded between uterine contractions. Periodic changes occur in association with uterine contractions, and episodic changes are those not obviously associated with uterine contractions.

Baseline Features

The baseline features of the heart rate are those predominant characteristics that can be recognized between uterine contractions. They are the *baseline rate* and the *variability* of the FHR.

BASELINE RATE

The definition of *baseline* as the rate recorded between contractions is adequate in most clinical settings. However, a rigidly described definition suitable for research programs and computer applications is as follows (NICHD, 1997). Baseline FHR is the approximate mean FHR rounded to 5 beats/min during a 10-minute segment, excluding the following:

1. Periodic or episodic changes
2. Periods of marked FHR variability
3. Segments of the baseline that differ by at least 25 beats/min

In any 10-minute window, the minimum baseline duration must be at least 2 minutes; otherwise, the baseline for that period is indeterminate. In this case, one may need to refer to the previous 10-minute segments to determine the baseline.

The normal baseline FHR is conventionally considered to be between 110 and 160 beats/min. Values below 110 beats/min are termed *bradycardia*; values above 160 beats/min are called *tachycardia*. Baseline bradycardia and tachycardia are quantified by the actual rate observed, in keeping with the above definition of baseline rate.

FETAL HEART RATE VARIABILITY

The FHR monitor tracing in most cases produces an irregular line. These irregularities demonstrate the FHR variability and represent a slight difference in time interval, and therefore in calculated FHR, from beat to beat. If all intervals between heart beats were identical, the line would be regular or smooth.

Baseline FHR variability is defined as fluctuations in the baseline FHR of 2 cycles per minute or greater. These fluctuations are irregular in amplitude and frequency. A pattern called *sinusoidal* differs from variability, in that it has a smooth sine wave of regular frequency and amplitude and is excluded from the definition of FHR variability. The above definition is adequate for clinical visual interpretation, although in fact two characteristics of FHR variability are recognized. First, *short-term variability* is considered to be the beat-to-beat fluctuation in heart rate that arises from the slight difference in the period between R waves of the electrocardiogram in the normal fetus. The second component, *long-term variability*, can be described as either amplitude excursions or frequency of the longer-term unidirectional changes of FHR that occupy a cycle of less than 1 minute. More rigidly stated definitions of variability suitable for research or computer applications are available (NICHD, 1997).

The most commonly accepted quantification of long-term variability in North America is the visually determined approximate amplitude range of the fluctuations in long-term variability. Frequency changes in long-term variability have gained little popularity in clinical practice.

Periodic Heart Rate Patterns

Periodic patterns are the alterations in FHR that are associated with uterine contractions. These are late decelerations, early decelerations, variable decelerations, and accelerations.

LATE DECELERATIONS

Late deceleration of the FHR is a visually apparent gradual decrease (onset of deceleration to nadir of at least 30 seconds) and a return to baseline FHR associated with a uterine contraction. The decrease is calculated from the most recently determined portion of the baseline. It is delayed in timing, with the nadir of the deceleration late in relation to the peak of the contraction. In most cases the onset, nadir, and recovery are all late in relation to the beginning, peak, and ending of the contraction, respectively.

EARLY DECELERATION

Early deceleration of the FHR is a visually apparent gradual decrease (onset of deceleration to nadir of at least 30 seconds) and a return to baseline FHR associated with a uterine contraction. The decrease is calculated from the most recently determined portion of the baseline. It is coincident in timing, with the nadir of the deceleration coincident to the peak of the contraction. In most cases the onset, nadir, and recovery are all coincident to the beginning, peak, and ending of the contraction, respectively.

VARIABLE DECELERATIONS

Variable deceleration is defined as a visually apparent abrupt decrease (onset of deceleration to beginning of nadir less than 30 seconds) in FHR from the baseline. The decrease is calculated from the most recently determined portion of the baseline. The decrease in FHR below the baseline is at least 15 beats/min, lasting (from baseline to baseline) at least 15 seconds and no more than 2 minutes. When variable decelerations are associated with uterine contractions, their onset, depth, and duration commonly vary with successive uterine contractions.

Prolonged deceleration is a visually apparent decrease in FHR below the baseline. The decrease is calculated from the most recently determined portion of the baseline. The decrease from the baseline is at least 15 beats/min and lasts no more than 2 minutes but less than 10 minutes from onset to return to baseline. Prolonged deceleration of at least 10 minutes is a *baseline change*.

ACCELERATIONS

Acceleration is defined as a visually apparent abrupt increase (defined as onset of acceleration to peak in less than 30 seconds) in FHR above the baseline. The increase is calculated from the most recently determined portion of the baseline. The acme is at least 15 beats/min above the baseline, and the acceleration lasts at least 15 seconds and less than 2 minutes from the onset to return to baseline. Before 32 weeks of gestation, accelerations are defined as having an acme of at least 10 beats/min above the baseline and a duration of at least 10 seconds. *Prolonged acceleration* is at least 2 minutes and less than 10 minutes in duration. Acceleration of at least 10 minutes' duration is a *baseline change*.

There is a close association between the presence of accelerations and normal FHR variability. At times it may be difficult to decide on whether a pattern is "acceleration" or a normal long-term variability complex. The final decision is not important, because both accelerations and normal variability have the same positive prognostic significance of normal fetal oxygenation.

QUANTIFICATION

Any deceleration is quantified by the depth of the nadir in beats per minute below the baseline (excluding transient spikes or electronic artifact). The duration is quantified in minutes and seconds from the beginning to the end of the deceleration. Acceleration is quantified similarly. Decelerations are defined as *recurrent* if they occur with more than 50% of uterine contractions in any 20-minute period. Bradycardia and tachycardia are quantified by the actual FHR in beats per minute or by the visually determined range if the FHR is not stable at one rate.

Normal Heart Rate Pattern

The normal FHR pattern (Fig. 22-1) is accepted as that with a predominant baseline heart rate of between 110 and 160 beats/min. The FHR variability amplitude is between 6 and 25 beats/min. No decelerative periodic changes occur, but there may be periodic or episodic accelerations.

It is widely accepted in clinical practice that the fetus born with this normal heart rate pattern is virtually always vigorous and normally oxygenated if delivery occurs when the normal heart rate pattern is traced (Paul et al., 1975; Krebs et al., 1979; Parer, 1997). This, of course, does not hold if there is a subsequent traumatic delivery or if there is a congenital anomaly inconsistent with extrauterine life.

In contrast to this high predictability of fetal normoxia and vigor in the presence of the normal pattern, most variant patterns are not as accurately predictive of fetal compromise. However, when these patterns are placed in the context of the clinical case, the progressive change in the patterns, and the duration of the variant patterns, one can make reasonable judgments about the likelihood of fetal decompensation. With this screening approach, impending intolerable fetal acidosis can be presumed or, in certain cases, ruled out by the use of ancillary techniques, such as the fetal stimulation test, vibroacoustic stimulation, or fetal blood sampling (see Chapter 23).

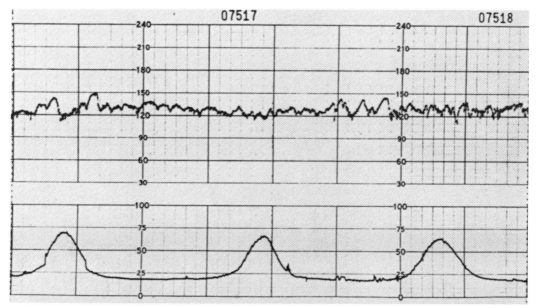

FIGURE 22-1 ■ Normal fetal heart rate pattern with normal rate (approximately 130 beats/min) and normal variability (amplitude range about 15 beats/min) and absence of periodic changes. This pattern represents a nonacidemic fetus without evidence of hypoxic stress. Uterine contractions are 2 to 3 minutes apart and about 60 to 70 mm Hg in intensity.

Variant Fetal Heart Rate Patterns

A number of FHR patterns, although different from the "normal" pattern described, are certainly not "abnormal." Most infants born after displaying these patterns have no evidence of immediate or long-term compromise. These patterns that are not normal are thus called "variant."

Baseline Rate

BRADYCARDIA

The initial response of the normal fetus to acute hypoxia or acidosis is bradycardia (Court and Parer, 1984). This statement is in contrast to some earlier beliefs whereby under acutely operated or anesthetized conditions, a fetal tachycardia was sometimes noted in response to acutely imposed hypoxia. Tachycardia has also been reported in experimental animals with very mild hypoxia, but clinically and experimentally the initial statement regarding bradycardia holds in most cases, because initially the vagal nerve activity is greater than the sympathetic activity.

A number of causes of bradycardia other than hypoxia and acidosis include the bradyarrhythmias (e.g., complete heart block), certain drugs (e.g., β-adrenergic blockers or "-caine" drugs), and hypothermia. Other fetuses have a heart rate below 110 beats/min but are otherwise totally normal and simply represent a normal variation outside our arbitrarily set limits of normal heart rate.

Bradycardia is arbitrarily distinguished from a deceleration, which is transient. As defined earlier, a bradycardia is considered to represent a decrease in heart rate below 110 beats/min for 10 minutes or longer. Prolonged deceleration or bradycardia is considered to represent a prolonged stepwise decrease in fetal oxygenation (Fig. 22-2). This may be a consequence of fetal hypoxia resulting from vagal activity (and later hypoxic myocardial depression), or the bradycardia may eventually result in fetal hypoxia because of the inability of the fetus to maintain a compensatory increase in stroke volume. As noted earlier, the hypoxic fetus has a certain ability to increase stroke volume in response to bradycardia, but this breaks down at severe decreases in heart rate, probably below 60 beats/min. Under these conditions, fetal cardiac output cannot be maintained, and therefore umbilical blood flow decreases. This results in insufficient oxygen transport from the fetal placenta to the fetal body and may result in eventual fetal hypoxic decompensation.

Reasons for the decreased heart rate include the following:

1. A stepwise drop in oxygenation, such as occurs with maternal apnea or amniotic fluid embolus
2. A decrease in umbilical blood flow, such as occurs with a prolapsed cord
3. A decrease in uterine blood flow, such as occurs with severe maternal hypotension

Specific bradycardias are reviewed later in this chapter.

TACHYCARDIA

Defined as a baseline of more than 160 beats/min, tachycardia is arbitrarily distinguished from an acceleration, or prolonged acceleration, in that its duration is at least 10 minutes. Tachycardia is seen in some cases of fetal hypoxia but virtually never alone during labor; that is, in the presence of normal FHR variability and absent periodic changes, tachycardia must be assumed to be a result of some other cause besides hypoxia. Tachycardia is sometimes seen on recovery from hypoxia or acidosis and probably represents catecholamine activity after sympathetic nervous or adrenal medullary activity in response to this stress and withdrawal of vagal activity when the hypoxia is relieved.

There are a number of nonhypoxic causes of tachycardia. The most common of these is maternal or fetal infection, especially chorioamnionitis. Some drugs cause tachycardia (e.g., β-mimetic agents and parasympathetic blockers such as atropine). Tachyarrhythmias occasionally occur, and at severe elevations of rate (greater than 240 beats/min) these may cause fetal cardiac failure with subsequent hydrops.

Baseline Variability

As noted earlier, in research and mathematical terms, normal FHR variability has two components: short-term and long-term variability. Usually, both are present and the baseline has a jagged appearance, with unpredictable movements of heart rate up or down. Clinically, no distinction is made between short-

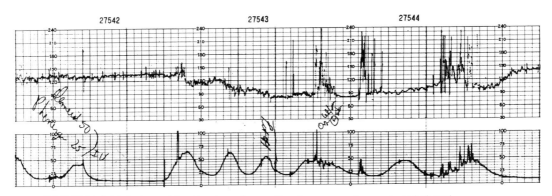

FIGURE 22-2 ■ Prolonged fetal bradycardia resulting from excessive oxytocin-induced hyperstimulation of the uterus after intravenous infusion of meperidine (Demerol) and promethazine (Phenergan) into the same tubing. The heart rate is returning to normal at the end of the tracing, after appropriate treatment (signified by the notes "Pit off," "O₂ 6L/min," and "side"). Note that fetal heart rate variability was maintained throughout this asphyxial stress, signifying adequate central oxygenation.

term and long-term variability, because in actual practice they are determined as a unit. Therefore, the definition of variability is based visually on the amplitude of the complexes, with the exclusion of the regular smooth sinusoidal pattern.

There is no consensus whether beat-to-beat variability alone is interpretable to the unaided eye, but quantification is possible with a number of computer techniques. Computer programs have also been used to quantify the amplitude range and frequency of the long-term complexes.

There are four basic classes of heart rate variability, visually quantified as the amplitude of the peak-to-trough (beats/min) as follows:

1. Amplitude range, undetectable: absent FHR variability
2. Amplitude range, greater than undetectable at no more than 5 beats/min: minimal FHR variability
3. Amplitude range, 6 to 25 beats/min: moderate FHR variability
4. Amplitude range, greater than 25 beats/min: marked FHR variability.

The source of FHR variability is complex, with inputs from many cycling physiologic phenomena, including respiratory arrhythmia, blood pressure fluctuations, and thermoregulation, at least in the adult. However, many of the observations are most consistent with the theory that the presence of normal variability requires integrity of the pathways responsible for the production and transmission of variability in the cerebral cortex, the mid-brain, the vagus nerve, and the cardiac conduction system (Parer, 1997).

Different fetuses have an intrinsic "quantity" of variability, and this can change with differences in fetal state (Nijhuis et al., 1982). The components used to describe fetal state can be altered by hypoxia or hypercapnia and by short periods of decreased uterine blood flow. Again, the presence of certain state variables can affect others; for example, during fetal breathing movements there is a respiratory arrhythmia, and during prelabor myometrial activity there is a change to the quiescent state in fetal sheep. One must be aware of such activities to make the appropriate distinction between hypoxic and nonhypoxic causes of decreased variability.

As described earlier, FHR variability was ascribed in the past to an interaction between two branches of the autonomic nervous system—parasympathetic and β-adrenergic—with different time constants. Because variability is primarily transmitted via the parasympathetic nerves in primates, this theory

is unlikely to be true in humans. Variability is more likely due to numerous sporadic inputs from various areas of the cerebral cortex and lower centers to the cardiac integratory centers in the medulla oblongata, which are then transmitted down the vagus nerve. Current theory suggests that these inputs decrease in the presence of cerebral hypoxia and acidosis and that variability thus decreases after failure of the fetal hemodynamic compensatory mechanisms to maintain cerebral oxygenation.

The key aspect of these clinical correlates is that if the FHR variability is normal, regardless of what other FHR patterns may be present, the fetus is not suffering cerebral tissue acidemia because it has been able to successfully centralize the available oxygen and is thus physiologically compensated. If excessive hypoxic stress is present, however, as evidenced by severe periodic changes or substantial prolonged bradycardia, this compensation may break down and the fetus may have progressive hypoxia in cerebral and myocardial tissues. In this case, it is theorized that FHR variability decreases and eventually is lost.

There are several possible nonhypoxic causes of decreased or absent FHR variability:

1. Absence of the cortex (anencephaly)
2. Narcotized or drugged higher centers (e.g., by morphine, meperidine, diazepam, magnesium sulfate) (Fig. 22-3)
3. Vagal blockade (e.g., by atropine or scopolamine)
4. Defective cardiac conduction system (e.g., complete heart block) (Fig. 22-4)

The essence of the art of intrapartum FHR interpretation is to note a decrease or disappearance of FHR variability in the presence of patterns that suggest hypoxia or acidemia. Fortunately, most fetuses in the beginning of labor have normal FHR variability, so changes can be followed. The ability of the human eye to quantify FHR variability clinically appears to be equal to the technology of a computer program (Knopf et al., 1992).

Fetal heart tracings that display unexplained virtual absence of FHR variability and no periodic changes occur in several settings:

1. Quiet fetal sleep state
2. Idiopathic reduced FHR variability, with no obvious explanation, but no evidence of hypoxia or compromised central nervous system
3. Centrally acting drugs
4. Congenital neurologic abnormality, as a result of a developmental central nervous system defect, or acquired from an

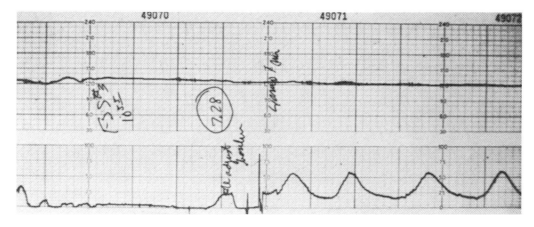

FIGURE 22-3 ■ No variability of fetal heart rate. The patient had severe preeclampsia and was receiving magnesium sulfate and narcotics. The normal scalp blood pH (7.28) ensures that the absence of variability is nonasphyxic in origin and that the fetus is not chronically asphyxiated and decompensating. The uterine activity channel has an inaccurate trace in the first half.

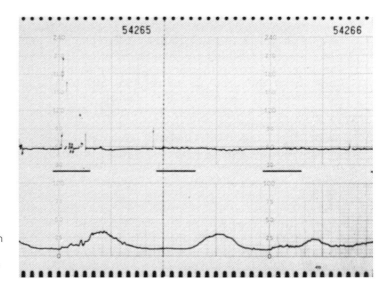

FIGURE 22-4 ■ Unremitting fetal bradycardia. This does not signify asphyxia, because this fetus had complete heart block, with a ventricular rate of about 55 beats/min. Note the absence of fetal heart rate variability. There were serious cardiac structural defects, and the fetus died shortly after birth.

in utero infection or hypoxic event (Nijhuis et al., 1990; Phelan and Ahn, 1994; Schifrin et al., 1994)

5. Profound acidemia with inability of the heart to manifest periodic changes

Clinical observations also suggest that some severely growth-restricted fetuses may have reduced or even absent FHR variability, even in the absence of obvious hypoxia. The mechanism of this depressed variability is not known. If the FHR variability is reduced or absent on initial placement of the monitor, the ability to determine whether progressive acidemia is present becomes difficult, or even impossible, without ancillary testing. Delivery is sometimes expedited to give the fetus the benefit of uncertainty, although there is no consensus that this is the correct approach.

Periodic Changes in Fetal Heart Rate

LATE AND EARLY DECELERATIONS

Late and early decelerations, already defined earlier, have the following characteristics (Hon and Quilligan, 1967) (Fig. 22-5):

1. They are smooth and rounded in configuration and are the mirror image of the contraction.
2. They are persistent, often occurring with each contraction.
3. Their onset, nadir, and recovery are generally delayed 10 to 30 seconds after the onset, apex, and resolution of the contraction.
4. The depth of the dip is related to the intensity of the contraction.

Late decelerations are of two varieties: *reflex* and *nonreflex* (Martin et al., 1979; Parer et al., 1980; Harris et al., 1982; Parer, 1997).

REFLEX LATE DECELERATION. Reflex late deceleration is sometimes seen when an acute insult (e.g., reduced uterine blood flow resulting from maternal hypotension) is superimposed on a previously normally oxygenated fetus in the presence of contractions. These late decelerations are caused by a decrease in uterine blood flow (with the uterine contraction) beyond the capacity of the fetus to extract sufficient oxygen. The relatively deoxygenated blood is carried from the fetal placenta through the umbilical vein to the heart and is distributed to the aorta, neck vessels, and head. Here, the low oxygen

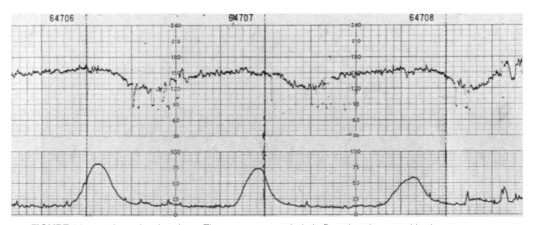

FIGURE 22-5 ■ Late decelerations. These were recorded via Doppler ultrasound in the antepartum period in a severely growth-restricted (1700-g) term infant born to a 32-year-old preeclamptic primipara. Delivery was by cesarean section because neither a direct fetal electrocardiogram nor fetal blood sample could be obtained because of a firm closed posterior cervix. The infant subsequently did well.

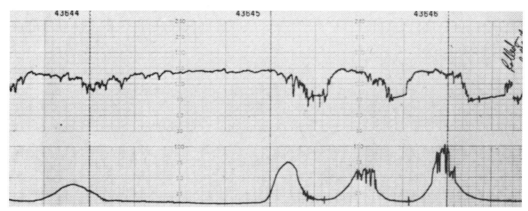

FIGURE 22-6 ■ Reflex late decelerations. The fetal heart rate pattern was previously normal, but late decelerations appeared after severe maternal hypotension (70/30 mm Hg) after sympathetic blockade caused by a caudal anesthetic agent.

tension is sensed by chemoreceptors, and neuronal activity results in a vagal discharge, which causes the transient deceleration. The deceleration is presumed to be "late" because of the circulation time from the fetal placental site to the chemoreceptors and because the progressively decreasing partial pressure of oxygen must reach a certain threshold before vagal activity occurs. There may also be baroreceptor activity causing the vagal discharge (Martin et al., 1979). Between contractions, oxygen delivery is adequate and there is no additional vagal activity, so the baseline heart rate is normal.

These late decelerations are accompanied by normal FHR variability and thus signify normal central nervous system integrity (i.e., the fetus is physiologically "compensated" in the vital organs) (Fig. 22-6). The periodic change, historically called "early deceleration," appears to simply be a variant of the reflex late deceleration (Fig. 22-7). It is not clear why the deceleration is not late, but early decelerations have been noted to evolve into late decelerations.

NONREFLEX LATE DECELERATION. The second type is a result of the same initial mechanism, except that the deoxygenated bolus of blood from the placenta is presumed to be insufficient to support myocardial action. Thus, for the period of the contraction, there is direct myocardial hypoxic depres-

sion (or failure) and vagal activity (Martin et al. 1979; Harris et al., 1982). This variety is seen without variability (Fig. 22-8), signifying fetal "decompensation" (i.e., inadequate fetal cerebral and myocardial oxygenation). It is seen most commonly in states of decreased placental reserve, for example, with preeclampsia or intrauterine growth restriction or after prolonged hypoxic stress, such as a long period of severe reflex late decelerations. The distinguishing feature between reflex and nonreflex late decelerations is therefore the presence of FHR variability in the former. Each category can be subdivided into two groups based on pH, with reflex late deceleration in the normal range of pH (Paul et al., 1975).

Further support for the two etiologic mechanisms of late decelerations comes from observations on chronically catheterized fetal monkeys in spontaneous labor during the course of intrauterine death (Murata et al., 1982). The animals were initially observed with normal blood gases, normal FHR variability, presence of accelerations, and no persistent periodic changes. After a variable period of time, they first demonstrated late decelerations and retained accelerations. This period was associated with a small decline in ascending aortic partial pressure of oxygen, from 28 to 24 mm Hg, and a normal acid-base state. These late decelerations were probably of the

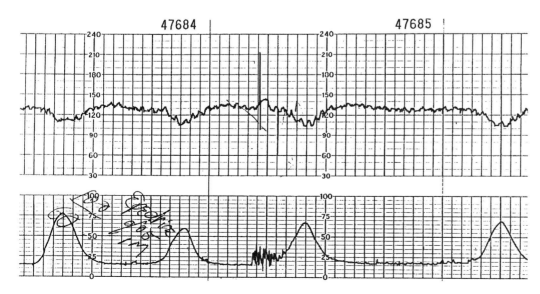

FIGURE 22-7 ■ Early decelerations.

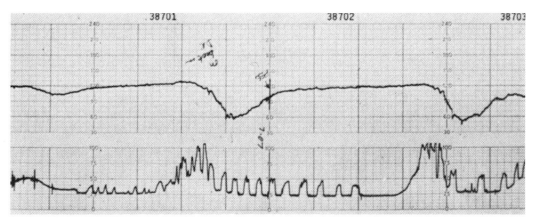

FIGURE 22-8 ■ Nonreflex late decelerations with virtual absence of fetal heart rate (FHR) variability. The decelerations represent transient asphyxic myocardial failure as well as intermittent vagal decreases in heart rate. The lack of FHR variability also signifies decreased cerebral oxygenation. Note the acidemia in fetal scalp blood (7.07). The infant, a 3340-g girl with Apgar scores of 3 (1 minute) and 4 (5 minutes), was delivered soon after this tracing. Cesarean section was considered to be contraindicated because of a severe preeclamptic coagulopathy.

vagal reflex type caused by chemoreceptor activity. At an average of more than 3 days after the onset of these reflex decelerations, accelerations were lost in the presence of worsening hypoxia (partial pressure of oxygen, 19 mm Hg) and acidemia (7.22). Fetal death followed an average of 36 hours of persistent late decelerations, and these latter decelerations without accelerations were presumed to be of the nonreflex myocardial depression type.

Severe late decelerations are those with a drop of more than 45 beats/min below the baseline. They may be seen with reflex or nonreflex late decelerations (Kubli et al., 1969). *Mild late decelerations* are those with a drop in heart rate of less than 15 beats/min, and moderate later decelerations are those with a drop in heart rate of greater than 15 and less than 45 beats/min below the baseline. The degree of academia is related to the severity of the decelerations when there is reduced FHR variability.

When late decelerations are present, one should make efforts to eliminate them by optimizing placental blood flow and maternal hyperoxia. Vagal late decelerations, which in most cases are a result of an acute hypoxemic episode, can generally be abolished. If not, the fetus may accumulate an oxygen debt, although usually not before 30 minutes in a normally grown fetus who was previously normoxic. Late decelerations caused by myocardial failure, however, usually are seen when placental reserve is surpassed and the intermittent decreases in uterine blood flow with each contraction can no longer be tolerated (Fig. 22-9). The abolition of such late decelerations is less likely.

VARIABLE DECELERATIONS

Variable decelerations, defined previously in the chapter (Fig. 22-10), have the following characteristics:

1. The appearance of the dip is variable in duration, depth, and shape from contraction to contraction.
2. They are usually abrupt in onset and cessation, sometimes falling 60 beats/min in one or several beats. They are thus neurogenic (vagal) in origin.
3. They are described as *severe* when the decelerations are less than 70 beats/min for more than 60 seconds. *Moderate* variable decelerations are defined as an FHR between 70 and 80

for greater than 60 seconds, or an FHR less than 70 beats/min for 30 to 60 seconds. All others are defined as *mild* (Kubli et al., 1969).

Decelerations more than 60 beats/min below the baseline heart rate have also been called severe, but this is not so clearly accepted, presumably because it may still be within the ability of the Frank-Starling mechanism to compensate.

These abrupt decelerations in heart rate represent the firing of the vagus nerve in response to certain stimuli such as umbilical cord compression in the first stage of labor or substantial head compression during pushing in the second stage of labor (Ingemarsson et al., 1980; Ball and Parer, 1992). Whether the fetus is still normoxic in the central tissues (i.e., physiologically compensated) can be determined by observations of the maintenance of FHR variability.

The clinical significance of variable decelerations is that they indicate a reduction of umbilical blood flow. It is obvious why this is so if they are caused by compression of the umbilical cord. If they are caused by intense vagal activity, the associated decrease in umbilical blood flow results from a drop in fetal cardiac output because of the relative inability of the fetus to maintain cardiac output at very low heart rates (e.g., less than 60 beats/min; see earlier).

When severe variable decelerations are present, efforts should be made to abolish them because it is likely that even the normally grown fetus with normal placental function eventually will decompensate, although usually not before 30 minutes. The normal fetus, however, can better tolerate mild or moderate variable decelerations for a prolonged period.

The theory that variable decelerations are caused by cord compression has given rise to the technique of *amnioinfusion* (Miyazaki and Nevarez, 1985). In this straightforward technique, sterile crystalloid is infused into the amniotic cavity through an intrauterine catheter, with an initial bolus of 250 to 1000 mL and a maintenance rate of about 2 to 3 mL/min. This technique results in a lowered incidence of severe variable decelerations and may allow a vaginal delivery instead of a cesarean section for presumed fetal acidemia (Strong et al., 1990). It also decreases the incidence of meconium aspiration when the meconium is thick, probably secondary to decreasing

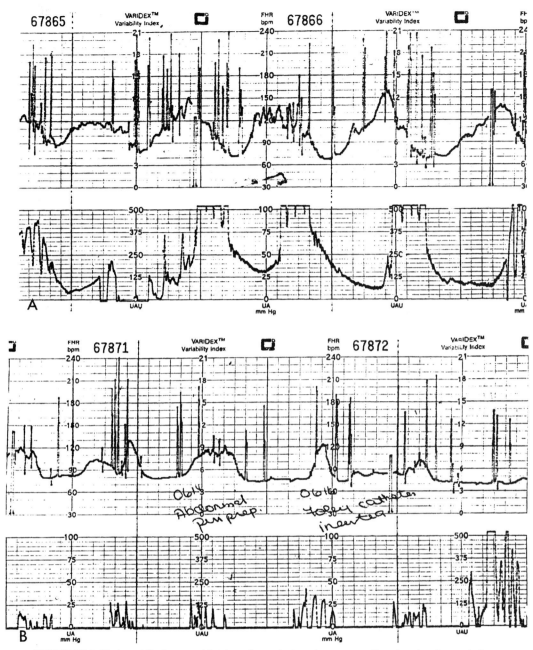

FIGURE 22-9 ■ **A** and **B**, A case of fetal cardiorespiratory decompensation showing the evolution of the smooth baseline over 30 minutes. In this case the asphyxial stress is manifested as late decelerations. Death occurred *in utero* 30 minutes later.

cord compression and fetal hypoxia (Spong et al., 1994). It does not appear to be as effective in the second stage of labor, consistent with the theory that second stage variable decelerations are due to head, not cord, compression.

ACCELERATIONS WITH CONTRACTIONS

Accelerations sometimes occur with uterine contractions and have no adverse prognostic significance. They are probably similar to the accelerations that are seen with fetal movement in the antepartum period and thus are indicative of a reactive and healthy fetus. Accelerations with contractions probably represent the net result of greater sympathetic activity than parasympathetic activity during contractions in the case of a particular fetus. "Shoulders" and the "overshoot pattern" probably represent a combination of sympathetic and vagal activity, with the sympathetic being predominant when the shoulders or overshoot occur. There is no sound evidence that they have any prognostic significance, and if they are seen in the absence of FHR variability, their presence is subservient to this observation.

Influence of *In Utero* Treatment

Fetal oxygenation can be improved, acidemia relieved, and variant FHR patterns abolished by certain modes of treatment. The events that result in fetal stress (recognized by FHR patterns) are presented in Table 22-2 together with the

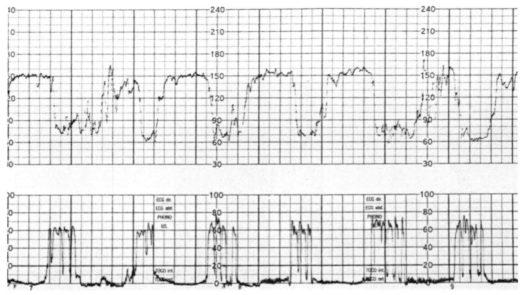

FIGURE 22-10 ■ Variable decelerations. Intrapartum recording using fetal scalp electrode and tocodynamometer. The spikes in the uterine activity channel represent maternal pushing efforts in the second stage of labor. The normal baseline variability between contractions signifies normal central oxygenation despite the intermittent hypoxic stress represented by the moderate variable decelerations.

recommended treatment maneuvers and presumed mechanisms for improving fetal oxygenation. These should be the primary maneuvers carried out; if the hypoxic event is acute and the fetus was previously normoxic, there is an excellent chance that the undesired FHR pattern will be abolished. Should late decelerations occur in such cases, they are likely to be the reflex type rather than a result of myocardial failure.

During labor, an FHR pattern with decreasing variability resulting from acidemia is virtually always preceded by a heart rate pattern signifying hypoxic stress, such as late decelerations, variable decelerations (usually severe), or a substantial prolonged bradycardia. However, in the antepartum period, before the onset of uterine contractions, this does not necessarily hold; decreasing or absent variability may develop

TABLE 22-2. INTRAUTERINE TREATMENT FOR VARIANT FETAL HEART RATE (FHR) PATTERNS

Causes	Possible Resulting FHR Patterns	Corrective Maneuver	Mechanism
Hypotension (e.g., supine hypotension, conduction anesthesia)	Bradycardia, late decelerations	Intravenous fluids, position change ephedrine	Return of uterine blood flow toward normal
Excessive uterine activity	Bradycardia, late decelerations	Decrease in oxytocin, lateral position	Same as above
Transient umbilical cord compression	Variable decelerations	Change in maternal position (e.g., left or right lateral, Trendelenburg) Amnioinfusion	Presumably removes fetal part from cord "Pads" the cord, protecting it from compression
Head compression, usually second stage	Variable decelerations	Push only with alternate contractions	Allows fetal respite
Decreased uterine blood flow associated with uterine contraction below limits of fetal oxygen needs	Late decelerations	Change in maternal position (e.g., left lateral or Trendelenburg) establishment of maternal hyperoxia	Enhancement of uterine blood flow toward optimum: increase in maternal–fetal oxygen gradient
		Tocolytic agents (e.g., ritodrine or terbutaline)	Decrease in contractions or uterine tonus, thus abolishing associated decrease in uterine blood flow
Prolonged asphyxia	Decreasing FHR variability*	Change in maternal position (e.g., left lateral or Trendelenburg) establishment of maternal hyperoxia	Enhancement of uterine blood flow to optimum; increase in maternal–fetal oxygen gradient

*During labor, this is virtually always preceded by a heart rate pattern signifying asphyxial stress (e.g., late decelerations, usually severe), severe variable decelerations, or a prolonged bradycardia. This is not necessarily so in the antepartum period, before the onset of uterine contractions.

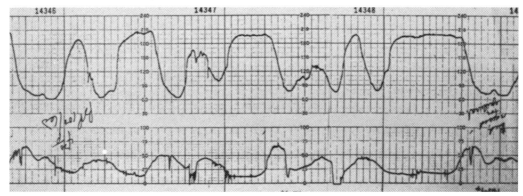

FIGURE 22-11 ■ Sinister heart rate pattern in a 28-week fetus (gestational age determined after delivery) with baseline tachycardia, absence of heart rate variability, and severe periodic changes. The scalp blood pH was 7.0, and the fetus died shortly after this tracing. Cesarean section was not performed because the fetus was believed to be previable, although in fact it weighed 1100 g. There is much artifact in the uterine activity channel.

without periodic or baseline FHR changes. In addition, the usual evolution from normal to decreased or absent variability sometimes occurs with relatively minor decelerations in cases of chorioamnionitis and dysmaturity.

If the FHR patterns cannot be improved (i.e., if the stress patterns indicative of peripheral tissue or central tissue hypoxia persist for a significant period), further diagnostic steps or delivery may be indicated. Certain patterns are of such a severe character that immediate delivery without ancillary testing, such as fetal scalp sampling, is warranted if they cannot rapidly be relieved. These patterns include those with undetectable variability and severe uncorrectable late or variable decelerations (Fig. 22-11) or those with a prolonged bradycardia below 60 beats/min with a smooth baseline. Such fetuses are either already acidemic or are likely to soon become so.

Other Patterns

A number of patterns do not easily fit into the category of basic patterns. They are less common, and their significance is generally more controversial.

Bradycardias

As noted previously, bradycardia is defined as a baseline heart rate below 110 beats/min in a 10-minute window. This is to distinguish it from *deceleration*, which refers to a decrease in FHR below 110 beats/min for less than 10 minutes. These criteria are necessarily somewhat arbitrary and have been developed primarily for communication, rather than based strictly on a physiologic foundation.

There are a number of clearly nonhypoxic causes of a persistent FHR below 110 beats/min (e.g., heart block, hypothermia). A number of labels have been placed on various bradycardias, reflecting their appearance, occurrence, or presumed etiology, for example, prolonged bradycardia, prolonged end-stage bradycardia, and postparacervical block bradycardia.

PROLONGED BRADYCARDIA (PROLONGED DECELERATION)

Moderate bradycardia, not below 100 beats/min, may represent continuous head compression and therefore vagal activity. The reason for the vagal response to head compression is uncertain, but the cause may be cerebral ischemia (Hon and Quilligan, 1967) or stimulation of the dura. If FHR variability is maintained, prolonged moderate bradycardia is not associated with fetal depression. Some fetuses with moderate bradycardia may simply have rates below the arbitrary level of 110 beats/min.

Prolonged deceleration or bradycardia generally refers to a sudden drop from a normal FHR to values below 110 beats/min, especially below 80 beats/min. As mentioned previously, bradycardia is the initial response of the fetus to acute hypoxia. It is probably a vagal response to peripheral or central chemoreceptor activity. The hypoxic stimulus may be caused by the following:

1. A decrease in maternal oxygen tension, such as during the apnea of a seizure
2. A decrease in uterine blood flow, such as during excessive uterine contractions or acute maternal hypotension
3. A decrease in umbilical blood flow, such as by cord compression (Fig. 22-12)
4. Loss of placental area, such as in abruptio placentae

The extent of the bradycardia depends on the degree of fetal hypoxia. There may also be a baroreceptor influence causing the bradycardia with prolongation of hypoxia. In rare cases, a prolonged bradycardia is the result of fetal hemorrhage, sometimes catastrophic, such as tearing of vasa previa or rupture of an anomalous fetal placental vessel. In such cases, the fetus may be born not only acidemia but in hemorrhagic shock.

Immediately on recognition of a bradycardia, the physician should attempt to optimize fetal oxygenation by maintaining maternal blood pressure and avoiding excessive uterine activity, position change, hydration, and (possibly) maternal hyperoxia (see Table 22-2). There is no need for grave concern if moderate bradycardia is not abolished. However, if the heart rate is below 100 beats/min, efforts should be made to alleviate it, even in the presence of good FHR variability. An acute drop in heart rate to below 60 beats/min usually results in fetal hypoxia and eventual decompensation, and it becomes an obstetric emergency to abolish it or deliver the baby before severe central acidemia occurs.

Fortunately, most sudden bradycardias resolve spontaneously or with various positional changes. However, they are of sufficient concern that many women whose infants exhibit several prolonged bradycardic episodes are brought to the

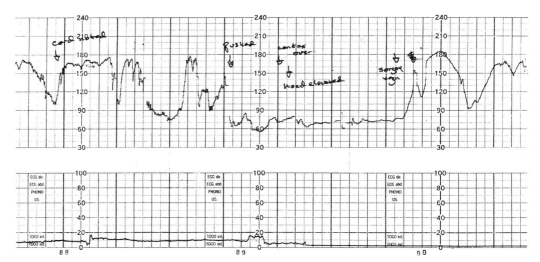

FIGURE 22-12 ■ Bradycardia resulting from cord prolapse. The infant was delivered by cesarean section and did well.

delivery room for labor, in case the FHR does not recover after one of them. On rare occasions the bradycardia does not resolve, and the infants may be deeply depressed because of acidemia. Such cases are seen more commonly in postdate pregnancies and, fortunately, are rare. The etiology of the bradycardia is not always apparent, and some have ascribed it to excessive vagal activity.

PROLONGED END-STAGE BRADYCARDIA

This term refers to a prolonged deceleration, most often in the second stage of labor, in the presence of an otherwise normal FHR tracing (Herbert and Boehm, 1981). This pattern is not uncommon and is seen more frequently if one adopts the practice of monitoring in the delivery room and continuing to monitor FHR until the time of delivery.

Prolonged end-stage bradycardia is likely to be a vagal response to head compression as the head traverses the depths of the pelvis. Compression may cause a decrease in cerebral blood flow and brief local ischemia, which could produce a vagal response. Alternatively, the vagal discharge may be caused by compression of the dura.

In the past, this pattern was usually managed by rapid termination of labor, either by forceps or by encouragement of the mother to push. As with the spontaneous prolonged bradycardias, however, the results of expectant management have not been well tested. Position change (which is somewhat limited in the second stage) and discouragement from pushing sometimes appear to result in resolution of prolonged bradycardia. Elevation of the fetal head may also be efficacious, but studies purporting to demonstrate the benefit of the maneuver suffer from the defect of having no equivalent untreated group.

The current recommendation is that if the bradycardia is persistent and FHR variability decreases, delivery should ensue as rapidly as possible. If variability is retained, efforts should be made to abolish the bradycardia or effect a spontaneous delivery. It is unusual for this pattern to lead to absence of FHR variability and fetal decompensation in less than 10 minutes as long as the FHR is above 60 beats/min.

POSTPARACERVICAL BLOCK BRADYCARDIA

The use of a paracervical block for labor has decreased concomitantly with the increased availability of epidural anesthesia for relief in labor; however, it is still used and thus is reviewed.

Bradycardia related to the placement of a paracervical block typically occurs 7 minutes after the block is administered and lasts 8 minutes. These time relationships, the degree of bradycardia, and the associated FHR abnormalities are all variable. The incidence of bradycardia varies from 0 to 56%, depending on drug, dosage, and definition; an average incidence is 15%. Fetal death has rarely been associated with paracervical block bradycardia (Ralston and Shnider, 1978).

Although the cause of bradycardia is controversial, the most likely is a direct fetal toxic reaction to the local anesthetic drug, not necessarily because of direct fetal injection but because of rapid uptake of the drug by the fetus, possibly via the uterine arteries. Fetal levels of such a drug can be quite high, although rarely higher than those of the mother. Another theory is that the local anesthetic agent causes spasm of the uterine arteries, resulting in decreased uterine blood flow and, hence, fetal hypoxia. Acidemia has been demonstrated by blood sampling in affected fetuses during episodes of bradycardia (Ralston and Shnider, 1978).

This undesirable side effect of a paracervical block can be decreased if minimal quantities of drugs are used. Careful technique to ensure that the drug is placed just submucosally avoids inadvertent fetal injection. Paracervical block is contraindicated if the fetus already has an abnormal heart rate pattern. If bradycardia does develop, supportive management (i.e., position change and maternal hyperoxia) is recommended until it resolves. If the pattern does resolve and the FHR returns to normal, no further evaluation is needed; however, subsequent paracervical injection should be avoided. Except in rare and profoundly abnormal cases, delivery should be avoided during the bradycardia because the fetus can eliminate the drug transplacentally more easily than detoxifying it postnatally.

Arrhythmias

A complete discussion of fetal arrhythmias is presented in Chapter 26.

Numerous fetal dysrhythmias have been observed *in utero*. These include complete heart block, premature atrial contractions, premature ventricular contractions, bigeminy, supraventricular tachycardia, paroxysmal atrial tachycardia, blocked atrial premature beats, atrial flutter, and asystole of variable duration. The FHR monitor detects and depicts the interval between beats and is thus a very sensitive dysrhythmia detector. Bradyarrhythmias are the most commonly reported. Complete heart block appears as an FHR of approximately 50 to 60 beats/min, with virtually absent FHR variability.

Bradycardias and tachycardias may be doubled or halved by the cardiotachometer, particularly in the Doppler mode. This artifact can almost always be ruled out by brief auscultation or ultrasound imaging. Dysrhythmias generally represent cardiac conduction defects that have an anatomic or functional basis. The persistent types appear to carry a worse prognosis than the intermittent ones, the latter often resolving in the newborn. An infant with heart block may have a mother with collagen-vascular disease, particularly systemic lupus erythematosus; such women should be screened appropriately (see Chapter 54).

Extreme tachycardia above 240 beats/min has sometimes been associated with hydrops, apparently because of intrauterine cardiac failure. Reports of *in utero* treatment with digoxin, β-adrenergic blocking agents, procainamide, or calcium channel blockers describe some success for *in utero* pharmacologic treatment (see Chapter 26).

In the past, much concern was experienced over the fetus with a dysrhythmia. It has become obvious that only rarely are early interventions required, and most of these infants can tolerate labor well. The most common dysrhythmia, intermittent premature beats, need no particular workup besides a routine sonogram. Echocardiography may be helpful in diagnosis and in determining whether there are any obvious structural abnormalities before birth in persistent dysrhythmia.

The major problem in the fetus with a persistent severe dysrhythmia generally appears in the newborn period. For such infants, delivery should be in a tertiary care center with immediate access to pediatric cardiology care. Infants with heart block may need cardiac pacing, and those with tachycardia may need drug therapy to prevent cardiac failure.

Sinusoidal Pattern

The sinusoidal pattern is a regular smooth sine wave–like baseline, with a frequency of approximately 3 to 6 cycles per minute and an amplitude range of up to 30 beats/min. The regularity of the waves distinguishes this pattern from long-term variability complexes, which are crudely shaped and irregular. Another distinguishing feature is the absence of beat-to-beat or short-term variability (Fig. 22-13).

The sinusoidal pattern was first described in a group of severely affected Rh-alloimmunized fetuses but has subsequently been noted in association with fetuses that are anemic for other reasons and in severely depressed infants. It has also been described in cases of normal infants born without depression or acid-base abnormalities, although in these cases there is dispute about whether the patterns are truly sinusoidal or whether, because of the moderately irregular pattern, they are variants of long-term variability. Such patterns, often called *pseudosinusoidal*, may also be seen after administration of narcotics to the mother. It is believed that an essential characteristic of the sinusoidal pattern is extreme regularity and smoothness.

Murata and colleagues (1985) implicated arginine vasopressin in the sinusoidal pattern. Sinusoidal FHR patterns and increased arginine vasopressin blood levels were produced in fetal lambs by hemorrhage and by arginine vasopressin infusion into vagotomized or atropinized fetuses. These authors proposed that the direct effect of arginine vasopressin on the sinus node may have affected calcium transfer, resulting in the pattern.

The presence of a sinusoidal pattern or variant of this in an Rh-sensitized patient usually suggests anemia with a fetal hematocrit value below 30%. The presence of hydrops in such a fetus suggests a fetal hematocrit of 15% or lower. Many severely anemic Rh-affected fetuses do not have a sinusoidal pattern but rather have a rounded blunted pattern, and accelerations are usually absent.

If a sinusoidal pattern is seen in an Rh-sensitized patient and severe hemolysis is confirmed (e.g., by peak systolic

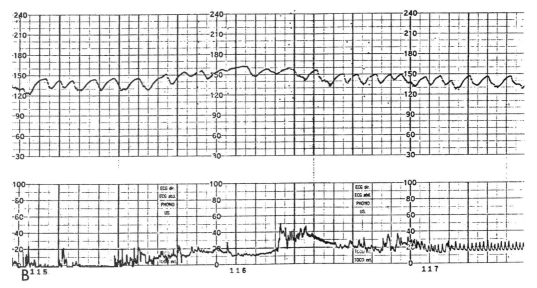

FIGURE 22-13 ■ Sinusoidal pattern in a term fetus with severe hemolysis caused by Rh disease. Cord hematocrit was 20%, and the infant, delivered by cesarean section, was subsequently normal. Recording by direct fetal electrode.

velocity measurement of flow in the middle cerebral artery of the fetus, cordocentesis, or the Δ optical density at 450 mμ determination by spectrophotometry of amniotic fluid), rapid intervention is needed. This step may take the form of delivery or intrauterine transfusion, depending on gestational age and the fetal status (see Chapter 30).

Management of a sinusoidal pattern in the absence of alloimmunization is somewhat more difficult to recommend. If the pattern is persistent, monotonously regular, and unaccompanied by short-term variability and cannot be abolished by the maneuvers just described, further workup and evaluation of adequacy of fetal oxygenation (e.g., contraction stress test, fetal stimulation test, biophysical profile, or fetal blood sampling) are indicated. Nonalloimmune sinusoidal patterns have been associated with severe fetal acidemia and with fetal anemia resulting from fetal-maternal bleeding. The latter diagnosis is supported by identification of fetal red blood cells in maternal blood, detected by the Kleihauer-Betke test. The presence of sinusoidal patterns in cases of fetal–maternal bleeding and the less striking blunted variant in alloimmunized infants have given rise to the view that an acute, rather than a gradual, onset of anemia seen in alloimmunization is required to produce a true sinusoidal pattern. As yet, there is little evidence for this theory; however, it is consistent with the hormonal causation of the pattern described above.

If the pattern is irregularly sinusoidal or pseudosinusoidal, intermittently present, and not associated with intervening periodic decelerations, fetal compromise is unlikely. Hence, immediate delivery is not warranted. The aforementioned ancillary tests may assist in confirming normality in such cases.

Saltatory Pattern

The saltatory pattern consists of rapid variations in FHR with a frequency of 3 to 6 cycles per minute and an amplitude range greater than 25 beats/min (Fig. 22-14). It is qualitatively described as marked variability, and the variations have a strikingly bizarre appearance.

The saltatory pattern was associated with low Apgar scores in early observations of FHR variability, but it was not possible to relate the time course of the pattern to the fetal depression

(Hammacher et al., 1968). That is, fetuses with the pattern in the intrapartum period tended to have low Apgar scores, but it was not clear whether the pattern was present immediately before delivery or whether it preceded an evolution to a more serious FHR pattern.

The saltatory pattern is almost invariably seen during labor rather than in the antepartum period. The etiology is uncertain, but it may be similar to that of the increased FHR variability seen in animal experiments with brief and acute hypoxia in the previously normoxic fetus. This increase is presumed to result from an increase in α-adrenergic activity, of which the primary function is to cause selective vasoconstriction of certain vascular beds. A secondary effect of this increased α-adrenergic activity may be excessive variability.

Because it is believed that the fetus with this pattern is hemodynamically compensated (although it may be mildly hypoxemic), we recommend that attempts be made to abolish it by maneuvers such as using a change to the lateral position, avoiding hypotension, avoiding excessive uterine activity, and perhaps maternal hyperoxia. The pattern is probably similar in significance to mild or moderate variable decelerations.

Premature Fetus

Comparison of the antepartum and intrapartum FHR patterns of the premature and their relationship to fetal blood acid-base status (Bowes et al., 1980; Zanini et al., 1980) has revealed that the same general criteria used in the term fetus can be used for the premature fetus. It had been stated that the premature fetus can quickly develop abnormal patterns and that these patterns may progress in severity much more rapidly than in the term fetus, but this is unconfirmed.

There are some commonly held and erroneous beliefs with regard to prematurity. The first is that the premature fetus normally has tachycardia. In fact, the average heart rate of the 28-week-old fetus is about 150 beats/min, with a range of about 130 to 170 beats/min (only slightly above that of the term fetus). The second is that premature heart rates have "flat" baselines. Most premature fetuses have normal FHR variability, and its disappearance or absence should be managed as for a term fetus. However, premature fetuses do tend to have a

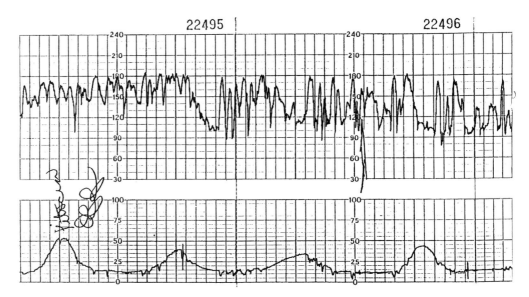

FIGURE 22-14 ■ Saltatory pattern showing excessive fetal heart rate variability of up to 60 beats/min in brief intervals, probably representing mild hypoxic stress.

smaller amplitude of variability and a lower amplitude of accelerations. They also tend to have more episodic, small, and variable decelerations.

The response of the premature fetus to vibroacoustic stimulation also differs from the response of the term fetus. The percentage of reactive nonstress tests after vibroacoustic stimulation is 90% or more above 26 weeks but only 20% or less below this gestational age (see Chapter 21).

Congenital Anomalies

Except as described for the dysrhythmias, most fetuses with congenital anomalies have normal FHR patterns and a response to hypoxia similar to those of the normal fetus. There are several exceptions (e.g., complete heart block and anencephaly). Thus, aneuploid fetuses, such as those with Down syndrome and trisomy 18, and fetuses with aplastic lungs, meningomyelocele, and hydrocephalus may give no FHR warning of defects. In one series, although there was no pathognomonic pattern in such fetuses, the rate of cesarean section for fetal distress was significantly increased (Garite et al., 1979).

An important exception is seen with *Potter syndrome*. Affected fetuses are generally recognized as growth restricted because of the oligohydramnios and in addition may have substantial variable decelerations, presumably for the same reason; that is, umbilical cord compression is more likely without the "padding" of adequate amniotic fluid. Before the widespread use of ultrasound imaging, a number of such fetuses were delivered by cesarean section because of "fetal distress," with the tragic outcome being rapid neonatal death resulting from hypoplastic lungs.

"Shoulders" and "Overshoot"

Shoulders and overshoot are terms used to describe transient increases in FHR, either preceding or immediately after a deceleration. They have an undeserved poor reputation. They simply represent the transient net result of dominance of sympathetic over parasympathetic activity. Others believe that shoulders may result from mild cord compression during which only the umbilical vein is compressed; this would produce a temporary fetal hypovolemia. We believe that the shoulders do *not* represent an hypoxic stress and that any fetal compromise results from the associated decelerations. As with all patterns, the significance of the presence or absence of shoulders is secondary to the retention of FHR variability. In Figure 22-11, shoulders would neither ameliorate nor add to the diagnosis of presumed severe fetal hypoxia because of the absence of variability in the tracing.

Infection

The presence of infection, particularly chorioamnionitis, is often associated with tachycardia. This is usually *uncomplicated*, meaning that the baseline FHR is greater than 160 beats/min but variability is normal, accelerations are usually present, and periodic changes are absent. However, variability tends to be concomitantly reduced with tachycardia. Anecdotal evidence suggests another disturbing aspect of some cases of fetal infection—an atypical evolution of FHR patterns. That is, the FHR pattern may evolve from a tachycardia with somewhat reduced FHR variability to one with mild late decelerations with reduced variability and, finally, a profound bradycardia without variability. As noted, this expected evolution normally follows deep late or variable decelerations or bradycardia.

Amnionitis caused by *Listeria monocytogenes* has also been seen with patterns normally associated with fetal acidemia (i.e., late decelerations without FHR variability) (Koh et al., 1980). It has been theorized that these patterns were produced not by global acidemia but by cardiogenic and septic shock resulting from overwhelming fetal sepsis. This same mechanism may well apply to abnormal patterns resulting from infections other than *L. monocytogenes*.

Infants with these patterns are sometimes depressed (i.e., low Apgar scores) but may only have moderate acidemia. Nevertheless, we believe that these infants will benefit from early delivery, so that extrauterine support can be instituted. The major management difficulty is timely recognition of the severity of the fetal condition despite the atypical evolution of the FHR pattern because we have no tool to determine the rare case of fetal sepsis.

MANAGEMENT OF VARIANT PATTERNS

Clinical Management

Over more than three decades have passed since the introduction of continuous FHR monitoring, and there have been numerous recommendations for action based on certain patterns. Algorithms, some more complete than others, can be found in several publications. Because of their wide variation, they are not reviewed here. In general, these protocols have evolved and matured over time, particularly because up to one in three infants has a variant (formerly called "abnormal" or "ominous") pattern, but this is many times higher than the incidence of severe acidemia, seizures, or cerebral palsy. Thus, dramatic intervention is in fact rarely required in such patterns to avoid the birth of a compromised fetus.

Here we include guidelines to avoid the rare case of hypoxia-acidemia–induced damage in a timely manner and to restrict potentially hazardous intervention (cesarean section or vaginal operative delivery) to appropriate cases.

Late Decelerations

If one examines any heart rate tracing, it is almost always possible to find at least one deceleration that fits the criteria of late deceleration. However, because an essential part of the definition is that they are persistent, the text covers only those that are either seen with every contraction or come in runs or families of late decelerations (see Figs. 22-5, 22-6, and 22-8).

Late decelerations with normal FHR variability (*reflex* late decelerations) can occur from first placement of the monitor or may appear during the course of labor. They may be in response to (1) lowered uterine blood flow resulting from a recognizable event, such as a small drop in blood pressure after activation of a regional anesthetic; (2) the onset of more frequent or stronger contractions; (3) the gradual onset of hypovolemia resulting from insufficient fluid intake in a laboring mother; or (4) a relatively minor manifestation of the supine hypotension syndrome.

In most of these examples, the decelerations can be abolished by conservative means. As noted, attempts should be made to abolish persistent late decelerations, because they may evolve into the nonreflex type, manifested by a reduction and finally loss of FHR variability. This latter pattern is assumed to represent acidemic decompensation and indicates the need for ancillary testing or delivery.

Most term normally grown fetuses tolerate at least 30 minutes of reflex late decelerations before decompensation, so this can be considered to be the time available for conservative management to abolish the decelerations or, if they cannot be abolished, to prepare for possible operative delivery. Because the specific preparations to be made are dependent on the institution, its staffing, and its facilities, no overall recommendations can be made for all cases.

An accepted evolution occurs from reflex to nonreflex decelerations during labor (see Fig. 22-9). There is a gradual deepening of the decelerations, then intermittent reduction of variability, and finally loss of variability with persistence of the decelerations. This is a general rule that applies in specific circumstances, namely, a gradual rather than sudden decrease in maternal placental function (specifically, a reduction in uterine blood flow, or oxygen flow), and the evolution from a normal pattern. There appear to be occasional exceptions to this pattern of evolution, although this is not well established. This may occur in some cases of chorioamnionitis and the postmaturity syndrome. In some cases, the evolution to reduced or absent FHR variability occurs with relatively minor late decelerations and, in chorioamnionitis, a relatively mild tachycardia.

Nonreflex late decelerations (persistent late decelerations without FHR variability) that cannot be abolished are an indication for delivery unless ancillary testing can be done without unduly delaying delivery, and the results exclude acidemia. Most fetuses with such late decelerations are either already acidemic or will soon become so, and rapid delivery will minimize exposure of the fetus to such acidemia. Admittedly, a small percentage may in fact not be deeply acidotic but simply may have reflex late decelerations accompanied by a nonhypoxic decrease in FHR variability. Although this can be determined by ancillary testing, such as stimulation testing or fetal blood sampling, the relatively small number of institutions where fetal blood sampling is available motivates the recommendation for rapid delivery if there is no response to stimulation testing.

Why might an infant have reflex late decelerations with an accompanying pattern showing nonhypoxic reduced variability? One possible reason is drugs (narcotics, sedatives, magnesium sulfate), although it is rare to have a total loss of variability after intake of such drugs. If the drug is given episodically rather than as an infusion, absent variability is usually transient.

Another reason for a nonhypoxic reduction of variability is a neurologic deficit, either developmental or acquired as a result of a prior global or regional hypoxic or ischemic event. If the event is acidemia from which the fetus has subsequently recovered its oxygenation, there may be reduced or absent FHR variability without late decelerations; if there is persistent cardiac hypoxia, associated late decelerations should be present. There is no simple rapid means of ruling in or out such prior damage in most cases without obtaining a high-quality ultrasound study and ancillary testing, that is, stimulation

testing (Smith et al., 1986a) or fetal blood sampling. Indeed, such neurologic damage may not be diagnosable on ultrasound imaging.

Further, despite late decelerations, absent FHR variability, and the theoretical mechanisms of loss of variability noted, there is no assurance that the infant will in fact have hypoxia-related neurologic damage. Thus, the recommendation for immediate delivery gives the infant the benefit of the uncertainty in diagnosis. Whether such an infant has in fact not suffered damage or is able to recover from neuronal damage by remodeling is unlikely to be known in any specific fetus.

Variable Decelerations

The description and presumed etiology of variable decelerations has been described. Variable decelerations may occur sporadically in the antepartum period, during the latent phase of labor, during the first-stage active phase of labor, or during the second stage. As noted, the etiology varies according to when they occur.

Variable decelerations in the latent phase of labor are usually of modest depth and duration, sometimes in the "mild to moderate" category. When variable decelerations occur with mild uterine activity early in labor, they are probably due to umbilical cord compression. The usual approach is to attempt to modify the depth and duration of the decelerations or abolish them by altering the position of the mother (to the lateral or another position). It is extremely unlikely that a fetus will develop inadequate oxygenation as a result of these mild to moderate variable decelerations; however, they may develop into *severe* variable decelerations, which may eventually result in compromise. Therefore, it is reasonable to attempt to abolish any such decelerations.

If the decelerations cannot be abolished by conservative means (e.g., a change in maternal position) and become deeper and more prolonged, an ultrasound examination may be performed to determine the adequacy of amniotic fluid. A low amniotic fluid index might well explain the decelerations, and amnioinfusion may be used to abolish them if the membranes are ruptured. A similar management scheme is appropriate for the first-stage active phase of labor in the presence of mild to moderate variable decelerations and a reactive FHR tracing. That is, attempts should be made to abolish the decelerations by conservative means. If they cannot be modified by position changes of the mother, the patient may be observed for progress of the decelerations or amnioinfusion may be carried out if the amniotic fluid index is low.

If it is not possible to modify or abolish such variable decelerations, no particular further management is necessary except to observe the decelerations for evolution to the more serious type. This implies continuous electronic monitoring and the ability to intervene or react in a reasonable period of time if such an evolution occurs.

If the variable decelerations evolve to the severe type, fetal hypoxic decompensation becomes a possibility, and amniotomy to allow amnioinfusion should be considered. Because such decompensation rarely occurs in less than 30 minutes in the normally grown term fetus, this time is available for planning potential intervention, which usually means cesarean section during the latent or first-stage active phase.

During severe variable decelerations, the heart rate pattern must be observed for an intermittent reduction in

FHR variability during and after the variable decelerations. Should this begin to occur and abolition of the decelerations still cannot be achieved by the means outlined above, delivery is recommended before the total loss of variability. This may signify hypoxic-acidemic decompensation and, indeed, must be presumed to do so unless it can be ruled out by ancillary methods.

Severe variable decelerations in the presence of frequent uterine activity may become confluent and may form a prolonged deceleration and, eventually, a bradycardia. Therefore, in the presence of persistent severe variable decelerations, it is prudent to attempt to maintain uterine contractions more than 2 minutes apart. This may be achieved by reducing or discontinuing the oxytocin dosage (if it is being used) or placing the mother in the lateral position, which sometimes results in spacing out of the contractions. If the severe variable decelerations evolve to a bradycardia, this is managed as described later for bradycardia.

Variable decelerations in the second stage of labor are managed somewhat differently. The incidence of variable decelerations increases in the second stage, and they are more likely to be caused by head compression (and subsequent dural stimulation) than by cord compression. Intervention by an operative vaginal delivery can often be carried out safely and is often chosen by some practitioners rather than tolerating persistent severe variable decelerations.

Bradycardia

Bradycardia is technically defined as a baseline heart rate below 110 beats/min with specific additional criteria. The lower the FHR, the more likely the possibility of fetal compromise. A heart rate below 60 beats/min without FHR variability (in the absence of heart block) is highly predictive of hypoxic compromise.

Management of bradycardia is described with the assumption that there was a normal FHR admission strip (e.g., a normal rate with normal variability and absence of persistent decelerations at arrival). Should this tracing evolve into a bradycardia with a heart rate between 100 and 110 beats/min with normal variability, most fetuses can probably tolerate this for essentially unlimited periods of time.

The same is likely true of bradycardia between 80 and 100 beats/min with normal variability; that is, there is no particular limit of time when this bradycardia will evolve into a decompensatory pattern, as signified by a decrease and finally loss of FHR variability. Nevertheless, most practitioners make some preparations for an emergency delivery in case decompensation should occur, even though they may not carry out the emergency delivery if the pattern resolves.

When a persistent bradycardia occurs with a rate between 60 and 80 beats/min, most practitioners attempt to abolish it; if it cannot be rapidly abolished, immediate preparation for delivery should be made. Delivery under these conditions would be called for if the bradycardia does not resolve and the variability declines. However, in the presence of retained variability, observation is acceptable. A persistent unresolvable heart rate below 60 beats/min in the absence of heart block is an obstetric emergency and delivery should be carried out, more emergently (if possible) in the absence of FHR variability. Because the management of bradycardia in the second stage includes the option of rapid emergency vaginal delivery

rather than cesarean section, a second stage bradycardia may sometimes be observed for a longer period before intervention than in the first stage.

EFFICACY, RISKS, AND RECOMMENDATIONS FOR USAGE

Efficacy of Fetal Heart Rate Monitoring

Randomized Controlled Trials

Until recently, controlled trials of electronic FHR monitoring have shown little or no beneficial effect compared with conventional management. This is not only puzzling but also of great concern to many clinicians who believe that electronic FHR monitoring is effective based on clinical observations and the physiologic basis of FHR patterns. Many obstetricians recall patients for whom the use of electronic FHR monitoring undoubtedly led to early intervention and a decreased duration of intrapartum acidemia for the fetus. Nonetheless, the trials have not consistently shown a beneficial effect and, in fact, have found a detrimental effect of increased cesarean section rates in the monitored group (Thacker, 1987).

One reason for this lack of consistent benefit is that in earlier trials patient numbers were inadequate to show a difference in mortality rates when the intrinsic rate is so low. Second, criteria used for diagnosis of fetal compromise were unsophisticated, bearing little relationship to modern criteria. In particular, there had been little or no recognition of the importance of FHR variability in the determination of fetal status. The largest trial contains no description whatsoever of the FHR indices used to determine "abnormalities of FHR" (Leveno et al., 1986). A further effect of unsophisticated FHR interpretation is the tendency to diagnose fetal compromise too frequently, especially in the presence of decelerations with normal FHR variability. This had the effect of elevating the cesarean section rate unnecessarily. Third, response times are rarely noted in the trials. Clearly, an acidemic fetus needs prompt delivery and resuscitation before damage occurs, not according to some predetermined, arbitrary, "standard" time, such as "a cesarean section performed within 30 minutes." Brain damage apparently can occur in approximately 10 minutes in the case of total cessation of oxygen delivery. If an obstetric facility cannot achieve delivery within this critical period, the fault does not rest with electronic FHR monitoring. Many of the intrapartum stillbirths in recent trials may well have been avoided with ideal response times, but such are either not discussed or are discussed in relation to a time frame that is more dependent on obstetric practicality than on biological (i.e., fetal) need.

The gold standard evidence for efficacy of a medical treatment (grade I quality of evidence of the U.S. Preventive Services Task Force, 1989) is demonstration of efficacy in at least one well-designed randomized controlled trial. The epidemiologic planning of the FHR monitoring trials cannot in general be faulted, but certainly the definitions of FHR patterns and algorithms for management have varied widely in the different publications. For this reason, a recommendation has been made for the standardization of FHR pattern interpretation (NICHD, 1997). Although this has been attempted numerous times before, definitions that are unambiguous, quantifiable, and computer compatible have not previously been agreed upon.

Paneth and coworkers (1993) suggested that the randomized controlled trials were conducted too soon, before three key conditions regarding monitoring were (and have yet to be) met:

1. *Reliability* of interobserver agreement regarding the identity and meaning of FHR patterns
2. *Validity* of an association between specific FHR patterns and the adverse neurologic outcome to be prevented
3. A *causal relationship* between specific FHR patterns and adverse outcome

Strength of agreement is measured by the kappa coefficient, which tests the null hypothesis that an observed agreement occurs by chance. Hence, a coefficient of 0 represents complete independence of two observations and a coefficient of 1 represents complete agreement. *Intra*observer reliability in FHR pattern interpretation in four studies averaged 0.7 (substantial agreement); in FHR case management, the average was 0.58 (moderate agreement). *Inter*observer agreement for FHR pattern interpretation averaged 0.40 (fair to moderate agreement) and for FHR case management, 0.37 (fair agreement). Although these numbers cannot be used to quantify agreement, they are disappointingly low and suggest a variation in both interpretation and management. They do at least demonstrate that the clinicians are specific, not random, in their decisions. These observations make a strong case for FHR nomenclature standardization.

The validity of FHR monitoring regarding the association between FHR patterns and neurodevelopmental outcome has been examined in relatively few studies, including about 800 patients (Paneth et al., 1993). With criteria dating back to 1980, the pooled relative risk for developmental handicap in children having "abnormal" tracings was about 2. Despite this modest correlation, most fetuses with "abnormal FHR patterns," as defined by these works, have a normal outcome.

The third factor (i.e., a causal relationship between FHR patterns and adverse outcomes) needs to be confirmed to prove that interventions prevent neurologic damage. The most recent cumulative meta-analysis of the randomized controlled trials supports this concept, in that the relative risk of neonatal seizures in the electronically monitored group was 0.5, compared with the group managed by FHR auscultation (Thacker et al., 1995). Though the link between neonatal seizures and long-term abnormal outcome could not be made in these studies, a reduced incidence of seizures is clearly a desirable outcome. Apart from the emotional impact of newborn seizures on the family, the cost of the medical evaluation and treatment of such infants is substantial. Clearly, the overall cost-to-benefit ratio of this reduction in seizures needs to be addressed.

The weaknesses in the randomized trials of monitoring make the significant and substantial reduction of seizures with FHR monitoring all the more optimistic, and one wonders whether even stronger results may not be obvious with standardized interpretation, giving reliable and consistent management.

Auscultation

Reports that electronic FHR monitoring, as practiced in the 1970s and 1980s, had doubtful benefit and some risk led to renewed interest in FHR auscultation as a form of surveillance.

However, there is no evidence from randomized controlled trials that auscultation is any more effective than no auscultation, and its risks have not been determined. In a large survey of nearly 25,000 pregnancies more than 30 years ago, Benson and colleagues (1968) concluded that FHR auscultation was not effective in detecting fetal ill health except in extreme degrees of bradycardia.

Auscultation is proposed as an appropriate means of surveillance, particularly in the "low-risk" patient by national organizations in both the United States and Canada. The American College of Obstetricians and Gynecologists (1995) considers intermittent auscultation to be equivalent to electronic fetal monitoring: "Well controlled studies have shown that intermittent auscultation of the FHR is equivalent to continuous electronic monitoring in assessing fetal condition when performed at specific intervals with a 1:1 nurse-to-patient ratio."

These recommendations and allusions to the efficacy of auscultation are quite extraordinary because the technique of auscultation has not been subjected to a trial of treatment in contrast to no auscultation, which is the appropriate trial to demonstrate efficacy (RCOG, 2001). We still await a trial of electronic monitoring versus auscultation versus no FHR assessment, using rigidly defined nomenclature, modern interpretation, a rigidly followed management algorithm, and sufficient numbers.

Risks of Fetal Heart Monitoring

Cesarean Section

The major risk associated with electronic FHR monitoring is an increase in cesarean section rates, and the risk in the earliest trials was often severalfold. The relative risk in the cumulative meta-analysis of nine studies from 1976 to 1993, with more than 18,000 patients, was 1.21, a gratifying decrease. The relative risk of total operative deliveries was 1.23 (Thacker et al, 1995).

Another approach to determining appropriate intervention was seen in a study of 17 British expert obstetricians when presented with 50 clinical cases (Keith et al., 1995). Most experts did not recommend operative delivery in actual cases when there was a normal delivery and outcome but did recommend operative intervention in 83% of cases when the newborns were acidemic, with umbilical arterial pH less than 7.05. In the same study, an intelligent decision-support computer system, using FHR pattern feature extraction and a database of more than 400 rules, performed at least as well as the clinicians. Such systems hold hope for more standardized management in the future.

Infectious and Other Morbidity

Fetal morbidity has most often occurred as infectious complications through either an increased risk of chorioamnionitis or direct fetal infection using the scalp electrode as a portal of entry. Case reports of herpes and group B streptococcal and gonococcal infections exist. There is concern as well about the potential risk of transmission of the human immunodeficiency virus with the direct fetal electrode. Current recommendations are to avoid techniques resulting in breaks in the fetal skin in the presence of such infectious agents.

Maternal infectious morbidity with monitoring devices has been difficult to demonstrate because of confounding features. That is, chorioamnionitis is more common in obstructed or desultory labor, which is when internal monitoring, especially the intrauterine pressure catheter, tends to be used. However, when correction has been attempted for such confounders, it is not clear whether there is an increase in maternal infection (Sweet and Gibbs, 1995). As in any aspect of medicine, the benefits of the use of monitoring in avoiding fetal morbidity must be weighed against any infectious morbidity.

Mechanical morbidity with the intrauterine pressure catheter is a rare but nevertheless important complication. Catheter insertion has been associated with uterine perforation, placental laceration, and abruption.

Intrusiveness

The use of a technologic device in one of the most intimate experiences of a couple's life presents a distinct hazard of interfering with family interaction and physician–patient interaction and of dehumanizing the birth process. For this reason, the monitor must never become the central focus of labor and delivery; it should be ancillary and subservient to the couple's experience. All attendants should maintain an appropriate social interaction with the patient and make it obvious that she is more important than the machine, for example, by making eye contact predominantly with her, not the record during examinations. Another way to minimize intrusiveness is to interpret knowledgeably, minimizing dramatic comments and activities.

Recommendations for Fetal Heart Rate Monitoring

The near dichotomy in regard to electronic FHR monitoring can make it difficult for the practicing obstetrician to take a stand. Based on current recommendations, physicians can opt for universal monitoring, monitoring only high-risk patients, or not using electronic monitoring at all. However, if obstetricians choose any of these courses, they must do so from a firm base of experience and knowledge of the literature on the subject. Few obstetricians opt for no electronic monitoring because they feel legally vulnerable. From the nursing care viewpoint, electronic monitoring is logistically easier than intermittent auscultation.

Reasonable current recommendations are as follows. On admission to rule out labor or in a patient in actual labor, an FHR record with either external or internal monitoring should be documented for approximately 20 minutes. This practice has been termed the "admission test," and though it is popular, there is no incontrovertible evidence of its efficacy to predict fetal safety throughout labor. It is sometimes coupled with vibroacoustic stimulation (Ingemarsson et al., 1988).

In the case of an at-risk patient, monitoring should continue throughout labor, although this need not be obsessively so in all cases. There are difficulties with the definition of "high risk"; suffice it to say that such a patient is one who has a condition listed in publications on the subject. Should the contractions be obvious and the FHR pattern be "normal" (normal rate, normal FHR variability, and absence of periodic changes except accelerations), the tocodynamometer does not need to be placed. The need for the tocodynamometer to measure contraction frequency or for the intrauterine pressure catheter to measure intrauterine pressure arises when labor progress is inappropriate.

For a low-risk patient who remains so, in that she does not demonstrate any abnormality of labor or have risk factors appearing subsequently, electronic FHR monitoring may be intermittent. In such cases, a short recorded strip of approximately 5 minutes every 30 minutes or in accordance with the hospital's policy or American College of Obstetricians and Gynecologists recommendation for frequency of evaluation of FHR should be sufficient. If equivocal changes in these short strips occur, continuous electronic FHR monitoring should be instituted until the condition of the fetus is resolved. During the second stage of labor, the frequency or recording needs to be increased in accordance with the hospital's auscultation protocol.

Perhaps the most difficult aspects of monitoring include recognition and prediction of the fetus who is at risk for hypoxic damage without overdiagnosis. The crucial step in this regard is projecting the potential for hypoxic decompensation. This requires a dynamic approach to FHR interpretation, with the recognition that oxygen levels in the fetus are continuously variable—from moment to moment, with contractions, and with longer cycles. Appropriate interpretation also requires an understanding of the evolution of FHR patterns in relation to progressive decreases in oxygenation, for example, in the initially normoxic fetus, the deepening of decelerations, the subsequent intermittent decrease or loss of variability, and, finally, the absence of variability.

With careful interpretation and conservative management, we believe that many of the rare cases of intrapartum acidemia developing during labor can be recognized and, in many cases, intervention can be carried out before damage occurs. This goal does not need to be achieved at the expense of excessive cesarean section and other potential morbidity.

FETAL PULSE OXIMETRY

FHR monitoring is intended to assess fetal oxygenation indirectly, as reflected in specific changes in heart rate. FHR monitoring is not a direct measure of fetal oxygenation, and it has insufficient specificity and sensitivity to correctly identify the fetus who is in oxygen debt. Continuous direct assessment of fetal oxygenation has been proposed as a technique to overcome the suboptimal specificity and sensitivity of continuous FHR monitoring. Ideally, a monitor that measures the fetal oxygenation or pH directly would be preferable to identify the physiologically compromised fetus. Efforts to develop instrumentation to measure fetal oxygenation or pH continuously have been limited by difficulty with fetal access, safety, and accuracy of the information generated (e.g., stasis of capillary blood in the fetal scalp during active labor).

Pulse oximetry has been a significant advance in the assessment of oxygenation status for adult and pediatric patients. Essentially all patients in surgery and intensive care units are now monitored continuously with a noninvasive transcutaneously applied pulse oximeter. Pulse oximetry provides a continuous source of reliable information about oxygen status in intraoperative and critically ill patients that has been shown to reduce the number of hypoxia-related anesthetic deaths (Johnson, 1991). Several obstacles prevented the use of this technology for intrapartum fetal assessment, including access to the fetus (ruptured membranes are required), an appropriate surface to apply the sensor (a stable surface is needed that will not change significantly during labor), and differences in fetal versus adult physiology (the fetal blood pressure is lower, whereas the pulse and hemoglobin are higher, and the oxyhemoglobin dissociation is different than the adult).

Adult and pediatric pulse oximetry uses *transmission oximetry* in which light is passed through tissue to a sensor on the opposite side of the patient's finger or earlobe. The noninvasive determination of oxygen saturation is founded upon the different absorption of red and infrared light by oxyhemoglobin and deoxyhemoglobin: less red light is absorbed by oxyhemoglobin than by deoxyhemoglobin, and more infrared light is absorbed by oxyhemoglobin than by deoxyhemoglobin. The ratio of these differences is used to measure the oxygen saturation during each arterial pulse.

Detection of oxygen saturation in the fetus has been difficult because the fetus has no body part that can be used for transmission oximetry. This technical problem has been addressed by the development of a sensor that remains stable when applied to the fetal cheek or back and that uses *reflectance oximetry*, in which light is emitted and then reflected to a photosensor located on the same probe by the underlying fetal tissue.

Studies have related the oxygen saturation as measured by reflectance pulse oximetry to fetal arterial oxygen saturation measured directly in fetal lambs (Nijiland et al., 1995) and to fetal scalp pH in humans (Kuhnert et al., 1998). Dildy and coworkers (1996) suggested that an arterial oxygen saturation of 30% is a reasonable threshold to detect acidemia. This conclusion was based on their analysis of 1101 paired umbilical artery and vein gases in which significant umbilical acidemia (arterial pH less than 7.13) occurred rarely (1.6%) when arterial oxygen saturation exceeded 30%; acidemia was more common (10.4%) when the arterial oxygen saturation is below 30%.

Other studies (Dildy et al., 1994; Bloom et al., 1999) investigated the duration required to produce metabolic acidosis in the human fetus in labor. They found that fetal acidemia did not occur unless the fetal pulse oximeter revealed a saturation below a critical threshold of 30% for more than 2 minutes.

Garite and colleagues (2000) applied fetal pulse oximetry to a population of more than 1000 laboring women who had FHR tracings that were worrisome but not sufficiently ominous to require immediate delivery, including (1) mild or moderate decelerations greater than 30 minutes, (2) a baseline 100 to 110 beats/min without accelerations, (3) a baseline below 100 or above 160 beats/min, (4) variability less than 5 or greater than 25 beats/min, (5) late decelerations, or (6) prolonged decelerations. Patients were randomly assigned to receive FHR monitoring alone or FHR plus fetal pulse oximetry. In those assigned to the latter group, if the FHR tracing was reassuring, labor was allowed to continue regardless of the fetal pulse oximetry level. If the FHR tracing was ominous, delivery was accomplished, again regardless of the fetal pulse oximetry data. The pulse oximetry data was used when the FHR tracing was nonreassuring: Labor was allowed to continue if the fetal oxygen saturation was greater than 30%, and delivery was recommended if the fetal oxygen saturation was below 30% for the entire interval between two contractions. The primary end point was the rate of cesarean section performed for fetal intolerance to labor. This rate was in fact significantly decreased, but the rate of cesarean delivery for dystocia was correspondingly increased; the overall cesarean section rate was not different in the FHR versus FHR plus pulse oximetry groups. An independent investigator concluded that biased or mislabeled indications for cesarean section did not explain the difference, but the results of this study have not been explained or duplicated. There was no evidence of fetal risk in the trial reported by Garite and coworkers. The American College of Obstetricians and Gynecologists Committee on Obstetric Practice did not endorse the adoption of this device "because of concerns that its introduction could further escalate the cost of medical care without necessarily improving clinical outcome" (American College of Obstetricians and Gynecologists, 2001).

REFERENCES

American College of Obstetricians and Gynecologists: Fetal Heart Rate Patterns: Monitoring, Interpretation, and Management. Washington, DC, ACOG Technical Bulletin No. 207, 1995.

American College of Obstetricians and Gynecologists Committee Opinion No. 258: Fetal pulse oximetry. Obstet Gynecol **98**:523, 2001.

Anderson PAW, Glick KL, Killam AP, et al: The effect of heart rate on *in utero* left ventricular output in the fetal sheep. J Physiol **372**:557, 1986.

Anderson PAW, Killam AP, Mainwaring RD, et al: In utero right ventricular output in the fetal lamb: The effect of heart rate. J Physiol **387**:297, 1987.

Ball RH, Parer JT: The physiological mechanisms of variable decelerations. Am J Obstet Gynecol **166**:1683, 1992.

Benson RC, Shubeck F, Deutschberger J, et al: Fetal heart rate as a predictor of fetal distress. Obstet Gynecol **32**:259, 1968.

Bloom SL, Swindle RG, McIntire DD, et al: Fetal pulse oximetry: duration of desaturation and intrapartum outcome. Obstet Gynecol **93**:1036, 1999.

Bowes WA, Gabbe SG, Bowes C: Fetal heart rate monitoring in premature infants weighing 1500 grams or less. Am J Obstet Gynecol **137**:791, 1980.

Brace RA: Current topic: Progress toward understanding the regulation of amniotic fluid volume: Water and solute fluxes in and through the fetal membranes. Placenta **16**:1, 1995.

Cohn HE, Sacks EJ, Heymann MA, et al: Cardiovascular responses to hypoxemia and acidemia in fetal lambs. Am J Obstet Gynecol **120**:817, 1974.

Court DJ, Parer JT: Experimental studies of fetal asphyxia and fetal heart rate interpretation. *In* Nathanielsz PW, Parer JT (eds): Research in Perinatal Medicine, vol I. New York, Perinatology Press, 1984, p. 113.

Dalton KJ, Phill D, Dawes GS, et al: The autonomic nervous system and fetal heart rate variability. Am J Obstet Gynecol **146**:456, 1983.

DeHaan J, Stolte LAM, Veth AFL, et al: The significance of short-term irregularity in the fetal heart rate pattern. *In* Dudenhausen JW, Saling E (eds): Perinatale Medezin, vol 4. Stuttgart, Thieme Verlag, 1973, p. 398.

Dildy GA, Thorp JA, Yeast JD: The relationship between oxygen saturation and pH in umbilical blood: Implications for intrapartum fetal oxygen saturation monitoring. Am J Obstet Gynecol **175**:682, 1996.

Dildy GA, van den Berg PP, Katz M: Intrapartum fetal pulse oximetry: fetal oxygen saturation trends during labor and relation to delivery outcome. Am J Obstet Gynecol **171**:679, 1994.

Fisher DS, Heymann MA, Rudolph AM: Fetal myocardial oxygen and carbohydrate consumption during acutely induced hypoxemia. Am J Physiol **242**:H657, 1982.

Garite TJ, Dildy GA, McNamara H, et al: A multicenter controlled trial of fetal pulse oximetry in the intrapartum management of non-reassuring fetal heart rate patterns. Am J Obstet Gynecol **183**:1049, 2000.

Garite TJ, Linzey EM, Freeman RK, et al: Fetal heart rate patterns and fetal distress in fetuses with congenital anomalies. Obstet Gynecol **53**:716, 1979.

Gill RW, Trudinger BJ, Garrett WJ, et al: Fetal umbilical venous flow measured in utero by pulsed Doppler and B-mode ultrasound. Am J Obstet Gynecol **139**:720, 1981.

Hammacher K, Huter KA, Bokelmann J, et al: Foetal heart rate frequency and perinatal condition of foetus and newborn. Gynaecologia (Basel) **166**:349, 1968.

Hanson MA: The importance of baro- and chemo-reflexes in the control of the fetal cardiovascular system. J Dev Physiol **10**:491, 1988.

Harris JL, Krueger TR, Parer JT: Mechanisms of late decelerations of the fetal heart rate during hypoxia. Am J Obstet Gynecol **144**:491, 1982.

Herbert CM, Boehm FM: Prolonged end-stage fetal heart rate deceleration: A reanalysis. Obstet Gynecol **57**:589, 1981.

Hon EH: An Atlas of Fetal Heart Rate Patterns. New Haven, Harty Press, 1968.

Hon EH, Quilligan EJ: The classification of fetal heart rate. Conn Med **31**:779, 1967.

Ingemarsson I, Arulkumaran S, Paul RH, et al: Fetal acoustic stimulation in early labor in patients screened with the admission test. Am J Obstet Gynecol **158**:70, 1988.

Ingemarsson E, Ingemarsson I, Solum T, et al: Influence of occiput posterior position on the fetal heart rate pattern. Obstet Gynecol **55**:301, 1980.

Johnson N: Development and potential of pulse oximetry. Contemp Rev Obstet Gynecol **3**:193, 1991.

Jones MD, Sheldon RE, Peeters LL, et al: Fetal cerebral oxygen consumption at different levels of oxygenation. J Appl Physiol **43**:1080, 1977.

Keith RDF, Beckley S, Garibaldi JM, et al: A multicentre comparative study of 17 experts and an intelligent computer system for managing labour using the cardiotocogram. Br J Obstet Gynaecol **102**:688, 1995.

Kenny J, Plappert T, Doubilet P, et al: Effects of heart rate on ventricular size, stroke volume, and output in the normal human fetus: A prospective Doppler echocardiographic study. Circulation **76**:52, 1987.

Klapholz H, Schifrin B, Myrick R: Role of maternal artifact in fetal heart rate pattern interpretation. Obstet Gynecol **44**:373, 1974.

Knopf K, Parer JT, Espinoza ME, et al: Comparison of mathematical indices of fetal heart rate variability with visual assessment in the human and sheep. J Dev Physiol **16**:367, 1992.

Koh KS, Cole TL, Orkin AJ: Listeria amnionitis as a cause of fetal distress. Am J Obstet Gynecol **136**:261, 1980.

Krebs HB, Petres RE, Dunn LJ, et al: Intrapartum fetal heart rate monitoring. I. Classification and prognosis of fetal heart rate patterns. Am J Obstet Gynecol **133**:762, 1979.

Kubli FW, Hon EH, Khazin AF, et al: Observations on heart rate and pH in the human fetus during labor. Am J Obstet Gynecol **104**:1190, 1969.

Kuhnert M, Seelback-Gobel B, Butterwegge M. Predictive agreement between the fetal arterial oxygen saturation and fetal scalp pH: Results of the German multicenter study. Am J Obstet Gynecol **178**:330, 1998.

Leveno KJ, Cunningham FG, Nelson S, et al: A prospective comparison of selective and universal electronic fetal monitoring in 34,995 pregnancies. N Engl J Med **315**:615, 1986.

Llanos AJ, Green JR, Creasy RK, et al: Increased heart rate response to parasympathetic and beta-adrenergic blockade in growth-retarded fetal lambs. Am J Obstet Gynecol **136**:808, 1980.

Low JA, Pancham SR, Worthington D, et al: The acid-base and biochemical characteristics of intrapartum fetal asphyxia. Am J Obstet Gynecol **121**:446, 1975.

Mann LI: Effects in sheep of hypoxia on levels of lactate, pyruvate, and glucose in blood of mothers and fetus. Pediatr Res **4**:46, 1970.

Mann LI, Tejani NA, Weiss RR: Antenatal diagnosis and management of the small-for-gestational-age fetus. Am J Obstet Gynecol **120**:995, 1974.

Martin CB Jr, DeHaan J, van der Wildt B, et al: Mechanisms of late decelerations in the fetal heart rate: A study with autonomic blocking agents in fetal lambs. Eur J Obstet Gynaecol Reprod Biol **9**:361, 1979.

Mendez-Bauer C, Poseirio JJ, Arellano-Hernandez G, et al: Effects of atropine on the heart rate of the human fetus during labor. Am J Obstet Gynecol **85**:1033, 1963.

Miyazaki FS, Nevarez F: Saline amnioinfusion for relief of repetitive variable decelerations: A prospective randomized study. Am J Obstet Gynecol **153**:301, 1985.

Murata Y, Martin CB, Ikenoue T, et al: Fetal heart rate accelerations and late decelerations during the course of intrauterine death in chronically catheterized rhesus monkeys. Am J Obstet Gynecol **144**:218, 1982.

Murata Y, Miyake Y, Yamamoto T, et al: Experimentally produced sinusoidal fetal heart rate patterns in the chronically instrumented fetal lamb. Am J Obstet Gynecol **153**:693, 1985.

Myers RE: Two patterns of brain damage and their conditions of occurrence. Am J Obstet Gynecol **112**:246, 1972.

National Institute of Child Health and Human Development Research Planning Workshop: Electronic fetal heart rate monitoring: Research guidelines for interpretation. Am J Obstet Gynecol **177**:1385, 1997.

Nijhuis JG, Crevels AJ, Van Dongen PWJ: Fetal brain death: The definition of a fetal heart rate pattern and its clinical consequences. Obstet Gynecol Surv **45**:229, 1990.

Nijhuis JG, Prechtl HFR, Martin CB Jr, et al: Are there behavioural states in the human fetus? Early Hum Dev **6**:177, 1982.

Nijiland R, Jongsma HW, Nijhuis JG: Arterial oxygen saturation in relation to metabolic acidosis in fetal lambs. Am J Obstet Gynecol **172**:810, 1995.

Paneth N, Bommarito M, Stricker J: Electronic fetal monitoring and later outcome. Clin Invest Med **16**:159, 1993.

Parer JT: The effect of acute maternal hypoxia on fetal oxygenation and the umbilical circulation in the sheep. Eur J Obstet Gynaecol Reprod Biol **10**:125, 1980.

Parer JT: Handbook of Fetal Heart Rate Monitoring, 2nd ed. Philadelphia, WB Saunders, 1997.

Parer JT, Krueger TR, Harris JL: Fetal oxygen consumption and mechanisms of heart rate response during artificially produced late decelerations of fetal heart rate in sheep. Am J Obstet Gynecol **136**:478, 1980.

Parer JT, Laros RK, Heilbron DC, et al: The roles of parasympathetic and beta-adrenergic activity in beat-to-beat fetal heart rate variability. In Kovach AGB, Monos E, Rubanyi G (eds): Cardiovascular Physiology—Heart, Peripheral Circulation and Methodology: Proceedings of the 28th International Congress of Physiological Sciences, Budapest, 1980. (Advances in Physiological Science, vol 8, p. 327). New York, Pergamon, 1981.

Paul RH, Suidan AK, Yeh S, et al: Clinical fetal monitoring. VII. The evaluation and significance of intrapartum baseline FHR variability. Am J Obstet Gynecol **123**:206, 1975.

Phelan JP, Ahn MO: Perinatal observations in forty-eight neurologically impaired term infants. Am J Obstet Gynecol **171**:424, 1994.

Ralston DH, Shnider SM: The fetal and neonatal effects of regional anesthesia in obstetrics. Anesthesiology **48**:34, 1978.

Reuss ML, Parer JT, Harris JL, et al: Hemodynamic effects of alpha-adrenergic blockade during hypoxia in fetal sheep. Am J Obstet Gynecol **142**:410, 1982.

Royal College of Obstetricians and Gynaecologists (RCOG): The Use of Electronic Fetal Monitoring. The Use and Interpretation of Cardiotocography in Intrapartum Fetal Surveillance. Evidence-Based Clinical Guideline No. 8. Clinical Effectiveness Support Unit. London, RCOG, 2001, p. 136.

Rudolph AM, Heymann MA: Control of the foetal circulation. In Comline KS, Cross KW, Dawes GS, et al (eds): Foetal and Neonatal Physiology. Proceedings of the Barcroft Centenary Symposium. Cambridge, Cambridge University Press, 1973.

Schifferli PY, Caldeyro-Barcia R: Effect of atropine and beta-adrenergic drugs on the heart rate of the human fetus. In Boreus L (ed): Fetal Pharmacology. New York, Raven Press, 1973.

Schifrin BS, Hamilton-Rubinstein T, Shields JR: Fetal heart rate patterns and the timing of fetal injury. J Perinatol **14**:174, 1994.

Smith CV, Nguyen HN, Phelan JP, et al: Intrapartum assessment of fetal well-being: A comparison of fetal acoustic stimulation with acid–base determinations. Am J Obstet Gynecol **155**:726, 1986a.

Smith CV, Phelan JP, Platt LD, et al: Fetal acoustic stimulation testing. II. A randomized clinical comparison with the non-stress test. Am J Obstet Gynecol **155**:131, 1986b.

Spong CY, Ogundipe OA, Ross MG: Prophylactic amnioinfusion for meconium stained amniotic fluid. Am J Obstet Gynecol **171**:931, 1994.

Strong TH, Hetzler G, Sarno AP, et al: Prophylactic intrapartum amnioinfusion: A randomized clinical trial. Am J Obstet Gynecol **162**:1370, 1990.

Sweet RL, Gibbs RS: Infectious Diseases of the Female Genital Tract, 3rd ed. Baltimore, Williams & Wilkins, 1995.

Thacker SB, Stroup DF, Peterson HB: Efficacy and safety of intrapartum electronic fetal monitoring: An update. Obstet Gynecol **86**:613, 1995.

Thacker SB: The efficacy of intrapartum electronic fetal monitoring. Am J Obstet Gynecol **156**:25, 1987.

U.S. Preventive Services Task Force: Guide to Clinical Preventive Services. No 39. Screening for Fetal Distress. Washington, DC, U.S. Preventive Services Task Force, 1989, p. 157.

Yaffe H, Parer JT, Block BS, et al: Cardiorespiratory responses to graded reductions of uterine blood flow in the sheep fetus. J Dev Physiol **9**:325, 1987.

Zanini B, Paul RH, Huey JR: Intrapartum fetal heart rate: Correlation with scalp pH in the preterm fetus. Am J Obstet Gynecol **136**:43, 1980.

Chapter 23
FETAL ACID-BASE BALANCE

Larry C. Gilstrap III, MD

PHYSIOLOGY

Normal metabolism in the fetus results in the production of both carbonic and organic acids. These acids in turn are buffered by various mechanisms resulting in the regulation of fetal pH within a very narrow range. Although the concentration of hydrogen ions is extremely low, changes in fetal pH as small as 0.1 unit can have profound effects on metabolic activity and on the cardiovascular and central nervous systems (CNS). Extreme changes in pH can even be fatal.

The maternal acid-base status can adversely affect fetal acid-base status. In normal pregnancies, the difference between maternal and fetal pH is usually 0.05 to 0.10 units (ACOG, 1995b).

Carbonic Acid

Carbonic acid is a volatile acid produced from the metabolism of glucose and fatty acids. During fetal oxidative metabolism (i.e., aerobic glycolysis or cellular respiration), the oxidation of glucose uses oxygen (O_2) and produces carbon dioxide (CO_2):

$$C_6H_{12}O_6 + 6O_2 \leftrightarrow 6CO_2 + 6H_2O$$

Hydration of carbon dioxide is facilitated by erythrocyte carbonic anhydrase according to the reaction

$$CO_2 + H_2O \leftrightarrow H_2CO_3 \leftrightarrow H^+ + HCO_3$$

From a practical standpoint, carbonic acid formation is equivalent to carbon dioxide generation, and most of the free hydrogen ion formed is buffered intracellularly. As blood passes through the placenta (or through the lung in the adult), bicarbonate reenters erythrocytes and combines with hydrogen ions to form carbonic acid, which then dissociates to carbon dioxide and water. The carbon dioxide thus formed in the fetus diffuses across the placenta and is excreted by the maternal lung. Carbon dioxide diffuses rapidly across the human placenta, so that even large quantities produced by the fetus can be eliminated rapidly if maternal respiration, uteroplacental blood flow, and umbilical blood flow are normal.

The rate of fetal carbon dioxide production expressed on a molar basis is roughly equivalent to the fetal oxygen consumption rate (James et al., 1972). In order for carbon dioxide to diffuse from fetus to mother, both a gradient between fetal umbilical blood and maternal uteroplacental blood PCO_2 must be maintained and adequate perfusion of both sides of the placenta must be preserved. Secondary to hyperventilation, the maternal arterial PCO_2 is reduced from a mean of 39 mmHg during nonpregnancy to a mean of 31 mmHg during pregnancy. Renal compensation, in turn, results in an increase in bicarbonate excretion, resulting in levels of 18 to 22 mEq/L during pregnancy (Landon, 1994).

Noncarbonic Acids

Anaerobic metabolism in the fetus results in the production of nonvolatile or noncarbonic acids. These acids are produced via two mechanisms in the fetus:

1. Use of nonsulfur-containing amino acids resulting in uric acid formation
2. Incomplete combustion of carbohydrates and fatty acids resulting in production of lactic acid and the ketoacids (e.g., beta-hydroxybutyric acid)

As a result of relatively immature renal function, the fetus is unable to handle excretion of these acids; they are thus transported to the placenta, where they diffuse slowly (in contradistinction to carbon dioxide) into the maternal circulation. The maternal kidney excretes noncarbonic acids produced by both maternal and fetal metabolism and thus helps regenerate bicarbonate. Because the maternal glomerular filtration rate (GFR) increases significantly during normal pregnancy, the maternal kidney filters and reabsorbs large quantities of bicarbonate daily.

The fetus does have the ability to metabolize accumulated lactate in the presence of sufficient oxygen; however, this is a slow process, and for practical purposes it is not thought to account for a large proportion of lactic acid elimination from the fetal compartment.

Buffers

Dramatic changes in pH are minimized via the action of buffers. The two major buffers are plasma bicarbonate and hemoglobin. Other quantitatively less important buffers include erythrocyte bicarbonate and inorganic phosphates (Blechner, 1993).

Terms that are used for the expression of buffering capacity include the following:

1. *Delta base*, a measure of "change" in the buffering capacity of bicarbonate
2. *Base deficits*, bicarbonate values below normal
3. *Base excess*, bicarbonate values above normal

Although the fetus has a limited ability to buffer an increase in acid production with bicarbonate and hemoglobin, the placental bicarbonate pool could also play a role in buffering the fetus against changes in maternal pH or blood gas status. Aarnoudse and colleagues (1984) studied bicarbonate permeability in the perfused human placental cotyledon model and found that acidification of the maternal circulation to pH 7.06 for 30 minutes did not significantly alter fetal pH. Instead, there was an efflux of total carbon dioxide from the placenta into the maternal circulation in the form of bicarbonate, which was not matched by an influx of total carbon dioxide from the fetal circulation. By this mechanism, bicarbonate transfer could take place between the placental tissue pool and the maternal circulation, while the transmission of maternal pH and blood gas changes to the fetal circulation would be minimized.

pH Determination

The pH is a measure of the acid-base status of various body fluids. Specifically, pH is the negative logarithm of the hydrogen ion concentration. It is directly related to concentration of bicarbonate (base), and inversely related to the concentration of carbonic acid (acid). The H_2CO_3 is calculated from the PCO_2. This relation is best illustrated by the Henderson-Hasselbach equations summarized next:

$$pH = pK + \log \frac{[base]}{[acid]}$$

$$pH = pK + \log \frac{HCO_3^-}{H_2CO_3}$$

$$pH = pK + \log \frac{HCO_3^- \, (mEq/L)}{PCO_2 \, (mm \, Hg)}$$

In simplest terms, the HCO_3^- represents the "metabolic" component, while the H_2CO_3 (or PCO_2) represents the "respiratory" component (Cunningham et al., 2001).

Terminology

Acidemia refers to an increase in hydrogen ions in the blood; *acidosis* refers to an increase in hydrogen ions in tissue. Similarly, *hypoxemia* is a decrease in oxygen content in blood; *hypoxia* is a decrease in oxygen content in tissue (Table 23-1).

Although an umbilical artery pH below 7.20 has traditionally been used to define newborn acidemia, most clinicians define academia as two standard deviations below the mean umbilical artery pH (7.10–7.18). The concept of clinically

TABLE 23-1. TERMINOLOGY

Acidemia	Increased concentration of hydrogen ions in blood
Acidosis	Increased concentration of hydrogen ions in tissue
Asphyxia	Hypoxia with metabolic acidosis
Base deficit	HCO_3^- concentration below normal
Base excess	HCO_3^- concentration above normal
Delta base	Measure of change in buffering capacity of bicarbonate
Hypoxemia	Decreased oxygen content in blood
Hypoxia	Decreased level of oxygen in tissue
pH	Negative logarithm of hydrogen ion concentration

Adapted from American College of Obstetrics and Gynecologists (ACOG): Umbilical artery blood acid-base analysis. Technical Bulletin No. 216, November 1995.

TABLE 23-2. TYPES OF ACIDEMIA*

Metabolic	Normal PCO_2 and decreased HCO_3^-
Respiratory	Increased PCO_2 and normal HCO_3^- (after correction of PCO_2)
Mixed	Increased PCO_2 and decreased HCO_3^-

* Umbilical artery pH <7.10.

significant or "pathologic" acidemia is discussed later in this chapter. The pH cutoff for defining fetal acidemia on the basis of scalp blood is closer to 7.20.

Acidemia in the newborn can be classified into three basic types: *metabolic*, *respiratory*, or *mixed*. The type is based primarily on the levels of HCO_3 and PCO_2 (Table 23-2). With marked elevations of the PCO_2, there is a compensatory increase of 1 mEq of HCO_3^-/liter for each 10 mm Hg increase in PCO_2 (Goldaber et al. 1991).

Factors Affecting Acid-Base Balance

With regard to acid-base balance in the fetus, the placenta acts as both "lungs" and "kidneys" by supplying oxygen and removing carbon dioxide and various metabolites. The pH in the fetus is thus controlled within a very tight range. Umbilical oxygen content and saturation and fetal arterial delta base depend primarily on uterine blood flow (Fig. 23-1). Oxygen supply, in turn, depends on the following:

- Adequate maternal oxygenation
- Blood flow to the placenta
- Transfer across the placenta
- Fetal oxygenation
- Delivery to fetal tissues

Removal of carbon dioxide depends on fetal blood flow to the placenta and transport across the placenta. Fixed-acid equilibrium depends on a continued state of balance between production and removal.

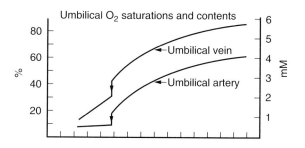

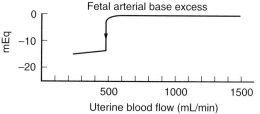

FIGURE 23-1 ■ Effect of decreasing uterine blood flow on umbilical oxygen saturations and contents and the base excess of fetal blood in a 3-kg sheep fetus. (From Battaglia FC, Meschia G: An Introduction to Fetal Physiology. Orlando, Academic Press, 1986.)

Respiratory Factors

Respiratory acidosis results from increased carbon dioxide tension and subsequent decreased pH. In the fetus, this picture is usually associated with a decrease in PO_2 as well. The most common cause of acute respiratory acidosis in the fetus is a sudden decrease in placental or umbilical perfusion. Umbilical cord compression, uterine hyperstimulation, and abruptio placentae are good examples, with transient cord compression being the most common factor (Williams et al., 2001).

Conditions associated with maternal hypoventilation or hypoxia can also result in respiratory acidosis in the fetus (and obviously, metabolic acidosis if severe enough). Coleman and Rund (1997) have reviewed the association of maternal hypoxia with nonobstetric conditions (such as asthma and epilepsy) during pregnancy. As these authors have pointed out aptly, the normal physiologic changes that occur during pregnancy may make the early recognition of maternal hypoxia difficult. For example, in a mother with asthma, a pH of less than 7.35 and a PCO_2 above 38 mm Hg could indicate respiratory compromise (Huff, 1989). To minimize the risk of hypoxemia in the fetus, Coleman and Rund (1997) recommend early intubation in these mothers who have borderline or poor blood gas values or respiratory compromise.

Other conditions can result in maternal hypoventilation (acute or chronic) during pregnancy. Induction of anesthesia or narcotic overdose can depress the medullary respiratory center. Hypokalemia, neuromuscular disorders (e.g., myasthenia gravis), and drugs that impair neuromuscular transmission (e.g., magnesium sulfate) can, in toxic doses, result in hypoventilation or even paralysis of the respiratory muscles. Finally, airway obstruction from foreign bodies can also result in maternal respiratory acidosis. Restoration of normal fetal acid-base balance depends on the reversibility of maternal etiologic factors.

Maternal respiratory alkalosis may occur when hyperventilation reduces the PCO_2 and subsequently increases pH. Severe anxiety, acute salicylate toxicity, fever, sepsis, pneumonia, pulmonary emboli, and acclimation to high altitudes are etiologic factors. As in respiratory acidosis, restoration of maternal acid-base balance by appropriate treatment of causative factors results in normalization of fetal blood gases.

Metabolic Factors

Fetal metabolic acidosis is characterized by loss of bicarbonate, high base deficit, and a subsequent fall in pH. This type of acidosis results from protracted periods of oxygen deficiency to a degree that results in anaerobic metabolism. The etiology can be fetal or maternal and usually implies the existence of a chronic metabolic derangement. Conditions such as growth restriction resulting from chronic uteroplacental hypoperfusion can be associated with fetal metabolic acidosis secondary to decreased oxygen delivery.

Maternal metabolic acidosis can also cause fetal metabolic acidosis and is classified according to the status of the anion gap. In addition to bicarbonate and chloride, the remaining anions required to balance the plasma sodium concentration are referred to as "unmeasured anions" or the *anion gap*. Reduced excretion of inorganic acids (as in renal failure) or accumulation of organic acids (as in alcoholic, diabetic, or starvation ketoacidosis and lactic acidosis) result in an increased anion gap metabolic acidosis. Bicarbonate loss, as seen in renal tubular acidosis, hyperparathyroidism, and diarrheal states and failure of bicarbonate regeneration, result in metabolic acidosis characterized by a normal anion gap. Fetal responses to these maternal conditions are manifested by a pure metabolic acidosis with normal respiratory gas exchange as long as placental perfusion remains normal.

Prolonged fetal respiratory acidosis, as seen in cord compression and abruptio placentae, can also result in accumulation of noncarbonic acids from anaerobic metabolism, characterized by blood gas measurements that reflect a mixed respiratory and metabolic acidosis.

ACID-BASE MONITORING IN LABOR

With each contraction during labor, uterine blood flow diminishes, placental perfusion is reduced, and transplacental gaseous exchange is impaired transiently. The intermittent nature of uterine contractions appears teleologically designed to allow periods of recovery and resumption of normal oxygen supply. Most fetuses tolerate labor without incident because they enter labor with adequate reserve; however, as labor progresses, there can be some reduction in fetal pH, PO_2, and bicarbonate level and an increase in PCO_2 and base excess. Fetal scalp blood values during labor are summarized in Table 23-3.

The *de novo* development of hypoxia in a normal-sized, full-term fetus that enters labor with normal placental function and reserve is unusual. When reserve is not adequate (e.g., in some cases of intrauterine growth restriction), uterine contractions can lead to a more rapid onset of fetal acidosis or can aggravate a preexisting degree of acidosis. In many cases, there are premonitory signs that may be noted only for the first time

■ TABLE 23-3. FETAL SCALP BLOOD VALUES IN LABOR*

	Early First Stage	Late First Stage	Second Stage
pH	7.33 ± 0.03	7.32 ± 0.02	7.29 ± 0.04
PCO_2 (mm Hg)	44.00 ± 4.05	42.00 ± 5.1	46.30 ± 4.2
PO_2 (mm Hg)	21.8 ± 2.6	21.3 ± 2.1	16.5 ± 1.4
Bicarbonate (mMol/liter)	20.1 ± 1.2	19.1 ± 2.1	17 ± 2
Base excess (mMol/liter)	3.9 ± 1.9	4.1 ± 2.5	6.4 ± 1.8

* Mean ± standard deviation.

From Huch R, Huch A: Maternal-fetal acid-base balance and blood gas measurement. *In* Beard RW, Nathanielsz PW (ed): Fetal Physiology and Medicine. New York, Marcel Dekker, 1984, p. 713.

in labor, such as a nonreassuring fetal heart rate pattern. Although preliminary efforts have been made to develop continuous tissue pH and PO_2 monitors for attachment to the fetal presenting part in labor, in practice, fetal acid-base status assessment requires a fetal blood sample.

Fetal Scalp Blood Sampling

Saling and Schneider (1967) introduced the technique of obtaining a sample of blood from the fetal presenting part to help evaluate fetal status during labor. A fetal blood sample may actually be obtained from either the scalp or buttocks when indicated. Unfortunately, there appears to be poor correlation between fetal heart rate patterns and abnormally low fetal blood sample values, although decreasing fetal blood pH is correlated with increasing severity of late decelerations (Paul et al., 1975) (Fig. 23-2). Low and colleagues (2001), in a study of 166 term pregnancies with fetal asphyxia (base deficit at delivery of greater than 12 mmol/L), have suggested that knowledge of the fetal heart rate pattern and fetal capillary blood assessment may be useful in preventing progression of "mild asphyxia to moderate or severe asphyxia in some cases."

Indications for Fetal Blood Sampling

Although fetal scalp blood sampling can provide useful information in some settings of nonreassuring fetal heart rate patterns, it is not generally used in obstetric practice in the United States (Clark and Paul, 1985; ACOG, 1995a). Moreover, in one study of more than 100,000 deliveries,

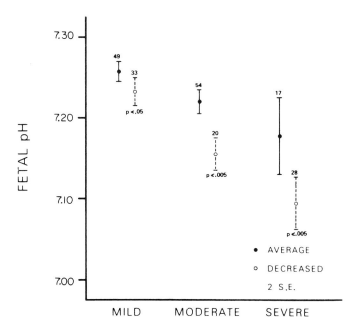

FIGURE 23-2 ■ Relationship between fetal blood pH and severity of late decelerations at time of blood sampling. Each fetal heart rate (FHR) classification is further divided into average (> 5 beats per minute) or decreased (< 5 beats per minute) fetal heart rate variability. (From Paul RH, Sudan AK, Yeh SY, et al: Clinical fetal monitoring: VII. The evaluation and significance of intrapartum baseline FHR variability. Am J Obstet Gynecol **123**:206, 1975.)

Goodwin and colleagues (1994) reported a decline in scalp blood sampling from approximately 1.8% for the first 3 years of the study to 0.03% in 1992 without an increase in cesarean delivery for fetal distress or an increase in "indicators of perinatal asphyxia."

In spite of the findings in the aforementioned study, in some situations fetal scalp blood sampling can provide clinically useful information. Probably one of the most useful indications is in decisions concerning the efficacy of cesarean delivery for the woman who presents in labor with a "straight-line" (i.e., absent variability) fetal heart rate pattern. Another indication is a nonreassuring fetal heart rate pattern and absent or decreased variability in a woman given medications which, in turn, may affect variability.

A woman with a nonreassuring fetal heart rate pattern who is within 1 to 2 hours of expected delivery may also benefit from scalp blood sampling for pH. This is especially true in the latter scenario if there is absence of fetal heart rate acceleration with fetal scalp stimulation or with vibroacoustic stimulation (ACOG, 1995a). For example, it has been reported that up to 50% of fetuses that do not demonstrate fetal heart acceleration with these two methods of stimulation will have acidosis (Clark et al., 1984; Smith et al., 1986; ACOG, 1995a). Others have reported a much lower rate (i.e., only 9%) of acidosis in fetuses without acceleration on stimulation (Spencer, 1991). Lin and colleagues (2001), in a study of 113 women in either the first or second stage of labor, reported that both the vibroacoustic stimulation test and fetal acidosis "have equal predictability for neonatal morbidity." Moreover, in a meta-analysis of intrapartum fetal stimulation test, Skupski and colleagues (2002) reported that the likelihood ratio of a negative (accelerations present) vibroacoustic test predicting the lack of acidemia was 0.20 (95% CI 0.11–0.37); for a positive test (absence of accelerations) predicting the presence of fetal acidemia, the likelihood ratio was 5.06 (95% CI 2.69–9.50).

Interpretation of Results

The pH of scalp blood is the same as that of capillary blood, which is lower than the pH of umbilical venous blood. Although the scalp blood pH is closer to that found in the umbilical artery, the values used for "abnormal" status differ between the two sources. For example, clinically significant or pathologic acidemia is defined as a pH of less than 7.00 when the umbilical artery is used and less than 7.20 when scalp blood is utilized. (Until recently, the cutoff value for an umbilical artery pH of less than 7.20 was also used to define acidemia.)

Most protocols for the interpretation of scalp blood pH results employ the ranges reported by Zalar and Quilligan (1979). In this protocol, a scalp blood pH of greater than 7.25 is considered normal, and labor may be allowed to continue. Values between 7.20 and 7.25 are considered borderline and warrant further sampling, usually within 30 minutes. Values below 7.20 are considered nonreassuring and, if they are confirmed, expedient delivery is recommended.

It is important to interpret results in the light of the complete clinical picture, with such factors as stage of labor, color and volume of amniotic fluid, estimated fetal weight, gestational age, and parity taken into account. Outcome in very-low-birth-weight fetuses may be related directly to acid-base balance at birth (Westgren et al., 1984); these small fetuses may not tolerate even the most benign episodes of intrapartum hypoxia without becoming acidotic. As with many intrapartum tests, however, low pH alone does not seem to predict subsequent development of cerebral palsy.

Frequency of Fetal Blood Sampling

There is no unanimity of opinion about when fetal blood sampling should be repeated. The decision basically depends on the clinical circumstances, which can change with the progress of labor. This is only one aspect of care of the fetus during labor and must be viewed in context. As a rule, a second sample should be obtained if the circumstances dictating the first sample do not resolve or if delivery is not expected within 30 to 40 minutes. The results of other tests of fetal well-being, such as scalp stimulation or vibroacoustic stimulation, also influence how often scalp blood testing should be performed.

Contraindications

Fetal blood sampling should not be performed when the fetus has a known or suspected blood dyscrasia (e.g., hemophilia or von Willebrand's disease). Fetal death because of excess blood loss has been reported in such cases (Ledger, 1978).

A potential disadvantage occurs with the use of the vacuum extractor after fetal blood sampling. Although this is not a contraindication to either procedure, one must be wary of using vacuum extraction on a fetus whose scalp has had numerous punctures for blood sampling. Amnionitis is considered a relative contraindication to fetal blood sampling because of the possibility of an increased risk of fetal scalp infection. If the mother is in early labor and frequent testing is mandated by a borderline value (i.e., 7.20–7.25), one should consider other, less invasive tests.

Fetal Complications

Fetal death from exsanguination after blood sampling, caused by unsuspected fetal coagulopathy, has been reported (Mondanlou and Linzey, 1978). In addition, there have been isolated case reports of neonatal scalp bleeding after fetal blood sampling, possibly because scalp vasoconstriction resulting from fetal hypoxia, which had previously prevented bleeding, resolved after delivery.

The incidence of scalp infections has been cited as less than 1% (Ledger, 1978), with the large majority requiring only local treatment (i.e., hair trimming, cleanliness). With the currently more common use of fetal heart rate monitoring via spiral electrodes, the incidence of fetal blood sampling complications is somewhat confused because fetal heart rate monitoring almost always precedes fetal blood sampling. Therefore, if the mortality rate resulting from coagulopathies is excluded, the infectious complications of fetal blood sampling are quantitatively minor.

Effects on Cesarean Delivery Rate

One of the major benefits of fetal scalp blood pH measurements has been reported to be a decrease in the cesarean delivery rate for fetal distress (Young et al., 1980; Grant, 1985). It has been suggested, however, that fetal scalp blood pH measurements have little effect on the cesarean delivery rate

(Goodwin et al., 1994). This latter observation could be due in part to the fact that other tests, such as scalp stimulation and the vibroacoustic stimulation test, are now being used more frequently than scalp blood pH measurements.

In summary, fetal scalp blood pH determinations appear to have a role in select cases, but their role may be limited.

UMBILICAL CORD BLOOD ACID-BASE ANALYSIS

Classically, the Apgar score has been used both as an assessment of newborn condition and as a major criterion in defining newborn asphyxia. The Committee on Obstetric Practice of the American College of Obstetricians and Gynecologists (ACOG) and the Committee on Fetus and Newborn of the American Academy of Pediatrics have stated the use of this score as the definition of asphyxia is "use and abuse of the Apgar score" (ACOG, 1996). Asphyxia implies hypercarbia, hypoxemia, and metabolic acidemia, which obviously is not measured by the Apgar score. The two organizations have suggested that terms such as *hypoxia* and *acidemia* (metabolic or respiratory) be used instead (ACOG, 1996). Another obvious problem with the Apgar scoring system is that several of its components are subjective. Moreover, many different factors unrelated to asphyxia—for example, maternal anesthesia and medications, gestational age, congenital malformations, infection, and the person assigning the score—can affect the score. The Apgar score should be used for what it was designed for—a quick method of assessing the immediate condition of the newborn. The Apgar score, however, would also appear to be a good predictor of neonatal survival, especially in term newborns. For example, in a recent review of 132,228 live-born singleton infants at term, the risk of neonatal death was eight times greater with a low 5-minute Apgar score (0–3) than with a low umbilical artery pH (7.0 or lower) (Casey and colleagues, 2001).

Umbilical cord blood acid-base analysis provides a more objective method of evaluating a newborn's condition, especially with regard to hypoxia and acidemia (ACOG, 1995b). Umbilical cord blood pH has become an important adjunct in defining hypoxia, "proximate to delivery that is severe enough to result in acute neurologic injury" (ACOG, 1996). Moreover, the technique is simple and relatively inexpensive.

Technique

A segment of cord (~10–20 cm) should be doubly clamped immediately after delivery in all women in the event that cord blood analysis is desired or deemed necessary. The cord is clamped immediately because a delay as short as 20 seconds can significantly alter the arterial pH and PCO_2 (Lievaart and de Jong, 1984). Specimens for analysis should generally be obtained from the umbilical artery, not the umbilical vein. The umbilical artery contains blood returning from the fetus to the placenta and thus should provide the most useful information on the acid-base status of the fetus (ACOG, 1996). Moreover, in cases such as cord prolapse, the umbilical artery pH may be extremely low, even in the presence of a normal umbilical vein pH (Riley and Johnson, 1993). In spite of this, some clinicians still prefer to use the umbilical vein, which is easier to access for drawing blood, especially in the very premature infant. In one study of

TABLE 23-4. NORMAL UMBILICAL CORD BLOOD pH AND BLOOD GAS VALUES IN TERM NEWBORNS (MEAN ± SD)

	Yeomans et al., 1985 (*n* = 146)	Ramin et al., 1989 (*n* = 1292)	Riley and Johnson, 1993 (*n* = 3520)	Thorp et al., 1989 (*n* = 1924)
Arterial Blood				*(n = 1694)*
pH	7.28 (0.05)	7.28 (0.07)	7.27 (0.07)	7.24 (0.07)
PCO$_2$ (mm Hg)	49.20 (8.4)	49.90 (14.2)	50.30 (11.1)	56.30 (8.6)
HCO$_3^-$ (mEq/L)	22.30 (2.5)	23.10 (2.8)	22.00 (3.6)	24.10 (2.2)
Base excess (mEq/L)	—	– 3.60 (2.8)	– 2.70 (2.8)	– 3.60 (2.7)
Venous Blood				*(n = 1820)*
pH	7.35 (0.05)	—	7.34 (0.06)	7.32 (0.06)
PCO$_2$ (mm Hg)	38.20 (5.6)	—	40.70 (7.9)	43.80 (6.7)
HCO$_3^-$ (mEq/L)	20.40 (4.1)	—	21.40 (2.5)	22.60 (2.1)
Base excess (mEq/L)	—	—	– 2.40 (2.0)	2.90 (2.4)

453 term infants, D'Souza and colleagues (1983) reported that umbilical venous and arterial blood pH are significantly related to each other and that umbilical venous pH measurements do provide useful information regarding newborn acidemia at birth.

It is easy to draw a blood sample from the artery on the surface of the placenta if the physician encounters difficulty in obtaining a sample from the umbilical cord (Riley and Johnson, 1993). The arteries always cross over the vein on the surface on the placenta.

Samples should be drawn in plastic or glass syringes that have been flushed with heparin (1000 U/mL). Commercial syringes (1–2 mL) containing lyophilized heparin are also available for obtaining specimens. Kirshon and Moise (1989) reported that the addition of 0.2 mL of 10,000 U/mL of heparin with 0.2 mL of blood significantly decreased the pH, PCO$_2$, and bicarbonate. Thus, any residual heparin (as well as air) should be ejected, and the needle should be capped.

A few practical points merit mention. First, it is not necessary to draw the sample from the umbilical artery immediately as long as the cord is clamped. Adequate specimens have been obtained from a clamped segment of cord for up to 60 minutes after delivery without significant changes in pH or PCO$_2$ (Duerbeck et al., 1992). Moreover, once the specimens have been drawn into the syringe, they are relatively stable at room temperature for up to 60 minutes and do not need to be transported to the laboratory on ice (Strickland et al., 1984). The same may not be true for specimens obtained from placental vessels, and the deterioration in acid-base status is greater in smokers than in nonsmokers (Meyer et al., 1994).

Chauhan and colleagues (1994) have prepared a mathematical model that allows for the calculation of the umbilical artery pH for up to 60 hours after delivery. This model permits the estimation of fetal pH at birth.

Normal Values

Although there is no consensus as to what the most appropriate umbilical artery pH cutoff should be to define acidemia, the mean pH values from four studies are shown in Table 23-4. The mean value for umbilical artery pH appears to be very close to 7.28. The subjects in the study reported by Riley and Johnson (1993) were from 3522 unselected women undergoing vaginal delivery.

The mean pH for umbilical venous blood has been reported to be 7.32 to 7.35 (see Table 23-4). In a study of umbilical venous blood pH, D'Souza and associates (1983) reported a mean venous pH of 7.34 (±0.07). Huisjes and Aarnoudse (1979) also reported good correlation between umbilical venous and arterial pH.

Although the Apgar scores for premature infants may be low because of immaturity, mean values for both arterial and venous pH and blood gas values are similar to those of the term infant. Mean values for almost 2000 premature infants are summarized in Table 23-5.

Pathologic Fetal Acidemia

What level of umbilical artery pH should be considered abnormal, "pathologic," or clinically significant? It has now been well established that using the classic pH cutoff of less than 7.20 to define significant acidemia is not appropriate (Goldaber and Gilstrap, 1993; ACOG, 1995b). Most newborns with an umbilical artery pH below 7.20 are born vigorous and without evidence of hypoxia. Recent evidence suggests that significant neonatal morbidity is more likely to occur in neonates with umbilical artery pH values below 7.00, especially if they are associated with a low Apgar score (i.e., less than or equal to 3). For example, in a study of 2738 term newborns, hypotonia, seizures, and need for intubation were significantly correlated with an umbilical artery pH of less than 7.00 and an Apgar score of less than or equal to 3 at 1 minute (Gilstrap et al., 1989). The authors concluded that the newborn must be severely depressed at birth for birth hypoxia to be implicated as the cause of seizures.

TABLE 23-5. NORMAL ARTERY BLOOD GAS VALUES FOR PREMATURE INFANTS (MEAN ± SD)

	Dickenson et al., 1992 (*n* = 949)	Riley and Johnson, 1993 (*n* = 1015)
pH	7.27 (0.07)	7.28 (0.089)
PCO$_2$ (mm Hg)	51.60 (9.4)	50.20 (12.3)
HCO$_3^-$ (mEq/L)	23.90 (2.1)	22.40 (3.5)
Base excess (mEq/L)	– 3.00 (2.5)	– 2.50 (3.0)

Winkler and colleagues (1991) reported similar findings in a study of 358 term newborns with an umbilical artery pH of less than 7.20. The only two neonates in this study with morbidity consistent with hypoxia had an umbilical artery pH of less than 7.00 and low Apgar scores. Sehdev and colleagues (1997) in a study of 73 neonates with an umbilical artery pH of < 7.00 at birth, reported that high base deficits and low 5-minute Apgar scores were the best predictors of neonatal morbidity in these infants.

Goldaber and co-workers (1991), in an attempt to better define the critical cutoff for defining pathologic fetal acidemia, studied the neonatal outcome of 3506 term newborns. The critical pH cutoff, as determined in this study, was 7.00 (Table 23-6). Many of the babies in this latter study, however, had no complications and went to the newborn nursery. In a follow-up study from the same institution, King and associates (1998) reported on 35 term newborns with an umbilical artery pH of greater than 7.00 who were triaged to the newborn nursery. These authors concluded that term newborns with this degree of acidemia at birth but with stable appearance in the delivery room (and without other complications) do not have evidence of hypoxia or ischemia in the 48 hours after birth. It has been reported that less than half of neonates with an umbilical artery pH of less than 7.00 actually have neonatal complications (Sehdev et al., 1997). Thus, the critical pH cutoff for neonatal morbidity may actually be even lower than 7.00. Data presented by Andres and colleagues (1999) would suggest a pH cutoff closer to 6.90. In a review of 93 neonates (greater than 34 weeks' gestational age) with an umbilical artery pH of greater than 7.00, the median pH for the group was 6.92 (range 6.62 to 6.99); however, the median pH was 6.75 for neonates with seizures (25th to 75th percentile, 6.72–6.88) compared with 6.93 for those without seizures ($P = .02$). The median pH for newborns with hypoxic-ischemic encephalopathy was also significantly lower (6.69; 25th to 75th percentile, 6.62–6.75) than for those without this diagnosis (6.93; 25th to 75th percentile, 6.85–6.97; $P = .03$). The median pH was also less than 6.90 in newborns who required intubation (6.83) or cardiopulmonary resuscitation (6.83) and was significantly lower (P less than .05) than in newborns without these complications It should also be noted that the median PCO_2 and base deficit were significantly higher in neonates with these morbidities (Andres et al., 1999).

Acute Neurologic Injury

As previously suggested, there is poor correlation between neurologic outcome and the 1- and 5-minute Apgar scores. The correlation does improve when the scores remain at 0 to 3 at 10, 15, and 20 minutes; however, many such babies will still be "normal" if they survive. Similarly, a low umbilical artery pH in and of itself also has poor correlation with adverse outcome. Both the ACOG and The American Academy of Pediatrics (ACOG, 1996) have established the following criteria, which indicate hypoxia proximate to delivery severe enough to be associated with acute neurologic injury:

1. pH less than 7.00 with a metabolic component
2. An Apgar score of 0 to 3 for longer than 5 minutes
3. Seizures, coma, and hypotonia
4. Multiorgan system failure

TABLE 23-6. NEONATAL MORBIDITY AND MORTALITY ACCORDING TO pH CUTOFF

pH	Neonatal Deaths	Seizures	Both
7.15–7.19 ($n = 2236$)	3 (0.1%)	2 (0.1%)	1 (0.05%)
7.10–7.14 ($n = 798$)	3 (0.4%)	1 (0.1%)	0 (0.00%)
7.05–7.09 ($n = 290$)	0 (0.0%)	0 (0.0%)	1 (1.1%)
7.00–7.04 ($n = 95$)	1 (1.1%)	1 (1.1%)	1 (1.1%)
<7.00 ($n = 87$)	7 (8.0%)*	8 (9.2%)*	2 (2.3%)

* $P < .05$.

From Goldaber KG, Gilstrap LC, Leveno KJ, et al: Pathologic fetal acidemia. Obstet Gynecol 78:1103, 1991.

Many of these infants will not survive to manifest long-term neurologic sequelae. A characteristic umbilical artery blood gas profile seen in such infants is shown next:

- pH, 6.89
- PCO_2, 120 (mm Hg)
- HCO_3^-, 13 (mEq/L)
- Base excess, –22 (mm)

In two publications, Low and associates (1994, 1997) reported on the association of severe or significant metabolic acidosis (as determined by the umbilical artery blood gas profile) and newborn complications. Low (1997) proposed a classification of intrapartum fetal asphyxia, the severity of which is based on newborn encephalopathy and other organ system dysfunction.

OTHER CLINICAL EVENTS AND UMBILICAL BLOOD ACID-BASE ANALYSIS

Beyond its use in assessing prematurity and neurologic injury, umbilical blood gas analysis has been used in a variety of clinical situations, such as acute chorioamnionitis, nuchal cords, meconium, prolonged pregnancy, fetal heart rate anomalies, operative vaginal delivery, breech delivery, and use of oxytocin (Goldaber and Gilstrap, 1993). Such analysis may also prove useful in assessing the interval to delivery in shoulder dystocia cases.

Acute Chorioamnionitis

In one study of 123 women with acute chorioamnionitis compared with more than 6000 noninfected women, Maberry and co-authors (1990) found no significant association between infection and fetal acidemia (Table 23-7). Hankins and colleagues (1991) found no association between acute chorioamnionitis and newborn acidemia. Meyer and colleagues (1992) however, reported an association of fetal sepsis with a decrease in umbilical artery pH compared with controls (7.21 versus 7.26).

Nuchal Cords

In a study of 110 newborns with nuchal cords, Hankins and colleagues (1987) reported that significantly more newborns with nuchal cords were acidemic (U_A pH less than 7.20) compared with controls (20% versus 12%; P less than .05);

TABLE 23-7. COMPARISON OF UMBILICAL ARTERY (U_A) pH AND ACUTE CHORIOAMNIONITIS

U_A pH	Chorioa (n = 123) (%)	Controls (n = 6769) (%)
<7.20	18 (15.0)	701 (10.0)
<7.15	4 (3.0)	242 (4.0)
<7.00	0 —	6 (0.1)
Metabolic acidemia	1 (0.8)	9 (0.1)

From Maberry MC, Ramin SM, Gilstrap LC, et al: Intrapartum asphyxia in pregnancies complicated by intraamniotic infection. Obstet Gynecol **76:**351, 1990. Reprinted with permission from the American College of Obstetricians and Gynecologists.

however, there were no significant differences in mean pH (7.25 versus 7.27); PCO_2 (49 versus 48), or HCO_3^- (20.5 versus 21.0).

Meconium

In one study of 53 term pregnancies with moderate to thick meconium, Mitchell and colleagues (1985) reported that approximately half of the newborns were acidemic, and that significantly more acidemic newborns had meconium below the cords compared with controls (32% versus 0%; *P* less than .05). These authors, however, used an umbilical artery pH cutoff of less than 7.25 to define acidemia.

In another report of 323 newborns with meconium by Yeomans and associates (1989), there was a significantly increased frequency of meconium below the cords in acidemic fetuses than in nonacademic fetuses (31% versus 18%; *P* less than .05). Meconium aspiration syndrome, however, was an uncommon event, occurring in only 3% of newborns. Ramin and colleagues (1996), in a study of meconium, reported that 55% of meconium aspiration syndrome cases occurred in newborns with an umbilical artery pH of greater than 7.20.

In a review of 4985 term neonates born to mothers with meconium-stained amniotic fluid, Blackwell and colleagues (2001) identified 48 cases of severe meconium aspiration syndrome who had umbilical artery pH measurements. Of these, 29 had an umbilical artery pH of 7.20 or greater and 19 had a pH of less than 7.20. There was no difference in the frequency of seizures between the two pH groups. These authors concluded that severe meconium aspiration syndrome occurred in the presence of normal acid-base status at delivery in many of the cases, suggesting that a "preexisting injury or a nonhypoxic mechanism is often involved."

Prolonged Pregnancy

In a study of 108 women with a prolonged pregnancy, Silver and colleagues (1988) reported a mean U_A pH of 7.25. Moreover, significantly more newborns who were delivered for fetal heart rate indications had acidemia than newborns who were not (45% versus 13%; *P* less than .05).

Fetal Heart Rate Abnormalities

Gilstrap and colleagues (1984a), in a study of 403 term newborns with fetal heart rate abnormalities in the second stage of labor compared with 430 control newborns, reported

TABLE 23-8. ASSOCIATION OF UMBILICAL ARTERY (U_A) ACIDEMIA AND SECOND-STAGE FETAL HEART RATE ABNORMALITIES (N = 403) COMPARED WITH NORMALS (N = 430)

FHR Pattern	UA pH <7.20
Tachycardia*	15%
Mild bradycardia*	18%
Moderate/marked bradycardia*	27%
Normal	4%

* *P* < .05 compared to normal.

From Gilstrap LC, Hauth JC, Toussaint S: Second stage fetal heart rate abnormalities and neonatal acidosis. Obstet Gynecol **63:**209, 1984. Reprinted with permission from the American College of Obstetricians and Gynecologists.

an association of abnormalities and acidemia (Table 23-8). This was confirmed in a follow-up study (Gilstrap et al., 1987). Honjo and Yamaguchi (2001) also reported a correlation between second-stage baseline fetal heart rate abnormalities and fetal acidemia at birth. Although there may be an association between fetal heart rate abnormalities and acidemia, the association with adverse long-term neurologic outcome is uncommon. For example, Nelson and colleagues (1996), in a population-based study of children with cerebral palsy and a birth weight of 2500 g or more, reported that specific fetal heart rate abnormalities (i.e., late deceleration and decreased beat-to-beat variability) were associated with an increased risk of cerebral palsy. The children with cerebral palsy and these abnormal fetal heart rate findings, however, represented only 0.19% of infants with these abnormal heart rate findings. Thus, the false-positive rate was 99.8%.

Operative Vaginal Delivery

Gilstrap and co-workers (1984b) found no significant difference in the frequency of newborn acidemia according to the method of delivery (Table 23-9). This was true even when the indication for delivery was fetal distress.

Breech Delivery

Although the mean umbilical artery pH was lower for infants delivered vaginally in breech presentations compared with cephalic presentations in two studies (Luterkort and Marsaál, 1987; Christian and Brady, 1991), pH levels were not

TABLE 23-9. METHOD OF DELIVERY AND FETAL ACIDEMIA (U_A pH < 7.20)

Method of Delivery	Acidemia
Spontaneous (n = 303)	7%
Elective outlet/low forceps (n = 177)	9%
Indicated outlet/low forceps (n = 293)	18%
Indicated midforceps (n = 234)	21%
Cesarean delivery (n = 111)	18%

From Gilstrap LC, Hauth JC, Shiano S, et al: Neonatal acidosis and method of delivery. Obstet Gynecol **63:**681, 1984. Reprinted with permission from the American College of Obstetricians and Gynecologists.

significantly low from a clinical standpoint (7.23 and 7.16, respectively). It seems unlikely that delivery of the breech presentations by the vaginal route is related to significant newborn acidemia.

Shoulder Dystocia

Most adverse outcomes associated with shoulder dystocia are due to actual physical injury to the brachial plexus (Gherman and colleagues, 1998) and not to acidemia or asphyxia (unless extreme protracted periods of time are needed to extract the fetus). In a review of 134 infants born following shoulder dystocia, Stallings and colleagues (2001) reported that this complication was associated with a "statistically significant but clinically insignificant" reduction in mean umbilical artery pH levels compared to their obstetric population (7.23 versus 7.27).

Oxytocin

In a study of 556 women who received oxytocin compared with 704 who did not, Thorp and colleagues (1988) found no significant difference in mean umbilical artery pH measurements (7.23 versus 7.24, respectively).

OTHER METHODS TO DETERMINE ACID-BASE BALANCE IN THE FETUS

Several other techniques have been used to assess fetal-acid base status. These include the following:

1. Continuous tissue acid-base measurements in labor
2. Fetal pulse oximetry
3. Percutaneous umbilical blood sampling

Continuous Tissue Acid-Base Measurement in Labor

There have been several reports of continuous fetal tissue pH measurements in labor (Boos et al., 1978; Young et al., 1979; Young, 1981). Technical difficulties, however, relating mainly to attachment of the electrode to the fetal scalp, have inhibited the widespread acceptance of this method, although with experience satisfactory recording can be obtained in many cases (Antoine et al., 1982; Boos et al., 1978; Flynn and Kelly, 1980).

Pulse Oximetry

Pulse oximetry has proved to be a most useful tool for assessing oxygenation in both adults and children. New technology has been developed for intrapartum fetal pulse oximetry. The device consists of a sensor that is placed transvaginally alongside the fetal face. Dildy and colleagues (1994) have evaluated this method during labor and its relation to newborn outcome. Both the device and its clinical efficacy are under investigation in several centers. One of the major technical problems encountered thus far is the inability to obtain reliable signal data 50% of the time (Jongsma et al., 1996). In the French Study Group on Fetal Pulse Oximetry, Goffinet and colleagues (1997) reported a mean reliable signal 65% of the time during the first stage of labor. It was also noted that physicians found it easy to place the sensor in 88% of cases compared with fetal blood sampling, which was felt to be easy in 79% of cases. These authors reported a mean fetal oxygen saturation of 42.2% (30% to 53% for the 10th to 90th percentile range) during the first stage of labor. A significant association was found between an oxygen saturation of less than 30% and poor newborn status.

Bloom and colleagues (1999), in a study of fetal pulse oximetry in 129 fetuses, reported that 53% of fetuses had at least one episode of oxygen saturation of less than 30% and that most of these fetuses had a normal outcome. There was, however, a significant increase in fetal compromise when the oxygen saturation fell below 30% for 2 minutes or longer.

In a multicenter trial conducted in nine centers, Garite and colleagues (2000) randomized 502 women to electronic fetal heart monitoring alone (controls) and 508 to electronic monitoring in combination with continuous fetal pulse oximetry (study group). These authors reported a reduction in the cesarean delivery rate for nonreassuring fetal heart rates in the pulse oximetry group (10.2% to 4.5%). Cesarean delivery was performed for "fetal distress" when the pulse oximetry values were less than 30% for the interval between two contractions; however, there was an increase in the cesarean delivery rate in the pulse oximetry group for dystocia (19% versus 9%). Thus, there was no significant difference in the overall cesarean delivery rates between the control group and the study group (26% versus 29%; P = .49).

In a recent study comparing fetal oxygen saturation obtained by pulse oximetry to that obtained by hemoximeter from fetal scalp blood sampling, Luttkus and colleagues (2002) reported good correlation between the two methods in acidemic fetuses (pH less than or equal to 7.16 and base excess less than or equal to –9.4 mmol/L). However, the authors also reported that compared with hemoximeter values, pulse oximetry tends to overestimate oxygen saturation.

In an update on fetal pulse oximetry, East and colleagues (2002) have aptly pointed out that this technique should not be used as the sole basis of fetal assessment and that the whole clinical picture must be considered. These authors also pointed out the ease of placing the sensor and that a randomized, multicenter clinical trial was underway in Australia. It should also be noted that the centers in the NICHD Maternal-Fetal Medicine Units Network are currently conducting a randomized clinical trial on the efficacy of pulse oximetry.

The Committee on Obstetric Practice of the American College of Obstetrician and Gynecologists (2001) has stated that it "cannot endorse the adoption of this device in clinical practice at this time because of concerns that its introduction could further escalate the cost of medical care without necessarily improving clinical outcome." This committee also calls for the study of this technology via randomized clinical trial.

Percutaneous Umbilical Blood Sampling

Fetal acid-base status can also be assessed during the antepartum period by insertion of a needle, under ultrasound control, into the umbilical artery or vein (cordocentesis) (see Chapter 21).

■ SUMMARY

The fetus maintains its pH in very limited ranges and is dependent on the placenta and the maternal circulation to maintain acid-base balance. Several methods for assessing fetal-newborn acid-base status have been described. Of these methods, umbilical blood gas analysis is probably the most useful and the easiest (and relatively the least expensive) to perform. Fetal pulse oximetry is a relatively new and promising technique that may allow for a method of continuous assessment of fetal oxygenation and acid-base status. Several randomized clinical trials regarding the efficacy of this technique are underway. The authors of one randomized clinical trial did find a decrease in cesarean delivery for nonreassuring fetal status with the use of pulse oximetry (Garite et al., 2000).

Should all newborns have umbilical blood gas analysis? There are few data to justify such a policy. In a survey of 133 universities in the United States, Johnson and Riley (1993) reported that approximately 27% of centers used cord blood for assessing newborn acid-base status in all deliveries. Two-thirds of the programs used them for tracing abnormal fetal heart rate or for low Apgar scores. The Royal College of Obstetricians and Gynecologists and the Royal College of Midwives (1999) recommend routine cord blood measurements for all cesarean deliveries and instrumental deliveries for fetal distress. They also state that "consideration should be given to measurement of cord gases following all deliveries." In a survey of 215 obstetric units in the United Kingdom, Waugh and colleagues (2001) reported that 181 (84%) units currently sampled cord blood gases but that 160 (74%) did so selectively. Interestingly, 54% performed both arterial and venous blood analysis and 54% performed a full blood gas analysis. Some clinicians recommend routine umbilical cord blood sampling for pH and blood gas analysis in all deliveries; others recommend sampling only in select cases. A protocol for select sampling is as follows:

1. *Double-clamp a segment of umbilical cord immediately after delivery on all births.*
2. *In a term newborn who is vigorous and crying and with a normal 5-minute Apgar score, discard the specimen.*
3. *Obtain umbilical artery blood (or blood from the surface of the placenta) in the following situations:*
   a. *All premature newborns*
   b. *Meconium-stained amniotic fluid*
   c. *Operative vaginal or abdominal delivery for nonreassuring fetal heart rate pattern*
   d. *Term newborns who are depressed at birth or who have 5-minute Apgar scores below 7*

REFERENCES

Aarnoudse JG, Deesley NP, Penfold P, et al: Permeability of the human placenta to bicarbonate: In vitro perfusion studies. Br J Obstet Gynaecol **91**:1096, 1984.

American College of Obstetricians and Gynecologists (ACOG): Fetal heart rate patterns: Monitoring, interpretations, and management. Technical Bulletin No. 207, July 1995a.

American College of Obstetricians and Gynecologists (ACOG): Umbilical artery blood acid-base analysis. Technical Bulletin No. 216, November 1995b.

American College of Obstetricians and Gynecologists (ACOG): Fetal pulse oximetry. Committee Opinion No. 258, September 2001.

American College of Obstetricians and Gynecologists (ACOG) Committee on Obstetric Practice: Use and abuse of the Apgar score. No. 174, July 1996.

Andres RL, Saade MD, Gilstrap LC, et al: Association between umbilical blood gas parameters and neonatal morbidity and death in neonates with pathologic fetal acidemia. Am J Obstet Gynecol **181**:867, 1999.

Antoine C, Silverman F, Young B: Current status of continuous fetal pH monitoring. Clin Perinatol **9**:409, 1982.

Blackwell SC, Moldenhauer J, Hassan SS, et al: Meconium aspiration syndrome in term neonates with normal acid-base status at delivery: is it different? Am J Obstet Gynecol **184**:1422, 2001.

Blechner JN: Maternal-fetal acid-base physiology. Clin Obstet Gynecol **36**:3, 1993.

Bloom SL, Swindle RG, McIntire DD, et al: Fetal pulse oximetry: Duration of desaturation and intrapartum outcome. Obstet Gynecol **93**:1036, 1999.

Boos R, Ruttgers H, Muliawan D, et al: Continuous measurement of tissue pH in the human fetus. Arch Gynecol **226**:183, 1978.

Casey BM, McIntire DD, Leveno KJ: The continuing value of the Apgar score for the assessment of newborn infants. N Engl J Med **344**:467, 2001.

Chauhan SP, Cowan BD, Meydrech EF, et al: Determination of fetal acidemia at birth from a remote umbilical arterial blood gas analysis. Am J Obstet Gynecol **170**:1705, 1994.

Christian SS, Brady K: Cord blood acid-base values in breech-presenting infants born vaginally. Obstet Gynecol **78**:778, 1991.

Clark SL, Gimovsky ML, Miller FC: The scalp stimulation test: A clinical alternative to fetal scalp blood sampling. Am J Obstet Gynecol **148**:274, 1984.

Clark SL, Paul RH: Intrapartum fetal surveillance: The role of fetal scalp blood sampling. Am J Obstet Gynecol **153**:717, 1985.

Coleman MT, Rund DA: Nonobstetric conditions causing hypoxia during pregnancy: Asthma and epilepsy. Am J Obstet Gynecol **177**:1, 1997.

Cunningham FGC, Gant NF, Leveno KJ, et al: The newborn infant. In Williams Obstetrics, 21st ed. New York, McGraw-Hill, 2001, p. 385.

Dickinson JE, Eriksen NL, Meyer BA, et al: The effect of preterm birth on umbilical cord blood gases. Obstet Gynecol **79**:575, 1992.

Dildy GA, van den Berg PP, Katz M, et al: Intrapartum fetal pulse oximetry: Fetal oxygen saturation trends during labor and relation to delivery outcome. Am J Obstet Gynecol **171**:679, 1994.

D'Souza SW, Black P, Cadman J, et al: Umbilical venous blood pH: A useful aid in the diagnosis of asphyxia at birth. Arch Dis Child **58**:15, 1983.

Duerbeck NB, Chaffin DG, Seeds JW: A practical approach to umbilical artery pH and blood gas determinations. Obstet Gynecol **79**:959, 1992.

East CE, Colditz PB, Begg LM, et al: Update on intrapartum on fetal pulse oximetry. Aust N Z J Obstet Gynaecol **42**:119, 2002.

Flynn AM, Kelly J: The continuous measurement of tissue pH in the human fetus during labour using a new application technique. Br J Obstet Gynaecol **87**:666, 1980.

Garite TJ, Dildy GA, McNamara H, et al: A multicenter controlled trial of fetal pulse oximetry in the intrapartum management of nonreassuring fetal heart rate patterns. Am J Obstet Gynecol **183**:1049, 2000.

Gherman RB, Ouzounian JG, Goodwin TM: Obstetric maneuvers for shoulder dystocia and associated fetal morbidity. Am J Obstet Gynecol **178**:1126, 1998.

Gilstrap LC, Hauth JC, Hankins GD, et al: Second-stage fetal heart rate abnormalities and type of neonatal acidemia. Obstet Gynecol **70**:191, 1987.

Gilstrap LC, Hauth JC, Schiano S, et al: Neonatal acidosis and method of delivery. Obstet Gynecol **63**:681, 1984.

Gilstrap LC, Hauth JC, Toussaint S: Second stage fetal heart rate abnormalities and neonatal acidosis. Obstet Gynecol **63**:209, 1984.

Gilstrap LC, Leveno KJ, Burris JB, et al: Diagnoses of birth asphyxia based on fetal pH, Apgar score and newborn cerebral dysfunction. Am J Obstet Gynecol **161**:825, 1989.

Goffinet F, Langer B, Carbonne B, et al: Multicenter study on the clinical value of fetal pulse oximetry. I. Methodologic evaluation. The French Study Group on Fetal Pulse Oximetry. Am J Obstet Gynecol **177**:1238, 1997.

Goldaber KG, Gilstrap LC III: Correlations between obstetric clinical events and umbilical cord acid-base and blood gas values. Clin Obstet Gynecol **36**:47, 1993.

Goldaber KG, Gilstrap LC, Leveno KJ, et al: Pathologic fetal acidemia. Obstet Gynecol **78**:1103, 1991.

Goodwin TM, Milner-Masterson L, Paul RH: Elimination of fetal scalp blood sampling on a large clinical service. Obstet Gynecol **83**:971, 1994.

Grant A: The Dublin randomized controlled trial of intrapartum fetal heart rate monitoring. D.M. Thesis. Oxford, England, University of Oxford, 1985.

Hankins GDV, Snyder RR, Hauth JC, et al: Nuchal cords and neonatal outcome. Obstet Gynecol **70**:687, 1987.

Hankins GDV, Snyder RR, Yeomans ER: Umbilical arterial and venous acid-base and blood gas values and the effect of chorioamnionitis on those values in a cohort of preterm infants. Am J Obstet Gynecol **164**:1261, 1991.

Honjo S, Yamaguchi M: Umbilical artery blood acid-base analysis and fetal heart rate baseline in the second stage of labor. J Obstet Gynaecol Res 27:249, 2001.

Huff RW: Asthma in pregnancy. Med Clin North Am 73:653, 1989.

Huisjes HJ, Aarnoudse JG: Arterial or venous umbilical pH as a measure of neonatal morbidity? Early Hum Dev 3:155, 1979.

James EJ, Raye JR, Gresham EL, et al: Fetal oxygen consumption, carbon dioxide production and glucose uptake in a chronic sheep preparation. Pediatrics 50:361, 1972.

Johnson JWC, Riley W: Cord blood gas studies: A survey. Clin Obstet Gynecol 36:99, 1993.

Jongsma HW, van den Berg PP, Menssen JJM, et al: The validity of intrapartum pulse oximetry: A quantitative analysis. Am J Obstet Gynecol 174:492, 1996.

King TA, Jackson GL, Josey AS, et al:The effect of profound umbilical artery acidemia in term neonates admitted to a newborn nursery. J Pediatr 132:624, 1998.

Kirshon B, Moise KJ: Effect of heparin on umbilical arterial blood gases. J Reprod Med 34:267, 1989.

Landon MB: Acid-base disorders during pregnancy. Clin Obstet Gynecol 37:16, 1994.

Ledger WJ: Complications associated with invasive monitoring. Semin Perinatol 2:187, 1978.

Lievaart M, de Jong PA: Acid-base equilibrium in umbilical cord blood and time of cord clamping. Obstet Gynecol 63:44, 1984.

Lin CC, Vassallo B, Mittendorf R. Is intrapartum vibroacoustic stimulation an effective predictor of fetal acidosis? J Perinat Med 29:506, 2001.

Low JA: Intrapartum fetal asphyxia: Definition, diagnosis, and classification. Am J Obstet Gynecol 176:957, 1997.

Low JA, Panagiotopoulos C, Derrick EJ, et al: Newborn complications after intrapartum asphyxia with metabolic acidosis in the term fetus. Am J Obstet Gynecol 170:1081, 1994.

Low JA, Pickersgill H, Killen H, et al. The prediction and prevention of intrapartum fetal asphyxia in term pregnancies. Am J Obstet Gynecol 184:724, 2001.

Luterkort M, Marsaál K: Umbilical cord acid-base state and Apgar score in term breech neonates. Acta Obstet Gynecol Scand 66:57, 1987.

Luttkus AK, Lubke M, Buscher U, et al: Accuracy of fetal pulse oximetry. Acta Obstet Gynecol Scand 81:417, 2002.

Maberry MC, Ramin SM, Gilstrap LC, et al: Intrapartum asphyxia in pregnancies complicated by intraamniotic infection. Obstet Gynecol 76:351, 1990.

Meyer BA, Dickinson JE, Chamber C, et al: The effect of fetal sepsis on umbilical cord blood gases. Am J Obstet Gynecol 166:612, 1992.

Meyer BA, Thorp JA, Cohen GR, et al: Umbilical cord blood gases: The effect of smoking on delayed sampling from the placenta (abstr No. 158). Am J Obstet Gynecol 170:320, 1994.

Mitchell J, Schulman H, Fleischer A, et al: Meconium aspiration and fetal acidosis. Obstet Gynecol 65:352, 1985.

Mondanlou HD, Linzey EM: An unusual complication of fetal blood sampling during labor. Obstet Gynecol 51:7s, 1978.

Nelson KB, Dambrosia JM, Ting TY, et al: Uncertain value of electronic fetal monitoring in predicting cerebral palsy. N Engl J Med 334:613, 1996.

Paul RH, Suidan AK, Yeh SY, et al: Clinical fetal monitoring: VII. The evaluation and significance of intrapartum baseline fetal heart rate variability. Am J Obstet Gynecol 123:206, 1975.

Ramin KD, Leveno KJ, Kelly MA, et al. Amniotic fluid meconium: a fetal environmental hazard. Obstet Gynecol 87:181, 1996

Ramin SM, Gilstrap LC, Leveno KJ, et al: Umbilical artery acid–base status in the preterm infant. Obstet Gynecol 74:256, 1989.

Riley RJ, Johnson JWC: Collecting and analyzing cord blood gases. Clin Obstet Gynecol 36:13, 1993.

Royal College of Obstetricians and Gynaecologists, Royal College of Midwives: Toward safer childbirth. Minimum standards for the organization of labour wards. Report of a joint working party. London: RCOG Press, 1999, p. 22.

Saling E, Schneider D: Biochemical supervision of the foetus during labour. J Obstet Gynaecol Br Commonw 74:799, 1967.

Sehdev HM, Stamilio DM, Macones GA, et al: Predictive factors for neonatal morbidity in neonates with an umbilical arterial pH less than 7.00. Am J Obstet Gynecol 177:1030, 1997.

Silver RK, Dooley SL, MacGregor SN, et al: Fetal acidosis in prolonged pregnancy cannot be attributed to cord compression alone. Am J Obstet Gynecol 159:666, 1988.

Skupski DW, Rosenberg CR, Eglinton GS. Intrapartum fetal stimulation tests: a meta-analysis. Obstet Gynecol 99:129, 2002.

Smith CV, Nguyen HN, Phelan JP, et al: Intrapartum assessment of fetal wellbeing: A comparison of fetal acoustic stimulation with acid-base determinations. Am J Obstet Gynecol 155:726, 1986.

Spencer JA: Predictive value of a fetal heart rate acceleration at the time of fetal blood sampling in labour. J Perinat Med 19:207, 1991.

Stallings SP, Edwards RK, Johnson JW. Correlation of head-to-body delivery intervals in shoulder dystocia and umbilical artery acidosis. Am J Obstet Gynecol 185:268, 2001.

Strickland DM, Gilstrap LC III, Hauth JC, et al: Umbilical cord pH and PCO_2: Effect of interval from delivery to determination. Am J Obstet Gynecol 148:191, 1984.

Thorp JA, Boylan PC, Parisi VM, et al: Effects of high-dose oxytocin augmentation on umbilical cord blood gas values in primigravid women. Am J Obstet Gynecol 159:670, 1988.

Thorp JA, Sampson JE, Parisi VM, et al: Routine umbilical cord blood gas determinations? Am J Obstet Gynecol 161:600, 1989.

Visser GHA, Sadovsky G, Nicolaides KH: Antepartum heart rate patterns in small-for-gestational-age third-trimester fetuses: Correlations with blood gas values obtained at cordocentesis. Am J Obstet Gynecol 162:698, 1990.

Waugh J, Johnson A, Farkas A: Analysis of cord blood gas at delivery: questionnaire study of practice in the United Kingdom. BMJ 323:727, 2001

Westgren M, Holmqvist P, Ingemarsson I, et al: Intrapartum fetal acidosis in preterm infants: Fetal monitoring and long-term morbidity. Obstet Gynecol 63:355, 1984.

Winkler CL, Hauth JC, Tucker JM, et al: Neonatal complications at term as related to the degree of umbilical artery acidemia. Am J Obstet Gynecol 164:637, 1991.

Yeomans ER, Gilstrap LC, Leveno KL, et al: Meconium in the amniotic fluid and fetal acid-base status. Obstet Gynecol 73:175, 1989.

Yeomans ER, Hauth JC, Gilstrap LC, et al: Umbilical cord pH, PCO_2 and bicarbonate following uncomplicated term vaginal deliveries. Am J Obstet Gynecol 151:798, 1985.

Young BK: Continuous fetal tissue pH monitoring in labor. J Perinat Med 9:189, 1981.

Young BK, Katz M, Klein SA: The relationship of heart rate patterns and tissue pH in the human fetus. Am J Obstet Gynecol 134:685, 1979.

Young DC, Gray JH, Luther ER, et al: Fetal scalp blood pH sampling: Its value in an active obstetric unit. Am J Obstet Gynecol 136:276, 1980.

Zalar RW, Quilligan EJ: The influence of scalp sampling on the cesarean section rate for fetal distress. Am J Obstet Gynecol 135:239, 1979.

Chapter 24

SIGNIFICANCE OF AMNIOTIC FLUID MECONIUM

J. Christopher Glantz, MD, MPH, and James R. Woods Jr., MD

Meconium is a term derived from the Greek *mekonion*, a word for poppy juice or opium. Aristotle is credited with having drawn the analogy between the presence of this substance in the amniotic fluid and the "sleepy" newborn. Although meconium may not be the most glamorous subject in maternal-fetal medicine, its significance and management continue to be topics of controversy and debate. Meconium-stained amniotic fluid has been associated with adverse perinatal outcome, but it is common in fetuses without apparent compromise.

Management recommendations for deliveries complicated by meconium range from amnioinfusion and aggressive neonatal suctioning to no intervention. Some authors have questioned whether *meconium aspiration syndrome* (MAS) even requires the presence of meconium or whether meconium is merely a marker for a previous asphyxic event. This chapter deals with the controversies regarding the clinical significance of meconium in the amniotic fluid.

FORMATION AND COMPOSITION OF MECONIUM

The gastrointestinal tract originates from both endoderm and splanchnic mesoderm by day 14 after fertilization and is lined by undifferentiated cuboidal cells by day 18 (Arey, 1974; Grand et al., 1976). Intestinal villi appear by 7 weeks, and active absorption of glucose and amino acids occurs at 10 weeks and 12 weeks, respectively. By 12 weeks' gestation, development of Meissner's and Auerbach's plexuses within the intestinal wall coincides with onset of peristalsis of the small intestine and colon. Meconium appears in the fetal intestine at approximately 70–85 days' gestation (Smith, 1976). High concentrations of intestinal enzymes are present in amniotic fluid early in gestation, followed by a decline that could be related to increased anal sphincter tone (Potier et al., 1978; Mulivor et al., 1979). Enzyme concentrations are lower when the anus is imperforate, implicating the lower intestinal tract as the portal of exit. The fetus swallows increasing amounts of amniotic fluid as pregnancy progresses (Pritchard, 1966), which may account in part for the clearance of meconium released into amniotic fluid (Kimble et al., 1999). Fetuses with impaired swallowing (e.g., esophageal atresia), however, do not necessarily have increased frequencies of meconium. Meconium clearance is incompletely understood and could be multifactorial.

Meconium is composed primarily of water (72%–80%). Large concentrations of bile pigments excreted by the biliary tract from the fourth month onward give meconium its green color. The principal components of term fetal meconium are listed in Table 24-1. The fetus lacks intestinal bacteria, which accounts for many of the differences in composition between meconium and adult stool.

MECONIUM IN AMNIOTIC FLUID

Physical Characteristics of Meconium

The degree to which tissues stain when exposed to meconium depends on the following:

1. Meconium concentration
2. Length of exposure
3. The nature of the exposed tissue

Vernix suspended in meconium stains yellow in 12–14 hours. Newborn fingernails stain yellow in 4–6 hours (Desmond et al., 1956). Miller and associates (1985) exposed placentas *in vitro* to meconium in varying concentrations and durations of exposure. Within 1 hour, surface staining was observed and was found to be proportional to the length of exposure and concentration of meconium. Pigment accumulation in macrophages within the placenta depended on length of exposure only, but it was visible in all placentas by 3 hours. Umbilical cord staining occurred at 1 hour with 5% meconium and at 15 minutes with 10% meconium. This information can be important postpartum in determining how long meconium has been present, especially in cases of meconium aspiration. Meconium in pulmonary macrophages suggests antepartum *in utero* aspiration.

Meconium could have direct vasoconstrictive effects on the umbilical vein that result in vasospasm and impaired fetal-placental blood flow (Altshuler and Hyde, 1989). In addition, meconium present for more than 16 hours occasionally induces umbilical cord ulceration and vascular necrosis, potentially compromising fetal oxygenation (Altshuler et al., 1992). These effects may be due to bile acids present in meconium, although the complex composition of meconium makes precise definition difficult.

Meconium concentrations exceeding 1% enhance the ability of amniotic fluid to sustain bacterial growth (Florman and Tuebner, 1969). The mechanism is uncertain; meconium

TABLE 24-1. COMPOSITION OF TERM FETAL MECONIUM

Cholesterol and sterol precursors	Lipid
Blood group substances	Bile acids and salts
Water	Enzymes
Mucopolysaccharides	Blood group substances
Cholesterol and sterol precursors	Squamous cells
Protein	Vernix caseosa

inhibits neutrophils in some reports (Clark and Duff, 1995) but activates them in others (Matsubara et al., 1999). Alterations in zinc concentrations related to meconium could favor bacterial growth (Hoskins et al., 1987; Usta et al., 2000). Several authors have reported increased rates of chorioamnionitis when amniotic fluid contains meconium (Romero et al., 1991; Mazor et al., 1995; Usta, Mercer, Sibai, 1995).

Meconium and Pulmonary Maturity Testing

The degree of influence of amniotic fluid meconium contamination on fetal maturity testing remains uncertain. Compounding the confusion are the multiple laboratory methods used to determine maturity, such as the lecithin-sphingomyelin (L/S) ratio and the phosphatidylglycerol (PG) level (Freer and Statland, 1981; Parker, 1981). The lecithin-sphingomyelin ratio is reported to increase (Kulkarni et al., 1972; Wagstaff et al., 1974) or decrease (Buhi and Spellacy, 1975) when meconium is added to amniotic fluid samples. Hill and Ellefson (1983) and Longo and associates (1998) reported that meconium has a variable and unpredictable effect on the lecithin-sphingomyelin ratio. Meconium could interfere with lipid extraction or contain moieties that migrate similarly to lecithin or sphingomyelin, confounding interpretation of results. Tabsch and coworkers (1981) concluded that, in the presence of meconium, lecithin-sphingomyelin ratios of less than 2.2 in the premature fetus (<35 weeks) or less than 2.5 in the fluid of term fetuses should not be considered "mature."

Phosphatidylglycerol analysis using thin-layer chromatography can be difficult, if not impossible, with heavily stained amniotic fluid. Phosphatidylglycerol determination, however, may be reliable in lightly stained amniotic fluid if the precipitated spot representing phosphatidylglycerol can be discerned adequately (Schmidt-Sommerfeld et al., 1982; Tsao and Zachman, 1982; Hill and Ellefson, 1983; Yambao et al., 1984). Phosphatidylglycerol values determined by immunologic (agglutination) techniques may be unaffected by meconium (Towers and Garite, 1989).

Such conflicting results suggest that one must take caution in interpreting fetal lung maturity tests from meconium-contaminated amniotic fluid, particularly in the case of the lecithin-sphingomyelin ratio.

Ultrasonographic Detection of Meconium-Stained Amniotic Fluid

Amniotic fluid that appears echogenic or particulate during sonography has been reported as consistent with *in utero* passage of meconium (Benacerraf et al., 1984). Unfortunately, vernix also could have this appearance (Hill and Breckle, 1986). In a small series, the positive predictive value of echogenic fluid on sonography for the antenatal detection of meconium was only 10% (Sherer et al., 1991). This is similar to the reported frequency of meconium at delivery and thus is equal to chance. Because this sonographic finding is not specific for meconium, it cannot be applied to management decisions.

Theories of Meconium Passage

In the adult, the processes of intestinal peristalsis and defecation are a complex interaction of hormonal, myogenic, and neurogenic factors (Davenport, 1971). Bowel activity is controlled primarily by local reflexes acting through intramural neural plexuses, but extrinsic innervation can modify intrinsic reflex activity. Stimulation of sympathetic innervation to the rectum inhibits rectal activity while causing constriction of the internal anal sphincter. Parasympathetic activity increases motor activity in the rectum while inhibiting constriction of the internal anal sphincter. The principal stimulus for peristalsis is increased intraluminal pressure and radial stretching of the bowel, which in turn activates two distinct neural pathways to produce contraction waves (Hirst, 1979). These descending contraction waves, which involve the longitudinal and circular muscles of the bowel, act through cholinergic excitation. Our knowledge of the mechanisms of bowel peristalsis and meconium passage in the fetus is not nearly as substantive as in the adult, but the mechanisms are assumed to be similar.

Maturation Theory

Because meconium seldom is observed preterm (Scott et al., 2001), its presence in amniotic fluid could reflect gastrointestinal maturity in late gestation (Matthews and Warshaw, 1979). Becker and coworkers (1940) first observed that meconium-stained amniotic fluid is a natural occurrence in certain species late in pregnancy. In these early experiments, researchers injected radiopaque dye into the amniotic cavity of pregnant guinea pigs in midgestation and took sequential radiographs until term. A progressive decrease occurred in the time the dye took to reach the small intestine. Many healthy fetuses routinely passed dye into the amniotic fluid in the last week of gestation, and some fetuses cleared the dye from the amniotic fluid by swallowing.

Transit time through the fetal small intestine decreases as gestation advances (McLain, 1963). Prolonged transit time in the preterm fetus has been attributed to poor gut musculature, but because peristalsis begins at 11–12 weeks in the human, this explanation seems unlikely. Immaturity of intrinsic and extrinsic innervation of the bowel could impair the ability of the premature fetus to pass meconium into the amniotic fluid. At autopsy, preterm neonates have more unmyelinated nerve trunks and fewer ganglion cells in the distal colon compared with term neonates. Furthermore, as the fetus matures, the intestinal tract becomes more responsive to sympathomimetic agents (Grand et al., 1976).

Fenton and Steer (1962) suggested that meconium passage is a normal maturational phenomenon that occurs before delivery in some fetuses. Although these maturational events do not explain why meconium is passed into the amniotic fluid by one fetus and not by another, they must be considered an integral part of this process.

Theory of Fetal Distress

The relationship of fetal hypoxia and intestinal peristalsis has been a consideration for many years. Fetal guinea pigs exposed to maternal hypoxia swallow more rapidly but manifest no significant increase in gastrointestinal motility (Becker et al., 1940). Moreover, brief episodes of maternal hypoxia failed to alter intestinal peristalsis in monkey fetuses (Speert, 1943). Walker (1954), however, demonstrated that meconium was released more frequently when the oxygen saturation of the umbilical vein was below 30% and that heavy meconium is associated with lower oxygen saturation more often than is light meconium. Hon (1963) suggested that meconium is passed in response to parasympathetic stimulation during cord compression, but Krebs and associates (1980) found no difference in the frequency of variable decelerations regardless of whether meconium was present. In fetal lambs, long-term single umbilical artery ligation causes passage of meconium only after significant chronic fetal wasting has occurred (Emmanouilides et al., 1968), a phenomenon analogous to chronic intrauterine stress and meconium passage in the severely dysmature human fetus. Umbilical cord erythropoietin concentrations are elevated in human pregnancies complicated by meconium-stained amniotic fluid, suggesting an association between chronic hypoxemia and meconium passage (Richey et al., 1995; Manchanda et al., 1999; Jazayeri et al., 2000). Manning and coworkers (1990) reported that amniotic fluid meconium was present more than twice as often if the last biophysical profile score was abnormal (6 or less) as opposed to normal (8 or 10). When scores were abnormal, however, there was no increase in meconium incidence with progressively lower biophysical profile scores. Interestingly, Ciftci and colleagues (1999) reported that in fetal rabbits, hypoxia impaired meconium clearance but had no effect on intestinal transport and defecation. Our understanding of the relationship of meconium passage to fetal distress is incomplete, and many deliveries complicated by fetal meconium passage are otherwise unremarkable.

Incidence, Associations, and Perinatal Outcome

Second-Trimester Passage of Meconium

The interpretation of "meconium-stained" amniotic fluid in the second trimester of pregnancy has become an issue as data emerge from large series of patients undergoing amniocentesis for genetic counseling. Discolored amniotic fluid is encountered in approximately 2% of genetic amniocenteses (Karp and Schiller, 1977; King et al., 1978; Svigos et al., 1981; Allen, 1985). In these reports, aggregate perinatal outcome was favorable in more than 90% of patients with discolored midtrimester amniotic fluid. In Allen's study (1985), there was no correlation between the degree of staining of fluid and fetal outcome, because all cases of heavy staining were associated with a normal birth. In addition, most patients with stained fluid during amniocentesis in this study had clear fluid by the time of delivery, indicating the transient nature of midtrimester discoloration.

A major problem in all studies of discolored second-trimester amniotic fluid is the inability of the clinician to distinguish meconium staining from blood pigment staining. Francoual and colleagues (1986) analyzed 78 amniotic samples in the third trimester by measuring both total hemoglobin and coproporphyrin concentrations, representing blood and meconium contamination, respectively. They found that simple visual observation by the obstetrician was not sufficient to distinguish meconium from old blood. Of 33 samples judged visually to be meconium-stained, only five were contaminated solely with meconium. Golbus and associates (1979), Legge (1981), Hankins and coworkers (1984), and Zorn and colleagues (1986) concluded that brown amniotic fluid from the second trimester nearly always was secondary to the presence of hemoglobin rather than meconium, suggesting intraamniotic hemorrhage. Hankins and associates (1984) reported no differences between the study group and matched controls in the incidence of spontaneous abortions, abnormal fetal karyotypes or anomalies, preterm labor, or cesarean section, whereas Zorn and coworkers (1986) reported a 9% spontaneous abortion rate in pregnancies complicated by stained fluid as opposed to a 1.6% miscarriage rate for the entire amniocentesis group. Of the women with discolored fluid in the latter report, 62% gave a history of bleeding prior to undergoing amniocentesis.

The composite conclusions from these studies suggest that green-stained or brown-stained second-trimester amniotic fluid usually contains degraded blood pigments rather than meconium. Accurate distinction requires biochemical or spectrophotometric analysis for hemoglobin or coproporphyrin. Even this exercise may be academic, because most of these pregnancies involving discolored fluid ultimately continue to term without significant morbidity or mortality, and the amniotic fluid often is cleared of the abnormal pigment.

Third-Trimester Passage of Meconium

With the use of third-trimester amnioscopy or amniocentesis, the incidence of antepartum meconium-stained amniotic fluid varies from 2% to 11%. Using amnioscopy, Lee (1972) documented meconium in 10% of 720 high-risk patients. Active intervention in the presence of meconium-stained amniotic fluid produced a perinatal mortality rate of four per 1000; for the population as a whole, the rate was 19 per 1000.

Mandelbaum (1973), employing serial amniocentesis in 272 patients during the last 10 weeks of gestation, detected antepartum meconium in 11% of patients, often in those with hypertensive conditions. He recommended active intervention because 26% of babies in this high-risk group died *in utero* and 42% had neonatal complications. Kaspar and colleagues (2000) reported that chronic meconium staining was associated with worse outcomes than was acute passage.

In another report of weekly amnioscopic examination of 508 patients, meconium was diagnosed infrequently before labor (2.2%) and by itself was not associated with low Apgar scores or fetal acidosis at delivery (Saldana et al., 1976). Once antepartum meconium is detected, proper management of the high-risk patient is controversial; however, it is apparent that the fetus should undergo additional antepartum evaluation if meconium is detected and delivery is not imminent.

Intrapartum Meconium

The approximate incidence of meconium at delivery at term is between 7% and 22%, although it approaches 40% in postterm gestations (Miller and Read, 1981; Katz and Bowes, 1992). Early reports related meconium passage to increased risk of perinatal morbidity and mortality, especially when accompanied by abnormal fetal heart rate (FHR) patterns (Fenton and Steer, 1962; Hobel, 1971; Miller et al., 1975; Krebs et al., 1980). If hypoxia during labor is associated with the presence of meconium, or if it is in fact the cause of intrapartum meconium passage, one may frequently expect to find ominous FHR tracings suggestive of hypoxia in pregnancies complicated by discolored amniotic fluid. Several groups have reported such associations (Starks, 1980; Nathan et al., 1994), and Krebs and colleagues (1980) and Meis and coworkers (1978) associated meconium with decreased baseline variability and fewer FHR accelerations. Late decelerations, however, are not necessarily found more often in the presence of meconium (Miller and Read, 1981).

The relationship of intrapartum meconium to low Apgar scores and acidosis remains controversial. A number of investigators associated low Apgar scores with meconium-stained fluid (Krebs et al., 1980; Starks, 1980; Cole et al., 1985; Steer et al., 1989; Nathan et al., 1994, Ziadeh and Sunna, 2000). In these studies, incidence of low 1- and 5-minute Apgar scores was approximately two times greater when meconium was present than when it was absent. Most authors did not control for FHR abnormalities, and the conclusions of those who did are inconsistent. For example, Steer and colleagues (1989) reported an independent effect of meconium on low Apgar scores, whereas Krebs and colleagues (1980) ascribed the association to accompanying FHR abnormalities. At least some of these Apgar score differences may have been due to vigorous endotracheal suctioning in meconium-affected babies resulting in neonatal depression on this basis alone. A number of reports have not found differences in Apgar scores between meconium-stained and non–meconium-stained fetuses (Meis et al., 1982; Mitchell et al., 1985; Dijxhoorn et al., 1986, 1987; Jazayeri et al., 2000). Dijxhoorn and associates (1986) could not correlate meconium in labor with neurologic status of the infants at 4 or 5 days of life.

The association between meconium-stained fluid and fetal acidosis during labor remains controversial. Some investigators have reported no association between meconium and either mean umbilical artery pH or frequency of acidosis (Abramovici et al., 1974; Krebs et al., 1980; Dijxhoorn et al., 1986; Richey et al., 1995; Jazayeri et al., 2000); others suggest a relationship between amniotic fluid meconium and fetal blood gas values (Starks, 1980; Miller and Read, 1981; Nathan et al., 1994; Ziadeh and Sunna, 2000).

Steer and coworkers (1989), controlling for FHR abnormalities, concluded that meconium was not an independent predictor of acidosis. Although the presence of meconium is not by itself an indication for fetal pH assessment (Baker et al., 1992), if meconium is thick and variability is decreased or spontaneous accelerations are absent, a lower threshold for obtaining fetal scalp pHs may be appropriate (Miller and Read, 1981; Shaw and Clark, 1988). In the absence of FHR abnor-

malities, meconium alone does not constitute fetal compromise and is not, in itself, a cause for intervention (Miller et al., 1975; Bochner et al., 1987; Baker et al., 1992).

Meconium Consistency and Fetal Hypoxemia, Acidemia, and Low Apgar Scores

Investigators have tried to correlate thick meconium with a higher incidence of poor fetal outcome compared with thin staining. When interpreting such studies, one must account for the subjective nature of assessing "thin" versus "thick" meconium. Thick meconium often is described as "pea-soup," particulate, viscous, and opaque, in contrast with watery, translucent, lightly stained thin meconium. Weitzner and colleagues (1990) proposed quantitating meconium concentration using a "meconium-crit," but this practice has not been adopted clinically. Given this caveat, Starks (1980) presented data that demonstrated lower Apgar scores and fetal scalp blood pH values when thick meconium was present. Meis and associates (1978) found that heavy meconium increased the risk of low Apgar scores, MAS, and death compared with light meconium. In addition, "early" passage of meconium (meconium passed before or during the active phase of labor) carried a greater risk than "late" passage of meconium (meconium passed during the second stage, after clear fluid had been noted). The risk of adverse perinatal outcomes was not greater in patients in the group with light meconium than in controls with clear fluid. Hobel (1971), Miller and coworkers (1975), Rossi and colleagues (1989), and Berkus and associates (1994) all found meconium thickness to be related to adverse perinatal outcome; however, Bochner and coauthors (1987) reported that even with thick meconium, perinatal morbidity was increased only when nonreassuring FHR patterns were present.

Conversely, Miller and colleagues (1975, 1981) could not conclusively demonstrate any difference in Apgar scores between fetuses exposed to thick versus thin meconium-stained fluid. Krebs and associates (1980) concluded that various thicknesses did not affect Apgar scores or FHR patterns. Abramovici and coworkers (1974) and Trimmer and Gilstrap (1991) could not differentiate meconium consistency by fetal scalp pH, Apgar scores, or ultimate fetal outcome. In a study by Yeomans and associates (1989), thick meconium was associated with low 1-minute Apgar scores but did not influence pH results. Such contradictory views about meconium thickness have not been resolved, although most obstetricians intuitively view thick meconium as a more ominous sign than thin meconium.

Because meconium-stained fluid is a common intrapartum finding, any striking associations between meconium and the usual parameters signifying fetal distress should be readily apparent. Investigators, however, have been unable to document consistent differences in Apgar scores, acidosis, and FHR patterns between meconium-stained infants and infants with clear amniotic fluid. Most authors do not control for abnormal FHR patterns and other confounding factors, which confuses the issue of whether meconium causes or simply is associated with adverse outcomes.

More than 40 years ago, Fenton and Steer (1962) questioned the grave significance of meconium-stained fluid when ominous FHR patterns were not present. In a review on meconium and adverse perinatal outcome, Katz and Bowes (1992) concluded that "when normal FHR patterns are found with meconium-stained fluid, the neonatal outcome is similar to that of neonates with clear fluid. Similarly, when infants with meconium have antepartum signs of distress . . . neonatal outcomes are similar to those of non–meconium-stained infants with similar FHR abnormalities." Current data appear to support this view, and the presence of meconium per se does not imply fetal distress during labor until other parameters support such a contention. Perhaps the most important clinical value of meconium-stained amniotic fluid is to alert the obstetrician to look further for signs of fetal compromise. When available, internal FHR monitoring should be considered when meconium is noted. Finally, the obstetrician should anticipate both suctioning the infant's oropharynx at delivery (see later) and the need to alert pediatric staff.

MECONIUM ASPIRATION SYNDROME AND ITS PREVENTION

The term "meconium aspiration" refers to the presence of meconium below the vocal cords and in the lungs. When amniotic fluid contains meconium, meconium is found below the vocal cords in approximately one-third of neonates (range, 21%–56%) (Gregory et al., 1974; Dooley et al., 1985; Falciglia, 1988; Rossi et al., 1989). Fetal breathing (gasping in particular) presumably leads to meconium entering the lungs. Although the net flow of fluid is out of the fetal lungs, deep respirations occur during normal pregnancy (Dawes et al., 1972).

Duenhoelter and Pritchard (1977) demonstrated inhalation of chromium-labeled red blood cells that had been injected into the amniotic fluid in humans. In term sheep fetuses, hypoxia elicited meconium aspiration (Dawes et al., 1972), and fetal hypoxia or acidosis induced gasping in monkeys (Martin et al., 1974; Manning et al., 1979). In baboons, acidosis with or without hypoxia resulted in meconium aspiration, but hypoxia alone did not (Block et al., 1981).

MAS develops in 2%–8% of infants delivered through meconium-stained amniotic fluid (Davis et al., 1985; Falciglia, 1988; Rossi et al., 1989); this condition is characterized by mild to severe respiratory distress at birth. In its mildest form, the disease could present with neonatal tachypnea associated with normal pH and low PCO_2, resolving within 2–3 days. In its more severe form, the syndrome can present with hypoxemia, acidosis, and respiratory failure within minutes to hours after birth. The sickest neonates could require extracorporeal membrane oxygenation (ECMO) to maintain oxygenation and prevent barotrauma until alveolar healing occurs and pulmonary function improves enough to meet baseline oxygen demands. The death rate from MAS is as high as 40% in affected neonates in some studies (Davis et al., 1985; Falciglia, 1988), although it is much lower in other studies (Wiswell et al., 1990; Wiswell at al., 2000)

The pathophysiology of MAS classically was thought to involve a combination of mechanical obstruction and chemical pneumonitis of small airways by particulate meconium inhaled at the time of the infant's first breath (Tyler et al., 1978; Tran et al., 1980; Perlman et al., 1989). Resultant pulmonary vascular spasm then would lead to pulmonary hypertension and right-to-left shunting through the patent foramen ovale or ductus arteriosus. Worsening hypoxia could lead to convulsions, renal

failure, disseminated intravascular coagulation, and heart failure (Brady and Goldman, 1986). Pulmonary function can be compromised further by displacement of pulmonary surfactant by free fatty acids in meconium (Clark et al., 1987), or by direct inhibition of surfactant's surface tension-reducing properties by meconium (Moses et al., 1991; Bae et al., 1998; Oh and Bae, 2000; Hertig et al., 2001).

DeLee and Tracheal Suctioning

Because of the belief that the pathophysiology of MAS centers on inhalation of meconium at delivery, suctioning of the infant's pharynx at the time of delivery, combined with visualization of the vocal cords and tracheal suctioning, has been proposed to minimize deep aspiration. Bulb suctioning of the infant's pharynx is performed routinely to clear secretions after delivery. Several studies over the years report increased frequency of tracheal meconium in neonates who develop MAS (Gregory et al., 1974; Wiswell et al., 2000; Meydanli et al., 2001). Carson and coworkers (1976) demonstrated that deep DeLee suctioning of the fetus immediately after delivery of the head and before delivery of the thorax, along with selective tracheal intubation and suctioning, effectively reduced the incidence and severity of MAS. Ting and Brady (1975) and Gregory and colleagues (1974) reported similar results with aggressive tracheal suctioning.

Gage and associates (1981), studying the effectiveness of suction techniques in fetal kittens, reported that catheter suctioning consistently removed larger quantities of meconium than bulb suctioning did. Pfenninger and coworkers (1984) also demonstrated that oropharyngeal suction is superior to nasal suctioning, and although both methods should be used in succession, oropharyngeal suctioning should be carried out first. These findings appeared to validate the concept that meconium aspiration occurs as the first breath is taken following delivery.

After these studies were published, DeLee suctioning was adopted to clear the oropharynx when meconium stains the amniotic fluid, with the neonate often undergoing laryngoscopic visualization of the vocal cords (with endotracheal suction if meconium is visible). Despite widespread acceptance of DeLee suctioning for meconium, subsequent studies have not found one form of suctioning to be superior to another (Hageman et al., 1988; Locus et al., 1990). Wiswell and colleagues (2000) found that oropharyngeal suctioning before delivery of the thorax decreased the incidence of MAS, but there was no difference between bulb suctioning and DeLee suctioning.

Unfortunately, even the most vigorous suctioning before the first breath does not remove meconium already aspirated into the lungs before birth and thus does not eliminate the occurrence of MAS (Davis et al., 1985; Byrne and Gau, 1987; Sunoo et al., 1989; Wiswell et al., 1990). Several investigators have documented *in utero* meconium aspiration (Manning et al., 1978; Turbeville et al., 1979; Brown and Gleicher, 1981). The evidence supporting this contention comes from autopsy studies showing meconium in the alveolar spaces both in stillborn infants and in newborns vigorously suctioned before the first breath. Researchers have used animal models to illustrate intrauterine meconium aspiration when the fetus is made hypoxic and acidotic experimentally (Block et al., 1981). Thus, MAS is not always preventable despite aggressive airway management at delivery. In fact, subsequent reports of aggressive suctioning policies have not demonstrated the same effectiveness as initial reports did. Dillard (1977) and Falciglia (1988) reported no differences in the incidence of meconium below the vocal cords or of MAS between infants born during years when suctioning was not performed in the presence of meconium and infants born during years when suctioning was routine. In a follow-up study, Falciglia and colleagues (1992) reported that DeLee suctioning before the first breath offered no advantage over suctioning performed after complete delivery.

Asphyxia, Pulmonary Artery Hypertrophy, and Meconium

Hypoxia, pulmonary hypertension, and persistent fetal circulation are the hallmarks of MAS. Pulmonary arteries constrict during episodes of hypoxia, increasing pulmonary vascular resistance and decreasing pulmonary artery blood flow and oxygenation. Prolonged hypoxia causes hypertrophy of the muscular pulmonary artery walls, leading to pulmonary hypertension (James and Rowe, 1957; Naeye and Letts, 1962). Gersony and associates (1976) reported that hypoxia in fetal sheep caused right-to-left shunting as a result of pulmonary vascular obstruction and hypothesized a vicious circle of hypoxia—pulmonary vasoconstriction—right/left shunting—hypoxia. Drummond and Bissonnette (1978) demonstrated that prolonged hypoxia caused pulmonary hypertension in third-trimester sheep fetuses. Medial hypertrophy of the vessel wall takes at least 3 days to develop (Meyrick and Reid, 1979, 1981) but has been reported in some neonates dying of reported MAS shortly after delivery (Murphy et al., 1984; Thureen et al., 1997), consistent with preexisting asphyctic pulmonary disease. In newborn guinea pigs with meconium pulmonary lavage, only asphyxiated pups showed histologic findings of intra-alveolar hemorrhage and wall destruction (Jovanovic and Nguyen, 1989). Neither acute asphyxia nor meconium instillation into the lungs of newborn baboons caused persistent pulmonary hypertension or histologic medial hypertrophy (Cornish et al., 1994). Lung disease in humans is profoundly worse when both asphyxia and meconium are present compared with either alone (Thibeault et al., 1984). Muscularization of the pulmonary arteries can be seen in infants regardless of whether there is meconium-stained amniotic fluid, and—in some cases in which amniotic fluid *is* meconium-stained—in the absence of evidence of meconium aspiration (Perlman et al., 1989). Meconium could be an association without direct pathological significance in these latter cases. Katz and Bowes (1992) questioned whether meconium is necessary for a reported diagnosis of MAS. This thesis was reiterated by Ghidini and Spong (2001), who recommended assiduously ruling out all other causes of neonatal respiratory compromise before making a diagnosis of MAS. They distinguished between mild and severe MAS as two separate entities: Mild MAS may follow from the classic theory of meconium inhalation, but severe instances appear to be multifactorial and to require hypoxia, with the presence of meconium optional.

Meconium is more common after 40 weeks' gestation, but so is oligohydramnios. Usher and coworkers (1988) reported that the incidence of MAS was increased eightfold in post-

term (compared with term) pregnancies, even though the incidences of meconium and fetal distress were increased only twofold. Meconium and oligohydramnios-related FHR abnormalities perhaps act synergistically under these circumstances. This idea has been supported in a report by Bochner and colleagues (1987) of post-term gestations with normal antepartum FHR patterns; such infants born in the presence of heavy meconium were at no greater risk for adverse perinatal outcome than low-risk infants with clear amniotic fluid.

Meconium is commonly present, yet MAS occurs in only a small fraction of newborns who aspirate meconium and is most likely when nonreassuring FHR patterns occur before or during labor. Abnormal chest radiographic findings are common in infants born through meconium, but most do not have respiratory distress (Gregory et al., 1974). Given these data, one interpretation is that meconium alone, although capable of causing chemical pneumonitis, rarely causes severe pulmonary disease in normally developed lungs. *In utero* hypoxia may cause fetal gasping, potentially increasing the volume of meconium inhaled before delivery. Lungs compromised by acute asphyxia or by *in utero* hypoxia-induced medial thickening may respond to meconium pneumonitis by exaggerated vascular constriction, resulting in pulmonary hypertension, right-to-left shunting through the ductus arteriosus (persistent fetal circulation), and worsening local and systemic hypoxia. These processes delay meconium clearance, prolong pulmonary inflammation, impair alveolar healing, and progressively cripple pulmonary function. MAS is best viewed not as derived from a single pathophysiologic mechanism, but as a multifactorial process involving varying contributions of hypoxic, mechanical, and inflammatory damage to the lungs. No single theory adequately accounts for all of the reported clinical characteristics.

Selective Suctioning Based on Risk Factors

Thickness of meconium and abnormal FHR patterns have been associated with a higher risk of MAS. Benny and associates (1987) and Wiswell and coworkers (2000) reported MAS to be more common when meconium was thick rather than thin. Rossi and colleagues (1989) found that 19% of infants with thick meconium had MAS, compared with 5% of those with moderate and 3% of those with thin meconium. Hernandez and coworkers (1993) reported no difference in MAS between neonates with thick and those with moderate meconium. Ghidini and Spong (2001) argue that, although there is evidence associating meconium thickness with MAS, evidence is lacking if only severe MAS is considered.

Rossi and associates (1989) found that the combination of fetal tachycardia and absent accelerations correlated with an increased risk of MAS, and Hernandez and colleagues (1993) confirmed an independent association between fetal tachycardia and MAS requiring mechanical ventilation. Benny and associates (1987) found MAS to be more common when late decelerations had been present; Ramin and coworkers (1996) reported FHR abnormalities in 68% of infants with MAS; and Fleischer and colleagues (1992) reported that the risk of neonatal respiratory complications in the presence of meconium was 2% when FHR patterns were normal and 12% when they were abnormal. Paz and associates (2001) found associations between MAS and higher fetal heart baseline rate, fewer accelerations, greater numbers of decelerations, and reduced variability. Wiswell and colleagues (2000) and Meydanli and associates (2001) both reported abnormal fetal heart tracings to be independently associated with risk of MAS.

Dooley and coworkers (1985) studied 58 infants with meconium below the vocal cords at delivery and compared their umbilical cord arterial blood gas values with those of 214 matched infants without meconium below the vocal cords. They detected no significant differences in mean pH, PCO_2, or base deficit between the two groups, but a rising FHR baseline and decreased variability were more common in infants who subsequently had meconium below the vocal cords. Yeomans and colleagues (1989) found that acidosis increased the incidence of meconium below the vocal cords but not the incidence of MAS. In a study by Mitchell and associates (1985), all cases of MAS occurred in acidotic infants, in contrast to studies by Blackwell and colleagues (2001) and Ramin and associates (1996), in which umbilical artery acidosis was present in less than 50% of infants with MAS.

Cesarean delivery is more common when meconium is present, but this probably is due to associated FHR abnormalities. There is no evidence that cesarean delivery itself protects against MAS when FHR patterns are normal. In fact, Wiswell and colleagues (2000) used multivariable analysis to demonstrate that cesarean section was an independent risk factor for MAS.

On the basis of these reports, several investigators decided to study selective suctioning and intubation according to either antecedent FHR abnormalities or the consistency of meconium. Linder and coworkers (1988) prospectively studied 572 vaginally delivered infants with meconium-stained amniotic fluid who had 1-minute Apgar scores of 9 or 10. All infants underwent DeLee suctioning immediately upon delivery of the head; 308 infants underwent endotracheal visualization and suctioning, and 264 infants underwent neither endotracheal visualization nor suctioning. There were no differences in neonatal outcome except for several cases of laryngeal stridor in the intubated group. Cunningham and colleagues (1990) proposed that oropharyngeal suctioning be routine and that endotracheal visualization and suctioning be reserved for depressed infants.

Yoder (1994) used a protocol that included routine oropharyngeal DeLee suctioning of all infants with meconium in the amniotic fluid but tracheal intubation only for depressed infants with moderate-to-thick meconium. In the presence of meconium of any thickness, vigorous infants who did not undergo tracheal intubation experienced outcomes similar to those having clear amniotic fluid.

Using a similar protocol on vigorous term infants delivered vaginally in the presence of meconium, Peng and associates (1996) reported no MAS in nonintubated infants. Wiswell and Henley (1992) used thin consistency, lack of hypopharyngeal meconium, and "apparent vigor" of the neonate as criteria for observing meconium-stained infants rather than performing tracheal intubation. They reported that 33% of the total cases of MAS occurred in the nonintubated group despite their "low-risk" characteristics. In a subsequent large (n = 2094) randomized trial, however, Wiswell and colleagues (2000) demonstrated no benefit to intubation and tracheal suctioning in vigorous infants born through amniotic fluid stained by any thickness of meconium. Using multivariable analysis to assess independent secondary effects, oropharyngeal suctioning was beneficial, and MAS was associated with oligohydramnios, abnormal fetal monitoring, meconium below the vocal cords, and cesarean delivery.

Because several studies have shown minimal increases in morbidity or mortality in vigorous newborns with meconium staining who underwent only DeLee suctioning, endotracheal procedures may not be necessary for all of these infants. Normal FHR patterns and lack of acidosis during labor make MAS unlikely, but the risk is not zero. Lung injury may have predated labor in some of these cases, making endotracheal procedures less likely to prevent respiratory compromise. There could still be a mechanical or inflammatory contribution of inhaled meconium, however, so that oropharyngeal suctioning to decrease residual volume of meconium has benefit. The American Academy of Pediatrics (2000) recommended early oropharyngeal suctioning (before delivery of the shoulders) of all infants in the presence of meconium and tracheal visualization and suctioning for neonates who are depressed or born through particulate meconium.

Amnioinfusion for Meconium

Amnioinfusion has been proposed as a way of diluting meconium and possibly decreasing the incidence of intrapartum MAS. In a randomized trial, Wenstrom and Parsons (1989) infused 1000 mL of saline through an intrauterine catheter into laboring women with thick meconium. They compared outcomes to those of women with thick meconium who received routine care. The amnioinfusion group experienced a sixfold decrease in the incidence of meconium visualized below the vocal cords. Although there were three cases of MAS in the control group and none in the amnioinfusion group, this difference was not statistically significant. Sadovsky and coworkers (1989) randomized laboring women with higher than trace levels of meconium to either an amnioinfusion or a control group. In the amnioinfusion group, 79% had thick meconium before infusion, decreasing to 5% after infusion. The rate of thick meconium in the control group was 62%. The incidence of meconium below the vocal cords was 29% in the control group compared with 0% in the amnioinfusion group, with no cases of MAS in either group.

Similar results have been reported by some authors (Macri et al., 1992; Lo and Rogers, 1993; Cialone et al., 1994; Eriksen et al., 1994), but not by others (Spong et al., 1994; Usta, Mercer, Aswad, et al., 1995). A meta-analysis by Glantz and Letteney (1996) concluded that amnioinfusion decreased the risk of meconium below the umbilical cords by 84%. Subsequent meta-analyses by Pierce and colleagues (2000) and Hofmeyr (2001) confirmed this and demonstrated reductions in MAS associated with amnioinfusion (relative risk approximately 0.25). It is possible that some of the benefit of amnioinfusion is not related to the meconium per se, but rather to alleviating umbilical cord compression and variable fetal heart decelerations by replacing amniotic fluid volume, thereby restoring normal fetal oxygenation. These results would improve Apgar scores, raise umbilical artery pH, and minimize *in utero* fetal gasping. Whatever the mechanism, amnioinfusion should be considered when thick meconium is noted, especially when FHR monitoring is abnormal.

■ SUMMARY

The significance and management of meconium passage in utero continue to challenge the obstetrician. Although the body of information concerning the pathophysiology of meconium-stained amniotic fluid is sizable, the practicing clinician must understand that these data are far from complete and often contradictory, and the salient features are surprisingly difficult to grasp. For a clinical entity so frequently encountered, meconium serves as a reminder to obstetricians of the limits of medical knowledge. From a practical standpoint, the discovery of meconium-stained fluid should alert the obstetrician to potential fetal and neonatal problems and encourage increased vigilance in managing such cases; however, the isolated presence of meconium-stained amniotic fluid should not compel the obstetrician to institute needless or harmful intervention.

REFERENCES

Abramovici H, Brandes JM, Fuchs K, et al: Meconium during delivery: A sign of compensated fetal distress. Am J Obstet Gynecol **118**:251, 1974.

Allen R: The significance of meconium in midtrimester genetic amniocentesis. Am J Obstet Gynecol **152**:413, 1985.

Altshuler G, Arizawa M, Molnar-Nadasdy G: Meconium-induced umbilical cord vascular necrosis and ulceration: A potential link between the placenta and poor outcome. Obstet Gynecol **79**:760, 1992.

Altshuler G, Hyde S: Meconium-induced vasoconstriction: A potential cause of cerebral and other fetal hypoperfusion and of poor pregnancy outcome. J Child Neurol **4**:137, 1989.

American Academy of Pediatrics/American Heart Association: Neonatal Resuscitation Manual, 4th ed., Elk Grove Village, Ill, 2000.

Arey LB: Developmental Anatomy. Philadelphia, WB Saunders, 1974.

Bae CW, Takahashi A, Chida S, et al: Morphology and function of pulmonary surfactant inhibited by meconium. Pediatr Res **44**:187, 1998.

Baker PN, Kilby MD, Murray H: An assessment of the use of meconium alone as an indication for fetal blood sampling. Obstet Gynecol **80**:792, 1992.

Becker RF, Windle WF, Barth EE, et al: Fetal swallowing, gastrointestinal activity and defecation in utero. Surg Gynecol Obstet **70**:603, 1940.

Benacerraf BR, Gatter MA, Ginsburgh F: Ultrasound diagnosis of meconium-stained amniotic fluid. Am J Obstet Gynecol **149**:570, 1984.

Benny PS, Malani S, Hoby MA, et al: Meconium aspiration: Role of obstetric factors and suction. Aust N Z Obstet Gynecol **27**:36, 1987.

Berkus MD, Langer O, Samueloff A, et al: Meconium-stained amniotic fluid: Increased risk for adverse neonatal outcome. Obstet Gynecol **84**:115, 1994.

Blackwell SC, Moldenhauer J, Hassan S, et al: Meconium aspiration syndrome in term neonates with normal acid-base status at delivery: Is it different? Am J Obstet Gynecol **184**:1422, 2001.

Block JC, Kallenberger DA, Kern JD, et al: In utero meconium aspiration by the baboon fetus. Obstet Gynecol **57**:37, 1981.

Bochner CJ, Medearis AL, Ross MG, et al: The role of antepartum testing in the management of postterm pregnancies with heavy meconium in early labor. Obstet Gynecol **96**:903, 1987.

Brady JP, Goldman SL: Management of meconium aspiration syndrome. *In* Thibeault DW, Gregory GA (eds): Neonatal Pulmonary Care. Norwalk Conn, Appleton-Century-Crofts, 1986, p. 483.

Brown BL, Gleicher N: Intrauterine meconium aspiration. Obstet Gynecol **57**:26, 1981.

Buhi WC, Spellacy WN: Effects of blood or meconium on the determination of the amniotic fluid lecithin/sphingomyelin ratio. Am J Obstet Gynecol **121**:321, 1975.

Byrne DL, Gau G: In utero meconium aspiration: An unpreventable cause of neonatal death. Br J Obstet Gynaecol **94**:813, 1987.

Carson BJ, Losey RW, Bowes WA, et al: Combined obstetric and pediatric approach to prevent meconium aspiration syndrome. Am J Obstet Gynecol **126**:712, 1976.

Cialone PR, Sherer DM, Ryan RM, et al: Amnioinfusion during labor complicated by particulate meconium-stained amniotic fluid decreases neonatal morbidity. Am J Obstet Gynecol **170**:842, 1994.

Ciftci AO, Tanyel FC, Bingöl-Kologlu M, et al: Fetal distress does not affect in utero defecation but does impair the clearance of amniotic fluid. J Pediatr Surg **34**:246, 1999.

Clark DA, Nieman GF, Thompson JE, et al: Surfactant displacement by meconium free fatty acids: An alternative explanation for atelectasis in meconium aspiration syndrome. J Pediatr **110**:765, 1987.

Clark P, Duff P: Inhibition of neutrophil oxidative burst and phagocytosis by meconium. Am J Obstet Gynecol **173**:1301, 1995.

Cole JW, Portman RJ, Lim Y, et al: Urinary beta-2-microglobulin in full-term newborns: Evidence for proximal tubular dysfunction in infants with meconium-stained amniotic fluid. Pediatrics **76**:958, 1985.

Cornish JD, Dreyer GL, Snyder GE, et al: Failure of acute perinatal asphyxia or meconium aspiration to produce persistent pulmonary hypertension in a neonatal baboon model. Am J Ostet Gynecol **171**:43, 1994.

Cunningham AS, Lawson EE, Martin RJ, et al: Tracheal suction and meconium: A proposed standard of care. J Pediatr **116**:153, 1990.

Davenport HW (ed): Physiology of the Digestive Tract, 3rd ed., Chicago, Year Book Medical Publishers, 1971.

Davis RO, Philips JB III, Harris BA, et al: Fetal meconium aspiration syndrome occurring despite airway management considered appropriate. Am J Obstet Gynecol **151**:731, 1985.

Dawes GS, Fox HE, Leduc BM, et al: Respiratory movements and rapid eye movement sleep in the foetal lamb. J Physiol **220**:119, 1972.

Desmond MM, Lindley JE, Moore J, et al: Meconium staining of newborn infants. J Pediatr **49**:540, 1956.

Dijxhoorn MJ, Visser GHA, Fidler VJ, et al: Apgar scores, meconium and acidaemia at birth in relation to neonatal neurological morbidity in term infants. Br J Obstet Gynaecol **93**:217, 1986.

Dijxhoorn MJ, Visser GHA, Touwen BCL, et al: Apgar score, meconium and acidaemia at birth in small-for-gestational age infants born at term, and their relation to neonatal neurological morbidity. Br J Obstet Gynaecol **94**:873, 1987.

Dillard RG: Neonatal tracheal aspiration of meconium-stained infants. J Pediatr **90**:163, 1977.

Dooley SL, Pesavento DJ, Depp R, et al: Meconium below the vocal cords at delivery: Correlation with intrapartum events. Am J Obstet Gynecol **153**:767, 1985.

Drummond WH, Bissonnette JM: Persistent pulmonary hypertension in the neonate: Development of an animal model. Am J Obstet Gynecol **131**:761, 1978.

Duenhoelter JH, Pritchard JA: Fetal respiration. Am J Obstet Gynecol **129**:326, 1977.

Emmanouilides GC, Townsend DE, Bauer RA: Effects of single umbilical artery ligation in the lamb fetus. Pediatrics **42**:919, 1968.

Eriksen NL, Hostetter M, Parisi VM: Prophylactic amnioinfusion in pregnancies complicated by thick meconium. Am J Obstet Gynecol **171**:1026, 1994.

Falciglia HS: Failure to prevent meconium aspiration syndrome. Obstet Gynecol **71**:349, 1988.

Falciglia HS, Henderschott C, Potter P, et al: Does DeLee suction at the perineum prevent meconium aspiration syndrome? Am J Obstet Gynecol **167**:1243, 1992.

Fenton AN, Steer CM: Fetal distress. Am J Obstet Gynecol **83**:354, 1962.

Fleischer A, Anyaegbunam A, Guidetti D, et al: A persistent clinical problem: Profile of the term infant with significant respiratory complications. Obstet Gynecol **79**:185, 1992.

Florman AL, Tuebner D: Enhancement of bacterial growth in amniotic fluid by meconium. J Pediatr **74**:111, 1969.

Francoual J, Lindenbaum A, Benattar C, et al: Importance of simultaneous determination of coproporphyrin and hemoglobin in contaminated amniotic fluid. Clin Chem **32**:877, 1986.

Freer DE, Statland BE: Measurement of amniotic fluid surfactant. Clin Chem **27**:1629, 1981.

Gage JE, Taeusch HW, Treves S, et al: Suctioning of upper airway meconium in newborn infants. JAMA **246**:2590, 1981.

Gersony WM, Morishima HO, Daniel SS, et al: The hemodynamic effects of intrauterine hypoxia: An experimental model in newborn lambs. J Pediatr **89**:631, 1976.

Ghidini A, Spong CY: Severe meconium aspiration syndrome is not caused by aspiration of meconium. Am J Obstet Gynecol **185**:931, 2001.

Glantz JC, Letteney DL: Pumps and warmers during amnioinfusion: Is either necessary? Obstet Gynecol **87**:150, 1996.

Golbus MS, Loughman WD, Epstein CJ, et al: Prenatal genetic diagnosis in 3000 amniocenteses. N Engl J Med **300**:157, 1979.

Grand RJ, Watkins JB, Torti FM: Progress in gastroenterology: Development of the human gastrointestinal tract. A review. Gastroenterology **70**:790, 1976.

Gregory GA, Gooding CA, Phibbs RH, et al: Meconium aspiration in infants—a prospective study. J Pediatr **85**:848, 1974.

Hageman JR, Conley M, Francis K, et al: Delivery room management of meconium staining of the amniotic fluid and the development of meconium aspiration syndrome. J Perinatol **8**:127, 1988.

Hankins GDV, Rowe J, Quirk JG, et al: Significance of brown and/or green amniotic fluid at the time of second trimester genetic amniocentesis. Obstet Gynecol **64**:3, 1984.

Hernandez C, Little BB, Dax JS, et al: Prediction of the severity of meconium aspiration syndrome. Am J Obstet Gynecol **169**:61, 1993.

Hertig E, Rauprich P, Stichtenoth G, et al: Resistance of different surfactant preparations to inactivation by meconium. Pediatr Res **50**:44, 2001.

Hill LM, Breckle R: Vernix in amniotic fluid: Sonographic detection. Radiology **158**:80, 1986.

Hill LM, Ellefson R: Variable interference of meconium in the determination of phosphatidylglycerol. Am J Obstet Gynecol **47**:339, 1983.

Hirst GDS: Mechanisms of peristalsis. Br Med Bull **35**:263, 1979.

Hobel CJ: Intrapartum clinical assessment of fetal distress. Am J Obstet Gynecol **110**:336, 1971.

Hofmeyr GJ: Amnioinfusion for meconium-stained liquor in labour. Cochrane Library Issue **2**:1, 2001.

Hon EH: Modern Trends in Human Reproductive Physiology, London, Butterworths, 1963.

Hoskins IA, Hemming VG, Johnson TR, et al: Effects of alterations of zinc-to-phosphorus ratios and meconium content on group B *Streptococcus* growth in human amniotic fluid in vitro. Am J Obstet Gynecol **157**:770, 1987.

James MB, Rowe RD: The pattern of response of pulmonary and systemic arterial pressures in newborn and older infants to short periods of hypoxia. J Pediatr **51**:5, 1957.

Jazayeri A, Politz L, Tsibris JCM, et al: Fetal erythropoietin levels in pregnancies complicated by meconium passage: Does meconium suggest fetal hypoxia? Am J Obstet Gynecol **183**:188, 2000.

Jovanovic R, Nguyen HT: Experimental meconium aspiration in guinea pigs. Obstet Gynecol **73**:652, 1989.

Karp LE, Schiller HS: Meconium staining of amniotic fluid in midtrimester amniocentesis. Obstet Gynecol **50**(S):47, 1977.

Kaspar HG, Abu-Musa A, Hannoun A, et al: The placenta in meconium staining: Lesions and early neonatal outcome. Clin Exp Obstet Gynecol **27**:63, 2000.

Katz VL, Bowes WA: Meconium aspiration syndrome: Reflections on a murky subject. Am J Obstet Gynecol **166**:171, 1992.

Kimble RM, Trudenger B, Cass D: Fetal defaecation: Is it a normal physiologic process? J Paediatr Child Health **35**:116, 1999.

King CR, Prescott G, Pernoll M: Significance of meconium in midtrimester diagnostic amniocenteses. Am J Obstet Gynecol **132**:667, 1978.

Krebs HB, Peters RE, Dunn LJ, et al: Intrapartum fetal heart rate monitoring: III. Association of meconium with abnormal fetal heart rate patterns. Am J Obstet Gynecol **137**:936, 1980.

Kulkarni BD, Bieniarz J, Burd L, et al: Determination of L/S ratio in amniotic fluid. Obstet Gynecol **40**:173, 1972.

Lee KH: Supervision of high-risk cases by amnioscopy. Am J Obstet Gynecol **112**:46, 1972.

Legge M: Dark brown amniotic fluid—identification of contributing pigments. Br J Obstet Gynaecol **88**:632, 1981.

Linder N, Aranda JV, Tsur M, et al: Need for endotracheal intubation and suction in meconium-stained neonates. J Pediatr **112**:613, 1988.

Lo KW, Rogers M: A controlled trial of amnioinfusion: The prevention of meconium aspiration in labour. Aust N Z J Obstet Gynecol **33**:51, 1993.

Locus P, Yeomans E, Crosby U: Efficacy of bulb versus DeLee suction at deliveries complicated by meconium stained amniotic fluid. Am J Perinatol **7**:87, 1990.

Longo SA, Towers CV, Strauss A, et al: Meconium has no lecithin or sphingomyelin but affects the lecithin/sphingomyelin ratio. Am J Obstet Gynecol **179**:1640, 1998.

Macri CJ, Schrimmer DB, Leung A, et al: Prophylactic amnioinfusion improves outcome of pregnancy complicated by thick meconium and oligohydramnios. Am J Obstet Gynecol **167**:117, 1992.

Manchanda R, Vora M, Gruslin A: Influence of postdatism and meconium on fetal erythropoietin. J Perinatol **19**:479, 1999.

Mandelbaum B: Gestational meconium in the high-risk pregnancy. Obstet Gynecol **42**:87, 1973.

Manning FA, Harman CR, Morrison I, et al: Fetal assessment based on fetal biophysical profile scoring: IV. An analysis of perinatal morbidity and mortality. Am J Obstet Gynecol **162**:703, 1990.

Manning FA, Martin CB, Murata Y, et al: Breathing movements before death in the primate fetus (Macaca mulata). Am J Obstet Gynecol **135**:71, 1979.

Manning FA, Schreiber J, Turkel SB: Fatal newborn aspiration "in utero": A case report. Am J Obstet Gynecol **132**:111, 1978.

Martin CB, Murata Y, Petrie RH, et al: Respiratory movements in fetal rhesus monkeys. Am J Obstet Gynecol **119**:939, 1974.

Matsubara S, Yamada T, Minakami H, et al: Meconium-stained amniotic fluid activates polymorphonuclear leukocytes. Eur J Histochem **43**:205, 1999.

Matthews TG, Warshaw JB: Relevance of the gestational age distribution of meconium passage in utero. Pediatrics **64**:30, 1979.

Mazor M, Furman B, Wiznitzer A, et al: Maternal and perinatal outcome of patients with preterm labor and meconium-stained amniotic fluid. Obstet Gynecol **86**:830, 1995.

McLain CR: Amniography studies of the gastrointestinal motility of the human fetus. Am J Obstet Gynecol **86**:1079, 1963.

Meis PJ, Hall M, Marshall JR, et al: Meconium passage: A new classification for risk assessment during labor. Am J Obstet Gynecol **131**:509, 1978.

Meis PJ, Hobel CJ, Ureda JR: Late meconium passage in labor—a sign of fetal distress? Obstet Gynecol **59**:332, 1982.

Meydanli MM, Dilbaz B, Caliskan S, et al: Risk factors for meconium aspiration syndrome in infants born through thick meconium. Int J Gynecol Obstet **72**:9, 2001.

Meyrick B, Reid L: Hypoxia and incorporation of 3H-thymidine by cells of the rat pulmonary and alveolar wall. Am J Pathol **96**:51, 1979.

Meyrick B, Reid L: The effect of chronic hypoxia on pulmonary arteries in young rats. Exp Lung Res **2**:257, 1981.

Miller FC, Read JA: Intrapartum assessment of the postdates fetus. Am J Obstet Gynecol **141**:516, 1981.

Miller FC, Sacks DA, Yeh SY, et al: Significance of meconium during labor. Am J Obstet Gynecol **122**:573, 1975.

Miller PW, Coen RW, Benirschke K: Dating the time interval from meconium passage to birth. Obstet Gynecol **66**:459, 1985.

Mitchell J, Schulman H, Fleischer A, et al: Meconium aspiration and fetal acidosis. Obstet Gynecol **65**:352, 1985.

Moses D, Holm BA, Spitale P, et al: Inhibition of pulmonary surfactant function by meconium. Am J Obstet Gynecol **164**(2):477, 1991.

Mulivor RA, Mennuti MT, Harris H: Origin of the alkaline phosphatases in amniotic fluid. Am J Obstet Gynecol **135**:77, 1979.

Murphy JD, Vawter GF, Reid LM: Pulmonary vascular disease in fetal meconium aspiration. J Pediatr **104**:758, 1984.

Naeye RL, Letts HW: The effects of prolonged neonatal hypoxemia on the pulmonary vascular bed and heart. Pediatrics **30**:902, 1962.

Nathan L, Leveno KJ, Carmody TJ, et al: Meconium: A 1990s perspective on an old obstetric hazard. Obstet Gynecol **83**:329, 1994.

Oh MH, Bae CW: Inhibitory effect on meconium on pulmonary surfactant function tested in vitro using the stable microbubble test. Eur J Pediatr **159**:770, 2000.

Parker SL: Laboratory variables in determining lecithin/sphingomyelin ratios. Am J Med Technol **47**:901, 1981.

Paz Y, Solt I, Zimmer EZ: Variables associated with meconium aspiration syndrome in labors with thick meconium. Eur J Obstet Gynecol Reprod Biol **94**:27, 2001.

Peng TCC, Gutcher GR, Van Dorsten P: A selective aggressive approach to the neonate exposed to meconium-stained amniotic fluid. Am J Obstet Gynecol **175**:296, 1996.

Perlman EJ, Moore W, Hutchins GM: The pulmonary vasculature in meconium aspiration. Hum Pathol **20**:701, 1989.

Pfenninger E, Dick W, Brecht-Krauss D, et al: Investigation of intrapartum clearance of the upper airway in the presence of meconium-contaminated amniotic fluid using an animal model. J Perinatol Med **12**:57, 1984.

Pierce J, Gaudier FL, Sanchez-Ramos L: Intrapartum amnioinfusion for meconium-stained fluid: Meta-analysis of prospective trials. Obstet Gynecol **95**:1051, 2000.

Potier M, Melancon SB, Dellaire L: Developmental patterns of disaccharidases in human amniotic fluid. Am J Obstet Gynecol **131**:73, 1978.

Pritchard JA: Fetal swallowing and amniotic fluid volume. Obstet Gynecol **28**:606, 1966.

Ramin KD, Leveno KJ, Kelly MA, et al: Amniotic fluid meconium: A fetal environmental hazard. Obstet Gynecol **87**:181, 1996.

Richey SD, Ramin SM, Bawdon RE, et al: Markers of acute and chronic asphyxia in infants with meconium-stained amniotic fluid. Am J Obstet Gynecol **172**:1212, 1995.

Romero R, Hanaoka S, Mazor M, et al: Meconium-stained amniotic fluid: A risk factor for microbial invasion of the amniotic cavity. Am J Obstet Gynecol **164**:859, 1991.

Rossi EM, Philipson EH, Williams TG, et al: Meconium aspiration syndrome: Intrapartum and neonatal attributes. Am J Obstet Gynecol **161**:1106, 1989.

Sadovsky Y, Amon E, Bade ME, et al: Prophylactic amnioinfusion during labor complicated by meconium: A preliminary report. Am J Obstet Gynecol **161**:613, 1989.

Saldana LR, Schulman H, Lin CC: Routine amnioscopy at term. Obstet Gynecol 47:521, 1976.

Schmidt-Sommerfeld E, Litmeyer H, Penn D: A rapid qualitative method for detecting PG in amniotic fluid. Clin Chim Acta 119:243, 1982.

Scott H, Walker M, Gruslin A: Significance of meconium-stained amniotic fluid in the preterm population. J Perinatol 21:174, 2001.

Shaw K, Clark S: Reliability of intrapartum fetal heart rate monitoring in the postterm fetus with meconium passage. Obstet Gynecol 72:886, 1988.

Sherer DM, Abramowicz JS, Smith SA, et al: Sonographically homogeneous echogenic amniotic fluid in detecting meconium-stained amniotic fluid. Obstet Gynecol 78:819, 1991.

Smith CA: Physiology of the digestive tract. In Smith CA, Nelson NW (eds): The Physiology of the Newborn Infant, Springfield, IL, Charles C Thomas, 1976, p. 459.

Speert H: Swallowing and gastrointestinal activity in the fetal monkey. Am J Obstet Gynecol 45, 1943.

Spong CY, Ogundipe OA, Ross MG: Prophylactic amnioinfusion for meconium-stained amniotic fluid. Am J Obstet Gynecol 171:931, 1994.

Starks GC: Correlation of meconium-stained amniotic fluid, early intrapartum fetal pH and Apgar scores as predictors of perinatal outcome. Obstet Gynecol 56:604, 1980.

Steer PJ, Eigbe F, Lissauer TJ, et al: Interrelationships among abnormal cardiotocograms in labor, meconium staining of the amniotic fluid, arterial cord blood pH and Apgar scores. Obstet Gynecol 74:715, 1989.

Sunoo C, Kosasa TS, Hale RW: Meconium aspiration syndrome without evidence of fetal distress in early labor before elective cesarean delivery. Obstet Gynecol 73:707, 1989.

Svigos JM, Steward-Rattray SF, Pridmore BR: Meconium-stained liquor at second trimester amniocentesis: Is it significant? Aust N Z J Obstet Gynecol 21:5, 1981.

Tabsch KMA, Brinkman CR III, Bashore R: Effect of meconium contamination on amniotic fluid L/S ratio. Obstet Gynecol 58:605, 1981.

Thibeault DW, Hall FK, Sheehan MB, et al: Postasphyxial lung disease in newborn infants with severe perinatal acidosis. Am J Obstet Gynecol 150:393, 1984.

Thureen PJ, Hall DM, Hoffenberg A, et al: Fatal meconium aspiration in spite of appropriate perinatal airway management: Pulmonary and placental evidence of prenatal disease. Am J Obstet Gynecol 176:967, 1997.

Ting P, Brady J: Tracheal suction in meconium aspiration. Am J Obstet Gynecol 22:767, 1975.

Towers CV, Garite TJ: Evaluation of the new Amniostat-FLM test for the detection of phosphatidylglycerol in contaminated fluids. Am J Obstet Gynecol 160:298, 1989.

Tran N, Lowe C, Sivieri EM, et al: Sequential effects of acute meconium obstruction on pulmonary function. Pediatr Res 14:34, 1980.

Trimmer KJ, Gilstrap LC: "Meconiumcrit" and birth asphyxia. Am J Obstet Gynecol 165:1010, 1991.

Tsao FHC, Zachman RD: Determination of PG in amniotic fluid by a simple one-dimensional thin-layer chromatography method. Clin Chim Acta 118:109, 1982.

Turbeville DF, McCaffree MA, Bloch MF, et al: In utero distal pulmonary meconium aspiration. South Med J 72:535, 1979.

Tyler DC, Murphy J, Cheney FW: Mechanical and chemical damage to lung tissue caused by meconium aspiration. Pediatrics 62:454, 1978.

Usher RH, Boyd ME, McLean FH, et al: Assessment of fetal risk in postdate pregnancies. Am J Obstet Gynecol 158:259, 1988.

Usta IM, Mercer BM, Aswad NK, et al: The impact of a policy of amnioinfusion for meconium-stained amniotic fluid. Obstet Gynecol 85:237, 1995.

Usta IM, Mercer BM, Sibai B: Risk factors for meconium aspiration syndrome. Obstet Gynecol 86:230, 1995.

Usta IM, Sibai BM, Mercer BM, et al: Use of maternal plasma level of zinc-coproporphyrin in the prediction of intrauterine passage of meconium. J Matern-Fetal Med 9:201, 2000.

Wagstaff TI, Whyley GA, Freedman G: Factors influencing the measurement of the L/S ratio in amniotic fluid. J Obstet Gynaecol Br Commonw 81:264, 1974.

Walker J: Fetal anoxia. Obstet Gynaecol Br Emp 61:162, 1954.

Weitzner JS, Strassner HT, Rawlins RG, et al: Objective assessment of meconium content of amniotic fluid. Obstet Gynecol 76:1143, 1990.

Wenstrom KD, Parsons MT: The prevention of meconium aspiration in labor using amnioinfusion. Obstet Gynecol 73:647, 1989.

Wiswell TE, Tuggle JM, Turner BS: Meconium aspiration syndrome: Have we made a difference? Pediatrics 85:715, 1990.

Wiswell TE, Gannon CM, Jacob J, et al: Delivery room management of the apparently vigorous meconium-stained neonate: Results of the multicenter, international collaborative trial. Pediatr 105:1, 2000.

Wiswell TE, Henley MA: Intratracheal suctioning, systemic infection, and the meconium aspiration syndrome. Pediatrics 89:203, 1992.

Yambao TJ, Tawwater B, Chuachingco J, et al: Effect of meconium on the detection of phosphatidylglycerol. Am J Obstet Gynecol 150:426, 1984.

Yeomans ER, Gilstrap LC, Leveno KJ, et al: Meconium in the amniotic fluid and fetal acid-base status. Obstet Gynecol 73:175, 1989.

Yoder BA: Meconium-stained amniotic fluid and respiratory complications: Impact of selective tracheal suction. Obstet Gynecol 83:77, 1994.

Ziadeh SM, Sunna E: Obstetric and perinatal outcome of pregnancies with term labour and meconium-stained amniotic fluid. Arch Gynecol Obstet 264:84, 2000.

Zorn EM, Hanson FW, Greve LC, et al: Analysis of the significance of discolored fluid detected at midtrimester amniocentesis. Am J Obstet Gynecol 154:1234, 1986.

Chapter 25

ASSESSMENT AND INDUCTION OF FETAL PULMONARY MATURITY

Brian M. Mercer, MD

Respiratory distress syndrome (RDS) results when immature lungs fail to produce adequate surface acting proteins and phospholipids to reduce alveolar surface tension and prevent alveolar collapse during expiration. Because the work necessary to open a collapsed alveolus is much more than that needed to expand an already open alveolus, the increased work of breathing leads to muscular exhaustion and mechanical respiratory failure. Alveolar collapse, fluid build-up in the immature alveolus, and diminished respiratory gas exchange lead to hypoxia, hypercarbia, and subsequently, acidosis. RDS is the most common major acute morbidity at any gestational age between viability and 36 weeks. Neonatal RDS and complications of its treatment are associated with an increased risk of serious acute and long-term morbidities, including intraventricular hemorrhage (IVH), patent ductus arteriosus (PDA), retinopathy of prematurity (ROP), and chronic lung diseases, including bronchopulmonary dysplasia. Although the frequency and severity of RDS tends to be worse when delivery occurs remote from term, RDS occurring near term can also lead to serious complications or even death.

When preterm delivery is inevitable, treatment is directed to optimizing the timing of delivery, newborn condition, and resources for neonatal care. When continuation of pregnancy is an option, the relative fetal and maternal risks of conservative management versus delivery must be considered. Because cardiopulmonary function is a principal requirement for neonatal survival, identification of fetuses at risk for RDS and methods to induce fetal maturity before preterm birth are important.

AMNIOTIC FLUID ASSESSMENT OF FETAL PULMONARY MATURITY

Invasive and noninvasive tests for prediction of fetal pulmonary maturity have been evaluated. The optimal test of maturity would provide clear discrimination between the mature fetus and the fetus likely to suffer RDS. Because central respiratory drive, muscular strength, infection, hypoxia, and hypotension can alter the clinical course also, antenatal pulmonary maturity testing cannot completely differentiate between the mature and the immature fetus. Currently, biochemical and biophysical analysis of the amniotic fluid offer the most accurate means to predict fetal pulmonary maturity. In general, the predictive value of a mature test is 97% to 100%. The risk of RDS after an immature test varies from 5% to nearly 100%, depending on the gestational age and the degree of immaturity predicted by the test.

Clinical tests to determine fetal pulmonary maturity from amniotic fluid specimens have been available since the early 1970s, when Gluck and co-workers first introduced the *lecithin/sphingomyelin ratio* (L/S ratio) (Gluck, 1971; Gluck et al., 1971). The relative proportion of lecithin (disaturated phosphatidylcholine) and sphingomyelin are stable until the mid-third trimester, at which time the pulmonary active phospholipid lecithin increases relative to the nonpulmonary sphingomyelin. An L/S ratio of at least 2:1 is considered indicative of fetal maturity. Determination of the L/S ratio requires thin-layer chromatography after initial centrifugation of cellular debris, extraction with methanol and chloroform, and cold acetone treatment. The time and technical expertise required limit the use of the test to large-volume laboratories and create considerable intra- and interobserver variability. The L/S ratio has in the past been considered the "gold standard" for assessment of fetal pulmonary maturity, but it is neither 100% sensitive nor specific. Despite its complexity and cost, L/S ratio determination continues to be performed in some labs. *Phosphatidylglycerol* (PG) is one of the last pulmonary phospholipids to become evident in the amniotic fluid. The detection of PG by thin-layer chromatography (Hallman et al., 1976; Hallman et al., 1977), enzymatic assays (Jones and Ashwood, 1994), or by slide agglutination (Garite et al., 1983; Lockitch et al., 1984; Halvorsen and Gross, 1985; O'Dwyer et al., 1988) is highly predictive of fetal pulmonary maturity. An advantage of PG determination is reliability in the presence of blood, meconium, or vaginal secretions; however, the test is usually immature when performed before 36 weeks gestation. Like the L/S ratio, the original PG assay is performed by thin-layer chromatography and requires considerable time and expertise. Recognizing that the relative proportions of the fetal pulmonary phospholipids change with increasing gestational age, Kulovich introduced the fetal "*lung profile*" in 1979 (Kulovich et al., 1979). The lung profile includes information obtained by two-dimensional thin-layer chromatography regarding the L/S ratio, the presence of PG, and the relative fractions of lecithin, PG, and phosphatidylinositol (PI), which generally rises to 35 weeks and then declines with the appearance of PG in the amniotic fluid. The lung profile was proposed to improve prediction of pulmonary maturity and to help determine the optimal timing of subsequent testing after an immature result.

Several functional tests of fetal pulmonary maturity were developed in the 1970s and 1980s. The "*shake test*" was initially described in 1972 (Clements et al., 1972). The presence of a stable foam ring 15 minutes after 15 seconds of shaking of amniotic fluid diluted with 95% ethanol is suggestive of fetal pulmonary maturity and is correlated to an L/S ratio of at least 1.5:1. The test is easy to perform and uses inexpensive reagents, but falsely immature results are common. Further, glassware contamination and ethanol evaporation make this test clinically impractical. The *Foam Stability Index* (FSI) was proposed in 1978 (Sher et al., 1978). After centrifugation to remove cellular debris, amniotic fluid is added to vials containing various ethanol dilutions and shaken for 30 seconds. No cases of RDS were found when a stable uninterrupted foam ring was seen at the meniscus with an ethanol volume fraction of 0.48 or higher. The test compares favorably to the L/S ratio and offers a graded scale to assess pulmonary maturity, but still relies on technical expertise. The *Lumadex-FSI* (Beckman Instruments, Carlsbad, CA) offered a standardized version of the Foam Stability Index and shake tests (Sher and Statland, 1983), but this is no longer available for clinical use in the United States. The "*tap test*," a rapid bedside test for assessing fetal pulmonary maturity, was first introduced by Socol and colleagues (1984). One mL of amniotic fluid is mixed in a test tube with one drop 6-Normal hydrochloric acid and 1.5 mL of diethyl ether. The tube is then tapped briskly three or four times to generate 200–300 bubbles within the ether layer. The specimen is considered mature if the bubbles disperse from the ether layer within 5 minutes, and a mature result is associated with a low likelihood of neonatal RDS. Like the other fetal pulmonary maturity assays, an immature tap test predicts an increased risk of RDS but carries a significant false immaturity rate: Forty-eight percent of "immature" infants did not develop RDS.

Developed in the late 1980s, the surfactant /albumin ratio (S/A ratio) is performed by evaluating competitive binding to surfactant and albumen by a ligand that exhibits fluorescence polarization (TDx FLM, Abbott Laboratories, Abbott Park, Illinois) (Russell et al., 1989; Herbert et al., 1993). The TDx FLM assay is simple to perform, rapid, highly accurate, reproducible, and independent of amniotic fluid volume. There is less intertest variability than is seen with thin-layer chromatography. Because the test can be performed with equipment generally found in clinical laboratories, no additional equipment is needed, and the requirement for technical expertise is limited. The TDx FLM assay and its subsequent modification, the TDx FLM II assay, have been compared favorably with the L/S ratio, shake test, Foam Stability Index, and PG test (Ashwood et al., 1986; Steinfeld et al., 1992; Bender et al., 1994; Bonebrake et al., 1997), and have been shown to reduce lab time significantly, to 30–45 minutes (Bonebrake et al., 1997). In a multicenter study, Russell and colleagues found sensitivity and specificity of 96% and 58%, respectively, with the TDx FLM using a cutoff of 50 mg/g (Russell et al., 1989). A TDx FLM value above 50 or 70 was similarly predictive of pulmonary maturity as the PG test and the L/S ratio. This test is among the most commonly used today.

Lamellar bodies are 1–5 μm diameter (1.28–6.4 fL) surfactant-containing particles secreted by type II pneumocytes (Dubin, 1989; Ashwood et al., 1990). The number of lamellar bodies found in the amniotic fluid increases with the onset of functional fetal pulmonary maturity. Because lamellar bodies are similar in size to platelets (2–20 fL), they can be counted

using an automated particle counter calibrated for platelet quantitation. Measurement in this manner leads to underestimation of total lamellar body number (~10%), as does centrifugation of the specimen. In a study of 833 women who delivered within 72 hours of testing, the lamellar body count (LBC) compared favorably with L/S ratio and PG test in the prediction of fetal pulmonary maturity (97.7% versus 96.8% and 94.7% predictive values for pulmonary maturity, respectively) (Neerhof, Haney, et al., 2001). In a recent attempt to introduce standardization in LBC testing, Neerhof and associates formed a consensus group (Neerhof, Dohnal, et al., 2001) that reached agreement on the following points:

1. Centrifugation is not required to remove cellular debris in the amniotic fluid and should be abandoned.
2. In the absence of centrifugation, a count greater than or equal to 50,000/μL should be considered mature, and a count less than or equal to 15,000/μL should be considered immature. A transitional count of 15,000–50,000/μL should lead to consideration of an additional test in order to clarify the result.
3. Because meconium can interfere with the cell counter and can reduce the count, either the LBC should not be performed in the presence of meconium, or clinical judgment should be exercised in interpretation of the results.
4. If there is bloody contamination, a hematocrit should be performed, and the clinician should be notified if the value is greater than 1% HCT.
5. Although vaginal pool specimens may be acceptable, such specimens should not be analyzed if there is evident mucous, as it can obstruct the counter channels.
6. Severe oligohydramnios can increase the LBC, while polyhydramnios could lead to a false immature result. Should centrifugation be performed, a cutoff of 30,000/μL has been suggested to be predictive of fetal pulmonary maturity (Fakhoury et al., 1994; Dalence et al., 1995).

Amniotic fluid density based on spectrophotometric absorbance at 650 nm for prediction of fetal pulmonary maturity reflects the presence of fetal squamous cells rather than amniotic fluid phospholipid content (Plauche et al., 1981), but it does not correlate well to other biochemical tests (Arias et al., 1978; Anceschi et al., 1996) and has a high false immaturity rate. In 1975, Hastwell found the presence of vernix in a fluid sample to correlate to an L/S ratio above 2:1 (and more than 4:1 in most cases) (Hastwell, 1975). Ninety-one percent of samples that were cloudy but without vernix also had an L/S ratio above 2:1, while 60% of those that were clear had an L/S ratio of 2:1 or less. Subsequently, Sbarra and colleagues found that visual assessment of amniotic fluid turbidity correctly classified 87.2% of amniotic fluid samples submitted for assessment of lung maturity by optical density, L/S ratio, and PG determination (Sbarra et al., 1991). Strong and coworkers found that when news print cannot be read through a test tube filled with amniotic fluid, the L/S ratio is at least 2:1, and PG is present in 97% of cases (Strong et al., 1992). Most recently, the presence of amniotic fluid turbidity was found to have a 91.8% positive predictive value and an 87% negative predictive value for a mature TDx FLM result (Adair et al., 1995)

Amniotic fluid prolactin, cholesterol palmitate, desmosine, surfactant apoproteins, fluorescent polarization microviscosity, and drop volume have also been related to fetal pulmonary maturity but are not commonly assessed in clinical practice.

NONINVASIVE ASSESSMENT OF FETAL PULMONARY MATURITY

Even when performed near term, amniocentesis is not without risk. Before ultrasound was used routinely to guide amniocentesis, invasive testing was associated with high rates of complications (19%), including tachycardia and bradycardia (1%), spontaneous membrane rupture (3%), bloody specimens (15%), and failure to obtain fluid (11%) (Sabbagha and Salvino, 1979). Although ultrasound guidance is associated with a much lower failure rate (1.6%), there remains a low but significant risk of complications in experienced hands, including a 0.7% risk of emergent delivery and a 6.6% risk of bloody fluid (Stark et al., 2000). Because of these concerns, noninvasive markers, including direct and ultrasonographic amniotic fluid visualization, placental grading, fetal biometry, and fetal lung imaging, have been studied for their predictive value regarding fetal pulmonary maturity.

In one study (Gross et al., 1985), ultrasonographic visualization of free-floating echogenic particles was correlated to the L/S ratio; the sensitivity of ultrasound to detect a mature L/S ratio was 35%. Others have found poor correlation between the presence of amniotic fluid particles and biochemical fetal pulmonary maturity testing (53% predictive value for a mature test result; 100% predictive value for an immature result) (Helewa et al., 1989). At term, free-floating particles on ultrasound correlate to the presence of fetal vernix caseosa (Brown et al., 1994), but such particles can be seen at any gestation, regardless of the presence of vernix (Parulekar, 1983). Before elective delivery at term, a grade III placenta has been correlated to a mature L/S ratio (Grannum et al., 1979; Ragozzino et al., 1983), but when preterm and term women are evaluated, placental grade correlates less well with the L/S ratio (7% immature) and PG test (25% absent), limiting the utility of this finding (Harman et al., 1982). First introduced as a potential marker for fetal pulmonary maturity in 1971, a biparietal diameter greater than 87 or 90 correlates poorly with the L/S ratio (Lee et al., 1971; Spellacy et al., 1978; Strassner et al., 1979). When assessed before elective cesarean delivery at term, the presence of a biparietal diameter of at least 92 mm or of a Grade III placenta was correlated to the lack of neonatal pulmonary complications (Golde et al., 1982; Petrucha et al., 1982; Golde et al., 1984). A biparietal diameter greater than 92 mm, however, was associated with a 9%–14% incidence of immature fetal pulmonary testing in other studies (Spellacy et al., 1978; Newton et al., 1983) and should not be used for women with unsure dating or anticipated preterm delivery. These restrictions severely limit the potential utility of biometric evaluation for assessment of fetal pulmonary maturity (Hadlock, 1982; Hadlock et al., 1985).

Noninvasive imaging of the fetal lung has been proposed to predict fetal pulmonary maturity. In evaluations of lung echogenicity, texture, and through transmission, Cayea and colleagues and Fried and associates found a poor correlation between ultrasound findings and mature amniotic fluid indices (Cayea et al., 1985; Fried et al., 1985). Lecithin has a characteristic magnetic resonance signal that may be amenable to assessment by magnetic resonance spectroscopy (Fenton et al., 2000) or by echoplanar magnetic resonance imaging (Moore et al., 2001). Although preliminary data is interesting, technical difficulties in these modalities remain to be resolved.

IMPACT OF GESTATIONAL AGE ON FETAL PULMONARY MATURITY TESTING

Because fetal pulmonary maturity is highly correlated to gestational age, the predictive value of a mature or an immature test result varies significantly with the gestation at which the test is performed (Fig. 25-1) (Tanasijevic et al., 1994). At term, the risk of RDS resulting from pulmonary immaturity is 1% or less. Although an immature test result is associated with RDS, the risk is low, and severe disease is unlikely in the absence of other complications. Alternatively, when a preterm infant is delivered remote from term, the risk of RDS is high if amniotic fluid testing suggests fetal pulmonary immaturity. Both at and near term, the likelihood of RDS is low after a mature result. On the other hand, Wigton and colleagues found significant risk of RDS (19.2%), severe IVH (8.1%), and necrotizing enterocolitis (4.8%) when preterm birth occurred before 34 weeks despite a mature L/S ratio or positive PG test (Wigton et al., 1993). Lauria and associates found a similar progressive increase in infant morbidity despite a mature L/S ratio or a positive PG test with decreasing gestational age at

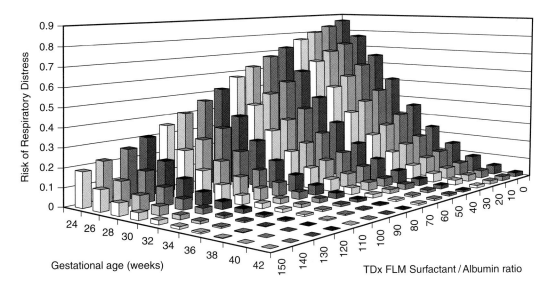

FIGURE 25-1 ■ Risk of neonatal respiratory distress based on gestational age and TDx FLM surfactant/albumin assay result (mg/g). (Adapted from Tanasijevic MJJ, Wybenga DR, Richardson D, et al: A predictive model for fetal lung maturity employing gestational age and test results. Am J Clin Pathol **102**:788, 1994.)

delivery and found a low (8.3%) risk of RDS after an immature result at term (Lauria et al., 1996).

ASSESSMENT OF FETAL PULMONARY MATURITY IN SPECIAL GROUPS

Because the predictive value of a test varies with the prevalence of the outcome studied, clinical conditions that affect the risk of RDS could also alter the predictive value of testing for fetal pulmonary maturity. Richardson, Berman, and colleagues found a lower incidence of RDS among African-American infants and found a lower risk of RDS among African-American infants at any cutoff for the TDx FLM assay (Richardson and Torday, 1994; Berman et al., 1996). Similarly, female fetuses appear to have higher L/S ratios and earlier appearance of PG and are more likely to have a mature test result than males at any given gestational age (Fleisher et al., 1985). When matched by gestational age at delivery, twin neonates have similar morbidity rates compared with singleton neonates (Nielson et al., 1997; Donovan et al., 1998), but twin fetuses could have accelerated TDx FLM results after 31 weeks (McElrath et al., 2000). It remains controversial whether Rh-isoimmunized pregnancies, growth-restricted fetuses, and those affected by preeclampsia have altered risk for RDS when compared with gestational age-matched controls delivering after preterm labor (Leveno et al., 1984; Horenstein et al., 1985; Quinlan et al., 1984; Schiff et al., 1993; Winn et al., 1992; Winn et al., 2000; Piazze et al., 1998).

Diabetes complicating pregnancy can alter the rate of fetal lung development and has been proposed to alter the validity of diagnostic tests for fetal pulmonary maturity. Gluck and Kulovich found a delay in pulmonary maturity based on L/S ratio in fetuses of women with Class A, B, and C diabetes mellitus (Gluck, 1973). Others have found an increased risk of RDS despite a mature L/S ratio of 2:1 (Cruz et al., 1976; Tabsh et al., 1982), and some have suggested an L/S ratio cutoff value of 3:1 in the setting of diabetes. Amniotic fluid from women with diabetes has been found to have lower fluorescence polarization at any gestation (Ashwood et al., 1986). The major factor that influences pulmonary maturation in diabetic progeny appears to be adequacy of blood glucose control, as those with good control do not appear to have delayed maturation (Curet et al., 1979; Dudley and Black, 1985). Hyperinsulinemia and hyperglycemia decrease incorporation of choline into phosphatidylcholine and disaturated phosphatidylcholine as well as PG production. Hyperinsulinemia prevents cortisol-induced phosphatidylcholine and disaturated phosphatidylcholine production by type II pneumocytes and appears to cause a delay in morphologic pulmonary maturation despite increased lung size related to fetal macrosomia (Smith et al., 1975; Lawrence et al., 1989). The increased risk of RDS despite a mature L/S ratio and delayed appearance of PG result could in part be due to increased levels of myoinositol with hyperglycemia (Hallman et al., 1982), which in turn enhances phosphatidylinositol production to the detriment of PG synthesis (Bourbon et al., 1986). PG appears later in poorly controlled diabetic pregnancies (Piper and Langer, 1993; Piper et al., 1998). The presence of PG, however, is reliable in prediction of fetal pulmonary maturity (Kulovich and Gluck, 1979). Women with more advanced diabetes (Class D, R, F) may demonstrate accelerated fetal maturation (Gluck and Kulovich, 1973), possibly related to vascular compromise leading to uteroplacental insufficiency and fetal growth restriction (Ferroni et al.,

1984). The fetal lung maturity (FLM) surfactant/albumin ratio, with a cutoff of 70 mg/g, is a reliable predictor of pulmonary maturity in women with diabetes (Tanasijevic et al., 1996), as is a mature LBC (Neerhof, Haney, et al., 2001). Because the impact of delayed fetal pulmonary maturation is resolved by 38 weeks' gestation, well dated pregnancies with good blood glucose control generally do not require assessment of fetal pulmonary maturity after 38 completed weeks (Berkowitz et al., 1997). When a term infant of a diabetic mother suffers RDS, other possible causes such as hypertrophic cardiomyopathy, cardiac malformations, and isolated ventricular septal hypertrophy should be considered.

IMPACT OF CONTAMINANTS ON FETAL PULMONARY TESTING RESULTS

Because of the presence of nonpulmonary phospholipids, contamination of amniotic fluid with blood can alter the results of nonspecific fetal pulmonary maturity tests for pulmonary phospholipids (Table 25-1). Buhi and Spellacy found maternal serum to have an intrinsic L/S ratio of 1.3:1–1.5:1, raising the possibility that significant blood contamination could falsely elevate an immature result and lower a mature result (Buhi and Spellacy, 1975). Similarly, Cotton and associates found maternal serum to have an L/S ratio of 1.8–1.9:1 (Cotton et al., 1984). A mature result should thus be reassuring, as an immature value could not be expected to increase to a mature level with blood contamination. Tabsh and colleagues found that meconium contamination increased the L/S ratio by 0.1–0.2 in preterm infants and by as much as 0.5 after 35 weeks. Because of the potential for a false mature result, the authors recommended cutoffs of 2.2:1 and 2.5:1 for preterm and term pregnancies, respectively, when meconium staining is present (Tabsh et al., 1981). The PG test is not affected by blood contamination. Blood contamination can falsely lower the TDx FLM assay result, but a mature result reliably predicts fetal pulmonary maturity (Carlan et al., 1997). Because red blood cell phospholipids may interfere with the TDx FLM result, some elect not to perform aTDx FLM II assay if there is blood in the specimen (Apple et al., 1994). Dubin suggested that the LBC is not affected by osmotically lysed blood (Dubin, 1989). Others, however, have suggested that blood contamination may alter the LBC in a biphasic manner, initially increasing the count as a result of the presence of platelets and subsequently decreasing the count as a result of sequestration of lamellar bodies with coagulation (Ashwood et al., 1993). As such, the LBC should be treated with caution if there is greater than 1% contamination with blood.

ASSESSMENT OF FETAL PULMONARY MATURITY FROM VAGINAL FLUID SPECIMENS

In some circumstances, vaginal pool specimens may be inappropriate for fetal pulmonary testing. Regardless of the method of fluid collection, blood and meconium have the potential to alter testing results as delineated in the foregoing discussion. Practically, if significant blood or meconium is present in a vaginal pool specimen, serious consideration should be given to expeditious delivery for fetal indication, rather than conservative management. Clinical studies support a role for vaginally collected amniotic fluid specimens after preterm premature

TABLE 25-1. SELECTED ANTENATAL TESTS FOR ASSESSMENT OF FETAL PULMONARY MATURITY: TECHNIQUE, PREDICTIVE VALUES, AND PREDICTED RELIABILITY BASED ON CONTAMINATION AND SOURCE

Test	Selected References	Technique	Cutoff	Impact of Contamination — Blood	Impact of Contamination — Meconium	Vaginal Pool Collection	Comments
Lecithin/sphingomyelin ratio (L/S ratio)	Gluck (1973) Buhi (1975) Cotton (1984)	Thin-layer chromatography	2.0:1	Mature result valid	Not valid	Valid*	Blood decreases mature and increases immature result. *Free flowing vaginal fluid may be valid if no blood or meconium.
Phosphatidyl-glycerol (PG)	Hallman (1976), Hallman (1977) Schumacher (1985)	Thin-layer chromatography	Present	Valid	Valid	Valid#	#Heavy genital bacterial contamination may yield false mature result due to bacterial phospholipid production.
Amniostat-FLM phosphatidyl-glycerol (PG)	Garite (1983), Halvorson (1985) Pastorek (1988)	Slide agglutination	Positive (>2%)	Valid	Valid	Valid#	Rapid test kit. Little technical expertise required. #Heavy bacterial contamination may yield false mature result.
Shake test	Clements (1972)	Ethanol dilution	Stable foam ring in 1:1 dilution	Not valid	False maturity	Not valid*	*Free-flowing vaginal fluid may be valid if no blood or meconium.
Tap test	Socol (1984)	Ether emulsification	< = 5 bubbles in ether layer	Unknown	Unknown	Unknown	Affected by contamination, evaporation.
Lumadex foam stability index (Lumadex-FSI)	Sher (1978) Sher (1983)	Ethanol dilution	Stable foam ring at > = 0.47	Unknown	Unknown	Valid	Simple standardized bedside test.
TDx FLM Surfactant/albumin ratio	Russell (1989) Steinfeld (1992) Tanasijevic (1994)	Fluorescent polarization	50–70 mg/g	Mature result valid	Not valid?	Valid*	*Free-flowing vaginal fluid may be valid if no blood or meconium. Blood decreases test result.
TDx FLM II Surfactant/albumin ratio	Carlan (1997)	Fluorescent polarization	55 mg/g	Mature result valid	Not valid?	Valid*	*Free-flowing vaginal fluid may be valid if no blood or meconium. Blood decreases test result.
Lamellar body count (uncentrifuged)	Neerhof (2001)	Cell counter	50,000/µL	Mature result valid	Reduces count	Valid^	Reliable if HCT <1%. Platelets initially increase count. Coagulation subsequently decreases count. ^Vaginal fluid may be valid if no blood, meconium, or mucous.
Lamellar body count (centrifuged)	Dalence (1995) Fakhoury (1994)	Cell counter	30,000/µL	Mature result valid	Reduces count	Valid^	Reliable if HCT <1%. Platelets initially increase count. Coagulation subsequently decreases count. ^Vaginal fluid may be valid if no blood, meconium, or mucous.
Amniotic fluid turbidity	Sbarra (1991) Strong (1992) Adair (1995)	Direct visualization	Unable to read newsprint through fluid	Unknown	Unknown	Unknown	Increased turbidity by blood and meconium might give false mature result. Use only if amniotic fluid analysis not available.
Amniotic fluid particles	Gross (1985) Helewa (1989) Parulekar (1983)	Ultrasound	Present	N/A	N/A	N/A	Use only if amniotic fluid analysis not available.
Biparietal diameter	Golde (1982) Newton (1983) Hadlock (1985)	Ultrasound	>92 mm	N/A	N/A	N/A	Use only if amniotic fluid analysis not available.
Placental grade	Grannum (1979) Harman (1982) Kazzi (1985)	Ultrasound	Grade III throughout placenta	N/A	N/A	N/A	Use only if amniotic fluid analysis not available.

rupture of the membranes (pPROM). Shaver and coworkers obtained amniotic fluid by amniocentesis and from the vaginal pool of women admitted with pPROM (Shaver et al., 1987). There was a close correlation between L/S ratios obtained from vaginal pool specimens and amniocentesis (r = 0.88) and an 89% concordance regarding fetal pulmonary maturity. The mean L/S ratio from vaginal pool specimens was not significantly higher than from amniocentesis (2.56 versus 2.3:1, P = 0.06). Similarly, the correlation coefficient for PG was 0.94, and all patients with a positive amniocentesis result also had PG present in the vaginal pool. In addition, phosphatidylinositol, phosphatidylethanolamine, and phosphatidylserine levels were similar between amniocentesis and vaginal pool specimens. Sbarra and associates found no evident lecithin or sphingomyelin in lavage fluid from the vagina; the L/S ratio was not affected by vaginal cervical saline washes (Sbarra et al., 1981). Phillippe found no differences in the L/S ratio or in the amounts of lecithin between vaginal and amniocentesis specimens (Phillippe et al., 1982). Although prolonged exposure to vaginal fluids has been suggested to yield inaccurate results because of bacterial degradation or phospholipid production (Schumacher et al., 1985; Pastorek et al., 1988), Golde found the L/S ratio, PG, and phosphatidylinositol levels to be similar when collected directly from the vagina or collected over a period of hours from perineal pads (Golde, 1983). Lewis also found no cases of RDS among infants delivered after a mature PG result from vaginal pool fluid (Lewis et al., 1993). In a further evaluation of 447 women with PROM, PG determinations from vaginal fluid collected via perineal pads were found to be highly predictive of fetal pulmonary maturity (97.8%) and similarly predictive of pulmonary immaturity (33.7%) to specimens collected by amniocentesis (Estol et al., 1992). In a study of 60 vaginally collected samples, no cases of RDS occurred after a mature L/S ratio, PG, or TDx FLM result greater than 50 mg/g (Russell et al., 1989). Regarding the vaginally collected fluid for TDx FLM II analysis, a mature surfactant/albumin ratio (greater than or equal to 55 mg/g) had a predictive value of 97.6% in a study of 153 women with pPROM at 30–36 weeks; 24.4% of infants with an immature result less than 40 mg/g suffered RDS (Edwards et al., 2000). The LBC could be falsely elevated by vaginal mucous, which also can block Coulter analyzer channels (Ashwood et al., 1993). In the absence of blood, mucous, or meconium, vaginally collected fluid yields similar results when analyzed for pulmonary phospholipids, L/S ratio,

and surfactant/albumin ratio. As such, it is reasonable to evaluate free-flowing vaginal fluid samples by L/S ratio, surfactant/albumin ratio, PG determination, and the LBC, provided there is no evident blood, meconium, or mucous. Perineal collection appears appropriate for L/S ratio and PG determination, but it is not known whether perineal pad collection is appropriate for TDx FLM II analysis or LBC.

INDUCTION OF FETAL PULMONARY MATURITY

Antenatal Corticosteroids—Physiologic and Clinical Benefits

First demonstrated to reduce RDS and neonatal death in 1972, antenatal corticosteroid administration is one of the most effective and cost-efficient prenatal interventions for preventing perinatal morbidity and mortality related to preterm birth (Liggins and Howie, 1972). Glucocorticoids act through reversible binding to the promoter region of genes that code for functional and structural proteins in various organs. In the lung, glucocorticoids induce lipogenic enzymes necessary for surfactant phospholipid synthesis and conversion of unsaturated to disaturated phosphatidylcholine, stimulate antioxidant and surfactant protein (SP A-D) production, and induce enzymes responsible for sodium and potassium channel ion and fluid flux (summarized by Ballard and Ballard, 1995). The physiologic effect of glucocorticoids on the lung include increased compliance and maximal lung volume, decreased vascular permeability, enhanced lung water clearance, parenchymal structural maturation, and improved respiratory function, in addition to an enhanced response to postnatal surfactant treatment (Ballard and Ballard, 1995). Glucocorticoids have demonstrated maturational effects in the brain, heart, skin, digestive system, and kidney through cytodifferentiation, enzyme induction, and protein synthesis. Betamethasone and dexamethasone are long-acting synthetic corticosteroids with similar glucocorticoid potency and negligible mineralocorticoid effects (Table 25-2) (Drug Facts and Comparisons, 1995). Because of differences in albumin binding, placental transfer, and glucocorticoid receptor affinity, substantially higher doses of cortisol, cortisone, hydrocortisone, prednisone, and prednisolone are

TABLE 25-2. RELATIVE GLUCOCORTICOID, MINERALOCORTICOID ACTIVITY AND EQUIVALENT DOSES OF NATURAL AND SYNTHETIC ADRENAL STEROIDS (DRUG FACTS AND COMPARISONS 1995)

Glucocorticoid	Approximate Equivalent Dose (mg)	Relative Anti-inflammatory (Glucocorticoid) Potency	Relative Mineralocorticoid Potency
Cortisone	25	0.8	2
Hydrocortisone	20	1	2
Prednisone	5	4	1
Prednisolone	5	4	1
Triamcinolone	4	5	0
Methylprednisolone	4	5	0
Dexamethasone	0.75	20–30	0
Betamethasone	0.65–0.75	20–30	0

From Drug Facts and Comparisons. St. Louis, Mo, Facts and Comparisons, 1995, p. 504.

required to reach dose equivalency to betamethasone and dexamethasone in the fetus. Women receiving corticosteroids other than betamethasone or dexamethasone should not be considered to have received an adequate dose to stimulate fetal pulmonary maturation. Although one study has suggested an increased protective effect of betamethasone regarding periventricular leucomalacia when compared with dexamethasone (Baud et al., 1999), a review of published trials reveals no apparent difference in efficacy with either agent regarding prevention of RDS (Crowley, 2002). Meta-analysis of more than 18 randomized clinical trials has confirmed that antenatal corticosteroids administered to women at risk for preterm birth reduce the incidences of RDS (odds ratio 0.53), IVH (odds ratio 0.38), and neonatal death (odds ratio 0.60) without increasing maternal or neonatal infection (Fig. 25-2) (Crowley, 2002). In this and a previous review, Crowley (1995) found antenatal corticosteroid administration to be effective regardless of infant gender, race, or the presence of pPROM. While this analysis supported the belief that the efficacy of antenatal corticosteroids persists for more than 7 days, the duration of effect is not ultimately known. Recent randomized clinical trials have evaluated antenatal corticosteroid administration with concurrent antibiotic treatment administration after pPROM (Lewis et al., 1995; Pattinson et al., 1999). Lewis and associates demonstrated less RDS (18.4% versus 43.6%, P = 0.03) and no obvious increase in perinatal infection (3% versus 5%, P = NS) with antenatal corticosteroids and antibiotics (Lewis et al., 1995). Women allocated to a single course of dexamethasone demonstrated no significant reduction in overall morbidity in the multicenter DEXIPROM trial (Pattinson et al., 1999). This study did, however, find a lower incidence of perinatal death (1.3% versus 8.3%, P = 0.05) in the subgroup delivering at least 24 hours after study entry. The most recent meta-analysis regarding this issue included data from Liggins's original trial and found antenatal corticosteroid administration after pPROM to reduce the risks of RDS substantially (20% versus 35.4%, odds ratio 0.56), IVH (7.5% versus 15.9%, odds ratio 0.47), and necrotizing enterocolitis (0.8% versus 4.6%, odds ratio 0.21), without significantly increasing the risks of maternal infection (9.2% versus 5.1%, odds ratio 1.95) or neonatal infection (7.0% versus 6.6%, odds ratio 1.05) (Harding et al., 2001). Although Liggins's original trial suggested that corticosteroids may increase the risk of fetal death in the setting of maternal hypertension, this was not confirmed in subsequent studies (Gamsu et al., 1989; Collaborative Group on Antenatal Steroid Therapy, 1981; Kari et al., 1994). In 1994, a National Institutes of Health (NIH) consensus panel reviewed the available literature and published guidelines regarding antenatal corticosteroid administration (Table 25-3) (National Institutes of Health, 1995). There is no advantage to administering glucocorticoids other than beta- or dexamethasone, nor to alternate routes of glucocorticoid administration. In fact, despite a similar pharmacokinetic profile to intramuscular injection, orally administered dexamethasone is not recommended because it has been associated with an increased risk of neonatal IVH and sepsis when compared with intramuscular injection (Egerman et al., 1997; Egerman et al., 1998). Because placental transfer of betamethasone and dexamethasone are rapid, there is no rationale for direct fetal administration.

Amniotic fluid testing for fetal pulmonary maturity identifies women with fetuses more likely to benefit from antenatal corticosteroids, thus reducing the number of women treated unnecessarily. The number of women who need to be treated to prevent one case of RDS varies with the risk of RDS in the population (Sinclair, 1995). In a population with an 80% risk, only three to four women need to be treated to prevent one case (Fig. 25-3). More than 50 women would need to be treated to prevent one case of RDS in a population at 5% risk. The Collaborative Group on Antenatal Steroid Therapy permitted enrollment of women beyond 34 weeks if an L/S ratio yielded an immature result and excluded those with a mature result at any gestational age (Collaborative Group on Antenatal Steroid Therapy, 1981). Infants born after an immature L/S ratio had a significant reduction in RDS with antenatal dexamethasone (8.7% versus 17.3%, P = 0.03). Because of these findings, antenatal corticosteroid administration is reasonable when an immature fetal pulmonary maturity test is discovered between 34 and 36 completed weeks' gestation.

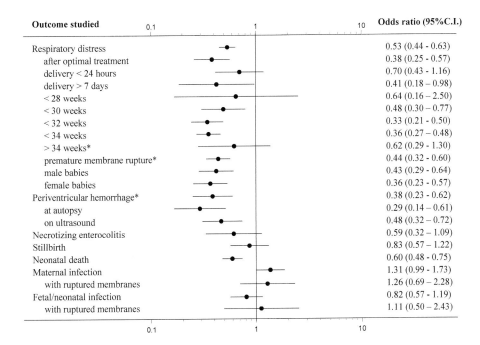

Outcome studied	Odds ratio (95%C.I.)
Respiratory distress	0.53 (0.44 - 0.63)
after optimal treatment	0.38 (0.25 - 0.57)
delivery < 24 hours	0.70 (0.43 - 1.16)
delivery > 7 days	0.41 (0.18 - 0.98)
< 28 weeks	0.64 (0.16 - 2.50)
< 30 weeks	0.48 (0.30 - 0.77)
< 32 weeks	0.33 (0.21 - 0.50)
< 34 weeks	0.36 (0.27 - 0.48)
> 34 weeks*	0.62 (0.29 - 1.30)
premature membrane rupture*	0.44 (0.32 - 0.60)
male babies	0.43 (0.29 - 0.64)
female babies	0.36 (0.23 - 0.57)
Periventricular hemorrhage*	0.38 (0.23 - 0.62)
at autopsy	0.29 (0.14 - 0.61)
on ultrasound	0.48 (0.32 - 0.72)
Necrotizing enterocolitis	0.59 (0.32 - 1.09)
Stillbirth	0.83 (0.57 - 1.22)
Neonatal death	0.60 (0.48 - 0.75)
Maternal infection	1.31 (0.99 - 1.73)
with ruptured membranes	1.26 (0.69 - 2.28)
Fetal/neonatal infection	0.82 (0.57 - 1.19)
with ruptured membranes	1.11 (0.50 - 2.43)

FIGURE 25-2 ■ Impact of antenatal corticosteroids before anticipated preterm birth on infant morbidity and mortality. (From Crowley PA: Antenatal corticosteroid therapy: A meta-analysis of the randomized trials, 1972 to 1994. Am J Obstet Gynecol **173:**322, 1995; Crowley PA: Prophylactic corticosteroids for preterm birth. The Cochrane database of systematic reviews, October 27, 1999, Cochrane Library **2:**2002.)

TABLE 25-3. NATIONAL INSTITUTES OF HEALTH CONSENSUS PANEL GUIDELINES (1995) REGARDING ANTENATAL CORTICOSTEROIDS FOR FETAL MATURATION.

The benefits of antenatal administration of corticosteroids to fetuses at risk of preterm delivery vastly outweigh the potential risks. These benefits include not only a reduction in the risk of respiratory distress syndrome but also a substantial reduction in mortality and intraventricular hemorrhage.

All fetuses between 24 and 34 weeks' gestation at risk of preterm delivery should be considered candidates for antenatal treatment with corticosteroids.

The decision to use antenatal corticosteroids should not be altered by fetal race or gender or by the availability of surfactant replacement therapy.

Patients eligible for therapy with tocolytics should also be eligible for treatment with antenatal corticosteroids.

Treatment consists of two doses of 12 mg of betamethasone given intramuscularly 24 hours apart or four doses of 6 mg of dexamethasone given intramuscularly 12 hours apart. Optimal benefit begins 24 hours after initiation of therapy and lasts at least 7–14 days.

Because treatment with corticosteroids for less than 24 hours is still associated with significant reductions in neonatal mortality, respiratory distress syndrome, and intraventricular hemorrhage, antenatal corticosteroids should be given unless immediate delivery is anticipated.

In preterm premature rupture of the membranes at less than 30–32 weeks' gestation in the absence of clinical chorioamnionitis, antenatal corticosteroid use is recommended because of the high risk of intraventricular hemorrhage at these early gestational ages.

In complicated pregnancies where delivery prior to 34 weeks' gestation is likely, antenatal corticosteroid use is recommended unless there is evidence that corticosteroids will have an adverse effect on the mother or delivery is imminent.

From National Institutes of Health Consensus Development Conference Statement. Effect of corticosteroids for fetal maturation on perinatal outcomes, February 28 to March 24, 1994. Am J Obstet Gynecol **173**:246, 1995.

Antenatal Corticosteroids— Maternal Consequences

Antenatal corticosteroid administration has been associated with a transient increase in maternal white blood cell count that becomes evident within 24 hours (Diebel et al., 1998). Maternal white blood cell count increases 4.4×10^3/mL on average but is not expected to rise above $20,000 \times 10^3$/mL. Glucose intolerance can occur, with transient maternal hyperglycemia in nondiabetic women and increasing insulin needs in diabetic women (Fisher et al., 1997; Bedalov and Balasubramanyam, 1997). Assessment for gestational diabetes is best delayed at least one week after corticosteroid administration. In Liggins's original trial, betamethasone transiently reduced plasma cortisol; levels returned to normal by the fourth day after administration (Liggins and Howie, 1972). In addition to a reduction in basal maternal cortisol (1.9 versus 26.5 µg/mL, $P < 0.001$), McKenna and colleagues demonstrated a decreased maternal response to corticotropin stimulation with antenatal corticosteroids (McKenna et al., 2000). Although betamethasone and dexamethasone have virtually no mineralocorticoid effects, it has been suggested that antenatal corticosteroid administration could predispose pregnant women to pulmonary edema (Elliott et al., 1979). This issue is confounded by concurrent administration of fluid boluses, tocolytic administration, and coexisting infection as a cause of preterm labor, all of which can lead to pulmonary edema. Current data does not support an independent role for antenatal treatment with either betamethasone or dexamethasone in the pathogenesis of maternal pulmonary edema.

Antenatal Corticosteroids— Fetal/Neonatal Consequences

Neonatal white blood cell counts are generally not affected by maternal glucocorticoid administration (Zachman et al., 1988). Sporadic case reports of neonatal Cushingoid syndrome and adrenal dysfunction have been reported with prolonged antenatal exposure to steroids (Grajwer et al., 1977; Bradley et al., 1994). Terrone and coworkers, however, found no significant decrease in cortisol levels with increasing antenatal

corticosteroid exposure after controlling for other variables (Terrone et al., 1997), and several studies have found normal neonatal responsiveness to adrenocorticotropic hormone (ACTH) stimulation after exposure to antenatal corticosteroids (Ohrlander et al., 1977; Teramo et al., 1980; Terrone et al., 1999). Isolated cases of neonatal hypertrophic cardiomyopathy, a known complication in infants of diabetic mothers and with postnatal corticosteroid exposure, have been reported after antenatal corticosteroid exposure in the absence of significant maternal glucose intolerance (Yunis et al., 1999). A direct cause-effect relationship and the biologic mechanism of this finding remain to be elucidated.

A number of clinical studies have been performed to determine the impact of antenatal corticosteroid exposure on fetal biophysical and heart rate activity (Dawes et al., 1994; Magee et al., 1997; Mulder et al., 1997; Senat et al., 1998; Rotmensch et al., 1999). In summary, these studies have found that both

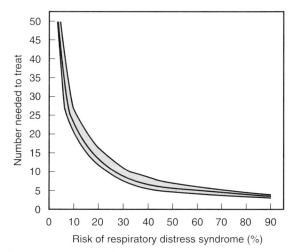

FIGURE 25-3 ■ Number of women who must be treated with antenatal corticosteroids to prevent one case of neonatal RDS based on the a-priori risk of respiratory distress. (From Sinclair JC: Meta-analysis of randomized controlled trials of antenatal corticosteroid for the prevention of respiratory distress syndrome: Discussion. Am J Obstet Gynecol **173**:335, 1995.

betamethasone and dexamethasone reduce fetal breathing and body movements (Magee et al., 1997; Mulder et al., 1997; Rotmensch et al., 1999) with no consistent effect on heart rate baseline (Magee, 1997; Mulder et al., 1997; Senat et al., 1998; Rotmensch et al., 1999). Data addressing the effect of antenatal corticosteroids on fetal heart rate reactivity are conflicting (Senat et al., 1998; Rotmensch et al., 1999). Overall, the fetal biophysical effects of betamethasone are more pronounced than those of dexamethasone and resolve within 4–7 days after administration (Mulder et al., 1997; Senat et al., 1998; Rotmensch et al., 1999). Although the physiologic implications of these findings are unclear, these data should be considered when a decrease in fetal activity occurs after a course of antenatal glucocorticoids.

Antenatal Corticosteroids—Repeated Courses

Review of published research in animals reveals a consistent improvement in lung function at the expense of decreased fetal growth and adverse effects on brain development with repeated courses of antenatal corticosteroids (Aghajafari et al., 2002). Jobe and coworkers found a single course and three weekly courses of antenatal betamethasone to cause a dose-dependent reduction in birth weight in preterm and term lambs. Weekly steroid administration is associated with decreased head size in term lambs (Jobe et al., 1998). Reduced brain growth, nerve growth, and myelination have been demonstrated after exposure to antenatal corticosteroids, particularly with repeated courses (Carlos et al., 1992; Dunlop et al., 1997; Huang et al., 1999; Quinlivan et al., 2000; Huang et al., 2001). Corticosteroid exposure has been linked to persistent forebrain abnormalities correlating to administration during peak mitotic activity (Carlos et al., 1992), dose-dependent reductions in the number of hippocampal neurons, perikarya, and dendritic degeneration (Uno et al., 1994), and higher basal and stress-induced cortisol levels compared with age-matched placebo controls at nine months (Uno et al., 1990). Postnatal cortisol exposure is associated with reduced total body weight (50%) and brain weight (30%), with a proportional reduction in cerebral (30%) and cerebellar (20%) cell number, suggesting a reduction in cell division during the first two weeks of life (Cotterrell et al., 1972).

Retrospective and observational studies in humans have revealed similar effects on fetal and brain growth with multiple courses of antenatal corticosteroids. In 2000, Abbasi found infants exposed to more than one course of antenatal steroids to have smaller head circumferences (28.1 versus 28.4 cm, $P = 0.01$), and a lower incidence of RDS (34.9 versus 45.2%, $P = 0.005$) (Abbasi et al., 2000). In an observational study of 447 infants born before 33 weeks' gestation, French and colleagues found a dose-dependent reduction in birthweight (122 grams, $P = 0.01$), and head circumference (1.02 cm, $P = 0.002$) with three or more courses of antenatal corticosteroids (French et al., 1999). In a post hoc analysis of 710 fetuses exposed to various doses of antenatal corticosteroids in a trial of antenatal thyrotropin-releasing hormone (TRH), exposure to more than one course of antenatal corticosteroids was associated with a 32-g decrease in birth weight for infants born before 32 weeks, and an 80-g reduction for infants born after 32 weeks' gestation (Banks et al., 1999). A review of retrospective and nonrandomized observational studies of antenatal corticosteroids in humans found that multiple courses were

associated with reduced RDS (odds ratio 0.79) and patent ductus arteriosus (odds ratio 0.56), but no differences in mortality, IVH, bronchopulmonary dysplasia, or necrotizing enterocolitis when compared with a single course (Aghajafari et al., 2001). Overall these studies reveal no consistent increase in the risk of neonatal sepsis or amnionitis with multiple courses, despite an increased rate of endometritis (odds ratio 3.22). Although postnatal systemic corticosteroid administration has been shown to reduce chronic lung disease and reduce ventilatory requirements, short-term peripartum treatment of preterm infants is also associated with hyperglycemia, hypertension, hypertrophic cardiomyopathy, and growth failure (Halliday and Ehrenkranz, 2002). Long-term data regarding the effects of antenatal corticosteroid exposure in humans are limited. The Collaborative Group on Antenatal Steroid Therapy followed infants exposed antenatally to dexamethasone for 3 years. Steroid-exposed infants were slightly (3%) heavier and taller ($P = 0.05$); the placebo group had more respiratory complications (3.5 versus 0.5%, $P = 0.02$), and heart murmurs (11.2% versus 5.6%, $P = 0.04$) (Collaborative Group on Antenatal Steroid Therapy, 1984). Head circumferences and neurologic outcomes were similar in the placebo and steroid groups. Infants evaluated 10–12 years after participating in a randomized placebo-controlled trial of antenatal betamethasone demonstrated more admissions for infections during the first years of life, but no differences in weight, height, head circumference, neurologic development, pulmonary function, or visual acuity (Smolders-de Haas et al., 1990). Long-term evaluation of the preterm infants followed by French and colleagues revealed catch-up growth after exposure to multiple courses of antenatal corticosteroids, with no differences in infant weight, length, or head circumference at 3 years (French et al., 1999).

Data are available from two prospective randomized clinical trials of antenatal corticosteroids in humans (Guinn et al., 2001; Mercer et al., 2001, a, b). Guinn and coworkers randomized 502 women to receive either weekly betamethasone to 34 weeks or no further treatment after an initial course of antenatal corticosteroids. Repeated antenatal corticosteroids did not significantly reduce composite morbidity (severe RDS, bronchopulmonary dysplasia, severe IVH, periventricular leucomalacia, sepsis, necrotizing enterocolitis, or death: 22.5% versus 28.0%, $P = 0.16$). Severe RDS, however, decreased (15.3% versus 24.1%, $P = 0.01$), and composite morbidity was decreased if delivery occurred between 24 and 27 weeks (77.4% versus 96.4%, $P = 0.03$) in those who received repeated doses. The relative risk of composite morbidity after repeated corticosteroids decreased with increasing gestational age at birth. There was no significant relationship between birth weight and repeated steroids (2009 versus 2139 grams, $P = 0.10$), but the effect size was similar to that previously described (French et al., 1999; Banks et al., 1999). Had the anticipated enrollment of 1000 participants been achieved without multiple interim analyses, and had the incidences of composite morbidity and birth weights in the two groups remained stable, this study might have demonstrated a reduction in composite morbidity and birth weight with repeated antenatal corticosteroid courses. Mercer and associates evaluated the practice of weekly corticosteroid administration versus rescue therapy for women at high risk for preterm birth. Women randomly allocated to receive weekly betamethasone through 34 weeks were twice as likely to receive corticosteroids within one week of birth before 35 weeks, with only 37% of those assigned to rescue therapy receiving corticosteroids in a timely fashion before early preterm birth ($P = 0.001$) (Mercer et al., 2001a). The practice of weekly corticosteroid administration was not associated with overall lower birthweights; however, multivariate analysis revealed a dose-dependent reduction in birthweight ($P < 0.02$) and length ($P = 0.045$) but not head circumference ($P = 0.38$) with increasing exposure to antenatal corticosteroids (Mercer et al., 2001b). Multicenter clinical trials are ongoing to evaluate the potential benefits and risks of repeated antenatal corticosteroid administration.

In response to the rapid adoption of the practice of routine repeated antenatal corticosteroid administration to women at high risk for preterm birth into clinical practice, and accumulating data suggesting potential risks associate with this practice, the National Institutes of Health reconvened the consensus panel to review the available literature regarding repeated corticosteroid administration in August, 2000. A second consensus statement was published, which reaffirmed the benefits of antenatal corticosteroid administration (National Institutes of Health, 2001). The panel also made the following recommendations:

1. All pregnant women between 24 and 34 weeks' gestation who are at risk of preterm delivery within 7 days should be considered candidates for antenatal treatment with corticosteroids.
2. There is no proof of efficacy of any regimen of antenatal corticosteroid administration other than a mixture of 6 mg of betamethasone phosphate and 6 mg of betamethasone acetate (total of 12 mg of betamethasone), given intramuscularly every 24 hours for two doses, or dexamethasone 6 mg given intramuscularly every 12 hours for four doses.
3. Because of insufficient scientific data from randomized clinical trials regarding efficacy and safety, repeated courses of corticosteroids should not be used routinely. In general, repeated courses should be reserved for patients enrolled in randomized controlled trials.

ALTERNATIVE APPROACHES TO ANTENATAL FETAL PULMONARY MATURATION

Prolactin, ambroxol, aminophylline, intralipid and beta-adrenergic agents, among others, have also been evaluated as potential treatments to enhance fetal pulmonary maturation but have not been consistently effective. Thyroxine has been shown to act directly on the type II pneumocyte to induce surfactant synthesis in animal and human models (Wu et al., 1973; Gonzales and Ballard, 1984). Because thyroxine crosses the placenta poorly, intra-amniotic thyroxine instillation with fetal ingestion would be necessary to achieve therapeutic fetal levels. Alternatively, thyrotropin-releasing hormone administered to the mother can cross the placenta to induce fetal thyroxine synthesis via thyroid-stimulating hormone production. Despite early encouraging results, a recent meta-analysis of this approach failed to demonstrate benefit of concurrent antenatal maternal thyrotropin-releasing hormone and corticosteroid administration (Crowther et al., 2002). In one study, adverse neurologic outcomes—including delayed motor and sensory

development as well as social delay—were seen with thyrotropin-releasing hormone exposure (ACTOBAT Study Group, 1995).

■ SUMMARY

The induction of fetal maturation through timely antenatal administration of betamethasone or dexamethasone is one of the most effective prenatal interventions available for reduction of perinatal morbidity and mortality related to preterm birth. Like many medications with strong effects, antenatal corticosteroids have the potential for significant side effects. The optimal timing and dosage of antenatal steroids before anticipated preterm birth is the subject of important ongoing research. In the meantime, unless delivery is imminent, a single course of antenatal corticosteroids should be considered when preterm birth before 34 completed weeks is anticipated, and repeated courses should not be administered routinely outside the setting of randomized clinical trials. Alternative techniques to promote fetal pulmonary maturation are not recommended. Fetal pulmonary maturity testing through amniotic fluid analysis can be helpful in determining the relative risks of neonatal complications. Whereas a mature amniotic fluid result can identify pregnancies that will not benefit from aggressive attempts at pregnancy prolongation for infant benefit, an immature result can identify those who may benefit from pregnancy prolongation for antenatal corticosteroid administration. Regardless, delivery should not be delayed for fetal maturation in the setting of nonreassuring fetal testing, suspected intrauterine infection, or worsening maternal condition.

REFERENCES

Abbasi S, Hirsch D, Davis J, et al: Effect of single versus multiple courses of antenatal corticosteroids on maternal and neonatal outcome. Am J Obstet Gynecol 182:1243, 2000.

ACTOBAT Study Group. Australian collaborative trial of antenatal thyrotropin-releasing hormone (ACTOBAT) for the prevention of neonatal respiratory disease. Lancet 345:877, 1995.

Adair CD, Sanchez-Ramos L, McDyer DL, et al: Predicting fetal lung maturity by visual assessment of amniotic fluid turbidity: Comparison with fluorescence polarization assay. South Med J 88:1031, 1995.

Aghajafari F, Murphy K, Matthews S, et al: Repeated doses of antenatal corticosteroids in animals: A systematic review. Am J Obstet Gynecol 186:843, 2002.

Aghajafari F, Murphy K, Willan A, et al: Multiple courses of antenatal corticosteroids: a systematic review and meta-analysis. Am J Obstet Gynecol 185:1073, 2001.

Anceschi MM, Piazze Garnica JJ, Unfer V, et al: A comparison of the shake test, optical density, L/S ratio (planimetric and stechiometric) and PG for the assessment of fetal lung maturity. J Perinat Med 24:355, 1996.

Apple FS, Bilodeau L, Preese LM, et al: Clinical implementation of a rapid, automated assay for assessing fetal lung maturity. J Reprod Med 39:883, 1994.

Arias F, Andrinopoulos G, Pineda J: Correlation between amniotic fluid optical density, L/S ratio, and fetal pulmonary maturity. Obstet Gynecol 51:152, 1978.

Ashwood ER, Oldroyd RG, Palmer SE: Measuring the number of lamellar body particles in amniotic fluid. Obstet Gynecol 75:289, 1990.

Ashwood ER, Tait JF, Foerder CA, et al: Improved fluorescence polarization assay for use in evaluating fetal lung maturity. III. Retrospective clinical evaluation and comparison with the lecithin/sphingomyelin ratio. Clin Chem 32:260, 1986.

Ashwood ER, Palmer SE, Taylor JS, et al: Lamellar body counts for rapid fetal lung maturity testing. Obstet Gynecol 81:619, 1993.

Ballard PL, Ballard RA: Scientific basis and therapeutic regimens for use of antenatal glucocorticoids. Am J Obstet Gynecol 173:254, 1995.

Banks BA, Cnaan A, Morgan MA, et al: Multiple courses of antenatal corticosteroids and outcome of premature neonates. North American Thyrotropin-Releasing Hormone Study Group. Am J Obstet Gynecol 181:709, 1999.

Baud O, Foix-L'Helias L, Kaminski M, et al: Antenatal glucocorticoid treatment and cystic periventricular leukomalacia in very premature infants. N Engl J Med 341:1190, 1999.

Bedalov A, Balasubramanyam A: Glucocorticoid-induced ketoacidosis in gestational diabetes: Sequela of the acute treatment of preterm labor. A case report. Diabetes Care 20:922, 1997.

Bender TM, Stone LR, Amenta JS: Diagnostic power of lecithin/sphingomyelin ratio and fluorescence polarization assays for RDS compared by relative operating characteristic curves. Clin Chem 40:541, 1994.

Berkowitz K, Reyes C, Saadat P, et al: Fetal lung maturation. Comparison of biochemical indices in gestational diabetic and nondiabetic pregnancies. J Reprod Med 42:793, 1997.

Berman S, Tanasijevic MJ, Alvarez JG, et al: Racial differences in the predictive value of the TDx fetal lung maturity assay. Am J Obstet Gynecol 175:73, 1996.

Bonebrake RG, Towers CV, Rumney PJ, et al: Is fluorescence polarization reliable and cost efficient in a fetal lung maturity cascade? Am J Obstet Gynecol 177:835, 1997.

Bourbon JR, Doucet E, Rieutort M, et al: Role of myo-inositol in impairment of fetal lung phosphatidylglycerol biosynthesis in the diabetic pregnancy: Physiological consequences of a phosphatidylglycerol-deficient surfactant in the newborn rat. Exp Lung Res 11:195, 1986.

Bradley BS, Kumar SP, Mehta PN, et al: Neonatal cushingoid syndrome resulting from serial courses of antenatal betamethasone. Obstet Gynecol 83:869, 1994.

Brown DL, Polger M, Clark PK, et al: Very echogenic amniotic fluid: Ultrasonography-amniocentesis correlation. J Ultrasound Med 13:95, 1994.

Buhi WC, Spellacy WN: Effects of blood or meconium on the determination of the amniotic fluid lecithin/sphingomyelin ratio. Am J Obstet Gynecol 121:321, 1975.

Carlan SJ, Gearity D, O'Brien WF: The effect of maternal blood contamination on the TDx-FLM II assay. Am J Perinatol 14:491, 1997.

Carlos RQ, Seidler FJ, Slotkin TA: Fetal dexamethasone exposure alters macromolecular characteristics of rat brain development: A critical period for regionally selective alterations? Teratology 46:45, 1992.

Cayea PD, Grant DC, Doubilet PM, et al: Prediction of fetal lung maturity inaccuracy of study using conventional ultrasound instruments. Radiology 155:473, 1985.

Clements JA, Platzker ACG, Tierney DF, et al: Assessment of the risk of respiratory distress syndrome by a rapid test for surfactant in amniotic fluid. N Engl J Med 286:1077, 1972.

Collaborative Group on Antenatal Steroid Therapy: Effect of antenatal dexamethasone administration on the prevention of respiratory distress syndrome. Am J Obstet Gynecol 141:276, 1981.

Cotterrell M, Balazs R, Johnson AL: Effects of corticosteroids on the biochemical maturation of rat brain: postnatal cell formation. J Neurochem 19:2151, 1972.

Cotton DB, Spillman T, Bretaudiere JP: Effect of blood contamination on lecithin to sphingomyelin ratio in amniotic fluid by different detection methods. Clin Chim Acta 137:299, 1984.

Crowley PA: Antenatal corticosteroid therapy: A meta-analysis of the randomized trials, 1972 to 1994. Am J Obstet Gynecol 173:322, 1995.

Crowley PA: Prophylactic corticosteroids for preterm birth. The Cochrane database of systematic reviews, 10/27/1999, The Cochrane Library 2:2002.

Crowther CA, Alfirevic Z, Haslam RR: Prenatal thyrotropin-releasing hormone for preterm birth. The Cochrane database of systematic reviews, 13-3-2001, The Cochrane Library 2:2002.

Cruz AC, Buhi WC, Birk SA, et al: Respiratory distress syndrome with mature lecithin/sphingomyelin ratios: diabetes mellitus and low Apgar scores. Am J Obstet Gynecol 126:78, 1976.

Curet LB, Olson RW, Schneider JM, et al: Effect of diabetes mellitus on amniotic fluid lecithin/sphingomyelin ratio and respiratory distress syndrome. Am J Obstet Gynecol 135:10, 1979.

Dalence CR, Bowie LJ, Dohnal JC, et al: Amniotic fluid lamellar body count: A rapid and reliable fetal lung maturity test. Obstet Gynecol 86:235, 1995.

Dawes GS, Serra-Serra V, Moulden M, et al: Dexamethasone and fetal heart rate variation. Br J Obstet Gynaecol 101:675, 1994.

Diebel ND, Parsons MT, Spellacy WN: The effects of betamethasone on white blood cells during pregnancy with pPROM. J Perinat Med 26:204, 1998.

Donovan EF, Ehrenkranz RA, Shankaran S, et al: Outcomes of very low birth weight twins cared for in the National Institute of Child Health and Human Development Neonatal Research Network's intensive care units. Am J Obstet Gynecol 179:742, 1998.

Drug Facts and Comparisons. St Louis, Mo, Facts and Comparisons, 1995, p. 504.

Dubin SB: Characterization of amniotic fluid lamellar bodies by resistive-pulse counting: Relationship to measures of fetal lung maturity. Clin Chem 35:612, 1989.

Dudley DK, Black DM: Reliability of lecithin/sphingomyelin ratios in diabetic pregnancy. Obstet Gynecol 66:521, 1985.

Dunlop SA, Archer MA, Quinlivan JA, et al: Repeated prenatal corticosteroids delay myelination in the ovine central nervous system. J Matern Fetal Med 6:309, 1997.

Edwards RK, Duff P, Ross KC: Amniotic fluid indices of fetal pulmonary maturity with preterm premature rupture of membranes. Obstet Gynecol 96:102, 2000.

Egerman RS, Mercer BM, Doss JL, et al: A randomized, controlled trial of oral and intramuscular dexamethasone in the prevention of neonatal respiratory distress syndrome. Am J Obstet Gynecol 179:1120, 1998.

Egerman RS, Pierce WF IV, Andersen RN, et al: A comparison of the bioavailability of oral and intramuscular dexamethasone in women in late pregnancy. Obstet Gynecol 89:276, 1997.

Elliott JP, O'Keeffe DF, Greenberg P, et al: Pulmonary edema associated with magnesium sulfate and betamethasone administration. Am J Obstet Gynecol 134:717, 1979.

Estol PC, Poseiro JJ, Schwarcz R: Phosphatidylglycerol determination in the amniotic fluid from a PAD placed over the vulva: A method for diagnosis of fetal lung maturity in cases of premature ruptured membranes. J Perinat Med 20:65, 1992.

Fakhoury G, Daikoku NH, Benser J, et al: Lamellar body concentrations and the prediction of fetal pulmonary maturity. Am J Obstet Gynecol 170:72, 1994.

Fenton BW, Lin CS, Ascher S, et al: Magnetic resonance spectroscopy to detect lecithin in amniotic fluid and fetal lung. Obstet Gynecol 95:457, 2000.

Ferroni KM, Gross TL, Sokol RJ, et al: What affects fetal pulmonary maturation during diabetic pregnancy? Am J Obstet Gynecol 150:270, 1984.

Fisher JE, Smith RS, Lagrandeur R, et al: Gestational diabetes mellitus in women receiving beta-adrenergics and corticosteroids for threatened preterm delivery. Obstet Gynecol 90:880, 1997.

Fleisher B, Kulovich MV, Hallman M, et al: Lung profile sex differences in normal pregnancy. Obstet Gynecol 66:327, 1985.

French NP, Hagan R, Evans SF, et al: Repeated antenatal corticosteroids: Size at birth and subsequent development. Am J Obstet Gynecol 180:114, 1999.

Fried AM, Loh FK, Umer MA, et al: Echogenicity of fetal lung relation to fetal age and maturity. Am J Roentgenol 145:591, 1985.

Gamsu HR, Mullinger BM, Donnai P, et al: Antenatal administration of betamethasone to prevent respiratory distress syndrome in preterm infants: Report of a UK multicentre trial. Br J Obstet Gynaecol 96:401, 1989.

Garite TJ, Yabusaki KK, Moberg LJ, et al: A new rapid slide agglutination test for amniotic fluid phosphatidylglycerol: Laboratory and clinical correlation. Am J Obstet Gynecol 147:681, 1983.

Gluck L: Biochemical development of the lung: Clinical aspects of surfactant development, RDS and the intrauterine assessment of lung maturity. Clin Obstet Gynecol 14:710, 1971.

Gluck L, Kulovich MV: Lecithin-sphingomyelin ratios in amniotic fluid in normal and abnormal pregnancy. Am J Obstet Gynecol 115:539, 1973.

Gluck L, Kulovich MV, Borer RC Jr, et al: Diagnosis of the respiratory distress syndrome by amniocentesis. Am J Obstet Gynecol 109:440, 1971.

Golde SH: Use of obstetric perineal pads in collection of amniotic fluid in patients with rupture of the membranes. Am J Obstet Gynecol 146:710, 1983.

Golde SH, Petrucha R, Meade KW, et al: Fetal lung maturity: The adjunctive use of ultrasound. Am J Obstet Gynecol 142:445, 1982.

Golde SH, Tahilramaney MP, Platt LD: Use of ultrasound to predict fetal lung maturity in 247 consecutive elective cesarean deliveries. J Reprod Med 29:9, 1984.

Gonzales LK, Ballard PL: Glucocorticoid and thyroid hormone stimulation of phosphatidylcholine synthesis in cultured human fetal lung. Pediatr Res 18:310A, 1984.

Grajwer LA, Lilien LD, Pildes RS: Neonatal subclinical adrenal insufficiency. Result of maternal steroid therapy. JAMA 238:1279, 1977.

Grannum PAT, Berkowitz RL, Hobbins JC: The ultrasonic changes in the maturing placenta and their relation to fetal pulmonic maturity. Am J Obstet Gynecol 133:915, 1979.

Gross TL, Wolfson RN, Kuhnert PM, et al: Sonographically detected free-floating particles in amniotic fluid predict a mature lecithin-sphingomyelin ratio. J Clin Ultrasound 6:405, 1985.

Guinn DA, Atkinson MW, Sullivan L, et al: Single vs weekly courses of antenatal corticosteroids for women at risk of preterm delivery: A randomized controlled trial. JAMA 286:1581, 2001.

Hadlock FP: Biparietal diameter and fetal lung maturity. Am J Obstet Gynecol 144:993, 1982.

Hadlock FP, Irwin JF, Roecker E, et al: Ultrasound prediction of fetal lung maturity. Radiology **155**:469, 1985.

Halliday HL, Ehrenkranz RA: Early postnatal (<96 hours) corticosteroids for preventing chronic lung disease in preterm infants. The Cochrane database of systematic reviews, 13-3-2001, The Cochrane Library 2:2002.

Hallman M, Feldman BH, Kirkpatrick E, et al: Absence of phosphatidylglycerol (PG) in respiratory distress syndrome in the newborn. Study of the minor surfactant phospholipids in newborns. Pediatr Res **11**:714, 1977.

Hallman M, Kulovich M, Kirkpatrick E, et al: Phosphatidylinositol and phosphatidylglycerol in amniotic fluid: Indices of lung maturity. Am J Obstet Gynecol **125**:613, 1976.

Hallman M, Wermer D, Epstein BL, et al: Effects of maternal insulin or glucose infusion on the fetus: Study on lung surfactant phospholipids, plasma myoinositol, and fetal growth in the rabbit. Am J Obstet Gynecol **142**:877, 1982.

Halvorsen PR, Gross TL: Laboratory and clinical evaluation of a rapid slide agglutination test for phosphatidylglycerol. Am J Obstet Gynecol **151**:1061, 1985.

Harding JE, Pang J, Knight DB, et al: Do antenatal corticosteroids help in the setting of preterm rupture of membranes? Am J Obstet Gynecol **184**:131, 2001.

Harman CR, Manning FA, Stearns E, et al: The correlation of ultrasonic placental grading and fetal pulmonary maturation in five hundred sixty-three pregnancies. Am J Obstet Gynecol **143**:941, 1982.

Hastwell GB: Amniotic fluid: Visual assessment of fetal maturity. Lancet. 1:349, 1975.

Helewa M, Manning F, Harman C: Amniotic fluid particles: Are they related to a mature amniotic fluid phospholipid profile? Obstet Gynecol **74**:893, 1989.

Herbert WN, Chapman JF, Schnoor MM: Role of the TDx FLM assay in fetal lung maturity. Am J Obstet Gynecol **168**:808, 1993.

Horenstein J, Golde SH, Platt LD: Lung profiles in the isoimmunized pregnancy. Am J Obstet Gynecol **153**:443, 1985.

Huang WL, Beazley LD, Quinlivan JA, et al: Effect of corticosteroids on brain growth in fetal sheep. Obstet Gynecol **94**:213, 1999.

Huang WL, Harper CG, Evans SF, et al: Repeated prenatal corticosteroid administration delays myelination of the corpus callosum in fetal sheep. Int J Dev Neurosci **19**:415, 2001.

Jobe AH, Wada N, Berry LM, et al: Single and repetitive maternal glucocorticoid exposures reduce fetal growth in sheep. Am J Obstet Gynecol **178**:880, 1998.

Jones GW, Ashwood ER: Enzymatic measurement of phosphatidylglycerol in amniotic fluid. Clin Chem **40**:518, 1994.

Kari MA, Hallman M, Eronen M, et al: Prenatal dexamethasone treatment in conjunction with rescue therapy of human surfactant: a randomized placebo-controlled multicenter study. Pediatrics **93**:730, 1994.

Kulovich MV, Gluck L: The lung profile. II. Complicated pregnancy. Am J Obstet Gynecol **135**:64, 1979.

Kulovich MV, Hallman MB, Gluck L: The lung profile. I. Normal pregnancy. Am J Obstet Gynecol **135**:57, 1979.

Lauria MR, Dombrowski MP, Delaney-Black V, et al: Lung maturity tests. Relation to source, clarity, gestational age and neonatal outcome. J Reprod Med **41**:685, 1996.

Lawrence S, Warshaw J, Nielsen HC: Delayed lung maturation in the macrosomic offspring of genetically determined diabetic (db/+) mice. Pediatr Res **25**:173, 1989.

Lee BO, Major FJ, Weingold AB: Ultrasonic determination of fetal maturity at repeat cesarean section. Obstet Gynecol **38**:294, 1971.

Leveno KJ, Quirk JG, Whalley PJ, et al: Fetal lung maturation in twin gestation. Am J Obstet Gynecol **148**:405, 1984.

Lewis DF, Fontenot MT, Brooks GG, et al: Latency period after preterm premature rupture of membranes: A comparison of ampicillin with and without sulbactam. Obstet Gynecol **86**:392, 1995.

Lewis DF, Towers CV, Major CA, et al: Use of Amniostat-FLM in detecting the presence of phosphatidylglycerol in vaginal pool samples in preterm premature rupture of membranes. Am J Obstet Gynecol **169**:573, 1993.

Liggins GC, Howie RN: A controlled trial of antepartum glucocorticoid treatment for prevention of the respiratory distress syndrome in premature infants. Pediatrics **50**:515, 1972.

Lockitch G, Wittmann BK, Mura SM, et al: Evaluation of the Amniostat-FLM assay for assessment of fetal lung maturity. Clin Chem **30**:1233, 1984.

Magee LA, Dawes GS, Moulden M, et al: A randomised controlled comparison of betamethasone with dexamethasone: Effects on the antenatal fetal heart rate. Br J Obstet Gynaecol **104**:1233, 1997.

McElrath TF, Norwitz ER, Robinson JN, et al: Differences in TDx fetal lung maturity assay values between twin and singleton gestations. Am J Obstet Gynecol **182**:1110, 2000.

McKenna DS, Wittber GM, Nagaraja HN, et al: The effects of repeat doses of antenatal corticosteroids on maternal adrenal function. Am J Obstet Gynecol **183**:669, 2000.

Mercer B, Egerman R, Beazley D, et al: Antenatal corticosteroids in women at risk for preterm birth: A randomized trial. Am J Obstet Gynecol **184**:S6, 2001a.

Mercer B, Egerman R, Beazley D, et al: Steroids reduce fetal growth: Analysis of a prospective trial. Am J Obstet Gynecol **184**:S6, 2001b.

Moore RJ, Strachan B, Tyler DJ, et al: In vivo diffusion measurements as an indication of fetal lung maturation using echo planar imaging at 0.5T. Magn Reson Med **45**:247, 2001.

Mulder EJ, Derks JB, Visser GH: Antenatal corticosteroid therapy and fetal behaviour: A randomised study of the effects of betamethasone and dexamethasone. Br J Obstet Gynaecol **104**:1239, 1997.

National Institutes of Health Consensus Development Conference Statement: Effect of corticosteroids for fetal maturation on perinatal outcomes, February 28–March 24, 1994. Am J Obstet Gynecol **173**:246, 1995.

National Institutes of Health Consensus Development Conference Statement, August 17–18, 2000: Antenatal corticosteroids revisited: Repeat courses. Obstet Gynecol **98**:144, 2001.

Neerhof MG, Dohnal JC, Ashwood ER, et al: Lamellar body counts: A consensus on protocol. Obstet Gynecol **97**:318, 2001.

Neerhof MG, Haney EI, Silver RK, et al: Lamellar body counts compared with traditional phospholipid analysis as an assay for evaluating fetal lung maturity. Obstet Gynecol **97**:305, 2001.

Newton ER, Cetrulo CL, Kosa DJ: Biparietal diameter as a predictor of fetal lung maturity. J Reprod Med **7**:480, 1983.

Nielson HC, Harvey-Wilkes K, MacKinnon B, et al. Neonatal outcome of very premature infants from multiple and singleton gestations. Am J Obstet Gynecol **177**:563, 1997.

O'Dwyer PG, MacGillivray AI, Whittle MJ, et al: A comparison of AmnioStat-FLM with three established methods of assessing fetal lung maturity. Eur J Obstet Gynecol Reprod Biol **27**:59, 1988.

Ohrlander S, Gennser G, Nilsson KO, et al: ACTH test to neonates after administration of corticosteroids during gestation. Obstet Gynecol **49**:691, 1977.

Parulekar SG: Ultrasonographic demonstration of floating particles in amniotic fluid. J Ultrasound Med **2**:107, 1983.

Pastorek JG II, Letellier RL, Gebbia K: Production of a phosphatidylglycerol-like substance by genital flora bacteria. Am J Obstet Gynecol **159**:199, 1988.

Pattinson RC, Makin JD, Funk M, et al: The use of dexamethasone in women with preterm premature rupture of membranes—a multicentre, double-blind, placebo-controlled, randomised trial. Dexiprom Study Group. S Afr Med J **89**:865, 1999.

Petrucha RA, Golde SH, Platt LD: The use of ultrasound in the prediction of fetal pulmonary maturity. Am J Obstet Gynecol **144**:931, 1982.

Phillippe M, Acker D, Torday J, et al: The effects of vaginal contamination on two pulmonary phospholipid assays. J Reprod Med **27**:283, 1982.

Piazze JJ, Maranghi L, Nigro G, et al: The effect of glucocorticoid therapy on fetal lung maturity indices in hypertensive pregnancies. Obstet Gynecol **92**:220, 1998.

Piper JM, Langer O: Does maternal diabetes delay fetal pulmonary maturity? Am J Obstet Gynecol **168**:783, 1993.

Piper JM, Xenakis EM, Langer O: Delayed appearance of pulmonary maturation markers is associated with poor glucose control in diabetic pregnancies. J Matern Fetal Med **7**:148, 1998.

Plauche WC, Faro S, Wycheck J: Amniotic fluid optical density: relationship to L:S ratio, phospholipid content, and desquamation of fetal cells. Obstet Gynecol **58**:309, 1981.

Quinlan RW, Buhi WC, Cruz AC: Fetal pulmonary maturity in isoimmunized pregnancies. Am J Obstet Gynecol **148**:787, 1984.

Quinlivan JA, Archer MA, Evans SF, et al: Fetal sciatic nerve growth is delayed following repeated maternal injections of corticosteroid in sheep. J Perinat Med **28**:26, 2000.

Ragozzino MW, Hill LM, Breckle R, et al: The relationship of placental grade by ultrasound to markers of fetal lung maturity. Radiology **148**:805, 1983.

Richardson DK, Torday JS: Racial differences in predictive value of the lecithin/sphingomyelin ratio. Am J Obstet Gynecol **170**:1273, 1994.

Rotmensch S, Liberati M, Vishne TH, et al: The effect of betamethasone and dexamethasone on fetal heart rate patterns and biophysical activities. A prospective randomized trial. Acta Obstet Gynecol Scand **78**:493, 1999.

Russell JC, Cooper CM, Ketchum CH, et al: Multicenter evaluation of TDx test for assessing fetal lung maturity. Clin Chem **35**:1005, 1989.

Sabbagha R, Salvino C: Report on third trimester amniocentesis at Prentice Women's Hospital of Northwestern University Medical School, Chicago,

Illinois. Antenatal diagnosis. NIH Consensus Statement. National Institutes of Health. Bethesda, Maryland 2:61. *In*: Stark (2000), 1979.

Sbarra AJ, Blake G, Cetrulo CL, et al: The effect of cervical/vaginal secretions on measurements of lecithin/sphingomyelin ratio and optical density at 650 nm. Am J Obstet Gynecol **139**:214, 1981.

Sbarra AJ, Chaudhury A, Cetrulo CL, et al: A rapid visual test for predicting fetal lung maturity. Am J Obstet Gynecol **165**:1351, 1991.

Schiff E, Friedman SA, Mercer BM, et al: Fetal lung maturity is not accelerated in preeclamptic pregnancies. Am J Obstet Gynecol **169**:1096, 1993.

Schumacher RE, Parisi VM, Steady HM, et al: Bacteria causing false positive test for phosphatidylglycerol in amniotic fluid. Am J Obstet Gynecol **151**:1067, 1985.

Senat MV, Minoui S, Multon O, et al: Effect of dexamethasone and betamethasone on fetal heart rate variability in preterm labour: A randomised study. Br J Obstet Gynaecol **105**:749, 1998.

Shaver DC, Spinnato JA, Whybrew D, et al: Comparison of phospholipids in vaginal and amniocentesis specimens of patients with premature rupture of membranes. Am J Obstet Gynecol **156**:454, 1987.

Sher G, Statland BE: Assessment of fetal pulmonary maturity by the Lumadex Foam Stability Index Test. Obstet Gynecol **61**:444, 1983.

Sher G, Statland BE, Freer DE, et al: Assessing fetal lung maturation by the foam index stability test. Obstet Gynecol **52**:673, 1978.

Sinclair JC: Meta-analysis of randomized controlled trials of antenatal corticosteroid for the prevention of respiratory distress syndrome: Discussion. Am J Obstet Gynecol **173**:335, 1995.

Smith BT, Giroud CJ, Robert M, et al: Insulin antagonism of cortisol action on lechithin synthesis by cultured fetal lung cells. J Pediatr **87**:953, 1975.

Smolders-de Haas H, Neuvel J, Schmand B, et al: Physical development and medical history of children who were treated antenatally with corticosteroids to prevent respiratory distress syndrome: A 10- to 12-year follow-up. Pediatrics **86**:65, 1990.

Socol ML, Sing E, Depp OR: The tap test: A rapid indicator of fetal pulmonary maturity. Am J Obstet Gynecol **148**:445, 1984.

Spellacy WN, Gelman SR, Wood SD, et al: Comparison of fetal maturity evaluation with ultrasonic biparietal diameter and amniotic fluid lecithin-sphingomyelin ratio. Obstet Gynecol **51**:109, 1978.

Stark CM, Smith RS, Lagrandeur RM, et al: Need for urgent delivery after third-trimester amniocentesis. Obstet Gynecol **95**:48, 2000.

Steinfeld JD, Samuels P, Bulley MA, et al: The utility of the TDx test in the assessment of fetal lung maturity. Obstet Gynecol **79**:460, 1992.

Strassner HT, Platt LD, Whittle M, et al: Amniotic fluid phosphatidylglycerol and real-time ultrasonic cephalometry. Am J Obstet Gynecol **135**:804, 1979.

Strong TH Jr, Hayes AS, Sawyer AT, et al: Amniotic fluid turbidity a useful adjunct for assessing fetal pulmonary maturity status. Int J Gynaecol Obstet **38**:97, 1992.

Tabsh KM, Brinkman CR III, Bashore R: Effect of meconium contamination on amniotic fluid lecithin: Sphingomyelin ratio. Obstet Gynecol **58**:605, 1981.

Tabsh KM, Brinkman CR III, Bashore RA: Lecithin:sphingomyelin ratio in pregnancies complicated by insulin-dependent diabetes mellitus. Obstet Gynecol **59**:353, 1982.

Tanasijevic MJ, Winkelman JW, Wybenga DR, et al: Prediction of fetal lung maturity in infants of diabetic mothers using the FLM S/A and disaturated phosphatidylcholine tests. Am J Clin Pathol **105**:17, 1996.

Tanasijevic MJ, Wybenga DR, Richardson D, et al: A predictive model for fetal lung maturity employing gestational age and test results. Am J Clin Pathol **102**:788, 1994.

Teramo K, Hallman M, Raivio KO: Maternal glucocorticoid in unplanned premature labor. Controlled study on the effects of betamethasone phosphate on the phospholipids of the gastric aspirate and on the adrenal cortical function of the newborn infant. Pediatr Res **14**:326, 1980.

Terrone DA, Rinehart BK, Rhodes PG, et al: Multiple courses of betamethasone to enhance fetal lung maturation do not suppress neonatal adrenal response. Am J Obstet Gynecol **180**:1349, 1999.

Terrone DA, Smith LG Jr, Wolf EJ, et al: Neonatal effects and serum cortisol levels after multiple courses of maternal corticosteroids. Obstet Gynecol **90**:819, 1997.

Uno H, Eisele S, Sakai A, et al: Neurotoxicity of glucocorticoids in the primate brain. Horm Behav **28**:336, 1994.

Uno H, Lohmiller L, Thieme C, et al: Brain damage induced by prenatal exposure to dexamethasone in fetal rhesus macaques. I. Hippocampus. Brain Res Dev Brain Res **53**:157, 1990.

Wigton TR, Tamura RK, Wickstrom E, et al: Neonatal morbidity after preterm delivery in the presence of documented lung maturity. Am J Obstet Gynecol **169**:951, 1993.

Winn HN, Klosterman A, Amon E, et al: Does preeclampsia influence fetal lung maturity? J Perinat Med **28**:210, 2000.

Winn HN, Romero R, Roberts A, et al: Comparison of fetal lung maturation in preterm singleton and twin pregnancies. Am J Perinatol **9**:326, 1992.

Wu B, Kikkaway, Orzalesi MM, et al: The effect of thyroxine on the maturation of fetal rabbit lungs. Biol Neonate **22**:161, 1973.

Yunis KA, Bitar FF, Hayek P, et al: Transient hypertrophic cardiomyopathy in the newborn following multiple doses of antenatal corticosteroids. Am J Perinatol **16**:17, 1999.

Zachman RD, Bauer CR, Boehm J, et al: Effect of antenatal dexamethasone on neonatal leukocyte count. J Perinatol **8**:111, 1988.

Chapter 26

FETAL CARDIAC ARRHYTHMIAS
Diagnosis and Therapy

Charles S. Kleinman, MD, Rodrigo Nehgme, MD, and Joshua A. Copel, MD

Most disturbances of fetal cardiac rhythm are due to isolated extrasystoles that are of little clinical import to the human fetus. On occasion, however, isolated extrasystoles precipitate sustained fetal tachycardias, which can have important clinical implications. Sustained cardiac arrhythmias can eventually lead to fetal heart failure, which manifests as nonimmune hydrops fetalis. In such cases, antiarrhythmic therapy may be required before delivery. Such therapy should be provided in a logical and well-planned fashion, based on an understanding of the electrophysiologic mechanism of the arrhythmia and an understanding of the pharmacokinetics and pharmacology of the fetus, placenta, and mother (Juchau et al., 1973; Krauer and Krauer, 1977; Levy, 1981; McKercher and Radde, 1985; Mattison et al., 1992; Pacifici and Nottoli, 1995; Ward, 1995). This understanding can then guide a logical selection of antiarrhythmic agents. Close monitoring of maternal and fetal hemodynamic responses is essential for any therapy to be provided safely.

This chapter reviews the application of fetal echocardiography for analysis of fetal cardiac arrhythmias and for monitoring transplacental antiarrhythmic therapy. The most commonly used antiarrhythmic agents are reviewed in the context of their use for fetal therapy, and a rationale is proposed for the management of clinically important fetal arrhythmias.

A fetal arrhythmia is defined as any irregularity of fetal cardiac rhythm or any regular rhythm that remains outside the general range of 100 to 160 beats per minute. These occur without association to uterine contractions, and periodic decelerations of the fetal heart rate are not included.

FREQUENCY

In most cases, the original reason for referral is the detection by the referring obstetrician or midwife of a fetal cardiac arrhythmia during routine auscultation. The most frequent finding is the impression of a skipped beat. In most cases, the "skipping" actually represents either a pause following an extrasystole or an extrasystole occurring early enough in the cardiac cycle to result in a stroke volume that is inadequate to produce a detectable Doppler signal. In rare instances, patients are referred because of sustained fetal tachyarrhythmias or bradyarrhythmias.

Of 1384 fetuses evaluated at our institution over the course of 20 years for fetal arrhythmias, 1213 (88%) had either

normal rhythm or isolated extrasystoles (Table 26-1). Most of these (1181) extrasystoles were supraventricular in origin, whereas the others had a ventricular or junctional origin. These arrhythmias resolved either later in the pregnancy or over the first several days after birth.

In a review of 595 patients referred because of irregular heart rhythms, it was noted that 55% had normal sinus rhythm by the time of their evaluation. There were isolated extrasystoles, overwhelmingly atrial in origin, in 43%. Clinically significant rhythm abnormalities were found in 1.6% before birth and in another 0.8% after birth. Significant structural heart disease was no more common than in the general population (0.3%, 95% confidence interval 0–0.7%). Extended evaluation of the fetal heart rate to detect significant tachycardias continues to be warranted, and intermittent auscultation on a weekly basis for affected fetuses with extrasystoles to exclude any new runs of tachycardia also seems prudent (Copel et al., 2000).

A total of 164 fetuses presented with sustained arrhythmias (Table 26-2). This number included 114 patients with sustained tachyarrhythmias; 69 with supraventricular tachycardia (SVT), 21 with atrial flutter, three with atrial fibrillation, four with chaotic atrial rhythms (tachyarrhythmias arising from three or more locations in the atrium), two with junctional tachycardia, eight with sinus tachycardia, and seven with ventricular tachycardia. Another 50 patients were seen with sustained bradyarrhythmias, including ten with second-degree AV block, two with sinus bradycardia, and 38 with complete heart block.

METHODS OF DIAGNOSIS

Echocardiographic Analysis of Fetal Cardiac Rhythm

The depolarization and repolarization of cardiac muscle cells result in electrical activity that can be recorded easily on the body surface as an electrocardiogram (ECG). Cardiac electrical activity, however, has its mechanical and dynamic translation in the motion of the heart walls and in flow across the atrioventricular (AV) and semilunar valves. Atrial depolarization —represented by the P wave on the surface ECG—results in atrial contraction, which forces flow across the AV (mitral and tricuspid) valves. Ventricular depolarization—represented by the QRS complex on the surface ECG—results in ventricular contraction, which closes the AV valves and pumps blood

TABLE 26-1. FETAL CARDIAC ARRHYTHMIAS
(n = 1384)

Isolated extrasystoles	1213
Supraventricular tachycardia	69
Atrial flutter	21
Atrial fibrillation	4
Chaotic atrial rhythm	4
Sinus tachycardia	8
Junctional tachycardia	2
Ventricular tachycardia	7
Second-degree atrioventricular block	10
Sinus bradycardia	2
Complete heart block	39

across the semilunar (aortic and pulmonic) valves. The T wave on the surface ECG represents ventricular electrical repolarization. Electrophysiologists use the surface ECG to analyze the normal cardiac rhythm and its disturbances. The ECG gives information about heart rate, the relationship between atrial and ventricular activity, cardiac intervals, and the origin and mechanisms of abnormal rhythms. The ECG also helps to evaluate the response to therapeutic interventions and to monitor potential proarrhythmic side effects of antiarrhythmic drugs.

Although it would be preferable to use high-quality recordings of the fetal ECG to analyze the fetal cardiac rhythm, the technology required to obtain such recordings against interference from the maternal ECG signal and the background noise of 60 Hz interference has not yet been fully developed. Fetal magnetocardiography (Quinn et al., 1994; Dorostkar et al., 1997) is a novel, noninvasive method for measuring the electrical activity of the heart with sufficient resolution to record P waves and QRS-T complexes as early as 20 weeks of gestation. The clinical applicability of fetal magnetocardiography and its correlation with the more standard techniques to assess fetal cardiac rhythm, however, have not been demonstrated. Its expense and lack of wide availability further limit its current clinical utility.

Analysis of the motion of the cardiac chambers and flow dynamics against time can also yield information about rate, AV relationship, and intervals. In fact, motion and flow dynamics are the almost simultaneous mechanical and dynamic translation of the electrical heart signals. In the absence of an adequate fetal ECG, M-mode echocardiographic recordings of cardiac motion or Doppler studies of cardiac flow against time serve as the cornerstones for the diagnosis and monitoring of fetal cardiac arrhythmias. One can actually consider them to be mechanical and dynamic ECG.

M-Mode Echocardiography

When real-time imaging techniques are used, an initial analysis of cardiac anatomy should be performed. The two-dimensional image is used to orient the position of the M-mode sampling line. M-mode echocardiographic recordings of cardiac motion against time are performed. These recordings, which are used to time electromechanical events in the fetal cardiac cycle, can be obtained by placing the sampling line to intercept both atrial and ventricular walls. These recordings can provide sufficient information to allow accurate timing of atrial and ventricular mechanical events in the cardiac cycle,

based on the presumption that cardiac mechanical events reflect preceding electrical events. A ladder-diagram analysis of the AV contraction sequence can then be constructed to provide accurate analysis of cardiac rhythm (Kleinman et al., 1980, 1983) (Fig. 26-1).

Pulsed-Doppler Echocardiography

Spectral Doppler echocardiography, using the two-dimensional image to orient the sample volume within the cardiac chambers or great vessels, provides information with regard to the timing of mechanical events and their influence on ventricular filling and great arterial flow. Sample volume placement is usually at the junction of ventricular inflow and outflow tracks (Kleinman et al., 1984, 1987). Placement overlapping a pulmonary vein and pulmonary artery (DeVore and Horenstein, 1993) or the inferior vena cava and aorta (Chan et al., 1990) has also been described, providing both venous filling and arterial ejection information simultaneously.

TABLE 26-2. FETAL TACHYARRHYTHMIAS

Supraventricular Tachycardia (n = 69)

Gestational age	16–40 weeks
Hydrops fetalis	44/69
Intermittent tachycardia	19
Incessant tachycardia	50
In utero therapy	47
In utero control	42/47
Postnatal control	5/47
Congenital heart disease	1/69
Deaths	4/69

Atrial Flutter (n = 21)

Gestational age	24–39 weeks
Hydrops fetalis	9/21
In utero therapy	19
In utero control	13/19
Postnatal control	4
Congenital heart disease	6/21
Deaths	4/21

Atrial Fibrillation (n = 4)

Gestational age	19–38 weeks
Hydrops fetalis	0
In utero therapy	4
In utero control	3
Postnatal control	1
Deaths	0

Ventricular Tachycardia (n = 7)

Gestational age	19–34 weeks
Hydrops fetalis	1
Intermittent tachycardia	5
Incessant tachycardia	2
Atrioventricular dissociation	6
In utero therapy	2
In utero control	2
Postnatal control	2
Persistent ventricular tachycardia	2
Arrhythmogenic RV	1
Deaths	0

From Kleinman CS, Donnerstein RL, Jaffe CC, et al: Fetal echocardiography: A tool for evaluation of in utero cardiac arrhythmias and monitoring of *in utero* therapy: Analysis of 71 patients. Am J Cardiol **51**:237, 1983.

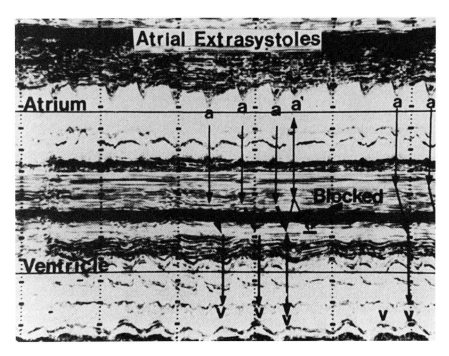

FIGURE 26-1. ■ Ladder diagram analysis of fetal cardiac rhythm using dual M-mode echocardiographic recording of atrial and ventricular activity. Upper tracing represents atrial wall motion. Regular atrial rhythm, denoted by a, is interrupted by early contraction, a', which represents an atrial extrasystole. Simultaneously recorded ventricular wall movement is shown lower with the letters "V." These occur following a slight delay of conduction in the atrioventricular node. The atrial extrasystole has occurred too soon after the last normally conducted sinus beat, resulting in block within the still refractory atrioventricular node and the absence of a ventricular response to the atrial beat.

Color-Encoded M-Mode Echocardiography

Color flow Doppler mapping has added a new modality to the two-dimensional imaging of fetal cardiac structure by providing flow information in color over the two-dimensional grayscale image of the fetal heart. This information provides important physiologic data, which, although rarely absolutely required to establish an anatomic diagnosis of congenital heart disease (Copel et al., 1991), may improve the accuracy of prenatal structural diagnosis by imparting simultaneous flow data. The major shortcoming of color flow mapping is the lack of temporal resolution. Postnatally, this shortcoming can be overcome with the simultaneous recording of an ECG, which adds temporal information. Without a fetal electrocardiographic signal, the use of color-encoded M-mode echocardiography can provide insight into the analysis of fetal cardiac rhythm disturbances. By superimposing color flow information on the M-mode echocardiogram, one can take advantage of the cardiac motion against time information of the M-mode echocardiogram. Therefore, these hard-copy simultaneous recordings of cardiac motion and cardiac flow over time can be used to analyze the electromechanical activity of the fetal heart.

Doppler Tissue Velocity Imaging

Using the newer techniques of Doppler Tissue Imaging, the motion of the myocardium at various locations in the fetal heart can provide information concerning the timing and activation sequence of electrical stimulation of various parts of the fetal heart. Rein and colleagues (2002), using stored digital scan-line data, constructed simultaneous tissue velocity imaging curves of segmental motion from 4 small regions of interest in the fetal heart (Fig. 26-2; Color Plate 15). Using these curves, a "ladder-diagram" type of temporal analysis of atrial and ventricular electromechanical events was performed (Fig. 26-3). This was termed the *fetal kinetocardiogram*. This technique promises to provide significant insights into the mode of initiation of fetal tachycardia and to allow assessment

of such variables as the effect of spontaneous bundle branch block on the persistence and rate of tachycardia. The technique could also permit identification of conduction abnormalities such as preexcitation and various degrees of AV block. In addition, by determining atrial activation sequence, this technique could allow identification of cases of fetal SVT that are particularly likely to lead to circulatory compromise and hydrops fetalis. As noted elsewhere in this chapter, atrial tachycardia that initiates left atrial contraction before right atrial contraction results in transient alteration of the atrial pressure relationships, favoring partial closure of the foramen ovale. This hemodynamic perturbation is likely to result in a greater increase of mean right atrial pressure at any given atrial rate than if the tachycardia were initiated on the right side of the atrial septum. Because fetal systemic venous hemodynamic versus oncotic pressure relationships are in a relatively precarious balance, even the slight increase in mean systemic pressure related to left atrial tachycardia makes such fetuses particularly prone to the development of hydrops fetalis, and thus candidates for early drug intervention, even in the absence of manifest fetal edema or fluid third-spacing.

Fetal Magnetocardiography

Using external leads affixed to the maternal abdomen, it is possible to detect weak magnetic fields that are caused by the electrical excitation of the fetal heart. These magnetic fields, in the range of 0.2 to 5 picotesla, are a miniscule fraction of the strength of the Earth's magnetic field. These magnetic field variations can be plotted against time, providing hardcopy representation of fetal atrial and ventricular activity from the second trimester onward. Such records provide information equivalent to the surface ECG. These studies can provide important information concerning QRS duration and morphology, which in turn would provide the necessary information to employ the algorithm presented in Figure 26-4 for determining the tachycardia mechanism. Fetal magnetocardiography has demonstrated usefulness for

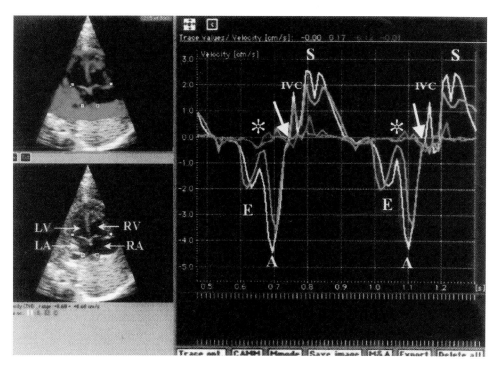

FIGURE 26-2 ■ Doppler tissue velocity imaging tracing demonstrating diphasic diastolic waves below the baseline (E and A), followed by systolic motion in the opposite direction (above baseline). Simultaneous tracings from the right and left atrial posterior walls and right and left AV valve rings are displayed. The electromechanical activation sequence can be discerned from these tracings. (Reproduced with permission from Rein AJJT, O'Donnell C, Geva T, et al: Use of tissue velocity imaging in the diagnosis of fetal cardiac arrhythmias. Circulation **106:**1827, 2002.) See Color Plate 15.

the detection of abnormalities of ventricular repolarization in fetuses with prolonged QT interval and for evaluating the nature of fetal cardiac rhythm disturbances (Fig. 26-5), including fetal atrial flutter and SVT (Menendez et al., 2001; Kariniem V, et al., 1974; Hamada et al., 1999; Horigome et al., 1999; Huirne et al., 1999; Van Leeuwen et al., 1999). Fetal magnetocardiography could represent the equivalent of a noninvasive fetal electrocardiogram. As this technology becomes more widely available, its reliability and ease of use will need to be defined.

ELECTROPHYSIOLOGY OF FETAL CARDIAC ARRHYTHMIAS

Tachyarrhythmias

Supraventricular Tachycardia

Postnatal experience in the analysis and management of SVT has demonstrated the importance of determining the electrophysiologic mechanism of SVT, and subsequently formulat-

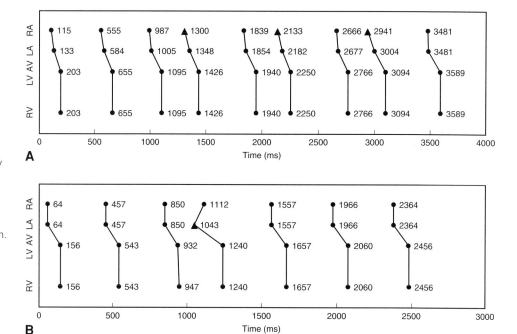

FIGURE 26-3 ■ Fetal kinetocardiogram constructed from Doppler tissue velocity imaging tracings. This is a ladder diagram, allowing analysis of the timing of events in the electromechanical activation sequence. **A,** Every third beat represents an atrial premature contraction arising within the right atrium. Note the delay imparted at the AV node. **B,** The fourth beat is a premature atrial beat arising in the left atrium. (Reproduced with permission from Rein AJJT, O'Donnell C, Geva T, et al: Use of tissue velocity imaging in the diagnosis of fetal cardiac arrhythmias. Circulation **106:**1827, 2002.)

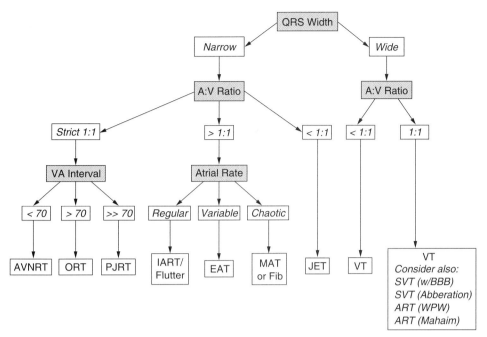

FIGURE 26-4 ■ Algorithm for determining the electrophysiologic mechanism of tachycardia based on evaluation of the ECG. Note that the initial step of this analysis requires evaluation of the morphology or duration of the QRS complex. Of the currently available techniques for fetal cardiac rhythm analysis, only fetal magnetocardiography provides a means of making this measurement. (ART, antidromic reciprocating tachycardia; AV, atrioventricular; AVNRT AV nodal reentrant tachycardia; BBB, bundle branch block; EAT, ectopic atrial tachycardia; IART, intra-atrial reentrant tachycardia; JET, junctional ectopic tachycardia; MAT, multifocal atrial tachycardia; ORT, orthodromic reciprocating tachycardia; PJRT, permanent junctional reciprocating tachycardia; SVT, supraventricular tachycardia; VA, ventriculoatrial interval; VT, ventricular tachycardia; WPW, Wolff-Parkinson-White). (Reproduced with permission from Walsh EP: Clinical approach to diagnosis and acute management of tachycardias in children. *In* Walsh EP, Saul JP, Treidman JK (eds): Cardiac Arrhythmias in Children and Young Adults with Congenital Heart Disease. Philadelphia, Lippincott Williams & Wilkins, 2001, p. 103.)

ing management strategy based on this information. Most frequently, but not always, the mechanism of the tachycardia can be surmised on the basis of a noninvasive assessment of the ECG. Occasionally, the mechanism and definitive treatment of arrhythmia requires electrophysiologic catheterization and radio frequency ablation. It should be no surprise, therefore, that despite the application of elaborate algorithms for the echocardiographic evaluation of fetal arrhythmias and aggressive treatment programs, some fetal arrhythmias remain unresponsive to medical treatment. In some cases this lack of response could be due to inaccurate identification of the nature of the arrhythmia, in other cases to inadequate fetal drug delivery, and, in some cases, to the existence of a particularly recalcitrant arrhythmia.

In his excellent review of the clinical approach to the diagnosis and management of tachycardias in children, Walsh (2001) emphasizes the importance of narrowing the possible underlying electrophysiologic mechanism of tachycardia from the nearly two dozen possible causes of tachycardia in childhood to the one or two most likely. This eliminative process is essential to guide safe and effective acute and chronic drug management (see Fig. 26-4). Note the fundamental inability of echocardiography to provide information concerning QRS duration. Of the techniques currently used for fetal cardiac rhythm analysis, only fetal magnetocardiography (see the following discussion) offers the potential for analysis of this variable. Note, as well, the lower left quadrant of this figure, in

which it is shown that demonstration of a 1:1 AV ratio of conduction is not sufficient to distinguish the etiology of the underlying SVT. The timing of retrograde (ventriculoatrial [VA]) activation of the atrium (less than, greater than, or equal to 70 msec) distinguishes between forms of tachycardia that are likely to be responsive to medical treatment (e.g., atrioventricular nodal reentry tachycardia [AVNRT] or orthodromic reciprocating tachycardia [ORT]) from SVT, which is likely to be recalcitrant to therapy (permanent junctional reciprocating tachycardia [PJRT]).

Using M-mode and pulsed-Doppler echocardiography, Jaeggi and colleagues demonstrated the feasibility of measuring the time intervals between atrial and ventricular activation in fetuses with SVT (Jaeggi et al., 1998) (Figs. 26-6 and 26-7). Using these techniques, the AV (antegrade) and VA (retrograde) time intervals of the electrical reentry circuit of SVT can be analyzed. In the most common form of fetal tachycardia (orthodromic reciprocating tachycardia [ORT]), the electrical pathway involves electrical activation of the ventricle by way of the normal AV node. AV node conduction is inherently slower than conduction through an accessory pathway (e.g., Kent bundle). When a patient has reentry tachycardia, there is one atrial depolarization for each ventricular depolarization (1:1 ratio). If the conduction down to the ventricle is via the AV node, the AV conduction time will be longer than the VA) conduction, up the fast-conducting accessory pathway, from ventricle to atrium. The ECG shows a QRS complex followed

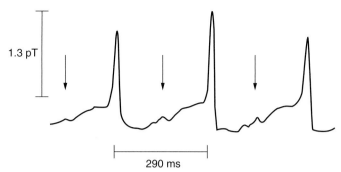

FIGURE 26-5 ■ Fetal magnetocardiogram from a fetus with SVT. Note the cycle length of 290 msec (heart rate ~207 per minute). This rate is not consistent with the "usual" heart rate of 240–260 beats per minute encountered in cases of fetal orthodromic reciprocating tachycardia. There is one atrial depolarization for each ventricular depolarization (A:V = 1:1). Note the relatively broad QRS complex and the long VA interval between the onset of the QRS complex and the subsequent retrograde P-wave. This is consistent with the permanent form of junctional reciprocating tachycardia (PJRT). (Reproduced from Menendez T, Achenbach S, Beinder E, et al: Usefulness of magneto-cardiography for the investigation of fetal arrhythmias. Am J Cardiol **88:**334, 2001.)

closely by a retrograde P wave (short VA time lag), with a longer time lag between that retrograde P wave and the subsequent QRS complex (long AV time, down the slow-conducting AV node). This "usual" type of AV reentry tachycardia (AVRT) will usually respond to "standard" treatments such as digoxin and propranolol. This form of tachycardia accounts for greater than or equal to 90% of fetal tachycardia. On the other hand, another form of reentry tachycardia, often called reciprocating junctional tachycardia (or PJRT for "permanent junctional reciprocating tachycardia") can, by its very name, be expected to represent a particularly recalcitrant reentry tachycardia. This tachycardia typically conducts backward, from ventricle to atrium, by way of the AV node (slow pathway), and it presents a long VA time (greater than 70 msec) and a shorter AV delay (AV time). This tachycardia rarely responds to digoxin or propranolol, and even postnatally, it requires treatment with agents such as flecainide, soltalol, or amiodarone, if drug therapy is to be successful at all. The failure of digoxin in such cases is not related to inadequate blood levels of drug, but to the unique nature of the underlying arrhythmia. In other words, simply determining that there is tachycardia, and noting that there is one atrial beat for each ventricular beat, provides information that is necessary, but not sufficient, to ascertain electrophysiologic mechanism and to predict therapeutic response.

Atrial Flutter and Fibrillation

The incidence of atrial flutter and fibrillation in the fetus is much lower than that of SVT. These patients often present with hydrops fetalis. The relatively high mortality rate in this subgroup of patients (see Table 26-2) attests to the difficulties encountered in controlling these arrhythmias *in utero* and is also related to the relatively high incidence of associated congenital cardiac malformations.

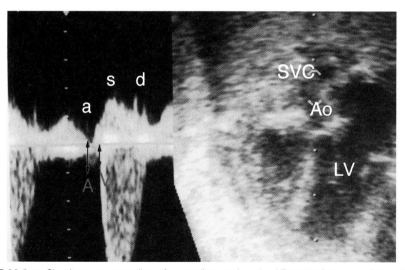

FIGURE 26-6 ■ Simultaneous recording of ascending aortic pulsed-Doppler flow waveform (above the baseline) and superior vena cava flow waveform (below the baseline). Superior vena cava flow is triphasic, consisting of prominent systolic forward flow (related to ventricular systole and suction of venous return into the fetal thorax), a secondary forward flow pulsation related to diastolic passive atrial filling, and a brief retrograde pulsation representing backflow associated with the active atrial contraction that follows the electrocardiographic P-wave. The distance from the onset of the atrial pulsation in the superior vena cava and the onset of the ejection into the ascending aorta (AV) represents the electromechanical delay between the onset of atrial activity and the mechanical ejection of left ventricular blood into the ascending aorta. This is an approximation (but not an exact measurement) of the electrocardiographic PR interval. The delay between the onset of ventricular ejection and the onset of the atrial pulsation (VA) represents the delay between ventricular activity and the onset of the subsequent atrial activation. In the presence of SVT, the measurement of the VA interval could provide valuable information for the differential diagnosis of the electrophysiologic mechanism of the arrhythmia. (Reprinted from Am J Cardiol, **88,** Andelfinger G, Fouron JC, Sonesson SE, et al, Reference values for time intervals between atrial and ventricular contractions of the fetal heart measured by two Doppler techniques, 1433, 2001, with permission from Excerpta Medica, Inc.)

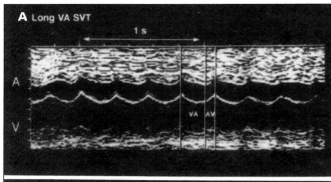

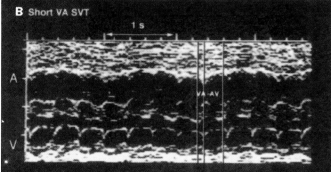

FIGURE 26-7 ■ M-mode echocardiographic tracings demonstrating atrial and ventricular wall motion during fetal SVT. **A,** This fetus has a heart rate of approximately 240 beats per minute, with an AV ratio of 1:1. The VA interval is greater than or equal to 70 msec. This is compatible with a diagnosis of permanent junctional reciprocating tachycardia (PJRT). This arrhythmia is likely to be resistant to antiarrhythmic therapy. **B,** This fetus also has a heart rate of approximately 240 beats per minute, with an AV ratio of 1:1. The VA interval is less than 70 msec. This is compatible with a diagnosis of orthodromic reciprocating tachycardia (ORT), which is likely to be responsive to digoxin therapy. (Reproduced with permission from Jaeggi E, Fouron JC, Fournier A, et al: Ventriculo-atrial time interval measured on M-mode echocardiography: A determining element in diagnosis, treatment, and prognosis of fetal supraventricular tachycardia. Heart **79**:582, 1998.)

Atrial flutter is also a reentry tachyarrhythmia requiring pathways with distinct electrophysiologic properties separated by electrically inactive tissue (fibrous or scar tissue within the atrium), but the reentry circuit is confined to the atrium. The AV node is not part of the circus movement mechanism and only transmits, with a variable degree of restriction or block, the atrial flutter waves to the ventricles. Slowing or blocking conduction through the AV node does not terminate the arrhythmia but does decrease the ventricular response rate. AV synchrony is not restored, and the potential for elevated atrial pressures still exists because atrial contractions occur against closed AV valves during ventricular systole.

The atrial rate in atrial flutter in the neonate is typically 300–360 beats per minute, whereas in the fetus, atrial flutter rates of 400–500 are seen (Fig. 26-8). Varying degrees of AV block can be seen in association with fetal atrial flutter, resulting in varying ventricular response rates, which can be either fixed (with fixed 2:1 or 3:1 AV block) or irregular (with varying degrees of AV block). In either case, the fetal heart rate does not change with fetal activity. The common presence of some degree of AV block is important evidence that this arrhythmia does not involve AV reentry through the AV

node as the underlying electrophysiologic mechanism (Johnson et al., 1987).

Clinical experience has demonstrated that digoxin, propranolol, or verapamil can increase the degree of AV block, resulting in a slower ventricular response rate. Unlike the experience with postnatal therapy of atrial flutter, in which decreasing the ventricular response rate could lead to a decrease in the degree of heart failure, control of the ventricular response rate in fetuses with severe hydrops secondary to atrial flutter has not improved the fetal hemodynamic status. This is likely attributable to the relatively restrictive ventricular myocardium and relatively volume-loaded right heart of the fetus and further suggests that much of the fetal cardiovascular decompensation that accompanies supraventricular tachyarrhythmias reflects diastolic rather than systolic dysfunction. Unless the atrial flutter is controlled, therefore, there will continue to be atrial contraction against a closed or partially closed AV valve, resulting in atrial pressure waves that elevate the mean venous pressure, retarding resolution of fetal edema and effusions.

The therapeutic end point in atrial flutter with hydrops fetalis must be restoration of normal sinus rhythm, with resumption of a 1:1 AV contraction sequence. This usually requires administration of either a type I antiarrhythmic agent such as flecainide or procainamide, or use of a type III agent such as amiodarone or sotalol. Because type I agents initially slow the flutter rate, which favors AV nodal conduction, this therapy is usually initiated after control of the ventricular response rate has been achieved with digoxin or propranolol. Verapamil is not used because of the relative dependence of immature myocardium on transmembrane calcium passage for contraction.

Atrial fibrillation is even more rare in the fetus than is atrial flutter. In this series, three patients with the arrhythmia responded to digoxin therapy alone; however, if the arrhythmia

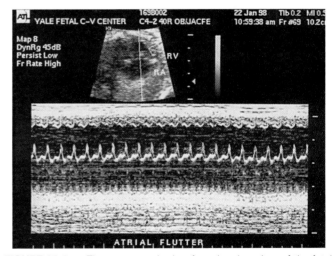

FIGURE 26-8 ■ The *upper portion* is a four-chamber view of the fetal heart, with the right ventricle (RV) and right atrium (RA) designated. The M-mode sample line runs through these two chambers. The *lower portion* shows the movement of the atria and ventricles. The lower chamber (atrium) can be seen to move at twice the rate of the upper chamber. The larger vertical marks on the time scale at the bottom represent 1 second, so that the eight atrial movements in each second give a calculated atrial rate of 480. The four corresponding ventricular movements in each second show the ventricular rate to be 240 (2:1 block).

had persisted despite control of the ventricular response rate in the presence of hydrops fetalis, a type I or type III antiarrhythmic agent would have been added, for the same reasons as for atrial flutter. The high mortality rate (4 of 21 cases) with atrial flutter reflects, in part, the difficulty encountered in controlling this arrhythmia and the association of congenital heart disease in the presence of the arrhythmia. In all cases of congenital heart disease (two with critical pulmonary outflow obstruction and tricuspid insufficiency, one with Ebstein's malformation of the tricuspid valve with severe tricuspid insufficiency, and one with AV septal defect with AV valve insufficiency and associated complete AV block), marked atrial dilation was associated with the development of atrial flutter. The four deaths in the series included three of the patients with associated congenital heart disease. It should be noted that only 1 of 69 cases of fetal SVT was associated with a congenital cardiac structural abnormality, characterized by premature closure of the foramen ovale (Buis-Liem et al., 1987); that fetus was one of four who died. That fetus and one other died despite restoration of normal sinus rhythm for several days before fetal death.

The association of congenital heart disease with sustained fetal cardiac arrhythmias and hydrops fetalis is an ominous one that imparts an extremely poor prognosis for survival, with or without vigorous *in utero* or postnatal therapy.

Ventricular Tachycardia

Our experience has included seven patients with fetal ventricular tachycardia (see Table 26-2). In each case, the heart rate during tachycardia did not fall into the usual range of 240–260 beats per minute encountered in fetuses with AV reciprocating SVT. The common denominator in this group of patients with ventricular tachycardia was the finding of AV dissociation (the lack of a 1:1 relationship between atrial and ventricular contractions) (Fig. 26–9).

AV dissociation can also be found in junctional tachycardia but is almost never seen in AV reciprocating SVT. The presence of AV dissociation, therefore, could be suggestive of the presence of ventricular tachycardia but is not sufficient to establish this as a certain diagnosis because junctional tachycardia can also be associated with AV dissociation. It is, therefore, impossible to rely solely on AV dissociation as the means of diagnosing ventricular tachycardia in the fetus.

Not all neonates with ventricular tachycardia are ill, and not all require antiarrhythmic therapy. All but one of the fetuses with ventricular tachycardia in this series was free of hydrops, all had normal cardiac anatomy, and only two were treated *in utero*. One of these neonates required antiarrhythmic therapy after birth.

If a diagnosis of ventricular tachycardia is suspected in a previable fetus with evidence of congestive cardiac failure, antiarrhythmic therapy should be considered (Lopes et al., 1996). Digoxin should be avoided, and direct umbilical venous infusion of lidocaine followed by maternal oral therapy with propranolol, mexiletine, quinidine, procainamide, amiodarone, or sotalol should be considered.

Sinus Tachycardia

Eight fetuses in the series had sinus tachycardia alone. These fetuses had baseline heart rates of approximately 180–190 beats per minute, with normal variations in rate around this baseline value, and associated normal fetal activity. In five fetuses, no explanation for the tachycardia was found, even after birth, despite careful monitoring and screening for abnormalities such as thyroid dysfunction and catecholamine levels. The fetuses remained well throughout the remainder of gestation and were

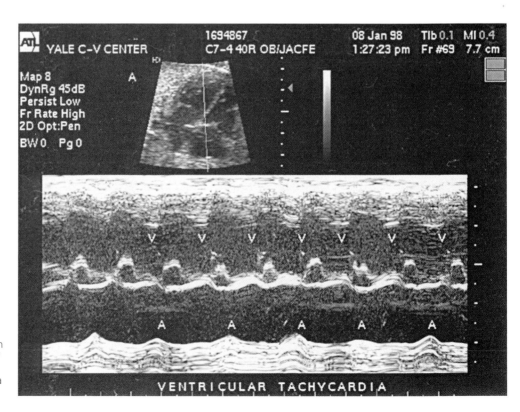

FIGURE 26-9 ■ M-mode echocardiogram of a fetus in ventricular tachycardia. The *upper portion* is an orienting four-chamber view showing the M-mode sample line going through the left ventricle and right atrium from upper to lower portions of the image. The M-mode portion shows ventricular beats (V) in the upper part and atrial beats (A) in the lower part. The ventricular beats can be seen occurring at a faster rate than the atrial beats and not in relation to the atrial beats. A similar pattern of atrial and ventricular rates may be seen in Junctional Ectopic Tachycardia (JET).

healthy neonates, despite baseline tachycardia after birth of between 155 and 165 beats per minute. Two of these fetuses were thought to have sinoatrial reentry tachycardia, and ultimately, progressive left ventricular dysfunction developed. One of the two fetuses responded well to digoxin therapy. Two fetuses with sinus tachycardia had goiters and were the offspring of mothers with poorly controlled thyrotoxicosis. Although the goiters tended to resolve as maternal thyroid function was better controlled with propylthiouracil, the sinus tachycardia persisted. Hydrops fetalis never developed in any of these fetuses.

Bradyarrhythmias

Sinus Bradycardia

Only two fetuses with sinus bradycardia have been seen by these authors during the last 20 years. Both of these fetuses had left atrial isomerism with normal AV conduction postnatally. Postnatally, they were found to have wandering supraventricular pacemakers without a dominant sinus node, which is normally located in the right atrium. None of these fetuses had associated hydrops fetalis. One of these patients required emergency systemic-to-pulmonary artery shunting in the neonatal period because of severe pulmonary outflow obstruction.

In the presence of normal cardiac structure and normal heart rate response to fetal activity and in the absence of hydrops fetalis, moderate (heart rate of 80–100 beats per minute) sinus bradycardia should not be an ominous finding.

Second-Degree Atrioventricular Block

Ten fetuses in the authors' experience have had second-degree AV block. These fetuses presented with irregular rhythms, which on auscultation gave the impression of skipped beats; however, the fetuses did not have premature beats with varying post-extrasystolic pauses but, rather, true skipped beats (i.e., regular sinus beats not conducted through the AV junction). The hallmark of this diagnosis is a regular atrial rhythm.

Prenatally, the fetuses had varying degrees of AV block. One of the fetuses remained in second-degree AV block. The others were born with varying degrees of Mobitz type I (Wenckebach) and Mobitz type II AV block, but complete heart block subsequently developed by 1 month of age. Two fetuses with second-degree heart block were treated *in utero* with dexamethasone, after high maternal anti-Ro or anti-La titers were documented, and heart block resolved (Copel et al., 1995). One of the patients with second-degree AV block had structural heart disease (Fig. 26-10), and eight of the mothers had anti-Ro and/or anti-La antibodies.

An example of intermittent second-degree heart block is seen in Figure 26-10.

Complete Heart Block

Clinical experience with fetal complete heart block suggests that these fetuses may be divided into two groups of relatively equal prevalence (Moodley et al., 1986; Schmidt et al., 1991). Either they have congenital complete heart block associated with complex congenital heart disease, or the cardiac structure is normal and the heart block appears to be the result of immune complex–related damage to the fetal conduction tissue secondary to maternal autoantibodies (Litsey et al., 1985; Taylor et al., 1986; Horsfall et al., 1991). An example of complete heart block is shown in Figure 26-11.

In one series of 55 fetuses with complete heart block (Schmidt et al., 1991), 27 had associated structural heart disease involving abnormalities of AV connection, such as ambiguous connections (in a setting of left atrial isomerism), discordant AV connections (congenitally corrected transposition of the great

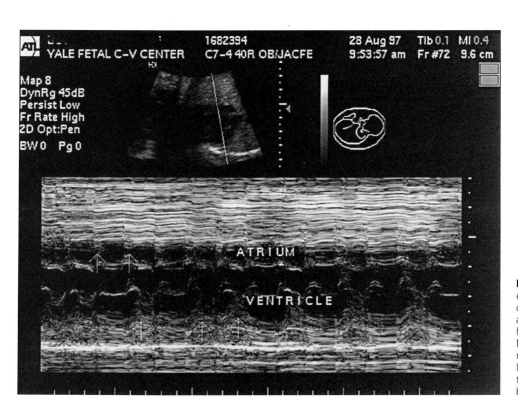

FIGURE 26-10 ■ M-mode echocardiogram of a fetus with corrected transposition of the great arteries and intermittent second-degree heart block. The upper chamber on the M-mode portion is labeled atrium, and regular beats *(arrows)* can be seen. The lower portion of the M-mode is taken through the ventricle. Only some atrial beats are conducted.

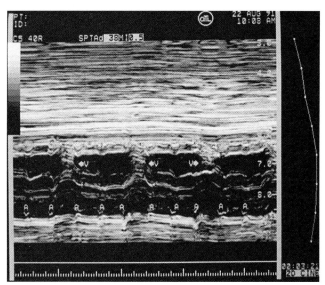

FIGURE 26-11 ■ M-mode echocardiogram of a fetus in complete heart block. The much slower ventricular rate and lack of constant time relationship between the atrial beats (A) and ventricular beats (V) can be readily appreciated.

arteries), or AV septal defect. The remaining patients in the series had no evidence of congenital heart disease. Twenty-one had anti-Ro and/or anti-La tests. Several mothers in the group entered the pregnancies with clinical diagnoses of Sjögren's syndrome or systemic lupus erythematosus (SLE). Several neonates required pacemaker insertion for a variety of clinical indications, including extreme bradycardia, ventricular arrhythmias, and congestive cardiac failure (Michaelson and Engle, 1972). Some studies have suggested a role for anti-SSA/Ro and anti-SSB/La antibodies in the development of fetal heart block by specifically damaging the function of calcium channels at the AV nodal level (Garcia et al., 1994; Boutjdir et al., 1997).

The association between maternal autoimmune disease and fetal congenital heart block has been well established (Taylor et al., 1986). Immunofluorescent stains demonstrate binding of immune complexes to His-Purkinje tissue as well as to fetal myocardium (Horsfall et al., 1991). These are associated with inflammatory infiltrates and fibrosis of the region of the AV node and bundle of His. The immune complex binding and inflammatory infiltration of fetal ventricular myocardium could account for the clinical finding of congestive cardiomyopathy.

Maternal administration of a beta agonist such as ritodrine or terbutaline may increase the fetal heart rate (Engelhardt, 1990; Groves et al., 1995) but does not lead to resolution of hydrops fetalis, with or without structural heart disease. This probably relates to the necessity of restoring a 1:1 AV contraction sequence in these fetuses. If systemic venous pressure is to be reduced sufficiently to allow resolution of hydrops fetalis, the cannon A-waves associated with atrial contraction against a closed AV valve must be ameliorated.

The data from the series by Schmidt and associates (Schmidt et al., 1991) suggest that fetuses with hydrops fetalis, associated congenital cardiac malformations, or ventricular escape rates of below 55 beats per minute carry a particularly poor prognosis.

An aggressive therapeutic approach should be taken in cases of complete heart block associated with fluid accumulation in

the fetus, especially when relatively normal heart rates have been documented by accurate observers within a week or 10 days of presentation with complete heart block (Buyon et al., 1987, 1995; Carreira et al., 1993; Copel et al., 1995; Groves et al., 1996). If these patients have high anti-Ro or anti-La titers, the use of fluorinated steroids that cross the placenta is worth considering. The optimal steroids are dexamethasone and betamethasone. The use of oral dexamethasone, 4 mg daily, resulted in improvement from complete heart block to second-degree block or sinus rhythm in five cases and resolution of second-degree block with associated antibodies to sinus rhythm in two other patients (Copel et al., 1995). Two other patients had no demonstrable response. Steroids are offered on an investigational basis only and are withheld if there are any specific contraindications to their use. A larger retrospective series, incorporating pregnancies reported to the Neonatal Lupus Registry, failed to show any change in the degree of heart block among those fetuses exposed to steroids, but did show a tendency toward improvement in fetal hydrops among those treated with steroids (Saleeb et al., 1999).

The postnatal treatment for complete heart block often includes pacemaker placement. In cases of heart block with severe hydrops, the possibility of fetal pacemaker placement has been considered. There have been two reports of such attempts, neither resulting in fetal survival (Carpenter et al., 1986; Walkinshaw et al., 1994). At this point, fetal pacemaker insertion does not appear to be a useful approach to complete heart block.

Patients incidentally identified to carry anti-Ro and anti-La antibodies will be concerned about the risk of developing fetal heart block, as are patients with previously affected children. Series of women entering pregnancy with these antibodies but no history of affected children suggest that the risk of heart block is about 1% (Brucato et al., 2001). Those with a previously affected child have about a 15% risk of recurrence (Buyon et al., 1998). Given these low rates and the uncertain value of steroid administration, prophylactic steroid use appears unwarranted. The time interval between atrial and ventricular systole should therefore correlate with the PR interval, and in normal fetuses this interval averages 120–130 milliseconds throughout the second and third trimesters. This interval should lengthen in first-degree heart block, which should precede complete heart block.

■ FETAL ANTIARRHYTHMIC AGENTS

Therapeutic Rationale

The existence of a technique for the accurate diagnosis of fetal cardiac rhythm disturbances is necessary, but not sufficient, to justify the administration of potent antiarrhythmic agents to pregnant women and their fetuses. An appropriate management scheme requires an understanding of the natural history of the underlying arrhythmia, a precise definition of the electrophysiologic mechanism of the arrhythmia, and a complete understanding of the pharmacology and pharmacokinetics of these antiarrhythmic agents in the mother and fetus. In short, a detailed common-sense risk-benefit analysis is in order.

The association of nonimmune hydrops fetalis with sustained fetal supraventricular tachyarrhythmias is well described (Kleinman et al., 1982). It is also evident in studies from many centers that the mortality rate for hydropic neonates is high, regardless of the underlying cause of the hydrops (Andersen et al., 1983). It seems reasonable, therefore, to assume that hydropic fetuses with sustained supraventricular tachyarrhythmias are at extremely high mortality risk and that vigorous efforts at *in utero* therapy may be warranted if they can be applied with a reasonable expectation of success and at an acceptably low risk to the mother. Even a moderate risk to the fetus could be acceptable in this setting, in light of the extremely poor prognosis for the neonate if the arrhythmia and the hydrops are unremitting. The risk to the fetus increases proportionately with the degree of prematurity and lung immaturity at the time of initial diagnosis.

The most reasonable approach to the fetus with sustained tachycardia in the absence of hydrops fetalis must be dictated by an estimation of the risk-benefit ratio, both to mother and fetus. For example, if the diagnosis of sustained tachycardia without hydrops fetalis is made at a gestational age when pulmonary maturity of the fetus is likely, or at an earlier age but with lung maturity documented by amniocentesis, delivery for postnatal therapy is advisable. At extremely premature gestational ages, immediate delivery may not be a viable option. In this setting, the decision with regard to administration of therapy must depend on multiple considerations, including the following:

1. Potential risk for the development of hydrops fetalis without intervention
2. Potential risk of antiarrhythmic therapy to both mother and fetus
3. Individual considerations, which may include the feasibility of providing medical follow-up to the mother and fetus, the mother's own perception of her desire to take such medications, and issues such as maternal autonomy versus fetal risk

The risks inherent in antiarrhythmic therapy depend largely on the electrophysiologic mechanism of the arrhythmia, because this determines which antiarrhythmic agents should be used, and on individual responses of mother and fetus to each agent. The latter places a responsibility on the treating team to monitor carefully the hemodynamic responses of both mother and fetus. The decision to treat fetal arrhythmias must be based on an understanding of the natural history of the rhythm disturbance and cannot be predicated simply on the basis of the presence of the arrhythmia or on the frequency of the episodes of fetal tachycardia.

Determining the likelihood of the development of hydrops fetalis in a patient may be difficult or impossible. In one series (Kleinman et al., 1983), 45 of 69 fetal patients with SVT were hydropic at the time of diagnosis and, therefore, warranted *in utero* therapy (see Table 26-2). Five additional patients with sustained tachycardia before the 34th week of gestation were observed without therapy for 24 to 48 hours after initial presentation. Fetuses usually received antiarrhythmic therapy only after pleural or pericardial effusions or ascites was detected. A total of 47 patients received *in utero* therapy. A few patients were treated with digoxin for SVT, even in the absence of hydrops fetalis. This medication was elected after an exhaustive discussion of the pros and cons of such therapy with the parents.

Not all fetuses with SVT develop nonimmune hydrops. The parallel circuitry of the fetal cardiovascular system could provide some protection against the development of hydrops fetalis. However, the unique properties of the fetal cardiovascular system make the fetus more, rather than less, susceptible to the development of systemic edema in response to a variety of hemodynamic disturbances. These differences include a physiologic volume overload of the right atrium and ventricle as well as the intrinsic reduced compliance of the fetal ventricular myocardium when compared with neonatal myocardium and the diminished systolic reserve of this myocardium compared to mature myocardium (Friedman, 1973). Kallfelz (1979) suggested that even a brief interlude of sinus rhythm interposed into incessant tachycardia provides the fetus with protection against the development of hydrops fetalis. It seems likely that there is some threshold beyond which heart failure will develop, but this threshold has not been identified, making blanket recommendations regarding medical therapy unjustifiable.

The site of origin of fetal SVT could play an important role in determining whether a particular fetus is at a higher risk for the development of systemic edema in the presence of SVT. When atrial depolarization appears to arise in the left rather than in the right atrium, the preexcitation of the left atrium appears to result in a reversal of the usual pressure gradient, which normally maintains a right-to-left shunt across the foramen ovale. This pressure differential favoring the left atrium results in complete or partial closure of the foramen ovale as a result of apposition of the atrial septum primum against the rim of the foramen ovale. This narrowing of the foramen ovale tends to trap volume in the right atrium, increasing the volume load of the right heart and consequently systemic venous pressure. In the presence of the restrictive physiology inherent in the fetal right ventricle, any sudden increase in right atrial volume would be expected to increase right atrial and systemic venous pressure.

Increases in hydrostatic pressure can result in increased transmural passage of fluid across the capillary bed. In addition, this increased venous pressure results in backflow of venous return into the inferior vena cava and hepatic venous system. This can also result in passive congestion of the liver, possibly leading to impaired protein synthesis. The consequent combination of increased hydrostatic pressure and decreased serum oncotic pressure related to diminished fetal serum protein concentration may precipitate the rapid and dramatic development of systemic edema and fluid third-spacing, which is seen in nonimmune hydrops fetalis.

Therapy for the fetus with sustained tachycardia, even in the absence of hydrops fetalis, may be warranted. This consideration is based, in part, on observations that the hydropic fetus and placenta tend to absorb maternally administered antiarrhythmic agents less well than the nonhydropic fetus (Younis and Granat, 1987; Weiner and Thompson, 1988).

The pharmacologic treatment of arrhythmias *in utero* involves the administration of potent cardiac antiarrhythmic medications to the mother. The treatment of this unique patient within a patient, therefore, involves moral, ethical, and even legal considerations in compromising the mother's autonomy and exposing her to the potential side effects of these agents.

The pharmacologic agents used to treat fetal arrhythmias, with their indicators, recommended doses, side effects, and efficacy, are summarized in Table 26-3.

TABLE 26-3. FETAL ANTIARRHYTHMIC AGENTS

Drug	Class	Arrhythmia	Dose	Metabolism	Side Effects and Precautions	PA (%)*	Clinical Experience
Procainamide	IA	Supraventricular tachyarrhythmias; ventricular tachyarrhythmias	IV: 100-mg bolus over 2 min; up to 25 mg/min to 1 g over 1st hour; maintenance 2–6 mg/min PO: 1 g: then up to 500 mg q3h	Hepatic metabolism to N-acetyl-procainamide; rapid renal elimination; $t_{1/2}$ 3.5 hr; therapeutic level 4–10 ng/mL.	Hypotension with IV; limit oral use to 3–6 mo (lupus), gastrointestinal symptoms; agranulocytosis; torsades de pointes rare; interacts with class III agents (torsades de pointes); fetal levels may exceed maternal	9–21	Rarely effective; frequency of oral dosing major limitation to compliance; gastrointestinal side effects often limit compliance
Disopyramide	IA	Supraventricular tachyarrhythmias; ventricular tachyarrhythmias	PO: loading dose, 300 mg; then 100–200 mg q6h	Hepatic 50%; renal excretion of unmetabolized drug 50%; $t_{1/2}$ 8 hr; therapeutic level 3–6 μg/mL; toxic >7 μg/mL	Hypotension; torsades de pointes; negative inotropic agent; vagolytic side effects; interacts with class III agents (torsades de pointes)	1–6	Rarely used in children; limited experience in fetus; side effects limit compliance; may worsen signs of CHF; may stimulate uterine contraction
Flecainide	IC	Supraventricular tachyarrhythmias; ventricular tachyarrhythmias	IV: Not available in USA PO: 100–400 mg bid	Hepatic 67%, 33% renally excreted as unmetabolized drug; $t_{1/2}$ 13–19 hr; therapeutic trough level <1 μg/mL	Narrow therapeutic range; visual disturbances; lightheadedness; nausea; important negative inotropic effect; proarrhythmia; increases mortality post-MI; interacts with many antiarrhythmics	4–33	Probably safe with structurally normal hearts; must monitor for proarrhythmia; contraindicated with cardiac pump failure
Propafenone	IC	Supraventricular tachyarrhythmias; ventricular tachyarrhythmias	IV: Not available in USA PO: 150–300 mg tid	Hepatic (cytochrome P-450) $t_{1/2}$ 2–10 hr, up to 32 hr in nonmetabolizers; therapeutic level 0.2–3.0 μg/mL	Increases digoxin level; prolongs QRS duration; negative inotropic effect; proarrhythmia; gastrointestinal side effects	5–15	Gastrointestinal side effects common
Propranolol	II	Supraventricular tachyarrhythmias; ventricular tachyarrhythmias	IV: 1–6 mg, slowly PO: 40–160 mg q6h	Hepatic $t_{1/2}$ 1–6 hr; serum levels not therapeutically useful	Bronchospasm; heart block; negative inotropic effect; drug interactions; CNS depression; may mask symptoms of hypoglycemia in diabetics; may impair glucose tolerance in non-insulin-dependent diabetics; contraindicated in Raynaud phenomenon; contraindicated in sick-sinus syndrome	?	May prefer longer acting β-blockers (Inderal LA; atenolol); may prefer more cardioselective agents (labetolol; atenolol; metoprolol); has been useful to suppress ectopy in fetuses with recurrent SVT; may depress respirations or cause hypoglycemia or bradycardia in neonate; possible association with low birthweight
Amiodarone	III	Supraventricular tachyarrhythmias; ventricular tachyarrhythmias	IV: 5 mg/kg over 20 min; 500–1000 mg over 24 hr, then oral PO: (loading) 1200–1600 mg/d in two divided doses for 7–14 days, then 400–800 mg qd for 1–3 wk; maintenance, 200–400 mg/d	Hepatic lipid soluble, distributes extensively throughout body; $t_{1/2}$ 25–110 days; therapeutic level 1.0–2.5 μg/mL	Increases digoxin level; interacts with type I agents to predispose to torsades de pointes; side effects fetal or maternal hypo- or hyperthyroidism; corneal microdeposits; photosensitivity; life-threatening pulmonary alveolitis (not dose-related); hepatitis; myopathy; neuropathy; nausea; rash; alopecia; tremor; insomnia; nightmares	4–30	Drug of last resort for fetal treatment; should not be used unless adequate doses of other antiarrhythmics are unsuccessful or poorly tolerated; adverse reactions require drug discontinuation in approximately 20% of patients; may be excreted in milk for several weeks

Drug	Class	Indication	Dosage	Metabolism/Pharmacokinetics	Adverse Effects	%*	Comments
Sotalol	III	Supraventricular tachyarrhythmias; ventricular tachyarrhythmias	IV: Not available in USA PO: 80–320 mg bid	Not metabolized; renal excretion of intact drug; $t_{1/2}$ 15–17 hr; therapeutic levels not measured	Torsades de pointes with hypokalemia; negative inotropic effect; sinus bradycardia; atrioventricular block; proarrhythmia more common in renal failure; proarrhythmia more common in females	10–16	Limited fetal experience; should probably be considered for early inclusion in treatment protocol for atrial flutter if β-blockade is not contraindicated
Verapamil	IV	Supraventricular tachyarrhythmias	IV: 5–10 mg over 30–60 sec PO: 80–160 mg tid	Renal 75%; gastrointestinal 25%; $t_{1/2}$ 3–7 hr; serum levels not clinically useful	Calcium-channel blocking agent; increases digoxin levels; depresses sinoatrial and atrioventricular node function; contraindicated in sinus node dysfunction; contraindicated with magnesium sulfate; interacts with β-blockers; may cause cardiovascular collapse if given to immature heart with CHF; may cause cardiovascular collapse if given to patient with ventricular tachycardia	18	Use of IV verapamil for supraventricular tachycardia with CHF in neonates considered contraindicated; use with caution, if at all, in fetuses
Adenosine	IV	Reentrant supraventricular tachycardia	IV: 100–200 μg/kg estimated fetal weight by rapid bolus into umbilical vein; fetal therapy by maternal IV administration not feasible PO: Not available	Metabolized throughout body by conversion to ATP; $t_{1/2}$ 10–30 sec; therapeutic levels not measured	Bronchospasm, especially in asthmatics; transient arrhythmias after conversion; briefly increases atrioventricular block	?	May be useful as diagnostic test to identify reentrant SVT; may break incessant SVT; does not prevent recurrent SVT
Digoxin	Cardiac glycoside	Supraventricular tachyarrhythmias	IV: 1 mg divided over 24 hr to load only PO: 0.25–1.0 mg daily in two divided doses	Most excreted unchanged in urine; approximately 30% nonrenal clearance, more in presence of renal failure; $t_{1/2}$ 36 hr; therapeutic levels 1–2 ng/mL	Toxicity results in arrhythmias, nausea, anorexia, vomiting, diarrhea, malaise, fatigue, confusion, facial pain, insomnia, depression, vertigo, colored vision; may be encountered at low drug serum levels with hypokalemia or hypomagnesemia; interacts with quinidine, verapamil, amiodarone, propafenone, erythromycin; dose should be adjusted downward in renal failure	?	Contraindicated with ventricular arrhythmias; Contraindicated in Wolff-Parkinson-White syndrome (impossible to detect in fetus prenatally; mother should have ECG prior to therapy); may be poorly absorbed by hydropic fetuses; should have frequent ECG monitoring for evidence of toxicity

* Percentage of patients reported to develop proarrhythmia when using this agent for postnatal antiarrhythmic therapy.

ATP, adenosine triphosphate; CHF, congestive heart failure; CNS, central nervous system; ECG, electrocardiogram; IV, intravenous; MI, myocardial infarction; PO, oral; SVT, supraventricular tachycardia.

From Kleinman CS, Copel JA, Nehgme R: The fetus with cardiac arrhythmia. In Harrison MR, Evans MI, Adzick NS, et al (eds): The Art and Science of Fetal Therapy, 3rd ed, Philadelphia, WB Saunders, 2001, pp. 430–431.

The treatment of arrhythmias is one of the most specialized disciplines of cardiology, and the management of these patients is often difficult, frustrating, and associated with significant morbidity and mortality. The availability of newer antiarrhythmic agents offers the promise of more rapid and effective control of arrhythmias, but only rarely have investigators demonstrated significant improvements in mortality risks after inclusion of newer antiarrhythmic agents in the treatment of potentially life-threatening arrhythmias.

To complicate matters, virtually none of the available antiarrhythmic agents is without significant potential risk of undesired side effects, particularly the risk of pro-arrhythmia—the tendency of a drug, through its electrophysiologic activity, to cause, rather than ameliorate, arrhythmias (Morganroth, 1987; Roden, 1994). Pro-arrhythmias could be of equal or greater potential risk to the patient than the arrhythmia being treated.

An example of this risk has been the use of flecainide in the treatment of fetal SVT(Wren and Hunter, 1988; Allan et al., 1990, 1991; Kofinas et al., 1991; Perry et al., 1991; Bourget et al., 1994; Frohn-Mulder et al., 1995). Initial enthusiasm for the use of flecainide and related agents was tempered by the ominous report of the Cardiac Arrhythmia Suppression Trial, a double-blinded placebo-controlled trial of prophylactic administration of these agents to suppress ventricular ectopy following myocardial infarction (CAST Investigators, 1989). The initial and long-term results of this trial demonstrated a significant increase in sudden arrhythmic death among postmyocardial infarction patients who received flecainide and/or encainide compared to a placebo-treated group. As a result, the Food and Drug Administration issued a warning to physicians, suggesting that type Ic antiarrhythmic agents be used only for the treatment of otherwise refractory, life-threatening ventricular arrhythmias. The fetus and mother are different from the study population in the CAST study—older, male patients, who had suffered myocardial infarctions. Nonetheless, concern over the potential of causing potentially dangerous arrhythmias in the mother or fetus via the pro-arrhythmic effects of flecainide must temper physicians' enthusiasm for therapy.

The potential for interaction between potent antiarrhythmic agents must also be considered. These medications exert their electrophysiologic effects by alterations in ion flux, and in most cases they function at the level of ion channels within the cell membrane. Rational antiarrhythmic therapy must be based on a complete understanding of the underlying electrophysiologic mechanism and the electrophysiologic and hemodynamic effects of the agents. The indiscriminate application of antiarrhythmic therapy with little consideration of the underlying electrophysiology and the potential hazards of additive therapy on basic cellular electrophysiology and pharmacokinetics could raise the risk of inadvertently precipitating a more dangerous situation secondary to pro-arrhythmia. It could also impair myocardial performance and interfere with metabolism of other medications, resulting in toxic accumulation of drugs or, in some circumstances, change an intermittent into an incessant, life-threatening arrhythmia (Blandon and Leandro, 1985).

The greatest initial successes have been achieved in the *in utero* treatment of fetal SVT. Although there have been isolated reports involving the use of many antiarrhythmic agents in this setting (Teuscher et al., 1978; Kerenyi et al., 1980; Lingman et al., 1980; Wolff et al., 1980; Dumesic et al., 1982; Given

et al., 1984; Spinnato et al., 1984; Bergmans et al., 1985; Golichowski et al., 1985; Lusson et al., 1985; Arnoux et al., 1987; Johnson et al., 1987; Allan et al., 1990; Hansmann et al., 1991; Azancot-Benisty et al., 1992), no single regimen has emerged as the ultimate therapy of choice.

M-mode or pulsed-Doppler echocardiography demonstration of sudden onset and sudden termination of episodes of tachycardia with induction of the arrhythmia by extrasystoles has been considered pathognomonic of reentrant SVT. The onset and termination of the arrhythmia may not be observed until after a trial of antiarrhythmic therapy has begun. If therapy aimed at slowing conduction and increasing refractoriness in the slow AV conduction pathways results in AV nodal block without termination of the arrhythmia, one can rule out AV node reentry or AV node reentry tachycardia (with the AV node serving as one limb of the reentrant circuit) as the mechanism for its arrhythmia. Further therapy should be directed by this information.

Specific Medications

It is beyond the scope of this chapter to review all of the available antiarrhythmic agents in detail. Selected information is summarized in Table 26-3. Digoxin is the first-choice drug for the treatment of fetal *in utero* SVT, but treatment with this or any other agent can be accomplished only with close collaboration between the obstetric and pediatric cardiology teams.

It is preferable not to consider the use of a second-line antiarrhythmic agent for a fetus with a tachyarrhythmia in the absence of hydrops fetalis because there is little information on which to base a risk-benefit analysis for the fetus and mother. Beta-blocking agents (type II antiarrhythmic agents), such as propranolol, have been used on occasion for treatment of neonatal or fetal SVT. These agents tend to slow AV conduction and to decrease the frequency of the triggering ectopic beats; they are well tolerated by mother and fetus. The broad therapeutic index of propranolol allows an increase in maternal dosage in efforts to attain therapeutic fetal drug levels without untoward maternal effects. The favorable risk-benefit ratio for the use of this agent makes it the second choice for the treatment of fetal SVT, despite the modest success observed with this agent alone or in combination with digoxin. The risks of maternal propranolol therapy have been well described, and the potential for causing low birth weight, hypoglycemia, and sinus node depression must be weighed against the therapeutic goal of conversion of *in utero* tachycardia (Wu et al., 1974; Gladstone et al., 1975; Habib and McCarthy, 1977; Rubin, 1981). For the fetus with multiple brief runs of tachycardia triggered by ectopic beats, oral propranolol should be considered as a possible first-line agent, especially because it can be safely initiated on an outpatient basis.

Suggested Protocol

In general, antiarrhythmic therapy, except for oral propranolol, should be initiated on an inpatient basis. External fetal cardiac monitoring is carried out for 12–24 hours to determine the proportion of time that the fetus spends in tachycardia. This helps determine the severity of the arrhythmia and whether the situation requires antiarrhythmic medications.

There can be no cookbook algorithm for the therapy of fetal arrhythmias. Arrhythmias do not respond in a predictable fashion postnatally. Occasional patients require aggressive

PLATE 15

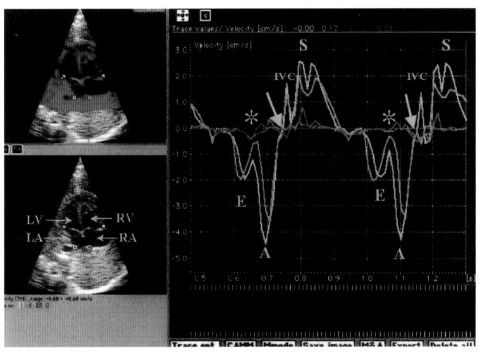

FIGURE 26-2 ■ Doppler tissue velocity imaging tracing demonstrating diphasic diastolic waves below the baseline (E and A), followed by systolic motion in the opposite direction (above baseline). Simultaneous tracings from the right and left atrial posterior walls and right and left AV valve rings are displayed. The electromechanical activation sequence can be discerned from these tracings. (Reproduced with permission from Rein AJJT, O'Donnell C, Geva T, et al: Use of tissue velocity imaging in the diagnosis of fetal cardiac arrhythmias. Circulation **106**:1827, 2002.)

multidrug therapy or even catheterization and radiofrequency ablation. It is naive to assume that a single "magic bullet" can be found that will successfully treat all forms of fetal tachycardia, or even all cases of reentrant tachycardia.

With this caveat, the following protocols for treatment of fetuses that present with fetal tachycardia can be considered. The accompanying algorithms refer to the use of individual antiarrhythmic agents. Information regarding specific agents and their dosages, routes of administration, maternal and fetal side effects, desired maternal serum levels, and, where known, information concerning relative maternal and fetal serum levels is found in Table 26-3. It is important to recognize the potential for drug interactions. The half-lives of these drugs must be borne in mind when changing medications and/or adding multiple drugs to the fetal treatment regimen.

Supraventricular Tachycardia

For the fetus documented to have what appears to be reentrant SVT, with a 1:1 relationship between atrial and ventricular activity; a fetal heart rate between 240 and 260 beats per minute, and either frequent episodes of tachycardia, incessant tachycardia in the extremely premature infant (less than 24 weeks' gestation), or the presence of hydrops fetalis, *in utero* therapy should be considered. When close to term, or even remote from term (32–35 weeks) with documented fetal lung maturity, expedited delivery for neonatal management of the arrhythmia is the most prudent approach. For fetuses with intermittent runs of SVT in the absence of hydrops, Simpson has demonstrated that observation alone is often sufficient (Simpson et al., 1997).

The mother is intravenously loaded with digoxin according to the protocol as outlined in Table 26-3. Continuous maternal electrocardiographic monitoring and daily 12-lead ECGs are obtained to search for electrocardiographic evidence of digoxin toxicity. The mother must be questioned daily concerning the potential signs and symptoms of clinical digoxin toxicity, as digoxin toxicity is a clinical diagnosis rather than one based on laboratory findings.

Before administration of digoxin, maternal serum electrolytes, blood urea nitrogen, creatinine, and ECG data should be obtained to determine baseline maternal health and to rule out any significant electrolyte imbalances such as hypokalemia, hypocalcemia, or hypomagnesemia that could conceivably be dangerous in light of a digoxin load. In addition, a diagnosis of maternal Wolff-Parkinson-White syndrome (WPW) should be ruled out, because it could lead to lethal maternal arrhythmias. It is emphasized to parents that it is impossible to detect Wolf-Parkinson-White syndrome in the fetus during tachycardia. In Wolff-Parkinson-White syndrome, administration of digoxin could precipitate malignant fetal arrhythmias.

If tachycardia resolves with digoxin, the drug is continued and no further therapy is initiated. Hydrops fetalis may take a number of days or even weeks to resolve, depending on its severity and duration before therapy. Under no circumstances are second-line agents considered unless severe hydrops fetalis is unremitting despite digoxin therapy.

If a second-line agent is required, propranolol is the drug of choice. The maternal ECG is carefully monitored for excessive maternal bradycardia, and maternal blood pressure is carefully monitored in both the supine and erect positions for evidence of orthostatic hypotension.

In the event of sustained fetal tachycardia despite the administration of digoxin and propranolol, third-line therapy can be considered with flecainide. Careful monitoring of maternal ECG for undue QRS prolongation and prolongation of the PT interval is necessary. There is a small but significant pro-arrhythmic danger to both the fetus and mother with the initiation of flecainide.

It is important to allow sufficient time for the patient to reach therapeutic trough levels of these agents before assuming that therapy is not successful. This therapeutic level could take five to six half-lives to attain (see Table 26-3). Only if a triple therapy is unsuccessful should a fourth-level agent be considered, such as maternal sotalol or amiodarone.

Prior to the use of sotalol, propranolol and flecainide must first be discontinued for 72 hours to allow clearance of these drugs from the system. Sotalol does not increase digoxin bioavailability, so digoxin doses do not need to be reduced.

If SVT persists, the next agent to consider is amiodarone, which should not be administered until sotalol has been discontinued for at least 96 hours. Digoxin bioavailability can be increased with concomitant amiodarone therapy, so the digoxin dose should be halved (Vlahot et al., 1987). Amiodarone treatment of the fetus is of concern because of the heavy iodine load of this drug and reports of neonatal hypothyroidism in treated fetuses (Laurent et al., 1987; Rovet et al., 1987; deWolf et al., 1988; Hijazi et al., 1992). Extensive discussion of risks and benefits should occur with the family before initiating this drug. Fortunately, the success rates of the other available drugs discussed previously make this a rare necessity.

Atrial Flutter

Treatment of fetuses with atrial flutter and associated hydrops is virtually identical to that for SVT. An initial load of intravenous digoxin is administered at the same dose after obtaining the same admission laboratory tests and fetal monitoring.

Digoxin is administered to slow the ventricular response rate to the atrial flutter. Rarely, atrial flutter can be controlled with the simple administration of digoxin. Once digoxin loading is completed and maintenance is initiated, a second agent, such as propranolol or sotalol, can be added. If these drugs fail to restore sinus rhythm, the second agent can be discontinued for at least 72 hours and amiodarone begun.

Ventricular Tachycardia

The fear that ventricular tachycardia can progress to ventricular fibrillation drives much of the aggressive therapeutic approach in the neonate and young infant. Many of these patients have normal cardiac structure and difficult-to-treat arrhythmias that appear to have a low risk of deterioration into unstable rhythms. For this reason, slow ventricular tachycardias (less than 200 beats per minute), unassociated with structural or functional heart disease, may not always require treatment in the newborn. The decision to treat or not to treat could be more difficult in the fetus because subtle abnormalities in the heart (right ventricular dysplasia or miniscule intramyocardial tumors) that are quite difficult to diagnose postnatally may be nearly impossible to diagnose in the fetus.

In the rare situation of a diagnosis of rapid ventricular tachycardia, ventricular tachycardia associated with structural heart disease, or ventricular tachycardia associated with myocardial failure (primary or secondary), *in utero* therapy can be considered. There is little experience with treatment of this arrhythmia; therapy is based on a common-sense approach, with emphasis on maternal well being.

Patients should be treated initially on an inpatient basis, and the fetal and maternal heart rates are monitored for at least 24 hours to characterize the frequency and duration of the fetal arrhythmia episodes. Mature fetuses should be delivered by cesarean section for postnatal evaluation and treatment. Without structural heart disease, one would observe the premature fetus for evidence of hemodynamic compromise before starting antiarrhythmic therapy unless the tachycardia rate was greater than 200–250 beats per minute.

The drug of first choice should be propranolol (see Table 26-3). If propranolol therapy is ineffective, one may consider direct umbilical venous administration of lidocaine. If this agent is successful in converting to sinus rhythm, chronic maintenance therapy with the lidocaine congener mexiletine should be considered.

■ SUMMARY

Most fetal cardiac arrhythmias relate to relatively benign fetal atrial premature beats. Most of these resolve spontaneously, either later in pregnancy or during the first few days after birth. Only rarely do extrasystoles precipitate persistent SVT that may be of clinical importance. Sustained fetal tachyarrhythmias or bradyarrhythmias are uncommon. They are rarely associated with congenital heart disease, but structural heart disease does occur, especially with atrial flutter and congenital complete heart block.

Only in cases of sustained tachycardia in extremely early gestation or in the presence of hydrops fetalis should the use of antiarrhythmic therapy be considered. Fetal antiarrhythmic therapy must be undertaken with great respect for the potential for catastrophic pro-arrhythmic effects on the mother or fetus. Caution with regard to the use of these medications singly and in combination must be exercised, especially in light of the potentially additive pro-arrhythmic or cardiac depressive effect of many such agents.

A common-sense approach to risk-benefit analysis must be made before antiarrhythmic therapy is offered; in particular, the presence or absence of hydrops fetalis and the fetal gestational age and possible pulmonary maturity must be considered. In the absence of hydrops fetalis, and especially when the fetus is likely to be mature enough for independent survival, the administration of antiarrhythmic agents to both mother and fetus is not warranted.

All therapy must be grounded in a firm understanding of the electrophysiologic nature of the arrhythmia and the pharmacology and pharmacokinetics of the antiarrhythmic agents in both mother and fetus as well as in the placenta.

Finally, therapy should be undertaken only with close collaboration between obstetricians, pediatric cardiologists, and informed parents.

REFERENCES

Allan L, Chita S, Maxwell D, et al: Use of flecainide in fetal atrial tachycardia. Br Heart J **64**:90, 1990.

Allan LD, Chita SK, Sharland GK, et al: Flecainide in the treatment of fetal supraventricular tachycardias. Br Heart J **65**:46, 1991.

Andelfinger G, Fouron JC, Sonesson SE, et al: Reference values for time intervals between atrial and ventricular contractions of the fetal heart measured by two Doppler techniques. Am J Cardiol **88**:1433, 2001.

Andersen HM, Drew JH, Beischer NA, et al: Non-immune hydrops fetalis: Changing contribution to perinatal mortality. Br J Obstet Gynaecol **90**:636, 1983.

Arnoux P, Seyral P, Llurens M, et al: Amiodarone and digoxin for refractory fetal tachycardia. Am J Cardiol **59**:166, 1987.

Azancot-Benisty A, Jacqz-Aigrain E, Guirguis NM, et al: Clinical and pharmacological study of fetal supraventricular tachyarrhythmias. J Pediatr **121**:608, 1992.

Bergmans MGM, Jonker GJ, Kock HCLV: Fetal supraventricular tachycardia: Review of the literature. Obstet Gynecol Surv **40**:61, 1985.

Blandon R, Leandro I: Fetal heart arrhythmia: Clinical experience with antiarrhythmic drugs. In Doyle EF, Engle MA, Gersony WM, et al (eds): Pediatric Cardiology: Proceedings of the Second World Congress. New York, Springer-Verlag, 1985, p. 483.

Bourget P, Pons JC, Delouis C, et al: Flecainide distribution, transplacental passage, and accumulation in the amniotic fluid during the third trimester of pregnancy. Ann Pharmacother **28**:1031, 1994.

Boutjdir M, Chen L, Zhang ZH, et al: Arrhythmogenicity of IgG and anti-52-KD SSA/Ro affinity-purified antibodies from mothers of children with congenital heart block. Circ Res **80**:354, 1997.

Brucato A, Frassi M, Franceschini F, et al: Risk of congenital complete heart block in newborns of mothers with anti-Ro/SSA antibodies detected by counterimmunoelectrophoresis: A prospective study of 100 women. Arthritis Rheum **44**:1832, 2001.

Buis-Liem TN, Ottenkamp J, Meerman RH, et al: The occurrence of fetal supraventricular tachycardia and obstruction of the foramen ovale. Prenat Diagn **7**:425, 1987.

Buyon JP, Hiebert R, Copel JA, et al: Autoimmune-associated congenital heart block: Demographics, mortality, morbidity and recurrence rates obtained from a national neonatal lupus registry. J Am Coll Cardiol **31**:1658, 1998.

Buyon JP, Swersky SH, Fox HE, et al: Intrauterine therapy for presumptive fetal myocarditis with acquired heart block due to systemic lupus erythematosus. Arthritis Rheum **30**:44, 1987.

Buyon JP, Waltuck J, Kleinman C, et al: In utero identification and therapy of congenital heart block. Lupus **4**:116, 1995.

Cardiac Arrhythmia Suppression Trial (CAST) Investigators: Preliminary report: Effect of encainide and flecainide on mortality in a randomized trial of arrhythmia suppression after myocardial infarction. N Engl J Med **321**:406, 1989.

Carpenter RJ, Strasburger JF, Garson A Jr, et al: Fetal ventricular pacing for hydrops secondary to complete atrioventricular block. J Am Coll Cardiol **8**:1434, 1986.

Carreira PE, Gutierrez-Larraya F, Gomez-Reino JJ: Successful intrauterine therapy with dexamethasone for fetal myocarditis and heart block in a woman with systemic lupus erythematosus. J Rheumatol **20**:2104, 1993.

Chan FY, Woo SK, Ghosh A, et al: Prenatal diagnosis of congenital fetal arrhythmias by simultaneous pulsed Doppler velocimetry of the fetal abdominal aorta and inferior vena cava. Obstet Gynecol **76**:200, 1990.

Copel JA, Buyon JP, Kleinman CS: Successful in utero therapy of fetal heart block. Am J Obstet Gynecol **173**:1384, 1995.

Copel JA, Liang R-I, Demasio K, et al: The clinical significance of the irregular fetal heart rhythm. Am J Obstet Gynecol **182**:813, 2000.

Copel JA, Morotti R, Hobbins JC, et al: The antenatal diagnosis of congenital heart disease using fetal echocardiography: Is color flow mapping necessary? Obstet Gynecol **78**:1, 1991.

DeVore GR, Horenstein J: Simultaneous Doppler recording of the pulmonary artery and vein: A new technique for the evaluation of a fetal arrhythmia. J Ultrasound Med **12**:669, 1993.

deWolf D, deSchepper J, Verhaaren H, et al: Congenital hypothyroid goiter and amiodarone. Acta Paediatr Scand **77**:616, 1988.

Dorostkar PC, Steiner P, Suda K, et al: Comparison of echocardiography and magnetocardiography for evaluation of fetal cardiac rhythms (abstr). J Am Coll Cardiol **29**:358A, 1997.

Dumesic DA, Silverman NH, Tobias S, et al: Transplacental cardioversion of fetal supraventricular tachycardia with procainamide. N Engl J Med **307**:1128, 1982.

Engelhardt W, Lehnen H, Grabitz R, et al: Diagnosis and therapy of fetal bradyarrhythmia. Z Geburtshilfe Perinatol **194**:153, 1990.

Friedman WF: The intrinsic physiologic properties of the developing heart. In Friedman WF, Lesch M, Sonnenblick EH (eds): Neonatal Heart Disease. New York, Grune and Stratton, 1973, p. 87.

Frohn-Mulder IM, Stewart PA, Witsenburg M, et al: The efficacy of flecainide versus digoxin in the management of fetal supraventricular tachycardia. Prenat Diagn **15**:1297, 1995.

Garcia S, Nascimento JH, Bonfa E, et al: Cellular mechanism of the conduction abnormalities induced by serum from Anti Ro/SSA positive patients in rabbit hearts. J Clin Invest 93:718, 1994.

Given BD, Phillippe M, Sanders SP, et al: Procainamide cardioversion of fetal supraventricular tachyarrhythmia. Am J Cardiol 53:1460, 1984.

Gladstone GR, Hordof A, Gersony WM: Propranolol administration during pregnancy: Effects on the fetus. J Pediatr 86:962, 1975.

Golichowski AM, Caldwell R, Hartsough A, et al: Pharmacologic cardioversion of intrauterine supraventricular tachycardia: A case report. J Reprod Med 30:139, 1985.

Groves AM, Allan LD, Rosenthal E: Therapeutic trial of sympathomimetics in three cases of complete heart block in the fetus. Circulation 92:3394, 1995.

Groves AM, Allan LD, Rosenthal E: Outcome of isolated congenital complete heart block diagnosed in utero. Heart 75:190, 1996.

Habib A, McCarthy JS: Effects on the neonate of propranolol administered during pregnancy. J Pediatr 91:808, 1977.

Hamada H, Horigome H, Asaka M, et al: Prenatal diagnosis of long QT syndrome using fetal magnetocardiography. Prenat Diagn 19:677, 1999.

Hansmann M, Gembruch U, Bald R, et al: Fetal tachyarrhythmias: Transplacental and direct treatment of the fetus. A report of 60 cases. Ultrasound Obstet Gynecol 1:162, 1991.

Hijazi ZM, Rosenfeld LE, Copel JA, et al: Amiodarone therapy of intractable atrial flutter in a premature, hydropic neonate. Pediatr Cardiol 13:227, 1992.

Horigome H, Takahashi MI, Asaka M, et al: Investigation of fetal premature cardiac contractions by magnetocardiography. In: Yoshimoto T (ed): Recent Advances in Biomagnetism. Sendai Japan, Tohoku University Press, 1999, p. 952.

Horsfall AC, Venables PJW, Taylor PV, et al: Ro and La antigens and maternal autoantibody idiotype in the surface of myocardial fibres in congenital heart block. J Autoimmune 4:165, 1991.

Huirne JAF, Krooshoop HJG, Quartero HWP, et al: The classification of foetal cardiac conduction disorders by means of magnetocardiography. In: Yoshimoto T (ed): Recent Advances in Biomagnetism. Sendai Japan, Tohoku University Press, 1999, p. 967.

Jaeggi E, Fouron JC, Fournier A, et al: Ventriculo-atrial time interval measured on M-mode echocardiography: A determining element in diagnosis, treatment, and prognosis of fetal supraventricular tachycardia. Heart 79:582, 1998.

Johnson WH Jr, Dunnigan A, Fehr P, et al: Association of atrial flutter with orthodromic reciprocating fetal tachycardia. Am J Cardiol 59:374, 1987.

Juchau MR, Pedersen MG, Fantel A, et al: Drug metabolism by placenta. Clin Pharmacol Ther 14:673, 1973.

Kallfelz HC: Cardiac arrhythmias in the fetus: Diagnosis, significance, and prognosis. In: Goodman MJ, Marquis RM (eds): Paediatric Cardiology, Vol 2. New York, Churchill Livingstone, 1979, p. 80.

Kariniem V, Ahopelto J, Karp PJ, et al: The fetal magnetocardiogram. J Perinat Med 2:214, 1974.

Kerenyi TD, Gleicher N, Meller J, et al: Transplacental cardioversion of intrauterine supraventricular tachycardia with digitalis. Lancet 2:393, 1980.

Kleinman CS, Copel JA, Hobbins JC: Combined echocardiographic and Doppler assessment of fetal congenital atrioventricular block. Br J Obstet Gynaecol 94:967, 1987.

Kleinman CS, Donnerstein RL, DeVore GR, et al: Fetal echocardiography for evaluation of in utero congestive heart failure: A technique for study of nonimmune fetal hydrops. N Engl J Med 306:568, 1982.

Kleinman CS, Donnerstein RL, Jaffe CC, et al: Fetal echocardiography. A tool for evaluation of in utero cardiac arrhythmias and monitoring of in utero therapy: Analysis of 71 patients. Am J Cardiol 51:237, 1983.

Kleinman CS, Hobbins JC, Jaffe CC, et al: Echocardiographic studies of the human fetus: Prenatal diagnosis of congenital heart disease and cardiac dysrhythmias. Pediatrics 65:1059, 1980.

Kleinman CS, Valdes-Cruz LM, Weinstein EM, et al: Two-dimensional Doppler echocardiographic analysis of fetal cardiac arrhythmias. Pediatr Res 18:124A, 1984.

Kofinas AD, Simon NV, Sagel H, et al: Treatment of fetal supraventricular tachycardia with flecainide acetate after digoxin failure. Am J Obstet Gynecol 165:630, 1991.

Krauer B, Krauer F: Drug kinetics in pregnancy. Clin Pharmacokinet 2:167, 1977.

Laurent M, Betremieux P, Biron Y, et al: Neonatal hypothyroidism after treatment by amiodarone during pregnancy (letter). Am J Cardiol 60:942, 1987.

Levy G: Pharmacokinetics of fetal and neonatal exposure to drugs. Obstet Gynecol 58:9S, 1981.

Lie KI, Duren DR, Cats VM, et al: Long-term efficacy of verapamil in the treatment of paroxysmal supraventricular tachycardias. Am Heart J 105:688, 1983.

Lingman G, Ohrlander S, Ohlin P: Intrauterine digoxin treatment of fetal paroxysmal tachycardia. Br J Obstet Gynaecol 87:340, 1980.

Litsey SE, Noonan JA, O'Connor WN, et al: Maternal connective tissue disease and congenital heart block: Demonstration of immunoglobulin in cardiac tissue. N Engl J Med 312:98, 1985.

Lopes LM, Cha SC, Scanavacca MI, et al: Fetal idiopathic ventricular tachycardia with nonimmune hydrops: Benign course. Pediatr Cardiol 17:192, 1996.

Lusson JR, Beytout M, Jacquetin B, et al: Traitement d'une tachycardie supraventriculaire foetale: Association digoxine-amiodarone. Coeur 15:315, 1985.

Mattison DR, Malek A, Cistola C: Physiological adaptations to pregnancy: Impact on pharmacokinetics. In: Yaffe SJ, Aranda JV (eds): Pediatric Pharmacology: Therapeutic Principles in Practice. Philadelphia, WB Saunders, 1992, p. 81.

McKercher HG, Radde IC: Placental transfer of drugs and fetal pharmacology. In: McLeon SM, Radde IC (eds): Textbook of Pediatric Clinical Pharmacology. Littleton, Mass, PSG Publishing, 1985, p. 293.

Menendez T, Achenbach S, Beinder E, et al: Usefulness of magnetocardiography for the investigation of fetal arrhythmias. Am J Cardiol 88:334, 2001.

Michaelson M, Engle MA: Congenital complete heart block: An international study of the natural history. Cardiovasc Clin 4:85, 1972.

Moodley TR, Baughan JE, Chuntarpursat I, et al: Congenital heart block detected in utero. A case report. S Afr Med J 70:433, 1986.

Morganroth J: Risk factors for the development of pro-arrhythmic events. Am J Cardiol 59:32E, 1987.

Pacifici GM, Nottoli R: Placental transfer of drugs administered to the mother. Clin Pharmacokinet 28:235, 1995.

Perry JC, Ayres NA, Carpenter RJ: Fetal supraventricular tachycardia treated with flecainide acetate. J Pediatr 118:303, 1991.

Quinn A, Weir A, Shahani U, et al: Antenatal fetal magnetocardiography: A new method for fetal surveillance? Br J Obstet Gynaecol 101:866, 1994.

Rein AJJT, O'Donnell C, Geva T, et al: Use of tissue velocity imaging in the diagnosis of fetal cardiac arrhythmias. Circulation 106:1827, 2002.

Roden DM: Risks and benefits of antiarrhythmic therapy. N Engl J Med 331:785, 1994.

Rovet J, Ehrlich R, Sorbac D: Intellectual outcome in children with fetal hypothyroidism. J Pediatr 110:700, 1987.

Rubin PC: Beta-blockers in pregnancy. N Engl J Med 305:1323, 1981.

Saleeb S, Copel J, Friedman D, et al: Comparison of treatment with fluorinated glucocorticoids to the naturael history of autoantibody-associated congenital heart block: Retrospective review of the Research Registry for Neonatal Lupus. Arthritis Rheum 42:2335, 1999.

Schmidt KG, Ulmer HE, Silverman NH, et al: Perinatal outcome of fetal congenital complete atrioventricular block: A multicenter experience. J Am Coll Cardiol 17:1360, 1991.

Simpson LL, Marx GR, D'Alton ME: Supraventricular tachycardia in the fetus: Conservative management in the absence of hemodynamic compromise. J Ultrasound Med 16:459, 1997.

Spinnato JA, Shaver DC, Flinn GS, et al: Fetal supraventricular tachycardia: In utero therapy with digoxin and quinidine. Obstet Gynecol 64:730, 1984.

Taylor PV, Scott JS, Gerlis LM, et al: Maternal antibodies against fetal cardiac antigens in congenital complete heart block. N Engl J Med 315:667, 1986.

Teuscher A, Bossi E, Imhof P, et al: Effect of propranolol on fetal tachycardia in diabetic pregnancy. Am J Cardiol 42:304, 1978.

Van Leeuwen P, Hailer B, Bader W, et al: Magnetocardiography in the diagnosis of fetal arrhythmia. Br J Obstet Gynaecol 106:1200, 1999.

Vlahot N, Morvan J, Bernard AM, et al: Tachycardie supraventriculaire foetale: Traitement antenatal par l'association digoxine-amiodarone. J Gynecol Obstet Biol Reprod (Paris) 16:393, 1987.

Walkinshaw SA, Welch CR, McCormack J, et al: In utero pacing for fetal congenital heart block. Fetal Diagn Ther 9:183, 1994.

Walsh EP: Clinical approach to diagnosis and acute management of tachycardias in children. In: Walsh EP, Saul JP, Treidman JK (eds): Cardiac Arrhythmias in Children and Young Adults with Congenital Heart Disease. Philadelphia, Lippincott Williams & Wilkins, 2001, p. 103.

Ward RM: Pharmacological treatment of the fetus: Clinical pharmacokinetic considerations. Clin Pharmacokinet 28:343, 1995.

Weiner CP, Thompson MIB: Direct treatment of fetal supraventricular tachy-cardia after failed transplacental therapy. Am J Obstet Gynecol **158:**570, 1988.

Wolff F, Breuker KH, Schlensker KH, et al: Prenatal diagnosis and therapy of fetal heart rate anomalies with a contribution on the placental transfer of verapamil. J Perinatol Med **8:**203, 1980.

Wren C, Hunter S: Maternal administration of flecainide to terminate and suppress fetal tachycardia. Br Med J **296:**249, 1988.

Wu D, Denes P, Dhingra R, et al: The effects of propranolol on induction of AV nodal re-entrant paroxysmal tachycardia. Circulation **50:**665, 1974.

Younis JS, Granat M: Insufficient transplacental digoxin transfer in severe hydrops fetalis. Am J Obstet Gynecol **157:**1268, 1987.

Chapter 27

FETAL THERAPY
Medical and Surgical Approaches

Alan W. Flake, MD

The primary impetus for *in utero* therapeutic intervention for fetal medical and surgical abnormalities arose from the clinical frustration of obstetricians, neonatologists, and pediatric surgeons involved in the treatment of abnormalities after birth. In many instances, it was apparent that the damage had already been done. A simple anatomic defect (e.g., posterior urethral valves or a diaphragmatic defect) in an otherwise normal newborn often led to devastating physiologic consequences prior to birth that resulted in death or irreversible organ failure after birth. Similarly, nonanatomic abnormalities (such as erythroblastosis fetalis) that could be easily treated *ex utero* resulted in intrauterine fetal demise or irreversible fetal injury. In these cases, the rationale for prenatal intervention was compelling and obvious.

Less obvious, but no less compelling, are abnormalities in the fetus which, although not lethal in the fetal or neonatal period, may be optimally treated before birth. Treatment of the fetus, in many instances, may offer an advantage over treatment of the neonate, child, or adult because of the unique aspects of fetal development or because of biological characteristics of the fetal environment. This chapter reviews specific medical and surgical interventions that are currently applicable to the fetus and discusses potential future fetal interventions that may prove effective.

FETAL THERAPY FOR MEDICAL DISEASE

The concept of the fetus as a patient has evolved from the prenatal diagnosis and serial observation of fetuses with anatomic abnormalities. This has resulted in increased clinical experience and knowledge of the natural history and pathophysiology of fetal disorders and the consequent consideration of the fetus as a patient. Rh isoimmunization provided the first successful example of medical intervention in the developing fetus and offers a model for medical treatment of other fetal diseases (see Chapter 30). In the early 1960s, Sir William Liley, a pioneer in fetal treatment, performed the first successful prenatal transfusion of a hydropic fetus affected with Rh isoimmunization, and the field of fetal therapy was born (Liley, 1963). Since that time, a number of other medical diseases have been treated successfully *in utero* either by direct treatment of the fetus or by transplacental treatment of the fetus via the mother. Fetal disorders for which medical therapy could be

appropriate are categorized in Table 27-1. Medical treatment of the fetus with cardiac dysrhythmias is addressed in detail in Chapter 26, and the prenatal induction of lung maturity is covered in detail in Chapter 25.

FUTURE DIRECTIONS IN PRENATAL MEDICAL THERAPY

Hematopoietic Stem Cell Transplantation

Although many diseases are potentially amenable to prenatal surgical or medical treatment, most are relatively rare and, even in summation, fetal treatment would be applicable to relatively few patients. In contrast, a large number of patients are affected by congenital hematologic diseases. These diseases, most of which can be diagnosed early in gestation, are partially listed in Table 27-2; they include the hemoglobinopathies, immunodeficiency diseases, and lysosomal storage diseases, among others. Many of these diseases can be treated by conventional postnatal bone marrow transplantation (BMT). Unfortunately, application of conventional BMT has serious limitations (Hoelzer and Gokbuget, 2000; Martin and Gajewski, 2001). Only 35% of candidates for BMT have a histocompatibility leukocyte antigen–identical (HLA-identical) donor available so that an optimal transplant can be performed. In addition, bone marrow conditioning (myeloablation) is usually required with its associated immunosuppression and risk of lethal infection. Rejection and graft-versus-host disease are constant threats, requiring further immunosuppressive therapy. By the time postnatal transplants are performed, most recipients have been ravaged by their underlying disease. Growth restriction, multiple transfusions, and recurrent infection result in a suboptimal clinical result. Finally, in many of the storage diseases, the neurologic damage begins before birth and is not entirely reversible by BMT (Krivit et al., 1998; Shapiro et al., 2000). In these fetuses, *in utero* treatment is not only advantageous but may be necessary to cure the disease. For all of these diseases, the morbidity and mortality of the disease and its treatment remain significant and, in many cases, prohibitive for application of postnatal BMT. For these disorders, the prenatal transplantation of multipotent hematopoietic stem cells (HSCs) could offer a number of advantages over postnatal BMT (Flake and Zanjani, 1999).

TABLE 27-1. NONANATOMIC FETAL ABNORMALITIES AMENABLE TO PRENATAL THERAPY

Disorder	Example	Treatment
Anemia	Rh isoimmunization	Transfusion: intraperitoneal or intravenous
	Other red blood cell antigens	Transfusion
Surfactant deficiency	Pulmonary immaturity	Glucocorticoids: transplacental
Biochemical defects	Multiple carboxylase deficiency	Biotin: transplacental
	Methylmalonic acidemia	Vitamin B_{12}: transplacental
	Menkes' kinky-hair syndrome	Copper: transplacental
	Galactosemia	Galactose restriction during pregnancy
Cardiac arrhythmias	Supraventricular tachycardia	Digitalis: transplacental
		Propranolol: transplacental
		Procainamide: transplacental
	Heart block	Beta mimetics: transplacental
Endocrine deficiency	Congenital adrenal hyperplasia	Corticosteroids: transplacental
	Hypothyroidism and goiter	Thyroxin: transamniotic

Rationale for Fetal Hematopoietic Stem Cell Transplantation

The rationale for prenatal HSC transplantation arises from aspects of normal immunologic and hematologic (Metcalf et al., 1971) ontogeny that are unique to fetal development. Early in gestation, the fetus is immunologically immature and susceptible to the induction of antigen-specific tolerance (Billingham et al., 1953; Blackman et al., 1990). In addition, during hematopoietic ontogeny, hematopoiesis migrates from the yolk sac to the fetal liver and, finally, to the bone marrow. There is a period prior to population of the bone marrow and prior to thymic processing of self-antigen, when the fetus should theoretically be receptive to engraftment of foreign HSC. Because of the unique fetal environment, prenatal HSC transplantation theoretically could avoid many of the current limitations of postnatal BMT (Flake and Zanjani, 1999). There would be no requirement for histocompatibility leukocyte antigen matching. Transplanted cells would not be rejected, which means that the need for toxic immunosuppressive and myeloablative drugs would be eliminated. The mother's uterus is the ultimate sterile isolation chamber, eliminating the high risk and costly 2 to 4 months of isolation required after postnatal BMT prior to immunologic reconstitution. Finally, prenatal transplantation would preempt the clinical manifestations of the disease, thus avoiding the recurrent infections, multiple transfusions, growth restriction, and other complications that cause immeasurable suffering for the patient and that often compromise postnatal treatment.

Experimental evidence supports the concept of *in utero* hematopoietic stem cell transplantation (IUHSCTx). Early gestational transplantation of allogeneic cells in the mouse, sheep, and monkey models (Fleischman and Mintz, 1979; Flake et al., 1986b; Harrison et al., 1989) have shown that long-term multilineage hematopoietic chimerism can be achieved across major histocompatibility barriers without evidence of rejection or the need for immunosuppression. The phenomenon of *fetal tolerance* also allows engraftment and long-term hematopoietic chimerism across xenogeneic barriers, the best example of which is the well-studied human sheep model (Zanjani et al., 1992). The hematopoietic chimerism created by *in utero* hematopoietic stem cell transplantation in the human sheep model has

been shown definitively to be secondary to the engraftment of true pluripotent HSC by repopulating studies in which stable multilineage hematopoietic chimerism has been created in second-generation fetal recipients (Zanjani et al., 1994).

TABLE 27-2. CONGENITAL HEMATOPOIETIC DISEASES POTENTIALLY AMENABLE TO *IN UTERO* HEMATOPOIETIC STEM CELLS

Disorders of Erythropoiesis

Thalassemia major
Sickle cell anemia
Diamond-Blackfan syndrome
Fanconi anemia

Disorders of Lymphopoiesis

Severe combined immunodeficiency syndrome
Bare lymphocyte syndrome

Disorders of Myelopoiesis

Chronic granulomatous disease
Chédiak-Higashi syndrome
Wiskott-Aldrich syndrome
Infantile agranulocytosis (Kostmann's syndrome)
Lazy leukocyte syndrome (neutrophil actin deficiency)
Neutrophil membrane GP-180 deficiency
Cartilage-hair syndrome

Metabolic Errors of Lysosomes of Reticuloendothelial Cells

Mucopolysaccharidoses
  Hurler's disease (MSP I) (α-iduronidase deficiency)
  Hurler-Scheie syndrome
  Hunter disease (MSP II) (iduronate sulfatase deficiency)
  Sanfilippo B (MSP IIIB) (α-glycosaminidase deficiency)
  Morquio (MSP IV) (hexosamine-6-sulfatase deficiency)
  Maroteaux-Lamy syndrome (MSP VI) (arylsulfatase B deficiency)
Mucolipidoses
  Fabry disease (α-galactosidase A deficiency)
  Gaucher disease (glucocerebrosidase deficiency)
  Krabbe disease (galactosylceramidase deficiency)
  Metachromatic leukodystrophy (arylsulfatase A deficiency)
  Niemann-Pick disease (sphingomyelinase deficiency)
  Adrenal leukodystrophy

Disorder of Osteoclast

Infantile osteopetrosis

Clinical Experience with Fetal Hematopoietic Stem Cell Transplantation

Current techniques of prenatal diagnosis and fetal transfusion make diagnosis and prenatal HSC transplantation feasible in humans well within the immunologic and hematopoietic window of opportunity. Mature T cells are not found in the fetal circulation until after 12 to 14 weeks' gestation, and the bone marrow remains relatively empty until 18 to 20 weeks' gestation.

More than 40 in utero hematopoietic stem cell transplants have been discussed in the literature since the initial report by Linch and co-authors in 1986 (Jones et al., 1996; Flake and Zanjani, 1997). With the exception of immunodeficiency disorders (Flake et al., 1996; Wengler et al., 1996), in which a competitive advantage exists for normal cells, no successful cases have been reported. This and analogous experimental data suggest that the primary barrier to in utero hematopoietic stem cell transplantation is competition from the host hematopoietic compartment. Therefore, in its current form, consideration of in utero hematopoietic stem cell transplantation should be limited to disorders in which a competitive advantage exists—either at a stem cell or progenitor level—or in which a very low level of engraftment may be curative. A list of such disorders is provided in Table 27-3. Such procedures should be performed only under strict experimental guidelines by multidisciplinary teams in centers with experience and expertise in both treatment of the target disorder and fetal therapy.

Future Approaches for in Utero Hematopoietic Stem Cell Transplantation

Unfortunately, the vast majority of target disorders have highly competitive hematopoietic biology. Thus, in order for in utero hematopoietic stem cell transplantation to fulfill its promise, new approaches that can overcome host hematopoietic competition will need to be developed. One such approach is prenatal tolerance induction for postnatal cellular therapy. We have documented the potential of such an approach in the previously engraftment-resistant allogeneic mouse model, and we now can achieve complete allogeneic chimerism without toxicity across full allogeneic barriers using a combination of prenatal tolerance induction and postnatal nonmyeloablative BMT (Hayashi et al., 2002; Peranteau et al., 2002). Other, more powerful approaches based on providing a competitive advantage to donor cells or specific immunotherapy should allow achievement of high levels of donor cell engraftment with a "single shot" in utero. If translatable to large animal systems, these approaches could significantly expand the application of in utero hematopoietic stem cell transplantation to any disorder that could be diagnosed early in gestation and cured by BMT.

Gene Therapy

Advances in molecular biology have made human gene therapy a clinical reality. There are a number of potential advantages to prenatal gene therapy (Yang, Flake, et al., 1999). The small size of the fetus compared to the adult recipient provides a stoichiometric advantage with respect to vector-to-target cell ratio, while favoring increased compartmental and hematogenous distribution of the vector. The early gestational environment is also uniquely proliferative and contains an increased frequency of stem cells that migrate to and seed developing organs. Thus, transduction of stem cells with their subsequent migration and expansion during the normal process of ontogeny could result in an amplification of therapeutic effect. Finally, the early gestational fetus is immunologically naïve, allowing the potential for development of tolerance to the viral vector or transgene-encoded proteins. This could be a significant advantage, as immune reactions have hampered postnatal clinical and experimental gene therapy efforts (Herzog and High, 1998).

The main challenge in fetal gene therapy, as in postnatal gene therapy, is the development of safe and effective gene transfer techniques that allow long-term, tissue-specific, regulated expression of the desired protein. In addition, there are appropriate concerns about fetal gene therapy regarding insertional mutagenesis, alteration of the germ line, and detrimental effects on normal development. Until these concerns are addressed, fetal gene therapy should remain preclinical. Nevertheless, rapid progress has been made in this field, and gene transfer technology has made sufficient progress to allow fetal gene therapy to be thoroughly assessed in experimental animal models. Limited studies to date support the theoretical biological advantages of the early gestational fetal environment. A number of studies in the fetal sheep, primate, and murine models document relatively efficient transduction, with long-term expression of transgene-encoded protein in various tissues using various gene transfer technologies (Yang, Kim, et al., 1999; Tran et al., 2000; Tarantal et al., 2001). In addition, limited evidence of primary immune response against foreign protein has been observed, and tolerance has been documented in some studies (Tran et al., 2001). Although these results are promising, many more studies are needed before clinical application can be considered.

Tolerance Induction for Organ Transplantation

Although organ transplantation is now a routine procedure in older children and adults, it remains a formidable challenge in the newborn (Webber, 1996; Durand et al., 2001). The long-term ramifications of neonatal and lifelong immunosuppression are unknown and disturbing (Gajarski et al., 1998). Tolerance

---

 TABLE 27-3. DISEASES POTENTIALLY AMENABLE TO IUHSCTx

Rationale = Selective Advantage for Donor Cells

SCID: X-linked*
    ZAP 70
    Jac 3
    ADA deficiency
Wiskott-Aldrich syndrome
Chromosomal breakage syndromes:
    Fanconi anemia
    Bloom syndrome

Rationale = Minimal Engraftment Requirement

    Hyper IgM syndrome
    Chronic granulomatous disease
    Leukocyte adhesion deficiency

---

* Has been successfully treated by IUHSCTx.
IUHSCTx, in utero hematopoietic stem cell transplantation.

induction for organ transplantation would reduce the need for lifelong immunosuppression. Since Billingham and colleagues' (1953) classic observations of "acquired" immunologic tolerance, the phenomenon of fetal tolerance has been relatively accepted. Evidence is now overwhelming that the fetal thymic microenvironment plays a primary role in determining self-recognition and a repertoire of response to foreign antigen. Pre-T-cells undergo positive and negative selection during a series of maturational steps in the fetal thymus that are controlled by thymic stromal cells (Schwartz, 1989; Blackman et al., 1990). The end result is deletion of T-cell clones with high affinity for self-antigen in association with self-major histocompatibility complex (MHC), and preservation of a T-cell repertoire against foreign antigen. Therefore, theoretically at least, introduction of foreign antigen prior to thymic processing should result in presentation of donor antigen in the thymus with clonal deletion of alloreactive T-cells. It is important to note, however, that the mechanism of central thymic tolerance has been defined primarily in T-cell antigen receptor–transgenic mice. In addition to deletional tolerance, there are other mechanisms of rejection, including NK or B-cell mediated responses that are relatively poorly understood. In fact, experimental efforts to induce tolerance by prenatal presentation of antigen have had inconsistent results. It has been documented recently that consistent tolerance based on deletional mechanisms is dependent on the level of engraftment following *in utero* hematopoietic stem cell transplantation and that consistent tolerance can be achieved across full allogeneic barriers if adequate levels of chimerism are attained (Kim et al., 1999; Hayashi et al., 2002). This tolerance is permissive for skin grafting and postnatal cellular transplantation and would undoubtedly be permissive of the less rigorous test of vascularized organ transplantation.

Fetal Therapy for Surgical Disease

The Fetus as a Surgical Patient

Correcting an anatomic malformation *in utero* with open fetal surgery jeopardizes the pregnancy and entails potential surgical risks to the mother as well as the fetus. Until risks of surgery, anesthesia, and preterm labor become relatively trivial, indications for open fetal surgery should remain limited to conditions which, if allowed to continue, would irreversibly interfere with fetal organ development but which, if alleviated, would allow normal development to proceed. Fetal surgery should be performed only in a limited number of centers with (at a minimum) the following expertise:

1. A maternal-fetal specialist experienced in perinatal intervention
2. A sonographer with extensive experience and skill in fetal diagnosis
3. A pediatric surgeon experienced in operating on tiny preterm infants
4. An environment that includes a high-risk obstetric unit associated with a tertiary intensive care nursery
5. A team approach that includes designated individuals from the specialties of genetics, anesthesia, neonatology, urology, neurosurgery, cardiology, and radiology, committed to counseling and intervention
6. An environment with high-level and informed oversight, including an Institutional Review Board and a Fetal Surgery Oversight Committee consisting of uninvolved professional colleagues and a qualified ethicist
7. An associated research laboratory capable of performing a high level of translational research in appropriate fetal animal models

It cannot be overemphasized that the creation of a Fetal Treatment Center with fetal surgical competence requires a major personal commitment by the individuals involved as well as a significant institutional commitment of facilities and support (Howell and Adzick, 1999).

Malformations that qualify for consideration of fetal surgery should satisfy the following prerequisites:

1. Prenatal diagnostic techniques should identify the malformation and exclude other lethal malformations with a high degree of certainty.
2. The defect should have a defined natural history and cause progressive injury to the fetus that is irreversible after delivery.
3. Repair of the defect should be feasible and should reverse or prevent the injury process.
4. Surgical repair must not entail excessive risk for the mother or her future fertility (Harrison, Golbus, Filly, et al., 1982b).

Table 27-4 lists the anatomic defects that theoretically may satisfy the requirements for open fetal surgery. This discussion is limited to those defects that have actually satisfied these authors' requirements and for which treatment *in utero* has been attempted.

TABLE 27-4. ANATOMIC MALFORMATIONS THAT INTERFERE WITH DEVELOPMENT AND THEORETICALLY MIGHT BENEFIT FROM SURGICAL RELIEF BEFORE BIRTH

Malformation	Effect on Development	
Urinary tract obstruction	→ Hydronephrosis/lung hypoplasia	→ Renal/respiratory failure
Cystic adenomatoid malformation	→ Low output cardiac failure/lung hypoplasia	→ Fetal hydrops/demise
Diaphragmatic hernia	→ Lung hypoplasia	→ Respiratory failure
Sacrococcygeal teratoma	→ High output cardiac failure	→ Fetal hydrops/demise
Myelomeningocele	→ Chiari malformation/cord injury	→ Hydrocephalus/neurologic deficit
Cardiac ventricular outflow obstruction	→ Ventricular and pulmonary vascular hypoplasia	→ Hypoplastic left heart/pulmonary hypertension
Cerebrospinal fluid obstruction	→ Hydrocephalus/brain injury	→ Neurologic deficit

The Fetus with Congenital Hydronephrosis

The approach to fetal hydronephrosis that has evolved in the last two decades is a paradigm for fetal treatment in general. A combination of clinical observation and experience along with simultaneous laboratory studies defined the natural history and pathophysiology of the disease and allowed formulation of appropriate selection criteria for fetal treatment. In addition, treatment has evolved from invasive open fetal surgical approaches to relatively minimal intervention, pointing out how technological innovation can dramatically influence fetal treatment. As a result of this experimental and clinical work, families can now be counseled on an individual basis about the prognosis and management options for their fetuses, including prenatal intervention for a few selected fetuses.

Development of an Experimental Model

To study the pathophysiology of fetal urethral obstruction and the efficacy and feasibility of correction *in utero*, it was first necessary to develop relevant animal models of obstructive uropathy. Harrison and colleagues (1983) created a model of severe bilateral hydronephrosis in the lamb by ligating the urachus and occluding the urethra with an ameroid constrictor or ligature at 95 to 105 days' gestation (full term = 145 days) and demonstrated correction of hydronephrosis and prevention of pulmonary hypoplasia by prenatal correction (Harrison, Nakayama, et al., 1982). This relatively late model of urinary obstruction, however, did not reproduce the typical cystic and dysplastic changes noted with severe human obstructive nephropathy.

To test whether earlier obstruction resulted in renal dysplasia, Glick and associates (Glick et al., 1983) performed complete unilateral ureteral obstruction in fetal lambs at the beginning of the second trimester (55 to 65 days' gestation). In this model, the renal changes were both hydronephrotic (with ureteral and caliceal dilatation proximal to the obstruction) and dysplastic when examined at term. Prenatal decompression prevented renal dysplasia, with the degree of dysplasia and functional impairment being proportional to the length of time the kidney was obstructed (Glick et al., 1984). Other studies have shown that oligohydramnios-induced pulmonary hypoplasia associated with urinary obstruction is similar to that seen in human fetuses and that decompression of the obstructed urinary tract permits restoration of amniotic fluid volume and allows lung growth (Adzick et al., 1987; Docimo et al., 1989).

Natural History of Congenital Hydronephrosis

The sonographic diagnosis of fetal lower urinary tract obstruction is suggested by the triad of a dilated and thickened bladder, hydronephrosis, and oligohydramnios. These findings in a male fetus are highly suggestive of posterior urethral valves. Other etiologic factors, however, such as urethral strictures or atresia, urethral agenesis, megalourethra, vesicoureteral reflux, and cloacal anomalies, may be present and may have a similar appearance on a sonogram. Detailed investigation of the anatomy by ultrasound and fetal magnetic resonance imaging can now resolve the differential diagnosis, and in particularly difficult cases, fetal vesicoscopy can define the etiology of obstruction definitively.

Unrelieved urinary tract obstruction interferes with fetal development. The severity of damage at birth depends on the type, degree, and duration of obstruction (Harrison, Filly, et al., 1981). Although children born with partial bilateral obstruction at birth may have only mild hydronephrosis (which is easily treated), long-standing obstruction can result in advanced renal dysplasia incompatible with life. In addition, oligohydramnios secondary to decreased fetal urine output can produce pulmonary hypoplasia, which often is fatal at birth.

Obviously, fetuses with unilateral obstruction do not develop oligohydramnios and are not candidates for prenatal treatment. The presence of oligohydramnios requires bilateral obstruction and is a critical determinant of death (Harrison, Golbus, Filly, et al., 1982a). In fetuses identified with oligohydramnios at first examination in the early second trimester, the mortality rate is nearly 100%. If oligohydramnios develops during serial ultrasonographic evaluations and before adequate pulmonary maturity for *ex utero* viability, morbidity and mortality are high. In addition, a subset of fetuses may sustain severe renal damage but maintain normal amniotic fluid throughout gestation. The major challenge in managing this situation is to determine which fetuses have severe enough obstruction to compromise renal and pulmonary function after birth yet still have adequate renal function for salvage by prenatal decompression.

Appropriate selection of fetuses with lower obstructive uropathy for prenatal intervention depends primarily on fetal urine analysis. The utility of analysis of urinary sodium, chloride, and osmolality on a single bladder aspiration was documented by retrospective and prospective analyses (Glick et al., 1985; Crombleholme et al., 1990) but can be misleading on occasion. The ultrasound appearance of the renal parenchyma is valuable in identifying fetuses with end-stage renal damage as manifested by increased echogenicity and cystic changes. Finally, Johnson and coworkers (Johnson et al., 1995) have documented the superiority of sequential bladder aspirations to avoid analysis of stagnant urine. Improvement of urine electrolytes into the favorable category (Table 27-5) on three sequential aspirations at 48- to 72-hour intervals is highly predictive of preserved renal parenchyma and good ultimate renal function. It should be emphasized that tubular function improves during gestation, and these values are not reliable prior to 20 weeks of gestation. The accuracy of any parameter for identification of fetuses with high-grade obstruction that maintain normal or near-normal amniotic fluid and that ultimately sustain severe renal damage resulting in renal failure after birth remains to be established; this is the current challenge in the treatment of fetal obstructive uropathy.

 TABLE 27-5. URINARY VALUES FOR ASSESSMENT OF FETAL RENAL FUNCTION ON SERIAL ANALYSIS*

Sodium (mg/dL)	≤ 100
Osmolality (mOsm/L)	≤ 200
Chloride (mg/dL)	≤ 90
Total protein (mg/dL)	≤ 20
Calcium (mg/dL)	≤ 8
β_2-microglobulin (mg/L)	≤ 4

* Values must fall with three serial bladder aspirates and ultimately be below these thresholds to be in the "good renal function" prognostic category.

Management of Congenital Hydronephrosis

The authors recommend the following general guidelines for management of the fetus with hydronephrosis, based on collective and cumulative clinical and laboratory experience (Fig. 27-1):

1. An initial ultrasonogram should be obtained to confirm the diagnosis, determine the anatomic level of obstruction, evaluate the volume of amniotic fluid, and rule out the presence of associated anomalies.
2. If no associated anomalies are present and the amniotic fluid volume is adequate, the fetus should be observed and followed up by serial ultrasonography.
3. If amniotic fluid volume remains adequate, the mother should receive routine obstetric care, and the fetus can be treated after term delivery.
4. If moderate-to-severe oligohydramnios develops, the fetus should undergo a complete prognostic evaluation to determine its potential for normal renal and pulmonary function after birth. This includes serial bladder aspiration for urinary electrolytes and protein analysis; some cases may require diagnostic vesicoscopy if the etiology of obstruction is unclear. For the fetus with predicted renal dysplasia, aggressive obstetric care or *in utero* decompression is not indicated.

For the fetus with predicted good renal function, management options depend on fetal lung maturity. If the lungs are mature, immediate delivery and *ex utero* decompression are recommended. If the lungs are immature, *in utero* decompression by vesicoamniotic shunting is recommended.

Shunts require frequent monitoring after placement and often require replacement for migration or obstruction.

Complications related to shunt placement have included iatrogenic gastroschisis with bowel herniation and compromise, vascular injury with secondary fetal demise, retroperitoneal urinoma or urinary ascites, and premature delivery. All of these potential complications emphasize the need for experience with these procedures.

Using the foregoing approach, it is clear that pulmonary hypoplasia can be prevented and that renal function can probably be preserved in a subset of highly selected fetuses with obstructive uropathy. The approach has been validated by documentation of good postnatal renal function in the "good prognosis" fetuses and of renal failure in a few fetuses that were predicted to have "poor prognosis." In the future, well-designed studies to identify the subset of fetuses at risk for renal failure despite normal amniotic fluid are needed. In addition, the experimental and clinical evaluation of more "physiologic" approaches to decompression—such as prenatal laser ablation of posterior urethral valves and the relative effects on postnatal bladder physiology and function—are needed.

The Fetus with Congenital Cystic Adenomatoid Malformation

Congenital cystic adenomatoid malformation (CCAM) represents a spectrum of disease characterized by cystic lesions of the lung. In most cases, CCAM becomes manifest after birth and is easily treated *ex utero* (Bond et al., 1990). These cases present as pulmonary masses causing either respiratory difficulty or recurrent pulmonary infections in infancy or childhood. The more severe end of the spectrum is a lesion that results in fetal hydrops, pulmonary hypoplasia, and fetal demise.

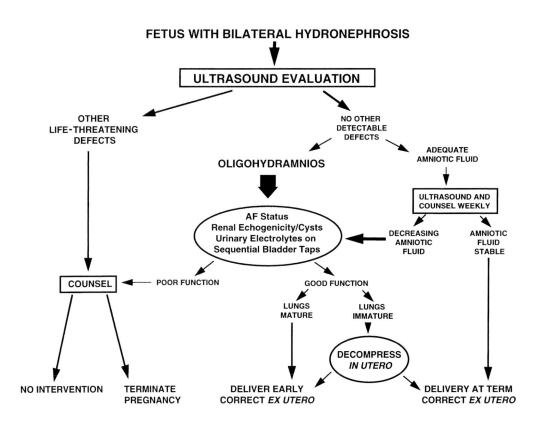

FIGURE 27-1 ■ Management scheme for the fetus with bilateral hydronephrosis. Note that the development of prognostic criteria based on the assessment of fetal renal function allows improved counseling and management. AF, amniotic fluid. (Modified from Glick PL, Harrison MR, Golbus MS, et al: Management of the fetus with congenital hydronephrosis: II. Prognostic criteria and selection for treatment. J Pediatr Surg **20**:376, 1985.)

Natural History of Congenital Cystic Adenomatoid Malformation

CCAMs can be divided into *macrocystic* or *microcystic* (solid) types, depending on the presence or absence of single or multiple cysts greater than 5 mm in diameter, respectively (Adzick, Harrison, Glick, et al., 1985a). In contrast to these authors' early experience, the classification of CCAM is of little value in predicting the probability of fetal hydrops. More important are the size and rate of growth of the lesion. A recently described parameter, the CAM volume ratio or CVR, is predictive of hydrops for microcystic CCAMs and has proven valuable in counseling patients.

The fatal outcome sometimes seen with large CCAMs is related to several factors, including development of hydrops, hypoplasia of the lung secondary to prolonged compression *in utero*, and, in some cases, lack of early diagnosis and immediate postnatal surgery. The pathophysiology of hydrops associated with CCAM has been reproduced in the lamb model (Rice et al., 1994). A slowly enlarging thoracic mass results in gradual shift of the mediastinum with compromise of cardiac venous return and increased central venous pressure with secondary hydrops. Decompression of the mass reverses the physiology and results in resolution of hydrops. These authors therefore postulated that prenatal resection of the pulmonary mass might reverse the hydrops and allow sufficient lung growth to permit survival in these selected severe cases. It has been demonstrated in the lamb model that *in utero* pulmonary resection is feasible and that compensatory growth of the opposite lung occurs (Adzick, Hu, et al., 1986).

Management of Congenital Cystic Adenomatoid Malformation

Patients with CCAM should undergo ultrasonography to confirm the diagnosis, evaluate for polyhydramnios or hydrops, determine the appearance of the lesion, and rule out other life-threatening anomalies. The majority of these patients have isolated small lesions without hydrops and are best treated by surgical resection after term delivery. In the early gestational fetus with a large CCAM, the probability of trouble is higher, and frequent serial sonography should be performed. The period of rapid growth of these tumors is between 20 and 28 weeks when growth frequently plateaus; this is, therefore, the period when maximal vigilance must be maintained. Recommendations for management depend on the size of the tumor (or CAM volume ratio) (Crombleholme, et al., 2002), the presence or absence of associated hydrops, and gestational age.

If pulmonary maturity is established and hydrops evolves, the fetus should be emergently delivered by the *ex utero* intrapartum treatment (EXIT) procedure, and the lesion should be resected while the neonate is on placental support (Bouchard et al., 2002). If significant ventilatory compromise is present after resection of the CCAM, the fetus can then be placed directly on extracorporeal membrane oxygenation (ECMO) support for salvage. Fetuses between 32 weeks and lung maturity with evolving hydrops should undergo an attempt at steroid-induced lung maturation followed by delivery by the *ex utero* intrapartum strategy, with surfactant administration and surgical resection. The immature fetus (32 weeks) with a large

CCAM and evolution of hydrops should be considered for immediate *in utero* resection of the tumor.

In utero therapy has been very successful in appropriately selected cases of CCAM (Adzick et al., 1998). The present authors have published an experience documenting 60% survival of hydropic fetuses with CCAM treated by open fetal surgery, and we currently have a greater than 80% survival of fetuses with macrocystic CCAMs and associated hydrops that have been treated by thoracoamniotic shunting.

The Fetus with Congenital Diaphragmatic Hernia

Congenital diaphragmatic hernia (CDH) is perhaps the ultimate example of a simple anatomic defect that has devastating physiologic consequences during fetal development. The diaphragmatic defect is easily repaired after birth, but many patients with CDH die of pulmonary insufficiency despite optimal postnatal care, because their lungs are too hypoplastic to support extrauterine life. Pulmonary hypoplasia secondary to CDH appears to be secondary to compression of the developing fetal lungs by herniated abdominal viscera. The rationale for prenatal intervention is to allow lung development *in utero* and prevent pulmonary hypoplasia.

Development of an Experimental Model of Congenital Diaphragmatic Hernia

The pathophysiologic rationale and feasibility of *in utero* surgery for CDH have been demonstrated in the fetal lamb model. Creation of a diaphragmatic hernia at 60 days' gestation results in severe pulmonary hypoplasia, which is morphometrically and functionally analogous to that seen in severe cases of human CDH (Harrison, Ross, et al., 1981; Adzick, Outwater, et al., 1985).

Repair of the CDH *in utero* prevents pulmonary hypoplasia, with severity of lung hypoplasia being directly related to the timing and volume of visceral herniation. More recently, prenatal tracheal occlusion has been demonstrated to be a potent stimulator of prenatal lung growth. The lungs are net producers of amniotic fluid, and normal lung development depends on the stenting pressures generated by lung fluid production and distal airway and glottic resistance. Tracheostomy, which bypasses the glottic mechanism and increases the egress of lung fluid, results in pulmonary hypoplasia; tracheal occlusion prevents the egress of lung fluid and results in lung growth. When applied to the lamb model of diaphragmatic hernia, tracheal occlusion results in rapid lung growth with reduction of herniated viscera from the chest (Wilson et al., 1993; Hedrick et al., 1994; DiFiore et al., 1994). The functional consequences of tracheal occlusion in lungs effected by CDH hernia-induced severe pulmonary hypoplasia remains an important question.

Natural History of Congenital Diaphragmatic Hernia

In general, the mortality rates associated with prenatally diagnosed CDH have been approximately 70–90% (Adzick, Harrison, Glick, et al., 1985b; Benacerraf and Adzick, 1987; Sharland et al., 1992). Harrison and associates (1994) reported on the natural history of CDH diagnosed before 24 weeks' gestation and without associated anomalies or fetal surgery; 48 of 83 died (seven were stillborn). Extracorporeal membrane oxygenation was required in 22 of 35 survivors, and in nine of these there was severe residual morbidity. The natural history of fetal CDH remains a moving target, however, as there have been significant advances in postnatal treatment of CDH that have improved upon the documented natural history. Nevertheless, there continues to be significant mortality and morbidity associated with severe CDH and there continues to be a compelling rationale for prenatal intervention in the most severe subset of fetuses.

A major remaining challenge is to define selection criteria that will reliably identify the most severely affected fetuses that would be the most likely to benefit from prenatal therapy. Herniation of the left lobe of the liver into the chest is one predictor of poor outcome (Metkus et al., 1996). The single most predictive criterion is the right lung two-dimensional area (measured at the level of the right atrium) to head circumference ratio or LHR (Lipshutz et al., 1997). Although for a time, experience with this parameter validated an approximately 90% mortality for an LHR of less than 1.0, recent experience in multiple centers has suggested a significantly higher survival rate. The LHR, however, remains a valuable predictor of severity, of the potential need for extracorporeal membrane oxygenation, and of the potential for short- and long-term morbidity in CDH infants.

Management of Congenital Diaphragmatic Hernia

Although techniques have been developed to repair the diaphragmatic defect *in utero*, direct repair of fetal CDH remains a technical *tour de force*. The physiologic obstacle of liver in the chest with distortion of the umbilical vein and ductus venosus has not been overcome. It has not been proven that this approach can improve on the natural history of CDH (Harrison et al., 1993). Although success has been, and can be, achieved in fetuses without liver herniation, these fetuses are more likely to do well with conventional postnatal therapy. These authors' management of fetuses with CDH has changed significantly since the previous edition of this text. Based on experience with both open fetal surgery to repair the defect, and later, prenatal tracheal occlusion, these authors no longer recommend fetal intervention for CDH. Although prenatal tracheal occlusion may ultimately have value for the most severe subset of fetuses with CDH, further research needs to be performed to determine the optimal application of this approach. The authors have performed open fetal surgery for tracheal occlusion in 15 fetuses with severe CDH (Flake et al., 2000). The survival rate was 33%, and survival was associated with significant morbidity resulting from a combination of poor lung function and prematurity. Despite the achievement of impressive lung growth in many of these fetuses, poor lung function that was not corrected by surfactant therapy remained the limiting factor. Of particular interest was the observation that those fetuses with the most impressive lung growth were also those that delivered the earliest, suggesting that rapid lung growth resulted in fetal distress and fetal-maternal signaling with secondary preterm labor. One potential approach is to employ temporary tracheal occlusion to achieve lung growth, with subsequent release of occlusion to prevent fetal distress

and permit lung maturation. Although intuitively appealing, this approach has not been proven experimentally. Significant interest remains in clinical application of balloon tracheal occlusion, but these authors feel it is important to validate the pathophysiologic rationale of this approach prior to further clinical application. In addition, prognostic criteria that are representative of the current survival of CDH infants with postnatal care need to be validated prospectively in centers planning fetal intervention for this anomaly.

The Fetus with Sacrococcygeal Teratoma

Sacrococcygeal teratoma (SCT) is the most common tumor of the newborn. The estimated incidence is 1 in 35,000 live births. Most patients remain asymptomatic *in utero*, and the diagnosis is confirmed after birth. Prenatal diagnosis is increasing and has allowed analysis of the natural history of SCT.

Natural History of Sacrococcygeal Teratoma

A review of 27 cases of prenatally diagnosed SCT revealed that five cases were terminated electively, with 15 of the 22 remaining fetuses dying *in utero* or soon after birth (Flake et al., 1986a). A more detailed study confirmed the high mortality rate asociated with SCT, with 22 of 42 fetuses dying *in utero* or at birth (Bond et al., 1990). When placentomegaly or hydrops occurred, 15 of 15 fetuses died precipitously *in utero*. Presentation after 30 weeks was a relatively good prognostic sign, with six of eight fetuses surviving; this was in contrast to 1 of 14 cases presenting prior to 30 weeks' gestation (Flake et al., 1986a). An additional prognostic indicator was that when a maternal indication for sonography was present, 22 of 32 fetuses died, whereas nine of ten fetuses detected by routine screening sonography survived. Although diagnosis prior to 30 weeks' gestation was associated with poor outcome, the incidental finding of SCT was favorable at any gestational age.

Death appears to result from secondary effects of SCT rather than from malignant invasion. Tumor mass and associated polyhydramnios frequently cause preterm labor and delivery, with fetal survival dependent on fetal lung maturity. Massive hemorrhage into the tumor with secondary fetal exsanguination can occur spontaneously *in utero* or can be precipitated by labor and delivery. Dystocia (secondary to tumor bulk) or tumor rupture can occur during vaginal delivery or cesarean section. In a few cases, placentomegaly and/or hydrops can occur, and high-output failure has been documented. The observation of fetal demise after the appearance of placentomegaly/hydrops in combination with confirmation of a vascular steal pathophysiology of hydrops, led to treatment by prenatal tumor resection. Subsequent experience has confirmed that prenatal tumor resection can reverse fetal hydrops and result in fetal survival (Adzick et al., 1997).

Management of Sacrococcygeal Teratoma

All fetuses with a diagnosis of SCT undergo detailed sonographic evaluation to confirm the diagnosis and to rule out associated (rare) anomalies. An assessment of placental size, type of SCT, and the presence or absence of hydrops should be made. If the diagnosis is serendipitous and the tumor is small, the outlook is optimistic, and the pregnancy can be followed with infrequent serial sonography to term vaginal delivery. If the tumor is large or if obstetric indications for sonography exist, a guarded prognosis should be given, and the pregnancy is followed by frequent sonography. Sonographic observation should include fetal echocardiography and Doppler blood flow assessments to observe for the evolution of high output failure. If no placentomegaly or hydrops evolves, the fetus should be delivered by elective cesarean section to avoid dystocia or tumor rupture and hemorrhage. If placentomegaly/ hydrops evolves after fetal pulmonary maturity is established, the fetus should be delivered by emergent cesarean section and treated *ex utero*. If placentomegaly/hydrops evolves before 32 weeks' gestation and the tumor is anatomically amenable to resection (APSA type I or II SCT) (Altman et al., 1974), *in utero* tumor resection should be considered. Another approach that has been described recently for fetal SCT is radiofrequency ablation of the blood supply. Unfortunately, the dissemination of energy with this technology is difficult to predict or control, and considerable morbidity has resulted from collateral damage to adjacent structures.

Clinical Experience with Sacrococcygeal Teratoma

Open fetal surgery for SCT has now been performed at two centers. At the Children's Hospital of Philadelphia, the authors have evaluated 26 fetuses with SCT since 1995. Of those, two fetuses were terminated, eight died *in utero*, 11 were delivered by cesarean section and underwent standard postnatal therapy, and one expired shortly after birth as a result of perinatal hemorrhage (no resection). In 1997, the authors reported the first successful fetal surgical resection of SCT (Adzick et al., 1997). Since that time, the authors have performed three additional resections for SCT with two survivors, for an overall survival rate of 75%.

The Fetus with Congenital Hydrocephalus

Although the rationale for prenatal decompression of congenital hydrocephalus remains compelling, a number of complicating factors limit clinical application. First, fetuses with isolated high-pressure hydrocephalus (which may benefit most from prenatal decompression) represent a minority of fetuses presenting with hydrocephalus. There is a high rate of associated central nervous system (CNS) anomalies and secondary hydrocephalus that would not be expected to benefit from prenatal intervention. Frequently, diagnostic uncertainty exists, making prediction of outcome difficult. In addition, the natural history of isolated congenital hydrocephalus has not been defined adequately in humans, and experimental end points are difficult. Although fetal magnetic resonance imaging (MRI) scanning has made detailed imaging of the central nervous system possible, future intervention for hydrocephalus will depend on the development of validated selection criteria.

The Fetus with Myelomeningocele

Myelomeningocele (MMC) is a form of spina bifida, defined as the protrusion of the spinal cord and meninges from the spinal canal because of a defect in the overlying vertebral arches, muscle tissue, and skin. Spina bifida affects about 1 of every 2000 children worldwide (Edmonds and James, 1990;

Lary and Edmonds, 1996) and causes lifelong disabilities including paraplegia, hydocephalus, sexual dysfunction, skeletal deformities, incontinence, and mental impairment. A growing body of evidence from both animal and human studies suggests that early gestational repair of MMC could help preserve neurological function that might otherwise be lost during gestation because of *in utero* mechanical and chemical trauma. The rationale behind fetal intervention in the treatment of MMC is to correct the structural defect at a time when significant neuronal damage has either not yet occurred or still has the potential to be reversed (Walsh et al., 2001).

Natural History of Myelomeningocele

The true natural history of untreated MMC in the modern era has not been defined prospectively. A recently published retrospective chart review of 297 patients treated and followed at the Children's Hospital of Philadelphia represents the most updated information on natural history of this anomaly (Rintoul et al., 2002). This study documented an overall rate of shunting of 81%, with the level of the lesion significantly effecting the incidence of shunting. In 86% of patients, the functional level was found to be equal to or higher (worse) than the radiologic level. In other studies, the infant death rate related to open spina bifida in the United States is estimated at 10% and remains 1% per year after one year of age (Hunt, 1997; Manning et al., 2000).

Management of Myelomeningocele

Because significant risk to the mother is justified only by clear and dramatic benefit to the fetus, fetal surgeons initially limited their target anomalies to those that were highly lethal. The extension of fetal surgery to repair of fetal MMC represents a significant new development in maternal-fetal intervention. Although few would argue that prenatal intervention to prevent severe disability that impairs a normal quality of life is a laudable goal, there are a number of reasons for concern with the application of this rationale to MMC. First and foremost is the absence of proven benefit for this procedure to offset the significant maternal risk involved. Proof of benefit is particularly complex for MMC because of the spectrum of disease severity, the imperfect correlation of anatomic level and level of neurologic defect, and the multiple potential therapeutic endpoints, some of which will take many years to define. It is much more difficult to quantify and compare degrees of disability than to compare percentage of survival. A second major concern is the significant likelihood that maternal-fetal surgery will increase mortality and that overall morbidity could be increased by the consequences of prematurity. The third fear is that this shift in paradigm might lead to the attempted treatment of other nonlethal anomalies, including cleft palate or other relatively minor defects. Treatment of such defects would be difficult to justify in the context of any significant maternal risk. For these reasons, it is imperative that the prenatal treatment of MMC be performed only in the context of a multicenter randomized clinical trial. Such a trial, sponsored by the National Institutes of Health, is now underway. The results of intervention for MMC accrued prior to the trial are encouraging. The intervention has uniformly reversed the hindbrain herniation associated with MMC and, at 1 year of follow-up, appears to have dramatically reduced the need for ventricular shunting (Sutton et al., 1999). The current authors therefore recommend that all pregnancies diagnosed prenatally with MMC receive appropriate information regarding the availability of the trial and, if interested, referral for counseling.

FUTURE DIRECTIONS IN PRENATAL SURGICAL THERAPY

Reduction in Maternal and Fetal Risk

The remaining challenges in open fetal surgery involve primarily reduction of maternal and fetal risk. It is unlikely that the list of anatomic diseases potentially amenable to fetal surgery (see Table 27-4) will expand significantly, given that most anatomic abnormalities can be treated adequately after birth. The full potential of prenatal anatomic correction has not been realized, however, because of prohibitive risk, and there could be benefit for prenatal correction of cleft lip and palate or other anomalies in order to take advantage of scarless fetal wound healing, advantageous fetal biology, or remodeling. If new surgical techniques, physiologic support systems, and tocolytic therapy can reduce the fetal and maternal risk to that of elective postnatal surgery, indications for fetal surgery may be liberalized.

Fetoscopic Approaches to Fetal Disease

The resurgence of interest in laparoscopic techniques has resulted in an explosion of new technology available for fetoscopic procedures, and the ability to perform major fetal surgery under direct vision through small puncture sites in the uterus has become a realistic possibility. A large number of fetal procedures are currently being performed or could be performed in the future by fetoscopic technique (Table 27-6), thus resulting in the potential for reduced maternal and fetal risk and reduced likelihood of preterm labor.

The most frequent procedures currently performed by fetoscopic technique are extrafetal procedures, such as laser ablation of communicating vessels in twin-to-twin transfusion (De Lia et al., 1999) and cord ligations—both for acardiac twins (Quintero et al., 1996) and complicated monochorionic multiple gestations. Fetal procedures, such as fetal cystoscopy with laser ablation of posterior urethral valves, are now technically possible (Quintero et al., 1995), although they have not yet been clinically successful. With improvements in current laparoscopic equipment and technique, clinical application of "minimally invasive" fetal surgery should continue to increase.

TABLE 27-6. ENDOSCOPIC FETAL INTERVENTIONS: POTENTIAL

Twin separations
Cord ligations
Laser ablation of posterior urethral valves
Tracheal occlusion
Ablation or embolization of fetal tumors
Sealing premature rupture of membranes
Coverage of spina bifida defects
In utero hematopoietic stem cell transplantation/fetal gene therapy

It should be emphasized, however, that fetoscopic procedures still entail significant risk, which is proportional to the size and number of trocars utilized and to the severity of the fetal pathophysiology being treated. In fact, it is remarkable that the only maternal deaths related to fetal surgery have occurred with fetoscopic procedures.

MATERNAL-FETAL MANAGEMENT AND RISK

Fetal surgery is unique because of its inherent risks to both the mother and the fetus. Although maternal safety is of overriding importance in any fetal surgical procedure, management of the maternal and fetal units is interdependent. Prior to human application, it was necessary to develop anesthetic, surgical, and tocolytic techniques and to establish maternal safety by performing multiple fetal procedures in the primate model (Harrison, Golbus, Filly, et al., 1982a; Nakayama et al., 1984). Since that time, the current authors have applied these techniques and have continuously developed others to improve maternal and fetal safety and to improve clinical outcome in approximately 400 open fetal surgical cases.

Clinical Experience: Operative Technique

Prior to open fetal surgery, mothers receive a 50-mg indomethacin suppository and undergo placement of an epidural catheter. After induction of isoflurane general anesthesia, the mother is positioned supine, with her right side elevated to avoid uterine caval compression. An arterial line and Foley catheter are placed for intraoperative and postoperative maternal monitoring.

A large, transverse lower abdominal incision is made. For most patients, flaps are raised, and a vertical incision in the midline fascia provides adequate exposure. If the placenta is anterior, necessitating a posterior hysterotomy, division of the rectus muscles may be required. Exposure is enhanced by placement of a large, circular fixed retraction system and exteriorization of the uterus. The level of isoflurane anesthesia is titrated to achieve adequate uterine relaxation prior to the uterine incision. Other tocolytic agents available in the operating room include magnesium sulfate, terbutaline, and nitroglycerin, which are used selectively for uncontrolled uterine contraction.

Once the position of the hysterotomy is decided, the physician maps the placental margin by tracing the margin of the placenta with ultrasonography and by marking the surface of the uterus with electrocautery. The hysterotomy should be placed at least 5 cm from the placental margin, and farther if possible. A modified uterine stapler is then passed through the uterus and fired once in each direction, hemostatically compressing and dividing the layers of the uterus (including the membranes) with each application. The appropriate fetal part is then exteriorized for the fetal procedure.

The authors' current fetal monitoring consists of real-time ultrasound monitoring of heart rate and cardiac function as well as fetal pulse oximetry. The fetus is kept warm by limited exposure and continuous perfusion of the amniotic space with warm Ringer's lactate solution. Additional fetal anesthesia is achieved by intramuscular injection of narcotic and a paralysis agent. Fetal intravenous access is obtained via a peripheral IV when needed. On completion of the fetal procedure, the fetus is returned to the uterine cavity, and the amniotic fluid is replaced by warm lactated Ringer's solution containing antibiotics. The uterus is meticulously closed in two layers of absorbable suture, with care taken to control the membranes, and an omental patch is secured over the hysterotomy to prevent amniotic fluid leak. Magnesium sulfate is initiated at completion of uterine closure prior to lightening the gaseous anesthetic agent.

In the postoperative period, the mother is monitored in the maternal-fetal intensive care unit. Tocolytic therapy is magnesium sulfate, supplemented by indomethacin and terbutaline as necessary. Uterine activity and fetal heart rate are continuously monitored by tocodynamometry, and fetal well-being is assessed by ultrasound twice per day and by fetal echocardiography once per day. The epidural catheter is an essential component of the maternal regimen, and these authors feel that its use has reduced the maternal stress response and the incidence of early preterm labor.

After the second postoperative day, the mother is transferred to the maternity ward. Usually, she can be discharged by the fourth postoperative day.

Maternal Outcome

In the entire series of more than 400 open fetal operations, there have been no maternal deaths and few major maternal complications. The most concerning complication in the mother has been postoperative noncardiogenic pulmonary edema. In two cases, this was an ongoing manifestation of the *maternal mirror syndrome*, which was evident preoperatively and necessitated discontinuation of tocolytic therapy and delivery of a previable fetus. In three other cases, it occurred unexpectedly, with no obvious etiologic mechanism, and mechanical ventilation was required prior to resolution. In one of the initial cases, a uterine rupture that might have been avoidable occurred during labor. Other complications, including membrane separations with amniotic fluid leaks, pseudomembranous colitis, and wound complications, have been relatively minor. It is understood by the mother prior to the procedure that all subsequent pregnancies must be delivered by cesarean section because of the high position of the hysterotomy performed for fetal surgery.

Effect on Reproductive Potential

In most instances, a procedure to save a defective fetus that would render the mother incapable of having future children would be unacceptable. Through retrospective analysis of detailed medical records maintained at the California Primate Research Center on 94 primates that had undergone fetal surgery, these authors found no reduction in fertility relative to colony controls (Adzick, Harrison, Flake, et al., 1985; Adzick, Harrison, et al., 1986). Although a complete analysis needs to be performed, it has been our experience that the majority of patients who desired future pregnancies have succeeded.

■ SUMMARY

In summary, prenatal diagnosis has dramatically changed the physician's perception of the fetus. The fetus is now appropriately considered a patient, and fetal therapy for a wide variety of prenatally diagnosed abnormalities can be offered. Medical treatment of the fetus is now the standard of care for a number of abnormalities and has potential for significant expansion. Its efficacy for many potential medical diseases that are amenable to therapy has yet to be established, and further experimental work and clinical experience are required. More invasive therapeutic maneuvers involve significant risk for both fetus and mother, raising difficult questions about their rights, risks, and potential benefits. Because of the current high risk of open fetal surgery, it is imperative that efficacy be established when possible by controlled clinical trials.

REFERENCES

Adzick N, Harrison M, Flake A, et al: Automatic uterine stapling devices in fetal surgery: Experience in a primate model. Surg Forum **36**:479, 1985.

Adzick NS, Crombleholme TM, Morgan MA, et al: A rapidly growing fetal teratoma. Lancet **349**:538, 1997.

Adzick NS, Harrison MR, Crombleholme TM, et al: Fetal lung lesions: Management and outcome. Am J Obstet Gynecol **179**:884, 1998.

Adzick NS, Harrison MR, Glick PL, et al: Fetal cystic adenomatoid malformation: Prenatal diagnosis and natural history. J Pediatr Surg **20**:483, 1985a.

Adzick NS, Harrison MR, Glick PL, et al: Diaphragmatic hernia in the fetus: Prenatal diagnosis and outcome in 94 cases. J Pediatr Surg **20**:357, 1985b.

Adzick NS, Harrison MR, Glick PL, et al: Fetal surgery in the primate. III. Maternal outcome after fetal surgery. J Pediatr Surg **21**:477, 1986.

Adzick NS, Harrison MR, and Hu L: Pulmonary hypoplasia and renal dysplasia in a fetal lamb urinary tract obstruction model. Surg Forum **38**:666, 1987.

Adzick NS, Hu LM, Davies P, et al: Compensatory lung growth after pneumonectomy in fetal lambs: A morphometric study. Surg Forum **37**:309, 1986.

Adzick NS, Outwater KM, Harrison MR, et al: Correction of congenital diaphragmatic hernia in utero. IV. An early gestational fetal lamb model for pulmonary vascular morphometric analysis. J Pediatr Surg **20**:673, 1985.

Altman RP, Randolph JG, and Lilly JR: Sacrococcygeal teratoma: American Academy of Pediatrics Surgical Section Survey—1973. J Pediatr Surg **9**:389, 1974.

Benacerraf BR and Adzick NS: Fetal diaphragmatic hernia: Ultrasound diagnosis and clinical outcome in 19 cases. Am J Obstet Gynecol **156**:573, 1987.

Billingham R, Brent L, and Medawar PB: Actively acquired tolerance of foreign cells. Nature **172**:603, 1953.

Blackman M, Kappler J, and Marrack P: The role of the T-cell receptor in positive and negative selection of developing T-cells. Science **248**:1335, 1990.

Bond SJ, Harrison MR, Schmidt KG, et al: Death due to high-output cardiac failure in fetal sacrococcygeal teratoma. J Pediatr Surg **25**:1287, 1990.

Bouchard S, Johnson MP, Flake AW, et al: The EXIT procedure: Experience and outcome in 31 cases. J Pediatr Surg **37**:418, 2002.

Crombleholme TM, Coleman B, Hedrick H, et al: Cystic adenomatoid malformation volume ratio predicts outcome in prenatally diagnosed cystic adenomatoid malformation of the lung. J Pediatr Surg **37**:331, 2002.

Crombleholme TM, Harrison MR, Golbus MS, et al: Fetal intervention in obstructive uropathy: Prognostic indicators and efficacy of intervention. Am J Obstet Gynecol **162**:1239, 1990.

De Lia JE, Kuhlmann RS, and Lopez KP: Treating previable twin-twin transfusion syndrome with fetoscopic laser surgery: Outcomes following the learning curve. J Perinat Med **27**:61, 1999.

DiFiore JW, Fauza DO, Slavin R, et al: Experimental fetal tracheal ligation reverses the structural and physiological effects of pulmonary hypoplasia in congenital diaphragmatic hernia. J Pediatr Surg **29**:248, 1994.

Docimo SG, Luetic T, Crone RK, et al: Pulmonary development in the fetal lamb with severe bladder outlet obstruction and oligohydramnios: A morphometric study. J Urol **142**:657, 1989.

Durand P, Debray D, Mandel R, et al: Acute liver failure in infancy: A 14-year experience of a pediatric liver transplantation center. J Pediatr **139**:871, 2001.

Edmonds LD and James LM: Temporal trends in the prevalence of congenital malformations at birth based on the birth defects monitoring program, United States, 1979–1987. Mor Mortal Wkly Rep CDC Surveill Summ **39**:19, 1990.

Flake A, Roncarolo MG, Puck J, et al: Treatment of X-linked severe combined immunodeficiency by in utero transplantation of paternal bone marrow. N Engl J Med **335**:1806, 1996.

Flake AW, Crombleholme TM, Johnson MP, et al: Treatment of severe congenital diaphragmatic hernia by fetal tracheal occlusion: Clinical experience with fifteen cases. Am J Obstet Gynecol **183**:1059, 2000.

Flake AW, Harrison MR, Adzick NS, et al: Fetal sacrococcygeal teratoma. J Pediatr Surg **21**:563, 1986a.

Flake AW, Harrison MR, Adzick NS, et al: Transplantation of fetal hematopoietic stem cells in utero: The creation of hematopoietic chimeras. Science **233**:776, 1986b.

Flake AW and Zanjani ED: In utero hematopoietic stem cell transplantation. A status report. Jama **278**:932, 1997.

Flake AW and Zanjani ED: In utero hematopoietic stem cell transplantation: Ontogenic opportunities and biologic barriers. Blood **94**:2179, 1999.

Fleischman R and Mintz B: Prevention of genetic anemias in mice by microinjection of normal hematopoietic cells into the fetal placenta. Proc Natl Acad Sci USA **76**:5736, 1979.

Gajarski RJ, Smith EO, Denfield SW, et al: Long-term results of triple-drug-based immunosuppression in nonneonatal pediatric heart transplant recipients. Transplantation **65**:1470, 1998.

Glick PL, Harrison MR, Adzick NS, et al: Correction of congenital hydronephrosis in utero IV: In utero decompression prevents renal dysplasia. J Pediatr Surg **19**:649, 1984.

Glick PL, Harrison MR, Golbus MS, et al: Management of the fetus with congenital hydronephrosis II: Prognostic criteria and selection for treatment. J Pediatr Surg **20**:376, 1985.

Glick PL, Harrison MR, Noall RA, et al: Correction of congenital hydronephrosis in utero III. Early mid-trimester ureteral obstruction produces renal dysplasia. J Pediatr Surg **18**:681, 1983.

Harrison MR, Adzick NS, Estes JM, et al: A prospective study of the outcome for fetuses with diaphragmatic hernia. Jama **271**:382, 1994.

Harrison MR, Adzick NS, and Flake AW: Congenital diaphragmatic hernia: An unsolved problem. Sem Pediatr Surg **2**:109, 1993.

Harrison MR, Filly RA, Parer JT, et al: Management of the fetus with a urinary tract malformation. Jama **246**:635, 1981.

Harrison MR, Golbus MS, Filly RA, et al: Fetal surgery for congenital hydronephrosis. N Engl J Med **306**:591, 1982a.

Harrison MR, Golbus MS, Filly RA, et al: Fetal surgical treatment. Pediatr Ann **11**:896, 1982b.

Harrison MR, Nakayama DK, Noall R, et al: Correction of congenital hydronephrosis in utero II. Decompression reverses the effects of obstruction on the fetal lung and urinary tract. J Pediatr Surg **17**:965, 1982.

Harrison MR, Ross NA, and de Lorimier AA: Correction of congenital diaphragmatic hernia in utero. III. Development of a successful surgical technique using abdominoplasty to avoid compromise of umbilical blood flow. J Pediatr Surg **16**:934, 1981.

Harrison MR, Ross N, Noall R, et al: Correction of congenital hydronephrosis in utero. I. The model: fetal urethral obstruction produces hydronephrosis and pulmonary hypoplasia in fetal lambs. J Pediatr Surg **18**:247, 1983.

Harrison MR, Slotnick RN, Crombleholme TM, et al: In-utero transplantation of fetal liver haemopoietic stem cells in monkeys. Lancet **2**:1425, 1989.

Hayashi S, Peranteau WH, Shaaban AF, et al: Complete allogeneic hematopoietic chimerism achieved by a combined strategy of in utero hematopoietic stem cell transplantation and postnatal donor lymphocyte infusion. Blood **100**:804, 2002.

Hedrick MH, Estes JM, Sullivan KM, et al: Plug the lung until it grows (PLUG): A new method to treat congenital diaphragmatic hernia in utero. J Pediatr Surg **29**:612, 1994.

Herzog RW and High KA: Problems and prospects in gene therapy for hemophilia. Curr Opin Hematol **5**:321, 1998.

Hoelzer D and Gokbuget N: Recent approaches in acute lymphoblastic leukemia in adults. Crit Rev Oncol Hematol **36**:49, 2000.

Howell LJ and Adzick NS: The essentials of a fetal therapy center. Semin Perinatol **23**:535, 1999.

Hunt GM: The median survival time in open spina bifida. Dev Med Child Neurol **39**:568, 1997.

Johnson MP, Corsi P, Bradfield W, et al: Sequential urinalysis improves evaluation of fetal renal function in obstructive uropathy. Am J Obstet Gynecol **173**:59, 1995.

Jones DR, Bui TH, Anderson EM, et al: In utero haematopoietic stem cell transplantation: Current perspectives and future potential. Bone Marrow Transplant **18**:831, 1996.

Kim HB, Shaaban AF, Milner R, et al: In utero bone marrow transplantation induces tolerance by a combination of clonal deletion and anergy. J Pediatr Surg **34**:726, 1999.

Krivit W, Shapiro EG, Peters C, et al: Hematopoietic stem-cell transplantation in globoid-cell leukodystrophy. N Engl J Med **338**:1119, 1998.

Lary JM and Edmonds LD: Prevalence of spina bifida at birth—United States, 1983–1990: A comparison of two surveillance systems. Mor Mortal Wkly Rep CDC Surveill Summ **45**:15, 1996.

Liley AW: Intrauterine transfusion of the foetus in haemolytic disease. Brit Med J **2**:1107, 1963.

Lipshutz GS, Albanese CT, Feldstein VA, et al: Prospective analysis of lung-to-head ratio predicts survival for patients with prenatally diagnosed congenital diaphragmatic hernia. J Pediatr Surg **32**:1634, 1997.

Manning SM, Jennings R, and Madsen JR: Pathophysiology, prevention, and potential treatment of neural tube defects. Ment Retard Dev Disabil Res Rev **6**:6, 2000.

Martin TG and Gajewski JL: Allogeneic stem cell transplantation for acute lymphocytic leukemia in adults. Hematol Oncol Clin North Am **15**:97, 2001.

Metcalf D, Moore MAS: Embryonic aspects of hemopoiesis. In Neuberger A, Tatum EL (eds): Frontiers of Biology—Hemopoietic Cells. Amsterdam, North Hollad, 1971, p. 172.

Metkus AP, Filly RA, Stringer MD, et al: Sonographic predictors of survival in fetal diaphragmatic hernia. J Pediatr Surg **31**:148, 1996.

Nakayama DK, Harrison MR, Seron-Ferre M, et al: Fetal surgery in the primate II. Uterine electromyographic response to operative procedures and pharmacologic agents. J Pediatr Surg **19**:333, 1984.

Peranteau WF, Hayashi S, Hsieh M, et al: High Level Allogeneic Chimerism Achieved by Prenatal Tolerance Induction and Postnatal Non-Myeloablative Bone Marrow Transplantation. Blood **100**: 2225, 2002.

Quintero RA, Johnson MP, Romero R, et al: In-utero percutaneous cystoscopy in the management of fetal lower obstructive uropathy. Lancet **346**:537, 1995.

Quintero RA, Romero R, Reich H, et al: In utero percutaneous umbilical cord ligation in the management of complicated monochorionic multiple gestations. Ultrasound Obstet Gynecol **8**:16, 1996.

Rice HE, Estes JM, Hedrick MH, et al: Congenital cystic adenomatoid malformation: A sheep model of fetal hydrops. J Pediatr Surg **29**:692, 1994.

Rintoul NE, Sutton LN, Hubbard AM, et al: A new look at myelomeningoceles: Functional level, vertebral level, shunting, and the implications for fetal intervention. Pediatrics **109**:409, 2002.

Schwartz R: Acquisition of Immunologic Self Tolerance. Cell **57**:1073, 1989.

Shapiro E, Krivit W, Lockman L, et al: Long-term effect of bone-marrow transplantation for childhood-onset cerebral X-linked adrenoleukodystrophy. Lancet **356**:713, 2000.

Sharland GK, Lockhart SM, Heward AJ, et al: Prognosis in fetal diaphragmatic hernia. Am J Ob Gynecol **166**:9, 1992.

Sutton LN, Adzick NS, Bilaniuk LT, et al: Improvement in hindbrain herniation demonstrated by serial fetal magnetic resonance imaging following fetal surgery for myelomeningocele. Jama **282**:1826, 1999.

Tarantal AF, Lee CI, Ekert JE, et al: Lentiviral vector gene transfer into fetal rhesus monkeys (Macaca mulatta): Lung-targeting approaches. Mol Ther **4**:614, 2001.

Tran ND, Porada CD, Almeida-Porada G, et al: Induction of stable prenatal tolerance to beta-galactosidase by in utero gene transfer into preimmune sheep fetuses. Blood **97**:3417, 2001.

Tran ND, Porada CD, Zhao Y, et al: In utero transfer and expression of exogenous genes in sheep. Exp Hematol **28**:17, 2000.

Walsh DS, Adzick NS, Sutton LN, et al: The rationale for in utero repair of myelomeningocele. Fetal Diagn Ther **16**:312, 2001.

Webber SA: Newborn and infant heart transplantation. Curr Opin Cardiol **11**:68, 1996.

Wengler G, Lanfranchi A, Frusca T, et al: In-utero transplantation of parental CD34 haematopoietic progenitor cells in a patient with X-linked severe combined immunodeficiency (SCIDX1). Lancet **348**:1484, 1996.

Wilson JM, DiFiore JW, and Peters CA: Experimental fetal tracheal ligation prevents the pulmonary hypoplasia associated with fetal nephrectomy: Possible application for congenital diaphragmatic hernia. J Pediatr Surg **28**:1433, 1993.

Yang EY, Flake AW, and Adzick NS: Prospects for fetal gene therapy. Semin Perinatol **23**:524, 1999.

Yang EY, Kim HB, Shaaban AF, et al: Persistent postnatal transgene expression in both muscle and liver after fetal injection of recombinant adenovirus. J Pediatr Surg **34**:766, 1999.

Zanjani ED, Flake AW, Rice H, et al: Long-term repopulating ability of xenogeneic transplanted human fetal liver hematopoietic stem cells in sheep. J Clin Invest **93**:1051, 1994.

Zanjani ED, Pallavicini MG, Flake AW, et al: Engraftment and long-term expression of human fetal hemopoietic stem cells in sheep following transplantation in utero. J Clin Invest **89**:1178, 1992.

Chapter 28
INTRAUTERINE GROWTH RESTRICTION

Robert Resnik, MD, and Robert K. Creasy, MD

Human pregnancy, similar to pregnancy in other polytocous animal species, can be affected by conditions that restrict the normal growth of the fetus. The growth-restricted fetus is at higher risk for perinatal morbidity and mortality, the risk rising with the severity of the growth restriction. This chapter reviews the various causes of fetal growth restriction and considers the methods of antepartum recognition and diagnosis along with clinical management. The term *intrauterine growth restriction* (IUGR), which we first introduced in the third edition of this text, is preferred over *intrauterine growth retardation*, which frequently connotes mental retardation to the patient.

DEFINITIONS

The World Health Organization (1969) classifies all newborns weighing less than 2500 g as having low birth weight. Although the majority of these low-birth-weight newborns are born preterm, many are born near term having sustained IUGR. Following the recognition that neonates could be born undernourished at term, with increased morbidity and mortality, Lubchenco and colleagues (1963) published detailed graphs comparing birth weights at different gestational ages. This led to the classification of low-birth-weight newborns into the following three groups (Battaglia, 1970; Yerushalmy, 1970):

1. *Preterm neonates*—newborns delivered before 37 completed weeks of gestation who are of appropriate size for gestational age (AGA)
2. *Preterm and growth-restricted neonates*—newborns delivered before 37 completed weeks of gestation who are small for gestational age (SGA)
3. *Term growth-restricted neonates*—newborns delivered after 37 completed weeks of gestation who are SGA (not all SGA neonates are growth restricted, however; some cases result from the normal distribution of neonatal weight among a normal base population)

The diagnosis of IUGR is in part dependent on an accurate evaluation of gestational age. The last menstrual period is a reliable index of gestational age if the mother is seen early in gestation, unless there is a history of irregular menstrual cycles or conception occurred soon after discontinuation of oral contraceptives. Because IUGR (particularly asymmetric IUGR) is rarely detected clinically before 22 to 24 weeks, uterine size should equate with gestational age up to that time (Murphy, 1969). Ultrasonographic evaluation is particularly useful in dating pregnancies if it is performed before biological variation begins to have a significant impact (i.e., before 22 weeks of gestation) (see Chapter 20).

Methods are also available to date the gestation retrospectively by physical and neurologic examination of the newborn (Dubowitz et al., 1970). Such methods rely on the development of various physical characteristics and responses throughout the latter part of gestation. Unfortunately, the usefulness of these characteristics for growth-restricted fetuses has not yet been verified. It is possible that the appearance of these various milestones of growth and maturation can be delayed or accelerated with different types of IUGR. For instance, skeletal maturation is delayed with severe growth restriction (Roord et al., 1978).

Different standards for fetal growth throughout gestation have been reported. These standards set the normal range, on the basis of statistical considerations, between two standard deviations of the mean (2.5th–97.5th percentile) or between the 10th and 90th percentiles for fixed gestational ages. The standards most widely used in the United States in the 1960s and 1970s were those developed in Denver, Colorado (Lubchenco et al., 1963; Battaglia and Lubchenco, 1967). The Denver standards, however, do not reflect the increase in median birth weights that has occurred over the last three decades or the birth weight standards for babies born at sea level. More contemporary standards are available from large geographic regions, such as the state of California, based on data from more than 2 million singleton births between 1970 and 1976 (Williams et al., 1982); from Canada, based on more than 1 million singleton births and more than 10,000 twin gestations between 1986 and 1988 (Arbuckle et al., 1993); and from 3.8 million births in the United States in 1991 (Alexander et al., 1996). A comparison of the 1991 national data with previous reports (Fig. 28-1) revealed that most of the previous reports underestimated fetal growth beginning at about 32 weeks. Thus, the use of the Colorado or California data bases would result in only 2.8% and 7.1% of births, respectively, being classified as below the 10th percentile compared with the 1991 data. The gender-specific 10th percentile values from 20 to 44 weeks are listed in Table 28-1.

The reliance on only gestational age and birth weight neglects the issue of body size and length and the clinical observations that there are two main clinical types of IUGR infants: (1) the infant who is of normal length for gestational age but whose weight is below normal (asymmetrically small) and (2) the infant whose length and weight are both below normal (symmetrically small).

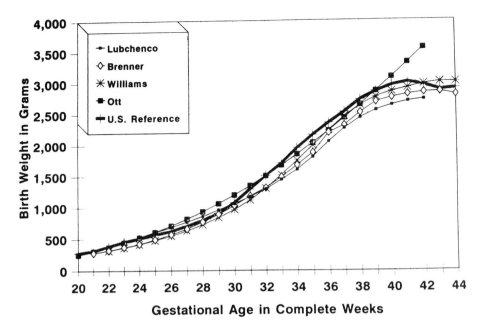

FIGURE 28-1 ■ Fetal weight as a function of gestational age by selected references. (From Alexander GR, Himes JH, Kaufman RB, et al: A United States national reference for fetal growth. Obstet Gynecol **87**:167, 1996. Reprinted with permission from the American College of Obstetricians and Gynecologists.)

One method used to evaluate this issue is the ponderal index (Miller and Hassanein, 1971; Daikoku et al., 1979), which is calculated by the formula:

birth weight (g)/crown-heel length (cm)^3 × 100

Infants with a ponderal index of less than the 10th percentile for gestational age or a crown-rump length less than the

TABLE 28-1. TENTH PERCENTILE OF BIRTH WEIGHT (g) FOR GESTATIONAL AGE BY GENDER: UNITED STATES, 1991, SINGLE LIVE BIRTHS TO RESIDENT MOTHERS

Gestational Age (Wk)	Male	Female
20	270	256
21	328	310
22	388	368
23	446	426
24	504	480
25	570	535
26	644	592
27	728	662
28	828	760
29	956	889
30	1117	1047
31	1308	1234
32	1521	1447
33	1751	1675
34	1985	1901
35	2205	2109
36	2407	2300
37	2596	2484
38	2769	2657
39	2908	2796
40	2986	2872
41	3007	2891
42	2998	2884
43	2977	2868
44	2963	2853

From Alexander GR, Himes JH, Kaufman RB, et al: A United States national reference for fetal growth. Obstet Gynecol **87**:167, 1996.

third percentile are defined as growth restricted. This index in term infants is not affected significantly by differences in race or sex. The disadvantage of this index is the potential error introduced by cubing the length. It is not clear whether asymmetric IUGR and symmetric IUGR are two distinct entities or are merely reflections of the severity of the growth restriction process (excluding chromosomal aberrations and infectious disease).

There is currently no acceptable means, except perhaps by the ponderal index, to classify a newborn whose weight is more than 2500 g as having IUGR. The newborn who weighs 2800 g at birth may be growth restricted if the mother has had three previous infants weighing more than 3700 g, but the classification systems would place such an infant in the normal growth category (Brar and Rutherford, 1988).

Maternal birth weights and birth weights of siblings also have a significant effect on birth weights. Standards for birth weight per gestational age percentiles can differ by more than 1 kg when the siblings' weights are used, and by up to 700 g when the maternal birth weights are utilized (Skjaerven et al., 2000). At present, then, there is no uniform consensus on which growth curve to use. It would appear reasonable to use a standard within a specific geographic area for all racial groups unless standards are also available by race.

RATE OF FETAL GROWTH

Data obtained from study of induced abortions and spontaneous deliveries indicate that the rate of fetal growth increases from 5 g/day at 14–15 weeks of gestation to 10 g/day at 20 weeks, and to 30–35 g/day at 32–34 weeks. Thus, the substrate needs of the fetus are relatively small in the first half of pregnancy, after which the rate of weight gain rises precipitously. The mean rate peaks at approximately 230–285 g/week at 32–34 weeks of gestation, after which it decreases, reaching zero weight gain, or even weight loss, at 41–42 weeks of gestation (Williams et al., 1982; Alexander et al., 1996) (Fig. 28-2). If growth rate is expressed as the percentage of increase in

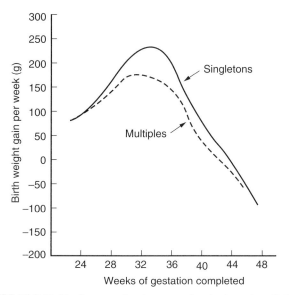

FIGURE 28-2 ■ Median growth rate curves for single and multiple births in California, 1970–1976. (From Williams RL, Creasy RK, Cunningham GC, et al: Fetal growth and perinatal viability in California. Obstet Gynecol **59**:624, 1982. Reprinted with permission from the American College of Obstetricians and Gynecologists.)

weight over the previous week, however, the maximum percentage of increase occurs in the first trimester and decreases steadily thereafter.

INCIDENCE OF INTRAUTERINE GROWTH RESTRICTION

The incidence of IUGR varies according to the population under examination, the geographic location, the standard growth curves used as reference, and the percentile chosen to indicate abnormal growth (i.e., the 3rd, 5th, 10th, or 15th). Traditionally, the 10th percentile is used. Approximately one fourth to one third of all infants weighing less than 2500 g at birth have sustained IUGR, and approximately 4%–8% of all infants born in developed countries and 6%–30% in developing countries are classified as growth restricted (Gruenwald, 1963; Scott and Usher, 1966; Galbraith et al., 1979; Kramer, 1987).

PERINATAL MORTALITY AND MORBIDITY

IUGR is associated with an increase in fetal and neonatal mortality and morbidity rates. Reports in the early 1980s indicated that despite overall advances in the preceding decade in perinatal medicine, the perinatal mortality rate was higher when IUGR was present. Infants weighing between 1500 and 2500 g near term (38–42 weeks) had a perinatal mortality rate 5–30 times that of infants between the 10th and 50th percentiles, and in infants weighing less than 1500 g near term, the perinatal mortality rate was increased 70–100 times (Williams et al., 1982). With birth weights below the 10th percentile, the fetal mortality rate increases as gestation advances

if the birth weight does not increase. For instance, the fetal mortality rate for an infant weighing 1250 g born at 38 weeks is greater than that of an infant of the same weight born at 32 weeks.

In general, fetal mortality rates for IUGR fetuses are 50% again higher than neonatal mortality rates, and male fetuses with IUGR have a higher mortality rate than female fetuses. Perinatal mortality and morbidity in the 1st to 10th percentiles in 1560 SGA fetuses is depicted in Figure 28-3 (Manning, 1995). A relatively marked increase in mortality and morbidity occurred below the 6th percentile, but mortality and morbidity are still elevated at the 10th percentile compared with appropriate-for-gestational-age infants (greater than 10 in Fig. 28-3). An increased odds ratio (1.9) of increased mortality between the 10th and 15th percentiles has also been reported (Seeds and Peng, 1998).

The 10%–30% increase in incidence of minor and major congenital anomalies associated with IUGR accounts for 30%–60% of the IUGR perinatal deaths (50% of stillbirths and 20% of neonatal deaths) (Scott and Usher, 1966; Ounsted et al., 1981). Infants with symmetric IUGR are more likely to die in association with anomalous development or infection. If, however, there is an absence of congenital abnormalities, chromosomal defects, and infection, then neonates with symmetric IUGR are probably not at increased risk of neonatal morbidity (Dashe et al., 2000). The incidence of mortality in the preterm newborn is higher if IUGR is also present (Teberg et al., 1988; Piper, Xenakais, et al., 1996). The incidence of intrapartum fetal distress with IUGR approximates 25%–50% (Low et al., 1972; Lin et al., 1991; Spinillo et al., 1995; Minior and Divon, 1998). SGA neonates with a low ponderal index have a significantly increased risk of numerous neonatal complications compared with SGA neonates who have an adequate ponderal index (Villar et al., 1990). Specific morbidities are discussed later in this chapter and in Chapter 60.

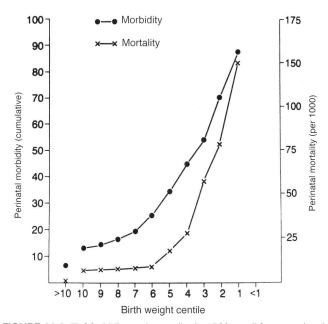

FIGURE 28-3 ■ Morbidity and mortality in 1560 small-for-gestational-age fetuses. (From Manning FA: Intrauterine growth retardation. *In* Fetal Medicine: Principles and Practice. Norwalk, Conn., Appleton & Lange, 1995, p. 312.)

Long-term sequelae of IUGR are discussed in greater detail at the end of this chapter, but lower intelligence quotients, increased mental retardation, and cerebral palsy have been reported (Blair and Stanley, 1990; Goldenberg et al., 1996; Wienerroither et al., 2001).

ETIOLOGY OF INTRAUTERINE GROWTH RESTRICTION

IUGR encompasses many different maternal and fetal entities. Some can be detected prior to birth, whereas others can be found only at autopsy. It is important to discern the cause of IUGR, as many etiologies can recur.

Genetic Factors

There has been much interest in determining the relative contribution of factors that produce birth weight variation, namely the maternal and fetal genetic factors and the environment of the fetus. Approximately 40% of total birth weight variation is due to the genetic contributions from mother and fetus (approximately half from each), and the other 60% is due to contributions from the fetal environment (Penrose and Penrose, 1961; Polani, 1974).

Although both parents' genes affect childhood growth and final adult size, the maternal genes have the main influence on birth weight. The classic horse-pony cross-breeding experiments demonstrated the important role of the mother (Walton and Hammond, 1938). Foals of the maternal horse and paternal pony are significantly larger than foals of the maternal pony and paternal horse, and foals of each cross are comparable in size to foals of the pure maternal breed. These results clearly demonstrate the maternally related constraint on fetal growth.

Similar conclusions are reached from family studies in humans. Low and high birth weights recur in families with seemingly normal pregnancies. Sisters of women with IUGR babies tend to have IUGR babies, a trend that is not seen in their brothers' babies (Johnstone and Inglis, 1974). There is also a greater similarity in birth weights of infants of maternal half siblings and full siblings than of paternal half siblings and full siblings (Morton, 1955). Mothers of IUGR infants frequently were growth restricted at birth themselves (Ounsted and Ounsted, 1966). Although the maternal phenotypic expression may affect fetal growth—particularly maternal height—the evidence for such an influence is not convincing. Social deprivation has also been associated with IUGR, a finding not explained by known physiologic or pathologic factors (Wilcox et al., 1995).

The one definite paternal influence on fetal growth and size at birth is through the contribution of a Y chromosome rather than an X chromosome. The male fetus grows more quickly than the female fetus and weighs approximately 150–200 g more than the female at birth (Karn and Penrose, 1951; Thomson et al., 1968). There is a suggestion that paternal size at birth can influence fetal growth (Klebanoff et al., 1998). Also, the greater the antigenic dissimilarity between parents, the larger the fetus.

Whether it is genetically determined or not, women who were SGA at birth have double the risk of reduced intrauterine growth of their fetuses (Klebanoff et al., 1997). In similar fashion, fetuses destined to deliver preterm have a higher inci-

dence of reduced fetal growth (Bukowski et al., 2001). The role that the genetic constitution of mother or fetus plays in these observations is not clear.

Specific maternal genotypic disorders can cause IUGR, an example of which is phenylketonuria (Saugstad, 1972). Infants born to homozygously affected mothers almost always have IUGR, but whether the reason is an abnormal amount of metabolite crossing from mother to fetus or an inherent problem in the fetus is unknown.

There is a significant association between IUGR and congenital malformations, as will be discussed shortly. Such abnormalities can be due to established chromosomal disorders or to various dysmorphic syndromes, such as various forms of dwarfism. Some of these are the expression of a specific gene abnormality with a known inheritance pattern, whereas others are only presumed to be the result of a gene mutation or an adverse environmental influence.

Birth weights in infants with trisomy 13, 18, and 21 are below normal (Chen et al., 1972; Peuschel et al., 1976), with the decrease in birth weight being less pronounced in trisomy 21. The frequency distribution of birth weights in infants with trisomy 21 is shifted to the left of the normal curve after 34 weeks of gestation, resulting in gestational ages 1–1.5 weeks less than normal, and birth weights and lengths are less than in control infants from 34 weeks until term. This effect is more marked after 37 weeks of gestation, but birth weights are still only approximately 1 standard deviation from mean weight. Birth weights in translocation trisomy 21 are comparable to those in primary trisomy 21. Birth weights of newborns who are mosaic for normal and 21-trisomic cells are lower than normal but higher than those of 21-trisomic infants (Polani, 1974). Although in some reports only 2%–5% of IUGR infants may have a chromosomal abnormality, the incidence rises to 20% if IUGR and mental retardation are both present (Chen et al., 1970; Anderson, 1976; Snijders et al., 1993). Newborns with other autosomal abnormalities, such as deletions (numbers 4, 5, 13, and 18) and ring chromosome structure alterations, also have had impaired fetal growth.

Although abnormalities of the female (X) and male (Y) sex chromosomes are frequently lethal (80%–95% result in first-trimester spontaneous abortions), they could be a cause of IUGR in a newborn (Polani, 1974; Manning, 1995). Infants with XO sex chromosomes have a lower mean birth weight than control infants (~85% of normal for gestational age) and are approximately 1.5 cm shorter at birth. Mosaics of 45,X and 46,XX cells are affected to a lesser degree. Although a paucity of reports prevents definite conclusions, it appears that the repressive effect on fetal growth is increased with the addition of X chromosomes, each of which results in a 200- to 300-g reduction of birth weight (Barlow, 1973).

There are numerous other dysmorphic syndromes—particularly those causing abnormal brain development—with which IUGR is associated (see Chapters 1 and 18).

The overall contribution that chromosomal and other genetic disorders make to human IUGR is estimated to be 5%–20%. Approximately 25% of fetuses with early-onset fetal growth restriction could have chromosomal abnormalities, and karyotyping via cordocentesis can be considered (Weiner and Williamson, 1989) (see Chapter 18). A genetic basis should be considered strongly when IUGR is encountered with associated neurologic impairment (Hill, 1978), or when there is associated early polyhydramnios (Sickler et al., 1997).

Congenital Anomalies

In a study of more than 13,000 anomalous infants, 22% were IUGR (Khoury et al., 1988). Newborns with cardiac malformations are frequently of low birth weight and length for gestation, with the possible exception of those with tetralogy of Fallot and transposition of the great vessels (Richards et al., 1955). The subnormal size of many infants with cardiac anomalies (as low as 50%–80% of normal weight with septal defects) is associated with a subnormal number of parenchymal cells in organs such as the spleen, liver, kidneys, adrenals, and pancreas (Naeye, 1965b). The anencephalic fetus is also usually growth restricted.

Approximately 25% of newborns with a single umbilical artery weigh less than 2500 g at birth, and some of these are born preterm (Froehlich and Fujikura, 1966). Abnormal umbilical cord insertions into the placenta are also occasionally associated with poor fetal growth (Shanklin, 1970; Feldman et al., 2002).

The presence of cord encirclements around the fetal body is also associated with IUGR (Sornes, 1995). Structural malformations, single umbilical artery, and monozygotic twins are relatively rare and probably account for no more than 1%–2% of all human instances of IUGR.

Infection

Infectious disease is known to cause IUGR, but the number of organisms having this effect is poorly defined. There is sufficient evidence for a causal relationship between infectious disease and IUGR for only two viruses—rubella and cytomegalovirus—and there is evidence for a possible relationship with varicella-zoster and human immunodeficiency virus (HIV) (Klein and Remington, 1990) (see Chapters 39 and 40).

With rubella infection, the infected cells usually remain viable for many months. IUGR is thought to arise as a result of capillary endothelial damage during organogenesis, resulting in a decreased number of cells with a cytoplasmic mass that is within normal range (Alford, 1976). In rubella-infected newborns, growth of the adrenals and thymus is particularly limited, and brain growth tends to be more restricted than in IUGR associated with poor uteroplacental perfusion.

Cytomegalovirus infection results in cytolysis and localized necrosis within the fetus. Affected newborns have various organs of subnormal size, owing mainly to a decrease in cell number, unlike newborns with IUGR resulting from maternal vascular disease (Naeye, 1967). The growth rate of various individual fetal organs is altered in an unpredictable fashion by cytomegalovirus.

There are no bacteria known to cause IUGR; however, histologic chorioamnionitis is strongly associated with IUGR. Symmetric IUGR between 28 and 36 weeks, and asymmetric IUGR after 36 weeks of gestation, are strongly associated with evidence of intrauterine infection (Williams et al., 2000).

Protozoan infections resulting from *Toxoplasma gondii*, *Plasmodium sp.*, or *Trypanosoma cruzi* reportedly can cause IUGR (Klein and Remington, 1990).

Although the incidence of maternal infections with various organisms may be as high as 15%, the incidence of congenital infections is estimated to be no more than 5%. It is believed that infectious disease can account for no more than 5%–10% of human IUGR.

Multiple Gestation

Multiple pregnancies are associated with a high progressive decrease in fetal and placental weight as the number of offspring increases in humans and various animal species (Barcroft and Kennedy, 1939; McKeown and Record, 1952) (see also Chapter 29). In both singleton and twin gestations, there is a relationship between total fetal mass and maternal mass. The increase in fetal weight in singleton gestations is linear from approximately 22–24 weeks until approximately 32–36 weeks of gestation (Gruenwald, 1966; Williams et al., 1982; Alexander et al., 1996). During the last weeks of pregnancy, the increase in fetal weight declines, actually becoming negative after 42 weeks in some pregnancies.

If nutrition is adequate in the neonatal period, the slope of the increase in neonatal weight parallels the increase in fetal weight seen before 34–38 weeks. The decline in fetal weight increase occurs when the total fetal mass approximates 3000–3500 g for either singleton or twin gestations. When growth rate is expressed incrementally, the weekly gain in singletons peaks at approximately 230–285 g/week at 32–34 weeks of gestation (see Fig 28-2). In individual twin fetuses, the incremental weekly gain peaks at 160–170 g/week at 28–32 weeks of gestation (Williams et al., 1982).

More recent studies in triplets indicate that growth of individual triplets may continue in a linear fashion well beyond a total combined weight of 3500 g (Jones et al., 1991). Others have reported that before 35 weeks gestation, triplets grow at about the 30th percentile for singletons, and by 38 weeks the average weight of each triplet is at the 10th percentile (Elster et al., 1991).

The decrease in weight of twin fetuses, frequently with mild IUGR, is usually due to decreased cell size; the exception is severe IUGR associated with monozygosity and vascular anastomoses, wherein cell number also may be decreased (Naeye, 1965a; Naeye et al., 1966). These changes in twins are similar to those seen in IUGR secondary to poor uterine perfusion or maternal malnutrition. Twins with mild IUGR have an acceleration of growth after birth, so that their weight equals the median weight of singletons by 1 year of age. This observation supports the thesis that the etiology of poor fetal growth in twin gestations is an inability of the environment to meet fetal needs, rather than an inherent diminished growth capacity of the twin fetus. The example of twin fetuses supports the thesis derived from normal singleton pregnancies that the human fetus seldom is able to express its full potential for growth.

Any one of the components of the environment can limit fetal growth, as will be described next. Twin-to-twin transfusion secondary to vascular anastomoses in monochorionic-monozygotic twins frequently results in IUGR of one twin, usually the donor (see Chapter 29). Maternal complications associated with IUGR occur more frequently in twins; the incidence of anomalies is almost twice that of singletons and monozygosity referred to previously. All such complications increase the probability of delivery of an IUGR fetus. The incidence of IUGR in twins is 15%–25% (Houlton et al., 1981; Secher et al., 1985; Arbuckle et al., 1993), and because the incidence of multiple gestations is less than 1%, these pregnancies probably account for less than 3% of all cases of human IUGR. The actual incidence could be closer to 5% because of the increase in multiple gestations secondary to assisted reproductive techniques.

Inadequate Maternal Nutrition

Numerous animal studies have demonstrated that undernutrition of the mother owing to protein or caloric restriction can affect fetal growth adversely (Dobbing, 1970; Brasel and Winick, 1972). Information from experiments using small animals, in which the fetomaternal mass is much greater than in human pregnancy and the fetal and neonatal growth rate reaches its maximum after birth, must be extrapolated with caution. Such animal studies, however, have engendered important concepts.

Winick (1971) reported three phases of fetal growth: cellular hyperplasia, followed by both hyperplasia and hypertrophy, and then predominantly hypertrophy. Thus, if there is a decrease in available substrate, the timing of the decrease is reflected in the type of IUGR observed. If the insult occurs early in pregnancy, the fetus is likely to be born with a decrease in cell number and cell size (such as might be observed with severe chronic maternal undernutrition or an inability to increase uteroplacental blood flow during gestation) and have symmetric IUGR. If, however, the insult occurs late in gestation, such as with twin gestation, the fetus is likely to have a normal cell number but a restriction of cell size (which can be returned to normal with adequate postnatal nutrition) and have asymmetric IUGR.

The importance of maternal nutrition in fetal growth and birth weight has, unfortunately, been demonstrated by studies in Russia and Holland, where women suffered inadequate nutrition during World War II. The population in Leningrad underwent a prolonged period of poor nutrition, during which both preconceptual nutritional status and gestational nutrition were poor and birth weights were reduced by 400–600 g (Antonov, 1947). In Holland, a 6-month famine created conditions that permitted evaluation of the effect of malnutrition during each of the trimesters of pregnancy in a group of women previously well nourished (Stein and Susser, 1975). Birth weights declined approximately 10%, and placental weights 15%, only when undernutrition occurred in the third trimester with caloric intake below 1500 g. The difference in severity of the IUGR in these two populations suggests the importance of prepregnancy nutritional status, an idea that has been substantiated (Love and Kinch, 1965; Kramer, 1987; Abrams and Newman, 1991). More recent studies show that inadequate weight gain in pregnancy (defined as less than 0.27 kg/week, or less than 10 kg at 40 weeks, or based on suggested weight gain for body mass indices) (see Chapter 11) is associated with an increased risk of IUGR. Weight gain in the second trimester appears to be particularly important (Abrams and Selvin, 1995). Adequate maternal weight gain by 24–28 weeks in multiple pregnancies correlates positively with good fetal growth (Harding, 1999; Luke et al., 2002).

It is still unclear whether generalized calorie intake reduction or specific substrate limitation (such as protein or key mineral restriction) or both is important in producing IUGR (see Chapter 11). Glucose uptake by the fetus is critical, as there is the suggestion that little glucogenesis occurs in the normal fetus. In the IUGR fetus, the maternal-fetal glucose concentration difference is increased as a function of the severity of the IUGR (Marconi et al., 1996). This concentration difference would facilitate glucose transfer across the small placenta. Decreases in zinc content of peripheral blood leukocytes correlate positively with IUGR (Meadows et al., 1981; Wells et al., 1987), and serum zinc concentrations of less than 60 µg/dL in the third trimester are associated with a fivefold increase in low-birth-weight newborns (Neggers et al., 1991). Similarly, an association between low serum folate levels and IUGR has been reported (Goldenberg, Tamura, et al., 1992). Although there is no convincing evidence that high-protein supplementation is beneficial (Stein et al., 1978; Rush et al., 1980), caloric supplementation can improve birth weights by 50–225 g, the largest increase being demonstrated when the net energy increment exceeds 430 kcal/day in an otherwise poorly nourished population (Prentice et al., 1983). Warshaw (1985), however, pointed out that, in a fetus receiving decreased oxygen delivery as a result of decreased uteroplacental perfusion and who has adapted by slowing metabolism and growth, it may not be advisable to increase substrate delivery. This important issue remains unresolved.

Another maternal nutrient that could be important to fetal growth is oxygen, which is probably a primary determinant of fetal growth. IUGR infants have a decrease in the partial pressure of oxygen and oxygen saturation values in the umbilical vein and artery (Lackman et al., 2001). The median birth weight of infants of women living more than 10,000 feet above sea level is approximately 250 g less than that of infants of women living at sea level (Lichty et al., 1957). Pregnancies complicated by maternal cyanotic heart disease usually result in IUGR, but it is unclear whether abnormal maternal hemodynamics or the reduction in oxygen saturation (by approximately 40% in the umbilical vein) accounts for poor fetal growth (Novy et al., 1968). The association between hemoglobinopathies and IUGR could be due to a decrease in either blood viscosity or fetal oxygenation (Pritchard et al., 1973). Patients with chronic pulmonary disease, such as poorly controlled asthma, cystic fibrosis, or bronchiectasis, or those with severe kyphoscoliosis may be at increased risk (Kopenhager, 1977; Palmer et al., 1983; Thaler et al., 1986).

Placental Factors

Although placental size does not necessarily equate with function, our inability to clinically evaluate human placental function properly has resulted in studies of the interrelationships of size, morphometry, and clinical outcome. In general, birth weight increases with increasing placental weight in both animals and humans (Aherne, 1966; Dawes, 1968). IUGR without other anomalies is usually associated with a small placenta. Chromosomally normal IUGR newborns have a 24% smaller placenta per gestational age (Heinonen et al., 2001). A small placenta is not always associated with an IUGR newborn, but the large infant from an otherwise normal pregnancy does not have a small placenta. Placental weight increases throughout normal gestation; in IUGR pregnancy, the placental weight plateaus after 36 weeks or earlier, and the placenta (after being trimmed of the membranes and cord) weighs less than 350 g (Molteni et al., 1978). As normal gestation advances, there is a greater increase in fetal weight than in placental weight. Thus, there is an increase in the fetal-placental weight ratio in large-for-gestational-age (LGA), appropriate-for-gestational-age, and SGA infants in the last half of gestation. In all three categories, when the fetal-placental weight ratio is greater than 10, there is an increased incidence of depressed newborns; this suggests that it is not only the IUGR fetus that can outgrow the capacity of the placenta to bring about adequate transfer of necessary nutrients (Molteni et al., 1978).

The villous surface area and the capillary surface area increase as normal gestation advances (Aherne and Dunnill, 1966). It is not known whether the relative villous surface area available for exchange can keep up with the metabolic needs of the enlarging fetus (Baur, 1977), but because the capillary vessels are closer to the periphery of the villi, the efficiency per unit may improve as gestation progresses (Aherne, 1975). In placentas of IUGR infants, the mean surface area and the capillary surface area are reduced, implying a diminished diffusing capacity (Aherne and Dunnill, 1966). Cytotrophoblastic hyperplasia, thickening of the basement membrane, placental infarction, and chorionic villitis are commonly present in placentas from pregnancies complicated by maternal vascular disease and IUGR (Fox, 1967; Salafia et al., 1992; Salafia et al., 1995). More recently, it has been reported that trophoblastic apoptosis is increased in IUGR, the mechanism being unknown (Ishihara et al., 2002; Levy et al., 2002).

The terminal villi are maldeveloped in IUGR pregnancies when absent end-diastolic flow is demonstrated, indicating that these morphologic changes are associated with increased vascular impedance (Krebs et al., 1996). Absent end-diastolic flow shows more occlusive lesions of the intraplacental vasculature than when end-diastolic flow is present (Salafia et al., 1997).

Information from cordocentesis studies reveals fetal hypoxemia, hypercapnia , acidosis, and hypoglycemia in severe IUGR (Soothill et al., 1986; Soothill et al., 1987). There is also a decrease in α-aminonitrogen, particularly branched-chain amino acids, in plasma of the IUGR fetus (Cetin et al., 1990). Recent work, however, indicates that placental metabolism rather than transport could be the abnormality. Perfused cotyledons of IUGR fetuses have increased oxygen and glucose consumption with increased lactate production (Challis et al., 1998).

Abnormal insertions of the cord, placental hemangiomas, abruptio placenta, and placenta previa are also associated with IUGR (Shanklin, 1970; Ananth and Wilcox, 2001; Ananth et al., 2001).

Maternal Vascular Disease

Substantial evidence from experimental animal studies suggests that alterations in uteroplacental perfusion affect the growth and status of the placenta as well as the fetus. Ligation of the uterine artery of one horn of the pregnant rat results in IUGR of those fetuses nearest the constriction (Wigglesworth, 1964). Fetal and placental weights in guinea pigs, mice, and rabbits are lowest in the middle of each uterine horn, where arterial perfusion is lowest (Dawes, 1968; Duncan, 1969). Repetitive embolization of the uterine vascular bed during the last one fourth of gestation in the sheep gives rise to localized hyalinization and fibrinoid changes in the placenta (Creasy et al., 1972) and results in a 40% reduction in placental weight and alterations in organ growth patterns similar to those observed in IUGR fetuses from pregnancies complicated by maternal hypertensive disease. In addition, umbilical blood flow is reduced, and fetal oxidative metabolism is decreased (Creasy et al., 1972; Clapp et al., 1980, 1981). Doppler umbilical artery flow-velocity wave-form studies also indicate a reduction of umbilical blood flow in human IUGR (Trudinger, 1987) (see Chapter 21).

That uteroplacental blood flow is decreased in pregnancies complicated by maternal hypertensive disease has been strongly suggested by results of various studies. The clearance of radioactive sodium, or xenon, from the intervillous space is reduced in preeclamptic patients (Browne and Veall, 1953; Dixon et al., 1963; Kaar et al., 1980). Dynamic scintigraphic studies also have revealed a decreased blood flow index in IUGR pregnancies (Lunell and Nylund, 1992). As maternal body mass and plasma volume are correlated, reduced plasma volume or prevention of plasma volume expansion could lead to decreased cardiac output and uterine perfusion and a resultant decrease in fetal growth (Daniel et al., 1989; Rosso et al., 1992; Duvekot et al., 1995).

Obstructive arterionecrosis, which can result in local ischemia of villi, is seen frequently in histologic examination of the implantation site in pregnancies complicated by preeclampsia and IUGR (Dixon and Robertson, 1961; Brosens et al., 1977). Similar obstructive lesions are not present in normotensive IUGR pregnancies, although there is frequently a reduction of the normal endovascular migration of trophoblast in such pregnancies, suggesting that even without hypertension, the vascular response at the implantation site is altered in some cases of IUGR (Robertson et al., 1976). There appears to be a continuous adverse relationship between fetal growth and maternal blood pressure (Churchill et al., 1997). Before term, IUGR in normotensive women generally results in higher perinatal mortality than in women with hypertension, but the reverse is true at term (Piper, Langer, et al., 1996).

Uteroplacental flow-velocity wave-form studies, using Doppler methods in pregnancies complicated by hypertension, have shown a higher incidence of IUGR in pregnancies in which abnormal wave-forms were recorded. These are thought to reflect abnormally increased resistance to blood flow (Fleischer et al., 1986; Campbell et al., 1987). High-resistance hypertension is associated with a marked decrease in fetal weight compared with low-resistance hypertension (Easterling et al., 1991). Increasing uteroplacental resistance, recorded with this methodology, has been positively correlated with fetal hypoxemia as determined by cordocentesis in IUGR fetuses (Soothill et al., 1986).

As discussed in Chapter 48, the antiphospholipid syndrome, caused by anticardiolipin and lupus anticoagulant antibodies, is strongly associated with IUGR. The syndrome involves a wide spectrum of disease, including early and late fetal loss, early-onset IUGR, and maternal hypertensive and thromboembolic disease (Lockwood and Rand, 1994).

The inherited thrombophilias—most commonly, the prothrombin gene mutation—have also been associated with IUGR (Kupferminc et al., 2000; Martinelli et al., 2001; von Kries et al., 2001; Alfirevic et al., 2002; Lockwood, 2002). This phenomenon may well be related to the increase in placental vascular thrombosis observed with these inherited disorders (Many et al., 2001). Not all investigators have observed a correlation, however. In a case-control study of 493 IUGR infants compared with 472 controls, Infante-Rivard and colleagues (2002) observed no increases in polymorphisms associated with thrombophilia among the mothers in the IUGR group.

There are only fragmentary suggestions relating abnormal maternal vascular anatomy and IUGR. IUGR may occur at a higher frequency when the pregnancy is in a unicornuate uterus, in which vascular abnormalities are likely but unproven (Andrews and Jones, 1982). Patients with two (rather than the usual one) ascending uterine arteries on each side of the uterus also have a higher rate of IUGR (Burchell et al., 1978). Pregnancy after bilateral ligation of the internal iliac and ovarian arteries, however, is not associated with IUGR (Mengert et al., 1969; Shinagawa et al., 1981).

Because exercise may affect uterine perfusion, this subject has been studied extensively, and the effects have been quite variable (Hall and Kaufman, 1987; Clapp and Capeless, 1990; Clapp et al., 1992). A moderate regimen of weight-bearing exercise in early pregnancy probably enhances fetal growth (Clapp et al., 2000). If there is an adverse effect, it appears to occur at high levels of exercise (greater than 50% of prepregnancy levels) in mid and late pregnancy and results mainly in a symmetrical reduction in fetal growth and neonatal fat mass (Clapp et al., 2002).

Recurrent antepartum hemorrhage from either premature separation of the placenta or placenta previa is associated with an increased incidence of IUGR (Hibbard and Jeffcoate, 1966; Varma, 1973) (see Chapter 37).

Clinical maternal vascular disease and the presumed decrease in uteroplacental perfusion can account for at least 25%–30% of IUGR infants. Undiagnosed decreased perfusion could also be the cause of IUGR in an otherwise normal pregnancy, such as with recurrent idiopathic fetal growth restriction. A previous low-birth-weight infant is significantly associated with a subsequent birth of decreased weight, decreased ponderal index, and decreased head circumference (Goldenberg, Hoffman, et al., 1992). This finding of symmetric growth restriction is in contrast to the asymmetric IUGR usually seen with maternal vascular disease.

Low-dose aspirin therapy directed against vascular disease has been used with conflicting results to prevent recurrent idiopathic IUGR (Wallenberg and Rotmans, 1987) and to improve fetal weight in patients with abnormal umbilical artery wave-forms (Trudinger et al., 1988). A meta-analysis of trials of low-dose aspirin for the prevention, rather than the treatment, of IUGR, particularly if treatment was begun before 17 weeks, decreased IUGR by 18% (Leitich et al., 1997). Two major prospective investigations using aspirin (low dose), however, did not confirm the beneficial effect of aspirin (Sibai et al., 1993; CLASP, 1994).

Vascular disease becomes more prevalent with advancing age. In one recent large study, controlled for confounding variables, the incidence of SGA births was increased more in nulliparous patients than in multiparous patients older than 30 years of age (Cnattingius et al., 1993).

Environmental Toxins

Maternal cigarette smoking decreases birth weight by approximately 135 to 300 g; the fetus is symmetrically smaller (Miller and Hassanein, 1974; Haworth et al., 1980; Wen et al., 1990; Cliver et al., 1995). If smoking is stopped before the third trimester, its adverse effect on birth weight is reduced (Rantakallo, 1978; Cliver et al., 1995). More disturbing is the recent report indicating a dose-response relationship between maternal smoking and both a head circumference below 32 cm and a value more than 2 standard deviations below that expected for gestational age (Kallen, 2000). The reason why not all women who smoke have IUGR infants could be due to maternal genetic susceptibility (Wang et al., 2002).

The mechanism by which cigarette smoking decreases fetal growth is not well established, but most interest centers on the increased carboxyhemoglobin concentrations in maternal and fetal blood and relative fetal hypoxemia (Longo, 1977). Erythropoietin, stimulated by hypoxia, is doubled in umbilical cord plasma with maternal smoking (Jasayeri et al., 1998). A reduction in exhaled carbon monoxide is associated with a decreased adverse effect on fetal weight (Secker-Walker et al., 1997).

Reduction in birth weight is also affected by maternal alcohol ingestion of one to two drinks per day (Mills et al., 1984). Cocaine use in pregnancy decreases birth weight, but the reduction of head circumference is more pronounced than the reduction in birth weight, which is similar to that caused by maternal alcohol ingestion (Little and Snell, 1991). Prolonged use of other drugs, such as steroids, phenytoin, warfarin, and heroin, has been implicated in IUGR (see Chapter 19).

Maternal and Fetal Hormones

In general, there is limited transfer of the various circulating maternal hormones into the fetal compartments (see Chapters 49–51).

Although the effects of hypothyroidism or hyperthyroidism on fetal size are not striking, studies in the subhuman primate indicate that when the mother and fetus are athyroid, there is retarded osseous development and reduced protein synthesis in the fetal brain (Holt et al., 1973; Thorburn, 1974).

Maternal diabetes without vascular disease is frequently associated with excessive fetal size (see Chapter 49). Although insulin does not cross the placenta, fetal hyperinsulinemia as well as hyperplasia of the pancreatic islet cells is seen frequently with maternal diabetes. These changes are thought to occur as a result of maternal hyperglycemia, which leads to fetal hyperglycemia and an increased response of the fetal pancreas.

Fetal hypoinsulinemia produced experimentally in the rhesus monkey results in IUGR (Hill et al., 1972), and infants have been born, although rarely, with severe IUGR and requiring insulin treatment at birth, suggesting hypoinsulinemia *in utero* (Liggins, 1974; Sherwood et al., 1974). If nutrient transfer becomes limited owing to placental disease secondary to maternal vascular disease, the fetus of the diabetic mother can sustain IUGR.

Even though human growth hormone is present early in gestation, there is minimal evidence that it regulates fetal weight, although a deficiency could retard skeletal growth (Liggins, 1974). Convincing evidence is also lacking that adrenal hormones have a role in producing IUGR in humans.

Several small polypeptides with *in vitro* growth-promoting activity have been purified. There is a correlation between birth weight and cord blood levels of insulin-like growth factor-I (IGF-I) but not IGF-II (Gluckman et al., 1983; Ashton et al., 1985; Bernstein et al., 1997). Concentrations of the maternal serum placenta growth factor are significantly increased in the first trimester in pregnancies resulting in IUGR (Ong et al., 2001). The exact role of these peptides as fetal growth factors and their relationship to IUGR are currently not understood.

Leptin (from Greek *leptos*: thin) is a polypeptide hormone discovered in 1994. It has been shown to moderate feeding behavior and adipose stores. It is produced predominantly by adipocytes but can also be produced by the placenta as neonatal levels fall dramatically after birth. Fetal plasma concentrations of leptin (but not maternal concentrations) correlate with fetal weight (Tamura et al., 1998). Reported concentrations in IUGR have varied, and the exact role that this interesting hormone plays in fetal growth remains to be clarified (for recent reviews, see Henson and Castracane, 2000; Sabogal and Munoz, 2001).

DIAGNOSIS OF INTRAUTERINE GROWTH RESTRICTION

Determination of Cause

An attempt should be made to determine the cause of fetal aberrant growth before delivery in order to provide appropriate counseling, perform ultrasonographic evaluation for both growth and delineation of anatomy, and obtain neonatal consultation.

Frequently, the cause is readily apparent. Among patients with significant chronic hypertensive disease, those who take prescribed medications known to be associated with prenatal growth deficiency, and those fetuses with congenital or chromosomal abnormalities, the diagnosis is easily established, and management plans can be made. At times, however, the causal factors can be more elusive. For example, growth restriction associated with preeclampsia may antedate the appearance of hypertension and/or proteinuria by several weeks. In many instances, a careful history, maternal examination, and ultrasound evaluation reveal the etiology.

History and Physical Examination

Clinical diagnosis of IUGR by physical examination alone is inaccurate; frequently, the diagnosis is not made until after delivery. Most clinical studies demonstrate that using physical examination alone, the diagnosis of IUGR is missed or incorrectly made almost half the time (Campbell and Thomas, 1977; Cnattingius et al., 1984).

Techniques such as tape measurement of the uterine fundus are helpful in documenting continued growth if performed repeatedly by the same observer, but they are not sensitive enough for accurate detection of most infants with IUGR (Beazley and Underhill, 1970). Experienced obstetricians attempting to estimate fetal size are accurate to within 450 g in 80% of cases, but their accuracy drops to only 40% for infants weighing less than 2270 g (Loeffler, 1967).

Despite the inaccuracy of such indicators, fetal assessment and specific aspects of the patient's risk factors increase the clinician's index of suspicion about suboptimal fetal growth, without which more definitive laboratory investigation might not be considered. As discussed earlier, maternal disease entities such as hypertension (in particular, severe preeclampsia and chronic hypertension with superimposed preeclampsia), chronic antepartum hemorrhage, uncorrected cyanotic congenital heart disease, and insulin-dependent diabetes with vascular disease carry a high incidence of IUGR. The diagnosis of

a multiple gestation suggests the likelihood of diminished fetal growth relative to gestational age, as well as preterm birth. Additional maternal risk factors include documented rubella and cytomegalovirus infections, heavy smoking, heroin and cocaine addiction, alcoholism, and poor nutritional status both before conception and during pregnancy combined with inadequate weight gain during pregnancy.

The obstetric history is also pertinent, inasmuch as correlation between weights of siblings is high (Billewicz and Thomson, 1973). The history can be significant if one considers a hypothetical situation in which a third-born infant weighs 2800 g and the two preceding siblings had birth weights exceeding 3700 g. Although the youngest may not meet strict weight criteria for the diagnosis of IUGR, it is likely that fetal growth did not reach full potential.

Ultrasonography

Currently, ultrasonographic evaluation of the fetus is the preferred and accepted modality for the diagnosis of inadequate fetal growth. It offers the advantages of reasonably precise estimations of fetal weight, determination of interval fetal growth, and measurement of several fetal dimensions to describe the pattern of growth abnormality. Use of these ultrasound measurements requires accurate knowledge of gestational age. Accordingly, if a patient is known to be at risk for a fetal growth abnormality, the crown-to-rump length should be determined during the first trimester. The application of ultrasound technology to fetal growth is reviewed extensively in Chapter 20, and only a few additional comments are made here.

Measurement of the biparietal diameter, the head and abdominal circumferences, and femur length allows the clinician to use accepted formulas to estimate fetal weight and to determine whether a fetal growth aberration represents an asymmetric, symmetric, or mixed pattern (Hadlock et al., 1984) (Fig. 28-4). As discussed previously, intrinsic fetal insults occurring early in pregnancy—for example, infection, exposure to certain drugs or other chemical agents, chromosomal abnormalities, and other congenital malformations—are likely to affect fetal growth at a time of development when cell division is the predominant mechanism of growth. Consequently, musculoskeletal dimensions and organ size may be adversely affected, and symmetric growth restriction is observed. Given this set of circumstances, one might expect to find that femur length and head circumference are low for a given gestational age, as are abdominal circumference and overall fetal weight, all of which are characterized as symmetric IUGR.

At the other end of the spectrum, an extrinsic insult occurring later in pregnancy, usually characterized by inadequate fetal nutrition, is more likely to result in asymmetric growth restriction. In this type, femur length and head circumference are spared, but abdominal circumference is decreased because of subnormal liver growth, and there is a paucity of subcutaneous fat. The most common disorders that limit fetal substrates for metabolism are the hypertensive complications of pregnancy, which are associated with decreased uteroplacental perfusion, and placental infarcts, which limit trophoblastic surface area for substrate transfer. In fact, a falloff in the interval growth of the abdominal circumference is one of the earliest findings in extrinsic or asymmetric IUGR; conversely,

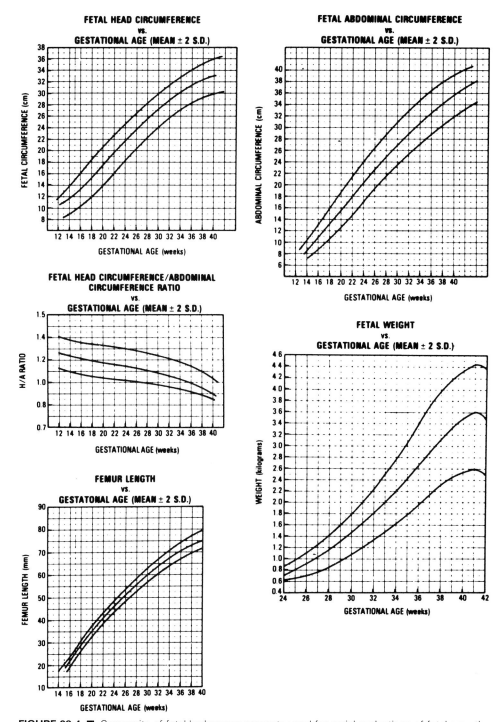

FIGURE 28-4 ■ Composite of fetal body measurements used for serial evaluations of fetal growth.

the finding of an abdominal circumference in the normal range for gestational age markedly decreases the likelihood.

Frequently, these patterns of growth abnormality merge, particularly after long-standing fetal nutritional deprivation. An example of this mixed pattern is seen in Figure 28-5, which demonstrates fetal growth in a patient with severe ulcerative colitis, in whom uteroplacental blood flow and placental function were presumably normal, but maternal caloric intake was profoundly decreased, resulting in suboptimal substrate availability.

Recently, considerable attention has been directed at the ultrasound assessment of uterine artery flow dynamics to predict the risk of IUGR. Utilizing transvaginal color Doppler at 23 weeks' gestation, Papageorghiou and colleagues (2001) observed that increases in uterine artery pulsatility index and "notching" were highly associated with subsequent devel-

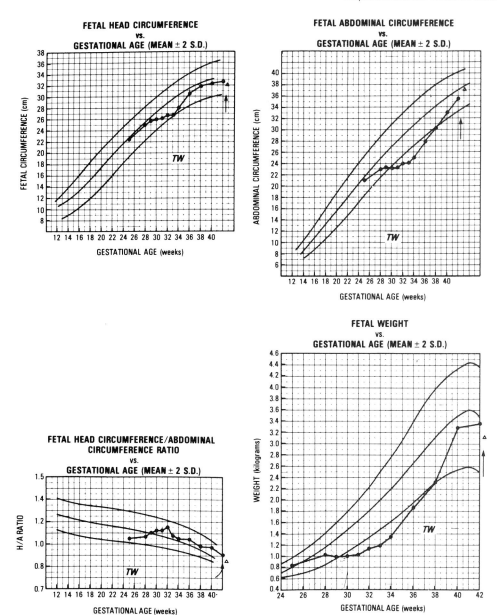

FIGURE 28-5 ■ Serial fetal body measurements in a mother with severe ulcerative colitis. Fetal growth begins to decrease markedly in midgestation but returns to normal after the initiation of central hyperalimentation at approximately 28 to 30 weeks.

opment of IUGR. The eventual role that uterine artery Doppler will play in the prediction of IUGR awaits more extensive testing.

MANAGEMENT OF PREGNANCY

Antepartum Fetal Testing

At present, when a pregnancy is complicated by abnormal fetal growth, most perinatal centers use the biophysical profile (BPP) or umbilical flow velocimetry (usually in combination) to evaluate fetal condition. These diagnostic modalities are covered in Chapter 21, but additional comment is pertinent here and worthy of reemphasis.

Biophysical Profile

The biophysical profile is appealing, inasmuch as it provides a multidimensional survey of fetal physiologic parameters. In particular, amniotic fluid volume (AFV) assessment is an important aspect of the profile because oligohydramnios is a frequent finding in the IUGR pregnancy. This is presumably due to diminished fetal blood volume, renal blood flow, and urinary output. Human fetal urinary production rates can be measured with considerable accuracy (Rabinowitz et al., 1989), and three separate studies have shown decreased urinary production rates in the presence of fetal growth restriction (Wladimiroff and Campbell, 1974; Kurjak et al., 1981; Nicolaides et al., 1990).

The significance of amniotic fluid volume with respect to fetal outcome has been well documented. Manning and coworkers (1981) reported the diagnostic value of amniotic fluid volume measurement in discriminating normal from aberrant fetal growth. Among 91 patients with normal amniotic fluid volume, 86 delivered infants whose birth weights were appropriate for gestational age. In contrast, 26 of 29 patients with decreased amniotic fluid volume delivered growth-restricted infants. The outcome of pregnancies with severe oligohydramnios is associated with a high risk of fetal compromise (Chamberlain et al., 1984; Bastide et al., 1986).

It is likely that the chronic hypoxic state frequently observed in the IUGR fetus is responsible for diverting blood flow from the kidney to other organs that are more critical during fetal life (see Chapters 13 and 15). Nicolaides and associates (1990) have observed reduced fetal urinary flow rates in the IUGR fetus, and the degree of reduction is well correlated with the degree of fetal hypoxemia as reflected by fetal blood PO$_2$ measured after cordocentesis.

The value of the biophysical profiles has been validated by several reports. In a study of 19,221 high-risk pregnancies, Manning and colleagues (1987) observed that the fetal death rate following a normal biophysical profile (score of 8 or higher) was 0.726 in 1000 births; only 14 fetuses died. Of the total patient population, approximately 4380 were pregnancies complicated by IUGR, and only four died following a normal test, yielding a false-negative test rate of less than 1 in 1000. In a subsequent analysis of perinatal morbidity and mortality among patients followed with the biophysical profile, a highly significant inverse correlation was observed for IUGR and last test score. When the last test score was 8 or higher, only 3.4% of 6500 high-risk patients had infants with IUGR. Conversely, when the last test score was 4 or 2, the incidence of IUGR increased to 29% and 41%, respectively (Manning et al., 1990).

Doppler Ultrasound Assessment of Fetal Blood Flow

ARTERIAL CIRCULATION

There has been great interest during the last few years in the roles of uterine and fetal vascular blood flow velocities to predict and evaluate fetal growth restriction as well as other fetal complications (see Chapter 21). As noted earlier in this chapter, there is considerable interest in evaluating the uterine circulation with color Doppler to predict the risk of IUGR (Papageorghiou et al., 2001). The utility of such measurements needs further evaluation.

In contrast, umbilical arterial velocimetry is of considerable value in predicting perinatal outcome in the IUGR fetus. A substantial pathologic correlation helps explain the increased vascular resistance in IUGR fetuses. Specifically, fetuses demonstrating an absence of end-diastolic flow exhibit maldevelopment of the placental terminal villous tree (Krebs et al., 1996). The correlation between placental pathology, abnormal umbilical artery velocimetry, and IUGR has been reviewed by Kingdom and coworkers (1997).

Several randomized controlled trials have been reported which, taken together, demonstrate a decrease in perinatal deaths when umbilical arterial velocimetry has been used in conjunction with other types of antenatal testing (Almstrom et al., 1992; Omtzigt et al., 1994; Pattison et al., 1994). A subsequent meta-analysis of 12 randomized controlled trials showed that clinical action guided by umbilical Doppler velocimetry reduces the odds of perinatal death by 38% (Alfirevic

and Neilson, 1995). Although the authors hypothesize that this beneficial effect depended on the incidence of absent end-diastolic velocity rather than simply decreased flow, the number of studies with sufficient data was inadequate to draw this conclusion. Thus, umbilical artery velocimetry now plays a significant role in the management of the growth-restricted fetus. Normal velocimetry in the suspect small fetus is usually indicative of a constitutionally small, otherwise normal baby (Ott, 2000). At the other end of the spectrum, the absence or reversal of end-diastolic flow is indicative of significant increases in perinatal morbidity and mortality and long-term poor neurologic outcome compared with those fetuses with continuing diastolic flow (Karsdorp et al., 1994; Valcamonico et al., 1994). The association of fetal hypoxia and acidosis, as measured by blood obtained at cordocentesis, is also clearly demonstrated (Nicolaides et al., 1988). This study reported that 88% of fetuses with absence of diastolic flow were hypoxic and acidotic. The relationship between umbilical cord blood gases in those fetuses with diminished but continuing diastolic flow, however, has not been consistent among studies. Furthermore, markedly abnormal or absent end-diastolic flow can be observed at very premature gestational ages, well before the biophysical profile demonstrates abnormalities. Consequently, abnormal umbilical velocimetry should be interpreted in conjunction with other tests of fetal well-being and in the context of the gestational age and fetal lung maturity, in order to determine fetal condition and delivery timing (Divon, 1996; ACOG Practice Bulletin, 1999).

There also has been interest in evaluation of middle cerebral artery flow, inasmuch as the normal adaptive response to hypoxia within the fetus is to increase cerebral blood flow. However, it is unclear from at least one randomized trial whether such measurements add additional benefit in making management decisions (Ott et al., 1998).

VENOUS CIRCULATION

In contrast to abnormalities in arterial circulation, abnormalities observed in the venous circulation presumably reflect central cardiac failure, and current studies suggest that specific aberrations of flow through the ductus venous, pulmonary, and umbilical veins could be indicative of imminent fetal demise. The temporal sequence of abnormalities in flow in the peripheral and central circulations of the IUGR fetus as measured by Doppler have recently been described (Ferrazzi et al., 2002). The severely IUGR fetus first demonstrates "early" changes in the umbilical and middle cerebral arteries. "Late" changes include reversal of flow through the umbilical artery as well as changes in the ductus venosus, aorta, and pulmonary outflow tracts. These changes and their pathophysiology have also been summarized in detail by Baschat and Harman (2001).

Cordocentesis

Fetal blood gases and other metabolic parameters measured from umbilical blood samples obtained by cordocentesis have also been used to aid in determining fetal condition in the growth-restricted fetus (see Chapter 23). Normative values have been reported at various gestational ages, and it is clear that, compared with the appropriate-for-gestational-age fetus, the SGA fetus is more frequently hypoxemic, hypercapneic, hyperlacticacidemic, and acidotic (Pardi et al., 1987; Nicolaides et al., 1988, 1989; Marconi et al., 1990). Furthermore, abnormal fetal heart rate patterns are more commonly observed when fetal hypoxemia or acidosis is present (Visser et al., 1990). Among 32 fetuses with absent umbilical end-diastolic flow, however, umbilical blood gas determinations did not discriminate between fetuses that would survive and those that would die (Nicolini et al., 1990). The use of antenatal umbilical blood pH and gas measurements is not required for most clinical situations involving the IUGR fetus.

Antepartum Therapy

Maternal hyperoxia has been shown to increase umbilical PO_2 and pH in the hypoxemic, acidotic, growth-restricted fetus (Nicolaides et al., 1987). Among surviving fetuses, there was also an improvement in mean velocity of blood flow through the thoracic aorta. In support of these findings, Battaglia and coworkers (1992) treated 17 of 36 women whose pregnancies were complicated by IUGR with maternal hyperoxia and confirmed improvement in both blood gases and Doppler flow. They also observed a significant improvement in perinatal mortality in the oxygen-treated patients. Evidence is inconclusive, however, regarding whether maternal oxygen therapy is of value, and any differences reported in outcome could be due to more advanced gestational age in oxygen-tested groups (Gulmezoglu and Hofmeyer, 2000).

The role of low-dose aspirin remains controversial. One meta-analysis, which included 13,234 women from 13 randomized studies, showed a significant reduction in the frequency of IUGR in women treated with aspirin before IUGR or preeclampsia was diagnosed (odds ratio, 0.43) (Leitich et al., 1997). The authors cautioned, however, that their data did not include a large RCT from Brazil, which had not yet been published. Subsequently, the Brazilian report, which evaluated

the pregnancy effects of low-dose aspirin, found no ameliorating effect on IUGR (ECPPA Collaborative Group, 1996).

Timing of Delivery

The prohibitive perinatal morbidity and mortality rates among IUGR infants have been discussed previously. Controversy continues with regard to the timing of delivery for such infants to ensure that intrauterine demise does not occur because of chronic oxygen deprivation. This problem is underscored by the fact that if deaths among congenitally infected and anomalous infants are excluded, the perinatal risk is still higher for growth-restricted infants than for appropriate-for-gestational-age newborns. Although opinions vary as to the role of preterm versus term delivery of the SGA infant, it is generally prudent to deliver the growth-restricted infant before term in the presence of maternal hypertensive disease, as soon as fetal lung maturity has been achieved, or if there is absence or reversal of the end-diastolic flow velocity of the umbilical artery wave-form.

The overall findings and guidelines for evaluation of the IUGR fetus are summarized in Table 28-2.

Intrapartum Management

That the growth-restricted infant is at risk of intrapartum asphyxia has been well documented by the second British Perinatal Mortality Survey, which demonstrated a fivefold increase in the intrapartum stillbirth rate of SGA infants compared with the rate in normally grown infants at a comparable gestational age (Butler and Alberman, 1969). It has long been recognized that lower Apgar scores and meconium aspiration, as well as other manifestations of poor oxygenation

TABLE 28-2. EVALUATION AND MANAGEMENT OF THE IUGR FETUS

	Constitutionally Small Fetus	Fetus with Structural and/or Chromosome Abnormality: Fetal Infection	Substrate Deprivation: Uteroplacental Insufficiency
Growth rate and pattern	Usually below but parallel to normal; symmetric	Markedly below normal: symmetric	Variable: usually asymmetric
Anatomy	Normal	Usually abnormal	Normal
Amniotic fluid volume	Normal	Normal or hydramnios: decreased in the presence of renal agenesis or urethral obstruction	Low
Additional evaluation	None	Karyotype; specific testing for viral DNA in amniotic fluid as indicated	Fetal lung maturity testing as indicated
Additional laboratory evaluation of fetal well-being	Normal BPP/UAV	BPP variable; normal UAV	BPP score decreases; UAV evidence of vascular resistance
Continued surveillance and timing of delivery	None: anticipate term delivery	Dependent upon etiology	BPP and UAV: delivery timing requires balance of gestational age and BPP/UAV findings: fetal lung maturity testing often helpful

BPP, biophysical profile; IUGR, intrauterine growth restriction; UAV, umbilical artery velocimetry.
From Resnik R: Intrauterine growth restriction. Obstet Gynecol **99**:490, 2002.

during labor, occur with greater frequency among IUGR infants. The problem of intrapartum asphyxia has been further elucidated by studies demonstrating the acid-base status of growth-restricted infants at the time of delivery. If moderate-to-severe metabolic acidosis is defined as an umbilical artery buffer base value of less than 37 mEq/L (normal = greater than 40 mEq/L), almost 50% of IUGR neonates show signs of acidosis at the time of delivery (Low et al., 1972). These findings document the problems of oxygenation during labor in such infants and emphasize that intensive fetal observation is required during this critical period.

Consequently, cesarean delivery should be considered seriously if there is evidence of deteriorating fetal status or an unripe cervix, or if there is any indication of additional fetal compromise during labor.

NEONATAL COMPLICATIONS AND LONG-TERM SEQUELAE

The growth-restricted fetus can experience numerous complications in the neonatal period related to the etiology of the growth insult as well as antepartum and intrapartum factors. These include neonatal asphyxia, meconium aspiration, hypoglycemia and other metabolic abnormalities, and polycythemia (see Chapter 60). Data by Low and colleagues (1992) show that fetal growth restriction has a deleterious effect on cognitive function, independent of other variables. With the use of numerous standardized tests to evaluate learning ability and by excluding those children with genetic or major organ system malformations, almost 50% (37 of 77) of SGA children had learning deficits at ages 9–11 years.

Blair and Stanley (1990) also reported a strong association between IUGR and spastic cerebral palsy in newborns born after 33 weeks. This association was highest in IUGR infants who were short, thin, and of small head size (Blair and Stanley, 1992). Newborns at or above the 10th percentile for weight but with abnormal ponderal indices were also at risk for spastic cerebral palsy. Other researchers (Paz et al., 2001; McCowan et al., 2002) have not found a marked increase in long-term neurological deficiencies to be associated with IUGR.

There is increasing evidence to suggest an association between IUGR and adult disease: the so-called "fetal origins of disease" hypothesis. Publication of the epidemiologic studies of Barker's group indicate that IUGR is a significant risk factor for the subsequent development of chronic hypertension, ischemic heart disease, type II diabetes, and obstructive lung disease (Barker and Robinson, 1992). In a recent study of individuals conceived during the Dutch famine in late World War II, there was an increased risk of developing heart disease in midlife if the pregnancy was in the first trimester during the famine, but not if it was in the second or third trimesters (Roseboom et al., 2000). They also suggest that the phenomenon of programming may be operable and that an adverse fetal environment during a critical period of fetal growth helps to promote these adult diseases.

More recently, Veening and associates (2002) demonstrated decreased insulin sensitivity among 9-year-old children who had been SGA at birth, compared with control appropriate-for-gestational-age children, particularly among those with catch-up growth and a high body mass index.

Maternal and fetal malnutrition seem to have both short- and long-term effects. The concept of programming during intrauterine life, however, needs to include a host of other factors such as genotype of both mother and her fetus, maternal size and obstetrical history, and postnatal and lifestyle factors.

REFERENCES

Abrams B, Newman V: Small-for-gestational-age birth: Maternal predictors and comparison with risk factors of spontaneous preterm delivery in the same cohort. Am J Obstet Gynecol **164:**785, 1991.

Abrams B, Selvin S: Maternal weight gain pattern and birth weight. Obstet Gynecol **86:**163, 1995.

Aherne W: A weight relationship between the human fetus and placenta. Biol Neonate **10:**113, 1966.

Aherne W: Morphometry. In Gruenwald P (ed): The Placenta and Its Maternal Supply Line. Baltimore, Md, University Park Press, 1975.

Aherne W, Dunnill MS: Quantitative aspects of placental structure. J Pathol Bacteriol **91:**123, 1966.

Alexander GR, Himes JH, Kaufman RB, et al: A United States national reference for fetal growth. Obstet Gynecol **87:**163, 1996.

Alfirevic Z, Neilson JP: Doppler ultrasonography in high-risk pregnancies: Systematic review with a meta-analysis. Am J Obstet Gynecol **172:**1379, 1995.

Alfirevic Z, Roberts D, Martlew V: How strong is the association between maternal thrombophilia and adverse pregnancy outcome? A systematic review. Eur J Obstet Gynecol Reprod Biol **101(1):**6, 2002.

Alford CA Jr: Rubella. In Remington JS, Klein JO (eds): Infectious Diseases of the Fetus and Newborn Infant. Philadelphia, WB Saunders, 1976.

Almstrom H, Axelsson O, Cnattingius S, et al: Comparison of umbilical artery velocimetry and cardiotacography for surveillance of small-for-gestational-age fetuses: A multicenter randomized controlled trial. Lancet **340:**936, 1992.

American College of Obstetricians and Gynecologists (ACOG) Practice Bulletin: Antepartum Fetal Surveillance 9:Oct 1999.

Ananth CV, Demissie K, Smulian JC, et al: Relationship among placenta previa, fetal growth restriction and preterm delivery: A population based study. Obstet Gynecol **98:**299, 2001.

Ananth CV, Wilcox AJ: Placental abruption and perinatal mortality in the United States. Am J Epidemiol **153:**332, 2001.

Anderson NG: A five-year study of small for dates infants for chromosomal abnormalities. Aust Paediatr J **12:**19, 1976.

Andrews MC, Jones HW Jr: Impaired reproductive performance of the unicornuate uterus: Intrauterine growth retardation, infertility, and recurrent abortion in five cases. Am J Obstet Gynecol **144:**173, 1982.

Antonov AN: Children born during siege of Leningrad in 1942. J Pediatr **30:**250, 1947.

Arbuckle TE, Wilkins R, Sherman GJ: Birth weight percentiles by gestational age in Canada. Obstet Gynecol **81:**39, 1993.

Ashton IK, Zapf J, Einschenk I, et al: Insulin-like growth factors (IGF) I and II in human foetal plasma and relationships to gestational age and fetal size during mid pregnancy. Acta Endocrinol **10:**558, 1985.

Barcroft J, Kennedy JA: The distribution of blood between the fetus and placenta in sheep. J Physiol **95:**173, 1939.

Barker DJP, Robinson RJ (eds): Fetal and Infant Origins of Adult Disease. London, British Medical Journal, 1992.

Barlow P: The influence of inactive chromosomes on human development: Anomalous sex chromosome complements and the phenotype. Hum Genet **17:**105, 1973.

Baschat AA, Harman CR: Antenatal assessment of the growth restricted fetus. Current Opinion. Obstet Gynecol **13:**161, 2001.

Bastide A, Manning FA, Harman C, et al: Ultrasound evaluation of amniotic fluid: Outcome of pregnancies with severe oligohydramnios. Am J Obstet Gynecol **154:**895, 1986.

Battaglia FC: Intrauterine growth retardation. Am J Obstet Gynecol **106:**1103, 1970.

Battaglia C, Artini PG, d'Ambrogio G, et al: Maternal hyperoxygenation in the treatment of intrauterine growth retardation. Am J Obstet Gynecol **167:**430, 1992.

Battaglia FC, Lubchenco LO: A practical classification of newborn infants by weight and gestational age. J Pediatr **71:**159, 1967.

Baur R: Morphometry of the placental exchange area. Adv Anat Embryol Cell Biol **53:**3, 1977.

Beazley JA, Underhill RA: Fallacy of the fundal height. Br J Med **4:**404, 1970.

Bernstein IM, Goran MI, Copeland KC: Maternal insulin sensitivity and cord blood peptides: Relationships to neonatal size at birth. Obstet Gynecol **90:**780, 1997.

Billewicz WZ, Thomson AM: Birth weights in consecutive pregnancies. Br J Obstet Gynaecol **80:**491, 1973.

Blair E, Stanley F: Intrauterine growth and spastic cerebral palsy. I. Association with birth weight for gestational age. Am J Obstet Gynecol **162:**229, 1990.

Blair E, Stanley F: Intrauterine growth and spastic cerebral palsy. II. The association with morphology at birth. Early Hum Dev **28:**91, 1992.

Brar HS, Rutherford SP: Classification of intrauterine growth retardation. Semin Perinatol **12:**2, 1988.

Brasel JA, Winick M: Maternal nutrition and prenatal growth: Experimental studies of effects of maternal undernutrition on fetal and placental growth. Arch Dis Child **47:**479, 1972.

Brosens I, Dixon HG, Robertson WB: Fetal growth retardation and the arteries of the placental bed. Br J Obstet Gynaecol **84:**656, 1977.

Browne JCM, Veall N: The maternal placental blood flow in normotensive and hypertensive women. J Obstet Gynaecol Br Emp **60:**141, 1953.

Bukowski R, Gahn D, Denning J, et al: Impairment of growth in fetuses destined to deliver preterm. Am J Obstet Gynecol **185:**463, 2001.

Burchell RC, Creed F, Rasoulpour M, et al: Vascular anatomy of the human uterus and pregnancy wastage. Br J Obstet Gynaecol **85:**698, 1978.

Butler NR, Alberman ED: In Butler NR (ed): Perinatal Problems: The Second Report of the British Perinatal Mortality Survey. Edinburgh, Churchill Livingstone, 1969.

Campbell S, Bewley S, Cohen-Overbeek T: Investigation of the uteroplacental circulation by Doppler ultrasound. Semin Perinatol **11:**362, 1987.

Campbell S, Thomas A: Ultrasound measurement of the fetal head to abdominal circumference ratio in the assessment of growth retardation. Br J Obstet Gynaecol **84:**165, 1977.

Cetin I, Corbetta C, Sereni LP, et al: Umbilical amino acid concentrations in normal and growth-retarded fetuses sampled in utero by cordocentesis. Am J Obstet Gynecol **162:**253, 1990.

Challis DE, Ritchie JWK, Tesoro AM, et al: Metabolism not transport is abnormal in perfused placental cotyledons of IUGR fetuses. Part 2 (Abstract No. 15). Am J Obstet Gynecol **178:**S7, 1998.

Chamberlain PF, Manning FA, Morrison I, et al: Ultrasound evaluation of amniotic fluid: I. The relationship of marginal and decreased amniotic fluid volume to perinatal outcome. Am J Obstet Gynecol **150:**245, 1984.

Chen ATL, Chan Y-K, Falek A: The effects of chromosome abnormalities on birth weight in man: II. Autosomal defects. Hum Hered **22:**209, 1972.

Chen ATL, Sergovich FR, McKim JS, et al: Chromosome studies on full term, low birth weight mentally retarded patients. J Pediatr **76:**393, 1970.

Churchill D, Perry IJ, Beevers DG: Ambulatory blood pressure in pregnancy and fetal growth. Lancet **349:**7, 1997.

Clapp JF, Capeless EL: Neonatal morphometrics after endurance exercise during pregnancy. Am J Obstet Gynecol **163:**1805, 1990.

Clapp JF, Kim H, Burciu B, et al: Beginning regular exercise in early pregnancy: Effect upon fetoplacental growth. Am J Obstet Gynecol **183:**1484, 2000.

Clapp JF, Kim H, Burciu B, et al: Continuing regular exercise during pregnancy: Effect of exercise volume on fetoplacental growth. Am J Obstet Gynecol **186:**142, 2002.

Clapp JF, Rokey R, Treadway JL, et al: Exercise in pregnancy. Med Sci Sports Exerc **24:**S294, 1992.

Clapp JF III, Szeto HH, Larrow R, et al: Umbilical blood flow response to embolization of the uterine circulation. Am J Obstet Gynecol **138:**60, 1980.

Clapp JF III, Szeto HH, Larrow R, et al: Fetal metabolic response to experimental placental vascular damage. Am J Obstet Gynecol **140:**446, 1981.

CLASP: A randomized trial of low-dose aspirin for the prevention and treatment of preeclampsia among 9364 pregnant women. Lancet **343:**619, 1994.

Cliver SP, Goldenberg RL, Cutter GR, et al: The effect of cigarette smoking on neonatal anthropometric measurements. Obstet Gynecol **85:**625, 1995.

Cnattingius S, Axelsson O, Lindmark G: Symphysis-fundus height measurements and intrauterine growth retardation. Acta Obstet Gynecol Scand **63:**335, 1984.

Cnattingius S, Forman MR, Poerendes HW, et al: Effect of age, parity and smoking on pregnancy outcome: A population based study. Am J Obstet Gynecol **168:**16, 1993.

Creasy RK, Barrett CT, de Swiet M, et al: Experimental intrauterine growth retardation in the sheep. Am J Obstet Gynecol **112:**566, 1972.

Daikoku NH, Johnson JWC, Graf C, et al: Patterns of intrauterine growth retardation. Obstet Gynecol **54:**211, 1979.

Daniel SS, James LS, Stark RI, et al: Prevention of the normal expansion of maternal plasma volume: A model for chronic fetal hypoxaemia. J Dev Physiol **11:**225, 1989.

Dashe JS, McIntire DD, Lucas MJ, et al: Effects of symmetric and asymmetric fetal growth on pregnancy outcomes. Obstet Gynecol **96:**321, 2000.

Dawes GS: The placenta and foetal growth. In Dawes GS (ed): Foetal and Neonatal Physiology. Chicago, Year Book Medical Publishers, 1968.

Divon MY: Umbilical artery velocimetry: Clinical utility in high-risk pregnancies. Am J Obstet Gynecol **174:**10, 1996.

Dixon HG, Browne JCM, Davey DA: Choriodecidual and myometrial blood flow. Lancet **2:**369, 1963.

Dixon HG, Robertson WB: Vascular changes in the placental bed. Pathol Microbiol **23:**262, 1961.

Dobbing J: Undernutrition and the developing brain. Am J Dis Child **120:**411, 1970.

Dubowitz LMS, Dubowitz V, Goldberg CG: Clinical assessment of gestational age of the newborn infant. J Pediatr **77:**1, 1970.

Duncan SLB: The partition of uterine blood flow in the pregnant rabbit. J Physiol **204:**421, 1969.

Duvekot JJ, Cheriex EC, Pieters FAA, et al: Maternal volume homeostasis in early pregnancy in relation to fetal growth restriction. Obstet Gynecol **85:**361, 1995.

Easterling TR, Benedetti TJ, Carlson KC, et al: The effect of maternal hemodynamics on fetal growth in hypertensive pregnancies. Am J Obstet Gynecol **165:**902, 1991.

ECPPA Collaborative Group: ECPPA: A randomized trial of low-dose aspirin for the prevention of maternal and fetal complications in high-risk pregnant women. Br J Obstet Gynaecol **103:**39, 1996.

Elster AD, Bleyl JL, Craven TE: Birth weight standards for triplets under modern obstetric care in the United States 1984–1989. Obstet Gynecol **77:**387, 1991.

Feldman DM, Borgida AF, Trymbulak WP, et al: Clinical implications of velamentous cord insertion in triplet gestations. Am J Obstet Gynecol **186:**809, 2002.

Ferrazzi E, Bozzo M, Rigano S, et al: Temporal sequence of abnormal Doppler changes in the peripheral and central circulatory systems of the severely growth-restricted fetus. Ultrasound Obstet Gynecol **19(2):**140, 2002.

Fleischer A, Schulman H, Farmakides G, et al: Uterine artery Doppler velocimetry in pregnant women with hypertension. Am J Obstet Gynecol **154:**806, 1986.

Fox H: The significance of placental infarction in perinatal morbidity and mortality. Biol Neonate **11:**87, 1967.

Froehlich LA, Fujikura R: Significance of a single umbilical artery. Am J Obstet Gynecol **94:**174, 1966.

Galbraith RS, Karchmar EJ, Piercy WM, et al: The clinical prediction of intrauterine growth retardation. Am J Obstet Gynecol **133:**281, 1979.

Gluckman PD, Barrett-Johnson JJ, Butler JH, et al: Studies of insulin like growth factor I and II by specific radiological assays in umbilical cord blood. Clin Endocrinol **19:**405, 1983.

Goldenberg RL, DuBard MB, Cliver SP, et al: Pregnancy outcomes and intelligence at age 5 years. Am J Obstet Gynecol **175:**1511, 1996.

Goldenberg RL, Hoffman HJ, Cliver SP, et al: The influence of previous low birth weight or birth weight, gestational age, and anthropometric measurement in the current pregnancy. Obstet Gynecol **79:**276, 1992.

Goldenberg RL, Tamura T, Cliver SP, et al: Serum folate and fetal growth retardation: A matter of compliance? Obstet Gynecol **79:**71, 1992.

Gruenwald P: Chronic fetal distress and placental insufficiency. Biol Neonate **5:**215, 1963.

Gruenwald P: Growth of the human fetus. I: Normal growth and its variation. Am J Obstet Gynecol **94:**1112, 1966.

Gulmezoglu AM, Hofmeyer GJ: Maternal oxygen administration for suspected and impaired fetal growth. Cochran Database Syst Rev **2000:**2: CD000137.

Hadlock FP, Harrist RB, Carpenter RD, et al: Sonographic estimation of fetal weight. Radiology **150:**535, 1984.

Hall DC, Kaufman DA: Effects of aerobic and strength conditioning on pregnancy outcomes. Am J Obstet Gynecol **157:**1199, 1987.

Harding J: Nutritional causes of impaired fetal growth and their treatment. J R Soc Med **92:**612, 1999.

Haworth JC, Ellestad-Sayed JJ, King J, et al: Fetal growth retardation in cigarette smoking mothers is not due to decreased maternal food intake. Obstet Gynecol **137:**719, 1980.

Heinonen S, Taipale P, Saarikoski S: Weights of placenta from small-for-gestational-age infants revisited. Placenta **86:**428, 2001.

Henson MC, Castracane VD: Leptin in pregnancy. Biol Reprod **63:**1219, 2000.

Hibbard BM, Jeffcoate TNA: Abruptio placentae. Obstet Gynecol **27:**155, 1966.

Hill DE: Physical growth and development after intrauterine growth retardation. J Reprod Med **21:**335, 1978.

Hill DE, Holt AB, Reba R, et al: Alterations in the growth pattern of fetal rhesus monkeys following the *in utero* injection of streptozotocin. Pediatr Res **6:**336, 1972.

Holt AB, Cheek DB, Kerr GR: Prenatal hypothyroidism and brain composition in a primate. Nature (London) **243:**413, 1973.

Houlton MCC, Marivate M, Philpott RH: The prediction of fetal growth retardation in twin pregnancy. Br J Obstet Gynaecol **88:**264, 1981.

Infante-Rivard C, Rivard GE, Yotov WV, et al: Absence of association of thrombophilia polymorphisms with intrauterine growth restriction. N Engl J Med **47:**19, 2002.

Ishihara N, Matsuo H, Murakoshi H, et al: Increased apoptosis in syncytiotrophoblast in human term placentas complicated by either preeclampsia or intrauterine growth retardation. Am J Obstet Gynecol **186:**158, 2002.

Jasayeri A, Tsibris JCM, Spellacy WN: Umbilical cord plasma erythropoietin levels in pregnancies complicated by maternal smoking. Obstet Gynecol **178:**433, 1998.

Johnstone F, Inglis L: Familial trends in low birth weight. Br Med J **3:**659, 1974.

Jones JS, Newman RB, Miller MC: Cross-sectional analysis of triplet birth weight. Am J Obstet Gynecol **164:**135, 1991.

Kaar K, Joupilla P, Kuikka J, et al: Intervillous blood flow in normal and complicated late pregnancy measured by means of an intravenous Xe133 method. Acta Obstet Gynecol Scand **59:**7, 1980.

Kallen K: Maternal smoking during pregnancy and infant head circumference at birth. Early Hum Dev **58:**197, 2000.

Karn MN, Penrose LS: Birth weight and gestation time in relation to maternal age, parity and infant survival. Ann Eugenics **16:**147, 1951.

Karsdorp VH, van Vugt JM, van Geijn HP, et al: Clinical significance of absent or reversed end-diastolic velocity waveforms in the umbilical artery. Lancet **334:**1664, 1994.

Khoury MJ, Erickson D, Cordero JE, et al: Congenital malformation and intrauterine growth retardation: A population study. Pediatrics **82:**83, 1988.

Kingdom JCP, Burrell SJ, Kaufmann P: Pathology and clinical implications of abnormal umbilical artery Doppler waveforms. Ultrasound Obstet Gynecol **9:**271, 1997.

Klebanoff MA, Mednick BR, Schulsinger C, et al: Father's effect on infant birth weight. Am J Obstet Gynecol **178:**1022, 1998.

Klebanoff MA, Schulsinger C, Mednick BR, et al: Preterm and small-for-gestational-age birth across generations. Am J Obstet Gynecol **176:**521, 1997.

Klein JO, Remington JS: Current concepts of infections of the fetus and newborn infant. In Remington JS, Klein JO (eds): Infectious Diseases of the Fetus and Newborn Infant, 3rd ed., Philadelphia, WB Saunders, 1990.

Kopenhager T: A review of 50 pregnant patients with kyphoscoliosis. Br J Obstet Gynaecol **84:**585, 1977.

Kramer MS: Determinants of low birth weight: Methodological assessment and meta-analysis. Bull WHO **65:**663, 1987.

Krebs C, Marca LM, Leiser RL, et al: Intrauterine growth restriction with absent end-diastolic flow velocity in the umbilical artery is associated with maldevelopment of the placental terminal villous tree. Am J Obstet Gynecol **175:**1534, 1996.

Kupferminc MJ, Peri H, Zwang E, et al. High prevalence of the prothrombin gene mutation in women with intrauterine growth retardation, abruptio placentae and second trimester loss. Acta Obstet Gynecol Scand **79:**963, 2000.

Kurjak A, Kirkinen P, Latin V, et al: Ultrasonic assessment of fetal kidney function in normal and complicated pregnancies. Am J Obstet Gynecol **141:**266, 1981.

Lackman F, Capewell V, Gagnon R, et al: Fetal umbilical cord oxygen values and birth to placental weight ratio in relation to size at birth. Am J Obstet Gynecol **185:**674, 2001.

Leitich H, Egarter C, Husslein P, et al: A meta-analysis of low dose aspirin for the prevention of intrauterine growth retardation. Br J Obstet Gynaecol **104:**450, 1997.

Levy R, Smith SD, Yusuf K, et al: Trophoblast apoptosis from pregnancies complicated by fetal growth restriction is associated with enhanced p53 expression. Am J Obstet Gynecol **186:**1056, 2002.

Lichty JA, Ting RY, Bruns PD, et al: Studies of babies born at high altitude. Am J Dis Child **93:**666, 1957.

Liggins GC: The influence of the fetal hypothalamus and pituitary on growth. In Elliot K, Knight J (eds): Size and Birth. Amsterdam, Associated Scientific Publishers, 1974.

Lin C-C, Su S-J, River LP: Comparison of associated high-risk factors and perinatal outcome between symmetric and asymmetric fetal intrauterine growth retardation. Am J Obstet Gynecol **164:**1535, 1991.

Little BB, Snell LM: Brain growth among fetuses exposed to cocaine in utero: Asymmetrical growth retardation. Obstet Gynecol **77:**361, 1991.

Lockwood CJ: Inherited thrombophilias in pregnant patients: Detection and treatment paradigm Obstet Gynecol **99:**333, 2002.

Lockwood CJ , Rand J: The immunobiology and obstetrical consequences of antiphospholipid antibodies. Obstet Gynecol Surv **49:**432, 1994.

Loeffler FE: Clinical fetal weight prediction. J Obstet Gynaecol Br Commonw **74:**675, 1967.

Longo LD: The biological effects of carbon monoxide on the pregnant woman, fetus and newborn infant. Am J Obstet Gynecol **129:**69, 1977.

Love EJ, Kinch RAH: Factors influencing the birth weight in normal pregnancy. Am J Obstet Gynecol **91:**342, 1965.

Low JA, Boston RW, Pancham SR: Fetal asphyxia during the antepartum period in intrauterine growth retarded infants. Am J Obstet Gynecol **113:**351, 1972.

Low JA, Handley-Derry MH, Burke SO, et al: Association of intrauterine fetal growth retardation and learning deficits at age 9 to 11 years. Am J Obstet Gynecol **167:**1499, 1992.

Lubchenco LO, Hansman C, Boyd E: Intrauterine growth as estimated from liveborn birth-weight data at 24 to 42 weeks of gestation. Pediatrics **32:**793, 1963.

Luke B, Nugent C, van de Ven C, et al: The association between maternal factors and perinatal outcome in triplet pregnancies. Am J Obstet Gynecol **187:** 752, 2002.

Lunell NO, Nylund L: Uteroplacental blood flow. Clin Obstet Gynecol **35:**108, 1992.

Manning FA: Intrauterine growth retardation. In Fetal Medicine: Principles and Practice. Norwalk, Conn, Appleton & Lange, 1995, p. 307.

Manning FA, Harman CR, Morrison I, et al: Fetal assessment based on fetal biophysical profile scoring. Am J Obstet Gynecol **162:**703, 1990.

Manning FA, Hill LM, Platt LD: Qualitative amniotic fluid volume determination by ultrasound: Antepartum detection of intrauterine growth retardation. Am J Obstet Gynecol **139:**254, 1981.

Manning FA, Morrison I, Harman CR, et al: Fetal assessment based on fetal biophysical profile scoring: Experience in 19,221 high-risk pregnancies. Am J Obstet Gynecol **157:**880, 1987.

Many A, Schreiber L, Rosner S, et al: Pathologic features of the placenta in women with severe pregnancy complications and thrombophilia. Obstet Gynecol **98:**1041, 2001.

Marconi AM, Cetin I, Ferrazzi E, et al: Lactate metabolism in normal and growth-retarded human fetuses. Pediatr Res **28:**652, 1990.

Marconi AM, Paolin C, Buscaglia M, et al: The impact of gestational age and fetal growth on the maternal-fetal glucose concentration differences. Obstet Gynecol **87:**937, 1996.

Martinelli P, Grandone E, Colaizzo D, et al: Familial thrombophilia and the occurrence of fetal growth restriction. Haematologia **86:**428, 2001.

McCowan LME, Pryor J, Harding JE: Perinatal predictors of neurodevelopmental outcome in small-for-gestational-age children at 18 months of age. Am J Obstet Gynecol **186:**1069, 2002.

McKeown T, Record RG: Observations on foetal growth in multiple pregnancy in man. J Endocrinol **8:**386, 1952.

Meadows NJ, Ruse W, Smith MF, et al: Zinc and small babies. Lancet **2:**1135, 1981.

Mengert WF, Burchell RC, Blumstein RW, et al: Pregnancy after bilateral ligation of the internal iliac and ovarian arteries. Obstet Gynecol **34:**664, 1969.

Miller HC, Hassanein K: Diagnosis of impaired fetal growth in newborn infants. Pediatrics **48:**511, 1971.

Miller HC, Hassanein K: Maternal smoking and fetal growth of full-term infants. Pediatr Res **8:**960, 1974.

Mills JL, Graubard BI, Harley EE, et al: Maternal alcohol consumption and birthweight. How much drinking during pregnancy is safe. JAMA **252:**1875, 1984.

Minior VK, Divon MY: Fetal growth restriction at term: Myth or Realty. Obstet Gynecol **92:**57, 1998.

Molteni RA, Stys SJ, Battaglia FC: Relationship of fetal and placental weight in human beings: Fetal/placental weight ratios at various gestational ages and birth weight distributions. J Reprod Med **21:**327, 1978.

Morton NE: The inheritance of human birth weight. Ann Hum Genet **20:**125, 1955.

Murphy PJ: The estimation of fetal maturity with retarded fetal growth. J Obstet Gynecol Br Commonw **76**:1070, 1969.

Naeye RL: Organ abnormalities in a human parabiotic syndrome. Am J Pathol **46**:892, 1965a.

Naeye RL: Unsuspected organ abnormalities associated with congenital heart disease. Am J Pathol **47**:905, 1965b.

Naeye RL: Cytomegalovirus disease: The fetal disorder. Am J Clin Pathol **47**:738, 1967.

Naeye RL, Benirschke K, Hagstrom JWC, et al: Intrauterine growth of twins as estimated from liveborn birth weight data. Pediatrics **37**:409, 1966.

Neggers YH, Cutter GR, Alvarez JO, et al: The relationship between maternal serum zinc levels during pregnancy and birthweight. Early Hum Dev **25**:75, 1991.

Nicolaides KH, Bilardo CM, Soothill PW, et al: Absence of end-diastolic frequencies in umbilical artery: A sign of fetal hypoxia and acidosis. Br Med J **297**:1026, 1988.

Nicolaides KH, Bradley RJ, Soothill PW, et al: Maternal oxygen therapy for intrauterine growth retardation. Lancet **1**:942, 1987.

Nicolaides KH, Economides DL, Soothill PW: Blood gases, pH, and lactate in appropriate and small-for-gestational-age-fetuses. Am J Obstet Gynecol **161**:996, 1989.

Nicolaides KH, Peters MT, Vyas S: Relation of rate of urine production to oxygen tension in small-for-gestational age fetuses. Am J Obstet Gynecol **162**:387, 1990.

Nicolini U, Nicolaidis P, Fisk NM, et al: Limited role of fetal blood sampling in prediction of outcome in intrauterine growth retardation. Lancet **336**:768, 1990.

Novy MJ, Peterson EN, Metcalfe J: Respiratory characteristics of maternal and fetal blood in cyanotic congenital heart disease. Am J Obstet Gynecol **100**:821, 1968.

Omtzigt AM, Reuwer PJ, Bruinse HW: A randomized controlled trial on the clinical value of umbilical Doppler velocimetry in antenatal care. Am J Obstet Gynecol **170**:625, 1994.

Ong CYT, Liao W, Cacho AM, et al: First trimester maternal serum levels of placenta growth factor as predictor of preeclampsia and fetal growth restriction. Obstet Gynecol **98**:608, 2001.

Ott WJ: Intrauterine growth restriction and Doppler ultrasonography. J Ultrasound Med **19**:661, 2000.

Ott WJ, Mora G, Arias F, et al. Comparison of the modified biophysical profile to a "new" biophysical profile incorporating the middle cerebral artery to umbilical artery velocity flow systolic/diastolic ratio. Am J Obstet Gynecol **178**:1346, 1998.

Ounsted M, Moar V, Scott WA: Perinatal morbidity and mortality in small-for-dates babies: The relative importance of some maternal factors. Early Hum Dev **5**:367, 1981.

Ounsted M, Ounsted C: Maternal regulations of intrauterine growth. Nature **187**:777, 1966.

Palmer J, Dillon-Baker C, Tecklin JS, et al: Pregnancy in patients with cystic fibrosis. Am Intern Med **99**:596, 1983.

Papageorghiou AT, Yu CK, Bindra R, et al: The Fetal Medicine Foundation Second Trimester Screening Group. Multicenter screening for preeclampsia and fetal growth restriction by transvaginal uterine artery Doppler at 23 weeks of gestation. Ultrasound Obstet Gynecol **18**:441, 2001.

Pardi G, Buscaglia M, Ferrazzi E, et al: Cord sampling for the evaluation of oxygenation and acid-base balance in growth-retarded human fetuses. Am J Obstet Gynecol **157**:1221, 1987.

Pattison RC, Norman K, Odendal HJ: The role of Doppler velocimetry in the management of high-risk pregnancies. Br J Obstet Gynaecol **101**:114, 1994.

Paz I, Laor A, Gale R, et al: Term infants with fetal growth restriction are not all at increased risk for low intelligence scores at 17 years. J Pediat **138**:87, 2001.

Penrose LS, Penrose LS (eds): Recent Advances in Human Genetics. London, Churchill Livingstone, 1961, p. 55.

Peuschel SM, Rothman KJ, Ogilvy JD: Birth weight of children with Down's syndrome. Am J Ment Defic **80**:442, 1976.

Piper JM, Langer O, Xenakis E M-J, et al: Perinatal outcome in growth restricted fetuses: Do hypertensive and normotensive pregnancies differ? Obstet Gynecol **88**:194, 1996.

Piper JM, Xenakais E M-J, McFarland M, et al: Do growth-retarded premature infants have different rates of perinatal morbidity and mortality than appropriately grown premature infants? Obstet Gynecol **87**:169, 1996.

Polani PE: Chromosomal and other genetic influences on birth weight variation. In Elliot K, Knight J (eds): Size at Birth. Amsterdam, Associated Scientific Publishers, 1974.

Prentice AM, Watkinson M, Whitehead RG, et al: Prenatal dietary supplementation of African women and birth weight. Lancet **1**:489, 1983.

Pritchard JA, Scott DE, Whalley PJ, et al: The effects of maternal sickle cell hemoglobinopathies and sickle cell trait on reproductive performance. Am J Obstet Gynecol **117**:662, 1973.

Rabinowitz R, Peters MT, Sanjay V, et al: Measurement of fetal urine production in normal pregnancy by real time ultrasonography. Am J Obstet Gynecol **161**:1264, 1989.

Rantakallo P: The effect of maternal smoking on birth weight and the subsequent health of the child. Early Hum Dev **2**:371, 1978.

Resnik R: Intrauterine growth restriction. Obstet Gynceol **99**:490, 2002.

Richards MR, Merrit KK, Samuels JH, et al: Congenital malformations of the cardiovascular system in a series of 6053 infants. Pediatrics **15**:12, 1955.

Robertson WB, Brosens I, Dixon G: Maternal uterine vascular lesions in the hypertensive complications of pregnancy. In Lindheimer MD, Katz AL, Zuspan FP (eds): Hypertension in Pregnancy. New York, John Wiley and Sons, 1976.

Roord JJ, Ramekers LHF, van Engelshoven JMA: Intrauterine malnutrition and skeletal retardation. Biol Neonate **34**:167, 1978.

Roseboom TJ, van der Meulen JHP, Osmond C, et al : Coronary heart disease after the prenatal exposure to the Dutch famine, 1944-45. Heart **84**:595, 2000.

Rosso P, Donoso E, Braun S, et al: Hemodynamic changes in underweight pregnant women. Obstet Gynecol **79**:908, 1992.

Rush D, Stein Z, Susser M: A randomized controlled trial of prenatal supplementation in New York City. Pediatrics **65**:683, 1980.

Sabogal JC, Munoz L: Leptin in Obstetrics and Gynecology: A review. Obstet Gynecol Surv **56**:225, 2001.

Salafia CM, Minior VK, Pezzullo JC, et al: Intrauterine growth restriction in infants of less than 32 weeks' gestation: Associated placental pathologic features. Am J Obstet Gynecol **173**:1049, 1995.

Salafia CM, Pezzullo JC, Minior VK, et al: Placental pathology of absent and reversed end-diastolic flow in growth restricted fetuses. Obstet Gynecol **90**:830, 1997.

Salafia CM, Vintzielos AM, Silberman L, et al: Placental pathology of idiopathic growth retardation at term. Am J Perinatol **9**:179, 1992.

Saugstad LF: Birth weights in children with phenylketonuria and in their siblings. Lancet **1**:809, 1972.

Scott KE, Usher R: Fetal malnutrition: Its incidence, causes and effects. Am J Obstet Gynecol **94**:951, 1966.

Secher NJ, Kaern J, Hansen PK: Intrauterine growth in twin pregnancies: Prediction of fetal growth retardation. Obstet Gynecol **66**:63, 1985.

Secker-Walker RH, Vacek PM, Flynn BS, et al: Smoking in pregnancy, exhaled carbon monoxide, and birth weight. Obstet Gynecol **89**:648, 1997.

Seeds JW, Peng T: Impaired fetal growth and risk of fetal death: Is the tenth percentile the appropriate standard? Am J Obstet Gynecol **178**:658, 1998.

Shanklin DR: The influence of placental lesions and the newborn infant. Pediatr Clin North Am **17**:25, 1970.

Sherwood WG, Chance GW, Hill DE: A new syndrome of pancreatic agenesis. Pediatr Res **8**:360, 1974.

Shinagawa S, Nomura Y, Kudoh S: Full-term deliveries after ligation of bilateral internal iliac arteries and infundibulopelvic ligaments. Acta Obstet Gynecol Scand **60**:439, 1981.

Sibai BM, Caritas SN, Thom E, et al: Prevention of pre-eclampsia with low dose aspirin in healthy, nulliparous pregnant women. N Eng J Med **329**:1213, 1993.

Sickler GK, Nyberg DA, Solaney R, et al: Polyhydramnios and fetal growth restriction: Ominous combination. J Ultrasound Med. **16**:609, 1997.

Skjaerven R, Gjessing HK, Bakketeig LS: New standards for birth weight by gestational age using family data. Am J Obstet Gynecol **183**:689, 2000.

Snijders RJM, Sherrod C, Gosden CM, et al: Fetal growth retardation: Associated malformations and chromosomal abnormalities. Am J Obstet Gynecol **168**:547, 1993.

Soothill PW, Nicolaides KH, Bilardo K, et al: Uteroplacental blood velocity index and umbilical venous PO_2, PCO_2, pH, lactate and erythroblast count in growth retarded fetuses. Fetal Ther **1**:174, 1986.

Soothill PW, Nicolaides KH, Campbell S: Prenatal asphyxia, hyperlactiacidemia, hypoglycemia and erythroblastosis in growth retarded fetuses. B Med J **294**:1046, 1987.

Sornes T: Umbilical cord encirclements and fetal growth restriction. Obstet Gynecol **86**:725, 1995.

Spinillo A, Capuzzo E, Egbe TO, et al: Pregnancies complicated by idiopathic intrauterine growth retardation. J Reprod Med **40**:209, 1995.

Stein Z, Susser M: The Dutch famine, 1944–1945, and the reproductive process: I. Effects on six indices at birth. Pediatr Res **9:**70, 1975.

Stein Z, Susser M, Rush D: Prenatal nutrition and birth weight: Experiments and quasi-experiments in the past decade. J Reprod Med **21:**287, 1978.

Tamura T, Goldenberg RL, Johnston KE, et al: Serum leptin concentrations during pregnancy and their relationship to fetal growth. Obstet Gynecol **91:**389,1998.

Teberg AJ, Walther FJ, Pena IC: Mortality, morbidity and outcome of the small-for-gestational-age infant. Semin Perinatol **11:**84, 1988.

Thaler I, Bronstein M, Rubin AE: The course and outcome of pregnancy associated with bronchiectasis. Br J Obstet Gynaecol **93:**1006, 1986.

Thomson AM, Billewicz WZ, Hytten FE: The assessment of fetal growth. J Obstet Gynaecol Br Commonw **75:**906, 1968.

Thorburn GD: The role of the thyroid gland and kidneys in fetal growth. *In* Elliot K, Knight J (eds): Size at Birth. Amsterdam, Associated Scientific Publishers, 1974.

Trudinger BJ: The umbilical circulation. Semin Perinatol **11:**311, 1987.

Trudinger BJ, Cook CM, Thompson RS, et al: Low-dose aspirin therapy improves fetal weight in umbilical placental insufficiency. Am J Obstet Gynecol **159:**681, 1988.

Valcamonico A, Danti L, Frusca T, et al: Absent end-diastolic velocity in umbilical artery: Risk of neonatal morbidity and brain damage. Am J Obstet Gynecol **170:**796, 1994.

Varma TR: Fetal growth. J Obstet Gynaecol Br Commonw **80:**311, 1973.

Veening MA, Van Weissenbruch MM, Delemarre-Van De Waal HA: Glucose tolerance, insulin sensitivity, and insulin secretion in children born small for gestational age. J Clin Endocrinol Metab **87:**4657, 2002.

Villar J, de Onis M, Kestler E, et al: The differential neonatal morbidity of the intrauterine growth retardation syndrome. Am J Obstet Gynecol **163:**151, 1990.

Visser GHA, Sadovsky G, Nicolaides KH: Antepartum heart rate patterns in small-for-gestational age third trimester fetuses: Correlations with blood gas values obtained at cordocentesis. Am J Obstet Gynecol **162:**698, 1990.

Von Kries R, Junker R, Oberle D, et al: Foetal growth restriction in children with prothrombotic risk factors. Thromb Haemost **86:**1012, 2001.

Wallenberg HCS, Rotmans N: Prevention of recurrent fetal growth retardation by low-dose aspirin and dipyridamole. Am J Obstet Gynecol **157:**1230, 1987.

Walton A, Hammond J: The maternal effects on growth and conformation in the Shire horse-Shetland pony crosses. Proc R Soc Biol **125:**311, 1938.

Wang X, Zuckerman B, Pearson C, et al : Maternal cigarette smoking, metabolic gene polymorphism and infant birth weight. JAMA **287:**195, 2002.

Warshaw JB: Intrauterine growth retardation: Adaptation or pathology? Pediatrics **76:**998, 1985.

Weiner CP, Williamson RA: Evaluation of severe growth retardation using cordocentesis—hematologic and metabolic alterations by etiology. Obstet Gynecol **73:**225, 1989.

Wells JL, James DK, Luxton R, et al: Maternal leukocyte zinc deficiency at start of third trimester as a predictor of fetal growth retardation. Br Med J **294:**1054, 1987.

Wen SW, Goldenberg RL, Cutter GR, et al: Smoking, maternal age, fetal growth and gestational age at delivery. Am J Obstet Gynecol **162:**53, 1990.

Wienerroither H, Steiner H, Tomaselli J, et al: Intrauterine blood flow and long term intellectual, neurologic and social development. Obstet Gynecol **97:**449, 2001.

Wigglesworth JS: Experimental growth retardation in the foetal rat. J Pathol Bacteriol **88:**1, 1964.

Wilcox MA, Smith SJ, Johnson IR, et al: The effect of social deprivation on birthweight, excluding physiologic and pathologic effects. Br J Obstet Gynaecol **102:**918, 1995.

Williams MC, O'Brien WF, Nelson RN, et al: Histologic chorioamnionitis is associated with fetal growth restriction in term and preterm infants. Am J Obstet Gynecol **183:**1094, 2000.

Williams RL, Creasy RK, Cunningham GC, et al: Fetal growth and perinatal viability in California. Obstet Gynecol **59:**624, 1982.

Winick M: Cellular changes during placental and fetal growth. Am J Obstet Gynecol **109:**166, 1971.

Wladimiroff JW, Campbell S: Fetal urine production rates in normal and complicated pregnancies. Lancet **2:**151, 1974.

World Health Organization: Prevention of perinatal morbidity and mortality. *In* Public Health Papers, 1969, p. 42.

Yerushalmy J: Relation of birth weight, gestational age, and the rate of intrauterine growth to perinatal mortality. Clin Obstet Gynecol **13:**107, 1970.

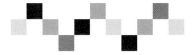

Chapter 29
MULTIPLE GESTATION
Clinical Characteristics and Management

Fergal D. Malone, MD, and Mary E. D'Alton, MD

The incidence of multiple gestation has increased significantly during the last 10 years, now accounting for 3% of all live births in the United States (Martin et al., 2002). As shown in Table 29-1, during the last decade there has been a 25% increase in the number of twin births, a 116% increase in triplets, a 149% increase in quadruplets, and a 250% increase in the number of quintuplet or higher order births. The two major factors accounting for these increases are the widespread availability of assisted reproductive technologies and increasing maternal age at childbirth. Given that perinatal and maternal morbidity and mortality are more common in multiple gestation, this increased incidence will have a significant impact on the practice of maternal-fetal medicine. Therefore, a demand exists for contemporary data on the outcome of twin and higher order multiple gestations and on the management options available for such pregnancies. In addition, when congenital abnormalities occur in multiple gestation, management decisions become complex because the fates of sibling fetuses are necessarily linked. For these reasons, it has been recommended that care of the gravida with a multiple gestation be provided under the supervision of an appropriately trained specialist (Newman and Ellings, 1995).

PERINATAL MORTALITY AND MORBIDITY

Prematurity, monochorionicity, and growth restriction pose the main risks to fetuses and neonates in multiple gestations. Although perinatal deaths may have decreased, the risk of prematurity does not appear to have changed significantly in more than 20 years (Alvarez and Berkowitz, 1990). The mean duration of twin gestations is 37 weeks and that of triplets and quadruplets is 33 and 31 weeks, respectively (Petrikovsky and Vintzileos, 1989; Minakami and Sato, 1996; Pons et al., 1996; Devine et al., 2001). The mean gestational age at delivery for multiple pregnancies can be misleading because it does not reveal the true incidence of extreme prematurity, which has greater clinical significance. Although the incidence of very premature delivery before 28 weeks for singletons in the United States is 0.7%, that incidence increases to 5% for twin and 14% for triplet gestations (Luke, 1994; Devine et al., 2001; Martin et al., 2002). The perinatal mortality rate for twins is at least threefold higher than that for singletons. In a single Swedish population database of over 2.2 million births, the fetal and infant mortality rates for singletons were 4.1 per 1000

and 5.0 per 1000 births, respectively, whereas those of twins were 12.0 per 1000 and 16.0 per 1000 births, respectively (Rydhstroem and Heraib, 2001). Mortality rates were significantly higher among same-sex twins when compared with unlike-sex twins. It therefore appears that the two most important factors explaining increased mortality in twin gestations are increased rates of prematurity and complications of monochorionicity. The risk that twins will weigh less than 1500 g at birth is 10 times the risk for singletons. These increased risks are more pronounced in male–male pairs, black infants, and infants of younger mothers (Powers and Wampler, 1996).

Most published data on perinatal outcome for higher order multiple gestations are limited by (1) noncontemporary study periods, (2) small sample size, (3) long duration of sample collection, (4) lack of control groups for comparison, and (5) accumulation of data from multiple centers with differing management practices. These limitations are even more pronounced for pregnancies with four or more fetuses. A summary of this limited neonatal outcome data for triplet pregnancies is presented in Table 29-2. This meta-analysis of studies of perinatal outcome of triplet gestations from the last 10 years shows a mean gestational age of delivery of 33 weeks but with a 13% incidence of delivery at less than 28 weeks and a perinatal mortality rate of 103 per 1000 births. In addition, spontaneous loss rate before 24 weeks for triplet pregnancies with confirmed cardiac activity may be as high as 20% (Lipitz et al., 1994). Some quadruplet pregnancy series have suggested perinatal mortality rates ranging from 0 to 67 per 1000 quadruplet births (Collins and Bleyl, 1990; Elliott and Radin, 1992). However, caution is needed when interpreting studies of higher order multiple gestations, because often only pregnancies reaching viability are included, thereby giving an overly positive view of perinatal outcome.

Perinatal morbidity is also more likely in multiple gestations. Although multiple gestation accounts for only 3% of all births in the United States, infants of multiple gestations comprise 23% of low-birth-weight infants (Martin et al., 2002). The incidence of severe handicap in neonatal survivors of multiple gestation is increased from 19.7 per 1000 singleton survivors to 34.0 and 57.5 per 1000 twin and triplet survivors, respectively (Luke and Keith, 1992). Twins account for between 5% and 10% of all cases of cerebral palsy in the United States (Scheller and Nelson, 1992). The risks of producing at least one infant with cerebral palsy from one pregnancy has been reported to be

TABLE 29-1. INCIDENCE OF MULTIPLE BIRTHS IN THE UNITED STATES

Year	Twins	Triplets	Quadruplets	Quintuplets and Higher Order
2000	118,916	6,742	506	77
1999	114,307	6,742	512	67
1998	110,670	6,919	627	79
1997	104,137	6,148	510	79
1996	100,750	5,298	560	81
1995	96,736	4,551	365	57
1994	97,094	4,233	315	46
1993	96,445	3,834	277	57
1992	95,372	3,547	310	26
1991	94,779	3,121	203	22

From Martin JA, Hamilton BE, Ventura SY, et al: Births: Final Data for 2000. National Vital Statistics Reports, vol 50, no 5. Hyattsville, Md., National Center for Health Statistics, 2002.

1.5% for twin, 8.0% for triplet, and 42.9% for quadruplet gestations (Yokoyama et al., 1995).

As a group, mean birth weight is significantly lower for twin neonates and triplet neonates compared with singletons, with a mean triplet birth weight of 1697 g, compared with 2362 g for twins and 3348 g for singletons in the United States (Martin et al., 2002). However, there is no evidence that twin or triplet neonates have outcomes different from gestational age-matched singletons. When matched by gestational age at delivery, twin and triplet neonates have similar birth weight, morbidity, and mortality when compared with singleton neonates (Kaufman et al., 1998).

MATERNAL MORTALITY AND MORBIDITY

Given that the maternal mortality rate is very low in developed countries today and that published series of multiple gestations are relatively small, it has not been possible to confirm an increased risk of maternal death in contemporarily managed multiple gestations. However, maternal morbidity is significantly increased in mothers with multiple gestations and seems to be related to the number of fetuses present. Twin pregnancies are associated with significantly higher risks of hypertension (2.5-fold), abruption (3-fold), anemia (2.5-fold), and urinary tract infections (1.5-fold) compared with singleton pregnancies (Spellacy et al., 1990).

The percentage of maternal morbidity associated with triplet pregnancies is summarized in Table 29-3. The most recent of these data suggests a 96% risk of antenatal complications and a 44% risk of postpartum complications (Devine et al., 2001). This includes a 78% incidence of preterm labor, 26% preeclampsia, 9% hemolysis, elevated liver enzymes, low platelets syndrome, 24% anemia, 24% preterm premature rupture of membranes, 14% gestational diabetes, 4% acute fatty liver, 16% chorioendometritis, and 9% postpartum hemorrhage. No differences in the frequency of complications were noted between spontaneous triplets or those arising from ovulation induction or *in vitro* fertilization. Data on quadruplets suggest an almost 100% risk of preterm labor and a 32% to 90% risk of gestational hypertension (Collins and Bleyl, 1990; Elliott and Radin, 1992). In addition, it appears that preeclampsia in higher order multiple gestations is frequently atypical, occurs at an earlier gestational age, and is more severe than preeclampsia in singleton gestations (Hardardottir et al., 1996; Devine et al., 2001).

TABLE 29-2. CONTEMPORARY TRIPLET NEONATAL OUTCOME DATA

Author	Year	*n*	Mean Gestational Age (wk)	Gestational Age at Delivery		PNM
				<32 wk	<28 wk	
Peaceman et al.	1992	15	35	67%	7%	22
Boulot et al.	1992	33	34	15%	3%	71
Jonas and Lumley	1993	133	33	32%	14%	108
Lipitz et al.	1993	106	34	24%	—	50
Santema et al.	1995	40	32	55%	28%	200
Albrecht and Tomich	1996	57	33	28%	7%	41
Skrablin et al.	2000	52	33	27%	14%	167
Devine et al.	2001	100	33	42%	14%	103
Summary		536	33	33%	13%	103

n, number of pregnancies; PNM, perinatal mortality rate per 1000 births.

TABLE 29-3. CONTEMPORARY TRIPLET MATERNAL MORBIDITY DATA

Author	Year	n	Preterm Labor	Preeclampsia	PPROM	Anemia	Endometritis	PPH
Seoud et al.	1992	15	92%	39%	15%	20%	—	—
Peaceman et al.	1992	15	60%	20%	20%	—	—	—
Santema et al.	1995	40	90%	22%	12%	38%	—	15%
Albrecht and Tomich	1996	57	86%	33%	18%	58%	14%	12%
Skrablin et al.	2000	52	79%	23%	6%	—	—	—
Devine et al.	2001	100	78%	26%	24%	24%	16%	9%
Summary		279	81%	27%	17%	35%	15%	13%

n, number of pregnancies; PPH, postpartum hemorrhage; PPROM, preterm premature rupture of membranes.

MATERNAL ADAPTATION

The normal maternal physiologic adaptation seen in singleton pregnancy is exaggerated in multiple gestation. These physiologic responses consist of both observed changes and expected changes extrapolated from singleton pregnancy physiology (Yeast, 1990; Gardner and Wenstrom, 1996). Serum levels of progesterone, estradiol, estriol, human placental lactogen, human chorionic gonadotropin (hCG), and α-fetoprotein (AFP) are all significantly higher in multiple than in singleton gestations.

Heart rate and stroke volume are significantly increased in gravidas with twins during the third trimester, leading to a significant increase in cardiac output and cardiac index compared with gravidas with singletons (Veille et al., 1985). These increases most likely occur secondary to increased myocardial contractility in the setting of multiple gestation. Systolic and diastolic blood pressures mirror the changes seen during singleton pregnancy, with an even greater drop in pressures noted during the second trimester in twin pregnancy. However, by the time of delivery mean blood pressures are significantly higher in multiple pregnancy compared with singletons (Campbell, 1986). Depending on the number of fetuses, plasma volume increases by 50% to 100%, which may lead to dilutional anemia.

During multiple gestation, uterine volume increases rapidly, with a 25-week twin gestation uterus equal in size to a term singleton uterus (Redford, 1982). Uterine blood flow increases significantly in a twin pregnancy and is related to both increased cardiac output and decreased uterine artery resistance (Rizzo et al., 1993). In multiple gestations, the normal increase in tidal volume and oxygen consumption is probably increased further, which may lead to an even more alkalotic arterial pH than that seen with singleton pregnancy. Similarly, the normal increase in glomerular filtration rate and size of the renal collecting system is probably more marked in women with multiple gestations.

Increased daily caloric intake to 2800 kcal/day is recommended in multiple gestations compared with 2400 kcal/day in singleton gestations (National Academy of Sciences, 1990). The recommended maternal weight gain for twin pregnancies is 1 to 1.5 pounds per week, for a total pregnancy weight gain of 35 to 45 pounds. Although specific recommendations have not been issued, ideal weight gain in higher order multiple gestations is likely to be significantly greater than in twin gestations. Some have suggested that optimal fetal growth in higher order multiple gestations can be achieved with maternal weight gain of at least 1.5 pounds per week during the first 24 weeks of pregnancy (Luke et al., 1995).

ULTRASONOGRAPHY

Routine prenatal ultrasonography has proved valuable in early detection of multiple gestation (LeFevre et al., 1993). It is only after diagnosis of a multiple gestation prenatally that steps can be taken to reduce the perinatal and maternal morbidity associated with the condition. Prenatal ultrasonography in multiple gestation is useful for the following:

- Confirming a diagnosis of multiple gestation
- Determining chorionicity
- Detecting fetal anomalies
- Guiding invasive procedures
- Evaluating fetal growth
- Measuring cervical length
- Confirming fetal well-being
- Assisting in delivery

Diagnosis of Multiple Gestation

Positive sonographic diagnosis of multiple gestation can be made by visualizing multiple gestational sacs with yolk sacs by 5 weeks of gestation and multiple embryos with cardiac activity by 6 weeks. If two gestational sacs are seen at early ultrasound, the chances of delivering twins are 57%, but this increases to 87% if two embryonic poles with cardiac activity are visualized (Dickey et al., 1990). If three gestational sacs are seen at early ultrasound, the chances of delivering triplets are 20%, but this increases to 68% if three embryonic poles with cardiac activity are visualized. In addition to twins, the early sonographic visualization of two intrauterine fluid collections may represent a singleton in a bicornuate uterus, a singleton with a subchorionic hemorrhage, or a vanishing twin, which can occur in 20% to 50% of cases of early multiple gestation diagnoses (Divon and Weiner, 1995).

Chorionicity

Because 20% of twins are monochorionic and such pregnancies are associated with up to a 26% risk of perinatal mortality, the establishment of chorionicity is crucial for clinical management in multiple gestation (D'Alton and Simpson, 1995). In most patients, sonographic assessment can determine

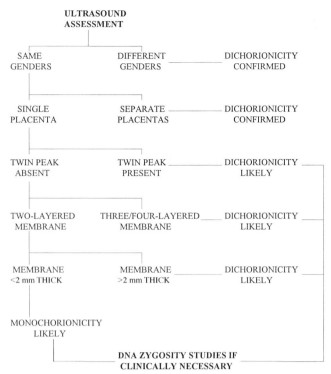

FIGURE 29-1 ■ Determining chorionicity in multiple gestation.

chorionicity (Fig. 29-1). Sonographic determination of chorionicity should be attempted in all multiple gestations and is best performed in the late first and early second trimesters. At less than 8 weeks' gestation, obvious separate gestational sacs each surrounded by a thick echogenic ring is suggestive of dichorionicity (Barss et al., 1985). If separate echogenic rings are not visible, monochorionicity is likely. In such situations, counting the number of yolk sacs may assist in establishing amnionicity. Two fetal poles with two yolk sacs in a monochorionic gestation suggests diamnionicity, whereas the presence of two fetal poles with only one yolk sac is consistent with a monoamniotic gestation (Bromley and Benacerraf, 1995). Later in gestation, when two placentas are visualized or when twins are discordant for gender, the gestation is confirmed with certainty as being dichorionic (Fig. 29-2). In the absence of these findings monochorionicity is possible, and other sonographic features should be assessed.

The visualization of only one placental mass has a positive predictive value for monochorionicity of only 42%, because many dichorionic gestations develop apparent fusion of separate placentas as pregnancy progresses (Scardo et al., 1995). Counting the number of layers in the dividing membrane, near its insertion into the placenta, is 100% predictive of dichorionicity but is not as reliable in predicting monochorionicity (D'Alton and Dudley, 1989; Vayssiere et al., 1996). When this method is used, it is assumed that if only two layers are present, the placentation is monochorionic and the presence of three or four layers suggests dichorionicity. The use of a membrane thickness cutoff value of 2 mm has also been reported to correctly assign chorionicity in more than 90% of cases, but the reproducibility of this measurement has been questioned (Stagiannis et al., 1995). Visualization of a triangular projection of placenta between the layers of the dividing membrane (known as the *twin-peak* or *lambda sign*) is also useful in diag-

nosis of dichorionicity, but its absence is not as reliable in the prediction of monochorionicity. Although each of these sonographic features individually has a poor positive predictive value for monochorionicity, use of a composite sonographic approach by combination of one placenta, gender concordance, thin dividing membrane, and absence of the twin-peak sign may yield a positive predictive value for monochorionicity of 92% (Scardo et al., 1995).

In certain clinical situations, such as the presence of fetal anomalies or of twins discordant for growth, management requires the reliable exclusion of monochorionicity. If monochorionicity cannot be reliably excluded by the presence of separate placentas or different genders, serious consideration should be given to invasive testing to assign chorionicity. This can be performed by DNA zygosity studies on amniocytes or, more recently, by injection of microbubble contrast angiography into the umbilical cord of one fetus (Denbow et al., 1997; Norton et al., 1997).

Detection of Fetal Anomalies

Because the risk of congenital anomalies is increased in multiple gestations, such pregnancies should be managed with careful sonographic surveys of fetal anatomy. The ability of ultrasonography to detect congenital fetal anomalies in multiple gestations has not been adequately studied because no large series of patients have been available for review. Several smaller series from single centers have tried to establish the predictive value of prenatal ultrasound in the detection of anomalies in multiple gestations. In one series of 24 fetuses with anomalies, it was found that serial ultrasonography in a specialist center achieved an 88% detection rate, with 100% specificity, in the prenatal diagnosis of anomalies in twin pregnancies (Edwards et al., 1995). It may also be possible to detect up to 88% of cases of Down syndrome in twin pregnancies by combining risks derived from maternal age and nuchal translucency thickness measurement at 10 to 14 weeks of gestation (Sebire et al., 1996). The finding of increased nuchal translu-

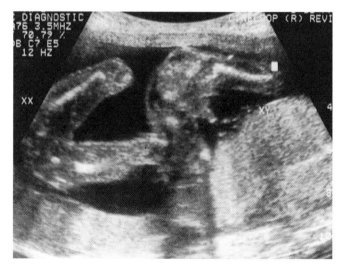

FIGURE 29-2 ■ A single ultrasound view demonstrates female external genitalia on the left and male external genitalia on the right, therefore confirming dichorionic twin gestation with certainty. (Courtesy of Sabrina Craigo, MD, New England Medical Center, Boston.)

cency in one fetus of a monochorionic pair may also presage the development of twin-to-twin transfusion syndrome (TTS).

Evaluation of Fetal Growth

Serial ultrasonography is the most accurate method to assess fetal growth in multiple gestation. Intrauterine growth for twins is similar to that of singletons until 30 to 32 weeks' gestation, when abdominal circumference measurements of twins begin to lag behind those of singletons (Grumbach et al., 1986). Composite assessments of fetal weight appear to be superior to individual biometric parameters, such as abdominal circumference and femur length, to predict growth discordance (Hill et al., 1994). Although the predictive value of all biometric assessments to identify growth discordance has been questioned, no other sonographic markers for discordance have yet been validated (Caravello et al., 1997).

Even though individual growth curves for twin and triplet gestations have been described, singleton fetal weight standards are still commonly used to assess growth in multiple gestation. In one prospective study of serial biometric measurements in twins, no significant differences in fetal growth were noted compared with measurements in singleton gestations (Reece et al., 1991). Because growth restriction is a dynamic process and sibling fetuses are immediately available for comparison, we consider it reasonable to assess growth in multiple gestation with serial evaluations, based on singleton growth curves, using as many biometric parameters as possible and comparing sibling estimated fetal weights for discordance. Typically, a 20% to 25% difference in estimated fetal weight between sibling fetuses, expressed as a percentage of the larger fetal weight, suggests clinically significant growth discordance (D'Alton and Mercer, 1990). In one study of 460 twin pregnancies, weight discordance of 25% or more was associated with a 6.5-fold increase in the rate of stillbirth compared with nondiscordant twins and an overall perinatal death rate of 9.7% (Erkkola et al., 1985). In another study of 1370 twin pregnancies in which weight discordance was stratified in 5% increments, a statistically significant increase in fetal death occurred only with weight discordance greater than 30% (Hollier et al., 1999).

It is unclear if adverse outcome seen with significant weight discordance is related to continuation of pregnancy within a hostile intrauterine environment or is related to iatrogenic prematurity. In general, we use the finding of significant weight discordance as an indication for close fetal surveillance rather than an indication for immediate delivery. Decisions regarding delivery are then made based on the results of tests of fetal well-being together with gestational age, rather than solely on the basis of significant weight discordance.

Measurement of Cervical Length

Ultrasound has an important role to play in the surveillance of multiple gestation for preterm labor and delivery. Transvaginal assessment of cervical length has been shown to be particularly effective in identifying multiple gestations at additional risk for preterm delivery. In the Maternal-Fetal Medicine Units Network Preterm Prediction Study of risk factors for preterm birth in twins, a transvaginal sonographic measurement of cervical length of less than or equal to 2.5 cm at 24 weeks' gestation was associated with a 6.9-fold increased

risk of delivery before 32 weeks' gestation (Goldenberg et al., 1996). A short cervix at 28 weeks' gestation was not a strong predictor of preterm birth. In another study of cervical length in 215 twin gestations, a length of 2.5 cm or less at 23 weeks' gestation had sensitivities for detecting preterm delivery at or before 28 weeks, 30 weeks, and 32 weeks of 100%, 80%, and 47%, respectively (Souka et al., 1999). Approximately 11% to 17% of all twin gestations can be expected to have cervical lengths less than or equal to 2.5 cm (Goldenberg et al., 1996; Souka et al., 1999). In a study of 66 triplet gestations, a cervical length cutoff of 2 cm at 24 weeks' gestation was significantly associated with preterm delivery (McElrath et al., 2001).

When evaluating cervical length with ultrasound, the maternal bladder should first be emptied. Transvaginal sonography is the preferred approach. Care must be taken to avoid pressure on the cervix from the ultrasound probe. A sagittal view should be obtained with an echogenic endocervical mucosa visible along the length of the cervical canal. Measurements should be taken between the v-shaped notch at the internal os and the triangular echolucent area at the external os. The optimal interval at which to perform sonographic assessments of cervical length during gestation is unclear. Our practice has been to measure cervical length every 2 weeks from 16 to 24 weeks in selected cases of multiple gestation deemed to be at highest risk for preterm delivery (e.g., those with higher order multiple gestations or those with prior preterm deliveries). For all other multiple gestations, we perform sonographic assessment of cervical length at the time of sonography for fetal anatomy or growth. Two studies have found that cervical length measurement of 3.5 cm or more at 24 weeks can identify twin pregnancies with a very low (3% to 4%) risk of preterm birth before 34 weeks (Imseis et al., 1997; Yang et al., 2000).

Confirmation of Fetal Well-Being

Ultrasonography is useful to confirm fetal well-being in multiple pregnancies. The use of non-stress testing in multiple gestation is discussed later under Antepartum Management: Fetal Surveillance. The biophysical profile may also be of benefit in multiple gestation whenever a non-stress test is not reassuring or in cases of higher order multiple gestation when non-stress tests can be impractical to perform.

Doppler velocimetry may also be used to evaluate fetal well-being in multiple gestations. Umbilical artery systolic-to-diastolic ratios are similar in singleton and twin gestations. A deterioration in this ratio may occur before the sonographic detection of growth restriction. Normal Doppler velocimetry indices of other fetal vessels, such as the middle cerebral artery and the descending aorta, are similar between singleton, twin, and triplet fetuses (Akiyama et al., 1999). An absolute difference of 0.4 (or 15%) or more in umbilical artery systolic-to-diastolic ratios between sibling fetuses identifies growth discordance as accurately as a difference in estimated fetal weight, presumably because such systolic-to-diastolic differences represent unequal fetoplacental perfusion (Divon and Weiner, 1995). We reserve Doppler velocimetry for multiple gestation complicated by significant growth restriction or discordance.

Sonographic measurement of amniotic fluid volume is an important tool to evaluate fetal well-being. In a dye-dilution study of diamniotic twin pregnancies, the amniotic fluid volume in each amniotic sac was noted to be independent of the volume in the neighboring sac and was similar to singleton fluid volumes (Magann et al., 1995). There is no agreement on the optimal sonographic method to assess amniotic fluid volume in multiple gestations. Methods in use include (Chau et al., 1996; Porter et al., 1996) the following:

1. A single overall amniotic fluid index without reference to the dividing membrane
2. Individual amniotic fluid indices for each sac
3. Largest two-diameter pocket in each sac
4. Subjective assessment of the relative distribution of fluid between sacs

No one method, however, has been shown to be optimal to predict perinatal outcome in multiple gestation.

PRENATAL DIAGNOSIS

Prenatal diagnosis and genetic counseling are important in the management of gravidas in multiple gestation inasmuch as such patients are at higher risk of fetal anomalies because of (1) the presence of a multiple gestation and (2) the positive association between twinning and maternal age.

In dizygotic twin pregnancies, each fetus has its own independent risk of aneuploidy; thus, the chance of at least one abnormal fetus is increased. In addition, monozygotic pregnancies are at increased risk for many structural anomalies. Monozygotic twins may not necessarily be concordant for chromosomal abnormalities because the phenomenon of postzygotic nondisjunction can result in heterokaryotypic twins. Because of this phenomenon and because the diagnosis of monochorionicity is rarely made with certainty, whenever invasive prenatal diagnosis is indicated, each gestation should be sampled separately.

The role of ultrasonography to detect fetal anomalies in multiple gestations has already been discussed.

Risks of Chromosomal Abnormalities

Risks for Down syndrome and other chromosomal aneuploidies have been calculated for twin gestations at various maternal ages (Rodis et al., 1990). In the population studied by Rodis and coworkers, the risk that one fetus in a twin pregnancy would have Down syndrome for a 33-year-old woman was similar to that of a 35-year-old woman with a singleton gestation. These specific risks do change, depending on the incidence of dizygotic twinning, which is dependent on the maternal age and race profiles of the study population. After correction for different rates of dizygosity based on maternal age and race, it has been suggested that invasive prenatal diagnosis be offered to women in the United States with twin gestations at age 31 and older (Table 29-4) (Meyers et al., 1997).

For triplets, the risk that a 28-year-old woman will have at least one fetus with Down syndrome may be similar to that of a 35-year-old woman with a single fetus. These alterations in risk assessment for chromosomal abnormalities are important because invasive prenatal diagnosis may be offered at an even earlier maternal age for gravidas with higher order multiple gestations.

TABLE 29-4. RISKS OF AT LEAST ONE CHROMOSOMAL ABNORMALITY IN WHITE SINGLETON AND TWIN GESTATIONS BASED ON MATERNAL AGE AT THE TIME OF AMNIOCENTESIS

Maternal Age (yr)	Singleton Gestation		Twin Gestation	
	Down Syndrome	**All Chromosomal Abnormalities**	**Down Syndrome**	**All Chromosomal Abnormalities**
25	1/885	1/1533	1/481	1/833
26	1/826	1/1202	1/447	1/650
27	1/769	1/943	1/415	1/509
28	1/719	1/740	1/387	1/398
29	1/680	1/580	1/364	1/310
30	1/641	1/455	1/342	1/243
31	1/610	1/357	1/324	1/190
32	1/481	1/280	1/256	1/149
33	1/389	1/219	1/206	1/116
34	1/303	1/172	1/160	1/91
35	1/237	1/135	1/125	1/71
36	1/185	1/106	1/98	1/56
37	1/145	1/83	1/77	1/44
38	1/113	1/65	1/60	1/35
39	1/89	1/51	1/47	1/27
40	1/69	1/40	1/37	1/21
41	1/55	1/31	1/29	1/17
42	1/43	1/25	1/23	1/13
43	1/33	1/19	1/18	1/10
44	1/26	1/15	1/14	1/8
45	1/21	1/12	1/11	1/6

From Meyers C, Adam R, Dungan J, et al: Aneuploidy in twin gestations: When is maternal age advanced? Obstet Gynecol **89**:248; 1997. Reprinted with permission from the American College of Obstetricians and Gynecologists.

Genetic Amniocentesis

Genetic amniocentesis in twins is most commonly performed with an ultrasound-guided double-needle approach (Wapner, 1995). After the first sac is entered and amniotic fluid is aspirated, several milliliters of the blue dye indigo carmine are instilled and the needle is removed. A new needle is then placed into the second sac, and aspiration of clear fluid confirms successful sampling of two different sacs. Methylene blue dye should not be used because of the risks of fetal hemolytic anemia, small intestinal atresia, and fetal demise. We successfully extended this procedure sequentially to perform triplet and quadruplet genetic amniocenteses.

Careful sonographic mapping of placentas and sacs is mandatory to assist in future management plans when karyotype results return, often as much as 2 weeks later. The rate of pregnancy loss after genetic amniocentesis in twins is considered similar to that seen with singletons (Ghidini et al., 1993). The initial appearance of a higher loss rate with amniocentesis in twins most likely reflects the higher spontaneous loss rate seen in twins (Wapner, 1995). No data exist on loss rates for amniocentesis with higher order multiple gestation or on loss rates for early amniocentesis (<14 weeks) with multiple gestations.

Chorionic Villus Sampling

Chorionic villus sampling (CVS) is usually performed in twin gestations at 10 to 13 weeks. It is considered an equally safe alternative to amniocentesis in twins (Wapner et al., 1993). One must take care to always keep the needle tip under constant sonographic visualization to ensure that both chorion frondosum sites have been separately sampled. Because as many as 4% of samples can show evidence of twin–twin contamination, the cytogenetic laboratory should be made aware that a twin CVS has been performed (Wapner, 1995).

Serum Screening for Down Syndrome

Screening for Down syndrome using maternal serum levels of AFP, hCG, and unconjugated estriol together with maternal age is commonly performed in the United States during the second trimester for singleton pregnancies. In twin pregnancies, experience with such screening is limited. Average levels of AFP, hCG, and unconjugated estriol are increased 2.04-fold, 1.93-fold, and 1.64-fold, respectively, in twin compared with singleton pregnancies (Wapner, 1995). In the only prospective evaluation of multiple serum marker screening in twins published to date, the screen-positive rate remained at 5%, but no cases of Down syndrome were detected in the study population (Neveux et al., 1996). Using statistical modeling and maintaining a 5% false-positive rate, these authors estimated that 73% of monozygotic twins and 43% of dizygotic twins with Down syndrome would be detected. In another series of 420 twin pregnancies, AFP and hCG levels were twice the levels seen in singletons (Spencer et al., 1995). The authors postulated that risk prediction from singletons could be extrapolated to twin gestations using a twin correction method, in which the multiple of the median (MoM) value would be divided by the mean MoM of the twin population. This process with AFP and hCG screening was predicted to yield a 51% Down syndrome detection rate at a 5% false-positive rate (Spencer et al., 1995).

However, in a larger review of serum samples from 4443 twin pregnancies, several inconsistencies in the serum marker increases were noted across twin populations (O'Brien et al., 1997). These authors suggested that use of a mathematical correction to convert singleton Down syndrome risks for multiple gestations may not be valid. Until more experience is reported, we are not routinely offering this investigation for aneuploidy screening with multiple gestation.

Screening for Neural Tube Defects

A second-trimester maternal serum AFP level greater than 2.5 MoM has been used to screen for neural tube defects in singleton gestation. Because the maternal serum AFP level is approximately doubled in normal twin pregnancy, different cutoffs are needed to interpret this test in multiple gestation. When a 2.5 MoM cutoff in twin pregnancy is used, 99% of cases of anencephaly and 89% of open neural tube defects are detected but generate a 30% false-positive rate (Cuckle et al., 1990). Raising the twin cutoff to 5.0 MoM decreases the false-positive rate to 3% but also decreases the detection of anencephaly to 83% and open neural tube defects to 39%.

We use a cutoff of 4.5 MoM, which has a detection rate of 50% to 85%, based on a 5% false-positive rate (Wapner, 1995). Amniotic fluid AFP and acetylcholinesterase levels in different amniotic sacs are independent of each other in dichorionic twins but are interdependent in monochorionic twins (Stiller et al., 1988). Because serum screening for fetal abnormalities in multiple gestation will always be limited by the inability to confirm which fetus is affected, many centers do not offer serum screening in multiple gestation even for neural tube defects. Whenever an increased maternal serum AFP value is obtained, sonographic evaluation will always be necessary for further evaluation. Therefore, it may be more straightforward to provide neural tube defect screening using sonography alone. Use of this approach relies on identifying either the neural tube defect along the fetal spine or the secondary intracranial effects, such as the Chiari malformation. These sonographic features include the "lemon" sign, representing scalloping of the frontal bones, and the "banana" sign, representing downward displacement of the cerebellum toward the foramen magnum.

First-Trimester Screening

With the availability of late first-trimester *multifetal reduction* procedures in higher order multiple gestations, there is now increasing interest in screening tests for fetal abnormalities in the first trimester. Although serum screening for Down syndrome with free β-hCG and pregnancy-associated plasma protein A has been reported in singletons, little is known about the performance of first-trimester serum screening in multiples. In one series of first-trimester serum samples from 67 twin pregnancies, average free β-hCG levels were 1.85 MoM and average pregnancy-associated plasma protein A levels were 2.36 MoM in chromosomally normal twin pregnancies (Niemimaa et al., 2002). However, free β-hCG levels were not as high as expected, with twin pregnancies secreting somewhat less free β-hCG than expected. Larger studies of serum screening in twin gestations, including those affected by Down syndrome, would be needed before true performance characteristics of first-trimester serum screening with twins could be established (Niemimaa et al., 2002).

At present, we use only increased nuchal translucency thickness to screen for aneuploidies in multiple gestations in the first trimester In one study of 448 twin gestations, this form of screening delivered an 88% detection rate for Down syndrome, with a 7.3% screen-positive rate (Sebire et al., 1996). In another series of 24 multiple gestations and 79 singleton control subjects, the distribution of nuchal translucency measurements, including 95th percentile values, was similar in all cases, implying that this form of screening could be implemented using established normative data from singleton populations (Maymon et al., 1999). If multifetal reduction is being planned, we incorporate the nuchal translucency measurement into consideration in deciding which fetus to target for reduction.

ANTEPARTUM MANAGEMENT

The incidence and range of antenatal complications, both maternal and fetal, seen in multiple gestation suggest that multiple pregnancies be managed under the supervision of an appropriately trained specialist (Newman and Ellings, 1995). In a nonrandomized study comparing the outcome of 67 triplet gestations managed by maternal-fetal medicine specialists with 24 triplet gestations managed by generalist physicians, significant increases in gestational age at delivery and birth weight were noted for cases managed by specialists (Meyer et al., 2001). Additionally, significant reductions in neonatal intensive care unit length of stay and cost were also noted for cases managed by specialists, compared with those managed by generalists. Interventions to improve outcome cannot reasonably be expected to work unless an early diagnosis of multiple gestation has been made. This supports our practice of offering routine ultrasonography to all pregnant patients. If ultrasound diagnosis is not offered, vigilance should be maintained for early clinical signs of multiple gestation, such as size greater than dates, excessive maternal weight gain, auscultation of more than one fetal heart rate, elevated maternal serum AFP levels, or unexplained severe anemia.

In addition to the standard prenatal care provided for singletons, antenatal management of multiple gestations necessitates watchfulness for the development of several maternal complications (see Table 29-3). This may best be achieved by frequent prenatal visits with an appropriate level of awareness regarding potential complications.

Preterm Labor and Delivery

Preterm labor occurs in more than 40% of twin and 75% of triplet gestations (Kovacs et al., 1989; Devine et al., 2001). Although patient education regarding the early signs of preterm labor in multiple gestations is important, surveillance for cervical change may also be helpful in predicting premature delivery. A cervical score based on digital examination (consisting of cervical length in centimeters minus internal os dilation in centimeters) has been proposed for predicting preterm delivery in twin gestation (Newman et al., 1991):

1. When the score is less than or equal to 0, there is a 75% positive predictive value for preterm delivery.
2. When the score is greater than 0, preterm labor occurred in only 3% of patients during the following week.

Other parameters used to predict preterm delivery in multiple gestations include sonographic assessment of cervical length and cervicovaginal assays for fetal fibronectin. As described previously under the role of ultrasound in multiple gestation, these factors were evaluated in a large multicenter prospective study of twin gestations (Goldenberg et al., 1996). When screened at 24 weeks, a cervical length less than or equal to 25 mm is significantly associated with preterm delivery before 32 weeks, with an odds ratio of 6.9. In the setting of such a short cervix, the rate of spontaneous preterm birth before 32 weeks is 27%, compared with 5% for twin gestation with normal cervical length. A positive cervicovaginal fetal fibronectin assay at 28 weeks is also significantly associated with preterm delivery before 32 weeks, with an odds ratio of 9.4. The rate of spontaneous preterm birth before 32 weeks in the setting of positive fetal fibronectin obtained at 28 weeks is 29%, compared with 4% for twin gestation with negative fetal fibronectin. No other risk factors for preterm delivery were found to be significantly associated with preterm delivery of twins (Goldenberg et al., 1996).

Interventions to prevent preterm labor in multiple gestations have been disappointing. There is no evidence that prophylactic cervical cerclage or prophylactic tocolytic agents have been beneficial (Keirse et al., 1989). A nonrandomized trial in which 128 twin pregnancies with cervical length less than 2.5 mm at 18 to 26 weeks' gestation were offered cervical cerclage revealed no benefit for any outcome measure after cerclage placement (Newman et al., 2002). Although this study might be criticized because the decision on whether or not to place cerclage was left entirely up to the patient, there are no well-designed randomized trials confirming a benefit to cerclage for a shortened cervix in multiple gestations. In one series of 16 triplet gestations receiving elective prophylactic cervical cerclage, compared with 52 triplet gestations who did not receive cerclage, no differences in outcome were noted, with mean gestational age at delivery of 34 weeks in both groups and perinatal mortality rates of 104 and 71 per 1000 births in the cerclage and no cerclage groups, respectively (Lipitz et al., 1989). In another nonrandomized series of 59 triplet gestations, 20 received prophylactic cervical cerclage and the remaining 39 were expectantly managed (Elimian et al., 1999). Although the authors suggested a decrease in the incidence of extreme low birth weight, there were no significant differences in mean gestational age at delivery or any other measure of neonatal outcome. We reserve cervical cerclage for women with multiple gestation in whom we strongly suspect cervical incompetence. Additionally, cerclage placement may be considered in cases of higher order multiple gestation in which sonographic surveillance of cervical length demonstrates progressive cervical shortening or funneling. However, no data exist at this time to confirm or exclude a benefit of such a practice in the setting of multiple gestation.

No methods of long-term maintenance tocolysis have proved effective in preventing prematurity in multiple gestation, including the oral administration of terbutaline or nifedipine, the rectal administration of indomethacin, or subcutaneous infusion of terbutaline. Caution is advised in the administration of tocolytics to patients with multiple gestation because of the significant potential for maternal cardiovascular and pulmonary morbidity. The combination of one or more tocolytic agents, corticosteroids, and intravenous fluid replacement in the setting of the increased blood volume of multiple gestation leads to a significant risk of pulmonary edema. We therefore reserve tocolysis, typically by means of intravenous magnesium sulfate or rectal indomethacin, only for cases of documented preterm labor, with a goal of delaying delivery so that there is time for transport to an appropriate medical center and for a 48-hour exposure to betamethasone. Betamethasone (12 mg intramuscularly, two doses, 24 hours apart) is given whenever there is a high risk of delivery between 24 and 34 weeks of gestation. The use of routine prophylactic corticosteroids on a weekly basis for multiple gestations has never been validated. Indeed, the most recent National Institutes of Health Consensus Development Conference on antenatal corticosteroids reaffirmed the lack of safety or efficacy data needed to support repeat or rescue dosing of corticosteroids in clinical practice (National Institutes of Health, 2000).

Bed rest, at home or in hospital, has not proved effective in preventing preterm labor or delivery (MacLennan et al., 1990). Initial nonrandomized retrospective studies supported the practice of routine hospitalization and bed rest for patients with multiple gestation, but subsequent prospective trials and meta-analyses have not supported this intervention. In a review of six randomized trials, involving over 600 multiple gestations, a trend toward a decrease in low-birth-weight infants was noted with inpatient bed rest (Crowther, 2001). However, there was no improvement in very-low-birth-weight infants, and in the group with uncomplicated twin pregnancies, inpatient bed rest was actually associated with an increased risk of delivery at less than 34 weeks' gestation. There have been no recent prospective trials evaluating the role of bed rest at home for patients with multiple gestation. Because it is extremely difficult to standardize home bed rest and consequently difficult to refute any potential benefit, we continue to recommend modified rest at home for higher order multiple gestations starting at approximately 20 weeks of gestation (Newman and Ellings, 1995). For example, one suggested activity modification algorithm for triplet gestation recommends lateral recumbent rest for 4 to 6 hours per day, beginning at 16 weeks' gestation, increasing to 6 to 8 hours per day by 20 weeks, and extending to rest for most of the day by 24 weeks (Adams et al., 1998). Others omit a recommendation for bed rest in women with multiple gestation when cervical sonography indicates a length greater than 35 mm at 24 weeks' (Imseis et al., 1997; Yang et al., 2000).

The role of home uterine activity monitoring to prevent preterm labor and delivery has been refuted for both singleton and multiple gestations (American College of Obstetricians and Gynecologists, 1998). A meta-analysis of six randomized trials showed no significant benefit of home uterine activity monitoring to reduce the risk of preterm birth in twin gestations (Colton et al., 1995). In a randomized trial of 2422 patients that included 844 twin gestations in which patients were randomized to weekly nurse contact, daily nurse contact, or daily nurse contact plus home uterine activity monitoring, there were no differences in preterm delivery before 35 weeks' gestation (Dyson et al., 1998). Specifically, there was no significant benefit in women with twin gestations. Whether home uterine activity monitoring may benefit patients who have undergone fetal reduction procedures in higher order multiple gestation or *in utero* fetal surgery is unknown.

Preeclampsia

The risk of gestational hypertension, or preeclampsia, has been reported to range from 10% to 20% in twins, 25% to 60% in triplets, and up to as much as 90% in quadruplet pregnancies (Kovacs et al., 1989; Spellacy et al., 1990; Elliott and Radin, 1992; Hardardottir et al., 1996; Devine et al., 2001). The incidence of preeclampsia with multiple gestation may be increased in pregnancies that follow assisted reproductive technologies, but it does not appear to be related to zygosity (Maxwell et al., 2001; Lynch et al., 2002). When preeclampsia occurs in higher order multiple gestations, it more often occurs earlier, is more severe, and is atypical (Hardardottir et al., 1996; Devine et al., 2001). A multicenter study of preeclampsia in 87 twin and 143 singleton gestations demonstrated lower gestational age at delivery, lower birth weight, and higher rates of cesarean delivery among twin gestations with preeclampsia when compared with singletons with preeclampsia (Sibai et al., 2000). These data emphasize the importance of specialist supervision of multiple gestations and regular monitoring for early signs and symptoms of preeclampsia. To date, however, no interventions (e.g., low-dose aspirin or calcium supplementation) have been shown to prevent or reduce the incidence of preeclampsia in these high-risk pregnancies. In the National Institutes of Health Maternal-Fetal Medicine Units Network randomized trial of aspirin to prevent preeclampsia, 688 patients with multiple gestation were randomized to low-dose aspirin or placebo between 13 and 26 weeks' gestation (Caritis et al., 1998). There was no difference in incidence of preeclampsia between the two groups, with rates of 12% and 16% for aspirin and placebo, respectively.

Other Maternal Complications

Daily supplementation with at least 60 mg of elemental iron and 1 mg of folic acid is recommended because of the increased risk of iron- and folate-deficiency anemia in multiple gestation. Surveillance for other potential maternal complications of higher order multiple gestations, including acute fatty liver of pregnancy, gestational diabetes, urinary tract infections, and intervertebral disk disease, is important as well (Devine et al., 2001). In particular, multiple gestation is a risk factor for the development of acute fatty liver of pregnancy, perhaps because of the increase in placental mass (Davidson et al., 1998). Acute fatty liver should be carefully considered in the differential diagnosis if hepatic dysfunction is found in a multiple gestation.

Fetal Surveillance

As described earlier, serial sonographic assessment of fetal growth is recommended for multiple gestations. We evaluate fetal weight and growth discordance every 3 to 4 weeks from approximately 18 weeks' gestation or every 2 weeks if growth restriction or growth discordance (>20%) is discovered. Although some obstetricians routinely monitor all multiple gestations using weekly non-stress tests or biophysical profiles from 34 weeks, this practice has not been validated by prospective studies. Surveillance with non-stress tests or biophysical profile is reserved for multiple pregnancies with the following indications:

- Significant growth restriction in either fetus
- Growth discordance

- Oligohydramnios
- Decreased fetal movement
- Maternal medical complications

Fetal testing for monoamniotic twins, twin-to-twin-transfusion syndrome, demise of one fetus, and anomalous twins is discussed later under Special Considerations in Management.

As soon as the diagnosis of significant growth discordance is confirmed, fetal testing should begin intensively. In our practice, this consists of twice weekly non-stress tests supplemented by biophysical profiles and umbilical artery Doppler velocimetry. If absent or reversed end-diastolic flow is discovered, delivery should be considered if gestational age is sufficiently advanced that the healthy twin would not be significantly compromised by delivery. Selecting the appropriate time for delivery is extremely difficult in such cases because an effort intended to save a twin that may already be significantly compromised may lead to iatrogenic morbidity in the healthy twin. Daily fetal testing should be performed in cases of absent or reversed end-diastolic flow until delivery is accomplished.

Assessment of fetal lung maturity is rarely needed for clinical management of multiple gestation. When amniocentesis for lung maturity is indicated, it is probably reasonable to sample only one sac, because lung maturity studies in most cases should be similar in each sac (Norman et al., 1983). In the case of preterm labor, ruptured membranes, diabetes mellitus, growth restriction, or growth discordance, it is difficult to predict which fetus will have higher lung maturity indices. In one series, 9 of 15 discordant twin pairs showed higher lung maturity indices in the larger twin, whereas theoretically the growth-restricted fetus would have been predicted to have more advanced lung maturity owing to stress responses (Leveno et al., 1984). Therefore, we believe each amniotic sac should be sampled in selected cases if lung maturity testing will affect management.

INTRAPARTUM MANAGEMENT

Preparations

All twin fetuses should be delivered by 40 weeks of gestation because of rising perinatal morbidity after that date. One recent study reported a rate of stillbirth for multiple gestations at 39 weeks that surpassed the risk for singleton gestations at greater than 42 weeks' gestation (Sairam et al., 2002). The use of prostaglandins for induction and oxytocin for induction or augmentation of labor is acceptable in the management of twin gestation. An attempt at vaginal birth after a previous low transverse cesarean delivery is considered by some to be an acceptable alternative to elective repeated cesarean section in twin gestation (Miller et al., 1996). However, it should be noted that no studies of adequate design and size are available to confirm the safety of vaginal birth after cesarean in the setting of multiple gestation. The absence of data describing adverse outcomes from vaginal birth after cesarean in multiple gestations should not be equated with confirmation of the safety of this approach.

Intrapartum management of the parturient with a multiple gestation requires multidisciplinary cooperation. Adequate obstetric and nursing staff, together with an anesthesiologist and at least one neonatologist or pediatrician, should be present for delivery. Intravenous access and prompt availability of blood products should be ensured.

As soon as possible after the patient enters the delivery unit, ultrasonography should be performed to confirm fetal presentations and size before a decision is made on mode of delivery. Electronic fetal heart monitoring should also be available. If a trial of labor is elected, continuous lumbar epidural anesthesia should be strongly recommended because it allows a full range of obstetric interventions to be performed rapidly if needed. Vaginal deliveries should be performed in an operating room because emergent cesarean section may be required for the second twin in a significant number of cases (Simpson and D'Alton, 1997). Before vaginal delivery of a second twin, ultrasonography should also be available in the operating room so that its presentation can be confirmed.

Vertex-Vertex Twins

The vertex-vertex presentation occurs in 40% to 45% of all twin pregnancies. In the absence of obstetric indications for cesarean delivery, vaginal birth should be planned regardless of gestational age (Simpson and D'Alton, 1997). Routine cesarean delivery for all vertex-vertex twins is not supported by the literature; no improvement in perinatal outcome has been found.

After delivery of the first twin, the cord should be clamped. No blood samples should be obtained until after delivery of the second twin. Unless the presentation is obviously vertex by clinical examination, ultrasonography should be performed to confirm presentation of the second twin and to exclude a funic presentation. With the availability of continuous electronic fetal heart monitoring, there is no absolute indication to deliver the second twin within a specified time limit. However, active intervention to complete the delivery (amniotomy, if safe, and oxytocin augmentation) is encouraged by studies that link length of delivery interval to fetal acid-base status. In one series of 118 cases of twin deliveries, significant negative correlations were noted between the length of delivery interval and umbilical cord pH and base excess (Leung et al., 2002). These authors demonstrated an increase in the rate of umbilical arterial pH of 7.00 or less from 0 when delivery interval was less than 15 minutes, to 6% for 16- to 30-minute interval, and to 27% for intervals greater than 30 minutes. Undue delay may also allow time for the fully dilated cervix to contract down, thereby limiting the range of options for urgent delivery of the second twin should a problem develop. The cesarean section rate for the second twin also increases with increasing delivery interval (Simpson and D'Alton, 1997).

Vertex-Nonvertex Twins

Vertex-breech or *vertex-transverse* presentation occurs in 35% to 40% of all twin pregnancies. Selection of mode of delivery depends on the following:

1. Size of the second twin
2. Presence of growth discordance
3. Availability of obstetric staff skilled in assisted breech delivery, internal podalic version, or total breech extraction

In the absence of an appropriately skilled obstetrician or if the second twin is significantly larger than the first, cesarean delivery is recommended.

Another option is *external cephalic version* of the second twin immediately after delivery of the first. This method can be successful in up to 70% of cases of vertex-nonvertex twins (Chervenak et al., 1983). Vaginal delivery is not always possible after successful external version of the second twin and may be associated with complications, such as cord prolapse, fetal distress, and placental abruption. Breech extraction, therefore, may be a better alternative, with success rates of more than 95% (Gocke et al., 1989).

Vaginal breech delivery of the second twin is possible and should be encouraged in appropriately selected cases. The worst perinatal outcome associated with twins is more likely to be related to prematurity or growth restriction and has not proved to be related to mode of delivery of the second twin (Simpson and D'Alton, 1997). Cesarean section cannot guarantee a good delivery outcome with twins, because birth trauma is still possible during the procedure. The use of a liberal cesarean delivery policy in relation to the nonvertex second twin has not been found to significantly improve perinatal outcome. Published reports of outcomes for fetuses with birth weights of 1500 g or more have shown no benefit from cesarean delivery over vaginal breech delivery for the nonvertex second twin. Data for fetuses with birth weight under 1500 g are insufficient to make such a firm conclusion; conversely, vaginal breech delivery of fetuses estimated to weigh less than 1500 g is not absolutely contraindicated. In a series of 141 twin deliveries in which the second twin was nonvertex, including 35 cases of vaginal delivery, there was no evidence of benefit from cesarean delivery when gestational age was greater than 24 weeks and when birth weight exceeded 1500 g (Winn et al., 2001). We currently offer vaginal breech delivery for the nonvertex second twin with estimated weight between 1500 and 3500 g, provided it is not significantly larger than the first twin and the head is not hyperextended.

If a vaginal breech delivery is planned for the second twin, the delivery of the presenting vertex twin is performed as previously described. If the second twin is in a *frank* or *complete breech presentation* and the fetal heart tracing is reassuring, membranes may be left intact until engagement of the presenting part and an assisted breech delivery can be performed.

If the second twin is in a transverse lie or a footling breech presentation or if fetal testing is not reassuring, membranes should be left intact until the feet can be secured in the pelvis, following which immediate amniotomy and total breech extraction should be performed (Simpson and D'Alton, 1997). Whenever total breech extraction is indicated, it should be performed as soon as possible after delivery of the first twin, while the cervix is still fully dilated.

Nonvertex First Twin

Breech-vertex or *breech-breech* presentations occur in 15% to 20% of all twin pregnancies. Such cases are almost always managed by cesarean delivery, mostly because of a concern that the heads in breech-vertex twins may interlock. This is an extremely rare complication, however, and has prompted some centers to offer vaginal delivery to breech-vertex twins that meet the same selection criteria as singleton vaginal breech deliveries. Among 239 vaginal deliveries in which the first twin was breech, there was no evidence of depressed Apgar scores or increased neonatal deaths when the first twin's weight was greater than 1500 g (Blickstein et al., 2000). However,

Apgar scores and neonatal deaths were significantly increased for first twins weighing less than 1500 g delivered vaginally from breech presentation.

External cephalic version of a breech presenting twin has also been described (Bloomfield and Philipson, 1997). In the absence of prospective studies validating these approaches, cesarean section for the nonvertex first twin may be the optimal delivery choice.

Higher Order Multiple Gestations

Although case series of successful vaginal delivery of triplets exist, there are no prospective series large enough to establish the safety of vaginal delivery over cesarean delivery (Thiery et al., 1988; Clarke and Roman, 1994; Dommergues et al., 1995). One center described a protocol for vaginal delivery of selected cases of triplet gestation in which 8 of 11 women with triplet gestations eligible for vaginal delivery were successfully delivered vaginally (Alamia et al., 1998). No increase in maternal or neonatal morbidity was noted. However, because of practical difficulties in adequately monitoring three or more fetuses in labor and through delivery, we recommend cesarean delivery under regional anesthesia for all patients with three or more live fetuses that are of a viable gestational age. There is no conclusive evidence to recommend one type of uterine incision over another in higher order multiple gestation.

Asynchronous Delivery

Asynchronous delivery, or delayed interval delivery, refers to delivery of one fetus in a multiple gestation that is not followed promptly by the delivery of the remaining fetus or fetuses. This is an extremely rare scenario and is acceptable only in the management of extreme prematurity, when the remaining fetuses are either previable or would be at very high risk for complications of prematurity if delivered. Clinical conditions that should generally contraindicate an attempt at asynchronous delivery include monochorionicity, intra-amniotic infection, placental abruption, and the coexistence of preeclampsia. Successful outcomes have been reported in carefully selected cases (Lavery et al., 1994). The largest series of delayed interval delivery from a single center described the outcome of 24 twin and triplet gestations that were candidates for this approach (Farkouh et al., 2000). A protocol of initial amniocentesis of the remaining sac to exclude infection, ligation of the cord of the delivered fetus with absorbable suture near the placenta, aggressive tocolysis, placement of a cerclage, broad-spectrum antibiotics for up to 7 days, bed rest, and close surveillance was instituted. These authors described a mean latency interval gained of 36 days, ranging from 3 to 123 days. However, only 16 of the 24 cases were previable (≤24 weeks' gestation) at the time of presentation, and of these, 10 (63%) reached viability, with the survival of 8 of 18 (44%) remaining infants (Farkouh et al., 2000). Given the limitations of these data, it is essential that careful counseling be provided and informed consent be obtained from the mother regarding risks to her health before attempting such management. Eligible patients should be followed closely for the development of chorioamnionitis or maternal sepsis. Cervical cerclage and tocolytic agents should be used with extreme caution and only after first excluding chorioamnionitis in the remaining gestations. Data are insufficient to comment on the role of prophylactic antibiotics in this setting.

SPECIAL CONSIDERATIONS IN MANAGEMENT

Twin-to-Twin Transfusion Syndrome

TTS occurs because of an imbalance in blood flow through vascular communications in the placenta, leading to overperfusion of one twin and underperfusion of its cotwin (Fig. 29-3). It occurs almost always in monochorionic twin pregnancies (Benirschke and Kim, 1973). The syndrome is estimated to occur in 5% to 15% of monochorionic twin pregnancies but has also been occasionally demonstrated in dichorionic twin gestations (Benirschke and Kim, 1973; Lage et al., 1989). The precise incidence of TTS is extremely difficult to define because the syndrome is associated with a wide spectrum of clinical presentations, ranging from the *vanishing-twin phenomenon* in the first trimester to *unexplained fetal demise* in the third trimester. There is even disagreement on terminology defining the syndrome. Some authors suggest that "twin oligohydramnios-polyhydramnios sequence" is a more precise term (Bruner and Rosemond, 1993; King et al., 1995).

The precise cause of TTS is unknown. Initial theories suggested that pregnancies affected by TTS demonstrate significantly fewer placental anastomoses than pregnancies unaffected by TTS, and in TTS the few anastomoses present are more likely to be deep than superficial (Bajoria et al., 1995). This theory implies that TTS is more likely the result of a paucity of placental anastomoses, which interferes with the placenta's ability to regulate blood flow equally between both twins. More recent work has demonstrated that it is the anatomic type of placental anastomoses, rather than simply their number, that underlies the pathophysiology of TTS. Arteriovenous (AV) anastomoses have been described on the placental surface as a single unpaired artery carrying blood from the donor twin to a placental cotyledon, together with a single unpaired vein carrying blood from that cotyledon back to the recipient twin (Machin et al., 2000). Although these vessels run along the surface of the placenta separately, they enter the same placental cotyledon. It is theorized that these AV anastomoses result in net transfusion of blood from the donor to the recipient fetus. However, such AV anastomoses are present in up to 70% of monochorionic placentas, whereas the clinical syndrome of TTS is far less common (5% to 15%) (De Lia et al., 2000). Therefore, a protective mechanism must be in place that prevents TTS from developing in the majority of monochorionic pregnancies. It has been suggested that arterioarterial anastomoses are bidirectional and that the presence of a large number of such arterioarterial anastomoses in a monochorionic placenta may compensate for unidirectional AV anastomotic flow, thereby preventing the appearance of TTS (De Lia et al., 2000). This theory is consistent with earlier studies suggesting that a lack of superficial placental anastomoses (presumably arterioarterial) together with the existence of a number of deep placental anastomoses (presumably AV) explains the pathophysiology of TTS (Bajoria et al., 1995).

The clinical features of TTS can be explained by these placental architecture findings. The donor fetus is relatively hypoperfused, demonstrating signs of intrauterine growth restriction and oligohydramnios. Eventually, anhydramnios develops, and this fetus attains the typical "stuck twin" appearance because of the inability to visualize the dividing membrane separate from the fetal body. Fetal blood sampling studies have demonstrated that this donor fetus has a significantly lower hematocrit than the recipient fetus (36% versus 47%, respectively) (Denbow et al., 1998). Echocardiographic studies have not shown any specific pattern of abnormal findings among donor fetuses (Fesslova et al., 1998; Simpson et al., 1998). By contrast, the recipient fetus is relatively hyperperfused, becomes hypertensive, and produces increasing amounts of atrial and brain natriuretic peptides in an effort to handle its larger blood volume (Bajoria et al., 2002). This results in significant polyhydramnios and increasing intrauterine pressure. Uterine overdistention and raised intrauterine pressure may then contribute to increased rates of preterm labor or preterm rupture of membranes, as well as exacerbating hypoperfusion of the donor fetus by compression effects. Echocardiographic features in the recipient twin include ventricular hypertrophy and dilation, tricuspid regurgitation, and cardiac failure (Fesslova et al., 1998; Simpson et al., 1998). Additionally, acquired progressive right ventricular

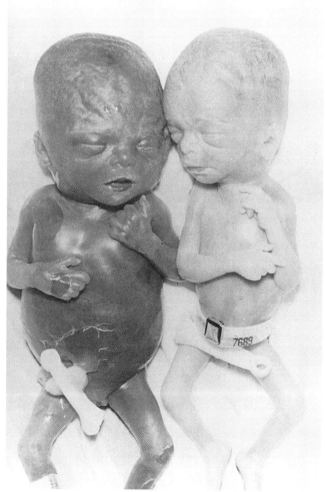

FIGURE 29-3 ■ Twin-to-twin transfusion syndrome resulting in pregnancy loss at 22 weeks' gestation, with the plethoric recipient twin on the left and the anemic donor twin on the right. (Courtesy of Steven Ralston, MD, New England Medical Center, Boston.)

outflow tract obstruction, possibly leading to right ventricular outflow atresia, has been described in up to 9% of recipient fetuses (Lougheed et al., 2001).

Prenatal diagnosis of TTS depends on a high degree of clinical suspicion in monochorionic pregnancies, together with the visualization of certain ultrasonographic criteria. These include the following (D'Alton and Simpson, 1995):

1. Presence of a single placenta
2. Gender concordance
3. Significant growth discordance (usually > 20%)
4. Discrepancy in amniotic fluid volume between the two amniotic sacs (usually oligohydramnios and polyhydramnios)
5. Discrepancy in size of the umbilical cords
6. Presence of fetal hydrops or cardiac dysfunction
7. Abnormal umbilical artery Doppler findings, such as absent end-diastolic flow in the donor fetus

Not all sonographic criteria need to be met to make the diagnosis of TTS, and none of the criteria is specific for TTS. The most important criterion appears to be discrepancy in amniotic fluid volume, with a maximum vertical pocket less than 2 cm expected around the donor fetus and a maximum vertical pocket greater than 8 cm around the recipient fetus. The differential diagnosis of significant growth discordance or *stuck twin phenomenon* includes uteroplacental insufficiency, structural or chromosomal fetal abnormalities, abnormal cord insertion, and intrauterine infection (e.g., cytomegalovirus infection).

Other methods of prenatal diagnosis of TTS have included fetal blood sampling to detect a difference in hemoglobin concentration between twins and transfusion of adult rhesus-negative red blood cells into the donor twin followed by Kleihauer detection in the recipient twin. Although fetal blood sampling studies have demonstrated significantly lower hematocrit values in donor compared with recipient fetuses, only some cases of TTS have sufficient hematocrit differences to be of diagnostic value (Denbow et al., 1998). Neonatal diagnosis of TTS also relies on significant birth-weight discordance and by the demonstration of a difference of at least 5 g/dL in initial neonatal hemoglobin levels. However, because weight and hemoglobin differences are common in most monochorionic gestations, with or without TTS, it is difficult to use these criteria alone for diagnosis (Wenstrom et al., 1992). Because great clinical variability exists in the appearance of TTS, sonographic criteria have been proposed to classify severity. The clinical value of scoring systems to improve fetal outcome has not yet been determined, but they may foster comparison of published treatment strategies. One system uses the following markers (Quintero et al., 1999):

Stage I: Donor twin bladder still visible, fetal Doppler values normal
Stage II: Donor twin bladder no longer visible, fetal Doppler values normal
Stage III: Donor twin bladder no longer visible, fetal Doppler values critically abnormal
Stage IV: Presence of hydrops
Stage V: Intrauterine death of one or both fetuses

Because the diagnosis of TTS is essentially one of exclusion, management first involves excluding other causes of significant growth discordance or stuck twin phenomenon. This requires careful sonographic assessment of fetal anatomy, cardiac function, and cord insertion together with the performance of amniocenteses on both sacs to exclude chromosomal anomaly or infection and, possibly, to provide fetal cells for zygosity studies. Expectant management is associated with high rates of perinatal mortality; if only one twin dies, there is a significant risk of profound neurologic handicap in the surviving twin as well (Weir et al., 1979). Medical management with maternal administration of digoxin has not been widely used, and administration of indomethacin is no longer practiced because of a high likelihood of intrauterine demise, presumably because of interference with fetal renal perfusion (Jones et al., 1993).

Therapy for TTS currently involves one of three possible management approaches: serial reduction amniocenteses, amniotic septostomy, or selective laser photocoagulation of placental anastomoses. The most common therapy is *serial reduction amniocentesis*, an effort to equilibrate amniotic fluid volume across the dividing membrane and to reduce overall intrauterine pressure, although the precise mechanism of action is unclear. With this technique, aggressive decompression amniocentesis is performed under ultrasound guidance. An 18-gauge needle is used to drain off as much fluid as possible, and as quickly as possible, from around the recipient twin. The procedure is repeated as often as necessary to maintain near-normal amniotic fluid volume around the recipient twin. The rationale for amnioreduction is that a decrease in uterine distension leads to reduced risk of preterm labor and preterm rupture of membranes, thereby prolonging gestation and improving perinatal outcome. However, an improvement in fetal condition has also been noted after reduction amniocentesis, which suggests that this therapy may also provide direct benefit for the fetus. Because amnioreduction does not affect the placental anastomoses that are the basis of TTS, it is difficult to elucidate a mechanism by which reduction amniocentesis improves the fetal condition. Possible mechanisms include a reduction in polyhydramnios and intrauterine pressure, which may improve circulation in superficial arterioarterial anastomotic placental vessels at the donor side, leading to increased donor fetal renal perfusion, formation of urine, and improvement in oligohydramnios.

Perinatal outcome with serial reduction amniocenteses as primary therapy for TTS has been mixed, with perinatal survival rates ranging from 37% to 83% and averaging approximately 62% overall survival (Malone and D'Alton, 2000). Explanations for the variability in reported performance of reduction amniocenteses include reporting bias, small study sizes, and significant variation in the timing and volume of fluid removed. An international registry of 223 twin pregnancies with TTS detected before 28 weeks' gestation and managed with reduction amniocenteses reported an overall survival rate of 78% (Mari et al., 2001). The median number of amnioreduction procedures performed was two, with a median of 1400 mL of amniotic fluid removed per procedure. Predictors of poor outcome included earlier gestational age at diagnosis, absent end-diastolic umbilical arterial blood flow in the donor fetus, and the presence of hydrops. Survival at 4 weeks of age was 60%, and approximately 25% of survivors had abnormal intracranial ultrasound findings (Mari et al., 2001). However, the prevalence of long-term neurologic abnormality may be lower than suggested by these sonographic data. In a series of 33 TTS pregnancies, in which surviving infants were followed to 2 years of age, there were only two cases (4.9%) of cerebral palsy, one of which was a surviving infant after an intrauterine demise of its cotwin, and the second was in an infant that also had cardiac malformations (Mari et al., 2000).

Amniotic septostomy involves deliberate perforation of the dividing membrane separating the stuck twin from its cotwin with polyhydramnios (Saade et al., 1995). The mechanism of action for this therapeutic approach is unclear but may involve equalization of fluid across the dividing membrane, resulting in a fluid bolus being ingested by the donor twin and thereby expanding its intravascular volume. However, such a theory has not been proven and does not explain the finding of TTS in monoamniotic twin pregnancies. In 12 patients managed with amniotic septostomy, an overall survival rate of 83% was achieved (Saade et al., 1998). In another observational report of 14 patients, 7 managed with serial reduction amniocentesis and 7 managed with amniotic septostomy, there was no difference in overall survival, but the septostomy patients had significantly greater pregnancy prolongation (Johnson et al., 2001). In another report of three cases of amniotic septostomy, all fetuses were lost within 5 days of the procedure (Pistorius and Howarth, 1999). Septostomy has been criticized because it may result in an iatrogenic monoamniotic twin pregnancy, with all the negative implications of this condition. Microseptostomy has also been advocated, in which a single needle perforation is made in the dividing membrane to reduce the likelihood of iatrogenic monoamnionicity. Comparison of amnioreduction versus septostomy is difficult because septostomy may inadvertently occur during amnioreduction and because many cases of septostomy are treated with amnioreduction as well.

The third management option for TTS is *selective photocoagulation* of the chorioangiopagus (AV anastomotic vessels in the placenta) using a fetoscopically placed neodymium-yttrium aluminum garnet laser. A 2- to 3-m fetoscope is placed into the polyhydramnios-recipient twin sac under ultrasound guidance, and the vessels on the surface of the placenta are inspected. AV anastomoses are easily identifiable as a single unpaired artery coming from the donor side entering a foramen on the placental surface, together with a single unpaired vein exiting the same area on the placental surface with blood flowing toward the recipient twin. Selective photocoagulation involves placement of a 0.4-mm neodymium-yttrium aluminum garnet laser fiber through the fetoscope and ablating all visible anastomoses. Debate continues as to the benefit of ablating all anastomoses or just the AV anastomoses (De Lia et al., 2000). It would appear to be preferable to ablate all vascular communications that connect the two fetal circulations, because this would prevent reverse fetal transfusion and neurologic injury if one fetus dies. Amnioreduction is also performed as part of the same procedure. An apparent advantage of selective photocoagulation is that it is the only therapy that directly addresses the underlying pathophysiology of TTS. By ablating AV anastomoses, the net transfusion of blood from donor to recipient can be reduced. Ablation of all placental anastomoses that connect the fetuses essentially makes the pregnancy dichorionic, thereby preventing neurologic injury in a survivor should demise of one twin occur.

Overall survival rates of 55%, 69%, 65%, and 57% have been reported from series of 144, 93, 200, and 72 TTS pregnancies, respectively (Ville et al., 1998; De Lia et al., 1999; Hecher et al., 2000; Quintero et al., 2001). The mean survival

for the 471 TTS cases in these series was 62%, with a 5% incidence of neurologic injury among survivors.

Minimal data are available to compare the outcomes with these three management options for TTS. A summary of studies of serial reduction amniocenteses suggests overall survival of 60%, whereas a summary of studies of laser photocoagulation suggests similar overall survival of 62%. However, these summaries also describe from 5% to 25% rates of neurologic injury among survivors after reduction amniocenteses compared with 5% neurologic injury after laser photocoagulation (Malone and D'Alton, 2000). In the only comparative study published to date, 73 patients treated with laser photocoagulation performed at one center were compared with 43 patients treated with reduction amniocenteses at another center; overall survival rates were similar (61% versus 51%, respectively) (Hecher et al., 1999). This study also suggested significantly lower neurologic injury among survivors after laser photocoagulation (6% versus 18%, respectively).

These data are still insufficient to support a definitive recommendation on the optimal management of TTS. Although laser photocoagulation may yield similar survival as reduction amniocenteses with lower neurologic morbidity, it is a significantly more invasive procedure, available only at a limited number of centers. Randomized trials are currently ongoing to compare these two forms of therapy for TTS. In the United States, a randomized trial of serial reduction amniocenteses versus laser photocoagulation organized by the National Institute of Child Health and Human Development is currently recruiting patients (www.fetalsurgery.chop.edu). A similar randomized trial is also currently recruiting patients in Europe and at selected other international centers (www.eurofetus.org). A third randomized trial is ongoing in the United States, in which patients are being randomized to either serial reduction amniocenteses or amniotic septostomy (Dorman et al., 2000).

When treating a patient with TTS, consideration should first be given to enrollment in one of these randomized trials. If enrollment is not possible, current management begins with an aggressive reduction amniocentesis using an 18-gauge or 20-gauge spinal needle, with the goal being a maximum vertical amniotic fluid pocket of less than 5 cm. Frequent sonographic follow-up is required. Reduction amniocentesis should be repeated if the maximum vertical fluid pocket around the recipient fetus exceeds 8 cm or if the donor fetus remains stuck or does not have a visible bladder. Intensive fetal surveillance should be performed when viability is reached. Betamethasone administration is recommended because of the high likelihood of early delivery. Delivery should be based on usual obstetric indications, although cesarean section is likely. Two neonatal resuscitation teams should be present at delivery. Surviving infants are at increased risk for long-term morbidity, including cardiomyopathy and periventricular leukomalacia (Cincotta et al., 1996). There have been no reports of recurrent TTS in subsequent pregnancies.

Monoamniotic Twins

Monoamniotic twinning results in a single amniotic sac containing both twins and occurs in approximately 1% of monozygotic gestations (D'Alton and Simpson, 1995). Prenatal diagnosis is established when a dividing membrane cannot be identified by an experienced sonographer in a twin gestation. The diagnosis is also confirmed after sonographic identification of entangled umbilical cords (Fig. 29-4); this feature has been reported in 70% to 100% of cases (Lee, 1992; Rodis et al., 1997). Cord entanglement has been diagnosed using color Doppler ultrasonography as early as 10 weeks' gestation (Arabin et al., 1999). It can be difficult to visualize the dividing membrane sonographically in certain situations, especially in the early first trimester. Other techniques used to diagnose monoamnionicity include sonographic visualization of only one yolk sac in a twin gestation at less than 10 weeks' gestation and amniography with iopamidol or indigo carmine–air mixture (Lavery and Gadwood, 1990; Tabsh, 1990; Bromley and Benacerraf, 1995).

Monoamniotic twins carry a higher risk of perinatal morbidity and mortality compared with diamniotic twins (54% perinatal mortality rate) (Carr et al., 1990). However, more recent series and reviews of prenatally diagnosed cases of monoamniotic twins suggest mortality rates ranging from 10% to 21% (Rodis et al., 1997; Allen et al., 2001). This risk may be secondary to premature delivery, growth restriction, congenital anomalies, vascular anastomoses between twins, and umbilical cord entanglement or cord accidents. Because umbilical cord accidents seem to be the primary cause of fetal death, most management protocols for monoamniotic twins emphasize intensive fetal surveillance. Such fetal surveillance should occur from the time of fetal viability, because intrauterine fetal demise has been documented in monoamniotic twins throughout gestation (Rodis et al., 1997; Arabin et al., 1999). Additionally, surveillance must be repeated frequently because fetal compromise and death have been documented despite twice-weekly fetal testing (Rodis et al., 1997). The only intervention described to reduce the incidence of cord accidents in monoamniotic twins is with maternal administration of the prostaglandin inhibitor sulindac, which results in decreased amniotic fluid volume, stabilizes fetal lie, and theoretically prevents cord compression (Peek et al., 1997). However, because of a lack of safety and efficacy evidence, such medical intervention should be considered experimental.

Because umbilical cord accidents are not predictable by our current methods of fetal surveillance and because continuous fetal heart monitoring throughout pregnancy is not feasible, we have managed monoamniotic twin gestations with daily non-stress tests from 26 weeks' gestation to evaluate for increasing frequency of variable decelerations. If variable decelerations increase in frequency, we perform continuous fetal heart monitoring and intervene with cesarean delivery if fetal heart testing becomes nonreassuring.

In the absence of nonreassuring fetal testing, the timing and mode of delivery of monoamniotic twins are controversial. In two series of 44 sets of monoamniotic twins, no fetal deaths occurred after 32 weeks, suggesting that prophylactic early delivery was not indicated (Carr et al., 1990; Tessen and Zlatnik, 1991). In an addendum to the Tessen and Zlatnik series, however, it was noted that a double fetal death occurred at 35 weeks' gestation in one monoamniotic twin set, therefore calling into question the safety of expectant management of monoamniotic twins beyond a gestational age at which neonatal morbidity is likely to be low. In these two series, vaginal delivery was achieved in more than 70% of cases, although in the series by Carr and coauthors the diagnosis of monoamniotic twins was made prenatally in only 21% of cases. Although vaginal delivery of monoamniotic twins is clearly possible, the incidence of cesarean delivery is high when fetal testing is nonreassuring. In addition, at delivery of the first twin's head, case reports have described cutting of a nuchal cord, which turned out to be the second twin's cord (McLeod and McCoy, 1981; Kantanka and Buchmann, 2001).

Because of these concerns about expectant management of monoamniotic twins, we electively perform cesarean delivery at 34 weeks' gestation after maternal administration of betamethasone. However, it is also reasonable to follow selected patients beyond this gestational age with careful fetal surveillance or to base timing of delivery on fetal lung maturity indices. Further, vaginal delivery may be acceptable if the patient has received continuous fetal heart monitoring and has been informed that an emergent cesarean delivery is possible.

Acardiac Twins

Acardiac twinning is a unique abnormality of multiple gestations in which one twin has an absent, rudimentary, or nonfunctioning heart. The incidence is estimated as 1% of monozygotic twin pregnancies, with birth estimates ranging from 1 in 35,000 to 1 in 150,000 births (D'Alton and Simpson, 1995). A more precise term may be *twin reversed arterial perfusion sequence*, which occurs because of the early development of arterial-to-arterial anastomoses between the umbilical arteries of two twin fetuses that share a fused placenta (Van Allen et al., 1983). Almost all cases occur in monochorionic twins, and previous theories of polar body fertilization to explain acardius in sex discordant twins have been excluded (Fisk et al., 1996).

The donor, or "pump twin," provides circulation for itself and for the recipient, or perfused, twin, through a direct umbilical arterial to umbilical arterial anastomosis at the placental surface. There is reversal of blood flow in the umbilical artery of the acardiac twin, with the artery bringing deoxygenated blood from the cotwin to the acardiac twin. This perfusion is usually asymmetrical in the recipient, or perfused, twin, with relative hypoperfusion of the upper part of the body, leading to

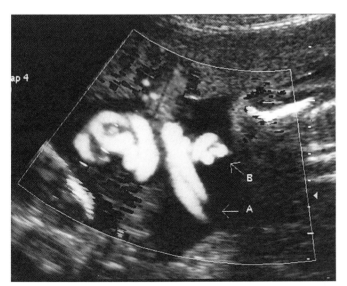

FIGURE 29-4 ■ Amplitude-based Doppler image of monoamniotic twins at 29 weeks' gestation demonstrates entangled umbilical cords. (Courtesy of Achilles Athanassiou, MD, New England Medical Center, Boston.)

significant structural anomalies in the perfused twin. A bizarre range of anomalies can be seen in the acardiac twin, including anencephaly, holoprosencephaly, absent limbs, absent lungs or heart, intestinal atresias, abdominal wall defects, and absent liver, spleen, or kidneys (Van Allen et al., 1983). Up to one third of the fetuses also have an abnormal karyotype, and 9% of pump twins have trisomy (Healey, 1994).

Prenatal diagnosis of acardiac twinning is based on the recognition of one normal-appearing fetus in a twin pregnancy, together with an additional profoundly abnormal-appearing fetus or amorphous mass of tissue. The pregnancy should be clearly monochorionic, and two thirds of cases demonstrate a single umbilical artery. The acardiac fetus may be unrecognizable as a fetus or may have an abnormally appearing head or trunk with no obvious heart. Sonographic signs of cardiac failure may be visible in the pump twin, including polyhydramnios, cardiomegaly, and tricuspid regurgitation. The differential diagnosis of acardiac twinning includes intrauterine fetal demise of one fetus and anencephaly. Doppler velocimetry of the umbilical cords demonstrating reversed direction of flow in the umbilical artery and vein may be helpful in confirming the diagnosis (Langlotz et al., 1991).

The goal of antepartum management of acardiac twin pregnancies is to maximize outcome for the structurally normal pump twin. The pump twin is at risk for development of hydrops or congestive cardiac failure, and this finding, factored with that of prematurity, results in a 55% perinatal mortality rate (Moore et al., 1990). In one series of 49 cases of acardiac twinning, the overall perinatal mortality rate for the pump twin was 55%, with polyhydramnios leading to prematurity being a major factor in prognosis (Moore et al., 1990). Prediction of prognosis for the pump twin depends on the ratio of perfused twin weight to weight of the pump twin, with a 30% chance of congestive cardiac failure when the ratio is greater than 0.70, compared with 10% when the ratio is less than 0.70. Because standard biometric parameters cannot be used to predict weight for the often grossly abnormal perfused twin, the following formula based on maximum linear measurement of the perfused twin is recommended (Moore et al., 1990):

$$Weight\ (g) = -1.66\ [length] + 1.21\ [length^2]$$

Management of acardiac twin gestations is controversial. In the absence of poor prognostic features (twin weight ratio > 0.70, congestive cardiac failure, polyhydramnios), expectant management with serial sonographic evaluation is reasonable (Malone and D'Alton, 2000). Serial weekly echocardiographic surveillance of the pump twin is recommended for early signs of cardiac failure, such as atrial or ventricular enlargement, tricuspid regurgitation, or decreased ventricular fractional shortening capacity. Rapid growth of the acardiac fetus may also be a sign of poor outcome (Brassard et al., 1999). Antenatal corticosteroid administration should be given if delivery is expected to occur between 24 and 34 weeks' gestation. Signs of cardiac decompensation after 32 to 34 weeks' gestation should prompt consideration for delivery. Antenatal intervention on behalf of the pump twin should be considered when such signs of cardiac failure are noted before 32 to 34 weeks' gestation. Medical management with maternal administration of digoxin or indomethacin has been reported, but no significant case series are available for review. More invasive management has included selective delivery by hysterotomy of

the acardiac recipient fetus, followed by successful interval delivery of the pump twin (Fries et al., 1992). This option now has only historic interest because of the availability of a range of less invasive percutaneous approaches to selective termination of the acardiac fetus.

Various percutaneous procedures have been described to interrupt the umbilical circulation in acardiac twins, including (1) insertion of a thrombogenic coil into the recipient twin's umbilical cord, (2) injection of silk soaked in alcohol into the cord, (3) injection of absolute alcohol into the cord, (4) fetoscopic ligation of the acardiac fetus's cord, (5) fetoscopic laser coagulation of the acardiac fetus's cord, (6) bipolar forceps cautery of the acardiac fetus's cord, (7) thermocoagulation of the aorta of the acardiac fetus (Porreco et al., 1991a; Holzgreve et al., 1994; Quintero et al., 1994; Sepulveda et al., 1995; Arias et al., 1998; Rodeck et al., 1998; Challis et al., 1999), or (8) radiofrequency thermablation (Tsao et al., 2002). Injection of coils or sclerosants is generally no longer performed because of unreliability in achieving complete occlusion. Fetoscopic cord ligation may be associated with a failure rate of 10% together with a 30% risk of preterm rupture of membranes (Challis et al., 1999). Laser and cautery options have the advantage of generally only requiring one access port in the uterus and therefore may be associated with less morbidity. No comparative studies are available, however, to suggest one optimal method of selective termination in this setting. The recurrence risk for acardiac twinning is estimated at 1 in 10,000 (Van Allen et al., 1983).

Conjoined Twins

Conjoined twins are a subset of monozygotic twin gestations in which incomplete embryonic division occurs 13 to 15 days after conception, resulting in varying degrees of fusion of the two fetuses. The estimated frequency of conjoined twinning is 1 in 50,000 births (D'Alton and Simpson, 1995). The prenatal diagnosis should be straightforward and is confirmed by failure to visualize two fetuses separately in what appears to be a single amniotic sac. Other sonographic features that assist in making the diagnosis include bifid appearance of the first-trimester fetal pole, more than three umbilical cord vessels, heads persistently at the same level and body plane, and failure of the fetuses to change position relative to each other over time (Van Den Brand et al., 1994). Prenatal diagnosis of conjoined twins has been made in the first trimester with the aid of three-dimensional sonography (Maymon et al., 1998). However, caution should be exercised in making a definite diagnosis of conjoined twins at less than 10 weeks' gestation, because false-positive diagnoses have been documented (Usta and Awaad, 2000).

By careful sonographic survey of the shared anatomy, it should be possible to classify conjoined twins into one of the following five types:

1. Thoracopagus, in which the two fetuses face each other, accounts for 75% of conjoined twins (Fig. 29-5). The fetuses usually have common sternum, diaphragm, upper abdominal wall, liver, pericardium, and gastrointestinal tract. Because 75% of thoracopagus twins have joined hearts, prognosis for surgical division is extremely poor.
2. Omphalopagus (or xiphopagus) is a rare subgroup of thoracopagus, in which there is an abdominal wall connection,

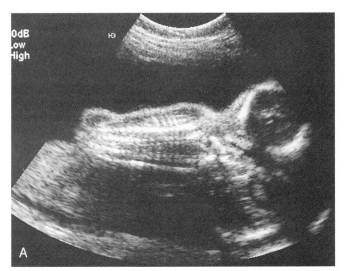

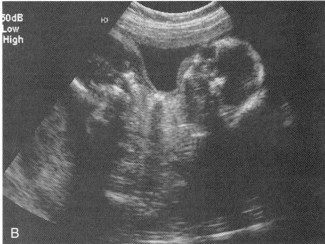

FIGURE 29-5 ■ Thoracopagus conjoined twins at 20 weeks' gestation demonstrating a single trunk containing two parallel spines (**A**) and leading to two separate heads (**B**).

often also with common liver. Because joined hearts are rare in omphalopagus, twins in this subgroup have a much better surgical prognosis than twins with other forms of thoracopagus.

3. Pygopagus accounts for 20% of cases, and because the twins share a common sacrum, they face away from each other. There is a single rectum and bladder, and prognosis for surgical separation is usually good.

4. Ischiopagus, in which the twins share a single common bony pelvis, accounts for 5% of conjoined twins. Surgical prognosis is good, although the remaining lower spines are often abnormal.

5. Craniopagus accounts for 1% of cases and is marked by partial or complete fusion of skull, meninges, and vascular structures. Surgical prognosis depends on the degree of fusion of vascular structures, in particular the presence of an adequate superior sagittal sinus to allow venous drainage (Van Den Brand et al., 1994).

Termination of pregnancy is commonly requested by parents of conjoined twins, especially in cases of thoracopagus with joined hearts. If expectant management is selected by parents, fetal echocardiography and possibly magnetic reso-

nance imaging should be used to delineate the exact extent of union and assist in neonatal surgical planning. In addition, a careful search must be made to exclude other anomalies that commonly coexist with conjoined twins. In one series of 14 sets of prenatally diagnosed conjoined twin pregnancies from a single center, the combination of prenatal ultrasonography, echocardiography, and magnetic resonance imaging accurately defined the anatomy in all cases (Mackenzie et al., 2002). In this series, 3 pregnancies were terminated, 1 resulted in intrauterine demise, and of the remaining 10 pregnancies delivered after viability, five individual fetuses survived. When expectant management is selected, cesarean section is the delivery method of choice to minimize maternal and fetal trauma (D'Alton and Simpson, 1995). Vaginal delivery is reasonable only in cases of extreme prematurity in which fetal survival is not an issue and maternal trauma should be less likely.

The surgical separation of conjoined twins, although beyond the scope of this chapter, has been summarized by Filler (1986). Tremendously complex moral and ethical debate can be expected in the neonatal period when trying to decide appropriate surgical options in cases of conjoined twins where only one twin has the potential of survival (Annas, 2001). We are unaware of any reported cases of recurrence after the diagnosis of conjoined twins.

Intrauterine Demise of One Fetus

Intrauterine demise of one fetus in a multiple gestation during the first trimester is common and has no established effect on the prognosis for the surviving fetus or fetuses. A "vanishing twin" was reported to occur in 21% of twin pregnancies, with no obvious detrimental effect on the remaining fetus (Landy et al., 1986). Intrauterine demise of one fetus in the second or third trimester is rarer (2% to 5% of twin pregnancies or 14% to 17% of triplet pregnancies) and has the potential for significant morbidity for the surviving fetus or fetuses (D'Alton and Simpson, 1995). The outcome of multiple gestations complicated by a single intrauterine demise is worse for monochorionic than for dichorionic gestations, with mean gestational ages at delivery of 30.6 and 32.9 weeks, respectively (Eglowstein and D'Alton, 1993).

The risk of significant neurologic morbidity is also increased after intrauterine demise of one fetus in a monochorionic, but not in a dichorionic, gestation. One of the most significant long-term complications, multicystic encephalomalacia leading to profound neurologic handicap, is estimated to occur in 12% of surviving fetuses after demise of a cotwin in a monochorionic gestation (D'Alton and Simpson, 1995). Neurologic morbidity has been reported after demise of a cotwin as early as 18 weeks of gestation (D'Alton and Simpson, 1995). In a review of birth certificate data from the United Kingdom, 434 gender-concordant twin pregnancies were found in which intrauterine demise of one fetus had occurred (Pharoah and Adi, 2000). The prevalence of cerebral palsy among surviving fetuses was 10.6% and the prevalence of other neurologic injury was 11.4%. The main limitation, however, of such birth certificate data is the inability to be sure of the prevalence of monochorionicity among the gender-concordant pairs. In a literature review of 119 monochorionic twin pregnancies complicated by single intrauterine fetal demise, 9% of surviving fetuses subsequently died *in utero*, a further 10% subsequently died in the neonatal period, and 24% had serious neonatal morbidity, including porencephaly, multicystic encephalomalacia, renal cortical necrosis, and small bowel atresia (Nicolini and Poblete, 1999).

Neurologic injury in the surviving fetus probably occurs because of significant hypotension at the time of demise of the cotwin. A previously proposed mechanism for this injury involving fetal disseminated intravascular coagulopathy as a result of fetal-to-fetal transfer of thromboplastic material from the dead fetus now appears unlikely. In a series of fetal blood sampling studies performed immediately before and after intrauterine demise of one twin, no evidence of fetal anemia was noted before fetal death, but all surviving fetuses were found to be anemic after death of the cotwin (Nicolini et al., 1998). This study is further evidence of acute blood loss from the surviving fetus into the dead fetus occurring at the time of fetal demise and suggests that subsequent obstetric intervention may not be able to influence eventual fetal outcome. Antenatal neurologic injury, such as multicystic encephalomalacia, may not be predictable by either ultrasound or cardiotocographic monitoring. The risk of neurologic morbidity is present from the moment of demise of one twin, and therefore expectant management may not be appropriate for monochorionic gestations in which one fetus appears to be in a premorbid condition (Malone and D'Alton, 1997). This 12% risk of multicystic encephalomalacia after demise of a cotwin must be weighed against the risk of complications of prematurity with a premorbid fetus in a monochorionic multiple gestation. If fetal demise has already occurred, close fetal surveillance for the surviving fetuses is recommended, although this may not prevent neurologic injury, which may already have occurred. Similarly, immediate delivery after diagnosis of the demise of one fetus in a monochorionic gestation may not protect the surviving fetus or fetuses from neurologic morbidity, most likely because of the instantaneous onset of such morbidity after demise of the cofetus. Delivery at 37 weeks, or after lung indices suggest maturity, is reasonable in such situations.

The maternal risks after intrauterine demise of one fetus have probably also been overestimated. Risk of maternal disseminated intravascular coagulopathy was once estimated at 25%, but in recent reviews of spontaneous fetal demise and selective termination in multiple gestations, no clinical cases of disseminated intravascular coagulopathy have been noted. Our practice has been to obtain a baseline set of coagulation indices after diagnosis of a demise of one fetus, and subsequent laboratory surveillance with coagulopathy studies is probably unnecessary (Malone and D'Alton, 1997).

Selective Termination of an Anomalous Fetus

When a multiple gestation is complicated by the discovery of a significant anomaly in one fetus, counseling of parents and management decisions are difficult. Factors to incorporate into the decision-making analysis include the following:

- Severity of the anomaly
- Chorionicity of the pregnancy
- Effect of the anomalous fetus on the normal cotwin or cotriplets
- Ethical beliefs of the parents

Three main choices are available (Malone and D'Alton, 1997), as follows:

- Expectant management
- Termination of the entire pregnancy
- "Selective termination" of the anomalous fetus

The term selective termination is used specifically to describe deliberate termination of a particular fetus in a multiple gestation, almost always in the second trimester, to optimize outcome for the normal fetus and to prevent delivery of an abnormal fetus. This differs from "multifetal reduction," a nonspecific reduction in the number of fetuses present in a higher order multiple gestation, almost always in the first trimester, to lower the risk of prematurity for the remaining fetuses (Berkowitz and Lynch, 1990).

Expectant management of a multiple gestation complicated by a single anomalous fetus is not without risks. These risks include an additional 20% increase in risk of preterm delivery attributable to the presence of an anomalous fetus and lower gestational age at delivery, lower birth weight, and higher cesarean delivery rate in twin pregnancies with anomalies compared with normal twins (Malone et al., 1996). In addition, expectant management of twins discordant for anencephaly is associated with an increased rate of intrauterine lethality for the normal cotwin in monochorionic gestations and with an increased rate of premature delivery, probably secondary to polyhydramnios, in both monochorionic and dichorionic gestations (Sebire et al., 1997). Amnioreduction to lessen the incidence of prematurity may therefore be reasonable when significant polyhydramnios develops in twins discordant for anencephaly.

The method of selective termination depends on the chorionicity (Malone and D'Alton, 1997). In dichorionic gestations, ultrasound-guided intracardiac injection of potassium chloride is the most common technique; in monochorionic gestations, complete ablation of the umbilical cord of the anomalous fetus is required to avoid death or neurologic injury in the normal fetus. Techniques used successfully to date include the following:

1. Hysterotomy (Fries et al., 1992)
2. Percutaneous injection of absolute alcohol or other occlusive materials into the umbilical cord or intrahepatic vein (Sepulveda et al., 1995)
3. Fetoscopic cord ligation (Quintero et al., 1994; Challis et al., 1999)
4. Fetoscopic laser ablation of umbilical vessels (Challis et al., 1999)
5. Bipolar forceps cautery of umbilical cord (Challis et al., 1999)
6. Fetoscopic transection of umbilical cord using ultrasonic harmonic scalpel (Lopoo et al., 2000)
7. Radiofrequency thermablation of umbilical cord (Tsao et al., 2002)

These selective termination procedures for monochorionic gestations are significantly more complicated than the potassium chloride injection procedure used for dichorionic gestations. Little data are available to counsel patients as to the safety and efficacy of each of these monochorionic techniques. Earlier procedures such as hysterotomy and injection of various sclerosants have largely been abandoned because of more recent development of less invasive and more effective techniques. Fetoscopic cord ligation may be associated with a 10% procedure failure rate and up to 30% risk of preterm rupture of membranes (Challis et al., 1999). In addition, reports of fetoscopic ligation of the cord of the normal fetus have also been described (Young et al., 2001). More recent procedures, such as bipolar cautery and aortic thermocoagulation, using single fetoscopic ports or single spinal needle access with sonographic guidance, may be safer. However, insufficient data exist at this time to recommend one of these procedures as the optimal choice for selective termination in monochorionic gestations.

Before performing the procedure, the physician must confirm that the targeted fetus has the anomaly in question. If the abnormal fetus has a structural anomaly, correct fetal identification is straightforward. If a chromosomal abnormality exists without structural markers and there is doubt about the position of the target fetus, repeated chromosomal analysis using rapid techniques (e.g., fetal blood sampling or fluorescence *in situ* hybridization) is required immediately before termination. The physician must be certain of the chorionicity of the pregnancy. Potassium chloride injection is contraindicated if dichorionicity cannot be confirmed with certainty. If such sonographic confirmation cannot be obtained, DNA zygosity studies on amniocytes may be required in excluding monochorionicity (Norton et al., 1997).

Results of selective termination from a large multicenter study of 402 cases of twins, triplets, quadruplets, and quintuplets demonstrated a 100% technical success rate, with an 8% rate of pregnancy loss before 24 weeks (5% if procedure performed before 12 weeks versus 9% if performed from 13 to 18 weeks and 7% if performed from 19 to 24 weeks) (Evans et al., 1999). All procedures used intracardiac potassium chloride injection. In addition, another 6% of patients delivered between 25 and 28 weeks, 8% between 29 and 32 weeks, and 17% between 33 and 36 weeks. There were no cases of laboratory or clinical coagulopathies or other complications in mothers (Evans et al., 1999).

A large series from a single center of 200 cases of twins, triplets, and quadruplets demonstrated increased risks of preterm delivery if the presenting twin was terminated and an increased risk of pregnancy loss among triplet pregnancies (Eddleman et al., 2001). The overall unintended pregnancy loss rate at this center was 4% but increased to 12.5% for selective termination in triplet gestation. Selective termination of a single anomalous fetus in a multiple gestation therefore seems to be a reasonable management option. These data should be used to counsel patients according to the unique circumstances of each case.

Multifetal Pregnancy Reduction

The goal of first-trimester multifetal pregnancy reduction (MFPR) is to reduce the number of fetuses in a higher order multiple gestation to decrease the chance of premature delivery and thereby to improve the outcome for the remaining fetuses. Higher order multiple gestations are associated with a significant risk of delivery before viability. Fetuses that reach viability have a significant risk of birth before 28 weeks, when serious long-term neonatal morbidity is likely.

The natural history of triplet gestation suggests a 7% to 8% risk of delivery from 24 to 28 weeks' gestation (Stone and Eddleman, 2000; Devine et al., 2001). The natural history of quadruplet gestation suggests a 14% risk of delivery before 28 weeks' gestation (Stone and Eddleman, 2000). The risk of spontaneous loss of a triplet pregnancy before 24 weeks' gesta-

tion is approximately 11% (Stone and Eddleman, 2000). The risk of losing the entire pregnancy before 20 or 24 weeks in quadruplet or higher gestations is unknown because generally only pregnancies that successfully reach 20 weeks' gestation are reported in the literature. In addition, the risks to maternal health of expectantly managed higher order multiple gestations are significant. All the risks just described should be carefully discussed with each couple during counseling before selecting a management plan in all cases of higher order multiple gestations.

The technique of transabdominal MFPR, as generally performed between 10 and 13 weeks, is straightforward (Berkowitz et al., 1996). The patient may receive an oral sedative agent and a single oral antibiotic dose (pentobarbital, 200 mg; dicloxacillin, 500 mg) immediately before the procedure. Ultrasonography is used to precisely map the location of all gestations within the uterus, and measurements are taken of crown-rump length and nuchal translucency thickness. If an abnormality is found or if these measurements are abnormal in a particular fetus, that fetus is targeted for reduction. Otherwise, the fetus or fetuses that are technically easiest to access are targeted, with the exception of the fetus overlying the internal os, which is rarely reduced. Under continuous ultrasound guidance and with sterile technique, a 22-gauge needle is placed into the thorax of the targeted fetus, followed by injection of 2 to 3 mEq of potassium chloride, and asystole is observed for at least 3 minutes. The procedure is then repeated for additional fetuses as required, with a different needle. Another ultrasound study is performed 1 hour after the procedure and again 1 week later to confirm demise of the targeted fetuses and viability of the remaining fetuses. Transvaginal MFPR is less commonly performed because it is associated with significantly higher loss rates when compared with the transabdominal approach (12% versus 5%, respectively) (Evans et al., 2001).

A current area of debate with MFPR is the role of prenatal diagnosis before or after the procedure. Options for prenatal diagnosis in this setting include amniocentesis for surviving fetuses 4 weeks after MFPR and CVS for some or all fetuses before MFPR. Amniocentesis after MFPR does not appear to further increase the risk of pregnancy loss (McLean et al., 1998). The main drawback of CVS is that if an abnormality is subsequently discovered, patients may have to consider yet another reduction procedure. CVS has also been shown to be safe when performed before MFPR, with success rates over 99% and with no obvious increase in the risk of pregnancy loss (Eddleman et al., 2000). Decisions on which placentas to sample are made based on starting fetal number, finishing fetal number, likely target fetuses, and ease of access to particular placentas. A sampling error rate of 1% to 2% can be expected.

The overall pregnancy loss rate before 24 weeks for transabdominal MFPR procedures is 5%, down from an earlier reported loss rate of 8%, probably reflecting a procedure-related learning curve (Evans et al., 2001). It is impossible to be certain how much of this loss is due to the spontaneous wastage seen with multiple gestations and how much is directly caused by the invasive procedure. The most recent international collaborative MFPR data from over 3500 pregnancies demonstrate that the loss rate before 24 weeks is directly related to both the starting and the finishing number of fetuses (Evans et al., 2001). This loss rate decreases from 22% to 15%, 12%, 6%, and 6% with six, five, four, three, and two fetuses

TABLE 29-5. SUMMARY OF EIGHT STUDIES COMPARING OUTCOME OF EXPECTANTLY MANAGED TRIPLET GESTATIONS, WITH TRIPLETS REDUCED TO TWINS, AND WITH NONREDUCED TWIN GESTATIONS

Pregnancy Type	Number of Pregnancies	Pregnancy Loss Rate <24 Wk (%)	Preterm Delivery Rate 24–28 Wk (%)	Gestational Age at Delivery (wk)	Birth Weight (g)	Perinatal Mortality Rate (per 1000)
Triplets, expectant	381	13	8	33.1	1879	80
Twins, reduced from triplets	412	7	3	35.4	2353	46
Twins, nonreduced	778	5	7	34.6	2187	35

From Porreco et al, 1991b; Melgar et al, 1991; Macones et al, 1993; Lipitz et al, 1994; Smith-Levitin et al, 1996; Yaron et al, 1999; Boulot et al, 2000; Leondires et al, 2000.

present, respectively, at the start of the procedure. In addition, the risk of very premature delivery at 25 to 28 weeks decreases from 6% to 6%, 4%, 3%, and 1% with six, five, four, three, and two fetuses present, respectively, at the start of the procedure. The optimal finishing number of fetuses appears to be twins, with a loss rate before 24 weeks of 9%, compared with 20% for triplets. Reflecting the importance of the learning curve, these authors demonstrated that the pregnancy loss rates for MFPR procedures performed most recently (1995 to 1998) were 4% for triplets reduced to twins and 7% for quadruplets reduced to twins (Evans et al., 2001).

For fetuses that reach viability after MFPR, 85% to 90% can be expected to be born at 32 weeks' gestation or later, with only 3% to 5% born between 25 and 28 weeks (Berkowitz et al., 1996). At this stage, MFPR is clearly associated with better outcomes for patients with quadruplet and higher gestations. When counseling such patients, the option of MFPR should be presented and patients should be informed that their best chance of delivering healthy surviving infants is by undergoing MFPR. Much debate still exists, however, on the role of MFPR for triplet gestation. Over the last decade, there have been eight studies published in which the outcome of expectantly managed triplet gestations has been compared with the outcome of triplet reduced to twin pregnancies and also compared with nonreduced twin pregnancies (Melgar et al., 1991; Porreco et al., 1991b; Macones et al., 1993; Lipitz et al., 1994; Smith-Levitin et al., 1996; Yaron et al., 1999; Boulot et al., 2000; Leondires et al., 2000). These data are summarized in Table 29-5. As can be seen from Table 29-5, for all measures of perinatal outcome, reduction of triplets to twins yields improvements, with overall outcomes similar to that expected for nonreduced twin gestations. Additionally, some data suggest that maternal complications can also be decreased when triplets are reduced to twins, with one study suggesting a 22% incidence of gestational diabetes among nonreduced triplet pregnancies, compared with 6% incidence among triplets reduced to twins (Sivan et al., 2002).

The data of published studies summarized in Table 29-5 may be a little misleading, however, particularly with reference to perinatal mortality rates. MFPR involves the obligate death of one fetus in a triplet gestation, so that the overall fetal mortality rate for triplets reduced to twins must be at least 333 per 1000. This may not be clear to patients if the perinatal mortality rates of 46 to 80 per 1000, as shown in Table 29-5, are presented. Additionally, no long-term outcome data for the survivors of reduced triplet pregnancies are available. We believe the available information does make a convincing argument to include MFPR in the counseling of all patients

with triplet gestations. For an individual patient to select MFPR with triplets, they must decide if the obligate death of one fetus, together with a 4% risk of procedure-related pregnancy loss, justifies a 500-g birth-weight increase, a 2-week gestational age increase, and a 50% reduction of the risk of delivery before 24 and 28 weeks' gestation. This decision should be individualized in all cases.

After the MFPR procedure, patients should be followed closely for the usual complications of multiple gestation. Surveillance of the pregnancy for appropriate fetal growth is recommended because there may be an increased risk of intrauterine growth restriction after MFPR (Depp et al., 1996). In addition, the psychological implications for mothers who have undergone MFPR can be significant. Seventy percent of these women demonstrate grief reactions, and 84% describe the procedure as very stressful (Schreiner-Engel et al., 1995).

In view of the complex issues involved, MFPR should not be considered a simple solution to the problems of higher order multiple gestations in this era of assisted reproductive technologies (Berkowitz et al., 1996). Instead, attention should be focused on prevention of the problem, which may be alleviated at least in part through careful supervision of assisted reproductive practices.

REFERENCES

Adams DM, Sholl JS, Haney EI, et al: Perinatal outcome associated with outpatient management of triplet pregnancy. Am J Obstet Gynecol **178**:843, 1998.

Akiyama M, Kuno A, Tanaka Y, et al: Comparison of alterations in fetal regional arterial vascular resistance in appropriate-for-gestational-age singleton, twin and triplet pregnancies. Hum Reprod **14**:2635, 1999.

Alamia V, Royek AB, Jaekle RK, et al: Preliminary experience with a prospective protocol for planned vaginal delivery of triplet gestations. Am J Obstet Gynecol **179**:1133, 1998.

Albrecht JL, Tomich PG: The maternal and neonatal outcome of triplet gestations. Am J Obstet Gynecol **174**:1551, 1996.

Allen VM, Windrim R, Barrett J, et al: Management of monoamniotic twin pregnancies: A case series and systematic review of the literature. Br J Obstet Gynaecol **108**:931, 2001.

Alvarez M, Berkowitz RL: Multifetal gestation. Clin Obstet Gynecol **33**:79, 1990.

American College of Obstetricians and Gynecologists: Special Problems of Multiple Gestation (Educational Bulletin No. 253). Washington, DC, American College of Obstetricians and Gynecologists, 1998.

Annas GJ: Conjoined twins—The limits of law at the limits of life. N Engl J Med **344**:1104, 2001.

Arabin B, Laurini RN, van Eyck J: Early prenatal diagnosis of cord entanglement in monoamniotic multiple pregnancies. Ultrasound Obstet Gynecol **13**:181, 1999.

Arias F, Sunderji S, Gimpelson R, et al: Treatment of acardiac twinning. Obstet Gynecol **91**:818, 1998.

Bajoria R, Ward S, Chatterjee R: Natriuretic peptides in the pathogenesis of cardiac dysfunction in the recipient fetus of twin-twin transfusion syndrome. Am J Obstet Gynecol 186:121, 2002.

Bajoria R, Wigglesworth J, Fisk NM: Angioarchitecture of monochorionic placentas in relation to the twin-twin transfusion syndrome. Am J Obstet Gynecol 172:856, 1995.

Barss VA, Benacerraf BR, Frigoletto FD: Ultrasonographic determination of chorion type in twin gestation. Obstet Gynecol 66:779, 1985.

Benirschke K, Kim CK: Multiple pregnancy. N Engl J Med 288:1276, 1973.

Berkowitz RL, Lynch L: Selective reduction: An unfortunate misnomer. Obstet Gynecol 75:873, 1990.

Berkowitz RL, Lynch L, Stone J, Alvarez M: The current status of multifetal pregnancy reduction. Am J Obstet Gynecol 174:1265, 1996.

Blickstein I, Goldman RD, Kupferminc M: Delivery of breech first twins: a multicenter retrospective study. Obstet Gynecol 95:37, 2000.

Bloomfield MM, Philipson EH: External cephalic version of twin A. Obstet Gynecol 89:814, 1997.

Boulot P, Hedon B, Pelliccia G, et al: Favorable outcome in 33 triplet pregnancies managed between 1985–1990. Eur J Obstet Gynaecol Reprod Biol 43:123, 1992.

Boulot P, Vignal J, Vergnes C, et al: Multifetal reduction of triplets to twins: A prospective comparison of pregnancy outcome. Hum Reprod 15:1619, 2000.

Brassard M, Fouron JC, Leduc L, et al: Prognostic markers in twin pregnancies with an acardiac fetus. Obstet Gynecol 94:409, 1999.

Bromley B, Benacerraf B: Using the number of yolk sacs to determine amnionicity in early first trimester monochorionic twins. J Ultrasound Med 14:415, 1995.

Bruner JP, Rosemond RL: Twin-to-twin transfusion syndrome: A subset of the twin oligohydramnios-polyhydramnios sequence. Am J Obstet Gynecol 169:925, 1993.

Campbell DM: Maternal adaptation in twin pregnancy. Semin Perinatol 10:14, 1986.

Caravello JW, Chauhan SP, Morrison JC, et al: Sonographic examination does not predict twin growth discordance accurately. Obstet Gynecol 89:529, 1997.

Caritis S, Sibai B, Hauth J, et al: Low-dose aspirin to prevent preeclampsia in women at high risk. N Engl J Med 338:701, 1998.

Carr SR, Aronson MP, Coustan DR: Survival rates of monoamniotic twins do not decrease after 30 weeks' gestation. Am J Obstet Gynecol 163:719, 1990.

Challis D, Gratacos E, Deprest JA: Cord occlusion techniques for selective termination in monochorionic twins. J Perinat Med 27:327, 1999.

Chau AC, Kjos SL, Kovacs BW: Ultrasonographic measurement of amniotic fluid volume in normal diamniotic twin pregnancies. Am J Obstet Gynecol 174:1003, 1996.

Chervenak FA, Johnson RE, Berkowitz RL, et al: Intrapartum external version of the second twin. Obstet Gynecol 62:160, 1983.

Cincotta R, Oldham J, Sampson A: Antepartum and postpartum complications of twin-twin transfusion. Aust N Z J Obstet Gynaecol 36:303, 1996.

Clarke JP, Roman JD: A review of 19 sets of triplets: The positive results of vaginal delivery. Aust N Z J Obstet Gynaecol 34:50, 1994.

Collins MS, Bleyl JA: Seventy-one quadruplet pregnancies: Management and outcome. Am J Obstet Gynecol 162:1384, 1990.

Colton T, Kayne HL, Zhang Y, et al: A meta-analysis of home uterine activity monitoring. Am J Obstet Gynecol 173:1499, 1995.

Crowther CA: Hospitalisation and bed rest for multiple pregnancy. Cochrane Database Syst Rev 1:CD000110, 2001.

Cuckle H, Wald N, Stevenson JD, et al: Maternal serum alpha-fetoprotein screening for open neural tube defects in twin pregnancies. Prenat Diagn 10:71, 1990.

D'Alton ME, Dudley DK: The ultrasonographic prediction of chorionicity in twin gestation. Am J Obstet Gynecol 160:557, 1989.

D'Alton ME, Mercer BM: Antepartum management of twin gestation: Ultrasound. Clin Obstet Gynecol 33:42, 1990.

D'Alton ME, Simpson LL: Syndromes in twins. Semin Perinatol 19:375, 1995.

Davidson KM, Simpson LL, Knox TA, et al: Acute fatty liver of pregnancy in triplet gestation. Obstet Gynceol 91:806, 1998.

De Lia J, Fisk N, Hecher K, et al: Twin-to-twin transfusion syndrome—Debates on the etiology, natural history and management. Ultrasound Obstet Gynecol 16:210, 2000.

De Lia JE, Kuhlmann RS, Lopez KP: Treating previable twin-twin transfusion syndrome with fetoscopic laser surgery: Outcomes following the learning curve. J Perinat Med 27:61, 1999.

Denbow M, Fogliani R, Kyle P, et al: Hematological indices at fetal blood sampling in monochorionic pregnancies complicated by feto-fetal transfusion syndrome. Prenat Diagn 18:941, 1998.

Denbow ML, Blomley MJK, Cosgrove DO, et al: Ultrasound microbubble angiography in monochorionic twin fetuses. Lancet 349:773, 1997.

Depp R, Macone GA, Rosenn MF, et al: Multifetal pregnancy reduction: Evaluation of fetal growth in the remaining twins. Am J Obstet Gynecol 174:1233, 1996.

Devine PC, Malone FD, Athanassiou A, et al: Maternal and neonatal outcome of 100 consecutive triplet pregnancies. Am J Perinatol 18:225, 2001.

Dickey RP, Olar TT, Curole DN, et al: The probability of multiple births when multiple gestational sacs or viable embryos are diagnosed at first trimester ultrasound. Hum Reprod 5:880, 1990.

Divon MY, Weiner Z: Ultrasound in twin pregnancy. Semin Perinatol 19:404, 1995.

Dommergues M, Mahieu-Caputo D, Mandelbrot L, et al: Delivery of uncomplicated triplet pregnancies: Is the vaginal route safer? Am J Obstet Gynecol 172:513, 1995.

Dorman K, Saade GR, Smith H, et al: Use of the world wide web in research: Randomization in a multicenter clinical trial of treatment for twin-twin transfusion syndrome. Obstet Gynecol 96:636, 2000.

Dyson DC, Danbe KH, Bamber JA, et al: Monitoring women at risk for preterm labor. N Engl J Med 338:15, 1998.

Eddleman K, Stone J, Lynch L, et al: Selective termination of anomalous fetuses in multiple pregnancies: 200 cases at a single center. Am J Obstet Gynecol 185:S79, 2001.

Eddleman KA, Stone JL, Lynch L, et al: Chorionic villus sampling before multifetal pregnancy reduction. Am J Obstet Gynecol 183:1078, 2000.

Edwards MS, Ellings JM, Newman RB, et al: Predictive value of antepartum ultrasound examination for anomalies in twin gestations. Ultrasound Obstet Gynecol 6:43, 1995.

Eglowstein MS, D'Alton ME: Single intra-uterine demise in twin gestation. J Maternal Fetal Med 2:272, 1993.

Elimian A, Figueroa R, Nigam S, et al: Perinatal outcome of triplet gestation: Does prophylactic cerclage make a difference? J Maternal Fetal Med 8:119, 1999.

Elliott JP, Radin TG: Quadruplet pregnancy: Contemporary management and outcome. Obstet Gynecol 80:421, 1992.

Erkkola R, Ala-Mello S, Piiroinen O, et al: Growth discordancy in twin pregnancies: A risk factor not detected by measurements of biparietal diameter. Obstet Gynecol 66:203, 1985.

Evans MI, Berkowitz RL, Wapner RJ, et al: Improvement in outcomes of multifetal pregnancy reduction with increased experience. Am J Obstet Gynecol 184:97, 2001.

Evans MI, Goldberg JD, Horenstein J, et al: Selective termination for structural, chromosomal and mendelian anomalies: International experience. Am J Obstet Gynecol 181:893, 1999.

Farkouh LJ, Sabin ED, Heyborne KD, et al: Delayed-interval delivery: Extended series from a single maternal-fetal medicine practice. Am J Obstet Gynecol 183:1499, 2000.

Fesslova V, Villa L, Nava S, et al: Fetal and neonatal echocardiographic findings in twin-twin transfusion syndrome. Am J Obstet Gynecol 179:1056, 1998.

Filler RM: Conjoined twins and their separation. Semin Perinatol 10:82, 1986.

Fisk NM, Ware M, Stanier P, et al: Molecular genetic etiology of twin reversed arterial perfusion sequence. Am J Obstet Gynecol 174:891, 1996.

Fries MH, Goldberg JD, Golbus MA: Treatment of acardiac-acephalus twin gestations by hysterotomy and selective delivery. Obstet Gynecol 79:601, 1992.

Gardner MO, Wenstrom KD: Maternal adaptation. In Gall SA (ed): Multiple Pregnancy and Delivery. Mosby, St. Louis, 1996, p. 99.

Ghidini A, Lynch L, Hicks C, et al: The risk of second-trimester amniocentesis in twin gestations: A case-control study. Am J Obstet Gynecol 169:1013, 1993.

Gocke SE, Nageotte MP, Garite T, et al: Management of the nonvertex second twin: Primary cesarean section, external version, or primary breech extraction. Am J Obstet Gynecol 161:111, 1989.

Goldenberg RL, Iams JD, Miodovnik M, National Institute of Child Health and Human Development Maternal-Fetal Medicine Units Network: The preterm prediction study: Risk factors in twin gestations. Am J Obstet Gynecol 175:1047, 1996.

Grumbach K, Coleman BG, Arger PH, et al: Twin and singleton growth patterns compared using ultrasound. Radiology 158:237, 1986.

Hardardottir H, Kelly K, Bork MD, et al: Atypical presentation of preeclampsia in high-order multifetal gestations. Obstet Gynecol 87:370, 1996.

Healey MG: Acardia: Predictive risk factors for the co-twin's survival. Teratology **50**:205, 1994.

Hecher K, Diehl W, Zikulnig L, et al: Endoscopic laser coagulation of placental anastomoses in 200 pregnancies with severe mid-trimester twin-to-twin transfusion syndrome. Eur J Obstet Gynaecol Reprod Biol **92**:135, 2000.

Hecher K, Plath H, Bregenze T, et al: Endoscopic laser surgery versus serial amniocenteses in the treatment of severe twin-twin transfusion syndrome. Am J Obstet Gynecol **180**:717, 1999.

Hill LM, Guzick D, Chenevey P, et al: The sonographic assessment of twin growth discordancy. Obstet Gynecol **84**:501, 1994.

Hollier LM, McIntire DD, Leveno KJ: Outcome of twin pregnancies according to intrapair birth weight differences. Obstet Gynecol **94**:1006, 1999.

Holzgreve W, Tercanli S, Krings W, et al: A simpler technique for umbilical-cord blockade of an acardiac twin. N Engl J Med **331**:56, 1994.

Imseis HM, Albert TA, Iams JD: Identifying twin gestations at low risk for preterm birth with a transvaginal ultrasonographic cervical measurement at 24–26 weeks' gestation. Am J Obstet Gynecol **177**:1149, 1997.

Johnson JR, Rossi KQ, O'Shaughnessy RW: Amnioreduction versus septostomy in twin-twin transfusion syndrome. Am J Obstet Gynecol **185**:1044, 2001.

Jonas HA, Lumley J: Triplets and quadruplets born in Victoria between 1982 and 1990. The impact of IVF and GIFT on rising birthrates. Med J Aust **158**:659, 1993.

Jones JM, Sbarra AJ, Delillo L, et al: Indomethacin in severe twin-to-twin transfusion syndrome. Am J Perinatol **10**:24, 1993.

Katanka KS, Buchmann EJ: Vaginal delivery of monoamniotic twins with umbilical cord entanglement. A case report. J Reprod Med **46**:275, 2001.

Kaufman GE, Malone FD, Harvey-Wilkes KB, et al: Neonatal morbidity and mortality associated with triplet pregnancy. Obstet Gynecol **91**:342, 1998.

Keirse MJNC, Grant A, King JF: Preterm labour. In Chalmers I, Enkin M, Keirse MJNC (eds): Effective Care in Pregnancy and Childbirth. Oxford University Press, New York, 1989, p. 644.

King AD, Soothill PW, Montemagno R, et al: Twin-to-twin blood transfusion in a dichorionic pregnancy without the oligohydramnios-polyhydramnios sequence. Br J Obstet Gynaecol **102**:334, 1995.

Kovacs BW, Kirschbaum TH, Paul RH: Twin gestations. 1. Antenatal care and complications. Obstet Gynecol **74**:313, 1989.

Lage JM, Vanmarter LJ, Mikhail E: Vascular anastomoses in fused, dichorionic twin placentas resulting in twin transfusion syndrome. Placenta **10**:55, 1989.

Landy HJ, Weiner S, Corson SL, et al: The "vanishing twin": Ultrasonographic assessment of fetal disappearance in the first trimester. Am J Obstet Gynecol **155**:14, 1986.

Langlotz H, Sauerbrei E, Murray S: Transvaginal Doppler sonographic diagnosis of an acardiac twin at 12 weeks' gestation. J Ultrasound Med **10**:175, 1991.

Lavery J, Gadwood KA: Amniography for confirming the diagnosis of monoamniotic twinning: A case report. J Reprod Med **35**:911, 1990.

Lavery JP, Austin RF, Schaefer DS, et al: Asynchronous multiple birth: A report of five cases. J Reprod Med **39**:55, 1994.

Lee CY: Management of monoamniotic twins diagnosed antenatally by ultrasound. Am J Gynecol Health **6**:25, 1992.

LeFevre ML, Bain RP, Ewigman BG, the RADIUS Study Group: A randomized trial of prenatal ultrasonographic screening: Impact on maternal management and outcome. Am J Obstet Gynecol **169**:483, 1993.

Leondires MP, Ernst SD, Miller BT, et al: Triplets: Outcomes of expectant management versus multifetal reduction for 127 pregnancies. Am J Obstet Gynecol **183**:454, 2000.

Leung TY, Tam WH, Leung TN, et al: Effect of twin-to-twin delivery interval on umbilical cord blood gas in the second twins. Br J Obstet Gynaecol **109**:63, 2002.

Leveno KJ, Quirk JG, Whalley PJ, et al: Fetal lung maturity in twin gestation. Am J Obstet Gynecol **148**:405, 1984.

Lipitz S, Reichman B, Paret G, et al: The improving outcome of triplet pregnancies. Am J Obstet Gynecol **161**:1279, 1989.

Lipitz S, Reichman B, Uval J, et al: A prospective comparison of the outcome of triplet pregnancies managed expectantly or by multifetal reduction to twins. Am J Obstet Gynecol **170**:874, 1994.

Lipitz S, Seidman DS, Alcalay M, et al: The effect of fertility drugs and in vitro methods on the outcome of 106 triplet pregnancies. Fertil Steril **60**:1031, 1993.

Lopoo JB, Paek BW, Maichin GA, et al: Cord ultrasonic transection procedure for selective termination of a monochorionic twin. Fetal Diagn Ther **15**:177, 2000.

Lougheed J, Sinclair BG, Fung Kee Fung K, et al: Acquired right ventricular outflow tract obstruction in the recipient twin in twin-twin transfusion syndrome. J Am Coll Cardiol **38**:1533, 2001.

Luke B: The changing pattern of multiple births in the United States: Maternal and infant characteristics, 1973 and 1990. Obstet Gynecol **84**:101, 1994.

Luke B, Bryan E, Sweetland C, et al: Prenatal weight gain and the birthweight of triplets. Acta Genet Med Gemell **44**:93, 1995.

Luke B, Keith LG: The contribution of singletons, twins and triplets to low birth weight, infant mortality and handicap in the United States. J Reprod Med **37**:661, 1992.

Lynch A, McDuffie R, Murphy J, et al: Preeclampsia in multiple gestations: the role of assisted reproductive technologies. Obstet Gynecol **99**:445, 2002.

Machin GA, Feldstein VA, Van Gemert MJ, et al: Dopler sonographic demonstration of arterio-venous anastomoses in monochorionic twin gestation. Ultrasound Obstet Gynecol **16**:214, 2000.

Mackenzie TC, Crombleholme TM, Johnson MP, et al: The natural history of prenatally diagnosed conjoined twins. J Pediatr Surg **37**:303, 2002.

MacLennan AH, Green RC, O'Shea R, et al: Routine hospital admission in twin pregnancy between 26 and 30 weeks' gestation. Lancet **335**:267, 1990.

Macones GA, Schemmer G, Pritts E, et al: Multifetal reduction of triplets to twins improves perinatal outcome. Am J Obstet Gynecol **169**:982, 1993.

Magann EF, Whitworth NS, Bass JD, et al: Amniotic fluid volume of third-trimester diamniotic twin pregnancies. Obstet Gynecol **85**:957, 1995.

Malone FD, Craigo SD, Chelmow D, et al: Outcome of twin gestations complicated by a single anomalous fetus. Obstet Gynecol **88**:1, 1996.

Malone FD, D'Alton ME: Management of multiple gestations complicated by a single anomalous fetus. Curr Opin Obstet Gynecol **9**:213, 1997.

Malone FD, D'Alton ME: Anomalies peculiar to multiple gestations. Clin Perinatol **27**:1033, 2000.

Mari G, Dett L, Oz U, et al: Long-term outcome in twin-twin transfusion syndrome treated with serial aggressive amnioreduction. Am J Obstet Gynecol **183**:211, 2000.

Mari G, Roberts A, Detti L, et al: Perinatal morbidity and mortality rates in severe twin-twin transfusion syndrome: Results of the International Amnioreduction Registry. Am J Obstet Gynecol **185**:708, 2001.

Martin JA, Hamilton BE, Ventura SJ, et al: Births: Final Data for 2000. National Vital Statistics Reports, vol. 50, No 5. Hyattsville, Md, National Center for Health Statistics, 2002.

Maxwell CV, Lieberman E, Norton M, et al: Relationship of twin zygosity and risk of preeclampsia. Am J Obstet Gynecol **185**:819, 2001.

Maymon R, Dreazen E, Tovbin Y, et al: The feasibility of nuchal translucency measurement in higher order multiple gestations achieved by assisted reproduction. Hum Reprod **14**:2102, 1999.

Maymon R, Halperin R, Weinraub Z, et al: Three-dimensional transvaginal sonography of conjoined twins at 10 weeks: a case report. Ultrasound Obstet Gynecol **11**:292, 1998.

McElrath T, Kaimal A, Benson C, et al: Gestational age at delivery of triplet pregnancies as a function of cervical length throughout gestation. Am J Obstet Gynecol **185**:S250, 2001.

McLean LK, Evans MI, Carpenter RJ, et al: Genetic amniocentesis following multifetal pregnancy reduction does not increase the risk of pregnancy loss. Prenat Diagn **18**:186, 1998.

McLeod FN, McCoy DR: Monoamniotic twins with an unusual cord complication. Br J Obstet Gynaecol **88**:774, 1981.

Melgar CA, Rosenfeld DL, Rawlinson K, et al: Perinatal outcome after multifetal reduction to twins compared with nonreduced multiple gestations. Obstet Gynecol **78**:763, 1991.

Meyer B, Elimian A, Royek A: Comparison of clinical and financial outcomes of triplet gestations managed by maternal-fetal medicine versus community physicians. Am J Obstet Gynecol **185**:S102, 2001.

Meyers C, Adam R, Dungan J, et al: Aneuploidy in twin gestations: When is maternal age advanced? Obstet Gynecol **89**:248, 1997.

Miller DA, Mullin P, Hou D, et al: Vaginal birth after cesarean section in twin gestations. Am J Obstet Gynecol **175**:194, 1996.

Minakami H, Sato I: Reestimating date of delivery in multifetal pregnancies. JAMA **275**:1432, 1996.

Moore TR, Gale S, Benirschke K: Perinatal outcome of forty-nine pregnancies complicated by acardiac twinning. Am J Obstet Gynecol **163**:907, 1990.

National Academy of Sciences: Nutrition During Pregnancy. Washington, DC, National Academy Press, 1990.

National Institutes of Health Consensus Statement: Antenatal Corticosteroids Revisited: Repeat Courses. National Institutes of Health, vol. 17, No. 2. Bethesda, Md, National Institutes of Health, 2000.

Neveux LM, Palomaki GE, Knight GJ, et al: Multiple marker screening for Down syndrome in twin pregnancies. Prenat Diagn **16**:29, 1996.

Newman RB, Ellings JM: Antepartum management of the multiple gestation: The case for specialized care. Semin Perinatol **19**:387, 1995.

Newman RB, Godsey RK, Ellings JM, et al: Quantification of cervical change: Relationship to preterm delivery in the multifetal gestation. Am J Obstet Gynecol 165:264, 1991.

Newman RB, Krombach RS, Myers MC, et al: Effect of cerclage on obstetric outcome in twin gestations with a shortened cervical length. Am J Obstet Gynecol 186:634, 2002.

Nicolini U, Pisoni MP, Cela E, et al: Fetal blood sampling immediately before and within 24 hours of death in monochorionic twin pregnancies complicated by single intrauterine death. Am J Obstet Gynecol 179:800, 1998.

Nicolini U, Poblete A: Single intrauterine death in monochorionic twin pregnancies. Ultrasound Obstet Gynecol 14:297, 1999.

Niemimaa M, Suonapaa M, Heinonen S, et al: Maternal serum human chorionic gonadotrophin and pregnancy-associated plasma protein A in twin pregnancies in the first trimester. Prenat Diagn 22:183, 2002.

Norman RJ, Joubert SM, Marivate M: Amniotic fluid phospholipids and glucocorticoids in multiple pregnancy. Br J Obstet Gynaecol 90:51, 1983.

Norton ME, D'Alton ME, Bianchi DW: Molecular zygosity studies aid in the management of discordant multiple gestations. J Perinatol 17:202, 1997.

O'Brien JE, Dvorin E, Yaron Y, et al: Differential increases in AFP, hCG, and uE₃ in twin pregnancies: Impact on attempts to quantify Down syndrome screening calculations. Am J Med Genet 73:109, 1997.

Peaceman AM, Dooley SL, Tamura RK, et al: Antepartum management of triplet gestations. Am J Obstet Gynecol 167:1117, 1992.

Peek MJ, McCarthy A, Kyle P, et al: Medical amnioreduction with sulindac to reduce cord complications in monoamniotic twins. Am J Obstet Gynecol 176:334, 1997.

Petrikovsky BM, Vintzileos AM: Management and outcome of multiple pregnancy of high fetal order: Literature review. Obstet Gynecol Surv 44:578, 1989.

Pharoah PO, Adi Y: Consequences of in-utero death in a twin pregnancy. Lancet 355:1597, 2000.

Pistorius LR, Howarth GR: Failure of amniotic septostomy in the management of 3 subsequent cases of severe previable twin-twin transfusion syndrome. Fetal Diagn Ther 14:337, 1999.

Pons JC, Nekhlyudov L, Dephot N, et al: Management and outcome of 65 quadruplet pregnancies: Sixteen years' experience in France. Acta Genet Med Gemellol 45:367, 1996.

Porreco RP, Barton SM, Haverkamp AD: Occlusion of umbilical artery in acardiac, acephalic twin. Lancet 337:326, 1991a.

Porreco RP, Burke S, Hendriz ML: Multifetal reduction of triplets and pregnancy outcome. Obstet Gynecol 78:335, 1991b.

Porter TF, Dildy GA, Blanchard JR, et al: Normal values for amniotic fluid index during uncomplicated twin pregnancy. Obstet Gynecol 87:699, 1996.

Powers WF, Wampler NS: Further defining the risks confronting twins. Am J Obstet Gynecol 175:1522, 1996.

Quintero RA, Bornick PW, Allen MH, et al: Selective laser photocoagulation of communicating vessels in severe twin-twin transfusion syndrome in women with an anterior placenta. Obstet Gynecol 97:477, 2001.

Quintero RA, Morales WJ, Allen MH, et al: Staging of twin-twin transfusion syndrome. J Perinatol 19:550, 1999.

Quintero RA, Reich H, Puder KS, et al: Brief report: Umbilical-cord ligation of an acardiac twin by fetoscopy at 19 weeks' gestation. N Engl J Med 330:469, 1994.

Redford DHA: Uterine growth in twin pregnancy by measurement of total intrauterine volume. Acta Genet Med Gemmellol 32:145, 1982.

Reece EA, Yarkoni S, Abdalla M, et al: A prospective study of growth in twin gestations compared with growth in singleton pregnancies. I. The fetal head. J Ultrasound Med 10:439, 1991.

Rizzo G, Arduini D, Romanini C: Uterine artery Doppler velocity waveforms in twin pregnancies. Obstet Gynecol 82:978, 1993.

Rodeck C, Deans A, Jauniaux E: Thermocoagulation for the early treatment of pregnancy with an acardiac twin. N Engl J Med 339:1293, 1998.

Rodis JF, Egan JFX, Craffey A, et al: Calculated risks of chromosomal abnormalities in twin gestations. Obstet Gynecol 76:1037, 1990.

Rodis JF, McIlveen PF, Egan JF, et al: Monoamniotic twins: improved perinatal survival with accurate prenatal diagnosis and antenatal surveillance. Am J Obstet Gynecol 177:1046, 1997.

Rydhstroem H, Heraib F: Gestational duration, and fetal and infant mortality for twins vs singletons. Twin Res 4:227, 2001.

Saade GR, Belfort MA, Berry DL, et al: Amniotic septostomy for the treatment of twin oligohydramnios-polyhydramnios sequence. Fetal Diagn Ther 13:86, 1998.

Saade GR, Olson G, Belfort MA, et al: Amniotomy: A new approach to the "stuck twin" syndrome. Am J Obstet Gynecol 172:429, 1995.

Sairam S, Costeloe K, Thilaganathan B: Prospective risk of stillbirth in multiple-gestation pregnancies: A population-based analysis. Obstet Gynecol 100:638, 2002.

Santema JG, Bourdrez P, Wallenburg HC: Maternal and perinatal complications in triplet compared with twin pregnancy. Eur J Obstet Gynaecol Reprod Biol 60:143, 1995.

Scardo JA, Ellings JM, Newman RB: Prospective determination of chorionicity, amnionicity, and zygosity in twin gestations. Am J Obstet Gynecol 173:1376, 1995.

Scheller JM, Nelson KB: Twinning and neurologic morbidity. Am J Dis Child 146:1110, 1992.

Schreiner-Engel P, Walther VN, Mindes J, et al: First-trimester multifetal pregnancy reduction: Acute and persistent psychologic reactions. Am J Obstet Gynecol 172:541, 1995.

Sebire NJ, Sepulveda W, Hughes KS, et al: Management of twin pregnancies discordant for anencephaly. Br J Obstet Gynaecol 107:216, 1997.

Sebire NJ, Snijders RJM, Hughes K, et al: Screening for trisomy 21 in twin pregnancies by maternal age and fetal nuchal translucency thickness at 10–14 weeks of gestation. Br J Obstet Gynaecol 103:999, 1996.

Seoud MA, Toner JP, Kruithoff C, et al: Outcome of twin, triplet and quadruplet in vitro fertilization pregnancies: The Norfolk experience. Fertil Steril 57:825, 1992.

Sepulveda W, Bower S, Hassan J, et al: Ablation of acardiac twin by alcohol injection into the intra-abdominal umbilical artery. Obstet Gynecol 86:680, 1995.

Sibai BM, Hauth J, Caritis S, et al: Hypertensive disorders in twin versus singleton gestations. Am J Obstet Gynecol 182:938, 2000.

Simpson LL, D'Alton ME: Multiple pregnancy. In Creasy RK (ed): Management of Labor and Delivery. Malden, Mass, Blackwell, 1997, p. 395.

Simpson LL, Marx GR, Elkadry EA, et al: Cardiac dysfunction in twin-twin transfusion syndrome: A prospective, longitudinal study. Obstet Gynecol 92:557, 1998.

Sivan E, Maman E, Homko CJ, et al: Impact of fetal reduction on the incidence of gestational diabetes. Obstet Gynecol 99:91, 2002.

Skrablin S, Kuvacic I, Pavicic D, et al: Maternal neonatal outcome in quadruplet and quintuplet versus triplet gestations. Eur J Obstet Gynaecol Reprod Biol 88:147, 2000.

Smith-Levitin M, Kowalik A, Birnholz J, et al: Selective reduction of multifetal pregnancies to twins improves outcome over nonreduced triplet gestations. Am J Obstet Gynecol 175:878, 1996.

Souka AP, Heath V, Flint S, et al: Cervical length at 23 weeks in twins in predicting spontaneous preterm delivery. Obstet Gynecol 94:450, 1999.

Spellacy WN, Handler A, Ferre CD: A case-control study of 1253 twin pregnancies from a 1982–1987 perinatal data base. Obstet Gynecol 75:168, 1990.

Spencer K, Salonen R, Muller F: Down's syndrome screening in multiple pregnancies using alpha-fetoprotein and free beta hCG. Prenat Diagn 15:94, 1995.

Stagiannis KD, Sepulveda W, Southwell D, et al: Ultrasonographic measurement of the dividing membrane in twin pregnancy during the second and third trimesters: A reproducibility study. Am J Obstet Gynecol 173:1546, 1995.

Stiller RJ, Lockwood CJ, Belanger K, et al: Amniotic fluid alpha-fetoprotein concentrations in twin gestations: Dependence on placental membrane anatomy. Am J Obstet Gynecol 158:1088, 1988.

Stone J, Eddleman K: Multifetal pregnancy reduction. Curr Opin Obstet Gynecol 12:491, 2000.

Tabsh K: Genetic amniocentesis in multiple gestation: A new technique to diagnose monoamniotic twins. Obstet Gynecol 75:296, 1990.

Tessen JA, Zlatnik FJ: Monoamniotic twins: A retrospective controlled study. Obstet Gynecol 77:832, 1991.

Thiery M, Kermans G, Derom R: Triplet and higher-order births: What is the optimal delivery route? Acta Genet Med Gemmell 37:89, 1988.

Tsao K, Feldstein VA, Albanese CT, et al: Selective reduction of acardiac twin by radiofrequency ablation. Am J Obstet Gynecol 187:635, 2002.

Usta IM, Awwad JT: A false positive diagnosis of conjoined twins in a triplet pregnancy: Pitfalls of first trimester ultrasonographic prenatal diagnosis. Prenat Diagn 20:169, 2000.

Van Allen MI, Smith SW, Shepard TH: Twin reversed arterial perfusion (TRAP) sequence: A study of 14 twin pregnancies with acardius. Semin Perinatol 7:285, 1983.

Van Den Brand SFJJ, Nijhuis JG, Van Dongen PWJ: Prenatal ultrasound diagnosis of conjoined twins. Obstet Gynecol Surv 49:656, 1994.

Vayssiere CF, Heim N, Camus EP, et al: Determination of chorionicity in twin gestations by high-frequency abdominal ultrasonography: Counting the layers of the dividing membrane. Am J Obstet Gynecol 175:1529, 1996.

Veille JC, Morton MJ, Burry KJ: Maternal cardiovascular adaptations to twin pregnancy. Am J Obstet Gynecol **153:**261, 1985.

Ville Y, Hecher K, Gagnon A, et al: Endoscopic laser coagulation in the management of severe twin-to-twin transfusion syndrome. Br J Obstet Gynaecol **105:**446, 1998.

Wapner RJ: Genetic diagnosis in multiple pregnancies. Semin Perinatol **19:**351, 1995.

Wapner RJ, Johnson A, Davis G: Prenatal diagnosis in twin gestations: A comparison between second trimester amniocentesis and first trimester chorionic villus sampling. Obstet Gynecol **82:**49, 1993.

Weir PE, Ratten GJ, Beischer NA: Acute polyhydramnios—A complication of monozygous twin pregnancy. Br J Obstet Gynaecol **86:**849, 1979.

Wenstrom KD, Tessen JA, Zlatnik FJ, et al: Frequency, distribution, and theoretical mechanisms of hematologic and weight discordance in monochorionic twins. Obstet Gynecol **80:**257, 1992.

Winn HN, Cimino J, Powers J, et al: Intrapartum management of nonvertex second-born twins: A critical analysis. Am J Obstet Gynecol **185:**1204, 2001.

Yang JH, Kuhlman K, Daly S, et al: Prediction of preterm birth by second trimester cervical sonography in twin gestations. Ultrasound Obstet Gynecol **15:**288, 2000.

Yaron Y, Bryant-Greenwood PK, Dave N, et al: Multifetal pregnancy reduction of triplets to twins: Comparisons with nonreduced triplets and twins. Am J Obstet Gynecol **180:**1268, 1999.

Yeast JD: Maternal physiologic adaptation to twin gestation. Clin Obstet Gynecol **33:**10, 1990.

Yokoyama Y, Shimizu T, Hayakawa K: Prevalence of cerebral palsy in twins, triplets and quadruplets. Int J Epidemiol **24:**943, 1995.

Young BK, Roque H, Abdelhak Y, et al: Endoscopic ligation of the umbilical cord at 19 weeks' gestation in monoamniotic monochorionic twins discordant for hypoplastic left heart syndrome. Fetal Diagn Ther **16:**61, 2001.

Chapter 30

HEMOLYTIC DISEASE OF THE FETUS AND NEWBORN

Kenneth J. Moise Jr., MD

RED CELL ALLOIMMUNIZATION IN PREGNANCY

Terminology

Maternal antibodies to red cell antigens can pass transplacentally, attach to fetal red cells, and lead to their destruction. Historically, the perinatal effects of these antibodies could not be assessed until after delivery, thus giving rise to the descriptive term *hemolytic disease of the newborn* (HDN). The advent of such diagnostic tools as ultrasound and fetal blood sampling (FBS) have allowed for the diagnosis of fetal anemia and hydrops fetalis before delivery. For this reason, the term *hemolytic disease of the fetus and newborn* (HDFN) is more appropriate to describe this disorder. Another historical term, *erythroblastosis fetalis*, was first used when neonatal studies revealed a large percentage of circulating erythroblasts in cases of severe HDFN. This represents a profound state of fetal anemia that probably occurs in only a small percentage of cases of HDFN. Thus, the term *erythroblastosis fetalis* should be replaced by *HDFN*. Finally, the maternal etiology of HDFN, namely the formation of antibodies to red cell antigens, should be called *red cell alloimmunization* instead of the older term of *red cell isoimmunization*.

Historical Perspectives

The first case of HDFN was probably described in 1609 in the French literature by a midwife (Bowman, 1998). The case was a twin gestation in which the first fetus was stillborn and the second twin developed jaundice and succumbed soon after birth. There is some suggestion that RhD HDFN may have played a role in the ultimate formation of the Anglican Church (Rosse, 1990). Henry VIII's first wife, Katherine of Aragon, conceived six children; five died in the perinatal period from presumed HDFN. Only one daughter, Mary Tudor, survived the union. The ultimate failure of Katherine to bear a viable male heir to the English throne resulted in a divorce that the Roman Pope would not grant. This led to Henry's declaration of the formation of the Church of England. The modern era of Rhesus disease probably began in 1939 when Levine and Stetson (1939) described an antibody in a woman who gave birth to a stillborn fetus. The patient experienced a severe hemolytic transfusion reaction after later receiving her husband's blood. One year later, Landsteiner and Weiner (1940) injected red cells from rhesus monkeys into guinea pigs. The antibody that was isolated from these was used to test human blood samples from whites, and agglutination was noted in 85% of individuals. One year later, Levine and associates (1941) were able to demonstrate a causal relationship between RhD antibodies in RhD-negative women and HDFN in their offspring.

The advent of therapy for HDFN began in 1945 with the description by Wallerstein (1946) of the technique of neonatal exchange transfusion. Later Bevis (1956) and then Liley (1961) proposed the use of amniotic fluid bilirubin assessment as an indirect measure of the degree of fetal hemolysis. Sir William Liley's (1963) major contribution to the story of rhesus disease was the introduction of the intraperitoneal fetal transfusion (IPT). He learned from a visiting geneticist who had returned from Africa that the infusion of red cells into the peritoneal cavity of neonates with sickle cell disease produced normal-appearing red blood cells on peripheral blood smear. Liley realized that he had previously inadvertently entered the peritoneal cavity of fetuses at the time of amniocentesis by the marked contrast in the yellow hue of the ascitic fluid as compared with amniotic fluid. He postulated that purposeful entry into the fetal peritoneal cavity could be accomplished. After three unsuccessful attempts that resulted in fetal demises, the fourth fetus was delivered at $34\frac{4}{7}$ weeks' gestation after undergoing two IPTs at $32\frac{1}{7}$ and $33\frac{4}{7}$ weeks (Liley, 1963). Several investigators made futile attempts to transfuse the fetus by direct access via hysterotomy using the fetal femoral artery, saphenous vein, and internal jugular vein (Freda and Adamsons, 1964; Asensio et al., 1966, 1968). Early attempts at IPT used fluoroscopy for needle guidance. With the introduction of real-time ultrasound in the early 1980s, IPTs became a safer procedure as fluoroscopy was abandoned. Rodeck and coworkers (1981) are credited with the first intravascular fetal transfusion (IVT) using a fetoscope to guide the transfusion needle into a placental plate vessel. Bang and coworkers (1982) performed the first ultrasound-guided IVT using the intrahepatic portion of the umbilical vein.

The 1990s saw the introduction of genetic techniques using amniocentesis to perform fetal red cell typing. With the dawn of the new millennium, the noninvasive detection of fetal anemia through Doppler ultrasound became a reality.

Incidence

The advent of the routine administration of antenatal and postpartum rhesus immune globulin (RhIG) resulted in a marked reduction in cases of red cell alloimmunization secondary to the RhD antigen. A report from surveillance hospitals of the Centers for Disease Control and Prevention noted in 1991 that 1 in every 1000 liveborn infants exhibited some effect from rhesus hemolytic disease (Chavez et al., 1991). Data from a 2000 review of the national registry of U.S. birth certificates indicated an incidence of 6.8 cases per 1000 live births (Martin et al., 2002). Although at first glance this would appear to indicate an increasing incidence, reporting bias in the latter study probably explains this difference.

Clearly, a shift to other red cell antibodies associated with HDFN has occurred as a result of the decreasing incidence of RhD alloimmunization. Geifman-Holtzman and coworkers (1997) evaluated 37,506 serum samples from female patients at two New York blood centers between the years of 1993 and 1995. Sixty percent of the women were of childbearing age. A positive screen for an antibody previously reported to be associated with HDFN was identified in 424 of the samples (1.1%). Rhesus antibodies were the most common, accounting for over half of significant antibodies with the RhD antibody and accounting for almost one fourth of all antibodies. Kell antibodies were next most frequent (29%), followed by Duffy (7%), MNS (6%), Kidd, and anti-U.

These authors compared their findings with previous investigations of antibody prevalence. As expected, secondary to the widespread adoption of RhIG prophylaxis, the incidence of RhD alloimmunization decreased from 43.3 per 1000 samples in 1967 to 2.6 per 1000 in 1996 (Fig. 30-1) (Queenan et al., 1969). Kell alloimmunization was higher in the 1996 series (3.2 per 1000) compared with studies of the U.S. population in 1967 (1.6 per 1000). The authors proposed that this increase could be related to enhanced detection of antibodies through improvement of blood banking techniques. Alternatively, increasing maternal age could result in a higher likelihood of exposure to blood transfusions that have the potential to result in red cell sensitization. Finally, these investigators noted important differences in the incidence of such antibodies as Kell when comparing the

U.S. population to similar populations in Australia (Pepperell et al., 1977) or Sweden (Filbey et al., 1995) (Kell incidence 3.2, 0.5, and 0.4 per 1000, respectively). These differences are likely explained by geographic variations in gene frequency, although specific national transfusion practices could also have an influence.

Pathophysiology

It is now well established that the fetal–maternal interface is not an absolute barrier because there is evidence that considerable trafficking of many types of cells occurs between the fetus and mother throughout gestation. In most cases, the antigenic load of a putative antigen on the fetal erythrocytes and erythrocytic precursors is insufficient to stimulate the maternal immune system. However, in the case of a large antenatal fetomaternal hemorrhage (FMH) or an FMH at delivery, B lymphocyte clones that recognize the foreign red cell antigen are established. The initial maternal IgM production is short-lived, with a rapid change to an IgG response. A human antiglobulin titer can usually be detected 5 to 16 weeks after the sensitizing event.

The anti-D immune response is the best characterized of the anti-red cell antibodies associated with HDFN. In one third of cases, only subclass IgG1 is produced; in the remainder of cases a combination of IgG1 and IgG3 subclasses are found (Pollock and Bowman, 1990). IgG3 anti-D is thought to promote monocyte–red cell interaction more efficiently than IgG1. A longer hinge region in its structure enables the IgG3 molecule to more easily bridge the gap between sensitized red cells and reticuloendothelial (RE) cells (Hadley and Kumpel, 1989). Anti-D IgG is a nonagglutinating antibody that does not bind complement.

After the initial antigenic exposure, memory B lymphocytes await the appearance of red cells containing the putative antigen in the subsequent pregnancy. If stimulated by fetal erythrocytes, these B lymphocytes differentiate into plasma cells that can rapidly proliferate and produce IgG antibodies and an increase in the maternal titer. Maternal IgG crosses the placenta and attaches to fetal erythrocytes that have expressed the paternal antigen. These cells are then sequestered by macrophages in the fetal spleen where they undergo extravascular hemolysis, producing fetal anemia. Fetal sex may play a significant role in the fetal response to maternal antibodies. Ulm et al. (1999) reported that the chance for hydrops fetalis was increased by 13-fold in RhD-positive male fetuses as compared with their female counterparts; the adjusted odds ratio for perinatal mortality was 3.38 in male fetuses.

Several important physiologic responses occur in fetuses secondary to this anemia. An enhanced bone marrow production of reticulocytes is noted when the fetal hemoglobin deficit exceeds 2 g/dL compared with norms for gestational age; erythroblasts from the fetal liver occur at a hemoglobin deficit of 7 g/dL or greater (Nicolaides, Thilaganathan, et al., 1988). Cardiac output increases, and 2,3-diphosphoglycerate levels are enhanced. Tissue hypoxia appears as anemia progresses. An increased umbilical artery lactate level occurs when the fetal hemoglobin falls below 8 g/dL, and increased venous lactate is noted with a hemoglobin below 4 g/dL (Soothill et al., 1987). Hydrops fetalis, a collection of fluid in serous compartments, heralds end-stage disease with

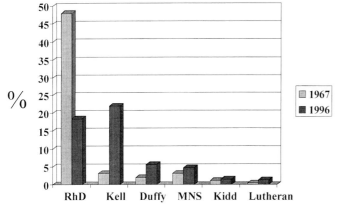

FIGURE 30-1 ■ Incidence of maternal anti-red cell antibodies associated with hemolytic disease of the fetus and newborn in women of reproductive age.

hemoglobin deficits of 7 g/dL or greater (Nicolaides, Thilaganathan, et al., 1988). It first presents as fetal ascites with later findings of pleural effusion and scalp edema. The exact pathophysiology of this condition is unknown. Lower serum albumin levels have been reported, presumably owing to depressed synthesis by the fetal liver that shifts to an erythropoietic function (Nicolaides et al., 1985). Colloid osmotic pressure appears to decrease (Moise et al., 1992). However, congenital analbuminemia is not associated with hydrops fetalis, and experimental removal of fetal plasma proteins does not produce hydrops (Cormode et al., 1975; Moise et al., 1991). An alternative hypothesis is that tissue hypoxia resulting from anemia enhances capillary permeability. In addition, iron overload resulting from ongoing hemolysis may contribute to free radical formation and endothelial cell dysfunction (Berger et al., 1990). Central venous pressures do appear elevated in the hydropic fetus with HDFN (Moise et al., 1992). This may cause a functional blockage of the lymphatic system at the level of the thoracic duct as it empties into the left brachiocephalic vein. This theory is supported by reports of poor absorption of donor red cells when infused into the intraperitoneal cavity in cases of hydrops (Lewis et al., 1973).

Several specific antibody situations probably affect the pathophysiology of HDFN. Spong and coworkers (2001) reported an increased degree of fetal anemia when multiple maternal antibodies associated with HDFN are present as compared with anti-D alone. Red cell sensitization to multiple antibodies was associated with a 1.8-fold increased need for intrauterine transfusions compared with patients with only anti-D. The body of *in vitro* and *in vivo* evidence would suggest that fetal anemia in cases of Kell (anti-K1) sensitization is secondary to two mechanisms: hemolysis and erythropoietic suppression. Vaughan and coworkers (1994) studied 11 anemic fetuses from pregnancies with Kell alloimmunization matched for gestational age and hematocrit to 11 anemic fetuses from pregnancies complicated by RhD alloimmunization. The anti-Kell group was noted to have a lower level of both reticulocytosis and erythroblastosis. Weiner and Widness (1996) compared 11 fetuses from Kell-sensitized pregnancies to 54 RhD-sensitized pregnancies. Like the previous investigators, the authors noted an inverse correlation between the fetal hemoglobin concentration and the reticulocyte count in the RhD fetuses; such a correlation could not be demonstrated in the Kell fetuses. Finally, Vaughan et al. (1998) undertook an *in vitro* analysis of erythroid progenitors to assess the impact of anti-K1 antibodies as compared with anti-D antibodies. Kell-negative and Kell-positive erythroid cell lines were established from umbilical cord blood. Serum from 22 women sensitized to Kell suppressed the growth of Kell-positive erythroid burst-forming and colony-forming units; no suppression occurred in Kell-negative cultures. Monoclonal anti-K1 antibody caused a dose-dependent suppression of growth in Kell-positive cells lines but not in Kell-negative cell lines. Monoclonal anti-RhD antibody exhibited no suppression in either cell line. The role of the Kell antigen in red cell physiology is unknown; however, the Kell protein has structural similarities to endopeptidases and therefore may be involved in protein regulation and cell growth in the erythroid cells. At this time, little is known as to whether other anti-red cell antibodies are associated with suppression of fetal erythropoiesis.

RHESUS ALLOIMMUNIZATION AND FETAL/NEONATAL HEMOLYTIC DISEASE OF THE NEWBORN

Genetics

Fisher and Race (1946) proposed the concept of three genes that encode for the three major Rh antigen groups—D, C/c, and E/e. Some 45 years later, the Rh locus was localized to the short arm of chromosome one (Cherif-Zahar et al., 1991). Only two genes were identified—an RhD gene and an RhCE gene. Each gene is 10 exons in length with 96% homology between the genes. This has led some to conclude that these genes represent a duplication of a common ancestral gene. Production of two distinct proteins from the RhCE gene probably occurs as a result of alternative splicing of messenger RNA (Le Van Kim et al., 1992). One nucleotide difference, cytosine to thymine, in exon 2 of the RhCE gene results in a single amino acid change of a serine to proline. This causes the expression of the C antigen as opposed to the c antigen (Carritt et al., 1997). A single cytosine to guanine change in exon 5 of the RhCE gene, producing a single amino acid change of a proline to alanine, results in formation of the e antigen instead of the E antigen (Avent, 2002).

The gene frequency found in different ethnic groups can be traced to the Spanish colonization in the 15th and 16th centuries. Native populations to certain land masses have less than a 1% incidence of RhD negativity—Eskimos, Native Americans, Japanese, and Chinese individuals. The Basque tribe in Spain is noted to have a 30% incidence of Rh negativity. This may well be the origin of the RhD gene deletion that is the most common genetic basis of the RhD-negative state in whites (Fig. 30-2). Whites of European descent exhibit a 15% incidence of RhD negativity, whereas an 8% incidence occurs in African Americans and Hispanics of Mexico and Central America. This latter incidence probably reflects ethnic diversity secondary to Spanish colonization of the New World.

Recently, an RhD pseudogene has been described in 69% of South African blacks and 24% of African Americans

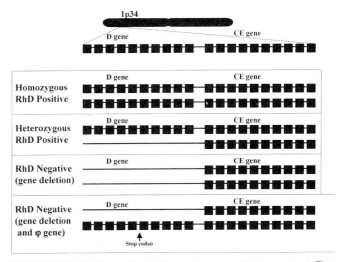

FIGURE 30-2 ■ Schematic of Rh gene locus on chromosome 1. The homozygous RhD-positive, heterozygous RhD-positive, typical RhD-negative, and RhD-negative with pseudogene genotypes are demonstrated.

(Singleton et al., 2000) (see Fig. 30-2). In this situation, all 10 exons of the RhD gene are present; however, translation of the gene into a messenger RNA product does not occur because of the presence of a stop codon in the intron between exons 3 and 4. Thus, no RhD protein is synthesized, and the patient is serologically RhD negative. The presence of this gene in an RhD-negative pregnant patient has important implications for the prenatal diagnosis of the fetal blood type using amniocentesis or chorion villus biopsy (see later).

Prevention of RhD Hemolytic Disease of the Fetus and Newborn

Most RhIG used in the United States is derived from human plasma that undergoes Cohn cold ethanol fractionation for purification. This method of preparation results in contamination with IgA and other plasma proteins. As a result, all such preparations must be given by intramuscular injection. Sepharose column isolation is used for one commercially available RhIG preparation, so this product can be given intravenously. Although once produced from the plasma of sensitized women, the decreasing prevalence of rhesus disease has necessitated the use of male donors that undergo repeated injections of RhD-positive red cells. In addition, concerns regarding Creutzfeldt-Jakob disease in the United Kingdom have resulted in only plasma from the United States being used as the source of antibody for RhIG preparation in that region at the current time. Occasional outbreaks of hepatitis C related to the administration of RhIG have been reported in Ireland (Yap, 1997) and Germany (Wiese et al., 2000) in the late 1970s, although none has occurred in the United States. Because RhIG is a blood derivative, patients who choose not to accept blood products secondary to religious beliefs should be informed of its source and give informed consent. Although most RhIG is issued from hospital blood banks, various manufacturers' products can be purchased by private physicians for use in their offices. A recent recall by one manufacturer warrants that careful records of lot numbers be documented in the patient's medical chart and a general clinic logbook.

Two monoclonal antibodies, BRAD-1 and BRAD-3, have been derived by immortalizing B lymphocyte cell lines from hyperimmunized donors with Ebstein-Barr virus (Kumpel, 2002). In male volunteers injected with ^{51}Cr-labeled RhD-positive red cells, the half-life of the circulating red blood cells was calculated after administration of BRAD-1, BRAD-3, and polyclonal anti-D. Half-lives for the red blood cells were 12.7, 5.9, and 5.0 hours as compared with a half-life of 31 days in the absence of any exogenous anti-D (Kumpel, 2002). Large-scale clinical trials to evaluate the efficacy of these monoclonal antibodies for the prevention of RhD alloimmunization are underway.

The exact mechanism by which RhIG prevents alloimmunization to the RhD antigen is unknown. Studies using intramuscular monoclonal anti-D have revealed that only about 20% of RhD antigenic sites are bound by anti-D antibody after injection (Kumpel and Judson, 1995). This would negate the theory that masking of antigenic sites is the explanation for the effectiveness of RhIG. Passive anti-K has been shown to prevent the formation of anti-D in K-negative RhD-negative patients exposed to K-positive RhD-positive red cells (Woodrow et al., 1975). This led Kumpel (2002) to theorize

that an Fc-dependent mechanism is involved in the effectiveness of RhIG. Downregulation of B lymphocytes probably occurs by coaggregation of both the B cell and FcγRIIb receptors by exogenous anti-D bound to red cells.

All pregnant patients should undergo an antibody screen at the first prenatal visit. Patients who are RhD-negative but determined to be *weak Rh positive* (previously *Du positive*) are not at risk for rhesus alloimmunization and therefore do not require RhIG. In these situations, the maternal red cells express a reduced number of RhD antigens on their surface. Therefore, recognition of the RhD antigen as foreign to the patient's immune system does not occur. If there is no evidence of anti-D alloimmunization in the RhD-negative woman, recommendations in North America include the intramuscular administration of 300 μg of RhIG at 28 weeks of gestation (ACOG, 1999). This practice has been reported to reduce the incidence of antenatal alloimmunization from 2% to 0.1% (Bowman, 1988). In the United Kingdom, an antenatal protocol of administering 100 μg (500 IU) of RhIG at 28 and 34 weeks is used (NICE, 2002). Limited resources have not allowed for extension of this protocol to all subsequent pregnancies. The American Association of Blood Banks recommends that a repeat antibody screen be obtained before antenatal RhIG, although the incidence of alloimmunization before 28 weeks is very low (Synder, 1998). The cost-effectiveness of this practice has been questioned by the American College of Obstetricians and Gynecologists (ACOG) (1999). If a repeat antibody screen is to be undertaken, a maternal blood sample can be drawn at the same office visit as the RhIG injection. Although the administration of the exogenous anti-D will eventually result in a weakly positive titer, this will not occur in the short interval of several hours because of the slow absorption from the intramuscular site. Some experts recommend that a second dose of RhIG be given if the patient has not delivered by 40 weeks' gestation.

Although not well studied, additional indications for the antepartum administration of RhIG include spontaneous abortion, elective abortion, ectopic pregnancy, genetic amniocentesis, chorion villous sampling, and FBS. A dose of 50 μg of RhIG is effective until 12 weeks' gestation because of the small volume of red cells in the fetoplacental circulation (ACOG, 1999). From a practical sense, most hospitals and offices do not stock this dose of RhIG; therefore, a standard dose of 300 μg is often given. The use of RhIG in other scenarios that breach the fetoplacental barrier is lacking. However, most experts agree that such events as hydatidiform mole, threatened abortion, fetal death in the second or third trimester, blunt trauma to the abdomen, and external cephalic version warrant strong consideration for the use of RhIG.

Because the half-life of RhIG is approximately 16 days, 15% to 20% of patients receiving it at 28 weeks will have a very low anti-D titer (usually 2 or 4) detected at the time of admission for labor at term (Goodrick et al., 1994). In North America, the recommendation is to administer 300 μg of RhIG within 72 hours of delivery if umbilical cord blood typing reveals an RhD-positive infant (ACOG, 1999). This is sufficient to protect from sensitization because of an FMH of 30 mL of fetal whole blood. In the United Kingdom, 100 μg is given at delivery (Synder, 1998). Approximately 1 in 1000 deliveries will be associated with an excessive FMH; risk factors will only identify 50% of these (Bowman, 1985; Ness et al., 1987). Routine screening of all women at the time of delivery for excessive

FMH should therefore be undertaken. A qualitative yet sensitive test for FMH, the rosette test, is first performed. Results return as positive or negative. A negative result warrants administration of a standard dose of RhIG. If the rosette is positive, a Kleihauer-Betke stain or fetal cell stain using flow cytometry is undertaken. The percentage of fetal blood cells is multiplied by a factor of 50 to estimate the volume of the FMH. Because this calculation includes an inaccurate estimation of the maternal blood volume, the blood bank will typically indicate that additional vials of RhIG should be administered over the calculated amount. No more than five units of RhIG should be administered by the intramuscular route in one 24-hour period. Should a large dose of RhIG be necessary, an alternative method would be to give the entire calculated dose using the intravenous preparation of RhIG that is now available. Should RhIG be inadvertently omitted after delivery, some protection has been proven with administration within 13 days; recommendations have been made to administer it as late as 28 days after delivery (Bowman, 1985). If delivery occurs less than 3 weeks from the administration of RhIG used for antenatal indications such as amniocentesis for fetal lung maturity or external cephalic version, a repeat dose is unnecessary unless a large FMH is detected at the time of delivery (ACOG, 1999). Despite the widespread acceptance of similar guidelines, studies from Scotland have revealed that two thirds of rhesus alloimmunized cases are secondary to antepartum sensitization, whereas an additional 13% are due to failure to administer RhIG for the usual obstetric indications (Hughes et al., 1994).

If a patient is undergoing initial blood typing at delivery and a *weak Rh-positive* result is obtained, this may be secondary to a large FMH causing a mixed field agglutination reaction and a false interpretation of the maternal blood type. A standard test for FMH should be performed. If none is detected, then the *weak Rh-positive* typing can be considered valid and RhIG is not required. The administration of RHIG after a postpartum tubal ligation is controversial. The possibility of a new partner in conjunction with the availability of *in vitro* fertilization would seem to make the use of RhIG in these situations prudent. RhIG is not effective once alloimmunization to the RhD antigen has occurred. Currently, prophylactic immune globulin preparations to prevent other forms of red cell alloimmunization such as anti-K1 do not exist.

Diagnostic Methods

Maternal Antibody Determination

The maternal titer is the first step in the evaluation of the RhD-sensitized patient. Previous methodologies using albumin or saline should no longer be practiced because they detect varying levels of IgM antibody. The pentamer structure of this class of antibody does not allow for transplacental passage; therefore, the contribution of IgM to the titer quantitation has no clinical relevance. The human antiglobulin titer (indirect Coombs) is used to determine the degree of alloimmunization as it measures the maternal IgG response. By convention, titer values are reported as the reciprocal of the last tube dilution with a positive agglutination reaction, that is, a titer of 16 is the equivalent of a dilution of 1:16. Variation in results between laboratories is not uncommon because many commercial laboratories use enzymatic treatment of red cells to prevent failure of detection of low titer samples. However, in the same laboratory the titer should not vary by more than one dilution if the two samples are run in tandem. Thus, an initial titer of 8 that returns at 16 may not represent a true increase in the amount of antibody in the maternal circulation. A critical titer is defined as the titer associated with a significant risk for fetal hydrops. When this is present, further fetal surveillance is required. This titer will vary with institution and methodologies; however, in most centers a critical value for anti-D between 8 and 32 is used.

In the United Kingdom, quantitation of anti-D is undertaken through the use of an automated technique using a device known as the autoanalyzer. Red cell samples are mixed with agents to enhance agglutination by the anti-D antibodies. Agglutinated cells are separated from nonagglutinated cells and then lysed. The amount of released hemoglobin is then compared with an international standard; results are reported as international units (IU) per milliliter. Levels of less than 4 IU/mL are rarely associated with HDFN. In one series of 42 fetuses undergoing serial FBS, a maternal anti-D level of less than 15 IU/mL was associated with only mild fetal anemia (Nicolaides and Rodeck, 1992). An increase in the maternal anti-D level of more than 15 IU/mL over a 2- to 3-week interval was associated with the development of moderate to severe fetal anemia in approximately 50% of cases.

In Vitro Tests

Because measurements of maternal anti-D have been poor predictors of HDFN, there has been considerable interest in *in vitro* assays that might better predict fetal disease by mimicking the red cell destruction that occurs in the fetus (Hadley, 1995). Typically, maternal serum containing anti-red cell antibodies is mixed with adult red cell heterozygous for the specific antigen. These sensitized red cells are then combined with various types of RE cells, such as macrophages, monocytes, or lymphocytes. The degree of red cell hemolysis or activation of the RE cells is then quantitated. The three tests most commonly used are the antibody-dependent cell-mediated cytotoxicity (ADCC) assay, the monocyte monolayer assay, and the monocyte chemiluminescence test. In the ADCC assay, the release of ^{51}Cr from sensitized red cells previously incubated with this isotope is used as a measure of the *in vitro* destruction caused by the monocytes. The percentage of total monocytes involved in adherence or phagocytosis of red cells is assessed by microscopic examination in the monocyte monolayer assay. The chemiluminescence assay uses the photoactivity of luminol, a compound that generates light as it reacts with oxygen-free radicals released from the activated monocytes.

Many of the original studies using these assays sought to predict the neonatal outcome of HDFN. In a multicenter trial using FBS to assess fetal disease, the percentage of phagocytosis in the monocyte monolayer assay was similar in antigen-negative, nonanemic, antigen-positive, and anemic antigen-positive fetuses (Moise et al., 1995), indicating that the monocyte monolayer assay was not useful to forecast the need for intrauterine transfusion. Zupanska and coworkers (2001) studied the ability of the chemiluminescence and ADCC assays to predict a fetal hemoglobin deficit of more than 3 g/dL, their threshold for IUT, in 37 pregnancies with anti-D sensitization. The chemiluminescence test was 89% predictive, whereas the ADCC was 78% predictive; the former was associated with fewer false positives. Negative tests for the assays always predicted that FBS was not necessary.

These assays do not enjoy widespread use in the United States, although countries such as Belgium routinely use the ADCC performed at one central location (Central Laboratory of the Netherlands Red Cross) to decide when to proceed with invasive testing in the fetus.

Amniocentesis for Fetal Blood Typing

First described in 1993, amniocytes have become the primary source used to test the fetal blood type in cases of a heterozygous paternal genotype (Bennett et al., 1993). In the 50% of cases where an RhD-negative fetus is found, further maternal and fetal testing is eliminated.

Because the RhC/c and E/e antigens are inherited in a closely linked fashion to RhD, anti-sera for these antigens can be used with gene frequency tables based on ethnicity to determine the paternal zygosity at the RhD locus. In addition, mathematic modeling should be used to modify the incidence of heterozygosity based on the paternal history of previous RhD-positive offspring (Kanter, 1992). As an example, a white partner who undergoes serologic testing with the results of anti-D positive, anti-C negative, anti-c positive, anti-E negative, and anti-e positive would be considered to have the genotype *Dce*. If there was no history of an RhD-positive progeny, then his chance of being heterozygous is 94% (Table 30-1). A history of repeated RhD-positive offspring would markedly decrease the chance of a heterozygous state. Ethnicity must be taken into account when calculating the likelihood of being heterozygous because disparate results can be noted with similar serologic findings. In the future, paternal zygosity testing will probably be performed with such techniques as quantitative polymerase chain reaction (PCR) (Chiu et al., 2001).

Amniocentesis to detect the fetal blood type actually assesses the fetal genotype instead of the fetal phenotype, the expression of the RhD antigen on the fetal red cells as determined by serology. Serologic fetal red cell typing can be performed on blood obtained by ultrasound-directed FBS, but this technique is associated with a fourfold or more rate of perina-

tal loss as compared with amniocentesis. Extensive experience with the use of amniocentesis for determining fetal blood type has revealed rare discrepancies. In the event of a DNA result that reveals an RhD-negative fetus when the fetus is RhD positive by serology, usual surveillance techniques would not be used and fetal loss can occur. In one series of 500 amniocenteses, this occurred in 1.5% of cases (Van den Veyver and Moise, 1996). The most likely etiology for this inconsistency is either erroneous paternity or a rearrangement at the paternal RhD gene locus. Such rearrangements have been documented in approximately 2% of individuals (Simsek et al., 1995). Checking paternal blood, the source of the fetal RhD gene, with the same PCR primers used on the amniotic fluid, verifies that a gene rearrangement is not a potential source of error. For this reason, most laboratories offering fetal red cell typing on amniotic fluid require an accompanying paternal blood sample. In addition, multiplex PCR that targets at least two different exons of the RhD gene is used by many centers to decrease the chance of nondetection of a gene rearrangement (Fig. 30-3).

In situations where paternity is not assured or there is no partner available to send a blood sample for confirmation of PCR primers, one must consider the result of an RhD-negative fetal blood type performed by amniocentesis suspect. Hopkins (1970) assessed serial titers in patients with RhD alloimmunization who subsequently delivered RhD-negative offspring and noted that serial maternal titers rose by fourfold in less than 2% of cases. In situations of questionable paternity, a repeat maternal anti-globulin titer should be obtained 4 to 6 weeks after the results of the amniocentesis as a confirmatory strategy (Fig. 30-4). If a fourfold rise in antibody titer is noted, then an RhD-negative PCR result on amniotic fluid should be questioned. Repeat amniocentesis to evaluate the spectral analysis of amniotic fluid at 450 nm (ΔOD_{450}) or FBS to determine the fetal RhD status using serologic techniques should be considered.

If the maternal ethnicity is black, then the presence of a maternal pseudogene must be excluded. In this situation, the pregnant patient would be RhD negative on serologic testing but the entire RhD gene is present. Because the fetus inherits one of its RhD genes from its mother, amniotic PCR testing would therefore yield a false-positive result, that is, the fetus is RhD positive by genotype testing but RhD negative by

TABLE 30-1. INCIDENCE OF PATERNAL HETEROZYGOSITY (%) BASED ON SEROLOGY, ETHNIC BACKGROUND, AND NUMBER OF PREVIOUS RhD-POSITIVE OFFSPRING

	White						Black						Hispanic					
	No. of RhD+ Infants						No. of RhD+ Infants						No. of RhD+ Infants					
	0	1	2	3	4	5	0	1	2	3	4	5	0	1	2	3	4	5
DCce	90	82	69	53	36.0	22.0	41	26.0	15.0	8.0	4.0	2.0	85	74.0	59.0	42.0	26.0	15.0
DCe	9	5	2	1	0.6	0.3	19	11.0	6.0	3.0	1.0	0.7	5	2.0	1.0	0.6	0.3	0.1
DCEe	90	82	69	53	36.0	22.0	37	23.0	13.0	7.0	4.0	2.0	85	74.0	59.0	42.0	26.0	15.0
DcE	13	7	4	2	0.9	0.5	1	0.5	0.3	0.1	0.1	0.0	2	0.9	0.5	0.2	0.1	0.1
DCcEe	11	6	3	2	0.8	0.4	10	5.0	3.0	1.0	0.7	0.3	12	6.0	3.0	2.0	0.8	0.4
Dce	94	89	80	66	50.0	33.0	54	37.0	23.0	13.0	7.0	4.0	92	85.0	74.0	59.0	42.0	26.0

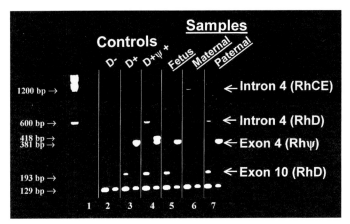

FIGURE 30-3 ■ Electrophoresis gel of maternal, paternal, and amniotic fluid analysis for fetal RhD testing using multiplex polymerase chain reaction. Intron 4 of the RhCE gene (internal control), intron 4 and exon 10 of the RhD gene, and exon 4 of the Rh pseudogene are used in the analysis. Lane numbers are indicated at bottom of figure. *Lane 1,* molecular weight ladder. *Lane 2,* RhD-negative control; 1200-base pair (bp) band noted indicating RhCE amplification as internal control. *Lane 3,* RhD-positive control; 1200-bp band for RhCE gene present. Additional bands of 600 bp (intron 4) and 193 bp (exon 10) also noted, indicating presence of RhD gene. *Lane 4,* RhD/pseudogene heterozygous control; 1200-bp (RhCE gene) as well as 600-bp and 193-bp bands noted (RhD gene). Additional bands noted at 418 *and* 381 bp, indicating presence of Rh pseudogene (ψ +). *Lane 5,* fetal sample = RhD positive; 1200 bp (RhCE gene), 600 and 193 bp (RhD gene), 381 bp only noted from exon 4, indicating absence of Rh pseudogene. *Lane 6,* maternal sample = RhD negative, no pseudogene present; only 1200-bp band noted (RhCE gene). No RhD or Rh pseudogene bands present. *Lane 7,* paternal sample = RhD positive; 1200 bp (RhCE gene), 600 and 193 bp (RhD gene), only 381 bp of exon 4, indicating absence of Rh pseudogene. (Courtesy of Daniel Bellissimo, PhD, Molecular Diagnostics Laboratory, The Blood Center of Southeastern Wisconsin, with permission.)

serology. This could lead to unnecessary intervention with its inherent risks. For this reason, a maternal blood sample should also accompany the amniotic fluid sent for fetal RhD testing in an effort to rule out the presence of a maternal RhD pseudogene. If the maternal sample is positive for this variant, then fetal testing for the gene should also be undertaken (see Fig. 30-4).

Chorion villus biopsy has been used for fetal red cell typing, but this technique should be discouraged in patients who wish to continue their pregnancy in the event that the fetus is found to be RhD positive. Disruption of the chorion villi during the procedure can result in FMH and a rise in maternal titer, thereby worsening the fetal disease (Moise and Carpenter, 1993).

Noninvasive fetal testing for the RhD gene should be routinely available in the near future. Sorting of maternal blood for fetal cells using flow cytometry has been reported to be successful in identifying the RhD-positive fetus (Geifman-Holtzman et al., 1996). More recently, free fetal DNA in the maternal serum has been used to detect RhD sequences in the case of an RhD-positive fetus (Lo et al., 1998). This methodology would appear to be preferable to the isolation of nucleated fetal cells because free fetal DNA is cleared from the maternal plasma within minutes after delivery, thereby reducing the chance of contamination from a previous gestation. In a series of 137 sensitized pregnancies, fetal typing using

DNA from maternal serum was 100% accurate in determining the RhD type in 94 RhD-positive and 43 RhD-negative cases (Finning et al., 2002).

Amniocentesis to Follow the Severity of Hemolytic Disease of the Fetus and Newborn

Since it was first introduced to clinical practice by Bevis (1956), the ΔOD_{450} has been used to measure the level of bilirubin, an indirect indicator of the degree of fetal hemolysis. Liley (1961) proposed a management scheme involving three zones based on gestational ages between 27 and 42 weeks. The Liley curve has proved useful for following alloimmunized pregnancies. Extrapolated Liley curves to gestational ages before 27 weeks have proven erroneous. Nicolaides and coworkers (1986) correlated fetal hematologic values in 59 RhD-sensitized pregnancies between 18 and 25 weeks' gestation with ΔOD_{450} values on a Liley curve extrapolated to 18 weeks' gestation. If intervention were reserved for fetuses with ΔOD_{450} values in zone 3, 70% of cases of fetal anemia would not be detected. Even if all cases of fetal hydrops were excluded, 56% of cases of fetal anemia would still have been misdiagnosed. For a brief period after this report, many centers used FBS exclusively in cases of severe red cell alloimmunization if fetal assessment was indicated before 27 weeks' gestation. A modified ΔOD_{450} curve for such situations was proposed by Queenan and coworkers (1993) from a series of 789 amniotic fluid samples obtained between 14 and 40 weeks' gestation (Fig. 30-5). In a prospective evaluation of this curve, Scott and Chan (1998) followed 35 pregnancies with 72 ΔOD_{450} determinations. Fifty percent of these were undertaken before 27 weeks. The Queenan curve was predictive of severely affected fetuses (more than 7 g/dL deficit in hemoglobin) with a sensitivity of 100% and a specificity of 79%. The sensitivity for detecting moderate anemia (hemoglobin deficit of 3 to 7 g/dL) was 83% with a specificity of 94%.

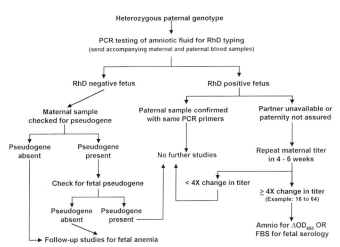

FIGURE 30-4 ■ Algorithm for fetal RhD testing in the case of a heterozygous paternal phenotype. Amnio, amniocentesis; FBS, fetal blood sampling; PCR, polymerase chain reaction. (With permission from Moise KJ: Diagnosis, management, and prevention of rhesus (Rh) alloimmunization. *In* UpToDate, Rose BD (ed): UpToDate, Wellesley, Mass, 2003. Copyright 2003 UpToDate, Inc. For more information, visit www.uptodate.com.)

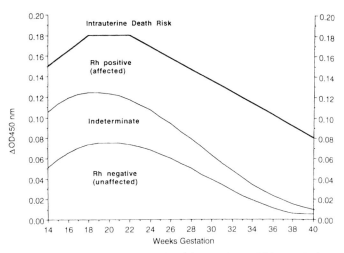

FIGURE 30-5 ■ Queenan curve for ΔOD_{450} values. (With permission from Queenan JT, Tomai TP, Ural SH, et al: Deviation in amniotic fluid optical density at a wavelength of 450 nm in Rh-immunized pregnancies from 14 to 40 weeks' gestation: A proposal for clinical management. Am J Obstet Gynecol **168**:1370, 1993. Mosby, Inc., copyright © 2001.)

If amniocentesis is used to monitor fetal disease, serial procedures are undertaken at 10-day to 2-week intervals and continued until delivery to follow trends in the ΔOD_{450} values. All attempts should be made to avoid transplacental passage of the needle because this can lead to FMH and a rise in maternal antibody titer. A rising or plateauing ΔOD_{450} value that reaches the 80th percentile of zone 2 of the Liley curve or a value that enters the *intrauterine transfusion* zone of the Queenan curve necessitates investigation by FBS. After 37 weeks' gestation, fetal lung maturity testing can be assessed because induction of labor with mature studies can be considered instead of undertaking subsequent amniocenteses. Fluorescence depolarization techniques (TDx-FLM, Abbott Laboratories, Abbot Park, IL) should not be used to assess fetal lung maturity because the value can be falsely elevated as a result of excess bilirubin; the lamellar body count or lecithin-to-sphingomyelin ratio is reliable because these assays are not affected by the excess bilirubin.

Fetal Blood Sampling

Ultrasound-directed FBS (also *percutaneous umbilical blood sampling*, *cordocentesis*, and *funipuncture*) allows direct access to the fetal circulation to obtain important laboratory values such as hematocrit, direct Coombs, fetal blood type, reticulocyte count, and total bilirubin. Serial FBS has been proposed as a primary method of fetal surveillance after a maternal critical titer is reached. Weiner, Williamson, and coworkers (1991) studied 128 red cell alloimmunized pregnancies and described four patterns to predict fetal anemia based on fetal values for hematocrit, direct Coombs, and reticulocyte counts (Table 30-2). FBS is associated with a 1% to 2% rate of fetal loss and up to a 50% risk for FMH with subsequent worsening of the alloimmunization (Weiner, Wenstrom, et al., 1991). For these reasons, it is usually reserved for patients with elevated ΔOD_{450} values or elevated peak middle cerebral artery (MCA) Doppler velocities (see later). However, if the fetal hematocrit is noted to be normal at the time of sampling, use of the direct Coombs and reticulocyte count may be of value to time subsequent procedures. Weiner (1992) also noted that a fetal umbilical venous total serum bilirubin more than 3 mg/dL was associated with the development of severe fetal anemia or postnatal hyperbilirubinemia in 94% of cases. If a transplacental approach has been used for FBS, a repeat maternal antibody titer should be repeated in 1 week. If a large increase is noted as a result of an anamnestic response, the interval to the next FBS should be reduced because the onset of fetal anemia can be rapid in these circumstances. When FBS is indicated by other first-line diagnostic modalities, blood should be immediately available for IVT if fetal anemia is detected (hematocrit less than 30% or less than 2 standard deviations for gestational age).

Ultrasound

Ultrasound plays a key role in the management of the alloimmunized pregnancy. It should be used early in the pregnancy to establish the correct gestational age because this parameter becomes important in determining such normative laboratory values as ΔOD_{450} levels and fetal hematologic values. Although hydrops fetalis can be easily detected with ultrasound, its presence represents the end-stage state of fetal

TABLE 30-2. FETAL BLOOD SAMPLING FOR SURVEILLANCE

Pattern	Hematocrit	Reticulocyte Count	Direct Coombs	Interval for Fetal Blood Sampling (wk)	Comments
1	Normal	Normal	Negative or trace	NA	Repeat sampling if initial maternal titer <128 and 2-fold increase noted in titer
2	Normal	Normal or <2.5th percentile	1+ or 2+	5–6	Do not repeat sampling after 32 weeks if fetal values unchanged; deliver at term
3	Normal	>97.5th percentile	3+ or 4+	2	Continue sampling through 34 weeks if fetal hematocrit stable; deliver at 37–38 weeks if not transfused
4	<2.5th percentile but <30%	Any	Any	1–2	Repeat as long as fetal hematocrit criteria fulfilled; deliver after documented fetal lung maturity

Modified with permission from Moise KJ, Schumacher B: Anaemia. *In* Fisk NM, Moise KJ (eds): Fetal Therapy: Invasive and Transplacental. Cambridge, Cambridge University Press, 1997, p. 149. Copyright © 1997.

anemia. Therefore, many investigators have sought alternative ultrasound parameters that could predict the early onset of anemia. In one large series, assessment of fetal abdominal circumference, head-to-abdomen circumference ratio, intraperitoneal volume, intrahepatic and extrahepatic umbilical vein diameter, and placental thickness was assessed in an effort to predict severe fetal anemia defined as a fetal hemoglobin less than 5 g/dL (Nicolaides, Fontanarosa, et al., 1988). Placental thickness and intraperitoneal volume detected only one fourth of cases, whereas other parameters detected approximately 10% or less of severe cases. Because the fetal liver is a site of extramedullary hematopoiesis in cases of severe fetal anemia, several authors have used ultrasound to measure the length of the right lobe as a measure of hepatomegaly (Vintzileos et al., 1986; Roberts et al., 2001). In one series, a liver length of more than the 95th percentile correctly predicted fetal anemia in 64 of 69 cases (93%). The spleen is also a site of extramedullary hematopoiesis and the destruction and sequestration of sensitized red cells in cases of severe HDFN. The measurement of the splenic perimeter (length + width × 1.57) has therefore been studied. In two series, a splenic perimeter of more than 2 standard deviations was predictive of severe fetal anemia in 94% and 100% of cases (Oepkes et al., 1993; Bahado-Singh et al., 1998). Despite these data, both hepatic length and splenic perimeter have not enjoyed widespread use for noninvasive surveillance in red cell alloimmunization.

Many investigations have attempted to use Doppler ultrasound to correlate blood velocities in various fetal vessels to the level of fetal hemoglobin. Sites of study have included the descending aorta (Rightmire et al., 1986), umbilical vein (Kirkinen et al., 1983), splenic artery (Bahado-Singh et al., 2000), and common carotid artery (Bilardo et al., 1989). The rationale for this approach is that decreasing fetal hemoglobin is associated with a lower blood viscosity that produces less shearing in blood vessels resulting in higher blood velocities. Alternatively, the increased cardiac output associated with fetal anemia may contribute to the higher blood velocities.

Vyas and coworkers (1990) were the first to report the use of the Doppler velocity in the MCA to detect fetal anemia. Using the intensity-weighted time-averaged mean velocity of the MCA, these authors found one of the best correlations with fetal hemoglobin reported to date (R = –0.77). However,

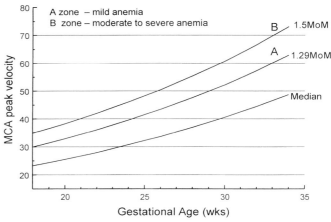

FIGURE 30-6 ■ Middle cerebral artery (MCA) Doppler peak velocities based on gestational age. Zone A, mild anemia; zone B, moderate to severe anemia. MoM, multiples of the median. (Reproduced with permission from Moise KJ: Modern management of Rhesus alloimmunization in pregnancy. Obstet Gynecol **100**:600, 2002. Elsevier Science Company, copyright © 2002.)

on closer analysis of their data, only 50% of the cases of fetal anemia were detected. Measurement of the peak systolic velocity in the fetal MCA has proven to be the most accurate Doppler method for the determination of fetal anemia. In the initial report by Mari and coworkers (2000), normative data for gestational age was established. Using receiver operating characteristic analysis, a threshold value of 1.5 multiples of the median (MoM) was used to predict moderate to severe anemia (less than 0.65 MoM for fetal hemoglobin) (Fig. 30-6). The authors calculated that more than 70% of invasive testing could be avoided using this modality to monitor alloimmunized pregnancies. Since this report, several other investigators (Teixeira et al., 2000; Delle Chiaie et al., 2001; Roberts et al., 2001; Deren and Onderoglu, 2002; Haugen et al., 2002; Zimmerman et al., 2002) have confirmed the accuracy of the MCA in detecting fetal anemia (Table 30-3).

A recent meta-analysis of noninvasive monitoring of the alloimmunized pregnancy reported that the diagnostic test with the highest methodologic quality was the peak MCA velocity (positive likelihood ratio, 8.45 [95% confidence interval, 4.7–15.6]; negative likelihood ratio, 0.02 [95%

TABLE 30-3. ACCURACY OF MCA DOPPLER STUDIES

Author	n	Definition of Fetal Anemia	Definition of Elevated MCA	Sensitivity	Specificity	PPV	NPV
Mari et al. (2000)	111	<0.65 MoM	>1.5 MoM	100%	88%	65%	100%
Roberts et al. (2001)	45	<90 gm/L	>95%	79%	100%	100%	87%
Teixeria et al. (2000)	26	<2 SD	>1 SD	64%	100%	100%	71%
		<3 SD		73%	93%	89%	82%
		<4 SD		83%	80%	56%	94%
Delle Chiaie et al. (2001)	30	≤0.84 MoM	>1.29 MoM	73%	82%	88%	63%
Deren and Onderoglu (2001)	52	≤0.60 MoM	≥1.35 MoM	100%	91%	—	—
Haugen et al. (2002)	35	≤2 SD	>95%	45%	100%	100%	80%
Zimmerman et al. (2002)	125	<0.65 MoM	>1.5 MoM	89%	89%	55%	99%
Mean values*	—	NA	NA	81%	89%	77%	87%

* Less than 4 standard deviations (SD) fetal hemoglobin used for Teixeria study.

MCA, middle cerebral artery; MoM, multiples of the median; NPV, negative predictive value; PPV, positive predictive value.

confidence interval, 0.001–0.25]) (Divakaran et al., 2001). In the first multicenter intent-to-treat prospective study, the peak MCA velocity proved accurate in detecting moderate to severe anemia in 98% of fetuses in which longitudinal measurements were obtained (Zimmerman et al., 2002). In the two cases of anemia that were not detected (neonatal hemoglobin of 5 and 8.2 g/dL), an interval of 17 and 21 days, respectively, had elapsed between the last Doppler study and delivery. The authors concluded that serial MCA Dopplers are optimally obtained on a weekly basis and that the accuracy is decreased after 35 weeks' gestation because of the high number of false-positive cases.

Finally, Detti and coworkers (2002) studied the trend in MCA velocities in detecting anemia (Fig. 30-7). After three consecutive Doppler determinations, a slope of the regression line more than 1.95 was more likely to be associated with the subsequent development of moderate to severe fetal anemia. These investigators proposed the following protocol for use of MCA Doppler:

- Perform Doppler studies weekly for three consecutive determinations.
- If the MCA peak velocity remains less than 1.5 MoM, calculate the slope of the increase between the three measurements (the slope of the line can be determined using the *SLOPE* function in Microsoft Excel).
- If the slope is less than 1.95, repeat studies at 10- to 14-day intervals.
- If the slope is at least 1.95, repeat studies at 7-day intervals.
- If the MCA velocity is found to be at least 1.5 MoM and there are other ultrasound findings consistent with fetal anemia, proceed with FBS with blood readied for IUT. If there are no ultrasound signs of anemia, repeat the MCA determination later that day or within 24 hours to confirm elevation; if persistent, proceed with FBS with blood readied for IUT.
- Do not use the MCA after 35 weeks' gestation.

The fetal MCA closest to the maternal skin should be evaluated using a minimal angle of insonation; angle correc-

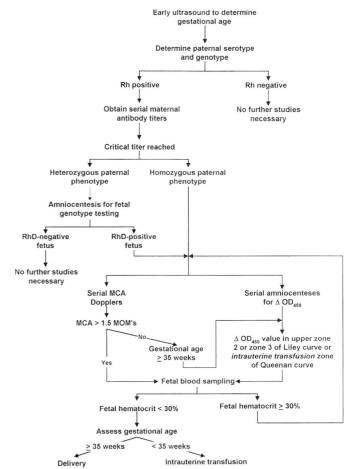

FIGURE 30-8 ■ Algorithm for overall clinical management of the red cell–sensitized gestation. MCA, middle cerebral artery; MOM, multiples of the median. (Modified with permission from Moise KJ: Diagnosis, management, and prevention of rhesus (Rh) alloimmunization. *In* UpToDate, Rose BD (ed): UpToDate, Wellesley, Mass, 2003. Copyright 2003 UpToDate, Inc. For more information visit www.uptodate.com.)

tion can be used if necessary. The Doppler gate is placed over the vessel just as it bifurcates from the carotid siphon. Placement of the gate on the more distal aspects of the MCA will result in a false depression of the real peak systolic velocity. Color Doppler aids in determining the correct location. Because a learning curve is associated with performing MCA Doppler, a center with minimal experience with this technique should perform these in conjunction with serial amniocenteses for ΔOD_{450}. MCA Doppler is proving to revolutionize the care of the RhD-sensitized pregnancy by potentially minimizing invasive diagnostic testing. In the near future, it will probably replace amniocentesis for ΔOD_{450}.

Summary of Clinical Management

The approach using the available diagnostic tools is based on the patient's past history of fetal or neonatal manifestations of HDFN (Fig. 30-8). As a general rule the patient's first RhD-sensitized pregnancy involves minimal fetal/neonatal disease; subsequent gestations are associated with a worsening degree of anemia.

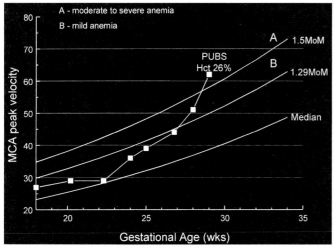

FIGURE 30-7 ■ Serial middle cerebral artery (MCA) Doppler studies. Hct, hematocrit; MoM, multiples of the median; PUBS, percutaneous umbilical blood sampling.

First Affected Pregnancy

Once sensitization to the RhD antigen is detected, maternal titers are repeated every month until approximately 24 weeks; titers are repeated every 2 weeks thereafter. Paternal blood is drawn to determine RhD status and zygosity. Once a critical titer is reached (usually 32), serial amniocenteses for ΔOD_{450} are initiated and repeated at 10-day to 2-week intervals. The first amniocentesis is rarely indicated before 24 to 26 weeks' gestation in the first affected pregnancy. In cases of a heterozygous paternal phenotype, an amniotic fluid sample along with maternal and paternal blood samples are sent to a DNA reference laboratory at the time of first amniocentesis to determine the fetal RhD status. In the case of an RhD-negative paternal blood type or fetal RhD-negative genotype at amniocentesis, further maternal and fetal monitoring is unwarranted as long as paternity is assured.

If there is evidence of an RhD-positive fetus (homozygous paternal phenotype or RhD-positive fetus by PCR testing on amniotic fluid), serial amniocenteses are continued. If a rising or plateauing ΔOD_{450} trend into the 80th percentile of zone 2 of the Liley curve or a value in the *intrauterine transfusion* zone of Queenan curve is noted, FBS is undertaken with blood readied for intrauterine transfusion if the fetal hematocrit is found to be less than 30%. If no rise in the ΔOD_{450} values is detected, the last amniocentesis should be performed at 37 weeks. If the lecithin-to-sphingomyelin ratio or lamellar body count indicates fetal maturity, then induction at 39 weeks' gestation would appear to be warranted.

If serial MCA Doppler assessments are used as the primary means of fetal surveillance once a critical maternal titer has been reached, one amniocentesis should be performed in the case of a heterozygous paternal phenotype to determine the fetal RhD status. If one notes a homozygous paternal phenotype or RhD-positive fetus by PCR testing, serial MCA testing should be continued every 1 to 2 weeks until 35 weeks' gestation. Because of the higher false-positive rate with the MCA at this gestation, a switch to amniocentesis for ΔOD_{450} should then be undertaken; fetal pulmonary studies at 37 weeks' gestation are in order. Again, induction at 39 weeks' gestation is indicated after documentation of fetal lung maturity.

Previously Affected Fetus or Infant

If there is a history of a perinatal loss related to HDFN, a previous need for intrauterine transfusion, or a previous need for neonatal exchange transfusion, the patient should be referred to a tertiary care center with experience in the management of the severely alloimmunized pregnancy. In these cases, maternal titers are *not* predictive of the degree of fetal anemia. In the case of a heterozygous paternal phenotype, an amniocentesis at 15 weeks' gestation to determine the fetal RhD status is indicated. Many centers are now using serial MCA Doppler measurements to monitor these pregnancies at risk for severe HDFN. Testing should begin at 18 weeks' gestation and repeated every 1 to 2 weeks. Alternatively, serial amniocenteses for measurement of ΔOD_{450} can be used with the Queenan curve for reference values. If a rising ΔOD_{450} value into the *intrauterine transfusion* zone of the Queenan curve or a rising value for peak MCA Doppler velocity greater than 1.5 MoM is found, an FBS is performed with blood readied for intrauterine transfusion if the fetal hematocrit is found to be less than 30%.

Intrauterine Transfusion

ACCESS SITE

The cord insertion proximate to the fetal umbilicus should be avoided because vagal innervation is thought to be present, increasing the likelihood of fetal bradycardia. Weiner, Wenstrom, and coworkers (1991) also noted that puncture of the mid-segment of the umbilical cord was associated with a 2.5-fold higher incidence of fetal bradycardia as compared with puncture at the placental insertion. Therefore, the cord insertion into the placenta is the preferred site for access. The vessel of interrogation should be the umbilical vein instead of one of the umbilical arteries. In one series of 750 diagnostic or therapeutic FBS, the incidence of fetal bradycardia was 21% with puncture of the umbilical artery as compared with 3% with umbilical venous puncture. (Weiner, Wenstrom, et al., 1991). Several authors conjectured that this may be due to spasm of the muscularis of the umbilical artery. Other centers have advocated the use of the intrahepatic portion of the umbilical vein in an effort to prevent fetal bradycardia. Nicolini and coworkers (1988) reported a 2.3% incidence of fetal bradycardia using this approach in 214 procedures. These authors proposed that the absence of the umbilical artery at the anatomic level of the intrahepatic vein explained their low incidence of fetal bradycardia. An additional advantage proposed by the authors was that blood loss from the cord puncture site would be minimized by absorption from the peritoneal cavity. Despite these theoretical advantages, IUTs using the intrahepatic vein have been reported to be associated with an increase in the fetal stress hormones of noradrenaline, cortisol, and beta-endorphin (Giannakoulopoulos et al., 1994, 1999). Similar changes were not detected in these levels when the cord placental insertion was used as the site of transfusion. Puncture of the intrahepatic vein is technically more challenging than using the placental insertion, predominantly because of fetal movement. In addition, the fetus must present with its spine toward the maternal back to allow access. Most centers in the United States therefore use the umbilical cord insertion into the placenta as the primary site of access for IUT. However, in cases of poor visualization, the use of the intrahepatic vein is a viable option.

Direct cardiac puncture has been reported as a method of access for IUT. It has been associated with a high rate of fetal death, and therefore its use cannot be advocated. In one series of 158 cases of diagnostic cardiocentesis for the prenatal diagnosis of hemoglobinopathies, the corrected fetal loss rate was 5.6%, significantly higher than 1% loss rate generally quoted for FBS (Antsaklis et al., 1992).

METHOD OF TRANSFUSION

Until the direct IVT was introduced in the mid-1980s, the IPT was the method of IUT for almost 20 years. With the advent of ultrasound-directed FBS, direct transfusion of cells into the umbilical circulation became the preferred method for IUT. Experience in the hydropic fetus indicated that the absorption of transfused red cells from the peritoneal cavity is compromised. Harman et al. (1990) compared the direct IVT and IPT techniques matching patients for severity of disease, placental location, and gestational age at the start of transfusions. Several important outcome differences were noted. When the fetuses were divided into nonhydropic and hydropic groups at the time of the first transfusion, a 13% increase in survival was noted in nonhydropic fetuses using IVT as

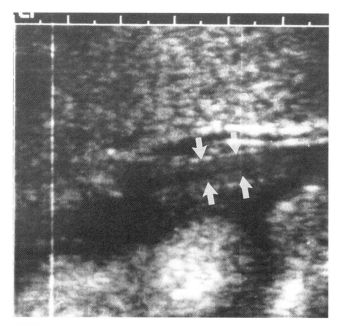

FIGURE 30-9 ■ Direct intravascular transfusion through the umbilical vein. *Arrows* indicate outer walls of the vein. Echoes in the vein are the result of the streaming of infused red blood cells. Placental cord insertion is seen to the left of the *arrows*.

compared with IPT. In hydropic fetuses, however, the rate of survival was almost doubled with IVT. IVT resulted in the need for fewer neonatal exchange transfusions compared with IPT and a shorter stay in the intensive care nursery. Direct IVT therefore has become the preferred method of transfusion of the anemic fetus (Fig. 30-9). Initial interest in performing the IVT by an exchange technique much like neonatal exchange transfusions waned after further experience with the direct IVT. It was soon realized that the fetus could tolerate large transfusion volumes because of the capacity of the placental vasculature to vasodilate. The IPT remains a practical method for delivering red cells to the nonhydropic fetus when there is difficulty with access to the umbilical cord or intrahepatic umbilical vein. Bowman (1978) proposed a formula for the intraperitoneal transfusion volume (mL) that has withstood the test of time. The volume of red cells to be infused is calculated by subtracting 20 from the gestational age in weeks and multiplying by 10. Blood in the peritoneal reservoir can be expected to be absorbed over a 7- to 10-day period.

Serial hematocrits from fetuses transfused with IVTs alone revealed a marked decline between procedures of approximately 1% per day (Berkowitz et al., 1986). To avoid this problem, we investigated whether a combined IPT–IVT technique would result in a more stable fetal hematocrit between intrauterine transfusions (Moise, Carpenter, et al., 1989). The technique involved administering enough packed red cells (hematocrit, 75% to 85%) by IVT to achieve a final fetal hematocrit of 35% to 40%; this was followed by a standard IPT. The hypothesis was that the intraperitoneal infusion of blood would serve as a reservoir, allowing the slow absorption of red cells between procedures and producing a more stable hematocrit. A combined direct IVT–IPT achieved a more stable fetal hematocrit compared with direct IVT alone, resulting in a decline in hematocrit of 0.01% per day between transfusions compared with a decline of 1.14% per day. Nicolini and coworkers (1989) compared 17 IVTs with 32 combined

IVT–IPT procedures. A final fetal hematocrit of 40% was targeted for the IVT portion of the procedure. Assuming complete absorption of the blood infused into the peritoneal cavity, a theoretical final hematocrit of 50% to 60% was used by these investigators to determine the volume for the IPT. Although the decline in hematocrit per day was identical for IVT and IVT–IPT, the combined procedure achieved a significantly longer interval between transfusions and also maintained a higher initial fetal hematocrit at subsequent transfusion. Although these data suggest several theoretical advantages to a combined transfusion technique, most centers exclusively use the direct IVT, citing the need for two punctures and prolonged procedure times as the disadvantages of a combined approach.

Reports of IUTs in twin gestations are limited to case reports. In one series of nine pregnancies complicated by RhD alloimmunization, five cases required IUT (Lepercq et al., 1999). Four of the five cases were noted to be dizygotic based on first-trimester ultrasound. In one case, only one fetus was RhD positive, illustrating the need to sample each fetus for antigen testing. In one case of monozygotic gestation, the IUT of one fetus was quickly followed by the movement of donor red cells through intraplacental anastomoses as illustrated by a positive K-B stain at the time of FBS of the second twin. In subsequent IUTs, the transfusion of only one member of the twin pair resulted in adequate levels of hemoglobin in both twins. Therefore, caution against over transfusion should be undertaken in the monozygotic gestation. In addition, the intrahepatic portion of the umbilical vein may be the preferred target for vascular access when transfusing a twin gestation when the corresponding placental cord insertions are difficult to identify.

AMOUNT TO TRANSFUSE

The end point for the completion of an intrauterine transfusion varies considerably. Most centers use a target hematocrit to decide when a transfusion is completed. Advocates of direct IVT often transfuse to a final hematocrit value of 50% to 65%. This allows a reasonable interval between procedures based on a projected decline in hematocrit of 1% per day. However, caution should be exercised in transfusing the fetus to nonphysiologic values for hematocrit. Welch and coworkers (1994) demonstrated that a marked rise in whole blood viscosity is associated with fetal hematocrits above 50%. Centers that use a combined technique usually choose a final target hematocrit of 35% to 40% for the intravascular portion of the procedure.

Several authors proposed formulas to calculate the volume of red blood cells to be transfused. The method of Mandelbrot and coworkers (1988) requires the calculation of the fetoplacental volume (mL) from the ultrasound estimate of the fetal weight by multiplying the weight in grams by a factor of 0.14. The volume of red cells in milliliters to be transfused is then calculated using the following formula:

$$V_{transfused} = \frac{V_{fetoplacental} \times (hematocrit_{final} - hematocrit_{initial})}{Hematocrit_{transfused\ blood}}$$

Giannina and coworkers (1998) proposed a simpler method of calculating the volume of packed red cells needed for IUT. Assuming a hematocrit of approximately 75% for the donor unit, a series of transfusion coefficients were determined for

TABLE 30-4. TRANSFUSION COEFFICIENT FOR CALCULATING TRANSFUSION VOLUME

Target Increase in Fetal Hematocrit (%)	Transfusion Coefficient
10	0.02
15	0.03
20	0.04
25	0.05
30	0.06

Reproduced with permission from Moise KJ, Whitecar PW: Antenatal therapy for haemolytic disease. *In* Hadley A, Soothill P (eds): Alloimmune Disorders of Pregnancy: Anaemia, Thrombocytopenia and Neutropenia in the Fetus and Newborn. Cambridge, Cambridge University Press, 2002, p. 182. Copyright © 2002.

raising the initial fetal hematocrit to a desired final value (Table 30-4). The operator simply multiplies the coefficient by the ultrasound estimation of fetal weight in grams to calculate the volume of the transfusion in milliliters needed to achieve the final desired fetal hematocrit. This practical approach is used exclusively at our center.

After the first IUT, subsequent procedures are scheduled at 14-day intervals until suppression of fetal erythropoiesis is noted on K-B stain or fetal cell stain using flow cytometry. This usually occurs by the third IUT. Thereafter, the interval for repeat procedures can be determined based on the decline in hematocrit for the individual fetus, usually a 3- to 4-week interval.

Recently, the peak MCA velocity has been studied for deciding upon the transfusion interval (Detti et al., 2001). In 64 fetuses that had undergone one IUT, a threshold for the MCA of 1.69 MoM yielded a sensitivity of 100% and a specificity of 94% for the prediction of severe fetal anemia (fetal hemoglobin less than 0.55 MoM) at the time of the second IUT. An MCA value of 1.32 MoM resulted in a sensitivity of 100% with a specificity of 63% in the ability to detect moderate anemia (fetal hemoglobin, 0.65 to 0.55 MoM). It appears that lower MCA thresholds for the detection of fetal anemia should be used once IUTs have been initiated. This may be related to the rheology of the mixture of fetal and adult hemoglobins as a result of the transfused red cells. There are no current data on the accuracy of the MCA for the prediction of fetal anemia after the second IUT.

The Severely Anemic Fetus

In our experience, the severely anemic fetus at 18 to 24 weeks' gestation is less able to adapt to the acute correction of its anemia by IVT, resulting in a higher perinatal mortality. An increase of greater than 10 mm Hg in the umbilical venous pressure at the conclusion of an IVT correctly predicted fetal death within 24 hours with a sensitivity of 80% (Hallak et al., 1992). This finding may be the result of cardiac failure in these fetuses resulting from the acute change in viscosity secondary to correction of the fetal hematocrit into the normal range. Radunovic and coworkers (1992) noted a 37% mortality within 72 hours of IVT in fetuses presenting with severe anemia and hydrops. Based on their data, these authors recommended that in the severely anemic fetus, the final post-transfusion hematocrit after IVT should not exceed a value of

25% or a fourfold increase from the pretransfusion value. When severe anemia occurs in the fetus at less than 24 weeks, a stepwise progression in the correction of the fetal hematocrit should be undertaken using the fourfold rule for increase in hematocrit at the time of the first procedure. A repeat IVT is performed within 48 hours to correct the fetal hematocrit into the normal range; the third procedure is scheduled in 7 to 10 days. Thereafter, repeat transfusions are undertaken based on fetal hematocrits and K-B stains. If a combined procedure is used, an IPT should not be undertaken until there is resolution of fetal hydrops owing to impaired absorption associated with this condition.

Adjunctive Measures

Another important development in fetal transfusion has been the use of fetal paralysis during the procedure. Before this modification, fetal movement often resulted in injury to fetal viscera during IPT or umbilical cord damage during IVT. Fetal paralysis was first introduced by de Crespigny and colleagues (1985) in Australia. Initial use in the United States involved the intramuscular injection of *d*-tubocurarine into the fetal thigh under ultrasound guidance (Moise et al., 1987). Later, pancuronium bromide was used intravascularly (Moise, Deter, et al., 1989). More recently, short-acting agents such as atracurium besylate and vecuronium bromide have been used (Bernstein et al., 1988; Daffos et al., 1988). These latter agents do not appear to cause the fetal tachycardia and loss of short-term heart rate variability associated with pancuronium (Pielet et al., 1988). A vecuronium dose of 0.1 mg/kg of the ultrasound-estimated fetal weight produces almost immediate cessation of fetal movement after intravascular injection at the start of the IUT. Fetal paralysis can be expected to last 1 to 2 hours. No untoward effects have been observed in neonates treated in this manner. In cases of anterior placentation, some centers do not routinely use fetal paralysis. Anecdotally, we have noted cord trauma resulting from fetal movement even in this scenario; therefore, we use vecuronium in all cases of IUT.

Prophylactic antibiotics have not been studied in association with IUT. Various centers have developed their own preferences. If they are to be used, a broad-spectrum cephalosporin with coverage that includes gram-positive skin flora would appear to be appropriate.

Source of Red Cells

Red cells used for IUT must undergo the same rigorous testing that occurs for any allogenic donation. In the United States, this includes a written questionnaire that inquires about illicit substance abuse, high risk sexual behavior, and travel outside of the continental United States. Serum testing for antibodies to syphilis, hepatitis B core antigen, human immunodeficiency viruses (types 1 and 2), hepatitis C virus, and human lymphotropic viruses (types I and II) as well as testing for the p24 antigen of the human immunodeficiency virus, hepatitis B surface antigen, and alanine aspartate transferase is undertaken. Additional testing by nucleic acid amplification for human immunodeficiency virus and hepatitis C virus is currently being performed on an investigational basis in the vast majority of donations collected in the United States. In the United Kingdom, all donors are screened for the hepatitis B surface antigen and antibodies against human immunodeficiency virus types 1 and 2, hepatitis C virus, and syphilis. In both countries, red cells to be used for IUT are often cytomegalovirus (CMV) seronegative or leukocyte reduced to decrease the risk of transmitting CMV. A fresh unit is preferred to stored blood to enhance the level of 2, 3-diphosphoglycerate. Standards in the United Kingdom require that red cells used for IUT have a shelf life of less than 5 days. A recent review noted that six cases of graft-versus-host reaction have been reported in infants who underwent IUT (Harte et al., 1997). Bohm and colleagues (1977) proposed that this was due to the induction of immune tolerance to engrafting lymphocytes that gain entry into the fetal circulation through large volumes of blood infused during IUTs. The British Blood Transfusion Task Force (1996) and the American Association of Blood Banks' standards (Vengelen-Tyler, 1999) require that red cell units for IUT undergo gamma irradiation using 25 Gy to prevent graft-versus-host reaction. In addition, leukodepletion is a requirement in the United Kingdom and, although not routinely practiced in the United States, is often used to reduce CMV risk and will likely be universally accepted in the near future.

Maternal blood donation is an excellent source of red cells for IUT. In a series of 21 patients, up to six units of blood per patient were harvested for intrauterine transfusion (Gonsoulin et al., 1990). No serious maternal or fetal effects were noted. Theoretical advantages to the use of maternal blood include a decreased risk for sensitization to new red cell antigens, a longer circulating half-life in the fetus because of the fresh source of cells, and a decreased risk for transmission of viral agents. Vietor and coworkers (1994) investigated the source of new red cell antibodies in 91 patients undergoing 280 IUTs. Twenty-six percent of the women developed new antibodies. In 14 cases, the source of the sensitizing antigen could be determined; in one fifth of the cases donor red cells carried the involved antigen. Thus, it appears that in 5% of cases, use of maternal blood as the source of red cells for IUT would theoretically prevent development of new anti-red cell antibodies.

Only one investigation has compared the fetal effects of maternal red cells versus unrelated donor red cells for IUT (el-Azeem et al., 1997). Seventy-six IUTs in which maternal blood was used were compared with 213 IUTs in which donor red cells were used. The fetal hematocrit did not decline as rapidly when maternal red cells were used for IUT; however, this difference did not manifest until after 33 weeks' gestation. In addition, infants who received maternal blood required fewer neonatal transfusions as compared with those who received unrelated donor cells. The authors conjectured that this finding could be related to an increased maternal reticulocytosis that probably occurs secondary to repeated blood donation. Such reticulocytosis would result in a younger population of red cells that would exhibit a longer half-life in the fetus. They concluded that maternal red cells were preferred over unrelated donor red cells because they offered the potential advantage of decreasing the total number of IUTs necessary for the treatment of a particular fetus. To date, no study has compared maternal versus unrelated donor red cells regarding the risk of fetal viral infection.

In a maternal blood donation program, if IUTs are likely, the patient can donate a unit of red cells after the first trimester. The unit can be separated into two smaller aliquots and refrigerated for up to 42 days. If not used by this time interval, the unit can then be frozen for use for up to 10 years.

Patients should be supplemented with iron therapy (324 mg ferrous sulfate twice daily) and folate (1 mg daily) in addition to prenatal vitamins. The left lateral recumbent position should be used during the donation; the donated volume should be replaced with isotonic intravenous fluids. Fetal monitoring during the procedure is unnecessary (Herbert et al., 1988). A standard volume of 450 ± 45 mL is taken because subsequent processing will markedly reduce the final volume available for IUT. The blood is washed several times to remove the offending antibody present in any contaminating plasma. The use of maternal blood in the CMV-seropositive patient is controversial. Dormant CMV virus is noted to reside in the polymorphonuclear leukocytes. Both leukoreduction and washing have been demonstrated to be effective mechanisms to prevent the transmission of CMV (Pamphilon et al., 1999). For this reason, use of maternal CMV-seropositive blood after careful counseling of the patient can be considered. Finally, the use of ABO-incompatible maternal red cells for IUT has raised concern. With fetal typing now available at the first FBS, situations may arise in which the patient is found to be type A or B and the fetus is typed as O. We have used maternal blood in two such cases with no deleterious effects noted in the fetus. Follow-up at 3 years of age in one of these infants revealed anti-A and anti-B titers that were appropriate for age.

Timing of Delivery

Until the introduction of the direct IVT, fetuses were routinely delivered by 32 weeks' gestation. Hyaline membrane disease and the need for neonatal exchange transfusions for the treatment of hyperbilirubinemia were common. As experience with IVT became widespread, several centers began to question this policy of premature delivery. Klumper and colleagues (2000) compared perinatal mortality for IUTs undertaken before and after 32 weeks' gestation. Perinatal loss occurred in 3.4% of the 409 early IUTs as compared with 1% in the 200 procedures performed after that gestation. Most experienced centers now perform the final IUT at up to 35 weeks' gestation, with delivery anticipated at 37 to 38 weeks. This practice allows maturation of the hepatic enzyme systems, which virtually eliminates the need for neonatal exchange transfusions. After a viable gestational age is attained, performing the transfusion in immediate proximity to the labor and delivery suite and allowing the patient nothing by mouth in the preoperative period appears prudent so that cesarean section can be undertaken if fetal distress should occur.

Outcome

Survival after intrauterine transfusion varies with center, experience, and the presence of hydrops fetalis. Overall survival in one review was 84%; up to one fourth fewer hydropic fetuses survive with IUT (70%) compared with fetuses who undergo their first IUT when they are not hydropic (survival, 92%) (Schumacher and Moise, 1996). The experience of a single treatment center with 213 fetuses receiving 599 IUTs was very similar. Survival with any degree of hydrops was 78% as compared with 92% for nonhydropic fetuses (van Kamp et al., 2001). The authors further classified hydrops into mild (only mild ascites) and severe (significant ascites with scalp edema, pericardial effusion or pleural effusion). Mild hydrops reversed in 88% of cases, whereas severe hydrops only reversed in 39%, a finding clearly linked to overall perinatal survival: 98% of fetuses survived after reversal of hydrops. With persistent hydrops, only 39% of fetuses survived; if the hydrops was severe and persisted, only one fourth survived.

Immediate follow-up studies of infants treated with IVTs *in utero* revealed a need for *top-up* transfusions in the early months of life. Typically, these infants are born with a virtual absence of reticulocytes with a red cell population consisting mainly of transfused red cells containing adult hemoglobin. Exchange transfusions for hyperbilirubinemia are rarely necessary. However, at 1 month of age these infants often require a simple transfusion because of symptoms associated with anemia. In our series of 36 infants that had undergone IUTs, 50% required top-up transfusions at a mean age of 38 days with a range of 20 to 68 days (Saade et al., 1993). Studies of these infants indicate erythroid hypoplasia of the bone marrow accompanied by low levels of circulating erythropoietin and reticulocytes (Koenig et al., 1989). This led Ovali and coworkers (1996) to study the use of exogenous erythropoietin in neonates after IUTs. Twenty infants were randomized to receive 200 U/kg of recombinant human erythropoietin or saline placebo administered subcutaneously three times a week between the 2nd and 8th week of life. Infants in the treatment group required a mean of 1.8 red cell transfusions compared with a mean of 4.2 transfusions in the placebo group. Recovery of the neonate's bone marrow occurred earlier in the treatment group as compared with control subjects.

Because of this phenomenon, neonatal hematocrit and reticulocyte determinations should be checked weekly until hematopoiesis recovers in infants who have undergone IUTs. Proposed criterion for transfusion of the infant vary and are usually described for premature infants. A more conservative approach is advocated by Maier and coworkers (1994). A threshold for transfusion is a hematocrit of less than 27% if the infant is asymptomatic and less than 32% with symptoms. Shannon and colleagues (1991) proposed a threshold value for hematocrit of less than 20% without symptoms or less than 30% in conjunction with symptoms. If erythropoietin is to be used, initiation in the 1st week of life in the infant with a persistent low circulating reticulocyte count may prove beneficial. Supplemental iron therapy is unnecessary because of the high levels of circulating iron in these infants secondary to ongoing hemolysis *in utero*. Supplemental folate therapy (0.5 mg/day) should be considered.

Investigations regarding the long-term neurologic evaluation of infants that have been treated with IUTs are limited. Hardyment and colleagues (1979) reported a series of fetuses transfused with IPT between 1966 and 1975 when survival was only 48%. Twenty-one of the 27 fetuses underwent evaluation, and evidence of cerebral palsy was found in 10% of cases. Advancements in treatment techniques suggest that more moribund and severely anemic fetuses now survive. Doyle and coworkers (1993) evaluated 38 surviving infants at 2 years of age. The authors noted one case of cerebral palsy, one case of mild disability with a mental developmental index of 72, and one case of severe developmental delay associated with seizures. Comparison with a group of 51 randomly selected infants of normal birth weight who underwent a similar assessment at 2 years of age yielded no significant differences in the incidence of sensorineural outcomes. Janssens and coworkers (1997) studied 69 infants for 6 months to 6 years of age. Seven

percent of the children exhibited some evidence of neurologic handicap; 4% were diagnosed with cerebral palsy. Sixteen percent of the children were noted to have developmental delay; six cases showed mild delay, whereas five additional cases exhibited severe delay. The overall 10% rate of disability in their group was comparable with a cohort of normal Dutch children with 6% disability and a cohort of high-risk children with 12% disability. We followed 40 surviving infants for up to 62 months of age. Only one case of spastic hemiplegia was detected. Gesell and McCarthy developmental scores were similar to norms for the general population (Hudon et al., 1998). Grab and colleagues (1999) followed 30 infants and noted mild sensorineural disabilities in 2. One infant exhibited delayed speech development at 24 months; the second had mild psychomotor developmental delay at 1 year of age that had resolved by 6 years of age.

Hearing loss in the neonate has been reported in association with high bilirubin levels. Because red cell destruction can lead to high levels of *in utero* bilirubin and elevated levels in neonatal life, HDFN could be associated with sensorineural hearing loss. Janssens and colleagues (1997) found that 14% of 58 children screened at 9 months had evidence of hearing loss. However, five cases were thought to be conductive in nature because of the association with middle ear or respiratory infection and the transient nature of the findings. Hudon and coworkers (1998) tested 21 infants just before discharge. Two infants had mild peripheral sensitivity loss with recovery noted in one at 5 months of age; the other child was lost to follow-up. A third child exhibited severe bilateral deafness. Based on these studies, it would appear that hearing loss is increased 5- to 10-fold over the general population in infants requiring *in utero* therapy for HDFN. Thus, careful follow-up of these infants is warranted.

The issue of enhanced survival of the hydropic fetus and the relationship to long-term outcome has been addressed in two investigations. Using a two-sample analysis, Janssens and coworkers (1997) found no correlation between either the presence of hydrops or the number of IUTs and poor neonatal neurologic outcome. Using a multivariate analysis, our group (Hudon et al., 1998) could find no relationship between global developmental scores and the number of IUTs, lowest fetal hematocrit, or presence of hydrops. These data are reassuring in counseling couples that present with a severely anemic fetus. A normal neurologic outcome can be expected in over 90% of surviving infants, even if hydrops fetalis is noted at the time of the first IUT.

Other Treatment Modalities

Plasmapheresis

Plasmapheresis has been relegated to a historical treatment modality for HDFN with the advent of modern IUT techniques. Most literature reports include single cases or relatively small case series. Many of the series use the historical control of the outcome of the patient's previous pregnancy to suggest a therapeutic effect. In addition, plasmapheresis is often combined with IUT or intravenous immune globulin (IVIG), making discernment of its beneficial effect more difficult. Despite these limitations, a review of the published cases reveals a perinatal survival of 69% (Moise and Whitecar, 2002). A randomized clinical trial was attempted by the

Canadian Apheresis study group in patients with severe red cell alloimmunization; unfortunately, insufficient enrollment necessitated premature termination of the study.

Reported protocols vary considerably, but all involve repeated procedures because of a rebound increase in antibody titer. In animal studies, Bystryn and coworkers (1970) experimentally lowered antibody levels by exchange transfusion. Antibody levels were noted to rebound to over 200% of the initial levels with the greatest increase of 50% to 80% seen in the first 48 hours. Using weekly plasmaphereses, Angela and coworkers (1980) noted three different patterns of antibody titer among their patients. Some patients were noted to have an initial suppression of their anti-RhD titer that remained low throughout gestation; a second group remained suppressed until 32 weeks' gestation, when a marked rise occurred. The titers in the third group remained high despite repeated procedures with a rapid rebound to pre-pheresis levels. Interestingly, all cases exhibited a dramatic rise in titer after delivery ranging from 66% to 1566% of baseline.

Most reports suggest starting plasmapheresis after 12 weeks' gestation. This approach seems reasonable in view of the documented transplacental passage of up to 60% of maternal IgG1 and 30% of IgG3 antibodies by this gestation (Schur et al., 1973). One school of thought advocates the removal of large volumes of plasma of 2 to 3 liters two to five times weekly, whereas others believe that smaller volumes of 500 mL to 1 liter removed once weekly produce less rebound in antibody titer (Graham-Pole et al., 1977; al-Omari, 1989). The plasma that is removed requires replacement; saline, plasma protein fraction, Rh-negative plasma, and albumin have all been used. With modern concerns regarding viral transmission through blood products, 5% albumin would seem to be the preferred fluid. Automated cell separators are now routinely used for the procedure, with citrate being used in the machine's extracorporeal circuit to prevent coagulation. Angela and coworkers (1980) reported a 15% incidence of complications in 261 procedures in pregnant women. These included delayed vertigo, headache, allergic reaction to plasma, peripheral edema, and syncope; 10 cases involved mild citrate toxicity. The latter is usually heralded by circumoral paresthesia and can be treated with oral calcium. In some cases intravenous calcium gluconate is required at the conclusion of the procedure.

Intravenous Immune Globulin

IVIG has been used effectively as the sole antenatal treatment for HDFN. In the largest series reported to date, Margulies and coworkers (1991) described the use of IVIG without IUTs in 24 patients with severe rhesus disease. The study population represented a high-risk group with over half the patients having experienced a fetal or neonatal death in a previous pregnancy and 12% of the previous pregnancies involving two or more perinatal losses. All patients in the series were noted to have an RhD-positive fetus, three having undergone FBS in the case of a heterozygous paternal genotype. Patients received a total dose of 2 g/kg IVIG administered over 4 consecutive days (400 mg/kg/day); the dose was repeated at 2- to 3-week intervals throughout the pregnancy. The patients were divided into three groups based on gestational age at the initiation of IVIG therapy: less than 20 weeks' gestation, 20 to 28 weeks' gestation, and more than 28 weeks' gestation. There was a total of three fetal losses in groups 1 and 2. All three

fetuses were noted to be hydropic at the start of therapy. There were no neonatal deaths, yielding a perinatal survival rate for the series of 88%. Half the neonates in group 1, one third in group 2, and 88% of group 3 required exchange transfusions, leading the authors to conclude that IVIG is not effective if initiated after 28 weeks' gestation. Interestingly, the maternal anti-D titers declined in all three groups, although this difference was not statistically significant in group 2.

In a follow-up case-control study of 69 patients, this same group of investigators compared the outcome of pregnancies that received IVIG before 20 weeks' gestation followed by IUT to the use of only IUTs after 20 weeks (Voto et al., 1997). Again the study group represented cases of severe rhesus alloimmunization in that 73% of the IVIG group and 56% of the IUT group had experienced previous perinatal losses. Significant differences were noted between the groups. Hydrops at the first IUT occurred in one fourth of the IVIG–IUT group as compared with three fourths of the IUT alone group. The first IUT was performed a median of 1.5 weeks later in the patients that had received IVIG. Fetal death was 2.5-fold more likely in the IUT only group (51% versus 20%). Neonatal death occurred in 8% of the IVIG–IUT group as compared with 21% in the IUT only group, although this difference did not achieve statistical significance.

The mechanism of action of IVIG in cases of severe HDFN is not well understood. At least three different theories for its effect have been postulated: decreased production of maternal anti-red cell antibodies, decreased placental transport of antibodies, and fetal RE blockade. Dooren and coworkers (1994) randomized 20 patients to receive either IVT alone or IVT in conjunction with the direct fetal infusion of IVIG. No significant differences in the transfusion requirement or clinical outcome could be demonstrated between the two groups. However, the average fetal IVIG dose of 85 mg/kg was fairly low compared with the 500-mg/kg dose usually used to treat neonatal HDFN (Rubo et al., 1992). In a case report, Alonso and coworkers (1994) used between 406 and 481 mg/kg of IVIG and administered this directly to the fetus on four occasions at the time of FBS. Fetal hematocrit increased and ΔOD_{450} values decreased with advancing gestation. To further elucidate the protective mechanism of IVIG, one investigation compared six pregnancies treated with maternal IVIG with seven control sensitized women that were only followed with serial FBS (Gottvall and Selbing, 1995). No obvious inhibitory effect on the transplacental passage of anti-D or the maternal anti-D production was noted. Finally, Besalduch and colleagues (1991) reported a case in which IVIG was used in a patient with early hydrops fetalis secondary to anti-E alloimmunization. These authors used a pepsin-treated preparation resulting in a purified IgG product with loss of Fc receptors. Fetal hydrops and hepatosplenomegaly were noted to resolve with repeated IVIG administration. The authors postulated that the effectiveness of the IVIG in their case was related to suppression of the maternal antibody levels because their product could not have crossed the placenta owing to the lack of the Fc receptors.

Yu and Lennon (1999) proposed a mechanism to explain the potential ability of IVIG to cause the accelerated catabolism of circulating anti-red cell antibodies. An intracellular Fc receptor abundant in endothelial cells normally binds the IgG that has entered the cell through pinocytosis and presents it back to the surface of the cell for release back into the microcirculation. In cases of excess circulating IgG secondary to IVIG, the protective intracellular Fc receptors become saturated, allowing the accelerated catabolism of free IgG molecules that enter the endothelial cells. These data would lead one to conclude that multiple mechanisms may contribute to the effectiveness of IVIG. Although the primary effect may be the suppression of the level of maternal antibody, a fetal RE blockade may also be involved.

Combined Plasmapheresis and Intravenous Immune Globulin

Berlin and coworkers (1985) used a combined plasmapheresis–IVIG approach when problems with continued venous access precluded continued plasmaphereses in a patient with severe anti-D alloimmunization. A total of 10 liters of plasma were exchanged over 4 days at 25 weeks' gestation. This was followed by an IVIG dose of 0.4 g/kg/day over 5 consecutive days. The patient's anti-D concentration became markedly reduced and did not return to pretreatment levels for 6 to 7 weeks. The infant was delivered at 35 weeks and was noted to have a cord hemoglobin of 12.5 g/dL. Currently, our center will offer a combination of plasmaphereses and IVIG to those patients with a previous fetal loss before 20 weeks' gestation. In these rare cases, the technical limitations of gaining access to the fetal circulation in conjunction with the inability of the very premature fetus to compensate for the acute cardiovascular changes that occur with IVT make this experimental approach a reasonable alternative. This approach is based on a randomized trial of 383 adult patients with Guillain-Barré syndrome (Plasma Exchange/Sandoglobulin Guillain-Barré Syndrome Trial Group, 1997). In this trial, patients received one of three therapies: plasmapheresis alone, IVIG alone, or plasmaphereses followed by IVIG. Patients in the latter group showed a trend toward more favorable outcome. In our protocol, a single volume of plasmapheresis is undertaken every other day for three procedures in the 12th week of gestation. Five percent albumin is used for volume replacement. Maternal titers can be expected to decline by several dilutions. The IgG pool is replaced after the third procedure by administering a 1-g/kg loading dose of IVIG diluted in normal saline. The patient is premedicated with 25 mg of intravenous diphenhydramine HCl. The 10% IVIG infusion is started at a rate of 60 mL/hr and increased by 30 mL/hr every 30 minutes to a maximum rate of 240 mL/hr. A second dose of 1 g/kg IVIG is given the following day. The patient is then treated with a weekly dose of 1 g/kg IVIG until 20 weeks' gestation. This dosing regimen gives plasma levels of IgG equivalent to the regimen of 0.4 g/kg daily for 5 days that has been previously used and is generally well tolerated. Further administration of IVIG is not undertaken because of the prohibitive cost.

Typical side effects encountered during IVIG administration include urticaria and severe headache. We have found that premedication with 1000 mg of oral acetaminophen several hours before the scheduled infusion can prevent this latter complication. In some situations, a change to a different manufacturer will produce fewer headaches in some patients. On occasion, patients will complain of a mild desquamation of the palmer surface of the hands; the etiology of this phenomenon is unknown.

In the case of a heterozygous paternal genotype, an amniocentesis is undertaken at 15 weeks' gestation using DNA techniques to determine the fetal red cell antigen status. If the fetus is found to be antigen negative, the IVIG is discontinued. Standard noninvasive or invasive fetal testing is used to determine the timing of the first IUT in the case of a homozygous paternal phenotype or an RhD-positive fetus by amniocentesis. In our experience, this approach is successful in deferring the need for the first IUT until approximately 24 to 26 weeks' gestation.

Oral Tolerance

Studies to date attempting oral desensitization to red cell antigens have revealed conflicting results. In 1979, Bierme and associates (1979) investigated the use of oral RhD antigen in seven severely alloimmunized women. All previous pregnancies had resulted in intrauterine death even though IUTs were used in four cases. RhD titers were noted to remain stable in all cases. In addition, in some cases a new anti-Rh class of antibody appeared of the IgM or IgA variety. In six of the seven treated cases, an RhD-positive infant was born at 35 weeks' gestation in good condition. In an attempt to duplicate these results, American investigators treated four patients with a history of severe HDN with oral erythrocytes using the method of Bierme and associates (Gold et al., 1983). All four cases resulted in either fetal or neonatal death; hydrops fetalis was noted in all cases. In a rebuttal letter to the editor, Bierme's group reported a larger series of 16 pregnancies with 12 live births using oral erythrocyte therapy in conjunction with oral promethazine (Parinaud et al., 1984). The authors proposed that a therapeutic trial should be undertaken.

Three years later, Barnes and coworkers (1987) conducted a scientific investigation to study the effects of oral erythrocyte membrane therapy in the nonpregnant patient. Six previously sensitized women were administered a 2-g/day dose of a lyophilized preparation of erythrocyte membranes for 4 weeks. Half the patients received an erythrocyte preparation made from RhD-negative red cells and half received RhD-positive red cell preparations. In three subjects there was no change in antibody levels, whereas in the remaining three there was a clear elevation in antibody titers. In this latter group, two of the three had received RhD-positive oral antigen. These findings led the authors to conclude that their oral preparation was not tolerogenic but in fact immunogenic. No further reports can be found in peer-reviewed literature regarding this therapy because it appears to have been abandoned as a potential treatment with the advent of more effective methods of IUT.

Chemotherapeutic Agents

In vitro, promethazine interferes with the ability of human fetal macrophages to phagocytize red cells coated with anti-RhD antibodies (Gusdon et al., 1976). This led several investigators to use this agent in an effort to ameliorate the effects of maternal anti-red cell antibodies in HDFN. Gusdon (1981) treated 72 patients with RhD alloimmunization with doses of 3.7 to 5.0 mg/kg/day divided in four doses beginning as early as 14 weeks' gestation. The lower dose was used in the patients with their first affected pregnancy, whereas the highest dose was used in patients with a history of previous IUTs or fetal death. When compared with previous pregnancy, there was a marked improvement in outcome. Three perinatal deaths occurred in the pregnancies treated with promethazine as compared with eight deaths in previous pregnancies. The infants in 28% of the treated pregnancies required neonatal exchange transfusion as compared with a 44% need for neonatal exchange transfusion in the previous pregnancies in these patients. A similar investigation in 21 pregnancies was undertaken (Stenchever, 1978), giving a general impression that promethazine was not beneficial in view of the continued need for IUTs. However, a therapeutic effect was possibly seen in some gestations with previous neonatal demise.

Steroids have been proposed as a treatment for HDFN, but no case series have been published (Caudle and Scott, 1982). Agents such as betamethasone and dexamethasone cross the placenta and have been associated with decreases in ΔOD_{450} (Caritis et al., 1977). However, these changes have not been associated with a decrease in the severity of HDFN but instead are probably related to alterations in fetal bilirubin metabolism (Caudle and Scott, 1982).

Sensitization to Paternal Leukocyte Antigens

In vitro data and clinical case reports suggest that maternal alloantibodies to paternal leukocytes may result in an Fc blockade, thereby protecting the fetal red cells from hemolysis in cases of RhD alloimmunization. Neppert and coworkers (1986) reported that human sera with human leukocyte antigen (HLA)-A, -B, -C, and -DR antibodies inhibited the binding activity and phagocytosis of monocytes. The authors proposed that this inhibitory effect of maternal anti-HLA antibodies on the fetal RE system may explain the lack of clinical disease in cases of HDFN with a strongly positive direct Coombs at birth (Neppert, 1987). Dooren and coworkers (1992) studied 12 cases of RhD alloimmunization in which the ADCC assay predicted severe fetal disease, but the neonatal clinical course was instead benign. When donor monocytes were replaced in the assay by paternal cells (monocytes that should share HLA antigens with the neonate), seven of the repeat assays revealed lack of lysis of the sensitized red cells. Six of the seven cases involved maternal monocyte-reactive antibodies of the paternal HLA-DR specificity. Three reports of clinical cases have appeared in the literature in which maternal HLA antibodies were thought to be the explanation for the mild clinical course in HDN (Dooren et al., 1993; Eichler et al., 1995). In two cases the specificity of the maternal antibody was HLA-DR, whereas in the remaining case the antibody was directed against the HLA-A10 and DR13 antigens. Data suggest that these alloantibodies prevent the binding of anti-D–sensitized fetal red cells to FcγR-bearing splenic phagocytes, thus reducing the severity of HDN (Shepard et al., 1996; Wiener et al., 1995).

We have shown in a rabbit model for HDFN that alloimmunization to paternal leukocytes produces fetal hemoglobin levels that approach normal in does that have been previously sensitized to red cells (Whitecar et al., 2002). Limitations of this method of treatment for severe red cell alloimmunization are substantial. In human trials, any contamination of the paternal leukocytes with paternal red cells could produce a substantial anamnestic effect in the maternal antibody titer. In addition, maternal sensitization to paternal HLA antigens could produce alloimmune thrombocytopenic purpura in the fetus or neonate.

HEMOLYTIC DISEASE OF THE FETUS AND NEWBORN OWING TO NON-RHD ANTIBODIES

More than 50 different red cell antigens have been reported to be associated with HDFN (Table 30-5). However, the antibodies frequently associated with severe HDFN appear to include anti-RhD, -Rhc, and -Kell (K1). In a series from Manitoba, Canada encompassing the years 1962 to 1988, 1022 cases of non-RhD alloimmunization were accumulated (Bowman, 1990). Only anti-c was associated with severe HDFN that ended in a hydropic stillbirth or necessitated intrauterine transfusion. Anti-c resulted in a twofold incidence and sevenfold incidence of hemolytic disease as compared with -K1 and -E antibodies, respectively. Anti-c and anti-K1 antibodies were equally likely to be associated with the need for neonatal exchange transfusion or phototherapy; anti-E was half as likely to require neonatal treatment. A select population of 22 patients was referred from outside Manitoba during the same time period (Bowman, 1990). The following antibodies were associated with the need for IUTs: -K1 ($n = 9$), -k (1), -c (7), -cE (1), -Fy^a (1), -Jk^a (1), -CC^w (1), and -E (1).

Kell

The Kell red cell antigen system includes 23 different members. Individual antigens in the system are designated by name, letter abbreviation, or number. Antibodies to at least nine of the antigens have been associated with HDFN. The most common of these is Kell (K, K1) and cellano (k, K2). Additional antibodies that have been reported to be causative for HDFN include -Penny (Kp^a, K3), -Rautenberg (Kp^b, K4), -Peltz (Ku, K5), -Sutter (Js^a, K6), -Matthews (Js^b, K7), -Karhula (Ul^a, K10), and -K22 (Daniels, 2002).

Anti-K (K1)

The K1 antigen is found on the red cells of 9% of whites and 2% of blacks with virtually all antigen-positive individuals being heterozygous (Table 30-6). Kell antibody was detected in 127 of 127,076 pregnancies in one series, yet because of the gene frequency only 13 cases resulted in Kell-positive fetuses (Caine and Mueller-Heubach, 1986). Hydrops fetalis was noted in four cases; three of these infants suffered *in utero* demise or neonatal death. Bowman and colleagues (1992) reported a 46-year experience of 459 Kell-alloimmunized pregnancies in 311 women. Fourteen percent of these pregnancies ended in spontaneous or induced abortions, 82% resulted in Kell-negative infants or infants with no recorded clinical disease, and the remaining 4% were affected. In these 20 infants, there was one neonatal death and three fetuses with hydrops that died *in utero*. In a referral series of 16 pregnancies that occurred between 1970 and 1985, the authors reported a perinatal mortality of 67% before the advent of IVT as compared with a rate of 10% after this technique began to be used.

Berkowitz and colleagues (1982) described a case of Kell alloimmunization with a maternal titer of 2048. Amniocenteses at 20 and 21 weeks revealed a declining trend in the ΔOD_{450} values; however, a hydropic fetal demise was noted at 24 weeks' gestation. Amniocentesis at that time revealed a lower ΔOD_{450} value as compared with the previous values.

TABLE 30-5. NON-RhD ANTIBODIES AND ASSOCIATED HDFN

Antigen System	Specific Antigen	Antigen System	Specific Antigen	Antigen System	Specific Antigen
		Frequently Associated with Severe Disease			
Kell	-K (K1)				
Rhesus	-c				
		Infrequently Associated with Severe Disease			
Colton	-Co^a	MNS	-Mt^a	Rhesus	-HOFM
	-Co3		-MUT		-LOCR
Diego	-ELO		-Mur		-Riv
	-Di^a		-M^v		-Rh29
	-Di^b		-s		-Rh32
	-Wr^a		-s^D		-Rh42
	-Wr^b		-S		-Rh46
Duffy	-Fy^a		-U		-STEM
Kell	-Js^a		-Vw		-Tar
	-Js^b	Rhesus	-Be^a	Other antigens	-HJK
	-k (K2)		-C		-JFV
	-Kp^a		-Ce		-JONES
	-Kp^b		-C^w		-Kg
	-K11		-C^x		-MAM
	-K22		-ce		-REIT
	-Ku		-D^w		-Rd
	-Ul^a		-E		
Kidd	-Jk^a		-E^w		
MNS	-En^a		-Evans		
	-Far		-e		
	-Hil		-G		
	-Hut		-Go^a		
	-M		-Hr		
	-Mi^a		-Hr$_o$		
	-Mit		-JAL		
		Associated with Mild Disease			
Dombrock	-Do^a	Gerbich	-Ge^2	Scianna	-Sc2
	-Gy^a		-Ge^3	Other	-Vel
	-Hy		-Ge^4		-Lan
	-Jo^a		-Ls^a		-At^a
Duffy	-Fy^b	Kidd	-Jk^b		-Jr^a
	-Fy^3		-Jk^3		

From Issitt PD, Anstee DJ: Hemolytic disease of the newborn. *In* Issitt PD, Anstee DJ (eds): Applied Blood Group Serology. Durham, NC, Montgomery Scientific Publications, 1998, p. 1045; Daniels G: Blood group antibodies in haemolytic disease of the fetus and newborn. *In* Hadley A, Soothill P (eds): Alloimmune Disorders in Pregnancy: Anaemia, Thrombocytopenia, and Neutropenia in the Fetus and Newborn. Cambridge, Cambridge University Press, 2002, p. 21.

These findings led the authors to conclude that ultrasound detection of fetal hydrops could be a better predictor of fetal deterioration than amniotic fluid bilirubin. Four years later, Caine and Mueller-Heubach (1986) reported three cases of poor perinatal outcome with fetal hydrops in two cases and one neonatal demise. ΔOD_{450} values 1 week before delivery were noted to be in upper zone 2 of the Liley curve. In a matched comparison, Vaughan and coworkers (1994) noted lower amniotic fluid bilirubin in Kell alloimmunization pregnancies as compared with pregnancies complicated by RhD alloimmunization. The authors suggested that serial amniocenteses were therefore not a reliable method of management of the Kell-alloimmunized pregnancy. In a similar matched comparison, Weiner and Widness (1996) noted that Kell-affected fetuses exhibited a lower total serum bilirubin as compared with their RhD counterparts. These authors suggested that serial FBS rather than ΔOD_{450} analysis would appear to be the preferred method for following the pregnancy complicated by Kell alloimmunization.

Bowman's group (1992) suggested that ΔOD_{450} values are still useful in the management of the Kell alloimmunized pregnancy. Twelve Kell-positive fetuses were followed with amniocenteses. Two cases involved hydropic losses at 21 and 24 weeks after a previous low or mid-zone 2 reading. Combining these results with the ΔOD_{450} values in the Kell-negative fetuses, these authors suggested an 83% to 89% accuracy for serial amniocenteses as compared with an accuracy of 95% cited for rhesus disease. The authors did recommend the use of a ΔOD_{450} value of greater than 0.15 before 20 weeks' gestation and a subsequent value in excess of the 65th percentile of zone 2 of the Liley curve as the threshold to initiate FBS. In addition, they suggested the use of a critical maternal titer of 8 instead of 16 or 32 as the threshold as to when to begin serial amniocenteses.

In their prospective study using the peak MCA velocity to detect fetal anemia, Mari and coworkers (2000) reported that 16% of the fetuses in their series were evaluated secondary to Kell alloimmunization. A subgroup analysis of the accuracy of

TABLE 30-6. GENE FREQUENCIES AND ZYGOSITY FOR OTHER RED CELL ANTIGENS ASSOCIATED WITH HEMOLYTIC DISEASE OF THE NEWBORN

	White		Black	
	Antigen + (%)	Heterozygous (%)	Antigen + (%)	Heterozygous (%)
K (K1)	9.0	97.8	2	100
k (K2)	99.8	8.8	100	2
M	78.0	64.0	70	63
N	77.0	65.0	74	60
S	55.0	80.0	31	90
s	89.0	50.0	97	29
U	100.0	—	99	—
Fy^a	66.0	26.0	10	90
Fy^b	83.0	41.0	23	96
Jk^a	77.0	36.0	91	63
Jk^b	72.0	32.0	43	21

From Vengelen-Tyler V (ed): Technical Manual of the American Association of Blood Banks. Bethesda, Md, American Association of Blood Banks, 1999.

this technique in these fetuses revealed no difference from the group as a whole (Mari, personal communication). Anecdotally, we have had the opportunity to evaluate several fetuses at risk for anemia as a result of maternal anti-K1 antibodies with serial MCA Dopplers and have found the technique to be very predictive of moderate to severe fetal anemia.

Management of the K1-sensitized pregnancy should entail paternal red cell typing and genotype testing. If the paternal typing returns K1 negative (kk) and paternity is assured, no further maternal testing is undertaken. If paternal testing reveals a positive result, maternal titers of less than 4 are followed monthly until a critical value of 8 is attained. At that time, if the paternal genotype is heterozygous, amniocentesis for DNA typing of the fetus is offered after 15 weeks' gestation because 50% of fetuses will be unaffected. Paternal blood should be studied simultaneously with amniotic fluid using the same PCR primers to assess for the accuracy of the technique. However, cases of gene rearrangements in the Kell gene have not been reported to date. If the fetus is found to be K1 negative, no further fetal or maternal testing is warranted. In the case of a homozygous paternal genotype or K1-positive fetus, serial MCA Dopplers are repeated every 1 to 2 weeks starting at 18 weeks' gestation. An elevated value of more than 1.50 MoM is followed by FBS with blood readied for intrauterine transfusion.

Anti-k (K2)

Bowman and colleagues (1989) reviewed 20 years of antibody screening of approximately 350,000 pregnancies in a Manitoba population and detected only one case of anti-k alloimmunization. Levine and colleagues (1949) reported the first case of HDN secondary to anti-k with a resulting mildly affected infant; this was followed by the report of a second mild case by Bryant (1965). Additional individual cases of HDN have required treatment with a single neonatal exchange transfusion, a single simple neonatal transfusion, and a simple neonatal transfusion followed by a top-up transfusion for delayed neonatal anemia (Kulich, 1967; Bowman et al., 1989;

Duguid and Bromilow, 1990). A sixth case referred to Bowman's group (1989) required three intrauterine transfusions beginning at 30 weeks' gestation The maternal titer was noted to be 16. In the second case reported from their institution, the maternal antiglobulin titer was 8. These findings led these investigators to surmise that anti-k antibody, analogous to anti-K1 antibody, may produce fetal erythropoietic suppression at lower maternal titers than are typically used for a critical value in cases of anti-RhD.

MNS

Anti-M

The MNS system consists of 40 red cell antigens, antibodies to the M, N, S, s, and U antigens representing the more common members of this group that have been associated with HDFN. The M and N antigens can be expressed simultaneously on the glycophorin A molecule or can be expressed alone. The S, s, and U antigens are expressed on the glycophorin B molecule in various combinations. In most cases, the paternal genotype will be positive for antigen with most genotypes being heterozygous (see Table 30-6).

Anti-M is a naturally occurring IgM antibody that typically presents as a cold agglutinin. An IgG type can occur rarely and can be associated with HDFN. A total of six patients with severe HDFN have been reported in the English literature. The first case involved a maternal anti-M albumin titer of 1000 in association with a hydropic fetal death in one twin and the need for exchange transfusions in the sibling (Stone and Marsh, 1959). A second patient with a titer of 2048 was noted to have a history of four fetal deaths (Macpherson and Zartman, 1965). Matsumoto and colleagues (1981) reported a patient that had experienced three fetal losses in conjunction with a maternal anti-M titer of 1024. Furukawa and coworkers (1993) reported a patient with a history of three perinatal losses. A successful outcome was achieved in a fourth pregnancy after intensive plasmapheresis to treat a titer of 4096; the infant required only phototherapy. Duguid and coworkers (1995) described a patient with a titer of 16 that gave birth to a child requiring phototherapy and exchange transfusion. Kanra and colleagues (1996) investigated a patient that had experienced seven pregnancies with losses occurring between 10 and 33 weeks' gestation secondary to in utero or neonatal deaths; five of these pregnancies were associated with hydrops fetalis. A maternal anti-M titer of 512 was detected, although little is available regarding the evaluation of the neonates.

De Young-Owens and colleagues (1997) reviewed a 26-year experience at their institution and noted an anti-M antibody in 115 pregnancies in 90 women. The authors noted a three- to sevenfold increased incidence of detection over the course of the study period; anti-M comprised 10% of all pregnant patients with a positive antibody screen. Explanations offered for the increasing frequency included a change in antibody screening technique from albumin to ethylene glycol and the addition of indicator red cells homozygous for the M antigen to their red cell screening panel. The antiglobulin titer was less than four in 90% of cases. In five cases there was more than a two-tube increase in titer; however, the fetuses were noted to be negative for the M antigen in four of the five cases; in the fifth case the M antigen status of the fetus was unknown. In 42 cases of antigen-positive fetuses, there was no increase in maternal titer. Clinical outcome for the fetuses revealed minimal disease. Of the 70 infants who tested positive for the M antigen, only 17% exhibited a positive direct Coombs at birth. Only one of these infants required phototherapy. In this case the maternal anti-M antibody titer was 1 and the finding of a neonatal three plus direct Coombs was believed to be related to an ABO incompatibility. Four additional infants required phototherapy; all had negative direct Coombs testing and were associated with a maternal titer of less than 2. The authors proposed that prematurity accounted for the need for phototherapy because all four infants were born at less than 36 weeks' gestation.

This data led De Young-Owens and coworkers (1997) to conclude that if there is no previous history of an affected pregnancy, an initial titer of 4 or less requires no further evaluation. If the titer is greater than 4 or there is a history of a previously affected fetus or infant, serial titers should be obtained. Bowman (1990) recommended amniocentesis for ΔOD_{450} assessment if the indirect Coombs titer is 64 or higher. At our center, we elected to follow serial maternal titers until a value of 32 is reached. Consultation with the transfusion service is then obtained to determine if the antibody class is predominantly IgM or a combination of IgM and IgG (Vengelen-Tyler, 1999). This can be accomplished by treating the serum with dithiothreitol or 2-mercaptoethanol. These agents disrupt the disulfide bonds between the components of the pentamer structure of the IgM molecule, thereby abolishing the agglutinating and complement-binding properties. Serum treated with dithiothreitol containing only an IgM antibody will exhibit a loss of reactivity and a subsequent negative titer. Serum containing a mixture of IgM and IgG antibody will exhibit a decrease in the original titer. Once the IgG component of the titer reaches 32, we proceed with serial amniocenteses for ΔOD_{450} assessment. In cases of a heterozygous paternal genotype, fetal typing using PCR techniques on amniotic fluid is available for the M antigen (M. J. Hessner, personal communication, The Blood Center of Southeastern Wisconsin) using a technique previously described by Corfield and colleagues (1993).

Anti-S

In one series of 175,000 pregnancies during a 5-year period in the Oxford region of England, anti-S antibody was detected in 22 pregnancies in 19 women (Mayne et al., 1990). Previous transfusions were believed to be the likely source of sensitization in 13 patients. A positive direct Coombs was noted in only four cases; one infant required exchange transfusions. Most cases of HDFN described in the literature involve mild neonatal disease (Feldman et al., 1973). Only three cases of severe disease have been described. The first case was reported in 1952 with the infant dying secondary to kernicterus at 60 hours of life (Levine et al., 1952). Griffith (1980) described a case of stillbirth at 41 weeks' gestation complicated by the finding of a maternal anti-S antibody and autopsy findings consistent with erythroblastosis fetalis. Finally, Mayne and coworkers (1990) reported a case of maternal anti-S alloimmunization that resulted in the birth of a neonate requiring three exchange transfusions and 5 days of phototherapy.

Anti-s

Three cases of severe HDFN and one case of mild HDN have been reported (Davie et al., 1972).

Anti-N

One case of mild HDFN requiring only phototherapy has been reported (Telischi et al., 1976). PCR typing of the fetus in amniotic fluid has proven problematic, particularly in the black race where there is up to 15% discordance between paternal serology and genotype (M. J. Hessner, personal communication, The Blood Center of Southeastern Wisconsin).

Anti-U

The U antigen is unique to the black race; the antigen is virtually never seen in the white population. Smith and colleagues (1998) reviewed six of their own cases of HDFN secondary to anti-U alloimmunization and an additional nine cases from peer-reviewed literature. The neonates in four cases managed at their institution required only phototherapy for treatment despite maternal antibody titers of as high as 4000 in conjunction with a strongly positive direct Coombs assay on cord blood. One patient delivered an infant that required six simple transfusions after birth. A subsequent pregnancy in this same patient was complicated by the need for four intrauterine transfusions. At birth, two additional exchange transfusions and three simple transfusions were necessary during the neonatal course. In the review of the nine cases reported in the literature, they noted one stillbirth at 35 weeks (Burki et al., 1964), three neonates requiring exchange transfusions (Austin et al., 1976; Dhandsa et al., 1981; Gottschall, 1981), one infant with late-onset of anemia at 3 weeks of age (Magaud et al., 1981), and four additional cases with minimal evidence of HDFN (Alfonso and de Alvarez, 1961; Tuck et al., 1982; Dopp and Isham, 1983). Based on the clinical course noted in these 15 cases, the authors recommended a threshold for a critical titer of 128 if there was no HDFN in a previous pregnancy. Experience in several of their cases indicated that amniocentesis for ΔOD_{450} was an accurate method of assessing the severity of fetal anemia.

In cases of anti-U alloimmunization requiring treatment with intrauterine transfusion, maternal blood should be strongly considered as the primary source of red cells because fresh U-negative blood is often not readily available because of the high frequency of this antigen in the white population, the primary source of the donor pool (Gonsoulin et al., 1990). Alternatively, maternal siblings or parents can be tested to determine whether they can serve as donors.

Duffy

The Duffy antigen system consists of two antigens, Fy^a and Fy^b. Inheritance is by codominant alleles that result in four possible phenotypes. Anti-Fy^b antibodies have only been associated with mild HDFN. A review of 19 cases of HDFN secondary to anti-Fy^a antibody between 1956 and 1975 revealed a neonatal mortality of 18%, with almost one third of cases requiring neonatal exchange transfusion (Weinstein and Taylor, 1975). Maternal titers as low as 8 were associated with moderate HDFN, necessitating exchange transfusion. PCR typing of the fetus through amniocentesis is available in cases of a heterozygous paternal genotype (Hessner et al., 1999).

Kidd

The Kidd antigen system consists of two antigens, Jk^a and Jk^b. Inheritance is by codominant alleles that produce four possible phenotypes, although the Jk^a– /Jk^b– genotype is extremely rare. Rare cases of mild hemolytic disease have been reported. PCR typing of the fetus through amniocentesis is available in cases of a heterozygous paternal genotype (Hessner et al., 1998).

■ SUMMARY

Irregular anti-red cell antibodies associated with HDFN will continue to challenge the practitioner because the development of these antibodies is often related to transfusion therapy. In addition, prophylactic immune globulins are unlikely to be developed because of the rarity of these situations. In Australia only K1-negative red cells are used for transfusion in female children and women of reproductive age in an effort to markedly decrease the incidence of Kell alloimmunization. Such policies should receive further consideration in other countries.

Guidelines for intervention in cases of irregular antibodies are limited by the bias of anecdotal reports in the literature in favor of severe cases of HDFN. Large published series of patients with anti-K1 or anti-M in which most fetuses and neonates are minimally affected or unaffected substantiate this bias. In general, principles used in the management of the RhD-alloimmunized patient should be followed in most cases of irregular anti-red cell antibodies. A notable exception is K1 or K2 alloimmunization. A lower maternal critical titer of 8 and a lower threshold value for ΔOD_{450} in midzone 2 of the LiIey curve or serial MCA Doppler studies should be used to decide when to proceed to FBS.

REFERENCES

Alfonso JF, de Alvarez RR: Maternal isoimmunization to the red cell antigen U. Am J Obstet Gynecol 81:45, 1961.

al-Omari WR: Improved fetal survival with small volume plasmapheresis in Rhesus disease. Int J Gynaecol Obstet 30:237, 1989.

Alonso JG, Decaro J, Marrero A, et al: Repeated direct fetal intravascular high-dose immunoglobulin therapy for the treatment of Rh hemolytic disease. J Perinat Med 22:415, 1994.

American College of Obstetricians and Gynecologists (ACOG): Prevention of RhD alloimmunization. ACOG Practice Bulletin 4:1999.

Angela E, Robinson E, Tovey LA: Intensive plasma exchange in the management of severe Rh disease. Br J Haematol 45:621, 1980.

Antsaklis AI, Papantoniou NE, Mesogitis SA, et al: Cardiocentesis: an alternative method of fetal blood sampling for the prenatal diagnosis of hemoglobinopathies. Obstet Gynecol 79:630, 1992.

Asensio SH, Figueroa-Longo JG, Pelegrina IA: Intrauterine exchange transfusion. Am J Obstet Gynecol 95:1129, 1966.

Asensio SH, Figueroa-Longo JG, Pelegrina IA: Intrauterine exchange transfusion: A new technic. Obstet Gynecol 32:350, 1968.

Austin TK, Finklestein J, Okada DM, et al: Hemolytic disease of newborn infant due to anti-U (letter). J Pediatr 89:330, 1976.

Avent ND: Fetal genotyping. In Hadley A, Soothill P (eds): Alloimmune Disorders in Pregnancy. Anaemia, Thrombocytopenia, and Neutropenia in the Fetus and Newborn. Cambridge, Cambridge University Press, 2002, p. 121.

Bahado-Singh R, Oz U, Deren O, et al: Splenic artery Doppler peak systolic velocity predicts severe fetal anemia in rhesus disease. Am J Obstet Gynecol 182:1222, 2000.

Bahado-Singh R, Oz U, Mari G, et al: Fetal splenic size in anemia due to Rh-alloimmunization. Obstet Gynecol 92:828, 1998.

Bang J, Bock JE, Trolle D: Ultrasound-guided fetal intravenous transfusion for severe rhesus haemolytic disease. Br Med J 284:373, 1982.

Barnes RM, Duguid JK, Roberts FM, et al: Oral administration of erythrocyte membrane antigen does not suppress anti-Rh(D) antibody responses in humans. Clin Exp Immunol 67:220, 1987.

BCSH Blood Transfusion Task Force: Guidelines on gamma irradiation of blood components for the prevention of transfusion-associated graft-versus-host disease. Transfus Med 6:261, 1996.

Bennett PR, Le Van Kim C, Colin Y, et al: Prenatal determination of fetal RhD type by DNA amplification. N Engl J Med 329:607, 1993.

Berger HM, Lindeman JH, van Zoeren-Grobben D, et al: Iron overload, free radical damage, and rhesus haemolytic disease. Lancet 335:933, 1990.

Berkowitz RL, Beyth Y, Sadovsky E: Death in utero due to Kell sensitization without excessive elevation of the delta OD_{450} value in amniotic fluid. Obstet Gynecol 60:746, 1982.

Berkowitz RL, Chitkara U, Goldberg JD, et al: Intrauterine intravascular transfusions for severe red blood cell isoimmunization: Ultrasound-guided percutaneous approach. Am J Obstet Gynecol 155:574, 1986.

Berlin G, Selbing A, Ryden G: Rhesus haemolytic disease treated with high-dose intravenous immunoglobulin. Lancet 1:1153, 1985.

Bernstein HH, Chitkara U, Plosker H, et al: Use of atracurium besylate to arrest fetal activity during intrauterine intravascular transfusions. Obstet Gynecol 72:813, 1988.

Besalduch J, Forteza A, Duran MA, et al: Rh hemolytic disease of the newborn treated with high-dose intravenous immunoglobulin and plasmapheresis. Transfusion 31:380, 1991.

Bevis DC: Blood pigments in haemolytic disease of newborn. J Obstet Gynaecol Br Emp 63:68, 1956.

Bierme SJ, Blanc M, Abbal M, et al: Oral Rh treatment for severely immunised mothers. Lancet 1:604, 1979.

Bilardo CM, Nicolaides KH, Campbell S: Doppler studies in red cell isoimmunization. Clin Obstet Gynecol 32:719, 1989.

Bohm N, Kleine W, Enzel U: Graft-versus-host disease in two newborns after repeated blood transfusions because of rhesus incompatibility. Beitr Pathol 160:381, 1977.

Bowman JM: The management of Rh-isoimmunization. Obstet Gynecol 52:1, 1978.

Bowman JM: Controversies in Rh prophylaxis. Who needs Rh immune globulin and when should it be given? Am J Obstet Gynecol 151:289, 1985.

Bowman JM: The prevention of Rh immunization. Transfus Med Rev 2:129, 1988.

Bowman JM: Treatment options for the fetus with alloimmune hemolytic disease. Transfus Med Rev 4:191, 1990.

Bowman JM: RhD hemolytic disease of the newborn. N Engl J Med 339:1775, 1998.

Bowman JM, Harman FA, Manning CR, et al: Erythroblastosis fetalis produced by anti-k. Vox Sang 56:187, 1989.

Bowman JM, Pollock JM, Manning FA, et al: Maternal Kell blood group alloimmunization. Obstet Gynecol 79:239, 1992.

Bryant LB: A case of anti-cellano (k) with review of the present status of the Kell blood group system. Bull South Central Assoc Blood Banks 8:4, 1965.

Burki U, Degan T, Rosenfield R: Stillbirth due to anti-U. Vox Sang 9:209, 1964.

Bystryn JC, Graf MW, Uhr JW: Regulation of antibody formation by serum antibody. II. Removal of specific antibody by means of exchange transfusion. J Exp Med 132:1279, 1970.

Caine ME, Mueller-Heubach E: Kell sensitization in pregnancy. Am J Obstet Gynecol 154:85, 1986.

Caritis SN, Mueller-Heuback E, Edelstone DI: Effect of betamethasone on analysis of amniotic fluid in the rhesus-sensitized pregnancy. Am J Obstet Gynecol 127:529, 1977.

Carritt B, Kemp TJ, Poulter M: Evolution of the human RH (rhesus) blood group genes: A 50 year old prediction (partially) fulfilled. Hum Mol Genet 6:843, 1997.

Caudle MR, Scott JR: The potential role of immunosuppression, plasmapheresis, and desensitization as treatment modalities for Rh immunization. Clin Obstet Gynecol 25:313, 1982.

Chavez GF, Mulinare J, Edmonds LD: Epidemiology of Rh hemolytic disease of the newborn in the United States. JAMA 265:3270, 1991.

Cherif-Zahar B, Mattei MG, Le Van Kim C, et al: Localization of the human Rh blood group gene structure to chromosome region 1p34.3-1p36.1 by in situ hybridization. Hum Genet 86:398, 1991.

Chiu RW, Murphy MF, Fidler C, et al: Determination of RhD zygosity: Comparison of a double amplification refractory mutation system approach and a multiplex real-time quantitative PCR approach. Clin Chem 47:667, 2001.

Corfield VA, Moolman JC, Martell R, et al: Polymerase chain reaction-based detection of MN blood group-specific sequences in the human genome. Transfusion 33:119, 1993.

Cormode EJ, Lyster DM, Israels S: Analbuminemia in a neonate. J Pediatr **86**:862, 1975.

Daffos F, Forestier F, MacAleese J, et al: Fetal curarization for prenatal magnetic resonance imaging. Prenat Diagn **8**:312, 1988.

Daniels G: Blood group antibodies in haemolytic disease of the fetus and newborn. *In* Hadley A, Soothill P (eds): Alloimmune Disorders in Pregnancy: Anaemia, Thrombocytopenia, and Neutropenia in the Fetus and Newborn. Cambridge, Cambridge University Press, 2002, p. 21.

Davie MJ, Smith DS, White UM, et al: An example of anti-s causing mild haemolytic disease of the newborn. J Clin Pathol **25**:772, 1972.

de Crespigny LC, Robinson HP, Quinn M, et al: Ultrasound-guided fetal blood transfusion for severe rhesus isoimmunization. Obstet Gynecol **66**:529, 1985.

Delle Chiaie L, Buck G, Grab D, et al: Prediction of fetal anemia with Doppler measurement of the middle cerebral artery peak systolic velocity in pregnancies complicated by maternal blood group alloimmunization or parvovirus B19 infection. Ultrasound Obstet Gynecol **18**:232, 2001.

Deren O, Onderoglu L: The value of middle cerebral artery systolic velocity for initial and subsequent management in fetal anemia. Eur J Obstet Gynaecol Reprod Biol **101**:26, 2002.

Detti L, Mari G, Akiyama M, et al: Longitudinal assessment of the middle cerebral artery peak systolic velocity in normal fetuses and in fetuses at risk for anemia. Am J Obstet Gynecol **187**:937, 2002.

Detti L, Oz U, Guney I, et al: Doppler ultrasound velocimetry for timing the second intrauterine transfusion in fetuses with anemia from red cell alloimmunization. Am J Obstet Gynecol **185**:1048, 2001.

De Young-Owens A, Kennedy M, Rose RL, et al: Anti-M isoimmunization: management and outcome at the Ohio State University from 1969 to 1995. Obstet Gynecol **90**:962, 1997.

Dhandsa N, Williams M, Joss V, et al: Haemolytic disease of the newborn caused by anti-U. Lancet **2**:1232, 1981.

Divakaran TG, Waugh J, Clark TJ, et al: Noninvasive techniques to detect fetal anemia due to red blood cell alloimmunization: a systematic review. Obstet Gynecol **98**:509, 2001.

Dooren MC, Kuijpers RW, Joekes EC, et al: Protection against immune haemolytic disease of newborn infants by maternal monocyte-reactive IgG alloantibodies (anti-HLA-DR). Lancet **339**:1067, 1992.

Dooren MC, van Kamp IL, Kanhai HH, et al: Evidence for the protective effect of maternal FcR-blocking IgG alloantibodies HLA-DR in Rh D-haemolytic disease of the newborn. Vox Sang **65**:55, 1993.

Dooren MC, van Kamp IL, Scherpenisse JW, et al: No beneficial effect of low-dose fetal intravenous gammaglobulin administration in combination with intravascular transfusions in severe Rh D haemolytic disease. Vox Sang **66**:253, 1994.

Dopp SL, Isham BE: Anti-U and hemolytic disease of the newborn. Transfusion **23**:273, 1983.

Doyle LW, Kelly EA, Rickards AL, et al: Sensorineural outcome at 2 years for survivors of erythroblastosis treated with fetal intravascular transfusions. Obstet Gynecol **81**:931, 1993.

Duguid JK, Bromilow IM: Haemolytic disease of the newborn due to anti-k. Vox Sang **58**:69, 1990.

Duguid JK, Bromilow IM, Entwistle GD, et al: Haemolytic disease of the newborn due to anti-M. Vox Sang **68**:195, 1995.

Eichler H, Zieger W, Neppert J, et al: Mild course of fetal RhD haemolytic disease due to maternal alloimmunisation to paternal HLA class I and II antigens. Vox Sang **68**:243, 1995.

el-Azeem SA, Samuels P, Rose RL, et al: The effect of the source of transfused blood on the rate of consumption of transfused red blood cells in pregnancies affected by red blood cell alloimmunization. Am J Obstet Gynecol **177**:753, 1997.

Feldman R, Luhby AL, Gromisch DS: Erythroblastosis fetalis due to anti-S antibody. J Pediatr **82**:88, 1973.

Filbey D, Hanson U, Wesstrom G: The prevalence of red cell antibodies in pregnancy correlated to the outcome of the newborn: A 12 year study in central Sweden. Acta Obstet Gynaecol Scand **74**:687, 1995.

Finning KM, Martin PG, Soothill PW, et al: Prediction of fetal D status from maternal plasma: Introduction of a new noninvasive fetal RhD genotyping service. Transfusion **42**:1079, 2002.

Fisher RA, Race RR: Rh gene frequencies in Britain. Nature **157**:48, 1946.

Freda VJ, Adamsons K: Exchange transfusion in utero. Report of a case. Obstet Gynecol **89**:817, 1964.

Furukawa K, Nakajima T, Kogure T, et al: Example of a woman with multiple intrauterine deaths due to anti-M who delivered a live child after plasmapheresis. Exp Clin Immunogenet **10**:161, 1993.

Geifman-Holtzman O, Bernstein IM, Berry SM, et al: Fetal RhD genotyping in fetal cells flow sorted from maternal blood. Am J Obstet Gynecol **174**:818, 1996.

Geifman-Holtzman O, Wojtowycz M, Kosmas E, et al: Female alloimmunization with antibodies known to cause hemolytic disease. Obstet Gynecol **89**:272, 1997.

Giannakoulopoulos X, Sepulveda W, Kourtis P, et al: Fetal plasma cortisol and beta-endorphin response to intrauterine needling. Lancet **344**:77, 1994.

Giannakoulopoulos X, Teixeira J, Fisk N, et al: Human fetal and maternal noradrenaline responses to invasive procedures. Pediatr Res **45**:494, 1999.

Giannina G, Moise KJ Jr, Dorman K: A simple method to estimate the volume for fetal intravascular transfusion. Fetal Diagn Ther **13**:94, 1998.

Gold WR Jr, Queenan JT, Woody J, et al: Oral desensitization in Rh disease. Am J Obstet Gynecol **146**:980, 1983.

Gonsoulin WJ, Moise KJ Jr, Milam JD, et al: Serial maternal blood donations for intrauterine transfusion. Obstet Gynecol **75**:158, 1990.

Goodrick J, Kumpel B, Pamphilon D, et al: Plasma half-lives and bioavailability of human monoclonal Rh D antibodies BRAD-3 and BRAD-5 following intramuscular injection into Rh D-negative volunteers. Clin Exp Immunol **98**:17, 1994.

Gottschall JL: Hemolytic disease of the newborn with anti-U. Transfusion **21**:230, 1981.

Gottvall T, Selbing A: Alloimmunization during pregnancy treated with high dose intravenous immunoglobulin. Effects on fetal hemoglobin concentration and anti-D concentrations in the mother and fetus. Acta Obstet Gynaecol Scand **74**:777, 1995.

Grab D, Paulus WE, Bommer A, et al: Treatment of fetal erythroblastosis by intravascular transfusions: outcome at 6 years. Obstet Gynecol **93**:165, 1999.

Graham-Pole J, Barr W, Willoughby ML: Continuous-flow plasmapheresis in management of severe rhesus disease. Br Med J **1**:1185, 1977.

Griffith TK: The irregular antibodies: A continuing problem. Am J Obstet Gynecol **137**:174, 1980.

Gusdon JP Jr: The treatment of erythroblastosis with promethazine hydrochloride. J Reprod Med **26**:454, 1981.

Gusdon JP Jr, Caudle MR, Herbst GA, et al: Phagocytosis and erythroblastosis. I. Modification of the neonatal response by promethazine hydrochloride. Am J Obstet Gynecol **125**:224, 1976.

Hadley AG: In vitro assays to predict the severity of hemolytic disease of the newborn. Transfus Med Rev **9**:302, 1995.

Hadley AG, Kumpel BM: Synergistic effect of blending IgG1 and IgG3 monoclonal anti-D in promoting the metabolic response of monocytes to sensitized red cells. Immunology **67**:550, 1989.

Hallak M, Moise KJ Jr, Hesketh DE, et al: Intravascular transfusion of fetuses with rhesus incompatibility: Prediction of fetal outcome by changes in umbilical venous pressure. Obstet Gynecol **80**:286, 1992.

Hardyment AF, Salvador HS, Towell ME, et al: Follow-up of intrauterine transfused surviving children. Am J Obstet Gynecol **133**:235, 1979.

Harman CR, Bowman JM, Manning FA, et al: Intrauterine transfusion—intraperitoneal versus intravascular approach: a case-control comparison. Am J Obstet Gynecol **162**:1053, 1990.

Harte G, Payton D, Carmody F, et al: Graft versus host disease following intrauterine and exchange transfusions for rhesus haemolytic disease. Aust N Z J Obstet Gynaecol **37**:319, 1997.

Haugen G, Husby H, Helbig AE, et al: Ultrasonographic monitoring of pregnancies complicated by red blood cell alloimmunization in a cohort with mild to moderate risk according to previous obstetric outcome. Acta Obstet Gynaecol Scand **81**:227, 2002.

Herbert WN, Owen HG, Collins ML: Autologous blood storage in obstetrics. Obstet Gynecol **72**:166, 1988.

Hessner MJ, Pircon RA, Johnson ST, et al: Prenatal genotyping of Jk(a) and Jk(b) of the human Kidd blood group system by allele-specific polymerase chain reaction. Prenat Diagn **18**:1225, 1998.

Hessner MJ, Pircon RA, Johnson ST, et al: Prenatal genotyping of the Duffy blood group system by allele-specific polymerase chain reaction. Prenat Diagn **19**:41, 1999.

Hopkins DF: Maternal anti-Rh(D) and the D-negative fetus. Am J Obstet Gynecol **108**:268, 1970.

Hudon L, Moise KJ Jr, Hegemier SE, et al: Long-term neurodevelopmental outcome after intrauterine transfusion for the treatment of fetal hemolytic disease. Am J Obstet Gynecol **179**:858, 1998.

Hughes RG, Craig JI, Murphy WG, et al: Causes and clinical consequences of Rhesus (D) haemolytic disease of the newborn: a study of a Scottish population, 1985–1990. Br J Obstet Gynaecol **101**:297, 1994.

Issitt PD, Anstee DJ: Hemolytic disease of the newborn. *In* Issitt PD, Anstee DJ (eds): Applied Blood Group Serology. Durham, NC, Montgomery Scientific Publications, 1998, p. 1045.

Janssens HM, de Haan MJ, van Kamp IL, et al: Outcome for children treated with fetal intravascular transfusions because of severe blood group antagonism. J Pediatr **131**:373, 1997.

Kanra T, Yuce K, Ozcebe IU: Hydrops fetalis and intrauterine deaths due to anti-M. Acta Obstet Gynaecol Scand **75**:415, 1996.

Kanter MH: Derivation of new mathematic formulas for determining whether a D-positive father is heterozygous or homozygous for the D antigen. Am J Obstet Gynecol **166**:61, 1992.

Kirkinen P, Jouppila P, Eik-Nes S: Umbilical vein blood flow in rhesus-isoimmunization. Br J Obstet Gynaecol **90**:640, 1983.

Klumper FJ, van Kamp IL, Vandenbussche FP, et al: Benefits and risks of fetal red-cell transfusion after 32 weeks' gestation. Eur J Obstet Gynaecol Reprod Biol **92**:91, 2000.

Koenig JM, Ashton RD, De Vore GR, et al: Late hyporegenerative anemia in Rh hemolytic disease. J Pediatr **115**:315, 1989.

Kulich V: Hemolytic disease of the newborn caused by anti-k antibody. Cesk Pediatr **22**:823, 1967.

Kumpel BM: On the mechanism of tolerance to the Rh D antigen mediated by passive anti-D (Rh D prophylaxis). Immunol Lett **82**:67, 2002.

Kumpel BM, Judson PA: Quantitation of IgG anti-D bound to D-positive red cells infused into D-negative subjects after intramuscular injection of monoclonal anti-D. Transfus Med **5**:105, 1995.

Landsteiner K, Weiner AS: An agglutinable factor in human blood recognized by immune sera for rhesus blood. Proc Soc Exp Biol Med **43**:223, 1940.

Le Van Kim C, Cherif-Zahar B, Raynal V, et al: Multiple Rh messenger RNA isoforms are produced by alternative splicing. Blood **80**:1074, 1992.

Lepercq J, Poissonnier MH, Coutanceau MJ, et al: Management and outcome of fetomaternal Rh alloimmunization in twin pregnancies. Fetal Diagn Ther **14**:26, 1999.

Levine P, Backer M, Wigod M: A human blood group property (Cellano) present in 99.8% of all bloods. Science **109**:464, 1949.

Levine P, Ferraro LR, Koch E: Haemolytic disease of the newborn due to anti-S. Blood **7**:1030, 1952.

Levine P, Katzin EM, Burham L: Isoimmunization in pregnancy: Its possible bearing on etiology of erythroblastosis foetalis. JAMA **116**:825, 1941.

Levine P, Stetson R: An unusual case of intragroup agglutination. JAMA **113**:126, 1939.

Lewis M, Bowman JM, Pollock J, et al: Absorption of red cells from the peritoneal cavity of an hydropic twin. Transfusion **13**:37, 1973.

Liley AW: Liquor amnii analysis in the management of pregnancy complicated by rhesus sensitization. Am J Obstet Gynecol **82**:1359, 1961.

Liley AW: Intrauterine transfusion of foetus in haemolytic disease. BMJ **2**:1107, 1963.

Lo YM, Hjelm NM, Fidler C, et al: Prenatal diagnosis of fetal RhD status by molecular analysis of maternal plasma. N Engl J Med **339**:1734, 1998.

Macpherson CR, Zartman ER: Anti-M antibody as a cause of intrauterine death: A follow-up. Am J Clin Pathol **43**:544, 1965.

Magaud JP, Jouvenceaux A, Bertrix F, et al: Perinatal hemolytic disease due to incompatibility in the U system. Arch Fr Pediatr **38**:769, 1981.

Maier RF, Obladen M, Scigalla P, et al: The effect of epoetin beta (recombinant human erythropoietin) on the need for transfusion in very-low-birth-weight infants. European Multicentre Erythropoietin Study Group. N Engl J Med **330**:1173, 1994.

Mandelbrot L, Daffos F, Forestier F, et al: Assessment of fetal blood volume for computer-assisted management of in utero transfusion. Fetal Ther **3**:1, 1988.

Margulies M, Voto LS, Mathet E: High-dose intravenous IgG for the treatment of severe rhesus alloimmunization. Vox Sang **61**:181, 1991.

Mari G, for the Collaborative Group for Doppler Assessment of the Blood Velocity of Anemic Fetuses: Noninvasive diagnosis by Doppler ultrasonography of fetal anemia due to maternal red-cell alloimmunization. N Engl J Med **342**:9, 2000.

Martin JA, Hamilton BE, Ventura SJ, et al: Births: Final data for 2000. Natl Vital Stat Rep **50**:1, 2002.

Matsumoto H, Tamaki Y, Sato S, et al: A case of hemolytic disease of the newborn caused by anti-M: serological study of maternal blood. Acta Obstet Gynaecol Jpn **33**:525, 1981.

Mayne KM, Bowell PJ, Green SJ, et al: The significance of anti-S sensitization in pregnancy. Clin Lab Haematol **12**:105, 1990.

Moise AA, Gest AL, Weickmann PH, et al: Reduction in plasma protein does not affect body water content in fetal sheep. Pediatr Res **29**:623, 1991.

Moise KJ Jr, Carpenter RJ Jr: Chorionic villus sampling for Rh typing: Clinical implications. Am J Obstet Gynecol **168**:1002, 1993.

Moise KJ Jr, Carpenter RJ Jr, Deter RL, et al: The use of fetal neuromuscular blockade during intrauterine procedures. Am J Obstet Gynecol **157**:874, 1987.

Moise KJ Jr, Carpenter RJ Jr, Hesketh DE: Do abnormal Starling forces cause fetal hydrops in red blood cell alloimmunization? Am J Obstet Gynecol **167**:907, 1992.

Moise KJ Jr, Carpenter RJ Jr, Kirshon B, et al: Comparison of four types of intrauterine transfusion: Effect on fetal hematocrit. Fetal Ther **4**:126, 1989.

Moise KJ Jr, Deter RL, Kirshon B, et al: Intravenous pancuronium bromide for fetal neuromuscular blockade during intrauterine transfusion for red-cell alloimmunization. Obstet Gynecol **74**:905, 1989.

Moise KJ Jr, Perkins JT, Sosler SD, et al: The predictive value of maternal serum testing for detection of fetal anemia in red blood cell alloimmunization. Am J Obstet Gynecol **172**:1003, 1995.

Moise KJ Jr, Whitecar PW: Antenatal therapy for haemolytic disease of the fetus and newborn. *In* Hadley A, Soothill P (eds): Alloimmune Disorders in Pregnancy: Anaemia, Thrombocytopenia and Neutropenia in the Fetus and Newborn. Cambridge, Cambridge University Press, 2002, p. 173.

National Institute For Clinical Excellence (NICE): Technology Appraised Guidance #41. Guidance on the use of routine antenatal anti-D prophylaxis for RhD-negative women. 1, 2002.

Neppert J: Rhesus-Du and -D incompatibility in the newborn without haemolytic disease: Inhibition of immune phagocytosis? Vox Sang **53**:239, 1987.

Neppert J, Pohl E, Mueller-Eckhardt C: Inhibition of immune phagocytosis by human sera with HLA A, B, C and DR but not with DQ or EM type reactivity. Vox Sang **51**:122, 1986.

Ness PM, Baldwin ML, Niebyl JR: Clinical high-risk designation does not predict excess fetal-maternal hemorrhage. Am J Obstet Gynecol **156**:154, 1987.

Nicolaides KH, Fontanarosa M, Gabbe SG, et al: Failure of ultrasonographic parameters to predict the severity of fetal anemia in rhesus isoimmunization. Am J Obstet Gynecol **158**:920, 1988.

Nicolaides KH, Rodeck CH: Maternal serum anti-D antibody concentration and assessment of rhesus isoimmunisation. BMJ **304**:1155, 1992.

Nicolaides KH, Rodeck CH, Mibashan RS, et al: Have Liley charts outlived their usefulness? Am J Obstet Gynecol **155**:90, 1986.

Nicolaides KH, Thilaganathan B, Rodeck CH, et al: Erythroblastosis and reticulocytosis in anemic fetuses. Am J Obstet Gynecol **159**:1063, 1988.

Nicolaides KH, Warenski JC, Rodeck CH: The relationship of fetal plasma protein concentration and hemoglobin level to the development of hydrops in rhesus isoimmunization. Am J Obstet Gynecol **152**:341, 1985.

Nicolini U, Kochenour NK, Greco P, et al: When to perform the next intrauterine transfusion in patients with Rh allo-immunization: combined intravascular and intraperitoneal transfusion allows longer intervals. Fetal Ther **4**:14, 1989.

Nicolini U, Santolaya J, Ojo OE, et al: The fetal intrahepatic umbilical vein as an alternative to cord needling for prenatal diagnosis and therapy. Prenat Diagn **8**:665, 1988.

Oepkes D, Meerman RH, Vandenbussche FP, et al: Ultrasonographic fetal spleen measurements in red blood cell-alloimmunized pregnancies. Am J Obstet Gynecol **169**:121, 1993.

Ovali F, Samanci N, Dagoglu T: Management of late anemia in Rhesus hemolytic disease: use of recombinant human erythropoietin (a pilot study). Pediatr Res **39**:831, 1996.

Pamphilon DH, Rider JR, Barbara JA, et al: Prevention of transfusion-transmitted cytomegalovirus infection. Transfus Med **9**:115, 1999.

Parinaud J, Bierme S, Fournie A, et al: Oral Rh treatment for severely immunized mother. Am J Obstet Gynecol **150**:902, 1984.

Pepperell RJ, Barrie JU, Fliegner JR: Significance of red-cell irregular antibodies in the obstetric patient. Med J Aust **2**:453, 1977.

Pielet BW, Socol ML, MacGregor SN, et al: Fetal heart rate changes after fetal intravascular treatment with pancuronium bromide. Am J Obstet Gynecol **159**:640, 1988.

Plasma Exchange/Sandoglobulin Guillain-Barré Syndrome Trial Group: Randomised trial of plasma exchange, intravenous immunoglobulin, and combined treatments in Guillain-Barré syndrome. Lancet **349**:225, 1997.

Pollock JM, Bowman JM: Anti-Rh(D) IgG subclasses and severity of Rh hemolytic disease of the newborn. Vox Sang **59**:176, 1990.

Queenan JT, Smith BD, Haber JM, et al: Irregular antibodies in the obstetric patient. Obstet Gynecol **34**:767, 1969.

Queenan JT, Tomai TP, Ural SH, et al: Deviation in amniotic fluid optical density at a wavelength of 450 nm in Rh-immunized pregnancies from 14 to 40 weeks' gestation: A proposal for clinical management. Am J Obstet Gynecol **168**:1370, 1993.

Radunovic N, Lockwood CJ, Alvarez M, et al: The severely anemic and hydropic isoimmune fetus: changes in fetal hematocrit associated with intrauterine death. Obstet Gynecol **79**:390, 1992.

Rightmire DA, Nicolaides KH, Rodeck CH, et al: Fetal blood velocities in Rh isoimmunization: Relationship to gestational age and to fetal hematocrit. Obstet Gynecol **68**:233, 1986.

Roberts AB, Mitchell JM, Lake Y, et al: Ultrasonographic surveillance in red blood cell alloimmunization. Am J Obstet Gynecol **184**:1251, 2001.

Rodeck CH, Kemp JR, Holman CA, et al: Direct intravascular fetal blood transfusion by fetoscopy in severe Rhesus isoimmunisation. Lancet 1:625, 1981.

Rosse WF. Clinical Immunohematology: Basic Concepts in Clinical Applications. Boston, Blackwell, 1990.

Rubo J, Albrecht K, Lasch P, et al: High-dose intravenous immune globulin therapy for hyperbilirubinemia caused by Rh hemolytic disease. J Pediatr 121:93, 1992.

Saade GR, Moise KJ, Belfort MA, et al: Fetal and neonatal hematologic parameters in red cell alloimmunization: Predicting the need for late neonatal transfusions. Fetal Diagn Ther 8:161, 1993.

Schumacher B, Moise KJ Jr: Fetal transfusion for red blood cell alloimmunization in pregnancy. Obstet Gynecol 88:137, 1996.

Schur PH, Alpert E, Alper C: Gamma G subgroups in human fetal, cord, and maternal sera. Clin Immunol Immunopathol 2:62, 1973.

Scott F, Chan FY: Assessment of the clinical usefulness of the "Queenan" chart versus the "Liley" chart in predicting severity of rhesus iso-immunization. Prenat Diagn 18:1143, 1998.

Shannon KM, Mentzer WC, Abels RI, et al: Recombinant human erythropoietin in the anemia of prematurity: results of a placebo-controlled pilot study. J Pediatr 118:949, 1991.

Shepard SL, Noble AL, Filbey D, et al: Inhibition of the monocyte chemiluminescent response to anti-D-sensitized red cells by Fc gamma RI-blocking antibodies which ameliorate the severity of haemolytic disease of the newborn. Vox Sang 70:157, 1996.

Simsek S, Faas BH, Bleeker PM, et al: Rapid Rh D genotyping by polymerase chain reaction-based amplification of DNA. Blood 85:2975, 1995.

Singleton BK, Green CA, Avent ND, et al: The presence of an RHD pseudogene containing a 37 base pair duplication and a nonsense mutation in Africans with the Rh D-negative blood group phenotype. Blood 95:12, 2000.

Smith G, Knott P, Rissik J, et al: Anti-U and haemolytic disease of the fetus and newborn. Br J Obstet Gynaecol 105:1318, 1998.

Soothill PW, Nicolaides KH, Rodeck CH, et al: Relationship of fetal hemoglobin and oxygen content to lactate concentration in Rh isoimmunized pregnancies. Obstet Gynecol 69:268, 1987.

Spong CY, Porter AE, Queenan JT: Management of isoimmunization in the presence of multiple maternal antibodies. Am J Obstet Gynecol 185:481, 2001.

Stenchever MA: Promethazine hydrochloride: Use in patients with Rh isoimmunization lyophilized preparation of erythrocyte membranes. Am J Obstet Gynecol 130:665, 1978.

Stone B, Marsh WL: Hemolytic disease of the newborn caused by anti-M. Br J Haemotol 5:344, 1959.

Synder EL: Prevention of hemolytic disease of the newborn due to anti-D. Prenatal/perinatal testing and Rh immune globulin administration. Am Assoc Blood Banks Bull 98-2, 1998.

Teixeira JM, Duncan K, Letsky E, et al: Middle cerebral artery peak systolic velocity in the prediction of fetal anemia. Ultrasound Obstet Gynecol 15:205, 2000.

Telischi M, Behzad O, Issitt PD, et al: Hemolytic disease of the newborn due to anti-N. Vox Sang 31:109, 1976.

Tuck SM, Studd JW, White JM: Sickle cell disease in pregnancy complicated by anti-U antibody. Case report. Br J Obstet Gynaecol 89:91, 1982.

Ulm B, Svolba G, Ulm MR, et al: Male fetuses are particularly affected by maternal alloimmunization to D antigen. Transfusion 39:169, 1999.

Van den Veyver IB, Moise KJ Jr: Fetal RhD typing by polymerase chain reaction in pregnancies complicated by rhesus alloimmunization. Obstet Gynecol 88:1061, 1996.

van Kamp IL, Klumper FJ, Bakkum RS, et al: The severity of immune fetal hydrops is predictive of fetal outcome after intrauterine treatment. Am J Obstet Gynecol 185:668, 2001.

Vaughan JI, Manning M, Warwick RM, et al: Inhibition of erythroid progenitor cells by anti-Kell antibodies in fetal alloimmune anemia. N Engl J Med 338:798, 1998.

Vaughan JI, Warwick R, Letsky E, et al: Erythropoietic suppression in fetal anemia because of Kell alloimmunization. Am J Obstet Gynecol 171:247, 1994.

Vengelen-Tyler V. (ed): Technical Manual of the American Association of Blood Banks. Bethesda, Md, American Association of Blood Banks, 1999.

Vietor HE, Kanhai HH, Brand A: Induction of additional red cell alloantibodies after intrauterine transfusions. Transfusion 34:970, 1994.

Vintzileos AM, Campbell WA, Storlazzi E, et al: Fetal liver ultrasound measurements in isoimmunized pregnancies. Obstet Gynecol 68:162, 1986.

Voto LS, Mathet ER, Zapaterio JL, et al: High-dose gammaglobulin (IVIG) followed by intrauterine transfusions (IUTs): A new alternative for the treatment of severe fetal hemolytic disease. J Perinat Med 25:85, 1997.

Vyas S, Nicolaides KH, Campbell S: Doppler examination of the middle cerebral artery in anemic fetuses. Am J Obstet Gynecol 162:1066, 1990.

Wallerstein H: Treatment of severe erythroblastosis by simultaneous removal and replacement of blood of the newborn infant. Science 103:583, 1946.

Weiner CP: Human fetal bilirubin levels and fetal hemolytic disease. Am J Obstet Gynecol 166:1449, 1992.

Weiner CP, Wenstrom KD, Sipes SL, et al: Risk factors for cordocentesis and fetal intravascular transfusion. Am J Obstet Gynecol 165:1020, 1991.

Weiner CP, Widness JA: Decreased fetal erythropoiesis and hemolysis in Kell hemolytic anemia. Am J Obstet Gynecol 174:547, 1996.

Weiner CP, Williamson RA, Wenstrom KD, et al: Management of fetal hemolytic disease by cordocentesis. I. Prediction of fetal anemia. Am J Obstet Gynecol 165:546, 1991.

Weinstein L, Taylor ES: Hemolytic disease of the neonate secondary to anti-Fya. Am J Obstet Gynecol 121:643, 1975.

Welch R, Rampling MW, Anwar A, et al: Changes in hemorrheology with fetal intravascular transfusion. Am J Obstet Gynecol 170:726, 1994.

Whitecar P, Farb R, Subramanyam L, et al: Paternal leukocyte alloimmunization as a treatment for hemolytic disease of the newborn/fetus in a rabbit model. Am J Obstet Gynecol 187:977, 2002.

Wiener E, Mawas F, Dellow RA, et al: A major role of class I Fc gamma receptors in immunoglobulin G anti-D-mediated red blood cell destruction by fetal mononuclear phagocytes. Obstet Gynecol 86:157, 1995.

Wiese M, Berr F, Lafrenz M, et al: Low frequency of cirrhosis in a hepatitis C (genotype 1b) single-source outbreak in Germany: A 20-year multicenter study. Hepatology 32:91, 2000.

Woodrow JC, Clarke CA, Donohow WT, et al: Mechanism of Rh prophylaxis: an experimental study on specificity of immunosuppression. Br Med J 2:57, 1975.

Yap PL: Viral transmission by blood products: A perspective of events covered by the recent tribunal of enquiry into the Irish Blood Transfusion Board. Ir Med J 90:84, 1997.

Yu Z, Lennon VA: Mechanism of intravenous immune globulin therapy in antibody-mediated autoimmune diseases. N Engl J Med 340:227, 1999.

Zimmerman R, Durig P, Carpenter R, et al: Longitudinal measurement of the peak systolic velocity in the fetal middle cerebral artery for monitoring pregnancies complicated by red cell alloimmunization—A prospective multi-center trial with intention to treat. Br J Obstet Gynaecol 109:746, 2002.

Zupanska B, Lenkiewicz B, Michalewska B, et al: The ability of cellular assays to predict the necessity for cordocenteses in pregnancies at risk of haemolytic disease of the newborn. Vox Sang 80:234, 2001.

Chapter 31
NONIMMUNE HYDROPS

Isabelle Wilkins, MD

Hydrops fetalis is the term used to describe generalized edema in the neonate. This edema is accompanied by collections of fluid in serous spaces. In the past, most cases of hydrops fetalis were due to severe erythroblastosis from Rh alloimmunization. Potter (1943) was the first to describe nonimmune hydrops fetalis in a group of infants without erythroblastosis whose mothers were Rh-positive.

Since first described 60 years ago, nonimmune hydrops (NIH) has become more common than hydrops from alloimmunization. Santolaya and associates (1992) reported a series of 76 hydropic fetuses of which 87% were nonimmune. Only 4 of 87, or 4.5% of cases assessed at a fetal medicine unit reported by Sohan and associates (2001) were because of red cell alloimminization, and Ismail and coworkers reported 63 prenatally detected cases in which 8 were immune, for a rate of 12.7% (2001). Graves and Baskett (1984) examined all babies born at their institution with hydrops and reported that 76% of cases were nonimmune.

The incidence of NIH at delivery in published accounts is approximately 1 in 1500 to 1 in 3800 (Hutchison et al., 1982; Graves and Baskett, 1984; Im et al., 1984). A large, unselected prenatal ultrasound screening clinic in Finland had a similar rate of 1 in 1700 (Heinonen et al., 2000). Reviews from ultrasonography referral centers, however, show an incidence between 1 in 150 and 1 in 244 sonographic examinations (Santolaya et al., 1992; Anandakumar et al., 1996).

NIH is a heterogeneous disorder with a large number of possible causes and associations. Overall, the prognosis is poor; a 52%–98% perinatal mortality rate is typical (McCoy et al., 1995; Heinonen et al., 2000; Ismail et al., 2001; Sohan et al., 2001). Elucidation of etiology is of primary importance because treatment and prognosis of this disorder are determined by the underlying fetal condition, but the task may be difficult. Most authors differentiate the rate of prenatal detection of etiology, which is lower than the rate following delivery or at autopsy. Both are important in counseling families and discussing recurrence risks, but only prenatal detection is useful in guiding management and therapy. In most series an etiology is found in approximately 51%–85% of cases before delivery but in up to 95% after delivery, depending in part on parental acceptance of autopsy and karyotype (McCoy et al., 1995; Anandakumar et al., 1996; Heinonen et al., 2000; Ismail et al., 2001; Sohan et al., 2001). It is clear that both success in determining etiology and survival statistics differ between early and late gestation, largely because of the different gestational ages at which the various etiologies present. In general, presentation before 24 weeks of gestation occurs in more-severe

cases, in which etiology is easier to ascertain but perinatal survival is worse (McCoy et al., 1995; Anandakumar et al., 1996; Heinonen et al., 2000; Ismail et al., 2001; Sohan et al., 2001).

PRESENTING SIGNS AND SYMPTOMS

Although NIH is a clinical diagnosis concerning the neonate, the condition can be determined antenatally by obstetric sonographic examination with a success rate of nearly 100%. The indication for ultrasonography varies in different series. In 1986, Watson and Campbell found that 63% of cases of NIH were discovered on routine ultrasonography, whereas another 30% of patients were referred because of suspected hydramnios. Graves and Baskett (1984) found that NIH was less commonly discovered on routine ultrasonography than on ultrasonography ordered for a specific indication. The most common indications in their population were hydramnios, size greater than dates, fetal tachycardia, and maternal pregnancy-induced hypertension. Other frequently cited indications for ultrasound evaluation have included decreased fetal movement and antenatal hemorrhage (Warsof et al., 1986).

Maternal complications of pregnancy are increased in NIH. Hydramnios, pregnancy-induced hypertension, severe anemia, postpartum hemorrhage, preterm labor, birth trauma, gestational diabetes, a retained placenta, or difficult delivery of the placenta are all frequently mentioned in large series (Macafee et al., 1970; Hutchison et al., 1982; Graves and Baskett, 1984; Castillo et al., 1986; McCoy et al., 1995).

An uncommon maternal complication of fetal hydrops is called *mirror syndrome*. This condition is rarely a presenting complaint and may develop during conservative management of such pregnancies. Patients generally experience edema, pulmonary edema, and possibly hypertension; they may be gravely ill and recover after delivery. The syndrome may also develop postpartum, as it did in two mothers in one series (McCoy et al., 1995). Although no series exist to direct management, most authors do not advise continuation of the pregnancy (Van Selm et al., 1991; Dorman and Cardwell, 1995).

ULTRASONOGRAPHY

Ultrasound examination is essential to the diagnosis of NIH, and criteria for definition of the disorder in the fetus are based exclusively on ultrasound parameters. The fluid that accumulates may include ascites, pleural effusions, pericardial effusions, and skin edema. Several definitions of fetal NIH have been proposed based on the quantity and distribution of excess fetal water. Variations in these definitions have made direct comparison among published series inexact. Mahony and coworkers (1984) defined hydrops as generalized skin edema with or without an associated serous effusion. Although others have also used this definition (Brown, 1986), NIH is more commonly defined as edema with one effusion or more, or effusions in at least two spaces—that is, two of the following must be present: ascites, pleural effusion, pericardial effusion, or skin edema (Platt and DeVore, 1982; Romero et al., 1988).

The degree or severity of hydrops is generally subjective. Hutchison and associates (1982) described a score based on total number of serous space effusions. Because the only requirement for the definition of NIH was edema, it was possible to have a score of zero (0) with no serous involvement. This score was not predictive of outcome in this series since the overall perinatal mortality rate was close to 100%. Saltzman and colleagues (1989) described a different scoring system in which each effusion was quantified. With this system, they were able to predict which cases were likely to be due to fetal anemia and which were from other causes. Although they included isoimmunized pregnancies in their series, other forms of anemia followed the same general pattern.

Fluid in one of these spaces may be an early finding in a fetus destined to develop hydrops. At the very least, a careful search for fluid in other serous sites is warranted. Such fetuses should undergo follow-up over time to ensure that hydrops is not developing.

■ FETAL FLUID ACCUMULATION

Ascites appears sonographically as an echolucent rim of varying size in the fetal abdomen (Fig. 31-1). A small rim of ascites may be hard to distinguish from a similarly located area

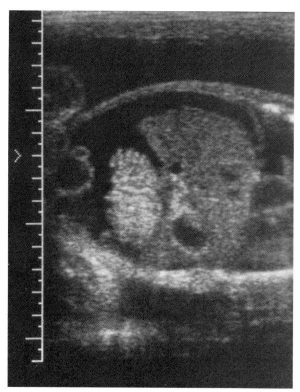

FIGURE 31-2 ■ Longitudinal image of the fetal abdomen with ascitic fluid outlining the liver and compressing the bowel.

of echo dropout common with normal fetuses (Platt and DeVore, 1982). One possible distinguishing feature is that a true rim of fluid should be visible all the way around the abdomen in transverse viewing plane. Longitudinally, the edge of the liver, bladder, or diaphragm may be outlined. When ascites is more marked, the entire liver is outlined and the bowel is compressed (Fig. 31-2). In these more extreme cases, the diagnosis is relatively easy. When one is trying to distinguish early ascites from a normal rim of echolucency, another useful sign is small amounts of fluid surrounding loops of bowel (Fig. 31-3). This was first described by Benacerraf and Frigoletto (1985) and mimics the radiographic signs of free peritoneal air on abdominal radiographs.

Pleural effusions may be unilateral or bilateral. Although the effusions may present as small rims of fluid outlining the pleural space and diaphragm, more commonly they are large and compress the lung (Figs. 31-4 and 31-5). It is uncommon for a unilateral effusion to shift the mediastinum. In such a case, an extrinsic fluid-filled mass, such as a diaphragmatic hernia or another space-occupying lesion, is likely to be present. Pulmonary hypoplasia is a frequent cause of death in neonates with NIH, and the size of pleural effusions may help to predict this complication (Castillo et al., 1987).

Pericardial effusions are smaller in total volume and are therefore more difficult to see than ascites or pleural effusions (Fig. 31-6). M-mode examination of the heart can also be useful in visualizing pericardial fluid (Fig. 31-7).

Some authors (Platt and DeVore, 1982) have proposed that pericardial effusions indicate cardiac decompensation and that this is the earliest sign of hydrops in fetuses with cardiac lesions. In a group of patients with mixed etiology, Carlson and colleagues (1990) found that the biventricular dimension, an

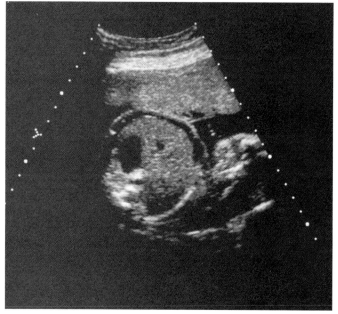

FIGURE 31-1 ■ Transverse image of the fetal abdomen at the level of the stomach. A small rim of ascites is seen within the abdominal wall.

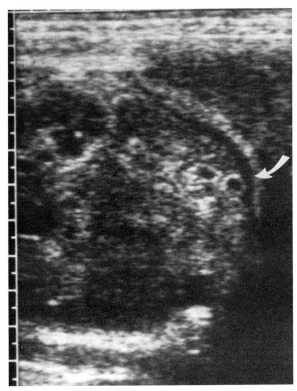

FIGURE 31-3 ■ Fetal abdomen with a small rim of ascites and loops of bowel separated by fluid (arrow).

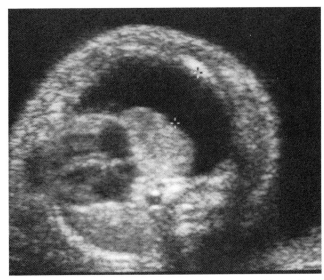

FIGURE 31-5 ■ Large pleural effusion with compressed lung. Also note skin edema overlying ribs.

indicator of overall cardiac size as measured on M-mode examination, was highly predictive of survival.

Skin edema is usually a generalized process, although it is easiest to see with ultrasonography over the chest wall or scalp, where soft tissue is typically thin and any thickness can be appreciated. The usual definition of edema is greater than 5 mm of subcutaneous tissue. This may be misleading if the fetus has redundant skin folds or is macrosomic.

Placental thickening is frequently considered a sign of hydrops as well. Abnormal thickening is generally defined as greater than 6 cm (Chitkara et al., 1988; Romero et al., 1988), although some authors have used a cutoff of 4 cm (Fleischer et al., 1981; Hoddick et al., 1985). With hydramnios, the

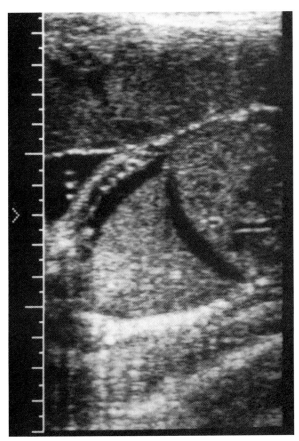

FIGURE 31-4 ■ Small pleural effusion.

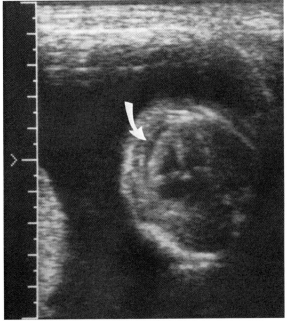

FIGURE 31-6 ■ Four-chamber view of the fetal heart with a pericardial effusion present (arrow).

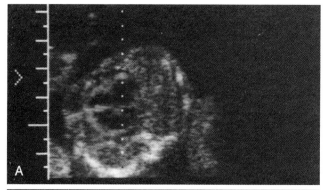

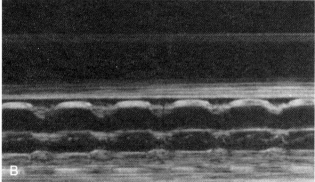

FIGURE 31-7 ■ **A,** Fetal pericardial effusion is seen by two-dimensional imaging. **B,** The M-mode cursor placed through the suspected effusion is seen more clearly.

placenta may appear compressed and instead be thin. When therapeutic amniocenteses are performed because of severe hydramnios, the placenta may "thicken" by the end of the procedure, and this occurrence implies that hydrostatic pressure was responsible for the thinned appearance (Elliott et al., 1991).

According to various authors, hydramnios is present in 40%–75% of cases of NIH. Although the definition of hydramnios differs among these series, when the condition is present, it is often severe and would therefore be detected by any quantifying technique (see Chapter 3). In some cases of fetal hydrops, oligohydramnios is present, and many authors consider this an ominous or late finding. Although oligohydramnios is generally associated with poor pregnancy outcome, its prognosis in NIH depends on the underlying cause rather than simply on this sonographic feature.

■ ETIOLOGY

One of the greatest challenges in the management of a fetus with NIH is ascertaining the cause of the disorder. Unfortunately, causes are numerous, and new associations continually appear in the literature. The causes may be divided into several broad categories, which are helpful in organizing an approach to this often-frustrating problem (Table 31-1).

Many of the conditions listed in Table 31-1 are placed into a category somewhat arbitrarily. For example, many anatomic cardiac lesions have a chromosomal basis. Similarly, viral syndromes that lead to NIH may be associated with fetal anemia, with fetal malformation complexes, or with myocarditis. It is also obvious from the table that some of these syndromes are extremely rare and others are more common. In addition,

many of these conditions represent congenital anomalies whereas others are acquired defects. Classifying these conditions differently may be helpful when considering particular problems such as management, recurrence risks, or possible fetal therapy.

Table 31-1 is not a list of etiologic factors but, rather, a list of conditions associated with NIH. The pathophysiology of NIH is well worked out in only a few cases. Furthermore, not all cases have the same pathophysiologic mechanism.

A review by Machin (1989) tried to elucidate some of these mechanisms. As he pointed out, hydrops is generally a common end stage for a variety of diseases reached by several pathways. He proposed five basic disease processes that lead to hydrops: cardiovascular failure, chromosomal abnormalities, thoracic compression, twinning, and fetal anemia. He believed that each of these has a common pathway for the development of hydrops. Furthermore, he suggested that most causes could be classified into one of these large groups.

Cardiovascular Causes

Fetal cardiac abnormalities are among the most common causes of hydrops in most series.

Congenital heart disease is a common problem with an incidence of 8 or 9 per 1000 liveborn infants. Malformations of the cardiovascular system are of varying degrees of complexity and seriousness, but it is not always clear why some of these fetuses experience hydrops whereas others are born in a well-compensated condition (McFadden and Taylor, 1989). No forms of congenital heart disease reliably lead to hydrops, although one would expect that more-minor abnormalities are less likely to cause the ultimate decompensation of the fetus. Overall, a structural malformation of the heart with associated fetal hydrops carries an extremely poor prognosis, with a mortality rate approaching 100% (Allan et al., 1986; Crawford et al., 1988).

Structural heart disease is diagnosed by means of ultrasonography, with either a targeted ultrasound examination or fetal echocardiography. In general, regardless of the presence of hydrops, cases of cardiac malformation that are diagnosed prenatally have a poor outcome. Crawford and coauthors (1988) found only a 17% survival rate in such fetuses. Copel and coworkers (1988) suggested that 30% of fetuses with prenatally diagnosed structural congenital heart disease have an abnormal karyotype. They therefore recommended that chromosomes be obtained whenever this diagnosis is made. Because of the poor prognosis associated with hydrops when an abnormal karyotype is involved, such fetuses generally are not considered candidates for in utero fetal therapy or for active intervention with early delivery and vigorous resuscitation.

Cardiac arrhythmias are also an important cause of hydrops, but the prognosis is entirely different from that for structural heart disease. Tachyarrhythmias associated with hydrops are usually associated with a better prognosis than are most other causes of NIH (Cameron et al., 1988; Romero et al., 1988). Arrhythmias may be of several types, including tachyarrhythmias, bradyarrhythmias, and dysrhythmias. If an arrhythmia is associated with underlying structural heart disease, the prognosis is as poor as for heart disease without arrhythmia, as described earlier (Shenker et al., 1987). The diagnosis and management of these disorders is discussed more fully in Chapter 26.

■ **TABLE 31-1.** CONDITIONS ASSOCIATED WITH NONIMMUNE HYDROPS

Cardiovascular	Malformation	Hematologic	Alpha-thalassemia
	Left heart hypoplasia		Fetomaternal transfusion
	A-V canal defect		Parvovirus B19 infection
	Right heart hypoplasia		*In utero* hemorrhage
	Closure of foramen ovale		G6PD deficiency
	Single ventricle		Red cell enzyme deficiencies
	Transposition of the great vessels	Thoracic	Congenital cystic adenomatoid
	VSD		malformation of lung
	ASD		Diaphragmatic hernia
	Tetralogy of Fallot		Intrathoracic mass
	Ebstein's anomaly		Pulmonary sequestration
	Premature closure of ductus		Chylothorax
	Truncus arteriosus		Airway obstruction
	Tachyarrhythmia		Pulmonary lymphangiectasia
	Atrial flutter		Pulmonary neoplasia
	Paroxysmal atrial tachycardia		Bronchogenic cyst
	Wolff-Parkinson-White	Infections	CMV
	Supraventricular tachycardia		Toxoplasmosis
	Bradyarrhythmia		Parvovirus B19 (fifth disease)
	Other arrhythmia		Syphilis
	High-output failure		Herpes
	Neuroblastoma		Rubella
	Sacrococcygeal teratoma	Malformation sequences	Congenital lymphedema, e.g., Noonan's
	Large fetal angioma	and genetic syndromes	syndrome
	Placental chorioangioma		Arthrogryposis
	Umbilical cord hemangioma		Multiple pterygia
	Cardiac rhabdomyoma		Neu-Laxova syndrome
	Other cardiac neoplasia		Pena-Shokeir syndrome
	Cardiomyopathy		Myotonic dystrophy
Chromosomal	45,X		Saldino-Noonan syndrome
	Trisomy 21	Metabolic	Gaucher's disease
	Trisomy 18		GM$_1$ gangliosidosis
	Trisomy 13		Sialidosis
	18q +		MPS IVa
	13q −	Urinary	Urethral stenosis or atresia
	45,X/46,XX		Posterior urethral valves
	Triploidy		Congenital nephrosis (Finnish type)
	Other		Prune belly syndrome
Chondrodysplasias	Thanatophoric dwarfism	Gastrointestinal	Midgut volvulus
	Short rib polydactyly		Malrotation of the intestines
	Hypophosphatasia		Duplication of the intestinal tract
	Osteogenesis imperfecta		Meconium peritonitis
	Achondrogenesis		Hepatic fibrosis
Twin pregnancy	Twin-twin transfusion syndrome		Cholestasis
	Acardiac twin		Biliary atresia
			Hepatic vascular malformations

ASD, atrial septal defect; A-V, atrioventricular; CMV, cytomegalovirus; G6PD, glucose-6-phosphate dehydrogenase; MPS, mucopolysaccharide; VSD, ventral septal defect.

Premature closure of the foramen ovale is generally idiopathic and can occur at any time during gestation. It can be diagnosed by careful ultrasound examination of the fetal heart, with Doppler studies and color Doppler studies as useful adjuncts to imaging. Generally, this diagnosis is made only after the onset of hydrops, and prognosis is therefore poor.

Premature closure or narrowing of the ductus arteriosus also has been associated with fetal hydrops (Harlass et al., 1989). In some cases, the mother was receiving indomethacin for the arrest of preterm labor (Mogilner et al., 1982). Moise and associates (1988) described narrowing of the ductus in response to maternal indomethacin ingestion but found it to be measurable and reversible. Vanhaesebrouck and colleagues (1988) described NIH with neonatal ileal perforation in fetuses exposed to indomethacin for the arrest of preterm labor.

A variety of cardiac abnormalities can lead to hydrops. For example, neoplasias such as rhabdomyomas may be present with hydrops. In such cases, one should seek a family history of tuberous sclerosis because this autosomal dominant disorder may present in this fashion (Ostor and Fortune, 1978).

Cardiac failure from myocarditis is responsible for at least some cases of hydrops in fetuses that have congenital infections (Naides and Weiner, 1989). Such cases have been documented with fetal parvovirus B19, with cytomegalovirus (CMV), and much more rarely with toxoplasmosis. These conditions are discussed later under infectious causes of hydrops.

Various noncardiac lesions can lead to high-output cardiac failure, a presumed mechanism of hydrops. Sacrococcygeal teratomas are large vascular tumors that act as arteriovenous shunts and may be associated with hydrops on this basis (Mostoufi-Zadeh et al., 1985; Langer et al., 1989). The majority of these tumors are well tolerated by the fetus, however, and do not lead to hydrops (Gross et al., 1987). Open fetal surgery with resection of the tumor has been attempted in cases associated with fetal hydrops, but only one success has been reported to date (Graf et al., 2000).

Placental tumors may lead to hydrops. These are most commonly chorioangiomas, which are vascular and likely act as arteriovenous shunts (Bauer et al., 1978; Maidman et al., 1980; Hutchinson et al., 1982; Hirata et al., 1993; Dorman and Cardwell, 1995; D'Ercole, 1996).

Other causes of presumed high-output failure associated with fetal hydrops include fetal adrenal neuroblastomas, multiple cases of which have been reported. These rare tumors most likely lead to heart failure based on increased catecholamine release, much as they would in a child with the same lesion. Other angiomas that may also lead to hydrops have been described in the cord (Seifer et al., 1985) and in a fetus in the angio-osteohypertrophy syndrome (Mor et al., 1988).

Chromosomal Abnormalities

Chromosomal abnormalities are fairly common in cases of fetal hydrops, and they may cause the disorder by any of several mechanisms (Machin, 1989). Among chromosomally abnormal fetuses with hydrops, cystic hygromas are common (Holzgreve et al., 1984). In fact, cystic hygromas are among the most common causes of hydrops, particularly among fetuses diagnosed prior to 20 weeks (Santolaya et al., 1992). The chromosomal abnormality most frequently seen in these fetuses is 45,X, or Turner's syndrome. On the other hand, fetuses with this phenotype may also have trisomy 21 or a normal karyotype (Cullen et al., 1990). Among fetuses with a 45,X karyotype, two common structural abnormalities can lead to the development of hydrops. Certainly one is cystic hygroma, but fetuses with this condition also frequently have a tubular coarctation of the aorta. There is some controversy about which of these is the more important mechanism for causing NIH (Machin, 1989).

Other chromosomal abnormalities have also been described in fetuses with hydrops. The most common are trisomy 21, trisomy 18, trisomy 13, and triploidy. Sex chromosome abnormalities that result in Turner's syndrome, such as 45,X/46,XX, have also been reported, as have a large number of more unusual autosomal rearrangements. Structural cardiac lesions are common in aneuploid fetuses and may be associated with hydrops. If no structural cardiac lesion is found, the pathophysiology for the development of hydrops in this situation is unclear. The myeloproliferative disorder common in neonates with Down syndrome has been described in four fetuses with Down syndrome and NIH (Smrcek et al., 2001).

Certainly, when the karyotype is abnormal, the prognosis is poor, and important information can be given to the parents about recurrence risk and diagnosis in future pregnancies. The overall rate of chromosome abnormality among fetuses with hydrops varies between 7% and 45%, with higher rates among those in whom hydrops is detected before 24 weeks (Holzgreve

et al., 1984; Landrum et al., 1986; Santolaya et al., 1992; McCoy et al., 1995; Anandakumar et al., 1996; Heinonen et al., 2000; Ismail et al., 2001; Sohan et al., 2001). Obtaining a fetal karyotype is an essential part of the workup of any fetus with hydrops.

Thoracic Abnormalities

Increases in intrathoracic pressure may lead to the development of hydrops by obstructing venous return and altering cardiovascular hemodynamics. Most of these conditions involve space-occupying lesions of the thorax.

Cystic adenomatoid malformation of the lung is divided into several different subtypes, depending on the size and distribution of the cysts. In most cases, if pulmonary hypoplasia is not life threatening, this lesion is amenable to surgery in the neonate. These fetuses may develop hydrops, however, and this markedly worsens the prognosis.

Most cases of cystic adenomatoid malformation of the lung associated with hydrops involve a single large cyst and a shift of the mediastinum. In several cases, continuous drainage of the solitary cyst by means of pleuroamniotic shunt placement or cyst aspiration has been successful (Clark et al., 1987; Blott et al., 1988; Bernaschek et al., 1994; Crombleholme et al., 2002). In cases in which cysts are microscopic or otherwise not amenable to shunt placement and hydrops is present, open fetal surgery has been performed. Although the outcomes have been poor, some of the fetuses have survived; left untreated, they would not have (Harrison et al., 1990; Crombleholme et al., 2002; Adzick et al., 1998). A substantial proportion of prenatally diagnosed cystic adenomatoid malformations resolve spontaneously or regress but do not entirely resolve. Hydrops has been absent in all reported cases of this nature.

Other types of masses or lesions in the chest may be associated with hydrops as well. These include diaphragmatic hernias, hamartomas or other neoplasms of the lung or chest, pulmonary extralobar sequestration syndrome, and various bronchogenic cysts. Diaphragmatic hernia is the most common of these lesions, but it is unusual for these fetuses to experience hydrops. Once again, *in utero* therapy has been attempted (see Chapter 27). Open fetal surgery with primary repair has largely been abandoned, and attempts at tracheal occlusion have produced mixed results (Morin et al., 1994; Kitano et al., 1999).

Unilateral hydrothorax may present as a space-occupying lesion in the chest and is frequently associated with hydrops. Bilateral hydrothorax may be indistinguishable from other causes of NIH because one of the features of hydrops is pleural effusion. In such cases, the effusions are the primary event and the hydrops a secondary problem. Many authors have considered unilateral or bilateral fetal hydrothorax to be analogous to neonatal chylothorax (Roberts et al., 1986; Booth et al., 1987). Because there are no chylomicrons in the fetus, this is not known with certainty, and in most cases after birth no particular surgery on the presumably abnormal lymphatic system is performed (Rodeck et al., 1988). Overall, these fetuses have a relatively poor prognosis because pulmonary hypoplasia is frequently present (Beischer et al., 1971; Castillo et al., 1987). In the neonate, isolated pleural effusion without hydrops has a much more favorable prognosis, with a 15% mortality rate (Chernick and Reed, 1970).

Many authors recommend diagnostic fetal thoracentesis when unilateral or bilateral hydrothorax is suspected. In cases of isolated hydrothorax, lymphocytes predominate in the fluid obtained, although Eddleman and coauthors (1991) have reported two cases in which this test was misleading. In one of their cases, a single thoracentesis and drainage of the space was sufficient; no effusion reaccumulated. However, in most cases reported, serial thoracenteses have been performed because of rapid reaccumulation of fluid. This has led some authors to propose placement of a pleuroamniotic shunt for continual drainage of this space. The results of such therapy have been mixed, but some successes have been reported (Booth et al., 1987; Rodeck et al., 1988; Bernaschek et al., 1994; Anandakumar et al., 1996; Sohan et al., 2001).

Because prediction of pulmonary hypoplasia *in utero* is difficult, selecting appropriate candidates for invasive procedures is also difficult. In Rodeck's series, the failures occurred at later gestational ages than did the successes, and these late cases presumably involved preexisting pulmonary hypoplasia. Various authors have attempted to measure chest size to predict pulmonary hypoplasia. Nimrod and coworkers (1988) believe that this technique is useful in patients with ruptured membranes but is not predictive in the presence of pleural effusions.

The rate of aneuploidy in association with fetal hydrothorax or isolated pleural effusion is high. Rodeck and associates (1988) placed shunts prior to the availability of a fetal karyotype, and one of eight fetuses had Down syndrome. Petrikovsky and colleagues (1991) reported three consecutive cases of pleural effusion, all of which involved aneuploid fetuses.

Twinning

When one of a set of twins is determined to have fetal hydrops, the differential diagnosis requires special considerations. If it is known that the twins are not monozygotic, the cause is probably unrelated to the twin pregnancy, and the diagnostic approach to the twin with hydrops should be similar to that for any other fetus with the condition. In the case of monozygotic twins, the hydrops is probably related to abnormal vessels in the placenta, resulting in *twin-to-twin transfusion syndrome*. Twin-to-twin transfusion syndrome and other abnormal aspects of twins are discussed in Chapter 29.

In the twin-to-twin transfusion syndrome, the fetus with hydrops may be either the donor or the recipient (Macafee et al., 1970). In the classic situation, the donor twin has growth restriction and oligohydramnios, and the recipient twin has plethora, hydramnios, and perhaps hydrops (Brown et al., 1989; Blickstein, 1990). Presumably, this scenario results from cardiac overload and congestive heart failure; however, it is also possible for the donor twin to have hydrops, in which case the pathophysiology is likely to be related to chronic anemia (Holzgreve et al., 1985).

Twin-to-twin transfusion syndrome carries a poor prognosis, particularly when it is found early in gestation or when hydrops is present (Shah and Chaffin, 1989; Gonsoulin et al., 1990). Various aggressive therapies have been proposed, including serial amniocenteses, *in utero* laser ablation of communicating placental vessels, and transabdominal needle septostomy of the dividing membrane (DeLia et al., 1990; Elliott et al., 1991; Johnson et al., 2001; Mari et al., 2001; Quintero et al., 2001).

In addition, there have been several reports of selective feticide of one twin. This was originally performed as delivery of one twin (Wittmann et al., 1986; Urig et al., 1988). More recently, a variety of techniques to ablate or to ligate the cord of one twin have been attempted (Taylor et al., 2002).

Fetal Anemia

Anemia is a well-known cause of fetal hydrops, and the model used to elucidate the pathophysiology of this condition is *alloimmunization*. Because immune hydrops has been extensively studied, this anemia is the best-understood mechanism for the development of NIH as well.

One of the most common causes of hydrops in patients from Asia or the eastern Mediterranean region is α-thalassemia (Nakayama et al., 1986; Anandakumar et al., 1996). This recessive disorder causes formation of abnormal tetramers of the beta chain of hemoglobin, which cannot carry oxygen (see Chapter 47). Thus, there is massive tissue hypoxia. Fetuses with this disorder commonly develop hydrops as early as 20 weeks' gestation. Because long-term survival of fetuses with homozygous α-thalassemia is extremely rare, there is no current recommendation for treatment. However, proper diagnosis is important for counseling and prenatal diagnosis in future pregnancies.

Fetomaternal hemorrhage is relatively common and, in rare instances, may be massive enough to cause fetal hydrops (Owen et al., 1989). In most cases, the etiology of the fetomaternal hemorrhage or transfusion is unknown. This diagnosis can be made by use of a Kleihauer-Betke stain to examine peripheral maternal blood for the presence of fetal cells. It is also possible to detect a fetomaternal bleed by an abnormally elevated maternal serum α-fetoprotein level. Although the hemorrhage may be self-limited, if a fetus has developed hydrops, many authors have advocated more-aggressive management because of the risk for demise. There have now been several case reports of fetuses that have undergone serial transfusions with resolution of hydrops and an ultimately good outcome (Cardwell, 1988; Rouse and Weiner, 1990; Thorp et al., 1992).

Fetal hemorrhage with subsequent anemia and hydrops formation has also been reported. This has usually been associated with an intracranial hemorrhage, and in the absence of a history of trauma, one should suspect a fetal coagulation deficiency such as alloimmune thrombocytopenia (Bose, 1978; Daffos et al., 1984).

Glucose-6-phosphate dehydrogenase deficiency is a common X-linked condition in African Americans and persons of Mediterranean heritage. This disorder is characterized by hemolytic crises, usually in response to various stimuli including sulfa drugs, aspirin, and fava beans. Female carriers are usually asymptomatic. There are two reports of affected male fetuses developing anemia and hydrops after maternal ingestion of these substances (Perkins, 1971; Mentzer and Collier, 1975).

A number of inherited erythrocyte enzyme deficiencies may cause fetal anemia and, in rare cases, fetal hydrops (Matthay and Mentzer, 1981; Ravindranath et al., 1987). Examples include glucose phosphate isomerase deficiency and pyruvate kinase deficiency. These conditions commonly lead to chronic hemolytic anemia, but rarely to severe anemia, in fetal life.

Congenital leukemia may cause anemia and hydrops, and leukemic infiltration of the myocardium has also been demonstrated (Gray et al., 1986). Transmission of maternal antibodies to erythroid precursors in a mother who had acquired red blood cell aplasia has been reported. Transfusions to the fetus reversed the hydrops and resulted in a healthy liveborn infant with a normal outcome (Oie et al., 1984).

Mari and associates (1995) predicted anemia in fetuses with immune hydrops, based on the velocity of blood flow in the middle cerebral artery. This has been substantiated in subsequent trials and is now widely accepted (Vyas et al., 1990; Mari et al., 2000; Teixeira et al., 2000). The same findings appear to be true in fetuses affected by anemia from other causes, including NIH. The most studied model is in parvovirus-induced anemia, described below (Delle Chiaie et al., 2001).

Infection

A great deal of literature concerns congenital infection as a cause of NIH. Although many different viruses, bacteria, and parasites cause congenital infection, the effects on the fetus are variable, and no infection predictably results in hydrops fetalis (see Chapter 39). In addition, although researchers have long believed anemia to be the common mechanism for the development of hydrops in these fetuses, myocarditis, hepatitis, or other pathways yet to be elucidated may also be involved.

Congenital syphilis is a well-known cause of fetal hydrops. One can confirm the diagnosis by obtaining a positive serologic test result in the mother. A dark-field examination of amniotic fluid may also be helpful (Wendel, 1988). A fetus with syphilis and hydrops faces a poor prognosis compared to one with a milder case of congenital syphilis. Management remains the same, however: treating the infection in the mother.

CMV is a common perinatally acquired infection (Demmler, 1991) (see Chapter 39). Rates of attack and of vertical transmission to the fetus are high, but the percentage of fetuses with symptoms is much smaller. Symptomatic fetuses frequently show growth restriction and may have hydrops (Demmler, 1991). In severe cases, findings at birth may include microcephaly, chorioretinitis, and intracerebral calcifications. Ideally, maternal infection is determined by documentation of seroconversion. Alternatively, rising titers of CMV immunoglobulin (IgG) antibody may be used. Primary infection causes prolonged viral shedding, and a positive maternal urine culture also may be helpful. Blood obtained from the fetus can be tested for CMV-specific IgM if the fetus is past 20 weeks' gestation and is capable of producing IgM; however, some authors have found this technique to be unreliable (Hogge et al., 1993; Revello et al., 1995). Determination of fetal IgG levels is unhelpful because these levels may merely reflect transplacental passage of maternal IgG.

A culture or polymerase chain reaction for CMV using amniotic fluid is the most reliable predictor of CMV infection in the fetus (Fadel and Ruedrich, 1988; Hogge et al., 1993; Van den Veyver et al., 1998). With amniotic fluid culture, gestational age at the time of sampling is important, because many false-negative results are obtained prior to 20 weeks. In addition, the time from infection to sampling is important. In the face of a presumptive clinical diagnosis, one should consider repeating amniocentesis, cordocentesis, or both if these have yielded negative results (Donner et al., 1993; Revello et al., 1995). At present, there is no *in utero* treatment for fetal CMV infection.

The most frequent manifestation of infection with parvovirus B19 is *fifth disease*, or erythema infectiosum (see Chapter 39). This common disorder may be acquired by a pregnant woman from an affected child. It causes a characteristic rash, flu-like symptoms, and arthralgias that may be mild. Fetal infections clearly occur, but the transmission rate is not established.

A large study in England and Wales by the Public Health Laboratory Service Working Party on Fifth Disease (1990) demonstrated a 33% transplacental infection rate with 9% fetal loss in pregnant women infected with the disease. Most fetal losses occurred during the second trimester, and only one case of fetal hydrops was recorded. The Centers for Disease Control (1989) published data from an ongoing study. Researchers there found that among 95 recently infected women, two had fetal losses; one of these fetuses had developed hydrops. By contrast, Rodis and associates (1988) found fetal hydrops in three of four women who acquired this infection during pregnancy.

Until the recent advent of polymerase chain reaction testing of amniotic fluid and serum, the diagnosis of human parvovirus infection in a fetus with hydrops was difficult (Gentilomi et al., 1998; Dieck et al., 1999). Data from older series were based on diagnoses made by isolating virus from fetal blood, detecting parvovirus-specific IgM in fetal serum, or demonstrating virus in fetal tissues (Samuels and Ludmir, 1990; Weiner et al., 1992). Viral particles can be detected by electron microscopy, polymerase chain reaction, or finding intranuclear inclusions on cytologic specimens (Porter, Khong, et al., 1988; Centers for Disease Control, 1989; Naides and Weiner, 1989; Iwa and Yutani, 1995). Fetal serology may be negative in some cases of fetal infection in which hydrops has developed (Carrington et al., 1987; Anderson et al., 1988; Peters and Nicolaides, 1990). Easier diagnosis has led to an appreciation of how common this infection is. In a recent review of published series (Von Kaisenberg and Jonat, 2001), it accounted for 27% of all cases of NIH. Human parvovirus infection may underlie a substantial portion of NIH cases previously labeled idiopathic (Porter, Khong, et al., 1988; Samuels and Ludmir, 1990).

A characteristic although nonspecific finding in fetuses with this infection and hydrops is elevated maternal serum α-fetoprotein (Anand et al., 1987). Data from Carrington and colleagues (1987) and from Bernstein and Capeless (1989) suggest that very elevated maternal serum α-fetoprotein is a useful marker because it may herald the onset of hydrops in an affected pregnancy. The usual mechanism for the development of hydrops in parvovirus infections is presumably anemia from an aplastic crisis. Parvovirus-infected fetuses undergoing percutaneous umbilical blood sampling have been found to be severely anemic (Carrington et al., 1987; Rodis et al., 1988). The virus has been shown to invade myocardium as well, however, and myocarditis may also account for hydropic changes, particularly in less-anemic fetuses (Porter, Quantril, et al., 1988; Naides and Weiner, 1989).

Because this virus is not known to be associated with congenital malformations or long-term sequelae, aggressive *in utero* supportive therapy has been attempted. Transfusions of packed cells to the fetus have resulted in some good outcomes (Peters and Nicolaides, 1990; Soothill, 1990; Sahakian et al.,

1991). Upon reviewing published descriptions of 705 confirmed cases of fetal parvovirus in which 230 fetuses received transfusions, Von Kaisenberg and Jonat (2001) concluded that aggressive therapy has a benefit over expectant management.

The transient nature of this infection and the absence of fetal demise have led many investigators to speculate that the virus may be a causative agent in cases of ascites or hydrops that spontaneously resolve *in utero* (Peters and Nicolaides, 1990; Morey et al., 1991).

Various other infectious agents have been related to hydrops in at least a few cases (Bain et al., 1956; Spahr et al., 1980; Robb et al., 1986; Gembruch et al., 1987; Ranucci-Weiss et al., 1998; Zornes et al., 1988). These include adenovirus, toxoplasmosis, herpes simplex, rubella, and *Listeria*. In some cases, an infectious process is suspected, but no causative organism can be identified (Zimmer et al., 1986). It is possible that coxsackievirus or certain influenza viruses or enteroviruses can produce fetal hydrops, either transiently or with subsequent fetal death (Van den Veyver et al., 1998). An interesting report by Robertson and coauthors (1985) describes a case in which multiple cultures were negative. Nonetheless, the infant showed continuing evidence of hepatitis for several weeks following delivery. Eventual outcome was good.

Metabolic Disease

A variety of genetic metabolic diseases, particularly lysosomal storage diseases, can cause hydrops in the fetus (Gillan et al., 1984). Gaucher's disease, generalized (GM_1) gangliosidosis, Salla's disease, sialidosis, mucopolysaccharidosis types IV and VII, Tay-Sachs disease, and others can all present in this manner (Abu-Dalu et al., 1982; Beck et al., 1984; Bonduelle et al., 1991; Tasso et al., 1996). Gaucher's disease is the most common of these disorders and has been reported the most frequently, but presentation with hydrops is rare (Ginsburg and Groll, 1973). These conditions can recur in subsequent pregnancies because they are typically inherited in an autosomal-recessive fashion. Establishing the correct diagnosis is therefore extremely important. This can be accomplished by analysis of oligosaccharides in fetal or neonatal urine or blood, enzyme analysis and carrier testing in the parents, or histologic examination of appropriate fetal tissues (Gillan et al., 1984; Piraud et al., 1996; Groener et al., 1999). Unfortunately, most of these tests are performed after a fetal or neonatal death, because the prognosis is poor.

Other Malformations

A variety of chondrodysplasias may present with fetal hydrops. Pretorius and coworkers (1986) found all such cases to be associated with fatal dwarfing syndromes. In these cases, the chest is compressed, and the neonates die of respiratory insufficiency. The most common skeletal dysplasias described with fetal hydrops are short-rib polydactyly syndrome, thanatophoric dysplasia, and achondrogenesis. One can diagnose skeletal dysplasia fairly easily with ultrasonography by measuring the extremities relative to head and abdominal size, but classifying the type of chondrodysplasia in a fetus by ultrasonography alone may be difficult. After birth, x-ray studies as well as examination of other pheno-

typic features of the neonate can be used to determine the specific type of chondrodysplasia. Because many of the lethal types are inherited in a recessive fashion, the recurrence rate is high. For several of these disorders, the gene responsible has been identified, and detection of the genetic abnormality on fetal or neonatal tissue specimens can therefore be accomplished.

A number of other genetic syndromes have also been associated with fetal hydrops. These include congenital myotonic dystrophy, arthrogryposis, multiple fetal pterygia, Neu-Laxova syndrome, and Pena-Shokeir type I (Holzgreve et al., 1984; Jauniaux et al., 1990; Afifi et al., 1992).

Urinary tract malformations have been described in conjunction with hydrops in numerous reports; however, close examination of these cases reveals that most involve isolated ascites with a urinary tract malformation. This condition, known as urinary ascites, is common, well described, and generally self-limited. It rarely progresses to hydrops.

Various intra-abdominal processes related to the gastrointestinal tract commonly present with ascites, but in rare cases they are associated with hydrops. These include meconium peritonitis, small bowel volvulus, and various intestinal atresias.

Other Causes

Diabetes is frequently cited as a cause of NIH, and several large series have included a few cases in which preexisting maternal diabetes was the only etiology (Poeschmann et al., 1991). It is not clear whether these fetuses were structurally normal. Other authors have found no association between maternal diabetes and NIH (Macafee et al., 1970).

The list of causes given above is certainly not complete. Numerous case reports describe other syndromes or malformations associated with fetal hydrops. In some of these cases, the association may not be causative or may be unproven, but in others it is more convincing. The literature is constantly being updated, not only with series but with case reports, and this discussion is therefore not exhaustive.

EXPERIMENTAL MANAGEMENT OF IDIOPATHIC CASES

Various management strategies have been attempted in cases of NIH of unknown etiology. Shimokawa and associates (1988) injected albumin on two occasions into the peritoneal cavity of a fetus with hydrops, and hydrops subsequently resolved. This group later published a series of 21 cases treated with a combination of red blood cell transfusions and serial albumin injections. Improvements occurred only in fetuses without pleural effusions, but within this group five of seven fetuses (72%) survived (Maeda et al., 1988).

Lingman and colleagues (1989) attempted direct intravascular albumin transfusion on five occasions in a fetus later found to have a lysosomal storage disease. Doppler studies and blood counts before and after the procedures indicated effective plasma expansion and peripheral vasodilatation.

Goldberg and associates (1986) placed a peritoneal-amniotic shunt in a second-trimester fetus with NIH of unknown etiology and massive ascites. Although the ascites resolved, other features of hydrops developed, and the fetus ultimately died.

DIAGNOSTIC APPROACH TO THE FETUS WITH HYDROPS

The workup of a patient with a diagnosis of fetal hydrops should be directed at possible causes. Because the diagnosis is confirmed with ultrasonography, this is frequently the first test performed. During a careful ultrasound examination, the known causes of NIH should be kept in mind. Many of the fetal conditions, congenital anomalies, and malformation sequences that are known causes of hydrops are found or eliminated on the initial ultrasound examination. Twins, cardiac arrhythmias, and hydrothorax are all examples of obvious ultrasonography-derived diagnoses. The blood-flow velocity of the middle cerebral artery may be assessed to screen for fetal anemia.

If the examination is unsatisfactory, it should be repeated later to delineate the fetal anatomy as well as possible. Although the underlying diagnosis is far more predictive of outcome than are any specific ultrasonographic parameters, the initial examination can be used to assess the severity of the hydrops and to initiate antenatal testing, if appropriate, depending on gestational age. Assessing the severity of the hydrops is particularly important if the fetus is observed for some length of time or if fetal therapy is attempted. Ultrasound parameters can be longitudinally followed to predict fetal decompensation or fetal response to *in utero* therapy.

A history should be taken, with particular attention to ethnic background and any family history of genetic diseases or congenital anomaly, consanguinity, and recent maternal infections or exposures. Once again, careful scrutiny of the listed causes of hydrops gives direction to the types of questions that should be asked of the mother and family.

The initial testing of the mother should include the elimination of immune causes of hydrops with blood typing and the indirect Coombs test. A screen for hemoglobinopathies, a Kleihauer-Betke test to look for fetal red blood cells in the maternal circulation, and titers for *toxoplasmosis, rubella, cytomegalovirus,* and *herpes* simplex (TORCH) are also useful at this time. Some of these tests may not be immediately available, but blood should be drawn and sent to the laboratory.

In addition to careful ultrasonography, fetal echocardiography may be helpful. A fetal karyotype should be obtained in most cases. With the availability of fluorescence in situ hybridization, rapid karyotype can be obtained from amniotic fluid. If infection is suspected, amniotic fluid can be sent for polymerase chain reaction testing or culture. Fetal blood can also be used for a rapid karyotype, and it can be sent for other tests, such as a complete blood count and platelet count, to rule out fetal anemia or thrombocytopenia. If blood is obtained, serologies and cultures can be performed on the specimen.

Fetal serum or amniotic fluid can be frozen or can be sent for other studies, such as screening for lysosomal storage diseases, if these are suspected. Although delta optical density 450 values are increased in many cases of NIH (Appelman et al., 1988), this is not clinically useful information, and therefore the study is not generally indicated. Amniotic fluid should be sent for lung-maturity studies when appropriate. A frozen sample of amniotic fluid may be useful for future viral DNA hybridization studies or oligosaccharide analysis if not ordered initially.

Because some test findings are not available promptly, numerous tests may need to be ordered before initial results are available. It is helpful to establish a connection with cooperative laboratory facilities or, if these are not available locally, with reference laboratories to which specimens can be sent.

MANAGEMENT

Management issues are difficult to generalize because they depend on prognosis, gestational age, and presenting signs and symptoms. Before the fetus becomes viable, the prognosis should be explained to the parents, who should be given the option of terminating the pregnancy. If the underlying etiology is amenable to fetal therapy, this should be frankly discussed with the family, but generally the parents should be warned that diagnostic error is always possible and that the overall prognosis in NIH is still grim.

Unfortunately, many cases of NIH are detected during the third trimester. If the patient presents in preterm labor or if symptomatic hydramnios exists, difficult decisions need to be made about whether to administer tocolytic medications or to allow labor to continue. In many cases, patients have presented in labor, and tocolysis has been initiated before the diagnosis of hydrops is made. I recommend continuing tocolysis, as long as the mother is stable, while the fetal workup is being pursued. If a potentially reversible cause of hydrops is found, every attempt should be made to prolong the pregnancy to maximize fetal survival and initiate *in utero* resuscitation.

If a fetal diagnosis with a poor prognosis seems fairly certain, however, a frank discussion with the family may lead to the discontinuation of tocolytic medication. Patients who present with or later show signs of maternal compromise, such as preeclampsia or antenatal hemorrhage, should be managed without regard to fetal outcome since it is so poor. Management decisions are particularly difficult in idiopathic cases because the prognosis is uncertain. Even though the overall prognosis is poor in idiopathic cases, every attempt should be made to prolong pregnancies that present during the third trimester to 32 or 34 weeks' gestation in order to maximize fetal survival, unless there are signs of fetal or maternal decompensation. If significant or symptomatic hydramnios is present, it may be treated with therapeutic amniocenteses, indomethacin, or, more conservatively, bed rest and conventional tocolytic therapy. Treatment of hydramnios is further discussed in Chapter 3.

Fetal decompensation may be difficult to measure, but the usual biophysical parameters are nonetheless useful. If a fetal reactive heart rate tracing becomes abnormal, this should be interpreted as a sign of acute decompensation. Similarly, oligohydramnios, a decrease in fetal movement, and poor fetal tone are all ominous signs. Unless there is evidence that hydrops is resolving or that treatment has otherwise been effective, there does not seem to be any reason to prolong a pregnancy past 34 weeks' gestation or the attainment of a mature lung profile.

RECURRENCE RISKS

After the delivery of a fetus with NIH, investigation of the cause should continue in the nursery, if necessary. If the fetus is stillborn or dies during the early neonatal period, every attempt should be made to obtain a postmortem examination directed at finding the underlying cause of the problem. Without this information, counseling the patient and her family about future pregnancies is frustrating. Overall, recurrent hydrops fetalis is unusual, and for most families the prognosis is good for a normal pregnancy in the future. However, there are numerous case reports of recurrent pregnancies with hydropic fetuses (Cumming, 1979; Etches and Lemons, 1979; Schwartz et al., 1981). One must therefore be wary of reassuring families that idiopathic hydrops is not going to recur, and future pregnancies should be carefully monitored.

■ DELIVERY CONSIDERATIONS

Delivery of a fetus with hydrops should be attended by an experienced pediatric team prepared to deal with a sick neonate. Some authors have recommended the liberal use of cesarean section to avoid asphyxia and birth trauma, although no objective data support this approach (Spahr et al., 1980). Predelivery thoracentesis or paracentesis has also been advocated to enable immediate postnatal resuscitation or, in the case of a large fetal abdominal girth, to facilitate vaginal delivery (deCrespigny et al., 1980; Holzgreve et al., 1985; Romero et al., 1988; Cardwell, 1996).

Immediate problems of the neonate are likely to center on respiratory support and fluid management. Virtually all neonates with hydrops require mechanical ventilation, and edema may make intubation difficult (Carlton et al., 1989; Stephenson et al., 1994).

Postnatal drainage of pleural or peritoneal fluid may be required to maintain oxygenation. Some authors reserve these procedures for extreme cases, whereas others propose a more liberal use of fluid drainage (Davis, 1982; Carlton et al., 1989; Ringer and Stark, 1989). Fluid restriction, careful management of electrolytes, judicious use of albumin and diuretics, correction of anemia, and continuous assessment of intravascular volume are all important issues in the first few days of life.

■ S U M M A R Y

Although there have been many advances in our understanding of the causes of fetal NIH, it remains a difficult clinical problem. Many conditions have been associated with fetal hydrops, but few shed light on the pathophysiology of its development. Once the diagnosis of NIH is established, a careful search for causative fetal pathology should be undertaken. Unfortunately, the results of such a search may not be available when difficult management decisions need to be made. Recent advances in fetal therapy have increased the number of fetal conditions for which treatment is possible. However, the overall rates of morbidity in mother and fetus, and of mortality in the fetus, remain high.

REFERENCES

Abu-Dalu KI, Tamary H, Livni N, et al: GM₁ gangliosidosis presenting as neonatal ascites. J Pediatr **100**:940, 1982.

Adzick NS, Harrison MR, Crombleholme TM, et al: Fetal lung lesions: Management and outcome. Am J Obstet Gynecol **179**:884, 1998.

Afifi AM, Bhatia AR, Eyal F: Hydrops fetalis associated with congenital myotonic dystrophy. Am J Obstet Gynecol **166**:929, 1992.

Allan LD, Crawford DC, Sheridan R, et al: Aetiology of non-immune hydrops: The value of echocardiography. Br J Obstet Gynaecol **93**:223, 1986.

Anand A, Gray ES, Brown T, et al: Human parvovirus infection in pregnancy and hydrops fetalis. N Engl J Med **316**:183, 1987.

Anandakumar C, Biswas A, Wong YC, et al: Management of non-immune hydrops: 8 years' experience. Ultrasound Obstet Gynecol **8**:196, 1996.

Anderson MJ, Khousam MN, Maxwell DJ, et al: Human parvovirus B19 and hydrops fetalis. Lancet **1**:535, 1988.

Appelman Z, Blumberg BD, Golabi M, et al: Nonimmune hydrops fetalis may be associated with an elevated delta OD₄₅₀ in the amniotic fluid. Obstet Gynecol **71**:1005, 1988.

Bain AD, Bowie JH, Flint WF, et al: Congenital toxoplasmosis disease stimulating haemolytic disease of the newborn. J Obstet Gynecol **63**:826, 1956.

Bauer CR, Fojaco RM, Bancalari E, et al: Microangiopathic hemolytic anemia and thrombocythemia in a neonate associated with a large placental chorioangioma. Pediatrics **62**:574, 1978.

Beck M, Bender SW, Reiter HL, et al: Neuraminidase deficiency presenting as non-immune hydrops fetalis. Eur J Pediatr **143**:135, 1984.

Beischer NA, Fortune DW, Macafee J, et al: Nonimmunologic hydrops fetalis and congenital abnormalities. Obstet Gynecol **38**:86, 1971.

Benacerraf BR, Frigoletto FD Jr: Sonographic sign for the detection of early fetal ascites in the management of severe isoimmune disease without intrauterine transfusion. Am J Obstet Gynecol **152**:1039, 1985.

Bernaschek G, Dentinger J, Hansmann M: Feto-amniotic shunting—report of the experience of four European centres. Prenat Diagn **14**:821, 1994.

Bernstein IM, Capeless EL: Elevated maternal serum alpha-fetoprotein and hydrops fetalis in association with fetal parvovirus B-19 infection. Obstet Gynecol **74**:456, 1989.

Blickstein I: The twin-twin transfusion syndrome. Obstet Gynecol **76**:714, 1990.

Blott M, Nicolaides KH, Greenough A: Pleuroamniotic shunting for decompression of fetal pleural effusions. Obstet Gynecol **71**:798, 1988.

Bonduelle M, Lissens W, Goossens A, et al: Lysosomal storage diseases presenting as transient or persistent hydrops fetalis. Genet Couns **2**:227, 1991.

Booth P, Nicolaides KH, Greenough A, et al: Pleuro-amniotic shunting for fetal chylothorax. Early Hum Dev **15**:365, 1987.

Bose C: Hydrops fetalis and in utero intracranial hemorrhage. J Pediatr **93**:1023, 1978.

Brown BS: The ultrasonographic features of nonimmune hydrops fetalis: A study of 30 successive patients. Can Assoc Radiol J **37**:164, 1986.

Brown DL, Benson CB, Driscoll SG, et al: Twin-twin transfusion syndrome: Sonographic findings. Radiology **170**:61, 1989.

Cameron A, Nicholson S, Nimrod C, et al: Evaluation of fetal cardiac dysrhythmias with two-dimensional, M-mode, and pulsed Doppler ultrasonography. Am J Obstet Gynecol **158**:286, 1988.

Cardwell MS: Successful treatment of hydrops fetalis caused by fetomaternal hemorrhage: A case report. Am J Obstet Gynecol **158**:131, 1988.

Cardwell MS: Aspiration of fetal pleural effusions or ascites may improve neonatal resuscitation. South Med J **89**:177, 1996.

Carlson DE, Platt LD, Medearis AL, et al: Prognostic indicators of the resolution of nonimmune hydrops fetalis and survival of the fetus. Am J Obstet Gynecol **163**:1785, 1990.

Carlton DP, McGillivray BC, Schreiber MD: Nonimmune hydrops fetalis: A multidisciplinary approach. Clin Perinatol **16**:839, 1989.

Carrington D, Whittle MJ, Gibson AAM, et al: Maternal serum alpha-fetoprotein—a marker of fetal aplastic crisis during intrauterine human parvovirus infection. Lancet **1**:433, 1987.

Castillo RA, Devoe LD, Falls G, et al: Pleural effusions and pulmonary hypoplasia. Am J Obstet Gynecol **157**:1252, 1987.

Castillo RA, Devoe LD, Hadi HA, et al: Nonimmune hydrops fetalis: Clinical experience and factors related to a poor outcome. Am J Obstet Gynecol **155**:812, 1986.

Centers for Disease Control (CDC): MMWR **38**:81, 1989.

Chernick V, Reed MH: Pneumothorax and chylothorax in the neonatal period. J Pediatr **76**:624, 1970.

Chitkara U, Wilkins I, Lynch L, et al: The role of sonography in assessing severity of fetal anemia in Rh- and Kell-isoimmunized pregnancies. Obstet Gynecol **71**:393, 1988.

Clark SL, Vitale DJ, Minton SD, et al: Successful fetal therapy for cystic adenomatoid malformation associated with second-trimester hydrops. Am J Obstet Gynecol **157**:294, 1987.

Copel JA, Cullen M, Green JJ, et al: The frequency of aneuploidy in prenatally diagnosed congenital heart disease: An indication for fetal karyotyping. Am J Obstet Gynecol **158**:409, 1988.

Crawford DC, Sunder KC, Allan LD: Prenatal detection of congenital heart disease: Factors affecting obstetric management and survival. Am J Obstet Gynecol **159**:352, 1988.

Crombleholme TM, Coleman B, Hedrick H, et al: Cystic adenomatoid malformation volume ratio predicts outcome in prenatally diagnosed cystic adenomatoid malformation of the lung. J Pediatr Surg 37:331, 2002.

Cullen MT, Gabrielli S, Green JJ, et al: Diagnosis and significance of cystic hygroma in the first trimester. Prenat Diagn 10:643, 1990.

Cumming DC: Recurrent nonimmune hydrops fetalis. Obstet Gynecol 54:124, 1979.

Daffos F, Forestier F, Muller JY, et al: Prenatal treatment of alloimmune thrombocytopenia. Lancet 2:632, 1984.

Davis CL: Diagnosis and management of nonimmune hydrops. J Reprod Med 27:594, 1982.

DeLia JE, Cruikshank DP, Keye WR: Fetoscopic neodymium: YAG laser occlusion of placental vessels in severe twin-twin transfusion syndrome. Obstet Gynecol 75:1046, 1990.

deCrespigny LC, Robinson HP, McBain JC: Fetal abdominal paracentesis in the management of gross fetal ascites. Aust N Z J Obstet Gynaecol 20:228, 1980.

Delle Chiaie L, Buck G, Grab D, et al: Prediction of fetal anemia with Doppler measurement of the middle cerebral artery peak systolic velocity in pregnancies complicated by maternal blood group alloimmunization or parvovirus B19 infection. Ultrasound Obstet Gynecol 18:232, 2001.

Demmler GJ: Summary of a workshop on surveillance for congenital cytomegalovirus disease. Rev Infect Dis 13:315, 1991.

D'Ercole C: Large chorioangioma associated with hydrops fetalis: Prenatal diagnosis and management. Fetal Diagn Ther 11:357, 1996.

Dieck D, Lothar Schild R, Hansmann, et al: Prenatal diagnosis of congenital parvovirus B19 infection: Value of serological and PCR techniques in maternal and fetal serum. Prenat Diagn 19:1119, 1999.

Donner C, Liesnard C, Brancart F, et al: Accuracy of amniotic fluid testing before 21 weeks' gestation in prenatal diagnosis of congenital cytomegalovirus infection. Prenat Diagn 14:1055, 1994.

Donner C, Liesnard C, Content J, et al: Prenatal diagnosis of 52 pregnancies at risk for congenital cytomegalovirus infection. Obstet Gynecol 82:481, 1993.

Dorman SL, Cardwell MS: Ballantyne syndrome caused by a large placental chorioangioma. Am J Obstet Gynecol 173:1632, 1995.

Eddleman KA, Levine AB, Chitkara U, et al: Reliability of pleural fluid lymphocyte counts in the antenatal diagnosis of congenital chylothorax. Obstet Gynecol 78:530, 1991.

Elliott JP, Urig MA, Clewell WH: Aggressive therapeutic amniocentesis for treatment of twin-twin transfusion syndrome. Obstet Gynecol 77:537, 1991.

Etches PC, Lemons JA: Nonimmune hydrops fetalis: Report of 22 cases including three siblings. Pediatrics 64:326, 1979.

Fadel HE, Ruedrich DA: Intrauterine resolution of nonimmune hydrops associated with cytomegalovirus infection. Obstet Gynecol 71:1003, 1988.

Fleischer AC, Killam AP, Boehm FH, et al: Hydrops fetalis: Sonographic evaluation and clinical implications. Radiology 141:163, 1981.

Gembruch U, Niesen M, Hansmann M, et al: Listeriosis: A cause of nonimmune hydrops fetalis. Prenat Diagn 7:277, 1987.

Gentilomi G, Zerbini M, Gallinella G, et al: B19 parvovirus induced fetal hydrops: Rapid and simple diagnosis by detection of B19 antigens in amniotic fluids. Prenat Diagn 18:363, 1998.

Gillan JE, Lowden JA, Gaskin K, et al: Congenital ascites as a presenting sign of lysosomal storage disease. J Pediatr 104:225, 1984.

Ginsburg SJ, Groll M: Hydrops fetalis due to infantile Gaucher's disease. J Pediatr 82:1046, 1973.

Goldberg JD, Mitty H, Dische MR, et al: Prenatal shunting of fetal ascites in nonimmune hydrops fetalis. Am J Perinatol 3:92, 1986.

Gonsoulin W, Moise KJ, Kirshon B, et al: Outcome of twin-twin transfusion diagnosed before 28 weeks of gestation. Obstet Gynecol 75:214, 1990.

Graf JL, Albanese CT, Jennings RW, et al: Successful fetal sacrococcygeal teratoma resection in a hydropic fetus. J Pediatr Surg 35:1489, 2000.

Graves GR, Baskett TF: Nonimmune hydrops fetalis: Antenatal diagnosis and management. Am J Obstet Gynecol 148:563, 1984.

Gray ES, Balch NJ, Kohler H, et al: Congenital leukaemia: An unusual cause of stillbirth. Arch Dis Child 61:1001, 1986.

Groener JEM, de Graaf FL, Poorthuis JHM, et al: Prenatal diagnosis of lysosomal storage diseases using fetal blood. Prenat Diagn 19:930, 1999.

Gross SJ, Benzie RJ, Sermer M, et al: Prenatal diagnosis and management. Am J Obstet Gynecol 156:393, 1987.

Harlass FE, Duff P, Brady K, et al: Hydrops fetalis and premature closure of the ductus arteriosus: A review. Obstet Gynecol Surv 44:541, 1989.

Harrison MR, Adzick NS, Jennings RW, et al: Antenatal intervention for congenital cystic adenomatoid malformation. Lancet 336:965, 1990.

Heinonen S, Ryynanen M, Kirkinen P: Etiology and outcome of second trimester non-immunologic fetal hydrops. Acta Obstet Gynecol Scand 79:15, 2000.

Hirata GI, Masaki D, O'Toole M, et al: Color flow mapping and Doppler velocimetry in the diagnosis and management of a placental chorioangioma associated with nonimmune fetal hydrops. Obstet Gynecol 81:850, 1993.

Hoddick WK, Mahony BS, Callen PW, et al: Placental thickness. J Ultrasound Med 4:479, 1985.

Hogge WA, Buffone GJ, Hogge JS: Prenatal diagnosis of cytomegalovirus (CMV) infection: A preliminary report. Prenat Diagn 13:131, 1993.

Holzgreve W, Curry CJ, Golbus MS, et al: Investigation of nonimmune hydrops fetalis. Am J Obstet Gynecol 150:805, 1984.

Holzgreve W, Holzgreve B, Curry CJR: Nonimmune hydrops fetalis: Diagnosis and management. Semin Perinatol 9:52, 1985.

Hutchison AA, Drew JH, Yu VYH, et al: Nonimmunologic hydrops fetalis: A review of 61 cases. Obstet Gynecol 59:347, 1982.

Im SS, Rizos N, Joutsi P, et al: Nonimmunologic hydrops fetalis. Am J Obstet Gynecol 148:566, 1984.

Ismail KM, Martin WL, Ghosh S, et al: Etiology and outcome of hydrops fetalis. J Matern Fetal Med 10:175, 2001.

Iwa N, Yutani C: Cytodiagnosis of parvovirus B19 infection from ascites fluid of hydrops fetalis. Diagn Cytopathol 13:139, 1995.

Jauniaux E, Van Maldergem L, De Munter C, et al: Nonimmune hydrops fetalis associated with genetic abnormalities. Obstet Gynecol 75:568, 1990.

Johnson JR, Rossi KQ, O'Shaughnessy RW: Amnioreduction versus septostomy in twin-twin transfusion syndrome. Am J Obstet Gynecol 185:1044, 2001.

Kitano Y, Flake AW, Crombleholme TM: Open fetal surgery for life-threatening fetal malformations. Semin Perinatol 23:448, 1999.

Landrum BG, Johnson DE, Ferrara B, et al: Hydrops fetalis and chromosomal trisomies. Am J Obstet Gynecol 154:1114, 1986.

Langer JC, Harrison MR, Schmidt KG, et al: Fetal hydrops and death from sacrococcygeal teratoma: Rationale for fetal surgery. Am J Obstet Gynecol 160:1145, 1989.

Lingman G, Stangenberg M, Legarth J, et al: Albumin transfusion in nonimmune fetal hydrops: Doppler ultrasound evaluation of the acute effects on blood circulation in the fetal aorta and the umbilical arteries. Fetal Ther 4:120, 1989.

Macafee CAJ, Fortune DW, Beischer NA: Non-immunological hydrops fetalis. J Obstet Gynaecol Br Commonw 77:226, 1970.

Machin GA: Hydrops revisited: Literature review of 1,414 cases published in the 1980s. Am J Med Genet 34:366, 1989.

Maeda H, Shimokawa H, Nakano H, et al: Effects of intrauterine treatment on nonimmunologic hydrops fetalis. Fetal Ther 3:198, 1988.

Mahony BS, Filly RA, Callen PW, et al: Severe nonimmune hydrops fetalis: Sonographic evaluation. Radiology 151:757, 1984.

Maidman JE, Yeager C, Anderson V, et al: Prenatal diagnosis and management of nonimmunologic hydrops fetalis. Obstet Gynecol 56:571, 1980.

Mari G, Abuhamad AZ, Uerpairojkit B, et al: Blood flow velocity waveforms of the abdominal arteries in appropriate- and small-for-gestational-age fetuses. Ultrasound Obstet Gynecol 6:15, 1995.

Mari G, Detti L, Oz U, et al: Long-term outcome in twin-twin transfusion syndrome treated with serial aggressive amnioreduction. Am J Obstet Gynecol 183:211, 2000.

Mari G, Roberts A, Detti L, et al: Perinatal morbidity and mortality rates in severe twin-twin transfusion syndrome: results of the International Amnioreduction Registry. Am J Obstet Gynecol 185:708, 2001.

Matthay KK, Mentzer WC: Erythrocyte enzymopathies in the newborn. Clin Haematol 10:31, 1981.

McCoy MC, Katz VL, Gould N, et al: Non-immune hydrops after 20 weeks' gestation: Review of 10 years' experience with suggestions for management. Obstet Gynecol 85:578, 1995.

McFadden DE, Taylor GP: Cardiac abnormalities and nonimmune hydrops fetalis: A coincidental, not causal relationship. Pediatr Pathol 9:11, 1989.

Mentzer WC, Collier E: Hydrops fetalis associated with erythrocyte G-6-PD deficiency and maternal ingestion of fava beans and ascorbic acid. J Pediatr 86:565, 1975.

Mogilner BM, Ashkenazy M, Borenstein R, et al: Hydrops fetalis caused by maternal indomethacin treatment. Acta Obstet Gynecol Scand 61:183, 1982.

Moise KJ, Huhta JC, Sharif DS, et al: Indomethacin in the treatment of premature labor: Effects on the fetal ductus arteriosus. N Engl J Med **319:**327, 1988.

Mor A, Schreyer P, Wainraub Z, et al: Nonimmune hydrops fetalis associated with angio-osteohypertrophy (Klippel-Trenaunay) syndrome. Am J Obstet Gynecol **159:**1185, 1988.

Morey AL, Nicolini U, Welch CR, et al: Parvovirus B19 infection and transient fetal hydrops. Lancet **337:**496, 1991.

Morin L, Crombleholme TM, D'Alton ME: Prenatal diagnosis and management of fetal thoracic lesions. Semin Perinatol **18:**228, 1994.

Mostoufi-Zadeh M, Weiss LM, Driscoll SH: Nonimmune hydrops fetalis: A challenge in perinatal pathology. Hum Pathol **16:**785, 1985.

Naides SJ, Weiner CP: Antenatal diagnosis and palliative treatment of nonimmune hydrops fetalis secondary to fetal parvovirus B19 infection. Prenat Diagn **9:**105, 1989.

Nakayama R, Yamada D, Steinmiller V, et al: Hydrops fetalis secondary to Bart hemoglobinopathy. Obstet Gynecol **67:**176, 1986.

Nimrod C, Nicholson S, Davies D, et al: Pulmonary hypoplasia testing in clinical obstetrics. Am J Obstet Gynecol **158:**277, 1988.

Oie BK, Hertel J, Seip M, et al: Hydrops foetalis in 3 infants of a mother with acquired chronic pure red cell aplasia: Transitory red cell aplasia in 1 of the infants. Scand J Haematol **33:**466, 1984.

Ostor A, Fortune DW: Tuberous sclerosis initially seen as hydrops fetalis. Arch Pathol Lab Med **102:**34, 1978.

Owen J, Stedman CM, Tucker TL: Comparison of predelivery versus postdelivery Kleihauer-Betke stains in cases of fetal death. Am J Obstet Gynecol **161:**663, 1989.

Perkins RP: Hydrops fetalis and stillbirth in a male glucose-6-phosphate dehydrogenase–deficient fetus possibly due to maternal ingestion of sulfisoxazole. Am J Obstet Gynecol **3:**379, 1971.

Peters MT, Nicolaides KH: Cordocentesis for the diagnosis and treatment of human fetal parvovirus infection. Obstet Gynecol **75:**501, 1990.

Petrikovsky BM, Shmoys SM, Baker DA, et al: Pleural effusion in aneuploidy. Perinatology **8:**214, 1991.

Piraud M, Froissart R, Mandon G, et al: Amniotic fluid for screening of lysosomal storage diseases presenting in utero (mainly as non-immune hydrops fetalis). Clin Chim Acta **248:**143, 1996.

Platt LD, DeVore GR: In utero diagnosis of hydrops fetalis: Ultrasound methods. Clin Perinatol **9:**627, 1982.

Poeschmann RP, Verheijen RHM, Van Dongen WJ: Differential diagnosis and causes of nonimmunological hydrops fetalis: A review. Obstet Gynecol Surv **46:**223, 1991.

Porter HJ, Khong TY, Evans MF, et al: Parvovirus as a cause of hydrops fetalis: Detection by in situ DNA hybridization. J Clin Pathol **41:**381, 1988.

Porter HJ, Quantril AM, Fleming KA: B19 parvovirus infection of myocardial cells. Lancet **1:**535, 1988.

Potter EL: Universal edema of the fetus unassociated with erythroblastosis. Am J Obstet Gynecol **46:**130, 1943.

Pretorius DH, Rumack CM, Manco-Johnson ML, et al: Specific skeletal dysplasias in utero: Sonographic diagnosis. Radiology **159:**237, 1986.

Public Health Laboratory Service Working Party on Fifth Disease: Prospective study of human parvovirus (B19) infection in pregnancy. BMJ **300:**1166, 1990.

Quintero RA, Bornick PW, Morales WJ, et al: Selective photocoagulation of communicating vessels in the treatment of monochorionic twins with selective growth retardation. Am J Obstet Gynecol **185:**689, 2001.

Ranucci-Weiss D, Uerpairojkit B, Bowles N, et al: Intrauterine adenoviral infection associated with fetal non-immune hydrops. Prenat Diagn **18:**182, 1998.

Ravindranath Y, Paglia DE, Warrier I, et al: Glucose phosphate isomerase deficiency as a cause of hydrops fetalis. N Engl J Med **316:**258, 1987.

Revello MG, Baldanti F, Furione M, et al: Polymerase chain reaction for prenatal diagnosis of congenital human cytomegalovirus infection. J Med Virol **47:**462, 1995.

Ringer SA, Stark AR: Management of neonatal emergencies in the delivery room. Clin Perinatol **16:**23, 1989.

Robb JA, Benirschke K, Mannino F, et al: Intrauterine latent herpes simplex virus infection: Latent neonatal infection. Hum Pathol **17:**1210, 1986.

Roberts AB, Clarson RM, Pattison NS, et al: Fetal hydrothorax in the second trimester of pregnancy: Successful intrauterine treatment at 24 weeks' gestation. Fetal Ther **1:**203, 1986.

Robertson L, Ott A, Mack L, et al: Sonographically documented disappearance of nonimmune hydrops fetalis associated with maternal hypertension. West J Med **143:**382, 1985.

Rodeck CH, Fisk NM, Fraser DI, et al: Long-term in utero drainage of fetal hydrothorax. N Engl J Med **319:**1135, 1988.

Rodis JF, Hovick TJ, Quinn DL, et al: Human parvovirus infection in pregnancy. Obstet Gynecol **72:**733, 1988.

Romero R, Pilu G, Jeanty P, et al: Other anomalies: Nonimmune hydrops fetalis. *In* Romero R, Pilu G, Jeanty P, et al (eds): Prenatal Diagnosis of Congenital Anomalies. Norwalk, Conn, Appleton & Lange, 1988, p. 403.

Rouse D, Weiner C: Ongoing fetomaternal hemorrhage treated by serial fetal intravascular transfusions. Obstet Gynecol **76:**974, 1990.

Sahakian V, Weiner CP, Naides SJ, et al: Intrauterine transfusion treatment of nonimmune hydrops fetalis secondary to human parvovirus B19 infection. Am J Obstet Gynecol **164:**1090, 1991.

Saltzman DH, Frigoletto FD, Harlow BL, et al: Sonographic evaluation of hydrops fetalis. Obstet Gynecol **74:**106, 1989.

Samuels P, Ludmir J: Nonimmune hydrops fetalis: A heterogeneous disorder and therapeutic challenge. Semin Roentgenol **25:**353, 1990.

Santolaya J, Alley D, Jaffe R, et al: Antenatal classification of hydrops fetalis. Obstet Gynecol **79:**256, 1992.

Schwartz SH, Viseskul C, Laxova R, et al: Idiopathic hydrops fetalis report of 4 patients including 2 affected sibs. Am J Med Genet **8:**59, 1981.

Seifer DB, Ferguson JE, Behrens CM, et al: Nonimmune hydrops fetalis in association with hemangioma of the umbilical cord. Obstet Gynecol **66:**283, 1985.

Shah DM, Chaffin D: Perinatal outcome in very preterm births with twin-twin transfusion syndrome. Am J Obstet Gynecol **161:**1111, 1989.

Shenker L, Reed KL, Anderson CF, et al: Congenital heart block and cardiac anomalies in the absence of maternal connective tissue disease. Am J Obstet Gynecol **157:**248, 1987.

Shimokawa H, Hara K, Fukuda A, et al: Idiopathic hydrops fetalis successfully treated in utero. Obstet Gynecol **71:**984, 1988.

Smrcek JM, Baschat AA, Germer U, et al: Fetal hydrops and hepatosplenomegaly in the second half of pregnancy: A sign of myeloproliferative disorder in fetuses with trisomy 21. Ultrasound Obstet Gynecol **17:**403, 2001.

Sohan K, Carroll SG, De La Fuente S, et al: Analysis of outcome in hydrops fetalis in relation to gestation age at diagnosis, cause and treatment. Acta Obstet Gynecol Scand **80:**726, 2001.

Soothill P: Intrauterine blood transfusion for non-immune hydrops fetalis due to parvovirus B19 infection. Lancet **336:**121, 1990.

Spahr RC, Botti JJ, MacDonald HM, et al: Nonimmunologic hydrops fetalis: A review of 19 cases. Gynaecol Obstet **18:**303, 1980.

Stephenson T, Zuccollo J, Mohajer M: Diagnosis and management of nonimmune hydrops in the newborn. Arch Dis Child **70:**F151, 1994.

Tasso MJ, Martinez-Gutierrez A, Carrascosa C, et al: GM$_1$-gangliosidosis presenting as nonimmune hydrops fetalis: A case report. J Perinat Med **24:**445, 1996.

Taylor MJ, Shalev E, Tanawattanacharoen S, et al: Ultrasound-guided umbilical cord occlusion using bipolar diathermy for Stage III/IV twin-twin transfusion syndrome. Prenat Diagn **22:**70, 2002.

Teixeira JM, Duncan K, Letsky E, et al: Middle cerebral artery peak systolic velocity in the prediction of fetal anemia. Ultrasound Obstet Gynecol **15:**205, 2000.

Thorp JA, Cohen GR, Yeast JD, et al: Nonimmune hydrops caused by massive fetomaternal hemorrhage and treated by intravascular transfusion. Perinatology **9:**22, 1992.

Urig MA, Simpson GF, Elliott JP, et al: Twin-twin transfusion syndrome: The surgical removal of one twin as a treatment option. Fetal Ther **3:**185, 1988.

Van den Veyver IB, Bowles N, Carpenter RJ, et al: Detection of intrauterine viral infection using the polymerase chain reaction. Mol Genet Metab **63:**85, 1998.

Van Selm M, Kanhai H, Gravenhorst B: Maternal hydrops syndrome: A review. Obstet Gynecol Surv **46:**785, 1991.

Vanhaesebrouck P, Thiery M, Leroy JG, et al: Oligohydramnios, renal insufficiency, and ileal perforation in preterm infants after intrauterine exposure to indomethacin. J Pediatr **113:**738, 1988.

Von Kaisenberg CS, Jonat W: Fetal parvovirus B19 infection. Ultrasound Obstet Gynecol **18:**280, 2001.

Vyas S, Nicolaides KH, Campbell S: Doppler examination of the middle cerebral artery in anemic fetuses. Am J Obstet Gynecol **162:**1066, 1990.

Warsof SL, Nicolaides KH, Rodeck C: Immune and non-immune hydrops. Clin Obstet Gynecol **29:**533, 1986.

Watson J, Campbell S: Antenatal evaluation and management in nonimmune hydrops fetalis. Obstet Gynecol **67:**589, 1986.

Weiner CP, Naides SJ, Pringle K: Fetal survival after human parvovirus B19 infection: Spectrum of intrauterine response in a twin gestation. Am J Perinatol **9:**66, 1992.

Wendel GD: Gestational and congenital syphilis. Clin Perinatol **15:**287, 1988.

Wittmann BK, Farquharson DF, Thomas WDS, et al: The role of feticide in the management of severe twin transfusion syndrome. Am J Obstet Gynecol **155:**1023, 1986.

Zimmer EZ, Gutterman E, Blazer S: Recurrent nonimmune hydrops. J Reprod Med **31:**193, 1986.

Zornes SL, Anderson PG, Lott RL: Congenital toxoplasmosis in an infant with hydrops fetalis. South Med J **81:**391, 1988.

Part III
MATERNAL COMPLICATIONS

Chapter 32

RECURRENT PREGNANCY LOSS

Joseph A. Hill, MD

Pregnancy loss is the most common complication of pregnancy (Wilcox et al., 1988). *Recurrent pregnancy loss*, defined historically as three or more spontaneous abortions before 20 weeks of gestation, occurs in 0.3% of pregnant women (Edmonds et al., 1982; Alberman, 1988). Recurrence risk is now understood to occur with two consecutive spontaneous abortions, and subsequent outcomes are similar for women having two and three prior losses (Regan, 1991; Hill, 1994). Approximately 1% of pregnant women have had at least two previous spontaneous abortions (Regan, 1991).

Data derived from epidemiologic studies indicate that the risk of subsequent pregnancy loss is approximately 24% after two clinical pregnancy losses, 30% after three, and 40% after four consecutive spontaneous abortions (Regan et al., 1989).

POTENTIAL ETIOLOGIC FACTORS

Many potential causes have been presumed for recurrent pregnancy loss (Table 32-1). The precise incidence of these is difficult to define because of physician referral bias and the different diagnostic tests used.

Genetic Factors

Chromosomal aneuploidy has been reported in 60% of first-trimester abortuses (Boue et al., 1975; Golbus, 1981; Stern et al., 1996). In a study of 545 abortuses successfully karyotyped and compiled by the author, 154 were first losses, with 45% found to have an abnormal karyotype. The incidence of aneuploidy was approximately 60% in abortuses of women having two to nine previous losses. Trisomies are the most common abnormality found in abortal tissue, with the descending order of prevalence being trisomy 16, 22, 21, 15, 18, and 13 (Warburton et al., 1986). Trisomy 16 accounts for approximately 26% of all pregnancy losses prior to 11 weeks of gestation. Monosomy X (45X) is the second most common single chromosome abnormality found in abortal tissue. Triploidy (69 chromosomes) is also common; while tetraploidy (92 chromosomes) occurs less frequently. The precise mechanism of loss in chromosomally abnormal embryos is unknown, but disordered timing of developmental gene regulation and hormonal regulation are speculated. Inborn chromosomal aberrations may be inherited, but more commonly arise de novo by spontaneous mutations during embryo development. Maternal age–related problems in oocyte spindle formation and meiotic division errors lead to chromosomal abnormalities involving trisomies (Hook et al., 1983; Battaglia et al., 1996). Monosomy X and polyploidies are not maternal age related. Recent evidence suggests that women with a history of recurrent pregnancy loss are more likely than age-matched controls to have chromosomally abnormal eggs. Paternal age greater than age 50 years may also be associated with a higher frequency of chromosomally abnormal sperm. One chromosomally abnormal spontaneous abortion increases the risk of a subsequent loss caused by a chromosomal abnormality (Golbus, 1981).

Inborn chromosomal abnormalities occur in 3% to 6% of couples experiencing recurrent pregnancy loss (Khudr, 1974; Stray-Pedersen and Stray-Pedersen, 1984; Hill, 1994; Clifford et al., 1994; Stephensen, 1996). Neither family nor reproductive history is sufficient to rule out a potential chromosomal abnormality in the couple. The most common parental chromosomal abnormality contributing to pregnancy loss is a translocation, which involves two chromosomes in a mutual exchange of broken-off fragments. A *Robertsonian translocation* is a special category of reciprocal translocation involving two acrocentric chromosomes; breakage occurs close to the centromere in the short arm of one chromosome and in the long arm of the other. One of the resulting chromosomes is smaller than normal and is lost in subsequent mitotic divisions. An individual having a balanced reciprocal translocation in which no genetic material has been lost will be normal phenotypically but may experience recurrent abortion. Depending upon the type of meiotic segregation the involved chromosomes undergo, the resulting zygote may be normal, a balanced translocation carrier like the parent, trisomic for part of a chromosome, or monosomic for part of a chromosome. The last two conditions often lead to pregnancy loss. Robertsonian translocations involving homologous chromosomes are rare (1 in 2500) but always result in aneuploidy.

Mathematically, the risk of aneuploidy resulting in a potential pregnancy loss in the couple with a chromosomal abnormality other than a Robertsonian translocation of homologous chromosomes would be approximately 50%. Clinically, however, the risk is approximately 10% that any given conception will be aneuploid if the woman has a translocation other than to homologous chromosomes, and only 8% if her partner has the abnormality (Simpson and Martin, 1970).

Other parental structural chromosome anomalies including mosaicism and potentially chromosome inversions may contribute to recurrent pregnancy loss (Wolf et al., 1994). Single gene disorders may be recognized through analysis of detailed family histories or by a particular pattern of anomalies that constitute a syndrome with a known pattern of inheritance. Genetic polymorphisms such as those affecting the estrogen receptor may also contribute to recurrent pregnancy loss

TABLE 32-1. ETIOLOGIC MECHANISMS HISTORICALLY PRESUMED FOR RECURRENT PREGNANCY LOSS

Genetic Factors	***Immunologic Factors***
1. Chromosomal	1. Autoimmune
2. Single-gene disorders	a. Antiphospholipid
3. Multifactorial	antibodies
Anatomic Factors	b. Other autoantibodies
1. Congenital	2. Alloimmune
2. Acquired	a. Th1 immunity
Endocrine Factors	(immunodystrophism)
1. Luteal phase insufficiency	b. Blocking antibody
2. Androgen disorders, including	deficiency
luteinizing hormone	***Miscellaneous Factors***
disorders	1. Environmental
3. Prolactin disorders	2. Stress
4. Thyroid disorders	3. Placental abnormalities
5. Diabetes mellitus	4. Medical illnesses
Infectious Factors	5. Male factors
1. Bacteria	6. Dyssynchronous
2. Viruses	fertilization
3. Parasites	7. Coitus
4. Zoonotics	8. Exercise
5. Fungal	

(Berkowitz et al., 1994). Rarely, X-linked disorders may result in recurrent abortion of approximately 50% of male conceptions. There is also an increased risk of neural tube defects in women with a history of recurrent pregnancy loss (Adam et al., 1995).

Skewed X-chromosome inactivation is maternally inherited and can cause preferential activation of the paternal X-chromosome, leading to recurrent pregnancy loss. A linkage study has localized this trait to Xq28, thus defining a specific locus for recurrent spontaneous abortion (Pegoraro et al., 1997).

Anatomic Factors

Anatomic distortion of the intrauterine cavity is found in 10% to 20% of women experiencing recurrent pregnancy loss (Hill et al., 1992; Stephensen, 1996; Probst and Hill, 2000). The range in prevalence is most likely due to selection bias. The causes of congenital müllerian anomalies, other than diethylstilbestrol (DES) exposure, are largely unknown. Failure of müllerian duct fusion, resulting in types II, III, and IV (unicornuate, didelphys, and bicornuate) anomalies (Buttram and Gibbons, 1979), is not generally associated with recurrent pregnancy loss, but incomplete caudal-to-cephalad septum reabsorption, type V (septate) anomalies are associated with recurrent abortion (Maneschi et al., 1995). Surgical correction of types II, III, and IV anomalies is probably not warranted (Acien, 1993), but resection of an intrauterine septum and cervical cerclage for women exposed *in utero* to DES have been advocated (Patton, 1994), based on retrospective and anecdotal case series. One study found a septum to be associated with a 60% chance of pregnancy loss (Buttram, 1983). Another study has found that a septum less than 1 cm in length is less likely than one that is larger to be associated with adverse reproductive events (Fedele et al., 1996).

Second-trimester losses attributable to congenital uterine anomalies may be due to limitation of space and an incompetent cervix (Treffers, 1990). First-trimester pregnancy loss may occur in women with type V anomalies as a result of inadequate vascularization of the septum contributing to poor placental growth and dyssynchronous hormonal and adhesion molecule responsiveness (Keller et al., 1979).

Incompetent cervix may result from congenital collagen abnormalities in the cervix or, more commonly, from prior cervical trauma or surgery (Shirodkar, 1955; MacDonald, 1963), including cervical conization (Bullter and Jones, 1982) (see Chapter 33). Women with a history of incompetent cervix do not have a higher incidence of first-trimester pregnancy loss.

Other acquired anatomic abnormalities associated with recurrent pregnancy loss include intrauterine adhesions, leiomyomas, adenomyosis, and endometrial polyps (Shafer, 1986; Fitzsimmons et al., 1987; Rice et al., 1989; March, 1995; Ouyang and Hill, 2002). Endometriosis is not a cause of recurrent pregnancy loss (Olive and Haney, 1986), and pregnancy outcome is not affected adversely by endometriosis following *in vitro* fertilization–embryo transfer (IVF-ET) (Garcia et al., 1991).

Leiomyoma-associated pregnancy loss involving submucosal fibroids may be due to distortion of the intrauterine cavity potentially compromising implantation, with resulting compromised placental development. Increased uterine irritability and contractility secondary to rapid fibroid growth and subsequent degeneration or alteration in oxytocinase activity may disrupt the normal progression of pregnancy. Compressive effects of leiomyomas may alter the endometrium directly or interfere with the growth of the conceptus mechanically (Ouyang and Hill, 2002).

Endocrine Factors

Endocrine problems have been found in 15% to 60% of women experiencing recurrent abortion, depending on the series (Fritz, 1988; Regan, 1991; Hill et al., 1992; Clifford et al., 1994; Stephensen, 1996). Luteal phase insufficiency, hyperprolactinemia, thyroid dysfunction, diabetes mellitus, and hyperandrogenic disorders including polycystic ovary syndrome (PCOS) have all been associated with recurrent pregnancy loss. Isolated progesterone receptor defects in the endometrium may be a rare cause of recurrent abortion (Keller et al., 1979).

Luteal phase insufficiency is controversial, as are the other potential causes of recurrent abortion (Balasch and Varnell, 1987). Luteal phase insufficiency may result from abnormal follicle-stimulating hormone secretion, abnormal gonadotropin-releasing hormone pulses, excess luteinizing hormone (LH) secretion as occurs in PCOS, and hyperandrogenic disorders (Soules et al., 1988; Soules, Clifton, et al., 1989; Regan et al., 1990; Baird et al., 1991; Balen et al., 1993). Premature ovulation may occur, and a hyperandrogenic environment may cause disordered resumption of meiosis, endometrial asynchrony, and impaired estrogen secretion, prostaglandin synthesis, and intraovarian growth factor regulation, although these potential mechanisms remain speculative (Bonney and Franks, 1990). Oligomenorrhea and delayed ovulation are associated with pregnancy loss, with the incidence of oligomenorrhea being inversely proportional to fetal size exclusively in abortions with normal fetal karyotypes (Hasegawa et al., 1996). Women over age 40 may be particularly prone to luteal phase insufficiency and thus pregnancy loss because progesterone production is significantly less in women over age 40 than in younger women.

Abnormal maternal thyroid function has also been implicated in pregnancy loss (Gilnoer et al., 1991). The incidence of antithyroid antibodies is reported to be higher in women with recurrent abortion than in those with successful reproductive histories; however, pregnancy outcome does not differ between women with and without antithyroid antibodies (Stagnaro-Green et al., 1990; Lejeune et al., 1983). In one study, antithyroid antibodies were associated with clinical pregnancy loss but not with biochemical pregnancy loss (Singh et al., 1995).

The incidence of spontaneous abortion is also not different between women with well-controlled diabetes mellitus and those without this disease. However, women with poorly controlled disease, as evidenced by elevated plasma glycosylated hemoglobin levels, have an increased incidence of fetal loss (Mills et al., 1988).

Infectious Factors

Bacterial, viral, parasitic, fungal, and zoonotic infections have been associated with recurrent pregnancy loss (Charles and Larsen, 1990), but evidence linking infection and recurrent pregnancy loss remains anecdotal. Chorioamnionitis resulting from an ascending infection is a common cause of second-trimester abortion, although hematogenous spread and other direct mechanisms may also be causative (Shaw et al., 1995). Infections may contribute indirectly to first-trimester or second-trimester pregnancy loss through activation of inflammatory cytokines and free oxygen radicals, causing cytotoxicity. Alternatively, they could theoretically contribute to loss through prostaglandin production, culminating in premature labor and delivery (Romero and Mazor, 1988; Dudley et al., 1996; Svinarich et al., 1996). Infections may also contribute to loss through elevation of core body temperature above 39°C, which can be teratogenic and embryocidal if occurring before 8 weeks of gestation (Milunsky et al., 1992).

Mycoplasma hominis (Sompolinsky et al., 1975) and *Ureaplasma urealyticum* (Kundsin et al., 1967; Kundsin et al., 1981) have been associated with recurrent abortion. Significantly higher colonization of the endometrium with T-strain *Mycoplasma* has been reported in women with a history of recurrent pregnancy loss than in normal controls, which was interpreted as implicating *Mycoplasma* as a cause of abortion (Stray-Pedersen et al., 1978). An alternative explanation may be that women who had spontaneous abortions had more intrauterine instrumentation, which may transfer this organism from the cervix to the uterus, because *Mycoplasma* is often found commensal in the cervix. Bacterial vaginitis/vaginosis (BV) is associated with preterm labor and delivery. BV may be more prevalent in women with recurrent pregnancy loss; however, the occurrence of subsequent spontaneous abortion in these women is no different than in women without evidence of BV.

The role of *Chlamydia* in endometritis and salpingitis leading to tubal pathology is well substantiated (Centers for Disease Control and Prevention, 1993), whereas its role in recurrent pregnancy loss remains speculative (Summers, 1994) but could be related to inciting immune cell activation leading to pregnancy loss (Witkin, 1995). BV has been associated with second-trimester pregnancy loss (Llahi-Camp et al., 1996),

chorioamnionitis, and preterm labor (Gravett et al., 1986; Gibbs, 1993; Hiller et al., 1995). However, the occurrence of subsequent spontaneous abortion in these women is not different than in women without evidence of BV. Group B β-hemolytic streptococci have also been associated with preterm birth and low birth weight (Regan et al., 1996) but not with early pregnancy loss directly.

Herpesvirus is associated with an increased risk of spontaneous abortion (Nahmias et al., 1971; Gronroos et al., 1983). A 34% spontaneous abortion rate in women with a history of genital herpes compared with a 10.6% abortion rate in controls has been reported (Nahmias et al., 1971), prompting the suggestion that reactivation of latent infection during pregnancy may culminate in pregnancy loss (Gronroos et al., 1983). This virus was reported to disrupt human leukocyte antigen (HLA)-G expression in the placental trophoblast, which may afford a potential mechanism for pregnancy loss in susceptible individuals (Schust, Hill, and Ploegh, 1996).

The obligate intracellular parasite *Toxoplasma gondii* can invade the placenta and fetus. Associations between toxoplasmosis and recurrent pregnancy loss have been based on antibody titers to this organism, but most studies suggest that it is not a significant factor for loss (Lolis et al., 1978; Sahwi et al., 1995).

Whether infection is a cause of recurrent loss remains speculative. An individual's immunologic susceptibility to an infectious organism may be the determining factor in whether pregnancy loss occurs. Other probable factors include primary exposure during early gestation, capability of the organism to cause placental infection, development of an infectious carrier state, and immunocompromise of the individual infected (Summers, 1994).

Immunologic Factors

The immune system evolved to protect the individual from non-self tissue. Immunity can be either innate or adaptive (also called acquired), depending upon the antigenic stimulus. Innate responses are the body's first line of immune defense against an immunologically "foreign" stimulus. They are rapid and are not antigen specific. The cell types and mechanisms involved in innate immunity include complement activation, macrophage phagocytosis, and natural killer (NK) cell lysis. T-cell receptor (TCR) γ, δ T cells may also be involved. In contrast, acquired immunity is antigen specific and is primarily mediated by T cells and B cells. Acquired immunity is further divided into primary responsiveness, which is associated with initial antigen contact, and secondary responsiveness, which is a quick-acting and strong amnestic response associated with repeat exposure to an offending antigen.

Antigen specificity is regulated by genes in the major histocompatibility complex (MHC), located on chromosome 6 in humans. MHC class I molecules include HLA-A, -B and -C) and are expressed on the surface of almost every cell in the human body. These surface-expressed molecules are important in the defense against intracellular pathogens, such as viruses and cancer-causing influences. MHC class I molecules act as ligands both for T-cell receptors on CD8+ cytotoxic/suppressor T cells and for a variety of receptors on NK cells. MHC class II molecules include HLA-DR, HLA-DP, and HLA-DQ. MHC class II molecules are present on many cells, enabling them to present antigens to the body's immune system. These cells include dendritic cells, macrophages, monocytes, B cells, and tissue-specific cells such as Langerhans cells in the skin and Hofbauer cells in the placenta. The molecules assist in immune defense against intracellular pathogens. The major ligand for MHC class II is the T-cell receptor on CD4 T-helper cells.

Immune tolerance is another important immunological concept that is applicable to human pregnancy. Bone marrow–derived T cells pass through the fetal thymus during early human development in a process referred to as "thymic education." During this process, T cells are chosen that express either the CD4 or the CD8 co-receptor and autoreactive T cells are eliminated, promoting T-cell tolerance. This allows selection and survival of only those T cells that can recognize nonself-tissues and not react against self-tissues.

Immune mechanisms operating in the peripheral circulation have been thoroughly investigated. The peripheral immune system components include the spleen and peripheral lymph nodes, and these are responsible for protecting the body against blood-borne pathogens. Pathogens entering via the lacrimal ducts, respiratory system, gastrointestinal tract, mammary ducts, and genitourinary tract encounter an immune environment that is distinctively different from the peripheral immune system. This mucosal immune system is responsible for initial protection against most exogenous pathogens. Appreciation of the immune nuances of the mucosal immune system has lagged behind understanding of the peripheral system.

Many of the immune theories proposed for recurrent pregnancy loss have arisen from attempts to define immune phenomena as they relate to the mucosa of the reproductive tract. Four fundamental questions outline the theoretical thinking involving the establishment and maintenance of pregnancy:

1. Which immune cells populate the reproductive tract specifically at the site of implantation?
2. How do these cells arrive there, and are they programmed or educated in the same way as those in the peripheral circulation?
3. What are the characteristics of antigen presentation at the maternal-fetal interface?
4. What regulatory mechanisms specifically affect immune cells within the reproductive tract?

Resident Cells

The human endometrium is populated by T cells, macrophages, and NK-like cells, but very few B cells and no plasma cells in the absence of infection (Kabawsat et al., 1985; Vince and Johnson, 2000). The relative numbers of these populations vary depending upon the menstrual cycle and pregnancy. During the luteal phase, in response to progesterone or a chemokine mediated by progesterone, a unique population of immune cells migrates to the human endometrium. These cells, variously termed decidual granular lymphocytes, large granular lymphocytes, and decidual NK cells, constitute up to 80% of the total lymphoid population of the endometrium at this time and express the CD56 phenotype. The implantation site represents the largest accumulation of NK cells in any state of human health or disease. The precise function of these cells remains speculative. Other immune cells with characteristics of both NK and T cells have been described in the peripheral circulation. Called NKT cell, they have been reported to play a role in pregnancy loss in animal models (Ito et al., 2000).

In the peripheral circulation, the majority of T cells express a T-cell receptor composed of an α and β heterodimer (TCRab+). In addition to these cells, the human reproductive tract also contains another subset of T cells with a distinctive T-cell receptor composed of the α-δ heterodimer (TCRgd+). The numbers of these cells increase in early pregnancy. Functions of TCRgd+ T cells, such as being able to respond directly via non-MHC-restricted recognition of antigens, may be distinct from those of TCRab+ T cells. Their precise role in pregnancy remains speculative.

A subset of macrophages, called "suppressor" macrophages, has also been found to be involved in pregnancy maintenance. These cells differ from typical macrophages in their ability to promote anti-inflammatory effects. These cells have been detected in murine placentae. The immune cells populating human decidua (NK, T, and NKT cells) and the activation status of these cells have been reported to be altered in women with a history of recurrent pregnancy loss.

Immune Cell Education and Homing to the Reproductive Tract

Since the human embryo contains paternally inherited gene products and its own unique differentiation antigens, it can be considered a semi-allograft. Precisely how the maternal immune system avoids rejection of the implanting hatched blastocyst and the early developing feto-placental unit remains a biological enigma, but the process must involve immune tolerance. How then are the immune effector cells migrating to the developing decidua recruited, educated, and maintained? Studies in animal models suggest that selection and maintenance of these cells in terms of their requirement for MHC recognition and their education within the thymus may be distinct from what occurs in the peripheral circulation or even at other mucosal sites. In the human, it is known that the concentrations of cells populating the early decidua are also distinct from those occurring in the peripheral circulation and at other mucosal sites. The education of TCRgd+ cells may occur outside the thymus and involve mechanisms modifying MHC interaction requirements. The cells recruited to the uterus do this through interactions of their cell surfaces mediated by integrins interacting with cell-surface-expressed molecules (selectins, vascular cell adhesion molecule [VCAM]) on the endothelial cells lining mucosal blood vessels. This cellular recruitment process is termed homing.

Antigen Presentation at the Maternal-Fetal Interface

Unlike most cells within the human body, placental trophoblast cells do not express the classical MHC class I HLA-A and HLA-B molecules. Instead, they express HLA-C and a unique form of class I, the nonclassical HLA-E and HLA-G molecules. These molecules are expressed on extravillous trophoblast cells that have invasive potential. They can also replace cells within the walls of decidual vessels (King et al., 2000).

It is not known why or how placental cells do not express HLA-A and HLA-B molecules, while extravillous trophoblast expresses HLA-C, HLA-E, and HLA-G molecules. Theories abound, however. Since NK cells do not require MHC recognition for killing, the complete downregulation of MHC on trophoblast could still render them susceptible to NK-mediated attack. One theory with some supportive experimental evidence is that extravillous trophoblast expression of HLA-C, -E, and -G may protect against NK cell lysis by modifying cytokine expression and release at the maternal-fetal interface and by masking NK-cell receptors. Soluble or secreted MHC products may aid in the development of maternal tolerance toward the placental allograft. Studies to date have not found an association between polymorphisms in these MHC products and recurrent pregnancy loss. Aberrant expression of class II MHC determinants or enhanced expression of MHC class I molecules on syncytiotrophoblast occurring in response to interferon-γ has been theorized to be a potential mechanism of immunologic spontaneous abortion by enhancing cytotoxic T-cell attack. This explanation appears improbable, however, because the expression of classical MHC antigenic molecules is not present on spontaneously aborted tissue from women with a history of recurrent pregnancy loss.

Regulation of Decidual Immune Cells

Interactions between immune effector cells within the decidua and the developing placenta may be affected by regulatory mechanisms involving alterations in T helper cell phenotypes, reproductive hormones, and tryptophan metabolism. CD4+ T cells are divided into two major classes, T helper 1 (TH1) cells and T helper 2 (TH2) cells.

These cells in turn secrete different cytokines with different functions. The production of these cell populations and their associated responses arise from the differentiation of CD4+ TH0 cells. In response to interferon (INF)-γ, TH0 cells will differentiate into TH1-type cells, and those exposed to interleukin (IL)-4 will differentiate into TH2-type cells. TH1-type cells are classically associated with inflammation primarily involving INF-γ, IL-12, IL-2, and tumor necrosis factor (TNF)-β. TH2-type cells are generally associated with antibody production and the cytokines IL-10, IL-4, IL-5, and IL-6. TNF-α can be secreted by both TH1 and TH2 cells, although it is most often associated with a TH1 type of response. A reciprocal regulating relationship exists between TH1 and TH2 cells and their associated cytokines, with one response supporting its own persistence while averting conversion to the other.

Maternal Tolerance

The concept that successful pregnancy requires maternal immune suppression is supported by experimental evidence that failure to downregulate maternal immunity to recall antigens such as tetanus toxoid and influenza was associated with poor pregnancy outcome among women with a history of recurrent pregnancy loss (Bermas and Hill, 1997). Cellular immunity can be suppressed by reproductive hormones such as progesterone (Siiteri et al., 1977). An immunosuppressed environment may be maintained by the high levels of progesterone attained at the maternal-fetal interface, which far exceed the levels attained in the peripheral circulation. *In vitro* studies have demonstrated that progesterone mediates suppression of T-cell effector function by altering membrane-resident potassium channels and cell membrane depolarization. This then affects intracellular calcium signaling cascades and gene expression, which may not be mediated through progesterone receptors. Progesterone at levels attained at the maternal-fetal interface has been shown to modify TH1 cytokine production (Piccini et al., 1998) and facil-

itate the development of TH2 immunity. Since a shift in the intrauterine immune environment from TH2 to TH1 has been associated with early pregnancy loss (Piccini et al., 1998), the elevated concentrations of progesterone characteristic of early pregnancy may promote a favorable environment for the maintenance of pregnancy. Progesterone can inhibit both mitogen-induced proliferation of and cytokine secretion by CD8+ T cells (Vassiliadou et al., 1999). Estrogens may also modify local immunity during pregnancy. Estrogens are capable of downregulating delayed-type hypersensitivity reaction and promoting the development of TH2-type immunity.

An additional regulatory mechanism proposed for the induction of maternal tolerance during pregnancy involves the amino acid tryptophan and its catabolizing enzyme, indolamine 2,3 dioxygenase. This hypothesis is based on the finding that T cells need tryptophan for activation and proliferation (Munn et al., 1998 and that local alterations in tryptophan metabolism at the maternal-fetal interface could either activate or fail to suppress maternal anti-fetal immunity (Mellor and Munn, 2000).

Studies in mice have shown that inhibition of indolamine 2,3 dioxygenase leads to loss of allogeneic but not syngeneic fetuses and that this effect is mediated by lymphocytes (Munn et al., 1998). In other animal studies, hamsters fed diets high in tryptophan have shown higher rates of pregnancy loss than control animals (Meier and Wilson, 1983). Although not fully substantiated in humans, demonstration of indolamine 2,3 dioxygenase expression in human decidua (Kamimura et al., 1991) and alterations in serum tryptophan levels with increasing gestational age during human pregnancy (Schrocksnadel et al., 1996) further support the hypothesis of indolamine 2,3 dioxygenase involvement with recurrent pregnancy loss.

■ IMMUNE MECHANISMS IMPLICATED IN RECURRENT PREGNANCY LOSS

Immunity against self is called *autoimmunity*, and immunity against non-self is termed *alloimmunity*. Both autoimmune and alloimmune mechanisms have been proposed for human pregnancy loss (see Table 32-1).

The conceptus is composed of both maternal and paternal antigens as well as its own unique differentiation antigens. As such, the conceptus is semiallogenic and should normally be expected to be rejected because it contains molecules genetically foreign to the maternal host. Therefore, mechanisms (Table 32-2) should be operative to protect the semiallogenic conceptus from immunologic attack.

Autoimmune Mechanisms

The immunologic theory that has fulfilled most of the criteria for causality is that involving antiphospholipid antibodies. However, controversial questions remain:

1. Are antiphospholipid antibodies causative, coincidental, or a consequence of reproductive dysfunction?
2. Which antiphospholipid antibodies are involved?
3. What is the incidence of their occurrence in women with reproductive failure?
4. By what precise mechanisms do they adversely affect pregnancy?

Thrombocytopenia and pregnancy loss generally occur after 10 weeks of gestation (Oshiro et al., 1996). The association of

TABLE 32-2. POTENTIAL MECHANISMS
PROTECTING THE SEMIALLOGENIC CONCEPTUS
FROM IMMUNOLOGIC REJECTION

Immune/inflammatory cells
Cytokines/growth factors/hormones
Absence of class I and class II major
    histocompatibility complex on
    trophoblast
Expression of human leukocyte
    antigen (HLA)-G on trophoblast
Expression of complement regulatory
    proteins on trophoblast
Fas ligand/Fas receptor system
Systemic immunosuppression

antiphospholipid antibodies with recurrent pregnancy loss (Branch et al., 1985) has been termed the *antiphospholipid syndrome* (Harris, 1986) (see Chapter 48).

The incidence of the antiphospholipid syndrome in women with recurrent abortion varies according to which antibodies are measured and the methods used to define a positive value. With well-defined clinical and laboratory criteria, the incidence is conservatively below 5% (Branch et al., 1992; Hill et al., 1992), although much higher estimates have been reported (Petri, 1997).

A number of hypotheses have been proposed for the pathophysiologic mechanisms potentially involved in antiphospholipid antibody–mediated pregnancy loss (Carreras and Vernylan, 1982; Harris et al., 1985; Dudley et al., 1990; Lockshin, 1994; Petri, 1997; Rand et al., 1997). Most of these mechanisms involve increased platelet aggregation, decreased endogenous anticoagulant activity, increased thrombosis, and decreased fibrinolysis, culminating in uteroplacental thrombosis and vasoconstriction resulting from immunoglobulin binding to both platelet and endothelial-membrane phospholipid.

Monoclonal antibodies against phosphatidylserine inhibit intercellular fusion of human trophoblast cell lines and cells *in vitro* (Adler et al., 1995; Katsuragawa et al., 1997) and can impair both trophoblast hormone production and trophoblast invasion *in vitro* (Katsuragawa et al., 1997). These data provide experimental evidence of a potential mechanism for antiphosphatidylserine-mediated pregnancy loss.

Autoimmunity other than to phospholipids has also been associated with recurrent pregnancy loss based on finding autoantibodies to various cell components and organ tissues in higher percentages of women with a history of recurrent pregnancy loss than women without a history of reproductive difficulty (Geva et al., 1997). Data such as these have led to speculation that in addition to phospholipids, autoimmunity to other cellular components and tissues is a cause of reproductive failure or that reproductive difficulty is the first manifestation of some undiagnosed autoimmune disorder (Christiansen, 1996). An alternative explanation is that these associations are either an epiphenomenon or an artifact related to a prior loss, because there are neither definitive data substantiating causality nor plausible mechanisms proposed as to how loss would occur as a result of these autoantibodies. The concept that autoimmunity is a cause of infertility is also unlikely, because infertility is not a compo-

nent of well-characterized autoimmune disorders such as systemic lupus erythematosus.

Alloimmune Mechanisms

The most recent alloimmune hypothesis proposed for some cases of reproductive difficulty is T helper 1 (TH1) immunodystrophism (Hill, 1991). The concept is that aberrant or inappropriate maternal immunostimulation may result in overproduction of certain cytokines (particularly TH1-type cytokines) that have deleterious effects on the conceptus.

A dichotomous TH1 and TH2 cytokine profile to trophoblast has been associated with human pregnancy loss and success, respectively (Hill, Anderson, et al., 1995; Marzi et al., 1996). TH1 cytokines include IL-2, TNF, and INF-γ, whereas TH2 cytokines include IL-4, -5, -6, and -10 and are secreted by activated T cells expressing the CD4 phenotype. NK cells expressing the CD56 phenotype can also produce these factors (Romagnani, 1991), as can certain endocrinologically responsive tissues (Hill and Anderson, 1990). This dichotomous TH1 and TH2 response during pregnancy to human trophoblast may explain why rheumatoid arthritis generally improves during pregnancy (Cecere and Persellin, 1981) and why the incidence of spontaneous abortion is lower in women with this condition than in those with systemic lupus erythematosus, because therapeutically administered antibodies directed against TNF-α can cause clinical improvement in rheumatoid arthritis (Rankin et al., 1995), and the absence of TNF and other TH1 cytokines is lower in women with successful reproductive histories (Hill, Anderson, et al., 1995). In contrast, diminished IL-2 production in response to recall antigens correlates with systemic lupus erythematosus disease activity (Bermas et al., 1994), which generally worsens during pregnancy and is associated with the increased incidence of pregnancy loss in women with this condition (Petri et al., 1991).

In animal models, downregulation of TH1 cytokines has been demonstrated in successful pregnancy (Wegman et al., 1993; Raghupathy, 1997). In approximately 35% to 50% of women with unexplained recurrent pregnancy loss, immune and inflammatory cell responsiveness to trophoblast is activated, as evidenced by increased proliferation (Yamada et al., 1994) and secretion of embryotoxic INF-γ (Hill et al., 1992; Hill, Anderson, et al., 1995). INF-γ and TNF have been reported to be toxic to both embryo development (Hill et al., 1987) and trophoblast growth (Berkowitz et al., 1988; Haimovici et al., 1991).

The human endometrium is replete with immune and inflammatory cells capable of cytokine secretion. Cytokines may affect reproductive events either directly or indirectly, depending on the specific cytokines secreted, their concentrations, and the differentiation stage of potential reproductive target tissues. TH1-type cytokines may be harmful to an implanting embryo (Hill et al., 1987). They may also be involved in some women with recurrent pregnancy loss through dysregulation of TH1-type immunity to reproductive antigens at the maternal-fetal interface. Depending upon the individual series, 20% to 50% of nonpregnant women with a history of otherwise unexplained recurrent pregnancy loss have been reported to have evidence of abnormal *in vitro* TH1 cellular immune responses, whereas fewer than 3% of nonpregnant women with normal reproductive histories have such evidence (Hill, Anderson, et al., 1995). On the contrary, most women with normal reproductive histories exhibit a TH2-type immune response to these same antigens (Hill, Anderson, et al., 1995).

Methods to test for potential cytokine dysregulation among women with recurrent pregnancy loss have varied among clinical investigators, but recent reports have confirmed such abnormalities within reproductive tissues (Lachapelle et al., 1996) and in cells isolated from the decidua (Hill, Melling, et al., 1995; Vassiliadou and Bulmer, 1998) of these patients. Others have historically used peripheral blood lymphocytes obtained from women with prior spontaneous pregnancy losses, stimulated *in vitro* with trophoblast-derived cell-surface antigens (Hill et al., 1992). Aberrant cytokine secretion has also been reported from peripheral blood mononuclear cells of women with a history of recurrent pregnancy loss, stimulated *in vitro* by HLA-G–bearing cells (Hamai et al., 1998). In another study, decidual and peripheral immune cells were noted to exhibit a shift toward a TH2-type phenotype when exposed to HLA-G (Kanai et al., 2001). Whether peripheral cytokine levels reflect T-helper cell dysregulation at the maternal-fetal interface or whether this dysregulation affects peripheral or local immunity during pregnancy remains controversial.

Polymorphism of cytokine genes influences cytokine production and may be associated with susceptibility to various clinical problems such as infections and inflammatory and autoimmune diseases. Cytokines in the IL-1 system are produced at the maternal-fetal interface during early human pregnancy (Von Wolff et al., 2000). The IL-1 system may be involved in the regulation of TH1/TH2 cytokine production, since IL-1 can function as a co-stimulator for TH2 cell generation in both rodents and humans (Oriss et al., 1997) and may influence INF-γ production mediated by NK and T cells (Hunter et al., 1995). Significant increases in frequencies of IL-1β promoter region variants IL-1β-511C and IL-1β-31T have been reported in women with a history of recurrent pregnancy loss. Increased frequencies of these two variants and their homozygotes were found only in cases having evidence of TH1 immunity to trophoblast. Significantly higher INF-γ production by peripheral blood mononuclear cells in response to trophoblast was correlated in the authors with variant IL1β-511C and its homozygosity in women with recurrent pregnancy loss, suggesting that variants -511C and -31T in the IL-1β promoter region confer risk for recurrent pregnancy loss associated with TH1 immunity to trophoblast antigens (Wang and Hill, personal communication).

Polymorphism of IL-1 could lead to alterations in IL-1 production affecting the balance of TH1/TH2 responsiveness involving either pregnancy success or failure by two potential mechanisms. First, since IL-1α and β are important co-stimulators for TH2 cell production, decidual IL-1 may influence TH2 cell generation. Conversely, low IL-1β production at the maternal-fetal interface may reduce TH2-type cytokine production and thus, in concert with elevated decidual IL-12 levels, favor a TH1-type response to the developing conceptus, which could contribute to early pregnancy failure. This potential mechanism is supported by recent data from our laboratory indicating a correlation between reduction of IL-1β and an elevated INF-γ/IL-10 ratio at the mRNA level in the decidua of women with a history of recurrent pregnancy loss who had another early loss of a chromosomally normal conceptus. Altered IL-1β production in the decidua may explain the defective production of TH2 cytokines by decidual T cells

recently reported in women with recurrent pregnancy loss (Piccini et al., 1998). Altered IL-1β production may also contribute to pregnancy loss by directly affecting trophoblast growth and invasion during early pregnancy. These mechanisms are distinct from those in other diseases associated with overproduction and pro-inflammatory effects of IL-1.

The frequency of HLA-DR6 alleles has also been found to be significantly increased in women with recurrent pregnancy loss who also have evidence of TH1 immunity to trophoblast. This phenomenon was associated with increased frequency of the HLA-DQ P9 pocket shared by the DQB1*0503,*0603,*0607 alleles. These observations suggest that this particular P9 pocket of DQ molecules may be involved in antigen presentation that may trigger a TH1-type cytokine response to trophoblast and thus confer susceptibility to recurrent pregnancy loss, since TH1 cytokines have been shown to interfere with many different reproductive processes associated with normal reproductive function.

Human CD46, a membrane cofactor protein of the complement system, is involved in protection of cells from complement-mediated lysis and in downregulation of TH1 immunity. Recent studies from our laboratory also suggest that polymorphism in intron 1 of the CD46 gene is associated with unexplained recurrent pregnancy loss attributable to TH1 immunity to trophoblast.

Another alloimmune hypothesis that has been proposed historically for recurrent abortion is the concept that blocking antibodies are necessary for successful pregnancy. This hypothesis (Rocklin et al., 1976) was based on suppositions that a maternal, antifetal, cellular immune response develops in all pregnancies and must be blocked by a factor measurable in serum. This serum factor was presumed to be an antibody, and in the absence of this maternal blocking factor, fetal loss was speculated to result. Such suppositions were never substantiated (Sargent et al., 1994). The investigators who originally proposed this hypothesis later retracted it (Rocklin et al., 1982) because 40% of normal women with successful reproductive histories do not produce these purported blocking factors (Amos and Kostyn, 1980). When blocking factors are produced, they generally occur only after 28 weeks of gestation, and they may disappear between normal pregnancies (Regan et al., 1981). The most compelling information disproving the blocking antibody hypothesis is that women incapable of antibody secretion can nevertheless achieve successful pregnancies (Rodger, 1985). Thus, the hypothesis that an immunoglobulin effector (i.e., blocking antibody) is necessary for successful pregnancy is not clinically valid.

Miscellaneous Factors

Environmental

The Occupational Safety and Health Administration issued standards of exposure for lead, mercury, ethylene oxide, ionizing radiation, and dibromochloropropane on the basis that these substances adversely affect reproduction, including the induction of spontaneous abortion (Polifka and Friedman, 1991). Additional reproductive concerns include occupational exposure to anesthetic gases and organic solvents (Paul and Kurtz, 1990). Adequately controlled prospective studies demonstrated that exposure to electromagnetic fields was not associated with an increased risk of pregnancy loss (Lindbohm et al., 1992).

Other agents implicated in spontaneous abortion include ethanol, caffeine, nicotine, and other metabolic products of cigarette smoking. Alcohol consumption of more than two drinks per day is associated with twice the risk of spontaneous abortion in non–alcohol-consuming controls (Harlop and Shiono, 1980). However, low-level alcohol consumption does not appear to be a significant risk factor for spontaneous fetal loss (Cavallo et al., 1995). The minimum threshold dose for increasing the risk of spontaneous abortion is 2 ounces of alcohol per week (Kline et al., 1980).

Smoking also has a dose-response relationship with spontaneous abortion (Ferguson et al., 1979). Women who smoked half a pack of cigarettes per day had a higher risk of having chromosomally normal spontaneous abortions than did women who did not smoke (Kline et al., 1980). There is also a dose-response effect with caffeine consumption, but only in doses higher than 300 mg per day (Dlugosz and Bracken, 1992).

Maternal core body temperature greater than 102°F for extended periods of time may also be embryocidal in early pregnancy (Smith et al., 1978).

Pregnant women whose occupation requires prolonged periods of standing and long working hours may be at increased risk for preterm birth and delivery of a low-birth-weight infant (Gabbe and Turner, 1997), but working women do not have an increased risk of spontaneous abortions, stillbirths, or intrauterine growth restriction (Klebanoff et al., 1990, 1991).

Mattison (1992) noted several issues to be considered before definitive conclusions can be made regarding environmental factors, including the following:

1. Gestational age at the time of exposure
2. Amount of toxin reaching the conceptus
3. Duration of exposures
4. Impact of other factors or agents to which the mother or the conceptus is simultaneously exposed
5. Physiologic status of mother and conceptus
6. Genetic differences
7. Interrelationship among frequency of exposures, frequency of effect, and recognizability of adverse outcome, such as spontaneous abortion

Placental Anomalies

Placental abnormalities have historically been associated with second-trimester losses caused by circumvallate placenta and placenta marginata (Torpin, 1955). Defective hemochorial placentation not necessarily linked with fetal chromosomal abnormalities has been noted, and the concept has been put forth that spontaneous abortions and pregnancies complicated by preeclampsia or intrauterine growth restriction may represent a continuum of disorders with similar placental-bed pathology related to limited depth of invasion (Kong et al., 1987). A delicate cytokine balance may exist, facilitating successful pregnancy through control of trophoblast invasion. In general, TH2-type cytokines and other growth factors such as colony-stimulating factor–1 and IL-3 may promote trophoblast invasion, whereas TH1-type cytokines may limit trophoblast invasiveness. Abnormalities in the delicate cytokine/growth factor balance, such as too much IL-12, transforming growth factor–β, or INF-γ may limit trophoblast invasion. If invasion is compromised, increased flow pressure in maternal spiral arteries may dislocate the thin tro-

phoblastic shell, and if detachment is widespread, pregnancy loss occurs (Jaffe et al., 1997).

Placental apoptosis increases significantly as pregnancy progresses, suggesting that it may play a role in normal placental development and placental aging (Runia et al., 1996). Premature induction of apoptosis may contribute to trophoblast dysfunction, resulting in early pregnancy loss (Lea et al., 1997). Dysregulation of trophoblast protein production (Johnson et al., 1993) may also lead to early pregnancy loss.

Maternal Illness

Chronic maternal illnesses, including severe cardiac, pulmonary, and renal disease, are associated with recurrent pregnancy loss. Vascular compromise is thought to be the major etiologic factor for loss. Inflammatory bowel disease has also been associated with recurrent pregnancy loss (Karnfeld et al., 1997). Obesity, defined as a body mass index greater than or equal to 30, is also associated with a higher chance of poor reproductive outcome, including infertility and pregnancy loss.

Rare conditions also associated with recurrent pregnancy loss include high copper levels found in Wilson disease (Schagen van Leeunen et al., 1991) and methionine intolerance related to hyperhomocystinemia (Wouters et al., 1993). Hematologic disorders rarely are found, but they often have high maternal mortality (Shafer, 1985; Mitus and Shafer, 1990). Hypercoagulability may contribute to pregnancy loss because of other concomitant medical conditions, such as the antiphospholipid syndrome.

Inherited Thrombophilias

The inherited abnormalities of coagulation, which are discussed in detail in Chapter 48, have been associated with an increased risk of certain adverse pregnancy outcomes, including second- and third-trimester fetal loss, and with recurrent pregnancy loss (Schved et al., 1989; Gris et al., 1990; Braulke et al., 1993; Rai et al., 1996; Dizon-Townson et al., 1997). Thrombocytosis and thrombocythemia (Rosner and Grunwald, 1988; Lishner et al., 1993) have also been associated with recurrent pregnancy loss, especially when associated with hyperhomocystenemia (Goddijn-Wessel et al., 1996).

Male Factors

Paternal factors contributing to recurrent pregnancy loss are largely unknown except for chromosomal abnormalities. Paternal alcoholism was associated with recurrent pregnancy loss even after correcting for maternal drinking (Halmesmaki et al., 1989). Whether this epidemiologic observation was due to maternal stress or teratogenic effects on spermatozoa is unknown. Men whose partners experience recurrent abortion do not have a higher incidence of morphologically abnormal sperm (Hill et al., 1994; Sbracia et al., 1996). However, it is not clear whether the partners of men with teratospermia, which is not associated with chromosomally abnormal sperm (Rosenbusch et al., 1992), have a higher frequency of pregnancy loss. Men whose partners have experienced recurrent pregnancy loss have been reported to have a higher concentration of chromosomally abnormal sperm than do men whose partners have had normal pregnancies. Leukocytospermia is also not associated with recurrent abortion, but a higher incidence of elevated T-lymphocyte concentrations was reported in semen from men whose partners had recurrent pregnancy loss and evidence of TH1 cellular immunity to sperm (Hill et al., 1994).

Dyssynchronous Fertilization

The timing of sexual intercourse may be critical for the establishment of a successful pregnancy in some couples. Preovulatory oocyte aging and postovulatory gamete aging may contribute to spontaneous abortion (Guerrero and Rojas, 1975), and nuclear degeneration and meiotic aberrations have been observed in human oocytes (Racowsky and Kaufman, 1992). Polyspermic fertilization leading to a triploid or tetraploid conceptus is also more likely to occur in aged oocytes as a result of a defective corticogranular reaction (Lopata et al., 1980). In addition, aged sperm have been noted to undergo chromosomal breakdown before losing their ability to fertilize (Martin-Deleon and Boice, 1982). An increased risk of spontaneous abortion because of chromosomal anomalies has been noted in humans when intercourse occurs remote from ovulation, as assessed with basal body temperature recordings (Boue and Boue, 1973), but there is no evidence that seasonal variations in conception influence the incidence of spontaneous abortion (Drugan et al., 1989).

Coitus

Large-scale studies among pregnant women without a history of recurrent pregnancy loss indicate that coitus during pregnancy is not associated with adverse outcome (Cohn, 1982). There have been no studies to date addressing this issue in women with recurrent pregnancy loss.

Exercise

There is no evidence that mild to moderate exercise during pregnancy in healthy women is associated with an increased risk of adverse outcome. The American College of Obstetricians and Gynecologists (1994) has published guidelines for women who exercise during pregnancy; contraindications to exercise do not include a history of previous spontaneous abortion, threatened abortion, or first-trimester vaginal bleeding.

■ EVALUATION

When to initiate the evaluation of the couple experiencing pregnancy loss is debatable. Investigation following three spontaneous abortions has been recommended historically. This suggestion was not based on evidence. Many have recommended a search for possible causes following two consecutive pregnancy losses. This recommendation was based on epidemiologic data indicating that the chance of a subsequent abortion as well as the potential of discovering a cause were equivalent for women experiencing two and three losses.

Data derived from cytogenetic studies of abortal tissues from women with and without recurrent spontaneous abortion warrant considering that these recommendations be further modified. Approximately 45% to 60% of first miscarriages involve chromosomal abnormality (Boue and Boue, 1975; Golbus, 1981). If the first pregnancy loss is due to chromoso-

mal abnormality, the second loss has a 75% chance of also being due to such an abnormality. If the fetus in the first loss is chromosomally normal, a 66% chance exists that the fetus in the next pregnancy loss will also be chromosomally normal (Golbus, 1981).

In a series of more than 500 cases of pregnancy loss where a karyotype was obtained of abortion tissue at Brigham and Women's Hospital in Boston, approximately 60% were found to be abnormal, regardless of the number of prior losses. These findings were maternal age–related. Women older than 35 years of age were more likely than younger women to have pregnancy loss associated with an abnormal karyotype. Based on these findings, consideration should be given to obtaining the karyotype in all pregnancy losses, especially in women older than 35 years, and recommending investigation of couples only if a normal karyotype in the abortus is found.

Preconception Assessment

A history obtained from both partners of the couple experiencing recurrent abortion should include their age and past medical, surgical, psychological, social, and genetic histories. Questions should be specific regarding chronic medical illnesses, presence of galactorrhea, previous pelvic infections, uterine instrumentation, and in utero DES exposure.

If a previous induced abortion occurred, it is important to reassure the couple that induced first-trimester abortions are not a cause of subsequent spontaneous losses (Daling and Emanuel, 1977). Menstrual cycle history may give clues regarding oligo-ovulation, PCOS, and dyssynchronous fertilization. Family history of recurrent pregnancy loss, stillbirths, and birth defects may be informative.

Current medications should be recorded, and information concerning "street" drugs, smoking, caffeine consumption, alcohol use, and potential occupational exposures should be ascertained. A descriptive sequence of all previous pregnancies, including age of gestation and fetal size (if known) when the loss occurred, may be informative since pregnancy losses within individuals tend to cluster around the same time in sequential pregnancies. Gestational age may not be as informative because fetal death often occurs several weeks before symptoms appear (Miller et al., 1980). The time required for conception should be recorded. Approximately one third of the more than 3500 couples with a history of recurrent pregnancy loss who were evaluated by this author also had a history of attempting conception for more than 1 year before achieving pregnancy. Difficulty in achieving conception may in some instances indicate subclinical (preimplantation) pregnancy loss.

Insight into possible genetic abnormalities may be provided by a history of malformed children, including those with neural tube defects. Knowledge of karyotypes of prior abortuses is also helpful. Information about a normal female karyotype should be interpreted cautiously, especially in cases in which fetal tissue was not identified grossly. A review of all histologic assessments of previous abortuses is rarely helpful but may, in a few cases, provide insight into potential causation (Doss et al., 1995).

Physical Examination

The physical examination should include height, weight, calculation of body mass index, blood pressure, and a general assessment for signs of metabolic illnesses. Body habitus should be defined, and the presence of hirsutism or other signs of hyperandrogenism should be noted. The breasts should be examined for galactorrhea, and the pelvic examination should look for signs of previous cervical trauma or DES exposure. The uterine size and shape should also be noted.

Laboratory Testing

Laboratory testing implies that the test being performed has predictive value for a potential etiology, the knowledge of which would affect clinical management. The test should have small inter- and intra-assay coefficients of variation and high positive and negative predictive values. Unfortunately, few tests fulfill these ideals. Testing for recurrent pregnancy loss has historically sought potential infections and genetic, anatomic, endocrinologic, and immunologic abnormalities (Table 32-3).

Genetic Assessment

Cytogenetic investigation of the couple with recurrent abortion is recommended. Determination of a balanced translocation would prompt the recommendation for *preimplantation genetic diagnosis*; a Robertsonian translocation of homologous chromosomes would necessitate donor gametes for the affected partner. Referral to a genetic counselor should be arranged if a cytogenetic anomaly is detected.

Anatomic Assessment

Hysteroscopy of the uterine cavity has largely replaced hysterosalpingography (Siegler, 1983) because of hysteroscopy's higher specificity and lower false-positive and false-negative rates (Valle, 1980; Raziel et al., 1994). Both hysteroscopy and *hysterosalpingography* are limited because they cannot differentiate between a class IV (bicornuate) and a class V (septate) uterus.

Laparoscopy has been used to differentiate between these two abnormalities, but the cost of this procedure and the risks involved limit its use. *Nuclear magnetic resonance imaging* may be useful (Fielding, 1996), although this procedure is associated with high cost. *Ultrasound* evaluation has also been reported by some, but not all, to be useful (Pellerito et al., 1992; Letterie et al., 1995).

Sonohysterography has been reported to be very sensitive and specific for the evaluation of müllerian anomalies (Bonilla-Musales et al., 1992; Keltz et al., 1997). *Sonohysterosalpingography* is able to distinguish class IV from class V uterine anomalies and can provide information about tubal patency for individuals who have subfertility in addition to recurrent pregnancy loss.

Endocrinologic Assessment

Various modalities are used to detect luteal phase insufficiency, including menstrual cycle history, basal body temperature determinations, reproductive hormone level assessment, and ultrasound monitoring. However, because of the characteristic endometrial changes caused by progesterone during the luteal phase (Noyes et al., 1950), the "gold standard" for assessing luteal phase adequacy is determining the effect of progesterone on the endometrium by biopsy (Jones, 1976).

 TABLE 32-3. TESTS POTENTIALLY USEFUL IN THE EVALUATION OF RECURRENT PREGNANCY LOSS

Parental and abortal karyotypes
Intrauterine cavity assessment
Luteal phase endometrial biopsy
Thyroid-stimulating hormone
Lupus anticoagulant
Anticardiolipin antibody IgG, IgM
Antiphosphatidylserine antibody IgG, IgM
Embryotoxic factor–lymphocyte assay
Platelet count

Ig, immunoglobulin.

The endometrial biopsy is associated with discomfort, is expensive, and is subject to both inter- and intra-observer variation. In addition, an isolated endometrial biopsy exhibiting evidence of an inadequate luteal phase (a lag of 3 or more days in endometrial development) has been reported in approximately 30% of presumably fertile women (Davis et al., 1989).

Timing of the biopsy is also controversial. Traditionally, the biopsy was obtained 2 days prior to anticipated menses, but a potentially more precise method is to perform the biopsy 10 days following the luteinizing hormone (LH) surge (Jones, 1976). The biopsy has also been performed during the implantation window. Concerns regarding interrupting pregnancy by a biopsy are valid but may be obviated by obtaining a sensitive pregnancy test before a scheduled biopsy (Herbert et al., 1990). Endometrial sampling should not be performed within two cycles of a prior pregnancy loss because 45% of women will have an out-of-phase biopsy during this time. Thus, presumed luteal phase insufficiency that may not be indicative of the patient's natural cycles but rather related to the prior loss (Nakajima et al., 1994). Couples should therefore be advised to avoid conception for two cycles following a loss. This recommendation can be modified if ovulation induction is required for conception. Successful pregnancies can occur even when they are conceived within two cycles of a prior loss and even in cases in which the endometrium was presumably out of phase, although the chances are presumably less than in otherwise-normal cycles (Wentz et al., 1986).

The best test for the prediction of low integrated progesterone is a single serum progesterone level less than 10 ng/mL (31.8 nmol/L) obtained during the midluteal phase or a sum of three random serum progesterone measurements that is less than 30 ng/mL (95.4 nmol/L) obtained during the luteal phase (Jordan et al., 1994). Low peripheral blood levels of progesterone have been correlated with out-of-phase endometrial biopsies (Babalioglu et al., 1996). However, biopsy specimens can be normal despite low levels of progesterone in peripheral serum (Li et al., 1991). Also, progesterone in peripheral blood is pulsatile (Soules et al., 1988) and levels in the peripheral circulation are not indicative of levels within the endometrium (Miles et al., 1994). Considerable overlap also exists between normal and abnormal levels in women having successful pregnancies (Azuma et al., 1993). Therefore, ascertainment of progesterone levels is not necessarily helpful in determining luteal phase insufficiency (Soules, McLachlan, et al., 1989).

When luteal phase insufficiency is suspected, serum prolactin, 17-hydroxyprogesterone, and androgen profiles may be warranted. PCOS is another diagnostic possibility that should be considered, especially if oligomenorrhea occurs (Yen, 1980). Preconception LH determinations and ultrasonographic examination have been suggested to facilitate the diagnosis of PCOS. A single determination of LH is problematic because, like progesterone, LH is pulsatile. However, an LH value greater than 20 mIU/mL during the early follicular and late luteal phase is clearly elevated. Ultrasonographic scanning may be the most sensitive method for diagnosis of PCOS in women with recurrent pregnancy loss. However, 22% of normal fertile women have polycystic ovaries by ultrasonographic criteria (Polson et al., 1980).

A glucose tolerance test is not necessary in the evaluation of recurrent pregnancy loss because there is no conclusive evidence that unsuspected diabetes, or even overt diabetes that is adequately controlled, is a cause of loss (Kalter, 1987). Serum should be assayed for thyroid-stimulating hormone with a sensitive assay because both hypothyroidism and hyperthyroidism are associated with a greater incidence of spontaneous abortion than is seen in euthyroid controls. Unlike patients with hypothyroidism, however, mild to moderately thyrotoxic women generally do not have reproductive dysfunction; severe thyrotoxicosis, however, is associated with an increased risk of early pregnancy loss (Mandel et al., 1994; Becks and Burrow, 1995) (see Chapter 50). Elevated thyroid peroxidase antibody titers have been reported in approximately 24% to 36% of women with recurrent pregnancy loss and 17% to fewer than 10% of women with normal reproductive histories (Stagnaro-Green et al., 1990; Pratt et al., 1993; Bussen and Steck, 1995). This association is no longer thought causal for loss, but it is a marker for subsequent thyroid dysfunction.

Infection Assessment

Cervical cultures are generally not helpful, but they should be considered if no other abnormalities are revealed or if there is a history of chorioamnionitis or premature rupture of membranes. In such cases, consideration should be given to culturing for group B β-hemolytic streptococci, *Mycoplasma*, *Ureaplasma*, and *Chlamydia*. Women with signs of bacterial vaginosis (BV) are no more likely to have pregnancy loss than individuals without BV, although BV is associated with premature rupture of membranes and preterm labor and birth. In the absence of clinical infection, TORCH (*t*oxoplasmosis, *r*ubella, *c*ytomegalovirus, and *h*erpes simplex) titers are neither revealing nor indicated (Sahwi et al., 1995). Detection of antibodies to other infections is also unnecessary (Rae et al., 1994).

Immunologic Assessment

Testing for lupus anticoagulant using either an activated partial thromboplastin time or the more informative Russell's viper venom time test and the IgG immunoglobulin (IgG) of anticardiolipin (aCL) and perhaps the IgM isotype of antiphosphatidylserine antibodies should be part of the clinical evaluation of recurrent pregnancy loss (see Chapter 48). Low or unsustained moderate positive values are clinically meaningless (Cowchock et al., 1997). Neither aCL nor antiphosphatidylserine serves as a substitute for the lupus anticoagulant test (Cowchock and Fort, 1994).

Antiphosphatidylserine is often found in the serum of women with the antiphospholipid syndrome who are seropositive for aCL (Branch et al., 1997), which may indicate autoantibody cross-activity in some cases (Charavi et al., 1987).

Assessment of antiphosphatidylserine (IgM) in addition to lupus anticoagulant and aCL (IgG) may be useful clinically because antiphosphatidylserine inhibits syncytial formation of placental trophoblast cell lines (Katsuragawa et al., 1997).

Testing for other antiphospholipid antibodies is not clinically justified, because women with recurrent pregnancy loss are no more likely than fertile controls to have elevated levels of these other antiphospholipid antibodies once lupus anticoagulant, the IgG isotype of aCL, and an obvious clinical history of autoimmune disease have been excluded (Branch et al., 1997).

In addition to tests for the autoantibodies mentioned previously, many other immunologic tests have been recommended historically but are of no clinical benefit (Table 32-4). Antinuclear antibody titers need not be obtained because these autoantibodies are heterogenous, occurring transiently and nonspecifically. The association between antinuclear antibody titers and reproductive difficulty has never been substantiated (Petri et al., 1987; Eroglu and Scopelitis, 1994). Other autoantibody associations with reproductive failure (Geva et al., 1997) have not differentiated between cause and effect of their occurrence and are often age related (Monlias et al., 1984).

Determining maternal antipaternal leukocyte antibodies by any method, including the leukocyte antibody detection assay (Stephenson et al., 1995), is unnecessary because antipaternal cytotoxic antibodies are rarely demonstrable before 28 weeks of gestation in women with successful reproductive histories and may disappear between normal pregnancies (Regan et al., 1981). They are also absent in approximately 40% of women having successful pregnancies (Amos and Kostyn, 1980).

Similarly, mixed lymphocyte culture reactivities between maternal responder and paternal stimulator cells are also unnecessary to obtain in couples with recurrent pregnancy loss because the blocking response of these uncharacterized serum factors is the consequence rather than the cause of pregnancy success (Coulam, 1992).

TABLE 32-4. IMMUNOLOGIC TESTS OF NO CLINICAL BENEFIT

Antinuclear antibodies
IgA isotype of anticardiolipin and antiphosphatidylserine
Antiphosphatidic acid
Antiphosphatidylcholine
Antiphosphatidylethanolamine
Antiphosphatidylglycerol
Antiphosphatidylinositol
Antihistones
Anti-DNA (SS DNA, DS DNA)
Rheumatoid factor
Complement
Smooth muscle antibodies
Antiovarian and antiendometrial antibodies
Antibodies to gonadotropins and gonadal steroids
Antipaternal cytotoxic antibodies (leukocyte antibody detection assay)
Mixed lymphocyte culture reactivities
Human leukocyte antigen (HLA) profiles, including HLA-DR, -DP, -DQ
Peripheral blood immunophenotypes, including CD56+ cells
Natural killer cell activity
Embryotoxicity of peripheral serum
Serum cytokines and adhesion molecules

DNA, deoxyribonucleic acid; DS, double-stranded; Ig, immunoglobulin; SS, single-stranded.

A significant deficit of HLA-DQA1–compatible liveborn offspring was observed in one study (Ober et al., 1993), suggesting that HLA-DQA1–compatible fetuses may be aborted early. In a follow-up study, this laboratory was unable to confirm an association between either HLA-DQA1 or HLA-DQB1 haplotypes and recurrent pregnancy loss (Steck et al., 1995). Others (Dizon-Townson et al., 1995; Wagenknecht et al., 1997) have confirmed that HLA-DQ genotyping is not helpful in the clinical management of recurrent pregnancy loss.

Human serum used in murine studies assessing embryotoxicity has been reported useful in predicting pregnancy outcome (Chavez and McIntyre, 1984). However, the use of human serum in assays involving murine embryos is not scientifically valid because of the presence of complement in serum and heterophilic antibodies in 40% of individuals (Haimovici et al., 1991).

Peripheral blood mononuclear cell activation by cell-surface-expressed protein on the human trophoblast cell line Jeg-3 has been reported to stimulate TH1-type cytokine secretion in some women with recurrent pregnancy loss. Supernatants from these stimulated cultures contained INF-γ, which was toxic to murine embryo development (Hill et al., 1992). This assay and modified versions of it were used extensively in the past in women with a history of recurrent pregnancy loss treated at Brigham and Women's Hospital. (Hill, Anderson, et al., 1995). Depending on the individual series, approximately 30% of women with otherwise unexplained recurrent pregnancy loss produced TH1-type cytokines in response to trophoblast stimulation. Fertile controls may produce INF-γ in response to trophoblast, but at significantly lower levels than women with otherwise-unexplained recurrent pregnancy loss. The diagnostic assay to detect the propensity of having TH1 immunity to trophoblast as a potential cause of recurrent pregnancy loss was changed from the above assays to the detection of the IL-1β polymorphism, which represented the first genetic test, other than karyotype assessment, for diagnosing a potential cause of recurrent pregnancy loss. However, this author no longer uses or recommends any assay to diagnose TH1 immunity to trophoblast, since the administration of immunosuppressive doses of progesterone (100 mg vaginally twice daily, beginning 3 days after detection of the LH surge) will block the production of TH1 cytokines to trophoblast.

◼ POSTCONCEPTION MONITORING

Close monitoring is advised once conception has occurred, not only for psychological well-being of the couple but also to confirm an intrauterine pregnancy (Coulam et al., 1991). The incidence of ectopic pregnancy in the 3500 couples evaluated in the author's Recurrent Pregnancy Loss Clinic was 2.5%. Complete molar gestations were also observed in 6 of the 3500 women. This is an unusually high occurrence of complete moles, since the expected incidence in the general population in the United States is 1 in 2000 pregnancies (Bagshawe, 1969). Therefore, recurrent pregnancy loss appears to be a risk factor for both ectopic pregnancy and complete molar gestation. Concerns that women with recurrent pregnancy loss are also at increased risk for intrauterine growth restriction, premature labor and delivery, low birth weight, and pregnancy-induced hypertension (Labarrere and Althabe, 1986) are not supported by this author's experience, unless they also have antiphospholipid syndrome.

The endocrinologic events associated with both normal pregnancy and pregnancy ending in loss have been well studied. Gonadotropins and gonadal steroids have not been found to be significantly different between conception cycles culminating in pregnancy loss and those ending in success (Stewart et al., 1993). Elevated alpha-fetoprotein levels in maternal serum have been associated with subsequent fetal loss (Maher et al., 1984) but are not definitive. Many clinicians routinely monitor serum progesterone levels in early pregnancy and recommend exogenous supplementation if the level is below a certain value. The clinical utility of such practice is dubious, since low levels of progesterone in early pregnancy are more indicative of an ectopic gestation than a pending intrauterine loss. Also, in cases of pending loss, a low progesterone value in the peripheral circulation may simply represent inadequate human chorionic gonadotropin (hCG) production or interaction with the corpus luteum. In such cases, progesterone replacement should not be expected to be of any benefit since it would not be able to compensate for dysfunctional trophoblast production of hCG. This scenario can occur even in the presence of seemingly adequate hCG levels, because the immunoactivity of this molecule could in some cases be different from its bioactivity.

Immunoreactive inhibin levels are not a prognostic indicator of pregnancy outcome, but subnormal hCG is a useful predictor of early pregnancy loss (France et al., 1996). Precisely when the β-subunit of hCG becomes detectable in maternal serum is unknown, but by the time implantation has occurred, β-hCG is detectable. Levels of β-hCG are expected to double every 48 hours for the first 10 weeks of pregnancy (Laird and Whittaker, 1990). An inadequate doubling time, although ominous, does not necessarily indicate that a loss will occur. Postconception LH levels have been compared with preconception levels, with postconception hypersecretion of LH associated more frequently with early loss (Regan et al., 1990), but no single hormone determination can predict subsequent pregnancy outcome following detection of fetal heart activity (Salem et al., 1984). Therefore, it is not clinically necessary to monitor hCG following ultrasound detection of fetal heart activity. Following pregnancy loss, hCG may not clear the maternal serum for up to 30 days (Steier et al., 1984). Thus, monitoring hCG concentrations every 10–14 days should be advised to rule out persistent trophoblastic disease and the need for methotrexate therapy.

In the normal population, once fetal cardiac activity has been detected with ultrasound monitoring, the chance of subsequent delivery is approximately 95%. In women with a history of two or more pregnancy losses, the chance of viable birth following ultrasound detection of fetal cardiac activity at 6 weeks of gestation is approximately 77% (Laufer et al., 1994). Fetuses with heart rates below 110 beats/minute at 7–8 weeks of gestation are more likely to die than are those with heart rates above this value (Doubilet and Benson, 1995).

Failure to detect a fetal pole and fetal cardiac activity by 7 weeks of gestation is diagnostic for an aembryonic pregnancy (Pennell et al., 1991). A gestational sac greater than 15 mm or crown-rump length greater than 5 mm without fetal cardiac activity is also diagnostic for an aembryonic pregnancy (Achiron et al., 1993). Rarely, even with well-timed intercourse and good dating, ultrasonographic findings may lag 4–9 days behind what dates and timing would otherwise indicate. These events suggest delayed implantation, and in such cases, repeating the ultrasound examination in 1 week is necessary to distinguish this situation from a true aembryonic pregnancy. Pregnancies occurring following delayed implantation are also more likely to end in loss.

Thyroid function studies have been reported to be useful in monitoring pregnancy by some (Mauro et al., 1992; Mazzaferri, 1997) but not all investigators (Ross et al., 1989). In women who are positive for thyroid peroxidase antithyroid antibodies, determining thyroid-stimulating hormone level during the first 6 to 8 weeks of pregnancy may be helpful, since 1% of individuals who are thyroid peroxidase–positive may not meet the increased demand and utilization of thyroid induced in early pregnancy. These women are also at increased risk for postpartum, postabortal, or postectopic autoimmune thyroiditis (Marqusee et al., 1997). It is not necessary to repeat thyroid peroxidase testing during pregnancy, nor is it necessary to determine antithyroid antibody status using hemagglutination techniques, because these have been reported to change during pregnancy and are not helpful for predicting subsequent pregnancy outcome (Amino et al., 1978).

The assessment of CD56 (the NK cell phenotype), CD16 (the Fc receptor, NK cell activation maker), and other immunophenotypes in peripheral blood has been advocated by some based on small, poorly controlled studies (Coulam, Goodman, et al., 1995; Kwak et al., 1995). Larger studies have not substantiated this position. One series, performed by the author, on 87 women with a history of recurrent spontaneous abortion (median 4, range 2 to 12 prior losses) who had peripheral blood obtained at 6 to 9 weeks of gestation after documentation of fetal cardiac activity on ultrasound, found 21 who subsequently aborted spontaneously, yet there were no differences in the percentages of CD56$^+$, CD16$^+$, or other NK- and T-cell regulatory activation markers between women who aborted and those who had a viable delivery. Thus assessment of immunophenotypes was not clinically useful in predicting pregnancy outcome in women with a history of recurrent spontaneous abortion. Similarly, the assessment of immunophenotypes is also not helpful in the care of women with infertility, including those with failed implantation following IVF-ET.

Assessment of TH1, TH2, or adhesion molecules in the peripheral serum of pregnant women with a history of reproductive failure is also not useful in predicting subsequent pregnancy outcome (Schust and Hill, 1996). Inflammatory cytokines may occur in the peripheral circulation at the time of an inevitable or missed abortion and most likely represent an inflammatory response to fetal demise.

Complement activation has been associated with pregnancy loss, and levels have been reported to fall prior to loss of fetal viability (Tichenor et al., 1995). The clinical implications of this study remain unclear, although this area warrants further investigation.

Assessment of TH1 immunity to trophoblast during early pregnancy was reported to be useful in predicting ultimate pregnancy outcome (Ecker et al., 1993). The proliferative response of peripheral blood leukocytes to influenza and tetanus (recall antigens) assessed at 6 weeks of gestation has also been reported to be predictive of pregnancy outcome, with loss of responsiveness associated with subsequent pregnancy success (Bermas and Hill, 1997).

My practice is to monitor women with a history of recurrent pregnancy loss weekly, or more frequently if needed, determining β-hCG from the day of the missed menstrual period until the level is 1000 to 5000 mIU/mL. At that time, a pelvic ultrasound is recommended to confirm an intrauterine gestation, and blood sampling is discontinued unless required for a specific research study protocol. Ultrasonographic examination is recommended every 2 weeks in conjunction with a physician or nurse visit and is continued at that frequency until the time of gestation when the woman had previously lost her pregnancies. This close monitoring provides a psychological advantage; furthermore, if absence of fetal cardiac activity is detected, intervention can be recommended so that tissue for karyotype assessment can be obtained. For some couples, this level of monitoring is too stressful, and it must therefore be modified to meet their individual needs. I do not monitor serum progesterone levels for reasons outlined earlier, and because preimplantation hormonal profiles neither consistently nor significantly differ between pregnancies ending in early loss and those proceeding to viability (Baird et al., 1991).

Assessment of the fetal karyotype should be considered not only for women older than 35 years of age (Hook et al., 1983), but also for all women who have had recurrent pregnancy loss, since these patients are potentially more likely than age-matched controls to have a subsequent aneuploid pregnancy (Drugan et al., 1990).

Assessment of fetal karyotype following pregnancy loss is both clinically useful and cost effective (Wolf and Harger, 1995). However, because fetal karyotyping following either spontaneous expulsion or evacuation is often unsuccessful, consideration should be given to performing a pre-termination procedure such as chorionic villus sampling after fetal demise is confirmed (Johnson et al., 1990; Kyle et al., 1996). When sending tissue for karyotype assessment, it is important to place it in a sterile collection container containing sterile media because villus material is difficult to differentiate from maternal decidual tissue without the use of magnification.

Phenotypic and histologic analysis is seldom helpful in providing predictive value for future pregnancies or providing the couple with a potential reason for their loss. Morphologic assessment is not a substitute for karyotyping, since neither decidual nor placental lesions are characteristic of an abnormal karyotype (Salafia et al., 1993). Histologic assessment of abortus material has been used to support an immunologic etiology for loss (Benirschke and Kaufmann, 1990), especially in cases of decidual vasculitis (Salafia and Burnes, 1989) and massive chronic intervillositis (Doss et al., 1995); however, even definitive proof of the antiphospholipid syndrome as evidenced by decidual vasculopathy and extensive placental infarction (DeWolf et al., 1982) often remains elusive (Out et al., 1991). Cause versus effect mechanisms cannot always be discerned because abnormal histologic findings may be the result of intrauterine fetal death and not necessarily the cause. Therefore, the clinical utility of routine microscopic assessment of abortal tissue is doubtful.

■ THERAPY

Although many therapies have been proposed (Table 32-5), there is no definitive agreement on the management for recurrent pregnancy loss because few properly designed studies have been performed. There are 12 study design criteria (Hill, 1997) that should be fulfilled in a study of therapeutic efficacy for

TABLE 32-5. PROPOSED THERAPIES

Gamete donation for Robertsonian translocation of homologous
    chromosomes
Synchronizing fertilization with ovulation
Supportive care
Oocyte donation for advanced maternal age
In vitro fertilization (IVF) and preimplantation genetic diagnosis (PGD)
Surgical correction of an intrauterine filling defect
Correction of luteal phase insufficiency
    Progesterone
    Ovulation induction with or without pituitary desensitization
Correction of hypothyroidism—thyroid replacement
Correction of hyperprolactinemia—bromocriptine
Eradication of infection, if detected
Aspirin and heparin for antiphospholipid syndrome
Other immunotherapies given historically
    Immunization—leukocytes, intravenous immune globulin
    Immunosuppression—corticosteroids, progesterone

recurrent pregnancy loss. A general outline of prognosis is given in Table 32-6.

Parental Chromosomal Factors

For the couple with an inborn chromosomal abnormality in one or both partners, genetic counseling is warranted. Prognosis for success is high (up to 90%) for synchronizing fertilization with conception, except in cases of a Robertsonian translocation involving homologous chromosomes. In such cases, either donor oocyte or donor sperm is indicated, depending upon which partner has this abnormality.

Anatomic Factors

Studies indicating that surgical correction of müllerian anomalies for recurrent pregnancy loss was of benefit (Goldenberg et al., 1995; Heinonen, 1997) failed to address the problem of regression to the mean (Forrow et al., 1995); other studies suggesting no benefit (Kirk et al., 1993; Colacurci et al., 1996) lacked sufficient power to address this issue definitively. No significant difference in pregnancy outcome was reported in one study following IVF-ET in women with congenital uterine malformations, although only five women with septate uterus (type V) were included (Marcus et al., 1996). None of the studies assessing pregnancy outcome after

surgery corrected for the size of the intrauterine abnormality. A residual septum of less than 1 cm following hysteroscopic resection has been reported not to influence reproductive outcome (Fedele et al., 1996).

The use of prophylactic antibiotics and postoperative hormonal therapy has been questioned for women undergoing hysteroscopic resection of intrauterine lesions (March and Israel, 1987). Postoperative estrogen supplementation, although controversial, may be of benefit following resection of intrauterine adhesions but is probably unnecessary following metroplasty (Vercellini et al., 1989). When hormonal preparations are used following surgery, 2.5 mg of conjugated estrogen is given daily for 30 days, for the last 10 days of which an oral progestin (10 mg) is added. Conception is attempted following withdrawal bleeding. Concomitant laparoscopy is not generally performed for correction of submucous myomas or a septum, because the rate of complications related to uterine perforation is less than 1%. If perforation inadvertently occurs, laparoscopy may be necessary to assess possible intra-abdominal injury, and conception should be avoided for at least three cycles.

Cervical cerclage has been recommended in women with a history of recurrent pregnancy loss, even in the absence of a typical history of incompetent cervix (Cromblehome et al., 1983) or in the presence of congenital müllerian anomalies (Abramovici et al., 1983). These retrospective studies did not address regression to the mean. Cervical cerclage is not a benign procedure (Charles and Edwards, 1981) and should not be performed except in cases of preexisting cervical incompetence or, perhaps, in cases of uterine anomalies as a result of DES exposure (Barth, 1994) (see Chapter 33).

Endocrine Factors

Luteal phase insufficiency is treated with progesterone, hCG, ovulation induction, or a combination of all three. The efficacy of progesterone therapy for luteal phase insufficiency has not been substantiated because of lack of uniform case definitions, failure to control for regression to the mean, and lack of randomized controlled trials of sufficient power to reach a definitive conclusion (Karamardian and Grimes, 1992). The appropriate dose, the route of administration, and when to initiate and discontinue therapy have not been standardized. Progesterone supplementation has been advocated (Soules et al., 1997) for mild luteal phase defects (3- to 4-day out-of-phase endometrial biopsy). I use 100-mg progesterone vaginal suppositories twice a day beginning 3 days after the LH surge,

TABLE 32-6. PROGNOSIS FOR VIABLE BIRTH*

Status	Intervention	Percent
Genetic factors	Timed intercourse and supportive care	20–90
Anatomic factors	Surgery and supportive care	60–90
Endocrine factors		
Luteal phase deficiency	Progesterone and/or ovulation induction with or without pituitary desensitization and supportive care	80–90
Hypothyroidism	Thyroid replacement and supportive care	80–90
Infections	Appropriate antibiotic and supportive care	70–90
Antiphospholipid syndrome	Aspirin, heparin, and supportive care	70–90
Th1 cellular immunity	Progesterone immunosuppression and supportive care	70–90
Unknown factors	Timed intercourse and supportive care	60–90

* Derived from more than 1000 cases by this author at Brigham and Women's Hospital.

as detected with a urine ovulation-predictor test kit, and continue this therapy until 10 weeks of gestation.

Concerns of potential teratogenicity have limited the use of synthetic progestins (Nora et al, 1978). The 21-carbon molecule progesterone, although not teratogenic, may cause minor side effects, including fatigue, fluid retention, and delayed menses. Progesterone may also facilitate the growth of leiomyomata and cause depression in some individuals. The route of administration should be vaginal rather than intramuscular or oral because of the higher progesterone levels achieved locally within the uterus following vaginal administration (Miles et al., 1994) as a result of direct transit into the uterus through a "first uterine pass effect" (Fanchin et al., 1997). Administration should begin before implantation but after ovulation (Jones, 1968). Care should also be exercised in the choice of pharmacy making this compounded agent, since regulations regarding compounding are not as stringent as those for manufactured pharmaceuticals. Therefore the potency of formulations compounded by different pharmacies may not be the same even for the same prescription because of differences in dosage, bioavailability, and stability of the compounded product containing progesterone.

Luteal function has also been stimulated by serial hCG injections. The efficacy of hCG for pregnancy loss was not substantiated in a placebo-controlled trial except for women with oligomenorrhea (Quenby and Farquharson, 1994).

Ovulation induction has been advocated in women with severe luteal phase insufficiency (endometrial biopsy more than 5 days out of phase) (Soules et al., 1997). Downregulation with gonadotropin-releasing hormone agonists to reduce the rate of pregnancy loss in women with PCOS (Homburg et al., 1993) was not substantiated in a randomized controlled trial in women following LH downregulation, ovulation induction, and luteal phase progesterone compared with women having spontaneous ovulation followed with or without progesterone supplementation (Clifford et al., 1996). Metformin may be of benefit in women with recurrent pregnancy loss associated with PCOS who have insulin resistance.

Laparoscopic ovarian diathermy has been reported to reduce the incidence of subsequent pregnancy loss in women with PCOS (Amar et al., 1993). Enthusiasm for this approach should be tempered until well-designed studies have been performed, because there is the potential of causing harm through the inherent risks of the laparoscopic procedure and the formation of ovarian adhesions following ovarian diathermy.

Hypothyroidism should be treated with thyroid replacement, with careful titration so that thyroid-stimulating hormone remains in the normal range. Close monitoring during early pregnancy is essential because of the increased demand and utilization of thyroid during the first trimester. Hyperprolactinemia should be treated to maintain normal prolactin levels.

Infections

In individuals with either *Mycoplasma hominis* or *U. urealyticum*, I treat the couple with 100 mg of doxycycline twice a day for 10 days. However, there are no randomized, double-blind, placebo-controlled studies substantiating this approach. Empirical antibiotic treatments are unwarranted in the absence of an identifiable infection. If a potentially infectious organism is documented, appropriate antibiotic therapy should be considered for both partners, with post-treatment

cultures to verify elimination of the infection prior to attempting pregnancy. Appropriately designed clinical trials are needed to substantiate an infectious etiology for recurrent pregnancy loss and to determine whether specific antibiotics are able to ameliorate subsequent pregnancy outcome.

Immunologic Factors

Antiphospholipid Syndrome

Placental damage resulting from thrombosis is thought to be the end result of autoimmunity to phospholipids, and therapeutic approaches have included prophylactic anticoagulation with aspirin and heparin (Farquarson et al., 1985; Gutenby et al., 1989; Branch et al., 1992; Kutteh, 1996; Rai et al., 1997) (see Chapter 48). Corticosteroids (prednisone, prednisolone) have also been used, but not substantiated (Lubba et al., 1983; Silver et al., 1993; Harger et al., 1995; Laskin et al., 1997), and the maternal side effects limit their use.

Heparin and aspirin are reported to be more effective than aspirin and corticosteroids for the antiphospholipid syndrome (Lockshin et al., 1989; Cowchock et al., 1992). Corticosteroids should not be used, especially concomitantly with heparin, because of the potentiation of osteoporosis with these agents, but the risk of osteoporosis appears to be lower with low-molecular-weight heparin. Use of low-molecular-weight heparin allows once per day dosing, and monitoring coagulation parameters is unnecessary (Weitz, 1997). Heparin is also reported to bind aCL *in vitro*, which may explain the decreased aCL levels reported with heparin (Ermel et al., 1995).

Because of the inherent side effects of anticoagulant therapy, the empirical use of heparin or aspirin is not justified for women without evidence of the antiphospholipid syndrome. The use of 81 mg of aspirin every day has not been shown to be of benefit in women with three or more first-trimester pregnancy losses. Similarly, treatment of pregnant women who have antiphospholipid antibodies of low titer or who are otherwise at low risk for loss, including those with infertility and those having *in vitro* fertilization, cannot be justified (Lockwood et al., 1989; Cowchock et al., 1997; Kutteh, Yetman, et al., 1997). Initiating heparin and aspirin before conception is potentially dangerous because of the risk of hemorrhage at the time of ovulation.

Therapeutic recommendations for the antiphospholipid syndrome include 81 mg of aspirin per day, followed by 10,000 to 20,000 units of subcutaneous heparin per day in divided doses (Rai et al., 1997) (see Chapter 48). Low-molecular-weight heparin (2500 to 5000 units/day) is an effective alternative for obstetric thromboprophylaxis (Nelson-Piercy et al., 1997). Combination therapy with aspirin and heparin may reduce pregnancy loss in women with antiphospholipid antibodies by 54% (Empson et al., 2002). Aspirin alone is not helpful for women with unexplained first-trimester pregnancy loss (Rai et al., 2000).

Alloimmune Recurrent Pregnancy Loss

Therapy for alloimmune reproductive failure largely remains anecdotal because of the lack of well-designed clinical trials. There is controversy not only on how to treat but also on how to diagnose alloimmune recurrent pregnancy loss (Hill, 1996, 1997; Kutteh, Stovall, et al., 1997).

TH1 immunity to trophoblast may best be treated with potentially immunosuppressive doses of progesterone vaginal suppositories (100 mg twice daily, beginning 3 days after ovulation). Progesterone has been called "nature's immunosuppressant" because concentrations at the maternal-fetal interface (10^{-5} mol/L) inhibit macrophage phagocytosis, lymphocyte proliferation, NK cell function, and cytotoxic T-cell activity (Siiteri et al., 1977; Hill et al., 1987). Evidence from our laboratory indicates that in women with TH1 immunity to trophoblast, progesterone can inhibit TH1 cytokine release and embryotoxic factor production *in vitro* (Choi et al., 2000). Although preliminary results indicate that this is efficacious (see Table 32-6), verification is still needed from properly designed clinical trials.

The immunotherapies originally proposed for the now-disproved blocking-antibody hypothesis continue to be promulgated by some. These immunotherapies include active immunization with either third-party or paternal allogenic peripheral blood mononuclear cells (leukocytes) and passive immunization with intravenous immune globulin (IVIG). Many anecdotal case series and inadequately designed trials have been published concerning leukocyte immunization (Taylor and Faulk, 1981; Beer et al., 1985; Mowbray et al., 1985; Carp et al., 1990; Christiansen et al., 1993; Gatenby et al., 1993). Meta-analyses (Fraser et al., 1993; Recurrent Miscarriage Immunotherapy Trialists Group, 1994) and reviews of these analyses (Scott, 1994; Jeng et al., 1995; Hill, 1996; Kutteh, Stovall, et al., 1997) have also been published. In summary, the efficacy of leukocyte immunization has never been substantiated (Jeng et al., 1995). In the largest clinical trial performed to date, individuals receiving leukocyte immunization had a significantly higher pregnancy loss rate than did saline controls (Ober et al., 1999). According to a recent review using the 95% confidence intervals from the largest meta-analysis to date (Recurrent Miscarriage Trialists Group, 1994), as few as 4 to as many as 167 women would need to receive leukocyte immunization to achieve a single additional live birth (Kutteh, Stovall, et al., 1997).

Adverse side effects caused by leukocyte immunization occur in 1 in 50 treated women (Recurrent Miscarriage Immunotherapy Trialists Group, 1994). These side effects, some of which can be life threatening, include transfusion reactions, autoimmunity, erythrocyte and platelet sensitization, difficulty in obtaining donor organs should they be needed, infections, intrauterine growth restriction, graft-versus-host disease, and thrombocytopenia leading to neonatal death (Hill and Andersen, 1986; Katz et al., 1992; Kutteh, Stovall, et al., 1997).

An alloimmune problem is suspected by some when an evaluation reveals no genetic, anatomic, or endocrinologic problems or antiphospholipid antibodies. However, because of the adverse publicity leukocyte immunization therapy has received (unsubstantiated efficacy, potential for adverse side effects), immunotherapists are currently promoting IVIG. IVIG has many potential immunomodulating effects (Dwyer, 1992). IVIG infusions (500 mg/kg) have been reported to downregulate CD56 and LFA-1 cells in the peripheral circulation of pregnant women with a history of recurrent spontaneous abortion (Rigal et al., 1994). IVIG (400 mg/kg) has also been reported to decrease peripheral blood NK activity in three of five pregnant women with a history of recurrent abortion who delivered successfully (Ruiz et al., 1996). The biological significance of these anecdotal data remains ill defined because clinical studies to date using IVIG for recurrent pregnancy loss have not substantiated efficacy (German

RSA/IVIG Group, 1994; Heine and Muller-Eckhardt, 1994; Christiansen et al., 1995; Coulam, Krysa, et al., 1995; Carp et al., 1996; Perino et al., 1997). The cost of this unsubstantiated therapy is estimated to be $7000 to $14,000. Hypotension, nausea, and headache are common side effects. Life-threatening anaphylaxis can occur in IgA-deficient individuals (Thorton and Bellow, 1993), and long-term effects of this therapy for pregnant women are unknown. Prion diseases, such as Creutzfeldt-Jakob and mad cow disease, are remote possibilities because blood from approximately 150 paid blood donors is needed to produce one vial of IVIG.

Other Therapeutic Considerations

IVF-ET following ovulation induction with gonadotropin-releasing hormone agonists and gonadotropins was reported useful in treating 12 women with unexplained recurrent abortion (Balasch et al., 1996b). In a study of 20 couples with unexplained recurrent abortion and secondary infertility subjected to a total of 42 IVF-ET cycles, the subsequent miscarriage rate was 50% for women with a history of recurrent pregnancy loss, indicating that IVF-ET was not beneficial therapy for recurrent pregnancy loss (Raziel et al., 1997).

Oocyte donation has also been reported to be efficacious in treating recurrent pregnancy loss (Remohi et al., 1996). Eight couples in which the woman was a low responder to gonadotropin stimulation with a history of recurrent abortion underwent a total of 12 oocyte donation cycles. Clinical pregnancy and delivery rates per cycle were 75% and 66%, respectively. The delivery rate per patient was 86%, and the miscarriage rate was 11%, suggesting that the oocyte may be the origin of reproductive difficulty in these women. This study questions the role of other maternal and paternal factors in recurrent loss (Remohi et al., 1996).

An alternative to oocyte donation in the treatment of women with recurrent pregnancy loss who have adequate ovarian reserve may include IVF, which allows preimplantation genetic diagnosis (PGD) to be performed prior to embryo transfer (Delhanty and Handyside, 1995; Munne and Wells, 2002). Preimplantation genetic diagnosis involves genetic testing on embryos before a clinical pregnancy is established. In most cases, single cells (blastomeres) are biopsied from embryos generated using assisted reproductive technologies. These are then analyzed for unbalanced chromosome arrangements and DNA mutations that cause single gene disorders. PGD may improve the overall pregnancy success rate, not only for women with a history of recurrent pregnancy loss, but for all women over age 35 having IVF (Roesler et al., 1989), since the majority of pregnancy losses following IVF are chromosomally abnormal. Alternatively, polar bodies may be biopsied from oocytes and subjected to similar tests. These tests usually involve fluorescence *in situ* hybridization (Lebo et al., 1992). This approach has been shown to improve successful pregnancy rates in women with recurrent pregnancy loss. Currently, probes for chromosomes X, Y, 13, 14, 15, 16, 21, and 22 are being used simultaneously, with the potential of detecting 70% of the aneuploidies found in spontaneous abortions (Munne et al., 1998). Another investigational technique, *comparative genomic hybridization* (Kallioniemi et al., 1994), may one day enable preimplantation genetic diagnosis of all chromosomes on a single blastomere (Reubinoff and Shusan, 1996).

There is a significant spontaneous pregnancy success rate in couples with recurrent pregnancy loss (see Table 32-6).

The spontaneous cure rate may be enhanced by synchronizing intercourse with ovulation followed by formalized supportive care (Stray-Pedersen and Stray-Pedersen, 1984; Liddell et al., 1991; Pruyn et al., 2002). Dedication to supportive care with and without pharmacologic or surgical intervention will facilitate successful pregnancy outcome (Clifford et al., 1997). Individual clinics have different success rates even when using the same intervention therapy and controlling for maternal age and number of prior losses, suggesting that the ability to offer supportive care is important in achieving pregnancy success (Cauchi et al., 1995).

Adoption of a caring, empathetic attitude by the physician and the entire health care team toward the couple experiencing recurrent pregnancy loss is imperative. Acknowledging the pain and suffering these couples experience because of their reproductive difficulty and the resulting stress within themselves and their relationships may act as a catharsis, enabling incorporation of their experience of loss into their lives rather than their lives into their experience of loss. Incorporation of self-help measures including healthful diet, meditation, yoga, or exercise may be helpful. Referrals to behavioral medicine specialists, psychologists, psychiatrists, and licensed social workers with an interest in the problems these couples encounter may also be of benefit.

■ SUMMARY

Recurrent pregnancy loss is emotionally difficult for couples experiencing such loss and is often a frustrating challenge for their physicians. This frustration often results in the recommendation of unsubstantiated tests and therapies of dubious efficacy. Recommendations regarding the routine clinical use of therapy for recurrent pregnancy loss should rely on level-one evidence from the outcome of well-designed clinical trials based on testable hypotheses and using diagnostic tests assessed by their performance on receiver operating characteristic curves (Beck and Schultz, 1986; Hanley and McNeil, 1992). Otherwise, we risk adding still more unsubstantiated tests and therapies to an already cumbersome therapeutic repertoire, resulting in further expansion of health care expenditures and the potential exploitation of couples seeking care (Hill, 1997).

The possibility of achieving a successful pregnancy for couples with recurrent pregnancy loss is high, depending on both maternal age and number of earlier losses. Potential causes and interventional choices may also affect the prognosis. Understanding the potential mechanisms involved in recurrent pregnancy loss together with a caring, empathetic attitude toward the couple will enable amelioration of the emotional distress these couples encounter and facilitate a rational, cost-effective evaluation leading to appropriate consultation and effective therapy.

REFERENCES

Abramovici H, Faktor JH, Pascal B: Congenital uterine malformations as indication for cervical suture (cerclage) in habitual abortion and premature delivery. Int J Fertil **28**:161, 1983.

Achiron R, Goldenberg M, Lipitz S, et al: Transvaginal duplex Doppler ultrasonography in bleeding patients suggested of having residual trophoblastic tissue. Obstet Gynecol **81**:507, 1993.

Acien P: Reproductive performance of women with uterine malformations. Hum Reprod **8**:122, 1993.

Adam Z, Poulin F, Papp Z: Increased risk of neural tube defects after recurrent pregnancy losses. Am J Med Genet **55**:512, 1995.

Adler RR, Ng AK, Rote RS: Monoclonal antiphosphatidylserine antibody inhibits intercellular fusion of the choriocarcinoma cell line JAR. Biol Reprod **53**:905, 1995.

Alberman E: The epidemiology of repeated abortion. *In* Beard RW, Bishop F (eds): Early Pregnancy Loss: Mechanisms and Treatment. New York, Springer-Verlag, 1988, p. 9.

Amar NA, Rachelin GC: Laparoscopic ovarian diathermy: An effective treatment for anti-estrogen resistant anovulatory infertility in women with the polycystic ovary syndrome. Br J Obstet Gynaecol **100**:161, 1993.

American College of Obstetricians and Gynecologists: Exercise during pregnancy and the postpartum period. Washington, DC, ACOG Technical Bulletin, No. 189, 1994.

Amino N, Kuro R, Tanizowa O, et al: Changes of serum antithyroid antibodies during and after pregnancy in autoimmune thyroid disease. Clin Exp Immunol **31**:30, 1978.

Amos DB, Kostyn DD: HLA: A central immunologic agency of man. Adv Hum Genet **10**:137, 1980.

Azuma K, Calderon I, Besanko M, et al: Is the luteo-placental shift a myth? Analysis of low progesterone levels in successful ART pregnancies. J Clin Endocrinol Metab **77**:195, 1993.

Babalioglu R, Varol FG, Ilhan R, et al: Progesterone profiles in luteal-phase defects associated with recurrent spontaneous abortions. J Assist Reprod Genet **13**:306, 1996.

Bagshawe KD: Choriocarcinoma. Baltimore, Williams & Wilkins, 1969, p. 32.

Baird DD, Weinberg CR, Wilcox AJ, et al: Hormonal profiles of natural conception cycle ending in unrecognized pregnancy loss. J Clin Endocrinol Metab **72**:793, 1991.

Balasch J, Crews M, Fabreques F, et al: In vitro fertilization treatment for unexplained recurrent abortion: A pilot study. Hum Reprod **11**:1579, 1996b.

Balasch J, Varnell J: Corpus luteum insufficiency and fertility: A matter of controversy. Hum Reprod **2**:557, 1987.

Balen AH, Tan SL, Jacobs HS: Hypersecretion of luteinizing hormones: A significant case of infertility and miscarriage. Br J Obstet Gynaecol **100**:1082, 1993.

Barth WH Jr: Cervical incompetence and cerclage: Unresolved controversies. Clin Obstet Gynecol **37**:831, 1994.

Battaglia DE, Goodwin P, Klein NA, Soules MR: Influence of maternal age on meiotic spindle assembly in oocytes from naturally cycling women. Hum Reprod **11**:2217, 1996.

Beck R, Schultz E: The use of receiver operating characteristics (ROC) curves in test performance and evaluation. Arch Pathol Lab Med **110**:13, 1986.

Becks GP, Burrow GN: Diagnosis and treatment of thyroid disease during pregnancy. *In* DeGroot LJ (ed): Endocrinology, 3rd ed. Philadelphia, WB Saunders, 1995, p. 799.

Beer AE, Semprini AE, Zho XY, et al: Pregnancy outcome in human couples with recurrent spontaneous abortions: HLA antigen profiles, HLA antigen sharing, female MLR blocking factors, and paternal leukocyte immunization. Exp Clin Immunogenet **2**:137, 1985.

Benirschke K, Kaufmann P: Abortion, placentas of trisomies and immunological considerations of recurrent reproductive failure. *In* Pathology of the Human Placenta. New York, Springer-Verlag, 1990, p. 754.

Berkowitz GS, Stone JL, Lehrer SP, et al: An estrogen receptor polymorphism and the risk of primary and secondary recurrent spontaneous abortion. Am J Obstet Gynecol **171**:1579, 1994.

Berkowitz RS, Hill JA, Kutz CB, et al: Effects of products of activated leukocytes (lymphokines and monokines) on the growth of malignant trophoblast cells in vitro. Am J Obstet Gynecol **158**:199, 1988.

Bermas BL, Hill JA: Proliferation responses to recall antigens are associated with pregnancy outcome in women with a history of recurrent spontaneous abortion. J Clin Invest **100**:1330, 1997.

Bermas BL, Petri M, Goldman D, et al: T helper cell dysfunction in systemic lupus erythematosus (SLE): Relation to disease activity. J Clin Immunol **14**:169, 1994.

Bonilla-Musales F, Simon C, Serra V, et al: An assessment of hysterosalpingography as a diagnostic tool for uterine cavity defects and tubal patency. J Clin Ultrasound **20**:175, 1992.

Bonney RC, Franks S: The endocrinology of implantation and early pregnancy. Baillieres Clin Endocrinol Metab **4**:207, 1990.

Boue J, Boue A: Increased frequency of chromosomal anomalies in abortions after induced ovulation. Lancet **7804**:679, 1975.

Boue J, Boue A, Laser P: Retrospective and prospective epidemiologic studies of 1,500 karyotyped spontaneous abortions. Teratology **11**:11, 1975.

Branch DW, Scott JR, Kochenour NK, et al: Obstetric complications associated with the lupus anticoagulants. N Engl J Med **313**:1322, 1985.

Branch DW, Silver R, Blackwell JL, et al: Outcome of treated pregnancies in women with antiphospholipid syndrome: An update of the Utah experience. Obstet Gynecol **80**:614, 1992.

Branch DW, Silver R, Dierangeli S, et al: Antiphospholipid antibodies other than lupus anticoagulant and anticardiolipin antibodies in women with recurrent pregnancy loss, fertile controls, and antiphospholipid syndrome. Obstet Gynecol **89**:549, 1997.

Braulke I, Pruggmayer M, Melloh P, et al: Factor XI (Hyaman) deficiency in women with habitual abortion: New subpopulation of recurrent aborters? Fertil Steril **59**:98, 1993.

Bullter RE, Jones HW: Pregnancy following conization of the cervix: Complication related to the cone sizes. Am J Obstet Gynecol **142**:506, 1982.

Bussen S, Steck T: Thyroid autoantibodies in euthyroid nonpregnant women with recurrent spontaneous abortus. Hum Reprod **10**:2938, 1995.

Buttram VC Jr: Mullerian anomalies and their management. Fertil Steril **40**:159, 1983.

Buttram VC Jr, Gibbons WE: Mullerian anomalies: A proposed classification (an analysis of 144 cases). Fertil Steril **32**:40, 1979.

Carp HJ, Ahirm R, Mashiach S, et al: Intravenous immunoglobulin in women with five or more abortions. Am J Reprod Immunol **35**:360, 1996.

Carp HJ, Toder V, Bzait E, et al: Immunization by paternal leukocytes for prevention of primary habitual abortion: Results of a matched control trial. Gynecol Obstet Invest **29**:16, 1990.

Carreras LO, Vernylan JG: Lupus anticoagulant and thrombosis: Possible role of inhibition of prostacyclin formation. Thromb Haemost **48**:38, 1982.

Cauchi MN, Coulam CB, Cowchuck S, et al: Predictive factors in recurrent spontaneous aborters: A multicenter study. Am J Reprod Immunol **33**:165, 1995.

Cavallo F, Russo R, Zotti C, et al: Moderate alcohol consumption and spontaneous abortion. Alcohol **30**:195, 1995.

Cecere FA, Persellin RH: The interaction of pregnancy and the rheumatic diseases. Clin Rheum Dis **7**:747, 1981.

Centers for Disease Control and Prevention: Recommendations for the prevention and management of *Chlamydia trachomatis* infections. MMWR Morb Mortal Wkly Rep **42**:1, 1993.

Charavi AE, Harris EN, Asherson RA, et al: Anticardiolipin antibodies: Isotope distribution and phospholipid specificity. Ann Rheumatol Dis **46**:1, 1987.

Charles D, Edwards WR: Infectious complications of cervical cerclage. Am J Obstet Gynecol **141**:1065, 1981.

Charles D, Larsen B: Spontaneous abortion as a result of infection. *In* Huisjes HJ, Lind T (eds): Early Pregnancy Failure. New York, Churchill Livingstone, 1990, p. 161.

Chavez DJ, McIntyre JA: Sera from women with histories of repeated pregnancy losses cause abnormalities in mouse periimplantation blastocyst. J Reprod Immunol **6**:273, 1984.

Choi BC, Polgar K, Xiao L, et al: Progesterone inhibits in vitro embryotoxic Th1 cytokine production to trophoblast in women with recurrent pregnancy loss. Hum Reprod **15**:46, 2000.

Christiansen OB: A fresh look at the causes and treatments of recurrent miscarriage, especially its immunological aspects. Hum Reprod Update **2**:271, 1996.

Christiansen OB, Mathiesen O, Husth M, et al: Placebo controlled trials of active immunization with third-party leukocytes in recurrent miscarriage. Acta Obstet Gynecol Scand **72**:1, 1993.

Christiansen OB, Mathiesen O, Husth M, et al: Placebo-controlled trial of treatment of unexplained secondary recurrent spontaneous abortions and recurrent late spontaneous abortions with IVF immunoglobulin. Hum Reprod **10**:2690, 1995.

Clifford K, Rai R, Regan L: Future pregnancy outcome in unexplained recurrent first trimester miscarriage. Hum Reprod **12**:387, 1997.

Clifford K, Rai R, Watson H, et al: An informative protocol for the investigation of recurrent miscarriage: Preliminary experience of 500 consecutive cases. Hum Reprod **9**:1328, 1994.

Clifford K, Rai R, Watson H, et al: Does suppressing luteinizing hormone secretion reduce the miscarriage rate? Results of a randomized controlled trial. BMJ **312**:1508, 1996.

Cohn SD: Sexuality in pregnancy: A review of the literature. Nurs Clin North Am **17**:91, 1982.

Colacurci N, De Placido G, Mollo A, et al: Reproductive outcome after hysteroscopic metroplasty. Eur J Obstet Gynecol Reprod Biol **66**:147, 1996.

Coulam CB: Immunological tests in the evaluation of reproductive disorders: A critical review. Am J Obstet Gynecol **167**:1844, 1992.

Coulam CB, Goodman C, Roussev RG, et al: Systemic CD56 cells can predict pregnancy outcome. Am J Reprod Immunol **33**:40, 1995.

Coulam CB, Johnson PM, Ramsden GH, et al: Occurrence of ectopic pregnancy among women with recurrent abortion. Am J Reprod Immunol **21**:105, 1991.

Coulam CB, Krysa L, Stern JJ, et al: Intravenous immunoglobulin for treatment of recurrent pregnancy loss. Am J Reprod Immunol **34**:33, 1995.

Cowchock FS, Fort JG: Can tests for IgA, IgG or IgM antibodies to cardiolipin or phosphatidyl serine substitute for lupus anticoagulant assays in screening for antiphospholipid antibodies? Autoimmunity **17**:119, 1994.

Cowchock FS, Reece EA: Do low-risk pregnant women with antiphospholipid antibodies need to be treated? Am J Obstet Gynecol **176**:109, 1997.

Cowchock FS, Reece EA, Balandon D, et al: Repeated fetal losses associated with antiphospholipid antibodies: A collaborative randomized trial comparing prednisone with low dose heparin treatment. Am J Obstet Gynecol **166**:1318, 1992.

Cromblehome WR, Minkoff HL, Delke I, et al: Cervical cerclage: An aggressive approach to threatened or recurrent pregnancy wastage. Am J Obstet Gynecol **146**:168, 1983.

Daling JR, Emanuel I: Induced abortion and subsequent outcome of pregnancy in a series of American women. N Engl J Med **297**:1241, 1977.

Davis OK, Berkeley AS, Naus GJ, et al: The incidence of luteal phase defect in normal fertile women, determined by serial endometrial biopsies. Fertil Steril **51**:582, 1989.

Delhanty JDA, Handyside AH: The origin of genetic defects in the human and their detection in the preimplantation embryo. Hum Reprod Update **1**:201, 1995.

DeWolf F, Carreras LO, Moerman P, et al: Decidual vasculopathy and extensive placental infarction in a patient with repeated thromboembolic accidents, recurrent loss and a lupus anticoagulant. Am J Obstet Gynecol **42**:829, 1982.

Dizon-Townson D, Meline L, Nelson LM, et al: Fetal carriers of the factor V Leiden mutation are prone to miscarriage and placental infarction. Am J Obstet Gynecol **177**:402, 1997.

Dizon-Townson D, Nelson L, Scott J Jr, et al: Human leukocyte antigens DQ alpha sharing is not increased in couples with recurrent miscarriage. Am J Reprod Immunol **34**:209, 1995.

Dlugosz L, Bracken MB: Reproductive effects of caffeine: A review and theoretical analysis. Epidemiol Rev **4**:83, 1992.

Doss BJ, Greene MF, Hill JA, et al: Massive chronic intervillositis associated with recurrent abortions. Hum Pathol **26**:1245, 1995.

Doubilet PM, Benson CB: Embryonic heart rate in the early first trimester: What rate is normal? J Ultrasound Med **14**:431, 1995.

Drugan A, Boltums SF, Johnson MP, et al: Seasonal variation in conception does not appear to influence the rates of prenatal diagnosis of nondisjunction. Fetal Diagn Ther **4**:195, 1989.

Drugan A, Koppitch FC III, Williams JC III, et al: Prenatal genetic diagnosis following recurrent early pregnancy loss. Obstet Gynecol **75**:381, 1990.

Dudley DJ, Collmer D, Mitchell MD, et al: Inflammatory cytokine mRNA in human gestational tissues: Implications for term and preterm labor. J Soc Gynecol Invest **3**:328, 1996.

Dudley DJ, Mitchell MD, Branch DW: Pathophysiology of antiphospholipid antibodies: Absence of prostaglandin-mediated effects on cultured endothelium. Am J Obstet Gynecol **162**:953, 1990.

Dwyer JM: Manipulating the immune system with immune globulin. N Engl J Med **326**:107, 1992.

Ecker JL, Laufer MR, Hill JA: Measurement of embryotoxic factors is predictive of pregnancy outcome in women with a history of recurrent spontaneous abortion. Obstet Gynecol **81**:84, 1993.

Edmonds DK, Lindsay KS, Miller JF, et al: Early embryonic mortality in women. Fertil Steril **38**:447, 1982.

Empson M, Lassere M, Craig JC, et al: Recurrent pregnancy loss with antiphospholipid antibody: A systemic review of therapeutic trials. Obstet Gynecol **99**:135, 2002.

Ermel LD, Marshburn PB, Kutteh WH: Interaction of heparin with antiphospholipid antibodies from the sera of women with recurrent pregnancy loss. Am J Reprod Immunol **33**:14, 1995.

Eroglu GE, Scopeliltis E: Antinuclear and antiphospholipid antibodies in healthy women with recurrent spontaneous abortion. Am J Reprod Immunol **31**:1, 1994.

Fanchin R, DeZiegler D, Bergeron C, et al: Transvaginal administration of progesterone. Obstet Gynecol **90**:396, 1997.

Farquharson R, Blown A, Compton A: The lupus anticoagulant: A plan for pregnancy treatment? Lancet **ii**:842, 1985.

Fedele L, Bianchi S, Marchini M, et al: Residual uterine septum of less than 1 cm after hysteroscopic metroplasty does not impair reproductive outcome. Hum Reprod **11**:727, 1996.

Ferguson DM, Horwood LJ, Shannon FT: Smoking during pregnancy. N Z Med J **89**:41, 1979.

Fielding JR: MR imaging of mullerian anomalies: Impact on therapy. Am J Roentgenol **167**:1491, 1996.

Fitzsimmons J, Stahl R, Gocial B, et al: Spontaneous abortion in women with endometriosis. Fertil Steril **47**:696, 1987.

Forrow L, Calkins DR, Allshouse K, et al: Evaluating cholesterol screening: The importance of controlling for regression to the mean. Arch Intern Med **155**:2177, 1995.

France JT, Keelan J, Sang L, et al: Serum concentrations of human chorionic gonadotropin and immunoreactive inhibin in early pregnancy and recurrent miscarriage: A longitudinal study. Aust N Z J Obstet Gynaecol **36**:325, 1996.

Fraser EJ, Grimes DA, Schultz KF: Immunization as therapy for recurrent spontaneous abortion: A review and meta-analysis. Obstet Gynecol **82**:854, 1993.

Fritz MA: Inadequate luteal function and recurrent abortion. Semin Reprod Endocrinol **6**:129, 1988.

Gabbe SG, Turner LP: Reproductive hazards of the American lifestyle: Work during pregnancy. Am J Obstet Gynecol **176**:826, 1997.

Garcia JE, Tran T, Smith RD, et al: Relationship of endometriosis staging and in vitro fertilization outcome. Hum Reprod **6**:74, 1991.

Gatenby PA, Cameron K, Simes RJ, et al: Treatment of recurrent spontaneous abortion by immunization with paternal lymphocytes: Results of a controlled trial. Am J Reprod Immunol **29**:88, 1993.

German RSA/IVIG Group: Intravenous immunoglobulin in the prevention of recurrent miscarriage. Br J Obstet Gynaecol **101**:1072, 1994.

Geva E, Amit A, Lerner-Gera L, et al: Autoimmunity and reproduction. Fertil Steril **67**:599, 1997.

Gibbs RS: Chorioamnionitis and bacterial vaginosis. Am J Obstet Gynecol **169**:460, 1993.

Gilnoer D, Soto MF, Bourdoux P, et al: Pregnancy in patients with mid thyroid abnormalities: Maternal and neonatal repercussion. J Clin Endocrinol Metab **73**:421, 1991.

Goddijn-Wessel TA, Wonters MG, Von de Molen EF, et al: Hyperhomocystenemia: A risk factor for placental abruption or infarction. Eur J Obstet Gynecol Reprod Biol **66**:23, 1996.

Golard R, Jozak S, Warren W, et al: Elevated levels of umbilical cord anticorticotropin releasing hormone in growth retarded fetuses. J Clin Endocrinol Metab **77**:1174, 1993.

Golbus MJ: Chromosome aberrations and mammalian reproduction. In Mastroianni L, Biggers J, Sadler W (eds): Fertilization and Embryonic Development in Vitro. New York, Plenum Press, 1981.

Goldenberg M, Sivan E, Sherabi Z, et al: Reproductive outcome following hysteroscopic management of intrauterine septum and adhesions. Hum Reprod **10**:2663, 1995.

Gravett MG, Nelson HP, DeRouen T, et al: Independent associations of bacterial vaginosis and *Chlamydia trachomatis* infection with adverse pregnancy outcome. JAMA **256**:1899, 1986.

Gris JC, Schved JF, Neven S, et al: Impaired fibrinolytic capacity and early recurrent spontaneous abortions. Br Med J **300**:1500, 1990.

Gronroos M, Honkonen E, Punnoren R: Cervical and serum IgA and serum IgG antibodies to *Chlamydia trachomatis* and herpes simplex virus in threatened abortion: A prospective study. Br J Obstet Gynaecol **90**:167, 1983.

Guerrero R, Rojas OI: Spontaneous abortion and aging of human ova and spermatozoa. N Engl J Med **293**:573, 1975.

Gutenby PA, Cameron K, Sherman RP: Pregnancy loss with phospholipid antibodies: Improved outcome with aspirin continuing treatment. Aust N Z J Obstet Gynaecol **29**:294, 1989.

Haimovici F, Hill JA, Anderson DJ: The effects of soluble products of activated lymphocytes and macrophages on blastocyte implantation events in vitro. Biol Reprod **44**:69, 1991.

Halmesmaki E, Valimak M, Roine R, et al: Maternal and paternal alcohol consumption and miscarriage. Br J Obstet Gynaecol **96**:188, 1989.

Hamai Y, Fujii T, Yamashita T, et al: Peripheral blood mononuclear cells from women with recurrent spontaneous abortion exhibit an aberrant reaction to release cytokines upon the direct contact of human leukocyte antigen G expressing cells. Am J Reprod Immunol **40**:408, 1998.

Hanley J, McNeil B: The meaning and use of the area under a receiver operating characteristic curve (ROC). Radiology **143**:29, 1992.

Harger JH, Laifer SA, Bontempo FA, et al: Low-dose aspirin and prednisone treatment of pregnancy loss caused by lupus anticoagulants. J Perinatol **15**:46, 1995.

Harlop S, Shiono PH: Alcohol, smoking, and incidence of spontaneous abortions in the first and second trimester. Lancet **2**:173, 1980.

Harris EN: Syndrome of the black swan. Br J Rheumatol **26**:324, 1986.

Harris EN, Asherson RA, Gharavi AE, et al: Thrombocytopenia in SLE and related disorders: Association with anticardiolipin antibodies. Br J Haemotol **59**:227, 1985.

Hasegawa I, Takakuwa K, Tanaka K: The roles of oligomenorrhoea and fetal chromosomal abnormalities in spontaneous abortions. Hum Reprod **11**:2304, 1996.

Heine O, Muller-Eckhardt G: Intravenous immune globulin in recurrent abortion. Clin Exp Immunol **97**(Suppl 1):39, 1994.

Heinonen PK: Reproductive performance of women with uterine anomalies after abdominal or hysteroscopic metroplasty or no surgical treatment. J Am Assoc Gynecol Laparosc **4**:311, 1997.

Herbert CM, Hill GA, Maxson WS, et al: Case of sensitive urine pregnancy before endometrial biopsies taken in the later luteal phase. Fertil Steril **53**:162, 1990.

Hill JA: Implications of cytokines in male and female sterility. In Chaouat GA, Mowbrary JF (eds): Cellular and Molecular Biology of the Maternal-Fetal Relationship. Paris, INSERM/John Libbey Eurotext, 1991, p. 269.

Hill JA: Sporadic and recurrent spontaneous abortion. Curr Probl Obstet Gynecol Fertil **17**:114–162, 1994.

Hill JA: Immunologic factors in spontaneous abortion. In Bronson AA, Alexander NJ, Anderson DJ, et al (eds): Reproductive Immunology. Cambridge, Blackwell Science, 1996, p. 433.

Hill JA: Immunotherapy for recurrent pregnancy loss: "Standard of care or buyer beware." J Soc Gynecol Investig **4**:267–273, 1997.

Hill JA, Abbott AF, Politch JA: Sperm morphology and recurrent abortion. Fertil Steril **61**:776, 1994.

Hill JA, Anderson DJ: Blood transfusions for recurrent abortion: Is the treatment worse than the disease? Fertil Steril **46**:152, 1986.

Hill JA, Anderson DJ: Evidence for the existence and significance of immune cells and their soluble products in reproductive tissues. Immunol Allergy Clin North Am **10**:1, 1990.

Hill JA, Anderson DJ, Polgar K: T helper 1–type cellular immunity to trophoblast in women with recurrent spontaneous abortion. JAMA **273**:1933, 1995.

Hill JA, Haimovici F, Anderson DJ: Products of activated lymphocytes and macrophages inhibit mouse embryo development in vitro. J Immunol **132**:2250, 1987.

Hill JA, Melling GC, Johnson PM: Immunohistochemical studies of human uteroplacental tissues from first trimester spontaneous abortion. Am J Obstet Gynecol **173**:90, 1995.

Hill JA, Polgar K, Harlow BL, et al: Evidence of embryo and trophoblast-toxic cellular immune response(s) in women with recurrent spontaneous abortion. Am J Obstet Gynecol **166**:1044, 1992.

Hiller SL, Nugent RP, Eschenbach DA, et al: Association between bacterial vaginosis and preterm delivery of a low-birth-weight infant. N Engl J Med **335**:1737, 1995.

Homburg R, Levy T, Berkowitz D, et al: Gonadotropin-releasing hormone agonist reduces the miscarriage rate for pregnancies achieved in women with polycystic ovarian syndrome. Fertil Steril **59**:527, 1993.

Hook EB, Cross PK, Schreinemachers DM: Chromosomal abnormality rates of amniocentesis and in live-born infants. JAMA **249**:2034, 1983.

Hunter CA, Chizzonite A, Remington JS: IL-1Bis required for IL-12 to induce production of IFN-gamma by NK cells. J Immunol **155**:4347, 1995.

Ito K, Karasawa M, Kawano T, et al: Involvement of decidual V alpha 14 NK T cells in abortion. Proc Natl Acad Sci USA **97**:740, 2000.

Jaffe R, Jauniaux E, Hustin J: Maternal circulation in the first-trimester human placenta: Myth or reality? Am J Obstet Gynecol **176**:695, 1997.

Jeng GT, Scott JR, Burmeister LF: A comparison of meta-analytic results using literature vs. individual patient data. JAMA **274**:830, 1995.

Johnson MP, Drugan A, Koppitch FC, et al: Postmortem chorionic villus sampling is a better method for cytogenetic evaluation of early fetal loss than culture of abortus material. Am J Obstet Gynecol **163**:1505, 1990.

Johnson MR, Riddle AF, Grudzinskas JG, et al: The role of trophoblast dysfunction in the aetiology of miscarriage. Br J Obstet Gynaecol **100**:353, 1993.

Jones CT: Luteal phase defects. In Behrman SJ, Kistner RW (eds): Progress in Infertility. Boston, Little, Brown & Co, 1968.

Jones GES: The luteal phase defect. Fertil Steril **27**:351, 1976.

Jordan J, Craig K, Clifton DK, et al: Luteal phase defect: The sensitivity and specificity of diagnostic methods in common clinical use. Fertil Steril **62**:54, 1994.

Kabawsat SE, Mostaouti-Zedeh M, Driscoll SG, et al: Implantation site in normal pregnancy: A study with monoclonal antibodies. Am J Pathol **118**:76, 1985.

Kallioniemi A, Kallioniemi OP, Piper J, et al: Detection and mapping of amplified DNA sequences in breast cancer by comparative genomic hybridization. Proc Natl Acad Sci USA **91**:2150, 1994.

Kalter H: Diabetes and spontaneous abortion: A historical review. Am J Obstet Gynecol **150**:1243, 1987.

Kamimura S, Eguchi K, Yonezawa M, et al: Localization and developmental change of indolamine 2,3-dioxygenase activity in human placenta. Acta Med Okayama **45**:135, 1991.

Kanai T, Fujii T, Unno N, et al: Human leukocyte antigen-G expressing cells differentially modulate the release of cytokines from mononuclear cells present in the decidua versus peripheral blood. Am J Reprod Immunol **45**:94, 2001.

Karamardian LM, Grimes DA: Luteal phase deficiency: Effects of treatment on pregnancy rates. Am J Obstet Gynecol **167**:1391, 1992.

Karnfeld D, Cnattingins S, Ekbom A: Pregnancy outcomes in women with inflammatory bowel disease: A population-based cohort study. Am J Obstet Gynecol **177**:942, 1997.

Katsuragawa H, Kanzaki H, Inoue T, et al: Monoclonal antibody against phosphatidylserine inhibits in vitro human trophoblast hormone production and invasion. Biol Reprod **56**:50, 1997.

Katz I, Fisch B, Amlt S, et al: Cutaneous graft-versus-host live reaction after paternal lymphocyte immunization for prevention of recurrent abortion. Fertil Steril **57**:927, 1992.

Keller DW, Wrest WH, Askin FB, et al: Pseudocorpus luteum insufficiency: A local defect of progesterone action on endometrial stroma. Fertil Steril **48**:127, 1979.

Keltz MD, Olive DL, Kim AH, et al: Sonohysterography for screening in recurrent pregnancy loss. Fertil Steril **67**:670, 1997.

Khudr G: Cytogenetics of habitual abortion. Obstet Gynecol Surv **29**:299, 1974.

King A, Hiby SE, Gardner L, et al: Recognition of trophoblast HLA class I molecules by decidual NK cell receptors: A review. Placenta Suppl A, Trophoblast Research, **14**:S81, 2000.

Kirk EP, Chuong CJ, Coulam CB, et al: Pregnancy after metroplasty for uterine anomalies. Fertil Steril **59**:1164, 1993.

Klebanoff MA, Shiono PH, Rhodes GG: Outcomes of pregnancy in a national sample of resident physicians. N Engl J Med **323**:1040, 1990.

Klebanoff MA, Shiono PH, Rhodes GG: Spontaneous and induced abortion among resident physicians. JAMA **265**:2821, 1991.

Kline J, Stein Z, Susser M, et al: Environmental influences in early reproductive loss in a current New York City study. *In* Porter IHM, Hook HB (eds): Human Embryonic and Fetal Death. New York, Academic Press, 1980.

Kong TY, Liddell R, Robertson WB: Detective haemochorial placentation as a cause of miscarriage: A preliminary study. Br J Obstet Gynaecol **94**:649, 1987.

Kundsin RB, Driscoll SC: Strain of mycoplasma associated with human reproductive failure. Science **157**:1573, 1967.

Kundsin RB, Driscoll SC, Pelletier PA: *Ureaplasma urealyticum* incriminated in perinatal morbidity and mortality. Science **213**:474, 1981.

Kutteh WH: Antiphospholipid antibody–associated recurrent pregnancy loss: Treatment with heparin and low-dose aspirin vs. superior to low-dose aspirin alone. Am J Obstet Gynecol **174**:1584, 1996.

Kutteh WH, Ermel LD: A clinical trial for the treatment of antiphospholipid antibody associated recurrent pregnancy loss with lower dose heparin and aspirin. Am J Reprod Immunol **35**:402, 1996.

Kutteh WH, Stovall DW, Scott JR: The immunologic diagnosis and treatment of recurrent pregnancy loss. Infertil Reprod Med Clin North Am **8**:267, 1997.

Kutteh WH, Yetman DL, Chantilis SJ, et al: Effect of antiphospholipid antibodies in women undergoing in vitro fertilization: Role of heparin and aspirin. Hum Reprod **12**:1171, 1997.

Kwak JY, Beaman KP, Gilman-Sachs A, et al: Up-regulated expression of CD56+, CD56+/CD16+, and DC19+ cells in peripheral blood lymphocytes in pregnant women with recurrent pregnancy loss. Am J Reprod Immunol **34**:93, 1995.

Kyle PM, Sepuleda W, Blunt S, et al: High failure rate of postmortem karyotyping after termination for fetal abnormality. Obstet Gynecol **88**:859, 1996.

Labarrere CA, Althabe OH: Hypothesis: Primary chronic abortion, preeclampsia, idiopathic intrauterine growth retardation, hydatidiform mole and choriocarcinoma: A unique concept. Am J Reprod Immunol **10**:156, 1986.

Lachapelle MH, Miron P, Hemmings R, et al: Endometrial T, B and NK cells in patients with recurrent spontaneous abortion: Altered profile and pregnancy outcome. J Immunol **156**:4027, 1996.

Laird T, Whittaker PG: The endocrinology of early pregnancy failure. *In* Huisjes HJ, Lind T (eds): Early Pregnancy Failure. New York, Churchill Livingstone, 1990, p. 39.

Laskin CA, Bombardier C, Hannah ME, et al: Prednisone and oral aspirin in women with autoantibodies and unexplained recurrent fetal loss. N Engl J Med **357**:148, 1997.

Laufer M, Ecker JL, Hill JA: Pregnancy outcome following ultrasound documented fetal cardiac activity in women with a history of multiple spontaneous abortions. J Soc Gynecol Invest **1**:138, 1994.

Lea RG, al-Sharekh N, Tulppala M, et al: The immunolocalization of bcl-2 at the maternal-fetal interface in healthy and failing pregnancies. Hum Reprod **12**:153, 1997.

Lebo RV, Flandermeyer RR, Diukman R, et al: Prenatal diagnosis with repetitive in situ hybridization probes. Am J Med Genet **43**:848, 1992.

Lejeune B, Grun JP, DeNager PA, et al: Antithyroid antibodies underlying thyroid abnormalities and miscarriage or pregnancy induced hypertension. Br J Obstet Gynaecol **100**:669, 1983.

Letterie GS, Haggerty M, Lindee G: A comparison of pelvic ultrasound and magnetic resonance imaging as diagnostic studies for müllerian tract abnormalities. Int J Fertil Menopausal Stud **40**:34, 1995.

Li TC, Dockery P, Cooke ID: Endometrial development in the luteal phase of women with various types of infertility: Comparison with women of normal fertility. Hum Reprod **6**:325, 1991.

Liddell HS, Pattison NS, Zanderigo A: Recurrent miscarriage: Outcome after supportive care in early pregnancy. Aust N Z J Obstet Gynaecol **31**:320, 1991.

Lindbohm MJ, Heitanen M, Kyyronen P, et al: Magnetic fields of video display terminals and spontaneous abortion. Am J Epidemiol **136**:1041, 1992.

Lishner M, Amato D, Frine D: Different outcomes of pregnancy in women with essential thrombocytosis. J Med Sci **29**:100, 1993.

Llhahi-Camp JM, Rai R, Ison C, et al: Association of bacterial vaginosis with a history of second trimester miscarriage. Hum Reprod **11**:1575, 1996.

Lockshin MD: Antiphospholipid antibody syndrome? Rheum Dis Clin North Am **20**:45, 1994.

Lockshin MD, Druzin ML, Qamar T: Prednisone does not prevent recurrent fetal death in women with antiphospholipid antibody. Am J Obstet Gynecol **160**:439, 1989.

Lockwood C, Romero R, Feinberg R, et al: The prevalence and significance of lupus anticoagulant and cardiolipin antibodies in a general obstetric population. Am J Obstet Gynecol **161**:369, 1989.

Lolis D, Tzigounis V, Michalas S, et al: Toxoplasma antibodies and spontaneous abortion. Int J Gynaecol Obstet **15**:229, 1978.

Lopata A, Sathanathan AH, McBain JC, et al: The ultrastructure of the preovulatory human egg fertilized in vitro. Fertil Steril **33**:12, 1980.

Lubba WF, Butler WS, Palmer SJ, et al: Fetal survival after prednisone suppression of maternal lupus anticoagulant. Lancet **1**:1361, 1983.

MacDonald IA: Incompetent cervix as a cause of recurrent abortion. J Obstet Gynaecol Br Commonw **70**:105, 1963.

Maher JE, Davis RO, Goldenberg RL, et al: Unexplained elevation in maternal serum alpha-fetoprotein and subsequent fetal loss. Obstet Gynecol **83**:138, 1984.

Mandel SJ, Brent GA, Larsen PR: Preview of antithyroid drug use during pregnancy and report of a case of aplasia cutis. Thyroid **4**:129, 1994.

Maneschi F, Zupi E, Marconi D, et al: Hysteroscopically detected asymptomatic mullerian anomalies: Prevalence and reproductive implications. J Reprod Med **40**:684, 1995.

March CM: Intrauterine adhesions. Obstet Gynecol Clin North Am **22**:491, 1995.

March CM, Israel R: Hysteroscopic management of recurrent abortion caused by septate uterus: With discussion. Am J Obstet Gynecol **156**:834, 1987.

Marcus S, Al Shawaf T, Brinsden P: The obstetric outcome of in vitro fertilization and embryo transfer in women with congenital uterine malformation. Am J Obstet Gynecol **175**:85, 1996.

Marqusee E, Hill JA, Mandel SJ: Thyroiditis after pregnancy loss. J Clin Endocrinol Metab **82**:2455, 1997.

Martin-Deleon PA, Boice ML: Sperm aging in the male and cytogenic anomalies: An animal model. Hum Genet **62**:70, 1982.

Marzi M, Vigano A, Trabattoni D, et al: Characterization of type 1 and type 2 cytokine production profile in physiologic and pathologic human pregnancy. Clin Exp Immunol **106**:127, 1996.

Mattison DR: Minimizing toxic hazards to fetal health. Contemp Ob Gyn **8**:81, 1992.

Mauro T, Katayama K, Matuso H, et al: The role of maternal thyroid hormones in maintaining early pregnancy in threatened abortion. Acta Endocrinol **127**:118, 1992.

Mazzaferri EL: Evaluation and management of common thyroid disorders in women. Am J Obstet Gynecol **176**:507, 1997.

Meier AH, Wilson JM: Tryptophan feeding adversely influences pregnancy. Life Sci **32**:1193, 1983.

Mellor AL, Munn DH: Immunology at the maternal-fetal interface: Lessons for T cell tolerance and suppression. Ann Rev Immunol **18**:367, 2000.

Miles RA, Paulson RJ, Lobo RA, et al: Pharmacokinetics and endometrial tissue levels of progesterone after administration by intramuscular and vaginal routes: A comparative study. Fertil Steril **62**:485, 1994.

Miller JF, Williamson E, Glue J, et al: Fetal loss after implantation: A prospective study. Lancet **2**:554, 1980.

Mills JL, Simpson JL, Driscoll SE, et al: Incidence of abortion among normal women and insulin-dependent diabetic women whose pregnancies were identified within 21 days of conception. N Engl J Med **319**:1617, 1988.

Milunsky A, Ulcickas M, Rothman KJ, et al: Maternal heat exposure and neural tube defects. JAMA **268**:882, 1992.

Mitus AJ, Schafer AI: Thrombocytosis and thrombocythemia. Hematol Oncol Clin North Am **4**:157, 1990.

Monlias R, Prost J, Wanga A: Age related increase in autoantibodies. Lancet **1**:1128, 1984.

Mowbray JF, Gibbings C, Liddell H, et al: Controlled trial of treatment of recurrent spontaneous abortion by immunostimulation with paternal cells. Lancet **2**:941, 1985.

Munn DH, Zhou M, Atwood JT, et al: Prevention of allogenic fetal rejection by tryptophan catabolism. Science **281**:1191, 1998.

Munne S, Magli C, Bahoe M, et al: Preimplantation diagnosis of the aneuploidies most commonly found in spontaneous abortions and live births: X,Y,13,14,15,16,18,21,22. Prenat Diag **18**:1459, 1998.

Munne S, Wells D. Preimplantation genetic diagnosis. Curr Opin Obstet Gynecol **14**:239, 2002.

Nahmias AJ, Josey WE, Naib ZM, et al: Perinatal risk associated with maternal genital herpes simplex virus infection. Am J Obstet Gynecol **110**:825, 1971.

Nakajima ST, Molloy MH, Oi KH, et al: Clinical evaluation of luteal function. Obstet Gynecol **84**:219, 1994.

Nelson-Piercy C, Letsky EA, de Swiet M: Low-molecular-weight heparin for obstetric thromboprophylaxis: Experience of sixty-nine pregnancies in sixty-one women at high risk. Am J Obstet Gynecol **176**:1062, 1997.

Nora JJ, Nora H, Blu J, et al: Exogenous progesterone and estrogen implicated in birth defects. JAMA **240**:837, 1978.

Noyes RW, Hertig AT, Rock J: Dating the endometrial biopsy. Fertil Steril **1**:3, 1950.

Ober C, Karrison T, Odem RR, et al: Mononuclear-cell immunization in prevention of recurrent miscarriages: A randomized trial. Lancet **354**:365, 1999.

Ober C, Steck T, Van der Van K, et al: MHC class II compatibility in abortal fetuses and term infants of couples with recurrent spontaneous abortion. J Reprod Immunol **25**:195, 1993.

Olive DL, Haney AF: Endometriosis-associated infertility: A critical review of therapeutic approaches. Obstet Gynecol Surv **50**:538, 1986.

Oriss TB, McCarthy SA, Morel BF, et al: Crossregulation between T helper cell (Th)1 and Th2: Inhibition of Th2 proliferation by IFN-gamma involves interference with IL-1. J Immunol **158**:3666, 1997.

Oshiro BT, Silver RM, Scott JR, et al: Antiphospholipid antibodies and fetal death. Obstet Gynecol **87**:489, 1996.

Out HJ, Kooijman CD, Bruinse HW, et al: Histopathological findings in placentae from patients with intrauterine fetal death and antiphospholipid antibodies. Eur J Obstet Gynecol Reprod Biol **41**:179, 1991.

Ouyang D, Hill JA: Leiomyomas, pregnancy and pregnancy loss. Infert Reprod Med Clin N Am **13**:325, 2002.

Patton PE: Anatomic uterine defects. Clin Obstet Gynecol **37**:705, 1994.

Paul M, Kurtz S: Reproductive Hazards in the Work Place. Worcester, Mass, University of Massachusetts Medical Center, Occupational and Environmental Reproductive Hazards Center, 1990.

Pegoraro E, Whitaker J, Mowery-Rushton P, et al: Familial skewed X inactivation: A molecular trait associated with high spontaneous-abortion rate maps to Xq28. Am J Hum Genet **61**:160, 1997.

Pellerito J, McCarthy S, Doyle M, et al: Diagnosis of uterine anomalies: Relative accuracy of MRI, endovaginal sonography, and hysterosalpingography. Genitourin Radiol **183**:795, 1992.

Pennell RG, Neederman L, Pajak T, et al: Prospective comparison of vaginal and abdominal sonography in normal early pregnancy. J Ultrasound Med **10**:63, 1991.

Perino A, Vassiliadis A, Vucetich A, et al: Short-term therapy for recurrent abortion using intravenous immunoglobulins: Results of a double-blind placebo-controlled Italian study. Hum Reprod **12**:2388, 1997.

Petri M: Pathogenesis and treatment of the antiphospholipid antibody syndrome. Med Clin North Am **81**:151, 1997.

Petri M, Golbus M, Anderson R, et al: Antinuclear antibody, lupus anticoagulant, and anticardiolipin antibody in women with idiopathic habitual abortion. Arthritis Rheum **30**:601, 1987.

Petri M, Howard D, Repke J: Frequency of lupus flare in pregnancy: The Hopkins Lupus Pregnancy Center experience. Arthritis Rheum **34**:1538, 1991.

Piccini MP, Boleni L, Liu C, et al: Defective production of both leukemia inhibiting factor and type 2 cytokine production by decidual T cells in unexplained recurrent abortion. Nat Med **4**:1020, 1998.

Polifka JE, Friedman JM: Environmental toxins and recurrent pregnancy loss. Infertil Reprod Med Clin North Am **2**:175, 1991.

Polson DW, Wedsworth J, Adams J, et al: Polycystic ovaries: A common finding in normal women. Lancet **2**:870, 1980.

Pratt D, Nowtry M, Kaberlein G, et al: Antithyroid antibodies and the association in nonspecific antibodies in recurrent pregnancy loss. Am J Obstet Gynecol **168**:837, 1993.

Probst AM, Hill JA: Anatomic factors associated with recurrent pregnancy loss. Semin Reprod Med **18**:341, 2000.

Pruyn Goldstein RR, Croughan MS, Robertson PA: Neonatal outcomes in immediate versus delayed conceptions after spontaneous abortion: A retrospective case series. Am J Obstet Gynecol **186**:1230, 2002.

Quenby S, Farquharson RG: Human chorionic gonadotropin supplementation in recurrent pregnancy loss: A controlled trial. Fertil Steril **62**:708, 1994.

Racowsky C, Kaufman ML: Nuclear degeneration and meiotic aberrations observed in human oocytes in vitro: Analysis by light microscopy. Fertil Steril **58**:750, 1992.

Rae R, Smith IW, Liston WA, et al: Chlamydial serologic studies and recurrent spontaneous abortion. Am J Obstet Gynecol **170**:782, 1994.

Raghupathy R, Makhseed M, Azizieh F, et al: Maternal Th1 and Th2 type reactivity to placental antigens in normal human pregnancy and unexplained recurrent spontaneous abortion. Cell Immunol **196**:122, 1999.

Rai R, Backos M, Baxter N, et al: Recurrent miscarriage—an aspirin a day? Hum Reprod **15**:2220, 2000.

Rai R, Cohen HR, Dave M, et al: Randomized controlled trial of aspirin and aspirin plus heparin in pregnant women with recurrent miscarriage associated with phospholipid antibodies (or antiphospholipid antibodies). BMJ **314**:253, 1997.

Rai R, Regan L, Hadley E, et al: Second-trimester pregnancy loss is associated with activated C resistance. Br J Haematol **92**:489, 1996.

Rand JH, Wu XX, Andre HAM, et al: Pregnancy loss in the antiphospholipid antibody syndrome—a possible thrombogenic mechanism. N Engl J Med **337**:154, 1997.

Rankin EC, Choy EH, Kassimos D, et al: The therapeutic effects of engineered human anti-tumor necrosis factor-alpha antibody (CDP571) in rheumatoid arthritis. Br J Rheumatol **34**:334, 1995.

Raziel A, Arieli S, Bukovsky I, et al: Investigation of the uterine cavity in recurrent aborters. Fertil Steril **62**:1080, 1994.

Raziel A, Harmon A, Stressburger D, et al: The outcome of in vitro fertilization in unexplained habitual aborters concurrent with secondary infertility. Fertil Steril **67**:88, 1997.

Recurrent Miscarriage Immunotherapy Trialists Group: Worldwide Collaborative Observational Study and meta-analysis on allogenic leukocyte immunotherapy for recurrent spontaneous abortion. Am J Reprod Immunol **32**:55, 1994.

Regan L: Recurrent miscarriage. BMJ **302**:543, 1991.

Regan L, Brande PR, Hill DP: A prospective study of the incidence, time of, appearance of, significance of anti-paternal lymphocytotoxic antibodies in human pregnancy. Hum Reprod **6**:294, 1981.

Regan L, Brande PR, Trembath PL: Influence of postreproductive performance on risk of spontaneous abortion. BMJ **299**:541, 1989.

Regan JA, Klebanoff MA, Nugent RP, et al: Colonization with group B streptococci in pregnancy and adverse outcome. Am J Obstet Gynecol **174**:1354, 1996.

Regan L, Owen EJ, Jacobs HS: Hypersecretion of luteinizing hormone, infertility and miscarriage. Lancet **336**:1141, 1990.

Remohi J, Gallardo E, Levy M, et al: Oocyte donation in women with recurrent pregnancy loss. Hum Reprod **11**:2048, 1996.

Reubinoff BE, Shushan A: Preimplantation diagnosis in older patients: To biopsy or not to biopsy? Hum Reprod 11:2071, 1996.

Rice JP, Kay HH, Mahony BS: The clinical significance of uterine leiomyomas in pregnancy. Am J Obstet Gynecol 160:1212, 1989.

Rigal D, Vermot-Desroches C, Heitz S, et al: Effects of intravenous immunoglobulins on peripheral blood B, NK, and T cell subpopulations in women with recurrent spontaneous abortions: Specific effects on LFA-1 and CD56 molecules. Clin Immunol Immunopathol 71:309, 1994.

Rocklin RE, Kitzmiller JL, Carpenter CB, et al: Maternal-fetal relation: Absence of an immunologic blocking factor from serum of women with chronic abortion. N Engl J Med 295:1209, 1976.

Rocklin RE, Kitzmiller JR, Garvey MR: Maternal-fetal relation: Further characterization of an immunologic blocking factor that develops during pregnancy. Clin Immunol Immunopathol 22:305, 1982.

Rodger C: Lack of a requirement for a maternal humoral immune response to establish and maintain successful allogenic pregnancy. Transplantation 40:372, 1985.

Roesler M, Wise L, Katayama UP: Karyotype analysis of blighted ova in pregnancies achieved by in vitro fertilization. Fertil Steril 51:1065, 1989.

Romagnani S: Human Th1 and Th2 subsets: Doubt no prose. Immunol Today 8:256, 1991.

Romero R, Mazor M: Infection and preterm labor. Clin Obstet Gynecol 31:553, 1988.

Rosenbusch B, Strehler E, Sterzik D: Cytogenetics of human spermatozoa: Correlation with sperm morphology and age of fertile men. Fertil Steril 58:1071, 1992.

Rosner F, Grunwald HW: Thrombocytosis and spontaneous abortion. Am J Hematol 27:233, 1988.

Ross HA, Exalto N, Kloppanberg PW, et al: Thyroid hormone binding in early pregnancy and the risk of spontaneous abortion. Eur J Obstet Gynecol Reprod Biol 32:129, 1989.

Ruiz JE, Kwak JY, Baum L, et al: Intravenous immunoglobulin inhibits natural killer cell activity in vivo in women with recurrent spontaneous abortion. Am J Reprod Immunol 35:370, 1996.

Runia R, Lockwood CJ, Ma Y, et al: Expression of Fas ligand by human cytotrophoblast: Implications in placentation and fetal survival. J Clin Endocrinol Metab 81:3119, 1996.

Sahwi SY, Zaki MS, Haiba NY, et al: Toxoplasmosis as a cause of repeated abortion. J Obstet Gynaecol 21:145, 1995.

Salafia C, Maier D, Vogel C, et al: Placental and decidual histology in spontaneous abortion: Detailed description and correlation with chromosome number. Obstet Gynecol 82:295, 1993.

Salafia CM, Burnes JP: The correlation of placental and decidual histology with karyotype and fetal viability. Teratology 39:478, 1989.

Salem HT, Ghoneimah SA, Shouber MM, et al: Prognostic value of biochemical tests in the assessment of fetal outcome in threatened abortion. Br J Obstet Gynaecol 91:382, 1984.

Sargent IL, Wilkins T, Redman CWG: Maternal immune responses to the fetus in early pregnancy and recurrent miscarriage. Lancet 2:1099, 1994.

Sbracia S, Cozza G, Grasso JA, et al: Sera parameters and sperm morphology in men in unexplained recurrent spontaneous abortion, before and during a 3 year follow-up period. Hum Reprod 11:117, 1996.

Schagen van Leeunen JH, Christians GCML, Googenrand TU: Recurrent abortion and the diagnosis of Wilson disease. Obstet Gynecol 78:547, 1991.

Schrocksnadel H, Baier-Bitterlich G, Dapunt O, et al: Decreased plasma tryptophan in pregnancy. Obstet Gynecol 88:47, 1996.

Schust D, Hill JA: Correlation of serum cytokine and adhesion molecule determinations with pregnancy outcome. J Soc Gynecol Invest 3:259, 1996.

Schust DJ, Hill AB, Ploegh HL: Herpes simplex virus blocks intracellular transport of HLA-G in placentally derived human cells. J Immunol 157:3375, 1996.

Schved J, Gris JC, Neven S, et al: Factor XII congenital deficiency and early spontaneous abortion. Fertil Steril 52:335, 1989.

Scott JR: Recurrent miscarriage: Overview and recommendations. Clin Obstet Gynecol 37:768, 1994.

Shafer AI: The hypercoagulable states. Ann Intern Med 102:814, 1985.

Shafer W: Role of uterine adhesions in the cause of multiple pregnancy losses. Clin Obstet Gynecol 29:912, 1986.

Shaw FM, Reinus JF, Leikin EL, et al: Recurrent chorioamnionitis and second-trimester abortion because of an enterouterine fistula. Obstet Gynecol 86:639, 1995.

Shirodkar VN: A new method of operative treatment for habitual aborters in the second trimester. Antiseptic 59:68, 1955.

Siegler AM: Hysterosalpingography. Fertil Steril 40:139, 1983.

Siiteri PK, Febres F, Clemens LE, et al: Progesterone and maintenance of pregnancy: Is progesterone nature's immunosuppressant? Ann NY Acad Sci 286:384, 1977.

Silver RK, MacGregor SW, Sholl JS, et al: A comparative trial of prednisone plus aspirin versus aspirin alone in the treatment of anticardiolipin antibody positive obstetric patients. Am J Obstet Gynecol 169:1411, 1993.

Simpson JL, Martin AO: Parental diagnosis of cytogenetic disorders. Clin Obstet Gynecol 19:841, 1970.

Singh A, Dentas ZN, Stone SC, et al: Presence of thyroid antibodies in early reproductive failure: Biochemical versus clinical pregnancies. Fertil Steril 62:277, 1995.

Smith DW, Clarren SK, Harvey MA: Hyperthermia as a possible teratogenic agent. J Pediatr 92:878, 1978.

Sompolinsky D, Solomon F, Elkina L, et al: Inactions with mycoplasma and bacteria in induced midtrimester and fetal loss. Am J Obstet Gynecol 121:610, 1975.

Soules MR, Clifton DK, Cohen NL, et al: Luteal phase deficiency: Abnormal gonadotropins and progesterone secretion patterns. J Clin Endocrinol Metab 69:813, 1989.

Soules MR, Clifton DK, Steiner RA, et al: The corpus luteum: Determinants of progesterone secretion in the normal menstrual cycle. Obstet Gynecol 71:659, 1988.

Soules MR, McLachlan RI, Ek M, et al: Luteal phase defect: Characteristics of reproductive hormones over the menstrual cycle. J Clin Endocrinol Metab 69:804, 1989.

Soules MR, Wiebe RH, Alesel S, et al: The diagnosis and therapy of luteal phase deficiency. Fertil Steril 28:1033, 1997.

Stagnaro-Green A, Roman SH, Colin RH, et al: Detection of at risk pregnancy by means of highly sensitive assays for thyroid autoantibodies. JAMA 264:1421, 1990.

Steck T, Van der Ven K, Kwak K, et al: HLA-DQA1 and HLA-DQB1 haplotypes in aborted fetuses and couples with recurrent spontaneous abortion. J Reprod Immunol 29:95, 1995.

Steier JA, Bergsijo P, Myking OL: Human chorionic gonadotropin in maternal plasma after induced abortion, spontaneous abortion and removed ectopic pregnancy. Obstet Gynecol 64:391, 1984.

Stephensen MD: Frequency of factors associated with habitual abortion in 197 couples. Fertil Steril 66:24, 1996.

Stephenson MD, Wu V, MacKinnon M, et al: Standardization of flow cytometric cross match (FCXM) for investigation of unexplained habitual abortion. Am J Reprod Immunol 33:1, 1995.

Stern JJ, Dorzman A, Gutiercz-Nagar AJ, et al: Frequency of abnormal karyotypes among abortuses from women with and without a history of recurrent spontaneous abortion. Fertil Steril 65:250, 1996.

Stewart DR, Overstreet JW, Nakajima ST, et al: Enhanced ovarian steroid secretion before implantation in early human pregnancy. J Clin Endocrinol Metab 76:1470, 1993.

Stray-Pedersen B, Eng J, Reikram TM: Uterine T-mycoplasma colonization in reproductive failure. Am J Obstet Gynecol 130:307, 1978.

Stray-Pedersen B, Stray-Pedersen S: Etiologies and subsequent reproductive performance in 195 couples with a prior history of habitual abortion. Am J Obstet Gynecol 148:140, 1984.

Summers PR: Microbiology relevant to recurrent miscarriage. Clin Obstet Gynecol 37:722, 1994.

Svinarich DM, Bitoni OM, Romero R, et al: Induction and posttranslational expression of cytokines in a first-trimester trophoblast cell line by lipopolysaccharide. Am J Obstet Gynecol 175:970, 1996.

Taylor C, Faulk MP: Preventing recurrent abortion with leukocyte transfusions. Lancet 40:372, 1981.

Taylor PJ, Cumming DC: Hysteroscopy in 100 patients. Fertil Steril 31:301, 1979.

Thellin O, Coumans B, Zorzi W, et al: Tolerance of the feto-placental "graft"; ten ways to support a child for nine months. Curr Opin Immunol 12:731, 2000.

Thorton CA, Bellow M: Safety of intravenous immunoglobulin. Arch Neurol 50:135, 1993.

Tichenor JR, Bledsoe LB, Opsahl MS, et al: Activation of complement in humans with a first-trimester pregnancy loss. Gynecol Obstet Invest 39:79, 1995.

Torpin R: Placenta circumvallata and placenta marginata. Obstet Gynecol 6:277, 1955.

Treffers PE: Uterine causes of early pregnancy failure: A critical evaluation. In Huisjes HJ, Lind T (eds): Early Pregnancy Failure. New York, Churchill Livingstone, 1990, p. 114.

Valle RF: Hysteroscopy in the evaluation of female infertility. Am J Obstet Gynecol 137:425, 1980.

Vassiliadou N, Bulmer JN: Characterization of endometrial T lymphocyte subpopulations in spontaneous early pregnancy loss. Hum Reprod **13**:44, 1998.

Vercellini P, Fedele L, Arcaini L, et al: Value of intrauterine device insertion and estrogen administration after hysteroscopic metroplasty. J Reprod Med **34**:447, 1989.

Vince GS, Johnson PM. Leukocyte populations and cytokine regulation in human uteroplacental tissues. Biochem Soc Trans **28**:191, 2000.

Von Wolff M, Thaler CJ, Strowitzki T, et al: Regulated expression of cytokines in human endometrium throughout the menstrual cycle: dysregulation in habitual abortion. Mol Hum Reprod **6**:627, 2000.

Wagenknecht DR, Green KM, McIntyre JA: Analysis of HLA-DQ alleles in recurrent spontaneous abortion couples. Am J Reprod Immunol **37**:1, 1997.

Warburton D, Kline J, Stein Z, Strobino B: Cytogenetic abnormalities in spontaneous abortions of recognized conceptions. *In* Porter IH, Hatcher N, Willey A (eds): Perinatal Genetics. New York, Academic Press, 1986, p. 23.

Wegman TG, Lin H, Gilbert L, et al: Bidirectional cytokine interactions in the maternal-fetal relationship: Is successful pregnancy a Th2 phenomena? Immunol Today **14**:353, 1993.

Weitz JI: Low-molecular-weight heparins. N Engl J Med **337**:688, 1997.

Wentz AC, Herbert CM III, Maxson WS, et al: Cycle of conception endometrial biopsy. Fertil Steril **46**:196, 1986.

Wilcox AJ, Weinberg CR, O'Connor JF, et al: Incidence of early loss of pregnancy. N Engl J Med **319**:188, 1988.

Witkin SS: Immune pathogenesis of asymptomatic *Chlamydia trachomatis* infections in the female genital tract. Infect Dis Obstet Gynecol **3**:169, 1995.

Wolf GC, Harger EO III: Indications for examination of spontaneous abortion specimens: A reassessment. Am J Obstet Gynecol **175**:1364, 1995.

Wolf GC, Mao J, Izquierdo L, et al: Paternal pericentric inversion of chromosome 4 as a cause of recurrent pregnancy loss. J Med Genet **31**:153, 1994.

Wouters MGAJ, Broers GHJ, Blom HJ, et al: Hyperhomocysteinemia: A risk factor in women with unexplained recurrent early pregnancy loss. Fertil Steril **60**:820, 1993.

Yamada H, Polgar K, Hill JA: Cell-mediated immunity to trophoblast antigens in women with recurrent spontaneous abortion. Am J Obstet Gynecol **170**:1339, 1994.

Yen SSC: The polycystic ovary syndrome. Clin Endocrinol (Oxf) **12**:177, 1980.

Yetman DL, Kutteh WH: Antiphospholipid antibody panels and recurrent pregnancy loss: Prevalence of anticardiolipin antibodies compared with other antiphospholipid antibodies. Fertil Steril **66**:540, 1996.

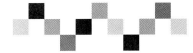

Chapter 33

ABNORMAL CERVICAL COMPETENCE

Jay D. Iams, MD

Few subjects in obstetrics generate as much controversy as does abnormal cervical competence, or *cervical incompetence*, a term that describes a presumed weakness of the cervix that causes loss of an otherwise healthy pregnancy, usually in the second trimester. Despite recent research, the definition, pathophysiology, clinical presentation, and management of this disorder remain controversial. An historical overview provides insight into the current state of knowledge.

Cole and Culpepper are credited with recognition of cervical incompetence as a clinical entity in 1658 in a text entitled *Practice of Physick*. They described cervical incompetence as a condition in which "the orifice of the womb is so slack that it cannot rightly contract itself to keep in the seed; which is chiefly caused by abortion, or hard labor and childbirth, whereby the fibers of the womb are broken in pieces one from another and they, and the inner orifice of the womb, overmuch slackened." This initial description attributed a physical injury to the "fibers of the womb" as the cause, with a corresponding physical, i.e., surgical, treatment. To the present day, treatment of cervical incompetence has been principally surgical rather than medical, based on the concept of a purely physical deficit in the strength of the cervical tissue that is either congenital or acquired. Reports of surgical repair appeared at the end of the nineteenth century. Palmer and La Comme (1948) and Lash and Lash (1950) reported surgical operations to repair anatomic defects in the nonpregnant cervix. Shirodkar (1955) and McDonald (1957) introduced methods of transvaginal cervico-isthmic repair, called *cerclage*, that remain the most commonly used procedures to treat cervical incompetence during pregnancy. In 1965, a transabdominal approach for the placement of a cerclage was described for patients in whom the transvaginal approach had failed, or in whom cervical scarring or congenital abnormality was so severe as to make the transvaginal approach technically impossible (Benson and Durfee, 1965). Modifications of these procedures and adjunctive therapy with antimicrobials and tocolytics have been proposed, but the basic techniques of surgical treatment have not changed.

Ongoing controversies surrounding both diagnosis and treatment derive from the inconsistent success of cerclage to correct the clinical syndrome of recurrent second-trimester pregnancy loss. This inconsistency is evident in both anecdote—the patient with a history of "cervical incompetence" who delivers at term without a cerclage is not rare—and research reports of conflicting results. Evidence of benefit for cerclage rests primarily on favorable anecdote and reports of comparisons of pregnancy outcomes before and after cerclage in women with a history of recurrent second-trimester delivery following painless cervical dilation. The randomized trials that have been conducted enrolled women with suspicious obstetrical histories and/or clinical and ultrasound evidence of early cervical effacement; these too have shown mixed outcomes. There has never been a randomized trial of cerclage versus no therapy or cerclage versus medical therapy (e.g., bed rest) in women with the classic history of painless dilation leading to recurrent second-trimester loss.

Given this background, controversy about the diagnosis and treatment of cervical incompetence is clearly due to an incomplete understanding of cervical function in pregnancy: Why and how does the cervix efface? Is the process the same at 20 weeks' as at 30 or 40 weeks' gestation? Recent clinical, biochemical, and ultrasound studies of the cervix have broadened our understanding of cervical performance as a continuous rather than a categorical variable, in which cervical effacement occurs more slowly than was previously thought, and in response to stimuli other than uterine contractions or physical weakness. Abnormal cervical competence is increasingly understood as a syndrome with several clinical presentations that lead to early preterm birth. This in turn has led to revised criteria for the diagnosis of reduced or absent cervical competence and to a reevaluation of the appropriate role of cerclage.

DEFINITION OF CERVICAL COMPETENCE

The task of the cervix is first to retain the conceptus until maturity and later to dilate sufficiently to allow delivery of the mature infant. The ability to perform these functions repeatedly in successive pregnancies is called cervical competence. Though now seen as incomplete, the earlier concept of competence as a categorical variable in which the cervix is either fully functional (competent) or nonfunctional (incompetent) has been the cornerstone of diagnosis. The diagnosis has traditionally been made and is still most confidently established by an obstetric history of recurrent passive and painless dilation of the cervix in the second trimester. This classic picture was once thought to be the only true presentation, distinct from other causes of early preterm delivery (such as preterm labor). The idea that cervical competence might function as a continuous variable was proposed by Parikh and Mehta (1961), who used digital examination to assess cervical dilation and length in women with a history of midtrimester birth. They ". . . wondered whether there can be any degrees in the incompetence of the internal os. If an incompetent os can cause abortion, is it possible that a lesser degree of incompetency . . . can lead to premature labour?" The results of digital cervical examination in 655 pregnant women led these authors to conclude that "A degree of incompetence of the internal os that would lead to a premature labour does not seem to exist." Two subsequent lines of inquiry, however, have overturned that conclusion.

The first was a reconsideration of whether the characteristic clinical presentation of incompetent cervix might be fortuitous, i.e., that some women with a passively dilated cervix could develop contractions, intra-amniotic infection, or membrane rupture *after* the cervix had dilated passively and thus present for care with an atypical chief complaint. To evaluate this hypothesis, women with a history of second-trimester delivery not typical of cervical incompetence were treated with prophylactic cerclage (Crombleholme et al., 1983), and benefit was inferred compared with historical controls. Neither of two subsequent randomized trials of cerclage in women with a history of preterm birth, however, found any benefit to cerclage (Lazar et al., 1984; Rush et al., 1984). In fact, the rate of complications was increased with cerclage. The Medical Research Council/Royal College of Obstetricians and Gynaecologists (MacNaughton et al., 1993) Working Party on Cervical Cerclage enrolled 1292 women whose physicians were not certain whether cerclage was indicated into a prospective randomized trial of prophylactic cerclage. Women with a history typical of cervical incompetence were not enrolled. There were significantly fewer births before 33 weeks in the cerclage group than in the control group (13% versus 17%) and fewer very-low-birth-weight infants (10% versus 13%), but there was no significant difference in the frequency of preterm births between 33 and 36 weeks, and the cerclage group experienced a higher incidence of pyrexia and medical complications. The MRC study confirmed the absence of benefit of cerclage for women with a prior preterm birth, but the suggestion of benefit for a few gave some credence to the idea that the clinical presentations of cervical incompetence might be diverse.

ULTRASOUND STUDIES OF THE CERVIX IN PREGNANCY

The second line of inquiry has come from ultrasound images of the cervix generated with transabdominal, transperineal, and endovaginal transducers. These studies caused a reassessment of the role of the cervix in premature birth in general (see Chapter 34) and of cervical incompetence in particular. Early studies used transabdominal sonography (Brook et al., 1981; Michaels et al., 1986), a technique that requires a full maternal bladder to visualize the cervix (Confino et al., 1986) and thus introduces unpredictable measurement artifact (Mason and Maresh, 1990; Andersen, 1991). These observations have been confirmed by the more reproducible images obtained with transvaginal and translabial ultrasound probes. Transvaginal imaging of the cervix is now considered to be the standard method (Laing et al., 2000). There is disagreement about the reproducibility of translabial imaging of the cervix (Kurtzman et al., 1998; Owen et al., 1999; Carr et al., 2000;

Hertzberg et al., 2001; Cicero et al., 2001). Translabial sonography is an alternative when endovaginal sonography is deemed unwise, e.g., in women with preterm premature rupture of fetal membranes (PROM) or bleeding. Figure 33-1 depicts the image that is generated by placing the endovaginal probe in the anterior vaginal fornix. The technique used to measure the cervix is important. The standard method used in most studies (Iams et al., 1996; Taipale and Hiilesmaa, 1998; Hibbard, Tart, et al., 2000) employs endovaginal sonography and the "shortest best" technique of cervical measurement, in which initial measurements are ignored until the same length is generated repeatedly with the least pressure applied to the cervix to obtain a good image of the endocervical canal (Iams et al., 1995; Yost et al., 1999). Use of alternate methods generates longer measurements that may not be reproducible (Gramellini et al., 2002).

Measurement of Cervical Length in Pregnancy

Normative values have been established for the length of the cervix in the second and third trimesters of pregnancy as measured by transvaginal ultrasonography (Kushnir et al., 1990; Andersen et al., 1990; Zorzoli et al., 1994; Zilianti et al., 1995; Iams et al., 1996; Taipale and Hiillesmaa, 1998; Hibbard, Tart, et al., 2000). Cervical length remains relatively stable in the late second and early third trimesters but shortens or effaces slightly with gestational age, with median cervical length falling from 35 to 40 mm at 24 and 28 weeks to 30 to 35 mm after 32 weeks. Between 22 and 32 weeks of pregnancy, the length of the cervix is described by a normal bell curve distribution, with the 50th percentile at about 35 mm and the 10th and 90th percentiles at 25 mm and 45 mm, respectively (see Chapter 34, Fig. 34-5). Studies conducted at 16 through 22 weeks (Taipale and Hiilesmaa, 1998; Hibbard, Tart, et al., 2000) report the 10th percentile to be about 30 mm, in contrast to measurements obtained at 22–24 and 26–29 weeks showing the 10th percentile as approximately 25 mm (Iams et al., 1996). Measurements of the cervix in the nonpregnant state and in the first trimester of pregnancy have not been useful to identify reduced function.

Three major findings have been reported consistently based on ultrasound evaluation of the cervix in pregnancy: (1) Cervical effacement begins at the internal cervical os and proceeds caudad, (2) the ultrasound changes in the cervix that precede both term and preterm delivery occur over a period of weeks rather than days, suggesting a chronic rather than an acute process, and (3) the risk of spontaneous preterm birth increases as the cervical length decreases between 16 and 32 weeks.

Cervical effacement begins at the internal cervical os and proceeds caudad. The relationship of the lower uterine segment to the axis of the cervical canal changes as effacement occurs over a period of weeks, according to the shape of the letters *T, Y, V, and U* (Zilianti et al., 1995) (Fig. 33-2 A and B; Color Plate 16). The process of effacement is seen with real-time ultrasound to be dynamic, i.e., the internal os is seen to open and close, giving the appearance of a funnel at the internal os. This can occur in the absence of palpable uterine contractions. Whether electromyographic evidence of contractions occurs with funneling is not known. Intermittent funneling may be observed normally in the second half of pregnancy and occurs

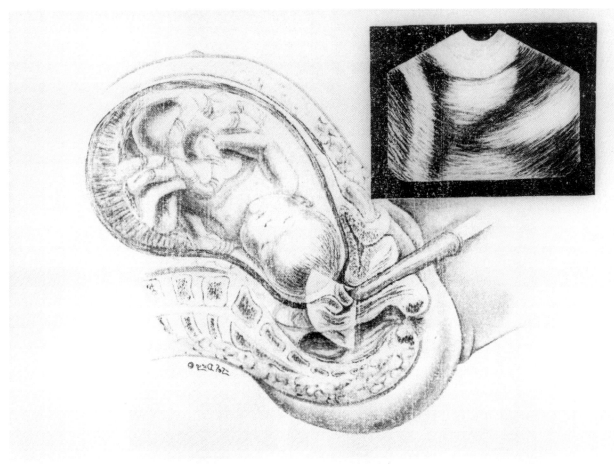

FIGURE 33-1 ■ Drawing of an endovaginal ultrasound probe placed into the anterior fornix to obtain the corresponding image of the cervix shown in the inset.

commonly after 32 weeks; however, a persistently short or funneled cervix that comprises approximately 40%–50% or more of the total cervical length (Okitsu et al., 1992; Berghella et al., 1997) is uncommon before 32 weeks and, together with a cervical length below the 10th (25 mm) to 25th (30 mm) percentile, is one of two findings that have been associated consistently with an increased risk of preterm birth. The knowledge that effacement begins at the internal os has explained the clinical anecdote of an extremely preterm birth within 24 hours of a digital pelvic examination in which the cervix was described as closed. Representative endovaginal ultrasound images of normal, short, and funneled cervixes are shown in Figures 33-3, 33-4, and 33-5, respectively.

The ultrasound changes in the cervix that precede both term and preterm delivery occur over a period of weeks rather than days, suggesting a chronic rather than an acute process. Ultrasound studies of the cervix indicate that the cervix begins to change normally at about 32–34 weeks in preparation for birth at term. These same changes, following the T-Y-V-U pattern, also precede spontaneous deliveries in the second and third trimesters, regardless of whether the clinical diagnosis at delivery is incompetent cervix, preterm labor, or preterm PROM, and often without much evidence of uterine contractions. Thus, a short or funneled cervix may be observed with ultrasound whenever the cervix is preparing for delivery, regardless

of gestational age, and regardless as well of the presumed mechanism—structural weakness, biochemically induced changes in the cervical stroma, or biophysical changes resulting from contractions.

The risk of spontaneous preterm birth increases as the cervical length decreases between 16 and 32 weeks. Multiple studies (Andersen et al., 1990; Iams et al., 1996; Taipale and Hiilesmaa, 1998, Hibbard, Tart, et al., 2000) have confirmed that cervical length measured by transvaginal ultrasound in the second and early third trimesters is inversely related to the risk of preterm delivery. (Fig. 33-6). The relationship between cervical length and preterm birth in these studies is not limited to women whose cervical length is below the tenth percentile, but rather extends throughout the range of length: The longer the cervix, the lower the risk of preterm birth, and the shorter the cervix, the greater the risk. Nevertheless, women with very short cervical length (e.g., below the third percentile) do not always deliver preterm without treatment; there is no threshold value below which the patient always presents with incompetent cervix. The association between cervical length and preterm birth is strongest in women with a prior preterm birth and especially strong when the prior preterm birth occurred before 32 weeks (Iams et al., 1995, 1998; Goldenberg et al., 1998; Owen et al., 2001).

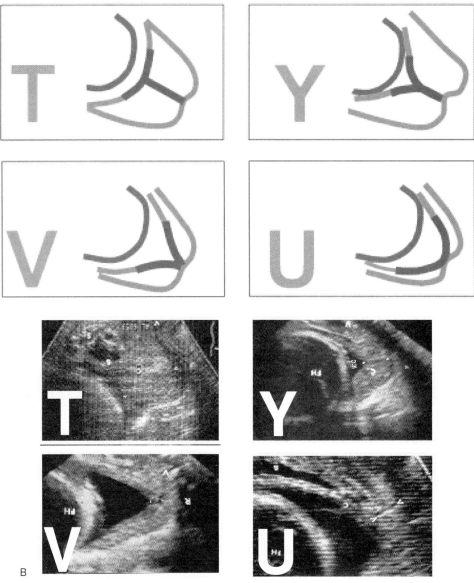

FIGURE 33-2 ■ **A,** Schematic presentation of the process of cervical effacement as it proceeds caudad from the internal os, as indicated by the letters T, Y, V, and U. (Modified from Zilianti M, Azuaga A, Calderon F, et al: Monitoring the effacement of the uterine cervix by transperineal sonography. J Ultrasound Med **14:**719, 1995.) **B,** Corresponding endovaginal ultrasound images showing the same process of cervical effacement. See Color Plate 16.

WHAT IS CERVICAL COMPETENCE?

The findings described thus far indicate that cervical competence functions not as an absolute variable but instead as a continuum in which the classic history of recurrent painless second-trimester pregnancy loss represents the clinical expression of the lowermost end of a bell curve. A corollary of the concept of cervical competence as a continuum is that competence is also relative to the circumstances of the pregnancy. The most obvious example is higher-order multiple gestation: Few women have sufficient cervical competence to carry a quadruplet gestation to 38 weeks, while some will carry triplets and many will carry twins to term without medical intervention. Ultrasound studies of the cervix in women with

multiple gestations have confirmed this hypothesis—women who carry twins and triplets to term without intervention have cervical length measurements above the 50th–75th percentile (35–40 mm) at 24–28 weeks' gestation (Imseis et al., 1997; Ramin et al., 1999; Souka et al., 1999).

Cervical length can be viewed as an indirect and imperfect marker of cervical competence or function. Keeping the concept of competence as relative in mind, reduced cervical competence may be defined as a congenital or acquired property of the cervix that is clinically manifest as repeated early preterm delivery of a singleton pregnancy. The definition is clinical (i.e., functional), based on obstetrical outcome rather than on the appearance or measured length of the cervix. Cervical length as a test to predict preterm birth is considered

PLATE 16

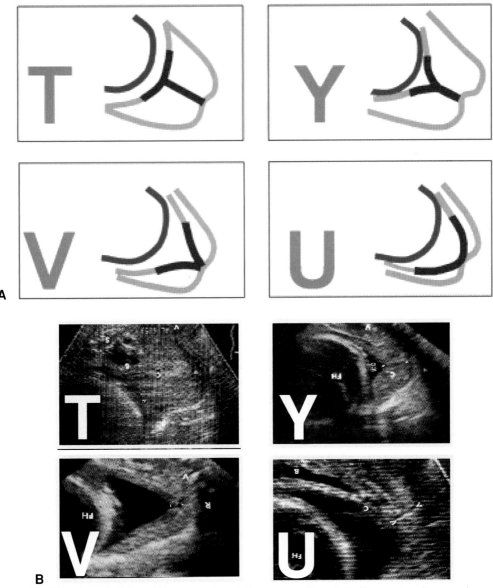

FIGURE 33-2 ■ A, Schematic presentation of the process of cervical effacement as it proceeds caudad from the internal os, as indicated by the letters T, Y, V, and U. (Modified from Zilianti M, Azuaga A, Calderon F, et al: Monitoring the effacement of the uterine cervix by transperineal sonography. J Ultrasound Med **14:**719, 1995.) **B,** Corresponding endovaginal ultrasound images showing the same process of cervical effacement.

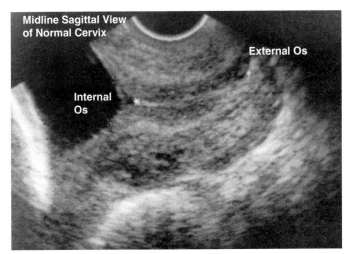

FIGURE 33-3 ■ Endovaginal ultrasound image of a normal cervix.

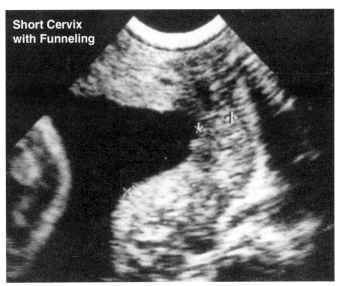

FIGURE 33-5 ■ Endovaginal ultrasound image of a funneled cervix.

in Chapter 34. The focus in this chapter is the identification of women whose cervical competence is at the lowest end of the spectrum and for whom cerclage may be an appropriate treatment.

ETIOLOGY OF REDUCED CERVICAL COMPETENCE

Anatomy of the Cervix

The uterine cervix and corpus are derived from fusion of the distal müllerian ducts and subsequent central atrophy (Crosby and Hill, 1962). The cervix is primarily fibrous tissue with some (10%–15%) smooth muscle (Danforth, 1947). The cervico-isthmic histologic transition from fibrous to muscular tissue varies from a narrow 1–2 mm zone to a relatively wide 5–10 mm zone (Danforth, 1947), whereas the proportion of cervical smooth muscle varies from 29% in the upper third to 6.4% in the lower third (Rorie and Newton, 1967). During

pregnancy, the muscular uterine isthmus distends and elongates between the 12th and 20th weeks of gestation, consistent with ultrasound studies of the cervix and lower segment at the same interval of gestation (Kushnir et al., 1990).

Congenital Factors

Primary disorders of the cervico-isthmic junction may result from abnormalities in the muscular isthmus and the upper cervix as well as from derangement of the cervical fibrous tissue, with a result of decreased cervical resistance. Higher concentrations of smooth muscle relative to collagen fibers in the cervixes of women with cervical incompetence have been found compared with women who have no history of preterm birth (Buckingham et al., 1965). Cervical biopsy specimens

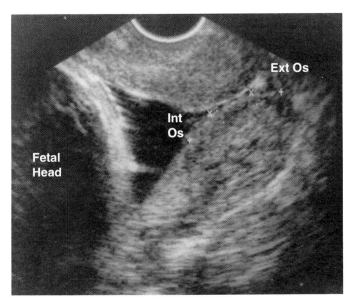

FIGURE 33-4 ■ Endovaginal ultrasound image of a short cervix. Int, internal; ext, external.

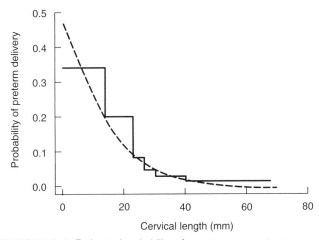

FIGURE 33-6 ■ Estimated probability of spontaneous preterm delivery before 35 weeks of gestation from the logistic-regression analysis (*dashed line*) and the observed frequency of spontaneous preterm delivery (*solid line*) according to cervical length measurement by transvaginal ultrasonography at 24 weeks. (From Iams JD, Goldenberg RL, Meis PJ, et al: The length of the cervix and the risk of spontaneous preterm delivery. N Engl J Med **334**:567, 1996.)

obtained from normal women after parturition (Rechberger et al., 1988) revealed a 12-fold decrease in mechanical strength, a 50% reduction in the concentrations of collagen and sulfated glycosaminoglycans, a 35% reduction in hyaluronic acid, an increase in collagen extractability, and a fivefold increase in collagenolytic activity compared with tissue obtained from normal non-pregnant women. In contrast, cervical biopsy specimens obtained in the second trimester from pregnant women with a history of cervical incompetence revealed normal collagen concentrations, but high collagen extractability and collagenolytic activity, higher than normal postpartum values (Rechberger et al., 1988). Furthermore, significantly lower concentrations and increased extractability of hydroxyproline were observed in cervical biopsies obtained from 10 nonpregnant women with a history of typical cervical incompetence in their first pregnancy compared with cervical tissue obtained from 31 normal parous controls (Petersen and Uldbjerg, 1996). This finding suggests that cervical connective tissue may be anatomically different in some women with the clinical syndrome of cervical incompetence.

Biological Variation

Perhaps the most prevalent "congenital factor" contributing to abnormal cervical competence may be the biological variation in cervical function implied by the increased risk of preterm birth for women whose cervical length falls in the lower quartile of the bell-curve distribution of cervical length measurements (Iams et al., 1996; Taipale and Hiilesmaa, 1998; Hibbard, Tart, et al., 2000). The risk of spontaneous preterm birth increases as the length declines, especially below the 10th percentile. To the extent that this occurs because of an inherently short cervix, any preterm birth, regardless of clinical presentation, in a woman with a cervical length below the median value can be said to be the result in part of a "congenitally" short or less competent cervix. Additional evidence derives from studies that link short cervical length to repetitive preterm birth. In one study, cervical length at 24 weeks' gestation was compared in 363 women to their obstetrical histories, categorized as (1) typical cervical incompetence, (2) preterm birth at or before 26 weeks' gestation, (3) preterm birth between 27 and 32 weeks' gestation, (4) preterm birth between 33 and 36 weeks' gestation, (5) birth at 37 weeks' gestation or greater (Iams et al., 1995).

Cervical length in the current pregnancy was directly related to the gestational age of the prior delivery: The earlier the gestational age of the previous birth, the shorter the cervix in the current pregnancy.

An observational study of risk factors for premature delivery in 3015 women found that a cervical length of less than 25 mm was the risk factor most strongly related to a history of preterm birth, again suggesting that a woman brings her own inherent level of cervical competence to each successive pregnancy (Goldenberg et al., 1998).

Uterine Anomalies

Congenital structural uterine abnormalities have been associated with an increased incidence of reproductive loss, some of which may relate to inadequate cervical competence. Case series describing pregnancy outcomes in women with uncorrected uterine anomalies consistently report three

findings (Ludmir et al., 1990; Seidman et al., 1991; Leibovitz et al., 1992; Surico et al., 2000; Woelfer et al., 2001):

1. Women with septate and bicornuate uteri have higher rates of preterm delivery than do those with didelphys or unicornuate uteri.
2. Several authors have described improved pregnancy outcome in women with uterine anomalies treated with cerclage compared with their prior pregnancies without cerclage.
3. Good pregnancy outcomes are not rare in women with untreated uterine anomalies, regardless of the type of anomaly.

Woelfer and colleagues (2001), using three-dimensional ultrasound, reported a twofold increase in the history of second-trimester miscarriage among women with untreated arcuate uteri (7.9%) compared with 3.6% for women with subseptate and 3.5% for women with normal uteri. The current authors follow women with uterine anomalies with serial sonography and find that few develop criteria for cerclage.

Diethylstilbestrol

Poor pregnancy outcome and structural genital tract abnormalities have been reported in women exposed to diethylstilbestrol (DES) *in utero* (Kaufman et al., 1977, 1980, 2000), due at least in part to cervical incompetence attributed to DES exposure (Goldstein, 1978). In the most recent and comprehensive report, Kaufman and associates (2000) reported a 4.25- to 5.84-fold increased risk of second trimester pregnancy loss in DES-exposed women (6.3%–7.1%) compared with unexposed controls (1.6%). Other possible causes for adverse pregnancy outcomes in DES progeny include upper genital tract abnormalities of uterine cavity shape (e.g., a T-shape) and intrauterine defects such as synechiae and diverticulae (Kaufman et al., 1984). As many as six million people could have been exposed to DES *in utero* before the U.S. Food and Drug Administration banned its use as a treatment for recurrent abortion (Robboy et al., 1983). As the cohort of exposed women ages, DES is now a less common cause of adverse pregnancy outcome. As for women with uterine anomalies, transvaginal sonography between 16 and 26 weeks' gestation in women exposed *in utero* to DES is an appropriate method to evaluate the need for cerclage.

Acquired Abnormalities of Cervical Competence

Cervical Trauma

Cervical incompetence attributed to trauma can occur during obstetric or gynecologic operative procedures or may follow a spontaneous obstetric injury during labor or delivery. The cervix may be lacerated, may heal poorly, or may be stretched beyond tolerance. Women delivered by cesarean section after an arrested second stage of labor can present in the next pregnancy with cervical incompetence. Cervical injury also can occur in the course of cesarean delivery should the incision extend vertically into the cervix.

Dilation and Curettage

Although mechanical dilation of the cervix before curettage for either diagnosis or therapeutic termination of pregnancy has been blamed for cervical incompetence (Hulka and

Higgins, 1961; Johnstone et al., 1976), most reports indicate that first-trimester termination of pregnancy presents little, if any, risk of cervical incompetence if it is performed by an experienced operator with the use of laminaria (Mandelson et al., 1992; Zhou et al., 2000; Henriet and Kaminski, 2001). Pregnancy termination in the second trimester requires more dilation than for first-trimester abortion and thus offers greater opportunity for cervical injury; pretreatment with laminaria may reduce this risk (Schuly et al., 1983).

Cervical Biopsy and Ablation of Neoplasia

Diagnosis and treatment of intraepithelial neoplasia could require cervical biopsy, laser ablation, loop electrosurgical excision procedure (LEEP), or cold knife conization. The literature on pregnancy outcome after cervical conization indicates that this procedure could contribute to cervical incompetence, the major risk factor being the extent of the cone biopsy (Leiman et al., 1980; Kristensen et al., 1993; Raio et al., 1997). Kristensen and associates (1993) reviewed pregnancy outcome in 170 women before and after conization among a Danish cohort study of 14,233 women. The risk of preterm birth was increased after conization. Women who underwent conization reported a higher rate of preterm birth in pregnancies even before the conization, a finding consistent with ultrasound studies showing that cervical length is an independent variable for preterm birth risk. Women with a cervical length below the 10th to 25th percentiles might then manifest an increased rate of preterm birth after conization, whereas women with a cervical length above the 50th percentile might tolerate conization without a clinically important increase in risk of preterm birth in subsequent pregnancy.

Raio and colleagues (1997) compared pregnancy outcome in 64 women who underwent laser conization with 64 control subjects matched for parity, smoking status, and history of prior preterm birth. The risk of preterm birth increased when the cone height was at least 10 mm.

The risk of cervical injury after loop electrosurgical excision procedure is controversial. Ferenczy and coworkers (1995) did not observe an increased rate of preterm birth in 53 women who had undergone a loop electrosurgical excision procedure for treatment of intraepithelial lesions of the cervix. Chwe and colleagues (1997) observed higher rates of preterm delivery and second-trimester pregnancy loss among 77 women with a history of loop electrosurgical excision procedure compared with 203 women with a history of cold knife conization. Althuisius and associates (2001) reached the opposite conclusion based on data from 52 women, wherein the mean duration of pregnancy was only slightly less than 40 weeks and no deliveries occurred before 32 weeks. A study of cervical length measured with endovaginal ultrasound before and after cervical loop excision in 20 women found that excision of the transformation zone had no significant effect on length, but obstetrical performance was not reported (Gentry et al., 2000).

Biochemical Influences on Cervical Competence

Biochemical changes in cervical function can occur as a result of endocrine or inflammatory factors. Although exploration of their roles in cervical function is just beginning, these two potential mechanisms are important because of the opposite effects that treatment with cerclage may produce in each case.

Relaxin

Relaxin is a peptide hormone secreted by the corpus luteum that causes connective tissue remodeling. Preterm births that include cases suggestive of incompetent cervix have been reported after superovulation (McElrath and Wise, 1997; Dhont et al., 1999; Schieve et al., 2002). It has been postulated that increased levels of relaxin such as occur following superovulation from multiple corpora lutea may account for these observations through an effect on cervical competence (Weiss et al., 1993). Relaxin levels are 140% higher in twins than in singleton gestations and 330% higher still in multiple gestations that follow induction of ovulation with menotropins. Twin gestations resulting from in vitro fertilization or gamete intrafallopian transfer have an additional 260% increase in relaxin compared with relaxin levels in spontaneous twin pregnancies (Haning et al., 1985; Haning, Canick, et al., 1996; Haning, Goldsmith, et al., 1996). Elevated serum relaxin in the midtrimester has been related to decreased cervical length (Eppel et al., 1999) and to early preterm birth (Vogel et al., 2001). Another study of serum relaxin levels and cervical length at 24 and 28 weeks in spontaneous twin pregnancies, however, found no relationship between relaxin levels and cervical length (Iams et al., 2001). Whether cervical length or competence is influenced by menotropin treatment or assisted reproductive techniques via other pathways remains to be determined.

Infection

Infection-related influences on cervical competence have been inferred by reports that relate changes in cervical length to infection. One study related cervical length to maternal bacterial vaginosis (Surbek et al., 2000), a finding disputed by another (Boomgaard et al., 1999). Studies summarized by Goldenberg and colleagues (2000) have suggested that microorganisms present in the upper genital tract before conception may give rise to an indolent inflammatory response at the chorioamniotic-decidual interface, which in turn leads to cervical effacement via biochemical mediators (e.g., cytokines and prostaglandins). It is likely that individual variation in immune response may influence the clinical manifestations of both upper- and lower-tract infection. A study from Denmark found differences in the HLA-DR-1 and HLA-DR-3 alleles in women whose recurrent midtrimester losses were treated unsuccessfully with cerclage (Mohapeloa et al., 1998). These two alleles have been associated with increased responsiveness to tumor necrosis factor-α.

DIAGNOSIS OF ABNORMAL CERVICAL COMPETENCE

It is difficult to identify a point on the continuum of competence that defines "incompetence" and thus indicates surgical intervention. The history remains the cornerstone of diagnosis, but the combination of an appropriate history supported by ultrasound images of the cervix is becoming the standard. In 1996, in recognition of the increasing contribution of ultrasound, the American College of Obstetricians and

Gynecologists listed both a history of painless dilation leading to recurrent midtrimester delivery and "sonographic evidence of cervical funneling in a patient with a prior history of midtrimester delivery" as indications for cerclage (ACOG, 1996). Currently, a history of recurrent second-trimester delivery in the absence of other causes is the only history sufficient to make the diagnosis. Any other clinical presentations should be supported by clinical or ultrasound evidence of advanced effacement before the diagnosis can be made. Similarly, ultrasound changes in the absence of an appropriate history are not sufficient to establish a diagnosis.

CLINICAL PRESENTATIONS OF ABNORMAL CERVICAL COMPETENCE

There are four clinical settings in which the diagnosis of abnormal cervical competence should be considered:

1. A history of recurrent midtrimester pregnancy loss in the absence of other causes
2. Acute presentation in the second trimester with advanced cervical effacement and dilation with few or no contractions
3. Observation by ultrasound of progressive cervical effacement in a patient whose obstetric or gynecologic history has suggested cervical incompetence
4. Incidental observation by ultrasound of cervical effacement and funneling (this is an increasingly common scenario for which no standard management protocol has been developed)

In each instance, the most important diagnostic tool is a careful history, remembering that "regardless of the cause of the pregnancy loss, the cervix always dilates before the conceptus emerges from the uterus. Cervical dilatation is . . . merely a final common pathway for many causes of pregnancy loss" (Harger, 1983).

History

The diagnosis of cervical incompetence is most securely established when there is a well-documented history of painless cervical dilation in the absence of contractions, bleeding, infection, ruptured membranes, fetal anomaly, or elevated maternal serum alpha-fetoprotein that may indicate significant fetomaternal or extraovular bleeding. Variations from this classic picture may suggest, but cannot establish, the diagnosis.

In taking a history of prior preterm births, much has been made of the presence or absence of contractions and the degree of pain described by the patient. Olah and Gee (1992) and Gee and associates (1988) observed that the compliance of the cervical stroma influences wall tension within the uterus and, with it, the pain of the contraction as well. Thus, a soft or compliant cervix may efface and dilate without development of significant intrauterine pressure. Variation in the apparent pain of labor is then a function not only of a woman's pain threshold but also of her cervical compliance. Contractions are more likely to be described as painful when the cervix is uneffaced, suggesting the acute onset of contractions such as might occur after trauma or abruption. Additional markers of reduced cervical resistance include a history of short labors, advanced dilation before the onset of labor, and progressively earlier deliveries in successive pregnancies.

Women with previously unsuspected cervical incompetence often present late, after significant effacement and dilation have occurred. Presenting complaints in these patients include mild contractions, ruptured membranes, amnionitis with intact membranes, and even occasional cases of bleeding in which placenta previa and abruption have been excluded. These patients presumably had asymptomatic effacement with exposure of membranes to the vagina until pressure, backache, amniorrhexis, amnionitis, or spotting brought them to attention. At this point, their terminal symptom, whether labor, ruptured membranes, or infection, becomes the diagnosis of record. Women who have a history of delayed atypical presentation should not, however, be determined to have an incompetent cervix and thus be treated automatically in subsequent pregnancies with a cerclage. Rather, they are candidates for close surveillance in future pregnancies.

Physical Examination

Serial digital and speculum examinations have been employed to follow patients with suspected cervical incompetence, but physical changes are often not evident until the cervix is well effaced. Digital and speculum examination of the cervix eventually reveal bulging membranes, a pink or tan discharge, or appreciable softening of the cervix and lower segment. Not surprisingly, a closed cervix does not exclude the diagnosis, as cervical effacement and dilation begin at the internal os. The feature of the digital examination most strongly correlated with early effacement is a soft, well-developed lower uterine segment. Digital examination is significantly less consistent than ultrasound to assess cervical length (Sonek, Iams, et al., 1990; Jackson et al., 1992; Phelps et al., 1995; Goldberg et al., 1997).

Diagnostic Tests

There are no specific tests or criteria to detect cervical incompetence outside of pregnancy. Although several techniques have been suggested (e.g., passage of dilators or hysterography), none has enjoyed much popularity because of inaccuracy and inconvenience.

Ultrasound

The ultrasound appearance of the cervix before conception and in early pregnancy does not offer any consistent evidence of subsequent incompetence. Serial ultrasound examination of the cervix to detect incompetent cervix was first reported in studies performed with transabdominal transducers (Sarti et al., 1979; Bernstine et al., 1981; Brook et al., 1981; Michaels et al., 1986; Ayers et al., 1988; Podobnik et al., 1988). These studies were confirmed by others using transvaginal probes (Ludmir, 1988; Andersen et al., 1990; Guzman et al., 1994, 1997) that produce a more consistent and accurate image of the cervix while avoiding the confounding effect of a full maternal bladder.

Although sonographic images may support a diagnosis of cervical incompetence, ultrasound findings alone are insufficient. Sonographic criteria that support the diagnosis in women with a history of midtrimester delivery include (1) cervical shortening to a length below the first (13 mm)

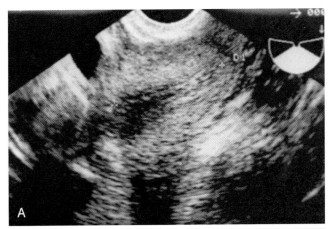

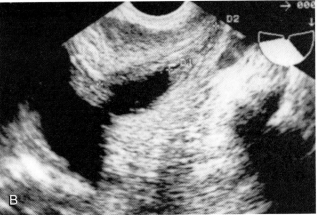

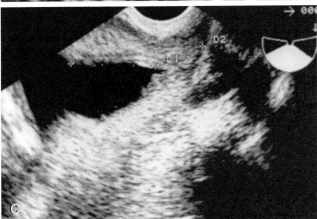

FIGURE 33-7 ■ Transvaginal ultrasound image of the cervix in a patient with incompetent cervix at 18 weeks' gestation showing progressive funneling in response to fundal pressure: without pressure (**A**), after fundal pressure (**B**), and four minutes after fundal pressure (**C**).

even a modest amount of excess pressure on the endovaginal probe and can be mimicked by contractions of the lower uterine segment above an otherwise normal cervix (Yost et al., 1999).

The period between 16 and 24 weeks' gestation is the optimal interval for surveillance. Changes suggestive of incompetence are rarely seen before 16 weeks and rarely begin after 24 weeks. When serial examinations are performed, the rate of decrease in cervical length can be helpful. Guzman, Mellon, and associates (1998) studied 61 women at risk for early preterm birth with serial ultrasound examinations between 15 and 24 weeks' gestation. Women who eventually displayed signs of incompetence (cervical length less than 20 mm with funneling) before 24 weeks' gestation had a mean decrease in canal length of at least 0.4 cm per week compared with women who never displayed such signs. MacDonald and coworkers (2001) studied 106 women with increased risk of preterm delivery with regular endovaginal sonography. When shortening or funneling occurred before 24 weeks, either at rest or in response to fundal pressure, the cervical length always decreased to less than 10 mm within 17 days or less. Andrews and associates (2000) followed 69 women with a prior history of preterm birth between 16 and 30 weeks' gestation with transvaginal sonography every two weeks. Among 53 who had an examination before 20 weeks' gestation that revealed either a length less than 22 mm (the 10th percentile) or significant funneling, 33% delivered within two weeks and 67% delivered within four weeks of the examination; 100% of women who met these criteria before 20 weeks' gestation delivered before 35 weeks' gestation.

Although ultrasound criteria have been used clinically in some centers, they have not been tested in a prospective blinded observational study in women with suspected abnormal cervical competence, nor has cerclage been shown to offer significant advantage over bed rest or other noninvasive therapy when such findings are observed. At present, these criteria are useful in clinical care to exclude the diagnosis of incompetence, but positive sonographic findings cannot be regarded as a certain indication for cerclage until a randomized trial has been completed that shows favorable results. Such trials are underway.

In 1999, the American College of Radiology (ACR) recommended that the cervix and lower uterine segment be imaged as part of every transabdominal obstetrical ultrasound examination in the second trimester to search for funneling and/or a short (less than 30 mm) cervix. Because of the poor reproducibility of transabdominal sonography of the cervix, the American College of Radiology recommends that a transabdominal cervical measurement of less than 30 mm be followed by a transvaginal ultrasound measurement with an empty maternal bladder. A measurement of greater than 25 mm in a patient without symptoms and a negative risk history allows the obstetrician to reassure the patient that the risk of preterm birth is not increased. There is no established protocol for care of women with an incidental finding of a short cervix. In the absence of data about how best to manage these pregnancies, education about the signs and symptoms of preterm labor, more frequent visits, and consideration of antenatal corticosteroids seems reasonable. Available data is insufficient to recommend a cerclage in this setting (see the upcoming discussion of Rust et al., 2001).

to the fifth (20 mm) percentile before 24 weeks and (2) funneling of the internal os that occupies at least 30%–40% of the total length of the cervix (funnel plus residual length), observed spontaneously or in response to fundal pressure (Figure 33-7 A–C; Sonek, Blumenfeld, et al., 1990; Guzman et al., 1994, 1997; Wong et al., 1997; MacDonald et al., 2001).

Of these two criteria, the residual cervical length measurement is much more reliable than observation of funneling because it is less subject to inter- and intra-operator variation and operator-induced artifact. Funneling can be obscured by

■ TREATMENT OF CERVICAL INCOMPETENCE

Treatment of incompetent cervix has traditionally been by surgical correction of the presumed physical deficit in tissue strength with an encircling or cerclage suture, placed electively between 12 and 15 weeks or urgently in the second trimester. As the concept of categorical incompetence has broadened to include variable degrees of competence, the role of cerclage has come under review. Disputes about the efficacy of cerclage procedures, already common when competence was thought to be categorical, are even more frequent now that the continuum of competence concept has muddied the waters still further. This situation has led to a reconsideration of both medical and surgical therapy for women with a history of recurrent midpregnancy loss. Proposed medical therapies include bed rest, progesterone supplementation, antibiotics, and anti-inflammatory drugs. Surgical options include various cerclage techniques performed transvaginally or transabdominally, before or during pregnancy. Two majors concerns limit any review of the efficacy of these treatments: (1) inadequate study design, with a preponderance of descriptive and observational studies, and (2) lack of uniform criteria for inclusion and cerclage placement.

Despite the prolonged controversy about the role of cerclage, a randomized trial of cerclage versus bed rest or no therapy in women with a typical history of incompetent cervix has not been reported. Reports to date include observational studies of women with typical histories and randomized trials conducted in women with atypical histories or other risk factors.

Most descriptive studies report success rates of 75%–90% but are flawed by comparing pregnancy outcome with previous pregnancies in the same woman (Harger, 1980; Treadwell et al., 1991). There is good evidence that repeated midtrimester pregnancy loss does not preclude successful outcome in subsequent untreated pregnancies. One hundred couples with a history of three consecutive pregnancy losses had a 71% chance of successful outcome if they had a normal karyotype and hysterosalpingogram (Tho et al., 1979). Harger and coworkers (1983) reported a pregnancy success rate of 73% after recurrent pregnancy loss in 155 couples studied.

Several randomized controlled trials evaluated the efficacy of cerclage before the advent of transvaginal sonography. A study of prophylactic cerclage versus no cerclage conducted in 50 women with twin pregnancies following ovulation induction found no difference in outcomes (Dor et al., 1982). Lazar and associates (1984) studied 506 women with low-to-moderate risk of preterm birth randomized to cerclage versus controls; they found no evidence to suggest that McDonald cerclage prolonged gestation or decreased perinatal mortality. Rush and associates (1984) performed a similar trial in 194 subjects and again found no advantage for McDonald cerclage.

In 1993, the Medical Research Council of the Royal College of Obstetricians and Gynaecologists (United Kingdom) reported results of a multicenter randomized trial of cervical cerclage in 1292 women with second-trimester loss or preterm delivery (71%) or previous cervical surgery (29%) (MacNaughton et al., 1993). Women with histories typical of incompetence were intentionally excluded. The cerclage group had statistically fewer deliveries at less than 33 weeks (13% versus 17%, $P = .03$), fewer infants weighing less than 1500 g at birth (10% versus 13%, $P = .05$), and fewer pregnancy losses including miscarriage, stillbirth, and neonatal death (9% versus 11%, $P = .06$). The percentage of deliveries occurring between 33 and 36 weeks was similar. The authors believed that the observed benefit was limited to a small number of women with histories of multiple previous pregnancy losses or preterm deliveries.

Transvaginal ultrasound would seem to offer an objective method to identify women who may benefit from cerclage among a group with historical risk factors. Initial retrospective series reported mixed results, summarized in Table 33-1, (Heath et al., 1998; Berghella et al., 1999; Hibbard, Snow, et al., 2000; Novy et al., 2001; Hassan et al., 2001; Owen et al., 2003). Some studies enrolled only women with historical risk, and others employed cervical length criteria regardless of history. All studies required ultrasound measurement of cervical length, but the threshold for cerclage placement ranged from 15 mm to 30 mm.

Two randomized trials of cerclage conducted in women chosen by sonography have subsequently been performed, both described in sequential reports (Althuisius et al., 2000; Althuisius et al., 2001; Rust et al., 2000; Rust et al., 2001). The trials differ mainly in their specific entry criteria. The cervical incompetence prevention randomized cerclage trial (CIPRACT) enrolled women with a history of preterm birth at less than 34 weeks (Althuisius et al., 2000); the final report also included women with a history of DES exposure, cold-knife conization, and uterine anomalies (Althuisius et al., 2001). Thirty-five women with risk factors were followed with sonography and randomized to cerclage or bed rest if the cervical length fell below 25 mm. The Lehigh Valley Hospital trial (Rust et al., 2000; Rust et al., 2001) enrolled 138 women found to have a cervical length of less than 25 mm or greater than 25% funneling of the internal os, regardless of their obstetrical or gynecological history. Amniocentesis was performed to exclude infection before randomization in this trial. Women in both trials were treated with perioperative antibiotics and indomethacin. In the cervical incompetence prevention randomized cerclage trial, women randomized to receive a cerclage had better outcomes: no births earlier than 34 weeks' gestation in the cerclage group versus 44% of births before 34 weeks' gestation in the bed rest group. In the Lehigh Valley trial, the rate of birth earlier than 34 weeks was about 35% in both groups. The two trials are contrasted in Table 33-2, modified from Rust and associates (2001). The most prominent differences are the entry criteria, sample size, and use of amniocentesis. Although many of the subjects in the Lehigh Valley study had risk factors for preterm birth, many (the exact number is not reported) had no risk factors for preterm birth.

This review does not leave the clinician with a clear protocol for clinical management. The contradictory results of the two recent trials support a conclusion that neither history nor cervical sonographic evidence alone is sufficient to determine who will benefit from a cerclage. When a history of recurrent early preterm birth is accompanied by sonographic evidence of substantial effacement before 24 weeks, cerclage may an appropriate choice. A multicenter randomized trial has recently

TABLE 33-1. COHORT SERIES AND RANDOMIZED TRIALS OF CERCLAGE FOR SONOGRAPHICALLY SUSPECTED CERVICAL INCOMPETENCE

1st Author, Yr	Population	N	Selection Criteria	GA	Outcome	Benefit
Retrospective Cohort Series						
Heath, 1998	Unselected	43	CL ≤5 mm	23 weeks	Preterm birth <32 wks: cerclage—5% vs. no cerclage—50%	Yes
Berghella, 1999	Risk factors	63	CL <25 mm or >25% funneling	14–24 weeks	Adjusted odds ratio for preterm birth <35 wks: 1.1 (0.3, 4.6)	No
Novy, 2001	Symptomatic and asymptomatic women with certain physical findings	35	CL <30 mm plus funneling and softening or <60% effaced and external os <2 cm dilated	18–27 weeks	Mean 4-wk increase in delivery gestational age: 29 vs. 25 wks	Yes
Hibbard, 2000	Risk factors, symptoms or physical findings	85	CL ≤30 mm	8–30 weeks	Mean 2-wk increase in delivery gestational age: 34 vs. 32 wks	Yes
Hassan, 2001	Unselected	70	CL ≤15 mm	14–24 weeks	Preterm birth <34 wks: cerclage—68% vs. no cerclage—53%	No
Randomized Clinical Trials						
Althuisius, 2001	High-risk history consistent with CI	35	CL <25 mm	<27 weeks	Preterm birth <34 wks: cerclage—0% vs. no cerclage—44%	Yes
Rust, 2001	Unselected, but many had risk factors	113	CL <25 mm or >25% funneling	16–24 weeks	Preterm birth <34 wks: cerclage—35% vs. no cerclage—36%	No

CL, cervical incompetence; CL, cervical length; GA, gestational age.

From Owen J, Iams JD, Hauth JC: Vaginal sonography and cervical incompetence. Am J Obstet Gynecol **188**:586, 2003.

begun. Until additional information is available, clinicians are challenged to make the best management decision for each patient based on her history and cervical examination. The criteria recommended by the American College of Obstetricians and Gynecologists as sufficient to recommend a cerclage remain appropriate: Women with either a typical history of recurrent midtrimester delivery in the absence of another diagnosis, or with an atypical history accompanied by significant cervical effacement (e.g., residual cervical length less than 20 mm between 16 and 24 weeks' gestation) should be offered treatment with cerclage, accompanied by an acknowledgment that its efficacy is unproven.

Cervical Cerclage Procedures

Surgery in the Nonpregnant State

Cerclage in the nonpregnant state is uncommon in clinical practice, but the occasional patient may benefit, especially if the cervix has a large traumatic defect. The major disadvantage of preconceptional cerclage placement is that it could complicate management of spontaneous first-trimester loss or the possibility of a genetically abnormal fetus.

Lash and Lash (1950) described a transvaginal procedure to correct a structural defect within the cervix. A transverse incision in the anterior cervical mucosa is made approximately 2 cm above the external os, and the bladder is reflected as

necessary. The observed defect is then plicated with interrupted sutures of 2–0 chromic catgut. The authors suggested that larger lesions be excised in an elliptical fashion before suture plication. Lash (1960) reported improved fetal survival rate after surgery compared with prior pregnancies, but fertility could be compromised (Lees and Sutherst, 1974). An alternate procedure has been described (Mann et al., 1961) to facilitate dissection of an abnormally shortened or scarred cervix with placement of the suture at the level of the internal os. The cervical mucosa is incised and dissected anteriorly and posteriorly to the level of the peritoneal reflection. A nonabsorbable suture is placed circumferentially at the level of the internal os, including the uterosacral ligaments and a small amount of cervical tissue both anteriorly and posteriorly in the suture. A second suture is placed 1 to 2 cm distal to the first.

Surgery during Pregnancy

The two most commonly performed procedures during pregnancy have been described by Shirodkar (1955) and McDonald (1957).

SHIRODKAR CERCLAGE

The procedure as described by Shirodkar (1955) used maternal fascia lata as the "suture" material and aneurysm needles to thread the fascia lata strip submucosally after first incising the

TABLE 33-2. COMPARISON OF TWO RANDOMIZED TRIALS OF CERCLAGE VERSUS NO CERCLAGE

	Rust et al., 2001	Althuisius et al., 2001
Sample size	113	35
Ethnic background	60% white, 30% Hispanic, 10% other	Not defined
Inclusion criteria	All patients with dilation of internal os and short cervix	Singleton, historic risk factor, and short cervix
Mean cervical length at enrollment (cm)	2.0	2.0
Gestational age (wk) at diagnosis (range and mean)	16–24 (21.4)	Up to 27 (20.7)
Preoperative amniocentesis to rule out infection	Yes	No
Precerclage therapy	All patients: preoperative antibiotic and indomethacin × 48–72 h, after operation × 24 h	All patients: perioperative antibiotics Cerclage patients: perioperative indomethacin
Cerclage technique	McDonald	McDonald
Suture material	Single permanent monofilament	Single braided tape
Neonatal death or serious morbidity (%)		
Cerclage	23.9	5.2
No cerclage	20.6	50.0
Statistical power	0.82	0.34

Modified from Rust OA, Atlas RO, Reed J, et al: Revisiting the short cervix detected by transvaginal ultrasound in the second trimester: Why cerclage therapy may not help. Am J Obstet Gynecol **185**:1098, 2001, table IV.

vaginal epithelium transversely both anteriorly and posteriorly, and reflecting the vesicovaginal and rectovaginal fascia to the level of the internal os. The "suture" was tied anteriorly, and the anterior and posterior incisions were closed with absorbable material. Since the original report, many modifications have been suggested, including tying the knot posteriorly, leaving the ends of the knot exposed for easier removal, and most commonly replacing fascia lata with either No. 2 or No. 5 polyester (Mersilene or Ethibond) or nylon or a 5-mm polyester band mounted on atraumatic needles. Instead of tunneling the suture submucosally, some obstetricians advocate inserting a long curved Allis clamp into the incisions both anteriorly and posteriorly and applying lateral traction on the submucosal tissue in order to place the cerclage next to the body of the cervix and medial to the uterine vessels. That is the technique used in these authors' institution with a 5-mm tape, with the knot tied anteriorly and tagged to facilitate later removal. Some surgeons anchor the Shirodkar suture anteriorly and posteriorly to avoid slippage or displacement. If a 5-mm tape is chosen, a permanent suture may be used to anchor the tape to the cervical tissue; if a No. 2 or No. 5 suture is used, the cerclage may be anchored directly if an extra bite of cervical tissue is taken both anteriorly and posteriorly.

McDONALD CERCLAGE

McDonald (1957) described a procedure that requires no submucosal dissection. The purse-string suture is begun anteriorly at the junction of the ectocervix and rugated vagina. Four to six bites of cervix are taken in a circumferential fashion well into the body of the cervix, avoiding entry into the endocervical canal. Care must be taken to place the suture high on the posterior aspect of the cervix, as this is the most likely site for suture displacement. The suture is tied anteriorly, and the ends are left long enough to facilitate removal at term or at the onset of labor. Variations include use of braided nylon or polyester or a 5-mm tape. The cervix may be reentered at the previous point of exit with successive bites to place the suture

entirely submucosally, or it may be placed so that it encompasses the cervical serosa.

Intraoperative Sonography

Intraoperative ultrasound is helpful in securing satisfactory placement of both Shirodkar and McDonald cerclage sutures (Wheelock et al., 1984; Ludmir et al., 1991). The current authors use endovaginal sonography after the sutures are placed but before the knots are tied. It has been helpful to judge the site of the suture relative to the internal os and to the maternal bladder and rectum. This immediate feedback allows removal and replacement of sutures that are too low or that impinge on adjacent structures. It also provides a starting point for comparison with subsequent examinations.

CLINICAL CONSIDERATIONS

A cerclage operation may be considered during pregnancy in four clinical settings:

1. The elective cerclage, placed at 11–15 weeks on the basis of a typical obstetric history
2. The urgent cerclage, placed when a diagnosis has been made by ultrasound in a patient with an atypical history or risk factors followed with ultrasound surveillance
3. The emergency or "heroic" cerclage placed when the patient presents with advanced cervical dilation, effacement, and membranes evident at the external os, usually between 16 and 24 weeks' gestation
4. The transabdominal cerclage, placed when the vaginal approach is either unlikely to succeed or when it has failed repeatedly in the past (see criteria by Benson and Durfee, 1965)

The perioperative management and choice of procedure are different in each scenario. Contraindications to cerclage placement at any time during pregnancy include ruptured membranes, evidence of cervical or intrauterine infection, major congenital anomalies of the fetus, vaginal bleeding of undetermined cause, and active labor regardless of etiology.

Prophylactic Cerclage versus Ultrasound Surveillance and Selective Cerclage

Although placement of a prophylactic cerclage at 12–15 weeks' gestation for women with a typical clinical history currently is within the standard of care, data from the cervical incompetence prevention randomized cerclage trial (Althuisius et al., 2000) attests to the safety and comparable efficacy of deferring a decision about placement of a cerclage in at-risk women until there is sonographic evidence of premature cervical effacement. The first cervical incompetence prevention randomized cerclage trial report provided data to allow comparison of preterm birth rates in women who were randomized to receive either a prophylactic cerclage (n = 23) or ultrasound surveillance with cerclage. The rate of preterm birth earlier than 34 weeks' gestation in the prophylactic cerclage arm was 13%, compared with 10% in women assigned to cerclage after a cervical length of less than 25 mm was noted. Notably, 26 of 44 women (59%) followed with transvaginal sonography every two weeks had cervical length measurements that remained above 25 mm; none were treated, and none delivered before 34 weeks' gestation. This impression is supported by recent observational reports (Fox et al., 1996; Guzman, Forster, et al., 1998; Cook and Ellwood, 2000; Kelly et al., 2001; To et al., 2002). These data suggest that a policy of prophylactic cerclage offers no advantage over ultrasound surveillance and could subject more than half of women treated with cerclage for historical criteria to an unnecessary procedure. Although a protocol of sonographic surveillance may not necessarily select women who will definitely benefit from cerclage, it appears that such surveillance can safely avoid consideration of cerclage for many women with uncertain obstetrical histories. Given the uncertainty in diagnosis of incompetent cervix, regardless of the criteria used, prophylactic cerclage may ultimately be replaced by frequent sonography between 16 and 24 weeks' gestation, with selective use of medical therapy and/or cerclage. Though prophylactic cerclage remains a choice for women with a typical history, it is not inappropriate to follow even these women with ultrasound instead of with the current custom of "once a cerclage, always a cerclage."

Women with uterine anomalies, a history of cervical ablative treatment for neoplasia, therapeutic abortion, or exposure to diethylstilbestrol are all candidates for ultrasound surveillance rather than elective cerclage. Cerclage is often recommended empirically for women with these risk factors, but the current authors have found transvaginal ultrasound between 16 and 26 weeks' gestation useful to reassure these women and their physicians of the safety of expectant management, thus averting many unnecessary cerclage procedures. In women with a history of conization, the vaginal cervix may be shorter than expected, but substantial cervical tissue is often visible on ultrasound that is not appreciated by inspection or palpation. A minority of women observed for these conditions display the ultrasound criteria for cerclage.

Elective Cerclage

When the obstetric history is diagnostic, a prophylactic cerclage suture in the late first or early second trimester is an appropriate option. Concerns about spontaneous abortion after cerclage and exposure of the fetus to medication during a first-trimester cerclage have been reduced by use of ultrasound confirmation of fetal viability and conduction anesthesia, respectively. For women who choose prenatal diagnosis because of a risk of chromosomal or genetic aberration, serum screening and/or chorionic villus sampling may be performed before 13 weeks' gestation, and the cerclage can be deferred until after the results are known. Alternately, an amniocentesis may be elected two or more weeks after the cerclage is placed.

Perioperative care for a woman undergoing an elective cerclage is minimal. At this early age and in the absence of cervical dilation or effacement, the benefit of adjunctive medications is doubtful. In the absence of data, the current authors prescribe perioperative antibiotics at the time of surgery but do not use any tocolytic or hormonal medications routinely. The patient is ordinarily ready to go home in several hours after her anesthetic has worn off, with instructions to expect mild abdominal cramping, spotting, and pain in the labia and vagina (from retraction during the procedure) for a few days. Pain is treated with nonsteroidal anti-inflammatory drugs or acetaminophen with codeine for 1–2 days.

Common choices for elective cerclage are the McDonald or Shirodkar sutures described previously. The choice of technique is largely a matter of individual experience, supplemented by such factors as whether a previous cerclage procedure was successful, the length of the vaginal portion of the cervix, and any previous vaginal or cervical surgery (e.g., cold-knife conization).

Urgent Cerclage

Placement of a cerclage after there is evidence of significant funneling can occur between 16 and 22 weeks' gestation, while a woman with a history of early preterm birth is being followed with sonography. Management algorithms for patients in this category are almost entirely empiric (Guzman et al., 1996).

Perioperative care for patients treated with an urgent cerclage includes empirical treatment with antibiotics and tocolytics (usually indomethacin) and a period of hospital observation before and after cerclage placement. The choice of which procedure to perform is an individual one, influenced by the degree of cervical effacement and dilation. The current authors' custom is preoperative evaluation for infection, fluid leakage and uterine activity, perioperative antibiotic prophylaxis, and 24 hours of treatment with a nonsteroidal anti-inflammatory drug such as indomethacin.

Emergency Cerclage

When reduced cervical competence presents unexpectedly, initial symptoms may include pelvic pressure, low backache, or premenstrual symptoms accompanied by increased vaginal discharge that may be light tan or streaked with blood. A speculum examination should always be performed to exclude ruptured membranes and to look for membranes at or below the external os. Sonography at this point usually reveals a large

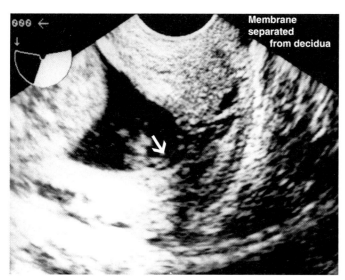

FIGURE 33-8 ■ Endovaginal image of the cervix showing membranes separated from underlying decidua at the internal cervical os.

funnel and substantial shortening, with or without dilation of the external os. Separation of the membranes can sometimes be seen with endovaginal sonography and is a poor prognostic sign (Fig. 33-8).

When the membranes are visible at the external os or bulge into the vagina, the prognosis for neonatal survival decreases significantly; however, a cerclage may still be placed if appropriate conditions are met. The patient should be placed in Trendelenburg position, and uterine activity should be monitored. Infection is a frequent complication; maternal temperature and white blood cell and differential counts should be determined and repeated as necessary to exclude infection. Amniocentesis to obtain amniotic fluid for infection with culture, Gram's stain, and glucose should be considered, based on reports that women who present with visible membranes often have positive amniotic fluid cultures and are unlikely to benefit from emergency cerclage (Romero et al., 1992; Mays et al., 2000). Ultrasonographic examination to assess fetal viability and to rule out major congenital anomalies is indicated. If abruptio placentae or chorioamnionitis is suspected, cerclage placement is contraindicated.

If infection, abruption, and progressive cervical change can be ruled out, prophylactic antibiotics and tocolytics are often employed despite the absence of studies to support their benefit. Most authors prescribe preoperative treatment with indomethacin, 25 mg orally every 6 hours and for 24 hours postoperatively, and broad spectrum perioperative antibiotic prophylaxis (Novy et al., 2001; Althuisius et al., 2001; Rust et al., 2001). Reports of candida amnionitis in women treated with antibiotics suggest that a limited duration of prophylaxis may be wise (Qureshi et al., 1998).

The McDonald cerclage is favored by most authors when the cervix is well dilated, but the Shirodkar and Wurm (nonabsorbable mattress sutures from 12 to 6 o'clock and from 3 to 9 o'clock) techniques have also been employed. Placement of a cervical cerclage of any type under these circumstances is difficult at best. Bulging or prolapsed membranes are easily ruptured intraoperatively. Careful inspection of the membranes to identify separation or loss of the chorion from the intact amnion should be routine. If only the amnion remains, pro-

longation of pregnancy beyond a few days is unlikely, and consideration should be given to abandoning the procedure. Visible membranes may be replaced into the uterus with gauze on a ring forceps covered by either a condom or a finger cot (Novy, 1985) or with a No. 16 French Foley catheter (Holman, 1973). The tip of the catheter is cut off, and the catheter is inserted through the external os. The balloon is inflated slowly and acts to keep the membranes from prolapsing through the cervix. Either a McDonald or a Shirodkar cerclage may then be placed and tied with the catheter in place. The balloon is deflated, and the catheter is withdrawn. Tsatsaris and colleagues (2001) recently described a technique to replace and protect the membranes within the uterus using a balloon device originally designed for endoscopic preperitoneal dissection. Transabdominal amniocentesis may temporarily reduce amniotic fluid volume and assist in spontaneous replacement of the membranes within the uterus (Locatelli et al., 1999). Other techniques that have been advocated include filling the maternal bladder with sufficient fluid to compress the lower uterine segment, thus returning a bulging amniotic sac into the uterus sufficiently to allow cerclage (Sheerer et al., 1987), and placement of the cerclage suture with the patient in the knee-chest position (Ogawa et al., 1999).

Preoperative dilation of the cervix was the factor most strongly associated with complications and fetal survival in a review of 482 cerclage procedures (Treadwell et al., 1991); others have reported the same association (Minimaki et al., 1999).

Reported success rates for emergency cerclage—defined as reaching "viability"—rose from 10% in 1980 (Harger, 1980) to 42% in a report from 1988 (Chryssikopoulos et al., 1988) and over 60% in 1995 (Aarts et al., 1995). Aarts and coworkers summarized data from 13 reports that described 249 patients treated with emergency cerclage procedures performed at a median gestational age of 22.8 weeks. The mean prolongation of pregnancy was 8.1 weeks, and the mean neonatal survival was 64% (range, 22%–100%). A French study (Benifla et al., 1997) of 34 pregnancies treated with emergency cerclage for cervical dilation after 20 weeks' gestation reported that 32 of 37 fetuses (86.5%) survived. An American review of 75 women treated with emergency cerclage between 1984 and 1994 at a mean gestational age of 19 weeks reported that 65% delivered after 28 weeks' and 49% after 34 weeks' gestation (Chasen and Silverman, 1998). Long-term outcomes were not reported in either study.

Often, the only alternative to emergency cerclage in patients with advanced dilation is hospital bed rest. Olatunbosun and associates (1995) compared pregnancy outcomes in 22 women treated with emergency cerclage with outcomes in 15 women who elected bed rest in a nonrandomized study. All patients were enrolled between 20 and 27 weeks of gestation, and all had cervical dilation greater than 4 cm. The perinatal mortality did not differ, but the cerclage group spent fewer days in the hospital.

There is no consensus about an upper gestational age limit for placement of a cerclage suture. As neonatal intensive care technology continues to improve and mortality statistics for very-low-birth-weight babies continue to fall, it seems reasonable to withhold cerclage placement at that gestational age when there is significant opportunity for fetal survival. In many centers, 24 weeks is a commonly chosen threshold based on current neonatal mortality data. After 24 weeks, the current authors treat most patients with hospital bed rest in the Trendelenburg position, accompanied by thromboembolism prophylaxis and a dietary and laxative regimen to produce a soft stool. This clinical setting is one of the few indications at our center for prophylactic use of tocolytic drugs to keep the uterus quiet. Whether this protocol is effective is unknown. The duration of hospitalization after an emergency cerclage must be individualized. These patients have a higher risk of postoperative complications, including infection, membrane rupture, and labor than after an elective or urgent cerclage and may require a prolonged stay if home care is limited.

Complications after Cerclage

Morbidity associated with cervical cerclage of all types includes complications related to the procedure itself (anesthetic risks, bleeding, maternal soft tissue injury, spontaneous suture displacement, PROM, and infection) and those related to subsequent delivery (cervical laceration and fistulae, increased incidence of cesarean section). Bleeding that requires transfusion is a rare complication of cerclage. In a report of 202 elective transvaginal procedures, Harger (1980) noted no blood loss greater than 150 mL. Benson and Durfee (1965) reported transfusion in 2 of 13 patients undergoing transabdominal cerclage. Premature rupture of membranes can occur in 1% to 40% of women treated with cerclage (Harger 1980; Treadwell et al., 1991). This risk increases with the degree of dilation and effacement and gestational age at placement (Treadwell et al., 1991).

Management of preterm PROM in a patient with a cerclage is controversial. Reports of an increased incidence of infectious complications and poor neonatal outcome when the cerclage was in left *in situ* after membrane rupture (Ludmir et al., 1994) have not been confirmed by two recent studies. In a retrospective report of 81 women with preterm PROM with cerclage who had no clinical signs of labor or infection at presentation, McElrath and associates (2000) found no differences in latency, gestational age at delivery, chorioamnionitis, or neonatal morbidity according to whether the suture was removed or left in place. Jenkins and colleagues (2000) reported outcomes for 79 women with cerclage and subsequent preterm PROM between 18 and 34 weeks' gestation managed with either immediate (less than 24 hours) or delayed (greater than 24 hours) suture removal after presentation with PROM. Seventeen were excluded (six with labor, nine who chose induction earlier than 24 weeks' gestation, and one each with chorioamnionitis and nonreassuring fetal testing); among the 62 remaining patients, women managed with delayed removal more often received prophylactic antibiotics and tocolytics; use of antenatal corticosteroids was not different. The delayed removal group had longer latency but no greater incidence of risk (chorioamnionitis) or benefit (birth weight, duration of neonatal intensive care unit stay, respiratory distress). Both studies examined retrospectively collected data, likely to be influenced by physician preferences for each patient. Nonetheless, the risk of leaving the cerclage in place may be acceptable, if only to allow sufficient time for antenatal corticosteroids. A 1999 review (O'Connor et al.) concluded that retention has acceptable risks when preterm PROM occurs early, but that the benefit-to-risk ratio declines as gestational age increases.

Chorioamnionitis resulting from cervical cerclage placement has been reported with varying frequency from 1% (Harger, 1980) to 6%–8% (Treadwell et al., 1991). The incidence of postoperative chorioamnionitis increases with the gestational age at cerclage placement (Charles and Edwards, 1981), no doubt related both to the increased participation of infection as a cause of premature cervical effacement and to the greater degree of cervical dilation when cerclage is performed after 20 weeks' gestation. In a review of 482 patients treated with cerclage, Treadwell and coworkers (1991) found that the rate of chorioamnionitis (6.6% overall) was significantly associated with cervical dilation (6.2% if the cervix was no more than 2 cm versus 41.7% if the cervix was greater than 2 cm) and with the timing of the procedure (5.2% if elective versus 14.4% if emergent).

Displacement of the cervical suture usually occurs posteriorly and is probably more common than was realized before the use of postoperative sonography (Rana et al., 1990). Most authors have found that ultrasound surveillance is a valuable adjunct to prenatal care of patients with cerclage (Rana et al., 1990; Andersen et al., 1994; Guzman et al., 1996). Surveillance with sonography is useful to guide advice about activity restriction and also offers an opportunity to place a second suture when the membranes are seen to protrude below the plane of the cerclage suture before 20–22 weeks' gestation (Fox et al., 1996).

Remote sequelae of cervical cerclage procedures include uterine rupture, excessive bleeding at the time of suture removal, cervical dystocia thought to be caused by scarring at the cerclage site, and cervical lacerations and fistulae. Lindberg (1979) reported uterine rupture when labor began before the suture could be removed. This is a particular concern in a patient with a prior cesarean delivery performed through a classic uterine incision. The cervix may not dilate normally in response to labor after a cerclage has been in place, despite its removal at the appropriate time (Kuhn and Pepperell, 1977; Harger, 1980).

Treadwell and coworkers (1991) reported an overall incidence of cesarean delivery of 31.8% in 482 patients. Cesarean section for cervical dystocia was more common after Shirodkar than after McDonald cerclage: 11.4% versus 2.6%, respectively (P < .005) in this series. Cervical lacerations at delivery thought to be related to cerclage have been reported (Harger, 1980; Treadwell et al., 1991). Treadwell and co-workers (1991) observed cervical lacerations in 6.2% of patients, more commonly when the cerclage was placed after 18 weeks' gestation. Other maternal morbidity associated with cerclage placement includes vesicovaginal and urethrovaginal fistulae (Bates and Cropley, 1977; Ulmsten, 1977) and ulceration of the trigone of the bladder from erosion of the knot of the cerclage (Hortenstine and Witherington, 1987).

Transabdominal Cervicoisthmic Cerclage

First described by Benson and Durfee (1965), the transabdominal approach to cerclage placement has been studied extensively and continually updated by Novy (1982, 1991) and others (Mahran, 1978; Wallenburg and Lotgering, 1987; Cammarano et al., 1995; Davis et al., 2000). The criteria recommended by Benson and Durfee and reaffirmed by Davis and associates (2000) include the following:

1. A congenitally short or amputated cervix
2. Previously unsuccessful cerclage with cervical scarring
3. Deeply notched, multiple cervical defects
4. Unhealed forniceal lacerations or subacute cervicitis

Suggested timing for abdominal cerclage is between 10 and 14 weeks of gestation so that uterine manipulation for visualization of both anterior and posterior leaves of the broad ligament can be accomplished easily, but the procedure is possible with a vertical incision up to 17 to 18 weeks' gestation.

The operation described by Benson and Durfee (1965) begins with either a Pfannenstiel or vertical abdominal incision. The peritoneal reflections are divided transversely, and the bladder is advanced carefully to avoid wide lateral dissection that may injure the massive vascular plexus present during pregnancy. At the level of the uterine isthmus, the space between the ascending and descending branches of the uterine artery is identified and developed by blunt dissection medial to the uterine arteries and veins, and lateral to the connective tissue of the uterine isthmus. Upward traction on the uterine fundus by an assistant exposes the region of the internal os, and the vessels are placed on traction.

After the tunnel has been developed in the vascular space bilaterally, the posterior leaf of the broad ligament is punctured bilaterally, and a 5-mm Mersilene tape is passed under direct vision to lie over the posterior peritoneum at the level of the insertions of the uterosacral ligaments. The Mersilene band is tied snugly anteriorly or posteriorly with a single square knot, and the cut ends are sutured to the band with fine, nonabsorbable sutures. The peritoneum and abdomen are then closed in routine fashion.

Mahran (1978) described a slightly different procedure in which the uterine vessels are retracted laterally with the operator's fingers while a synthetic 5-mm tape is placed around the cervix from anterior to posterior at the level of the isthmus. The suture is anchored in the cervical tissue both anteriorly and posteriorly (and laterally in Mackenrodt's ligament) and is tied posteriorly. Mahran preferred a vertical midline incision for the operation performed at 10–14 weeks' gestation but found this incision to be suitable for use well into the second trimester. The principal advantage of this technique is that it minimizes the opportunity for injury to the dilated parametrial venous plexus. This is the technique used by Davis and associates (2000) and in the hospital of the current authors. Davis and colleagues reported a retrospective comparison of transvaginal and transabdominal cerclage in women with grossly normal cervical anatomy who had a previous "failed" transvaginal cerclage; failure was defined as delivery before 33 weeks' gestation. Delivery before 35 and 33 weeks' gestation was less common (18% versus 42%, $P = .04$, and 10% versus 38%, $P = .01$, respectively) in women treated with transabdominal cerclage ($n = 40$) than with transvaginal cerclage ($n = 24$). Mean gestational age at delivery was correspondingly longer; the principal difference was a marked reduction in the frequency of preterm ruptured membranes—8% in the transabdominal group versus 29% in those treated with a transvaginal procedure ($P = .03$). Figure 33-9 shows an endovaginal image of the cervix from a woman treated with a transabdominal cerclage. The cerclage is seen near the internal os, at a level rarely achieved with a transvaginal procedure.

Risks unique to the transabdominal procedure include the need for laparotomy for cerclage placement and again for

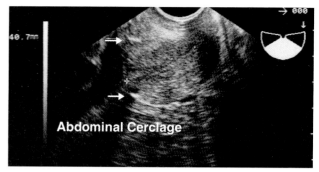

FIGURE 33-9 ■ Endovaginal ultrasound image of the cervix in a woman with a transabdominal cerclage. *Arrows* point to the 5-mm tape used for the procedure.

cesarean section. Emergency removal of the suture can sometimes be accomplished by posterior colpotomy but can be accompanied by substantial hemorrhage from tearing of the intensely vascular parametrial venous plexus. Most physicians leave the cerclage in place and perform elective cesarean section before labor. A well-placed cerclage rarely causes symptoms between pregnancies if future childbearing is planned.

POSTOPERATIVE CARE

Postoperative care varies according to the circumstances that led to the cerclage, including especially the gestational age and the degree of cervical dilation at the time of cerclage. An elective procedure at 10–14 weeks' gestation performed with an undilated cervix is an outpatient procedure. A 2- to 5-day rest period is recommended, depending on the patient's work requirements and any operative complications, after which intercourse, prolonged standing (greater than 90 minutes), and heavy lifting are avoided. For urgent and emergent cerclage patients, a longer period of hospital care for bed rest and observation is usually recommended, with discharge to home individualized according to the availability of family or others for home care.

Postoperative assessment of suture location as well as pregnancy management and outcome can be improved with ultrasonographic assessment of the cervix (Parulekar and Kiwi, 1982; Rana et al., 1990; Andersen et al., 1994; Guzman et al., 1996; Fox et al., 1996). Both the nylon and Ethibond sutures commonly used in the McDonald procedure and the 5-mm Mersilene tape used in the Shirodkar procedure (Fig. 33-10) can be seen easily with transvaginal ultrasound. The length of the cervix from the plane of the suture to both the internal and external os can be measured.

Andersen and associates (1994) studied 32 women after elective cerclage with serial endovaginal sonography. One of 20 patients who maintained a cervical length of more than 10 mm above the level of the cerclage until 30 weeks of gestation delivered before 34 weeks. In contrast, six of the 12 patients whose cervical length above the suture was less than or equal to 10 mm delivered before 34 weeks. Guzman and associates (1996) performed preoperative and postoperative transvaginal ultrasound examinations in 29 women who received an emergency cerclage between 16 and 26 weeks of pregnancy and found correlations between good perinatal outcome and the immediate postoperative sonographic appearance of the cervix, including increased cervical length above and below the stitch and decreased funnel width. In this study, all subjects eventually displayed an upper cervical length less than 10 mm by 28 weeks, reflecting the advanced effacement at the time of cerclage in the population. In a study of 20 women with endovaginal sonography after cerclage, half did not display a funnel when the cerclage was removed in the third trimester (Quinn, 1992), suggesting that the diagnosis of incompetence was incorrect and that sonographic surveillance would be a better choice in future pregnancies.

When the cerclage sutures remain within the middle or upper third of the cervix without the development of a funnel and the length of the cervix is at least 25 mm, the current authors allow normal physical activity except for coitus, standing more than 90 minutes, and weight-bearing exercise. Placement of a second cerclage when the first appears to be failing, as indicated by protrusion of the membranes past the plane of the cerclage, can be considered if observed before 20–22 weeks' gestation. Patients in whom membrane protrusion is noted with ultrasound after 22–24 weeks' gestation are placed on bed rest, usually in the hospital if the membranes are seen to extend below the level of the cerclage with transvaginal sonography (Fig. 33-11).

Removal can usually be accomplished in the office or clinic without anesthesia if good lighting is provided. Most women expect labor to begin immediately, but that is the exception. An interval of days between removal and the onset of labor does not mean the diagnosis was incorrect but instead typifies the different etiologies of abnormal cervical competence.

NONSURGICAL THERAPY

Through the years, several nonsurgical approaches to the management of patients with supposed cervical incompetence have been attempted, although none has gained widespread

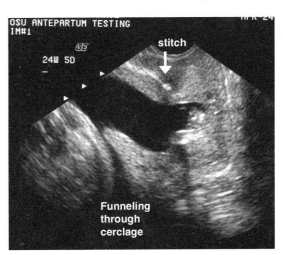

FIGURE 33-11 ■ Endovaginal ultrasound image of the cervix in a woman with membranes funneled past the level of a cerclage suture. *Arrow* points to the suture. Note the echogenic material (debris) within the funnel. Its origin is unclear, but it is often seen with preterm cervical effacement.

acceptance or proved efficacious in a controlled trial. Various types of vaginal pessaries have been used in an attempt to change the axis of the cervical canal and prevent alleged gravitational forces from causing cervical dilation and subsequent delivery (Oster and Javert, 1966). Newcomer (2000) reviewed the use of pessaries and concluded that there was insufficient evidence to exclude the possibility of benefit.

■ SUMMARY

The clinical syndrome of incompetent cervix results in early, often recurrent preterm birth in the second trimester. Advanced cervical dilation and effacement with minimal uterine activity is the most typical presentation, but not an exclusive one. The syndrome is the result of the interaction of many factors that affect the strength of the cervix, including biological variation, obstetrical and gynecological injuries, and inflammation-mediated changes. Diagnosis is difficult and should be based on both the obstetrical history and ultrasound evidence of premature effacement. The most effective treatment has not been established. Treatment with cerclage is considered when both historical and ultrasound criteria are met.

REFERENCES

Aarts JM, Brons JTJ, Bruinse HW: Emergency cerclage: A review. Obstet Gynecol Surv **50:**459, 1995.

Althuisius SM, Dekker GA, Hummel P, et al: Final results of the cervical incompetence prevention randomized cerclage trial (CIPRACT): Therapeutic cerclage with bed rest versus bed rest alone. Am J Obstet Gynecol **185:**1106, 2001.

Althuisius SM, Dekker GA, van Geijn HP, et al: Cervical incompetence prevention randomized cerclage trial (CIPRACT): Study design and preliminary results. Am J Obstet Gynecol **183:**823, 2000.

Althuisius SM, Schornagel IJ, Dekker GA, et al: Loop electrosurgical excision procedure of the cervix and time of delivery in subsequent pregnancy. Int J Gynaecol Obstet **72:**31, 2001.

American College of Obstetricians and Gynecologists Committee on Quality Assessment. Criteria Set 18, October 1996.

American College of Radiology: ACR Appropriateness Criteria: Expert Panel on Women's Imaging. Premature cervical dilatation. American College of Radiology, Reston, Va, 1999. Available at *http://www.acr.org.*

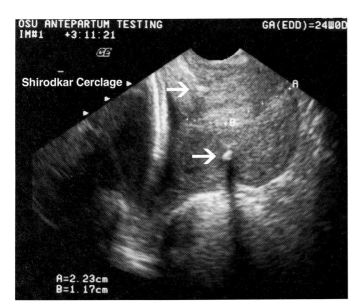

FIGURE 33-10 ■ Endovaginal ultrasound image of the cervix in a woman with a transvaginal cerclage. *Arrows* point to the 5-mm tape used for the procedure.

Andersen HF: Transvaginal and transabdominal ultrasonography of the uterine cervix during pregnancy. J Clin Ultrasound **19**:77, 1991.

Andersen HF, Karimi A, Sakala EP, et al: Prediction of cervical cerclage outcome by endovaginal sonography. Am J Obstet Gynecol **171**:1102, 1994.

Andersen HF, Nugent CE, Wanty SD, et al: Prediction of risk for preterm delivery by ultrasonographic measurement of cervical length. Am J Obstet Gynecol **163**:859, 1990.

Andrews WW, Copper RL, Hauth JC, et al: Second-trimester cervical ultrasound: Associations with increased risk for recurrent early spontaneous delivery. Obstet Gynecol **95**:222, 2000.

Ayers JWT, DeGrood RM, Compton AA, et al: Sonographic evaluation of cervical length in pregnancy: Diagnosis and management of preterm cervical effacement in patients at risk for premature delivery. Obstet Gynecol **71**:939, 1988.

Bates JL, Cropley T: Complications of cervical cerclage. Lancet **2**:1035, 1977.

Benifla JL, Goffinet F, Darai E, et al: Emergency cervical cerclage after 20 weeks' gestation: A retrospective study of six years' practice in 34 cases. Fetal Diagn Ther **5**:274, 1997.

Benson RC, Durfee RB: Transabdominal cervicouterine cerclage during pregnancy for the treatment of cervical incompetency. Obstet Gynecol **25**:145, 1965.

Berghella V, Daly SF, Tolosa JE, et al: Prediction of preterm delivery with transvaginal ultrasonography of the cervix in patients with high-risk pregnancies: Does cerclage prevent prematurity? Am J Obstet Gynecol **181**:809, 1999.

Berghella V, Kuhlman K, Weiner S, et al: Cervical funneling: Sonographic criteria predictive of preterm delivery. Ultrasound Obstet Gynecol **10**:161, 1997.

Bernstine RL, Lee SH, Crawford WL, et al: Sonographic evaluation of incompetent cervix. J Clin Ultrasound **9**:417, 1981.

Boomgaard JJ, Dekker KS, van Rensburg E, et al: Vaginitis, cervicitis, and cervical length in pregnancy. Am J Obstet Gynecol **181**:964, 1999.

Brook I, Feingold M, Schwartz A, et al: Ultrasonography in the diagnosis of cervical incompetence in pregnancy: A new diagnostic approach. Br J Obstet Gynecol **88**:640, 1981.

Buckingham JC, Buethe RA, Danforth DN: Collagen-muscle ratio in clinically normal and clinically incompetent cervices. Am J Obstet Gynecol **91**:231, 1965.

Cammarano CL, Herron MA, Parer JT: Validity of indications for transabdominal cervicoisthmic cerclage for cervical incompetence. Am J Obstet Gynecol **172**:1871, 1995.

Carr DB, Smith K, Parsons L, et al: Ultrasonography for cervical length measurement: Agreement between transvaginal and translabial techniques. Obstet Gynecol **96**:554, 2000.

Charles D, Edwards WR: Infectious complications of cervical cerclage. Am J Obstet Gynecol **141**:1065, 1981.

Chasen ST, Silverman NS: Mid-trimester emergent cerclage: A ten year single institution review. J Perinatol **18**:338, 1998.

Chryssikopoulos A, Botsis D, Vitoratos N, et al: Cervical incompetence: A 24-year review. Int J Gynecol Obstet **26**:245, 1988.

Chwe M, Raynor B, Graves W: The effect of conization method on subsequent pregnancy outcome (Abstract No. 17). Am J Obstet Gynecol **176**:S8, 1997.

Cicero S, Skentou C, Souka A, et al: Cervical length at 22–24 weeks of gestation: Comparison of transvaginal and transperineal-translabial ultrasonography. Ultrasound Obstet Gynecol **17**:335, 2001.

Confino E, Mayden KL, Giglia RV, et al: Pitfalls in sonographic imaging of the incompetent uterine cervix. Acta Obstet Gynecol Scand **65**:593, 1986.

Cook CM, Ellwood DA: The cervix as a predictor of preterm delivery in "at-risk" women. Ultrasound Obstet Gynecol **15**:109, 2000.

Crombleholme WR, Minkoff HL, Delke I, et al: Cervical cerclage: An aggressive approach to threatened or recurrent pregnancy wastage. Am J Obstet Gynecol **146**:168, 1983.

Crosby WM, Hill EC: Embryology of the müllerian duct system. Obstet Gynecol **20**:507, 1962.

Danforth DN: The fibrous nature of the human cervix and its relation to the isthmic segment in gravid and nongravid uteri. Am J Obstet Gynecol **53**:541, 1947.

Davis G, Berghella V, Talucci M, et al: Patients with a prior failed transvaginal cerclage: A comparison of obstetrics outcomes with either transabdominal or transvaginal cerclage. Am J Obstet Gynecol **183**:836, 2000.

Dhont M, DeSutter P, Ruyssinck G, et al: Perinatal outcome of pregnancies after assisted reproduction: A case-control study. Am J Obstet Gynecol **181**:688, 1999.

Dor J, Shaley J, Mashiach S, et al: Elective cervical suture of twin pregnancies diagnosed ultrasonically in the first trimester following induced ovulation. Gynecol Obstet Invest **13**:55, 1982.

Eppel W, Kucera E, Bieglmayer C: Relationship of serum levels of endogenous relaxin to cervical size in the second trimester and to cervical ripening at term. Br J Obstet Gynaecol **106**:917, 1999.

Ferenczy A, Choukroun D, Falcone T, et al: The effect of cervical loop electrosurgical excision on subsequent pregnancy outcome. Am J Obstet Gynecol **172**:1246, 1995.

Fox R, James M, Tuohy J, et al: Transvaginal ultrasound in the management of women with suspected cervical incompetence. Br J Obstet Gynaecol **103**:921, 1996.

Gee H, Taylor EW, Hancox R: A model for the generation of intrauterine pressure in the human parturient uterus which demonstrates the critical role of the cervix. J Theor Biol **133**:281, 1988.

Gentry DJ, Baggish MS, Brady K, et al: The effects of loop excision of the transformation zone on cervical length. Am J Obstet Gynecol **182**:516, 2000.

Goldberg J, Newman RB, Rust PF: Interobserver reliability of digital and endovaginal ultrasonographic cervical length measurements. Am J Obstet Gynecol **177**:853, 1997.

Goldenberg RL, Hauth JC, Andrews WW: Intrauterine infection and preterm delivery. N Engl J Med **342**:1500, 2000.

Goldenberg RL, Iams JD, Mercer BM, et al. The preterm prediction study: The value of new vs. standard risk factors in predicting early and all spontaneous preterm births. Am J Public Health **88**:233, 1998.

Goldstein DP: Incompetent cervix in offspring exposed to diethylstilbestrol in utero. Obstet Gynecol **52**:S735, 1978.

Gramellini D, Fieni S, Molina E, et al: Transvaginal sonographic cervical length changes during normal pregnancy. J Ultrasound Med **21**:227, 2002.

Guzman EJ, Forster JK, Vintzeleos AM, et al: Pregnancy outcomes in women treated with elective versus ultrasound-indicated cerclage. Ultrasound Obstet Gynecol **12**:323, 1998.

Guzman ER, Houlihan C, Vintzileos A, et al: The significance of transvaginal ultrasonographic evaluation of the cervix in women treated with emergency cerclage. Am J Obstet Gynecol **175**:471, 1996.

Guzman ER, Mellon C, Vintzeleos AM, et al. Longitudinal assessment of endocervical canal length between 15 and 24 weeks' gestation in women at risk for pregnancy loss or preterm birth. Obstet Gynecol **92**:31, 1998.

Guzman ER, Pisatowski DM, Vintzileos M, et al: A comparison of ultrasonographically detected cervical changes in response to transfundal pressure, coughing, and standing in predicting cervical incompetence. Am J Obstet Gynecol **177**:660, 1997.

Guzman ER, Rosenberg JC, Houlihan C, et al: A new method using vaginal ultrasound and transfundal pressure to evaluate the asymptomatic incompetent cervix. Obstet Gynecol **83**:248, 1994.

Haning RV Jr, Canick JA, Goldsmith LT, et al: The effect of ovulation induction on the concentration of maternal serum relaxin in twin pregnancies. Am J Obstet Gynecol **174**:227, 1996.

Haning RV Jr, Goldsmith LT, Seifer DB, et al: Relaxin secretion in in vitro fertilization pregnancies. Am J Obstet Gynecol **174**:233, 1996.

Haning RV Jr, Steinetz B, Weiss G: Elevated serum relaxin levels in multiple pregnancy after menotropin treatment. Obstet Gynecol **66**:42, 1985.

Harger JH: Comparison of success and morbidity in cervical cerclage procedures. Obstet Gynecol **56**:543, 1980.

Harger JH: Cervical cerclage: Patient selection, morbidity and success rates. Clin Perinatol **10**:321, 1983.

Harger JH, Archer DF, Marchese SM, et al: Etiology of recurrent pregnancy losses and outcome of subsequent pregnancies. Obstet Gynecol **62**:574, 1983.

Hassan SS, Romero R, Maymon E, et al. Does cervical cerclage prevent preterm delivery in patients with a short cervix? Am J Obstet Gynecol **184**:1325, 2001.

Heath VCF, Souka AP, Erasmus I, et al: Cervical length at 23 weeks' gestation: The value of Shirodkar suture for the short cervix. Ultrasound Obstet Gynecol **12**:318, 1998.

Henriet L, Kaminski M: Impact of induced abortions on subsequent pregnancy outcome: The 1995 French national perinatal survey. Br J Obstet Gynaecol **108**:1036, 2001.

Herman GE: Notes on Emmet operation as a prevention of abortion. J Obstet Gynaecol Br Commonw **2**:256, 1902.

Hertzberg BS, Livingston E, DeLong DM, et al: Ultrasonographic evaluation of the cervix: Transperineal versus endovaginal imaging. J Ultrasound Med **20**:1071, 2001.

Hibbard JU, Snow J, Moawad AH: Short cervical length by ultrasound and cerclage. J Perinatol **3**:161, 2000.

Hibbard JU, Tart M, Moawad AH: Cervical length at 16–22 weeks' gestation and risk for preterm delivery. Obstet Gynecol **96**:972, 2000.

Holman MR: An aid for cervical cerclage. Obstet Gynecol **42**:478, 1973.

Hortenstine JS, Witherington R: Ulcer of the trigone: A late complication of cervical cerclage. J Urol **137**:109, 1987.

Hulka JF, Higgins G: Trauma to the internal cervical os during dilatation for diagnostic curettage. Am J Obstet Gynecol **82**:913, 1961.

Iams JD, Goldenberg RL, Meis PJ, et al: The length of the cervix and the risk of spontaneous preterm delivery. N Engl J Med **334**:567, 1996.

Iams JD, Goldenberg RL, Mercer BM, et al: The preterm prediction study: Recurrence risk of spontaneous preterm birth. Am J Obstet Gynecol **178**:1035, 1998.

Iams JD, Johnson FF, Sonek J, et al: Cervical competence as a continuum: A study of ultrasonographic cervical length and obstetric performance. Am J Obstet Gynecol **172**:1097, 1995.

Iams JD for the NICHD MFMU Network, Goldsmith LT, Weiss G: The preterm prediction study: Maternal serum relaxin, sonographic cervical length, and spontaneous preterm birth in twins. J Soc Gynecol Investig **8**:39, 2001.

Imseis HM, Albert TA, Iams JD: Identifying twin gestations at low risk for preterm birth with a transvaginal ultrasonographic cervical measurement at 24 to 26 weeks' gestation. Am J Obstet Gynecol **177**:1149, 1997.

Jackson GM, Ludmir J, Bader TJ: The accuracy of digital examination and ultrasound in the evaluation of cervical length. Obstet Gynecol **79**:214, 1992.

Jenkins TM, Berghella V, Shlossman PA, et al: Timing of cerclage removal after preterm premature rupture of the membranes: Maternal and neonatal outcomes. Am J Obstet Gynecol **183**:847, 2000.

Johnstone FD, Beard RJ, Boyd IE, et al: Cervical diameter after suction termination of pregnancy. Br Med J **1**(6001):68, 1976.

Kaufman RH, Adam E, Binder GL, et al: Upper genital tract changes and pregnancy outcome in offspring exposed in utero to diethylstilbestrol. Am J Obstet Gynecol **137**:299, 1980.

Kaufman RH, Adam E, Hatch EE, et al: Continued follow-up of pregnancy outcomes in diethylstilbestrol-exposed offspring. Obstet Gynecol **96**:483, 2000.

Kaufman RH, Binder GL, Gray PM, et al: Upper genital tract changes associated with exposure in utero to diethylstilbestrol. Am J Obstet Gynecol **128**:51, 1977.

Kaufman RH, Noller K, Adam E, et al: Upper genital tract abnormalities and pregnancy outcome in diethylstilbestrol-exposed progeny. Am J Obstet Gynecol **148**:973, 1984.

Kelly S, Pollock M, Maas B, et al: Early transvaginal ultrasonography versus early cerclage in women with an unclear history of incompetent cervix. Am J Obstet Gynecol **184**:1097, 2001.

Kristensen J, Langhoff-Roos J, Kristensen FB: Increased risk of preterm birth in women with cervical conization. Obstet Gynecol **81**:1005, 1993.

Kuhn RJP, Pepperell RJ: Cervical ligation: A review of 242 pregnancies. Aust N Z J Obstet Gynaecol **17**:79, 1977.

Kurtzman JT, Goldsmith LJ, Gall SA, et al: Transvaginal versus transperineal ultrasonography: A blinded comparison in the assessment of cervical length at midgestation. Am J Obstet Gynecol **179**:852, 1998.

Kushnir O, Vigil DA, Izquierdo L, et al: Vaginal ultrasonographic assessment of cervical length changes during normal pregnancy. Am J Obstet Gynecol **162**:991, 1990.

Laing F, Mendelson E, Bohm-Velez M, et al: Premature cervical dilatation. American College of Radiology. ACR Appropriateness Criteria Radiology **215**:939, 2000.

Lash AF: Fertility and reproduction following repair of the incompetent internal os of the cervix. Fertil Steril **11**:531, 1960.

Lash AF, Lash SR: Habitual abortion: The competent internal os of the cervix. Am J Obstet Gynecol **59**:68, 1950.

Lazar P, Guegen S, Dreyfus J, et al: Multicentred controlled trial of cervical cerclage in women at moderate risk of preterm delivery. Br J Obstet Gynaecol **91**:731, 1984.

Lees DH, Sutherst JR: The sequelae of cervical trauma. Am J Obstet Gynecol **120**:1050, 1974.

Leibovitz Z, Levitan,{AU: first initial of Levitan?} Aharoni A, et al: Cervical cerclage in uterine malformations. Int J Fertil **37**:214, 1992.

Leiman G, Harrison NA, Rubin A: Pregnancy outcome following conization of the cervix: Complications related to cone size. Am J Obstet Gynecol **136**:14, 1980.

Lindberg BS: Maternal sepsis, uterine rupture, and coagulopathy complicating cervical cerclage. Acta Obstet Gynecol Scand **58**:317, 1979.

Locatelli A, Vergani P, Bellini P, et al: Amnioreduction in emergency cerclage with prolapsed membranes: Comparison of two methods for reducing the membranes. Am J Perinatol **16**:73, 1999.

Ludmir J: Sonographic detection of cervical incompetence. Clin Obstet Gynecol **31**:101, 1988.

Ludmir J, Bader T, Chen L, et al: Poor perinatal outcome associated with retained cerclage in patients with premature rupture of membranes. Obstet Gynecol **84**:823, 1994.

Ludmir J, Jackson M, Samuels P: Transvaginal cerclage under ultrasound guidance in cases of severe cervical hypoplasia. Obstet Gynecol **78**:1067, 1991.

Ludmir J, Samuels P, Brooks S, et al: Pregnancy outcome of patients with uncorrected uterine anomalies managed in a high risk setting. Obstet Gynecol **75**:906, 1990.

MacDonald R, Smith P, Vyas S: Cervical incompetence: the use of transvaginal sonography to provide an objective diagnosis. Ultrasound Obstet Gynecol **18**:211, 2001.

MacNaughton MC, Chalmers IG, Dubowitz V, et al. Final report of the Medical Research Council/Royal College of Obstetrics and Gynaecology multicentre randomised trial of cervical cerclage. Br J Obstet Gynaecol **100**:516, 1993.

Mahran M: Transabdominal cervical cerclage during pregnancy. Obstet Gynecol **52**:502, 1978.

Mandelson MT, Maden CB, Daling JR: Low birth weight in relation to multiple induced abortions. Am J Public Health **82**:391, 1992.

Mann EC, McLaren WD, Hoyt OB: The physiology and clinical significance of the uterine isthmus. Am J Obstet Gynecol **81**:209, 1961.

Mason GC, Maresh MJA: Alterations in bladder volume and the ultrasound appearance of the cervix. Br J Obstet Gynaecol **97**:457, 1990.

Mays JK, Figueroa R, Shah J, et al: Amniocentesis for selection before rescue cerclage Obstet Gynecol **95**:652, 2000.

McDonald IA: Suture of the cervix for inevitable miscarriage. J Obstet Gynaecol Br Commonw **64**:346, 1957.

McElrath TF, Norwitz ER, Lieberman ES, et al: Management of cervical cerclage and preterm premature rupture of the membranes: Should the stitch be removed? Am J Obstet Gynecol **183**:840, 2000.

McElrath TF, Wise PH: Fertility therapy and the risk of very low birth weight. Obstet Gynecol **90**:600, 1997.

Michaels WH, Montgomery C, Karo J, et al: Ultrasound differentiation of the competent from the incompetent cervix: Prevention of preterm delivery. Am J Obstet Gynecol **154**:537, 1986.

Minakami H, Matsubara S, Izumi A, et al: Emergency cervical cerclage: relation between its success, preoperative serum level of C-reactive protein and WBC count, and degree of cervical dilation. Gynecol Obstet Invest **47**:157, 1999.

Mohapeloa H, Christiansen OB, Grunnet N: HLA-DR typing of women with recurrent late spontaneous abortion and unsuccessful cerclage. Hum Reprod **13**:1079, 1998.

Newcomer J: Pessaries for the treatment of incompetent cervix and premature delivery. Obstet Gynecol Surv **55**:443, 2000.

Novy MJ: Transabdominal cervicoisthmic cerclage for the management of repetitive abortion and premature delivery. Am J Obstet Gynecol **143**:44, 1982.

Novy MJ: Combating recurrent abortion and premature delivery with cervical cerclage. Special issue. Contemp Obstet Gynecol **25**:113, 1985.

Novy MJ: Transabdominal cervicoisthmic cerclage: A reappraisal 25 years after its introduction. Am J Obstet Gynecol **164**:1635, 1991.

Novy MJ, Gupta A, Wothe DD, et al: Cervical cerclage in the second trimester of pregnancy: A historical cohort study. Am J Obstet Gynecol **184**:1447, 2001.

O'Connor S, Kuller JA, McMahon MJ: Management of cervical cerclage after preterm premature rupture of membranes. Obstet Gynecol Surv **54**:391, 1999.

Ogawa M, Sanada H, Tsuda A, et al: Modified cervical cerclage in pregnant women with advanced bulging membranes: Knee-chest positioning. Acta Obstet Gynecol Scand **78**:779, 1999.

Okitsu O, Mimura T, Nakayama T, et al: Early prediction of preterm delivery by transvaginal ultrasonography. Ultrasound Obstet Gynecol **2**:402, 1992.

Olah KS, Gee H: The prevention of prematurity: Can we continue to ignore the cervix? Br J Obstet Gynaecol **99**:278, 1992.

Olatunbosun OA, al-Nuaim L, Turnell RW: Emergency cerclage compared with bedrest for advanced cervical dilatation during pregnancy. Int Surg **80**:170, 1995.

Oster S, Javert CT: Treatment of the incompetent cervix with the Hodge pessary. Obstet Gynecol **28**:206, 1966.

Owen J, Iams JD, Hauth JC: Vaginal sonography and cervical incompetence. Am J Obstet Gynecol **188**:586, 2003.

Owen J, Neely C, Northen A: Transperineal versus endovaginal ultrasonographic examination of the cervix in the midtrimester: A blinded comparison. Am J Obstet Gynecol **181**:780, 1999.

Owen J, Yost N, Berghella V, et al: Mid-trimester endovaginal sonography in women at high risk for spontaneous preterm birth. JAMA **286:**1340, 2001.

Palmer R, LaComme JL: La beáance de l'orifice interne, cause d'avortment a repetition une observation de dechirure cervico-isthmique repare chirurgicalement, avec gestation a term consecutive. Gynecol Obstet (Paris) **47:**905, 1948.

Parikh MN, Mehta AC: Internal cervical os during the second half of pregnancy. J Obstet Gynaecol Br Commonw **68:**818, 1961.

Parulekar SG, Kiwi R: Ultrasound evaluation of sutures following cervical cerclage for incompetent cervix uteri. J Ultrasound Med **1:**223, 1982.

Petersen LK, Uldbjerg N: Cervical collagen in non-pregnant women with previous cervical incompetence. Eur J Obstet Gynecol Reprod Biol **67:**41, 1996.

Phelps JY, Higby K, Smyth MH, et al: Accuracy and intraobserver variability of simulated cervical dilatation measurements. Am J Obstet Gynecol **173:**942, 1995.

Podobnik M, Bulic M, Smiljanic N, et al: Ultrasonography in the detection of cervical incompetency. J Clin Ultrasound **13:**383, 1988.

Quinn MJ: Vaginal ultrasound and cervical cerclage: A prospective study. Ultrasound Obstet Gynecol **2:**410, 1992.

Qureshi F, Jacques SM, Bendon RW, et al: Candida funisitis: A clinicopathologic study of 32 cases. Pediatr Dev Pathol. **1:**118, 1998.

Raio L, Ghezzi F, Di Naro E, et al: Duration of pregnancy after carbon dioxide laser conization of the cervix: Influence of cone height. Obstet Gynecol **90:**978, 1997.

Ramin KD, Ogburn PL, Mulholland TA, et al. Ultrasonographic assessment of cervical length in triplet pregnancies. Am J Obstet Gynecol **180:**1442, 1999.

Rana J, Davis SE, Harrington JT: Improving the outcome of cervical cerclage by sonographic follow-up. J Ultrasound Med **9:**275, 1990.

Rechberger T, Uldbjerg N, Oxlund H: Connective tissue changes in the cervix during normal pregnancy and pregnancy complicated by cervical incompetence. Obstet Gynecol **71:**563, 1988.

Robboy SJ, Noller KJ, Kaufman RT, et al: An Atlas of Findings in the Human Female After Intrauterine Exposure to Diethylstilbestrol. Washington, DC, U.S. Department of Health and Human Services, National Institutes of Health, 1983.

Romero R, Gonzalez R, Sepulveda W, et al: Infection and labor VIII. Microbial invasion of the amniotic cavity in patients with suspected cervical incompetence. Am J Obstet Gynecol **167:**1086, 1992.

Rorie DK, Newton M: Histological and chemical studies of the smooth muscle in human cervix and uterus. Am J Obstet Gynecol **99:**466, 1967.

Rush RW, Issacs S, McPherson K, et al: A randomized controlled trial of cervical cerclage in women at high risk of spontaneous delivery. Br J Obstet Gynaecol **91:**724, 1984.

Rust OA, Atlas RO, Jones KJ, et al: A randomized trial of cerclage versus no cerclage among patients with ultrasonographically detected second-trimester preterm dilatation of the internal os. Am J Obstet Gynecol **183:**830, 2000.

Rust OA, Atlas RO, Reed J, et al: Revisiting the short cervix detected by transvaginal ultrasound in the second trimester: Why cerclage therapy may not help. Am J Obstet Gynecol **185:**1098, 2001.

Sarti DA, Sample WF, Hobel CJ, et al: Ultrasonic visualization of a dilated cervix during pregnancy. Radiology **130:**417, 1979.

Schieve LA, Meikle SF, Ferre C, et al: Low and very low birth weight in infants conceived with the use of assisted reproductive technology. N Engl J Med **346:**731, 2002.

Schuly KF, Grimes DA, Cates W Jr: Measures to prevent cervical injury during suction curettage abortion. Lancet **1:**1182, 1983.

Seidman DS, Ben-Rafael Z, Bider D, et al: The role of cervical cerclage in the management of uterine anomalies. Surg Gynecol Obstet **173:**384, 1991.

Sheerer LJ, Lam L, Katz M: A New Technique for Cervical Cerclage in the Presence of Prolapsed Fetal Membranes. Orlando, Fla, Society for Perinatal Obstetricians, 1987.

Shirodkar VN: A new method of operative treatment for habitual abortions in the second trimester of pregnancy. Antiseptic **52:**299, 1955.

Shirodkar VN: Long-term results with the operative treatment of habitual abortion. Triangle **8:**123, 1967.

Sonek J, Blumenfeld M, Foley M, et al: Cervical length may change during ultrasonographic examination. Am J Obstet Gynecol **162:**1355, 1990.

Sonek JD, Iams JD, Blumenfeld M, et al: Measurement of cervical length in pregnancy: Comparison between vaginal ultrasonography and digital examination. Obstet Gynecol **76:**172, 1990.

Souka AP, Heath V, Flint S: Cervical length at 23 weeks in twins in predicting spontaneous preterm delivery. Obstet Gynecol **94:**540, 1999.

Surbek DV, Hoelsi IM, Holzgreve W: Morphology assessed by transvaginal ultrasonography differs in patients in preterm labor with vs. without bacterial vaginosis. Ultrasound Obstet Gynecol **15:**242, 2000.

Surico N, Ribaldone R, Arnulfo A, et al: Uterine malformations and pregnancy losses: Is cervical cerclage effective? Clin Exp Obstet Gynecol **27:**147, 2000.

Taipale P, Hiilesmaa V: Sonographic measurement of uterine cervix at 18–22 weeks' gestation and the risk of preterm delivery. Obstet Gynecol **92:**902, 1998.

Tho PT, Byrd JR, McDonough PG: Etiologies and subsequent reproductive performance in 100 couples with recurrent abortion. Fertil Steril **32:**389, 1979.

To MS, Palaniappan V, Skentou C, et al: Elective cerclage vs. ultrasound-indicated cerclage in high risk pregnancies. Ultrasound Obstet Gynecol **19:**475, 2002.

Treadwell MC, Bronsteen RA, Bottoms SF: Prognostic factors and complication rates for cervical cerclage: A review of 482 cases. Am J Obstet Gynecol **165:**555, 1991.

Tsatsaris V, Senat MV, Gervaise A, et al: Balloon replacement of fetal membranes to facilitate emergency cervical cerclage. Obstet Gynecol **98:**243, 2001.

Ulmsten U: Complication of cervical cerclage. Lancet **2:**1350, 1977.

Vogel I, Salvig JD, Secher NJ, et al: Association between raised serum relaxin levels during the eighteenth gestational week and very preterm delivery. Am J Obstet Gynecol **184:**390, 2001.

Von Maillot KV, Zimmermann BK: The solubility of collagen of the uterine cervix during pregnancy and labour. Arch Gynaekol **220:**275, 1976.

Wallenburg HCS, Lotgering FK: Transabdominal cerclage for closure of the incompetent cervix. Eur J Obstet Reprod Biol **25:**121, 1987.

Weiss G, Goldsmith L, Sachdev R, et al: Elevated first trimester serum relaxin concentrations in pregnant women following ovarian stimulation predict prematurity risk and preterm delivery. Obstet Gynecol **82:**821, 1993.

Wheelock JB, Johnson TRB, Graham D, et al: Ultrasound-assisted cervical cerclage. J Clin Ultrasound **12:**307, 1984.

Woelfer B, Salim R, Banerjee S, et al: Reproductive outcomes in women with congenital uterine anomalies detected by three-dimensional ultrasound screening. Obstet Gynecol **98:**1009, 2001.

Wong G, Levine D, Ludmir J: Maternal postural challenge as a functional test for cervical incompetence. J Ultrasound Med **16:**169, 1997.

Yost NP, Bloom SL, Twickler DM, et al: Pitfalls in ultrasonic cervical length measurement for predicting preterm birth. Obstet Gynecol **93:**510, 1999.

Zhou W, Sorenson HT, Olsen J. Induced abortion and low birthweight in the following pregnancy. Int J Epidemiol **29:**100, 2000.

Zilianti M, Azuaga A, Calderon F, et al: Monitoring the effacement of the uterine cervix by transperineal sonography. J Ultrasound Med **14:**719, 1995.

Zorzoli A, Soliani A, Perra M, et al: Cervical changes throughout pregnancy as assessed by transvaginal sonography. Obstet Gynecol **84:**960, 1994.

Chapter 34
PRETERM LABOR AND DELIVERY

Jay D. Iams, MD, and Robert K. Creasy, MD

Preterm delivery and congenital malformations are the two most common causes of perinatal morbidity and mortality. About 40% of preterm births follow preterm labor and another 30% from preterm ruptured membranes, a related condition (see Chapter 38). Although refinements in perinatal care have improved outcome for preterm infants, the incidence of low-birth-weight and preterm newborns has not improved. Despite renewed efforts to reduce preterm birth, the rate has actually increased in the last decade.

DEFINITIONS

A *preterm birth* is any delivery, regardless of birth weight, that occurs before 37 completed weeks from the first day of the last menstrual period. The lower limits of gestational age at which the phrase *preterm labor and delivery* can be used is not well defined. Pregnancies ending before 20 completed weeks of gestation have traditionally been termed "spontaneous abortions," while pregnancies ending after 20 weeks have been termed "deliveries." In this chapter, we use the traditional definition of *preterm delivery* as beginning at 20 weeks and ending at 36 and 6/7ths weeks' gestation, recognizing that the 20-week distinction is arbitrary and can lead to misunderstanding about the cause of the delivery unless a careful history is taken and the exact duration of pregnancy is noted.

Newborns who weigh under 2500 g at birth were once classified as "premature," but as many as one-third of such neonates are born near term but restricted in growth (see Chapter 28). Infants who weigh under 2500 g at birth, regardless of gestational age, are designated as low birth weight (LBW); those who weigh under 1500 g are classified as very low birth weight (VLBW).

INCIDENCE OF PRETERM AND LOW-BIRTH-WEIGHT INFANTS

Preterm Birth

Assessment of the true incidence of preterm delivery has been compromised by difficulty in differentiating growth-restricted from preterm infants. The incidence of preterm birth before 37 weeks in the United States was 9.4% in 1981 but has risen since then to 10.6% in 1990, 11.6% in 2000, and 11.9% in 2001. These figures include both singleton and multiple gestations (Martin et al., 2002b). Significant racial differences in the rates of preterm and low birth weight remain largely unexplained. Rates of preterm birth in singleton gestations before 32 weeks', between 32 and 36 weeks', and before 37 weeks' gestation for non-Hispanic whites, non-Hispanic blacks, and Hispanics for 1990, 1995, 2000, and 2001 are shown in Table 34-1.

Rates of preterm birth rose between 1990 and 2001 for both non-Hispanic whites and Hispanics but fell significantly for non-Hispanic blacks. Nevertheless, the incidence of preterm birth among African-Americans is still nearly double that of non-Hispanic whites and Hispanics. In 2000, non-Hispanic black women accounted for 37.7% of early preterm births before 28 weeks' gestation (Martin et al., 2002a).

Low Birth Weight

The rate of low birth weight (under 2500 g) for singleton and multiple gestations of all races was 7.7% in 2001, representing an increase from 6.8% in the mid-1980s. The same ethnic disparity noted for preterm birth is also evident for low birth weight. For singleton births, the rate in 2001 was 6.04% for all women, 4.96% for non-Hispanic whites, 11.19% for non-Hispanic blacks, and 5.40% for Hispanics (Martin et al., 2002b).

VLBW (under 1500 g) deliveries increased from 1.16% of births in 1981 to 1.27% in 1990 and 1.44% in 2001, caused primarily by a substantial increase in multiple gestations (Table 34-2; Martin et al., 2002b). In 2000, 23% of low-birth-weight infants were born in a twin, triplet, or higher-order multiple gestation (Martin et al., 2002a). This trend is evident in all ethnic groups but is most pronounced in whites. The increase is mainly due to increased use of assisted reproductive technology (ART) and to a lesser degree to deferred child-bearing. The rate of triplet and higher-order multiple gestations has slowed somewhat with improved ART practices, but the increase in twin deliveries has continued. For singleton gestations, the most common maternal diagnoses that precede the birth of an infant whose weight is below 1 kg are preterm labor and preterm ruptured membranes (Fig. 34-1) (Bottoms et al., 1997; Iams and Mercer 2003). These two diagnoses also include women whose primary diagnosis was abnormal cervical competence.

The Effect of Multiple Gestation on Preterm Delivery and Birth Weight

The frequency of multiple gestation has a direct effect on rates of preterm and low-birth-weight deliveries. In 2001, 57% of twins and 92% of triplets were born before 37 weeks'

TABLE 34-1. RATE OF PRETERM BIRTH AMONG SINGLETONS BY RACE AND HISPANIC ORIGIN OF MOTHER, UNITED STATES: 1990, 1995, 2000, AND 2001

Group	2001	2000	1995	1990*
Total, All Races, Origins†		*Percent*		
Fewer than 32 weeks	1.57	1.58	1.61	1.69
32–36 weeks	8.81	8.54	8.21	8.01
Total, fewer than 37 weeks	10.38	10.12	9.82	9.70
Non-Hispanic White				
Fewer than 32 weeks	1.15	1.14	1.13	1.11
32–36 weeks	7.83	7.55	6.99	6.43
Total, fewer than 37 weeks	8.98	8.69	8.12	7.54
Non-Hispanic Black				
Fewer than 32 weeks	3.52	3.58	3.83	4.22
32–36 weeks	12.49	12.29	12.70	13.63
Total, fewer than 37 weeks	16.01	15.87	16.53	17.85
Hispanic‡				
Fewer than 32 weeks	1.45	1.48	1.48	1.52
32–36 weeks	9.04	8.82	8.64	8.77
Total, fewer than 37 weeks	10.49	10.30	10.12	10.29

* Data by race and Hispanic origin exclude data for New Hampshire and Oklahoma, which did not require reporting of Hispanic origin of mother.
†Includes births among races not shown.
‡Includes persons of Hispanic origin of any race.

Martin JA, Hamilton BE, Ventura SE, et al: Births: Final data for 2001, National Vital Statistics Reports, Vol. 51, No. 2, Table F. Hyattesville, Md, National Center for Health Statistics, 2002.

gestation, compared with 10% of singletons. The mean gestational ages at delivery and birth weight for singletons, twins, and higher-order multiple gestations are shown in Table 34-3 (Martin et al., 2002b). Notably, the rates of VLBW, with the attendant increased risk of mortality and morbidity, are strikingly higher for multiple gestations than for singletons. More than 10% of twins, 30% of triplets, and 70% of higher-order multiple gestations result in VLBW infants; by comparison, just 1.6% of singletons had birth weights below 1500 g. A study of 1997 higher-order (triplet or greater number) births estimated that 43% resulted from ART and 38% were the result of ovulation-inducing drugs; only 20% were conceived spontaneously (Centers for Disease Control and Prevention, 2000).

INFANT MORTALITY AND MORBIDITY

The leading causes of infant mortality (deaths from birth to one year of age) in 2000 were congenital malformations (142.2 per 100,000 live births) and prematurity-related conditions (130.5 per 100,000 live births) (Minino and Smith, 2001). For black infants, prematurity-related diagnoses were the leading causes of infant mortality (340.5 per 100,000 live births, compared with 171.8 per 100,000 for congenital malformations) (Demissie et al., 2001). As noted in the National Vital Statistics report for births in 2000, despite the decrease in recent years in mortality among infants born too early, preterm newborns—especially those born before 32 weeks' gestation—have a substantially increased risk of long-term disability and death (Minino and Smith, 2001). For 2000, 18% of very

preterm infants (fewer than 32 weeks' gestation) died within the first year of life, compared with 1% of moderately preterm infants (32–36 weeks' gestation) and 0.03% of infants delivered at term (37–41 weeks' gestation) (Mathews et al., 2002).

Perinatal Mortality

A perinatal death is one that occurs at any time after 22 weeks' gestation (or above 500 g if gestational age is not known) through 28 days after delivery. The perinatal mortality rate is the sum of fetal (stillbirths) and neonatal deaths (American College of Obstetricians and Gynecologists, 1995). Perinatal mortality and morbidity are inversely related to both gestational age and birth weight. Preterm birth is the leading cause of perinatal morbidity and neonatal mortality.

In 2003, the majority of infants born at 25 weeks' gestation or more will survive, and most of the survivors born at 26 weeks' gestation or later will survive without major disability (MacDonald and the Committee on Fetus and Newborn, 2002). These rates are substantially higher than in 1970, when infants born at 28 weeks' gestation or who weighed under 1 kg were not expected to survive. Current survival rates at 30 weeks' gestation approach 90% in most perinatal centers, a figure far higher than the public and many health care personnel appreciate (Morse et al., 2000). Figure 34-2 shows survival and mortality rates from a population-based cohort of 8523 infants born in 1997 and 1998 at both community and tertiary-level hospitals (Mercer, 2003). The "threshold of viability" can be seen to lie between 22 and 25 weeks' gestation, after which the majority of infants survive to hospital discharge.

Recent mortality data for VLBW infants born in the National Institute of Child Health and Human Development Neonatal Network are shown in Figures 60-2, 60-3, and 60-4 in Chapter 60 according to their gestational age and weight at birth. Data from Canada is similar to data from the United

TABLE 34-2. NUMBERS OF TWIN, TRIPLET, QUADRUPLET, AND QUINTUPLET AND OTHER HIGHER ORDER MULTIPLE BIRTHS: UNITED STATES, 1989–2000

Year	Twins	Triplets	Quadruplets	Quintuplets and Other Higher Order Multiples*
2000	118,916	6,742	506	77
1999	114,307	6,742	512	67
1998	110,670	6,919	627	79
1997	104,137	6,148	510	79
1996	100,750	5,298	560	81
1995	96,736	4,551	365	57
1994	97,064	4,233	315	46
1993	96,445	3,834	277	57
1992	95,372	8,547	310	26
1991	94,779	3,121	203	22
1990	93,865	2,830	185	13
1989	90,118	2,529	229	40

*Quintuplets, sextuplets, and higher order multiple births are not differentiated in the national data set.

Martin JA, Hamilton BE, Ventura SJ, et al: Births: Final data for 2000. National Vital Statistics Reports, Vol. 50, No. 5, Table H from page 19. Hyattsville, Md, National Center for Health Statistics, 2002.

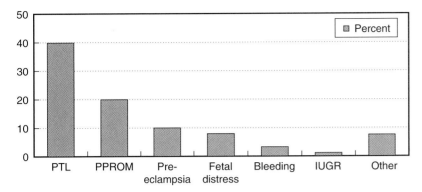

FIGURE 34-1 ■ Maternal diagnoses preceding births of infants weighing less than 1 kg. (Data from Bottoms SF, Paul RH, Iams JD, et al: Obstetric determinants of neonatal survival: Influence of willingness to perform cesarean delivery on survival of extremely low-birth-weight infants. Am J Obstet Gynecol **176**:960, 1997; Iams JD, Mercer BM for the National Institute of Child Health and Human Development Maternal-Fetal Medicine Units Network: Antenatal prediction of neonatal morbidity and mortality: The Obstetric Determinants of Neonatal Survival Study. Seminars in Perinatology **27**:199, 2003.

States. In a study of every live-born singleton infant born at 24 and 25 weeks' gestation at 13 of Canada's 17 tertiary perinatal centers from 1991 through 1996 (Effer et al., 2002), birth weights for 406 babies born at 24 weeks ranged from 627 to 725 grams; 56.1% survived to discharge. In the 454 babies born at 25 weeks, birth weights ranged from 698 to 832 grams, and 68% survived to discharge from the hospital.

Several factors can influence the likelihood of survival for VLBW and extremely-low-birth-weight (ELBW, under 1 kg) infants. Risk factors associated with lower mortality rates for very-low-birth-weight infants include greater birth weight (odds ratio [OR], 0.38; 95% CI, 0.29–0.49), female gender (OR, 0.42; 95% CI, 0.29–0.61), small-for-gestational-age designation (OR, 0.58; 95% CI, 0.38–0.88), antenatal treatment with corticosteroids (OR, 0.52; 95% CI, 0.36–0.76), and neonatal treatment with surfactant (Tyson et al., 1996; Effer et al., 2002). Intrauterine infection has an adverse influence on both survival and morbidity.

Rates of neonatal mortality and morbidity for live-born twins do not differ significantly from those for singletons born at the same gestational age (Donovan et al., 1998). Survival and morbidity rates are known to vary significantly across neonatal intensive care units, despite apparently similar care protocols (Horbar et al., 1988). The expectations of physicians and nurses who provide care during labor, delivery, and neonatal intensive care about the possibility of survival also exert an important influence on survival for extremely-low-birth-

weight infants (Bottoms et al., 1997; Morse et al., 2000; Shankaran et al., 2002).

Perinatal Morbidity

Improved survival for preterm infants has been accompanied by concern about the morbidity attendant to preterm birth and the quality of survival. Common causes of perinatal morbidity in premature infants include respiratory distress syndrome, intraventricular hemorrhage (IVH), bronchopulmonary dysplasia, patent ductus arteriosus, necrotizing enterocolitis, sepsis, apnea, retinopathy of prematurity, hyperbilirubinemia and jaundice, hypoglycemia, nutritional difficulties, apnea, and thermal instability (see also Chapter 60). Rates of respiratory distress, sepsis, and necrotizing enterocolitis have declined from those reported for preterm infants born between 1982 and 1986, but the rate of IVH has not changed appreciably (Robertson et al., 1992). In the NICHD Network of tertiary care neonatal intensive care units, the rate of major morbidity (defined as chronic lung disease, Grades 3 and 4 IVH, and/or necrotizing enterocolitis) declined between 1988 and 1994 for infants in all birth weight categories between 501 and 1500 g (Stevenson et al, 1998) but did not decline further between 1991 and 1996 (Lemons et al., 2001). The incidence of major morbidity was more than 60% for infants with birth weights between 501 and 750 g and approached 50% for infants weighing between 751 and 1000 g who were born

TABLE 34-3. GESTATIONAL AGE AND BIRTHWEIGHT CHARACTERISTICS BY PLURALITY: UNITED STATES, 2001

	Twins	Triplets	Quadruplets	Quintuplets	Singletons
Number	121,246	6,885	501	85	3,897,216
Percent very preterm*	11.8	36.7	64.5	78.6	1.6
Percent preterm[†]	57.4	92.4	97.8	91.7	10.4
Mean gestational age (weeks) standard deviation	35.4(3.7)	32.0(4.0)	29.6(4.1)	29.1(3.9)	38.8(2.5)
Percent very low birthweight[‡]	10.2	34.8	68.4	77.4	1.1
Percent low birthweight[§]	54.9	94.0	98.4	91.7	6.04
Mean birthweight (grams) standard deviation	2,353(647)	1,678(574)	1,290(549)	1,269(676)	3,339(573)

* Very preterm is fewer than 32 completed weeks of gestation.
[†] Preterm is fewer than 37 completed weeks of gestation.
[‡] Very low birthweight is under 1,500 grams.
[§] Low birthweight is under 2,500 grams.

Martin JA, Hamilton BE, Ventura SJ, et al: Births: Final data for 2001. National Vital Statistics Reports, Vol. 51, No. 2, Table H from page 21. Hyattsville, Md, National Center for Health Statistics, 2002.

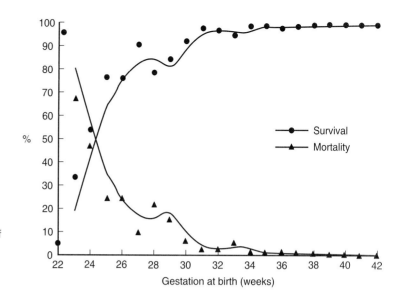

FIGURE 34-2 ■ Survival by gestational age among live-born resuscitated infants. Results of a community-based evaluation of 8523 deliveries, 1997–1998, Shelby County, Tennessee. Curves smoothed by 2-point average. (From Mercer BM: Preterm premature rupture of the membranes. Obstet Gynecol **101**(1):178, 2003, Fig. 1.)

between 1991 and 1996 (Lemons et al., 2000). These rates may not be representative of morbidities for preterm infants born at hospitals without neonatal intensive care capabilities. Typical rates for the most common neonatal morbidities are shown in Figure 34-3, from the same population-based dataset of 8523 infants born in 1997–1998 at community and tertiary centers (Mercer, 2003). The frequencies of major morbidity are clearly related to gestational age.

Prediction of Outcome for Very-Low-Birth-Weight Infants

Estimation of perinatal, neonatal, and infant mortality and short- and long-term morbidity are particularly important when counseling and caring for pregnant women at risk of preterm births before 28 weeks' gestation. Data on which to base counseling and clinical decisions are reported from both obstetrical datasets based on gestational age (Wood et al., 2000; Mercer, 2003) and from neonatal datasets based on birth weight (Lemons et al., 2001; Effer et al., 2002). Because the former include all living fetuses at entry to the obstetrical suite, while the latter include only newborns admitted to the nursery,

rates of survival and morbidity at the same gestational age and/or birth weight are somewhat higher in the neonatal datasets. Antenatal counseling and decisionmaking are appropriately based on information available before delivery. Another important feature of both perinatal and neonatal data is the nature of the patient population described. Population-based data includes all data from a geographic region (e.g., a county or state). Data collected from a site of care such as a tertiary perinatal/neonatal center describes a referral population that could be skewed by including or excluding infants who did or did not survive long enough to be transferred.

The contrast in data can be seen in two recent publications—one a population-based obstetrical dataset, the other a neonatal tertiary referral dataset from the NICHD Neonatal Network. Wood and colleagues (2000) reported data from a population-based study of infants born to all women who presented for delivery between 20 and 25 weeks' gestation in the United Kingdom and Ireland during a 10-month period in 1995. In this report, 24 weeks was the gestational age at which an upturn in the rates of survival and survival without major morbidity was first evident (Table 34-4). Outcome at 30 months of age for survivors born at 22–25 weeks are shown

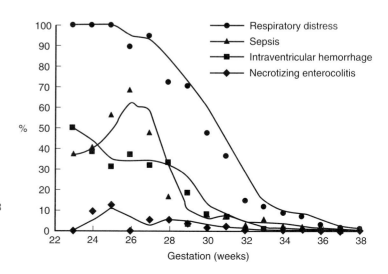

FIGURE 34-3 ■ Acute morbidity by gestational age among surviving infants. Results of a community-based evaluation of 8523 deliveries, 1997–1998, Shelby County, Tennessee. Curves smoothed by 2-point average. (From Mercer BM: Preterm premature rupture of the membranes. Obstet Gynecol **101**(1):178, 2003, Fig. 2.)

TABLE 34-4. SUMMARY OF OUTCOMES AMONG INFANTS BORN ALIVE AT 22 THROUGH 25 WEEKS OF GESTATION*

Outcome	22 W (*N* = 138)	23 W (*N* = 241)	24 W (*N* = 382)	25 W (*N* = 424)
	Number (Percent)			
Died in delivery room	116 (84)	110 (46)	84 (22)	67 (16)
Admitted to NICU	22 (16)	131 (54)	298 (78)	357 (84)
Died in NICU	20 (14)	105 (44)	198 (52)	171 (40)
Survived to discharge	2 (1)	26 (11)	100 (26)	186 (44)
Died after discharge	0	1 (0.4)	2 (0.5)	3 (0.7)
Lost to follow-up	0	0	1 (0.3)	1 (0.2)
Had severe disability at 30 mo	1 (0.7)	8 (3)	24 (6)	40 (9)
Had other disabilities at 30 mo	0	6 (2)	28 (7)	44 (10)
Survived without overall disability at 30 mo				
As a percentage of live births	1 (0.7)	11 (5)	45 (12)	98 (23)
As a percentage of NICU admissions	1 (5)	11 (8)	45 (15)	98 (27)

* Three infants, all of whom died, were admitted at less than 22 weeks of gestational age. For infants who died in the delivery room, gestational age was based on the estimate used in the delivery room. For infants who were admitted to the NICU, gestational age was confirmed postnatally.

NICU, neonatal intensive care unit.

From Wood NS, Marlow N, Costeloe K, et al: Neurologic and developmental disability after extremely preterm birth. EPICure Study Group. N Engl J Med **343**(6):378, 2000, Table 1.

in Figure 34-4 (Wood et al., 2000). Because these data include all infants born at any site within a geographic region regardless of their antenatal, intrapartum, and immediate neonatal care, they best reflect the baseline outcomes for these early preterm births. Lemons and associates (2001) reported data from a population of 4633 VLBW infants born at tertiary perinatal centers in the NICHD Neonatal Network between 1995 and 1996. Approximately 70% received antenatal corticosteroids, 60% received antenatal antibiotics, 50% were delivered by cesarean section, 25% were born after preterm premature rupture of membranes (PROM), 20% were from a multiple gestation, and 20% were under the 10th percentile for gestational age. The duration of infant follow-up is also important. Outcomes at hospital discharge are not as predictive as an examination at two to three years of age. Outcomes at hospital discharge from these two studies are contrasted in Table 34-5 from MacDonald and the Committee on Fetus and Newborn (2002).

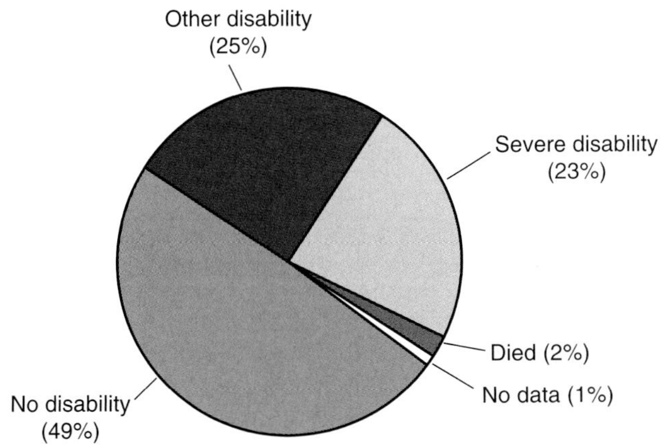

Long-Term Outcomes for Low-Birth-Weight Infants

Concerns about long-term morbidity are focused on long-term neurological functions such as mental retardation, cerebral palsy, sensory perception, school performance, and overall quality of life, all of which have been reported to be compromised in some VLBW survivors. An increasing number of reports of long-term outcomes for VLBW infants have been published as more reach school age and adolescence. In one study of school-age outcomes, rates of cerebral palsy, severe visual impairment, and reduced head size and height for children with birth weights below 750 g were greater than for children with birth weights between 750 g and 1499 g and children born at term (Hack et al., 1994). Abnormal cognitive, academic, visual motor, gross motor, and adaptive performance were also more frequent among children with birth weights below 750 g.

Factors significantly associated with neurodevelopmental disability among extremely-low-birth-weight infants (under 1 kg) born in 1993 and 1994 who survived to 18 to 22 months included chronic lung disease, grades 3-4 IVH and periventricular leukomalacia, necrotizing enterocolitis, male gender, lower maternal education, and nonwhite race (Vohr et al., 2000).

Hack and colleagues (2002) investigated adolescent outcomes in a cohort of 242 survivors with birth weights under 1500 g (mean birth weight = 1179 g; mean gestational age at birth = 29.7 weeks' gestation) born between 1977 and 1979 who were compared with 233 matched controls of normal birth weight. Very-low-birth-weight infants who survived had

FIGURE 34-4 ■ Summary of outcome with respect to overall disability at 30 months for 314 children born at 22 through 25 weeks of gestation. (From Wood NS, Marlow N, Costeloe K, et al: Neurologic and developmental disability after extremely preterm birth. EPICure Study Group. N Engl J Med **343**(6):378, 2000.)

TABLE 34-5. NEONATAL SURVIVAL/MORBIDITY BY GESTATIONAL AGE AND BIRTH WEIGHT

Factor	Mean Survival Rates (%)		Moderate or Severe Disability (%)	
	Wood et al.	NICHD	Wood et al.	NICHD
Gestational age (wk)				
23	11	30	56	–
24	26	52	53	–
25	54	76	46	–
Weight (g)				
401–500		11	–	*
501–600		27	–	29
601–700		63	–	30
701–800		74	–	28

* Too few infants in study to assess.
NICHD National Institute of Child Health and Human Development.

The Wood et al. paper is Wood NS, Marlow N, Costeloe K, et al: Neurologic and developmental disability after extremely preterm birth. N Engl J Med **343**:378, 2000. The NICHD paper is Lemons J A, Bauer CR, Oh W, et al: Very low birth weight outcomes of the National Institute of Child Health and Human Development Neonatal Research Network, January 1995 through December 1996. Pediatrics **107**:1, 2000.

lower IQ scores (87 versus 92), were less likely to have graduated from high school, and had higher rates (10% versus less than 1%) of neurosensory impairment, defined as cerebral palsy, blindness, deafness, and shunted hydrocephalus. VLBW survivors also were more likely to be of subnormal height (10% versus 5%). A meta-analysis of cognitive and behavioral outcomes in school-aged children who were born preterm found reduced cognitive function that was directly proportional to the degree of prematurity, and increased rates of attention deficit/hyperactivity disorder (Bhutta et al., 2002).

Saigal and coworkers (2002) reported self-described quality of life among 132 adolescents born between 1977 and 1982 who weighed under 1 kg at birth (extremely low birth weight). Comparisons were made with 127 sociodemographically matched controls. Although 24% of the extremely-low-birth-weight adolescents reported sensory deficits, they reported no difference in self-perception of global self worth, scholastic or job competence, or social acceptance.

The Causes of Morbidity in Prematurely Born Children

The relationship between prematurity and neonatal morbidity is increasingly understood as caused not only by immature organ systems but also in part by an underlying indolent intrauterine infection that precedes as many as 40% of preterm births, especially those before 32 weeks, when morbidity is the greatest (Gomez et al., 1998). Recent clinical and pathologic studies have linked chorioamnionitis to both cerebral palsy and bronchopulmonary dysplasia. Amniotic fluid cytokines have been related to neonatal brain lesions (e.g., IVH and periventricular leukomalacia) that are thought to be precursors for cerebral palsy (Yoon et al., 1995; Yoon, Jun, et al., 1997), to the development of cerebral palsy (Yoon, Jun, et al., 1997; Yoon et al., 2000), and to bronchopulmonary dysplasia (Yoon, Romero, et al., 1997; Yoon et al., 1999). Umbilical cord blood levels of interleukin-6 obtained at delivery are elevated in infants born to mothers with clinical chorioamnionitis, indicating a fetal response to intrauterine infection (Chaiworapongsa et al., 2002).

THE EPIDEMIOLOGY OF PRETERM BIRTH

Preterm birth is often called "multifactorial" because of the numerous and diverse maternal risk factors and clinical diagnoses that precede it. Preterm labor, preterm ruptured membranes, multiple gestation, preeclampsia, abruptio placenta, placenta previa, vaginal bleeding, fetal growth retardation, excessive or inadequate amniotic fluid volume, fetal anomalies, amnionitis, incompetent cervix, and medical problems such as diabetes, connective tissue disorders, hypertension, systemic infections, pyelonephritis, and drug abuse all can lead to preterm delivery. Maternal characteristics associated with preterm delivery include maternal race (incidence among blacks higher than among nonblacks), a history of previous preterm birth, low socioeconomic status, poor nutrition, periodontal disease, low prepregnancy weight, absent or inadequate prenatal care, age under 18 years or over 35 years, strenuous work, high personal stress, anemia, cigarette smoking, bacteriuria, genital colonization or infection, cervical injury or abnormality (e.g., *in utero* exposure to diethylstilbestrol, a history of cervical conization or second-trimester induced abortion), uterine anomaly or fibroids, excessive uterine contractility, and premature cervical dilation of greater than 1 cm or effacement greater than 80%. These various conditions and risk factors have been organized by Meis and colleagues (Meis et al., 1987; Meis, Michielutte, et al., 1995; Meis et al., 1998) into two broad categories—spontaneous and indicated—that facilitate an appreciation of the relative importance of various causes of prematurity.

Indicated preterm deliveries follow medical or obstetric disorders that place the mother and/or fetus at risk—for example, maternal hypertension, diabetes, placenta previa or abruption, and intrauterine growth restriction. These preterm births account for about 25% of births before 37 weeks and 1%–4% of all births in developed nations. In a study of more than 2900 births (Meis et al., 1998), the most common diagnoses that accompanied an indicated preterm birth before 37 weeks were preeclampsia (42.5%), fetal distress (26.7%), intrauterine growth restriction (10%), placental abruption (6.7%), and fetal demise (6.7%). Other factors associated with indicated preterm birth were maternal proteinuria (OR, 5.7), chronic hypertension (OR, 4.9), müllerian duct fusion anomaly (OR, 4.8), hospitalization for preterm labor (OR, 4.2), a prior preterm birth (OR, 3.6), age over 30 years (OR, 3.0), nulliparity (OR, 2.9), maternal pulmonary disease (OR, 2.6), and a history of stillbirth (OR, 2.2). Illicit drug use in pregnancy, especially cocaine ingestion, was associated with preterm birth in early but not subsequent studies (Cherukuri et al., 1988; Shiono et al., 1995). Maternal asthma has been linked to preterm birth in the past; however, a prospective cohort study of 1811 women with asthma and 928 women without asthma showed no relationship between asthma of any severity and preterm birth before 32 or 37 weeks' gestation, preterm ruptured membranes, or birth weight (Dombrowski, 2000).

Spontaneous preterm births occur when the parturitional process begins in the absence of overt maternal or fetal illness. Spontaneous preterm birth usually follows preterm labor, preterm ruptured membranes, or related diagnoses such as incompetent cervix or amnionitis. The clinical risk factors most often associated with spontaneous preterm birth are genital tract infection, nonwhite race, multiple gestation, bleeding in the second trimester, low prepregnancy weight, and a history of previous preterm birth (Mercer et al., 1996, 1999). Approximately 75% of preterm births fall into the spontaneous category (Meis et al., 1987; Meis, Michielutte, et al., 1995; Meis et al., 1998), in which the process leading to preterm birth is incompletely understood.

Categorizing preterm births as being either spontaneous or indicated recognizes that some preterm births are beneficial for the mother and/or fetus, while others are not. Apparently spontaneous preterm labor or preterm PROM, however, could be the only sign of fetal stress or compromise. Poor intrauterine growth has been reported in infants born after spontaneous preterm labor in the absence of apparent maternal disease (Ott, 1993; Hediger et al., 1995). Decidual and placental vascular lesions and increased impedance in the uterine arteries have been found in women who delivered after preterm labor (Salafia et al., 1991; Arias et al., 1993; Strigini et al., 1995) or ruptured membranes (Arias et al., 1997). Maternal and fetal stress have also been associated with spontaneous preterm birth in several studies (Copper et al., 1996; Lockwood, 1999; Hobel et al., 1999; Challis and Smith, 2001). This relationship may be mediated by endocrine pathway resulting from increased activity of the fetal hypothalamic-pituitary-adrenal axis (Challis and Smith, 2001). Cortisol, derived from the fetal adrenal in cases of intrauterine compromise or from the maternal adrenal in response to stress, or generated locally from cortisone in choriodecidual trophoblasts, could lead to increased production of prostaglandins by fetal membranes and the decidua via up-regulation of prostaglandin synthase and down-regulation of prostaglandin dehydrogenase. Abnormalities in the regulation of corticotropin-releasing hormone (CRH) could also influence the production of inflammatory cytokines (Dudley, 1999). (See also Chapter 6.) These data serve to remind clinicians that abnormalities of fetal oxygenation could lead to preterm labor, and that occult fetal compromise should always be considered in the evaluation of apparently idiopathic preterm labor.

The relative strength of the associations between common risk factors with spontaneous and indicated preterm birth is summarized from several studies (Meis, Michielutte, et al., 1995; Meis et al., 1998; Goldenberg et al., 1998) in Table 34-6. This chapter will focus on spontaneous preterm birth.

Spontaneous Preterm Birth

The pathogenesis of spontaneous preterm birth is complex. Epidemiological studies of spontaneous preterm birth reveal two related patterns of preterm birth according to the gestational age at delivery and the risk of recurrent preterm birth in subsequent pregnancy (Goldenberg et al., 1998). Early preterm births before 32 weeks are much more frequently accompanied by clinical or subclinical evidence of infection, occur more commonly in African-Americans, are more often followed by long-term morbidity for the infant, and are more likely to recur in subsequent pregnancies. Spontaneous preterm births after 32 weeks are often associated with increased frequency of uterine contraction and increased uterine volume resulting from hydramnios or multiple gestation, and they are less likely to be complicated by infection.

TABLE 34-6. CLINICAL RISK FACTORS FOR SPONTANEOUS AND INDICATED PRETERM BIRTH

Spontaneous Preterm Birth	Odds Ratio	Indicated Preterm Birth	Odds Ratio
Multiple gestation	6		
History of PTD	4	Proteinuria	5
2nd trimester bleeding	2 or >	High blood pressure	4
Genitourinary tract infection	2	History of stillbirth	3.5
African-American	2	Lung diseases	2.5
Age < 18	2	Age > 30	2.4
Low BMI	2	Bacteriuria	2
Cigarette smoking	1.5		
Frequent contractions	1.5		

Meis PJ, Michielutte R, Peters TJ, et al: Factors associated with preterm birth in Cardiff, Wales: II. Indicated and spontaneous preterm birth. Am J Obstet Gynecol **173**:597, 1995; Meis PJ, Goldenberg RL, Mercer BM, et al: The preterm prediction study: Risk factors for indicated preterm birth. Am J Obstet Gynecol **178**:562, 1998; Goldenberg RL, Iams JD, Mercer BM, et al: The preterm prediction study: The value of new vs. standard risk factors in predicting early and all spontaneous preterm births. Am J Public Health **88**:233, 1998.

TABLE 34-7. RISK OF PRETERM BIRTH IN SUBSEQUENT BIRTHS

First Birth	Second Birth	Subsequent Preterm Birth (%)
Not preterm		4.4
Preterm		17.2
Not preterm	Not preterm	2.6
Preterm	Not preterm	5.7
Not preterm	Preterm	11.1
Preterm	Preterm	28.4

From Bakketeig LS, Hoffman HJ: Epidemiology of preterm birth: Results from a longitudinal study of births in Norway. *In* Elder MG, Hendricks CH (eds): Preterm Labor. London, Butterworths, 1981, p. 17.

Obstetrical History

A history of preterm birth confers an increased risk of early delivery in subsequent pregnancies. In the classic study of obstetric history and outcome in subsequent pregnancies, the risk of a subsequent preterm birth rose as the number of prior preterm births increased, and the risk declined with each birth that was not preterm (Bakketeig and Hoffman, 1981) (Table 34-7). Note the markedly decreased recurrence risk in the third pregnancy for women whose first birth was preterm and whose second birth was at term, compared with women who experienced two successive preterm deliveries. There are somewhat different risk profiles for women with recurrent versus nonrecurrent preterm births. Risk factors for nonrecurrent spontaneous preterm birth include second-trimester bleeding, abnormal amniotic fluid volume, multiple gestation, substance abuse, and trauma. Premature contractions or membrane rupture can result from decidual hemorrhage with thrombin generation, which in turn may stimulate uterine contractions and proteases that affect membrane integrity (Elovitz et al., 2001). Excessive uterine volume, which can occur with polyhydramnios or multiple gestation, is another pathway to increased uterine activity via increased formation of gap junctions, oxytocin receptors, and production of prostaglandin and collagenase.

Recurrent preterm birth has been linked to maternal ethnicity, genitourinary infection, and especially to the gestational age of the first preterm birth—the earlier the birth, the greater the likelihood of recurrence (Mercer et al., 1999). This tendency is strongly associated with maternal cervical length measured by transvaginal ultrasound (Goldenberg et al., 1998; Iams et al., 1998).

Cervical Length

Cervical length as measured by transvaginal ultrasonography is inversely and continuously related to the risk of preterm birth in both singleton (Andersen et al., 1990; Iams et al., 1996) and multiple gestations (Goldenberg, Iams, et al., 1996) (see also Chapter 33). The risk of spontaneous prematurity rises as the cervical length at 18–28 weeks' gestation declines (Andersen et al., 1990; Iams et al., 1996; Taipale and Hiilesmaa, 1998). This relationship holds throughout the entire range of cervical length: Women whose cervical length is at the median (about 35 mm for 24–28 weeks' gestation)

have a greater risk of preterm birth than do women whose cervical length exceeds the 75th percentile (about 40 mm) (Fig. 34-5). Cervical length may, therefore, be viewed as a surrogate for cervical competence, which in turn functions along a continuum (see Chapter 33).

A cervical length of 25 mm or less (10th percentile) as measured by transvaginal ultrasound conferred a 6.5-fold relative risk (95% CI, 4.5, 9.3) of preterm birth before 35 weeks' gestation and a 7.7-fold relative risk (95% CI, 4.5, 13.4) of preterm birth before 32 weeks' gestation in the Preterm Birth Prediction Study (Iams et al., 1996). Cervical length is strongly related to a history of spontaneous preterm birth, especially before 32 weeks' gestation. In one study, the gestational age at delivery in prior pregnancies was studied in relation to cervical length in subsequent pregnancy: The earlier the gestational age at delivery, the shorter the cervix in the next pregnancy (Iams, Johnson, et al., 1995). Cervical length is also related to the risk of recurrent preterm birth (Iams et al., 1998; Andrews et al., 2000). For women with a prior preterm birth, the likelihood of recurrent preterm birth before 35 weeks fell from 31% when the cervical length at 24 weeks was 25 mm or less, to 16% when the cervical length was 26–35 mm, and to just 8% when the cervical length was 36 mm or more (35 mm = the 50th percentile). In contrast, among women whose only prior birth(s) were at term, the rate of birth earlier than 35 weeks' gestation was 8% when the cervix was 25 mm or less, 4% when it was 26–35 mm, and 2% when it was 36 mm or more (Iams et al., 1998). This relationship persists when other factors such as maternal ethnicity and presence of genitourinary tract infection are controlled. These data indicate that cervical function or competence is an independent variable that affects a woman's risk for preterm delivery in each pregnancy. The inherent length of the cervix can also be influenced in any given pregnancy by exogenous factors such as infection or contractions.

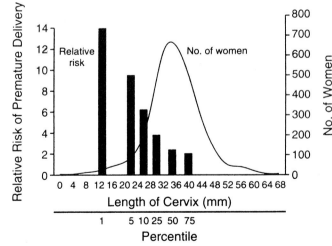

FIGURE 34-5 ■ Distribution of subjects among percentiles for cervical length measured by transvaginal ultrasonography at 24 weeks of gestation (solid line) and relative risk of spontaneous preterm delivery before 35 weeks of gestation according to percentiles for cervical length (bars). The risks among women with values at or below the 1st, 5th, 10th, 25th, 50th, and 75th percentiles for cervical length are compared with the risk among women with values above the 75th percentile. (From Iams JD, Goldenberg RL, Meis PJ, et al: The length of the cervix and the risk of spontaneous preterm delivery. N Engl J Med **334**:567, 1996.)

Infection

There is epidemiological, microbiological, and clinical evidence of an association between infection and preterm birth (Hillier et al., 1988; Romero, Sirtori, et al., 1989; Watts et al., 1992; Andrews et al., 2000; Goldenberg, Hauth, et al., 2000). Both maternal and neonatal infections are more common after preterm than term birth, with increasing risk as gestational age decreases. Most bacteria found in the uterus in association with preterm labor are of vaginal origin (Krohn et al., 1995). In women in spontaneous preterm labor with intact membranes, the most commonly identified bacteria are vaginal organisms of low virulence: *Ureaplasma urealyticum, Mycoplasma hominis, Gardnerella vaginalis, Peptostreptococci* sp., and *Bacteroides* sp. Microorganisms such as *Chlamydia trachomatis, Trichomonas* sp., *E. coli*, and group B *Streptococcus*, are less commonly recovered. The strength of the association between both clinical infection and histologic amnionitis increases as the gestational age at delivery decreases, especially before 30–32 weeks. Positive cultures of fetal membranes were found in more than 70% of births before 30 weeks' gestation, compared with 20% at term (Hillier et al., 1988). Positive amniotic fluid cultures have been reported in 20%–30% of women with preterm labor, especially before 30 weeks' gestation (Watts et al., 1992). The frequency of positive cultures increased as gestational age decreased, to 60% at 23–24 weeks' gestation. Infection is much less common after 34 weeks.

Bacterial vaginosis (BV)—an alteration of the maternal vaginal flora in which normally predominant lactobacilli are largely replaced by gram-negative anaerobic bacteria such as *Gardnerella vaginalis, Bacteroides* sp., *Prevotella* sp., *Mobiluncus* sp., and *Mycoplasma* sp.—has been associated with a twofold increased risk of spontaneous preterm birth (Krohn et al., 1991; Hillier et al., 1995; Meis, Goldenberg, et al., 1995). The association between BV and preterm birth is stronger when BV is detected early in pregnancy (Riduan et al., 1993). Rates of preterm birth were decreased by antibiotic treatment in women who had a history of preterm birth and BV in two studies (Hauth et al., 1995; McDonald et al., 1997). There was no effect, however, on the rate of preterm birth in women treated with metronidazole in a larger, placebo-controlled trial of 1900 women with asymptomatic BV (Carey et al., 2000). In this study, the rates of birth before 37, 35, and 32 weeks' gestation were not reduced by treatment, nor were the rates of low-birth-weight or VLBW infants reduced. Analysis of subsets of women according to their obstetric history of preterm birth, race, gestational age at initiation of treatment, eradication of BV, and prepregnancy weight did not reveal any subgroup in which treatment improved perinatal outcome.

The relationship between infection with vaginal microorganisms and prematurity is more complex than can be explained by ascent of organisms from the lower to the upper genital tract during pregnancy (Goldenberg and Andrews, 1996). If ascending infection were the predominant pathway, a more even distribution of infection-related births throughout pregnancy would be expected, with an increased occurrence in the third trimester as the cervix effaces and dilates. The predominance of infection-related preterm births before 30 weeks' gestation is thus not consistent with a theory of ascending infection. Colonization with microorganisms and markers of inflammatory response have been reported in amniotic fluid obtained in the second trimester and correlated with an increased rate of preterm delivery occurring weeks later (Horowitz et al., 1995; Ghidini et al., 1996; Wenstrom et al., 1998). There is further evidence that microorganisms associated with preterm birth could colonize the endometrial cavity before conception and exert their influence by eliciting a maternal and/or fetal response that leads to hormonal, cytokine, and prostaglandin production and ultimately to cervical ripening, weakening of the membranes, and uterine contractions (Goldenberg, Hauth, et al., 2000). The pathways by which intrauterine infection may lead to spontaneous preterm birth are indicated in Figure 34-6 (Goldenberg, Hauth, et al., 2000). Bacterial colonization of the choriodecidual interface induces production of cytokines, including tumor necrosis factor alpha, interleukin-1 alpha, interleukin-1ß (beta), interleukin-6, interleukin-8, and granulocyte colony-stimulating factor, leading to prostaglandin synthesis and release, neutrophil activation, and synthesis and release of metalloproteases. The prostaglandins stimulate uterine contractions; the metalloproteases weaken the chorioamniotic membranes and remodel and soften cervical collagen (Goldenberg, Hauth, et al., 2000).

Infections outside the genital tract have also been related to preterm birth, most commonly urinary tract and intra-abdominal infections such as pyelonephritis and appendicitis (Romero, Oyarzun, et al., 1989). Maternal periodontal infections have also been associated with increased risk of spontaneous preterm birth (Offenbacher et al., 1996, 1998, 2001). This novel association persists after other confounding covariables are controlled and may be mediated by systemic induction of cytokines in response to chronic inflammation. Host factors, such as maternal cervical length and the maternal and fetal immune response, could also be important in the genesis of preterm labor and preterm membrane rupture. Immune response could be influenced by chronic extragenital infections such as periodontal disease or by variations in cytokine response resulting from maternal or fetal polymorphisms in matrix metalloproteinase or cytokine (e.g., tumor necrosis alpha gene) expression (Roberts et al., 1999; Amory et al., 2001; Fujimoto et al., 2002).

Maternal Race

The association of black race with preterm birth is well known but remains unexplained. Despite decreases since 1990, African-American women still have a rate of preterm delivery before 37 weeks' gestation that is twice that for women of other races, and their rate of preterm birth before 32 weeks is three times higher than that for whites (see Table 34-1). For singleton births in 2001, 3.52% of non-Hispanic black women delivered before 32 completed weeks' gestation, compared with 1.45% for Hispanic women and 1.15% of non-Hispanic white women.

Socioeconomic factors apparently do not entirely explain the higher rate of preterm birth in U.S.-born African-American women. Although the rate of preterm birth decreases with advancing education among African-Americans, it is still higher than the rate for non-black women at all educational levels (Kogan and Alexander, 1998). Another study of 1029 black and 462 white parous indigent women in Alabama found that black women delivered preterm and low-birth-weight infants more frequently than white women, even though white indigent women in the population studied had greater sociodemographic risk (Goldenberg,

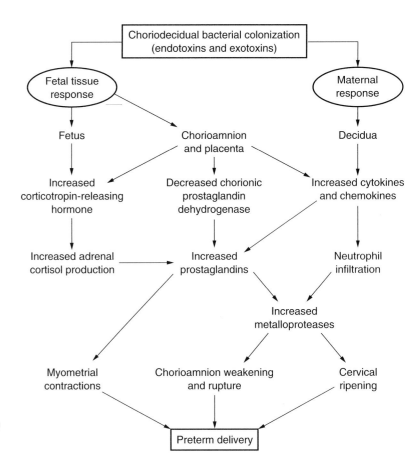

FIGURE 34-6 ■ Potential pathways from choriodecidual bacterial colonization to preterm delivery. (From Goldenberg RL, Hauth JC, Andrews WW: Intrauterine infection and preterm delivery. N Engl J Med **342:**1500, 2000, Fig. 3.)

Cliver, et al., 1996). Finally, black women born outside the U.S. have a lower risk of preterm delivery than those born within the 50 states and the District of Columbia (14% versus 17.8% in 2000) (Cabral et al., 1990; Martin et al., 2000b).

BV is more common among African-American women than among other races and has thus been studied as a possible explanation for the higher rate of preterm birth. A large observational study of vaginal microflora in pregnancy found organisms associated with BV more often in black women, even when differences in health behaviors were controlled (Goldenberg, Klebanoff, et al., 1996). In the NICHD Preterm Prediction Study, the relation between preterm birth before 32 weeks' gestation and BV was significant only in black women, where the population-attributable risk for BV was 40% for births before 32 weeks' gestation (Goldenberg et al., 1998). The rate of preterm birth, however, was increased in BV-positive African-American women only when the fetal fibronectin test (see the later section in this chapter under Pathways to Preterm Birth) was positive. The presence of fetal fibronectin in the vagina and cervix is a marker for disruption of the chorioamnion and the decidua; a positive test is an indicator of infection or inflammation in the upper genital tract. Thus, BV may be only an indirect marker for upper-tract inflammation indicated by fibronectin positivity.

An increased prevalence of cytokine polymorphisms has also been suggested to explain the increased preterm births in various ethnic groups, including African-American women. Genc and colleagues (2002) found that fetal carriage of certain IL-1 alleles was associated with spontaneous preterm delivery in women of African (IL-1 Beta+3953) and non-African

Hispanic (IL1RN*2) descent. This line of inquiry has been supported by some (Roberts et al., 1999; Macones, Parry, et al., 2001) but not by all (Ferriman et al., 2001) studies. The association of preterm birth with fetal carriage of the polymorphism for IL-1 β signifies the complexity of the relationship between host response to inflammation and preterm delivery.

Bleeding

Vaginal bleeding during pregnancy is a risk factor for preterm birth even when it is not caused by placenta previa or abruption (Meis, Michielutte, et al., 1995; Yang and Savitz, 2001). Ekwo and coauthors (1992) observed an association between second-trimester bleeding, PROM (RR, 15.1; 95% CI, 2.8–81), and preterm labor (RR, 19.7; 95% CI, 2.1–186). An unexplained increase in maternal serum alpha-fetoprotein, a marker of feto-maternal bleeding, is often seen in women with vaginal bleeding and is associated as well with an increased incidence of preterm birth (Burton, 1988), suggesting that occult placental hemorrhage could eventually lead to preterm delivery. The relationship between decidual hemorrhage and preterm labor may be the result of the uterotonic effect of activated thrombin (Elovitz et al., 2001).

Uterine Factors

The relationship between preterm birth and cervical length was discussed earlier in this section and in Chapter 33. Uterine anomalies, contraction frequency, and distention have all been related to preterm birth risk.

UTERINE ANOMALIES

Preterm births are reported in 25%–50% of women with uterine malformations (Raga et al., 1997). Uterine anomalies are associated with an increased chance of preterm birth through mechanisms that could be either "indicated" or "spontaneous." Müllerian fusion anomalies could include the cervix, thus predisposing the patient to an increased risk of preterm labor via abnormal cervical function. Abnormalities of placental implantation associated with a uterine septum could also lead to preterm birth via antenatal placental separation and hemorrhage, with or without clinical signs of abruption. In addition, the T-shaped uterus that may be present in women exposed *in utero* to diethylstilbestrol is associated with an increased risk of preterm labor and birth (Kaufman et al., 2000).

UTERINE CONTRACTIONS

Uterine activity, whether indicated by self-reported detection (Mercer et al., 1996) or measured by intermittent tocodynamometry (Nageotte et al., 1988; Iams et al., 2002), has been associated with an increased incidence of preterm delivery. Self-reported contractions were associated with preterm delivery before 35 weeks' gestation in both nulliparous (RR, 2.41; CI, 1.47–3.94; $P < .001$) and parous (RR, 1.62; CI, 1.20–2.18; $P = .002$) women (Mercer et al., 1996). Uterine contraction frequency was measured in 306 women (274 with and 46 without risk factors for preterm birth) for two or more hours a day at least twice weekly between 22 and 37 weeks' gestation (Iams et al., 2002). A total of 34,908 hours of contraction data were recorded. Contraction frequency was unrelated to maternal risk status but was significantly greater in women who delivered before 35 weeks' gestation when compared with women who delivered after 35 weeks. Contractions increased significantly with gestational age and between 4 PM and 4 AM regardless of gestational age at delivery (Iams et al., 2002) (Fig. 34-7). The difference, though statistically significant, was too small to be clinically useful (see later in this chapter under Prediction of Spontaneous Preterm Birth).

Multiple Gestation

The association between multiple gestation and preterm birth is well known. As the incidence of multiple gestation has increased with assisted reproductive techniques (Wilcox et al., 1996; Centers for Disease Control and Prevention, 2000), the proportion of preterm births caused by multiple gestation inevitably has increased (Martin et al., 2002b) (see Table 34-2).

The higher rate of preterm birth in multiple gestations is probably due in part to overdistention of the uterus, as the rate of preterm birth approaches 100% for quadruplets. Fetal anomalies associated with twinning could also lead to polyhydramnios and preterm labor. Both spontaneous and indicated preterm births are increased in multiple gestation. Gardner and associates (1995) found that 22% of preterm births in twins were indicated, with 44% resulting from maternal hypertension, 33% for fetal compromise, and 9% for abruption. Though only 2.6% of neonates were twins, they accounted for 12.2% of all preterm infants, 15.6% of all neonatal deaths, and 9.5% of fetal deaths in this data base. Newman and Luke calculated the contribution of multiple gestation to the incidence of perinatal mortality and various categories of perinatal morbidity (Fig. 34-8). Though multiple gestations account for just 2.9% of all births (3.0% in 2001), multiple birth was associated with 13% of perinatal deaths, 16% of neonatal deaths, 10% of fetal deaths, and 15% of cases of cerebral palsy.

Cervical length is the strongest risk factor for spontaneous preterm birth in twins. In the Preterm Prediction Study, a short cervix assessed by transvaginal ultrasonography (under 25 mm, or the 10th percentile) was the only factor at 24 weeks' gestation associated with preterm birth at fewer than 32 weeks' gestation (OR, 6.9; 95% CI, 2.0–24.2), before 35 weeks (OR, 3.2; 95% CI, 1.3–7.9), and before 37 weeks (OR, 2.8; 95% CI, 1.1–7.7) (Goldenberg, Iams, et al., 1996).

Assisted Reproductive Technology

Preterm and low-birth-weight deliveries occur more commonly in pregnancies conceived after ovulation induction and ART, such as *in vitro* fertilization (IVF) and gamete and zygote intrafallopian transfer, frozen embryo transfer, and donor embryo transfer (Schieve et al., 2002). A study by the Centers for Disease Control and Prevention (CDC) (Wilcox et al., 1996) found that ART pregnancies contributed 22% of all higher-order multiple gestations in 1990 and 1991. A study of 1997 higher-order (triplet or greater) births estimated that 43% resulted from ART and 38% were the result of ovulation-inducing drugs; only 20% were conceived spontaneously (Centers for Disease Control and Prevention, 2000).

The increase in preterm birth after ovulation induction and ART has been attributed primarily to the increase in the incidence of multiple gestation, but the rate of preterm and low-birth-weight singleton deliveries is increased as well (FIVNAT, 1995; Schieve et al., 2002). Of 42,463 infants born after ART in a large U.S. study, 43% were singletons, 43% were twins, 12% were triplets, and 1% were quadruplets or greater (Schieve et al., 2002). Preterm low birth weight was increased 1.4-fold, and VLBW was increased 1.8-fold. Other studies have found an increase in preterm (a 3.5-fold increase

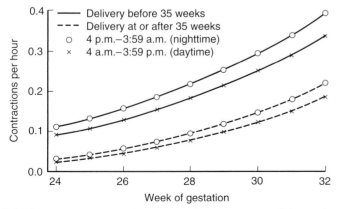

FIGURE 34-7 ■ Relation of the week of gestation, time of day, and timing of delivery (before 35 weeks of gestation or at 35 weeks or more of gestation) to the frequency of contractions between 24 and 32 weeks. (From Iams JD, Newman RB, Thom EA, et al: Frequency of uterine contractions and the risk of spontaneous preterm delivery. N Engl J Med **346**:250, 2002, Fig. 1.)

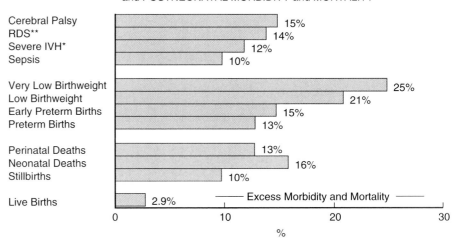

CONTRIBUTION of MULTIPLE BIRTHS to PERINATAL
and POSTNEONATAL MORBIDITY and MORTALITY

FIGURE 34-8 ■ Contribution of multiple births to perinatal and postneonatal morbidity and mortality. (Graph from Newman R, Luke B: Multifetal Pregnancy. Philadelphia, Lippincott Williams and Wilkins, 2001, p. 244. Data from Ventura SJ, Martin JA, Curtin SC, et al: Births: Final data for 1998. National Vital Statistics Reports **48**:1, 2000; Ventura SJ, Martin JA, Curtin SC, et al: Report of final natality statistics 1996. Monthly Vital Statistics Report **46**:1, 1998. Provided courtesy of Roger Newman.)

* IVH is intraventricular hemorrhage
* RDS is respiratory distress syndrome

in a Dutch study [Dhont et al., 1999]) and VLBW births (a 2.6-fold increase in a U.S. study [McElrath and Wise, 1997]) in women who conceive after fertility treatment. Interestingly, the U.S. study also found an increased rate of VLBW infants (1.4-fold) in women who were candidates for but did not receive fertility therapy.

These observations suggest that the difference in preterm birth rates associated with ovulation induction and *in vitro* fertilization are not fully explained by the increased frequency of multiple pregnancy. Increased production of relaxin induced by superovulation is one proposed explanation (Weiss et al., 1993; Vogel et al., 2001).

Lifestyle and Risk of Preterm Birth

Reported behavioral risk factors for preterm birth include maternal cigarette smoking, sexual practices, maternal stress, and the duration and intensity of work. Smoking is important because of its high prevalence in the population and because it is associated with an increase in preterm ruptured membranes (Savitz et al., 2001). A population-based study from Sweden of more than 300,000 singleton births found a dose-related association between smoking and spontaneous preterm birth (OR, 1.7 for more than 10 cigarettes per day) (Kyrklund-Blomberg and Cnattingius, 1998). Information about a possible relationship between sexual activity and preterm birth is indirect, limited to observations of increased contraction frequency following coitus (Moore et al., 1994) and to sexual activity as an opportunity to acquire genital-tract infections that could influence preterm birth risk. Stress has been related to preterm birth, as noted earlier in this chapter. The duration and intensity of work was related to the risk of preterm birth by Mamelle and colleagues (1984). These data have been supplemented by more recent reports that support a modest relationship (ORs, 1.22–1.6 with confidence intervals [CIs] that do not cross 1) between physically demanding work and preterm birth (Luke et al., 1995; Mozurkewich et al., 2000; Escriba-Aguir et al., 2001; Newman et al., 2001).

PATHWAYS TO PRETERM BIRTH

Making sense of the multiple risk factors and clinical diagnoses that lead to preterm birth is an ongoing process. Decades ago, preterm birth was viewed simply as the common endpoint of numerous separate complications of pregnancy, and the morbidity of prematurity was seen as the result of being born too soon. Based on information accumulated over the last two decades, a more complicated picture has emerged to explain most instances of spontaneous preterm labor and birth. Figure 34-9 summarizes this information in terms of four broad pathologic pathways that occur within a maternal-fetal environment of endogenous (immutable, e.g., maternal and fetal inflammatory response, endocrine milieu, cervical length) and exogenous, potentially mutable characteristics (e.g., periodontal infection, genital tract microflora, lifestyle choices regarding work, smoking, and so on). More than one pathway may operate to initiate preterm parturition in a given pregnancy. These pathways represent avenues to a final common hypothesized pathway in which the decidua and membranes are "activated" to initiate labor, membrane rupture, or both.

Premature activation of the usual physiologic maternal/fetal hypothalamic pituitary axis can occur under conditions that increase maternal or fetal stress, mediated by increased corticotropin-releasing hormone and increased levels of estrogen. Excessive uterine distention can occur when the normal uterine capacity is exceeded by increased uterine volume because of multifetal gestation or hydramnios, or when a uterine abnormality restricts uterine expansion. Decidual hemorrhage has gained increased attention as the uterotonic effect of thrombin has been documented (Elovitz et al., 2001). Abruption is an obvious source of decidual hemorrhage, but lesser degrees of bleeding at the maternal-fetal interface could explain reported relationships between vaginal bleeding and elevated maternal serum alpha-fetoprotein in the second trimester and subsequent preterm birth (Williams et al., 1992; Krause et al., 2001; Moawad et al., 2002).

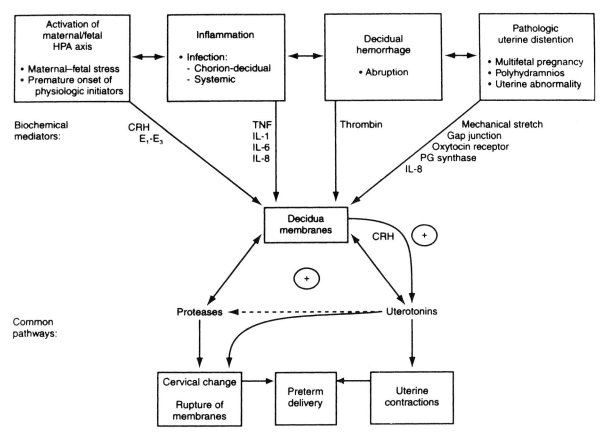

FIGURE 34-9 ■ Major pathogenic pathways of preterm delivery resulting in preterm rupture of membranes, preterm labor, or both. CRH, corticotropin-releasing hormone; E_1, estrone; E_3, estriol; HPA, hypothalamic-pituitary-adrenal; IL-1, IL-6, and IL-8, interleukins-1ß, -6, and -8, respectively; PG, prostaglandin; TNF, tumor necrosis factor. *Activation of the maternal and/or fetal HPA axis:* Maternal and fetal stress lead to increased expression of placental-amniochorion-decidual CRH and placental estrogen expression. CRH enhances PG production in placental-amniochorion-decidual cells, while estrogens activate the myometrium. *Inflammation:* Ascending genital tract and severe systemic infections lead to activation of genital tract cytokine networks generating IL-1 and TNF-1, which enhance production of myometrial-decidual-amniochorionic-cervical uterotonins (i.e., prostaglandins, endothelins, leukotrienes) and proteases (e.g., matrix metalloproteinases-collagenases, plasmin). These proparturition effects are amplified by IL-1-TNF-mediated induction of (a) IL-6, which further enhances PG production; and (b) IL-8, a granulocyte chemotactant and activator, which causes the release of elastases and collagenases. *Decidual hemorrhage:* Abruptions lead to local generation of thrombin, which binds to cellular receptors in the deciduas to enhance local protease and PG production. *Pathologic uterine distention:* Multifetal gestation, hydramnios, and uterine abnormalities resulting from diethylstilbestrol exposure and congenital müllerian duct defects promote excessive stretching of the fetal membranes, the myometrium, or both, which causes myometrial activation (enhanced gap junctions, oxytocin receptors, $PGF_{2\alpha}$ synthase) and fetal membrane cytokine (IL-8) production. *Final common pathway:* Each of these four pathogenic mechanisms has a unique set of biochemical initiators but shares a final common pathway; enhanced expression of fetal membrane, decidual, and cervical proteases and uterotonins (e.g., prostaglandins). This leads to membrane rupture, cervical change and progressive uterine contractions, and preterm delivery. (From American College of Obstetricians and Gynecologists: Preterm labor and delivery. *In* Lockwood CJ (ed): Precis: Obstetrics, 2nd ed. Washington, DC, p. 198, © ACOG, 1999.)

Infection has been said to account for 20%–40% of spontaneous preterm births based on traditional markers such as cultures or histology. The proportion may be higher than that, especially for early preterm births, when the infection-driven pathway is understood to occur as a product of the immune response mounted by both mother and fetus to the presence of microorganisms at the decidual-membrane interface. Ascent of vaginal microorganisms through a dilated or shortened cervix during pregnancy to infect the decidua and chorioamnion was the initial explanation for the association between genital-tract infection and prematurity. Understanding of the relation between infection and preterm birth, however, has been enhanced by studies of fetal fibronectin in the cervicovaginal secretions in the second and third trimesters. Fibronectin is an extracellular matrix protein that acts as an adhesive between the fetal membranes and decidua. It is commonly present in cervical secretions in the first half of pregnancy but is uncommon thereafter until term, when it reappears as labor approaches (Feinberg et al., 1991). Its presence in the cervical mucus between 22 and 34 weeks' gestation is thought to indicate a disruption or injury to the maternal-fetal interface. Studies have linked the presence of fetal fibronectin in cervical mucus between 13 and 28 weeks to an increased risk of preterm birth, especially within 4 weeks of a positive test, and to infectious morbidity in the mother and infant occurring months later (Goldenberg, Mercer, et al., 1996; Goldenberg, Thom, et al., 1996; Goldenberg et al., 1998; Goldenberg, Klebanoff, et al., 2000). In the Preterm Prediction study, women with a positive fibronectin who delivered before 32 weeks' gestation all had histological evidence of chorioamnionitis and were 16 times more likely to have clinical chorioamnionitis; their infants were six times more likely to have neonatal sepsis (Goldenberg, Thom, et al., 1996).

When fibronectin is included in analyses that relate BV to preterm birth, BV is associated with preterm birth only when fibronectin is present in the vaginal fluid (Goldenberg et al., 1998), suggesting that upper rather than lower genital-tract colonization with BV is important in the pathogenesis of preterm birth. Goldenberg and Andrews (1996) have therefore argued that microorganisms resident in the vagina may colonize the upper genital tract before conception and lead to a subclinical infection that becomes manifest in pregnancy as a decidual injury marked by a positive fibronectin. In this model, most women with microorganisms in the upper tract resolve the infection without initiating sufficient inflammation to induce preterm birth or neonatal morbidity. The occurrence of preterm birth and neonatal morbidity could be the consequence of variations in exogenous (physical or sexual activity, smoking) and/or endogenous (e.g., cervical length or polymorphisms of the immune response) factors.

When information about fibronectin, cervical length, and second-trimester amniotic fluid cytokines are considered with the data about intrauterine infection and neonatal morbidity, a model of early preterm birth as an indolent rather than an acute process emerges: In response to a chronic intrauterine inflammatory insult (usually infectious but possibly related to decidual hemorrhage), and influenced by maternal and fetal immune response (Gomez et al., 1998) and by infection-induced activation of the fetal hypothalamic-pituitary-adrenal axis (Gravett et al., 2000), the fetal membranes and decidua produce cytokines (tumor necrosis factor alpha, interleukins-1, -6, and -8, and matrix metalloproteinase 8), which in turn initiate labor or ruptured membranes as shown in Figure 34-9.

There is increasing evidence that intrauterine exposure to infection as detected by positive amniotic fluid cultures or, more commonly, by the presence of inflammatory markers such as tumor necrosis factor alpha, interleukins -6 or -8, or matrix metalloproteinase 8, are linked not only to early preterm labor but also to infant morbidities including respiratory distress, IVH, periventricular leukomalacia, bronchopulmonary dysplasia, and necrotizing enterocolitis (Hitti et al., 2001; Maymon et al., 2001; Gibbs, 2001; Yoon et al., 2001).

PREDICTION OF SPONTANEOUS PRETERM BIRTH

An effort to predict or screen for preterm birth presumes that women with increased risk can be treated to improve pregnancy outcome. Prophylaxis of preterm birth has been attempted for women with risk factors such as a prior preterm birth or positive risk score (Collaborative Group on Preterm

Birth Prevention, 1993), genital-tract infection (Eschenbach et al., 1991; Carey et al., 2000; Klebanoff et al., 1995, 2001), increased uterine contractions (Collaborative Home Uterine Monitoring Study Group, 1995; Dyson et al., 1998), multiple gestation (Dyson et al., 1991), social disadvantage (Olds et al., 1986; Spencer et al., 1989), suspected cervical incompetence and/or short cervix assessed by ultrasound (MacNaughton et al., 1993; Althuisius et al., 2000; Rust et al., 2001), and a positive cervicovaginal fetal fibronectin test (Andrews et al., 2003), all without much success. Recently, however, two reports of successful prevention of preterm birth in women with a prior preterm delivery have been published; in both, the intervention was supplemental progesterone (da Fonseca et al., 2003; Meis et al., 2003). The success reported in these trials will renew the search for sensitive and specific tests to predict preterm birth risk in order to apply progesterone supplementation appropriately.

Clinical Risk Assessment

Risk assessment based on clinical risk factors has a sensitivity ranging from 20%–60% at best to predict preterm birth (Creasy et al., 1980; Mercer et al., 1996). Factors such as low prepregnancy weight (body mass index less than 19.8), African-American ethnicity, and BV have significant attributable risk conferred by their prevalence in the population but have only modest effect in an individual pregnancy (relative risk less than twofold). Major clinical risk factors are multiple gestation (relative risk five- to sixfold), a history of preterm birth (relative risk three- to fourfold), and vaginal bleeding (relative risk threefold). Of these, a history of preterm birth is more important than is generally realized. A population-based cohort study of births in the state of Georgia found that about a third of preterm births between 20 and 31 weeks' gestation occurred in women with a prior preterm delivery (Adams et al., 2000). The earlier the prior preterm birth, the greater is the likelihood that preterm delivery will recur (Mercer et al., 1999).

Cervical Assessment

Cervical dilation, effacement, and softening of the lower uterine segment have been associated with a three- to 13-fold increase in the risk of preterm birth (Copper et al., 1995; Mercer et al., 1996). Nevertheless, their sensitivity to predict preterm birth has been low, even when combined as composite scores of cervical readiness for labor. Despite relative risks for birth before 35 weeks' gestation of 5.3 (95% CI, 3.4, 8.5) for the Cervical Score (defined as cervical length in centimeters minus cervical dilation in centimeters), and 3.5 (95% CI, 2.4, 5.0) for the Bishop score, the sensitivity for both scores at 24 weeks' gestation to predict preterm birth in a general obstetrical population was low: 13.4% and 27.6%, respectively (Newman, 1997; Iams et al., 1996).

A cervical length of 25 mm or less assessed by endovaginal ultrasound measurement at 24 weeks' gestation in the same study was more strongly associated with an increased risk of preterm birth than was digital exam (relative risk of 6.19 [95% CI, 3.84, 9.97]), but sensitivity was still only 37% (Iams et al., 1996, 2001). In a study of 3694 women with low risk of preterm birth (0.8% fewer than 35 weeks' gestation), the relative risk of preterm birth was increased eightfold when the cervical length at 18–22 weeks' gestation was under 29 mm, but the sensitivity and positive predictive value were only 19% and 6%, respectively (Taipale and Hiilesmaa, 1998). In a study of tests to predict risk of preterm delivery in women with risk factors, a cervical length of under 25 mm was the strongest test, yet had sensitivity and predictive value of just 47% and 37%, respectively, at 22–24 weeks' gestation to predict preterm birth at fewer than 35 weeks' gestation (Iams et al., 2002) (Table 34-8). Cervical length has been the strongest predictor of preterm birth risk remote from delivery, an observation that derives from the understanding that cervical ripening precedes preterm birth at any gestational age by weeks or more (see also Chapter 33).

Frequency of Uterine Contraction

Uterine activity has been studied extensively to identify women who will enter preterm labor. In 109 normal women monitored for contraction frequency for 24 hours twice weekly for the last half of pregnancy, contraction frequency increased throughout gestation with a diurnal rhythm; peak uterine activity occurred at night (Fig. 34-10) (Moore et al., 1994).

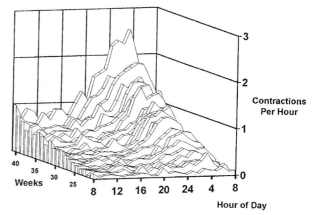

FIGURE 34-10 ■ Contractions per hour (CPH) as a function of gestational age (weeks) and time of day in normal singleton pregnancy. (Reprinted from Obstet Gynecol **83,** Moore TM, Iams JD, Creasy RK, et al: Diurnal and gestational patterns of uterine activity in normal human pregnancy, 517–523, 1994, with permission from American College of Obstetrics and Gynecology.)

There was significant individual variability in contraction frequency in normal pregnancy, an observation that has confounded efforts to use monitored contractions as a screen for preterm labor. A study of contraction frequency in 254 high-risk and 52 low-risk women found that although uterine contractions were significantly more frequent in women who would ultimately deliver preterm, the difference was not sufficient to be clinically useful (Iams et al., 2002). Sensitivity and positive predictive value of contraction frequency were quite low at 22–24, 27–28, and 31–32 weeks' gestation (see Table 34-8), even in high-risk populations. This observation may explain the lack of benefit found when this technology was employed in prematurity prevention programs (Dyson et al., 1998).

Biochemical Markers

Moawad and colleagues (2002) reported analyses of multiple markers in maternal blood obtained at 24 weeks' gestation, including alkaline phosphatase, alpha-fetoprotein, beta-2-microglobulin, CRH, C-reactive protein, ferritin, IL-6, and intracellular adhesion molecule-1 (ICAM-1). Of these, elevated alkaline phosphatase and alpha-fetoprotein levels at 24 and 28 weeks' gestation had significant associations with spontaneous preterm birth before 32 and 35 weeks' gestation, and elevated CRH levels at 28 weeks' gestation was associated with preterm birth at fewer than 35 weeks' gestation. Despite ORs approximating four for both alkaline phosphatase and alpha-fetoprotein at 24 weeks' gestation, the sensitivities were low (15% and 35%, respectively); the positive predictive values were 81% and 72%. Maternal plasma granulocyte colony stimulating factor (GCSF) has also been related to risk of preterm birth, but it performed poorly as a clinical test for preterm birth risk (Goldenberg, Andrews, et al., 2000). At 24 weeks' gestation, the sensitivity of an elevated plasma granulocyte colony-stimulating factor value to predict spontaneous preterm birth within four weeks was 54%, but the positive predictive value was just 2.2%. At 28 weeks' gestation, an elevated plasma granulocyte colony-stimulating factor value had a sensitivity of 37% and a positive predictive value of 7%.

TABLE 34-8. VALUE OF TESTS IN PREDICTING SPONTANEOUS DELIVERY BEFORE 35 WEEKS

Test	Week of Gestation at Time of Testing		
	22–24	27–28	31–32
	Percent		
Maximal nighttime contraction frequency ≥ 4/hr			
Sensitivity	8.6	28.1	27.3
Specificity	96.4	88.7	82.0
Positive predictive value	25.0	23.1	11.3
Negative predictive value	88.3	91.1	93.0
Maximal daytime contraction frequency ≥4/hr			
Sensitivity	0	12.9	13.6
Specificity	98.4	93.9	84.9
Positive predictive value	0	20.0	7.1
Negative predictive value	87.0	90.2	92.1
Cervicovaginal fibronectin ≥50 ng/mL			
Sensitivity	18.9	21.4	41.2
Specificity	95.1	94.5	92.5
Positive predictive value	35.0	30.0	30.4
Negative predictive value	89.4	91.6	95.2
Cervical length ≤25 mm			
Sensitivity	47.2	53.6	82.4
Specificity	89.2	82.2	74.9
Positive predictive value	37.0	25.0	20.9
Negative predictive value	92.6	94.1	98.1
Bishop score ≥4			
Sensitivity	35.1	46.4	82.4
Specificity	91.0	77.9	61.8
Positive predictive value	35.1	18.8	14.7
Negative predictive value	91.0	92.9	97.8

From Iams JD, Newman RB, Thom EA, et al. Frequency of uterine contractions and the risk of spontaneous preterm delivery. N Engl J Med **346:**250, 2002, Table 3.

Cervicovaginal secretions have been tested as screening tests for preterm birth in asymptomatic women; secretions tested include fetal fibronectin (Goldenberg, Mercer, et al., 1996; Goldenberg et al., 1998), interleukins 6 and 8 (Goepfert et al., 2001; Kurkinen-Raty et al., 2001), ferritin (Ramsey et al., 2002), and human chorionic gonodotropin (Bernstein et al., 1998). Fibronectin has been shown in crosssectional studies to be present in cervicovaginal secretions in 3%–4% of pregnant women between 21 and 37 weeks' gestation (Lockwood et al, 1991; Goldenberg, Mercer, et al., 1996). In a study of women with historical risk factors for preterm delivery, a positive fibronectin test had a sensitivity of 93%, a specificity of 52%, a positive predictive value of 46%, and a negative predictive value of 94% for preterm delivery before 34 weeks' gestation (Nageotte et al., 1994) but the sensitivity and positive predictive value observed in this report were lower in subsequent reports (Goldenberg, Mercer, et al., 1996; Iams et al., 2002). When fibronectin was evaluated as a screen for spontaneous preterm birth before 35 weeks' gestation in asymptomatic women with low to moderate historical risk who were tested at 24, 26, 28, and 30 weeks' gestation, the sensitivity ranged between 20% and 29%, and the positive predictive value decreased as gestational age advanced (Goldenberg, Mercer, et al., 1996). In this study, the sensitivity of the test at 24 weeks' gestation for births within the four weeks after testing (63%) was conducted in a predominantly indigent population.

Because half of preterm births occur in women without clinical risk factors, a simplified screening process for low-risk pregnancy has been sought through attempts to improve sensitivity and predictive value by combining some of the tests just described, either at one time or in sequence. Goldenberg and associates (2001) studied fetal fibronectin, cervical sonography, serum alkaline phosphatase, alpha-fetoprotein, and plasma granulocyte colony stimulating factor. The combination of any two positive tests had a sensitivity of 43% with a false positive rate of 6% for delivery before 35 weeks of gestation. In an analysis limited to women without clinical risk factors, sequential use of fibronectin or Bishop Score followed by cervical sonography had a sensitivity of only 15% for preterm birth before 35 weeks' gestation (Iams et al., 2001).

Monitored contraction frequency, digital and ultrasound assessment of the cervix, and fetal fibronectin were compared as predictors of preterm birth in a prospective cohort study conducted in women with increased risk of preterm birth (Iams et al., 2002). As can be seen in Figure 34-11 and Table 34-8, sonographic and digital examination of the cervix were superior to fetal fibronectin and uterine contraction monitoring, but no test had both high sensitivity and positive predictive value. In this study population, in which 35% were delivered before 37 weeks' gestation, 16% before 35 weeks' gestation, and 6% before 32 weeks' gestation, a sonographic cervical length of 25 mm or less at 22–24 weeks' gestation had a sensitivity of 47% and a positive predictive value of 37% for preterm birth prior to 35 weeks' gestation.

The foregoing review of risk factors to predict preterm birth emphasizes the important distinction between association and prediction. Despite significant associations with preterm birth, none of the clinical or laboratory tests described predict preterm birth well—that is, none has both high sensitivity and positive predictive value (see Chapter 17). This finding is a function of the prevalence of positive test results in women

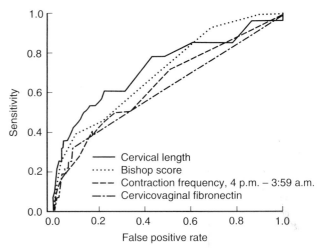

FIGURE 34-11 ■ Receiver-operating-characteristic curves for cervical length, Bishop score, frequency of contractions between 4 PM and 3:59 AM, and presence or absence of fetal fibronectin in cervicovaginal secretions at 27–28 weeks in the prediction of spontaneous preterm delivery (fewer than 35 weeks). (From Iams JD, Newman RB, Thom EA, et al: Frequency of uterine contractions and the risk of spontaneous preterm delivery. N Engl J Med **346:**250, 2002.)

who will deliver at term (e.g., contractions), the interval between testing and preterm birth (e.g., fibronectin), and the multiple pathways that lead to preterm birth (see under Pathways to Preterm Birth). That cervical length is the most accurate test reflects the chronic, indolent process that leads to most preterm births.

Risk Assessment in Women with Clinical Risk Factors

Although women with risk factors are often advised to limit their activities or to undergo treatment or surveillance for preterm birth, the likelihood of preterm birth varies widely according to cervical length and fibronectin in women with a preterm birth history (Iams et al., 1998) and with cervical length in women with twins (Goldenberg, Iams, et al., 1996; Imseis et al., 1997). The risk of recurrent preterm birth varies considerably by fibronectin status and cervical length, from less than 10% when the cervix is longer than 35 mm and the fibronectin is negative, to more than 60% when the cervix is shorter than 25 mm and the fibronectin is positive (Table 34-9). A cervical length greater than 35 mm after 24 weeks' gestation in twin pregnancies identifies women with a low risk of preterm birth (Imseis et al., 1997). These assessments could be useful to avoid unnecessary and expensive interventions.

■ PREVENTION OF PRETERM BIRTH

The ultimate benchmark of prematurity prevention is a reduction in neonatal morbidity and mortality. Prevention of preterm birth is only a surrogate obstetrical endpoint. Efforts to prevent preterm birth have targeted two groups of pregnant women: those with clinical risk factors for preterm birth (e.g., multiple gestations or a history of preterm birth) and women with a positive test result (e.g., frequent contractions, BV, fibronectin, or short cervix). The interventions applied have focused either on eradication of a specific risk factor (e.g.,

TABLE 34-9. PROBABILITY OF SPONTANEOUS PRETERM BIRTH BEFORE 35 WEEKS IN PAROUS WOMEN ACCORDING TO OBSTETRIC HISTORY (PRETERM VERSUS TERM BIRTH), FIBRONECTIN STATUS, AND CERVICAL LENGTH BY TRANSVAGINAL ULTRASONOGRAPHY AT 24 WEEKS

| | Previous Birth | |
Probability Based on	Preterm	Term
Ob history only	.15	.03
Ob history and fibronectin		
Positive	.48	.13
Negative	.13	.02
Ob history and cervical length		
≤25 mm	.31	.08
26–35 mm	.16	.04
>35 mm	.08	.02
Ob history, FFN negative, and cervical length		
≤25 mm	.25	.06
26–35 mm	.14	.03
>35 mm	.07	.01
Ob history, FFN positive, and cervical length		
≤25 mm	.64	.25
26–35 mm	.45	.14
>35 mm	.28	.07

FFN, cervicovaginal fetal fibronectin; positive = ≥50 ng/dL; Ob, obstetric; ob history, history of prior preterm birth before 37 weeks.

Adapted from Iams JD, Goldenberg RL, Mercer BM, et al: The Preterm Prediction Study: Recurrence risk of spontaneous preterm birth. Am J Obstet Gynecol **178:**1035, 1998.

antimicrobial therapy for BV or on a more global effort to reduce risk by behavioral or pharmacologic intervention.

Treatment for Infection

Preterm birth has been associated with infection of the upper and lower genital tracts. Interest in antibiotic prophylaxis of prematurity was stimulated by a report of fewer preterm births in women who were randomly assigned to receive tetracycline treatment compared with controls in a trial of prophylaxis of bacteriuria (Elder et al., 1971). Antibiotic treatment, however, had no effect on the rate of preterm birth in randomized placebo-controlled trials conducted in women colonized with *Chlamydia*, *Ureaplasma*, and group B streptococci (Eschenbach et al., 1991; Klebanoff et al., 1995).

The association between BV and preterm birth led to studies of screening and treatment of BV for women with high-risk pregnancies and for all pregnant women. In a placebo-controlled trial of metronidazole and erythromycin in women with a previous preterm birth, there was a reduced rate of preterm birth (49% versus 31%) only in the subset of women treated with antibiotics who also had BV (Hauth et al., 1995). The baseline rate of preterm birth (49%) in the control group, however, was higher than expected, and antibiotic treatment for women without BV was associated with an increase in the rate of preterm birth (13.4% versus 4.8%; P < .02). In a randomized trial conducted in women with BV, there was no benefit for treatment with metronidazole except in the subset of women who also had a history of preterm birth (McDonald et al., 1997).

Carey and coauthors (2000) randomly assigned 1953 women at 16 to 24 weeks of pregnancy to receive two 2-g doses of metronidazole or placebo. BV resolved in 78% of the metronidazole group and in 37% of the placebo group, but there was no difference in the rate of preterm delivery (12.2% in the metronidazole group versus 12.5% in the placebo group). Treatment had no effect on the incidence of preterm deliveries that resulted from spontaneous labor or spontaneous rupture of the membranes, nor did it prevent delivery before 32 weeks' gestation. Treatment with metronidazole did not reduce the occurrence of preterm labor, intra-amniotic or postpartum infections, neonatal sepsis, or admission of the infant to the neonatal intensive care unit. In contrast to previous reports (Hauth et al., 1995; McDonald et al., 1997), there was no reduction in preterm birth among women treated with antibiotics who had a history of preterm birth; in fact, there was a trend toward increased rates of preterm birth for women with a prior preterm birth. Though only a trend in the study by Carey and associates, significant increases in preterm births in women treated with antibiotics for genital-tract infection have been reported in other trials, conducted in the following groups:

1. Women without BV (Hauth et al., 1995)
2. Women with asymptomatic *Trichomonas vaginalis* (Klebanoff et al., 2001)
3. Women with a history of preterm birth who also had a positive fibronectin (Andrews et al., 2003)

Because a positive fibronectin test has been associated with upper genital-tract infection, antibiotic prophylaxis with metronidazole and erythromycin for women with a positive fetal fibronectin test between 20 and 25 weeks' gestation was studied in a randomized placebo-controlled trial (Andrews et al., 2003). Antibiotic treatment did not influence the rate of overall or spontaneous preterm birth before 37, 35, or 32 weeks' gestation. Among a subgroup of women with a prior preterm birth who had a positive test for fibronectin, the rate of preterm birth before 37 weeks' gestation actually increased in women treated with antibiotics (46.7 versus 23.9%, P = 0.04) (Fig. 34-12). In contrast, an analysis of data from six randomized trials, in which antibiotic prophylaxis was administered during the second or third trimester of pregnancy, found a decreased rate of preterm PROM in treated women (OR, 0.32; CI, 0.14, 0.73) (Thinkhamrop et al., 2002). The same group analyzed five trials of antibiotic treatment for BV and found insufficient evidence to support screening and treatment of all pregnant women but left open the question of whether women with a history of preterm birth should be screened routinely and treated for BV (Brocklehurst et al., 2002). Screening and treatment for BV is not recommended for all pregnant women but can be considered for women with a history of preterm birth. If treatment is chosen, oral rather than topical therapy is preferred, based on reports showing no effect on preterm birth rate with vaginal treatment (Joesoef et al., 1995; Kekki et al., 2001).

Antimicrobial prophylaxis with cefetamet-pivoxil, an oral third-generation cephalosporin active against a broad range of both gram-positive and gram-negative organisms, was studied in a placebo-controlled trial in high-risk women in Kenya (Gichangi et al., 1997). The antibiotic group had

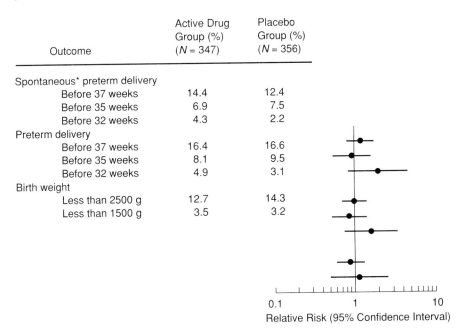

Outcome	Active Drug Group (%) (N = 347)	Placebo Group (%) (N = 356)
Spontaneous* preterm delivery		
Before 37 weeks	14.4	12.4
Before 35 weeks	6.9	7.5
Before 32 weeks	4.3	2.2
Preterm delivery		
Before 37 weeks	16.4	16.6
Before 35 weeks	8.1	9.5
Before 32 weeks	4.9	3.1
Birth weight		
Less than 2500 g	12.7	14.3
Less than 1500 g	3.5	3.2

FIGURE 34-12 ■ Rates of preterm and spontaneous preterm delivery before 32, 35, and 37 weeks' gestation and low birth weight and VLBW by treatment group in fibronectin-positive women enrolled in a randomized trial of antibiotic vs. placebo. (From Andrews WW, Sibai BM, Thom EA, et al for the National Institute of Child Health and Human Development Maternal-Fetal Medicine Units Network: Randomized clinical trial of metronidazole plus erythromycin to prevent spontaneous preterm delivery in fetal fibronectin-positive women. Obstet Gynecol **101**:847, 2003.)

*Due to spontaneous onset of preterm labor or spontaneous preterm permature rupture of membranes

fewer low-birth-weight babies (19% versus 33%), but there was no difference in gestational age at delivery, raising some question about the applicability of this treatment in more developed nations. A randomized trial of periodontal therapy (dental planing) for women with periodontal disease was conducted in 400 pregnant women (Lopez et al., 2002). Therapy for periodontal disease before 28 weeks' gestation was associated with a significant decline in the incidence of preterm or low-birth-weight infants (1.84% versus 10.11% before 37 weeks' gestation; OR, 5.49; 95% CI, 1.65, 18.22; $P > 0.001$). These reports indicate that the relationship between infection and preterm birth is not simply mediated by the ascent of organisms from the lower to upper genital tract during pregnancy. Maternal and fetal immune response to the various genital (Genc et al., 2002) and oral (Madianos et al., 2001) flora involved with preterm birth, as well as maternal dietary intake of antioxidants and omega-3 fatty acids (to be discussed shortly), have been suggested as cofactors. Although new data about periodontal disease is promising, similar hopes for antibiotic prophylaxis of preterm birth have not been fulfilled. At present, antibiotic prophylaxis of preterm birth cannot be recommended. Reports of increased preterm birth in women treated with antibiotic prophylaxis are as yet unexplained.

Screening and Treatment for Short Cervix

A randomized controlled study of routine digital cervical examination to prevent prematurity found no benefit (Buekens et al., 1994). Cerclage for women found to have a short cervix and/or a history of preterm birth is discussed in Chapter 33. Despite the strong association between a short or funneled cervix and preterm birth, the etiology of short cervix is not necessarily addressed by placement of a cerclage (Rust et al., 2001).

Detection and Suppression of Uterine Contractions

Daily monitoring of uterine activity in women with increased risk has been studied as a method to prevent preterm birth on the assumption that subclinical contractions could be detected and arrested with early initiation of tocolytic drugs.

Early trials (Katz et al., 1986; Morrison et al., 1987) found a decrease in preterm births in women followed with home monitors, but subsequent larger trials did not repeat these findings (Collaborative Home Uterine Monitoring Study Group, 1995; Dyson et al., 1998). The largest trial enrolled 2422 high-risk women, including 844 with twins, into a three-armed trial to receive weekly contact with a nurse, daily contact with a nurse, or daily contact with a nurse and a uterine contraction monitor (Dyson et al., 1998). There were no significant differences among the three groups in the rate of preterm delivery before 35 weeks' gestation, in mean cervical dilation at the time of preterm labor diagnosis, or in neonatal outcomes. Women who received daily contact with a nurse and a monitor had more visits and were treated with prophylactic medication significantly more often than women who were contacted only once a week. These results are not surprising, as uterine contraction frequency performs poorly as a screening test for preterm labor (Iams et al., 2002). Suppression of uterine contractions with oral or subcutaneous terbutaline has been advocated to prevent preterm birth in high-risk women (Lam et al., 1998), but there was no evidence of benefit in randomized placebo-controlled trials of oral (summarized by Macones et al., 1995) or subcutaneous terbutaline (Wenstrom et al., 1997; Guinn et al., 1998). Together, these studies indicate that monitoring and suppression of uterine activity in high-risk women does not reduce the frequency of preterm birth.

Enhanced Prenatal Care

Multidisciplinary programs to prevent preterm birth have been developed to address the social, educational, and nutritional problems prevalent in women who experience preterm labor. Many women with preterm labor present for care only after cervical dilation and effacement are advanced or membranes have ruptured, unaware of the subtlety of the early symptoms and/or unable to get to the hospital (Zlatnik, 1972). A multicenter randomized trial of education about the early symptoms and signs of preterm labor provided in a special clinic revealed marked heterogeneity among centers, but no consistent benefit (Collaborative Group on Preterm Birth Prevention, 1993).

Nutritional Supplements

Calcium supplementation was studied to prevent preeclampsia and/or prematurity in two randomized trials conducted in nulliparous women. An Australian trial of 456 women reported fewer preterm births in calcium-treated women (Crowther et al., 1999), but an American study of 4589 women found no effect of calcium on preterm birth rates (Levine et al., 1997). Magnesium supplementation has also been studied without evidence of benefit (Makrides and Crowther, 2001). Supplemental intake of the antioxidant vitamins C and E to prevent preterm birth resulting from preterm PROM by reducing free radicals (Woods et al., 2001) and increased intake of omega-3 fatty acids (e.g., fish oil supplements) to modify host immune response have been proposed as supplements capable of reducing the occurrence of preterm birth. These novel approaches await larger studies before they can be recommended.

Hormonal Supplements

The hypothesis that preterm labor could be initiated by a decrease in progesterone (Csapo et al., 1974) has led to studies testing the possibility that administration of progesterone or a similar compound may prevent preterm labor and delivery. A meta-analysis of five randomized controlled trials of injections of 17α-hydroxyprogesterone caproate to prevent preterm labor and delivery revealed a significant decrease in preterm birth (OR, 0.50; 95% CI, 0.30–0.85) (Keirse et al., 1989). This approach has been studied in two prospective random trials, both conducted in women with a history of preterm birth. A placebo-controlled trial of supplemental progesterone vaginal suppositories, 100 mg once daily between 24 and 34 weeks' gestation, was conducted in 142 women (da Fonseca et al., 2003). Rates of preterm birth were significantly reduced by progesterone supplementation: 2.7% for progesterone versus 18.6% for placebo at 34 weeks' gestation, and 13.8% versus 28.5% at 37 weeks' gestation. A multicenter randomized trial of weekly injections of 250 mg of 17 α-hydroxyprogesterone caproate versus placebo was conducted in 459 women. Progesterone-treated women were significantly less likely to deliver before 37 (36.3% versus 54.9%; RR, 0.66; 95% CI, 0.54–0.93), 35 (20.6% versus 30.7%; RR, 0.67; 95% CI, 0.48–0.93), and 32 (11.4% versus 19.6%; RR, 0.58; 95% CI, 0.37–0.91) weeks' gestation in this study (Meis et al., 2003). Infants of women treated with 17-OH-progesterone had significantly lower rates of IVH (1.3% versus 5.2%), necrotizing enterocolitis (0 versus 2.6%), need for supplemental oxygen (14.9% versus 23.8%), and birth weight below 2500 g (27.2% versus 41.1%). The benefit of progesterone was observed for both early and later preterm births and in both African-American and non–African-American women. There were no adverse side effects reported.

Behavioral Changes

Advice regarding behavior and preterm birth risk abounds despite (or perhaps because of) the paucity of scientific reports to support or refute the benefit or risk of work, rest, stress, and sex. Although there are reports that link the duration and intensity of physical work to preterm birth risk (Mozurkewich et al., 2000; Escriba-Aguir et al., 2001; Newman et al., 2001), there are no corresponding reports of reduced rates of preterm birth in women for whom bed rest was prescribed. Uterine activity does decrease following a rest period in normal singleton pregnancies (Moore et al., 1994), but a review of bed rest as a strategy to decrease preterm birth (Goldenberg et al., 1994) revealed no benefit. Four controlled trials of in-hospital bed rest in women with twin pregnancies found no reduction in preterm birth (Hartikainen-Sorri and Jouppila, 1984; Saunders et al., 1985; Crowther et al., 1989; MacLennan et al., 1990), a conclusion supported by two recent reviews (Goldenberg and Rouse, 1998; Crowther, 2003). Similarly, stress has been related to preterm birth risk (see earlier in this chapter), but successful interventional programs based on stress reduction have not been described.

An association between coitus and preterm labor has been theorized, based on stimulation of uterine activity resulting from female orgasm or semen deposition, or increased risk of intrauterine infection. No reports of reduced preterm birth in couples who abstain have been described. The use of condoms may alleviate postcoital contractions for some patients, and cessation of coitus between 20 and 36 weeks in very-high-risk patients may be considered. Benign coitus-induced increases in uterine activity return to normal within two to three hours (Moore et al., 1994).

DIAGNOSIS OF PRETERM LABOR

Clinical Assessment of Women with Possible Preterm Labor

Clinical management of preterm labor is based on a careful assessment of the risks for mother and infant of continuing the pregnancy versus delivery. Evaluation of possible preterm labor begins with a search for the underlying cause and an assessment of fetal well being. The cause of preterm labor may also cause fetal compromise (e.g., when preterm labor accompanies placental abruption or oligohydramnios). A decision to prolong pregnancy requires assurance that intrauterine growth and maturity will continue in a safe intrauterine environment. Preterm labor associated with infection or ischemia is more likely to result in perinatal morbidity than preterm labor for which no cause is found (Germain et al., 1999). Evaluation of fetal growth and well being should accompany any effort to prolong pregnancy, as fetal growth restriction has been reported in infants delivered after preterm labor or preterm PROM, even in otherwise uncomplicated pregnancies

(Hediger et al., 1995). After fetal well being and possible causes of preterm labor have been evaluated, the next consideration is gestational age. The effort to delay delivery is inversely related to the expected neonatal morbidity and mortality: the earlier the gestational age, the greater the risk of prematurity-related problems for the newborn. Care for women with preterm labor focuses on assessment of risks for the infant, but maternal health must also be considered.

Diagnosis of Preterm Labor

The diagnosis of preterm labor is traditionally made when persistent uterine contractions are accompanied by dilation and/or effacement of the cervix detected by digital examination (Gonik and Creasy, 1986). Symptoms are often nonspecific and are not necessarily those of labor at term. Women treated for preterm labor report symptoms of pelvic pressure, increased vaginal discharge, backache, and menstrual-like cramps, all of which can occur in normal pregnancy. Contractions may be painful or painless and are distinguished from the benign contractions of normal pregnancy primarily by their persistence. The accuracy of these criteria has been questioned by studies suggesting poor sensitivity and specificity for each of the criteria. The symptoms and signs of early preterm labor occur often in normal pregnancy (Copper et al., 1990; Iams, Johnson, et al., 1994; Iams, 2000), and the digital examination of the cervix is imprecise until significant dilation and effacement have occurred. Although digital assessment of cervical dilation of 3 cm or more is straightforward, the reproducibility of digital examination when dilation is greater than 3 cm and/or effacement is greater than 80% is low (Jackson et al., 1992). Uterine contraction frequency varies considerably in normal pregnancy according to gestational age, time of day, and maternal activity (see Fig. 34-10). Moore and coauthors (1994) studied uterine contractions. Uterine activity was monitored continuously for 24 hours twice weekly from 20 weeks until delivery in 109 normal women who delivered at term. There was substantial variation in contraction frequency according to gestational age and time of day. Contractions were more common at night and after 28 weeks' gestation. The night-to-day ratio of contractions per hour was 1.8:1 at 21–24 weeks', 2.3:1 at 28–32 weeks', and 2.0:1 at 38–40 weeks' gestation ($P < .001$). Contractions decreased in the hours following maternal rest and increased after coitus.

In symptomatic women, the best clinical signs of preterm delivery within a week of presentation include an initial cervical dilation greater than 3 cm or effacement of 80% or more, vaginal bleeding, and ruptured membranes (Hueston, 1998; Macones et al., 1999a, 1999b). Considered alone as a criterion for diagnosis, contraction frequency of four or more contractions per hour has low sensitivity and low positive predictive value for preterm birth within 7 to 14 days of presentation (Iams, Casal, et al., 1995; Peaceman et al., 1997). The practice of initiating tocolytic drugs for contraction frequency without additional diagnostic criteria results in unnecessary treatment of women who do not actually have preterm labor (Hueston, 1998). Thus, women with symptoms of preterm labor whose cervical dilation is under 2 cm and/or whose effacement is less than 80% present a diagnostic challenge.

Transvaginal sonography to measure cervical length and the presence of fetal fibronectin in cervicovaginal fluid have been studied as methods to improve the accuracy of preterm labor

diagnosis by reducing the number of false-positive diagnoses. Endovaginal sonography provides satisfactory and consistent images of the cervix in more than 95% of patients regardless of maternal body habitus. Five studies have indicated that the accuracy of diagnosis is improved with this technique compared with digital examination (Murakawa et al., 1993; Gomez et al., 1994; Iams, Paraskos, et al., 1994; Timor-Tritsch et al., 1996; Crane et al., 1997). In each study, transvaginal ultrasound imaging was superior to digital examination in predicting preterm birth in women with acute preterm labor signs and symptoms. A cervical length of 30 mm or greater has been consistently observed to have a very high negative predictive value for preterm birth in studies of symptomatic women (Leitich, Brumbauer, et al., 1999). Transabdominal sonography has poor reproducibility for cervical measurement and should not be used clinically without confirmation by a transvaginal ultrasound (Andersen, 1991; Mason and Maresh, 1990). An ultrasound image of the cervix in a woman with preterm labor is shown in Figure 34-13. Note the "Y" relationship of the cervical canal to the uterus, and see Figure 33-3 to compare with the appearance of a normal cervix. Care must be taken to perform the examination in a reproducible manner. Criteria for a reproducible examination include a flat or triangular internal os, a view of the entire cervical canal, a symmetric image of the external os, and an equal distance from the endocervical canal to the anterior and posterior external margins of the cervix (Burger et al., 1997).

The fetal fibronectin test can also be used to improve the accuracy of diagnosis of preterm labor. A positive test result in a patient with contractions and cervical dilation of under 3 centimeters has better sensitivity (90%) and negative predictive value (97%) for delivery within 7–14 days than standard clinical markers, but the positive predictive value for preterm birth within 7–14 days is less than 20% in most studies (Iams, Casal, et al., 1995; Peaceman et al., 1997; Leitich, Egarter, et al., 1999). It is thus a better test for excluding than for establishing the diagnosis. Two studies of the impact of the fibronectin test on clinical care algorithms have been reported. Joffe and colleagues (1999) noted fewer admissions for preterm labor, shorter hospital stays, and less use of tocolytic drugs without an adverse effect on neonatal outcome. Giles et al. (2000) found no benefit when the test was used in women

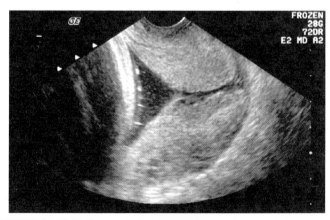

FIGURE 34-13 ■ Transvaginal ultrasound image of the cervix in a woman with preterm labor. Note the "Y"-shaped relationship of the cervical canal to the lower uterine segment. (From Iams JD: Prediction and early detection of preterm labor. Obstet Gynecol **101**:402, 2003.)

whose cervical dilation was 3 cm or greater; a negative test in women without significant dilation led to a 90% reduction in maternal transfer to a tertiary care facility. To be clinically useful in the acute management of preterm labor, the test must be rapidly available, and the clinician must be willing to act on a negative test result by not initiating treatment. Combined use of fibronectin and cervical sonography in the evaluation of symptomatic women has been evaluated in two studies. One found that the tests were complimentary in improving the accuracy of diagnosis (Rizzo et al., 1996); the other found that the combination was not superior to either one alone (Rozenberg et al., 1997).

To summarize, the diagnosis of preterm labor can be difficult, and the treatment is not always benign. The goal of the initial evaluation of a patient who may have preterm labor should be sensitivity, but the goal of evaluation in labor and delivery should be specificity. Any patient complaining of possible symptoms should be evaluated with contraction monitoring and a cervical examination. Severity of symptoms bears little relation to their clinical significance.

Cervical effacement of 80% or more, dilation of more than 2 cm, change in dilation of 1 cm or more, a sonographic cervical length under 30 mm, or a positive fibronectin level should be documented before the diagnosis of preterm labor is accepted. In a patient with persistent contractions who does not meet these criteria, a cervical length measurement of greater than or equal to 30 mm assessed by transvaginal sonography may be used to exclude the diagnosis. The range of contraction frequency in normal pregnancy is wide, especially in the afternoon and evening. The incidental observation of frequent contractions noted during a routine visit is not sufficient to initiate treatment in the absence of other signs or symptoms.

MANAGEMENT OF PRETERM LABOR

Before considering the use of a tocolytic agent, one must establish the diagnosis, search for treatable conditions that may be triggering preterm labor, and decide whether there are any maternal or fetal contraindications to attempting inhibition of labor.

The patient thought to be at risk for preterm labor should initially be placed at bed rest in the lateral decubitus position, and external tocographic and fetal heart rate recording should be instituted. If the membranes are intact, a careful evaluation of the cervix is then performed. If the physician decides to withhold drug therapy and await confirmation of the diagnosis in the form of progressive cervical change, frequent digital examination may be required so that the patient does not pass unidentified to an advanced stage of cervical dilation. A diagnosis of preterm labor is established if the criteria outlined earlier are met.

Owing to the frequent association of preterm labor and urinary tract infections, a urinary microscopic examination and culture are warranted, and antibiotic and antipyretic treatment should be instituted as appropriate. No information is yet available to prove that cultures of the cervix are useful in regard to treatment of preterm labor (Gibbs et al., 1992). If the labor is progressive or the membranes rupture, however, culture evidence of herpes, *Chlamydia*, or hemolytic streptococci could alter subsequent perinatal management. The cost effectiveness of routine cervical cultures remains to be determined.

A more worrisome infection causing preterm labor is chorioamnionitis. If fever is present and its source is obscure, amniocentesis to search for infection is indicated. Chorioamnionitis also can occur with intact membranes but without maternal signs or symptoms other than preterm labor, especially when it occurs before 30 weeks' gestation (Duff and Kopelman, 1987).

Amniotic fluid cultures may be positive in 0%–24% of patients (Gibbs et al., 1992). A study of 264 women in preterm labor with intact membranes revealed positive amniotic fluid cultures in 9.1% overall, but 22% in those progressing to preterm delivery (Romero, Sirtori, et al., 1989). Routine amniocentesis to rule out an infectious cause of preterm labor in an otherwise asymptomatic patient, however, has not proved effective. Amniocentesis may be of value in refractory preterm labor. Because culture results are not immediately available, if amniocentesis is performed, glucose concentrations in the amniotic fluid may provide further insight. Amniotic fluid glucose concentrations below 14 mg/dL have a sensitivity of 87%, a positive predictive value of 63%, and a negative predictive value of 98% in the detection of a positive culture (Romero et al., 1990). Yoon and associates (2001) have argued that cultures fail to detect more than half of cases of infection-related preterm labor, which may be better detected by an elevated amniotic fluid level of interleukin-6 (greater than 2.6 ng/mL) as confirmed after delivery by infection-related morbidity or histologic examinations. In the absence of a clinically available test for interleukin-6, this information reminds clinicians that a negative culture does not necessarily exclude an infectious cause for preterm labor.

In an effort to treat possible underlying infection, there have been a number of trials of the combined use of antibiotics and tocolytic agents conducted in women in preterm labor with intact membranes. The largest and most recent was the ORACLE II trial, in which 6295 women in spontaneous preterm labor with intact membranes were randomized to receive amoxicillin plus clavulanic acid, erythromycin, both, or placebo (Kenyon et al., 2001). The primary outcome—a composite of neonatal mortality and morbidity—occurred with equal frequency in all four study arms. There was no benefit for supplemental antibiotic therapy. Among three reviews of reported trials, two concluded that there was no benefit for adjunctive antibiotic treatment (Gibbs and Eschenbach, 1997; King and Flenady, 2002), and the third found only a small prolongation of pregnancy (gestational age gain of approximately 4 days), but no evidence of a beneficial effect on morbidity and mortality of the neonates (Thorp et al., 2002). Prophylaxis to prevent group B streptococcal infection, however, is recommended for women with preterm labor before 37 weeks' gestation who have unknown or positive vaginal or anal cultures for group B streptococcus (see Fig. 34-14 for an algorithm of care offered by the Centers for Disease Control and Prevention; Schrag et al., 2002) (see also Chapter 39). In the setting of preterm labor, then, supplemental antibiotics should be used only to treat a specific pathogen, e.g. *Treponema pallidum* (syphilis) or *N. gonorrhea*, or as prophylaxis against group B streptococci.

Contraindications for Tocolysis

Tocolytic treatment is contraindicated for a variety of obstetric and medical reasons (Table 34-10). Many conditions are relative contraindications, wherein tocolysis can be

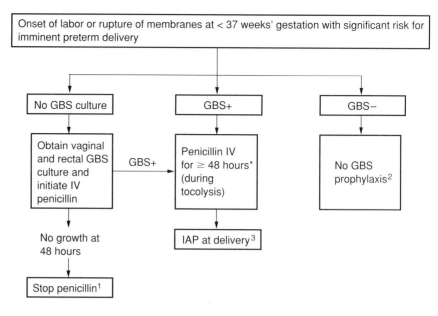

FIGURE 34-14 ■ Sample algorithm for intrapartum antibiotic prophylaxis of group B streptococcal infection for women with preterm labor. (From Schrag S, Gorwitz R, Fultz-Butts K, et al. Prevention of perinatal group B streptococcal disease; Revised guidelines from CDC. MMWR **51**(RR11):1, 2002.)

[1] Penicillin should be continued for a total of at least 48 hours, unless delivery occurs sooner. At the physician's discretion, antibiotic prophylaxis may be continued beyond 48 hours in a GBS culture-positive woman if delivery has not yet occurred. For women who are GBS culture positive, antibiotic prophylaxis should be reinitiated when labor likely to proceed to delivery occurs or recurs.

[2] If delivery has not occurred within 4 weeks, a vaginal and rectal GBS screening culture should be repeated and the patient should be managed as described, based on the result of the repeat culture.

[3] Intrapartum antiobiotic prophylaxis.

attempted if the risks of preterm birth and associated morbidity and mortality are high but intensive monitoring of mother and fetus is necessary. Maternal medical conditions such as diabetes mellitus may be adversely affected by some tocolytic agents, such as beta-adrenergic drugs. Such agents can be used if

TABLE 34-10. CONTRAINDICATIONS TO TOCOLYTIC INHIBITION OF PRETERM LABOR

Contraindications

Absolute contraindications
Severe pregnancy-induced hypertension
Severe abruptio placentae
Severe bleeding from any cause
Chorioamnionitis
Fetal death
Fetal anomaly incompatible with life
Severe fetal growth retardation
Relative contraindications
Mild chronic hypertension
Mild abruptio placentae
Stable placenta previa
Maternal cardiac disease
Hyperthyroidism
Uncontrolled diabetes mellitus
Fetal distress
Fetal anomaly
Mild fetal growth retardation
Cervix >5 cm dilated

resources for close glycemic observation and control are available. Minor degrees of vaginal bleeding or spotting are often seen in association with preterm labor owing to cervical change but could also represent a minor abruption. In such cases, if the fetus is not in distress and uterine tonus is normal, tocolytic treatment can be used with continued close observation.

If the cervix is dilated more than 4–5 cm when tocolytic treatment is begun, the chance of prolonging the gestation for a significant period is low. Occasionally, however, such a patient is observed whose uterine activity is highly sensitive to initial treatment. If the gestation is between 22 and 26 weeks, delay of delivery for 1–2 weeks could alter perinatal outcome significantly, and use of tocolysis can be considered, particularly for multiple gestations. Thus, the severity of any associated disease, individualization of patient care, and the tocolytic agent available must all be considered in the decision to inhibit the preterm labor process.

PHARMACOLOGIC TREATMENT OF PRETERM LABOR

There is little evidence to support the use of sedatives or narcotics as tocolytic agents; however, the use of mild sedation could be beneficial to allay the significant anxiety and fear so frequently seen in the patient in preterm labor. Bed rest and hydration are of no benefit in the treatment of preterm uterine contractions (Guinn et al., 1997; Maxwell and Amankwah, 2001).

The mechanisms of smooth muscle and uterine contraction are described in Chapters 5 and 6. The pharmacologic agents currently in use in various hospitals and countries for preterm labor tocolysis are discussed next. They include the following:

■ Magnesium sulfate
■ Prostaglandin synthesis inhibitors
■ Calcium antagonists
■ Beta-adrenergic agonists

Magnesium Sulfate

Magnesium sulfate has been used extensively in obstetrics for the treatment of preeclampsia, but as a tocolytic for only the past two decades. Although magnesium is known to have a depressant effect on myometrial contractility, the precise mechanism of action remains unknown, with several pathways being proposed. Elevated concentrations of magnesium have a central depressant effect, altering nerve transmission by affecting acetylcholine release and sensitivity at the motor end-plate (Saris et al., 2000). Magnesium also suppresses contractility of isolated myometrial strips *in vitro* in a dose-dependent manner, suggesting a direct cellular action (Harbert et al., 1969). In addition, magnesium has been reported to have its effect through an increase in cyclic adenosine monophosphate (AMP). Magnesium could also have a competitive antagonist role with calcium, decreasing the intracellular free calcium that is necessary for the actin-myosin interaction of smooth muscle contractility (see Chapter 5).

Pharmacology

Myometrial contractility is inhibited when maternal serum levels of magnesium are 5–8 mg/dL (Harbert et al., 1969; Petrie, 1981; Gordon and Iams, 1995; Taber et al., 2002). Deep tendon reflexes may be lost when concentrations reach 9–13 mg/dL, and respiratory depression defects occur at 14 mg/dL or higher. Magnesium is excreted almost entirely by the kidney, with at least 75% of the infused dose of magnesium (for the treatment of preeclampsia) excreted during the infusion and at least 90% excreted within 24 hours (Cruikshank et al., 1981; Idama and Lindow, 1998). As magnesium is reabsorbed in the loop of Henle by a transport-limited mechanism, the glomerular filtration rate (GFR) affects excretion significantly. Increases in maternal serum magnesium also result in maternal hypocalcemia (the total calcium level falling by approximately 25% [Cruikshank et al., 1981; Green et al., 1983]) and an increase in parathyroid hormone but no change in maternal phosphate or calcitonin level (Cruikshank et al., 1979).

Hypocalcemia results from increased urinary excretion. It is usually asymptomatic, although symptoms have been reported (Savory and Monif, 1971). Magnesium ions cross the placenta rapidly, with fetal and newborn levels increasing proportionately with maternal levels (Cruikshank et al., 1979). Total calcium levels in the fetus or newborn are unchanged or minimally reduced (Savory and Monif, 1971; Cruikshank et al., 1979). The mean half-life of neonatal hypermagnesemia secondary to maternal therapy is reported to be more than 40 hours (Dangman and Rosen, 1977).

Magnesium sulfate effects on the cardiovascular system have been studied in patients with severe pregnancy-induced hypertension (Cotton, Gonik, et al., 1984). Under these circumstances, an intravenous bolus of 4 g over 15 minutes resulted in a mild transient lowering of mean arterial blood pressure, no depression of myocardial work, and no effect on oxygen consumption or transport or pulmonary capillary wedge pressure.

Clinical Efficacy

Magnesium sulfate has been evaluated as a tocolytic agent against a placebo in three trials and against beta-adrenergics and other agents in at least 10 trials (Ramsey and Rouse, 2001). In the two randomized placebo-controlled trials, there was no demonstrable benefit for women treated with magnesium (Cotton, Strasner, et al., 1984; Cox et al., 1990). Efficacy is comparable to the beta-adrenergic agents but with fewer adverse maternal side effects seen with magnesium. Most reviews have not supported magnesium as a tocolytic drug, even for short-term delay of preterm labor (Higby et al., 1993; Keirse, 1995; Ramsay and Rouse, 2001). Another recent meta-analysis, however, suggested that magnesium offered small improvements in prolongation of pregnancy without any demonstrable effect on the neonate (Evidence Report, 2000).

Maternal Effects

Flushing, a sense of warmth, headache, nystagmus, nausea, dizziness, dryness of the mouth, and lethargy can be observed in up to 45% of patients, particularly during the intravenous loading dose (Hollander et al., 1987; Cox et al., 1990). Blurred vision or diplopia occurs in more than 75% of patients (Dirge et al., 1990). Ghia and colleagues (2000) reported that magnesium tocolysis decreases attention and working memory without effect on long-term memory. Transient ischemia (Sherer et al., 1992), urticarial eruption (Thorp et al., 1989), maternal hypothermia (Rodis et al., 1987), osteoporosis with spontaneous calcaneal fractures with treatment over 60 days (Levav et al., 1998), and neuromuscular blockade in conjunction with nifedipine tocolysis have been the subjects of isolated reports. If renal function is impaired (and magnesium excretion thus reduced), hypermagnesemia leading to respiratory (and thus cardiac) impairment is possible. Theoretically, high serum magnesium concentrations could alter the amount of muscle relaxant needed during general anesthesia. In addition, it should be used only with extreme caution (if ever) in patients with myasthenia gravis. Pulmonary edema has also been reported in patients receiving both magnesium and corticosteroid therapy.

Serum concentrations of both ionized and nonionized calcium decrease during magnesium infusions, with urinary output of calcium significantly elevated (Smith et al., 1992). Serum phosphorus and parathyroid hormone levels increase. These changes can lead to decreased bone density at 1–11 weeks postpartum if magnesium treatment is prolonged.

If either beta-adrenergic treatment or magnesium sulfate treatment is unsuccessful as an initial tocolytic, a combination of the two may be more effective (Hatjis et al., 1987). A study of 1000 patients treated with magnesium sulfate and terbutaline revealed a relatively low incidence of side effects (Kosasa et al., 1994). Others, however, have reported a worrisome increase in severe maternal side effects when ritodrine was used with magnesium (Ferguson et al., 1984; Ogburn et al., 1985; Wilkins et al., 1988).

Fetal and Neonatal Effects

Maternal magnesium sulfate treatment is used frequently in the presence of maternal hypertensive disease, which by itself could increase the risks of neonatal depression. In addition, many different regimens of maternal magnesium treatment, with varying periods of treatment, make interpretation of reports difficult.

Green and associates (1983) found no significant alterations in neurologic state or Apgar scores with mean umbilical cord magnesium concentrations of 3.6 mg/dL. Stone and Pritchard (1970) observed no correlation between cord magnesium levels, Apgar scores, and depression in newborns whose mothers had received intramuscular magnesium therapy for preeclampsia. Respiratory and motor depression, however, have been observed in infants with umbilical cord magnesium concentrations between 4 and 11 mg/dL (Lipshitz and English, 1967; Savory and Monif, 1971). Petrie (1981) reported decreased muscle tone and drowsiness in newborns whose mothers were given magnesium for tocolysis with maternal serum levels of 4–7 mg/dL. Fetal heart rate variability has been reported to be unchanged, increased, or decreased. At plasma concentrations of 6–8 mg/dL for 24 hours, 50% of fetuses have a nonreactive nonstress test, and only 20% have sustained respiratory movements affecting the biophysical profile interpretation (Peaceman et al., 1989).

Dual tocolysis with magnesium sulfate and indomethacin has been reported to increase the incidence of grades 3 and 4 IVH (Iannucci et al., 1996) (see the discussion on indomethacin later in this chapter). Magnesium therapy for more than seven days can potentially result in demineralization of long bones in more than 50% of fetuses (Holcomb et al., 1991), and congenital rickets has been reported (Lamm et al., 1988).

In 1995, Nelson and Grether published information from a case-controlled study demonstrating that magnesium sulfate therapy was associated with a decreased incidence of cerebral palsy. Grether and colleagues (2000), however, reported data from another case-controlled study, which concluded that magnesium tocolysis was not associated with a reduced incidence of cerebral palsy in preterm infants. Boyle and associates (2000) also reported no overall association between magnesium tocolysis and cerebral palsy. The data suggested a possible protective effect in neonates weighing under 1500 g, but an increase in risk in neonates above that weight threshold. In contrast, increased neonatal mortality was reported in association with magnesium therapy in 85 newborns who received magnesium, compared with 51 infants whose mothers received other tocolytics and 29 who received no tocolysis (Mittendorf et al., 1997). This analysis is flawed, however, by post-hoc creation of a composite outcome, by double-counting of infants who experienced more than one of the composite outcomes (i.e., death and grade 1 IVH in the same infant = two outcomes in the composite post hoc analysis), and by the inclusion of perinatal deaths resulting from congenital anomalies and complications of monochorionic twins in the analysis (Rouse et al., 2003). Nevertheless, the report prompted a thorough review by the Data and Safety Monitoring Committee of an ongoing National Institutes of Health (NIH) sponsored randomized trial of perinatal magnesium versus placebo to reduce neurologic morbidity in preterm infants (Rouse et al., 2003). As of October 2002, this committee found no reason to interrupt the trial after reviewing morbidity and mortality for more than 1400 infants delivered within the trial, half of whom received antenatal magnesium.

Dosage and Administration

An initial loading dose of 4–6 g administered intravenously over 20 minutes has been recommended (Petrie, 1981; Spisso et al., 1982), followed by a maintenance dose of 1–4 g/hour. The relation between serum magnesium concentration and tocolysis success is poorly established (Madden et al., 1990). Individual titration is strongly recommended, according to response and side effects, up to 8 mg/dL. Intravenous therapy is continued for approximately 12 hours after contractions reduce to fewer than 4–6/hour.

Because pulmonary edema has been observed with magnesium sulfate treatment (Elliott et al., 1979), it is prudent to maintain careful observation of intake and output and, perhaps, to restrict total fluid intake as with beta-adrenergic treatment to under 1500–2500 mL daily. Constant monitoring of deep tendon reflexes is indicated, and serum magnesium and calcium levels should be obtained if there is concern about toxicity. Calcium gluconate should be readily available to reverse any untoward toxic effects of magnesium.

It had previously been suggested that continuing oral magnesium, given as a gluconate (or oxide), may be effective in doses of 500 mg–2 g every 2–4 hours, even though serum levels of magnesium are only in the 2.5 mg/dL range with 1 g every 4 hours (Martin et al., 1987). This regimen did not prevent the initiation of preterm labor in high-risk patients (Martin et al., 1992).

Magnesium Tocolysis Summary

Magnesium sulfate tocolysis has not been proven to have either short- or long-term effectiveness but is a relatively safe agent for the mother and, despite current concerns, is probably safe for the infant as well.

Prostaglandin Synthesis Inhibitors

Because prostaglandins have a significant stimulatory role in established labor, there naturally has been interest in prostaglandin synthesis inhibitors to treat preterm labor. Various nonsteroidal compounds, such as indomethacin, naproxen, and fenoprofen, depress synthesis of prostaglandins by inhibiting the cyclooxygenase enzyme necessary for the conversion of arachidonic acid to prostaglandin G, the precursor of prostaglandins E and F (see Chapter 6).

Pharmacology

Indomethacin, a nonspecific cyclooxygenase inhibitor, is absorbed after oral and rectal administration, with plasma concentrations in maternal serum peaking 1–2 hours after oral administration and somewhat sooner with the rectal route (Alvan et al., 1976). The half-life is approximately 4–5 hours. The drug is extensively protein-bound and is eliminated unchanged in pregnant women. Indomethacin readily passes across the placenta, and umbilical artery serum concentrations equilibrate with maternal concentrations by 5 hours after oral administration. Unlike aspirin, the drug binds in a reversible manner to cyclooxygenase, resulting in inhibition that lasts only until the drug is excreted, rather than the lifespan of the platelet. The half-life in the full-term neonate is approximately 15 hours; it is almost half again longer in preterm neonates (Bhat et al., 1979). More than 90% of the drug is protein bound in the neonate.

CLINICAL EFFICACY

In an observational trial of indomethacin, Zuckerman and colleagues (1974) reported that tocolysis was achieved in 40 out of 50 patients. In a small, prospective, randomized, controlled trial, preterm delivery occurred within 24 hours in one of 15 patients treated with indomethacin versus nine of 15 controls (Niebyl et al., 1980). In another trial, indomethacin was superior to placebo in delaying delivery for 48 hours (95% versus 23%) (Zuckerman et al., 1984a, 1984b). One week after treatment, 83% of the indomethacin group was undelivered, versus 16% of the control group. In another small ($n = 34$) placebo-controlled trial, 81% of indomethacin-treated subjects were undelivered after 48 hours versus 56% of the controls, a non–statistically significant difference (Panter et al., 1999). Dudley and Hardie (1985) reported their observations of 167 patients treated with indomethacin for tocolysis, usually for only 24–48 hours. Delivery was delayed for more than 72 hours in 79% of patients. Comparison trials with beta-adrenergic agents reveal at least comparable tocolytic effectiveness (Besinger et al., 1991) and fewer maternal side effects.

MATERNAL EFFECTS

Prostaglandins mediate several physiologic functions, and thus inhibition of prostaglandin synthesis potentially can lead to a number of side effects. Nevertheless, serious maternal side effects are infrequent. Although indomethacin has a reversible effect on cyclooxygenase, one report associated it with postpartum hemorrhage (Reiss et al., 1976). Lunt and colleagues (1994) reported that indomethacin tocolysis, although having no impact on prothrombin or activated partial thromboplastin times, essentially doubled bleeding times. Gastrointestinal side effects can also be seen, but they may be kept to a minimum if the drug is taken with meals. Prolonged administration could be associated with headaches, dizziness, depression, and psychosis (Tepperman et al., 1977), but these latter effects have not been reported during brief tocolytic treatment, and the incidence of these side effects is not well defined. In general, this agent should not be used in patients with drug-induced asthma, coagulation disorders, hepatic or renal insufficiency, or peptic ulcer disease.

FETAL AND NEONATAL EFFECTS

One of the major concerns with prostaglandin inhibition has been the possibility of serious adverse fetal effects, in particular constriction of the fetal ductus arteriosus, neonatal pulmonary hypertension, IVH, and oligohydramnios.

Studies in the pig have revealed the cyclooxygenase-1 (COX-1)-dependent prostaglandins to be the main mediators of ductal arteriosus patency in utero (Guerguerian et al., 1998). Indomethacin inhibits both COX-1 and COX-2 enzymes and readily crosses the placenta. Moise and coworkers (1988), with serial fetal echocardiography, brought attention to antenatal indomethacin treatment potentially causing ductal arteriosus constriction, the constriction resolving within 24 hours of dis-

continuing treatment. In another study of 53 fetuses during indomethacin tocolysis, ductal constriction was observed in 61% at 31–34 weeks, in 43% between 27 and 30 weeks, and in none under 27 weeks (Tulzer et al., 1992). In another report, by 31 weeks of gestation, 70% of fetuses had demonstrated constriction of the ductus if exposed to indomethacin (Vermillion et al., 1997). These findings are the basis for the suggestion that indomethacin tocolysis be limited to fewer than 32 weeks of gestation. There is also the suggestion that fetal echocardiography be performed to evaluate for possible ductus arteriosus constriction if indomethacin treatment is used for more than 48–72 hours (Vermillion and Landen, 2001). In addition, although the normal fetus may tolerate transient partial ductal narrowing, if it occurs in a growth-restricted fetus, with decreased umbilical blood flow and attendant increased dependence on ductal flow, partial constriction of the ductus could become problematic.

Prolonged diversion of blood away from the ductus arteriosus and toward the pulmonary vasculature has been suggested as the etiology of reports of neonatal primary pulmonary hypertension (Manchester et al., 1967; Csaba et al., 1978; Besinger et al., 1991). Most of these cases involved indomethacin treatment for longer than 48 hours. In addition, it has been suggested that antenatal indomethacin exposure could be associated with postnatal ductus arteriosus patency that is refractory to medical closure therapy (Suarez et al., 2002).

Fetal exposure to indomethacin has been linked to the incidence of IVH when this therapy is used after other agents have failed (Norton et al., 1993), or when it is used in combination with magnesium sulfate (Iannucci et al., 1996). Other authors have been unable to show any increased incidence of IVH with indomethacin exposure (Vermillion and Newman, 1999; Suarez et al., 2001). Reports also conflict regarding a potential association of treatment with necrotizing enterocolitis (Norton et al., 1993; Major et al., 1994; Vermillion and Newman, 1999; Parilla et al., 2000). Long-term exposure (up to at least 5 weeks) has also been associated with anuria, renal microcystic lesions, and neonatal mortality (Van der Heijden et al., 1994).

Various authors have indicated that the incidence of fetal death and perinatal morbidity may be no higher in those patients treated for 24–72 hours before 34 weeks than in those treated with placebo or beta-adrenergics, or not treated at all (Zuckerman et al., 1984a, b; Amy and Thiery, 1985; Dudley and Hardie, 1985; Niebyl and Witter, 1986; Vermillion and Newman, 1999). Confounding by indication may explain some of the adverse reports, in that those who received indomethacin were at early gestational ages, had refractory labor, and thus were more likely to have had in utero infection (Macones, Marder, et al., 2001). Recent information about the inflammatory causes of morbidities in extremely premature infants thus suggests that the morbidities attributed to indomethacin may in fact result from the factors that led to preterm labor. Large studies in which these factors can be controlled may ultimately resolve the question of safety.

Indomethacin treatment has been associated with the development of oligohydramnios secondary to decreased fetal urine production. This occurrence is somewhat unpredictable and is reversible on cessation of treatment. It developed in 10% of patients in one study on maintenance therapy (Vermillion et al., 1997). Oligohydramnios has been observed in human pregnancies in which indomethacin has been given for a number of days (Cantor et al., 1980; Itskovitz et al., 1980). Symptomatic polyhydramnios has also been treated successfully with indomethacin (Cabrol et al., 1987; Kirshon et al., 1990). In summary, indomethacin could lead to oligohydramnios, particularly after long-term use, but its onset is not predictable.

DOSAGE AND ADMINISTRATION

Most reports have used either a 50-mg or 100-mg rectal suppository of indomethacin, or 50 mg orally as a loading dose, followed by 25–50 mg orally every 6 hours depending upon response. Rectal suppositories are no longer supplied by the manufacturer but can be compounded by a hospital pharmacy.

It is suggested that tocolysis with indomethacin be limited to women before 32 weeks of gestation whose fetuses have no evidence of growth restriction and whose amniotic fluid volume is normal. Most clinicians treat for only 48–72 hours. Evaluation of both amniotic fluid volume and the ductus arteriosus should be considered if treatment is continued for a longer period of time.

Prostaglandin Inhibition Tocolysis Summary

Indomethacin is effective in delaying delivery for at least 48 hours, if not longer. Serious side effects for the mother are relatively infrequent. The potential serious adverse effects for the fetus are also probably relatively infrequent with short-term (under 48 hours) tocolysis treatment before 32 weeks of gestation. More selective prostaglandin inhibitors may be of benefit. Specific COX-2 inhibitors such as celecoxib are only beginning to be evaluated for safety and efficacy as potential tocolytic drugs (Stika et al., 2002).

Calcium Channel Blockers

Owing to the central role that cytoplasmic free calcium plays in smooth muscle contractility, interest has arisen in the use of the newer calcium channel blockers as off-label tocolytic drugs. Agents such as nifedipine are believed to act by inhibiting the influx of calcium ions through the cell membrane, primarily by affecting the voltage-dependent calcium channels (Fleckenstein, 1977; McDonald et al., 1994).

Pharmacology

Both nifedipine and nicardipine have been evaluated as tocolytic agents. Plasma concentrations of nifedipine peak in 30–60 minutes after oral administration, but sublingual administration can result in more rapid increases in the blood (Forman et al., 1981; Ferguson et al., 1989). The half-life is 1–2 hours, with elimination through the kidney and gut. Calcium channel blockade is reversible after discontinuation of the drug. Nifedipine has been shown to cross the placenta (Ferguson et al., 1989), but the kinetics of the transfer and metabolism within the fetus are largely unreported.

Clinical Efficacy

In the original observational trial, nifedipine abolished uterine activity and prevented delivery for 3 days in all of ten patients treated (Ulmsten et al., 1980). No randomized placebo-controlled trial of any calcium channel blocker has been reported. Prospective randomized trials of the calcium channel blockers (usually nifedipine) have been made in comparison with other tocolytic agents, mainly the beta-adrenergic drugs. Individual studies (Read and Welby, 1986; Ferguson et al, 1990; Papatsonis et al., 1997) have revealed that nifedipine is equal or superior to the beta-adrenergic ritodrine in suppressing contractions and delaying delivery for at least 48 hours. A meta-analysis of 13 trials revealed nifedipine to be superior to beta-adrenergic agents in terms of delaying delivery for 48 hours, reaching 34 weeks of gestation, the incidence of respiratory distress syndrome of the newborn, and neonatal intensive care admissions (Tsatsaris et al., 2001). A study comparing nicardipine and magnesium revealed similar efficacy for both drugs (Larmon et al., 1999).

Maternal Effects

Calcium antagonists cause vasodilation. Flushing is frequent, possibly accompanied by short-lasting headache and/or nausea. A transient tachycardia and mild decreases in blood pressure are common, with occasional significant hypotension (Ferguson et al., 1989). Modest increases in blood glucose also have been reported. Isolated hepatotoxicity has been observed during tocolysis (Sawaya and Robertson, 1992), and adjunctive treatment with magnesium can result in neuromuscular blockade (Ben-Ami et al., 1994). Using data from the tocolytic comparison trials, the meta-analyses revealed that side effects were more common with the beta-adrenergics and with magnesium (two trials), and that discontinuation of the tocolytic was less frequent with the calcium channel blockers (Tsatsaris et al., 2001).

Fetal Effects

Clinical studies of efficacy are limited in number, and the interpretation is frequently complicated by use of other tocolytic beta-adrenergic drugs. A concern has been raised by animal studies. Significant decreases in fetal arterial PO_2 and pH were reported following maternal administration of nicardipine in the rhesus monkey, probably as a result of decreased uterine blood flow (Ducsay et al., 1987). Similar fetal acidemic responses, including fetal demise, have been seen with maternal administration of nicardipine or nifedipine in sheep (Harake et al., 1987; Parisi et al., 1989). Doppler studies during nifedipine treatment in humans, however, have not shown abnormal fetal or uteroplacental circulations (Mari et al., 1989). Other observational reports in humans have not revealed any alarming incidence of low Apgar scores or core pH (Murray et al., 1992; Ray et al., 1994).

Dosage and Administration

A loading dose of 10 mg of oral nifedipine is usually used, to be repeated after 20 minutes if contractions persist and perhaps repeated in another 20 minutes. The use of sublingual administration has been discontinued because of potential hypotension. Oral therapy is then continued with 10–20 mg every 4–6 hours. The duration of treatment has not been established.

Calcium Channel Blockade Summary

Nifedipine appears to be as effective as or superior to the beta-adrenergics and magnesium in delaying delivery for 48–72 hours; it also appears to have a relatively low incidence of significant adverse reactions for the mother and fetus. It should not be used together with the beta-adrenergics or magnesium sulfate. As with the other tocolytic agents, it remains to be proven whether the calcium channel blockers can decrease morbidity and mortality associated with preterm labor and birth. Further large studies are needed to fully assess efficacy and safety.

Beta-Adrenergic Agonists

The beta-adrenergic agonists, used as tocolytics for three decades, include isoxsuprine, hexoprenaline, fenoterol, orciprenaline, ritodrine, salbutamol, and terbutaline. These agents are derivatives of epinephrine that have been formulated to maximize the beta$_2$-adrenergic effects on the uterus, although all have some beta$_1$-adrenergic activity. Their action is mediated via adenyl cyclase-induced increase in cyclic adenosine monophosphate, which inhibits myosin light-chain kinase and thus inhibits uterine contraction (see Chapter 6).

Pharmacology

Most of the clinically utilized beta-adrenergic agonists are excreted unaltered, or are excreted as conjugates by the kidney. Although minimal information is available concerning placental transfer, it is known that some agents (e.g., ritodrine, terbutaline) cross into the fetus; others (e.g., fenoterol, hexoprenaline) probably cross to a lesser degree.

The concentration of ritodrine in maternal serum increases with increasing infusion rates but can vary by more than 100% from patient to patient at low infusion rates (Caritis, Venkataramanan, Darby, et al., 1990). Intravenous administration of either ritodrine or terbutaline results in peak plasma concentration within 10 minutes, which is similar to intramuscular ritodrine and subcutaneous terbutaline (Gonik et al., 1988; Caritis, Venkataramanan, Cotroneo, et al., 1990). The half life of ritodrine is approximately 2 hours, and of terbutaline, approximately 3–4 hours. The therapeutic blood concentrations of these agents are not established, in part because of the degree of uterine activity and cervical change that may be present and in part because of differences between patients in plasma clearance. These factors may explain some of the negative efficacy reports of studies wherein a rigid protocol rather than individualization of treatment is followed.

Myometrial beta-adrenergic receptors are reduced in pregnant women treated with beta-agonist drugs (Berg et al., 1985). The continuous exposure to beta-adrenergic stimulation leads to a reduction of inhibition of oxytocin-stimulated contractility in sheep (Caritis et al., 1987), whereas intermittent administration of ritodrine revealed no change in the myometrial beta-adrenergic receptors or adenylcyclase activity and maintenance of inhibition of oxytocin-induced contractility (Caritis et al., 1991).

Clinical Efficacy

The effectiveness of the different beta-adrenergic drugs used clinically for tocolysis is comparable. There is little consistent evidence that supports the superiority of one agent over another. Beta-adrenergic therapy can delay delivery for 3 days, but its effect on preterm birth remains controversial (Creasy and Katz, 1984; King et al., 1988; Leveno et al., 1990; Canadian Preterm Labor Investigators Group, 1992; Higby et al., 1993). The Canadian study, although complicated by inclusion of women with ruptured membranes (27%), reported fewer patients in the ritodrine group who delivered within 7 days (difference of –9.0; 95% CI, –14.8, 3.2); the study also found a nonsignificant difference in favor of ritodrine of delivery at fewer than 32 weeks (–9.2; 95% CI, –18.6, 0.2). There were also fewer neonatal deaths at 24–27 weeks that did not reach significance (–7.2; 95% CI, –19.1, 4.7). Overall, these agents have the ability to inhibit uterine activity rapidly and delay delivery for 3–7 days, but without proven benefit to the neonate.

Oral administration of the drugs has not proven useful in the near or long term, with meta-analyses failing to demonstrate any improvement in prevention of preterm birth, interval to delivery, or recurrence of preterm labor (Macones et al., 1995).

Maternal Effects

Although formulated to maximize their uterine effects and minimize extrauterine effects, the beta-adrenergic drugs can influence maternal cardiovascular and metabolic physiology significantly. Table 34-11 summarizes the tissue responses to beta-adrenergic stimulation that are the basis for the potential adverse maternal effects. Most of these are relatively mild, but some are serious enough to have the potential for maternal mortality. Of all the tocolytic agents, the beta-adrenergic drugs have the highest rate of serious adverse maternal effects (Evidence Report, 2000).

TABLE 34-11. RESPONSE OF VARIOUS TISSUES TO BETA-ADRENERGIC RECEPTOR ACTIVITY

Beta$_2$-Adrenergic Responses

↑ Bronchiolar tone

Beta$_1$-Adrenergic Responses

Cardiac
↑ Heart stroke
↑ Stroke volume
Bowel
↓ Motility
Metabolic
↑ Lipolysis
↑ Intracellular K$^+$

Beta$_2$-Adrenergic Responses

Smooth muscle
↓ Vascular tone
↓ Uterine activity
↓ Bronchiolar tone
Kidney
↑ Renin
↓ Urinary output
Metabolic
↑ Glycogenolysis
↑ Insulin release

Cardiovascular Effects

The more serious side effects of beta-adrenergic agents include hypotension, cardiac arrhythmias, myocardial ischemia, and pulmonary edema; the reported incidence of these serious complications varies between 0.3% and 5% of treated patients. Intravenous administration of ritidrine has been associated with mild palpitations in at least one-third of patients, with flushing in 10%–15% (Merkatz et al., 1980), and with chest pain in 8% (Canadian Preterm Labor Investigators Group, 1992). These effects could necessitate discontinuing treatment in as many as 7%–10% of patients (Tsatsaris et al., 2001).

Cardiac arrhythmias are usually asymptomatic and include premature nodal and ventricular contractions that commonly respond quickly to cessation of treatment (Benedetti, 1983). Myocardial ischemia has been reported with several different agents (Katz et al., 1981; Ying and Tejani, 1982; Benedetti, 1983). The severity of the myocardial ischemia seems to occur mainly at high heart rates (greater than 120–130 beats/minute). Maternal deaths have been reported in association with beta-adrenergic therapy, especially in women with unrecognized cardiac disease or myocarditis (Barden et al., 1980; Benedetti, 1983). Known or suspected cardiac disease is thus a contraindication to beta-adrenergic tocolysis.

Pulmonary edema is the most common serious side effect. Cessation of the beta-adrenergic treatment and institution of appropriate treatment with diuretics usually results in prompt improvement (Katz et al., 1981). If not recognized and addressed quickly, however, adult respiratory distress syndrome could result. Predisposing factors are twin gestations (approximately 50% of reported cases), in which mean plasma volume expansion is greater than in singletons; persistent heart rate over 130 beats/minute; anemia below 9 g/dL; maternal infection (Hatjis and Swain, 1988); and iatrogenic fluid overload. The beta-adrenergic drugs stimulate the renin-aldosterone system, decrease urinary output, and decrease colloid osmotic pressure by approximately 20% after 24 hours of infusion (Lammintausta and Erkkola, 1979; Armson et al., 1992) (see Chapter 45). All these factors predispose the patient to volume overload over time, particularly if the colloid osmotic pressure drops below 15 mm Hg. Most reported cases of pulmonary edema occur 30–60 hours after initiation of treatment, regardless of whether treatment is ongoing.

The concomitant use of beta-adrenergic tocolytics and corticosteroids to induce fetal lung maturity in women with pulmonary edema has prompted concern that corticosteroids could be a predisposing factor. The incidence of corticosteroid therapy in these patients, however, is similar to that in the overall preterm labor population who receive tocolytics, a fact suggesting that corticosteroids are not a factor in the pathogenesis of the beta-adrenergic–associated pulmonary edema (Robertson et al., 1981). With the recognition of fluid dynamics and recognition of the importance of close observation of intake and output and observance of fluid restriction, the incidence of pulmonary edema has been reported to be low (e.g., just 0.3% in the large Canadian trial).

Metabolic Effects

There is an increase in hepatic glycogenolysis and maternal hyperglycemia with beta-adrenergic agents. The elevation in maternal glucose level begins to decrease after the peak, which occurs within 3 hours of initiation of intravenous treatment

and is still elevated at 24 hours. Modest hyperglycemia persists for an indeterminate period of time (Young et al., 1983). The risk of abnormal carbohydrate metabolism is increased by the concomitant use of corticosteroids (Fisher et al., 1997). The acute alterations in carbohydrate metabolism are usually not of consequence in the normal patient but have been associated with ketoacidosis in the insulin-dependent diabetic patient (Miodovnik et al., 1985) and rarely, in nondiabetic populations (Leopold and McEvoy, 1977). These effects on carbohydrate metabolism make other tocolytics the first-line choices in women with diabetes mellitus.

Concomitant with the hyperglycemia is the development of hypokalemia (Smith and Thompson, 1977; Young et al., 1983). Although plasma potassium concentrations are reduced at first, they return to near normal by 24 hours. Urinary excretion of potassium is not increased. There is no evidence to support the need for exogenous potassium treatment during the acute hypokalemia. No changes are known to occur in serum magnesium, calcium, or phosphate concentration.

It is not rare for patients to experience some nausea and occasional emesis in addition to some restlessness and general agitation during beta-adrenergic tocolysis. Paralytic ileus, pruritis, and dermatitis occur rarely (Robertson et al., 1981).

Fetal and Neonatal Effects

Most beta-adrenergic drugs (except perhaps hexoprenaline) cross the placenta, but little is known about the kinetics of transfer in human pregnancy. In the human, there are no changes in fetal heart rate at low infusion rates. Mild fetal tachycardia and increases in beat-to-beat variability can occur with higher doses. One echocardiographic study of neonates exposed to beta-adrenergic drugs reported interventricular septal thickening; the effect was related to duration of exposure and was absent at follow-up (Nuchpuckdee et al., 1986).

Neonatal hypoglycemia, hypocalcemia, ileus, and hypotension were more common in a retrospective review of infants born to mothers who delivered within 48 hours of treatment with isoxsuprine (Brazy and Pupkin, 1979). Similar findings were reported with use of terbutaline, isoxsuprine, and fenoterol (Epstein et al., 1979).

The incidence of periventricular-IVH in preterm neonates exposed to beta-adrenergic agents was reported to be increased in two reports (Dolfin et al., 1984; Groome et al., 1992), but this finding has not been observed by others (Levene et al., 1982; Van de Bor et al., 1986; Laros et al., 1991). In fact, a marked protective effect of beta-adrenergic exposure has been reported (Ment et al., 1995).

Follow-up studies by Freysz and associates (1977) of children exposed in utero to beta-adrenergic agents show normal growth and development at 2 years of age. Studies of children aged 6 years after exposure found no significant alterations in anthropometric measurement, neurologic tests, or general behavior but did show decreased school performance, as evaluated by teachers (Hadders-Algra et al., 1986).

Dosage and Administration

The beta-adrenergic agents may be administered intravenously, intramuscularly, subcutaneously, or orally. Treatment with ritodrine or terbutaline may be initiated by intravenous infusion using a calibrated infusion pump, or by the intramuscular route with ritodrine, or by the subcutaneous route with terbutaline. Before treatment, the patient is placed in the lateral tilt or decubitus position so that supine hypotension can be avoided. Intake and output are recorded, and the total recommended intake is between 1500 and 2500 mL. The lungs should be auscultated every 4–8 hours for evidence of early pulmonary edema.

Ritodrine is usually initiated intravenously at the rate of 0.05–0.10 mg/min and is increased by 0.05 mg/min at 10- to 30-minute intervals to a potential maximum rate of 0.350 mg/min. Terbutaline can also be administered intravenously, beginning at a rate of 0.01 mg/min and increased by 0.01 mg/min at 10–30-minute intervals to a maximum rate of 0.08 mg/min. The infusion rate is adjusted according to uterine activity or until adverse maternal effects are noted. The infusion rate should not be increased further if maternal pulse rate reaches 130 beats per minute or if systolic pressure falls below 80–90 torr.

Once tocolysis is achieved, some physicians continue the infusion for another 6–24 hours. On the other hand, one author (Caritis et al., 1983; Caritis, 1988) has recommended that once labor is halted, the infusion rate should be reduced slowly until the lowest inhibitory rate is established; the maintenance rate should then be continued for 12 hours.

Owing to the potential for desensitization with prolonged use, there has been interest in intermittent bolus administration of beta-adrenergic drugs. Terbutaline is frequently initiated by the subcutaneous route, using 0.25 mg, with repeated doses at 3–4-hour intervals. Another approach suggested is the use of a pump to administer a very low dose of terbutaline (0.3–0.5 mg/hour) with intermittent boluses of approximately 0.25 mg at times of peak activity (Lam et al., 1988). In general, this approach appears to be associated with the need for less agonist, fewer side effects, and less recurrent preterm labor (Allbert et al., 1994; Perry et al., 1995). Two randomized placebo-controlled trials, however, found no advantage for subcutaneous infusion of terbutaline by pump (Wenstrom et al., 1997; Guinn et al., 1998). Adverse anecdotal reports prompted the FDA to issue a warning about this form of treatment (U.S. Food and Drug Administration, 1998).

Beta-Adrenergic Tocolysis Summary

The beta-adrenergic drugs, once the first choice for tocolysis, have been replaced by other drugs with better maternal side effect profiles and similar or improved efficacies. On the other hand, short-term use of terbutaline or ritodrine intravenously, or of terbutaline subcutaneously, is a relatively easy and effective method to obtain short-term delay of delivery to allow time for maternal transfer, corticosteroid treatment, and group B streptococcus prophylaxis. Maintenance treatment with oral agents does not appear to be warranted. The use of beta-adrenergic agents, as with other tocolytics, has not been associated with a decrease in overall perinatal morbidity and mortality resulting from preterm labor and birth.

Miscellaneous Tocolytic Drugs

Oxytocin antagonists have been proposed as tocolytic agents, potentially being of value by blockade of oxytocin receptors. Their potential appeal is the apparent lack of significant side effects. Two noncontrolled studies of short-

term infusions of one oxytocin antagonist resulted in inhibition of premature labor in all 13 patients in one study and in nine of 12 patients in the other (Akerlund et al., 1987; Andersen et al., 1989). The oxytocin antagonist atosiban was studied in a placebo-controlled trial in which women whose contractions continued after the first hour of placebo or atosiban therapy could then be treated with another tocolytic agent, thus confounding comparisons (Romero et al., 2000). Seventy-three percent of women in the atosiban group (versus 58% in the control group) were undelivered after 24 hours without alternate tocolysis. For unknown reasons, there were more neonatal deaths in the treatment arm. There was no benefit in patients between 20 and 28 weeks' gestation. There was no difference in efficacy in a multicenter trial of atosiban versus ritodrine (Moutquin et al., 2000).

Lees and associates (1999) compared the nitric oxide donor glycerol trinitrate with ritodrine for tocolysis with no differences in efficacy. A comparison of intravenous nitroglycerin with magnesium sulfate in 31 patients revealed more tocolytic failures in the nitroglycerin group, and in one fourth of this latter group, treatment was stopped because of hypotension (El-Sayed et al., 1999).

Summary of Pharmacologic Treatment of Preterm Labor

A number of agents can suppress smooth muscle contractility, but all of these tocolytic drugs appear to have drawbacks and potential adverse effects. In addition, their use necessitates close observation of the patient under controlled circumstances. Their success depends on use early in the course of preterm labor, but they should not be given until the diagnosis of preterm labor is relatively secure. That they can delay delivery for a few days appears to be well established, but their ability to decrease the incidence of preterm birth and its attendant neonatal morbidity remains to be proved.

As of this writing, the use of beta-adrenergic agents for tocolysis has decreased in the United States with magnesium sulfate, prostaglandin synthesis inhibitors, or the calcium channel blockers being the preferred choices for tocolysis at different centers. Further controlled trials of the latter two classes of agents not only are warranted on the basis of current clinical information but also are indicated and needed. New agents are also desired.

■ MANAGEMENT OF PROGRESSIVE PRETERM LABOR

There are numerous situations in which attempts to inhibit preterm labor are not indicated, tocolytic therapy is unlikely to succeed for many days, or, indeed, tocolytic therapy may fail. Decisions must be made about whether any other therapy is indicated, how the labor and delivery should be managed, and where delivery should take place.

The delivery of small preterm newborns is best accomplished in a specialized perinatal center. Preterm infants born in an intensive care setting have a greater chance for survival and less short-term and long-term morbidity than infants who are transferred after birth for specialized neonatal care (McCormick et al., 1985; Yeast et al., 1998; Towers et al., 2000). Short-term tocolytic therapy frequently can delay delivery sufficiently to allow administration of steroids, group B streptococcal prophylaxis, and transfer of the mother and fetus to a center with appropriate facilities and staff. The regionalization of perinatal care can make available the appropriate level of care through cost-effective use of resources (American Academy of Pediatrics and American College of Obstetricians and Gynecologists, 2002). Survival and morbidity have been addressed earlier in this chapter and are also discussed in Chapter 60. The key to management is coordination of intrapartum and neonatal care through effective communication between the parents and both obstetrical and pediatric caregivers.

Fetal Age and Size

Neonatal survival and morbidity are based on both gestational age and birth weight, so both are important issues for clinical management. As neonatal and perinatal care has improved, the lower limit of "viability" has been a progressively earlier gestational age. Because the likelihood of survival and morbidity is influenced by the expectations and aggressiveness of the perinatal care team, and because survival and morbidity are often underestimated by medical personnel (Haywood et al., 1994; Bottoms et al., 1997; Morse et al.,

2000) (Fig. 34-15 A and B), assessment of fetal size and gestational age are extremely important. For example, a study of 66 infants with birth weights between 500 and 749 g found that after controlling for birth weight and gestational age, fetuses who were considered by the perinatal care team to be "viable" (i.e., likely to survive) were 18 times more likely to survive than fetuses who were deemed "previable" (Reuss and Gordon, 1995). Another study of 713 infants who weighed less than 1 kg at birth found that aggressive attempts to save very premature fetuses as indicated by willingness to perform a cesarean birth for fetal indications resulted in a greater chance of survival and intact survival but with a significant increased probability of serious morbidity (Bottoms et al., 1997). Before delivery, the best predictor of survival is the "best obstetrical gestational age," a composite of a thorough history of obstetrical milestones supplemented by ultrasound measurement of the fetus. It is important that the latest information about rates of survival and morbidity be available when judgments about intrapartum care are being made (see Table 34-4, Table 34-5, Fig. 34-4, and Chapter 60). It is also important to recognize that parents and medical professionals often do not share the same beliefs about the quality of life and potential for intact survival in premature infants (Saigal et al., 1999).

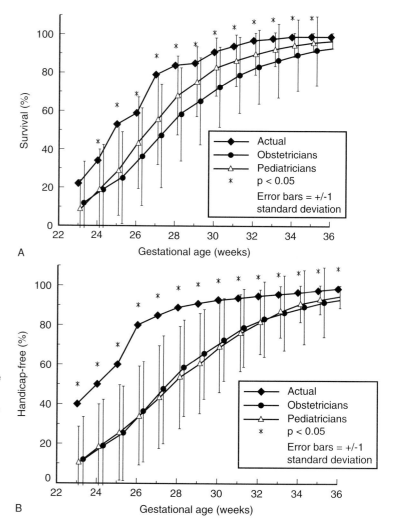

FIGURE 34-15 ■ **A,** Survival. Comparison of estimates of pediatricians and obstetricians of survival rates to actual survival rates obtained from national data. Estimates of pediatricians were significantly lower than actual survival rates at each gestational age from 24 to 35 weeks. Estimates for obstetricians were significantly lower than actual survival rates from 23 to 36 weeks' gestation. **B,** Freedom from handicap. Comparison of estimates of pediatricians and obstetricians of rates of freedom from handicap to actual handicap-free rates. Estimates of both pediatricians and obstetricians were significantly lower than actual handicap-free rates at each gestational age from 23 to 36 weeks. (From Morse SB, Haywood JL, Goldenberg RL, et al: Estimation of neonatal outcome and perinatal therapy use. Pediatrics **105:**1046, 2000.)

Antenatal Treatment to Reduce Perinatal Morbidity and Mortality

Three decades ago, on the basis of the observation in sheep that glucocorticoid administration to the fetus resulted in accelerated fetal lung maturation, the results of the first trial of antenatal glucocorticoid therapy in humans was reported (Liggins and Howie, 1972; Liggins, 1977). Since that time, multiple trials have shown that antenatal glucocorticoid therapy decreases neonatal mortality as well as morbidities that include respiratory distress syndrome, IVH, and necrotizing enterocolitis. Antenatal glucocorticoid therapy is the standard of care and has become a model for other attempts to improve neonatal outcome through antenatal treatment. It is discussed in detail in Chapter 25.

Antenatal treatment with thyrotropin releasing hormone was proposed as a means of reducing neonatal respiratory disease, but it has been found to be ineffective (Crowther et al., 2000). Intra-amniotic injection of thyroxine has also been studied as a means of reducing neonatal respiratory distress syndrome. Benefit was reported only in infants who weighed 1000–1500 g and received more than one dose, thus limiting the clinical utility of this approach (Reyes et al., 1997). Other treatments studied include antenatal treatment with phenobarbital or vitamin K and intrapartum magnesium sulfate as possible methods to reduce the incidence of IVH. In a randomized controlled trial, Thorp and coworkers (1995) compared phenobarbital and vitamin K versus placebo in 372 patients and found no difference in the rates of grade 3 and grade 4 intracranial hemorrhages in newborns fewer than 34 weeks' gestation. The Cochrane Review found that preliminary evidence of a reduction in IVH attributed to phenobarbital disappeared as additional higher-quality studies were incorporated into their database (Crowther and Henderson-Smart, 2003a). The same reviewers concluded that vitamin K does not reduce IVH (Crowther and Henderson-Smart, 2003b). Antenatal treatment with magnesium sulfate is now under study as a treatment to reduce the occurrence of intraventricular bleeding based on reports of a decreased risk of cerebral palsy in very-low-birth-weight infants born to women treated with $MgSO_4$ for preterm labor or preeclampsia (see the discussion earlier in this chapter).

Fetal Heart Rate Monitoring

The preterm fetus may tolerate labor poorly, and the cause of the preterm birth may create additional intrapartum risk. Perinatal asphyxia is a risk factor for short-term and long-term sequelae in the preterm infant as well as in the term infant. In a study of 30 preterm newborns with metabolic acidosis at delivery matched with 60 preterm infants for birth weight but without acidosis, neonatal mortality was higher in the acidotic newborns (23% versus 3%), and the incidence of major neurologic deficits at 12 months was also higher (8/30 versus 8/60) (Low et al., 1992). Apgar scores also reflect gestational age, and thus umbilical cord blood analysis is important to determine the presence of newborn acidosis (see Chapters 22 and 23).

Although the value of continuous fetal heart rate monitoring in normal term infants is controversial (see Chapter 22), this modality is indicated in the preterm infant during labor. Careful fetal surveillance with continuous monitoring has been associated with a reduction in neonatal mortality and morbidity rates in fetuses weighing under 1500 g (Paul and Hon, 1974; Neutra et al., 1978). When fetal heart rate recordings are normal, there are few neonatal deaths; however, severe variable or late decelerations and decreased baseline variability are associated with increased neonatal morbidity and mortality. In addition, deep variable decelerations with normal baseline variability or decreased variability without prolonged deceleration is not often associated with neonatal mortality or acidosis in the very-low-birth-weight fetus (Bowes et al., 1980; Zanini et al., 1980).

Delivery

Analgesia and Anesthesia

Analgesia and anesthesia of choice for labor and delivery of the preterm infant are not well established. Epidural anesthesia, by relaxation of the pelvic floor, should offer less soft-tissue impact on the presenting part and, therefore, presumably may result in less trauma. Epidural anesthesia can cause maternal hypotension, however, leading to potential fetal distress. Central nervous system depressant drugs are usually avoided, but if they are needed and neonatal resuscitation is available, the depression can be dealt with as if the newborn had been given these drugs for a surgical procedure.

Episiotomy

Episiotomy is usually advised for vaginal deliveries to help bring about controlled delivery, reduce resistance, and reduce the length of the second stage of labor, but there is minimal significant information on the benefit of routine episiotomy to the preterm neonate.

Forceps

Low forceps deliveries have been suggested in the past with the idea of protecting the head of the premature fetus, but there is no data to support this opinion (Barrett et al., 1983; Schwartz et al., 1983; Tejani et al., 1987). Standard intrapartum care is appropriate.

Route of Delivery

The recommended route of delivery remains a controversial issue for the very small preterm infant, particularly if the fetus is in a breech presentation. There is no convincing evidence to support the concept that vaginal delivery should not be the mode of delivery when all of the following conditions are met:

1. The presentation is cephalic.
2. Labor is progressing normally.
3. The fetal heart rate is within normal limits.

This approach assumes the capability to respond quickly to an ominous event by immediate cesarean section and available neonatal intensive care. Although some reports have suggested benefit of cesarean delivery for very small fetuses, this possibility is lost after one adjusts for confounding variables. An analysis of 1765 newborns weighing under 1500 g at birth could find no protective effect of cesarean birth relative to mortality or IVH (Malloy et al., 1991). Grant and associates (1996) reviewed six trials that addressed immediate neonatal and maternal morbidities after vaginal versus cesarean delivery for infants born between 24 and 36 weeks' gestation and found modest but nonsignificant trends in favor of elective cesarean birth.

The effect of labor and route of delivery on periventricular-IVH has been particularly difficult to evaluate. A prospective study of 230 newborns weighing under 1750 g has been reported wherein sonographic examinations of the head were performed within 30 minutes of birth and serially until 7 days of life (Shaver et al., 1992). The incidence of hemorrhage was not influenced by the route of delivery. Early hemorrhage (detected in the first hour after birth) was less frequent after cesarean birth than after vaginal delivery but no less frequent than after vaginal delivery with forceps. Late hemorrhage was more common after abdominal delivery regardless of duration of labor. Grade 3 and 4 hemorrhages were highest after vaginal delivery without forceps or abdominal delivery after the active phase of labor. Umbilical cord blood acid-base status was similar in infants with no hemorrhage or with early or late hemorrhage. A comparison of outcomes according to route of delivery and presence of labor among 278 singleton live-born infants who weighed between 750 and 1500 g found no association between respiratory distress, grade 3 or 4 IVH, sepsis, seizures, or death relative to these factors (Alexander et al., 1999). In the past, data about IVH and route of delivery were often based on an assumption that physical trauma during the labor process was the most common etiology of hemorrhage. Hansen and Leviton (1999) performed an extensive analysis of data from 1588 very-low-birth-weight infants (under 1.5 kg), including labor and delivery characteristics (duration of labor, interval between membrane rupture and delivery, and route of delivery) and results of neonatal cranial ultrasound assessments. Although vaginal delivery was the only obstetric characteristic associated with intracranial hemorrhage and white matter disease, the relationship was no longer significant when placental inflammation was accounted for in the analysis. This report is consistent with date presented earlier in this chapter showing a strong relationship between chronic intrauterine inflammation, early preterm birth, and neonatal morbidity including IVH.

Retrospective studies strongly support abdominal delivery as the method of choice for a preterm breech presentation (Lee et al., 1998; Effer et al., 2002). The reduction in neonatal mortality (birth to 28 days) of abdominal delivery was threefold, from 233 per 1000 vaginal births to 72 per 1000 cesarean births, for infants with birth weights between 1250 and 1500 g (Lee et al., 1998). Prospective randomized trials have not been done to confirm this concept. Experience with external cephalic version in preterm infants in early labor is insufficient to evaluate its safety. Vaginal delivery of the second twin is discussed in Chapter 29. The incidence of congenital anomalies may be as high as 20% when the preterm fetus is in breech presentation, so a careful ultrasound examination is mandatory.

REFERENCES

Adams MM, Elam-Evans LD, Wilson HG, et al: Rates of and factors associated with recurrence of preterm delivery. JAMA **283**:1591, 2000.

Akerlund M, Strömberg P, Hauksson A, et al: Inhibition of uterine contractions of premature labour with an oxytocin analogue: Results from a pilot study. Br J Obstet Gynaecol **94**:1040, 1987.

Alexander JM, Bloom SL, McIntire DD, et al: Severe preeclampsia and the very low birth weight infant: is induction of labor harmful? Obstet Gynecol **93**:485, 1999.

Allbert JR, Johnson C, Roberts WE, et al: Tocolysis for recurrent preterm labor using a continuous subcutaneous infusion pump. J Reprod Med **39**:614, 1994.

Althuisius SM, Dekker GA, van Geijn HP, et al: Cervical incompetence prevention randomized cerclage trial (CIPRACT): Study design and preliminary results. Am J Obstet Gynecol **183**:823, 2000.

Alvan G, Orne M, Bertilsson L, et al: Pharmacokinetics of indomethacin. Clin Pharmacol Ther **18**:364, 1976.

American Academy of Pediatrics and American College of Obstetricians and Gynecologists: Guidelines for Perinatal Care, 5th ed, Washington, DC, American Academy of Pediatrics and American College of Obstetricians and Gynecologists, 2002, p. 6.

American College of Obstetricians and Gynecologists Committee on Obstetric Practice, Clinical Opinion 167: Perinatal and Infant mortality statistics, Washington, DC, American College of Obstetricians and Gynecologists, 1995.

Amory JH, Hitti J, Lawler R, et al: Increased tumor necrosis factor-α production after lipopolysaccharide stimulation of whole blood in patients with previous preterm delivery complicated by intra-amniotic infection or inflammation. Am J Obstet Gynecol **185**:1964, 2001.

Amy JJ, Thiery M: The prevention of preterm labour. Prostaglandin Perspect **1**:9, 1985.

Andersen HF: Transvaginal and transabdominal ultrasonography of the uterine cervix during pregnancy. J Clin Ultrasound **19**:77, 1991.

Andersen HF, Nugent CE, Wanty SD, et al: Prediction of risk of preterm delivery by ultrasonographic measurement of cervical length. Am J Obstet Gynecol **163**:859, 1990.

Andersen LF, Lyndrup J, Akerlund M, et al: Oxytocin receptor blockade: A new principle in the treatment of preterm labor? Am J Perinatol **6**:196, 1989.

Andrews WW, Goldenberg RL, Mercer BM, et al: The preterm prediction study: Association of second trimester genitourinary Chlamydia infection with subsequent spontaneous preterm birth. Am J Obstet Gynecol **183**:662, 2000.

Andrews WW, Sibai BM, Thom EA, et al for the National Institute of Child Health and Human Development Maternal-Fetal Medicine Units Network: Randomized clinical trial of metronidazole plus erythromycin to prevent spontaneous preterm delivery in fetal fibronectin positive-women. Obstet Gynecol **101**:847, 2003.

Arias F, Rodriguez L, Rayne SC, et al: Maternal placental vasculopathy and infection: Two distinct subgroups among patients with preterm labor and preterm ruptured membranes. Am J Obstet Gynecol **168**:585, 1993.

Arias F, Victoria A, Cho K, et al: Placental histology and clinical characteristics of patients with preterm premature rupture of membranes. Obstet Gynecol **89**:265, 1997.

Armson BA, Samuels P, Miller F, et al: Evaluation of maternal fluid dynamics during tocolytic therapy with ritodrine hydrochloride and magnesium sulfate. Am J Obstet Gynecol **167**:758, 1992.

Bakketeig LS, Hoffman HJ: Epidemiology of preterm birth: Results from a longitudinal study of births in Norway. In Elder MG, Hendricks CH (eds): Preterm Labor. London, Butterworths, 1981, p. 17.

Barden TP, Peter JB, Merkatz IR: Ritodrine hydrochloride: A beta-mimetic agent for use in preterm labor. Obstet Gynecol **56**:1, 1980.

Barrett J, Boehm F, Vaughn W: The effect of type of delivery on neonatal outcome in singleton infants of birth weight of 1000 grams or less. JAMA **250**:625, 1983.

Ben-Ami M, Giladi Y, Shalev E: The combination of magnesium sulfate and nifedipine: A cause of neuromuscular blockade. Br J Obstet Gynaecol **101**:262, 1994.

Benedetti TJ: Maternal complications of parenteral betasympathomimetic therapy for premature labor. Am J Obstet Gynecol **145**:1,1983.

Berg G, Anderson R, Ryder G: α-Adrenergic receptors in human myometrium during pregnancy: Changes in the number of receptors after α-mimetic treatment. Am J Obstet Gynecol **151**:392, 1985.

Bernstein PS, Stern R, Lin N, et al: α-Human chorionic gonodotropin in cervicovaginal secretions as a predictor of preterm delivery. Am J Obstet Gynecol **179**:870, 1998.

Besinger R, Niebyl J, Keyes WG, et al: Randomized comparative trial of indomethacin and ritodrine for the long-term treatment of preterm labor. Am J Obstet Gynecol **164**:981, 1991.

Bhat R, Vidyasager D, Vadapalli MO, et al: Disposition of indomethacin in preterm infants. J Pediatr **95**:313, 1979.

Bhutta AT, Cleves MA, Casey PH, et al: Cognitive and behavioral outcomes of school-aged children who were born preterm. JAMA **288**:728, 2002.

Bottoms SF, Paul RH, Iams JD, et al: Obstetric determinants of neonatal survival: Influence of willingness to perform cesarean delivery on survival of extremely low-birth-weight infants. Am J Obstet Gynecol **176**:960, 1997.

Bowes WA, Gabbe SG, Bowes C: Fetal heart rate monitoring in premature infants weighing 1500 grams or less. Am J Obstet Gynecol **137**:791, 1980.

Boyle CA, Yeargin-Allsopp M, Schendel DE, et al: Tocolytic magnesium sulfate exposure and risk of cerebral palsy among children with birth weights less than 1750 grams. Am J Epidemiol **152**:120, 2000.

Brazy JE, Pupkin MJ: Effects of maternal isoxsuprine administration on preterm infants. J Pediatr **94**:444, 1979.

Brocklehurst P, Hannah M, McDonald H: Interventions for treating bacterial vaginosis in pregnancy (Cochrane Review). In The Cochrane Library, Issue 4. Oxford, Update Software, 2002.

Buekens P, Alexander S, Boutsen M, et al: Randomised controlled trial of routine cervical examinations in pregnancy. Lancet **344**:841, 1994.

Burger M, Weber-Rossler T, Willman M: Measurement of the pregnant cervix by transvaginal sonography: An interobserver study and new standards to improve the interobserver variability. Ultrasound Obstet Gynecol **9**:188, 1997.

Burton BK: Elevated maternal serum alpha-fetoprotein: Interpretation and follow-up. Clin Obstet Gynecol **31**:293, 1988.

Cabral H, Fried LE, Levenson S, et al: Foreign-born and US-born black women: Differences in health behaviors and birth outcomes. Am J Public Health **80**:70, 1990.

Cabrol D, Landersman R, Mueller J, et al: Treatment of polyhydramnios with prostaglandin synthetase inhibitor (indomethacin). Am J Obstet Gynecol **157**:422, 1987.

Canadian Preterm Labor Investigators Group: The treatment of preterm labor with beta-adrenergic agonist ritodrine. N Engl J Med **327**:308, 1992.

Cantor B, Tyler T, Nelson RM, et al: Oligohydramnios and transient neonatal anuria: A possible association with the use of prostaglandin synthetase inhibitors. J Reprod Med **24**:220, 1980.

Carey JC, Klebanoff MA, Hauth JC, et al: Metronidazole to prevent preterm delivery in pregnant women with asymptomatic bacterial vaginosis. N Engl J Med **342**:534, 2000.

Caritis SN: A pharmacologic approach to the infusion of ritodrine. Am J Obstet Gynecol **158**:380, 1988.

Caritis SN, Chiao JP, Kridgen P: Comparison of pulsatile and continuous ritodrine administration: Effects on uterine contractility and beta-adrenergic receptor cascade. Am J Obstet Gynecol **164**:1005, 1991.

Caritis SN, Chiao JP, Moore JJ, et al: Myometrial desensitization after ritodrine infusion. Am J Physiol **253**:E410, 1987.

Caritis SN, Lin LS, Toig G, et al: Pharmacodynamics of ritodrine in pregnant women during preterm labor. Am J Obstet Gynecol **147**:752, 1983.

Caritis SN, Venkataramanan R, Cotroneo M, et al: Pharmacokinetics and pharmacodynamics of ritodrine after intramuscular administration to pregnant women. Am J Obstet Gynecol **162**:1215, 1990.

Caritis SN, Venkataramanan R, Darby MJ, et al: Pharmacokinetics of ritodrine administered intravenously: Recommendations for changes in the current regimen. Am J Obstet Gynecol **162**:429, 1990.

Centers for Disease Control and Prevention. Contribution of assisted reproductive technology and ovulation-inducing drugs to triplet and higher-order multiple births—United States, 1980–1997. MMWR **49**:535, 2000.

Chaiworapongsa T, Romero R, Kim JC, et al: Evidence for fetal involvement in the pathologic process of clinical chorioamnionitis. Am J Obstet Gynecol **186**:1178, 2002.

Challis JR, Smith SK: Fetal endocrine signals and preterm labor. Biol Neonate **79**:163, 2001.

Cherukuri R, Minkoff H, Hansen RL, et al: A cohort study of alkaloidal cocaine ("crack") in pregnancy. Obstet Gynecol **72**:147, 1988.

Collaborative Group on Preterm Birth Prevention: Multicenter randomized controlled trial of a preterm birth prevention program. Am J Obstet Gynecol **169**:352, 1993.

Collaborative Home Uterine Monitoring Study (CHUMS) Group: A multicenter randomized trial of home uterine activity monitoring. Am J Obstet Gynecol **172**:253, 1995.

Copper RL, Goldenberg RL, Das A, et al: The preterm prediction study: Maternal stress is associated with spontaneous preterm birth at less than thirty-five weeks' gestation. Am J Obstet Gynecol **175**:1286, 1996.

Copper RL, Goldenberg RL, Davis RO, et al: Warning symptoms, uterine contractions and cervical examination findings in women at risk of preterm delivery. Am J Obstet Gynecol **152**:748, 1990.

Copper RL, Goldenberg RL, DuBard MB, et al: Cervical examination and tocodynamometry at 28 weeks' gestation: Prediction of spontaneous preterm birth. Am J Obstet Gynecol **172**:666, 1995.

Cotton DB, Gonik B, Dorman KF: Cardiovascular alterations in severe pregnancy-induced hypertension: Acute effects of intravenous magnesium sulfate. Am J Obstet Gynecol **148**:162, 1984.

Cotton DB, Strasner HT, Hill LM: Comparison of magnesium sulfate, terbutaline and a placebo for inhibition of preterm labor. J Reprod Med **29**:92, 1984.

Cox SM, Sherman LM, Leveno KY: Randomized investigation of magnesium sulfate for prevention of preterm birth. Am J Obstet Gynecol **163**:767, 1990.

Crane JMG, Van den Hof M, Armson BA, et al: Transvaginal ultrasound in the prediction of preterm delivery: Singleton and twin gestations. Obstet Gynecol **90**:357, 1997.

Creasy RK, Gummer BA, Liggins GC: A system for predicting spontaneous preterm birth. Obstet Gynecol **55**:692, 1980.

Creasy RK, Katz M: Beta-adrenergic tocolytics: Basic research and clinical experience in the United States. In Fuchs F, Stubblefield PG (eds): Preterm Birth: Causes, Prevention and Management. New York, Macmillan, 1984, p. 150.

Crowther CA: Hospitalisation and bed rest for multiple pregnancy (Cochrane Review). In The Cochrane Library, Issue 1. Oxford, Update Software, 2003.

Crowther CA, Alfirevic Z, Haslam RR: Prenatal thyrotropin-releasing hormone for preterm birth. Cochrane Database Syst Rev 2000 (2):CD000019.

Crowther CA, Henderson-Smart DJ: Phenobarbital prior to preterm birth for preventing neonatal periventricular haemorrhage (Cochrane Review). In The Cochrane Library, Issue 1. Oxford, Update Software, 2003a.

Crowther CA, Henderson-Smart DJ: Vitamin K prior to preterm birth for preventing neonatal periventricular haemorrhage (Cochrane Review). In The Cochrane Library, Issue 1. Oxford, Update Software, 2003b.

Crowther CA, Hiller JE, Pridmore B, et al: Calcium supplementation in nulliparous women for the prevention of pregnancy-induced hypertension, preeclampsia and preterm birth: An Australian randomized trial. FRACOG and the ACT Study Group. Aust N Z J Obstet Gynaecol **39**:12, 1999.

Crowther CA, Neilson JP, Verkuyl DA, et al: Preterm labour in twin pregnancies: Can it be prevented by hospital admission? Br J Obstet Gynaecol **96**:850, 1989.

Cruikshank DP, Pitkin RM, Donnelly E, et al: Urinary magnesium, calcium and phosphate excretion during magnesium sulphate infusion. Obstet Gynecol **58**:430, 1981.

Cruikshank DP, Pitkin RM, Reynolds WA, et al: Effects of magnesium sulphate treatment on perinatal calcium metabolism: I. Maternal and fetal responses. Am J Obstet Gynecol **134**:243, 1979.

Csaba IF, Sulyok E, Ertl T: Clinical note: Relationship of maternal treatment with indomethacin to persistence of fetal circulation syndrome. J Pediatr **92**:484, 1978.

Csapo A, Pohanka O, Kaihola HL: Progesterone deficiency and premature labour. Br Med J **1**:137, 1974.

da Fonseca EB, Bittar RE, Carvalho MHB, et al: Prophylactic administration of progesterone by vaginal suppository to reduce the incidence of spontaneous preterm birth in women at increased risk: A randomized placebo-controlled double-blind study. Am J Obstet Gynecol **188**:419, 2003.

Dangman BC, Rosen TS: Magnesium levels in infants of mothers treated with magnesium sulfate. Pediatr Res **11**:415, 1977.

Demissie K, Rhoads GG, Ananth CV, et al: Trends in preterm birth and neonatal mortality among blacks and whites in the United States from 1989 to 1997. Am J Epidemiol **154**:307, 2001.

Dhont M, De Sutter P, Ruyssinck G, et al: Perinatal outcome of pregnancies after assisted reproduction: A case control study. Am J Obstet Gynecol **181**:688, 1999.

Dirge KB, Varner MW, Schiffman JS: Neuroophthalmologic effects of intravenous sulfate. Am J Obstet Gynecol **163**:1848, 1990.

Dolfin T, Skidmore MB, Fong KW, et al: Perinatal factors that influence the incidence of subependymal and intraventricular hemorrhage in low-birth-weight infants. Am J Perinatol **1**:107, 1984.

Dombrowski MP for the NICHD MFMU Network: An observational cohort study to evaluate the effects of asthma on perinatal outcome. Am J Obstet Gynecol **182**:542, 2000.

Donovan EF, Ehrenkranz RA, Shankaran S, et al: Outcomes of very low birth weight twins cared for in the National Institute of Child Health and Human Development Neonatal Research Network's intensive care units. Am J Obstet Gynecol **179**:742, 1998.

Ducsay CA, Thompson JS, Wu AT, et al: Effects of calcium entry blocker (nicardipine) tocolysis in rhesus macaques: Fetal plasma concentrations and cardiorespiratory changes. Am J Obstet Gynecol **157**:1482, 1987.

Dudley DKL, Hardie MJ: Fetal and neonatal effects of indomethacin used as a tocolytic agent. Am J Obstet Gynecol **151**:181, 1985.

Dudley DJ: Immunoendocrinology of preterm labor: The link between corticotropin-releasing hormone and inflammation. Am J Obstet Gynecol **180**:S251, 1999.

Duff P, Kopelman JN: Subclinical intra-amniotic infection in asymptomatic patients with refractory preterm labor. Obstet Gynecol **69**:756, 1987.

Dyson DC, Crites YM, Ray DA, et al: Prevention of preterm birth in high-risk patients: The role of education and provider contact versus home uterine monitoring. Am J Obstet Gynecol **154**:756, 1991.

Dyson DC, Danbe KH, Bamber JA, et al: Monitoring women at risk for preterm labor. N Engl J Med **338**:15, 1998.

Effer SB, Moutquin JM, Farine D, et al: Neonatal survival rates in 860 singleton live births at 24 and 25 weeks' gestational age. A Canadian multicentre study. Br J Obstet Gynecol **109**:740, 2002.

Ekwo EE, Gosselink CA, Moawad A: Unfavorable outcome in penultimate pregnancy and premature rupture of membranes in successive pregnancy. Obstet Gynecol **80**:166, 1992.

Elder HA, Santamarina BAG, Smith S, et al: The natural history of asymptomatic bacteriuria during pregnancy: The effect of tetracycline on the clinical course and outcome of pregnancy. Am J Obstet Gynecol **111**:441, 1971.

Elliott JP, O'Keeffe DF, Greenberg P, et al: Pulmonary edema associated with magnesium sulfate and betamethasone administration. Am J Obstet Gynecol **134**:717, 1979.

Elovitz MA, Baron J, Phillippe M: The role of thrombin in preterm parturition. Am J Obstet Gynecol **185**:1059, 2001.

El-Sayed YY, Riley ET, Holbrook RH Jr, et al: Randomized comparison of intravenous nitroglycerin and magnesium sulfate for treatment of preterm labor. Obstet Gynecol **93**:79, 1999.

Epstein MF, Nichols E, Stubblefield PG: Neonatal hypoglycemia after beta-sympathomimetic tocolytic therapy. J Pediatr **94**:440, 1979.

Eschenbach DA, Nugent RP, Rao VR, et al: A randomized placebo-controlled trial of erythromycin for the treatment of *Ureaplasma urealyticum* to prevent premature delivery. Am J Obstet Gynecol **164**:734, 1991.

Escriba-Aguir V, Perez-Hoyos S, Saurel-Cubizolles MJ: Physical load and psychological demand at work during pregnancy and preterm birth. Int Arch Occup Environ Health **74**:583, 2001.

Evidence Report/Technology Assessment No 18: Management of Preterm Labor. AHRQ Publication No 01-E021, October 2000. Access at www.ahrq.gov.clinic/epix.htm.

Feinberg RF, Kleiman HJ, Lockwood CJ: Is oncofetal fibronectin a trophoblast glue for human implantation? Am J Pathol **138**:537, 1991.

Ferguson JE, Dyson DC, Schutz T, et al: A comparison of tocolysis with nifedipine or ritodrine: Analysis of efficacy and maternal, fetal and neonatal outcome. Am J Obstet Gynecol **163**:105, 1990.

Ferguson JE, Hensleigh PA, Kredenster D: Adjunctive use of magnesium with ritodrine for preterm tocolysis. Am J Obstet Gynecol **148**:66, 1984.

Ferguson JE, Schutz T, Perske R, et al: Nifedipine pharmacokinetics during preterm labor tocolysis. Am J Obstet Gynecol **161**:1485, 1989.

Ferriman E, Simpson N, Reid J, et al: Fetal carriage of IL-1 is not associated with premature membrane rupture and preterm delivery [abstract]. Am J Obstet Gynecol **184**:536, 2001.

Fisher JE, Smith RS, Lagrandeur R, et al: Gestational diabetes in women receiving beta-adrenergics and corticosteroids for threatened preterm delivery. Obstet Gynecol **90**:880,1997.

FIVNAT: Pregnancies and births resulting from in vitro fertilization: French national registry, analysis of data 1986 to 1990. Fertil Steril **64**:746, 1995.

Fleckenstein A: Specific pharmacology of calcium in myocardium, cardiac pacemakers, and vascular smooth muscle. Ann Rev Pharmacol Toxicol **17**:149, 1977.

Forman A, Anderson K-E, Ulmsten U: Inhibition of myometrial activity by calcium antagonists. Semin Perinatol **5**:288, 1981.

Freysz H, Willard D, Lehr A, et al: A long-term evaluation of infants who receive a beta-mimetic drug while *in utero*. J Perinat Med **5**:94, 1977.

Fujimoto T, Parry S, Urbanek M, et al: A single nucleotide polymorphism in the matrix metalloproteinase-1 (MMP-1) promoter influences amnion cell MMP-1 expression and risk for preterm premature rupture of the fetal membranes. J Biol Chem **277**:6296, 2002.

Gardner MO, Goldenberg RL, Cliver SP, et al: The origin and outcome of preterm twin pregnancies. Obstet Gynecol **85**:553, 1995.

Genc MR, Gerber S, Nesin M, et al: Polymorphism in the interleukin-1 gene complex and spontaneous preterm delivery. Am J Obstet Gynecol **187**:157, 2002.

Germain AM, Carvajal J, Sanchez M, et al: Preterm labor: Placental pathology and clinical correlation. Obstet Gynecol **94**:284, 1999.

Ghia N, Spong CY, Starbuck VN, et al: Magnesium sulfate therapy affects attention and working memory in patients undergoing preterm labor. Am J Obstet Gynecol **183**:940, 2000.

Ghidini A, Eglinton GS, Spong CY, et al: Elevated midtrimester amniotic fluid tumor necrosis alpha levels: A predictor of preterm delivery (Abstr. No. 14). Am J Obstet Gynecol **174**:307, 1996.

Gibbs RS: The relationship between infections and adverse pregnancy outcomes: A review. Ann Periodontol **6**:153, 2001.

Gibbs RS, Eschenbach DA: Use of antibiotics to prevent preterm birth. Am J Obstet Gynecol **177**:375, 1997.

Gibbs RS, Romero R, Hillier SL, et al: A review of premature birth and subclinical infection. Am J Obstet Gynecol **166**:1515, 1992.

Gichangi PB, Ndinya-Achola JO, Ombete J, et al: Antimicrobial prophylaxis in pregnancy: A randomized, placebo-controlled trial with cefetamet-pivoxil in pregnant women with a poor obstetric history. Am J Obstet Gynecol **177**:680, 1997.

Giles W, Bisits A, Knox M, et al: The effect of fetal fibronectin testing on admissions to a tertiary maternal-fetal medicine unit and cost savings. Am J Obstet Gynecol **182**:439, 2000.

Goepfert AR, Goldenberg RL, Andrews WW, et al for the National Institute of Child Health and Human Development Maternal-Fetal Medicine Units Network. The Preterm Prediction Study: Association between cervical interleukin 6 concentration and spontaneous preterm birth. Am J Obstet Gynecol **184**:483, 2001.

Goldenberg RL, Andrews WW: Intrauterine infection and why preterm prevention programs have failed (editorial). Am J Public Health **86**:781, 1996.

Goldenberg RL, Andrews WW, Mercer BM, et al: The preterm prediction study: Granulocyte colony-stimulating factor and spontaneous preterm birth. Am J Obstet Gynecol **182**:625, 2000.

Goldenberg RL, Cliver SP, Bronstein J, et al: Bed rest in pregnancy. Obstet Gynecol **84**:131, 1994.

Goldenberg RL, Cliver SP, Mulvihill XP, et al: Medical, psychosocial and behavioral risk factors do not explain the increased risk for low birth weight among black women. Am J Obstet Gynecol **175**:1317, 1996.

Goldenberg RL, Hauth JC, Andrews WW: Intrauterine infection and preterm delivery. N Engl J Med **342**:1500, 2000.

Goldenberg RL, Iams JD, Mercer BM, et al: The preterm prediction study: The value of new vs. standard risk factors in predicting early and all spontaneous preterm births. Am J Public Health **88**:233, 1998.

Goldenberg RL, Iams JD, Mercer BM, et al: The Preterm Prediction Study: Toward a multiple-marker test for spontaneous preterm birth. Am J Obstet Gynecol **185**:643, 2001.

Goldenberg RL, Iams JD, Miodovnik M, et al: The preterm prediction study: Risk factors in twin gestations. Am J Obstet Gynecol **175**:1047, 1996.

Goldenberg RL, Klebanoff M, Carey JC, et al: Vaginal fetal fibronectin measurements from 8 to 22 weeks' gestation and subsequent spontaneous preterm birth. Am J Obstet Gynecol **183**:469, 2000.

Goldenberg RL, Klebanoff MA, Nugent R, et al for the Vaginal Infections in Pregnancy Study Group: Bacterial colonization of the vagina in four ethnic groups. Am J Obstet Gynecol **174**:1618, 1996.

Goldenberg RL, Mercer BM, Meis PJ, et al: The preterm prediction study: Fetal fibronectin testing and spontaneous preterm birth. Obstet Gynecol **87**:643, 1996.

Goldenberg RL, Rouse DJ: Prevention of premature birth. N Engl J Med **339**:313, 1998.

Goldenberg RL, Thom E, Moawad AH, et al: The preterm prediction study: Fetal fibronectin, bacterial vaginosis, and peripartum infection. Obstet Gynecol **87**:656, 1996.

Gomez R, Galasso M, Romero R, et al: Ultrasonographic examination of the cervix is better than cervical digital examination as a predictor of preterm delivery in patients with preterm labor and intact membranes. Am J Obstet Gynecol **171**:956, 1994.

Gomez R, Romero R, Ghezzi F, et al: The fetal inflammatory response syndrome. Am J Obstet Gynecol **179**:194, 1998.

Gonik B, Benedetti T, Creasy RK, et al: Intramuscular versus intravenous ritodrine hydrochloride for preterm labor management. Am J Obstet Gynecol **159**:323, 1988.

Gonik B, Creasy RK: Preterm labor: its diagnosis and management. Am J Obstet Gynecol **154**:3, 1986.

Gordon MC, Iams JD: Magnesium sulfate. Clin Obstet Gynecol **38**:706, 1995.

Grant A, Penn ZJ, Steer PJ: Elective or selective cesarean delivery of the small baby? A systematic review of the controlled trials. Br J Obstet Gynecol **103**:1197, 1996.

Gravett MG, Hitti J, Hess DL, et al: Intrauterine infection and preterm delivery: Evidence for activation of the fetal hypothalamic-pituitary-adrenal axis. Am J Obstet Gynecol **182**:1404, 2000.

Green KW, Key TC, Coen R, et al: The effects of maternally administered magnesium sulfate on the neonate. Am J Obstet Gynecol **146**:29, 1983.

Grether JK, Hoogstrate J, Selvin S, et al: Magnesium sulfate tocolysis and risk of neonatal death. Am J Obstet Gynecol **178**:1, 1998.

Grether JK, Hoogstrate J, Walsh-Greene E, et al: Magnesium sulfate tocolysis and risk of spastic cerebral palsy in premature children born to women without preeclampsia. Am J Obstet Gynecol **183**:717, 2000.

Groome LJ, Goldenberg RL, Cliver SP, et al: Neonatal periventricular-intraventricular hemorrhage after maternal beta-sympathomimetic tocolysis. Am J Obstet Gynecol **167**:873, 1992.

Guerguerian AM, Hardy P, Bhattacharya M, et al: Expression of cyclooxygenases in ductus arteriosus of fetal and newborn pigs. Am J Obstet Gynecol **179**:1618, 1998.

Guinn DA, Goepfert AR, Owen J, et al: Management options in women with preterm uterine contractions: A randomized trial. Am J Obstet Gynecol **177**:814, 1997.

Guinn DA, Goepfert AR, Owen J, et al: Terbutaline pump maintenance therapy for prevention of preterm delivery: A double blind trial. Am J Obstet Gynecol **179**:874, 1998.

Hack M, Flannery DJ, Schluchter M, et al: Outcomes in young adulthood for very low birth weight infants. N Engl J Med **346:**149, 2002.

Hack M, Taylor HG, Klein N, et al: School-age outcomes in children with birth weights under 750 g. N Engl J Med **331**:753, 1994.

Hadders-Algra M, Touwen BCL, Huisjes HJ: Long-term follow-up of children prenatally exposed to ritodrine. Br J Obstet Gynaecol **93**:156, 1986.

Hansen A, Leviton A: Labor and delivery characteristics and risks of cranial ultrasonographic abnormalities among very low birth weight infants. The Developmental Epidemiology Network Investigators. Am J Obstet Gynecol **181**:997, 1999.

Harake B, Gilbert RD, Ashwal S, et al: Nifedipine: Effects on fetal and maternal hemodynamics in pregnant sheep. Am J Obstet Gynecol **157**:1003, 1987.

Harbert GM, Cornell GW, Thornton WN: Effect of toxemia therapy on uterine dynamics. Am J Obstet Gynecol **105**:94, 1969.

Hartikainen-Sorri AL, Jouppila P: Is routine hospitalization needed in antenatal care of twin pregnancy? J Perinat Med **12**:31, 1984.

Hatjis CG, Swain M: Systemic tocolysis for premature labor is associated with an increased incidence of pulmonary edema in the presence of maternal infection. Am J Obstet Gynecol **159**:723, 1988.

Hatjis CG, Swain M, Nelson LH, et al: Efficacy of combined administration of magnesium sulfate and ritodrine in the treatment of preterm labor. Obstet Gynecol **69**:317, 1987.

Hauth JC, Goldenberg RL, Andrews WW, et al: Reduced incidence of preterm delivery with metronidazole and erythromycin in women with bacterial vaginosis. N Engl J Med **333**:1732, 1995.

Haywood JL, Goldenberg RL, Bronstein J, et al: Comparison of perceived and actual rates of survival and freedom from handicap in premature infants. Am J Obstet Gynecol **171**:432, 1994.

Hediger ML, Scholl TO, Schall JI, et al: Fetal growth and the etiology of preterm delivery. Obstet Gynecol **85**:175, 1995.

Higby K, Xenakis EM-J, Pauerstein CJ: Do tocolytic agents stop preterm labor? A critical and comprehensive review of efficacy and safety. Am J Obstet Gynecol **168**:1247, 1993.

Hillier SL, Martius J, Krohn M, et al: A case-control study of chorioamniotic infection and histologic chorioamnionitis in prematurity. N Engl J Med **319**:972, 1988.

Hillier SL, Nugent RP, Klebanoff MA, et al: Association between bacterial vaginosis and preterm delivery of a low birthweight infant. N Engl J Med **333**:1737, 1995.

Hitti J, Tarczy-Hornoch P, Murphy J, et al: Amniotic fluid infection, cytokines, and adverse outcome among infants at 34 weeks' gestation or less. Obstet Gynecol **98**:1080, 2001.

Hobel CJ, Dunkel-Schetter C, Roesch SC, et al: Maternal plasma corticotropin-releasing hormone associated with stress at 20 weeks' gestation in pregnancies ending in preterm delivery. Am J Obstet Gynecol **180**:S257, 1999.

Holcomb WL Jr, Shackelford GD, Petrie RH: Magnesium tocolysis and neonatal bone abnormalities: A controlled study. Obstet Gynecol **78**:611, 1991.

Hollander DI, Nagey DA, Pupkin MJ: Magnesium sulfate and ritodrine hydrochloride. A randomized comparison. Am J Obstet Gynecol **156**:631, 1987.

Horbar JD, McAuliffe TL, Adler SM, et al: Variability in 28-day outcomes for very low birth weight infants: An analysis of 11 neonatal intensive care units. Pediatrics **82**:554, 1988.

Horowitz S, Mazor M, Romero R, et al: Infection of the amniotic cavity with *Ureaplasma urealyticum* in the midtrimester of pregnancy. J Reprod Med **40**:375, 1995.

Hueston WJ: Preterm contractions in community settings: I. Treatment of preterm contractions. Obstet Gynecol **92**:38, 1998.

Iams JD, Casal D, McGregor JA, et al: Fetal fibronectin improves the accuracy of diagnosis of preterm labor. Am J Obstet Gynecol **173**:141, 1995.

Iams JD, Goldenberg RL, Meis PJ, et al: The length of the cervix and the risk of spontaneous preterm delivery. N Engl J Med **334**:567, 1996.

Iams JD, Goldenberg RL, Mercer BM, et al: The Preterm Prediction Study: Recurrence risk of spontaneous preterm birth. Am J Obstet Gynecol **178**:1035, 1998.

Iams JD, Goldenberg RL, Mercer BM, et al: The Preterm Prediction Study: Can low-risk women destined for spontaneous preterm birth be identified? Am J Obstet Gynecol **184**:652, 2001.

Iams JD, Johnson FF, Parker M: A prospective evaluation of the signs and symptoms of preterm labor. Obstet Gynecol **84**:227, 1994.

Iams JD, Johnson FF, Sonek J, et al: Cervical competence as a continuum: A study of ultrasonographic cervical length and obstetric performance. Am J Obstet Gynecol **172**:1097, 1995.

Iams JD, Mercer BM for the National Institute of Child Health and Human Development Maternal-Fetal Medicine Units Network: What we have learned about antenatal prediction of neonatal morbidity and mortality. Semin Perinatol **27**:247, 2003.

Iams JD, Newman RB, Thom EA, et al: Frequency of uterine contractions and the risk of spontaneous preterm delivery. N Engl J Med **346**:250, 2002.

Iams JD, Paraskos J, Landon MB, et al: Cervical sonography in preterm labor. Obstet Gynecol **84**:40, 1994.

Iams JD for the NICHD MFMU Network: Self perceived symptoms to predict preterm birth. Am J Obstet Gynecol **182**:S32, 2000.

Iannucci TA, Besinger RE, Fisher SG, et al: Effect of dual tocolysis on the incidence of severe intraventricular hemorrhage among extremely low-birth-weight infants. Am J Obstet Gynecol **175**:1043, 1996.

Idama TO, Lindow SW: Magnesium sulfate: A review of clinical pharmacology applied to obstetrics. Br J Obstet Gynaecol **105**:260, 1998.

Imseis HM, Albert TA, Iams JD: Identifying twin gestations at low risk for preterm birth with a transvaginal ultrasonographic cervical measurement at 24 to 26 weeks' gestation. Am J Obstet Gynecol **177**:1149, 1997.

Itskovitz J, Abramovici H, Brandes JM: Oligohydramnios, meconium and perinatal death concurrent with indomethacin treatment in human pregnancy. J Reprod Med **24**:137, 1980.

Jackson GM, Ludmir J, Bader TJ: The accuracy of digital examination and ultrasound in the evaluation of cervical length. Obstet Gynecol **79**:214, 1992.

Jeffcoat MK, Geurs NC, Reddy MS, et al: Periodontal infection and preterm birth. JADA **132**:875, 2001.

Joesoef MR, Hillier SL, Wiknjosastro G, et al. Intravaginal clindamycin treatment for bacterial vaginosis: Effects on preterm delivery and low birth weight. Am J Obstet Gynecol **173**:1527, 1995.

Joffe GM, Jacques D, Bemis-Hayes R, et al: Impact of the fetal fibronectin assay on admissions for preterm labor. Am J Obstet Gynecol **180**:581, 1999.

Katz M, Gill PJ, Newman RB: Detection of preterm labor by ambulatory monitoring of uterine activity: A preliminary report. Obstet Gynecol **68**:773, 1986.

Katz M, Robertson PA, Creasy RK: Cardiovascular complications associated with terbutaline treatment for preterm labor. Am J Obstet Gynecol **139**:605, 1981.

Kaufman RH, Adam E, Hatch EE, et al: Continued follow-up of pregnancy outcomes in diethylstilbestrol-exposed offspring. Obstet Gynecol **96**:483, 2000.

Keirse MJNC: Magnesium sulphate in preterm labor. *In* Keirse MJNC, Renfrew MJ, Neilson JP et al (eds): Pregnancy and Childbirth Module. *In* The Cochrane Collaboration. The Cochrane Pregnancy and Childbirth Database, Issue # 2. Oxford, Update Software, 1995.

Keirse MJNC, Grant A, King JF: Preterm labour. *In* Chalmers I, Enkin M, Keirse MJNC (eds): Effective Care in Pregnancy and Childbirth. New York, Oxford University Press, 1989, p. 694.

Kekki M, Kurki T, Pelkonen J, et al: Vaginal clindamycin in preventing preterm birth and peripartal infections in asymptomatic women with bacterial vaginosis: A randomized, controlled trial. Obstet Gynecol **97**:643, 2001.

Kenyon SL, Taylor DJ, Tarnow-Mordi W for the ORACLE Collaborative Group: Broad-spectrum antibiotics for spontaneous preterm labour: The ORACLE II randomised trial. Lancet **357**:989, 2001.

King J, Flenady V: Prophylactic antibiotics for inhibiting preterm labour with intact membranes (Cochrane Review). *In* The Cochrane Library, Issue 4. Oxford, Update Software, 2002.

King JF, Grant A, Keirse MJNC: Beta-mimetics in preterm labour: An overview of the randomized controlled trials. Br J Obstet Gynaecol **95**:211, 1988.

Kirshon B, Mari G, Moise KJ Jr: Indomethacin therapy in the treatment of symptomatic polyhydramnios. Obstet Gynecol **75**:202, 1990.

Klebanoff MA, Carey JC, Hauth JC, et al: Failure of metronidazole to prevent preterm delivery among pregnant women with asymptomatic *Trichomonas vaginalis* infection. N Engl J Med **345**:487, 2001.

Klebanoff MA, Regan JA, Rao VR, et al: Outcome of the Vaginal Infections and Prematurity Study: Results of a clinical trial of erythromycin among pregnant women colonized with group B streptococci. Am J Obstet Gynecol **172**:1540, 1995.

Kogan MD, Alexander GR: Social and behavioral factors in preterm birth. Prenat Neonat Med **3**:29, 1998.

Kosasa TS, Busee R, Wahl N, et al: Long term tocolysis with combined terbutaline and magnesium sulfate: A ten year study of 1000 patients. Obstet Gynecol **84**:369, 1994.

Krause TG, Christens P, Wohlfahrt J, et al: Second-trimester maternal serum alpha-fetoprotein and risk of adverse pregnancy outcome. Obstet Gynecol **97**:277, 2001.

Krohn MA, Hillier SL, Lee ML, et al: Vaginal *Bacteroides* are associated with an increased rate of preterm delivery among women in preterm labor. J Infect Dis **164**:88, 1991.

Krohn MA, Hillier SL, Nugent RP, et al: The genital flora of women with intra-amniotic infection. J Infect Dis **171**:1475, 1995.

Kurkinen-Raty M, Ruokonen A, Vuopala S, et al: Combination of cervical interleukin-6 and -8, phosphorylated insulin-like growth factor-binding protein-1 and transvaginal cervical ultrasonography in assessment of the risk of preterm birth. BJOG **108**:875, 2001.

Kyrklund-Blomberg NB, Cnattingius S: Preterm birth and maternal smoking: Risks related to gestational age and onset of delivery. Am J Obstet Gynecol **179**:1051, 1998.

Lam F, Elliott J, Jones JS, et al: Clinical issues surrounding the use of terbutaline sulfate for preterm labor. Obstet Gynecol Survey **53**:S85, 1998.

Lamm CI, Norton KI, Murphy RJC, et al: Congenital rickets associated with magnesium sulfate infusion for tocolysis. J Pediatr **113**:1078, 1988.

Lammintausta R, Erkkola R: Effect of long-term salbutamol treatment on renin-aldosterone system in twin pregnancy. Acta Obstet Gynecol Scand **58**:447, 1979.

Larmon JE, Ross BS, May WL, et al: Oral nicardipine versus intravenous magnesium sulfate for the treatment of preterm labor. Am J Obstet Gynecol **181**:1432, 1999.

Laros RK Jr, Kitterman JA, Heilbron D, et al: Outcome of very-low-birthweight infants exposed to beta-sympathomimetics *in utero*. Am J Obstet Gynecol **164**:1657, 1991.

Lee KS, Khoshnood B, Sriram S, et al: Relationship of cesarean delivery to lower birth weight-specific neonatal mortality in singleton breech deliveries in the United States. Obstet Gynecol **92**:769, 1998.

Lees CC, Lojacono A, Thompson C, et al: Glyceryl trinitrate and ritodrine in tocolysis: An international multicenter randomized study. GTN Preterm Labour Investigation Group. Obstet Gynecol **94**:403, 1999.

Leitich H, Brumbauer M, Kaider A, et al: Cervical length and dilation of the internal os detected by vaginal ultrasonography as markers for preterm delivery: A systematic review. Am J Obstet Gynecol **181**:1465, 1999.

Leitich H, Egarter C, Kaider A, et al: Cervicovaginal fetal fibronectin as a marker for preterm delivery: A meta-analysis. Am J Obstet Gynecol **180**:1169, 1999.

Lemons JA, Bauer CR, Oh W, et al: Very low birth weight outcomes of the National Institute of Child Health and Human Development Neonatal Research Network, January 1995 through December 1996. Pediatrics **107**:1, 2000.

Leopold D, McEvoy A: Salbutamol-induced ketoacidosis. Br Med J **2**:1152, 1977.

Levav AL, Chan L, Wapner RJ: Long-term magnesium sulfate tocolysis and maternal osteoporosis in a triplet pregnancy: A case report. Am J Perinatol **15**:43, 1998.

Levene MI, Fawer CL, Lamont RF: Risk factors in the development of intraventricular hemorrhage in the preterm neonate. Arch Dis Child **57**:410, 1982.

Leveno KJ, Little BB, Cunningham FG: The national impact of ritodrine hydrochloride for inhibition of preterm labour. Obstet Gynecol **76**:12, 1990.

Levine RJ, Hauth JC, Curet LB, et al: Trial of calcium to prevent preeclampsia. N Engl J Med **337**:69, 1997.

Liggins GC: Prenatal glucocorticoid treatment: Prevention of respiratory distress syndrome. *In* Moore TD (ed): Report of the 70th Ross Conference on Pediatric Research. Columbus OH, Ross Laboratories, 1977.

Liggins GC, Howie RN: A controlled trial of antepartum glucocorticoid treatment of the respiratory distress syndrome in premature infants. Pediatrics **50**:515, 1972.

Lipshitz J, English IC: Hypermagnesemia in the newborn infant. Pediatrics **40**:856, 1967.

Lockwood CJ: Stress-associated preterm delivery: The role of corticotropin-releasing hormone. Am J Obstet Gynecol **180**:S264, 1999.

Lockwood CJ, Senjei AE, Dische MR, et al: Fetal fibronectin in cervical and vaginal secretions as a predictor of preterm delivery. N Engl J Med **325**:669, 1991.

Lopez NJ, Smith PC, Gutierrez J: Periodontal therapy may reduce the risk of preterm low birth weight in women with periodontal disease: A randomized controlled trial. J Periodontol **73**:911, 2002.

Low JA, Galbraith RS, Muir DW, et al: Mortality and morbidity after intrapartum asphyxia in the preterm fetus. Obstet Gynecol **80**:57, 1992.

Luke B, Mamelle N, Keith L, et al: The association between occupational factors and preterm delivery: a United States nurses' study. Am J Obstet Gynecol **173**:849, 1995.

Lunt CC, Satin AJ, Barth WH Jr, et al: The effect of indomethacin tocolysis on maternal coagulation status. Obstet Gynecol **84**:820, 1994.

MacDonald H and the Committee on Fetus and Newborn: Perinatal care at the threshold of viability. American Academy of Pediatrics Clinical Report. Pediatrics **110**:1024, 2002.

MacLennan AH, Green RC, O'Shea R, et al: Routine hospital admission in twin pregnancy between 26 and 30 weeks' gestation. Lancet **335**:267, 1990.

MacNaughton MC, Chalmers IG, Dubowitz V, et al. Final report of the Medical Research Council/Royal College of Obstetrics and Gynaecology multicentre randomised trial of cervical cerclage. Br J Obstet Gynaecol **100**:516, 1993.

Macones G, Parry S, Marder S, et al: Evidence of a gene-environment interaction in the etiology of spontaneous preterm birth [abstract]. Am J Obstet Gynecol **184**:53, 2001.

Macones GA, Berlin M, Berlin JA: Efficacy of oral beta-agonist maintenance therapy in preterm labor: A meta-analysis. Obstet Gynecol **85**:313, 1995.

Macones GA, Marder SJ, Clothier B, et al: The controversy surrounding indomethacin for tocolysis. Am J Obstet Gynecol **184**:264, 2001.

Macones GA, Segel SY, Stamilo DM, et al: Predicting delivery within 48 hours in women treated with parenteral tocolysis. Obstet Gynecol **93**:432, 1999a.

Macones GA, Segel SY, Stamilo DM, et al: Prediction of delivery among women with early preterm labor by means of clinical characteristics alone. Am J Obstet Gynecol **181**:1414, 1999b.

Madden C, Owen J, Hauth JC: Magnesium tocolysis: Serum levels versus success. Am J Obstet Gynecol **162**:1177, 1990.

Madianos PN, Lieff S, Murtha AP, et al: Maternal periodontitis and prematurity. Part II: Maternal infection and fetal exposure. Ann Periodontol **6**:175, 2001.

Major CA, Lewis DF, Harding JA, et al: Tocolysis with indomethacin increases the incidence of necrotizing enterocolitis in the low-birth-weight neonate. Am J Obstet Gynecol **170**:102, 1994.

Makrides M, Crowther CA: Magnesium supplementation in pregnancy. Cochrane Database Syst Rev 2001;(4):CD000937.

Malloy MH, Oustad L, Wright E: The effect of cesarean delivery on birth outcome in very-low-birthweight infants. Obstet Gynecol **77**:498, 1991.

Mamelle N, Laumon B, Lazar P: Prematurity and occupational activity during pregnancy. Am J Epidemiol **119**:309, 1984.

Manchester D, Margolis HS, Sheldon RE: Possible association between maternal indomethacin therapy and primary pulmonary hypertension of the newborn. Am J Obstet Gynecol **126**:467, 1967.

Mari G, Kirshon B, Moise KJ, et al: Doppler assessment of the fetal and uteroplacental circulation during nifedipine therapy for preterm labor. Am J Obstet Gynecol **161**:1514, 1989.

Martin JA, Hamilton BE, Ventura SJ, et al: Births: Final data for 2000. National Vital Statistics Reports **50**:1, 2002a.

Martin JA, Hamilton BE, Ventura SJ, et al: Births: Final data for 2001. National Vital Statistics Reports **51**:1, 2002b.

Martin RW, Gaddy DK, Martin JN, et al: Tocolysis with oral magnesium. Am J Obstet Gynecol **156**:433, 1987.

Martin RW, Perry KG, Hess LW, et al: Oral magnesium and the prevention of preterm labor in a high-risk group of patients. Am J Obstet Gynecol **166**:144, 1992.

Mason GC, Maresh MJA: Alterations in bladder volume and the ultrasound appearance of the cervix. Br J Obstet Gynecol **97**:457, 1990.

Mathews TJ, Menacker F, MacDorman MF: Infant mortality statistics from the 2000 period linked birth/infant death data set. National Statistics Reports **50**:12, 2002.

Maxwell CV, Amankwah KS: Alternative approaches to preterm labor. Sems Perinatol **25**:310, 2001.

Maymon E, Romero R, Chairworapongsa T, et al: Amniotic fluid matrix metalloproteinase-8 in preterm labor with intact membranes. Am J Obstet Gynecol 185:1149, 2001.

McCormick MC, Shapiro S, Starfield BH: The regionalization of perinatal services: Summary of the evaluation of a national demonstration program. JAMA 253:799, 1985.

McDonald HM, O'Loughlin JA, Bigneswaran R, et al: Impact of metronidazole treatment in women with bacterial vaginosis flora (*Gardnerella vaginalis*): A randomised, placebo controlled trial. Br J Obstet Gynecol 104:1391, 1997.

McDonald TF, Pelzer S, Trautwein W, et al: Regulation and modulation of calcium channels in cardiac, skeletal and smooth muscle cells. Physiol Rev 74:365, 1994.

McElrath TF, Wise PH: Fertility therapy and the risk of very low birth weight. Obstet Gynecol 90:600, 1997.

Meis PJ, Ernest JM, Moore ML, et al: Regional program for prevention of premature birth in northwestern North Carolina. Am J Obstet Gynecol 157:550, 1987.

Meis PJ, Goldenberg RL, Mercer BM, et al: The preterm prediction study: Significance of vaginal infections. Am J Obstet Gynecol 173:1231, 1995.

Meis PJ, Goldenberg RL, Mercer BM, et al: The preterm prediction study: Risk factors for indicated preterm birth. Am J Obstet Gynecol 178:562, 1998.

Meis PJ, Klebanoff M, Thom E, et al for the National Institute of Child Health and Human Development Maternal-Fetal Medicine Units Network: Prevention of recurrent preterm birth by 17 alpha-hydroxyprogesterone caproate. N Engl J Med 348:2379, 2003.

Meis PJ, Michielutte R, Peters TJ, et al: Factors associated with preterm birth in Cardiff, Wales: II. Indicated and spontaneous preterm birth. Am J Obstet Gynecol 173:597, 1995.

Ment L, Oh W, Ehrenkrantz RA, et al: Antenatal steroids, delivery mode and intraventricular hemorrhage in preterm infants. Am J Obstet Gynecol 172:795, 1995.

Mercer BM: Preterm premature rupture of the membranes. Obstet Gynecol 101:178, 2003.

Mercer BM, Goldenberg RL, Das A, et al: The preterm prediction study: A clinical risk assessment system. Am J Obstet Gynecol 174:1885, 1996.

Mercer BM, Goldenberg RL, Moawad A, et al: The preterm prediction study: Effect of gestational age and cause of preterm birth on subsequent obstetric outcome. Am J Obstet Gynecol 181:1216, 1999.

Merkatz IR, Peter JB, Borden TP: Ritodrine hydrochloride: A beta-mimetic agent for use in preterm labor: II. Evidence of efficacy. Obstet Gynecol 56:7, 1980.

Minino AM, Arias E, Kochanek MA, et al: Deaths: Final data for 2000. National Vital Statistics Report 50:8, 2001.

Miodovnik M, Peros N, Holroyde JC, et al: Treatment of premature labor in insulin-dependent diabetic women. Obstet Gynecol 65:621 1985.

Mittendorf R, Covert R, Boman J, et al: Is tocolytic magnesium sulfate associated with increased total paediatric mortality? Lancet 350:1517, 1997.

Moawad AH, Goldenberg RL, Mercer B, et al for the NICHD MFMU Network: The Preterm Prediction Study: the value of serum alkaline phosphatase, alpha-fetoprotein, plasma corticotropin-releasing hormone, and other serum markers for the prediction of spontaneous preterm birth. Am J Obstet Gynecol 186:990, 2002.

Moise KJ, Huhta JC, Dawood S, et al: Indomethacin in the treatment of preterm labor: Effects on the human fetal ductus arteriosus. N Engl J Med 319:327, 1988.

Moore TM, Iams JD, Creasy RK, et al: Diurnal and gestational patterns of uterine activity in normal human pregnancy. Obstet Gynecol 83:517, 1994.

Morrison JC, Martin JN, Martin RW, et al: Prevention of preterm birth by ambulatory assessment of uterine activity: A randomized study. Am J Obstet Gynecol 156:536, 1987.

Morse SB, Haywood JL, Goldenberg RL, et al: Estimation of neonatal outcome and perinatal therapy use. Pediatrics 105:1046, 2000.

Moutquin JM, Sherman D, Cohen H, et al: Double-blind, randomized, controlled trial of atosiban and ritodrine in the treatment of preterm labor: A multicenter effectiveness and safety study. Am J Obstet Gynecol 182:1191, 2000.

Mozurkewich EL, Luke B, Avni M, et al: Working conditions and adverse pregnancy outcome: a meta-analysis. Obstet Gynecol 95:623, 2000.

Murakawa H, Utumi T, Hasegawa I, et al: Evaluation of threatened preterm delivery by transvaginal ultrasonographic measurement of cervical length. Obstet Gynecol 82:829, 1993.

Murray C, Haverkamp AD, Orleans M, et al: Nifedipine for the treatment of preterm labor. Am J Obstet Gynecol 167:52, 1992.

Nageotte MP, Casal D, Senyei AE: Fetal fibronectin in patients at increased risk for premature birth. Am J Obstet Gynecol 170:20, 1994.

Nageotte MP, Dorchester W, Porto M, et al: Quantitation of uterine activity preceding preterm, term, and post-term labor. Am J Obstet Gynecol 158:1254, 1988.

Nelson KB, Grether JK: Can magnesium sulfate reduce the risk of cerebral palsy in very-low birthweight infants? Pediatrics 95:263, 1995.

Neutra R, Feinberg S, Greenland S, et al: Effect of fetal monitoring on neonatal death rates. N Engl J Med 299:324, 1978.

Newman RB for the NICHD Maternal-Fetal Medicine Network: The Preterm Prediction Study: Comparison of the cervical score and Bishop score for the prediction of spontaneous preterm birth (Abstract No. 293). J Soc Gynecol Invest 4:152A, 1997.

Newman RB, Goldenberg RL, Moawad AH, et al: Occupational fatigue and preterm premature rupture of membranes. Am J Obstet Gynecol 184:438, 2001.

Niebyl JR, Blake DA, White RD, et al: The inhibition of premature labor with indomethacin. Am J Obstet Gynecol 136:1014, 1980.

Niebyl JR, Witter FR: Neonatal outcome after indomethacin treatment for preterm labor. Am J Obstet Gynecol 155:747, 1986.

Norton ME, Merrill J, Cooper BA, et al: Neonatal complications after the administration of indomethacin for preterm labor. N Engl J Med 329:1602, 1993.

Nuchpuckdee P, Brodskyr N, Porat R, et al: Ventricular septal thickness and cardiac function in neonates after *in utero* ritodrine exposure. J Pediatr 109:687, 1986.

Offenbacher S, Jared HL, O'Reilly PG, et al: Potential pathogenic mechanisms of periodontitis associated pregnancy complications. Ann Periodontal 3:233, 1998.

Offenbacher S, Katz V, Fertik G, et al: Periodontal infection as a possible risk factor for preterm low birth weight. J Periodontol 67(10 Suppl):1103, 1996.

Offenbacher S, Lieff S, Boggess KA, et al: Maternal periodontitis and prematurity. Part I: Obstetric outcome of prematurity and growth restriction. Ann Periodontol 6:164, 2001.

Ogburn PL, Hansen CA, Williams PP, et al: Magnesium sulfate and β-mimetic dual-agent tocolysis in preterm labor after single agent failure. J Repro Med 30:583,1985.

Olds DL, Henderson CR, Tatelbaum R, et al: Improving the delivery of prenatal care and outcomes of pregnancy: a randomized trial of nurse home visitation. Pediatrics 77:16, 1986.

Ott WJ: Intrauterine growth retardation and preterm delivery. Am J Obstet Gynecol 168:1710, 1993.

Panter KR, Hannah ME, Amankkwah KS, et al: The effect of indomethacin tocolysis in preterm labour on perinatal outcome: A randomized placebo-controlled trial. Br J Obstet Gynaecol 1106:467, 1999.

Papatsonis DNM, van Geijn HP, Ader HJ, et al: Nifedipine and ritodrine in the management of preterm labor: A randomized multicenter trial. Obstet Gynecol 90:230, 1997.

Parilla BV, Grobman WA, Holtzman RB, et al: Indomethacin tocolysis and risk of necrotizing enterocolitis. Obstet Gynecol 96:120, 2000.

Parisi VM, Salinas J, Stockan EJ: Fetal vascular responses to maternal nicardipine administration in the hypertensive ewe. Am J Obstet Gynecol 161:1035, 1989.

Paul RH, Hon EH: Clinical fetal monitoring: V. Effect on perinatal outcome. Am J Obstet Gynecol 118:529, 1974.

Peaceman AM, Andrews WW, Thorp JM, et al: Fetal fibronectin as a predictor of preterm birth in patients with symptoms: A multicenter trial. Am J Obstet Gynecol 177:13, 1997.

Peaceman AM, Meyer BA, Thorp JA, et al: The effect of magnesium sulfate tocolysis on the fetal biophysical profile. Am J Obstet Gynecol 161:771, 1989.

Perry KG, Morrison JC, Rust O, et al: Incidence of adverse cardiopulmonary effects with low-dose continuous terbutaline infusion. Am J Obstet Gynecol 173:1273, 1995.

Petrie RH: Tocolysis using magnesium sulfate. Semin Perinatol 5:266, 1981.

Raga F, Bauset C, Remohi J, et al: Reproductive impact of congenital Müllerian anomalies. Hum Reprod 12:2277, 1997.

Ramsey PS, Rouse DJ: Magnesium sulfate as a tocolytic agent. Semin Perinatol 25:236, 2001.

Ramsey PS, Tamura T, Goldenberg RL, et al: The preterm prediction study: elevated cervical ferritin levels at 22 to 24 weeks of gestation are associated with spontaneous preterm delivery in asymptomatic women. Am J Obstet Gynecol 186:458, 2002.

Ray D, Dyson D, Crites Y: Nifedipine tocolysis and neonatal acid-base status at delivery. Am J Obstet Gynecol 170:387, 1994.

Read MD, Wellby DE: The use of a calcium antagonist (nifedipine) to suppress preterm labour. Br J Obstet Gynaecol **93**:933, 1986.

Reiss U, Atad J, Rubinstein I, et al: The effect of indomethacin in labour at term. Int J Gynaecol Obstet **14**:369, 1976.

Reuss ML, Gordon HR: Obstetrical judgments of viability and perinatal survival of extremely low birth weight infants. Am J Pub Health **85**:362, 1995.

Reyes G, Romaguera J, Zapata R, et al: Effect of prenatal T4 treatment in neonatal morbidity. P R Health Sci J **16**:5, 1997.

Riduan JM, Hillier SL, Utomo B, et al: Bacterial vaginosis and prematurity in Indonesia: Association in early and late pregnancy. Am J Obstet Gynecol **169**:175, 1993.

Rizzo G, Capponi A, Arduini D, et al: The value of fetal fibronectin in cervical and vaginal secretions and of ultrasonographic examination of the uterine cervix in predicting premature delivery for patients with preterm labor and intact membranes. Am J Obstet Gynecol **175**:1146, 1996.

Roberts AK, Monzon-Bordonaba F, Van Deerlin PG, et al: Association of polymorphism within the promoter of the tumor necrosis factor alpha gene with increased risk of preterm premature rupture of the fetal membranes. Am J Obstet Gynecol **180**:1297, 1999.

Robertson PA, Herron M, Katz M, et al: Maternal morbidity associated with isoxsuprine and terbutaline tocolysis. Eur J Obstet Gynecol Reprod Biol **11**:317, 1981.

Robertson PA, Sniderman SH, Laros RK Jr, et al: Neonatal morbidity according to gestational age and birth weight from five tertiary centers in the United States, 1983 through 1986. Am J Obstet Gynecol **166**:1629, 1992.

Rodis JF, Vintzileos AM, Campbell WA, et al: Maternal hypothermia: An unusual complication of magnesium sulfate therapy. Am J Obstet Gynecol **156**:435, 1987.

Romero R, Kimenez C, Lokda AK, et al: Amniotic fluid glucose concentration: A rapid and simple method for the detection of intraamniotic infection in preterm labor. Am J Obstet Gynecol **163**:968, 1990.

Romero R, Oyarzun E, Mazor M, et al: Meta-analysis of the relationship between asymptomatic bacteriuria and preterm delivery/low birth weight. Obstet Gynecol **73**:576, 1989.

Romero R, Sibai BM, Sanchez-Ramos L, et al: An oxytocin receptor antagonist (atosiban) in the treatment of preterm labor. A randomized double-blind, placebo controlled trial with tocolytic rescue. Am J Obstet Gynecol **182**:1171, 2000.

Romero R, Sirtori M, Oyarzun E, et al: Infection and labor: V. Prevalence, microbiology, and clinical significance of intraamniotic infection in women with preterm labor and intact membranes. Am J Obstet Gynecol **16**:817, 1989.

Rouse DJ, Hirtz DG, Thom E: Association between use of antenatal magnesium sulfate in preterm labor and adverse health outcomes in infants. Am J Obstet Gynecol **188**:295, 2003.

Rozenberg P, Goffinet F, Malagrida L, et al: Evaluating the risk of preterm delivery: A comparison of fetal fibronectin and transvaginal ultrasonographic cervical length. Am J Obstet Gynecol **176**:196, 1997.

Rust OA, Atlas RO, Reed J, et al: Revisiting the short cervix detected by transvaginal ultrasound in the second trimester: Why cerclage therapy may not help. Am J Obstet Gynecol **185**:1098, 2001.

Saigal S, Lambert M, Russ C, et al: Self-esteem of adolescents who were born prematurely. Pediatrics **109**:429, 2002.

Saigal S, Stoskopf BL, Feeny D, et al: Differences in preferences for neonatal outcomes among health care professionals, parents and adolescents. JAMA **281**:1991, 1999.

Salafia CM, Vogel CA, Vintzileos AM, et al: Placental pathologic findings in preterm birth. Am J Obstet Gynecol **165**:934, 1991.

Saris NE, Mervaala E, Karppanen H, et al: Magnesium: An update on physiological, clinical and analytical aspects. Clin Chim Acta **294**:1, 2000.

Saunders MC, Dick JS, Brown IM, et al: The effects of hospital admission for bed rest on the duration of twin pregnancy: A randomised trial. Lancet **2**:793, 1985.

Savitz DA, Dole N, Terry JW, et al: Smoking and pregnancy outcome among African American and white women in central North Carolina. Epidemiology **12**:636, 2001.

Savory J, Monif G: Serum calcium levels in cord sera of the progeny treated with magnesium sulfate for toxemia of pregnancy. Am J Obstet Gynecol **110**:556, 1971.

Sawaya GF, Robertson PA: Hepatotoxicity with the administration of nifedipine for treatment of preterm labor. Am J Obstet Gynecol **167**:512, 1992.

Schieve LA, Meikle SF, Ferre C, et al. Low and very low birth weight in infants conceived with use of assisted reproductive technology. N Engl J Med **346**:731, 2002.

Schrag S, Gorwitz R, Fultz-Butts K, et al. Prevention of perinatal group B streptococcal disease; Revised guidelines from CDC. MMWR **51**(RR11):1, 2002.

Schwartz D, Miodovnik M, Lavin J: Neonatal outcome among low birth weight infants delivered spontaneously or by low forceps. Obstet Gynecol **62**:283, 1983.

Shankaran S, Fanaroff AA, Wright LL, et al: Risk factors for early death among extremely low birth weight infants. Am J Obstet Gynecol **186**:796, 2002.

Shaver DC, Bada HS, Korones SB, et al: Early and late intraventricular hemorrhage: The role of obstetric factors. Obstet Gynecol **80**:831, 1992.

Sherer DM, Cialone PR, Abramowicz JS, et al: Transient symptomatic subendocardial ischemia during intravenous magnesium sulfate tocolytic therapy. Am J Obstet Gynecol **166**:33, 1992.

Shiono PH, Klebanoff MA, Nugent RP, et al: The impact of cocaine and marijuana use on low birth weight and preterm birth: A multicenter study. Am J Obstet Gynecol **172**:19, 1995.

Smith LG Jr, Burns PA, Schanler RJ: Calcium homeostasis in pregnant women receiving long-term magnesium sulfate therapy for preterm labor. Am J Obstet Gynecol **167**:45, 1992.

Smith SK, Thompson D: The effects of intravenous salbutamol upon plasma and urinary potassium during premature labour. Br J Obstet Gynaecol **84**:344, 1977.

Spencer B, Thomas H, Morris J: A randomized controlled trial of the provision of a social support service during pregnancy: The South Manchester Family Worker Project. Br J Obstet Gynaecol **96**:281, 1989.

Spisso KR, Harbert GM, Thiagoriajah S: The use of magnesium sulfate as the primary tocolytic agent to prevent delivery. Am J Obstet Gynecol **142**:840, 1982.

Stevenson DK, Wright LL, Lemons JA, et al: Very low birth weight outcomes of the National Institute of Child Health and Human Development Neonatal Research Network, January 1993 through December 1994. Am J Obstet Gynecol **179**:1632, 1998.

Stika CS, Gross GA, Leguizmon G, et al: A prospective randomized safety trial of celecoxib for treatment of preterm labor. Am J Obstet Gynecol **187**:653, 2002.

Stone SR, Pritchard JA: Effect of maternally administered magnesium sulfate on the neonate. Obstet Gynecol **35**:574, 1970.

Strigini FA, Lencioni G, De Luca G, et al: Uterine artery velocimetry and spontaneous preterm delivery. Obstet Gynecol. **85**(3):374, 1995.

Suarez RD, Grobman WA, Parilla BV: Indomethacin tocolysis and intraventricular hemorrhage. Obstet Gynecol **97**:921, 2001.

Suarez VR, Thompson LL, Jain V, et al: The effect of in utero exposure to indomethacin on the need for surgical closure of a patent ductus in the neonate. Am J Obstet Gynecol **187**:886, 2002.

Taber EB, Tan L, Chao CR, et al: Pharmacokinetics of ionized versus total magnesium in subjects with preterm labor and preeclampsia. Am J Obstet Gynecol **186**:1017, 2002.

Taipale P, Hiilesmaa V: Sonographic measurement of the uterine cervix at 18–22 weeks' gestation and the risk of preterm delivery. Obstet Gynecol **92**:902, 1998.

Tejani N, Verma U, Hameed C, et al: Method and route of delivery in the low birth weight vertex presentation correlated with early periventricular intraventricular hemorrhage. Obstet Gynecol **69**:1, 1987.

Tepperman HM, Beydoun SN, Abdul-Karim RW: Drugs affecting myometrial contractility in pregnancy. Clin Obstet Gynecol **20**:423, 1977.

Thinkhamrop J, Hofmeyr GJ, Adetoro A, et al: Prophylactic antibiotic administration in pregnancy to prevent infectious morbidity and mortality (Cochrane Review). In The Cochrane Library, Issue 4. Oxford, Update Software, 2002.

Thorp JA, Ferrette-Smith D, Gaston LA, et al: Combined antenatal vitamin K for preventing intracranial hemorrhage in newborns less than 34 weeks' gestation. Obstet Gynecol **86**:1, 1995.

Thorp JM Jr, Hartmann KE, Berkman ND, et al: Antibiotic therapy for the treatment of preterm labor: A review of the evidence. Am J Obstet Gynecol **186**:587, 2002.

Thorp JM Jr, Katz VL, Campbell D, et al: Hypersensitivity to magnesium sulfate. Am J Obstet Gynecol **161**:889, 1989.

Timor-Tritsch I, Boozarjomehri F, Masakowski Y, et al: Can a snapshot sagittal view of the cervix by transvaginal ultrasonography predict active preterm labor? Am J Obstet Gynecol **174**:990, 1996.

Towers CV, Bonebrake R, Padilla G, et al: The effect of transport on the rate of severe intraventricular hemorrhage in very low birth weight infants. Obstet Gynecol **95**:291, 2000.

Tsatsaris V, Papasonis D, Goffinet F, et al: Tocolysis with nifedipine or beta-adrenergic agonists: A meta-analysis. Obstet Gynecol **97**:840, 2001.

Tulzer G, Gudmundsson S, Tews G, et al: Incidence of indomethacin-induced fetal ductal constriction. J Maternal Fetal Invest **1**:267, 1992.

Tyson JE, Younes N, Verter J, et al: Viability, morbidity, and resource use among newborns of 501- to 800-g birth weight. National Institute of Child Health and Human Development Neonatal Research Network. JAMA **276**(20):1645, 1996.

Ulmsten U, Anderson K-E, Wingerup L: Treatment of premature labor with the calcium antagonist nifedipine. Arch Gynecol **229**:1, 1980.

U.S. Food and Drug Administration (FDA): Warning on use of terbutaline sulfate for preterm labor. JAMA **279**:9, 1998.

Van de Bor M, van Bel F, Lineman R, et al: Perinatal factors of periventricular-intraventricular hemorrhage in preterm infants. Am J Dis Child **140**:1125, 1986.

Van der Heijden BJ, Carlus C, Narcy F, et al: Persistent anuria, neonatal death, and renal microcystic lesions after prenatal exposure to indomethacin. Am J Obstet Gynecol **171**:617, 1994.

Vermillion ST, Landen CN Jr: Prostaglandin inhibitors as tocolytic agents. Sems Perinatol **25**:256, 2001.

Vermillion ST, Newman RB: Recent indomethacin tocolysis is not associated with neonatal complications in preterm infants. Am J Obstet Gynecol **181**:1083, 1999.

Vermillion ST, Scardo JA, Lashus AG, et al: The effect of indomethacin tocolysis of fetal ductus arteriosus constriction with advancing gestational age. Am J Obstet Gynecol **177**:256, 1997.

Vogel I, Salvig JD, Secher NJ, et al: Association between raised serum relaxin levels during the eighteenth gestational week and very preterm delivery. Am J Obstet Gynecol **184**:390, 2001.

Vohr BR, Wright LL, Dusick AM, et al: Neurodevelopmental and functional outcomes of extremely low birth weight infants in the National Institutes of Child Health and Human Development Neonatal Research Network, 1993–94. Pediatrics **105**:1216, 2000.

Watts DH, Krohn MA, Hillier SI, et al: The association of occult amniotic fluid infection with gestational age and neonatal outcome among women in preterm labor. Obstet Gynecol **79**:351, 1992.

Weiss G, Goldsmith LT, Sachdev R, et al: Elevated first-trimester serum relaxin concentrations in pregnant women following ovarian stimulation predict prematurity risk and preterm delivery. Obstet Gynecol **82**:821, 1993.

Wenstrom KD, Andrews WW, Hauth JC, et al: Elevated second-trimester amniotic fluid interleukin-6 levels predict preterm delivery. Am J Obstet Gynecol **178**:546, 1998.

Wenstrom KD, Weiner CP, Merrill D, et al: A placebo controlled randomized trial of the terbutaline pump for prevention of preterm delivery. Am J Perinatol **14**:87, 1997.

Wilcox LS, Kiely JL, Melvin CL, et al: Assisted reproductive technologies: Estimates of their contribution to multiple births and newborn hospital days in the United States. Fertil Steril **65**:361, 1996.

Wilkins IA, Lynch L, Mehalek KE, et al: Efficacy and side effects of magnesium sulfate and ritodrine as tocolytic agents. Am J Obstet Gynecol **159**:685, 1988.

Williams MA, Hickok DE, Zingheim RW, et al: Low birth weight and preterm delivery in relation to early-gestation vaginal bleeding and elevated maternal serum alpha-fetoprotein. Obstet Gynecol **80**:745, 1992.

Wood NS, Marlow N, Costeloe K, et al: Neurologic and developmental disability after extremely preterm birth. N Engl J Med **343**:378, 2000.

Woods JR Jr, Plessinger MA, Miller RK: Vitamins C and E: Missing links in preventing preterm premature rupture of membranes? Am J Obstet Gynecol **185**:5, 2001.

Yang J, Savitz DA: The effect of vaginal bleeding during pregnancy on preterm and small-for-gestational-age births: US National Maternal and Infant Health Survey, 1988. Paediatr Perinat Epidemiol. **15**:34, 2001.

Yeast JD, Poskin M, Stockbauer JW, et al: Changing patterns in regionalization of perinatal care and the impact on neonatal mortality. Am J Obstet Gynecol **178**:131, 1998.

Ying YK, Tejani NA: Angina pectoris as a complication of ritodrine hydrochloride therapy in premature labor. Obstet Gynecol **60**:385, 1982.

Yoon BH, Jun JK, Romero R, et al: Amniotic fluid inflammatory cytokines (interleukin-6, interleukin-1β, and tumor necrosis factor-α) and neonatal brain white matter lesions and cerebral palsy. Am J Obstet Gynecol **177**:19, 1997.

Yoon BH, Romero R, Jun JK, et al: Amniotic fluid cytokines (interleukin-6, tumor necrosis factor-α, interleukin 1-β) and the risk for the development of bronchopulmonary dysplasia. Am J Obstet Gynecol **177**:825, 1997.

Yoon BH, Romero R, Kim CJ, et al: Amniotic fluid interleukin-6; A sensitive test for antenatal diagnosis of acute inflammatory lesions of preterm placenta and prediction of perinatal morbidity. Am J Obstet Gynecol **172**:9960, 1995.

Yoon BH, Romero R, Kim KS, et al: A systemic fetal inflammatory response and the development of bronchopulmonary dysplasia. Am J Obstet Gynecol **181**:773, 1999.

Yoon BH, Romero R, Moon JB, et al: Clinical significance of intra-amniotic inflammation in patients with preterm labor and intact membranes. Am J Obstet Gynecol **185**:1130, 2001.

Yoon BH, Romero R, Park JS, et al: Fetal exposure to an intra-amniotic inflammation and the development of cerebral palsy at the age of three years. Am J Obstet Gynecol **182**:675, 2000.

Young DC, Toofanian A, Leveno KJ: Potassium and glucose concentrations without treatment during ritodrine tocolysis. Am J Obstet Gynecol **145**:105, 1983.

Zanini B, Paul R, Huey J: Intrapartum fetal heart rate: Correlation with scalp pH in the preterm fetus. Am J Obstet Gynecol **136**:43, 1980.

Zlatnik FJ: The applicability of labor inhibition to the problem of prematurity. Am J Obstet Gynecol **113**:704, 1972.

Zuckerman H, Reiss U, Rubinstein I: Inhibition of human premature labor by indomethacin. Obstet Gynecol **44**:787, 1974.

Zuckerman H, Shalev E, Gilad G, et al: Further study of the inhibition of premature labor by indomethacin: Part I. J Perinat Med **12**:19, 1984a.

Zuckerman H, Shalev E, Gilad G, et al: Further study of the inhibition of premature labor by indomethacin: Part II. J Perinatol Med **12**:25, 1984b.

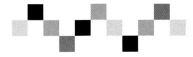

Chapter 35
POST-TERM PREGNANCY

Jamie L. Resnik, MD, and Robert Resnik, MD

In 1902, Ballantyne described the problem of the post-term pregnancy for the first time in modern obstetric terms. Although the language used to describe the entity in early 20th-century Scotland was different from that of today, Ballantyne's words clearly reflected current thinking when he said, "The postmature infant . . . has stayed too long in intra-uterine surroundings; he has remained so long *in utero* that his difficulty is to be born with safety to himself and his mother. The problem of the . . . postmature infant is intranatal."

During the ensuing years, the issue of post-term pregnancy, its risks, and its management have generated great controversy. An abundance of older as well as more recent data, however, has firmly established that although the fetal risk associated with a prolonged pregnancy is small, it is real. Consequently, the pregnancy that continues beyond 42 weeks requires careful surveillance.

EPIDEMIOLOGY

By definition, a term gestation is one completed in 38–42 weeks. Pregnancy is considered prolonged, or post-term, when it exceeds 294 days or 42 weeks. The frequency of this occurrence has been reported to range from 4%–14%, with those completing 43 weeks, 2%–7%. The chances that parturition will occur precisely at 280 days after the first day of the last menstrual period (40 weeks) is only 5%.

One of the major problems in delineating the extent of risk beyond term has been related to the limited reliability of the last menstrual period (LMP) as a basis for accurately predicting gestational age. Until a decade ago, most epidemiologic studies pertaining to fetal and neonatal risks of delayed parturition were based on the LMP. More recently, the more precise technology of ultrasound biometry has been applied to the issue of pregnancy dating for the post-term gestation, and the data confirm that the LMP is a relatively poor predictor of true gestational age. For example, the incidence of post-term gestation fell from 7.5% when based on menstrual dating to 2.6% when based on early ultrasound examination, and to 1.1% when the diagnosis required menstrual and ultrasound dates to reach 294 days or more (Boyd et al., 1988). In a more recent study by Gardosi and colleagues (1997), the post-term delivery rate among women dated by LMP was 9.5%, but it decreased to 1.5% if ultrasound dating was used. In fact, 71.5% of "post-term" inductions as dated by LMP were not post-term according to ultrasound. In this study population, using ultrasound dating, the incidence of post-term pregnancy was only 2.2%.

This is consistent with the observations of Taipale and Hiilermaa (2001), who performed ultrasound between 8 and 16 weeks' gestation in 17,221 women. When they used ultrasound biometric criteria rather than the LMP to determine gestational age, the number of post-term pregnancies fell from 10.3% to 2.7%.

Nevertheless, virtually all reports up to the present time, even given their inherent limitations, suggest an increase in perinatal morbidity and mortality when pregnancy goes beyond 42 weeks' gestation. One of the earliest and most frequently cited studies was provided by the National Birthday Trust of Britain in 1958, when a detailed analysis was undertaken to examine more than 17,000 births in the United Kingdom from March 3 to March 9 of that year (Butler and Alberman, 1969). Figure 35-1 demonstrates that the perinatal mortality rate begins to increase after 42 weeks' gestation, doubling at about 43 weeks, and that it is four to six times higher at 44 weeks than at term. Numerous other reports since that time have confirmed this increase in risk (Nakano, 1972; Sachs and Friedman, 1986; Eden et al., 1987). More recently, Alexander and associates (2000) retrospectively evaluated outcomes of more than 27,000 pregnancies at 41 and 42 weeks' gestation, compared with approximately 29,000 born at 40 weeks' gestation. The length of labor, incidence of prolonged second-stage labor, forceps use, and cesarean delivery were all increased with the longer gestation period. It is not clear, however, whether the observed increase in complications was due to prolonged gestation, routine use of induction at 42 weeks, or both.

Another source of controversy has resulted from a widely quoted publication by Clifford (1954). In his classic description of the undernourished postmature infant, Clifford suggested that the risk of postmaturity was limited to the primigravid pregnancy. It has now been clearly established that although the perinatal mortality rate in the multigravid pregnancy after 42 weeks is lower than for primigravidae, some degree of risk remains.

ETIOLOGY

Our knowledge of the mechanism of parturition is increasing rapidly, and the pertinent biochemical and physiologic findings have been reviewed in Chapter 6. Although it is not known specifically why some pregnancies are abnormally prolonged, clues exist from observation of unknown natural occurrences in normal labor, as well as from interesting

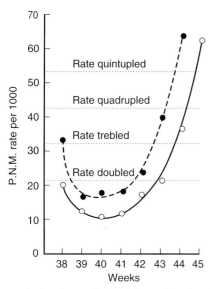

FIGURE 35-1 ■ Perinatal mortality (PNM) rate for all prolonged pregnancies (solid line), which increases markedly after 42 weeks' gestation, and for prolonged pregnancies with superimposed toxemia (hatched line). (From McClure-Browne JC: Post-maturity. Am J Obstet Gynecol **85**:573, 1963.)

observations of aberrant timing of labor in humans and other species.

It appears that the production of prostaglandins E_2 and F_2 alpha in the amnion and deciduas, respectively, represent the final common pathway triggering myometrial contractility. The initiation of prostaglandin synthesis could result from a complex chain of events occurring within the fetus, which require normal and appropriate release of hormones within the fetal brain, pituitary and adrenal glands, and placenta. For example, it has long been known that fetal pituitary defects in Holstein cattle could lead to failure of normal delivery timing (Holm, 1967). In humans, congenital primary fetal adrenal hypoplasia and placental sulfatase deficiency leading to low estrogen production could result in delayed onset of labor and failure of normal cervical ripening (France and Liggins, 1969; Fliegner et al., 1972).

Reduced to its simplest terms, labor consists of myometrial contractions, which cause effacement and dilation of the cervix to allow expulsion of the fetus. For normal pregnancy and labor, the myometrium and cervix must act in concert with one another. Prior to the onset of labor, a transition occurs in the structure of the cervix, during which the cervix undergoes significant alterations in its shape and consistency. Before the seminal contribution of Danforth (1947), which established that the cervix was essentially a connective tissue structure, clinicians and investigators had assumed that it was composed of smooth muscle and indeed behaved as a muscular sphincter. It is now recognized that the cervix is composed predominantly of fibrous connective tissue, with an extracellular matrix consisting of collagen with elastin and proteoglycans, and a cellular portion including smooth muscles cells and fibroblasts. In their review, Ludmir and Sehdev (2000) describe the process of cervical ripening, which involves an increase in the water content of the cervix, a decrease in the collagen concentration, and a remodeling of the collagen. These processes are undertaken as pregnancy progresses. Collagenases are involved in remodeling the collagen fibers, and as this

occurs, hyaluronic acid (a glycosaminoglycan) is secreted by fibroblasts, bringing about an increase in the water concentration of the cervix. This increased water, in turn, causes the cervix to soften, as is appreciated clinically. While collagenases and degradative enzymes are allowing the remodeling and dispersal of the extracellular matrix, the cellular component of the cervix is undergoing physiologic cell death. This causes invasion of the cervix by neutrophils and macrophages, thereby increasing the concentration of inflammatory mediators, which further augments the concentration of degradative enzymes while also increasing the amount of hyaluronic acid.

Thus, pregnancy could be prolonged because the pregnancy, cervix, or both are defective in some way that leads not only to delayed labor and cervical ripening, but also to impaired efficiency of labor.

DIAGNOSIS

When one considers the rapidly accelerating risk of fetal morbidity and mortality between 42 and 43 weeks' gestation and again at 43–44 weeks' gestation (see Figure 35-1), it becomes apparent that no historically derived or laboratory measurement of fetal age provides the precision required in the management of the post-term pregnancy. As previously mentioned, the rate of post-term pregnancy can vary from 1.5% to 9.5% depending on whether a given pregnancy is dated by the LMP or by ultrasound measurements (Gardosi et al., 1997). Traditional landmarks, such as LMP, uterine size, and first auscultation of fetal heart tones, could be miscalculated by 2 weeks or more in terms of accurate determination of gestational age. Even sensitive sonographic determinations, such as crown-to-rump length in the first trimester, demonstrate a range of several days. In fact, in any given gestation, the actual fetal age is known only when the time of ovulation and conception have been studied, as in the case of the infertile couple who undergo ovulation induction and/or *in vitro* fertilization.

Because the diagnosis of "post-term pregnancy" is often uncertain or can vary depending on the dating criteria used, it can be difficult at times to identify those pregnancies that are truly post-term and therefore at risk for increased perinatal morbidity. In these instances, it can be helpful to perform an assessment of the amniotic fluid, as the amniotic fluid volume is known to decrease in some post-term gestations. Furthermore, the risks to the fetus of post-term pregnancies may well be related to the degree of oligohydramnios. Diminished amniotic fluid volume is associated with higher rates of intrapartum fetal distress and cesarean section (Leveno et al., 1984). Bochner and coworkers (1987) observed an almost 24-fold increase in cesarean section for the indication of fetal distress when the maximum vertical amniotic fluid pocket depth was less than 3 cm. The incidence of meconium-stained amniotic fluid in the post-term gestation was 37% in those women with adequate amniotic fluid volume but increased to 71% when the amniotic fluid volume was decreased (Phelan et al., 1984). Consequently, if there is a question of the accuracy of dates, the finding of normal amniotic fluid volume is reassuring, while the finding of oligohydramnios may encourage the practitioner to manage a given pregnancy more actively.

The amniotic fluid index (AFI) shown in Figure 35-2 is a useful clinical tool in defining the adequacy of amniotic fluid

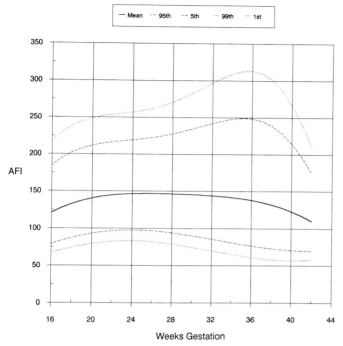

AMNIOTIC FLUID INDEX

FIGURE 35-2 ■ The mean and various percentiles for amniotic fluid index (AFI). Data obtained from 768 patients. (Adapted from Moore TR, Cayle JE: Amniotic fluid index in normal human pregnancy. Am J Obstet Gynecol **162**:1168, 1990.)

volume. When the volume decreases sharply over time or falls below 5 cm, oligohydramnios becomes a concern. Debate exists about whether oligohydramnios is better defined by an amniotic fluid index of less than 5 cm or by the absence of a single vertical pocket greater than or equal to 3 cm (see Chapters 20 and 21). The presence of oligohydramnios, however, is generally recognized as a sign of placental insufficiency, which is often associated with post-term pregnancies.

FETAL COMPLICATIONS

Aberrations in Fetal Growth

Since the report of Clifford (1954) and his description of the postmature-dysmature neonate with wasting of subcutaneous tissue, meconium staining, and peeling of skin, many have focused their attention on the problems of the undernourished post-term fetus. In fact, only 10%–20% of true post-term fetuses exhibit any of the findings described by Clifford. Macrosomia is actually a far more common complication because, under most circumstances, the fetus continues to grow *in utero*. Twice as many post-term fetuses weigh more than 4000 g compared with term infants (Zwerdling, 1967; Eden et al., 1987), and birth injuries can occur as a result of difficult forceps deliveries and shoulder dystocia. Morbidity also includes cephalohematomas, fractures, and brachial plexus palsy (Usher et al., 1988). Study of fetal growth characteristics in 7000 post-term infants confirms a gradual shift toward higher birth weights and greater head circumference between 273 and 300 days of gestational age (McLean et al., 1991).

These findings are further reinforced by a study of 519 pregnancies beyond 41 weeks, in which 23% of the newborns weighed more than 4000 g and 4% weighed more than 4500 g (Pollack et al., 1992).

Although the majority of post-term infants are appropriately grown or macrosomic, the risk of a small-for-gestational-age (SGA) infant is also increased in post-term pregnancy. In a population-based study of 510,029 singleton pregnancies from the Swedish Birth Registry, the rate of small-for-gestational-age infants increased from 2.2% in term infants to 3.8% in post-term infants (Clausson et al., 1999).

Meconium Staining and Pulmonary Aspiration

Virtually all studies of post-term gestation report a markedly higher incidence of meconium-stained amniotic fluid, and the greater risk of meconium aspiration syndrome in these infants is well recognized (Eden et al., 1987). In infants defined by ultrasound-estimated fetal growth curves to be appropriately sized for gestational age (AGA), post-term infants had a threefold higher incidence of meconium aspiration compared with term appropriate-for-gestational-age infants, and a doubled risk of Apgar scores less than 4 at 5 minutes (Clausson et al., 1999). The presence of oligohydramnios further complicates the risks of meconium staining owing to the lack of fluid to dilute the meconium, resulting in thicker, more tenacious material in the oropharynx and lower in the respiratory tract.

FETAL EVALUATION AND MANAGEMENT

It is generally accepted that careful antepartum and intrapartum fetal monitoring can virtually eliminate fetal post-term mortality and reduce fetal morbidity (Hauth et al., 1980; Freeman et al., 1981; Eden et al., 1982; Phelan et al., 1984; Johnson et al., 1986). A careful evidence-based literature analysis, however, has concluded that data are insufficient to determine whether routine antenatal surveillance prior to 42 weeks' gestation improves outcome or which type of monitoring and frequency is most appropriate (American College of Obstetricians and Gynecologists, 1997). Nevertheless, most obstetricians initiate antenatal testing at 41–42 weeks' gestation and repeat the testing twice weekly.

In a study of 307 women whose pregnancies had proceeded beyond 294 days, a normal twice-weekly biophysical profile (BPP) that included normal amniotic fluid volume resulted in no perinatal mortalities, and morbidity was equivalent to a comparison group undergoing elective labor induction with a favorable cervix (Johnson et al., 1986). Based on a cumulative experience with 19,221 high-risk pregnancies, the same investigative group recommended delivery if amniotic fluid volume decreased (Manning et al., 1987).

Other studies, however, have not confirmed the correlation between any critical AFI measurement and suboptimal neonatal outcome. A cohort study done in Sweden showed no correlation between an AFI below 5 cm and adverse outcome (Montan and Malcus, 1995). Similarly, Divon and associates (1995), in a longitudinal assessment of AFI in 139 post-term women, found an increased frequency of abnormal fetal heart rate tracings and meconium staining but no other significant adverse fetal outcome. Consequently, although a normal amount of amniotic fluid should be considered as a favorable prognostic finding, less is known about the dynamic changes of amniotic fluid volume in the lower ranges. Consequently, the ability of such measurements to predict adverse outcome remains controversial.

If a measurement of amniotic fluid volume is used, there is also disagreement about whether the AFI or the maximum vertical pocket depth is preferable. Each technique has its proponents (Manning et al., 1987; Moore and Cayle, 1990). In an analysis of 198 women at 40 weeks' gestation or beyond who were studied with AFI and largest vertical pocket measurements, Fischer and coauthors (1993) found that a single vertical pocket threshold of 2.7 cm was the most accurate parameter in defining abnormal perinatal outcome. Alfirevic and colleagues (1997) compared both methods with respect to pregnancy intervention in post-term pregnancies and found more frequent abnormal AFIs than abnormal vertical pocket depths, leading to more inductions and fetal monitoring but no difference in perinatal outcomes. This finding confirmed a previous study by the same group (Alfirevic and Walkinshaw, 1995), who showed that the use of a modified biophysical profile (with AFI) led to more interventions than did the non-stress test (NST) and maximum amniotic fluid pool depth, but without differences in neonatal outcome after 42 weeks' gestation.

There does not appear to be any value in monitoring Doppler flow velocity in fetal vessels, inasmuch as there is no correlation between the findings and outcome (Guidetti et al., 1987). Zimmerman and associates (1995) demonstrated that the sensitivity of umbilical artery velocimetry for predicting poor outcome was 7%.

Fetal Monitoring Versus Induction of Labor

Even though antenatal monitoring can virtually eliminate perinatal mortality in the post-term gestation, morbidity—including meconium staining, increased cesarean delivery for a diagnosis of fetal distress, and macrosomia with its associated complications—still exists. The continuing concern regarding morbidity has been addressed by an alternative approach—that of cervical ripening with prostaglandin gel or misoprostol, followed by induction at 41 weeks' gestation.

Recent randomized controlled trials comparing outcomes following serial fetal monitoring and induction have yielded inconclusive results. Hannah and coauthors (1992) studied 3407 women with uncomplicated pregnancies at 41 or more weeks' duration, randomly assigned to either elective induction after cervical ripening with PGE_2 gel or serial antenatal monitoring (fetal kicks, non-stress test, amniotic fluid). In the monitored group, labor was induced only if there was evidence of compromised fetal status. The authors observed a lower cesarean delivery rate for a diagnosis of fetal distress in the induction group but no significant difference between the two groups in fetal mortality or morbidity. The same investigative group subsequently reported that routine induction was more cost-effective than serial antenatal monitoring (Goeree et al., 1995).

The Maternal-Fetal Medicine Network prospectively evaluated 440 patients, comparing induction with serial monitoring (National Institute of Child Health and Development, 1994). They observed no fetal deaths in either group, and rates of neonatal morbidity and cesarean delivery were similar.

These combined trials led to the conclusion that neither approach has substantive advantage over the other.

Nevertheless, it is clear that medical induction rates have increased sharply in the United States. Between 1980 and 1996, the rate of induction doubled (from 12.9% to 25.8%), the most common indication being that of the post-term pregnancy (Yawn et al., 2001). The evidence obtained from recent population-based studies and meta-analyses suggest that the use of routine induction at 41 weeks' gestation decreases the still birth rate without increasing the rate of cesarean deliveries (Sue-A-Quan et al., 1999; Crowley, 2000).

Management Summary

It seems appropriate to recommend the following steps to evaluate and manage the post-term gestation:

1. Although there is insufficient evidence because of the low-risk nature of either approach, current obstetric practice dictates that labor be induced between 41 and 42 weeks' gestation in the presence of a favorable cervix.
2. If the cervix is unfavorable, alternate approaches include cervical ripening followed by induction of labor, or twice-weekly fetal monitoring. Delivery should be accomplished with evidence of fetal compromise.
3. It is prudent to use the biophysical profile, or some modification of the biophysical profile, to determine antenatal fetal condition.

Methods of Labor Induction

Because normal labor depends on efficient myometrial contractions acting on a compliant cervix to efface and dilate it, methods of labor induction must take account of both components of the uterus. If the cervix is already soft, effaced, and partially dilated, intravenous infusion of oxytocin may be sufficient to stimulate contractions. Conventional practice would require amniotomy to be performed as a first step, as this procedure maximizes the effectiveness of oxytocin. If the cervix is unripe, oxytocin will not cause it to ripen, and amniotomy is inappropriate. Although labor contractions can be stimulated by oxytocin, such a result is futile, because many hours of such contractions are required to produce any sort of change in the cervix, and the ensuing prolonged labor can lead to an increase in obstetrical morbidity, including a significant risk of postpartum hemorrhage and an increased risk of cesarean delivery.

The Bishop score (Bishop, 1964), or some suitable modification of it, can be used as a guide to select the most appropriate induction technique. This is especially true in primigravid women. If the Bishop score is below 5, amniotomy and oxytocin infusion are associated with an unacceptably high incidence of fetal and maternal complications (Calder and Greer, 1992). In these circumstances, cervical ripening should be undertaken before provoking uterine contractions. Given the rapidly increasing use of transvaginal ultrasound (TVUS) to assess cervical length and dilatation, and its usefulness in the diagnosis of preterm labor, it is not unreasonable to attempt applying this technology to cervical assessment in post-term pregnancy. One recent study of 240 women, comparing transvaginal ultrasound to digital cervical examination utilizing ROC curves, demonstrated that a cervical length of

28 mm was a better predictor of induction success (vaginal delivery within 24 hours) than the Bishop score (Pandis et al., 2001). Conflicting findings, however, have been reported by Chandra and associates (2001).

A popular method of achieving cervical ripening is to use PGE_2 in an aqueous gel either vaginally (Prostin E_2 gel) or endocervically (Prepidil) or, alternatively, as a sustained-release vaginal suppository (Cervidil). These compounds are highly effective in ripening the cervix and reducing the problems associated with prolonged pregnancy, including the need for labor induction (Hannah et al., 1992). In one study, it was shown that in pregnancies beyond 41 weeks' gestation with unfavorable cervices, the daily placement of a PGE_2 gel (Prepidil) caused a decrease in the incidence of induction at 42 weeks' gestation for post-term pregnancies to 20%, compared with an induction rate of 63% when no intervention was undertaken (Magann et al., 1998). In a similar study, placement of Prepidil gel at the time of routine antenatal testing (approximately every 3 days) decreased the induction rate in the patient population having Bishop scores between 3 and 6. In those patients with unfavorable cervices, however, the induction rate was not affected by the application of PGE_2 gel (Lien et al., 1998).

More recently, misoprostol (Cytotec) has gained favor as an effective cervical ripening agent. Misoprostol is a PGE_1 analog that has been used primarily for the treatment of peptic ulcer disease. Although it is used "off label," it has been shown to be safe and effective for cervical ripening. A recent Cochrane database review concludes that the use of vaginal misoprostol is more effective than conventional methods of cervical ripening and labor induction. Compared with placebo, oxytocin, or intracervical or vaginal PGE_2, misoprostol use results in increased cervical ripening, decreased use of oxytocin, and increased rate of vaginal delivery. Misoprostol, however, also causes an increased rate of uterine hyperstimulation (Hofmeyr and Gulmezoglu, 2003). Additionally, misoprostol use is contraindicated in patients who have previously undergone cesarean delivery because of a possible increased risk of uterine rupture.

The increased rate of uterine hyperstimulation seen with misoprostol as compared with dinoprostone appears to be dose dependent. Thus, a review of the literature to assess safety and efficacy is difficult because the dosage used in various studies ranges from 25-μg to 200 μg, and the frequency of administration ranges from every 3 to every 6 hours. Although the optimal dose of misoprostol is still a subject of debate, a recent American College of Obstetrics and Gynecology Committee Opinion (1999) recommends an initial vaginal dose of 25 μg.

Also still under investigation is the optimal route of administration for misoprostol. Currently, vaginal administration is used most commonly, but this involves serial vaginal examinations, which can be uncomfortable to patients. Multiple randomized controlled trials have been performed comparing oral to vaginal misoprostol, with the findings varying depending on the dosage used and the frequency of administration. In two studies using a 50-μg dosage administered every 6 hours either vaginally or orally, it was observed that vaginal administration resulted in a faster interval from induction to delivery than did oral administration (Kwon et al., 2001; Le Roux et al., 2002). When this same dosage was administered every 4 hours, the vaginal study group had a shorter interval until delivery and less oxytocin requirements than the oral group but also had a

higher rate of uterine hyperstimulation and fetal distress (Shetty et al., 2001). Therefore, vaginal misoprostol in dosages equivalent to oral misoprostol is shown to be more effective but with the caveat of increased uterine hyperstimulation. In these studies, however, the effective vaginal dose is higher because vaginally administered misoprostol is absorbed through mucus membranes, thereby bypassing the first-pass liver metabolism that occurs with oral administration. The oral dosages have been shown to have decreased bioavailability compared with vaginal absorption (Zieman et al., 1997), so safety and efficacy regarding route of administration cannot truly be compared using the same dosage. In studies comparing a higher oral dosage of 200 μg compared with 50 μg administered vaginally, the oral treatment group has been shown to experience an efficacy similar to vaginal treatment, but also an increased rate of uterine hyperstimulation (Carlan et al., 2001; Adair et al., 1998).

In summary, when the effective dose is similar, vaginal administration appears to be a safer route, although less convenient than oral. Alternative routes are currently being investigated. These include sublingual—which has been shown to be more effective than oral misoprostol (Shetty et al., 2002)—and buccal, which has been shown to have similar efficacy to oral administration but with a higher incidence of uterine hyperstimulation (Carlan et al., 2002).

DEVELOPMENTAL EFFECTS OF POST-TERM GESTATION

Studies on subsequent development of children from prolonged pregnancies are difficult to evaluate because investigators have not separated neonates asphyxiated in utero and growth-retarded (dysmature) post-term neonates from otherwise normally born neonates. A study of neonatal behavior among 106 postmature infants revealed an increased number of illnesses and sleep disorders as well as diminished social competence during the first year of life (Vineland Social Maturity Scale). Also, and not unexpectedly, the incidence of fetal distress was high, and those babies who were asphyxiated in utero had a higher incidence of abnormal neurologic signs in the neonatal period (Lovell, 1973). All infants had signs of desquamation of skin and wasting of subcutaneous tissue, however, and the group of children studied was not compared with any post-term children who did not have these physical findings at birth.

Field and coworkers (1977) studied a group of 40 postmature offspring, all of whom had parchment-like skin and long, thin bodies. At birth, their Brazelton interaction and motor scores were lower than term controls, and at 4 months they scored lower on the Denver Developmental Scale. By 8 months, the Bayley motor scores of the post-term subjects were equivalent to those of control infants, but the mental scores were slightly lower. This study differs in at least one significant way from that of Lovell (1973): The Apgar scores at 5 minutes in the two groups were identical, thus partially correcting for in utero asphyxia.

In a large retrospective review, Zwerdling (1967) observed that post-term infants weighing less than 2500 g had a neonatal mortality rate seven times that for post-term infants as a whole. This figure confirmed the additional risk of the occasionally observed abnormal growth pattern (dysmaturity) in some post-term infants. This increase in mortality rate was observed up to 2 years of age. Data on growth and intelligence in Zwerdling's study population, however, revealed no differences between prolonged-gestation and normal-gestation children at age 5 years. These findings are confirmed in a more recent prospective study, in which 129 children born of prolonged pregnancy were compared with 184 term controls (Shime et al., 1986). At 1 year and again at 2 years of age, there were no differences between the two groups with respect to intelligence scores, physical milestones, and intercurrent illnesses.

It is clear that the child of a post-term gestation must be evaluated in follow-up studies in relation to the presence or absence of antepartum or intrapartum asphyxia and of the dysmaturity syndrome (long fingernails, skin desquamation, and decreased subcutaneous tissue). It is entirely possible that later development is normal in the absence of these factors.

REFERENCES

Adair CD, Weeks JW, Barrilleaux S, et al: Oral or vaginal misoprostol administration for induction of labor: A randomized double-blind trial. Obstet Gynecol **92**:810, 1998.

Alexander JM, McIntire DD, Leveno UJ: Forty weeks and beyond: Pregnancy outcomes by week of gestation. Obstet Gynecol **96**:291, 2000.

Alfirevic Z, Luckas M, Walkinshaw SA, et al: A randomized comparison between amniotic fluid index and maximum pool depth in the monitoring of postterm pregnancy. Br J Obstet Gynaecol **104**:207, 1997.

Alfirevic Z, Walkinshaw SA: A randomised controlled trial of simple compared with complex antenatal fetal monitoring after 42 weeks of gestation. Br J Obstet Gynaecol **102**:638, 1995.

American College of Obstetricians and Gynecologists: ACOG Practice Patterns: Management of Postterm Gestation. No. 6, October 1997.

American College of Obstetricians and Gynecologists: ACOG Committee Opinion: Induction of Labor with Misoprostol. No. 228, November 1999.

Ballantyne JW: The problem of the postmature infant. J Obstet Gynaecol Br Emp **2**:36, 1902.

Bishop EH: Pelvic scoring for elective induction. Obstet Gynecol **24**:266, 1964.

Bochner CJ, Medearis AI, Davis J, et al: Antepartum predictors of fetal distress in post-term pregnancy. Am J Obstet Gynecol **157**:353, 1987.

Boyd ME, Usher RH, McLean FH, et al: Obstetric consequences of postmaturity. Am J Obstet Gynecol **158**:334, 1988.

Butler NR, Alberman ED: The Second Report of the 1958 British Perinatal Mortality Survey. Edinburgh, E & S Livingstone, 1969, p. 327.

Calder AA, Greer CA: Cervical Physiology and Induction of Labor: Recent Advances in Obstetrics and Gynecology. No. 17. Edinburgh, Churchill Livingstone, 1992.

Caldeyro-Barcia R: Uterine contractility in obstetrics. Proceedings of the Second International Congress of Gynecology and Obstetrics, Montreal, **1**:65, 1958.

Carlan SJ, Blust D, O'Brien WF: Buccal versus intravaginal misoprostol administration for cervical ripening. Am J Obstet Gynecol **186**:229, 2002.

Carlan SJ, Bouldin S, Blust D, et al: Safety and efficacy of misoprostol orally and vaginally: A randomized trial. Obstet Gynecol **98**:107, 2001.

Chandra S, Crane JMG, Hutchens D, et al: Transvaginal ultrasound and digital examination in predicting successful labor induction. Obstet Gynecol **98**:2, 2001.

Clausson B, Cnattingius S, Axelsson O: Outcomes of post-term births: The role of fetal growth restriction and malformations. Obstet Gynecol **94**:758, 1999.

Clifford SH: Postmaturity—with placental dysfunction. J Pediatr **44**:1, 1954.

Crowley P: Interventions for preventing or improving the outcome of delivery at or beyond term. Cochrane Database Syst Rev 2:2000, CD000170.

Danforth DN: The fibrous nature of the human cervix, and its relation to the isthmic segment in gravid and nongravid uteri. Am J Obstet Gynecol **53**:541, 1947.

Divon M, Marks AD, Henderson CE: Longitudinal measurement of amniotic fluid index in postterm pregnancies and its association with fetal outcome. Am J Obstet Gynecol **172**:142, 1995.

Eden R, Gergely RZ, Schifrin BS, et al: Comparison of antepartum testing schemes for the management of the postdate pregnancy. Am J Obstet Gynecol **144**:683, 1982.

Eden R, Seifert L, Winegar A, et al: Perinatal characteristics of uncomplicated post-date pregnancies. Obstet Gynecol **69**:296, 1987.

Field TM, Dabiri C, Hallock N, et al: Developmental effects of prolonged pregnancy in the postmaturity syndrome. J Pediatr **90**:836, 1977.

Fischer RL, McDonnell M, Biarculli KW, et al: Amniotic fluid volume estimation in the postdate pregnancy: A comparison of techniques. Obstet Gynecol **81**:698, 1993.

Fliegner JRH, Schindler I, Brown JB: Low urinary oestriol excretion during pregnancy associated with placental sulphatase deficiency or congenital adrenal hypoplasia. J Obstet Gynaecol Br Commonw **79**:810, 1972.

France JT, Liggins GC: Placenta sulfatase deficiency. J Clin Endocrinol **29**:138, 1969.

Freeman RK, Garite TJ, Modanlou H, et al: Postdate pregnancy: Utilization of contraction stress testing for primary fetal surveillance. Am J Obstet Gynecol **140**:128, 1981.

Gardosi J, Vanner T, Francis A: Gestational age and induction of labour for prolonged pregnancy. Br J Obstet Gynaecol **104**:792, 1997.

Goeree R, Hannah ME, Hweson S: Cost-effectiveness of induction of labor versus serial antenatal monitoring in the Canadian Multicentre Postterm Pregnancy Trial. Canadian Med Assoc **152**:1445, 1995.

Guidetti DA, Divon MY, Cavalieri RL, et al: Fetal umbilical artery flow velocimetry in post-date pregnancies. Am J Obstet Gynecol **157**:1521, 1987.

Hannah ME, Hannah WJ, Hellmann J, et al: Induction of labor as compared with serial antenatal monitoring in post-term pregnancy. N Engl J Med **326**:1587, 1992.

Hauth JC, Goodman MT, Gilstrap LC III, et al: Post-term pregnancy. J Obstet Gynecol **56**:467, 1980.

Hofmeyr GJ, Gulmezoglu AM: Vaginal misoprostol for cervical ripening and induction of labour (Cochrane Review). The Cochrane Library 1:2003, CD000941.

Holm LW: Prolonged pregnancy. Adv Vet Sci **11**:159, 1967.

Johnson JM, Harman CR, Lange IR, et al: Biophysical profile scoring in the management of the post-term pregnancy. Am J Obstet Gynecol **154**:269, 1986.

Kwon JS, Davies GA, Mackenzie VP: A comparison of oral and vaginal misoprostol for induction of labour at term: A randomized trial. Br J Obstet Gynaecol **108**:23, 2001.

Le Roux PA, Olarogun JO, Penny J, et al: Oral and vaginal misoprostol compared with dinoprostone for induction of labor: a randomized controlled trial. Obstet Gynecol **99**:201, 2002.

Leveno KJ, Quirk JG, Cunningham FG, et al: Prolonged pregnancy: I. Observations concerning the causes of fetal distress. Am J Obstet Gynecol **150**:465, 1984.

Lien JM, Morgan MA, Garite TJ, et al: Antepartum cervical ripening: applying prostaglandin E2 gel in conjunction with scheduled nonstress tests in postdate pregnancies. Am J Obstet Gynecol **179**:453, 1998.

Lovell KE: The effect of postmaturity on the developing child. Med J Austr **1**:13, 1973.

Ludmir J, Sehdev HM: Anatomy and physiology of the uterine cervix. Clin Obstet Gynecol **43**:433, 2000.

Magann EF, Chauhan SP, Nevils BG, et al: Management of pregnancies beyond forty-one weeks' gestation with an unfavorable cervix. Am J Obstet Gynecol **178**:1279, 1998.

Manning FA, Morrison I, Harman CR, et al: Fetal assessment based on fetal biophysical profile scoring: Experience in 19,221 referred high risk pregnancies: II. An analysis of false negative deaths. Am J Obstet Gynecol **157**:880, 1987.

McClure-Browne JC: Post-maturity. Am J Obstet Gynecol **85**:573, 1963.

McLean FH, Boyd ME, Usher RH: Post-term infants: Too big or too small? Am J Obstet Gynecol **164**:619, 1991.

Montan S, Malcus P: Amniotic fluid index in prolonged pregnancy. J Matern Fetal Invest **5**:4, 1995.

Moore TR, Cayle JE: Amniotic fluid index in normal human pregnancy. Am J Obstet Gynecol **162**:1168, 1990.

Nakano R: Post-term pregnancy: A five year review from Osaka National Hospital. Acta Obstet Gynecol Scand **51**:217, 1972.

National Institute of Child Health and Development (NICHD) Network of Maternal-Fetal Medicine Unit: A clinical trial of induction of labor versus expectant management in postterm pregnancy. Am J Obstet Gynecol **170**:716, 1994.

Pandis GU, Papageorghiou AJ, Ramanathan JG, et al: Preinduction sonographic measurement of cervical length in the prediction of successful induction of labor. Ultrasound Obstet Gynecol **18**:623, 2001.

Phelan JP, Platt LP, Yeh S-Y, et al: The role of ultrasound assessment of amniotic fluid volume in the management of the post-date pregnancy. Am J Obstet Gynecol **151**:304, 1984.

Pollack RN, Hauer-Pollack G, Divon MY: Macrosomia in post-dates pregnancy: The accuracy of routine ultrasonographic screening. Am J Obstet Gynecol **167**:7, 1992.

Sachs BP, Friedman EA: Results of an epidemiological study of post-date pregnancy. J Reprod Med **31**:162, 1986.

Shetty A, Danielian P, Templeton A: A comparison of oral and vaginal misoprostol tablets in induction of labour at term. Br J Obstet Gynaecol **108**:238, 2001.

Shetty A, Danielian P, Templeton A: Sublingual misoprostol for the induction of labor at term. Am J Obstet Gynecol **186**:72, 2002.

Shime J, Librach CL, Gare DJ, et al: The influence of prolonged pregnancy on infant development at one and two years of age: A prospective controlled study. Amer Obstet Gynecol **154**:341, 1986.

Sue-A-Quan AK, Hannah ME, Cohen MM, et al: Effect of labour induction on rates of stillbirth and cesarean section in post-term pregnancies. CMAJ **160**:1145, 1999.

Taipale P, Hiilermaa V: Predicting delivery date by ultrasound and last menstrual period on early gestation. Obstet Gynecol **97**:189, 2001.

Usher RH, Boyd ME, McLean FH, et al: Assessment of fetal risk in post-date pregnancies. Am J Obstet Gynecol **158**:259, 1988.

Wenstrom KD, Parsons MT: The prevention of meconium aspiration in labor using amnioinfusion. Obstet Gynecol **73**:647, 1989.

Yawn BP, Wollan P, McKeon K, et al: Temporal changes in rates and reasons for medical induction of term labor, 1980–1996. Am J Obstet Gynecol **184**:611, 2001.

Zieman M, Fong SK, Benowitz NL, et al: Absorption kinetics of misoprostol with oral or vaginal administration. Obstet Gynecol **90**:88, 1997.

Zimmerman P, Alback T, Koskinen J, et al: Doppler flow velocimetry of the umbilical artery, uteroplacental arteries and fetal middle cerebral artery in prolonged pregnancy. Ultrasound Obstet Gynecol **5**:189, 1995.

Zwerdling MA: Factors pertaining to prolonged pregnancy and its outcome. Pediatrics **40**:202, 1967.

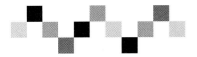

Chapter 36

CLINICAL ASPECTS OF NORMAL AND ABNORMAL LABOR

Watson A. Bowes Jr., MD, and John M. Thorp Jr., MD

NORMAL LABOR AND ITS LIMITS

The proper management of labor and delivery depends on a thorough understanding of the anatomy and physiology of normal labor. Moreover, the recognition and management of labor abnormalities require a knowledge of the limits of labor and of the physiologic response of both the mother and the fetus to the stresses of labor and delivery.

The uterus contracts throughout normal pregnancy. These contractions are irregular in timing and intensity, discoordinate in distribution, and, for the most part, entirely painless. Such uterine activity continues in normal pregnancy until late in the third trimester, when the contractions become more frequent, of greater and more consistent intensity, and more coordinated. Also, during the latter part of the third trimester, effacement (shortening) and dilation of the cervix begin. The beginning of clinical labor has been described as the onset of painful uterine contractions associated with effacement and dilation of the cervix.

The precise onset of this combination of events frequently cannot be ascertained, and for practical purposes clinicians must rely on the patient's best estimate of when her contractions began or when they became regular in consistency and intensity. The specific onset of cervical effacement and dilation can rarely be documented in cases of spontaneous onset of labor, and not uncommonly, both effacement and dilation occur late in the third trimester prior to the onset of regular or noticeable uterine contractions. The precise onset of labor is difficult to determine, and much of what is written about false labor, prodromal labor, and the latent phase of labor is influenced by this uncertainty.

Hendricks and colleagues (1970), who reported the findings of serial cervical examinations of 303 patients in the third trimester, studied these prelabor changes of the cervix. Cervical dilation began earlier and was of greater magnitude in multiparas than in primiparas. Cervical effacement, on the other hand, began earlier and was of greater magnitude in primiparas than in multiparas. These authors introduced the concept of the "cervical coefficient," which is the product of cervical dilation (in centimeters) and the percentage of effacement. They found that at any point in prelabor, the cervical coefficient is relatively the same for all patients regardless of parity. The mean cervical dilation during the last three days prior to the onset of labor is 1.8 cm for nulliparas and 2.2 cm for multiparas. Their study stressed the importance of the

prelabor preparation of the cervix and its influence on the duration of labor. It also pointed out the difficulty of using a specific time for onset of labor if it is defined as the beginning of cervical dilation.

It has been the convention to divide labor into three stages:

1. *First stage:* from onset of labor to full dilation of the cervix
2. *Second stage:* from full dilation of the cervix to delivery of the infant
3. *Third stage:* from delivery of the infant to delivery of the placenta

Pritchard and MacDonald (1980) described a fourth stage of labor as the hour following the delivery of the placenta.

One of the most thorough evaluations of the first stage of labor is that by Friedman (1978), conveniently summarized in a monograph. His graphostatistical analysis of labor in term patients (1955, 1978) depicted the relationship between the duration of labor and dilatation as a sigmoid curve reflecting its exponential nature. He divided the first stage of labor into two major phases:

1. *Latent phase:* from the onset of regular uterine contractions to the beginning of the active phase
2. *Active phase:* from the time the rate of cervical dilation begins to change rapidly to full dilation (the active phase usually begins at about 3–4 cm of dilation)

Data from several thousand patients, in whom cervical dilation and the station of the presenting fetal part were documented throughout labor, were used to establish normal limits of labor for nulliparous and multiparous patients. A group of nulliparas and a group of multiparas were selected in whom there were no apparent complications of labor and who delivered normal infants. From these cases, the norms for ideal labor were determined (Table 36-1). Descent of the fetal head in relationship to the ischial spines was found to begin well before the second stage. The rate of descent increased late in the first stage and continued linearly into the second stage of labor until the perineal floor was reached. Data for the maximum rate of descent and the length of the second stage of labor in all patients are given in Table 36-1.

Friedman formulated a series of definitions that have been incorporated into routine obstetrical care. For example, he defined no cervical dilation for 2 hours as an arrest of active phase and a rate of dilation in the active phase of 1.2 cm/hour as a protracted active phase. His work has helped generations

TABLE 36-1. CHARACTERISTICS OF LABOR IN NULLIPARAS AND MULTIPARAS*

Characteristic	Nulliparas		Multiparas	
	All Patients	**Ideal Labor**	**All Patients**	**Ideal Labor**
Duration of first stage (hr)				
Latent phase	6.4 (±5.1)	6.10 (±4.0)	4.80 (±4.9)	4.50 (±4.2)
Active phase	4.6 (±3.6)	3.40 (±1.5)	2.40 (±2.2)	2.10 (±2.0)
Total	11.0 (±8.7)	9.50 (±5.5)	7.20 (±7.1)	6.60 (±6.2)
Maximum rate of descent (cm/hr)	3.3 (±2.3)	3.60 (±1.9)	6.60 (±4.0)	7.00 (±3.2)
Duration of second stage (hr)	1.1 (±0.8)	0.76 (±0.5)	0.39 (±0.3)	0.32 (±0.3)

* All values given are ±1 SD.

Data from Friedman EA: Labor: Clinical Evaluation and Management, 2nd ed. New York, Appleton-Century-Crofts, 1978.

of obstetricians conceptualize progress in labor and provided a standardized model for intervention.

Are Friedman's labor curve and definitions applicable to populations a half century later? Numerous studies done in the last decade indicate that the pattern of labor progression is different from what was observed in the 1950s (Kilpatrick and Laros, 1989; Albers et al., 1996; Rinehart et al., 2000; Impey et al., 2000; Kelly et al., 2000) and that clinical cut points for intervention and the duration of those interventions derived from Friedman's work are no longer clinically useful (Rouse et al., 1999, 2000). Zhang, Troendle, and Yancey (2002), in a landmark paper using statistical information unavailable to Friedman, demonstrated how different contemporary labor progression is from that described in earlier years. Differences include a gradual rather than an abrupt transition from latent to active-phase labor, an active length of 5.5 hours rather than the 2.5 hours described by Friedman, no deceleration phase, the common occurrence of at least 2 hours elapsing in the active phase without cervical dilation, and the 5th percentile of rate of dilation being less than 1 cm/hour.

The findings of Zhang, Troendle, and Yancey (2002) appear in Table 36-2 and Figure 36-1. The figure allows the reader to compare Friedman's labor curves to those generated from contemporary practice. Rouse and colleagues (2000) have incorporated this finding of slower rates of progression in modern labor into a demonstration, which shows that extending the minimum period of oxytocin augmentation for active-phase labor arrest from 2 to at least 4 hours was both effective and safe.

The intelligent management of labor depends on an understanding of its mechanism as well as the norms and limits of its progress. One of the most important and helpful studies for understanding the mechanism of labor was that of Caldwell and associates (1935). This report was the culmination of a study of more than 1000 radiographic examinations of the pelvis and fetal head performed before, during, or after labor, in relation to the known details of delivery and the facts ascertained by vaginal examination. Many of the findings of this and later studies by the same authors (Caldwell et al., 1940) are incorporated in a monograph by Steer (1959).

Although a complete review of these important works is beyond the scope of this text, a study of these contributions will substantially increase one's understanding of the influence of the pelvic architecture on normal and abnormal labor.

Several of the important findings of these studies are worth reemphasizing.

With a gynecoid or android type of pelvis, the fetal head engages in the transverse position 60%–70% of the time. The anthropoid pelvis predisposes to engagement in the occiput anterior or posterior position. After the fetal head enters the pelvis in the transverse position, it is carried downward and backward until it impinges on the sacrum low in the midpelvis. It is at this point that internal rotation begins.

Internal rotation usually occurs in the midpelvis. Anterior rotation of the fetal head is practically complete when the head makes contact with the lower aspects of the pubic rami.

The common occurrence of engagement and descent predominantly in the posterior pelvis is usually associated with a normal progress of labor and spontaneous delivery; when engagement and descent occur predominantly in the forepelvis, however, there is a higher incidence of abnormal progress of labor and a higher rate of operative delivery. If the fetal head is descending in the posterior pelvis, the cervix usually is felt posteriorly in the vagina. If the cervix is palpated in a forward position, closer to the symphysis than to the sacrum, engagement and descent in the forepelvis must be suspected.

TABLE 36-2. EXPECTED TIME INTERVAL AND RATE OF CHANGE AT EACH STAGE OF CERVICAL DILATION

Cervical Dilation (cm)		Time Interval (hr)*	Rate of Cervical Dilation (cm/hr)*
To	**From**		
2	3	3.2 (0.6, 15.0)	0.3 (0.1, 1.8)
3	4	2.7 (0.6, 10.1)	0.4 (0.1, 1.8)
4	5	1.7 (0.4, 6.6)	0.6 (0.2, 2.8)
5	6	0.8 (0.2, 3.1)	1.2 (0.3, 5.0)
6	7	0.6 (0.2, 2.2)	1.7 (0.5, 6.3)
7	8	0.5 (0.1, 1.5)	2.2 (0.7, 7.1)
8	9	0.4 (0.1, 1.3)	2.4 (0.8, 7.7)
9	10	0.4 (0.1, 1.4)	2.4 (0.7, 8.3)

* Median (5th and 95th percentiles).

Data from Zhang J, Troendle J, Yancey MK: Reassessing the labor curve in nulliparous women. Am J Obstet Gynecol **187:**824, 2002. Printed with permission from CV Mosby.

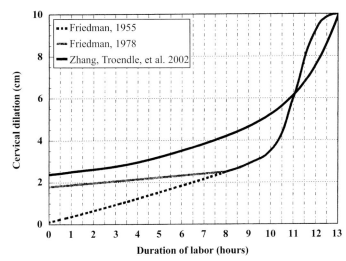

FIGURE 36-1 ■ Comparison between Friedman labor curves and the pattern of cervical dilation. (Data from Zhang J, Troendle J, Yancey MK: Reassessing the labor curve in nulliparous women. Am J Obstet Gynecol **187**:824, 2002. Printed with permission from CV Mosby.)

The increasing use of the vacuum extractor and the cesarean operation for delivery of second-stage arrest of labor has contributed to the lessening of emphasis on knowledge about pelvic types and their influence on descent and rotation of the fetal head. The relationship between pelvic architecture and the position of the fetal head, however, often allows useful prediction or explanation of abnormal labor, especially in the descent phase.

A careful clinical examination frequently discloses the essential dimensions and shape of the pelvis. In general, the characteristics of the anterior segment of the inlet correspond to the anterior portion of the lower pelvis:

- A subpubic arch with a well-rounded apex and ample space between the ischial tuberosities is associated with a gynecoid anterior segment at the inlet.
- A subpubic arch with a narrow angle and straight rami, convergent sidewalls, and prominent spines is associated with a narrowed, android anterior segment at the inlet.
- A narrow subpubic arch with straight sidewalls is characteristic of an anthropoid anterior segment at the inlet.
- A wide subpubic arch with straight or divergent sidewalls and a wide interspinous diameter is associated with a flat anterior segment at the inlet.

The posterior segment can best be characterized by palpation of the sacrospinous ligament and the sacrosciatic notch. A narrow notch, associated with a short sacrosciatic ligament (<2 fingerbreadths), suggests an android posterior segment. A sacrosciatic ligament length of 2–3 fingerbreadths suggests a gynecoid posterior segment. If the ligament is directed backward and the spines are close together, the posterior segment of the inlet is probably anthropoid. If the ligament is directed laterally and the spines are far apart, the posterior segment of the inlet is likely to be flat.

The pelvic configuration can be assessed at the time of a pelvic examination when the patient is admitted to the labor unit, or it can be part of the initial examination when the patient registers for prenatal care. The advantages of perform-

ing the assessment when the patient is hospitalized in labor are the increased relevance of the information at that time and the probability that the individual performing the examination will incorporate the results into a comprehensive assessment of the labor.

One of the most important aspects of the management of labor is accurate and thorough documentation of the progress of labor or the lack of it. Most authorities agree that a graphic display of intrapartum data that allows a prompt visualization of the status and progress of cervical dilation and, in some cases, descent of the presenting part is an essential adjunct to intrapartum patient monitoring. This can be accomplished with a simple record of cervical dilation plotted against time on ruled graph paper or by a more comprehensive recording of all intrapartum data related in graphic form to the progress of cervical dilation.

If the data about effacement and dilation of the cervix and station and position of the presenting part are recorded only in narrative form, early and significant abnormalities of labor may not be recognized as soon as if a more visual display of labor progress were available. This is especially important if more than one attendant follows the patient, as frequently occurs in a labor that is longer than normal or a labor that overlaps a change of shift in the hospital. Tabular and graphic displays of intrapartum data are entirely in keeping with the concept that labor and delivery are worthy of intensive surveillance and afford a convenient method of reviewing labor events in situations of an untoward fetal or maternal outcome.

The compulsiveness, form, and orderliness of documenting labor events need not interfere with compassionate, family-centered care of a woman in labor. In fact, the challenge of modern obstetrics is to manage a pregnancy with the least interference and yet maintain the capability of recognizing and correcting incipient complications at the earliest possible moment.

■ MANAGEMENT OF LABOR ABNORMALITIES

Abnormalities of the First Stage

Pursuant to the foregoing discussion of the problems extending Friedman's (1955, 1978) work into contemporary obstetrics when women have longer normal labors, the modern obstetrician is trapped in a conundrum of definitions, the applicability to patients of which he or she cannot be certain. Other than the recommendations of Rouse and colleagues (2000) to prolong augmentation in the face of second-stage arrest, we know of no new clinical guidelines for obstetricians to use. Moreover, Friedman's management suggestions were made without experimental verification of the hypotheses underlying his thinking. Until such desperately needed investigations are completed, Friedman's framework (1978)—in which he described labor abnormalities, identified associated problems, detailed the prognosis for the mother and fetus, and recommended a course of management—remains clinically useful.

Friedman (1978, p. 69) reported that abnormalities of the first stage of labor occurred in 8% of parturients, with a much higher incidence among primiparas than among nulliparas. Philpott and Castle (1972a) found that 11% of primiparas

TABLE 36-3. FACTORS ASSOCIATED WITH FAILURE TO PROGRESS IN THE FIRST STAGE OF LABOR

Factor	Odds Ratio	95% Confidence Interval
Premature rupture of membranes	3.8	3.2–4.5
Nulliparity	3.8	3.3–4.3
Labor induction	3.3	2.9–3.7
Maternal age > 35 years	3.0	2.6–3.6
Fetal weight > 4 kg	2.2	1.8–2.7
Hypertensive disorder	2.1	1.8–2.6
Hydramnios	1.9	1.5–2.3
Fertility treatment	1.8	1.4–2.4

Modified from Sheiner E, Levy A, Feinstein O, et al.: Risk factors and outcomes of failure to progress during the first stage of labor: A population-based study. Acta Obstet Gynecol Scand **81**(3):224, 2002, table IV. Printed with permission from Blackwell Munksgaard.

experienced abnormal labor progress in the first stage and required oxytocin augmentation. In a population-based study of 92,918 women, Sheiner and associates (2002) found that failure to progress complicated 1.3% of all labors and resulted in abdominal deliveries. Independent risk factors are listed in Table 36-3.

Prolonged Latent Phase

On the basis of the 95th percentile limit of the distribution of latent-phase duration in the primiparous population, 20 hours is considered the definition of an abnormal latent phase. For multiparas, 14 hours is the corresponding definition of prolonged latent phase. Sometimes it is difficult to ascertain the difference between a prolonged latent phase and so-called "false" labor. Friedman (1978, pp. 80–82) found that prolongation of the latent phase was associated with excessive sedation, prematurely administered epidural anesthesia, unfavorable cervical status, or myometrial dysfunction.

Although early studies suggested that prolongation of the latent phase was not associated with increased perinatal mortality and was not the harbinger of other abnormalities of labor (Friedman, 1967), subsequent studies have shown otherwise. In a study of 10,979 patients in San Francisco, Chelmow and colleagues (1993) found that prolonged latent phase of labor, defined as longer than 12 hours for nulliparous patients and longer than 6 hours for multiparous patients, was associated with an increased risk for subsequent labor abnormalities, cesarean delivery, low Apgar scores, and need for neonatal resuscitation. These risks for adverse outcomes remained significantly elevated even when the data were controlled for other labor abnormalities, prolonged rupture of membranes, meconium-stained amniotic fluid, parity, and epidural use. In addition to the increased risk of cesarean delivery, these authors found that a prolonged latent phase of labor in patients who delivered vaginally was associated with an approximately twofold increased incidence of third-degree and fourth-degree lacerations, febrile morbidity, and intrapartum blood loss.

One of the major problems with the evaluation and management of the latent phase of labor is knowing at what hour labor began. For this reason, some authorities have used the time of admission to the hospital as a convenient starting point for judging when to intervene in the progress of labor (Beazley and Kurjak, 1972; Philpott and Castle, 1972a; O'Driscoll and Meagher, 1980). Friedman (1978, p. 22), however, regarded the onset of regular contractions as the beginning of labor and recommended intervention when the duration of the latent phase of labor reached 20 hours in the primipara. He found that either adequate sedation ("therapeutic narcosis") or oxytocin augmentation resulted in the resumption of normal cervical dilation. Because most patients are exhausted after 20 hours of labor, Friedman preferred therapeutic narcosis over oxytocin augmentation. For narcosis, he recommended morphine sulfate, 15–20 mg, with 10–15 mg more if the first dose has not made the patient somnolent and therefore inhibited uterine contractions. The obvious advantage of this therapy is that the patient awakens rested and refreshed and prepared for the active phase of labor.

Critics of this approach, especially O'Driscoll and Meagher (1980), argued that waiting out 20 hours of latent phase before considering the labor abnormal only promotes exhaustion and discourages the patient. They advocated an active management of labor, which has been practiced and evaluated at the National Maternity Hospital in Dublin. This involves several important features:

1. Patients are admitted to the labor unit only when they are experiencing painful uterine contractions as well as complete effacement of the cervix, ruptured membranes, or passage of blood-stained mucus.
2. Amniotomy is performed soon after admission for patients who have intact membranes.
3. Oxytocin augmentation of labor is performed if progress of labor is less than 1 cm/hour over a 2-hour period. Oxytocin infusion is begun at 4 mU/minute and is increased by 6 mU/minute every 15 minutes until there are seven contractions per 15 minutes. The oxytocin infusion rate does not exceed 40 mU/minute.
4. Continuous electronic fetal heart rate monitoring is used only if there is meconium-stained amniotic fluid and after fetal scalp pH has been performed to rule out fetal acidosis.
5. A nurse-midwife is in constant attendance with the patient throughout labor.
6. The patient is assured that if her labor exceeds 12 hours, cesarean delivery will probably be performed.
7. The progress of labor is documented on a simple graphic form, and the senior obstetrician in charge of the unit reviews all cases daily.
8. This approach to the management of labor is confined to nulliparas.

The active management protocol, with minor modifications, has been evaluated in several obstetric services in the United States as well as in other countries. These studies have consistently demonstrated a small but significant shortening of labor associated with active management. Although most of these studies have also demonstrated a decrease in the incidence of cesarean delivery for dystocia (Akoury et al., 1988; Turner et al., 1988; Boylan et al., 1991; Lopez-Zeno et al., 1992), the largest prospective and best-designed controlled trial showed no difference in the incidence of cesarean delivery for dystocia (Frigoletto et al., 1995), but did show shortened labor and decreased maternal infection with the active management protocol.

Holmes and associates (2001) clearly demonstrated that women who present to the hospital at less than 3-cm dilation are more likely to undergo cesarean section or operative vaginal delivery than women presenting with more advanced dilation. Interestingly, they found that women presenting at less than 3-cm dilation had spent less time at home (2.0 versus 4.5 hours) since the onset of painful uterine contractions. Their results imply that women who present with reduced cervical dilation could have intrinsically different labors than those who present with more advanced dilation. Murphy and coworkers (1998) and Falzone and colleagues (1998) made similar observations, noting that nulliparous women presenting in labor with unengaged and particularly floating (above minus 3 station) fetal heads had higher risks for obstetrical intervention.

Protraction Disorders

Protraction disorders are those in which progress of cervical dilation and descent of the fetal head occur at a slower than normal rate in the active phase of labor. The rate of cervical dilation for nulliparas should be 1.2 cm or more per hour; for multiparas, it should be 1.5 cm or more. For descent of the fetal head, the rate for nulliparas should be 1.0 cm or more per hour; for multiparas, it should be 2.0 cm per hour.

Friedman (1978, pp. 89–101) found protraction disorders in primiparas to be associated frequently with cephalopelvic disproportion (CPD), use of conduction anesthesia, and fetal malposition. Whether these factors are related in a cause-and-effect manner is not known. Moreover, he found oxytocin augmentation and therapeutic narcosis of little value in these cases. Friedman also noted unusually high neonatal mortality and morbidity rates when this labor abnormality was terminated by mid-forceps delivery; however, the diagnosis of a primary dysfunctional labor (i.e., persisting at a cervical dilation rate of less than 1.2 cm/hour) is usually made in retrospect after oxytocin augmentation has been used and found not to increase the dilation rate.

The experiences of Beazley and Kurjak (1972) and O'Driscoll and Meagher (1980) suggest that an early, more active use of oxytocin, as described in the active management of labor, effectively corrects most protraction disorders, although these authors do not specifically separate the protraction disorders from the arrest disorders. Those who advocate the active management of labor explain that the use of x-ray pelvimetry is unnecessary in the nulliparous patient because rupture of the uterus does not occur with the recommended oxytocin augmentation. Therefore, in nulliparous patients with suboptimal progress of labor of any source, it is safe to use a trial of oxytocin to determine whether labor will progress to completion.

Ganström and associates (1991) have demonstrated significant differences in the collagen content and collagen remodeling in the cervix and lower uterine segment in patients with protracted labors compared with those having normal labors. This finding may explain why some patients with protracted labor do not respond to oxytocin augmentation.

Arrest Disorders

Friedman (1978, p. 102) defines an arrest disorder as the cessation of either cervical dilation or the descent of the fetal head in the active phase of labor for more than 2 hours. In their pure form, arrest disorders differ from protraction abnormalities in that prior to the arrest of progress, the rate of cervical dilation or descent of the fetal head is normal. The arrest of progress can also complicate a protraction disorder. In either situation, Friedman (1978, p. 108) found that 45% of the cases of arrest disorder were associated with CPD. Philpott and Castle (1972b) also found that patients whose labor progress crossed the "action line" (i.e., those with protraction or arrest disorders) had smaller pelvic measurements and more often required cesarean delivery for CPD.

Because of the frequent association between arrest disorders and CPD, Friedman (1978, pp. 374–377) recommended radiographic cephalopelvimetry followed by cesarean delivery for those who have CPD and oxytocin augmentation for the remainder. He found that 80% of women with arrest disorders who did not have CPD delivered following oxytocin augmentation. Philpott and Castle (1972b) and O'Driscoll and Meagher (1980) found that radiographic studies are not required, especially in primiparas, and that a trial of oxytocin augmentation is indicated in all protraction and arrest disorders. If mother and fetus are carefully monitored and if the augmentation is discontinued when there is no progress in 4–6 hours, patients are not in danger. This is the approach of most, if not all, obstetric services in the United States; and radiographic cephalopelvimetry is seldom used in the management of abnormal labor in vertex presentations (O'Brien and Cefalo, 1982; Parsons and Spellacy, 1985; Floberg et al., 1987).

A notable exception is the use of the fetal-pelvic index by Thurnau and Morgan (1988). This technique combines ultrasound measurement of the fetal head circumference (HC) and abdominal circumference (AC) and radiographic measurement of the maternal pelvic inlet circumference (IC) and midpelvic circumference (MC). The fetal-pelvic index is the sum of the two greatest positive circumference differences (HC–IC, HC–MC, AC–IC, AC–MC, respectively). A positive fetal-pelvic index value indicates the presence of fetal-pelvic disproportion, and a negative fetal-pelvic index value indicates the absence of fetal-pelvic disproportion. This index had a 94% positive predictive value for cesarean delivery of patients with abnormal labor patterns. These authors also found the fetal-pelvic index useful in predicting the success of induction of labor (Morgan and Thurnau, 1988) and the success of women attempting vaginal birth after previous cesarean delivery (Thurnau et al., 1991). Ferguson and colleagues (1998) were not able to confirm the efficacy of the fetal-pelvic index, and the method is not widely used.

Using labor progression guidelines based on the slower labor curves characteristic of modern parturients, Rouse and colleagues (1999) demonstrated the effectiveness of a new protocol to treat arrest disorders. Their protocol has three principal elements:

- An intent to achieve a sustained uterine contraction pattern of greater than 200 Montevideo units as measured by an intrauterine pressure catheter
- A minimum of 4 hours of oxytocin-augmented labor arrest with a contractions pattern of greater than 200 Montevideo units before proceeding to abdominal delivery for active phase arrest, which is more liberal than the original Friedman (1978, p. 102) cutoff of 2 hours
- For patients who cannot achieve a sustained uterine contraction pattern of greater than 200 Montevideo

units, administration of a minimum of 6 hours of oxytocin augmentation before proceeding to cesarean delivery for active-phase labor arrest

The researchers demonstrated not only the effectiveness (92% vaginal delivery rate) but also the safety of this approach, with no serious adverse maternal or perinatal effects. The only cost of liberalization of the minimums was an increased risk of maternal infection, with the risks proportional to the time elapsed.

Several authors have evaluated the effect of ambulation on the progress of labor. Flynn and coworkers (1978) found that patients who ambulated had more rapid labor with fewer instances of fetal distress than a similar number of patients who labored in bed. Williams and associates (1980), studying 48 ambulated patients, could find no differences in duration of labor or frequency of fetal distress compared with control patients. Read and colleagues (1981) studied 14 patients whose labors were regarded as requiring augmentation because of lack of progress attributed to inadequate contractions. In eight patients who were randomized to an ambulation study protocol, progress of labor was as rapid as in six control patients whose labors were augmented with oxytocin.

These studies suggest that ambulation is not detrimental to the progress of labor or the well-being of the fetus. It has not been established, however, whether ambulation is clearly beneficial or a substitute for pharmacological augmentation of labor in cases of abnormal progress.

Abnormalities of the Second Stage

Abnormalities of Rotation and Descent

Textbooks of obstetrics traditionally have discussed the first and second stages of labor as if they were separate clinical and biological entities, which, in fact, they are not. Descent and rotation of the fetal head frequently occur prior to complete dilation of the cervix, a phenomenon that is clear to most clinicians and that is confirmed by the studies of Friedman (1978, pp. 37–44). In addition to showing slower rates of cervical dilation than did Friedman, the contemporary data of Zhang, Troendle, and Yancey (2002) show a slower rate of fetal head descent. As demonstrated in Table 36-4 and Figure 36-2, it can take up to 3 hours to descend from +1/3 to +3/3 station and an additional 30 minutes for delivery. Again, there is a clear need for practice guidelines to incorporate these new data.

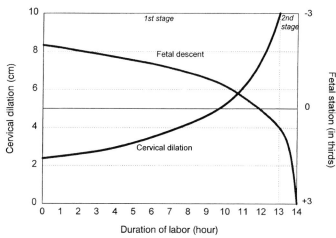

FIGURE 36-2 ■ Patterns of cervical dilation (left scale) and fetal descent (right scale) in nullipara. (From Zhang J, Troendle J, Yancey MK: Reassessing the labor curve in nulliparous women. Am J Obstet Gynecol **187**:824, 2002. Printed with permission from CV Mosby.)

Arrest of descent and rotation, whether it occurs before or after complete dilation of the cervix, is a matter of concern and requires evaluation. Arbitrary limits on the duration of the second stage of labor probably resulted from the misinterpretation of the data presented by Hellman and Prystowsky (1952). In that study, patients whose second stage of labor was longer than 2 hours were at increased risk for perinatal and maternal morbidity. This observation was interpreted by many clinicians to mean that delivery of the fetus should be accomplished, by whatever means, before 2 hours of the second stage had elapsed. This interpretation occasionally resulted in traumatic mid-forceps operations or unnecessary cesarean deliveries, not to mention the overzealous use of the vacuum extractor.

Cohen (1977) demonstrated that if patients with fetal distress or traumatic delivery are excluded, the duration of the second stage bears no relationship to perinatal outcome. If there are no serious fetal heart rate abnormalities, if the mother is well hydrated and reasonably comfortable, and if there is some progress of descent or rotation of the fetal head (regardless of how slow), there is no need for operative delivery. Similarly, Menticoglou and associates (1995) confirmed that the duration of the second stage of labor is in itself not related to untoward outcomes. Hansen and coauthors (2002), in a trial of active versus passive pushing in the second stage, found that second-stage lengths of up to 4–9 hours had no

---

TABLE 36-4. EXPECTED TIME INTERVAL AND RATE OF DESCENT AT EACH STAGE OF STATION

| Station (in Thirds) | | 1st and 2nd Stages | | 2nd Stage Only | |
From[†]	To	Time Interval (hr)*	Rate (cm/hr)*[†]	Time Interval (hr)*	Rate (cm/hr)*
−2	−1	7.9 (0.9, 65)	0.2 (0.03, 1.8)	—	—
−1	0	1.8 (0.1, 23)	0.9 (0.07, 12)	—	—
0	+1	1.4 (0.1, 13)	1.2 (0.12, 12)	—	—
+1	+2	0.4 (0.04, 3.8)	4.4 (0.44, 42)	0.27 (0.02, 2.93)	6.2 (0.57, 3.9)
+2	+3	0.1 (0.02, 0.9)	12.8 (1.9, 83)	0.11 (0.02, 0.63)	15.2 (2.6, 83)

* Median (5th and 95th percentiles).
† Measurement has been converted from thirds to fifths.

Data from Zhang J, Troendle J, Yancey MK: Reassessing the labor curve in nulliparous women. Am J Obstet Gynecol **187**:824, 2002. Printed with permission from CV Mosby.

harmful effects. Moreover, delayed pushing was better tolerated by patients and was associated with fewer fetal heart rate decelerations.

After the cervix is dilated more than 7 cm, descent or rotation of the fetal head can be expected. If this does not occur, uterine contractions, if they are not adequate, should be augmented with oxytocin. Manual examination to determine the position of the fetal head and the dimensions and shape of the pelvis often helps at this point. Posterior presentation, brow presentation, marked degrees of asynclitism, and very large infants are associated with longer labors, even with adequate contractions.

The Mueller-Hillis maneuver also may help. With one hand, the obstetrician applies pressure to the uterine fundus and with the examining finger in the vagina detects descent of the fetal head. If the fetal head descends 1 cm or more with fundal pressure, the prognosis for vaginal delivery is good; if no descent occurs, the prognosis for delivery is poor (March et al., 1996). This maneuver is not predictive of outcome if performed early in labor (Thorp et al., 1993), but it is helpful late in the first or in the second stage of labor (March et al., 1996).

Shoulder Dystocia

Shoulder dystocia occurs in 0.24%–2.00% of vaginal deliveries (Acker et al., 1986; Gross et al., 1987; Nocon et al., 1993; Basket and Allen, 1995). The cause is impingement of the biacromial diameter of the fetus against the symphysis pubis anteriorly and the sacral promontory posteriorly. Why the shoulders do not descend in the oblique diameters of the pelvis is unclear, although sometimes the fetus is simply too large. Although the risk of shoulder dystocia rises with increasing birth weight, 40%–50% of cases occur in infants whose birth weight is below 4000 g.

Risk factors for shoulder dystocia (Benedetti and Gabbe, 1978; Acker et al., 1986; Smith et al., 1994; Lewis et al., 1995) include the following:

- Fetal macrosomia
- Diabetes
- A history of shoulder dystocia in a previous birth
- Prolonged second stage of labor

Other factors that have been inconsistently reported as increasing the risk (Nocon et al., 1993; Basket and Allen, 1995; McFarland et al., 1995) include a history of the following:

- Macrosomia
- Post-term pregnancy
- Multiparity
- Obesity
- Operative vaginal delivery from the midpelvis

About 50% of patients with shoulder dystocia have no risk factors.

Maternal morbidity from shoulder dystocia includes postpartum hemorrhage and fourth-degree perineal lacerations. The morbidity for the infant is attributable to asphyxia from delay in delivery or to trauma from the maneuvers used to deliver the fetus. Infant morbidity related to trauma includes brachial plexus and phrenic nerve injuries and fractures of the humerus and clavicle (Al-Najashi et al., 1989). The most serious traumatic morbidity is brachial plexus injury (Erb palsy), which occurs in 10%–20% of infants born following shoulder dystocia (Al-Najashi et al., 1989; Nocon et al., 1993). When recognized early, 80%–90% of brachial plexus injuries recover completely with proper physical therapy and, in some situations, neurosurgical management (Sloof, 1995).

Most brachial plexus injuries resulting from shoulder dystocia involve the arm and shoulder that are in the anterior pelvis at the time of delivery. The brachial plexus is subject to injury when excessive downward traction and lateral extension of the fetal head and neck occur in the attempt to deliver the anterior shoulder (Basket and Allen, 1995); however, there are exceptions to this cause of brachial plexus injury. Some infants with brachial plexus injuries were born by vaginal delivery in which there was no evidence of shoulder dystocia (Jennet et al., 1992). Also, brachial plexus palsy can involve the arm that was in the posterior pelvis at the time of delivery (Hankins and Clark, 1995). Furthermore, Erb palsy has occurred in infants born by cesarean delivery (McFarland et al., 1986; Morrison et al., 1992). Finally, several reports describe brachial plexus injuries in newborns in whom other physical findings and electromyographic tests confirmed that the lesions occurred prior to the onset of labor (Dunn and Engle, 1985; Koenigsberger, 1980). It is postulated that these injuries resulted from chronic nerve compression from malposition *in utero* (Sandmire and DeMott, 2002; Gherman et al., 1999).

Prevention of shoulder dystocia by prophylactic induction of labor is not effective (Gonen et al., 1997). Primary cesarean delivery can prevent shoulder dystocia in a small proportion of patients when several predisposing factors are present, such as multiparity, gestational diabetes, and an estimated fetal weight in excess of 4500 g. Rouse and Owen (1999), using decision analytic techniques, concluded that prophylactic cesarean delivery for sonographically detected fetal macrosomia to prevent shoulder dystocia was a "Faustian bargain." Using either a 4000 g or 4500 g threshold as the cutoff for abdominal delivery would require over 1000 cesarean sections to prevent one permanent injury to the brachial plexus. Also, if arrest of descent of the fetal head occurs in labor along with other risk factors for shoulder dystocia, operative vaginal delivery should be avoided.

The most effective treatment includes promptly recognizing that delivery of the shoulders will be difficult and avoiding excessive downward traction on the fetal head in an attempt to deliver the anterior shoulder. Retraction of the fetal head immediately on its delivery (turtle sign) is an early warning that delivery of the shoulders will be difficult. Studies using simulated models of the fetus and pelvis demonstrated that obstetricians frequently underestimate the amount of traction they apply to the fetal head (Allen et al., 1991; Allen et al., 1994).

Several maneuvers have been useful in resolving shoulder dystocia. Hyperflexion of the mother's thighs, known as the McRoberts maneuver, flattens the lumbosacral curve, thereby removing the sacral promontory as an obstruction to the inlet (Gonik et al., 1983, 1989). The knee-chest position tends to accomplish the same end. Suprapubic pressure can be applied in conjunction with the McRoberts maneuver.

Rubin (1964) described the rotation of the fetal shoulders into the oblique position by inserting the fingers of one hand vaginally behind the most accessible shoulder (usually the posterior) and pushing the shoulder towards the fetal chest. This is a substantial improvement on the commonly described Woods maneuver, which involves pushing the shoulder toward the fetal back (Woods, 1943).

If these maneuvers are not successful, the posterior arm of the fetus can be delivered if the obstetrician inserts one hand posteriorly, grasps the elbow, and draws the arm across the chest of the fetus (Barnum, 1949). This maneuver may result in fracture of the humerus or the clavicle, which is a consistently remedial injury and preferable to a brachial plexus injury of the opposite arm. Finally, replacement of the fetal head in the uterus followed by cesarean delivery—the Zavanelli maneuver—could be necessary in rare instances (O'Leary, 1993).

Although the soft tissue of the perineum does not contribute to shoulder dystocia, many protocols recommend a wide episiotomy to facilitate performing one or more of the described maneuvers.

The successful management of shoulder dystocia is a matter of considerable obstetric judgment and skill. There is an inverse relationship between the incidence of brachial plexus injuries from shoulder dystocia and the experience of the obstetrician (Acker et al., 1988).

Abnormalities of the Third Stage

Placental Separation and Control of Uterine Bleeding

The third stage of labor is defined as the time from delivery of the infant to delivery of the placenta. For all practical purposes, one should include the hour after the delivery of the placenta in the third stage of labor because it is during this time that the patient is at greatest risk for postpartum hemorrhage.

After the infant is born, the uterus contracts, and placental separation occurs by cleavage along the plane of the decidua basalis. Placental separation usually is complete by the time two contractions have occurred, although several additional contractions may be necessary to accomplish expulsion of the placenta from the uterus. Large venous sinuses are exposed following separation of the placenta, and control of bleeding from these sinuses depends primarily on contraction of uterine muscle and only secondarily on coagulation and thrombus formation in the placental site. The average blood loss during a normal vaginal delivery is about 600 mL (Pritchard, 1965). In the young, healthy parturient, acute blood loss is well tolerated because of the increased blood volume of pregnancy and the decrease in vascular volume that occurs with the reduction of the uteroplacental circulation at the time of birth.

Management of the placenta in the third stage is a matter of debate among qualified obstetricians. Elective manual removal of the placenta, if performed promptly, has been associated with no increase in puerperal morbidity. Advantages include immediately identifying retained placental fragments and intrauterine extensions of cervical lacerations and shortening the time of placental removal (Thomas, 1963; Blanchette, 1977). Manual removal, however, is not a painless procedure in the unanesthetized patient and is unnecessarily invasive in most cases. Gentle massage of the uterine fundus encourages uterine contractions and helps one to detect changes in the shape of the uterus that signal placental separation. Vigorous fundal massage accomplishes nothing, is painful, and, when combined with excessive traction on the umbilical cord of a placenta implanted in the fundus of the uterus, could promote uterine inversion.

The prophylactic administration of a uterotonic medication to reduce blood loss, either immediately after delivery of the infant or after delivery of the placenta, is a generally accepted practice, and prospective trials show that such use decreases blood loss and reduces the need for therapeutic oxytocics (Elbourne et al., 2002). These trials also found no difference in effectiveness of ergot preparations compared with oxytocin, although there were nonsignificant trends for an increase in the need for manual removal of the placenta and blood transfusions and an increase in blood pressure associated with the use of ergot alkaloids. Intravenous oxytocin is the drug of choice on most obstetric services. The prophylactic administration of the thermostable prostaglandin E_1 analog, misoprostol, has been used to reduce bleeding in the third stage of labor (Walley et al, 2000; Ng et al., 2001; Gulmezoglu et al., 2001; Lokugamage et al., 2001).

If the placenta has not been delivered with gentle umbilical cord traction and uterine massage after 30 minutes, it should be removed manually under general anesthesia or after a tocolytic drug has been given intravenously in combination with sufficient parenteral analgesia. Nitroglycerin is particularly useful in this situation as a tocolytic (DeSimone et al., 1990). It may be given by translingual spray (400 µg/metered spray, 1–2 sprays repeated every 3–5 minutes for a maximum of three doses in 15 minutes) or by intravenous injection (50–150 µg, repeated in 30–60 seconds if blood pressure is stable).

In rare instances, placental retention could be due to placenta accreta, the result of defective decidua basalis. It is characterized by the attachment and growth of chorionic villi directly into the myometrium. If the placenta cannot be removed manually and placenta accreta is suspected, hysterectomy is usually required to avoid catastrophic hemorrhage. The etiology of placenta accreta is not known, but there is a strong association with implantation of the placenta in the lower uterine segment, placenta previa, and prior cesarean delivery.

A report of 22 cases of placenta accreta by Read and coworkers (1980) suggests that in cases of focal or partial placenta accreta without excessive blood loss, conservative management may be successful. The conservative approach includes curettage of the retained placenta or suturing of the bleeding site (in cases of cesarean delivery) and should be considered only when the preservation of fertility is of utmost importance and with the awareness that hysterectomy will be necessary if the conservative approach does not promptly control the blood loss. Descargues and associates (2001) described the role of prophylactic, selective embolization of the uterine arteries in cases of abnormal placentation diagnosed prior to delivery.

The episiotomy and vaginal or cervical lacerations are also sources of blood loss in the third stage of labor. Careful inspection of the vagina and cervix immediately after delivery allows one to identify lacerations of these structures so that they can be repaired promptly. Prompt repair also facilitates the management of an unexpected hemorrhage in the immediate recovery period by allowing the obstetrician to promptly attend to uterine atony.

In the event of an immediate postpartum hemorrhage, the patient's vital signs should be monitored frequently, adequate intravenous lines should be established promptly, adequate fluid replacement should be started with lactated Ringer's infusion, and preparations should be made for blood transfusion. Thereafter, a prompt review of possible sources of hemorrhage should be accomplished, including the following:

- Uterine atony
- Cervical, vaginal, or uterine lacerations
- Coagulopathies (spontaneous or iatrogenic)
- Adherent placenta (accreta)
- Uterine inversion

Real-time ultrasound scan is helpful in identifying retained portions of placenta or residual blood clots within the uterus.

Because the usual source of hemorrhage is uterine atony, intravenous oxytocin should be given in amounts adequate to compensate for the decreased sensitivity of the postpartum uterus to this drug (Hendricks, 1962). Usually, 20–30 units of oxytocin in 1000 mL of fluid given at an infusion rate not to exceed 100 mU/minute suffices. Because this amount of oxytocin far exceeds the threshold for its maximum antidiuretic effect (Munsick, 1970), it must be recognized that fluid overloading is a potential danger in these patients. Bolus injections of oxytocin could cause hypotension and should be avoided, especially in patients who are at risk of volume depletion from hemorrhage (Hendricks and Brenner, 1970). Methylergonovine or ergonovine maleate, given in doses of 0.2 mg intramuscularly, is often effective in maintaining uterine tonus, but such drugs should not be given intravenously because of the danger of hypertension, central nervous system vasospasm, and hemorrhage (Browning, 1974).

Increasingly, the 15-methyl analog of prostaglandin $F_{2\alpha}$ (carboprost tromethamine) is being used to treat uterine atony if oxytocin infusion is not successful (Buttino and Garite, 1986). The recommended dose is 250 μg intramuscularly, which can be repeated within a few minutes if the first injection does not suffice. Prostaglandin, particularly prostaglandin $F_{2\alpha}$, should be used with great caution, if at all, in patients with cardiovascular disease or obstructive lung disease (asthma).

Based on its demonstrated effectiveness as a prophylactic measure against hemorrhage when given in the third stage of labor equivalent to oxytocin and methergine, misoprostol has been used to manage severe postpartum hemorrhage. Abdel-Aleem and colleagues (2001) gave 1000 μg of misoprostol rectally, and Adekanmi and associates (2001) administered 800 μg of misoprostol into the uterus transvaginally to control hemorrhage. Both authors report successes after failure of conventional pharmacotherapy.

In some cases, uterine atony and uterine hemorrhage persist in spite of all measures taken to enhance uterine contractions and after other possible sources of vaginal or cervical hemorrhage have been excluded. In these situations, exploratory laparotomy is often necessary (see also Chapter 45).

During preparation for laparotomy, one can take several measures that may adequately control the hemorrhage and avoid an operative procedure:

1. A large Foley catheter balloon as a tamponade to halt bleeding from a low placental implantation site (Bowen and Beeson, 1985)
2. Packing of the uterine cavity with sterile gauze (although no well-designed study has been undertaken to prove that packing is effective, retrospective evidence indicates that this measure can control hemorrhage resulting from atony in some cases [Hester, 1975])

3. For some patients, selective embolization of pelvic vessels to control hemorrhage adequately in hospitals where the necessary facilities and personnel are available (Vedantham et al., 1997)

If all of these procedures have been tried in vain, laparotomy is performed with one or more of the following goals:

- To identify any sources of occult intra-abdominal bleeding, such as unexpected uterine laceration
- To control the bleeding by appropriate arterial ligations
- In the most extreme and refractory cases, to perform hysterectomy

When laparotomy is performed for postpartum hemorrhage, the patient should be placed in semilithotomy position. Sterile drapes should be applied in such a way that one observer can, with a sterile speculum, examine the vagina and cervix to determine when the bleeding has ceased. If major uterine lacerations are not found, the uterine arteries should be ligated by the method described by O'Leary and O'Leary (1974) (see Chapter 45). If this measure does not control uterine bleeding, the hypogastric arteries should be ligated. In 1997, B-Lynch and colleagues described a "brace" suturing technique that results in closure of the uterine blood supply. Other authors have confirmed the effectiveness of this uterine-conserving technique in small case series (Ferguson et al., 2000; Hayman et al., 2002).

Burchell (1968) described the pelvic vascular supply and demonstrated that the transient decreases in blood pressure and blood flow through regional vessels that occur at the time of internal iliac artery ligation are responsible for the control of hemorrhage. Because of the ample collateral circulation, there appear to be no long-term consequences of hypogastric artery ligation, and women have delivered normal infants in pregnancies following this procedure. Occasionally, a patient complains of mild bladder dysfunction and buttock pain in the immediate postoperative period, but these symptoms are transient.

In cases of extensive postpartum hemorrhage, the use of a central venous pressure line or a Swan-Ganz catheter facilitates more accurate monitoring of the cardiovascular status of the patient and avoids serious errors of hydration and pulmonary edema (Swan, 1975; Berkowitz and Rafferty, 1980) (see Chapter 45).

Inversion of the Uterus

Inversion of the uterus, a rare but dramatic complication of the third stage of labor and the immediate puerperium, must be recognized and corrected promptly to avoid serious long-term morbidity (Watson et al., 1980). Uterine inversion is probably related to fundal implantation of the placenta, which results in thinning of the uterine wall in the area of implantation. Fundal implantation occurs in only 10% of all pregnancies but has been found in virtually all reported cases of acute puerperal uterine inversion in which the site of placental implantation has been recorded (McCullagh, 1925; Watson et al., 1980). The thin fundal area of the myometrium invaginates as the placenta separates, whereupon the inversion proceeds, with the uterus virtually delivering itself inside out. With this scenario in mind, one can easily imagine that vigorous fundal pressure or excessive cord traction could contribute to the tendency to inversion in the uterus predisposed by fundal implantation of the placenta.

Complete uterine inversion occurs when the inverted fundus extends beyond the cervix, usually looking like a beefy-red mass at the vaginal introitus. Incomplete inversions occur when the inverted fundus has not extended beyond the external cervical os. These cases are not as obvious and may be detected only by bimanual or visual examination of the cervix. In cases of postpartum hemorrhage in which the uterine fundus cannot be palpated abdominally, incomplete uterine inversion should be suspected.

Tocolytic drugs, including magnesium sulfate (Grossman, 1981), beta-mimetic compounds (Catanzarite et al., 1986), and nitroglycerin (Altabef et al., 1992) have been used to assist in the reinversion of the uterus. Because of the extensive blood loss and shock that often are associated with uterine inversion, however, an anesthesiologist should be summoned as soon as the diagnosis is recognized so that general anesthesia will be available if reinversion using tocolysis fails.

The technique of reinversion is the same whether accomplished with intravenous tocolysis or general anesthesia. The uterus is reinverted with gentle but firm and persistent pressure applied on the fundus to elevate it into the vagina (Johnson, 1949). In most cases, this technique, which presumably results in reinversion by indirect traction on the round ligaments when the uterus is elevated into the abdomen, is successful. Authorities disagree about whether the placenta, which is often attached to the inverted fundus, should be removed prior to attempts to reinvert the fundus. The practical matter is that the Johnson technique for reinversion is easier if the placenta is not in place.

If the diagnosis is made and reinversion is accomplished promptly, there are no long-term sequelae. If the complication is unrecognized and reinversion is delayed, tissue edema magnifies the constriction of the cervix around the inverted fundus, making reinversion difficult. Tissue necrosis and damage to the bladder or urethra could ensue.

If the Johnson method of reinversion is not successful, laparotomy should be performed. The first step is to grasp the round ligaments about 1 inch into the inverted uterus and to exert traction while an assistant elevates the uterus with a hand in the vagina. This procedure, described by Huntington (1921), may fail because the inverted fundus is too tightly trapped below the cervical ring, in which case the Haultain (1901) procedure may be performed. In the Haultain procedure, a longitudinal incision is made posteriorly through the inverted fundus that allows ample room to reinvert the fundus. The incision is then closed, leaving the equivalent of a classic cesarean incision on the posterior surface of the uterus. If uterine inversion is recognized and treated promptly, an operative procedure is rarely necessary to accomplish reinversion.

The third stage of labor and the immediate puerperal recovery period are a crucial time for the parturient. Occasionally, uterine hemorrhage goes undetected or, when recognized, is treated inadequately. Acute tubular necrosis, pituitary necrosis, and adult respiratory distress syndrome—all recognized complications of puerperal shock and hypoxia—can be avoided by careful observation of all patients during this time and by deliberate and aggressive management of hemorrhage if it occurs.

■ INDUCTION OF LABOR

Induction of labor is elective (i.e., performed for the convenience of the patient or professional staff) or is indicated for medical, obstetric, or fetal complications of pregnancy.

Between 1989 and 1998 in the United States, there was an increase in the incidence of induction of labor from 9% to 19% of all births (Fig. 36-3) (Zhang, Yancey et al., 2002; MacDorman et al., 2002). In 1998, the incidence of induction of labor varied widely from region to region, from 10.9% in Hawaii to 41.6% in Wisconsin. Also, the increase in indicated induction was significantly smaller than the overall increase (70% to 100% increase), suggesting that the rate of elective induction increased more rapidly than did the rate of indicated induction.

Elective Induction

Elective induction of labor is usually justified on one or more of the following grounds:

- To assure the patient that the physician with whom she has good rapport will be present during delivery
- To ensure that labor will occur when maximum physician, nursing, and support personnel coverage is available in case of labor complications
- To enable the patient to plan for care of her home and other children and allow her partner to make suitable arrangements to be with her during labor and delivery

The studies by Keettel at the University of Iowa between 1957 and 1966 established the safety of elective induction of labor in patients who were at term and the cervix partially effaced and dilated at least 2 cm (Keettel, 1968). Subsequent studies confirmed this salutary experience (Cole et al., 1975; Tylleskär et al., 1979). Long-term follow-up studies of children as long as 8 years found no evidence of neurodevelopmental abnormalities related to elective induction of labor (Black and McBride, 1979; Friedman et al., 1979).

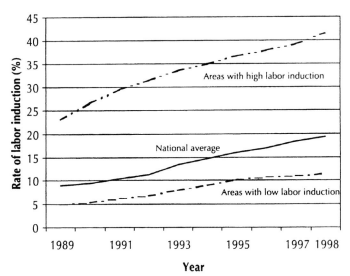

FIGURE 36-3 ■ Rate of labor induction in the United States, 1989–1998. (From Zhang J, Yancey MK, Henderson CE: U.S. national trends in labor induction, 1989–1998. J Reprod Med **47**(2):121, 2002. Printed with permission from the Journal of Reproductive Medicine.)

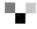

TABLE 36-5. PELVIC SCORING TABLE FOR SELECTION OF PATIENTS FOR ELECTIVE INDUCTION*

Factor	Points Assigned			
	0	1	2	3
Dilation (cm)	0	1–2	3–4	5–6
Effacement (%)	0–30	40–50	60–70	80
Station	–3	–2	–1 or 0	+1 or +2
Consistency	Firm	Medium	Soft	
Position	Posterior	Mid	Anterior	

* Total pelvic score is obtained by adding the points for each factor.

Adapted from Bishop EH: Pelvic scoring for elective induction. Obstet Gynecol 24:266, 1964.

There are two major risks of elective induction of labor: an increased risk for cesarean delivery and an increased risk for neonatal respiratory morbidity. Elective induction of labor at term is associated with a twofold increase in the incidence of cesarean delivery compared with spontaneous labor (Maslow and Sweeny, 2000; Seyb et al., 1999). The increase in the cesarean delivery rate related to elective induction of labor is confined almost entirely to nulliparous women and, more specifically, to those in whom the induction of labor is attempted when the cervix is not well effaced and somewhat dilated (Dublin et al., 2000; Heinberg et al., 2002). This risk can be minimized by restricting elective induction of labor to patients with a favorable or ripe cervix.

An objective classification for selection of patients who are "favorable" for induction of labor (Bishop, 1964) is shown in Table 36-5. Bishop found that a pelvic score of 9 or more, in the term multipara, was associated with no failed inductions of labor in his series and that the average duration of labor was 4 hours. Although the criteria for successful induction of labor as described by Bishop applied to multiparous women, subsequent studies have shown the usefulness of Bishop's scoring system in nulliparous patients (Macer et al., 1992). There is a 50% risk of failed induction of labor in nulliparous women at term, for whom the Bishop pelvic score is 5 or less. Lange and colleagues (1982), in a study of induction of labor in 808 patients, found that of the five components in the Bishop score, dilatation was the most important and recommended that it be given twice the value given by Bishop. Most experienced obstetricians would agree with this. Transvaginal ultrasound examination of the cervix does not improve upon the Bishop score in predicting the success of induction of labor (Ware and Raynor, 2000; Watson et al., 1996). The presence of fetal fibronectin (fFN) in cervical and vaginal secretions is an additional means for predicting success of induction of labor (Garite et al., 1996; Bailit et al., 2002). The role that vaginal fFN will play in selecting patients for elective induction of labor has yet to be determined.

Amniotomy is often successful in inducing labor in patients who have a favorable cervix, although the mechanism of action is not entirely clear. Mitchell and associates (1977) showed that artificial rupture of the membranes is followed by a substantial increase in plasma prostaglandins. In one of the largest studies of elective induction of labor, Keettel (1968), at the University of Iowa, found that in patients at term with a vertex presentation, the fetal vertex engaged in the pelvis, and

the cervix at least 2 cm dilated and partially effaced, only 3.4% required oxytocin infusion following amniotomy to induce labor successfully. If the use of oxytocin is necessary, it should be given by intravenous infusion, preferably by constant infusion pump, with monitoring of the fetal heart rate, uterine contractions, and maternal vital signs. Whether for elective or indicated induction of labor, adequate stimulation of uterine contractions is important in reducing the incidence of failed induction of labor. Rouse and associates (2000) showed the effectiveness of requiring a minimum of 12 hours of oxytocin stimulation after membrane rupture before failed labor induction is diagnosed.

The second major risk of elective induction of labor is neonatal respiratory morbidity (Maisels et al., 1977; Madar et al., 1999). Part of this problem is surfactant deficiency caused by unexpected delivery of a premature infant. Consequently, scrupulous attention to confirmation of gestational age is necessary. The following criteria should be fulfilled before a patient is considered a candidate for induction:

- A well-established ovulation date, which can be determined by one of the following:
  - A regular menstrual history prior to the last menstrual period. The last menstrual period should not be considered normal if it occurred following cessation of oral contraceptive use
  - Basal body temperature chart demonstrating a biphasic rise
  - Clomiphene induction of ovulation followed by early confirmation of ovulation in pregnancy
  - Artificial insemination or *in vitro* fertilization and embryo transfer
- Examination of the patient by the 14th week of pregnancy in which the uterine size was consistent with estimated gestational dates
- Sonographic estimation of fetal weight performed prior to 20 weeks' gestation
- Bishop pelvic score of 6 or more

Using these criteria, the patient should be considered for elective induction of labor 40 weeks (280 days plus or minus 3 days) after the last menstrual period (if the menstrual interval is 28 days), or 266 days plus or minus 3 days after the suspected ovulation date.

For some infants who develop respiratory morbidity after elective induction of labor, the cause is that birth takes place before the occurrence of the normal events associated with parturition that prepare the fetus for the transition to extrauterine life (Gluckman et al., 1999). One of the critical transition phenomena is a decrease in fetal lung fluid associated with the spontaneous onset of labor (Bland, 1988; McCray and Bettencourt, 1993). If this does not occur, the most common manifestation in the newborn is "wet lung syndrome" that clears spontaneously in a few hours. In some infants, the respiratory morbidity may be more serious, involving persistence of the fetal circulation and requiring mechanical ventilation (Wax et al., 2002).

Waiting until the pregnancy is at 40 weeks' gestation and the cervix is well effaced and partially dilated before induction of labor can minimize the risks of cesarean delivery and neonatal respiratory morbidity.

If an obstetrics service concludes that elective induction of labor is permissible, the professional staff, including physicians and nurses from labor and delivery and the nursery, should collectively agree on criteria for patient selection and draw up a protocol for the labor induction procedure. After such guidelines of care are established, elective induction of labor should undergo periodic review to determine the degree of compliance with the guidelines and to identify any related maternal or perinatal morbidity.

Indicated Induction

Induction of labor is indicated when prolongation of pregnancy is dangerous for either the mother or the fetus and there are no contraindications to amniotomy or the augmentation of uterine contractions. Maternal indications include the following:

- Severe pregnancy-induced hypertension
- Fetal death
- Chorioamnionitis

Fetal indications for pregnancy termination include any condition in which a variety of fetal tests demonstrate significant fetal jeopardy in any of the following complications of pregnancy:

- Diabetes mellitus
- Post-term pregnancy, especially in association with oligohydramnios
- Hypertensive complications of pregnancy
- Intrauterine growth restriction
- Isoimmunization
- Chorioamnionitis
- Premature rupture of the membranes with established fetal maturity

Induction of labor is contraindicated any time that spontaneous labor and delivery would be more dangerous for the mother or fetus than abdominal delivery. Such conditions include:

- Acute severe fetal distress
- Shoulder presentation
- Floating fetal presenting part
- Uncontrolled hemorrhage
- Placenta previa
- Previous uterine incision that would preclude a trial of labor

The following are relative contraindications to induction of labor:

- Grand multiparity (five or more previous pregnancies beyond 20 weeks' gestation)
- Multiple pregnancy
- Suspected CPD
- Breech presentation
- Inability to adequately monitor the fetal heart rate throughout labor

The relative contraindications are all controversial, and there are mitigating circumstances under which induction of labor might be attempted in any of them.

If the cervical status is favorable and the vertex is well engaged (Bishop pelvic score of 6 or more), the preferred method of labor induction is amniotomy followed, when necessary, by a closely monitored oxytocin infusion. If the cervical status is not favorable, as is common when delivery is indicated

for maternal or fetal complications, several methods may improve cervical effacement and dilatation.

Danforth (1947) was among the first to study the effect of pregnancy on the cervix and to describe the histology of cervical softening and effacement. The cervix is composed largely of connective tissue including Types I, III, and IV collagen and only 10%–15% smooth muscle (Leppert, 1995). Prior to the onset of labor, the collagen content of the cervix decreases by 30%–50% as the content of water and noncollagen and nonelastin proteins increases. The process of cervical ripening involves the production of cytokines (TNF-alpha, IL-1 beta, IL-6, IL-8) and the extravasation of neutrophils into the cervical stroma. Degranulation of the neutrophils releases proteases that are involved in the modification of cervical collagen (Winkler and Rath, 1999). The proteolytic enzymes are responsible for degrading cross-linked, newly synthesized collagen, thereby contributing to the rearrangement of collagen cells that is a hallmark of cervical softening. Apoptosis of smooth muscle cells in the cervix may also contribute to cervical ripening (Allaire et al., 2001). That this process is a genetically determined timed event may explain the length of gestation. Although the specific endocrine and biomolecular mechanisms of cervical ripening (including the role of prostaglandins) are not fully understood, the result of this phenomenon is softening, thinning, and early dilation of the cervix.

Multiple drugs and devices have been used to enhance cervical ripening: oxytocin, estrogen, corticosteroids, hyaluronidase, breast stimulation, sexual intercourse, relaxin, castor oil, prostaglandin E_1 (PGE$_1$) and E_2 (PGE$_2$), mefipristone, hydrophilic cervical inserts, balloon catheters, and extra-amniotic saline infusion. Systematic reviews of the studies of most of these methods are included in the Cochrane Database. Table 36-6 lists methods that have been found to be ineffective, unsafe, or for other reasons not commonly used. Table 36-7 summarizes the findings of the systematic reviews in the Cochrane Database regarding methods of cervical ripening that are presently in common use and for which there is some evidence of both efficacy and safety. The end points of the studies on cervical ripening include changes in the effacement and dilatation of the cervix, the time of delivery after the medication or devices is applied, and the incidence of cesarean delivery. Vaginal applications of PGE$_2$, available in the United States as dinoprostone (Prepedil and Cervidil) have been shown to be effective in promoting cervical ripening (Kelly et al., 2002c).

Misoprostol (PGE$_1$), originally approved for use in preventing NSAID-induced gastric ulcers, has proven to be an effective cervical ripening agent when applied intravaginally in doses of 25 or 50 mcg. A meta-analysis by Hofmeyr and Gulmezoglu (2002) found that misoprostol was more effective in cervical ripening and induction of labor than intravaginal or intracervical PGE$_2$. Although intravaginal misoprostol in doses of 25 mcg compared with 50 mcg results in greater need for oxytocin augmentation, there is less uterine hyperstimulation; therefore, 25 mcg doses repeated every 4 hours is the most commonly recommended regimen. In April 2002, the manufacturer of misoprostol (Cytotec) revised the drug labeling information to acknowledge the use of the medication for cervical ripening and induction of labor, although the FDA has not formally approved the drug for this use.

A systematic review of the studies of various cervical inserts, including laminaria tents and balloon catheters, found that the cervical inserts (compared with intravaginal PGE$_2$)

TABLE 36-6. CERVICAL RIPENING—METHODS EITHER INEFFECTIVE OR NOT IN COMMON USE

Method of Cervical Ripening	On-Line Source(s)	Number of Trials in the Review	Major Findings
Oxytocin	Kelly and Tan, 2002	58	Less effective than intracervical or intravaginal PGE_2
Estrogen	Thomas et al., 2002	6	Insufficient data to determine efficacy
Corticosteroids	Kavanagh et al., 2002b	2	Insufficient data to determine efficacy; not recommended for clinical practice
Hyaluronidase	Kavanagh et al., 2002c	8	Insufficient data to determine efficacy
Breast stimulation	Kavanagh et al., 2002a	6	Effective in increasing incidence of women in labor within 72 hours, but safety issues not fully evaluated
Sexual intercourse	Kavanagh et al., 2002d	6	Insufficient data to determine efficacy
Castor oil	Kelly et al., 2002a	1	No reduction in cesarean delivery rate; high incidence of side effects
Relaxin	Kelly et al., 2002b	4	Improves cervical softening and effacement but does not increase success of induction of labor; not clinically useful
Extra-amniotic prostaglandin	Hutton and Mozurkewich, 2002	10	Compared with intravaginal or intracervical PGE_2 or Foley catheter: No difference in outcomes
Intravenous prostaglandin	Luckas and Bricker, 2002	13	No more effective than IV oxytocin and has more side effects and uterine hyperstimulation
Stripping (sweeping) membranes	Boulvain, Stan, et al., 2002	17	Does not produce clinically important benefits; safe but associated with patient discomfort
Mefipristone	Neilson, 2002	7	Insufficient data to determine efficacy
Oral PGE_1	Alfirevic, 2002	13	No evidence for great efficacy than intravaginal PGE_1; doses of 100 mcg or more increase the incidence of side effects and uterine hyperstimulation
Oral PGE_2	French, 2002	19	No more effective than IV oxytocin and has more side effects

From Cochrane Database of Systemic Reviews. Available at: *http://gateway2.ovidweb.cgi.*

achieved a lower rate of delivery within 24 hours, resulted in no difference in cesarean delivery rate, and were less likely to cause uterine hyperstimulation (Boulvain, Kelly, et al., 2002). Small studies found that the use of the Foley catheter compares favorably with intravaginal PGE_1 (misoprostol) for cervical ripening (Sciscione et al., 2001), but larger prospective trials are needed to confirm this impression.

Although randomized trials have shown that prostaglandins in general and misoprostol specifically result in cervical ripening as manifest in a significant increase in the Bishop pelvic score, they have not shown a significant decrease in the incidence of failed induction of labor or a decrease in the risk of cesarean delivery following induction of labor in nulliparous patients. This suggests that failed

TABLE 36-7. CERVICAL RIPENING—METHODS COMMONLY USED

Method of Cervical Ripening	On-line Source(s)	Number of Trials in the Review	Major Findings
Mechanical methods (laminaria Foley catheter)	Boulvain, Kelly et al., 2002	45	Compared with intravaginal and intracervical PGE_2: No reduction in cesarean delivery rate, lower incidence of uterine hyperstimulation
Intravaginal and intracervical PGE_2	Kelly et al., 2002c	52	Compared with placebo: Increased incidence of vaginal delivery within 24 hours, but no decrease in cesarean delivery
Intravaginal PGE_1	Hofmeyr and Gulmezoglu, 2002	45	Compared with vaginal or cervical PGE_2: increased incidence of vaginal delivery within 24 hours, no difference in cesarean delivery rate, higher incidence of uterine hyperstimulation

From Cochrane Database of Systemic Reviews. Available at: http://gateway2.ovidweb.cgi.

induction of labor could be the result of several incomplete mechanisms of parturition, of which cervical ripening is but one manifestation.

ABNORMAL PRESENTATIONS

Breech Presentation

Breech presentation occurs in approximately 3%–4% of all deliveries. Its incidence decreases with advancing gestation. Weisman (1944), using periodic radiographic examination throughout pregnancy, found that at 18–22 weeks of gestation, 24% of fetuses were in breech presentation; at 28–30 weeks, 8%; at 34 weeks, 7%; and at 38–40 weeks, 2.8%. It is generally agreed that higher rates of neonatal morbidity and mortality are associated with breech presentation than with cephalic presentation at all gestational ages and birth weights (Brenner et al., 1974). There is less agreement as to what can be done to eliminate the risk for the infant in breech presentation at the time of delivery.

Part of the problem could be inherent in the etiology of breech presentation itself. Term breech presentation is associated with fundal-cornual implantation of the placenta, which occurs in only 7% of all pregnancies (Stevenson, 1950). This association suggests that breech presentation often is related to a space problem in the uterus, and that given the fundal-placental implantation, an otherwise normal fetus finds it more comfortable to assume a breech position. Other studies have suggested that breech presentation could result from abnormal motor ability or diminished muscle tone in the fetus.

Braun and colleagues (1975), reporting from a dysmorphology clinic, showed that the expected incidence of breech presentation (corrected for gestational age) was higher in a variety of congenital disorders. Specifically, infants with neuromuscular disorders had an inordinately high rate of breech presentation at delivery (Axelrod et al., 1974; Ralis, 1975). Furthermore, McBride and associates (1979) found that 100 children delivered in a breech presentation at term and studied at 5 years of age scored less well on motor skills than children delivered in cephalic presentations, regardless of the method by which the breech delivery was accomplished. These studies suggest that, at least in some cases, the fetus remains in a breech position because it is less capable of movement within the uterus. If these concepts are accurate, the outcome for the fetus in a breech presentation could depend to a great extent on the reason it is in the breech position rather than on the actual mode of delivery.

Some risks to the fetus inherent in breech presentation during labor and delivery include the following:

- Prolapse of the umbilical cord (especially in the footling breech)
- Trapping of the after-coming head by the incompletely dilated cervix (particularly in preterm infants weighing less than 1500 g), CPD
- Trauma resulting from extension of the head or nuchal position of the arms

Wright (1959) was the first to suggest that a policy of cesarean delivery for all breech presentations would result in the lowest possible perinatal morbidity and mortality rates. Nevertheless, most patients with a term breech presentation were delivered vaginally until the mid-1970s, when the cesarean delivery rate began to increase as the result of the concern for fetal well being. At one university center, the rate of cesarean delivery for term breech presentation abruptly increased from 13% in the years 1970–1975 to 54% in the years 1976–1977 (Bowes et al, 1979). In that study, a detailed analysis of the eight perinatal deaths that occurred in patients with a term breech presentation who delivered vaginally after having documented criteria for safe vaginal delivery found that six of the deaths would have been prevented by planned cesarean delivery. After 1975, the rate of cesarean delivery for breech presentation increased among most obstetric services in the United States. Data combined largely from retrospective cohort studies comparing vaginal with cesarean birth for patients with term breech presentations showed a small but statistically significant increase in risk of perinatal mortality and morbidity in patients who had vaginal deliveries (Bingham and Lilford, 1987; Cheng and Hannah, 1993; Hannah and Hannah, 1996).

In 2000, Hannah and colleagues published the results of a large multicenter, randomized controlled trial comparing planned vaginal delivery with planned cesarean delivery in patients with a breech presentation at term. This study of 2088 subjects was terminated when an independent data monitoring committee found statistically significant evidence that perinatal morbidity and mortality were greater with planned vaginal delivery without any significant differences in maternal mortality or serious morbidity. There were several limitations to this study:

- Less than 10% of women underwent x-ray pelvimetry (thought by many authorities to be essential in screening patients for safe vaginal delivery).
- The frequency and use of oxytocin for induction or augmentation of labor were not controlled for in the regression analyses.
- Most important, 22% of patients who delivered vaginally were not attended by an obstetrician, whereas this occurred in only one of the patients who were born by cesarean section (Hauth and Cunningham, 2002; Somerset, 2002; Keirse, 2002).

These and other limitations notwithstanding, the results of this study confirmed the mounting evidence from most of the retrospective studies that even with careful screening of patients for a trial of labor, the risk of perinatal death and serious morbidity is slightly but significantly greater for planned vaginal delivery than for planned cesarean delivery. In light of these findings, the ACOG (2001) recommends that, if external version is not successful in a woman with a breech presentation at term, the patient should be advised to undergo a planned cesarean delivery. This recommendation does not apply to patients with a second twin that is a breech presentation.

Long-term developmental outcome (5 years) of surviving infants delivered vaginally in a breech presentation does not differ significantly from those infants delivered by cesarean because of breech presentation (McBride et al., 1979; Danielian et al., 1996; Munstedt et al., 2001).

Some authorities still take the position that in the presence of a qualified obstetrician, a patient who fulfills criteria for safe vaginal delivery of a breech presentation can be offered this option (Irion et al., 1998; Kayem et al., 2002; Hauth and

Cunningham, 2002). And there may be patients in these circumstances who, with thorough knowledge of the risks and benefits, will request a trial of labor. Because of the declining frequency of breech delivery, fewer obstetricians are acquiring the requisite skills to safely allow a trial of labor and vaginal delivery for patients with breech presentations. Criteria for allowing a trial of labor in a breech presentation are as follows:

- Frank or complete breech presentation
- Estimated fetal weight of 2000–3800 g
- Normal gynecoid pelvis with adequate measurements
- Flexed fetal head

Safe vaginal delivery of a breech presentation depends, to a great extent, on the experience, judgment, and skill of the obstetrician. If an obstetrician is unsure about his or her skills for vaginal delivery with a breech presentation, a cesarean delivery is the preferred method of delivery.

Most authorities agree that radiographic pelvimetry has a place in selecting patients for a trial of labor when there is a breech presentation. Potter and coworkers (1960) studied 13 term infants without congenital defects who died of intracranial injury as a result of vaginal breech delivery. In seven of the 13 mothers, pelvic radiographs (five of which were obtained in the puerperium) revealed diminished pelvic capacity. In the remaining six patients, radiographs were not obtained.

Beischer (1966) reviewed the outcome of term breech radiographs. Thirteen patients were delivered by cesarean section; all infants survived. In the 51 infants delivered vaginally, there were four deaths, three of which were due to tentorial tears. That study, together with the report of Todd and Steer (1963) of 1006 term breech deliveries, suggests that the following are radiographic pelvic measurements below which vaginal delivery of a breech is not safe:

- Anteroposterior diameter of the inlet: 11 cm
- Widest transverse of the inlet: 12 cm
- Interspinous diameter: 9 cm

Any other encroachment on the space below the inlet also contraindicates vaginal delivery. Pelvimetry performed with computed tomography (CT) exposes the fetus to substantially less radiation and is performed with greater facility in most hospitals than conventional x-ray pelvimetry (Kopelman et al., 1986; Christian et al., 1990). Also, pelvimetry by magnetic resonance imaging (MRI) has been used for breech presentation, but the cost and the greater time required for this procedure make it less practical than pelvimetry via computed tomography (Van Loon et al., 1990).

Not uncommonly, patients are found to be in labor with an unexpected breech presentation. This will continue to occur despite the increasing practice of planned cesarean delivery for all patients with a term breech presentation. In a study by Zatuchni and Andros (1967), clinical screening of patients with breech presentations at term identified mothers who safely accomplished a vaginal delivery. Screening criteria did not include radiographic pelvimetry. On admission to the hospital in labor, patients were evaluated according to a "diagnostic index" (Table 36-8). In a prospective study of 139 patients with term breech presentations, which excluded patients with a prolapsed umbilical cord, severe congenital anomaly, or uterine bleeding, the authors found that perinatal mortality and morbidity occurred only in patients with an index of 3 or

TABLE 36-8. PROGNOSTIC INDEX FOR VAGINAL BREECH DELIVERY*

Factor	Points Assigned		
	0	**1**	**2**
Parity	0	>1	—
Gestational age (weeks)	39	38	37
Estimated fetal weight	>8 lb (3630 g)	7 lb1 oz to 7 lb 15 oz (3176–3629 g)	<7 lb (3175 g)
Previous breech deliveries (birth weight > 2500 g)	0	1	2
Dilation (cm)	2	3	4
Station	–3 or higher	–2	–1 or lower

* Index is obtained by adding the points for each factor.

Adapted from Zatuchni GI, Andros GJ: Prognostic index for vaginal delivery in breech presentation at term. Prospective study. Am J Obstet Gynecol **98**:854, 1967.

lower and that cesarean delivery of all patients with such an index would have resulted in an abdominal delivery rate of 21.5%.

The method of pain control for a vaginal breech delivery is another controversial issue. Conduction anesthesia has been used with good results (Crawford, 1974), and a case can be made that it prevents the mother from pushing uncontrollably in the second stage and allows for an easier and more comfortable application of the Piper forceps to the after-coming head. In a study of 643 single term breech presentations, however, epidural analgesia was associated with longer duration of labor, increased need for augmentation of labor with oxytocin, and a significantly higher cesarean delivery rate in the second stage of labor (Chadha et al., 1992). An anesthesiologist can be of great assistance if there is difficulty in delivery of nuchal arms or the after-coming head.

Fetal monitoring is essential during labor with a breech presentation. Because the fetal abdomen and the insertion of the umbilical cord will be in the lower uterine segment during the late first stage and the second stage of labor, significant variable decelerations are more likely to be encountered than with cephalic presentation. For this reason, membranes should be left intact as long as possible to provide some hydraulic protection against umbilical cord compression. Vaginal breech deliveries are more often associated with significant fetal acidosis than cephalic presentations (Hill et al., 1976). Therefore, one must exercise careful judgment as to when to intervene for "fetal distress." Fetal blood samples can be obtained from the buttock when there is a suspected or ominous fetal heart rate pattern, and if the pH obtained between contractions is below 7.20 early in the second stage, abdominal delivery should be considered.

The use of oxytocin for induction of labor or augmentation of abnormal labor in a breech presentation is controversial. In the randomized controlled trial by Hannah and associates (2000), a disproportionate number (64%) of the perinatal deaths in the intended vaginal delivery arm occurred in labors that were induced or augmented with oxytocin. If oxytocin is used, it must be with extraordinary caution.

Skillful, atraumatic delivery of the infant regardless of the route of birth is essential in keeping infant morbidity to a minimum. Milner (1975) showed that application of forceps to the after-coming head was associated with a reduced rate of neonatal mortality from breech delivery. The well-illustrated publication by Piper and Bachman (1929), describing the use of the forceps designed by Piper and presenting in detail the method of breech delivery, should be standard reading for all physicians planning to assist in the vaginal delivery of a breech presentation. Even when the delivery is cesarean, forceps should be available (use of Piper forceps is not necessary) and should be applied through the uterine incision to the after-coming head if there is any difficulty with its extraction. Calvert (1980) found that infants in breech presentation born by cesarean section have a higher incidence of birth asphyxia than a comparable group of infants in cephalic presentation born by cesarean. A uterine incision does not ensure an atraumatic delivery of an infant, especially a breech presentation.

External version substantially reduces the incidence of term breech presentation (Zhang et al., 1996; Hofmeyr and Kulier, 2002). When the procedure is performed at 36 weeks' gestation, the success rate is approximately 65%. Complications that require immediate delivery—including placental separation and umbilical cord compression—occur in 1%–2% of patients. The procedure is performed late in gestation and with cesarean delivery capability available so that prompt delivery can be accomplished if persistent umbilical cord compression or premature separation of the placenta occurs. Tocolytic medications have been used in most series to prevent uterine contractions during the procedure, and the evidence shows that their use improves the success rate of external version (Hofmeyr, 2002). Some have found that the use of epidural analgesia, either with the initial attempt or after a first attempt has failed, improves the success rate of external version, but the extant studies are not large enough to determine the safety of this practice or the cost effectiveness (Schorr et al., 1997; Neiger et al., 1998; Rozenberg et al., 2000).

Overall, in patients who undergo external version of a breech presentation at 36 weeks' gestation, the risk of cesarean delivery is reduced by 50%. In addition to a reduced morbidity risk for mother and infant, cost savings are substantial when external version is performed in patients with breech presentations near term (Mauldin et al., 1996). Chan and coauthors (2002) compared delivery outcomes in pregnancies that had undergone successful external cephalic version for breech presentation with deliveries in singleton vertex presentations that had not had external version. Patients following successful external version had significantly higher rates of instrumental delivery and emergency cesarean delivery. The higher risk of operative delivery was the result of an increase in several major indications: fetal heart rate abnormalities, failure of labor to progress, and failed induction of labor. It is apparent that external cephalic version, even when successful, does not eliminate all of the risks inherent in breech presentation.

Contraindications to external version include the following:

- Uterine anomalies
- Third-trimester bleeding
- Multiple gestation
- Oligohydramnios
- Evidence of uteroplacental insufficiency
- A nuchal cord as identified by ultrasonography
- Previous cesarean delivery or other significant uterine surgery
- Obvious CPD

Primiparity, maternal obesity, advanced gestation, anterior implantation of the placenta, and excessive fetal weight have been associated with decreased success of external version but are not in themselves contraindications.

The procedure should be performed in the hospital in which cesarean delivery can be accomplished if unrelenting fetal distress occurs. A real-time ultrasonographic scan is performed to confirm the breech presentation; to detect multiple gestation, oligohydramnios, or fetal abnormalities; and to measure fetal dimensions.

Following a reactive non-stress test, a tocolytic drug is administered (terbutaline sulfate, 0.25 mg subcutaneously). (Some obstetricians may first prefer to attempt version without tocolysis, and if this is unsuccessful, they proceed with external version under tocolysis.) When the uterus relaxes, the version is attempted. One person can elevate and laterally displace the breech while a second person manipulates the fetal head in the opposite direction. Mineral oil on the abdomen facilitates movement of the hands during the procedure. A forward roll is attempted, and if this is unsuccessful, a backward roll is tried. The fetal heart rate should be monitored intermittently with Doppler or with real-time scanning. Fetal bradycardia occurs in about 20% of cases but almost always subsides when the manipulation ceases. External fetal heart rate monitoring is continued for one hour, after which the patient is discharged.

Patients who are Rh-negative and who have a negative antibody titer should be given 1 unit (300 µg) of Rh immune globulin because of the risk of fetal-maternal transfusion associated with version (6%–28%) (Marcus et al., 1975; Gjode et al., 1980).

Transverse Lie (Shoulder Presentation)

Transverse lie occurs in approximately one in 300 deliveries (Seeds and Cefalo, 1982). Cruikshank and White (1973), reporting on 118 shoulder presentations, found that prematurity (38%) and high parity (87% had already borne three or more infants) were the two most frequently associated conditions. Premature rupture of membranes (30%) and placenta previa (10%) are also more common in transverse lie than in longitudinal presentation. The high perinatal mortality rates of 3.9%–24% associated with transverse lie (Seeds and Cefalo, 1982) are almost surely due to the high prevalence of low-birth-weight infants in shoulder presentations, although prolapse of the umbilical cord occasionally results in perinatal death of a term infant in transverse lie. These accidents usually happen most unexpectedly, when spontaneous rupture of the membranes occurs outside the hospital setting. In such cases, the patient is usually admitted to the hospital with a severely asphyxiated or dead fetus.

The diagnosis can usually be made by palpation of the abdomen. Not infrequently, the patient notes that the fetus is in an unusual position and draws this fact to the physician's attention. The fetal position can be confirmed by real-time ultrasonography.

Management of the patient with a confirmed diagnosis of transverse lie depends on the following factors:

1. Length of gestation
2. Size of the fetus
3. Position of the placenta
4. Whether the membranes have ruptured

If the patient is in labor with a transverse lie and the expected fetal weight and gestational age are below those compatible with a reasonable (10%) chance of survival, no intervention is necessary beyond attempts to stop labor in the interest of gaining fetal weight and maturity. A fetus of this size (usually less than 600 g) eventually is delivered vaginally in shoulder presentation (*conduplicato corpore*) without undue trauma to the mother. If the gestational age or expected fetal weight is such that the chance for neonatal survival, in the absence of severe asphyxia or trauma, is greater than 10%, cesarean delivery is usually necessary, especially if the membranes are ruptured or placenta previa is present.

The role of external version in the management of transverse lie is highly controversial. Before 36–37 weeks' gestation in patients who are not in labor, external version should not be attempted because of the danger of cord entanglement or placental trauma and the difficulty of maintaining the normal axial lie following version. Moreover, there is the possibility that spontaneous version to a longitudinal lie will occur with additional growth and maturity of the fetus or with the onset of contractions. When a transverse lie is identified at or beyond 36–37 weeks' gestation with intact membranes, however, and CPD and placenta previa are not present, external version often results in a longitudinal lie and a normal vaginal delivery.

Edwards and Nicholson (1969) demonstrated the benefits of a policy of admitting to the hospital all patients beyond 37 weeks' gestation in whom "unstable lie" is diagnosed. Their protocol in such patients was to search for etiologic factors and, in those in whom CPD and placenta previa were excluded, to perform external version followed by induction of labor after 38 weeks' gestation. In 102 patients so managed, 86 delivered vaginally with only one case of cord prolapse and no perinatal deaths. In 50 cases of unstable lie at or beyond 37 weeks' gestation in which the onset of spontaneous labor was awaited, there were 10 cases of prolapsed cord and four perinatal deaths. Their experience suggests that when a transverse or oblique lie is identified at or beyond 37 weeks' gestation, thorough etiologic evaluation and admission to the hospital should be considered.

If fetal mobility is restricted by well-advanced labor or the absence of amniotic fluid or if placenta previa or CPD is detected, abdominal delivery of transverse lie is mandatory. Most authorities advise a low vertical or classic uterine incision in such cases, although Cruikshank and White (1973) found an extraordinarily high maternal morbidity rate (21% severe intraperitoneal infection and 8.3% maternal death) to be associated with classic incisions for delivery of patients with shoulder presentations. The low transverse incision often suffices in cases of a back-up transverse lie, and the high transverse incision described by Durfee (1972) can be used in cases of a back-down shoulder presentation.

Finally, a technique of intra-abdominal version to allow use of a low transverse incision has been described (Pelosi et al., 1979). Using the transverse rather than a vertical incision decreases the overall maternal morbidity of cesarean delivery by reducing acute puerperal complications associated with vertical incisions and by allowing the option of subsequent pregnancies to be managed with a trial of labor and vaginal delivery. Uterine incision, however, should always be chosen with the primary purpose of abdominal delivery in mind (i.e., to avoid fetal trauma and asphyxia).

Deflection Abnormalities

Brow and face presentations are manifestations of different degrees of deflection of a cephalic presentation and, therefore, they can be considered together. Seeds and Cefalo (1982) reviewed the literature regarding brow and face presentations. Brow and face presentations each occur with a frequency of about one in 500 deliveries, although the incidence would likely be higher if all fetal presentations were assessed carefully early in labor. About 50% of such diagnoses are not made until the second stage of labor; many of the deflection problems detected early in labor correct themselves spontaneously as labor progresses.

With the exception of anencephaly, which almost always results in a face presentation, fetal anomalies do not seem to account for deflection problems in labor. Commonly reported etiologic factors in brow and face presentations include these:

- CPD
- Increased parity
- Prematurity
- Premature rupture of membranes

Apart from prematurity and anencephaly, the major problem associated with deflection presentations is dysfunctional labor in brow presentations. Friedman (1978, pp. 174–178) found that face presentation, contrary to generally held clinical impressions, did not appear to affect the course of labor significantly in either nulliparas or multiparas.

Brow presentation, in contrast, was associated with abnormalities of descent and longer second stage of labor compared with vertex presentation in matched controls. This is not surprising, in light of the fact that with brow presentation the largest dimension of the head—the mento-occipital diameter—must negotiate the inlet of the pelvis. Consequently, successful descent, rotation, and delivery of a brow presentation in the term infant depend on conversion to either a face or a vertex presentation. Moreover, it is often the delay in labor associated with this conversion that results in a more careful assessment of fetal position and the recognition of a brow presentation. Perinatal mortality rates for brow and face presentations are higher than for vertex presentations, but the increase can be accounted for by fetal anomalies (anencephaly), prematurity, and asphyxia and trauma associated with manipulation during vaginal delivery.

Management begins with recognition of the abnormality. An emphasis on careful vaginal examination and a description of the position and characteristics of the presenting fetal part as an essential element in labor monitoring enhance one's awareness and diagnosis of deflection problems. If on vaginal examination the lambdoid sutures and the posterior fontanelle cannot be easily identified as occupying a central position in the pelvis, an abnormal presentation or deflection of a cephalic presentation must be suspected. Palpation of the anterior fontanelle or one of the orbits clearly identifies a deflection problem. Furthermore, in cases of abnormal descent or prolonged second stage of labor, deflection of the fetal head should be considered one of the possible causes, and the patient should be reevaluated with this in mind.

When deflection of the fetal head is identified in association with abnormal progression of labor, CPD must be suspected. Friedman (1978, pp. 178–181) found that 10.9% of patients with brow presentation had clinical and radiographic evidence of CPD, compared with 2.7% of controls with vertex presentations. If progress of labor is arrested and CPD is suspected, cesarean delivery is indicated. If labor progresses and there is evidence of resolution of a brow presentation to either a face or vertex presentation, labor should be managed with the expectation of vaginal delivery. If labor is arrested and there are poor uterine contractions in the absence of CPD, the use of a carefully monitored course of oxytocin augmentation may be warranted. Seeds and Cefalo (1982) suggest that radiographic pelvimetry be considered in these situations to exclude CPD.

Most brow presentations convert spontaneously to either face or vertex presentations, and 70%–90% of face presentations result in spontaneous delivery. If the brow presentation fails to convert or the face presentation rotates to a persistent mentum posterior, cesarean delivery is required. If uncorrectable fetal distress occurs, labor should be terminated by abdominal delivery. It is generally agreed that rotating the fetal head or converting its deflection position either manually or with forceps is excessively dangerous to fetus and mother.

Compound Presentation

A compound presentation exists if an extremity is adjacent to the presenting part. This complication of labor occurs in approximately one in 1000 deliveries and is associated with high rates of prematurity (31%–61%) and fetal mortality (16%–22%) (Breen and Wiesmeier, 1968; Cruikshank and White, 1973; Weissberg and O'Leary, 1973). Cord prolapse, which occurs in 11%–20% of cases, is the most common intrapartum complication (Seeds and Cefalo, 1982). The vertex-arm combination is the most common among the compound presentations and has the best prognosis.

Management includes early diagnosis and fetal monitoring, with retraction of the presenting extremity and normal vaginal delivery occurring in the majority of patients. If fetal distress or cord prolapse occurs or labor progress ceases, abdominal delivery should be accomplished promptly. Stimulation or manipulation of the presenting extremity to encourage retraction within the uterus is controversial.

Cruikshank and White (1973) found that in 16 of 32 compound presentations the presenting extremity could be manually replaced, 15 of which resulted in uneventful vaginal deliveries. On the other hand, Seeds and Cefalo (1982), in their review of the literature regarding compound presentation, advise against manipulation of the prolapsed part. Indeed, spontaneous retraction of the extremity occurs so frequently that attempts to replace it may not be necessary and, in certain cases, may encourage prolapse of the umbilical cord.

OPERATIVE DELIVERY

Cesarean Delivery

The evolution of cesarean delivery as a safe procedure with extraordinarily low maternal and fetal mortality rates is one of the most important developments in modern perinatal medi-

cine. Maternal mortality rates from cesarean operations in the 19th century were 85% or greater, with the operation being performed only in the most extraordinary circumstances to save the life of the mother (Eastman, 1932). By the early decades of the 20th century, several important innovations in surgical care had occurred: aseptic technique, reliable anesthesia, and the control of hemorrhage by proper suturing of tissue planes as well as ligation of severed blood vessels. Specifically for the cesarean operation, introduction of the low-segment incision, which allows exclusion of the uterine wound from the peritoneal cavity, dramatically decreased the risk of postoperative peritonitis as a complication of puerperal endometritis (Frank, 1907).

The later additions of blood transfusion and antibiotic therapy further reduced the morbidity and mortality of cesarean delivery to the extent that in 1950 D'Esopo published a remarkable study reporting 1000 consecutive cesarean deliveries without a single maternal death. The decrease in maternal morbidity of cesarean delivery made the operation a reasonable alternative for delivery of the fetus at increased risk for asphyxia or trauma from labor and vaginal delivery. This decrease, together with more sophisticated methods of detecting chronic and acute fetal distress—including ultrasonography, continuous fetal heart monitoring, and fetal scalp blood sampling—changed the indications for and frequency of cesarean section for delivery.

Prior to 1960, cesarean deliveries generally constituted less than 5% of births and were performed primarily for maternal indications such as placenta previa, radiographically documented cephalopelvic disproportion (CPD), failure of induction of labor in severe preeclampsia, and repeat cesarean delivery (Smith and MacDonald, 1953). After 1960, with the emergence of fetal diagnostic and monitory techniques, cesarean delivery rates gradually increased worldwide as cesarean deliveries were more commonly performed for fetal indications (Notzon et al., 1987; Notzon, 1990). The rate and duration of the increase varied from one country to another; in the United States the rate of cesarean delivery reached a high of 23.5% in 1988 (Curtin et al., 2000). Four indications were found to account for 90% of the increase in the United States: dystocia, repeat cesarean delivery, breech presentation, and "fetal distress" (Rosen, 1981). Although new indications for cesarean delivery, such as fetal spinal or abdominal wall abnormalities and prevention of vertical transmission of certain infectious diseases, played a small role in this increase, a more important effect was a lowered threshold for the standard indications (Leitch and Walker, 1998). The fear of litigation also played a role in the rise in cesarean delivery rates, not only in the United States but also in the United Kingdom (Notzon et al., 1994). Although it has been suggested that the rate of cesarean delivery is linked to physician reimbursement, the increase in cesarean delivery rates in countries (such as Australia) that have global obstetrical fees suggest that the financial incentive alone cannot account for the rise in cesarean delivery rates (Walker et al., 2002).

In some countries, such as Brazil and Chile, the increase in the cesarean delivery rate has been well beyond that which could be accounted for by obstetrical or medical indications (Belizan et al., 1999; Potter et al., 2001). In these countries, the increase in cesarean delivery rates occurred largely as a result of an increase in prelabor elective cesarean delivery, presumably for the convenience of patients or doctors. This phenomenon has occurred primarily, though not exclusively, among women in upper income levels. There is debate as to whether this has resulted from a patient population that is well educated in the risks and benefits of vaginal versus cesarean delivery and exercising their right of patient autonomy or a patient population that has been overly influenced and biased by healthcare providers to choose cesarean delivery (Béhague et al., 2002).

In the 1990s, interest emerged in the role of cesarean delivery to prevent pelvic floor dysfunction that has been variously attributed to vaginal birth. The risk of urinary incontinence at 6 months postpartum is twofold greater for women who have a spontaneous vaginal delivery compared with those who have a cesarean delivery (Farrell et al., 2001). In a large, multicenter, prospective controlled trial of planned prelabor cesarean delivery compared with planned vaginal delivery in women with a term breech presentation, urinary incontinence was less common at 3 months postpartum in women randomized to planned cesarean delivery (RR, 0.62; 95% CI, 0.41–0.93 [Hannah et al., 2002]). The long-term effects of vaginal delivery on urinary continence are less clear-cut. Buchsbaum and colleagues (2002) found no significant difference in the incidence of urinary incontinence in nulliparous and parous postmenopausal women. In a large population-based study in Australia, MacLennan and associates (2000) found that long-term pelvic floor dysfunction, including urinary incontinence, was greater in women who had operative vaginal deliveries compared with those who had cesarean deliveries. There was, however, no difference in the incidence of pelvic floor dysfunction between those women who had cesarean deliveries and those who had spontaneous vaginal deliveries.

Sultan and colleagues (1993) found that forceps delivery and episiotomy were risk factors for anal sphincter lacerations, whereas vacuum-assisted deliveries and cesarean delivery were protective (Sultan et al., 1993). Other studies have found that cesarean deliveries were associated with a reduced incidence of fecal incontinence if they were performed before onset of the second stage of labor (Fynes et al., 1998). Associations between the method of delivery and long-term anal sphincter function are less clear. Nygarrd and associates (1997), in a 30-year follow-up study of anal incompetence, found that the aging process was as important as obstetrical events.

Notwithstanding the mounting evidence of an untoward effect of vaginal delivery (especially forceps delivery) on postpartum pelvic floor dysfunction, prospective randomized trials with adequate follow-up are necessary to adequately evaluate the effect of various methods of delivery on long-term pelvic floor function. There is currently insufficient evidence to recommend elective cesarean delivery to prevent long-term urinary or anal incontinence.

Another factor that tends to increase the cesarean delivery rate is the waning enthusiasm for a trial of labor in women who have had a previous cesarean delivery. This has occurred as a result of the increase in the number, if not the incidence, of untoward fetal and maternal consequences of uterine rupture. In the 1980s, the incidence of vaginal delivery after a previous cesarean (vaginal birth after cesarean, VBAC) increased following initiatives to control the rising cesarean delivery rate. As the incidence of VBAC increased, so did the number of physicians who had one or more experiences with a uterine rupture, even though the incidence of symptomatic scar separation remained constant at about 0.5%. Relatively large population-based retrospective studies have found the overall risk of serious maternal complications (uterine rupture, hys-

terectomy, etc.) to be from two- to threefold higher for a trial of labor after a previous cesarean compared with a repeat elective cesarean delivery (McMahon et al., 1996; Lydon-Rochelle et al., 2001c). These concerns about maternal complications related to VBAC are compounded by the results of a large population-based study from Scotland comparing perinatal outcomes (not related to congenital abnormalities) for women who had a trial of labor after a previous cesarean delivery with those who had an elective repeat cesarean delivery (Smith et al., 2002). The risk of delivery-related perinatal death in women who underwent a trial of labor (12.9/10,000) was 11 times greater than in those who had a repeat cesarean.

Finally, a number of the common risk factors for cesarean delivery—fetal macrosomia, advanced maternal age, increased maternal body mass index, gestational diabetes, multiple pregnancy, and dystocia in nulliparous women—are all increasing in frequency, especially in developed countries.

Cesarean delivery rates vary widely worldwide, from as low as 5% in Bolivia to as high as 40% in Chile (Walker et al., 2002). In the United States, the rate of cesarean deliveries declined 8% between 1991 and 1996 but has steadily increased thereafter, primarily because of a decline in vaginal births after previous cesarean deliveries (Ventura et al., 2001). It seems unlikely that the cesarean delivery rate in the United States or in most developed countries will ever be as low as 15%, which is the goal of the World Health Organization (WHO, 1985). The cesarean delivery rate will not reach this level and is likely to increase gradually for the following reasons:

- There is a heightened sensitivity to and lowered threshold for using cesarean delivery for the traditional indications.
- There is an increased proportion of pregnant women whose pregnancies are complicated by the conditions for which cesarean delivery is necessary.
- There are evolving new indications for cesarean delivery, albeit indications that are variously supported by reliable evidence.
- Emphasis on patient autonomy in making decisions about method of delivery will result in women being vulnerable to bias and non-evidenced-based information about the relative risks and benefits of cesarean delivery.
- The benefits of a trial of labor for women with a previous cesarean delivery are equivocal.
- Fear of litigation will persist in the absence of tort reform.

Complications

MATERNAL COMPLICATIONS

Although cesarean delivery is a reasonably safe surgical procedure, it is generally regarded as associated with higher risks of morbidity and mortality than vaginal delivery. Data from the Professional Activities Survey of the Commission of Professional and Hospital Activities for the year 1978, which include about 1 million births and 100,000 cesarean deliveries, showed the rates of maternal death per 100,000 births to be 9.8 for vaginal deliveries, 40.0 for all cesarean deliveries, and 18.4 for "repeat" cesarean deliveries (Rosen, 1981). Others have documented lower risks for cesarean delivery.

Sachs and colleagues (1988), reviewing cesarean delivery–related mortality in Massachusetts in the period 1954–1985, found that the rate of death directly related to cesarean birth was 5.8 per 100,000 procedures. Previously, Frigoletto and coworkers (1980) reported on 10,231 consecutive cesarean deliveries at Boston Hospital for Women between 1968 and 1978 without a single maternal death. Varying definitions of maternal mortality and failure to control for the confounding influences of parity, maternal age, and medical and obstetric complications account for some of the differences in maternal mortality rates associated with cesarean delivery. In a study of 250,000 deliveries, Lilford and associates (1990) found a sevenfold relative risk of death associated with cesarean compared with vaginal delivery when preexisting medical conditions were excluded. The same authors found that the relative risk of dying from a nonelective cesarean birth compared with an elective cesarean birth when preexisting medical conditions were excluded was 1.5. A population-based study in Washington State (1987–1997) that controlled for parity, maternal age, severe preeclampsia, and deaths unrelated to pregnancy found no significant increase in maternal mortality related to cesarean delivery (Lydon-Rochelle et al., 2001a).

It is apparent that the risks of morbidity and mortality of cesarean delivery are influenced by the associated medical complications in the patient requiring abdominal delivery and the skill of the medical team performing the procedure. Serious intra-operative complications occur in approximately 2% of cesarean deliveries and include the following (Neilsen and Hökgäard, 1984):

- Anesthesia accidents (e.g., problems with intubation, drug reactions, aspiration pneumonitis)
- Hemorrhage
- Bowel or bladder injury
- Amniotic fluid embolism
- Air embolism

Frequently, cesarean delivery must be performed under emergency conditions soon after the patient is admitted to the hospital. Patient anxiety, obesity, an incompletely emptied stomach, acute hemorrhage from a placental accident, a low blood volume and constricted vascular space in association with pregnancy-induced hypertension, and hypotension secondary to vena caval and aortic compression by the pregnant uterus are just a few of the problems frequently encountered in patients requiring emergency cesarean delivery. These problems challenge even the most skilled anesthesiologist. Emergency cesarean deliveries must often be performed with such haste that on some occasions sterile and surgical technique is compromised. Urinary tract injuries, which occur in 1–2 deliveries per thousand, are ten times more common in cesarean deliveries than in operative vaginal deliveries (Rajasekar and Hall, 1997). Most of the injuries that occur with cesarean delivery are simple bladder lacerations that are promptly identified and repaired without sequelae. Bowel injuries are often associated with intra-abdominal adhesions from previous cesarean deliveries or other abdominal surgery. Some intraoperative complications, such as amniotic fluid embolus syndrome and air embolus, are extremely rare and usually not preventable.

The following are postpartum maternal complications associated with cesarean delivery:

- Atelectasis
- Endomyometritis
- Urinary tract infection
- Abdominal wound hematoma formation, dehiscence, infection, or necrotizing fasciitis
- Thromboembolic disease
- Bowel dysfunction—adynamic ileus, pseudo-obstruction of the cecum (Ogilvie syndrome) and sigmoid vovulus

Duff (1987) found that with the use of prophylactic antibiotics, the rate of febrile puerperal complications for cesarean delivery was 5%–10% in a University obstetric service (see Chapter 39). Watson and colleagues (1997) found that febrile morbidity occurred in only 2.3% of high-risk private patients who underwent cesarean delivery. The rate of febrile morbidity in cesarean delivery patients without labor was only 0.5%. These studies emphasize that low socioeconomic status and labor are important risk factors for postpartum febrile morbidity following cesarean delivery. Postcesarean endomyometritis is a polymicrobial infection characterized by abdominal pain, malaise, anorexia, fever, uterine tenderness, and malodorous lochia. Prompt diagnosis and proper selection of antibiotic therapy for patients who become symptomatic with endomyometritis is important. In a systematic review of 47 trials comparing various antibiotic regimens for treatment of puerperal endometritis, French and Smaill (2002) found that the combination of clindamycin and gentamycin administered intravenously was more effective than other regimens. Regimens with activity against penicillin-resistant anaerobic bacteria were superior to those without. Furthermore, they found that once the clinical signs indicate improvement, oral follow-up treatment is not necessary.

Postcesarean bacteriuria occurs in approximately 11% of patients and is related largely to routine urethral catheterization (Buchholz et al., 1994). Studies have shown that the risk of urinary tract infections after cesarean delivery can be reduced substantially by eliminating catheterization or by using intermittent rather than indwelling catheterization (Tangtrakul et al., 1994; Barnes, 1998).

Wound hematomas are usually caused by faulty hemostasis and respond to drainage of the hematoma. The use of prophylactic antibiotics has substantially decreased the incidence of postcesarean abdominal wound infections, which now occur in 3% or less of cesarean deliveries (Emmons et al., 1988; Roberts et al., 1993). Cesarean deliveries performed in the second stage of labor are at greater risk for wound infection; and obesity and the use of suprafascial drains are also risk factors. Obese women are at increased risk for developing necrotizing fasciitis, one of the most serious and potentially fatal consequences of wound infection (Gallup et al., 2002). Twenty-five to 30% of wound infections are caused by *Staphylococcus aureus*, organisms that do not usually originate from wound contamination from the endometrium. For this reason, attention to sterile technique and proper wound care are essential for patients undergoing cesarean delivery.

Puerperal deep-vein thrombosis occurs in 1%–2% of patients delivered by cesarean (Bergqvist et al., 1979). Although pulmonary embolism is rare, it is one of the major causes of maternal mortality. Obesity, prolonged operative procedures, endometritis, and any inherited thrombophilia are risk factors. Treatment is intravenous heparinization followed by treatment with oral anticoagulants, the duration of which depends upon the severity of the disease and whether the patient is found to have an inherited thrombophilia. Postoperative pelvic thrombophlebitis is a diagnosis made by exclusion when puerperal fever does not respond to antibiotic therapy and the fever resolves when the patient is treated with heparin. Ovarian vein thrombosis can be recognized in patients with postoperative abdominal pain and a palpable tender mass extending from the lower quadrant into the flank, usually on the right side. Prophylactic heparinization is commonly used in the United Kingdom and Europe for both elective and emergency cesarean deliveries, but in the United States it is used only in patients at high risk for thromboembolism (Stirrup et al., 2001; Tulley et al., 2002). There is no consensus as to whether an evaluation for inherited thrombophilia should be recommended for all patients with postcesarean deep-vein thrombosis or pulmonary embolism. Clearly, such testing is in order if there is a family history of thromboembolism.

Postoperative adynamic ileus is not uncommon after cesarean section, especially if the bowel has been manipulated during the surgery. Kammen and colleagues (2000), in a study of 21 patients who had abdominal radiographs because of obstructive symptoms following cesarean delivery, found that there were radiographic signs of distal colonic obstruction in 15 of the patients. All of the 21 patients had rapid clinical and radiographic improvement on conservative management confirming the eventual diagnosis of transient postoperative ileus. A more serious problem is postcesarean pseudocolonic obstruction with marked dilation of the cecum (Ogilvie syndrome). Although the etiology and pathogenesis of this syndrome is not clear-cut, early recognition and surgical decompression are necessary to avoid rupture of the cecum (Ravo et al., 1983).

Prophylactic antibiotics, regional anesthesia, early ambulation, and intermittent rather than indwelling urethral catheterization all have contributed to reducing the incidence of postcesarean febrile complications.

The incidence of long-term complications of cesarean delivery is more difficult to document. These complications include the following:

- Cesarean delivery in a subsequent pregnancy
- Uterine rupture in a subsequent pregnancy
- Placenta previa and placenta accreta in a subsequent pregnancy
- Ectopic pregnancy
- Infertility
- Bowel obstruction resulting from intra-abdominal adhesions

In the United States, the incidence of repeat cesarean delivery is over 75%. Among women who have a trial of labor after a previous cesarean delivery in which a low-transverse uterine incision was used, the risk of uterine rupture is 0.5 to 1.0% (Flamm et al., 1994). This risk has remained remarkably constant for decades. The risk is substantially increased for the classical (i.e., fundal) cesarean incision. Ananth and associates (1997), in a systematic review of 36 studies published from 1950 through 1996, found that women who had a cesarean delivery were at two- to threefold greater risk of having a placenta previa in the subsequent pregnancy compared with women who had a vaginal delivery, and the risk increased with the number of prior cesarean deliveries (see Chapter 37).

A more recent population-based retrospective study of births in the state of Washington found a somewhat lower, but statistically significant risk of placenta previa (OR, 1.4; 95% CI, 1.1, 1.6) for the next pregnancy following a first-birth cesarean (Lydon-Rochelle et al., 2001b). Some authors also have found an association between previous cesarean delivery and placenta accreta in subsequent pregnancies, but this association is more difficult to document because of the rarity of placenta accreta (Clark et al., 1985) (see Chapter 37). Although there is controversy as to whether there is an increased risk of ectopic pregnancy following cesarean delivery, there are a number of reports of ectopic pregnancies occurring in the uterine incision (Kendrick et al., 1996; Hemminki and Meriläinen, 1996; Haimov-Kochman et al., 2002). Somewhat less controversial is the increased risk of infertility for patients delivered by cesarean (Hemminki, 1996). Postcesarean infertility is not explained by increased maternal age or by voluntary infertility, but it may be related to fallopian tube damage from postpartum infection.

Cesarean delivery also incurs added risks for infants of future pregnancies, including fetal death resulting from antepartum rupture of uterine incisions and neonatal respiratory disease associated with subsequent elective cesarean delivery as discussed next.

NEONATAL COMPLICATIONS

It appears that the safest, most atraumatic method of delivery for an infant is by cesarean section, and the increase in cesarean delivery rates after 1960 undoubtedly was, in part, the result of concerns about the dangers to the fetus of labor and vaginal delivery in certain situations. Nevertheless, abdominal delivery is also associated with uncommon but significant dangers to the infant, including the following:

- Fetal asphyxia resulting from uteroplacental hypoperfusion induced by conduction anesthesia or maternal position
- Neonatal respiratory morbidity
- Scalpel lacerations

Maternal hypotension and its deleterious effect on uteroplacental perfusion are well-known dangers of the supine position. Conduction anesthesia, by blocking vasoconstriction in the lower extremities through the sympathetic nervous system, can further reduce cardiac output and further compromise uterine blood flow. Corke and associates (1982) have demonstrated that even brief (2 minutes) episodes of hypotension result in umbilical blood gas values consistent with metabolic acidosis.

Cesarean delivery has long been recognized to be associated with an increase in neonatal respiratory morbidity at all gestational ages (Clifford, 1934; Usher et al., 1964; van den Berg et al., 2001). The frequency of this complication, its specific etiology and pathophysiology, and the mortality rate associated with it are all matters of dispute. The incidence of severe respiratory morbidity in infants born by elective cesarean delivery at term is inversely related to gestational age. Wax and colleagues (2002) found that infants born by elective cesarean delivery at 37 and 38 weeks' gestation were at 38-fold and 13-fold increased risk of severe respiratory morbidity requiring mechanical ventilation, respectively, compared with those born at 39 or 40 weeks' gestation. This syndrome could be due to a number of problems, without a clear-cut and similar pathophysiology in each case, but the common denominator is cesarean delivery, especially those performed in the absence of labor. Morrison and coauthors (1995), in a study of 33,289 deliveries at or after 37 weeks of gestation, found that the incidence of neonatal respiratory morbidity was significantly higher for the group delivered by cesarean section before labor (35.5/1000) compared with cesarean section during labor (12.2/1000) (OR, 2.9; 95% CI, 1.9, 4.4).

Some cases of respiratory morbidity following cesarean delivery are due to true iatrogenic prematurity, in which inaccurate gestational dates result unexpectedly in a premature infant. Even careful attention to the duration of pregnancy and the use of amniotic fluid tests of fetal lung maturity have not completely eliminated the problem, however. Schreiner and colleagues (1979) and Heritage and Cunningham (1985) suggest that neonatal respiratory disease following elective repeat cesarean delivery—usually manifested as mild transient tachypnea of the newborn (*wet lung syndrome*)—is, in its most severe form, persistence of the fetal circulation. These observations, together with the studies of Boon and associates (1981) demonstrating the reduced air volume in the lungs of infants delivered by cesarean compared with those delivered vaginally, suggest that the neonatal respiratory disease following cesarean delivery is due to incomplete adaptation of the fetal lung to extrauterine respiration. The specific sequence and timing for this adaptation to extrauterine cardiorespiratory status are unknown; nor is it known whether the physiologic and mechanical events of labor and delivery are necessary to complete pulmonary adaptation. The higher incidence of neonatal respiratory morbidity associated with repeat cesarean delivery in patients not in labor compared with those who are in labor suggests that labor is the signal that crucial physiologic changes have occurred to prepare a fetus for extrauterine life.

Accidental lacerations of the fetus occur in 1%–2% of cesarean deliveries (Gerber, 1974; Smith et al., 1997). The frequency of these accidents appears to be related to the experience of the surgeon, the most common situation being a well-thinned-out lower uterine segment in a patient who has ruptured membranes; in these cases, the uterus at the incision site may be only 2 mm or 3 mm thick. Usually, these inadvertent scalpel lacerations of the fetus are of only cosmetic importance, but these authors know of one infant who died as a result of a thrombosis of the sagittal sinus secondary to a scalpel incision incurred during cesarean delivery.

Indications

Reducing the frequency of maternal and neonatal complications of cesarean delivery begins with a proper respect for the dangers of the procedure and careful selection of patients to be delivered in this manner. In general, cesarean delivery is indicated any time delivery must be accomplished and when induction of labor, a trial of labor, additional labor, or vaginal delivery of the fetus is deemed to be of greater risk to the mother or the fetus than abdominal delivery. This straightforward generalization, although constituting a more rational approach than a simple list of absolute indications for the operation, does not do justice to the complexities of the decision in each case.

As the fetal indications for cesarean delivery have multiplied, so have the dilemmas of balancing the benefits and risks of operation for the two patients involved. For example, in placenta previa, vaginal delivery subjects both mother and fetus to unacceptable risks of exsanguination, and cesarean delivery is clearly in the best interests of both patients. In the case of a difficult mid-forceps delivery for fetal distress or failure of progress in the second stage of labor, however, the fetus will most certainly benefit from an expeditious abdominal delivery, and the mother's risks from the two procedures are a matter of serious debate. At the other end of the spectrum is the case of a footling breech presentation or genital herpes simplex infection, in which the operation is performed entirely for the benefit of the fetus with no advantages to the mother apart from the reassurance that it may help her infant. Countless other situations could be used as examples of the difficult decision that faces both physician and mother when evaluating the proper method of delivery. One of the most recent examples, ironically, is the interest in nulliparous patients being considered as candidates for elective cesarean delivery in the absence of the usual indications for abdominal delivery. Studies that have linked postpartum urinary and anal incontinence to vaginal delivery have encouraged some women, especially nulliparas, and their obstetricians to consider elective cesarean delivery at term to reduce the risk of pelvic floor dysfunction. Harer (2002) summarized the reasons in support of such a practice. As noted earlier in this chapter, however, there is insufficient evidence from adequate prospective trials to determine the long-term consequences of alternative methods of delivery on pelvic floor function or to support a recommendation for elective cesarean delivery to reduce the risk of urinary and anal sphincter incontinence.

The Consensus Development Statement on Cesarean Childbirth (Rosen, 1981) did much to clarify the indications for cesarean delivery and to draw attention to specific situations in which the need for cesarean delivery can be reduced by thorough evaluation of patient and facility.

The problem of dystocia, which includes both proven CPD and the less well-defined problem of "failure of labor to progress," was found to account for 30% of the increase in cesarean delivery rates in the United States. Studies by Silbar (1986) and Seitchik and colleagues (1986) found that the increase in cesarean birth rate for dystocia was due, in part, to an increased incidence of large infants causing an absolute increase in fetal-pelvic disproportion. Continuous electronic fetal heart rate monitoring contributed to the increase in cesarean delivery for "dystocia." Haverkamp and associates (1979), in a prospective controlled study of fetal heart rate monitoring, found that cesarean delivery was more often performed for dystocia in the group of patients for whom the continuous labor-fetal monitoring data were available to the physicians than in the group of patients in whom a nurse at the bedside was documenting uterine contractions and fetal heart rate data by palpation and auscultation. In the absence of data about absolute intrauterine pressure values and subtle fetal heart rate decelerations, it is tempting to speculate that there is longer and more vigorous oxytocin augmentation of desultory labors before cesarean section is considered. Or perhaps the nurse at the bedside allays anxiety and thereby contributes to a normal labor pattern and less fetal distress.

The diagnosis of fetal distress, which accounted for 10%–15% of the increase in cesarean delivery rate, is often made in the context of a labor that is not progressing normally. Zalar and Quilligan (1979) found that the use of fetal scalp blood sampling substantially reduced the number of cesarean deliveries performed for presumed fetal distress. Moreover, as experience is gained with reading fetal monitoring tracings, one is less likely to perform operative deliveries for abnormal but not necessarily ominous fetal heart rate changes. Consequently, judicious interpretation of continuous fetal heart rate monitoring data and persistent attention to factors that will improve the fetal environment often allow the additional time needed for successful labor and vaginal delivery. Garite et al. (2000) found that continuous fetal pulse oximetry in labor resulted in a 50% reduction in the number of cesarean deliveries for nonreassuring fetal status compared with controls undergoing continuous electronic fetal heart rate monitoring. Additional multicenter prospective trials of this technology, which currently are being conducted, will establish the place of fetal pulse oximetry in the conduct of labor.

The waning enthusiasm for mid-pelvic forceps deliveries has contributed to the increased number of cesarean deliveries in the "dystocia" category.

Before 1980, subsequent cesarean delivery accounted for 25%–30% of the increase in cesarean delivery rate (Rosen, 1981); however, previous cesarean delivery performed through a low transverse uterine incision for a nonrecurring indication (presumed CPD not included) need not be an indication for a subsequent cesarean delivery. In hospitals with appropriate facilities (i.e., services and staff for prompt emergency cesarean birth), a patient who has undergone previous cesarean delivery can be allowed a trial of labor.

In a meta-analysis of 31 studies that included 11,417 patients with a trial of labor after a previous low-transverse cesarean delivery, Rosen and associates (1991) found that maternal febrile morbidity was significantly lower after a trial of labor than after an elective repeat cesarean. Although the rate of rupture or dehiscence (combined) of the uterine wound was the same in patients with a trial of labor as for those with elective repeat cesareans, the odds ratio for perinatal death in all patients with a trial of labor compared with those who had undergone elective cesarean delivery was 2.1 (95% confidence interval [CI], 1.3–3.4). The intended route of delivery, the presence of an unknown type of scar, and the use of oxytocin made no difference in the rate of uterine wound dehiscence.

In a study of 6138 patients with one previous low-transverse cesarean birth, McMahon and colleagues (1996) found that major maternal complications defined as need for hysterectomy, uterine rupture, or serious operative injury occurred more often in women with a trial of labor than in those who delivered by repeat elective cesarean (odds ratio, 1.8; 95% CI, 1.1–3.0). All of the major complications occurred in women with unsuccessful vaginal birth.

Consequently, the way to decrease the overall risk associated with a trial of labor after a previous cesarean delivery is to select women who have a high probability (greater than 80%) of successful vaginal delivery. Women likely to have a successful vaginal birth after a cesarean delivery (VBAC) are those who are younger than 35 years of age, whose fetus weighs less than 4000 g, and whose previous cesarean delivery was performed for a reason other than failure of descent in the second stage of labor.

Small series of patients have addressed the question of the safety of VBAC in patients with breech presentation (Sarno et al., 1989), twin gestation (Strong et al., 1989), and postterm pregnancy (Yeh et al., 1984). Although each of these reports has noted no greater incidence of complications compared with VBAC with a vertex, term, singleton pregnancy, the small number of patients in each series demands continued caution in recommending VBAC for such patients.

Intrapartum rupture of a low transverse uterine scar, which occurs in 0.5%–1% of women who undertake a trial of labor after a cesarean delivery, is a serious emergency and can result in perinatal death (Scott, 1991). Furthermore, serious puerperal morbidity is more common in women who undergo cesarean delivery after a trial of labor than for those who undergo a repeat elective abdominal delivery (McMahon et al., 1996). After being fully informed about the risks and benefits of a trial of labor and vaginal birth after cesarean delivery, women are not universally enthusiastic. More than 25% choose to undergo another elective cesarean delivery if given the chance (Joseph et al., 1991).

Breech presentation as an indication for cesarean delivery has already been discussed. It is unlikely that the incidence of abdominal delivery for breech presentation will fall below 60%, even among obstetricians who are convinced that there is still a place in modern obstetrics for vaginal delivery of a breech presentation in selected patients.

Reducing Morbidity of Cesarean Delivery

When cesarean delivery must be performed, the following measures ensure the lowest morbidity and mortality risks for mother and infant:

- Anesthesia administered by a skilled anesthesiologist
- Attention to maternal position and blood volume in the peripartum period
- Prophylactic antibiotics
- Use of a transverse uterine incision whenever possible
- Awaiting the onset of labor whenever possible in cases of repeat cesarean delivery
- Presence of a person skilled in newborn resuscitation

Equally good neonatal and maternal outcomes from cesarean delivery can be obtained with spinal, epidural, or general anesthesia or with local infiltration, provided that it is administered by a skilled person fully aware of the unique physiologic problems of the pregnant patient and her fetus (Datta and Alper, 1980; Reisner, 1980; Abboud et al., 1985). There are, however, maternal and fetal risks associated with each method of anesthesia.

SPINAL ANESTHESIA

Spinal anesthesia is associated with the highest incidence of hypotension and should always be accompanied by uterine displacement, maternal prehydration, and (more controversially) prophylactic ephedrine administration. Lindblad and associates (1988) used Doppler ultrasound to estimate fetal aortic and umbilical blood flow in women during cesarean delivery with intrathecal anesthesia. They found that if maternal blood pressure was maintained within the normal range with preload infusion of lactated Ringer's solution and ephedrine, fetal blood flow was unaffected for 30 minutes after induction. After this time, the pulsatility index in the fetal vessels decreased. Most important for the obstetrician is the awareness that with spinal anesthesia, the time from onset of anesthesia to delivery of the infant is directly related to the degree of fetal metabolic acidosis resulting from uteroplacental hypoperfusion

(Crawford, 1965). Simply because the patient is alert is no reason to procrastinate in delivering the infant. There is perhaps as much, if not more, need for prompt delivery of the infant following spinal anesthesia as there is with general anesthesia.

EPIDURAL ANESTHESIA

Epidural anesthesia is associated with maternal hypotension less often than is spinal anesthesia. Jouppila and colleagues (1978), however, found that epidural anesthesia was associated with a decreased clearance of xenon 133, especially when hypotension occurs. The authors presume that xenon 133 clearance reflects uteroplacental perfusion. One major disadvantage of epidural block for cesarean delivery is the time required for the onset of operative anesthesia, which could preclude its use in many emergency situations. The study of Quinn and Kilpatrick (1994) of fetal outcomes in 212 consecutive cesarean deliveries demonstrated that regional anesthesia is satisfactory for urgent cesarean deliveries provided that delivery is not required within 20 minutes. Inhalation anesthesia was needed when the time interval from decision to delivery was less than 20 minutes.

GENERAL ANESTHESIA

General anesthesia, which has the advantage of rapid onset, is also associated with decreased uteroplacental perfusion during induction of the anesthesia (Jouppila et al., 1979). Pulmonary aspiration of gastric contents (Mendelson's syndrome) is always a major threat with general anesthesia, and this risk is accentuated by the delayed gastric emptying in patients in labor; Cohen (1982) reviewed this subject. There is evidence that the particulate antacids, which are commonly used preoperatively to neutralize gastric acidity, may themselves cause pulmonary damage if aspirated, and their use has not eliminated Mendelson's syndrome. A nonparticulate antacid such as sodium citrate, given 10–45 minutes before anesthesia, alone or in combination with an H_2 receptor blocker such as ranitidine, should significantly decrease the risk of aspiration without contributing added hazard (Stuart et al., 1996). Perhaps the most important safeguard against the aspiration syndrome is skillful intubation while cricoid pressure is applied.

In patients managed with general anesthesia as well as those managed with conduction anesthesia, prompt delivery of the infant is important, the crucial time being that from the incision of the uterus to delivery (Crawford et al., 1973). Delivery of the infant within 90 seconds of making the uterine incision reduces the risk of fetal hypoxemia from altered uteroplacental and umbilical blood flow.

When regional anesthesia is used, adequate volume replacement is important in preventing hypotension. Prehydration with 1000 mL of saline or lactated Ringer's injection frequently compensates for vasodilation following onset of anesthesia. The supine position is a well-known but frequently neglected danger in all pregnant women in the third trimester (Marx and Bassell, 1982). Often, during the preparation for surgery and administration of the anesthetic agent, the patient is placed flat on her back. Appropriate wedges, left lateral tilt of the table, and even operating with the patient in the lateral position have been shown to prevent supine hypotension and reduce fetal asphyxia.

In addition to the use of regional anesthesia and early ambulation, the widespread use of prophylactic antibiotics for patients undergoing a cesarean delivery has reduced the risk of puerperal morbidity (see Chapter 39). The use of prophylactic antibiotics for cesarean delivery is the subject of two extensive systematic reviews. Smaill and Hofmeyr (2002) reviewed 81 trials of women treated with prophylactic antibiotics for cesarean delivery and found a significant reduction of puerperal endometritis and wound infection compared with women who did not receive such treatment. Hopkins and Smaill (2002 reviewed 47 trials comparing various antibiotic regimens used as prophylaxis for cesarean delivery. Both ampicillin and first-generation cephalosporins were equally effective in reducing puerperal endometritis. Multiple-dose regimens were of no greater efficacy than single-dose treatment, and there was no significant difference in outcome between systemic and lavage administration. Also, there was no advantage found for using antibiotics with a broader range of activity. Although there is no conclusive evidence regarding optimal timing of administration, most obstetricians administer the medication after the umbilical cord is clamped in the interest of avoiding unnecessary exposure of the infant to an antibiotic. Finally, antibiotic prophylaxis reduces morbidity in elective cesarean delivery as well as in cesarean delivery performed in labor.

In the past, the extraperitoneal approach to cesarean delivery was used when chorioamnionitis was suspected (Hanson, 1978; Perkins, 1980). It appears that this operative technique is no longer widely taught or used, and the risks and benefits of this approach versus the standard intraperitoneal approach have not been delineated.

The advantages of the transverse over the vertical uterine incision for cesarean delivery were first recognized by Kerr (1926), who showed that low vertical incisions almost always extend into the thicker muscle layers of the fundus and are more frequently complicated by improper healing and subsequent rupture. Also, when the entire uterine incision can be covered by the bladder peritoneum, the risk of postoperative ileus, peritonitis, and subsequent adhesions and bowel obstruction is reduced.

The advantages of awaiting the onset of labor before performing a subsequent cesarean delivery are to eliminate iatrogenic prematurity and to reduce the risk of neonatal respiratory illness. Awaiting the onset of labor also results in thinning of the lower uterine segment, which decreases blood loss and facilitates development of the bladder flap during the procedure.

Finally, the presence of a professional skilled in neonatal resuscitation is essential, especially when cesarean delivery is performed for fetal distress. It is not only courteous but also often vitally important to inform the pediatrician or nursery personnel as early as possible of an impending cesarean delivery. Special equipment, drugs, and blood products may need to be assembled for a sick neonate. It is a disservice to a mother to perform a major operation in the interest of the fetus and not to follow up with the most expert care of the newborn.

Cesarean hysterectomy is occasionally lifesaving, especially in cases of uncontrolled hemorrhage from the site of a placenta previa, placenta accreta, or ruptured uterus. Cesarean hysterectomy could also be the treatment of choice in women with chorioamnionitis who desire sterilization and in whom cesarean delivery is indicated. For other indications, however, such as cervical intraepithelial neoplasia and a request for sterilization with a subsequent cesarean delivery, the operation is associated with sufficient morbidity to make its usefulness in these situations doubtful.

In a review of cesarean hysterectomy including 3913 operations, Park and Duff (1980) found the following complication rates: maternal mortality, 0.71%; bladder injury, 3%; vesicovaginal fistula, 0.4%; ureteral injury, 0.25%; and intraperitoneal bleeding requiring reoperation, 0.97%. Supracervical cesarean hysterectomy is justified in cases of life-threatening hemorrhage when the patient's vital signs are unstable. Complete removal of the cervix is one of the most difficult and time-consuming aspects of the cesarean hysterectomy procedure, especially when there has been substantial effacement and dilation of the cervix.

Obstetric Forceps Delivery

Obstetric forceps were first used by members of the Chamberlen family in the 17th century but were not widely accepted until 100 years later (Graham, 1951). William Smellie was the first to systematically teach the principles of forceps deliveries. It is clear that he also was fully aware of the potential dangers of the instruments; in the introduction to Volume II of *Treatise on the Theory and Practice of Midwifery* (Johnstone and Smellie, 1952), he wrote, "If these expedients (forceps) are used prematurely when the nature of the case does not absolutely require such assistance, the mischief that may ensue will often over balance the service for which they were intended and this consideration is one of my principal motives for publishing this second volume."

In 1988, the American College of Obstetricians and Gynecologists (ACOG) issued a Committee Opinion establishing new definitions for obstetric forceps. These definitions, which were incorporated in the ACOG Technical Bulletin entitled Operative Vaginal Delivery (1991), are as follows:

Outlet forceps:

- Scalp is visible at the introitus without separating labia.
- Fetal skull has reached pelvic floor.
- Sagittal suture is in anteroposterior diameter or right or left occiput anterior or posterior position.
- Fetal head is at or on perineum.
- Rotation does not exceed 45 degrees.

Low forceps:

- Leading point of fetal skull is at station greater than or equal to +2 cm and not on the pelvic floor.
    - Rotation is less than or equal to 45 degrees (left or right occiput anterior to occiput anterior or left or right occiput posterior to occiput posterior).
    - Rotation is greater than 45 degrees.

Mid-forceps:

- Station is above +2 cm but head is engaged.

This classification reflects what has been widely recognized among practicing obstetricians; that is, there are two types of forceps deliveries: low-forceps deliveries, which are usually simple and uncomplicated for both mother and infant, and mid-forceps deliveries, which sometimes are difficult and could cause substantial trauma to either patient.

Hagadorn-Freathy and colleagues (1991) prospectively evaluated forceps deliveries comparing outcomes as designated by the old (ACOG, 1965) and the more recent (ACOG, 1988) classifications. When the 1965 classification was used, there was no difference in outcome comparing outlet forceps deliveries with mid-forceps deliveries. When the deliveries were reclassified according to the 1988 criteria, mid-forceps deliveries were associated with lower cord pH values and a higher incidence of fetal injury compared with outlet or low-forceps deliveries. In a review of operative vaginal delivery, Bowes and Katz (1994) found that serious short-term maternal and perinatal morbidity are increased in forceps delivery when the vertex is above +2 station in the pelvis as opposed to when the vertex is at +2 station or below.

A retrospective, population-based study of 583,340 liveborn singleton infants in California found that for patients in labor for whom spontaneous vaginal delivery did not occur, there was no statistically significant difference in the incidence of neonatal intracranial hemorrhage between delivery by vacuum extraction, by forceps, or by cesarean (Towner et al., 1999). Another important finding of this study was that the incidence of serious neonatal morbidity was significantly greater when cesarean delivery followed a failed attempt at vaginal delivery with either forceps or vacuum extractor, compared with cesarean delivery after a trial of operative vaginal delivery. There were multiple limitations to this study, including the lack of information about the level of experience of those who performed the operative deliveries. Such limitations notwithstanding, this study suggests that, if spontaneous delivery cannot be accomplished safely for the mother or infant and the circumstances are not favorable for a relatively easy operative vaginal delivery, the patient should be delivered by cesarean. This contention is supported by evidence that many modern residency-training programs in obstetrics and gynecology are not providing sufficient skill in the safe use of forceps (Robson and Pridmore, 1999).

Few studies of long-term follow-up of infants delivered with forceps have been published. Friedman and colleagues (1984) published results from a collaborative perinatal project in which children delivered by mid-forceps demonstrated lower intelligence quotient (IQ) scores and a higher prevalence of suspected speech, language, and hearing abnormalities than did children born spontaneously. McBride and coworkers (1979) studied 700 5-year-old children, all of whom were born at term, 175 by mid-forceps delivery. Using a variety of neurologic, hearing, visual acuity, and development tests, these authors found no differences related to the method of delivery among the children who had been born in cephalic presentation. Dierker and associates (1986) compared 110 children 2 years of age or older who had been delivered by mid-forceps with a similar number of children of the same age delivered by cesarean section. They found five cases of abnormal development in the children delivered by mid-forceps and seven cases among those delivered by cesarean.

Seidman and coauthors (1991) related obstetric interventions to medical examinations and intelligence tests performed on more than 32,000 17-year-old men and women inducted into the Israeli Defense Forces. The mean intelligence scores for those delivered by forceps and vacuum extractor were not statistically different from those delivered spontaneously or by cesarean section.

In a retrospective study of 3417 children, Wesley and coworkers (1993) found no association of forceps deliveries (compared with spontaneous deliveries) with decreased IQ scores at 5 years of age. The studies that demonstrated no untoward long-term effect of operative vaginal delivery are those in which the infants were born after 1970. A more conservative attitude about obstetric force, which has characterized the period since the late 1970s, may have been responsible for the salutary outcomes noted in recent studies of both short-term and long-term effects of operative vaginal delivery.

Mid-forceps deliveries, as defined by the 1991 ACOG criteria, should be undertaken with caution and with a willingness to abandon the procedure in favor of cesarean delivery if there is difficulty with proper application of the instrument or if the head does not easily descend or rotate. The use and teaching of midforceps delivery under the appropriate circumstances and by an adequately trained individual is in accord with recommendations of the ACOG (2000).

Vacuum Extraction

Malmström introduced the vacuum extractor into modern obstetrics in 1954. Since that time, it has largely replaced the use of obstetric forceps in Scandinavia and continental Europe, and it is used with increasing frequency in the United States (Bofill et al., 1996). Bowes and Katz (1994) reviewed the use of the vacuum extractor for obstetric delivery. The indications for delivery with the vacuum extractor are virtually the same as those for the use of forceps:

- Arrest of labor in the second stage
- Maternal indication for shortening of the second stage of labor (e.g., cardiovascular or cerebrovascular disease, maternal exhaustion)
- Fetal distress
- Elective low pelvic delivery

Contraindications for use of the vacuum extractor include the following:

- CPD
- Face or brow presentation
- Breech presentation
- Unengaged fetal head
- Premature infant
- Incompletely dilated cervix

Maternal complications of vacuum extractor delivery, including cervical and vaginal trauma, are generally less frequent and less severe than those of forceps delivery; this is one of the major advantages of the instrument. Minor fetal complications include cephalohematomas and retinal hemorrhages, which are usually benign and self-limited. More serious complications, such as subgaleal hemorrhage (4%) and intracranial hemorrhage (2.5%), are usually associated with prolonged labor and fetal asphyxia but are probably less common than in forceps deliveries performed under the same circumstances.

Johanson and Menon (2002b) performed a systematic review of nine randomized, controlled trials comparing the vacuum extractor with forceps for assisted vaginal delivery. The authors concluded that the vacuum extractor failed to deliver the infant more often than the forceps. They also found that the vacuum extractor was associated with significantly less maternal pelvic trauma but with a greater risk for neonatal cephalhematomas and retinal hemorrhages. A 5-year follow-up study of 278 infants who were involved in a randomized, controlled trial of vacuum extraction versus forceps delivery found no statistical difference in long-term untoward effects between the methods (Johanson

et al., 1999). Almost all studies have found a substantial increase in risk of maternal and fetal morbidity when failure to deliver with the vacuum extractor is followed by an attempt to deliver with forceps. For example, Towner and colleagues (1999) found that the rate of intracranial hemorrhage was 7.4 times greater when both vacuum extraction and forceps were used compared with spontaneous delivery, and 3.4 times higher when compared to the use of the vacuum extractor as the sole instrument. Also, Gardella and associates (2001) compared 3741 combined vacuum and forceps deliveries with the same number of vacuum deliveries and forceps deliveries. These authors found that there was a significant increase in both neonatal and maternal injury with sequential use of the instruments. A recommendation to avoid the combination of vacuum extractor followed by forceps is in accord with guidelines on operative vaginal delivery published by ACOG (2002).

Two major advantages of the vacuum extractor are the ease with which it can be applied and the need for less anesthesia than is required for forceps delivery. Moreover, it is far easier to teach and to learn the appropriate skill required to use the vacuum extractor safely than to acquire a similar level of skill with forceps delivery. Many of the studies that established the comparative effectiveness and safety of the vacuum extractor compared with obstetric forceps were conducted with the Malmström metal cup or the Bird modification of the Malmström device. Currently, a variety of both rigid and soft polyethylene or silicone vacuum cups are the preferred instruments for vacuum extraction and the ones most commonly used in residency training programs in the United States (Bofill et al., 1996). Randomized trials of soft versus rigid vacuum extractor cups show that soft cups have lower success rates than rigid cups, but they are less likely to cause maternal and fetal trauma (Johanson and Menon, 2002a).

The collective evidence of the comparative efficacy and safety of vacuum extraction versus forceps has led some authorities to recommend the vacuum extractor as the instrument of first choice for operative vaginal delivery (Chalmers and Chalmers, 1989).

ANALGESIA AND ANESTHESIA FOR LOW-RISK LABOR AND VAGINAL DELIVERY

An interesting monograph by Caton (1999) and a shorter account by Caton and colleagues (2002) chronicle the history of pain relief for childbirth during the past two centuries. It is safe to say that the plight of women in labor has improved dramatically since the sixteenth century, when Eufame MacLayne, a woman of some station, was tried by due process, convicted of an act contrary to divine law, chained to a stake atop Castle Hill, and burned. Her only crime was having received "a certain medicine for the relief of pain in childbirth" (Atkinson, 1956). Until the eighteenth century, labor was conducted without the use of effective analgesia or anesthesia. The birth process was simply acknowledged to be a painful, traumatic, and often frightening experience that was to be endured with the aid of only crude and unproven potions. James Simpson, who held the Chair of Midwifery at the University of Edinburgh, was the first to administer chloroform to a woman in labor and became a champion of obstetrical anesthesia (Speert, 1996). His work, and especially his care of

Queen Victoria, who enjoyed the birth of one of her many children with the assistance of chloroform, changed both public and professional attitudes about the benefits of providing pain relief for women during labor. Modern obstetrical units, many with the service of full-time obstetrical anesthesiologists, provide a wide range of options for pain management including psycho-physiological methods, parenteral analgesia, and regional analgesia.

One of the most important assets of a modern facility offering a full range of perinatal services is the presence of a qualified obstetric anesthesiologist. The physiologic changes that characterize pregnancy result in metabolic, respiratory, and cardiovascular phenomena not encountered in the nonpregnant state. These changes, together with the presence of the fetus *in utero*, are a challenge for the anesthesiologist. Furthermore, high-risk obstetric patients frequently have fetal or maternal problems that further complicate the already difficult task of administering anesthesia to two patients simultaneously (see Chapter 59).

The choice of drug and anesthetic technique for labor and delivery depends on the skill and experience of the person who performs the procedure, the progress of labor, other complications of pregnancy or labor, and the desires of the patient. With proper antenatal psychological preparation, many patients require minimal, if any, analgesia or anesthesia throughout labor, and healthy infants are born in most of these cases. Nothing should be done to discourage such a practice. Furthermore, everything should be done to facilitate birthing in quiet, pleasant, and friendly surroundings in which a friend or family members accompany the parturient. There is considerable evidence that a supportive birth attendant (*doula*) reduces the need for analgesia and anesthesia and, in some populations, reduces the incidence of dystocia (Kennell et al., 1991; Zhang et al., 1996).

Analgesia

Sedatives and narcotic analgesics are frequently administered alone or in combination in the first stage of labor. There is increasing evidence that opioids given systemically do not relieve the pain of labor (Olofsson et al., 1996a, 1996b). These drugs do reduce anxiety and result in sedation. All drugs of this type rapidly appear in the fetal circulation when administered to the mother. Predictably, there will be some sedation of the infant, depending on the specific drug given, the amount, the time, and the route of administration.

The drug most commonly used for pain is meperidine in doses of 50–100 mg intramuscularly or 25–50 mg intravenously. To enhance its effect, provide additional sedation, and prevent nausea, physicians may prescribe a phenothiazine such as promethazine, 25 mg, as well.

The half-life of meperidine is increased and is more variable in pregnant women than in nonpregnant subjects. Furthermore, fetal hypoxia reduces clearance of meperidine from fetal blood (Barrier and Sureau, 1982). If the neonate appears depressed as the result of the administration of meperidine to the mother, injection of the narcotic antagonist naloxone may be indicated (0.1 mg/kg intravenously or intramuscularly). Other analgesics, such as butorphanol, nalbuphine, and fentanyl, all of which cause less respiratory depression, are used frequently for intrapartum pain control (Podlas and Breland, 1987; Atkinson et al., 1994; Rayburn et al., 1989).

Systematic reviews of parenteral opioids for relief of labor pain published by Elbourne and Wiseman (2002) and Bricker and Lavender (2002) include 48 trials comparing a variety of parenteral opioids with placebo, with each other, and with regional analgesia. These reviews conclude that epidural analgesia provides more effective pain relief than does parenteral analgesia. There is no clear evidence, however, that among the various drugs used for parenteral analgesia there is one medication or one method of administration that is superior to another. Long-term effects of parenteral opioids used during labor have not been studied extensively, although there is some concern about genetic imprinting at birth for later self-destructive behavior and drug addiction (Nyberg et al., 2000).

Paracervical Block

Paracervical block was a popular form of anesthesia for the first stage of labor until it was implicated in several fetal deaths and was shown to be associated with fetal bradycardia in 25%–35% of cases (Rosefsky and Petersiel, 1968; Goddard, 1971; Freeman et al., 1972). In some cases, death was related to direct injection of large doses of local anesthetic agents into the fetus, whereas the fetal bradycardia was probably a response to rapid uptake of the drug from the highly vascular paracervical space.

Although not advocated with enthusiasm by most authorities, this form of anesthesia is still used, especially in hospitals in which epidural anesthesia is not available. If paracervical block is used wisely in low-risk patients, it is safe and effective for the first stage of labor (Rosen, 2002). The anesthetic should be administered with great care to avoid direct fetal injection, with the smallest amount of drug possible. Chloroprocaine (1%–2%) rather than lidocaine or mepivacaine should be used if repeated doses will be required (Freeman and Arnold, 1975). Anyone using paracervical block anesthesia should read the excellent account of this method by Chestnut (1994).

Pudendal Block

Pudendal block is a common form of anesthesia used for vaginal delivery. When successful, it provides adequate pain relief for episiotomy, spontaneous delivery, forceps or vacuum extraction delivery from a low pelvic station, and repair of perineal, vaginal, or cervical lacerations. Because the local anesthetic agent is injected well away from the parauterine vasculature, uteroplacental blood flow and fetal heart rate are not affected to the same degree as in paracervical block. Occasionally, vaginal hematomas can be caused by pudendal nerve block, but the most dreaded complication is a retropsoas or pelvic abscess (Wenger and Gitchell, 1973; Svancarik et al., 1977). It is surprising that this complication does not occur more frequently, inasmuch as the injection is made through a nonsterile field. The infrequency of infections in Alcock's canal is probably due to the prolonged compression of the paravaginal tissues by the fetal head, which prevents hematoma formation.

The success of pudendal nerve block depends on a clear understanding of the anatomy of the pudendal nerve and surrounding structures. The anatomic study by Klink (1953) clarifies the course of the pudendal nerve, describes the variations of the nerve and its branches, and discusses the anatomy in relation to the performance of successful regional anesthesia. This article, with its helpful illustrations, is an excellent resource.

Spinal Anesthesia

Low spinal anesthesia, often called *saddle block*, is an effective means of anesthesia. It is relatively simple to perform and provides prompt, reliable pain relief that is adequate for spontaneous delivery or instrument delivery from the low pelvic or midpelvic station. It usually consists of 4 mg of tetracaine administered in a hyperbaric solution at the L4-L5 interspace with the patient sitting.

Although this technique is intended to anesthetize only the "saddle region," the level of anesthesia sometimes is as high as the T10 dermatome. Because of the ease of administration and the reliability of this form of anesthesia, it has been a favorite of obstetricians practicing in hospitals in which anesthesiologists are available only for cesarean delivery or other emergencies. As a result of the profound sympathetic block that occurs with spinal anesthesia, however, saddle block can be associated with profound hypotension and a decrease in uteroplacental perfusion. Furthermore, it could interfere with voluntary abdominal pushing effort far more than epidural anesthesia, frequently resulting in delivery of the infant by forceps. The popularity of this form of obstetric anesthesia is waning because it is being replaced by epidural anesthesia and because many patients insist on unmedicated, natural delivery.

Epidural Analgesia and Anesthesia

Epidural anesthesia is being used with increasing frequency, especially in hospitals where anesthesiologists are available to patients in labor 24 hours a day. In experienced hands, epidural anesthesia has an excellent safety record (Leighton and Halpern, 2002). Although it is the most difficult form of anesthesia to administer, it has the advantage of providing excellent pain relief for the first and second stages of labor and for delivery without altering the consciousness of the mother. Bupivacaine and chloroprocaine are the drugs most commonly used, the former providing more prolonged anesthesia but a greater delay in onset. The use of combinations of local anesthetics and narcotics also provides excellent analgesia with less motor blockade (Lysak et al., 1990).

Continuous lumbar epidural anesthesia has been associated with late decelerations in fetal heart rate suggestive of decreased uteroplacental perfusion in as many as 20% of cases. This is more common with bupivacaine than with chloroprocaine or lidocaine (Abboud et al., 1982). Also, the use of oxytocin to augment labor in cases in which continuous epidural anesthesia is used has been reported to increase the frequency of late decelerations noted on fetal monitoring (McDonald et al., 1974). When uterine hypertonus or maternal hypotension is associated with the augmentation of contractions in patients with epidural anesthesia, fetal heart rate patterns indicating uteroplacental insufficiency occur in as many as 70% of cases (Schifrin, 1972). Prehydration of the mother and avoidance of the supine position (Collins et al., 1978) can reduce the incidence of uteroplacental insufficiency with epidural anesthesia. The use of drug mixtures of local anesthetics and analgesics resulting in less motor block allows women who have epidural to be more mobile during labor and less likely to be confined to the supine position.

Thorp and Breedlove (1996) have reviewed the benefits and risks of epidural analgesia for labor and delivery. Both retrospective and prospective controlled trials have found that patients managed with epidural analgesia had longer labors and a higher incidence of operative vaginal delivery and cesarean delivery than did patients whose labors were managed with intravenous analgesia. Some studies have suggested that the untoward effect of epidural analgesia on labor is primarily in patients in whom the epidural is placed when the cervix is dilated less than 5 cm (Thorp et al., 1991); however, controlled trials by Chestnut and coauthors (1994a, 1994b) found that time of onset of epidural analgesia did not affect length of labor or method of delivery. In a retrospective case-controlled study, Thompson and colleagues (1998) showed evidence that those patients who had abnormal labor progress after epidural analgesia often had abnormal labor curves prior to placement of the epidural block.

Zhang and associates (2001) used a unique approach to determine whether epidural analgesia prolongs labor and increases the risk of cesarean delivery. A natural experiment occurred wherein the incidence of labor epidural anesthesia was suddenly increased from 1% to 84% in a brief period of time while other conditions remained unchanged. There was no resultant change in the overall abdominal delivery rates, abdominal delivery rates for dystocia, instrumental delivery rates, and the length of the first stage of labor. The second stage of labor was prolonged by a mean of 25 minutes. Moreover, on-demand epidural analgesia did not increase the risk of fetal head malposition (Yancey et al., 2001). Their work confirms the important studies of others (Bofill et al., 1997; Sharma et al., 1997; Ramin et al., 1995) in finding that labor epidural analgesia does not increase the risk of cesarean delivery or the use of oxytocin or operative vaginal delivery. The only consistent effect of epidural analgesia is prolongation of the second stage of labor. Thus, fear of increasing the risk of dystocia should not be used to limit patients' access to this effective analgesic technique.

The relationship between epidural analgesia for labor and delivery and chronic back pain following delivery is controversial. Retrospective studies have found an association between epidural analgesia for labor and chronic back pain (MacArthur et al., 1990). A more recent prospective study, however, in which women were followed for one year after delivery, found no statistically significant difference in the incidence of persistent back pain among women who had epidural analgesia during labor compared with a group of women who did not receive epidural analgesia (Macarthur et al., 1997).

Another problem encountered with epidural analgesia or anesthesia for labor is an increased incidence of intrapartum fever (Fusi et al., 1989). Fever occurs in approximately 30% of laboring patients after 4–5 hours of continuous epidural anesthesia. The specific cause of the febrile response is not known, although it could be related to the autonomic block that occurs with epidural anesthesia. Nevertheless, a clinical dilemma occurs in differentiating a "benign" febrile response to the epidural from intra-amniotic infection. As a consequence, most patients who develop a fever in labor are treated with antibiotics, and their infants are evaluated and treated for suspected sepsis (Lieberman et al., 1997). At present, there is no clear-cut way to avoid this problem.

An additional benefit of epidural anesthesia for patients undergoing cesarean delivery is that opioids can be injected into the epidural space to provide prolonged postoperative analgesia (Cousins and Mather, 1984). The rare occurrence of serious respiratory depression (1 in 1200) appears to be the only major complication. Transient nausea, urinary retention, and pruritus have also been reported in patients treated with epidural opioids.

Lieberman and O'Donoghue (2002), in a comprehensive systematic review of the unintended effects of epidural analgesia during labor, draw attention to the many unanswered questions that remain despite the large number of studies that has been performed. Because many such studies lack proper randomization to eliminate selection bias, there is a need for trials comparing epidural analgesia with other forms of analgesia wherein randomization occurs during pregnancy rather than after labor begins. Nevertheless, Lieberman and O'Donoghue contend that the current evidence supports the recommendation that women (especially nulliparous women) considering epidural analgesia for labor should be told the following:

- They are less likely to have a spontaneous vaginal delivery.
- The duration of their labor is likely to be longer.
- They will have an increased risk of having an instrument-assisted delivery, which is associated with an increased risk for serious perineal laceration.
- They are at greater risk of developing a fever during labor, which could lead to an evaluation and treatment of their infant for suspected sepsis.

There is evidence that the use of epidural anesthesia for pain control in labor is related to the size of the delivery service in hospitals in the United States (Marmor and Krol, 2002). In 1997, the use of epidural analgesia in labor was 50% among obstetric services with more than 1500 births per year, compared with 21% among obstetric units with fewer than 500 births per year. Clearly, this must reflect the more frequent availability of 24-hour coverage by anesthesiologists on the obstetric units of the larger hospitals. Proposed solutions to increase the availability of epidural anesthesia for women in labor include certified registered nurse anesthetists (CRNAs) or adequately trained obstetricians being allowed to perform epidural. Both of these possible solutions have economic and medico-legal ramifications that must be considered.

LABOR MONITORING

The term *fetal monitoring* has become almost synonymous with continuous electronic fetal monitoring (see Chapter 22). The more comprehensive term *labor monitoring* means the conduct and management of the labor event from its onset to its completion. The primary goal of labor monitoring is to achieve delivery of a healthy infant from a healthy mother with as little trauma as possible. A secondary goal is to accomplish this delivery in a manner that is not degrading to the mother and that enhances and strengthens family relationships in a way that is consistent with the cultural and personal expectations of the patient. In a narrower context, this latter goal has been defined as "reducing bonding failure" (Ounsted et al., 1982). Certainly, a healthy and supportive family unit augments the growth and development of the newborn. To accomplish these goals requires attention to all the details of

the labor and delivery process as they relate to a specific patient's medical, obstetric, and psychosocial situation.

One of the paradoxes of modern obstetric care is that the technologic advances that have contributed substantially to the identification and correction of the pathophysiologic abnormalities of labor may depersonalize the labor event and even introduce phenomena that alter maternal and fetal physiology and create substantial maternal and family anxiety. The outcry against such depersonalization has come from many quarters and has resulted in reexamination of the management of labor and delivery. Indeed, it has been found that many of the traditional hospital obstetric practices, such as the perineal shave, enemas, and isolation of the patient from her family and friends, are not beneficial. More liberal use of ambulation and positions of comfort in labor and delivery have been found to be physiologically beneficial. Furthermore, the presence of family members or supportive friends may decrease anxiety, shorten the duration of labor, and reduce the need for medications.

Perhaps the most important figure in this entire scenario is the bedside nurse in the labor and delivery unit. The nurse's role is to bridge the gap between the most sophisticated obstetric technology and the expectations and needs of the patient and her family. The nurse must thoroughly understand the physiology and pathophysiology of labor; must be able to collect, record, and interpret the data throughout the labor; and must anticipate both maternal and fetal problems. Furthermore, the nurse must provide timely communications to the physicians responsible for the patient's care and frequently must intelligibly and compassionately help to interpret the course of labor to the patient and her family. This implies a one-to-one nurse-patient ratio for patients in active labor. All of these goals should be accomplished in a facility in which there can be an immediate response to a fetal or maternal emergency in the form of prompt delivery or resuscitation when necessary.

REFERENCES

Abboud TK, Khoo SS, Miller F, et al: Maternal, fetal, and neonatal responses after epidural anesthesia with bupivacaine, 2-chloroprocaine, or lidocaine. Anesth Analg **61**:638, 1982.

Abboud TK, Nagappala S, Murakawa K, et al: Comparison of the effects of general and regional anesthesia for cesarean section on neonatal neurologic and adaptive capacity scores. Anesth Analg **64**:996, 1985.

Abdel-Aleem H, Nashar I, Abdel-Aleem A: Management of severe postpartum hemorrhage with misoprostol. Int J Gynecol Obstet **72**:75, 2001.

Acker DB, Gregory KD, Sachs BP, et al: Risk factors for Erb-Duchenne palsy. Obstet Gynecol **71**:389, 1988.

Acker DB, Sachs BP, Friedman EA: Risk factors for shoulder dystocia in the average infant. Obstet Gynecol **67**:614, 1986.

Adekanmi O, Purmessur S, Edwards G, et al: Intrauterine misoprostol for the treatment of severe recurrent atonic secondary postpartum haemorrhage. Brit J Obstet Gynaecol **108**:541, 2001.

Akoury HA, Brodie G, Caddick R, et al: Active management of labor and operative delivery in nulliparous women. Am J Obstet Gynecol **158**:255, 1988.

Albers LL, Schiff M, Gorwoda JG: The length of active labor in normal pregnancies. Obstet Gynecol **87**:355, 1996.

Alfirevic A: Oral misoprostol for induction of labour. Cochrane Database of Systematic Reviews. Available at *http://gateway2.ovidweb.cgi*. Accessed June 15, 2002.

Allaire AD, D'Andrea N, Truong P, et al: Cervical stroma apoptosis in pregnancy. Obstet Gynecol **97**:399, 2001.

Allen R, Sorab J, Gonik B: Risk factors for shoulder dystocia: An engineering study of clinician-applied forces. Obstet Gynecol **77**:352, 1991.

Allen RH, Bankoski BR, Butzin CA, et al: Comparing clinician applied leads for routine, difficult, and shoulder dystocia deliveries. Am J Obstet Gynecol **171**:1621, 1994.

Al-Najashi S, Al-Suleiman SA, El-Yahai A, et al: Shoulder dystocia—A clinical study of 56 cases. Aust N Z J Obstet Gynaecol **29**:129, 1989.

Altabef KM, Spencer JT, Zinberg S: Intravenous nitroglycerin for uterine relaxation of an inverted uterus. Am J Obstet Gynecol **166**:1237, 1992.

American College of Obstetricians and Gynecologists (ACOG): Manual of Standards in Obstetric-Gynecologic Practice, 2nd ed. Washington, DC, ACOG, 1965.

American College of Obstetricians and Gynecologists (ACOG): Obstetrics forceps. ACOG Committee Opinion 59. Washington, DC, ACOG, 1988.

American College of Obstetricians and Gynecologists (ACOG): Operative vaginal delivery. ACOG Technical Bulletin 152. Washington, DC, ACOG, 1991.

American College of Obstetricians and Gynecologists (ACOG): Operative vaginal delivery. ACOG Practice Bulletin 17. Washington, DC, ACOG, 2000.

American College of Obstetricians and Gynecologists (ACOG): Mode of term singleton breech delivery, ACOG Committee Opinion 265. Washington, DC, ACOG, 2001.

Ananth CV, Smulian JC, Vintzileous AM: The association of placenta previa with history of cesarean delivery and abortion. Am J Obstet Gynecol **177**:1071, 1997.

Atkinson BD, Truitt LJ, Rayburn WF, et al: Double-blind comparison of intravenous butorphanol (Stadol) and fentanyl (Sublimaze) for analgesia during labor. Am J Obstet Gynecol **171**:993, 1994.

Atkinson DT: Magic, Myth and Medicine. Cleveland, World Publishing, 1956, p. 271.

Axelrod FB, Leistner HL, Porges RF: Breech presentation among infants with familial dysautonomia. J Pediatr **84**:107, 1974.

Bailit JL, Downs SM, Thorp JM: Reducing the cesarean delivery risk in elective inductions of labor: a decision analysis. Paediatr Perinatal Epidemiol **16**:90, 2002.

Barnes JS: Is it better to avoid urethral catheterization at hysterectomy and caesarean section? Aust NZ J Obstet Gynaecol **38**:315, 1998.

Barnum CG: Dystocia due to the shoulders. Am J Obstet Gynecol **50**:439, 1949.

Barrier G, Sureau C: Effects of anaesthetic and analgesic drugs on labour, fetus, and neonate. Clin Obstet Gynaecol **9**:351, 1982.

Basket TF, Allen AC: Perinatal implications of shoulder dystocia. Obstet Gynecol **86**:14, 1995.

Beazley JM, Kurjak A: The influence of a partograph on the active management of labour. Lancet **2**:348, 1972.

Béhague DP, Victoria CG, Barros FC: Consumer demand for caesarean sections in Brazil: Population based birth cohort study linking ethnographic and epidemiological methods. BMJ **324**:942, 2002.

Beischer NA: Pelvic contraction in breech presentation. J Obstet Gynaecol Br Commonw **73**:421, 1966.

Belizan JM, Althabe F, Barros FC, et al: Rates and implications of cesarean sections in Latin America ecological study. BMJ **319**:1397, 1999.

Benedetti TJ, Gabbe SG: Shoulder dystocia: A complication of fetal macrosomia and prolonged second stage of labor with midpelvic delivery. Obstet Gynecol **52**:526, 1978.

Bergqvist A, Bergqvist D, Hallbooki T: Acute deep vein thrombosis (DVT) after cesarean section. Acta Obstet Gynecol Scand **58**:473, 1979.

Berkowitz RL, Rafferty TD: Pulmonary artery flow-directed catheter use in the obstetric patient. Obstet Gynecol **55**:507, 1980.

Bingham P, Lilford RJ: Management of the selected term breech presentation: Assessment of the risks of selected vaginal delivery versus cesarean section for all cases. Obstet Gynecol **69**:965, 1987.

Bishop EH: Pelvic scoring for elective induction. Obstet Gynecol **24**:266, 1964.

Black BP, McBride WG: Children born after elective induction of labour. Med J Aust **2**:362, 1979.

Blanchette H: Elective manual exploration of the uterus after delivery: A study and review. J Reprod Med **19**:13, 1977.

Bland RD: Lung liquid clearance before and after birth. Sem Perinatol **12**:124, 1988.

B-Lynch C, Coker A, Lawal A, et al: The B-Lynch surgical technique for the control of massive postpartum haemorrhage: an alternative to hysterectomy? Five cases reported. Brit J Obstet Gynaecol **104**:372, 1997.

Bofill JA, Rust OA, Perry KG Jr, et al: Forceps and vacuum delivery: A survey of North American residency programs. Obstet Gynecol **88**:622, 1996.

Bofill JA, Vincent RD, Ross EL, et al: Nulliparous active labor, epidural analgesia, and cesarean delivery for dystocia. Am J Obstet Gynecol **177**:1465, 1997.

Booker PD, Wilkes RG, Beddard J: Obstetric pain relief using epidural morphine. Anaesthesia **35**:377, 1980.

Boon AW, Milner AD, Hopkin IE: Lung volumes and lung mechanics in babies born vaginally and by elective and emergency lower segmental cesarean section. J Pediatr **98**:812, 1981.

Boulvain M, Kelly A, Lohse C, et al: Mechanical methods for induction of labour. Cochrane Database of Systematic Reviews. Available at *http://gateway2.ovidweb.cgi*. Accessed May 2002.

Boulvain M, Stan C, Irion O: Membrane sweeping for induction of labour. Cochrane Database of Systematic Reviews. Available at *http://gateway2.ovidweb.cgi*. Accessed June 15, 2002.

Bowen LW, Beeson JH: Use of a large Foley catheter balloon to control postpartum hemorrhage resulting from a low placental implantation. A report of two cases. J Reprod Med **30**:623, 1985.

Bowes WA Jr, Katz VL: Operative vaginal delivery: Forceps and vacuum extractor. Curr Prob Obstet Gynecol Fertil **17**:83, 1994.

Bowes WA Jr, Taylor ES, O'Brien M, et al: Breech delivery: Evaluation of the method of delivery on perinatal results and maternal morbidity. Am J Obstet Gynecol **135**:965, 1979.

Boylan P, Frankowski R, Rountree R, et al: The effect of active management of labor on the incidence of caesarean section for dystocia in nulliparae. Am J Perinatol **8**:373, 1991.

Braun FHT, Jones KL, Smith DW: Breech presentation as an indicator of fetal abnormality. J Pediatr **86**:419, 1975.

Breen JL, Wiesmeier E: Compound presentations: A survey of 131 patients. Obstet Gynecol **32**:419, 1968.

Brenner WE, Bruce RD, Hendricks CH: The characteristics and perils of breech presentation. Am J Obstet Gynecol **118**:700, 1974.

Bricker L, Lavender T: Parenteral opioids for labor pain relief: A systematic review. Am J Obstet Gynecol **186**:S94, 2002.

Browning DJ: Serious side effects of ergometrine and its use in routine obstetric practice. Med J Aust **1**:957, 1974.

Buchholz NP, Daly-Grandeau E, Huber-Buchholz M-M: Urological complications associated with caesarean section. Eur J Obstet Gynecol **56**:161, 1994.

Buchsbaum GM, Chin M, Glantz C, et al: Prevalence of urinary incontinence and associated risk factors in a cohort of nuns. Obstet Gynecol **100**:226, 2002.

Burchell RC: Physiology of internal iliac artery ligation. J Obstet Gynaecol Br Commonw **75**:642, 1968.

Buttino L Jr, Garite TJ: The use of 15 methyl F2 alpha prostaglandin (Prostin 15M) for the control of postpartum hemorrhage. Am J Perinatol **3**:241, 1986.

Caldwell WE, Moloy HC, D'Esopo DA: Further studies on the mechanism of labor. Am J Obstet Gynecol **30**:763, 1935.

Caldwell WE, Moloy HC, D'Esopo DA: The more recent conceptions of the pelvic architecture. Am J Obstet Gynecol **40**:558, 1940.

Calvert JP: Intrinsic hazard of breech presentation. Br Med J **281**:1319, 1980.

Catanzarite VA, Moffitt KD, Baker ML, et al: New approaches to the management of acute uterine inversion. Obstet Gynecol **68**:78, 1986.

Caton D: What a Blessing She Had Chloroform. The Medical and Social Response to the Pain of Childbirth from 1800 to the Present. New Haven, Yale University Press, 1999.

Caton D, Frölich MA, Euliano TY: Anesthesia for childbirth: Controversy and change. Am J Obstet Gynecol **186**:S25, 2002.

Chadha YC, Mahmood TA, Dick MJ, et al: Breech delivery and epidural analgesia. Br J Obstet Gynecol **99**:96, 1992.

Chalmers I, Campbell H, Turnbull AC: Use of oxytocin and incidence of neonatal jaundice. Br Med J **2**:116, 1975.

Chalmers JA, Chalmers I: The obstetric vacuum extractor is the instrument of first choice for operative vaginal delivery. Br J Obstet Gynaecol **96**:505, 1989.

Chan LY-S, Leung TY, Fok WY, et al.: High incidence of obstetric interventions after successful external cephalic version. BJOG **109**:627, 2002.

Chelmow D, Kilpatrick SJ, Laros RK Jr: Maternal and neonatal outcomes after prolonged latent phase. Obstet Gynecol **81**:486, 1993.

Cheng M, Hannah M: Breech delivery at term: A critical review of the literature. Obstet Gynecol **82**:605, 1993.

Chestnut DH: Alternative regional anesthetic techniques: Paracervical block, lumbar sympathetic block, pudendal block, and perineal infiltration. In Chestnut DH (ed): Obstetric Anesthesia: Principles and Practice. St. Louis, Mosby, 1994, pp. 420–425.

Chestnut DH, McGrath JM, Vincent RD Jr, et al: Does early administration of epidural analgesia affect obstetric outcome in nulliparous women who are in spontaneous labor? Anesthesiology 80:1201, 1994.

Chestnut DH, Vincent RD Jr, McGrath JM, et al: Does early administration of epidural analgesia affect obstetric outcome in nulliparous women who are receiving intravenous oxytocin? Anesthesiology 80:1193, 1994.

Christian SS, Brady K, Read JA, et al: Vaginal breech delivery: A five-year prospective evaluation of a protocol using computed tomographic pelvimetry. Am J Obstet Gynecol 163:848, 1990.

Clark SL, Koonings PP, Phelan JP: Placenta previa/accreta and prior cesarean section. Obstet Gynecol 66:89, 1985.

Clifford SH: A consideration of the obstetrical management of premature labor. N Engl J Med 210:570, 1934.

Cohen S: The aspiration syndrome. Clin Obstet Gynaecol 9:235, 1982.

Cohen WR: Influence of the duration of second stage of labor on perinatal outcome and puerperal morbidity. Obstet Gynecol 49:266, 1977.

Cole RA, Howie PW, MacNaughton MC: Elective induction of labour: A randomized prospective trial. Lancet 1:767, 1975.

Collins KM, Bevan DR, Beard RW: Fluid loading to reduce abnormalities of fetal heart rate and maternal hypotension during epidural analgesia in labour. Br Med J 2:1460, 1978.

Corke BC, Datta S, Ostheimer GW, et al: Spinal anesthesia for cesarean section: The influence of hypotension on neonatal outcome. Anaesthesia 37:658, 1982.

Cousins ML, Mather LE: Intrathecal and epidural administration of opioids. Anesthesiology 61:276, 1984.

Crawford JS: Maternal and cord blood at delivery: II. Parameters of respiratory exchange: Elective cesarean section. Am J Obstet Gynecol 93:37, 1965.

Crawford JS: Appraisal of lumbar epidural blockade in patients with singleton fetus presenting by breech. J Obstet Gynaecol Br Commonw 81:867, 1974.

Crawford JS: Some maternal complications of epidural analgesia for labour. Anaesthesia 40:1219, 1985.

Crawford JS, Burton M, Davies P: Anaesthesia for section: Further refinements of a technique. Br J Anaesth 45:726, 1973.

Cruikshank DP, White CA: Obstetric malpresentations: Twenty years' experience. Am J Obstet Gynecol 116:1097, 1973.

Curtin SC, Kozak LJ, Gregor KD: U.S. cesarean and VBAC rates stalled in the mid-1990s. Birth 27: 2000.

Danforth DN: The fibrous nature of the cervix and its relation to the isthmic segment in gravid and nongravid uteri. Am J Obstet Gynecol 53:541, 1947.

Danielian PJ, Wang J, Hall MH: Long-term outcome by method of delivery of fetuses in breech presentation at term: Population based follow up. Br Med J 312:1451, 1996.

Datta S, Alper MH: Anesthesia for cesarean section. Anesthesiology 53:142, 1980.

Descargues G, Douvrin F, Degre S, et al: Abnormal placentation and selective embolization of the uterine arteries. European J Obstet Gynecol 99:47, 2001.

DeSimone CA, Norris MC, Leighton BL: Intravenous nitroglycerin aids manual extraction of retained placenta. Anesthesiology 73:787, 1990.

D'Esopo DA: A review of cesarean section at Sloan Hospital for Women 1942–1947. Am J Obstet Gynecol 59:77, 1950.

Dierker LJ Jr, Rosen MG, Thompson K, et al: Midforceps deliveries: Long-term outcome of infants. Am J Obstet Gynecol 154:764, 1986.

D'Souza SW, Black P, Macfarlane T, et al: The effect of oxytocin in induced labour on neonatal jaundice. Br J Obstet Gynaecol 86:133, 1979.

Dublin S, Lydon-Rochelle M, Kaplan RC, et al: Maternal and neonatal outcomes after induction of labor without an identified indication. Am J Obstet Gynecol 183:986, 2000.

Duff P: Prophylactic antibiotics for cesarean delivery: A simple cost-effective strategy for prevention of postoperative morbidity. Am J Obstet Gynecol 157:794, 1987.

Dunn DW, Engle WA: Brachial plexus palsy: Intrauterine onset. Pediatr Neurol 1:365, 1985.

Durfee RB: Low classical cesarean section. Postgrad Med 51:219, 1972.

Eastman NJ: The role of Frontier America in the development of cesarean section. Am J Obstet Gynecol 24:919, 1932.

Edwards RL, Nicholson HO: The management of the unstable lie in late pregnancy. J Obstet Gynaecol Br Commonw 76:713, 1969.

Elbourne D, Wiseman RA: Types of intra-muscular opioids for maternal pain relief in labour. Cochrane Database of Systematic Reviews. Available at http://gateway2.ovidweb.cgi. Accessed June 20, 2002.

Elbourne DR, Prendiville WJ, Carroli G, et al: Prophylactic use of oxytocin in the third stage of labour. Cochrane Database of Systematic Reviews. Available at http://gateway2.ovidweb.cgi. Accessed June 20, 2002.

Emmons SL, Krohn M, Jackson M, et al: Development of wound infections among women undergoing cesarean section. Obstet Gynecol 72:559, 1988.

Falzone S, Chauhan S, Mobley J, et al: Unengaged vertex in nulliparous women in active labor. J Reprod Med 43:676, 1998.

Farrell SA, Allen VM, Baskett TF: Parturition and urinary incontinence in primiparas. Obstet Gynecol 97:350, 2001.

Ferguson JE, Bourgeois FJ, Underwood P: B-Lynch suture for postpartum hemorrhage. Obstet Gynecol 95:1020, 2000.

Ferguson JE, Newberry YG, DeAngelis GA, et al: The fetal-pelvic index has minimal utility in predicting fetal-pelvic disproportion. Am J Obstet Gynecol 179:1186, 1998.

Flamm BL, Goings JR, Liu Y, et al: Elective repeat cesarean delivery versus trial of labor: A prospective multicenter study. Obstet Gynecol 83:927, 1994.

Floberg J, Belfrage P, Ohlsen H: Influence of pelvic outlet capacity on labor: A prospective pelvimetry study of 1429 unselected primiparas. Acta Obstet Gynaecol Scand 66:121, 1987.

Flynn AM, Kelly J, Hollins G, et al: Ambulation in labor. Br Med J 2:591, 1978.

Frank F: Suprasymphyseal delivery and its relation to other operations in the presence of contracted pelvis. Arch Gynaecol 81:46, 1907.

Freeman DW, Arnold NI: Paracervical block with low doses of chloroprocaine: Fetal and maternal effects. JAMA 231:56, 1975.

Freeman RK, Gutierrez NA, Ray ML, et al: Fetal cardiac response to paracervical block anesthesia: I. Obstet Gynecol 113:583, 1972.

French L: Oral prostaglandin E2 for induction of labour. Cochrane Database of Systematic Reviews. Available at http://gateway2.ovidweb.cgi. Accessed June 15, 2002.

French L, Smaill FM: Antibiotic regimens for endometritis after delivery. Available at http://gateway2.ovidweb.cgi. Accessed June 15, 2002.

Friedman EA: Primigravid labor: a graphicostatistical analysis. Obstet Gynecol 6:567, 1955.

Friedman EA: Labor: Clinical Evaluation and Management. New York, Appleton-Century-Crofts, 1967.

Friedman EA: Labor: Clinical Evaluation and Management, 2nd ed. New York, Appleton-Century-Crofts, 1978.

Friedman EA, Sachtleben MR, Wallace BA: Infant outcome following labor induction. Am J Obstet Gynecol 133:718, 1979.

Friedman EA, Sachtleben-Murray MR, Dahrouge D: Long-term effects of labor and delivery on offspring: A match-pair analysis. Am J Obstet Gynecol 150:941, 1984.

Frigoletto FD, Leiberman E, Lang JM, et al: A clinical trial of active management of labor. N Engl J Med 333:485, 1995.

Frigoletto FD Jr, Ryan KJ, Phillippe M: Maternal mortality rate associated with cesarean section: An appraisal. Am J Obstet Gynecol 136:969, 1980.

Fusi L, Steer PJ, Maresh MJA, et al: Maternal pyrexia associated with the use of epidural analgesia in labour. Lancet 1:1250, 1989.

Fynes M, Donnelly VS, O;Connell PR, et al: Cesarean delivery and anal sphincter injury. Obstet Gynecol 92:496, 1998.

Gallup DG, Freedman MA, Meguiar RV, et al: Necrotizing fasciitis in gynecologic and obstetric patients: A surgical emergency. Am J Obstet Gynecol 187:305, 2002.

Ganstrom L, Ekman G, Malmstrom A: Insufficient remodeling of the uterine connective tissue in women with protracted labour. Br J Obstet Gynaecol 98:1212, 1991.

Gardella C, Taylor M, Benedetti T, et al: The effect of sequential use of vacuum and forceps for assisted vaginal delivery on neonatal and maternal outcomes. Am J Obstet Gynecol 185:896, 2001.

Garite T, Casal D, Garcia-Alonso A, et al: Fetal fibronectin: a new tool for the prediction of successful induction of labor. Am J Obstet Gynecol 175:1516, 1996.

Garite TJ, Dildy GA, McNamara H, et al: A multicenter controlled trial of fetal pulse oximetry in the intrapartum management of nonreassuring fetal heart rate patterns. Am J Obstet Gynecol 183:1049, 2000.

Gerber AH: Accidental incision of the fetus during cesarean delivery. Int J Gynaecol Obstet 12:46, 1974.

Gherman R, Ouzounian J, Goodwin T: Brachial plexus palsy: An in utero injury? Am J Obstet Gynecol 180:1303, 1999.

Gjode P, Rasmussen TB, Jorgenson J: Feto-maternal bleeding during attempts at external version. Br J Obstet Gynaecol 87:571, 1980.

Gluckman PD, Sizonenko SV, Bassett NS: The transition from fetus to neonate—an endocrine perspective. Acta Paediat Suppl 88:7, 1999.

Goddard WB: Fetal monitoring in a private hospital: Observations of fetal bradycardia following paracervical block anesthesia. Am J Obstet Gynecol 109:1145, 1971.

Gonen O, Rosen DJD, Dolfin Z, et al: Induction of labor versus expectant management in macrosomia: A randomized study. Obstet Gynecol 89:913, 1997.

Gonik B, Allen R, Sorab J: Objective evaluation of the shoulder dystocia phenomenon: Effect of maternal pelvic orientation of force reduction. Obstet Gynecol 74:44, 1989.

Gonik B, Stringer CA, Held B: An alternate maneuver for management of shoulder dystocia. Am J Obstet Gynecol 145:882, 1983.

Graham H: Eternal Eve. The History of Gynaecology and Obstetrics. Garden City, NY, Doubleday, 1951, pp. 171–213.

Gross SJ, Shime J, Farine D: Shoulder dystocia: Predictors and outcome: A five-year review. Am J Obstet Gynecol 156:1408, 1987.

Grossman RA: Magnesium sulfate for uterine inversion. J Reprod Med 26:261, 1981.

Gulmezoglu A, Villar J, Ngoc N, et al: WHO multicentre randomised trial of misoprostol in the management of the third stage of labour. Lancet 358:689, 2001.

Hagadorn-Freathy AS, Yeomans ER, Hankins GDV: Validation of the 1988 ACOG forceps classification system. Obstet Gynecol 77:356, 1991.

Haimov-Kochman R, Sciaky-Tamir Y, Yancii N, et al: Conservative management of two ectopic pregnancies implanted in previous uterine scars. Ultrasound in Obstet Gynecol 19:616, 2002.

Hankins GDV, Clark SL: Brachial plexus palsy involving the posterior shoulder at spontaneous vaginal delivery. Am J Perinatol 14:44, 1995.

Hannah M, Hannah W: Cesarean section or vaginal birth for breech presentation at term. Br Med J 312:1451, 1996.

Hannah ME, Hannah WJ, Hewson SA, et al: Planned caesarean section versus planned vaginal birth for breech presentation at term: a randomized multicentre trial. Lancet 356:1375, 2000.

Hannah ME, Hannah WJ, Hodnett ED, et al: Outcomes at 3 months after planned cesarean vs planned vaginal delivery for breech presentation at term. The International Randomized Term Breech Trial. JAMA 287:1822, 2002.

Hansen S, Clark S, Foster J: Active pushing versus passive fetal descent in the second stage of labor: A randomized controlled trial. Obstet Gynecol 99:29, 2002.

Hanson H: Revival of the extraperitoneal cesarean section. Am J Obstet Gynecol 130:102, 1978.

Harer WB Jr: A guest editorial: Quo vadis cesarean delivery? Obstet Gynecol Surv 57:61, 2002.

Haultain FWN: The treatment of chronic uterine inversion by abdominal hysterotomy with a successful case. Br Med J 2:974, 1901.

Hauth JC, Cunningham FG: Vaginal breech delivery is still justified. Obstet Gynecol 99:1115, 2002.

Haverkamp AD, Orleans M, Langendoerfer S, et al: A controlled trial of the differential effects of intrapartum fetal monitoring. Am J Obstet Gynecol 134:399, 1979.

Hayman RG, Arulkumaran S, Steer PJ: Uterine compression sutures: Surgical management of postpartum hemorrhage. Obstet Gynecol 99:502, 2002.

Heinberg EM, Wood RA, Chambers RB: Elective induction of labor in multiparous women. Does it increase the risk of cesarean section? J Reprod Med 47:399, 2002.

Hellman LM, Prystowsky H: Duration of the second stage of labor. Am J Obstet Gynecol 63:1223, 1952.

Hemminki E: Impact of caesarean section on future fertility—A review of cohort studies. Paediatr Perinat Epidemiol 10:366, 1996.

Hemminki E, Meriläinen J: Long-term effects of cesarean sections: Ectopic pregnancies and placental problems. Am J Obstet Gynecol 174:1569, 1996.

Hendricks CH: Uterine contractility at delivery and in the puerperium. Am J Obstet Gynecol 83:890, 1962.

Hendricks CH, Brenner WE: Cardiovascular effects of oxytocic drugs used postpartum. Am J Obstet Gynecol 108:751, 1970.

Hendricks CH, Brenner WE, Kraus G: The normal cervical dilatation pattern in late pregnancy and labor. Am J Obstet Gynecol 106:1065, 1970.

Heritage CK, Cunningham MD: Association of elective repeat cesarean delivery and persistent pulmonary hypertension of the newborn. Am J Obstet Gynecol 152:627, 1985.

Hester JD: Postpartum hemorrhage and re-evaluation of uterine packing. Obstet Gynecol 45:501, 1975.

Hill JG, Eliot BW, Campbell AJ, et al: Intensive care of the fetus in breech labor. Br J Obstet Gynaecol 83:271, 1976.

Hofmeyr GJ: Interventions to help external cephalic version for breech presentation. Cochrane Database of Systematic Reviews. Available at http://gateway2.ovidweb.cgi. Accessed June 15, 2002.

Hofmeyr GJ, Gulmezoglu AM: Vaginal misoprostol for cervical ripening and induction of labor. Cochrane Database of Systematic Reviews. Available at http://gateway2.ovidweb.cgi. Accessed June 15, 2002.

Hofmeyr GJ, Kullier R: External cephalic version for breech presentation at term. Cochrane Database of Systematic Reviews. Available at http://gateway2.ovidweb.cgi. Accessed May 15, 2002.

Holmes P, Oppenheimer L, Wen S: The relationship between cervical dilatation at initial presentation in labour and subsequent intervention. Br J Obstet Gynaecol 108:1120, 2001.

Hopkins L, Smaill F: Antibiotic prophylaxis regimens and drugs for cesarean section. Cochrane Database of Systematic Reviews. Available at http://gateway2.ovidweb.cgi. Accessed June 20, 2002.

Huntington JL: Acute inversion of the uterus. Boston Med Surg J 15:376, 1921.

Hutton E, Mozurkewich E: Extra-amniotic prostaglandin for induction of labour. Cochrane Database of Systematic Reviews. Available at http://gateway2.ovidweb.cgi. Accessed June 15, 2002.

Impey L, Hobson J, O'Herligy C: Graphic analysis of actively managed labor: Prospective computation of labor progression in 500 consecutive nulliparous women in spontaneous labor at term. Am J Obstet Gynecol 183:438, 2000.

Irion O, Almagbaly PH, Morabia A: Planned vaginal delivery versus elective caesarean section: A study of 705 singleton term breech presentations. Br J Obstet Gynaecol 105:710, 1998.

Jennet RJ, Tarby TJ, Kreinick CJ: Brachial plexus palsy: An old problem revisited. Am J Obstet Gynecol 166:1673, 1992.

Johanson RB, Heycock E, Carter J, et al: Maternal and child health after assisted vaginal delivery: Five-year follow-up of a randomized controlled study comparing forceps and ventouse. Br J Obstet Gynaecol 106:544, 1999.

Johanson R, Menon V: Soft versus rigid vacuum extractor cups for assisted vaginal delivery. Cochrane Database of Systematic Reviews. Available at http://gateway2.ovidweb.cgi.Accessed June 22, 2002a.

Johanson RB, Menon V: Vacuum extraction versus forceps for assisted vaginal delivery. Cochrane Database of Systematic Reviews. Available at http://gateway2.ovidweb.cgi. Accessed June 22, 2002b.

Johnson AB: A new concept in the replacement of the inverted uterus and a report of nine cases. Am J Obstet Gynecol 57:557, 1949.

Johnstone RW, William Smellie: The Master of British Midwifery. London, E & S Livingstone, 1952.

Joseph GF Jr, Steman CM, Robichaux AG: Vaginal birth after cesarean section: The impact of patient resistance to a trial of labor. Am J Obstet Gynecol 164:1441, 1991.

Jouppila P, Kuikka J, Jouppila R, et al: Effect of induction of general anesthesia for cesarean section on intervillous blood flow. Acta Obstet Gynecol Scand 58:249, 1979.

Jouppila R, Jouppila P, Kuikka J, et al: Placental blood flow during cesarean section under lumbar extradural anesthesia. Br J Anaesth 50:275, 1978.

Kammen BF, Sevine MS, Rubesin SE, et al: Adynamic ileus after cesarean section mimicking intestinal obstruction: findings on abdominal radiographs. Br J Radiol 73:951, 2001.

Kavanagh J, Kelly AJ, Thomas J: Breast stimulation for cervical ripening and induction of labour. Cochrane Database of Systematic Reviews. Available at http://gateway2.ovidweb.cgi. Accessed June 15, 2002a.

Kavanagh J, Kelly AJ, Thomas J: Corticosteroids for induction of labour. Cochrane Database of Systematic Reviews. Available at http://gateway2.ovidweb.cgi. Accessed June 15, 2002b.

Kavanagh J, Kelly AJ, Thomas J: Hyaluronidase for cervical priming and induction of labour. Cochrane Database of Systematic Reviews. Available at http://gateway2.ovidweb.cgi. Accessed June 15, 2002c.

Kavanagh J, Kelly AJ, Thomas J: Sexual intercourse for cervical ripening and induction of labour. Cochrane Database of Systematic Reviews. Available at http://gateway2.ovidweb.cgi. Accessed June 15, 2002d.

Kayem G, Goffinet F, Clèment D, et al: Breech presentation at term: Morbidity and mortality according to the type of delivery at Port Royal Maternity Hospital from 1993 through 1999. Eur J Obstet Gynecol Reprod Biol 102:137, 2002.

Keettel WC: Inducing labor by rupturing membranes. Postgrad Med 44:199, 1968.

Keirse MJNC: Evidence-based childbirth only for breech babies? Birth 29:55, 2002.

Kelly AJ, Kavanagh J, Thomas J: Castor oil, bath and/or enema for cervical priming and induction of labour. Cochrane Database of Systematic Reviews. Available at http://gateway2.ovidweb.cgi. Accessed June 15, 2002a.

Kelly AJ, Kavanagh J, Thomas J: Relaxin for cervical ripening and induction of labour. Cochrane Database of Systematic Reviews. Available at *http://gateway2.ovidweb.cgi.* Accessed June 15, 2002b.

Kelly AJ, Kavanagh J, Thomas J: Vaginal prostaglandin (PGE2 and PGF2a) for induction of labour at term. Cochrane Database of Systematic Reviews. Available at *http://gateway2.ovidweb.cgi.* Accessed June 15, 2002c.

Kelly AJ, Tan B: Intravenous oxytocin alone for cervical ripening and induction of labour. Cochrane Database of Systematic Reviews. Available at *http://gateway2.ovidweb.cgi.* Accessed June 15, 2002.

Kelly G, Peaceman AM, Colangelo L, et al: Normal nulliparous labor: Are Friedman's definitions still relevant? (Abstract) Am J Obstet Gynecol 182:S129, 2000.

Kendrick JS, Tierney EF, Lawson HW, et al: Previous cesarean delivery and the risk of ectopic pregnancy. Obstet Gynecol 87:297, 1996.

Kennell J, Klaus M, McGrath S, et al: Continuous emotional support during labor in a US Hospital. JAMA 265:2197, 1991.

Kerr JMM: The technic of cesarean section with special reference to the lower uterine segment incision. Am J Obstet Gynecol 12:729, 1926.

Kilpatrick SJ, Laros RK Jr: Characteristics of normal labor. Obstet Gynecol 74:85, 1989.

Klink EW: Perineal nerve block: An anatomic and clinical study in the female. Obstet Gynecol 1:137, 1953.

Koenigsberger MR: Brachial plexus palsy at birth: Intrauterine or due to birth trauma? Ann Neurol 8:228, 1980.

Kopelman JN, Duff P, Karl RT, et al: Computed tomographic pelvimetry in the evaluation of breech presentation. Obstet Gynecol 68:455, 1986.

Lange AP, Secher NJ, Westergaard JG, et al: Prelabor evaluation of inducibility. Obstet Gynecol 60:137, 1982.

Leighton BL, Halpern SH: The effects of epidural analgesia on labor, maternal, and neonatal outcomes: A systematic review. Am J Obstet Gynecol 186:S69, 2002.

Leitch CR, Walker JJ: The rise in cesarean section rate: The same indications but a lower threshold. Br J Obstet Gynaecol 105:621, 1998.

Leppert PC: Anatomy and physiology of cervical ripening. Clin Obstet Gynecol 38:267, 1995.

Lewis DF, Raymond RC, Perkins MB, et al: Recurrence rate of shoulder dystocia. Am J Obstet Gynecol 172:1369, 1995.

Lieberman E, Lang JM, Frigoletto F Jr, et al: Epidural analgesia, intrapartum fever, and neonatal sepsis evaluation. Pediatrics 99:415, 1997.

Lieberman E, O'Donoghue C: Unintended effects of epidural analgesia during labor: A systematic review. Am J Obstet Gynecol 186:S31, 2002.

Lilford RJ, Van Coeverden De Groot HA, Moore PJ, et al: The relative risks of caesarean section (intrapartum and elective) and vaginal delivery: A detailed analysis to exclude the effects of medical disorders and other acute pre-existing physiological disturbance. Br J Obstet Gynaecol 97:883, 1990.

Lindblad A, Bernow J, Marsal K: Fetal blood flow during intrathecal anaesthesia for elective caesarean section. BJA 61:376, 1988.

Lokugamage A, Sullivan K, Niculescu I, et al: A randomized study comparing rectally administered misoprostol versus Syntometrine combined with an oxytocin infusion for the cessation of primary postpartum hemorrhage. Acta Obstet Gynecol Scand 80:835, 2001.

Lopez-Zeno JA, Peaceman AM, Adashek JA, et al: A controlled trial of a program for the active management of labor. N Engl J Med 326:450, 1992.

Luckas M, Bricer L: Intravenous prostaglandin for induction of labour. Cochrane Database of Systematic Reviews. Available at *http://gateway2.ovidweb.cgi.* Accessed June 15, 2002.

Lydon-Rochelle M, Holt V, Easterling TR, et al: Cesarean delivery and postpartum mortality among primiparas in Washington State, 1987–1996. Obstet Gynecol 97:169, 2001a.

Lydon-Rochelle M, Holt VL, Easterling TR, et al: First-birth cesarean and placental abruption or previa at second birth. Obstet Gynecol 97:765, 2001b.

Lydon-Rochelle M, Holt VL, Easterling TR, et al: Risk of uterine rupture during labor among women with a prior cesarean delivery. N Engl J Med 345:3, 2001c.

Lysak SZ, Eisenach JC, Dobson CE II: Patient-controlled epidural analgesia during labor: A comparison of three solutions with a continuous infusion control. Anesthesiology 72:44, 1990.

Macarthur AJ, Macarthur C, Weeks SK: Is epidural anesthesia in labor associated with chronic low back pain? A prospective cohort study. Anesth Analg 85:1066, 1997.

MacArthur C, Lewis M, Knox EG, et al: Epidural anaesthesia and long term backache after childbirth. Br Med J 301:9, 1990.

MacDorman MF, Mathews TJ, Martin JA, et al: Trends and characteristics of induced labour in the United States, 1989–98. Paediatr Perinat Epidemiol 16:263, 2002.

Macer JA, Macer CL, Chan LS: Elective induction versus spontaneous labor: A retrospective study of complications and outcome. Am J Obstet Gynecol 166:1690, 1992.

MacLennan AH, Taylor AW, Wilson DH, et al: The prevalence of pelvic floor disorders and their relationship to gender, age, parity and mode of delivery. BJOG 107:1460, 2000.

Madar J, Richmond S, Hey E: Surfactant-deficient respiratory distress after elective delivery at "term." Acta Paediatr 88:1244, 1999.

Maisels MJ, Rees R, Marks K, et al: Elective delivery of the term fetus: An obstetrical hazard. JAMA 238:2036, 1977.

Malmström T: Vacuum extractor: An obstetrical instrument. Acta Obstet Gynecol Scand 33:S1, 1954.

March MR, Adair CD, Veille J-C, et al: The modified Mueller-Hillis maneuver in predicting abnormalities in second stage of labor. Int J Gynaecol Obstet 55:105, 1996.

Marcus RG, Crewe-Brown H, Krawitz S, et al: Fetomaternal hemorrhage following successful and unsuccessful attempts at external version. Br J Obstet Gynaecol 82:578, 1975.

Marmor TR, Krol DM: Labor pain management in the United States: Understanding patterns and the issues of choice. Am J Obstet Gynecol 186:S173, 2002.

Marx GF, Bassell GM: Hazards of the supine position in pregnancy. Clin Obstet Gynaecol 9:255, 1982.

Maslow AS, Sweeny A: Elective induction of labor as a risk factor for cesarean delivery among low-risk women at term. Obstet Gynecol 95:917, 2000.

Mauldin JG, Mauldin PD, Feng T, et al: Determining the clinical efficacy and cost savings of successful external cephalic version. Am J Obstet Gynecol 175:1639, 1996.

McBride WG, Black BP, Brown CJ, et al: Method of delivery and developmental outcome at five years of age. Med J Aust 1:301, 1979.

McCray PB Jr, Bettencourt JD: Prostaglandins stimulate fluid secretion in human lung fluid. J Develop Physiol 19:29, 1993.

McCullagh WM III: Inversion of the uterus: A report of three cases and an analysis of 223 recently recorded cases. J Obstet Gynaecol Br Emp 32:280, 1925.

McDonald JS, Bjorkman LL, Reed EC: Epidural analgesia for obstetrics: A maternal, fetal, and neonatal study. Am J Obstet Gynecol 120:1055, 1974.

McFarland LV, Raskin M, Daling J, et al: Erb/Duchenne's palsy: A consequence of fetal macrosomia and method of delivery. Obstet Gynecol 68:784, 1986.

McFarland M, Hod M, Piper JM, et al: Are labor abnormalities more common in shoulder dystocia? Am J Obstet Gynecol 173:1211, 1995.

McMahon MJ, Luther ER, Bowes WA Jr, et al: Comparison of a trial of labor with an elective second cesarean section. N Engl J Med 335:689, 1996.

Menticoglou SM, Manning F, Harman C, et al: Perinatal outcome in relation to second-stage duration. Am J Obstet Gynecol 173:906, 1995.

Milner RDG: Neonatal mortality of breech deliveries with and without forceps to the after-coming head. Br J Obstet Gynaecol 82:783, 1975.

Mitchell MD, Flint APF, Bibby J, et al: Rapid increases in plasma prostaglandin concentrations after the vaginal examination and amniotomy. Br Med J 2:1183, 1977.

Morgan MA, Thurnau GR: Efficacy of the fetal-pelvic index in patients requiring labor inductions. Am J Obstet Gynecol 159:621, 1988.

Morrison JC, Sanders JR, Magann EF, et al: The diagnosis and management of dystocia of the shoulder. Surg Gynecol Obstet 175:515, 1992.

Morrison JJ, Rennie JM, Milton PJ: Neonatal respiratory morbidity and mode of delivery at term: Influence of timing of elective caesarean section. Br J Obstet Gynaecol 102:101, 1995.

Munsick RA: Renal hemodynamic effects of oxytocin in antepartal and postpartal women. Am J Obstet Gynecol 108:729, 1970.

Munstedt K, von Georgi R, Reucher S, et al: Term breech and long-term morbidity—cesarean section versus vaginal delivery. Eur J Obstet Gynecol Reprod Biol 96:163, 2001.

Murphy K, Shah L, Cohen W: Labor and delivery in nulliparous women who present with an unengaged fetal head. J Perinatol 18:122, 1998.

Neiger R, Hennessy MD, Patel M: Reattempting failed external cephalic version under epidural anesthesia. Am J Obstet Gynecol 179:1136, 1998.

Neilsen TF, Hökegård K-H: Cesarean section and intraoperative surgical complications. Acta Obstet Gynecol Scand 63:103, 1984.

Neilson JP: Mifepristone for induction of labour. Cochrane Database of Systematic Reviews. Available at *http://gateway2.ovidweb.cgi.* Accessed June 15, 2002.

Ng PS, Chan A, Sin WK, et al: A multicentre randomized controlled trial of oral misoprostol and i.m. syntometrine in the management of the third stage of labour. Hum Reprod 16:31, 2001.

Nocon JJ, McKenzie DK, Thomas LJ, et al: Shoulder dystocia: An analysis of risks and obstetric maneuvers. Am J Obstet Gynecol **168**:1732, 1993.

Notzon FC: International differences in the use of obstetric interventions. JAMA **263**:3286, 1990.

Notzon FC, Cnattingius S, Bergsjø P, et al: Cesarean section delivery in the 1980s: International comparison by indication. Am J Obstet Gynecol **170**:495, 1994.

Notzon FC, Placek PJ, Taffels M: Comparison of national cesarean-section rates. N Engl J Med **316**:386, 1987.

Nyberg K, Buka SL, Lipsitt LD: Perinatal medication as a potential risk factor for adult drug abuse in a North American cohort. Epidemiology **11**:715, 2000.

Nygaard IE, Rao SS, Dawson JD: Anal incontinence after anal sphincter disruption: A 30-year retrospective cohort study. Obstet Gynecol **89**:896, 1997.

O'Brien WF, Cefalo RC: Evaluation of x-ray pelvimetry and abnormal labor. Clin Obstet Gynecol **25**:157, 1982.

O'Driscoll K, Meagher D: Active Management of Labour. Philadelphia, WB Saunders, 1980.

O'Leary JA: Cephalic replacement for shoulder dystocia: Present status and future role of the Zavanelli maneuver. Obstet Gynecol **82**:847, 1993.

O'Leary JL, O'Leary JA: Uterine artery ligation for control of postcesarean section hemorrhage. Obstet Gynecol **43**:849, 1974.

Olofsson CH, Ekblom A, Ekman-Ordeberg G, et al: Analgesic efficacy of intravenous morphine in labour pain: A reappraisal. Int J Obstet Anesth **5**:176, 1996a.

Olofsson CH, Ekblom A, Ekman-Ordeberg G, et al: Lack of analgesic effect of systemically administered morphine or pethidine on labour pain. Br J Obstet Gynaecol **103**:968, 1996b.

Ounsted C, Roberts JS, Gordon M, et al: Fourth goal of perinatal medicine. Br Med J **284**:879, 1982.

Park RC, Duff WP: Role of cesarean hysterectomy in modern obstetric practice. Clin Obstet Gynecol **23**:601, 1980.

Parsons MT, Spellacy WN: Prospective randomized study of x-ray pelvimetry in the primigravida. Obstet Gynecol **66**:76, 1985.

Pelosi MA, Apuzzio J, Fricchione D, et al: The intra-abdominal version technique for delivery of transverse lie by low segment cesarean section. Am J Obstet Gynecol **136**:1009, 1979.

Perkins RP: Role of extraperitoneal cesarean section. Clin Obstet Gynecol **25**:583, 1980.

Philpott RH, Castle WM: Cervicographs in the management of labour in primigravidae. I. The alert line for detecting abnormal labor. J Obstet Gynaecol Br Commonw **79**:592, 1972a.

Philpott RH, Castle WM: Cervicographs in the management of labour in primigravidae: II. The action line and treatment of abnormal labor. J Obstet Gynaecol Br Commonw **79**:599, 1972b.

Piper EB, Bachman C: The prevention of fetal injuries in breech delivery. JAMA **92**:217, 1929.

Podlas J, Breland BD: Patient-controlled analgesia with nalbuphine during labor. Obstet Gynecol **70**:202, 1987.

Potter JE, Berquó E, Perpétuo IHO, et al: Unwanted caesarean sections among public and private patients in Brazil: prospective study. BMJ **323**:1155, 2001.

Potter MG, Heaton CH, Douglas GW: Intrinsic fetal risk in breech delivery. Obstet Gynecol **15**:158, 1960.

Pritchard JA: Changes in the blood volume during pregnancy and delivery. Anesthesiology **26**:393, 1965.

Pritchard JA, MacDonald PC (eds): Williams' Obstetrics, 16th ed. New York, Appleton Century Crofts, 1980, p. 426.

Quinn AJ, Kilpatrick A: Emergency caesarean section during labour: Response time and type of anaesthesia. Eur J Obstet Gynecol Reprod Biol **54**:25, 1994.

Rajasekar D, Hall M: Urinary tract injuries during obstetric intervention. BJOG **104**:731, 1997.

Ralis ZA: Traumatizing effect of breech delivery on infants with spina bifida. J Pediatr **87**:613, 1975.

Ramin SM, Gambling DR, Lucas MJ: Randomized trial of epidural versus intravenous analgesia during labor. Obstet Gynecol **86**:783, 1995.

Ravo B, Pollane M, Ger R: Pseudo-obstruction of the colon following cesarean section. A review. Dis Colon Rectum **26**:440, 1983.

Rayburn WF, Smith CV, Parriott JE, et al: Randomized comparison of meperidine and fentanyl during labor. Obstet Gynecol **74**:604, 1989.

Read JA, Cotton DB, Miller FC: Placenta accreta: Changing clinical aspects and outcome. Obstet Gynecol **56**:31, 1980.

Read JA, Miller FC, Paul RH: Randomized trial of ambulation versus oxytocin for labor enhancement: A preliminary report. Am J Obstet Gynecol **139**:669, 1981.

Reisner LS: Anesthesia for cesarean section. Clin Obstet Gynecol **23**:517, 1980.

Rinehart BK, Terrone DA, Hudson C, et al: Lack of utility of standard labor curves in the prediction of progression during labor induction. Am J Obstet Gynecol **182**:1520, 2000.

Roberts S, Maccato M, Faro S, et al: The microbiology of post-cesarean wound morbidity. Obstet Gynecol **81**:383, 1993.

Robson S, Pridmore B: Have Kielland forceps reached their "use by" date? Aust NZ J Obstet Gynaecol **39**:301, 1999.

Rosefsky JB, Petersiel ME: Perinatal deaths associated with mepivacaine paracervical-block anesthesia in labor. N Engl J Med **278**:530, 1968.

Rosen M: Paracervical block for labor analgesia: A brief historic review. Am J Obstet Gynecol **186**:D127, 2002.

Rosen MG (Chairman): Consensus Task Force on Cesarean Childbirth. National Institutes of Health, NIH Publication No. 82-2067, 1981.

Rosen MG, Dickinson JC, Westhoff CL: Vaginal birth after cesarean: A meta-analysis of morbidity and mortality. Obstet Gynecol **77**:465, 1991.

Rouse DJ, Owen J: Prophylactic cesarean delivery for fetal macrosomia diagnosed by means of ultrasonography—A Faustian bargain? Am J Obstet Gynecol **181**:332, 1999.

Rouse DJ, Owen J, Hauth JC: Active-phase labor arrest: Oxytocin augmentation for at least 4 hours. Obstet Gynecol **93**:323, 1999.

Rouse DJ, Owen J, Hauth JC: Criteria for failed labor induction: Prospective evaluation of a standardized protocol. Obstet Gynecol **96**:671, 2000.

Rouse DJ, Owen J, Savage KG, et al: Active phase labor arrest: Revisiting the 2-hour minimum. Obstet Gynecol **98**:550, 2001.

Rozenberg P, Goffinet F, de Spirlet M, et al: External cephalic version with epidural anaesthesia after failure of a first trial with beta-mimetics. BJOG **107**:406, 2000.

Rubin A: Management of shoulder dystocia: JAMA **188**:835, 1964.

Sachs BP, Yeh J, Acker D, et al: Cesarean section-related maternal mortality in Massachusetts, 1954–1985. Obstet Gynecol **71**:385, 1988.

Sandmire H, DeMott R: Erb's Palsy causation: A historical perspective. Birth **29**:52, 2002.

Sarno AP, Phelan JP, Ahn MO, et al: Vaginal birth after cesarean delivery: Trial of labor in women with breech presentation. J Reprod Med **34**:831, 1989.

Schifrin BS: Fetal heart rate patterns following epidural anaesthesia and oxytocin infusion during labour. J Obstet Gynaecol Br Commonw **79**:332, 1972.

Schorr SJ, Speights SE, Ross EL, et al: A randomized trial of epidural anesthesia to improve external cephalic version success. Am J Obstet Gynecol **177**:1133, 1997.

Schreiner RL, Stevens DC, Smith WL, et al: Etiology of the respiratory distress following elective cesarean section (Abstract 107). Pediatr Res **13**:505, 1979.

Sciscione AC, Nguyen L, Manley J, et al : A randomized comparison of transcervical Foley catheter to intravaginal misoprostol for preinduction cervical ripening. Obstet Gynecol **97**:603, 2001.

Scott JR: Mandatory trial of labor after cesarean delivery: An alternative viewpoint. Obstet Gynecol **77**:881, 1991.

Seeds JW, Cefalo RC: Malpresentations. Clin Obstet Gynecol **25**:145, 1982.

Seidman DS, Laor A, Gale R, et al: Long-term effects of vacuum and forceps deliveries. Lancet **337**:1583, 1991.

Seitchik J, Holden AEC, Castillo M: Amniotomy and oxytocin treatment of functional dystocia and route of delivery. Am J Obstet Gynecol **155**:585, 1986.

Seyb ST, Berka RJ, Socol ML, et al: Risk of cesarean delivery with elective induction of labor at term in nulliparous women. Obstet Gynecol **94**:600, 1999.

Sharma SK, Sidawi JE, Ramin SM, et al: Cesarean delivery: A randomized trial of epidural versus patient-controlled meperidine analgesia during labor. Anesthesiology **87**:487, 1997.

Sheiner E, Levy A, Feinstein U, et al: Risk factors and outcome of failure to progress during the first stage of labor: A population-based study. Acta Obstet Gynecol Scand **81**:222, 2002.

Silbar EL: Factors related to the increasing cesarean section rates for cephalopelvic disproportion. Am J Obstet Gynecol **154**:1095, 1986.

Sims DG, Neligan GA: Factors affecting the increasing incidence of severe nonhaemolytic neonatal jaundice. Br J Obstet Gynaecol **82**:863, 1975.

Sloof ACJ: Obstetric brachial plexus lesions and their neurosurgical treatment. Microsurgery **16**:30, 1995.

Smaill F, Hofmeyr GJ: Antibiotic prophylaxis for cesarean section. Cochrane Database of Systematic Reviews. Available at *http://gateway2.ovidweb.cgi*. Accessed June 20, 2002.

Smith EF, MacDonald FA: Cesarean section. An evaluation of current practice in the New York Lying-In Hospital. Obstet Gynecol 6:593, 1953.

Smith GC, Cameron AD, Dobbie R: Risk of perinatal death associated with labor after previous cesarean delivery in uncomplicated term pregnancies. JAMA 287:2684, 2002.

Smith JF, Hernandez C, Wax JR: Fetal laceration injury at cesarean delivery. Obstet Gynecol 90:344, 1997.

Smith RB, Lane C, Pearson JF: Shoulder dystocia: What happens at the next delivery? Br J Obstet Gynaecol 101:713, 1994.

Somerset D: Term breech trial does not provide unequivocal evidence. BMJ 324:50, 2002.

Speert H: Obstetric and Gynecologic Milestones, Illustrated. New York, Parthenon, 1996, p. 498.

Steer CM (ed): Moloy's Evaluation of the Pelvis in Obstetrics. Philadelphia, WB Saunders, 1959.

Stevenson CS: The principal cause of breech presentation in single term pregnancies. Am J Obstet Gynecol 60:41, 1950.

Stirrup CA, Lucas DN, Cox MC, et al: Maternal anti-factor Xa activity following subcutaneous unfractionated heparin after caesarean section. Anaesthesia 56:855, 2001.

Strong TH, Whelan JP, An MO, et al: Vaginal birth after cesarean delivery in twin gestation. Am J Obstet Gynecol 161:29, 1989.

Stuart HC, An AF, Rubidium SJ, et al: Acid aspiration prophylaxis for emergency caesarean section. Anaesthesia 51:415, 1996.

Sultan AH, Kamm MA, Hudson CN, et al: Anal-sphincter disruption during vaginal delivery. N Engl J Med 329:1905, 1993.

Svancarik W, Cairina O, Schaefer G Jr, et al: Retropsoas and subgluteal abscesses following paracervical and pudendal anesthesia. JAMA 237:892, 1977.

Swan HJC: Balloon flotation catheters: Their use in hemodynamic monitoring in clinical practice. JAMA 233:865, 1975.

Tangtrakul S, Taechaiya S, Suthutvoravat S: Post-caesarean section urinary tract infection: A comparison between intermittent and indwelling catheterization. J Med Assoc Thailand 77:244, 1994.

Thomas J, Kelly AJ, Kavanagh J: Oestrogens alone or with amniotomy for cervical ripening or induction of labour. Cochrane Database of Systematic Reviews. Available at http://gateway2.ovidweb.cgi. Accessed June 15, 2002.

Thomas WO: Manual removal of the placenta. Am J Obstet Gynecol 86:600, 1963.

Thompson TT, Thorp JM Jr, Mayer D, et al: Does epidural anesthesia cause dystocia? J Clin Anesth 70:58, 1998.

Thorp JA, Breedlove G: Epidural analgesia in labor: An evaluation of risks and benefits. Birth 23:63, 1996.

Thorp JA, Eckert LO, Ang MS, et al: Epidural analgesia and cesarean section for dystocia: Risk factors in nulliparas. Am J Perinatol 8:402, 1991.

Thorp JA, Hu DH, Albin RM, et al: The effect of intrapartum epidural analgesia on nulliparous labor: A randomized, controlled, prospective trial. Am J Obstet Gynecol 169:851, 1993.

Thorp JM, Pahel-Short L, Bowes WA Jr: The Mueller-Hillis maneuver: Can it be used to predict dystocia? Obstet Gynecol 82:519, 1993.

Thurnau GR, Morgan MA: Efficacy of the fetal-pelvic index as a predictor of fetal-pelvic disproportion in women with abnormal labor patterns that require labor augmentation. Am J Obstet Gynecol 159:1168, 1988.

Thurnau GR, Scates DH, Morgan MA: The fetal-pelvic index: A method of identifying fetal-pelvic disproportion in women attempting vaginal birth after previous cesarean delivery 165:353, 1991.

Todd WD, Steer CM: Term breech: Review of 1006 term breech deliveries. Obstet Gynecol 22:583, 1963.

Towner D, Castro MA, Eby-Wilkens E, et al: Effect of mode of delivery in nulliparous women on neonatal intracranial injury. N Engl J Med 341:1709, 1999.

Tulley L, Gates S, Brocklehurst P: Surgical techniques used during cesarean section operations: Results of a national survey of practice in the UK. Eur J Obstet Gynecol Reprod Biol 102:120, 2002.

Turner MJ, Brassil M, Gordon H: Active management of labor associated with a decrease in the cesarean section rate in nulliparas. Obstet Gynecol 71:150, 1988.

Tylleskär J, Finnstrom O, Leijon I, et al: Spontaneous labor and elective induction—A prospective randomized study: I. Effects on mother and fetus. Acta Obstet Gynecol Scand 58:513, 1979.

Usher R, McLean F, Maughan GB: Respiratory distress syndrome in infants delivered by cesarean section. Am J Obstet Gynecol 88:806, 1964.

Van den Berg A, Van Elberg RM, van Geijn HP, et al: Neonatal respiratory morbidity following elective caesarean section in term infants. A 5-year retrospective study and review of the literature. Eur J Obstet Gynecol Reprod Biol 98:9, 2001.

Van Loon AJ, Mantinoh A, Thiun CJ, et al: Pelvimetry by magnetic resonance imaging in breech presentation. Am J Obstet Gynecol 163:1256, 1990.

Vedantham S, Goodwin SC, McLucas B, et al: Uterine artery embolization: An underused method of controlling hemorrhage. Am J Obstet Gynecol 176:938, 1997.

Ventura SJ, Martin JA, Curtin SC, et al: Births: final data for 1999. Natl Vital Stat Rep 49:1, 2001.

Walker R, Turnbull D, Wilkinson C: Strategies to address global cesarean section rates: A review of the evidence. Birth 29:28, 2002.

Walley R, Wilson J, Crane J, et al: A double-blind placebo controlled randomised trial of misoprostol and oxytocin in the management of the third stage of labour. Brit J Obstet Gynecol 107:1111, 2000.

Ware V, Raynor BD: Transvaginal ultrasonographic cervical measurement as a predictor of successful labor induction. Am J Obstet Gynecol 182:1030, 2000.

Watson P, Besch N, Bowes WA Jr: Management of acute and subacute puerperal inversion of the uterus. Obstet Gynecol 55:12, 1980.

Watson WJ, George RJ, Welter S, et al: High-risk obstetric patients: Maternal morbidity after cesareans. J Reprod Med 42:267, 1997.

Watson WJ, Stevens D, Welter S, et al: Factors predicting successful labor induction. Obstet Gynecol 88:990, 1996.

Wax JR, Herson V, Carignan E, et al: Contribution of elective delivery to severe respiratory distress at term. Am J Perinatol 19:81, 2002.

Weisman AI: An antepartum study of fetal polarity and rotation. Am J Obstet Gynecol 48:550, 1944.

Weissberg SM, O'Leary JA: Compound presentation of the fetus. Obstet Gynecol 41:60, 1973.

Wenger DR, Gitchell RG: Severe infections following pudendal block anesthesia: Need for orthopedic awareness. J Bone Joint Surg 55:202, 1973.

Wesley BD, van den Berg BJ, Reece EA: The effect of forceps delivery on cognitive development. Am J Obstet Gynecol 169:1091, 1993.

Williams RM, Thom MH, Studd JW: A study of the benefits and acceptability of ambulation in spontaneous labour. Br J Obstet Gynaecol 87:122, 1980.

Winkler M, Rath W: Changes in the cervical extracellular matrix during pregnancy and parturition. J Perinat Med 27:45, 1999.

Woods CE: A principle of physics as applicable to shoulder dystocia. Am J Obstet Gynecol 45:796, 1943.

World Health Organization: Appropriate technology for birth. Lancet 2:436, 1985.

Wright RC: Reduction of perinatal mortality and morbidity in breech delivery through routine use of cesarean delivery. Obstet Gynecol 14:758, 1959.

Yancey M, Zhang J, Schweitzer D, et al: Epidural analgesia and fetal head malposition at vaginal delivery. Obstet Gynecol 97:608, 2001.

Yeh S, Huang X, Whelan JP: Postterm pregnancy after previous cesarean section. J Reprod Med 29:41, 1984.

Zalar RW, Quilligan EJ: The influence of scalp sampling on the cesarean section rate for fetal distress. Am J Obstet Gynecol 135:239, 1979.

Zatuchni GI, Andros GJ: Prognostic index for vaginal delivery in breech presentation at term. Prospective study. Am J Obstet Gynecol 98:854, 1967.

Zhang J, Bernask JW, Leybovich E, et al: Continuous labor support from labor attendant for primiparous women: A meta-analysis. Obstet Gynecol 88:739, 1996.

Zhang J, Bowes WA Jr, Fortney JA: Efficacy of external cephalic version: a review. Obstet Gynecol 82:306, 1993.

Zhang J, Troendle J, Yancey MK: Reassessing the labor curve in nulliparous women. Am J Obstet Gynecol 187:824, 2002.

Zhang J, Yancey MK, Henderson CE: U.S. national trends in labor induction, 1989–1998. J Reprod Med 47:120, 2002.

Zhang J, Yancey M, Klebanoff M, et al. Does epidural analgesia prolong labor and increase risk of cesarean delivery? A natural experiment. Am J Obstet Gynecol 185:128, 2001.

Chapter 37
PLACENTA PREVIA AND ABRUPTIO PLACENTAE

Steven L. Clark, MD

Hemorrhage from placenta previa, placental abruption, and, rarely, vasa previa has traditionally been classified as third-trimester bleeding. However, the principles discussed in this chapter apply, in general, to bleeding beyond 20 weeks' gestation. Such bleeding complicates about 6% of all pregnancies (Ananth, Savitz, Luther, 1996). Placenta previa is ultimately documented in 7% of cases, and evidence of significant placental abruption is found in 13%. In the remaining 80% of cases, the bleeding can be ascribed either to early labor or local lesions of the lower genital tract, or no source can be identified (Ananth, Savitz, Luther, 1996). These latter cases probably represent small degrees of placental separation as well and should be treated as such. In cases of placenta previa, as well as those involving significant premature placental separation (abruption), the clinical consequences of hemorrhage may be life-threatening to both the mother and fetus. Bleeding from vasa previa may also be rapidly fatal to the fetus. Thus, any amount of bleeding in the second half of pregnancy mandates a thorough evaluation.

PLACENTA PREVIA

Definition and Classification

Recent advances in the precision of sonographic diagnosis of placenta previa and an increased understanding of the changing relationship between the placenta and the internal cervical os as pregnancy advances have rendered traditional definitions and classifications of placenta previa obsolete. This statement is based on several observations.

First, in the past, difficulty in defining the exact lower margin of the placenta in relation to the internal cervical os and the critical clinical importance of not missing a placenta that did encroach upon the os led to the classification of a *low-lying placenta* as a type of placenta previa. This ambiguous term is of limited clinical utility because, until recently, there has been no generally accepted definition of how low the placenta must be to mandate cesarean delivery or double set-up examination. Given our present ability to precisely define the distance between the lowest edge of the placenta and the internal cervical os using high-resolution transvaginal sonography, such ambiguity is unnecessary. Investigators have documented no increased risk of intrapartum hemorrhage when the distance from the lower margin of the placenta to the internal os is at least 2 to 3 cm (Timor-Tritsch and Monteagudo, 1993).

Second, because the normal prelabor internal os is essentially dimensionless, the distinction between a placenta that partially covers the os (traditional *partial placenta previa*) and one that completely covers the os (traditional *complete placenta previa*) is clearly artificial. Thus, the term partial placenta previa is ill defined and of limited clinical utility.

Finally, even with the most sophisticated ultrasound equipment available, most placentas that appear to cover the cervical os in the second trimester will not cover the os at term (Fig. 37-1). Thus, the diagnosis of placenta previa should be made with great caution in the asymptomatic patient during the second trimester.

The previous considerations suggest the following classifications: *placenta previa*, when the placenta covers the internal os in the third trimester, and *marginal placenta previa*, when the placenta lies within 2 to 3 cm of the internal os but does not cover it. With this classification scheme, the term *low-lying placenta* should be reserved for cases in which the exact relationship of the placenta to the os has not been determined or for cases of apparent placenta previa before the third trimester.

Incidence and Etiology

The incidence of placenta previa at the time of delivery varies widely in published series but averages approximately 0.5% of births (Iyasu et al., 1993; Love and Wallace, 1996). The incidence of this condition appears to be increasing (Fredricksen et al., 1999). A number of factors appear to increase the risk of placenta previa, including advancing age, multiparity, African or Asian ethnic background, smoking, cocaine use, prior placenta previa, one or more previous cesarean births, prior suction curettage for spontaneous or induced abortion, and male fetal gender (Zhang and Savitz, 1993; Handler et al., 1994; Taylor et al., 1994; Thomas et al., 1994; Herschkowitz et al., 1995; Monica and Lilja, 1995; Ananth, Savitz, Luther, 1996; Ananth, Wilcox, et al., 1996; Andres, 1996; Chelmow et al., 1996; Hemminki and Merilainen, 1996; Demissie et al., 1999; Mortensen et al., 2001). Relative risks for these factors are described in Table 37-1.

The strong association between placenta previa and parity, previous cesarean delivery, and suction curettage suggests that

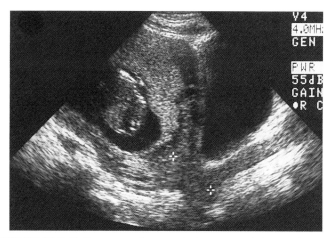

FIGURE 37-1 ■ Sonogram of apparent placenta previa in a patient during the second trimester. At term, the placenta did not encroach upon the cervical os, and the patient underwent uneventful vaginal delivery. (Courtesy of Dr. Paula Woodward, University of Utah.)

endometrial damage is an etiologic factor. Presumably, each pregnancy damages the endometrium underlying the implantation site, rendering the area unsuitable for implantation. Subsequent pregnancies are more likely to become implanted in the lower uterine segment by a process of elimination. This effect is most clearly seen with prior term pregnancies, but multiple early pregnancy terminations may also be related to an increased incidence of placenta previa. Histopathologic investigation of the placental implantation site in women with placenta previa demonstrate increased invasion of trophoblastic giant cells into the decidua, myometrium, and myometrial spiral arteries and increased inflammatory cell infiltration compared with women with normal implantation (Biswas et al., 1999). Such findings may relate to the association between placenta previa and smoking, but the details of this association remain poorly understood.

It is important to recognize that these statistics relate to *symptomatic* placenta previa and the few asymptomatic cases discovered incidentally late in pregnancy by pelvic examination. Low implantations are much more common early in pregnancy, but most of these "resolve" and never become symptomatic (Wexler and Gottesfeld, 1979) (see Fig. 37-1).

  TABLE 37-1. RISK FACTORS AND RELATIVE RISK OF PLACENTA PREVIA

Risk Factor	Increased Risk
Previous placenta previa	8× (Monica and Lilja, 1995)
Previous cesarean section	1.5–15× (Herschkowitz et al., 1995; Hemminki and Merilainen, 1996)
Previous suction curettage for abortion	1.3× (Taylor et al., 1994)
Age >35 years	4.7× (Iyasu et al., 1993)
Age >40 years	9× (Ananth, Wilcox, et al., 1996)
Multiparity	1.1–1.7× (Williams and Mittendorf, 1993)
Non-white (all)	0.3× (Iyasu et al., 1993)
Asian	1.9×
Cigarette smoking	1.4–3× (Handler et al., 1994; Ananth et al., 1996a; Chelmow et al., 1996)

"Resolution" may not be an entirely appropriate term, because a high rate of other complications has been observed in women with early placenta previa, despite apparent resolution in 97% (Newton et al., 1984). Forty-five percent of these women had significant antenatal complications, including antepartum hemorrhage, abruptio placentae, and suspected intrauterine growth restriction. Statistically significant increases in prematurity and perinatal mortality were also seen in this group.

At most, 10% of placenta previa diagnosed in the second trimester are actually found to be such at the time of delivery. The term *placental migration* has been used to describe this phenomenon, but this is a misnomer; no evidence exists that the process of chorionic villus invasion on both sides of the internal os is a reversible process. Rather, such "migration" appears to reflect an inability to precisely determine which placentas do cross the cervical os in early pregnancy, coupled with differential growth of the relatively adynamic lower uterine segment compared with the rapid hypertrophy of myometrial cells in the fundus. Thus, those placentas that in early pregnancy were mistakenly believed to be implanted on both sides of the internal os are drawn cephalad relative to the actual internal os by the growth of their underlying myometrium.

Diagnosis

The hallmark of placenta previa is the sudden onset of painless bleeding in the second or third trimester of pregnancy. The absence of abdominal pain and uterine contractions has classically been considered an important distinguishing feature between placenta previa and abruptio placentae. Because painful labor may precipitate bleeding from a placenta previa, however, this diagnosis must be excluded by sonography in all cases of bleeding during the second half of pregnancy. The initial episode of bleeding has a peak incidence in the early third trimester; one third of cases become symptomatic before the 30th week and one third after the 36th week (Crenshaw et al., 1973). Bleeding may begin without an obvious inciting cause or after pelvic examination, intercourse, or the onset of labor. Absence of bleeding before term does not rule out placenta previa. In approximately 10% of cases, bleeding begins only with the onset of labor.

Sonographic localization of the placenta is a necessary step in the evaluation of the patient with bleeding, except when the bleeding is heavy enough to mandate immediate surgical intervention irrespective of the source (Fig. 37-2). Transabdominal sonography is highly accurate but not infallible, because there are no markers to locate the internal cervical os precisely. As a consequence, both false-positive and false-negative results have been reported. False-negative reports are particularly worrisome because they can lead to a potentially catastrophic management plan. The rate of false-negative results with transabdominal sonography was earlier reported to be as high as 7% (Cotton et al., 1980). The most common reasons for missing placenta previa are positioning of the fetal head that obscures the region of the cervix and failure to scan the *lateral* uterine walls (Laing, 1981). In addition, the presence of blood in the area of the cervix can create the illusion that amniotic fluid is present, falsely ruling out placenta previa. In an asymptomatic patient with a posterior placenta or accessory lobe, even properly performed transabdominal sonography may occasionally miss placenta previa, especially if the patient is obese. However, when the diagnosis is suspected clinically

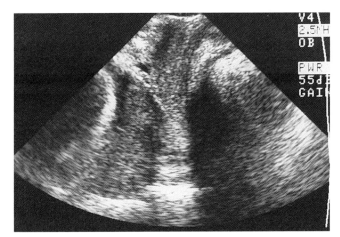

FIGURE 37-2 ■ Sonogram of a placenta previa at term; delivery by cesarean section was necessary. (Courtesy of Dr. Paula Woodward, University of Utah.)

and the scan is performed for this indication, false-negative diagnoses should not occur; if the exact relationship of the placenta to the internal cervical os is uncertain, transvaginal scanning should be performed.

False-positive results are harder to define unless the absence of placenta previa is confirmed immediately by digital examination or at the time of cesarean section. More often, there is a variable interval between the sonogram and the event that confirms or rules out the diagnosis. Overfilling of the bladder can result in a false-positive diagnosis because of compression of the lower uterine segment. The diagnosis should be reported only if the condition appears to persist after the bladder is emptied.

In the past several years, *transvaginal sonography* has been increasingly used for placental localization. Multiple reports attest both to its safety and diagnostic superiority over standard *transabdominal scanning* in the diagnosis and to exclusion of placenta previa (Timor-Tritsch and Monteagudo, 1993; Rosati and Guariglia, 2000; Becker et al., 2001; Oppenheimber et al., 2001). Despite the potential for probe-induced trauma to the placenta, this approach is safe in experienced hands. Indeed, Timor-Tritsch and Yunis (1993) demonstrated that the angle between the cervix and the vaginal probe is sufficient to prevent the probe from inadvertently entering the cervix.

The transvaginal approach offers superior definition of the spatial relationship of the lower placental margin to the internal cervical os. In one series, transvaginal sonography was 100% sensitive in the diagnosis of placenta previa (Farine et al., 1990). False-positive and false-negative results have only rarely been reported (Leerentveld et al., 1990). Ideally, these two approaches should be considered complementary. Generally, a transabdominal scan is performed first. If the placenta is obviously fundal in location or if a placenta previa is clearly seen, the transvaginal examination is unnecessary. When the exact relationship of the lower placental margin to the internal cervical os remains in doubt after transabdominal sonography, a transvaginal or translabial scan may provide useful information. This is especially true when technical difficulties (such as an overfilled or underfilled bladder, a low presenting part, posterior placental location, or maternal obesity) prevent optimal transabdominal examination.

Because of the high rate of spontaneous resolution of placenta previa diagnosed before the third trimester, those women who remain asymptomatic do not need to undergo any special measures or restriction of activity (including intercourse) until 26 to 28 weeks' gestation, at which time another sonogram should be obtained. If the condition persists at this examination, it is more likely that it will be present at the time of delivery. Nevertheless, even when asymptomatic placenta previa is present into the late second trimester, there remains a significant chance of resolution by term depending on the degree of overlap. If the placenta overlaps the internal os by 25 mm or more at 20 to 23 weeks, as ascertained by careful transvaginal sonography, vaginal delivery is unlikely (Becker et al., 2001). Overlap more than 20 mm beyond 26 weeks has similarly been reported as incompatible with subsequent resolution and vaginal delivery (Oppenheimer et al., 2001).

The probability of resolution has not been established for women with symptomatic placenta previa, but it is probably lower. Periodic ultrasonographic examinations should be performed in women being managed expectantly, and a final diagnostic sonogram should be obtained shortly before elective delivery by cesarean section if persistence remains in doubt.

Management

Two major factors have been responsible for the dramatic reduction in both maternal and perinatal mortality rates in patients with placenta previa over the past 40 years: the expectant management approach and the liberal use of cesarean section rather than vaginal delivery. As a result, the maternal mortality rate has fallen from approximately 25% to less than 1%. The perinatal mortality rate has fallen from about 60% to under 10% during the same time period.

General Measures

Any woman with bleeding in the late second trimester or the third trimester should be evaluated immediately. In the patient who is actively bleeding, this evaluation is best performed in the hospital; a secure intravenous line should be established, a complete blood count should be obtained, and crossmatched blood should be made available. If the mother's condition is unstable from a cardiovascular standpoint, adequate fluid and blood replacement are the first priorities. The fetal condition can generally be simultaneously evaluated with electronic fetal heart rate monitoring. Only when the conditions of both the mother and fetus are stable and ongoing hemorrhage is not worrisome should attention be directed to establishing the diagnosis by ultrasonography. If the diagnosis of placenta previa is confirmed, a plan for the timing and method of delivery is outlined with the patient.

Timing of Delivery

The principal fetal risk of placenta previa is the need for preterm delivery because of maternal hemorrhage. Thus, the goal of management for placenta previa is to obtain the maximum fetal maturation possible while minimizing the risk to both fetus and mother. Since the 1940s, an expectant approach has been increasingly advocated as one that optimizes this goal. The basis for this approach is that most episodes of bleeding are usually self-limited and not of immediate danger to either the fetus or the mother. Under carefully controlled conditions, delivery of the fetus may be safely delayed to a more advanced stage of maturity in a significant proportion of cases.

Such delay allows the administration of corticosteroids in appropriate patients. An additional advantage to this approach is that a small proportion of cases, particularly those discovered early with lesser degrees of placenta previa, resolve to an extent permitting vaginal delivery at term.

Once the diagnosis is established, the clinician must decide whether the patient is a suitable candidate for expectant management. If the pregnancy has reached 37 weeks or more at the time of initial bleeding or if lung maturity has been documented by amniocentesis, cesarean delivery is indicated. Delivery should also be undertaken in the presence of life-threatening maternal hemorrhage at any gestational age or beyond 24 weeks' gestation in the presence of fetal distress. Cesarean delivery is also indicated for the laboring patient with placenta previa beyond 32 to 34 weeks' gestation. When the fetus is premature and the bleeding is not life-threatening, the volume of hemorrhage tolerated by the clinician before delivery will be inversely related to gestational age and may also be affected by the level of available facilities for neonatal care. Consultation with maternal-fetal medicine and neonatology may be useful in deciding between conservative management, active tocolysis, delivery, or maternal transport.

In a study by Cotton and associates (1980), approximately 20% of patients lost in excess of 500 mL of blood at the initial episode, yet half of these women were managed expectantly, with a mean gain of 16.8 days. Fourteen patients in labor at the time of the initial bleeding episode, including 5 with initial blood loss estimated in excess of 1000 mL, were treated with tocolytics. In this group, there was a mean gain of 3.4 weeks, with no perinatal deaths. Love and Wallace (1996) demonstrated a median gestational age at the time of the first bleeding episode of 29 weeks, with a median age at delivery in this group of 36 weeks. In a similar manner, Magann and colleagues (1993) described a first bleeding episode at a mean gestational age of 29 weeks, with a mean age at delivery of 34 weeks.

With expectant management, there is no sharp peak in the incidence of deliveries at any given week of gestation but rather a steady rise as the pregnancy advances (Brenner et al., 1978). The probability that the pregnancy will be maintained for 1, 2, or 4 more weeks is a function of the gestational age already attained (Fig. 37-3). It can be seen, for example, that the fetus at 32 weeks has an 80% probability of achieving 36 weeks *in utero*, with potentially significant gains in maturity. Conversely, the fetus at 36 weeks has only slightly better than a 50–50 chance of gaining an additional 2 weeks *in utero*, with considerably less significant gain in maturity.

For patients with placenta previa before 34 weeks in whom bleeding is secondary to uterine activity, tocolysis may be safely undertaken if the maternal or fetal condition does not mandate delivery (Towers et al., 1999). Although magnesium sulfate is associated with fewer potential hemodynamic alterations than β-mimetic agents, both have been used safely (Besinger et al., 1995). The actual risks of inducing clinically significant hemodynamic instability with judiciously administered β-mimetic agents in an otherwise stable patient without active bleeding are small and, at present, remain theoretical.

Several retrospective analyses and one prospective randomized clinical trial have documented the safety of outpatient management for carefully selected patients with placenta previa whose initial episode of bleeding stops (Droste and Keil, 1994; Mouer, 1994; Rosen and Peek, 1994; Love and Wallace, 1996; Wing et al., 1996). In one study, such management was

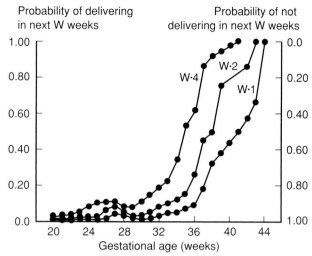

FIGURE 37-3 ■ Graph showing the probability that pregnancy in a patient with placenta previa can be maintained for some time longer (1, 2, or 4 weeks). The fetus at 32 weeks has an 80% chance of remaining in utero for 4 weeks; the fetus at 36 weeks, however, has only a 50% chance of gaining 2 additional weeks of gestation. (From Brenner WE, Edelman DA, Hendricks CH: Characteristics of patients with placenta previa and results of "expectant management." Am J Obstet Gynecol **132**:180, 1978.)

associated with a medical cost savings of more than $15,000 per patient (Wing et al., 1996). Patients considered for such outpatient management should be clinically stable without bleeding, able to maintain bed rest at home, and within a reasonable distance from the hospital, with emergency transportation available 24 hours a day. For such patients, outpatient management, with readmission as necessary for bleeding, is standard in most centers in the United States. There appears to be little benefit to autologous blood donation in patients managed conservatively before term (Dinsmoor and Hogg, 1995).

Delivery

Cesarean section should be performed for all patients in whom the placenta covers the internal os at the time of delivery. In cases of marginal placenta previa in which the placenta is 2 to 3 cm from the os, the risk of intrapartum bleeding remains significant (Timor-Tritsch and Monteagudo, 1993; Dawson et al., 1996). However, such patients may be allowed to labor as long as personnel and facilities are available for emergency operative delivery, should this become necessary. In many cases, the fetal head will tamponade the lower margin of the placenta as it descends, and vaginal delivery may be safely accomplished without significant hemorrhage.

Although the placenta may sometimes be incised during cesarean delivery if a low transverse uterine incision is made in a patient with placenta previa, placenta previa is not a recognized indication for routine vertical uterine incision. Indeed, some degree of placental disruption is commonly necessary for low transverse cesareans performed in the presence of a normally implanted anterior placenta. In such circumstances, fetal blood loss may be kept to a minimum by rapidly going through the placenta or, if possible, by pushing it to one side and expediting delivery of the fetus. Blood loss may also continue after delivery of the placenta. Normally, the blood vessels supplying the intervillous space are occluded by myometrial contractions. The lower uterine segment is only weakly contractile and may be ineffective in occluding such bleeding vessels. Major bleeding vessels can sometimes be controlled by suturing or the direct injection of methylergonovine maleate (Methergine) or 15-methyl prostaglandin $F_{2\alpha}$ into the bleeding area. Systemic administration of these agents may also be effective. Packing of the bleeding area may be useful as a temporizing measure but is rarely sufficient by itself. Ultimately, total abdominal hysterectomy may be necessary, as with frank placenta accreta. Regional anesthesia is often appropriate for such patients and in one study was associated with less blood loss than general anesthesia (Fredricksen et al., 1999).

Complications

Placenta Accreta

One of the most serious complications of placenta previa is the development of placenta accreta. This condition involves trophoblastic invasion beyond the normal boundary established by Nitabuch fibrinoid layer. When invasion extends into the myometrium, the term *placenta increta* is used; placental invasion beyond the uterine serosa (at times involving the bladder or other pelvic organs and vessels) is termed *placenta percreta*. Histologic examples of normal placental implantation and placenta accreta are shown in Figure 37-4.

Placenta accreta is associated positively with advanced maternal age and parity, but the strongest recognized association is with placenta previa and prior uterine surgery. In patients with placenta previa, the risk of accreta is 10% to 25% with one prior cesarean section and exceeds 50% in women with two or more prior cesareans (Clark et al., 1985; Chattopadhyay et al., 1993; Lira Plascencia et al., 1995). Prevalence appears to be the same in women with these risk factors undergoing second-trimester pregnancy termination (Rashbaum et al., 1995).

The diagnosis of placental invasion of the myometrium may be made by abdominal or transvaginal ultrasound, and magnetic resonance imaging has also been used to confirm the diagnosis or better delineate the presence or extent of accreta. Magnetic resonance imaging is useful particularly in the presence of a posterior placenta and in the assessment of deep myometrial, parametrial, and bladder involvement (Levine et al, 1997; Maldjian et al., 1999). The ultrasound appearance of a normal placental attachment site as imaged with ultrasound is shown in Figure 37-5. Normal attachment is characterized by a hypoechoic boundary between the placenta and the bladder that represents the myometrium and the normal retroplacental myometrial vasculature. Placental invasion is associated with the loss of the normal hypoechoic boundary, and there are usually intraplacental sonolucent spaces adjacent to the involved uterine wall. Color-flow and power Doppler sonography have also been reported to facilitate the diagnosis (Lerner et al., 1995; Twickler et al., 2000; Chou et al., 2001). Chou and associates (2001) evaluated 80 women with placenta previa to determine the accuracy of color-flow Doppler in distinguishing between uncomplicated placenta previa and accreta. Using their criteria, the antepartum diagnosis of accreta was made in 16 of the 80 women studied and confirmed histopathologically in 14. The sensitivity and specificity for diagnosis were 82% and 97%, respectively. Although it is clear that larger numbers of patients will need to be studied by these various modalities to more accurately determine the sensitivity

and specificity of diagnosis, various types of ultrasound diagnosis and magnetic resonance imaging appear promising in making or excluding the diagnosis in most cases.

It is important if at all possible to make the diagnosis before delivery, because hemorrhage may be massive intraoperatively. In an effort to diminish blood loss, it is recommended that delivery be accomplished through a fundal incision followed by clamping of the cord. The placenta is allowed to remain in situ, while the surgeons then proceed to a total abdominal hysterectomy. This may require very complex surgical technique and planning, and a pelvic surgeon capable of wide resection of the lower uterine segment and parametrial areas should be available, as well as ample transfusion capability.

Although published reports are not extensive, it has been suggested that balloon occlusion of the aorta or internal iliac vessels may help to prevent excessive blood loss during resection of the lower uterine segment. This involves preoperative placement of balloon-tipped catheters retrograde through the femoral arteries immediately before surgery. The catheters are

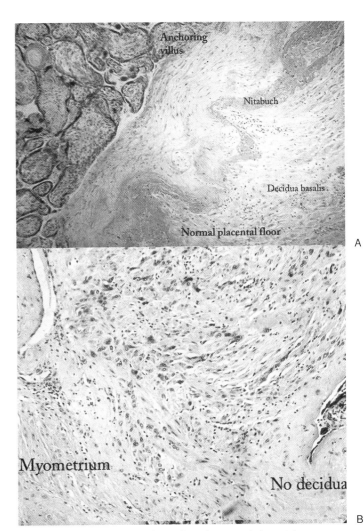

FIGURE 37-4 ■ A, Histologic section of a normal placental attachment site. Trophoblastic tissue with anchoring villi encroach but do not go through the Nitabuch membrane. **B,** Representative histologic section of placenta accreta, demonstrating invasion of trophoblast into the myometrial tissue.

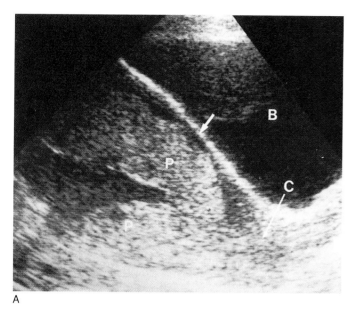
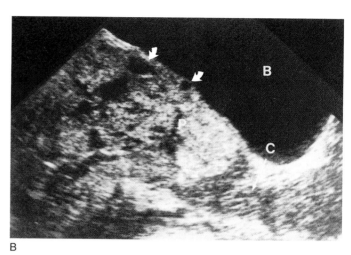

FIGURE 37-5 ■ **A,** Ultrasound appearance of a normal placental attachment in an anterior placenta previa. A hypoechoic area separates the bladder wall and the placental tissue, representing myometrium and myometrial vasculature. B, bladder; C, cervix; P, placenta. **B,** Characteristic ultrasound appearance of placenta accreta. Note the lack of a hypoechoic area, as well as obliteration of the well-delineated bladder wall. In addition, there are intraplacental sonolucent spaces adjacent to the involved uterine wall.

guided under fluoroscopic direction into the internal iliac arteries and inflated during the dissection.

A few reports have suggested a conservative approach, that is, leaving the uterus and placenta in situ and using methotrexate postoperatively (Jaffe et al., 1994; Matthews et al., 1996; Mussalli et al., 2000). However, the numbers of reported cases are very few, and hemorrhagic and infectious complications have resulted. Consequently, a definitive surgical approach to this serious obstetric complication is strongly recommended.

Intrauterine Growth Restriction and Congenital Abnormalities

Varma (1973) reported a 16% rate of fetal growth restriction in association with placenta previa and found a good correlation between the occurrence of such restriction and multiple episodes of antepartum bleeding. On the other hand, Brenner and colleagues (1978) described normal growth in fetuses with placenta previa managed expectantly. Nearly all reports confirm an approximate doubling of the rate of serious congenital malformations in cases of placenta previa, the most common being major anomalies of the central nervous system, cardiovascular system, respiratory tract, and gastrointestinal tract.

A detailed fetal anatomic survey at initial sonographic diagnosis and serial sonographic evaluation of fetal growth should be performed in all cases. An increase in neurodevelopmental abnormalities has been reported at 2-year follow-up in the infants of women with antepartum bleeding secondary to placenta previa and likely represents subtle degrees of fetal hypoxia not detectable or preventable by present means (Spinillo et al., 1994). Although one study suggested acceler-

ated fetal neurologic maturation in the presence of placenta previa, this finding remains of uncertain clinical relevance (Reubinoff et al., 1995).

Sudden Infant Death Syndrome

Li and Wi (1999) presented data linking placenta previa and abruption to an increased risk of sudden infant death syndrome (odds ratio 2.1) and postulated that impaired fetal development resulting from placental abnormality may predispose to infant death.

▪ VASA PREVIA

Vasa previa is uncommon, occurring in about 1 in 3000 deliveries, but it is among the most lethal fetal conditions. It is defined as a velamentous insertion of the cord in the lower uterine segment so that the cord vessels course unsupported through the membranes in advance of the fetal presenting part and often across the cervical os. The unsupported fetal vessels are prone to tearing, especially at the time of spontaneous or artificial rupture of the membranes, with resultant fetal exsanguination, leading to death in at least 75% of cases. Membrane rupture is not invariably the proximate cause of tearing of the vessels (Pent, 1979). Furthermore, the perinatal loss even in the absence of bleeding from torn fetal vessels approaches 50% to 60% because of compression of the vessels by the presenting part and extreme compromise of the placental circulation.

Making the diagnosis in time to save the fetus requires a high index of suspicion. It is rare for this diagnosis to be made before delivery. In most cases, emergency cesarean delivery takes place on the basis of severe variable decelerations (reflecting umbilical cord compression or acute fetal hemorrhage), often with the presumptive diagnosis of placental abruption. Unfortunately, because of the nonspecific nature of variable decelerations, their generally benign clinical course, and the rapidity with which fetal exsanguination occurs (total fetal blood volume = 80 to 100 mL/kg), fetal death or profound neurologic injury is the rule, rather than the exception, despite appropriate management. On rare occasions, vasa previa has been detected by color-flow Doppler techniques (Hata et al., 1994; Catanzarite et al., 2001). However, such a diagnosis is generally fortuitous—routine obstetric sonography would not be expected to detect this condition in most cases.

ABRUPTIO PLACENTAE

Definition

The term abruptio placentae denotes separation of a normally implanted placenta before the birth of the fetus. The diagnosis is most commonly made in the third trimester, but the term may be used after the 20th week of pregnancy when the clinical and pathologic criteria are met. This is a uniquely dangerous condition to both the mother and the fetus because of its potentially serious pathologic sequelae.

Pathophysiology

Abruptio placentae is initiated by bleeding into the decidua basalis. In most cases, the source of the bleeding is small arterial vessels in the basal layer of the decidua that are pathologically altered and prone to rupture. In some cases, the bleeding may be initiated from fetal–placental vessels. The resultant hemorrhage splits the decidua, leaving a thin layer attached to the placenta. As the decidual hematoma grows, there is further separation. Compression by the expanding hematoma leads to obliteration of the overlying intervillous space. Ultimately, there is destruction of the placental tissue in the involved area. This area may sometimes be identified on gross inspection of the placenta by an organized clot lying within a cup-shaped depression on the maternal surface. From the standpoint of the fetus, this occurrence represents a loss of surface area for exchange of respiratory gases and nutrients.

In some cases, the process may be self-limited and of no further consequence to the pregnancy. Often, however, bleeding continues, and the blood under pressure will seek the path of least resistance. If the initial point of separation is toward the center of the placenta, there may be continued dissection and separation in the decidua as well as extravasation into the myometrium and through to the peritoneal surface. This results in the so-called *Couvelaire uterus*. Once the blood reaches the edge of the placenta, it may continue to dissect between the decidua and the fetal membranes and gain access to the vagina through the cervix. It may pass through the membranes into the amniotic sac, causing the port wine discoloration that is almost pathognomonic of abruption. The amount of blood that eventually finds its way through the cervix is often only a small portion of that lost from the circulation and is never a reliable indication of the severity of the condition.

Incidence and Etiology

The reported incidence of abruptio placentae varies widely in published series according to the population studied and the diagnostic criteria applied. Knab (1978) found a range of 0.49% to 1.29% in the series he reviewed, with a mean incidence of 0.83%, or 1 per 120 deliveries. Abruption severe enough to kill the fetus is less common, being found only once in 420 deliveries (Pritchard et al., 1970). However, with the recent rise in cocaine use (a major risk factor for placental abruption), this complication is now seen with increasing frequency in some populations. Between 1967 and 1991, perinatal mortality from abruption decreased from 2.5 per 1000 births to 0.9 per 1000 births in a population in Norway (Rasmussen et al., 1996a). This decline was seen in all age groups and was attributed to improvements in obstetric and neonatal care.

Numerous factors have been suggested to play a causal role in abruptio placentae, but a unifying etiologic concept is still lacking. Underlying disease of the decidua and uterine blood vessels seems to explain best the diversity of associated factors that have been described. For pregnancies culminating in abruption, there is often evidence of a long-standing pathologic fetal–maternal relationship, in that 81% of infants born at less than 36 weeks' gestation are below the mean birth weight for gestational age (Hibbard and Jeffcoate, 1966). Similar findings were confirmed by Rasmussen and colleagues (1996b). Thus, abruptio placentae is usually the final dramatic expression of a long-standing placental disorder. Indeed, histologic evidence of old bleeding is noted frequently in the placentas of women giving birth prematurely without evidence of current placental abruption (Salafia et al., 1995). In addition, systemic immunologic deviations toward suppressed immune response have been documented in patients with placental abruption, although it is not established whether this finding represents cause or effect (Matthiesen et al., 1995). This phenomenon may also account for the increased incidence of sudden infant death syndrome seen in newborns who suffered placental abruption as a fetus (Li and Wi, 1999). A detailed discussion of potential etiologic factors may be found elsewhere (Preucel et al., 1981). Some common factors that play an etiologic role in the development of abruptio placentae are discussed next.

Trauma

Although trauma is clearly related to severe abruption, it accounts for only a few cases. Nevertheless, with significant maternal trauma, especially motor vehicle accidents, a high index of suspicion should be maintained. Most cases associated with trauma evolve within 24 hours of the precipitating event. Even in the absence of vaginal bleeding, close observation and continuous monitoring of the fetus are warranted after significant abdominal trauma in late pregnancy.

In the presence of uterine activity, 24 hours of continuous electronic fetal monitoring is recommended after serious abdominal trauma, because clinical manifestations may be delayed (Kettle et al., 1988) (Fig. 37-6). In the absence of uterine contractions, and with a reassuring fetal heart rate

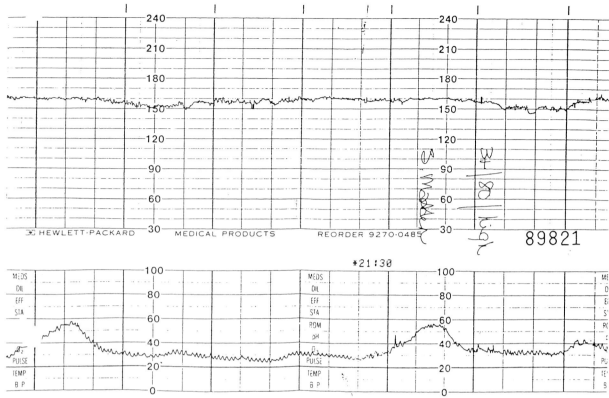

FIGURE 37-6 ■ Late decelerations occurring 18 hours after admission in a 36-week fetus whose mother was involved in a motor vehicle accident. At the time of delivery, a 30% abruption was demonstrated. The infant did well.

tracing, monitoring for as little as 4 to 6 hours is probably sufficient (Dahmus and Sibai, 1993; Towery et al., 1993).

Uterine or Umbilical Cord Anomaly

Extreme shortening of the umbilical cord, sudden decompression of the uterus (at the time of membrane rupture or after delivery of a first twin), and the presence of a uterine anomaly or myoma at the implantation site may be occasionally implicated in abruptio placentae.

Maternal Hypertension

Maternal hypertension, both chronic and pregnancy induced, is a major risk factor for placental abruption (Morgan et al., 1994; Ananth, Savitz, Williams, 1996; Kramer et al., 1997). Mild abruption is not associated with clinically apparent hypertension. However, nearly 50% of cases of abruption sufficiently severe to kill the fetus are associated with maternal hypertension, about half chronic and half pregnancy related (Pritchard et al., 1970); this rate represents a fivefold increase over the rate of hypertension in patients without abruption. Golditch and Boyce (1970) found the incidence of toxemia with abruption to be 13.9% in mild abruption, 25.7% in moderate abruption, and 52.1% in severe abruption. These observations are consistent with the hypothesis that underlying maternal vascular disease is etiologic in both the hypertension and the abruption and that abruption may be an even more sensitive indicator of vascular pathology than hypertension.

Cigarette Smoking

Maternal cigarette smoking is associated with the finding of decidual necrosis on pathologic examination of the placenta. It is therefore not surprising that both a dramatically increased incidence of abruption and an increase in fetal deaths caused by abruption are seen among women who smoke (Cnattingius, 1997; Kramer et al., 1997; Ananth, 1999, 2001; Castles et al., 1999). Furthermore, among women with abruption, smokers have an increased perinatal mortality rate (relative risk 2.5) compared with nonsmokers, a risk that increases by 40% for each pack per day smoked (Raymond and Mills, 1993). Ananth and colleagues (2001) and Kyrklund-Blomberg and coworkers (2001) demonstrated a dose-response relationship between number of cigarettes smoked daily and placental abruption. There is also an increased risk of abruption even in women who smoke before pregnancy; for each year of prepregnancy smoking, Misra and Ananth (1999) demonstrated a 40% increased risk of abruption. This is one potential etiologic factor that is an appropriate target for preventive measures.

Maternal Age and Parity

Abruptio placentae has long been known to occur more frequently in older women, but this increase probably reflects the effect of increased parity (Hibbard and Jeffcoate, 1966; Ananth, Wilcox, et al., 1996; Kramer et al., 1997). The incidence is less than 1% among primigravidas and rises to about 2.5% among grand multiparas. This finding may reflect permanent damage to the endometrium, as with the association between placenta previa and parity. The incidence of abruptio placentae has declined in some studies, perhaps reflecting the effects of widely available family planning and limitation of family size.

Cocaine Abuse

Cocaine-related abruption has been seen with increased frequency over the past several years. Although the complete pathophysiology of cocaine-induced fetal damage and abruption has not been determined, such effects appear to be related, at least in part, to cocaine-induced vasoconstriction. The risk of fetal damage and abruption with cocaine use is substantial, particularly with free-base ("crack") cocaine (Dusick et al., 1993; Emery et al., 1995; Lampley et al., 1996, Addis et al., 2001). As many as 10% of women using cocaine in late gestation have pregnancies that terminate with abruption (Hoskins et al., 1991).

Other Risk Factors

The risk of placental abruption is increased significantly in women with premature rupture of the membranes (Major et al., 1995; Ananth, Savitz, Williams, 1996; Kramer et al., 1997). This observation suggests the need for heightened surveillance in women with this condition. The sonographic identification of subchorionic hemorrhage early in pregnancy is also a risk factor for the later development of placental abruption (Ball et al., 1996). A cesarean delivery in the preceding pregnancy increases the risk of abruption (Hemminki and Merilainen, 1996). Case reports also exist of abruption temporally related to placement of an intrauterine pressure catheter (Handwerker and Selick, 1995). On the other hand, low-dose aspirin, administered for the prevention of pregnancy-induced hypertension, does not increase the risk of abruption (Hauth et al., 1995). Oxytocin does not cause abruption. The thrombophilia are addressed in detail in Chapter 48.

Recent studies have demonstrated an association between maternal hyperhomocystinemia and placental abruption (deVries et al., 1997; Eskes, 2001). The combination of hyperhomocystinemia and thrombophilias such as factor V Leiden increases the risk of abruption by three- to sevenfold (Eskes, 2001). Other conditions such as antiphospholipid syndrome, which give rise to endothelial dysfunction and thrombosis, may also initiate the sequence of pathophysiologic events culminating in placental abruption.

Recurrence

Abruptio placentae is clearly not an acute event in many cases but, instead, an expression of a pathologic process of long duration. This phenomenon probably relates to an increased risk of recurrent abruption in subsequent pregnancies (Ananth, Savitz, Williams, 1996; Misra and Ananth, 1999). The risk of recurrence has been reported to be 5.5% to 16.6%, as much as 30 times the incidence in the general population. Pritchard and coworkers (1970) noted that 7% of women with abruption severe enough to kill the fetus will have the same outcome in a subsequent pregnancy. After two consecutive abruptions, the risk of a third rises to 25%. It is not clear what effect elimination of risk factors (such as pharmacologic control of hypertension or smoking cessation) has on this recurrence risk.

Perinatal Outcome

The overall perinatal mortality rate attributable to placental abruption may be declining because of improvements in obstetric and neonatal care. In 1977, Naeye and associates reported a perinatal mortality rate of 4 per 1000 for abruption in the United States. Rasmussen and colleagues (1996a) reported a rate of 2.5 per 1000 in a series from Norway. By 1991, the rate in the latter population had declined to 0.9 per 1000; this decrease was seen across all birth weights. An increased risk of perinatal asphyxia (Perlman and Risser, 1996; Rasmussen et al., 1996b), cerebral palsy (Spinillo et al., 1993, 1994), periventricular leukomalacia, and intraventricular hemorrhage (Gibbs and Weindling, 1994) is also seen with placental abruption. In many cases, it is difficult to distinguish adverse effects secondary to abruption-related asphyxia from those related to premature delivery necessitated by the abruption.

Diagnosis

The classic symptoms and signs of abruptio placentae are vaginal bleeding, abdominal pain, uterine contractions, and uterine tenderness. The clinician must be aware that not all of these are always present and that the absence of one or more does not exclude the diagnosis or necessarily suggest a mild form. Although vaginal bleeding is the hallmark of abruptio placentae, about 10% of affected women present with only concealed hemorrhage. When the initial point of separation is in the center of the implantation site, a large portion of the placenta may separate before retroplacental blood gains access to the space between the membranes and the decidua and ultimately to the vagina. The observed amount of bleeding thus may give little or no indication of the total loss from the maternal circulation and cannot be used to gauge the severity of the problem or to guide replacement therapy.

Abdominal pain is a less constant presenting symptom than vaginal bleeding, being found in some series in only slightly over half of cases at admission. Its presence probably indicates extravasation of blood into the myometrium or painful hypertonic uterine contractions induced by the abruption. In mild cases, the pain may be intermittent and difficult to distinguish from the pain of labor. In severe cases, the pain may be sharp, sudden in onset, and severe. The initial episode may subside, only to be followed by an intermittent crampy pain or a persistent dull pain in the lower abdomen or back. There may be associated nausea and vomiting.

Uterine contractions are present in most cases but may be difficult to appreciate clinically. They are characteristically of high frequency but low amplitude, and if the baseline uterine tonus is elevated, they may not be palpable and may not register reliably on an external tocodynamometer. A case of total placental abruption that demonstrates some of these points is illustrated in Figure 37-7. In severe cases, the uterus may become so rigid that outlining the fetus is difficult or impossible. Uterine tenderness may be generalized or localized to the site of placental detachment. When it is localized, the point of maximal tenderness often corresponds to the area in which the patient's pain is perceived. Especially when the placenta is implanted posteriorly, uterine tenderness may be absent and the pain is often in the lower back.

Ultrasonography, although useful to exclude placenta previa, is not sufficiently sensitive to reliably either diagnose

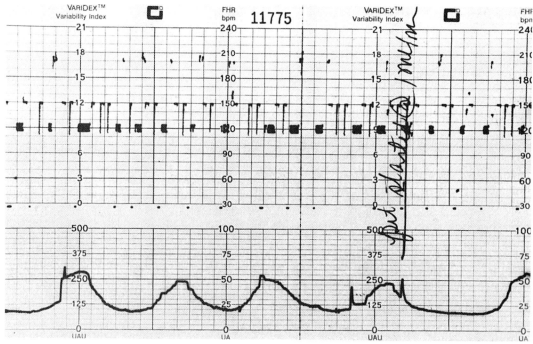

FIGURE 37-7 ■ Internal monitor tracing from a case of severe abruption. The *upper panel* shows artifact only; the fetus is dead. The *lower panel*, derived from a calibrated internal pressure transducer, shows modest elevation of the baseline tonus and uterine tachysystole. Five contractions occurred in a 7-minute period.

or exclude abruptio placentae. However, a spectrum of sonographic findings may occasionally be found that supports the diagnosis. Acute hemorrhage is characteristically hyperechoic or isoechoic compared with the placenta and may therefore be misinterpreted as an abnormally thick placenta (Nyberg et al., 1987). Resolving hematomas become hypoechoic within 1 week and sonolucent within 2 weeks. Prospective use of ultrasonography is rarely helpful in guiding the decision for expectant management as opposed to delivery. It must be emphasized that valuable time should not be lost performing a sonogram in the presence of obvious fetal distress or an unstable maternal condition or in one requiring continuous electronic fetal heart rate monitoring.

In most cases, the diagnosis of abruption is a tentative one, based on a constellation of clinical findings; decisions regarding timing and mode of delivery will generally be made on the basis of electronic fetal heart rate monitoring. Several studies have shown the Kleihauer-Betke test for fetal hemoglobin to be of no value in the general workup of patients with placental abruption (Dahmus and Sibai, 1993; Towery et al., 1993; Emery et al., 1995). In a similar manner, although CA-125 appears to be elevated in abruption, it has no apparent clinical utility (Williams et al., 1993).

Management

General Measures

Any patient with suspected abruptio placentae should be hospitalized immediately. If the fetus is alive and at or near term on admission, delay in instituting an effective plan for delivery may have dire consequences. In Knab's (1978) series, 22% of all perinatal deaths occurred after hospitalization but before delivery, 30% of these within 2 hours of

admission. A rapid evaluation of the mother's condition is initially made. A blood pressure reading in the normal range may be misleading because an underlying hypertensive condition may be revealed only after intravascular volume is restored. The vital signs are obtained frequently. An external fetal monitor is placed, and evidence of fetal distress is sought. After maternal and fetal conditions have been determined to be stable, real-time ultrasound may be performed to exclude placenta previa if this has not already been accomplished during the course of prenatal care.

A large-bore intravenous line is placed, through which the initial blood samples for the laboratory may be drawn. The initial infusate generally consists of crystalloid solution. If there is evidence of maternal hypovolemia, at least two such lines should be placed and secured well, because subsequent attempts at intravenous placement may become progressively more difficult. An indwelling Foley catheter may assist in monitoring urine output. The initial hematocrit readings may be falsely reassuring, especially if the patient's symptoms are of recent onset. Baseline electrolyte, renal function, and coagulation studies may be useful for later comparison if massive transfusion is required as well as for later detection of renal complications. Depending on the initial hematocrit level and overall clinical condition of the patient, blood may be typed and screened or crossmatched.

Method and Timing of Delivery

Once the diagnosis is established, a rational plan for effecting delivery of the fetus must be established. This is the single most important therapeutic goal. The method and timing of delivery depend on the condition and gestational age of the fetus, the condition of the mother, and the status of the cervix.

If the fetus is immature and the abruption is judged to be mild, an expectant approach may be followed. Indeed, it is impossible in some cases to distinguish between idiopathic preterm labor and mild abruptio placentae. In the absence of fetal distress or maternal complications, a trial of tocolytic treatment may be undertaken. Delivery should be accomplished, however, if the abruption is adversely affecting maternal or fetal condition.

If the fetal heart rate tracing is normal and the uterus relaxes well between contractions, an attempt at vaginal delivery may be considered. Even before the introduction of electronic fetal monitoring, there was no increase in the perinatal mortality rate with mild abruption, irrespective of the interval from diagnosis to delivery, as long as the auscultated heart rate was normal (Golditch and Boyce, 1970). A report by Manolitsas and coworkers (1994) validated the general approach of basing delivery decisions principally on the fetal heart rate pattern. This finding has been validated by widespread clinical practice since that time and is standard practice today. In some cases, the use of intravenous oxytocin is required to augment uterine activity. Caution must be exercised because the uterine response may be erratic. No specific time limit may be rationally applied as long as intensive fetal and maternal surveillance reveals no significant advancement in abruption severity and the labor is progressing.

When delivery is planned, amniotomy allows placement of a fetal scalp electrode for heart rate monitoring and an intra-amniotic catheter. Careful calibration of the pressure transducer gives a reliable measure of resting baseline tonus and the contraction pattern. A resting tonus higher than 15 to 25 mm Hg may be associated with deficits of uterine blood flow, compounding the deleterious effects of the reduced exchange area and frequent contractions. In such cases, the prospect for vaginal delivery of a healthy infant is small unless the labor is far advanced, and early resort to cesarean section may be necessary.

Although vaginal delivery is appropriate for many fetuses with ongoing placental abruption, it is important to keep in mind that fetal condition may deteriorate rapidly. Thus, the threshold for operative intervention based on an abnormal fetal heart rate pattern should be lower in such cases than in the laboring woman without evidence of abruption. Because disseminated intravascular coagulopathy (DIC) is uncommon with a living fetus, its presence rarely interferes with decisions regarding operative delivery.

Complications

Hemorrhagic Shock

Shock is characterized by tissue hypoperfusion. Various compensatory physiologic mechanisms allow the mother to remain hemodynamically stable until the volume of blood loss exceeds 25% of her total blood volume (approximately 1500 mL). Beyond this point, additional unreplaced blood loss results in rapid hemodynamic deterioration (Clark et al., 1997). Rational therapy should be aimed at restoring effective perfusion by restoring effective circulating blood volume. This restoration is necessary to avoid major complications, such as ischemic necrosis of the kidneys, and often requires massive amounts of blood product replacement. A urine output of 0.5 mL/kg suggests that peripheral perfusion is adequate. If oliguria persists after volume expansion, however, other methods for monitoring effective circulating volume are necessary. The use of central monitoring techniques is more commonly required when severe preeclampsia complicates replacement therapy, because there is no definable "end point" for blood pressure and because intrinsic renal disease may render urine output a false indicator of effective circulating volume.

Crystalloid solution can be infused until crossmatched blood is available. If there is clear evidence of massive hemorrhage on admission, the initial use of type and screened or type-specific blood may be necessary. Initial crystalloid therapy should consist of volumes two to three times in excess of the actual hemorrhage because most shock states are associated with significant fluid shifts from the intravascular to the extravascular compartment (Clark et al., 1997). Subsequent fluid therapy is aimed at maintaining an adequate circulating blood volume and hematocrit.

Massive transfusion may be defined as transfusion in excess of 1 to 1.5 times the patient's estimated circulating blood volume (approximately 8 units). Several problems may be encountered in this situation. The first is dilutional coagulopathy that may be confused with the diagnosis of DIC in abruptio placentae. Banked blood is generally fractionated into packed red blood cells and plasma; administration of the former alone does not replace the procoagulants lost with the patient's own blood. In the absence of overt coagulopathy, the prophylactic replacement of platelets and other clotting factors is usually unnecessary. Blood samples may be taken for coagulation analysis after 6 to 8 units of packed cells have been administered. A platelet count lower than 30,000/mm³ in a bleeding patient indicates the need for platelet transfusion. Each bag of platelet concentrate administered can be expected to raise the count by 8000 to 10,000/mm³ (Clark et al., 1997). Similarly, a fibrinogen level less than 100 mg/dL may indicate the need for replacement with fresh frozen plasma. Banked blood is also characterized by loss of potassium from red blood cells and can raise the serum potassium to dangerous levels in the massively transfused patient. The serum potassium level should be checked after each 4 to 6 units infused, and continuous monitoring by electrocardiogram is highly desirable.

Disseminated Intravascular Coagulation

Disorders of coagulation are discussed comprehensively in Chapters 45 and 47, but it is pertinent to review here the pathophysiology and management of DIC with abruptio placentae. Clinically significant coagulopathy is encountered in only about 10% of cases of abruption, but it is much more common in severe abruption marked by death of the fetus or massive hemorrhage. Proper management of this disorder demands an understanding of its pathophysiology and correct interpretation of various laboratory tests of hemostasis and blood coagulation.

A general outline of the clotting and fibrinolytic systems is shown in Figure 37-8. Thrombus formation is initiated by platelets, which adhere to the site of blood vessel injury. The process makes available platelet factor 3, which interacts with factors XI, XII, and XIII to form the intrinsic activator complex. Alternately, the extrinsic pathway involves the interaction of tissue thromboplastins released at the site of injury and factor VII, leading to the formation of the extrinsic activator complex. Either the intrinsic or extrinsic activator complex

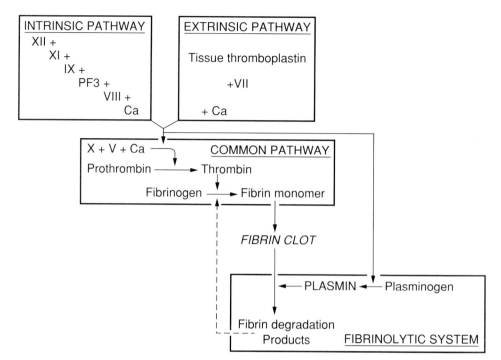

FIGURE 37-8 ■ General outline of coagulation and fibrinolytic systems. *Solid lines* indicate stimulation; *broken lines* indicate inhibition.

can interact with factors X and V in the common pathway, resulting in the generation of thrombin. A proteolytic enzyme, thrombin acts on fibrinogen to cause the formation of fibrin monomer, which spontaneously polymerizes to form fibrin polymer. This unstable product is stabilized in the presence of factor XIII, resulting in the formation of the fibrin clot.

The extraordinary potency of the clotting mechanism is illustrated by the fact that sufficient potential thrombin exists in 10 mL of blood to clot 2500 mL of plasma. Thus, the unimpeded action of thrombin can result in total coagulation of the circulating blood volume in the absence of equally potent counterbalancing factors, the most important of which is the *fibrinolytic system*. Circulating plasminogen (profibrinolysin) is converted to plasmin (fibrinolysin) by a variety of plasminogen activators. Plasmin is a proteolytic enzyme that can cleave a variety of substrates. When plasmin acts on fibrinogen and fibrin, fragments are produced that are collectively termed *fibrin degradation products*. Certain of these fragments serve as antithrombins, both by competing with fibrinogen for available thrombin and by forming nonclottable complexes with fibrin monomer. Thus, the fibrinolytic system is a potent anticoagulation mechanism. Normal hemostatic function depends on the critical balance between the coagulation and fibrinolytic systems to maintain the fluid state of the vascular system while allowing the local formation of clots at various sites of injury. This balance is clearly disturbed in a number of cases of abruptio placentae.

The pathophysiology of DIC is illustrated in Figure 37-9. Entry of thromboplastins into the circulation from the site of placental injury is the inciting event. This process does not appear to be intrinsically different from that causing DIC in the more serious *amniotic fluid embolus syndrome*; indeed, abruption is a relatively common antecedent to this condition (Clark et al., 1995). The thromboplastins initiate widespread intravascular activation of the clotting cascade. Clotting factors are consumed in the process. It is unusual, in the absence of severe shock, to see clinical evidence of intravascular coagulation per

se, such as plugging of vascular beds with end-organ infarction. Lack of such is evidence of the secondary activation of the fibrinolytic system, which may be viewed as a protective mechanism in this clinical setting. The costs of maintaining the fluid state of the blood are the further depletion of fibrinogen

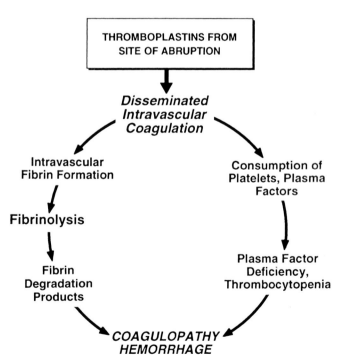

FIGURE 37-9 ■ Pathogenesis of the coagulation disorder in abruptio placentae. The entry of thromboplastic materials from the site of placental injury causes a widespread intravascular initiation of the clotting cascade. It is rare to observe evidence of intravascular thrombus formation because the fibrinolytic system rapidly dissolves the clot. Activation of the fibrinolytic system, in concert with consumption of procoagulants (especially fibrinogen), is responsible for the coagulopathy seen with severe abruption.

(through the proteolytic action of fibrinolysin) and the production of fibrin (and fibrinogen) split products, which are potent thrombin inhibitors. The result of this process is a coagulation disorder characterized by severe hypofibrinogenemia, moderate to severe depletion of other procoagulants and platelets, and the presence of circulating anticoagulants.

The *diagnosis* of DIC is sometimes obvious, with bleeding from needle puncture sites or uncontrollable hemorrhage at surgery. Nevertheless, a significant coagulation disorder can exist without obvious clinical signs as long as the physical integrity of the vascular system is maintained. The advantage in earlier diagnosis is that the need for blood component therapy may be anticipated. The tests that are most helpful in establishing the diagnosis are listed in Table 37-2.

In the absence of markedly abnormal values, a trend toward the abnormal range on serial testing can be helpful in establishing the presence of significant coagulopathy; however, commonly used tests of coagulation, such as prothrombin time and partial thromboplastin time, are insensitive indicators of the intravascular consumption/fibrinolysis process; more than 50% of clotting factors must be consumed before such tests become abnormal. The whole blood clotting time is also insensitive because it will remain essentially normal even with a moderate coagulation disorder. Nevertheless, it is a valuable bedside test if performed serially. If blood fails to clot within 8 minutes, a significant coagulopathy is present, and one need not await confirmatory tests before ordering appropriate replacement products. The fibrinogen level is a sensitive indicator of the process on serial testing, but an initially normal result does not rule out DIC. The serum fibrinogen level increases in normal pregnancy and generally exceeds 400 mg/dL. The platelet count often falls in concert with fibrinogen levels, but there are sometimes striking differences in magnitude. In almost all such cases, the degree of fall in the fibrinogen level exceeds that in the platelet count.

The most sensitive laboratory test for diagnosis of abruption-related coagulopathy is the determination of fibrin-fibrinogen degradation products by one of a variety of techniques, including assays for D-dimer. Their presence at abnormal levels confirms the presence of a coagulopathy but gives only qualitative information as to the severity of the process.

Delivery of the fetus and placenta is the ultimate treatment of DIC with abruptio placentae. Clear evidence of spontaneous resolution after delivery has been presented by Pritchard and Brekken (1967). With removal of the placenta, fibrinogen levels rise by an average of 9 mg/dL/hour. Even in the most severe cases, it is uncommon for clinically evident coagulopathy to persist beyond 12 hours after delivery. The postpartum rise in the platelet count is delayed because of the time required for maturation and release of new platelets by the bone marrow. Therefore, the platelet count may not fully normalize until several days postpartum. The only clear indication for clotting factor replacement in patients with DIC is severe coagulopathy (fibrinogen level less than 100 mg/dL, platelet count less than 30,000 cells/mm³) in a patient who requires cesarean section. In such a patient, perioperative administration of plasma and other procoagulants may be necessary.

The various blood replacement products commonly used are shown in Table 37-3. Fresh whole blood is rarely available and should not be viewed as offering any advantage over component therapy in most cases. Fibrinogen is the specific procoagulant most often needed. Approximately 4 g is necessary to raise the concentration by 100 mg/dL. It may be administered as fresh frozen plasma if there is a concurrent need for volume expansion. Alternatively, fibrinogen may be administered as cryoprecipitate, which contains 3 to 10 times the fibrinogen per unit volume as plasma. The fibrinogen content of a bag of cryoprecipitate is variable but averages 0.25 g. Platelet

TABLE 37-2. COAGULATION TESTS IN DIAGNOSIS OF ABRUPTIO PLACENTAE

Test	What It Measures	Normal Value	Value in Abruption
Bleeding time	Vascular integrity and platelet function	1–5 min	Usually normal; test of little clinical use in diagnosing abruption
Whole blood clotting time	Platelet function Fibrinolytic activity	Clot formation: 4–8 min	Clot formation abnormality indicates severe deficiency
		Clot retraction: <1 hr Clot lysis: none in 24 hr	Abnormal retraction with thrombocytopenia
Fibrinogen	Fibrinogen level	400–650 mg/100 mL	Usually decreased (see text)
Platelet count	Number of platelets	>140,000/mm³	Usually decreased (see text)
Fibrin degradation products	Fibrin and fibrinogen degradation products	<10 µg/mL	Nearly always elevated; most sensitive test
Euglobulin clot lysis time	Fibrinolytic activity	None in 2 hr	Difficult to interpret with low fibrinogen levels
Prothrombin time	Factors II, V, VII, X	10–12 sec	Normal to prolonged
Partial thromboplastin time	Factors II, V, XIII, IX, X, XI	24–38 sec	Normal to prolonged
Thrombin time	Factors I, II Circulating split products Heparin effect	16–20 sec	Parallels fall in fibrinogen; good marker of abruption severity
Red blood cell (RBC) morphology	Microangiopathic hemolysis	Absence of RBC distortion or fragmentation	Presence of distortion or fragmentation is uncommon but indicates risk of renal cortical necrosis

TABLE 37-3. BLOOD REPLACEMENT PRODUCTS

Component	Volume/Unit*	Factors Present	Effect Unit
Fresh whole blood	500	Red blood cells; all procoagulants	Increase hematocrit 3%
Packed red blood cells	200	Red blood cells only	Increase hematocrit 3%
Fresh frozen plasma	200–400	All procoagulants; no platelets	Increase fibrinogen 25 mg/dL
Cryoprecipitate	20–50	Fibrinogen; factors VIII and XIII	Increase fibrinogen 15%–25%
Platelet concentrate	35–60	Platelets; small amounts of fibrinogen; factors V and VIII	Increase platelet count by about 8000/mm³

* Volume depends on individual blood bank.

concentrates are indicated when the platelet count is less than 30,000 cells/mm³ in a patient undergoing surgery. Each bag can be expected to raise the platelet count by 8000 to 10,000 cells/mm³ (Clark et al., 1997). The need for subsequent replacement is guided by serial coagulation tests.

Once delivery is accomplished, further replacement is often unnecessary because the process usually resolves fairly rapidly. Formation of a normal clot signals that frequent coagulation tests are no longer required. The use of either heparin or antifibrinolytic agents is generally not indicated in abruption-induced DIC.

Ischemic damage to the kidneys is among the most severe maternal complications of abruptio placentae. The damage takes the form of either acute tubular necrosis or bilateral cortical necrosis and is caused by hypoxia resulting from hemorrhagic shock or microvascular obstruction by fibrin deposition. Both forms are characterized in the early phase by oliguria or anuria, and they may be impossible to distinguish. Acute tubular necrosis tends to appear somewhat late in the clinical course and is usually reversible with time. Renal cortical necrosis tends to occur early in the course of abruption and leads to death from uremia within 1 to 2 weeks unless chronic dialysis is initiated.

The key to prevention of either of these complications is vigorous blood and fluid therapy to combat hypovolemic shock. Renal cortical necrosis has not been observed in more than 300 consecutive cases of severe abruption treated with this approach (Pritchard et al., 1970). In addition to the kidneys, hypoxic damage has been observed in the liver, adrenal glands, and pituitary gland. Anterior pituitary necrosis (*Sheehan syndrome*) may lead to later symptoms of hypopituitarism.

Fetal Complications

Because abruptio placentae is probably the result of a long-standing pathologic process, it is not surprising that there is a high incidence of growth restriction and congenital abnormalities. Abnormal neurologic development may occur despite timely delivery of a nonasphyxiated infant. Birth weight in about 80% of infants born before 36 weeks' gestation is below the mean for gestational length (Hibbard and Jeffcoate, 1966). In addition, there is a threefold increase in the rate of major malformations, mostly involving the central nervous system. There may be significant fetal bleeding in rare cases of abruption, with a resultant neonatal anemia. Abnormal neurologic development at 2-year follow-up has been noted in infants of women with antepartum hemorrhage caused by either placenta previa or placental abruption (Spinillo et al., 1994).

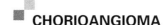

CHORIOANGIOMA

Placental chorioangiomas (hemangiomas) are the most common benign tumors of the placenta. One study suggested an increased incidence of this condition at high altitude (Reshitnikova et al., 1996). Although small chorioangiomas are relatively common, they are of little consequence. Multiple and large tumors (>5 cm) are associated with a variety of complications, including polyhydramnios, hydrops fetalis, preeclampsia, preterm labor, fetomaternal transfusion, abruptio placentae, abnormal presentation, and elevated amniotic fluid alpha-fetoprotein. The diagnosis should be considered in the investigation of all cases of polyhydramnios (Hirata et al., 1993). In many cases, however, the diagnosis is made as an incidental finding on ultrasonographic examination. Chorioangiomas characteristically appear as complex masses

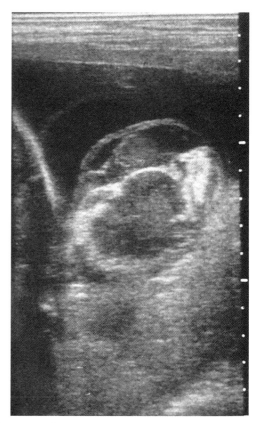

FIGURE 37-10 ■ Sonogram of placental chorioangioma. The appearance of such tumors is highly variable.

on the fetal surface of the placenta, and their vascular nature can be demonstrated with Doppler studies (Grundy et al., 1986) (Fig. 37-10). In some cases, however, they may be multiple and distributed throughout the placental substance (O'Malley et al., 1981). In these cases, they may be difficult to differentiate from other causes of placental thickening. A high incidence of fetal death (up to 30%) has been reported with large tumors that are associated with polyhydramnios or, occasionally, with oligohydramnios (Engel et al., 1981). Frequent antenatal surveillance should be carried out in patients with chorioangiomas (Hurwitz et al., 1983).

REFERENCES

Addis A, Moretti ME, Ahmed SF, et al: Fetal effects of cocaine: An updated meta-analysis Reprod Toxicol **15**:341, 2001.

Ananth CV, Savitz DA, Luther ER: Maternal cigarette smoking as a risk factor for placental abruption, placenta previa, and uterine bleeding in pregnancy. Am J Epidemiol **144**:881, 1996.

Ananth CV, Savitz DA, Williams MA: Placental abruption and its association with hypertension and prolonged rupture of membranes: A methodologic review and meta-analysis. Obstet Gynecol **88**:309, 1996.

Ananth CV, Smulian JC, Demisssie K, et al: Placental abruption among singleton and twin births in the United States: Risk factor profiles. Am J Epidemiol **153**:771, 2001.

Ananth CV, Smulian JC, Vintzileos AM: Incidence of placental abruption in relation to cigarette smoking and hypertensive disorders during pregnancy: A meta-analysis of observational studies. Obstet Gynecol **93**:622, 1999.

Ananth CV, Wilcox AJ, Savitz DA, et al: Effect of maternal age and parity on the risk of uteroplacental bleeding disorders in pregnancy. Obstet Gynecol **88**:511, 1996.

Andres RL: The association of cigarette smoking with placenta previa and abruptio placentae. Semin Perinatol **20**:154, 1996.

Ball RH, Ade CM, Schoenborn JA, et al: The clinical significance of ultrasonographically detected subchorionic hemorrhages. Am J Obstet Gynecol **174**:996, 1996.

Becker RH, Vonk R, Mende BC, et al: The relevance of placental location at 20–23 gestational weeks for prediction of placenta previa at delivery: Evaluation of 8650 cases. Ultrasound Obstet Gynecol **17**:496, 2001.

Besinger RE, Moniak CW, Paskiewicz LS, et al: The effect of tocolytic use in the management of symptomatic placenta previa. Am J Obstet Gynecol **172**:1770, 1995.

Biswas R, Sawhney H, Dass R, et al: Histopathological study of placental bed biopsy in placenta previa. Acta Obset Gynaecol Scand **78**:173, 1999.

Brenner WE, Edelman DA, Hendricks CH: Characteristics of patients with placenta previa and results of "expectant management." Am J Obstet Gynecol **132**:180, 1978.

Castles A, Adams EK, Melvin CL, et al: Effects of smoking during pregnancy. Five meta-analyses. Am J Prev Med **16**:208, 1999.

Catanzarite V, Maida C, Thomas W, et al: Prenatal sonographic diagnosis of vasa previa: Ultrasound findings and obstetric outcome in ten cases. Ultrasound Obstet Gynecol **18**:109, 2001.

Chattopadhyay SK, Kharif H, Sherbeeni MM: Placenta previa and accreta after previous cesarean section. Eur J Obstet Gynaecol Reprod Biol **52**:151, 1993.

Chelmow D, Andrew DE, Baker ER: Maternal cigarette smoking and placenta previa. Obstet Gynecol **87**:703, 1996.

Chou MM, Tseng JJ, Ho ES, et al: Three dimensional color power Doppler imaging in the assessment of uteroplacental neovascularization in placenta previa increta/percreta. Am J Obstet Gynecol **185**:1257, 2001.

Clark SL, Cotton DB, Hankins GDV, et al: Critical Care Obstetrics, 3rd ed. Cambridge, Mass, Blackwell, 1997.

Clark SL, Hankins GDV, Dudley DA, et al: Amniotic fluid embolism: Analysis of the national registry. Am J Obstet Gynecol **172**:1159, 1995.

Clark SL, Koonings PP, Phelan JP: Placenta previa/accreta and prior cesarean section. Obstet Gynecol **66**:89, 1985.

Cnattingius S: Maternal age modifies the effect of maternal smoking on intrauterine growth retardation but not on late fetal death and placental abruption. Am J Epidemiol **145**:319, 1997.

Cotton DB, Read JA, Paul RH, et al: The conservative aggressive management of placenta previa. Am J Obstet Gynecol **137**:687, 1980.

Crenshaw C, Jones DED, Parker RT: Placenta previa: A survey of twenty years experience with improved perinatal survival by expectant therapy and cesarean delivery. Obstet Gynecol Surv **28**:461, 1973.

Dahmus MA, Sibai BM: Blunt abdominal trauma: Are there any predictive factors for abruptio placentae or maternal-fetal distress? Am J Obstet Gynecol **169**:1054, 1993.

Dawson WB, Dumas MD, Romano WM, et al: Translabial sonography and placenta previa. J Ultrasound Med **15**:441, 1996.

DeVries JI, Dekker GA, Huijens PC, et al: Hyperhomocysteinaemia and protein S deficiency in complicated pregnancies. Br J Obstet Gynaecol **104**:1248, 1997.

Dinsmoor MJ, Hogg BB: Autologous blood donation with placenta previa: Is it feasible? Am J Perinatol **12**:382, 1995.

Droste S, Keil K: Expectant management of placenta previa: Cost-benefit analysis of outpatient treatment. Am J Obstet Gynecol **175**:1254, 1994.

Dusick AM, Covert RF, Schreiber MD, et al: Risk of intracranial hemorrhage and other adverse outcomes after cocaine exposure in a cohort of 323 very low birth weight infants. J Pediatr **122**:438, 1993.

Emery CL, Morway LF, Chung-Park M, et al: The Kleihauer-Betke test: Clinical utility, indication, and correlation in patients with placental abruption and cocaine use. Arch Pathol Lab Med **119**:1032, 1995.

Engel K, Haln T, Karschnia R: Sonographic diagnosis of a placental tumour with high-grade intrauterine foetal development deficiency, increasing anhydramnia and subsequent foetal death. Geburtshilfe Frauenheilkd **41**:570, 1981.

Eskes TK: Clotting disorders and placental abruption: homocysteine—A new risk factor. Eur J Obstet Gynaecol Reprod Biol **95**:206, 2001.

Farine D, Peisner DB, Timor-Tritsch IE: Placenta previa: Is the traditional diagnostic approach satisfactory? J Clin Ultrasound **18**:328, 1990.

Fredricksen MC, Glassenberg R, Stika CS: Placenta previa: A 22-year analysis. Am J Obstet Gynecol **180**:1432, 1999.

Gibbs JM, Weindling AM: Neonatal intracranial lesions following placental abruption. Eur J Pediatr **153**:195, 1994.

Golditch IM, Boyce NE: Management of abruptio placentae. JAMA **212**:288, 1970.

Grundy HU, Byersa L, Walton S, et al: Antepartum ultrasonographic evaluation and management of placental chorioangioma: A case report. J Reprod Med **31**:520, 1986.

Handler AS, Mason ED, Rosenberg DL, et al: The relationship between exposure during pregnancy to cigarette smoking and cocaine use and placenta previa. Am J Obstet Gynecol **170**:884, 1994.

Handwerker SM, Selick AM: Placental abruption after insertion of catheter tip intrauterine pressure transducers: A report of four cases. J Reprod Med **40**:845, 1995.

Hata K, Hata T, Fujiwake R, et al: An accurate antenatal diagnosis of vasa previa with transvaginal color Doppler ultrasound. Am J Obstet Gynecol **171**:265, 1994.

Hauth JC, Goldenberg RL, Parker CR, et al: Low-dose aspirin: Lack of association with an increase in abruptio placentae or perinatal mortality. Obstet Gynecol **85**:1055, 1995.

Hemminki E, Merilainen J: Long-term effects of cesarean sections: Ectopic pregnancies and placental problems. Am J Obstet Gynecol **174**:1569, 1996.

Herschkowitz R, Fraser D, Mazor M, et al: One or multiple previous cesarean sections are associated with similar increased frequency of placenta previa. Eur J Obstet Gynaecol Reprod Biol **62**:185, 1995.

Hibbard BM, Jeffcoate TNA: Abruptio placentae. Obstet Gynecol **27**:155, 1966.

Hirata GI, Masaki DI, O'Toole M, et al: Color flow mapping and Doppler velocimetry in the diagnosis and management of placental chorioangioma associated with non-immune hydrops. Obstet Gynecol **81**:850, 1993.

Hoskins IA, Friedman DA, Frieden FJ, et al: Relationship between antepartum cocaine abuse, abnormal umbilical artery Doppler velocimetry and placental abruption. Obstet Gynecol **78**:279, 1991.

Hurwitz A, Milwidsky A, Yarkoni S, et al: Severe fetal distress with hydramnios due to chorioangioma. Acta Obstet Gynecol Scand **62**:633, 1983.

Iyasu S, Saftlas AK, Rowley DL, et al: The epidemiology of placenta previa in the United States, 1979 through 1987. Am J Obstet Gynecol **168**:1424, 1993.

Jaffe R, DuBeshter B, Sherer DM, et al: Failure of methotrexate treatment for term placenta percreta. Am J Obstet Gynecol **171**:558, 1994.

Kettle LM, Branch DW, Scott JR: Occult abruption after maternal trauma. Obstet Gynecol **71**:449, 1988.

Knab DR: Abruptio placentae: An assessment of the time and method of delivery. Obstet Gynecol **52**:625, 1978.

Kramer MS, Usher RH, Pollack R, et al: Etiologic determinants of abruptio placentae. Obstet Gynecol **89**:221, 1997.

Kyrklund-Blomberg NB, Gennser G, Cnattingius S: Placental abruption and perinatal death. Paediatr Perinat Epidemiol **15**:290, 2001.

Laing FC: Placenta previa: Avoiding false-negative diagnoses. J Clin Ultrasound 9:109, 1981.

Lampley EC, Williams S, Myers SA: Cocaine-associated rhabdomyolysis causing renal failure in pregnancy. Obstet Gynecol 87:804, 1996.

Leerentveld RA, Gilberts EC, Arnold MJ, et al: Accuracy and safety of transvaginal placental localization. Obstet Gynecol 76:759, 1990.

Lerner JP, Deane S, Timor-Tritsch IE: Characterization of placenta accreta using transvaginal sonography and color Doppler imaging. Ultrasound Obstet Gynecol 5:198, 1995.

Levine D, Hulka CA, Ludmir J, et al: Placenta accreta. Evaluation with color Doppler US, Power Doppler US, and MI imaging. Radiology 205:773, 1997.

Li DK, Wi S: Maternal placental abnormality and the risk of sudden infant death syndrome. Am J Epidemiol 149:608, 1999.

Lira Plascencia J, Ibarguengoitia Ochoa F, et al: Placenta praevia/accreta and previous cesarean section: Experience of five years at the Mexico National Institute of Perinatology. Gynecol Obstet Mex 63:337, 1995.

Love CD, Wallace EM: Pregnancies complicated by placenta previa: What is appropriate management? Br J Obstet Gynaecol 103:864, 1996.

Magann EF, Johnson CA, Gookin KS, et al: Placenta previa: Does uterine activity cause bleeding? Aust N Z J Obstet Gynaecol 33:22, 1993.

Major CA, de Veciana M, Lewis DF, et al: Preterm premature rupture of membranes and abruptio placentae: Is there an association between these pregnancy complications? Am J Obstet Gynecol 172:672, 1995.

Maldjian C, Adam R, Pelosi M, et al: MRI appearance of placenta percreta and placenta accreta. Magn Reson Imaging 17:965, 1999.

Manolitsas T, Wein P, Beischer NA, et al: Value of cardiotocography in women with antepartum hemorrhage: Is it too late for cesarean section when the cardiotocograph shows ominous features? Aust N Z J Obstet Gynaecol 34:403, 1994.

Matthews NM, McCowan LM, Patten P: Placenta previa accreta with delayed hysterectomy. Aust N Z J Obstet Gynaecol 36:476, 1996.

Matthiesen L, Berg G, Ernerudh J, et al: Lymphocyte subsets and autoantibodies in pregnancies complicated by placental disorders. Am J Reprod Immunol 33:31, 1995.

Misra DP, Ananth CV: Risk factor profiles of placental abruption in first and second pregnancies: Heterogeneous etiologies. J Clin Epidemiol 52:453, 1999.

Monica G, Lilja C: Placental previa, maternal smoking and recurrence risk. Acta Obstet Gynaecol Scand 74:341, 1995.

Morgan MA, Berkowitz KM, Thomas SG, et al: Abruptio placentae: Perinatal outcome in normotensive and hypertensive patients. Am J Obstet Gynecol 170:1595, 1994.

Mortensen JT, Thulstrup AM, Larsen H, et al: Smoking, sex of the offspring, and risk of placental abruption, placenta previa, and preeclampsia: a population-based cohort study. Acta Obstet Gynaecol Scand 80:894, 2001.

Mouer JR: Placenta previa: Antepartum conservative management, inpatient versus outpatient. Am J Obstet Gynecol 170:1683, 1994.

Mussalli GM, Shah J, Berch DJ, et al: Placenta accreta and methotrexate therapy: three case reports. J Perinatal 20:331, 2000.

Naeye RL, Haskness WL, Utts J: Abruptio placentae and perinatal death. Am J Obstet Gynecol 128:740, 1977.

Newton ER, Barss V, Cetrulo CL: The epidemiology and clinical history of asymptomatic midtrimester placenta previa. Am J Obstet Gynecol 148:743, 1984.

Nyberg DA, Cyr DR, Mack LA, et al: Sonographic spectrum of placental abruption. AJR Am J Roentgenol 148:161, 1987.

O'Malley BP, Toi A, deSa DJ, et al: Ultrasound appearances of placental chorioangioma. Radiology 138:159, 1981.

Oppenheimer L, Holmes P, Simpson N, et al: Diagnosis of low lying placenta: Can migration in the third trimester predict outcome? Ultrasound Obstet Gynecol 18:100, 2001.

Pent D: Vasa previa. Am J Obstet Gynecol 134:151, 1979.

Perlman JM, Risser R: Can asphyxiated infants at risk for neonatal seizures be rapidly identified by current high-risk markers? Pediatrics 97:456, 1996.

Preucel RW, Lavin JP, Colman RW: Placental abruption and premature separation. In Sciarra JJ (ed): Gynecology and Obstetrics, vol 2. New York, Harper & Row, 1981.

Pritchard J, Mason R, Corley M, et al: Genesis of severe placental abruption. Am J Obstet Gynecol 108:22, 1970.

Pritchard JA, Brekken AL: Clinical and laboratory studies on severe abruption placenta. Am J Obstet Gynecol 97:681, 1967.

Rashbaum WK, Gates EJ, Jones J, et al: Placenta accreta encountered during dilation and evacuation in the second trimester. Obstet Gynecol 85:701, 1995.

Rasmussen S, Irgens LM, Bergsjo P, et al: Perinatal mortality and case fatality after placental abruption in Norway 1967–1991. Acta Obstet Gynaecol Scand 75:229, 1996a.

Rasmussen S, Irgens LM, Bergsjo P, et al: The occurrence of placental abruption in Norway 1967–1991. Acta Obstet Gynaecol Scand 75:222, 1996b.

Raymond EG, Mills JL: Placental abruption: Maternal risk factors and associated fetal conditions. Acta Obstet Gynaecol Scand 72:633, 1993.

Reshitnikova OS, Burton GJ, Milovanov AP, et al: Increased incidence of placental chorioangioma in high altitude pregnancies: Hypobaric hypoxia as a possible etiologic factor. Am J Ostet Gynecol 174:557, 1996.

Reubinoff BE, Weinstein D, Langer O, et al: Antenatal bleeding and fetal heart rate. Gynecol Obstet Invest 39:19, 1995.

Rosati P, Guariglia L: Clinical significance of placenta previa detected at early routine transvaginal scan. J Ultrasound Med 19:581, 2000.

Rosen DM, Peek MJ: Do women with placenta previa without antepartum hemorrhage require hospitalization? Aust N Z J Obstet Gynaecol 34:130, 1994.

Salafia CM, Lopez-Zeno JA, Sherer DM, et al: Histologic evidence of old intrauterine bleeding is more frequent in prematurity. Am J Obstet Gynecol 173:1065, 1995.

Spinillo A, Fazzi E, Stronati M, et al: Severity of abruptio placentae and neurodevelopmental outcome in low birth weight infants. Early Hum Dev 35:45, 1993.

Spinillo A, Fazzi E, Stronati M, et al: Early morbidity and neurodevelopmental outcome in low-birthweight infants born after third trimester bleeding. Am J Perinatol 11:85, 1994.

Taylor VM, Kramer MD, Vaughan TL, et al: Placenta previa and prior cesarean delivery: How strong is the association? Obstet Gynecol 84:55, 1994.

Thomas AG, Alvarez M, Friedman F Jr, et al: The effect of placenta previa on blood loss in second-trimester pregnancy termination. Obstet Gynecol 84:58, 1994.

Timor-Tritsch IE, Monteagudo A: Diagnosis of placenta previa by transvaginal sonography. Ann Med 25:279, 1993.

Timor-Tritsch IE, Yunis RA: Confirming the safety of transvaginal sonography in patients suspected of placenta previa. Obstet Gynecol 81:742, 1993.

Towers CV, Pircon RA, Heppard M: Is tocolysis safe in the management of third trimester bleeding? Am J Obstet Gynecol 180:1572, 1999.

Towery R, English TP, Wisner D: Evaluation of pregnant women after blunt injury. J Trauma 35:731, 1993.

Twickler DM, Lucas MJ, Balis AB, et al: Color flow mapping for myometrial invasion in women with a prior cesarean delivery. J Matern Fetal Med 9:330, 2000.

Varma TR: Fetal growth and placental function in patients with placenta praevia. J Obstet Gynaecol Br Commonw 80:311, 1973.

Wexler P, Gottesfeld KR: Early diagnosis of placenta previa. Obstet Gynecol 54:231, 1979.

Williams MA, Hickok DE, Zingheim RW, et al: Maternal serum CA 125 levels in the diagnosis of abruptio placentae. Obstet Gynecol 82:808, 1993.

Williams MA, Mittendorf R: Increasing maternal age as a determinant of previa: More important than increasing parity? J Reprod Med 38:425, 1993.

Wing DA, Paul RH, Millar LK: Management of the symptomatic placenta previa: A randomized controlled trial of inpatient versus outpatient expectant management. Am J Obstet Gynecol 175:806, 1996.

Zhang J, Savitz DA: Maternal age and placenta previa: A population-based, case-control study. Am J Obstet Gynecol 168:641, 1993.

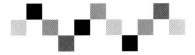

Chapter 38

PREMATURE RUPTURE OF THE MEMBRANES

Thomas J. Garite, MD

Premature rupture of the fetal membranes (PROM), or *amnior-rhexis*, is one of the most common and controversial problems facing the obstetric clinician. The fetal membranes and the amniotic fluid they encase have functions that are critical for normal fetal protection, growth, and development. The fluid environment allows full fetal movement, enhancing normal muscle development and growth. Fetal swallowing and urination are integral to normal fetal fluid balance and to the development of the gastrointestinal and urinary systems. The amniotic fluid provides a column of fluid within the fetal tracheal–bronchial tree, which during normal fetal inspiratory and expiratory movements allows development of the fetal lungs. The amniotic fluid also protects the fetus from traumatic injury and by allowing the umbilical cord to float freely, protects it from compression during fetal movement or uterine contractions.

Besides encasing the amniotic fluid, the membranes also serve as an important barrier that separates the sterile fetus and the amniotic fluid from a bacteria-laden vaginal canal and preventing prolapse of any intra-amniotic contents through the cervix, which often dilates somewhat before the onset of labor. Finally, the membranes also function as a repository for substrates for many critical biochemical processes, including storage of phosphoglycerolipids, which release the precursors for prostaglandins. Thus, any disruption in the integrity of the amniotic cavity may potentially interrupt or interfere with any or all of these important functions.

DEFINITION AND INCIDENCE

PROM is defined as rupture of the chorioamniotic membranes before the onset of labor. The definition is independent of gestational age, and PROM before term is correctly termed *preterm* PROM (PPROM). Because there is often confusion over the meaning of "premature" rupture of membranes (ROMs) (i.e., before labor versus preterm), recently authors are using the term "prelabor rupture of membranes" to mean ROMs before the onset of labor and "preterm prelabor rupture of membranes" for the premature gestations. The interval between PROM and the onset of labor is referred to as the *latency period*. Although some authors impose an arbitrary latency period for the definition of PROM, varying from 1 to 12 hours, most define PROM simply as ROM before the onset of contractions. Traditionally, pediatricians are concerned with

the duration of ROM, especially in the term gestation—hence the term *prolonged* ROM, usually referring to ROM for more than 24 hours.

The reported incidence of PROM varies between 3% and 18.5% (Gunn et al., 1970). This wide variation is attributed to differences in definition (with or without a latency period) and by variation in the incidence of PROM in differing populations. Approximately 8% to 10% of patients at term present with ROM before the onset of labor. PPROM accounts for 25% of all cases of PROM and is responsible for about 30% of all premature deliveries (Kaltreider and Kohl, 1980). The contribution of PPROM to premature delivery is greater in populations of lower socioeconomic status and those with higher rates of sexually transmitted diseases.

ETIOLOGY

Normal fetal membranes are extremely strong early in pregnancy, to the extent that they withstand rupture from nearly all acute nonpenetrating forces (Artal et al., 1976; Parry-Jones and Priya, 1976). As term approaches, the fetal membranes are subjected to forces that cause them to become progressively weakened (Artal et al., 1976; Parry-Jones and Priya, 1976; Lavery and Miller, 1979; Skinner et al., 1981; Lavery et al., 1982). The combination of stretching of the membranes with uterine growth and the frequent strain caused by normal uterine contractions and fetal movements may contribute to the weakening of this membrane. In addition, significant biochemical changes occur in the membranes near term, including a substantial decrease in the collagen content. Thus, at term PROM may be a physiologic variant rather than a pathologic event. Because membranes are so strong in the preterm gestation, it is likely that either a pathologic intrinsic weakness or extrinsic factors are responsible for PPROM. Studies examining membranes from patients with PPROM do not show a difference in membrane strength except near the site of rupture (Artal et al., 1976). This local difference suggests an exogenous source of weakening.

In at least a substantial number of cases, local infection ascending from the vagina appears to be responsible for membrane weakening and rupture (Lonky and Hayashi, 1988). Patients in early gestation who are carriers of one or more sexually transmitted organisms (e.g., gonococci, group B streptococci, *Chlamydia*, *Trichomonas*, and *Gardnerella vaginalis*) have substantially increased incidences of PROM (Edwards et al., 1978; Regan et al., 1981; Martin et al., 1982; Minkoff et al., 1984). Although data on some of these organisms are inconsistent, studies uniformly show increased risks of PPROM in patients who are carriers of group B streptococci, gonococci, and G. *vaginalis*. Histologic chorioamnionitis is much more prevalent with preterm than with term PROM (Naeye, 1979). Studies evaluating amniotic fluid and fetal cord blood immunoglobulins suggest that many patients with PPROM are infected before ROM (Cederqvist et al., 1979). Patients with PPROM are much more likely than their term counterparts to have clinical chorioamnionitis and endometritis (Daikoku et al., 1982; Garite and Freeman, 1982), even when frequency is corrected for differences in other clinical variables (e.g., duration of membrane rupture and number of pelvic examinations).

Studies have shown that bacteria, which attach to fetal membranes, elaborate substances such as proteases, which cause membrane weakening and likely ROM (McGregor et al., 1986). Recent studies implicate the matrix metalloproteinase, particularly matrix metalloproteinase-9, as being the specific enzymes involved in membrane rupture in those cases caused by infection (Athayde et al., 1998; Fortunato et al., 2001). Thus, in many cases bacteria ascending from the vagina are probably responsible for membrane weakening and subsequent rupture. It is not clear, however, why some patients who harbor similar organisms do not have PPROM or preterm labor. Therefore, it is obvious that some as yet undefined host factor or environmental cofactor must be involved.

Occasionally, other etiologic mechanisms can be identified. PPROM is more commonly seen in the setting of polyhydramnios or incompetent cervix or after such procedures as cervical cerclage or amniocentesis. In most cases, the cause is undefined.

Few epidemiologic factors are consistently associated with an increased risk of PROM (Kaltreider and Kohl, 1980; Naeye, 1982). Smoking has been incriminated in some studies. Multiple gestation, abruptio placentae, cocaine, previous PPROM, and previous cervical operations or lacerations usually are correlated with increased risk of PROM. In addition, occupational fatigue and long working hours (Newman et al., 2001) and vitamin C and E deficiencies (Woods et al., 2001) have also been implicated. No relationship has been shown between PROM and maternal age, parity, maternal weight or weight gain, trauma, or meconium.

◾ COMPLICATIONS

PROM may lead to a number of complications, and the risk of these complications varies significantly with gestational age. The lack of agreement over the relative contribution of each of these complications to perinatal morbidity and mortality is responsible for much of the controversy that exists over management. Complications associated with PROM include the following:

- Maternal and fetal or neonatal infections
- Premature labor and delivery
- Hypoxia and asphyxia secondary to umbilical cord compression and/or coincident abruptio placentae
- Increased rates of cesarean section
- Fetal deformation syndrome

Premature Labor

Once membranes rupture, the onset of labor usually follows within a relatively short time. The duration of the latency period varies inversely with gestational age. At term, labor follows PROM within 24 hours in 90% of cases (Gunn et al., 1970). When PROM occurs between 28 and 34 weeks, 50% of patients are in labor within 24 hours and 80% to 90% within 1 week (Mead, 1980; Garite et al., 1981). Before 26 weeks, approximately 50% of the patients begin labor within 1 week (Taylor and Garite, 1984).

Obviously, labor at term is a desirable sequel to PROM, and only when labor does not spontaneously begin within a short time is there any need for concern. When PPROM occurs, subsequent delivery and the resultant complications of prematurity are the most common causes of perinatal mortality and morbidity with this diagnosis. In addition to being associated with the onset of labor, PROM also influences the duration and course of labor. Generally, there is a moderate shortening of the first stage but no effect on the duration of the second stage with ROMs in contrast to labor with intact membranes (Schwarz et al., 1974). It is not clear whether dystocia occurs more frequently in patients with PROM when spontaneous labor ensues; however, among patients with PROM, although results are inconsistent, some show a higher rate of cesarean section for failure to progress in labor that has been induced than with spontaneous labor after PROM (Duff et al., 1984; Hannah et al., 1996).

Infection

Both mother and fetus are at increased risk for infection when membranes rupture before the onset of labor. Maternal infection is termed *chorioamnionitis*. Fetal infection may occur as septicemia, pneumonia, or urinary tract infection or as a local infection, such as omphalitis or conjunctivitis. Generally, maternal chorioamnionitis precedes such fetal infections; however, serious fetal sepsis may occur before chorioamnionitis is clinically evident in the mother. This is explained by preclinical infection, which occurs when the amniotic sac becomes colonized with virulent bacteria but before there are clinically evident signs of maternal infection. To clarify this apparent discrepancy, some authors have used the term *intra-amniotic infection* to include both preclinical and clinical chorioamnionitis (Gibbs et al., 1982; Yoder et al., 1983).

The incidence of chorioamnionitis, in association with PROM, varies according to population type. For all pregnancies, the incidence is 0.5% to 1%. In prolonged ROM, the rate of occurrence has been 3% to 15%. Chorioamnionitis appears to be more common in PPROM, with reported frequencies of 15% to 25% (Ledger, 1976; Garite and Freeman, 1982; Gibbs et al., 1982). The rate and severity increase even more with very early, or previable, gestational ages. The frequency of chorioamnionitis is more than 40% with PROM before 24 weeks.

The impact of PROM and chorioamnionitis on fetal or neonatal infection also varies with populations and gestational age. The incidence of neonatal sepsis at term is about 1 in 500 infants. With prolonged ROM, this is increased several-fold, and with chorioamnionitis, the incidence rises to 3% to 5% (Yoder et al., 1983). With PPROM, perinatal infections are much more common than at term. Major neonatal infec-

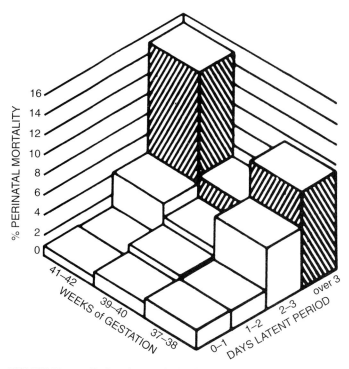

FIGURE 38-1 ■ Perinatal mortality by duration of latent period for term infants. The cross-hatching indicates that the observed perinatal mortality is significantly higher than that noted among infants of the same gestational age with latent periods under 1 day. (Reprinted with permission from the American College of Obstetricians and Gynecologists [Johnson JWC, Daikoku NH, Niebyl JR, et al: Premature rupture of the membranes and prolonged latency. Obstetrics and Gynecology, 1981, **57,** 547.])

specific study populations (Kappy et al., 1979; Schreiber and Benedetti, 1980; Garite et al., 1981; Stedman et al., 1981; Varner and Galask, 1981; Barrett and Boehm, 1982; Daikoku et al., 1982; Wilson et al., 1982; Morales, 1987). In most cases, perinatal mortality consequent to PPROM arises from complications of prematurity, such as respiratory distress syndrome (RDS), intraventricular hemorrhage, and necrotizing enterocolitis. Combining all gestational ages into one category for the purpose of this analysis, however, may lead to oversimplified conclusions. In the 26-week gestation, for example, the relative contribution of prematurity to the risks of perinatal morbidity and mortality far outweigh any risks from infection, and thus all efforts at prolonging gestation to decrease the complications of prematurity seem warranted. In a fetus at 34 weeks' gestation, at which point perinatal mortality is not substantially different from that for the fetus at term and complications of morbidity are minor, the contribution of infection becomes much more important.

Studies by Garite and Freeman (1982) and by Morales (1987) have shown that the risks of serious neonatal infections and of RDS increase severalfold with chorioamnionitis in the preterm pregnancy. In addition, long-term neurologic complications are increased in fetuses delivered after the onset of maternal infection (Hardt et al., 1985). Yoon, Romero, and coworkers (1999, 2000) introduced the term "fetal inflammatory response syndrome" to describe the phenomenon of fetal infection that precedes clinically apparent chorioamnionitis and results in central nervous system damage to the fetus. This

tions occur in about 5% of all cases of PPROM and in 15% to 20% of those with chorioamnionitis that has developed before term (Ledger, 1976; Gibbs et al., 1980; Garite and Freeman, 1982). The preterm infant is much more likely to die of infectious complications than is its term counterpart.

It is conventional teaching that the incidence of infection after PROM increases as the duration of the latency period increases. The proposed explanation is that with increasing duration of ROM, the likelihood of ascending infection from vaginal bacteria increases. A detailed analysis of this problem, however, reveals that this is probably true only in the term gestation (Figs. 38-1 and 38-2). In PPROM, the incidences of both chorioamnionitis and perinatal infections are not changed with increasing duration of ROM (Johnson et al., 1981). This is probably explained by the fact that many preterm patients are already infected at the time of membrane rupture. It is also suggested that in most cases increased infection rates with prolonged ROM may correlate more closely with the timing of the first digital cervical examination than with the interval between ROM and the onset of infection (Adoni et al., 1990; Lewis et al., 1992). It should be noted that not all studies have observed a correlation between a single digital examination and an increased likelihood of infection (Alexander et al., 2000).

With PPROM, the relative contributions of prematurity and perinatal infections to perinatal mortality are responsible for much of the controversy that exists regarding management of patients with this diagnosis. Table 38-1 presents a comparison of studies describing the causes of perinatal mortality in

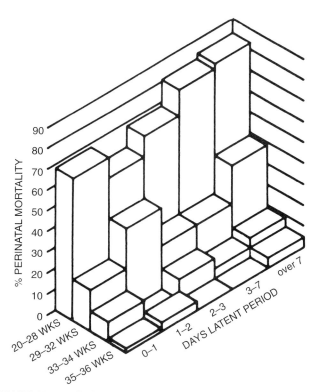

FIGURE 38-2 ■ Perinatal mortality by duration of latent period for preterm deliveries. Within each gestational age group, no significant differences were noted for the various latent period lengths. (Reprinted with permission from the American College of Obstetricians and Gynecologists [Johnson JWC, Daikoku NH, Niebyl JR, et al: Premature rupture of the membranes and prolonged latency. Obstetrics and Gynecology, 1981, **57,** 547.])

TABLE 38-1. PERINATAL OUTCOME WITH EXPECTANT MANAGEMENT OF PRETERM LABOR

| | | | Cause of Death | | |
Study	No. of Patients	PND	RDS/Prematurity	Infection	Other
Kappy et al., 1979	45	10	4	1	5
Garite et al., 1981	80	5	3	0	2
Stedman et al., 1981	55	3	2	1	0
Varner and Galask, 1981	115	4	3	1	0
Daikoku et al., 1982	203	28	8	4	16
Schreiber and Benedetti, 1980	90	12	4	1	7
Wilson et al., 1982	143	22	10	4	8
Barrett and Boehm, 1982	53	7	5	1	1
Total	784	91	39 (43%)	13 (14%)	39 (43%)

PND, perinatal deaths; RDS, respiratory distress syndrome.

is manifested in periventricular white matter lesions (leukomalacia) mediated through an intense fetal central nervous system inflammatory response, with cytokines leading to the damage. These lesions and the subsequent development of cerebral palsy at age 3 have been correlated with elevated intra-amniotic leukocyte concentrations and levels of interleukin-6 and the presence of funisitis. These studies and others are contributing to the mounting evidence that many, if not most, cases of cerebral palsy, particularly in prematurely delivering newborns, are the result of intra-amniotic infection. This further raises the question of the wisdom of expectant management when the risk of such infection may exceed the risk of prematurity and will undoubtedly be the subject of future investigation into the management of patients with PPROM. The issue of chorioamnionitis is also addressed from a microbiologic and treatment perspective in Chapter 39.

Hypoxia and Asphyxia

It is well known that umbilical cord prolapse occurs more frequently when ROM occurs before the onset of labor (incidence 1.5%), because the presenting fetal part is less likely to occupy the pelvis (Gunn et al., 1970). The combination of PROM and malpresentation further increases the frequency of this complication.

It has also become apparent that umbilical cord compression, even without prolapse, is more common with PROM secondary to oligohydramnios (Gabbe et al., 1976; Rutherford et al., 1987). This may occur before labor or during labor. In preterm patients in labor after PROM, Moberg and Garite (1987) reported a high incidence of fetal distress, mostly from cord compression, in 8.5% of patients with PROM compared with only 1.5% of those in premature labor with intact membranes (Moberg et al., 1984).

Series of expectantly managed patients with PPROM frequently reveal increased incidences of stillbirth, unexplained by infection, of up to 3% (Miller et al., 1978; Johnson et al., 1981; Wilson et al., 1982). Studies of antepartum testing in patients with PPROM suggest a high incidence of antepartum fetal distress requiring intervention for fetal heart rate (FHR) patterns consistent with umbilical cord compression occurring even before the onset of labor (Moberg and Garite, 1987). Vintzileos and coworkers (1985b) showed a good correlation between the severity of oligohydramnios and the frequency of severe variable decelerations.

Fetal Deformation Syndrome

The final naturally occurring major complication that may result from PROM is the fetal deformation syndrome. As in fetuses with Potter syndrome, PROM that occurs very early in gestation can lead to growth restriction, compression malformations of the fetal face and limbs, and, most important, pulmonary hypoplasia. Prolonged and early oligohydramnios seems to be the cause of all these problems. Bain and associates (1964) described 16 such cases in which there was a maternal history of PROM of 3 to 19 weeks' duration.

The incidence of this syndrome is not clearly defined. Retrospective case series in patients with PROM before 26 weeks revealed a combined frequency of 3.5% (Taylor and Garite, 1984; Moretti and Sibai, 1988; Bengston and Van Marter, 1989; Major and Kitzmiller, 1990); however, these tend to underestimate the frequency. The largest prospective series that specifically addressed the issue of lethal pulmonary hypoplasia showed a rate of 20%, increasing to nearly 50% with severe oligohydramnios (Kilbride et al., 1996). These differences in the incidence of this syndrome, particularly pulmonary hypoplasia, undoubtedly are not only due to differences in the criteria used to define this entity but also due to differences in populations included in their studies, including gestational age at rupture, degree of oligohydramnios, and duration of latency, which all profoundly affect the frequency of this syndrome (Winn et al., 2000).

PATIENT EVALUATION

Management of the patient with PROM depends on a number of variables. Therefore, the initial evaluation of the patient who presents with a history suggestive of PROM must result in a basic data base that includes the following:

1. Confirming the diagnosis
2. Determining gestational age
3. Evaluating for the presence of maternal and/or fetal infection
4. Establishing the onset of labor
5. Ruling out fetal distress

Only when all these factors are known, in addition to a complete review of the patient's obstetric and past medical history, can decisions be made regarding management.

Diagnosis

Obviously, making the correct diagnosis of PROM is essential. A patient's history, consisting of a large gush of clear fluid from the vagina followed by persistent leakage, is accurate in 90% of cases (Friedman and McElin, 1969). Other explanations for such a history include urinary leakage, excessive vaginal discharge, or, rarely, bloody show. A watery vaginal discharge is also a common presenting symptom in patients with premature cervical dilation (incompetent cervix), even in the absence of ROM.

The diagnosis of premature ROM is established by aseptic speculum vaginal examination. The physician should make an effort, in the process of examining the patient, to avoid introducing infection. The physician should avoid digital intracervical examination altogether when the patient is not in labor and when immediate induction is not planned. Such examinations add little needed information and probably increase the risk of complications from infection (Wagner et al., 1989). Several studies have shown that patients with PROM who have digital intracervical infection have shorter latency periods, and most, but not all, have shown increased risks of neonatal sepsis (Schutte et al., 1983; Wagner et al., 1989; Adoni et al., 1990; Lewis et al., 1992; Alexander et al., 2000). Confirmation of the diagnosis by speculum examination includes the identification of a pool of fluid in the posterior fornix (pooling). Prolonged ROM may result in loss of most fluid, and occasionally vaginal mucosa appears only moist. In such cases, either the Valsalva maneuver or pressure on the uterine fundus during speculum examination allows visualization of leakage from the endocervical canal.

The next test for confirmation of amniorrhexis is the use of Nitrazine, a pH-sensitive paper strip that changes color from yellow-green to dark blue at a pH above 6.0 to 6.5. The pH of the vagina in pregnancy is usually 4.5 to 6.0, and amniotic fluid has a pH of 7.1 to 7.3. Hence, testing for this alkaline pH usually confirms the presence of amniotic fluid. Nitrazine may cause a false-positive result from contamination with blood, semen, or alkaline antiseptics (Friedman and McElin, 1969). Vaginal infections may raise the pH of the vagina. Occasionally, alkaline urine may cause a false-positive result. If pooling and Nitrazine are not both positive, a swab of the posterior vaginal fornix should be taken, smeared on a slide, allowed to dry, and examined under a microscope for the presence of a typical *ferning* appearance (Kovacs, 1962) (Fig. 38-3). Although a swab inadvertently taken from the endocervical canal may cause a false-positive picture of ferning, the ferns seen from cervical mucus are not the typical lush and elaborate pattern seen with amniotic fluid.

Finally, oligohydramnios seen on ultrasonography is usually confirmatory. When the diagnosis remains unclear, as with concomitant bleeding and oligohydramnios, an alternative invasive method may be applied whereby amniocentesis is done and a dye, such as Evans Blue or fluorescein, is injected; the cervix can then be visualized for leakage of dye (Atlay and Sutherst, 1970; Smith, 1976).

At the time of speculum examination, other information is also obtained. The cervix should be visualized to ascertain that no fetal extremity or umbilical cord prolapses through the os. An impression of cervical dilation and effacement can be ascertained with a moderate degree of reliability with visual examination alone. Endovaginal ultrasound can also be used to assess cervical dilation and effacement, and at least one study

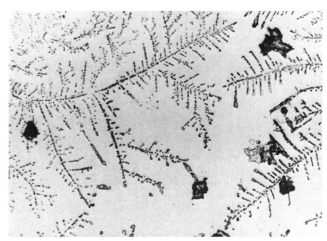

FIGURE 38-3 ■ Typical "ferning" appearance as seen with a swab from the posterior vaginal fornix, smeared on a slide and allowed to dry, from a patient with premature rupture of membranes.

evaluating this modality in patients with PROM showed no increased risk of infection (Carlan et al., 1997). Cultures of the cervix and vagina can be taken for gonococci, group B streptococci, and *Chlamydia*. Culturing for other organisms adds little clinically useful information. In certain premature gestations, a sample of amniotic fluid from the posterior fornix can be aspirated and submitted for maturity testing; the presence of phosphatidylglycerol (PG) is the most reliable indicator of maturity (Stedman et al., 1981).

Establishing Gestational Age from Fetal Maturity

Menstrual dating, prenatal examinations, and previous ultrasonograms should all be reviewed to carefully establish gestational age because the most critical factor in determining management of the patient with PROM is fetal age. If any doubt exists, ultrasonography should be performed. In patients with PROM or oligohydramnios from any cause, compression may cause alteration in measurements of biparietal diameter or abdominal circumference (O'Keeffe et al., 1985). Careful biometric evaluation of all routinely measured fetal parameters should be compared to eliminate this potential cause of error. Because cervical examination usually is to be avoided in patients with PROM and who are not in labor, ultrasonography also is useful in confirming the presentation of the fetus.

Ruling Out Chorioamnionitis

All patients with premature ROM, regardless of gestational age and uterine activity, must be evaluated carefully for signs of infection. (Chapter 39 describes the diagnosis and management of chorioamnionitis.) However, patients with PPROM should be evaluated for signs of infection, including fever, leukocytosis, maternal and fetal tachycardia, uterine tenderness, or malodorous vaginal discharge. In early or less severe cases, any or all of these signs may be missing. The diagnosis of chorioamnionitis, to be based on clinical signs and symptoms alone, must include a fever (100.4°F) in the setting of ROM and in the absence of any other explanation for the elevated temperature.

Cervicovaginal specimens for group B streptococci, *Chlamydia*, and gonococci are obtained for culture principally for the purpose of screening the uninfected patients and providing prophylactic antibiotics to prevent perinatal transmission. Because antibiotics will be used in patients with chorioamnionitis anyway and one cannot be assured that the organism isolated from the vagina is actually the organism causing the intra-amniotic infection, a more general cervicovaginal culture is of little value.

Other laboratory tests also have limited utility. Maternal white blood cell count and C-reactive protein elevations may indicate impending infection, but these determinations are relatively nonspecific, are increased in patients in early labor, and must be interpreted along with all other clinical parameters (Ohlsson and Wong, 1990).

In cases of suspected chorioamnionitis when the diagnosis cannot be clinically confirmed, amniocentesis may be of value and can be performed in most patients with PROM. A further discussion of amniocentesis for the purpose of screening for occult intra-amniotic infection follows in this chapter, but for the purposes of ruling out infection in the patient with subtle but inconclusive signs, this is a place where amniocentesis may have its greatest value. Amniotic fluid from patients with chorioamnionitis should have evidence of bacteria on Gram stain and, by the time evidence of infection is clinically present, should also demonstrate some white blood cells on Gram stain.

Ruling Out Labor

The patient who is having regular and painful uterine contractions in the presence of ROM generally is found to be in active labor. Because digital examinations generally should be avoided until one is certain of labor, preliminary speculum examination and/or endovaginal ultrasound may be used to determine whether cervical dilation is present. Patients who have PROM often experience contractions that stop spontaneously. External electronic fetal monitors may be applied to determine the presence and frequency of contractions and to allow early diagnosis of labor in most cases. In the very early preterm gestation, uterine activity may be difficult to detect on external monitors and frequently variable decelerations of the FHR will be the first sign of labor (Moberg and Garite, 1987).

Ruling Out Fetal Distress

As previously noted, PROM increases the risk of umbilical cord prolapse and cord compression from oligohydramnios. Continuous FHR monitoring should be included in the initial evaluations of all patients with this diagnosis if the fetus is of a viable gestational age (i.e., at least 24 weeks). Besides variable decelerations, late decelerations may reveal a coexistent abruption (Major et al., 1995) or uteroplacental pathology, and loss of FHR accelerations (loss of reactivity) and/or fetal tachycardia may suggest fetal sepsis.

CONTROVERSIES IN MANAGEMENT

Even though much investigation has been reported (including many prospective randomized trials) regarding the management of patients with PROM at varying gestational ages, this topic remains one of the most controversial and enigmatic clinical problems that the obstetrician must face. In a survey of maternal-fetal medicine specialists by Capeless and Mead (1987), it was evident that many important issues (e.g., the use of corticosteroids, tocolytic therapy, amniocentesis, and several other diagnostic and therapeutic modalities) could not be agreed on to any degree approaching a consensus. In many areas, however, information is more clear, and agreement on management does exist. A patient with a history suggestive of PROM should be brought to the hospital immediately and evaluated to confirm or to rule out the diagnosis of PROM. Those in whom the diagnosis is confirmed should be hospitalized and, in most cases, should remain in the hospital until delivery. An exception would be the patient with PROM in whom the gestational age is below that of likely neonatal viability; in these patients, fetal status is not an immediate issue and outpatient expectant management may be appropriate. In some patients, leakage stops, and reaccumulation of normal amniotic fluid has been noted on ultrasonography; their prognosis seems to be similar to that of patients who have never had ROM, and they can be safely discharged from the hospital once resealing of the membranes is confirmed (Johnston et al., 1990).

Delivery is obviously urgent for patients with advanced active labor, clinical chorioamnionitis, and irreversible fetal distress. Otherwise, management depends principally on gestational age. In the patient with PROM who is not in labor, and without evidence of infection or fetal distress, especially in premature gestational ages, a great deal of controversy remains regarding management.

Tocolysis

Because premature labor is an expected sequela of PROM and prematurity is the leading cause of perinatal morbidity and mortality in such cases, the appeal of agents to prevent or stop premature labor is obvious. It is clear from all studies of tocolytic therapy, regardless of the agent used, that patients with intact membranes are more likely to experience successful cessation of labor than those with ROM.

Several prospective, randomized, controlled trials of tocolytic agents in patients with PPROM have been conducted (Christensen et al., 1980; Garite et al., 1987; Weiner et al., 1988) (Table 38-2). One study showed prolongation of pregnancy of up to 24 hours in patients with tocolytic therapy (Christensen et al., 1980); however, the other two showed no difference, and none showed any prolongation of pregnancy beyond that point or any difference in any index of perinatal mortality or morbidity measured. Two randomized trials of prophylactic oral tocolytics also failed to show pregnancy prolongation (Levy and Warsof, 1985; Dunlop et al., 1986). In the past, some have been concerned about increasing the risk of infection by attempts to prolong pregnancy in patients with PROM; however, none of these studies showed any difference. Of course, one would not expect a difference in studies that did not show any prolongation of pregnancy.

Corticosteroids

Liggins and Howie (1972) first demonstrated that when betamethasone was given to mothers about to deliver prematurely, the incidence and severity of RDS in the premature

TABLE 38-2. STUDIES EVALUATING TOCOLYTICS TO PROLONG PREGNANCY WITH PRETERM PREMATURE RUPTURE OF MEMBRANES

Author	No.		Delivery >24°	Delivery >48°	Delivery >7 days	Respiratory Distress Syndrome	Mortality
Christensen et al., 1980	30	Rx	14/14	7/14	3/14	2/14	1/14
		Control	10/16*	7/16	1/16	1/16	0/16
Garite et al., 1987	79	Rx	35/39	30/39	12/39	20/39	6/39
		Control	36/40	30/40	13/40	23/40	2/40
Weiner et al., 1988	75	Rx	31/33	29/33	Not stated	15/33	5/33
		Control	39/42	32/42	Not stated	22/40	3/40

* *P* <.05; all others not significant.

neonates were substantially reduced. Many subsequent randomized trials have uniformly confirmed the benefit. Because PROM is an obvious prelude to premature delivery, this seems an ideal circumstance for the application of corticosteroids. In the past, some studies have shown some acceleration of fetal lung maturity from ROM alone after 24 to 48 hours. Therefore, one would not necessarily be able to apply the data showing benefit of corticosteroids in patients with preterm labor to the situation of PPROM. In fact, there are now a large number of prospective randomized controlled trials of corticosteroids with PPROM, and most of these trials, unlike the unanimity with preterm labor, have not shown a reduction in the rate or severity of RDS in treated patients (Block et al., 1977; Papageorgiou et al., 1979; Taeusch et al., 1979; Young et al., 1980; Collaborative Group, 1981; Garite et al., 1981; Iams et al., 1985; Nelson et al., 1985; Simpson and Harbert, 1985; Morales et al., 1986) (Table 38-3). Five of these 10 studies also showed an increase in the risk of maternal and/or neonatal infections in the patients randomized to the corticosteroid group.

Two meta-analyses, combining the data of all these trials, resulted in conflicting conclusions. One included all studies and concluded that the use of corticosteroids in patients with PROM resulted in a decrease in both the incidence and severity of RDS without any increase in the likelihood of infectious complications (Crowley et al., 1990). Conversely, the other analysis, which only included studies judged by Ohlsson (1989) to meet more stringent criteria of appropriate studies used for a meta-analysis, suggested minimal reduction in the incidence of RDS with corticosteroids in PROM and confirmed a statistically increased risk of infectious complications.

In 1994, the National Institutes of Health (NIH) held a consensus conference (National Institute of Child Health and Human Development, 1994), which concluded that "the use of corticosteroids to reduce infant morbidity in the presence of PPROM remains controversial." Although concluding that steroids reduced the overall incidence of RDS in this situation, the committee also acknowledged that the magnitude of this reduction was not as great as when membranes are intact. On the basis of this reduction and the observation of a reduction in intraventricular hemorrhage seen in infants younger than 30 to 32 weeks, they recommended that antenatal corticosteroid use is appropriate in the absence of chorioamnionitis.

Two important studies may have resolved some of the controversy. Both included prophylactic antibiotics and showed more dramatic reductions in RDS comparable with that seen with intact membranes (Morales et al., 1989; Lewis et al., 1996). It may well be that, with the elimination of the excess increase in infectious morbidity seen with corticosteroids (particularly neonatal pneumonia), steroid therapy may be allowed to achieve its maximal benefit.

TABLE 38-3. EFFECT OF CORTICOSTEROIDS ON RESPIRATORY DISTRESS SYNDROME (RDS) IN PRETERM PREMATURE RUPTURE OF MEMBRANES (RANDOMIZED CONTROLLED STUDIES ONLY)

Author	No. of Patients		Effect on RDS
	Steroids	**Control**	
Block et al., 1977	43	26	No difference
Taeusch et al., 1979	17	24	No difference*
Papageorgiou et al., 1979	17	19	Decreased
Young et al., 1980	38	37	Decreased
Garite et al., 1981	80	80	No difference*
Collaborative Group, 1981	153	135	No difference
Iams et al., 1985	38	35	No difference*
Nelson et al., 1985	22	46	No difference*
Simpson and Harbert, 1985	112	105	More RDS in steroid group*
Morales et al., 1986	121	124	Decreased

* Studies also suggesting an increased incidence of maternal and/or neonatal infection in the steroid group.

TABLE 38-4. COMBINED FREQUENCY OF ORGANISMS CULTURED FROM AMNIOTIC FLUID OBTAINED BY AMNIOCENTESIS IN PATIENTS WITH PRETERM PREMATURE RUPTURE OF MEMBRANES (SEVEN STUDIES)

Group B streptococci	20%
Gardnerella vaginalis	17%
Peptostreptococcus/peptococcus	11%
Fusobacteria	10%
Bacteroides fragilis	9%
Other streptococci	9%
Bacteroides sp.	5%

More recently, the NIH convened a second consensus conference on antenatal steroids to specifically address the issue of multiple doses (NIH Consensus Statement, 2000). Although this group did not specifically revisit the issue of steroids with PPROM, it did conclude that because there was mounting evidence of harmful effects of multiple doses of antenatal corticosteroids and little evidence of increased efficacy, that only a single course should be used except in research protocols. Subsequently, two studies have reported a substantial increase in maternal and neonatal infection and shorter latency periods in patients with PPROM receiving multiple courses as opposed to a single course (Vermillion et al., 1999; Lee et al., 2001).

Therefore, corticosteroids should be used in the earlier gestational ages (less than 30 to 32 weeks) where maximum benefit for RDS, intraventricular hemorrhage, and mortality will be achieved in conjunction with antibiotics, and only a single course should be given regardless of the duration of the latency period.

Prophylactic Antibiotics

The use of prophylactic antibiotics in patients with PPROM is theoretically appealing from two standpoints: (1) Maternal and perinatal risks of infection would be reduced and (2) the interval between PROM and delivery might be prolonged (because occult infection is a probable cause of PPROM and subsequent preterm labor).

The first large prospective trial was undertaken in the 1960s and showed no benefit from prophylactic antibiotics (Lebherz et al., 1980). Unfortunately, these authors had little to choose from in the way of broad-spectrum antibiotics and the drug used—tetracycline—has poor amniotic fluid penetration and probably a poor spectrum of activity for the organisms involved. Table 38-4 presents the most commonly identified organisms from amniotic fluid obtained by amniocentesis in patients with PPROM (Garite et al., 1979; Miller et al., 1980; Cotton et al., 1984; Zlatnick et al., 1984; Broekhuizen et al., 1985; Gonik and Cotton, 1985; Romero et al., 1988). The predominance of anaerobes and group B streptococci indicates a need for antibiotics effective against both types of organisms.

A number of randomized controlled trials of prophylactic antibiotics in patients with PPROM show a great deal of promise. Most of these studies (Table 38-5) show a prolongation of latency period by an average of 5 to 7 days, and some also show a reduction in the incidence of maternal amnionitis, neonatal sepsis, or both (Amon et al., 1988; Morales et al., 1989; Johnson et al., 1990; McGregor et al., 1991; Christmas et al., 1992; Blanco et al., 1993; Lockwood et al., 1993; Mercer et al., 1993, 1997; Owen et al., 1993; Lovett, et al., 1997).

The first large multicenter randomized trial was done by the NIH Maternal-Fetal Medicine Collaborative Group (Mercer et al., 1997). The authors randomized more than 600 patients to ampicillin and erythromycin versus placebo. All major neonatal morbidities, including sepsis, pneumonia, RDS, and necrotizing enterocolitis, were reduced in the antibiotic group. A subsequent multinational study, termed the "Oracle I Randomised Trial" (Kenyon et al., 2001), involving 4826 women with prolonged ROM confirmed the benefit of antibiotics in prolonging latency and reducing major pulmonary and infectious neonatal morbidity. They further found that erythromycin alone was equivalent to ampicillin/clavulanic

TABLE 38-5. ANTIBIOTIC PROPHYLAXIS IN PREMATURE RUPTURE OF MEMBRANES

Author	No.	Antibiotic	Outcome
Amon et al., 1988	82	Ampicillin IV/PO	PR LAT/<NN INF
Morales et al., 1989	165	Ampicillin IV	<IAI/<NN INF
Johnston et al., 1990		Mezlocillin	PR LAT/<NN INF
		Ampicillin IV/PO	<IAI
McGregor et al., 1991	54	Erythromycin	PR LAT
Christmas et al., 1992	56	Ampicillin	PR LAT
		Gentamicin	
		Clindamycin	
Mercer and Arheart, 1995	220	Erythromycin base	PR LAT
Lockwood et al., 1992	75	Piperacillin	PR LAT
Blanco et al., 1993	306	Cefizox	<NN INF
Owen et al., 1993	117	Ampicillin,	<IAI
		Erythromycin base	
Lovett et al., 1997	112	Unasyn	PR LAT, <RDS
			<NN INF, <NND
Mercer et al., 1997	614	Ampicillin/erythromycin	<NN INF, <RDS
			<PNEUMONIA, <NEC

IAI, intra-amniotic infection (chorioamnionitis); IV, intravenous; NEC, necrotizing enterocolitis; NN INF, neonatal infection; NND, neonatal death; PO, orally; PR LAT, prolonged latency; RDS, respiratory distress syndrome.

acid in efficacy but that the latter was associated with an increase in neonatal necrotizing enterocolitis.

Mercer and Arheart (1995) published a comprehensive review of this topic. They concluded that the use of prophylactic antibiotics in patients with PPROM resulted in a longer latent period and in reductions in maternal infections, including both chorioamnionitis and endometritis. Fetal and neonatal benefit is also seen, including lower rates of sepsis, pneumonia, and intraventricular hemorrhage.

Clearly, there is no uniformity in antibiotics chosen or in duration of therapy. Many questions remain, including the following:

- Do all these studies apply to all populations?
- What is the best antibiotic, including route and duration of therapy?
- Can therapy be reserved for a specific group of patients at higher risk?

Given such uniformity of benefit in many prospective randomized trials, it appears that prophylactic antibiotics are a reasonable choice. This recommendation can be made particularly in patients at less than 30 to 32 weeks' gestation where prolongation of pregnancy by a week and reduction in many of the major complications seen in these gestational ages are likely to be of major benefit.

As discussed in Chapter 39, it is always necessary to use prophylactic antibiotics for group B streptococcal infection in patients with preterm ROM or prolonged ROM at term if the patient is a known carrier or if there has been insufficient time to obtain culture results for the presence or absence of *Streptococcus*. The purpose of this therapy is to prevent perinatal transmission of this devastating organism to the newborn, and many trials now show that intrapartum treatment is effective in significantly reducing the risk of this complication (Regan et al., 1981; Boyer et al., 1983).

Ruling Out Occult Intra-Amniotic Infection

A significant controversy exists over the issue of identifying occult intra-amniotic infection. Clearly, once chorioamnionitis occurs, the incidence of neonatal morbidity and mortality is significantly aggravated (Garite and Freeman, 1982). It seems logical therefore that a method to detect occult or early intra-amniotic infection and to treat this subgroup of patients selectively, with either delivery or antibiotics or with both, would have the potential for improving the outcome in this group. Thus, the controversy surrounds two questions, as follows:

- What is the best way to identify such early or occult infection?
- Is there indeed any benefit in detecting occult intra-amniotic infection before it becomes clinically apparent?

Table 38-6 lists the many reported tests for detecting occult intra-amniotic infection. Clinical signs and symptoms are often nonspecific. Maternal laboratory test findings, including the white blood cell count and erythrocyte sedimentation rate, are particularly nonspecific unless counts are unusually high (Ohlsson and Wong, 1990).

Much debate has surrounded the issue of C-reactive protein. This nonspecific maternal serum marker has been reported to be elevated in patients destined to have intraamniotic infection before delivery. However, results of a large

TABLE 38-6. REPORTED TESTS FOR THE PRECLINICAL DIAGNOSIS OF INTRA-AMNIOTIC INFECTION

Clinical Tests

C-reactive protein
White blood cell count
Erythrocyte sedimentation rate

Amniotic Fluid Tests

Culture
Gram stain
Gas-liquid chromatography
Lemulus lysate
Fibronectin
Glucose
Leukocyte esterase
Cytokines

Biophysical

Biophysical profile
Amniotic fluid volume
Non-stress test

number of studies attempting to evaluate this question have been conflicting, with most of the studies showing inadequate sensitivity and specificity to act on this marker alone (Ohlsson and Wong, 1990).

Amniocentesis, with the Gram stain and subsequent culture, was one of the first described attempts at specifically addressing the problem of intra-amniotic infection (Garite et al., 1979). Many other methods of analyzing the amniotic fluid have subsequently been described.

According to a careful analysis of all the available methods for analyzing amniotic fluid by Romero and associates, the Gram stain on spun or unspun amniotic fluid and the amniotic fluid glucose determination (with positive values less than 15 mg/dL) are probably the best combination of methods for amniotic fluid analysis to detect occult infection (Romero, 1991). Amniotic fluid interleukin-6 is even more accurate but not generally available (Romero et al., 1993). Matrix metalloproteinase 9 may prove to be the most specific and sensitive test ultimately for both maternal and neonatal infections (Angus et al., 2001; Park et al., 2001; Harirah, et al., 2002). The Gram stain generally reveals the presence of bacteria that have a high specificity for subsequent development of chorioamnionitis. If the Gram stain is positive but chorioamnionitis does not develop, the patient generally delivers within a short time and thus has not had sufficient opportunity to mount an inflammatory response and systemic reaction that would result in a clinical syndrome of chorioamnionitis. However, the sensitivity of the Gram stain is somewhat low, especially when colony counts are low. Colony counts of approximately 10^5 or greater are generally necessary to bring about a positive Gram stain. Similarly, amniotic fluid glucose levels, when low, have a relatively high specificity but fairly poor sensitivity.

Much attention has been given to the use of various fetal biophysical parameters to detect signs of infection. Vintzileos and coworkers (1985a) first introduced the concept of the biophysical profile (BPP) for detecting occult intra-amniotic and/or fetal infection. Initial results showed a high degree of sensitivity and specificity for detecting either or both types of

■ **TABLE 38-7.** ANALYSIS OF BIOPHYSICAL PROFILE OF 16 INFECTED CASES (GROUP 1)

Case No.	NST	FBM	FM	FT	AF	PL	Total Score	Diagnosis
1	2	0	2	2	2	2	10	Amnionitis
2	0	0	2	1	1	2	6	Amnionitis
3	0	0	2	2	1	2	7	Possible neonatal sepsis
4	0	0	2	2	0	2	6	Possible neonatal sepsis
5	0	0	2	2	0	2	6	Possible neonatal sepsis
6	0	0	2	2	1	2	7	Amnionitis—possible neonatal sepsis
7	1	0	0	1	2	2	6	Amnionitis—possible neonatal sepsis
8	0	0	2	2	0	2	6	Amnionitis—possible neonatal sepsis
9	0	0	0	1	0	1	2	Amnionitis—possible neonatal sepsis
10	0	0	1	2	1	2	6	Neonatal sepsis
11	1	0	2	0	2	0	5	Neonatal sepsis
12	0	0	0	0	0	2	2	Neonatal sepsis
13	0	0	0	2	0	2	4	Amnionitis—neonatal sepsis
14	0	0	1	1	0	2	4	Amnionitis—neonatal sepsis
15	0	0	0	2	0	1	3	Amnionitis—neonatal sepsis
16	0	0	0	1	0	2	3	Amnionitis—neonatal sepsis

AF, amniotic fluid; FBM, fetal breathing movements; FM, fetal movements; FT, fetal tone; NST, non-stress test; PL, placental grading.

From Vintzileos AM, Campbell WA, Nochimson DJ, et al: The fetal biophysical profile in patients with premature rupture of the membranes: An early predictor of fetal infection. Obstet Gynecol **152:**510, 1985.

infection. In analyzing the various parameters of the BPP that may detect infection, there is some debate over whether the loss of reactivity or loss of fetal breathing movements provides the better single marker (Vintzileos et al., 1986). In a review of 14 patients from the initial study of Vintzileos et al. (1985a) (Table 38-7), one can see that when the FHR was reactive (three cases), the remainder of the BPP was normal. When the BPP score was low, the FHR was always nonreactive.

Therefore, based on these data and other studies looking specifically at FHR as a predictor of infection, it appears that the evaluation of FHR reactivity is a good screening tool for fetal infection. If heart rate accelerations are absent, the more complete BPP can be used as a backup test. In all series evaluating these biophysical parameters, testing was done on a daily basis, and it appears that this frequency is necessary to provide adequate fetal evaluation. Not all analyses of the use of the BPP for the evaluation of infection have been as supportive of its value as those in the Vintzileos study (Miller et al., 1990).

Further analysis of the literature evaluating the detection of infection by the BPP reveals that this modality reveals fetal infection much more accurately than it detects maternal infection—the loss of reactivity, fetal movement, tone, and breathing being similar to the nonspecific signs seen with sepsis in the newborn nursery. The simple presence of bacteria in the amniotic fluid may or may not lead to depressed fetal responses, although it is speculated that release of prostaglandins associated with bacterial invasion has an impact on such biophysical parameters as fetal breathing (Vintzileos et al., 1986).

Lewis et al. (1999) compared the BPP and the non-stress test in a randomized trial as the initial daily screening test in patients with PPROM. They concluded that at gestational ages beyond 28 weeks, the non-stress test was equivalent and less costly than the BPP and that neither had good sensitivity for detecting infectious complications. Before 28 weeks, because the fetus was often nonreactive because of prematurity alone, they advocated using the daily BPP as the primary screening evaluation.

It appears that some initial form of careful maternal and fetal assessment on admission, followed by daily evaluation, is necessary to detect early infection. Because fetal infection sometimes may occur in the absence of maternal infection, the use of a fetal evaluation technique is also important. After the initial clinical evaluation on admission, a daily non-stress test and/or a daily BPP would be appropriate adjuncts to the daily clinical examination. In the absence of reactivity, the fetus should be evaluated with a BPP and if a markedly abnormal result is found, delivery will be required, presumably on the basis of fetal sepsis.

The clinical utility of amniocentesis for ruling out infection remains controversial. In a multivariate analysis, one study suggested that of all clinical parameters, a fetal tachycardia or a nonreactive non-stress test was the most predictive indicator of a positive amniotic fluid culture (Asrat et al., 1990). Therefore, when infection is suspected on the basis of such FHR changes or other nonspecific indicators of infection, amniocentesis may be beneficial in ruling in or out intraamniotic infection.

Fetal Lung Maturity Testing

Another important debate regarding the management of PROM involves the question of whether fetal lung maturity testing should be incorporated into the management algorithm. The protocol involves taking patients of selected gestational ages in whom some reasonable likelihood of fetal lung maturity exists (e.g., ≥32 weeks) and selectively managing these patients on the basis of lung maturity. An early description of this protocol by Garite (1982) reported that amniotic fluid was successfully obtained by amniocentesis in 50% of patients with PPROM, and approximately 50% had lecithin-to-sphingomyelin ratios consistent with fetal lung maturity. There were 63 such deliveries with two cases of mild RDS, one case of fetal pneumonia resulting in neonatal death, and no other major complications of prematurity in mature patients. Subsequently, Stedman and colleagues (1981) tested amniotic fluid obtained from the posterior vaginal fornix for the presence or absence of PG and reported similar results. Because amniotic fluid obtained from the vagina may be contaminated by substances present there, the PG test is the only fetal maturity test that is reliable. A significant number of fetuses, however, have lung maturity in the absence of PG, and PG generally indicates maturity a week or more later than other tests, such as the lecithin-to-sphingomyelin ratio. Therefore, it is advisable to use the PG obtained from the vaginal pool as an initial screening test and to follow with amniocentesis if PG is absent. Amniotic fluid analysis for lung maturity is discussed in detail in Chapters 16 and 25.

Two randomized studies have subjected such a management scheme to careful scrutiny. Spinnato and coworkers (1987) studied 46 patients, all of whom had fetal lung maturity as documented by amniotic fluid tests. These patients were categorized according to either delivery or expectant management. For patients who delivered immediately, the incidence of chorioamnionitis was lower overall than for patients who were managed expectantly. Similarly, Mercer and colleagues (1993) found that patients with mature amniotic fluid indices managed with delivery, as opposed to expectant management, had lower rates of chorioamnionitis. This resulted in shorter hospital stays for both mother and newborn.

Although there were no differences in the incidence of neonatal sepsis or other newborn complications in either study, the sample sizes were not large enough to sufficiently answer this question. We may infer, however, that if maternal infection rates are higher in the expectantly managed group, the rate of neonatal complications is likely to increase.

PATIENT MANAGEMENT

As stated, the management of patients with PROM remains one of the most controversial problems in obstetrics. All patients who present with symptoms suggestive of PROM should be brought to the hospital and evaluated. For women who are not in advanced active labor, the obstetrician should perform a speculum examination to confirm the diagnosis and to evaluate the status of the cervix. For patients who are in advanced active labor, delivery is obviously indicated regardless of gestational age and cesarean section is performed for the usual obstetric indications. Patients who have clinical chorioamnionitis need to be treated with antibiotics, and delivery is indicated regardless of gestational age.

Although there are a few cases in the obstetric literature in which patients with chorioamnionitis in very early gestational ages were treated with antibiotics and not delivered (Monif, 1983), in many more cases serious maternal infectious complications developed as a result of such management (Webb, 1967). Labor should be induced in patients without other indications for cesarean section and a reasonable trial of labor allowed, because chorioamnionitis in and of itself is not an indication for cesarean section regardless of gestational age. In cases of irreversible fetal distress, usually associated with variable decelerations of heart rate in the face of PROM, delivery is indicated. The management of patients who do not exhibit advanced labor, clinical infection, or fetal distress is based primarily on gestational age on admission.

Term Premature Rupture of Membranes

At 36 weeks and beyond, the goal of management of PROM is delivery. Patients in active labor should be allowed to progress, and management is the same as for any other term patient. Most of the remaining patients go into labor within 24 hours after PROM. Because the risk of neonatal infection increases as the duration of ROM becomes prolonged, however, many clinicians have aggressively managed term patients by inducing labor with oxytocin shortly after PROM in an effort to shorten the interval between rupture and delivery.

Over the past decade, studies evaluating the question of immediate induction of labor versus delayed induction or expectant management have shown conflicting results. Some have suggested that an aggressive approach with oxytocin induction only serves to increase the cesarean section rate, usually for failed induction or failure to progress in labor, and is not effective in lowering the infection rate (Kappy et al., 1979; Duff et al., 1984). In these studies, because cesarean section rates were increased with induction, there were higher rates of postpartum endometritis; however, not all studies have confirmed this finding (Wagner et al., 1989).

The largest study to evaluate this question was performed by an international collaborative group in which more than 5000 patients were randomized (Hannah et al., 1996). They compared immediate induction of labor with either oxytocin or prostaglandin E_2 gel versus expectant management of up to 4 days. There were no differences in the rates of cesarean section or neonatal sepsis among the groups. However, chorioamnionitis and postpartum fever were less likely in the group managed with immediate induction with oxytocin. In addition, in evaluating patient reaction to their management, the authors concluded that patients viewed immediate induction of labor more positively than they viewed expectant management.

Although the large collaborative study did not find any advantage to using prostaglandin E_2 for preinduction cervical ripening over oxytocin alone, other studies have suggested a benefit to this approach. A randomized trial by Ray and Garite (1992) compared three management schemes: (1) immediate oxytocin induction, (2) placebo prostaglandin (expectant management), and (3) prostaglandin using 3-mg vaginal suppositories, two doses, 6 hours apart, followed by induction for those patients not in labor. The shortest intervals between admission and delivery were found in the oxytocin and prostaglandin groups. The lowest cesarean section rates were found in the prostaglandin and expectant management groups, and the lowest rate of overall infection was seen in the prostaglandin group. Other nonrandomized studies have described such a protocol with similarly encouraging results (Magos et al., 1983).

Another common controversy is the optimal time period one should wait before beginning oxytocin when delayed induction is chosen. In a randomized trial of 200 patients with PROM at term, delay of 24 hours as opposed to 12 hours resulted in a 30% decrease in necessity for induction (47% versus 17%) without any increase in infection rate (Hjertberg et al., 1996).

Preterm Premature Rupture of Membranes

As previously noted, the major risks to the infant after PPROM are related to complications of prematurity. Therefore, management is aimed at prolonging gestation for the patient who is not in labor, not infected, and not experiencing fetal distress. However, based on the previously described controversies and the individual clinician's interpretation of these data, several possible alternative management schemes can be developed.

The most commonly accepted management scheme for the patient at less than 36 weeks with PROM but with a viable fetus is expectant management in the hospital. This measure basically consists of careful observation for signs of infection, labor, or fetal distress in an effort to gain time for fetal growth and maturation. On admission, the diagnosis is confirmed by speculum examination. Patients are initially evaluated by prolonged monitoring of FHR and uterine contractions (i.e., for 12 to 24 hours). If labor begins and infection or fetal distress develops, delivery is warranted; in other cases, patients may be transferred to a regular hospital room for observation. This measure includes daily clinical evaluation, frequent nonstress tests, and BPP evaluation. Patients in early labor are transferred immediately to the labor and delivery suite for careful fetal evaluation and supervision of labor. Although most of these patients do go into labor, some patients do reach term and the timing of delivery must be decided. When the patient reaches 36 or 37 weeks' gestation, delivery is indicated; documented fetal lung maturity may permit a somewhat earlier delivery.

Another management plan involves the use of selective expectant management. In this algorithm, patients are evaluated on admission for fetal lung maturity, and delivery is indicated if this maturity can be documented. It is reasonable to assume that lung maturity is unlikely at less than 31 weeks' gestation, and this group of patients can be managed expectantly. At 32 weeks or more, examination of vaginal pool fluid for PG by means of the rapid slide agglutination test yields an answer in a short time. In patients with PG-negative results, amniocentesis can be considered, and if any test of amniotic fluid documents fetal lung maturity, labor can be induced. Fluid obtained at amniocentesis should be submitted to Gram stain examination and glucose level determination. The discovery of occult infection is an indication for delivery and antibiotic treatment. The immature fetal lung and absence of occult infection are indications for expectant management.

Recently, several studies have evaluated the option of immediate delivery for all patients above a certain premature gestational age (e.g., 30 or 34 weeks). In their inner city populations, immediate delivery resulted in no increase in neonatal mortality or morbidity as compared with expectant management (Cox and Leveno, 1995; Naef et al., 1998).

Finally, many clinicians have varying views regarding tocolysis and corticosteroid treatment. Although prolonged tocolytic therapy has not been supported in clinical trials, many clinicians elect to continue this therapy with oral tocolytics in an effort to prolong gestation. Based on the NIH consensus conference (National Institute of Child Health and Human Development, 1994) and on the encouraging results of many randomized trials of prophylactic antibiotics, a more rational middle ground can be recommended. Patients at 24 to 30 or 32 weeks' gestation, who are most likely to benefit by corticosteroids and the 5 to 7 days that antibiotics can gain, should be considered for such therapy. Broad-spectrum parenteral antibiotics with good amniotic fluid penetration can be given in conjunction with the corticosteroids. Several questions remain, however, including (1) What is the optimal duration of antibiotic therapy? (2) Does 48 hours of tocolytic therapy add any benefit?

One of the main arguments for keeping patients in the hospital is that once labor begins, there is a high incidence of fetal distress, especially from umbilical cord compression. As has been described (Westgren et al., 1983), fetal distress in the very preterm gestation can be quite different from distress in the term gestation. These fetuses progress from mild to severe variable decelerations more rapidly, FHR variability is lost more rapidly, and there is better correlation between such abnormal heart rate patterns and depressed Apgar scores, umbilical cord acidosis, and neonatal complications (Fig. 38-4). Therefore, it is necessary to promptly evaluate fetal well-being once the patient goes into labor and to bring about quick delivery if fetal distress develops.

Another important issue is the use of *amnioinfusion* for the prevention of fetal distress. Because the incidence of fetal distress in association with PPROM is so high and because this fetal distress is caused most often by umbilical cord compression, this group of patients is ideally suited to amnioinfusion. Nageotte and coworkers (1985) randomly assigned patients with PPROM who were in active labor to either prophylactic amnioinfusion or none. Patients given prophylactic amnioinfusion demonstrated a lower rate and severity of variable decelerations, higher Apgar scores and umbilical cord pH values, and a lower incidence of fetal distress requiring cesarean section. The advantage of prophylactic amnioinfusion over waiting for abnormal FHR patterns and then instituting amnioinfusion in these patients is that once fetal distress develops in the very preterm gestation, there is insufficient time for the amnioinfusion to work before operative intervention is necessary.

Previable and Preterm Premature Rupture of Membranes

PROM that occurs very early in pregnancy (e.g., less than 25 weeks) presents a special set of problems, as previously described. In these patients there is a relatively low probability (25% to 40%) that a viable gestational age will be achieved and that the patient will deliver a surviving infant. There are real maternal risks (e.g., infection, abruption) associated with the process of waiting. A review of available retrospective series (Taylor and Garite, 1984; Moretti and Sibai, 1988; Bengtson and Van Marter, 1989; Major and Kitzmiller, 1990) reveals substantial maternal morbidity and a rather dismal outlook for the fetus, including a high rate of serious neurologic morbidity, in those that are managed expectantly (Table 38-8). Not only are maternal chorioamnionitis rates much higher than at later preterm gestational ages (39%), but other serious maternal complications (e.g., need for blood transfusions, serious maternal sepsis) and even death from sepsis have been described in these series.

There is increasing interest in the problem of the *fetal deformation syndrome* in patients with very early and prolonged ROM. This syndrome includes growth restriction, compression deformities, and pulmonary hypoplasia. The most serious complication, pulmonary hypoplasia, occurs relatively infrequently (approximately 20%) (Kilbride et al., 1996) but has the most devastating impact. Many efforts have been made to detect pulmonary hypoplasia by means of various sonographic parameters. Measurements used to assess this problem include fetal chest circumference, which can be compared with normograms for gestational age, and various ratios (e.g., fetal chest

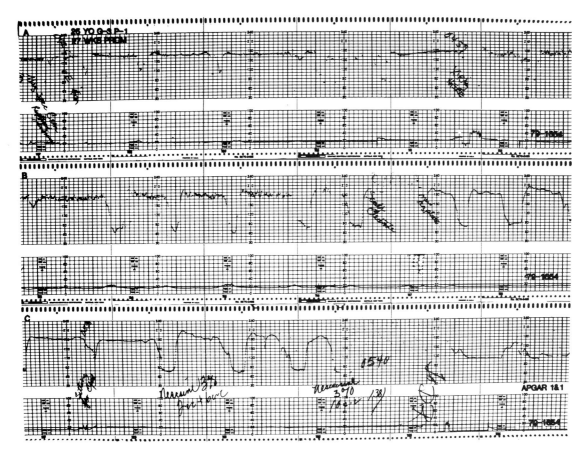

FIGURE 38-4 ■ Rapid progression in depth and duration of variable decelerations in a patient with preterm premature rupture of membranes and oligohydramnios. This is characteristic of the very premature fetus.

circumference-to-abdominal circumference or fetal chest circumference-to-cardiac circumference). Unfortunately, all these parameters have shown limited sensitivity and specificity and are far too unreliable for clinical use in making any management decision (Vintzileos et al., 1989).

Management of these patients consists of initial evaluation and, if labor or clinical infection is present, delivery. For the remainder, there are essentially two options: expectant management and termination. It is crucial, with such a high maternal risk and poor prognosis for good fetal outcome, that the patient be involved in this decision process. In many cases, the patient is admitted to the hospital before she is presented with

these options so that should she elect to terminate her pregnancy this can be carried out immediately. If the patient chooses expectant management, this can be carried out at home, because there is little benefit of hospitalization. The mother is discharged and instructed to maintain bed rest, avoid intercourse, check her temperature regularly, and await contractions. Once the patient reaches a viable gestational age (e.g., 25 to 26 weeks), she can be admitted to the hospital for daily fetal evaluation and prompt intervention should labor occur. For patients who elect termination, several methods are available: High-dose oxytocin or 20-mg prostaglandin E_2 suppositories every 4 hours are reasonable options. The diagnosis

TABLE 38-8. OUTCOME WITH PREMATURE RUPTURE OF MEMBRANES IN PREVIABLE GESTATIONS (ALL STUDIES < 26 WEEKS)

Study	No. of Mothers	Chorioamnionitis	No. of Infants	Newborn Survivors	Normal Neurologic Development
Taylor and Garite, 1984	53	13 (25%)	60	13 (22%)	38%
Major and Kitzmiller, 1990	70	30 (43%)	71	46 (65%)	31%
Moretti and Sibai, 1988	118	46 (39%)	124	40 (32%)	33%
Bengston and Van Marter, 1989	59	27 (46%)	63	32 (51%)	16%
Overall	300	116 (39%)	318	131 (41%)	30%

of incompetent cervix as a cause of PROM in such patients should be considered in the planning of a subsequent pregnancy.

Some exciting possibilities for more definitive treatment involving surgical resealing of the membranes are being developed. Preliminary studies involving laboratory models or very small human case series describe sealing of membranes with substances ranging from collagen grafts (Quintero et al., 2002), platelets and cryoprecipitate (Quintero et al., 1999), and fibrin and/or thrombin (Reddy et al., 2001; Sciscione et al., 2001) to gelatin sponge (O'Brien et al., 2001). One other experimental option being evaluated for patients with previable PROM involves serial transabdominal amnioinfusion. Preliminary results are encouraging, but the safety of this technique is not yet established and should still be considered experimental (Locatelli et al., 2000).

PRETERM PREMATURE RUPTURE OF MEMBRANES WHEN A CERVICAL CERCLAGE IS IN PLACE

One particularly perplexing management dilemma occurs when a preterm patient with a cervical cerclage presents with PROM. When the cerclage is removed immediately, there is evidence that these patients are not different from other patients with PPROM at similar gestational ages and can then be managed similarly (Yeast and Garite, 1988). Two questions remain unanswered that are critical to deciding on whether it is reasonable not to remove the cerclage. Does leaving the cerclage in place result in a longer interval to delivery and does leaving the cerclage in place increase the infectious risk to mother and/or infant? The first question is unanswered with studies concluding no difference (Yeast and Garite, 1988; McElrath et al., 2000), a prolonged latency with cerclage retention (Ludmir et al., 1994; Jenkins et al., 2000), and one study that showed a shortened latency with cerclage retention (Moore-Goldman et al., 1990). From these same studies it is also unclear whether infection is increased with cerclage retention, but most show either an increase in chorioamnionitis and/or sepsis or a strong trend in that direction. Our current practice is to remove the cerclage when a patient presents with PROM and proceed with management as one would with patients of similar gestational ages; a multicenter randomized trial to answer this question is needed.

RISK OF RECURRENCE

Very little information exists regarding the risk of recurrence in patients with PPROM. Asrat and coworkers (1991) evaluated this issue and looked at subsequent pregnancy outcome in patients who had been managed with PPROM in the index pregnancy. Of these patients, 32% had recurrent PPROM at an average of 2 weeks later in the subsequent pregnancy. Therefore, these patients should be counseled regarding the high risk of recurrence of this complication; unfortunately, little can be said at this point about prevention.

■ SUMMARY

The management of the patient with PROM is a common and perplexing problem. Despite many efforts, little progress has been made obstetrically toward reducing complications of this problem, especially from prematurity. Primary goals of management of PROM include making the diagnosis promptly without increasing the risk of infection in the process and evaluating the patient for signs of infection, fetal distress, and impending labor. Because prematurity accounts for most of the perinatal mortality and morbidity with PPROM, management designed to minimize complications of prematurity is appropriate. Complications from infection and asphyxia do occur, however, and efforts to avoid and minimize these problems are necessary.

REFERENCES

Adoni A, Chetrit AB, Zacut D, et al: Prolongation of the latent period in patients with premature rupture of the membrane by avoiding digital vaginal examination. Int J Gynecol Obstet **32**:19, 1990.

Alexander JM, Mercer BM, Miodovnik M: The impact of digital cervical examination on expectantly managed preterm rupture of membranes. Am J Obstet Gynecol **183**:1003, 2000.

Amon E, Lewis SV, Sibai B, et al: Antibiotic prophylaxis in preterm PROM: A prospective randomized study. Am J Obstet Gynecol **159**:539, 1988.

Angus SR, Segel SY, Hsu CD, et al: Amniotic fluid matrix metalloproteinase-8 indicates intra-amniotic infection. Am J Obstet Gynecol **185**:1232, 2001.

Artal JP, Sokol RJ, Neuman M, et al: The mechanical properties of prematurely and non-prematurely ruptured membranes. Am J Obstet Gynecol **125**:655, 1976.

Asrat T, Lewis DF, Garite TJ, et al: Rate of recurrence of preterm PROM in consecutive pregnancies. Am J Obstet Gynecol **165**:1111, 1991.

Asrat T, Nageotte MP, Garite TJ, et al: Gram stain results from amniocentesis in patients with preterm premature rupture of membranes: Comparison of maternal and fetal characteristics. Am J Obstet Gynecol **163**:887, 1990.

Athayde N, Edwin SS, Romero R, et al: A role for matrix metalloproteinase-9 in spontaneous rupture of the fetal membranes. Am J Obstet Gynecol **179**:1248, 1998.

Atlay RD, Sutherst JR: Premature rupture of the fetal membranes confirmed by intra-amniotic injection of dye (Evans blue T-1824). Am J Obstet Gynecol **108**:993, 1970.

Bain AD, Smith II, Gould IK: Newborn after prolonged leakage of liquor amnii. Br Med J **2**:598, 1964.

Barrett JM, Boehm FH: Comparison of aggressive and conservative management of premature rupture of fetal membranes. Am J Obstet Gynecol **144**:12, 1982.

Bengston JM, Van Marter LJ: Pregnancy outcome after premature rupture of the membranes at or before 26 weeks' gestation. Obstet Gynecol **73**:921, 1989.

Blanco J, Iams J, Artal R, et al: Multicenter double-blind prospective random trial of ceftizoximes: Placebo in women with preterm premature ruptured membranes. Am J Obstet Gynecol **168**:378, 1993.

Block MF, Kling OR, Crosby WM: Antenatal glucocorticoid therapy for the prevention of respiratory distress syndrome in the premature infant. Obstet Gynecol **50**:186, 1977.

Boyer KM, Gadzala CA, Kelly PD, et al: Selective intrapartum chemoprophylaxis of neonatal group B streptococcal early onset disease. II. Predictive value of prenatal cultures. J Infect Dis **148**:802, 1983.

Broekhuizen FF, Gilman M, Hamilton PR: Amniocentesis for Gram stain and culture in preterm premature rupture of the membranes. Obstet Gynecol **66**:316, 1985.

Capeless EL, Mead PB: Management of preterm premature rupture of membranes: Lack of a national consensus. Am J Obstet Gynecol **157**:11, 1987.

Carlan SJ, Richmond LB, O'Brien WF: Randomized trial of endovaginal ultrasound in preterm premature rupture of membranes. Am J Obstet Gynceol **89**:458, 1997.

Cederqvist LL, Zervoudakis IA, Ewool LC, et al: The relationship between prematurely ruptured membranes and fetal immunoglobulin production. Am J Obstet Gynecol **134**:784, 1979.

Christensen KK, Ingemarsson I, Leideman T, et al: Effect of ritodrine on labor after premature rupture of membranes. Obstet Gynecol 55:187, 1980.

Christmas JT, Cox SM, Gilstrap LC, et al: Expectant management of preterm ruptured membranes: Effects of antimicrobial therapy. Obstet Gynecol 80:759, 1992.

Collaborative Group on Antenatal Steroid Therapy: Effect of antenatal dexamethasone administration on the prevention of respiratory distress syndrome. Am J Obstet Gynecol 141:276, 1981.

Cotton DB, Hill LM, Strassner HT, et al: Use of amniocentesis in preterm gestation with ruptured membranes. Obstet Gynecol 63:38, 1984.

Cox SM, Leveno KJ: Intentional delivery versus expectant management with preterm ruptured membranes at 30–34 weeks' gestation. Obstet Gynecol 86:875, 1995.

Crowley P, Chalmers I, Keirse MJNC: The effects of corticosteroid administration before preterm delivery: An overview of the evidence from controlled trials. Br J Obstet Gynaecol 97:11, 1990.

Daikoku NH, Kaltreider F, Khozami VA, et al: Premature rupture of membranes and spontaneous preterm labor: Maternal endometritis risks. Obstet Gynecol 59:13, 1982.

Duff P, Huff RW, Gibbs RS: Management of PROM and unfavorable cervix in term pregnancy. Obstet Gynecol 63:697, 1984.

Dunlop PDM, Crowley PA, Lamont RF, et al: Preterm ruptured membranes, no contractions. J Obstet Gynecol 7:92, 1986.

Edwards LE, Barrada MI, Haaman AA, et al: Gonorrhea in pregnancy. Am J Obstet Gynecol 132:637, 1978.

Fortunato SJ, Menon R: Distinct molecular events suggest different pathways for preterm labor and premature rupture of membranes. Am J Obstet Gynecol 184:1399, 2001.

Friedman ML, McElin TW: Diagnosis of ruptured fetal membranes: Clinical study and review of the literature. Am J Obstet Gynecol 104:544, 1969.

Gabbe SG, Ettinger BB, Freeman RK, et al: Umbilical cord compression associated with amniotomy: Laboratory observations. Am J Obstet Gynecol 126:353, 1976.

Garite TJ: What's the best care in preterm PROM? Contemp Obstet Gynecol 19:178, 1982.

Garite TJ, Freeman RK: Chorioamnionitis in the preterm gestation. Obstet Gynecol 54:539, 1982.

Garite TJ, Freeman RK, Linzey EM, et al: The use of amniocentesis in patients with premature rupture of membranes. Obstet Gynecol 54:226, 1979.

Garite TJ, Freeman RK, Linzey EM, et al: Prospective randomized study of corticosteroids in the management of premature rupture of the membranes and the premature gestation. Am J Obstet Gynecol 141:508, 1981.

Garite TJ, Keegan KA, Freeman RK, et al: A randomized trial of ritodrine tocolysis vs. expectant management in patients with preterm PROM at 25 to 30 weeks. Am J Obstet Gynecol 157:388, 1987.

Gibbs RS, Blanco JD, St. Clair PJ, et al: Quantitative bacteriology of amniotic fluid from patients with clinical intra-amniotic infection at term. J Infect Dis 145:1, 1982.

Gibbs RS, Castillo MS, Rodgers PJ: Management of acute chorioamnionitis. Am J Obstet Gynecol 136:709, 1980.

Gonik B, Cotton DB: The use of amniocentesis in preterm premature rupture of membranes. Am J Perinatol 2:21, 1985.

Gunn GC, Mishell DR, Morton DG: Premature rupture of the fetal membranes: A review. Am J Obstet Gynecol 106:469, 1970.

Hannah M, Ohlsson A, Farine D, et al: Induction of labor compared with expectant management for prelabor rupture of membranes at term. N Eng J Med 334:1005, 1996.

Hardt NS, Kostenbauder M, Ogborn M, et al: Influence of chorioamnionitis on long-term prognosis in low birth weight infants. Obstet Gynecol 65:5, 1985.

Harirah H, Donia SE, Hsu CD: Amniotic fluid matrix metalloproteinase-9 and interleukin-6 in predicting intra-amniotic infection. Obstet Gynecol 99:80, 2002.

Hjertberg R, Hammarstrom M, Moberger B, et al: Premature rupture of the membranes (PROM) at term in nulliparous women with a ripe cervix. Acta Obstet Gynaecol Scand 75:48, 1996.

Iams JD, Talbert ML, Barrows H, et al: Management of preterm prematurely ruptured membranes: A prospective randomized comparison of observation versus use of steroids and timed delivery. Am J Obstet Gynecol 151:32, 1985.

Jenkins TM, Berghella V, Shlossman, PA, et al: Timing of cerclage removal after preterm premature rupture of membranes: Maternal and neonatal outcomes. Am J Obstet Gynecol 183:847, 2000.

Johnson JWC, Daikoku NH, Niebyl JR, et al: Premature rupture of the membranes and prolonged latency. Obstet Gynecol 57:547, 1981.

Johnson JWC, Egerman RS, Moorhead J: Cases with ruptured membranes that "reseal." Am J Obstet Gynecol 163:1024, 1990.

Johnston MM, Sanchez-Ramos L, Vaughn AJ, et al: Antibiotic therapy in preterm PROM: A randomized prospective double blind trial. Am J Obstet Gynecol 163:743, 1990.

Kaltreider DF, Kohl S: Epidemiology of preterm delivery. Clin Obstet Gynecol 23:17, 1980.

Kappy KA, Cetrulo CL, Knuppel RE, et al: Premature rupture of the membranes: A conservative approach. Am J Obstet Gynecol 134:655, 1979.

Kenyon SL, Taylor DJ, Tarnow-Mordi W: Broad-spectrum antibiotics for preterm, prelabour rupture of fetal membranes: the ORACLE I randomized trial. Lancet 356:979, 2001.

Kilbride HW, Yeast J, Thibeault DW: Defining limits of survival: Lethal pulmonary hypoplasia after midtrimester premature rupture of membranes. Am J Obstet Gynecol 175:675, 1996.

Kovacs D: Crystallization test for the diagnosis of ruptured membranes. Am J Obstet Gynecol 83:1257, 1962.

Lavery JP, Miller CE: Deformation and creep in the human chorioamniotic sac. Am J Obstet Gynecol 134:366, 1979.

Lavery JP, Miller CE, Knight RD: The effect of labor on the rheologic response of chorioamniotic membranes. Obstet Gynecol 60:87, 1982.

Lebherz TB, Hellman LP, Madding R, et al: Double blind study of premature rupture of the membranes. N Engl J Med 303:769, 1980.

Ledger WJ: Amnionitis, endometritis and premature rupture of membranes. *In* Current Concepts. Kalamazoo, Mich, The Upjohn Co., 1976.

Lee M, Davies J, Atkinson MW, et al: Efficacy of weekly courses of antenatal corticosteroids (ACS) in preterm premature rupture of the membranes. Abstract presented at the Society for Maternal Fetal Medicine, Feb 5, 2001, Reno, Nev.

Levy DL, Warsof SL: Oral ritodrine and preterm premature rupture of membranes. Obstet Gynecol 66:621, 1985.

Lewis DF, Adair D, Weeks JW, et al: A randomized clinical trial of daily nonstress testing versus biophysical profile in the management of preterm premature rupture of membranes. Am J Obstet Gynecol 181:1495, 1999.

Lewis DF, Brody K, Edwards MS, et al: Preterm premature ruptured membranes: A randomized trial of steroids after treatment with antibiotics. Obstet Gynecol 88:801, 1996.

Lewis DF, Major CA, Towers CV, et al: Effects of digital vaginal examinations on latency period in preterm premature rupture of membranes. Obstet Gynecol 80:630, 1992.

Liggins GC, Howie RN: A controlled trial of antepartum glucocorticoid treatment for the prevention of respiratory distress syndrome in premature infants. Pediatrics 50:515, 1972.

Locatelli A, Vergani P, DiPirro G, et al: Role of amnioinfusion in the management of premature rupture of the membranes at < 26 weeks' gestation. Am J Obstet Gynecol 183:878, 2000.

Lockwood CJ, Costigan K, Ghidine A, et al: Double blind placebo-controlled trial of piperacillin prophylaxis in preterm membrane rupture. Am J Obstet Gynecol 169:970, 1993.

Lonky NM, Hayashi RH: A proposed mechanism for premature rupture of membrane. Obstet Gynecol Surv 43:22, 1988.

Lovett SM, Weiss JD, Diogo MJ, et al: A prospective, double-blind, randomized, controlled clinical trial of ampicillin-sulbactam for preterm premature rupture of membranes in women receiving antenatal corticosteroid therapy. Am J Obstet Gynecol 176:1070, 1997.

Ludmir J, Bader T, Chen L, et al: Poor perinatal outcome associated with retained cerclage in patients with premature rupture of membranes. Obstet Gynecol 84:823, 1994.

Magos AL, Nobem MCB, Wong Ten Yuen A, et al: Controlled study comparing vaginal prostaglandin E$_2$ pessaries with intravenous oxytocin for the stimulation of labour after spontaneous rupture of the membranes. Br J Obstet Gynaecol 90:726, 1983.

Major CA, deVeciana M, Lewis DF, et al: Preterm premature rupture of membranes and abruptio placentae: Is there an association between these pregnancy complications? Am J Obstet Gynecol 172:672, 1995.

Major CA, Kitzmiller JL: Perinatal survival with expectant management of midtrimester rupture of membranes. Am J Obstet Gynecol 163:838, 1990.

Martin DH, Koutsky L, Eschenbach DA, et al: Prematurity and perinatal mortality in pregnancies complicated by maternal *Chlamydia trachomatis* infections. JAMA 247:1585, 1982.

McElrath TF, Norwitz ER, Lieberman ES, et al: Management of cervical cerclage and preterm premature rupture of the membranes: Should the stitch be removed? Am J Obstet Gynecol 183:840, 2000.

McGregor JA, French JI, Seo K: Antimicrobial therapy in preterm premature rupture of the membranes: Results of a prospective, double-blind, placebo-controlled trial of erythromycin. Am J Obstet Gynecol 165:632, 1991.

McGregor JA, Lawellin D, Franco-Buff A, et al: Protease production by microorganisms associated with reproductive tract infection. Am J Obstet Gynecol 154:109, 1986.

Mead PB: Management of the patient with premature rupture of the membranes. Clin Perinatol 7:243, 1980.

Mercer BM, Arheart KL: Antimicrobial therapy in expectant management of preterm premature rupture of the membranes. Lancet 346:1271, 1995.

Mercer BM, Crocker LG, Boe NM, et al: Induction versus expectant management in premature rupture of the membranes with mature amniotic fluid at 32 to 36 weeks: A randomized trial. Am J Obstet Gynecol 169:775, 1993.

Mercer BM, Miodovnik M, Thurnau GR, et al: Antibiotic therapy for reduction of infant morbidity after preterm premature rupture of the membranes: A randomized controlled trial. JAMA 278:989, 1997.

Miller JM, Hill GB, Welt S, et al: Bacterial colonization of amniotic fluid in the presence of ruptured membranes. Am J Obstet Gynecol 137:451, 1980.

Miller JM, Pupkin MJ, Crenshaw C: Premature labor and premature rupture of the membranes. Am J Obstet Gynecol 132:1, 1978.

Miller JM Jr, Kho MS, Brown HL, et al: Clinical chorioamnionitis is not predicted by an ultrasonic biophysical profile in patients with premature rupture of membranes. Obstet Gynecol 76:1051, 1990.

Minkoff H, Grunebaum AN, Schwarz RH, et al: Risk factors for prematurity and premature rupture of membranes: A prospective study of vaginal flora in pregnancy. Am J Obstet Gynecol 150:965, 1984.

Moberg LJ, Garite TJ: Antepartum fetal heart rate testing in preterm PROM. Presented at the Seventh Annual Meeting of the Society of Perinatal Obstetricians, Feb 5–7, 1987, Lake Buena Vista, Fla.

Moberg LJ, Garite TJ, Freeman RK: Fetal heart rate patterns and fetal distress in patients with preterm premature rupture of membranes. Obstet Gynecol 64:60, 1984.

Monif GRG: Recurrent chorioamnionitis and maternal septicemia. A case of successful in utero therapy. Am J Obstet Gynecol 146:334, 1983.

Moore-Goldman J, Greene MF, Harlow BL, et al: Outcome of expectant management in preterm premature rupture of membranes with cervical cerclage in place. Abstract presented at the Society of Perinatal Obstetricians, Jan 23–27, 1990, Houston, Tex.

Morales W, Angel J, O'Brien W, et al: Use of ampicillin and corticosteroids in PROM: A randomized study. Obstet Gynecol 73:721, 1989.

Morales WJ: The effect of chorioamnionitis on developmental outcome of preterm infants at one year. Obstet Gynecol 70:183, 1987.

Morales WJ, Diebel ND, Lazar AJ, et al: The effect of antenatal dexamethasone on the prevention of respiratory distress syndrome in preterm gestations with premature rupture of membranes. Am J Obstet Gynecol 154:591, 1986.

Moretti M, Sibai BM: Maternal and perinatal outcome of expectant management of premature rupture of membranes in the midtrimester. Am J Obstet Gynecol 159:390, 1988.

Naef RW, Allbert JR, Ross EL, et al: Premature rupture of membranes at 34–37 weeks' gestation: Aggressive versus conservative management. Am J Obstet Gynecol 178:126, 1998.

Naeye RL: Coitus and associated amniotic fluid infections. N Engl J Med 22:1198, 1979.

Naeye RL: Factors that predispose to premature rupture of the fetal membranes. Obstet Gynecol 69:93, 1982.

Nageotte MP, Freeman RK, Garite TJ, et al: Prophylactic intrapartum amnioinfusion in patients with preterm premature rupture of membranes. Am J Obstet Gynecol 153:557, 1985.

National Institute of Child Health and Human Development: Report of the Consensus Development Conference on the Effect of Corticosteroids for Fetal Maturation on Perinatal Outcomes (NIH Publication No. 95-3784). Bethesda, Md, National Institutes of Health, 1994.

National Institutes of Health Consensus Statement: Antenatal Corticosteroids Revisited: Repeat Courses (NIH Consensus Statement 17(2)). Bethesda, Md, National Institutes of Health, 2000.

Nelson LH, Meis PJ, Hatjis CG, et al: Premature rupture of membranes: A prospective, randomized evaluation of steroids, latent phase and expectant management. Obstet Gynecol 66:55, 1985.

Newman RB, Goldenberg RL, Moawad AH, et al: Occupational fatigue and preterm premature rupture of membranes. Am J Obstet Gynecol 184:438, 2001.

O'Brien JM, Mercer BM, Barton JR, et al: An in vitro model and case report that used gelatin sponge to restore amniotic fluid volume after spontaneous premature rupture of the membranes. Am J Obstet Gynecol 185:1094, 2001.

Ohlsson A: Treatments of preterm premature rupture of membranes: A meta-analysis. Am J Obstet Gynecol 160:890, 1989.

Ohlsson A, Wong E: An analysis of antenatal tests to detect infection in preterm PROM. Am J Obstet 162:809, 1990.

O'Keeffe DF, Garite TJ, Elliott JP, et al: The accuracy of estimated gestational age based on ultrasound measurement of the biparietal diameter in preterm premature rupture of the membranes. Am J Obstet Gynecol 151:309, 1985.

Owen J, Gromme LJ, Hauth JC: Randomized trial of prophylactic antibiotic therapy after preterm amnion rupture. Am J Obstet Gynecol 169:976, 1993.

Papageorgiou AN, Desgranges MF, Masson M, et al: The antenatal use of betamethasone in the prevention of respiratory distress syndrome: A controlled double-blind study. Pediatrics 63:73, 1979.

Park JS, Romero R, Yoon BH, et al: The relationship between amniotic fluid matrix meetalloproteinase-8 and funisitis. Am J Obstet Gynecol 185:1156, 2001.

Parry-Jones E, Priya S: A study of elasticity and tension of fetal membranes and of the relation of the area of the gestational sac to the area of the uterine cavity. Br J Obstet Gynaecol 83:205, 1976.

Quintero RA, Morales WJ, Allen M, et al: Treatment of iatrogenic previable premature rupture of membranes with intra-amniotic injection of platelets and cryoprecipitate (amniopatch): Preliminary experience. Am J Obstet Gynecol 181:744, 1999.

Quintero RA, Morales WJ, Bornick PW, et al: Surgical treatment of spontaneous rupture of membranes: The amniograft—First experience. Am J Obstet Gynecol 186:155, 2002.

Ray DR, Garite TJ: Prostaglandin E2 for induction of labor in patients with PROM at term. Am J Obstet Gynecol 166:836, 1992.

Reddy UM, Shah SS, Nemiroff RL, et al: In vitro sealing of punctured fetal membranes: Potential treatment for midtrimester premature rupture of membranes. Am J Obstet Gynecol 185:1090, 2001.

Regan TA, Chao S, James LS: Premature rupture of membrane, preterm delivery and group B streptococcal colonization of mothers. Am J Obstet Gynecol 141:184, 1981.

Romero R: Infectious etiology of preterm labor. Presented at the World Symposium of Perinatal Medicine, Oct 31, 1991, San Francisco.

Romero R, Emamian M, Quintero R, et al: The value and limitations of the Gram stain examination in the diagnosis of intra-amniotic infection. Am J Obstet Gynecol 159:114, 1988.

Romero R, Yoon BH, Mazor M, et al: A comparative study of the diagnostic performance of amniotic fluid glucose, white blood cell count, interleukin-6, and Gram stain in the detection of microbial invasion in patients with preterm premature rupture of membranes. Am J Obstet Gynecol 169:839, 1993.

Rutherford SE, Phelan JP, Smith CV, et al: The four-quadrant assessment of amniotic fluid volume: An adjunct to antepartum fetal heart rate testing. Obstet Gynecol 70:353, 1987.

Schreiber J, Benedetti T: Conservative management of preterm premature rupture of the fetal membranes in a low socioeconomic population. Am J Obstet Gynecol 136:92, 1980.

Schutte MF, Treffers PE, Kloosterman GI, et al: Management of premature rupture of membranes: A risk of vaginal examination to the infant. Am J Obstet Gynecol 146:395, 1983.

Schwarz R, Belizan JM, Nieto F, et al: Third progress report on the Latin American Collaborative Study on the effects of late rupture of membranes on labor and the neonate. In Gluck L (ed): Modern Perinatal Medicine. Chicago, Year Book, 1974.

Sciscione AC, Manley JS, Pollock M, et al: Intracervical fibrin sealants: A potential treatment for early preterm premature rupture of the membranes. Am J Obstet Gynecol 184:368, 2001.

Simpson GL, Harbert GM: Use of betamethasone in management of preterm gestation with premature rupture of membranes. Obstet Gynecol 66:168, 1985.

Skinner SJM, Campos GA, Higgins GC: Collagen content of human amniotic membranes: Effect of gestational length and premature rupture. Obstet Gynecol 57:487, 1981.

Smith RP: A technic for the detection of rupture of the membranes. Obstet Gynecol 48:172, 1976.

Spinnato JA, Shaver DC, Bray E, et al: Preterm premature rupture of the membranes with fetal pulmonary maturity present: A prospective study. Obstet Gynecol 69:196, 1987.

Stedman CM, Crawford S, Staten E, et al: Management of preterm premature rupture of membranes: Assessing amniotic fluid in the vagina for phosphatidyl glycerol. Am J Obstet Gynecol 140:34, 1981.

Taeusch HW, Frigoletto F, Kitzmiller J, et al: Risk of respiratory distress syndrome after prenatal dexamethasone treatment. Pediatrics 63:64, 1979.

Taylor J, Garite TJ: Premature rupture of membranes before fetal viability. Obstet Gynecol 4:615, 1984.

Varner MW, Galask RP: Conservative management of premature rupture of the membranes. Am J Obstet Gynecol **140**:39, 1981.

Vermillion ST, Soper DE, Chasedunn-Roark J: Neonatal sepsis after betamethasone administration to patients with preterm premature rupture of membranes. Am J Obstet Gynecol **181**:320, 1999.

Vintzileos AM, Campbell WA, Nochimson DJ, et al: The fetal biophysical profile in patients with premature rupture of the membranes: An early predictor of fetal infection. Obstet Gynecol **152**:510, 1985a.

Vintzileos AM, Campbell WA, Nochimson DJ, et al: Degree of oligohydramnios and pregnancy outcome in patients with premature rupture of the membranes. Obstet Gynecol **66**:162, 1985b.

Vintzileos AM, Campbell WA, Nochimson DJ, et al: Fetal breathing as a predictor of infection in premature rupture of the membranes. Obstet Gynecol **67**:813, 1986.

Vintzileos AM, Campbell WA, Rodis JF, et al: Comparison of six different ultrasonographic methods of predicting lethal fetal pulmonary hypoplasia. Am J Obstet Gynecol **161**:606, 1989.

Wagner MV, Chin VP, Peters CJ, et al: A comparison of early and delayed induction of labor with spontaneous rupture of membranes at term. Obstet Gynecol **74**:93, 1989.

Webb GA: Maternal death associated with premature rupture of the membranes: An analysis of 54 cases. Am J Obstet Gynecol **98**:594, 1967.

Weiner CP, Renk K, Klugman M: The therapeutic efficacy and cost effectiveness of aggressive tocolysis for premature labor associated with PROM. Am J Obstet Gynecol **159**:216, 1988.

Westgren LM, Holmquist P, Svenningsen NW, et al: Intrapartum fetal monitoring in preterm deliveries: Prospective study. Obstet Gynecol **90**:726, 1983.

Wilson JC, Levy DC, Wilds PL: Premature rupture of membranes prior to term: Consequences of non-intervention. Obstet Gynecol **60**:601, 1982.

Winn HN, Ghen M, Amon E, et al: Neonatal pulmonary hypoplasia and perinatal mortality in patients with midtrimester rupture of amniotic membranes—A critical analysis. Am J Obstet Gynecol **182**:1638, 2000.

Woods JR, Plessinger MA, Miller RK: Vitamins C and E: Missing links in preventing preterm premature rupture of membranes. Am J Obstet Gynecol **185**:5, 2001.

Yeast JD, Garite TJ: The role of cervical cerclage in the management of preterm premature rupture of the membranes. Am J Obstet Gynecol **158**:106, 1988.

Yoder PR, Gibbs RS, Blanco JD, et al: A prospective, controlled study of maternal and perinatal outcome after intra-amniotic infection at term. Am J Obstet Gynecol **145**:695, 1983.

Yoon BH, Romero R, Kim KS, et al: A systemic fetal inflammatory response and the development of bronchopulmonary dysplasia. Am J Obstet Gynecol **181**:773, 1999.

Yoon BH, Romero R, Park JS, et al: Fetal exposure to an intra-amniotic inflammation and the development of cerebral palsy at the age of three years. Am J Obstet Gynecol **182**:675, 2000.

Young BK, Klein SA, Katz M, et al: Intravenous dexamethasone for prevention of neonatal respiratory distress: A prospective controlled study. Am J Obstet Gynecol **138**:203, 1980.

Zlatnick FJ, Cruikshank DP, Petzold CR, et al: Amniocentesis in the identification of inapparent infection in preterm patients with premature rupture of the membranes. J Reprod Med **29**:656, 1984.

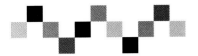

Chapter 39

MATERNAL AND FETAL INFECTIOUS DISORDERS

Ronald S. Gibbs, MD, Richard L. Sweet, MD, and W. Patrick Duff, MD

Since the last edition of this book, new advances have continued to occur in our knowledge of the pathogenesis, diagnosis, prevention, and management of maternal-fetal infections. Highlights include development of consensus guidelines for the prevention of early-onset neonatal infection with group B streptococci (GBS), strategies to decrease perinatal transmission of human immunodeficiency virus (HIV) infection, strategies to prevent infection-associated preterm premature rupture of membranes and preterm birth, and refinements in prenatal diagnosis of congenital infections.

Within the last 25 years, infection and immunology have become central issues in the study of the pregnant woman and her fetus. In practice, clinical infectious disease problems are both common and potentially severe. They involve a wide range of organisms, including group A and B streptococci, *Listeria monocytogenes*, *Escherichia coli*, the anaerobes, HIV, herpesvirus, rubella virus, hepatitis viruses (see Chapter 53), cytomegaloviruses, *Mycoplasma* spp., *Chlamydia* spp., treponemes, and *Toxoplasma gondii*. They span a range of diseases and situations: premature rupture of the membranes (PROM), endometritis and consequent sepsis, pyelonephritis, pneumonia, and sexually transmitted diseases. They also lead to a variety of effects—for example, abortion, malformation, congenital diseases, growth restriction, stillbirth, prematurity, sepsis, and shock. Of major importance is the link between immunology and infection on the one hand and two fundamental issues on the other: (1) the very existence of the fetus in the mother and (2) the pathogenesis of premature birth.

BACTERIAL INFECTIONS

Urinary Tract Infections

Urinary tract infections (UTIs) are the most common medical complications of pregnancy. Moreover, they are a major public health problem in women, accounting for 7–8 million office visits and 100,000 hospitalizations annually at a cost of $1.3 billion (Patton et al., 1991; Stamm and Hooten, 1993). They may be either asymptomatic (asymptomatic bacteriuria of pregnancy) or symptomatic (cystitis, acute pyelonephritis). Although the majority of UTIs in pregnancy are asymptomatic, asymptomatic bacteriuria (ASB) places the fetus at increased risk for preterm delivery and low birth weight (Romero et al., 1989; Meis et al., 1995).

UTIs are 14 times more common in females than in males. It has been suggested that this predominance is due to the following: (1) a shorter urethra in the female; (2) continuous contamination of the external third of the urethra by pathogenic bacteria from the vagina and rectum; (3) the high probability that females do not empty their bladders as completely as males; and (4) movement of the bacteria into the female bladder during sexual intercourse. In addition, the normal physiologic changes associated with pregnancy predispose the pregnant woman with ASB to the development of acute pyelonephritis, with its associated significant morbidity.

Symptomatic and Asymptomatic Urinary Tract Infections

Although obstetricians have long recognized the serious nature of symptomatic UTIs in pregnancy, it was not until in the early 1960s that Kass demonstrated that significant bacteriuria can occur in the absence of symptoms or signs of UTIs (Kass, 1960a, 1960b, 1973; Kass and Zinner, 1969, 1973). He established quantitative bacteriology as the indispensable laboratory aid for the diagnosis, follow-up, and confirmation of cure of UTI. From these studies evolved the commonly accepted definition of ASB: the presence of 10^5 or more colonies of a bacterial organism per milliliter of urine on two consecutive clean, midstream-voided specimens in the absence of signs or symptoms of UTI. Persistent ASB was identified in 6% of pregnant patients. Acute pyelonephritis developed in 40% of patients with the disorder who received a placebo; when bacteriuria was eliminated, pyelonephritis did not occur. Kass and Zinner also noted that rates of neonatal death and prematurity rates were two to three times greater in bacteriuric women receiving placebo than in nonbacteriuric women or bacteriuric women whose infection was eliminated by antibiotics. Kass concluded that detection of maternal bacteriuria would identify patients at risk for pyelonephritis and premature delivery and maintained that pyelonephritis in pregnancy could be prevented by detection and treatment of bacteriuria in early pregnancy. Moreover, Kass estimated that 10% of premature births would be prevented by such a program.

Symptomatic UTI is more often found in pregnant women than in nonpregnant women. This suggests that some factors present during gestation allow bacteria to replicate in the urine and ascend to the upper urinary tract. Several findings support this view. The normal female urinary tract undergoes dramatic physiologic and anatomic changes during pregnancy (see Chapters 8 and 44). Briefly, a decrease in ureteric muscle tone and activity results in a lower rate of passage of urine throughout the urinary collecting system. The upper ureters and renal pelvises become dilated, resulting in a physiologic hydronephrosis of pregnancy. These changes are caused by the effects of progesterone on muscle tone and peristalsis and, more important, by mechanical obstruction of the enlarging uterus. Vesicle changes also occur in pregnancy, including decreased tone, increased capacity, and incomplete emptying, all of which predispose to vesicoureteric reflux. Hypotonia of the vesicle musculature, vesicoureteric reflux, and dilatation of the ureters and renal pelvises result in static columns of urine in the ureters, facilitating the ascending migration of bacteria to the upper urinary tract after bladder infection is established. The hypokinetic collecting system reduces urine flow, and urinary stasis occurs, predisposing to infection.

It is also possible that alterations in the physical and chemical properties of urine during pregnancy exacerbate bacteriuria, further predisposing to ascending infection. Because of the increased excretion of bicarbonate, urinary pH rises, encouraging bacterial growth. Glycosuria, which is common in pregnancy, may favor an increase in the rate of bacterial multiplication. The increased urinary excretion of estrogens may also be a factor in the pathogenesis of symptomatic UTI during pregnancy. In animal experiments, estrogen can enhance the growth of strains of E. coli that cause pyelonephritis and predispose to renal infection. In addition, the renal medulla is particularly susceptible to infection because its hypertonic environment inhibits leukocyte migration, phagocytosis, and complement activity. The cumulative effect of these physiologic factors is an increased risk that infection in the bladder may ascend to the kidneys.

Pathogenic characteristics of microorganisms such as E. coli are major determinants of UTI. These include pili (adherence), K antigen (antiphagocytic activity), hemolysin (cytotoxicity), and antimicrobial resistance. Host susceptibility factors include anatomic or functional abnormalities of the urinary tract; uroepithelial and vaginal epithelial cells with increased attachment of uropathogenic E. coli; and nonsecretor status, which uncovers receptors for E. coli in uroepithelial and vaginal cells.

Most cases of ASB of pregnancy are detected at the initial prenatal visit, and relatively few pregnant women acquire bacteriuria after the initial visit. Thus bacteriuria antedates the pregnancy. The prevalence of asymptomatic bacteriuria in schoolgirls is approximately 1%. There is a considerable increase in the rate of ASB once a woman begins sexual activity. The prevalence of bacteriuria rises to 3.5% in females aged 15 to 19 years old and increases thereafter at a rate of about 1% for each decade of life.

Several studies have shown that the incidence of ASB in nonpregnant women is comparable to the incidence in pregnant women in the same locale. It appears that most women in whom bacteriuria is first discovered during pregnancy have acquired ASB earlier in life, the incidence of infection having increased as a result of sexual activity. Although pregnancy *per se* does not cause any major increase in incidence of bacteriuria, it does predispose to the development of acute pyelonephritis in bacteriuric patients.

It is generally accepted that untreated ASB during pregnancy often leads to acute pyelonephritis. For this reason, it is important that the presence of bacteriuria be identified. Other claims, however, such as that ASB predisposes the patient to anemia, preeclampsia, and chronic renal disease, are controversial and unproven. Until recently, controversy existed over claims for an association of bacteriuria with prematurity and low birth weight.

More-recent studies (including a meta-analysis) demonstrate an association between ASB and low birth weight (Romero et al., 1989; Schieve et al., 1994; Meis et al., 1995). With recognition that ASB increases the risk for developing acute pyelonephritis and preterm delivery and low birth weight, the American College of Obstetricians and Gynecologists (ACOG) and the U.S. Preventive Services Task Force recommend screening to detect ASB in pregnancy (ACOG, 1988; U.S. Preventive Services, 1989).

The prevalence of ASB in pregnant women ranges from 2% to 11%, with the majority of investigations reporting 4% to 7%. An increased prevalence of bacteriuria in females has been associated with the presence of sickle cell trait, lower socioeconomic status, lower availability of medical care, and increased parity. Escherichia coli is the predominant pathogen isolated in each study of asymptomatic bacteriuria and is cultured in 60% to 90% of cases. The next most common organisms are Proteus mirabilis, Klebsiella pneumoniae, and the enterococci. Group B β-hemolytic streptococci and Staphylococcus saprophyticus are also potential pathogens in the urinary tract during pregnancy. These uropathogens are similar to those recovered from pregnant women with symptomatic UTI (cystitis or pyelonephritis).

BACTERIURIA AND PYELONEPHRITIS

Acute pyelonephritis is a serious threat to maternal and fetal well-being. An association between acute pyelonephritis in pregnancy and premature delivery was recognized in the pre-antibiotic era, with prematurity rates of 20% to 50% reported. Studies made after the advent of antibiotics have confirmed this association between acute pyelonephritis and an increased risk of premature delivery. A variety of bacterial products stimulate the immune system to release cytokines such as interleukin-1, interleukin-6, tumor necrosis factor, and platelet activating factor, which in turn trigger prostaglandin production.

A significant factor in understanding the pathogenesis of pyelonephritis was the concept of quantitative urine culture, which made it possible to diagnose ASB. Early studies identified the presence of ASB as the most significant factor associated with the development of acute pyelonephritis of pregnancy. As mentioned, Kass (1960b) noted that in 20% to 40% of pregnant women with ASB who were receiving a placebo, pyelonephritis subsequently developed. When the bacteriuria was treated and eliminated with antimicrobial agents, however, pyelonephritis did not occur. Subsequent studies have confirmed that pregnant women with untreated ASB are at high risk (13.5% to 65%) for development of acute pyelonephritis during pregnancy. Detection and treatment of ASB significantly reduce the risk of pyelonephritis. A small proportion of women without bacteriuria at the first antenatal visit do acquire pyelonephritis. In pregnant women whose bacteriuria is treated, the reported incidence of pyelonephritis ranges from 0% to 5.3%, with an average of 2.9%. In addition, pyelonephritis may develop in women with ASB prior to their initial prenatal visit and thus before screening attempts. Detection and eradication by treatment of bacteriuria early in pregnancy should prevent pyelonephritis in at least 70% to 80% of cases. Widespread screening for GBS in pregnancy has been demonstrated to reduce the incidence of pyelonephritis in pregnancy significantly (Harris, 1979; Smaill, 1995; Gratacos et al., 1994). Recent cost-effectiveness and cost-benefit analysis noted that screening for and treatment of ASB to prevent acute pyelonephritis in pregnancy is cost-beneficial (Rouse et al., 1995).

BACTERIURIA AND HYPERTENSION

An increased incidence of hypertensive disease of pregnancy has been alleged to exist in pregnant women with ASB. Some investigations have confirmed the association, but most studies have not documented any relationship between bacteriuria and hypertension (Whalley et al., 1975; Whalley, 1967).

BACTERIURIA AND CHRONIC RENAL DISEASE

Although UTIs are related to renal disease, the factors that determine their frequency in the etiology of chronic renal disease have not been defined. It has been estimated that 10% to 15% of bacteriuric pregnant women are destined to have evidence of chronic pyelonephritis 10 to 12 years after delivery (Zinner and Kass, 1971). Renal failure ultimately develops in one of every 3000 pregnant women with bacteriuria. Because persistent bacteriuria, abnormal renal function, and radiologic evidence of chronic pyelonephritis are found so commonly in follow-up studies of patients with ASB of pregnancy, long-term follow-up of women who have bacteriuria is essential.

BACTERIURIA AND PRETERM DELIVERY AND LOW BIRTH WEIGHT

That acute pyelonephritis during pregnancy is associated with a significantly increased rate of prematurity is well documented. In contrast, the relationship of ASB to premature delivery, babies who are small for gestational age, and fetal mortality has been controversial. Kass (1973) initially reported an association between ASB and prematurity and noted that eradication of bacteriuria with antimicrobial therapy significantly reduces the rate of preterm delivery. He proposed that early detection and treatment of bacteriuria would prevent 10% to 20% of prematurity (<2500 g). Subsequently, numerous studies have demonstrated conflicting results regarding bacteriuria and prematurity. Kincaid-Smith and Bullen (1965) first suggested the hypothesis that underlying renal disease was the major cause of the excessive risk of prematurity or low birth weight among bacteriuric pregnant women. The many different definitions for prematurity used in the literature have contributed to the confusion, although the majority of authors base their definitions on birth weight of less than 2500 g.

Bacteriuria is only one of many factors that may influence the onset of premature labor. Because the incidence of pregnancy bacteriuria as well as of prematurity increases inversely with socioeconomic status, any relationship between bacteriuria and gestational length and birth weight may be complex and difficult to establish. In an attempt to resolve this controversy, Romero and colleagues (1989) used the technique of meta-analysis to assess the relationship between ASB and preterm delivery and/or low birth weight. Although only 5 of the 17 studies included in the analysis demonstrated a statistically significant increase in low-birth-weight infants among patients with bacteriuria, meta-analysis confirmed a statistically significant increased risk for low-birth-weight infants among bacteriuric women. Similarly, this study demonstrated a significant association between bacteriuria and preterm delivery, although only two of four accepted studies demonstrated a statistically significant risk. Finally, this meta-analysis showed a statistically significant reduction in low birth weight among bacteriuric women treated in eight placebo-controlled treatment trials.

Meis and colleagues (1995) demonstrated in a multivariate analysis that bacteriuria significantly increased the occurrence of preterm birth (relative risk, 2.03; 95% confidence interval [CI], 1.50 to 2.75). Moreover, Smaill (1995) reported a meta-analysis of treatment versus placebo trials for ASB in pregnancy, which demonstrated a one-third reduction in the rate of low-birth-weight infants (from 15% to 10%) in women whose bacteriuria was treated. Thus, it appears that maternal ASB is a risk factor for preterm delivery and low birth weight, and this risk can be reduced by screening and treatment of ASB in pregnant women (Mittendorf et al., 1992).

DIAGNOSIS

Although the diagnosis of ASB was originally based on obtaining two consecutive midstream urine cultures containing at least 100,000 CFU/mL of a uropathogen, clinically a single positive urine specimen is used (Millar and Cox, 1997; Sweet and Gibbs, 2002). Urine cultures are relatively expensive and require 24 to 48 hours for results. Inexpensive, rapid, office-based screening tests have therefore undergone clinical testing (Millar and Cox, 1997). These include microscopic urinalysis, nitrite dipstick, Gram stain, Uricult dip slide, Cult-Dip Plus, and Uristat test (Millar and Cox, 1997; Sweet and Gibbs, 2002). However, although more costly than rapid tests, urine culture remains the screening test of choice for detecting ASB in pregnancy (Rouse et al., 1995; Hooten and Stamm, 1997; Millar and Cox, 1997; Sweet and Gibbs, 2002).

TREATMENT

Detection and treatment of ASB give the obstetrician an opportunity to prevent a significant medical complication of pregnancy. Screening at the original antenatal visit, appropriate treatment, and eradication of bacteriuria lead to the prevention of antenatal acute pyelonephritis in 70% to 80% of cases. Such a reduction, with its attendant decline in risk to mother and fetus, is itself sufficient justification for such a screening program. In addition, as discussed earlier, screening and treatment of ASB may also significantly reduce the risk for preterm delivery and low-birth-weight infants.

Treatment should be designed to maintain sterile urine throughout pregnancy, utilizing the shortest possible course of antimicrobial agents in order to minimize the toxic effects of these drugs in mother and fetus. Most antibacterial agents are excreted by glomerular filtration; as a result, therapeutic concentrations are readily achieved in the urine. In fact, the concentration of these drugs in the urine greatly exceeds that required for the treatment of most UTIs. Even drugs that do not reach therapeutic concentrations in serum, such as nitrofurantoin, are present in significant concentrations in urine.

Short courses of treatment (1 to 3 weeks) with sulfonamides, ampicillin, or nitrofurantoin are as effective as continuous therapy and eliminate the bacteriuria in 70% to 90% of patients. No single agent seems better than any other. At present, it is generally accepted that short courses of treatment are preferable because (1) the duration of initial therapy does not affect the recurrence rate, (2) a short course minimizes the adverse drug effects in mother and fetus, (3) emergence of resistant bacteria is discouraged, and (4) costs are kept to a minimum.

Although a 3-day course of antibiotic therapy is recommended for the treatment of uncomplicated UTI in nonpregnant women, a 7-day course is preferred for pregnant women (Stamm and Hooten, 1993). A wide variety of antimicrobial agents have successfully been used for management of ASB in pregnancy (Table 39-1). These include β-lactam antibiotics such as ampicillin and cephalosporins, which do not pose any significant risk to the fetus. Other commonly used antibiotics include short-acting sulfonamides, nitrofurantoin, and trimethoprim-sulfamethoxazole. The quinolone group of antimicrobial agents are not approved for use during pregnancy because of concerns regarding their teratogenic effect on fetal cartilage. In addition, sulfonamides should be used with caution during pregnancy because sulfa competes with bilirubin for binding on albumin. This is a theoretical risk that has not been clearly demonstrated clinically with use of short-acting sulfonamides. Ampicillin or amoxicillin use has been questioned for treatment of UTIs because the predominant etiologic organism is *E. coli*, and resistance rates of *E. coli* to ampicillin in the United States are 30% (Stamm and Hooten, 1993). Resistance to antimicrobial agents has increased among uropathogens (Stamm and Hooten, 1993; Hooten and Stamm, 1997; Gupta et al., 1999). Of concern is the decreased susceptibility of *E. coli*, the most common uropathogen, to trimethoprim-sulfamethoxazole, ranging from 5% to 15% in different geographic areas (Stamm and Hooten, 1993; Hooten and Stamm, 1997; Gupta et al., 1999; Warren et al., 1999).

TABLE 39-1. ANTIMICROBIAL TREATMENT OF ASYMPTOMATIC BACTERIURIA AND ACUTE CYSTITIS DURING PREGNANCY

Antimicrobial Agent	Regimen
Therapeutic	
Amoxicillin*	500 mg t.i.d. for 7 d
Sulfisoxazole*	Initial 2-g dose and then 1 g q.i.d. for 7 d
Trimethoprim-sulfamethoxazole*	160/800 mg b.i.d. for 7 d
Nitrofurantoin	100 mg q.i.d. for 7 d
Cefixime	400 mg q24h for 7 d
Cefpodoxime proxetil	100 mg q12h for 7 d
Suppressive Therapy	
Nitrofurantoin	100 mg h.s.
Trimethoprim-sulfamethoxazole	160/800 mg h.s.

* Only in geographic areas with low levels of resistance to *E. coli.*

b.i.d., twice daily; h.s., at bedtime; q, every; q.i.d., four times daily; t.i.d., three times daily.

When short courses of therapy are prescribed for ASB during pregnancy, continuous surveillance for recurrent bacteriuria by repeated urine cultures is essential. Persistent ASB may necessitate continuous antimicrobial therapy for the duration of pregnancy. A single daily dose of nitrofurantoin, 100 mg, preferably after the evening meal, is recommended. Alternatively, short-acting sulfonamide preparations may be prescribed.

It is appropriate to treat patients with recurrent ASB with antimicrobial agents on the basis of the microorganism's sensitivities for the remainder of the pregnancy and for 2 weeks following delivery. The duration of therapy for UTIs remains a subject of considerable debate, but studies favor the continued use of the standard 7-day course for treatment of ASB in pregnancy.

Cystitis in Pregnancy

Acute cystitis is a distinct syndrome characterized by urinary urgency and frequency, dysuria, and suprapubic discomfort, in the absence of systemic symptoms such as fever and costovertebral angle tenderness. Gross hematuria may be present; the urine culture is invariably positive for bacterial growth, with more than 100,000 colonies/mL. Stamm and co-workers (1982) have suggested that a urine culture positive for bacterial growth with more than 100 colonies/mL, in combination with symptoms of dysuria and frequency, is sufficient to confirm the diagnosis of cystitis.

The reported incidence of acute cystitis among pregnant women ranges from 0.3% to 1.3% (Harris and Gilstrap, 1974; Stenquist et al., 1987). Harris and Gilstrap (1974) reported a recurrence rate of 1.3% for cystitis during pregnancy. Although the increase in diagnosis and treatment of ASB reduced the incidence of pyelonephritis at their institution, the incidence of acute cystitis remained constant. On initial screening urine cultures, 64% of the patients who ultimately developed cystitis had negative cultures, in contrast to the patients with ASB and acute pyelonephritis, only a minority of whom had negative cultures. The authors noted that the recurrence pattern in patients with acute cystitis was also different from that in patients with either bacteriuria or acute pyelonephritis. Disease recurred in 75% of patients with acute pyelonephritis who were not given suppressive antimicrobial therapy compared to only 17% of patients with acute cystitis.

In nonpregnant women, the diagnosis of acute uncomplicated cystitis relies on symptoms of dysuria, urgency, and frequency plus evidence of pyuria (microscopic or dipstick). In pregnancy culture, however, confirmation is suggested (Stamm and Hooten, 1993). Once cystitis is suspected in pregnancy, either a catheterized specimen or a clean-catch midstream specimen for urinalysis and culture should be obtained prior to treatment with antibiotic therapy. Because of the symptomatology of acute cystitis and the danger of upward extension of the infection to the kidney, it is not possible to await the results of culture. The constellation of symptoms and demonstration by urinalysis of white blood cells and bacteria should be sufficient grounds for beginning therapy.

Pregnant women with acute cystitis should receive immediate therapy with an antibiotic agent. The organisms most commonly isolated in acute cystitis are *E. coli*, other gram-negative facultative organisms, and GBS. The duration of therapy in cystitis is 7 days. The antimicrobial agents utilized to treat cystitis in pregnancy are similar to those for ASB and are summarized in Table 39-1.

Acute Pyelonephritis in Pregnancy

The most common serious urinary tract complication that occurs during pregnancy is acute pyelonephritis. The overall incidence is reported to be 1% to 2.5% of all obstetric patients; in addition, recurrence occurs in 10% to 18% of patients during the same pregnancy (Millar and Cox, 1997; Sweet and Gibbs, 2002). Symptoms and signs of pyelonephritis include shaking chills, fever, flank pain, nausea and vomiting, urinary frequency and urgency, dysuria, and costovertebral angle tenderness. Laboratory tests reveal pyuria and bacteriuria. The pregnant woman with pyelonephritis generally has clear-cut signs and symptoms that allow one to make the diagnosis easily; most (85%) have chills and documented fever and complain of back pain. A significant number (40%) have symptoms of lower urinary tract infection (e.g., dysuria and frequency). Fever is universal, and the diagnosis should be only tentative in its absence.

Pyelonephritis not only is a serious risk for preterm labor and delivery but also poses a serious threat to maternal well-being. The adverse effects of pyelonephritis on pregnant women are primarily the result of endotoxin-mediated tissue damage (Millar and Cox, 1997). Therefore, multiple organ system involvement is common. Fortunately, although bacteremia accompanies pyelonephritis in 10% to 15% of pregnant women, full-blown septic shock occurs infrequently (Fein and Duvivier, 1992). The traditional approach has been to hospitalize affected patients for vigorous treatment with intravenous fluids and antimicrobial agents and close monitoring of renal function. Nausea, vomiting, anorexia, and pyrexia frequently result in severe dehydration.

Cunningham and co-workers (1987) reported that acute pyelonephritis of pregnancy may be complicated by adult respiratory distress syndrome. A report by Towers and colleagues (1991) identified several risk factors for pulmonary injury in antepartum pyelonephritis: elevated maternal heart rate (in excess of 110 beats per minute); use of a tocolytic agent; use of ampicillin alone; temperature of 103°F during the first 24 hours; and fluid overload.

According to these studies, respiratory insufficiency develops in 2% to 8% of pregnant women with acute pyelonephritis. This clinical situation should be suspected in patients presenting with dyspnea, tachypnea, hypoxemia, or a chest radiograph suggestive of pulmonary edema or adult respiratory distress syndrome. Moreover, approximately 20% of affected women have transient renal dysfunction, as documented by decreased creatinine clearance (Gilstrap et al., 1981). This latter complication is especially important when the antimicrobial agent used is nephrotoxic or is eliminated by the kidney. For this reason, aminoglycosides should be used with caution.

Also associated with pyelonephritis are hematologic and hemodynamic dysfunction, manifested by thrombocytopenia and hypotension. Important management points include (1) hydration and lowering of the elevated temperature, (2) monitoring of renal function with meticulous attention to intake and output, and (3) close observation for early indications of shock that may occur in gram-negative infections. Aggressive fluid resuscitation is critical in the management of patients demonstrating evidence of sepsis. Vasopressors may be necessary if fluid resuscitation alone is not successful (see Chapter 45). Cox and Cunningham (1993) reported that up to 25% of pregnant women with severe pyelonephritis have evidence of multiorgan dysfunction.

Administration of aminoglycosides requires particular caution and is not recommended for pregnant patients with pyelonephritis unless the identified microorganism is resistant to other antimicrobials or the patient has had an allergic reaction to them. The one exception is the patient who appears septic, with possibility of septic shock. In these patients, aminoglycosides should be used to cover the more resistant organisms and provide bactericidal activity. The most common microorganisms associated with acute pyelonephritis are *E. coli*, organisms of the *Klebsiella* and *Enterobacter* groups, and *Proteus* species. Dunlow and Duff (1990) studied 121 pregnant women with pyelonephritis and noted that the most frequent pathogens were *E. coli* (80%), *K. pneumoniae* (7.4%), *Staphylococcus aureus* (6%), and *P. mirabilis* (2%). In the past, therapy with ampicillin, 1 to 2 g intravenously every 6 hours, was sufficient; however, in 30% of hospitals, even community-acquired *E. coli* may be resistant to ampicillin. In the study by Dunlow and Duff, 26% of the uropathogens were ampicillin-resistant, but only 4% were resistant to first-generation cephalosporins (e.g., cefazolin). Thus, cephalosporins have replaced ampicillin as the choice for single-agent therapy for acute pyelonephritis in pregnancy. Currently, we utilize ceftriaxone for empiric therapy of acute pyelonephritis in pregnancy (Sweet and Gibbs, 2002). This third-generation cephalosporin is active against the major uropathogens (except enterococcus) and is administered once daily, thus facilitating home parenteral therapy and lowering costs. Sanchez-Ramos and colleagues (1995), in a prospective randomized clinical trial, reported that daily single-dose intravenous ceftriaxone is as effective as multiple-dose cefazolin in the treatment of acute pyelonephritis in pregnancy.

In cases of clinical sepsis, the combination of either ampicillin or a cephalosporin with an aminoglycoside such as gentamicin is usually indicated. The dosage recommended for aminoglycosides is 3–5 mg/kg/24 hours in three divided doses. Serum levels in pregnant women receiving aminoglycosides may be monitored selectively to ensure adequate dosage and prevent toxicity. Recently, single-dose gentamicin has been effective and has reduced the rate of adverse events associated with aminoglycosides.

With intravenous antimicrobial therapy, 85% of patients become afebrile within 48 hours, and 97% within 4 days. If resolution does not occur and the fever continues, the possibilities of resistant organisms and obstructive uropathy must be considered. A change of antibiotics, on the basis of microorganism sensitivities found on urine culture, may be necessary. The appropriate antibiotics for treatment are shown in Table 39-2.

The need to hospitalize all patients with acute pyelonephritis in pregnancy has been questioned. Angel and co-workers (1990) suggested that outpatient oral antimicrobial therapy was an acceptable alternative to inpatient parenteral therapy; however, 13 (14%) of the 90 patients had bacteremia, and no clinical finding at presentation was predictive of bacteremia. If the bacteremic patients are included in the analysis, oral therapy was successful in only 71% of cases, which is unacceptable with pyelonephritis, with its associated risk for preterm labor and delivery and septic shock.

TABLE 39-2. TREATMENT OF ACUTE PYELONEPHRITIS IN PREGNANCY

Drug	Dose
Ceftriaxone	1–2 g IV q24h
Trimethoprim-sulfamethoxazole	160/800 mg IV q12h
Ampicillin	1–2 g IV q6h plus gentamicin 1 mg/kg q8h
Cefazolin	1–2 g IV q8h plus gentamicin 1 mg/kg q8h*

* Some authors use cefazolin as a single agent.
IV, intravenously.

Millar and associates (1995) similarly proposed that outpatient parenteral therapy is an acceptable alternative to hospitalization for management of selected cases of acute pyelonephritis in pregnancy. Specifically, intramuscular ceftriaxone on an ambulatory basis was as effective as intravenous cefazolin in hospitalized patients. However, this randomized controlled trial included only women at less than 24 weeks' gestation who were observed in the emergency room for up to 24 hours to verify that they were stable and able to tolerate oral fluids. Such an approach also requires close follow-up for documenting patient compliance and clinical response (Millar and Cox, 1997). More recently, others assessed the efficacy of outpatient (two 1-g intramuscular doses of ceftriaxone 24 hours apart, followed by oral cephalexin 500 mg four times daily for 10 days) compared with inpatient treatment (two 1-g intramuscular doses of ceftriaxone 24 hours apart, and then oral cephalexin until the patients had been afebrile for 48 hours, at which point they were discharged home to complete a 10-day course). There were no significant differences reported for clinical response or birth outcomes among the patients completing their protocol. However, 30% of the outpatient group did not complete their protocol. In addition, most women with acute pyelonephritis were excluded from outpatient therapy because of suspected sepsis (blood pressure less than 90/50 mm Hg, temperature above 39.8°C, or sustained tachycardia at or above 110 beats per minute), signs of adult respiratory distress syndrome, serious underlying medical conditions (e.g., diabetes, systemic lupus), renal or urologic disorders, or inability to tolerate oral intake. Because of concerns mentioned in the previously discussed investigations, pregnant women with acute pyelonephritis at any gestational age should be hospitalized, with initiation of antimicrobial therapy, aggressive rehydration, and close monitoring for maternal complications of sepsis, preterm labor, and fetal well-being. Once patients have been stabilized and remain afebrile for 24 to 48 hours, they may be discharged on oral antimicrobial therapy to complete a 10-day course of treatment.

Acute pyelonephritis is reported to recur during the same gestation in 10% to 18% of patients. In a retrospective analysis, Harris and Gilstrap (1974) reported that for patients with acute pyelonephritis who did not receive suppressive antimicrobial therapy for the remainder of gestation, the rate of recurrence was 60% and rehospitalization was required. The incidence of recurrence and rehospitalization in patients who received suppressive antimicrobial therapy for the duration of the gestation was 2.7%. Suppression is accomplished with 100 mg of nitrofurantoin each night at bedtime. Alternatively, trimethoprim-sulfamethoxazole 160/800 mg can be given at bedtime. An acceptable alternative to suppressive therapy is the continued examination every 2 weeks of urine cultures for bacteriuria, with prompt treatment if it is found. Lenke and co-workers (1983) reported that recurrent or persistent bacteriuria was more common in the group followed with sequential cultures.

Intra-amniotic Infection

Bacterial infection of the amniotic cavity is an important cause of perinatal mortality and maternal morbidity. Indeed, just in the last few years, intriguing relationships have been reported between clinical infection and long-term neurologic development in the newborn, including cerebral palsy (see Chapter 61). A number of terms for this infection have been used, including "clinical chorioamnionitis," "amnionitis," "intrapartum infection," "amniotic fluid infection," and "intra-amniotic infection" (IAI). IAI is used to distinguish this clinical syndrome from asymptomatic bacterial colonization of amniotic fluid and from histologic inflammation of the placenta. Clinically evident IAI occurs in 0.5% to 10% of pregnancies (Gibbs and Duff, 1991).

Pathogenesis

With the onset of labor or with rupture of membranes, bacteria from the lower genital tract commonly ascend into the amniotic cavity. This is the most common pathway for development of IAI. Occasional cases of IAI in the absence of membrane rupture or labor support a presumed hematogenous or transplacental route of infection. For example, fulminant IAI with intact membranes may be caused by *L. monocytogenes*. Less commonly, IAI may develop as a consequence of obstetric procedures, such as cervical cerclage, diagnostic amniocentesis, intrauterine transfusion, or percutaneous umbilical blood sampling. The absolute risk is small with all of these procedures; IAI develops in 2% to 8% of patients after cerclage, in up to 1% after amniocentesis, and in up to 5% after intrauterine transfusion. Bacteria may also reach the uterine cavity from extragenital sources such as the urinary tract or periodontal tissue.

Epidemiology

Clinical IAI is a leading risk factor for neonatal sepsis. Yancey and co-workers (1996) found this infection had the highest odds ratio ([OR], 25) by far for suspected or proved neonatal sepsis compared with other obstetric risk factors, such as preterm delivery, rupture of membranes more than 12 hours, postpartum endometritis, or maternal carriage of GBS.

Risk factors for clinical IAI itself have largely been obstetric factors found in patients with difficult labor. These factors include the following:

Low parity
Long labor
Long period of membrane rupture
Multiple vaginal examinations in labor
Internal fetal monitoring
Long duration of monitoring

In addition, maternal bacterial vaginosis (BV) has been associated with clinical IAI (Newton et al., 1989, 1997; Soper et al., 1989, 1996; Gibbs, 1993).

Microbiology

As with many other pelvic infections, IAI is often polymicrobial in origin. In a controlled study, Gibbs and colleagues (1982) collected amniotic fluid from patients with clinical IAI. The most common organisms found were *Bacteroides* species (25%), *Gardnerella vaginalis* (24%), GBS (12%), other aerobic streptococci (13%), *E. coli* (10%), and other aerobic gram-negative rods (10%).

A role for genital mycoplasmas has been suggested by case reports isolating them in amniotic fluid of clinically infected patients and by a controlled study reporting that 35% of fluid specimens from patients with IAI yielded *Mycoplasma hominis*, whereas only 8% of matched control fluids had this organism ($P < .001$) (Blanco et al., 1983). The predominant organisms in IAI (anaerobes, genital mycoplasmas, and *G. vaginalis*) are precisely the same as those found in genital secretions of women with BV. Indeed, BV has been associated with development of IAI. (See the section Bacterial Vaginosis) Present evidence suggests a small role, if any, for *Chlamydia trachomatis* in amniotic fluid infections. This organism is rarely isolated from amniotic cells in cases of IAI, and no significant antibody changes to *C. trachomatis* have been noted in sera of women with IAI. Pregnant women with cervical *C. trachomatis* infections have not been found to have higher rates of intrapartum fever (Sweet et al., 1987).

Diagnosis

The diagnosis of intra-amniotic infection requires a high index of suspicion. Usual laboratory indicators of infection, such as positive stains for organisms or leukocytes and positive cultures, are found much more frequently than in clinically evident infection. Diagnosis is usually based on maternal fever, maternal or fetal tachycardia, uterine tenderness, foul odor of the amniotic fluid, and leukocytosis. In patients with fever, two sets of blood specimens should be drawn for culture, but bacteremia occurs in only 10%. Because peripheral blood leukocytosis occurs commonly in normal labor, this result is not always indicative of infection.

Direct examination of the amniotic fluid may provide important diagnostic information. Samples can be collected by aspiration through an intrauterine pressure catheter in 50% of cases. Positive amniotic fluid Gram stains for bacteria or leukocytes occur significantly more often in women with IAI than in matched controls (Gibbs et al., 1982). In patients with suspected amnionitis, low amniotic fluid glucose levels are a good predictor of a positive amniotic fluid culture but a poorer predictor of clinical IAI. When amniotic fluid glucose is above 20 mg/dL, the likelihood of a positive culture is less than 2%. When the glucose level is below 5 mg/dL, the likelihood of a positive culture rises to approximately 90% (Kiltz et al., 1991; Romero et al., 1993).

Maternal fever is recognized as a high-risk factor for neonatal sepsis. Immediately after birth, however, making the diagnosis of neonatal septicemia is difficult. The neonate's response to infection is impaired and often nonspecific.

Management

In broad principle, investigators agree that in this situation, delivery of the fetus is necessary for treatment with antibiotics; however, specific points of management are unresolved.

Regarding the timing of delivery, in recent studies excellent maternal-neonatal outcome has been reported without use of arbitrary time limits. Cesarean delivery was performed for standard obstetric indications and not for IAI alone. The mean time from diagnosis of IAI to delivery was between 3 and 5 hours. No critical interval from diagnosis of amnionitis to delivery could be identified. Cesarean section rates are higher among patients with IAI, running two to three times greater than in the general population.

Three comparative studies have demonstrated a significant advantage of *intrapartum* over immediate *postpartum* antibiotic treatment (Table 39-3). In a nonrandomized trial, Sperling and co-workers (1987) reported a lower incidence of neonatal sepsis when antibiotic treatment was begun during delivery than when treatment was begun immediately after delivery. Gilstrap and colleagues (1988) found a nearly fourfold reduction in neonatal sepsis with use of intrapartum treatment (5.7% versus 1.5%, $P = 0.06$). In a randomized trial, Gibbs and colleagues (1988) used ampicillin (2 mg intravenously every 6 hours) plus gentamicin (1.5 mg/kg every 8 hours), initiating treatment either intrapartum or immediately postpartum. In addition, clindamycin was used after umbilical cord clamping if cesarean delivery was performed because of the high failure rate of ampicillin and gentamicin alone. Maternal outcome was improved and confirmed neonatal sepsis was decreased by intrapartum treatment. Other initial regimens employing an extended-spectrum, cephalosporin-type antibiotic (ampicillin plus a cephalosporin) or other agents with similar activity may be equally effective, but no comparative trials have been performed.

Pharmacokinetic studies in early pregnancy show that ampicillin concentrations in maternal and fetal sera are comparable 120 minutes after administration. In late pregnancy, gentamicin also crosses the placenta rapidly; however, peak fetal levels may be low, especially since maternal levels are often subtherapeutic. An initial gentamicin dose of 1.5 to 2.0 mg/kg is indicated. As an alternative, use of a newer penicillin or cephalosporin with excellent aerobic gram-

TABLE 39-3. NEONATAL SEPSIS IS DECREASED BY INTRAPARTUM ANTIBIOTIC TREATMENT IN CASES OF INTRA-AMNIOTIC INFECTION

	Neonatal Sepsis Rate		
Study	Intrapartum Treatment (%)	*p*	Neonatal Treatment (%)
Sperling et al., 1987 (*n* = 257)	2.8	.001	19.6
Gibbs et al., 1988 (*n* = 45)	0	.03	21
Gilstrap et al., 1988 (*n* = 273)	1.5	.06	5.7

negative activity might be suggested, but there is little reported experience with these antibiotics in IAI. For ampicillin and aminoglycosides, levels in amniotic fluid are usually below fetal serum levels, and peak amniotic concentrations may be attained only after 2 to 6 hours.

SHORT-TERM OUTCOME. Since 1979, reports have provided systematically collected data on the outcome for mothers and neonates in pregnancies complicated by intra-amniotic infection. These studies have generally shown a vastly improved perinatal outcome compared with that in older studies. Maternal outcome was excellent, with no deaths, few cases of septic shock, and rare pelvic abscesses. The cesarean delivery rate was increased in all studies, usually because of dystocia. Nearly all abdominal deliveries were by the transperitoneal approach. Perinatal mortality is increased in cases of IAI, but little of the excess mortality can be attributed to infection per se. Among term infants born after IAI, perinatal mortality is less than 1%.

Yoder and colleagues (1983) provided a case-controlled study of 67 patients with microbiologically confirmed IAI at term. There was only one perinatal death (unrelated to infection). Cerebrospinal fluid cultures were negative in all 49 infants sampled, and there was no clinical evidence of meningitis. Chest radiographs were interpreted as "possible" pneumonia in 20% and as unequivocal pneumonia in only 4%. Neonatal bacteremia was documented in 8%. There was no significant difference in the frequency of low Apgar scores between the IAI and control groups.

Preterm neonates born to mothers with IAI experience a higher frequency of complications than do those born to mothers without this disorder. Garite and Freeman (1982) noted that the perinatal death rate was significantly higher in 47 preterm neonates with IAI than in 204 uninfected neonates with similar birth weights. The group with IAI also included a significantly higher number with respiratory distress syndrome and infection (13% versus 3%, P < .05). Similar results were reported by Morales (1987) in a larger study.

Patients with IAI are more likely to have a cesarean delivery. Women with IAI (or with high-virulence bacteria in amniotic fluid) often have uterine dysfunction, a poorer response to oxytocin, and abnormal cervical dilatation even when uterine activity is adequate. It is likely that these abnormal labor characteristics are the reason for the higher cesarean section rate. Thus, intra-amniotic infection has a significant adverse effect on the mother and the neonate, but vigorous antibiotic therapy and reasonably prompt delivery result in an excellent prognosis in most cases, especially for the mother and the term neonate. When the combination of prematurity and amnionitis occurs, the risk of serious sequelae in the neonate is increased.

LONG-TERM OUTCOME. There is increasing evidence that exposure to intrauterine infection is associated with an increased risk of cerebral palsy or its histologic precursor (periventricular leukomalacia) and an increased risk of respiratory distress syndrome. The unifying hypothesis is that intrauterine infection leads to fetal infection and to an over-exuberant fetal production of cytokines. In turn, this leads to cell damage. The fetal response syndrome has been likened to the systemic inflammatory response syndrome in adults. Several studies have linked maternal infection with cerebral palsy in preterm and in term infants and with cystic necrosis of the white matter. Recently, intrauterine exposure to maternal

TABLE 39-4. CHORIOAMNIONITIS AS A RISK FACTOR FOR CEREBRAL PALSY: META-ANALYSIS

Preterm Infants	
Cerebral Palsy	**RR**
Clinical chorio (n = 11)	1.9 (95% CI, 1.4–2.5)
Histologic chorio (n = 5)	1.6 (95% CI, 0.9–2.7)
Cystic PVL	**RR**
Clinical chorio (n = 6)	3.0 (95% CI, 2.2–4.0)
Histologic chorio (n = 7)	2.1 (95% CI, 1.5–2.9)

Term Infants	
Cerebral Palsy	**RR**
Clinical chorio (n = 2)	4.7 (95% CI, 1.3–16.2)
Histologic chorio (n = 1)	8.9 (95% CI, 1.9–40)

Chorio, chorioamnionitis; CI, confidence interval; PVL, periventricular leukomalacia; RR, relative risk.

Data from Grether JK, Nelson KB: Maternal infection and cerebral palsy in infants of normal birth weight. JAMA **278**:207, 1997; Wu YW, Colford JM Jr: Chorioamnionitis as a risk factor for cerebral palsy: A meta-analysis. JAMA **284**:1417, 2000.

infection was also found to be associated with an increased risk of otherwise-unexplained cerebral palsy (OR, 9.3) in infants of normal birth weight (Grether and Nelson, 1997). The results of a recent meta-analysis are summarized in Table 39-4. In addition, levels of inflammatory cytokines, interleukin-1b, interleukin-6, and tumor necrosis factor in the amniotic fluid are higher in preterm infants with periventricular leukomalacia than in those without such lesions (Yoon et al., 1996). Finally, additional work in a rabbit model has shown an increase in periventricular leukomalacia, an important histologic correlate of cerebral palsy, after experimental intrauterine infection with *E. coli* (Yoon et al., 1997). These issues are also addressed in Chapter 61.

Among preterm infants, respiratory distress syndrome has been significantly associated with high levels of tumor necrosis factor in amniotic fluid, with positive cultures of amniotic fluid, and with severe histologic chorioamnionitis, even after adjustment for birth weight, infant gender, race, and mode of delivery. These observations collectively have aroused renewed interest in the long-term effects of intrauterine infection, as well as in strategies to avoid their serious complications (Hitti et al., 1997).

Prevention

Numerous approaches have been tested as preventive techniques. Chlorhexidine vaginal washes in labor (Rouse et al., 1997; Sweeten et al., 1997) and selected infection-control measures (Soper et al., 1996) have been ineffective. Antepartum treatment of BV has not been shown to decrease IAI (Carey et al., 2000). Use of broad-spectrum antibiotics in patients with preterm labor but intact membranes appears ineffective overall in decreasing IAI (Egarter, Leitich, Husslein, et al., 1996). It is unclear whether intrapartum prophylaxis to prevent GBS neonatal sepsis may possibly decrease IAI. Three strategies, however, do appear effective. These are (1) active management of labor (López-Zeno et al., 1992); (2) induction of labor (compared with expectant management), after PROM, at term (Mozurkewich and Wolf, 1997); and (3) use of antibiotics in selected patients with PROM (Mercer and Arheart, 1995; Egarter, Leitich, Kara, et al., 1996; Mercer, et al., 1997; Kenyon et al., 2001a).

Postpartum Infection

Many studies have reported the incidence of "standard puerperal morbidity," which is defined by the U.S. Joint Committee on Maternal Welfare as "a temperature of 100.4° F (38.0° C), the temperature to occur in any two of the first 10 days postpartum, exclusive of the first 24 hours, and to be taken by mouth by a standard technique at least four times daily." Yet, the full criteria of the original definition can no longer be applied because of early patient discharge practices.

Low-grade fever occurs commonly in the postpartum period and often resolves spontaneously. When fever is caused by infection, the genital tract is the most common source in most reports, but the urinary tract may also be involved. Less-common sources of bacterial infection are the breasts and lungs.

At present, the rate of postpartum infection rarely exceeds 3% after vaginal delivery, but it is five to ten times higher after cesarean section. Although the absolute risk of death from postpartum infection is extremely low, infection continues to account for 7% of maternal deaths after live birth in the United States and is the fourth leading cause of death following delivery.

Puerperal Endometritis

EPIDEMIOLOGY

Endometritis (also termed endomyometritis) occurs in association with approximately 1% to 3% of vaginal deliveries. It is much more common following cesarean delivery, affecting approximately 15% to 20% of patients having unscheduled cesarean delivery and 5% to 10% of those having a scheduled elective cesarean prior to the onset of labor. In women who do not receive prophylactic antibiotics at the time of cesarean delivery, the frequency of infection is about 50% to 60% higher. The principal risk factors for puerperal endometritis are abdominal delivery, low socioeconomic class, prolonged labor, prolonged rupture of membranes, multiple vaginal examinations, internal fetal monitoring, and preexisting infection of the lower genital tract (GBS infection, BV) (Duff, 1986).

Endometritis is a polymicrobial bacterial infection caused by multiple aerobic and anaerobic microbes. The major pathogens are aerobic gram-positive cocci such as GBS and enterococci; aerobic gram-negative bacilli such as *E. coli, Klebsiella pneumoniae,* and *Proteus* species; anaerobic gram-positive cocci; and anaerobic gram-negative bacilli such as *Bacteroides* species and *Prevotella* species. Mycoplasmas (*Mycoplasma hominis* and *Ureaplasma urealyticum*) can be isolated from the endometrium of patients with puerperal endometritis. However, these organisms typically are found in association with other, more highly virulent bacteria and, by themselves, usually do not cause a serious infection. *Chlamydia trachomatis,* although an important cause of pelvic inflammatory disease and late-onset puerperal endometritis, is not a common cause of infection immediately following delivery (Duff, 1986).

CLINICAL PRESENTATION AND DIAGNOSIS

Patients with endometritis typically develop a fever in the range of 37.5° to 39.5° C 24 to 48 hours after delivery. Other common clinical manifestations include tachycardia, tachypnea, lower abdominal pain and tenderness, and malodorous lochia.

In the initial evaluation of a patient with a postpartum fever, several major diagnoses should be considered: endometritis, atelectasis, pyelonephritis, and appendicitis. Distinction among these entities is usually possible on the basis of physical examination and a few selected laboratory tests (Duff, 1986).

Patients with postpartum fever should be evaluated with a white blood cell count, which usually is elevated in the range of 13,000 to 15,000/mm^3. A chest x-ray is indicated only if pneumonia or extensive atelectasis is suspected. Similarly, a urine culture should be obtained only if there is a clinical suspicion of acute pyelonephritis. Blood cultures are indicated only if the patient is immunocompromised, is at high risk of developing bacterial endocarditis, or fails to respond appropriately to initial antibiotic therapy. Except in these situations, routine blood cultures rarely affect clinical decision-making and simply add to patient expense.

TREATMENT

When choosing among different antibiotics for the treatment of endometritis, the issues of spectrum of activity, safety profile, and cost must be considered. Several broad-spectrum cephalosporins and penicillins have extensive activity against the multiple pelvic pathogens and can be used as single agents for treatment of endometritis. Of the cephalosporins, cefotetan (2 g intravenously every 12 hours), cefepime (2 IV g every 12 hours), and ceftizoxime (2 g intravenously every 8 to 12 hours) are probably the most cost-effective selections. Of the extended-spectrum penicillins, ticarcillin-clavulanic acid (3.1 g intravenously every 6 hours) and ampicillin-sulbactam (3 g intravenously every 6 hours) are also effective and inexpensive selections. The carbapenem antibiotics, imipenem-cilastatin and meropenem, are excellent broad-spectrum agents, but they are too expensive for use as routine therapy in patients with endometritis (Duff, 1997, 2002).

Combination chemotherapy with generic formulations of antibiotics is also a highly effective method of treatment for endometritis. The regimen of clindamycin (900 mg intravenously every 8 hours) plus gentamicin (7.5 mg/kg of ideal body weight intravenously every 24 hours) has been studied extensively and provides excellent cure rates. The alternate combination of metronidazole (500 mg intravenously every 12 hours) plus gentamicin (7.5 mg/kg intravenously every 24 hours) plus penicillin (5 million units intravenously every 6 hours) or ampicillin (2 g intravenously every 6 hours) is also an excellent, inexpensive regimen for treating puerperal endometritis (Duff, 1997).

As a general rule, patients with endometritis should be treated with parenteral antibiotics until they have been afebrile for approximately 24 hours. At this point, antibiotics can usually be discontinued. Except in unusual circumstances, extended courses of oral antibiotics following the patient's discharge from the hospital are unnecessary (Milligan et al., 1992).

With any of the antibiotic regimens outlined above, 90% to 95% of patients will defervesce within 48 to 72 hours.

Approximately 5% of patients will continue to have a fever despite initiation of antibiotic therapy. The two most common causes of persistent postpartum fever are resistant microorganism and wound infection. For patients being treated with extended-spectrum cephalosporins, the most likely resistant organisms are enterococci, some aerobic gram-negative bacilli, and some anaerobic gram-negative bacilli. For those receiving extended-spectrum penicillins, the most likely resistant pathogens are some aerobic and anaerobic gram-negative bacilli. Enterococci are the most likely resistant organisms in women receiving clindamycin plus gentamicin. The triple combination of metronidazole (or clindamycin) plus gentamicin plus penicillin (or ampicillin) should provide virtually perfect coverage against all of the common pelvic pathogens and should be used when microbial resistance is suspected (Duff, 1986, 1997).

The diagnosis of wound infection (incisional abscess or wound cellulitis) is best made by physical examination. Incisional abscesses require drainage. Cellulitis can usually be managed by adding a specific antistaphylococcal antibiotic to the treatment regimen.

Other unusual conditions that must be considered in the differential diagnosis of refractory postpartum fever are septic pelvic vein thrombophlebitis, pelvic abscess, epidural abscess, recrudescence of connective tissue disease, and drug fever. Physical examination, ultrasound, and computed tomographic scanning are the best methods for identifying a pelvic abscess. Postcesarean abscesses are typically located in the anterior or posterior cul-de-sac or in the leaves of the broad ligament. With rare exceptions, such abscesses require surgical drainage. Septic pelvic vein thrombophlebitis is best diagnosed by computed tomographic scan or magnetic resonance imaging and has traditionally been treated by a short course of intravenous heparin (7 to 10 days) combined with broad-spectrum antibiotics.

Computed tomographic scanning or magnetic resonance imaging is the most useful test for identifying an epidural abscess. Measurement of serum complement or antinuclear antibody titers is helpful in assessing patients with suspected connective tissue disorders. Detection of a peripheral blood eosinophilia is suggestive of drug fever. The diagnosis is confirmed if the patient defervesces promptly after antibiotics are discontinued.

PREVENTION OF ENDOMETRITIS: PROPHYLACTIC ANTIBIOTICS

There are no prospective randomized clinical trials demonstrating that prophylactic antibiotics are of value in preventing endometritis after vaginal delivery. However, quite the contrary is true with respect to cesarean delivery. Multiple well-designed investigations have shown that prophylactic antibiotics are highly effective in reducing the frequency of postcesarean endometritis. The antibiotics that have been tested most extensively in this clinical situation are the limited-spectrum cephalosporins such as cefazolin. As a general rule, a single intravenous dose of cefazolin (1 g), administered immediately after the infant's umbilical cord is clamped, is sufficient to provide prophylaxis. Regimens for prophylaxis begun after cord clamping are as effective as those begun preoperatively and may help avoid otherwise-unneeded "septic workups" of the neonate. For patients who have an immediate hypersensitivity reaction to β-lactam antibiotics, a single dose of clindamycin (900 mg intravenously) plus gentamicin (1.5 mg/kg intravenously) is an appropriate alternative (Duff, 1987).

Antibiotic prophylaxis is of particular value in high-risk patients having cesarean delivery after an extended period of labor and ruptured membranes. However, even in patients having a scheduled cesarean before the onset of labor or rupture of membranes, prophylaxis is a cost-effective means of reducing the rate of postcesarean endometritis. In most investigations, antibiotic prophylaxis has reduced the rate of postcesarean infection by 50% to 60%, mainly because of decreases in uterine and wound infections (Sweet and Gibbs, 2002). Patients who develop infection despite receiving prophylaxis do not appear to be at increased risk for more-complicated infections (Duff, 1987). In rare instances, death has occurred from anaphylaxis or antibiotic-associated colitis after the administration of prophylactic antibiotics.

Potent or potentially toxic antibiotics that are required for the treatment of severe infection (e.g., clindamycin, chloramphenicol, and aminoglycosides) should not be used for prophylaxis. Studies have demonstrated that first-generation cephalosporin (cefazolin) is as effective as second- or third-generation cephalosporin (cefoxitin, moxalactam). Patients with fever or other signs of infection after prophylaxis need careful evaluation, cultures to rule out resistant organisms, and appropriate therapeutic antibiotics.

Septic Pelvic Thrombophlebitis

This condition was first recognized more than 35 years ago in autopsies of patients with puerperal sepsis. More recently, it has been described as "obscure" or "enigmatic" fever persisting despite long-term therapy with multiple antibiotics. Patients characteristically appear nontoxic, having either no pain or mild, poorly localized discomfort despite wide swings in temperature. Abdominal and pelvic findings are minimal and vague. Frank septic pulmonary emboli are rare complications.

In most cases, the diagnosis has been presumptive and has been based on rapid defervescence (within 48 to 72 hours) after initiation of heparin therapy. In some cases, however, the response to heparin is clouded by the concomitant response to a change of antibiotic. In some reports, the incidence of septic pelvic thrombophlebitis has been 0% to 2% of infected patients. Before heparin therapy became popular, laparotomy with ligation of the inferior vena cava and ovarian vessels was recommended, but surgical intervention is now rarely necessary.

Blood cultures may be helpful; positive culture results have been reported in approximately 25% of cases. Organisms include aerobic and anaerobic streptococci, S. aureus, E. coli, and Bacteroides spp. A computed tomographic scan may help to detect an occult abscess or may even depict the thrombus. The required duration of anticoagulant therapy (heparin either alone or followed by Coumadin) is not entirely clear, but 10 days of full anticoagulation with heparin has been widely used. It is possible that shorter periods of anticoagulation, such as 7 days, are also adequate.

Septic Shock

A thorough discussion of septic shock is beyond the scope of this review (see Chapter 45), but a few points deserve emphasis. First, the most likely causative organism is

E. coli, although other gram-negative aerobes as well as *Clostridium* and *Bacteroides* spp. should be considered. Appropriate antibiotic coverage must therefore be directed at all likely pelvic organisms. Second, although the reported incidence of death from septic shock is about 65% in large series, many of the patients who die have underlying debilitating diseases. In obstetric patients, the overall mortality rate would appear to be much lower. Third, vigorous supportive therapy (including, in some cases, Swan-Ganz catheter measurements) is necessary until the definitive therapy can take effect. Finally, one must consider the need for surgical treatment. If conservative treatment fails to bring about a response, surgery is indicated.

Unlike shock accompanying septic abortion, septic shock with term delivery usually involves infection extending beyond the uterine cavity. Therefore, curettage may be performed first, but unless large amounts of necrotic placental tissue are unexpectedly recovered, an abdominal hysterectomy and often bilateral salpingo-oophorectomy with drainage will be the procedure of choice.

Mastitis

EPIDEMIOLOGY

Puerperal mastitis occurs in two forms: *epidemic* mastitis and *endemic* mastitis (Ripley, 1999). Epidemic mastitis has been reported in hospitalized women in association with nursery epidemics of staphylococcal infection, but this form of mastitis is relatively uncommon today. Endemic mastitis occurs sporadically among nonhospitalized women who are nursing their infants. Endemic mastitis now is the most commonly encountered form of this disease, occurring in approximately 5% of all lactating women. In women with epidemic mastitis, the most common pathogen is *Staphylococcus aureus*. In women with endemic mastitis, *S. aureus* still is the most common pathogen, but other organisms include group A and group B streptococci, *Hemophilus influenzae,* and *Hemophilus parainfluenzae* (Niebyl et al., 1978; Ripley, 1999).

CLINICAL PRESENTATION

Endemic mastitis may occur at any time beyond the 2nd to 3rd week postpartum. The most common clinical manifestations are malaise, chills, fever (38° to 40° C), and localized

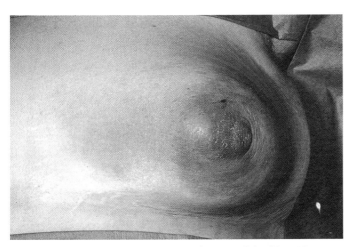

FIGURE 39-1 ■ Acute mastitis. See also Color Plate 17.

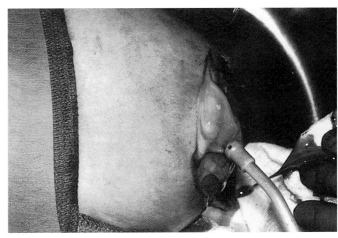

FIGURE 39-2 ■ Breast abscess complicating acute mastitis. See also Color Plate 17.

pain, erythema, and tenderness in the affected breast (Fig. 39-1; Color Plate 17). Many patients indicate that they feel as if they were "developing the flu" but then subsequently note localized changes in the breast. If a patient fails to seek prompt treatment for this condition, an actual breast abscess can develop (Fig. 39-2; Color Plate 17). A breast abscess, in turn, may be associated with bacteremia and even septic shock (Ripley, 1999).

DIAGNOSIS

The diagnosis of mastitis is best established by physical examination. In problematic cases, milk can be expressed from the affected breast and evaluated for white blood cell concentration and the presence of microorganisms. In women with mastitis, the leukocyte count in breast milk usually exceeds 10^6/mL, and bacterial counts exceed 10^3 colonies/mL. In patients with a breast abscess, purulent fluid may be aspirated for Gram stain and culture.

TREATMENT

Patients with mastitis usually can be treated successfully with oral antibiotics. Because *S. aureus,* the most common pathogen, is likely to be resistant to penicillin and ampicillin, patients should be treated with a specific antistaphylococcal antibiotic. Appropriate choices include sodium dicloxacillin, 500 mg every 6 hours, or cephalexin, 500 mg every 6 hours. These antibiotics have a similar safety profile and dosing interval, and both are relatively inexpensive. Antibiotics should be continued for approximately 7 to 10 days, depending upon the patient's clinical response (Duff, 2002).

Patients who have an actual breast abscess should be hospitalized for treatment with intravenous antistaphylococcal antibiotics. In addition, they require surgical incision and drainage to effect a cure. Blood cultures should be obtained in severely ill patients who are immunocompromised or who are at particular risk for bacterial endocarditis. In these select individuals, extended courses of antibiotics may be necessary to prevent serious sequelae related to the primary staphylococcal infection (Ripley, 1999; Duff, 2002).

In addition to antibiotic therapy, adjunctive measures such as ice packs, breast support, and analgesics may be helpful. With rare exceptions, the mother with mastitis may continue to nurse from both breasts. In fact, regular drainage of the infected breast is helpful in preventing milk stasis and possible abscess formation.

Wound Infection after Cesarean Section

Abdominal wound infection following cesarean section is a frequent occurrence, complicating up to 5% of primary cesarean sections. Prospective studies have suggested an increased incidence of wound infection if membranes have been ruptured for longer than 6 hours before delivery.

The two major factors that determine whether a wound will become infected are the dose of bacterial contamination and the resistance of the patient. Bacterial contamination is either endogenous (from the patient's own microbial flora) or exogenous (from the environment). The influence of endogenous contamination is readily documented by the progressive increase of the infection rate from 1% to 2% in clean wounds, to 10% in clean-contaminated wounds, to 20% in contaminated wounds, to 30% in dirty wounds (National Academy of Sciences, 1964; Cruse and Ford, 1973).

In general, the source of endogenous bacteria in post–cesarean section abdominal wound infections is the flora of the vagina and cervix. With labor, rupture of membranes, and delivery, the microorganisms from the lower genital tract gain access to the amniotic fluid. At the time of cesarean section, the uterine and abdominal wounds are exposed to the amniotic fluid containing these organisms. The most prevalent bacteria present in infected wounds after cesarean delivery are *Ureaplasma* spp., coagulase-negative staphylococci, enterococci, *Mycoplasma* spp., anaerobes, aerobic gram-negative rods, *S. aureus,* and GBS (Roberts et al., 1993). Clostridial organisms have also been noted as part of the normal lower genital tract flora. Because the normal flora is composed of aerobic and anaerobic bacteria, endogenous infections are often of the mixed aerobic and anaerobic, or polymicrobic, type. A relatively large number of bacteria are required to produce an infection, 10^5 bacteria per milliliter or gram being the crucial inoculum. The presence of a foreign body, such as suture material, reduces the required inoculum by a factor of 10,000.

Exogenous contamination is the key factor in the clean wound infection rate. Surveillance studies have identified factors that adversely affect this rate, including the following:

Razor-shaving the operative site
Use of the electrosurgical knife
Use of Penrose drains (especially if brought out through the skin incision)
Prolonged preoperative hospitalization
Nighttime or emergency surgery—for example, for fetal distress (three- to fourfold rate increase)
Increasing duration of the surgical procedure

In modern operating rooms, exogenous contamination is less important than the endogenous source of organisms from the patient's vagina or cervix. If general host resistance or local resistance is reduced, however, a smaller inoculum of bacteria can gain a foothold and exogenous contamination may become a significant cause of wound infection.

The patient's general resistance is an important detriment to infection. Increases in wound infection rate are associated with advancing age, diabetes, malnutrition, obesity, corticosteroid therapy, and immunosuppressed states. The condition of the wound is important in determining local resistance and

is, to a large extent, a reflection of surgical technique. Gentle tissue handling, complete hemostasis, debridement of devitalized tissue, adequate blood supply, obliteration of dead space, and closing of the wound without tension are commonly recognized principles of good surgical technique. The presence of hematomas or foreign bodies in the wound predisposes to the development of infection. Hemoglobin interferes with leukocyte migration and phagocytosis. An inadequate blood supply leads to a lower oxygen tension and acidosis in the wound, with a resultant inability of macrophages to kill bacteria.

EARLY-ONSET WOUND INFECTION

Early-onset wound infection occurs within the first 48 hours after operation. The first signs are elevated temperature and an alteration in appearance of the abdominal wall or the wound; this alteration may be a spreading cellulitis or discoloration of the skin in association with an advancing margin of active infection. Early wound infection is usually caused by a single bacterial pathogen, most commonly group A β-hemolytic streptococci or *Clostridium perfringens.* GBS may also be the cause of early-onset wound infection. A Gram stain of material aspirated from the active margin of infection is diagnostic. Gram-positive rods are strongly suggestive of clostridia, and gram-positive cocci indicate the probable presence of group A β-hemolytic streptococci. Infection resulting from group A streptococci should be suspected if a diffuse cellulitis or systemic illness, or both, develops. In clostridial infection, cellulitis of the skin and subcutaneous tissue is associated with a watery discharge. This is followed by the characteristic bronze appearance of the skin and crepitation in the vicinity of the wound.

Treatment of early wound infection consists of antibiotic therapy and excision of necrotic tissue. Penicillin is the antibiotic of choice for both clostridia and group A streptococci; alternatives include ampicillin, cephalosporins, cefoxitin, erythromycin, and chloramphenicol. Extensive debridement and excision of necrotic tissue may be required. It is crucial that all nonviable tissue be removed. Failure to treat an early-onset wound infection aggressively exposes the patient to the risk of necrotizing fasciitis, bacteremia, and disseminated intravascular coagulation.

A rare but potentially lethal condition is *toxic shock syndrome* associated with *S. aureus* wound infection. Patients with this condition have the classic findings of TSS:

1. Hypotension or syncope
2. Erythematous rash
3. Vomiting and/or diarrhea
4. Involvement of at least three major organ systems

Management of toxic shock syndrome requires early diagnosis, massive volume replacement, use of necessary life support systems, and antistaphylococcal antibiotic therapy.

LATE-ONSET WOUND INFECTION

Late-onset wound infections occur at about 4 to 8 days postoperatively. They manifest as fever and a swollen, erythematous, draining wound. Following a clean operation, such as an elective subsequent cesarean section with intact membranes and no labor, *S. aureus* is often the pathogen. In clean-contaminated cases in which membranes have been ruptured and labor has occurred, the pathogens are the endogenous bacteria from the vagina and cervix (i.e., mixed aerobes and anaerobes), and multiple bacteria are the rule.

The diagnosis is made clinically with the presence of purulent drainage. The basic treatment for late-onset wound infection is incision and drainage. Antibiotics are not generally required unless there is extensive coexistent cellulitis. Once the wound has been opened and drained and nonviable tissue has been excised, the patient should rapidly become afebrile, usually within 12 hours. If response does not occur within this time, broad-spectrum antibiotic therapy aimed at mixed aerobic and anaerobic bacteria should be instituted, and the possibility of a more extensive infection process, such as *necrotizing fasciitis*, must be considered. The diagnosis of this latter serious complication is based on the presence of edema and necrosis with partial liquefaction of the fascia adjacent to the wound site and the presence of thrombosed microvasculature in the tissue. Necrotizing fasciitis is a polymicrobic infection; its bacterial isolates include such anaerobes as peptostreptococci, peptococci, and *Bacteroides fragilis*, as well as such facultative bacteria as *E. coli, Klebsiella* sp., *Proteus* sp., and *S. aureus*.

Although necrotizing fasciitis is a rare clinical entity after cesarean section, the necessity for early recognition, extensive surgical debridement, aerobic and anaerobic cultures, and antimicrobial therapy is well documented. Clinical signs and symptoms suggesting this diagnosis are deep pain, toxicity and shock, edema that is unilateral or crosses tissue planes, and black or bluish bullae. Treatment must be aggressive and must include prompt, extensive debridement and administration of appropriate antibiotics, as indicated by the Gram stain and cultures, in high dosage as adjunctive therapy. In view of the mixed (aerobic-anaerobic) nature of these infections, appropriate antimicrobial regimens include (1) clindamycin with aminoglycoside, (2) metronidazole with aminoglycoside, (3) cefoxitin, and (4) one of the third-generation cephalo-sporins, such as imipenem, or (5) one of the extended-action penicillins such as piperacillin or mezlocillin.

Episiotomy and Other Pelvic Infections

Although episiotomy with repair of perineal lacerations is performed commonly, infection is an infrequent complication of this operation. Shy and Eschenbach (1979) have classified episiotomy infections according to the extent of the structures involved (Fig. 39-3).

SIMPLE EPISIOTOMY INFECTION

A localized infection may involve only the skin and subcutaneous tissue (including Camper fascia of the perineum) adjacent to the episiotomy. Signs are local edema and erythema with exudate; more-extensive findings should raise the suspicion of a deeper infection. Treatment consists of opening, exploration, and debridement of the perineal wound. Drainage alone is usually adequate, but appropriate antibiotics would be indicated if there is marked superficial cellulitis or isolation of group A streptococci. The episiotomy incision should not be resutured at this time. Most wounds heal by granulation. Wounds involving the sphincter muscle or rectal mucosa may be repaired when the field is free of infection.

More recently, there has been considerable interest directed at early repair of an episiotomy dehiscence. This involves prompt and meticulous debridement at the time of diagnosis, followed by antibiotics and frequent cleansing. When the tissue appears healthy (usually about 1 week or more), a bowel prep is given (for fourth-degree lacerations) and a definitive repair is done. This has been a viable option and is preferable to the 2 to 3 months patients have had to wait for repair by

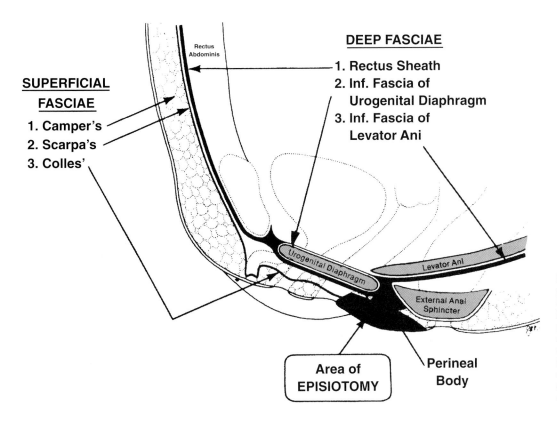

SUPERFICIAL FASCIAE
1. Camper's
2. Scarpa's
3. Colles'

Rectus Abdominis

DEEP FASCIAE
1. Rectus Sheath
2. Inf. Fascia of Urogenital Diaphragm
3. Inf. Fascia of Levator Ani

Urogenital Diaphragm

Levator Ani

External Anal Sphincter

Area of EPISIOTOMY

Perineal Body

FIGURE 39-3 ■ Paramedian sagittal section of the fascial layers of the perineum. (From Shy KK, Eschenbach DA: Fatal perineal cellulitis from an episiotomy site. Obstet Gynecol **54**:292, 1979. Reprinted with permission of the American College of Obstetricians and Gynecologists.)

traditional teaching (Hauth et al., 1986; Hankins et al., 1990; Ramin et al., 1992; Ramin and Gilstrap, 1994).

NECROTIZING FASCIITIS

Both layers of the superficial perineal fasciae (i.e., Camper and Colles fasciae) become necrotic, and infection spreads along the fascial planes to the abdominal wall, thigh, or buttock. Typically, the deep perineal fascia (i.e., inferior fascia of the urogenital diaphragm) is not involved. Skin findings are variable but initially include edema and erythema without clear borders. Later, there is progressive, brawny edema of the skin. The skin becomes blue or brown, and bullae or frank gangrene may occur. As the infection progresses, there may be loss of sensation or hyperesthesia.

Associated findings include marked hemoconcentrations, although often after fluid replacement the patient is anemic. Hypocalcemia may also develop owing to saponification of fatty acids. Traditionally, this infection has been associated with group A streptococci, but anaerobic bacteria also play an important role.

For therapy to be effective, appropriate antibiotics must be combined with adequate debridement. Indications for surgical exploration may include the following:

Extension beyond the labia
Unilateral or markedly asymmetric edema
Signs of systemic toxicity or deterioration
Failure of the infection to resolve within 24 to 48 hours

At surgery, necrotizing fasciitis may be recognized by separation of the skin from the deep fascia, absence of bleeding along incision lines, and a serosanguineous discharge. Dissection must be wide enough to remove all necrotic tissue.

MYONECROSIS

Myonecrosis is an infection that involves the muscle beneath the deep fascia. It is often the result of a mycotoxin elaborated by *C. perfringens,* but it may occasionally result from an extension of necrotizing fasciitis. Onset may be early and is typically accompanied by severe pain. Treatment of this form is also extensive debridement and high-dose antibiotics, including penicillin when clostridia are suspected.

Not all puerperal vulvar edema signifies serious perineal infection. Indeed, in most cases, vulvar edema results from less serious causes, such as hematoma, prolonged bearing down in labor, generalized edema from toxemia, allergic reactions, or trauma without serious infection. In these instances, however, the edema is usually bilateral, does not extend to the buttock and abdominal wall, and is not accompanied by signs of systemic toxicity.

Group B Streptococcal Infection

The hemolytic streptococci cause a variety of infectious syndromes and are significant causes of perinatal morbidity and mortality. In 1933, Lancefield used serologic techniques to subdivide β-hemolytic streptococci into specific groups, designated A, B, C, D, and E. Only groups A, B, and D are commonly involved in human disease.

Group A β-hemolytic streptococcus (*Streptococcus pyogenes*) has long been recognized as a major pathogen in perinatal sepsis (Gardner et al., 1979). Several case series have documented fulminant puerperal infection, with multisystem dysfunction, resulting from group A streptococci (Silver et al., 1992).

The group B streptococci (*Streptococcus agalactiae*) are serologically classified into five major serotypes on the basis of antigenic structure. They were virtually ignored as human pathogens until 1964, when their role in perinatal infections first became apparent. Today, GBS are among leading organisms in perinatal sepsis and have become the focus of national prevention strategies. In 1995, in surveillance areas set up by the CDC, the rate of perinatal sepsis was 1.3 per 1000 liveborns (CDC, 1997), accounting for an estimated 7000 to 8000 cases per year in the United States (ACOG, 1997). Outcome has improved dramatically in recent years, but morbidity is still substantial, particularly in preterm infants. One data set showed an overall case fatality rate of 4%, 2% in term infants but 16% in preterm infants.

GBS have been reported to cause 1% to 5% of UTIs in pregnancy. In addition, a characteristic early onset of puerperal endomyometritis has been associated with these organisms.

EPIDEMIOLOGY

Asymptomatic rectovaginal colonization with GBS occurs in approximately 20% of pregnant women. The choice of culture medium is a crucial determinant of the prevalence of GBS. The highest yield occurs when a selective medium, such as Todd-Hewitt broth with sheep blood, nalidixic acid, and gentamicin, is used. When selective media are not used, genital tract yield for GBS is significantly reduced.

The risk of a newborn being colonized with GBS increases if the mother is colonized. The transmission rate from mother to baby at birth approximates 75% (Silver et al., 1990). Also, 16% to 45% of nursery personnel are carriers of GBS infection, and nosocomial acquisition in newborns is common. There is an association between heavy growth of GBS in the maternal genital tract and the development of GBS sepsis in neonates. Yet, a large number of neonates with GBS sepsis (perhaps 25%) are born to women with light colonization. Thus, focusing solely on heavily colonized women in preventive approaches is inadequate.

The documented colonization rate for GBS has been far higher than the attack rate in terms of neonatal infection. Overall, sepsis develops in only 1% of infants of colonized mothers. The following are risk factors for GBS neonatal sepsis (CDC, 1996):

- Prematurity (or low birth weight as its surrogate)
- Maternal intrapartum fever (membrane rupture for longer than 12 to 18 hours)
- A previous infant infected with GBS disease
- GBS bacteriuria in this pregnancy

Because of the preponderance of term infants overall, 79% of cases in the United States occur in infants born after 36 weeks' gestation (CDC, 1997). Approximately 77% of cases are early in onset, with 23% late. The most common diagnosis with early-onset disease is bacteremia (89%), with meningitis but not bacteremia in 10%, and both bacteremia and meningitis in 1% (CDC, 1997).

CLINICAL MANIFESTATIONS IN THE NEONATE

Two clinically distinct neonatal GBS infections have been identified (Baker, 1977): early- and late-onset disease.

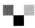

TABLE 39-5. EARLY-ONSET GBS DISEASE, BY GESTATIONAL AGE, 1993–1998

Gestational Age (Wk)	% of Cases	Case Fatality Rate (%)
≤33	9	30
34–36	8	10
≥37	83	2

Data from Schrag SJ, Zywicki S, Farley MM, et al: Group β streptocrocol disease in the era of intrapartum antibiotic prophylaxis. *N Engl J Med* **342**:15, 2000.

EARLY-ONSET INFECTION. Early-onset infection appears within the 1st week of life, usually within 48 hours. It is characterized by rapid clinical deterioration and a high mortality rate. Gestational age of cases of early-onset GBS infection is shown in Table 39-5. In the most fulminant form, early-onset GBS infection manifests as septic shock accompanied by respiratory distress, leading to death within several hours despite appropriate antibiotic therapy. In less severe disease, the clinical findings are similar to those seen in respiratory distress syndrome. Although pulmonary disease predominates in early-onset disease, meningitis may be present in 10% to 30% of cases. Overall, the case fatality rate for early-onset disease is now at 4.5% (CDC, 1997). Current nationwide prevention strategies have decreased the number of cases of early-onset GBS sepsis by an estimated 3900 per year and the number of deaths by 200 per year (Schrag et al., 2000).

LATE-ONSET INFECTION. Late-onset infection with GBS occurs more insidiously, usually after the 1st week of life. In the majority of infants, meningitis is the predominant clinical manifestation. Although the mortality rate in late-onset GBS infection is lower (2%) than with early-onset, up to 50% of babies with meningitis subsequently demonstrate neurologic sequelae. Late-onset disease may result in localized infections involving middle ears, sinuses, conjunctiva, breasts, lungs, bones, joints, or skin. Meningitis appears to be related to the serotype of GBS. More than 80% of early-onset GBS infections with meningitis present are due to type-III organisms, and in late-onset disease, 95% of meningitis is attributable to this subtype.

Although early-onset disease is acquired mainly via transmission from the mother's genital tract either prior to or during parturition, such a route of transmission is less common in late-onset disease. Nosocomial transmission of GBS can occur in the nursery from colonized nursing staff or from other infants. Current prevention strategies have not decreased the number of cases of late-onset GBS disease in newborns (Schrag et al., 2000).

CLINICAL MANIFESTATIONS IN THE MOTHER

GBS are a major cause of puerperal infection. Features of GBS puerperal infection are the development of a high fever within 12 hours of delivery, tachycardia, abdominal distention, and endomyometritis or endomyoparametritis. Some patients have no localizing signs early in the course of the infection.

DIAGNOSIS

The diagnosis of maternal asymptomatic genitourinary or gastrointestinal colonization with GBS can be confirmed only by culture, preferably with a selective medium. The symptoms of maternal genitourinary tract infection may include fever, chills, uterine tenderness, dysuria, urgency, and pyuria. Because none of these is specific for GBS, the diagnosis must be confirmed by isolation of the organism from culture.

Several rapid diagnostic tests are available for detection of GBS from maternal sources, but most methods suffer from insufficient sensitivity. Deoxyribonucleic acid (DNA) probes appear more sensitive but are not rapidly available in a clinical setting (Yancey et al., 1992).

Most colonized neonates are asymptomatic. None of the clinical manifestations of neonatal infection is sufficient for diagnosis in the absence of a positive culture. The diagnosis should be suspected when the clinical manifestations occur in association with a Gram stain of amniotic fluid or gastric aspirate that reveals a predominance of gram-positive cocci.

TREATMENT

Penicillin G remains the drug of choice for symptomatic GBS infection in mother or neonate if the infecting organism has been identified. The combination of penicillin with an aminoglycoside may eradicate the GBS faster. In most instances, however, treatment must be initiated prior to the availability of culture results. In these instances, a broad-spectrum approach for empirically treating the mother with chorioamnionitis or puerperal sepsis and the neonate with sepsis is required. Ampicillin is frequently used in such situations and provides adequate treatment for GBS infection. Alternative drugs for use in patients with a contraindication to penicillin are a cephalosporin in patients not at risk for immediate penicillin hypersensitivity or vancomycin in patients at risk (such as those with immediate urticaria or bronchospasm as manifestations of penicillin allergy). Because of rising resistance, clindamycin and erythromycin can no longer be relied upon to treat GBS infection unless susceptibility to these antibiotics has previously been demonstrated for a given isolate.

PREVENTION

Because of the severity of early-onset and late-onset GBS neonatal infection, major efforts have been directed to prophylactic administration of antibiotics to gravid women whose genital tracts are colonized with GBS. Strategies can be classified as antepartum, intrapartum, neonatal, and immunologic.

ANTEPARTUM STRATEGIES. Antepartum strategies to reduce maternal carrier rates have generally been unsuccessful owing to recolonization and are therefore not recommended.

INTRAPARTUM STRATEGIES. Intrapartum strategies have been the most attractive to date from both clinical and cost-effectiveness perspectives.

To standardize a national approach, in 1996 the CDC first published recommendations that were endorsed by the American College of Obstetricians and Gynecologists. These recommendations have been widely disseminated and have resulted in dramatic decreases in cases of early-onset neonatal GBS sepsis (Schrag et al., 2000). In 2002, these guidelines were revised, based upon several studies including a large case-control series (Schrag et al., 2002). The main changes in the 2002 Guidelines are the recommendation of the screen-based approach only, a change in recommended alternative antibiotics for penicillin-allergic patients, and provision of more-specific recommendations for selected clinical scenarios. These guidelines are summarized here (see Fig. 39-4):

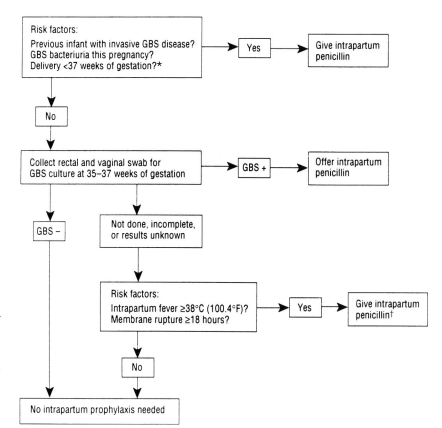

FIGURE 39-4 ■ Algorithm for prevention of early-onset group B streptococcal (GBS) disease in neonates, with prenatal screening at 35 to 37 weeks.
* If membranes rupture before 37 weeks' gestation and the mother has not begun labor, collect GBS culture and either (a) administer antibiotics until cultures are completed and the results are negative, or (b) begin antibiotics only when positive cultures are available.
† Broader-spectrum antibiotics may be considered at the physician's discretion, based on clinical indications.

(From Centers for Disease Control and Prevention [CDC]: Prevention of perinatal group B streptococcal disease: A public health perspective. MMWR Morb Mortal Wkly Rep **45**[RR-7]:1, 1996.)

1. All pregnant women should be screened at 35 to 37 weeks' gestation for vaginorectal GBS colonization. Intrapartum chemoprophylaxis (IPC) should be given at the time of labor or rupture of membranes to those identified as GBS carriers. GBS colonization in a previous pregnancy does not obviate need for screening in subsequent pregnancies; colonization in a previous pregnancy is not an indication for IPC in subsequent deliveries.
2. GBS bacteriuria: Give IPC to women with GBS in urine in any concentration.
   a. Prenatal screening at 35 to 37 weeks is not necessary in these patients.
   b. Treat bacteriuria by usual standards of care.
3. Women with previous birth of infant with GBS disease should receive IPC; prenatal screening is not necessary for these women.
4. If the result of the GBS culture is not known at the time of labor, give IPC under any of the three following circumstances:
   a. Less than 37 weeks' gestation
   b. Rupture of membranes at least 18 hours earlier
   c. Temperature at or above 100.4° F (38.0° C)
5. Onset of labor or rupture of membranes earlier than 37 weeks with "significant risk for imminent preterm delivery":
   a. If the patient is positive for GBS in this pregnancy, give penicillin for 48 hours or longer IPC at delivery.
   b. If the patient is negative for GBS in this pregnancy, IPC is not indicated.
   c. If there is no GBS culture at admission, culture and initiate penicillin IV; if the culture is negative, stop penicillin.

6. Specimens
   Collection
   a. Collect specimen from distal vagina and anorectum.
   b. It may be collected by patient or provider.
   c. Do not use a speculum.
   d. Transport medium is acceptable.
   e. Label the specimen "GBS culture."
   Laboratory processing
   f. Inoculate into selective broth medium (e.g., LIM or Trans-Vag)
   g. Methods have been provided for susceptibility to clindamycin/erythromycin for GBS from penicillin-allergic women.
   h. Labs "should report results to site of delivery and provider."
7. Inform patients of results and recommended intervention.
   a. In the absence of GBS bacteriuria, do not treat GBS genital colonization before the intrapartum period.
8. For cesarean delivery before rupture of membranes and before labor, GBS IPC is not indicated.
9. Penicillin G is the drug of choice.
   a. The recommended dose for penicillin G is 5 million units initially, then 2.5 million units every 4 hours intravenously until delivery.
   b. Ampicillin remains an alternative.
   c. When ampicillin is used, the dose is 2 g intravenously initially, followed by 1 g every 4 hours until delivery.
   d. For penicillin allergy, clindamycin/erythromycin are no longer the drugs of choice, unless susceptibility has been documented.
10. Patients with penicillin allergy:

a. If not at high risk for anaphylaxis, the dose is cefazolin, 2 g intravenously, then 1 g every 8 hours until delivery.
b. If at high risk for anaphylaxis:
   i. GBS susceptible: The dose is clindamycin, 900 mg intravenously every 8 hours *or* erythromycin, 500 mg intravenously 6 hours.
   ii. GBS resistant to clindamycin and erythromycin or of unknown susceptibility: The dose is vancomycin, 1 g every 12 hours.
11. Routine use of prophylaxis for newborns whose mothers received IPC is not recommended.
    a. Use for infants suspected clinically of having sepsis.
12. Other items:
    a. Consider establishing surveillance.
    b. Improve laboratory protocols for isolation and reporting.
    c. Ensure communication.
    d. Educate staff.

NEONATAL STRATEGIES. Measures to prevent GBS infection in the newborn have focused on the reports of decreases in neonatal early-onset disease when penicillin is given at birth. Although initial reports were encouraging, most trials in low-birth-weight infants have not found this approach to be effective. These results are not surprising in view of Boyer and Gotoff's observation (1986) that up to 40% of neonates in whom GBS sepsis has developed are already bacteremic at birth, suggesting that this approach of single-dose penicillin may be "too little and too late."

IMMUNOLOGIC STRATEGIES. The immunologic approach is appealing, but a vaccine has not yet been developed. Such a vaccine would need to be polyvalent to cover all serotypes involved in early-onset sepsis. One limitation of this approach is that it would not be optimally protective for infants born before 32 weeks of gestation, because of modest placental transfer of maternal antibody before that time. Thus, the most vulnerable infants would be left with minimal protection. Nevertheless, it is estimated that a vaccine approach would prevent up to 90% of cases of neonatal GBS infection (Coleman et al., 1992).

SUMMARY. No current approach is foolproof. It is estimated that with full application of these approaches, approximately 70% to 85% of cases would be prevented (CDC, 1996).

Listeriosis

Listeriosis is an infection caused by *L. monocytogenes*, a motile non–spore-forming, gram-positive rod. Although seven species of *Listeria* are recognized, *L. monocytogenes* is the principal human pathogen. Patients who are immunocompromised and pregnant women and their newborns are particularly susceptible to infection with *L. monocytogenes*. Of concern to the obstetrician is the association between maternal listerial infection, and stillbirths, preterm labor, and fetal infection. High perinatal morbidity and mortality rates have been reported for listerial infection in pregnancy (Ahlfors et al., 1977; Gellin and Broome, 1989; McLauchlin, 1990; Cherubin et al., 1991; Bortolussi and Schlech, 2001).

As is the case with GBS infection, neonatal listeriosis has been divided into two serologically and clinically distinct types: *Early-onset* disease associated with serotypes Ia and IVb takes the form of a diffuse sepsis with multi-organ involvement, including the lungs, liver, and central nervous system (CNS). Early-onset listeriosis is associated with a high stillbirth rate and a high neonatal mortality rate. It appears to occur more frequently in low-birth-weight infants. *Late-onset* listeriosis presents as meningitis, usually in term infants born to mothers with uneventful perinatal courses. Neurologic sequelae, such as hydrocephaly and mental retardation, are common with late-onset disease. In addition, a mortality rate approaching 40% is reported.

Charles (1990) proposed that an ascending route of infection from cervical colonization with *L. monocytogenes* (even across intact membranes) plays a role in the pathogenesis of neonatal infection. However, the more important and common route of infection arises from maternal infection, which spreads to placental infection and then to fetal septicemia and multi-organ involvement in the fetus.

Human listeriosis presents in both epidemic and sporadic forms. The *epidemic* form is associated with contamination of food and food products. Several major outbreaks of listeriosis have occurred over the last 2 decades, clearly demonstrating the role of food-borne transmission in epidemic listeriosis (Schlech et al., 1983; Fleming et al., 1985; Bula et al., 1988; Linnan et al., 1988). In a Nova Scotia outbreak, 34 perinatal cases and 7 adult nonpregnant cases occurred, with a case fatality rate for liveborn infants of 27%; in addition there were 19 intrauterine deaths (Schech et al., 1983). Although illness in a Massachusetts epidemic occurred predominantly in immunocompromised adults, the case fatality rate among infants with perinatal listeriosis was 29% (Fleming et al., 1985). In Los Angeles, from January 1 to August 15, 1985, 142 cases of human listeriosis were reported in association with ingestion of cheese contaminated by *L. monocytogenes* (Linnan et al., 1988). Two thirds of the infections occurred in pregnant women or their offspring, and 30 of the 48 deaths in this epidemic occurred in fetuses or neonates. In Switzerland 122 cases occurred during an epidemic in 1988 (Bula et al., 1988). Of these, 64 (53%) were perinatal, with a case fatality rate of 28%. In a report from Finland, a mortality rate of 30% was noted in the neonates infected with *L. monocytogenes*. Among the six pregnant women with listerial infection, five had fetal complications: three spontaneous abortions and two preterm deliveries (Skogberg et al., 1992). Interestingly, all healthy nonimmunocompromised nonpregnant patients survived the infection. Cherubin and colleagues (1991) reviewed more than 120 cases of listeriosis. They identified pregnancy and neonatal status as two of the major risk factors for listeriosis. Indeed, the mortality associated with listeriosis occurred predominantly among premature and stillborn infants delivered to infected pregnant women. Moreover, the earlier the stage of gestation when infection presented, the higher the risk of fetal death. These studies demonstrate that listerial infection tends to adversely affect immunocompromised adults and fetuses or neonates with immature immune systems.

The *sporadic* form of listeriosis occurs more commonly than the epidemic form. The CDC estimates that in 1986 1700 cases of listeriosis occurred in the United States, for an annual incidence of 7.1 cases per million population (Gellin and Broome, 1989). The attack rate was 12.4 cases per 100,000 live births in perinatal cases compared to 5.4 cases per million in nonpregnant adults.

Many pregnant women with listeriosis remain asymptomatic. When symptomatic, they present with a flu-like syndrome characterized by fever, chills, malaise, myalgia, back pain, and upper respiratory complaints. Such symptoms occur in two thirds of cases (Boucher and Yonekura, 1986). This prodrome characterizes the bacteremic stage of listeriosis, and Gellin and Broome (1989) suggest that it is probably the time when the placenta and fetus are seeded with *L. monocytogenes*. Maternal infection tends to be mild and is not associated with significant morbidity. On occasion, diffuse sepsis may occur. Unfortunately, no specific clinical manifestations have been demonstrated that help to distinguish listeriosis from other infections that may occur during pregnancy. Thus, pregnant women presenting with these symptoms in the late second or early third trimester should be evaluated for possible listeriosis.

Early-onset neonatal listeriosis occurs in infants infected in utero, often prior to the start of labor. Early-onset disease manifests itself during the first few hours to few days of life. Late-onset neonatal listeriosis occurs in term infants who appear healthy at birth and manifest infection several days to several weeks after delivery (Gellin and Broome, 1989). Meningitis is more common than sepsis with late-onset disease. Either intrapartum transmission or nosocomial transmission following delivery may occur (Gellin and Broome, 1989).

Because of the high mortality rate associated with both early- and late-onset neonatal listerial infection, it is crucial that the obstetrician maintain a high index of suspicion that any febrile illness in pregnancy may be due to *L. monocytogenes*. In such patients, cervical and blood cultures should be obtained for *L. monocytogenes* as soon as possible. Because colonies of *L. monocytogenes* may be mistaken on the Gram stain for diphtheroids and thus ignored, it is important to inform the microbiologist that listerial infection is a concern. In febrile pregnant women, a Gram stain revealing gram-positive pleomorphic rods with rounded ends is highly suggestive of, and should be presumed to be, *L. monocytogenes*.

Penicillin G and ampicillin are effective *in vivo* against *L. monocytogenes*. Current opinion holds that optimum therapy includes a combination of ampicillin plus an aminoglycoside. Maternal treatment consists of ampicillin (1 to 2 g intravenously every 4 to 6 hours) and gentamicin (2 mg/kg intravenously every 8 hours). For the newborn, the ampicillin dosage is 200 mg/kg/day in four to six divided doses. The duration of treatment is generally 1 week. A single case report has suggested that following documentation by amniocentesis of intrauterine listerial infection, antibiotic treatment without immediate delivery may be successful and result in a normal healthy fetus (Kalstone, 1991). An earlier study (Katz and Weinstein, 1982) also suggested that rapid diagnosis and aggressive antibiotic management of the antenatal patient with listeriosis may reduce the complications of this illness. In addition, these authors reviewed reported cases of listerial septicemia and antepartum antibiotic use. There was one maternal death, and 16 of 20 infants survived. These rates compared favorably to the 33% to 73% perinatal mortality noted in untreated maternal disease.

Lyme Disease

Lyme disease has emerged as an important infection since its initial description in 1977. The number of reported cases has grown steadily (CDC, 2001). This upsurge reflects not only a true rise in incidence but also increased recognition and reporting of Lyme disease. In 1999, 16,273 cases of Lyme disease were reported to the CDC (overall incidence, 6.0 per 100,000 population), representing a 40% increase from 1995, when 11,603 cases were reported. The highest numbers of cases were reported from the northeastern, north-central, and mid-Atlantic regions. Lyme disease is the most commonly reported vector-borne disease in the United States and accounts for 90% of vector-borne infections reported to the CDC.

Lyme disease, a tick-borne infection caused by the spirochete *Borrelia burgdorferi*, is a multisystem illness characterized by a distinct lesion, erythema chronicum migrans (ECM), which is often followed by neurologic, cardiac, and/or arthritic manifestations (Steere, Malawista, Hardin, et al., 1977; Steere, Malawista, Snydman, et al., 1977; Steere, 1989). The Lyme disease spirochete is transmitted by *Ixodes* ticks. The most common vector is the deer tick, *Ixodes dammini*, whose distribution coincides with endemic areas of the disease in the northeastern United States. In the western United States, *Ixodes pacificus*, the black-legged deer tick, is responsible for transmission of the disease. The white-footed mouse is host for the larval and nymph stage of the tick; white-tail deer are the preferred hosts for the adult stage. Most Lyme disease infections occur from May through August, coinciding with the height of both nymphal-stage activity and outdoor human activity (Steere, 1989).

Lyme disease generally occurs in stages, each of which is characterized by different clinical manifestations (Steere, 1989). The initial manifestation is ECM, which is followed several weeks or months later by meningitis or Bell's palsy and subsequently, months or years thereafter, by arthritis. Asbrink and Hovmark (1988) suggested a classification, based on the system used in syphilis, whereby Lyme disease is divided into "early" and "late" infection. *Early* infection consists of stage I (localized ECM), followed within days or weeks by stage II (disseminated infection), and within weeks or months by intermittent symptoms. *Late* infection, or stage III (persistent infection), generally begins a year or more after the initial disease presentation. Recently, Shapiro and colleagues (1992) attempted to assess the risk of infection with *B. burgdorferi* following exposure to deer-tick bites. Of interest, only 15% of the 344 deer ticks tested were infected with *B. burgdorferi*. These authors also assessed the efficacy of prophylactic and antimicrobial therapy following a deer-tick bite and noted that ECM occurred in only two patients, both in the placebo group. Overall the risk of infection among the placebo group was low: 1.2% (95% CI, 0.1% to 4.1%).

Following transmission of *B. burgdorferi*, ECM develops in approximately 60% to 80% of individuals. This lesion begins as a small erythematous papular macule, followed by a gradual centrifugal expansion over 3 to 4 weeks. The initial skin lesion is often accompanied by systemic symptoms, including fever and flu-like symptoms, with migratory arthralgias, myalgias, headaches, and regional lymphadenopathy (Steere, 1989). Even without treatment, ECM usually fades within 3 to 4 weeks.

Disseminated infection (Stage II early infection) occurs within days or weeks of transmission. It is often associated with characteristic symptoms involving the skin, nervous system, or musculoskeletal system. Secondarily annular skin lesions resembling primary ECM lesions develop in nearly 50% of patients. However, these are usually smaller and migrate less. Severe headaches and mild stiffness of the neck commonly occur in short attacks. Researchers utilizing a polymerase chain reaction (PCR) assay for *Borrelia*-specific DNA have demonstrated the presence of *B. burgdorferi* in the CNS during acute disseminated infection (Luft et al., 1992). The musculoskeletal pain associated with Lyme disease is migratory in nature, lasting only hours or days in any given location. During the disseminated stage, patients frequently have severe malaise and fatigue. As the infection begins to localize, 15% to 20% of patients experience frank neurologic involvement.

The classic triad of neurologic Lyme disease includes meningitis, cranial nerve palsies, and peripheral radiculopathies. The predominant symptoms of Lyme meningitis are severe headaches and mild neck stiffness, which fluctuate for several weeks. Leukocyte pleocytosis, slightly increased protein, and normal glucose levels are seen in the cerebral spinal fluid. Nearly half the cases of meningitis have an associated mild encephalitis that leads to loss of concentration, emotional lability, lethargy, sleep disturbances, or focal cerebral dysfunction. In addition, several late syndromes of the CNS have now been described. These include progressive encephalomyelitis (Ackerman et al., 1988), subacute encephalitis, and a syndrome suggestive of dementia. The most commonly affected cranial nerve is the seventh, leading to Bell's palsy. One third of the patients with Bell's palsy have bilateral involvement. Peripheral radiculopathies are characterized by severe neuritic pain, dysesthesias, focal weakness, and areflexia.

Within several weeks from the onset of disease, 5% to 10% of patients develop cardiac involvement. Fluctuating degrees of atrioventricular block are the most common abnormalities; this ranges from first-degree to complete heart block. Rarely, acute myopericarditis, mild left ventricular dysfunction, cardiomegaly, or fatal pancarditis occurs. The duration of cardiac abnormalities is usually between 3 days and 6 weeks.

Approximately 6 months after the onset of disease, about 60% of patients in the United States begin to have brief attacks of asymmetric, oligoarticular arthritis, primarily in the large joints, especially the knee. Stage III or late infection is characterized by episodes of arthritis, often lasting longer during the 2nd and 3rd year of the illness, or a chronic arthritis. With use of PCR technology, *B. burgdorferi* DNA has been detected in the synovial fluid of patients with Lyme arthritis; nearly all specimens from untreated patients contained *B. burgdorferi* DNA (Nocton et al., 1994). Several late-presenting syndromes involving the CNS have also been described (Ackerman et al., 1988). These include progressive encephalomyelitis, subacute encephalitis, dementia, and a syndrome suggesting demyelination.

Concern has arisen because other spirochetes such as *Treponema pallidum* cross the placenta and produce adverse effects on the fetus or neonate. Experience with Lyme disease during pregnancy is rather limited (Smith et al., 1991). In 1985, the first case of transplacental transmission of *B. burgdorferi* was documented by identification of the spirochete in multiple organs of an infant who died of congenital heart disease shortly after birth (Schlesinger et al., 1985). Subsequently, Weber and co-workers (1988) isolated the organism from the brain and liver of an infant who died within the first 24 hours of life. Both of these infants had been born to mothers who had ECM during the first trimester. Three cases of stillbirth with

recovery of *B. burgdorferi* from multiple organs subsequently were reported in the literature (MacDonald, 1986, 1987; Markowitz et al., 1986).

The CDC has assessed the effect of Lyme disease during pregnancy (Markowitz, 1986). In a retrospective study, five adverse outcomes in fetuses born to 19 women with Lyme disease were identified (Markowitz et al., 1986). Among the adverse outcomes noted were prematurity, cortical blindness, fetal demise, and syndactyly and rash in the neonate. However, no teratogenic pattern was observed, and a reduction in fetal morbidity was not observed among the mothers appropriately treated for Lyme disease. In a prospective study, 17 women with documented first-trimester Lyme infection were evaluated. Only two of these pregnancies were abnormal; one ended in a spontaneous abortion at 13 weeks, and in the second, the infant had syndactyly. In a survey of cord blood sera from 421 infants born in an area endemic for *B. burgdorferi*, Williams and colleagues (1988) demonstrated no relationship between congenital malformation and the presence of antibody to Lyme disease.

In a European study, 0.85% of umbilical cord blood samples obtained from more than 1400 pregnancies demonstrated elevated titers to *B. burgdorferi* (Nadl et al., 1989). Of these, only one patient had clinical disease during her pregnancy; her infant had a ventricular septal defect without other anomalies. In the remaining 11 infants with elevated immunoglobulin G (IgG) cord titers, six had an abnormal neonatal course: two had hyperbilirubinemia, one had macrocephaly, one had intrauterine growth restriction, and one had supraventricular extrasystoles. At an average follow-up of 9 months, however, all six infants were normal. Thus, any relationship between positive IgG titers and abnormalities in the fetus or neonate are inconclusive. Strobino and colleagues (1993) prospectively followed nearly 2000 pregnant women to determine whether prenatal exposure to Lyme disease was associated with an increased risk of adverse pregnancy outcome. The women were screened for antibody to *B. burgdorferi* at their first prenatal visit and at delivery. Neither maternal Lyme disease nor an increased risk of exposure to Lyme disease was associated with fetal death, decreased birth weight, or gestational age at delivery. Bites from infected ticks around the time of conception were not associated with congenital malformation. Tick bites within 3 years before conception were significantly associated with congenital malformation; the authors suggested that this reflected reporting differences between exposed and unexposed women (Strobino et al., 1993).

The diagnosis of Lyme disease is complicated by the various manifestations of the disorder. The culture of *B. burgdorferi* from patients' specimens is difficult, as is direct visualization, and thus serology has been the only practical laboratory diagnosis available. An indirect fluorescent antibody test and an enzyme-linked immunosorbent assay (ELISA) are the most commonly used diagnostic tests for Lyme disease. ELISA is the preferred method because of its greater sensitivity and specificity. It is important to recognize that false-positive serologic testing for Lyme disease can occur with other spirochetal diseases, infectious mononucleosis, autoimmune disorders, and Rocky Mountain spotted fever. Thus, an indirect screening test to rule out syphilis should be done in all patients testing positive for spirochetal disease. False-negative serologic results may be seen early in the disease (i.e., during the first 2 weeks), when infection is localized to the skin, or if antibiotics have been given, before an immune response can be mounted. Consequently, a two-test approach for the serologic diagnosis of Lyme disease is utilized by most laboratories. As an initial screening test, specimens are assessed with the more sensitive ELISA or indirect fluorescent antibody test. Specimens that are positive (or equivocal) are confirmed by the more specific IgG and IgM Western blot. However, the sensitivity and specificity of the ELISA and Western blot vary, depending upon the timing in the disease process of specimen acquisition. Thus, clinical and exposure history are critical components for interpreting serologic results.

Because laboratory diagnosis is uncertain, the following case definition has been developed to aid in the recognition of Lyme disease: (1) the occurrence of ECM no more than 30 days following exposure in an endemic area, or (2) the involvement of at least one of the three commonly affected organ systems, producing neurologic, cardiovascular, or arthritic symptoms, in conjunction with either a positive serologic result or isolation of *B. burgdorferi*, or (3) ECM or positive serology without a history of exposure. PCR has identified the presence of *B. burgdorferi* DNA in the cerebrospinal fluid (CSF) of patients with Lyme disease meningitis and the synovial fluid or tissue in Lyme disease arthritis (Persing et al., 1990; Luft et al., 1992; Nishi et al., 1993). In summary, the diagnosis of Lyme disease is based primarily on the presence of characteristic clinical findings, exposure in an endemic area, and an elevated antibody response to *B. burgdorferi* (Nadal et al., 1989).

Steere and colleagues (1993), in a Lyme disease clinic, analyzed the diagnoses, serologic test results, and treatment results of patients evaluated for Lyme disease. Active Lyme disease was confirmed in 180 (23% of 788 patients), usually manifested as arthritis, encephalopathy, or polyneuropathy. An additional 156 patients (20%) had evidence of prior Lyme disease, and the remaining 452 patients (57%) did not have the condition. Among those without Lyme disease, 45% had had positive serologic test results for Lyme disease in other laboratories. Most important, the primary explanation for failure to respond to antibiotic treatment of suspected Lyme disease was an incorrect diagnosis, as was determined in 322 (79%) of 409 patients who had been treated prior to referral to the Lyme disease clinic. Serologic testing for Lyme disease is hindered by a lack of standardization, with both false-negative and more commonly false-positive results occurring (Hedberg et al., 1987; Bakken et al., 1992). Thus, misdiagnosis—particularly overdiagnosis—and unreliable serologic testing are important issues for clinicians and patients dealing with Lyme disease.

Treatment of Lyme disease is most successful when it is commenced early in the disease process. Guidelines for the treatment of Lyme disease have been published by the Infectious Diseases Society of America (Kaslow, 1992) and are listed in Table 39-6. Oral amoxicillin (500 mg three times daily) or doxycycline (100 mg twice daily) for 14 to 28 days is the recommended treatment of early localized or early disseminated disease associated with ECM, in the absence or neurological involvement or third-degree heart block. In pregnant patients doxycycline is contraindicated. For patients unable to take amoxicillin or doxycycline (i.e., pregnant women allergic to penicillin), 500 mg of cefuroxime axetil orally twice per day is an alternative. Although ceftriaxone is effective, it is not superior to the oral agents and is not recommended as a first-line agent for treatment of Lyme disease in the absence of

TABLE 39-6. ANTIMICROBIAL TREATMENT OF LYME DISEASE IN ADULTS

Recommendation	Adult Dosage
Preferred Oral Agent	
Amoxicillin	500 mg t.i.d. for 14–28 d
Doxycycline*	100 mg b.i.d. for 14–28 d
Alternative Oral Agent	
Cefuroxime axetil	500 mg b.i.d. for 14–28 d
Preferred Parenteral Agent	
Ceftriaxone	2 g IV d for 14–28 d
Alternative Parenteral Agent	
Penicillin G	18–24 million units IV d divided into doses given every 4 h for 14–28 d
Cefotaxime	2 g IV t.i.d for 14–28 d

* Contraindicated in pregnancy.
b.i.d., twice daily; IV, intravenously; t.i.d., three times daily.

neurologic involvement or third-degree heart block (Kaslow, 1992).

For early disease with neurological involvement (e.g., meningitis or radiculopathy), 2 g of ceftriaxone intravenously once per day for 14 to 28 days is recommended (Kaslow, 1992). Intravenous penicillin G (18 to 24 million units daily, with equal doses administered every 4 hours) is an alternative choice. Patients with third-degree heart block should be hospitalized in addition to receiving antibiotic treatment similar to that for patients with neurologic involvement. Lyme arthritis is usually treated successfully with antimicrobial agents administered orally or intravenously (see Table 39-6) as recommended for patients without clinical manifestations of neurologic involvement. Doxycycline (contraindicated during pregnancy) or amoxicillin for 28 days is recommended in patients without neurologic disease. For patients with arthritis and neurologic involvement, 2 g of ceftriaxone once daily or 18 to 24 million units penicillin G daily for 28 days is recommended.

The role of primary antimicrobial prophylaxis to prevent Lyme disease following tick bites is controversial. Recent reports demonstrate that routine prophylaxis is neither indicated (Kaslow, 1992; Shapiro, 1992) nor successful (Shapiro et al., 1992).

Recently two Lyme disease vaccines using recombinant DNA technology have been tested (Sigal et al., 1998; Steere et al., 1998). Both vaccines have been demonstrated to be safe and efficacious.

VIRAL INFECTIONS

Rubella

Epidemiology

Rubella is caused by a ribonucleic acid (RNA) virus. Rubella infection develops primarily in young children and adolescents and is most common in the springtime. Major epidemics of rubella occurred in the United States in 1935 and 1964; minor sporadic epidemics occurred approximately every 7 years until the late 1960s. With licensure of an effective vaccine in 1969, the frequency of rubella has declined by almost 99%. However, a small number of cases still occur each year. Persistence of this infection appears to be due to failure to vaccinate susceptible individuals rather than to lack of immunogenicity of the vaccine (ACOG, 1992).

The rubella virus is spread by respiratory droplets. From the upper respiratory tract, the virus travels quickly to the cervical lymph nodes and is then disseminated hematogenously throughout the body. The incubation period is approximately 2 to 3 weeks. The virus is present in blood and nasopharyngeal secretions for several days before appearance of the characteristic rash and continues to be shed from the nasopharynx for several days after appearance of the exanthem. Therefore, the patient may be contagious for a period of 7 to 10 days (ACOG, 1992).

Antibody against rubella does not normally appear in the serum until after the rash has developed. Acquired immunity to rubella usually lasts for life. Second infections have occurred after both natural infections and vaccination, but recurrent infections generally are not associated with serious illness, viremia, or congenital infection.

Clinical Presentation

Most individuals with rubella have mild constitutional symptoms such as malaise, headache, myalgias, and arthralgias. The principal clinical manifestation of rubella is a widely disseminated nonpruritic, erythematous, maculopapular rash. Postauricular adenopathy and mild conjunctivitis also are common. These clinical manifestations usually are short lived and typically resolve within 3 to 5 days.

Diagnosis

The differential diagnosis of rubella includes rubeola, roseola, other viral exanthems, and drug reaction. Rubella usually can be distinguished from these other conditions on the basis of the characteristic rash and serologic testing. Serum IgM antibody concentration reaches a peak 7 to 10 days after the onset of illness and then declines over a period of 4 weeks. The serum concentration of IgG rises more slowly, but antibody levels persist throughout the lifetime of the individual. Several antibody detection tests are available, including indirect immunofluorescence, enzyme immunoassay, and latex agglutination. The latter two assays are the most rapid and convenient methods for testing (ACOG, 1992; Sautter et al., 1994).

Congenital Rubella Infection

Because of the success of rubella vaccination campaigns, the incidence of congenital rubella syndrome (CRS) in the United States has declined dramatically over the past 25 years. In recent years, fewer than 50 cases of congenital rubella have occurred each year. Unfortunately, approximately 10% to 20% of women in the United States remain susceptible to rubella, and their fetuses are therefore at risk for serious injury should infection occur during pregnancy (CDC, 1990).

Rubella virus crosses the placenta by hematogenous dissemination, and the frequency of congenital infection is critically dependent on the time of exposure to the virus. Approximately 50% of infants exposed to the virus within 4 weeks of conception will manifest signs of congenital infection. When maternal infection occurs in weeks 5 to 8 after conception, approximately 25% of fetuses will be infected; when it develops in weeks 9 to 12, about 10% of fetuses will be infected; when it occurs beyond this point in time, less than 1% of fetuses are affected (Miller et al., 1982; Munro et al., 1987).

The four most common anomalies associated with CRS are deafness (affecting 60% to 75% of fetuses), eye defects (10% to 30%), CNS defects (10% to 25%), and cardiac malformations (10% to 20%). The most common cardiac abnormality is patent ductus arteriosus, although supravalvular pulmonic stenosis is perhaps the most pathognomonic. Other possible abnormalities include microcephaly, mental retardation, pneumonia, intrauterine growth restriction, hepatosplenomegaly, hemolytic anemia, and thrombocytopenia (Miller et al., 1982; Munro et al., 1987; McIntosh and Menser, 1992; CDC, 1994).

A variety of tests have been proposed for the diagnosis of CRS. Cordocentesis can determine the total serum IgM concentration in fetal blood and detect viral-specific antibody. However, cordocentesis is technically difficult prior to 20 weeks' gestation, and fetal immunoglobulins usually cannot be detected before 22 to 24 weeks. Viral antigen can be identified in culture of placental tissue by RNA-DNA hybridization techniques, and amniotic fluid can be cultured for rubella virus. Unfortunately, although these tests can demonstrate that rubella virus is present in the fetal compartment, they do not indicate the degree of fetal injury. Accordingly, detailed ultrasound examination is the best test to determine if serious fetal injury has occurred as a result of maternal rubella infection. Possible anomalies detected by ultrasound include intrauterine growth restriction, microcephaly, CNS abnormalities, and cardiac malformations.

The prognosis for infants with CRS is guarded. Approximately 50% of affected individuals have to attend schools for the hearing-impaired. An additional 25% require at least some special schooling because of hearing impairment, and only 25% are able to attend mainstream schools. The estimated lifetime cost of caring for a child with CRS is approximately $200,000 to $300,000 (McIntosh and Menser, 1992).

Prevention of Rubella Infection

Ideally, women of reproductive age should have a preconception appointment when they are contemplating pregnancy. At this time, they should be evaluated for immunity to rubella. If serologic testing demonstrates that they are susceptible, they should be vaccinated with rubella vaccine prior to conception. When preconception counseling is not possible, patients should have a test for rubella at the time of their first prenatal appointment. Women who are susceptible to rubella should be counseled to avoid exposure to other individuals who may have viral exanthems.

If a susceptible patient is subsequently exposed to rubella, serologic tests should be obtained to determine whether acute infection has occurred. If acute infection is documented by identification of IgM antibody, the patient should be counseled about the risk of CRS. The diagnostic tests for detection of congenital infection should be reviewed, and the patient should be offered the option of pregnancy termination, depending upon the assessed risk of serious fetal injury.

Pregnant women who are susceptible to rubella should be vaccinated immediately postpartum. The present rubella vaccine is the RA 27/3 preparation, and it is available in monovalent, bivalent (measles-rubella), and trivalent (measles-mumps-rubella) forms. Approximately 95% of patients who receive rubella vaccine seroconvert, and antibody levels persist for at least 18 years in more than 90% of vaccinees.

Adverse effects of vaccination are minimal, even in adults. Fewer than 25% of patients experience mild constitutional symptoms such as low-grade fever and malaise. Fewer than 10% have arthralgias, and fewer than 1% develop frank arthritis. In susceptible adult women, joint symptoms are more common and tend to be more severe than in children. Other complaints, such as pain and paresthesias, have been rare. Women who have received the vaccine cannot transmit infection to susceptible contacts, such as younger children in the home. Therefore, vaccinated women still may breast-feed their infants. In addition, the vaccine can be administered in conjunction with other immunoglobulin preparations such as Rh immune globulin (CDC, 1990, 1994).

Women who receive rubella vaccine should practice secure contraception for at least 1 month after vaccination. For a number of years, the CDC maintained a registry of women who received the rubella vaccine within 3 months of conception. That registry included approximately 400 patients, and, fortunately, there were no instances in which CRS resulted from vaccination. The maximum theoretical risk of congenital rubella resulting from rubella vaccine in early pregnancy is 1% to 2% (Bart et al., 1985).

To decrease the occurrence of rubella, recommended policy includes vaccinating all children aged 12 to 15 months or older and all adolescents and adults not known to be immune, unless they are pregnant or have other contraindications to vaccination. Also, all prenatal patients should be screened as early as possible in pregnancy (ACOG, 1992). Contraindications to vaccination include febrile illnesses, immunosuppression, and pregnancy. Precautions are necessary in the rare individual with neomycin allergy.

Cytomegalovirus

Epidemiology

Cytomegalovirus (CMV) is a double-stranded DNA virus. Humans are its only known host. Like herpes simplex virus, CMV may remain latent in host cells after the initial infection. Recurrent infection usually is due to reactivation of endogenous latent virus rather than reinfection with a new strain of virus.

CMV is not highly contagious, and therefore close personal contact is required for infection to occur. *Horizontal transmission* may result from transplant of an infected organ or blood, from sexual contact, or from contact with contaminated saliva or urine. *Vertical transmission* may occur as a result of transplacental infection, exposure to contaminated genital tract secretions during delivery, or breast-feeding (Brown and Abernathy, 1998; Duff, 1994). The incubation period of the virus ranges from 28 to 60 days, with a mean of 40 days.

Among young children, the most important risk factor for infection is close contact with playmates, particularly in the setting of day care. Infected children clearly pose a risk of transmitting virus to adult day-care workers. Small children also pose a risk to members of their own family (Adler, 1989). In addition to acquiring infection from young children, adolescents and adults may develop infection as a result of sexual contact. CMV infection is endemic among homosexual men and heterosexual men and women with multiple partners. Additional risk factors for infection include lower socioeconomic status, history of abnormal cervical cytology, birth outside of North America, first pregnancy at less than 15 years, and coinfection with other sexually transmitted diseases such as trichomoniasis (Duff, 1994).

Clinical Presentation

Most children who acquire CMV infection are asymptomatic. When clinical manifestations are present, they include malaise, fever, lymphadenopathy, and hepatosplenomegaly. Similarly, most immunocompetent adults with primary or recurrent CMV are asymptomatic or have mild symptoms suggestive of mononucleosis. Severe respiratory infection, esophagitis, colitis, and chorioretinitis may occur in patients with immunodeficiency disorders such as HIV infection.

Diagnosis

The diagnosis of CMV infection can be confirmed by isolation of virus in tissue culture. The highest concentration of CMV is usually present in urine, seminal fluid, saliva, and breast milk. Techniques such as immunofluorescent staining and PCR permit identification of viral antigen within 24 hours of inoculation of the tissue culture.

Serologic methods also are helpful in establishing the diagnosis of CMV. In the acute phase of infection, virus-specific IgM antibody is present in serum. IgM titers usually decline rapidly over a period of 30 to 60 days but can remain elevated for many months. There is no absolute IgG titer that clearly differentiates acute from recurrent infection. However, a fourfold or greater change in the IgG titer is consistent with recent acute infection (Duff, 1994).

Antenatal (Congenital) CMV Infection

Antepartum (congenital) infection poses the greatest risk to the fetus and results from hematogenous dissemination of virus across the placenta. Dissemination may occur with both primary and recurrent (reactivated) infection but is much more likely in the former setting (Fowler et al., 1992; Boppana et al., 2001). Approximately 1% to 4% of uninfected women seroconvert during pregnancy. In women who acquire *primary* infection, 40% to 50% of the fetuses will be infected. The overall risk of congenital infection is greatest when maternal infection occurs in the third trimester, but the probability of severe fetal injury is highest when maternal infection occurs in the first trimester (Stagno et al., 1982; Chandler et al., 1985).

Of fetuses with congenital infection resulting from primary maternal infection, 5% to 18% are overtly symptomatic at birth. The most common clinical manifestations are hepatosplenomegaly, intracranial calcifications, jaundice, growth restriction, microcephaly, chorioretinitis, and hearing loss. The most frequent laboratory abnormalities are thrombocytopenia, hyperbilirubinemia, and elevated serum transaminase concentrations. Approximately 30% of severely infected infants die. Eighty percent of the survivors have major morbidity such as mental retardation, ocular abnormalities, or sensorineural hearing loss.

Approximately 85% to 90% of infants delivered to mothers with primary infection are asymptomatic at birth. Ten to 15% subsequently develop hearing loss, chorioretinitis, or dental defects within the first 2 years of life (Adler, 1992; Dobbins et al., 1992; Duff, 1994).

Pregnant women who experience *recurrent or reactivated* CMV infection are much less likely to transmit infection to their fetus. In a recent survey, Fowler and colleagues (1992), studied 125 women with serologic evidence of primary infection and 64 with recurrent infection. In the former group, 18% of infants were symptomatic at birth; an additional 7% developed at least one major sequela within the 5 years of follow-up. Two percent died, 15% had sensorineural hearing loss, and 13% had an IQ less than 70. In contrast, none of the infants delivered to mothers with recurrent infection were symptomatic at birth. During the period of surveillance, 8% had at least one sequela, but none had multiple defects. The most common sequela was hearing loss.

Identification of virus in amniotic fluid by culture or PCR is the most sensitive and specific means of diagnosing congenital infection. It is superior even to umbilical blood sampling and can be performed earlier in gestation, when cordocentesis is not possible. However, it does not necessarily delineate the severity of fetal injury, an issue that is obviously of great importance in counseling parents about the prognosis for their infant. Fortunately, sonography is invaluable in providing information about severity of fetal impairment. The principal sonographic findings suggestive of serious fetal injury include microcephaly, ventriculomegaly, intracerebral calcifications, hydrops, growth restriction, and oligohydramnios. Other unusual findings that also may indicate a severely infected infant include fetal heart block, echogenic bowel, renal dysplasia, and isolated serious effusions. Ultrasound examination may be normal early in the course of fetal infection. Therefore, fetuses at risk should have repeat examinations to determine if anomalies are apparent (Donner et al., 1993).

Intrapartum and Postpartum Infection

Perinatal CMV infection may occur during delivery as a result of exposure to infected genital tract secretions. At the time of delivery, up to 10% of pregnant women may shed CMV in cervical secretions or urine. Twenty percent to 60% of exposed fetuses subsequently shed virus in their pharynx or urine. The incubation period for this form of infection ranges from 7 to 12 weeks, with an average of 8 weeks. Fortunately, infected infants rarely have serious sequelae of infection acquired during delivery. In addition, infants who acquire CMV infection as a result of breast feeding are very unlikely to sustain serious injury (Adler, 1992; Duff, 1994).

Prevention of CMV Infection

At the present time, a vaccine for CMV is not available. Antiviral agents such as ganciclovir and foscarnet have moderate activity against CMV, but their use is limited primarily to treatment of severe infections in immunocompromised patients. Accordingly, obstetrician-gynecologists should focus attention on educating patients about preventive measures.

One of the most important interventions is helping patients to understand that CMV infection can be a sexually transmitted disease and that sexual promiscuity significantly increases an individual's risk of acquiring the infection. Individuals who have multiple sex partners should be counseled that latex condoms provide an effective barrier to transmission of CMV. Another important intervention is educating health-care workers, day-care workers, elementary school teachers, and mothers of young children about the importance of simple infection control measures such as hand-washing and proper cleansing of environmental surfaces. Obstetricians and pediatricians must consistently be aware of the importance of transfusing only CMV-free blood products to fetuses, neonates, pregnant women, and immunocompromised patients and of screening potential donors of organs and semen for CMV infection. Finally, health-care workers must adhere to the principles of universal precautions when treating patients and handling potentially infected body fluids.

For several reasons, routine prenatal screening for CMV infection is not recommended. First, laboratory resources could be overwhelmed if all pregnant women were screened. Second, if laboratories do not ensure a high level of quality control, the interpretation of serologic tests may be confusing and may lead to incorrect, and irreversible, interventions such as pregnancy termination. Third, neither antiviral chemotherapy nor immunoprophylaxis is available to protect the fetus or neonate. Accordingly, screening should be limited to women who have symptoms suggestive of acute CMV infection, who have had definite occupational exposure to CMV, or who are immunocompromised (Duff, 1994).

Varicella Zoster (Chickenpox)

The varicella zoster virus (VZV), a member of the herpesvirus family, is a DNA virus. Varicella, commonly known as *chickenpox,* is the acute primary disease. Herpes zoster, commonly known as *shingles,* is the recurrent form of infection.

Varicella (chicken pox) is a common childhood disease usually marked by typical skin lesions, which progress from macules and papules to vesicles and pustules (Gershon, 2001). A highly contagious disorder, varicella is acquired by approximately 90% of persons in the United States before reproductive age and is generally self-limited. Among women who do not recall a history of varicella, 70% to 90% have detectable antibodies (CDC, 1996). The incubation period has a mean of 15 days, with extremes of 10 to 21 days. In adults who contract the disease, constitutional and pulmonary symptoms may be more severe. Special problems for the obstetrician include a possible increase in severity of the disease in the pregnant woman and the effects on the fetus and newborn. Availability of varicella vaccine in the United States has resulted in a dramatic decrease in new cases of varicella (CDC, 2002).

Zoster (shingles) results when the latent virus is reactivated. Generally, zoster occurs in older adults or immunocompromised populations. The frequency of zoster increases with age. Characteristically, zoster manifests as painful vesicular lesions that occur along segmental dermatomes.

Maternal Varicella

Varicella is an uncommon infection among adults and appears to occur with no greater frequency among pregnant women. The estimated incidence of varicella in pregnancy is 0.7 per 1000 patients (Balducci et al, 1992). While adults are at increased risk of developing varicella pneumonia, this risk is not greater among pregnant women (Gershon, 2001; Sweet and Gibbs, 2002).

In 1965 Harris and Rhoades (1965) reviewed the literature and reported mortality in 41% of pregnant women with varicella pneumonia compared to 11% in nonpregnant women with the same illness. However, subsequent reports suggested that the mortality rate for varicella pneumonia in pregnancy ranges from 0% to 25%, which is similar to the rate seen in nonpregnant women (Paryani and Arvin, 1986; Smego and Asperilla, 1991). Gershon (2001), in a recently updated review of the literature on varicella pneumonia in pregnancy (Table 39-7), noted that varicella pneumonia occurred in 57 (28%) of 198 cases of chickenpox in pregnant women. There were 16 deaths, all among the patients with pneumonia, for a pneumonia mortality rate of 28% (overall mortality rate for varicella was 10%). Although pneumonia was previously associated with a significant mortality rate, it is an uncommon complication of varicella. Moreover, our ability to manage severe respiratory distress and failure has significantly improved, and acyclovir in high doses is effective against VZV (Smego and Asperilla, 1991). On the other hand, uncomplicated varicella does not appear to pose a severe risk to pregnant women.

Despite improved survival in women with varicella pneumonia during pregnancy following the availability of high-dose acyclovir, mortality remains a concern (Sweet and Gibbs, 2002). Thus, clinicians need to have a high index of suspicion that pneumonia may complicate varicella during pregnancy. Pulmonary symptoms begin on the 2nd to 6th day after appearance of the rash. Symptoms usually consist of a mild nonpro-

ductive cough. If the disease is more severe, there may also be pleuritic chest pain, hemoptysis, dyspnea, and frank cyanosis. Physical examination reveals fever, rales, and wheezes. A chest x-ray characteristically demonstrates a diffuse nodular or miliary pattern, particularly in the perihilar regions. Pregnant women should be warned to contact their physician immediately if even mild pulmonary symptoms develop. Hospitalization with full respiratory support, if necessary, and high-dose acyclovir should be initiated.

Smego and Asperilla (1991) reported on their use of acyclovir for the management of severe varicella (e.g., pneumonia) during pregnancy. They reviewed 21 patients, of whom 12 required intubation and mechanical ventilation. The mortality rate was 14% (3 deaths), all in the third trimester. The dosage recommended for acyclovir treatment of severe varicella is 10 to 15 mg/kg intravenously three times daily for 7 days. The equivalent oral dose is 800 mg five times per day. No adverse drug effects were noted.

The significant morbidity and mortality associated with varicella infection in pregnancy requires that prevention of varicella among susceptible exposed pregnant women be optimized. Following exposure to varicella, pregnant women with a past history of chickenpox or varicella vaccination should be assured that they are immune. Those with a negative history should be tested for antibody indicative of prior varicella infection (fluorescent antibody to membrane antigen test or ELISA). Susceptible women should receive varicella-zoster immune globulin (VZIG) within 96 hours of exposure. When submitting the specimen, it is critical to inform the laboratory that the test is from a pregnant woman exposed to varicella in order to ensure that results are available prior to the 96-hour limit. Although VZIG prevents and/or ameliorates maternal disease, it is unclear that such passive immunization prevents fetal infection (Sweet and Gibbs, 2002). The recommended dose of VZIG is 125 units per 10 kg of body weight up to a maximum of 625 units (5 vials) intramuscularly.

TABLE 39-7. MATERNAL MORTALITY ASSOCIATED WITH VARICELLA DURING PREGNANCY

Study	No. of Cases	No. with Pneumonia	No. of Deaths
Harris and Rhoades, 1965*	17	17	7
Siegal and Fuerst, 1966	11	0	0
Geeves et al., 1971	1	1	0
Paryani and Arvin, 1986	43	4	1
Esmonde et al., 1989	3	3	1
Cox et al., 1990	5	5	1
Broussard et al., 1991	1	1	0
Smegmo and Asperilla, 1991	21	21	3
Baren et al., 1996	28	1	0
Figueroa-Damian and Arrendondo-Garcia, 1997	22	0	0
Total	150	53 (35%)	13 (25%)†

* Includes review of the literature prior to 1963.
† All mortality among cases with pneumonia.

Modified from Gershon AA: Chickenpox, measles and mumps. *In* Remington JS, Kelin JO (eds): Infectious diseases of the fetus and newborn. Philadelphia: WB Saunders, 2001, p. 683.

VARICELLA IN EARLY PREGNANCY

Maternal varicella infection has been associated with spontaneous abortion, stillbirth, and congenital anomalies (Siegel and Fuerst, 1966; Brunell, 1983; Gershon, 2001). Congenital anomalies resulting from varicella in early pregnancy were not recognized until the mid-1970s. It is now appreciated that maternal varicella infection in the first 4 months of pregnancy *rarely* produces a congenital varicella syndrome, which consists of cutaneous scars, limb hypoplasia, rudimentary digits, and occasionally eye and CNS abnormalities, including cerebral cortical atrophy and mental retardation. In Table 39-8, the risk for developing the congenital varicella syndrome following first-trimester maternal varicella is summarized. Overall, approximately 1% of infants exposed to VZV early in pregnancy developed congenital varicella, with a range of 0% to 9%.

Higa and Manabe (1987) hypothesized that congenital malformations related to VZV may not be caused by varicella of the fetus, but rather can be ascribed to sequelae of herpes zoster infection *in utero*. In particular, recurrent zoster infection would explain the cutaneous and limb abnormalities, whereas acute varicella is responsible for the CNS or neurologic lesions.

Paryani and Arvin (1986) demonstrated that although varicella during pregnancy was associated with evidence of fetal infection in 25% of cases (immunologic evidence), zoster was not. More-recent evidence has also confirmed that congenital varicella infection is most unlikely in infants whose mothers had herpes zoster in pregnancy. There was no serologic evidence of intrauterine infection in more than 300 infants of mothers with zoster in pregnancy (Enders et al., 1994).

Although the risk of the congenital varicella syndrome is small, administration of VZIG is recommended to susceptible pregnant women who have not previously had varicella. This should occur as soon as possible, but within 96 hours of exposure, in the hope of protecting the fetus during the viremia. No clinical trials have been conducted to establish the benefit of this approach. However, treatment with VZIG is safe and does decrease maternal clinical manifestations.

Varicella in the Newborn

Acquisition of maternal antibody usually protects the fetus, but if an infant is born after the maternal viremia but before a maternal antibody response has developed, it is at high risk for life-threatening neonatal varicella infection. Infants are at risk if the mother has contracted varicella between 5 days before and 2 days after delivery. Congenital varicella infection has been reported in 17% of term infants born to mothers who have varicella within 4 to 5 days of delivery, and the case fatality rate is 31% (4 of 13) (DeNicola and Hanshaw, 1979). VZIG can prevent or moderate clinical varicella in susceptible individuals if it is given shortly after exposure. VZIG can be obtained from regional offices of the American Red Cross. Infants born to mothers who develop varicella between 5 days before and 2 days after delivery should receive at least 125 units of VZIG. In England, no deaths attributable to varicella occurred among 91 VZIG-treated seronegative infants whose mothers had acute varicella up to 2 weeks after delivery (Miller et al., 1989). Interestingly, two thirds of the infants had evidence of varicella infection, and one half of those infected had symptomatic disease. Thus, although VZIG may ameliorate the infection, it does not universally prevent varicella in the neonate.

In utero diagnosis of varicella infection has been demonstrated with ultrasonography, amniocentesis, chorionic villus biopsy, and cordocentesis (Scharf et al., 1990; Isada et al., 1991; Pretorius et al., 1992; Mouly et al., 1997). Although cordocentesis, by 19 to 22 weeks, can detect varicella-specific IgM antibody, amniocentesis can demonstrate VZV (PCR), and testing of placental tissue can reveal VZV (*in situ* hybridization), detection of virus or antibody fails to document the severity of fetal infection. Thus ultrasound appears to be the best available technique for assessing the severity of varicella fetal infection and determining whether intervention is a potential option. Pretorius and colleagues (1992) demonstrated that among a group of women with confirmed first-trimester varicella, all five fetuses with sonographic abnormalities had varicella embryopathy documented at neonatal examination or autopsy. The ultrasound findings included polyhydramnios, hydrops fetalis, and multiple hypoechogenic foci within the liver. Ultrasound may also demonstrate abnormal limb development in fetuses with varicella infection. These authors reported that 14 of 17 fetuses with hypoplastic limbs had concomitant brain damage or died in early infancy. More recently, utilization of PCR technology demonstrated the presence of VZV in 9 (8.4%) of 107 pregnant women with varicella infection prior to 24 weeks' gestation (Mouly et al., 1997). All three cases of congenital varicella syndrome were PCR-positive. In addition, two had abnormal ultrasound findings at 21 to 22 weeks; the third infant had bilateral microphthalmia despite a supposed normal ultrasound at 24 weeks.

The CDC (1996) has issued recommendations for prevention of varicella. An attenuated virus vaccine (Varivax) was approved in the United States in 1995. Because this preparation involves a live attenuated virus, it is recommended that pregnant women or those attempting to get pregnant should not be vaccinated (CDC, 1996). Nonpregnant women who are vaccinated should avoid becoming pregnant for 1 month after each injection. Inadvertent vaccination within 1 month before or during pregnancy should lead to counseling. Initial results from the Varivax Pregnancy Registry demonstrated that among 371 women vaccinated during pregnancy or within 3 months before, no cases of congenital varicella were reported (95% CI, 0.0 to 0.01). The risk from vaccine virus should be even less than from wild virus. This finding combined with the 1% risk of congenital varicella among

TABLE 39-8. RISK OF SYMPTOMATIC INTRAUTERINE VARICELLA-ZOSTER INFECTION AFTER FIRST-TRIMESTER MATERNAL VARICELLA

Study	No. of Infants Exposed	No. of Infants with Congenital Varicella
Siegal, 1973	27	2 (7.4%)
Paryani and Arvin, 1986	11	1 (9%)
Balducci et al., 1992	35	0
Enders et al., 1994	472	2 (0.4)
Pastuszak et al., 1994	49	1 (2)
TOTAL	594	6 (1%)

infants born to women who developed varicella in early pregnancy (see Table 39-8) led to the CDC recommending that in most circumstances, the decision to terminate a pregnancy should not be based on exposure to varicella vaccine (CDC, 1996). In addition, because the vaccine virus is not transmissible, presence of a pregnant woman in the household does not contraindicate vaccination of a susceptible household member.

Herpes Simplex

In the past few years, important new information has become available regarding perinatal herpes that has improved our understanding of its pathogenesis and has led to changes in treatment recommendations.

Herpes simplex virus (HSV) may infect the adult, the newborn, or on rare occasions, the fetus. In the adult, typical lesions are vesicular or ulcerative, involving only the skin and mucous membranes. More-widespread infection involving the CNS is an extremely unusual adult complication, most often developing in people with debilitating disease. On the other hand, because of an incompletely developed immune system, the newborn is subject to systemic, and frequently lethal, disease.

In adults, the virus commonly causes infection of the oral cavity, skin, and lower genital tract. In the past, HSV type 1 (HSV-1) was said to be responsible for infection of the mouth and of the skin above the waist, and type 2 virus (HSV-2) for infection of the genitalia and of the skin below the waist. Approximately 90% of cases still follow the pattern, but either type may cause infection at either site.

In surveys of adult females, herpesvirus has been isolated from the genitalia of 0.02% to 1%. Among pregnant women, one survey found positive cultures in 0.6% of asymptomatic women. The disease does not appear to be more severe or more protracted in pregnancy. Serologic surveys with a reliable antibody test for HSV-2 revealed a seroprevalence of 25% among females in the United States (Fleming et al., 1997).

Clinically, there are three herpetic syndromes in adults:

1. *First-episode primary genital herpes* is the clinical presentation in a patient without antibodies to either HSV-1 or HSV-2. Its clinical manifestations include severe local symptoms, with lesions lasting 2 to 3 weeks, regional adenopathy, constitutional symptoms, and in a small percentage of cases, viral meningitis. However, it should be noted that as many as two thirds of women with HSV-2 antibodies have acquired the infection asymptomatically (Kulhanjian et al., 1992). This observation represents a major change from previous concepts.
2. *First-episode nonprimary infection* is the initial clinical episode with either HSV-1 or HSV-2 in a patient with antibodies to the other viral serotype. It is more similar in presentation to recurrent episodes.
3. *Recurrent genital herpes infections* are much milder and shorter, with viral shedding lasting an average of only 3 to 5 days.

When primary genital herpes occurs in pregnancy, there is a high risk of fetal and neonatal involvement, but mainly with infection late in pregnancy. Brown and co-workers (1987) found that serious morbidity occurred in 6 of 15 infants born to women with primary infections in pregnancy and in 4 of

5 with primary infection in the third trimester. Overall, maternal seroconversion to HSV-2 in pregnancy does not result in greater risks of low birth weight, lower gestational age, growth restriction, stillbirth, or neonatal death (Brown et al., 1997).

Transplacental infection of the fetus resulting in congenital infection is a rare sequel to maternal infection, presumably arising from primary infections with viremia. Only a few such documented cases have been reported (Hutto et al., 1987).

When episodes recur in pregnancy, there appears to be no increase in abortion or low-birth-weight infants (Kulhanjian et al., 1992). When nonprimary first episodes occur in pregnancy, the clinical course is variable from mild, resembling recurrent episodes (Brown et al., 1987), to severe, resembling primary infection (Hensleigh et al., 1997). The likelihood of perinatal acquisition has also been reported as variable (Brown et al., 1987, 1991). One report shows that recent acquisition of genital HSV, whether primary or nonprimary first episode, is associated with a high rate of perinatal infection (Brown et al., 1997).

A major perinatal problem is neonatal herpes infection. Exact estimates of its frequency are subject to error, because up to 50% of infants with culture-proven fatal disease may not show typical lesions on the skin or mucous membranes. In addition, recent treatment recommendations have probably decreased the incidence of neonatal disease.

Neonatal herpes is acquired perinatally from an infected lower maternal genital tract, most commonly during vaginal delivery. Only those women with very recent infection (i.e., presence of virus in the genital tract, but without development of type-specific antibody) had infected infants (Brown et al., 1997). Here the risk is high (four of nine cases). The risk is considerably lower among women with recurrent clinically evident infection. In these women, the risk is probably now best estimated as being in the range of 1% to 2%. In one study, the risk to infants born vaginally to women with asymptomatic recurrent infection was 0 of 34 (Prober et al., 1987). Asymptomatically infected patients can give birth to seriously infected neonates. In a referral nursery, 70% of mothers of infected infants had asymptomatic infections. Among infants with disseminated herpes, the risk of death or serious sequelae is about 50%. Thus, maternal antibodies do not offer complete protection to the neonate (Nahmias et al., 1971; Amstey and Monif, 1974).

Diagnosis

The clinical diagnosis of genital herpes is based on typical, painful crops of vesicles and ulcers in various stages of progression. With primary infection, there is apt to be regional lymphadenopathy, fever, and other more marked constitutional symptoms. Primary genital herpes lesions usually last 2 to 3 weeks. Clinically detectable recurrences are variable, but about 50% of patients have recurrent disease within 6 months. Recurrences are milder, with fewer lesions, fewer constitutional symptoms, and a shorter course (usually 10 to 14 days). However, there is great individual variation, and proper classification of first episodes of genital HSV infection in pregnancy cannot be made correctly on clinical criteria alone (Hensleigh et al., 1997).

One third of women with genital herpes do not have typical lesions. Although herpes infection may be suggested by rather typical changes seen in Papanicolaou smears (intranuclear inclusion bodies and multinucleated giant cells), the 20% to 25% rate of false-negative results is too high for this to be used with diagnostic accuracy. The "gold standard" diagnostic test to detect the presence of herpesvirus infection has been the viral culture, but even the culture has a recognized false-negative rate. For clinical use, it is fortunate that this virus grows rapidly, with most positive cultures being identifiable at 48 to 72 hours. Rapid diagnostic tests are currently available, including a monoclonal antibody test and ELISA. As with rapid techniques for other genital infections, these methods have their best performance in high-prevalence populations. They may be reliable (compared to culture) in patients with vesicular or ulcerative genital lesions. As with other infectious agents, HSV can now also be detected by PCR, which is more sensitive than standard culture techniques and is becoming more widely available.

Neonatal herpes infection may be limited to the skin, or it may be systemic with or without cutaneous involvement. Typically, clinical disease begins at the end of the 1st week of life. Because the findings depend on the organ system involved, the presentation may include skin lesions, cough, cyanosis, tachypnea, dyspnea, jaundice, seizures, and disseminated intravascular coagulation. In infants at risk for, or suspected of having, neonatal herpes, the only reliable diagnostic test is the viral culture.

A few infants have been described with congenital (transplacental) herpes infection. Congenital infection has been manifested by typical cutaneous lesions apparent within 24 to 48 hours of life; fetal infection presumably occurs a few days before birth. In other cases, there have been less-specific clinical signs (microcephaly and spasticity), but serologic evidence of infection is present. Transplacental infection presumably results from maternal viremia, which occurs only with primary maternal infection (Hutto et al., 1987).

In the individual patient, most commercially available serologic techniques have little utility. Cross-reactivity of antibodies to serotypes 1 and 2 preclude differentiation. One use of these commercial tests is to rule out previous genital herpes in a patient with an unconfirmed or equivocal history by demonstrating absence of antibodies to both HSV-1 and HSV-2. A reliable antibody test to distinguish type 2 from type 1 is available through specialty research laboratories. Type-specific antibody to type 2 glycoprotein G is used (Kulhanjian et al., 1992). The test requires 1 mL of serum, and turn-around time is usually 3 to 5 days. Although IgG antibodies usually develop in a few weeks, it may take longer (12 to 16 weeks) for the full antibody response to develop.

Treatment

During clinically evident episodes, treatment consists of supportive measures such as analgesics, hygiene, and good topical anesthetics. Secondary infections such as *Monilia* should also be treated. Many women find that frequent bathing, followed by thorough drying of the affected area with a hair dryer, provides temporary relief.

Acyclovir, an antiviral agent with excellent activity against herpes infection, is a specific inhibitor of viral thymidine kinase. It is available in topical, oral, and intravenous preparations. In nonpregnant individuals, all of the forms have been of value in decreasing the duration of symptoms and of viral shedding in primary genital infection. In immunocompetent persons, the oral form is also effective in shortening some recurrences significantly (400 mg orally three times daily for 5 days) and in suppressing frequent recurrences (400 mg orally twice daily for 2 years or more). The safety of using of acyclovir during pregnancy has not been established, but a registry has not shown an increase in major birth defects (Reiff-Eldridge, et al., 2000). A prospective randomized trial of acyclovir (400 mg three times daily) from 36 weeks of gestation until delivery was carried out in women with first-episode genital herpes in pregnancy (Scott et al., 1996). No serologic testing was performed to distinguish maternal primary from nonprimary first-episode infections. There was a significant reduction in maternal infection at delivery and in cesarean delivery because of genital herpes infection ($P = 0.002$ for each). Another study was also supportive of suppressive acyclovir in pregnancy (Brocklehurst et al., 1998).

For treatment of genital herpes, famciclovir (Famvir), and valacyclovir (Valtrex) have the advantage of a better absorption and a longer half-life than acyclovir, and both are indicated for the treatment of recurrent genital herpes. Both have been classified as class B by the Food and Drug Administration, but experience with use in pregnancy is very limited (CDC, 2002).

Pregnancy Management

Because of the severity of neonatal herpes infection and the lack of satisfactory therapy, the only current means of preventing neonatal infection is to avoid contact between the fetus and the infected maternal lower genital tract by means of cesarean section. Accordingly, cesarean section is recommended when typical herpes lesions are present at labor, regardless of duration since membrane rupture (ACOG, 1988; Gibbs et al., 1988; CDC, 2002). Although the cost effectiveness of this approach has been questioned (Randolph et al., 1993), the practitioner is advised to follow the 1988 guidelines until new data are available (Gibbs et al., 1993). Asymptomatic pregnant women with positive viral cultures (recurrent herpes) are at low risk for perinatal infant transmission.

In 1986, Arvin and colleagues reported HSV cultures in a series of 515 pregnant women with recurrent herpes infection. Seventeen had positive antepartum cultures, but none was positive at delivery. Of 354 asymptomatic mothers, 5 (1.4%) had positive results at delivery, but none had positive antepartum cultures. The likelihood of asymptomatic shedding at delivery was 1.3%. Later, the same group reported a series of 34 neonates born vaginally to women with asymptomatic infection. None became infected, leading to a maximum theoretical risk of 8% (Prober et al., 1987).

Over the past years, some recommendations have changed:

1. The obstetrician should ask all pregnant women about a history of genital herpes.
2. If the diagnosis of genital herpes has not previously been confirmed by culture or PCR, specimens should be obtained during an active episode of apparent HSV infection.
3. Serial cultures beginning at 34 to 36 weeks are *not* recommended for *asymptomatic women* with a history of herpes infection.
4. The patient with a history of genital herpes should be instructed to come to the hospital early in labor or immediately

if PROM has occurred. Also, the patient should be informed of the low risk of asymptomatic infection at delivery (1%) and the low risk of neonatal infection after delivery through an asymptomatically infected genital tract.

5. When the patient arrives in labor with membrane rupture, a careful pelvic examination should be performed. If no lesions are present, the delivery can be managed normally. If lesions are observed, cesarean section is recommended to prevent neonatal herpes.

Newborns of mothers with nongenital herpes do not require any special precautions during labor and delivery. After the mother has contact, however, the possibility of herpes should be considered in the neonate, and management should proceed as just described.

Specimens should be obtained for culture from infants thought to have herpes and examined closely. If the parents are reliable, it is not necessary to delay the infant's discharge. Rather, the parents may be informed of signs and symptoms of possible neonatal infection and may then be contacted regularly by telephone.

Because the mother with nongenital herpes at delivery may also infect the newborn, many of the precautions advised for control of genital herpes are recommended. These include gown and glove precautions and proper disposal of linen and dressings. After the lesions have become encrusted, the mother may handle and feed her infant, provided that precautions used for women with genital herpes are followed.

Human Parvovirus Infection

Epidemiology

Human parvovirus B_{19} is a single-stranded DNA virus. It is distributed worldwide, and infection may occur in both a sporadic and an epidemic form. Humans are the only known host for the B_{19} virus. The organism is transmitted by respiratory droplets and infected blood components, and the incubation period is 4 to 20 days. Mothers of young children and school teachers are at particular risk for exposure to infection (Gillespie et al., 1990; Cartter et al., 1991). Serum and respiratory secretions become positive for the virus several days before clinical symptoms develop. Once symptoms appear, respiratory secretions and serum are usually free of the virus, and the patient is no longer contagious. Prevalence of antibody to parvovirus increases with age. Approximately 2% to 15% of preschool children are seropositive; in adolescents and adults, the seroprevalence increases to more than 60% (CDC, 1989; Public Health Laboratory Service Working Party on Fifth Disease, 1990).

Clinical Presentation

The most common clinical presentation of parvovirus infection is *erythema infectiosum* or *fifth disease*. This illness typically occurs in children in the late winter and early spring. Affected individuals have low-grade fever, malaise, adenopathy, polyarthritis, an erythematous "slapped cheek" rash on the face, and a finely reticulated erythematous rash on the trunk and extremities. The rash may wax and wane over a period of several months in response to stress, exercise, sunlight, or bathing. Erythema infectiosum is a self-limited illness, and complete recovery is the norm.

A second major clinical presentation is *transient aplastic crisis*. This disorder occurs primarily in individuals who have an underlying hemoglobinopathy and results from viral infection of the bone marrow. Affected patients have prodromal symptoms similar to those seen in erythema infectiosum. One to 7 days after the onset of the prodrome, signs of anemia develop. Patients with transient aplastic crisis usually do not have a skin rash. Given appropriate supportive care, full recovery without sequelae is the usual outcome.

Diagnosis

The best means of diagnosing maternal infection is detection of serum IgM and IgG antibody. Antibody to parvovirus can be measured by enzyme immunoassays, immunofluorescent assays, and Western blots. Assays that use a baculovirus-based vector appear to have greater sensitivity and specificity than do *E. coli*-based assays. IgM-specific antibody is usually positive by the 3rd day after symptoms develop. IgM typically disappears within 30 to 60 days but may persist for up to 120 days. IgG antibody is detectable by the 7th day of illness and usually persists for life. Recurrent and persistent parvovirus infection has been documented, but such cases are extremely rare.

Congenital Parvovirus Infection

Following a documented exposure to parvovirus, the mother should immediately have a serologic test to determine if she is immune or susceptible to the virus. If pre-existing IgG antibody is present, the patient can be reassured that second infections are extremely unlikely and that her fetus is not at risk. If the patient is susceptible, she should have a repeat serologic test in approximately 3 weeks to determine whether she has seroconverted. If seroconversion is detected, serial ultrasound examinations should be performed to evaluate fetal well-being. The incubation period for congenital parvovirus infection may be longer than in a child or adult. Approximately 85% of cases of severe fetal infection become apparent within 10 weeks of exposure (Rodis et al., 1990).

Fetal hydrops is the most ominous manifestation of congenital parvovirus infection. Hydrops results primarily from viral infection of fetal erythroid stem cells, which leads to aplastic anemia and heart failure. The virus specifically targets the erythrocyte P antigen. Cardiac failure may also result from direct infection of the myocardium by the virus as well as from hepatitic injury, which leads to impaired protein synthesis and decreased colloid oncotic pressure. Hydrops occurs in up to 10% of cases when maternal infection develops in the first 20 weeks of pregnancy. The risk of serious fetal injury declines to less than 5% when maternal infection occurs after 20 weeks' gestation.

If fetal hydrops is documented by ultrasound, cordocentesis should be performed if technically feasible (Peters and Nicolaides, 1990). Although case reports have described spontaneous resolution of hydrops in infected fetuses, criteria predictive of such a good outcome are not well established (Humphrey et al., 1991; Pryde et al., 1992). Therefore, if severe anemia is present, intrauterine transfusion is indicated. If intravascular transfusion is impossible because of gestational age, intraperitoneal transfusion may be feasible.

Fairly and colleagues (1995) recently reported the outcome of 66 fetuses with hydrops resulting from maternal parvovirus infection. In 26 cases the fetus was dead at the time of initial assessment, and in 2 cases, therapeutic abortion was performed. Twelve of the 38 fetuses who were alive at the time hydrops was diagnosed had intrauterine transfusions; 3 of the 12 died. Twenty-six fetuses did not undergo transfusion, and 13 died. After adjustment for severity of hydrops and gestational age, the odds ratio for death in the fetuses that had transfusions was 0.14 (95% CI, 0.02 to 0.96). In a similar but larger survey, Rodis and co-workers (1998) also demonstrated that transfusion improved fetal outcome. In their analysis, 30% of hydropic fetuses that were not transfused died compared to 16% of fetuses that received transfusions.

Although most infants with congenital parvovirus infection have had normal long-term growth and development, a few adverse outcomes have been reported. Conry and coworkers (1993) described three children with persistent neurologic morbidity following a maternal parvovirus infection at 21 to 24 weeks' gestation. Neurologic abnormalities included hypotonia, arthrogryposis, motor developmental delay, infantile spasms, intracranial calcifications, and ventriculomegaly. One child died on the 6th day of life. Brown and colleagues (1994) described three infants with persistent severe anemia following intrauterine transfusion for parvovirus infection. One of the infants died, and autopsy demonstrated widespread viral infection.

In the largest epidemiology survey yet reported, Rodis and coworkers (1998) evaluated 113 infants delivered to mothers with acute parvovirus infection. A group of 99 infants delivered to mothers with prior infection served as controls. The frequency of developmental delays was similar in the two groups (7.4% versus 7.2%). Two infants in the study group had cerebral palsy compared to none in the control group (NS). However, even this relatively large study had only a 30% power to detect a doubling of the frequency of developmental delay from 7.5% to 15%. Accordingly, clinicians should be cautious in counseling parents about the long-term prognosis for infected neonates.

Influenza

Epidemiology

Influenza is a highly contagious acute respiratory infection that is of major clinical importance both in the United States and worldwide. In the United States, the disease causes 10,000 to 40,000 excess deaths and more than 150,000 excess hospitalizations annually (Patriarca and Strikas, 1995). Influenza is caused by an RNA virus belonging to the *Orthomyxoviridae* family. This family has two major serotypes, A and B, that are responsible for the vast majority of cases of influenza (Patriarca and Strikas, 1995).

The virus is transmitted primarily by respiratory droplets and, to a limited extent, by direct contact. The incubation period is relatively short—1 to 5 days. Influenza occurs most commonly in the late fall and winter, and epidemics recur with regularity because the virus mutates in important ways from year to year. Thus, immunity to the strains that caused infection in one year does not necessarily provide protection against strains that circulate in subsequent years.

Clinical Manifestations

Influenza can range in severity from a mild respiratory infection to a life-threatening pneumonia. The illness typically begins abruptly with prodromal symptoms of malaise, myalgia, and headache in association with fever. Subsequently, the patient develops a dry, nonproductive cough, coryza, mild dyspnea, and sore throat. On physical examination, the temperature is elevated and the pharynx is inflamed; auscultation of the chest discloses rales and rhonchi. In some patients, a secondary bacterial pneumonia may develop, and their cough then becomes productive of purulent sputum (Carlan and Knuppel, 1994).

Diagnosis

The presence of the clinical manifestations outlined above is highly suggestive of influenza. The diagnosis can be confirmed by culturing the virus from respiratory secretions and by documenting characteristic rises in serum antibody to influenza A and B. Chest x-ray also may be of great value in assessing the severity of the pulmonary infection (Carlan and Knuppel, 1994).

Complications of Influenza in Pregnancy

Influenza virus has not been associated with an increased risk of spontaneous abortion, stillbirth, or congenital anomalies. However, an infant delivered to an acutely infected patient may develop neonatal influenza as a result of close personal contact with its mother after delivery. In addition, mothers with severe respiratory infections may have an increased risk of preterm labor. In previous reports of influenza pandemics, pregnant women have experienced increased risk of morbidity and mortality compared to nonpregnant patients.

Preventive Measures

The key to the prevention of influenza is vaccination. Immunization is 70% to 90% effective in either preventing influenza or diminishing the severity of illness (Patriarca and Strikas, 1995).

The composition of the influenza vaccine changes each year. The World Health Organization has a global network that tracks influenza-related morbidity. This surveillance network now includes more than 100 national laboratories in more than 80 countries. Investigators at these centers recommend changes in the vaccine to try to match the viral strains most likely to circulate in the current year.

Influenza vaccine is definitely indicated for all high-risk patients (Table 39-9). The optimal time for administration of the vaccine is from late October through January. For adults and children over the age of 3 years, a single intramuscular 0.5-mL dose is sufficient (Anonymous, 2001). Although the vaccine is an inactivated agent and should be safe for administration at any time during pregnancy, the CDC currently recommends deferring vaccination of pregnant women until beyond the first trimester. Delay is not warranted if the patient has a high-risk medical disorder or if the flu season will be over before completion of the first trimester.

In addition to the individuals listed in Table 39-9, published evidence also supports the value of immunizing even healthy

TABLE 39-9. RECOMMENDATIONS FOR INFLUENZA VACCINE

1. Pregnant aged ≥ 50 years
2. Pregnant women who will be in the 2nd or 3rd trimester of pregnancy during the influenza season
3. Residents of nursing homes and other chronic care facilities that house persons of any age who have chronic medical conditions
4. Adults and children who required medical follow-up or who were hospitalized during the preceding year because of diabetes mellitus, renal dysfunction, hemoglobinopathies, or immunosuppression
5. Adults and children with chronic disorders of the pulmonary or cardiovascular system, including asthma
6. Children and adolescents who are receiving long-term aspirin therapy and therefore might be at risk for developing Reye syndrome after influenza infection
7. Health-care workers

From Centers for Disease Control and Prevention (CDC): Prevention and control of influenza: Recommendations of the Advisory Committee on Immunization Practice (ACIP). MMWR Morb Mortal Wkly Rep **49**(RR-3), 2000.

adults. In a recent investigation, Nichol and colleagues (1995) conducted a randomized trial of vaccination in 841 healthy adults. Patients in the treatment arm of the study had significant reductions in rates of illness, use of sick leave, and visits to physicians' offices. The net savings per person vaccinated were approximately $47.00. On the basis of this investigation, the CDC now recommends that the influenza vaccination be provided to any healthy adult or child upon request.

Antiviral chemotherapy also can be used to prevent influenza in persons who were not vaccinated or who were vaccinated within 2 weeks of a community outbreak. For a number of years, amantadine and rimantadine have been used as prophylactic agents. Each of these drugs is approximately 70% to 90% effective in preventing clinical illness resulting from influenza A in healthy young adults. However, these drugs are ineffective against influenza B. In addition, they may cause prominent CNS toxicity and are not well tolerated by all patients, particularly the elderly. Moreover, amantadine should not be used during pregnancy because of concern about teratogenicity.

Two new drugs have recently been approved for prophylaxis against influenza A and B (Anonymous, 1999, 2001; Cox and Hughes, 1999). Both are neuraminidase inhibitors and exert their effect by decreasing the release of virus from infected cells. Zanamivir is administered as a dry powder by inhalation in a 10-mg dose twice daily. In a 4-week trial, Monto and co-workers (1999) observed that the drug was 67% effective in preventing illness and 84% effective in preventing "febrile influenza." Oseltamivir is administered orally in a dose of 75 mg twice daily. In a 6-week trial, Hayden and associates (1999) noted a significant reduction in the incidence of influenza in patients who received oseltamivir compared to those who received placebo (4.8% versus 1.2%).

Treatment

Pregnant women who develop influenza despite vaccination (or in the absence of vaccination) should be advised to remain at home and rest. They should maintain hydration and use acetaminophen (650 mg orally every 4 to 6 hours, maximum 4 g/24 hours) as needed to lower their temperature and reduce discomfort from headache and myalgias. They should be reevaluated immediately if signs of worsening pneumonia or preterm labor develop. In addition, if they have disabling symptoms, they should be offered treatment with either zanamivir (10 mg twice daily for 5 days) or oseltamivir (75 to 150 mg orally twice daily for 5 days) (Anonymous, 1999).

Rubeola

Epidemiology

The measles virus is a single-stranded RNA paramyxovirus that is closely related to the canine distemper virus. The wild virus is pathogenic only for primates, and humans are the only natural host.

The virus is spread by respiratory droplets and is highly contagious. Seventy-five to 90% of susceptible contacts become infected after exposure. Before a measles vaccine was available, essentially all children developed a natural measles infection. Since licensure of the first measles vaccine in 1963, however, the incidence of infection has decreased by almost 99%. As expected, children less than 10 years of age have shown the greatest decline in incidence. During the mid-1980s, almost 60% of reported cases affected children greater than 10 years of age compared with only 10% during the period from 1960 to 1964 (National Vaccine Advisory Committee, 1991).

In recent years, two major types of measles outbreaks have occurred in the United States. One type has developed among unvaccinated preschoolers, including children less than 15 months of age. Another has occurred among previously vaccinated school-age children and college students. Approximately one third of the cases in the latter type of outbreak have been in individuals who were previously vaccinated. Presumably, these cases result from either *primary failure* to respond to the first vaccine or *secondary failure*, a situation in which an adequate serologic response develops initially, with waning of immunity over time (National Vaccine Advisory Committee, 1991; Hersh et al., 1992).

The clinical manifestations of measles usually appear within 10 to 14 days of exposure. The most common are fever, malaise, coryza, sneezing, conjunctivitis, cough, photophobia, and Koplik spots (blue-gray specks on a red base that develop on the buccal mucosa opposite the second molars). All patients typically develop a generalized nonpruritic maculopapular rash that begins on the face and neck and then spreads to the trunk and extremities. It usually lasts for approximately 5 days and subsequently recedes in the order in which it appeared. The duration of illness is approximately 7 to 10 days. Patients are contagious from 1 to 4 days before the onset of coryza until several days after appearance of the rash. Immunity to measles should be lifelong following wild virus infection and is mediated by both humoral and cell-mediated mechanisms.

Although measles is typically a minor illness, some patients develop serious sequelae. Otitis media occurs in 7% to 9% of infected patients; bronchiolitis and pneumonia affect 1% to 6%. A severe form of hepatitis may also occur. In a recent report by Atmar and associates (1992), 7 of 13 pregnant women (54%) with measles developed hepatitis.

Encephalitis occurs in approximately 1 in 1000 cases of measles. It results from both viral infection of the CNS and a hypersensitivity reaction to the systemic viral infection. Measles encephalitis may lead to permanent neurologic impairment, including mental retardation; the mortality rate from this complication is approximately 15% to 33%. Another unusual, but extremely serious, complication of measles is subacute sclerosing panencephalitis. This complication occurs in 0.5 to 2 cases per 1000. It usually develops about 7 years after the acute measles infection and is more common in children who had measles before the age of 2 years. The disorder is characterized by progressive neurologic debilitation and a virtually uniformly fatal outcome (National Vaccine Advisory Committee, 1991; Atmar et al., 1992).

A final complication is *atypical measles*. This disorder is a severe form of measles reinfection that affects young adults previously vaccinated with the formalin-inactivated killed measles vaccine that was distributed in the United States from 1963 to 1967. Affected patients have extremely high antibody titers to measles, and they experience high fever, pneumonitis, pleural effusion, and a coarse maculopapular, hemorrhagic, or urticarial rash. Although the disease is usually self-limited, atypical measles can lead to hepatic, cardiac, and renal failure. Interestingly, affected patients are not contagious to others (National Vaccine Advisory Committee, 1991; Atkinson et al., 1992).

Five clinical criteria should be present to establish the diagnosis of measles: fever of 38.3° C or higher, characteristic rash lasting longer than 3 days, cough, coryza, and conjunctivitis. Although the virus can be cultured, the mainstay of diagnostic tests is detection of antibody to measles. The hemagglutination inhibition assay and ELISA are the most useful serologic tests for determination of a patient's susceptibility to measles and for confirmation of infection. The serologic confirmation of acute measles virus infection is based on detection of IgM-specific antibody or a fourfold change in the IgG titer in acute and convalescent sera. The acute titer for IgG antibody should be obtained within 3 days of the onset of the rash, and the convalescent titer, 10 to 20 days later.

A variety of other infections should be considered in the differential diagnosis of rubeola, including rubella, scarlet fever, Rocky Mountain spotted fever, toxoplasmosis, enterovirus infection, mononucleosis, meningococcemia, and serum sickness. Differentiation among these conditions usually is possible on the basis of physical examination and serologic testing.

Obstetric Considerations

Several reports have documented an increase in maternal mortality associated with measles infection during pregnancy; most fatalities have been due to pulmonary complications. In one of the earliest investigations, Christensen and colleagues (1953), described an epidemic of measles in Greenland in 1951. Four of 83 pregnant women (4.8%) who developed measles died. An unspecified number of these women also had active tuberculosis. In the report by Atmar et al. (1992), one of 13 pregnant women (8%) with measles died because of severe respiratory infection. In a more recent publication, Eberhart-Phillips and co-workers (1993) evaluated 58 pregnant women with measles. Thirty-five (60%) required hospitalization, 15 (26%) developed pneumonia, and 2 (3%) died.

Reports have also described a slight increase in the frequency of preterm delivery and spontaneous abortion among women who develop measles during pregnancy. In the study by Eberhart-Phillips and colleagues (1993), 13 of 50 women (26%) with continuing pregnancies delivered preterm. Fortunately, the frequency of congenital anomalies is not increased significantly in women who contract measles during pregnancy.

Although congenital anomalies are rare, infants of mothers who are acutely infected at the time of delivery are at risk for *neonatal measles*. This infection typically develops within the first 10 days of life and results from transplacental transmission of the virus. The mortality in preterm and term infants with neonatal measles has been as high as 60% and 20%, respectively (Stein and Grinspoon, 1991).

Preventive Measures

Ideally, all women of reproductive age should have evidence of immunity to measles before attempting pregnancy. Originally, public health officials thought that a single injection of live measles vaccine when a child was approximately 15 months of age provided lifelong immunity. As noted previously, however, several recent outbreaks of measles have been due to secondary vaccine failures. Accordingly, the Advisory Committee on Immunization Practices now recommends that all individuals who have not been infected with the live virus receive a second dose of the vaccine at 4 to 6 years of age. If this second dose is not administered in childhood, it should be administered before a woman plans her first pregnancy. There are only three contraindications to use of the live measles vaccine: pregnancy, severe febrile illness, and history of anaphylactic reaction to egg protein or neomycin (Stein and Grinspoon, 1991).

If a susceptible pregnant woman is exposed to measles, she should immediately receive passive immunoprophylaxis with immune globulin, 0.25 mL/kg intramuscularly, up to a maximum dose of 15 mL. If she develops measles despite immunoprophylaxis, she should be observed for evidence of serious complications such as otitis media, hepatitis, encephalitis, and pneumonia. Secondary bacterial infections should be treated promptly with antibiotics. Administration of aerosolized ribavirin may be of benefit to patients with severe viral pneumonitis (CDC, 1992).

The affected patient should be counseled that the risk of injury to her fetus is very low. The most effective method for evaluating the fetus for *in utero* infection is detailed ultrasound examination. Findings suggestive of *in utero* infection include microcephaly, growth restriction, and oligohydramnios. Neonates delivered to a mother who has developed measles within 7 to 10 days of delivery should receive intramuscular immunoglobulin in a dose of 0.25 mg/kg. These infants should subsequently receive the live measles vaccine when they are 15 months of age (CDC, 1989, 1992).

Mumps

Mumps, which is an acute generalized nonexanthematous infection with a predilection for the parotid and salivary glands, may also affect the brain, pancreas, and gonads. The mumps virus is a member of the paramyxovirus family and is thus an RNA virus. It is transmitted by saliva and droplet contamination and has been recovered from salivary and respiratory secretions from 7 days prior to the onset of parotitis until 9 days afterward. The usual incubation period is 14 to 18 days.

The prodrome of mumps consists of fever, malaise, myalgia, and anorexia. Parotitis occurs within 24 hours and is characterized by a swollen and tender parotid gland. The orifice of Stensen duct is usually red and swollen. In most cases parotitis is bilateral. The submaxillary glands are involved less often and almost never without parotid gland involvement. The sublingual glands are rarely affected. Although mumps is generally a self-limited and complication-free disease, it can be a significant cause of morbidity. It may cause aseptic meningitis, pancreatitis, mastitis, thyroiditis, myocarditis, nephritis, and arthritis.

Mumps in pregnant women is generally benign and no more severe than in nonpregnant patients. Aseptic meningitis in pregnant patients is neither more common nor more severe. Mortality in association with mumps is extremely rare in both pregnant and nonpregnant patients.

Retrospective studies have suggested that mumps during the first trimester is associated with a twofold increase in the incidence of spontaneous abortion. No significant association between maternal mumps infection and prematurity, intrauterine growth restriction, or perinatal mortality has been demonstrated (Monif, 1974).

The role of mumps virus in congenital disease remains controversial (Gershon, 1990). Despite animal studies in which mumps virus induced congenital malformations, definitive evidence of a teratogenic potential for mumps virus in humans has not been reported. Siegal (1973) has noted that the rate of congenital malformation in infants born to women who had mumps during pregnancy (2 of 117) was essentially the same rate as in infants born to uninfected mothers (2 of 123). The predominant concern has been the postulated association between maternal mumps infection and the development of subsequent congenital cardiac abnormalities, specifically endocardial fibroelastosis (St. Geme et al., 1966). The issue remains unresolved.

The treatment of mumps is symptomatic in pregnant as well as in nonpregnant patients. Analgesics, bed rest, and application of cold or heat to the parotids are useful. Maternal mumps is not an indication for termination of pregnancy. The live-attenuated mumps vaccine has been effective in preventing primary mumps. Ninety-five percent of vaccinated susceptible subjects develop antibodies without clinically adverse reactions. The duration of protection afforded by immunization is not known.

Although mumps vaccine virus has been recovered from the fetal placental tissue in susceptible women vaccinated during pregnancy, there is no evidence that the vaccine virus is teratogenic in humans. Nevertheless, immunization with the mumps live-virus vaccine in pregnancy is contraindicated on the theoretical grounds that the developing fetus might be harmed. Although the risk to the fetus seems negligible, the innocuous nature of mumps in pregnancy suggests that vaccination is unwarranted. Live mumps vaccine, when given with rubella, should not be administered to women known to be pregnant or considering becoming pregnant in the next 3 months. Women vaccinated with monovalent mumps vaccine should not become pregnant for at least 1 month. Vaccination with mumps vaccine in pregnancy should not be considered an indication for pregnancy termination, however.

Echoviruses

The echoviruses, along with polio and coxsackieviruses, are classified as enteroviruses. Echoviruses are responsible for a variety of illnesses, including respiratory disease, rash, gastroenteritis, conjunctivitis, aseptic meningitis, and pericarditis.

Many neonatally acquired infections caused by echoviruses have been reported. The clinical findings associated with neonatal echovirus infection include fever with splenomegaly and lymphadenopathy, macular rashes, diarrhea and vomiting, pneumonitis, otitis media, jaundice, coryza with cough, and septic meningitis.

This infection in pregnancy has not been associated with abortions, premature delivery, stillbirths, or congenital malformations; however, congenital echovirus infection can produce significant disease in the neonate. For example, echovirus 14 has been reported to be the cause of a febrile illness that developed at 3 days of life and progressed to cyanotic episodes, hypothermia, hepatomegaly, bradycardia, and purpura, and to death at 7 days of life (Hughes et al., 1972). Echovirus 19 has been reported to be the cause of hepatic necrosis and massive hemorrhage in three infants (Philip and Larsen, 1973).

Most infections are acquired in the immediate perinatal period, with 63% of cases having onset between the 3rd and 5th days of life (Modlin, 1986). Nearly 70% of the affected mothers have an acute illness within 1 week of delivery. Of the 61 reported cases of neonatal echovirus infection, 43 (70%) were due to echovirus 11.

No treatment or vaccine is available for echovirus infections.

Coxsackieviruses

Coxsackieviruses are RNA viruses of the enterovirus group. They are divided into group A (23 types) and group B (6 types). Those in group A do not cause significant perinatal illness except in rare cases.

The viruses in group B can cause pleurodynia, meningoencephalitis, and myocarditis. Hepatitis and pneumonia are infrequent but severe manifestations of group B coxsackievirus infection. Transplacental transmission has been demonstrated, but the magnitude of risk to the fetus has not been defined. Most maternal group B coxsackievirus infections result in no demonstrable adverse effects on the fetus.

Diagnosis is based on virus isolation from throat or rectum and serologic evidence of increasing antibody titer during the convalescent period. Hemagglutination inhibition or complement fixation tests may be performed.

No treatment or vaccination is available for the coxsackie viruses.

SEXUALLY TRANSMITTED DISEASES

Syphilis

Syphilis is a chronic systemic infectious process resulting from the spirochete *Treponema pallidum*. It has been recognized for several centuries that primary, secondary, and early latent syphilis in pregnant women cause infection of the fetus, with resultant stillbirths, congenital abnormalities, and active disease at birth. Because of this significant morbidity, great emphasis has been placed on routine screening of all pregnant women for syphilis. Acquisition is generally through sexual contact.

Epidemiology

With the introduction of penicillin in the 1940s, the total number of cases of syphilis, including congenital syphilis, in the United States progressively decreased. This trend then reversed, and the number of reported cases of primary and secondary syphilis (the best indicator of incidence trends) began steadily increasing, reaching a peak of 14.6 cases per 100,000 population in 1982, in large part because of increases among homosexual and bisexual men. Subsequently, a decrease of syphilis was again noted, due in large part to a decrease among homosexual males with the advent of the acquired immunodeficiency syndrome epidemic.

In the late 1980s, an increased incidence of primary and secondary syphilis was again seen in the United States (Rolfs and Nakoshima, 1990). Coincident with this rise was a dramatic increase in reported cases of congenital syphilis (CDC, 1988; Ricci et al., 1989). Following a low of 108 cases of congenital syphilis in 1978, there were 350 cases reported in 1986 and 3850 cases reported in 1992, with an incidence rate of 100 per 100,000 live births. Nearly 90% of congenital syphilis cases were among blacks or Hispanics, and 50% occurred among mothers receiving no prenatal care.

Reasons for this dramatic upsurge include exchange of drugs (e.g., "crack" cocaine) for sex, decreased funding for syphilis control, treatment of penicillinase-producing *Neisseria gonorrhoeae* with spectinomycin, which does not treat incubating syphilis, and the use of revised reporting guidelines for congenital syphilis, which were introduced in 1989. This latest epidemic of syphilis peaked in 1990, with 18.4 cases per 100,000 persons and more than 112,000 reported cases of primary and secondary syphilis. By 2000, this figure was reduced to less than 6000 reported cases, a rate of 2.2 cases of primary and secondary syphilis per 100,000 population.

Clinical Manifestations

After exposure, there is an incubation period ranging from 10 to 90 days (average, 21 days) before the *primary lesion* appears. The chancre is a painless, ulcerated lesion with a raised border and an indurated base. Painless inguinal lymphadenopathy is frequently present. Chancres on the external genitalia are easily recognized; more commonly, however, the lesion is on the cervix or in the vagina and is therefore not detected. Without treatment, the primary chancre spontaneously resolves in 2 to 6 weeks.

Following this, the patient enters the *secondary*, or *bacteremic*, stage of syphilis. The clinical manifestations of secondary syphilis include a generalized maculopapular rash involving the palms and soles, mucous patches, condylomata lata, and generalized lymphadenopathy. Syphilis always disseminates during the secondary stage, and thus any organ, including the CNS, can be affected. During the secondary stage, the CNS is invaded by spirochetes in 40% of cases (Lukehart et al., 1988).

These findings spontaneously clear within 2 to 6 weeks, and the *latent stage* of syphilis ensues, in which there is no apparent clinical disease. In about 25% of patients, the *early latent phase*

(< 1 year's duration) may be associated with an exacerbation of secondary syphilis in which the mucocutaneous lesions are infectious. The *late latent stage* (> 1 year's duration) is not infectious by sexual transmission, but the spirochete may still be transmitted transplacentally to the fetus.

If treatment for primary, secondary, or latent syphilis is not provided, *tertiary syphilis* develops in one third of patients, with involvement of the cardiovascular, central nervous, or musculoskeletal system or involvement of various organ systems by gummas (*late benign tertiary syphilis*).

Congenital Syphilis

Following the dramatic surge in cases of primary and secondary syphilis in the late 1980s and early 1990s, there was a subsequent rapid rise in cases of congenital syphilis. This epidemic peaked in 1991, when nearly 4500 cases of congenital syphilis occurred in the United States (CDC, 1999). Fortunately, by 2000 only 529 cases were reported to the CDC. According to the CDC (1996a), over 80% of reported congenital syphilis cases occur because of inadequate or no treatment of mothers infected with syphilis; in addition, 35.8% of cases were seen in infants delivered to mothers who received no prenatal care.

Research has documented that *T. pallidum* can be transferred across the placenta and can infect the fetus as early as 6 weeks of gestation (Harter and Benirschke, 1976). Clinical manifestations are not apparent until after 16 weeks of gestation, when fetal immunocompetence develops. Thus, the risk to the fetus is present throughout pregnancy, and the degree of risk is related to the quantity of spirochetes in the maternal bloodstream. Transmission may also occur intrapartum via contact with active genital lesions in the mother (Hollier and Cox, 1993). Women with primary or secondary syphilis are more likely to transmit infection to their offspring than are women with latent disease. Maternal primary syphilis and secondary syphilis are associated with a 50% probability of congenital syphilis and a 50% rate of perinatal death; maternal early latent syphilis, with a 40% risk of congenital syphilis and a 20% mortality rate; and maternal late syphilis, with a 10% risk of congenital syphilis (Fiumara et al., 1952; Fiumara and Lessel, 1970). Ingraham (1951) also reported high rates of morbidity and mortality among the infants of mothers with untreated syphilis of less than 4 years' duration. He noted a perinatal death rate of 43% (29% were stillborn, and 14% died during the neonatal period); among liveborn infants, 41% had congenital syphilis.

More-recent experience has confirmed that untreated syphilis is associated with significant and frequent adverse effects on pregnancy. Ricci and associates (1989) reported that among 56 cases of congenital syphilis, 19 (35%) were stillbirths, and the perinatal mortality was 464 per 1000 live births. Preterm labor and delivery were significantly more common, infants with congenital syphilis had significantly lower birth weights, and 21% had intrauterine growth restriction. McFarlin and coworkers (1994) reviewed 253 cases of maternal syphilis in Detroit. They reported a preterm delivery rate of 28%, and 10 of 72 cases (13.9%) of congenital syphilis were stillbirths. In addition, the manifestations of congenital syphilis are usually less severe in association with long-standing maternal disease than with early syphilis (less than 1 year's duration). Coles and colleagues (1995), in a review of

322 cases of congenital syphilis from 1989 to 1992, reported that 31 (10%) stillbirths and 59 (19%) newborns with clinical evidence of congenital syphilis were documented. Factors believed to contribute to development of congenital syphilis included infection late in pregnancy, treatment less than 30 days before delivery, misdiagnosis or inappropriate treatment of the mother, and no serologic testing during pregnancy.

The clinical spectrum in congenital syphilis infection includes stillbirth, neonatal death, clinically apparent congenital syphilis during the early months of life (early congenital syphilis), and development of the classic stigmata of late congenital syphilis. The characteristic manifestations of early congenital syphilis include a maculopapular rash that may progress to desquamation or formation of vesicles and bullae, snuffles (a flu-like syndrome associated with a nasal discharge), mucous patches in the oropharyngeal cavity, hepatosplenomegaly, jaundice, lymphadenopathy, chorioretinitis, iritis, and pseudoparalysis of Parrot resulting from osteochondritis. Both cutaneous and mucous lesions contain spirochetes that can be seen on dark-field microscope examination of specimens.

If early congenital syphilis is untreated or incompletely treated, the classic manifestations of late congenital syphilis appear. These include Hutchinson teeth, mulberry molars, interstitial keratitis, eighth nerve deafness, saddle nose, rhagades, saber shins, cardiovascular stigmata, neurologic manifestations (mental retardation, hydrocephalus, general paresis, optic nerve atrophy, and Clutton joints) (Ingall and Norins, 1976).

Diagnosis

The most definitive methods for diagnosis of early syphilis are dark-field microscope examination or direct fluorescent antibody tests of lesion exudate or tissue. Presumptive diagnosis can be made using serologic testing (CDC, 1997). The serologic tests are classified into two types: *nonspecific* tests for reagin-type antibodies and *specific* antitreponemal antibody tests.

Nonspecific antibody tests include the Venereal Disease Research Laboratory (VDRL) test and the rapid plasma reagin test. These are used for screening. All pregnant women should be screened at the initial prenatal visit. High-risk patients should be rescreened at 28 weeks of gestation. In areas with high rates of congenital syphilis, rescreening at admission in labor has been recommended. The CDC (1997) recommends that any woman who delivers a stillborn after 20 weeks of gestation should be screened for syphilis. In addition, it is recommended that no infant should leave the hospital without the maternal serostatus for syphilis having been assessed at some time in pregnancy.

Treponema-specific tests are employed for confirming the diagnosis of syphilis in patients who have reactive VDRL or rapid plasma reagin results. These tests include the *T. pallidum* immobilization test, the fluorescent treponemal antibody absorption test, and the microhemagglutination test for *T. pallidum*.

The pregnant woman with a positive nontreponemal test result should promptly be given a quantitative nontreponemal test (usually the VDRL) and a confirmatory treponemal test such as the fluorescent treponemal antibody absorption test. False-positive reactions can occur with all of these tests but are uncommon with the specific treponemal tests. False-positive results in nontreponemal tests are most often only weak or borderline reactions. Nontreponemal test antibody titers usually correlate with disease activity, and results should be reported quantitatively (CDC, 1997). Usually the nontreponemal result becomes nonreactive after treatment. In some patients, a low titer may persist for a long time, in some cases for life. Once reactive, specific treponemal tests usually remain positive for life. In pregnancy, it is best to consider all fluorescent treponemal antibody absorption test or microhemagglutination test results to be truly positive in order to maximize treatment of the fetus at risk (Jones and Harris, 1979).

It is critical to recognize that when the syphilitic chancre first appears, both the nonspecific treponemal test results and the treponemal-specific test results may be nonreactive. Thus, lesions suspicious for syphilitic chancres should be sampled for detection of spirochetes (dark-field examination or fluorescent-antibody staining).

Although the CNS is involved in nearly half of patients with early syphilis, less than 10% of untreated syphilis progresses to symptomatic late neurosyphilis, and few patients treated appropriately for early syphilis develop neurosyphilis. The CDC has stated that unless clinical signs or symptoms of neurologic involvement are present, lumbar puncture is not recommended for routine evaluation in primary or secondary syphilis. In patients with latent syphilis, prompt CSF examination should be performed for the following:

1. Neurologic or ophthalmologic signs or symptoms
2. Evidence of active tertiary syphilis (e.g., aortitis, gummas, iritis)
3. Treatment failure
4. HIV infection with latent syphilis or syphilis of unknown duration

No single test is adequate to diagnose neurosyphilis among all patients (CDC, 2002a). Thus, the diagnosis is based on various combinations of tests, including reactive serologic tests, abnormal CSF cell count, elevated protein, or a reactive VDRL-CSF (with or without clinical manifestations). CSF demonstrating pleocytosis, elevated protein levels, and a reactive VDRL-CSF is diagnostic of neurosyphilis (CDC, 2002a). On occasion, however, results may be nonreactive when neurosyphilis is present.

The diagnosis of reinfection or persistence of active syphilis can be made in patients previously known to have syphilis by following the titer of the quantitative VDRL. With successful therapy, the VDRL titer should decrease and become negligible within 6 to 12 months in early syphilis and 12 to 24 months in late syphilis of more than 1 year's duration. A rising titer would indicate a need for further diagnostic measures, such as a spinal tap, and appropriate treatment.

The diagnosis of congenital syphilis is easily confirmed in the clinically apparent case in which a jaundiced, hydropic baby with florid disease and a large, edematous placenta are delivered and laboratory studies confirm the presence of the disease. However, most infected newborns are asymptomatic at birth, but the cord blood gives a positive nonspecific test result for syphilis. Any infant with a positive VDRL result but no clinical evidence of syphilis should be given serial monthly quantitative VDRL tests for at least 9 months. A rising titer indicates active disease and the need for therapy. Infected infants may be asymptomatic and the serum VDRL result normal if maternal infection occurred late in pregnancy. In

TABLE 39-10. CONGENITAL SYPHILIS CASE DEFINITION

Confirmed Case

Infant in whom *Treponema palladium* is identified by dark-field microscopy, fluorescent antibody, or other specific stains in specimens from lesions, placenta, umbilical cord, or autopsy material

Presumptive Case

1. Any infant whose mother had untreated* or inadequately treated syphilis at delivery, regardless of signs or symptoms†
   OR
2. Any infant or child who has a reactive treponemal test for syphilis and any one of the following:
   a. Evidence of congenital syphilis on physical examination
   b. Evidence of congenital syphilis on long-bone x-ray
   c. Reactive CSF VDRL
   d. Elevated CSF cell count or protein‡
   e. Reactive test for FTA-ABS-195-IgM antibody

---

* On penicillin therapy of penicillin given <30 days before delivery.
† Clinical signs in an infant include hepatosplenomegaly, characteristic skin rash, condyloma lata, snuffles, jaundice, pseudoparalysis, anemia, thrombocytopenia, or edema. Stigmata in children older than 2 years include interstitial keratitis, nerve deafness, anterior bowing of shins, frontal bossing, mulberry molars, Hutchinson teeth, saddle nose, rhagades, or Clutton joints.
‡ White blood cell count, >5/mm³; protein concentration, >50 mg/dL.

CSF, cerebrospinal fluid; FTA-ABS, fluorescent Treponema antibody absorption; IgM, immunoglobulin M; VDRL, Venereal Disease Research Laboratory.

From Centers for Disease Control and Prevention (CDC): Congenital Syphillis Case Definition. 1998.

1991 the CDC implemented a new case definition for congenital syphilis surveillance (Table 39-10). A diagnosis of congenital syphilis can be confirmed by identifying spirochetes in suspicious lesions, body fluids, or tissues with dark-field microscopy, silver staining, immunofluorescence, or PCR for *T. pallidum* DNA (Genest et al., 1996). Several new laboratory tests have been introduced to facilitate the diagnosis of congenital syphilis. These include (1) the IgMb, Western blot for 47-KD protein, (2) the PCR, and (3) the rabbit infectivity test (RIT).

Treatment

All pregnant women who have a history of sexual contact with a person with documented syphilis, dark-field microscope confirmation of the presence of spirochetes, or serologic evidence of syphilis via a specific treponemal test should be treated. In addition, patients in whom the diagnosis cannot be ruled out with certainty or those who have been previously treated but now show evidence of reinfection, such as dark-field microscope confirmation or a fourfold rise in titer on a quantitative nontreponemal test, should receive appropriate treatment.

Treatment schedules for syphilis recommended by the CDC in 2002 are shown in Table 39-11. Penicillin is the preferred treatment. Secondary drugs are tetracycline and erythromycin. Tetracycline should not be used during pregnancy. Because the efficacy of erythromycin treatment of syphilis in pregnancy is inadequate, this agent is no longer recommended as an alternative for pregnant women with syphilis. In pregnancy, penicillin is effective for preventing transmission to the fetus and

for treating established fetal infection with syphilis. The CDC recommends that treatment during pregnancy should be the penicillin regimen appropriate for the patient's stage of syphilis. Parenteral penicillin G is the only agent with documented efficacy for the treatment of neurosyphilis or syphilis in pregnancy. Those who are allergic to penicillin should be treated with penicillin after being desensitized (CDC, 2002b). In nonpregnant patients the CDC recently suggested that ceftriaxone (1 g daily for 8 to 10 days) may be considered an alternative for the treatment of primary and secondary syphilis (CDC, 2002b). However, no data are available for this drug in pregnant women with syphilis. Parenteral penicillin G has been demonstrated to achieve local cure (healing of lesions and prevention of sexual transmission) and to prevent tertiary syphilis when used in the treatment of primary and secondary syphilis (CDC, 2002b).

Syphilis can involve the CNS during any stage of disease (CDC, 2002b). Thus, any patient with syphilis who demonstrates clinical evidence of neurologic involvement should have a spinal tap to assess the CSF for evidence of neurosyphilis. Patients with neurosyphilis should be treated with high doses of aqueous penicillin G as noted in Table 39-11.

Concern has been raised as to whether the recommended regimens of penicillin are optimal in pregnancy (CDC, 2002b). Several recent reports have demonstrated worrisome levels of failure to treat mother or prevent transmission and congenital infection (McFarlin et al., 1994; Sanchez and Wendel, 1997). A high maternal VDRL titer at the time of diagnosis, unknown duration of infection, treatment within 4 weeks of delivery, and ultrasound signs of fetal syphilis (e.g., hepatomegaly, fetal hydrops, or placentomegaly) were associated with failure to prevent congenital syphilis (McFarlin et al., 1994; Sanchez and Wendel, 1997; CDC, 2002b).

Because of these reports demonstrating a high failure rate for treatment of syphilis in pregnancy, some experts have recommended additional therapy (CDC, 2002b). Thus, a second dose of benzathine penicillin (2.4 million units intramuscularly) may be given 1 week after the initial dose for pregnant women with primary, secondary, or early latent syphilis.

TABLE 39-11. CENTERS FOR DISEASE CONTROL AND PREVENTION 2002: RECOMMENDED TREATMENT OF SYPHILIS DURING PREGNANCY

1. Primary, secondary, and early latent syphilis (<1 y)
   Benzathine penicillin G, 2.4 million units IM in a single dose
2. Late latent (>1 y) and tertiary syphilis
   Benzathine penicillin G, 7.2 million units total, administered as 3 doses of 2.4 million units IM at 1-wk intervals
3. Neurosyphilis
   Aqueous crystalline penicillin G, 18–24 million units d, administered as 3–4 million units IV every 4 hr for 10–14 d
      OR
   Procaine penicillin, 2.4 million units IM daily, plus probenecid 500 mg PO q.i.d., both for 10–14 d
4. Penicillin-allergic
   Pregnant women with a history of penicillin allergy should have allergy confirmed and then be desensitized

---

IM, intramuscularly; IV, intravenously; PO, orally; q.i.d., four times daily.

Modified from Centers for Disease Control and Prevention (CDC): Sexually transmitted diseases treatment guidelines 2002. MMWR Morb Mortal Wkly Rep **51**:18, 2002.

Obstetric caregivers should be aware that women treated for syphilis during the second half of pregnancy are at risk for preterm labor or fetal distress if the Jarisch-Herxheimer reaction occurs. The Jarisch-Herxheimer reaction occurs commonly during the treatment of early syphilis; among 33 pregnant women, the reaction complicated therapy in 100% and 60% of patients treated for primary or secondary syphilis, respectively (Klein et al., 1990). The Jarisch-Herxheimer reaction characteristically presents with fever, chills, myalgia, headache, hypotension, and transient worsening of cutaneous lesions (Brown, 1976). It commences within several hours following treatment and resolves by 24 to 36 hours. Among pregnant women, the most frequent findings include fever (73%), uterine contractions (67%), and decreased fetal movement (67%) (Klein et al., 1990). Transient late decelerations were observed in 30% of monitored fetuses (Klein et al., 1990). Because of these findings, sonographic assessment of the fetus prior to initiating therapy for early syphilis in the last half of pregnancy has been recommended (Hollier and Cox, 1993). If the results are normal, ambulatory treatment may be initiated. With abnormal findings suggesting fetal infection, hospitalization for treatment and fetal monitoring is recommended. Sanchez and Wendel (1977) demonstrated that in the presence of severe fetal compromise prior to treatment, early delivery with treatment of the mother and neonate following delivery may yield an improved outcome.

The recommendation for neurosyphilis is 18 to 24 million units of aqueous crystalline penicillin G, administered intravenously in doses of 3 to 4 million units every 4 hours for 10 to 14 days. An alternative regimen (if outpatient compliance can be ensured) is 2.4 million units of aqueous procaine penicillin G intramuscularly per day plus 500 mg of probenecid orally four times per day, both for 10 to 14 days. Both regimens can be followed by benzathine penicillin G, 2.4 million units intramuscularly, to provide a comparable total duration of therapy. For neurosyphilis patients with a history of allergy to penicillin, allergy should be confirmed and hospitalization for penicillin desensitization and treatment should follow.

Therapy should be monitored with monthly quantitative VDRL titers during pregnancy and then at 3, 6, 9, and 12 months after therapy for early syphilis. For patients with syphilis of more than 1 year's duration, titers should be measured at 18 and 24 months after therapy. Patients who show a fourfold rise should be treated again.

Congenital syphilis is unusual if the mother received adequate treatment with penicillin during pregnancy. It is recommended that infants should be treated for presumed congenital syphilis if they were born to mothers in the following categories:

1. Mothers who have untreated syphilis at delivery
2. Mothers who have serologic evidence of relapse or reinfection after treatment (i.e., a rise in titre by at least fourfold).
3. Mothers who were treated for syphilis during pregnancy with nonpenicillin regimens
4. Mothers who were treated for syphilis less than 1 month prior to delivery
5. Mothers who do not have a well-documented history of treatment of syphilis
6. Mothers who do not demonstrate an adequate response (fourfold decrease) of nontreponemal antibody titers despite appropriate penicillin treatment

7. Mothers who were treated for syphilis appropriately before pregnancy but had insufficient serologic follow-up to ensure response to treatment

Any child with symptomatic congenital syphilis should undergo a spinal tap, a complete blood count, and long-bone x-rays prior to treatment. If these results are normal, a single intramuscular dose of benzathine penicillin G (50,000 units/kg) should be given. With abnormal results or when compliance is not ensured, the infant should be given a 10-day course of either aqueous crystalline penicillin G (50,000 units/kg intravenously every 12 hours for the first 7 days of life, and then every 8 hours for the next 3 days) or procaine penicillin (50,000 units/kg intramuscularly per day) (CDC, 2002b).

Gonorrhea

Over 350,000 new infections with *N. gonorrhoeae* occur each year in the United States, ranking gonorrhea as the second most commonly reported communicable disease in the nation (CDC, 2002a). Infection with *N. gonorrhoeae* in pregnancy is a major concern. Gonococcal ophthalmia neonatorum has long been recognized as a major consequence of maternal infection. More recently, an association has been recognized between maternal gonococcal infection and disseminated gonococcal infection, amniotic infection syndrome, and perinatal complications such as PROM, chorioamnionitis, prematurity, intrauterine growth restriction, neonatal sepsis, and postpartum endometritis.

Epidemiology

The incidence of gonorrhea in pregnancy has been reported to range from 0.5% to 7%. This frequency depends on the socioeconomic status of the population and the number of sites cultured. Risk factors for the acquisition of *N. gonorrhoeae* infection include young age, numerous sex partners, use of nonbarrier contraceptive methods, and risk-taking behavior patterns.

Transmission of gonorrhea is almost entirely by sexual contact. The risk of transmission from an infected male to an exposed female is 50% to 90%. The incubation time is 3 to 5 days.

Clinical Manifestations

Gonococcal infections in pregnant patients are most commonly asymptomatic. When symptoms develop, they usually include vaginal discharge and dysuria. On examination, endocervicitis may be present, with erythema and a mucopurulent discharge.

Disseminated gonococcal infection is the most common clinical presentation of gonorrhea in pregnancy. Pregnant women, especially during the second and third trimesters, appear to be at increased risk for disseminated infection, which has two stages. The *early, bacteremic stage* is characterized by chills, fever, and typical skin lesions. The lesions appear initially as small vesicles, which become pustules and develop a hemorrhagic base. The center becomes necrotic. Such lesions can occur on any body region but are most frequently present on the volar aspects of the arms, hands, and fingers. They fade without residual scarring. Blood cultures are positive for *N. gonorrhoeae* in 50% of patients in whom culture is done during the bacteremic stage. Bacterial endocarditis occasionally ensues. Joint symptoms are frequently present during this stage, as well as in the *second, septic arthritis phase* (Holmes et al., 1971). This stage is characterized by a purulent synovial effusion. The knees, ankles, and wrists are most commonly involved. Blood culture specimens during this stage are usually sterile. Gonococci may be isolated from the septic joints during the second stage.

Neonatal Gonococcal Ophthalmia

Gonococcal ophthalmia neonatorum has been recognized since 1881. Introduction of routine prophylaxis with silver nitrate resulted in a rapid reduction in this complication. However, the resurgence of gonorrhea in the 1960s and 1970s led to a reappearance of neonatal gonococcal conjunctivitis, the most common clinical manifestation of *N. gonorrhoeae* infection in the newborn.

Most newborns who have gonorrhea acquire it during passage through an infected cervical canal. Gonococcal ophthalmia is usually observed within 4 days after birth, but incubation periods up to 21 days have been reported. A frank purulent conjunctivitis occurs, usually affecting both eyes. Untreated gonococcal ophthalmia can rapidly progress to corneal ulceration, resulting in corneal scarring and blindness.

Gonococcal Infection in Pregnancy and the Neonate

The effects of gonorrheal infection on both mother and fetus have not been fully appreciated until recently (Sarrel and Pruett, 1968; Handsfield et al., 1973; Amstey and Steadman, 1976). These studies have identified an association between untreated maternal endocervical gonorrhea and perinatal complications, including an increased incidence of PROM, preterm delivery, chorioamnionitis, neonatal sepsis, and maternal postpartum sepsis.

The *amniotic infection syndrome* is an additional manifestation of gonococcal infection in pregnancy. This entity manifests as placental, fetal membrane, and umbilical cord inflammation that occurs after PROM and is associated with infected oral and gastric aspirate, leukocytosis, neonatal infection, and maternal fever. The syndrome is characterized by PROM, premature delivery, and a high rate of infant morbidity (Handsfield et al., 1973).

Diagnosis

The diagnosis of these infections depends on sampling potentially infected sites. Methods include Gram stain, culture, immunochemical detection, or molecular diagnostic techniques. Ideally, a specimen should be obtained for identification of *N. gonorrhoeae* from every woman during her initial prenatal visit. In patients at high risk for gonorrheal infection, cultures should be repeated in the third trimester. In settings where routine screening of pregnant women for gonorrhea is not performed, high-risk patients should be screened. These include the following:

1. Partners of men with gonorrhea or urethritis
2. Patients known to have other sexually transmitted diseases
3. Patients with multiple sex partners
4. Young unmarried inner-city women
5. Intravenous drug users
6. Women with symptoms or signs of lower genital tract infection

The major site of primary infection in pregnant women is in the endocervix. The anal canal, urethra, and pharyngeal cavity are important sites to consider as well. Unfortunately, microscopic examination of a Gram-stained specimen from the infected site produces a diagnosis in only 60% of infected women compared with 95% of men. In women, making the diagnosis requires isolation of the organism by culture. Clinical isolation is best performed by use of Thayer-Martin medium for *N. gonorrhoeae*. Following inoculation, the medium should be placed in a carbon dioxide incubator or candle jar to provide an adequate concentration of carbon dioxide. Transgrow medium, a modification of the Thayer-Martin medium, is available to clinicians in a bottle sealed under carbon dioxide tension.

Several reliable nonculture assays for detection of *N. gonorrhoeae* have become available and are increasingly being utilized (Hook and Handsfield, 1999). These include non-amplified DNA probe tests (PACE 2 system by Gen-Probe) and nucleic acid amplification techniques (e.g., polymerase chain reaction, ligase chain reaction). These newer technologies compare favorably to culture with selective media (Hook and Handsfield, 1999).

Treatment

The treatment of pregnant women with gonococcal infection is similar to that of nonpregnant women, with the exception that tetracycline should not be used for concomitant chlamydial infection. Both asymptomatic and symptomatic infections should be treated. The treatment of gonococcal infection in the United States has been influenced by two factors.

First, there has been increasing prevalence and spread of infections because of antibiotic-resistant *N. gonorrhoeae* such as penicillinase-producing *N. gonorrhoeae*, tetracycline-resistant *N. gonorrhoeae,* and chromosomally mediated *N. gonorrhoeae*, which is resistant to multiple antibiotics. Currently more than 10% of gonorrheal isolates in the United States are resistant to penicillin (Cates and Hinman, 1991). In an investigation at public clinics for sexually transmitted diseases in Seattle, Brooklyn, Baltimore, and Denver, 39% of 303 gonococcal isolates demonstrated one or more types of antimicrobial resistance (Handsfield et al., 1991).

Second, there is a high frequency (20% to 50%) of co-existing chlamydial infection in women infected with *N. gonorrhoeae*. Current CDC recommendations for treatment of *N. gonorrhoeae* are listed in Table 39-12.

All patients treated for gonorrhea should receive concomitant therapy for *C. trachomatis* because 20%–50% of women with gonorrhea are also infected with *Chlamydia*. During pregnancy, amoxicillin is the drug of choice for *C. trachomatis*. In pregnant women allergic to β-lactam agents, spectinomycin, 2.0 g intramuscularly, is recommended. Quinolone agents (ciprofloxacin, ofloxacin) should not be used during pregnancy.

TABLE 39-12. CENTERS FOR DISEASE CONTROL AND PREVENTION RECOMMENDED TREATMENT OF GONORRHEA IN PREGNANT WOMEN, 2002

Uncomplicated Gonorrhea (Cervix, Urethra, Rectum)

Recommended regimens

Cefixime 400 mg PO as a single dose
OR
Ceftriaxone 125 mg IM in a single dose
PLUS
Azithromycin 1 g PO as a single dose
OR
Amoxicillin 500 mg t.i.d. for 7 d

Alternative regimens

Spectinomycin 2 g IM as a single dose
OR
Single-dose cephalosporins such as ceftizoxime 500 mg IM,
    cefotaxime 500 mg IM, cefotetan 1 g IM, or cefoxitin 2 g IM with
    probenecid 1 g PO

Disseminated Gonococcal Infection

Recommended initial regimen

Ceftriaxone 1 g IM or IV every 24 hr

Alternative initial regimens

Cefotaxime 1 g IV every 8 hr
OR
Ceftizoxime 1 g IV every 8 hr
OR
Spectinomycin 2 g IM every 12 hr
All regimens continued for 24–48 hr after improvement begins, at
    which time therapy may be switched to the following to complete
    a full wk of therapy
Cefixime 400 mg PO b.i.d.

b.i.d., twice daily; IM, intramuscularly; IV, intravenously; PO, orally; t.i.d., three times daily.

Data from Centers for Disease Control and Prevention (CDC): Recommended Treatment of Gonorrhea in Pregnant Women, 2002.

With use of recommended treatment, follow-up cultures to document eradication of gonorrhea are no longer recommended. Instead, reculturing in 2 to 3 months to identify reinfection is suggested. If other antimicrobial agents are used for the treatment of *N. gonorrhoeae*, follow-up assessment is suggested. Follow-up cultures should be obtained from the infected site 3 to 7 days after completion of treatment. In women, follow-up specimens must be obtained from the anal canal as well as the endocervix; failure to obtain a specimen from the anal canal results in missing 50% of resistant *N. gonorrhoeae* strains. With nucleic acid amplification tests, repeat testing should be performed 3 weeks after treatment.

The treatment of choice for ophthalmia neonatorum caused by *N. gonorrhoeae* is ceftriaxone 25 to 50 mg/kg intravenously or intramuscularly in a single dose, not to exceed 125 mg.

Prevention

The increasing frequency of asymptomatic gonorrheal infection in women makes screening for *N. gonorrhoeae* during the antepartum period an important aspect of preventing the perinatal morbidity associated with this organism. Instillation of a prophylactic agent into the eyes of all newborn infants is recommended to prevent gonococcal ophthalmia neonatorum.

The recommended regimens include erythromycin (0.5%) ophthalmic ointment, tetracycline (1%) ophthalmic ointment, or silver nitrate (1%) aqueous solution.

Condylomata Acuminata (Genital Warts)/Genital Human Papillomavirus Infection

Condylomata acuminata, often called genital warts, are very common. The disease is sexually transmitted, and the etiologic agent has been identified as a type of human papillomavirus (HPV). More than 100 types of HPV have been identified, of which 35 primarily affect the epithelium of the genital tract. Risk factors associated with HPV infection include early onset of sexual activity, multiple sex partners, cigarette smoking, and long-term use of oral contraception.

An estimated 24 million Americans are infected with HPV, and between 500,000 and 1 million new cases of HPV-induced genital warts occur annually in the United States (CDC, 1996a; Institute of Medicine, 1997; Beutner et al., 1998).

HPV infection may result in either clinically apparent, grossly visible disease or subclinical disease requiring magnification or acetic acid for visualization. The common genital HPV types can be divided into two major categories based on their oncogenic potential. HPV types in the low oncogenic risk group include 6, 11, 42, 43, and 44, which are associated with genital warts, condylomata, and some cases of low-grade squamous intraepithelial lesions. The high oncogenic risk group includes HPV types 16, 18, 20, 31, 45, 54, 55, 56, 64, and 68. These high-risk types are frequently detected in women with high-grade squamous intraepithelial neoplasia and invasive cancers (Sweet and Gibbs, 2002). Most HPV infections are asymptomatic, subclinical, or unrecognized (CDC, 1997). The majority of the clinically apparent lesions are the classic condyloma acuminatum. Condylomata acuminata are most commonly caused by low-risk HPV types 6 and 11; other HPV types associated with condylomata acuminata are 42, 43, 44, and 54. In addition, HPV may remain present in a latent form within cells. Application of PCR to amplify and detect the DNA or HPV has revealed that approximately 40% of sexually active women carry HPV in the genital tract.

Genital warts predominantly affect the young. Prevalence is highest among the 16- to 25-year age group, which is also the age group with the highest rate of pregnancy. The warts grow more rapidly during pregnancy and may involve the cervix, vagina, or vulva so extensively that vaginal delivery is precluded. The reason for the increase in size and number of lesions is not known but has been postulated to be the decrease in cell-mediated immunity that occurs during pregnancy.

These lesions occur in the urogenital and anorectal areas, which offer a warm, moist environment for viral replication. The risk of acquiring the virus by sexual contact with an infected partner is very high. An infection rate of approximately 65% has been documented, and the incubation period ranges from 3 weeks to 8 months, with an average of 2.8 months.

Condylomata acuminata are pedunculated lesions varying in size from a pinhead to large masses covering the entire vulva. Most warts are so characteristic in appearance that the diagnosis is obvious on physical examination alone. If lesions look atypical and are isolated, a specimen should be obtained for biopsy to rule out carcinoma *in situ*.

Management of these lesions in pregnancy presents difficult problems. Currently available therapy for genital warts during pregnancy includes trichloroacetic acid, dichloroacetic acid, cryotherapy, and surgical excision. None of these therapies has been shown to be superior to the others. Podophyllin, podofilox, and imiquimod should not be used during pregnancy. The best approach to treatment during pregnancy may be the excision of the lesions by cautery or the use of cryosurgery. Care must be taken to prevent extensive scarring or sloughing of tissue. Intralesional and parenteral injections of interferon have been successfully used to treat nonpregnant patients with recurrent condylomata. Interferon has not been studied in pregnancy for either efficacy or safety, however.

Respiratory papillomatosis (laryngeal papilloma) is a rare disease in the neonate caused by HPV 6 and 11. Laryngeal papillomas can be particularly troublesome because they may produce respiratory distress secondary to obstruction and because recurrence following treatment is common. Potential routes of vertical transmission of HPV include transplacental, intrapartum in the birth canal, and contact during the neonatal period, but the route of transmission is not completely understood (Cook et al., 1973; CDC, 2002a).

The risk for transmission of the virus from maternal condylomata acuminata to the neonate has not been established. Because genital papillomavirus infection is so common and respiratory papillomatosis is rare, the risk of intrapartum transmission is low, perhaps on the order of one case of juvenile respiratory papillomatosis per several hundred or per thousand children born to infected mothers (Shah et al., 1986; Watts et al., 1998; Kashima et al., 1999). Of interest is the prospective cohort study by Watts and colleagues (1998) that demonstrated the risk of transmission for any given mother-infant pair to be small. These authors reported that among 151 pregnant women evaluated for HPV by clinical, colposcopic, and PCR at less than 20 weeks, 34 weeks, and 36 weeks, 112 (74%) had evidence of HPV. However, HPV was detected in only 3 (4%) of 80 infants born to women with HPV detected at 34 to 36 weeks' gestation, and in 5 (8%) of 63 infants born to women in whom HPV DNA was not detected. Tenti and coworkers (1999) also demonstrated that pregnant women with latent HPV infection have a low potential for transmitting the virus to the oropharyngeal mucosa of their newborns. Although these authors reported that HPV DNA was detected in 11 neonates born vaginally to HPV-positive women (vertical transmission rate, 30%; 95% CI, 15.9% to 47%), by 5 weeks after birth, all infants tested negative and remained so throughout the 18-month follow-up. These findings suggest that the infants who were HPV-positive at birth were contaminated and not infected (Tenti et al., 1999). HPV is present in maternal blood and can be transmitted transplacentally to the fetus. Accordingly, cesarean section for prevention of transmission of HPV infection to the newborn is not indicated (CDC, 2002a). In rare circumstances, cesarean section may be indicated for women whose genital warts obstruct the birth canal or might result in excessive bleeding.

Chlamydial Infection

C. trachomatis is the most common sexually transmitted bacterial disease organism in the United States, where at least 4 million new chlamydial infections occur each year. The estimated annual cost of chlamydial infections exceeds $2.4 billion (CDC, 1993; CDC, 1996; CDC, 1997; Mangione-Smith et al, 1999; Schachter, 1999; Stamm, 1999; Sweet and Gibbs, 2002).

C. trachomatis causes significant disease in both men and women. In addition, investigations have documented the consequences to infants of perinatal exposure to the organism. Although inclusion conjunctivitis of the newborn has been studied for 60 years, the importance of extraocular chlamydial infections in infants was not appreciated until the mid-1970s (Beem and Saxon, 1977). Prior to widespread prenatal chlamydial screening, inclusion conjunctivitis of the newborn was the most common form of conjunctivitis seen in the 1st month of life, and chlamydia was a common cause of pneumonia in the first 6 months of life.

The chlamydiae are obligate intracellular bacteria separated into their own order, Chlamydiales, on the basis of a unique growth cycle that distinguishes them from all other microorganisms. This cycle involves infection of the susceptible host cell by a chlamydia-specific phagocytic process, so that these organisms are preferentially ingested. After attachment and ingestion, the chlamydiae remain in a phagosome throughout the growth cycle, but surface antigens of chlamydiae appear to inhibit phagolysosomal fusion. These two virulence factors—enhanced ingestion and inhibition of phagolysosomal fusion—attest to an exquisitely adapted parasitism.

Once in the cell, the chlamydial elementary body, which is the infectious particle, changes to a metabolically active replicating form called the reticulate body, which synthesizes its own macromolecules and divides by binary fission. The chlamydiae are energy parasites that do not synthesize their own adenosine triphosphate; thus, energy-rich compounds must be supplied to them by the host cell. By the end of the growth cycle (approximately 48 hours), most reticulate bodies have reorganized into elementary bodies, which are released as the result of mechanical disruption of the host cell to initiate new infectious cycles.

Chlamydiae are unique bacteria that do not stain with the Gram stain. In many respects, they are similar to other bacteria: They contain DNA and RNA, are susceptible to certain antibiotics, have a rigid cell wall similar in structure and content to those of gram-negative bacteria, and multiply by binary fission. However, they differ from other bacteria and resemble viruses in being obligate intracellular parasites. They may be regarded as bacteria that have adapted to an intracellular environment. They need viable cells for multiplication and survival.

The characteristics of the species that make up the genus *Chlamydia* are presented in Table 39-13. *Chlamydia psittaci* is the causative agent of psittacosis, a common pathogen in avian species and lower mammals. *C. pneumoniae* is a human pathogen that is a common cause of upper respiratory tract infections. *Chlamydia trachomatis* seems to be a specifically human pathogen (except for a few strains of rodent origin).

Although all chlamydiae share a common genus-specific antigen, *C. trachomatis* may be further differentiated on a serologic basis. There are currently 15 recognized serotypes. Three of these serotypes (L1, L2, L3) represent the agents causing lymphogranuloma venereum. The other serotypes of *C. trachomatis* represent the agents causing endemic blinding trachoma (A, B, Ba, and C) and the sexually transmitted *C. trachomatis* strains (D through K), which cause inclusion

TABLE 39-13. CHLAMYDIAE: TAXONOMY AND ASSOCIATION WITH HUMAN DISEASE

Organism	Origin	Serotype	Disease
Chlamydia psittaci	Common pathogen in birds and lower mammals	Many	Psittacosis
Chlamydia pneumoniae	Respiratory tract infections in humans	TWAR	
Chlamydia trachomatis	Mostly of human origin	A, B, Ba, C	Hyperendemic binding trachoma
		D, E, F, G, H, I, J, K	Inclusion conjunctivitis, nongonococcal urethritis, cervicitis, salpingitis, proctitis, epididymitis, pneumonia of newborn
		L^1, L^2, L^3	Lymphogranuloma venereum

conjunctivitis, newborn pneumonia, urethritis, cervicitis, endometritis, pelvic inflammatory disease, and the acute urethral syndrome.

Epidemiology and Transmission

C. trachomatis has long been recognized as the causative agent of trachoma, a chronic conjunctivitis affecting hundreds of millions of people in developing countries and resulting in millions of cases of blindness. However, the child-to-child and intrafamilial infection patterns that predominate in endemic areas have not been proved to cause disease in newborns. Studies that focus on the role of *C. trachomatis* in diseases of individuals living in industrialized countries have documented that the major method of transmission of chlamydial infections in these populations is sexual. These chlamydial infections, like other sexually transmitted diseases, have reached epidemic levels.

In the female, a number of clinical conditions can be attributed to *Chlamydia*, among them mucopurulent cervicitis, acute urethral syndrome, urethritis, and salpingitis. The cervix is the primary site for chlamydial infections in women. Unfortunately, many chlamydial infections of the cervix are clinically inapparent. Thus, asymptomatic and clinically inapparent infections occur in both women and men. They are usually discovered during routine screening procedures or as a result of contact tracing from symptomatic patients. Approximately one half to two thirds of women with chlamydial cervicitis have no signs or symptoms of their infection.

Brunham and coworkers (1984) have proposed that mucopurulent cervicitis, which is often due to *Chlamydia*, is the female equivalent of nongonococcal urethritis in men. Paavonen and co-authors (1982) described the characteristics associated with mucopurulent endocervicitis and ascribed the majority of such infections to *C. trachomatis*. More-recent studies in the general population have failed to confirm this, with positive predictive values of 11% to 54% (Sweet and Gibbs, 2002).

As seen in Table 39-14, the prevalence of *C. trachomatis* infection among pregnant women can vary broadly, with a reported range of 2% to 37%. The general consensus is that the national average in the United States for chlamydial infection of the cervix is 2% to 3% in sexually active women, although high-risk populations can be readily identified. A number of studies have shown that the same populations at high risk for other sexually transmitted infections are at highest risk for chlamydial infections. Among pregnant women, risk factors for chlamydial infection include the following:

1. Unmarried status
2. Age under 25 years
3. Multiple sex partners
4. New sex partner in past 3 months
5. Presence of another sexually transmitted disease
6. Partners with nongonococcal urethritis
7. Presence of mucopurulent endocervicitis
8. Sterile pyuria (acute urethral syndrome)
9. Resident of socially disadvantaged community
10. Late or no prenatal care

Detection rates as high as 25% to 30% have been reported in screening and prospective studies of such populations.

Infants born to women with a chlamydial infection of the cervix are at a 60% to 70% risk of acquiring the infection during passage through the birth canal (Sweet and Gibbs, 2002). Approximately 25% to 50% of exposed infants acquire conjunctivitis in the first 2 weeks of life, and 10% to 20% acquire pneumonia within 3 or 4 months. *In utero* transmission is not known to occur. Infants born by cesarean section are not at risk for chlamydial infection unless the membranes have ruptured prematurely.

Clinical Spectrum of Perinatal Infection

CONJUNCTIVITIS

Acute conjunctivitis of the newborn (inclusion conjunctivitis of the newborn, inclusion blennorrhea) was initially described in the 1st decade of the 20th century. It was recognized that the agent that caused inclusion conjunctivitis of the newborn was also present in the genital tract of the mother; intracytoplasmic inclusion bodies similar to those produced by trachoma were seen in scrapings from the conjunctiva of infants with conjunctivitis and in those from the cervices of their mothers. It is now recognized as the most common conjunctivitis in the 1st month of life.

The disease often starts with a watery eye discharge that rapidly and progressively becomes purulent. The eyelids are usually markedly swollen. The conjunctivae become reddened and somewhat thickened throughout. The mucopurulent conjunctivitis generally develops more than 5 days after birth. Thus, it is rarely diagnosed accurately because the infant will have left the hospital when the disease develops.

In severe cases, the diagnosis is readily made by demonstration of the typical inclusion bodies by Giemsa staining of conjunctival scrapings. Chlamydiae are also easily obtained from the eye for culture. Serologic diagnosis is not helpful

TABLE 39-14. PREVALENCE OF *CHLAMYDIA TRACHOMATIS* CERVICAL INFECTION IN PREGNANT WOMEN

Study	Location	Prevalence of Maternal Infection (%)
Chander et al., 1977	Seattle	13
Frommell et al., 1979	Denver	9
Hammerschlag et al., 1979	Boston	2
Hammerschlag et al., 1979	Seattle	12
Schachter et al., 1979	San Francisco	5.0
Mardh et al., 1980	Lund (Sweden)	9
Harrison et al., 1983	Tucson	7
Harrison et al., 1983	Gallup, NM	24
Hardy et al., 1984	Baltimore	37
Ismail et al., 1985	Chicago	21
Khurana et al., 1988	Manila	17
Fitz-Simmons et al., 1986	Philadelphia	15
Gravett et al., 1986	Seattle	9
Schachter, Grossman, et al., 1986	San Francisco	4.7
Baselski et al., 1987	Memphis	21
Sweet et al., 1987	San Francisco	4.5
Cohen et al., 1990	Cleveland	5.75
Ryan et al., 1990	Memphis	21

because of the presence of maternally transmitted chlamydial IgG antibody and because of the uncertain appearance of IgM in this disease. Chlamydial infections are unaffected by silver nitrate prophylaxis, and it thus seems reasonable to recommend a regimen active against both chlamydiae and gonococci for neonatal eye prophylaxis. Erythromycin ointment can prevent the development of inclusion conjunctivitis of the newborn.

PNEUMONIA

Until 1975, it was assumed that chlamydial infection in the infant was restricted to the conjunctiva. Beem and Saxon (1977) published a series of retrospective and prospective cases of chlamydial pneumonia in young infants. This report was followed by studies from other centers, and the clinical entity of chlamydial pneumonia became well defined. Following recognition, it became clear that this disease is very common indeed, and probably one of the three most common pneumonias seen in infancy.

The vast majority of infants manifest the disease between the 4th and 11th weeks of life; virtually all are symptomatic before the 8th week. Initially, they have respiratory symptoms. Usually, the infant is afebrile or has only a low-grade fever. The upper respiratory tract symptoms are congestion and obstruction of the nasal passages without significant discharge. The finding of abnormal, bulging eardrums is common, occurring in more than 50% of the cases described. The history or presence of conjunctivitis can be elicited in 50% of cases. Lower respiratory tract symptoms consist of tachypnea and a very prominent "staccato" cough. Some infants have apneic periods, and on occasion the infection is severe enough to warrant intubation. Crepitant inspiratory rales are commonly heard, but expiratory wheezes are uncommon. The cough, which often interferes with sleeping and feeding, may be disturbing to the infant and the parents. For the same reason, food intake drops and the infant fails to gain weight.

X-rays reveal hyperexpansion of the lungs, with bilateral symmetric interstitial infiltrates. The effects of hyperexpansion on the diaphragm may render the liver and spleen easily palpable.

Laboratory findings include a normal white blood cell count and an increase in eosinophils. Blood gas analysis usually indicates a mild or moderate degree of hypoxia. Levels of serum immune globulins, both the IgG and IgM varieties, are generally elevated.

ADVERSE PREGNANCY OUTCOME

Much more controversial is the question of whether maternal cervical C. trachomatis infection is associated with adverse pregnancy outcome. Some studies have demonstrated an association of cervical chlamydial infection with PROM, preterm labor and delivery, low birth weight, increased perinatal mortality, and late-onset postpartum endometritis. Other equally carefully designed studies have not demonstrated such an association.

Martin and associates (1982) were the first to demonstrate that Chlamydia-infected pregnant women screened prior to 19 weeks of gestation had a significantly shorter mean duration of pregnancy (35.9 versus 39.4 weeks), a significantly higher rate of birth weight less than 2500 g (28% versus 8%), and a tenfold increase in neonatal death (33% versus 3.4%). However, Harrison and coworkers (1983) and Sweet and colleagues (1987) demonstrated that although cervical infection with C. trachomatis did not increase the risk of low birth weight, abortion, stillbirth, prematurity, or PROM, the subgroup of IgM-seropositive Chlamydia-infected women had significantly more low-birth-weight infants and a significantly increased incidence of PROM and preterm birth. They postulated that IgM seropositivity reflected recent chlamydial acquisition and that such patients were at high risk for adverse pregnancy outcome.

In additional attempts to address the role of *C. trachomatis* in adverse pregnancy outcome, researchers have undertaken treatment studies of chlamydial infection in pregnant women. Ryan and colleagues (1990), in a high-prevalence population (21% positive), reported that untreated *Chlamydia*-infected pregnant women had significant increases in occurrences of PROM and low birth weight and decreased perinatal survival compared with treated women or those not infected with *Chlamydia*. Similarly, Cohen and coworkers (1990) reported that treatment of chlamydial infection resulted in decreased rates for preterm delivery, PROM, preterm labor, and fetal growth restriction; however, there were experimental design flaws or limitations in both studies.

The role of cervical chlamydial infection in producing postpartum endometritis is also highly controversial. Early studies in the ophthalmology literature demonstrated an association between newborns with inclusion conjunctivitis (chlamydial conjunctivitis) and an increased risk for postpartum infection in their mothers (Thygeson and Mengert, 1936). Subsequently, Wager and colleagues (1980), in a prospective study, demonstrated that pregnant women with chlamydial cervical infection at their initial prenatal visit were at significant increased risk for late-onset endometritis following vaginal delivery. Several more-recent reports confirmed this increased risk for endometritis following vaginal delivery in chlamydia-infected women (Ismail et al., 1985; Hoyme et al., 1986; Plummer et al., 1987). However, multiple studies have failed to confirm such an association (Harrison et al., 1983; Blanco et al., 1985; Berman et al., 1987; Sweet et al., 1987; McGregor et al., 1990).

Diagnosis

Schachter and Dawson (1977) have suggested that the principles for diagnosing chlamydial infections are essentially the same as those for any other microbial infection. The agent may be demonstrated by cytologic examination of clinical specimens, by serologic demonstration of rising antibody titers to chlamydial antigens, by isolation from culture of the patient's tissues, or by antigen detection methods such as fluorescein-conjugated monoclonal antibody smears or enzyme immunoassay (Amortegui and Meyer, 1985). More recently, the use of DNA probes and nucleic acid amplification techniques (PCR or ligase chain reaction [LCR]) have become available clinically. Cytologic identification of chlamydial infection was the only available diagnostic tool prior to 1957. Direct staining of epithelial cell scrapings with Giemsa or iodine identified the characteristic inclusion bodies of *C. trachomatis*. Although it is simple and inexpensive, standard cytology has little practical use as a diagnostic tool in genital tract infection. Compared with culture or antigen-detection methods, Papanicolaou smear has poor sensitivity and specificity.

Until recently, the optimum diagnostic test for chlamydial infection was culture. However, culture requires cold chain storage, waiting up to a week for results, and substantial technical expertise; in addition, it is expensive and, with the advent of nucleic acid amplification tests, has been shown to be relatively insensitive (65% to 85%).

Prior to the introduction of nucleic acid amplification tests, antigen-detection methods were widely used. Availability of antigen-detection tests simplified screening for chlamydia and allowed widespread clinical applicability. From a practical clinical perspective, two such methods are currently available: fluorescein-conjugated monoclonal antibody staining of a direct smear and enzyme immunoassay. Both of these antigen-detection methods have been demonstrated to be highly sensitive and specific. In a low-prevalence population (i.e., 2% to 3% chlamydial infection), the positive predictive value drops to about 50%; this means that there will be false-positive results. Of these two methods, the monoclonal antibody system has the advantage of rapid processing time and has a built-in quality control for assessing the adequacy of a clinical specimen (i.e., presence of epithelial cells). Compared to culture, antigen-detection methods have several advantages: they are less costly, do not require cold chain storage, are more rapid, and are more widely available to clinicians. A review by Stamm (1987) contains details regarding antigen-detection methods.

DNA amplification tests such as PCR and LCR, recently been introduced into clinical practice, are powerful tools for identifying infectious microorganisms. These tests have been very effective in the diagnosis of chlamydial genital tract infection (Loeffelholz et al., 1992; Bass et al., 1993; Bauwens et al., 1993; Wiesenfeld et al., 1994; Vogels et al., 1994; Lee et al., 1995; Schachter et al., 1995; van Doornum et al., 1995). In these studies, PCR or LCR has been more sensitive and specific and has had greater positive predictive value than culture or antigen-detection tests. With cervical or urethral swabs, PCR and LCR identify approximately 30% more cases of chlamydial genital tract infection. Most probably, this results from the ability of DNA-amplification tests to identify the presence of small numbers of organisms (i.e., small inocula), especially in asymptomatic infection.

Of great interest has been the use of PCR and LCR for population-based screening of asymptomatic persons. LCR assay of urine has been demonstrated to be an effective means of diagnosing genital tract infection with chlamydiae in women (as well as men) (Lee et al., 1995; Schachter et al., 1995). As a result, investigators have suggested that LCR assay of urine be utilized as a noninvasive screening test for chlamydial infection in asymptomatic women. More recently, it has been shown that PCR testing of vaginal introital swabs obtained by health-care providers or self-collected by patients is an excellent screening method for chlamydial infection of the cervix and urethra (Wiesenfeld et al., 1996). The latter approach provides significant logistic advantages over urine screening.

The question of which women should be screened for *C. trachomatis* has been controversial. Ideally, all sexually active women should be screened, especially during pregnancy. The most recent guidelines for the treatment of sexually transmitted diseases (CDC, 2002) recommend that all pregnant women be screened for chlamydial infection in the first trimester and that patients at high risk be rescreened in the third trimester.

Serologic diagnosis has not been useful as a test for the routine clinical determination of genital chlamydial infection; however, chlamydia serology is a helpful epidemiologic tool in large populations and can identify patients who have had previous chlamydial infection. The microimmunofluorescence test is the most commonly used serologic test for detecting IgG and IgM antibodies against *C. trachomatis*.

PLATE 17

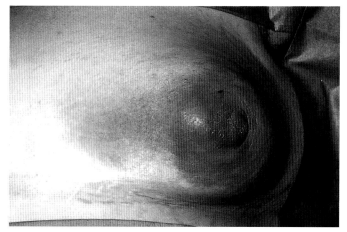

FIGURE 39-1 ■ Acute mastitis.

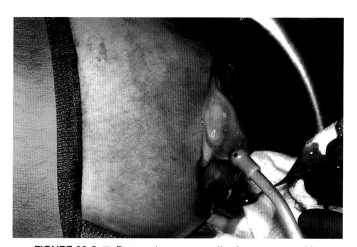

FIGURE 39-2 ■ Breast abscess complicating acute mastitis.

Treatment

Topical therapy alone is inadequate for chlamydial conjunctivitis because it is associated with a high failure rate and does not prevent chlamydial pneumonia. Thus, erythromycin 50 mg/kg/day orally divided into four doses for 10 to 14 days is the recommended therapy for ophthalmia neonatorum caused by *C. trachomatis* (CDC, 2002). A similar regimen is recommended for chlamydial pneumonia of the newborn.

Pregnant women who have proven infection with *C. trachomatis* should receive treatment. The recommended treatment for chlamydial infection in pregnancy is presented in Table 39-15. Erythromycin base and amoxicillin are the agents of choice for chlamydial infection during pregnancy. Doxycycline and ofloxacin, which are recommended for chlamydial treatment in nonpregnant patients, are contraindicated for pregnant women. The safety and efficacy of azithromycin among pregnant and lactating women have not been established. Thus, azithromycin is not recommended for routine use in pregnant women but can be an alternative, especially for patients who are allergic to amoxicillin or intolerant of erythromycin.

Several studies have documented the efficacy of erythromycin treatment in the third trimester for eradication of maternal cervical chlamydial infection and prevention of vertical transmission of *C. trachomatis* to neonates (Schachter, Sweet, et al., 1986; Alger and Lovchik, 1991; Magat et al., 1993; Alary et al., 1994; Bush and Rosa, 1994; Silverman et al., 1994; Edwards et al., 1996; Adair et al., 1998; Wehbeh et al., 1998). However, erythromycin is associated with substantial gastrointestinal side effects (range, 25% to 49%), which often results in poor compliance.

Consequently, investigators evaluated the efficacy and safety of alternative agents for the treatment of chlamydial infection in pregnancy. Crombleholme and coworkers (1990) initially reported that treatment of pregnant women with amoxicillin, 500 mg three times daily for 7 days, was well tolerated. This therapy resulted in eradication of cervical chlamydiae in 98.6% of infected women, and 95.6% of infants had negative cultures and serologic studies for *C. trachomatis*. Such

TABLE 39-15. TREATMENT RECOMMENDATIONS FOR CHLAMYDIAL INFECTION IN PREGNANT WOMEN

Recommended Regimens

Amoxicillin 500 mg PO t.i.d. for 7 d
OR
Erythromycin base 500 mg PO q.i.d. for 7 d

Alternative Regimens

Azithromycin 1 g PO as a single dose
OR
Erythromycin base 250 mg PO q.i.d. for 14 d
OR
Erythromycin ethylsuccinate 800 mg PO q.i.d. for 7 d
OR
Erythromycin ethylsuccinate 400 mg PO q.i.d. for 14 d

PO, orally; q.i.d., four times daily; t.i.d., three times daily.

Data from Centers for Disease Control and Prevention (CDC): Sexually transmitted diseases treatment guidelines 2002. MMWR Morb Mortal Wkly Rep **51**:32, 2002.

figures compared favorably with results for the erythromycin-treated group. In addition, only 2% of the amoxicillin-treated group stopped therapy compared to 13% in the erythromycin-treated group. More recently, other studies have confirmed the safety and efficacy of amoxicillin in the treatment of pregnant women with chlamydial infection (Magat et al., 1993; Alary et al., 1994; Silverman et al., 1994). In addition, a meta-analysis showed that the relative risk of success was significantly increased in the amoxicillin group compared to erythromycin (relative risk, 1.11; 95% CI, 1.05 to 1.18; $P < 0.01$). Azithromycin has been assessed for efficacy and safety during pregnancy in a limited number of studies (Bush and Rosa, 1994; Edwards et al., 1996; Adair et al., 1998; Wehbeh et al., 1998). Although small, these studies have demonstrated that azithromycin is an effective and well-tolerated agent for the treatment of chlamydial infection in pregnant women.

OTHER INFECTIONS

Mycoplasmal Infection

The mycoplasmas are a unique group of microorganisms that commonly inhabit the mucosal surfaces of the respiratory and genital tracts. To date, many antigenically distinct species that are infectious in humans have been characterized. These can be divided into *respiratory* mycoplasmas, mainly *Mycoplasma pneumoniae*, the agent responsible for atypical pneumonia, and *genital* mycoplasmas. The most common genital mycoplasmas are *M. hominis* and *U. urealyticum* (formerly T-mycoplasmas or T strains). *Mycoplasma genitalium* has been implicated in pelvic inflammatory disease.

Phylogenetically, mycoplasmas fall between bacteria and viruses. All mycoplasmas share certain characteristics:

1. Absence of cell walls
2. Growth in cell-free media
3. Dependence on the availability of sterols for adequate growth (except for species of Acholeplasma)
4. Inhibition of growth by specific antibody
5. Susceptibility to antimicrobial agents that inhibit protein synthesis
6. Resistance to agents that affect synthesis of cell walls

Mycoplasmas are the smallest known free-living organisms. They differ from bacteria because they have no cell walls but, rather, a nonrigid triple-layered membrane enclosing each cell. They differ from viruses in that they contain both DNA and RNA and can grow in cell-free media.

Mycoplasma hominis can be distinguished from *U. urealyticum* by differences in colonial morphology, metabolic characteristics, and susceptibility to antibiotics (Table 39-16). *Mycoplasma hominis* is recognizable as forming a "fried-egg" colony. The organism converts arginine or ornithine with the liberation of ammonia; this reaction has an easily recognized color change when an appropriate pH indicator is incorporated into a broth medium containing arginine. *Ureaplasma urealyticum* is a microaerophilic organism characterized by small colony size and the ability to hydrolyze urea. Urea is an essential substrate for growth and is converted to ammonia. This reaction can be detected by addition of a pH indicator to the broth or agar medium containing urea.

TABLE 39-16. CHARACTERISTICS OF GENITAL TRACT MYCOPLASMAS

Characteristic	Ureaplasma Urealyticum	Mycoplasma Hominis
Colony morphology	Small, granular	Large, "fried egg"
Colony size	20–30 μm	200–300 μm
Metabolic substrate	Urea	Arginine
Antibiotic susceptibility		
Tetracycline	+	+
Erythromycin	+	–
Lincomycin	–	+
Clindamycin	–	+
Penicillin	–	–
Cephalosporins	–	–
Aerobic growth	–	+

Epidemiology

Infants become colonized with genital mycoplasmas during the birth process. Presumably, the organisms are acquired from a contaminated cervix or vagina, since infants delivered by cesarean section are less frequently colonized with mycoplasmas than are those delivered vaginally. Genital mycoplasmas are uncommon in prepubertal girls. After puberty, colonization with genital mycoplasmas occurs primarily through sexual contact. The organism recovery rate increases dramatically with the onset of sexual intercourse. A wide range in the recovery rate has been reported for *U. urealyticum* (from 40% to 95%) and for *M. hominis* (from 15% to 72% among sexually active women).

Genital mycoplasmas are commonly isolated from gravid women at approximately the same rate as from nonpregnant women with the same degree of sexual activity. Genital mycoplasmas have been recovered more frequently from women of lower socioeconomic classes than from private patients and from African-American women than from white women.

Spontaneous Abortion and Stillbirth

Investigators have reported the isolation of genital mycoplasmas from the chorion, amnion, and decidua in spontaneous abortions, although a causal relationship has not been established. One issue is whether contamination occurs when the products of conception pass through the cervix and vagina. Another is whether the relationship was due, in fact, to other organisms not investigated.

The mycoplasmas isolated from abortuses and stillbirths cannot be explained completely by contamination; these organisms have been isolated from the lungs, brain, heart, and viscera. However, none of these observations provides an answer to the question of whether abortion occurs because mycoplasmas invade the fetus and cause its death or because the fetus dies from another cause, with subsequent invasion of necrotic tissue by the mycoplasmas (Taylor-Robinson and McCormack, 1980).

Fetal loss, if caused by these organisms, might be prevented by appropriate antimicrobial therapy. Kundsin and coworkers (1967) reported successful pregnancies after antibiotic therapy in women who were colonized by *Ureaplasma* and had a history of frequent spontaneous abortions. Stray-Pederson and associates (1978) used doxycycline to treat women who had had repeated spontaneous abortions, many of whom subsequently had normal pregnancies. These findings have led to the concept that subclinical mycoplasmal infection is an important cause of spontaneous abortion, especially repeated abortions. However, these studies have not assessed other microorganisms (especially *C. trachomatis* and anaerobes). Most significantly, the effectiveness of antibiotics in preventing spontaneous abortion remains controversial because all the antibiotic trials have been uncontrolled.

In summary, the evidence linking the genital mycoplasmas to spontaneous abortion and stillbirth is mainly anecdotal. Establishment of a causal relationship will require large-scale investigations that assess other potential pathogens and include placebo-controlled trials of antibiotics in patients who have had repeated spontaneous abortions.

Histologic Chorioamnionitis, Intra-amniotic Infection, and Neonatal Infection

Shurin and colleagues (1975) isolated *U. urealyticum* twice as frequently from neonates whose mothers had histologically severe chorioamnionitis as from newborns whose mothers had less severe or no disease. The histologic chorioamnionitis might be due to any of the other microorganisms that could gain entry to the amniotic cavity at the same time. These data are significant because they accounted for duration of membrane rupture and still revealed a statistically significant association between chorioamnionitis and ureaplasma infection.

As noted earlier, *M. hominis* is found much more often in the amniotic fluid of women with IAI than in matched controls, and there is a significant association between symptomatic IAI and a rise in maternal antibodies to *M. hominis*. *Ureaplasma urealyticum* is found equally in both groups (Gibbs et al., 1986). Among patients with PROM, *U. urealyticum* has been isolated as the only organism in 21% of cases and together with other organisms in an additional 9%. Isolation of *U. urealyticum* is associated with robust elaboration of inflammatory cytokines (Yoon et al., 1998). *Ureaplasma urealyticum* has been the most common isolate in membrane culture of placentas with histologic chorioamnionitis. *Mycoplasma hominis* has been isolated less commonly (Hillier et al., 1988; Eschenbach, 1994).

Genital mycoplasmas acquired by the infant during labor generally have not been associated with serious neonatal infection.

Low Birth Weight

Klein and associates (1969), in the first systematic study of the effects of mycoplasmas on infants, reported that 22% of infants weighing less than 2500 g were colonized with *M. hominis* or *U. urealyticum*, a rate significantly higher than the 12% seen among infants weighing more than 2500 g. In a multicenter study, however, antepartum cultures for *U. urealyticum* in 4934 women did not correlate with low-birth-weight infants, preterm labor, or preterm birth after adjustment for sociodemographic factors (Carey et al., 1991). This large, powerful study concluded that antepartum culture for *Ureaplasma* to predict pregnancy outcome is not justified on a routine basis.

Postpartum Infection

Like other organisms of the lower genital tract microflora, mycoplasmas can be recovered transiently in the bloodstream shortly after delivery. However, genital mycoplasmas are seldom recovered from the blood of postpartum women who are not febrile, whereas they are commonly found in the blood of febrile postpartum women (Lamey et al., 1982). Both genital mycoplasmas are isolated commonly in the endometrium of women with endometritis (see Watts [1990], Postpartum Infection).

The frequency with which endometritis resulting from *M. hominis* occurs without bloodstream invasion and the percentage of endometritis cases caused by M. *hominis* are not clear. Studies suggest that M. *hominis* is a common cause of postpartum infection (McCormack et al., 1973), but there is an excellent response of endometritis to antibiotics such as cefoxitin and broad-spectrum penicillins, therapies without notable activity against the mycoplasmas.

Neonatal Infection

Genital mycoplasmas appear to be an uncommon cause of sepsis or meningitis in young infants (up to 3 months of age) (Likitnukel et al., 1986). Among preterm newborns, however, genital mycoplasmas have been isolated more commonly in the CSF (8 per 100 for *U. urealyticum;* 5 per 100 for M. *hominis*) (Waites et al., 1988).

Diagnosis

The diagnosis of mycoplasmal infection is based on isolation of the organism from a site of infection and demonstration of a rise in antibody titer. For optimal isolation of mycoplasmas, specimens should be inoculated immediately into medium, kept at 4° C, and transported to the laboratory as soon as possible. The basic medium is a beef-heart–infusion broth, available commercially as pleuropneumonia-like organism broth, supplemented with fresh yeast extract and horse serum. Antibacterial agents are added to inhibit bacterial growth.

Various procedures including ELISA and metabolic inhibition have been used to detect serologic response to the genital mycoplasmas.

Treatment

The antimicrobial agents that inhibit protein synthesis, including the aminoglycosides, tetracyclines, and lincomycins as well as chloramphenicol and erythromycin, are active against most mycoplasmas. Tetracyclines are effective against both M. *hominis* and *U. urealyticum. Mycoplasma hominis* is sensitive to lincomycin but resistant to erythromycin. Ureaplasmas, on the other hand, are sensitive to erythromycin but not to lincomycin. In addition, M. *hominis* is highly sensitive and ureaplasmas are moderately sensitive to clindamycin. The penicillins, the cephalosporins, and vancomycin are ineffective.

On the basis of Kass's early controlled antibiotic trials with tetracycline in bacteriuric women, it has been suggested that antimicrobial treatment of microorganisms such as the mycoplasmas in the lower genital tract would decrease the risk of premature delivery. Kass and coworkers (1981) reported that erythromycin given in the third trimester significantly reduced the risk of premature, low-birth-weight infants in a group of 245 low-income pregnant women at the Boston City Hospital who were found at the initial antenatal visit to have mycoplasmal infections. These investigators used a double-blind protocol in which patients received placebo or erythromycin, 1 g per day for 6 weeks. They reported that the excess prematurity rate associated with mycoplasmal infection accounted for half of the birth-weight differences noted in their study; however, the antibiotic therapy may have acted on other infectious agents as well.

In 1991, Eschenbach and coworkers performed a large treatment trial attempting to resolve the role of *Ureaplasma* in preterm birth and excluding patients (in this part of their work) with C. *trachomatis.* In this multicenter, double-blind, randomized trial, pregnant women with *U. urealyticum* were treated with erythromycin base or placebo during the third trimester. Erythromycin did not eliminate *U. urealyticum* from the lower genital tract, and there was no association between erythromycin treatment and improved pregnancy outcome. The role of infectious agents in preterm labor is addressed in Chapter 34.

Treatment should be restricted to clinical situations in which mycoplasmas have been isolated from a body fluid or a focus of infection and appear to be significantly related to the disease process. Thus, erythromycin treatment of pregnant patients for the purpose of resolving repeated abortions, unexplained infertility, and poor late pregnancy outcome should be limited to formal research situations.

Candidiasis (Monilial Vaginitis)

Candida albicans is a saprophytic yeast that exists as part of the endogenous flora of the vagina. The organism is present in the vagina of approximately 25% of sexually active women. It may become an opportunistic pathogen, especially when host defense mechanisms are compromised. Systemic candidiasis is a rare event in gravid patients, occurring only when disease entities causing significant debilitation, such as sepsis and malignancy, are present. Candidal vulvovaginitis is a much more common infection. *Candida albicans* is the second most common cause of vaginitis after BV. Other yeasts, such as *Candida glabrata,* account for approximately 5% to 15% of yeast vaginitis.

Symptomatic candidal vulvovaginitis affects 15% of pregnant women. It is thought that the hormonal environment of pregnancy, in which high levels of estrogen produce an increased concentration of vaginal glycogen, accounts for the frequency of symptomatic infection in gravid patients. In addition, suppression of cell-mediated immunity in pregnancy may decrease the ability to limit fungal proliferation.

The clinical manifestations in pregnancy are similar to those in the nonpregnant state; they include pruritus and burning, dysuria, dyspareunia, excoriations with secondary infection, and pruritus ani. The vaginal discharge is frequently thick, white, and curdlike.

A presumptive diagnosis of candidiasis is best made by microscopic examination of vaginal secretions using 10% potassium hydroxide to facilitate identification of fungus. Because patients with yeast vulvovaginitis may have negative potassium hydroxide smears, the diagnosis may be confirmed by cultures on selective media such as Sabouraud's or Nickerson's. Yeast vulvovaginitis has not been associated with preterm birth, preterm labor, low birth weight, or PROM (Cotch et al., 1990). Epidemiology and outcomes are associated with moderate to heavy colonization by *Candida* during pregnancy.

The clinical manifestations of congenital candidiasis range from superficial skin infections to systemic disease with hemorrhage and necrosis of the heart, lungs, kidneys, and other organs. The most common route of infection is by direct contact during delivery through an infected vagina, and oropharyngeal candidiasis of the neonate (thrush) is the most common problem.

Nystatin was previously used for candidal vulvovaginitis. Topical drugs for therapy of candidiasis (e.g., miconazole, clotrimazole, terconazole, and butoconazole) have the advantages of somewhat greater efficacy and a shorter course of therapy. Although data on use of such drugs in the first trimester are not extensive, the use of miconazole and clotrimazole especially (the oldest of these preparations) later in pregnancy has not been accompanied by adverse effects on the fetus. The oral antifungal fluconazole (Diflucan) is a class C drug regarding use in pregnancy. The CDC recommends only topical azoles, for 7 days, for treating candidal infection in pregnancy (CDC, 2002).

Bacterial Vaginosis

Formerly called nonspecific vaginitis, *Gardnerella vaginalis* vaginitis, and *Haemophilus vaginalis* vaginitis, "bacterial vaginosis" is the preferable term in view of recent progress regarding pathophysiology. The condition is marked by a major shift in vaginal flora from the normal predominance of lactobacilli to a predominance of anaerobes, which are increased 100-fold compared with normal secretions. *Gardnerella vaginalis* is present in 95% of cases but is also present in 30% to 40% of normal women when selective media are used. *Mycoplasma hominis* in vaginal secretions is significantly increased in cases of BV.

Clinically, the primary symptoms are discharge and odor. Itching is not usually prominent. Diagnosis of BV is based upon presence of three of the following four clinical features: (1) an amine-like or fishy odor that may be accentuated after addition of potassium hydroxide or after coitus (owing to the alkaline pH of semen); (2) a milky or creamy discharge; (3) an elevated pH (4.5 or higher); and (4) on wet mount, true "clue" cells (squamous epithelial cells so heavily stippled with bacteria that the borders are obscured). Typically in BV, clue cells account for over 20% of epithelial cells, and there are few leukocytes. An experienced observer will also note an increase in numbers and kinds of bacteria and a reduction in numbers of lactobacilli. A Gram stain of vaginal secretions also demonstrates the shift in bacteria and clue cells.

BV is the most common type of infectious vaginitis. Approximately 15% of pregnant women fulfill the criteria, but half are asymptomatic.

Evidence has consistently associated BV with an increase in premature birth (Gravett, Hummel, et al., 1986; Gravett, Preston-Nelson, et al., 1986; Martius et al., 1988; Hillier et al., 1995), intra-amniotic infection (Silver et al., 1989), endometritis (Newton et al., 1990), and histologic chorioamnionitis (Hillier et al., 1988). The risk for preterm birth

among women with BV has varied (OR, 1.4 to 8) but has been significant in all populations studied.

In nonpregnant women, the most consistent cure rates (90%) have been achieved with metronidazole (e.g., 500 mg twice a day for 7 days). Lower cure rates (60% to 80%) are observed with a single 2.0-g dose of metronidazole. Oral clindamycin (300 mg twice a day for 7 days) is effective in treating nonpregnant patients and appears to be safe in pregnancy. Vaginal clindamycin creams (2%) have also been effective in nonpregnant women. The vaginal dose is 140 mg daily, with very little being absorbed. Metronidazole gel, 0.75%, one applicator-full (5 g) intravaginally twice daily for 5 days, is also effective in nonpregnant women. The preferred regimens in pregnancy are shown in Table 39-17. There is no longer an exclusion for use of metronidazole in any trimester of pregnancy. A recent meta-analysis showed no evidence of teratogenesis (Caro-Paton et al., 1997; see also Piper et al., 1993; Burtin et al., 1995; CDC, 2002).

In view of the consistent association of BV with adverse pregnancy outcomes, clinical treatment trials have been undertaken. Three trials, all conducted in high-risk patients (on the basis of either a previous preterm birth or other high-risk demographic features), have revealed improvement in outcome with prenatal treatment of BV (Table 39-18). In a group of women who experienced preterm birth or PROM during a previous pregnancy, treatment of BV with metronidazole led to a significant reduction in preterm birth, low birth weight, and PROM ($P < .05$ for each) (Morales et al., 1994). In a prospective, two-phased trial among 1260 women, treatment of BV significantly decreased preterm birth ($P < .05$) (McGregor et al., 1995). Finally, in women at risk because of previous preterm birth or low maternal weight, a combination of metronidazole and erythromycin significantly improved pregnancy outcome compared to placebo in patients who had BV ($P < 0.006$). In patients without BV pregnancy outcome was not improved (Hauth et al., 1995).

In a treatment trial of women at low risk, metronidazole (twice daily for 2 days at 24 weeks, with repeat treatment, if needed, at 29 weeks) led to no reduction in preterm birth overall but produced a significant reduction in women with previous preterm birth (McDonald et al., 1997). In the Maternal-Fetal Medicine Network treatment trial of women with asymptomatic BV, the treatment regimen was also short (two 2.0-gram doses at 16 to 24 weeks and again at 24 to 30 weeks, with the repeat treatment at least 14 days after the initial doses). Using metronidazole in this regimen led to no significant improvement either overall or in any subgroup (such as those with previous preterm birth) (Carey et al.,

TABLE 39-17. 2002 CDC RECOMMENDED REGIMEN FOR TREATING BACTERIAL VAGINOSIS IN PREGNANCY

Metronidazole 250 mg PO t.i.d. *for 7 d
OR
Clindamycin 300 mg PO b.i.d. for 7 d

* Some specialists recommend 500 mg b.i.d.
b.i.d., twice daily; PO, orally; t.i.d., three times daily.

Data from Centers for Disease Control and Prevention (CDC): Sexually transmitted diseases treatment guidelines 2002. MMWR Morb Mortal Wkly Rep **51:** 44, 2002.

TABLE 39-18. STUDIES OF BACTERIAL VAGINOSIS IN PREGNANCY IN PATIENTS AT HIGH RISK FOR PRETERM DELIVERY

Study	Design	Study Population	Preterm Birth		Significance (*P*)
			Antibiotic Treatment (%)	No Treatment, or Placebo (%)	
Morales et al., 1994	Randomized, placebo-controlled	80 women with previous preterm birth or PPROM, in Florida	18	39	< 0.05
Hauth et al., 1995	Randomized, placebo-controlled	258 inner-city women with previous preterm birth or low maternal weight, Birmingham, Ala	31	49	0.006
McGregor et al., 1995	Nonrandomized, two-phase trial	126 women in inner-city Denver hospital with 15% preterm birth rate	9.8	18.8	0.02

PPROM, preterm premature rupture of membranes.

Modified from Gibbs RS, Eschenbach DA: Use of antibiotics to prevent preterm birth. Am J Obstet Gynecol **177**:375, 1997.

2000). These studies are summarized in Figure 39-5. In view of these disparate results, the ACOG (2001) has concluded, "Currently, there are insufficient data to suggest screening and treating women at either low or high risk will reduce the overall rate of preterm birth." However, Goldenberg and colleagues (2000) have concluded differently, taking into consideration the metronidazole regimen used. We agree with their recommendation of treatment with oral metronidazole for at least 7 days, beginning in the second trimester, in women at high risk (e.g., those with previous preterm birth). Recommendations for managing BV in pregnancy are presented in Table 39-19.

Toxoplasmosis

Epidemiology

Toxoplasma gondii is a protozoan that exists in three stages: trophozoite, cyst, and oocyst. The life cycle of *T. gondii* is dependent on wild and domestic cats, which are the only host for the oocyst. The oocyst is formed in the cat's intestine and subsequently excreted in the feces. Mammals, such as cows, then ingest the oocyst, which is disrupted in the animal's intestine, releasing the invasive trophozoite. The trophozoite then is disseminated throughout the animal's body, ultimately forming cysts in brain and muscle. Human infection occurs when infected meat is ingested or when food is contaminated by cat feces—for example by flies, cockroaches, or fingers. Infection rates are highest in areas of poor sanitation and crowded living conditions. Stray cats and domestic cats that eat raw meat are most likely to carry the parasite (Krick and Remington, 1978; Egerman and Beazley, 1998).

Approximately 40% to 50% of adults in the United States have antibody to this organism, with highest prevalence in populations of lower socioeconomic status. The frequency of seroconversion during pregnancy is 5% or less, and approximately 3 infants per 1000 show evidence of congenital infection. Clinically significant congenital toxoplasmosis occurs in approximately 1 in 8000 pregnancies. Toxoplasmosis is more common in Western Europe, particularly France (Daffos et al., 1988).

Most infections in immunocompetent persons are asymptomatic. When symptoms are present, they are similar to those associated with mononucleosis. In immunosuppressed patients, however, toxoplasmosis can be a devastating infection. Because immunity to *T. gondii* is cell mediated, patients with HIV infection and those treated with chronic immunosuppressive therapy after organ transplantation are particularly susceptible to new or reactivated infection. In these patients, CNS dysfunction is the most common manifestation of infection. Findings typically include encephalitis, meningoencephalitis, and intracerebral mass lesions. Pneumonitis, myocarditis, and generalized lymphadenopathy are also common (MMWR, 1997).

Diagnosis

The diagnosis of toxoplasmosis can be confirmed by serologic and histologic methods. Serologic tests indicative of an acute infection include detection of IgM-specific antibody, demonstration of an extremely high IgG antibody titer, and documentation of IgG seroconversion from negative to positive. Clinicians should be aware that serologic assays for toxoplasmosis are not well standardized. When initial laboratory tests appear to indicate that an acute infection has occurred, repeat serology should be performed in an experienced reference laboratory. The best tissue for identification of *T. gondii* is a lymph node or brain biopsy specimen. Histologic

Study	Effect	
	Lowering of preterm birth	Increasing of preterm birth
Morales, 1994		
McGregor, 1995		
Hauth, 1995		
McDonald, 1997 (overall)		
(previous PTB)		
Carey, 2000 (overall)		
(previous PTB)		

FIGURE 39-5 ■ Summary of treatment trials of bacterial vaginosis in pregnancy to prevent preterm birth.

TABLE 39-19. RECOMMENDATIONS FOR MANAGING BACTERIAL VAGINOSIS IN PREGNANCY

- Symptomatic pregnant women with BV can be safely treated in any trimester
- Routine screening and treatment of BV in asymptomatic women at low risk for preterm birth CANNOT be endorsed (USPTF: D recommendation)
- Screening for BV may be considered in women at high risk for preterm birth, such as those with previous preterm birth
- In these high-risk women, treatment should be initiated in second trimester, with oral metronidazole for 1 wk or more
- In high-risk women, vaginal treatment should not be used
- The value of rescreening and retreating is unclear

BV, bacterial vaginosis; USPTF, U.S. Preventive Services Task Force.

preparations can be examined by light or electron microscopy. For light microscopy, specimens should be stained with either Giemsa or Wright stain (Krick and Remington, 1978).

Congenital Toxoplasmosis

Congenital infection can occur if a woman develops *acute* toxoplasmosis during pregnancy. *Chronic* or *latent* infection is unlikely to cause fetal injury except perhaps in an immunosuppressed patient. Approximately 40% of neonates born to mothers with *acute primary* toxoplasmosis show evidence of infection. Congenital infection is most likely to occur when maternal infection develops in the third trimester. Less than half of affected infants are symptomatic at birth. The major clinical manifestations of congenital toxoplasmosis include rash, hepatosplenomegaly, ascites, fever, chorioretinitis, periventricular calcifications, ventriculomegaly, seizures, mental retardation, and uveitis (Daffos et al., 1988).

The most valuable tests for antenatal diagnosis of congenital toxoplasmosis are ultrasound and amniocentesis. Cordocentesis should be reserved for cases in which ultrasound and amniocentesis are not definitive. Ultrasound findings suggestive of infection include ventriculomegaly, intracranial calcifications, microcephaly, ascites, hepatosplenomegaly, and growth restriction. Hohlfeld and colleagues (1994) have identified a specific gene of *T. gondii* in amniotic fluid using a PCR test. In their investigation, 34 of 339 infants had congenital toxoplasmosis confirmed by serologic testing or autopsy. All amniotic fluid samples from affected pregnancies were positive by PCR, and test results were available within 1 day of specimen collection. In a subsequent report, Romana and coworkers (2001) evaluated the performance of PCR in a series of 270 previous patients with proven primary toxoplasmosis. Seventy-five of the infants had congenital infection. The overall sensitivity of PCR in amniotic fluid specimens was 64%. The specificity and positive predictive value were 100%. The negative predictive value was 88%. The sensitivity of the assay was greatest for maternal infections that occurred in weeks 17 to 21.

When acute toxoplasmosis occurs during pregnancy, treatment of the mother is imperative to reduce the risk of congenital infection and decrease the late sequelae of infection. Pyrimethamine, one of the drugs of choice in nonpregnant

patients, is not recommended for use during the first trimester of pregnancy because of possible teratogenicity. Sulfonamides such as sulfadiazine can be used alone, but single-agent therapy appears to be less effective than combination therapy. In Europe, spiramycin, a macrolide antibiotic, has been employed extensively in pregnancy with excellent success. It is available for use in the United States upon special request through the CDC (Daffos et al., 1988; Hohlfeld et al., 1994).

The largest series of pregnancies at risk for congenital toxoplasmosis was reported by Daffos and colleagues (1988). These authors followed 746 pregnant women who had serologically confirmed primary toxoplasmosis. Infection was diagnosed antenatally in 39 fetuses by umbilical blood sampling. All mothers were treated during pregnancy with spiramycin. Mothers who had an infected fetus were also treated with pyrimethamine plus either sulfadoxine or sulfadiazine. Twenty-four of the 39 pregnancies were terminated. Of the 15 pregnancies carried to term, 13 neonates were clinically well during a 3-month observation period, and 2 infants had chorioretinitis.

Early aggressive treatment of the infected neonate is an alternative to *in utero* therapy. Guerina and coworkers (1994) recently reported the results of a large screening project for neonatal toxoplasmosis in Massachusetts and New Hampshire. Over 600,000 infants were tested, and congenital infection was confirmed in 52. Detailed physical examination in 48 children showed abnormalities of the CNS in 19 (40%). After the infants were treated with combinations of pyrimethamine, sulfadiazine, and leucovorin for 1 year, only one child had a persistent neurologic defect (hemiplegia). Subsequently, at ages 1 to 6, four other children were found to have ophthalmologic abnormalities. One child had a macular lesion, and three had minor retinal scars. Thus, early treatment reduces, but does not completely eliminate, the late sequelae of congenital toxoplasmosis.

In the management of the pregnant patient, prevention of acute toxoplasmosis is of paramount importance. Pregnant women should be advised to avoid contact with stray cats or cat litter. They should be instructed to wash their hands after preparing meat for cooking and never to eat raw or rare meat. Specifically, they should be told to cook their meat until the juices are "clear" rather than "bloody." Fruits and vegetables also should be carefully washed to remove possible contamination by oocysts (Egerman and Beazley, 1998).

Trichomoniasis

Trichomonas vaginalis is a common cause of vaginitis, with infection often characterized by intense pruritus, strong odor, and dysuria. Physical examination typically shows a malodorous, yellow-green, frothy discharge, but variations of the gross appearance occur in approximately 50% of cases. The diagnosis may be confirmed by a microscopic examination of a smear of the discharge diluted with saline. The examination reveals many leukocytes and bacteria; trichomonads are recognized by their size (slightly larger than leukocytes) and active flagella. Cultures for *Trichomonas* are more sensitive than the smear. Recent commercially available systems have facilitated culture of this parasite.

Trichomonas vaginalis vaginitis occurs in less than 10% up to 50% of pregnant women, depending on sexual activity and socioeconomic status. Consequently, it has been difficult to establish whether the incidence of this vaginal infection is truly increased in pregnant women. Premature rupture of membranes (PROM) at term has also been associated with positive cultures for *T. vaginalis* (27.5% with versus 12.8% without; *P* < 0.03) (Minkoff et al., 1984). In the large National Institutes of Health infection and prematurity study, *T. vaginalis* infection at mid-pregnancy was significantly associated with low birth weight (OR, 1.3; 95% CI, 1.1 to 1.5), preterm delivery (OR, 1.3; 95% CI, 1.1 to 1.4), and PROM (OR, 1.4; 95% CI, 1.1 to 1.6), even after adjustment for confounding factors and other microbes (Cotch et al., 1997).

In nonpregnant women with symptomatic trichomoniasis, treatment consists of oral metronidazole, with the preferred regimen being 2.0 g orally in a single dose and the alternative being 500 mg orally twice a day for 7 days (CDC, 2002). Pregnant women may be treated with 2 g of metronidazole orally in a single dose. No consistent association has been demonstrated between use of metronidazole in pregnancy and teratogenesis or mutagenesis in infants (Burtin et al., 1995). Topical agents are often unsuccessful in relieving symptoms or in eradicating this protozoon. Among women with asymptomatic trichomoniasis in pregnancy, treatment in the second trimester (2.0-g doses 48 hours apart at 16 to 23 weeks, repeated at 24 to 29 weeks) did not result in better pregnancy outcomes than did placebo. Indeed, those given metronidazole had significantly greater rates of prematurity (Klebanoff et al., 2001). Accordingly, although symptomatic women with trichomoniasis should be treated in pregnancy to relieve symptoms, routine screening and treatment is not recommended.

ANTIBIOTICS IN PREGNANCY

This section reviews the antibiotics that are most commonly used in perinatal medicine for treatment of bacterial infections. Special attention is devoted to spectrum of activity, toxicity, practical application, and cost of therapy. For ease of reference, the drugs are listed in alphabetical order. Drugs that are potentially teratogenic and are therefore contraindicated in pregnancy (e.g., doxycycline, fluoroquinolones, and tetracycline) are not discussed.

Aminoglycosides (Pregnancy Category D)

Three aminoglycosides commonly are used in clinical practice: amikacin, gentamicin, and tobramycin. They act by inhibiting bacterial protein synthesis. They function most effectively in tissues in which the pH and oxygen tension are normal and do not penetrate well into abscess cavities.

The principal strength of activity of the aminoglycosides is against aerobic gram-negative bacilli. Amikacin provides slightly better coverage of drug-resistant pathogens such as *Pseudomonas*, *Serratia*, and *Enterobacter* species. Aminoglycosides also provide effective coverage for *Neisseria gonorrhoeae* and staphylococci species; they are not active against streptococcal organisms or anaerobes.

The two major side effects of the aminoglycosides are nephrotoxicity and ototoxicity, and the three drugs are comparable in their potential for causing such reactions. Both adverse effects are rare in patients who have no underlying medical illnesses, who are not receiving other nephrotoxic drugs, and who require treatment for limited periods of time. The concern about the teratogenicity of the aminoglycosides

is based on reports of fetal ototoxicity in patients receiving streptomycin for extended periods of time for treatment of tuberculosis. With gentamicin, tobramycin, and amikacin, fetal injury is extremely unlikely when the drugs are administered for short periods of time (3 to 7 days) for treatment of pyelonephritis or chorioamnionitis.

The aminoglycosides are available in intramuscular and intravenous formulations but are usually administered by the latter route. Two dosing regimens have been developed for intravenous administration—multi-dose and single daily dose. The single daily dosing regimen is preferred in postpartum patients because it is more effective, less toxic, more convenient, and less expensive than the multi-dose regimen (Nicolau et al., 1995). There is limited information at present about the safety of single-dose therapy when the fetus still is *in utero*.

The appropriate multi-dose regimen for gentamicin and tobramycin is 1.0 to 1.5 mg/kg actual weight every 8 hours. The corresponding single-dose regimen is 7 mg/kg ideal body weight every 24 hours. For amikacin the appropriate multi-dose regimen is 5.0 mg/kg actual weight every 8 hours or 7.5 mg/kg actual weight every 12 hours. The single-daily dose is 15 mg/kg ideal body weight (Duff, 1997, 2002).

Aminoglycosides have two major applications in obstetrics. First, they may be used to treat pyelonephritis in patients who are allergic to β-lactam antibiotics or who are infected by microorganisms that are resistant to β-lactam antibiotics. Second, they may be used in combination with agents such as clindamycin or metronidazole plus penicillin or ampicillin to treat puerperal endometritis.

Gentamicin is available in generic formulation, and the cost of one day's treatment is usually less than $15. Both tobramycin and amikacin tend to be several times more expensive. Accordingly, as a general rule, gentamicin is the aminoglycoside of choice in obstetrics. Amikacin should be reserved for special situations to treat particularly virulent and resistant pathogens (Duff, 2002).

Amoxicillin-Clavulanate (Pregnancy Category B)

Amoxicillin is an oral β-lactam antibiotic that inhibits cell wall synthesis; clavulanate is a β-lactamase inhibitor that, when combined with amoxicillin, significantly expands the spectrum of activity of the latter. Compared to ampicillin or amoxicillin, amoxicillin-clavulanate has enhanced activity against staphylococcal species, *Hemophilus influenzae*, and anaerobic organisms. The drug is excreted largely unchanged in the urine and has a toxicity profile similar to those of ampicillin and amoxicillin.

Amoxicillin-clavulanate has two major applications in obstetrics. It is an excellent drug for treatment of lower urinary tract infections caused by resistant organisms and for outpatient therapy of mild pyelonephritis in a stable patient who is in the first half of pregnancy. For these indications, the drug should be administered in a dose of amoxicillin (875 mg) plus clavulanate (125 mg), twice daily for 7 to 10 days. Amoxicillin-clavulanate also has a sufficiently broad spectrum of activity that it can be used for treatment of patients with mild postoperative infections (endometritis or wound infection) that develop after initial discharge from the hospital. For these indications, the proper dose of amoxicillin-clavulanate is amoxicillin (875 mg) plus clavulanate (125 mg), twice daily until the patient has been afebrile and asymptomatic for 24 to 48 hours (Duff, 2002).

Unlike ampicillin and amoxicillin, amoxicillin-clavulanate is not available in generic formulation. Accordingly, it is quite expensive. A 7-day course of the antibiotic may cost between $60 and $70. Therefore, amoxicillin-clavulanate should be used only when less expensive antibiotics are not likely to be effective.

Amoxicillin and Ampicillin (Pregnancy Category B)

Like penicillin, amoxicillin and ampicillin are β-lactam antibiotics that inhibit bacterial cell wall synthesis. Their spectrum of activity is almost identical and includes the same organisms listed previously for penicillin. In addition, they have activity against many strains of *Hemophilus influenzae*, most strains of enterococci, and many aerobic gram-negative bacilli. However, because of the widespread use of amoxicillin and ampicillin over many years, a growing number of strains of coliform organisms have become resistant to these antibiotics (Dunlow and Duff, 1990).

Amoxicillin and ampicillin are excreted largely unchanged in the urine. Their two most common side effects are allergic reaction and drug-induced diarrhea. Pseudomembranous enterocolitis also may occur as a consequence of exposure to these agents.

Amoxicillin and ampicillin have four major uses in obstetrics. First, they are the drugs of choice for confirmed enterococcal UTI. For treatment of an enterococcal lower urinary tract infection, the appropriate oral dose of amoxicillin is 250 mg three times daily; the corresponding oral dose of ampicillin is 250 mg four times daily. For an initial infection, 3 days of treatment is usually sufficient. For recurrent infections, a 7- to 10-day course should be administered (Duff, 1994).

Ampicillin is an appropriate drug for intrapartum prophylaxis against GBS infection. In this clinical situation, the appropriate intravenous dose of ampicillin is 2 g initially, then 1 g every 4 hours until delivery. In a recent report, Edwards and colleagues (2002) showed that, when used for prophylaxis, ampicillin was no more likely than penicillin to select for resistant gram-negative bacilli.

When used in combination with gentamicin, ampicillin is suitable for treatment of chorioamnionitis. The appropriate intravenous dose of ampicillin is 2 g every 6 hours. This same combination regimen also may be used to provide prophylaxis against endocarditis in selected patients with heart disease who are undergoing obstetric procedures (Duff, 2002).

Like penicillin, ampicillin and amoxicillin are produced in generic formulations by several pharmaceutical companies. Accordingly, they are relatively inexpensive when compared to other antibiotics.

Azithromycin and Erythromycin (Pregnancy Category B)

Azithromycin and erythromycin are macrolide antibiotics that exert their antibacterial effect by inhibiting bacterial protein synthesis. Both drugs are highly effective against *Streptococcus pneumoniae*, *S. pyogenes*, *S. agalactiae*, most strains of staphylococci, and *Chlamydia trachomatis*. Azithromycin is more active than erythromycin against *Hemophilus influenzae*, *Moraxella catarrhalis*, and *Mycoplasma pneumoniae* (McCarty, 1996).

Both antibiotics are well absorbed when administered orally and are metabolized by the liver. Compared to erythromycin, azithromycin achieves sustained concentrations in intracellular and interstitial tissue compartments even though serum concentrations are low. Azithromycin is also better concentrated in phagocytes.

The most common side effects of erythromycin are nausea, vomiting, and diarrhea. In contrast, azithromycin is usually much better tolerated. Accordingly, in most situations, patients will demonstrate better compliance with a shorter course of azithromycin than to more-conventional regimens of erythromycin.

The principal application of azithromycin in obstetrics is for treatment of lower genitourinary tract infections caused by chlamydia (McCarty, 1996). In this clinical setting, azithromycin powder should be prescribed in a single 1-g dose. This drug is currently the only single-dose treatment for chlamydia and, as such, markedly increases patient compliance. When azithromycin is ordered in the powder formulation, the cost is relatively modest (approximately $20 to $25).

Aztreonam (Pregnancy Category B)

Aztreonam is a monobactam antibiotic that inhibits cell wall synthesis. Its principal strength of activity is against aerobic gram-negative bacilli, similar to the aminoglycosides. The drug may be administered intravenously or intramuscularly, and it is eliminated primarily by renal excretion. Toxicity is uncommon and is usually manifested by reversible increases in the serum transaminase concentrations and by allergic reactions. There is some crossover in reactivity to aztreonam and β-lactam antibiotics (Simmons and Lee, 1985).

In obstetrics, aztreonam may be used as a single agent for treatment of acute pyelonephritis. The appropriate intravenous dose is 500 mg to 1 g every 8 to 12 hours, depending upon the severity of the infection. The drug also may be used in combination with clindamycin or metronidazole plus penicillin or ampicillin for treatment of puerperal endometritis. In this situation, the appropriate intravenous dose is 1 to 2 g every 8 to 12 hours. Aztreonam is several times more expensive than gentamicin; it should therefore be reserved for patients who have a contraindication to use of an aminoglycoside (Duff, 2002).

Carbapenems (Pregnancy Categories B and C)

Carbapenems are parenteral β-lactam antibiotics that are relatively resistant to hydrolysis by bacterial β-lactamases. The first carbapenem introduced in the United States was imipenem-cilastatin (pregnancy category C). Imipenem is the active drug. Cilastatin inhibits the renal metabolism of imipenem by dehydropeptidase I, thus reducing the risk of nephrotoxicity and slowing the rate of renal excretion. Two other carbapenems, meropenem (pregnancy category B), and ertapenem (pregnancy category B) are now commercially available. Unlike imipenem, the latter drugs are not metabolized by dehydropeptidase and thus can be given without cilastatin (Anonymous, 1996, 2002).

The carbapenems inhibit bacterial cell wall synthesis and are active against the broad range of pelvic pathogens. Meropenem is slightly more active against aerobic gram-negative bacilli; imipenem-cilastatin is more effective against gram-positive bacteria. Ertapenem lacks effective coverage against *Pseudomonas aeruginosa* and *Acinetobacter* species. None of the three is effective against methicillin-resistant staphylococci or *Enterococcus faecium*, either of which may be implicated in soft-tissue pelvic or wound infections.

The principal adverse effects of the carbapenems are allergic reaction, diarrhea, nausea and vomiting, seizures and reversible increases in serum aminotransferases. Another possible, but rare, adverse effect of the carbapenems is induction of β-lactamase synthesis by the infecting bacteria. This effect has been of principal concern in immunocompromised patients who have infections caused by *Pseudomonas* species (Anonymous, 1996, 2002). There is some degree of cross reactivity between carbapenems and other β-lactam antibiotics. Accordingly, the drugs should be administered with extreme caution to patients who have a history of an immediate hypersensitivity reaction to penicillins.

The carbapenems are of greatest value in obstetrics as single agents for the treatment of polymicrobial infections such as chorioamnionitis or puerperal endometritis, especially in patients who have a contraindication to combination therapy that includes an aminoglycoside. Compared to other antibiotics commonly used in obstetrics, the carbapenems are very expensive.

Cephalosporins (Pregnancy Category B)

Cephalosporins are β-lactam antibiotics that inhibit bacterial cell wall biosynthesis. They vary widely in their spectrum of activity and can be divided into three categories: limited spectrum, intermediate spectrum, and extended spectrum.

The prototype of the limited-spectrum cephalosporins is cefazolin, which is available in intramuscular and intravenous formulations. The oral equivalent of cefazolin is cephalexin. The limited-spectrum cephalosporins have excellent activity against GBS, staphylococci, and anaerobic gram-positive cocci. They have good activity against aerobic gram-negative bacilli and only fair activity against anaerobic gram-negative bacilli. They are not effective against enterococci (Donowitz et al., 1988a,b).

The intermediate-spectrum cephalosporins include drugs such as cefonicid, cefoperazone, ceforanide, ceftazidime, and ceftriaxone. These agents are available in intramuscular and intravenous formulations. Their oral equivalent is cefixime. Compared to the limited-spectrum cephalosporins, these antibiotics have improved coverage against aerobic and anaerobic gram-negative bacilli and *Neisseria gonorrhoeae*, equivalent coverage of GBS, and decreased activity against staphylococci. Like the limited-spectrum agents, these drugs have no activity against enterococci (Donowitz et al., 1988a,b; Duff, 2002).

The extended-spectrum cephalosporins include cefepime, cefotaxime, cefotetan, cefoxitin, and ceftizoxime. They are available in intramuscular and intravenous formulations. Compared to limited- and intermediate-spectrum agents, these antimicrobials have expanded coverage against aerobic and anaerobic gram-negative bacilli and equivalent coverage of GBS. However, their coverage of staphylococci is not as effective, and they, too, lack activity against the enterococci (Donowitz et al., 1988a,b; Duff, 2002).

The cephalosporins are eliminated from the body primarily by renal excretion. Their principal adverse effect is an allergic reaction. Up to 15% of patients who are allergic to penicillin will also be allergic to cephalosporins. Other side effects include thrombophlebitis at the site of intravenous injection, pain at the site of intramuscular administration, diarrhea, and induction of β-lactamases. Some of the cephalosporins have also been associated with a bleeding diathesis resulting from platelet dysfunction and/or hypoprothrombinemia (Duff, 2002).

The limited-spectrum cephalosporins have four major applications in obstetrics. Intravenous cefazolin, 1 g every 8 hours, is an excellent treatment for acute pyelonephritis in pregnant women. In the same dosage regimen, cefazolin is an excellent treatment for a surgical wound infection. Cefazolin is a particularly good selection for surgical prophylaxis in patients having cesarean delivery; the appropriate dose is 1 g immediately after the umbilical cord is clamped. Finally, oral cephalexin (500 mg every 6 hours) is one of the drugs of choice for puerperal mastitis (Duff, 1997, 2002).

The principal application of the intermediate-spectrum cephalosporins in obstetrics is for treatment of gonorrhea. For gonococcal infections of the lower genitourinary tract, one of the drugs of choice is ceftriaxone, 125 mg administered intramuscularly in a single dose. An equally effective, and significantly less expensive, treatment is oral cefixime, 400 mg in a single dose (CDC, 1998).

The extended-spectrum cephalosporins are best used as single agents for treatment of polymicrobial pelvic infections such as chorioamnionitis or puerperal endometritis. For this indication, however, they may be more expensive than combinations of generic antibiotics. The extended-spectrum agents should not be used routinely for prophylaxis for cesarean delivery or for pyelonephritis in pregnancy because they are no more effective than cefazolin and are much more expensive.

Clindamycin (Pregnancy Category B)

Clindamycin is a macrolide antibiotic and exerts its antibacterial effect by acting on the bacterial ribosome and preventing the transcription of RNA into protein. Clindamycin has excellent activity against staphylococci, GBS, and anaerobic organisms. It is not effective against enterococci or aerobic gram-negative bacilli. The drug is metabolized in the liver. Its most common side effect is diarrhea, which occurs in up to 10% of patients. The most serious side effect is pseudomembranous enterocolitis, which fortunately is extremely rare.

In obstetrics, clindamycin has three primary uses. First, it is an acceptable agent for treatment of mastitis in patients who are allergic to β-lactam antibiotics. For this purpose, the drug should be administered orally, in a dose of 300 mg, four times daily for 5 to 7 days. Second, in either oral or topical form, clindamycin is an effective, but relatively expensive, treatment for BV. The appropriate dose of 2% clindamycin vaginal cream is one applicator-full daily for 7 days. The recommended oral dose of clindamycin for treatment of BV is 300 mg, twice daily, for 7 days. The third, and perhaps most important, use of clindamycin is in combination with other drugs such as gentamicin, or gentamicin plus penicillin or ampicillin, for treatment of polymicrobial infections such as chorioamnionitis or puerperal endometritis. The appropriate dose of clindamycin in these clinical situations is 900 mg intravenously every 8 hours until signs and symptoms of infection have resolved (Duff, 2002).

Extended-Spectrum Penicillins (Pregnancy Category B)

The extended-spectrum penicillins include two single agents (mezlocillin and piperacillin) and three combination antibiotics (ampicillin-sulbactam, ticarcillin-clavulanate, and piperacillin-tazobactam). Mezlocillin, piperacillin, ampicillin, and ticarcillin are β-lactam antibiotics that inhibit bacterial cell wall synthesis. Sulbactam, clavulanate, and tazobactam are β-lactamase inhibitors that negate the ability of bacterial β-lactamase enzymes to inactivate β-lactam antibiotics. The addition of these inhibitors significantly expands the spectrum of activity of ampicillin, mezlocillin, and piperacillin (Duff, 1997, 2002).

The extended-spectrum penicillins have excellent activity against aerobic and anaerobic streptococci, including enterococci species. They have very good activity against aerobic and anaerobic gram-negative bacilli and fair to good activity against staphylococci. These five drugs differ somewhat in their coverage of *Pseudomonas* species, but at least in immunocompetent patients, the differences in activity are not of major clinical importance.

Extended-spectrum penicillins are excreted largely unchanged in the urine. Their principal side effects are allergic reaction and diarrhea. They may also induce β-lactamase production by bacteria and impair platelet function (Duff, 1997, 2002).

In obstetrics, these drugs are of greatest value as single agents for treatment of polymicrobial infections such as chorioamnionitis and puerperal endometritis. Unfortunately, because the patents on these drugs are still intact, the cost of any of these single agents usually exceeds the cost of combination therapy with generic formulations of antibiotics.

Linezolid (Pregnancy Category C)

Linezolid is an oxazolidine antibiotic and acts on the bacterial ribosome to inhibit protein synthesis. Its spectrum of activity includes enterococci, staphylococci, and *Streptococcus pneumoniae*. It is effective against strains of these organisms that are resistant to antibiotics such as methicillin, penicillin, and vancomycin.

Linezolid is available in both oral and intravenous formulations. The drug is partly metabolized in the liver and then excreted in the urine. The most common adverse effects are diarrhea, nausea, and vomiting. Reversible thrombocytopenia, leukopenia, and hepatic-enzyme elevation are uncommon reactions. Severe hypertension may occur if the drug is ingested with large amounts of foods that contain tyramine.

Because of its unique spectrum of activity, linezolid should be reserved for treatment of serious infections caused by enterococci or staphylococci that are resistant to other antibiotics. The appropriate oral and intravenous dose of the drug is 600 mg every 12 hours. The wholesale cost of one 600-mg tablet is approximately $53. The 600-mg intravenous vial costs about $72 (Anonymous, 2000).

Metronidazole (Pregnancy Category B)

Metronidazole inhibits bacterial protein synthesis. The drug is metabolized in the liver and excreted largely in the urine. Its interest to obstetricians stems from its excellent activity against several genital tract pathogens, namely anaerobic organisms and *Trichomonas vaginalis*. Metronidazole is also active against *Clostridium difficile*, the causative organism of pseudomembranous enterocolitis. Metronidazole is not effective against aerobic gram-positive organisms or aerobic gram-negative bacilli (Robbie and Sweet, 1983).

The principal adverse effects of metronidazole are nausea, vomiting, diarrhea, and skin rash. In addition, the drug exerts a disulfiram-like effect when taken concurrently with alcohol. In experimental models, metronidazole has been mutagenic in bacteria and carcinogenic in animals. Fortunately, these same effects have not been documented in humans (Duff, 2002).

Metronidazole has several specific applications in obstetrics. It is the treatment of choice for trichomoniasis. For this indication, one of two oral dosing regimens may be used: a single 2-g dose or 250 mg three times daily for 7 days. Oral metronidazole is also the most cost-effective treatment for BV. In pregnant women, the recommended dose is 250 mg three times daily for 7 days. For noncompliant patients, a single 2-g dose may be used, but it is not quite as effective as the multi-dose regimen. Along with vancomycin, metronidazole is highly effective for the treatment of pseudomembranous enterocolitis. For this clinical indication, the appropriate dose is 500 mg orally every 6 hours until clinical improvement occurs. A final important use for metronidazole in obstetrics is in combination with penicillin or ampicillin plus gentamicin for treatment of puerperal endometritis. When used in this situation, metronidazole should be administered intravenously in a dose of 500 mg every 12 hours (Duff, 2002).

Nitrofurantoin (Pregnancy Category B)

Nitrofurantoin is a bactericidal antibiotic that is specific for UTIs. It inhibits bacterial synthesis of protein and cell walls. The drug is eliminated from the body primarily by renal excretion. Nitrofurantoin is highly active against most of the common uropathogens: *E. coli*, *Klebsiella* species, *Staphylococcus saprophyticus*, *S. aureus*, and *Enterococcus faecalis*. It is not active against most strains of *Proteus*, *Serratia*, or *Pseudomonas*.

As a general rule, nitrofurantoin is very well tolerated. The most frequent adverse effects are nausea, headache, and flatulence. Collectively, these effects occur in less than 15% of patients. Rare but potentially serious reactions include pulmonary hypersensitivity, hepatitis, peripheral neuropathy, and anemia resulting from glucose-6-phosphate dehydrogenase deficiency. The drug exerts minimal effect on the normal bowel or vaginal flora and is therefore unlikely to cause antibiotic-induced diarrhea or vulvovaginal moniliasis.

The unique applications of nitrofurantoin in obstetrics are for treatment of UTI and prophylaxis against recurrent UTI (Gupta et al., 1999; Jamie et al., 2002). The drug is available in two oral formulations: nitrofurantoin macrocrystals and nitrofurantoin monohydrate macrocrystals. The latter formulation is preferred because of its more convenient dosing schedule. For the initial treatment of an uncomplicated lower urinary tract infection, the appropriate dose of nitrofurantoin monohydrate macrocrystals is 100 mg orally twice daily for 3 days. For recurrent lower urinary tract infections, a dose of 100 mg orally twice daily for 7 to 10 days is indicated. This same dose could also be used for therapy of pyelonephritis once the patient has responded to the initial intravenous antibiotic treatment. For prophylaxis against recurrent infection, the drug may be given in an oral dose of 100 mg daily at bedtime.

Nitrofurantoin costs about twice as much as a comparable course of ampicillin or amoxicillin and about 25% to 30% more than trimethoprim-sulfamethoxazole. However, its excellent activity against almost all uropathogens (except *Proteus* species) and its excellent tolerability make it a valuable oral agent for treatment of UTI (Duff, 2002).

Penicillin (Pregnancy Category B)

Penicillin is a β-lactam antibiotic that inhibits bacterial cell wall synthesis. It has excellent activity against group A and group B β-hemolytic streptococci, *Streptococcus pneumoniae,* anaerobic gram-positive cocci, *Neisseria meningitidis,* and *Treponema pallidum.* It is effective against some anaerobic gram-negative bacilli, some strains of staphylococci, and many but not all strains of *N. gonorrhoeae.* By itself, it is not active against enterococci, but it may be effective in combination with an aminoglycoside. Penicillin has no activity against aerobic gram-negative bacilli.

Penicillin is excreted essentially unchanged in the urine. The best-known adverse effect of penicillin is an allergic reaction. This reaction may range from a mild morbilliform rash to anaphylaxis. In extremely high doses, penicillin can also cause neuromuscular excitability, seizures, and potassium excess (Duff, 2002).

In obstetrics, penicillin has several important uses. In combination with gentamicin, it provides excellent intrapartum treatment for chorioamnionitis. For this indication, the appropriate dose of aqueous penicillin G is 5 million units every 6 hours. Penicillin is an effective agent for intrapartum prophylaxis in parturients who are colonized with group B streptococci. The intravenous dosing regimen for prophylaxis is 5 million units initially, then 2.5 million units every 4 hours until delivery.

Penicillin is also the drug of choice for syphilis. In pregnancy, it is the only antibiotic that has been consistently effective in preventing congenital syphilis. For treatment of syphilis, penicillin is usually administered in an intramuscular repository formulation as benzathine penicillin G. The appropriate dose for primary, secondary, and early latent syphilis is 2.4 million units in a single dose (1.2 million units in each buttock). For late latent or tertiary syphilis, the dose is 2.4 million units weekly for 3 weeks. For neurosyphilis, the drug should be administered as aqueous crystalline penicillin G (18 to 24 million units intravenously per day in four to six divided doses for 10 to 14 days) or as procaine penicillin G (2.4 million units intramuscularly per day plus 500 mg of oral probenecid four times per day, both for 10 to 14 days (Duff, 2001).

Quinupristin/Dalfopristin (Pregnancy Category B)

Quinupristin and dalfopristin are streptogramin antibiotics that are marketed in a 30:70 combination as Synercid. They act synergistically on the bacterial ribosome to interfere with protein synthesis. The combination of drugs is active against *Enterococcus faecium,* methicillin-resistant *Staphylococcus aureus* and *S. epidermidis,* and penicillin-resistant strains of *Streptococcus pneumonia.* The combination is also effective against *Neisseria meningitides, Moraxella catarrhalis, Legionella pneumophila, Mycoplasma pneumoniae,* and *Clostridium perfringens.* Quinupristin/dalfopristin is not active against *Enterococcus faecalis.*

Quinupristin/dalfopristin is available only in an intravenous formulation. Both component drugs are metabolized in the liver and excreted mainly in the bile; their elimination half-life is approximately 1 hour. Their principal adverse effect of this drug combination is a reaction at the infusion site. Other possible adverse effects include arthralgias, myalgias, and hyperbilirubinemia. Quinupristin/dalfopristin is also a potent inhibitor of CYP3A4 and will increase the serum concentration of drugs that are substrates of 3A4 (e.g., nifedipine, midazolam, cyclosporine).

The principal indications for quinupristin/dalfopristin are for treatment of bacteremia and other life-threatening infections caused by vancomycin-resistant *Enterococcus faecium* and for treatment of complicated skin infections caused by *S. aureus* and *Streptococcus pyogenes.* The appropriate intravenous dose of quinupristin/dalfopristin (30:70 ratio) is 7.5 mg/kg every 8 hours. The wholesale pharmacy cost of a single day's treatment is approximately $300 (Anonymous, 1999).

Trimethoprim-Sulfamethoxazole (Pregnancy Category C)

Trimethoprim-sulfamethoxazole is a combination antibiotic that inhibits sequential steps in the biosynthesis of folic acid. It is available in both intravenous and oral formulations. Obstetricians are more likely to use the oral form.

Trimethoprim-sulfamethoxazole has excellent activity against most aerobic gram-negative bacilli, which are the usual pathogens responsible for UTIs. The drug also has activity against *Hemophilus influenzae, Streptococcus pneumoniae, and Pneumocystis carinii* (Rubin and Swartz, 1980).

Trimethoprim-sulfamethoxazole is metabolized in the liver and excreted in the urine. The most common adverse effects are nausea, vomiting, anorexia, and allergic reactions. The latter range from a simple morbilliform rash to life-threatening reactions such as the Stevens-Johnson syndrome, toxic epidermal necrolysis, and anaphylaxis. Trimethoprim-sulfamethoxazole has not been linked definitively with teratogenic effects in humans. However, in the neonate it may displace bilirubin from protein-binding sites. Therefore, as a general rule, it should not be used near the time of delivery (Duff, 2002).

In obstetrics, trimethoprim-sulfamethoxazole is used primarily for treatment of UTIs. For an initial episode of asymptomatic bacteriuria or acute cystitis, the appropriate oral dose is one double-strength tablet (160 mg of trimethoprim plus 800 mg of sulfamethoxazole) twice daily for 3 days. For recurrent infections, a 7- to 10-day course should be used. The latter regimen is also indicated for outpatient therapy of pyelonephritis after an initial course of intravenous antibiotics (Stamm and Hooton, 1993).

Trimethoprim-sulfamethoxazole is now available in generic formulation. The cost of one double-strength tablet is approximately $1.00, which makes this agent a highly cost-effective choice for treating UTIs in pregnancy.

REFERENCES

Bacterial Infections

Urinary Tract Infections

American College of Obstetricians and Gynecologists: Antimicrobial therapy for obstetric patients. Am Coll Obstet Gynecol Bull **17**:1, 1988.

Angel JL, O'Brien WF, Finan MA, et al: Acute pyelonephritis in pregnancy: A prospective study of oral versus intravenous antibiotic therapy. Obstet Gynecol **76**:28, 1990.

Cox SM, Cunningham FG: Urinary tract infection. In Charles D, Glover R (eds): Current Therapy in Obstetrics. Toronto, Ont, Dekker, 1993, p. 209.

Cunningham FG, Lucas MJ, Hankins GDV: Pulmonary injury complicating antepartum pyelonephritis. Am J Obstet Gynecol **156**:797, 1987.

Dunlow DP, Duff P: Prevalence of antibiotic-resistant uropathogens in obstetric patients with acute pyelonephritis. Obstet Gynecol **76**:241, 1990.

Fein AM, Duvivier R: Sepsis in pregnancy. Clin Chest Medicine **13**:709, 1992.

Gilstrap LC, Cunningham FG, Whalley PJ: Acute pyelonephritis in pregnancy: An anteroprospective study. Obstet Gynecol **57**:409, 1981.

Gratacos E, Torres PJ, Vila J, et al: Screening and treatment of asymptomatic bacteriuria in pregnancy prevents pyelonephritis. J Infect Dis **169**:1390, 1994.

Gupta K, Scholes D, Stamm WE: Increasing prevalence of antimicrobial resistance among uropathogens causing uncomplicated acute cystitis. JAMA **281**:736, 1999.

Harris RE: The significance of eradication of bacteriuria during pregnancy. Obstet Gynecol **53**:71, 1979.

Harris RE, Gilstrap LC: Prevention of recurrent pyelonephritis during pregnancy. Obstet Gynecol **44**:637, 1974.

Hooten TM, Stamm WE: Diagnosis and treatment of uncomplicated urinary tract infection. Infect Dis Clin North Am **11**:551, 1997.

Kass EH: Bacteriuria and pyelonephritis of pregnancy. Arch Intern Med **205**:194, 1960a.

Kass EH: The role of asymptomatic bacteriuria in the pathogenesis of pyelonephritis. In Quinn EL, Kass EH (eds): Biology of Pyelonephritis. Boston, Little, Brown, 1960b.

Kass EH: Pregnancy, pyelonephritis and prematurity. Clin Obstet Gynecol **13**:239, 1973.

Kass EH, Zinner SH: Bacteriuria and renal disease. J Infect Dis **120**:27, 1969.

Kass EH, Zinner SH: Bacteriuria and pyelonephritis in pregnancy. In Charles D, Finland M (eds): Obstetric and Perinatal Infections. Philadelphia, Lea & Febiger, 1973.

Kincaid-Smith P, Bullen M: Bacteriuria in pregnancy. Lancet **1**:395, 1965.

Lenke RR, VanDorsten, Schifrin BS: Pyelonephritis in pregnancy: A prospective randomized trial to prevent recurrent disease evaluating suppressive therapy with nitrofurantoin and close surveillance. Am J Obstet Gynecol **146**:953, 1983.

Meis PJ, Michielute R, Peters TJ, et al: Factors associated with preterm birth in Cardiff, Wales: II. Indicated and spontaneous preterm birth. Am J Obstet Gynecol **173**:597, 1995.

Millar LK, Cox SM: Urinary tract infections complicating pregnancy. Infect Dis Clin North Am **11**:13, 1997.

Millar LK, Wing DA, Paul RH, et al: Outpatient treatment of pyelonephritis in pregnancy: A randomized controlled trial. Obstet Gynecol **86**:560, 1995.

Mittendorf R, Williams MA, Kass EH: Prevention of preterm delivery and low birth weight associated with asymptomatic bacteriuria. Clin Infect Dis **14**:927, 1992.

Patton JP, Nash DB, Abrutyn E: Urinary tract infection: Economic considerations. Med Clin North Am **75**:495, 1991.

Romero R, Oyarzum E, Mazur M, et al: Meta-analysis of the relationship between asymptomatic bacteriuria and preterm delivery/low birth weight. Obstet Gynecol **73**:576, 1989.

Rouse DJ, Andrews WW, Goldenberg RL, et al: Screening and treatment of asymptomatic bacteriuria of pregnancy to prevent pyelonephritis: A cost-effectiveness and cost-benefit analysis. Obstet Gynecol **86**:119, 1995.

Sanchez-Ramos L, McAlpine KJ, Adair CD, et al: Pyelonephritis in pregnancy: Once a day ceftriaxone versus multiple doses of cefazolin: A randomized double-blind trial. Am J Obstet Gynecol **172**:129, 1995.

Schieve LA, Handler A, Hershow R, et al: Urinary tract infection during pregnancy: Its association with maternal morbidity and perinatal outcome. Am J Public Health **84**:405, 1994.

Smaill F: Antibiotic versus no treatment for asymptomatic bacteriuria. In Pre-Cochrane Reviews: The Cochrane Pregnancy and Childbirth Database. Issue 2. Oxford, BMJ Publishing Group, 1995.

Stamm WE, Counts GW, Running KR, et al: Diagnosis of coliform infection in acutely dysuric women. N Engl J Med **307**:463, 1982.

Stamm WE, Hooton TM: Management of urinary tract infections in adults. N Engl J Med **329**:1328, 1993.

Stenquist K, Sanberg G, Lidin-Janson F, et al: Virulence factors of E. coli in urinary isolates from pregnant women. J Infect Dis **156**:870, 1987.

Sweet RL, Gibbs RS: Infectious Diseases of the Female Genital Tract. 4th ed. Philadelphia, Lippincott–Williams & Wilkins, 2002.

Towers CV, Kaminskas CM, Garite TJ, et al: Pulmonary injury associated with antepartum pyelonephritis: Can patients at risk be identified? Am J Obstet Gynecol **164**:974, 1991.

U.S. Preventive Services Task Force: Guide to clinical preventative services: An assessment of the effectiveness of 169 interventions. Baltimore, Williams & Wilkins, 1989, p. 155.

Warren JW, Abrutyn E, Hebel JR, et al: Guidelines for antimicrobial treatment of uncomplicated acute bacterial cystitis and pyelonephritis in women. Clin Infect Dis **29**:745, 1999.

Whalley P: Bacteriuria of pregnancy. Am J Obstet Gynecol **97**:723, 1967.

Whalley P, Martin F, Peters P: Significance of symptomatic bacteriuria detected during pregnancy. JAMA **193**:879, 1975.

Zinner SH, Kass EH: Long-term (10–14 years) follow-up of bacteriuria of pregnancy. N Engl J Med **285**:820, 1971.

Intra-amniotic Infection

Blanco JD, Gibbs RS, Malherbe H, et al: A controlled study of genital mycoplasmas in amniotic fluid from patients with intra-amniotic infection. J Infect Dis **147**:650, 1983.

Carey JC, Klebanoff MA, Hauth JC, et al: Metronidazole to prevent preterm delivery in pregnant women with asymptomatic bacterial vaginosis. N Engl J Med **342**:534, 2000.

Egarter C, Leitich H, Husslein P, et al: Adjunctive antibiotic treatment in preterm labor and neonatal morbidity: A meta-analysis. Obstet Gynecol **88**:303, 1996.

Egarter C, Leitich H, Kara H, et al: Antibiotic treatment in preterm premature rupture of membranes and neonatal morbidity: A meta-analysis. Am J Obstet Gynecol **174**:589, 1996.

Garite TJ, Freeman RK: Chorioamnionitis in the preterm gestation. Obstet Gynecol **59**:539, 1982.

Gibbs RS: Chorioamnionitis and bacterial vaginosis. Am J Obstet Gynecol **169**:460, 1993.

Gibbs RS, Blanco JD, St. Clair PJ, et al: Quantitative bacteriology of amniotic fluid from patients with clinical intra-amniotic infection at term. J Infect Dis **145**:1, 1982.

Gibbs RS, Dinsmoor MJ, Newton ER, et al: A randomized trial of intrapartum vs. immediately postpartum treatment of intra-amniotic infection. Obstet Gynecol **72**:823, 1988.

Gibbs RS, Duff P: Progress in pathogenesis and management of clinical intra-amniotic infection. Am J Obstet Gynecol **164**:1317, 1991.

Gilstrap LC, Leveno KJ, Cox SM: Intrapartum treatment of acute chorioamnionitis: Impact on neonatal sepsis. Am J Obstet Gynecol **159**:579, 1988.

Grether JK, Nelson KB: Maternal infection and cerebral palsy in infants of normal birth weight. JAMA **278**:207, 1997.

Hitti J, Krohn MA, Patton D, et al: Amniotic fluid tumor necrosis factor-α and the risk of respiratory distress syndrome among preterm infants. Am J Obstet Gynecol **177**:50, 1997.

Kenyon SL, Taylor DJ, Tarnow-Mordi W, et al: Broad-spectrum antibiotics for spontaneous preterm labour: The ORACLE II randomised trial. Lancet **357**:989, 2001a.

Kiltz RJ, Burke MS, Porreco RP: Amniotic fluid glucose concentration as a marker for intra-amniotic infection. Am J Obstet Gynecol **78**:619, 1991.

Lopèz-Zeno JA, Peaceman AM, Adashek JA, et al: A controlled trial of a program for the active management of labor. N Engl J Med **326**:450, 1992.

Mercer BM, Arheart KL: Antimicrobial therapy in expectant management of preterm premature rupture of the membranes. Lancet **346**:1271, 1995.

Mercer BM, Miodovnik M, Thurnau G, et al: Antibiotic therapy for reduction of infant morbidity after preterm premature rupture of the membranes. JAMA **278**:989, 1997.

Morales WJ: The effect of chorioamnionitis and developmental outcome of preterm infants at one year. Obstet Gynecol **70**:183, 1987.

Mozurkewich EL, Wolf FM: Premature rupture of membranes at term: A meta-analysis of three management schemes. Am J Obstet Gynecol **89**:1035, 1997.

Newton ER, Piper J, Peairs W: Bacterial vaginosis and intraamniotic infection. Am J Obstet Gynecol **175**:672, 1997.

Newton ER, Prihoda TJ, Gibbs RS: Logistic regression analysis of risk factors for intra-amniotic infection. Obstet Gynecol **73**:571, 1989.

Romero R, Yoon BH, Mazor M, et al: The diagnostic and prognostic value of amniotic fluid white blood cell count, glucose, interleukin-6, and Gram stain in patients with preterm labor and intact membranes. Am J Obstet Gynecol **169**:805, 1993.

Rouse DJ, Hauth JC, Andrews WW, et al: Chlorhexidine vaginal irrigation for the prevention of peripartal infection: A placebo-controlled randomized clinical trial. Am J Obstet Gynecol **176**:617, 1997.

Soper DE, Mayhall CG, Dalton HP: Risk factors for intraamniotic infections: A prospective epidemiologic study. Am J Obstet Gynecol **161**:562, 1989.

Soper DE, Mayhall G, Froggatt JW: Characterization and control of intra-amniotic infection in an urban teaching hospital. Am J Obstet Gynecol **175**:304, 1996.

Sperling RS, Ramamurthy S, Gibbs RS: A comparison of intrapartum versus immediate postpartum treatment of intra-amniotic infection. Obstet Gynecol **70**:861, 1987.

Sweet RC, Landers DV, Walker C, et al: *Chlamydia trachomatis* infection and pregnancy outcome. Am J Obstet Gynecol **156**:9829, 1987.

Sweeten KM, Eriksen NJ, Blanco JD: Chlorhexidine versus sterile water vaginal wash during labor to prevent peripartum infection. Am J Obstet Gynecol **176**:426, 1997.

Wu YW, Colford JM Jr: Chorioamnionitis as a risk factor for cerebral palsy: A meta-analysis. JAMA **284**:1417, 2000.

Yancey MK, Duff P, Kubilis P, et al: Risk factors for neonatal sepsis. Am J Obstet Gynecol **87**:188, 1996.

Yoder RP, Gibbs RS, Blanco JD, et al: A prospective controlled study of maternal and perinatal outcome after intra-amniotic infection at term. Am J Obstet Gynecol **145**:695, 1983.

Yoon BH, Kim CJ, Romero R, et al: Experimentally induced intrauterine infection causes fetal brain white matter lesions in rabbits. Am J Obstet Gynecol **177**:797, 1997.

Yoon BH, Romero R, Yang SH, et al: Interleukin-6 concentrations in umbilical cord plasma are elevated in neonates with periventricular white matter lesions associated with periventricular leukomalacia. Am J Obstet Gynecol **174**:1433, 1996.

Postpartum Infection

Puerperal endometritis

Duff P: Pathophysiology and management of postcesarean endomyometritis. Obstet Gynecol **67**:269, 1986.

Duff P: Prophylactic antibiotics for cesarean delivery: A simple cost-effective strategy for prevention of postoperative morbidity. Am J Obstet Gynecol **157**:794, 1987.

Duff P: Antibiotic selection in obstetric patients. Infect Dis Clin North Am **11**:1, 1997.

Duff P: Antibiotic selection in obstetrics: Making cost-effective choices. Clin Obstet Gynecol **45**:59, 2002.

Milligan DA, Brady K, Duff P: Short-term parenteral antibiotic therapy for puerperal endometritis. J Mat Fetal Med **1**:60, 1992.

Mastitis

Duff P: Antibiotic selection in obstetrics: Making cost-effective choices. Clin Obstet Gynecol **45**:59, 2002.

Niebyl JR, Spence MR, Parmley TH: Sporadic (nonepidemic) puerperal mastitis. J Reprod Med **20**:97, 1978.

Ripley D: Mastitis. Prim Care Update **6**:88, 1999.

Wound infection after cesarean section

Cruse PJE, Ford R: A five-year prospective study of 23,649 surgical wounds. Arch Surg **107**:206, 1973.

National Academy of Sciences–National Research Council, Division of Medical Sciences, Ad Hoc Committee on Trauma: Postoperative wound infections: The influence of ultraviolet irradiation of the operative room and of various other factors. Ann Surg **160**(Suppl 2):1, 1964.

Roberts S, Maccato M, Faro S, et al: The microbiology of post-cesarean wound morbidity. Obstet Gynecol **81**:383, 1993.

Episiotomy and other pelvic infections

Hankins GDV, Hauth JC, Gilstrap LC III, et al: Early repair of episiotomy dehiscence. Obstet Gynecol **75**:48, 1990.

Hauth JC, Gilstrap LC III, Ward SC, et al: Early repair of an external sphincter ani muscle and rectal mucosal dehiscence. Obstet Gynecol **67**:806, 1986.

Ramin SM, Gilstrap LC III: Episiotomy and early repair of dehiscence. Clin Obstet Gynecol **37**:816, 1994.

Ramin SM, Ramus RM, Little BB, et al: Early repair of episiotomy dehiscence associated with infection. Am J Obstet Gynecol **167**:1104, 1992.

Shy KK, Eschenbach DA: Fatal perineal cellulitis from an episiotomy site. Obstet Gynecol **54**:292, 1979.

Group B streptococcal infection

American College of Obstetricians and Gynecologists: Prevention of early-onset group B streptococcal disease in newborns. ACOG Tech Bull **173**, 1996.

Baker CJ: Summary of the workshop on perinatal infections due to group B streptococcus. J Infect Dis **136**:137, 1977.

Boyer KM, Gotoff SP: Prevention of early-onset neonatal group B streptococcal disease with selective intrapartum chemoprophylaxis. N Engl J Med **314**:1665, 1986.

Centers for Disease Control and Prevention (CDC): Prevention of perinatal group B streptococcal disease: A public health perspective. MMWR Morb Mortal Wkly Rep **45**(RR-7):1, 1996.

Centers for Disease Control and Prevention (CDC): Decreasing incidence of perinatal group B streptococcal disease—United States, 1993–1995. MMWR Morb Mortal Wkly Rep **46**:473, 1997.

Coleman RT, Sherer DM, Maniscalco WM: Prevention of neonatal group B streptococcal infections: Advances in maternal vaccine development. Obstet Gynecol **80**:301, 1992.

Gardner SW, Yow MD, Leeds LJ, et al: Failure of penicillin to eradicate group B streptococcal colonization in the pregnant woman. Am J Obstet Gynecol **135**:1062, 1979.

Schrag, SJ, Zell ER, Lynfield R, et al: A population-based comparison of strategies to prevent early-onset group B streptococcal disease in neonates. N Engl J Med **347**:233, 2002.

Schrag SJ, Zywicki S, Farley MM, et al: Group B streptococcal disease in the era of intrapartum antibiotic prophylaxis. N Engl J Med **342**:15, 2000.

Silver HM, Gibbs RS, Gray BM, et al: Risk factors for perinatal group B streptococcal disease after amniotic fluid colonization. Am J Obstet Gynecol **163**:19, 1990.

Silver RM, Heddleston LN, McGregor JA, et al: Life-threatening puerperal infection due to group A streptococci. Obstet Gynecol **79**:894, 1992.

Yancey MK, Armer T, Clark P, et al: Assessment of rapid identification tests for genital carriage of group B streptococci. Obstet Gynecol **80**:1038, 1992.

Listeriosis

Ahlfors C, Goertzman BW, Holsted CC, et al: Neonatal listeriosis. Am J Dis Child **131**:405, 1977.

Bortolussi R, Schlech WF: Listeriosis. *In* Remington JS, Klein JO (eds): Infectious Diseases of the Fetus and Newborn Infant. Philadelphia, WB Saunders, 2001, p. 1157.

Boucher M, Yonekura ML: Perinatal listeriosis (early onset): Correlation of antenatal manifestations and neonatal outcome. Obstet Gynecol **68**:593, 1986.

Bula C, Bille J, Mean F, et al: Epidemic food-borne listeriosis in western Switzerland. Paper presented at the 28th Interscience Conference on Antimicrobial Agents and Chemotherapy, Oct 26, 1988, Los Angeles.

Cherubin CE, Appleman MD, Heseltine PN, et al: Epidemiologic spectrum and current treatment of listeriosis. Rev Infect Dis **13**:1180, 1991.

Fleming D, Cochi S, McDonald K, et al: Pasteurized milk as a vehicle of infection in an outbreak of listeriosis. N Engl J Med **312**:404, 1985.

Gellin BG, Broome CV: Listeriosis. JAMA **261**:1313, 1989.

Kalstone C: Successful antepartum treatment of listeriosis. Am J Obstet Gynecol **164**:571, 1991.

Katz VL, Weinstein L: Antepartum treatment of *Listeria monocytogenes* septicemia. South Med J **75**:1353, 1982.

Linnan MJ, Mascola L, Dong LX, et al: Epidemic listeriosis associated with Mexican-style cheese. N Engl J Med **319**:823, 1988.

McLauchlin J: Human listeriosis in Britain, 1967–85. A summary of 722 cases: I. Listeriosis during pregnancy and in the newborn. Epidemiol Infect **104**:181, 1990.

Schech WF, Lavigne PM, Bortolusse R, et al: Epidemic listeriosis: Evidence for transmission by food. N Engl J Med **308**:203, 1983.

Skogberg K, Syrjanen J, Jahkola M, et al: Clinical presentation and outcome of listeriosis in patients with and without immunosuppressive therapy. Clin Infect Dis **14**:815, 1992.

Lyme disease

Ackerman R, Rehse-Klupper B, Gallmer E, et al: Chronic neurologic manifestations of erythema migrans borreliosis. Ann N Y Acad Sci **539**:16, 1988.

Asbrink E, Hovmark A: Early and late cutaneous manifestations of *Ixodes*-borne borreliosis (erythema migrans borreliosis, Lyme borreliosis). Ann N Y Acad Sci **539**:4, 1988.

Bakken LL, Case KL, Callster SM, et al: Performance of 45 laboratories participating in a proficiency program for Lyme disease serology. JAMA **268**:891, 1992.

Centers for Disease Control and Prevention (CDC): Lyme disease—United States, 1999. MMWR Morb Mortal Wkly Rep **50**:181, 2001.

Hedberg CW, Osterhold MT, MacDonald KL, et al: An interlaboratory study of antibody to *Borrelia burgdorferi*. J Infect Dis **155**:1325, 1987.

Kaslow RA: Current perspective on Lyme borreliosis. JAMA **267**:1381, 1992.

Luft BJ, Steinman CR, Neimark HC, et al: Invasion of the central nervous system by *Borrelia burgdorferi* in acute disseminated infection. JAMA **267**:1364, 1992.

MacDonald A: Human fetal borreliosis, toxemia of pregnancy, and fetal death. Zentralbl Bakteriol **263**:189, 1986.

MacDonald AB, Benach JL, Burgdorfer W: Stillbirth following Lyme disease. N Y J Med **8**:615, 1987.

Markowitz LE, Steere AC, Benach JL, et al: Lyme disease during pregnancy. JAMA **255**:3394, 1986.

Nadl D, Hunziker VA, Bucher HV, et al: Infants born to mothers with antibodies against *Borrelia burgdorferi* at delivery. Eur J Pediatr **148**:426, 1989.

Nishi MJ, Liebling MR, Rodriguez A, et al: Identification of *Borrelia burgdorferi* using interrupted polymerase chain reaction. Arthritis Rheum **36**:665, 1993.

Nocton JJ, Dressler F, Rutledge BF, et al: Detection of *Borrelia burgdorferi* DNA by polymerase chain reaction in synovial fluid from patients with Lyme disease. N Engl J Med **330**:229, 1994.

Persing DH, Rys PN, Van Blaricom G, et al: Multitarget detection of *B. burgdorferi* associated DNA sequences in synovial fluid of patients with arthritis. Arthritis Rheum **33**:836, 1990.

Schlesinger PA, Duray PH, Burke BA, et al: Maternal-fetal transmission of the Lyme disease spirochete, *Borrelia burgdorferi*. Ann Intern Med **103**:67, 1985.

Shapiro ED, Gerber MA, Holabrid NB, et al: A controlled trial of antimicrobial prophylaxis for Lyme disease after deer-tick bites. N Engl J Med **237**:1769, 1992.

Sigal LH, Zahradnik JM, Levin P: A vaccine consisting of recombinant *Borrelia burgdorferi* outer membrane surface protein A to prevent Lyme disease. N Engl J Med **339**:216, 1998.

Smith LG Jr, Pearlman M, Smith LG, et al: Lyme disease: A review with emphasis on the pregnant woman. Obstet Gynecol Surv **46**:125, 1991.

Steere AC: Lyme disease. N Engl J Med **321**:586, 1989.

Steere AC, Malawista SE, Hardin JA, et al: Erythema chronicum migrans and Lyme arthritis: The enlarging clinical spectrum. Am Intern Med **86**:685, 1977.

Steere AC, Malawista SE, Snydman DR, et al: Lyme arthritis in children and adults in three Connecticut communities. Arthritis Rheum **20**:7, 1977.

Steere AC, Sikand VK, Meurice F, et al: Vaccination against Lyme disease with recombinant *Borrelia burgdorferi* outer surface lipoprotein A with adjuvant. N Engl J Med **339**:209, 1998.

Steere AC, Taylor E, McHugh GI, et al: The overdiagnosis of Lyme disease. JAMA **269**:1812, 1993.

Strobino BA, Williams CL, Abid S, et al: Lyme disease and pregnancy outcome: A prospective study of two thousand prenatal patients. Am J Obstet Gynecol **169**:367, 1993.

Weber K, Bratzke HJ, Neubert U, et al: *Borrelia burgdorferi* in a newborn despite oral penicillin for Lyme borreliosis during pregnancy. Pediatr Infect Dis J **7**:286, 1988.

Williams CL, Benach JL, Curran AS, et al: Lyme disease during pregnancy: A cord blood serosurvey. Ann N Y Acad Sci **539**:504, 1988.

Viral Infections

Rubella

American College of Obstetricians and Gynecologists: Rubella and pregnancy. ACOG Tech Bull **171,** 1992.

Bart SW, Stetler HC, Preblud SR, et al: Fetal risk associated with rubella vaccine: An update. Rev Infect Dis **7**:S95, 1985.

Centers for Disease Control and Prevention (CDC): Rubella prevention: Recommendations of the Immunization Practices Advisory Committee (ACIP). MMWR Morb Mortal Wkly Rep **39**:1, 1990.

Centers for Disease Control and Prevention (CDC): Rubella and congenital rubella syndrome—United States, January 1, 1991–May 7, 1994. MMWR Morb Mortal Wkly Rep **43**:391, 1994.

McIntosh EDG, Menser MA: A fifty-year follow-up of congenital rubella. Lancet **340**:414, 1992.

Miller E, Cradock-Watson JE, Pollock TM: Consequences of confirmed maternal rubella at successive stages of pregnancy. Lancet **2**:781, 1982.

Munro ND, Smithells RW, Sheppard S, et al: Temporal relations between maternal rubella and congenital defects. Lancet **2**:201, 1987.

Sautter RL, Crist AE, Johnson LM, et al: Comparison of five methods for the determination of rubella immunity. Infect Dis Obstet Gynecol **1**:188, 1994.

Cytomegalovirus

Adler SP: Cytomegalovirus and child day care. N Engl J Med **321**:1290, 1989.

Adler SP: Cytomegalovirus and pregnancy. Curr Opin Obstet Gynecol **4**:670, 1992.

Boppana SB, Rivera LB, Fowler KB, et al: Intrauterine transmission of cytomegalovirus to infants of women with preconceptional immunity. N Engl J Med **344**:1366, 2001.

Brown HL, Abernathy MP: Cytomegalovirus infection. Semin Perinatol **45**:260, 1998.

Chandler SH, Alexander ER, Holmes KK: Epidemiology of cytomegaloviral infection in a heterogeneous population of pregnant women. J Infect Dis **152**:249, 1985.

Dobbins JG, Stewart JA, Demmler GJ: Surveillance of congenital cytomegalovirus disease, 1990–1991. MMWR Morb Mortal Wkly Rep **41**:35, 1992.

Donner C, Liesnard C, Content J, et al: Prenatal diagnosis of 52 pregnancies at risk for congenital cytomegalovirus infection. Obstet Gynecol **82**:481, 1993.

Duff P: Cytomegalovirus infection in pregnancy. Infect Dis Obstet Gynecol **2**:146, 1994.

Fowler KB, Stagno S, Pass RF, et al: The outcome of congenital cytomegalovirus infection in relation to maternal antibody status. N Engl J Med **326**:663, 1992.

Stagno S, Pass RF, Dworsky ME, et al: Congenital cytomegalovirus infection. N Engl J Med **306**:995, 1982.

Varicella Zoster (Chickenpox)

Balducci J, Rodis JF, Rosengren S, et al: Pregnancy outcome following first-trimester varicella infection. Obstet Gynecol **79**:5, 1992.

Broussard OF, Payne DK, George RB: Treatment with acyclovir of varicella pneumonia in pregnancy. Chest **99**:1045, 1991.

Brunell PA: Fetal and neonatal varicella-zoster infections. Semin Perinatol **7**:47, 1983.

Centers for Disease Control and Prevention (CDC): Prevention of varicella: Recommendations of the Advisory Committee on Immunization Practices (ACIP). MMWR Morb Mortal Wkly Rep **45**(RR-11)**, 1996.

Centers for Disease Control and Prevention (CDC): Summary of notifiable diseases, United States 2000. MMWR Morb Mortal Wkly Rep **49**:3, 2002.

Cox SM, Cunningham FG, Luby J: Management of varicella pneumonia complicating pregnancy. Am J Perinatol **7**:300, 1990.

DeNicola LK, Hanshaw JB: Congenital and neonatal varicella [editorial]. J Pediatr **94**:175, 1979.

Enders G, Miller E, Cradock-Watson J, et al: Consequences of varicella and herpes zoster in pregnancy: Prospective study of 1739 cases. Lancet **343**:1548, 1994.

Esmonde TF, Herdman G, Anderson G: Chickenpox pneumonia: An association with pregnancy. Thorax **44**:812, 1989.

Figueroa-Damian R, Arrendondo-Garcia JL: Perinatal outcome of pregnancies complicated with varicella infection during the first 20 weeks of gestation. Am J Perinatol **14**:411, 1997.

Gershon AA: Chicken pox, measles, and mumps. In Remington JS, Klein JO (eds): Infectious Diseases of the Fetus and Newborn Infant. Philadelphia, WB Saunders, 2001, p. 683.

Harris RE, Rhoades ER: Varicella pneumonia complicating pregnancy: Report of a case and review of the literature. Obstet Gynecol **25**:734, 1965.

Higa K, Don K, Manabe H: Varicella-zoster virus infections during pregnancy: Hypothesis concerning the mechanisms of congenital malformations. Obstet Gynecol **69**:214, 1987.

Isada NB, Paar DP, Johnson MP, et al: In utero diagnosis of congenital varicella zoster virus infection by chorionic villus sampling and polymerase chain reaction. Am J Obstet Gynecol **165**:1727, 1991.

Miller E, Cradock-Watson JE, Ridehalgh MK: Outcome in newborn babies given anti-varicella zoster immune globulin after perinatal maternal infection with varicella zoster virus. Lancet **2**:301, 1989.

Mouly F, Miriesse V, Meritet JF, et al: Prenatal diagnosis of fetal varicella-zoster virus infection with polymerase chain reaction of amniotic fluid in 107 cases. Am J Obstet Gynecol **177**:894, 1997.

Paryani SG, Arvin AM: Intrauterine infection with varicella-zoster virus after maternal varicella. N Engl J Med **314**:1542, 1986.

Pastuszak AL, Levy M, Schick B, et al: Outcome after maternal varicella infection in the first 20 weeks of pregnancy. N Engl J Med **330**:901, 1994.

Pretorius DH, Hayward I, Jones KL, et al: Sonographic evaluation of pregnancies with maternal varicella infection. J Ultrasound Med **11**:459, 1992.

Scharf A, Scherr O, Enders et al: Virus detection in the fetal tissue of a premature delivery with congenital varicella syndrome. J Perinatal Med **18**:317, 1990.

Siegel M: Congenital malformations following chickenpox, measles, mumps, and hepatitis: Results of a chart study. JAMA **226**:1521, 1973.

Siegel M, Fuerst HT: Low birth weight and maternal virus diseases. JAMA **197**:88, 1966.

Smego RA, Asperilla MO: Use of acyclovir for varicella pneumonia during pregnancy. Obstet Gynecol **78**:1112, 1991.

Sweet RL, Gibbs RS: Perinatal infections. In Infectious Diseases of the Female Genital Tract. Philadelphia, Lippincott–Williams & Wilkins, 2002, p. 461.

Herpes Simplex

American College Obstetricians and Gynecologists: Perinatal herpes simplex infections. ACOG Tech Bull **22, 1988.

Amstey MS, Monif GRG: Herpes virus in pregnancy. Obstet Gynecol **44**:394, 1974.

Arvin AM, Hensleigh PA, Prober CG, et al: Failure of antepartum maternal cultures to predict the infant's risk of exposure to herpes simplex virus at delivery. N Engl J Med **315**:796, 1986.

Brocklehurst P, Kinghorn G, Carney O, et al: A randomized placebo controlled trial of suppressive acyclovir in late pregnancy in women with recurrent genital herpes infection. Br J Obstet Gynaecol **105**:275, 1998.

Brown ZA, Selke S, Zeh J, et al: The acquisition of herpes simplex virus during pregnancy. N Engl J Med **337**:509, 1997.

Brown ZA, Vantuer LA, Benedetti J, et al: Effects on infants of a first episode of genital herpes in pregnancy. N Engl J Med **317**:1246, 1987.

Brown ZA, Vantuer LA, Benedetti J, et al: Neonatal herpes simplex virus infection in relation to asymptomatic maternal infection at the time of labor. N Engl J Med **324**:1247, 1991.

Centers for Disease Control and Prevention (CDC): Pregnancy outcomes following systemic prenatal acyclovir exposure—June 1, 1984–June 30, 1993. MMWR Morb Mortal Wkly Rep **42**:806, 1993.

Centers for Disease Control and Prevention (CDC): Sexually transmitted diseases treatment guidelines 2002. MMWR Morb Mortal Wkly Rep **51**(RR-6)**, 2002.

Fleming DT, McQuillan GM, Johnson RE, et al: Herpes simplex virus type 2 in the United States, 1976–1994. N Engl J Med **337**:1105, 1997.

Gibbs RS, Amstey MS, Lezotte DC: Role of cesarean delivery in preventing neonatal herpes virus infection. JAMA **270**:95, 1993.

Gibbs RS, Amstey MS, Sweet RS, et al: Management of genital herpes infection in pregnancy. Obstet Gynecol **71**:779, 1988.

Hensleigh PA, Andrews WW, Brown Z, et al: Genital herpes during pregnancy: Inability to distinguish primary and recurrent infections clinically. Obstet Gynecol **89**:891, 1997.

Hutto C, Arvin A, Jacobs R, et al: Intrauterine herpes simplex virus infections. Pediatrics **110**:97, 1987.

Kulhanjian JA, Soroush V, Au DS, et al: Identification of women at unsuspected risk of primary infection with herpes simplex virus type 2 during pregnancy. N Engl J Med **326**:916, 1992.

Nahmias A, Josey WE, Naib ZM, et al: Perinatal risk associated with maternal genital herpes simplex infection. Am J Obstet Gynecol **110**:825, 1971.

Prober CG, Sullender WM, Yasukawa LL, et al: Low risk of herpes simplex virus infections in neonates exposed to the virus at the time of vaginal delivery to mothers with recurrent genital herpes simplex virus infections. N Engl J Med **316**:240, 1987.

Randolph AG, Washington AE, Prober CG: Cesarean delivery for women presenting with genital herpes lesions. JAMA **270**:77, 1993.

Reiff-Eldridge RA, Heffner CR, Ephross SA, et al: Monitoring pregnancy outcomes after prenatal drug exposure through prospective pregnancy registries: A pharmaceutical company commitment. Am J Obstet Gynecol **182**:159, 2000.

Scott LL, Sanchez PJ, Jackson GL, et al: Acyclovir suppression to prevent cesarean delivery after first-episode genital herpes. Obstet Gynecol **87**:69, 1996.

Human Parvovirus Infection

Brown KE, Green SW, deMayolo JA, et al: Congenital anaemia after transplacental B_{19} parvovirus infection. Lancet **343**:895, 1994.

Cartter ML, Farley TA, Rosengren S, et al: Occupational risk factors for infection with parvovirus B_{19} among pregnant women. J Infect Dis **163**:282, 1991.

Centers for Disease Control and Prevention (CDC): Risks associated with human parvovirus B_{19} infection. MMWR Morb Mortal Wkly Rep **38**:81, 1989.

Conry JA, Torok T, Andrews I: Perinatal encephalopathy secondary to in utero human parvovirus B-19 (HPV) infection [abstract]. Neurology **43**:A346, 1993.

Fairly CK, Smoleniec JS, Caul OE, et al: Observational study of effect of intrauterine transfusions on outcome of fetal hydrops after parvovirus B_{19} infection. Lancet **346**:1335, 1995.

Gillespie SM, Cartter ML, Asch S, et al: Occupation risk of human parvovirus B_{19} infection for school and daycare personnel during an outbreak of erythema infectiosum. JAMA **263**:2061, 1990.

Humphrey W, Magoon M, O'Shaughnessy R: Severe nonimmune hydrops secondary to parvovirus B_{19} infection: Spontaneous reversal in utero and survival of a term infant. Obstet Gynecol **78**:900, 1991.

Peters MT, Nicolaides KH: Cordocentesis for the diagnosis and treatment of human fetal parvovirus infection. Obstet Gynecol **75**:501, 1990.

Pryde PG, Nugent CE, Pridjian G, et al: Spontaneous resolution of nonimmune hydrops fetalis secondary to human parvovirus B_{19} infection. Obstet Gynecol **79**:859, 1992.

Public Health Laboratory Service Working Party on Fifth Disease: Prospective study of human parvovirus (B_{19}) infection in pregnancy. BMJ **300**:1166, 1990.

Rodis JF, Quinn DL, Gary W, et al: Management and outcomes of pregnancies complicated by human B_{19} parvovirus infection: A prospective study. Am J Obstet Gynecol **163**:1168, 1990.

Rodis JF, Rodner C, Hansen AA, et al: Long-term outcome of children following maternal human parvovirus B_{19} infection. Obstet Gynecol **91**:125, 1998.

Influenza

Anonymous: Two neuraminidase inhibitors for treatment of influenza. Med Lett Drugs Ther **41**:91, 1999.

Anonymous: Influenza prevention 2001–2002. Med Lett Drugs Ther **43**:81, 2001.

Carlan SJ, Knuppel RA: Specific intra-amniotic viral infections. In Pastorek JG (ed): Obstetric and Gynecologic Infectious Disease. New York, Raven Press, 1994.

Centers for Disease Control and Prevention (CDC): Prevention and control of influenza: Recommendations of the Advisory Committee on Immunization Practice (ACIP). MMWR Morb Mortal Wkly Rep **49**(RR-3)**,** 2000.

Cox NJ, Hughes JM: New options for the prevention of influenza. N Engl J Med **341**:1387, 1999.

Hayden FG, Atmar RL, Schilling M, et al: Use of the selective oral neuraminidase inhibitor oseltamivir to prevent influenza. N Engl J Med **341**:1336, 1999.

Monto AS, Robinson DP, Herlocher ML, et al: Zanamivir in the prevention of influenza among healthy adults: A randomized controlled trial. JAMA **282**:31, 1999.

Nichol KL, Lind A, Margolis, et al: The effectiveness of vaccination against influenza in healthy, working adults. N Engl J Med **333**:389, 1995.

Patriarca PA, Strikas RA: Influenza vaccine for healthy adults. N Engl J Med **333**:933, 1995.

Rubeola

Atkinson WL, Hadler SC, Redd SB, et al: Measles surveillance—United States, 1991. MMWR Morb Mortal Wkly Rep **41**:1, 1992.

Atmar RL, Englund JA, Hammill H: Complications of measles during pregnancy. Clin Infect Dis **14**:217, 1992.

Centers for Disease Control and Prevention (CDC): Measles prevention: Recommendations of the Immunization Practices Advisory Committee (ACIP). MMWR Morb Mortal Wkly Rep **38**:1, 1989.

Centers for Disease Control and Prevention (CDC): Measles prevention: Supplementary statement. MMWR Morb Mortal Wkly Rep **38**:11, 1992.

Christensen PE, Schmidt H, Bang HO, et al: An epidemic of measles in southern Greenland, 1951. Acta Med Scand **144**:430, 1953; **148**:430, 1953.

Eberhart-Phillips JE, Frederick PD, Baron RC, et al: Measles in pregnancy: A descriptive study of 58 cases. Obstet Gynecol **82**:797, 1993.

Hersh BS, Markowitz LE, Maes EF, et al: The geographic distribution of measles in the United States, 1980 through 1989. JAMA **267**:1936, 1992.

National Vaccine Advisory Committee: The measles epidemic: The problems, barriers, and recommendations. JAMA **266**:1547, 1991.

Stein SJ, Greenspoon JS: Rubeola during pregnancy. Obstet Gynecol **78**:925, 1991.

Mumps

Gershon A: Chickenpox, measles and mumps. In Remington JS, Klein JO (eds): Infectious Diseases of the Fetus and Newborn Infant. Philadelphia, WB Saunders, 1990.

Monif GRG: Maternal mumps infection during gestation: Observations in the progeny. Am J Obstet Gynecol **119**:549, 1974.

Siegal M: Congenital malformations following chickenpox, measles, mumps, and hepatitis: Results of a chart study. JAMA **226**:1521, 1973.

St. Geme JW Jr, Noren GR, Adams P: Proposed embryopathic relationship between mumps virus and primary endocardial fibroelastosis. N Engl J Med **275**:339, 1966.

Echoviruses

Hughes JR, Wilfert CM, Moore M, et al: Echovirus 14 infection associated with fatal neonatal hepatic necrosis. Am J Dis Child **123**:61, 1972.

Modlin JF: Perinatal echovirus infection: Insights from a literature review of 61 cases of serious infection and 16 outbreaks in nurseries. Rev Infect Dis **8**:918, 1986.

Philip AGS, Larsen EJ: Overwhelming neonatal infection with echo 19 virus. J Pediatr **82**:391, 1973.

Sexually Transmitted Diseases

Syphilis; Gonorrhea; Condylomata Acuminata (Genital Warts)/ Genital Human Papillomavirus Infection

Amstey MS, Steadman KT: Symptomatic gonorrhea and pregnancy. J Am Vener Dis Assoc **3**:14, 1976.

Beutner KR, Reitano MV, Richwald GA, et al: External genital warts: Report of the American Medical Association Conference. Clin Infect Dis **27**:796, 1998.

Brown ST: Adverse reactions in syphilis therapy. J Am Vener Dis Assoc **3**:172, 1976.

Cates W Jr, Hinman AR: Sexually transmitted diseases in the 1990s. N Engl J Med **325**:1368, 1991.

Centers for Disease Control and Prevention (CDC): Syphilis and congenital syphilis—United States, 1985–1988. MMWR Morb Mortal Wkly Rep **37**:486, 1988.

Centers for Disease Control and Prevention (CDC): Sexually transmitted disease surveillance, 1995. Rockville, Md, US Department of Health and Human Services, 1996a.

Centers for Disease Control and Prevention (CDC): Summary of notifiable diseases, United States, 1995. MMWR Morb Mortal Wkly Rep **44**: 1996b.

Centers for Disease Control and Prevention (CDC): Contraceptive practices before and after an intervention promoting condom use to prevent HIV infection and other sexually transmitted diseases among women— selected US sites, 1993–1995. MMWR Morb Mortal Wkly Rep **46**:373, 1997.

Centers for Disease Control and Prevention (CDC): Congenital syphilis— United States, 1998. MMWR Morb Mortal Wkly Rep **48**:757, 1999.

Centers for Disease Control and Prevention (CDC): Summary of notifiable diseases—United States, 2000. MMWR Morb Mortal Wkly Rep **49**, 2002a.

Centers for Disease Control and Prevention (CDC): 2002 Guidelines for treatment of sexually transmitted diseases. MMWR Morb Mortal Wkly Rep **51**:1, 2002b.

Coles FB, Hipps SS, Silberstein GS, et al: Congenital syphilis surveillance in upstate New York, 1989–1992: Implications for prevention and clinical management. J Infect Dis **171**:732, 1995.

Cook TA, Cohn AM, Brunchwig JP, et al: Wart viruses and laryngeal papillomas. Lancet **1**:782, 1973.

Fiumara NJ, Fleming WL, Downing JG, et al: The incidence of prenatal syphilis at the Boston City Hospital. N Engl J Med **247**:48, 1952.

Fiumara NJ, Lessel S: Manifestations of late congenital syphilis. Arch Dermatol **102**:78, 1970.

Genest DR, Choi-Hang, Tate JE, et al: Diagnosis of congenital syphilis from placental examination: Comparison of histopathology, silver stain, and polymerase chain reaction for *Treponema pallidum* DNA. Hum Pathol **27**:366, 1996.

Handsfield HH, Hodson A, Holmes KK: Neonatal gonococcal infection: I. Orogastric contamination with *Neisseria gonorrhoeae*. JAMA **225**:697, 1973.

Handsfield HH, McCormack WM, Hook EW III, et al: A comparison of single-dose cefixime with ceftriaxone as treatment for uncomplicated gonorrhea. N Engl J Med **325**:337, 1991.

Harter CA, Benirschke K: Fetal syphilis in the first trimester. Am J Obstet Gynecol **124**:705, 1976.

Hollier LM, Cox SM: Syphilis. Semin Perinatol **22**:323, 1993.

Holmes KK, Counts LW, Beaty HN: Disseminated gonococcal infection. Ann Intern Med **74**:979, 1971.

Hook EW, Handsfield HH: Gonococcal infections in adults. In Holmes KK, Sparling PF, Mardh PA, et al (eds): Sexually Transmitted Diseases. New York, McGraw-Hill, 1999, p. 451.

Ingall D, Norins L: Syphilis. In Remington JS, Klein JO (eds): Infectious Diseases of the Fetus and Newborn Infant. Philadelphia, WB Saunders, 1976.

Ingraham NR: The value of penicillin alone in the prevention and treatment of congenital syphilis. Acta Derm Venereol Suppl (Stockh) **31**:60, 1951.

Institute of Medicine, Committee on Prevention and Control of Sexually Transmitted Diseases: The hidden epidemic: Confronting sexually transmitted diseases. Washington, DC, National Academy Press, 1997.

Jones JE, Harris RE: Diagnostic evaluation of syphilis during pregnancy. Obstet Gynecol **54**:611, 1979.

Kashima H, Shah K, Mounts P: Recurrent respiratory papillomatosis. In Holmes KK, Sparling PF, Mardh PA, et al (eds): Sexually Transmitted Diseases. New York, McGraw-Hill, 1999, p. 1213.

Klein VR, Cox SM, Mitchell MD, et al: The Jarisch-Herxheimer reaction complicating syphilotherapy in pregnancy. Obstet Gynecol **75**:375, 1990.

Lukehart SA, Hook EW III, Baker-Zander SA, et al: Invasion of the central nervous system by *Treponema pallidum*: Implications for diagnosis and treatment. Ann Intern Med **109**:855, 1988.

McFarlin BL, Bottoms SF, Dock BS, et al: Epidemic syphilis: Maternal factors associated with congenital infection. Am J Obstet Gynecol 170:535, 1994.

Ricci JM, Fojaco RM, O'Sullivan MJ: Congenital syphilis. The University of Miami/Jackson Memorial Medical Center experience, 1986–88. Obstet Gynecol 74:687, 1989.

Rolfs RT, Nakoshima AK: Epidemiology of primary and secondary syphilis in the United States, 1981 through 1989. JAMA 264:1432, 1990.

Sanchez PJ, Wendel GD: Syphilis in pregnancy. Clin Perinatol 24:71, 1997.

Sarrel PM, Pruett KA: Symptomatic gonorrhea during pregnancy. Obstet Gynecol 32:670, 1968.

Shah K, Ashima H, Polk BF, et al: Rarity of cesarean delivery in cases of juvenile-onset respiratory papillomatosis. Obstet Gynecol 68:795, 1986.

Sweet RL, Gibbs RS: Infectious Diseases of the Female Genital Tract. 4th ed. Philadelphia, Lippincott–Williams & Wilkins, 2002.

Tenti P, Zappatore R, Migliora P, et al: Perinatal transmission of human papillomavirus from gravidas with latent infections. Obstet Gynecol 3:475, 1999.

Watts DH, Koutsky LA, Holmes KK, et al: Low risk of perinatal transmission of human papillomavirus: Results of a prospective cohort study. Am J Obstet Gynecol 178:365, 1998.

Chlamydial Infection

Adair CD, Gunter M, Stovall TG, et al: Chlamydia in pregnancy: A randomized trial of azithromycin and erythromycin. Obstet Gynecol 91:165, 1998.

Alary M, Jolly JR, Moutquin JM, et al: Randomized comparison of amoxicillin and erythromycin treatment of genital chlamydial infection in pregnancy. Lancet 344:1461, 1994.

Alger L, Lovchik JC: Comparative efficacy of clindamycin versus erythromycin in eradication of antenatal Chlamydia trachomatis. Am J Obstet Gynecol 165:375, 1991.

Amortegui AJ, Meyer MP: Enzyme immunoassay for detection of Chlamydia trachomatis from the cervix. Obstet Gynecol 65:523, 1985.

Baselski VS, McNeely SG, Ryan G, et al: A comparison of non-culture-dependent methods for detection of Chlamydia trachomatis infections in pregnant women. Obstet Gynecol 70:47, 1987.

Bass CA, Jungkind DL, Silverman NS, et al: Clinical evaluation of a new polymerase chain reaction assay for detection of Chlamydia trachomatis in endocervical specimens. J Clin Microbiol 31:2648, 1993.

Bauwens JE, Clark AM, Stamm WE: Diagnosis of Chlamydia trachomatis endocervical infections by a commercial polymerase chain reaction assay. J Clin Microbiol 31:3023, 1993.

Beem MO, Saxon EM: Respiratory tract colonization and a distinctive pneumonia syndrome in infants infected with Chlamydia trachomatis. N Engl J Med 296:306, 1977.

Berman SM, Harrison HR, Boyce WT, et al: Low birth weight, prematurity and postpartum endometritis: Association with prenatal cervical Mycoplasma hominis and Chlamydia trachomatis infection. JAMA 257:1189, 1987.

Blanco JD, Diaz KC, Lipscomb KA, et al: Chlamydia trachomatis isolation in patients with endometritis after cesarean section. Am J Obstet Gynecol 152:278, 1985.

Brunham RC, Paavonen J, Stevens CE, et al: Mucopurulent cervicitis: The ignored counterpart in women of urethritis in men. N Engl J Med 311:1, 1984.

Bush MR, Rosa C: Azithromycin and erythromycin treatment of cervical chlamydial infection during pregnancy. Obstet Gynecol 84:61, 1994.

Centers for Disease Control and Prevention (CDC): Recommendation for the prevention and management of Chlamydia trachomatis infection. MMWR Morb Mortal Wkly Rep 41:1, 1993.

Centers for Disease Control and Prevention (CDC): Ten leading nationally notifiable infectious diseases—United States, 1995. MMWR Morb Mortal Wkly Rep 45:883, 1996.

Centers for Disease Control and Prevention (CDC): Chlamydia trachomatis genital infections—United States, 1995. MMWR Morb Mortal Wkly Rep 46:193, 1997.

Centers for Disease Control and Prevention (CDC): Sexually transmitted diseases treatment guidelines 2002. MMWR Morb Mortal Wkly Rep 51:32, 2002.

Chandler JW, Alexander ER, Pheiffer TH, et al: Ophthalmia neonatorum associated with maternal chlamydial infections. Trans Am Acad Ophthalmol Otolaryngol 83:302, 1977.

Cohen I, Veille C, Calkins BM, et al: Improved pregnancy outcome following successful treatment of chlamydial infection. JAMA 263:3160, 1990.

Crombleholme WR, Schachter J, Grossman M, et al: Amoxicillin therapy for Chlamydia trachomatis in pregnancy. Obstet Gynecol 75:752, 1990.

Edwards MS, Newman RB, Carter SG, et al: Randomized clinical trial of azithromycin vs. erythromycin for the treatment of chlamydia cervicitis in pregnancy. Infect Dis Obstet Gynecol 4:333, 1996.

Fitz-Simmons J, Callahan C, Shanahan B, et al: Chlamydial infections in pregnancy. J Reprod Med 31:19, 1986.

Frommell GT, Rothenberg R, Wang S-P, et al: Chlamydia infection of mothers and their infants. J Pediatr 95:28, 1979.

Gravett MG, Nelson HP, DeRonent, et al: Independent associations of bacterial vaginosis and Chlamydia trachomatis. JAMA 256:1899, 1986.

Hammerschlag MR, Anderka M, Semine DZ, et al: Prospective study of maternal and infantile infection with Chlamydia trachomatis. Pediatr 64:142, 1979.

Hardy PH, Hardy JB, Nell EE, et al: Prevalence of six sexually transmitted disease agents among inner-city adolescents and pregnancy outcome. Lancet 2:333, 1984.

Harrison HR, Alexander ER, Weinstein L, et al: Cervical Chlamydia trachomatis and mycoplasmal infections in pregnancy. JAMA 250:1721, 1983.

Hoyme UB, Kiviat N, Eschenbach DA: Microbiology and treatment of late postpartum endometritis. Obstet Gynecol 68:226, 1986.

Ismail MA, Chandler AE, Beem MO, et al: Chlamydial colonization of the cervix in pregnant adolescents. J Reprod Med 30:549, 1985.

Khurana CM, Deddish PA, delMundo F: Prevalence of Chlamydia trachomatis in the pregnant cervix. Obstet Gynecol 66:241, 1988.

Lee HH, Chernesky MA, Schachter J, et al: Diagnosis of Chlamydia trachomatis genitourinary infection in women by ligase chain reaction assay of urine. Lancet 345:213, 1995.

Loeffelholz MJ, Lewinski CA, Silver SR, et al: Detection of Chlamydia trachomatis in endocervical specimens by polymerase chain reaction. J Clin Microbiol 30:2847, 1992.

Magat AH, Alger LS, Nagey DA, et al: Double-blind randomized study comparing amoxicillin and erythromycin for the treatment of Chlamydia trachomatis in pregnancy. Obstet Gynecol 81:745, 1993.

Mangione-Smith R, O'Leary J, McGlynn EA: Health and cost benefits of Chlamydia screening in young women. Sex Transm Dis 26:309, 1999.

Mardh P-A, Helin I, Bobeck S, et al: Colorization of pregnant and pueperal women and neonates with Chlamydia trachomatis. Br J Vener Dis 56:96, 1980.

Martin DH, Koutsky L, Eschenbach DA, et al: Prematurity and perinatal mortality in pregnancies complicated by maternal Chlamydia trachomatis infections. JAMA 247:1585, 1982.

McGregor JA, French JL, Richter R, et al: Antenatal microbiologic and maternal risk factors associated with prematurity. Am J Obstet Gynecol 1990.

Paavonen J, Brunham R, Kiviat N, et al: Cervicitis: Etiologic, clinical and histopathologic findings. In Mårdh PA, Holmes KK, Oriel JD, et al (eds): Chlamydial Infections. Amsterdam, Elsevier-Biomedical Press, 1982, p. 141.

Plummer FA, Laga M, Brunham RC, et al: Postpartum upper genital tract infections in Nairobi, Kenya: Epidemiology, etiology and risk factors. J Infect Dis 156:92, 1987.

Ryan GM, Abdella TN, McNeeley SG, et al: Chlamydia trachomatis infection in pregnancy and effect of treatment on outcome. Am J Obstet Gynecol 162:34, 1990.

Schachter J: Infection and disease epidemiology. In Stephens RS (ed): Chlamydia: Intracellular Biology, Pathogenesis and Immunity. Washington, DC, American Society for Microbiology, 1999, p. 139.

Schachter J, Dawson CR: Comparative efficiency of various diagnostic methods for chlamydial infection. In Holmes KK, Hobson D (eds): Nongonococcal Urethritis and Related Conditions. Washington, DC, American Society for Microbiology, 1977.

Schachter J, Grossman M, Sweet RL, et al: Prospective study of perinatal transmission of Chlamydia trachomatis. JAMA 255:3374, 1986.

Schachter J, Holt J, Goodner E, et al: Prospective study of chlamydial infection in neonates. Lancet 2:377, 1979.

Schachter J, Moncada J, Whidden R, et al: Noninvasive tests for diagnosis of Chlamydia trachomatis infection: Application of ligase chain reaction to first-catch urine specimens of women. J Infect Dis 172:1411, 1995.

Schachter J, Sweet RL, Grossman M, et al: Experience with the routine use of erythromycin for chlamydial infections in pregnancy. N Engl J Med 314:276, 1986.

Silverman NS, Sullivan M, Hochman M, et al: A randomized, prospective trial comparing amoxicillin and erythromycin for the treatment of *Chlamydia trachomatis* in pregnancy. Am J Obstet Gynecol 170:829, 1994.

Stamm WE: Diagnosis of *Chlamydia trachomatis* genitourinary infections. Ann Intern Med 108:710, 1987.

Stamm WE: *Chlamydia trachomatis* infections of the adult. *In* Holmes KK, Sparling PF, Mardh PA, et al (eds): Sexually Transmitted Diseases. New York, McGraw-Hill, 1999, p. 407.

Sweet RL, Gibbs RS: Chlamydial infections. *In* Sweet RL, Gibbs RS: Infectious Diseases of the Female Genital Tract. 4th ed. Philadelphia, Lippincott–Williams & Wilkins, 2002, p. 57.

Sweet RL, Landers DV, Walker C, et al: *Chlamydia trachomatis* infection and pregnancy outcome. Am J Obstet Gynecol 156:824, 1987.

Thygeson P, Mengert WE: The virus of inclusion conjunctivitis: Further observations. Arch Ophthalmol 377, 1936.

van Doornum GJ, Buimer M, Prins M, et al: Detection of *Chlamydia trachomatis* infection in urine samples from men and women by ligase chain reaction. J Clin Microbiol 33:2042, 1995.

Vogels VHM, Vader PC, Schorder FP: *Chlamydia trachomatis* infection in a high risk population: Comparison of polymerase chain reaction and cell culture for diagnosis and follow-up. J Clin Microbiol 31:1103, 1994.

Wager GP, Martin DH, Koutsky L, et al: Puerperal infectious morbidity: Relationship to route of delivery and to antepartum *Chlamydia trachomatis* infection. Am J Obstet Gynecol 138:1028, 1980.

Wehbeh HA, Ruggierio RM, Shahem S, et al: Single-dose azithromycin for *Chlamydia* in pregnant women. J Reprod Med 43:509, 1998.

Wiesenfeld HC, Heine RP, Rideout A, et al: The vaginal introitus: A novel site for *Chlamydia trachomatis* testing in women. Am J Obstet Gynecol 174:1542, 1996.

Wiesenfeld HC, Uhrim M, Dixon MW, et al: Rapid polymerase chain reaction–based test for the detection of female urogenital chlamydial infections. J Infect Dis Obstet Gynecol 1:182, 1994.

Other Infections

Mycoplasmal Infection

Carey JC, Blackwelder WC, Nugent RP, et al: Antepartum cultures for *Ureaplasma urealyticum* are not useful in predicting pregnancy outcome. Am J Obstet Gynecol 164:728, 1991.

Eschenbach DA: *Ureaplasma urealyticum* and premature birth. Clin Infect Dis 17(Suppl 1): S100, 1994.

Eschenbach DA, Nugent RP, Ra AV, et al: A randomized placebo-controlled trial of erythromycin for the treatment of *Ureaplasma urealyticum* to prevent premature delivery. Am J Obstet Gynecol 164:734, 1991.

Gibbs RS, Cassel GH, Davis JK, et al: Further studies on genital mycoplasmas in intra-amniotic infection: Blood cultures and serologic response. Am J Obstet Gynecol 154:717, 1986.

Hillier SL, Joachim M, Krohn M, et al: A case-control study of chorioamnionic infection and histologic chorioamnionitis in prematurity. N Engl J Med 319:972, 1988.

Kass EH, McCormack WM, Lin JS, et al: Genital mycoplasmas as a cause of excess premature delivery. Trans Assoc Am Physicians 94:261, 1981.

Klein JO, Buckland D, Finland M: Colonization of newborn infants by mycoplasmas. N Engl J Med 280:1025, 1969.

Kundsin RB, Driscoll SG, Ming PL: Strains of mycoplasma associated with human reproductive failure. Science 157:1573, 1967.

Lamey JR, Eschenbach DA, Mitchell SH, et al: Isolation of mycoplasmas and bacteria from the blood of postpartum women. Am J Obstet Gynecol 143:104, 1982.

Likitnukel S, Kusmiesz H, Nelson JD, et al: Rate of genital mycoplasmas in young infants with suspected sepsis. J Pediatr 109:971, 1986.

McCormack WM, Lee YH, Lin JS, et al: Genital mycoplasmas in postpartum fever. J Infect Dis 127:193, 1973.

Shurin PA, Alpert S, Rosner B, et al: Chorioamnionitis and colonization of the newborn infant with genital mycoplasmas. N Engl J Med 293:5, 1975.

Stray-Pederson B, Erg J, Reikuan TM: Uterine T-mycoplasma colonization in reproductive failure. Am J Obstet Gynecol 130:307, 1978.

Taylor-Robinson D, McCormack WM: The genital mycoplasmas. N Engl J Med 302:1003, 1980.

Waites KB, Rudd PT, Course PT, et al: *U. urealyticum* and M. *hominis* infection of central nervous system in preterm infants. Lancet 1:17, 1988.

Yoon BH, Romero R, Park JS, et al: Microbial invasion of the amniotic cavity with *Ureaplasma urealyticum* is associated with a robust host response in fetal, amniotic and maternal compartments. Am J Obstet Gynecol 179:1254, 1998.

Candidiasis (Monolilial Vaginitis)

Centers for Disease Control and Prevention (CDC): Sexually transmitted diseases treatment guidelines 2002. MMWR Morb Mortal Wkly Rep 51(RR-6), 2002.

Cotch MF, Eschenbach DA, Martin D, et al: NIH C. *trachomatis* trial. Paper presented at the 30th Interscience Conference on Antimicrobial Agents and Chemotherapy, October 21–24, 1990, Atlanta.

Bacterial Vaginosis

American College of Obstetricians and Gynecologists: Assessment of Risk Factors for Preterm Birth. ACOG Practice Bull 31, 2001.

Burtin P, Taddio A, Ariburnu O, et al: Safety of metronidazole in pregnancy: A meta-analysis. Am J Obstet Gynecol 172:525, 1995.

Carey JC, Klebanoff MA, Hauth JC, et al: Metronidazole to prevent preterm delivery in pregnant women with asymptomatic bacterial vaginosis. N Engl J Med 342:534, 2000.

Caro-Paton T, Carvajal A, Martin de Diego I, et al: Is metronidazole teratogenic? A meta-analysis. Br J Clin Pharmacol 44:179, 1997.

Centers for Disease Control and Prevention (CDC): Sexually transmitted diseases treatment guidelines 2002. MMWR Morb Mortal Wkly Rep 51(RR-6), 2002.

Gibbs RS, Eschenbach DA: Use of antibiotics to prevent preterm birth. Am J Obstet Gynecol 177:375, 1997.

Goldenberg RL, Hauth JC, Andrews WW: Intrauterine infection and preterm delivery. N Engl J Med 342:1500, 2000.

Gravett MG, Hummel D, Eschenbach DA, et al: Preterm labor associated with subclinical amniotic fluid infection and with bacterial vaginosis. Obstet Gynecol 67:229, 1986.

Gravett MG, Preston-Nelson HP, DeRouen T, et al: Independent associations of bacterial vaginosis and *Chlamydia trachomatis* infection with adverse pregnancy outcome. JAMA 256:1899, 1986.

Hauth JC, Goldenberg RL, Andrews WW, et al: Reduced incidence of preterm delivery with metronidazole and erythromycin in women with bacterial vaginosis. N Engl J Med 333:1732, 1995.

Hillier SL, Martius J, Kohn M, et al: A case-control study of chorioamnionic infection and histology of chorioamnionitis in prematurity. N Engl J Med 319:972, 1988.

Hillier SL, Nugent RP, Eschenbach DA, et al: Association between bacterial vaginosis and preterm delivery of a low-birth-weight infant. N Engl J Med 333:2737, 1995.

Martius J, Krohn MA, Hillier SL, et al: Relationships of vaginal *Lactobacillus* species, cervical *Chlamydia trachomatis*, and bacterial vaginosis to preterm birth. Obstet Gynecol 71:89, 1988.

McDonald HM, O'Loughlin JA, Vigneswaran R, et al: Impact of metronidazole therapy on preterm birth in women with bacterial vaginosis flora (*Gardnerella vaginalis*): A randomised, placebo controlled trial. Br J Obstet Gynaecol 104:1391, 1997.

McGregor JA, French JI, Parker R, et al: Prevention of premature birth by screening and treatment for common genital tract infections: Results of a prospective controlled evaluation. Am J Obstet Gynecol 173:157, 1995.

Morales WJ, Schorr S, Albritton J: Effect of metronidazole in patients with preterm birth in preceding pregnancy and bacterial vaginosis: A placebo-controlled, double-blind study. Am J Obstet Gynecol 171:345, 1994.

Newton ER, Prihoda TJ, Gibbs RS: A clinical and microbiologic analysis of risk factors for puerperal endometritis. Obstet Gynecol 75:402, 1990.

Piper JM, Mitchel EF, Ray WA: Prenatal use of metronidazole and birth defects: No association. Obstet Gynecol 82:348, 1993.

Silver HM, Sperling RS, St Clair PJ, et al: Evidence relating bacterial vaginosis to intraamniotic infection. Am J Obstet Gynecol 161:808, 1989.

Toxoplasmosis

MMWR: 1997 USPHS/IDSA guidelines for the prevention of opportunistic infections in persons infected with human immunodeficiency virus. MMWR Morb Mortal Wkly Rep (Suppl) 46:1, 1997.

Daffos F, Forestier F, Capella-Pavlovsky M, et al: Prenatal management of 746 pregnancies at risk for congenital toxoplasmosis. N Engl J Med 318:271, 1988.

Egerman RS, Beazley D: Toxoplasmosis. Semin Perinatol 22:332, 1998.

Guerina NG, Hsu HW, Meissner HC, et al: Neonatal serologic screening and early treatment for congenital *Toxoplasma gondii* infection. N Engl J Med 330:1858, 1994.

Hohlfeld P, Daffos F, Costa JM, et al: Prenatal diagnosis of congenital toxoplasmosis with a polymerase-chain reaction test on amniotic fluid. N Engl J Med 331:695, 1994.

Krick JA, Remington JS: Toxoplasmosis in the adult—an overview. N Engl J Med **298**:550, 1978.

Romana S, Wallon M, Franck J, et al: Prenatal diagnosis using polymerase chain reaction on amniotic fluid for congenital toxoplasmosis. Obstet Gynecol **97**:296, 2001.

Trichomoniasis

Burtin P, Taddio A, Ariburnu O, et al: Safety of metronidazole in pregnancy: A meta-analysis. Am J Obstet Gynecol **172**:525, 1995.

Centers for Disease Control and Prevention (CDC): Sexually transmitted diseases treatment guidelines 2002. MMWR Morb Mortal Wkly Rep **51**(RR-6)**,** 2002.

Cotch MF, Pastorek JG II, Nugent RP, et al: *Trichomonas vaginalis* associated with low birth weight and preterm delivery: The Vaginal Infections and Prematurity Study Group. Sex Transm Dis **24**:353, 1997.

Klebanoff MA, Carey JC, Hauth JC, et al: Failure of metronidazole to prevent preterm delivery among pregnant women with asymptomatic *Trichomonas vaginalis* infection. New Engl J Med **345**:487, 2001.

Minkoff H, Grunebaum AN, Schwarz RH, et al: Risk factors for prematurity and premature rupture of membranes: A prospective study of the vaginal flora in pregnancy. Am J Obstet Gynecol **150**:965, 1984.

Antibiotics in Pregnancy

Anonymous: Meropenem—a new parenteral broad-spectrum antibiotic. Medical Lett Drugs Ther **38**:88, 1996.

Anonymous: Quinupristin/dalfopristin. Medical Lett Drugs Ther **41**:109, 1999.

Anonymous: Linezolid (Zyvox). Medical Lett Drugs Ther **42**:45, 2000.

Anonymous: Ertapenem (Invanz)—a new parenteral carbapenem. Medical Lett Drugs Ther **44**:25, 2002.

Centers for Disease Control and Prevention (CDC): 1998 Guidelines for treatment of sexually transmitted diseases. MMWR Morb Mortal Wkly Rep (Suppl) **47**:1, 1998.

Donowitz GR, Mandell GL: Beta-lactam antibiotics. Part I. N Engl J Med **318**:419, 1988a.

Donowitz GR, Mandell GL: Beta-lactam antibiotics. Part II. N Engl J Med **318**:490, 1988b.

Duff P: Urinary tract infections. Prim Care Update OB/GYNs **1**:12, 1994.

Duff P: Antibiotic selection in obstetric patients. Infect Dis Clin North Am **11**:1, 1997.

Duff P: Maternal and perinatal infections. *In* Gabbe SG, Niebyl JR, Simpson JL (eds): Obstetrics: Normal and Problem Pregnancies (4th ed). New York, Churchill Livingstone, 2001.

Duff P: Antibiotic selection in obstetrics: Making cost-effective choices. Clin Obstet Gynecol **45**:59, 2002.

Dunlow SG, Duff P: Prevalence of antibiotic-resistant uropathogens in obstetric patients with acute pyelonephritis. Obstet Gynecol **76**:241, 1990.

Edwards R, Clark P, Duff P: Intrapartum antibiotic prophylaxis 2: Positive predictive value of antenatal group B streptococci cultures and antibiotic susceptibility of clinical isolates. Obstet Gynecol **100**:590, 2003.

Gupta K, Scholes D, Stamm WE: Increasing prevalence of antimicrobial resistance among uropathogens causing acute uncomplicated cystitis in women. JAMA **281**:736, 1999.

Jamie W, Edwards R, Duff P: Antimicrobial susceptibility of gram-negative uropathogens isolated from obstetric patients. Infect Dis Obstet Gynecol **10**:123, 2002.

McCarty JM: Azithromycin (Zithromax®). Infect Dis Obstet Gynecol **4**:215, 1996.

Nicolau DP, Freeman CD, Belliveau PP, et al: Experience with a once-daily aminoglycoside program administered to 2184 adult patients. Antimicrob Agents Chemother **39**:650, 1995.

Robbie MO, Sweet RL: Metronidazole use in obstetrics and gynecology: A review. Am J Obstet Gynecol **145**:865, 1983.

Rubin RH, Swartz MN: Trimethoprim-sulfamethoxazole. New Engl J Med **303**:426, 1980.

Simmons WJ, Lee TJ: Treatment of gram-negative infections with aztreonam. Am J Med **78**(Suppl 2A):27, 1985.

Stamm WE, Hooton TM: Management of urinary tract infections in adults. N Engl J Med **329**:1328, 1993.

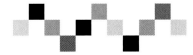

Chapter 40

HUMAN IMMUNODEFICIENCY VIRUS

Howard L. Minkoff, MD

In the 22 years since acquired immunodeficiency syndrome (AIDS) was first reported, the course of the human immunodeficiency virus (HIV) epidemic has progressed along two distinct paths. In the developed world, rapid advances in our understanding of the virology and natural history of HIV have led to the development of interventions that, though often toxic and expensive, have transformed a disease that was inexorably and rapidly progressive and uniformly lethal to one that can be controlled for long periods of time. Concomitantly, rates of opportunistic infections, of hospitalizations, and of mother-to-child transmission of HIV have plummeted. In the developing world, similar advances have not been witnessed. Indeed, the number of deaths and AIDS orphans is more staggering than ever. The disparity between regions was best described by Farmer (2001), who noted that "excellence without equity looms as the major human rights dilemma of health care in the 21st century." Although global efforts will be required to close the gap between countries, American providers will continue to face their own set of challenges. To ensure American women who are infected with HIV of the benefits of the medical advances of the last several years, obstetricians must be familiar with a rapidly evolving array of complex medications and interventions that have become part of the standard of care. This chapter briefly reviews the scope of the HIV epidemic, as well as the virology and pathophysiology of HIV, but focuses primarily on the steps obstetricians must take to optimize the care of HIV-infected pregnant women.

EPIDEMIOLOGY

Within months of the first reported incidence of AIDS in men in June 1981, the Centers for Disease Control and Prevention (CDC) reported the first cases of AIDS in women (CDC, 1981). By the end of the 1980s the disease had become the sixth leading cause of death in women aged 25 to 44 years and by 1998 was the fifth leading cause of death in that age group overall and the third leading cause among black women (CDC, 1990, 2001). During the 1990s the number of persons living with AIDS increased as a result of the expanded AIDS case definition that was introduced in 1993 and, more recently, improved survival as a result of increasingly effective therapies. At the same time, women were becoming an increasing proportion of persons living with AIDS. In 1992, women accounted for 14% of adults/adolescents living with AIDS, and 7 years later they accounted for 20% of cases. By 1999 32% of new HIV infections were being reported among women (CDC, 1999).

Demographic shifts have also been seen among infected women. The expansion of the epidemic in women has been most dramatic among women of color. African-American and Hispanic women together represent less than one fourth of all U.S. women, yet they account for more than three-fourths (78%) of AIDS cases among women reported to date. Geographic shifts have occurred as well. The epidemic was initially centered among drug-using women in the Northeast. More recently, there has been an increasing percentage of new infections occurring in the South, among women with heterosexual sex as their risk factor, and among black women (Hader et al., 2001). The South has long been a region with one of the highest rates of sexually transmitted infections in the nation.

Heterosexual spread of HIV had surpassed intravenous drug use as a mode of acquisition among women by 1995. In 2000, 38% of women reported with AIDS were infected through heterosexual exposure to HIV, whereas injection drug use accounted for 25% of cases. However, in addition to the direct risks associated with drug injection, drug use also contributes to the heterosexual spread of HIV. A large number of women infected heterosexually are infected through sex with an injection drug user. Many HIV/AIDS-infected women initially deny any known risk, suggesting that they may be unaware of their partners' risk factors. Ultimately, more than two thirds of AIDS cases among women initially reported without identified risk are reclassified as heterosexual transmission, and just over one fourth are attributed to injection drug use.

An important issue of concern is that younger women are disproportionately at risk. It is estimated that between one fourth and one half of HIV-infected women who acquire their infection heterosexually do so in their teens or twenties (Neal et al., 1997). As with other infections tracked by the National Health and Nutrition Evaluation Survey, such as herpes, women tend to become infected at younger ages than do men (Fleming et al., 1997). That fact might reflect American dating patterns, with younger women tending to date older men. Clinicians should be aware of the relatively young age at which women are first at sexual risk of HIV infection and use that information in establishing standards for educating women about those risks within their practices.

VIROLOGY AND PATHOGENESIS

HIV-1 and HIV-2 are members of the lentivirus subfamily of Retroviridae and are the only lentiviruses known to infect humans. These organisms are single-stranded RNA-enveloped viruses that have the ability to become incorporated into cellular DNA. The lentiviruses are slower acting than viruses that cause acute infection (e.g., influenza virus) but are not as slow acting as other retroviruses. The features of acute primary infection with HIV (an acute mononucleosis-like syndrome) resemble those of more classic acute infections. The characteristic chronicity of HIV disease is consistent with the designation lentivirus (Fauci and Lane, 2001).

HIV preferentially infects cells with the CD4 antigen, particularly helper lymphocytes, but also macrophages, cells of the central nervous system, and, according to some evidence, cells of the placenta (Maury et al., 1989). At least two other cell surface molecules help HIV to enter the cells. These coreceptors for HIV, called CXCR4 and CCR5, are receptors for chemokines (Levy, 1996). It has also been reported that individuals who are homozygous for a 32-base pair deletion at the CCR5 gene are less likely to acquire HIV, whereas those who are heterozygous for the deletion progress less rapidly if infected. Once the virus is internalized, its RNA is released from the nucleocapsid and is reverse transcribed into proviral DNA. The provirus is inserted into the genome and then transcribed into RNA, the RNA is translated, and virions assemble and are extruded from the cell membrane by budding. Viral RNA molecules then have one of three fates: They are exported to the cytoplasm, where they are packaged as the viral RNA in infectious viral particles; they are spliced to form the message for the envelope polyprotein; or they are translated into Gag and Pol proteins. The virus is composed of core (p18, p24, and p27) and surface (gp120 and gp41) proteins, genomic RNA, and the reverse-transcriptase enzyme surrounded by a lipid bilayer envelope. The virion contains three structural genes (*gag*, *pol*, and *env*) and a complex set of regulatory genes, including *tat*, *vif*, *nef*, *vpu*, and *ref*, that control the rate of virion production.

HIV infection leads to progressive debilitation of the immune system, rendering infected individuals susceptible to opportunistic infections (e.g., *Pneumocystis carinii* pneumonia and central nervous system toxoplasmosis) and neoplasias (e.g., Kaposi sarcoma) that rarely afflict patients with intact immune systems. For an HIV-infected patient with one of several specific opportunistic infections, neoplasia, dementia encephalopathy, or wasting syndrome, the diagnosis of AIDS is assigned. The diagnosis can be made in the absence of laboratory evidence of infection if the patient has no other known cause of immune deficiency and has the definitive diagnosis of one of a number of indicator diseases (Liu et al., 1996). In 1993, the CDC changed the case definition to include all individuals with HIV infection whose CD4 counts drop below 200 CD4 lymphocytes/mm^3 and HIV-infected individuals with advanced cervical cancer, pulmonary tuberculosis, and recurrent pneumonia (CDC, 1992).

At the time of initial infection there may be no symptoms, or an acute mononucleosis-like syndrome, sometimes accompanied by aseptic meningitis, may develop. There is an immediate viremia of substantive proportions (up to a billion viral particles turned over per day) and an equally impressive immune response with similar levels of T-cell turnover (Ho et al., 1995). After the initial viremia, the level of virus returns to a "set point." The level of virus in the plasma at that time can provide an estimate of the probability that an individual, if left untreated, will develop AIDS within 5 years. Antibodies are usually detectable 1 month after infection and are almost always detectable within 3 months. After seroconversion has

occurred, an asymptomatic period of variable length usually follows. The median clinical latency in the pre–highly active antiretroviral therapy (HAART) era was estimated at approximately 11 years with only a few (less than 5%) developing AIDS within 3 years (Hessol et al., 1989; Lemp et al., 1990).

Evidence of immune dysfunction may be followed by clinical conditions ranging from fever, weight loss, malaise, lymphadenopathy, and central nervous system dysfunction to infections such as herpes simplex virus or oral candidiasis. These nonspecific conditions are usually progressive and are a prelude to an opportunistic infection that is diagnostic of AIDS. Studies of infected individuals have noted that 5 years after infection was confirmed, up to 35% had progressed to AIDS (Lifson et al., 1988; Goedert et al., 1989). A study of subjects with hemophilia demonstrated that the incidence rate of AIDS after seroconversion was 2.67 per 100 person-years and was directly related to age (AIDS developed in younger individuals at a slower rate) (Goedert et al., 1989). It should be noted that all these statistics antedate the use of new, more powerful antiretroviral agents that have been shown to have a significant effect on surrogate markers of disease progression and on rates of opportunistic infections and hospitalizations.

HUMAN IMMUNODEFICIENCY VIRUS INFECTION IN PREGNANCY: NATURAL HISTORY AND DETERMINANTS OF TRANSMISSION

Interactions between Human Immunodeficiency Virus and Pregnancy

Since early in the HIV epidemic, the possibility that pregnancy might cause immune alterations has raised concerns about the possibility of an accelerated course of immune deterioration among HIV-infected pregnant women. In the mid-1980s, reports of adverse outcomes among pregnant HIV-infected women lent credence to those suppositions. The first five women with AIDS in pregnancy who were reported in the medical literature, each of whom had opportunistic infections, all had poor outcomes (Wetli et al., 1983; Jensen et al., 1984; Minkoff et al., 1986). However, the limited diagnostic tests available and the absence of effective therapies for HIV at the time of those reports limited the conclusions that could reasonably be drawn from those data. However, despite their shortcomings, those works contributed to concerns regarding the safety of pregnancy among HIV-infected women.

As a consequence of those reports, as well as beliefs about the potential effect of pregnancy on immune status, it was suggested that an interaction between pregnancy and HIV disease was a theoretic risk that HIV-infected women should be informed of by clinical staff (Lifson et al., 1988), and several researchers chose to initiate studies addressing the issue. In the last decade a large number of reports on the subject have been published (Wetli et al., 1983; Jensen et al., 1984; Minkoff et al., 1986, 1987; Berrebi et al., 1990; MacCallum et al., 1988; Schaefer et al., 1988; Biggar et al., 1989; Goedert et al., 1989; Holman et al., 1989; Hocke et al., 1995; Alliegro et al., 1997; Kumar et al., 1997; Bessinger et al., 1998; French and Brocklehurt, 1998; Weisser et al., 1998; Saada et al., 2000). One of the earliest studies reported that among 34 HIV-positive mothers followed for a mean of 27.8 ± 21.6 months,

15 developed AIDS or AIDS-related complex (Minkoff et al., 1987), a higher than expected rate suggesting that pregnancy could accelerate women's illness. However, because the mothers were identified through the birth of a child who developed AIDS, the findings may have been representative only of women with advanced immunocompromise. Indeed, evidence suggests that the course of illness in a child relates to the stage of maternal illness, with the infant's risk of death correlated inversely with the mother's CD4 count (Blanche et al., 1994).

Subsequently, most authors have found slight or no effect. Schaeffer and associates (1988) followed 32 HIV-positive women and 40 HIV-negative women during pregnancy and for 6 months after delivery and observed no clinical progression of illness during pregnancy among seropositive women, although 9% of patients developed signs of clinical deterioration during postpartum observation. In a follow-up of 88 postpartum patients, MacCallum and coworkers (1988) were unable to demonstrate any adverse effect of pregnancy on the course of HIV disease. Similarly, in a study of 23 pregnant patients followed for 2 years after delivery, compared with matched seropositive nonpregnant control subjects, no significant differences were observed in the number of opportunistic infections between the two groups (MacCallum et al., 1988; Liu et al., 1996). In a prospective study from Bordeaux, France, 57 women who completed a pregnancy during the course of their HIV infection were compared with 114 HIV-infected women who never conceived (Hocke, 1995). The two groups were matched on CD4 lymphocyte count, age, and year of HIV diagnosis. The main outcome measures were death, occurrence of a first AIDS-defining event, and a drop of the CD4 below 200/mm^3. No significant difference was observed in the two groups with regard to the different end points studied, even after adjustment for other prognostic variables. Adjusted hazards ratio (pregnant/nonpregnant) were 0.92 for death (95% confidence interval, 0.40–2.12), 1.02 for occurrence of a first AIDS-defining event (95% confidence interval, 0.48–2.18), and 1.20 for drop in CD4 to less than 200/mm^3 (95% confidence interval, 0.63–2.27). In contrast, in a study from India (Kumar et al., 1997), where mortality was much higher overall, 32 pregnant women had greater maternal and fetal mortality than 38 age, parity, and CD4 matched nonpregnant women.

French and Brocklehurst (1998), in a review of this subject, believed there was an apparent consensus that pregnancy is not a major determinant of survival among HIV-infected women. However, they also noted several limitations of the studies upon which this consensus was based, including inappropriate control subjects (uninfected pregnant women), small sample sizes (in their meta-analysis the average number of the pregnant patients in each study was 42, range 15 to 85), and a failure of reviews in the area to be systematic. After performing their review they concluded the following:

> Studies measuring the association between HIV infection and maternal outcome have involved relatively small numbers and will have been unable to detect modest differences in survival or disease progression. This review . . . is still unable to determine with any certainty the effect of pregnancy on HIV disease progression. . . . There is a need for further large observational cohorts of pregnant and non-pregnant women infected with HIV to be undertaken which include long-term follow-up.

Around the time of French and Brocklehurst's review, HAART became available. Thereafter, biological factors became only one mechanism whereby pregnancy could effect the course of HIV disease. Pregnancy could also result in the less aggressive use of therapies, though recent studies have not found dramatic differences in access based on pregnancy status in the United States (Minkoff et al., 2001). Additionally, treatments designed to reduce mother-to-child transmission have the potential to predispose to the development of resistant strains of HIV that might not respond as rapidly to some agents in subsequent pregnancies. Finally, caring for an infant might make compliance with complex therapeutic regimens more difficult for new mothers.

Several additional studies of the interaction between pregnancy and disease progression have been reported since French's meta-analysis. They seem to confirm an ongoing absence of effect. Saada and colleagues (2000), using a cohort with known dates of seroconversion, compared 241 women who delivered after HIV infection with 124 women who did not become pregnant while HIV infected. They found no effect of pregnancy on the risk of developing AIDS. In another study of women with known time of seroconversion (within 2 years), the 69 women who had a pregnancy (including 45 term pregnancies) were not more likely to progress to AIDS or to have a CD4 count less than 100/mm^3 than the 262 women who had no pregnancy (Alliegro et al., 1997). The median follow-up was 5.5 years. The authors controlled for age, CD4 count, and use of therapy. Bessinger and colleagues (1998) also found no difference between 192 women with term pregnancies and 162 women without. They noted, as did we in a recent study including the largest cohort studied to date (Minkoff et al., in press), that women who became pregnant were younger and healthier at baseline. Finally, in a Swiss study 32 women with term pregnancies and follow-up at 6 months were not more likely to progress than 416 control subjects matched for CD4 count and age at entry (Weisser et al., 1998).

Although there is scant evidence that pregnancy has a substantial deleterious effect on the natural history of HIV disease, investigators continue to assess the converse, that is, whether HIV infection has a significant impact on pregnancy outcomes such as rates of preterm birth or low birth weight. The conclusions of these investigations seem to vary with the settings in which they take place. In the United States most investigators have found that HIV-infected women do not have substantively higher rates of adverse outcomes than uninfected women once they control for confounders such as drug and alcohol use (Minkoff et al., 1990). However, there have been a few authors whose results are in conflict, but in those instances the differences, though statistically significant, did not occur at a time when HAART therapy was routinely available. In countries in which women might be anticipated to have more advanced and/or untreated disease, the differences between infected and uninfected women have been more noteworthy. Anemia, low birth weight, and prolonged labor are among the complications that have been reported (Chamiso, 1996; Leroy et al., 1998). These findings may be explained by cofactors such as advanced maternal disease or poor nutrition.

Determinants of Transmission: Viral Load and Antiretroviral Therapy

Several factors that increase the risk of mother-to-child transmission of HIV have been described. The most consistently reported factors are those that correlate with maternal disease stage, with more advanced disease being linked with higher transmission rates. More advanced disease can be measured clinically (AIDS defining conditions), immunologically (lower CD4 counts or percents), or virologically (maternal p24 antigenemia or high plasma HIV RNA levels). Other associated factors include placental inflammation and sexually transmitted diseases (European Collaborative Study, 1992; Sutton et al., 1999; Wabwire-Mangen et al., 1999). Less consistently reported factors include preterm birth, maternal illicit drug use, vitamin A deficiency, and female gender of the infant (Burns et al., 1994, 1999; Semba et al., 1994; Temmerman et al., 1995; Rodriguez et al., 1996).

Viral factors have been most carefully studied. Studies from both untreated and treated cohorts of pregnant women have consistently demonstrated an association between maternal HIV RNA levels and risk of transmission (Dickover et al., 1996; Sperling et al., 1996; Thea et al., 1997; Mofenson et al., 1999). In untreated women, transmission rates increased from about 10% (range, 0% to 22%) among women with HIV RNA levels near delivery of less than 1000 copies/mL, to 17% (range, 0% to 67%) with levels of 1000 to 10,000 copies/mL, and to 33% (range, 22% to 64%) with levels above 10,000 copies/mL (Watts and Minkoff, 2003). Additionally, the characteristics of the virus also plays a role with recent reports noting an association between nonsyncytium-forming virus and rates of transmission (LaRussa et al., 2002). Nonsyncytium-forming viruses are more likely to infect those cells that may have a greater proclivity to cross the placenta. However, regardless of these factors, antiretroviral medications reduce transmission rates (Cooper et al., 2002). When loads are reduced to undetectable levels, transmission becomes an extremely uncommon event. In the original PACTG 076 study, which first highlighted the utility of zidovudine (ZDV) in reducing rates of mother-to-child transmission of HIV, among women receiving antiretroviral therapy, predominantly ZDV monotherapy, transmission rates increased from 1% (range, 0% to 7%) with HIV RNA levels below 1000 copies/mL, to 6% (range, 0% to 12%) with levels of 1000 to 10,000 copies/mL, and to 13% (range, 9% to 29%) with levels above 10,000 copies/mL. Treatment lowered the transmission rate among women in each viral load group, even among women with low or undetectable HIV RNA levels, suggesting that the effects of treatment are not all related to decreasing maternal plasma HIV RNA levels but may also be related to decreasing genital tract HIV levels and pre- and postexposure prophylaxis of the infant. These same findings have been replicated among women on several agents and most recently among those on HAART (see later) (Cooper et al., 2002). Although transmission rates are low among women with HIV RNA levels below 1000 copies/mL, there is not a threshold below which the absence of transmission can be assured (Ioannidis et al., 2001).

More recent observational data suggest that transmission rates are reduced even further, to 2% or lower, by the use of maternal combination antiretroviral therapy (Cooper et al., 2002). Four small studies reported one transmission (0.6%) among a total of 160 infants born to women on two or more antiretrovirals during pregnancy (Lorenzi et al., 1998; McGowan et al., 1999; Clarke et al., 2000; Morris et al., 2000). Similarly, low transmission rates have been reported from the Women and Infants Transmission Study, which found a trans-

mission rate of 3.8% among 186 women on dual therapy and 1.2% among 250 women on HAART (Cooper et al., 2002). However only 16 of the former and 21 of the latter had HIV-1 RNA levels greater than 30,000 copies. These data suggest that highly active antiretroviral regimens indicated for HIV-infected women for their own health are also beneficial in reducing the risk of perinatal transmission.

Determinants of Transmission: Obstetric Factors

Although the mother's virologic, immunologic, and clinical statuses are the primary predictors of transmission rate, obstetric factors can modify the rate. The first hint that intrapartum interventions could potentially have a role in reducing rates of transmission derived from studies detailing the timing of transmission. Although transmission may occur during the antepartum or postpartum period, in non–breast-feeding populations only about one third (20% to 40%) appears to occur *in utero* (antepartum), with the remaining two thirds (40% to 80%) occurring during labor and delivery (Blanche et al., 1990; European Collaborative Study, 1991; Luzuriaga et al., 1993; McIntosh et al., 1994). Several types of evidence have been cited in support of intrapartum transmission, including the lag between delivery and the detection of HIV by culture, antigen detection, or DNA in the neonate (Luzuriaga et al., 1993; McIntosh et al., 1994). Additionally, newborns have a delayed onset of clinical symptoms (European Collaborative Study, 1991), and there is a significantly higher transmission rate in first-born compared with second-born twins (Duliege et al., 1995). Several authors have also reported an association of higher transmission rates with increasing duration of ruptured membranes in labor (Minkoff et al., 1995; Landesman et al., 1996). These data support the thesis that interventions directed at late pregnancy, delivery, and the neonate may substantially reduce transmission. As a consequence, investigators began to assess the role of cesarean delivery in reducing transmission rates.

Cesarean delivery had already been shown to influence the rate of mother-to-child transmission of several other viral agents. Perhaps most well known is the report of Amstey and Monif in 1974 of a protective effect of cesarean delivery in the setting of herpes simplex virus lesions. Their report led to the "4-hour rule" that, for more than a decade, guided the timing of surgery after rupture of membranes in the setting of an active herpes simplex virus lesion (Amstey and Monif, 1974). Other researchers have linked the use of cesarean delivery to lower rates of transmission of hepatitis C virus (Gibb et al., 2000), hepatitis B virus (Lee et al., 1988), and human papillomavirus (Shah et al., 1986), fueling speculation, early in the HIV epidemic, of a similar effect in regard to HIV. Recent reports have confirmed a protective effect of surgery.

Those data come from observational studies, randomized clinical trials, and meta-analyses. The first direct evidence of a protective effect from elective cesarean delivery came from two prospective cohort studies, the French Perinatal Cohort (Mandelbrot et al., 1998) and the Swiss Neonatal HIV Study Group (Kind et al., 1998), both of which demonstrated reduced rates of perinatal HIV-1 transmission among women who received ZDV and underwent elective cesarean delivery. The French reported on 872 HIV-infected women who received ZDV and found that the transmission rate of HIV for mothers delivering by elective cesarean delivery, emergency cesarean delivery, and vaginal delivery were 0.8%, 11.4%, and 6.6%, respectively ($P = .02$). The Swiss study included 414 children with known infection status and found that the overall infection rate was 16.2% (95% confidence interval, 13.0–18.5), whereas the rate among women undergoing elective cesarean delivery with intact membranes was 6% (odds ratio, 0.29; 95% confidence interval, 0.12–0.70; $P = .006$). In both studies an interaction was found between ZDV use and cesarean delivery, with their combined use being associated with a significantly lower transmission rate.

Confirmatory data came from a primary data set meta-analysis by Read and colleagues who took advantage of access to individual patient data from 15 cohort studies to assess more than 7800 mother–child pairs. Her results were similar to those in the studies cited above (International Perinatal HIV Group, 1999). The rate of perinatal HIV-1 transmission in women undergoing elective cesarean delivery was 8.2% in the group not receiving antiretrovirals and 2% in those receiving ZDV. The rate in both groups was significantly decreased compared with those seen among women delivered by either nonelective cesarean or vaginal delivery. Finally, a European randomized trial of cesarean delivery was reported in 1999 (European Mode of Delivery Collaboration, 1999). The results paralleled those found by Read. In that trial, HIV-infected women between 34 and 36 weeks of gestation were randomly assigned to undergo an elective cesarean delivery at 38 weeks or to have a vaginal delivery. Three (1.8%) of 170 infants born to women assigned cesarean delivery were infected compared with 21 (10.5%) of 200 born to women assigned to vaginal delivery ($P < .001$). Seven (3.4%) of 203 infants of women who actually gave birth by cesarean delivery were infected compared with 15 (10.2%) of 167 born vaginally ($P = .009$). Unfortunately, the number of participants was not adequate to allow for a separate analysis of the benefit of cesarean delivery in the setting of antiretroviral therapy. Additionally, HAART use was not reported from the cohort. Despite those limitations, the results suggest that among women who were not optimally treated with HAART, cesarean delivery could have an important effect on reducing rates of mother-to-child transmission of HIV. In sum, the above-cited studies strongly suggest that compared with other types of delivery, cesarean delivery performed before the onset of labor and before rupture of membranes (elective or scheduled cesarean) significantly reduces the rate of perinatal HIV-1 transmission.

MANAGEMENT OF HUMAN IMMUNODEFICIENCY VIRUS INFECTION IN PREGNANCY

Human Immunodeficiency Virus Testing

Although a variety of highly effective regimens is now available for the treatment of HIV-infected women, before those therapies can be initiated a woman's HIV status must be known. It is not uncommon for HIV serostatus to be determined for the first time during pregnancy. It is the responsibility of all clinicians charged with the care of pregnant women to be certain that serostatus is determined as early in pregnancy as possible through the establishment and vigorous performance of a counseling and testing program within their

practice or institution. The evolution in our understanding of this virus and in the development of therapies has been paralleled by an evolution in, and proliferation of, testing algorithms. The CDC in its treatment guidelines for sexually transmitted diseases recommends that all pregnant women be offered voluntary HIV testing at the first prenatal visit and that testing is reoffered to those who initially refuse testing (CDC, 2002). They go on to suggest that women at particular risk (e.g., partners of HIV-infected males or intravenous drug users) should be retested in the third trimester. The Institute of Medicine proposed an approach to testing that is both simple and practical and should ensure continued respect for patient autonomy. In its report, the Institute of Medicine's National Research Council (1999) recommended an informed right of refusal approach to testing. Although such an approach would require that a prenatal patient be informed that she was going to be tested for the virus that causes AIDS and that she had the right to refuse such a test, a written affirmative consent would not be required. Thereby, the HIV test would still be offered with more consideration than that applied to the panel of other prenatal tests for which the "general care" consent generally suffices. However, the process of testing would not be so onerous as to dissuade physicians from offering it or to convey the sense that the test is reserved for women who in some way were perceived to be at special risk.

Even if routine testing is performed in clinics, because approximately 15% of HIV-infected women receive no or minimal care and 20% do not initiate care until the third trimester, a number of women will still arrive in labor and delivery suites with unknown serostatus. In some circumstances, despite early care women will not have been offered the test. Compelling evidence suggests that intrapartum and early neonatal prophylaxis, even in the absence of antepartum therapy, can reduce the risk of mother-to-child transmission (Wade et al., 1998), and the CDC recommends that women who have not received prenatal counseling should be encouraged to be tested for HIV infection at delivery. Although the current generation of rapid tests (often using a single enzyme-linked immunosorbent assay) are not as reliable as the standard approach used for prenatal testing (one or two enzyme-linked immunosorbent assays followed by a confirmatory Western blot), they are still sufficiently sensitive to identify women who should be offered therapy while confirmatory tests are pending. Patients should be informed that if the confirmatory tests turn out to be negative (which they frequently will in low prevalence communities), treatment of the infant would be discontinued at that time.

Monitoring: Viral Load, CD4, and Resistance Testing

Viral load testing and CD4 testing are complementary ways of monitoring a woman's status, with the latter determining how far advanced the illness is and the former suggesting how rapidly the woman is likely to progress. During pregnancy the viral load status should be determined every month until the virus is no longer detectable. Viral load should drop by approximately 1 to 2 logs per month if effective therapy is being used. Once the virus in no longer detectable, testing can be reduced to once every 3 months. The higher the viral load, the longer it will take to become undetectable. However, in all circumstances the viral load should become undetectable within

6 months of starting therapy. The CD4 count can be used to decide when it is necessary to institute prophylaxis for opportunistic infections. No such medications are required if the CD4 count is higher than 200/mm³. If such therapy is begun at a lower count but the CD4 count rises back above 200/mm³ consequent to HAART, the prophylaxis can be discontinued once the count has remained over that threshold for 6 months. As is discussed below, the viral load and CD4 count can also be used to determine when HAART should be started.

Additionally, along with viral load testing and CD4, testing is often required to help in choosing optimal therapy because of drug resistance. The life cycle of HIV predisposes to mutations and hence resistance because of the combination of the rapid turnover of HIV (10^7 to 10^8 rounds of replication/day) and the high error rate of reverse transcriptase when replicating the nearly 10,000 nucleotides present in the HIV genome. When incompletely suppressive drug regimens are used, they provide the evolutionary pressure that selects those mutations that cause resistance to antiretroviral agents. The number of mutations required to cause a clinically relevant effect varies with the agent in question. Thus, the rate at which resistance develops will depend on the number of mutations necessary to create a significant change in susceptibility.

Although obstetricians have often used culture and sensitivity testing to choose appropriate antimicrobials, antiviral resistance testing can be a bit more complicated. However, evidence suggests that it is worth mastering this facet of HIV care. A few randomized trials have demonstrated that those assigned to study arms with access to resistance test results have a greater reduction in viral load after the initiation of salvage therapy, though follow-up has generally been short (Durant et al., 1999). Currently, two types of testing are available, genotypic and phenotypic, each with distinct advantages and disadvantages (Minkoff, 2003).

Phenotypic testing is a measure of the activity of the virus under a particular set of conditions, whereas genotyping provides a molecular biological snapshot of the viral structure. Phenotypic tests compare the ability of the virus to replicate in various concentrations of an antiretroviral drug with its ability to replicate in the absence of the drug (Watts and Minkoff, 2003). As such, these tests are somewhat analogous to bacterial sensitivity tests with which most physicians are familiar. Results are usually expressed as the amount of drug required to inhibit viral production *in vitro* by 50%, although other levels such as 90% or 95% inhibition can be used. Resistance is related to the ability of the virus to overcome treatments aimed at viral activities needed for replication (i.e., reverse transcription and at the protease gene). Accordingly, phenotypic testing uses recombinant assays, in which the reverse transcriptase and protease genes from the patient's plasma HIV are amplified by reverse transcriptase-coupled polymerase chain reaction and inserted into an HIV-1 clone lacking these genes. The recombinant HIV ensures that the envelope and accessory genes are the same in all assays, with only the reverse transcriptase and protease genes varied, thereby minimizing interassay variability and focusing on those aspects of replication that are the targets of antiviral therapy. In general, if the amount of drug required to inhibit viral production by 50% is fourfold or greater for the patient's virus than the control strain, then the patient's strain is considered resistant.

Genotypic testing seeks to detect mutations in the genes that encode reverse transcriptase and protease formation by the virus. These tests establish the nucleotide sequence (ergo the amino acid sequence) of the portion of the viral genome coding for reverse transcriptase and protease. Point mutations in the virus result in the substitution of amino acids in the proteins produced (i.e., reverse transcriptase or protease). The significance of these point mutations is determined by correlating specific mutations with phenotypic resistance as measured by viral susceptibility assays and correlation with clinical response to therapy.

Primary mutations effect the binding of the drug to its target site, thus increasing the amount of drug necessary to inhibit the enzyme activity. However, mutant strains are often less "fit," that is, less able to replicate in the host and to induce immunologic compromise. Other secondary mutations make the mutant virus more pathogenic. Although those secondary changes do not cause an increase in the level of drug necessary to inhibit the enzyme by themselves, they work by improving the ability of the virus with primary mutations to replicate and cause immunologic damage (i.e., they restore fitness).

Certain limitations are present for both genotypic and phenotypic assays. Both types of assays require a plasma HIV RNA level above 1000 copies/mL to allow reverse transcriptase-polymerase chain reaction amplification of the reverse transcriptase and protease genes for further testing. In addition, because most HIV-infected persons have several circulating viral quasi-species, the assays may not detect resistant species that constitute 20% or less of the population. This issue may be especially important for evaluating resistance to drugs that a person took in the past but is no longer receiving because wild-type virus, being more fit, may have overgrown the mutant strain in the interim. It also means that resistance testing is more useful for ruling out, rather than for ruling in, therapies to be used in a given patient. That is because the absence of resistance may merely reflect the reemergence of that wild-type strain. In that circumstance the assays will not detect the minority mutant strain. However, if the patient is re-exposed to the offending agent, the resistant strain may again attain dominance.

Currently, genotypic assays are more widely available commercially than phenotypic assays. Genotypic assays can usually be performed more rapidly, with results available in 1 to 2 weeks, compared with phenotypic assays that still require several weeks for results despite use of recombinant assays. Although all resistance testing is expensive, genotypic assays are usually cheaper than phenotypic testing (Hader et al., 2001). Genetic mutations that confer resistance may be detected before a change in susceptibility is detectable on phenotypic assays. However, the genetic basis for resistance must be understood before the impact of a specific mutation can be predicted. In addition, mutational interactions may make prediction of phenotype (i.e., susceptibility) difficult when multiple mutations are present. Prediction of cross-resistance to other drugs within a class such as protease inhibitors (PIs) can be difficult to predict based only on genotype. In clinical practice most clinicians will rely on algorithms developed by panels of experts or to online databases. Obstetricians should interpret and act on these results in consultation with an expert in the field.

There are several defined circumstances in which clinicians should use these tests. The most common indication for testing is treatment failure. Treatment failure is defined as the failure to attain an undetectable level of virus or the persistent presence of virus after it had become undetectable. If it has been determined that failure has occurred, resistance testing should be performed *before* the failing regimen is discontinued. This is to prevent the overgrowth of wild-type strain that might occur after the regimen is discontinued, such that resistant strains would not be detected even though they would be "lying in wait" for the reinstitution of some components of the regimen. Resistance testing can also be helpful in the setting of an individual who has recently seroconverted. It has been reported that a substantial percentage of new infections are with organisms that are resistant (Hirsch et al., 2000). If testing can be performed before a wild-type virus overgrows the infecting strain, the clinician will have an opportunity to choose an initial regimen that will have a high probability of success against the infecting virus.

It has also been suggested that all HIV-infected pregnant women will benefit from HIV testing, but a few caveats are necessary in that regard. The goal in pregnancy is always to maintain a viral load under 1000 because that would both allow a vaginal delivery and minimize the mother-to-child transmission rate. If a regimen were successful in dropping the load to or below that level, it would be impossible to perform resistance testing in any case. If the regimen is unsuccessful, then resistance testing is warranted regardless of the patent's pregnancy status. That said, there are considerations unique to pregnancy and they relate to the fitness of resistance virus for mother-to-child transmission of HIV, that is, there is an open question as to whether resistant viruses are more or less likely to be transmitted. In general, ZDV and other resistance mutations have not been associated with an increased risk of perinatal transmission. However, in one study detection of ZDV resistance was associated with transmission when adjustment was made for duration of ruptured membranes and total lymphocyte count (Welles et al., 2000). Although perinatal transmission of resistant virus has been reported (Johnson et al., 2001), it appears to be unusual, and it is not clear that the mutant strains are more likely to be transmitted. In a multisite study of HIV-infected pregnant women (Women and Infants Transmission Study), it was reported that when a transmitting mother had a mixed viral population of wild-type and low-level resistant virus, only the wild-type virus was found in the infant, suggesting that virus with low-level ZDV resistance may be less transmissible (Colgrove et al., 1998).

Drug Therapy for Maternal Human Immunodeficiency Virus Disease in Pregnancy

A philosophic cornerstone of care laid early in the AIDS epidemic was that pregnant women should not, *a priori*, be treated differently from other HIV-infected individuals. With nonpregnant individuals, treatment initiation is recommended when the CD4 count falls below 350/mm^3 or when plasma HIV RNA levels exceed 30,000 copies/mL (bDNA assay) or 55,000 copies/mL (reverse transcriptase-polymerase chain reaction assay). When that threshold has been crossed, the standard for treatment of HIV is HAART. In pregnancy the landmarks for starting therapy are reached somewhat earlier in the course of disease. That is because in addition to attempting to optimize maternal health, both the woman and her obstetrician have an additional goal—minimizing rates of mother-to-child transmission of HIV. Those rates are linked to viral

loads, and they start to climb well before viral loads of 55,000 copies are reached. As discussed later, the American College of Obstetricians and Gynecologists (ACOG) currently recommends cesarean delivery for women whose viral loads exceed 1000 copies. For both those reasons there are justifiable reasons to initiate HAART whenever a pregnant woman's viral load is above 1000 copies. Even women whose counts are below 1000 will have lower rates of transmission if they take antiretroviral therapy during gestation, though in that circumstance the advantage of HAART over the simpler PACTG 076 ZDV regimen is less clear. However, even in that circumstance, HAART might lower the likelihood (already relatively low in women with undetectable virus) of development of resistance. A clearer understanding of the relative advantage of HAART over monotherapy in that setting will await trials of HAART versus ZDV.

HAART regimens are those that result in a sustained virologic response. Although a large and expanding number of drug regimens have been shown to achieve that goal, a few general categories of HAART can be described. The first regimens described included dual nucleoside therapy accompanied by a PI. Currently, there are seven nucleoside reverse transcriptase inhibitors (NRTIs), three non-NRTIs (NNRTIs), seven PIs, and one fusion inhibitor approved for therapy, so theoretically a large number of choices within these categories exist. However, certain of these medications should not be used in combination. For example, ZDV and stavudine have overlapping toxicities, dideoxyinosine and dideoxycytidine in combination have diminished efficacy, and dideoxyinosine and stavudine have recently been linked to several fatal cases of mitochondrial toxicity in pregnancy (Bristol-Myers Squibb, 2001).

Choosing an initial regimen is one of the most important decisions a clinician will be called upon to make, bearing in mind that choosing an appropriate second-line regimen is even more difficult than choosing an initial course of therapy. Therefore, the initial choice should reflect an understanding of the fact that adherence to therapy is crucial and should always include a consideration of the possible need to deal with the failure of that regimen.

In regard to the first factor, adherence is the *sine qua non* of successful therapy. Haphazard or intermittent compliance with a drug regimen is a formula for the development of resistant virus. Even very brief drug holidays have been associated with the replacement of wild-strain virus with mutant strains that are resistant to therapeutic agents. Therefore, it is essential that time and effort be expended by providers to educate patients about the need to start treatment only after they are ready to commit to sustained life-long adherence to complex regimens. Providers must also assist patients in developing the tools that will aid them in maintaining successful regimens.

Because of the very real possibility that a time will come when provider and patient will have to confront a failing or poorly tolerated regimen, it is useful for the clinician to choose an initial regimen that "spares" one class of antiretroviral agent. Thus, a regimen should spare PIs or NNRTIs or both. In fact, increasingly popular regimens use three nucleosides alone. When those regimens are used, the patient is assured that if resistance develops, there are classes of drugs available to which the virus has not yet been exposed and to which they are unlikely to have resistance. However, recent evidence suggests that three nucleoside regimens are not as effective.

The public health service maintains a frequently updated website (*www.AIDSinfo.nih.gov*) that is designed to assist providers in staying abreast of the rapidly evolving standards for the care of HIV-infected adults. The panel that authors those guidelines "strongly recommends" HAART regimens that include a PI or an NNRTI in combination with one of several NRTI combinations. The latter approach is supported by a great deal of clinical outcome data (Gulick et al., 1997). Some of the PIs, such as ritonavir, are less often used as first-line therapy because of the difficulty many patients have in tolerating standard doses and because of the drug's many interactions. Other PIs create difficulties because of the large pill burden associated with their use. However, if a patient is first seen in pregnancy already successfully using one of these agents, there is no requirement to switch her off, provided she is tolerating it and the regimen is effective. If a nonpregnant woman who is on HAART is contemplating pregnancy, then a decision must be made as to the appropriateness of maintaining therapy throughout the first trimester. If the patient's clinical and virologic status is not ominous, a decision to discontinue therapy until the second trimester is reasonable. However, all therapy should be stopped at the same time, lest the individual be exposed to a suboptimal regimen that would facilitate the development of resistant virus.

As noted above, a critical factor to remember is that there are often less than ideal responses to antiretroviral regimens that are instituted after virologic failure with another regimen. That fact should sensitize the clinician to the reality that the first regimen affords the best opportunity for long-term control of viral replication. Because the genetic barrier to resistance is greatest with PIs, some experts would consider a PI plus two NRTIs to be the preferred initial regimen. Alternatively, efavirenz (an NNRTI) plus two NRTIs appears to be at least as effective as a PI and two NRTIs in suppressing plasma viremia and increasing $CD4^+$ T-cell counts. Other experts have suggested that such a regimen is the preferred initial regimen because it may spare the toxicities of PIs for a considerable time (Staszewski et al., 1999). However, concerns about teratogenicity that have been demonstrated in animal models and neural tube defects in humans make this a poor choice for use in early pregnancy. Abacavir and two NRTIs, a triple NRTI regimen, has been used with some success as well but may have short-lived efficacy when the baseline viral load is more than 100,000 copies/mL, and recent studies have found this regimen to be less effective. Certain individuals may have a genetic predisposition to a rash associated with abacavir, a rash that can be a harbinger of a fatal reaction (Mallal et al., 2002). In all circumstances, a rash signals the need to immediately discontinue therapy. Dual therapy with NRTIs is less likely to persistently suppress viremia to below detectable levels than HAART regimens and should be used only if more potent treatment is not possible. Use of antiretroviral agents as monotherapy is contraindicated, except when there are no other options or in pregnant women with very low viral loads when it is being used solely to reduce perinatal transmission as noted later.

When women become pregnant, the approach to antiretroviral therapy undergoes subtle modification. Although the goal is still to use a combination of highly active agents to slow progression of disease, the choice of agents and the point of initiation are altered. In regard to agents, the first principle at the moment is to include ZDV as a component of the HAART regimen whenever possible. Although recent evidence suggests that HAART *per se* may be more effective than ZDV, ZDV's benefits have been demonstrated by a wealth of empiric data. The current standard ZDV dosing regimen is 300 mg twice daily. Because the mechanism by which ZDV reduces perinatal transmission is not known, it is theoretically possible that that dosing regimen may not have equivalent efficacy to that observed in PACTG 076 when 100 mg five times daily was used. However, a twice-daily regimen has the advantage of probable enhanced adherence.

The choice of regimen in pregnancy is influenced not only by ZDV's track record but by the safety profile of other agents as well. NRTIs were the first class of drug used for treatment of HIV, and there is a greater experience with their use than with other classes of drug. Almost all that experience has been reassuring (Culnane et al., 1999)—NRTIs have been generally well tolerated and have not been demonstrated to be teratogenic in humans. However, concerns have been raised about potential adverse effects in both mothers and infants related to the avidity of these drugs for mitochondria (Shiramizu et al., 2003). By binding to mitochondrial gamma DNA polymerase and interfering with replication, these drugs can induce mitochondrial dysfunction (Brinkman et al., 1998). Dideoxycytidine demonstrates the greatest inhibition of mitochondrial gamma DNA polymerase, followed in order by dideoxyinosine, stavudine, lamivudine, ZDV, and abacavir. In the mother, clinical disorders associated with mitochondrial toxicity include neuropathy, myopathy, cardiomyopathy, pancreatitis, hepatic steatosis, and lactic acidosis.

Several cases of lactic acidosis, three of which were fatal and two of which were accompanied by pancreatitis, have been reported among pregnant or recently delivered women who had been on dideoxyinosine and stavudine therapy along with a variety of third agents since before conception (Bristol-Myers Squibb, 2001). Two cases of fatal liver failure in pregnant women on ZDV, lamivudine, and nelfinavir have also been reported. These cases developed in late pregnancy, and in several cases the presentation was similar to that seen with acute fatty liver of pregnancy, a condition that itself has been linked to mitochondrial fatty oxidation disorders in the fetus (homozygotic) and mother (heterozygotic) (Ibday et al., 2000). This has led to speculation that the metabolic changes of late pregnancy may enhance susceptibility to complications of nucleoside agents, especially those with greater inhibition of mitochondrial gamma DNA polymerase. Although these serious morbidities appear to be rare, providers caring for HIV-infected women receiving nucleoside analogue agents should be aware of the risk and monitor accordingly. One approach would be to monitor hepatic enzyme levels during the last trimester and to aggressively investigate all new symptoms. Women with substantial elevations in transaminase levels above baseline or other new abnormalities, in the absence of other explanations, such as preeclampsia, for the abnormalities, should have their nucleoside agents discontinued, either with substitution of agents from another class of antiretrovirals or discontinuation of all antiretrovirals. In view of the reports of maternal deaths and toxicity associated with prolonged use of stavudine and dideoxyinosine in pregnancy, this combination should be used in pregnancy with caution and only if other nucleoside agents cannot be used because of resistance or toxicity.

Mitochondrial toxicity may also pose a risk to neonates. A French group reported eight cases of HIV-uninfected infants with abnormalities potentially related to mitochondrial dysfunction that developed after prophylactic nucleoside therapy (both antenatal and neonatal) among 1754 exposed fetuses (Blanche et al., 1999). Two infants had progressive neurologic symptoms and died several months after completing *in utero* and neonatal courses of ZDV–lamivudine. Three other infants had mild to moderate symptoms, and three had asymptomatic laboratory abnormalities. Although mitochondrial abnormalities were not proven to be the cause of the abnormalities, investigators from several large U.S. cohort studies responded to these data by reviewing all 353 deaths among more than 20,000 children born to HIV-infected women. They found no deaths similar to those in the French cohort, although only 6% of the children had been exposed to the combination of ZDV–lamivudine (Perinatal Safety Review Working Group, 2000). Review of data on living children from these cohorts for diagnoses or conditions suggestive of mitochondrial dysfunction is ongoing.

Other concerns that have been raised in regard to NRTIs. These have included preterm births, mutagenesis, and febrile seizures. A putative association with prematurity was raised by a small European study (European Collaborative Study and The Swiss Mother+Child HIV Cohort Study, 2000). Larger American studies have not yielded similar findings. In the largest assessment of the risks of medications to date, Tuomala and colleagues (2002) reported on 2123 HIV-infected women enrolled in seven clinical studies who received antiretroviral therapy. The data was generally quite reassuring. Those on no therapy and those on therapy had similar rates of low Apgar scores, premature births, and low-birth-weight infants. After adjustment for multiple risk factors, combination antiretroviral therapy was not associated with an increased risk of premature or low-birth-weight delivery as compared with monotherapy. Seven women (5%) whose combination regimen included a PI had a very-low-birth-weight infant (less than 1500 g) compared with nine (2%) women whose combination did not include a protease. Although those differences were statistically significant, the numbers in both groups were quite small.

Concerns about potential mutagenicity arose on the basis of studies conducted on small animal models at the National Cancer Institute. Those studies suggested that mice exposed to high doses of ZDV *in utero* had both high rates of malignancies of the skin, lung, liver, and genital tract and a higher number of tumors among those with malignancies (Olivero et al., 1997). These findings occurred in the same mouse model that had demonstrated transplacental carcinogenicity with diethylstilbestrol. Based on these findings the NIH convened a blue ribbon panel to review the findings. That panel concluded that even if the adverse outcomes seen in the animals did signal a risk from *in utero* exposure, the demonstrated benefits of the medication was such that the routine use of the PACTG 076 protocol should continue. Finally, in regard to nucleosides, the French collaborative study recently reported on first febrile seizures among 4426 HIV-uninfected children and found a significantly increased risk for those infants who had been perinatally exposed to nucleoside therapy compared with unexposed (P = .0198) (French Perinatal Cohort Study, 2002).

Finally, as previously noted, when an NNRTI is chosen to be a component of a woman's HAART regimen, if she is pregnant, efavirenz should not be used in the first trimester. There have been reported teratogenic effects in monkey models and

reports of myelomeningoceles in humans (Fundarao et al., 2002). Among the proteases, indinavir may predispose to nephrolithiasis and hyperbilirubinemia, although evidence of harm to neonates has not been forthcoming. Proteases in general have been linked to abnormal glucose metabolism, but problems particular to pregnancy in this regard have not been noted. Despite these concerns, pregnant women in the United States tend to receive HAART therapy as often as other women with similar immunologic status (Minkoff et al., 2001). All pregnant women on antiretroviral therapy should have regular monitoring of liver functions and blood counts to detect toxicity as early as possible.

Obstetric Interventions

On the basis of the data summarized previously, regarding the protective role of cesarean delivery, ACOG published a committee opinion in August 1999 that concluded that HIV-infected women should be offered scheduled cesarean delivery to reduce the rate of transmission beyond that which could be achieved with ZDV alone (ACOG Committee on Obstetric Practice, 1999). That report also noted that data were insufficient to demonstrate a benefit for women with viral loads less than 1000 copies/mL of plasma, because the rate of transmission below that level was extremely low independent of the mode of delivery. They suggested that scheduled cesarean deliveries should be performed at 38 weeks of gestation to minimize the risk of labor and/or ruptured membranes before the procedure. They went on to counsel against amniocentesis to avoid contamination of the amniotic cavity with viral antigen from maternal blood.

Although ACOG believed there was no proven benefit of cesarean delivery with low viral loads (less than 1000 copies/mL), some data do exist that speak to risks in that particular subgroup. Although not as compelling as other data cited previously, there is some evidence that cesarean delivery could be beneficial even in the setting of viral loads under 1000 copies (Ioannidis et al., 2001). Those data come from a meta-analysis of studies that focused exclusively on women who had viral loads less than 1000 copies. Among those women, antiretroviral therapy still played a major role in reducing transmission, dropping rates from approximately 10% to approximately 1%. Although cesarean delivery apparently dropped the rate from 6% to 1.5%, there was no control in that analysis for the use of antiretroviral therapy. However, among those women who underwent elective cesarean deliveries and received antiretroviral therapy (n = 270), there were no cases of mother-to-child transmission of HIV compared with a 1.8% transmission rate among women who received therapy and had a vaginal delivery (n = 396).

Although there are circumstances in which the role of cesarean delivery is clear, there are other clinical situations in which its role has not been as clearly delineated (Minkoff, 2003). For example, if a patient who had been scheduled for cesarean delivery ruptures her membranes before delivery, the physician must balance the potential benefit of shortening the period between rupture and delivery against the risks of surgery. The longer the time since the membranes ruptured, the greater the percentage of eventual transmissions that will have occurred before a surgical procedure can be undertaken. However, if the interval has been relatively short and the viral load is high, there is still probably sufficient benefit to justify the increased morbidity. Another difficult clinical situation involves the woman with preterm premature rupture of membranes remote from term. In that circumstance the balance that must be struck is between the risks to the neonate from extreme prematurity and the risk from acquisition of HIV while the mother is managed expectantly. Although the former risks can be roughly quantified by reviewing institutional data related to prematurity, there is less empiric data on which to base estimates of the risk of acquisition of HIV in the setting of prolonged ruptured membranes and HAART. Obviously, the closer the patient is to term the greater the advantage to rapid delivery.

Operative Morbidity

In the European randomized trial of cesarean delivery, there were few postpartum complications and no serious morbidity was noted in either the cesarean or the vaginal delivery group (International Perinatal HIV Group, 1999). However, several other authors who assessed the morbidity of a cesarean delivery noted increased risk both by mode of delivery and by HIV serostatus. A French study found that, as with HIV-uninfected individuals, operative deliveries were associated with more morbidity than vaginal deliveries (Marcollet et al., 2002). In a multivariate analysis that adjusted for CD4 count, the relative risk of any complication increased by 1.85 (1.00 to 3.39) after elective cesarean delivery and by 4.17 (2.37 to 7.49) after emergency cesarean delivery compared with vaginal delivery.

In assessing the impact of HIV serostatus, Grubert and colleagues (2002) found marked differences between HIV-infected and -uninfected women in a report on postoperative complications among 235 HIV-infected women who underwent obstetric and gynecologic procedures and HIV-uninfected age-matched women undergoing the same procedures. They reported significantly higher postoperative complication rates after abdominal surgery (odds ratio, 3.6, P = .001) and noted that the risk of complications was associated with immune status. An American case-control study focused more narrowly on women undergoing cesarean delivery and reported that HIV-infected women were significantly more likely to have minor postoperative complications (Rodriquez et al., 2001). They found no significant difference in major morbidities, but their power to detect differences was somewhat attenuated. These reports support ACOG, whose recommendations for performing elective cesarean delivery included the suggestion that prophylactic antibiotics be used because of concerns of heightened risks of postoperative infectious morbidity.

Although the data supporting a heightened risk for postoperative morbidity among HIV-infected women undergoing elective surgery is not robust, the evidence that all women undergoing an operative delivery face a greater risk of infectious morbidity is overwhelming. The liberal use of antibiotics in the setting of cesarean delivery and HIV infection as suggested by ACOG guidelines would therefore seem reasonable.

CONCLUSION

The ability of powerful new drug regimens and improved obstetric care to dramatically alter the natural history of HIV infection in women and to markedly reduce rates of mother-to-child transmission of HIV has been clearly and irrefutably demonstrated. Indeed, and unfortunately, the ongoing contrast in outcomes between infected women in developed and in developing parts of the world provides an ongoing coda to the published proof of efficacy. Although the details of the management that has wrought these remarkable advances are complex and will undoubtedly become more so as new agents reach the market, the general approach to care remains eloquently simple. Obstetricians must identify all HIV-infected women as early in pregnancy as possible and reduce the fetus's and neonate's exposure to HIV to the greatest degree possible through a combination of powerful antiretroviral agents and appropriate use of cesarean delivery. With the input of consultants with expertise in the interactions and risks of various agents, the benefits of 21st century care can be purchased with the lowest possible cost in maternal and infant morbidity.

REFERENCES

ACOG Committee on Obstetric Practice: Scheduled Cesarean Delivery and the Prevention of Vertical Transmission of HIV Infection. Committee Opinion. Washington, DC, American College of Obstetricians and Gynecologists, 1999.

Alliegro MB, Dorrucci M, Phillips AN, et al: Incidence and consequences of pregnancy in women with known duration of HIV infection. Italian Seroconversion Study Group. Arch Intern Med **157**:2585, 1997.

Amstey MS, Monif GR: Genital herpes virus infection in pregnancy. Obstet Gynecol **44**:394, 1974.

Berrebi A, Kobuch WE, Puel J, et al: Influence of pregnancy on human immunodeficiency virus disease. Eur J Obstet Gynecol Reprod Biol **37**:211, 1990.

Bessinger R, Clark R, Kissinger P, et al: Pregnancy is not associated with the progression of HIV disease in women attending an HIV outpatient program. Am J Epidemiol **147**:434, 1998.

Biggar RJ, Pahava S, Minkoff HL, et al: Immunosuppression in pregnant women infected with human immunodeficiency virus. Am J Obstet Gynecol **161**:1239, 1989.

Blanche S, Mayaux MJ, Rouzioux C, et al: Relation of the course of HIV infection in children to the severity of the disease in their mothers at delivery. N Engl J Med **330**:308, 1994.

Blanche S, Tardieu M, Duliege A-M, et al: Longitudinal study of 94 symptomatic infants with perinatally acquired human immunodeficiency virus infection: Evidence for a bimodal expression of clinical and biological symptoms. Am J Dis Child **144**:1210, 1990.

Blanche S, Tardieu M, Rustin P, et al: Persistent mitochondrial dysfunction and perinatal exposure to antiretroviral nucleoside analogues. Lancet **354**:1084, 1999.

Brinkman K, Ter Hofstede HJM, Burger DM, et al: Adverse effects of reverse transcriptase inhibitors: Mitochondrial toxicity as common pathway. AIDS **12**:1735, 1998.

Bristol-Myers Squibb. Dear Health Care Provider letter. January 5, 2001. Available at *www.fda.gov/medwatch/safety/2001/zerit&videx_letter.htm*.

Burns DN, Fitzgerald G, Semba R, et al: Vitamin A deficiency and other nutritional indices during pregnancy in human immunodeficiency virus infection: Prevalence, clinical correlates, and outcome. Women and Infants Transmission Study Group. Clin Infect Dis **29**:328, 1999.

Burns DN, Landesman S, Muenz LR, et al: Cigarette smoking, premature rupture of membranes and vertical transmission of HIV-1 among women with low CD4+ levels. J Acquir Immune Defic Syndr **7**:718, 1994.

Centers for Disease Control: Follow-up on Kaposi's sarcoma and *Pneumocystis* pneumonia. MMWR Morb Mortal Wkly Rep **30**:409, 1981.

Centers for Disease Control: AIDS in women—United States. MMWR Morb Mortal Wkly Rep **39**:845, 1990.

Centers for Disease Control and Prevention: 1993 Revised classification system for HIV infection and expanded surveillance case definition for AIDS among adolescents and adults. MMWR Morb Mortal Wkly Rep **41**:1, 1992.

Centers for Disease Control and Prevention: HIV/AIDS Surveillance Report, vol 11. Atlanta, Ga: U.S. Dept. of Health and Human Services, Public Health Service, Centers for Disease Control and Prevention, 1999.

Centers for Disease Control and Prevention: Mortality L285 slide series (through 1998). Available at *www.cdc.gov/hiv/graphics/mortalit.htm*. Accessibility verified February 6, 2001.

Centers for Disease Control and Prevention: Sexually transmitted diseases treatment guidelines 2002. MMWR Morb Mortal Wkly Rep **51**:1, 2002.

Chamiso D: Pregnancy outcomes in HIV-1 positive women in Ghandi Memorial Hospital Addis Ababa Ethiopia. East Afr Med J **73**:805, 1996.

Clarke SM, Mulcahy F, Healy CM, et al: The efficacy and tolerability of combination antiretroviral therapy in pregnancy: Infant and maternal outcome. Int J STD AIDS **11**:220, 2000.

Colgrove RC, Pitt J, Chung PH, et al: Selective vertical transmission of HIV-1 antiretroviral resistance mutations. AIDS **12**:2281, 1998.

Cooper ER, Chaurat M, Mofenson L, et al: Combination antiretroviral strategies for the treatment of pregnant HIV-1 infected women and prevention of perinatal HIV-1 transmission. J AIDS **29**:484, 2002.

Culnane M, Fowler M, Lee SS, et al: Lack of long-term effects of in utero exposure to zidovudine among uninfected children born to HIV-infected women. Pediatric AIDS Clinical Trials Group Protocol 219/076 Teams. JAMA **281**:151, 1999.

Dickover RE, Garratty EM, Herman SA, et al: Identification of levels of maternal HIV-1 RNA associated with risk of perinatal transmission: Effect of maternal zidovudine treatment on viral load. JAMA **275**:599, 1996.

Duliege A-M, Amos CI, Felton S, et al: Birth order, delivery route, and concordance in the transmission of human immunodeficiency virus type 1 from mothers to twins. J Peditar **126**:625, 1995.

Durant J, Clevenbergh P, Halfon P, et al: Drug-resistance in HIV-1 therapy: The VIRADAPT randomized control trial. Lancet **353**:2195, 1999.

European Collaborative Study: Children born to women with HIV-1 infection: Natural history and risk of transmission. Lancet **337**:253, 1991.

European Collaborative Study: Risk factors for mother-to-child transmission of HIV-1. Lancet **339**:1007, 1992.

European Collaborative Study and the Swiss Mother+Child HIV Cohort Study. Combination antiretroviral therapy and duration of pregnancy. AIDS **14**:2913, 2000.

European Mode of Delivery Collaboration: Elective cesarean section versus vaginal delivery in prevention of vertical HIV-1 transmission: A randomized clinical trial. Lancet **353**:1035, 1999.

Farmer P: The major infectious diseases in the world—To treat or not to treat? N Engl J Med **345**:208, 2001.

Fauci AS, Lane HC: Human immunodeficiency virus (HIV) disease: AIDS and related disorders. *In* Brunwald E, Fauci As, Isselbecher KJ, et al (eds): Harrison's Textbook of Medicine. New York, McGraw-Hill, 2001.

Fleming D, McQuillan G, Johnson R, et al: Herpes simplex virus type 2 in the United States, 1976 to 1994. N Engl J Med **337**:1105, 1997.

French Perinatal Cohort Study: Risk of early febrile seizures with perinatal exposure to nucleoside analogues. Lancet **359**:583, 2002.

French R, Brocklehurst P: The effect of pregnancy on survival in women infected with HIV: A systemic review of the literature and meta-analysis. Br J Obstet Gynaecol **105**:827, 1998.

Fundarao C, Genovese O, Rendeli C, et al: Myelomeningocele in a child with intrauterine exposure to efavirnez. AIDS **16**:299, 2002.

Gibb DM, Goodall RL, Dunn DT, et al: Mother-to-child transmission of hepatitis C virus: Evidence for preventable peripartum transmission. Lancet **356**:904, 2000.

Goedert JJ, Kessler CM, Aledort LM, et al: A prospective study of human immunodeficiency virus type 1 infection and the development of AIDS in subjects with hemophilia. N Engl J Med **321**:1141, 1989.

Grubert TA, Reindelle D, Kastner R, et al: Rates of postoperative complications among human immunodeficiency virus-infected women who have undergone obstetric and gynecologic surgical procedures. Clin Infect Dis **34**:822, 2002.

Gulick RM, Mellors JW, Havlir D, et al: Treatment with indinavir, zidovudine, and lamivudine in adults with human immunodeficiency virus infection and prior antiretroviral therapy. N Engl J Med **337**:734, 1997.

Hader SL, Smith DK, Moore JS, et al: HIV infection in women in the United States: Status at the Millennium. JAMA **285**:1186, 2001.

Hessol NA, Lifson AR, O'Malley PM, et al: Prevalence, incidence, and progression of human immunodeficiency virus infection in homosexual and bisexual men in hepatitis B vaccine trials, 1978–1988. Am J Epidemiol **130**:1167, 1989.

Hirsch MS, Brun-Vezinet F, D'Auila RT, et al: Antiretroviral drug resistance testing in adult HIV-1 infection: Recommendations of an international AIDS Society-USA Panel JAMA **283**:2417, 2000.

Ho DD, Neumann AU, Perelson AS, et al: Rapid turnover of plasma virons and CD4 lymphocytes in HIV-1 infection. Nature **373**:123, 1995.

Hocke C, Morlat P, Chene G, et al: Prospective cohort study of the effect of pregnancy on the progression of human immunodeficiency virus infection. Obstet Gynecol **86**:886, 1995.

Holman S, Sunderland A, Berthaud M, et al: Prenatal HIV counseling and testing. Clin Obstet Gynecol **32**:445, 1989.

Ibday JA, Yang Z, Bennett MJ: Liver disease in pregnancy and fetal fatty acid oxidation defects. Mol Genet Metab **71**:182, 2000.

Institute of Medicine National Research Council: Reducing the Odds: Preventing Perinatal Transmission of HIV in the United States. Washington, DC, National Academy Press, 1999.

Ioannidis JPA, Abrams EJ, Ammann A, et al: Perinatal transmission of human immunodeficiency virus type 1 by pregnant women with RNA virus loads <1000 copies/ml. J Infect Dis **183**:539, 2001.

Jensen LP, O'Sullivan MJ, Gomez-del-rio M, et al: Acquired immune deficiency syndrome in pregnancy. Am J Obstet Gynecol **148**:1145, 1984.

Johnson VA, Woods C, Hamilton CD, et al: Vertical transmission of multidrug-resistant human immunodeficiency virus type 1 (HIV-1) and continued evolution of drug resistance in an HIV-1-infected infant. J Infect Dis **183**:1688, 2001.

International Perinatal HIV Group: The mode of delivery and the risk of vertical transmission of human immunodeficiency virus type 1—A meta-analysis of 15 prospective cohort studies. N Engl J Med **340**:977, 1999.

Kind C, Rudin C, Siegrisi CA, et al: Prevention of vertical HIV transmission: additive protective effect of elective cesarean section and zidovudine prophylaxis. AIDS **12**:205, 1998.

Kumar RM, Uduman SA, Khurrana AK: Impact of pregnancy on maternal AIDS. J Reprod Med **42**:429, 1997.

Landesman SH, Kalish LA, Burns DN, et al: Obstetrical factors and the transmission of human immunodeficiency virus type 1 from mother to child. N Engl J Med **334**:1617, 1996.

LaRussa P, Magder LS, Pitt J, et al: Association of HIV-1 viral phenotype in the MT-2 assay with perinatal HIV transmission. J AIDS **30**:88, 2002.

Lee SD, Lo KJ, Tsai YT, et al: Role of caesarean section in prevention of mother-infant transmission of hepatitis B virus. Lancet **2**:833, 1988.

Lemp GF, Payne SF, Rutherford GW, et al: Projections of AIDS morbidity and mortality in San Francisco. JAMA **263**:1497, 1990.

Leroy V, Ladner J, Nyiraziraje M, et al: Effect of HIV-q1 infection on pregnancy outcome in women in Kigali, Rwanda 1992–1994. Pregnancy and HIV study group. AIDS **12**:643, 1998.

Levy JA: Infection by human immunodeficiency virus: CD4 is not enough. N Engl J Med **335**:1528, 1996.

Lifson AR, Rutherford GW, Jaffe HW: The natural history of human immunodeficiency virus infection. J Infect Dis **158**:1360, 1988.

Liu R, Paxton WA, Choe S, et al: Homozygous defect in HIV-1 coreceptor accounts for resistance for some multiply-exposed individuals to HIV-1 infection. Cell **86**:367, 1996.

Lorenzi P, Spicher VM, Laubereau B, et al: Antiretroviral therapies in pregnancy: Maternal, fetal and neonatal effects. Swiss HIV Cohort Study, the Swiss Collaborative HIV and Pregnancy Study, and the Swiss Neonatal HIV Study. AIDS **12**:241, 1998.

Luzuriaga K, McQuilken P, Alimenti A, et al: Early viremia and immune responses in vertical human immunodeficiency virus type 1 infection. J Infect Dis **167**:1008, 1993.

MacCallum LR, France AJ, Jones ME, et al: The effects of pregnancy on the progression of HIV disease. Abstract No. 4041. Abstract presented at the Fourth International Conference on AIDS, 1988, Stockholm.

Mallal S, Nolan D, Witt C, et al: Association between presence of HLA-B*5701, HLA-DR7, and HLA-DQ3 and hypersensitivity to HIV-1 reverse-transcriptase inhibitor abacavir. Lancet **359**:727, 2002.

Mandelbrot L, Le Chenadec J, Berrebi A, et al: Perinatal HIV-1 transmission: Interaction between zidovudine prophylaxis and mode of delivery in the French Perinatal Cohort. JAMA **280**:55, 1998.

Marcollet A, Goffinet F, Firtion G, et al: Differences in postpartum morbidity in women who are infected with human immunodeficiency virus after elective cesarean delivery, emergency cesarean delivery or vaginal delivery. Am J Obstet Gynecol **186**:784, 2002.

Maury W, Potts BJ, Rabson AB: HIV-1 infection of the first-trimester and term human placental tissue: A possible mode of maternal-fetal transmission. J Infect Dis **160**:583, 1989.

McGowan JP, Crane M, Wiznia AA, et al: Combination antiretroviral therapy in human immunodeficiency virus-infected pregnant women. Obstet Gynecol **94**:641, 1999.

McIntosh K, Pitt J, Brambilla D, et al: Blood culture in the first 6 months of life for the diagnosis of vertically transmitted human immunodeficiency virus infection. J Infect Dis **170**:996, 1994.

Minkoff H: HIV infections in pregnancy. Obstet Gynecol **101**:797, 2003.

Minkoff H, Ahdieh L, Watts DH, et al: The relationship of pregnancy to the use of highly active antiretroviral therapy. Am J Obstet Gynecol **184**:1221, 2001.

Minkoff H, Burns DN, Landesman S, et al: The relationship of the duration of ruptured membranes to vertical transmission of human immunodeficiency virus. Am J Obstet Gynecol **173**:585, 1995.

Minkoff H, DeRegt RH, Landesman S, et al: *Pneumocystis carinii* pneumonia associated with acquired immunodeficiency syndrome in pregnancy: A report of three maternal deaths. Obstet Gynecol **67**:284, 1986.

Minkoff H, Henderson C, Mendez H, et al: Pregnancy outcomes among mothers infected with HIV and uninfected control subjects. Am J Obstet Gynecol **163**:1598, 1990.

Minkoff H, Hershow R, Watts H, et al: The relationship of pregnancy to HIV disease progression. Am J Obstet Gynecol. In press.

Minkoff H, Nanda D, Menez R, et al: Pregnancies resulting in infants with acquired immunodeficiency syndrome or AIDS related complex. Obstet Gynecol **69**:285, 1987.

Mofenson LM, Lambert JS, Stiehm ER, et al: Risk factors for perinatal transmission of human immunodeficiency virus type 1 in women treated with zidovudine. N Engl J Med **341**:385, 1999.

Morris AB, Cu-Uvin S, Harwell JI, et al: Multicenter review of protease inhibitors in 89 pregnancies. J Acquir Immune Defic Syndr **25**:306, 2000.

Neal JJ, Fleming PL, Green TA, et al: Trends in heterosexually acquired AIDS in the United States 1988–1995. J Acquir Immune Defic Syndr **14**:465, 1997.

Olivero OA, Anderson LM, Diwan BA, et al: Transplacental effects of 3′-azido-2′3′-dideoxythymidine (AZT): Tumorigenicity in mice and genotoxicity in mice and monkeys. J Natl Cancer Inst **89**:1602, 1997.

Perinatal Safety Review Working Group: Nucleoside exposure in the children of HIV-infected women receiving antiretroviral drugs: Absence of clear evidence for mitochondrial disease in children who died before 5 years of age in five United States cohorts. J Acquir Immune Defic Syndr **25**:261, 2000.

Rodriquez EJ, Spann C, Jamieson D, et al: Postoperative morbidity associated with cesarean delivery among human immunodeficiency virus-seropositive women. Am J Obstet Gynecol **184**:1108, 2001.

Rodriguez EM, Mofenson LM, Chang B-H, et al: Association of maternal drug use during pregnancy with maternal HIV culture positivity and perinatal HIV transmission. AIDS **10**:273, 1996.

Saada M, Le Chenedec J, Berrebi A, et al: Pregnancy and progression to AIDS: Results of the French prospective cohorts. SEROGEST and SEROCO study groups. AIDS **14**:2355, 2000.

Schaefer A, Grosch-Woerner Friedman I, et al: The effect of pregnancy on the natural course of HIV disease. Abstract No. 4039. Abstract presented at the Fourth International Conference on AIDS, 1988, Stockholm.

Semba RD, Miotti PG, Chiphangwi JD, et al: Maternal vitamin A deficiency and mother-to-child transmission of HIV-1. Lancet **343**:1593, 1994.

Shah K, Kashima H, Polk BF, et al: Rarity of cesarean delivery in cases of juvenile-onset respiratory papillomatosis. Obstet Gynecol **68**:795, 1986.

Shiramizu B, Shikuma KM, Kamemoto L, et al: Brief report: Placenta and cord blood mitochondria DNA toxicity in HIV-infected women receiving nucleoside reverse transcriptase inhibitors in pregnancy. J Acquir Immune Defic Syndr **32**:370, 2003.

Sperling RS, Shapiro DE, Coombs RW, et al: Maternal viral load, zidovudine treatment, and the risk of transmission of human immunodeficiency virus type 1 from mother to infant. N Engl J Med **335**:1621, 1996.

Staszewski S, Morales-Ramirez J, Tashima KT, et al: Efavirenz plus zidovudine and lamivudine, efavirenz plus indinavir, and indinavir plus zidovudine and lamivudine in the treatment of HIV-1 infection in adults. N Engl J Med **341**:1865, 1999.

Sutton MY, Sternberg M, Nsuami M, et al: Trichomoniasis in pregnant human immunodeficiency virus-infected and human immunodeficiency virus-uninfected women: Prevalence, risk factors, and association with low birth weight. Am J Obstet Gynecol **181**:656, 1999.

Temmerman M, Nyong'o A, Bwayo J, et al: Risk factors for mother-to-child transmission of human immunodeficiency virus-1 infection. Am J Obstet Gynecol **172**:700, 1995.

Thea DM, Steketee RW, Pliner V, et al: The effect of maternal viral load on the risk of perinatal transmission of HIV-1. AIDS **11**:437, 1997.

Tuomala RE, Shapiro DE, Mofenson LM, et al: Antiretroviral therapy in pregnancy and the risk of an adverse outcome. N Engl J Med **346**:1863, 2002.

Wabwire-Mangen F, Gray RH, Mmiro FA, et al: Placental membrane inflammation and risks of maternal-to-child transmission of HIV-1 in Uganda. J Acquir Immune Defic Syndr **22**:379, 1999.

Wade N, Birkhead GS, Warren BL, et al: Abbreviated regimens of zidovudine prophylaxis and perinatal transmission of human immunodeficiency virus. N Engl J Med **339**:1409, 1998.

Watts H, Minkoff H: Managing pregnant patients. *In* Dolin R, Masur H, Saag M (ed): AIDS Therapy, 2nd ed. New York, Churchill Livingstone. In press.

Weisser M, Rudin C, Battegay M, et al: Does pregnancy influence the course of HIV infection? Evidence from two large Swiss cohort studies. J Acquir Immune Defic Syndr Hum Retrovirol **17**:404, 1998.

Welles SL, Pitt J, Colgrove R, et al: HIV-1 genotypic zidovudine drug resistance and the risk of maternal-infant transmission in the Women and Infants Transmission Study Group. AIDS **14**:263, 2000.

Wetli CV, Roldan EO, Fujaco RM: Listeriosis as a cause of maternal death: An obstetric complication of acquired immune deficiency syndrome. Am J Obstet Gynecol **147**:7, 1983.

Chapter 41

CARDIAC DISEASES

Daniel G. Blanchard, MD, FACC, and Ralph Shabetai, MD

DIAGNOSIS OF HEART DISEASE IN PREGNANCY

Pregnant women with heart disease are at higher risk for cardiovascular complications during pregnancy and also have a higher incidence of neonatal complications (Siu et al., 2002). The significant hemodynamic changes that accompany pregnancy, however, make the diagnosis of certain forms of cardiovascular disease difficult. During normal pregnancies, women frequently experience dyspnea, orthopnea, easy fatigability, dizzy spells, and, occasionally, even syncope. On physical examination, dependent edema, rales in the lower lung fields, visible neck veins, and cardiomegaly are commonly found. Systolic murmurs occur in more than 95% of pregnant women, and internal mammary flow murmurs and venous hums are common. Certain findings, however, indicate heart disease in pregnancy and should suggest the presence of a significant cardiovascular abnormality. The symptoms include severe dyspnea, syncope with exertion, hemoptysis, paroxysmal nocturnal dyspnea, and chest pain related to exertion. Physical signs of organic heart disease include cyanosis, clubbing, diastolic murmurs, sustained cardiac arrhythmias, and loud harsh systolic murmurs.

If there is a strong suspicion of heart disease during pregnancy, confirmatory diagnostic tests should be initiated. The changes of normal pregnancy must be recognized so that the findings are not misinterpreted. For example, nonspecific ST segment and T-wave abnormalities and shifts in the electrical axis can occur (Oram and Holt, 1961; Boyle and Lloyd-Jones, 1966; Schwartz and Schamroth, 1979). Pregnancy also produces changes in the echocardiogram, including alterations in cardiac dimensions and performance. The internal dimensions of all the cardiac chambers are increased, and slight regurgitation through the four valves is frequently observed. The ejection fraction and stroke volume are concomitantly larger, and the cardiac output is increased (Rubler et al., 1977). A small pericardial effusion can be a normal finding in pregnant women (Haiat and Halphen, 1984). Both radiographic and radionuclide diagnostic procedures should be avoided during pregnancy unless the procedure is deemed essential for the health and safety of the mother.

PRECONCEPTION COUNSELING

If a woman plans to become pregnant but knows that she has heart disease, she and her physicians must be fully aware of several fundamental principles. The cardiovascular system undergoes specific adaptations to meet the increased demands of the mother and fetus during pregnancy. The most important of these are increases in blood volume, cardiac output, and heart rate. These adaptations exacerbate the symptoms and clinical signs of heart disease and may necessitate significant escalation in treatment.

Cardiac risk varies among specific forms of heart disease and with its severity. During prepregnancy counseling, the physician should describe the nature of the heart disease in terms comprehensible to prospective parents. The risk to the woman, which may vary from negligible to prohibitive, should be spelled out as clearly as possible. On this basis, the patient may be advised that the contemplated pregnancy is safe, will be uncomfortable and will necessitate treatment, carries a significantly increased risk, or would be extremely dangerous and should not be undertaken.

In the case of a cardiac condition that can be completely or virtually cured, the patient should be strongly advised to undergo the necessary treatment before pregnancy and allow several months to elapse before becoming pregnant. Examples in this category include the following:

- The secundum type of atrial septal defect (ASD)
- Patent ductus arteriosus (PDA)
- Some cases of coarctation of the aorta

In other cases, the heart condition can be ameliorated but not cured. Examples include the following:

- Mitral stenosis and regurgitation
- Aortic stenosis
- Tetralogy of Fallot
- Ventricular septal defect (VSD) with mild or moderate pulmonary hypertension
- Pulmonary stenosis
- Various congenital malformations and acquired heart diseases

Again, it is imperative that the palliative procedure be carried out *before* pregnancy is undertaken and that a year or so elapse before pregnancy occurs. Flexibility in clinical judgment, however, is necessary. A woman with moderately severe valvular disease may require a prosthetic valve in the future. In such a case, the patient should be advised to have her family before valve replacement—with its associated anticoagulant risk—is required (Born et al., 1992) (see Pregnancy in Patients with Artifical Heart Valves, later).

As previously noted, some cardiac disorders are so serious in nature that the physiologic changes of a superimposed pregnancy pose prohibitive risks to the mother and carry such a high maternal mortality risk that pregnancy is contraindicated. In such circumstances, patients must be strongly cautioned against becoming pregnant. If such a patient is seen for the first time when she is already pregnant, termination of the pregnancy is recommended. The most serious of the cardiac disorders are those involving pulmonary hypertension, particularly associated with a right-to-left shunt in cardiac blood flow (*Eisenmenger syndrome*). Low cardiac output states and entities in which there is an increased risk of aortic dissection (*Marfan syndrome*) also represent an extraordinarily high risk of maternal mortality. These high-risk maternal cardiovascular disorders are listed in Table 41-1.

In some women with specific dangerous cardiovascular diseases, pregnancy is contraindicated because of the substantial risk of maternal death. Examples include the following:

- Dilated cardiomyopathy
- Primary pulmonary hypertension
- Eisenmenger syndrome
- Marfan syndrome with aortic root dilation

If the patient with one of these disorders presents when she is already pregnant, she should be strongly urged to consider termination. A carefully planned suction curettage before 13 weeks' gestation would place such a patient at minimal risk. Termination of pregnancy beyond this stage increases the risk to the mother, because many of the cardiovascular alterations occurring in pregnancy have taken place. The use of prostaglandins E_2 and $F_{2\alpha}$ and their analogues is successful in evacuating the uterus during the second trimester, but all these agents have significant cardiovascular side effects and should be used with caution. In experienced hands, and with knowledgeable anesthetic consultation, dilation and evacuation performed up to 22 weeks' gestation may be an appropriate alternative.

Infective endocarditis often causes rapid and serious deterioration of the cardiac status, posing a major threat to the life and health of the mother and, therefore, of the fetus as well. Scrupulous attention to prophylaxis against endocarditis is critical during pregnancy. Pregnant women must pay meticulous attention to their dental health; if they have cardiac lesions susceptible to infective endocarditis, neglect of antibacterial prophylaxis may have dire consequences.

The prospective parents will want to know not only about the risk to the health and life of the future mother but also about the fetal risks. One of the most important questions is whether the mother's heart disease is hereditary and, if so, what is the risk that the infant will be born with the same defect. A detailed family cardiac history must be obtained before pregnancy, especially if the prospective mother has heart disease.

Some of the cardiomyopathies, especially hypertrophic, may be inherited in a mendelian manner (Bjarnason et al., 1982). Familial dilated cardiomyopathy has also been described (Mestroni et al., 1990). Approximately 20% of idiopathic dilated cardiomyopathy is inherited (McMinn and Ross, 1995). The genetic basis is currently the subject of intense investigation. Patients with this disorder should be made aware of this fairly recent development.

There is a strong familial tendency in certain congenital malformations, such as PDA (Burman, 1961) and ASD (Johansson and Sievers, 1967). Additionally, mothers with congenital heart disease may have children with unrelated congenital malformations (Corone et al., 1983). Also, pregnant women with advanced heart disease, especially those with low cardiac output or severe hypoxia, experience a greatly increased incidence of spontaneous abortion, stillbirths, and small or deformed children (Cannell and Vernon, 1963).

Today's prospective mother wants to know about the risks to her fetus of drugs that must be given to treat heart disease and that other treatments, such as electrical cardioversion, are safe. Echocardiography poses no threat to the fetus, but radiation incurred with radionuclide angiography, cardiac catheterization with contrast angiography, and computed tomography may pose a potential hazard to the fetus. When these studies are required, they should be performed before pregnancy occurs; they should be repeated thereafter only when mandated for the safety of the mother and then with pelvic shielding.

Maternal infection with the virus of German measles (rubella) is associated with a high risk of congenital malformation of the fetal heart as well as PDA. If the patient has not had German measles as a child and has never been inoculated against it and her antibody titer confirms the absence of immunity, she should be vaccinated some months before becoming pregnant.

Every pregnant woman known or thought to have heart disease should, at a minimum, be evaluated once by a cardiologist who understands the cardiovascular adaptations to pregnancy. The cardiologist will prescribe necessary diagnostic studies and treatment and, of equal importance, will not allow unnecessary ones. The effects of heart disease can often be ameliorated by correcting coexisting medical problems, such as anemia, chronic infection, anxiety, thyroid dysfunction, hypertension, and arrhythmia.

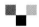

TABLE 41-1. HIGH-RISK MATERNAL CARDIOVASCULAR DISORDERS

Disorder	Maternal Mortality Rate* (%)
Aortic valve stenosis	10–20
Coarctation of the aorta	5
Eisenmenger syndrome	30–70
Marfan syndrome	25–50 (estimated)
Mitral stenosis with atrial fibrillation	14–17
Peripartum cardiomyopathy	15–60
Primary pulmonary hypertension	50
Tetralogy of Fallot	12

* These figures, compiled from 18 references, represent different study periods and disorders of varying severity; therefore, they must be regarded as approximations.

Modified from Ueland K: Cardiovascular disease complicating pregnancy. Clin Obstet Gynecol **21**:429, 1978.

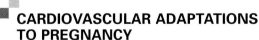

CARDIOVASCULAR ADAPTATIONS TO PREGNANCY

Increased Blood Volume

The cardiovascular alterations observed in pregnancy are reviewed extensively in Chapter 8. However, it is worthwhile to reconsider and emphasize some of the most important cardiovascular changes that occur during pregnancy, because they may significantly alter the course of cardiac disease or may themselves be influenced by a specific disorder.

Blood volume and cardiac output increase during pregnancy (Sullivan and Ramanathan, 1985). The uterus hypertrophies, endometrial vascularization is greatly increased, and the placenta becomes a highly vascular structure that functions to some extent as an arteriovenous shunt. In addition, generalized arteriolar dilation develops, mediated most probably by estrogen. These mechanisms combine to lower systemic vascular resistance. The total blood volume increases steadily during the first trimester and is increased by almost 50% by the 30th week, remaining more or less constant thereafter (Ueland et al., 1973; Elkayam and Gleicher, 1990). Several mechanisms are responsible for increasing blood volume in pregnancy, including steroid hormones of pregnancy, elevated plasma renin activity, and elevated plasma aldosterone levels. Human placental lactogen, atrial natriuretic factor, and other peptides may also play significant roles in governing changes of blood volume in pregnancy. Hypervolemia also occurs with trophoblastic disease, indicating that a fetus is not essential for its development. Heart rate increases by 10 to 20 beats/min. Blood pressure does not increase normally, because the increased intravascular volume is balanced by decreased peripheral vascular resistance mediated by the placenta. Plasma volume tends to increase more than the red blood cell mass, accounting for a "physiologic" anemia that is common in pregnancy (Hytten and Thompson, 1968). Treatment with iron corrects the anemia that, if untreated, may be significant (hematocrit as low as 33 and hemoglobin 11 g/dL).

Cardiac Output

Cardiac output rises during the first few weeks of pregnancy and is 30% to 45% above the nonpregnant level by the 20th week, remaining there until term (Sullivan and Ramanathan, 1985). The increase in cardiac output in the first trimester begins rapidly and peaks around the 20th to 26th week. Early in pregnancy, the dominant factor is elevated stroke volume; later, increased heart rate predominates (Metcalfe and Ueland, 1974). In late pregnancy, the enlarged uterus partially impedes venous return by compressing the inferior vena cava, accounting for lower cardiac output (Ueland and Hansen, 1969). This is one reason why some obstetricians prefer to manage labor with the patient in the Sims (left decubitus) position.

Cardiac Performance

Echocardiographic studies have shown increases in left ventricular fiber shortening velocity and ejection fraction (Perloff, 1988). These changes do not necessarily indicate increased myocardial contractility but may simply be the result of decreased peripheral vascular resistance and increased preload. In any case, stroke volume is increased and cardiac output is further augmented by the 10% to 15% increase in heart rate that characterizes normal pregnancy (Katz et al., 1978).

Demands on the cardiovascular system increase significantly during labor and delivery. Pain increases sympathetic tone, and uterine contractions induce wide swings in the systemic venous return. With placental separation, autotransfusion of at least 500 mL takes place, placing an acute load on the diseased heart, unless offset by blood loss. These large shifts in blood volume can precipitate, on the one hand, shock and,

on the other, pulmonary edema in women with severe heart disease.

When a chest radiograph is obtained in the pregnant woman, the cardiac silhouette often appears slightly enlarged owing to the combined effects of volume overload and elevation of the diaphragm. Routine echocardiographic studies have demonstrated that a small silent pericardial effusion is quite common (Haiat and Halphen, 1984).

Electrocardiogram

The mean QRS axis may shift to the left (Carruth et al., 1981) as a result of the elevated diaphragm. In later pregnancy, the axis may shift to the right when the fetus descends into the pelvis. Minor ST (Boyle and Lloyd-Jones, 1966) and T-wave changes may be observed, usually in lead 3 but sometimes aVF as well. Less often, T inversions may appear transiently in the left precordial leads. Occasionally, small Q waves may accompany T-wave inversion in leads 3 and aVF. These changes are seldom of sufficient magnitude to raise the question of ischemic heart disease, which in any case is relatively uncommon in pregnancy, especially when the mother is young and free from symptoms. Extrasystoles and supraventricular tachycardia are more common during pregnancy. Symptoms of palpitations are common during pregnancy but only rarely signify the presence of organic heart disease.

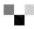

GENERAL GUIDELINES TO MANAGEMENT

During treatment of all pregnant patients with heart disease, priority must be given to maternal health, but all possible therapeutic measures should also be taken to protect the developing fetus. The aspects of management are outlined in Table 41-2.

Because pregnancy increases the demands on the heart, physical exertion frequently must be restricted, especially if it causes symptoms. Some women with certain forms of cardiac disease, such as significant mitral stenosis and cardiomyopathy, tolerate pregnancy poorly and cannot endure physical exertion. They may require strict bed rest for the duration of the pregnancy, particularly during the last trimester. Women with heart disease have a limited ability to increase cardiac output

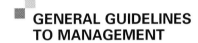

TABLE 41-2. CARDIAC DISEASE IN PREGNANCY: ASPECTS OF MANAGEMENT

Activity restriction
Diet modification
Team approach for medical care
Infection control
   Immunizations
   Prophylaxis against bacterial endocarditis
   Prophylaxis against rheumatic fever
Interruption of pregnancy
Counseling
Contraception or sterilization
Cardiovascular surgery
Cardiovascular drugs

to meet increased metabolic demands and should minimize the demands placed on the heart from physical activity.

Cardiovascular Drugs

Some of the drugs commonly used in the management of patients with cardiovascular disease have potential harmful effects on the developing embryo and fetus. For example, there is no question that oral anticoagulants are potential teratogens when administered in the first trimester (see also Chapter 19 and later in this chapter). The "warfarin embryopathy syndrome," consisting of nasal hypoplasia, optic atrophy, digital abnormalities, and mental impairment, may occur in as many as 15% to 25% of cases (Hall et al., 1980; Stevenson et al., 1980). The fetal risks continue beyond the first trimester, because these drugs increase the possibility of both fetal and intrauterine bleeding.

Anticoagulation presents a significant practical problem in managing pregnant patients with atrial fibrillation, systemic or pulmonary embolism, thrombophlebitis, and pulmonary hypertension. The most vexing problem arises in the case of prosthetic heart valves (Born et al., 1992), which is discussed later in this chapter. In the case of mechanical valve prostheses, warfarin appears to be superior to heparin in preventing valvular thrombosis. Although heparin is safer for the fetus, there is likely an increased risk to the mother (Salazar et al., 1996). This is a complex medical issue, and a randomized trial to determine the optimal anticoagulant therapy for women with a prosthetic valve has not been conducted. Therefore, recommendations are based on smaller studies and on clinical judgment (Elkayam, 1996). No single regimen is likely to be applicable to all such cases, because the issue is complicated by the type and generation of the prosthetic valve, the cardiac rhythm, and the size and contractility of the cardiac chambers.

β-Adrenergic blocking agents, used for the treatment of hypertension and tachyarrhythmia, have been associated with neonatal respiratory depression, sustained bradycardia, and hypoglycemia when administered late in pregnancy or just before delivery. When used judiciously in selected cases (e.g., in women with cardiomyopathy and heart failure), however, beta-blockers are usually well tolerated.

The thiazide diuretics are another class of drugs that can produce harmful effects on the fetus—especially when used in the third trimester or for extended periods—and may impair normal expansion of plasma volume. Rarely, severe neonatal electrolyte imbalance, jaundice, thrombocytopenia, liver damage, and even death have been reported.

There have been numerous reports of fetal and neonatal renal complications after the use of angiotensin-converting enzyme inhibitors during pregnancy (Rosa et al., 1989; Scott and Purohit, 1989). These complications suggest a profound and deleterious effect on fetal renal function, leading to decreased renal function and oligohydramnios, as well as neonatal renal failure. Angiotensin-converting enzyme inhibitors are absolutely contraindicated during pregnancy. Another class of antihypertensive drugs, the angiotensin receptors blockers, also may affect fetal renal function and are therefore absolutely contraindicated in pregnancy.

The indications and possible adverse effects of commonly prescribed cardioactive drugs during pregnancy are summarized in Table 41-3.

Team Approach to Medical Care

Medical care for pregnant women with heart disease is best provided through the cooperative efforts of a cardiologist familiar with the hemodynamic changes of pregnancy and an obstetrician. Frequent visits to both specialists along with open consultations can provide the patient with consistent advice and reassurance and can circumvent the worry and anxiety created by confusing and conflicting information. In addition, the anesthesiologist needs to be consulted during the antepartum period to outline the anticipated approach to intrapartum management, a time of maximum risk for most of these women.

◼ CONGENITAL HEART DISEASE

A number of simple congenital malformations are compatible with a normal or nearly normal pregnancy. Congenital malformations previously associated with high maternal morbidity and mortality and fetal wastage now frequently end with a satisfactory outcome because of palliative or corrective surgery.

The care of adults with congenital heart malformation is an important and growing branch of cardiology (Skorton et al., 1995; Warnes, 1995) that requires the cooperative efforts of medical and pediatric cardiologists, cardiac surgeons, and, in the case of pregnancy, obstetricians and anesthesiologists (Perloff, 1991).

Left-to-Right Shunt

Atrial Septal Defect

ASD may be undiscovered before pregnancy because symptoms are often absent and the physical findings are not blatant. Other causes of left-to-right shunt, such as PDA and VSD, are more likely to be discovered and treated in infancy or childhood. Physicians should be alert to the higher possibility of uncorrected defects in women who have immigrated from an undeveloped country.

Surgical closure of uncomplicated ostium secundum ASD is straightforward and safe and usually is curative. The operation should therefore be done before pregnancy. In addition, many ASDs can now be closed percutaneously, using a "clamshell" or "umbrella" device inserted via a transvenous catheter (Aeschbacher et al., 2000). If the patient is unwilling to undergo ASD closure, she can be advised that the lesion is unlikely to complicate pregnancy and labor, providing that pulmonary hypertension is not present (Neilson et al., 1970; Perloff, 1988).

Metcalfe and colleagues (1986) reported one maternal death in 219 pregnancies in 113 women with ASD. Peripheral vasodilation, if anything, reduces the left-to-right shunt (Metcalfe and Ueland, 1974). Because ASD in young women is not associated with heart failure, diuretics and extreme limitation of intravenous infusion are not warranted. A small percentage of patients with ASD have atrial flutter or fibrillation, which usually is paroxysmal. This arrhythmia can be managed along conventional lines, often with digoxin if necessary. The prospective mother should be informed that surgical closure of the defect does not prevent arrhythmia.

TABLE 41-3. INDICATIONS FOR AND POSSIBLE ADVERSE EFFECTS OF COMMONLY PRESCRIBED CARDIOACTIVE DRUGS ON MOTHER AND FETUS

Agent: Maternal	Indication	Adverse Effects: Fetal (FDA Pregnancy Category)	Adverse Effects: Maternal
Digitalis (digoxin, digitoxin)	Heart failure, arrhythmia, especially atrial fibrillation	Fetal toxicity and neonatal death have been reported with overdosage. Animal studies have not demonstrated teratogenic effects (category C)	Arrhythmias, conduction disturbances, anorexia, nausea, vomiting
Newer inotropic drugs IV milrinone IV amrinone	Not FDA approved Acute heart failure, cardiogenic shock Approved for intravenous use Do not prescribe for pregnant women	Animal studies conflicting (category C)	Gastrointestinal symptoms, headache, reversible thrombocytopenia, hypotension
Diuretics Loop diuretics (furosemide, bumetanide)	Heart failure, hypertension, constrictive pericarditis	Growth restriction No adequate well-controlled studies (category C)	Electrolyte disturbances (hyponatremia, hypokalemia), hypotension, increased creatine and urea nitrogen levels
Thiazides (hydrochlorothiazide)	Hypertension	Neonatal jaundice, thrombocytopenia, hemolytic anemia, hypoglycemia (category C)	Same as loop diuretics but less potent
Metolazone	Hypertension, heart failure	(category B)	Same as loop diuretics but more potent
Potassium sparing Spironolactone	Excessive edema, hypokalemia	Chronic administration in rats has shown it to be mutagenic. Feminization occurs in male rat fetuses (category C)	Gastrointestinal disturbance, amenorrhea, hirsutism, deepening of voice, hyperkalemia
Triamterene	Excessive edema, hypokalemia	No adequate well-conducted studies done on pregnant women (category B)	Gastrointestinal disturbance, hyperkalemia
Vasodilators (directly acting) Hydralazine, isosorbide	Heart failure, hypertension, pulmonary hypertension, angina	Teratogenic in animals, thrombocytopenia, leukopenia reported in newborns (category C)	Hypotension, nausea, diarrhea, headache, systemic lupus erythematosus
Vasodilators (ACE inhibitors) Captopril Enalapril Benazapril Fosinopril Quinapril Lisinopril	Heart failure, hypertension; contraindicated in pregnancy	Renal failure in fetus and neonate (category D)	May worsen renal function, cough, hypotension, hyperkalemia, angioedema (1–2%)
Vasodilators (angiotensin receptor blockers) Losartan Valsartan Candesartan Irbesartan	Heart failure, hypertension; contraindicated in pregnancy	Potential renal failure in fetus and neonate (category D)	May worsen renal function, but side effects are generally very rare
Vasodilators (α-antagonist) Prazosin Terazosin Doxazosin	Hypertension	No well-controlled studies (category C) (category C) (category B)	First dose syncope, nasal congestion, headache, drowsiness
β-Adrenergic antagonists Propranolol Metoprolol	Angina, hypertrophic cardiomyopathy, hypertension, mitral valve prolapse, arrhythmia	During delivery: bradycardia, hypotension, oliguria, hypoglycemia (category C)	Uterine contraction, bradycardia, hypotension, bronchospasm

Category B: Animal studies have not demonstrated a risk to the fetus, but there are no adequate studies in pregnant women.
Category C: Animal studies have shown no adverse effect on the fetus, but there are no adequate studies in humans; benefits may be acceptable despite potential risks.
Category D: Absolutely contraindicated.
ACE, angiotensin-converting enzyme; IV, intravenous.

Adapted from Food and Drug Administration (FDA) Pregnancy Categories, February 1991.

TABLE 41-3. INDICATIONS FOR AND POSSIBLE ADVERSE EFFECTS OF COMMONLY PRESCRIBED CARDIOACTIVE DRUGS ON MOTHER AND FETUS—Cont'd

Agent: Maternal	Indication	Adverse Effects: Fetal (FDA Pregnancy Category)	Adverse Effects: Maternal
Calcium channel blockers Diltiazem, nifedipine, verapamil	Angina, hypertension, arrhythmia (verapamil)	Teratogenicity in small animals No controlled human studies (category C)	Constipation (verapamil), bradycardia, conduction disturbances, negative inotrope, hypotension
Antiarrhythmics Quinidine	Arrhythmia	Neonatal thrombocytopenia reported (category C)	Thrombocytopenia, cinchonism, gastrointestinal, life-threatening arrhythmia
Procainamide	Arrhythmia	Quinidine preferred due to more experience	Gastrointestinal disturbance, SLE
Disopyramide	Arrhythmia	(category C)	Arrhythmia
Lidocaine	Arrhythmia	(category C)	Anticholinergic
Mexiletine	Arrhythmia	(category B)	Epilepsy, drowsiness, confusion
Propafenone	Arrhythmia	(category C)	Gastrointestinal disturbance, tremor, lightheadedness, arrhythmia
Flecainide	Arrhythmia	Embryotoxic in animals (category C)	
Moricizine	Arrhythmia	Teratogenic in rabbits (category C)	Gastrointestinal disturbance, dizziness, AV block, arrhythmia
Amiodarone	Arrhythmia	(category B)	Gastrointestinal disturbance, dizziness, headache, arrhythmia
		Growth restriction in rats (category C)	Dizziness, nausea, arrhythmia Pulmonary fibrosis, thyroid abnormalities, photosensitivity
Anticoagulants Coumadin	Valve disease, prosthetic valves, hypercoagulable states, atrial fibrillation, intracardiac thrombus	Fetal hemorrhage, prematurity, stillbirth, congenital malformations (category X)	Hemorrhage
Heparin	Same as Coumadin		Hemorrhage Loss of bone density, thrombocytopenia
Corticosteroids	Myocarditis, recurrent pericarditis, immunosuppression for cardiac transplant recipients	Cleft palate (category C) in laboratory animals; not in humans	Multiple fluid and electrolyte disturbances, osteoporosis, peptic ulcer, mental disturbance
Cyclosporine	Cardiac transplant recipients, myocarditis?	Embryotoxic in animals (category C)	Impaired immunity, hypertension, renal disease, hirsutism, tremor

Category X: Studies demonstrate fetal risk or abnormalities. Risks outweigh potential benefits.
AV, atrioventricular; SLE, systemic lupus erythematosus.

ASD can be difficult to diagnose during pregnancy. The murmur associated with ASD may be inconspicuous, being a pulmonary ejection systolic murmur and therefore not unlike the physiologic murmur of pregnancy. However, the second heart sound is widely split and may be fixed throughout the respiratory cycle, a distinctly abnormal finding. The electrocardiogram (ECG) shows incomplete right bundle branch block and, in the case of the much more common ostium secundum defect, right axis deviation. In the less common ostium primum defect, marked left axis deviation accompanies incomplete right bundle branch block. The chest x-ray shows right atrial and right ventricular enlargement, prominent pulmonary arteries, and plethoric lung fields. Echocardiography establishes or confirms the diagnosis (Fig. 41-1; Color Plate 18), obviating the need for cardiac catheterization in many cases.

Complicated Atrial Septal Defect

When atrial arrhythmias recur frequently—and especially when the heart rate is difficult to control—catheter ablation is successful in restoring normal sinus rhythm without the need for antiarrhythmic drugs. Generally, this procedure should not be done until after delivery because of the extensive radiation exposure that is needed. In rare instances, labor may be associated with a paradoxical systemic embolus resulting from preferential flow from the inferior vena cava to the left atrium (Somerville et al., 1973).

In the uncommon event that the patient is over 35 years old and has an uncorrected large ASD, the likelihood of chronic atrial fibrillation, right ventricular dysfunction, and pulmonary hypertension rises significantly. Pregnancy is not advised if any of these sequelae are present. If the patient insists on going through with the pregnancy, prolonged bed rest will be required, and vigorous treatment of heart failure may be needed. The maternal risk will be increased, and there will be significant risk of fetal loss. Although warfarin is generally recommended for chronic atrial fibrillation, its use is best avoided (especially in the first trimester); aspirin would be a reasonable compromise. Severe pulmonary hypertension is an uncommon feature of an ostium secundum ASD but is a contraindication to pregnancy. The ostium primum ASD, which is associated with Down syndrome and poses a risk of

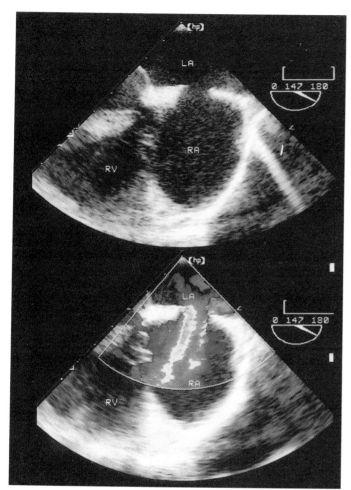

FIGURE 41-1 ■ Transesophageal echocardiographic image of atrial septal defect (ostium secundum). In the *upper panel*, a large defect in the interatrial septum is present. In the *lower panel*, the blue/yellow color represents blood flow from the left atrium (LA) into the right atrium (RA). RV, right ventricle. See Color Plate 18.

endocarditis, is more often associated with severe pulmonary hypertension.

Infective endocarditis rarely if ever complicates a simple ostium secundum ASD; therefore, prophylaxis during labor is not warranted.

Ventricular Septal Defect

The clinical spectrum and risk of VSD may range from so mild that it has little or no effect on pregnancy to so high that maternal or fetal death can occur. Small defects in the muscular ventricular septum frequently close spontaneously during childhood. However, these defects occasionally persist, allowing a small left-to-right shunt manifest by a loud pansystolic murmur along the left sternal border accompanied by a coarse thrill. The chest radiograph is often normal, as is the ECG. The echocardiogram is usually diagnostic (Fig. 41-2; Color Plate 19). These findings constitute the *maladie de Roger*. Prophylaxis against infective endocarditis is indicated, but otherwise this lesion has no effect on pregnancy or labor.

When the defect is in the membranous septum, the left-to-right shunt is larger than in *maladie de Roger*, and spontaneous closure is rare. In the absence of significant pulmonary vascu-

lar disease, the same pansystolic murmur and thrill that characterize *maladie de Roger* are found. Because the shunt is larger, however, the lung fields are plethoric on chest radiography and the heart and pulmonary arteries are enlarged. The classic ECG shows a pattern of biventricular hypertrophy. In such cases, flow through the pulmonary vascular bed is usually at least twice the systemic cardiac output. Patients with a relatively large uncomplicated left-to-right shunt through a VSD tolerate pregnancy well and, in this respect, are comparable with patients with ASD. However, prophylaxis against endocarditis is essential in cases of VSD.

Here it is appropriate to detour from clinical description to pathophysiology. Pulmonary vascular resistance is calculated as the pressure drop across the pulmonary vascular bed divided by the flow through it:

$$R_{\text{Wood units}} = \text{MPAP} - \text{MPCWP (mm Hg)}/Q_{\text{pulmonary}} \text{ (liters/min)}$$

where R is pulmonary vascular resistance, MPAP and MPCWP are the mean pulmonary arterial and capillary wedge pressures, respectively, and $Q_{\text{pulmonary}}$ is total flow through the right heart and pulmonary circulation (i.e., cardiac output plus left-to-right shunt).

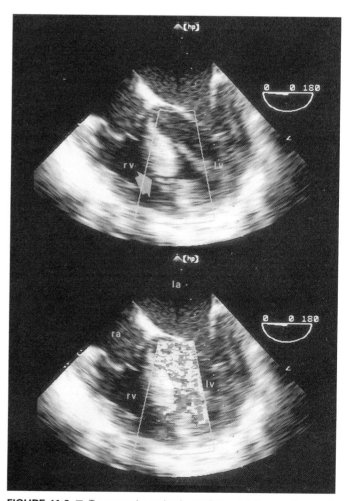

FIGURE 41-2 ■ Transesophageal echocardiographic image of a small muscular ventricular septal defect. In the upper panel, a small communication is seen (*arrow*) between the right ventricle (rv) and left ventricle (lv). In the lower panel, color imaging confirms blood flow between the two chambers. la, left atrium; ra, right atrium. See Color Plate 19.

Resistance can be described in Wood units or in dyne/cm•sec^{-5}. The Wood unit has the merit of simplicity and is derived from clinical units of pressure and flow. The more fundamental but less friendly dyne/cm•sec^{-5} can be obtained by multiplying Wood units by 80. Normal pulmonary vascular resistance is 0.5 to 1.5 Wood units. When a clinician is faced with a pregnant woman with pulmonary hypertension, the key to her risk during pregnancy lies in the pulmonary vascular resistance. High flow *per se* can be the mechanism for pulmonary hypertension without resistance being dangerously elevated. This mechanism can be appreciated by rewriting the resistance equation to read

$$P = Q \times R$$

where P is the pressure drop and Q is the flow across the pulmonary vascular bed.

A patient at one extreme may have a large shunt with pulmonary flow at 20 liters/min and pulmonary vascular resistance at 3 units, yielding a mean pulmonary artery pressure of 55 mm Hg, assuming a normal pulmonary wedge pressure of 5 mm Hg. At the other extreme, a patient with pulmonary vascular disease may have a pulmonary blood flow of 7 liters/min and a pulmonary vascular resistance of 7 units, yielding a pulmonary arterial mean pressure of 44 mm Hg (49 − 5). The higher the pulmonary vascular resistance, the greater the maternal risk. The risk is prohibitive when the pulmonary vascular resistance reaches the systemic level (around 15 Wood units). In borderline cases (e.g., patients with pulmonary vascular resistance between 5 and 8 units), a pulmonary arteriolar vasodilating agent is sometimes administered to determine whether the increased pulmonary vascular resistance is partially reversible or completely irreversible. Mild increase in pulmonary vascular resistance is in the range of 3 to 4 units, moderate 5 to 7 units, and severe above 8 units, sometimes up to 15 or 20 units.

VSD may be associated with considerable increase in pulmonary vascular resistance, reflecting occlusive disease of the small pulmonary arteries and arterioles. This development, if it is to occur, usually does so in childhood and, unless corrected, leads to the Eisenmenger syndrome (see later). However, a small number of adults may survive with VSD and pulmonary vascular resistance that is significantly elevated but falls short of the Eisenmenger syndrome. Such patients are at high risk for death during pregnancy or labor, and there is a high risk of fetal impairment or loss (Neilson et al., 1971). The patient should be told that, in the first trimester, therapeutic abortion would be the safest and wisest option and that later pregnancy would be hazardous and require intensive care. Physical exercise would be strictly curtailed, and prolonged bed rest would be enforced. The combination of decreased physical activity, pulmonary hypertension, and pulmonary vascular disease would constitute sound reasons for instituting anticoagulation, another reason why pregnancy is better avoided or terminated.

Some authorities strongly advise delivery prematurely by means of cesarean section and urge sterilization at the same operation. The dangers must be thoroughly understood by women in this category who insist on continuing pregnancy.

Patent Ductus Arteriosus

The loud *continuous* or *machinery* murmur of typical PDA with a large left-to-right shunt and no pulmonary vascular disease is so striking that the lesion is almost invariably detected and corrected in infancy or childhood. Occasionally, however, women of childbearing age or pregnant women from underprivileged communities may present with a PDA. If the left-to-right shunt is large, the circulation is hyperdynamic with a wide arterial pulse pressure, low arterial diastolic pressure, and hyperactive precordium. The heart may be somewhat enlarged to clinical and radiologic examination, and the ECG may be normal or show left ventricular hypertrophy. The echocardiogram is useful for demonstrating a shunt between the two great vessels (Fig. 41-3; Color Plate 19). The signs of hyperdynamic circulation because of the PDA are exaggerated by pregnancy.

The murmur of PDA is systolic–diastolic and is thus commonly referred to as a "continuous" murmur, although it usually peaks late in systole. Because of its characteristics, the murmur is also referred to as a "machinery" murmur. It is maximal in the left infraclavicular region. It must be distinguished from a *venous hum*, which is loudest in the neck rather than the infraclavicular area. Venous hum is common in pregnant women (Hardison, 1968), and changes dramatically with changes in the position of the head.

Division or occlusion of the PDA should be accomplished before pregnancy is undertaken. Currently, most cases of PDA can be closed by the insertion of a coil delivered via a percutaneous intravascular catheter (Rashkind et al., 1987). If a patient does become pregnant before PDA occlusion, uncomplicated left-to-right shunt can be managed safely, similarly to ASD or VSD. Endocarditis is a risk in patients with PDA and requires antibiotic prophylaxis. Embolic complications of infective endocarditis and endarteritis secondary to PDA may take the form of infected pulmonary emboli. The patient becomes febrile with respiratory symptoms, and the chest radiogram shows multiple opacities and infiltrates.

The leading cause of Eisenmenger syndrome is a large VSD, although a large PDA also may increase pulmonary vascular resistance, sometimes to the extent of Eisenmenger pathophysiology. As with VSD, individuals with PDA may sustain severe increases in pulmonary vascular resistance with the corresponding pulmonary hypertension and right ventricular

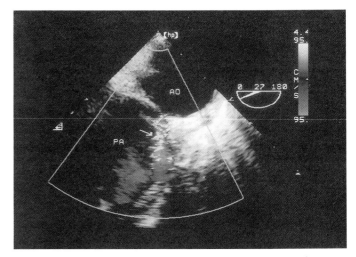

FIGURE 41-3 ■ Transesophageal echocardiographic image of a patent ductus arteriosus. A communication is present between the proximal portion of the descending aorta (AO) and the pulmonary artery (PA). Color imaging (*arrow*) confirms blood flow from the aorta into the pulmonary artery. See Color Plate 19.

hypertrophy yet fall short of Eisenmenger physiology. The maternal risk during pregnancy is high, similar to that encountered in VSD with equivalent pathophysiology. Treatment is the same as VSD with Eisenmenger syndrome. When the pulmonary pressure rises, aortopulmonary shunt decreases and the murmur becomes progressively quieter and shorter until it finally disappears.

The woman with uncomplicated PDA tolerates pregnancy well. If pulmonary hypertension supervenes, the risk to the mother becomes significant. If indeed pulmonary hypertension is suspected and documented, termination of pregnancy is strongly recommended.

Eisenmenger Syndrome

Eisenmenger syndrome is characterized by a congenital communication between the systemic and pulmonary circulations and increased pulmonary vascular resistance, either to systemic level (so there is no shunt across the defect) or with pulmonary vascular resistance exceeding systemic (allowing right-to-left shunt). The most common underlying defect is a large VSD, followed in prevalence by a large PDA. Eisenmenger pathophysiology is less common in ASD (Craig and Selzer, 1968). Occasionally, this type of pathophysiology develops in other less common defects. By the time the syndrome is fully developed, it is often difficult clinically to diagnose the underlying defect. For this discussion, the VSD serves as a good model (Fig. 41-4).

Eisenmenger pathophysiology develops only when the defect is large and is not restrictive, resulting in equal systolic pressure in the two ventricles. It is more common in girls and develops at a young age. Therefore, when increased pulmonary vascular resistance is detected in a child with a large VSD, operative closure must be done as soon as possible to prevent the development of Eisenmenger pathophysiology. Once this has appeared, pulmonary hypertension is irreversible and the VSD therefore is inoperable.

The major clues that pulmonary vascular resistance is increasing are (1) diminution of evidence of a left-to-right shunt and (2) the appearance of progressively severe pulmonary hypertension. The pansystolic murmur of VSD or the continuous murmur of PDA is replaced by a short ejection systolic murmur. The lungs are no longer plethoric but show large central pulmonary arteries and small peripheral arteries characteristic of severe pulmonary hypertension. Because the shunt has disappeared, the radiographic cardiothoracic ratio returns to normal but the main pulmonary segment is prominent. There is usually a striking right ventricular heave, a loud and palpable pulmonary valve closure sound, and an ejection sound in early systole. When concentric ventricular hypertrophy gives way to dilatation and right heart failure, evidence of tricuspid regurgitation appears. Until then, the mean venous pressure is normal but the amplitude of the a wave may be increased, reflecting decreased right ventricular diastolic compliance. When pulmonary vascular resistance is significantly higher than systemic levels, right-to-left shunting of blood occurs and causes cyanosis and clubbing of the fingers and toes. This shunting of deoxygenated blood into the systemic circulation leads to hypoxemia and triggers a reactive erythrocytosis as the system attempts to increase peripheral oxygen delivery. This erythrocytosis consequently increases blood viscosity and can cause sludging and decreased flow of blood,

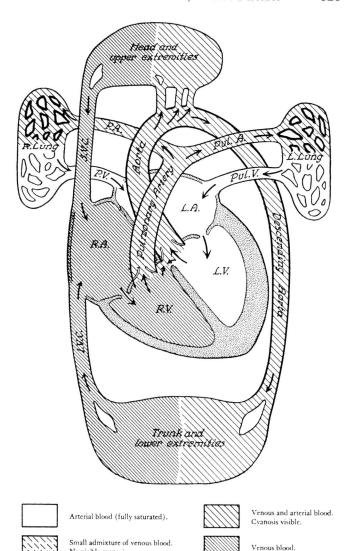

FIGURE 41-4 ■ Eisenmenger complex. Here the cause of right-to-left shunt across the ventricular septal defect is increased pulmonary vascular resistance arising in the small pulmonary arteries and arterioles. I.V.C., interior vena cava; L.A., left atrium; L.V., left ventricle; P.A., Pul. A., pulmonary artery; P.V., Pul. V., pulmonary vein. (Reprinted by permission of the publisher. From Taussig HB: Congenital Malformations of the Heart. Cambridge, Mass, Harvard University Press, 1960. Copyright © 1960 by the Commonwealth Fund by the President and Fellows of Harvard College.)

especially in small vessels. A high hematocrit value, however, is not an automatic indication for serial phlebotomy, because this can lead to iron deficiency and microcytosis. Tissue hypoxia may then actually worsen, a particularly undesirable result in pregnancy. Phlebotomy is reserved for patients without evidence of iron deficiency on laboratory testing who have symptoms of hyperviscosity, including headache, dizziness, visual disturbance, myalgia, and bleeding diathesis. Quantitative volume replacement is necessary during phlebotomy.

Attempting surgical correction of a congenital cardiac shunt after Eisenmenger syndrome is present usually results in the death of the patient (Wood, 1958). Many patients ultimately die of right heart failure, pulmonary hypertension, or pulmonary hemorrhage (Haroutunian and Neill, 1972).

The woman with Eisenmenger syndrome must be informed that pregnancy carries a mortality risk of about 50% (Gleicher et al., 1979). Even if the woman survived, the outcome for the fetus is likely to be poor, because fetal mortality exceeds 50% in cyanotic women with Eisenmenger syndrome (Young and Mark, 1971). Sudden death may occur at any time, but labor, delivery, and the early puerperium seem to be the most dangerous periods (Pitts et al., 1977; Spinnato et al., 1981). Any significant fall in venous return, regardless of etiology, impairs the ability of the right heart to pump blood through the high fixed pulmonary vascular resistance. Hypotension and shock can occur quickly and are often unresponsive to medical therapy.

The major physiologic difficulty in pulmonary hypertension is maintenance of adequate pulmonary blood flow. Anything that decreases venous return, such as vasodilation on the systemic side of the circulation from epidural anesthesia or pooling of blood in the lower extremities from vena caval compression, decreases preload to the right ventricle and pulmonary blood flow. Therefore, management during pregnancy centers on the maintenance of pulmonary blood flow. If the patient insists on maintaining the pregnancy, limitation of physical activity is essential, as is the use of pressure-graded elastic support hose, low-flow home oxygen, and monthly monitoring of platelet counts. Because of the precarious physiologic balance, a planned delivery should be performed with intensive care monitoring, including a Swan-Ganz catheter and provisions for skilled obstetric anesthesia care (Nelson et al., 1983). Anesthetic considerations for this entity are discussed in Chapter 59.

A later report (Avila et al., 1995) struck a more optimistic note. The authors reported on 13 pregnancies in 12 women with Eisenmenger syndrome who elected not to accept advice to terminate pregnancy. Mean systolic pulmonary arterial pressure was 113 mm Hg. Three spontaneous abortions, one premature labor, and two maternal deaths occurred. The seven patients who reached the end of the second trimester were hospitalized until term, treated with oxygen and heparin, and delivered by cesarean section. One patient died a month after delivery. Most of the infants were small, and one died. Despite this better than average outcome, pregnancy should not be encouraged in women with Eisenmenger syndrome or with a systemic level of pulmonary hypertension of any cause.

Primary Pulmonary Hypertension

Severe idiopathic ("primary") pulmonary hypertension, like the Eisenmenger syndrome, carries a high risk in pregnancy, and therefore the same principles apply to its management. Pregnancy is not advised in women with this condition, because the mortality rate approaches 50% (McCaffrey and Dunn, 1964).

Severe pulmonary hypertension can result from taking appetite-suppressing drugs. The fenfluramine–phentermine regimen ("fen-phen") was a notorious culprit (Abenhaim et al., 1996) and therefore has been withdrawn from the market. Treatment strategies include vasodilators, sometimes by chronic intravenous infusion, and nitric oxide inhalation. In some 25% of cases, pulmonary arterial pressure is lowered by prostacyclin infusion (Barst et al., 1996). This response predicts a favorable response to chronic oral nifedipine administration and a good prognosis. Balloon atrial septostomy

(Rothman et al., 1993; Thanopoulos et al., 1996) through the foramen ovale or via transseptal puncture can, in extreme cases, be used to relieve right heart pressure, usually as a bridge to transplantation.

CONGENITAL OBSTRUCTIVE LESIONS

Some congenital cardiac malformations are characterized by obstruction to left or right ventricular outflow. The more frequent examples include pulmonary stenosis, aortic stenosis, and coarctation of the aorta. The hypoplastic left heart syndrome seldom allows survival to the childbearing age, but when it does, there has usually been a major palliative procedure, such as construction of a ventriculoaortic conduit with a prosthetic valve, which would constitute a strong contraindication to pregnancy.

Mitral Stenosis

Congenital mitral stenosis is a rare malformation. When associated with an ASD, it constitutes the *Lutembacher syndrome*. Survival to childbearing age is usual. Both lesions tend to promote atrial fibrillation. Ideally, the mitral valve and the atrial defect should be repaired before pregnancy.

Aortic Stenosis

See also the later section on aortic stenosis under Aortic Valve Disease.

Bicuspid aortic valve is one of the more common congenital malformations that may lead to aortic stenosis, regurgitation, or both (Fig. 41-5). Aortic stenosis is often not present during early life but progresses over time because of valve calcification and gradual restriction in leaflet motion. The bicuspid valve may occur as an isolated defect or in combination with other congenital anomalies, most commonly aortic coarctation. Congenital aortic stenosis, on the other hand, can be a quite severe at birth and may cause severe left ventricular hypertrophy that limits the ability of the heart to respond to demands for increased cardiac output.

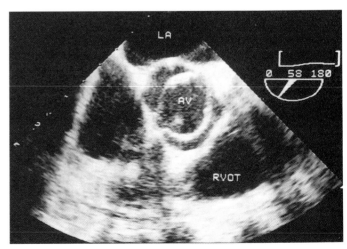

FIGURE 41-5 ■ Transesophageal echocardiographic image of a bicuspid aortic valve. During systole, only two aortic valve (AV) leaflets are seen. LA, left atrium; RVOT, right ventricular outflow tract.

In the syndrome of severe congenital aortic stenosis, the pulses are of slow upstroke and diminished amplitude. Unlike adults with acquired aortic stenosis, children and young adults with congenital aortic stenosis have an abnormally loud aortic valve closure sound. Left ventricular ejection is prolonged, so that the aortic valve closure sound may occur after the pulmonary valve closure sound. Therefore, splitting of the second heart sound is paradoxical and heard in expiration instead of inspiration. Often a loud ejection sound is heard in early systole. The duration of the ejection murmur and the time to its peak intensity increase with worsening severity of aortic stenosis.

The ECG shows severe left ventricular hypertrophy. The chest radiograph is characterized by poststenotic dilatation of the aorta. Although some patients may complain of dyspnea, chest pain, and syncope, others remain asymptomatic. The lesion can be recognized and its severity assessed by Doppler echocardiography.

Critical calcific aortic stenosis is usually treated by aortic valve replacement in older patients, but aortic valve repair is often possible in younger women of childbearing age with congenital aortic stenosis. If aortic stenosis is severe—and especially when it is symptomatic—the woman should be advised against becoming pregnant. She should be advised that if the aortic valve must be replaced, pregnancy and labor would be difficult and dangerous because of the need for anticoagulant treatment if a mechanical prosthesis is implanted. Maternal mortality rates as high as 17% have been reported (Arias and Pineda, 1978), though more recent data suggest a somewhat lower risk. These studies, however, also emphasize the adverse effects of severe maternal aortic stenosis on fetal outcomes, including increased rates of preterm delivery and intrauterine growth restriction (Hameed et al., 2001). If aortic stenosis is moderate in severity, the patient should be advised to undergo pregnancy before the aortic valve is replaced. Labor can be managed in such cases without a high maternal or fetal risk (Neilson et al., 1970).

Strict limits on physical exertion and prolonged periods of bed rest may be required. Left ventricular failure may appear and may necessitate the use of diuretic agents and digitalis. Rarely, even in the presence of severe aortic stenosis, heart failure may be due to another cause (e.g., peripartum cardiomyopathy) (Purcell and Williams, 1995). Prophylaxis against bacterial endocarditis at delivery is recommended.

Vasodilators, helpful in patients with heart failure of other etiology, are dangerous in patients with aortic stenosis because the impeded left ventricle may not be able to fill the dilated peripheral vascular bed. It should be remembered that the lowered systemic vascular resistance of pregnancy adversely affects aortic stenosis. The obstructed left ventricle is limited in its ability to fill the dilated peripheral bed, a situation that can lead to syncope or more serious manifestations of limited relatively fixed cardiac output.

Pulmonary Stenosis

The murmur of pulmonary stenosis is loud and long and is often accompanied by a thrill. The lesion, therefore, is usually detected in early childhood and is thus likely to have been corrected before the childbearing age. Expectant mothers who have not had adequate health supervision in childhood may have unrecognized pulmonary stenosis.

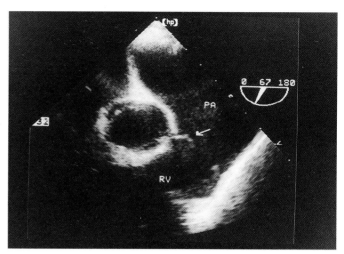

FIGURE 41-6 ■ Transesophageal echocardiographic image of pulmonic stenosis. The pulmonic valve leaflets exhibit characteristic doming (*arrow*). PA, pulmonary artery; RV, right ventricle.

The diagnosis is suggested by a long harsh systolic murmur over the upper left sternal border that is usually preceded by an ejection sound. The venous pressure is normal, but there are striking a waves in the jugular venous pulse. The pulmonary valve closure sound is usually too soft to hear when pulmonary stenosis is severe. Severe pulmonary stenosis causes massive concentric right ventricular hypertrophy manifested by a left parasternal heave and by tall R waves and deeply inverted T waves in the right precordial leads of the ECG. Tall pointed P waves are also present, denoting right atrial enlargement.

Right ventricular enlargement and poststenotic dilatation of the main and left pulmonary arteries are seen on the chest radiograph, which also may show slightly diminished peripheral pulmonary vasculature. Echocardiography demonstrates limited opening of the pulmonic valve leaflets (Fig. 41-6), right ventricular hypertrophy, and abnormally high velocity of blood flow in the pulmonary artery. Doppler echocardiography also allows calculation of the right ventricular pressure and the systolic pressure gradient across the valve. These pressures can also be measured directly in the hemodynamics laboratory (Fig. 41-7).

Mild or *moderate* pulmonary stenosis is well tolerated so that neither pregnancy nor labor poses a significant threat. Prophylaxis against infective endocarditis is necessary. More severe pulmonary stenosis requires treatment. Unlike aortic stenosis, however, critical pulmonary stenosis does not require valve replacement or open repair. Most cases are treated successfully with transvenous balloon valvuloplasty (Stanger et al., 1990). Ideally, this should be carried out before pregnancy is undertaken; if a woman does become pregnant, however, the procedure can still be safely performed, although at some risk to the fetus. *Extreme* pulmonary stenosis (right ventricular systolic pressure more than 150 mm Hg) is a contraindication to pregnancy until the lesion has been adequately treated.

Right-to-Left Shunt without Pulmonary Hypertension (Tetralogy of Fallot)

The congenital cyanotic heart diseases discussed so far have been associated with a communication between the pulmonary and systemic circulations and pulmonary vascular resistance

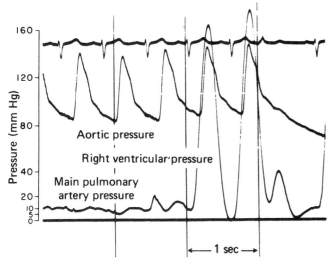

FIGURE 41-7 ■ Pressure tracings in severe pulmonary stenosis. Pulmonary pressure is extremely low and appears damped. Right ventricular pressure is suprasystemic. (From Shabetai R, Adolph RJ: Principles of cardiac catheterization. *In* Fowler NO (ed): Cardiac Diagnosis and Treatment. Hagerstown, Md, Harper & Row, 1980, p. 106.)

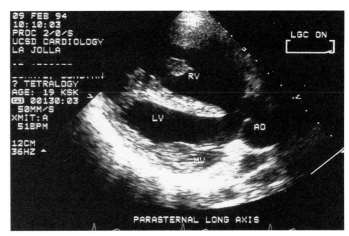

FIGURE 41-9 ■ Transthoracic echocardiographic image of tetralogy of Fallot. A large ventricular septal defect is present, and the aorta (AO) overrides the interventricular septum. LV, left ventricle; MV, mitral valve; RV, right ventricle.

sufficiently high to cause a right-to-left shunt. However, cyanosis occurs in other congenital malformations that have a defect between the right and left sides of the heart but also right ventricular outflow obstruction (Figs. 41-8 and 41-9). Examples include the tetralogy of Fallot and tricuspid atresia.

Tetralogy of Fallot is used to illustrate this class of congenital malformation of the heart because it is by far the most common form of cyanotic congenital heart disease encountered in pregnancy. Moreover, the hereditary risk of this combination of anomalies, if one parent has congenital heart disease, is between 2% and 13% (Nora et al., 1981; Whittemore et al., 1982; Morris and Menashe, 1985). The syndrome includes (1) a large defect high in the ventricular septum; (2) pulmonary stenosis, which may be at the valve itself but more commonly is in the infundibulum of the right ventricle; (3) dextroposition of the aorta so that the aortic orifice sits astride the VSD and overrides, at least in part, the

right ventricle; and (4) right ventricular hypertrophy (Fig. 41-10).

A wide spectrum of clinical presentations may be present, depending on the relative size of the VSD and the degree of right ventricular outflow obstruction that diverts blood flow through the VSD. In the typical case, right and left ventricular systolic pressures are equal but the pulmonary artery pressure is exceedingly low. A loud long systolic murmur is audible along the left sternal border. The murmur is caused by an abnormal flow pattern through the obstructed right ventricular outflow tract. The pulmonary valve closure sound is usually inaudible. Patients are usually cyanotic and often have significant clubbing of the fingers and toes. The hematocrit value is greatly elevated because of the severe erythremia. Phlebotomy is not indicated to treat the hematocrit level *per se* but is indicated when symptoms of hyperviscosity occur. Ignoring this important therapeutic principle induces a microcytic anemia that further complicates pregnancy. The ECG shows severe right ventricular hypertrophy. The chest radiograph is characterized by a normal-sized heart and a concavity in the region where the pulmonary artery should be (Fig. 41-11). As in all malformations of this general type, the lung fields are oligemic, showing small vessels throughout.

Most adults born with the tetralogy of Fallot and lesions with similar pathophysiology will have undergone prior surgical treatment before reaching young adulthood. Children raised in undeveloped countries are an important exception. Many will have had surgery to close the VSD and relieve the pulmonary stenosis, constituting virtual "total repair," rendering them potentially safe candidates for pregnancy and delivery. The operation, however, is not curative. Significant arrhythmia and conduction defects that may eventually lead to the need for electronic cardiac pacing or implantable defibrillators may occur years after an apparently successful operation. Other sequelae and residua include only partial relief of the right ventricular outflow obstruction and/or pulmonary regurgitation. This latter problem is usually well tolerated early but may lead to late right-sided heart failure.

The cyanotic patient with tetralogy of Fallot has special problems during pregnancy. The reduced systemic vascular resistance of pregnancy causes more blood to shunt from right

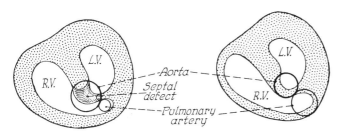

FIGURE 41-8 ■ Tetralogy of Fallot. The anatomic pathology (*left*) compared with normal (*right*). Note the ventricular septal defect, the aorta (which overrides the defect), the pulmonary stenosis, and right ventricular hypertrophy. L.V., left ventricle; R.V., right ventricle. (Reprinted by permission of the publisher. From Taussig HB: Congenital Malformations of the Heart. Cambridge, Mass, Harvard University Press, 1960. Copyright © 1960 by the Commonwealth Fund by the President and Fellows of Harvard College.)

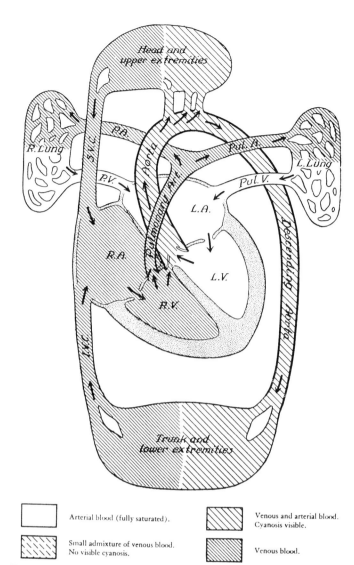

Arterial blood (fully saturated).

Venous and arterial blood. Cyanosis visible.

Small admixture of venous blood. No visible cyanosis.

Venous blood.

FIGURE 41-10 ■ In the tetralogy of Fallot, cyanosis is present because blood shunts from left to right through the ventricular septal defect because its flow to the lungs is impeded by pulmonary stenosis. L.A., left atrium; L.V., left ventricle; P.A., Pul. A., pulmonary artery; P.V., Pul. V., pulmonary vein. (Reprinted by permission of the publisher. From Taussig HB: Congenital Malformations of the Heart. Cambridge, Mass, Harvard University Press, 1960. Copyright © 1960 by the Commonwealth Fund by the President and Fellows of Harvard College.)

to left, leaving less to flow to the pulmonary circulation. This intensifies hypoxemia and can lead to syncope or death. Maintenance of venous return is crucial. The most dangerous times for these women are late pregnancy and the early puerperium, because venous return is impeded by the large gravid uterus near term and by peripheral venous pooling after delivery. Pressure-graded elastic support hose are recommended. Blood loss during labor may compromise venous return, and blood volume must be promptly and adequately restored. Anesthetic considerations during delivery are discussed in detail in Chapter 59. Antibiotic prophylaxis should be used in these susceptible patients at delivery.

Because of the combined high maternal risk and the high incidence of fetal loss, pregnancy is discouraged in women with uncorrected tetralogy of Fallot. The prognosis is particularly bleak in women with a history of repeated syncopal

episodes, a hematocrit level above 60%, or right ventricular systolic pressure above 120 mm Hg.

If a young woman with untreated tetralogy of Fallot requests prepregnancy counseling, she should be advised to undergo surgical correction before pregnancy. Pregnancy does not represent a significantly increased risk for patients in whom the VSD has been patched and the pulmonary infundibular stenosis corrected.

Coarctation of the Aorta

Coarctation of the aorta is a congenital defect in the area of the aorta where the ligamentum arteriosum and the left subclavian artery insert (the distal portion of the aortic arch). The malformation may be simple or complex, and it is either isolated or associated with PDA and other malformations, notably aortic stenosis and aortic regurgitation secondary to a bicuspid aortic valve. It may also be found in association with the Turner XO syndrome. The lesion should be detected and treated surgically or by balloon dilatation in infancy or childhood, but it may be present in women who are, or want to become, pregnant.

Typical features include the following:

■ Upper extremity hypertension but lower extremity hypotension
■ Visible and palpable collateral arteries in the scapular area
■ A late systolic murmur usually loudest over the interscapular region
■ Femoral pulses that lag behind the carotid pulses and are of diminished amplitude
■ Notching of the inferior rib borders seen on the chest radiogram and resulting from erosion by arterial collaterals that bridge the coarctation

Electrocardiographic evidence of severe left ventricular hypertrophy strongly suggests associated aortic stenosis. Surgical grafting or percutaneous intravascular balloon dilation reduces the upper extremity hypertension, but blood pressure does not always return to normal—and hypertension may recur in later life.

Whenever possible, the operation should be performed before pregnancy; otherwise, the maternal mortality rate is 3% (Deal and Wooley, 1973). Coarctation is associated with congenital berry aneurysm of the circle of Willis and hemorrhagic stroke. The risk of stroke may increase during labor because of transient elevations in blood pressure. Patients are at risk for aortic dissection and infective endocarditis involving an abnormal aortic valve; these risks increase during pregnancy (Deal and Wooley, 1973; Barash et al., 1975). Hypertension will often worsen as well (Beauchesne et al., 2001). Operation does not require cardiopulmonary bypass and can be carried out with safety for the mother and with less fetal risk than accompanies open heart surgery with cardiopulmonary bypass. Although transvascular balloon dilatation of aortic coarctation is a viable option for children and infants with coarctation, it is not generally used in adults (Ovaert et al., 2000)

If delivery must be undertaken in cases of unoperated coarctation, blood pressure can be titrated with α-adrenergic–stimulating and α-adrenergic–blocking agents delivered by intravenous drip.

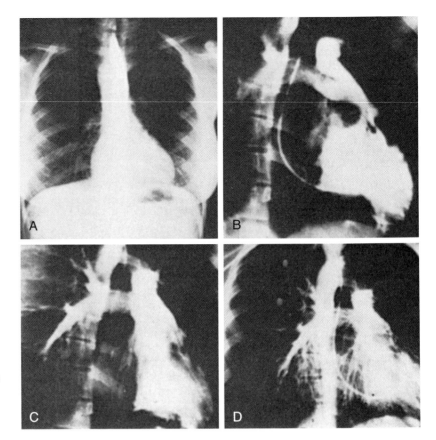

FIGURE 41-11 ■ Tetralogy of Fallot. **A,** Chest radiograph. Note concavity in the area of the pulmonary artery, oligemic lungs, and right aortic arch. **B,** Right ventriculogram. Note narrow right ventricular outflow tract. **C,** Further clarification of the pulmonary arteries. The left ventricle is slightly opacified via the ventricular septal defect. **D,** The associated right-sided aortic arch is now visible. (From Shabetai R, Adolph RJ: Principles of cardiac catheterization. In Fowler NO (ed): Cardiac Diagnosis and Treatment. Hagerstown, Md, Harper & Row, 1980, p. 106.)

OTHER CONGENITAL CARDIAC MALFORMATIONS

Ebstein Anomaly

Ebstein anomaly is a malformation of the tricuspid valve in which the septal leaflet is displaced apically and the anterior leaflet is abnormally large in size. The deformed tricuspid valve apparatus may be significantly incompetent or stenotic, depending on the location of the anomalously placed cusps of the valve. In some cases, the malformation causes impediment to right ventricular outflow.

The clinical features are easily recognized by a cardiologist, and the echocardiogram is characteristic and reliable (Fig. 41-12). This syndrome is frequently associated with anomalous atrioventricular conduction pathways and the *Wolff-Parkinson-White syndrome*. Patients may also have an ASD with right-to-left shunting and cyanosis. Supraventricular arrhythmias are also common.

The most favored treatment is reconstruction of the tricuspid valve, for which satisfactory techniques have now been developed. The operation should be performed before pregnancy is undertaken. Interruption of anomalous conduction pathways also can be performed during surgery.

The Mayo Clinic group (Connolly and Warnes, 1994) reported on 111 pregnancies in 44 women with Ebstein anomaly resulting in 95 live births, although most of the infants had low birth weight. Vaginal delivery was performed in 89% and cesarean section in 9%; 23 deliveries were premature. Nineteen pregnancies ended with spontaneous abortion, and 7 ended with therapeutic abortion. Congenital heart disease occurred in 6% of the children of mothers with Ebstein anomaly and in 1% of fathers with Ebstein anomaly.

Congenital Atrioventricular Block

Congenital atrioventricular block differs somewhat from heart block in adults. The ventricular pacemaker is usually higher, and therefore the QRS complex is normal or only

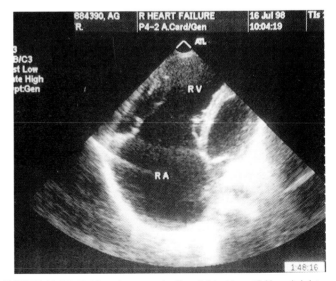

FIGURE 41-12 ■ Ebstein anomaly. The right atrium (RA) and right ventricle (RV) are markedly dilated, and the tricuspid valve is displaced toward the cardiac apex.

slightly widened and the ventricular rate is more rapid than in acquired atrioventricular block. Although these patients appear to do well during childhood and young adulthood, the lesion is associated with an unexpectedly high mortality rate. Therefore, treatment with a pacemaker is indicated in many of the cases (Reid et al., 1982). The pacemaker used should be dual chamber and rate responsive so that normal cardiovascular dynamics at rest and exercise will be preserved. Patients who are untreated or have received a pacemaker are at slight or no increased risk during pregnancy.

Additional Malformations

A number of other malformations may be present in women of childbearing age, including the following:

- Other left-to-right or right-to-left shunts
- Transposition of the great vessels
- Truncus arteriosus
- Single-ventricle double-outlet right ventricle
- Various obstructive lesions

The malformations may be multiple and complex. Survival to adulthood depends on at least partial correction, which may have been furnished by surgical operation or may be part of the malformation. For example, in D-type transposition of the great vessels, the aorta arises from the right ventricle and the pulmonary artery from the left. Survival requires a shunt at some level (e.g., ASD, VSD, or PDA) so oxygenated blood can enter the systemic circulation.

Some of these women with untreated and delicately balanced lesions bear children, but usually this is not wise. Transposition of the great vessels is now treated by anastomosis of the aorta to the morphologic right (anatomic left) ventricle and the pulmonary artery to the morphologic left (anatomic right) ventricle. Lesions such as single ventricle may be palliated by the Fontan procedure, in which venous return is connected directly to the pulmonary circulation, bypassing the right heart. Neither procedure constitutes a cure, but successful pregnancy can occur.

In summary, patients should be evaluated and tracked by a cardiologist experienced in congenital heart disease and an obstetrician with special knowledge and experience in managing women with congenital cardiac lesions (Sciscione and Callan, 1993).

RHEUMATIC HEART DISEASE

Rheumatic Fever

Rheumatic fever is now distinctly uncommon in the United States, Western Europe, and Great Britain but is still prevalent in less economically developed countries. Many young women emigrate to the Western world and constitute a large proportion of the patients with a history of rheumatic fever. Women with such a history should take daily penicillin or, if they are allergic, its equivalent throughout pregnancy to prevent a recurrence. Acute rheumatic fever or acute streptococcal throat infection mandates a full bactericidal dose for 10 days. Acute rheumatic heart disease can present with pericarditis, symptoms of heart failure, cardiac murmurs, and/or enlargement of the heart.

Chronic Rheumatic Heart Disease

In the United States, acute rheumatic fever with carditis has been uncommon for many years, and chronic rheumatic heart disease, which presents years to decades after the episode of acute rheumatic fever, is becoming uncommon among the native childbearing population. Control of rheumatic fever has largely shifted the burden of rheumatic heart disease from teenagers to women in the third and fourth decades of life.

The characteristic lesion of rheumatic heart disease is mitral stenosis, and the next most common is the combination of mitral stenosis with aortic regurgitation. The mitral valve may become both stenotic and incompetent, and the valve may calcify. Pure mitral regurgitation is almost always nonrheumatic, except in young people with acute carditis. Similarly, aortic valve disease without mitral involvement is seldom rheumatic. Tricuspid regurgitation is a late secondary manifestation secondary to pulmonary hypertension and right ventricular enlargement.

Mitral Stenosis

The principal features are enlargement of the left atrium and right ventricle, a diastolic murmur at the cardiac apex, and pulmonary hypertension. Inflow to the left ventricle is impeded by the narrowed valve and can be accomplished only by an increased level of pressure in the left atrium (Figs. 41-13 and 41-14). The faster the heart rate, the less time in diastole, and therefore the less time for ventricular filling. Left atrial pressure therefore is further elevated by tachycardia. Atrial fibrillation eventually supervenes, causing a fall in cardiac output and escalation of left atrial hypertension, especially if the ventricular rate is not controlled. Atrial fibrillation substantially increases the probability of thrombus in the left atrial appendage and the threat of a subsequent embolic stroke.

Effect of Pregnancy

Pregnancy drastically stresses the circulation in women with severe mitral stenosis. The increased blood volume, heart rate, and cardiac output raise left atrial pressure to a level that causes severe pulmonary congestion, leading to progressive exertional dyspnea, orthopnea, paroxysmal nocturnal dyspnea, and pulmonary edema. Women who have not been receiving antenatal care often present initially with severe pulmonary edema during pregnancy. In long-standing cases, severe right heart failure develops. Infective endocarditis, pulmonary embolism, and massive hemoptysis may also occur. The maternal risk for death is highest in the third trimester and in the puerperium (Szekely et al., 1973).

Significant Mitral Stenosis without Heart Failure

Patients should be advised to undergo percutaneous balloon mitral valvuloplasty and to postpone pregnancy until after full recovery from the procedure. If they do not follow this advice and do become pregnant, one reasonable course for some individuals in the first trimester may be therapeutic abortion, followed by mitral valve operation and subsequent pregnancy planning. If this is not acceptable, the patient can be advised to remain under frequent close supervision by the cardiologist

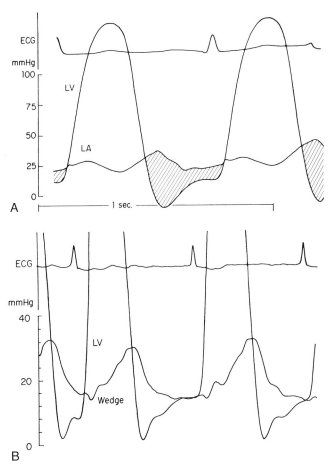

FIGURE 41-13 ■ Hemodynamics of mitral valve disease. **A,** Mitral stenosis. The diastolic pressure gradient (*shaded*) between the left atrium (LA) and left ventricle (LV) persists to end-diastole. **B,** Mitral regurgitation. Note the large systolic pressure wave of the pulmonary wedge pressure tracing. The diastolic pressure gradient is limited to early diastole. ECG; electrocardiogram.

and obstetrician and to accept long periods of rest, prohibition of strenuous activity, salt restriction, and diuretic treatment. When this type of regimen is followed closely and is expertly supervised, maternal mortality is low (Szekely et al., 1973). Atrial fibrillation signals the need for digitalis, a β-adrenergic blocking agent, or a calcium channel blocking agent to maintain a normal heart rate. More than one of these drugs may be needed to achieve the desired result without side effects. For patients with atrial fibrillation and significant mitral stenosis, anticoagulant treatment is required. The problems with warfarin have been discussed (Hall et al., 1980).

Depending on her course, the woman may have to spend many weeks in bed and should be admitted to the hospital well in advance of labor. The supine posture should be avoided as much as possible, and delivery in the Sims position is desirable. The lithotomy position, with the patient on her back and her feet elevated in stirrups, is an invitation to pulmonary edema. The crisis of pulmonary edema may appear despite good management. Sedation to drop the heart rate and promote cardiac filling and output and diuretic treatment must then be followed by prompt delivery if the fetus is viable.

Percutaneous balloon valvuloplasty is a nonsurgical means to dilate mitral stenosis and is the current treatment of choice for most patients with symptomatic mitral stenosis (Kaplan

et al., 1987; McKay, Lock, et al., 1987; Esteves et al., 1991; Kalra et al., 1994; Lefevre et al., 1991). The procedure can be done during pregnancy if heart failure is severe and appears to be safer for the fetus than open mitral commissurotomy (de Souza et al., 2001). Obviously, lead shielding should be used, because fluoroscopy is required to guide the balloon into the mitral orifice. If at all possible, the procedure should be put off at least until after the first trimester. Patients with confirmed mitral stenosis and right heart failure with severe pulmonary congestion should avoid pregnancy until after the valvular disease is corrected, because the risk of maternal mortality is high.

MITRAL VALVE PROLAPSE

A degree of prolapse of the mitral valve used to be considered so prevalent in the general population (Devereux et al., 1976), particularly among young women, that authorities differed as to whether mitral valve prolapse (MVP) should be considered a normal variant or abnormal. More exacting echocardiographic criteria yield more realistic and much lower estimates of the prevalence (Wann et al., 1983; Levine et al., 1989).

True MVP occurs because portions of the mitral valve apparatus are redundant and therefore the leaflets balloon into the left atrium during systole. The leaflets may remain coapted during systole or may separate, causing a variable degree of mitral regurgitation. More severe prolapse may be caused by myxomatous degeneration of the mitral leaflets. These abnormalities of connective tissue may be isolated to the mitral valve or may be a part of *Marfan syndrome* (see later). MVP (and sometimes tricuspid valve prolapse) may be associated with congenital malformations, notably ASD.

Mitral regurgitation may be absent, intermittent, or permanent and may be of any degree of severity. Severe mitral regurgitation greatly enlarges the left atrium (Fig. 41-15) and ventricle and eventually leads to left ventricular failure and pulmonary hypertension, the latter less severe than with mitral stenosis.

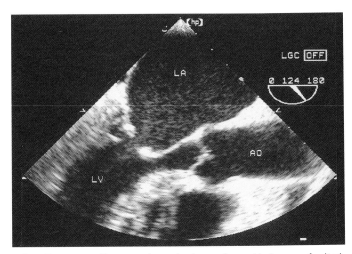

FIGURE 41-14 ■ Transesophageal echocardiographic image of mitral stenosis. During diastole, opening of the mitral valve is restricted by scarring and fusion of the leaflet tips. Characteristic doming of the leaflet is also present. AO, aorta; LA, left atrium; LV, left ventricle.

PLATE 18

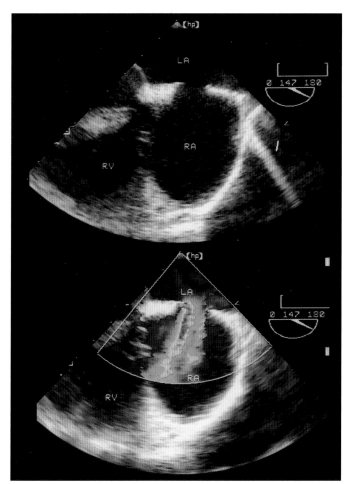

FIGURE 41-1 ■ Transesophageal echocardiographic image of atrial septal defect (ostium secundum). In the *upper panel*, a large defect in the interatrial septum is present. In the *lower panel*, the blue/yellow color represents blood flow from the left atrium (LA) into the right atrium (RA). RV, right ventricle.

PLATE 19

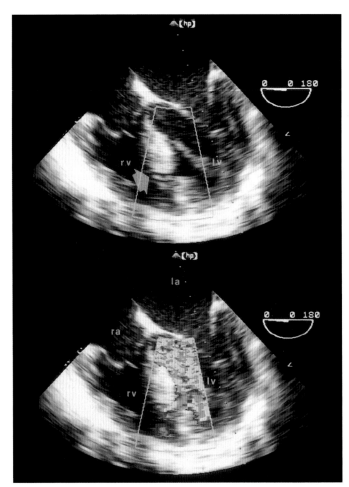

FIGURE 41-2 ■ Transesophageal echocardiographic image of a small muscular ventricular septal defect. In the upper panel, a small communication is seen (*arrow*) between the right ventricle (rv) and left ventricle (lv). In the lower panel, color imaging confirms blood flow between the two chambers. la, left atrium; ra, right atrium.

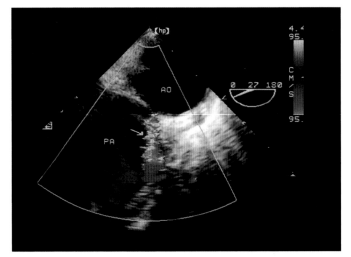

FIGURE 41-3 ■ Transesophageal echocardiographic image of a patent ductus arteriosus. A communication is present between the proximal portion of the descending aorta (AO) and the pulmonary artery (PA). Color imaging (*arrow*) confirms blood flow from the aorta into the pulmonary artery.

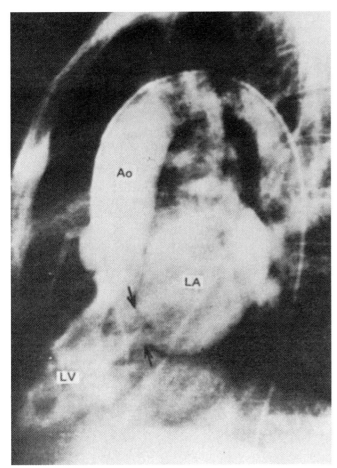

FIGURE 41-15 ■ Mitral regurgitation. Contrast was injected into the left ventricle (LV). There is massive opacification of the enlarged left atrium (LA). Ao, aorta. (From Shabetai R, Adolph RJ: Principles of cardiac catheterization. *In* Fowler NO (ed): Cardiac Diagnosis and Treatment. Hagerstown, Md, Harper & Row, 1980, p. 106.)

Past reports have associated MVP with a number of disorders, including stroke, dysautonomia, panic attacks, anxiety, and transient ischemic attacks (Coghlan et al., 1979; Hartman et al., 1982; Perloff et al., 1986), but more recent studies (Freed et al., 1999; Gilon et al., 1999) have largely discounted these associations. The syndrome of myxomatous mitral valve degeneration with prolapse and mitral regurgitation is relatively uncommon, and many women who were diagnosed with MVP more than 10 years ago do not have any actual pathology. For this reason, it may be prudent to order an echocardiogram in any woman diagnosed with MVP a number of years ago if she has no symptoms or signs of mitral regurgitation. This may prevent needless and repeated exposure to antibiotics before dental procedures and the like.

Some women with MVP complain of chest pain, which can be suggestive of angina pectoris. Although the coronary arteriogram is normal, T-wave inversions, especially in leads 2, 3, and aVF, are found in a small proportion, and the treadmill exercise test may induce ST segment depression, indistinguishable from ischemia (Butman et al., 1982).

In most cases, the diagnosis of MVP is made by the physician providing preconception counseling and antenatal care. The examination reveals a systolic click occurring between the first and second heart sounds. The click may or may not be followed by a mid- or late systolic murmur. The click and murmur

vary with the patient's posture and hydration status. In most patients, no other abnormality is found on clinical examination. Unless significant mitral regurgitation is present, the patient should be told that pregnancy, labor, and delivery will be safe and unaffected by the prolapse. Antibiotic prophylaxis for MVP is needed only when mitral regurgitation is present and/or the mitral valve is clearly thickened and myxomatous on echocardiographic examination.

Patients with MVP and significant mitral regurgitation are far fewer in number than those with simple prolapse. The murmur is louder, longer, and more consistent and may become pansystolic. Clinical and laboratory evidence of enlargement of the left atrium and ventricle increases with increasing severity and duration of regurgitation. Volume overload of the heart is well tolerated for many years, with the enlarged left ventricle maintaining full compensation. However, the inevitable eventual onset of deterioration of left ventricular function is subtle because resistance to regurgitant flow to the pulmonary venous bed is far less than resistance to flow through the systemic arterioles. This low impedance leak is one of the mechanisms that preserves the pumping function of the left ventricle, even after myocardial damage has occurred as a consequence of the longstanding volume overload (Eckberg et al., 1973).

Even modest impairment of left ventricular function, especially when progressive, indicates that pregnancy may well precipitate heart failure and cannot be lightly undertaken. More obvious left ventricular dysfunction (e.g., ejection fraction less than 35%) indicates that the woman should be strongly advised to avoid pregnancy. She should then be referred for complete cardiologic evaluation (Ross, 1981) and surgery to address the mitral regurgitation. In most cases of MVP, the valve can be repaired rather than replaced. It is important to appreciate that left ventricular function deteriorates after mitral valve replacement but may improve after mitral valve repair (Bach and Bolling, 1995). Thereafter, if the result is good and ventricular function is significantly improved, pregnancy may be undertaken successfully.

Chest pain and arrhythmias are best managed with β-adrenergic blockers such as atenolol or metoprolol. When symptoms are unusually pronounced, thyroid function tests should be checked as well.

Because the gravid uterus and vasodilation may add to postural hypotension, the patient should be informed that during pregnancy she may experience lightheadedness, dizziness, or fainting during prolonged standing. Although there may be a familial tendency toward MVP, the condition is not serious enough to counsel against considering pregnancy (Shell et al., 1969).

Mitral Regurgitation Not Caused by Prolapse

In younger women, mitral regurgitation may result from rheumatic or congenital disease. In older women, mitral regurgitation is more often a manifestation of hypertension, ischemia, idiopathic myocardial disease, or infective endocarditis.

Most of the information regarding mitral regurgitation in prolapse also applies here. In older women, the valve is more likely to be calcified; fewer of the valves are amenable to repair and must be replaced. The problems posed by prosthetic valves in pregnant women have been discussed; the hemodynamics are illustrated in Figure 41-13 and angiography is illustrated in Figure 41-15.

In patients with far advanced left ventricular dysfunction or failure who have severe mitral regurgitation, it can be difficult to determine which is the cause and which the result. In either case, the patient with a greatly enlarged grossly hypokinetic ventricle must be advised against becoming pregnant. Most of the pregnancy would be spent in bed, the course would be punctuated by episodes of uncompensated congestive heart failure (any of which could prove fatal or require therapeutic abortion), and the risk to the fetus would exceed 50%.

Patients with *mild* or *moderate* mitral regurgitation can be managed safely with a conservative regimen of reduced physical activity, salt restriction, and low doses of a diuretic agent. Low-dose digoxin may be helpful if atrial fibrillation supervenes. As mentioned previously, severe mitral regurgitation indicates a need for repair or replacement of the valve when symptoms and/or *early* evidence of declining ventricular function appear (Otto, 2001). Clearly, surgical treatment is best undertaken before pregnancy. If the woman is already pregnant, the physician should make every effort to help her to carry the pregnancy to term using strict medical measures. This course is particularly important when clinical, radiologic, and echocardiographic criteria suggest that the valve is irreparable and would require replacement.

AORTIC VALVE DISEASE

Aortic Stenosis

See also the previous section on aortic stenosis under Congenital Obstructive Lesions.

The etiology of aortic stenosis commonly is degeneration, often of a congenitally bicuspid valve. The problem may be encountered in women a decade or more older than those with rheumatic or congenital aortic valve disease. The combination of aortic and mitral stenosis is usually due to rheumatic heart disease. Critical aortic stenosis leads to severe left ventricular hypertrophy and, eventually, to left ventricular failure. Even before the advent of overt heart failure, syncope or even sudden death may occur.

The characteristic findings include an ejection systolic murmur—harsher, longer, and peaking later than the normal ejection murmur of pregnancy. It is usually loudest at the second right intercostal space. When aortic stenosis is severe, the pulse upstroke is slow and left ventricular hypertrophy is evident on the ECG. The echocardiogram is a more sensitive and more specific marker of left ventricular hypertrophy. Doppler echocardiographic measurement of the blood flow velocity through the aortic valve permits reliable estimation of the systolic pressure drop across the valve, as well as calculation of the valve area. The hemodynamics are illustrated in Figure 41-16. The left ventricle in women remodels differently than in men. The concentric hypertrophy is more pronounced, the cavity is smaller, and systolic function is supranormal.

The left ventricle does not dilate until the ventricle fails, and so a dilated ventricle in aortic stenosis is an ominous sign that calls for rapid intervention. In general, aortic valve replacement is preferred to percutaneous balloon aortic valvuloplasty, but open heart surgery presents a high risk to the fetus. Therefore, some have advised balloon aortic valvuloplasty for treatment of aortic stenosis during pregnancy (Banning et al.,

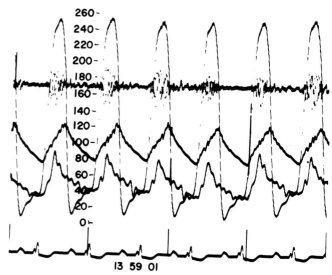

FIGURE 41-16 ■ Hemodynamic data in aortic stenosis. Left ventricular pressure is 250/40 mm Hg (normal 120/10 mm Hg). Aortic systolic pressure is 130 mm Hg lower than left ventricular and shows a slow upstroke and vibrations representing the systolic thrill. The record above the aortic pressure tracing is a phonocardiogram showing the systolic murmur. Also shown is the pulmonary wedge pressure (lowest pressure tracing), which is elevated to equal the left ventricular diastolic pressure. The bottom tracing is the electrocardiogram. (From Shabetai R, Adolph RJ: Principles of cardiac catheterization. *In* Fowler NO (ed): Cardiac Diagnosis and Treatment. Hagerstown, Md, Harper & Row, 1980, p. 106.)

1993), but valve replacement will almost certainly have to be done soon after delivery. When heart failure is severe, the wisest option is to deliver the fetus abdominally if possible and replace the aortic valve.

Absolute contraindications to pregnancy in women with uncorrected critical aortic stenosis (Arias and Pineda, 1978) include the following:

- Heart failure (past or present)
- Syncope
- A previous episode of cardiac arrest

Pregnancy in women with a mechanical aortic valve replacement is not advised, because continuous anticoagulation is necessary (see later section under Pregnancy in Patients with Artificial Heart Valves).

Aortic Regurgitation

The etiologic mechanism is commonly rheumatic heart disease, in which case mitral stenosis often coexists. Other diseases, such as Marfan syndrome, bicuspid aortic valve, infective endocarditis, and systemic lupus erythematosus, also may cause severe aortic regurgitation. This valvular lesion imposes a volume rather than pressure overload on the heart and as such is usually well tolerated in pregnancy and labor (Sullivan and Ramanathan, 1985).

The diagnosis is usually based on the typical high-pitched blowing diastolic murmur and can be quantified by Doppler echocardiography. Both pregnancy and aortic regurgitation contribute to hypervolemia and peripheral vasodilatation. A prolonged course without decompensation is characteristic of chronic aortic regurgitation; once heart failure appears, however, the course may progress rapidly downhill.

Traditionally, aortic valve replacement is not recommended until symptoms of heart failure (most notably exertional dyspnea) occur or left ventricular dysfunction/enlargement is seen on echocardiography. Repair of aortic regurgitation is much less successful than repair of mitral regurgitation. For a woman who is contemplating pregnancy, the need for aortic valve replacement constitutes the grounds on which the medical advisor must recommend against pregnancy and make the patient fully understand the consequences of choosing otherwise. When left ventricular dysfunction and heart failure are absent, carefully supervised pregnancy is in order and the woman should be encouraged to complete her family before cardiac dysfunction and the need for valve replacement arise.

In many cases, the cause of aortic regurgitation is unclear. Special care must be taken to rule out aortic aneurysm or dissection, especially when associated with Marfan syndrome or coarctation of the aorta, because these conditions may result in aortic rupture and constitute strong reasons to advise against pregnancy.

DRUG-INDUCED VALVULAR HEART DISEASE

A recently recognized cause of deformity and regurgitation of the cardiac valves is the ingestion of fenfluramine-phentermine. This led to withdrawal of this drug combination from the market several years ago. The mechanism of the effect of these drugs is unclear, and fortunately there is evidence that valvular lesions may sometimes gradually improve after discontinuation of the drugs (Mast et al., 2001). In some cases, however, valve surgery has been necessary (Connolly et al., 1997).

CARDIOMYOPATHY

Cardiomyopathy is a disorder of myocardial structure or function. A number of forms exist, and we discuss several types that are seen in pregnant women.

Dilated Cardiomyopathy

In this condition, the cardiac chambers are severely dilated and the left ventricle is diffusely hypokinetic. Left ventricular wall tension is increased, and systolic pump function progressively declines. Consequently, cardiac output falls and filling pressures increase; both changes cause progressive dyspnea, edema, and fatigue. Serious ventricular arrhythmia develops in most cases.

The 5-year prognosis for survival is less than 50%, and during that time heart failure becomes less and less responsive to treatment (Clemens et al., 1982). In some cases, however, improvement or even return to normal has been noted. Both angiotensin-converting enzyme inhibitors and β-adrenergic blocking agents (most notably carvedilol and long-acting metoprolol) have been shown to slow the deterioration of left ventricular function in patients with congestive heart failure and occasionally actually improve the left ventricular ejection fraction (ACC/AHA Guidelines, 2001). In addition, some of the patients who recover may have had unrecognized myocarditis that did not progress to cardiomyopathy. Dilated cardiomyopathy may be the outcome of an autoimmune response to a myocardial injury, most commonly viral myocarditis. The exact role of alcohol is unclear, but it is at least a major aggravating factor in some cases.

Patients may have symptoms and signs of heart failure for which no cause can be found on clinical and laboratory examination. Weight is increased, the jugular venous pressure is elevated, and the heart is enlarged. A third heart sound gallop is often present, frequently accompanied by the murmurs of mitral and tricuspid regurgitation, which develop as a consequence of cardiac dilatation. The ECG is usually grossly abnormal, often showing left ventricular hypertrophy or left bundle branch block. Echocardiography shows enlargement and hypocontractility of the ventricles. The patients are subject to mural thrombus in the cardiac chambers and therefore to the risk of stroke or pulmonary embolism. Established dilated cardiomyopathy, even when heart failure is compensated, is a contraindication to pregnancy.

It was formerly thought that dilated cardiomyopathy was sporadic and not familial (Shabetai and Shine, 1973), but inherited cases have now been observed (Mestroni et al., 1990). It is now known that 20% of cases are genetic in origin (McMinn and Ross, 1995). Therefore, if an extensive family history of heart failure is present, the prospective mother and father should be informed of the potential risk of genetic transmission.

In a young woman with severe dilated cardiomyopathy, manifested by greatly impaired ventricular function and drastically reduced exercise capacity, cardiac transplantation should be considered. Eventually, such women may have children with reasonable safety (Kossoy et al., 1988; Key et al., 1989).

Peripartum Cardiomyopathy

Peripartum cardiomyopathy is a form of dilated cardiomyopathy that occurs in the last month of pregnancy or the first 5 months after delivery, in the absence of previous heart disease (Pearson et al., 2000). The incidence in America is 1 case per 3000 to 4000 live births. Additional diagnostic criteria include a left ventricular ejection fraction of less than 45% and—most importantly—the absence of other identifiable causes of heart failure (Hibbard et al., 1999). Whether the peripartum or postpartum state somehow constitutes the original myocardial insult or is an aggravating factor in individuals susceptible to cardiomyopathy for other reasons is not known (Cunningham et al., 1986; O'Connell et al., 1986). It has been suggested that some cases are caused by active myocarditis (Van Hoeven et al., 1993), but other investigators have reported that the incidence of myocarditis is the same in idiopathic and peripartum cardiomyopathy (Rezeq et al., 1994). It is also possible that the stress of pregnancy may "unmask" an underlying cardiomyopathic process that may have otherwise presented later in life (Lampert et al., 1997). Tragically, this devastating disease may affect previously healthy young women and may cause unexpected sudden death (McIndor et al., 1995).

The clinical course of peripartum cardiomyopathy is frustratingly variable and difficult to predict (Reimold and Rutherford, 2001). About 20% have a dramatic and fulminant downhill course and can be saved only with cardiac transplantation. Others, perhaps 30% to 50%, have partial recovery with persistence of some degree of cardiac dysfunction. The rest show remarkable recovery (Van der Leeuw-Harmsen et al., 1985). Apparently, the initial degree of left ventricular dysfunction does not predict the long-term outcome (Cole et al., 1987). Women who recover from peripartum cardiomyopathy must be informed that cardiomyopathy may recur with a subsequent pregnancy. For some time, this risk has been believed to be 50% (Cole et al., 1987). However, one report of four women who had peripartum cardiomyopathy with a previous pregnancy but whose hearts remained normal clinically and by echocardiography in a subsequent pregnancy indicated that the risk may be less (St. John Sutton et al., 1991). The largest study to date of patients with a history of peripartum cardiomyopathy who subsequently became pregnant (Elkayam et al., 2001) showed that heart failure recurred in 20% of patients whose ejection fractions had normalized after the previous pregnancy. None of these patients died during the study period. However, heart failure recurred in 40% of the patients with persistent left ventricular dysfunction after the previous pregnancy, and maternal mortality was 19%. Therefore, the risk of recurrent heart failure is high in women with peripartum cardiomyopathy, especially in those who do not have complete recovery of left ventricular function.

Treatment is similar to that of other patients with heart failure. Because angiotensin-converting enzyme inhibitors are contraindicated during pregnancy, hydralazine is the vasodilator of choice. If cardiac dysfunction is severe, anticoagulation is generally recommended, given the prothrombic tendency of pregnancy. Low-molecular-weight heparin is probably preferred over unfractionated heparin (warfarin is not advertised) (Reimold and Rutherford, 2001).

Idiopathic Hypertrophic Cardiomyopathy

Usually inherited as an autosomal dominant trait with variable penetrance but sometimes caused by a spontaneous mutation, hypertrophic cardiomyopathy is being recognized with increasing frequency. The phenotypes vary greatly, so that left ventricular outflow tract obstruction may or may not be present and the hypertrophy may be either symmetrical or asymmetrical. The chief symptoms are angina, dyspnea, arrhythmia, and syncope. Sudden death is a feature mostly confined to patients in whom the diagnosis is established in childhood or youth, patients with a history of syncope or ventricular arrhythmia, and patients with a family history of hypertrophic cardiomyopathy and sudden death. Recent research has shown that certain specific genetic defects place patients at great risk for sudden death.

When the disease is first detected in older adults, the course is more benign and sudden death is rare. Left ventricular hypertrophy is often apparent on clinical examination and ECG and is invariably present on the echocardiogram. The echocardiographic findings are often diagnostic and include marked thickening of the ventricular septum, usually with less thickness of the other walls of the left ventricle (asymmetrical hypertrophy), and abnormal systolic anterior movement of the mitral valve (Fig. 41-17). The internal dimensions of the left ventricle are normal or small, and its contractility is increased.

An important feature in many cases is obstruction of the space between the ventricular septum and the anterior leaflet of the mitral valve. This space constitutes the left ventricular outflow tract. Outflow obstruction by the anterior mitral valve leaflet is worsened by increased inotropy, decreased heart size,

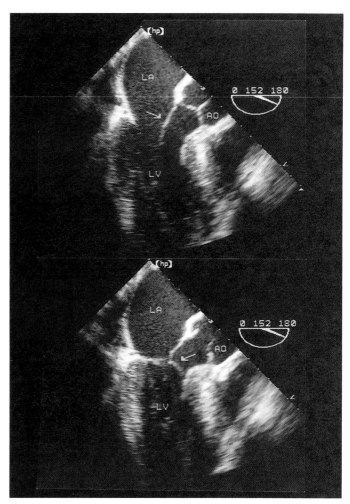

FIGURE 41-17 ■ Transesophageal echocardiographic images of hypertrophic cardiomyopathy. During diastole (*upper frame*), the anterior leaflet of the mitral valve (*arrow*) is a normal position. During systole, however (*lower frame*), the leaflet (*arrow*) is pulled by Venturi forces into the left ventricular outflow tract, causing obstruction to outflow. AO, aorta; LA, left atrium; LV, left ventricle.

and diminished peripheral vascular resistance. The normal fall in peripheral vascular resistance accompanying pregnancy tends to increase outflow tract obstruction, although this effect may be compensated for by the physiologic increase in blood volume. In addition, vena caval obstruction in late pregnancy and blood loss at delivery, both of which may result in hypotension, may have a similar deleterious effect. Outflow tract obstruction may also be worsened by the increases in circulating catecholamine levels frequently encountered during labor and delivery.

Straining during the second stage means frequently performing the Valsalva maneuver, which greatly diminishes heart size and increases outflow tract obstruction. Despite all these problems, however, most pregnant women with hypertrophic cardiomyopathy do tolerate labor and delivery (Oakley et al., 1979).

There is a complex interplay between the hemodynamics of the cardiomyopathy and those of pregnancy, neither of which is constant. Exacerbation of symptoms (Kolibash et al., 1975; Tessler et al., 1990) and even sudden death (Pelliccia et al., 1992) have been reported during pregnancy in women with obstructive cardiomyopathy. Treatment is aimed at avoiding hypovolemia, maintaining venous return, and diminishing the force of myocardial contraction by avoiding anxiety, excitement, and strenuous activity.

Because left ventricular diastolic compliance can be greatly reduced in this disease, excessive or too rapid volume repletion can induce pulmonary edema. β-Adrenergic blockade is generally considered first-line pharmacologic therapy for symptomatic hypertrophic cardiomyopathy and can be continued or instituted in pregnancy. The dose should be the minimal effective to avoid excessive slowing of the fetal heart.

Esmolol can be given intravenously if the patient first presents with severe symptoms. Volume replacement and vasopressor therapy may be needed along with β-adrenergic blockers. Calcium channel blockers, such as verapamil, have been shown to be effective in reducing symptoms (Lorell et al., 1982), but they must be used cautiously because they can cause pulmonary edema in severe cases. Nifedipine, because of its vasodilator properties, is best avoided.

Vaginal delivery is almost always appropriate in the absence of an obstetric indication for abdominal delivery. Impaired venous return is highly undesirable in hypertrophic cardiomyopathy and can be ameliorated by managing the second stage with the patient in the left lateral decubitus position.

Acquired Immunodeficiency Syndrome

Myocarditis or cardiomyopathy is frequently discovered when patients with acquired immunodeficiency syndrome (AIDS) are examined postmortem (Bestetti, 1989; Lewis, 1989). Symptomatic myocardial disease, although considerably less common, is observed with increasing frequency. If patients with AIDS are screened for cardiac involvement (e.g., by echocardiography), cardiac or pericardial involvement is found in almost 75% of the cases (Raffanti et al., 1988). In some cases, these abnormalities are transient (Blanchard et al., 1991). Myocarditis is usually caused by opportunistic infection, but in some cases hybridization studies have proved direct AIDS infection. Clinical findings range from occult ventricular dysfunction to severe uncompensated heart failure. Rarely, even Kaposi sarcoma has been detected in the heart or pericardium. Pericardial effusion, often occult, is one of the more common cardiac manifestations and suggests a worse prognosis (Heidenreich et al., 1995). Malignant lymphoma involving the myocardium and endocardium has been reported frequently.

Cardiac failure ranks low on the list of problems faced by the physician managing pregnancy complicated by AIDS. Nevertheless, physicians need to be on guard lest severe dilated cardiomyopathy, myocarditis, or cardiac tamponade develop, and the family must be prepared for a child with human immunodeficiency virus (see also Chapter 40.)

■ CORONARY ARTERY DISEASE

Because premenopausal women enjoy substantial protection against coronary atherosclerosis (Sullivan and Ramanathan, 1985), ischemic heart disease is rarely relevant to obstetric practice. However, coronary artery disease may be found in women of childbearing age when other risk factors, such as insulin-dependent diabetes, overwhelm the natural protection they should normally enjoy. Lupus erythematosus, especially

when treated with steroidal agents, may precipitate premature coronary artery disease (Meller et al., 1975). Coronary atherosclerosis appears in a significant proportion of patients who have received a cardiac transplant (Johnson et al., 1991) and may be found in familial lipid disorders. In the latter instance, the exact nature of the lipid disorder must be defined by detailed analysis of the patient's lipid chemistry and lipoproteins to enable the physician to provide an accurate forecast of the risk that the infant would inherit the lipid disorder and premature coronary artery disease. In women with coronary artery disease or severe dyslipidemia, oral contraceptives may be detrimental (Ratnoff and Kaufman, 1982). In addition, spasm of anatomically normal coronary arteries leading to myocardial infarction has been reported (Maekawa et al., 1994).

Spontaneous coronary artery dissection is quite rare and occurs chiefly in young women during or soon after pregnancy (Klutstein et al., 1997; Vilke et al., 1998). Treatment has included placement of a stent, emergency coronary bypass operation, and thrombolysis (Kearney et al., 1993; Efstratiou and Singh, 1994; Porras and Gill, 1998; Thistlethwaite et al., 1998). Although very uncommon, the diagnosis of coronary artery dissection is extremely important to consider whenever a woman presents with severe chest pain in the peripartum period. If the coronary artery dissection is undetected, massive myocardial infarction and even death can occur. If the diagnosis is made expediently, however, outcome appears to be quite good, and long-term survival is expected (Koul et al., 2001).

Management of Stable Angina Pectoris

Patients with coronary artery disease who experience angina pectoris with moderate to high levels of exertion may require treatment with nitrates, calcium channel blocking drugs, or β-adrenergic blocking drugs, but otherwise this condition should have no major effect on pregnancy, labor, or delivery. Similarly, if a woman had previously sustained a myocardial infarction but recovered without heart failure, significant left ventricular dysfunction, or unstable angina pectoris, she too can be advised that her pregnancy and labor should be relatively uncomplicated.

The major indications that pregnancy and labor would pose a significant risk to women with ischemic heart disease include the presence of overt heart failure, significant enlargement and/or dysfunction of the left ventricle, and ischemia at rest or provoked by mild exertion.

Severe Myocardial Ischemic Syndromes: Unstable Angina

The diagnosis of severe ischemia may be confirmed when angina occurs at rest or with mild exertion. This *unstable* angina frequently, but not necessarily, follows a period of classic *stable* angina pectoris. Unstable angina is a reliable symptom of severe extensive myocardial ischemia and thus is a clear warning of the imminence of a major ischemic event, such as acute myocardial infarction or a fatal ventricular arrhythmia. Starting a pregnancy under these circumstances is not advisable.

In some women with advanced heart disease, the clinical picture is less dramatic, but a treadmill exercise test demonstrates that profound and dangerous ischemia can be precipitated by minimal exertion. Thus, if the treadmill test provokes an abnormal response at a low level of exercise, and particularly if this response is accompanied by either angina pectoris or a fall in blood pressure, the woman is at high risk for a serious and possibly fatal myocardial ischemic event and must not undertake pregnancy unless the myocardium can be revascularized.

Patients with unstable angina or severe ischemia must be referred to a cardiology center where the acute problem can be stabilized and the patient can be assessed for revascularization of the myocardium by coronary bypass graft operation or transluminal coronary angioplasty. If the outcome is satisfactory, the patient may then bear children.

Pregnant women who have severe unstable ischemia require aspirin, heparin, and intravenous nitroglycerin in an intensive care unit. If the ischemia proves intractable or if the syndrome progresses to infarction, coronary angioplasty or bypass operation is indicated, depending on the result of the preceding arteriogram. The coronary bypass operation should be performed without cardiopulmonary bypass to help decrease the risk to the fetus (Silberman et al., 1996).

Myocardial Infarction

Acute myocardial infarction complicates about 1 in 10,000 pregnancies (Mabie and Freire, 1995). The highest incidence appears to occur in the third trimester and in older (more than 33 years) multigravidas. The maternal mortality rate is high (about 20%), and death usually occurs at the time of infarction or during labor and delivery (Roth and Elkayam, 1996). Coronary angiography in this population has shown atherosclerosis in about 40% of cases, coronary thrombosis without atherosclerosis in 20%, and coronary dissection in 16%. Interestingly, 30% had normal coronary arteries (Roth and Elkayam, 1996). Treatment of acute myocardial infarction during pregnancy should include use of heparin and beta-blockers (unless acute heart failure is present). The use of thrombolytics in pregnancy is controversial, because there is increased risk of maternal hemorrhage. Therefore, direct percutaneous coronary angioplasty (often with coronary stenting) is probably the procedure of choice. Obviously, this exposes the fetus to radiation; extensive lead shielding should be used.

A *remote* myocardial infarction, followed by recovery without angina, major left ventricular dysfunction, or heart failure, should have little influence on pregnancy or labor. Patients should wait a year after an infarction before undertaking pregnancy. In many cases, coronary arteriography should be done first so that if critical coronary stenoses are found, myocardial revascularization can be done. Severe left ventricular damage and heart failure are relative contraindications to pregnancy and, when far advanced, absolute contraindications.

Patients with ischemic heart disease may experience episodic myocardial ischemia without angina. Patients should therefore undergo objective tests, such as treadmill exercise tolerance and myocardial perfusion imaging, at rest and after peak exercise. Similarly, myocardial infarction may lead to severe depression of left ventricular function, which may or may not be accompanied by evidence of heart failure. Left ventricular function testing by echocardiography or determination of the left ventricular ejection fraction should be carried out, preferably before pregnancy or, failing that, shortly thereafter.

For remote myocardial infarction without evidence of ischemia, heart failure, or severe left ventricular dysfunction, simple electrocardiographic monitoring suffices during labor. If a large myocardial infarction has occurred during pregnancy, then arterial blood pressure, central venous pressure, pulmonary arterial and pulmonary wedge pressure, and cardiac output should be monitored invasively. Cardiac function can also be assessed via transesophageal echocardiography. Monitoring should be continued until after the completion of labor because, with birth, maternal preload abruptly increases, after which substantial loss of blood accompanies delivery of the placenta.

HEART FAILURE

Chronic heart failure is a syndrome that develops when the heart cannot meet the metabolic requirements of the normally active individual. It may be defined as ventricular dysfunction causing dyspnea, fatigue, and sometimes arrhythmia. The lesion may be an intrinsic myocardial abnormality. Examples include myocarditis, the various cardiomyopathies, ischemic heart disease, other specific myocardial disorders (e.g., amyloidosis), and metabolic abnormalities (e.g., myxedema). The myocardial response to chronic pressure overload is concentric hypertrophy with increased thickness of the ventricular walls; the response to chronic volume overload is dilatation (eccentric hypertrophy). Eventually, with either type of overload, contractile power is diminished, resulting in decreased pump function of the heart. Causes include valvular disease, systemic and pulmonary hypertension, and congenital malformations. The clinical manifestations are due in part to the abnormal loading conditions and in part to the damaged myocardium.

Manifestations

The principal manifestations of heart failure are caused by increased left and right ventricular diastolic pressure, which engenders pulmonary and systemic congestion, and reduced cardiac output (in severe cases at rest or in less severe cases, only during exercise). The combined effects of inadequate cardiac output and congestion are dyspnea, fatigue, and edema. In the later stages of heart failure, these changes lead to progressive dysfunction of vital organs, principally the liver and kidneys. The prognosis of severe uncorrectable heart failure is less than 50% survival after 5 years.

The critical clinical features that enable physicians to diagnose and follow the course of heart failure are body weight, jugular venous pressure, the third heart sound, cardiac size, radiologic evidence of pulmonary congestion, pulmonary rales, and peripheral edema—usually in this order. Echocardiography is an extremely useful tool for evaluating left ventricular function and prognosis in heart failure (Xie et al., 1994) and should be performed without delay when heart failure is suspected. Circulating B-type natriuretic peptide (BNP) is increased in congestive heart failure. Serum B-type natriuretic peptide levels provide an effective, inexpensive, and quickly available test for heart failure. The degree of BNP increase correlates with the severity of heart failure (Maisel et al., 2002).

The presence of heart failure greatly limits physical activity and warrants several or all of the following treatments:

- Continuous, usually escalating courses of diuretic drugs
- β-Adrenergic receptor blockers
- Angiotensin-converting enzyme inhibitors (or if not well tolerated, angiotensin receptor blockers)
- Salt restriction
- Digoxin

Pregnancy imposes a powerful, often intolerable, additional load on the failing heart. Once it is clear that no remediable cause of heart failure exists, pregnancy is contraindicated.

Symptoms and Treatment

The chief symptoms associated with heart failure are dyspnea and fatigue. These symptoms are exacerbated by pregnancy, which often induces edema, orthopnea, nocturnal dyspnea, and pulmonary edema. Five-year survival is less than 50% in patients with severe heart failure (Foster et al., 1981), and the course is likely to be progressively downhill. For all these reasons, such women should be advised against becoming pregnant.

If heart failure is first discovered during pregnancy, episodes of cardiac decompensation that do not respond to adjustment of orally administered medicine necessitate admission to an intensive care unit. There, the effects of treatment on cardiac output, pulmonary arterial pressure, systemic venous pressure, and pulmonary wedge pressure along with the maternal and fetal ECGs can be monitored. When the hemodynamic parameters and clinical condition indicate continuing deterioration despite maximal medical therapy, emergency abdominal delivery may be necessary. In general, patients with heart failure should receive diuretics, a salt-restricted diet, beta-blockers, digoxin, and angiotensin-converting enzyme inhibitors (though this last drug class is contraindicated in pregnancy).

Left Ventricular Dysfunction

There is a remarkable lack of correlation between symptoms of heart failure and objective evidence of left ventricular dysfunction (Engler et al., 1982). Patients with chronic heart disease after myocardial infarction, for example, may have a considerably enlarged and extremely hypokinetic ventricle and yet be relatively free from symptoms. For this reason, any woman who has sustained myocardial damage should have left ventricular function assessed by a radionuclide ventriculogram, an echocardiogram, or sometimes both before deciding on pregnancy. A left ventricular ejection fraction in the range of 20% calls for advice basically the same as that given to patients with overt heart failure, because pregnancy may be the event that transforms the clinical picture from that of compensated left ventricular dysfunction to overt congestive heart failure. Moderately impaired left ventricular systolic function, for instance, as documented by a left ventricular ejection fraction in the range of 40%, is compatible with safe pregnancy and delivery, if the patient remains under meticulous care from a cardiologist and obstetrician and is prepared to follow a strict regimen throughout pregnancy.

Cardiac Transplantation

Some fortunate women with advanced heart failure may become successful recipients of a cardiac transplant. Successful pregnancy and delivery in patients with cardiac transplanta-tion have been reported (Kossoy et al., 1988; Key et al., 1989). Posttransplant medical treatment is complex because of the immunosuppressive drug regimen, the frequent endomyocardial biopsies, and the uncertain long-term prognosis. Nevertheless, it is likely that more women will desire pregnancy after heart and, perhaps, heart-lung transplantation. Women should delay pregnancy for at least 1 year after cardiac transplantation, by which time the risk of acute rejection and the intensity of immunosuppression and biopsy surveys are considerably less.

DISTURBANCES OF CARDIAC RHYTHM

Isolated supraventricular and ventricular extrasystoles are very common, and no treatment is necessary. Preconception counseling is simplified by a clear appreciation of several general principles.

Arrhythmia that occurs in the absence of organic heart disease is almost always benign and is therefore not an indication for pharmacologic treatment unless the woman finds palpitation intolerable. Reassuring her of the benign nature of this symptom is often all that is required. It has not been proven that drug treatment of unsustained asymptomatic arrhythmia can prevent death, even when organic heart disease is present. Therefore, the need for pharmacologic treatment is disputed.

Sustained symptomatic arrhythmia, however, requires treatment, which can be pharmacologic or procedural (e.g., transcatheter ablation of an anomalous conduction pathway or insertion of an implantable cardiac defibrillator).

Pregnancy and labor should be safe except in the group with sustained ventricular arrhythmia, with its attendant risk of cardiac arrest and need for vigorous treatment. Pharmacologic treatment for serious arrhythmia is likely to include newly introduced agents, such as amiodarone, for which there is at best limited knowledge of potentially unfavorable effects on the fetus. Ideally, pregnancy should be postponed until the arrhythmia has been eliminated or at least controlled, preferably by nonpharmacologic means. If antiarrhythmic drugs must be used, whenever possible they should be those that have been used for several decades, allowing prediction of the fetal risk.

High-grade atrioventricular conduction disturbance, especially when symptomatic, is treated by artificial pacing, which should not influence pregnancy, labor, or the fetus. Electrical cardioversion or defibrillation of the mother's heart does not disturb or damage the fetal heart (Schroeder and Harrison, 1971).

It is clearly desirable to evaluate disturbances of cardiac rhythm and conduction before pregnancy, proceeding when indicated to full electrophysiologic testing. This plan avoids antiarrhythmic agents that are potentially toxic to the fetus and protects against the radiation associated with electrophysiologic investigation.

MARFAN SYNDROME

Marfan syndrome is variably expressed and inherited as an autosomal dominant trait. Left untreated, life expectancy is reduced by half in those who exhibit the classic syndrome

(Murdoch et al., 1972). The basic defect is one of connective tissue, and connective tissue weakness in the aorta causes the dangerous complications, most notably aortic dissection (Pyeritz and McKusick, 1979).

Symptoms and signs, when present, may include dyspnea and chest pain, an aortic diastolic murmur, and a mid-systolic click. The best diagnostic test and apparently the most critical for determining the outcome of pregnancy is the echocardiogram. More than 90% of patients have evidence of MVP, whereas 60% have echocardiographic evidence of aortic root dilatation (Brown et al., 1975).

Pregnancy is particularly dangerous for patients with this syndrome because there appears to be a higher risk of aortic rupture and dissection, especially if dilatation of the aortic root is present (Elkayam et al., 1995). Women with an aortic diameter exceeding 40 mm are at greatest risk of death during pregnancy (Pyeritz, 1981). If the woman exhibits all the manifestations of Marfan syndrome, it would be prudent to avoid becoming pregnant altogether. The physician should also make sure the woman understands the 50% risk of genetic transmission to her children.

Deficiency of elastic tissue is the cause of myxomatous degeneration of the aortic and mitral valves and cystic medial necrosis of the aorta (Figs. 41-18 and 41-19). This abnormality translates to large aneurysms of the aortic root, multiple aneurysms elsewhere along the course of the aorta and great vessels, and severe aortic and mitral regurgitation with resulting heart failure. Surgery is indicated for rapidly expanding aneurysm or if dissection is evident. Pregnancy is poorly tolerated under these conditions, and labor may precipitate rupture of an aneurysm, aortic dissection, or heart failure.

If a woman with Marfan syndrome chooses to become pregnant, therapy is directed at markedly limiting physical activity, preventing hypertensive complications, and decreasing the pulsatile forces on the aortic wall with the use of a beta-blocker. Long-acting beta-blockers are indicated before, during, and after pregnancy in women with Marfan syndrome and aortic root enlargement (Shores et al., 1994). Once aortic root diameter reaches 50 to 55 mm, most authorities recommend prophylactic aortic valve and root replacement, because the risk of aortic dissection is quite high.

PREGNANCY IN PATIENTS WITH ARTIFICIAL HEART VALVES

This is one of the most complex and challenging areas where cardiology and obstetrics intersect and could be the topic of an entire chapter itself. The discussion here, however, is brief and covers three basic groups of patients: (1) Women contemplating pregnancy who will likely need a valve replacement in the medium- to long-term future (e.g., women with moderate aortic or pulmonic stenosis, severe but asymptomatic mitral or aortic regurgitation with normal myocardial function, or mild to moderate mitral stenosis); (2) women who wish to become pregnant but have severe valve disease that must be addressed expediently (e.g., severe aortic or mitral stenosis, severe mitral regurgitation with cardiac dysfunction, or severe aortic regurgitation with cardiac dysfunction); and (3) women with mechanical valve replacements who become pregnant.

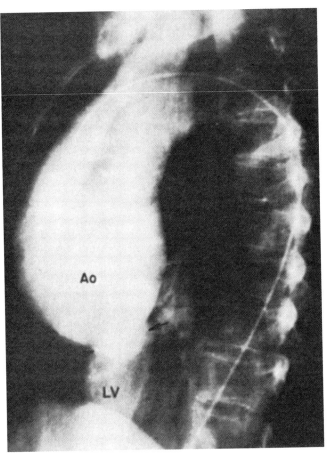

FIGURE 41-18 ■ Aortogram showing an aneurysm of the ascending aorta (Ao) with regurgitation of contrast through an incompetent aortic valve into the left ventricle (LV). (From Shabetai R, Adolph RJ: Principles of cardiac catheterization. *In* Fowler NO (ed): Cardiac Diagnosis and Treatment. Hagerstown, Md, Harper & Row, 1980, p. 106.)

The only group where no management controversy exists is the first (Oakley, 1995). Without question, women who will likely need valve surgery in several years should be strongly encouraged to complete their childbearing as quickly as possible—so they will not become members of the second or third groups.

Women in the second group require valve replacement before pregnancy. In most instances (but *excluding* women who wish to become pregnant), mechanical prosthetic valves are favored over biological prostheses in adults less than 70 to 75 years old because biological valves have a shorter life span and deteriorate much more quickly than mechanical valves. This difference appears even more pronounced in younger patients. It was thought that pregnancy itself hastened biological valve deterioration, but this does not appear to be true (Salazar et al., 1999). Therefore, young patients with biological valves will almost certainly require repeat surgery. The "down side" of a mechanical valve, however, is the requirement for life-long anticoagulation and the resultant small increase in risk of bleeding. It is important to note that the anticoagulant of choice with a mechanical valve is warfarin, not heparin. Although heparin is clearly safer for the fetus (Ginsberg et al., 1989), it is *not* equivalent in efficacy to warfarin (especially during the prothrombic state of preg-

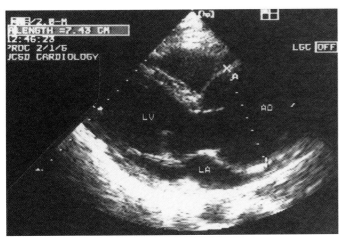

FIGURE 41-19 ■ Marfan syndrome. The echocardiogram shows a markedly dilated aortic root, measuring 7.4 cm in diameter (normal is up to 3.5 cm). AO, aorta; LA, left atrium; LV, left ventricle.

nancy) and is associated with a higher thromboembolic risk. This has been shown in several studies and appears to be most striking in the case of tilting-disk mechanical prostheses (Salazar et al., 1996; Born et al., 1992). Therefore, most experts agree that women requiring valve surgery before pregnancy should receive a bioprosthetic valve—even though repeat surgery will be necessary in the future—because these valves have a much lower thromboembolic risk and do not generally require systemic anticoagulation (Kloster, 1979). Women with normally functioning biological valve replacements tolerate pregnancy well.

Management of the last group (i.e., women with mechanical cardiac valves who become pregnant) is the most difficult. A woman with a mechanical prosthetic heart valve should be counseled strongly that pregnancy is dangerous and not recom-

mended. Unfortunately, pregnancies still do occur and must be managed. As mentioned above, warfarin is superior to heparin for preventing thromboemboli with mechanical valves. However, warfarin is teratogenic and carries a 5% to 10% risk of warfarin embryopathy (Ayhan et al., 1991; Chan et al., 2000). This risk appears to be dose dependent as well (Vitale et al., 1999). Therefore, the manufacturer of Coumadin (warfarin) in America states that the drug is absolutely contraindicated during pregnancy. Although warfarin is used during pregnancy in Europe (after the first 12 weeks) and is recommended until the 35th week of pregnancy, American physicians face a particularly difficult dilemma because of the manufacturer's contraindication (even though this contradicts guidelines from acknowledged expert panels [Elkayam, 1996; Bonow et al., 1998]). In addition, many pregnant women would prefer to put themselves rather than the fetus at risk (although a risk to themselves usually *is* a risk to the fetus). Thus, subcutaneous or intravenous heparin is used during pregnancy in most American women with mechanical heart valves, even though thromboembolic risk is higher (Evans et al., 1997; Chan, 2000). There is some evidence that low-molecular-weight heparin may be superior to unfractionated heparin in patients with mechanical prostheses (Montalescot et al., 2000), and this has been used successfully in a number of pregnant patients (Arnaout et al., 1998; Elkayam, 1999). However, because randomized trials have not been performed, more information is needed before low-molecular-weight heparin can be recommended over unfractionated heparin (Shapira et al., 2002).

Figure 41-20 shows a currently accepted protocol for anticoagulation in pregnant women with mechanical heart valves. This general method has been validated, and the risk of warfarin embryopathy appears low even if it is started during the first trimester (Sareli et al., 1989). Most authorities, however, would recommend using heparin through the first trimester unless the patient has a first-generation tilting-disk prosthesis in the mitral position (Elkayam, 1999). Consultation and close

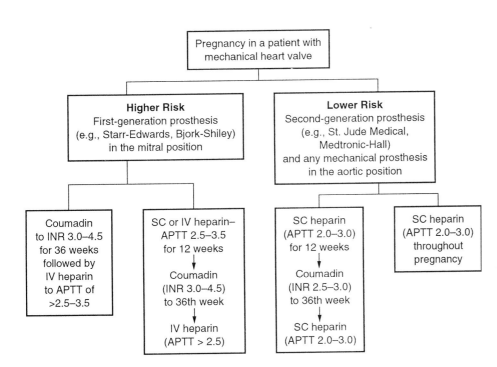

FIGURE 41-20 ■ Recommendations for anticoagulation in pregnant women with mechanical heart valves. APTT, activated partial thromboplastin time; INR, International Normalized Ratio; IV, intravenous; SC, subcutaneous. (From Elkayam U: Pregnancy through a prosthetic heart valve. J Am Coll Cardiol **33**:1642, 1999, used with permission.)

follow-up during pregnancy with an experienced cardiologist is strongly recommended, as well as obsessive attention to blood coagulation testing. Because premature labor occurs frequently in this group (Salazar et al., 1996), warfarin should be substituted with therapeutic doses of heparin at the 35th or 36th week of gestation. If labor occurs while a patient is taking warfarin, cesarean section is recommended to avoid fetal cerebral hemorrhage during vaginal delivery (Elkayam, 1996).

All patients with prosthetic heart valves require antibiotic prophylaxis for dental and surgical procedures and at delivery. Prevention of prosthetic valve endocarditis is essential, because mortality can reach 40%. The patient who experiences endocarditis with a prosthetic valve must receive aggressive antibiotic therapy and often will require valve replacement. Obviously, the risk to the fetus is exorbitant.

CARDIAC SURGERY DURING PREGNANCY

Whenever possible, any woman requiring cardiac surgery should undergo the procedure before becoming pregnant. Nevertheless, as explained previously, in rare instances a patient may require surgery during pregnancy. Valvular surgery has been performed successfully during pregnancy for many years, and patients have also undergone coronary artery bypass surgery and emergency aortic dissection repair (Becker, 1983). Cardiac surgery during pregnancy does not appear to increase maternal mortality risk (Strickland et al., 1991; Pomini et al., 1996). There is, however, a 10% to 15% risk of fetal mortality because of the nonpulsatile blood flow and hypotension associated with conventional cardiopulmonary bypass. Therefore, whenever possible, cardiac surgery should be performed without cardiopulmonary bypass. In addition, hypothermia should be avoided, because this appears to be especially dangerous to the fetus. In one study, fetal mortality was halved when normothermic was compared with hypothermic perfusion (Pomini et al., 1996). Hypothermia stimulates uterine contractions and impairs oxygen delivery to the fetus, mandating careful monitoring of the uterus and the fetal heart. The deleterious effect of hypothermia on umbilical blood flow has been documented by transvaginal ultrasound (Goldstein et al., 1995).

Experimental studies suggest that fetal survival can be improved by the use of pulsatile perfusion, but results are not yet clear. If bypass is required for cardiac surgery at an immature gestational age, high-flow high-pressure normothermic perfusion should be instituted (Parry and Westaby, 1996). If possible, surgery should be postponed until the third trimester, when the fetal risk is considerably reduced. Fetal bradycardia is often seen during surgery and may require rapid treatment, usually with intravenous nitroprusside. In addition, preterm labor occurs more frequently in women undergoing cardiac surgery.

During surgery and the immediate postoperative period, these patients should be monitored very closely. In general, use of intra-arterial and Swan-Ganz catheters and electrocardiographic monitoring of the woman and the fetus are recommended. Transesophageal echocardiography is also helpful in some cases and provides direct assessment of valvular and ventricular function. Maintenance of acceptable arterial oxygen levels and normal blood pressure, plus avoidance of hypothermia, are of utmost importance to the fetus.

REFERENCES

Abenhaim L, Moride Y, Brenot F, et al: Appetite suppressant drugs and the risk of primary pulmonary hypertension. N Engl J Med **335**:609, 1996.

ACC/AHA Guidelines for the evaluation and management of chronic heart failure in the adult: Executive summary. J Am Coll Cardiol **38**:2101, 2001.

Aeschbacher BC, Chatterjee T, Meier B: Transesophageal echocardiography to evaluate success of transcatheter closure of large secundum atrial septal defects in adults using the buttoned device. Mayo Clin Proc **75**:913, 2000.

Arias F, Pineda J: Aortic stenosis in pregnancy. J Reprod Med **20**:229, 1978.

Arnaout MS, Kazma H, Khalil A, et al: Is there a safe anticoagulation protocol for pregnant women with prosthetic valves? Clin Exp Obstet Gynecol **25**:101, 1998.

Avila WS, Grinberg M, Snitcowsky R, et al: Maternal and fetal outcome in pregnant women with Eisenmenger's syndrome. Eur Heart J **16**:460, 1995.

Ayhan A, Yapar EG, Yuce K, et al: Pregnancy and its complications after cardiac valve replacement. Int J Gynaecol Obstet **35**:117, 1991.

Bach DS, Bolling SF: Early improvement in congestive heart failure after correction of secondary mitral regurgitation in end-stage cardiomyopathy. Am Heart J **129**:1165, 1995.

Banning AP, Pearson JF, Hall RJ: Role of balloon dilatation of the aortic valve in pregnant patients with severe aortic stenosis. Br Heart J **70**:544, 1993.

Barash PG, Hobbins JC, Hook R, et al: Management of coarctation of the aorta during pregnancy. J Thorac Cardiovasc Surg **69**:781, 1975.

Barst RJ, Rubin LJ, Long WA, et al: A comparison of continuous intravenous epoprostenol (prostacyclin) with conventional therapy for primary pulmonary hypertension: The Primary Pulmonary Hypertension Study Group [see comments]. N Engl J Med **334**:296, 1996.

Beauchesne LM, Connolly HM, Ammash NM, et al: Coarctation of the aorta: Outcome of pregnancy. J Am Coll Cardiol **38**:1728, 2001.

Becker RM: Intracardiac surgery in pregnant women. Ann Thorac Surg **36**:453, 1983.

Bestetti RB: Cardiac involvement in the acquired immune deficiency syndrome. Int J Cardiol **22**:143, 1989.

Bjarnason I, Jonsson S, Hardarson T: Mode of inheritance of hypertrophic cardiomyopathy in Iceland. Br Heart J **47**:122, 1982.

Blanchard DG, Hagenhoff C, Chow L, et al: Reversibility of cardiac abnormalities in human immunodeficiency virus (HIV)-infected individuals: a serial echocardiographic study. J Am Coll Cardiol **17**:270, 1991.

Bonow RO, Carabello B, DeLeon AC, et al: ACC/AHA Guidelines for the management of patients with valvular heart disease. J Am Coll Cardiol **32**:1486, 1998.

Born D, Martinez EE, Almeid PAM, et al: Pregnancy in patients with prosthetic heart valves: The effects of anticoagulation on mother, fetus and neonate. Am Heart J **124**:413, 1992.

Boyle DM, Lloyd-Jones RL: The electrocardiographic ST segment in pregnancy. J Obstet Gynaecol Br Commonw **73**:986, 1966.

Brown OR, DeMots H, Kloster FE, et al: Aortic root dilatation and mitral valve prolapse in Marfan's syndrome: An echocardiographic study. Circulation **52**:651, 1975.

Burman D: Familial patent ductus arteriosus. Br Heart J **23**:603, 1961.

Butman S, Chandraratna PA, Milne N, et al: Stress myocardial imaging in patients with mitral valve prolapse: Evidence of a perfusion abnormality. Cathet Cardiovasc Diagn **8**:243, 1982.

Cannell DE, Vernon CP: Congenital heart disease and pregnancy. Am J Obstet Gynecol **85**:744, 1963.

Carruth JE, Mivis SB, Brogan DR, et al: The electrocardiogram in normal pregnancy. Am Heart J **102**:1075, 1981.

Chan WS, Anand S, Ginsberg JS: Anticoagulation of pregnant women with mechanical heart valves. Arch Intern Med **160**:191, 2000.

Clemens JD, Horwitz RI, Jaffe CC, et al: Controlled evaluation of the risk of bacterial endocarditis in persons with mitral valve prolapse. N Engl J Med **307**:776, 1982.

Coghlan HC, Phares P, Cowley M, et al: Dysautonomia in mitral valve prolapse. Am J Med **67**:236, 1979.

Cole P, Cook F, Plappert T: Longitudinal changes in left ventricular architecture and function in peripartum cardiomyopathy. Am J Cardiol **60**:811, 1987.

Connolly HM, Crary JL, McGoon MD, et al: Valvular heart disease associated with fenfluramine-phentermine. N Engl J Med **337**:581, 1997.

Connolly HM, Warnes CR: Ebstein's anomaly: Outcome of pregnancy. J Am Coll Cardiol **23**:1194, 1994.

Corone P, Bonaiti C, Feingold J, et al: Familial congenital heart disease: How are the various types related? Am J Cardiol **51**:942, 1983.

Craig RJ, Selzer A: Natural history and prognosis of atrial septal defect. Circulation 37:805, 1968.

Cunningham FG, Pritchard JA, Hankins GD, et al: Peripartum heart failure: Idiopathic cardiomyopathy or compounding cardiovascular events? Obstet Gynecol 67:157, 1986.

Deal K, Wooley CF: Coarctation of the aorta and pregnancy. Ann Intern Med 78:706, 1973.

de Souza JAM, Martinez EE, Ambrose JA, et al: Percutaneous balloon mitral valvuloplasty in comparison with open mitral valve commissurotomy for mitral stenosis during pregnancy. J Am Coll Cardiol 37:900, 2001.

Devereux RB, Perloff JK, Reichek N, et al: Mitral valve prolapse. Circulation 54:3, 1976.

Eckberg DL, Gault JH, Bouchard RL, et al: Mechanics of left ventricular contraction in chronic severe mitral regurgitation. Circulation 47:1252, 1973.

Efstratiou A, Singh B: Combined spontaneous postpartum coronary artery dissection and pulmonary embolism with survival. Cathet Cardiovasc Diagn 31:29, 1994.

Elkayam U: Anticoagulation in pregnant women with prosthetic heart valves: A double jeopardy. J Am Coll Cardiol 27:1704, 1996.

Elkayam U: Pregnancy through a prosthetic heart valve. J Am Coll Cardiol 33:1642, 1999.

Elkayam U, Gleicher N: Hemodynamics and cardiac function during normal pregnancy and the puerperium. In Elkayam U, Gleicher N (eds): Cardiac Problems in Pregnancy. New York, Liss, 1990.

Elkayam U, Ostrzega E, Shotan A, et al: Cardiovascular problems in pregnant women with the Marfan syndrome. Ann Intern Med 123:117, 1995.

Elkayam U, Tummala PP, Rao K, et al: Maternal and fetal outcomes of subsequent pregnancies in women with peripartum cardiomyopathy. N Engl J Med 344:1567, 2001.

Engler R, Ray R, Higgins CB, et al: Clinical assessment and follow-up of functional capacity in patients with chronic congestive cardiomyopathy. Am J Cardiol 49:1832, 1982.

Esteves CA, Ramos AIO, Braga SLN, et al: Effectiveness of percutaneous balloon mitral valvotomy during pregnancy. Am J Cardiol 68:930, 1991.

Evans W, Laifer SA, McNanley TJ, et al: Management of thromboembolic disease associated with pregnancy. J Matern Fetal Med 6:21, 1997.

Foster V, Gersh BJ, Giuliani ER, et al: The natural history of idiopathic dilated cardiomyopathy. Am J Cardiol 47:525, 1981.

Freed LA, Levy D, Levine RA, et al: Prevalence and clinical outcome of mitral-valve prolapse. N Engl J Med 341:1, 1999.

Gilon D, Buananno FS, Leavitt M, et al: Lack of evidence of an association between mitral-valve prolapse and stroke in young patients. N Engl J Med 341:8, 1999.

Ginsberg JS, Hirsh J, Turner DC: Risks to the fetus of anticoagulant therapy during pregnancy. Thromb Haemost 61:197, 1989.

Gleicher N, Midwall J, Hochberger D, et al: Eisenmenger's syndrome and pregnancy. Obstet Gynecol Surv 34:721, 1979.

Goldstein I, Jacobi P, Gutterman E, et al: Umbilical artery flow velocity during maternal cardiopulmonary bypass. Ann Thorac Surg 60:1116, 1995.

Haiat R, Halphen C: Silent pericardial effusion in late pregnancy: A new entity. Cardiovasc Intervent Radiol 7:267, 1984.

Hall JG, Pauli RM, Wilson KM: Maternal and fetal sequelae of anticoagulation during pregnancy. Am J Med 68:122, 1980.

Hameed A, Karaalp IS, Tummala PP, et al: The effect of valvular heart disease on maternal and fetal outcome. J Am Coll Cardiol 37:893, 2001.

Hardison JE: Cervical venous hum: A clue to the diagnosis of intracranial arteriovenous malformations. N Engl J Med 278:587, 1968.

Haroutunian LM, Neill CA: Pulmonary complications of congenital heart disease: Hemoptysis. Am Heart J 84:540, 1972.

Hartman N, Kramer R, Brown T, et al: Panic disorder in patients with mitral valve prolapse. Am J Psychiatry 139:669, 1982.

Heidenreich PA, Eisenberg MJ, Kee LL, et al: Pericardial effusion and AIDS: incidence and survival. Circulation 92:3229, 1995.

Hibbard JU, Lindheimer M, Lang RM: A modified definition for peripartum cardiomyopathy and prognosis based on echocardiography. Obstet Gynecol 94:311, 1999.

Hytten FE, Thompson AM: Maternal physiologic adjustments. In Assali NS (ed): Biology of Gestation. New York, Academic Press, 1968.

Johansson BW, Sievers J: Inheritance of atrial septal defect. Lancet 1:1224, 1967.

Johnson, DE, Alderman EL, Schroeder JS, et al: Transplant coronary artery disease: Histopathologic correlation with angiographic morphology. J Am Coll Cardiol 17:449, 1991.

Kalra GS, Arora R, Khan JA, et al: Percutaneous mitral commissurotomy for severe mitral stenosis during pregnancy. Cathet Cardiovasc Diagn 33:28, 1994.

Kaplan JD, Isner JM, Karas RH, et al: In vitro analysis of mechanisms of balloon valvuloplasty of stenotic mitral valves. Am J Cardiol 59:318, 1987.

Katz R, Karliner JS, Resnik R: Effects of a natural volume overload state (pregnancy) on left ventricular performance in normal human subjects. Circulation 58:434, 1978.

Kearney P, Singh H, Hutter J, et al: Spontaneous coronary artery dissection: A report of three cases and review of the literature. Postgrad Med J 69:940, 1993.

Key TC, Dittrich H, Reisner L, et al: Successful pregnancy following cardiac transplantation. Am J Obstet Gynecol 160:367, 1989.

Kloster FE: Complications of artificial heart valves. JAMA 241:2201, 1979.

Klutstein MW, Tzivoni D, Bitran D, et al: Treatment of spontaneous coronary artery dissection: Report of three cases. Cathet Cardiovasc Diag 40:372, 1997.

Kolibash AJ, Ruiz DE, Lewis RP: Idiopathic hypertrophic subaortic stenosis in pregnancy. Ann Intern Med 82:791, 1975.

Kossoy LR, Herbert CM, Wentz AC: Management of heart transplant recipients: Guidelines for the obstetrician-gynecologist. Am J Obstet Gynecol 159:490, 1988.

Koul AK, Hollander G, Moskovits N, et al: Coronary artery dissection during pregnancy and the postpartum period: two case reports and a review of the literature. Cathet Cardiovasc Intervent 52:88, 2001.

Lampert MB, Weinert L, Hibbard J, et al: Contractile reserve in patients with peripartum cardiomyopathy and recovered left ventricular function. Am J Obstet Gynecol 176:189, 1997.

Lefevre T, Bonan R, Serra A, et al: Percutaneous mitral valvuloplasty in surgical high risk patients. J Am Coll Cardiol 17:348, 1991.

Levine RA, Handschumacher MD, Sanfilippo AJ, et al: Three-dimensional echocardiographic reconstruction of the mitral valve, with implications for the diagnosis of mitral valve prolapse. Circulation 80:589, 1989.

Lewis W: AIDS: Cardiac findings from 115 autopsies. Progr Cardiovasc Dis 32:207, 1989.

Lorell BH, Paulus WJ, Grossman W, et al: Modification of abnormal left ventricular diastolic properties by nifedipine in patients with hypertrophic cardiomyopathy. Circulation 65:499, 1982.

Mabie WC, Freire MV: Sudden chest pain and cardiac emergencies in the obstetric patient. Obstet Gynecol Clin North Am 22:19, 1995.

Maekawa K, Ohnish H, Hirase T, et al: Acute myocardial infarction during pregnancy caused by coronary artery spasm. J Intern Med 235:489, 1994.

Maisel AS, Krishnaswany P, Nowalk RM, et al: Rapid measurement of B-type natriuretic peptide in the emergency diagnosis of heart failure. N Engl J Med 347:161, 2002.

Mast ST, Jollis JG, Ryan T, et al: The progression of fenfluramine-associated valvular heart disease assessed by echocardiography. Ann Intern Med 134:261, 2001.

McCaffrey RM, Dunn LJ: Primary pulmonary hypertension in pregnancy. Obstet Gynecol Surv 19:567, 1964.

McIndor AK, Hammond EJ, Babington PCB: Peripartum cardiomyopathy presenting as a cardiac arrest at induction of anaesthesia for emergency caesarean section. Br J Anaesth 75:97, 1995.

McKay RG, Safian RD, Lock JE, et al: Assessment of left ventricular and aortic valve function after aortic balloon valvuloplasty in adult patients with critical aortic stenosis. Circulation 75:192, 1987.

McMinn TR, Ross J Jr: Hereditary dilated cardiomyopathy. Clin Cardiol 18:7, 1995.

Meller J, Conde CA, Deppisch LM, et al: Myocardial infarction due to coronary atherosclerosis in three young adults with systemic lupus erythematosus. Am J Cardiol 35:309, 1975.

Mestroni L, Miani D, Di Lenarda A, et al: Clinical and pathologic study of familial dilated cardiomyopathy. Am J Cardiol 65:1449, 1990.

Metcalfe J, McAnulty JH, Ueland K: Cardiac Disease and Pregnancy: Physiology and Management. Boston, Little, Brown, 1986, p. 223.

Metcalfe J, Ueland K: Maternal cardiovascular adjustments to pregnancy. Progr Cardiovasc Dis 16:363, 1974.

Montalescot G, Polle V, Collet JP, et al: Low molecular weight heparin after mechanical heart valve replacement. Circulation 101:1083, 2000.

Morris CD, Menashe VD: Recurrence of congenital heart disease in offspring of parents with surgical correction. Clin Res 33:68A, 1985.

Murdoch JL, Walker BA, Halpern BL, et al: Life expectancy and causes of death in the Marfan syndrome. N Engl J Med 286:804, 1972.

Neilson G, Galea EG, Blunt A: Congenital heart disease and pregnancy. Med J Aust 1:1086, 1970.

Neilson G, Galea EG, Blunt A: Eisenmenger's syndrome and pregnancy. Med J Aust 1:431, 1971.

Nelson DM, Main E, Crafford W: Peripartum heart failure due to primary pulmonary hypertension. Obstet Gynecol 62:58s, 1983.

Nora JJ, Nora AH, Wexler P: Hereditary and environmental aspects as they affect the fetus and newborn. Clin Obstet Gynecol 24:851, 1981.

Oakley CM: Anticoagulants in pregnancy. Br Heart J 74:107, 1995.

Oakley GDG, McGarry K, Limb DG, et al: Management of pregnancy in patients with hypertrophic cardiomyopathy. Br Med J 1:1749, 1979.

O'Connell JB, Costanzo-Nordin MR, Subramanian R, et al: Peripartum cardiomyopathy: Clinical, hemodynamic, histologic and prognostic characteristics. J Am Coll Cardiol 8:52, 1986.

Oram S, Holt M: Innocent depression of the S-T segment and flattening of the T-wave during pregnancy. J Obstet Gynaecol Br Commonw 68:765, 1961.

Otto CM: Evaluation and management of chronic mitral regurgitation. J Engl J Med 345:740, 2001.

Ovaert C, McCrindle BW, Nykanen D, et al: Balloon angioplasty of native coarctation: Clinical outcomes and predictors for success. J Am Coll Cardiol 35:988, 2000.

Parry AJ, Westaby S: Cardiopulmonary bypass during pregnancy. Ann Thorac Surg 61:1865, 1996.

Pearson GD, Veille JC, Rahimtoola S, et al: Peripartum cardiomyopathy: NHLBI/NIH workshop recommendations and review. JAMA 283:1183, 2000.

Pelliccia F, Cianfroca C, Gaudio C, et al: Sudden death during pregnancy in hypertrophic cardiomyopathy. Eur Heart J 13:421, 1992.

Perloff JK: Pregnancy and cardiovascular disease. In Braunwald E (ed): A Textbook of Cardiovascular Disease, 3rd ed. Philadelphia, Saunders, 1988.

Perloff JK: Special facilities for the comprehensive care of adults with congenital heart disease. In Perloff JK, Child JS (eds): Congenital Heart Disease in Adults. Philadelphia, Saunders, 1991, p. 7.

Perloff JK, Child JS, Edwards JE: New guidelines for the clinical diagnosis of mitral valve prolapse. Am J Cardiol 57:1124, 1986.

Pitts JA, Crosby WM, Basta LL: Eisenmenger's syndrome in pregnancy: Does heparin prophylaxis improve the maternal mortality rate? Am Heart J 93:321, 1977.

Pomini F, Mercogliano D, Cavalletti C, et al: Cardiopulmonary bypass in pregnancy. Ann Thorac Surg 61:259, 1996.

Porras MC, Gill JZ: Intracoronary stenting for postpartum coronary artery dissection. Ann Intern Med 128:873, 1998.

Purcell IF, Williams DO: Peripartum cardiomyopathy complicating severe aortic stenosis. Int J Cardiol 52:163, 1995.

Pyeritz RE: Maternal and fetal complications of pregnancy in Marfan syndrome. Am J Med 71:784, 1981.

Pyeritz RE, McKusick VA: The Marfan syndrome: Diagnosis and management. N Engl J Med 300:772, 1979.

Raffanti SP, Chiaramida AJ, Sen P, et al: Assessment of cardiac function in patients with the acquired immunodeficiency syndrome. Chest 93:592, 1988.

Rashkind WJ, Mullins CE, Hellenbrand WE, et al: Nonsurgical closure of patent ductus arteriosus: Clinical application of the Rashkind PDA Occluder System. Circulation 75:583, 1987.

Ratnoff OD, Kaufman R: Arterial thrombosis in oral contraceptive users. Arch Intern Med 142:447, 1982.

Reid JM, Coleman EN, Doig W: Complete congenital heart block: Report of 35 cases. Br Heart J 48:236, 1982.

Reimold SC, Rutherford JD: Peripartum cardiomyopathy. N Engl J Med 344:1629, 2001.

Rezeq MN, Rickenbacher PR, Fowler MB, et al: Incidence of myocarditis in peripartum cardiomyopathy. Am J Cardiol 74:474, 1994.

Rosa FW, Bosco LA, Graham CF, et al: Neonatal anuria with maternal angiotensin-converting enzyme inhibition. Obstet Gynecol 74:371, 1989.

Ross J Jr: Left ventricular function and the timing of surgical treatment in valvular heart disease. Ann Intern Med 94:498, 1981.

Roth A, Elkayam U: Acute myocardial infarction associated with pregnancy. Ann Intern Med 125:751, 1996.

Rothman A, Beltran D, Kriett JM, et al: Graded balloon dilation atrial septostomy as a bridge to lung transplantation in pulmonary hypertension. Am Heart J 125:1763, 1993.

Rubler S, Damani PM, Pinto ER: Cardiac size and performance during pregnancy estimated with echocardiography. Am J Cardiol 40:534, 1977.

Salazar E, Espinola N, Roman L, et al: Effect of pregnancy on the duration of bovine pericardial bioprostheses. Am Heart J 137:714, 1999.

Salazar E, Izaguirre R, Verdejo J, et al: Failure of adjusted doses of subcutaneous heparin to prevent thromboembolic phenomena in pregnant patients with mechanical cardiac valve prostheses. J Am Coll Cardiol 27:1698, 1996.

Sareli P, England MJ, Berk MR: Maternal and fetal sequelae of anticoagulation during pregnancy in patients with mechanical heart valve prostheses. Am J Cardiol 63:1462, 1989.

Schroeder JS, Harrison DC: Repeated cardioversion during pregnancy: Treatment of refractory paroxysmal atrial tachycardia during 3 successive pregnancies. Am J Cardiol 27:445, 1971.

Schwartz DB, Schamroth L: The effect of pregnancy on the frontal plane QRS axis. J Electrocardiol 12:279, 1979.

Sciscione AC, Callan NA: Pregnancy and contraception: Congenital heart disease in adolescents and adults. Cardiol Clin 11:701, 1993.

Scott AA, Purohit DM: Neonatal renal failure: A complication of maternal antihypertensive therapy. Am J Obstet Gynecol 160:1223, 1989.

Shabetai R, Shine I: Heritable and familial aspects of myocardial diseases. In Fowler ND (ed): Myocardial Diseases. New York, Grune & Stratton, 1973.

Shapira Y, Sagie A, Battler A: Low-molecular-weight heparin for the treatment of patients with mechanical heart valves. Clin Cardiol 25:323, 2002.

Shell WE, Walton JA, Clifford ME, et al: The familial occurrence of the syndrome of mid-late systolic click and late systolic murmur. Circulation 39:327, 1969.

Shores J, Berger KR, Murphy EA, et al: Progression of aortic dilatation and the benefit of long-term beta-adrenergic blockade in Marfan's syndrome. N Engl J Med 330:1335, 1994.

Silberman S, Fink D, Berko RS, et al: Coronary artery bypass surgery during pregnancy. Eur J Cardiothorac Surg 10:925, 1996.

Siu SC, Colman JM, Sorensen S, et al: Adverse neonatal and cardiac outcomes are more common in pregnant women with cardiac disease. Circulation 105:2179, 2002.

Skorton DJ, Cheitlin MD, Freed MD, et al: Guidelines for training in adult cardiovascular medicine: Core Cardiology Training Symposium (COCATS). J Am Coll Cardiol 25:31, 1995.

Somerville J, Khaliq SU, Brewer AC, et al: Clinical pathologic conference: Atrial septal defect with paradoxical embolism. Am Heart J 86:822, 1973.

Spinnato JA, Kraynack BJ, Cooper MW: Eisenmenger's syndrome in pregnancy: Epidural anesthesia for elective cesarean section. N Engl J Med 304:1215, 1981.

St. John Sutton M, Cole P, Plappert M: Effects of subsequent pregnancy on left ventricular function in peripartum cardiomyopathy. Am Heart J 121:1776, 1991.

Stanger P, Cassidy SC, Girod DA, et al: Balloon pulmonary valvuloplasty: Results of the valvuloplasty and angioplasty register. Am J Cardiol 65:775, 1990.

Stevenson RE, Burton M, Ferlanto GJ, et al: Hazards of oral anticoagulant during pregnancy. JAMA 243:1549, 1980.

Strickland RA, Oliver WC Jr, Chantigian RC, et al: Anesthesia, cardiopulmonary bypass, and the pregnant patient. Mayo Clin Proc 66:411, 1991.

Sullivan JM, Ramanathan KB: Management of medical problems in pregnancy: Severe cardiac disease. N Engl J Med 313:304, 1985.

Szekely P, Turner R, Snaith L: Pregnancy and the changing pattern of rheumatic heart disease. Br Heart J 35:1293, 1973.

Tessler MJ, Hudson R, Naugler-Colville MA, et al: Pulmonary oedema in two parturients with hypertrophic obstructive cardiomyopathy (HOCM). Can J Anaesth 37:469, 1990.

Thanopoulos BD, Georgakopoulos D, Tsaousis GS, et al: Percutaneous balloon dilatation of the atrial septum: Immediate and midterm results. Heart 76:502, 1996.

Thistlethwaite PA, Tarazi RY, Giordano FJ, et al: Surgical management of spontaneous left main coronary artery dissection. Ann Thorac Surg 66:258, 1998.

Ueland K, Hansen JM: Maternal cardiovascular dynamics. II. Posture and uterine contractions. Am J Obstet Gynecol 103:1, 1969.

Ueland K, Novy MJ, Metcalfe J: Cardiorespiratory responses to pregnancy and exercise in normal women and patients with heart disease. Am J Obstet Gynecol 115:4, 1973.

Van der Leeuw-Harmsen L, de Graaff J, Chappin JJ: Peripartal cardiomyopathy. Eur J Obstet Gynaecol Reprod Biol 19:59, 1985.

Van Hoeven KH, Kitsis RN, Katz SD, et al: Peripartum versus idiopathic dilated cardiomyopathy in young women—A comparison of clinical, pathologic and prognostic features. Int J Cardiol 40:57, 1993.

Vilke GM, Mahoney G, Chan TC: Postpartum coronary artery dissection. Ann Emerg Med 32:260, 1998.

Vitale N, De Feo M, De Santo LS, et al: Dose-dependent fetal complications of warfarin in pregnant women with mechanical heart valves. J Am Coll Cardiol 33:1637, 1999.

Wann LS, Grove JR, Hess TR, et al: Prevalence of mitral prolapse by two dimensional echocardiography in healthy young women. Br Heart J **49**:334, 1983.

Warnes C: Establishing an adult congenital heart disease clinic. Am J Card Imaging **9**:11, 1995.

Whittemore R, Hobbins JC, Engle MA: Pregnancy and its outcome in women with and without surgical treatment of congenital heart disease. Am J Cardiol **50**:641, 1982.

Wood P: The Eisenmenger syndrome or pulmonary hypertension with reversed central shunt. Br Med J **701**:755, 1958.

Xie G-Y, Berk MR, Smith MD, et al: Prognostic value of Doppler transmitral flow patterns in patients with congestive heart disease. J Am Coll Cardiol **24**:132, 1994

Young D, Mark H: Fate of the patient with the Eisenmenger syndrome. Am J Cardiol **28**:658, 1971.

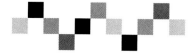

Chapter 42
THROMBOEMBOLIC DISEASE

Russell K. Laros Jr., MD, MSc

Thromboembolic disease is the leading obstetric cause of postpartum maternal mortality (MacKay et al., 2001). Fortunately, it is also a disease in which early recognition and proper treatment can improve the outcome dramatically. The pregnant patient is unique in that she is actually two patients; consequently, the usual diagnostic and therapeutic maneuvers must be modified so as not to affect the fetus adversely.

■ INCIDENCE AND PATHOPHYSIOLOGY

Incidence

Although thrombophlebitis is serious because of its potentially fatal consequences, it is, fortunately, rare in young women. Thromboembolism is reported to occur during pregnancy with a frequency of 0.5 to 3 per thousand. Events occur with equal frequency during the antepartum and postpartum periods. Although earlier studies suggested a postpartum predominance, these were probably influenced by prolonged bed rest and hospitalization after both vaginal delivery and cesarean section (Barbour and Pickard, 1995). The frequent use of high-dose estrogen for lactation suppression also may have influenced postpartum events.

The incidence of pulmonary embolism depends on whether or not deep venous thrombosis (DVT) is adequately treated. Untreated, as many as 24% of patients with antenatal DVT will have pulmonary embolism, with a mortality rate of approximately 15% (Wessler, 1976a). If patients are treated with anticoagulants, embolization occurs in only 4.5%, with a mortality rate of less than 1% (Villasanta, 1965). The importance of proper treatment with anticoagulation is clear.

Pathophysiology

More than a century ago, Virchow described a triad of factors that play an essential role in the initiation of intravascular coagulation:

1. Injury to the vessel wall
2. Stasis
3. Changes in local clotting factors

During pregnancy, thrombosis can occur without any known abnormality of the endothelium. During the first trimester, however, vein distensibility increases (McCausland et al., 1961); by the third trimester, the velocity of venous flow in the lower extremities is reduced by half, in part because the gravid uterus provides a mechanical impediment to venous return (Wright et al., 1950). This tendency toward stasis is augmented if the patient requires periods of prolonged bed rest, as in preeclampsia, threatened abortion, or premature labor.

Todd and associates (1965) have shown that fibrinogen, factor VIII, and other vitamin K–dependent clotting factors increase during pregnancy. There is evidence of decreased fibrinolytic activity with reduced levels of available circulating plasminogen activator as well (Nilsson and Kullander, 1967). Bleeding time, however, is unaffected by pregnancy (Berge et al., 1993). The risk of thromboembolism is enhanced by the following factors:

- Thrombophilia
- Lupus anticoagulant
- Cesarean section (a ninefold increase over vaginal delivery)
- Instrument delivery
- Advanced maternal age
- Increased parity
- Suppression of lactation by estrogens

Other risk factors reported (Rickles and Edwards, 1983) include the following:

- Varicosities
- Trauma or infection
- Obesity
- Blood type other than type O
- Congestive heart failure
- Dehydration
- Shock
- Disseminated cancer
- Dysproteinemia
- Polycythemia vera
- Anemia (especially sickle cell)

Additionally, a history of a prior thrombotic event in the absence of a predisposing cause or a family history of thromboembolism suggests the possibility of a defect in the physiologic antithrombotic mechanisms. Congenital defects in antithrombin III, protein C, protein S, factor V Leiden, prothrombin 20210, methylene tetrahydrofolate reductase deficiency (MTHFR), and plasminogen, as well as the presence of lupus anticoagulant, all predispose to thromboembolic events (Mueh et al., 1980; Taberino et al., 1991; Florell and Rogers, 1997). Table 42-1 outlines the various inherited thrombotic disorders and their prevalence in patients with thromboembolism.

TABLE 42-1. A CLASSIFICATION OF INHERITED THROMBOTIC DISORDERS

Deficiency	Inheritance	Prevalence (Patients with Thromboses)	Clinical Features
Plasma Factors			
ATIII	AD	1–2%	VTE
Protein C	AD	1–5%	VTE
Protein S	AD	1–5%	VTE
Factor V Leiden	AD	20–30%	VTE
Prothrombin mutation	AD	5–10%	VTE and arterial T
High factor VIII levels	?	20–25%	Recurrent VTE
High factor IX levels	?	–10%	VTE
High factor X levels	?	?	VTE
High factor XI levels	?	–10%	VTE
Impaired Clot Lysis			
Dysfibrinogenemia	AR	1–2%	Venous T > Arterial T
Plasminogen deficiency	AD and AR	1–2%	VTE
TPA deficiency	AD	?	VTE
Metabolic Defects			
Homocysteinemia (CBS)	AR	1/300,000	VTE and arterial T
Methelene tetrahydrofolate			
Reductase deficiency	AR	0–25%	VTE and arterial T (homozygous)

AD, autosomal dominant, AR, autosomal recessive; T, thrombosis; VTE, venous thromboembolism.

Adapted from Robetorye RS, Rodgers GM: Update on selected inherited venous thrombotic disorders. Am J Hematol **68**:256, 2001.

Whether or not patients hospitalized and placed at strict bed rest because of premature labor are at an increased risk for venous thromboembolism (VTE) is an area of debate. There is a single publication that reports an incidence of VTE in premature labor patients at bed rest of 15.6 cases per 1,000, compared with 0.8 cases per 1,000 in the remainder of their pregnant population (Kovacevich et al., 2000). Review of our own data over the past 25 years has not shown increased risk for patients hospitalized with premature labor.

Overall, the risk during pregnancy and postpartum is 5.5 times greater than that for nonpregnant controls (Hathaway and Bonnar, 1987). With the availability of effective contraceptives, more women are delaying childbearing, and a concomitant increase in the incidence of VTE can be expected because of the increase in maternal age.

DIAGNOSIS

It is as important to diagnose thromboembolism as it is difficult. Anticoagulation, although an invaluable therapeutic tool, is not without hazard. Therefore, the physician should be certain of this diagnosis before committing a patient to a lengthy course of treatment.

Deep Venous Thrombosis

The signs and symptoms most commonly used in the diagnosis of deep venous thrombosis (DVT) are listed in Table 42-2. Leg swelling is a measured difference between leg circumferences of greater than 2 cm. A positive Homans sign is pain in the calf when the great toe is passively dorsiflexed. Unfortunately, many of the complaints listed occur as normal physiologic changes of pregnancy. In a study by Haeger (1969),

not only were none of these symptoms or signs specific but their presence in limbs with and without thrombosis also occurred with almost equal frequency. Of patients thought to have clinically certain DVT, 45% had an entirely normal venous system by venography. Conversely, venograms in patients with pulmonary emboli have demonstrated clots in a totally asymptomatic limb (Cranley et al., 1976). In only 10% of patients is the diagnosis of DVT made before the occurrence of fatal pulmonary embolism (Coon, 1976). It appears that the more symptomatic the thrombus, the more tightly adherent it is to the vessel wall.

The diagnosis of septic pelvic thrombophlebitis may be even more difficult to confirm, and the only signs may be chills and a hectic febrile course (Duff and Gibbs, 1983). Pelvic examination is frequently unrevealing, and the diagnosis is usually made on the basis of failure to respond to a 48- to 72-hour regimen of adequate antibiotic therapy including coverage of anaerobes.

Doppler Ultrasonography

Doppler ultrasound technique has become the diagnostic study of choice in cases of suspected proximal vein occlusion

TABLE 42-2. SIGNS AND SYMPTOMS OF DEEP VENOUS THROMBOSIS

Muscle pain
Palpable deep linear cord
Tenderness
Swelling
Homans sign
Dilated superficial veins

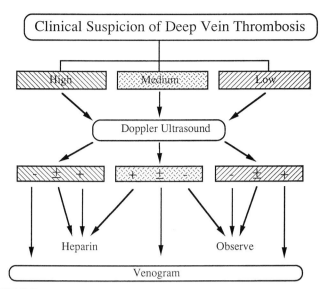

FIGURE 42-1 ■ Diagnostic algorithm for suspected deep vein thrombosis in pregnancy.

(Cronan, 1991). A 5 MHz transducer is placed over the vein. Venous flow produces a characteristic low-pitched sound that is abolished by venous occlusion. Concomitant evaluation of venous anatomy, flow, augmentation (increased flow with muscular activity in the calf), and compression (elimination of residual lumen by firm pressure with the transducer probe using one hand) yields a correct diagnosis with a high degree of sensitivity and specificity compared with venography (Lensing et al., 1989). The sensitivity and specificity in the evaluation of popliteal and femoral vein thromboses are 91% and 99%, respectively. Doppler flow studies are less effective in calf vein thrombosis, with a sensitivity and specificity of 36% and 95%, respectively (Polak and Wilkinson, 1991).

When DVT below the popliteal vein is suspected, serial measurements are necessary to rule out propagation of a clot. In a comparative study of 985 outpatients, Doppler flow studies were superior to impedance plethysmography in detecting DVT (Heijboer et al., 1993). The algorithm used by the authors to evaluate pregnant women thought to have a DVT is shown in Figure 42–1.

Venography

For years, venography has been the reference standard against which all other methods are compared. Although venography is the most specific, it has limitations—it is invasive, expensive, and difficult to interpret unless all of the deep veins are filled adequately. It cannot be used to demonstrate the pelvic venous plexus. The procedure cannot be repeated frequently, and the contrast material can cause chemical phlebitis. Venography has not often been used during pregnancy because of possible hazards to the fetus, but it is a useful tool when results of other studies are equivocal. The radiation to the fetus is only 0.0005 Gy (Ginsberg et al., 1989).

Impedance Plethysmography

This technique utilizes temporary occlusion of venous return by inflation of a thigh cuff. The occlusion causes an increase in the venous volume of the calf. Release of the cuff results in a rapid decrease in volume as the blood drains proximally. If venous obstruction is present, the rate of outflow is diminished. These changes in blood volume can be detected by measurement of electrical resistance in the calf (Toy and Schrier, 1978).

Clarke-Pearson and Jelovsek (1981) documented the reliability of this technique in the gynecologic patient and suggested that it could also be a sensitive and specific test during pregnancy; however, only a few cases of documented DVT during pregnancy have been studied with this technique, and its ultimate place in the diagnostic armamentarium remains unclear.

Ginsberg and colleagues (1989) demonstrated that the combination of Doppler ultrasound and photoplethysmography are more reliable than either study alone in predicting the presence or absence of proximal DVT. Unfortunately, pregnant patients were not included in their series.

Blood Tests for Thrombosis

Hirsh (1981) summarized several tests that reflect the formation of intravascular fibrin. Results are invariably positive when thrombosis has occurred. Unfortunately, the findings are also positive in the presence of hematomas or inflammatory exudates containing fibrin. The assay for fibrinopeptide A and the fibrin degradation product, D-dimer, are the most sensitive. The finding of a normal level of either of these essentially rules out DVT.

Pulmonary Embolism

Clinical Signs and Symptoms

Although small emboli may go unrecognized by the patient, the hallmark of pulmonary embolism is dyspnea. The major sign is tachypnea. Table 42-3 shows the signs and symptoms most frequently encountered (Sasahara et al., 1983). Small emboli become lodged more peripherally and can produce infarction accompanied by pleural signs that include cough, hemoptysis, pleuritic chest pain with splinting, and a friction rub, although for many patients, emboli infarction and its associated symptoms are absent. Leg discomfort and shortness of breath can be the result of uterine enlargement in the third trimester but may also indicate multiple small emboli. Also, multiple small emboli can mimic a major embolus. Massive pulmonary embolism, defined for clinical purposes as occlusion

TABLE 42-3. SIGNS AND SYMPTOMS OF PULMONARY EMBOLISM

Tachypnea	89*
Dyspnea	81
Pleuritic pain	72
Apprehension	59
Cough	54
Tachycardia	43
Hemoptysis	34
Temperature >37°C	34

* Percentage of patients with proven pulmonary embolism having these findings.

From Sasahara AA, Sharma GVRK, Barsamian EM, et al.: Pulmonary thromboembolism. JAMA **249**:2945, 1983. Copyright 1988, American Medical Association.

of at least 50% of the pulmonary arterial circulation, can cause symptoms suggestive of myocardial infarction, including hypotension and, occasionally, syncope or convulsions.

Tachycardia or a few atelectatic rales may be the only finding on physical examination. Massive emboli, however, can produce right-sided heart failure with jugular venous distention, an enlarged liver, a left parasternal heave, and fixed splitting of the second heart sound. Cardiac auscultation during normal pregnancy could reveal a variety of "functional" murmurs or an increase in the pulmonic second heart sound; thus, these findings are valuable only if they are clearly new.

Laboratory Studies

ELECTROCARDIOGRAM

Although the electrocardiogram (ECG) is abnormal in 90% of patients, tachycardia alone is the most common abnormality. Nonspecific T-wave inversion is found in 40%, and the classic right axis shift with strain pattern $(S_1Q_3T_3)$ is observed in those patients with extensive embolization.

ARTERIAL PaO$_2$

An arterial partial pressure of oxygen (PaO$_2$) of greater than 80 mm Hg with the patient breathing room air makes pulmonary embolism unlikely. In one study, 11.5% of patients with proven pulmonary embolism had a PaO$_2$ of between 80 and 90 mm Hg (Sasahara et al., 1983). Although a PaO$_2$ of 90 mm Hg makes the diagnosis of pulmonary embolism unlikely, if the signs and symptoms persist, additional studies are needed to better define the diagnosis.

LUNG SCANNING AND PULMONARY ARTERIOGRAPHY

Because pulmonary embolism is a diagnosis of such consequence, if it cannot be excluded on the basis of a normal PaO$_2$, a lung scan should be done. The agent of choice is microspheres of macroaggregates labeled with technetium (^{99m}Tc), which has a half-life of 6 hours. Because a 1-millicurie (mCi) dose given to the mother yields a fetal dose of only about 2 mrad, a perfusion scan is a safe procedure during pregnancy. The radiation doses yielded by the radionuclides commonly used are listed in Table 42-4. The likelihood of a pulmonary embolus depends on the nature of the scan abnormality observed. The specificity of the lung scan is significantly improved if it is coupled with a ventilation study. This is especially true if the perfusion defects are not typical of embolization or if they are accompanied by chest film abnormalities suggesting consolidation (Hull et al., 1983).

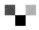

TABLE 42-4. RADIATION DOSES PRODUCED BY VARIOUS RADIONUCLIDES USED IN LUNG SCANNING

Radionuclide	Half-Life	Usual Dose (mCi)	Whole Body Radiation Dose (Gy)
^{99m}Tc	6.0 hr	3	0.0002
^{133}Xe	5.3 days	10–20	0.0044
^{127}Xe	36.4 days	5–10	0.0001
^{125}I	8.1 days	0.3	0.03
^{127}I	60.2 days	0.1–0.3	0.001

A prospective study of more than 900 patients with acute pulmonary embolism (PIOPED Investigators, 1990) showed that nearly all patients with an embolus had an abnormal ventilation-perfusion quotient ratio (V/Q) scan (high, intermediate, or low probability). Unfortunately, so did most patients without emboli (sensitivity, 98%; specificity, 10%). The sensitivity of the V/Q scan was 41% for high-probability scans, 82% for intermediate- or high-probability scans, and 98% for low-, intermediate-, or high-probability scans. The specificities were 97%, 52%, and 10%, respectively. The diagnostic algorithm that we currently use (Fig. 42-2) combines several diagnostic studies, including pulmonary arteriography. Pulmonary angiography is indicated if surgical intervention is contemplated. In attempting to assess anticoagulation failures requiring caval interruption, this method is the only one capable of reliably distinguishing between recurrent embolism and fragmentation and distal migration of the original clot.

SPIRAL COMPUTED TOMOGRAPHY

Spiral computed tomography (CT) angiography is being used with increasing frequency for the evaluation of patients thought to have a pulmonary embolism. At this author's institution, it has largely replaced the ventilation/perfusion lung scan in the diagnostic algorithm used.

Spiral CT achieves angiogram-like views of the pulmonary circulation and can be acquired with a single breath hold. The sensitivity for diagnosis of pulmonary embolism at the segmental pulmonary artery level is approximately 95%, and the specificity is 98% (Van Erkel et al., 1996; Van Rossum et al., 1996). Sensitivity is lower when obstruction is at the subsegmental level; however, the specificity of spiral CT for and the clinical significance of such emboli is thus far unclear.

OTHER LABORATORY STUDIES

A preliminary study suggests that magnetic resonance angiography (MRA) with gadolinium shows high sensitivity and specificity compared with conventional pulmonary angiography (Meaney et al., 1997). Laboratory examinations are typically unrevealing, although the white blood cell count, serum lactate dehydrogenase (LDH), bilirubin, and erythrocyte sedimentation rate (ESR) may be elevated.

As discussed, fibrin split products are always present; however, they can be found in uncomplicated pregnancy and in most postoperative patients. Their absence, however, essentially excludes the possibility of embolism (Hirsh, 1981).

When a family history of repeated thromboembolism is encountered, the levels of antithrombin III, protein C, protein S, and factor V Leiden, prothrombin 20210, and methylenetetrahydrofolate reductase deficiency (MTHFR) should be studied (Mackie et al., 1978; Griffin et al., 1981; Comp and Esmon, 1984; Rosendaal, 1997; Florell and Rogers, 1997). Lupus anticoagulant can also cause venous thrombosis (Hallak et al., 1997). Because of the approximately 50% prevalence, studies for these factors should be done as part of the evaluation of a parturient with thromboembolism.

MANAGEMENT OF THROMBOEMBOLIC DISEASE

Anticoagulation therapy (discussed later in this chapter) is the mainstay of therapy for deep thrombophlebitis with or

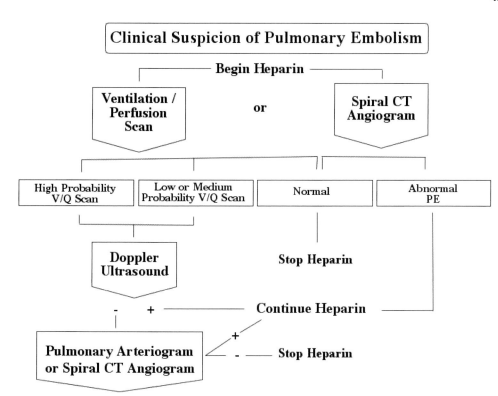

Clinical Suspicion of Pulmonary Embolism

Begin Heparin

Ventilation / Perfusion Scan   or   Spiral CT Angiogram

High Probability V/Q Scan | Low or Medium Probability V/Q Scan | Normal | Abnormal PE

Doppler Ultrasound

Stop Heparin

−   + — Continue Heparin —

Pulmonary Arteriogram or Spiral CT Angiogram — + − Stop Heparin

FIGURE 42–2 ■ Diagnostic algorithm for suspected pulmonary embolism in pregnancy. (Adapted from Hull RD, Hirsh J, Carter CJ, et al: Pulmonary angiography, ventilation lung scanning, and venography for clinically suspected pulmonary embolism with abnormal perfusion lung scan. Ann Intern Med **98**:891, 1983.)

without pulmonary embolism. For both entities, however, a number of additional modalities can help achieve symptomatic relief.

Deep Venous Thrombosis

Bed rest with elevation of the involved extremity is valuable initially because it promotes venous return and decreases edema. The Trendelenburg position, which involves elevating the foot of the bed by approximately 8 inches, is preferable to using pillows, which can impede femoral flow because they flex the hip. The patient may be supplied with a foot board and instructed in the performance of hourly flexion and extension exercises of both lower extremities. As soon as symptoms permit, however, the patient should be encouraged to ambulate, as bed rest itself can enhance venous stasis. There is no evidence that bed rest will prevent embolus detachment. Sitting with legs dependent is contraindicated. Application of moist heat to involved areas can be beneficial. Although moist heat is more effective than dry heat, it is useless unless hot packs are replaced as frequently as they cool. Analgesic drugs may be required, but those that affect platelet function (e.g., aspirin) must be avoided while anticoagulants are being used. Anti-inflammatory drugs, although useful agents, are generally contraindicated during pregnancy.

When correctly designed, elastic stockings increase the velocity of venous flow. The pressure gradient should decrease from ankle to thigh without a constricting garter at the top. Certain brands designed for ambulatory patients can be overly compressive if one is in the recumbent position. Elastic bandages, once in vogue, are best avoided because they are easily wrapped incorrectly with the greatest pressure ending at the top, thus impeding venous return.

Pulmonary Embolism

If an embolic source can be traced to the lower extremities, the aforementioned measures can be employed. In addition, specific treatment of the embolus is required. Oxygen therapy is particularly important during pregnancy because even if the mother survives, the fetus could die or be damaged secondary to maternal hypoxia. The maternal PaO_2 should be maintained above 70 mm Hg. Positive pressure administration could be required if pulmonary edema is present. Meperidine or morphine may be used for pain and apprehension. Bed rest is indicated for at least 5 to 7 days, allowing time for the initial organization of the clot. Straining at stool is best avoided, and stool softeners may prove helpful.

A vasoactive amine, such as isoproterenol or dopamine, is indicated for treatment of shock. The objective is to increase the mean arterial pressure and the flow through the pulmonary vasculature. Isoproterenol (1 mg mixed in 500 mL of normal saline yielding 2 µg/mL) is given at 2 to 8 µg/minute, and dopamine (200 mg in 500 mL of normal saline yielding 400 µg/mL) is started at 200 µg/minute. Administration of both fluids and vasoactive amines should be monitored via a Swan-Ganz catheter measuring pulmonary artery and wedge pressure (see Chapter 45).

Aminophylline and digoxin may also be useful. Aminophylline decreases reflex bronchospasm and has a diuretic action that is particularly useful if pulmonary edema is present. Digoxin can be administered if heart failure is present but is rarely of benefit. Aminophylline (250 mg in 500 mL of normal saline yielding 500 µg/mL) is infused rapidly over 20 minutes to give a dose of 4–5 mg/kg of body weight. The infusion is then slowed to 12 to 15 µg/kg/minute). The dosage is adjusted to achieve a serum concentration of 10 to 20 mg/mL. Antibiotics are not indicated unless a septic embolus is suspected.

Anticoagulation

Currently, three major types of therapeutic agents are available for treating thrombosis. Each is directed at a different portion of the coagulation process. They consist of the following:

1. Agents that interfere with platelet adhesion and aggregation
2. Agents that interfere with fibrin formation
3. Agents that facilitate clot lysis

Although it is agreed that proximal DVT should be treated by anticoagulation, the need for treatment of thrombosis below the level of the popliteal fossa remains in dispute. Because approximately 20% of lower leg DVTs extend proximally and heparin can prevent this spread, many believe that treatment is required (Bentley et al., 1980). An alternative is frequent Doppler flow studies or impedance plethysmography to document that extension has not occurred. In essence, one must balance the risks of anticoagulation with the benefits of preventing proximal extension.

Agents that interfere with fibrin formation are by far the most important in treating thromboembolism, and in the United States they are heparin and the coumarin derivatives. Heparin is the preferred agent in the initial treatment of thromboembolism, but for long-term management in the nonpregnant state, conversion to a coumarin derivative is usually ideal. For reasons to be discussed shortly, this author believes that heparin should be the preferred drug throughout pregnancy with the exception of those patients with mechanical heart valve prostheses or with antithrombin III deficiency.

Heparin

UNFRACTIONATED HEPARIN

Heparin is a naturally occurring mucopolysaccharide organic base found within mast cells of most mammals. In plasma, it combines with an alpha-globulin, known as antithrombin III (AT-III), to become a potent inhibitor of thrombin (thus preventing conversion of fibrinogen to fibrin) and to increase the circulating level of activated factor X (Xa) inhibitor (Rosenberg, 1987). Heparin has only a minimal antiplatelet effect and does not stimulate fibrinolysis or directly lyse thrombi (Wessler and Gitel, 1979). Commercial preparations of unfractionated heparin are heterogeneous, with molecular weights from 3000 to 30,000 (mean molecular weight = 15,000).

Because of its large size and negative charge, heparin does not cross the placenta or appear in breast milk; both features are advantageous when anticoagulation is required during pregnancy or lactation. If necessary, heparin effects can be reversed rapidly with protamine sulfate in a dose of 1 mg/100 units of administered heparin. (When constant infusion methods are used, twice the amount necessary to neutralize the hourly dose should be sufficient.) No more than 50 mg should be given over any 10-minute period because protamine itself can cause bleeding. Heparin is used primarily to prevent either initiation or propagation of venous thromboembolism.

THERAPEUTIC DOSE THERAPY

There is evidence that monitoring the dose of heparin affects the recurrence rate of thrombotic events (Hirsch, 1991a). Lack of adequate anticoagulation increases the risk of

recurrence by 11- to 15-fold. Optimal anticoagulation is obtained with an activated partial thromboplastin time (aPTT) of 1.5 to 2.5 times control (60–80 seconds). Spontaneous hemorrhage frequently occurs if the aPTT exceeds 135 seconds for periods longer than 12 hours. The circulating level of heparin is a balance between input of new drug, rapid metabolism, and excretion either directly by the kidneys or indirectly by diffusion into extravascular spaces. Before heparin is initiated, a complete blood count (CBC), platelet count, prothrombin time (PT), aPTT, and urinalysis are obtained. Heparin should not be used except in extraordinary circumstances if the platelet count is below 50×10^9/liter.

The initial loading dose for patients with a pulmonary embolus is 150 units/kg. For patients with uncomplicated DVT, the loading dose is 100 units/kg, with a minimum of 5000 units. The half-life of heparin is approximately 1.5 hours. Following the loading dose, the initial infusion rate should be 15–25 units/kg/hour. An aPTT should be obtained 4 hours after the loading dose and after each dosage change, and adjustments should be made according to the scheme outlined in Table 42-5. Once a steady state has been achieved, aPTT should be obtained daily.

A useful method for administering a heparin infusion is to mix 15,000 units of heparin in 250 mL of 5% dextrose in water, yielding a concentration of 60 units/mL. When a very large amount of thrombus is present, heparin resistance is created by release of large amounts of platelet factor IV. The level of circulating heparin should be decreased under circumstances of recent bleeding, hematologic disorders associated with bleeding, previous antithrombotic therapy, or surgery within the previous 10 days.

Continuous intravenous heparin should be administered for 3–5 days for active thromboembolic disease or until symptoms have resolved and there is no evidence of recurrence (Hull et al., 1990). At this point, the patient may be switched to subcutaneous heparin or oral coumarin if long-term anticoagulation is indicated. If warfarin is to be used, it should be started as soon as possible. Heparin is well absorbed after subcutaneous administration and should never be administered intramuscularly because of the high incidence of hematoma formation. When an intermittent subcutaneous regimen is used for chronic therapy, the total daily dose should be divided by two or three and administered every 8–12 hours. Once a stable dose of subcutaneous heparin has been achieved, aPTT monitoring can be decreased to a weekly and, eventually, a monthly basis. The dose will change throughout the course of pregnancy as the blood volume changes (Whitfield et al., 1983).

Treatment for DVT or pulmonary embolism should last for 4–6 months. One study has shown a twofold increase in the rate of recurrence in patients treated for 6 weeks compared with 6 months (Schulman et al., 1995). When a second recurrence has occurred, indefinite anticoagulation is associated with a much lower rate of another episode (Schulman et al., 1997). There could be an increased risk of serious hemorrhage with indefinite anticoagulation, however.

When the first episode of DVT occurs during pregnancy, an adjusted dose regimen of heparin should be used for 4–6 months; this is followed by a prophylactic dose for the remainder of pregnancy, labor, and delivery and for 6–12 weeks postpartum. If a pulmonary embolism has occurred, therapy with an adjusted-dose regimen should be extended to 6 months. Similarly, therapy should be extended for patients

TABLE 42-5. DOSAGE ADJUSTMENTS FOR CONTINUOUS HEPARIN INFUSION

aPTT (sec)	Bolus (U/kg)	Hold Infusion (min)	Rate Change (U/hr)	Repeat aPTT (hr)
<50	70	0	+200	4–5
50–59	0	0	+100	4–5
60–80	0	0	0	next A.M.
81–99	0	0	−100	4–5
>100	0	60	−200	4–5

A.M., morning; aPTT, activated partial thromboplastin time.

Adapted from American College of Obstetricians and Gynecologists: ACOG Educational Bulletin No. 234, March 1997.

with iliofemoral venous thrombosis and recurrent DVT. An adjusted dose heparin regimen is accomplished by administration of the drug subcutaneously every 12 hours and adjustment of the dose to achieve an aPTT of 1.5 times control at 6 hours (40–60 seconds). This regimen is as effective as full-dose warfarin therapy in preventing recurrent DVT (Hull et al., 1982).

PROPHYLACTIC DOSE THERAPY

Minidose heparin is effective in preventing thromboembolism. The rationale for using small doses centers on the concept that a critical concentration of factor Xa (activated factor X) is required for thrombus formation. Heparin markedly enhances the action of the major inhibitor of Xa (AT-III). It takes much less heparin to inhibit factor Xa than to prevent clotting once thrombin has been formed. A standard minidose regimen employs only 5000 U of heparin subcutaneously every 12 hours. This dose is insufficient to do more than minimally prolong the aPTT. An alternative regimen is 5000 U every 12 hours during the first trimester, 7500 U every 12 hours during the second trimester, and 10,000 U every 12 hours during the third trimester (Kakkar et al., 1975; Barbour and Pickard, 1995). Although this increased dose is required to achieve the same level of Xa inhibition, no data have confirmed increased prophylactic benefit. Consequently, there is no need to monitor dosage and no increase in hemorrhagic complications. The only adverse effect reported is a slight increase in the number of wound hematomas when the regimen is used during the perioperative period. Multiple studies confirm that minidose heparin prophylaxis in patients undergoing abdominothoracic surgery markedly decreases the incidence of DVT (Gallus et al., 1973; Wessler, 1976b; Consensus Conference, 1986). In one multicenter trial, the incidence of fatal pulmonary embolism was also reduced (Kakkar et al., 1995).

If the previous thromboembolic event did not occur during a pregnancy, therapy is used for 6–12 weeks postpartum. If the thromboembolic event occurred during an earlier pregnancy, prophylaxis is started at an early gestational age and continued for 4–6 weeks postpartum. In the latter circumstance, it is useful to administer heparin peripartally and to then switch to warfarin during the puerperium. These and other clinical situations are covered with possible approaches in Table 42-6. Few or no data are available to guide therapy in most situations, and many approaches are acceptable. A recent study by Gerhardt and associates (2000), however provides the best available data to help clinicians in making the risk-benefit decision of whether or not to prophylactically anticoagulate a patient with thrombophilia (Table 42-7).

A recent multicenter study of 125 women with a single episode of thromboembolism withheld antepartum heparin (Brill-Edwards et al., 2000). Anticoagulation with minidose heparin and warfarin was begun within 24 hours of delivery, and the dose of warfarin was adjusted to achieve an international normalization ratio of 2.0–3.0. There were three antepartum and three postpartum episodes of recurrent thromboembolism. Three of the six were found to have factor V Leiden deficiency, two had protein S deficiency, and one had no thrombophilic state. Had all patients been screened for thrombophilia, the antepartum recurrence risk would have been 1 of 125 or 0.8%. This author believes that this treatment option should be discussed with patients who have been screened appropriately for thrombophilia. Patients who choose not to be treated will eventually provide additional data on the risk of recurrence in women with absolutely no risk factors.

The major risk of heparin therapy is hemorrhage. The incidence is approximately 4% in properly monitored, nonsurgical patients receiving heparin via the intravenous route (Basu et al., 1972). Heparin also causes osteoporosis when administered in doses greater than 15,000 units/day for more than 6 months (Griffith et al., 1965). This can be a problem during pregnancy (De Swiet et al., 1983). A prospective study found radiologic evidence of osteoporosis in 17% of 25 pregnant patients on full-dose heparin (Dahlman et al., 1990). This side effect can be diminished by administration of adequate amounts of calcium and vitamin D.

Other rare effects of heparin include hypotension, alopecia, allergic reactions, pain at the injection site, and thrombocytopenia. Thrombocytopenia can be caused either by an immune reaction or by heparin-associated platelet aggregation and agglutination. The mild form of thrombocytopenia relating to aggregation and agglutination is self-limiting, and no therapy is necessary. A review of studies of patients treated with porcine heparin revealed only a 3% incidence of thrombocytopenia (Chong, 1995).

The severe form of thrombocytopenia is due to heparin-dependent immunoglobulin-G (IgG) antiplatelet antibodies and necessitates cessation of heparin therapy. Low-molecular-weight heparin (LMWH) has been tolerated in patients experiencing severe thrombocytopenia with standard heparin preparations (Warkentin et al., 1995). Thrombocytopenia is more frequent with bovine lung heparin than with heparin derived from porcine gut. Because of the risk of thrombocytopenia, a platelet count should be obtained periodically for the first 3 weeks of therapy regardless of which heparin dosing regimen is used.

TABLE 42-6. ACCEPTABLE REGIMENS FOR ANTICOAGULATION

Clinical Situation	Anticoagulation Regimen
Varicosities	None; monitor for other VTE risks
Superficial thrombophlebitis	None
Hypercoagulable states with previous VTE	
Antithrombin III deficiency	Therapeutic
Protein C deficiency or factor V Leiden plus prothrombin mutation	Prophylactic starting 4–6 weeks before gestational age of prior event and for 12 weeks postpartum
Prothrombin 20210 or factor V Leiden alone	Postpartum only
Homozygous methelene tetrahydrofolate reductase deficiency	Postpartum only
Hypercoagulable states without previous venous thromboembolism	None, monitor for other VTE risks or postpartum only
Previous deep VTE without any hypercoagulable state	Prophylactic or postpartum only
Antiphospholipid antibody syndrome	
With previous venous thromboembolism	Therapeutic
Without previous venous thromboembolism or fetal loss	None; monitor for other VTE risks
Recurrent VTE on chronic anticoagulation	Therapeutic
Recurrent VTE not anticoagulated	Prophylactic
VTE in current pregnancy	Therapeutic until 4–6 months postpartum or therapeutic for 4–6 months and prophylactic until 6–12 weeks postpartum
Artificial heart valves	Therapeutic heparin for 1st 12 weeks, warfarin from 12 through 35 weeks, and therapeutic heparin thorough delivery

VTE, venous thromboembolism.

Adapted from American College of Obstetricians and Gynecologists: ACOG Educational Bulletin No. 234, March 1997; American College of Obstetricians and Gynecologists: ACOG Practice Bulletin No. 19, August 2000; McColl MD, Walker ID, Greer IA: The role of inherited thrombophilia in venous thromboembolism associated with pregnancy, Br J Obstet Gynaecol **106**:756, 1999.

LOW-MOLECULAR-WEIGHT HEPARIN

In recent years, there has been a great deal of interest in LMWH (Hirsh and Levine, 1992; Sturridge and Letsky, 1994; Nelson-Piercy et al., 1997). LMWHs consist of a portion of the various sized molecules that make up standard heparin. Those molecules having fewer than 18 saccharide moieties (molecular weight less than 5400) are unable to bind AT-III and thrombin simultaneously. Thus, they are able to catalyze the inhibition of factor Xa by AT-III but not the accelerated inactivation of thrombin by AT-III. This property should allow LMWHs to produce less microvascular bleeding while retaining an equivalent antithrombotic effect with standard heparin. Additionally, LMWHs have a longer plasma half-life, and their anticoagulant response to weight-adjusted doses is less variable. The incidence of severe thrombocytopenia and osteoporosis is lower than for unfractionated heparin. The major disadvantage is the tenfold price excess over standard heparin.

TABLE 42-7. PROBABILITY OF VENOUS THROMBOEMBOLISM DURING PREGNANCY FOR WOMEN WITH SELECTED THROMBOPHILIA

Diagnosis	Probability (%)	95% Confidence Interval (%)
No risk factors	0.03	0.02–0.04
Factor V Leiden	0.25	0.20–0.30
Prothrombin G20210A	0.50	0.30–0.80
ATIII (<80% of normal)	0.40	0.30–0.60
Protein C (<75% of normal)	0.10	0.04–0.13
Factor V Leiden plus prothrombin G20210A	4.60	2.60–8.20

Adapted from Gerhardt A, Scharf RE, Beckman MW, et al.: Prothrombin and factor V mutations in women with a history of thrombosis during pregnancy and the puerperium. N Engl J Obstet Gynecol **342**:374, 2000.

Three preparations of LMWH are currently available in the United States. Characteristics of the various preparations, including therapeutic and prophylactic dosages, are summarized in Table 42-8. To date, the greatest published experience is with enoxaperin, which has been shown to be an effective and safe alternative to unfractionated heparin (Nelson-Piercy et al., 1997; Ellison et al., 2000; Eldor, 2001; Lepercq et al., 2001).

Two areas of uncertainty are proper therapeutic dosing during pregnancy and how to avoid the risk of subdural hematoma when conduction anesthesia is used in a patient receiving LMWH. There is clear data showing that the pharmokinetics of enoxaparin during pregnancy differs for the same women when not pregnant (Casele et al., 1999). During early and late pregnancy, the maximum concentration and the plasma activity versus time are significantly lower. This is thought to be due to increased renal clearance during pregnancy. Until more data become available, this author's practice has been to obtain an anti-Xa activity level after initiating a therapeutic regimen of enoxaparin and to repeat the level periodically every two to three months. Anti-Xa levels should also be monitored in women with morbid obesity and significant renal disease. The therapeutic target is a level of 0.5 to 1.5 IU/mL 4 hours after a dose (Busby et al., 2001). Table 42-9 outlines a regimen for correcting the dose of enoxaparin.

The second issue is the risk of intraspinal hematoma formation. Prior to the availability of LMWHs, intraspinal hematoma formation was a very rare complication of conduction anesthesia. The Society of Regional Anesthesia recommends that patients receiving a therapeutic dose of LMWH not receive epidural or spinal anesthesia for at least 24 hours after the last dose of LMWH (American Society of Regional Anesthesia, 1998). This author's approach is to switch patients to unfractionated heparin at 36 to 38 weeks' gestation using dosing as outlined previously.

TABLE 42-8. CHARACTERISTICS OF LOW-MOLECULAR-WEIGHT HEPARIN

Characteristics	Agent		
	Enoxaparin	Tinzaperin	Dalteparin
Molecular Weight (Daltons)			
<2,000	≤20%	<10%	3–15%
2,000–8,000	≥68%	60–72%	65–78%
> 8,000	≤15%	22–36%	14–26%
Half-Life	4.5 hours	3.9 hours	2.5 hours
Pregnancy			
Teratogenicity	Category B	Category B	Category X
Dosage			
Therapeutic	1 mg/kg q12h or 1.5 mg/kg q24h	175 IU/kg q24h	Not approved
Prophylactic	40 mg q24h	Not approved	2,500 IU q24h

Adapted from Sifton DW, Murray L, Kelly GL (eds): Physicians' Desk Reference. Montvale, NJ, Medical Economics Company, Inc., 2002.

Coumarin Agents

Of the various coumarin derivatives available, sodium warfarin (Coumadin) is the most widely used in managing thromboembolic disease. Its therapeutic efficacy lies in its ability to inhibit the actions of vitamin K. Vitamin K functions in the liver as a cofactor in the synthesis of four essential clotting factors: factor VII, factor IX, factor X, and prothrombin (Hirsh, 1991b).

As a small molecule loosely bound to albumin, warfarin easily crosses the placenta and is excreted in breast milk (Wessler and Gitel, 1984). For these reasons, its use during pregnancy can be extremely hazardous. If warfarin is administered during the first trimester (especially the fourth through eighth weeks), a syndrome that phenotypically resembles the Conradi-Hunermann type of chondrodysplasia punctata can result (Shaul and Hall, 1977). These children are born with multiple congenital anomalies, including nasal cartilage hypoplasia, stippling of bones, slight intrauterine growth retardation (IUGR), and brachydactyly. Warfarin can cause birth defects even if it is first administered in the second and third trimesters. Three children with microcephaly, bifrontal narrowing, mental retardation, and ophthalmologic abnormalities are known (Stevenson et al., 1980). It is postulated that the first-trimester anomalies could be secondary to either a direct teratogenic effect, use of warfarin, or a vitamin K deficiency effect, whereas second-trimester and third-trimester defects may result from fetal hemorrhage.

The primary problem of warfarin administration during the last two trimesters has been fetal and placental hemorrhage resulting in fetal demise. In a collected series of 214 patients, 25 fetuses died—a fetal mortality rate of 11.7% (Laros, 1975). Most such events, however, appear to be secondary to the trauma of delivery itself (Bloomfield, 1970). In a prospective study of 23 women with heart valve prostheses who conceived 40 times, the fetal wastage exceeded 80% (Lutz et al., 1978).

Although most investigators believe that coumarin therapy is contraindicated during pregnancy, Hall and associates (1980) state that two thirds of pregnancies exposed to coumarin derivatives resulted in normal infants and that heparin was not a clearly superior alternative. We disagree and think that coumarin derivatives should be used during pregnancy only in patients who are unable to master self-administration of heparin, who exhibit allergic reactions, who have a mechanical heart valve prosthesis *in situ*, or in cases of antithrombin III deficiency. In these cases, heparin should be used for the acute episode and until 14 weeks of gestation, at which point warfarin should be substituted. Warfarin should be stopped and heparin substituted well in advance of labor. The patient should be fully informed of the potential risks of using coumarin (and all other vitamin K antagonists) during pregnancy.

Evidence suggests that the antithrombotic effect of warfarin is largely related to reduction in circulating levels of factors IX and X, whereas untoward bleeding seems more closely related to the level of factor VII. Large loading doses tend to greatly depress factor VII (which has a half-life of only 6 hours) and produce bleeding. Thus, a good therapeutic dosage schedule aims at a smooth reduction in circulating levels of all of these factors. The usual anticoagulating dose of warfarin is 5 mg daily until a therapeutic prolongation of the PT is achieved. An appropriate International Normalized Ratio (INR) for either prevention or treatment of DVT or for an *in situ* tissue cardiac valve is 2.0–3.0. If a mechanical cardiac valve is present, the dose should be adjusted to achieve an INR of 3.0–4.5. The

TABLE 42-9. ADJUSTING ENOXAPARIN DOSAGE BASED ON ANTI-Xa LEVELS

Anti-Xa Level (IU/ml)	Dose	Repeat
<0.35	Increase 25%	24 hours to 1 week
0.35–0.49	Increase 10%	24 hours to 1 week
0.5–1.0	No change	q week to month
1.1–1.5	Decrease 20%	24 hours to 1 week
1.6–2.0	Decrease 30%	24 hours to 1 week
>2.0	None; restart when <0.5, restart at 40% original	24 hours

Adapted from Busby LT, Weyman A, Rodgers GM: Excessive anticoagulation in patients with mild renal insufficiency receiving long-term therapeutic enoxaparin. Am J Hematol **67**:54, 2001.

INR, rather than simply the PT, should be used because it corrects for variations in the potency of the thromboplastins used by different laboratories. Thereafter, a maintenance dose of 3–20 mg daily is utilized. Initially, the PT is monitored daily for 5–7 days, then twice weekly for 1 to 2 weeks, and then weekly for several months, depending on the stability of the response. During the first 5–7 days of warfarin therapy, heparin is continued. Because heparin can prolong PT by 2–4 seconds, the PT should be at least 2.5 times the control value by the time heparin is discontinued. Alternatively, heparin can be withdrawn in gradual decrements.

A number of drugs affect the activity of the coumarin derivatives (Koch-Weser and Sellers, 1971). Agents increasing the activity of warfarin include salicylates, phenothiazines, phenylbutazone, and antibiotics; ethyl alcohol and barbiturates decrease its activity. Fever, diarrhea, and a change in the intake of leafy green vegetables also have an effect.

As mentioned, warfarin is discontinued and heparin therapy is resumed well in advance of labor. The average half-life for disappearance of the drug is 44 hours (Wessler and Gitel, 1984). It is not known exactly how long it takes for the effects of oral anticoagulation on the fetus to wear off, but it could be between 3 and 14 days (Pridmore et al., 1975). If spontaneous labor occurs while the patient is still taking warfarin, its effects can be reversed by administering vitamin K and fresh frozen plasma. A single dose of 5 mg of vitamin K_3, given orally or subcutaneously, begins to normalize the prothrombin time within 6 hours. Higher doses (e.g., 25–50 mg) normalize the PT slightly more rapidly but also render the patient refractory to reanticoagulation for 10 days to 2 weeks. Because there is some experimental and clinical evidence that vitamin K crosses the placenta, its administration could enhance the rate of return of fetal clotting factors as well (Hirsh et al., 1972). Immediately after delivery, the infant is given 1 mg of vitamin K intramuscularly. If the newborn shows signs of bleeding, if it is younger than 35 weeks of gestation, or if a difficult instrument delivery took place, fresh frozen plasma, 5 mL/kg, may be required as well.

Many surgeons and cardiologists are concerned that the literature has not documented that heparin is as effective as warfarin at preventing thromboses on prosthetic heart valves. Several case reports of heparin failure have heightened their concerns. An alternative proposed by Lee and associates (1986) is a switch to adjusted-dose heparin as soon as pregnancy is confirmed. Heparin therapy is continued throughout the first trimester and reinstituted 3 weeks before term. Warfarin is used throughout the second trimester and most of the third.

Because the relative risks of these alternative approaches are unknown, this author believes that patients already taking coumarin agents and desiring to conceive (e.g., patients with prosthetic heart valves) should be switched to heparin prior to conception. Patients who inadvertently receive oral agents during the first trimester (for longer than the first 14–21 days after conception) must be advised of the risks involved and given the option of terminating the pregnancy.

Intrapartum, Intraoperative, and Postpartum Anticoagulation

Selected patients (i.e., those with recent pulmonary embolization, recent iliofemoral thrombosis, and heart valve prostheses) should be continued on a medium-dose heparin regimen during delivery or surgery. When hospitalized, these patients are switched to a regimen of continuous intravenous heparin. The dose should be adjusted to achieve an aPTT 1–1.5 times control during labor and delivery. Continuing this regimen does not increase the incidence of postpartum hemorrhage in a normal delivery; however, there is a slight increase in the incidence of episiotomy hematoma, and it could contribute to blood loss in patients with uterine atonia or retained placenta (Pridmore et al., 1975). Conduction anesthesia is contraindicated in these patients and in patients who have received LMWH within the prior 24 hours.

Full doses of heparin with LMWH should be reinstituted 6 hours after delivery or surgery. Warfarin may be started as soon as the patient resumes oral intake. Heparin is then discontinued 5–7 days later, as described previously. Oral agents should be continued for 4–6 months postpartum, depending on the seriousness of the condition. Clotting factors tend to return to normal approximately 8 weeks after delivery (Lee et al., 1986).

Warfarin can be monitored successfully on an outpatient basis, as described by Davis and coworkers (1977). In 263 patients followed over 5 years by means of serial hematocrit studies, PTs, and urinalyses, major bleeding episodes developed in only 4% and minor bleeding in another 4%.

A study of 68 patients with DVTs indicated that the administration of therapeutic doses of warfarin was superior to long-term administration of minidose heparin at preventing new episodes of thromboembolism (Hull et al., 1979). As already discussed, however, adjusted-dose heparin has been equivalent to warfarin at preventing recurrent DVT and is associated with a lower risk of bleeding.

Controversy exists regarding the safety of allowing women to take warfarin while nursing. Two studies of warfarin suggest that it does not pose a major risk to breast-fed infants (De Swiet and Lewis, 1977; Orme et al., 1977). Other vitamin K antagonists, however, do appear in the breast milk in large quantities and can lead to hemorrhagic complications (Bramel and Hunter, 1950; Illingworth and Finch, 1959). Estrogen suppression of lactation is contraindicated because of a tenfold increase in venous thrombosis in mothers over age 25 years (Daniel et al., 1967).

Alternative Therapy

Fibrinolytic Agents

Fibrinolytic agents can provide a more rapid return to the normal physiologic state and diminish long-term disability. They should be considered an adjunct to rather than a substitute for anticoagulant therapy. The challenge for the clinician is proper selection of the patient who will benefit from fibrinolytic therapy and will not have a major hemorrhagic complication.

Two first-generation fibrinolytic agents, streptokinase (SK) and urokinase (UK), have undergone extensive trials and are now available for clinical use. Both agents act to increase plasmin formation and thus the rate of clot lysis (Porter and Goodnight, 1977). In acute DVT, SK produces total clot lysis in 30%–50% of patients. Both SK and UK produce rapid resolution of pulmonary emboli evident on angiography, as noted by improvement in pulmonary hemodynamics (Urokinase

Pulmonary Embolism Trial, 1970, 1974). There are only a few case reports of use during pregnancy, and thus conclusions as to safety must be withheld (Ludwig, 1973; Delclos and Davilla, 1986; Kramer et al., 1995). Because of severe postpartum hemorrhage from the placental site, these agents should not be used for the first 10 postpartum days. UK should not be used in patients who have undergone anticoagulation therapy, and SK must be used with extreme caution, as the combination greatly enhances the risk of overanticoagulation and bleeding.

A group of second-generation and third-generation fibrinolytic agents is also undergoing clinical investigation. The second-generation agents include recombinant tissue plasminogen activator (tPA), acylated plasminogen, SK activator complex, and single-chain urokinase. The third-generation agents are polyethylene glycol-derived, antibody-directed, tailor-made recombinant forms, and hybrid complexes. The thrust of development of these newer agents is to make them more fibrin-specific.

Antiplatelet Agents

Antiplatelet drugs may play a role in arterial thromboembolism, but there is no definitive evidence that they are effective in the treatment or prophylaxis of venous thromboembolism (Genton et al., 1975).

Surgical Intervention

Surgery is reserved for patients in whom anticoagulants are contraindicated or for patients who have not responded after an adequate course. Lower-extremity thrombectomy is justified only if the patient is threatened by impending gangrene resulting from phlegmasia cerulea dolens (Lee et al., 1986). The procedure does not reduce subsequent chronic venous insufficiency because the majority of vessels so treated do not remain patent on long-term follow-up.

A randomized study of 400 patients with proximal deep-vein thrombosis, whose physicians felt them to be at high risk for pulmonary embolism, were treated by low-molecular-weight or unfractionated heparin with or without placement of a caval filter (Decousus et al., 1998). Outcome data showed that the initial beneficial effect of vena caval filters for preventing pulmonary embolism was counterbalanced by an increased occurrence of recurrent deep-vein thrombosis. Significantly, there was no difference in mortality between the two groups.

Indications for vena caval interruption or insertion of an intracaval device are the following:

1. Recurrent pulmonary emboli despite adequate anticoagulation
2. Pulmonary embolization or iliofemoral thrombosis in a patient with an absolute contraindication to anticoagulation
3. Development of hemorrhagic complications of anticoagulation
4. Following embolectomy (Hux et al., 1986; Kempczinski, 1986)

Inferior vena caval ligation, plication, clipping, or insertion of an umbrella is not indicated unless recurrent life-threatening embolization persists despite adequate anticoagulation.

A minor recurrence is observed in approximately 10% of patients during the first few days of heparin therapy and should not be considered a failure of therapy. Bilateral ligation of the femoral veins is not fully protective because of the frequent involvement during pregnancy of the pelvic and gluteal veins, which drain into the iliacs above the inguinal ligament. If a pelvic source of embolism is suspected, ligation of the left ovarian vein may also be required.

Pulmonary embolectomy could be lifesaving but should be considered only in patients with angiographically demonstrated massive embolization to the main pulmonary artery with persistent inadequate cardiac output refractory to appropriate measures. In such situations, the maternal outcome is of primary concern. Evans and colleagues (1968) described a patient who underwent interruption of the inferior vena cava, pulmonary angiography, peripheral venography, laparotomy, and thoracotomy on cardiopulmonary bypass with subsequent delivery of a normal baby.

▓ SPECIAL PROBLEMS

Septic Pelvic Thrombophlebitis

Septic thrombophlebitis is a serious complication of pyogenic pelvic infections. Findings on pelvic examination often are not diagnostic. Recognition depends on a high index of suspicion in postpartum, postabortal, and postoperative patients who demonstrate a spiking fever that persists despite adequate antibiotic therapy (Ledger and Peterson, 1970; Cohen et al., 1983; Duff and Gibbs, 1983). When a presumptive diagnosis of septic thrombophlebitis is made, a medium-dose heparin regimen is initiated. If the diagnosis is correct, the fever should decrease within 12–36 hours. Thus, heparin is both a diagnostic and a therapeutic tool. In the absence of a significant temperature response, a reassessment of the cause of the fever is indicated.

Although there is general agreement regarding initiation of therapy, there are no data on how long to continue therapy. It has been this author's practice to treat these patients similarly to those with acute, uncomplicated DVT. Thus, a medium-dose heparin regimen is started, and a coumarin agent is substituted and continued for a total course of anticoagulation of 3–6 weeks.

Ovarian Vein Thrombosis

Puerperal ovarian vein thrombosis is a difficult diagnosis to make. The diagnosis was made by laparotomy in 80% of cases (Munsick and Gillanders, 1981). Fever, pain, and a lateral pelvic mass are present in 50% of patients. In the experience of this author and in that of others, computed tomography has been helpful in confirming diagnosis without the need for surgery in some cases (Angel and Knuppel, 1984; Dunnihoo et al., 1991). The diagnosis of ovarian vein thrombosis can be confirmed by ultrasound, CT scan, or magnetic resonance imaging (Smith et al., 2002; Nagayama M, 2002).

R E F E R E N C E S

American College of Obstetricians and Gynecologists: Postpartum Hemorrhage. ACOG Educational Bulletin No. 234, 1997.
American College of Obstetricians and Gynecologists: Thromboembolism in Pregnancy. ACOG Practice Bulletin No. 19, 2000.
American Society of Regional Anesthesia: Recommendations for neuroaxial anesthesia and anticoagulation. Chicago, American Society of Regional Anesthesia, 1998.

Angel JL, Knuppel RA: Computed tomography in diagnosis of puerperal ovarian vein thrombosis. Obstet Gynecol 63:61, 1984.

Barbour LA, Pickard J: Controversies in thromboembolic disease during pregnancy: A critical review. Obstet Gynecol 86:621, 1995.

Basu D, Gallus A, Hirsach J, et al: A prospective study of the value of monitoring heparin treatment with the activated partial thromboplastin time. N Engl J Med 287:324, 1972.

Bentley PG, Kakkar VV, Scully MF, et al: An objective study of alternative methods of heparin administration. Thromb Res 18:177, 1980.

Berge LN, Lyngmo V, Svensson B, et al: The bleeding time in women: An influence of sex hormones? Acta Obstet Gynecol Scand 72:423, 1993.

Bloomfield DK: Fetal deaths and malformations associated with the use of coumarin derivatives in pregnancy. Am J Obstet Gynecol 107:883, 1970.

Bramel CE, Hunter RE: Effect of dicumarol on the nursing infant. Am J Obstet Gynecol 59:1153, 1950.

Brill-Edwards P, Ginsberg JS, Gent M, et al.: Safety of withholding heparin in women with a history of venous thromboembolism. N Engl J Med 343:1493, 2000.

Busby LT, Weyman A, Rodgers GM: Excessive anticoagulation in patients with mild renal insufficiency receiving long-term therapeutic enoxaparin. Am J Hematol 67:54, 2001.

Casele HL, Laifer SA, Woelkers DA, et al.: Changes in the pharmokinetics of the low-molecular-weight heparin enoxaparin sodium during pregnancy. Am J Obstet Gynecol 181:1113, 1999.

Chong BH: Heparin-induced thrombocytopenia. Br J Haematol 89:431, 1995.

Clarke-Pearson DL, Jelovsek FR: Alterations of occlusive cuff impedance plethysmography results in the obstetric patient. Surgery 89:594, 1981.

Cohen MB, Pernoll ML, Gevirtz CM, et al: Septic pelvic thrombophlebitis: An update. Obstet Gynecol 62:83, 1983.

Comp PC, Esmon CT: Recurrent venous thromboembolism in patients with partial deficiency of protein S. N Engl J Med 311:1525, 1984.

Consensus Conference: Prevention of venous thromboembolism. JAMA 256:744, 1986.

Coon WW: The spectrum of pulmonary embolism: Twenty years later. Arch Surg 111:398, 1976.

Cranley JJ, Canos AJ, Sull WJ: The diagnosis of deep venous thrombosis— fallibility of clinical symptoms and signs. Arch Surg 111:34, 1976.

Cronan JJ: Contemporary venous imaging. Cardiovasc Intervent Radiol 14:87, 1991.

Dahlman T, Lindvall N, Hellgren M: Osteopenia in pregnancy during long-term heparin treatment: A radiologic study postpartum. Br J Obstet Gynaecol 97:221, 1990.

Daniel DG, Campbell H, Turnbull AC: Puerperal thromboembolism and suppression of lactation. Lancet 2:287, 1967.

Davis FB, Estruch MT, Samson-Corvera EB, et al: Management of anticoagulation in outpatients. Arch Intern Med 137:197, 1977.

De Swiet M, Lewis PJ: Excretion of anticoagulants in breast milk. N Engl J Med 297:1471, 1977.

De Swiet M, Ward PD, Fidler J, et al: Prolonged heparin therapy in pregnancy causes bone demineralization. Br J Obstet Gynaecol 90:1129, 1983.

Decousus H, Leizorovicz A, Parent F, et al: A clinical trial of vena cava filters in the prevention of pulmonary embolism in patients with proximal deep-vein thrombosis. N Engl J Med 338:409, 1998.

Delclos GL, Davilla F: Thrombolytic therapy for pulmonary embolism in pregnancy. Am J Obstet Gynecol 155:375, 1986.

Duff P, Gibbs RS: Pelvic vein thrombophlebitis: Diagnostic dilemma and therapeutic challenge. Obstet Gynecol Surv 38:365, 1983.

Dunnihoo DR, Gallaspy JW, Wise RB, et al: Postpartum ovarian vein thrombophlebitis: A review. Obstet Gynecol Surv 46:415, 1991.

Eldor A: Unexplored territories in the nonsurgical patient: A look at pregnancy. Semin Hematol 38:39, 2001.

Ellison J, Walker ID, Greer IA: Antenatal use of enoxaparin for prevention and treatment of thromboembolism in pregnancy. Br J Obstet Gynaecol 107:1116, 2000.

Evans GL, Dalen JE, Dexter L: Pulmonary embolism during pregnancy. JAMA 206:320, 1968.

Florell SR, Rogers GM: Inherited thrombotic disorders: Update. Am J Hematol 54:53, 1997.

Gallus AS, Hirsh J, Tuttle RJ, et al: Small subcutaneous doses of heparin in prevention of venous thrombosis. N Engl J Med 288:545, 1973.

Genton E, Gent M, Hirsh J, et al: Platelet-inhibiting drugs in the prevention of clinical thrombotic disease. N Engl J Med 293:1296, 1975.

Gerhardt A, Scharf RE, Beckman MW, et al.: Prothrombin and factor V mutations in women with a history of thrombosis during pregnancy and the puerperium. N Engl J Obstet Gynecol 342:374, 2000.

Ginsberg JS, Hirsh J, Rainbow AJ, et al: Risk to the fetus of radiologic procedure used in the diagnosis of maternal venous thromboembolic disease. Thromb Haemost 61:189, 1989.

Griffin JH, Evatt B, Zimmerman TS, et al: Deficiencies in protein C in congenital thrombotic disease. J Clin Invest 68:1370, 1981.

Griffith GC, Nichols G, Asher JD, et al: Heparin osteoporosis. JAMA 193:185, 1965.

Haeger K: Problems of acute deep venous thrombosis. Angiology 20:219, 1969.

Hall JG, Pauli RM, Wilson KM: Maternal and fetal sequelae of anticoagulation during pregnancy. Am J Med 68:122, 1980.

Hallak M, Senderowicz J, Cassel A, et al: Activated protein C resistance (factor V Leiden) associated with thrombosis in pregnancy. Am J Obstet Gynecol 176:889, 1997.

Hathaway WE, Bonnar J: Thrombotic disorders in pregnancy and the newborn. In Hemostatic Disorders of the Pregnant Woman and Newborn Infant. New York, Elsevier Scientific Publishing, 1987.

Heijboer H, Bullerr HR, Lensing AWA, et al: A comparison of real-time compression ultrasonography with impedance plethysmography for the diagnosis of deep-vein thrombosis in symptomatic out-patients. N Engl J Med 329:1365, 1993.

Hirsh J: Blood tests for the diagnosis of venous and arterial thrombosis. Blood 57:1, 1981.

Hirsh J: Heparin. N Engl J Med 324:1565, 1991a.

Hirsh J: Oral anticoagulant drugs. N Engl J Med 324:1865, 1991b.

Hirsh J, Cade JF, Gallus AS: Anticoagulants in pregnancy: A review of indications and complications. Am Heart J 83:301, 1972.

Hirsh J, Levine MN: Low molecular weight heparin. Blood 79:1, 1992.

Hull R, Delmore T, Carter C, et al: Adjusted subcutaneous heparin versus warfarin sodium in the long-term treatment of venous thrombosis. N Engl J Med 306:189, 1982.

Hull R, Delmore T, Genton E, et al: Warfarin sodium versus low-dose heparin in the long-term treatment of venous thrombosis. N Engl J Med 301:855, 1979.

Hull RD, Hirsh J, Carter CJ, et al: Pulmonary angiography, ventilation lung scanning, and venography for clinically suspected pulmonary embolism with abnormal perfusion lung scan. Ann Intern Med 98:891, 1983.

Hull RD, Raskob GE, Rosenbloom D, et al: Heparin for 5 days as compared with 10 days in the initial treatment of proximal deep-venous thrombosis. N Engl J Med 322:1260, 1990.

Hux CH, Wapner RJ, Chayen B, et al: Use of the Greenfield filter for thromboembolic disease in pregnancy. Am J Obstet Gynecol 155:734, 1986.

Illingworth RS, Finch E: Ethyl biscoumacetate in human milk. J Obstet Gynaecol Br Commonw 66:487, 1959.

Kakkar VV, Corrigan TP, Fossard DP: Prevention of fatal postoperative pulmonary embolism by low doses of heparin: An international multicentre trial. Lancet 2:45, 1975.

Kempczinski RF: Surgical prophylaxis of pulmonary embolism. Chest 89:384s, 1986.

Koch-Weser J, Sellers EM: Drug interactions with coumarin anticoagulants. N Engl J Med 285:547, 1971.

Kovacevich GJ, Gaich SA, Lavin JP, et al: The prevalence of thrombolic events among women with extended bed rest prescribed as part of the treatment for premature labor or preterm rupture of membranes. Am J Obstet Gynecol 182:1089, 2000.

Kramer WB, Belfort M, Saade GR, et al: Successful urokinase treatment of massive pulmonary embolism in pregnancy. Obstet Gynecol 86:660, 1995.

Laros RK Jr: Anticoagulants: Indications and use. Contemp Obstet Gynecol 5:67, 1975.

Ledger WJ, Peterson EP: The use of heparin in the management of pelvic thrombophlebitis. Surg Gynecol Obstet 131:1115, 1970.

Lee PK, Wang RYC, Chow JSF, et al: Combined use of warfarin and adjusted subcutaneous heparin during pregnancy in patients with artificial heart valve. J Am Coll Cardiol 8:221, 1986.

Lensing AWA, Prandoni P, Brandjes D, et al: Detection of deep-vein thrombosis by real-time B-mode ultrasonography. N Engl J Med 320:342, 1989.

Lepercq J, Conard J, Borel-Derlon A, et al.: Venous thromboembolism during pregnancy: A retrospective study of enoxaperin safety in 624 pregnancies. Br J Obstet Gynaecol 108:1134, 2001.

Ludwig H: Results of streptokinase therapy in deep vein thrombosis during pregnancy. Postgrad Med J 8:65, 1973.

Lutz DJ, Noller KL, Spittell JA, et al: Pregnancy and its complications following cardiac valve prostheses. Am J Obstet Gynecol 131:460, 1978.

MacKay AP, Berg CJ, Atrash HK: Pregnancy-related mortality from preeclampsia and eclampsia. Obstet Gynecol 97:533, 2001.

Mackie M, Bennett B, Ogston D, et al: Familial thrombosis: Inherited deficiency of antithrombin III. Br Med J 1:136, 1978.

McCausland AM, Hyman C, Winsor T, et al: Venous distensibility during pregnancy. Am J Obstet Gynecol 81:472, 1961.

Meaney LFM, Weg JG, Chenevert TL, et al: Diagnosis of pulmonary embolism with magnetic resonance angiography. N Engl J Med 336:1422, 1997.

Mueh JR, Herbst KD, Rapaport SI: Thrombosis in patients with lupus anticoagulant. Ann Intern Med 92:156, 1980.

Munsick RA, Gillanders LA: A review of the syndrome of puerperal ovarian vein thrombophlebitis. Obstet Gynecol Surv 36:57, 1981.

Nagayama M, Watanabe Y, Okumura A, et al.: Fast MR Imaging in Obstetrics. Radiographics 22:563, 2002.

Nelson-Piercy C, Letsky EA, De Swiet M: Low-molecular-weight heparin for obstetric thromboprophylaxis: Experience of sixty-nine pregnancies in sixty-one women at high risk. Am J Obstet Gynecol 176:1062, 1997.

Nilsson I, Kullander S: Coagulation and fibrinolytic studies during pregnancy. Acta Obstet Gynecol Scand 46:273, 1967.

Orme MLE, de Swiet M, Serlin MJ, et al: May mothers given warfarin breast-feed their infants? Br Med J 1:1564, 1977.

PIOPED Investigators: Value of the ventilation/perfusion scan in acute pulmonary embolism. JAMA 263:2753, 1990.

Polak JF, Wilkinson DL: Ultrasonographic diagnosis of symptomatic deep venous thrombosis in pregnancy. Am J Obstet Gynecol 165:625, 1991.

Porter JM, Goodnight SH: The clinical use of fibrinolytic agents. Am J Surg 134:217, 1977.

Pridmore BR, Murray KH, McAllen PM: The management of anticoagulant therapy during and after pregnancy. Br J Obstet Gynaecol 82:740, 1975.

Rickles FR, Edwards RL: Activation of blood coagulation in cancer. Blood 62:14, 1983.

Rosenberg RD: The heparin-antithrombin system: A natural anticoagulant mechanism. In Colman RW, Hirsh J, Marder VJ, et al. (eds): Hemostasis and Thrombosis: Basic Principles and Clinical Practice, 2nd ed. Philadelphia, JB Lippincott, 1987, p. 1373.

Rosendaal FR: Risk factors for venous thrombosis: Prevalence, risk and interaction. Semin Hematol 34:171, 1997.

Sasahara AA, Sharma GVRK, Barsamian EM, et al: Pulmonary thromboembolism. JAMA 249:2945, 1983.

Schulman S, Granqvist S, Holmstrom M, et al: The duration of oral anticoagulant therapy after a second episode of venous thromboembolism. N Engl J Med 336:393, 1997.

Schulman S, Rhedin AS, Lindmarker P, et al: A comparison of six weeks with six months of oral anticoagulant therapy after a first episode of venous thromboembolism. N Engl J Med 332:1661, 1995.

Shaul WL, Hall JG: Multiple congenital anomalies associated with oral anticoagulants. Am J Obstet Gynecol 127:191, 1977.

Sifton DW, Murray L, Kelly GL: Physicians' Desk Reference, Montvale, NJ, Medical Economics Company, Inc., 2002, p. 746.

Smith MD, Felker RE, Emerson DS, at al.: Sonographic visualization of ovarian veins during the puerperium: An assessment of efficacy. Am J Obstet Gynecol 186:893, 2002.

Stevenson RE, Burton OM, Ferlauto GJ, et al: Hazards of oral anticoagulants during pregnancy. JAMA 243:1549, 1980.

Sturridge F, Letsky E: The use of low-molecular-weight heparin for thromboprophylaxis in pregnancy. Br J Obstet Gynaecol 101:69, 1994.

Taberino MD, Tomas JF, Alberca I, et al: Incidence and clinical characteristics of hereditary disorders associated with venous thrombosis. Am J Hematol 36:249, 1991.

Todd ME, Thompson JH, Bowie EJW, et al: Changes in blood coagulation during pregnancy. Mayo Clin Proc 40:370, 1965.

Toy PTCY, Schrier SL: Occlusive impedance plethysmography. West J Med 129:89, 1978.

Urokinase Pulmonary Embolism Trial Study Group: Urokinase pulmonary embolism trial: Phase 1. JAMA 214:2163, 1970.

Urokinase Pulmonary Embolism Trial Study Group: Urokinase pulmonary embolism trial: Phase 2. JAMA 229:1606, 1974.

Van Erkel AR, van Rossum AB, Bloem J, et al: Spiral CT angiography for suspected pulmnonary embolism: A cost–effectiveness analysis. Radiology 201:29, 1996.

Van Rossum AB, Treurniet FE, Kieft G, et al: Role of spiral volumetric computed tomographic scanning in the assessment of patients with clinical suspicion of pulmonary embolism and an abnormal ventilation/perfusion lung scan. Thorax 51:23, 1996.

Villasanta U: Thromboembolic disease in pregnancy. Am J Obstet Gynecol 93:142, 1965.

Warkentin TE, Levine MN, Hirsh J, et al: Heparin-induced thrombocytopenia in patients treated with low-molecular-weight heparin or unfractionated heparin. N Engl J Med 332:1330, 1995.

Wessler S: Medical management of venous thrombosis. Ann Rev Med 27:313, 1976a.

Wessler S: Heparin as an antithrombotic agent: Low-dose prophylaxis. JAMA 236:389, 1976b.

Wessler S, Gitel SN: Heparin: New concepts relevant to clinical use. Blood 53:525, 1979.

Wessler S, Gitel SN: Warfarin. N Engl J Med 311:645, 1984.

Whitfield LR, Lele AS, Levy G: Effect of pregnancy on the relationship between concentration and anticoagulant action of heparin. Clin Pharmacol Ther 34:23, 1983.

Wright HP, Osborn SB, Edmonds DG: Changes in the rate of flow of venous blood in the leg during pregnancy, measured with radioactive sodium. Surg Gynecol Obstet 90:481, 1950.

Chapter 43
PREGNANCY-RELATED HYPERTENSION

James M. Roberts, MD

CLASSIFICATION AND DEFINITIONS

The hypertensive disorders of pregnancy challenge the medical and obstetric skills of the health care team. Decisions as to the possible use and appropriate choice of pharmacologic agents require not only an understanding of the pathophysiology of the hypertensive disorders and a recognition of the pharmacokinetic changes occurring during pregnancy but also an appreciation of the possible fetal effects of such therapeutic agents. Obstetric management demands meticulous maternal observation and use of tests of fetal-placental function and fetal maturity in order to weigh maternal risks and the risks to the infant of intrauterine versus extrauterine existence.

The management of elevated blood pressure (BP) and the impact of the disorder on the mother and fetus depend on whether hypertension antedated the pregnancy or appeared as the marker of pregnancy-specific vasospastic syndrome. An attempt to distinguish between the two has led to several systems of nomenclature and classification. The hypertensive disorders of pregnancy were for many years called *toxemias of pregnancy*, a term that originally included even hyperemesis gravidarum and acute yellow atrophy of the liver. This term reflected the opinion that these disorders had, as a common etiology, circulating toxins. Failure to identify these toxins did not lead to a revision of this terminology, a circumstance which is indicative of the continuing confusion that has plagued the taxonomy of these disorders. This archaic terminology, which neither describes the disorders nor clarifies their etiology, has rightly been abandoned.

One of the difficulties in interpreting studies of the hypertensive disorders of pregnancy is the inconsistency of terminology (Rippman, 1969). Several systems of nomenclature are in use around the world. The system prepared by the National Institutes of Health (NIH) working group on hypertension in pregnancy (Gifford et al., 2000a) although as imperfect as all such systems, has the advantage of clarity and is available in published form to investigators throughout the world. This classification is as follows:

- Chronic hypertension
- Preeclampsia-eclampsia
- Preeclampsia superimposed upon chronic hypertension
- Gestational hypertension

The various classifications are explained in the following discussion.

Chronic Hypertension

Chronic hypertension is defined as hypertension that is present and observable prior to pregnancy or that is diagnosed before the 20th week of gestation. Hypertension is defined as a blood pressure greater than 140/90 mm Hg. Hypertension for which a diagnosis is confirmed for the first time during pregnancy, and which persists beyond the 84th day postpartum, is also classified as chronic hypertension.

Preeclampsia and Eclampsia

The diagnosis of preeclampsia is determined by increased blood pressure accompanied by proteinuria.. Diagnostic blood pressure increases are either a systolic blood pressure of greater than or equal to 140 mm Hg or a diastolic blood pressure of greater than or equal to 90 mm Hg. Diastolic blood pressure is determined as Krotkoff V (disappearance of sounds). It is recommended that gestational blood pressure elevation be defined on the basis of at least two determinations. The repeat blood pressure should be performed in a manner that will reduce the likelihood of artifact and/or patient anxiety (Gifford et al., 2000b). Absent from the diagnostic criteria is the former inclusion of an increment of 30 mm Hg systolic or 15 mm Hg diastolic blood pressure, even when absolute values are below 140/90 mm Hg. This definition was excluded because the only available evidence shows that women in this group are not likely to suffer increased adverse outcomes (North et al., 1999; Zhang et al., 2001). Nonetheless, women who have a rise of 30 mm Hg systolic or 15 mm Hg diastolic blood pressure warrant close observation, especially if proteinuria and hyperuricemia (uric acid [UA] greater than or equal to 6 mg/dL) are also present (Gifford et al., 2000b).

Proteinuria is defined as the urinary excretion of 0.3 g protein or greater in a 24-hour specimen. This will usually correlate with 30 mg/dL ("1+ dipstick") or greater in a random urine determination. Because of the discrepancy between random protein determinations and 24-hour urine protein in preeclampsia (which can be either higher or lower) (Abuelo, 1992; Kuo et al., 1992; Meyer et al., 1994), it is recommended that the diagnosis be based on a 24-hour urine specimen if at all possible or, if this is not feasible, it should be based on a timed collection corrected for creatinine excretion (Gifford et al., 2000b).

Preeclampsia occurs as a spectrum but is arbitrarily divided into mild and severe forms. This terminology is useful for descriptive purposes but does not indicate specific diseases, nor should it indicate arbitrary cutoff points for therapy. The diagnosis of severe preeclampsia is confirmed when the following criteria are present:

1. Systolic blood pressure of 160 mm Hg or greater, or diastolic pressure of 110 mm Hg or greater
2. Proteinuria of 2 g or more in 24 hours (2- or 3-plus on qualitative examination)
3. Increased serum creatinine (greater than 1.2 mg/dL unless known to be previously elevated)
4. Persistent headache or cerebral or visual disturbances
5. Persistent epigastric pain
6. Platelet count less than 100,000/mm³ and/or evidence of microangiopathic hemolytic anemia (with increased lactic acid dehydrogenase)

Eclampsia is the occurrence of seizures in a preeclamptic patient that cannot be attributed to other causes.

Edema occurs in too many normal pregnant women to be discriminant and has been abandoned as a marker in preeclampsia by the National High Blood Pressure Education Program (NHBPEP) and by other classification schemes (Brown et al., 2001; Helewa et al., 1997; Practice, 2002).

Preeclampsia Superimposed on Chronic Hypertension

There is ample evidence that preeclampsia can occur in women who are already hypertensive and that the prognosis for mother and fetus is much worse for these women than with either condition alone. Distinguishing superimposed preeclampsia from worsening chronic hypertension tests the skills of the clinician. For clinical management, the principles of high sensitivity and unavoidable overdiagnosis are appropriate. The suspicion of superimposed preeclampsia mandates close observation, with delivery indicated by the overall assessment of maternal-fetal well being rather than by any fixed endpoint. The diagnosis of superimposed preeclampsia is highly likely with the following findings:

1. In women with hypertension and no proteinuria early in pregnancy (prior to 20 weeks' gestation) and new-onset proteinuria, defined as the urinary excretion of 0.3 g protein or more in a 24-hour specimen
2. In women with hypertension and proteinuria prior to 20 weeks' gestation:
   a. A sudden increase in proteinuria—urinary excretion of 0.3 g protein or more in a 24-hour specimen, or two dipstick-test results of 2+ (100 mg/dL), with the values recorded at least 4 hours apart, with no evidence of urinary tract infection
   b. A sudden increase in blood pressure in a woman whose blood pressure has previously been well controlled
   c. Thrombocytopenia (platelet count lower than 100,000/mm³)
   d. An increase in ALT or AST to abnormal levels (Gifford et al., 2000b)

Gestational Hypertension

The woman who has blood pressure elevation detected for the first time during pregnancy, without proteinuria, is classified as having gestational hypertension. This nonspecific term includes women with preeclampsia syndrome who have not yet manifested proteinuria as well as women who do not have the syndrome. The hypertension may be accompanied by other signs of the syndrome, which will influence management. The final differentiation that the woman does not have preeclampsia syndrome is made only postpartum. If preeclampsia has not developed and blood pressure has returned to normal by 12 weeks postpartum, the diagnosis of *transient hypertension* of pregnancy can be assigned. If blood pressure elevation persists, the woman is diagnosed as having chronic hypertension. Note that the diagnosis of gestational hypertension is used during pregnancy only until a more specific diagnosis can be assigned postpartum (Gifford et al., 2000b).

Problems with Classification

The degree of blood pressure elevation that constitutes gestational hypertension is controversial. Because average blood pressure in women in their teens to 20s is 120/60 mm Hg, the standard definition of hypertension—blood pressure greater than 140/90 mm Hg—is judged by some investigators to be too high (Vartran, 1966). This has resulted in the suggestion in the NHBPEP report that women with increased BP greater than 30 mm Hg systolic or 25 mm Hg diastolic be observed closely even if absolute blood pressure has not exceeded 140/90.

There are also problems inherent in the use of blood pressures measured in early pregnancy to diagnose chronic hypertension. Blood pressure usually decreases early in pregnancy, reaching its nadir at about the stage of pregnancy at which women usually present for obstetric care (Fig. 43-1). The decrease averages 7 mm Hg for diastolic and systolic readings. In some women, obviously, blood pressure decreases more than 7 mm Hg; in others, the early decline and subsequent return of blood pressure to prepregnant levels in late gestation are sufficient for a diagnosis of preeclampsia. Women who have hypertension prior to pregnancy actually experience a greater decrease in blood pressure in early pregnancy than do normotensive women (Chesley and Annitto, 1947) and thus are

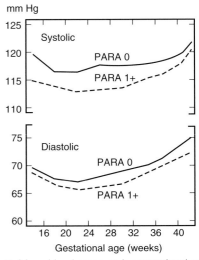

FIGURE 43-1 ■ Mean blood pressure by gestational age in 6000 Caucasian women 25–34 years of age who delivered singleton term infants. (From Christianson R, Page EW: Studies on blood pressure during pregnancy: Influence of parity and age. Am J Obstet Gynecol **125**:509, 1976. Courtesy of the American College of Obstetricians and Gynecologists.)

TABLE 43-1. RENAL BIOPSY FINDINGS IN PATIENTS WITH CLINICAL DIAGNOSIS OF PREECLAMPSIA

Biopsy Findings	Primigravidas (*N* = 62)	Multigravidas (*N* = 152)
Glomeruloendotheliosis	70%	14% (with or without nephrosclerosis)
Normal histologic appearance	5%	53%
Chronic renal disease (chronic GTN, chronic pyelonephritis)	25%	21%
Arteriolar nephrosclerosis	0	12%

GTN, gestational trophoblastic neoplasia.

Modified from McCartney CP: Pathological anatomy of acute hypertension of pregnancy. Circulation 30(Suppl II):37, 1964, by permission of the American Heart Association, Inc.

even more likely to be misdiagnosed as preeclamptic according to blood pressure criteria.

Also, the diagnosis of chronic hypertension based on the failure of blood pressure to return to normal by 84 days postpartum can be in error. In a long-range prospective study by Chesley (1956), many women who remained hypertensive 6 weeks postpartum were normotensive at long-term follow-up. Even the proteinuria and hypertension are nonspecific signs, and their presence in pregnancy could be due to conditions other than preeclampsia.

Renal biopsy specimens from women with a diagnosis of preeclampsia (blood pressure increase and proteinuria) demonstrate these diagnostic difficulties (Table 43-1) (McCartney, 1964). Of 62 women with a diagnosis of preeclampsia in their first pregnancies, 70% had a glomerular lesion believed to be characteristic of the disorder; 24%, however, had evidence of chronic renal disease that had not been suspected previously. Renal biopsy specimens of multiparous women with a clinical diagnosis of superimposed preeclampsia also demonstrates the difficulty in diagnosis. Of 152 subjects, only 3% had the characteristic glomerular lesion, but 43% had evidence of preexisting renal or vascular disease.

Preeclampsia has a clinical spectrum ranging from mild to severe forms and then potentially to eclampsia. Affected patients do not "catch" eclampsia or the severe forms of preeclampsia but rather progress through this spectrum. In most cases, progression is slow, and the disorder may never proceed beyond mild preeclampsia. In others, the disease can progress more rapidly, changing from mild to severe over days to weeks. In the most serious cases, progression can be fulminant, with mild preeclampsia evolving to severe preeclampsia or eclampsia over hours to days.

In a series of eclamptic women analyzed by Chesley (1978), 25% had evidence of only mild preeclampsia in the days preceding convulsions. Thus, for purposes of clinical management, we must accept the fact that we are overdiagnosing the condition because, as discussed later, a major goal in managing preeclampsia is the prevention of the serious complications of preeclampsia and eclampsia, primarily through timing of delivery. It is also evident, however, that studies of preeclampsia will be confounded by inclusion of women who have been given a diagnosis of preeclampsia but who actually have another cardiovascular or renal disorder.

HELLP

It is quite evident that the pathophysiological changes of preeclampsia can be present in the absence of hypertension and proteinuria. This should not be surprising, as these diagnostic criteria are of historical rather than pathophysiological relevance. Hypertension and proteinuria were the first signs recognized as predicating preeclampsia (Chesley, 1978). Understanding this historical evolution presents a challenge to clinicians and dictates a high index of suspicion in managing pregnant women with signs and symptoms that could be explained by reduced organ perfusion. One clear setting in which this occurs is the HELLP syndrome; the acronym stands for *H*emolysis, *E*levated liver enzymes, and *L*ow *P*latelets. This series of findings defines a reasonably consistent syndrome that has now been studied for over twenty years (Weinstein, 1982). Although for management purposes it is appropriate to consider HELLP as a variant of preeclampsia, there are differences in several features of preeclampsia and HELLP that suggest they could be different entities. Women with HELLP tend to be older and are more likely to be Caucasian and multiparous than preeclamptic women; in many cases, they are not hypertensive (Egerman and Sibai, 1999). From a pathophysiological perspective, changes in the renin-angiotensin system characteristic of preeclampsia are not present in HELLP (Bussen et al., 1998). Nonetheless, the progression of the disease and its termination with delivery argue for an observation and management strategy similar to that for preeclampsia. The serendipitous observation that women who had received antepartum steroids appeared to evidence improvement in the HELLP syndrome (Magann et al., 1993) stimulated several retrospective and observational studies (Magann and Martin, 1995; Martin et al., 1997; O'Brien et al., 2000; O'Brien et al., 2002; Tompkins and Thiagarajah, 1999; Yalcin et al., 1998). These studies and a small randomized controlled trial (Magann et al., 1994) suggest improvement in laboratory findings as well as prolongation of pregnancy. The determination of appropriate dosing and whether the benefit of therapy exceeds risks await larger, randomized controlled trials.

PREECLAMPSIA AND ECLAMPSIA

In spite of the difficulty of making a clinical diagnosis of preeclampsia, there is no question that a disorder exists that is unique to pregnancy, characterized by poor perfusion of many vital organs (including the fetoplacental unit), and completely reversible with the termination of pregnancy. Pathologic, pathophysiologic, and prognostic findings clearly indicate that this condition, preeclampsia, is not merely an unmasking of preexisting, underlying hypertension. Although this fact has been well documented for many years, problems still arise owing to approaches in the management of preeclampsia that are based solely on principles useful in managing hypertension in nonpregnant individuals. The successful management of preeclampsia requires an understanding of the pathophysiologic changes in this condition and the recognition that the signs of preeclampsia—increased blood pressure and proteinuria—are only signs, not causal abnormalities.

The etiology of preeclampsia-eclampsia is not completely understood; however, as Zuspan (1978) pointed out more than 20 years ago, we can manage the condition successfully using the information we do have about its pathophysiology, prognosis, and natural history.

It is tempting to use a new "label" to define this vasospastic syndrome in pregnancy. Because there are already too many labels, however, and because the diagnosis of this pregnancy-related condition can be made only retrospectively (i.e., when physiologic functions, including blood pressure, return to normal after pregnancy), the term *preeclampsia* is appropriate if its limitations are recognized.

Clinical Presentation

The "Typical" Preeclamptic Patient

Preeclampsia occurs in about 4% of pregnancies not terminating in first-trimester abortions. It would be useful to be able to identify the women at greatest risk. In preeclampsia, as with all diseases, there are no truly "typical" patients. Epidemiologic findings do indicate, however, that certain characteristics are more common in women who develop preeclampsia. The most important is nulliparity. Preeclampsia is primarily a disease of the first pregnancy. At least two thirds of cases occur in women during the first pregnancy not terminating in a first-trimester loss.

Preeclampsia is thought to be more common among women of lower socioeconomic status. In his study of pregnant women in Aberdeen, Scotland, nearly all of whom delivered in hospitals, Nelson (1955) found no relationship of preeclampsia-eclampsia to socioeconomic status. In similar studies in Finland (Vara et al., 1965) and Jerusalem (Davies et al., 1970), no relationship was established between this factor and the incidence of preeclampsia. It remains the current clinical impression of most individuals caring for pregnant women in the United States that preeclampsia is a disease of lower-income women. This impression may be accurate, but it is undoubtedly confounded by the relationship of preeclampsia to age, race, and parity.

Eclampsia, in contrast, is clearly a disease of women of lower socioeconomic status (Nelson, 1955; Vara et al., 1965; Davies et al., 1970). Eclampsia is preventable by careful obstetric observation and prompt delivery when severe preeclampsia is present. Therefore, the lack of availability and use of good-quality obstetric care to indigent women is undoubtedly a major factor in the increased incidence of eclampsia. It is interesting to note that in past years, the clinical impression was that preeclampsia-eclampsia was a disease of women of higher socioeconomic status (Chesley, 1978).

There is a relationship between the extremes of childbearing age and the incidence of eclampsia and preeclampsia. Because most pregnancies, particularly the first, occur in young women, most cases of preeclampsia-eclampsia occur in this age group. However, studies of entire populations in Aberdeen, Jerusalem, and Finland do not indicate an increased incidence of preeclampsia in young women if parity is considered. In all of

these studies, a higher incidence of preeclampsia not dependent on parity was found in older women. The information from the Collaborative Study in the United States (Vollman, 1970) does suggest a higher incidence of preeclampsia in younger women, although Davies (1971) has pointed out the deficiencies in this study. It is possible that the incidence of preeclampsia may be greater in young women in the United States but not in other parts of the world; however, even if this is true, the increased incidence among the youngest age groups in the Collaborative Study is not nearly as great as that of older patients.

The relationship of preeclampsia and eclampsia to race is equally difficult to evaluate. Data from both the United States Collaborative Study and the Jerusalem study indicate a relationship (Vollman, 1970; Davies et al., 1970). The Jerusalem study revealed the strong correlation of race and age during pregnancy. In the Collaborative Study, the incidence of preeclampsia was higher in blacks, in whom hypertension is generally more common. This finding raises the question of whether the incidence of preeclampsia is truly race-related or whether the finding is an example of the difficulty in differentiating preeclampsia from unrecognized preexisting chronic hypertension. In a case-control study of carefully defined preeclampsia, black race was a significant risk factor (odds ratio [OR] 12.3) but only in nulliparous women (Eskenazi et al., 1991). Several other studies support the increased risk in African-American women (Mittendorf et al., 1996; Knuist et al., 1998). In contrast, Chesley has stated that there is no difference in incidence of preeclampsia between blacks and Caucasians (unpublished observation cited by Davies, 1971). Analysis of subjects from a National Institutes of Health (NIH) study of aspirin prophylaxis for low-risk pregnancies also failed to identify race as a risk factor (Sibai et al., 1995).

A characteristic of preeclampsia-eclampsia that is frequently overlooked is the tendency of the condition to occur in daughters and sisters of women with a history of preeclampsia. In Aberdeen, the incidence of proteinuric preeclampsia was found to be four times higher among sisters of women who had preeclampsia in their first pregnancy than among sisters of women who did not (Adams and Finlayson, 1961). In one study of the same population, the incidence of preeclampsia was 15% in mothers but only 4% in mothers-in-law of preeclamptic women (Sutherland et al., 1981).

Chesley and Cooper (1986) evaluated preeclampsia in the first pregnancy of sisters, daughters, granddaughters, and daughters-in-law of women who had been eclamptic. The incidence of preeclampsia in sisters was 37%; in daughters, 26%; in granddaughters, 16%; but in daughters-in-law, only 6%. Reviewing these and other family studies, Arngrimsson and colleagues (1995) concluded that the inheritance pattern was not best explained by simple mendelian inheritance. Instead, the available data, although limited, was more consistent with either a dominant gene with reduced penetrance or multifactorial inheritance. There is also a contribution of the fetal genome to preeclampsia. Men who have fathered preeclamptic pregnancies are more likely to father preeclamptic pregnancies with new partners than are men who have never been fathers in preeclamptic pregnancies (Lie et al., 1998). In addition, men born in preeclamptic pregnancies are more likely to be fathers in preeclamptic pregnancies than are men who are born in nonpreeclamptic pregnancies (Esplin et al., 2001).

What is inherited in preeclampsia? Possibilities include immunologic differences, features that compromise implantation, and an increased sensitivity to respond to the systemic insult caused by reduced placental perfusion. Examinations of candidate genes thus far support all possibilities. In some populations, certain human leukocyte antigen (HLA) types are more common in the mother and the fetus from preeclamptic pregnancies (Johnson et al., 1990; Kilpatrick et al., 1990). Interestingly, a variant of the angiotensinogen gene—reported to be more common in some but not all studies (Arngrimsson et al., 1993; Ward et al., 1993; Wilton et al., 1995)—is speculated to influence not blood pressure but rather spiral artery remodeling (Morgan et al., 1997). Gene variants potentially leading to aberrations of endothelial function are more common in preeclamptic women (Arngrimsson et al., 1997; Grandone et al., 1997; Sohda et al., 1997). Mutations leading to increased risk factors for later-life cardiovascular disease, including function perturbing mutations of lipoprotein lipase genes (Hubel et al., 1999) and methylene tetrahydrofolate reductase (MTHFR, an enzyme abnormality associated with increased circulating homocysteine) (Grandone et al., 1997) are associated with preeclampsia. With all of these genetic polymorphisms, the results are inconsistent, being associated in some but not other populations (Roberts and Cooper, 2001). Nonetheless, these and other contemporary strategies (Harrison et al., 1997) support the heterogeneity of preeclampsia (Ness and Roberts, 1996).

Certain medical disorders also predispose to preeclampsia. For example, diabetes is frequently complicated by preeclampsia, with the incidence stated to be as high as 50% of diabetic pregnancies (Chesley, 1978). Preeclampsia is also more common in women with hypertension antedating pregnancy. In several studies, the reported incidence is approximately 20% (Caritis et al., 1998).

Obesity is also a risk factor. Eskenazi and coworkers (1991) and Stone and colleagues (1994) found prepregnancy obesity an independent risk factor for well-defined preeclampsia. In the NIH study of aspirin for low-risk pregnancies, a dose-response relationship of obesity and preeclampsia was present (Sibai et al., 1995). The incidence of preeclampsia increased with the magnitude of obesity. The mechanism of the increased risk could be related to increased insulin resistance, as preeclampsia is also more common in another setting of increased insulin resistance, gestational diabetes (Roach et al., 2000).

The relationships among obesity, insulin resistance, and preeclampsia are part of an interesting relationship of preeclampsia to the metabolic or insulin resistance syndrome (Barden et al., 1999). This syndrome predisposes to cardiovascular disease in later life and consists of obesity, hypertension, dyslipidemia (increased LDL cholesterol, decreased HDL cholesterol, and increased triglycerides), and increased uric acid. All of these changes are present in women with preeclampsia (Barden et al., 1999). Other conditions predisposing to later-life cardiovascular disease—including elevated homocysteine (Powers et al., 1998), evidence of androgen excess including polycystic ovarian syndrome (Fridstrom et al., 1999), elevated testosterone (Acromite et al., 1999), male fat distribution (increased waist-to-hip ratio) (Sattar et al., 2001), and lipoprotein lipase mutations (Hubel et al., 1999)—also increase the risk of preeclampsia.

Certain conditions of pregnancy also increase the risk of preeclampsia. The incidence is approximately 30% in women with twin pregnancies and is increased regardless of parity (Caritis et al., 1998). In a study by Bulfin and Lawler (1957), the incidence was 70% in primipara and 20% in multipara twin gestations. Preeclampsia is also present in 70% of women with large, rapidly growing hydatidiform moles and occurs earlier than usual in gestation (Page, 1939). In fact, in cases of preeclampsia occurring before 24 weeks' gestation, hydatidiform mole should be suspected and sought.

An interesting variant of preeclampsia occurs with fetal hydrops, although not with erythroblastosis uncomplicated by hydrops; the incidence is high (~50%), and preeclampsia is not confined to hydrops secondary to isoimmunization, occurring in one series in nine of 11 infants with hydrops of nonimmune etiology (Scott, 1958). This condition could present early in pregnancy and with severe signs and symptoms of preeclampsia. Proteinuria is massive, and blood pressure elevation and edema are marked. In spite of this severity, eclampsia is a rare complication.

Preeclampsia is also reported to be more common in pregnancies complicated by polyhydramnios; however, if the association of polyhydramnios with diabetes and multiple pregnancies is accounted for, the relationship is not present (Jeffcoate and Scott, 1959).

Signs of Preeclampsia

The diagnostic signs of preeclampsia usually antedate symptoms. The usual sequence of the appearance of the signs is increased blood pressure followed by proteinuria; however, signs can appear in any order (Chesley, 1978).

Edema

Despite the elimination of edema as a diagnostic criteria for preeclampsia, and the fact that rapid weight gain can occur in normal pregnancy, in one group of women who becme eclamptic, 10% manifested rapid weight gain (Chesley, 1978). Edema of the hands and face occurs in 10%–15% of women whose blood pressure remains normal throughout pregnancy (Thomson et al., 1967). Edema, however, can be massive in severe preeclampsia, rendering the patient virtually unrecognizable (Fig. 43-2).

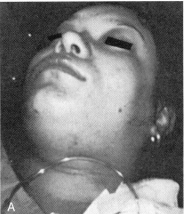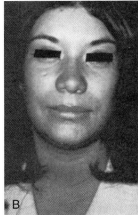

FIGURE 43-2 ■ Facial edema in severe preeclampsia. Markedly edematous facies of this severely preeclamptic woman **(A)** is especially evident when compared with her appearance 6 weeks postpartum **(B)**.

Blood Pressure Change

An increase in blood pressure is required for the diagnosis of preeclampsia. As discussed previously, however, the changes in blood pressure associated with normal pregnancy can lead to misdiagnosis. In clinical practice, the possible impact of preeclampsia on mother and fetus warrants such overdiagnosis. From a pathophysiologic viewpoint, of primary importance is poor tissue perfusion secondary to vasospasm, which is revealed more clearly by blood pressure changes than by absolute blood pressure levels. Thus, although a diagnosis of preeclampsia is not made without absolute blood pressure increases to 140 or 90, the woman who arrives at this level from a low early pregnancy value likely manifests more vasospasm than the woman in whom 140 or 90 is a lesser increase. Even the relative increase of blood pressure, however, does not always correlate well with decreased tissue perfusion and subsequent damage.

Serious complications of preeclampsia, eclampsia, and maternal or fetal death can occur in the patient who experiences only modest blood pressure elevation. In two series, 20% of women with eclampsia never had a systolic blood pressure exceeding 140 mm Hg (Chesley, 1978; Dieckman, 1952). Conversely, a woman with a substantial increase in blood pressure (greater than 160 mm Hg systolic or 100 mm Hg diastolic even without proteinuria) has increased risk for herself and her infant compared with women with lesser degrees of hypertension (Buchbinder et al., 2002).

Proteinuria

Among the diagnostic signs of preeclampsia, proteinuria accompanied by hypertension is the most reliable indicator of fetal jeopardy. In two studies of preeclampsia, the perinatal mortality rate tripled in women with proteinuria (MacGillivray, 1958), and the amount of proteinuria correlated with increased perinatal mortality rate and the number of growth-restricted infants (Tervila et al., 1973). If only eclampsia is considered—thus excluding cases of chronic hypertension misdiagnosed as preeclampsia—the relationship of proteinuria to perinatal mortality is even more striking. In the series reported by Nelson (1955) from Aberdeen, there were 15 neonatal deaths in 52 proteinuric women and no neonatal deaths in 17 women who became eclamptic but did not have proteinuria.

In spite of the specificity and fetal prognostic significance of proteinuria, however, eclampsia can occur without proteinuria. In one series of 298 eclamptic patients, 41% did not have proteinuria (Naidoo and Moodley, 1980), and in a series of eclamptic patients reviewed by Chesley (1978), 26 of 199 had either trace (16) or no (10) proteinuria prior to seizures. Also, as discussed previously, very high blood pressure without proteinuria is associated with increased fetal and maternal risk (Buchbinder et al., 2002).

Retinal Changes

Important and consistent signs in preeclamptic patients are retinal vascular changes on funduscopic examination. Localized or generalized changes occur in retinal arterioles in at least 50% of women with preeclampsia. These retinal vascular changes are the clinical sign that best correlates with renal biopsy changes of preeclampsia (Pollak and Nettles,

1960). Localized retinal vascular narrowing is visualized as segmental spasm, and the generalized narrowing is indicated by a decrease in the ratio of arteriolar-venous diameter from the usual 3:5 to 1:2 or even 1:3. It can occur in all vessels or, in early stages, in single vessels (Jaffe and Shatz, 1986). Preeclampsia does not cause chronic arteriolar changes; thus, the presence of arteriolar sclerosis detected by increased light reflex, copper wiring, or arteriovenous nicking indicates preexisting vascular disease.

Finnerty (1956) described a characteristic "retinal sheen" in preeclamptic patients. In the present author's experience, this finding is present in many young patients, pregnant and nonpregnant, male and female, and has not been a useful sign.

Hyperreflexia

Hyperreflexia is a sign that is given a great deal of clinical attention. Deep tendon reflexes are increased in many women prior to seizures; however, seizures can occur in the absence of hyperreflexia (Sibai et al., 1981), and many young subjects are consistently hyperreflexic without being preeclamptic. Changes, or lack of changes, in deep tendon reflexes are not part of the diagnosis of preeclampsia.

Other Signs

Other signs that occur less commonly in preeclampsia are indicators of involvement of specific organs of the preeclamptic process. Thus, patients with marked edema may have ascites and hydrothorax, and those in congestive heart failure have the usual signs—increased neck vein distention, gallop rhythm, and pulmonary rales. Hepatic capsular distention, manifested by hepatic enlargement and tenderness, is particularly ominous, as is disseminated intravascular coagulation (DIC) sufficient to result in petechiae or generalized bruising and bleeding.

Symptoms of Preeclampsia

It is important to remember that most women with early preeclampsia are asymptomatic. This lack of symptoms is, in fact, an important part of the rationale for frequent obstetric visits in late gestation. In most cases, increased blood pressure, increasing edema, and proteinuria antedate overt symptoms.

The multitude of symptoms that can occur secondary to preeclampsia—especially preeclampsia of increasing severity—are listed in Table 43-2. Because preeclampsia is a disease of poor perfusion to essentially all tissues, the occurrence of symptoms related to many organ systems is not surprising. Tightness of hands and feet and paresthesias secondary to medial or ulnar nerve compression occur because of fluid retention. Although these are of concern to the patient, who may be quite uncomfortable, they are not of prognostic significance. Certain symptoms, however, are indicators of the severity of the disease. Symptoms of hepatic capsular distention are particularly ominous. These include epigastric pain, "stomach upset," and pain penetrating to the back. Headache and mental confusion indicate poor cerebral perfusion and could be precursors of convulsions. Visual symptoms ranging from scotomata to blindness indicate retinal arterial spasm and edema. In evaluation of the patient with preeclampsia, these signs of poor perfusion are as important indicators of the severity of the disease as the easily quantifiable signs. Other symptoms, such

TABLE 43-2. SIGNS AND SYMPTOMS
OF PREECLAMPSIA-ECLAMPSIA

Cerebral	Headache
	Dizziness
	Tinnitus
	Drowsiness
	Change in respiratory rate
	Tachycardia
	Fever
Visual	Diplopia
	Scotomata
	Blurred vision
	Amaurosis
Gastrointestinal	Nausea
	Vomiting
	Epigastric pain
	Hematemesis
Renal	Oliguria
	Anuria
	Hematuria
	Hemoglobinuria

as congestive heart failure and abruptio placentae, may also be present secondary to the complications of preeclampsia.

Laboratory Findings

Proteinuria is, by strict definition, not a sign of preeclampsia-eclampsia. It is a laboratory finding. Because it is a diagnostic feature of the disorder, however, proteinuria has already been discussed. Major changes revealed by laboratory studies occur in severe preeclampsia and eclampsia. In the patient with mild preeclampsia, changes in most of these indicators may be minimal or absent.

Renal Function Studies

SERUM URIC ACID CONCENTRATION AND URATE CLEARANCE

Uric acid is the most sensitive laboratory indicator of preeclampsia available to clinicians. A decrease in uric acid clearance precedes a measurable decrease in glomerular filtration rate (GFR) (Gallery and Győry, 1979b). Also, serum uric acid levels were actually a better predictor of perinatal outcome than blood pressure (Redman et al., 1976a). Although it is widely held that increased serum uric acid is due to altered renal function, an alternative view favors increased production secondary to oxidative stress (Many et al., 1996). Table 43-3 shows normal uric acid levels during gestation and levels associated with preeclampsia.

SERUM CREATININE CONCENTRATION AND CREATININE CLEARANCE

Creatinine clearance is decreased in most patients with severe preeclampsia but can be normal in patients with milder forms of the disease. Serum creatinine determinations, if obtained serially, may reflect this decrease in clearance, but unless values are very elevated, they are not helpful because of the wide range of normal single values. The serum creatinine varies as a geometric function of creatinine clearance. Thus, an increase from 0.6 to 1.2 mg/dL indicates a halving of creatinine clearance. Interpretation of more subtle variations of serum creatinine concentration depends on the ability to differentiate between small changes in creatinine resulting from functional changes and those resulting from variations in laboratory technique. Thus, smaller changes in glomerular filtration are best determined by measurements of creatinine clearance.

BLOOD UREA NITROGEN AND UREA CLEARANCE

Changes in urea clearance and blood urea nitrogen (BUN) mirror the changes in creatinine clearance. One must take the same caution as with creatinine serum concentrations as well as understand that BUN concentration is also influenced by protein intake and liver function. BUN sometimes increases in hospitalized patients in spite of unchanging serum creatinine concentrations, probably owing to an improved diet.

URINARY SEDIMENT

Pollak and Nettles (1960) reported urinary sediment changes in cases of severe preeclampsia. Unfortunately, there was no control group, and there is evidence of increased urinary excretion of formed elements in normal pregnancy (Elden and Cooney, 1935). Urinary sediment analysis is probably not a useful aid to differential diagnosis except in individuals with urinary changes pathognomonic of other renal diseases who have clinical signs of mild preeclampsia.

Hematologic Changes

In patients with severe preeclampsia, reduction in plasma volume could be indicated by a rapid increase in hematocrit level over values obtained in the preceding week. Hematocrit

TABLE 43-3. PLASMA URATE CONCENTRATIONS IN NORMOTENSIVE AND HYPERTENSIVE PREGNANT WOMEN

Weeks Gestation	Normotensive Patients			Hypertensive Patients		
	mMol/liter	*	mg/dL	mMol/liter	*	mg/dL
24–28	0.18	(20%)	3.02	0.24	(20%)	4.03
29–32	0.18	(35%)	3.02	0.28	(25%)	4.7
33–36	0.20	(30%)	3.36	0.30	(20%)	5.04
37–40	0.26	(20%)	4.4	0.31	(23%)	5.28
41–42	0.25	(24%)	4.2	0.32	(12%)	5.38

* Numbers in parentheses are standard deviation as percentage of the mean values shown. Values for hypertensive and normotensive women are statistically different at all gestational ages ($P < .05$).

Modified from Shuster E, Weppelman B: Plasma urate measurements and fetal outcome in preeclampsia. Gynecol Obstet Invest **12:**162, 1981.

decreases postpartum or with volume expansion (Dieckman, 1952). In cases of mild preeclampsia, the hematocrit level is usually not elevated.

Liver Function Tests

The results of laboratory tests of liver function have been reviewed extensively by Chesley (1978). In reviewing published results of bilirubin, alkaline phosphatase, serum aspartate transaminase (AST), and alanine aminotransferase (ALT) determinations along with several older tests of liver function in preeclampsia, he concluded that none of these tests is useful prognostically or as a gauge of severity of the disease. The association, however, between microangiopathic anemia and elevations in AST and ALT carries an especially ominous prognosis for the mother and baby (Weinstein, 1982; Martin et al., 1991). These findings usually correlate with severity of disease and, when associated with hepatic enlargement, are an ominous sign of impending hepatic rupture.

Coagulation Factors

In approximately 20% of patients with severe preeclampsia, the usual laboratory evidence of consumption of procoagulants is present (Pritchard et al., 1976). The average platelet count in the patient with mild preeclampsia does not differ from the platelet count in normal pregnant women (Galton et al., 1971); however, careful platelet counts performed sequentially in individual patients may reveal decreased platelets in many patients (Redman et al., 1978). Highly sensitive indicators of activation of the clotting system, reduced serum concentrations of antithrombin III (Weiner and Brandt, 1982), a decrease in the ratio of factor VIII bioactivity to factor VIII antigen (Redman, Denson, et al., 1977), and subtle indicators of platelet dysfunction, including alteration of turnover (Inglis et al., 1982), activation (Janes et al., 1995), size (Hutt et al., 1994), and content (Douglas et al., 1982) are present in even mild preeclampsia and could, in fact, antedate clinically evident disease.

Lipid Changes in Preeclampsia

Striking changes occur in circulating lipids in normal pregnancy (Knopp, 1991), and these are accentuated in preeclampsia (Hubel and Roberts, 1999). Triglycerides and fatty acid levels are elevated, and these changes antedate clinically evident disease by weeks to months (Lorentzen et al., 1994; Hubel et al., 1996). Levels of the cardioprotective lipoprotein—high-density lipoprotein (HDL) cholesterol—are reduced in preeclamptic women (Rosing et al., 1989), whereas levels of a variant of low-density lipoprotein (LDL)—small dense LDL, which is strongly associated with cardiovascular disease—are increased (Sattar et al., 1997; Hubel et al., 1998). These changes all revert toward normal shortly after delivery.

Pathologic Changes in Preeclampsia

The pathologic changes found in organs of women dying of eclampsia and in biopsy specimens from women with preeclampsia provide strong evidence that preeclampsia is not merely an unmasking of essential hypertension or a variant of malignant hypertension. These findings also indicate that the elevation of blood pressure is probably not of primary pathogenetic importance.

Brain

Cerebral edema was once thought to be a common finding in women dying of eclampsia. Sheehan and Lynch (1973), on the basis of postmortem examinations performed within 2 to 3 hours of death, concluded that the findings previously reported were primarily postmortem changes and that cerebral edema was actually a rare complication. Studies using computed tomography (CT) have once again raised the possibility that cerebral edema is an important pathophysiologic event in some patients with preeclampsia (Naheedy et al., 1985). Recent noninvasive determinations of cerebral blood flow and resistance are providing new insights that suggest vascular barotrauma and loss of cerebral vascular autoregulation as keys in the pathogenesis of cerebral vascular changes of preeclampsia/eclampsia (Belfort et al., 2002).

Liver

Gross lesions of the liver are visible in about 60% of women dying of eclampsia, and one-third of the remaining livers are microscopically abnormal. Many early investigators thought that the hepatic changes were pathognomonic of eclampsia (Schmorl, 1901). Similar changes, however, have been described in women dying of abruptio placentae (Sheehan, 1950).

The most extensive account of the hepatic changes has been provided by Sheehan and Lynch (1973). They describe two types of lesions, which they consider temporally and etiologically distinct. Initially, the hepatic changes are most consistent with hemorrhage into the hepatic cellular columns, with dislocation and deformation of the hepatocytes in their stromal sleeves (Fig. 43-3). These changes are interpreted as hemorrhage secondary to vasodilatation of arterioles. Later,

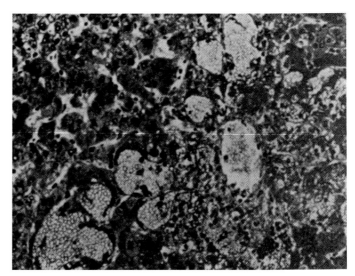

FIGURE 43-3 ■ Hemorrhagic hepatic lesions in eclampsia. Hemorrhage into periportal area with crescentic compression of liver cells. (From Sheehan HL, Lynch JB: Pathology of Toxemia in Pregnancy. London, Churchill Livingstone, 1973.)

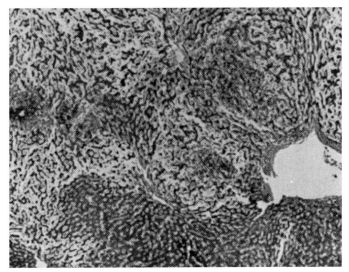

FIGURE 43-4 ■ Hepatic infarction in eclampsia. (From Sheehan HL, Lynch JB: Pathology of Toxemia in Pregnancy. London, Churchill Livingstone, 1973.)

signs of hepatic infarction are present. These changes range from small to large areas of infarction beginning near the sinusoids but eventually extending into the area adjacent to portal vessels (Fig. 43-4). These changes are believed to be secondary to intense vasospasm. Hemorrhagic changes are present in 66% and necrotic changes in 40% of eclamptic women and in about half as many preeclamptic women. Several authors have described hyalinization and thrombosis of hepatic vessels and have cited this finding as evidence of DIC, although it could represent a later stage of the hemorrhagic phenomenon.

Kidney

Pathologic renal changes in preeclamptic and eclamptic women are clearly different from the morphologic changes seen in other hypertensive or renal disorders. Glomerular, tubular, and arteriolar changes have been described. Of these, the most characteristic and consistent is the glomerular lesion, which is considered by some investigators to be pathognomonic of preeclampsia-eclampsia. Identical changes could be present, however, in kidneys of women who have placental abruption without evident preeclampsia (Thomson et al., 1972); this change is not seen in any other form of hypertension.

GLOMERULAR CHANGES

A number of characteristic changes are seen by light microscopy in glomeruli of preeclamptic women (Pollak and Nettles, 1960). There is a slight decrease in glomerular size, and the glomerular tuft protrudes into the proximal tubule. The diameter of the glomerular capillary lumen is decreased and contains few blood cells. The endothelial-mesangial cells, which are indistinguishable on light microscopy, are larger as a result of an increase in cytoplasmic volume and can contain lipoid droplets (Fig. 43-5).

Electron microscopic examination of glomeruli provides a more precise picture (Fig. 43-6). From both examinations, it is evident that the primary pathologic change occurs in endothelial cells. These cells, which line the glomerular capillaries, are greatly increased in size and can occlude the capillary lumen;

their cytoplasm contains electron-dense material (Spargo et al., 1959). The basement membrane bordering the epithelial cell may be slightly thickened and also contains electron-dense material. The epithelial cell podocytes are not altered. On the basis of these pathologic findings, the lesion has been termed "glomerular capillary endotheliosis."

Faith and Trump (1966) believed that the endothelial changes are secondary to phagocytosis of blood-borne materials by these cells, the nature of this material being a matter of controversy. It was originally reported on the basis of immunofluorescent staining studies that immune globulins were not present but that the material had the antigenic characteristics of fibrinogen (Vassali et al., 1963). In other studies using more specific anti-immunoglobulin, IgG, IgM, and complement have been demonstrated (Petruccho et al., 1974). Fibrin is also found in the glomeruli. Petruccho and colleagues (1974) have suggested that fibrin is present secondary to an immunologic reaction. Other investigators have not consistently found immunoglobulins or fibrin-like material in renal biopsy specimens (Spargo et al., 1976).

It is possible that differences can be accounted for by methodology. Kincaid-Smith and coworkers, using fixing techniques designed to maintain antigenicity of the deposits, demonstrated deposition of fibrinogen, IgA, IgG, IgM, complement, and albumin (Kincaid-Smith, 1991). Other investigators believe these changes to be nonspecific (Gaber et al., 1994).

The glomerular lesion, although not pathognomonic, is highly characteristic of preeclampsia. The more likely the diagnosis of preeclampsia, the more common the glomerular lesion. As stated above, characteristic glomerular changes are present in 70% of primiparas but in only 14% of multiparas given a diagnosis of preeclampsia (McCartney, 1964). In addition, as the clinical condition worsens, the magnitude of the glomerular lesion increases. The glomerular lesions are reversible after delivery and are not present in subsequent biopsy specimens obtained 5 to 10 weeks later (Pollak and Nettles, 1960).

The glomerular changes described correlate more consistently with proteinuria than with hypertension, suggesting that the proteins identified immunohistochemically may

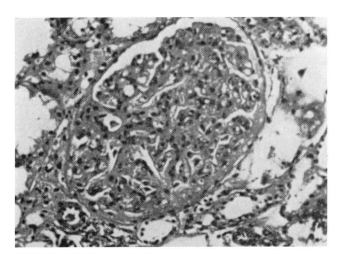

FIGURE 43-5 ■ Glomerular changes in preeclampsia by light microscopy. The enlarged glomerulus completely fills Bowman's capsule. Diffuse edema of the glomerular wall is indicated by the vacuolated appearance. The visible capillary loops are extremely narrow, and there are virtually no red blood cells in the capillary tuft.

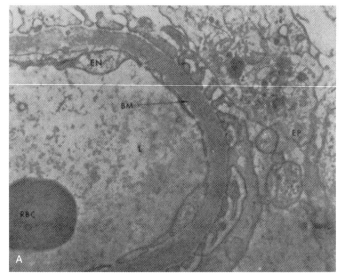

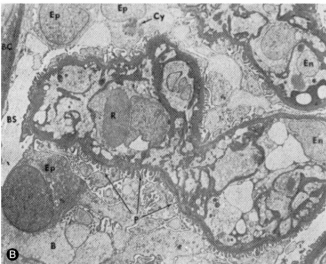

FIGURE 43-6 ■ Electron photomicrographs of renal glomeruli. **(A)** Normal anatomy. BM, basement membrane; EN, capillary endothelial cells that line the glomeruli; Ep, renal epithelial cells; L, the capillary lumen containing red blood cell (RBC). **(B)** Biopsy specimen from a preeclamptic woman. Endothelial cells (En) are markedly enlarged, obstruct the capillary lumen, and contain electron-dense inclusions. The basement membrane is slightly thickened with inclusions, but the epithelial foot processes (P) are normal. BS, Bowman's space; Cy, cytoplasmic inclusions; P, podocytes; R, red blood cell. (From McCartney CP: Pathological anatomy of acute hypertension of pregnancy. Circulation **30**[Suppl II]:37, 1964. By permission of the American Heart Association, Inc.)

simply be trapped in the glomerulus. These staining patterns, however, are not characteristic of findings in other renal disorders in which proteinuria is present.

NONGLOMERULAR CHANGES

Pathologic changes in renal tubules are less consistently or less frequently described than those in glomeruli. Changes described by several investigators include dilatation of proximal tubules with thinning of the epithelium (Sheehan and Lynch, 1973), tubular necrosis (Pollak and Nettles, 1960), enlargement of the juxtaglomerular apparatus (Altchek et al., 1968), and hyaline deposition in renal tubules (Sheehan

and Lynch, 1973). Fat deposition in women with prolonged heavy proteinuria has been reported by Sheehan and Lynch (1973). Altchek and coauthors (1968) described necrosis of the loop of Henle, a change that correlates with the degree of hyperuricemia and is also present in biopsy specimens from people with gout. It is possible that several of the other tubular changes described could also be secondary to the glomerular pathophysiology.

Thickening of renal arterioles is also present in some patients with preeclampsia and is more common in women with a known history of hypertension. Unlike the glomerular lesion, it does not regress postpartum (Pollak and Nettles, 1960), suggesting that the arteriolar change is due to coincident disease, not to preeclampsia.

Vascular Changes in the Placental Site

The characteristic changes in the decidual vessels supplying the placental site in normal pregnancy are depicted in Figure 43-7. In normal pregnancy, the spiral arteries (Fig. 43-8) increase greatly in diameter (Ramsey and Harris, 1966). Morphologically, the endothelium is replaced by trophoblast, and the internal elastic lamina and smooth muscle of the media are replaced by both trophoblast and an amorphous matrix containing fibrin (Brosens et al., 1972) (see Fig. 43-8). These changes occur originally in the decidual portion of the spiral arteries but extend into the myometrium as pregnancy advances and can even involve the distal portion of the uterine radial artery. The basal arteries are not affected. These morphologic changes are considered to be a vascular reaction to trophoblast, either directly or humorally, that results in increased perfusion of the placental site.

In placental site vessels of women with preeclampsia, the normal physiologic changes do not occur or are limited to the decidual portion of the vessels; myometrial segments of spiral arteries in myometrium retain the nonpregnant component of intima and smooth muscle, and the diameter of these arteries is about 40% that of vessels in normal pregnancy (Khong et al., 1986). In addition, some spiral arterioles in decidua and myometrium and some basal and radial arterioles are affected by a change termed *acute atherosis* (Zeek and Assali,

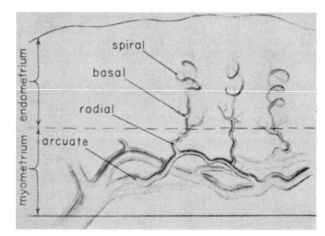

FIGURE 43-7 ■ Schematic representation of uterine arteries. (From Okkels H, Engle ET: Studies of the finer structure of the uterine vessels of the Macacus monkey. Acta Pathol Microbiol Scand **15**:150, 1938.)

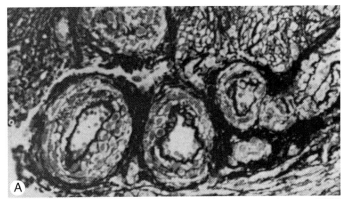

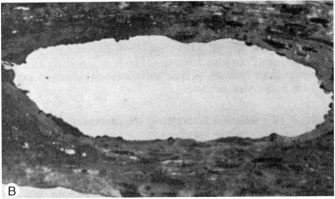

FIGURE 43-8 ■ Spiral arterial changes in normal pregnancy.
(A) Section of spiral arterioles at the junction of endometrium and myometrium in a nonpregnant individual. Note inner elastic lamina and smooth muscle. **(B)** Section of spiral arteriole in the same scale and from the same location during pregnancy. Note markedly increased diameter and absence of inner elastic lamina and smooth muscle. (From Sheppard BL, Bonnar J: Uteroplacental arteries and hypertensive pregnancy. *In* Bonnar J, MacGillivray I, Symonds G [eds]: Pregnancy Hypertension. Baltimore, University Park Press, 1980, p. 205.)

1950) (Fig. 43-9). The affected vessels are necrotic, and the usual components of the vessel wall are replaced by amorphous material and "foam cells." This lesion is best seen in basal arteries because these arteries do not undergo the normal changes of pregnancy. It is also present in decidual and myometrial spiral arteries and can progress to vessel obliteration. The obliterated vessels correspond to areas of placental infarction.

Although some believe that this change occurs only in preeclampsia, others hold that it is present in placental site vessels in pregnancies with fetal growth restriction and without clinical evidence of preeclampsia. Similar changes occur in decidual vessels of some diabetic women (Kitzmiller et al., 1981) as well as in about one-third of women who experience preterm labor (Arias et al., 1993). Thus, it appears that abnormal invasion may be necessary but is not sufficient to cause preeclampsia.

Investigators have reported changes characteristic of preeclampsia in the decidual vessels of approximately 14% of primiparous women and in a lower percentage of multiparous women at the time of first-trimester abortion (Nadji and Sommers, 1973; Lichtig et al., 1985). This finding indicates that preeclampsia is a disorder of placentation and that characteristic pathologic changes have preceded the clinical pres-

entation of this disorder. The etiology of the decidual vascular lesions is not known. The appearance of these vessels is somewhat similar to that of vessels in transplanted kidneys that have undergone rejection. This suggestion of an immunologic etiology is supported by the finding of Kitzmiller and Benirschke (1973), who demonstrated components of complement (C3) in decidual vessels with the lesion.

Recent advances have increased our understanding of the implantation process in humans considerably (Cross et al., 1994). The expression of adhesion molecules and their receptors that characterizes implantation is abnormal in preeclampsia (Zhou et al., 1993). Also, whereas the trophoblast that line the decidual vessels of normal pregnant women begin to express molecules usually present only on endothelium (Zhou, Fisher, et al., 1997), this does not occur in preeclampsia (Zhou, Damsky, et al., 1997). The mechanisms responsible for the normal and abnormal expression of these crucial molecules are only beginning to be understood. Current candidate molecules are decidually produced cytokines (Bass et al., 1994; Librach et al., 1994; Caniggia et al., 1999) and local oxygen tension (Genbacev et al., 1996, 1997; Caniggia et al., 2000).

Placental Pathologic Changes

Ultrastructural examination of placentas from women with preeclampsia provides details about the pathologic changes. The syncytiotrophoblast is abnormal, containing areas of cell death and degeneration. Viable-appearing syncytiotrophoblast is also abnormal, with decreased density of microvilli, dilated endoplasmic reticulum, and evidence of decreased pinocytotic and secretory activity. The cells of the villous cytotrophoblast cells are increased in number and have higher mitotic activity. The basement membrane of the trophoblast is irregularly thickened, with fine fibrillary inclusions (Jones and Fox, 1980).

The etiology of these anatomic changes is speculative. Similar syncytiotrophoblastic changes are present in placental segments maintained under hypoxic conditions *in vitro* (Fox, 1970). The cytotrophoblastic alterations are also consistent with hypoxia. The cytotrophoblast comprises the stem cells of the trophoblast and responds to damage by proliferation.

Although most of the findings are consistent with hypoxia secondary to poor perfusion as the cause of placental change, at least one finding suggests that other factors may be involved. Even though the cytotrophoblastic cells in most instances proliferate, there are also areas in which cytotrophoblast, resistant to hypoxia *in vitro*, is seen to be degenerating adjacent to normal syncytiotrophoblast, which is very susceptible to hypoxia. This evidence suggests either the absence of a factor other than oxygen that is required more by cytotrophoblast than by syncytiotrophoblast or the presence of factors specifically toxic to cytotrophoblast.

Pathologic Changes in Other Organs

Subendocardial hemorrhages are present in more than 50% of women who die of eclampsia. These hemorrhages are located primarily on the left side of the intraventricular septum. Hemorrhage rarely extends into myocardial tissue (Sheehan and Lynch, 1973). In character and location, these hemorrhages are identical to those found in patients dying of hypovolemic shock.

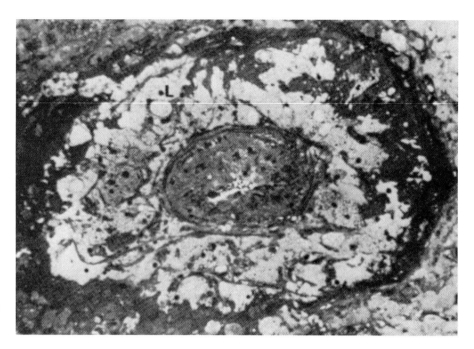

FIGURE 43-9 ■ Atherosis: Numerous lipid-laden cells (L) and fibrin deposition (F) are present in the media of this occluded decidual vessel. (From Sheppard BL, Bonnar J: Uteroplacental arteries and hypertensive pregnancy. *In* Bonnar J, MacGillivray I, Symonds G [eds]: Pregnancy Hypertension. Baltimore, University Park Press, 1980, p. 205.)

Histologic changes in adrenal tissue obtained inadvertently at percutaneous renal biopsy reveal areas of necrosis and hemorrhage. This observation is in keeping with the changes in adrenals of women dying of eclampsia as described by Sheehan and Lynch (1973), who noted ischemic cortical changes in approximately 50% of cases.

Summary of Pathological Changes in Preeclampsia

Structural changes associated with preeclampsia-eclampsia lead to two important conclusions: First, preeclampsia is not merely an alternate form of malignant hypertension. The renal changes in preeclamptic and eclamptic women and the structural changes in other organs of women dying of eclampsia differ from the alterations caused by malignant hypertension. Second, the pathologic findings indicate that the pathogenetic factor of primary importance is not blood pressure elevation but poor tissue perfusion. The histologic data support the clinical impression that the poor perfusion is secondary to profound vasospasm, which also increases total peripheral resistance and blood pressure.

Pathophysiologic Changes in Preeclampsia

As emphasized in the discussion of signs and symptoms, preeclampsia can cause changes in virtually all organ systems. Several organ systems are consistently and characteristically involved. They are discussed in detail, as they have been extensively studied and provide insight into the pathophysiologic changes in all organ systems.

Cardiovascular Changes

Blood pressure is the product of cardiac output (CO) and total peripheral resistance (TPR). Cardiac output is increased by up to 50% in normal pregnancy, yet blood pressure does not usually increase. As mentioned previously, blood pressure is, in fact, lower during the first half of pregnancy than in the postpartum period, when cardiac output subsides toward nonpregnant levels (see Fig. 43-1). During normal pregnancy, therefore, TPR decreases. There is interesting data that a subset of women destined to develop preeclampsia actually have higher cardiac outputs prior to clinically evident disease. Cardiac output, however, is reduced to usual levels with the onset of clinical preeclampsia (Easterling et al., 1990; Bosio et al., 1999). Although there is some controversy about the status of cardiac output in women with severe preeclampsia, with some authors suggesting increased cardiac output (Mabie et al., 1989), most studies of untreated preeclamptic women indicate that cardiac output is normal or slightly reduced (Wallenburg, 1988). Therefore, increased TPR must account for the increase in blood pressure in clinical preeclampsia.

There is considerable direct evidence that arteriolar narrowing occurs in preeclampsia. Changes in the caliber of retinal arterioles correlate with the clinical severity of the disorder and with renal biopsy diagnosis of preeclampsia (Pollak and Nettles, 1960). Similar findings are present in vessels of the nail bed and conjunctiva. Measurements of forearm blood flow indicate higher resistance in preeclamptic than in normal pregnant women (Spetz, 1965; Duncan et al., 1968). It is unlikely that this effect is determined by the autonomic nervous system. Although normal pregnant women are exquisitely sensitive to interruption of autonomic neurotransmission by ganglionic blockade and high spinal anesthesia, preeclamptic women are actually less sensitive (Assali and Prystowsky, 1950). This finding suggests that the arteriolar constriction of preeclampsia is not maintained by the autonomic nervous system, and humoral factors are implicated. Recent findings of increased sympathetic activity in preeclampsia, however, have raised questions about these older findings (Schobel and Grassi, 1998).

Assays of concentrations of recognized endogenous vasoconstrictors are limited to determinations of catecholamines and angiotensin II. Results suggest minimal, if any, change in catecholamines, whereas circulating angiotensin II concentrations are lower in preeclamptic women (Hanssens et al., 1991).

Levels of endothelin-1, a vasoconstrictor produced by endothelial cells, are increased in the blood of preeclamptic women (Taylor, Varma, et al., 1990). Concentrations present in these women, however, are much lower than those necessary to stimulate vascular smooth muscle contraction *in vitro*. Whether these circulating concentrations reflect endothelial production sufficient to stimulate vasoconstriction at the site of production or whether low concentrations of endothelin may potentiate contractile responses to other agonists in preeclampsia is speculative.

As indicated by the older term *toxemia*, early investigators suspected that preeclampsia was caused by circulating humors. Several investigators have reported finding pressor substances in blood, decidual extracts, placental extracts, and amniotic fluid of preeclamptic patients, but the results of their studies have been inconsistent and unreproducible. The explanation for the pressor effects was, in some studies, normal endogenous pressors; in others, the explanation was faulty methodology and failure to recognize the immunologic difference between the source of the extract and the animals tested. In other experiments, no defect is obvious. In contemporary thinking, probably appropriately, the hypothesis that arteriolar constriction of preeclampsia is caused by new circulating pressors has largely been abandoned (Chesley, 1978).

An alternative explanation for vasospasm in preeclampsia is a greater response to normal concentrations of endogenous pressors. Women with preeclampsia have higher sensitivity to all endogenous pressors thus far tested. They are exquisitely sensitive to vasopressin (Dieckman and Michel, 1937; Chesley and Valenti, 1958). Vasopressin can elicit marked blood pressure elevation, seizures, and oliguria in some patients (Dieckman and Michel, 1937). Sensitivity to epinephrine (Zuspan et al., 1964) and norepinephrine (Talledo et al., 1968) is also increased (Fig. 43-10). The most striking difference is seen in the sensitivity of the preeclamptic woman to angiotensin II. Normal pregnant women are less sensitive to angiotensin II than nonpregnant women, requiring approximately 2.5 times as much angiotensin to raise the blood pressure by a similar increment (Schwarz and Retzke, 1971). Preeclamptic women are much more sensitive to angiotensin II than are normal pregnant and nonpregnant women (Talledo

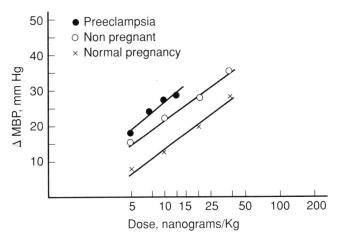

FIGURE 43-11 ■ Mean dose-response lines to angiotensin. (From Talledo OE, Chesley LC, Zuspan FP: Renin-angiotensin system in normal and toxemic pregnancies: III. Differential sensitivity to angiotensin II and norepinephrine in toxemia of pregnancy. Am J Obstet Gynecol **100**:218, 1968. Courtesy of the American College of Obstetricians and Gynecologists.)

et al., 1968), demonstrating a striking difference in dose response (Fig. 43-11).

In a classic study by Dallas-based investigators, angiotensin II sensitivity was reported to increase many weeks before the development of elevated blood pressure (Fig. 43-12) (Gant et al., 1973). Although resistance to angiotensin II does not decrease to nonpregnant levels until 32 weeks' gestation, as early as 14 weeks there are significant differences in sensitivity between women who later become hypertensive and those who remain normotensive. A large study in a British population did not confirm this classic finding (Kyle et al., 1995). This could be another example of the heterogeneity of preeclampsia (Ness and Roberts, 1996).

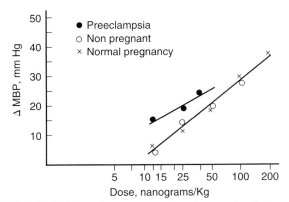

FIGURE 43-10 ■ Mean dose-response lines to norepinephrine. (From Talledo OE, Chesley LC, Zuspan FP: Renin-angiotensin system in normal and toxemic pregnancies: III. Differential sensitivity to angiotensin II and norepinephrine in toxemia of pregnancy. Am J Obstet Gynecol **100**:218, 1968. Courtesy of the American College of Obstetricians and Gynecologists.)

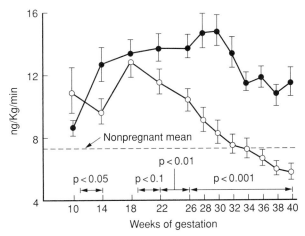

FIGURE 43-12 ■ Angiotensin sensitivity throughout pregnancy: comparison of the dose of angiotensin II necessary to increase diastolic blood pressure 20 mm Hg in women who developed elevated blood pressure in late pregnancy (○) and those who remained normotensive (●) demonstrates that a significantly lower dose was required in the former group as early as 10–14 weeks of gestation. (From Gant NF, Daley GL, Chand S, et al: A study of angiotensin II pressor response throughout primigravid pregnancy. J Clin Invest **49**:82, 1973. With permission of the American Society for Clinical Investigation.)

The decreased sensitivity of normal pregnant women to angiotensin II and the lower TPR in normal pregnancy suggest that arteriolar narrowing in preeclamptic women could be the result of decreased vasodilator substances, either circulating or local, rather than of increased circulating pressors. This attractive hypothesis, however, is not consistent with the unchanged sensitivities to norepinephrine, epinephrine, and vasopressin in normal pregnancy (Dieckman and Michel, 1937; Zuspan et al., 1964; Talledo et al., 1968).

Coagulation Changes

The syndrome of DIC occurs in preeclampsia and has been suggested as a primary pathogenetic factor (McKay, 1972) (also see Chapter 47). The activation of the coagulation system is manifested as the intravascular disappearance of procoagulants, the intravascular appearance of degradation products of fibrin, and end-organ damage secondary to the formation of microthrombi (Bell, 1980). In the most advanced form of DIC, procoagulants—especially fibrinogen and platelets—decrease to a degree sufficient to produce spontaneous hemorrhage. In milder forms, only highly sensitive indicators of clotting system activation are present. Decreasing platelet concentrations is such a sign but is usually evident in early cases only if the platelet count has been observed serially. An elevated level of fibrin degradation products is a sensitive indicator of intravascular coagulation. This and other sensitive indicators of intravascular coagulation, such as increased platelet turnover (Inglis et al., 1982), volume (Hutt et al., 1994), activation (Janes et al., 1995), reduced platelet content (Douglas et al., 1982), increased platelet content in plasma (Socol et al., 1985), reduced levels of antithrombin III (Weiner and Brandt, 1982), and a reduced ratio of factor VIII activity to factor VIII antigen (Denson, 1977), are frequently present when concentrations of procoagulants remain normal.

Abnormalities of blood coagulation sufficient to make the diagnosis of DIC are present in approximately 10% of patients with severe preeclampsia or eclampsia (Roberts and May, 1976). Levels of procoagulants are normal in the majority of patients with preeclampsia, which suggests that coagulation changes are secondary, rather than primary, pathogenetic factors (Pritchard et al., 1976). Results of highly sensitive assays of coagulation activation suggest, however, that abnormalities of the coagulation system are present in many patients with mild to moderate preeclampsia.

Some authors have reported that fibrin degradation products in plasma are a common occurrence in mild to moderate preeclampsia (Henderson et al., 1970; McKillop et al., 1976; Beller et al., 1979), but others (Gordon et al., 1976) have not reported this finding. The differing results probably reflect different assay specificities and sensitivities.

Redman and colleagues (1978) performed serial platelet counts in women at risk for preeclampsia and found a decrease in platelets coinciding with the appearance of clinical signs of the disease. Similarly, subtle signs of platelet dysfunction (Douglas et al., 1982; Inglis et al., 1982; Socol et al., 1985; Hutt et al., 1994; Janes et al., 1995), reduced antithrombin III (Weiner and Brandt, 1982), and reduction in the ratio of factor VIII bioactivity to factor VIII antigen (Redman, Denson, et al., 1977) are present in mild preeclampsia and may precede its clinical signs. Whether even the early appearance of coagulation changes indicates that activation of the clotting system is a primary pathogenetic factor has not been established because another early sign of preeclampsia—increased serum uric acid—may precede any measurable change in coagulation (Redman et al., 1978).

The etiology of the change in coagulation factors is a matter of controversy. Vascular damage secondary to vasospasm could initiate DIC (Pritchard et al., 1976). Although this phenomenon probably plays a role in intensifying the activation of the clotting system in severe preeclampsia, its effect is less likely in the early changes preceding the occurrence of vasospasm sufficient to elevate blood pressure. Signs of endothelial dysfunction also antedate clinical disease (Roberts, 1998), and activation of platelets and other components of the coagulation cascade is a well-recognized consequence of endothelial dysfunction (Nachman, 1995). It is also possible that vascular changes in the implantation site that appear to antedate blood pressure elevation could be pathogenetically important.

Whether coagulation changes measured in preeclamptic patients are true DIC or a localized consumption of procoagulants in the intervillous space is not clear. Microthrombi and the presence of fibrin antigen have been demonstrated in liver, placenta, and kidney by some investigators (Vassali et al., 1963; Arias and Muncilla-Jimenez, 1976; Matter and Faulk, 1980) but not by others (Sheehan and Lynch, 1973). The early coagulation changes—factor VIII activity-antigen ratios and platelet count—correlate better with fetal outcome as measured by mortality and growth restriction rates than with clinical severity of preeclampsia. Identical coagulation changes are present in normotensive women with growth-restricted fetuses (Whigham et al., 1980). These findings suggest that localized coagulation in the intervillous space could be of major importance. Consistent with this theory is the finding of an increased concentration of fibrin antigen in the placentas of preeclamptic patients (Matter and Faulk, 1980).

Endothelial Cell Changes (Endothelial Dysfunction)

An increasing body of information indicates endothelial dysfunction as a pathophysiologic component of preeclampsia (Roberts et al., 1989; Roberts and Redman, 1993; Roberts, 1998). As cited, alterations of glomerular endothelial cells are a consistent feature of preeclampsia. In addition, cellular fibronectin (Lockwood and Peters, 1990; Taylor, Crombleholme, et al., 1991), growth factors (Taylor, Heilbron, et al., 1990), VCAM-1 (Krauss et al., 1997), factor VIII antigen, and peptides released from injured endothelial cells are increased in preeclamptic women prior to the appearance of clinical disease (Redman, Denson, et al., 1977). Endothelial function of vessels of preeclamptic women is also impaired when examined *in vitro* (Knock and Poston, 1996; Cockell and Poston, 1997).

It is now evident that endothelium is a complex tissue with many important functions. Two of these (prevention of coagulation and modulation of vascular tone) have special relevance to preeclampsia. Intact vascular endothelium is resistant to thrombus formation (Rodgers et al., 1983). With vascular injury, endothelial cells can initiate coagulation either by the intrinsic pathway (contact activation) (Wiggins et al., 1980) or by the extrinsic pathway (tissue factor) (Maynard et al., 1987). Platelet adhesion can also occur after injury with exposure of subendothelial components, such as collagen (Baumgartner and Hardenschild, 1977) and microfibrils.

Endothelium also profoundly influences the response of vascular smooth muscle to vasoactive agents. The response to some agents (Furchgott, 1983) can change from dilator to constrictor with the removal of endothelium. Prostacyclin, a highly potent vasodilator, is produced by endothelium. Vessels from preeclamptic women and the umbilical vessels of their neonates generate less prostacyclin than similar vessels from normal pregnant women (Bussolino et al., 1980; Remuzzi et al., 1980; Dadak et al., 1982). If potent inhibitors preventing the synthesis of all prostaglandins (including prostacyclin) are administered to pregnant women, the usual resistance to the vasoconstrictor effect of angiotensin II is abolished (Everett et al., 1978). Conversely, if aspirin is used as an inhibitor of prostaglandin synthesis in a manner determined to specifically reduce contractile prostanoids (thromboxane A_2) much more than prostacyclin, the increased angiotensin II sensitivity of preeclamptic women is reduced (Sanchez-Ramos et al., 1987).

Nitric oxide (NO) is another bioactive material produced by normal endothelium (Moncada et al., 1991). Its release is stimulated by several hormones and neurotransmitters as well as by hydrodynamic shear stress. NO is quite labile and acts synergistically with prostacyclin as a local vasodilator and inhibitor of platelet aggregation. Current thinking favors NO as an endogenous vasodilator of pregnancy. Administration of inhibitors of NO synthesis reduces blood flow much more strikingly in pregnant than in nonpregnant women (Williams et al., 1997). Production of NO is reduced with endothelial cell injury. Information is conflicting (Seligman et al., 1994; Curtis et al., 1995; Davidge et al., 1996; Silver et al., 1996; Smarason et al., 1997; Pathak et al., 1999), in part because of the use of blood concentrations of nitric oxide metabolites to determine production in the setting of the reduced renal function of preeclampsia (Roberts, 1997). Nonetheless, two studies have documented reduced urinary NO excretion in preeclampsia (Begum et al., 1996; Davidge et al., 1996), while another found increased excretion (Ranta et al., 1999). Perhaps the most compelling data is from estimates of the tissue concentrations of nitrotyrosine (the product of the interaction of NO and superoxide). Nitrotyrosine residues are increased in the placenta (Myatt et al., 1996) and vessels (Roggensack et al., 1999) of women with preeclampsia. It is posited that the placenta either directly or indirectly produces factors that alter endothelial function. Candidate molecules include the following:

1. Cytokines (Greer et al., 1994)
2. Placental fragments (syncytiotrophoblast microvillous membranes) (Smarason et al., 1993)
3. Free radicals
4. Reactive oxygen species (Hubel et al., 1989)

The latter hypothesis—that oxidative stress is the genesis of endothelial dysfunction—is especially interesting in view of the similarities of the lipid changes of preeclampsia to those of atherosclerosis (Hubel et al., 1996), an endothelial disorder in which oxidative stress is thought to play a key role (Witztum, 1994).

The information available today indicates that endothelial cell dysfunction can alter both vascular responses and intravascular coagulation in a manner consistent with the pathophysiological abnormalities present in preeclampsia. Thus,

evidence is accumulating that endothelial injury could play a central role in the pathogenesis of preeclampsia.

Renal Function Changes

Renal function changes are consistent and characteristic in women with preeclampsia-eclampsia. Glomerular function changes, manifested by decreased GFR and proteinuria, are common findings. Tubular handling of certain substances is abnormal, although other materials apparently are handled normally. Changes in components of the renin-angiotensin system probably differ from those seen in normal pregnancy. Sodium excretion is decreased, resulting in fluid retention and edema.

GLOMERULAR FUNCTIONAL CHANGES

GLOMERULAR FILTRATION RATE. Decreased glomerular filtration frequently, but not inevitably, complicates preeclampsia. The decreased GFR is explained only partially by decreased renal plasma flow (RPF), and thus the filtration fraction, GFR/RPF, is decreased (Chesley, 1978). It is possible that the change in the filtration fraction is due to intrarenal redistribution of blood flow, which unfortunately is difficult to test (Hollenberg et al., 1968). A more obvious explanation is that the change is due to glomeruloendotheliosis, in which the occlusion of glomerular capillaries by swollen endothelial cells probably renders many glomeruli nonfunctional.

PROTEIN "LEAKAGE." The pathogenesis of proteinuria in preeclampsia involves primarily glomerular changes. The normal absence of protein from urine is due both to a relative impermeability of glomeruli to large protein molecules and to the tubular resorption of smaller proteins that cross the glomeruli. As glomerular damage occurs, permeability to proteins increases. As damage increases, so does the size of the protein molecule that can cross the glomerular membrane. This increase in permeability results in a decrease in selectivity; that is, with minimal glomerular damage or tubular dysfunction, only small protein molecules are excreted, but with greater damage, both large and small proteins are present in urine.

In patients with preeclampsia, selectivity is low, indicating increased permeability and glomerular damage (Katz and Berlyne, 1974). It is a familiar clinical observation, however, that proteinuria increases and decreases in preeclamptic women. The pattern was quantitated by Chesley (1938), who found that there was a great variability from hour to hour in the creatinine:protein ratio in urine of women with preeclampsia that was not present in the urine of individuals with other diseases causing proteinuria.

Because structural glomerular changes are obviously constant, proteinuria in preeclamptic women must depend, in part, on a varying functional cause (e.g., a variation in the intensity of the renal vascular spasm). That vascular spasm can cause proteinuria has been demonstrated by measuring urinary excretion of protein in individuals subjected to the cold pressor test. Immersing a patient's hand in ice water for 60 seconds increases blood pressure more than 16 mm Hg systolic and diastolic, and an increase in protein excretion almost invariably also occurs (Chesley et al., 1939).

RENAL TUBULAR FUNCTIONAL CHANGES

URIC ACID CLEARANCE. Three separate processes are involved in the renal excretion of urate. Urate is completely filtered at the glomerulus. It is not bound to plasma proteins under physiologic conditions (Farrell, 1974), and glomerular urate concentration is equal to renal arterial plasma concentration. Urate is both secreted and reabsorbed by renal tubules. Most urate (98%) is reabsorbed, and about 80% of excreted urate is accounted for by urate secretion. Both of these processes occur predominantly in the proximal tubule. Reabsorption occurs to a greater extent than secretion, and urate clearance is thus about 10% of creatinine clearance (Emmerson, 1974).

Abnormalities of uric acid clearance have long been recognized as a consistent phenomenon in preeclampsia (Stander and Cadden, 1934) and have been regarded as a function of decreased glomerular filtration (Schaffer et al., 1943). Several studies have demonstrated the discrepancy between uric acid clearance and both inulin clearance and creatinine clearance (Seitchik, 1953; Hayashi, 1956). Serial studies also reveal that decreased uric acid clearance precedes decreases in GFR (Gallery and Györy, 1979a).

The etiology of the tubular change that results in decreased uric acid clearance is attributed to the lactic acidosis believed to be present in preeclamptic patients (Handler, 1960). Lactic acid infusion decreases uric acid clearance (Yu et al., 1957), but the clearance of uric acid is frequently decreased in preeclamptic women who have normal acid-base balance and normal lactate levels (Fadel et al., 1976). Urate clearance is also decreased by hypovolemia, presumably as a result of nonspecific stimulation of proximal tubular reabsorption (Suki et al., 1967). Plasma volume depletion is coincident with urate clearance changes (Gallery et al., 1980), suggesting that volume change could account for the abnormality in urate clearance. The correlation between the degree of volume depletion and the decrease in urate clearance, however, is poor (Gallery et al., 1980).

Angiotensin II infusion decreases urate clearance even in the presence of normal blood volume (Ferris and Gordon, 1968). The increase in angiotensin II sensitivity seen in preeclampsia may account for the change in renal function. Local effects of angiotensin II may also be important because this substance can be produced locally (Sokabe, 1974), unassociated with increased circulating angiotensin II. Furthermore, although circulating lactate concentration cannot explain changes in uric acid excretion, local changes in lactate could be involved. Lactate concentration is greater in the renal medulla than in the renal cortex, presumably owing to greater anaerobic metabolism (Dell and Winters, 1967). The gradient of increasing lactate from cortex to medulla is matched by an increasing gradient of uric acid (Cannon et al., 1970). Renal ischemia increases renal medullary lactic acid and may thus explain changes in urate clearance without associated changes in circulating lactic acid levels.

In summary, uric acid clearance changes earlier in preeclamptic pregnancy than does GFR, suggesting a tubular rather than a glomerular functional explanation. Furthermore, although the exact mechanism for the urate clearance change is not established, the common feature in the suggested mechanisms is decreased renal perfusion; however, increased production by poorly perfused tissue cannot be excluded (Parks and Granger, 1986; Many et al., 1996).

URINARY CONCENTRATING CAPACITY. Although there are some problems with studies of increased urinary osmolality in response to water restriction during pregnancy, several investigations have concluded that tubular concentrating capacity is

unchanged in normal pregnancy (Kaitz, 1961). Assali and associates (1953) suggested that urinary concentrating ability is decreased in hypertensive women. The limitations of these studies include the failure to account for parallel changes in concentrating capacity and GFR (Steele et al., 1969) and the use of specific gravity—an unreliable estimate of osmolality—as the measure of concentration (Chesley, 1978).

In one study evaluating the response to vasopressin administration, normal pregnant women were found to have decreased capacity to concentrate urine (measured as osmolar concentration and corrected for GFR); this decrease was similar to that seen in pregnant women who either were or were destined to become hypertensive (Gallery and Györy, 1979b). Differences between these findings and those of other studies suggesting that tubular concentrating capacity is normal in normal pregnancy probably reflect the failure in other studies to correct for the increased GFR of normal pregnancy, which concomitantly increases concentrating capacity (Steele et al., 1969).

EXCRETION OF PHENOLSULFONPHTHALEIN (PSP). There are few studies that directly assay tubular function. PSP is secreted by proximal tubular cells, and its excretion can be used as a sensitive indicator of proximal tubular function (Gallery and Györy, 1979a). This technique has a number of potential limitations. PSP excretion is altered independently of tubular secretory capacity with increased (Ochwadt and Pitts, 1956) or decreased (Heidland and Reidl, 1968) renal plasma flow or reduced GFR (Healy et al., 1964), and with increased urinary dead space (an especially pertinent problem in pregnancy). When these factors are carefully controlled, reduced PSP excretion indicating abnormal proximal tubular function precedes both changes in GFR and clinically evident disease (Gallery and Györy, 1979a).

RENIN-ANGIOTENSIN-ALDOSTERONE SYSTEM. The renin-angiotensin-aldosterone system is an important factor in pressure and volume regulation in normal pregnancy (Ehrlich and Lindheimer, 1972). The components of this system in normal pregnancy (Fig. 43-13) have been examined extensively. The components, as evaluated by various assays, are presented in Table 43-4.

Dramatic changes occur in the renin-angiotensin system during pregnancy (Brown et al., 1997). The following components are increased:

- Angiotensinogen (renin substrate)
- Plasma renin activity (PRA) (Weir et al., 1971)
- Plasma renin concentration (PRC)

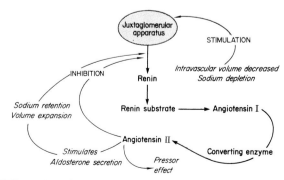

FIGURE 43-13 ■ Schematic representation of the renin-angiotensin system.

TABLE 43-4. EVALUATION OF RENIN-ANGIOTENSIN SYSTEM

Test	Method*	Results Determined by Endogenous Concentrations of the Following
Plasma renin activity (PRA)	Incubate plasma and angiotensinase inhibitors	Renin, angiotensinogen activators, inhibitors
Plasma angiotensinogen (PRS)	Incubate plasma, angiotensinase inhibitors, and excess exogenous renin	Renin substrate, activators, inhibitors
Plasma renin concentration (PRC)	Incubate plasma, angiotensinase inhibitors, and excess exogenous substrate	Renin, activators, inhibitors

* All tests use generated angiotensin I or II as the end point.

- Angiotensin II concentration (Weir et al., 1971; Gordon et al., 1973)
- Aldosterone (Bay and Ferris, 1979)

The theory that abnormalities of the renin-angiotensin system could be causal factors in preeclampsia is suggested by the following (Langford and Pickering, 1965):

1. The potent vasoconstrictor effect of angiotensin II
2. The effect of angiotensin II on aldosterone secretion and consequent sodium retention
3. The finding that large doses of the substance can cause proteinuria

This etiologic possibility is further supported by the observation that myometrium and chorion have the capacity to synthesize renin, which is stimulated in experimental animals by uterine ischemia (Ferris et al., 1972).

Most (though not all) authors agree that angiotensinogen remains elevated in preeclampsia (Weir et al., 1971; Tapia et al., 1972). PRA and PRC are reduced in preeclampsia compared with normal pregnancy (Nicholson et al., 1988). In a prospective study of chronic hypertension, PRA was lower in women in whom superimposed preeclampsia developed (diagnostic blood pressure increase and proteinuria) than in chronic hypertensive women without superimposed preeclampsia or in normal pregnant women. It is of interest that values were similar in early pregnancy in all groups and decreased only slightly prior to the increase in blood pressure (August et al., 1990).

The reduced renin activity in preeclampsia suggests suppression of renin release. This is puzzling, in view of the reduced plasma volume that is characteristic of preeclampsia. It does not appear that there is a "nonphysiologic" suppression of renin activity, as usual physiologic perturbations result in reduced and increased PRA. Thus, renin is increased with upright posture and head-up tilt (Brown et al., 1990) and falls with volume expansion (Brown et al., 1988). It is possible that, despite the reduced content of the vascular compartment in preeclampsia, the intense vasoconstriction characteristic of the condition results in a physiologic perception of overfill suppressing renin release.

As predicted, the reduced renin activity in preeclampsia results in reduced angiotensin II (Hanssens et al., 1991) and aldosterone concentrations (Brown et al., 1992) compared with levels in normal pregnancy.

Attempts to test the role of the renin-angiotensin system by using angiotensin II antagonists or by converting enzyme inhibitors have not, as yet, clarified this point. Administration of the angiotensin antagonist (1-Sar 8 Ile angiotensin II) to pregnant hypertensive women increases blood pressure (Saruta et al., 1981), and because this antagonist is a partial agonist, the increase in blood pressure may perhaps reflect the increased angiotensin sensitivity of hypertensive pregnant women. The administration of either the angiotensin antagonist saralasin (Pipkin et al., 1980) or the converting enzyme inhibitor SQ 20,881 (Sullivan et al., 1978) in the postpartum period has not had significant effects on blood pressure in a mixed group of women with hypertension.

Recently, interest in the role of the renin-angiotensin system (RAS) has increased with the recognition of effects of angiotensin on responses other than blood pressure (Wolf, 2000). The activation of NADPH oxidase in several tissues by angiotensin 2 can generate oxidative stress (Jaimes et al., 1998; Griendling and Ushio-Fukai, 2000; Wolf, 2000). In addition, the hypoxia-inducing factors (HIFs) induce molecules responsible for many of the responses to hypoxia. These factors are up-regulated in the placenta of women with preeclampsia (Rajakumar et al., 2001) and can also be activated by angiotensin II (Richard et al., 2000). Furthermore, antibodies to angiotensin II that activate angiotensin receptors and likely increase the sensitivity of these receptors to angiotensin II are present in women with preeclampsia (Wallukat et al., 1999).

Studies of the renin-angiotensin system indicate that no simple relationship exists between components of the renin-angiotensin system and preeclampsia. The significance, however, of reduced PRA, PRC, and angiotensin II level on blood pressure and sodium excretion in this group of women—who show apparent volume constriction and who are exquisitely sensitive to angiotensin II—requires and deserves elucidation. In addition, it is likely that recognition of the role of angiotensin in other important responses and its importance to preeclampsia will be deciphered.

ATRIAL NATRIURETIC FACTOR. Atrial natriuretic factor (ANF) is a peptide produced primarily in response to atrial stretch with hypervolemia, which regulates intravascular volume by several mechanisms. Among other functions, ANF increases sodium excretion and the egress of fluid from the intravascular compartment. Although the reduced plasma volume of preeclampsia predicts reduced ANF concentration, the concentration is increased (Irons et al., 1997), and this increase precedes clinical disease (Malee et al., 1992). The stimulus for this increase is unclear; however, the paradoxical finding of increased circulating ANF and reduced renin concentration with reduced plasma volume in preeclamptic women raises the possibility that this reduced plasma volume is actually increased relative to the constricted vascular compartment.

CHANGES IN SODIUM EXCRETION. Sodium retention has long been considered an integral part of the pathophysiology of preeclampsia. Women with eclampsia and severe preeclampsia have very little chloride and sodium in the urine (Zangmeister, 1903). After delivery, however, chloride excretion increases dramatically. Infusion of hypertonic saline into preeclamptic women results in excretion of the infused sodium at about one-half the rate seen in normal pregnant women (Chesley, Valenti, et al., 1958). Similar results are obtained in women with a renal biopsy diagnosis of glomeruloendotheliosis (Sarles et al., 1968). Most studies of exchangeable sodium have indicated an increase in total body sodium in preeclamptic patients (Dieckman and Pottinger, 1957; Chesley, 1966).

The etiology of sodium retention in preeclamptic women is difficult to determine because of the enormous number of factors that influence sodium excretion in normal pregnancy and, in part, to the many demonstrated anomalies of renal function in preeclampsia that could cause sodium retention (Table 43-5). Any or all of the demonstrated changes in plasma volume, angiotensin sensitivity, and renal function could act on several of the factors listed in Table 43-5 to cause sodium retention.

Several investigators have considered the increased sodium retention to be a primary factor inciting the pathogenetic changes in preeclampsia. Although this possibility

cannot be definitely excluded on the basis of sequential studies currently available, it is not likely for several reasons:

1. Angiotensin sensitivity precedes obvious fluid retention by months.
2. Sequential studies of thiocyanate space, which is proportional to sodium space, have not indicated that an increase in this space is a valuable predictor of preeclampsia (Chesley and Chesley, 1943).
3. Attempts to prevent preeclampsia by restricting dietary sodium or by increasing sodium excretion with diuretics have had no salutary effect on the occurrence of preeclampsia (Flowers et al., 1962; Weseley and Douglas, 1962; Kraus et al., 1966).

SUMMARY OF RENAL FUNCTION CHANGES. Renal function changes in preeclampsia are consistent and characteristic. Recent investigations indicate that changes in tubular function precede the more widely appreciated changes in glomerular function. It appears that these functional changes return completely to normal within weeks to months after the termination of pregnancy. Prospective sequential studies of renal function indicate that at least some of these changes antedate the clinical diagnosis of preeclampsia. They do not consistently antedate other sensitive indicators of preeclampsia, such as changes in coagulation and plasma volume, and they are thus unlikely to be causal abnormalities. Although the etiologies of these renal functional changes have not been precisely elucidated, they may all be explained by abnormalities of renal perfusion, either general or regional.

Immunologic Changes and Activation of Inflammatory Responses

Observed changes in components of the immune system and epidemiological observations have suggested that immunologic changes have a pathogenetic role, and that perhaps fetal-maternal immunologic interactions are etiologically important in the development of preeclampsia. The predominance of preeclampsia in first pregnancies and the protective effect even of miscarriage suggest a beneficial effect of maternal exposure to fetal antigen. The protective effect of previous pregnancy may be lost if the father is not the same man who fathered the prior pregnancy (Need, 1975; Trupin et al., 1996). Recent data indicates that the increased risk of preeclampsia with a new father is also determined by the interpregnancy interval, which tends to be longer in pregnancies with new fathers. This finding is also compatible with an immune-protective effect of antigen exposure, which is lost when antigen exposure is minimal for a prolonged period of time (Basso et al., 2001). In addition, the exposure to the paternal components of fetal antigen through increased sexual activity preceding the first pregnancy also reduces the risk of preeclampsia (Marti and Herrman, 1977; Robillard and Hulsey, 1996). The pathologic changes in decidual vessels at the placental site are similar to the vascular changes of acute immunological rejection (Kitzmiller and Benirschke, 1973).

Several immunological mechanisms have been suggested (Redman, 1980; Dekker and Sibai, 1999). Preeclampsia could be an immune complex disease. There is an efflux of fetal antigen into the maternal circulation during pregnancy. If the maternal antibody response is adequate, the complexes are cleared by the reticuloendothelial system, and no damage

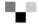

TABLE 43-5. FACTORS AFFECTING SODIUM BALANCE IN NORMAL PREGNANCY

Factors affecting glomerular filtration	Blood pressure in critical areas of the kidney
	Relative tonus of afferent and efferent glomerular arterioles
	Plasma oncotic pressure
	Intrarenal redistribution of blood flow
	Central nervous system effects
Factors affecting tubular reabsorption	Aldosterone
	Progesterone (an aldosterone antagonist)
	Renal vascular resistance
	Perfusional pressure in peritubular capillaries
	Oncotic pressure in peritubular capillaries
	Nonreabsorbable anions in the filtrate
	Velocity of flow in tubules
	Reabsorptive capacity of tubules
	Estrogens (stimulate sodium reabsorption, possibly indirectly, through effects on vascular permeability)
	Plasma sodium concentration
	Hematocrit (viscosity effects)
	Changes of plasma volume
	Angiotensin
	Sympathetic nervous system
	Possibly a natriuretic hormone ("third factor")

Modified from Chesley LC: Hypertensive Disorders in Pregnancy. New York, Appleton-Century-Crofts, 1978.

occurs. If the antibody response or clearance mechanisms are inadequate, the pathologic immune complexes thus formed would cause vasculitis, glomerular damage, and activation of the coagulation system. The postulated inadequacy of response may be due to an inadequate maternal antibody response, such as may, for example, occur in first pregnancies. The maternal antibody system may also be overwhelmed by an excess of fetal antigen, a condition compatible with the increased incidence of preeclampsia associated with increased amounts of trophoblastic tissue, as seen with twins, hydatidiform mole, and hydropic placenta. The data supporting this concept are few. The possibility that inadequate maternal antibody response could play a role in preeclampsia-eclampsia is indicated by HLA typing, which demonstrates an increased concordance of the major histocompatibility antigens in maternal-paternal pairs that result in preeclamptic pregnancies (Redman, 1980). The fact that preeclampsia is less common in consanguineous marriages, however, is incompatible with this concept (Stevenson, 1971).

Actual measurements of immune complexes are inconsistent because of widely differing methodologies, and although some studies have not demonstrated circulating immune complexes in preeclamptic pregnancy (Knox et al., 1978), other studies do indicate the presence of these complexes (Stirrat et al., 1978). Changes consistent with deposition of immune complex in the arterioles of the kidney (Petruccho et al., 1974), liver (Arias and Muncilla-Jimenez, 1976), and the uteroplacental bed (Kitzmiller and Benirschke, 1973) are described by some researchers. The evidence for increased consumption of complement, which would be predicted if preeclampsia were an immune complex disease, is also equivocal (Kitzmiller et al., 1973).

Another hypothesis of immunologic etiology is that the vascular changes in the spiral arterioles of the placental implantation site in preeclampsia are a consequence of an allograft rejection between mother and fetus. The question is, who is rejecting whom (Redman, 1980)? Should the spiral arteries lined with trophoblast be thought of as fetal vessels, with the fetus rejecting the mother, or as maternal vessels, with the mother rejecting the fetus?

If preeclampsia represents a rejection of the fetus by the mother, the epidemiologic evidence of the protective effect of previous exposure to antigen would indicate that the preeclamptic mother has a deficit of blocking antibodies or of suppressor cell function. The recognition of a unique HLA antigen, HLA-G, on trophoblast (Kavats et al., 1990) raises other possible causes of rejection of the fetus. HLA-G is a class 1 antigen present almost exclusively on cytotrophoblast. Thus far, there has been minimal heterogeneity noted in the HLA-G antigen. Therefore, unlike classic HLA antigens, which exhibit numerous epitopes, fetal HLA-G in trophoblast is likely to be identical in most (all) fetuses, and that of the fetus would be the same as that expressed by the mother during her fetal life. Because an immune cell found in maternal decidua in high numbers (the natural killer cell) is postulated to destroy cells not bearing HLA antigens, a reduced level of HLA-G could render the fetus a target for these cells. Also, unusual epitopes of HLA-G could also activate maternal immune defenses. Although there are suggestions that polymorphisms of HLA-G may be more common in preeclampsia (O'Brien et al., 2001), data is minimal thus far, and findings are not universally agreed upon (Aldrich et al., 2000).

If preeclampsia represents a rejection of the mother by the fetus, the preeclamptic mother would have to be deficient in the capacity to destroy fetal immune cells.

These alternative hypotheses—one requiring active intervention and the other passive intervention by the maternal immune system—should give disparate results in *in vitro* testing of maternal immune function. The experimental evidence currently available is not consistent enough to confirm or to contradict either hypothesis.

Recent information indicates a role of the innate immune response system (Sacks et al., 1999). Normal pregnancy is associated with an activation of inflammatory response that is nearly equivalent to that seen in sepsis. This is further increased in preeclampsia (Sacks et al., 1998). The hypothesis is advanced that materials released from the placenta—perhaps microvillus particles associated with apoptosis—interact with maternal immune cells to lead to inflammatory activation (Redman et al., 1999). An increased release of these materials in preeclampsia is posited to augment the immune response with secondary pathogenetic effects of this inflammatory activation.

The hypothesis of an immunologic cause of preeclampsia is consistent with much that is known about the disorder. The increased delineation of the changes in the immunologic activity in preeclampsia could well provide insight into the etiology of both preeclampsia and normal fetal-maternal compatibility during pregnancy.

Oxidative Stress

Oxidative stress is an excess of active oxygen products over the buffering mechanisms, antioxidants, and antioxidant enzymes. This phenomenon can occur with an excess of production of these reactive oxygen products or with a deficiency of antioxidant mechanisms, as reactive oxygen species are a product of normal mitochondrial mechanisms (Hubel, 1999). These reactive oxygen products are toxic and can damage proteins, lipids, and DNA, with endothelium particularly vulnerable. At least 20 years ago, lipid markers of oxidative stress were found to be increased in women with preeclampsia (Sekiba and Yoshioka, 1979; Maseki et al., 1981). These results have been confirmed and extended since that time (Hubel, 1999). In addition to numerous findings of increased lipid oxidation products, protein products of oxidation, protein carbonyls (Zusterzeel et al., 2001), and nitrotyrosine are present in the circulation, blood vessels (Roggensack et al., 1999), and placenta (Myatt et al., 1996) of preeclamptic women and their babies. Reduced antioxidants (Hubel et al., 1997; Magdy et al., 1994) and evidence of antibodies to oxidized LDL (Branch et al., 1994) are also present in excess in women with preeclampsia. These do not seem likely to be simply the result of preeclampsia, as reduced antioxidants and increased lipid peroxidation products are present in women destined to develop preeclampsia (Chappell, Seed, Briley, et al., 2002; Chappell, Seed, Kelly, et al., 2002). There are several origins for excess oxidative species that are relevant to preeclampsia. Transition metals, such as iron, catalyze the formation of reactive oxygen species, and free iron is increased in the blood of women with preeclampsia (Entman et al., 1982). Reduced perfusion of tissues sufficient to result in hypoxia that is followed by restored perfusion and reoxygenation results in the formation of reactive oxygen species (Many and Roberts, 1997). This mechanism would seem especially relevant to pregnancy and preeclampsia. Uterine (and, hence, placental) blood flow is not privileged and will be reduced with shunting of blood to other organs with exercise, eating, and so forth. Also, in late pregnancy, uterine and placental blood flow are reduced profoundly by postural effects on uterine perfusion. All of these changes are reversible and will be followed by restored perfusion. Although this is a setting in which reactive oxygen species may be generated, this does not happen in normal pregnancy. This indicates that in most cases, any reduction in oxygen delivery with the reduced placental perfusion is not sufficient to generate free radicals. With the reduced placental perfusion of preeclampsia, however, it is proposed (and evidence supports) that free radicals are generated in the intervillous space (Myatt et al., 1996; Many et al., 2000). The importance of this finding is that it could explain how reduced placental perfusion could result in a maternal systemic disease as products of oxidative stress are transferred to the maternal circulation (Roberts and Hubel, 1999). Oxidative stress is currently a target for therapy to prevent preeclampsia by the use of antioxidants (Chappell et al., 1999; Poston and Chappell, 2001).

Prognosis for Mother and Infant in Preeclampsia

Perinatal Mortality Rate

The perinatal mortality rate is higher for infants of preeclamptic women (Plouin et al., 1986). Causes of perinatal death are placental insufficiency and abruptio placentae (Naeye and Friedman, 1979)—which cause intrauterine death prior to or during labor—and prematurity. As one would expect, the mortality rate is higher in infants of women with more severe forms of the disorder. At any level of disease severity, the perinatal mortality rate is greatest in women with preeclampsia superimposed on preexisting vascular disease (Lopez-Llera and Horta, 1972).

Growth restriction is more common in infants born to preeclamptic women (see Chapter 28). As with perinatal mortality, intrauterine growth restriction (IUGR) is more common in infants of women with superimposed preeclampsia (Lopez-Llera and Horta, 1972). The dramatic decrease in perinatal mortality rate among infants of preeclamptic women in recent years results from more appropriate medical and obstetric management (specifically, avoiding the use of profound maternal, and hence neonatal, sedation) and from the ability to assess fetal well being in the antepartum and intrapartum periods. The primary impact on perinatal mortality rate, however, comes from improvements in neonatal care.

Although neonatal survival rates have improved dramatically, delivery before 34 weeks' gestation continues to be associated with an increased risk of long-range neurologic disability (see Chapter 34). The best obstetric management demands a decision for delivery that balances the risks of maternal and fetal mortality and long-range morbidity.

Maternal Mortality and Morbidity

MORTALITY

Maternal death in association with preeclampsia is due predominantly to complications of abruptio placentae, hepatic rupture, and eclampsia. The mortality rate of eclamptic women has been affected most dramatically by reduction of iatrogenic complications resulting from overmedication and overzealous approaches to vaginal delivery. In several series reported from the late 19th century, during which period immediate delivery was the practice, the mortality rate of eclamptic women was 20%–30%. The advent of expectant management with profound maternal sedation with narcotics and hypnotics in the early 20th century was associated with a 10%–15% mortality rate. In the 1920s and 1930s, the change to magnesium as the exclusive agent resulted in maternal mortality of 5%. Although magnesium undoubtedly had a salutary effect, perhaps more important to the improvement was the decreased use of sedatives, as the protocols for magnesium administration in some series would have minimally increased serum magnesium concentration (Chesley, 1978).

The combination of timely delivery and use of magnesium sulfate ($MgSO_4$) and hydralazine as sole pharmacologic agents has been associated with a maternal mortality rate of virtually zero (Pritchard and Pritchard, 1975; Sibai et al., 1981), owing to an appreciation of the profound pathophysiologic abnormalities of preeclampsia and to careful cardiopulmonary monitoring. It is important to realize, however, that the greatest improvement in survival can be attributed not to what was done but, rather, to what was not done.

LATER CONSEQUENCES

Women with the clinical diagnosis of preeclampsia during one pregnancy have an increased risk for development of hypertension in subsequent pregnancies and fixed hypertension in later life. This is not surprising, as this diagnostic group includes women with preexisting renal or cardiovascular disease. Two questions important for clinical management must be answered, however:

1. Is the risk of recurrence of preeclampsia in subsequent pregnancies high enough and would the recurrence be severe enough to influence the decision for future pregnancies?
2. Is there evidence that a hypertensive pregnancy adversely affects the long-range health of the mother? More specifically, does pregnancy accelerate the progression of underlying hypertensive or renal vascular disease, and does preeclampsia in women with normal cardiovascular and renal function cause damage leading to an increased incidence of cardiovascular morbidity (including hypertension) in later years?

RECURRENCE IN SUBSEQUENT PREGNANCIES

The recurrence of preeclampsia in a subsequent pregnancy is influenced by the certainty of the clinical diagnosis in the first pregnancy. Of 225 women with hypertension during pregnancy chosen for study without regard to parity, 70% experienced recurrence in their next pregnancy (Berman, 1930). In a study of primiparas with severe preeclampsia, the recurrence rate was 45% (Sibai et al., 1986). Because the diagnosis in both of these studies was based solely on clinical findings, these groups undoubtedly included patients with unrecognized preexisting blood pressure elevation or underlying renal or cardiovascular disease.

Chesley (1980), in an attempt to minimize confusion of prognosis by conditions other than preeclampsia, observed 270 women with eclampsia for more than 40 years, only two of whom were lost to follow-up. Twenty women with eclampsia as multiparas had recurrent hypertension in 50% of subsequent pregnancies. Among 187 women who had eclampsia in their first pregnancies, only 33% had some hypertensive disorder in any subsequent pregnancy. In the majority of women, the condition was not severe in subsequent pregnancies; however, 5% did experience a recurrence of eclampsia.

Thus, the woman with a clinical diagnosis of preeclampsia is at increased risk for a hypertensive disorder in subsequent pregnancies. The chances of recurrence decrease as the likelihood of true preeclampsia increases. If the condition does recur, it will usually not be worse, and if preeclampsia truly arose de novo, it probably will be less severe in subsequent pregnancies. Some women, however, are normotensive between pregnancies but have recurrent preeclampsia. The risk of such recurrence is increased when preeclampsia occurs in the late second or early third trimester (Sibai et al., 1991). The recurrence of severe preeclampsia or eclampsia in one pregnancy predicts its likely recurrence in subsequent pregnancies.

FUTURE HYPERTENSION AND CARDIOVASCULAR MORBIDITY

Several observations indicate that it is extremely unlikely that hypertensive disorders during pregnancy accelerate the progression of preexisting—perhaps unrecognized—hypertension or that they cause cardiovascular morbidity or hypertension in normal women. For women eclamptic in the first pregnancy with subsequent hypertensive pregnancies, the incidence of hypertension is greater, and the age of its appearance is earlier. When taken as a group, however, women who are eclamptic in first pregnancy show the same incidence of hypertension as an appropriate control group of unselected women. Interestingly, women who are normotensive in all pregnancies have a lower rate of hypertension than an unselected population of groups of women who were never pregnant (Chesley, 1980). The findings suggest that pregnancy, with or without eclampsia, does not accelerate hypertension but rather unmasks hypertension in women who either were not recognized as hypertensive in early pregnancy or who are destined to have hypertension in later life.

Many investigators have noted a correlation of preeclampsia with an increased risk of hypertension in later life. Some investigators use this correlation as evidence that residual damage from the preeclamptic process predisposes women to cardiovascular morbidity and mortality (Schreier et al., 1955; Epstein, 1964). There are serious flaws in many of these studies. All are compromised by the uncertainty of the clinical diagnosis of preeclampsia. In some, inappropriate control groups have been used (i.e., not corrected for age and race). Also, as noted earlier, the use of women who are normotensive in all pregnancies as controls is inappropriate. In all of these studies, as the likelihood that the clinical diagnosis was preeclampsia increased, the incidence of hypertension in later life decreased.

If women with preeclampsia in their first pregnancies are observed over time, the incidence of hypertension in later life is seen to be lower than in women with preeclampsia as multiparas. In women with proteinuria, the incidence of hypertension in later life is one-half that in women with a confirmed diagnosis of preeclampsia but without proteinuria (Berman, 1930). In a 15- to 20-year follow-up of women with preeclampsia in their first pregnancies, the incidence of diastolic blood pressures greater than 90 mm Hg was 60% in women who had not had proteinuria, 40% in those who had, and 35% in women who were never pregnant (Adams, Cantab, et al., 1961).

The definitive information about the long-range impact of preeclampsia-eclampsia comes from the masterful study by Chesley and associates (1976). In women with eclampsia in their first pregnancies who were followed up for more than 40 years, there was no excess rate of hypertension (Fig. 43-14) and no increase in cardiovascular mortality or in death rate in general. The follow-up results for women with eclampsia as multiparas supports the concept that preeclampsia rarely arises de novo in multiparous women. The incidence of hypertension is greater in these women, as are rates of death from all causes and, specifically, cardiovascular death.

The dramatic difference between the prognostic implications of eclampsia for primiparous and multiparous women is indicated in a survey of survival rates (Fig. 43-15). On the basis of this information, it seems reasonable to conclude that preeclampsia does not cause permanent damage or predispose to chronic hypertension. The increased incidence of hypertension in later life for women with preeclampsia indicates either misdiagnosis or the unmasking of potential for development of hypertension regardless of the pregnancy. The latter possibility seems quite likely and should be generalized to all cardiovascular disease. In a study of later-life cardiovascular disease, women with a history of preeclampsia had an increased risk of myocardial infarction, which occurred primarily among women with recurrent pregnancy hypertension (Jonsdottir et al., 1995). Even among women with preeclampsia in first pregnancies, follow up indicates an excess of metabolic and physiological findings associated with cardiovascular disease in later life, including insulin resistance (Laivuori et al., 1996), abnormal endothelial function (Chambers et al., 2001), elevated homocysteine (Dekker et al., 1995), and dyslipidemia (Hubel et al., 2000).

An alternative explanation also deserves careful scrutiny. The duration of preeclampsia in pregnancy could dictate outcome. It is possible that women with mild preeclampsia are

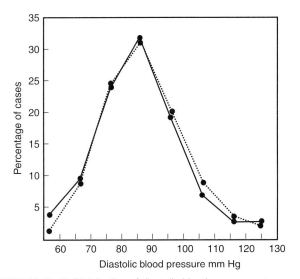

FIGURE 43-14 ■ Distribution of diastolic blood pressures at more than 20 years of follow-up of women with eclampsia in their first pregnancy *(solid line)* compared with women from an appropriate control group *(broken line)*. (From Chesley LC, Annitto JE, Cosgrove RA: Long-term follow-up study of eclamptic women: Fifth periodic report. Am J Obstet Gynecol **101**:886, 1968. Courtesy of the American College of Obstetricians and Gynecologists.)

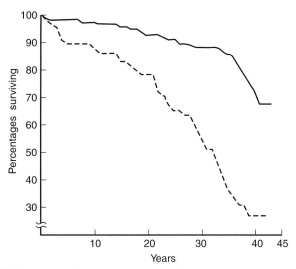

FIGURE 43-15 ■ Survivals of women with eclampsia in the first pregnancy *(solid line)* and those with eclampsia in a later pregnancy *(broken line)*. Survival of women with first-pregnancy eclampsia was not different from survival of a control group. (From Chesley LC, Annitto JE, Cosgrove RA: The remote prognosis of eclamptic women: Sixth periodic report. Am J Obstet Gynecol **124**:446, 1976. Courtesy of the American College of Obstetricians and Gynecologists.)

less likely to have expeditious deliveries than women with severe preeclampsia or eclampsia. The women who are mildly affected, therefore, are preeclamptic for a longer time and hence may face a higher risk of hypertension in later life (Schreier et al., 1955; Epstein, 1964). Examination of pathophysiologic changes in preeclampsia, however, indicates that these changes are present long before symptoms appear in all patients (whether mildly preeclamptic or eclamptic) and that the clinical stigmata of preeclampsia are present long before those of eclampsia.

If one uses the renal biopsy finding of glomeruloendotheliosis to increase the accuracy of the diagnosis of preeclampsia, incidences of hypertension are similar. In 53 women with this renal change, the incidence of hypertension was no higher than expected at follow-up, an average of 6 years after the hypertensive pregnancy (Fisher et al., 1981). Once again in this study, women who have been pregnant and never developed preeclampsia have a lower risk of hypertension than women in the general population.

Management of Preeclampsia

General Considerations

PHILOSOPHY OF MANAGEMENT

On the basis of the pathologic and pathophysiologic changes and the prognosis of preeclampsia, it is possible to formulate a philosophy of management, as follows.

1. DELIVERY IS ALWAYS APPROPRIATE THERAPY FOR THE MOTHER BUT MAY NOT BE SO FOR THE FETUS. Because we do not yet understand the etiology of preeclampsia, attempts to prevent it by conventional medical approaches have been understandably unsuccessful. In terms of maternal health, the goal of therapy is to prevent eclampsia. Preeclampsia is the precursor of eclampsia, and for this reason, careful antepartum observation can identify the woman at risk. Preeclampsia is completely reversible and begins to abate with delivery. Thus,

if only maternal well being were considered, delivery of all preeclamptic women, regardless of severity of process or stage of gestation, would be appropriate. When the fetus is considered, however, delivery for mild preeclampsia in a woman whose infant is immature and without evidence of fetal distress does not make sense.

There are two important corollaries of this statement. First, any therapy for preeclampsia other than delivery must have as its successful endpoint the reduction of perinatal mortality and morbidity. Second, the cornerstone of obstetric management of preeclampsia is based on a decision as to whether the infant is more likely to survive *in utero* or in the nursery.

2. THE SIGNS AND SYMPTOMS OF PREECLAMPSIA ARE NOT OF PATHOGENETIC IMPORTANCE. The pathologic and pathophysiologic changes of preeclampsia indicate that poor perfusion, most probably secondary to vasospasm, is the major factor leading to the derangement of maternal physiologic function and to increased perinatal mortality and morbidity rates. This same abnormality also causes increased total peripheral resistance, with subsequent elevation of blood pressure and decreased renal perfusion leading to sodium retention and edema. The proteinuria of preeclampsia is at least partially explained by vasospasm and also by reversible glomerular damage resulting from phagocytosis of abnormal circulating proteins by glomerulocapillary endothelial cells.

Attempts to treat preeclampsia by natriuresis or by the lowering of blood pressure do not alleviate the important pathophysiologic changes. In fact, natriuresis could be counterproductive and could adversely affect fetal outcome because plasma volume is already reduced in preeclamptic women.

3. THE PATHOGENETIC CHANGES OF PREECLAMPSIA ARE PRESENT LONG BEFORE CLINICAL CRITERIA LEADING TO THE DIAGNOSIS ARE MANIFESTED. Studies indicate that changes in vascular reactivity, plasma volume, and renal function antedate—in some cases by months—the increases in blood pressure, protein excretion, and sodium retention. These findings suggest that irreversible changes affecting fetal well being could be present prior to the clinical diagnosis. This possibility probably explains why dietary, pharmacologic, and postural therapy instituted after the recognition of clinical disease have not been successful when avoidance of perinatal morbidity and mortality is taken as the endpoint. If there is a rationale for modes of therapy other than delivery, it would be to palliate the maternal condition in order to allow fetal maturation. Even this rationale, however, is controversial.

INDICATIONS FOR DELIVERY

FETAL INDICATIONS. For the reasons already cited, the major consideration in decisions for delivery should usually be fetal well being. Therefore the indications are as follows:

1. If the maternal condition is stable, delivery is indicated by signs of abnormal fetal function.
2. If fetal growth and well being remain normal, pregnancy should proceed to spontaneous labor.
3. If the maternal condition is deteriorating rapidly, delivery is indicated for fetal well being.

With maternal deterioration, a reflection of increasingly poor perfusion of brain, kidney, and liver, uteroplacental blood flow is also likely to be compromised. In addition, the predictive value of all tests of fetal well being is invalidated by rapid changes in maternal (and hence, fetal) condition.

MATERNAL INDICATIONS. Although fetal considerations usually dictate the timing of delivery, there are important exceptions. In the rare case in which a choice is made to palliate maternal signs and symptoms in order to allow fetal growth or maturation, such efforts must be abandoned if the maternal condition worsens. Also, a potentially lethal complication of preeclampsia, hepatic rupture, cannot be prevented by any mode of therapy other than delivery; the mortality rate is 65%. Thus, for the woman with hepatic capsular distention manifested by hepatomegaly, liver tenderness, and abnormal liver function values, delivery is warranted regardless of fetal well being or maturity.

ROUTE OF DELIVERY. For the woman with preeclampsia, vaginal delivery is preferable to cesarean delivery. It is desirable, if possible, to avoid the added stress of surgery because of multiple physiologic abnormalities. Palliation for several hours should not increase maternal risk if the procedure is performed appropriately. In addition, several investigators have demonstrated that with postural manipulations and fluid infusion for volume expansion, many fetuses, even those with positive contraction stress test results, can tolerate labor.

Once the decision for delivery is made, induction should be carried out aggressively and expeditiously. In gestations remote from term and complicated by severe preeclampsia, consideration may be given to glucocorticoid treatment to accelerate fetal lung maturation. Although there is evidence that glucocorticoids may be used safely in preeclamptic women (Ricke et al., 1980), fetal or maternal indications for delivery frequently contraindicate 24–36 hours of delay to allow such drugs to be effective. The aggressive approach to induction indicates that amniotomy be performed as soon as possible and that a clear endpoint be formulated at the initiation of therapy. The cervical condition is generally predictive of the likelihood of successful induction. Many authors point out, however, that in individual preeclamptic women the success of induction could be greater than would be predicted by the cervical examination (Zuspan et al., 1968). A trial of induction is warranted regardless of cervical condition. Obviously, if vaginal delivery cannot be accomplished within the predetermined time frame, cesarean delivery should be performed.

Cesarean delivery should be reserved for the usual obstetric indications, with the following exceptions. Because the probability of fetal compromise in preeclampsia is high, it is mandatory in all vaginal deliveries that the fetus be monitored adequately. Internal monitoring is preferable in order to allow determination of beat-to-beat variability; however, external monitoring, if technically good, is adequate until internal monitoring is feasible. Periodic changes or inadequate long-range variability requires assessment by internal fetal heart rate monitoring. Cesarean delivery is indicated if internal monitoring is not possible. Magnesium sulfate may decrease beat-to-beat variability (Stallworth et al., 1981), but especially if normal variability was never evident, fetal scalp blood sampling should confirm that decreased variability is not secondary to asphyxia. For the woman with marked hepatic capsular distention, cesarean delivery is indicated if vaginal delivery is not imminent. Even several extra hours could be life-threatening, and no one palliative therapeutic method prevents liver rupture.

Regional anesthesia offers its usual advantages for vaginal and cesarean delivery but does carry the possibility of extensive sympatholysis with consequent decreased cardiac output, hypotension, and impairment of already compromised utero-placental perfusion. This problem can be avoided by meticulous attention to anesthetic technique and volume expansion. Regional anesthesia is not a rational means of lowering blood pressure because it does so at the expense of cardiac output. Similarly, although analgesia with narcotics is not contraindicated and should be used when necessary, attempting to manage or prevent eclampsia with profound maternal sedation has been dangerous and ineffective.

MONITORING OF MOTHER AND FETUS

MATERNAL MONITORING. There are two goals for antepartum monitoring of the mother:

1. Recognizing the condition early, because infants of mothers with even mild preeclampsia are at increased risk
2. Gauging the rate of progression of the condition, both to prevent eclampsia by delivery and to determine whether fetal well being can be monitored safely by the usual intermittent observations

Ideally, identification of early changes would allow intervention prior to the advent of clinical symptoms. Hemodynamic, volume, and biochemical changes appear to antedate the diagnostic clinical signs of preeclampsia. In the past, lability of blood pressure, which is a feature of preeclampsia, was suggested as a predictor; however, neither stimulation of sympathetic response by the cold pressor test (Chesley and Valenti, 1958) nor second-trimester blood pressure "spikes" (Browne, 1933) were specific enough as predictors.

More recently, higher early second-trimester blood pressures were measured in groups of women destined to have diagnostic blood pressure increases in later pregnancy (Gallery et al., 1977). The overlap of blood pressure levels between these women and women who remained normotensive, however, was too large to regard this value as a useful predictor for individual women. The increased blood pressure response to angiotensin II (Gant et al., 1973; Oney and Kaulhausen, 1982; Nakamura et al., 1986) in women destined to have elevated blood pressure in late pregnancy has been the gold standard against which other predictors are judged, but the test is neither simple enough nor safe enough for extensive clinical use. In addition, a large study failed to confirm the predictive value of the test (Kyle et al., 1995). Changes in renal function, serum urate, and PSP clearance (Gallery and Györy, 1979a) precede clinical signs of preeclampsia. Also, it appears that decreased plasma volume (Arias, 1975) and subtle coagulation changes are also predictors (Redman, Denson, et al., 1977). Abnormal uterine artery Doppler velocimetry in the second trimester has been found to predict adverse pregnancy outcome, including preeclampsia. The positive predictive value for preeclampsia is about 20%. These approaches are useful for research identification of subjects, but the sensitivity and positive predictive value do not render them useful for modifying clinical care (Chien et al., 2000).

The usefulness of these values as clinical predictors in patient management remains to be confirmed. Several other markers have been suggested as useful, but their confirmation awaits more extensive testing (Myatt and Miodovnik, 1999).

At present, clinical management is dictated by the overt clinical signs of preeclampsia. Unfortunately, because proteinuria—the most valid clinical indicator of preeclampsia—is often a late change, sometimes even preceded by seizures, it is not a useful sign for early recognition. Although rapid weight increase and hand and face edema indicate the fluid and sodium retention characteristic of preeclampsia, they are neither universally present nor uniquely characteristic of preeclampsia. These signs are, at most, a reason for closer observation of blood pressure and monitoring of urinary protein. Early recognition of preeclampsia is based primarily on diagnostic blood pressure increases in the late second and early third trimesters in relation to early pregnancy. Using blood pressure changes without evidence of proteinuria as an indicator does, undoubtedly, result in the close observation of some normal women as well as in some with underlying renal or vascular disease. Because the goal of early diagnosis is to identify patients requiring more careful observation, however, overdiagnosis is preferable to underdiagnosis.

Once blood pressure changes diagnostic of preeclampsia appear, laboratory assessment should be carried out to determine multiorgan involvement. Thus, a 24-hour urine specimen (or at least a timed collection) should be collected (Adelberg et al., 2001) regardless of findings on urine dip-stick evaluation. There is ample evidence that in preeclampsia—probably related to the hectic protein excretion characteristic of the disorder (Chesley, 1939)—24-hour urine collections may reveal greater than 300 mg of protein excretion, even with trace proteinuria on dip-stick evaluation (Meyer et al., 1994). In addtion, determination of platelet count and liver enzymes is recommended (Gifford et al., 2000a). To rule out fulminant progression, office examination is mandatory within 24 hours; or with selected patients, blood pressure and urinary protein must be checked at home. Frequency of subsequent observations is determined by these initial observations and the ensuing clinical progression. If the condition appears stable, weekly observations may be appropriate. If it appears to be accelerating, more frequent observations, perhaps in the hospital, are required. The initial appearance of proteinuria is an especially important sign of progression and dictates frequent observation.

If an increasing rate of deterioration is noted, as determined by laboratory findings, symptoms, and clinical signs, the decision to continue the pregnancy is determined day by day. Important clinical signs are blood pressure, urinary output, and fluid retention as evidenced by daily weight increase.

Laboratory studies are performed at intervals of no more than 48 hours. These tests include the following:

1. Examination for possible activation of the coagulation system as determined by platelet count and fibrin split products
2. Evaluation of renal function as measured by urinary protein excretion and serum creatinine and urate levels
3. Determination of hepatic dysfunction as evidenced by increasing ALT and AST

In addition, subjective evidence of central nervous system involvement—for example, headache, disorientation, and visual symptoms—and the presence of hepatic distention as indicated by abdominal pain and liver tenderness are equally important indicators of worsening preeclampsia.

FETAL OBSERVATION. Tests to assess fetal well-being provide information for determining whether the infant is safer in the uterus or outside after delivery (see Chapters 20 and 21). With the diagnosis of gestational hypertension, fetal assessment for size by sonography and function by non-stress testing is indicated. If the disease does not progress, these need not be repeated. Once the diagnosis of preeclampsia is made, it is mandatory to monitor the fetal condition. If the maternal condition is stable, weekly monitoring of the fetus appears to be adequate.

The etiology of fetal demise is apparently placental insufficiency. Thus, biophysical assessment of fetal oxygenation by observations of periodic changes in fetal heart rate and activity and contraction-stress testing are direct and accurate indicators of fetal condition (see Chapter 21).

Unfortunately, no test of fetal well-being is predictive when the mother's condition is rapidly deteriorating. The management of the fetus with IUGR, a common complication of preeclampsia, is discussed in Chapter 28. Assessment of amniotic fluid for determination of lung maturity aids in the decision to deliver the fetus with severe IUGR. Jeopardy of fetal well being rather than lung maturity is the fetal criterion for determining delivery in a pregnancy with preeclampsia that is remote from term.

Prophylaxis for Preeclampsia

Since the preeclamptic syndrome was first recognized, numerous approaches have been used to attempt prevention of preeclampsia. These strategies, which include restriction and supplementation of various nutrients and sodium, have been unsuccessful (Chesley, 1978). Several studies of women at high risk for preeclampsia indicate a beneficial effect of low-dose (60–80 mg/day) aspirin or calcium prophylaxis to prevent preeclampsia and IUGR (Imperiale and Petrulis, 1991).

Although meta-analysis (Imperiale and Petrulis, 1991) suggested that aspirin is beneficial when administered from early gestation onward, subsequent studies have not supported this conclusion. In large studies conducted by the NIH (Sibai et al., 1993; Caritis et al., 1998) and the CLASP group (CLASP, 1994), aspirin showed no benefit in reducing the occurrence of preeclampsia in women at low risk (CLASP, 1994; Sibai et al., 1993) or high risk (diabetes, hypertension, multiple gestation, or previous preeclampsia) for the disorder (Caritis et al., 1998). Part of the ineffectiveness in these studies may be explained by compliance. In a single-center study in which compliance was assessed biochemically, the incidence of preeclampsia was lower, especially in patients with objective evidence of compliance (Hauth et al., 1993). In the approximately 32,000 women tested in the several large trials of aspirin, there is a small (14%) reduction in perinatal mortality. Based on the confidence intervals, however, it could be necessary to treat as many as 10,000 women to prevent one perinatal death (Knight et al., 2000).

Calcium supplementation to prevent preeclampsia was initiated with similar enthusiasm. Based on studies, primarily outside of the United States, and subsequently supported by meta-analysis (Bucher et al., 1996), calcium was tested in a large, randomized controlled trial in the United States (Levine et al., 1997). The conclusion of this study was unequivocal. There was no evidence that 2 g of supplemental calcium administered to pregnant women from early gestation onward reduced the incidence of preeclampsia, altered blood pressure, or affected fetal weight. There was also no effect on preterm labor. This finding was independent of previous calcium intake.

Oxidative stress has been suggested as important in preeclampsia, and a recent trial tested whether treating women at high risk for preeclampsia with antioxidants (vitamin C, 1000 mg and vitamin E, 400 IU) from early pregnancy onward would reduce evidence of endothelial activation. The study was an intent-to-treat trial. Most women were determined as high risk by abnormal uterine artery velocimetry at 16–22 and 24 weeks' gestation. They were randomized based on the first study, and if the results of the 24 weeks' study were not abnormal, the assigned medication was stopped. With this intent-to-treat design, the 140 women assigned to treatment had reduced evidence of endothelial activation but also 50% lower incidence of preeclampsia. In the 78 women who actually took the vitamins, treatment was also effective. Whether these results will be maintained in larger cohorts and—more important—whether this therapy is safe for the fetus must be tested in larger studies (which are currently in progress) before this therapy is adopted clinically.

The results of these studies raise several important points:

1. Randomized clinical trials of appropriate population and size to result in sufficient power must guide clinical management. Nonetheless, the success of small trials and the failures of large multicenter trials could also be secondary to the heterogeneity of preeclampsia (Ness and Roberts, 1996). Perhaps therapy would be effective in a specific subset of women. This suggestion is especially relevant to calcium supplementation studies, in which success is present in developing countries with low average calcium intake but not in the United States.
2. In a disorder such as preeclampsia, in which the diagnosis is based on signs that are usually of minimal pathophysiological significance, it is important that the prophylactic therapy not merely treat one of the signs. As with all therapy for preeclampsia, efficacy is most appropriately judged by effects on perinatal outcome.
3. On a more optimistic note, the success of aspirin in single centers with compliant patients suggests that the model of beginning therapy before clinically evident disease manifests may be successful if rational therapy can be directed to appropriate subjects.

Antepartum Management in Preeclampsia

There is little evidence that therapeutic efforts alter the underlying pathophysiology of preeclampsia. Therapeutic intervention for clinically evident preeclampsia is palliative. At best, it may slow the progression of the condition, but it is more likely to merely allow continuation of the pregnancy. Bed rest is a usual and reasonable recommendation for the woman with mild preeclampsia, although its efficacy is not clearly established (Mathews, 1977). Prophylactic hospitalization with increased bed rest may reduce the incidence of preeclampsia for women at high risk, as identified by increased angiotensin sensitivity (Hauth et al., 1976). It is unclear, however, which of the several behavioral modifications involved in hospital residence is important. Anecdotal reports of clinical improvement with bed rest must be tempered by the recognition of the unpredictable course of preeclampsia.

Strict sodium restriction or diuretic therapy plays no role in the prevention or therapy of preeclampsia. In women with marked sodium retention as manifested by significant edema, modest sodium restriction may not alter the course of the disease but could reduce discomfort. Diuretics should not be given because these patients already have decreased plasma volume, and further volume depletion could affect the fetus adversely. Attempts to modify the progression of the disease by volume expansion are not conclusive and require more complete evaluation before they can be considered part of routine antepartum management (Goodlin et al., 1978).

Prolonged expectant antepartum management of women with severe preeclampsia is not practiced in most centers. With improvements in neonatal care, many investigators regard delivery of women with severe preeclampsia beyond 30 weeks' gestation to be in the best interests of not only the mother but also the fetus. Acute antihypertensive therapy is not used because it masks one important clinical sign of disease progression, and blood pressure control does not improve fetal well being. Diastolic pressure of 110 mm Hg and higher, which puts the mother at increased risk for cerebrovascular accident, is an indication for delivery with control of blood pressure.

When gestational age is critical (at 25–30 weeks), one might consider control of maternal blood pressure along with meticulous observation of maternal and fetal condition. Delivery is then indicated by worsening maternal symptoms, laboratory evidence of end-organ dysfunction, or deterioration of fetal condition. Whether this plan of action can bring about a decrease in perinatal morbidity and mortality rates after 30 weeks' gestation is not clear. The use of this approach with even very immature fetuses may only replace a nonviable neonate with an extremely premature one, with the attendant risks of long-range neurologic disability. Such an approach, therefore, should be attempted only in centers equipped to provide meticulous maternal observation and daily assessment of fetal and maternal condition.

Intrapartum Management in Preeclampsia

The intrapartum management of women with preeclampsia tests the obstetric and medical skills of the health care team. The patient with severe preeclampsia or eclampsia is acutely ill, with functional derangements of many organ systems. An appreciation of this situation and the availability of methods of accurate maternal monitoring have reduced mortality rates from 5% in earlier series to 1% or less in recent series. Failure to recognize and appropriately manage this grave condition probably accounts for most deaths. In addition, even mildly preeclamptic women can experience an acceleration of the process during labor.

Delivery terminates the preeclamptic process, and it is tempting to institute immediate delivery, frequently by cesarean section. Unfortunately, physiologic abnormalities are not immediately corrected by delivery, and adding surgical stress to the abnormal physiologic state is not desirable. It is possible to partially correct many of these abnormalities, and it is imperative to attempt to do so prior to imposing surgical stress. If the fetus can be monitored, several hours' palliation with vaginal delivery is preferable to the added maternal stress of operative delivery.

Baseline information should be obtained to determine renal function, coagulation status, and liver function. Determination of serum protein concentration indicates the choice of appropriate fluid administration. Some investigators advocate the use of intensive cardiovascular monitoring, preferably with Swan-Ganz catheters or with central venous pressure catheters in all women with severe preeclampsia and eclampsia (see Chapter 45). Such a practice is certainly indicated in oliguric patients whose urinary output does not improve with a modest fluid challenge. The major problems to be managed are those of high blood pressure, intravascular volume, and convulsions. Less commonly, patients with DIC and myocardial dysfunction require treatment.

ANTICONVULSANTS

PROPHYLAXIS. Most seizures occur during the intrapartum and postpartum periods, the times during which the preeclamptic process is most likely to accelerate. The Magpie study, in which 10,000 preeclamptic women were randomized to magnesium or placebo, demonstrated the efficacy of magnesium to prevent eclamptic seizures (Duley et al., 2002).

Even with the Magpie study, it is difficult to determine in which preeclamptic women the risks of seizure exceed the risk of magnesium. In this study, treatment was effective and safe even in developing countries. It appears, however, that most of these women had more than mild preeclampsia. Twenty-five percent were defined as having severe preeclampsia, and 75% required antihypertensive therapy. Nonetheless, a review of eclamptic patients from a major U.S. center indicates the problems with selecting the preeclamptic woman with disease severe enough to warrant therapy (Sibai et al., 1981). None of the clinical signs and symptoms considered to be prognostic of seizures was absolutely reliable. Seventeen percent of women who had seizures did not have headache, 80% did not have epigastric pain, and 20% had normal deep tendon reflexes (Table 43-6). The lack of absolute correlation with proteinuria is consistent with the observations by Chesley and Chesley (1943) more than 50 years ago that 24% of patients do not have proteinuria prior to seizure.

The prophylactic use of anticonvulsant therapy, which is the approach strongly recommended by most U.S. investigators, can protect most women at risk for seizures only if therapy is elected for all women with a blood pressure elevation diagnostic of preeclampsia whether or not other signs and symptoms, including proteinuria, are present. It is likely that this approach will include women for whom the risk of treatment exceeds the risks from seizures. Thus, the first requirement for anticonvulsant prophylaxis is that the agent and its dosage must be extremely safe for the mother. Magnesium, if used carefully and in moderate doses (1 g/hour) may satisfy this

requirement, although there is currently no data to support this contention. The other obvious requirement is safety for the infant, not only as a fetus but also when, as a neonate with appreciable blood levels of the drug, he or she begins the complex adaptation to extrauterine life.

In the past, a staggering array of drugs and combinations of drugs have been used as therapeutic and prophylactic agents for convulsions (Studd, 1977). Zuspan (1978), and Pritchard and Pritchard (1975), among others, have demonstrated the value of simplifying therapy by reducing the number of agents administered. Both reports advocate the use of magnesium sulfate—clearly the drug of choice for obstetricians in the United States—for anticonvulsant prophylaxis. Other anticonvulsant agents—primarily benzodiazepine derivatives and phenytoin—have been used in other parts of the world. There is now compelling evidence from a randomized controlled trial that magnesium is more effective than phenytoin as prophylaxis against eclampsia (Lucas et al., 1995a). On the basis of this finding, magnesium appears to be the drug of choice for prophylaxis of eclampsia. Investigators worldwide agree with the principle of simplifying therapy by avoiding polypharmaceutical regimens (Studd, 1977).

MAGNESIUM SULFATE. Magnesium sulfate offers considerable advantages for prophylaxis in women with preeclampsia. Its pharmacokinetic processes during pregnancy are well established, as are its efficacy and safety for mother and fetus.

PHARMACOKINETICS, MECHANISM OF ACTION, AND MATERNAL SIDE EFFECTS. The volume of distribution of magnesium is greater than that of sucrose, indicating that the distribution of this ion goes beyond extracellular fluid, also entering bones and cells (Chesley, 1979). Magnesium circulates largely unbound to protein and is almost exclusively excreted in urine. It is reabsorbed in the proximal tubule by a process limited by transport maximum (T_{max}), and its excretion increases as filtered load increases above the transport maximum (Massey, 1977). In patients with normal renal function, the half-time for excretion is about 4 hours (Chesley, 1979). Because excretion depends on delivery of a filtered load of magnesium that exceeds the T_{max}, the half-time of excretion is prolonged in women with decreased GFR.

The clinically significant results of elevated serum magnesium levels are related primarily to its membrane effects. Magnesium slows or blocks neuromuscular and cardiac conducting system transmission, decreases smooth muscle contractility, and depresses central nervous system irritability. The results include a desired anticonvulsant effect and, potentially, undesirable effects such as decreased uterine and myocardial contractility, depressed respirations, and interference with cardiac conduction. These effects occur at different serum magnesium concentrations (Table 43-7). Doses of magnesium sulfate sufficient for anticonvulsant therapy cause little change in blood pressure.

Because the depression of deep tendon reflexes occurs at serum concentrations lower than those associated with adverse cardiac and respiratory effects, the presence of deep tendon reflexes indicates that serum magnesium concentration is not dangerously high. If deep tendon reflexes are lost, serum magnesium concentration could be greater than 10 mEq/L; however, any attempt to control magnesium therapy by eliminating deep tendon reflexes is irrational and dangerous, as is the assumption that brisk deep tendon reflexes signify inadequate magnesium dosage.

TABLE 43-6. FREQUENCY OF SYMPTOMS PRECEDING ECLAMPSIA

Symptom	Patients in Whom It Is Present (%)
Headache	83
Hyperreflexia	80
Proteinuria	80
Edema	60
Clonus	46
Visual signs	45
Epigastric pain	20

Adapted from Obstetrics and Gynecology **57**, Sibai BM, Lipshitz J, Anderson GD, et al.: Reassessment of intravenous MgSO₄ therapy in preeclampsia-eclampsia, 199, 1981, with permission from *American College of Obstetricians and Gynecologists*.

TABLE 43-7. EFFECTS ASSOCIATED WITH VARIOUS SERUM MAGNESIUM LEVELS

Effect	Serum Level (mEq/liter)
Anticonvulsant prophylaxis	4–6
Electrocardiographic changes	5–10
Loss of deep tendon reflexes	10
Respiratory paralysis	15
General anesthesia	15
Cardiac arrest	>25

DOSAGE. Two regimens have been used extensively. Pritchard and Pritchard (1975) reported the use of a combination of intramuscular and intravenous magnesium (MgSO$_4$•7H$_2$O), with impressive results (Table 43-8); 2–4 g is given intravenously over 2–4 minutes, and 10 g is concomitantly administered intramuscularly. The intravenous dosage results in immediate elevation of serum magnesium, which falls rapidly. As the serum magnesium level from intravenous injection decreases, the absorption of intramuscular magnesium results in a relatively consistent serum concentration. The range of magnesium concentration attained in patients with differing renal functions and body sizes is indicated in Figure 43-16. Serum magnesium levels after initial administration are determined by volume of distribution, not by renal function (Chesley, 1979).

The initial dose can be administered safely without knowledge of renal function. It is recommended that 5 g of MgSO$_4$•7H$_2$O be readministered intramuscularly every 4 hours. The serum concentration of magnesium after subsequent doses is influenced by renal function, and if the patient is not excreting more than 40 mL/hour of urine, the dosage must be reduced as determined by serum magnesium levels. Prior to the administration of subsequent doses, deep tendon reflexes must be present, and the respiratory rate must be normal.

Because intramuscular administration of large volumes of MgSO$_4$•7H$_2$O is painful, many investigators advocate the use of a continuous intravenous infusion, in which 2–4 g of MgSO$_4$•7H$_2$O is given over 5 minutes, followed by controlled continuous infusion of 1 g/hour. Magnesium is administered by

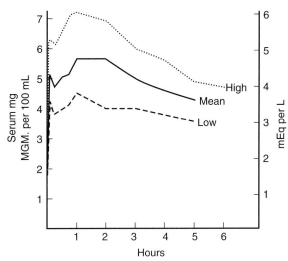

FIGURE 43-16 ■ Serum magnesium concentrations resulting from the concurrent administration of 3 g magnesium sulfate IV and 10 g IM. (From Chesley C, Tepper I: Plasma levels of magnesium attained in magnesium sulfate therapy for preeclampsia and eclampsia. Surg Clin North Am **37**:353, 1957.)

continuous infusion because intermittent bolus infusions result in only transient elevations of magnesium level. To ensure consistent infusion and to avoid inadvertent administration of large doses of magnesium, mechanically controlled infusion is mandatory. The rate of infusion is modified for patients with compromised renal function, in whom magnesium levels should be measured. If overdosage, especially with apnea, does occur, calcium gluconate (10 mL of a 10% solution injected intravenously over 3 minutes) is an effective antidote.

Both of these approaches have been tested clinically for more than 40 years and are effective and extremely safe for the mother (Table 43-9). It should be emphasized that the "therapeutic concentrations" of magnesium have been empirically determined and are the levels attained with dosages found to be usually effective. No study has yet compared magnesium concentrations in patients either successfully or unsuccessfully treated with MgSO$_4$•7H$_2$O. Also, magnesium is not a perfect anticonvulsant, and some women have convulsions even with high serum concentrations (Chesley and Tepper, 1957).

Attempts to modify this modality, which has been found effective and safe even though liberally administered to many women who do not need the therapy, must be made with caution. There is now extensive experience with the intravenous administration of magnesium at doses up to 2 g/hour,

TABLE 43-8. RESULTS OF STANDARDIZED TREATMENT OF PREECLAMPSIA USING MAGNESIUM SULFATE*

Fetuses dead when eclampsia diagnosed	7
Fetuses alive when eclampsia diagnosed	115
Intrapartum death	1†
Live births	114
Neonatal deaths	4‡
Survivors	100
Total fetuses	122

* Includes only fetuses weighing 1000 g or more at birth, at Parkland Memorial Hospital, 1955 to 1975.
† Weighed 1200 g.
‡ All weighed less than 1800 g. All 100 fetuses weighing 1800 g (4 pounds) or more and alive when eclampsia was diagnosed survived.

Modified from Pritchard JA, Pritchard SA: Standardized treatment of 154 consecutive cases of eclampsia. Am J Obstet Gynecol **123**:543, 1975.

TABLE 43-9. SAFETY AND EFFICACY OF INTRAVENOUS MAGNESIUM SULFATE THERAPY

Treated	1870
Seizures	11 (0.6%)
Seizure morbidity	1 (0.05%)
Treatment morbidity	0

Adapted from Obstetrics and Gynecology **57**, Sibai BM, Lipshitz J, Anderson GD, et al; Reassessment of intravenous MgSO$_4$ therapy in preeclampsia-eclampsia, 199, 1981, with permission from *American College of Obstetricians and Gynecologists.*

which appear to be safe for the patient with normal renal function. In the Magpie study, doses of 1 g/hour given intravenously were effective and even in a developing world setting had no serious complications in 5000 treated women. Based on this finding, it is difficult to justify higher dosing (Duley et al., 2002). If larger doses are chosen, however, these must be guided by deep tendon reflexes and serum magnesium concentrations monitored at least every 2 hours until a steady state has been reached.

FETAL AND NEONATAL EFFECTS. A major advantage of magnesium sulfate therapy is that at effective anticonvulsant doses, it is very safe for the fetus and neonate (see Table 48-8). Neonatal serum magnesium concentrations are nearly identical to those of the mother (Pritchard, 1955). Although amniotic fluid magnesium concentrations increase with prolonged infusion as a result of fetal renal excretion of the substance, fetal serum magnesium levels do not increase, and there is no evidence of cumulative effects of prolonged magnesium administration on the neonate.

In a study of 118 infants of mothers treated with magnesium sulfate, the average serum magnesium concentration was 3.7 mEq/L, and there was no correlation of magnesium level with Apgar scores (Pritchard and Stone, 1967). It is controversial whether the administration of magnesium to the mother may have additional beneficial effects for the fetus (see Chapter 34).

PHENYTOIN. Phenytoin is an effective anticonvulsant with pharmacologic effects that would not be predicted to adversely affect the fetus *in utero* or the physiologic events necessary for perinatal adaptation. In several small studies, there were no obvious adverse fetal or maternal effects (Crowther, 1990; Appleton et al., 1991). Although phenytoin is not as effective as magnesium for prophylaxis or treatment of eclampsia seizure (Eclampsia Trial Collaborative Group, 1995; Lucas et al., 1995b), it can be used safely in settings in which magnesium is associated with increased risk, such as with myasthenia gravis or markedly compromised renal function. Phenytoin nonetheless does have potential severe adverse effects, which are magnified by the fact that obstetric personnel are usually not familiar with its use.

ANTICONVULSANT THERAPY. Magnesium is a more effective treatment than phenytoin or benzodiazepam for eclamptic seizures (Eclampsia Trial Collaborative Group, 1995). If treatment with magnesium has not been given, 4 g can be administered safely intravenously, and intramuscular or intravenous MgSO$_4$ can be initiated, as described previously, to maintain serum magnesium levels. If the patient is already receiving magnesium, it is safer to terminate seizures with another anticonvulsant agent, such as diazepam (Valium), 5 mg, or a short-acting barbiturate, such as pentobarbital, 125 mg given intravenously.

Once seizures are terminated, serum magnesium concentration can be determined, and the rate of magnesium infusion can be adjusted accordingly. Because most seizures terminate spontaneously within 1–2 minutes, the most important measures for any seizure, which should be taken before pharmacologic therapy is initiated, are prevention of injury and protection of the airway to prevent aspiration.

ANTIHYPERTENSIVE THERAPY. Antihypertensive agents are not administered routinely to women with preeclampsia. There is no evidence that the acute administration of these agents has beneficial fetal effects. The suggestion that lowering blood pressure reduces the risk of seizures has not been tested. Therapy is reserved for women in whom blood pressure is elevated to a degree that may be associated with intracranial bleeding.

Treatment is recommended for women with diastolic blood pressure persistently greater than 105 mm Hg. The goal of blood pressure control is not to attain normal blood pressure but merely to reduce blood pressure to a level that will provide a margin of maternal safety (95–100 mm Hg) without compromising adequate uterine perfusion. These patients have elevated blood pressure with reduced plasma volume, and overly aggressive treatment will lower maternal cardiac output and uterine perfusion and could result in iatrogenic fetal distress.

A number of agents available for reducing blood pressure rapidly are listed in Table 43-10. Not listed in this table are potent diuretic agents that lower blood pressure rapidly by depleting plasma volume, because the use of these agents in the plasma volume-depleted patient would result in reduced maternal cardiac output and uterine perfusion.

HYDRALAZINE. The agent most widely used to reduce blood pressure in severe preeclampsia is hydralazine. A direct vasodilator, it offers two major advantages. Vasodilation with

 TABLE 43–10. DRUGS FOR TREATMENT OF HYPERTENSIVE EMERGENCIES

	Time Course of Action					Interval between Doses	
Drug	Onset	Maximum	Duration	IM	Dosage IV		Mechanism of Action
Hydralazine	10–20 min	20–40 min	3–8 hr	10–50 mg	5–25 mg	3–6 hr	Direct dilatation of arterioles
Sodium nitroprusside	$\frac{1}{2}$–2 min	1–2 min	3–5 min	—	IV solution, 0.01 g/liter; IV infusion rate, 0.2 to 0.8 mg/min		Direct dilatation of arterioles and veins
Labetalol	1–2 min	10 min	6–16 hr	—	20–50 mg	3–6 hr	Alpha- and beta-adrenergic blocker
Nifedipine	5–10 min	10–20 min	4–8 hr	—	10 mg orally	4–8 hr	Calcium channel blocker

hydralazine results in a reflex increase in cardiac output, which in animal studies leads to the first advantage—increased uterine blood flow. A more important advantage is that the increase in cardiac output blunts the hypotensive effect and makes it difficult to overdose the patient. The important side effects of hydralazine are headache and epigastric pain, which may be confused with worsening preeclampsia.

The pharmacokinetics of hydralazine are outlined in Table 43-10. The onset of action is 10 to 20 minutes, and peak action occurs 20 minutes after administration, even when the agent is given intravenously. The duration of action is 3 to 8 hours.

On the basis of these facts, the use of continuous intravenous infusions of hydralazine is not sensible because minute-to-minute control cannot be attained. An alternative approach is to administer the drug as a bolus infusion, repeated at 20-minute intervals until the desired control is attained and then repeated as necessary. A test dose of 1 mg is given over 1 minute, and blood pressure is determined to avoid idiosyncratic hypotensive effects; 4 mg is then infused over 2–4 minutes. After 20 minutes, the blood pressure is determined and the following criteria for action are taken into account:

- If there was no effect, the dose is repeated.
- If a suboptimal effect was obtained, a lower dose is given.
- If diastolic blood pressure is between 90 and 100 mm Hg, therapy is not repeated until diastolic blood pressure increases to 105 mm Hg.

OTHER DRUGS. In rare instances, hydralazine may not effectively lower blood pressure to the desired level. If blood pressure control is not adequate after the administration of 20 mg of hydralazine, other hypotensive agents must be used.

The calcium entry blocker nifedipine has also been used in doses of 10 mg orally after 30 minutes to lower blood pressure rapidly. It is quite effective and well tolerated (Greer et al., 1989). The mixed alpha-adrenergic and beta-adrenergic antagonist, labetalol, is also useful for reducing blood pressure acutely. It is given intravenously as a bolus infusion beginning with 20 mg, followed by doses of 10–50 mg repeated every 10 minutes as needed for blood pressure control (Mabie et al., 1987). The major reservation with the use of labetalol is that, unlike the vasodilators hydralazine and nifedipine, it does not reduce afterload. Thus, there are theoretical disadvantages with labetalol in managing cardiac failure associated with the hypertension of preeclampsia.

Although alpha-methyldopa is a safe and well-tested drug, its delayed onset of action (4–6 hours), even when administered intravenously, limits its usefulness for hypertensive emergencies.

Sodium nitroprusside is a potent, short-acting, direct vasodilator that allows excellent moment-to-moment blood pressure control. In experimental animals, there are reports of elevated concentrations of serum cyanide, sometimes to toxic levels, in the fetus (Naulty et al., 1981).

Diazoxide is a thiazide analog that has no diuretic effect, but it is an extremely potent antihypertensive agent, acting as a direct vasodilator. It is rarely used because of effects on maternal and fetal carbohydrate metabolism and its profound and slowly reversible effect on blood pressure.

On the basis of side effects and experience, the drug of first choice when hydralazine is ineffective is nifedipine or labetalol.

MANAGEMENT OF OLIGURIA. In preeclamptic women, oliguria can be of prerenal or renal origin (see Chapters 44 and 45). Even though it is agreed that plasma volume is decreased in preeclamptic patients, the use of fluids is controversial. Excessive fluid infusion could lead to congestive heart failure and perhaps cerebral edema (Benedetti and Quilligan, 1980); nevertheless, oliguria can be corrected in many patients by fluid infusion.

In order to avoid complications, the physician should not prescribe hypotonic fluids because they would worsen dilutional decreases in serum osmolality that may occur with any of the following:

1. Oliguria from renal causes
2. Elevated antidiuretic hormone (ADH) secondary to stress
3. Oxytocin treatment

Fluids must be administered with the consideration that oliguria could be of renal origin and that the patient is at risk for fluid overloading. Because acute renal failure resulting in permanent renal damage is extremely rare in pregnancy (whereas pulmonary edema is an almost monthly event on many obstetric services), oliguria should be defined conservatively, 20–30 mL/hr for 2 hours.

If there are no clinical signs or history of congestive heart failure, 1000 mL of isotonic crystalloid can safely be infused in 1 hour. If urine output increases, fluid infusion is maintained at 100 mL/hour of isotonic crystalloids. If the oliguria does not resolve, further fluid infusion should be guided by central venous or, preferably, pulmonary wedge pressures (see Chapter 45).

In addition, relatively small amounts of intrapartum and postpartum blood loss can result in profound hypovolemia and shock in those patients who already have compromised blood volumes. A large peripheral line should be in place at all times in case rapid replacement of blood volume becomes necessary.

MANAGEMENT OF LESS COMMON PROBLEMS

DISSEMINATED INTRAVASCULAR COAGULATION. Evidence of DIC is an important indicator of severity and progression of preeclampsia. DIC is measurable by the usual clinical tests in 20% of severely preeclamptic and eclamptic women and is sufficient to cause coagulation problems in less than 10%.

The definitive therapy of DIC is the removal of the inciting factor. In preeclampsia, whether the etiology of the coagulation disorder is endothelial cell damage, release of thromboplastic materials, vasospasm with attendant microangiopathic changes, or local consumption of procoagulants in the choriodecidual space, the inciting factor is clearly pregnancy-related, and definitive therapy is termination of the pregnancy. The long-range follow-up of women with preeclampsia indicates that all organ system functions return to normal. Thus, it is unlikely that occlusion of the microvasculature by thrombi in mild forms of DIC causes permanent damage.

Evidence of early DIC is not by itself an absolute indication for immediate delivery. With rapidly deteriorating renal or hepatic function or DIC complicated by spontaneous hemorrhage, however, delivery should be expeditious.

The experience with heparin anticoagulation, either to maintain pregnancies in women with symptomatic DIC or as a prophylactic measure to prevent DIC, indicates that these approaches are not effective (Howie et al., 1975). The use of heparin during labor in women in whom DIC necessitates delivery has not been studied extensively. The experiences already cited, however, indicate that it is unlikely that the benefits outweigh the risks.

If procoagulants decrease to a level associated with spontaneous hemorrhage, appropriate procoagulant therapy should be given prior to delivery, whether the anticipated mode of delivery is vaginal or cesarean (see Chapter 47). The choice of mode of delivery is based on other considerations and is not influenced by the presence or absence of DIC. Thus, with a decrease in procoagulants, vaginal delivery does not necessarily prevent hemorrhage, which may be apparent or may manifest less obviously as vulvar or vaginal hematomas.

PULMONARY EDEMA. Pulmonary edema occurs in a small number of women with preeclampsia. In past years, this complication was associated with high maternal mortality rates. The pathogenesis of pulmonary edema is frequently iatrogenic fluid overload but can also be cardiogenic or involve transudation of fluid into alveolae. The noncardiogenic variety is secondary either to decreased colloid oncotic pressure or to a pulmonary vascular leakage and can occur in the antepartum, intrapartum, or postpartum period. Delayed onset of pulmonary edema requires special awareness because the edema usually occurs during postpartum diuresis, when most concerns about the complications of preeclampsia are lessening.

The management of pulmonary edema requires intensive monitoring, with the capability to assess pulmonary and cardiac function accurately and to perform mechanical ventilation as needed (see Chapter 45). With accurate assessment of cardiopulmonary function and aggressive treatment, the mortality resulting from pulmonary edema in preeclampsia has been greatly reduced (Cotton and Benedetti, 1980).

Postpartum Management in Preeclampsia

Delivery does not immediately reverse the pathophysiologic changes of preeclampsia, and it is necessary to continue palliative therapy for variable lengths of time. Some of the constraints on therapy, however, are eliminated by delivery of the fetus. Approximately one-third of convulsions occur in the postpartum period, most within 24 hours and virtually all within 48 hours, although there are rare exceptions. Most physicians advocate continuing anticonvulsant therapy for 24 hours postpartum. For simplicity, magnesium sulfate therapy is usually continued, although (because there is no need to consider fetal effects) any safe anticonvulsant regimen is reasonable at this time.

Anticonvulsant efficacy rather than sedation is the goal, however, and barbiturate anticonvulsants in usual therapeutic doses will require days to achieve effective levels. Similarly, phenytoin must be administered intravenously in large doses to achieve therapeutic levels within hours, with the attendant dangers of cardiac arrhythmia. Serum magnesium concentrations decrease with increased urinary output, and with puerperal diuresis it is extremely unlikely that serum magnesium concentration is therapeutic at usual doses. In spite of this

drawback, with either the intravenous or intramuscular dosage regimen usually used, convulsions rarely occur in the postpartum period, suggesting that rapid diuresis indicates resolution of the preeclamptic process and that therapy may no longer be required.

On the basis of these considerations, it appears reasonable to discontinue magnesium sulfate therapy when diuresis occurs before 24 hours postpartum. Some authors recommend continuing magnesium sulfate administration for longer than 24 hours in selected patients, but it is difficult to determine the basis on which this selection can be made (see Table 43-6).

Hypertension may take considerably longer than 24–48 hours to resolve. Women who are hypertensive 6 weeks postpartum may be normotensive at long-term follow-up (Chesley et al., 1976). The indications for therapy are similar to those for the antepartum period. The patient with diastolic blood pressure greater than 105 mm Hg postpartum should be treated, and the fetus no longer influences therapeutic choices. If rapid blood pressure control is necessary, sodium nitroprusside is more effective and better tolerated than hydralazine. Also, diuretics and conventional oral antihypertensive agents can be started to achieve smooth control. The woman who remains hypertensive (greater than 100 mm Hg diastolic pressure) should be sent home with continued antihypertensive therapy.

Patients with lesser elevations require no therapy. The choice of drugs is based on the usual step method of antihypertensive therapy. It is important that the patient sent home with a therapeutic regimen be warned of symptoms of hypotension and that she be seen at weekly intervals, as the need for therapy diminishes rapidly in some cases.

Follow-up in Preeclampsia

Although it is evident from the studies cited that preeclampsia does not cause higher cardiovascular risk or hypertension in later life, the correlation between a clinical diagnosis of preeclampsia and hypertension in later life is also well proven. Because the early recognition and treatment of significant blood pressure elevation reduce morbidity, all women with a clinical diagnosis of preeclampsia deserve long-range follow-up. Decisions for evaluation and treatment should be deferred until 12 weeks postpartum because some women who are hypertensive at 6 weeks are normotensive years later. The woman who is normotensive 12 weeks after delivery should be advised of her slightly increased risk for hypertension and should be counseled to have her blood pressure checked at least yearly.

■ CHRONIC HYPERTENSION

The differentiation of the pregnant woman with chronic hypertension from the woman with preeclampsia is complex but important. Even more important is the difficult discrimination between the exacerbation of preexisting hypertension and the onset of superimposed preeclampsia. The rate of progression and the effect on mother and baby of these conditions differ in the two diseases. Management of the woman with hypertension in early pregnancy requires early recognition of blood pressure elevation, baseline testing to aid in the later diagnosis of superimposed preeclampsia, and meticulous maternal and fetal observation. If a decision is made to use antihypertensive therapy, antihypertensive drugs must be chosen on the basis of considerations specific to pregnancy.

Effects of Chronic Hypertension on the Mother

Blood pressure elevation during pregnancy without the superimposition of preeclampsia has the same impact as blood pressure increases in any other 10-month period. That is, if diastolic blood pressure exceeds 105 mm Hg, morbid events can occur over even this short time, whereas at diastolic pressures of 95–100 mm Hg, morbidity is extremely unlikely. This is not the case with superimposed preeclampsia, which occurs in 20% of hypertensive women, in contrast to a 4% incidence of preeclampsia in women who previously were normotensive. In addition, maternal morbidity and mortality rates are greater in superimposed preeclampsia than in preeclampsia arising *de novo*. Blood pressure elevation is also greater, increasing the possibility of intracranial bleeding. Whereas two-thirds of cases of eclampsia occur in first pregnancies, two-thirds of maternal deaths occur in pregnancies other than the first pregnancy, in which underlying hypertension is a common disposing factor (Neutra and Neff, 1975).

Effects of Chronic Hypertension on the Fetus

The perinatal mortality rate is higher in infants born to hypertensive mothers, increasing along with rising maternal blood pressure (Tervila et al., 1973). Prior to the advent of antihypertensive therapy, a woman with a systolic pressure of 200 mm Hg or a diastolic pressure of 120 mm Hg had only a 50% chance of bearing a living infant. The perinatal mortality rate is strikingly higher in hypertensive women with proteinuria, indicating the impact of superimposed preeclampsia on the fetus.

The perinatal mortality rate for infants of women with superimposed preeclampsia is greater than for infants of women in whom the condition arises *de novo* (Lin et al., 1982). There are two explanations for this difference.

First, the decidual vessels of women with even mild preexisting hypertension demonstrate vascular changes very similar to the changes in renal arterioles that occur in women with long-standing hypertension (Robertson et al., 1967). Decreased uteroplacental perfusion secondary to this change is probably at least additive and perhaps synergistic with the decidual vascular changes of preeclampsia. The decidual vascular changes also probably explain the higher incidence of abruptio placentae in women with superimposed preeclampsia.

Second, preeclampsia appears earlier in pregnancies of hypertensive women than in those of normotensive women. IUGR is also common in infants of hypertensive women and increases in frequency and severity with increasing maternal blood pressure (Tervila et al., 1973).

Some investigators suggest that hypertension without preeclampsia has no adverse effect on the fetus (Redman, 1980; Sibai et al., 1983a). In a study by Rey of almost 300 pregnancies in women with chronic hypertension, the only perinatal deaths were growth-restricted babies. (Rey and Couturier, 1994). It seems likely that in the absence of preeclampsia and fetal growth restriction, there is little if any increase in perinatal mortality in pregnancies of women with chronic hypertension.

Antihypertensive Therapy in the Reduction of Maternal and Fetal Morbidity and Mortality

Antihypertensive therapy reduces maternal mortality as effectively during pregnancy as at any other time. Lowering of markedly elevated blood pressure (greater than 100 mm Hg diastolic pressure) can reduce the risk of morbid events even over 10 months, whereas the impact of such reduction on the minimal morbidity associated with less elevated pressures is unlikely.

A major benefit of antihypertensive therapy to mother and fetus would be reduction of the incidence of superimposed preeclampsia. Unfortunately, such a reduction has not been evident in large studies of antihypertensive therapy administered during pregnancy. On the basis of findings that pathologic and pathophysiologic changes are present as early as 14 weeks' gestation, it is possible that in these studies, in which patients were identified and treated as late in gestation as 28 weeks, therapy was begun too late to be effective. In reports of series of women in whom therapy was begun early in pregnancy, it has been suggested that antihypertensive therapy prevented or delayed the appearance of superimposed preeclampsia (Arias and Zamora, 1979).

The ability of antihypertensive therapy to reduce rates of perinatal mortality and morbidity is controversial. Agreement as to the effect of antihypertensive agents on uterine perfusion in experimental animals is lacking (Ladner et al., 1970; Brinkman and Assali, 1976). In all clinical studies, however, antihypertensive therapy has not increased perinatal mortality rates (Roberts and Perloff, 1977; Naden and Redman, 1985). Thus, if therapy is indicated for maternal considerations (diastolic pressure greater than 100 mm Hg), it is safe for the fetus if the choice of drug is appropriate (Kincaid-Smith et al., 1966).

Controlled studies have shown lower perinatal mortality rates for infants of mildly hypertensive women given antihypertensive agents (Table 43-11). There was, however, an excess of second-trimester losses in the control group (a complication not usually ascribed to hypertension) in the studies reported by Redman and coworkers (1976b) and Leather and colleagues (1968). This first group has proposed that the reduction of perinatal mortality with alpha-methyldopa therapy may be the result of some other, nonhypertensive effect of the drug.

TABLE 43-11. FETAL OUTCOME WITH MATERNAL ANTIHYPERTENSIVE THERAPY

Study		No. of Pregnancies	Total Fetal Deaths	Third-Trimester Fetal Deaths
Redman et al., 1976b	Control	125	9	5
	Treated	127	1	1
Leather et al., 1968	Control	24	5	2
	Treated	23	0	0
Sibai et al., 1990	Control	90	1	1
	Treated	174	2	1

If cases of premature labor and incompetent cervix are excluded, however, there does appear to be a relationship between hypertension and second-trimester losses (Silverstone et al., 1980). In a more recent well-designed and controlled study (Sibai et al., 1990), no difference in perinatal mortality, perinatal morbidity as indicated by growth restriction, or low Apgar scores was seen in a group of women untreated or treated with alpha-methyldopa or labetalol. Thus, the impact of antihypertensive therapy in mild hypertension to improve fetal outcome remains unproven and controversial.

Summary: Therapy for Hypertension in Pregnancy

Antihypertensive therapy can be used safely when indicated according to maternal condition. Therapy reduces the maternal risks of markedly elevated pressures. It is unclear whether therapy can delay or prevent preeclampsia if it is begun early in pregnancy or whether it can reduce rates of perinatal mortality and morbidity. The decision to use antihypertensive therapy is based on these considerations.

If therapy is chosen for fetal indications, it should be used in all women with persistent diastolic blood pressure elevation to greater than 90 mm Hg in early pregnancy. Attempts should be made to document that blood pressure is persistently elevated—perhaps with home blood pressure determinations—as early in pregnancy as possible. The vascular changes in decidual vessels in cases of hypertension described by Robertson and associates (1967), as well as the presence of demonstrable physiologic changes in preeclamptic women in early pregnancy, argue for early initiation of therapy. There is no evidence that antihypertensive therapy begun after 30 weeks' gestation has any beneficial fetal effect.

If one concludes that antihypertensive therapy does not reduce perinatal mortality and morbidity rates, such therapy is reserved for women with diastolic pressure above 100 mm Hg. In addition, women using hypertensive therapy when they become pregnant, regardless of pretreatment blood pressure, would best be served by continuation of therapy. There is no evidence that antihypertensive therapy presents a risk to the fetus, and it is very possible that discontinuation of therapy could adversely affect long-range compliance with drug therapy, clearly increasing the risk to the mother.

Choice of Antihypertensive Agents

EFFECT ON THE FETUS

The presence of a fetus necessitates special considerations in the choice of antihypertensive agents. Of great concern is the possible teratogenic effect of such drugs. None of the currently available antihypertensive agents has been associated with morphologic teratogenic effects. Because development obviously does not end with gross organ development, however, the ultimate test of drug safety depends on long-range follow-up. At present, information from careful long-range follow-up is available only for alpha-methyldopa. Children of mothers treated with this agent during pregnancy showed no signs of neurologic or somatic abnormalities in a $7\frac{1}{2}$-year follow-up (Ounsted et al., 1983).

It is important to remember that maternal drug therapy also "treats" the fetus. In animal studies, maternal treatment with propranolol reduces fetal as well as maternal cardiac output

(Oakes et al., 1976). Because of the potential pharmacokinetic differences between mother and fetus, appropriate dosage for the mother could be excessive for the fetus (Rane and Tomson, 1980). Also, drug effects of minimal importance to mother and fetus could be of great importance to the infant as a neonate.

EFFECT ON UTERINE BLOOD FLOW

Another important consideration is the effect of drugs on uterine blood flow. This issue is especially pertinent with antihypertensive drugs, which lower blood pressure by reducing either cardiac output or total peripheral resistance, with consequent changes in blood flow distribution. Making a rational drug choice requires avoiding agents that reduce uterine and, hence, uteroplacental blood flow. Agents that reduce cardiac output are best avoided because they almost inevitably reduce uterine blood flow. Antihypertensive drugs that lower blood pressure through effects on total peripheral resistance can increase, decrease, or not change uterine perfusion, depending on the pattern of blood flow redistribution.

Unfortunately, there is little reliable information on the effects of antihypertensive drugs on human uterine blood flow. Data on potential effects of these drugs are based on studies of pregnant animals in which it was assumed that humans and sheep respond identically or in which blood flow to the kidney—an exquisitely autoregulated organ that usually receives 10% of cardiac output—was compared with blood flow to the uterus, an organ whose perfusion increases 500-fold over several months. Within these limitations, Table 43-12 outlines the available information about antihypertensive agents currently used in pregnancy.

USE OF DRUGS

A few drugs warrant special comment. The use of the two common classes of drugs for antihypertensive therapy—diuretics and beta-adrenergic blockers—is especially controversial during pregnancy.

DIURETICS. The indiscriminate use of diuretic agents during pregnancy has appropriately been condemned. In an epidemiologic assessment of 8000 pregnancies, a small but significant increase in perinatal mortality rate was demonstrated in women receiving continued or intermittent diuretic therapy for nonmedical indications, especially when the drug was begun late in pregnancy (Christianson and Page, 1976). Also, lack of expansion of intravascular volume during pregnancy has adverse prognostic significance (Arias, 1975; Soffronoff et al., 1977). In women taking diuretics from early pregnancy onward, plasma volume does not expand as much as in normal pregnancy (Sibai et al., 1983b, 1984). Because of this, several investigators recommend that diuretics not be used during pregnancy (Feitelson and Lindheimer, 1972; Redman, 1980). In the United States, however, diuretics are used frequently for antihypertensive therapy in nonpregnant patients, and their efficacy, safety, and infrequency of side effects are extensively documented (Jandhyala et al., 1974). The combination of diuretics with other antihypertensive drugs allows the use of lower doses of the other agents by preventing sodium retention.

In spite of the theoretical concerns, when continuous diuretic therapy is begun before 24–30 weeks' gestation, there is no evidence of increased perinatal mortality rate or decreased neonatal weight (Flowers et al., 1962; Kraus et al., 1966). However, diuretic therapy should never be instituted if

TABLE 43–12. ANTIHYPERTENSIVE AGENTS IN PREGNANCY

Agent	Mechanism of Action	Cardiac Output	Renal Blood Flow	Side Effects	
				Maternal	**Neonatal**
Thiazide	*Initial:* decreased plasma volume and cardiac output	Decreased	Decreased	Electrolyte depletion, serum uric acid increase, thrombocytopenia, hemorrhagic pancreatitis	Thrombocytopenia
	Later: decreased TPR	Unchanged	Unchanged or increased		
Methyldopa	False neurotransmission, CNS effect	Unchanged	Unchanged	Lethargy, fever, hepatitis, hemolytic anemia, positive Coombs' test result	
Hydralazine	Direct peripheral vasodilation	Increased	Unchanged or increased	Flushing, headache, tachycardia, palpitations, lupus syndrome	
Prazosin	Direct vasodilator and cardiac effects	Increased or unchanged	Unchanged	Hypotension with first dose; little information on use in pregnancy	
Clonidine	CNS effects	Unchanged or increased	Unchanged	Rebound hypertension; little information on use in pregnancy	
Propranolol	Beta-adrenergic blockade	Decreased	Decreased	Increased uterine tone with possible decrease in placental perfusion	Depressed respiration
Labetalol	Alpha- and beta-adrenergic blockade	Unchanged	Unchanged	Tremulousness, flushing, headache	See Propranolol
Reserpine	Depletion of norepinephrine from sympathetic nerve endings	Unchanged	Unchanged	Nasal stuffiness, depression, increased sensitivity to seizures	Nasal congestion, increased respiratory tract secretions, cyanosis, anorexia
Enalapril	Angiotensin converting enzyme inhibitor	Unchanged	Unchanged	Hyperkalemia, dry cough	Neonatal anuria
Nifedipine	Calcium channel blocker	Unchanged	Unchanged	Orthostatic hypotension, headache, tachycardia	None demonstrated in humans

CNS, central nervous system; TPR, total peripheral resistance.

there is any evidence of reduced uteroplacental perfusion, as is the case with fetal growth restriction or preeclampsia. Another problem with diuretic therapy is the resultant increase in uric acid that renders serum uric acid determinations invalid for determination of superimposed preeclampsia.

BETA-ADRENERGIC ANTAGONISTS. Beta-adrenergic antagonists are the initial antihypertensive agents for non-pregnant patients in many settings. These agents lower blood pressure by reducing cardiac output and perhaps by interfering with renin release. They are especially valuable adjuncts to hydralazine therapy, increasing the efficacy of this vasodilator by reducing the reflex increase in cardiac output. Despite earlier concerns (Reed et al., 1974; Gladstone et al., 1975), although a review of the use of beta antagonists during pregnancy (Rubin, 1981) mentioned no increase in perinatal mortality or growth restriction, a more recent trial by the same group (Butters et al., 1989) indicated that infants of mothers receiving the beta antagonist atenolol weighed 500 g less than infants of control mothers.

Of course, not all beta-adrenergic antagonists are identical. Some of these agents are beta$_1$-adrenergic subtype-specific (e.g., metoprolol and atenolol) and as such should have less effect on beta$_2$ receptors in myometrium. In addition, variations in lipid solubility of these drugs results in different effects on the central nervous system and probably on

placental transfer. Also, some of the beta-adrenergic antagonists, such as oxprenolol, actually have beta-agonist effects as well.

LABETALOL. Labetalol, in addition to its beta-adrenergic antagonist effects, is an alpha-adrenergic antagonist. The decision, both theoretical and empirical, about the safety and efficacy of these drugs requires evaluation of the pharmacologic characteristics of each drug rather than consideration of them as a class.

HYDRALAZINE. Although hydralazine seems to be an ideal antihypertensive drug for pregnant women, side effects (such as headache and palpitations) caused by reflex increase in cardiac output usually prevent its use in effective dosages.

ALPHA-METHYLDOPA. Alpha-methyldopa, the drug used in the largest study and the only drug whose safety for infants has been demonstrated in long-range follow-up, is the benchmark of antihypertensive therapy. It frequently causes drowsiness, however, especially when used in the large doses necessary when diuretics are not used concomitantly, and occasionally to a degree that is incapacitating, particularly for ambulatory patients (Redman, Beilin, et al., 1977). In the original examination of infants whose mothers received alpha-methyldopa, there was a small but statistically significant decrease in head circumference, although this effect was not found in follow-up studies (Ounsted et al., 1983).

NEWER DRUGS. Several other antihypertensive drugs are available that may offer theoretical advantages for use in pregnancy. The widespread use of these drugs during pregnancy, however, requires clinical testing of efficacy and immediate and long-range safety.

One agent that is widely used in nonpregnant patients is the angiotensin-converting enzyme (ACE) inhibitor enalapril. Animal studies with another ACE inhibitor, captopril, suggested caution in the use of this drug in pregnancy. There was unexplained fetal death when pregnant ewes and rabbit does were treated (Pipkin et al., 1982). These concerns have been borne out by clinical experience. Although there are no reports of fetal death, a number of infants have been born with neonatal renal dysfunction which, in some cases, has been permanent (Rosa et al., 1989). Thus, the drug should be discontinued during pregnancy. There are case reports of teratogenic effects, largely renal agenesis. It is clearly not established whether these are cause-and-effect relationships. This and the fact that this abnormality, if it should occur, can be diagnosed sonographically by absence of amniotic fluid at a time when termination is still feasible, suggests reassurance for the woman who becomes pregnant while using ACE inhibitors (Burrows and Burrows, 1998).

Pharmacologic Recommendations

On the basis of the preceding information, a plan for the pharmacologic management of hypertension in pregnancy can be advanced. The use of ganglionic blockers—rare in current practice—should be discontinued because of the extreme sensitivity of pregnant women to these agents and the potential fetal risk of meconium ileus. ACE inhibitors should also be discontinued during pregnancy. No other drugs are absolutely contraindicated.

The drug regimens suggested in the following paragraphs are preferred because of currently available information regarding efficacy, side effects, and long-term follow-up. If a woman has established excellent blood pressure control, however, especially after unsuccessful trials of other agents, she should continue the successful regimen on becoming pregnant. This is especially pertinent to beta-adrenergic antagonist use. Women receiving atenolol should switch if possible to another beta-adrenergic antagonist of equivalent efficacy.

The use of diuretic therapy is associated with few acute adverse effects and potentiates other drug effects. Although the use of diuretics from early pregnancy onward appears safe (Flowers, 1962; Weseley and Douglas, 1962; Kraus et al., 1966), theoretical concerns raised by the effects of these agents on plasma volume militate against their use as initial therapy. Diuretics are also contraindicated for women with evidence of decreased uterine perfusion manifested as IUGR or preeclampsia. Furthermore, there is no evidence that after 30 weeks of gestation diuretics do not adversely affect survival or growth. Another major consideration in the use of diuretics is the fact that they render uric acid determination invalid as an indicator of superimposed preeclampsia.

Aldomet is the drug of choice for the initiation of antihypertensive therapy in pregnancy. The initial dosage is 250 mg at night and then 250 mg twice daily, increasing to a maximum of 1 g twice daily. If side effects prevent the use of maximal doses or if 2 g daily does not sufficiently control blood pressure, another agent should be added (not substituted). The use of

small doses of diuretic usually dramatically increases the efficacy of Aldomet. If the pregnancy is less than 30 weeks of gestation, these drugs appear safe in spite of theoretical concerns. The initial dose should be 25 mg of hydrochlorothiazide equivalent, increasing at 2- to 4-day intervals to 50 mg/day. In view of the vagaries of electrolyte balance during pregnancy, it is prudent to supplement dietary potassium and, more important, to avoid stringent sodium restriction.

If this addition does not achieve adequate blood pressure control or if diuretics are contraindicated, nifedipine or labetolol may be substituted. Although the most experience has been with hydralazine during pregnancy, side effects associated with other agents are usually fewer. If hydralazine is chosen, dosage is begun at 10 mg daily, increasing to a maximum of 100 mg twice daily. Prazosin can be initiated at 1 mg daily, increasing to 10 mg twice daily. The woman should take the first dose at bedtime and be warned of the orthostatic hypotension that could accompany the first dose of prazosin. Nifedipine can be started as a 30-mg long-acting tablet. Labetalol is begun at 100 mg twice a day and the dosage increased incrementally to a maximum of 2400 mg/day.

Obstetric Management in Chronic Hypertension

Obstetric management of the woman with chronic hypertension comprises the following measures:

- Recognizing superimposed preeclampsia early in the pregnancy
- Monitoring fetal well-being
- Ruling-out pheochromocytoma

Early in pregnancy, studies of renal function (creatinine clearance and 24-hour protein excretion), serum urate determination, and a platelet count should be performed. These studies serve as a baseline to aid in the diagnosis of superimposed preeclampsia later in pregnancy. These baseline studies are especially helpful in determining whether increased blood pressure in later pregnancy is due to exaggeration of the usual blood pressure changes of pregnancy or to the superimposition of preeclampsia. Because preeclampsia occurs earlier in pregnancy in hypertensive women, these patients should be seen every other week beginning at 26 weeks' gestation and weekly beginning at 30 weeks'.

Ultrasonographic evaluation of the fetus between 18 and 24 weeks' gestation allows accurate dating and also provides a baseline to determine incremental growth in suspicion of growth retardation.

Most hypertensive pregnant women have essential hypertension. Thorough evaluation for most secondary forms of hypertension is best reserved for the postpartum period because of the obfuscation of many of these forms by physiologic changes of pregnancy and because of the risks of diagnostic procedures to mother and fetus.

Pheochromocytoma is a potentially lethal complication, especially during the intrapartum period. This condition can be simply, accurately, and inexpensively diagnosed in many individuals with fixed hypertension by determination of serum or urinary catecholamine concentration. Hypertensive women in whom this parameter has not been measured in the past should undergo this determination in early pregnancy.

Coarctation of the aorta, a rare cause of hypertension in women of reproductive age, can be detected readily by determination of a lag between radial and femoral pulses, which should be sought as part of the physical examination of hypertensive patients.

Because of the controversy about effects of hypertension uncomplicated by preeclampsia on perinatal mortality, and because the origin of the increased mortality of this condition is placental insufficiency, extensive fetal surveillance should be reserved for infants with evidence of growth restriction or whose mothers are preeclamptic.

REFERENCES

Abuelo JG: Validity of dipstick analysis as a method of screening for proteinuria in pregnancy. Am J Obstet Gynecol **167**:1654, 1992.

Acromite MT, Mantzoros CS, Leach RE, et al: Androgens in preeclampsia. Am J Obstet Gynecol **180**:60, 1999.

Adams EM, Cantab MA, Aberd MD, et al: Long-term effect of pre-eclampsia on blood pressure. Lancet **2**:1373, 1961.

Adams EM, Finlayson A: Familial aspects of preeclampsia and hypertension in pregnancy. Lancet **2**:1357, 1961.

Adelberg AM, Miller J, Doerzbacher M, et al: Correlation of quantitative protein measurements in 8-, 12-, and 24-hour urine samples for the diagnosis of preeclampsia. Am J Obstet Gynecol **185**:804, 2001.

Aldrich C, Verp MS, Walker MA, et al: A null mutation in HLA-G is not associated with preeclampsia or intrauterine growth retardation. Journal of Reproductive Immunology **47**:41, 2000.

Altchek A, Allbright NL, Sommers C: The renal pathology of toxemia of pregnancy. Obstet Gynecol **31**:595, 1968.

Appleton MP, Kuehl TJ, Raebel MA, et al: Magnesium sulfate versus phenytoin for seizure prophylaxis in pregnancy-induced hypertension. Am J Obstet Gynecol **165**:907, 1991.

Arias F: Expansion of intravascular volume and fetal outcome in patients with chronic hypertension and pregnancy. Am J Obstet Gynecol **123**:610, 1975.

Arias F, Muncilla-Jiminez R: Hepatic fibrinogen deposits in preeclampsia. N Engl J Med **295**:578, 1976.

Arias F, Rodriguez L, Rayne SC, et al: Maternal placental vasculopathy and infection: Two distinct subgroups among patients with preterm labor and preterm ruptured membranes. Am J Obstet Gynecol **168**:585, 1993.

Arias F, Zamora J: Antihypertensive treatment and pregnancy outcome in patients with mild chronic hypertension. Obstet Gynecol **53**:489, 1979.

Arngrimsson R, Bjornsson H, Geirsson RT: Analysis of different inheritance patterns in preeclampsia/eclampsia syndrome. Hypertens Pregnancy **14**:27, 1995.

Arngrimsson R, Hayward C, Nadaud S, et al: Evidence for a familial pregnancy-induced hypertension locus in the eNOS-gene region. Am J Hum Genet **61**:354, 1997.

Arngrimsson R, Purandare S, Connor M, et al: Angiotensinogen: A candidate gene involved in preeclampsia? Nat Genet **4**:114, 1993.

Assali NS, Kaplan SA, Fomon SJ, et al: Renal function studies in toxemia of pregnancy: Excretion of solutes and renal hemodynamics during osmotic diuresis in hydropenia. J Clin Invest **32**:44, 1953.

Assali NS, Prystowsky H: Studies on autonomic blockade: I. Comparison between the effects of tetraethylammonium chloride (TEAC) and high selective spinal anesthesia on blood pressure of normal and toxemic pregnancy. J Clin Invest **29**:1354, 1950.

August P, Lenz T, Ales KL, et al: Longitudinal study of the renin-angiotensin-aldosterone system in hypertensive pregnant women: Deviations related to the development of superimposed preeclampsia. Am J Obstet Gynecol **63**:1612, 1990.

Barden AE, Beilin LJ, Ritchie L, et al: Does a predisposition to the metabolic syndrome sensitize women to develop pre-eclampsia? J Hypertens **17**:1307, 1999.

Bass KE, Morrish D, Roth I, et al: Human cytotrophoblast invasion is up-regulated by epidermal growth factor: Evidence that paracrine factors modify this process. Dev Biol **164**:1, 1994.

Basso O, Christensen K, Olsen J: Higher risk of pre-eclampsia after change of partner. An effect of longer interpregnancy intervals? Epidemiology **12**:624, 2001.

Baumgartner HR, Hardenschild C: Adhesion of platelets to subendothelium. Ann N Y Acad Sci **201**:22, 1977.

Bay WH, Ferris TF: Factors controlling plasma reinin and aldosterone during pregnancy. Hypertension **1**:410, 1979.

Begum S, Yamasaki M, Mochizuki M: Urinary levels of nitric oxide metabolites in normal pregnancy and preeclampsia. J Obstet Gynaecol Res **22**:551, 1996.

Belfort MA, Varner MW, Dizon-Townson DS, et al: Cerebral perfusion pressure, and not cerebral blood flow, may be the critical determinant of intracranial injury in preeclampsia: A new hypothesis. Am J Obstet Gynecol **187**:626, 2002.

Bell WR: Disseminated intravascular coagulation. Johns Hopkins Med J **146**:289, 1980.

Beller FK, Ebert CH, Dame WR: High molecular fibrin derivatives in preeclamptic and eclamptic patients. Eur J Obstet Gynecol Reprod Biol **9**:105, 1979.

Benedetti TJ, Quilligan EJ: Cerebral edema in severe pregnancy-induced hypertension. Am J Obstet Gynecol **137**:861, 1980.

Berman S: Observations in the toxemic clinic, Boston Lying-In Hospital, 1923–1930. Obstet Gynecol **203**:361, 1930.

Bosio PM, McKenna PJ, Conroy R, et al: Maternal central hemodynamics in hypertensive disorders of pregnancy. Obstet Gynecol **94**:978, 1999.

Branch DW, Mitchell MD, Miller E, et al: Pre-eclampsia and serum antibodies to oxidised low-density lipoprotein. Lancet **343**:645, 1994.

Brinkman CR, Assali NS: Uteroplacental hemodynamic response to antihypertensive drugs in hypertensive pregnant sheep. In Ludheimer GD, Katz AI, Zuspan FP (eds): Hypertension in Pregnancy. New York, John Wiley and Sons, 1976.

Brosens IA, Robertson WB, Dixon HG: The role of the spiral arteries in the pathogenesis of preeclampsia. Obstet Gynecol Annu **1**:171, 1972.

Brown MA, Gallery ED, Ross MR, et al: Sodium excretion in normal and hypertensive pregnancy: A prospective study. Am J Obstet Gynecol **159**:297, 1988.

Brown MA, Lindheimer MD, de Swiet M, et al: The classification and diagnosis of the hypertensive disorders of pregnancy: Statement from the International Society for the Study of Hypertension in Pregnancy (ISSHP). Hypertens Pregnancy **20**:ix, 2001.

Brown MA, Wang JA, Whitworth JA: The renin-angiotensin-aldosterone system in pre-eclampsia. Clin Exp Hypertens **19**:713, 1997.

Brown MA, Zammit VC, Adsett D: Stimulation of active renin release in normal and hypertensive pregnancy. Clin Sci **79**:505, 1990.

Brown MA, Zammit VC, Mitar DA, et al: Renin-aldosterone relationships in pregnancy-induced hypertension. Am J Hypertens **5**:366, 1992.

Browne FJ: The early signs of preeclampsia toxaemia, with special reference to the order of their appearance, and their interrelation. J Obstet Gynaecol Br Emp **40**:1160, 1933.

Buchbinder A, Sibai BM, Caritis S, et al: Adverse perinatal outcomes are significantly higher in severe gestational hypertension than in mild preeclampsia. Am J Obstet Gynecol **186**:66, 2002.

Bucher HC, Guyatt GH, Cook RJ, et al: Effect of calcium supplementation on pregnancy-induced hypertension and preeclampsia. JAMA **275**:113, 1996.

Bulfin MJ, Lawler PE: Problems associated with toxemia in twin pregnancies. Am J Obstet Gynecol **73**:37, 1957.

Burrows RF, Burrows EA: Assessing the teratogenic potential of angiotensin-converting enzyme inhibitors in pregnancy. Aust N Z J Obstet Gynaecol **38**:306, 1998.

Bussen SS, Sutterlin MW, Steck T: Plasma renin activity and aldosterone serum concentration are decreased in severe preeclampsia but not in the HELLP-Syndrome. Acta Obstet Gynecol Scand **77**:609, 1998.

Bussolino F, Benedetto C, Massobrio M, et al: Maternal vascular prostacyclin activity in pre-eclampsia (letter). Lancet **2**:702, 1980.

Butters L, Kennedy S, Rubin P: Atenolol and fetal weight in chronic hypertension during pregnancy (abstr). Clin Exp Hypertens (A)**BA**:468, 1989.

Caniggia I, Grisaru-Gravnosky S, Kuliszewsky M, et al: Inhibition of TGF-beta 3 restores the invasive capability of extravillous trophoblasts in preeclamptic pregnancies. J Clin Invest **103**:1641, 1999.

Caniggia I, Winter J, Lye SJ, et al: Oxygen and placental development during the first trimester: Implications for the pathophysiology of pre-eclampsia. Placenta **21**:S25, 2000.

Cannon PJ, Svahn DS, DeMartini FE: The influence of hypertonic saline infusion upon the fractional reabsorption of urate and other ions in normal and hypertensive man. Circulation **41**:97, 1970.

Caritis S, Sibai B, Hauth J, et al: Low-dose aspirin to prevent preeclampsia in women at high risk. National Institute of Child Health and Human Development Network of Maternal-Fetal Medicine Units [see comments]. N Engl J Med **338**:701, 1998.

Chambers JC, Fusi L, Malik IS, et al: Association of maternal endothelial dysfunction with preeclampsia. JAMA **285**:1607, 2001.

Chappell LC, Seed PT, Briley AL, et al: Effect of antioxidants on the occurrence of pre-eclampsia in women at increased risk: A randomised trial. Lancet **354**:810, 1999.

Chappell LC, Seed PT, Briley A, et al: A longitudinal study of biochemical variables in women at risk of preeclampsia. Am J Obstet Gynecol **187**:127, 2002.

Chappell LC, Seed PT, Kelly FJ, et al: Vitamin C and E supplementation in women at risk of preeclampsia is associated with changes in indices of oxidative stress and placental function. Am J Obstet Gynecol **187**:777, 2002.

Chesley LC: Renal function tests in the differentiation of Bright's disease from so-called specific toxemia of pregnancy. Surg Gynecol Obstet **67**:481, 1938.

Chesley LC: The variability of proteinuria in the hypertensive complications of pregnancy. J Clin Invest **18**:617, 1939.

Chesley LC: Toxemia of pregnancy in relation to chronic hypertension. West J Surg Obstet Gynecol **64**:284, 1956.

Chesley LC: Sodium retention and preeclampsia. Am J Obstet Gynecol **95**:127, 1966.

Chesley LC: Hypertensive Disorders in Pregnancy. New York, Appleton-Century-Crofts, 1978.

Chesley LC: Parenteral magnesium sulfate and the distribution, plasma levels, and excretion of magnesium. Am J Obstet Gynecol **133**:1, 1979.

Chesley LC: Hypertension in pregnancy: Definitions, familial factor, and remote prognosis. Kidney Intl **18**:234, 1980.

Chesley LC, Annitto JE: Pregnancy in the patient with hypertensive disease. Am J Obstet Gynecol **53**:372, 1947.

Chesley LC, Annitto JE, Cosgrove RA: Long-term follow-up study of eclamptic women: Fifth periodic report. Am J Obstet Gynecol **101**:886, 1968.

Chesley LC, Annitto JE, Cosgrove RA: The remote prognosis of eclamptic women: Sixth periodic report. Am J Obstet Gynecol **124**:446, 1976.

Chesley LC, Chesley ER: An analysis of some factors associated with the development of preeclampsia. Am J Obstet Gynecol **45**:748, 1943.

Chesley LC, Cooper DW: Genetics of hypertension in pregnancy: Possible single-gene control of pre-eclampsia and eclampsia in the descendants of eclamptic women. Br J Obstet Gynaecol **93**:898, 1986.

Chesley LC, Markowitz I, Wetchler BB: Proteinuria following momentary vascular constriction. J Clin Invest **18**:51, 1939.

Chesley LC, Tepper I: Plasma levels of magnesium attained in magnesium sulfate therapy for preeclampsia and eclampsia. Surg Clin North Am **37**:353, 1957.

Chesley LC, Valenti C: The evaluation of tests to differentiate preeclampsia from hypertensive disease. Am J Obstet Gynecol **75**:1165, 1958.

Chesley LC, Valenti C, Rein H: The excretion of sodium loads by nonpregnant and pregnant normal, hypertensive and preeclamptic women. Metabolism **7**:575, 1958.

Chien PFW, Arnott N, Gordon A, et al: How useful is uterine artery Doppler flow velocimetry in the prediction of pre-eclampsia, intrauterine growth retardation and perinatal death? An overview. Br J Obstet Gynaecol **107**:196, 2000.

Christianson R, Page EW: Diuretic drugs and pregnancy. Obstet Gynecol **48**:647, 1976.

Christianson RE: Studies on blood pressure during pregnancy: 1. Influence of parity and age. Am J Obstet Gynecol **125**:509, 1976.

CLASP Collaborative Group: CLASP: A randomized trial of low-dose aspirin for the prevention and treatment of pre-eclampsia among 9364 pregnant women. Lancet **343**:619, 1994.

Cockell AP, Poston L: Flow mediated vasodilatation is enhanced in normal pregnancy but reduced in preeclampsia. Hypertension **30**:247, 1997.

Cotton DB, Benedetti TJ: Use of the Swan-Ganz catheter in obstetrics and gynecology. Obstet Gynecol **56**:641, 1980.

Cross JC, Werb Z, Fisher SJ: Implantation and the placenta: Key pieces of the development puzzle (review). Science **266**:1508, 1994.

Crowther C: Magnesium sulfate versus diazepam in the management of eclampsia: A randomized controlled trial. Br J Obstet Gynaecol **97**:110, 1990.

Curtis NE, Gude NM, King RG, et al: Nitric oxide metabolites in normal human pregnancy and preeclampsia. Hypertens Pregnancy **14**:339, 1995.

Dadak C, Kefalides A, Sinzinger H, et al: Reduced umbilical artery prostacyclin formation in complicated pregnancies. Am J Obstet Gynecol **144**:792, 1982.

Davidge S, Stranko C, Roberts J: Urine but not plasma nitric oxide metabolites are decreased in women with preeclampsia. Am J Obstet Gynecol **174**:1008, 1996.

Davies AG: Geographical Epidemiology of the Toxemias of Pregnancy. Springfield, Ill, Charles C Thomas, 1971.

Davies AM, Czaczkes JW, Sadovsky E, et al: Toxemia of pregnancy in Jerusalem: I. Epidemiological studies of a total community. Isr J Med Sci **6**:253, 1970.

Dekker GA, Devries JIP, Doelitzsch PM, et al: Underlying disorders associated with severe early-onset preeclampsia. Am J Obstet Gynecol **173**:1042, 1995.

Dekker GA, Sibai BM: The immunology of preeclampsia. Semin Perinatol **23**:24, 1999.

Dell RB, Winters RW: Lactate gradients in the kidney of the dog. Am J Physiol **213**:301, 1967.

Denson KWE: The ratio of factor VIII–related antigen and factor VIII biological activity as an index of hypercoagulability and intravascular clotting. Thromb Res **10**:107, 1977.

Dieckman WJ: The Toxemias of Pregnancy, 2nd ed. St Louis, CV Mosby, 1952.

Dieckman WJ, Michel HL: Vascular-renal effects of posterior pituitary extracts in pregnant women. Am J Obstet Gynecol **33**:131, 1937.

Dieckman WJ, Pottinger RE: Total exchangeable sodium and space in normal and preeclamptic patients determined with sodium[22]. Am J Obstet Gynecol **74**:816, 1957.

Douglas JT, Shah M, Lowe GDO, et al: Plasma fibrinopeptide and beta-thromboglobulin in pre-eclampsia and pregnancy hypertension. Thromb Haemost **47**:54, 1982.

Duley L, Farrell B, Spark P, et al: Do women with pre-eclampsia, and their babies, benefit from magnesium sulphate? The Magpie Trial: A randomised placebo-controlled trial. Lancet **359**:1877, 2002.

Duncan SLB, Ginsburg J, Bernard AG: Arteriolar distensibility in hypertensive pregnancy. Am J Obstet Gynecol **100**:222, 1968.

Easterling TR, Benedetti TJ, Schmucker BC, et al: Maternal hemodynamics in normal and preeclampsia pregnancies: A longitudinal study. Obstet Gynecol **76**:1061, 1990.

Eclampsia Trial Collaborative Group: Which anticonvulsant for women with eclampsia? Evidence from the collaborative eclampsia trial. Lancet **345**:1445, 1995.

Egerman RS, Sibai BM: HELLP syndrome. Clin Obstet Gynecol **42**:381, 1999.

Ehrlich EN, Lindheimer MD: Sodium metabolism, aldosterone and the hypertensive disorders of pregnancy (editorial). J Reprod Med **8**:106, 1972.

Elden CA, Cooney JW: The Addis sediment count and blood urea clearance test in normal pregnant women. J Clin Invest **14**:889, 1935.

Emmerson BT: Effect of drugs on the renal handling of urate. In Edwards DK (ed): Drugs and the Kidney (Progr Biochem Pharmacol Vol 9). Basel, S Karger, 1974.

Entman SS, Moore RM, Richardson LD, et al: Elevated serum iron in toxemia of pregnancy. Am J Obstet Gynecol **143**:398, 1982.

Epstein FH: Late vascular effects of toxemia of pregnancy. N Engl J Med **271**:391, 1964.

Eskenazi B, Fenster L, Sidney S: A multivariate analysis of risk factors for preeclampsia. JAMA **266**:237, 1991.

Esplin MS, Fausett MB, Fraser A, et al: Paternal and maternal components of the predisposition to preeclampsia. N Engl J Med **344**:867, 2001.

Everett RB, Worley RJ, McDonald PC, et al: Effect of prostaglandin synthetase inhibitors on pressor response to angiotensin II in human pregnancy. J Clin Endocrinol Metab **46**:1007, 1978.

Fadel HE, Northrop G, Misenheimer HR: Hyperuricemia in preeclampsia: A reappraisal. Am J Obstet Gynecol **125**:640, 1976.

Faith GC, Trump BF: The glomerular capillary wall in human kidney disease: Acute glomerulonephritis, systemic lupus erythematosus, and preeclampsia-eclampsia. Lab Invest **15**:1682, 1966.

Farrell PC: Protein binding of urate ions in vitro and in vivo. In Edwards DK (ed): Drugs and the Kidney (Progr Biochem Pharmacol Vol 9). Basel, S Karger, 1974.

Feitelson PJ, Lindheimer MD: Management of hypertensive gravidas. J Reprod Med **8**:111, 1972.

Ferris TF, Gordon P: Effect of angiotensin and norepinephrine upon urate clearance in man. Am J Med **44**:359, 1968.

Ferris TF, Stein JH, Kauffman J: Uterine blood flow and uterine renin secretion. J Clin Invest **51**:2827, 1972.

Finnerty FA: Toxemia of pregnancy as seen by an internist: An analysis of 1,081 patients. Ann Intern Med **44**:358, 1956.

Fisher KA, Luger A, Spargo BH, et al: Hypertension in pregnancy: Clinical-pathological correlations and remote prognosis. Medicine **60**:267, 1981.

Flowers CE, Grizzle JE, Easterling WE, et al: Chlorothiazide as a prophylaxis against toxemia of pregnancy: A double-blind study. Am J Obstet Gynecol **84**:919, 1962.

Fox H: Effect of hypoxia on trophoblast in organ culture. Am J Obstet Gynecol 107:1058, 1970.

Fridstrom M, Nisell H, Sjoblom P, et al: Are women with polycystic ovary syndrome at increased risk of pregnancy-induced hypertension and/or preeclampsia? Hypertens Pregnancy 18:73, 1999.

Furchgott RF: Role of endothelium in the response of vascular smooth muscle. Circ Res 53:558, 1983.

Gaber LW, Spargo BH, Lindheimer MD: Renal pathology in preeclampsia (review). Baillieres Clin Obstet Gynecol 8:443, 1994.

Gallery EDM, Györy AZ: Glomerular and proximal renal tubular function in pregnancy-associated hypertension: A prospective study. Eur J Obstet Gynec Reprod Biol 9:3, 1979a.

Gallery EDM, Györy AZ: Urinary concentration, white blood cell excretion, acid excretion, and acid-base status in normal pregnancy: Alterations in pregnancy-associated hypertension. Am J Obstet Gynecol 135:27, 1979b.

Gallery EDM, Hunyor SN, Ross M, et al: Predicting the development of pregnancy-associated hypertension: The place of standardised blood-pressure measurement. Lancet 1:1273, 1977.

Gallery EDM, Saunders DM, Boyce ES, et al: Relation between plasma volume and uric acid in the development of hypertension in pregnancy. In Bonnar MA, MacGillivray I, Symonds MS (eds): Pregnancy Hypertension. Baltimore, University Park Press, 1980, p. 175.

Galton M, Merritt K, Veller FK: Coagulation studies on the peripheral circulation of patients with toxemia of pregnancy: A study for the evaluation of disseminated intravascular coagulation in toxemia. J Reprod Med 6:78, 1971.

Gant NF, Daley GL, Chand S, et al: A study of angiotensin II pressor response throughout primigravid pregnancy. J Clin Invest 52:2682, 1973.

Genbacev O, Joslin R, Damsky CH, et al: Hypoxia alters early gestation human cytotrophoblast differentiation/invasion in vitro and models the placental defects that occur in preeclampsia. J Clin Invest 97:540, 1996.

Genbacev O, Zhou Y, Ludlow JW, et al: Regulation of human placental development by oxygen tension. Science 277:1669, 1997.

Gifford R, August P, Cunningham G, et al: The national high blood pressure education program working group on high blood pressure in pregnancy. Bethesda, National Institutes of Health and National Heart, Lung and Blood Institute, 2000a.

Gifford RW, August PA, Cunningham G, et al: Report of the National High Blood Pressure Education Program Working Group on High Blood Pressure in Pregnancy. Am J Obstet Gynecol 183:S1, 2000b.

Gladstone GR, Hordof A, Gersony WM: Propranolol administration during pregnancy: Effects on the fetus. J Pediatr 86:962, 1975.

Goodlin RC, Cotton DB, Haesslein HC: Severe edema-proteinuria-hypertension gestosis. Am J Obstet Gynecol 132:595, 1978.

Gordon RD, Symonds EM, Wilmhurst EG, et al: Plasma renin activity, plasma angiotensin and plasma and urinary electrolytes in normal and toxaemic pregnancy, including a prospective study. Clin Sci Molec Med 45:115, 1973.

Gordon YB, Ratky SM, Baker LRI, et al: Circulating levels of fibrin/fibrinogen degradation fragment E measured by radioimmunoassay in preeclampsia. Br J Obstet Gynaecol 83:287, 1976.

Grandone E, Margaglione M, Colaizzo D, et al: C > T MTHFR polymorphism and genetic susceptibility to preeclampsia. Thromb Haemost 77:1052, 1997.

Greer IA, Lyall F, Perera T, et al: Increased concentrations of cytokines interleukin-6 and interleukin-1 receptor antagonist in plasma of women with preeclampsia: A mechanism for endothelial dysfunction? Obstet Gynecol 84:937, 1994.

Greer IA, Walker JJ, Bjornsson S, et al: Second line therapy with nifedipine in severe pregnancy induced hypertension. Clin Exp Hypertens B8:277, 1989.

Griendling KK, Ushio-Fukai M: Reactive oxygen species as mediators of angiotensin II signaling. Regulatory Peptides 91:21, 2000.

Handler JS: The role of lactic acid in the reduced excretion of uric acid in toxemia of pregnancy. J Clin Invest 39:1526, 1960.

Hanssens M, Keirse MJ, Spitz B, et al: Angiotensin II levels in hypertensive and normotensive pregnancies. Br J Obstet Gynecol 98:155, 1991.

Harrison GA, Humphrey KE, Jones N, et al: A genome-wide linkage study of preeclampsia/eclampsia reveals evidence for a candidate region on 4q. Am J Hum Genet 60:1158, 1997.

Hauth JC, Cunningham FG, Whalley PJ: Management of pregnancy-induced hypertension in the nullipara. Am J Obstet Gynecol 48:253, 1976.

Hauth JC, Goldenberg RL, Parker CR, et al: Low-dose aspirin therapy to prevent preeclampsia. Am J Obstet Gynecol 168:1083, 1993.

Hayashi T: Uric acid and endogenous creatinine clearance studies in normal pregnancy and toxemias of pregnancy. Am J Obstet Gynecol 71:859, 1956.

Healy JK, Edwards KDG, Whyte HM: Simple tests of renal function using creatinine, phenolsulfonphthalein and pitressin. J Clin Pathol 17:557, 1964.

Heidland A, Reidl E: Klinisch-experimentelle Untersuchung uber den renalen Phenolsulfonphthalein-Transport. Arch Klin Med 214:163, 1968.

Helewa ME, Burrows RF, Smith J, et al: Report of the Canadian Hypertension Society Consensus Conference: 1. Definitions, evaluation and classification of hypertensive disorders in pregnancy. Can Med Assoc J 157:715, 1997.

Henderson AH, Pugsley DJ, Thomas DP: Fibrin degradation products in preeclamptic toxaemia and eclampsia. Br Med J 3:545, 1970.

Hollenberg NK, Epstein M, Rosen SM, et al: Acute oliguric renal failure in man: Evidence for preferential renal cortical ischemia. Medicine 47:455, 1968.

Howie PW, Prentice CRM, Forbes CD: Failure of heparin therapy to affect the clinical course of severe preeclampsia. Br J Obstet Gynecol 82:711, 1975.

Hubel CA: Oxidative stress in the pathogenesis of preeclampsia. Proc Soc Exp Biol Med 222:222, 1999.

Hubel CA, Kagan VE, Kisin ER, et al: Increased ascorbate radical formation and ascorbate depletion in plasma from women with preeclampsia—Implications for oxidative stress. Free Radic Biol Med 23:597, 1997.

Hubel CA, McClaughlin MK, Evans RW, et al: Fasting serum triglycerides, free fatty acids, and malondialdehyde are increased in preeclampsia, are positively correlated, and decrease within 48 hours post partum. Am J Obstet Gynecol 174:975, 1996.

Hubel CA, Roberts J: Lipid metabolism and oxidative stress. In Lindheimer M, Roberts J, Cunningham F (eds): Chesley's Hypertensive Disorders in Pregnancy. Stamford, Conn, Appleton and Lange, 1999, p. 453.

Hubel CA, Roberts JM, Ferrell RE: Association of pre-eclampsia with common coding sequence variations in the lipoprotein lipase gene. Clin Genet 56:289, 1999.

Hubel CA, Roberts JM, Taylor RN, et al: Lipid peroxidation in pregnancy: New perspectives on preeclampsia. Am J Obstet Gynecol 161:1025, 1989.

Hubel CA, Shakir Y, Gallaher MJ, et al: Low-density lipoprotein particle size decreases during normal pregnancy in association with triglyceride increases. J Soc Gynecol Investig 5:244, 1998.

Hubel CA, Snaedal S, Ness RB, et al: Dyslipoproteinaemia in postmenopausal women with a history of eclampsia. Br J Obstet Gynaecol 107:776, 2000.

Hutt R, Ogunniyi SO, Sullivan HF, et al: Increased platelet volume and aggregation precede the onset of preeclampsia. Obstet Gynecol 83:146, 1994.

Imperiale TF, Petrulis AS: A meta-analysis of low-dose aspirin for the prevention of pregnancy-induced hypertensive disease. JAMA 266:261, 1991.

Inglis TCM, Stuart J, George AJ, et al: Haemostatic and rheological changes in normal pregnancy and pre-eclampsia. Br J Haematol 50:461, 1982.

Irons DW, Baylis PH, Butler TJ, et al: Atrial natriuretic peptide in preeclampsia: Metabolic clearance, sodium excretion and renal hemodynamics. Am J Physiol 273:F483, 1997.

Jaffe G, Schatz H: Ocular manifestations of preeclampsia. Am J Ophthalmol 103:309, 1986.

Jaimes EA, Galceran JM, Raij L: Angiotensin II induces superoxide anion production by mesangial cells. Kidney Int 54:775, 1998.

Jandhyala BS, Clarke DE, Buckley JP: Effects of prolonged administration of certain antihypertensive agents. J Pharm Sci 63:1497, 1974.

Janes SL, Kyle PM, Redman C, et al: Flow cytometric detection of activated platelets in pregnant women prior to the development of pre-eclampsia. Thromb Haemost 74:1059, 1995.

Jeffcoate TNA, Scott JS: Some observations on the placental factor in pregnancy toxemia. Am J Obstet Gynecol 77:475, 1959.

Johnson N, Moodley J, Hammond MG: HLA status of the fetus born to African women with eclampsia. Clin Exp Hypertens Pregnancy B9:311, 1990.

Jones CJP, Fox H: An ultrastructural and ultrahistochemical study of the human placenta in maternal preeclampsia. Placenta 1:61, 1980.

Jonsdottir LS, Arngrimsson R, Geirsson RT, et al: Death rates from ischemic heart disease in women with a history of hypertension in pregnancy. Acta Obstet Gynecol Scand 74:772, 1995.

Kaitz AL: Urinary concentrating ability in pregnant women with asymptomatic bacteriuria. J Clin Invest 40:1331, 1961.

Katz M, Berlyne GM: Differential renal protein clearance in toxaemia of pregnancy. Nephron 13:212, 1974.

Kavats S, Main EK, Librach C, et al: Class I antigen, HLA-G, expressed in human trophoblasts. Sci 248:220, 1990.

Khong TY, De Wolf F, Robertson WB, et al: Inadequate maternal vascular response to placentation in pregnancies complicated by preeclampsia and by small-for-gestational age infants. Br J Obstet Gynaecol 93:1049, 1986.

Kilpatrick DC, Gibson G, Livingston J, et al: Preeclampsia is associated with HLA-DR4 sharing between mother and fetus. Tissue Antigens 35:178, 1990.

Kincaid-Smith P: The renal lesion of preeclampsia revisited. Am J Kidney Dis **144**:148, 1991.

Kincaid-Smith P, Bullen M, Mills J: Prolonged use of methyldopa in severe hypertension in pregnancy. Br Med J **1**:274, 1966.

Kitzmiller JL, Benirschke K: Immunofluorescent study of placental bed vessels in pre-eclampsia. Am J Obstet Gynecol **115**:248, 1973.

Kitzmiller JL, Stoneburner L, Yelenosky PF, et al: Serum complement in normal pregnancy and pre-eclampsia. Am J Obstet Gynecol **117**:312, 1973.

Kitzmiller JL, Watt N, Driscoll SG: Decidual arteriopathy in hypertension and diabetes in pregnancy: Immunofluorescent studies. Am J Obstet Gynecol **141**:773, 1981.

Knight M, Duley L, Henderson-Smart DJ, et al: Antiplatelet agents for preventing and treating pre-eclampsia. Cochrane Database of Systematic Reviews: CD000492, 2000.

Knock GA, Poston L: Bradykinin-mediated relaxation of isolated maternal resistance arteries in normal pregnancy and preeclampsia. Am J Obstet Gynecol **175**:1668, 1996.

Knopp RH: Lipid Metabolism in Pregnancy. New York, Springer-Verlag, 1991.

Knox GE, Stagno S, Volanakis JE, et al: A search for antigen-antibody complexes in pre-eclampsia: Further evidence against immunologic pathogenesis. Am J Obstet Gynecol **132**:87, 1978.

Knuist M, Bonsel GJ, Zondervan HA, et al: Riskfactors for preeclampsia in nulliparous women in distinct ethnic Groups—A prospective cohort study. Obstet Gynecol **92**:174, 1998.

Kraus GW, Marchese JR, Yen SSC: Prophylactic use of hydrochlorothiazide in pregnancy. JAMA **198**:1150, 1966.

Krauss T, Kuhn W, Lakoma C, et al: Circulating endothelial cell adhesion molecules as diagnostic markers for the early identification of pregnant women at risk for development of preeclampsia. Am J Obstet Gynecol **177**:443, 1997.

Kuo VS, Koumantakis G, Gallery ED: Proteinuria and its assessment in normal and hypertensive pregnancy [see comments]. Am J Obstet Gynecol **167**:723, 1992.

Kyle PM, Buckely RN, Kissane J, et al: The angiotensin sensitivity test and low-dose aspirin are ineffective methods to predict and prevent hypertensive disorders in nulliparous pregnancy. Am J Obstet Gynecol **173**:865, 1995.

Ladner CN, Weston PV, Brinkman CR, et al: Effects of hydralazine on uteroplacental and fetal circulations. Am J Obstet Gynecol **108**:375, 1970.

Laivuori H, Tikkanen MJ, Ylikorkala O: Hyperinsulinemia 17 years after preeclamptic first pregnancy. J Clin Endocrinol Metabol **81**:2908, 1996.

Langford HG, Pickering GW: The action of synthetic angiotensin on renal function in the unanesthetized rabbit. J Physiol (London) **177**:161, 1965.

Leather HM, Humphreys DM, Baker P, et al: A controlled trial of hypotensive agents in hypertension in pregnancy. Lancet **2**:488, 1968.

Levine RJ, Hauth JC, Curet LB, et al: Trial of calcium to prevent preeclampsia. N Engl J Med **337**:69, 1997.

Librach CL, Feigenbaum SL, Bass KE, et al: Interleukin-1B regulates human cytotrophoblast metalloproteinase activity and invasion in vitro. J Biol Chem **269**:17125, 1994.

Lichtig C, Deutsch M, Brandes J: Immunofluorescent studies of endometrial arteries in the first trimester of pregnancy. Am J Clin Pathol **83**:633, 1985.

Lie RT, Rasmussen S, Brunborg H, et al: Fetal and Maternal Contributions to Risk Of Pre-Eclampsia—Population Based Study. Br Med J **316**:1343, 1998.

Lin CC, Lindheimer MD, River P, et al: Fetal outcome in hypertensive disorders of pregnancy. Am J Obstet Gynecol **142**:255, 1982.

Lockwood CJ, Peters JH: Increased plasma levels of ED1+ cellular fibronectin precede the clinical signs of preeclampsia. Am J Obstet Gynecol **162**:358, 1990.

Lopez-Llera M, Horta JLH: Perinatal mortality in eclampsia. J Reprod Med **8**:281, 1972.

Lorentzen B, Endresen MJ, Clausen T, et al: Fasting serum free fatty acids and triglycerides are increased before 20 weeks of gestation in women who later develop preeclampsia. Hypertens Pregnancy **13**:103, 1994.

Lorentzen B, Endresen MJ, Haug THE, et al: Sera from preeclamptic women increase the content of triglycerides and reduce the release of prostacyclin in cultured endothelial cells. Thromb Res **363**:372, 1991.

Lucas MJ, Leveno KJ, Cunningham FG: A comparison of magnesium sulfate with phenytoin for the prevention of eclampsia. N Engl J Med **333**:201, 1995a.

Lucas MJ, Leveno KJ, Cunningham FG: Magnesium sulfate versus phenytoin for the prevention of eclampsia—reply. N Engl J Med **333**:1639, 1995b.

Mabie WC, Gonzalez AR, Sibai BM, et al: A comparative trial of labetalol and hydralazine in the acute management of severe hypertension complicating pregnancy. Obstet Gynecol **170**:328, 1987.

Mabie WC, Ratts TE, Sibai BM: The central hemodynamics of severe preeclampsia. Am J Obstet Gynecol **161**:1443, 1989.

MacGillivray I: Some observations on the incidence of preeclampsia. J Obstet Gynaecol **65**:536, 1958.

Magann EF, Bass D, Chauhan SP, et al: Antepartum corticosteroids: disease stabilization in patients with the syndrome of hemolysis, elevated liver enzymes, and low platelets (HELLP) [see comments]. Am J Obstet Gynecol **171**:1148, 1994.

Magann EF, Martin JN Jr: Complicated postpartum preeclampsia-eclampsia. Obstet Gynecol Clin N Am **22**:337, 1995.

Magann EF, Martin RW, Isaacs JD, et al: Corticosteroids for the enhancement of fetal lung maturity: Impact on the gravida with preeclampsia and the HELLP syndrome. Aust N Z J Obstet Gynaecol **33**:127, 1993.

Magdy SM, Akolisa A, David G, et al: Preeclampsia and antioxidant nutrients: Decreased plasma levels of reduced ascorbic acid, a-tocopherol, and beta-carotene in women with preeclampsia. Am J Obstet Gynecol **171**:150, 1994.

Malee MP, Malee KM, Azuma SD, et al: Increases in plasma atrial natriuretic peptide concentration antedate clinical evidence of preeclampsia. J Clin Endocrinol Metab **74**:1095, 1992.

Many A, Hubel CA, Fisher SJ, et al: Invasive cytotrophoblasts manifest evidence of oxidative stress in preeclampsia. Am J Pathol **156**:321, 2000.

Many A, Hubel CA, Roberts JM: Hyperuricemia and xanthine oxidase in preeclampsia revisited. Am J Obstet Gynecol **174**:288, 1996.

Many A, Roberts JM: Increased xanthine oxidase during labour—Implications for oxidative stress. Placenta **18**:725, 1997.

Marti JJ, Herrman U: Immunogestosis: A new concept of "essential" EPH gestosis, with special consideration of the primigravid patient. Am J Obstet Gynecol **128**:489, 1977.

Martin JN, Blake PG, Pery KG, et al: The natural history of HELLP syndrome: Patterns of disease progression and regression. Am J Obstet Gynecol **164**:1500, 1991.

Martin JN, Perry KG, Blake PG, et al: Better maternal outcomes are achieved with dexamethasone therapy for postpartum HELLP (hemolysis, elevated liver enzymes, and thrombocytopenia) syndrome. Am J Obstet Gynecol **177**:1011, 1997.

Maseki M, Nishigaki I, Hagihara M, et al: Lipid peroxide levels and lipids content of serum lipoprotein fractions of pregnant subjects with or without pre-eclampsia. Clin Chim Acta **115**:155, 1981.

Massey SG: Pharmacology of magnesium. Annu Rev Pharmacol Toxicol **17**:67, 1977.

Mathews DD: A randomized controlled trial of bed rest and sedation or normal activity and non-sedation in the management of nonalbuminuric hypertension in late pregnancy. Br J Obstet Gynaecol **84**:108, 1977.

Matter L, Faulk WP: Fibrinogen degradation products and factor VIII consumption in normal pregnancy and preeclampsia: Role of the placenta. In Bonnar MA, MacGillivray I, Symonds MS (eds): Pregnancy Hypertension. Baltimore, University Park Press, 1980, p. 327.

Maynard JR, Dreyer BE, Stemerman MB, et al: Tissue factor coagulant activity of cultured human endothelial and smooth muscle cells and fibroblasts. Blood **50**:387, 1987.

McCartney CP: Pathological anatomy of acute hypertension of pregnancy. Circulation **30**(S2):37, 1964.

McKay DG: Hematologic evidence of disseminated intravascular coagulation in eclampsia. Obstet Gynecol Surv **27**:399, 1972.

McKillop C, Howie PW, Forbes CD, et al: Soluble fibrinogen/fibrin complexes in preeclampsia. Lancet **1**:56, 1976.

Meyer NL, Mercer BM, Friedman SA, et al: Urinary dipstick protein: A poor predictor of absent or severe proteinuria. Am J Obstet Gynecol **170**:137, 1994.

Mittendorf R, Lain KY, Williams MA, et al: Preeclampsia. A nested, case-control study of risk factors and their interactions. J Reprod Med **41**:491, 1996.

Moncada S, Palmer RMJ, Higgs EA: Nitric oxide: Physiology, pathophysiology, and pharmacology. Pharmacol Rev **43**:109, 1991.

Morgan T, Craven C, Nelson L, et al: Angiotensinogen T235 expression is elevated in decidual spiral arteries. J Clin Invest **100**:1406, 1997.

Myatt L, Miodovnik M: Prediction of preeclampsia [Review]. Semin Perinatol **23**:45, 1999.

Myatt L, Rosenfield RB, Eis AL, et al: Nitrotyrosine residues in placenta. Evidence of peroxynitrite formation and action. Hypertension **28**:488, 1996.

Nachman RL: The 1994 Runme Shaw Memorial Lecture: Thrombosis and atherogenesis-molecular connections. Ann Acad Med Singapore **24**:281, 1995.

Naden RP, Redman CWG: Antihypertensive drugs in pregnancy. Clin Perinatol **12**:521, 1985.

Nadji P, Sommers SC: Lesions of toxemia in first trimester pregnancies. Am J Clin Pathol **59**:344, 1973.

Naeye RL, Friedman EA: Causes of perinatal death associated with gestational hypertension and proteinuria. Am J Obstet Gynecol **133**:8, 1979.

Naheedy MH, Biller J, Schiffer M, et al: Toxemia of pregnancy: Cerebral findings. J Comput Assist Tomogr **9**:497, 1985.

Naidoo DV, Moodley J: A survey of hypertension in pregnancy at the King Edward VIII Hospital, Durban. S Afr Med J **58**:556, 1980.

Nakamura T, Ito M, Matsui K, et al: Significance of angiotensin sensitivity test for prediction of pregnancy-induced hypertension. Obstet Gynecol **67**:388, 1986.

Naulty J, Cefalo RC, Lewis PE: Fetal toxicity of nitroprusside in the pregnant ewe. Am J Obstet Gynecol **139**:708, 1981.

Need JA: Pre-eclampsia in pregnancies by different fathers: Immunological studies. Br Med J **1**:548, 1975.

Nelson TR: A clinical study of preeclampsia. Parts I and II. J Obstet Gynaecol Br Emp **62**:48, 1955.

Ness RB, Roberts JM: Heterogeneous causes constituting the single syndrome of preeclampsia: A hypothesis and its implications (review). Am J Obstet Gynecol **175**:1365, 1996.

Neutra R, Neff R: Fetal death in eclampsia: II. The effect of nontherapeutic factors. Br J Obstet Gynaecol **82**:390, 1975.

Nicholson E, Gallery E, Brown M, et al: Renin activation in normal and hypertensive human pregnancy. Clin Exp Hypertens B **6**:435, 1988.

North RA, Taylor RS, Schellenberg JC: Evaluation of a definition of pre-eclampsia [see comments]. Br J Obstet Gynaecol **106**:767, 1999.

Oakes GK, Walker AM, Ehrenkranz RA, et al: Effect of propranolol infusion on the umbilical and uterine circulations of pregnant sheep. Am J Obstet Gynecol **126**:1038, 1976.

O'Brien JM, Milligan DA, Barton JR: Impact of high-dose corticosteroid therapy for patients with HELLP (hemolysis, elevated liver enzymes, and low platelet count) syndrome. Am J Obstet Gynecol **183**:921, 2000.

O'Brien JM, Shumate SA, Satchwell SL, et al: Maternal benefit of corticosteroid therapy in patients with HELLP (hemolysis, elevated liver enzymes, and low platelet count) syndrome: Impact on the rate of regional anesthesia. Am J Obstet Gynecol **186**:475, 2002.

O'Brien M, McCarthy T, Jenkins D, et al: Altered HLA-G transcription in pre-eclampsia is associated with allele specific inheritance: possible role of the HLA-G gene in susceptibility to the disease. Cell Mol Life Sci **58**:1943, 2001.

Ochwadt B, Pitts RF: Disparity between phenol red and Diodrast clearances in the dog. Am J Physiol **187**:318, 1956.

Okkels H, Engle ET: Studies of the fever structure of the uterine vessels of the Macacus monkey. Acta Pathol Microbiol Scand **15**:150, 1938.

Oney T, Kaulhausen H: The value of the angiotensin sensitivity test in the early diagnosis of hypertensive disorders in pregnancy. Am J Obstet Gynecol **142**:17, 1982.

Ounsted M, Cockburn J, Moar VA, et al: Maternal hypertension with super-imposed preeclampsia: Effects on child development at 7¹/₂ years. Br J Obstet Gynaecol **90**:644, 1983.

Page EW: The relation between hydatid moles, relative ischemia of the gravid uterus, and placental origin of eclampsia. Am J Obstet Gynecol **37**:291, 1939.

Parks DA, Granger DN: Xanthine oxidase: Biochemistry, distribution and physiology. Acta Physiol Scand Suppl **584**:87, 1986.

Pathak N, Sawhney H, Vasishta K, et al: Estimation of oxidative products of nitric oxide (nitrates, nitrites) in preeclampsia. Aust N Z J Obstet Gynaecol **39**:484, 1999.

Petruccio OM, Thomson NM, Lawrence JR, et al: Immunofluorescein studies in renal biopsies in preeclampsia. Br Med J **1**:473, 1974.

Pipkin FB, Oats JJ, Symonds EM: The effect of a specific AII antagonist (saralasin) on blood pressure in the immediate puerperium. In Bonnar MA, MacGillivray I, Symonds MS (eds): Pregnancy Hypertension. Baltimore, University Park Press, 1980, p. 75.

Pipkin FB, Symonds EM, Turner SR: The effect of captopril (SQ 14,225) upon mother and fetus in the chronically cannulated ewe and in the pregnant rabbit. J Physiol **323**:415, 1982.

Plouin PF, Chatellier G, Breart G, et al: Frequency and perinatal consequences of hypertensive disease of pregnancy. Adv Nephrol **57**:69, 1986.

Pollak VE, Nettles JB: The kidney in toxemia of pregnancy: A clinical and pathologic study based on renal biopsies. Medicine **39**:469, 1960.

Poston L, Chappell LC: Is oxidative stress involved in the aetiology of pre-eclampsia? Acta Paediatr **90**:3, 2001.

Powers RW, Evans RW, Majors AK, et al: Plasma homocysteine concentration is increased in preeclampsia and is associated with evidence of endothelial activation. Am J Obstet Gynecol **179**:1605, 1998.

Pritchard JA: The use of the magnesium ion in the management of eclamptogenic toxemias. Surgery **100**:131, 1955.

Pritchard JA, Cunningham FG, Mason RA: Coagulation changes in eclampsia: Their frequency and pathogenesis. Am J Obstet Gynecol **124**:855, 1976.

Pritchard JA, Pritchard SA: Standardized treatment of 154 consecutive cases of eclampsia. Am J Obstet Gynecol **123**:543, 1975.

Pritchard JA, Stone SR: Clinical and laboratory observations on eclampsia. Am J Obstet Gynecol **99**:754, 1967.

Rajakumar A, Whitelock KA, Weissfeld LA, et al: Selective overexpression of the hypoxia-inducible transcription factor, HIF-2 alpha, in placentas from women with preeclampsia. Biol Reprod **64**:499, 2001.

Ramsey EM, Harris HWS: Comparison of uteroplacental vasculature and circulation in the rhesus monkey and man. Contributions to Embryology. No. 261. Carnegie Institution of Washington **38**:59, 1966.

Rane A, Tomson G: Prenatal and neonatal drug metabolism in man. Eur J Clin Pharmacol **18**:9, 1980.

Ranta V, Viinikka L, Halmesmaki E, et al: Nitric oxide production with preeclampsia. Obstet Gynecol **93**:442, 1999.

Redman CWG: Treatment of hypertension in pregnancy. Kidney Int **18**:267, 1980.

Redman CWG, Beilin LJ, Bonnar J: Treatment of hypertension in pregnancy with methyldopa: Blood pressure control and side effects. Br J Obstet Gynaecol **84**:419, 1977.

Redman CWG, Beilin LJ, Bonnar J, et al: Plasma urate measurements in predicting fetal death in hypertensive pregnancy. Lancet **1**:1370, 1976a.

Redman CWG, Beilin LJ, Bonnar J, et al: Fetal outcome in trial of antihypertensive treatment in pregnancy. Lancet **2**:753, 1976b.

Redman CWG, Bonnar J, Beilin L: Early platelet consumption in preeclampsia. Br Med J **1**:467, 1978.

Redman CWG, Denson KWE, Beilin LJ, et al: Factor-VIII consumption in preeclampsia. Lancet **2**:1249, 1977.

Redman CW, Sacks GP, Sargent IL: Preeclampsia: An excessive maternal inflammatory response to pregnancy. Am J Obstet Gynecol **180**:499, 1999.

Reed RL, Cheney CB, Fearon RE, et al: Propranolol therapy throughout pregnancy: A case report. Anesth Analg Curr Res **53**:214, 1974.

Remuzzi G, Marchesi D, Zoja C, et al: Reduced umbilical and placental vascular prostacyclin in severe preeclampsia. Prostaglandins **20**:105, 1980.

Rey E, Couturier A: The prognosis of pregnancy in women with chronic hypertension. Am J Obstet Gynecol **171**:410, 1994.

Richard DE, Berra E, Pouyssegur J: Nonhypoxic pathway mediates the induction of hypoxia-inducible factor 1 alpha in vascular smooth muscle cells. J Biol Chem **275**:26765, 2000.

Ricke PS, Elliott JP, Freeman RK: Use of corticosteroids in pregnancy-induced hypertension. Obstet Gynecol **55**:206, 1980.

Rippman ET: Pra-eklampsie oder Schwangerschaftsspatgestose? Gynaecologia **167**:478, 1969.

Roach VJ, Hin LY, Tam WH, et al: The incidence of pregnancy-induced hypertension among patients with carbohydrate intolerance. Hypertens Pregnancy **19**:183, 2000.

Roberts JM: Plasma nitrites as an indicator of nitric oxide production: Unchanged production or reduced renal clearance in preeclampsia? [letter]. Am J Obstet Gynecol **176**:954, 1997.

Roberts JM: Endothelial dysfunction in preeclampsia. Semin Reprod Endocrinol **16**:5, 1998.

Roberts JM, Cooper DW: Pathogenesis and genetics of pre-eclampsia. Lancet **357**:53, 2001.

Roberts JM, Hubel CA: Is oxidative stress the link in the two-stage model of pre-eclampsia? [letter; comment]. Lancet **354**:788, 1999.

Roberts JM, May WJ: Consumptive coagulopathy in severe preeclampsia. Obstet Gynecol **48**:163, 1976.

Roberts JM, Perloff DL: Hypertension and the obstetrician-gynecologist. Am J Obstet Gynecol **127**:316, 1977.

Roberts JM, Redman CWG: Pre-eclampsia: More than pregnancy-induced hypertension. Lancet **341**:1447, 1993.

Roberts JM, Taylor RN, Musci TJ, et al: Preeclampsia: An endothelial cell disorder. Am J Obstet Gynecol **161**:1200, 1989.

Robertson WB, Brosens I, Dixon HG: The pathological response of the vessels of the placental bed to hypertensive pregnancy. J Pathol Bacteriol **93**:581, 1967.

Robillard PY, Hulsey TC: Association of pregnancy-induced hypertension pre-eclampsia, and eclampsia with duration of sexual cohabitation before conception. Lancet **347**:619, 1996.

Rodgers GM, Greenberg CS, Shuman MA: Characterization of the effects of cultured vascular cells on the activation of blood coagulation. Blood **61**:1155, 1983.

Roggensack AM, Zhang Y, Davidge ST: Evidence for peroxynitrite formation in the vasculature of women with preeclampsia. Hypertension **33**:83, 1999.

Rosa FW, Bosco LA, Graham CF, et al: Neonatal anuria with maternal angiotensin-converting enzyme inhibition. Obstet Gynecol **74**:371, 1989.

Rosing U, Samsioe G, Olund A, et al: Serum levels of apolipoprotein A-I, A-II, and HDL-cholesterol in second half of normal pregnancy and in pregnancy complicated by pre-eclampsia. Horm Metab Res **21**:376, 1989.

Rubin PC: Beta-blockers in pregnancy. N Engl J Med **305**:1323, 1981.

Sacks GP, Sargent I, Redman C: An innate view of human pregnancy [see comments]. Immunol Today **20**:114, 1999.

Sacks GP, Studena K, Sargent IL, et al: Normal pregnancy and preeclampsia both produce inflammatory changes in peripheral blood leukocytes akin to those of sepsis. Am J Obstet Gynecol **179**:80, 1998.

Sanchez-Ramos L, O'Sullivan MJ, Carrido-Calderon J: Effects of low-dose aspirin on angiotensin II pressor response in human pregnancy. Am J Obstet Gynecol **156**:193, 1987.

Sarles HE, Hill SS, LeBlanc AL, et al: Sodium excretion patterns during and following intravenous sodium chloride loads in normal and hypertensive pregnancies. Am J Obstet Gynecol **102**:1, 1968.

Saruta T, Nakamura R, Nagahama S, et al: Effects of angiotensin II analog on blood pressure, renin and aldosterone in women on oral contraceptives and toxemia. Gynecol Obstet Invest **12**:11, 1981.

Sattar N, Bendomir A, Berry C, et al: Lipoprotein subfraction concentrations in preeclampsia: Pathogenic parallels to atherosclerosis. Obstet Gynecol **89**:403, 1997.

Sattar N, Clark P, Holmes A, et al: Antenatal waist circumference and hypertension risk. Obstet Gynecol **97**:268, 2001.

Schaffer NK, Dill LV, Cadden JF: Uric acid clearance in normal pregnancy and preeclampsia. J Clin Invest **22**:201, 1943.

Schmorl G: Zur pathologischen Anatomie Untersuchung uber Puerperal-Eklampsie. Verhandl Dtsch Gesellsch Gyneakol **9**:303, 1901.

Schobel HP, Grassi G: Hypertensive disorders of pregnancy—A dysregulation of the sympathetic nervous system. J Hypertens **16**:569, 1998.

Schreier PC, Adams JQ, Turner HB, et al: Toxemia of pregnancy as an etiological factor in hypertensive vascular disease. JAMA **159**:105, 1955.

Schwarz R, Retzke U: Cardiovascular response to infusion of angiotensin II in pregnant women. Obstet Gynecol **38**:714, 1971.

Scott JR, Beer AA: Immunologic aspects of pre-eclampsia. Am J Obstet Gynecol **125**:418, 1976.

Scott JS: Pregnancy toxaemia associated with hydrops foetalis, hydatidiform mole and hydramnios. J Obstet Gynaecol Br Emp **65**:689, 1958.

Seitchik J: Renal tubular reabsorption of uric acid: I. Normal pregnancy and abnormal pregnancy. Am J Obstet Gynecol **65**:981, 1953.

Sekiba K, Yoshioka T: Changes of lipid peroxidation and superoxide dismutase activity in the human placenta. Am J Obstet Gynecol **135**:368, 1979.

Seligman SP, Buyon JP, Clance RM, et al: The role of nitric oxide in the pathogenesis of preeclampsia. Am J Obstet Gynecol **171**:944, 1994.

Sheehan HL: Pathologic lesions in the hypertensive toxaemias of pregnancy. In Hammond J, Browne FJ, Wolstenholm GEW (eds): Toxaemias of Pregnancy, Human and Veterinary. Philadelphia, Blakiston, 1950, p. 16.

Sheehan HL, Lynch JB: Pathology of Toxemia in Pregnancy. London, Churchill Livingstone, 1973.

Sheppard BL, Bonnar J: Uteroplacental arteries and hypertensive pregnancy. In Bonnar J, MacGillivray I, Symonds G (eds): Pregnancy Hypertension. Baltimore, University Park, 1980, p. 205.

Shuster E, Weppelman B: Plasma urate measurements and fetal outcome in preeclampsia. Gynecol Obstet Invest **12**:162, 1981.

Sibai BM, Abdella TLN, Anderson GD: Pregnancy outcome in 211 patients with mild chronic hypertension. Obstet Gynecol **61**:571, 1983a.

Sibai BM, Abdella TN, Anderson GD, et al: Plasma volume findings in pregnant women with mild hypertension: Therapeutic considerations. Am J Obstet Gynecol **15**:539, 1983b.

Sibai BM, Caritis SN, Thom E, et al: The National Institute of Child Health and Human Development Network of Maternal-Fetal Medicine Units: Prevention of preeclampsia with low-dose aspirin in healthy, nulliparous pregnant women. N Engl J Med **329**:1213, 1993.

Sibai BM, El-Nazer A, Gonzales-Ruiz A: Severe preeclampsia-eclampsia in young primigravid women: Subsequent pregnancy outcome and remote prognosis. Am J Obstet Gynecol **155**:1011, 1986.

Sibai BM, Gordon T, Thom E, et al: Risk factors for preeclampsia in healthy nulliparous women: A prospective multicenter study. The National Institute of Child Health and Human Development Network of Maternal–Fetal Medicine Units. Am J Obstet Gynecol **172**:642, 1995.

Sibai BM, Grossman RA, Grossman HG: Effects of diuretics on plasma volume in pregnancies with long-term hypertension. Am J Obstet Gynecol **150**:831, 1984.

Sibai BM, Mabie WC, Shamsa F, et al: A comparison of no medication versus methyldopa or labetalol in chronic hypertension during pregnancy. Am J Obstet Gynecol **162**:960, 1990.

Sibai BM, McCubbin JH, Anderson GD, Lipshitz J, Dilts PV: Eclampsia: I. Observation from 67 recent cases. Obstet Gynecol **58**:609, 1981.

Sibai BM, Mercer B, Sarinoglu C: Severe preeclampsia in the second trimester: Recurrent risk and long-term prognosis. Am J Obstet Gynecol **165**:1408, 1991.

Silver RK, Kupferminc MJ, Russell TL, et al: Evaluation of nitric oxide as a mediator of severe preeclampsia. Am J Obstet Gynecol **175**:1013, 1996.

Silverstone A, Trudinger BJ, Lewis PJ, et al: Maternal hypertension and intrauterine fetal death in midpregnancy. Br J Obstet Gynaecol **87**:457, 1980.

Smarason AK, Allman KG, Young D, et al: Elevated levels of serum nitrate, a stable end product of nitric oxide in women with pre-eclampsia. Br J Obstet Gynecol **104**:538, 1997.

Smarason AK, Sargent IL, Starkey PM, et al: The effect of placental syncytiotrophoblast microvillous membranes from normal and pre-eclamptic women on the growth of endothelial cells in vitro. Br J Obstet Gynecol **100**:943, 1993.

Socol ML, Weiner CP, Louis G, et al: Platelet activation in preeclampsia. Am J Obstet Gynecol **151**:494, 1985.

Soffronoff EC, Kaufmann BM, Connaughton JF: Intravascular volume determinations and fetal outcome in hypertensive diseases of pregnancy. Am J Obstet Gynecol **127**:4, 1977.

Sohda S, Arinami T, Hamada H, et al: Methylenetetrahydrofolate reductase polymorphism and pre-eclampsia. J Med Genet **34**:525, 1997.

Sokabe H: Phylogeny of the renal effects of angiotensin. Kidney Int **6**:263, 1974.

Spargo BH, Lichtig C, Luger AM, et al: The renal lesion in preeclampsia: Examination by light-, electron- and immunofluorescence-microscopy. In Lindheimer MD, Katz AI, Zuspan FP (eds): Hypertension in Pregnancy. New York, John Wiley and Sons, 1976, p. 453.

Spargo BH, McCartney CP, Winemiller R: Glomerular capillary endotheliosis in toxemia of pregnancy. AMA Arch Pathol **68**:593, 1959.

Spetz S: Peripheral circulation in pregnancy complicated by toxaemia. Acta Obstet Gynecol Scand **44**:243, 1965.

Stallworth JC, Yeh SY, Petrie RH: The effect of magnesium sulfate on fetal heart rate variability and uterine activity. Am J Obstet Gynecol **140**:702, 1981.

Stander HJ, Cadden JF: Blood chemistry in preeclampsia and eclampsia. Am J Obstet Gynecol **28**:856, 1934.

Steele TW, Györy AZ, Edwards KDG: Renal function in analgesic nephropathy. Br Med J **2**:231, 1969.

Stevenson AC, Davison BCC, Say B, et al: Contribution of fetal/maternal incompatibility to aetiology of preeclamptic toxaemia. Lancet **2**:1286, 1971.

Stirrat GM, Redman CWG, Levinsky RJ: Circulating immune complexes in pre-eclampsia. Br Med J **1**:1450, 1978.

Stone J, Lockwood C, Berkowitz G, et al: Risk factors for severe preeclampsia. Obstet Gynecol **83**:357, 1994.

Studd J: Pre-eclampsia. Br J Hosp Med **18**:52, 1977.

Suki WN, Hull AR, Rector FC Jr, et al: Mechanism of the effect of thiazide diuretics on calcium and uric acid. J Clin Invest **46**:1121, 1967.

Sullivan JM, Palmer EI, Schoeneberger AA, et al: SQ 20,811: Effect on eclamptic-preeclamptic women with postpartum hypertension. Am J Obstet Gynecol **131**:707, 1978.

Sutherland A, Cooper DW, Howie PW, et al: The incidence of severe preeclampsia amongst mothers and mothers-in-law of preeclamptics and controls. Br J Obstet Gynaecol **88**:785, 1981.

Talledo OE, Chesley LC, Zuspan FP: Renin-angiotensin system in normal and toxemic pregnancies: III. Differential sensitivity to angiotensin II and norepinephrine in toxemia of pregnancy. Am J Obstet Gynecol **100**:218, 1968.

Tapia HR, Johnson CE, Strong CG: Renin-angiotensin system in normal and in hypertensive disease of pregnancy. Lancet **2**:847, 1972.

Taylor RN, Crombleholme WR, Friedman SA, et al: High plasma cellular fibronectin levels correlate with biochemical and clinical features of preeclampsia but cannot be attributed to hypertension alone. Am J Obstet Gynecol **165**:895, 1991.

Taylor RN, Heilbron DC, Roberts JM: Growth factor activity in the blood of women in whom preeclampsia develops is elevated from early pregnancy. Am J Obstet Gynecol **163**:1839, 1990.

Taylor RN, Varma M, Teng NNH, et al: Women with preeclampsia have higher plasma endothelin levels than women with normal pregnancies. J Clin Endocrinol Metab **71**:1675, 1990.

Tervila L, Goecke C, Timonen S: Estimation of gestosis of pregnancy (EPH-gestosis). Acta Obstet Gynecol Scand **52**:235, 1973.

Thomson AM, Hytten FE, Billewicz WZ: The epidemiology of oedema during pregnancy. J Obstet Gynaecol Br Commonw **74**:1, 1967.

Thomson D, Paterson WG, Smart GE, et al: The renal lesions of toxemia and abruptio placentae studies by light and electron microscopy. J Obstet Gynaecol Br Commonw **79**:311, 1972.

Tompkins MJ, Thiagarajah S: HELLP (hemolysis, elevated liver enzymes, and low platelet count) syndrome: The benefit of corticosteroids. Am J Obstet Gynecol **181**:304, 1999.

Trupin LS, Simon LP, Eskenazi B: Change in paternity: A risk factor for preeclampsia in multiparas. Epidemiology **7**:240, 1996.

Vara P, Timonen S, Lokki O: Toxaemia of late pregnancy: A statistical study. Acta Obstet Gynecol Scand **44**(S):3, 1965.

Vartran CK: Hypertension in pregnancy: A new look. Proc R Soc Med **59**:841, 1966.

Vassali P, Morris RH, McCluskey RI: The pathogenic role of fibrin deposition in the glomerular lesions of toxemia of pregnancy. J Exp Med **118**:467, 1963.

Vollman RF: Rates of toxemia by age and parity. *In* Die Spat gestose (E and H-Gestose). Basel, Schwabe, 1970, p. 338.

Waisman GD, Mayorga LM, Camera MI, et al: Magnesium plus nifedipine: Potentiation of hypotensive effect in preeclampsia? Am J Obstet Gynecol **159**:308, 1988.

Wallenburg HCS: Hemodynamics in hypertensive pregnancy. *In* Rubin PC (ed): Hypertension in Pregnancy (Handbook of Hypertension, Vol 10). Amsterdam, Elsevier, 1988, p. 66.

Wallukat G, Homuth V, Fischer T, et al: Patients with preeclampsia develop agonistic autoantibodies against the angiotensin AT1 receptor. J Clin Invest **103**:945, 1999.

Ward K, Hata A, Jeunemaitre X, et al: A molecular variant of angiotensinogen associated with preeclampsia. Nat Genet **4**:59, 1993.

Weiner CP, Brandt J: Plasma antithrombin III activity: An aid in the diagnosis of preeclampsia-eclampsia. Am J Obstet Gynecol **142**:275, 1982.

Weinstein L: Syndrome of hemolysis, elevated liver enzymes, and low platelet count: A severe consequence of hypertension in pregnancy. Am J Obstet Gynecol **142**:159, 1982.

Weir RJ, Paintin DB, Brown JJ, et al: A serial study in pregnancy of the plasma concentrations of renin, corticosteroids, electrolytes and proteins; and haemotocrit and plasma volume. J Obstet Gynecol Br Commonw **78**:590, 1971.

Weseley AC, Douglas GW: Continuous use of chlorothiazide for prevention of toxemias of pregnancy. Obstet Gynecol **19**:355, 1962.

Whigham KAE, Howie PW, Shah MM, Prentice CRM: Factor VIII related antigen/coagulant activity ratio as a predictor of fetal growth retardation: A comparison with hormone and uric acid measurements. Br J Obstet Gynaecol **87**:797, 1980.

Wiggins RC, Loskutoff DJ, Cochrane CG, et al: Activation of rabbit Hageman factor by homogenates of cultured rabbit endothelial cells. J Clin Invest **65**:197, 1980.

Williams DJ, Vallance PJ, Neild GH, et al: Nitric oxide–mediated vasodilation in human pregnancy. Am J Phys **272**:H748, 1997.

Wilton AM, Kaye JA, Guo G, et al: Is angiotensinogen a good candidate gene for preeclampsia? Hypertens Pregnancy **14**:251, 1995.

Witztum J: The oxidation hypothesis of atherosclerosis. Lancet **344**:793, 1994.

Wolf G.: Free radical production and angiotensin. Current Hypertens Rep **2**:167, 2000.

Yalcin OT, Sener T, Hassa H, et al: Effects of postpartum corticosteroids in patients with HELLP syndrome. Int J Gynecol Obstet **61**:141, 1998.

Yu TF, Sirota JH, Berger L, et al: Effect of sodium lactate infusion on urate clearance in man. Proc Soc Exp Biol (NY) **96**:809, 1957.

Zangmeister W: Untersuchungen uber die Blutbeschaffenheit und die Harnsekretion bei Eklampsie. Z Geburtschilfe Gynaekol **50**:385, 1903.

Zeek PM, Assali NS: Vascular changes in the decidua associated with eclamptogenic toxemia. Am J Clin Pathol **20**:1099, 1950.

Zhang J, Klebanoff MA, Roberts JM: Prediction of adverse outcomes by common definitions of hypertension in pregnancy. Obstet Gynecol **97**:261, 2001.

Zhou Y, Damsky CH, Chiu K, et al: Cytotrophoblast expression of integrin extracellular matrix receptors is altered in preeclampsia. *In* Soares M, Handwerger S, Talamantes F (eds): Trophoblast Cells: Pathways for Maternal-Embryonic Communication. New York, Springer-Verlag, 1993, p. 109.

Zhou Y, Damsky CH, Fisher SJ: Preeclampsia is associated with failure of human cytotrophoblasts to mimic a vascular adhesion phenotype—One cause of defective endovascular invasion in this syndrome? J Clin Invest **99**:2152, 1997.

Zhou Y, Fisher SJ, Janatpour M, et al: Human cytotrophoblasts adopt a vascular phenotype as they differentiate: Strategy for successful endovascular invasion? (see comments). J Clin Invest **99**:2139, 1997.

Zuspan FP: Problems encountered in the treatment of pregnancy-induced hypertension. Am J Obstet Gynecol **131**:591, 1978.

Zuspan FP, Nelson GH, Ahlquist RP: Epinephrine infusions in normal and toxemic pregnancy: I. Nonesterified fatty acids and cardiovascular alterations. Am J Obstet Gynecol **90**:88, 1964.

Zuspan FP, Talledo E, Rhodes K: Factors affecting delivery in eclampsia. Am J Obstet Gynecol **100**:672, 1968.

Zusterzeel PL, Rutten H, Roelofs HM, et al: Protein carbonyls in decidua and placenta of pre-eclamptic women as markers for oxidative stress. Placenta **22**:213, 2001.

Chapter 44

RENAL DISORDERS

John M. Davison, MD, and Marshall D. Lindheimer, MD

Among the physiologic alterations that occur in normal pregnancy, few are as striking as those affecting the urinary system. These changes and various diagnostic pitfalls for the unwary clinician have already been discussed in Chapter 8. Improvements in our knowledge of background physiology, in prenatal care, in technology for fetal surveillance, and in neonatal intensive care have meant improved outcomes for women with renal problems and their newborns.

This chapter describes the natural history of pregnant women with renal disorders, focusing on urinary tract infection (UTI), chronic renal disease, and acute renal failure. Especially updated since the last edition is progress in the management of pregnancy in patients with a kidney allograft and those undergoing dialysis.

INFECTION OF THE URINARY TRACT

Definitions and Pathogenesis

Urinalysis during pregnancy is more likely to be contaminated with bacteria originating from the urethra, vagina, or perineum. This problem can be overcome by suprapubic aspiration of bladder urine, but the rather inconvenient procedure is distasteful to many patients and obstetricians. A more practical approach is to obtain a fresh mid-stream urine specimen. Nurse-supervised multiple vulvar washings give reproducible cultures more than 95% of the time. With the suprapubic technique, all growth is significant; with mid-stream urine specimens, true bacteriuria is traditionally defined as the presence of more than 100,000 bacteria/mL of urine of the same species in two consecutive mid-stream specimens. Some investigators suggest that lower colony counts may still represent active infection (Stamm et al., 1991). A number of presumptive tests based on changes in chemical indicators exist, but these are not considered reliable (Bachman et al., 1993; Shelton et al., 2001).

Asymptomatic or covert bacteriuria designates true bacteriuria in the absence of symptoms or signs of acute urinary infection. When there is symptomatic UTI, two clinical syndromes are recognized: lower UTI or cystitis and upper UTI or acute pyelonephritis. It must be remembered, however, that pregnant women often complain of or admit to frequency of micturition, dysuria, urgency, and nocturia, singly or in combination, and such symptoms are not in themselves diagnostic of UTI.

Bacteria probably originate from the large bowel and colonize the urinary tract transperineally. By far, the most common infecting organism is *Escherichia coli*, which is responsible for 75% to 90% of bacteriuria during pregnancy. The pathogenic virulence of this organism, which is not the most plentiful in feces, appears to involve a number of factors, including resistance to vaginal acidity, rapid division in urine, the presence of Dr operons coding for Dr adhesions (Goluszko et al., 2001), allowing adherence to uroepithelial cells, and production of chemicals that decrease ureteric peristalsis and inhibit phagocytosis. Other organisms frequently responsible for UTI include *Klebsiella*, *Proteus*, and *Pseudomonas* spp. and coagulase-negative staphylococci.

The stasis associated with ureteropelvic dilatation and partial ureteric obstruction (see Chapter 8), increased nutrient content of the urine, and the presence of potential pathogens are characteristic of most pregnant women, yet bacteriuria develops in only a few. Susceptible women may differ immunologically from those who resist infection; they are less likely to express antibody to the O antigen of *E. coli* on the vaginal epithelium and may display less effective leukocyte activity against the organism.

Finally, urinary sediments may be misleading in pregnancy. Although urine replete with white blood cells, casts, and bacteria is informative, cultures have been positive when fewer than five white blood cells were present in the sediment.

Asymptomatic Bacteriuria

Covert bacteriuria is a heterogeneous entity. Several methods have been used to try to differentiate between upper and lower urinary tract bacteriuria (e.g., ureteral catheterization, bladder washout tests, urinary concentration tests, serum antibody tests, and even renal biopsy). Biopsy and ureteral catheterization are too invasive for clinical practice, and the remainder are insufficiently precise to confidently localize infection.

The reservoir of young women with covert bacteriuria acquired during childhood is about 5%, but only 1.2% are infected at any one time (McGladdery et al., 1992). The incidence increases after puberty and is approximately equal in both the pregnant and nonpregnant populations (2% to 10%) but is two to three times more common in gravidas with diabetes mellitus or a renal transplant. The 16th gestational week is the optimal time for a single screening for bacteriuria.

During pregnancy, approximately 40% of those infected, if untreated, develop acute symptomatic UTI. Thus, treating patients with covert bacteriuria should prevent as much as 70% of all potential cases of symptomatic UTI infection in pregnancy (Pedler and Orr, 2000). However, acute infection develops in about 1.5% of women with initial negative cultures, and this accounts for the remaining 30% to 40% of acute symptomatic UTI in pregnancy.

Asymptomatic and untreated bacteriuria has been alleged to be associated with several complications of pregnancy, such as low birth weight, intrauterine death, preeclampsia, and maternal anemia. Several of these apparent correlations may have resulted from inaccuracies in matching case subjects and control subjects. There is also a view that underlying chronic pyelonephritis in some of the cases may be responsible for the reported increased incidences of preeclampsia, prematurity, and fetal loss (Graham et al., 2001). Furthermore, when evidence of previous damage is present, there may be a greater propensity to hypertension (McGladdery et al., 1992).

Not all untreated bacteriuric women develop symptoms of acute UTI during pregnancy; by the same token, women who have sterile urine when screened antenatally contribute substantially to the pool of those who eventually develop symptomatic infection. It has therefore been argued that screening programs are not cost effective (Pedler and Orr, 2000). Interestingly, it has been suggested that it is the women with a history of previous UTI as well as current bacteriuria who are 10 times more likely to develop symptoms during pregnancy. Women with renal scarring and persistent reflux constitute another group where acute pyelonephritis is more likely to develop (Martinelli et al., 1990).

Management in Pregnancy

Most obstetricians treat asymptomatic bacteriuria despite the screening controversy, an approach we favor. The agent chosen not only must be effective against the organism identified but also must be acceptable for use during pregnancy. The *Physicians' Desk Reference* now lists pregnancy risk factors for all medications (see also Chapters 19 and 39 and tables in Pedler and Orr, 2000).

Ampicillin and the cephalosporins are commonly prescribed, but short-acting sulfonamides may be equally effective. Sulfonamides should be avoided during the last few weeks of pregnancy, however, because they competitively inhibit the binding of bilirubin to albumin and may increase the risk of neonatal hyperbilirubinemia. Nitrofurantoin, with its common side effect of nausea, may not be readily tolerated in pregnancy. Furthermore, it should be avoided during late pregnancy because of the risk of hemolysis resulting from deficiency of erythrocyte phosphate dehydrogenase in the newborn. The tetracyclines are contraindicated during pregnancy because of problems of dental staining in the child.

A 2-week course of therapy is usually adequate (Pedler and Orr, 2000). Recurrent infections are noted in about 30% of bacteriuric women; after a second course about 15% continue to have positive urinary cultures. Recurrence may be caused by relapse, when the same organism is found within 6 weeks of the initial infection, or by reinfection, when a different organism is detected more than 6 weeks after treatment. Persistent infections may merit continuous treatment to the time of delivery. Finally, there is still controversy regarding very short (especially single high-dose) courses in pregnancy (Wing et al., 1999).

Long-Term Prognosis

In the longer term, there is little evidence that treatment during pregnancy affects the subsequent prevalence of bacteriuria (Dempsey et al., 1992) or that persistent bacteriuria in women with a normal urinary tract contributes to the development of chronic renal disease. About 20% of bacteriuric women have some abnormality of the urinary tract, but in most cases the abnormality is minor and not clearly related to the disease. Postpartum evaluation, such as intravenous urography or renal ultrasound, is probably therefore best reserved for bacteriuric women with a history of acute symptomatic infections before or during pregnancy and the puerperium and those in whom bacteriuria is difficult to eradicate.

Acute Cystitis

Acute cystitis occurs in about 1% of pregnant women, of whom 60% have a negative initial screening. The symptoms are often difficult to distinguish from those resulting from pregnancy itself. Features indicating a true infection include hematuria, dysuria, and suprapubic discomfort as well as a positive urine culture. The bacteriology is the same as in women with covert bacteriuria (Pedler and Orr, 2000). Similar treatment is recommended, with the aims of abolishing symptoms and preventing occurrence of acute pyelonephritis.

Acute Pyelonephritis

Acute pyelonephritis is the most common urinary tract complication of pregnancy, occurring in approximately 2% of all pregnancies (Gilstrap and Ramin, 2001). Its presentation in pregnant women is similar to that in nonpregnant women, with fever, flank pain, nausea, and vomiting with or without frequency, urgency, and dysuria. Clinical assessment usually confirms the presence of pyrexia and flank tenderness on the affected side. Causative organisms are similar to those in the general population, with P-fimbriated *E. coli* representing approximately 75%. At least 25% of patients experience a transient decrease in glomerular filtration rate (GFR) and a rise in blood creatinine. Ultrasonographic examination of the renal tract in gravidas with pyelonephritis has revealed significantly increased pelvicaliceal dilatation compared with normal physiologic dilatation during pregnancy, but because treatment did not produce a consistent decrease, their anomaly may antedate the acute infection (Twickler et al., 1994).

Acute pyelonephritis may or may not play a role in the etiology of hypertension and intrauterine deaths, but upper tract infections certainly may mimic or precipitate preterm labor. Bacteremia occurs in approximately 10% to 20% of all cases. Pregnant women are more vulnerable to endotoxins (lipopolysaccharide) than nonpregnant women, which is one reason they tolerate acute pyelonephritis poorly. Septic shock (on occasion in association with instrumentation of the infected urinary tract), adult respiratory distress syndrome, or anemia may develop, all probably a result of lipopolysaccharide-induced cell membrane damage (Cox et al., 1991). In such cases, prompt recognition and appropriate respiratory support may be necessary to prevent severe hypoxemia that may result in fetal death.

Management in Pregnancy

Treatment of acute pyelonephritis requires early hospitalization and adequate intravenous hydration (see Chapter 39, Tables 39-1 and 39-2). After appropriate specimens for culture are obtained, broad-spectrum intravenous antibiotics should be started, although advocates for once-a-day therapy (Sanchez-Ramos et al., 1995) are beginning to appear. More data on the latter approach are needed, cautioning that the *raison d'être* of most "long-acting" drugs is decreased renal excretion. Antibiotic therapy should be adjusted to organism sensitivities when known (Pedler and Orr, 2000). Most patients treated appropriately respond clinically within 48 hours. Lack of clinical improvement by 72 hours suggests inadequate or improper antibiotic use, an underlying anatomic urinary tract problem (e.g., obstruction by stone), and a need to reconsider the diagnosis (Hart et al., 2001). The overall recurrence rate is around 20%.

After resolution of an episode of acute pyelonephritis, the patient should be treated for at least 3 weeks and then followed with frequent urine cultures. Continuous antimicrobial suppression with close follow-up until term may be used in the noncompliant patient or when an underlying urinary tract abnormality is present or suspected, if assessment of this can be safely postponed until the puerperium.

It should not be forgotten that there is an association between UTI and postperinatal adverse outcomes. The difficulty of performing controlled studies in humans has promoted the development of animal models. In a murine model of urinary infection there was invariably evidence of metritis, which is important in terms of uterine activity because until now this was thought to be associated with systemically mediated "toxic" mechanisms (Mussalli et al., 2000).

Urinary infections in pregnancy may also influence cognitive development in the offspring. In a recent cohort study, 41,090 Medicaid-linked maternal and infant records were analyzed together with collected and noncollected prescriptions. In the 23% of gravidas without antibiotics there was a significant association between maternal urinary infection and mental retardation in childhood. Furthermore, the fetal death rate was 5.2% compared with no deaths in the group whose antibiotics were taken (McDermott et al., 2000).

Differential Diagnosis

Hematuria during Pregnancy

Spontaneous gross or microscopic hematuria can have a variety of causes. If associated with congenital anomalies, UTI can be difficult to eradicate and may predispose to hematuria. Rupture of small veins around the dilated renal pelvis may also cause bleeding; indeed, such hematuria may recur in subsequent pregnancies. Rarely, hematuria may be secondary to complications such as acute glomerulonephritis, calculi, neoplasm, hemangiomas, and fungal diseases. Endometriosis, inflammatory bowel lesions, leukoplakia, and granulomas may involve the urinary tract and may also produce hematuria. A bleeding ureteral stump after a nephrectomy (for either benign or malignant disease) can also occur.

Ultrasound and magnetic resonance imaging can be used in pregnancy, occasionally combined with a single abdominal radiograph. Until recently the general consensus was that in the absence of any demonstrable cause, hematuria could be designated idiopathic, with recurrences unlikely in subsequent pregnancy. It has been suggested, however, that hematuria is associated with an increased likelihood of adverse maternal outcomes, including preterm labor and preeclampsia (Stehman-Breen et al., 2000). From a retrospective case-controlled study, such gravidas had an eightfold increased risk of preeclampsia and the mean duration from dipstick detection of hematuria to diagnosis was about 11 weeks.

Acute Hydronephrosis and Hydroureter

There is an entity labeled "overdistention syndrome" that is not to be confused with the substantial ureteric and renal pelvic dilatation (and slight reduction in cortical width) that can occasionally occur in normal pregnancy without ill effect (Brown, 1990). With the overdistention syndrome, dilatation may be massive and there are definite symptoms; some women have transient mild flank pain, whereas others have recurrent episodes of severe flank or lower abdominal pain radiating to the groin (Fig. 44-1). There are also functional abnormalities characterized by increments in serum creatinine levels and occasionally hypertension (Satin et al., 1993), but urinalysis

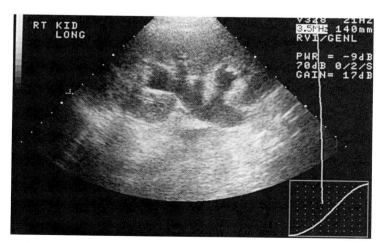

FIGURE 44-1 ■ Renal sonogram showing a grossly dilated right-sided pelvic caliceal system. Original diagnosis was acute right-sided pyelonephritis, which was unresponsive to antibiotics, with worsening loin pain radiating into the groin. Cystoscopy and ureteral stent immediately resolved the situation. The stent was removed 4 weeks after normal delivery with no residual urinary tract problems.

contains few or no red blood cells and repeated mid-stream specimens are sterile. Women who have had surgery for vesicoureteric reflux in childhood (especially bilaterally) can develop distal ureteral obstruction even in early gestation, which can masquerade as preeclampsia and/or severe renal insufficiency (Thorp et al., 1999).

The variations in symptoms with changes in posture and position are hallmarks of this condition. The diagnosis can be confirmed by limited excretory urography or sonar scanning (Delakas et al., 2000). Positioning of the patient in lateral recumbency or the knee–chest position often gives relief. If this fails, placement of ureteral stents or sonographically guided percutaneous nephrostomy may be necessary, so that surgery is delayed until the postpartum period (Fainaru et al., 2002).

Nontraumatic Rupture of the Urinary Tract

The intrusion of unremitting pain and hematuria upon the course of pyelonephritis or the overdistention syndrome suggests rupture of the urinary tract. Furthermore, this complication can masquerade as other obstetric and surgical abdominal catastrophes, including appendicitis, pelvic abscess, cholecystitis, stone disease (see later), and abruptio placentae. Prompt recognition may prevent extension or expansion or both of a small tear and urine leak, treatable by postural or tube drainage (Nielson and Rasmussen, 1998). Rupture of the renal parenchyma, with hemorrhagic shock, formation of a flank mass, or dissection of urinary tract contents intraperitoneally, compels prompt surgical intervention, usually with nephrectomy.

CHRONIC RENAL DISEASE

The majority view is that, with the exception of certain specific disease entities such as systemic lupus erythematosus (SLE), renal polyarteritis nodosa, and scleroderma, obstetric outcome is usually successful, provided renal function is at most moderately compromised and hypertension is absent or minimal, both before conception. Furthermore, pregnancy does not appear to adversely affect the natural history of the renal disease. There are also entities about which controversy exists, such as immunoglobulin (Ig) A nephropathy, membranoproliferative glomerulonephritis, focal glomerular sclerosis, and reflux nephropathy, but it is generally agreed that for all pathologies that as functional loss progresses, especially when hypertension is also present, risk to both mother and fetus increases substantially (Lindheimer et al., 2001).

Renal Function and Obstetric Considerations

Normal Pregnancy and Renal Assessment

The GFR, measured as 24-hour creatinine clearance, increases shortly after conception. Serum levels of creatinine and urea N, which average 70 µmol/liter (0.8 mg/dL) and 5 mmol/liter (13 mg/dL), respectively, in nonpregnant women, decrease to mean values of 50 µmol/liter (0.6 mg/dL) and 3 mmol/liter (9 mg/dL) in pregnant women. Near term, a 15% to 20% decrement in GFR occurs, which affects serum creatinine levels minimally (Milne et al., 2002).

Values of creatinine of 80 µmol/liter (0.9 mg/dL) and urea N of 6 mmol/liter (14 mg/dL), which are acceptable in nonpregnant subjects, are suspect in pregnancy. However, one should use caution in assessing renal function by serum creatinine levels alone, especially when some decrease in GFR has accrued. This is because creatinine is both filtered and secreted by the kidney, the ratio of creatinine-to-inulin clearance normally falling between 1.1 and 1.2. As renal disease progresses, a greater portion of urinary creatinine is formed as a result of secretion (clearance ratios rising to 1.4 to 1.6 when serum creatinine is 1.4). Therefore, the GFR may be considerably overestimated.

Formulas that use serum creatinine in relation to age, height, and weight to calculate GFR (e.g., the Crockroft-Gault formula) are best not used in pregnancy because of changing body weight. Ideally, evaluation of renal function in pregnancy should be based on the clearance of creatinine rather than its serum concentration. Creatinine levels may increase by up to 17 µmol/liter (0.15 mg/dL) shortly after ingestion of cooked meat (because cooking converts preformed creatine into creatinine), and the timing of the blood sample during a clearance period must take into account meals and their content.

Renal Dysfunction and Preconception Counseling

Conceiving and sustaining pregnancy are basically related to the degree of functional impairment. Fertility is diminished as renal function falls. When preconception serum creatinine exceeds 280 µmol/liter (3 mg/liter), corresponding to GFR less than 25 mL/min, normal pregnancy is unusual; however, such women do conceive and require appropriate preconception counseling. One should also note that successful outcomes have been documented in women with moderate to severe disease who conceived, including patients receiving dialysis, either from end-stage renal disease or for accelerated maternal renal deterioration (Abe, 1996; Jungers and Chauveau, 1997). These problems are discussed further later.

Ideally, pregnancy is probably best restricted to women with preconception serum creatinine levels below 180 µmol/liter (2 mg/dL) and diastolic blood pressure of 90 mm Hg or less. Some physicians extend this limit to 250 µmol/liter (2.8 mg/dL), and others believe it should be no higher than 140 µmol/liter (1.5 mg/dL); *we tend to favor the lower number* (Lindheimer et al., 2001). Whatever level is used, one should recognize that degrees of impairment not causing symptoms or disrupting homeostasis in nonpregnant individuals certainly can jeopardize pregnancy (Parmar, 2002). Additionally, if hypertension requires more than one medication for control, then prognosis becomes poorer (Jungers and Chauveau, 1997).

The question has to be asked: Is pregnancy advisable? If a woman with chronic renal disease wishes to have a family, the sooner she starts the better. In some of these patients, renal function continues to decline with time. Women are not always counseled before conception. A patient with suspected or known renal disease may present already pregnant, and the question then becomes whether to continue the pregnancy.

Renal Dysfunction and Impact of Pregnancy

Obstetric and remote prognoses differ in relation to the various degrees of renal insufficiency. The potential impact of pregnancy is best considered by categories of functional renal

TABLE 44-1. CATEGORIES OF PREPREGNANCY
FUNCTIONAL RENAL STATUS

Category	Serum Creatinine (μmol/liter [mg/dL])
Preserved/mildly impaired renal function	≤125 (≤1.4)
Moderate renal insufficiency	125–250 (1.4–2.8)
Severe renal insufficiency	>250 (>2.8)

status before conception. Based on the literature, weighted to that occurring during the last decade, we give advice for three functional categories (Tables 44-1 to 44-3).

PRESERVED OR MILDLY IMPAIRED RENAL FUNCTION AND MINIMAL HYPERTENSION

Women with chronic renal disease but with normal or only mildly decreased renal function at conception (serum creatinine less than 125 μmol/liter [1.4 mg/dL]) usually have a successful obstetric outcome, and pregnancy does not appear to adversely affect the course of their disease (Jungers and Chauveau, 1997; Lindheimer and Katz, 1999; Lindheimer et al., 2001). Although this holds true for most patients, there are exceptions. Most authors strongly advise against pregnancy in women with scleroderma and periarteritis nodosa. Others express reservations when the underlying renal disorder is lupus nephropathy, membranoproliferative glomerulonephritis, and perhaps IgA and reflux nephropathies.

Most women whose prepregnancy creatinine is no more than 1.4 mg/dL (no more than 125 μmol/liter) manifest increments in GFR but less than those of normal pregnant women. Increased proteinuria is common, occurring in 50% of pregnancies (although this is unusual in women with chronic pyelonephritis) and exceeding the nephrotic range (3 g in 24 hours) in 50% of gravidas. Perinatal outcome is said to be jeopardized by the presence of uncontrolled hypertension and for some when nephrotic range proteinuria is already present in early pregnancy (Jungers and Chauveau, 1997). In one study where creatinine clearances were available, a value below 70 ml/min before conception was associated with poorer outcomes, even when serum levels were in the "minimal dysfunction" range (Abe, 1996). Finally, gestation does not appear to influence the natural history of the renal disease when preconception renal function is only minimally impaired.

MODERATELY AND SEVERELY IMPAIRED RENAL FUNCTION

Prognosis is more guarded when renal function is moderately impaired (serum creatinine 125 to 250 μmol/liter [1.4 to 2.5 mg/dL]) before pregnancy and is very definitely affected with severe renal dysfunction (serum creatinine more than 250 μmol/liter [2.8 mg/dL]). These women do, however, become pregnant. Before 1996, there were few reports, all of limited size, in these women. Of particular interest is a study that assessed maternal and fetal outcomes of 82 pregnancies in 62 women (Jones and Hayslett, 1996), all of whom had serum creatinine levels exceeding 125 μmol/liter (1.4 mg/dL). The incidence of hypertension increased from 28% at the baseline to 48% by the third trimester, and the presence of significant proteinuria (urinary protein excretion more than 3 g in

24 hours) increased from 23% to 41%. Forty-three percent of the pregnancies were associated with a deterioration in renal function, at times rapid and substantial, and in 10% of these instances the deterioration did not reverse postpartum. Although the infant survival rate was high (93%), rates of premature delivery (59%) and growth restriction (37%) underscored the very high potential for obstetric complications in these women (Table 44-4).

The results reported by Jones and Hayslett actually confirm the previous reports of limited size in which one third to one half of gravidas with moderate to severe renal insufficiency experienced functional loss more rapidly than would have been expected from the natural course of their renal disease (Cunningham et al., 1990). A surprising observation from Jones and Hayslett was that good blood pressure control did not guarantee the preservation of maternal renal function, data that require confirmation.

Another study (Jungers et al., 1997) remained optimistic. Awareness of progress in obstetric and neonatal care means that more women with impaired renal function will contemplate pregnancy and anticipate a good obstetric outcome. It is suggested that this view holds as long as the serum creatinine level is below 200 μmol/liter (less than 2.3 mg/dL). Once creatinine levels exceed 250 μmol/liter (2.8 mg/dL), however, there is a substantial risk of both an unsuccessful fetal outcome and accelerated loss of maternal renal function (see Table 44-4). Also, we lack reliable and convincing data allowing prediction of which women will experience a rapid loss of renal function, and when function starts to decrease, terminating the pregnancy does not necessarily reverse the decline.

These messages from the 1980s and 1990s continue to be reiterated. A recent single-center experience (Bar et al., 2000) documented short- and long-term outcomes in 38 patients in 46 pregnancies. Successful outcome was defined as a live healthy infant without handicap by 2 years of age. This was the case in 96% of pregnancies from gravidas with diabetic nephropathy and 89% from those with transplants. Again, poorly controlled preexisting hypertension was the harbinger of poor outcome. The influences of serum creatinine and of proteinuria were more variable, but in general, a worse outcome and poorer renal prognosis occurred in those with the moderate and severe renal dysfunction.

Dialysis has also been instituted prophylactically during pregnancy to increase the chances of successful outcome

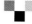

TABLE 44-2. PREGNANCY AND RENAL DISEASE: FUNCTIONAL RENAL STATUS AND PROSPECTS*

| Prospects | Category† | | |
	Mild	Moderate	Severe
Pregnancy	26%	47%	86%
Successful obstetric outcome	96% (85)‡	90% (59)	51% (19)
Long-term sequelae	<3% (9)	25% (71)	53% (92)

* Estimates are based on data from 2370 women in 3495 pregnancies (1973–1995) and do not include collagen diseases (see Davison and Baylis, 1998).
† See Table 49-1.
‡ Numbers in parentheses denote prognosis (%) when complications developed before 28 weeks' gestation.

TABLE 44-3. RENAL DISEASE AND PREGNANCY: IMPROVEMENTS IN PERINATAL OUTCOMES (%) OVER SIX DECADES*

Renal Disease	Pregnancy Outcome	1950s	1960s	1970s	1980s	1990s	2000s
Mild	Preterm delivery	8%	10%	19%	25%	25%	25%
	Perinatal mortality	18%	15%	7%	<5%	<3%	<2%
Moderate	Preterm delivery	15%	21%	40%	52%	57%	60%
	Perinatal mortality	58%	45%	23%	12%	10%	9%
Severe	Preterm delivery	~100%	~100%	~100%	~100%	~100%	~100%
	Perinatal mortality	100%	91%	58%	53%	50%	35%

* Estimates are based on data from 3090 women in 5370 pregnancies (from 1954 to 2001). Collagen diseases are excluded.

(Bagon et al., 1998; Chan et al., 1998; Okundaye et al., 1998). Obviously, "buying time" for fetal maturation in this way is independent of the inexorable further declines in renal function ultimately to end-stage failure. Nevertheless, extreme prematurity and/or disturbing life-threatening maternal problems are still commonplace, and we believe that such additional health risks for these gravidas should not be taken. The aim should be to preserve what little renal function remains and to achieve renal rehabilitation via dialysis and transplantation, after which the question of pregnancy can be considered if appropriate. Some women, however, will be prepared to take a chance and even seek assisted conception in the face of their infertility. This obsessional pursuit of pregnancy and the issues surrounding the clinician's obligation to accede to (or refute) care that poses a risk to the woman's health are discussed in detail elsewhere (Stotland and Stotland, 1997).

Finally, and of utmost importance to this discussion, the literature that forms the basis of our views is primarily *retrospective*. Most patients described had only mild dysfunction, women with greater dysfunctional disease being limited in number. Thus, confirmation of our guidelines requires adequate prospective observational trials.

Antenatal Strategy and Decision-Making

Patients should be seen at least biweekly until 32 weeks' gestation, after which assessment should be weekly. Routine serial antenatal observations should be supplemented with the following:

1. Evaluation of renal function preferably by 24-hour creatinine clearance and protein excretion on approximately a monthly basis
2. Careful monitoring of blood pressure for early detection of hypertension and then assessment of its severity
3. Early detection of superimposed preeclampsia (after mid-trimester)

4. Biophysical assessment of fetal size, development, and well-being
5. Early detection of asymptomatic bacteriuria or confirmation of UTI

Renal Function

If renal function deteriorates, reversible causes should be sought, such as UTI, subtle dehydration, or electrolyte imbalance, occasionally precipitated by inadvertent diuretic therapy. Near term, a 15% to 20% decrement in function, which affects serum creatinine levels minimally, is permissible. Failure to detect a reversible cause of a significant decrement is reason to end the pregnancy by elective delivery. When proteinuria occurs and persists but blood pressure is normal and renal function is preserved, the pregnancy can be allowed to continue.

Blood Pressure

Most of the specific risks of hypertension are mediated through superimposed preeclampsia (see Chapter 43). There is, however, controversy about the incidence of preeclampsia in those women with preexisting renal disease because the diagnosis cannot be made with certainty on clinical grounds alone. This is because hypertension and proteinuria may be manifestations of the underlying renal disease (Report of the National High Blood Pressure Education Program Working Group, 2000). Treatment of hypertension in pregnancy is considered in Chapter 43.

High blood pressure in the presence of an underlying kidney disorder is treated more aggressively than are other hypertensive complications of pregnancy. This is because such actions preserve function longer. Therefore, although diastolic levels no more than 100 mm Hg may be permissible in many pregnant women with underlying essential hypertension, a diastolic goal of no more than 90 mm Hg should be set for patients with renal disease (Tables 44-5 and 44-6).

It should be borne in mind that renal artery stenosis in pregnancy may present as chronic hypertension or as recurrent

TABLE 44-4. PREGNANCY PROSPECTS FOR WOMEN WITH MODERATE AND SEVERE CHRONIC RENAL DISEASE

Problems in Pregnancy (%)	Successful Obstetric Outcome (%)	Problems in Long Term (%)	End-Stage Renal Failure within 1 Year (%)
90 (81–97)	84 (65–93)	50 (30–57)	15 (10–23)

Values are means, with ranges in parentheses. Date are from 107 women in 125 pregnancies from Jones DC, Hayslett JP: Outcome of pregnancy in women with moderate or severe renal insufficiency. N Engl J Med **335**:226, 1996; Jungers P, Chauveau D: Pregnancy in renal disease. Kidney Int **52**:871, 1997.

TABLE 44-5. EFFECT OF BLOOD PRESSURE ON PREGNANCY COMPLICATIONS (%)

	Intrauterine Growth Retardation (%)	Preterm Delivery	Renal Deterioration (%)
Normotension	4	12	3
Hypertension	16	20	15

Estimated from Cunningham et al., 1990; Abe, 1996; Jones and Hayslett, 1996; Jungers et al., 1996, 1997; Jungers and Chauveau, 1997.

isolated preeclampsia (Heybourne et al., 1991). The diagnosis is further confounded because hypertension associated with renal artery stenosis and chronic parenchymal disease may both be difficult to control requiring multiple drug therapy. Renal angiography is the most sensitive and specific diagnostic technique, and concomitant therapeutic percutaneous transluminal angioplasty and/or stenting may be undertaken (Easterling et al., 1991).

Fetal Surveillance and Timing of Delivery

Serial assessment of fetal well-being is essential because renal disease can be associated with intrauterine growth restriction, and when complications do arise, the judicious moment for intervention is influenced by fetal status. Current technology should minimize the risk of intrauterine fetal death as well as neonatal morbidity and mortality. Regardless of gestational age, most infants weighing 1200 g or more are better off in a special care nursery than in a hostile intrauterine environment. Deliberate preterm delivery may be necessary if renal function deteriorates substantially or for the usual maternal and fetal causes, such as uncontrollable hypertension, and signs adduced by monitoring of fetal jeopardy.

Problems Associated with Specific Renal Disease

Table 44-7 lists specific diseases associated with pregnancy, the information having been derived from publications over the past 10 years. The crucial balance between obstetric outcome and long-term renal prognosis depends on prepregnancy renal functional status, the absence or presence of hypertension (and its management), and the kidney lesion itself, as well as better fetal surveillance, more timely delivery, and enhanced neonatal care (Lindheimer et al., 2000).

Acute and Chronic Glomerulonephritis

Acute poststreptococcal glomerulonephritis is a very rare complication of pregnancy, and if it occurs late in pregnancy, it can be mistaken for preeclampsia. With chronic glomerulonephritis, one view warns of aggravation because of the hypercoagulable state accompanying pregnancy, with patients more prone to superimposed preeclampsia or hypertensive crises earlier in pregnancy. The consensus, however, is that if renal function is stable and hypertension is absent, most pregnancies are successful.

Complications do develop more frequently in women who already have some dysfunction or hypertension in early pregnancy. In 25% there is *de novo* hypertension or worsening of preexisting hypertension usually reverting after delivery, suggesting superimposed preeclampsia, a diagnosis that is not easy to confirm in this group of patients. In 10%, however, hypertension persists after delivery, especially in focal and segmental glomerulosclerosis, membranoproliferative glomerulonephritis, and IgA nephropathy. The higher rates of fetal loss observed in these gravidas can be accounted for by the greater prevalence of severe hypertension and renal insufficiency.

The recent literature endorses these messages. For example, (1) pregnancy is well tolerated without effect on the course of the disease if blood pressure is normal and GFR is above 70 ml/min before conception, and (2) with hypertension the rate of live births is lower if it exists before pregnancy or if it is not well controlled during gestation (Abe, 1996; Jungers and Chanveau, 1997).

Hereditary nephritis, an uncommon disorder, may first become manifested or exacerbated during pregnancy, but most gestations succeed. Of interest is a variant of hereditary nephritis, involving disordered platelet morphology and function. In these cases, pregnancy has been successful but at times complicated by bleeding problems, especially at delivery.

TABLE 44-6. EFFECT OF BLOOD PRESSURE AND RENAL DETERIORATION (ALONE OR TOGETHER) ON NONSUCCESSFUL OBSTETRIC OUTCOME (I.E., FETAL MORTALITY) (%)

	Hypertension	Renal Deterioration	Both
Absent throughout pregnancy	6	7	7
Present at some time during pregnancy	12	12	19
Present and managed from first trimester	10	—	13
Present from first trimester and not managed	50	40	55
Present only during third trimester	8	9	10

Estimated from Cunningham et al., 1990; Abe, 1996; Jones and Hayslett, 1996; Jungers et al., 1996, 1997; Jungers and Chauveau, 1997.

TABLE 44-7. CHRONIC RENAL DISEASE AND PREGNANCY

Renal Disease	Effects
Chronic glomerulonephritis and focal glomerular sclerosis (FGS)	Increased incidence of high blood pressure late in gestation but usually no adverse effect if renal function is preserved and hypertension is absent before gestation. Some disagree, believing coagulation changes in pregnancy exacerbate disease, especially immunoglobulin A (IgA) nephropathy, membranoproliferative glomerulonephritis, and FGS.
IgA nephropathy	Some cite risks of sudden escalating or uncontrolled hypertension and renal deterioration. Most note good outcome when renal function is preserved.
Chronic pyelonephritis (infectious tubulointerstitial disease)	Bacteriuria in pregnancy and may lead to exacerbation.
Reflux nephropathy	In the past, some emphasized risks of sudden escalating hypertension and worsening of renal function. Consensus now is that results are satisfactory when preconception function is only mildly affected and hypertension is absent. Vigilant screening for urinary tract infections is necessary.
Urolithiasis	Ureteral dilatation and stasis do not seem to affect natural history, but infections can be more frequent. Stents have been successfully placed and sonographically controlled ureterostomy has been performed during gestation.
Polycystic kidney disease	Functional impairment and hypertension are usually minimal in childbearing years.
Diabetic nephropathy	No adverse effect on the renal lesion. Increased frequency of infections, edema, or preeclampsia.
Systemic lupus erythematosus	Prognosis is most favorable if disease is in remission 6 or more months before conception. Some authorities increase steroid dosage in immediate postpartum period.
Periarteritis nodosa	Fetal prognosis is poor. Associated with maternal death. Therapeutic abortion should be considered.
Scleroderma	If onset during pregnancy, there can be rapid overall deterioration. Reactivation of quiescent scleroderma can occur during pregnancy and postpartum.
Previous urologic surgery	Depending on original reason for surgery, there may be other malformations of the urogenital tract. Urinary tract infection is common during pregnancy, and renal function may undergo reversible decrease. No significant obstructive problem, but cesarean section might be necessary for abnormal presentation or to avoid disruption of the continence mechanism if artificial sphincters or neourethras are present.
After nephrectomy, solitary and pelvic kidneys	Pregnancy is well tolerated. Might be associated with other malformations of the urogenital tract. Dystocia rarely occurs with a pelvic kidney.

Chronic Pyelonephritis (Tubulointerstitial Disease)

Tubulointerstitial disease in pregnancy may be either infectious or noninfectious. The prognosis in pregnancy is similar to that for patients with glomerular disease, in that outcome is best in patients with adequate renal function and normal blood pressure. Compared with nonpregnant women, pregnant women have a higher frequency of symptomatic infections, but these patients may have a more benign antenatal course than do women with glomerular disease. Of interest is a report suggesting that women who develop frank pyelonephritis manifest greater degrees of pelvicaliceal dilatation in pregnancy that may not regress after delivery, underscoring the need for postpartum investigation of this population (Twickler et al., 1994).

Reflux Nephropathy

The term reflux nephropathy is used to describe renal morphologic and functional changes that relate to past (and usually present) vesicoureteric reflux, often complicated by recurrent infection. Opinions were once controversial, but with preserved renal function and no hypertension, both fetal and maternal outcomes appear to be excellent (Jungers et al., 1996). Vigilance is still necessary to detect and treat UTIs in these patients. Unfortunately, reflux nephropathy is often associated with hypertension and moderate or severe renal dysfunction by the time these patients reach childbearing age; as discussed earlier, such a scenario adversely affects pregnancy outcome. Specific obstetric concerns in affected patients include severe fetal intrauterine growth restriction and the risk of sudden rapid worsening of hypertension and renal function with accelerated progression to renal failure.

Urolithiasis

The prevalence of urolithiasis in pregnancy is 0.03% to 0.35% (Butler et al., 2000). Renal and ureteric calculi are common causes of nonuterine abdominal pain severe enough to necessitate hospital admission during pregnancy. Most calculi are the more benign calcium types (oxalate and brushite), but occasionally the more malicious struvite stones (e.g., infected and staghorn) are seen. Uric acid and cystine stones are much more infrequent.

All stone patients should be evaluated frequently for asymptomatic UTIs and rapidly treated when such complications are diagnosed. Management of stone symptoms should be conservative initially, with adequate hydration, appropriate antibiotic therapy, and pain relief with systemic analgesics (Evans and Wollin, 2001). The use of continuous segmental (T-11 to

L-2) epidural block has been advocated, as in nonpregnant patients with ureteric colic, and may even favorably influence spontaneous passage of the stones, especially as the ureter is dilated during gestation. With good pain relief, patients micturate without difficulty, move without assistance, and are less at risk from thromboembolic problems than if they are drowsy, nauseated, and bedridden with pain.

Pregnancy should not be a deterrent to intravenous urography, especially when there are complications that might require surgical intervention. The absence of ureteric jets may be significant if urolithiasis is suspected (Asrat et al., 1998). Specific clinical criteria suggested before a limited intravenous urography is done are microscopic hematuria, recurrent urinary tract symptoms, and sterile urine culture when pyelonephritis is suspected. The presence of two of these criteria indicates a diagnosis of calculi in a substantial percentage of women (Bucholz et al., 1998). Ultrasonography may be useful, but it is less efficient in detecting very small calculi (less than 5 mm diameter) and/or in defining the degree or site of obstruction (Shokeir et al., 2000).

Obstruction of the ureters by calculi can be treated by the cystoscopic placement of an internal ureteral tube, or stent, between the bladder and kidney under local anesthesia, a procedure that has been successfully used in pregnant women for decades with little or no reports of excess morbidity. The stent retains its position because it has a pigtail or J-like curve at each end (double J) and can be changed every 8 weeks to prevent encrustation. Early empirical use for presumed stone obstruction in pregnant women with flank pain is recommended, by some (Butler et al., 2000) especially when hydration, analgesia, and antibiotics do not resolve pain or fever, and when the pregnancy is over, the usual x-ray evaluation is obtained and standard management is resumed.

Sonographically guided percutaneous nephrostomy is another effective method of treating gravidas with ureteric colic or symptomatic obstructive hydronephrosis (Van Sonnenberg et al., 1992). The procedure is rapid, requires minimal anesthesia, and is perhaps a preferable alternative to retrograde stenting or more invasive surgery. Information on lithotripsy during pregnancy is limited. Until more is known the procedure is best avoided (Algari et al., 1999).

As noted, the relatively benign history of stone disease relates to patients with uncomplicated calcium stones, whereas anecdotally those with struvite (infected) stones do worse, in part because of functional loss and severe infections. Unfortunately, the pregnancy literature on struvite stones is sparse, and such women require close management with stone specialists. Finally, in patients with cystinuria, assiduous maintenance of high fluid intake is the mainstay of management. Although D-penicillamine appears relatively safe, it should be used only for severe cases, when urinary cystine excretion is known to be very high.

Autosomal Dominant Polycystic Kidney Disease

Autosomal dominant polycystic kidney disease is the most frequent genetic renal disorder, affecting 1 in 400 to 1000 persons, but may remain undetected during pregnancy (Gabow, 1993). Careful questioning for a history of familial problems and the use of ultrasonography may lead to earlier detection. Patients do well when functional impairment is minimal and hypertension is absent, as is often the case in

childbearing years (Morgan and Grünfeld, 1998); they do, however, have an increased incidence of hypertension late in pregnancy and a higher perinatal mortality compared with that in pregnancies of sisters unaffected by this autosomal dominant disease.

Women with advanced renal failure are best advised against pregnancy, although use of prophylactic dialysis has been advocated, despite lack of controlled studies, for just this type of patient (Okundaye et al., 1998). If one or the other prospective parent has evidence of polycystic renal disease, the couple may seek genetic counseling. There is a 50% chance of transmitting the disease to the offspring. DNA probe techniques (Calvet and Grantham, 2001) are now being developed so that antenatal diagnosis is possible by chorionic villus sampling, allowing women to undergo selective termination of pregnancy.

Diabetic Nephropathy

Because many patients have had diabetes since childhood, they probably already have microscopic changes in the kidneys (Hayslett and Reece, 1994; Ekban et al., 2001). During pregnancy, diabetic women have an increased prevalence of covert bacteriuria (and may be more susceptible to symptomatic UTI), peripheral edema, and preeclampsia (Jungers and Chauveau, 1997).

The consensus is that most women with diabetic nephropathy only nominal demonstrate normal GFR increments (and perhaps significant proteinuria), and pregnancy does not accelerate renal deterioration. There is, however, a report of diabetic women with moderate renal dysfunction (serum creatinine above 125 μmol/liter [at least 1.4 mg/dL]) whose renal function permanently deteriorated in pregnancy in comparison with the changes before and afterward (Purdy et al., 1996). Such changes occurred despite good metabolic control and might have been related to hypertension, which often accelerates in the third trimester. However, one uncontrolled report suggested that the best predictor of renal and pregnancy outcome is proteinuria, less than 1 g per 24 hours having better outcomes (Gordon et al., 1996).

Aggressive treatment of high blood pressure is extremely important in diabetic care, and pregnancy is no exception; even mild hypertension should be treated (Leguizaman and Reece, 2000). Diabetic gravidas frequently are prescribed angiotensin-converting enzyme inhibitors or angiotensin receptor blockers before conception. These medications, define by the U.S. Food and Drug Administration as safety class D, are considered X (contraindicated) by us and should be discontinued before conception. They cause fetopathies and neonatal anuria with renal failure, but their association with malformations is less certain. Thus, when women taking these medications present after conception, stopping the drug is usually all that is necessary (Hod et al., 1995).

Systemic Lupus Erythematosus

SLE has a predilection for women of childbearing age. Its coincidence with pregnancy poses complex clinical problems because of the profound disturbance of the immunologic system, multiple organ involvement, and complicated immunology of pregnancy itself (Jungers and Chauveau, 1997). Transient improvements, no change, and a tendency to relapse have all been reported (see Chapter 54).

Decisions regarding the status of the disease and the importance of having a baby to the patient and her partner should be made on an individual basis. Most pregnancies succeed, especially when the maternal disease has been in complete clinical remission for 6 months before conception and any renal dysfunction minimal, even if there were marked pathologic changes in the original renal biopsy and heavy proteinuria in the early stages of the disease (Hayslett, 1992). Continued signs of disease activity or increasing renal dysfunction reduces the likelihood of an uncomplicated pregnancy and the clinical course thereafter. Obviously, prepregnancy counseling must take account of the actual form of lupus nephritis (mild versus aggressive) and the medications used, either separately or in combination, for example, glucocorticoids, cyclophosphamide, azathioprine, and today mycophenolate mofetil (CellCept) (Falk, 2000).

The effects of gestation on SLE activity and on the course of lupus nephritis have long been debated. Taking into account both extrarenal manifestations and renal changes, at least 50% of women show some change in clinical status, often called "lupus flare" (Petri, 1994). Admittedly, increments in proteinuria or blood pressure could be due to preeclampsia. From recent reviews (Lockshin and Sammaritane, 2000; Le Thi Huong et al., 1994, 2001), however, it appears that as many as 20% (progressive in 8%) and 40% experience decrements in GFR and worsening hypertension, respectively. These reviews, however, tend to group together women with mild and more severe renal dysfunction, and here we must emphasize that the figures certainly become worse if renal insufficiency (serum creatinine more than 125 μmol/liter [more than 1.4 mg/dL]) antedates the pregnancy.

Lupus nephropathy may sometimes become manifest during pregnancy and, when accompanied by hypertension and renal dysfunction, may be mistaken for preeclampsia. Some patients tend to experience relapse, occasionally severely in the puerperium; therefore, some clinicians prescribe or increase steroids at this time (Le Thi Huong et al., 2001). Rarely, a particularly severe postpartum syndrome may develop, consisting of pleural effusion, pulmonary infiltration, fever, electrocardiogram abnormalities, and even cardiomyopathy, with extensive IgG, IgM, IgA, and C3 deposition in the myocardium. Of note, the disturbing complications above, especially that of a "stormy puerperium," are disputed. In fact, many now observe postpartum patients and do not institute or increase steroid therapy unless signs of increased disease activity are noted.

SLE sera may contain a bewildering array of autoantibodies (lupus serum factor) against nucleic acids, nucleoproteins, cell-surface antigens, and phospholipids. Antiphospholipid antibodies exert a complicated effect on the coagulation system (Cowchock et al., 1992). This led to the rather enigmatic definition of a lupus anticoagulant, found in 5% to 10% of patients with SLE (see Chapter 48). Because treatment with low-molecular-weight heparin and aspirin may lead to successful pregnancies, it is important to screen for lupus anticoagulant in women with SLE and perhaps in those with a history of recurrent intrauterine death or thrombotic episodes to identify this particular cohort. A decision to use prophylactic aspirin, however, must be weighed with the knowledge that this drug may cause decreases in GFR in lupus patients.

An increased incidence of congenital cardiac anomalies in the offspring of women with SLE, and particularly in patients with anti-Ro (SS-A) antibodies, is discussed in Chapter 54.

Periarteritis Nodosa

In contrast to lupus nephropathy where most outcomes are successful, the course of pregnancy in women with renal involvement resulting from periarteritis nodosa is very guarded, largely because of the associated hypertension, frequently malignant. The literature, however, is anecdotal, comprising selective case reports, but many of them involved maternal demise. Nevertheless, a few successful pregnancies have been reported. Still, in the absence of new data we recommend early therapeutic termination because of maternal risk.

Systemic Sclerosis

Scleroderma is a term that includes a heterogeneous group of limited and systemic conditions causing hardening of the skin. Systemic sclerosis implies involvement of both skin and other sites, particularly certain internal organs. Renal involvement is thought to occur in about 60% of these patients, usually within 3 to 4 years of diagnosis. The presentation may take one of three forms: sudden onset of malignant hypertension, rapidly progressive renal failure, or slowly increasing azotemia (Steen, 1999).

The combination of systemic sclerosis and pregnancy is infrequent because the disease occurs most often in the fourth and fifth decades and affected patients are usually infertile. When disease onset is during pregnancy, there appears to be a greater tendency for deterioration. Here, too, data are from selective case reports, some where patients with scleroderma and no evidence of renal involvement before conception have developed severe kidney disease in gestation. There are also instances in which pregnancy has been uneventful and successful but marked reactivation occurred unexpectedly in the puerperium. Most maternal deaths involve rapidly progressive scleroderma with severe pulmonary complications, infections, hypertension, and renal failure (Steen, 1999).

The extent of systemic involvement is probably more important than the duration of the disease, and limited mild disease carries a better prognosis. Sclerosis usually spares the abdominal wall skin, but theoretically thickened skin and decreased abdominal wall compliance could be troublesome.

Wegener Granulomatosis

Information on the outcome of pregnancy in women with granulomatosis is scarce. Proteinuria (with or without hypertension) is common from early in pregnancy (Auzary et al., 2000), and reports to date have described both complicated and uneventful pregnancies (Dayoan et al., 1998). Experience with cyclophosphamide (Cytoxan) in pregnancy is limited, and the risks to the embryo and fetus must be weighed in relation to the course of the disease if such therapy were to be withheld from the mother (Harber et al., 1999).

Previous Urinary Tract Surgery

Permanent urinary diversion is still used in the management of patients with congenital lower urinary tract defects, but its use for neurogenic bladder has declined since the introduction of self-catheterization. The most common complication of pregnancy is urinary infection. Premature labor occurs in 20%; the use of prophylactic antibiotics throughout pregnancy may reduce its incidence. Decline in renal function may occur, invariably related to infection or intermittent obstruction or both. With an ileal conduit or augmentation cystoplasty, elevation and compression by the expanding uterus can cause outflow obstruction, whereas with a ureterosigmoid anastomosis, actual ureteral obstruction may occur (Hill et al., 1990). The changes usually reverse after delivery.

The mode of delivery is dictated by obstetric factors. Abnormal presentation accounts for a cesarean section rate of 25%. Vaginal delivery is safe, but because the continence of a ureterosigmoid anastomosis depends on an intact anal sphincter, this area must be protected with a mediolateral episiotomy.

During the past decade, urinary tract reconstruction by means of augmentation cystoplasty, with or without artificial genitourinary sphincter, has become more commonplace. Deterioration of renal function as well as urinary tract obstruction or infection can occur at any time in pregnancy. Delivery by cesarean section is recommended for these gravidas because of the potential for disruption of the continence mechanism.

Solitary Kidney

Some patients have either a congenital absence of one kidney or marked unilateral renal hypoplasia. Most, however, have had a previous nephrectomy because of pyelonephritis (with abscess or hydronephrosis), unilateral tuberculosis, congenital abnormalities, a tumor, or, today, kidney donation (Wrenshall et al., 1996). It is important to know the indication for and the time elapsed since nephrectomy. In patients with an infectious or a structural renal problem, sequential prepregnancy investigation is needed to detect any persistent infection.

It makes no difference whether the right or left kidney remains, as long as it is located in the normal anatomic position. If function is normal and stable, women with this problem seem to tolerate pregnancy well despite the superimposition of GFR increments on already hyperfiltering nephrons. The rare occurrence of acute renal failure in pregnancy resulting from obstruction is most often associated with the presence of a single kidney.

Ectopic kidneys (usually pelvic) are more vulnerable to infection and are associated with decreased fetal salvage, probably because of associated malformations of the urogenital tract. If infection occurs in a solitary kidney during pregnancy and does not quickly respond to antibiotics, termination may have to be considered for preservation of renal function.

Nephrotic Syndrome

The most common cause of nephrotic syndrome in late pregnancy is preeclampsia that may have a poorer fetal prognosis than preeclampsia with less heavy proteinuria. The other most frequent cause is diabetic nephropathy, and next comes a host of glomerular disorders, including proliferative or membranoproliferative glomerulonephritis, minimal change disease, lupus nephropathy, rarely hereditary nephritis, and amyloidosis. Many of these diseases do not respond to steroids, and these drugs have side effects, emphasizing the importance of a tissue diagnosis before steroid therapy is begun (Uribe et al., 1991). In addition, the sudden appearance of nephrotic syndrome with any of these disorders should precipitate an evaluation for renal vein thrombosis given the hypercoagulable state of pregnancy.

If renal function is adequate and hypertension is absent, there should be few complications during pregnancy, although several physiologic changes occurring during pregnancy may mimic aggravation or exacerbation of the disease (Davison, 1998b). For example, increments in renal hemodynamics and increases in renal vein pressure may enhance protein excretion. Serum albumin levels usually decrease by 0.5 to 1.0 g/dL during normal pregnancy, and further decreases because of a nephrotic syndrome may enhance the tendency toward fluid retention. Because of decreased intravascular volume, diuretics may compromise uteroplacental perfusion or aggravate the increased tendency to thrombotic episodes. This recommendation, however, is relative, because in some nephrotic patients avid salt retention results in massive edema and even volume-induced hypertension. For example, when managing nephrotic syndrome resulting from diabetic nephropathy, some believe the judicious use of saluretic drugs prevents the development or aggravation of hypertension after mid-pregnancy and helps avoid early termination of the gestation (Hayslett and Reece, 1994). Finally, prophylactic anticoagulation has been suggested when such patients require hospitalization and/or prolonged bed rest. Obviously, these latter issues, diuretics and anticoagulation, require further investigation.

Human Immunodeficiency Virus with Associated Nephropathy

The worldwide pandemic of human immunodeficiency disease appears to involve greater numbers of pregnant women (Frassetto et al., 1991). This disease has a renal component, including nephrotic syndrome and severe renal impairment. Human immunodeficiency virus with associated nephropathy may be seen in human immunodeficiency virus–seropositive patients, patients with acquired immunodeficiency syndrome, or patients with acquired immunodeficiency syndrome-related complex. The condition is characterized by severe proteinuria and rapid progression to end-stage renal disease, possibly slowed down by the use of an angiotensin-converting enzyme inhibitor (a drug that cannot be used in pregnancy) and steroids. The distinctive features seen on histologic evaluation of renal biopsy are glomerulosclerosis, visceral epithelial cell hypertrophy, and variable tubulointerstitial nephritis (Winston et al., 1998). We are unaware of any literature on human immunodeficiency virus with associated nephropathy (HIVAN) in pregnancy but, given the ravages of this epidemic, note that the disease should be considered when nephritic proteinuria appears suddenly, especially in patients who have not been screened for the virus. Human immunodeficiency virus and HIVAN are discussed further and extensively elsewhere (Rao, 2000) and in Chapter 40.

Precis

The problems associated with the specific disorders discussed in this section are summarized in Table 44-7. In general, the view we continually repeat for emphasis is that preserved renal function and the absence of hypertension and other comorbidities before conception predict successful fetal outcome and few maternal complications, regardless of the nature of the disorder. Exceptions include several collagen disorders associated anecdotally with serious maternal problems. There is some controversy between authorities regarding four specific diseases (see Table 44-7), and we are with the optimists. *Finally, we reiterate that these conclusions are based on poorly controlled retrospective data, underscoring the need for registries and for prospectively acquired data.*

Remote Prognosis

Pregnancy does not adversely affect the natural history of the renal lesion if kidney dysfunction is minimal and hypertension is absent at conception, with the exception of certain collagen disorders; however, there is still debate concerning IgA and reflux nephropathies (Jungers and Chauveau, 1997; Lindheimer et al., 2000). An important factor in the eventual outcome of any debate on remote prognosis is the sclerotic effect that hyperfiltration during gestation might bestow in the residual (intact) glomeruli of kidneys of patients with renal insufficiency. Theoretically, further progressive loss of renal function can ensue in pregnancy, but it is encouraging that this is not the case in animals when pregnancy is superimposed on experimental glomerulonephritis (Baylis, 1994). In humans, the literature is primarily *retrospective*, and most data concern patients who had but mild functional impairment (Lindheimer et al., 2001). Clearly, large *prospective* studies are needed because patients with renal disease can have unpredicted, accelerated, and irreversible renal decline in pregnancy or immediately afterward, and the mechanisms are unknown.

The superimposition of pregnancy hyperfiltration on the compensatory changes already present in a single kidney could lessen the life span of the kidney. The crux of this hypothesis is the implication that increases in glomerular pressure or glomerular plasma flow cause sclerosis of capillaries within the glomerulus and that in pregnancy further physiologic hyperfiltration and intravascular coagulation changes could augment the damage. In health, it seems unlikely that there are long-term renal sequelae (Baylis, 1994).

■ HEMODIALYSIS PATIENTS AND PREGNANCY

It has been several decades since the first description of conception and successful delivery in a patient receiving chronic hemodialysis, and further case reports (some of successive pregnancies) and registry data have been published since then (Malik et al., 1997; Davison and Baylis, 1998; Okundaye et al., 1998). Any optimism must be tempered by the thought that clinicians are reluctant to publish failures or disasters, and consequently the true incidence of unsuccessful pregnancies in women on dialysis cannot be determined. The high therapeutic abortion rate in these patients, although decreased from 40% in 1989 to 18% today, still indicates that those who become pregnant do so accidentally, probably because they are unaware that pregnancy is a possibility.

Counseling and Early Pregnancy Assessment

Despite irregular or absent menstruation and impaired infertility, women receiving dialysis should use contraception if they wish to avoid pregnancy (Schmidt and Holley, 1998). The introduction of recombinant human erythropoietin (r-HuEPO)

for the treatment of women with renal failure appears to be associated in some cases with return of normal menses (and ovulation), probably because of correction of hyperprolactinemia or improved overall health (Braga et al., 1996).

There are substantial arguments against pregnancy, not the least of which are the risks to the patient (severe hypertension, cardiac failure, maternal death) and the fact that even when therapeutic termination of pregnancy is excluded, there is at best only a 40% to 50% likelihood of successful outcome (Hou and Firanek, 1998). If only data since the late 1990s are considered, outcomes seem to be improving, with fetal survival occurring in 50% to 70%, although maternal risk remains formidable (Romão et al., 1998; Toma et al., 1999).

Early diagnosis of pregnancy is difficult. A missed period is usually ignored. The mistake the clinician may make is failure to consider the possibility of pregnancy, and currently many of these patients have not been given contraception counseling. Resistance to r-HuEPO or progression of anemia (hematocrit decrease by 8% of prepregnancy levels) can be a useful clue to early diagnosis of pregnancy (Maruyama and Arakawa, 1997). Urine pregnancy tests can be unreliable, and definitive diagnosis and estimation of gestational age are best accomplished by sonar technology.

Antenatal Strategy and Decision-Making

For a successful outcome, scrupulous attention must be paid to blood pressure control, fluid balance, increased hours of dialysis, and provision of good nutrition (Hou, 1997; Bagon et al., 1998; Chan et al., 1998).

Dialysis Policy

Some patients demonstrate apparent increments in GFR even though the level of renal function is too poor to sustain life without hemodialysis, whereas other women remain completely anuric (Castillo et al., 1999). Women with some residual renal function and satisfactory daily urine volumes, in whom dialysis control is easier, are more likely to become pregnant (Hou and Firanek, 1998).

The planning of dialysis strategy should have the following seven aims:

1. Maintain serum urea at less than 20 mmol/liter (60 mg/dL), although some would argue lower (e.g., 15 mmol/liter [less than 45 mg/dL]). Intrauterine death is more likely if levels are much in excess of 20 mmol/liter, but occasional success has been achieved despite levels of 28 μmol/liter [84 mg/dL] for many weeks (Hou and Firanek, 1998)
2. Avoid hypotension during dialysis, which could be damaging to the fetus. In late pregnancy, the gravid uterus and the supine posture may aggravate this by decreasing venous return.
3. Ensure good control of blood pressure.
4. Ensure minimal fluctuations in fluid balance and limit volume changes.
5. Scrutinize carefully for preterm labor, because dialysis or uterine contractions with or without significant changes in fetal hemodynamics are associated (Oosterhof et al., 1993).
6. Watch calcium levels closely and avoid hypercalcemia (calciferol doses often must be reduced).
7. Limit interdialysis weight gain to about 1 kg until late pregnancy. After mid-pregnancy, one should take the

classic 0.5 kg/wk weight gain into account when considering dry weight. This should mean a 50% increase in hours and frequency of dialysis. Frequent dialysis renders dietary management and control of weight gain much easier.

Anemia

Patients with severe renal insufficiency are usually anemic. This anemia is aggravated further in pregnancy; therefore, increased erythropoietin therapy and even blood transfusion may be needed, especially before delivery. Caution is necessary because erythropoietin therapy or transfusion may exacerbate hypertension and impair the ability to control circulatory overload, even with extra dialysis. Fluctuations in blood volume can be minimized if packed red cells are transfused during dialysis.

It appears that genetically engineered erythropoietin (r-HuEPO) is well tolerated in pregnancy (Braga et al., 1996). In particular, the theoretical risks of hypertension, alluded to previously, and thrombotic complications have not been cited so far. Invariably, the r-HuEPO requirements to maintain a target hematocrit of 30% increase until delivery (Vora and Gruslin, 1998). Finally, no adverse effects have been noted in neonates in whom hematologic indices and erythropoietin concentrations are normal for gestational age, suggesting that r-HuEPO does not have significant transplacental effects.

Unnecessary blood sampling should be avoided when there is anemia or lack of venipuncture sites. The protocol for various tests usually performed in a particular unit should be followed strictly, with no more blood removed per venipuncture than is absolutely necessary (Hou and Firanek, 1998).

Hypertension

Because patients with hypertension may have abnormal lipid profiles and possibly accelerated atherogenesis, it is difficult to predict the cardiovascular capacity to tolerate pregnancy. Diabetic women receiving dialysis who have become pregnant are those in whom cardiovascular problems are most evident. In these and other women with renal disease, a normotensive state at conception is reassuring. Unfortunately, blood pressure tends to be labile and hypertension is a common problem, although it may be possible to help control it by dialysis.

Nutrition

Despite more frequent dialysis, relatively free dietary intake should be discouraged. A daily oral intake of 70 g protein, 1500 mg calcium, 50 mM potassium, and 80 mM sodium is advised, with supplements of dialyzable vitamins. Vitamin D supplements can be difficult to judge in patients who have had parathyroidectomy. In addition, the placenta produces hydroxy-vitamin D, which is one reason why oral supplementation may have to be curtailed. All of this poses risks for fetal nutrition, plus the fact that the exact impact of the uremic environment is difficult to assess. The use of parenteral nutrition supplementation in pregnancy in these gravidas has been advocated (Brookhyser and Wiggins, 1998).

Fetal Surveillance and Timing of Delivery

What has been said with regard to chronic renal disease applies here as well. Cesarean section should be necessary only for purely obstetric reasons. It could be argued, however, that

elective cesarean section in all cases might minimize potential problems during labor. In fact, preterm labor is generally the rule and may commence during hemodialysis (Blowey and Warady, 1998). The role of cesarean section in this situation needs to be carefully considered.

Peritoneal Dialysis Patients and Pregnancy

Since 1976, continuous ambulatory peritoneal dialysis and continuous cycling peritoneal dialysis have been used more frequently in the management of patients with all forms of renal insufficiency (Castillo et al., 1999). Several features of peritoneal dialysis make it an attractive approach for the management of renal failure in pregnancy:

1. Maintenance of a more stable environment for the fetus in terms of fluid and electrolyte concentrations
2. Avoidance of episodes of abrupt hypotension, a frequent occurrence during hemodialysis, which can cause fetal distress
3. Continuous allowance for extracellular fluid volume control so that blood pressure control is augmented
4. Refraining from systemic heparin use
5. Achievement of better maternal nutrition by allowing less restricted diet
6. Better blood sugar control in patients with diabetes mellitus via intraperitoneal insulin
7. Theoretically permitting safe use of intraperitoneal magnesium, facilitating prevention and treatment of premature labor and possibly preeclampsia

Nevertheless, a recent report failed to detect any differences in outcome because of mode of renal replacement therapy (hemodialysis versus peritoneal dialysis) and even suggests greater infertility in patients receiving continuous ambulatory peritoneal dialysis (Okundaye et al., 1998).

Finally, peritonitis, which can be a severe complication of continuous ambulatory peritoneal dialysis, accounts for most therapy failures in nonpregnant populations. Peritonitis superimposed on a pregnancy can present a confusing diagnostic picture and a whole series of treatment problems.

RENAL TRANSPLANT PATIENTS AND PREGNANCY

After transplantation, renal and endocrine functions return rapidly, and normal sexual activity can ensue (Hou, 1999). About 1 in 50 women of childbearing age with a functioning renal transplant becomes pregnant. Of the conceptions, 40% do not go beyond the initial trimester because of spontaneous or therapeutic abortion. More than 90% of pregnancies that continue past the first trimester end successfully (Davison and Baylis, 1998; Armenti et al., 2002) (Table 44-8).

Transplants have been undertaken with the surgeons unaware that the recipient was in early pregnancy (Pergola et al., 2001). Obstetric success in such cases does not negate the importance of contraception counseling for all patients with renal failure and the exclusion of pregnancy before transplantation.

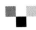

TABLE 44-8. PROSPECTS FOR PREGNANCY IN RENAL TRANSPLANT PATIENTS*

Problems in Pregnancy	Successful Obstetric Outcome	Problems in the Long Term
49%	95% (75%)†	12% (25%)

* Estimates are based on data from 5670 women in 7510 pregnancies that attained at least 28 weeks' gestation (from 1961 to 2001).
† Numbers in parentheses refer to implications when complications developed prior to 28 weeks' gestation.

Counseling and Early Pregnancy Assessment

A woman should be counseled from the time the various treatments for renal failure and the potential for optimal rehabilitation are discussed. Information regarding potential reproductive capacity must be included. Even after transplantation, stress will still be a major factor in everyday life, which will always have a "baseline of uncertainty." Couples who want a child should be encouraged to discuss all the implications, including the harsh realities of maternal prospects of survival (European Best Practice Guidelines, 2002).

Preconception Guidelines

Individual centers have their own specific guidelines (Armenti et al., 1998). In most, a wait of 18 months to 2 years after transplantation is advised. This has turned out to be good advice, because by then the patient will have recovered from the major surgery and any sequelae, graft function will have stabilized, and immunosuppression will be at maintenance levels (Jungers and Chauveau, 1997). If function is well maintained at 24 months, there also is a high probability of allograft survival at 5 years.

A suitable set of guidelines follows, but the criteria are only relative:

1. Good general health for about 2 years since transplantation
2. Stature compatible with good obstetric outcome
3. No or minimal proteinuria
4. Absence of hypertension
5. No evidence of graft rejection
6. Absence of pelvicaliceal distention on a recent intravenous urogram
7. Stable renal function with serum creatinine of 180 μmol/liter (2 mg/dL) or less, preferably less than 125 μmol/liter (1.4 mg/dL) (Table 44-9)

TABLE 44-9. RENAL TRANSPLANT PATIENTS: PROSPECTS FOR PREGNANCY AND RENAL STATUS*

Renal Status	Problems in Pregnancy	Successful Obstetric Outcome	Problems in Long Term
S$_{cr}$ ≤125 μmol/liter (1.4 mg/dL)	30%	97%	7%
S$_{cr}$ >125 μmol/liter (1.4 mg/dL)	82%	75%	27%

* Estimates are based on data from 5370 women in 7110 pregnancies (from 1961 to 2000) that attained at least 28 weeks' gestation.

S$_{cr}$, nonpregnant serum creatinine.

8. Drug therapy reduced to maintenance levels: prednisone, 15 mg/day or less, and azathioprine, 2 mg/kg/day or less, cyclosporine 2 to 4 mg/kg/day or less (experience is limited for the more recently introduced immunosuppressive drugs)

Ectopic Pregnancy

Ectopic pregnancy occurs in at least 0.5% of all conceptions. The diagnosis can be difficult because irregular bleeding and amenorrhea accompany deteriorating renal function or even an intrauterine pregnancy. Patients may be at higher risk of ectopic pregnancy because of pelvic adhesions from previous urologic surgery, peritoneal dialysis, pelvic inflammatory disease, or overzealous use of intrauterine contraceptive devices. The main clinical problem is that symptoms secondary to genuine pelvic pathology may erroneously be attributed to the transplant.

Antenatal Strategy and Decision-Making

Patients must be monitored as high-risk cases by both an obstetrician and an experienced transplant nephrologist. Management requires attention to serial assessment of renal function, diagnosis and treatment of rejection, blood pressure control, early diagnosis or prevention of anemia, treatment of any infection, and meticulous assessment of fetal well-being.

Antenatal visits should be every 2 weeks up to 32 weeks and weekly thereafter. The following tests should be undertaken monthly:

1. Complete blood count, including platelets
2. Blood urea nitrogen
3. Creatinine level
4. Electrolytes
5. Urate levels
6. 24-Hour creatinine clearance and protein excretion
7. Mid-stream urine specimens for microscopy and culture

Liver function tests, plasma protein, and calcium and phosphate levels should be checked at 6-week intervals. Tests for cytomegaloviruria and *Herpesvirus hominis* should be performed during each trimester if the initial findings are negative. Although immunosuppressive therapy is usually maintained at prepregnancy levels, adjustments may be needed if there are decreases in the maternal white blood cell and platelet counts. Hematinic agents should be prescribed if the various hematologic indices show deficiency. Of significance, even a well-functioning graft in pregnancy may not be able to increase production of erythropoietin to meet increased gestational demands, such that consideration should be given to treatment with r-HuEPO (Magee et al., 2000).

Allograft Function

Serial data on renal function are needed to supplement routine antenatal observations (see earlier). The anatomic changes (Baylis and Davison, 1998) and the increased and then sustained GFR characteristic of early pregnancy are evident, even though the allograft is ectopic, denervated, potentially damaged by previous ischemia, and immunologically different from both recipient and fetus. The better the prepregnancy GFR, the greater the increment in pregnancy. For example, in one series the stable problem-free group had a mean prepregnancy serum creatinine of 80 μmol/liter (0.9 mg/dL) in contrast to 212 μmol/liter (2.4 mg/dL) in the group with gestational problems (Nojima et al., 1996). Furthermore, in a single-center analysis of 33 pregnancies in 29 women, all those with serum creatinine more than 200 μmol/liter (more than 2.25 mg/dL) had progression of renal impairment and required dialysis within 2 years of delivery (Crowe et al., 1999).

Transient reductions in GFR can occur during the third trimester and usually do not represent a deteriorating situation with permanent impairment. In 15% of patients, significant renal functional impairment develops during pregnancy and may persist after delivery (see Table 44-8). Because a gradual decline in function is common in nonpregnant patients, however, it is difficult to delineate a specific effect of pregnancy.

Subclinical chronic rejection with declining renal function may occur after an episode of acute rejection or if immunosuppression becomes suboptimal. Increases in proteinuria, often to abnormal levels, occur near term in 40% of patients; this regresses postpartum and, in the absence of hypertension, is not significant. Whether cyclosporine is more nephrotoxic in pregnancy, compared with the blunting of augmentation in GFR in the nonpregnant patient, is not known (Armenti et al., 1998). Consequently, advice to switch to standard immunosuppressive regimens in pregnant women is based purely on clinical anecdote, and evaluations are urgently needed in pregnancy.

Allograft Rejection

Serious rejection episodes occur in 5% of pregnant allograft recipients. Although this incidence of rejection is no greater than that expected for nonpregnant transplant patients, it is unusual because it has been assumed that the privileged immunologic state of pregnancy would be beneficial. Rejection also occasionally occurs during pregnancy in women who have had years of stable function before conception. Rejection can occur in the puerperium and may be caused by return to a normal immune state (despite immunosuppression) or, possibly, a rebound effect from the altered immunoresponsiveness of pregnancy.

Chronic rejection may be a problem in all recipients, having a progressive subclinical course. Whether a pregnancy influences the course of subclinical chronic rejection is unknown. No factors consistently predict which patients will experience allograft rejection during pregnancy. Some have hypothesized a nonimmune contribution to chronic graft failure owing to the damaging effect of hyperfiltration through remnant nephrons, perhaps even exacerbated during pregnancy. From the clinical viewpoint, several points are impor-

tant. Because rejection is difficult to diagnose, when any of the clinical hallmarks are present (e.g., fever, oliguria, deteriorating renal function, renal enlargement, tenderness), the diagnosis should be considered. Although ultrasonography may prove helpful in the nonpregnant setting (Baxter and Rodger, 1997), in the pregnant state without renal biopsy, rejection cannot be distinguished from acute pyelonephritis, recurrent glomerulopathy, possibly severe preeclampsia, and even cyclosporine nephrotoxicity. Renal biopsy is indicated before aggressive antirejection therapy is begun.

Immunosuppression

Immunosuppressive therapy is usually maintained at prepregnancy levels, but adjustments may be needed if the maternal leukocyte or platelet count decreases. When white blood cell counts are maintained within physiologic limits for pregnancy, the neonate usually is born with a normal blood count. Azathioprine liver toxicity has been noted occasionally during pregnancy and responds to dose reduction.

There are many encouraging reports of (noncomplicated) pregnancies in patients taking cyclosporine (Armenti et al., 2000; Lessan-Pezeshki, 2002). Currently, the National Transplantation Pregnancy Registry (maintained by Vincent T. Armenti, MD, at Thomas Jefferson University, Philadelphia) is accruing data (Ahlswede et al., 1992; Armenti et al., 1994, 1998, 2000, 2002; Gaughan et al., 1996). A U.K. Registry has also been established as part of an international effort to coordinate data collection (Davison and Redman, 1997), and efforts are underway in Japan to audit pregnancies (Toma et al., 1998).

Numerous adverse effects are attributed to cyclosporine in nonpregnant transplant recipients, including renal toxicity, hepatic dysfunction, chronic hypertension, tremor, convulsions, diabetogenic effects, hemolytic uremic syndrome, and neoplasia (Gaughan et al., 1996). In pregnancy, some of the maternal adaptations that normally occur may theoretically be blunted or abolished by cyclosporine, especially plasma volume expansion and renal hemodynamic augmentation. A new cyclosporine preparation, Neoral, claimed to improve drug bioavailability and have more stable pharmacokinetics, is in use and in nonpregnant renal transplant patients appears to permit easier maintenance of trough blood drug concentrations in the therapeutic range. Data from the U.S. National Transplantation Pregnancy Registry suggest that patients treated with cyclosporine may have more hypertension and smaller infants, but it is still too premature for definitive conclusions.

Finally, newer agents such as tacrolimus (FK506 or Prograf), mycophenolate mofetil (CellCept), antithymocytic globulin (Atgam), and orthodione (OKTS) are being prescribed more frequently for transplant recipients (Newstead, 1997; Kainz et al., 2000), but there is minimal information about these agents in pregnancy (Ghandour et al., 1998). Some of these newer agents were originally considered to have a "rescue role" only in kidney and kidney–pancreas transplants, but today they can be used as primary immunosuppressive agents (Shapiro, 2000).

Hypertension and Preeclampsia

The appearance of hypertension in the third trimester, its relationship to deteriorating renal function, and the possibility of chronic underlying pathology and preeclampsia as well as cyclosporine dosage are diagnostic problems. Hypertension, particularly before 28 weeks' gestation, is associated with adverse perinatal outcome (Sturgiss and Davison, 1991), which may be due to covert cardiovascular changes that accompany or are aggravated by chronic hypertension. Pre-eclampsia is diagnosed clinically in about 30% of pregnancies. When eclampsia supervenes, its development may be rapid. Antihypertensive medication(s) can be used, as discussed in Chapter 43.

Infections

Patients should be carefully monitored for all types of infection throughout pregnancy (Lessan-Pezeshki, 2002). Prophylactic antibiotics must be given before any surgical procedure, however trivial.

Diabetes Mellitus

Because the results of renal transplantation have improved in those women whose renal failure was caused by juvenile-onset diabetes mellitus, pregnancies are now being reported in these women. Pregnancy complications occur with at least twice the frequency seen in the nondiabetic patient, and this may be due to the presence of generalized cardiovascular pathology (Davison and Baylis, 1998), which is part of the "metabolic risk factor syndrome" (Dimeny and Fellström, 1997). Successful pregnancies have been reported after confirmed pancreas-kidney allograft (Wilson et al., 2001).

Fetal Surveillance and Timing of Delivery

The points given for chronic renal disease are equally applicable for renal transplants. Preterm delivery is common (45% to 60%) because of intervention for obstetric reasons and the common occurrence of preterm labor or premature rupture of membranes. Preterm labor frequently is associated with poor renal function (Armenti et al., 1998). In some, it has been postulated that long-term steroid therapy may weaken connective tissues and contribute to the increased incidence of premature rupture of membranes.

Vaginal delivery should be the aim, and usually there is no mechanical injury to the transplant. Unless there are specific obstetric problems, spontaneous onset of labor can be awaited (Hussey and Pombar, 1998).

Management During Labor

Careful monitoring of maternal fluid balance, cardiovascular status, and temperature is essential; aseptic technique is important for every procedure. Surgical induction of labor (amniotomy) and episiotomy warrant antibiotic coverage. Pain relief is conducted as for healthy women. Augmentation of steroids is necessary to cover delivery.

Role of Cesarean Section

The kidney does not usually obstruct the birth canal, so cesarean section is necessary for the usual obstetric reasons. Several factors are important when one is choosing the deliv-ery route. Transplant patients may have pelvic osteodystrophy related to previous renal failure (and dialysis) or prolonged steroid therapy, particularly before puberty. Antenatal diagnosis of these problems is important and permits the planning of elective cesarean delivery.

If there is a question of disproportion or kidney compression, simultaneous intravenous pyelography and x-ray pelvimetry could be performed (with limitation of the intravenous urogram to one to three films) at 36 weeks' gestation. When a cesarean section is performed, a lower segment approach is usually feasible, although previous urologic surgery or peritonitis may make this difficult.

Pediatric Management
Immediate Problems

More than 50% of live births have no neonatal problems. Preterm delivery is common (45% to 60%), small-for-gestational-age infants are delivered in 30% to 50% of cases, and occasionally the two factors coexist (Little et al., 2000). Although management is the same as in neonates of other mothers, some specific problems exist (Table 44-10). Adrenocortical insufficiency resulting from the maternal steroid therapy potentially increases the risk of overwhelming neonatal infection. Finally, there are anecdotal data associating tacrolimus with oligoanuria and hypokalemia in the neonate (Blowey and Warady, 1998).

Breast-Feeding

There are substantial benefits to breast-feeding. It could be argued that because the infant has been exposed to azathioprine and its metabolites in pregnancy, breast-feeding should not be allowed. However, little is known about the quantities of azathioprine and its metabolites in breast milk and whether the levels are biologically trivial or substantial. Even less is known about cyclosporine in breast milk except that levels are usually greater than those in a simultaneously taken blood sample. Until the many uncertainties are resolved, breast-feeding should not be encouraged (Nyberg et al., 1998).

TABLE 44-10. NEONATAL PROBLEMS IN OFFSPRING OF RENAL TRANSPLANT PATIENTS

Preterm delivery or small for gestational age
Respiratory distress syndrome
Depressed hematopoiesis
Lymphoid and thymic hypoplasia
Adrenocortical insufficiency
Septicemia
Cytomegalovirus infection
Hepatitis B surface antigen carrier state
Congenital abnormalities
Immunologic problems
Reduced lymphocyte passive hemagglutination assay reactivity
Reduced T lymphocyte levels
Reduced immunoglobulin levels
Chromosome aberrations in leukocytes

Long-Term Assessment

Azathioprine can cause abnormalities in the chromosomes of leukocytes, which may take almost 2 years to disappear spontaneously. In tissues not yet studied, however, these anomalies may not be as temporary. The sequelae could be eventual development of malignant tumors in affected offspring, autoimmune complications, and/or abnormalities in the reproductive performance in the next generation (Scott et al., 2002). This latter effect must be initiated in the offspring when *in utero*. It is unlikely that such damage would be eliminated or repaired, as seems to happen in somatic cells, because synthesis of DNA stops when the germ cells are arrested in the prophase of the first meiotic division *in utero* and no new DNA is synthesized until after fertilization (see Chapter 1).

Any child exposed to immunosuppressants *in utero* must have evaluation of the immune system and pediatric follow-up. To date, information about general progress in early childhood has been good (Willis et al., 2000). A study evaluated 175 children from 133 gravidas on cyclosporin at 4 months to 12 years (mean, 4.4 years) (Stanley et al., 1999) who at birth had a mean gestational age of 36 weeks and mean birth weight of 2.49 kg. Twenty-nine children (16%) had "delays" or needed educational support; a much higher incidence of preterm delivery was also present in this group. Amongst U.S. children, 11% in state schools had special educational needs.

Maternal Follow-Up after Pregnancy

The ultimate measure of transplant success is the long-term survival of the patient and the graft. Because it is only 30 years since this procedure became widely used in the management of end-stage renal failure, few long-term data from sufficiently large series exist from which to draw conclusions. Furthermore, the long-term results for renal transplants relate to a period when many aspects of management would be unacceptable by present-day standards. Average survival figures of large numbers of patients worldwide indicate that about 87% of recipients of kidneys from related living donors are alive 5 years after transplantation (Andrews, 2002). With cadaver kidneys, the figure is approximately 50%. If renal function was normal 2 years after transplant, survival increased to about 80%. This is why women are counseled to wait about 2 years before considering a pregnancy.

A major concern is that the mother may not survive or remain well enough to rear the child she bears. Pregnancy occasionally and sometimes unpredictably causes irreversible declines in renal function. However, the consensus is that pregnancy has no effect on graft function or survival (First et al., 1995; Sturgiss and Davison, 1995; Nojima et al., 1996). Also, repeated pregnancies do not adversely affect graft function or fetal development, provided that renal function is well preserved at the time of conception (Ehrich et al., 1996; Owda et al., 1998).

Despite continuing improvement, there is still substantial early mortality and debilitating morbidity in transplant populations. Nevertheless, many women will choose parenthood in an effort to reestablish a normal life and possibly in defiance of the sometimes negative attitudes of the medical establishment. Psychiatrists are now asking the questions why women in such circumstances get pregnant and why there is such overwhelming maternalism. As mentioned earlier in relation to chronic renal disease, the so-called burning building syndrome defines this maternal obsession and tries to differentiate between healthy and pathologic levels of assumed risk (Stotland and Stotland, 1997).

Contraception

It is unwise to offer the option of sterilization at the time of transplantation; this decision should not take place at this time. Oral contraceptives may cause or aggravate hypertension or thromboembolism and can produce subtle changes in the immune system, but this does not necessarily contraindicate their use. Low-dose estrogen preparations or progesterone-only preparations can be used. Careful surveillance is important.

An intrauterine contraceptive device may aggravate menstrual problems, which in turn may obscure signs and symptoms of abnormalities of early gestation, such as threatened abortion and ectopic pregnancy. The increased risk of pelvic infection associated with the intrauterine device in an immunosuppressed patient makes this method worrisome. Indeed, because insertion or replacement of an intrauterine device can be associated with bacteremia of vaginal origin, antibiotic coverage is essential at this time. The efficacy of the intrauterine device may be reduced by immunosuppressive and anti-inflammatory agents, possibly because of modification of the leukocyte response. Careful counseling and follow-up are essential.

Gynecologic Problems

There is a danger that symptoms secondary to genuine pelvic pathology may be erroneously attributed to the transplant because of its location near the pelvis. Patients might be at slightly higher risk for ectopic pregnancy because of pelvic adhesions resulting from previous urologic surgery, pelvic inflammatory disease, or the overzealous use of the intrauterine device. Diagnosis can be overlooked because irregular bleeding and amenorrhea may be associated with deteriorating renal function and intrauterine pregnancy.

Transplant recipients receiving immunosuppressive therapy have a malignancy rate estimated to be 100 times greater than normal, and the female genital tract is no exception (Newstead, 1998). This association is probably related to factors such as loss of immune surveillance, chronic immunosuppression allowing tumor proliferation, and prolonged antigenic stimulation of the reticuloendothelial system. Therefore, regular gynecologic assessment is essential. Management should be on conventional lines, with the outcome unlikely to be influenced by stopping or reducing immunosuppression.

ACUTE RENAL FAILURE PARTICULAR TO PREGNANCY

Acute renal failure severe enough to require dialysis occurs in fewer than 1 in 20,000 gestations (Lindheimer et al., 1993), although complications with transient decrements in GFR of a mild to moderate degree probably occur in 1 in 8000 deliveries (Krane and Cuccazella, 1995; Nzerue et al., 1998). This section emphasizes specific problems in obstetric practice (Table 44-11) and focuses on avoidance of diagnostic errors that can further compound this serious obstetric emergency.

TABLE 44-11. OBSTETRIC ACUTE RENAL FAILURE

Volume contraction or hypotension	Antepartum hemorrhage due to placenta previa; postpartum hemorrhage from uterus; extensive soft tissue trauma; abortion; hyperemesis gravidarum; and adrenocortical failure (usually failure to augment steroids to cover delivery in patient receiving long-term therapy)
Volume contraction or hypotension and coagulopathy	Antepartum hemorrhage due to abruptio placentae; preeclampsia/eclampsia; amniotic fluid embolism; incompatible blood transfusion; drug reactions; acute fatty liver of pregnancy; and hemolytic uremic syndrome
Volume contraction or hypotension, coagulopathy, and infection	Septic abortion; chorioamnionitis; pyelonephritis; and puerperal sepsis
Urinary tract obstruction	Polyhydramnios; damage to ureters during cesarean section or repair of cervical/vaginal lacerations; pelvic hematoma; broad ligament hematoma; and calculus or clot in ureters primarily of single kidney

Usually, acute renal failure occurs in women with previously healthy kidneys, but it can complicate the course of patients with preexisting renal disease (Pertuiset and Grünfeld, 1994; Gaber and Lindheimer, 1999; Lindheimer and Katz, 2001).

Table 44-12 suggests an approach to patients with sudden decrements in urinary volumes, focusing on tests to differentiate acute tubular necrosis from prerenal failure. Before anuria or oliguria is ascribed to acute renal failure, obstruction to renal outflow must be excluded. Hydronephrosis leading to acute renal failure in late pregnancy can be due to obstruction, a situation that is resolvable (Khanna and Nguyen, 2001). If

delivery is not appropriate, ultrasound-guided percutaneous nephrostomy is safe and reliable (Van Sonnenberg et al., 1992). Furthermore, the urinary tract may be unwittingly damaged when surgery is performed for obstetric emergencies such as postpartum hemorrhage, which can themselves be the cause of acute renal failure.

Septic Abortion

Acute renal failure is associated with septic abortion for many reasons. Its incidence has declined markedly in areas of the world where sterile early pregnancy terminations are readily available, but it remains a major problem where such procedures are illegal or not easily obtainable as in many developing countries. Dehydration and hypotension can lead to considerable renal ischemia. Soap and some disinfectants (e.g., Lysol), common abortifacients, may have specific nephrotoxic effects. However, the marked hemolysis caused by some bacteria and chemical abortifacients is sufficient to provoke the renal shutdown. Most pregnancy sepsis is due to gram-negative bacteria, and although clostridia are responsible for only 0.5% of cases in which shock develops, it is *Clostridium* sp. that is responsible for one of the most devastating syndromes complicating gestation.

Presentation can be dramatic, with an abrupt rise in temperature (to 40° C), often associated with myalgias, vomiting, and diarrhea, the latter occasionally bloody. Once symptoms begin, hypotension, tachypnea, and progression to frank shock occur rapidly. The patient usually has jaundice, with the bronze-like color characteristic of the association of jaundice with cutaneous vasodilation, cyanosis, and pallor. Despite the presence of fever, the extremities are often cold and display purplish areas that may be precursors of small patches of necrosis on the toes, fingers, and nose. Generalized muscular pains, often most intense in the thorax and abdomen, may lead to confusion with intra-abdominal inflammatory processes; this is especially true when a history of provoked abortion is denied or not sought, because heavy vaginal bleeding is often not a prominent feature (see Chapter 45).

TABLE 44-12. DIFFERENTIAL DIAGNOSIS OF OLIGURIA

	Prerenal Failure	Acute Tubular Necrosis
History	Vomiting, diarrhea, other causes of dehydration	Dehydration, ischemic insult, ingestion of nephrotoxin; no specific history in 50% of cases
Physical examination	Decreased blood pressure, increased pulse rate, poor skin turgor	May have signs of dehydration, but physical examination often normal
Urinalysis	Concentrated urine; few formed elements on sediment, but many hyaline cases	Isosthenuria; sediment contains renal tubular cells and pigmented casts, but may be normal
Urinary sodium	<20 mEq/liter; most <10 mEq/liter	≥25, usually >60 mEq/liter
Urine-plasma (U/P) ratios	High	Low
Osmolality	Often ≥1.5	<1.1
Urea	≥20	≤3
Creatinine	>40	<15
Fractional sodium excretion ($U/P_{Na}/U/P_{creatinine}$)	<1%	>1%
Renal failure index ($U/P_{Na}/U/P_{creatinine}$)	<1	>1

From Lindheimer MD, Grünfeld J-P, Davison JM: Renal disorders. *In* Barron WM, Lindheimer MD (eds): Medical Disorders during Pregnancy. 3rd ed. St. Louis, Mosby Year Book, 2000, p. 48, with permission.

Acute Renal Failure and Preeclampsia

Preeclampsia is accompanied by a characteristic renal lesion in which the glomeruli enlarge and become ischemic because of swelling of the intracapillary cells—glomerular endotheliosis and mesangiosis. Most preeclamptic patients experience moderate decreases in GFR (Irons et al., 1997), but occasionally this decrease is accompanied by acute renal failure. The kidney failure is usually due to acute tubular necrosis, but acute cortical necrosis may also occur. It is possible that acute tubular necrosis is the obligatory outcome of glomerular cell swelling and loss of anionic change along with complete obliteration of the capillary lumen (Naicker et al., 1997) (see Chapter 43). This might be aggravated by inappropriate drug therapy, abruptio placentae, or hemorrhage in the antenatal and peripartum periods (Brown et al., 1990). If the renal failure is related solely to preeclampsia without chronic hypertension, renal disease, or both before pregnancy, long-term normal renal function is evident in about 80% of cases (Suzuki et al., 1997). Underlying chronic problems reduce this to 20%, with the rest needing long-term dialysis (Sibai et al., 1990), and perinatal mortality is increased to 40% (Drakeley et al., 2002).

Treatment should follow the standard approach (Lieberthal, 1997) (see later), with intensive hemodynamic intervention. Recently, more specific therapies for this group of patients have been tested, such as prostacyclin infusion. Interestingly, in the recent series of Drakeley and associates (2002) only 10% required temporary dialysis and there were no cases of end-stage renal failure needing permanent dialysis or renal transplant, contrasting with higher figures quoted by others, for example, 80% and 7%, respectively (Selcuk et al., 2000).

The syndrome of hemolysis, elevated liver enzymes, and low platelets (HELLP) was originally thought to be a rare complication of severe preeclampsia, but as more attention is paid to liver and hematologic functions it is now diagnosed more often (Gaber and Lindheimer, 1999). The incidence of acute renal failure with the HELLP syndrome seems to be considerably higher for that with preeclampsia in general, but this may reflect the experience of tertiary care centers that receive the most complicated cases in transfer. In one recent series of 72 women with a median maximum serum creatinine of 340 μmol/liter (3.85 mg/dL), 50% had HELLP syndrome (Drakeley et al., 2002), and in another of 39 women with renal failure (median serum creatinine of 496 μmol/liter [5.6 mg/dL]), 36% had HELLP syndrome (Selcuk et al., 2000). It is not clear, however, whether acute renal failure is a specific component of the HELLP syndrome itself or a complication of a particularly severe multisystem condition. Certainly it may occur without hemolysis (referred to by some as ELLP syndrome) (Sibai and Ramadan, 1993; Sibai et al., 1994).

Acute Renal Failure and Pyelonephritis

In the absence of complicating features, such as obstruction, calculi, papillary necrosis, and analgesic nephropathy, it is extremely rare for acute pyelonephritis to cause acute renal failure in nonpregnant subjects; however, this association appears to be more frequent in pregnant women. It is known that acute pyelonephritis in pregnancy is accompanied by decrements in GFR in contrast to test results in nonpregnant patients. It has been suggested that the vasculature in pregnancy may be more sensitive to the vasoactive effect of bacterial endotoxins.

Acute Fatty Liver of Pregnancy

Acute fatty liver of pregnancy, also called "obstetric pseudoacute yellow atrophy," is a rare complication of late pregnancy or the early postpartum period, occurring in approximately 1 in 13,000 deliveries (see Chapter 53). It is characterized by jaundice, severe hepatic dysfunction, including coma, and varying degrees of renal failure (Usta et al., 1994). It may also be associated with hypertension and with coagulation and platelet abnormalities that lead to diagnostic confusion with preeclampsia (Pertuiset and Grünfeld, 1994). In the past, tetracycline usage was associated with this condition. In addition, reversible urea cycle enzyme deficiencies (ornithine transcarbamylase and carbamoyl phosphate synthetase) resembling those seen in Reye syndrome have been described. More recently there have been reports noting that patients with acute fatty liver of pregnancy harbor a long-chain 3-hydroxy acyl-coenzyme A dehydrogenase deficiency or carry mutations of the enzyme's gene, resulting in deficiencies in the fetus (Ibdah et al., 1999). The only definitive therapy seems to be delivery, but irreversible forms still occur, and orthotopic liver transplantation may be life-saving (Ockner et al., 1990).

Idiopathic Postpartum Renal Failure

Idiopathic postpartum renal failure is also called postpartum malignant nephrosclerosis, irreversible postpartum renal failure, and postpartum hemolytic-uremic syndrome. It is a rare and frequently fatal syndrome, characterized by the onset of renal failure 3 to 10 weeks into the puerperium after the patient has had an uneventful pregnancy and delivery. The patient develops marked azotemia and severe hypertension, frequently associated with microangiopathic hemolytic anemia and platelet aggregation with formation of microthrombi in the terminal portions of the renal vasculature (Pertuiset and Grünfeld, 1994).

There is uncertainty concerning the management of this condition. The literature documents that in the past many of these patients succumbed despite treatment with dialysis, plasmapheresis, exchange transfusion, immunosuppression, heparin, streptokinase, dipyridamole, aspirin, or corticosteroids alone or combined. Others survived but required dialysis or transplantation. This literature, however, is rather dated, and mortality may be less now (Lindheimer et al., 1993). Previously, the pathology was reported as mixed kidney lesions, noted by some to resemble hemolytic uremic syndrome and by others, scleroderma kidney. It is now believed the latter is an end-stage picture of the former. Etiology remains obscure, but current thoughts relate to all theories of what causes thrombotic microangiopathies. The older literature focused on deficiencies in circulating prostacyclin, a powerful vasodilator and potent endogenous inhibitor of platelet aggregation, which may be counteracted by exchange transfusion or even plasma infusion alone. Prolonged prostacyclin infusions have been tried with the aim of restoring the deficiency, thus controlling the hypertension and reversing the platelet consumption, but such therapy remains to be proven effective. It has been argued that disseminated intravascular coagulation is significant (with placental thromboplastin being released during labor) and that antithrombin III may have a protective effect. Again, such claims are anecdotal.

Cortical Necrosis in Pregnancy

Renal cortical necrosis is an extremely rare complication that at one time seemed to be more common in pregnant than in nonpregnant populations. Most recently, its incidence during gestation has decreased to below 1 in 80,000 (Lindheimer et al., 1993). This pathologic entity is characterized by tissue death throughout the cortex, with sparing of the medullary portions. Acute cortical necrosis may develop in patients with disseminated intravascular coagulation or overwhelming septicemia, but most cases present in the third trimester or the puerperium. Multigravidas beyond age 30 years are more likely to develop cortical necrosis. The condition tends to be associated with specific obstetric complications, mainly placental abruption, unrecognized long-standing intrauterine death, and occasionally preeclampsia (Pertuiset and Grünfeld, 1994).

Although cortical necrosis may involve the entire renal cortex, resulting in irreversible renal failure, it is the "patchy" variety that occurs more often in pregnancy. This is characterized by an initial episode of severe oliguria, which lasts much longer than in uncomplicated acute tubular necrosis, followed by a variable return of function and stable period of moderate renal insufficiency (Chugh et al., 1994). Years later, for reasons still obscure, renal function may decrease again, often leading to end-stage renal failure.

Miscellaneous Causes

Acute renal failure can occur during pregnancy in a variety of situations similar to those causing sudden renal dysfunction in nonpregnant patients. These situations include (1) primary renal diseases (i.e., acute nephritis, sarcoidosis, lymphoma, and Goodpasture syndrome); (2) diseases related to systemic illnesses, such as endocarditis; (3) the ingestion of nephrotoxins; (4) incompatible transfusions; and (5) diseases in which structural infiltration of the kidneys is secondary to an extrarenal disease (Lindheimer et al., 1993; Pertuiset and Grünfeld, 1994).

The literature suggests that in some gravidas with underlying renal disease but well-preserved GFR, acute tubular necrosis can develop when pregnancy is complicated by severe superimposed preeclampsia with its intense vasoconstriction, hypovolemia, and generalized endothelial dysfunction (Sibai and Ramadan, 1993; Friedman et al., 1995). Certainly, in women with moderate to severe renal disease (serum creatinine more than 180 μmol/liter [2 mg/dL]), gestational exacerbation of renal dysfunction is common, with 10% of gravidas progressing to end-stage renal failure within a year of delivery (Jones and Hayslett, 1996). In some of the more severe cases, dialysis has to be introduced during pregnancy to "buy" time for the fetus (Jungers et al., 1997).

◼ MANAGEMENT

Treatment of sudden renal failure resembles that in nonpregnant populations and aims at retarding the appearance of uremic symptomatology, acid-base and electrolyte disturbances, and volume problems (i.e., overhydration when the patient is oliguric and dehydration during the polyuric phase) (Drakeley et al., 2002). One must also be aware of the propensity of patients with acute renal failure to acquire infection, a complication that can be serious in pregnant women. Many of the aforementioned problems respond to judicious conserv-ative management, but if such an approach is unsuccessful, dialysis will be necessary.

Dialysis in patients with acute renal failure is prescribed "prophylactically" (i.e., before the appearance of electrolyte, acidemic, or uremic symptoms). Such prophylactic dialysis appears even more necessary in prepartum patients with an immature fetus and in whom temporization is desired (Jungers and Chauveau, 1997; Hou and Firanek, 1998). Problems during dialysis peculiar to pregnancy were discussed in detail earlier.

Peritoneal dialysis is effective and safe as long as the catheter is inserted high in the abdomen under direct vision through a small incision. In fact, as discussed earlier, chronic ambulatory peritoneal dialysis may become the preferred dialysis approach in the prepartum woman because it minimizes rapid metabolic perturbations. Volume shifts during hemodialysis should be minimized to avoid impairment of uteroplacental blood flow.

Controlled anticoagulation with heparin (preferably including monitoring to verify that activated clotting time is maintained between 150 and 180 seconds) is desirable during hemodialysis. Observation for vaginal bleeding is also important.

As discussed previously, premature contractions or the onset of labor frequently occurs during or immediately after dialysis. Therefore, when possible, early delivery (as dictated by fetal maturity) should be undertaken. Blood losses should be replaced quickly to the point of overtransfusing slightly, because in the pregnant patient uterine bleeding may be concealed and thus underestimated. When delivery is imminent, nursery personnel should be advised that the neonate could be subject to rapid dehydration because of increased fetal levels of urea and other solutes that precipitate an osmotic diuresis shortly after birth.

◼ SUMMARY

Changes in the urinary tract during normal pregnancy are so marked that norms in the nonpregnant state cannot be used for obstetric management. Awareness of all alterations is essential if kidney problems in pregnancy are to be suspected or detected and then handled correctly.

Most women with mild and moderate renal disease tolerate pregnancy well and have a successful obstetric outcome without adverse effect on the natural history of the underlying renal lesion. Crucial determinants are renal functional status at conception, the presence or absence of hypertension, and the type of renal disease. There have been disagreements regarding pregnancy outcome in the presence of focal glomerular sclerosis, IgA nephropathy, mesangioproliferative glomerulonephritis, and reflux disease, although again the evidence seems to trend in favor of the functional status before pregnancy approach. Patients with certain collagen disorders (especially periarteritis nodosa and scleroderma) do poorly. In general, prognosis is good if renal dysfunction is minimal and hypertension is absent. We reiterate, however, that these guidelines are based primarily on retrospective evidence, there being a crucial need for prospective data.

Pregnancy in women receiving dialysis treatment can be excessively complicated. Increased frequency and duration of dialysis are needed. There is high fetal wastage at all stages of pregnancy.

In the absence of severe maternal problems, the hazards of pregnancy in renal transplant patients are minimal, and successful obstetric outcome is the rule. Acute obstetric renal failure can occur in women with previously healthy kidneys. Pathology peculiar to pregnancy must always be considered.

REFERENCES

Note: Citations here are focused on the literature appearing after 1990, often other more focused reviews. The reader may refer to previous editions of this book as well as Lindheimer MD, Katz AI: Renal physiology and disease in pregnancy. In Seldin DW, Giebisch G (eds): The Kidney: Pathology and Pathophysiology, 3rd ed. Philadelphia, Lippincott Williams & Wilkins, 1999, p. 2597, for more extensive citations and a guide to the older literature.

Abe S: Pregnancy in glomerulonephritic patients with decreased renal function. Hypertens Pregn **15**:305, 1996.

Ahlswede KM, Armenti VT, Morkritz MJ: Premature births in female transplant recipients: Degree and effect of immunosuppressive regimen. Surg Forum **443**:524, 1992.

Algari MA, Sararinejad MR, et al: Extracorporeal shock wave lithotripsy of renal calculi during early pregnancy. Br J Urol **84**:615, 1999.

Andrews PA: Renal transplantation. BMJ **324**:530, 2002.

Armenti VT, Ahlswede KM, Ahlswede BA, et al: National Transplantation Pregnancy Registry—Outcome of 154 pregnancies in cyclosporine-treated female kidney transplant recipients. Transplant **57**:502, 1994.

Armenti VT, Moritz MJ, Davison JM: Medical management of the pregnant transplant recipient. Adv Ren Replace Ther **5**:14, 1998.

Armenti VT, Moritz MJ, Radomski JS, et al: Pregnancy and transplantation. Graft **3**:59, 2000.

Armenti VT, Radomski JS, Moritz MJ, et al: Report from the National Transplantation Pregnancy Registry (NTPR): Outcomes of pregnancy after transplantation. In Cecka JM, Terasaki PI (eds): Clinical Transplants. Los Angeles, UCLA Immunogenetics Center, 2002, p. 97.

Asrat T, Roossin MC, Miller EI: Ultrasonographic detection of ureteral jets in normal pregnancy. Am J Obstet Gynecol **178**:1194, 1998.

Auzary C, Le Thi Huong D, Wechsler B, et al: Pregnancy in patients with Wegener's granulomatosis: Report of 5 cases in 3 women. Ann Rheum Dis **59**:800, 2000.

Bachman JW, Heise RH, Naessens JM: A study of various tests to detect asymptomatic urinary tract infections in an obstetric population. JAMA **270**:1971, 1993.

Bagon JA, Vernaeve H, De Muylder X, et al: Pregnancy and dialysis. Am J Kidney Dis **31**:756, 1998.

Bar J, Ben-Rafael Z, Padoa A, et al: Prediction of pregnancy outcome in subgroups of women with renal disease. Clin Nephrol **53**:437, 2000.

Baxter GM, Rodger RSC: Doppler ultrasound in renal transplantation. Nephrol Dial Transplant **12**:2449, 1997.

Baylis C: Glomerular filtration and volume regulation in gravid animal models. Baillieres Clin Obstet Gynaecol **1**:789, 1994.

Baylis C, Davison JM: The normal renal physiological changes which occur during pregnancy. In Davison AM, Cameron JS, Grünfeld, J-P, et al (eds): Oxford Textbook of Clinical Nephrology, 2nd ed. Oxford, Oxford University Press, 1998, p. 2297.

Blowey DL, Warady BA: Neonatal outcome in pregnancies associated with renal replacement therapy. Adv Ren Replace Ther **5**:45, 1998.

Braga J, Marques R, Blanco A, et al: Maternal and perinatal implications of the use of recombinant erythropoietin. Acta Obstet Gynaecol Scand **75**:449, 1996.

Brookhyser J, Wiggins K: Medical nutrition in pregnancy and kidney disease. Adv Ren Replace Ther **5**:53, 1998.

Brown MA: Urinary tract dilation in pregnancy. Am J Obstet Gynecol **164**:641, 1990.

Brown MA, Child RP, O'Connor M, et al: Pregnancy-induced hypertension and renal failure: Clinical importance of diuretics, plasma volume and vasospasm. Aust N Z J Obstet Gynaecol **30**:230, 1990.

Bucholz N-P, Biyabani MR, et al: Urolithiasis in pregnancy—A clinical challenge. Eur J Obstet Gynaecol Reprod Biol **80**:25, 1998.

Butler EL, Cox SM, Eberts EG, et al: Symptomatic nephrolithiasis complicating pregnancy. Obstet Gynecol **96**:753, 2000.

Calvet JP, Grantham JJ: The genetics and physiology of polycystic kidney disease. Semin Nephrol **21**:107, 2001.

Castillo AA, Lew SQ, Smith AM: Women's issues in female patients receiving peritoneal dialysis. Adv Renal Repl Ther **6**:327, 1999.

Chan WS, Okun N, Kjellstrand CM: Pregnancy in chronic dialysis: A review of the literature. Int J Artif Organs **21**:259, 1998.

Chapman AB, Johnson AM, Gabow PA: Pregnancy outcome and its relationship to progression of renal failure in autosomal dominant polycystic renal disease. J Am Soc Nephrol **5**:1178, 1994.

Chugh KS, Singhal PC, Kher VK: Acute renal cortical necrosis: A study of 113 patients. Ren Fail **16**:37, 1994.

Cowchock FS, Reece EA, Bulasan D, et al: Repeated fetal losses associated with antiphospholipid antibodies: A collaborative randomized trial comparing prednisone with low dose heparin treatment. Am J Obstet Gynecol **166**:1318, 1992.

Cox SM, Shelburne P, Mason RA, et al: Mechanisms of hemolysis and anemia associated with acute antepartum pyelonephritis. Am J Obstet Gynecol **164**:587, 1991.

Crowe AV, Rustom R, Gradden C, et al: Pregnancy does not adversely affect renal transplant function. Q J Med **92**:631,1999.

Cunningham FG, Cox SM, Harstad TW, et al: Chronic renal disease and pregnancy outcome. Am J Obstet Gynecol **163**:453, 1990.

Davison JM: Renal complications in pregnancy. In Zuspan FP, Quilligan EJ (eds): Handbook of Obstetrics, Gynecology and Primary Care. St. Louis, Mosby, 1998a, p. 358.

Davison JM: Renal complications that may occur in pregnancy. In Davison AM, Cameron JS, Grünfeld J-P, et al (eds): Oxford Textbook of Clinical Nephrology, 2nd ed. Oxford, Oxford University Press, 1998b, p. 2317.

Davison JM: Renal disorders in pregnancy. Curr Opin Obstet Gynecol **13**:19, 2001.

Davison JM, Baylis C: Pregnancy in patients with underlying renal disease. In Davison AM, Cameron JC, Grunfeld J-P, et al (eds): Oxford Textbook of Clinical Nephrology, 2nd ed. Oxford, Oxford University Press, 1998, p. 2327.

Davison JM, Redman CWG: Pregnancy post-transplant: The establishment of a U.K. Registry. Br J Obstet Gynaecol **104**:1106, 1997.

Dayoan ES, Diman LL, Boylen CT: Successful treatment of Wegener's granulomatosis during pregnancy: A case report and review of the medical literature. Chest **113**:836, 1998.

Delakas D, Karyotis I, Loumbakis P: Ureteral drainage by double-J-catheters during pregnancy. Clin Exp Obstet Gynecol **27**:200, 2000.

Dempsey C, Harrison RF, Maloney A: Characteristics of bacteriuria in a homogenous maternity hospital population. Eur J Obstet Gynaecol Reprod Biol **44**:189, 1992.

Dimeny E, Fellström B: Metabolic abnormalities in renal transplant recipients: Risk factors and prediction of graft dysfunction? Nephrol Dial Transplant **12**:21, 1997.

Drakeley AJ, Le Roux PA, Anthony J, et al: Acute renal failure complicating severe preeclampsia requiring admission to an obstetric intensive care unit. Am J Obstet Gynecol **186**:253, 2002.

Easterling TR, Brateng D, Goldman ML, et al: Renal vascular hypertension during pregnancy. Obstet Gynecol **78**:921, 1991.

Ehrich JHH, Loirat C, Davison JM, et al: Repeated successful pregnancies after kidney transplantation in 102 women. Nephrol Dial Transplant **11**:1312, 1996.

Ekban P, Damm P, et al: Pregnancy outcome in Type 1 diabetic women with microalbuminuria. Diabet Care **24**:1739, 2001.

European Best Practice Guidelines for Renal Transplantation: Pregnancy. Nephrol Dial Transpl **17**(Suppl 4):50, 2002.

Evans H, Wollin TA: The management of urinary calculi in pregnancy. Curr Opin Urol **11**:379,2001.

Fainaru O, Almog B, Gamzu R, et al: The management of symptomatic hydronephrosis. Brit J Obstet Gynaecol **109**:1385, 2002.

Falk RJ: Treatment of lupus nephritis. N Engl J Med **343**:1182, 2000.

First MR, Combs CA, Weiskittel P, et al: Lack of effect of pregnancy on renal allograft survival or function. Transplantation **59**:472, 1995.

Frassetto L, Schoenfeld PY, Humphreys MH: Increasing incidence of human immuno-deficiency virus-associated nephropathy at San Francisco Hospital. Am J Kidney Dis **18**:655, 1991.

Friedman SA, Schiff E, Emeis JJ, et al: Biochemical corroboration of endothelial involvement in severe preeclampsia. Am J Obstet Gynecol **172**:202, 1995.

Gaber LW, Lindheimer MD: Pathology of the kidney, liver and brain. In Lindheimer MD, Roberts JM, Cunningham FG (eds): Chesley's Hypertensive Disorders in Pregnancy, 2nd ed. Stamford, Conn, Appleton & Lange, 1999, p. 231.

Gabow PA: Autosomal dominant polycystic kidney disease. N Engl J Med **329**:332, 1993.

Gaughan WJ, Moritz MJ, Radomski JS, et al: National Transplantation Pregnancy Registry: Report on outcomes in cyclosporine-treated female kidney recipients with an interval from transplant to pregnancy of greater than 5 years. Am J Kidney Dis **28**:266, 1996.

Ghandour FZ, Knauss TC, Hricik DE: Immunosuppressive drugs in pregnancy. Adv Ren Replace Ther **5**:31,1998.

Gilstrap LS, Ramin SM: Urinary tract infections during pregnancy. Obstet Gynecol Clin **28**:581, 2001.

Goluszko P, Niesel D, Nowicki B, et al: Dr operon-associated invasiveness of *Escherichia coli* from pregnant patients with pyelonephritis. Infect Immun **69**:4678, 2001.

Gordon M, Landon MB, Samuels P, et al: Perinatal outcome and long term follow up associated with modern management of diabetic nephropathy. Obstet Gynecol **87**:401, 1996.

Graham JC, Leathart JBS, Keegan SJ, et al: Analysis of *Escherichia coli* strains causing bacteriuria during pregnancy: Selection for strains that do not express type 1 fimbriae. Infect Immun **69**:794, 2001.

Harber MA, Tso A, et al: Wegener's granulomatosis in pregnancy—The therapeutic dilemma. Nephrol Dial Transplant **14**:1789, 1999.

Hart A, Nowicki BJ, Reisner B, et al: Ampicillin-resistant *Escherichia coli* in gestational pyelonephritis: Increased occurrence and association with the colonization faction Dr adhesin. J Infect Dis **183**:1526, 2001.

Hayslett JP: The effect of systemic lupus erythematosus on pregnancy and pregnancy outcome. Am J Reprod Immunol **28**:199, 1992.

Hayslett JP, Reece EA: Managing diabetic patients with nephropathy and other vascular complications. Baillieres Clin Obstet Gynaecol **8**:405, 1994.

Heybourne KD, Schultz MF, Goodlin RC, et al: Renal artery stenosis during pregnancy: A review. Obstet Gynecol Surv **46**:509, 1991.

Hill DE, Chantigan PM, Kramer SA: Pregnancy after augmentation cystoplasty. Surg Gynecol Obstet **170**:485, 1990.

Hod M, van Dijk DJ, Karp M, et al: Diabetic nephropathy and pregnancy: The effect of ACE inhibitors prior to pregnancy on fetomaternal outcome. Nephrol Dial Transplant **10**:2328, 1995.

Hou S: Pregnancy in women treated with dialysis. Saudi J Kid Dis Transplant **8**:3, 1997.

Hou S: Pregnancy in chronic renal insufficiency and end stage renal disease. Am J Kidney Dis **32**:235, 1999.

Hou S, Firanek C: Management of the pregnant dialysis patient. Adv Ren Replace Ther **5**:24, 1998.

Hussey MJ, Pombar X: Obstetric care for renal allograft recipients or for women treated with hemodialysis or peritoneal dialysis during pregnancy. Adv Ren Replace Ther **5**:3, 1998.

Ibdah JA, Bennett MJ, et al: A fetal fatty-acid oxidation disorder as a cause of liver disease in pregnant women. N Engl J Med **340**:1723, 1999.

Irons DW, Baylis PH, Butler TJ, et al: Atrial natriuretic peptide in preeclampsia: Metabolic clearance, sodium excretion and renal hemodynamics. Am J Physiol **273**:F483, 1997.

Jones DC, Hayslett JP: Outcome of pregnancy in women with moderate or severe renal insufficiency. N Engl J Med **335**:226, 1996.

Jungers P, Chauveau D: Pregnancy in renal disease. Kidney Int **52**:871, 1997.

Jungers P, Chauveau G, Choukroun, et al: Pregnancy in women with impaired renal function. Nephrol **47**:281, 1997.

Jungers P, Houillier P, Chauveau D, et al: Pregnancy in women with reflux nephropathy. Kidney Int **50**:593, 1996.

Kainz A, Harabacz I, Cowlrick IS, et al: Analysis of 100 pregnancy outcomes in women treated systemically with tacrolimus. Transpl Int **13**:S299, 2000.

Khanna N, Nguyen H: Reversible acute renal failure in association with bilateral ureteral obstruction and hydronephrosis in pregnancy. Am J Obstet Gynecol **184**:239, 2001.

Krane K, Cuccazella A: Acute renal insufficiency in pregnancy: A review of 30 cases. J Matern Fetal Med **4**:12, 1995.

Le Thi Huong D, Wechsler B, Piette JC, et al: Pregnancy and its outcome in systemic lupus erythematosus. Q J Med **87**:721, 1994.

Le Thi Huong D, Wechsler B, Vauthier-Brouzes D, et al: Pregnancy in past or present lupus nephritis: A study of 32 pregnancies from a single center. Ann Rheum **60**:599, 2001.

Leguizaman G, Reece EA: Effect of medical therapy on progressive nephropathy: Influence of pregnancy, diabetes and hypertension. J Matern Fetal Med **9**:70, 2000.

Lessan-Pezeshki M: Pregnancy after renal transplantation: points to consider. Nephrol Dial Transplant **17**:703, 2002.

Lieberthal W: Biology of acute renal failure: Therapeutic implications. Kidney Int **52**:1102, 1997.

Lindheimer MD, Davison JM, Katz AI: The kidney and hypertension in pregnancy: twenty exciting years. Semin Nephrol **21**:173, 2001.

Lindheimer MD, Grünfeld J-P, Davison JM: Renal disorders. *In* Barron WM, Lindheimer MD (eds): Medical Disorders During Pregnancy, 2nd ed. St. Louis, Mosby, 2000, p. 39.

Lindheimer MD, Katz AI: Gestation in women with kidney disease: Prognosis and management. Baillieres Clin Obstet Gynecol **8**:387, 1994.

Lindheimer MD, Katz AI: Renal physiology and disease in pregnancy. *In* Seldin DW, Giebisch G (eds): The Kidney: Pathology and Pathophysiology, 3rd ed. Philadelphia, Lippincott, Williams & Wilkins, 1999, p. 281.

Lindheimer MD, Katz AI: The normal and diseased kidney in pregnancy. *In* Disease of the Kidney. 7th ed. Schrier RW (ed): Philadelphia, Lippincott, Williams & Wilkins 2001, p. 2129.

Lindheimer MD, Katz AL, Ganeval D, et al: Acute renal failure in pregnancy. *In* Brenner BM, Lazarus JM (eds): Acute Renal Failure, 3rd ed. New York, Churchill Livingstone, 1993.

Lindheimer MD, Roberts JM, Cunningham FG: Chesley's Hypertensive Disorders in Pregnancy, 2nd ed. Stamford, Conn, Appleton & Lange, 1999.

Little MA, Abraham KA, Kavanagh J, et al: Pregnancy in Irish renal transplant recipients. I. The cyclosporine era. Ir J Med Sci **169**:19, 2000.

Lockshin MD, Sammaratino LR: Rheumatic disease. *In* Barron WM, Lindheimer MD (eds): Medical Disorders During Pregnancy, 2nd ed. St. Louis, Mosby, 2000, p. 355.

Lockwood GM, Ledger WL, Barlow DH: Successful pregnancy outcome in a renal transplant patient following in-vitro fertilization. Hum Reprod **10**:1528, 1995.

Magee LA, van Dadeszen P, Darley J, et al: Erythropoiesis and renal transplant pregnancy. Clin Transplant **14**:127, 2000.

Malik GH, Al-Wakeel JS, Shaikh JF, et al: Three successive pregnancies in a patient on haemodialysis. Nephrol Dial Transplant **12**:144, 1997.

Martinell J, Jodal U, Lidiu-Janson G: Pregnancies in women with and without renal scarring after urinary infections in childhood. Br Med J **300**:840, 1990.

Maruyama H, Arakawa M: Diagnostic clue in haemodialysis patients: Progressive anaemia resistant to erythropoetin. J Am Soc Nephrol **8**:A1130, 1997.

McDermott S, Callaghan W, Szwejbka L, et al: Urinary tract infections during pregnancy and mental retardation and developmental delay. Obstet Gynecol **96**:113, 2000.

McGladdery SL, Aparicio S, Verrier-Jones K: Outcome of pregnancy in an Oxford-Cardiff cohort of women with previous bacteriuria. Q J Med **83**:533, 1992.

Milne JEC, Lindheimer MD, Davison JM: Glomerular heteroporous membrane modeling in third trimester and post partum before and during amino acid infusion. Am J Physiol **282**:F170, 2002.

Morgan SH, Grünfeld JP (eds): Inherited Disorders of the Kidney. Oxford, Oxford University Press, 1998.

Mussalli GM, Callaghan W, Szwejbka L, et al: Preterm delivery in mice with renal abscess. Obstet Gynecol **95**:453, 2000.

Naicker T, Randeree IGH, Moodley J, et al: Correlation between histological changes and loss of anionic change of the glomerular basement membrane in early onset pre-eclampsia. Nephron **75**:201, 1997.

Newstead CG: Tacrolimus in renal transplantation. Nephrol Dial Transplant **12**:1342, 1997.

Newstead CG: Assessment of risk of cancer after renal transplantation. Lancet **351**:610, 1998.

Nielson FR, Rasmussen PE: Hydronephrosis during pregnancy: 4 cases of hydronephrosis causing symptoms during pregnancy. Eur J Obstet Gynaecol Reprod Biol **3**:245, 1998.

Nojima M, Ihana H, Ichikawa Y, et al: Influence of pregnancy on graft function after renal transplantation. Transplant Proc **28**:1582, 1996.

Nyberg G, Haljamee M, et al: Breast feeding during treatment with cyclosporin. Transplantation **65**:253, 1998.

Nzerue CM, Hewan-Lowe K, Nwawka C: Acute renal failure in pregnancy: A review of clinical outcomes at an inner city hospital from 1986–1996. J Natl Med Assoc **90**:486, 1998.

Ockner SA, Brunt EM, Cohen SM: Fulminant hepatic failure caused by acute fatty liver of pregnancy treated by orthoptic liver transplantation. Hepatology **11**:59, 1990.

Okundaye IB, Abrinko P, Hou SH: Registry of pregnancy in dialysis patients. Am J Kidney Dis **31**:766, 1998.

Oosterhof H, Navis CJ, Go JG, et al: Pregnancy in patients on haemodialysis: Fetal monitoring by Doppler velocimetry of the umbilical artery. Br J Obstet Gynaecol **100**:1140, 1993.

Owda AK, Abdalla AH, Al-Sulaiman MH, et al: No evidence of functional deterioration of renal graft after repeated pregnancies—A report on 3 women with 17 pregnancies. Nephrol Dial Transplant **13**:1281, 1998.

Parmar MS: Chronic renal disease. BMJ **325**:85, 2002.

Pedler SJ, Orr KE: Bacterial, fungal and parasitic infections. *In* Barron WM, Lindheimer MS (eds): Medical Disorders during Pregnancy, 3rd ed. St. Louis, Mosby, 2000, p. 411.

Pergola PE, Kancharla A, Riley DJ: Kidney transplantation during the first trimester of pregnancy: Immunosuppression with mycophenolate mofetil, tacrolimus and prednisone. Transplantation **71**:994, 2001.

Pertuiset N, Grünfeld J-P: Acute renal failure in pregnancy. Baillieres Clin Obstet Gynaecol **8**:333, 1994.

Petri M: Systemic lupus erythematosus and pregnancy. Rheum Dis Clin North Am **20**:87, 1994.

Purdy LP, Hantsch CE, Molitch ME, et al: Effect of pregnancy on renal function in patients with moderate-to-severe diabetic renal insufficiency. Diabetes Care **19**:1067, 1996.

Rao TK: Human immunodeficiency virus infection and renal failure. Infect Dis Clin North Am **15**:833,2001.

Reeders ST, Zerres K, Jal A, et al: Prenatal diagnosis of autosomal dominant polycystic kidney disease with a DNA probe. Lancet **327**:6, 1986.

Report of the National High Blood Pressure Education Program Working Group on high blood pressure in pregnancy. Am J Obstet Gynecol **183**:S1, 2000.

Romão JE, Luders C, Kahhale S, et al: Pregnancy in women on chronic dialysis. Nephron **78**:416, 1998.

Sanchez-Ramos L, McAlpine KJ, Adair D, et al: Pyelonephritis in pregnancy: Once-a-day ceftriaxone versus multiple doses of cefazolin. Am J Obstet Gynecol **172**:129, 1995.

Satin SA, Seikin GL, Cunningham FG: Reversible hypertension in pregnancy caused by obstructive uropathy. Obstet Gynecol **81**:823, 1993.

Schmidt RJ, Holley JL: Fertility and contraception in end-stage renal disease. Adv Ren Replace Ther **5**:38, 1998.

Scott JR, Branch DW, Holman J: Autoimmune and pregnancy complications in the daughter of a kidney transplant patient. Transplantation **73**:815, 2002.

Selcuk, Odbas AR, Cetinkaya R, et al: Outcome of pregnancies with HELLP syndrome complicated by acute renal failure (1989–1999). Renal Failure **22**:319, 2000.

Shapiro R: Tacrolimus in renal transplantation—A review. Graft **3**:64, 2000.

Shelton SD, Boggess KA, et al: Urinary interleukin-8 with asymptomatic bacteriuria in pregnancy. Obstet Gynecol **97**:583, 2001.

Shokeir AA, Makran MR, Abdulmaaboud M: Renal colic in pregnancy women: role of renal resistive index. Urology **55**:344, 2000.

Sibai BM, Kusterman L, Velasco J: Current understanding of severe preeclampsia, pregnancy-associated hemolytic uremic syndrome, thrombotic thrombocytopenic purpura, hemolysis, elevated liver enzymes and low platelet syndrome and postpartum acute renal failure: Different clinical syndromes or just different names. Curr Opin Nephrol Hypertens **3**:436, 1994.

Sibai BM, Ramadan M: Acute renal failure in pregnancies complicated by hemolysis, elevated liver enzymes and low platelets. Am J Obstet Gynecol **168**:1682, 1993.

Sibai BM, Villar MA, Mabie BC: Acute renal failure in hypertensive disorders of pregnancy: Pregnancy outcome and remote prognosis in 31 consecutive cases. Am J Obstet Gynecol **162**:777, 1990.

Stamm WE, McKevitt M, Roberts PL, et al: Natural history of recurrent urinary tract infections in women. Rev Infect Dis **13**:77, 1991.

Stanley CW, Gottlieb R, Zager J, et al: Developmental well-being in offspring of women receiving cyclosporine post-renal transplant. Transplant Proc **31**:241, 1999.

Steen VD: Pregnancy in women with systemic sclerosis. Obstet Gynecol **94**:15, 1999.

Stehman-Breen C, Miller L, et al: Preeclampsia and premature labour among pregnant women with haematuria. Paediatr Perinatal Epidemiol **14**:136, 2000.

Stotland NL, Stotland NE: The mother and the burning building. Obstet Gynecol Surv **53**:1, 1997.

Sturgiss SN, Davison JM: Perinatal outcome in renal allograft recipients: Prognostic significance of hypertension and renal function before and during pregnancy. Obstet Gynecol **78**:573, 1991.

Sturgiss SN, Davison JM: Effect of pregnancy on long-term function of renal allografts. Am J Kidney Dis **26**:54, 1995.

Suzuki S, Gejyo F, Ogino S, et al: Post-partum renal lesions in women with pre-eclampsia. Nephrol Dial Transplant **12**:2488, 1997.

Szczech LA, Gange SJ, Van der Horst C, et al: Predictors of proteinuria and renal failure among women with HIV infection. Kidney Int **61**:195, 2002.

Thorp JA, Davis BE, Klingele C: Severe early onset pre-eclampsia secondary to bilateral ureteral obstruction reversed by stenting. Obstet Gynecol **94**:806, 1999.

Toma H, Tanabe K, Tokumoto T, et al: A nationwide survey on pregnancies in women on renal replacement therapy in Japan. Nephrol Dial Transplant **13**:A163, 1999.

Twickler D, Little BB, Satin AJ, et al: Renal pelvicalyceal dilatation in antepartum pyelonephritis: Ultrasonographic findings. Am J Obstet Gynecol **165**:1115, 1994.

Uribe LG, Thakur VD, Krane NK: Steroid-responsive nephrotic syndrome with renal insufficiency in the first trimester of pregnancy. Am J Obstet Gynecol **164**:568, 1991.

Usta IM, Barton JR, Amon EA, et al: Acute fatty liver of pregnancy: An experience in the diagnosis and management of fourteen cases. Am J Obstet Gynecol **171**:1342, 1994.

Vora M, Gruslin A: Erythropoietin in obstetrics. Obstet Gynecol Surv **53**:500, 1998.

Willis FR, Findlay CA, et al: Children of renal transplant recipient mothers. J Paediatr Child Health **36**:230, 2000.

Wilson GA, Coscia LA, McGrory CH, et al: National Transplantation Pregnancy Registry: Postpregnancy graft loss among female pancreas-kidney recipients. Transplant Proc **33**:1667, 2001.

Wing DA, Hendershott CM, Debuque L, et al: Outpatient treatment of acute pyelonephritis in pregnancy after 24 weeks. Obstet Gynecol **94**:683, 1999.

Wolf MC, Hollander JB, Salisz JA: A new technique of ureteral stent placement during pregnancy using endoluminal ultrasound. Surg Gynecol Obstet **175**:575, 1992.

Wrenshall LE, McHugh L, Felton P, et al: Pregnancy after donor nephrectomy. Transplantation **62**:1934, 1996.

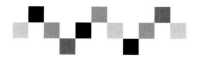

Chapter 45

INTENSIVE CARE MONITORING OF THE CRITICALLY ILL PREGNANT PATIENT

Bernard Gonik, MD, and Michael Raymond Foley, MD

As the field of obstetrics and gynecology continues to develop, physicians have become more aware of the need for a better understanding of critical care medicine as it applies to obstetrics (Mabie and Sibai, 1990). This issue is not based on the fact that maternal mortality is increasing in the United States or Europe, because demographic statistics demonstrate dramatic decreases in maternal mortality over the past 50 years. Neither does this approach advocate the exclusion of other traditional health care providers in the area of critical care medicine. However, it does point out that the gravid patient who becomes critically ill is best served by individuals who appreciate both maternal and fetal physiology, in addition to those needs associated with the acute medical or surgical pathologic condition at hand.

This chapter addresses basic critical care monitoring in obstetrics and specifically discusses conditions in which more intensive care management of the pregnant patient may be indicated.

MATERNAL MORTALITY

Maternal mortality is defined as the number of maternal deaths (direct and indirect) per 100,000 live births. Direct obstetric deaths result primarily from hypertensive disorders of pregnancy, hemorrhage, sepsis, and thromboembolic phenomenon. Indirect obstetric deaths arise from preexisting medical conditions including, but not limited to, diabetes, systemic lupus erythematosus, asthma, and heart disease aggravated by the physiologic changes of pregnancy. This vital statistic is periodically surveyed by various local, state, and national agencies. Because these maternal mortality committees frequently use death certificates as their only database, some have suggested that these numbers underestimate this mortality rate by as much as 20% to 50% (Kaunitz et al., 1985; Atrash et al., 1995). Variations in the definition of "maternal" death, medicolegal concerns, and physicians untrained in the proper completion of death certificates further confuse these investigations. To address these concerns, the Division of Reproductive Health at the Centers for Disease Control and Prevention, in collaboration with the American College of Obstetricians and Gynecologists (ACOG) and state health departments, began in 1987 to systematically collect these data in the Pregnancy-Related Mortality Surveillance System.

Mortality rates have declined in the United States over the last two decades (Fig. 45-1) (Atrash et al., 1990). Although this is true for all races, wide discrepancies still exist between white and nonwhite populations. These differences have been attributed mainly to socioeconomic factors limiting adequacy of health care for minority groups (Centers for Disease Control and Prevention, 1995). Geographic differences also appear to exist in maternal mortality. Rates are highest in the South and lowest in the Western states. Here again, racial differences within each region of the United States appear to be the factor influencing these discrepancies. More recently, Berg and colleagues (1996) reported a modest rise in maternal mortality from 1987 to 1990. They attributed some of this increase to better ascertainment of data collected prospectively and to the use of multiple source documents. The currently reported overall maternal mortality rate for the United States is 7.7 per 100,000 (5.3 per 100,000 for whites, 19.6 per 100,000 for African Americans) (Centers for Disease Control and Prevention, 1999).

Advanced maternal age is a recognized risk factor for death. This phenomenon appears to be a result of the increased age-associated incidence of chronic illnesses, such as hypertension, diabetes, and obesity, rather than age alone. In addition, advancing age is usually accompanied by increasing parity, which is associated with an increased incidence of abruptio placentae, placenta previa, and uterine rupture.

Variables related to health care delivery systems, such as hospital size, have also been correlated with maternal mortality. Both very large delivery services and very small obstetric units are associated with higher maternal death rates compared with medium-sized institutions. The underlying reasons for these discrepancies in mortality rates are distinctly different. For larger hospitals, patients tend to come from higher risk groups (i.e., African Americans, tertiary care referrals, and so on). As for smaller hospitals, less sophisticated blood banking facilities and limited intensive care technology make them less able to handle acute life-threatening conditions.

Figure 45-2 demonstrates cause-specific pregnancy-related mortality ratios for two time periods (Berg et al., 1996). As can be seen, the most commonly identified causes of death were obstetric hemorrhage, embolism, hypertensive disease, and infection. Although most causes declined between the two study periods, ratios for deaths because of infection and cardiomyopathy increased by approximately 36% and 70%, respectively.

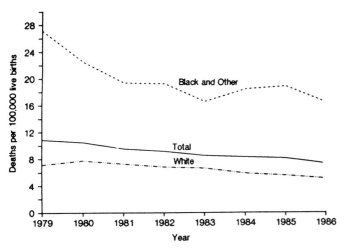

FIGURE 45-1 ■ Maternal mortality rates in the United States, 1979–1986. (From Atrash HK, Koonin LM, Lawson HW, et al: Maternal mortality in the United States, 1979–1986. Obstet Gynecol **76:**1055, 1990.)

CRITICAL CARE FACILITIES ON AN OBSTETRIC UNIT

Recent advances in critical care medical knowledge and instrumentation have influenced many directors of obstetric services to develop full cardiovascular hemodynamic monitoring capabilities within their labor and delivery suites or in nearby special care units. Because these special facilities are located on the obstetric ward, one is able to provide intensive fetal surveillance in addition to maternal care equivalent to that of most medical or surgical intensive care units. Precise information regarding which patients would most benefit from admission to these units has yet to be established (Mabie and Sibai, 1990).

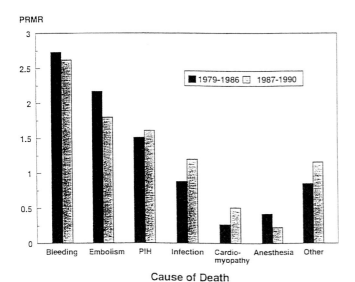

FIGURE 45-2 ■ Cause-specific pregnancy-related mortality ratios (per 100,000 live births). (From Berg CJ, Atrash HK, Koonin LM, et al: Pregnancy related mortality in the United States, 1987–1990. Obstet Gynecol **88:**161, 1996.)

The overall dimensions of a room designated for this purpose need to be large to accommodate large pieces of monitoring equipment, along with the expectation that many members of the management team may be in the room at any given time. In addition, it is necessary that capabilities be available within the room or nearby for emergency cesarean section. If a vaginal delivery is anticipated, this should be performed within the intensive care room itself to minimize the need for switching monitors or transporting the critically ill patient.

The basic monitoring equipment should preferably include a hemodynamics unit, oscilloscope, pressure transducers, electrocardiograph module, a cardiac output (CO) computer, and a pulse oximeter. Although direct oscilloscopic or digital display readings are usually adequate, a hard-copy chart recorder may be desirable for evaluating complex pressure tracings or for times when a patient's respiratory efforts add too much variation to the displayed values. The fetal surveillance equipment should include capabilities for both external and internal heart rate monitoring along with pressure transducer tracings. A hand-held or desktop computer can be programmed to calculate extrapolated hemodynamic variables. A pH/blood gas analyzer, co-oximeter, and oncometer are also preferred to complete the hemodynamic requirements of the unit. Most often, these latter pieces of equipment do not need to be individually purchased if the institution has an established emergency laboratory facility.

The most important component to the successful operation of a critical care unit is adequate health care provider training. Nursing supervisory staff should designate individuals from each work shift interested in working in these units. Training should include critical care patient management, Swan-Ganz data interpretation, and equipment maintenance. Frequently, this requires periodic assignments to the surgical or medical intensive care units of the hospital. Refresher courses to maintain these skills should also be planned at regular intervals, depending on the amount of utilization of the facility.

INVASIVE HEMODYNAMIC MONITORING

Indications for Pulmonary Artery Catheterization

Current indications for the use of invasive pulmonary artery catheterization in obstetrics are based on individual experiences and empirical thinking. Controlled trials evaluating this new technology in the management of the critically ill pregnant woman have yet to be carried out. These comparisons may never be made because of the limited clinical exposure to these types of patients in obstetrics and because too many confounding variables exist to make meaningful comparisons possible. Robin (1985) pointed out that invasive monitoring should be used in the clinical setting only when the data obtained will specifically influence acute management; too often this tenet is not followed.

The lack of clearly supportive literature mandates caution and selective application; however, the following include suggested indications for invasive monitoring of the obstetric patient (ACOG, 1992):

1. Hypovolemic shock that is unresponsive to initial volume resuscitation attempts
2. Septic shock when vasopressor therapy is needed

3. Pregnancy-induced hypertension complicated by unresponsive oliguria
4. Ineffective intravenous antihypertensive therapy
5. Adult respiratory distress syndrome requiring ventilatory support.
6. Cardiac disease, class 3 or 4, in labor or requiring surgery
7. Anaphylactoid syndrome of pregnancy (amniotic fluid embolism)
8. Isolated primary or secondary pulmonary hypertension in labor or during surgery (selective application)
9. Pulmonary edema, from any etiology, that is unresponsive to initial therapy

Central venous pressure (CVP) monitoring should not be considered equivalent to pulmonary artery catheter monitoring. Data evaluating the relationship between serial CVP measurements and pulmonary capillary wedge pressure (PCWP) readings in severe pregnancy-induced hypertension are shown in Figure 45-3 (Cotton et al., 1985a). Although statistically a linear relationship was noted, there was large variation in PCWP between patients for a given CVP measurement. For instance, a CVP reading of 8 mm Hg might be associated with a PCWP of between 8 and 21 mm Hg. Thus, from a clinical perspective, CVP measurement would not appear to be as satisfactory a measure of left atrial filling pressure as PCWP. Whether this holds true for pregnant women with critically ill disease states other than pregnancy-induced hypertension remains unknown.

Pulmonary Artery Catheterization

Description and Insertion Technique

In 1970, Swan and associates first described the use of a balloon-tipped pulmonary artery catheter that allowed invasive serial hemodynamic measurements. The original instru-

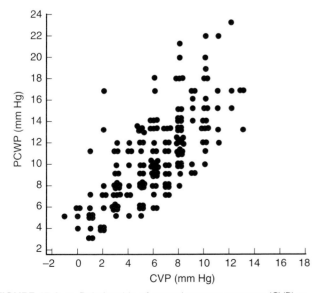

FIGURE 45-3 ■ Relationship of central venous pressure (CVP) to pulmonary capillary wedge pressure (PCWP) in severe pregnancy-induced hypertension. (From Cotton DB, Gonik B, Dorman K, et al: Cardiovascular alterations in severe pregnancy-induced hypertension: Relationship of central venous pressure to pulmonary capillary wedge pressure. Am J Obstet Gynecol **151**:762, 1985.)

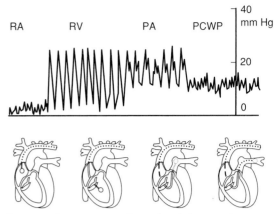

FIGURE 45-4 ■ Pressure wave forms in relation to pulmonary artery (PA) catheter position. PCWP, pulmonary capillary wedge pressure; RA, right artery; RV, right ventricle. (From Hankins GDC: Principles of invasive hemodynamic monitoring. *In* Cotton DB, Clark SL (eds): Clinics in Perinatology. Philadelphia, Saunders, 1986.)

ment has undergone numerous modifications and improvements. It is now commercially available through several suppliers in the United States and abroad. The Swan-Ganz catheter, a no. 7 French polyvinyl chloride multilumen device, is capable of directly measuring right atrial pressure (CVP), pulmonary artery pressure, and PCWP. CO and mixed venous oxygen saturation can be measured in the conventional manner by thermodilution and direct distil port aspiration, respectively, or by newer fiberoptic technology that allows continuous monitoring of CO and mixed venous oxygen saturation.

By percutaneous insertion, the catheter is directed into place via the internal or external jugular, subclavian, basilic, or femoral vein. Some of the more peripheral access sites make catheter positioning more difficult but may be preferred when a coagulopathy is present. Characteristic oscilloscopic pressure waveforms (Fig. 45-4) are used to establish the catheter's location when it is advanced.

Simultaneous continuous electrocardiographic monitoring is needed to identify catheter-related arrhythmias. These arrhythmias tend to be transient and generally do not require intervention except for withdrawal of the catheter. Inflation of the balloon assists in positioning of the catheter because the device is carried through the heart's chambers by established venous and cardiac flow patterns. Once the inflated balloon reaches the pulmonary artery, a dampened tracing (PCWP) usually indicates that the balloon is situated in the proper "wedged" position. When it is deflated, return of an identifiable pulmonary artery systolic and diastolic pressure tracing should occur. Periodic manipulation of the catheter may be needed to maintain accurate readings and to avoid permanent wedging of the catheter. A portable chest x-ray can be used to verify appropriate catheter positioning.

Complications of Pulmonary Artery Catheters

Recognized complications associated with insertion and maintenance of a pulmonary artery catheter are listed in Table 45-1. The initial complications seem to be most closely correlated with the technical skills and experience of the clinician. Many of the later complications can be minimized by

TABLE 45-1. POTENTIAL PULMONARY ARTERY CATHETER COMPLICATIONS

At Insertion	After Placement
Pneumothorax	Pulmonary infarction
Thrombosis	Pulmonary artery rupture
Arterial puncture	Infection
Air embolization	Balloon rupture
Catheter knotting	Endocardial/valvular
Cardiac arrhythmias	damage
(transient, sustained)	

having available ancillary health care personnel familiar with the catheter and its functioning.

As indicated earlier, cardiac arrhythmias are most often transient in nature, although fatal ventricular fibrillation has been reported. Their overall incidence during insertion has been reported to be between 15% and 50% (Swan et al., 1970; Sprung et al., 1982). The occurrence of a significant arrhythmia is more common when underlying cardiac disease is present or when metabolic disturbances are left uncorrected. Additional specific risk factors include hypocalcemia, hypokalemia, hypoxemia, and acidosis. With these latter two factors, some have noted a greater than 80% risk for ventricular tachyarrhythmias (Sprung et al., 1982). One should therefore have available lidocaine hydrochloride and amiodarone in case bolus administration is needed when attempting catheter placement. In addition, appropriate resuscitation equipment should be at hand for acute cardiopulmonary complications should they occur.

Pulmonary infarction may occur as a result of direct catheter tip occlusion of a pulmonary artery tributary or from thrombus dislodgment and embolization around the catheter. The diagnosis is typically confirmed by radiographic findings of a wedge-shaped infiltrate distal to the catheter tip. Although originally thought to occur in 35% of catheter placements, pulmonary infarction is a much less common event today, with a suggested incidence of 1.3% to 7.2% (Boyd et al., 1983). This probably relates to an overall better understanding of invasive monitoring techniques and the routine use of a continuous heparin flush.

Sepsis from continuous catheter usage occurs approximately 2% to 8% of the time (Boyd et al., 1983). One must distinguish between true infection and catheter tip contamination (or colonization), which can occur in up to 35% of catheter insertions. These two entities are distinguished by clinical evidence of septicemia with the same blood-identified and catheter-identified organisms, in the first case, and organism-positive catheter cultures only for the latter case. Risk factors for sepsis include underlying infection, prolonged catheter usage (more than 3 days), and nonsterile repositioning of the catheter after initial placement. This event has been minimized by the recent introduction of a sterile/clean catheter sheath system that allows catheter advancement under more aseptic conditions.

The other potential complications of using a pulmonary artery catheter occur infrequently (see Table 45-1). Pneumothorax risks (incidence, 1% to 6%) can be minimized by using an alternate site for insertion rather than the subclavian approach. Catheter knotting can be avoided during placement if the operator remains aware of the centimeter markings on the advancing catheter. As a general rule, the right ventricle is almost always reached when the catheter has

been inserted 25 to 30 cm from the jugular vein site. Few patients require more than 50 cm of catheter to reach the pulmonary artery. Inflated catheter balloons should be checked before insertion to reduce the risk of air leakage and balloon rupture. In addition, overinflation of the balloon with air (more than 1.5 mL) should be avoided. A pressure-release balloon has been recently described that limits overinflation and thereby minimizes pulmonary vessel injury. Pulmonary artery rupture (generally a fatal complication) is uncommon (incidence, 0.2%); the major risk factor is existing pulmonary artery hypertension with distal migration of the catheter. Valvular damage can occur from chronic catheter irritation or during insertion when the catheter balloon is not deflated before retrograde movement.

Hemodynamic Variables

With a pulmonary artery catheter, the following hemodynamic variables can be *directly measured* in the patient:

- Heart rate (beats/min)
- CVP (mm Hg)
- Pulmonary artery systolic and pulmonary artery diastolic pressures (mm Hg)
- PCWP (mm Hg)
- CO (liters/min)
- Mixed venous oxygen saturation

By use of a sphygmomanometer or by peripheral artery catheterization, direct measurements of systemic arterial pressures can also be obtained. Mean pressure values for both the arterial and pulmonary circulations can be calculated by the following formula:

$$MAP = \frac{\text{systolic pressure } + \text{ 2 (diastolic pressure)}}{3}$$

Other *calculated* hemodynamic variables, along with their respective formulas, are as follows:

$$SV = \frac{CO}{HR} \text{ mL/beat}$$

$$SVR = \frac{MAP - CVP}{CO} \times 80 \text{ (dyne} \times \text{sec} \times \text{cm}^{-5})$$

$$PVR = \frac{PAP - PCWP}{CO} \times 80 \text{ (dyne} \times \text{sec} \times \text{cm}^{-5})$$

$$LVSW = SV \times MAP \times 0.0144 \text{ (g} \times M/M^2)$$

where MAP is the mean arterial pressure, SV is the stroke volume, SVR is the systemic vascular resistance, PVR is the pulmonary vascular resistance, PAP is the pulmonary artery pressure, and LVSW is the left ventricular stroke work.

Many times these hemodynamic parameters are expressed in an "indexed" fashion (i.e., cardiac index). To do this, the original nonindexed CO value must be divided by body surface area. Because standard body surface area calculations have never been established specifically for pregnancy, this traditional way of expressing hemodynamic data is somewhat controversial in obstetrics. Those who argue for its use point out that indexing allows direct comparison of hemodynamic parameters for pregnant women of different sizes, a critical issue when interpreting these values.

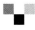

TABLE 45-2. NORMAL CENTRAL HEMODYNAMIC PARAMETERS IN HEALTHY NONPREGNANT AND PREGNANT PATIENTS

	Nonpregnant	Pregnant
Cardiac output (L/min)	4.3 ± 0.9	6.2 ± 1.0
Heart rate (beats/min)	71 ± 10	83 ± 10
Systemic vascular resistance (dyne × cm × sec^{-5})	1530 ± 520	1210 ± 266
Pulmonary vascular resistance (dyne×cm×sec^{-5})	119 ± 47	78 ± 22
Colloid oncotic pressure (mm Hg)	20.8 ± 1.0	18.0 ± 1.5
Colloid oncotic pressure–pulmonary capillary wedge pressure (mm Hg)	14.5 ± 2.5	10.5 ± 2.7
Mean arterial pressure (mm Hg)	86.4 ± 7.5	90.3 ± 5.8
Pulmonary capillary wedge pressure (mm Hg)	6.3 ± 2.1	7.5 ± 1.8
Central venous pressure (mm Hg)	3.7 ± 2.6	3.6 ± 2.5
Left ventricular stroke work index (gm × m × m^{-2})	41 ± 8	48 ± 6

From Clark SL, Cotton DB, Lee W, et al: Central hemodynamic assessment of normal term pregnancy. Am J Obstet Gynecol **161**:1439, 1989.

Mean hemodynamic measurements for pregnant and nonpregnant patients are presented in Table 45-2. These are paired data from 10 healthy subjects, taken between 36 and 38 weeks' gestation and between 11 and 13 weeks after delivery (Clark et al., 1989). Using the noninvasive technique of M-mode echocardiography, Capeless and Clapp (1989) demonstrated that many of these physiologic alterations in hemodynamics begin in the early phases of pregnancy. Clark and associates (1991) demonstrated that position changes late in pregnancy significantly influenced central hemodynamic stability. The standing position resulted in a 50% increase in pulse, a 21% fall in left ventricular stroke work index, and a 54% rise in pulmonary vascular resistance. It is interesting that the pregnant state compared with the nonpregnant state seemed to result in a *buffering* of orthostatic-related hemodynamic changes. The authors speculated that the increased intravascular volume during pregnancy accounted for this stabilizing effect.

Hemodynamic Considerations for Specific Conditions

This part of the chapter deals specifically with hemodynamic considerations for various pathologic conditions in the pregnant woman. A complete discussion of these conditions can be found in various chapters of this text.

Mitral Valve Stenosis

The principal hemodynamic problem associated with severe mitral valve stenosis in pregnancy relates to an obstruction in left ventricular filling (see Chapter 41). The resultant fixed CO limits the parturient's ability to tolerate large fluctuations in intravascular volume. During the intrapartum and postpartum periods, shunted blood returning to the heart may easily overload the cardiovascular system. The immediate clinical implication is the development of pulmonary congestion and edema. Other factors, such as increases in heart rate, can also limit ventricle diastolic filling and therefore can precipitate pulmonary edema more easily in patients with this condition. Management goals center on the prophylactic maintenance of a relatively non-overloaded or slightly constricted (for pregnancy) intravascular volume in anticipation of fluid shifts known to occur during the peripartum period. Adequate analgesia and anesthesia during labor and delivery also reduce excessive cardiac demands associated with pain and anxiety.

The other important hemodynamic consideration in the patient with mitral valve stenosis relates to the potential for misinterpretation of the invasive monitoring data. Because of the stenotic mitral valve, PCWP readings do not accurately reflect left ventricular diastolic pressure. In some instances, very high PCWP values are recorded (and are needed to maintain an adequate CO). Overt pulmonary edema is usually not associated with these high readings. Therefore, during attempts at maintaining a relatively "constricted" intravascular volume, CO should be concomitantly monitored and maintained. For each individual patient, optimal PCWP and CO values should be determined (i.e., those values that maintain blood pressure and tissue perfusion).

Aortic Stenosis

The major problem encountered with aortic stenosis centers on the patient's potential inability to maintain CO (see Chapter 41). Factors that cause a reduction in blood flow to the heart can trigger sudden decreases in CO and death. Hypotension from conduction anesthesia, positioning changes, and acute blood loss are particularly hazardous to the laboring woman. Unlike mitral stenosis, aortic valve stenosis requires that attempts be made to maintain the patient in a relatively hypervolemic state. Conduction anesthesia should be used cautiously because of the associated risks for hypotension.

Pulmonary Hypertension

Maternal mortality rates for patients with pulmonary hypertension have been reported to be as high as 50% to 80%. Despite advances in technology, the mortality rate has remained relatively unchanged in recent times (Sheude et al., 1994). The underlying problem in patients with this condition is obstruction to right ventricular outflow caused by a fixed and elevated pulmonary vascular resistance. When SVR is reduced, there is a tendency for right-to-left shunting of deoxygenated blood with resultant hypoxemia. In addition, reductions in blood return to the heart can decrease right ventricular preload so that the pulmonary vasculature is hypoperfused. The resultant hypoxemia has been associated with sudden death. Intrapartum management requires maintenance of a relatively "hypervolemic" state, with any interventions that would lead to significant preload reduction specifically avoided.

Anaphylactoid Syndrome of Pregnancy (Amniotic Fluid Embolism)

Confusion exists about the hemodynamic events associated with amniotic fluid embolization. In part, this relates to discrepancies between experimental animal data and a limited amount of anecdotal human observation. In an attempt to reconcile these differences, Clark, Montz, and coworkers (1985) postulated that a biphasic hemodynamic response pattern exists. First, an initial transient period of intense pulmonary vasospasm leads to acute right ventricular failure and hypoxemia. This initial event may explain the 50% occurrence of maternal deaths during the acute episode. Subsequently, however, the predominant feature is one of left ventricular heart failure with only mild to moderate elevations in pulmonary artery pressure. Characteristically, in this phase an elevated PCWP and a reduction in left ventricular stroke work are seen.

Treatment should be directed toward the latter hemodynamic response, with optimization of CO using crystalloid fluids to replenish intravascular volume depletion and vasopressor therapy for acute hypotension and congestive heart failure. Previous therapeutic recommendations aimed at selective reductions in pulmonary artery vasospasm do not appear to be helpful unless this finding is specifically identified by hemodynamic monitoring. Some reports have demonstrated the recovery of squamous epithelial cells from the pulmonary artery in a variety of conditions *not* associated with amniotic fluid embolism, including septic shock, pregnancy-induced hypertension, and severe cardiac disease (Clark et al., 1986). Therefore, this finding is not pathognomonic for amniotic fluid embolism, and other differential diagnoses need to be considered. An analysis of the data from the National Amniotic Fluid Embolism Registry (Clark et al., 1995) revealed marked similarities between the hemodynamic, clinical and hematologic manifestations of amniotic fluid embolism and both anaphylactic and septic shock. The authors postulated that although the conditions are not identical, a similar pathophysiologic mechanism may be responsible. All three of these conditions result from the intravascular access of a foreign substance (bacterial endotoxin or specific antigen) that results in the release of various primary and secondary endogenous mediators, leading to significant pathophysiologic derangements. The authors recommended that the term "amniotic fluid embolism" be discarded and replaced by the more descriptive designation of "anaphylactoid syndrome of pregnancy."

Pregnancy-Induced Hypertension

Thus far, most of the clinical hemodynamic monitoring studies in obstetrics have taken place in patients with pregnancy-induced hypertension. From a purely clinical perspective, clear indications for this invasive technology have not been established. Arguments for its use center on reports demonstrating a broad and variable spectrum of hemodynamic findings in this group of patients. For patients identified to be relatively hypovolemic, optimizing intravascular volume status should improve uteroplacental perfusion, reduce SVR, and blunt hypotensive complications associated with conduction anesthesia and antihypertensive therapy. Oliguria (particularly if unresponsive to fluid therapy) and refractory pulmonary edema, both recognized complications of severe pregnancy-induced hypertension, may also be better defined and managed with invasive monitoring.

Vasospasm is a central feature of pregnancy-induced hypertension. Empirically, one would assume that an elevated SVR is a constant finding with this disease state. Interestingly, Phelan and Yurth (1982) examined several clinical reports in the literature in which SVR data were available and found a

wide range of values. These observations, unfortunately, were marred by several critical factors. Many of the study patients were pretreated with a variety of antihypertensive agents, magnesium sulfate, and intravenous fluids before catheter insertion. These treatments have been shown to influence the hemodynamic status of preeclamptic patients (Cotton et al., 1984, 1985b; Hankins et al., 1984). It is of interest that Visser and Wallenburg (1991) presented hemodynamic data in 51 untreated preeclamptic patients that again suggests a uniform picture of an elevated SVR. In all likelihood, pregnancy-induced hypertension represents an overall vasoconstrictive condition that is frequently influenced by underlying disease processes such as chronic hypertension, duration and severity of illness, and various therapeutic modalities.

Unlike SVR, relatively uniform agreement exists regarding cardiac function in pregnancy-induced hypertension. Using ventricular function curves that correlate PCWP (preload) with left ventricular stroke work index (myocardial contractility), investigators found that most preeclamptic and eclamptic patients fall into a relatively hyperdynamic range (Benedetti et al., 1980; Hankins et al., 1984; Esterling et al., 1990). The values shown in Figure 45-5 are superimposed on ventricular function graphs derived from nonpregnant subjects. Therefore, the preeclamptic patient probably has at least a normal, and probably a somewhat hyperdynamic, functioning heart for pregnancy. As expected, this cardiac function, as estimated by CO, appears to be inversely related to SVR.

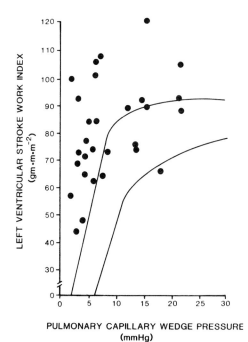

FIGURE 45-5 ■ Ventricular function in pregnancy-induced hypertensive patients. (Combined data from Benedetti TJ, Cotton DB, Read JC, et al: Hemodynamic observations in severe pre-eclampsia with a flow-directed pulmonary artery catheter. Am J Obstet Gynecol **136**:465, 1980; Hankins GDV, Wendel GP, Cunningham FG, et al: Longitudinal evaluation of hemodynamic changes in eclampsia. Am J Obstet Gynecol **15**:506, 1984; Phelan JP, Yurth DA: Severe preeclampsia. I. Peripartum hemodynamic observations. Am J Obstet Gynecol **144**:17, 1982; and Rafferty TD, Berkowitz RL. Hemodyamics in patients with severe toxemia during labor and delivery. Am J Obstet Gynecol **138**:263, 1980.)

Some investigators have recommended that patients with pregnancy-induced hypertension be classified by different hemodynamic subsets so that management protocols can be tailored to individual patient needs. Clark and coworkers (1988) first reported the use of this approach for dealing with the oliguric preeclamptic patient. They noted that these patients either had low PCWP values (hypovolemic) and showed severe vasoconstriction (elevated SVR) or were volume replete with normal to elevated vascular resistances. A third group had markedly elevated PCWP and SVR readings with depressed cardiac function. Management of these groups of oliguric patients would be varied. In the first subset, patients respond favorably to volume expansion therapy. Conversely, the next two groups of patients are best managed with vasodilators and aggressive afterload reduction therapy.

Another important clinical issue in the oliguric patient with pregnancy-induced hypertension relates to the use of standard urinary diagnostic indices, such as urine-to-plasma ratios of osmolality, urea nitrogen, and creatinine or fractional excretion of sodium. Although these urinary parameters are routinely used in nonobstetric patients to differentiate prerenal and renal causes of oliguria, they have proved to be unreliable in patients with preeclampsia (Lee et al., 1987). In preeclampsia complicated by oliguria, urinary diagnostic indices have suggested a prerenal picture despite a true functional intravascular volume, which is normal by invasive pressure measurement determinations. From a physiologic standpoint, it is postulated that the kidney misinterprets local renal artery vasospasm to indicate a volume-depleted state.

β-Adrenergic Agonist Tocolytic Therapy

There is concern for major cardiovascular side effects associated with the use of β-adrenergic agonist tocolysis for preterm labor (Katz et al., 1981; Robertson et al., 1981). The most significant side effect, by virtue of its frequency and severity, is pulmonary edema. Very limited hemodynamic data are available that help clarify the etiology of this untoward complication. Presented in Table 45-3 are available data examining hemodynamic changes associated with β-adrenergic agonist therapy. It is noteworthy that these findings are relatively uniform across different experimental animal species and in human subjects. In particular, the consistent rise seen in PCWP over time may be a crucial finding when one is extrapolating a cardiogenic cause for pulmonary edema. This PCWP rise occurs despite marked elevations in CO. Therefore, the fluid retention known to occur with β-adrenergic agonist therapy may be a dominant factor leading to fluid overload in a hyperdynamic functioning cardiovascular system (Hankins et al., 1983). Anecdotal clinical experiences with fluid restriction during intravenous tocolytic therapy support these conclusions, in that apparent reductions in the incidence of pulmonary edema have been noted.

One cannot, however, ignore two other factors as they relate to pulmonary edema and β-adrenergic agonist therapy. First, myocardial ischemia has been reported in association with β-agonist therapy. Although the underlying etiologic mechanism is unknown, it has usually been attributed to high output demands on the heart. The possibility of a direct catecholamine-induced cardiac muscle necrosis suggested by *in vitro* work (Haft, 1974) has not been supported to date by *in vivo* data (Zebe et al., 1982). Second, some preterm labor

TABLE 45-3. SPECIES DIFFERENCES IN HEMODYNAMIC RESPONSES TO β-ADRENERGIC AGONIST THERAPY*

	Baboon[†]	Sheep[‡]	Human[§]
HR	↑	↑ (50%)	↑ (18%)
MAP	↑	Slight ↓	Slight ↓
PAP	NC	↑	↑ (72%)
PCWP	↑ (282%)	↑	↑ (57%)
CO	↑ (60%)	↑ (40%)	↑ (50%)
SVR	↓ (35%)	↓ (70%)	—
PVR	NC	↓ (15%)	↓ (15%)

* Data expressed as increased (↑), decreased (↓), or no change (NC). When available, maximal percentage change (%) from control or baseline measurements is given.
† From Hankins GD, Hauth JC, Kuehl TJ, et al: Ritodrine hydrochloride infusion in pregnant baboons. II. Sodium and water compartment alterations. Am J Obstet Gynecol **147:**254, 1983.
‡ From Kleinman G, Nuwayhid B, Rudelstorfer R, et al: Circulatory and renal effects of β-adrenergic-receptor stimulation in pregnant sheep. Am J Obstet Gynecol **149:**865, 1984.
§ From Wolff F, Carstens V, Behrenbeck D, et al: The effect of fenoterol and betamethasone on pulmonary circulation—Results of intensive monitoring of pregnant women using cardiac catheter for prevention of pulmonary edema. *In* Jung H, Lamberti G (eds): Betamimetic Drugs in Obstetrics and Perinatology. New York, Thieme-Stratton, 1982.
CO, cardiac output: HR, heart rate; MAP, mean arterial pressure; PAP, pulmonary arterial pressure; PCWP, pulmonary capillary wedge pressure; PVR, pulmonary vascular resistance; SVR, systemic vascular resistance.

patients who experience pulmonary edema during β-mimetic therapy have normal or low PCWP readings, supporting a noncardiogenic etiology. Benedetti (1986) suggested that incipient or overt infection may induce transient injury to pulmonary capillary beds leading to increased permeability and edema. This mechanism of pulmonary injury has been supported by studies of pyelonephritis and associated pulmonary disease in pregnancy (Cunningham et al., 1987).

Septic Shock

"Septic shock" is a widely used generic term describing the systemic inflammatory response syndrome associated with infection, hypotension, and hypoperfusion despite adequate fluid resuscitation. Although septic shock has been well described in the nonobstetric literature, only anecdotal reports are available for obstetric patients. A paucity of clinical data is as yet available regarding hemodynamic parameters in this same critically ill obstetric population. Lee and colleagues (1988) studied the hemodynamic profiles of 10 obstetric patients, at various gestational ages, identified to have septic shock and requiring invasive monitoring. Prolonged rupture of membranes with the subsequent development of chorioamnionitis or postpartum endometritis were risk factors that commonly preceded the diagnosis of septic shock in these patients.

Figure 45-6 schematically describes the wide range of hemodynamic alteration seen in a subset of six of these patients, studied serially (Gonik et al., 1987). With successful therapy, SVR and CO are shown to be restored to more intermediate and normal ranges. Additionally, consistent improvements in cardiac function (Fig. 45-7) are demonstrated for those subjects who survived. These findings, and those of other investigators, suggest that, depending on duration and severity, septic shock in the pregnant woman can involve a wide variety of hemodynamic alterations (Mabie et al., 1997). Patients may

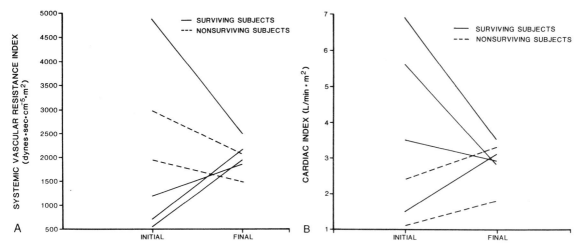

FIGURE 45-6 ■ **A,** Serial measurements of systemic vascular resistance index for pregnant women in septic shock. *Initial measurements:* taken at time of pulmonary artery insertion. *Final measurements:* taken just before catheter removal (*n* = 4) or immediately before profound alterations associated with rapid decompensation and death (*n* = 2). **B,** Serial measurements of cardiac index for gravidas in septic shock. (From Gonik B, Lee W, Giebel R, et al: Septic shock in obstetrics: Clinical perspective and hemodynamic observations. Abstract presented at the Infectious Disease Society for Obstetrics and Gynecology, July 6, 1987, Glasgow, Scotland.)

benefit from pharmacologic interventions in which these marked initial differences in cardiovascular hemodynamics are specifically taken into account. With the use of a bedside-generated cardiac function curve, one should be able to serially monitor patient status and predict outcome.

Myocardial Infarction

Although considered a rare condition associated with pregnancy, with national trends reporting delayed childbearing and with the increasing use of illicit substances, myocardial infarction may become a more frequently observed pregnancy complication. In the most recent comprehensive review of acute myocardial infarction associated with pregnancy, 125 cases of myocardial infarction in 123 pregnancies were identified (Roth and Elkayam, 1996). Myocardial infarction occurred predomi-

nantly in the third trimester of pregnancy in multigravidas older than 33 years of age. Maternal death occurred most often at the time of the infarct or within 2 weeks of the infarct, often associated with labor and delivery. The authors speculated that the increasing cardiovascular demands late in pregnancy and during labor seriously compromised women with ischemic heart disease.

From a hemodynamic standpoint, efforts should be directed as follows:

1. Limit myocardial oxygen consumption by bed rest, sedation, and pain relief during labor.
2. Avoid, if possible, delivery within 2 weeks of the acute myocardial infarction.
3. Recognize and treat any associated congestive heart failure.

Oxytocin, in dilute concentrations, is not specifically contraindicated during labor. Nitrate therapy for angina has been used in a very limited fashion during pregnancy without apparent adverse fetal effects. One case report (Schumacher et al., 1997) described the successful use of tissue plasminogen activator at 21 weeks' gestation after acute myocardial infarction.

■ NONINVASIVE HEMODYNAMIC AND VENTILATORY MONITORING

The noninvasive evaluation of cardiovascular hemodynamics in the pregnant woman has been explored. Using M-mode echocardiography in combination with electrocardiography and phonocardiography, Mashini and associates (1987) demonstrated the ability to measure or calculate heart rate, stroke volume (as a function of left ventricular dimensional changes during systole and diastole), CO, pulmonary vascular resistance, and PCWP. Although some of these noninvasively extrapolated hemodynamic parameters have been closely correlated to concomitant invasive determinations in the nonpregnant subject (Abdulla et al., 1980; Askenazi et al., 1981), minimal data are available in the pregnant woman to validate this new technology.

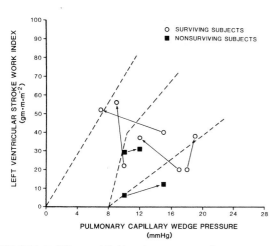

FIGURE 45-7 ■ Effects of fluid and vasopressor therapy on ventricular function in gravidas with septic shock. (From Gonik B, Lee W, Glebel R, et al: Septic shock in obstetrics: Clinical perspectives and hemodynamic observations. Abstract presented at the Infectious Disease Society for Obstetrics and Gynecology, July 6, 1987, Glasgow, Scotland.)

Easterling and colleagues (1987) reported on the use of Doppler ultrasonography to measure CO in both healthy pregnant women and those with pregnancy-induced hypertension. As a part of their study, 12 patients underwent concomitant pulmonary artery catheterization with thermodilutionally determined measurements of CO. In this pilot study, the noninvasive Doppler technique accurately estimated CO with a high degree of correlation. More recent studies focused on sonographic or bioimpedance technology to successfully estimate CO in both pregnant and nonpregnant patients (Clark et al., 1994; Ensing et al., 1994; Weiss et al., 1995; Belfort et al., 1996). These techniques certainly have value; however, the practicality of these methods outside of the research setting may be limiting.

Since its introduction into clinical medicine in the early 1980s, the pulse oximeter has gained widespread acceptance in the critical care area. As a noninvasive alternative to arterial blood gas sampling, the pulse oximeter is capable of providing rapid and continuous determinations of maternal blood oxygen saturation. The instrument consists of a sensor, a miniature computer, and a connecting cable. The sensor can be attached to any pulsatile tissue bed (e.g., fingertip). It transmits rapidly alternating beams of red and infrared light through the tissue bed to a photoelectric cell. The oxygen saturation is calculated by means of an algorithm based on the differential absorption of the two colors of light during pulsation of arterial blood through the tissue. The clinical issues that may impact the accuracy of pulse oximetry readings include the degree of peripheral vasoconstriction, inspired oxygen concentration, hemoglobulin concentration, and CO.

Previous studies have shown that the pulse oximeter accurately reflects oxygenation status in both healthy and decompensated subjects (Yelderman and New, 1983). Studies in pregnancy have shown this noninvasive device to be useful in the early detection of amniotic fluid embolization (Quance, 1988) and in describing the effects of labor and delivery (Deckardt et al., 1987) and conduction anesthesia on oxygen saturation during cesarean section (Brose and Cohen, 1989). The clinician is advised to not rely on the pulse oximeter as the sole means of monitoring respiratory function. Although pulse oximetry may accurately reflect "oxygenation," blood gas analysis and arterial carbon dioxide pressure determination is necessary to assess adequacy of "ventilation."

COLLOID OSMOTIC PRESSURE

Definitions and Determinations

Colloid osmotic pressure (COP) describes the ability of the intravascular (or interstitial) space to retain fluid by the presence of large molecules that, by virtue of their inability to traverse the semipermeable endothelial membrane, set up an "osmotic" gradient. Although COP is discussed separately here, one should recognize this separation as artificial in that COP is intimately associated with hydrostatic pressure (PCWP) as originally defined by Starling (1896) as follows:

$$Q = K (P_c - P_i) - k (\pi_c - \pi_i)$$

where Q is the fluid flux, K is the filtration coefficient, P is the hydrostatic pressure in the capillary vascular bed (P_c) and the interstitium (P_i), k is the reflection coefficient, and π is the

osmotic pressure in the plasma (π_c) and the interstitium (π_i). Thus, PCWP is a clinical determinant of P_c and COP is a clinical measure of π_c in the equation.

Albumin and globulin are the major components in plasma that influence COP. This close relationship to plasma proteins (TP) is sometimes used to indirectly calculate COP by the following equation:

$$COP = 2.1 (TP) + 0.16 (TP)^2 + 0.009 (TP)^3$$

More often, COP can be directly measured by use of an oncometer. This device is in essence a two-chambered instrument divided by a semipermeable membrane. Prepared clinical specimens can be directly injected into the first chamber, establishing an osmotic gradient that draws isotonic fluid from the second chamber. This net flux is electronically calculated and digitally displayed.

Predicting Pulmonary Edema: The Colloid Osmotic Pressure-to-Pulmonary Capillary Wedge Pressure Gradient

In the presence of a normal COP, PCWP readings around 18 mm Hg are usually associated with early evidence of pulmonary congestion. Between 20 and 25 mm Hg, congestion becomes more overt; beyond 25 mm Hg, frank pulmonary edema occurs. On the basis of Starling's equation and clinical experience (Stein et al., 1974), we can say that pulmonary edema will occur at lower PCWP readings if COP is reduced. Rackow and coauthors (1977) suggested that a COP-to-PCWP gradient of less than 4 mm Hg substantially increases the risk of pulmonary edema in critically ill nonpregnant patients. These same observations have been reported in the obstetric population as well (Benedetti et al., 1985; Cotton et al., 1985a). One should recognize this as a simplified approach to the understanding of pulmonary edema. Other critical factors, such as alterations in pulmonary capillary permeability and changes in interstitial fluid components (via changes in lymph flow), can equally influence the development of pulmonary edema. The utility of the COP-to-PCWP gradient concept centers on the fact that these are the only clinically measurable forces in the Starling relationship.

Colloid Osmotic Pressure in Obstetrics

Mean (± SD) COP values of 25.4 ± 2.3 mm Hg have been reported for nonpregnant ambulatory adults. Prolonged supine positioning reduces this value slightly because of redistribution of compartmental fluids. Several investigators have studied COP alterations in pregnancy with consistent findings of a steady decline until approximately 36 weeks' gestation (Wu et al., 1983). Mean values at term are reported to be 22.4 ± 0.5 mm Hg.

With delivery, a more substantial decrease in COP has been noted. In addition to fluid redistribution, other intrapartum factors, such as acute blood loss and aggressive intravenous crystalloid administration, have been suggested as causes of this decline (Cotton et al., 1984; Gonik and Cotton, 1984). Postpartum values of 15.4 ± 2.1 mm Hg have been reported (Cotton et al., 1984). Interestingly, no differences are seen between patients undergoing vaginal delivery and those delivered by cesarean section. These COP reductions are also noted to be independent of type of anesthesia used. Follow-up studies

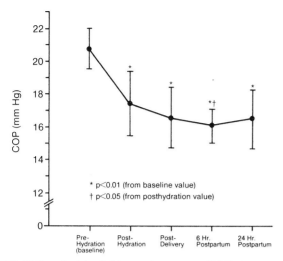

FIGURE 45-8 ■ Serial colloid osmotic pressure (COP) determinations during the peripartum period. (From Gonik B, Cotton DB, Spillman T, et al: Peripartum colloid osmotic changes: Effects of controlled fluid management. Am J Obstet Gynecol **151**:812, 1985.)

demonstrate that nadir values are reached by 6 hours postpartum (Gonik et al., 1985a) (Fig. 45-8). Fluid restriction, under these same circumstances, significantly moderates these reductions in COP, suggesting that overzealous intravenous hydration is an important component to these observed puerperal COP declines (Gonik and Cotton, 1984). Although none of the aforementioned studies reported clinical findings consistent with pulmonary edema in these otherwise healthy parturients, others have shown frequent incipient evidence of pulmonary interstitial fluid leakage during the postpartum period (Hughson et al., 1982).

Under certain pathologic conditions in obstetrics, COP changes should be more carefully evaluated. Pulmonary edema is a recognized complication of pregnancy-induced hypertension and of tocolytic therapy in preterm labor patients, both conditions occasionally being associated with fluid retention in the pregnant woman. In addition, traditional peripartum management strategies for these conditions may cause marked reductions in COP (Benedetti and Carlson, 1979; Gonik et al., 1985a).

Benedetti and Carlson (1979) reported mean COP values of 17.9 ± 0.7 and 13.7 ± 0.5 mm Hg during the antepartum and postpartum periods, respectively, in patients with pregnancy-induced hypertension. One can best appreciate the potential significance of these observations in COP by examining PCWP alterations during this same time period. In patients with severe preeclampsia, from delivery and continuing into the postpartum period, PCWP measurements may rise to levels as high as 23 mm Hg (Rafferty and Berkowitz, 1980). These acute hemodynamic changes in the patient with pregnancy-induced hypertension can result in a narrowing of the previously described critical PCWP–COP gradient; therefore, they increase the potential for pulmonary edema.

Again, minimal data are available for COP fluctuations during tocolytic therapy. Our group prospectively studied nine preterm labor patients undergoing parenteral ritodrine hydrochloride tocolysis, serially measuring COP changes (Gonik et al., 1985b). In this study, maintenance intravenous and oral fluids were restricted to less than 2500 mL/24 hours.

Over the ensuing 24-hour study period, mean COP levels progressively fell to a low of 16.8 ± 2.0 mm Hg (Fig. 45-9). This represented an overall 18% decline from baseline values. The cause of this drop in COP is most likely related to alterations in renal sodium and water retention known to occur potentially with this class of tocolytic agents (Hankins et al., 1983).

Use of Colloid Osmotic Pressure Determinations

The appropriate clinical use of COP determinations in obstetrics remains controversial. From the previous discussions, significant alterations do occur under certain clinical conditions and management protocols may benefit from this additional perspective. Controlled studies to demonstrate the clinical value and role in obstetric patients of COP measurement are currently lacking. Empirically, the following are examples of clinical circumstances that may benefit from COP monitoring.

1. *In conjunction with peripartum invasive hemodynamic monitoring of the severely preeclamptic patient.* Here, serial assessments of the COP-to-PCWP gradient may reduce risks for pulmonary edema, because PCWP can be clinically altered by preload or afterload reduction. Whether one should administer colloid fluids in an attempt to improve COP status is controversial. Although COP can be artificially increased with the use of these colloid solutions (i.e., albumin, hetastarch), arguments against their use are based on the transient nature of these improvements and the inability to predict subsequent capillary "leakage," thus potentially prolonging interstitial fluid accumulation.

2. *During intravenous β-adrenergic agonist tocolytic therapy, in particular when it is anticipated that baseline COP values are low (i.e., multiple gestation or after previous unknown amounts of intravenous hydration).* On occasion, β-mimetic tocolysis has been empirically decreased or discontinued on the basis of an extremely low (less than 12 mm Hg) COP alone. The other possibility might be to use invasive hemodynamic monitoring in those preterm labor patients with initial low COP values (less than 15 mm Hg) when use of aggressive tocolytic therapy is unavoidable. Under these unusual cir-

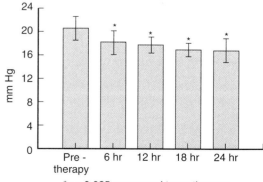

FIGURE 45-9 ■ Colloid osmotic pressure changes during ritodrine therapy in preterm labor subjects (*n* = 9). (From Gonik B, Creasy RK, Chambers SL: Colloid osmotic pressure alterations with ritodrine hydrochloride therapy. Abstract presented at the Eighth Annual Midwestern Conference in Perinatal Research, 1985.)

cumstances, pulmonary artery catheterization data would be available to calculate COP to PCWP relationships and to confirm an adequate, yet not overexpanded, intravascular volume status.

SHOCK

Pathogenesis

The term "shock" represents a morbid condition in which the patient's functional intravascular blood volume is below that of the capacity of the body's vascular bed. This pathologic state results in a lowering of blood pressure and decreased tissue perfusion. If the condition is left untreated, resulting cellular acidosis and hypoxia lead to end-organ tissue dysfunction and death.

Types of shock include the following:

- Hypovolemic and hemorrhagic shock, conditions associated with acute blood volume loss
- Cardiogenic shock, related to pump failure
- Neurogenic shock, caused by a loss of sympathetic control of resistance vessels

When the inciting cause stems from an infectious focus, the term *septic shock* is usually applied. With septic shock, a combination of both hypovolemic and cardiogenic shock frequently coexists. Because hemorrhagic shock and septic shock make up the overwhelming majority of cases identified in the obstetric patient, the remainder of the discussion focuses on these two entities. However, with the increasing use of conduction anesthesia, neurogenic shock may become a more prominent iatrogenic cause in the future. Similarly, the rare development of severe myocardial ischemia reported to occur with both β-adrenergic agonist tocolytics and illicit stimulant drugs such as cocaine may result in cardiogenic shock, related to myocardial dysfunction.

The central issue in shock relates to a deficiency in effective tissue perfusion. This is thought to occur as a direct result of physiologic homeostatic responses in the patient, leading to prolonged generalized vasoconstriction. In the case of experimentally induced hemorrhagic shock in the dog preparation, both amount of blood loss and time elapse until replacement begins critically influence the degree of vasoconstriction, via α-adrenergically mediated mechanisms (Lillehei et al., 1964). Until approximately 20% to 25% of total blood volume is lost, localized nonessential areas of vasoconstriction along with heart rate increases can maintain effective perfusion pressure. In pregnancy, this is particularly interesting, because this would suggest that the patient's normally expanded blood volume will allow for a much larger absolute blood loss before clinical evidence of shock (hypotension) appears. Beyond this amount, generalized intense vasoconstriction involving both essential and nonessential organ systems develops in response to hypotension.

As indicated earlier, rapid intervention in the experimental animal also influences the overall vasoconstrictive symphatho-adrenal response. Hemorrhagic shock, and its subsequent vasoconstriction, is best reversed if retransfusion occurs within 2 hours (Lillehei et al., 1964). Beyond 4 hours, even with adequate retransfusion, irreversible sympathetic-induced cellular changes have led to animal demise 80% of the time.

In the patient with septic shock, a more complex series of events leads to the aforementioned vasoconstrictive responses. With gram-negative sepsis, endotoxin appears to be the critical factor mediating the initial pathophysiologic derangements of shock (Sugerman et al., 1981). Endotoxin is a complex lipopolysaccharide present in the cell wall of aerobic gram-negative bacteria, which is released when the organism is destroyed. For gram-positive sepsis, similar events are thought to be initiated by the release of a variety of exotoxins produced within the organism (Kwann and Weil, 1969). Most of our current knowledge of septic shock is derived from studies using endotoxin-induced septic shock models.

Endotoxin-induced activation of the complement cascade leads to leukocyte migration and release of a variety of vasoactive substances, such as histamine, serotonin, and bradykinin (Fearon et al., 1975). These, in turn, increase capillary permeability, induce endothelial damage, and promote vasodilatation. Phagocytosis and killing of the bacteria by leukocytes potentiate two further events: an increased release of endotoxin and generalized systemic exposure to intracellular toxins such as superoxide free radials, lysosomes, and hydrogen peroxide. These local vasodilatory events then induce intact reflex sympathetic responses to produce profound vasoconstriction, as discussed earlier.

At a cellular level, intense vasoconstriction further worsens local capillary leakage and intravascular fluid loss. In addition, resultant reductions in tissue perfusion potentiate cellular hypoxia and acidosis. Individual cells become metabolically inadequate, losing their ability to use available oxygen supplies. The result of this pathologic sequence leads to a loss of cellular control of capillary vessel responsiveness, marked reductions in peripheral resistance, and extensive capillary pooling of blood. As the number of dilated capillary beds increases, an increasing disparity between effective intravascular volume and intravascular space develops. Tissue perfusion continues to deteriorate, as does venous return to the heart. This latter event again reduces CO. In addition, some have suggested that a circulating substance, myocardial depressant factor, is released from ischemic tissue, which further attenuates cardiac function (Lefer et al., 1967). Endogenous opiates, endorphins, are also released and are believed to cause a profound reduction in blood pressure (Holaday and Faden, 1978). The overall end-stage clinical complex is usually termed "secondary shock" and is considered irreversible regardless of intervention strategy.

Septic Shock

Incidence in Obstetrics

Although both lower and upper genital tract infections are commonly identified on an obstetric service, septic shock in the obstetric patient tends to be an uncommon event (ACOG, 1995). When an obstetric patient has clinical evidence of local sepsis, the incidence of bacteremia appears to be low (approximately 8% to 10%) (Ledger et al., 1975; Blanco et al., 1981; Bryan et al., 1984). More striking is the fact that overt septic shock rarely develops in obstetric patients with bacteremia. Ledger and associates (1975) identified only a 4% rate of shock in parturients with bacteremia. This value is in agreement with other investigators, who reported a 0% to 12% incidence of septic shock in bacteremic obstetric and gynecologic subjects

TABLE 45-4. INCIDENCE OF BACTERIAL INFECTIONS IN THE OBSTETRIC PATIENT

	Incidence (%)
Postpartum endometritis	
After cesarean section	15–87
After vaginal delivery	1–4
Urinary tract infections (lower tract)	1–4
Pyelonephritis	1–2
Septic abortion	1–2
Chorioamnionitis	0.5–1
Necrotizing fasciitis (postoperative)	<1
Toxic shock syndrome	<1

(Chow and Guze, 1974; Ledger et al., 1975; Blanco et al., 1981; Bryan et al., 1984).

Table 45-4 lists the types of bacterial infections, by incidence, specifically identified in the obstetric patient and associated with the development of septic shock. Of those listed, the use of prophylactic antimicrobial agents has dramatically reduced the incidence of postcesarean section endometritis; septic abortion has also become a less common event since the legalization of elective pregnancy termination.

Mortality Associated with Septic Shock

The mortality rate in medical and surgical specialty fields is extremely high in the face of septic shock but tends to be low in obstetrics. The incidence of death from sepsis is estimated at 0% to 28% in obstetric patients as compared with 10% to 81% in nonobstetric patients (Ledger et al., 1975; Blanco et al., 1981; Lee et al., 1988; Mabie et al., 1997). Suggested reasons for these improved outcomes include the following:

1. Younger age group
2. Transient nature of the bacteremia
3. Type of organisms involved
4. Primary site of infection (pelvis) more amenable to both surgical and medical intervention
5. Lack of other underlying disease that might negatively influence the prognosis for recovery

The last factor is supported by investigators who have demonstrated increased mortality when patients had significant underlying diseases in addition to their sepsis (Freid and Vosti, 1968).

Regardless of these optimistic perspectives, sepsis still constitutes a major source of obstetric maternal deaths because mortality in the gravida from all causes is very uncommon (Berg et al., 1996).

Endotoxin-Induced Septic Shock in Pregnancy

In the experimental animal model using endotoxin-induced septic shock, pregnant animals have a much more pronounced metabolic acidosis in response to fixed doses of lipopolysaccharide than do nonpregnant controls, with earlier cardiovascular collapse (Beller et al., 1985). These findings are in agreement with those of other investigators, who demonstrated an increased susceptibility to the harmful effects of endotoxin during pregnancy in several animal species at term (Bech-

Jansen et al., 1972; Morishima et al., 1978; O'Brian et al., 1985). It is interesting that the fetus and newborn are much more resistant to the direct deleterious effects of endotoxin in the experimental setting.

Bech-Jansen and associates (1972) demonstrated that the fetus and the immediate neonate are capable of tolerating doses 10 times greater than those proving to be lethal in the adult pregnant sheep. They hypothesized that these altered effects related to the immature status of the vasoactive response in the fetus (and newborn). Conversely, Morishima and coworkers (1978) demonstrated profound asphyxia and rapid deterioration in the fetuses of pregnant baboons administered endotoxin. These effects are thought to be mediated by maternal factors such as hypotension and increased myometrial activity, both of which contribute to a reduction in placental perfusion.

Clinical Manifestations

In the early phase of septic shock, bacteremia is typically heralded by a shaking chill, sudden rise in temperature, tachycardia, and warm extremities. Although the patient may appear "infected," the diagnosis of septic shock may be somewhat deceptive until blood pressure readings are ascertained. In addition, patients may initially present with nonspecific complaints, such as nausea, vomiting, and at times profuse diarrhea. Abrupt alterations in behavior may also herald the onset of septic shock; this symptom has been attributed to reductions in cerebral blood flow. Tachypnea and shortness of breath may be present, with minimal physical examination findings. This may represent a direct effect of endotoxin on the respiratory center or may immediately precede the development of adult respiratory distress syndrome.

Laboratory findings are variable during the early stages of septic shock. The white blood cell count may, at first, be ironically depressed; soon afterward, a marked leukocytosis is usually evident. Although there is a transient increase in blood glucose levels secondary to catecholamine release and tissue underutilization, hypoglycemia may later prevail as a reduction in gluconeogenesis occurs from hepatic dysfunction. Early evidence of disseminated intravascular coagulation (DIC) may be represented by decreased platelet count, decreased fibrinogen, elevated fibrin split products, and an elevation in prothrombin time. Initial arterial blood gases may show a transient respiratory alkalosis. These parameters later reflect an increasing metabolic acidosis as tissue hypoxia and lactic acid levels increase. Table 45-5 presents a list of laboratory studies that may be helpful in initial diagnosis.

As the septic process continues, generalized vasoconstriction leads to more typical findings of shock, which include cold extremities, oliguria, and peripheral cyanosis. Profound metabolic acidosis, electrolyte imbalances, and generalized DIC should now be anticipated. Terminally, CO will be markedly depressed and a generalized peripheral vasodilatation picture is reflected by a low SVR. Multiple end-organ failure usually becomes evident before coma and death.

Management

Initial intervention modalities in the patient with septic shock should be directed at the following goals:

1. Improvement in functional circulating intravascular volume

TABLE 45-5. INITIAL LABORATORY AND RADIOGRAPHIC STUDIES IN PATIENTS WITH SUSPECTED SEPTIC SHOCK

Computed blood count with differential and platelet count
Coagulation profile (PT, PTT, FSP, fibrinogen, TT)
Arterial blood gases
Electrolytes, creatinine, blood urea nitrogen, glucose
Colloid osmotic pressure
Urinalysis and culture
Blood cultures, Gram stain
Cultures of suspected infectious foci (aerobic and anaerobic)
Chest x-ray
Abdominal series and pelvic x-ray if suspected source of infection
Special radiographic studies if needed to help localize infectious focus (e.g., ultrasound, CT)

CT, computed tomography; FSP, fibrinogen split product; PT, prothrombin time; PTT, partial thromboplastin time; TT, thrombin time.

2. Establishment and maintenance of an adequate airway to facilitate management of respiratory failure
3. Initiation of diagnostic evaluations to determine septic focus
4. Use of empiric antimicrobial therapy to eradicate most likely pathogens

If the patient is pregnant, regardless of gestational age, priorities should be focused toward maternal concerns even in the face of the suggested deleterious effects of septic shock on the fetus. Because the fetus appears to be compromised mainly from maternal cardiovascular decompensation, improvements in the maternal status should also have a positive effect on the fetus. Furthermore, attempts at delivery in this tenuous situation may lead to increased risks of fetal distress and the need for more aggressive obstetric management. In a mother who is already partially decompensated, these iatrogenic insults can precipitate adverse results. This, of course, is presuming that the fetal compartment is not the source of sepsis, in which case appropriate therapy would mandate removal of the infected focus.

FLUID MANAGEMENT

The mainstay of immediate management of septic shock centers on volume expansion to correct for either an absolute or a relative hypovolemia (Hawkins, 1980; Packman and Rackow, 1983; Rackow and Astiz, 1991). Correction of this pathologic event is almost always needed in these patients and correlates closely with improvement in CO, oxygen delivery, and survival (Weil and Nishijima, 1978). At times, considerable quantities of fluid are needed to maintain effective tissue perfusion because of profound vasodilatation, increased capillary permeability, and extravasation of fluid into extravascular spaces. The best practical means of monitoring this crucial component of therapy is the use of a flow-direct pulmonary artery catheter (i.e., Swan-Ganz catheter) (Swan et al., 1970).

One method of monitoring the "fluid challenge" administered to the patient has been suggested by Shubin and associates (1977), who recommended administering 5 to 20 mL/min of intravenous fluid over 10 minutes. If the PCWP increases by more than 7 mm Hg (from the starting value), the next fluid bolus should be withheld. If after this 10-minute test period the PCWP does not exceed 3 mm Hg, another challenge should be administered. The optimal range for the PCWP is 10

to 12 mm Hg. An elevated PCWP may reflect an overexpanded intravascular space or a reduction in left ventricular function or both. Calculation of the left ventricular stroke work index and construction of a ventricular function curve can help one to differentiate between these possibilities (Shoemaker et al., 1983). Preload and afterload reduction therapy or inotropic support—separately or in combination—can then be instituted as indicated.

INOTROPIC SUPPORT

At times, fluid resuscitation proves inadequate in restoring optimal cardiovascular function. Under these circumstances, the use of vasopressor agents is indicated. The most widely used initial agent in this regard is dopamine hydrochloride, a drug with dose-dependent α-adrenergic and β-adrenergic effects (Goldberg, 1974). In lower doses (less than 10 μg/kg/min), the predominant effect increases myocardial contractility and CO without increasing myocardial oxygen consumption. In addition, a selective increase in mesenteric and renal blood flow occurs. As the dosage is increased (exceeding 20 μg/kg/min) alpha effects predominate, with marked vasoconstriction leading to further reductions in peripheral tissue perfusion. Dopamine is administered as a continuous infusion starting at 2 to 5 μg/kg/min and titrated according to clinical and hemodynamic responses.

Interestingly, Rolbin and colleagues (1979) demonstrated that dopamine decreases uterine blood flow in the hypotensive pregnant sheep. Therefore, dopamine may actually compromise the fetal status while improving the maternal condition. This adds support to the need for external fetal monitoring in the gestationally viable fetus during initial maternal resuscitation attempts. Table 45-6 lists other commonly used vasopressor agents along with their recommended dosages and hemodynamic effects.

ADULT RESPIRATORY DISTRESS SYNDROME

Special mention should be made of adult respiratory distress syndrome because this complication is common in septic shock. The diagnosis is made on the basis of progressive hypoxemia, a normal PCWP, diffuse infiltrates on chest x-ray, and decreased pulmonary compliance (Sugerman et al., 1981). These findings are consistent with a pathophysiologic state in which an increase in capillary permeability leads to extensive extravasation of fluid into the pulmonary interstitium. The cornerstone of therapy involves intubation and ventilatory support to maintain

TABLE 45-6. INOTROPIC DRUGS FOR MANAGEMENT OF SHOCK

Agent	Dose	Hemodynamic Effect
Dopamine		
Low dose	<10 μg/kg/min	↑ CO, vasodilation of renal arteries
High dose	10–20 μg/kg/min	↑ CO, ↑ SVR
Dobutamine	2.5–15 μg/kg/min	↑ CO, ↓ SVR or ↑ SVR
Phenylephrine	40–180 μg/min	↑ SVR
Norepinephrine	2–12 μg/min	↑ CO, ↑ SVR
Isoproterenol	0.5–5 μg/min	↓ CO, ↑ SVR

CO, cardiac output; SVR, systemic vascular resistance.

adequate gas exchange at nontoxic levels of fraction of inspired oxygen. Positive end-expiratory pressure is often necessary to accomplish this goal, and serial monitoring of arterial blood gases is essential. Even in the face of overt pulmonary capillary leakage, intravenous hydration must be continued, as outlined earlier, to promote the desired increase in systemic perfusion. In addition, when interpreting hemodynamic values, one must remember that positive end-expiratory pressure may artificially increase PCWP measurements. Therefore, momentary discontinuation of positive end-expiratory pressure support may be needed to record PCWP readings accurately.

EVALUATION OF SEPSIS AND ANTIMICROBIAL THERAPY

In concert with attempts at restoring normal cardiovascular function, one must initiate a careful investigation into the underlying etiology of the sepsis. Because the course of septic shock can be short and fulminant, this must be carried out without delay so that empiric antimicrobial therapy can be started. Microbiologic specimens from blood, sputum, urine, wound, and any other site of suspected infection should be collected. Even though mixed flora are usually identified in transvaginal cultures, a careful sampling of the endometrial cavity should be carried out if this is the suspected source of infection (Duff et al., 1983). In patients thought to have chorioamnionitis, transabdominal amniocentesis or culture specimens taken from a free-flowing internal pressure transducer catheter are useful (Gibbs, 1982).

Because empiric therapy in the obstetric patient should include coverage for a wide variety of both aerobic and anaerobic bacteria, we prefer to use a combination of intravenous aqueous penicillin (5,000,000 units/6 hours), gentamicin (1.5 mg/kg/8 hours), and clindamycin (900 mg/8 hours). Single daily dosing of the aminoglycoside component has been advocated (Del Priore et al., 1996). This approach ensures a high peak concentration and low trough levels, thus reducing the risk of nephrotoxicity while improving antimicrobial effectiveness (gentamicin 7 mg/kg/24 hours). Alternatively, imipenem-cilastatin (500 mg intravenously/6 hours) or meropenem (1g/8 hours) can be given as single agents.

If *Staphylococcus aureus* is a suspected pathogen, a semisynthetic penicillin should be substituted for aqueous penicillin. In patients who have received previous cephalosporin prophylaxis or therapy, empiric coverage for enterococcus may be warranted. Enterococcus is not uncommonly identified as part of the vaginal flora in the infected parturient, although its pathogenicity is still somewhat controversial.

Few, if any, antimicrobial agents are absolutely contraindicated in the critically ill obstetric patient. Tetracycline has been demonstrated to cause growth and color abnormalities in developing bone and teeth and therefore should be avoided during the period of fetal organogenesis in pregnancy. Aminoglycosides have been associated with fetal and maternal nephrotoxicity and ototoxicity, although this is rarely used as an argument for withholding this class of agents in the critically ill pregnant patient. If aminoglycosides are used, however, careful monitoring of peak (6 to 10 mg/mL) and trough (less than 2 mg/mL) levels is indicated.

A new class of antimicrobial agents, the quinolones, have excellent gram-negative coverage. However, these agents should not be used in pregnancy because of reported cartilage formation abnormalities seen in experimental animals.

SURGICAL APPROACH

Most clinicians would agree that in a life-threatening condition such as septic shock, extirpation of infected tissues may be needed, even in the face of a compromised or debilitated host, to ensure survival. In patients with septic abortion, surgical attempts at evacuating the uterus should begin promptly after antibiotics have been started and after initial attempts have been made to stabilize the patient's condition. Septic shock in association with chorioamnionitis and a gestationally viable fetus is best treated by expeditious evacuation of the uterus; this can be accomplished by the vaginal route if maternal hemodynamic parameters are stable. If this is not the case, the ethical decision of performing a cesarean section is perhaps weighted toward this more aggressive surgical approach, given the increased chance of survival of the fetus and the uncertain risks to the mother if the nidus for infection is not removed rapidly. Antibiotic therapy should be initiated before delivery. The protective effect to the fetus of intrapartum antibiotic therapy for maternal sepsis has never been carefully evaluated. However, Bray and associates (1966) demonstrated measurable levels of ampicillin in amniotic fluid and fetal blood when that drug was administered intravenously to the mother.

In the postpartum patient, hysterectomy may be needed if microabscess formation is identified within the myometrial tissues or if there is clinical evidence of deterioration in the patient's condition with appropriate antibiotic therapy. When the diagnosis of septic pelvic thrombophlebitis is entertained, treatment with heparin in combination with broad-spectrum antibiotics is appropriate. If this proves unsuccessful, again a surgical approach with ligation of the involved vessels is the treatment of choice (Collins, 1970).

CONTROVERSIAL THERAPEUTIC MODALITIES

A variety of adjuvant therapeutic modalities has also been suggested in the treatment of septic shock. Corticosteroids can theoretically exert a beneficial effect by stabilization of cellular membranes, inhibition of inflammatory responses, and improvements in myocardial performance. However, given the difficulty in evaluating this isolated variable in the clinical arena, numerous conflicting reports exist (Sprung et al., 1984). Current recommendations limit the use of systemic steroids in septic shock patients to those who have demonstrable diminished adrenal reserve.

Investigators have used prostaglandin synthetase inhibitors with some success in blunting the prostaglandin-related pathophysiologic responses of sepsis in experimental animals (Cefalo et al., 1980; O'Brian et al., 1981; Rao et al., 1981; Makabali et al., 1983). Antilipopolysaccharide immunoglobulin has also been used in preliminary clinical trials to reduce both morbidity and mortality in the obstetric and gynecologic septic shock patient (Lachman et al., 1984). In a much larger clinical trial involving nonobstetric subjects, adjunctive therapy with a human monoclonal antibody against endotoxin similarly reduced mortality in those with gram-negative sepsis (Ziegler et al., 1991). Studies have suggested that beta-endorphin, an opiate-like substance produced in the central nervous system, may have a deleterious effect on the outcome of septic shock (Holaday and Faden, 1978). Unfortunately, few if any of these modalities have proven to be clearly beneficial.

Several anecdotal reports now exist suggesting that narcotic antagonists, such as naloxone, can reverse these effects. This finding is particularly interesting in regard to the obstetric patient, in whom beta-endorphin levels are known to progressively increase throughout gestation (Genazzani et al., 1981). The efficacy and safety of recombinant human-activated protein C for severe sepsis has also been recently proposed. Bernard and associates (2000) conducted a randomized, double-blind, placebo-controlled, multicenter trial on 1690 nonpregnant patients (840 in placebo group and 850 in treatment group). They concluded that treatment significantly reduced mortality in patients with severe sepsis (reduction in relative risk of 19.4%) but may be associated with an increased risk of bleeding complications (3.5% versus 2%). This therapy may hold future promise for the obstetric population.

ADDITIONAL SUPPORTIVE MEASURES

Additional measures that require the attention of the clinician include management of electrolyte imbalances, correction of metabolic acidosis, stabilization of coagulation defects, and monitoring of renal function. Patients in septic shock may have either hypokalemia (secondary to losses from the alimentary canal) or hyperkalemia (secondary to acute cation shifts). Lactic acidosis from anaerobic metabolism should be monitored by serial arterial blood gas determinations and serum lactate levels. Normal saline infusions with one to two ampules of sodium bicarbonate per liter can be periodically administered to help correct these alterations. Serum glucose levels may be elevated, normal, or depressed.

Laboratory coagulation abnormalities tend to reflect a generalized picture similar to that of DIC. Unless the patient has clinical evidence of bleeding or requires surgical intervention, aggressive attempts at correcting these defects (see Chapters 37 and 47) should not be undertaken because spontaneous improvement will occur when the overall clinical picture improves.

Renal function is best monitored by an indwelling catheter and with serial creatinine and blood urea nitrogen determinations. Although acute tubular necrosis most often presents with oliguria, occasionally a high output picture can be seen. Regardless, tests of tubular function demonstrate increased fractional excretion of sodium and an impaired concentrating ability. In addition, serum creatinine determinations should be monitored when the course of acute tubular necrosis is being followed. Provided that irreversible damage has not occurred, correction of the hemodynamic and perfusion deficits should result in restoration of renal function.

Hemorrhagic Shock

Incidence and Etiology

Obstetric hemorrhage continues to be one of the leading causes of maternal mortality. Excluding pregnancies associated with abortive outcomes, postpartum hemorrhage accounts for more than 50% of these hemorrhagic deaths (Berg et al., 1996). Although lack of adequate blood banking facilities does contribute to some of these maternal deaths, most are due to lack of anticipation of excessive bleeding or gross underestimation of blood loss. The diagnosis and management of the various causes of intrapartum and postpartum hemorrhage have been already discussed in Chapter 37.

Some of the more common peripartum causes and approximate incidences of hemorrhage are presented in Table 45-7. As can be appreciated from this table, most often evidence of hemorrhage is obvious. Concealed types of hemorrhage, however, such as those that may occur with pelvic fracture or

TABLE 45-7. ETIOLOGY OF OBSTETRIC HEMORRHAGE*

	Incidence per Delivery
Late Pregnancy	
Abruptio placentae	1:120
Placenta previa	1:200
Toxemia associated	1:20
Delivery and Postpartum Period	
Cesarean section	1:6
Obstetric lacerations	1:8
Uterine atony	1:20
Retained placenta	1:160
Uterine inversion	1:2300
Placenta accreta	1:7000

* Obstetric hemorrhage is usually defined as an acute blood loss in excess of 500 mL.

Modified from American College of Obstetricians and Gynecologists (ACOG): Hemorrhagic shock. ACOG Technical Bulletin 82, 1984, p. 1.

with abruptio placentae, can also result in unrecognized extremely large blood losses and hemodynamic instability. Although the causes of obstetric hemorrhage—arbitrarily defined as an estimated blood loss of more than 500 mL—and their incidences have been frequently reported, information is lacking regarding the actual incidence of obstetric hemorrhagic shock.

Clinical Staging of Hemorrhage

Traditional signs of hypovolemic shock in the pregnant subject do not become evident until approximately 20% to 25% of total blood volume is lost (Baker, 1997). Table 45-8 outlines the clinical manifestations of hemorrhagic shock, depending on severity. Although shock is most often clinically identified by the finding of hypotension in a previously normotensive individual, this is too simplistic an approach. Most of the significant aberrations of shock relate to inadequate tissue oxygenation and perfusion. Therefore, a broader observational base, including an evaluation of mental status, respiratory rate, peripheral perfusion, and urinary output, is indicated.

Management

The two basic goals in the management of hemorrhagic shock are (1) restoration of blood volume and oxygen-carrying capacity and (2) definitive treatment of the underlying disorder causing hemorrhage. Ideally, stabilization of the patient should take priority before definitive therapy is begun. This is frequently impractical because of the degree of obstetric hemorrhage encountered. A minimum of laboratory diagnostics is needed before initial resuscitation attempts. These include a sample of blood for type and cross-matching and hematocrit determination and a red-topped tube to evaluate gross blood-clotting capabilities. This latter bedside diagnostic evaluation is a modification of the Lee-White whole blood clotting time test, which crudely estimates clot formation and platelet retraction. Although an established protocol is not available detailing the methodology for this test, by convention a tube of blood is collected and observed for clot formation, which should occur within 6 to 8 minutes.

TABLE 45-8. CLINICAL STAGING OF HEMORRHAGIC SHOCK BY VOLUME OF BLOOD LOSS

Severity of Shock	Findings	Blood Loss (%)	Volume (mL)*
None	None	Up to 20	Up to 900
Mild	Tachycardia (<100 beats/min) Mild hypotension Peripheral vasoconstriction	20–25	1200–1500
Moderate	Tachycardia (100–120 beats/min) Hypotension (80–100 mm Hg) Restlessness Oliguria	30–35	1800–2100
Severe	Tachycardia (>120 beats/min) Hypotension (<60 mm Hg) Altered consciousness Anuria	>35	>2400

* Based on an average blood volume of 6000 mL at 30 weeks' gestation.

VOLUME REPLACEMENT THERAPY

In the case of hemorrhagic shock, the best agent for intravascular volume replacement is blood. Unfortunately, acute management frequently must be initiated before the availability of type-specific or cross-matched or type O negative blood. Large-gauge intravenous access lines should be secured, and rapid crystalloid (approximately 2 to 3 mL per 1 mL estimated blood loss) or colloid fluid boluses should be administered.

As suggested for septic shock, a useful means of evaluating fluid replacement therapy is based on PCWP responses to intermittent fluid challenges. It should be anticipated that if crystalloids are used, two to three times the volume will be needed as would be with colloid solutions (Rackow and Weil, 1983). Colloids in the form of 5% albumin or 67% hetastarch have been recommended by some investigators (Rackow and Weil, 1983). Fresh frozen plasma should not be used for volume replacement alone (National Institutes of Health Consensus Conference, 1985). This relates to its excessive costs, its greater need in other more critical conditions such as for specific blood factor deficiencies, and the low but recognized risk of infectious disease transmission.

BLOOD COMPONENT THERAPY

Various blood components available for clinical use along with suggested indications are given in Table 45-9 (see Chapters 37 and 47). If hemorrhage is massive, fresh whole blood is preferable but usually is not readily available. Packed red blood cells can be exchanged for whole blood if one recognizes that additional components, such as fresh frozen plasma, may be needed concomitantly for dilutional coagulopathies. In this regard, there is no evidence that prophylactically administered fresh frozen plasma in the massively transfused patient is of any benefit. Therefore, transfusion protocols should not arbitrarily include this component after every 4 to 6 units of packed red blood cells (ACOG, 1994).

As indicated in Table 45-9, fresh frozen plasma should be reserved for identifiable coagulation defects or the need for specific blood factor replacement. Similarly, platelet packs should not be used for thrombocytopenia that is otherwise asymptomatic. The two exceptions to this statement are when the patient is scheduled for surgery with a preoperative platelet count of less than 50,000 or any time the platelet count is less

than 20,000. In the first case, hemostasis is more easily achieved intraoperatively when a more adequate number of platelets are available. Because the life span of these previously frozen platelets is limited, transfusion should be given within 6 to 12 hours of the planned surgery. Spontaneous pulmonary hemorrhage has been reported when platelet counts are below 20,000.

Transfusion reactions can be grouped into two categories: minor reactions, in which case the blood being administered may be continued, depending on circumstances, and major reactions, which mandate immediate discontinuation of the transfusion. Included in the first category are allergic reactions and low-grade febrile responses. Allergic reactions occur in approximately 4% of all recipients of whole blood or packed red blood cells. This is caused by passive transfer of donor antigens to a sensitive recipient. Symptoms may include fever, chills, urticaria, and hives. Low-grade febrile reactions (incidence, 2%) are caused by leukocyte or platelet agglutinins present in the donor blood. The usual approach to these two minor reactions includes continuation of the transfusion, diphenhydramine 50 mg by parenteral administration, and antipyretics.

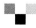 **TABLE 45-9.** INDICATIONS FOR BLOOD COMPONENT REPLACEMENT THERAPY

Blood Component	Indication for Use
Whole blood	Active bleeding and >25% blood volume loss or active bleeding and >4 units RBC used
Red blood cells (RBC)	Hypovolemia and decreased oxygen-carrying capacity or >15% blood volume loss or hematocrit <24%
Platelets	<20,000 or surgery and <50,000
Fresh frozen plasma (FFP)	Coagulation deficiencies with PTT >60, PT >16, or specific factor deficiency
Cryoprecipitate	Hemophilia A, von Willebrand disease, decreased fibrinogen, or factor XIII deficiency

PT, prothrombin time; PTT, partial thromboplastin time.

TABLE 45-10. TRANSFUSION-RELATED RISKS*

Hepatitis B	1/140,000
Hepatitis C	1/90,000
HIV-1, HIV-2	1/700,000
Bacterial contamination (red cells)	1/500,000
Bacterial contamination (platelets)	1/12,000
Acute hemolytic reaction	1/600,000
Delayed hemolytic reaction	1/1000

* Risk reported per unit of donated and screened blood (Dodd, 1992; Schreiber et al., 1996; Goodnough et al., 1999).

HIV, human immunodeficiency virus.

Severe reactions are less common, with acute hemolysis from administration of grossly incompatible blood occurring in 1 in 600,000 units of red cells transfused and bacteremia (usually because of cold-growing organisms) in less than 1 in 500,000 per unit (Table 45-10). These more serious reactions can be seen within the first few moments after the transfusion has been initiated or may be delayed for several hours to days. Symptoms can include acute decompensation with shock, DIC, fever, and renal failure. Delayed responses may be suspected only when jaundice develops distant from the transfusion period. Treatment involves discontinuation of the transfusion and supportive care. A blood sample from the recipient and the transfusion bag should be immediately sent to the laboratory for another cross-matching.

One is frequently questioned about the risks of hepatitis, acquired immunodeficiency syndrome, bacterial contamination, and transfusion reactions with a blood transfusion. Table 45-10 summarizes the approximate risks associated with blood product transfusion, including viral infections, bacterial contaminations, and hemolytic reaction.

It is expected that transfusion-related transmission rates for both hepatitis and human immunodeficiency virus will continue to further decline. Factors associated with this expectation include the following:

1. More judicious use of blood components
2. Further availability of genetically engineered products (e.g., factor VIII)
3. Development of better and more specific diagnostic screening tools for viral antigen (e.g., human immunodeficiency virus p24), surrogate markers (e.g., transaminases), and new viruses (e.g., hepatitis C and D).

ADDITIONAL MEASURES

Certain basic resuscitation maneuvers should be instituted concomitantly with blood volume replacement therapy. Blood loss not only reduces circulating volume but also significantly impairs the body's oxygen-carrying capabilities. Therefore, supplemental oxygen should always be administered by face mask. In addition, simple methods of autotransfusion, such as elevation of the lower extremities and use of the Trendelenburg position, can increase perfusion to more vital organs until blood volume replacement is accomplished.

A more sophisticated means of autotransfusion involves the use of antishock trousers (Gunning, 1983). This device, popularized in wartime applications, has two beneficial features. One is the ability to redistribute approximately 500 to 1000 mL of blood from the lower extremities to the central vasculature. The other is the ability to induce external pressure tamponade of actively bleeding pelvic and intra-abdominal structures. Actual experience with this unit is limited in obstetrics (Sandberg and Pelligra, 1983). In all likelihood, its primary use will be in those situations in which inadequate hospital facilities mandate patient transfer or when emergency medical personnel on a "scene" are unable to control hemorrhage locally. There are no data on use of antishock trousers during pregnancy because of the presumed deleterious effects on uteroplacental perfusion.

Specific guidelines should be followed in the use of antishock trousers. The device typically has three separate inflatable compartments. After each lower extremity compartment is inflated individually, the abdominal compartment should be inflated. Starting pressures should be in the range of 5 mm Hg, increasing in increments of 5 mm Hg until the desired effect is achieved. The average pressure needed to control hemorrhage ranges between 20 and 25 mm Hg. The antishock trousers can be left inflated for up to 12 hours. When the chambers are decompressed, deflation should take place over at least 30 minutes, with chamber pressures decreased by 5 mm Hg increments. Complications associated with antishock trousers usually occur at higher pressures and include peripheral metabolic acidosis and impairment of renal function.

Rebarber and colleagues (1998) studied the safety of intraoperative autologous blood collection and autotransfusion during cesarean section. In this report, blood salvage was initiated after delivery of the infant and removal of amniotic fluid from the operative field. Autotransfused volumes ranged from a median of 500 mL to approximately 11,000 mL in one patient. When compared with a control group of patients transfused donor blood under similar operative conditions, there were no differences in the rates of infections, coagulation abnormalities, or respiratory problems. This technology may be particularly valuable in patients that have the potential for severe blood loss and/or have religious preferences mandating the avoidance of transfused blood products.

DEFINITIVE THERAPY FOR HEMORRHAGIC SHOCK

The approach to definitive therapy for hemorrhagic shock must take into account individual circumstances. In the case of immediate postpartum hemorrhage, conventional methods to control bleeding (e.g., uterine massage, direct compression) are the first lines of treatment. One useful maneuver is to manually elevate the uterine fundus above the symphysis pubis for easier continual uterine massage. Confirmation that the uterine cavity is adequately clean of residual placental fragments should be undertaken without hesitation.

Pharmacologic agents useful in controlling hemorrhage from an atonic uterus are listed in Table 45-11. Oleen and Mariano (1990) reported a 95% success rate in the use of these agents for the control of refractory atonic postpartum hemorrhage. The physician should also check for a bleeding diathesis (as a cause or result of hemorrhage).

At times a surgical approach to severe hemorrhage is needed. Careful examination of the lower genital tract after delivery can disclose significant vaginal or cervical lacerations requiring repair. For uterine hemorrhage that is unresponsive to medical management, several approaches have been advocated. Ligation of the ascending branches of the uterine arteries is perhaps the easiest of procedures to perform from a technical perspective. O'Leary (1980) reported significant success using this technique in more than 100 patients with

TABLE 45-11. PHARMACOLOGIC AGENTS USEFUL FOR CONTROLLING UTERINE ATONY

Agent	Dose	Considerations/Side Effects
Oxytocin	10–20 units/L IV drip	Avoid IV bolus—may result in premature ventricular contractions and hypotension.
Methergine	0.2 mg IM (q 2–4 hours up to 5 doses)	Increased systemic vascular resistance, increased mean arterial blood pressure, and increased central venous pressure. Side effects include pulmonary edema, seizures, intracranial hemorrhage, retinal detachment, and coronary vasospasm. Avoid in patients with hypertension.
Prostaglandin 15-methyl $F_{2\alpha}$	0.25 mg IM (q 15–90 min up to 2 mg total)	Diarrhea. Bronchoconstriction. Increased cardiac output, increased heart rate, and increased right heart pressure. Increased pulmonary vascular resistance. Decreased systemic vascular resistance. Decreased coronary artery perfusion. Avoid in patients with asthma.
Prostaglandin E_2	20 mg per rectum, or vagina	Diarrhea, nausea, vomiting. Tachypnea, pyrexia, tachycardia. Decreased systemic vascular resistance. Decreased mean arterial pressure. Increased cardiac output.
Misoprostol (prostaglandin E_1) (O'Brien et al., 1998)	1000 micrograms per rectum (one dose)	Diarrhea, vomiting. Abdominal pain. Headache.

IM, intramuscularly; IV, intravenous.

postcesarean hemorrhage. The uterine arteries are usually identified anteriorly near the vesicouterine peritoneal reflection. A suture ligature with no. 0 chromic suture is passed through the broad ligament, around the uterine artery, and then into 2 to 3 cm of adjacent myometrium (Fig. 45-10).

Another approach is to displace the uterus anteriorly out of the pelvis so that the uterine vessels can be visualized coursing through the broad ligament from the posterior view. The individual vessels should not be divided. Recanalization is reported to occur, and subsequent pregnancies are apparently unaffected by this procedure (O'Leary, 1980). As an extra measure, if necessary, some investigators have suggested that an additional suture be placed beneath the ovarian ligament at its junction

with the uterus (Clark, Phelan, et al., 1985). This ligature should further reduce blood flow to the uterus by occluding ovarian artery anastomoses.

Hypogastric artery ligation is technically more difficult to perform compared with direct ligation of the uterine vessels. The success of this procedure depends on an overall decrease in pulse pressure to the uterus and is best accomplished by a bilateral approach. Access to the retroperitoneal space is obtained by division of the round ligament and gentle dissection of the loose areolar tissue along the pelvic side wall (Fig. 45-11). The ureter should always be identified beneath the medial margins of the peritoneum and retracted away. A right-angle clamp is placed below and lateral to the hypogastric artery approximately 2 to 3 cm distal to the bifurcation of the common iliac artery. The surgeon must take care to avoid injury to the hypogastric vein, which lies posterior and medial to the artery. Although some have suggested that ligation should take place below the posterior division of the hypogastric artery (superior gluteal artery) to prevent gluteal muscle ischemia, this area frequently cannot be easily identified. Two zero silk ties should be placed around the vessel and doubly ligated (see Fig. 45-11). The artery should not be surgically divided.

Clark, Phelan, and colleagues (1985) reviewed the effectiveness of hypogastric artery ligation for control of obstetric hemorrhage and found this procedure to be effective in controlling bleeding in only 42% of the cases studied. The remainder of patients required subsequent hysterectomy to control hemorrhage. Additionally, there was an increased incidence of complications, including cardiac arrest and ureteral injury, in patients requiring hysterectomy for intractable bleeding after attempted hypogastric artery ligation. Clark's group concluded that this procedure should be reserved for hemodynamically

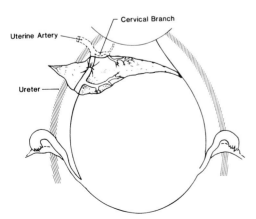

FIGURE 45-10 ■ Uterine artery ligation technique (anterior approach) for postpartum obstetric hemorrhage.

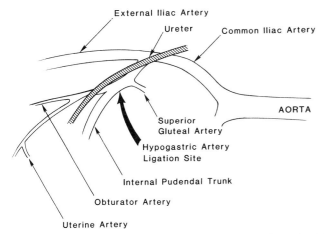

FIGURE 45-11 ■ Localization of the hypogastric artery along the right pelvic sidewall.

stable patients of low parity in whom future childbearing potential is of concern.

The incidence of emergency hysterectomy for obstetric hemorrhage ranges between 0.02% and 0.7% (Clark et al., 1984). This procedure is more commonly needed after cesarean section than vaginal delivery. Uterine atony is the most common indication cited in some reports (Plauche et al., 1981; Clark et al., 1984). Other indications for emergency hysterectomy in a large obstetric population are listed in Table 45-12 (Clark et al., 1984). In this study, the estimated blood loss averaged 3575 mL, substantially more than the 1400 mL reported by Pritchard (1965) in cases involving elective hysterectomy. Much of this difference was attributed to intraoperative attempts at conservative management before proceeding with hysterectomy.

Other complications encountered during emergency hysterectomy after delivery are summarized in Table 45-13. The choice between total and subtotal hysterectomy should be based on patient stability and availability of blood components; however, if hysterectomy is being performed for placenta accreta occurring in the lower uterine segment, adequate hemostasis may not be achieved with a subtotal procedure. Under these circumstances, the source of bleeding may be the cervical branch of the uterine artery.

PELVIC ARTERY EMBOLIZATION

Within the field of radiology, arteriography has become a well-accepted and refined tool for both diagnostic and therapeutic purposes. Internal iliac artery embolization using this new technology has already proved effective in the management of pelvic hemorrhage resulting from malignancy and trauma. It is therefore surprising that only a few isolated cases have been reported in the obstetric population with regard to arteriographic control of postpartum hemorrhage (Pais et al., 1980; Rosenthal and Colapinto, 1985; Chin et al., 1989).

In a small series of 10 patients reported by Gilbert and coinvestigators (1992), the angiographically directed embolization procedure was 100% successful in controlling hemorrhage. Absorbable gelatin sponge (Gelfoam) or another type of particulate material has been used for embolization, as have a variety of pharmacologic vasoconstrictive agents, with varying success. Precise catheter placement and manipulation require fluoroscopic imaging with optimal resolution. The femoral artery is usually chosen as the access route to the pelvic vessels.

After diagnostic arteriography is used to demonstrate dye extravasation, the involved artery is selectively catheterized and the embolic material is injected. Placement of the material into the target vessel can be fluoroscopically monitored. The contralateral hypogastric artery should be examined arteriographically as well after the successful embolization to make certain that no other sites of hemorrhage exist. Pelvic arteriography and embolization can often be completed within 2 hours from the start of the procedure.

Reported complications include excess ischemia or tissue necrosis and contrast medium–associated nephrotoxicity. It should be recognized that failure of this approach does not preclude a subsequent surgical attempt at hemorrhage control. Conversely, once hypogastric artery ligation is performed, successful arteriographic embolization is much more difficult to achieve.

OTHER APPROACHES

Several reports reintroduced the use of uterine (Irani and Penkar, 1990) and vaginal (Robie et al., 1990; Hallak et al., 1991) pressure packs to control life-threatening postpartum hemorrhage. In these reports, other more conventional approaches were first exhausted before these techniques were used. In each case, the pack was removed vaginally approximately 24 to 48 hours later, with good hemostasis noted. No rebleeding was reported in these selected cases, and no pack-related morbidity was identified. Use of these techniques stabilized the patient and reversed any consumptive coagulopathy that was severely hampering attempts to attain hemostasis.

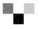

TABLE 45-12. OBSTETRIC HEMORRHAGE INDICATIONS FOR EMERGENCY HYSTERECTOMY

Uterine atony	43%
Placenta accreta	30%
Uterine rupture	13%
Incision extension	10%
Fibroid uterus	3%

Modified from Clark SL, Sze-Ya Y, Phelan JP: Emergency hysterectomy for obstetric hemorrhage. Obstet Gynecol **64**:376, 1984.

TABLE 45-13. COMPLICATIONS OF EMERGENCY HYSTERECTOMY FOR OBSTETRIC HEMORRHAGE

Blood transfusion	96%
Febrile morbidity	50%
Wound infection	12%
Coagulopathy	6%
Uretheral injury	4%
Cardiac arrest	4%
Septic pelvic thrombophlebitis	3%
Maternal death	1%

Modified from Clark SL, Sze-Ya Y, Phelan JP: Emergency hysterectomy for obstetric hemorrhage. Obstet Gynecol **64**:376, 1984. Reprinted with permission from the American College of Obstetricians and Gynecologists.

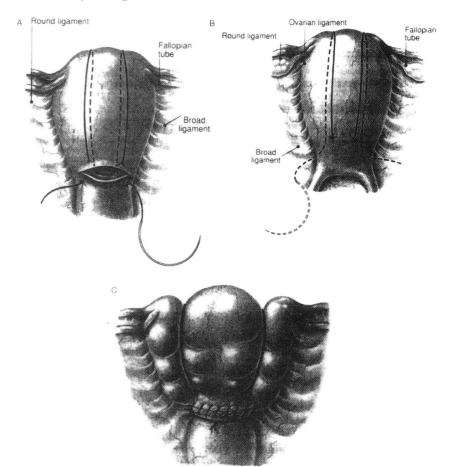

FIGURE 45-12 ■ B-Lynch surgical technique. **A,** Anterior view of the B-Lynch stitch placement. **B,** Posterior view of the B-Lynch stitch placement. **C,** Anterior view of completed procedure. (B-Lynch C, Coker A, Lawal AH, et al: The B-Lynch surgical technique for the control of massive postpartum haemorrhage: An alternative to hysterectomy? Five cases reported. Br J Obstet Gynaecol **104:**372, 1997. Reprinted with permission.)

The use of uterine compression sutures was reported to be helpful in controlling postpartum hemorrhage. B-Lynch and colleagues (1997) and Hayman and associates (2002) reported success using uterine compression sutures as the initial surgical step to control hypotonic uterine bleeding when routine uterotonic medications failed or were contraindicated. The authors used heavy absorbable suture to achieve hemostasis. Figure 45-12 illustrates the surgical approach to the placement of the B-Lynch stitch.

■ TRAUMA IN PREGNANCY

Epidemiology

Trauma continues to be a leading cause of death in women of childbearing age (Fildes et al., 1992). For the pregnant woman, accidental injury has been estimated to occur in 6% to 7% of all pregnancies (Peckham and King, 1963). According to one report from a large regional medical center, three to four women per 1000 giving birth sustained injuries sufficiently severe to require hospitalization (Lavin and Polsky, 1983). With regard to types of trauma, motor vehicle accidents are the leading cause of severe maternal trauma and death (Bremer and Cassata, 1986; Weiss et al., 2001). This is followed by violent assaults and suicide (Poole et al., 1996). These figures will probably continue to rise in the future because of (1) the tendency for women to remain actively employed during pregnancy, (2) an increase in jobs for women that are considered more hazardous, and (3) the trend toward a more violent society.

Influence of Physiologic Alterations on Trauma in Pregnancy

Pregnancy is accompanied by a variety of physiologic and anatomic alterations. Many of these changes can specifically influence both patterns of injuries and host responses (Pearlman et al., 1990b). Near term, the pregnant patient has a 35% to 40% increase in total blood volume. Because clinical signs of shock tend to present as a function of percentage of total blood loss, the pregnant patient will have an increased absolute amount of blood loss, compared with her nonpregnant counterpart, for the same clinically determined degree of shock (see previous section, Hemorrhagic Shock). It should therefore be anticipated that a large volume of blood and fluid will be needed during urgent resuscitation attempts. Additionally, the pregnant patient at term at times is able to temporarily maintain hemodynamic stability in the face of acute volume depletion only at the expense of the fetal status. Reflex vasoconstrictive responses can significantly decrease uteroplacental perfusion, thereby insidiously compromising the fetal compartment.

Several other hemodynamic alterations in pregnancy may potentially confuse the picture of shock. For example, although CO is increased by 40% near term, supine positioning can significantly decrease blood return to the heart, leading to overt hypotension and loss of consciousness. Simple maneuvers, such as lateral displacement of the uterus, may dramatically improve this event. Pulse rate increases by approximately 15% and maternal blood pressure falls in the mid-trimester; both findings may signal early signs of shock in the nonpregnant subject but are physiologic in pregnancy.

From an anatomic viewpoint, the genitourinary tract is the most significantly affected organ system in pregnancy as it pertains to trauma. The uterus, which in early pregnancy is a pelvic organ well protected by bony structures, becomes a prominent abdominal organ beyond 12 weeks' gestation. This results in an overall increase in risk of injury to the uterus and fetus as pregnancy advances. A parallel increase in blood supply to the uterus adds the additional risk of significant hemorrhage in the event of injury to this organ. Similarly, the urinary bladder is more prone to injury as a result of its proximity to the enlarging uterus. The ureters and renal pelvis are actually somewhat protected by the uterus later in pregnancy. However, the radiologist who is unfamiliar with these principles may misinterpret normal physiologic dilatation of these structures as abnormal.

The enlarging uterus also has profound influences on the gastrointestinal tract; the bowel is pushed into the upper abdominal cavity late in pregnancy. It is not surprising, therefore, that upper abdominal trauma frequently involves injury to both the small and large bowel. For this same reason, most investigators would agree that paracentesis or peritoneal lavage is more risky in pregnancy and is of limited value. Others, however, have advocated this diagnostic procedure in pregnancy, using a modified approach (Rothenberger et al., 1977; Stuart et al., 1980). It is controversial as to whether there is decreased gastrointestinal motility in pregnancy (see Chapter 52). However, as with any patient requiring general anesthesia, there is a risk of aspiration.

Several hematologic factors regarding the pregnant patient should be kept in mind. First, pregnancy represents a hypercoagulable state that may increase risks of thrombosis after injury. Because DIC is a common component of severe trauma, one should recall that the normal fibrinogen level in pregnancy ranges between 350 and 400 mg/dL. Values ranging from 80 to 180 mg/dL may be normal in the nonpregnant patient but may indicate early DIC in pregnancy. Careful screening for sepsis is also a routine part of the management of the traumatized patient. Pregnancy is frequently manifested by an associated mild leukocytosis, probably caused by demargination of peripheral leukocytes in the circulation. Therefore, the diagnosis of sepsis should not be made on the basis of a moderately elevated white blood cell count alone.

Effects of Trauma on the Fetus

As suggested earlier, during the first trimester the developing fetus is well protected from external forces by the bony pelvis, the fluid-filled amniotic sac, and soft tissues surrounding the pelvis. In a review of 240 noncatastrophic trauma cases in *early* pregnancy, no differences were apparent between the traumatized subjects and pregnant control subjects in terms of pregnancy losses (Fort and Harlin, 1970). There are some uncommon but recognized traumatic causes for fetal loss in the first trimester. Direct causes include severe pelvic fractures and penetrating injuries to the lower abdomen and lower genital tract. Potential indirect etiologic factors for early pregnancy

loss include generalized sepsis, maternal shock, and iatrogenic causes, such as excessive radiation exposure.

Later in pregnancy, the fetal compartment extends beyond the protective pelvis, becoming more vulnerable to injury. Penetrating trauma can result in membrane rupture or direct fetal injury. Blunt trauma can induce inertial types of fetal injury, including skull fracture and intracranial hemorrhage. Disruption of uteroplacental exchange by premature separation of the placenta has also been reported. Nonfatal injuries to the fetus may heal *in utero* and potentially lead to later recognized sequelae, such as neurologic deficits. Because these are recognized remote from the traumatic event, a cause-and-effect relationship is difficult to establish. With regard to fetal death, this event is most often the result of maternal death. If there is fetal death with maternal survival, placental abruption has been implicated as the most frequent cause. With traumatic rupture of the uterus, fetal mortality approaches 100%.

Blunt Abdominal Trauma

The protuberant abdomen of a pregnant patient is a common target site for injury. Most instances of mild to moderate blunt trauma to the abdomen are well tolerated by the fetus and mother; however, more severe blunt trauma has adverse consequences in pregnancy. It appears that automobile-associated trauma is the most common cause of severe blunt injury in pregnant women (Bremer and Cassata, 1986; Weiss et al., 2001). Maternal deaths occurring as a direct result of motor vehicle accidents are primarily attributed to head trauma and intra-abdominal hemorrhage. In support of this finding, Rothenberger and coworkers (1978) reviewed 103 cases of blunt trauma and noted that hemorrhagic shock was a consistent feature of all maternal deaths. Pathophysiologically, an acute deceleration phenomenon is thought to occur, which would lead to the shearing of intracranial and intra-abdominal blood vessels. A similar proposal has been suggested by Crosby (1986) regarding uteroplacental vasculature injuries leading to abruptio placentae.

The safety of seatbelt use in pregnancy has been questioned. Crosby's (1986) experimental work on pregnant baboons in automobile accidents demonstrated profound alterations in intrauterine pressure after collisions equivalent to a decelerative force of 20 G (35 miles/hr, head-on collision). Use of seatbelt restraints significantly improved both maternal and fetal outcomes, although lack or improper use minimizes these potential benefits (Pearlman and Philips, 1996). It is recommended that pregnant women wear three-point restraint seatbelts during automobile travel (ACOG, 1991), taking care to place the lower portion of the seat belt across the lap and not over the dome of the uterus.

Pelvic fracture is also a commonly reported injury in the bluntly traumatized pregnant woman. Several significant points should be emphasized. First, pelvic fracture is often associated with extensive hidden blood losses owing to the rich vasculature of the pelvic structures during pregnancy. Additionally, pelvic fracture has been associated with a 10% to 15% incidence of lower urinary tract injury. Finally, the decision to allow vaginal delivery after pelvic fracture should be based on timing and stability of the fracture. Well-healed fractures do not specifically prohibit vaginal delivery unless clear anatomic compromise, suggestive of cephalopelvic disproportion, is demonstrated by clinical and radiologic studies.

Penetrating Abdominal Trauma

Penetrating injuries to the abdomen in pregnancy are encountered less frequently than blunt trauma. As in the nonpregnant subject, the prognosis depends on the type of instrument used to create the injury and the number of organs injured. It is of interest that the mortality rate in these patients is thought to be lower (0 to 9%) than in nonpregnant counterparts because the uterus acts as a shield for vital abdominal structures during penetrating trauma. Buchsbaum (1968) reported only a 19% incidence of injury to intra-abdominal organs, other than the uterus, after gunshot wounds to the abdomen in pregnancy. Unfortunately, the fetus fares less well, with a reported injury rate of 59% to 80% and a perinatal mortality rate of 41% to 71%.

Management

The acute management of trauma in pregnancy differs little from that in the nonpregnant state. Use of various trauma scoring systems (e.g., Glasgow Coma Scale, Revised Trauma Score) are helpful in triaging the mother but do not seem to be predictive of subsequent adverse pregnancy outcome or the need for prolonged fetal monitoring (Biester et al., 1997).

As suggested previously, stabilization of the mother's condition is the most critical issue and results in improved maternal and fetal survival. Critical care management and fluid and blood replacement therapy have already been discussed. Several salient features involving the care of the traumatized pregnant woman are still worthy of comment. During acute resuscitative attempts, prolonged supine positioning should be avoided. Placement of a wedge along the right side of the patient to achieve lateral displacement of the uterus should be routine. One should anticipate the need for large fluid requirements for the patient in shock, as suggested earlier. If dopamine or other vasoactive agents are used for hemodynamic stability, it should be recognized that uteroplacental vasoconstriction may lead to fetal compromise.

With regard to the fetus, an attempt at establishing an accurate gestational age should be undertaken as soon as possible. One group of investigators suggested that a biparietal diameter of 54 mm or more was the best predictive means of emergently determining the potential for fetal survival (Smith and Bottoms, 1993). In the gestationally viable fetus, constant external monitoring is recommended. Electronic fetal and uterine monitoring is recommended for a minimum of 4 hours after trauma. The presence of frequent uterine contractions or fetal heart rate abnormalities should prompt extended monitoring for 24 hours (Pearlman et al., 1990b). Because abruptio placentae is a common sequela of trauma to the abdomen, one should monitor for classic features of this complication. This would include marking the top of the uterine fundus and serially measuring for evidence of change. Pepperell and coauthors (1977) reported that only 6 of 16 cases of placental abruption severe enough to cause fetal death involved vaginal bleeding.

There are no clear rules related to the management of the gravid uterus if laparotomy is needed after abdominal trauma.

Under no circumstances should the enlarged uterus be allowed to compromise the surgical exploration. Conversely, laparotomy is not an automatic indication for hysterotomy. If the uterus has not been significantly injured and the fetus is dead, vaginal delivery after exploratory surgery is an appropriate approach. Management of the live fetus under these same circumstances should be handled in a much more individualized fashion. If uterine injury has occurred and the fetus has reached a viable gestational age, delivery during the laparotomy procedure is probably indicated. Similarly, if it is expected that the maternal condition may continue to deteriorate, more aggressive fetal intervention would be warranted.

Few diagnostic procedures or therapeutic modalities used in the care of traumatized patients are absolutely contraindicated during pregnancy. Real-time ultrasonography to assess the fetus and Betke-Kleihauer stain analysis to assess fetal–maternal hemorrhage are certainly recommended procedures. Radiographic studies should be carefully selected, in particular during the first trimester, and pelvic and abdominal shielding should be used whenever possible. As mentioned earlier, the use of paracentesis or peritoneal lavage in pregnancy remains controversial. Indications for diagnostic lavage include unexplained abdominal signs or symptoms, altered sensorium, unexplained shock, major thoracic injury, and multiple major orthopedic injuries. If these are used, Rothenberger and associates (1977) recommend surgical opening of the peritoneum and insertion of a peritoneal dialysis catheter in the direction of the pelvis. Interpretations of peritoneal lavage findings are summarized in Table 45-14.

Choice of antibiotics for the infected patient should be modified according to known teratogenic factors and pharmacokinetic alterations that occur in pregnancy (see previous section, Septic Shock). Tetanus toxoid prophylaxis should be used for the same indications as in the nonpregnant patient.

TABLE 45-14. INTERPRETATION OF DIAGNOSTIC PERITONEAL LAVAGE FINDINGS AFTER BLUNT TRAUMA*

Positive[†]
   Grossly bloody lavage fluid
   RBC count >100,000/mm³
   WBC count >175/dL
   Amylase >175/dL
   Lavage fluid identified in Foley catheter
Indeterminate[‡]
   RBC count >50,000 but <100,000/mm³
   WBC count >100 but <500/mm³
   Amylase >75 but <175/dL
Negative
   RBC count <50,000/mm³
   WBC count <100/mm³
   Amylase <75/dL

* Peritoneal lavage is performed with 1 liter of Ringer lactated solution.
† Positive lavage (any one criterion) suggests the need for surgical exploration.
‡ Recommendations are to repeat lavage.
RBC, red blood cell; WBC, white blood cell.

Modified from Rothenberger DA, Quattlesbaum FW, Zabel J, et al.: Diagnostic peritoneal lavage for blunt trauma in pregnant women. Am J Obstet Gynecol **129:**479, 1977.

RhoGAM administration may be needed in the case of the traumatized Rh-negative woman if laboratory work reveals a fetomaternal hemorrhage. Under these circumstances, when RhoGAM is administered, blood bank personnel should be aware of this therapy so that confusion can be avoided during subsequent blood typing.

Duration of fetal monitoring after blunt trauma remains controversial. Although earlier reviews empirically suggested continuous fetal monitoring for longer than 24 hours, more recent studies (Goodwin and Breen, 1990; Pearlman et al., 1990a) support a shorter observation interval—*if* the patient does not have significant uterine activity or tenderness, vaginal bleeding, a worrisome fetal heart rate monitor pattern, or a positive Betke-Kleihauer stain. This last test may not be necessary in the Rh-positive gravida without other signs of abruptio placenta (Connolly et al., 1997).

BURNS IN PREGNANCY

Epidemiology and Definitions

Each year, approximately 75,000 people in the United States require hospitalization for significant burn injuries (Smith et al., 1983). Approximately 4% to 7% of the reproductive-age women in this group are pregnant (Matthews, 1982a; Smith et al., 1983). When these women are compared with nonpregnant women, limited data demonstrate that pregnancy does not increase the incidence or change the cause of burn injuries.

The approach to management of the burn victim depends on two basic issues: depth of the burn and size of the area involved. *Partial-thickness* burns are those in which sufficient numbers of epithelial cells allow for spontaneous reepithelialization after injury. These were previously classified as "first-degree" and "second-degree" burns. *Full-thickness* burns, formerly called "third-degree" burns, are those in which total destruction of the skin does not allow for regeneration of the epithelial surface.

"Minor" burns are usually defined as partial-thickness injuries covering less than 10% of the total body surface. "Major" burns are partial-thickness or full-thickness injuries covering more than 10% of body surface. These major burns can be further subclassified as "moderate" (10% to 19%), "severe" (20% to 39%), and "critical" (at least 40%). The term "major" can also be used in less extensive injuries if the host is significantly debilitated or when accompanying injuries are significant enough to be life-threatening.

Table 45-15 demonstrates one method of rapidly determining the percentage of total body surface burned. This represents estimates for the nonpregnant patient; a similar chart has not been established for the pregnant patient.

Effect on Pregnancy

Severe burns are morbid events with significant short-term and long-term consequences. Pregnancy (or gestational age) does not appear to have any direct influence on maternal prognosis after burn injury. As should be anticipated, maternal survival is most dependent on the severity of the burn itself (Table 45-16). Similarly, a favorable fetal outcome is primarily

TABLE 45-15. ESTIMATING AREA OF BURN WOUND INJURY

Anatomic Area	Body Surface Area (%)
Head	9
Upper extremity (each)	9
Lower extremity (each)	18
Anterior trunk	18
Posterior trunk	18
Neck	1

determined by maternal survival (Akhtar et al., 1994). However, one investigator (Matthews, 1982a) advocated prompt delivery of the second-trimester and third-trimester fetus, in the mother's interest, if the burn exceeds 50% of the body surface area. Matthews analyzed only a limited number of cases during pregnancy, in a retrospective fashion, and compared these results with previously published data in nonpregnant patients. Although this recommendation has been propagated through the literature (Rayburn et al., 1984), it appears that the existing data are insufficient to firmly support this management approach.

Management

As with most critical conditions in pregnancy, the management of a severe burn differs little from treatment of the nonpregnant patient (Monafo, 1996). A detailed description of burn wound management is beyond the scope of this chapter.

Basically, management in pregnancy can be divided into three components. Management in the *acute phase* (Nguyen et al., 1996) centers on the following:

1. Providing fluid and electrolyte therapy
2. Establishing hemodynamic and ventilatory stability
3. Evaluating fetal well-being when the fetus has reached a viable gestational age

Stillbirth or preterm delivery usually occurs within the first few days after injury and is most often associated with instability of the mother's condition. If fetal compromise can be minimized during this acute phase, prognosis is much improved.

Frequently, the question of tocolytic therapy is raised during this acute management period because of the common occurrence of preterm labor. Burns are uniformly associated with elevated prostaglandin levels. No ideal approach to therapy has been established. Clearly, burn patients are at high risk for β-agonist tocolytic complications owing to their high output state, extensive fluid requirements, and capillary permeability

TABLE 45-16. CRUDE MORTALITY RATES AFTER MATERNAL BURN INJURIES

Body Surface Injured (%)	Maternal Mortality (%)	Perinatal Mortality (%)
20–39	3	11–27
40–59	27–50	45–53
>60	92–100	100

problems. Magnesium sulfate therapy may also be dangerous in this setting because of the known vasodilatory effects of this drug and the already existing electrolyte disturbances related to the burn injury. This leaves few therapeutic alternatives.

In the near-term fetus, perhaps the best approach is expectant management. Gestational age cutoffs for this nonintervention approach should be based on each individual institution's perinatal mortality statistics. In the very preterm infant, there may be success if delivery is delayed with indomethacin therapy for 48 to 72 hours. After this point, if the patient's condition stabilizes, tocolytic therapy can be altered to more traditional agents or discontinued completely.

During the convalescent recovery period, careful monitoring for sepsis is critical. As burn areas demarcate healthy from devitalized tissues, serial debridements as well as grafting procedures are necessary. Topical agents, such as silver sulfadiazine, are typically used to dress the burn wounds; these are not specifically contraindicated in pregnancy. Early ambulation is especially important in the pregnant patient to reduce risks of thromboembolic disease. Route of delivery should be based on obstetric considerations.

Only a limited amount of information is available concerning remote consequences of severe burn injuries. By most reports, after severe abdominal burns the abdominal wall is able to expand sufficiently in subsequent pregnancies to allow for normal uterine enlargement and fetal growth (Rai and Jackson, 1975; Matthews, 1982b). Daw and Mohandas (1983), however, observed 11 pregnant patients with scarring from previous severe burns, noting frequent complaints of itching and painful abdominal tightness with advancing gestation. In 6 of 11 patients, delivery was prematurely induced because of these complaints. Others described surgical decompression procedures during pregnancy for abdominal scarring (Webb et al., 1995).

Electrical Shock

Electrical injuries are uncommonly reported during pregnancy, with a total of 21 electrical and 11 lightning-related events identified in the literature (Leiberman et al., 1986; Fatovich, 1993; Einarson et al., 1997). Although maternal death is rare, fetal mortality is disproportionately high.

Injury can be *thermal* or *conductive* in nature. Thermal injuries occur at the site of contact as well as internally along the path of the current. This has the potential to result in unsuspected deep tissue necrosis, cardiac injury, and rhabdomyolysis. Electrical current passing through the mother can also lead to arrhythmias, respiratory arrest, and tetanic muscle contractions with skeletal fractures. Amniotic fluid offers a low resistance path for electrical current to flow, thus explaining the vulnerability of the fetus. Severity of maternal injury is not predictive of fetal outcome, with *in utero* cardiac arrest presumed to be a common cause of death. Of interest, fetal growth restriction can be a late consequence of electrical thermal injury to the placenta (Rosati et al., 1995).

PERIMORTEM CESAREAN SECTION

Perimortem cesarean section represents a new and somewhat empiric approach to the care of a gestationally viable fetus when immediate maternal survival is in question. *Postmortem* delivery has been previously recognized to have limited success

in terms of fetal survival. Katz and coauthors (1986) reviewed these data and raised several crucial issues that need to be readdressed in modern obstetrics. In particular, the authors noted that the causes of maternal mortality have shifted from more chronic forms of illness to acute situations such as anesthetic complications, embolic disease, and cerebrovascular accidents. Under these circumstances, it is anticipated that more often the mother can be saved with aggressive intervention. In addition, it is less likely that the fetus has been chronically compromised before the acute events that lead to the maternal cardiopulmonary arrest.

The benefit of earlier attempts at delivery of the fetus have been argued from the perspectives of *both* the mother and the fetus. Successful cardiopulmonary resuscitation (CPR) depends on maintaining an adequate CO by chest compression. In the best of circumstances, CPR in the nonpregnant patient can generate only 30% of the normal CO. Supine positioning in pregnancy near term further reduces blood return to the heart as a result of vena caval occlusion (Lee et al., 1986). In the absence of supportive data, therefore, it would be expected that CPR in the term pregnant patient would be significantly less effective. However, anecdotal case reports have suggested more successful outcomes with CPR after emptying of the uterus (DePace et al., 1982; Marx, 1982).

From the infant's perspective, survival seems to be dependent on the timing of the operation. Few cases of surviving healthy infants have been reported for those born beyond 10 minutes after CPR was initiated. Clinical experience and laboratory experimentation suggest that an intact fetus can usually be delivered if total asphyxia is limited to 4 to 6 minutes (Windle, 1968; Katz et al., 1986).

On the basis of these perspectives, some authorities suggest that appropriate management during a perimortem event include the following principles:

1. Attempts at delivery of the gestationally viable fetus should be begun within 4 minutes after maternal cardiac arrest.
2. CPR should be continued during and after the procedure in cases in which the potential for maternal survival exists.
3. Staff should not waste time preparing a sterile field.
4. Because there have been isolated reports of infant survival well beyond the 4- to 6-minute time limit, attempts at delivery usually should be undertaken at any time after maternal death if signs of fetal life are present.

No data are yet available to document whether this approach actually improves maternal or fetal outcome. Comprehensive assessment of this approach needs to be carried out in future analyses, and at present each case must be individualized.

Three additional points need to be emphasized:

1. Cesarean delivery is associated with significant blood loss, and this may further compromise maternal stability unless blood volume is replaced.
2. Cesarean section should not be performed in an unstable patient because of anticipated cardiac arrest. Under these tenuous circumstances, this iatrogenic insult will precipitate a poorer outcome.
3. If a patient undergoes successful CPR before an attempt is made to deliver the infant, this operative procedure should not be performed because successful *in utero* resuscitation is likely.

Brain Death during Pregnancy

Maternal brain death, without apparent fetal compromise at nonviable gestational ages, has been reported on rare occasions (Dillon et al., 1982; Field et al., 1988; Bernstein et al., 1989; Catanzarite et al., 1997). Prolonging gestation in an attempt to salvage neonatal survival is possible, but aggressive maternal hemodynamic, respiratory, metabolic, and tocolytic support is required. Previous reports have described the initial moribund event at 15 to 25 weeks' gestation, with 24 to 107 days' prolongation of pregnancy. Delivery was required secondary to sepsis, maternal hypotension, and fetal distress. All four neonates survived. The complex ethical issues surrounding the family and health care provider decisions under these circumstances mandate individualized considerations.

REFERENCES

Abdulla AM, Kavouras T, Rivas F, et al: Determination of mean pulmonary capillary pressure by a noninvasive technique. JAMA **243**:1539, 1980.

Akhtar MA, Mulawkar PM, Kulkami HR: Burns in pregnancy: Effect on maternal and fetal outcomes. Burns **20**:351, 1994.

American College of Gynecologists and Obstetricians (ACOG): Automobile passenger restraints for children and pregnant women. ACOG Technical Bulletin **151**:1, 1991.

American College of Gynecologists and Obstetricians (ACOG): Invasive hemodynamic monitoring in obstetrics and gynecology. ACOG Technical Bulletin **175**:1, 1992.

American College of Gynecologists and Obstetricians (ACOG): Blood component therapy. ACOG Technical Bulletin **199**:1, 1994.

American College of Gynecologists and Obstetricians (ACOG): Septic shock. ACOG Technical Bulletin **204**:1, 1995.

Askenazi J, Koenigsberg DI, Ziegler JA, et al: Echocardiographic estimates of pulmonary artery wedge pressure. N Engl J Med **305**:1566, 1981.

Atrash HK, Alexander S, Berg CJ: Maternal mortality in developed countries: Not just a concern of the past. Obstet Gynecol **86**:700, 1995.

Atrash HK, Koonin LM, Lawson HW, et al: Maternal mortality in the United States, 1979–1986. Obstet Gynecol **76**:1055, 1990.

Baker R: Hemorrhage in obstetrics. Obstet Gynecol Annu **6**:295, 1997.

Bech-Jansen P, Brinkman CR, Johnson GH, et al: Circulatory shock in pregnant sheep. Am J Obstet Gynecol **112**:1084, 1972.

Belfort MA, Mares A, Saade GR, et al: A re-evaluation of the indications for pulmonary artery catheters in obstetrics: The role of 2-D echocardiography and Doppler ultrasound. Am J Obstet Gynecol 1996; **174**:331.

Beller FK, Schmidt EH, Holzfreve W, et al: Septicemia during pregnancy: A study in different species of experimental animals. Am J Obstet Gynecol **151**:967, 1985.

Benedetti TJ: Life-threatening complications of betamimetic therapy for preterm labor inhibition. Clin Perinatol **13**:843, 1986.

Benedetti TJ, Carlson RW: Studies of colloid osmotic pressure in pregnancy-induced hypertension. Am J Obstet Gynecol **135**:308, 1979.

Benedetti TJ, Cotton DB, Read JC, et al: Hemodynamic observations in severe preeclampsia with a flow-directed pulmonary artery catheter. Am J Obstet Gynecol **136**:465, 1980.

Benedetti TJ, Kates R, Williams V: Hemodynamic observations of severe preeclampsia complicated by pulmonary edema. Am J Obstet Gynecol **152**:330, 1985.

Berg CJ, Atrash HK, Koonin LM, et al: Pregnancy related mortality in the United States, 1987–1990. Obstet Gynecol **88**:161, 1996.

Bernard GR, Vincent JL, Pierre-Francois L, et al: Efficacy and safety of recombinant human activated protein C for severe sepsis. N Engl J Med **344**:699, 2000.

Bernstein IM, Watson M, Simmons GM, et al: Maternal brain death and prolonged fetal survival. Obstet Gynecol **74**:434, 1989.

Biester EM, Tomich PG, Esposito TJ, et al: Trauma in pregnancy: Normal revised trauma score in relation to other markers of maternal fetal status—A preliminary study. Am J Obstet Gynecol **176**:1206, 1997.

Blanco JD, Gibbs RS, Castaneda YS: Bacteremia in obstetrics: Clinical course. Obstet Gynecol **58**:621, 1981.

B-Lynch C, Coker A, Lawal AH, et al: The B-Lynch surgical technique for the control of massive postpartum haemorrhage: An alternative to hysterectomy? Five cases reported. Br J Obstet Gynaecol **104**:372, 1997.

Boyd KD, Thomas SJ, Gold J, et al: A prospective study of complications of pulmonary artery catheterizations in 500 consecutive patients. Chest **84**:245, 1983.

Bray RE, Boe RW, Johnson WL: Transfer of ampicillin into fetus and amniotic fluid from maternal plasma in late pregnancy. Am J Obstet Gynecol **96**:938, 1966.

Bremer C, Cassata L: Trauma in pregnancy. Nurs Clin North Am **21**:705, 1986.

Brose WG, Cohen SE: Oxyhemoglobin saturation following cesarean section in patients receiving epidural morphine, PCA, or IM meperidine analgesia. Anesthesiology **70**:948, 1989.

Bryan CD, Reynolds KL, Moore EE: Bacteremia in obstetrics and gynecology. Obstet Gynecol **64**:155, 1984.

Buchsbaum HJ: Accidental injury complicating pregnancy. Am J Obstet Gynecol **102**:752, 1968.

Capeless EL, Clapp JF: Cardiovascular change in early phase of pregnancy. Am J Obstet Gynecol **161**:1449, 1989.

Catanzarite VA, Wilms DC, Holdy KE, et al: Brain death during pregnancy: Tocolytic therapy and aggressive maternal support on behalf of the fetus. Am J Perinatol **14**:431, 1997.

Cefalo RC, Lewis PE, O'Brian WF, et al: The role of prostaglandins in endotoxemia: Comparisons in response in the nonpregnant, maternal, and fetal models. Am J Obstet Gynecol **137**:53, 1980.

Centers for Disease Control: Epidemiologic notes and reports: Human immunodeficiency virus infection in transfusion recipients and their family members. March 1987.

Centers for Disease Control and Prevention: Differences in maternal mortality among black and white women—United States, 1990. MMWR Morb Mortal Wkly Rep **44**:6, 1995.

Centers for Disease Control and Prevention: Differences in maternal mortality among black and white women—United States 1987–1996. MMWR Morb Mortal Wkly Rep **48**:492, 1999.

Chin HG, Scott DR, Resnik R, et al: Angiographic embolization of intractable puerperal hematomas. Am J Obstet Gynecol **160**:434, 1989.

Chow AW, Guze LB: Bacteroidaceae bacteremia: Clinical experience with 112 patients. Medicine **53**:93, 1974.

Clark SL, Cotton DB, Lee W, et al: Central hemodynamic assessment of normal term pregnancy. Am J Obstet Gynecol **161**:1439, 1989.

Clark SL, Cotton DB, Pivarnik JM, et al: Position change and central hemodynamic profile during normal third-trimester pregnancy and post partum. Am J Obstet Gynecol **164**:883, 1991.

Clark SL, Greenspoon J, Aldahl D, et al: Severe preeclampsia with persistent oliguria: Management of hemodynamic subsets. Am J Obstet Gynecol **159**:604, 1988.

Clark SL, Hankins GDV, Dudley DA, et al. Amniotic fluid embolism: Analysis of a national registry. Am J Obstet Gynecol **172**:1158, 1995.

Clark SL, Montz FJ, Phelan JP: Hemodynamic alterations associated with amniotic fluid embolism: A reappraisal. Am J Obstet Gynecol **15**:617, 1985.

Clark SL, Pavova Z, Horenstein J, et al: Squamous cells in the maternal pulmonary circulation. Am J Obstet Gynecol **154**:104, 1986.

Clark SL, Phelan JP, Sze-Ya Y: Hypogastric artery ligation for obstetric hemorrhage. Obstet Gynecol **66**:353, 1985.

Clark SL, Southwick J, Pivarnik JM, et al. A comparison of cardiac index in normal term pregnancy using thoracic electrical bioimpedance and oxygen extraction (Fick) technique. Obstet Gynecol **83**:669, 1994.

Clark SL, Sze-Ya Y, Phelan JP: Emergency hysterectomy for obstetric hemorrhage. Obstet Gynecol **64**:376, 1984.

Collins CG: Suppurative pelvic thrombophlebitis. Am J Obstet Gynecol **108**:681, 1970.

Connolly AM, Kate VL, Bash KL, et al: Trauma and pregnancy. Am J Perinatal **14**:331, 1997.

Cotton DB, Gonik B, Dorman K, et al: Cardiovascular alterations in severe pregnancy-induced hypertension: Relationship of central venous pressure to pulmonary capillary wedge pressure. Am J Obstet Gynecol **151**:762, 1985a.

Cotton DB, Gonik B, Dorman K: Cardiovascular alterations in severe pregnancy-induced hypertension: Acute effects of intravenous hydralazine bolus. Surg Gynecol Obstet **16**:240, 1985b.

Cotton DB, Gonik B, Spillman T, et al: Intrapartum to postpartum changes in colloid osmotic pressure. Am J Obstet Gynecol **149**:174, 1984.

Crosby W: Trauma in the pregnant patient. Conn Med **50**:251, 1986.

Cunningham FG, Lucas MJ, Hankins GDV: Pulmonary injury complicating antepartum pyelonephritis. Am J Obstet Gynecol **156**:797, 1987.

Daw E, Mohandas I: Pregnancy in patients after severe abdominal burns. Br J Obstet Gynaecol 90:69, 1983.

Deckardt R, Fembacher PM, Schneider KTM, et al: Maternal arterial oxygen saturation during labor and delivery: Pain-dependent alterations and effects in the newborn. Obstet Gynecol 70:21, 1987.

Del Priore G, Jackson-Stone M, Shim EK, et al: A comparison of once-daily and 8 hour gentamicin dosing in the treatment of postpartum endometritis. Obstet Gynecol 87:994, 1996.

DePace NL, Betesh SS, Kotter MN: "Postmortem" cesarean section with recovery of both mother and offspring. JAMA 248:971, 1982.

Dillon WP, Lee RV, Tronolone MJ, et al: Life support and maternal brain death during pregnancy. JAMA 248:1089, 1982.

Dodd RY: The risk of transfusion transmitted infection. N Engl J Med 327:419, 1992.

Duff P, Gibbs RS, Blanco JD, et al: Endometrial culture techniques in puerperal patients. Obstet Gynecol 61:217, 1983.

Easterling TR, Benedetti TJ, Schmucker BC, et al: Maternal hemodynamics in normal and preeclamptic pregnancies: A longitudinal study. Obstet Gynecol 76:1061, 1990.

Easterling TR, Watts DH, Schmucker BC, et al: Measurement of cardiac output during pregnancy: Validation of Doppler technique and clinical observations in preeclampsia. Obstet Gynecol 69:845, 1987.

Einarson A, Bailey B, Inocencion G, et al: Accidental electric shock in pregnancy: A prospective cohort study. Am J Obstet Gynecol 176:678, 1997.

Ensing G, Seward J, Darragh R, et al: Feasibility of generating hemodynamic pressure curves from noninvasive Doppler echocardiographic signals. J Am Coll Cardiol 23:434, 1994.

Fatovich DM: Electric shock in pregnancy. J Emerg Med 11:175, 1993.

Fearon DT, Ruddy S, Schur PH, et al: Activation of the properdin pathway of complement in patients with gram-negative bacteremia. N Engl J Med 292:937, 1975.

Field DR, Gates EA, Creasy RK, et al: Maternal brain death during pregnancy. Medical and ethical issues. JAMA 260:816, 1988.

Fildes J, Reed L, Jones N, et al: Trauma: The leading cause of maternal death. J Trauma 32:643, 1992.

Fort AT, Harlin RS: Pregnancy outcome after noncatastrophic maternal trauma during pregnancy. Obstet Gynecol 35:912, 1970.

Freid MA, Vosti KL: The importance of underlying disease in patients with gram-negative bacteremia. Arch Intern Med 121:418, 1968.

Genazzani AR, Facchinetti F, Parrini D: β-Lipotrophin and β-endorphin plasma levels during pregnancy. Clin Endocrinol 14:409, 1981.

Gibbs RS: Quantitative bacteriology of amniotic fluid. J Infect Dis 145:1, 1982.

Gilbert WM, Moore TR, Resnik R, et al: Angiographic embolization in the management of hemorrhagic complications of pregnancy. Am J Obstet Gynecol 166:493, 1992.

Goldberg LI: Dopamine—Clinical uses of an endogenous catecholamine. N Engl J Med 291:707, 1974.

Gonik B, Cotton DB: Peripartum colloid osmotic pressure changes: Influence of intravenous hydration. Am J Obstet Gynecol 150:99, 1984.

Gonik B, Cotton DB, Spillman T, et al: Peripartum colloid osmotic changes: Effects of controlled fluid management. Am J Obstet Gynecol 151:812, 1985a.

Gonik B, Creasy RK, Chambers SL: Colloid osmotic pressure alterations with ritodrine hydrochloride therapy. Abstract presented at the Eighth Annual Midwestern Conference on Perinatal Research, September 10, 1985b, Osage Beach, Mo.

Gonik B, Lee W, Giebel R, et al: Septic shock in obstetrics: Clinical perspectives and hemodynamic observations. Abstract presented at the Infectious Disease Society for Obstetrics and Gynecology, July 6, 1987, Glasgow, Scotland.

Goodnough LT, Ali S, Despotis M, et al. Transfusion medicine: blood transfusion. N Engl J Med 340:438, 1999.

Goodwin TM, Breen MT: Pregnancy outcome and fetomaternal hemorrhage after noncatastrophic trauma. Am J Obstet Gynecol 162:665, 1990.

Gunning JE: For controlling intractable hemorrhage: The gravity suit. Contemp Gynecol Obstet 22:23, 1983.

Haft JI: Cardiovascular injury induced by sympathetic catecholamines. Prog Cardiovasc Dis 17:73, 1974.

Hallak M, Dildy GA, Hurley TJ, et al: Transvaginal pressure pack for life threatening pelvic hemorrhage secondary to placenta accreta. Obstet Gynecol 78:938, 1991.

Hankins GD, Hauth JC, Kuehl TJ, et al: Ritodrine hydrochloride infusion in pregnant baboons. II. Sodium and water compartment alterations. Am J Obstet Gynecol 147:254, 1983.

Hankins GD, Wendel GD Jr, Cunningham FG, et al: Longitudinal evaluation of hemodynamic changes in eclampsia. Am J Obstet Gynecol 150:506, 1984.

Hankins GD, Wendel GD Jr, Leveno KJ, et al: Myocardial infarction during pregnancy: A review. Obstet Gynecol 65:139, 1985.

Hawkins DF: Management and treatment of obstetric bacteremia shock. J Clin Pathol 33:895, 1980.

Hayman RG, Arulkumaran S, Steer PJ: Uterine compression sutures: Surgical management of postpartum hemorrhage. Obstet Gynecol 99:502, 2002.

Holaday JW, Faden AI: Naloxone reversal of endotoxin hypotension suggests role of endorphins in shock. Nature 275:450, 1978.

Hughson WG, Friedman PJ, Feigin DS, et al: Postpartum pleural effusion: A common radiologic finding. Ann Intern Med 97:856, 1982.

Irani SA, Penkar SJ: Packing of uterus at cesarean section for refractory postpartum haemorrhage: Revival of a time tested technique. J Obstet Gynecol India 40:72, 1990.

Katz M, Robertson PA, Creasy RK: Cardiovascular complications associated with terbutaline treatment for preterm labor. Am J Obstet Gynecol 139:605, 1981.

Katz VL, Dotters DJ, Droegemueller W: Perimortem cesarean delivery. Obstet Gynecol 68:571, 1986.

Kaunitz AM, Hughes JM, Grimes DA: Causes of maternal mortality in the United States. Obstet Gynecol 65:605, 1985.

Kwann HM, Weil MH: Differences in the mechanism of shock caused by bacterial infections. Surg Gynecol Obstet 1:37, 1969.

Lachman E, Pitsoe SB, Gaffin SL: Anti-lipopolysaccharide immunotherapy in management of septic shock of obstetric and gynaecologic origin. Lancet 1:981, 1984.

Lavin JP, Polsky SS: Abdominal trauma during pregnancy. Clin Perinatol 10:423, 1983.

Ledger WJ, Norman M, Gee C, et al: Bacteremia on an obstetric-gynecologic service. Am J Obstet Gynecol 121:205, 1975.

Lee RV, Rodgers BD, White LM, et al: Cardiopulmonary resuscitation of pregnant women. Am J Med 81:311, 1986.

Lee W, Clark SL, Cotton DB, et al: Septic shock during pregnancy. Am J Obstet Gynecol 159:410, 1988.

Lee W, Gonik B, Cotton DB: Urinary diagnostic indices in preeclampsia-associated oliguria: Correlation with invasive hemodynamic monitoring. Am J Obstet Gynecol 156:100, 1987.

Lefer AM, Cowgill R, Marshall FF, et al: Characterization of a myocardial depressant factor present in hemorrhagic shock. Am J Physiol 213:492, 1967.

Leiberman JR, Mazor M, Molcho J, et al: Electrical accidents during pregnancy. Obstet Gynecol 67:861, 1986.

Lillehei RC, Longerbeam JK, Bloch JH, et al: The nature of irreversible shock: Experimental and clinical observations. Ann Surg 160:682, 1964.

Mabie WC, Barton JR, Sibai BM: Septic shock in pregnancy. Obstet Gynecol 90:553, 1997.

Mabie WC, Sibai BM: Treatment in an obstetric intensive care unit. Am J Obstet Gynecol 162:1, 1990.

Makabali GL, Mandal AK, Morris JA: An assessment of the participatory role of prostaglandins and serotonin in the pathophysiology of endotoxic shock. Am J Obstet Gynecol 145:439, 1983.

Marx GF: Cardiopulmonary resuscitation of late-pregnant women [letter]. Anesthesiology 56:156, 1982.

Mashini IS, Albazzaz SJ, Fadel HE, et al: Serial noninvasive evaluation of cardiovascular hemodynamics during pregnancy. Am J Obstet Gynecol 156:1208, 1987.

Matthews RN: Obstetric implications of burns in pregnancy. Br J Obstet Gynecol 89:603, 1982a.

Matthews RN: Old burns and pregnancy. Br J Obstet Gynaecol 89:610, 1982b.

Monafo WW: Initial management of burns. N Engl J Med 335:1581, 1996.

Morishima HO, Niemann WH, James LS: Effects of endotoxin on the pregnant baboon and fetus. Am J Obstet Gynecol 131:899, 1978.

National Institutes of Health Consensus Conference: Fresh frozen plasma. JAMA 253:551, 1985.

Nguyen TT, Gilpin D, Meyer NA, et al: Current treatment of severely burned patients. Ann Surg 223:14, 1996.

O'Brian WF, Cefalo RC, Lewis PE, et al: The role of prostaglandins in endotoxemia and comparisons in response in the nonpregnant, maternal, and fetal models. Am J Obstet Gynecol 139:535, 1981.

O'Brian WF, Golden SM, Davis SE, et al: Endotoxemia in the neonatal lamb. Am J Obstet Gynecol 151:671, 1985.

O'Brien P, El-Rafaey H, Gordon A, et al: Rectally administered misoprostol for the treatment of postpartum hemorrhage unresponsive to oxytocin and ergometrine: A descriptive study. Obstet Gynecol 92:212, 1998.

O'Leary JA: Pregnancy following uterine artery ligation. Obstet Gynecol **55**:112, 1980.

Oleen MA, Mariano JP: Controlling refractory atonic postpartum hemorrhage with Hamabate sterile solution. Am J Obstet Gynecol **162**:205, 1990.

Packman MI, Rackow EC: Optimum left heart filling pressure during fluid resuscitation of patients with hypovolemic and septic shock. Crit Care Med **11**:165, 1983.

Pais SO, Glickman M, Schwartz P, et al: Embolization of pelvic arteries for control of postpartum hemorrhage. Obstet Gynecol **55**:754, 1980.

Pearlman MD, Philips ME: Safety belt use during pregnancy. Obstet Gynecol **88**:1026, 1996.

Pearlman MD, Tintinalli JE, Lorenz RP: A prospective controlled study of outcome after trauma during pregnancy. Am J Obstet Gynecol **162**:1502, 1990a.

Pearlman MD, Tintinalli JE, Lorenz RP: Blunt trauma in pregnancy. N Engl J Med **323**:1609, 1990b.

Peckham CH, King RW: A study of intercurrent conditions observed during pregnancy. Am J Obstet Gynecol **87**:609, 1963.

Pepperell RJ, Rubinstein E, MacIssac IA: Motor-car accidents during pregnancy. Med J Aust **1**:203, 1977.

Phelan JP, Yurth DA: Severe preeclampsia. I. Peripartum hemodynamic observations. Am J Obstet Gynecol **144**:17, 1982.

Plauche WC, Gruich FG, Bourgeois MO: Hysterectomy at the time of cesarean section: Analysis of 108 cases. Obstet Gynecol **58**:459, 1981.

Poole GV, Martin JN, Perry KG, et al: Trauma in pregnancy: The role of interpersonal violence. Am J Obstet Gynecol **174**:1873, 1996.

Pritchard J: Changes in blood volume during pregnancy and delivery. Anesthesiology **26**:393, 1965.

Quance D: Amniotic fluid embolism: Detection by pulse oximetry. Anesthesiology **68**:951, 1988.

Rackow EC, Astiz ME: Pathophysiology and treatment of septic shock. JAMA **266**:548, 1991.

Rackow EC, Fein IA, Leppo J: Colloid osmotic pressure as a prognostic indicator of pulmonary edema and mortality in the critically ill. Chest **72**:709, 1977.

Rackow EC, Weil MH: Recent trends in diagnosis and management of septic shock. Curr Surg **40**:181, 1983.

Rafferty TD, Berkowitz RL: Hemodynamics in patients with severe toxemia during labor and delivery. Am J Obstet Gynecol **138**:263, 1980.

Rai YS, Jackson DM: Childbearing in relation to the scarred abdominal wall from burns. Burns **1**:167, 1975.

Rao PS, Cavanagh D, Gaston LW: Endotoxic shock in the primate: Effects of aspirin and dipyridamole administration. Am J Obstet Gynecol **140**:914, 1981.

Rayburn W, Smith B, Feller I, et al: Major burns during pregnancy: Effects on fetal well-being. Obstet Gynecol **63**:392, 1984.

Rebarber A, Lonser R, Jackson S, et al: The safety of intraoperative autologous blood collection and autotransfusion during cesarean section. Am J Obstet Gynecol **179**:715, 1998.

Robertson PA, Herron M, Katz M, et al: Maternal morbidity associated with isoxsuprine and terbutaline tocolysis. Eur J Obstet Gynaecol Reprod Biol **11**:317, 1981.

Robie GF, Morgan MA, Payne GC, et al: Logothetopulos pac for the management of uncontrollable postpartum hemorrhage. Am J Perinatol **7**:327, 1990.

Robin ED: The cult of the Swan-Ganz catheter. Ann Intern Med **103**:445, 1985.

Rolbin SH, Levinson G, Shnider DM, et al: Dopamine treatment of spinal hypotension decreases uterine blood flow in the pregnant ewe. Anesthesiology **51**:36, 1979.

Rosati P, Exacoustos C, Puggioni CF, et al: Growth retardation in pregnancy: Experimental model in the rabbit employing electrically induced thermal placental injury. Int J Exp Pathol **76**:179, 1995.

Rosenthal DM, Colapinto R: Angiographic arterial embolization in the management of postoperative vaginal hemorrhage. Am J Obstet Gynecol **151**:227, 1985.

Roth A, Elkayam U: Acute myocardial infarction associated with pregnancy. Ann Intern Med **125**:751, 1996.

Rothenberger D, Quattlebaum FW, Perry JF, et al: Blunt maternal trauma: A review of 103 cases. J Trauma **18**:173, 1978.

Rothenberger DA, Quattlebaum FW, Zabel J, et al: Diagnostic peritoneal lavage for blunt trauma in pregnant women. Am J Obstet Gynecol **129**:479, 1977.

Sandberg EC, Pelligra R: The medical antigravity suit for management of surgically uncontrollable bleeding associated with abdominal pregnancy. Am J Obstet Gynecol **146**:519, 1983.

Schreiber GB, Busch MP, Kleinman SH, et al: The risk of transmission related viral infections. N Engl J Med **337**:1685, 1996.

Schumacher B, Belfort MA, Card RJ: Successful treatment of acute myocardial infarction during pregnancy with tissue plasminogen activator. Am J Obstet Gynecol **176**:716, 1997.

Sheude K, Raab R, Lee P: Decreasing the risk of pulmonary artery rupture with a pressure relief balloon. J Cardiothorac Vasc Anesth **8**:30, 1994.

Shoemaker WC, Appel PL, Bland R, et al: Clinical trial of an algorithm for outcome prediction in acute circulatory failure. Crit Care Med **11**:165, 1983.

Shubin H, Weil MH, Carlson RW: Bacterial shock. Am Heart J **94**:112, 1977.

Smith BK, Rayburn WF, Feller I: Burns and pregnancy. Clin Perinatol **10**:383, 1983.

Smith RS, Bottoms SF: Ultrasonographic prediction of neonatal survival in extremely low-birth-weight infants. Am J Obstet Gynecol **169**:490, 1993.

Sprung CL, Caralis PV, Marcial EH, et al: The effects of high-dose corticosteroids in patients with septic shock. N Engl J Med **311**:1137, 1984.

Sprung CL, Pozen RG, Rozanski JJ, et al: Advanced ventricular arrhythmias during bedside pulmonary artery catheterization. Am J Med **72**:203, 1982.

Starling EH: On the absorption of fluids from the connective tissue spaces. J Physiol **19**:312, 1896.

Stein L, Bernard J, Cavanilles J, et al: Pulmonary edema during fluid infusion in the absence of heart failure. JAMA **229**:65, 1974.

Stuart GC, Harding PG, Davies EM: Blunt abdominal trauma in pregnancy. Can Med Assoc J **122**:901, 1980.

Sugerman HJ, Peyton JWR, Greenfield LJ: Gram-negative sepsis. In Thal A (ed): Current Problems in Surgery. Chicago, Year Book, 1981.

Swan HJ, Ganz W, Forrester J, et al: Catheterization of the heart in man with use of a flow-directed balloon-tipped catheter. N Engl J Med **283**:447, 1970.

Visser W, Wallenburg HCS: Central hemodynamic observations in untreated preeclamptic patients. Hypertension **17**:1072, 1991.

Webb JC, Baack BR, Osler TM, et al: A pregnancy complicated by mature abdominal burns scarring and its surgical solution: A case report. J Burn Care Rehabil **16**:276, 1995.

Weil MH, Nishijima H: Cardiac output in bacterial shock. Am J Med **64**:920, 1978.

Weiss HB, Songer TJ, Fabio A: Fetal deaths related to maternal injury. JAMA **286**:1863, 2001.

Weiss S, Calloway E, Cairo J, et al: Comparison of cardiac output measurements by thermodilution and thoracic electrical bioimpedance in critically ill vs noncritically ill patients. Am J Emerg Med **13**:62, 1995.

Windle WF: Brain damage at birth. JAMA **206**:1967, 1968.

Wu PYK, Udani V, Chan L, et al: Colloid osmotic pressure: Variations in normal pregnancy. J Perinatol **11**:193, 1983.

Yelderman M, New W: Evaluation of pulse oximetry. Anesthesiology **59**:349, 1983.

Zebe H, Roth V, Lorenz U, et al: Investigations into the effect on myocardial function of chronic intravenous tocolysis using non-invasive test methods. In Jung H, Lamberti G (eds): Betamimetic Drugs in Obstetrics and Perinatology. New York, Thieme-Stratton, 1982.

Ziegler EJ, Fisher CJ, Sprung CL, et al: Treatment of gram-negative bacteremia and septic shock with HA-1A human monoclonal antibody against endotoxin. N Engl J Med **324**:429, 1991.

Chapter 46
RESPIRATORY DISEASES IN PREGNANCY

Janice E. Whitty, MD, and Mitchell P. Dombrowski, MD

Pulmonary disease may frequently complicate pregnancy. The occurrence of pulmonary disease during pregnancy may result in increased morbidity and/or mortality for both the mother and her fetus. Depending on the diagnosis encountered, pregnancy may have either an adverse or positive impact on the pulmonary function of the gravida. Proper functioning of the cardiorespiratory system is imperative to achieve adequate oxygenation of maternal and fetal tissues. The maternal cardiorespiratory system undergoes significant changes during gestation to optimize oxygen delivery to the fetus and maternal tissues. In this chapter, we briefly review the physiologic adaptations of the respiratory system that occur during gestation. Specific respiratory diseases that occur in pregnancy and the potential impact of the disease on pregnancy as well as pregnancy on the disease will then be discussed. It is important for the obstetrician to realize that most diagnostic tests that need to be carried out to evaluate pulmonary function during gestation are not harmful to the fetus and, if indicated, should be performed. Likewise, most medications used to treat respiratory disease in pregnancy will also be well tolerated by the fetus. Therefore, with few exceptions the diagnostic and treatment algorithms for respiratory disease will closely resemble those used in a nonpregnant woman.

PHYSIOLOGIC CHANGES OF THE RESPIRATORY SYSTEM

Because there is no increase in respiratory rate, the increase in maternal minute ventilation is secondary to an increase in tidal volume (Prowse and Gaensler, 1965). The increase in tidal volume occurs at the expense of an 18% decrease in the functional residual capacity. This hyperventilation of pregnancy results in a compensated respiratory alkalosis (arterial partial pressure of carbon dioxide [$PaCO_2$] $\leq$ 30 mm Hg) and an increase in arterial oxygenation tension (101 to 104 mm Hg) in the third trimester (Templeton and Kelman, 1976). The $PaCO_2$ decreases early in pregnancy in parallel with the change in ventilation; however, a further progressive decrease in $PaCO_2$ may occur (Boutourline-Young and Boutourline-Young, 1956). The decrease in $PaCO_2$ is even greater in altitudes where the mother is hyperventilating in an attempt to maintain the arterial partial pressure of oxygen as high as possible. Additionally, the decrease in $PaCO_2$ is matched by an equivalent increase in renal excretion of and decrease in plasma bicarbonate concentration; therefore, arterial pH is not altered from the normal nonpregnant level of about 7.4.

It has been suggested that the hyperventilation of pregnancy results primarily from progesterone acting as a respiratory stimulant (Skatrud et al., 1978). Because hyperventilation has been observed during the luteal phase of the menstrual cycle and progesterone can produce similar changes in nonpregnant women, it is likely that this phenomenon results from progestational influences (Goodland and Pommerenke, 1952; Lyons and Huang, 1968). The $PaCO_2$ has been shown to be linearly and inversely related to the log of the progesterone concentration (Machida, 1981). Wilbrand and colleagues (1959) reported that progesterone lowers the CO_2 threshold of the respiratory center. In addition, during pregnancy the sensitivity of the respiratory center increases (Lyons and Antonio, 1959) so that an increase in $PaCO_2$ of 1 mm Hg increases ventilation by 6 liters/min in pregnancy, compared with 1.5 liters/min in the nonpregnant state (Prowse and Gaensler, 1965; Eng et al., 1975; Pernoll et al., 1975). It is also possible that progesterone acts as a primary stimulant to the respiratory center independently of any change in CO_2 sensitivity or threshold (Skatrud et al., 1978). In addition to stimulating ventilation, progesterone may also increase levels of carbonic anhydrase B in the red blood cell (Paciorek and Spencer, 1980). Schenker and associates (1972) reported that carbonic anhydrase levels increase in pregnant patients and in women taking oral contraceptives. An increase in the carbonic anhydrase level facilitates CO_2 transfer and tends to decrease $PaCO_2$ independently of any change in ventilation. This respiratory stimulant effect of progesterone has been used in the treatment of respiratory failure and emphysema (Cullen et al., 1959; Lyons and Huang, 1968; Sutton et al., 1975).

During gestation, ventilation is increased by the rise in tidal volume from about 500 to 700 mL in each breath (Cugell et al., 1953; Prowse and Gaensler, 1965; Lehmann and Fabel, 1973a; Puranik et al., 1994). Because there is no change in respiratory rate, minute ventilation rises from about 7.5 to 10.5 liters/min (Lehmann and Fabel, 1973a; Knuttgen and Emerson, 1974; Pernoll et al., 1975). Minute ventilation increases in the first trimester and remains at that level throughout pregnancy. The physiologic dead space is increased by about 60 mL in pregnancy. This may be secondary to dilation of the small airways (Pernoll et al., 1975). In addition, residual volume is reduced by about 20% (Cugell et al., 1953), from 1200 to 1000 mL (Gazioglu et al., 1970; Lehmann and Fabel, 1973b; Milne, 1979). The *vital capacity*, which is the maximum volume of gas that can be expired after a maximum inspiration, does not change in pregnancy (Cugell et al., 1953; Heidenreich et al., 1971; Lehmann and Fabel, 1973b; Sims et al., 1976; Alaily and Carrol, 1978; Milne, 1979).

ANATOMIC CHANGES OF THE RESPIRATORY SYSTEM

The observed changes in the configuration of the chest during pregnancy are in keeping with the findings of no change in vital capacity and a reduction in residual volume. The effect of pregnancy on pulmonary mechanics has been compared with the effect of a pneumoperitoneum. In both situations, the residual lung volume is decreased but ventilation remains unimpaired. Radiologic studies performed early in pregnancy have shown that the subcostal angle increases from 68 to 103 degrees before there is any mechanical pressure from the enlarging uterus (Thomson and Cohen, 1938). The level of the diaphragm rises by about 4 cm, and the transverse diameter of the chest increases by 2 cm (Klaften and Palugyay, 1926, 1927; Mobius, 1961). These changes account for the decrease in residual volume because the lungs are relatively compressed during forced expiration; however, the excursion of the diaphragm in respiration increases by about 1.5 cm in pregnancy compared with the nonpregnant state (McGinty, 1938; Mobius, 1961).

OXYGEN DELIVERY AND CONSUMPTION

Oxygen Delivery

All tissues require oxygen for the combustion of organic compounds to fuel cellular metabolism. The cardiopulmonary system serves to deliver a continuous supply of oxygen and other essential substrates to tissues. Oxygen delivery is dependent on oxygenation of blood in the lungs, oxygen-carrying capacity of the blood, and cardiac output (Barcroft, 1920). Under normal conditions, oxygen delivery exceeds oxygen consumption by about 75% (Cain, 1983). The amount of oxygen delivered is determined by the cardiac output (CO, liters/min) times the arterial oxygen content (CaO_2, $mL/O_2/min$):

$$Oxygen\ delivery = CO \times CaO_2 \times 10\ (700\ to\ 1400\ mL/min)$$

Arterial oxygen content (CaO_2) is determined by the amount of oxygen that is bound to hemoglobin (arterial blood saturation with oxygen, SaO_2) and by the amount of oxygen that is dissolved in plasma (arterial partial pressure of oxygen, $PaO_2 \times 0.0031$):

$$CaO_2 = (hemoglobin \times 1.34 \times SaO_2) + (PaO_2 \times 0.0031)$$
$$(16\ to\ 22\ mL\ O_2/dL)$$

It is clear from this formula that the amount of oxygen dissolved in plasma is negligible, and therefore the arterial oxygen content is dependent largely on hemoglobin concentration and arterial oxygen saturation. Oxygen delivery can be impaired by conditions that affect either arterial oxygen content, cardiac output (flow), or both. Anemia leads to low arterial oxygen content because of a lack of hemoglobin binding sites for oxygen. Carbon monoxide poisoning likewise will decrease oxyhemoglobin because of blockage of binding sites for oxygen. The patient with hypoxemic respiratory failure will not have sufficient oxygen available to saturate the hemoglobin molecule. In addition, it has been demonstrated that desaturated hemoglobin is altered structurally in such a fashion as to have a diminished affinity for oxygen (Bryan-Brown et al., 1973). It must be kept in mind that the amount of oxygen actually available to tissues also is affected by the affinity of the hemoglobin molecule for oxygen. Thus, the oxyhemoglobin dissociation curve (Fig. 46-1) and those conditions that influence the binding of oxygen either negatively or positively must be considered when attempts are made to maximize oxygen delivery (Perutz, 1978). An increase in the plasma pH level or a decrease in temperature or 2,3-diphosphoglycerate will increase hemoglobin affinity for oxygen, shifting the curve to the left and resulting in diminished tissue oxygenation. If the plasma pH level, temperature, or 2,3-diphosphoglycerate increases, hemoglobin affinity for oxygen will decrease and more oxygen will be available to tissues (Perutz, 1978) (see Fig. 46-1).

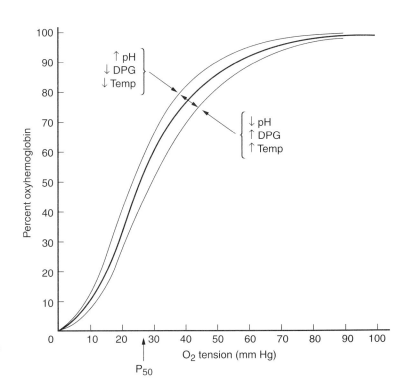

FIGURE 46-1 ■ The oxygen binding curve for human hemoglobin A under physiologic conditions (*dark curve*). The affinity is shifted by changes in pH, diphosphoglycerate (DPG) concentration, and temperature, as indicated. P_{50} represents the oxygen tension at half saturation.

In certain clinical conditions, such as septic shock and adult respiratory distress syndrome, there is maldistribution of flow relative to oxygen demand, leading to diminished delivery and consumption of oxygen. The release of vasoactive substances is hypothesized to result in the loss of normal mechanisms of vascular autoregulation, producing regional and microcirculatory imbalances in blood flow (Rackow and Astiz, 1991). This mismatching of blood flow with metabolic demand causes excessive blood flow to some areas, with relative hypoperfusion of other areas, limiting optimal systemic use of oxygen (Rackow and Astiz, 1991). The patient with diminished cardiac output secondary to hypovolemia or pump failure is unable to distribute oxygenated blood to tissues. Therapy directed at increasing the volume with normal saline, or with blood if the hemoglobin level is less than 10 g/dL, increases delivery of oxygen in the hypovolemic patient. The patient with pump failure may benefit from inotropic support and afterload reduction in addition to supplementation of intravascular volume.

Relationship of Oxygen Delivery to Consumption

Oxygen consumption is the product of the arteriovenous oxygen content difference ($C_{a-v}O_2$) and cardiac output (CO). Under normal conditions, oxygen consumption is a direct function of the metabolic rate (Shoemaker et al., 1989):

$$\text{Oxygen consumption} = C_{(a-v)}O_2 \times CO \times 10$$
$$(180 \text{ to } 280 \text{ mL/min})$$

The oxygen extraction ratio is the fraction of delivered oxygen that actually is consumed:

$$\text{Oxygen extraction ratio} = \text{oxygen consumption/oxygen delivery } (0.25)$$

The normal oxygen extraction ratio is about 25%. A rise in the oxygen extraction ratio is a compensatory mechanism used when oxygen delivery is inadequate for the level of metabolic activity. A subnormal value suggests flow maldistribution, peripheral diffusion defects, or functional shunting (Shoemaker et al., 1989). As the supply of oxygen is reduced, the fraction extracted from blood increases and oxygen consumption is maintained. If a severe reduction in oxygen delivery occurs, the limits of O_2 extraction are reached, tissues are unable to sustain aerobic energy production, and consumption decreases. The level of oxygen delivery at which oxygen consumption begins to decrease has been termed the "critical oxygen delivery" (Shibutani et al., 1983) (Fig. 46-2). At the critical oxygen delivery, tissues begin to use anaerobic glycolysis, with resultant lactate production and metabolic acidosis (Shibutani et al., 1983). If the oxygen deprivation continues, irreversible tissue damage and death ensue.

Mixed Venous Oxygenation

The mixed venous oxygen tension and mixed venous oxygen saturation ($S\overline{v}O_2$) are parameters of tissue oxygenation (Shibutani et al., 1983). The mixed venous oxygen tension is 40 mm Hg with a saturation of 73%. Saturations less than 60% are abnormally low. These parameters can be measured directly by obtaining a blood sample from the distal port of the pulmonary artery catheter. The $S\overline{v}O_2$ also can be measured con-

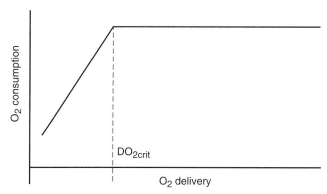

FIGURE 46-2 ■ Relationship of oxygen consumption (VO_2) to oxygen delivery (DO_2).

tinuously with special pulmonary artery catheters equipped with fiberoptics. Mixed venous oxygenation is a reliable parameter in the patient with hypoxemia or low cardiac output, but findings must be interpreted with caution. When the $S\overline{v}O_2$ is low, oxygen delivery can be assumed to be low. However, normal or high $S\overline{v}O_2$ does not guarantee that tissues are well oxygenated. In conditions such as septic shock and adult respiratory distress syndrome, the maldistribution of systemic flow may lead to abnormally high $S\overline{v}O_2$ in the face of severe tissue hypoxia (Rackow and Astiz, 1991). As mentioned before, the oxygen dissociation curve must be considered when interpreting the $S\overline{v}O_2$ as an indicator of tissue oxygenation (Bryan-Brown et al., 1973). Conditions that result in a left shift of the curve cause the venous oxygen saturation to be normal or high, even when the mixed venous oxygen content is low. The $S\overline{v}O_2$ is useful for monitoring trends in a particular patient, because a significant decrease will occur when oxygen delivery has decreased secondary to hypoxemia or a decrease in cardiac output.

Oxygen Delivery and Consumption in Pregnancy

The physiologic anemia of pregnancy results in a reduction in the hemoglobin concentration and arterial oxygen content. Oxygen delivery is maintained at or above normal despite this because of the 50% increase that occurs in cardiac output. It is important to remember, therefore, that the pregnant woman is more dependent on cardiac output for maintenance of oxygen delivery than is the nonpregnant patient (Barron and Lindheimer, 1991). Oxygen consumption increases steadily throughout pregnancy and is greatest at term, reaching an average of 331 mL/min at rest and 1167 mL/min with exercise (Pernoll et al., 1975). During labor, oxygen consumption increases by 40% to 60% and cardiac output increases by about 22% (Gemzell et al., 1957; Ueland and Hansen, 1969). Because oxygen delivery normally far exceeds consumption, the normal pregnant patient usually is able to maintain adequate delivery of oxygen to herself and her fetus, even during labor. When a pregnant patient has a low oxygen delivery, however, she very quickly can reach the critical oxygen delivery during labor, compromising both herself and her fetus. The obstetrician therefore must make every effort to optimize oxygen delivery before allowing labor to begin in the compromised patient.

PNEUMONIA IN PREGNANCY

Pneumonia is a rare complication of pregnancy, occurring in 1 per 118 to 2288 deliveries (Oxhorn, 1955; Madinger et al., 1989). However, pneumonia contributes to considerable maternal mortality and is reportedly the most common nonobstetric infection to cause maternal mortality in the peripartum period (Kaunitz et al., 1985). Maternal mortality was as high as 24% before the introduction of antibiotic therapy (Finland and Dublin, 1939). Research reports have documented a dramatic decrease in maternal mortality from 0% to 4% with modern management and antibiotic therapy (Benedetti et al., 1982; Madinger et al., 1989; Berkowitz and LaSala, 1990). Preterm delivery is a significant complication of pneumonia, complicating pregnancy. Even with antibiotic therapy and modern management, preterm delivery continues to occur in 4% to 43% of gravidas who have pneumonia (Benedetti et al., 1982; Madinger et al., 1989; Berkowitz and LaSala, 1990).

The incidence of pneumonia in pregnancy may be increasing primarily as a reflection of the declining general health status of certain segments of the childbearing population (Berkowitz and LaSala, 1990). In addition, the epidemic of human immunodeficiency virus (HIV) infection has increased the number of potential mothers who are at risk for opportunistic lung infections. HIV infection is also associated with increased risks of invasive pneumococcal disease (odds ratio, 41.8) and Legionnaire disease (odds ratio, 41.8) (Koonin, 1989). HIV infection further predisposes the pregnant woman to the infectious complications of the acquired immunodeficiency syndrome (Dinsmoor, 1989; Koonin et al., 1989). Women with medical conditions that increase the risk of pulmonary infection, such as cystic fibrosis (CF), are living to childbearing age more frequently than in the past. This disorder also contributes to the increased incidence of pneumonia in pregnancy.

Pneumonia can complicate pregnancy at any time during gestation and may be associated with preterm birth, poor fetal growth, and perinatal loss. In an early report, 17 of 23 patients developed pneumonia between 25 and 36 weeks' gestation (Hopwood, 1965). In that series, seven gravidas delivered during the course of their acute illness, and there were two maternal deaths. Another report described 39 cases of pneumonia in pregnancy (Benedetti et al., 1982). Sixteen gravidas presented before 24 weeks' gestation, 15 between 25 and 36 weeks' gestation, and 8 after 36 weeks' gestation. Twenty-seven patients in this series were followed to completion of pregnancy; only two required delivery during the acute phase of pneumonia. Of these 27 patients, 3 suffered a fetal loss and 24 delivered live fetuses, although there was one neonatal death resulting from prematurity. Madinger and associates (1989) reported 25 cases of pneumonia occurring among 32,179 deliveries and observed that fetal and obstetric complications were much more common than in earlier studies. Preterm labor complicated 11 of 21 gestations. Pneumonia was present at the time of delivery in 11 patients. Preterm delivery was more likely in those women who had bacteremia, needed mechanical ventilation, and had a serious underlying maternal disease. In addition to the complication of preterm labor, there were three perinatal deaths in this series. Berkowitz and LaSala (1990) reported 25 patients with pneumonia complicating pregnancy; full-term delivery occurred in 14 women, 1 delivered preterm, 3 had a voluntary termination of pregnancy, 3 had term deliveries of growth-restricted

babies, and 4 were lost to follow-up. Birth weight was significantly lower in the study group in this series (2770 ± 224 versus 3173 ± 99 g in the control group; $P < .01$). In this series, pneumonia complicated 1 per 367 deliveries. The authors attributed the increase in the incidence of pneumonia in this population to a decline in general health status, including anemia, a significant incidence of cocaine use (52% versus 10% in the general population) and HIV positivity (24% versus 2% of the general population) in the study group.

Bacteriology

Most series describing pneumonia complicating pregnancy used incomplete methodologies to diagnose the etiologic pathogens for pneumonia, relying primarily on cultures of blood and sputum. In most cases no pathogen was identified; however, pneumococcus and *Haemophilus influenza* remain the most common identifiable causes of pneumonia in pregnancy (Benedetti et al., 1982; Madinger et al., 1989; Berkowitz and LaSala, 1990). Because comprehensive serologic testing has rarely been done, the true incidence of viral pneumonia, *Legionella*, and mycoplasma pneumonia in pregnancy is difficult to estimate. The data presented by Benedetti, Madinger, Berkowitz, and their respective colleagues all support pneumococcus as the predominant pathogen causing pneumonia in pregnancy, with *H. influenza* being the second most common organism (Benedetti et al., 1982; Madinger et al., 1989; Berkowitz and LaSala, 1990). In the series of Berkowitz and LaSala (1990), one patient had *Legionella* species.

Several unusual pathogens have been reported to cause pneumonia in pregnancy, including mumps, infectious mononucleosis, swine influenza, influenza A, varicella, coccidioidomycosis, and other fungi (Rodrigues and Niederman, 1992). Varicella pneumonia will complicate primary varicella infections in 5.2% to 9% (Harger et al., 2002) of infections in pregnancy, as compared with 0.3% to 1.8% in the nonpregnant population (Haake et al., 1990). Influenza A has a higher mortality in pregnancy than in nonpregnant patients (McKinney et al., 1990). The increase in virulence of viral infections reported in pregnancy may be secondary to the alterations in maternal immune status that characterize pregnancy, including reduced lymphocyte proliferation response, reduced cell-mediated cytotoxicity by lymphocytes, and a decrease in the number of helper T lymphocytes (McKinney et al., 1990; American College of Obstetricians and Gynecologists [ACOG], 1996). Viral pneumonias can also be complicated by superimposed bacterial infection, particularly pneumococcus.

Aspiration Pneumonia

Mendelson syndrome describes chemical pneumonitis resulting from the aspiration of gastric contents in pregnancy. Chemical pneumonitis can be super-infected with pathogens present in the oropharynx and gastric juices, primarily anaerobes and gram-negative bacteria (Rodrigues and Niederman, 1992). Mendelson's original report of aspiration (Mendelson, 1946) consisted of 44,016 nonfasted obstetric patients between 1932 and 1945, of whom more than half received "operative intervention" with ether by mask without endotracheal intubation. He described aspiration in 66 cases (1:667). Although several of the patients were critically ill from their aspirations, most recovered within 24 to 36 hours and only two died from this complication (1:22,008). A review described 37,282 vaginal deliveries of which 85% were performed with general anesthesia by mask and without intubation; 65% to 75% had ingested liquids or solid food within 4 hours of onset of labor (Krantz and Edwards, 1973). The authors noted five mild cases of aspiration (1:7456) with no sequelae (Krantz and Edwards, 1973). Another report noted one occurrence of "mild aspiration" without adverse outcome in 1870 women undergoing nonintubated peripartum surgery with intravenous ketamine, benzodiazepines, barbiturates, and/or fentanyl (Ezri et al., 2000). Soreide and colleagues (1996) observed four episodes of aspiration each during 36,800 deliveries and 3600 cesarean sections with no mortality. Based on the above data, most hospitals permit free intake of clear liquids during labor. Therefore, the risk of aspiration, pneumonia, and death from general anesthesia appears to be very low. This may be secondary to modern techniques and the use of therapy to reduce gastric pH.

Bacterial Pneumonia

Streptococcus pneumonia (pneumococcus) is the most common bacterial pathogen to cause pneumonia in pregnancy, with *H. influenza* being the next most common. These pneumonias typically present as an acute illness accompanied by fever, chills, purulent productive cough, and a lobar pattern on the chest radiograph. Streptococcal pneumonia produces a "rusty" sputum, with gram-positive diplococci on Gram stain, and demonstrates asymmetrical consolidation with air bronchograms on chest radiograph (ACOG, 1996). *H. influenza* is a gram-negative coccobacillus that produces consolidation with air bronchograms, often in the upper lobes (ACOG, 1996). Less frequent bacterial pathogens include *Klebsiella* pneumonia, which is a gram-negative rod and causes extensive tissue destruction with air bronchograms, pleural effusion, and cavitation noted on chest radiograph. Patients with *Staphylococcus aureus* pneumonia present with pleuritis, chest pain, purulent sputum, and consolidation without air bronchograms noted on chest radiograph (ACOG, 1996).

Patients infected with atypical pneumonia pathogens, such as *Mycoplasma* pneumonia, *Legionella* pneumonia, and *Chlamydia* pneumonia (TWAR agent), present with gradual onset, a lower fever, appear less ill, have a mucoid sputum, and have a patchy or interstitial infiltrate on chest radiograph. In general, the severity of the findings on chest radiograph are out of proportion to the mild clinical symptoms. *Mycoplasma* pneumonia is the most common organism responsible for atypical pneumonia and is best detected by the presence of cold agglutinins in about 70% of cases.

The normal physiologic changes in the respiratory system associated with pregnancy result in a loss of ventilatory reserve. This, coupled with the immunosuppression that accompanies pregnancy, put the mother and fetus at great risk from respiratory infection. Therefore, any gravida suspected of having pneumonia should be managed aggressively. The pregnant patient should be admitted to the hospital and a thorough investigation undertaken to determine the pathologic etiology. Workup should include physical examination, arterial blood gases, chest radiograph, sputum Gram stain and culture, and blood cultures. Cold agglutinins and *Legionella* titers may also be useful. Empiric antibiotic coverage should be started, usually with a third-generation cephalosporin such as ceftriax-

one or cefotaxime. *Legionella* pneumonia has a high mortality and sometimes presents with consolidation, mimicking pneumococcal pneumonia. Therefore, it is recommended that a macrolide, such as azithromycin, be added to the empiric therapy. Once the results of the sputum culture, blood cultures, Gram stain, and serum studies are obtained and a pathogen has been identified, antibiotic therapy can be directed toward the identifiable pathogen. The third-generation cephalosporins are effective agents for most pathogens causing a community-acquired pneumonia. They are also effective against penicillin-resistant streptococcus pneumonia. In addition to antibiotic therapy, oxygen supplementation should be given. Frequent arterial blood gas measurements should be obtained to maintain partial pressure of oxygen at 70 mm Hg, a level necessary to ensure adequate fetal oxygenation. Arterial saturation can be monitored with pulse oximetry as well. When the gravida is afebrile for 48 hours and has signs of clinical improvement, an oral cephalosporin can be started and intravenous therapy discontinued. A total of 10 to 14 days of treatment should be completed.

Pneumonia in pregnancy can be complicated by respiratory failure requiring mechanical ventilation. Should this occur, team management should include the obstetrician, maternal-fetal medicine specialist, and intensivist. In addition to meticulous management of the gravida's respiratory status, the patient should be maintained in the left lateral recumbent position to improve uteroplacental perfusion. The viable fetus should be monitored with continuous fetal monitoring. If positive end-expiratory pressure greater than 10 cm H_2O is required to maintain oxygenation, central monitoring with a pulmonary artery catheter should be instituted to adequately monitor volume status and maintain maternal and uteroplacental perfusion. There is no evidence documenting that elective delivery results in an overall improvement in respiratory function (Tomlinson et al., 1998). Therefore, elective delivery should be reserved for the usual obstetric indications. However, if there is clear evidence of fetal compromise or profound maternal compromise and impending demise, delivery should be accomplished.

Viral Pneumonias

Influenza

There are an estimated 4 million cases of pneumonia and influenza annually in the United States, making it the sixth leading cause of death (National Center for Health Statistics, 1992). In contrast to the general population, pregnant women seem to be at higher risk for influenza pneumonia (Kort et al., 1986; Mullooly et al., 1986). Epidemiologic data from the 1918 to 1919 influenza A pandemic revealed a maternal mortality rate that approached 50% for pregnant women with influenza pneumonia (Harris, 1919; Freeman and Barno, 1959). Three types of influenza virus can cause human disease, A, B, and C, but most epidemic infections are due to influenza A (Rodrigues and Niederman, 1992). Influenza A typically has an acute onset after a 1- to 4-day incubation period and first manifests as high fever, coryza, headache, malaise, and cough. In uncomplicated cases the chest examination and chest radiograph remain clear (Rodrigues and Niederman, 1992). If symptoms persist longer than 5 days, especially in a pregnancy, complications should be suspected. Pneumonia may complicate influenza as the result of either secondary bacterial infection or viral infection of the lung parenchyma (Rodrigues and Niederman, 1992). In the epidemic of 1957, autopsies demonstrated that pregnant women died most commonly from fulminant viral pneumonia, whereas nonpregnant patients died most often from secondary bacterial infection (Hollingsworth et al., 1989). Primary influenza pneumonia is characterized by rapid progression from a unilateral infiltrate to diffuse bilateral disease. The gravida may develop fulminant respiratory failure requiring mechanical ventilation and positive end-expiratory pressure. Aggressive therapy is indicated when pneumonia complicates influenza in pregnancy. Therefore, antibiotics should be started, directed at the likely pathogens that can cause secondary infection, including S. aureus, pneumococcus, H. influenza, and certain enteric gram-negative bacteria. Antiviral agents, such as amantadine and ribavirin, should also be considered (Kirshon et al., 1988). It has been recommended that the influenza vaccine be given routinely to gravidas in the second and third trimester of pregnancy to prevent the occurrence of influenza and the development of pneumonia.

Varicella

Varicella zoster is a DNA virus that usually causes a benign self-limited illness in children but may infect up to 2% of all adults (Cox et al., 1990). Varicella infection occurs in 0.7 of every 1000 pregnancies (Esmonde et al., 1989). Pregnancy may increase the likelihood of varicella pneumonia complicating the primary infection (Haake et al., 1990). A recent report documents a 5.2% incidence of varicella pneumonia in gravidas with varicella-zoster infection. The authors also reported that gravidas who smoke or manifest more than 100 skin lesions are more likely to develop pneumonia (Harger et al., 2002). Varicella pneumonia occurs most often in the third trimester, and the infection is likely to be severe (Esmonde et al., 1989; Haake et al., 1990; Smego and Asperilla, 1991). The maternal mortality from varicella pneumonia may be as high as 35% to 40% as compared with 11% to 17% in nonpregnant individuals (Haake et al., 1990; Smego and Asperilla, 1991). Although one review reported a decreased mortality with only three deaths in 28 women with varicella pneumonia (Esmonde et al., 1989), another study documented a maternal mortality of 35% (Haake et al., 1990). However, a more recent report documented 100% survival in 18 gravidas with varicella pneumonia who were treated with acyclovir (Harger et al., 2002). In this report, there was one intrauterine fetal death at 25 weeks of gestation in a woman with varicella. However, the 17 other infants were delivered beyond 36 weeks, and there was no evidence of neonatal varicella (Harger et al., 2002).

Varicella pneumonia usually presents 2 to 5 days after the onset of fever, rash, and malaise and is heralded by the onset of pulmonary symptoms, including cough, dyspnea, pruritic chest pain, and hemoptysis (Haake et al., 1990). The severity of the illness may vary from asymptomatic radiographic abnormalities to fulminant pneumonitis and respiratory failure (Harris and Rhades, 1965; Haake et al., 1990). All gravidas with varicella pneumonia should be aggressively treated with antiviral therapy and admitted to the intensive care unit for close observation or intubation if indicated. Acyclovir, a DNA polymerase inhibitor, should be started. The early use of acyclovir was associated with an improved hospital course after the 5th day and a lower mean temperature, lower respiratory rate, and improved oxygenation (Haake et al., 1990). Treatment with acyclovir is safe in pregnancy. Among 312 pregnancies there was no increase in the number of birth defects and no consistent pattern of congenital abnormalities (Andrews et al., 1992). A dose of 7.5 mg/kg intravenously every 8 hours has been recommended (Brown and Baker, 1989).

Pneumocystis carinii

Infection with the HIV virus significantly increases the risk of pulmonary infection. Streptococcus pneumoniae and H. influenza are the most commonly isolated organisms (Pickard, 1968). A recent report also identified Pseudomonas aeruginosa as a significant cause of bacterial pneumonia in HIV-infected individuals (Afessa and Green, 2000). Pneumocystis carinii pneumonia (PCP) is the most frequent of the serious opportunistic infections in pregnant individuals infected with HIV (Minkoff et al., 1986; Armstrong, 1988). P. carinii is the number one cause of pregnancy-associated acquired immunodeficiency syndrome deaths in the United States (Stratton et al., 1992). Initial reports of PCP in pregnancy presented a 100% maternal mortality rate (Jensen et al., 1984; Antoine et al., 1986; Minkoff et al., 1986; Koonin et al., 1989; Kell et al., 1991). However, in a recent review of 22 cases of PCP in pregnancy, the mortality rate was 50% (11 of 22 patients). This is an improvement over the 100% mortality previously reported. However, the mortality rate is still higher than that reported for HIV-infected nonpregnant individuals (Ahmad et al., 2001). In that series, respiratory failure developed in 13 patients (59% required mechanical ventilation). The survival rate of gravidas requiring mechanical ventilation was 31%. In this series, maternal and fetal outcomes were better in cases of PCP that occurred during the third trimester of pregnancy.

A high index of suspicion is necessary when gravidas who are at risk for HIV infection present with symptoms such as weight loss, fatigue, fever, tachypnea, dyspnea, and nonproductive cough (Minkoff et al., 1986). The onset of disease can be insidious, including normal radiographic findings, and can then proceed to rapid deterioration (Minkoff et al., 1986). When the chest x-ray is positive, it is noted to have bilateral alveolar disease in the perihilar regions and lower lung fields, which can progress to include the entire parenchyma (Minkoff et al., 1986). Diagnosis can be accomplished via sputum silver stains, bronchial aspiration, or bronchoscope-directed biopsy (Clinton et al., 1992). Lung biopsy is recommended for definitive diagnosis (Jensen et al., 1984).

Because the diagnosis of PCP during pregnancy is associated with an increased mortality rate, prophylaxis should be started during the antepartum period. Initiation of therapy during the antepartum period can also prevent the rare occurrence of perinatally transmitted PCP (Bardeguez, 1996). Therapy for PCP in pregnancy includes trimethoprim-sulfamethoxazole (TMP-SMX), which is a category C drug. Gravidas with a history of PCP, a CD4 lymphocyte count of less than 200/mm^3, or oral pharyngeal candidiasis should receive prophylaxis (Hicks et al., 1990). TMP-SMX is the drug of choice and may provide cross protection against toxoplasmosis and other bacterial infections (Bardeguez, 1996). The usual dose is one double-strength tablet (150 mg/m^2 TMP, 750 mg/m^2 SMX three times a week). Adverse reactions such as drug allergy, nausea, fever, neutropenia, anemia, thrombocytopenia, and elevated transaminase have been reported in 20% to 30% of nonpregnant individuals receiving TMP-SMX therapy (Bardeguez, 1996). Complete blood count with differential and liver function tests should be obtained every 6 to 8 weeks to monitor for toxicity. Other regimens used for prophylaxis for individuals with an intolerance to TMP-SMX include aerosolized pentamidine (300 mg every month via Respigard II nebulizer) or dapsone (100 mg once daily). In a report by Hussain and colleagues (2001), it was noted that the survival rate of patients treated with SMX alone was 71% (5 of 7 patients) and with SMX and steroids was 60% (3 of 5 patients); an overall survival rate in both groups was 66.6% (8 of 12 patients). The authors concluded that PCP has a more aggressive course during pregnancy, with increased morbidity and mortality. However, treatment with SMX compared with other therapies may result in improved outcome. They also caution that withholding appropriate PCP prophylaxis may adversely affect maternal and fetal outcomes.

PCP is a devastating opportunistic infection in pregnant women who are HIV infected. The maternal mortality is extremely high, and therefore prophylaxis with TMP-SMX is indicated during the antepartum period in individuals with a CD4 count less than 200/mm^3 and/or a history of oropharyngeal candidiasis, as well as those individuals with a previous history of PCP infection. When a gravida is demonstrating symptoms consistent with a possible infection, a diligent search should be conducted to quickly identify PCP as the cause of pneumonia. When PCP is untreated, maternal mortality can approach 100%.

TUBERCULOSIS IN PREGNANCY

Tuberculosis kills more than 1 million women per year, and it is estimated that 646 million women and girls worldwide are already infected with tuberculosis. In women aged 15 to 44 years in developing countries, tuberculosis is the third most common cause of morbidity and mortality combined, and tuberculosis kills more women than any other infectious disease, including malaria and acquired immunodeficiency syndrome. Case-notification rates from countries with a high prevalence of tuberculosis suggest that tuberculosis may be less frequent among females (Diwan and Thorson, 1999).

Epidemiologic information shows differences between men and women in prevalence of infection, rate of progression from infection to disease, incidence of clinical disease, and mortality resulting from tuberculosis. Seventy percent more smear-positive males than female tuberculosis patients are diagnosed every year and reported to the World Health Organization (Diwan and Thorson, 1999). Differences between males and females have also been shown in the development and outcome of active disease, with female cases having a higher progression from infection to disease and a higher case-fatality rate (Holmes et al., 1998). The conclusion of a research workshop on gender and tuberculosis was that a combination of biological and social factors is responsible for these differences (Diwan and Thorson, 1999).

The incidence of tuberculosis in the United States began to decline in the early part of the 20th century and fell steadily until 1953, when the introduction of isoniazid led to a dramatic decrease in the number of cases, from 84,000 cases in 1953 to 22,255 cases in 1984 (MMWR, 1993). However, since 1984 there have been significant changes in tuberculosis mor-

bidity trends. From 1985 through 1991, reported cases of tuberculosis increased by 18%, representing approximately 39,000 more cases than expected had the previous downward trend continued. This increase is due to many factors, including the HIV epidemic, deterioration in the health care infrastructure, and more cases among immigrants (Frieden et al., 1993; MMWR, 1993). Between 1985 and 1992, the number of tuberculosis cases in women of childbearing age increased by 40% (Cantwell et al., 1994). One report noted tuberculosis-complicated pregnancies in 94.8 cases per 100,000 deliveries between 1991 and 1992 (Margono et al., 1994).

The emergence of drug-resistant tuberculosis has also become a serious concern. In New York City, in 1991, 33% of tuberculosis cases were resistant to at least one drug, and 19% were resistant to both isoniazid and rifampin. Multidrug resistance is an additional problem. Many centers advocate directly observed therapy in the treatment of multidrug-resistant disease. Pregnancy complicates treatment of multidrug-resistant tuberculosis for the following reasons:

- Several antimycobacterial drugs are contraindicated during gestation.
- Patients and physicians may fear the effects of chest radiography on the fetus.
- Untreated infectious multidrug-resistant tuberculosis may be vertically and laterally transmitted (Nitta and Milligan, 1999).

In one report (Nitta and Milligan, 1999), three patients had disease resulting from multidrug-resistant *Mycobacterium tuberculosis* and one had disease resulting from multidrug-resistant *Mycobacterium bovis*. Only one patient began retreatment during pregnancy, because her organism was susceptible to three antituberculosis drugs that were considered nontoxic to the fetus. Despite concern over teratogenicity of the second-line antituberculosis medications, careful timing of treatment initiation resulted in clinical cure for the mothers, despite some complications because of chronic tuberculosis and/or therapy. In this series, all infants were born healthy and remained free of tuberculosis (Nitta and Milligan, 1999).

Diagnosis

Most gravidas diagnosed with tuberculosis in pregnancy will be asymptomatic. All gravidas at high risk for tuberculosis (Table 46-1) should be screened with subcutaneous administration of intermediate-strength purified protein derivative (PPD). If anergy is suspected, control antigens such as candida, mumps, or tetanus toxoids should also be placed (Centers for Disease Control and Prevention, 1990). The sensitivity of the PPD is 90% to 99% for exposure to tuberculosis. The tine test should not be used for screening because of its low sensitivity.

The onset of the recent tuberculosis epidemic stimulated the need for rapid diagnostic tests using molecular biology methods to detect M. *tuberculosis* in clinical specimens. Two direct amplification tests have been approved by the U.S. Food and Drug Administration, the *Mycobacterium tuberculosis* Direct test (Gen-Probe, San Diego, CA) and the Amplicor *Mycobacterium tuberculosis* test (Roche Diagnostic Systems, Inc., Branchburg, NJ). Both tests amplify and detect M. *tuberculosis* 16S ribosomal DNA (Griffith, 1998). When testing acid-fast stain smear-positive respiratory specimens, each test has a sensitivity of greater than 95% and a specificity of essentially 100% for

TABLE 46-1. HIGH-RISK FACTORS FOR TUBERCULOSIS

Human immunodeficiency virus infection
Close contact with persons known or suspected to have tuberculosis
Medical risk factors known to increase risk of disease if infected
Birth in a country with high tuberculosis prevalence
Medically underserved status
Low income
Alcohol addiction
Intravenous drug use
Residency in a long-term care facility (e.g., correctional institutions, mental institutions, nursing homes and facilities)
Health professionals working in high-risk health care facilities

detecting the M. *tuberculosis* complex (American Thoracic Society Workshop, 1997; Barnes, 1997). When testing acid-fast stain smear-negative respiratory specimens, the specificity remains greater than 95%, but the sensitivity ranges from 40% to 77% (American Thoracic Society Workshop, 1997; Barnes, 1997). To date, these tests are U.S. Food and Drug Administration-approved only for testing acid-fast stain smear-positive respiratory specimens obtained from untreated patients or those who have received no more than 7 days of antituberculosis therapy. The PPD remains the most commonly used screening test for tuberculosis.

Immigrants from areas where tuberculosis is endemic may have received the bacillus Calmette-Guérin vaccine. Such individuals will likely have a positive response to the PPD. However, this reactivity should wane over time. Therefore, the PPD should be used to screen these patients for tuberculosis unless their skin tests are known to be positive (Centers for Disease Control, 1990). If the bacillus Calmette-Guérin vaccine was given 10 years earlier and the PPD is positive with a skin test reaction of 10 mm or more, that individual should be considered infected with tuberculosis and managed accordingly (Centers for Disease Control, 1990).

Women with a positive PPD skin test must be evaluated for active tuberculosis with a thorough physical examination for extrapulmonary disease and a chest radiograph once they are beyond the first trimester (ACOG, 1996). Symptoms of active tuberculosis include cough (74%), weight loss (41%), fever (30%), malaise and fatigue (30%), and hemoptysis (19%) (Good et al., 1981). Individuals with active pulmonary tuberculosis may have radiographic findings, including adenopathy, multinodular infiltrates, cavitation, loss of volume in the upper lobes, and upper medial retraction of hilar markings. The finding of acid-fast bacilli in early morning sputum specimens confirms the diagnosis of pulmonary tuberculosis. At least three first-morning sputum samples should be examined for the presence of acid-fast bacilli. If sputum cannot be produced, sputum-induction, gastric washings, or diagnostic bronchoscopy may be indicated.

Extrapulmonary tuberculosis occurs in up to 16% of cases in the United States; however, in patients with acquired immunodeficiency syndrome the pattern may occur in 60% to 70% of all patients (American Thoracic Society, 1987). Extrapulmonary sites include lymph nodes, bone, kidneys, intestine, meninges, breasts, and endometrium. Extrapulmonary tuberculosis appears to be rare in pregnancy (Hamadeh and Glassroth, 1992). Extrapulmonary tuberculo-

sis that is confined to the lymph nodes has no effect on obstetric outcomes, but tuberculosis at other extrapulmonary sites does adversely affect the outcome of pregnancy (Jana et al., 1999). Jana and colleagues (1999) documented that tuberculosis lymphadenitis did not affect the course of pregnancy or labor or the perinatal outcome. However, as compared with control women, the 21 women with tubercular involvement of other extrapulmonary sites had higher rates of antenatal hospitalization (24% versus 2%, P < .0001), infants with low Apgar scores (no more than 6) soon after birth (19% versus 3%, P = .01), and low-birth-weight (less than 2500 g) infants (33% versus 11%, P = .01). Rarely, mycobacteria invade the uteroplacental circulation, and congenital tuberculosis results (Hopwood, 1965; Vallejo and Starke, 1992; Cantwell et al., 1994). The diagnosis of congenital tuberculosis is based on one of the following factors (Cantwell et al., 1994):

1. Demonstration of primary hepatic complex or cavitating hepatic granuloma by percutaneous liver biopsy at birth
2. Infection of the maternal genital tract or placenta
3. Lesions noted in the 1st week of life
4. Exclusion of the possibility of postnatal transmission by a thorough investigation of all contacts, including attendants

Prevention

Most gravidas with a positive PPD in pregnancy will be asymptomatic with no evidence of active disease and therefore classified as infected without active disease. The risk of progression to active disease is highest in the first 2 years of conversion. It is important to prevent the onset of active disease while minimizing maternal and fetal risk. An algorithm for management of the positive PPD is presented in Figure 46-3 (Riley, 1997). In women with a known recent conversion (2 years) to a positive PPD and no evidence of active disease, the recommended prophylaxis is isoniazid, 300 mg/day, starting after the first trimester and continuing for 6 to 9 months (ACOG, 1996). In one recent report under base-case assumptions, the fewest cases of tuberculosis within the cohort occurred with antepartum treatment (1400 per 100,000) compared with no treatment (3300 per 100,000) or postpartum treatment (1800 per 100,000) (Boggess et al., 2000). Antepartum treatment resulted in a marginal increase in life expectancy because of the prevented isoniazid-related hepatitis and deaths, compared with no treatment or postpartum treatment. In addition, antepartum treatment was the least expensive (Boggess et al., 2000). Isoniazid should be accompanied by pyridoxine (vitamin B_6) supplementation, 50 mg/day, to prevent the peripheral neuropathy that is associated with isoniazid treatment. Women with an unknown or prolonged duration of PPD positivity (more than 2 years) should receive isoniazid, 300 mg/day, for 6 to 9 months after delivery. Isoniazid prophylaxis is not recommended for women older than 35 years of age who have an unknown or prolonged PPD positivity in the absence of active disease. The use of isoniazid is discouraged in this group because of an increased risk of hepatotoxicity. Isoniazid is associated with hepatitis in both pregnant and nonpregnant adults. However, monthly monitoring of liver function tests may prevent this adverse outcome. Among individuals receiving isoniazid, 10% to 20% will develop mildly elevated liver function tests. These changes resolve once the drug is discontinued (Robinson and Rose, 1999).

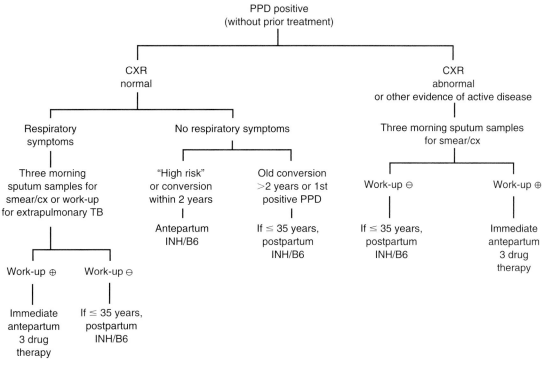

FIGURE 46-3 ■ Algorithm for management of positive purified protein derivative (PPD). B6, pyridoxine; cx, culture; CXR, chest x-ray; INH, isoniazid; TB, tuberculosis.

Treatment

The gravida with active tuberculosis should be treated initially with isoniazid, 300 mg/day, combined with rifampin, 600 mg/day (Table 46-2) (Fox and George, 1992). Resistant disease results from initial infection with resistant strains (33%) or can develop during therapy (Van Rie et al., 2000).

The development of resistance is more likely in individuals who are noncompliant with therapy. If resistance to isoniazid is identified or anticipated, 2.5 g/day of ethambutol should be added and the treatment period should be extended to 18 months (Fox and George, 1992). Ethambutol is teratogenic in animals; however, this has not been noted in humans. The most common side effect of ethambutol therapy is optic

 TABLE 46-2. ANTITUBERCULOSIS DRUGS

Drug	Dosage Forms	Daily Dose	Weekly Dose	Major Adverse Reactions
First Line Drugs (for Initial Treatment)				
Isoniazid	PO, IM	10 mg/kg up to 300 mg	15 mg/kg up to 900 mg	Hepatic enzyme elevation, peripheral neuropathy hepatitis, hypersensitivity
Rifampin	PO	10 mg/kg up to 600 mg	10 mg/kg up to 600 mg	Orange discoloration of secretions and urine; nausea, vomiting, hepatitis, febrile reaction, purpura (rare)
Pyrazinamide	PO	15–30 mg/kg up to 2 g	50–70 mg/kg, twice	Hepatotoxicity, hyperuricemia, arthralgias, skin rash, gastrointestinal upset
Ethambutol	PO	15 mg/kg up to 2.5 g	50 mg/kg	Optic neuritis (decreased red-green color discrimination, decreased visual acuity), skin rash
Streptomycin	IM	15 mg/kg up to 1 g	25–30 mg/kg up to 1 g	Ototoxicity, nephrotoxicity
Second Line Drugs (Daily Therapy)				
Capreomycin	IM	15–30 mg/kg up to 1 g		Auditory, vestibular, and renal toxicity
Kanamycin	IM	15–30 mg/kg up to 1 g		Auditory and renal toxicity, rare vestibular toxicity
Ethionamide	PO	15–20 mg/kg up to 1 g		Gastrointestinal disturbance, hepatotoxicity, hypersensitivity
Para-amino-salycylic acid	PO	150 mg/kg up to 1 g		Gastrointestinal disturbance, hypersensitivity, hepatotoxicity, sodium load
Cycloserine	PO	15–20 mg/kg up to 1 g		Psychosis, convulsions, rash

IM, intramuscularly; PO, orally.

neuritis. Streptomycin should be avoided during pregnancy because it is associated with eighth nerve damage in neonates (Robinson and Cambion, 1964). Antituberculous agents not recommended for use in pregnancy include ethionamide, streptomycin, capreomycin, kanamycin, cycloserine, and pyrazinamide (ACOG, 1996).

Women who are being treated with antituberculous drugs may breast-feed. Only 0.75% to 2.3% of isoniazid and 0.05% of rifampin are excreted into breast milk. Ethambutol excretion into breast milk is also minimal. However, if the infant is concurrently taking oral antituberculous therapy, excessive drug levels may be reached in the neonate, and breast-feeding should be avoided. Breast-fed infants of women taking isoniazid therapy should receive a multivitamin supplement, including pyridoxine (ACOG, 1996). Neonates of women taking antituberculous therapy should have a PPD skin test at birth and again at 3 months of age. Infants born to women with active tuberculosis at the time of delivery should receive isoniazid prophylaxis (10 mg/kg/day) until maternal disease has been inactive for 3 months as evidenced by negative maternal sputum cultures (ACOG, 1996). Infants of women with multidrug-resistant tuberculosis should probably be placed with an alternative caregiver until there is no evidence of active disease in the mother. The newborn should also receive bacille Calmette-Guérin (BCG) and isoniazid prophylaxis (Nitta and Milligan, 1999). Active tuberculosis in the neonate should be treated appropriately with isoniazid and rifampin immediately upon diagnosis or with multiagent therapy should drug-resistant organisms be identified. Infants and children who are at high risk of intimate and prolonged exposure to untreated or ineffectively treated persons should receive the bacillus Calmette-Guérin vaccine (Rendig, 1969).

Summary

High-risk gravidas should be screened for tuberculosis and treated appropriately with isoniazid prophylaxis for infection without overt disease and with dual antituberculous therapy for active disease. In addition, the newborn should be screened for evidence of tuberculosis as well. Proper screening and therapy will lead to a good outcome for mother and fetus in most cases.

ASTHMA IN PREGNANCY

Asthma is probably the most common potentially serious medical complication of pregnancy (Schatz et al., 1990). Approximately 4% of women of childbearing age have a history of physician-diagnosed asthma, but up to 10% of the population appears to have nonspecific airway hyper-responsiveness (National Asthma Education Program [NAEP], 1993). In general, the prevalence, morbidity, and morality from asthma are increasing. Asthma is characterized by chronic airway inflammation with acute airway obstruction to a variety of stimuli.

The effects of pregnancy on asthma and asthma on pregnancy are controversial. Published studies have had conflicting results in regards to many obstetric outcomes, including preeclampsia, cesarean delivery, prematurity, intrauterine growth restriction, and perinatal mortality rate. A recent prospective study of 900 subjects with moderate or severe asthma, 900 with mild asthma, and 900 control subjects did not find adverse perinatal outcomes (Dombrowski, 2000).

Patients with asthma have increased frequencies of chronic hypertension (Schatz et al., 1995) and maternal smoking (Dombrowski et al., 1986), which may also contribute to adverse pregnancy outcomes. Ethnicity may be a particularly important confounding factor in assessing the relationship between asthma and pregnancy outcomes, because African Americans are five times more likely to die and are twice as likely to be hospitalized because of asthma compared with whites (NAEP, 1991). Asthma has been associated with considerable maternal morbidity, with over 40% requiring hospitalization during pregnancy for asthma exacerbations (Mabie et al., 1992; Perlow et al., 1992).

In 1993, the NAEP working group defined mild, moderate, and severe asthma according to symptoms (wheezing, cough, and/or dyspnea) and objective tests of pulmonary function. The most commonly used objective parameters were peak expiratory flow rate (PEFR) and forced expiratory volume in 1 second after a maximal inspiration (FEV_1). The NAEP guidelines did not list the need for regular medications to be a factor for classifying asthma severity during pregnancy. In a recent prospective observational study of 1800 pregnant women with asthma, those with mild asthma but who required regular medications (ß-agonist, theophylline, or inhaled corticosteroids) were similar to subjects with moderate asthma in respect to prevalence of asthma exacerbations (Dombrowski, 2000). Patients with moderate asthma requiring regular systemic corticosteroids were similar to those with severe asthma in respect to asthma exacerbations. See Table 46-3 for modified NAEP asthma severity criteria. Studies have shown that patients with more severe asthma may have the greatest risk for exacerbations (Dombrowski, 2000) and complications during pregnancy (Greenberger and Patterson, 1988; Perlow et al., 1992).

Management

The ultimate goal of asthma therapy is prevention of hypoxic episodes in the mother and fetus. Optimal management of asthma during pregnancy relies on the following four integral components:

1. *Objective measures for assessment and monitoring.* Subjective assessments of lung function by the patient and physician

TABLE 46-3. MODIFIED NAEP ASTHMA SEVERITY CLASSIFICATION

Mild Asthma

Brief (<1 h) symptomatic exacerbations ≤ twice/week
PEFR ≥ 80% of personal best
FEV_1 ≥ 80% of predicted when asymptomatic

Moderate Asthma

Symptomatic exacerbations > twice/week
Exacerbations affect activity levels
Exacerbations may last for days
PEFR, FEV_1 range from 60% to 80% of predicted
Regular medications necessary to control symptoms

Severe Asthma

Continuous symptoms/frequent exacerbations limit activity levels
PEFR, FEV_1 < 60% of expected, and are highly variable
Regular oral corticosteroids necessary to control symptoms

FEV_1, forced expiratory volume in 1 second; PEFR, peak expiratory flow rate.

TABLE 46-4. MINIMIZING ASTHMA TRIGGERS

Use plastic mattress and pillow covers
Weekly washing of bedding in hot water
Animal dander control
　　Weekly bathing of the pet
　　Keeping pets out of the bedroom
　　Remove the pet from the home
Cockroach control
Hardwood flooring
Avoid tobacco smoke
Inhibit mite and mold growth by reducing humidity
Do not be present when home is vacuumed

are not reliable indicators of airway responsiveness, inflammation, and asthma severity. The FEV_1 is the single best measure of pulmonary function but requires a spirometer. PEFR correlates well with the FEV_1 and has the advantage that it can be measured with inexpensive, disposable, portable peak flowmeters. Patient self-monitoring of PEFR assesses circadian variation in pulmonary function and helps detect early signs of deterioration so that timely therapy can be instituted to mitigate or prevent an asthma exacerbation.

2. *Avoidance or control of asthma triggers.* Irritants and allergens can provoke acute symptoms and increase airway inflammation and hyper-responsiveness. Avoiding or controlling such triggers can reduce the need for medical therapy, an important benefit during pregnancy. Up to 75% to 85% of patients with asthma have positive skin tests to common allergens, including animal dander, house dust mites, cockroach antigens, pollens, and molds. Common nonimmunologic triggers include tobacco smoke, strong odors, air pollutants, exercise, food additives such as sulfites, and certain drugs, including aspirin and beta-blockers. For many patients, exercise-induced asthma can be avoided with inhalation of β_2-agonist, 5 to 60 minutes before the activity. Specific measures for avoiding asthma triggers are listed in Table 46-4. Limiting environmental triggers is especially important for controlling asthma during pregnancy.

3. *Patient education.* The gravida should know that controlling asthma during pregnancy is especially important for the well-being of the fetus. She should understand how she could reduce asthma triggers. The patient should have a basic understanding of the medical management during pregnancy, including self-monitoring of PEFRs and the correct use of inhalers. She should understand that it is safer to be treated with asthma medications than it is to have asthma exacerbations.

4. *Pharmacologic therapy.* The goals of medical therapy are to relieve bronchospasm, protect the airways from irritant stimuli, prevent the pulmonary and inflammatory response to an allergen exposure, and resolve the inflammatory process in the airways leading to improved pulmonary function with reduced airway hyper-responsiveness. Step-care therapy tailors the choice of medication to asthma severity.

Pharmacotherapy

Although it is assumed that asthma medications are as effective during pregnancy, differences in maternal physiology and pharmacokinetics may affect their absorption, distribu-

tion, metabolism, and clearance. Changes during pregnancy include elevations in free plasma cortisol, possible tissue refractoriness to cortisol (Nolten and Reuckert, 1981), and changes in cellular immunity (Bailey et al., 1985). Human studies have not consistently found asthma medications to be associated with an increased risk of birth defects (Briggs et al., 2002). Potential adverse effects of oral or high-dose inhaled corticosteroids include adrenal suppression, weight gain, impaired fetal growth, hypertension, diabetes, cataracts, and osteoporosis.

Current medical therapy emphasizes the treatment of airway inflammation for moderate and severe asthma. In the United States, three classes of inhaled anti-inflammatory asthma medications are available: inhaled corticosteroids, nedocromil sodium, and cromolyn sodium. In separate controlled studies of nongravid subjects, use of inhaled corticosteroids or cromolyn sodium led to improvement in asthma symptoms, pulmonary function, nonspecific bronchial hyperactivity, emergency room visits, and hospitalizations. Typical dosages of commonly used asthma medications are listed in Table 46-5.

Inhaled Corticosteroids

Inhaled corticosteroids have been associated with a marked reduction in fatal and near-fatal asthma among nonpregnant patients (Ernst et al., 1992). In addition to their anti-inflammatory effect, corticosteroids increase the effectiveness of ß-adrenergic drugs. Inhaled corticosteroids produce clinically important improvements in bronchial hyper-responsiveness that are dose related, occur as early as a few weeks but take months to attain maximal effect, and include prevention of increased bronchial hyper-responsiveness to allergens (Lowhagen and Rak, 1985; Kraan et al., 1988; Woolcock et al., 1988; Woolcock and Jenkins, 1990). Inhaled corticosteroids are more effective than ß-agonists, theophylline, nedocromil sodium, and cromolyn sodium in reducing airway hyper-responsiveness (Dutoit et al., 1987; Svendsen et al., 1987; Haahtela, 1991; Groot et al., 1992). In a prospective observational study of 504 pregnant subjects with asthma, 177 patients not initially treated with either inhaled budesonide or inhaled beclomethasone (Stenius-Aarniala et al., 1996) had a 17% acute exacerbation rate compared with a 4% exacerbation rate

TABLE 46-5. TYPICAL DOSAGES OF COMMON ASTHMA MEDICATIONS

Medication	Dose
Cromolyn sodium	Two inhalations qid
Beclomethasone	Two to five inhalations bid-qid
Triamcinolone	Two inhalations tid-qid or four inhalations bid
Budesonide	Two to four inhalations bid
Fluticasone	88–220 µg bid
Flunisolide	Two to four inhalations bid
Theophylline	Maintain serum levels of 8–12 µg/mL
	Decrease dosage by half if treated with erythromycin or cimetidine
Prednisone	1 week 40 mg/day burst for active symptoms followed by 1-week taper
Albuterol	Two inhalations q3–4h
Montelukast	10 mg orally each evening
Zafirlukast	20 mg bid

among those treated with inhaled corticosteroids from the start of pregnancy.

Inhaled corticosteroids can cause adrenal suppression and changes in bone metabolism in nonpregnant patients. The potential effects of inhaled corticosteroids on fetal adrenal function and bone development are unknown. There is concern they impair growth in children as measured by height or lower leg growth (Tinkelman et al., 1993; Thomas et al., 1994; Doull et al., 1995). Only about 10% to 20% of the inhaled dose of corticosteroid reaches the lungs, approximately 50% is deposited in the oropharynx (Lipworth, 1996). The use of spacers can increase delivery to the lungs. The use of spacers and mouth rinsing after inhalation will decrease oral absorption, thereby reducing the incidence of oral thrush and hoarseness.

In 1993 the NAEP working group recommended inhaled beclomethasone during pregnancy because most clinical studies had been conducted with beclomethasone. Since then, limited data during pregnancy and data from nonpregnant subjects have found that other inhaled corticosteroids may have therapeutic advantages compared with beclomethasone. Therefore, it seems reasonable to continue either triamcinolone acetonide, budesonide, fluticasone propionate, or flunisolide during pregnancy in a patient who is on one of these drugs and who is well controlled. All the inhaled corticosteroids are currently labeled U.S. Food and Drug Administration pregnancy class C.

Inhaled beclomethasone has not been associated with an increased risk of fetal malformations (Greenberger and Patterson, 1983; Fitzsimmons et al., 1986; Wendel et al., 1996). In a randomized study of 84 pregnant patients, inhaled beclomethasone was associated with a reduced readmission rate for asthma exacerbations (Wendel et al., 1996). In a study of 12,301 nonpregnant subjects, Ernst and associates (1992) reported that use of beclomethasone for at least 1 year resulted in a significantly lower risk of fatal and near-fatal asthma compared with therapies not including an inhaled corticosteroid. Betamethasone is known to effectively cross to the fetus. Beclomethasone is identical to betamethasone except for having a chlorine instead of a fluorine at the 9-alpha position.

Data on inhaled triamcinolone use during pregnancy are limited to a single retrospective analysis of 15 women treated with inhaled triamcinolone and 14 treated with inhaled beclomethasone (Dombrowski et al., 1996). There was a significantly lower incidence of hospital admissions for asthma exacerbations among gravidas receiving inhaled triamcinolone (33%) compared with those treated with inhaled beclomethasone cohort (79%; $P < .05$); this finding may be due to confounding factors in this small retrospective study. Triamcinolone has been shown to have minimal systemic absorption after oral administration via metered dose inhalers with spacers (Zaborny et al., 1992).

In a study from the Swedish Medical Birth Registry, in 2014 mothers who used inhaled budesonide in early pregnancy, their infants had a 3.8% (95% confidence interval, 2.9 to 4.6) frequency of congenital malformations, which was similar to the general population rate of 3.5% (Kallen et al., 1999). Budesonide and theophylline may have synergistic effects. In a double-blind placebo-controlled trial of nongravid subjects with moderate asthma, high-dose budesonide (800 μg) was compared with low-dose budesonide (400 μg) with theophylline at serum concentrations below the recommended therapeutic range (Evans et al., 1997). The low-dose budesonide with theophylline regimen resulted in significantly improved FEV_1, and serum cortisol concentrations were significantly reduced in the group treated with high-dose budesonide, but not the low-dose theophylline group.

Fluticasone propionate and flunisolide are potent anti-inflammatory corticosteroids. In a randomized double-blind study of nonpregnant adults and adolescents, inhaled fluticasone propionate was found to be significantly more effective than theophylline in the treatment of mild to moderate asthma (Galant et al., 1996). There are no published studies of their use during human pregnancy. In contrast to inhaled beclomethasone, inhaled fluticasone propionate therapy was not found to be associated with a decrease in growth velocity in children (Tinkelman et al., 1993; Allen et al., 1999).

Cromolyn Sodium and Nedocromil Sodium

Currently, cromolyn sodium and nedocromil sodium are the only approved nonsteroidal anti-inflammatory medications. Nedocromil sodium, a pyranoquinolone, exerts a number of anti-inflammatory effects *in vivo* and *in vitro* (Brogden and Sorokin, 1993). Cromolyn sodium blocks both the early- and late-phase pulmonary response to allergen challenge and prevents the development of airway hyper-responsiveness (Cockcroft and Murdock, 1987). Cromolyn sodium does not have any intrinsic bronchodilator or antihistaminic activity. Compared with inhaled corticosteroids, the time to maximal clinical benefit is longer for cromolyn sodium, 4 weeks versus 2 weeks. Nedocromil sodium and cromolyn sodium appear to be less effective than inhaled corticosteroids in reducing objective and subjective manifestations of asthma but have no significant side effects.

Bronchodilators

THEOPHYLLINE

Theophylline has been used for many decades with no known teratogenic effects. Serum theophylline concentrations should be maintained at 8 to 12 μg/mL during pregnancy (NAEP, 1993). Subjective symptoms of adverse theophylline effects, including insomnia, heartburn, palpitations, and nausea, may be difficult to differentiate from typical pregnancy symptoms. High doses have been observed to cause jitteriness, tachycardia, and vomiting in mothers and neonates. Other drugs can decrease theophylline clearance and result in toxicity. Two commonly used drugs are cimetidine, which can cause a 70% increase, and erythromycin, which causes a 35% increase in theophylline serum levels (Hendeles et al., 1995).

The main advantage of theophylline is the long duration of action, 10 to 12 hours with the use of sustained-release preparations, which is especially useful in the management of nocturnal asthma (Joad et al., 1987). Theophylline should be as an additional therapy when ß-agonists and inhaled anti-inflammatory agents do not adequately control symptoms. Theophylline is only indicated for chronic therapy and is not effective for the treatment of acute exacerbations during pregnancy (Wendel et al., 1996). Theophylline has anti-inflammatory actions (Pauwels et al., 1985) that may be mediated from inhibition of leukotriene production and its capacity to stimulate prostaglandin E_2 production (Juergens et al., 1999). In general, theophylline is now considered a second-line drug to be used to supplement inhaled corticosteroids when control is not achieved (NAEP, 1993). However, a randomized trial of inhaled beclomethasone versus theophylline for asthma during pregnancy found similar rates of asthma exacerbations requiring medical interventions (Dombrowski, 2001).

INHALED ß-AGONISTS

The greatest advantage of ß-agonists is their rapid onset of bronchodilation via smooth muscle relaxation. ß-Agonists are used with all degrees of asthma during pregnancy (Schatz et al., 1988; NAEP, 1991). They can be used before exercise to prevent bronchospasm. Before allergen exposure, they effectively block the pulmonary response but are of insufficient duration of action to prevent the late-phase pulmonary response unless administered in high doses (Twentyman et al., 1991). They have a relatively short duration of only 4 to 6 hours (Joad et al., 1987).

β_2-Agonists frequently cause tremor, tachycardia, and palpitations. Chronic reliance on ß-agonists has been associated with an increased risk of death (Sears et al., 1990; Spitzer et al., 1992). They do not block the development of airway hyperresponsiveness (Cockcroft and Murdock, 1987) and have even been implicated in the development of hyper-responsiveness (Haahtela et al., 1991).

Leukotriene Pathway Moderators

Leukotrienes are arachidonic acid metabolites that have been implicated in transducing bronchospasm, mucous secretion, and increased vascular permeability (Knorr et al., 1998). Treatment with leukotriene receptor antagonist montelukast has been shown to significantly improve pulmonary function as measured by FEV_1 (Knorr et al., 1998). The leukotriene receptor antagonists zafirlukast (Accolate) and montelukast (Singulair) are rated pregnancy category B, and 5-lipoxygenase inhibitor zileuton (Zyflo) is rated category C. It should be noted that there are no data regarding the efficacy or safety of these agents during human pregnancy. It has been our experience that montelukast and zafirlukast are very effective in controlling asthma exacerbations during pregnancy, even when inhaled corticosteroids have been ineffective.

Step Therapy

Especially during pregnancy, the least number of medications needed to control asthma symptoms should be used. The step-care therapeutic approach increases the number and frequency of medications with increasing asthma severity (Table 46-6). Systemic corticosteroids are indicated for exacerbations not responding to initial ß-agonist therapy regardless of asthma severity. Additionally, patients who require increasing inhaled β_2-agonist therapy (more than 12 puffs per day) to control their symptoms may benefit from a course of oral corticosteroids (oral prednisone, 40 to 60 mg/day for 1 week followed by 7 to 14 days of taper).

Antenatal Management

The first prenatal visit should include a detailed medical history with attention to medical conditions that could complicate the management of asthma, including diabetes, hypertensive disorders, cardiac disease, adrenal disease, hyperthyroidism, HIV, hemoglobinopathies, hepatic disease, and active pulmonary disease (e.g., CF, bronchiectasis, tuberculosis, sarcoidosis, recurrent sinopulmonary infections, bronchi-

TABLE 46-6. STEP THERAPY MANAGEMENT

Mild

Inhaled (β_2-agonist as needed)*

Moderate

Inhaled (β_2-agonist as needed)*
Inhaled corticosteroids (or cromolyn)
Theophylline for nocturnal asthma or increased symptoms

Severe

Inhaled (β_2-agonist as needed)*
Inhaled corticosteroids (or cromolyn)
Theophylline for nocturnal asthma or increased symptoms
Oral systemic corticosteroids

*Peak expiratory flow rate or forced expiratory volume in 1 second < 80%, asthma exacerbations, or exposure to exercise or allergens (oral corticosteroid burst if inadequate response to β_2-agonist regardless of asthma severity).

tis). An asthma history should include questions about the presence and severity of symptoms, episodes of nocturnal asthma, the number of days of work missed because of asthma exacerbations, history of acute asthma emergency care visits, and smoking history. The type and amount of asthma medications used each day should be recorded. Asthma severity should be determined (see Table 46-2).

Gravida with mild well-controlled asthma may receive routine prenatal care. Those with moderate and severe asthma will need more frequent prenatal visits based on clinical judgment. In addition to routine care, each antenatal visit should include an evaluation of asthma severity and symptom frequency, nocturnal asthma, PEFR or FEV_1, medications (assess compliance and dosage), emergency visits, and hospital admissions for asthma exacerbations. Patients should be instructed on proper dosing and administration of their asthma medications.

Patients should determine PEFR before taking medications, in the morning and after dinner. At each of these times the patient should make the measurement while standing, to take a maximum inspiration and to record the reading on the instrument. Personal best PEFR should be established and personalized green, yellow, and red zones should be established and explained (Table 46-7). Those with moderate to severe asthma should be instructed to maintain an asthma diary containing daily assessment of asthma symptoms, including morning and evening peak flow measurements, symptoms and activity limitations, indication of any medical contacts initiated, and a record of regular and as-needed medications taken.

Mitigating asthma triggers (see Table 46-4) is particularly important in pregnancy because pharmacologic control of asthma potentially has adverse fetal effects. Avoidance of

TABLE 46-7. INDIVIDUALIZED PEAK EXPIRATORY FLOW RATE (PEFR) ZONES

Establish "personal best" PEFR, then calculate:
1. Green zone > 80% of personal best PEFR
2. Yellow zone 50% to 80% of personal best PEFR
3. Red zone < 50% of personal best PEFR
(Typical PEFR = 380–550 liters/min)

TABLE 46-8. HOME MANAGEMENT OF ACUTE ASTHMA EXACERBATIONS

Use inhaled albuterol two to four puffs and check PEFR in 20 minutes
If PEFR < 50% predicted or symptoms are severe, obtain emergency care
If PEFR is 50%–70% predicted:
    Repeat albuterol treatment, check PEFR in 20 minutes
    If PEFR remains <70% predicted:
        Contact caregiver or go for emergency care
If PEFR > 70% predicted:
    Continue inhaled albuterol (two to four puffs q3–4h for 6–12 h as needed)
If decreased fetal movement:
    Contact caregiver or go for emergency care

PEFR, peak expiratory flow rate.

asthma triggers may result in a reduction of, or even an elimination of, the need for daily medications. Specific recommendations should be made for appropriate environmental controls, based on the patient's history of exposure and, when available, demonstrated skin test reactivity.

Gravida with moderate or severe asthma require additional fetal surveillance in the form of ultrasound examinations and antenatal fetal testing. Because asthma has been associated with intrauterine growth restriction and preterm birth, it is critical to accurately establish pregnancy dating. Repeat ultrasound examinations are recommended for patients with suboptimally controlled asthma and after asthma exacerbations to evaluate fetal activity, growth, and amniotic fluid volume. The intensity of antenatal fetal surveillance should be based on the severity of the asthma. All patients should be instructed to be attentive to fetal activity and keep a record of fetal kick counts.

Home Management of Asthma Exacerbations

An asthma exacerbation that causes minor problems for the mother may have severe sequelae for the fetus. An abnormal fetal heart rate tracing may be the initial manifestation of an asthmatic exacerbation. A maternal partial pressure of oxygen less than 60 or hemoglobin saturation less than 90% may be associated with profound fetal hypoxia. Therefore, asthma exacerbations in pregnancy must be aggressively managed.

Patients should be able to recognize signs and symptoms of early asthma exacerbations such as coughing, chest tightness, dyspnea, wheezing, or by a 20% decrease in their PEFR. This is important so that prompt home rescue treatment may be instituted to avoid maternal and fetal hypoxia. Patients should be given an individualized guide for decision-making and rescue management. In general, patients should use inhaled albuterol two to four puffs every 20 minutes up to 1 hour. A good response is characterized by symptoms that are resolved or become subjectively mild, the ability to resume normal activities, and PEFR more than 70% of personal best. The patient should seek further medical attention if the response is incomplete or if fetal activity is decreased (Table 46-8).

Hospital and Clinic Management

The prevention of hypoxia is the principal goal. Continuous electronic fetal monitoring should be initiated when there is potential fetal viability. Albuterol should be

delivered by nebulizer (2.5 mg = 0.5 mL albuterol in 2.5 mL normal saline) driven with oxygen; treatments should be given every 20 minutes (Nelson et al., 1983). Occasionally, nebulized treatment is not effective because the patient is moving air poorly; in such cases, terbutaline 0.25 mg can be administered subcutaneously every 15 minutes for three doses. The patient should be assessed for pulse rate, use of accessory muscles, wheezing, and FEV_1 and/or PEFR before and after each bronchodilator treatment. Measurement of oxygenation via pulse oximeter or arterial blood gases is essential. Arterial blood gases should be obtained if oxygen saturation remains less than 95%. Chest x-rays should not be routinely obtained. Guidelines for the management of asthma exacerbations are presented in Table 46-9.

Labor and Delivery Management

Asthma medications should be continued during labor and delivery. Although asthma is usually quiescent during labor, consideration should be given to assessing PEFRs upon admission and at 12-hour intervals. The patient should be kept hydrated and should receive adequate analgesia to decrease the risk of bronchospasm. If systemic corticosteroids have been used in the previous 4 weeks, then hydrocortisone (100 mg intravenously every 8 hours) should be administered during labor and for the 24-hour period after delivery to prevent maternal adrenal crisis (NAEP, 1993).

It is rarely necessary to deliver a fetus via cesarean for an acute exacerbation; usually, maternal and fetal distress can be managed by optimal medical management. Occasionally, delivery may improve the respiratory status of a patient with unstable asthma who is near term. Prostaglandin E_2 or E_1 can be used for cervical ripening, the management of spontaneous or induced abortions, or postpartum hemorrhage; 15-methyl prostaglandin $F_{2\alpha}$ and methylergonovine can cause bronchospasm.

TABLE 46-9. EMERGENCY ASSESSMENT AND MANAGEMENT OF ASTHMA EXACERBATIONS

1. Initial evaluation

History, examination, PEFR, oximetry
Fetal monitoring if potentially viable

2. Initial treatment

Inhaled β_2-agonist (3 doses over 60–90 min)
O_2 to maintain saturation > 95%
If no wheezing and PEFR or FEV_1 > 70% baseline, discharge with follow-up

3. If oximetry < 90%, FEV_1 < 1.0 liter, or PEFR < 100 liters/min upon presentation

Continue nebulized albuterol
Start intravenous corticosteroids
Obtain arterial blood gases
Admit to intensive care unit
Possible intubation

4. If PEFR or FEV_1 > 40% but <70% baseline after ß₂-agonist

Obtain arterial blood gases
Continue inhaled (β₂-agonist every 1–4 h
Start intravenous corticosteroids in most cases
Hospital admission in most cases

FEV_1, forced expiratory volume in 1 second; PEFR, peak expiratory flow rate.

Magnesium sulfate, which is a bronchodilator, can be used to treat preterm labor, but indomethacin can induce bronchospasm in the aspirin-sensitive patient. There are no reports of the use of calcium channel blockers for tocolysis among patients with asthma.

Epidural analgesia has the benefit of reducing oxygen consumption and minute ventilation during labor (Hägerdal et al., 1983). Meperidine causes histamine release but rarely causes bronchospasm during labor. A 2% incidence of bronchospasm has been reported with regional anesthesia (Fung, 1985). Communication between the obstetric, anesthetic, and pediatric caregivers is important for optimal care.

Breast-Feeding

Prednisone, theophylline, antihistamines, beclomethasone, ß-agonists, and cromolyn are not considered to be contraindications for breast-feeding (American Academy of Pediatrics Committee on Drugs, 1989; NAEP, 1993). However, among sensitive individuals, theophylline may cause toxic effects in the neonate, including vomiting, feeding difficulties, jitteriness, and cardiac arrhythmias.

■ RESTRICTIVE LUNG DISEASE IN PREGNANCY

Restrictive ventilatory defects occur when lung expansion is limited because of alterations in the lung parenchyma or because of abnormalities in the pleura, chest wall, or the neuromuscular apparatus (West, 1978). These conditions are characterized by a reduction in lung volumes and an increase in FEV_1 to forced vital capacity (King, 1992). The interstitial lung diseases include idiopathic pulmonary fibrosis, sarcoidosis, hypersensitivity pneumonitis, pneumomycosis, drug-induced lung disease, and connective tissue disease. Additional conditions that cause a restrictive ventilatory defect include pleural and chest wall diseases and extrathoracic conditions such as obesity, peritonitis, and ascites (King, 1992). Restrictive lung disease in pregnancy has not been well studied. Consequently, little is known about the effects of restrictive lung disease on the outcome of pregnancy or the effects of pregnancy on the disease process itself. A recent study presented data on nine pregnant women who were prospectively managed with interstitial and restrictive lung disease (Boggess et al., 1995). Diagnoses included idiopathic pulmonary fibrosis, hypersensitivity pneumonitis, sarcoidosis, kyphoscoliosis, and multiple pulmonary emboli. Three of the gravidas had severe disease characterized by a vital capacity no more than 1.5 liters (50% of predicted) or a diffusing capacity no more than 50% of predicted. Five of the patients had exercise-induced oxygen desaturation, and four patients required supplemental oxygen. Of the group, one patient had an adverse outcome and was delivered at 31 weeks. She subsequently required mechanical ventilation for 72 hours. All other patients were delivered at or beyond 36 weeks with no adverse intrapartum or postpartum complications. All infants were at or above the 30th percentile for growth (Boggess et al., 1995). The authors concluded that restrictive lung disease was well tolerated in pregnancy. However, exercise intolerance was common, and patients may require early oxygen supplementations (Boggess et al., 1995).

Sarcoidosis

Sarcoidosis is a systemic granulomatosis disease of undetermined etiology that often affects young adults. Pregnancy outcome for most patients with sarcoidosis is good (Agha et al., 1982; Haynes, 1987). In one study, 35 pregnancies in 18 patients with sarcoidosis were evaluated retrospectively (Agha et al., 1982). In nine patients there was no effect of the disease process during pregnancy, in six patients improvement was demonstrated, and in three patients there was a worsening of the disease. During the postpartum period, no relapse was noted in 15 patients; however, in 3 women, a progression of the disease continued. Another retrospective study presented 15 pregnancies complicated by maternal sarcoidosis over a 10-year period (Haynes, 1987). Eleven of these patients remained stable, 2 experienced disease progression, and 2 died because of complications of severe sarcoidosis. In this group, factors indicating a poor prognosis reportedly included parenchymal lesions on chest radiograph, advanced roentgenologic staging, advanced maternal age, low inflammatory activity, requirement for drugs other than steroids, and the presence of extrapulmonary sarcoidosis (Haynes, 1987). Both patients who succumbed during gestation had severe disease at the onset of pregnancy. The overall cesarean section rate was 40%, and in addition, 4 of 15 infants (27%) weighed under 2500 g. None of the patients developed preeclampsia. One possible explanation for the commonly observed improvement in sarcoidosis may be the increased concentration of circulating corticosteroids during pregnancy. However, because sarcoidosis improves spontaneously in many nonpregnant patients, the improvement may be coincident with but not because of pregnancy.

Maycock and associates (1957) reported on 16 pregnancies in 10 patients with sarcoidosis. Eight of these patients showed improvement in at least some of the manifestations of sarcoidosis during the antepartum period. In two patients no effect was noted. A recurrence of the abnormal findings was observed in the postpartum period within several months after delivery in approximately half of the patients. In addition, some had new manifestations of sarcoidosis not previously noted. Another study examined 17 pregnancies in 10 patients and concluded that pregnancy had no consistent effect on the course of the disease (Reisfield, 1958). Scadding (1967) separated patients into three categories based on characteristic patterns of their chest radiograph x-rays. When the chest radiograph had resolved before pregnancy, the normal radiograph persisted throughout gestation. In women with radiographic changes before pregnancy, resolution continued throughout the prenatal period. Patients with inactive fibrotic residual disease had stable chest radiographs and those with active disease tended to have partial or complete resolution of those changes during pregnancy. Most patients in this later group, however, experienced exacerbation of the disease within 3 to 6 months after delivery.

Patients with pulmonary hypertension complicating restrictive lung disease may suffer a mortality of as much as 50% during gestation. These patients need close monitoring during the labor, delivery, and postpartum periods. Invasive monitoring with a pulmonary artery catheter may be indicated to optimize cardiorespiratory function. Gravidas with restrictive lung disease including pulmonary sarcoidosis may benefit from early institution of steroid therapy for evidence of worsening pulmonary status. Individuals with evidence of severe disease will need close monitoring and may require supplemental oxygen therapy during gestation as well.

During labor, consideration should be given to early use of epidural anesthesia if not contraindicated. The early institution of pain management in this population will minimize pain, decrease sympathetic response, and therefore decrease oxygen consumption during labor and delivery. The use of general anesthesia should be avoided if possible because these patients may develop pulmonary complications after general anesthesia, including pneumonia and difficulty weaning from the ventilator. In addition, close fetal surveillance throughout gestation is indicated because impaired oxygenation may lead to impaired fetal growth and the development of fetal heart rate abnormalities during labor and delivery.

An additional consideration is the need to counsel all women with restrictive lung disease about the potential for continued impairment of their respiratory status during pregnancy, particularly if their respiratory status is deteriorating when they conceive. Certainly the individual with clinical signs consistent with pulmonary hypertension and/or severe restrictive disease should be cautioned about the possibility of maternal mortality resulting from worsening pulmonary function during gestation.

In summary, although the literature on restrictive lung disease in pregnancy is limited, it supports the conclusion that most patients with restrictive lung disease complicating pregnancy, including those with pulmonary sarcoidosis, will have a favorable pregnancy outcome. However, the clinician should keep in mind that patients with restrictive lung disease can have worsening of their clinical condition and may succumb during gestation.

CYSTIC FIBROSIS IN PREGNANCY

CF involves the exocrine glands and epithelial tissues of the pancreas, sweat glands, and mucous glands in the respiratory, digestive, and reproductive tracts. Chronic obstructive pulmonary disease, pancreatic exocrine insufficiency, and elevated sweat electrolytes are present in most patients with CF (Hilman et al., 1996). The disease is genetically transmitted with an autosomal recessive pattern of inheritance. The CF gene was identified and cloned in 1989. The gene is localized to chromosome 7, and the molecular defect accounting for most cases has been identified (Kerem et al., 1989; Riordan et al., 1989; Rommens et al., 1989). In the United States approximately 4% of the white population is heterozygous carriers of the CF gene. The disease occurs in 1 in 3000 white live births (Kotloff et al., 1992). Morbidity and mortality in CF is usually secondary to progressive chronic bronchial pulmonary disease. Pregnancy and the attendant physiologic changes can stress the pulmonary, cardiovascular, and nutritional status of women with CF. The purpose of this section is to familiarize the obstetrician/gynecologist with the physiologic effects of this complex disease and the impact of the disease on pregnancy and the impact of pregnancy on the disease. Additional factors that need to be addressed are the genetics of this disorder and the implications for the newborn, as well as social issues, including who will raise the child should the mother succumb to her disease.

Survival for patients with CF has increased dramatically since 1940. According to the Cystic Fibrosis Foundation's Patient Registry, survival in 1992 had increased to 29.6 years (Hilman et al., 1996). Females had a slightly lower median age of survival (27.3 years) as compared with males (29.6 years). The reasons for sex differences in mortality are unclear. This increase in survival of patients with CF is likely secondary to earlier diagnosis and intervention and also to advances in antibiotic therapy and nutritional support. Therefore, more women with CF are entering reproductive age. In contrast to males with CF who, for the most part, are infertile, women with CF are more often fertile. Infertility in women with CF may occasionally be due to anovulatory cycles and secondary amenorrhea, which result from significant malnutrition, associated with advanced disease. A more common reason for infertility appears to result from alteration in the physiologic properties of cervical mucus (Kopito et al., 1973).

The first case of CF complicating pregnancy was reported in 1960, and a total of 13 pregnancies in 10 patients with CF were reported in 1966 (Siegel and Siegel, 1960; Grand et al., 1966). Cohen and colleagues (1980) conducted a survey of 119 CF centers in the United States and Canada and identified a total of 129 pregnancies in 100 women by 1976. Hillman and colleagues (1996) surveyed 127 CF centers in the United States, between 1976 and 1982. A total of 191 pregnancies were reported during this period in women with CF, ranging in age from 16 to 36 years, with a mean age of 22.6 years (Hilman et al., 1996). The annual number of CF pregnancies reported to the Cystic Fibrosis Patient Registry doubled between 1986 and 1990, with 52 pregnancies reported in 1986, compared with 111 pregnancies reported in 1990. Because the number of women with CF achieving pregnancy is steadily increasing, it is imperative that the obstetrician be familiar with the disease.

Effect of Pregnancy on Cystic Fibrosis

The physiologic changes associated with pregnancy are well tolerated by healthy gravidas; however, those with CF may adapt poorly. During pregnancy there is an increase in resting minute ventilation, which at term may approach 150% of control values (Weinberger et al., 1980). This increase in minute ventilation occurs secondary to increased oxygen consumption and increased carbon dioxide burden that occur during pregnancy. An additional impact occurs secondary to circulating progesterone, which stimulates the respiratory drive. Enlargement of the abdominal contents and upward displacement of the diaphragm leads to a decrease in functional residual volume and a decrease in residual volume (Weinberger et al., 1980). Pregnancy is also accompanied by subtle alterations in gas exchange with widening of the alveolar-arterial oxygen gradient that is most pronounced in the supine position (Weinberger et al., 1980). These alterations in pulmonary function are of little consequence in the normal pregnant woman. However, in the gravida with CF, these changes may contribute to respiratory decompensation that can lead to increase in morbidity and mortality for the mother and the fetus as well.

During normal pregnancy, blood volume increases by an average of 50%. Cardiac output increases as well, reaching a plateau in mid-pregnancy (McAnulty et al., 1988). During labor, blood volume rises acutely, in large part because of the release of blood from the contracting uterus and is additionally increased after delivery, secondary to augmented venous return with the release of caval obstruction. Women with CF and advanced lung disease may suffer from pulmonary hypertension with high pulmonary artery pressures. Whatever the cause, pulmonary hypertension is associated with unacceptable maternal risk during pregnancy and is considered to be a contraindication to pregnancy (McAnulty et al., 1988). Women with significant pulmonary hypertension may develop cardiovascular collapse at the time of labor and delivery, with a maternal mortality exceeding 25% (Gleicher et al., 1979). Additionally, patients with pulmonary hypertension may not be able to adequately increase cardiac output during pregnancy and therefore suffer uteroplacental insufficiency, leading to intrauterine growth restriction and stillbirth (Kotloff et al., 1992).

Nutritional requirements are increased during pregnancy, with approximately 300 kcal/day in additional fuel being needed to meet the requirements of mother and fetus (Rush et al., 1988). Most patients with CF have pancreatic exocrine insufficiency. As a result, digestive enzymes and bicarbonate ions are diminished, resulting in maldigestion, malabsorption, and malnutrition (Rush et al., 1988). Gastrointestinal manifestations of CF include steatorrhea, abdominal pain, distal intestinal obstruction syndrome, and rectal prolapse. Gastroesophageal reflux, peptic ulcer disease, acute pancreatitis, and intussusception also occur to different degrees in patients with CF. Partial or complete obstruction of the gastrointestinal tract in older children and adults is known as distal obstruction syndrome. It can be precipitated by dehydration, change in eating habits, change in enzyme brand or dose, or immobility and is treated with a combination of laxatives and enemas. Patients with CF are encouraged to eat a diet that provides 120% to 150% of the recommended energy intake of normal age- and sex-matched control subjects. However, this is only a guideline, because in practice the energy requirement for a patient with CF is that of their ideal body weight when malabsorption has been minimized. Research done by the United Kingdom Dieticians Cystic Fibrosis Interest Group found that women with CF who received preconception counseling had a significantly greater mean maternal weight gain and significantly heavier infants than did those women who had not received preconception advice (Dowsett, 2000).

Grand and colleagues (1966) reported 13 pregnancies in 10 women with CF. Of these, five women had a progressive decline in their pulmonary function, two of whom died of cor pulmonale in the immediate postpartum period. Pregnancy was well tolerated in 5 of 10 women, 2 of whom went on to have subsequent pregnancies that were similarly well tolerated (Grand et al., 1966). In this study, the pregravid pulmonary status of the patient was the most important predictor of outcome. However, there was no quantification of pulmonary function. A case report by Novy and colleagues (1967) described in detail the pulmonary function and gas exchange in a pregnant woman with CF. The patient had severe disease as evidenced by a vital capacity of only 0.72 liters and an arterial partial pressure of oxygen of 50 mm Hg at presentation. The patient suffered a progressive increase in residual volume and decline in vital capacity that was accompanied by worsening hypoxemia and hypercapnia, resulting in respiratory distress and right-sided heart failure in the early postpartum period (Novy et al., 1967). Based on the experience with this patient and a review of the literature, the authors recommended therapeutic abortion in any patient demonstrating progressive pulmonary deterioration and hypoxemia despite maximal medical management (Novy et al., 1967). In 1980, Cohen and

associates described 100 patients and a total of 129 pregnancies. Ninety-seven pregnancies (75%) were completed, and 89% delivered viable infants. Twenty-seven percent of these fetuses were delivered preterm. There were 11 perinatal deaths and no congenital anomalies. In this study, 65% of patients required antibiotic therapy before delivery. In 1983, Palmer and colleagues retrospectively reviewed the pre-pregnancy status of eight women with CF who subsequently completed 11 pregnancies. They found that five women tolerated pregnancy without difficulty, but three had irreversible deterioration in their clinical status. She identified four maternal factors that were predictive of outcome: clinical status (Shwachman score), nutritional status (percent of predicted weight for height), the extent of chest radiologic abnormalities (assessed by the Brasfield chest roentgenogram score), and the magnitude of pulmonary function impairment. Women with good clinical studies, good nutritional status (within 15% of their predicted ideal body weight for height), with nearly normal chest radiographs and only mild obstructive lung disease tolerated pregnancy well without deterioration (Palmer et al., 1983).

Several reports suggest that patients with mild CF, good nutritional status, and less impairment of lung function tolerate pregnancy well. However, those with poor clinical status, malnutrition, hepatic dysfunction, and/or advanced lung disease are at increased risk from pregnancy (Corkey et al., 1981; Canny et al., 1991; Kent and Farquharson, 1993). Kent and Farquharson (1993) reviewed the literature and reported 217 pregnancies. In this series, the frequency of preterm delivery was 24.3%, and the perinatal death rate was 7.9%. Poor outcomes were associated with a maternal weight gain of less than 4.5 kg and a forced vital capacity of less than 50% of that predicted. Edenborough and colleagues (1995) also reported on pregnancies in women with CF. There were 18 live births (81.8%), one third of which were preterm deliveries, and 18.2% of patients had abortions. There were four maternal deaths within 3.2 years after delivery. In this series, lung function was available predelivery, immediately after delivery, and after pregnancy. They demonstrated a decline of 13% in FEV_1 and 11% in forced vital capacity during pregnancy. Most patients returned to baseline pulmonary function after pregnancy. Although most of the women in this series tolerated pregnancy well, those with moderate to severe lung disease, an FEV_1 of less than 60% of predicted, more often had preterm infants and had increased loss of lung function compared with those with milder disease (Edenborough et al., 1995). In two series, pre-pregnancy FEV_1 was found to be the most useful predictor of outcomes in pregnant women with CF (Edenborough et al., 1995; Olson, 1997). In addition, there was also a positive correlation of pre-pregnancy FEV_1 and maternal survival. From the 72 pregnancies identified, the outcomes were known for 69; there were 48 live births (70%) of which 22 were premature (46%); 14 therapeutic abortions (20%); and 7 miscarriages (10%). There were no stillbirths, neonatal, or early maternal deaths. Three major fetal anomalies were seen, but no infant had CF. Another report documented the outcome of 72 pregnancies with CF (Edenborough et al., 2000).

Pulmonary involvement in CF includes chronic infection of the airways and bronchiectasis. There is selective infection with certain microorganisms, such as *Staphylococcus aureus*, *Haemophilus influenza*, *Pseudomonas aeruginosa*, and *Burkholderia cepacia*. In one report, three of four deaths during pregnancy occurred in gravidas colonized with *B. cepacia* (Tanser et al.,

2000). Gilljam and associates (2000) reported outcome in a cohort of pregnancies for women with CF from 1963 to 1998. There were 92 pregnancies in 54 women. There were 11 miscarriages and seven therapeutic abortions. Forty-nine women gave birth to 74 children. The mean follow-up time was 11 ± 8 years. One patient was lost to follow-up shortly after delivery, and one was lost after 12 years. The overall mortality rate was 19% (9 of 48 patients). Absence of *B. cepacia* ($P < .001$), pancreatic sufficiency ($P = .01$), and pre-pregnancy FEV_1 more than 50% predicted ($P = .03$) were associated with better survival rates. When adjusted for the same parameters, pregnancy did not affect survival compared with the entire adult female CF population. The decline in FEV_1 was comparable with that in the total CF population. Three women had diabetes mellitus, and seven developed gestational diabetes. There were six preterm infants and one neonatal death. CF was diagnosed in two children. Gilljam and coworkers concluded that the maternal and fetal outcome is good for most women with CF. Risk factors for mortality are similar to those for nonpregnant CF population. Pregnancies should be planned so that there is opportunity for counseling and optimization of the medical condition. Good communication between the CF team and the obstetrician is important (Gilljam et al., 2000).

P. aeruginosa is the most frequent pathogen (Hilman et al., 1996). Parenteral antibiotics are the mainstays of treatment of these acute infections. However, pregnancy and CF-associated alterations in pharmacokinetics can have grave consequences for these patients. It is well known that pregnant subjects have lower serum levels and higher urine levels of antibiotics than nonpregnant subjects. The lower levels in plasma are attributed to the increase in volume of distribution and an increase in glomerular filtration and renal clearance of the drugs (Heikkila and Erkkola, 1994). Cloxacillin, dicloxacillin, ticarcillin, and methicillin are cleared more rapidly in patients with CF (Jusko et al., 1975; Yaffe et al., 1977; Spino et al., 1984). Plasma ceftazidime and gentamicin are likewise decreased in patients with CF (De Groot and Smith, 1987).

Counseling Patients with Cystic Fibrosis in Pregnancy

Several factors must be considered when counseling a woman who has CF and is considering pregnancy, including the possibility that her fetus will have CF. Approximately 4% of the white population in the United States is heterozygous carriers of the CF gene. The disease occurs in 1 in 3000 white births. When the mother has CF and the proposed father is white with an unknown genotype, the risk of the fetus having CF is 1 in 50, as compared with 1 in 3000 in the general white population. If the prospective father is a known carrier of a CF mutation, the risk to the fetus increases to 1 in 2. If, however, DNA testing does not identify a CF mutation in the prospective father, it is still possible that the father is a carrier of an unidentified CF mutation, making the risk to the offspring 1 in 492 (Lemna et al., 1990).

It is important that the woman with CF be advised about the potential adverse affects of pregnancy on maternal health status. Factors that may predict poor outcome include pre-pregnancy evidence of poor nutritional status, significant pulmonary disease with hypoxemia, and pulmonary hypertension. Liver disease and diabetes mellitus are also poor prognostic factors. Gravidas with poor nutritional status, pulmonary

hypertension (cor pulmonale), and deteriorating pulmonary function early in gestation should consider therapeutic abortion, because the risk of maternal mortality may be unacceptably high.

The woman with CF who is considering pregnancy should also give consideration to the need for strong psychosocial and physical support after delivery. The rigors of child-rearing may add to the risk of maternal deterioration during this period. Her family should also be willing to provide physical and emotional support and should be aware of the potential for deterioration in the mother's health and the potential for maternal mortality. In addition, the need for care of a potentially preterm growth restricted neonate with all of its attendant morbidities and potential mortality should be discussed. Long term, the woman and her family should also consider the fact that her life expectancy may be shortened by CF, and plans should be made for rearing of the child in the event of maternal death.

Management of the Pregnancy Complicated by Cystic Fibrosis

Care of the gravida with CF should be a coordinated team effort. Physicians familiar with CF and its complications and management should be included, as well as a maternal-fetal medicine specialist and neonatal team. The gravida should be assessed for potential risk factors such as severe lung disease, pulmonary hypertension, poor nutritional status, pancreatic failure, and liver disease, preferably before attempting gestation but certainly during the early months of pregnancy. Gravidas should be advised to be 90% of ideal body weight before conception if possible. A weight gain of 11 to 12 kg is recommended (Hilman et al., 1996). Frequent monitoring of weight, blood glucose, hemoglobin, total protein, serum albumin, prothrombin time, and fat-soluble vitamins A and E is suggested (Hilman et al., 1996). At each visit the history of caloric intake and symptoms of maldigestion and malabsorption should be taken, and pancreatic enzymes should be adjusted if needed. Patients who are unable to achieve adequate weight gain through oral nutritional supplements may be given nocturnal enteral nasogastric tube feeding. In this situation, the risk of aspiration should be considered, especially in patients with a history of gastroesophageal reflux, which is common in CF (Hilman et al., 1996). If malnutrition is severe, parenteral hyperalimentation may be necessary for successful completion of the pregnancy (Cole et al., 1987). Baseline pulmonary function should be assessed, preferably before conception. Assessment should include forced vital capacity, FEV_1, lung volumes, pulse oximetry, and arterial blood gases if indicated. These values should be serially monitored during gestation, and deterioration in pulmonary function addressed immediately. An echocardiogram can assess the patient for pulmonary hypertension and cor pulmonale. If pulmonary hypertension (cor pulmonale) is diagnosed, the gravida should be advised of the high maternal risk.

Early recognition and prompt treatment of pulmonary infections is important in the management of the pregnant woman with CF. Treatment includes intravenous antibiotics in the appropriate dose, keeping in mind the increased clearance of these drugs secondary to pregnancy and CF. Plasma levels of aminoglycosides should be monitored and adjusted as indicated. Chest physical therapy and bronchial drainage are also important components of the management of pulmonary infections in CF. Because *P. aeruginosa* is the most frequently isolated bacteria associated with chronic endobronchitis and bronchiectasis, antibiotic regimens should include coverage for this organism.

If the patient with CF has pancreatic insufficiency and diabetes mellitus, careful monitoring of blood glucose and insulin therapy are indicated. As previously mentioned, pancreatic enzymes may need to be replaced to optimize the patient's nutritional status. Because of malabsorption of fats and frequent use of antibiotics, the CF patient is prone to vitamin K deficiency. Therefore, prothrombin time should be checked regularly, and parenteral vitamin K should be administered if the prothrombin time is elevated.

It is imperative when managing pregnancy in a woman with CF to recognize that the fetus is at risk for uteroplacental insufficiency and intrauterine growth restriction. The maternal nutritional status and weight gain during pregnancy will likewise impact fetal growth. Therefore, fundal height should be measured routinely, and serial ultrasound evaluations of fetal growth and amniotic fluid volume should be made. Maternal kick counts may be useful for monitoring fetal status starting at 28 weeks. Nonstress testing should be started at 32 weeks or sooner, if there is evidence of fetal compromise. If there is evidence of severe fetal compromise, such as no interval fetal growth, persistent decelerations, or poor biophysical profile scoring, delivery should be accomplished. Likewise, evidence of profound maternal deterioration, such as a marked and sustained decline in pulmonary function, development of right-sided heart failure, refractory hypoxemia, and progressive hypercapnia and respiratory acidosis, may be maternal indications for early delivery. If the fetus is potentially viable, the administration of betamethasone may be beneficial. Vaginal delivery should be attempted when possible.

Labor, delivery, and the postpartum period can be particularly dangerous for the patient with CF. The augmentation in cardiac output stresses the cardiovascular system and can lead to cardiopulmonary failure in the patient with pulmonary hypertension and cor pulmonale. These patients are also more likely to develop right-sided heart failure. Heart failure should be treated with aggressive diuresis and supplemental oxygen. Management may be optimized by insertion of a pulmonary artery catheter to monitor right- and left-sided filling pressures. Pain control will reduce the sympathetic response to labor and tachycardia. This will benefit the patient who is demonstrating pulmonary or cardiac compromise. In the patient with a normal partial thromboplastin time, insertion of an epidural catheter for continuous epidural analgesia may be beneficial. This is also useful in the event a cesarean delivery is indicated because general anesthesia and its possible effects on pulmonary function can be avoided. If general anesthesia is needed, preoperative anticholinergic agents should be avoided because they tend to promote drying and inspissation of airway secretions. Close fetal surveillance is also extremely important, because the fetus may have been suffering from uteroplacental insufficiency during gestation and will be more prone to develop evidence of fetal compromise during labor. Delivery by cesarean section should be reserved for the usual obstetric indications.

In summary, more women with CF are living to childbearing age and are capable of conceiving. Clinical experience thus far has demonstrated that pregnancy in women with CF and mild disease is well tolerated. Women with severe disease have an associated increase in maternal and fetal morbidity

and mortality. The potential risk to any one individual with CF desirous of pregnancy should be assessed and discussed with the patient and her family in detail.

REFERENCES

Afessa B, Green B: Bacterial pneumonia in hospitalized patients with HIV infection. The pulmonary complications, ICU support, and prognostic factors of hospitalized patients with HIV (PIP) study. Chest 117:1017, 2000.
Agha FP, Vade A, Amendola MA, et al: Effects of pregnancy on sarcoidosis. Surg Gynecol Obstet 155:817, 1982.
Ahmad H, Mehta NJ, Manikal VM, et al: *Pneumocystis carinii* pneumonia in pregnancy. Chest 120:666, 2001.
Alaily AB, Carrol KB: Pulmonary ventilation in pregnancy. Br J Obstet Gynaecol 85:518, 1978.
Allen DB, Bronsky EA, LaForce CF, et al: Growth in asthmatic children treated with fluticasone propionate. Fluticasone propionate asthma study group. J Pediatr 132:472, 1999.
American Academy of Pediatrics Committee on Drugs: Transfer of drugs and other chemicals into human milk. Pediatrics 84:924, 1989.
American College of Obstetricians and Gynecologists: Pulmonary disease in pregnancy. ACOG Technical Bulletin 224. Washington, DC: ACOG, 1996.
American Thoracic Society Workshop: Rapid diagnostic tests for tuberculosis— What is the appropriate use? Am J Respir Crit Care Med 155:1804, 1997.
American Thoracic Society: Mycobacteriosis and the acquired immunodeficiency syndrome. Am Rev Respir Dis 136:492–496, 1987.
Andrews EB, Yankaskas BC, Cordero JF, et al: Acyclovir in pregnancy registry: Six years' experience. Obstet Gynecol 79:7, 1992.
Antoine C, Morris M, Douglas G: Maternal and fetal mortality in acquired immunodeficiency syndrome. New York State Journal of Medicine 86:443–445, 1986.
Armstrong D: Aerosol pentamidine. Ann Intern Med 109:852, 1988.
Bailey K, Herrod H, Younger R, et al: Functional aspects of T-lymphocyte subsets in pregnancy. Obstet Gynecol 66:211, 1985.
Barcroft J: On anoxemia. Lancet 11:485, 1920.
Bardeguez AD: Management of HIV infection for the childbearing age woman. Clin Obstet Gynecol 39:344, 1996.
Barnes PF: Rapid diagnostic tests for tuberculosis, progress but no gold standard. Am J Respir Crit Care Med 155:1497, 1997.
Barron W, Lindheimer M: Medical Disorders During Pregnancy, 1st ed. St. Louis, Mosby, 1991, p. 234.
Benedetti TJ, Valle R, Ledger W: Antepartum pneumonia in pregnancy. Am J Obstet Gynecol 144:413, 1982.
Berkowitz K, LaSala A: Risk factors associated with the increasing prevalence of pneumonia during pregnancy. Am J Obstet Gynecol 163:981, 1990.
Bertina RM: Factor V Leiden and other coagulation factor mutations affecting thrombotic risk. Clin Chem 43:1678, 1997.
Boggess KA, Easterling TR, Raghu G: Management and outcome of pregnant women with interstitial and restrictive lung disease. Am J Obstet Gynecol 173:1007, 1995.
Boggess KA, Myers ER, Hamilton CD: Antepartum or postpartum isoniazid treatment of latent tuberculosis infection. Obstet Gynecol 96:757, 2000.
Bonnar J: Venous thromboembolism and pregnancy. In Stallworthy J, Bourne G (eds): Recent Advances in Obstetrics and Gynaecology. London, Churchill Livingstone, 1979, p. 173.
Boutourline-Young H, Boutourline-Young E: Alveolar carbon dioxide levels in pregnant, parturient and lactating subjects. J Obstet Gynaecol Br Emp 63:509, 1956.
Briggs GG, Freeman RK, Yaffe SJ: Drugs in Pregnancy and Lactation, 6th ed. Baltimore, Williams & Wilkins, 2002.
Brogden RN, Sorokin EM: Nedocromil sodium: An updated review of its pharmacological properties and therapeutic efficacy in asthma. Drugs 45:693, 1993.
Brown ZA, Baker DA: Acyclovir therapy during pregnancy. Obstet Gynecol 73:526, 1989.
Bryan-Brown CW, Baek SM, Makabali G, et al: Consumable oxygen: Oxygen availability in relation to oxyhemoglobin dissociation. Crit Care Med 1:17, 1973.
Cain SM: Peripheral uptake and delivery in health and disease. Clin Chest Med 4:139, 1983.
Canny GJ, Corey M, Livingstone RA, et al: Pregnancy and cystic fibrosis. Obstet Gynecol 77:850, 1991.
Cantwell MF, Shehab AM, Costello AM: Brief report: Congenital tuberculosis. N Engl J Med 330:1051, 1994.

Centers for Disease Control: The use of preventive therapy for tuberculosis infection in the United States. MMWR Morb Mortal Wkly Rep **39**:9, 1990.

Chong BH: Heparin-induced thrombocytopenia. Br J Haematol **89**:431, 1995.

Clinton M, Niederman M, Matthay R: Maternal pulmonary disorders complicating pregnancy. In: Reece EA, Hobbins JC, Mahoney MJ, et al (eds): Medicine of the Fetus and Mother. Philadelphia, Lippincott, 1992, p. 317.

Cockcroft DW, Murdock KY: Comparative effects of inhaled salbutamol, sodium cromoglycate, and beclomethasone dipropionate on allergen-induced early asthmatic responses, last asthmatic responses, and increased bronchial responsiveness to histamine. J Allergy Clin Immunol **79**:734, 1987.

Cohen LF, di Sant' Agnese PA, Friedlander J: Cystic fibrosis and pregnancy: A national survey. Lancet **2**:842, 1980.

Cole BN, Seltzer MH, Kassabian J, et al: Parenteral nutrition in a pregnant cystic fibrosis patient. JPEN **11**:205, 1987.

Conard J, Horellou MH, van Dreden P, et al: Pregnancy and congenital deficiency in antithrombin III or protein C. Thromb Haemost **58**:39, 1987.

Cox SM, Cunningham FG, Luby J: Management of varicella pneumonia complicating pregnancy. Am J Perinatol **7**:300, 1990.

Cugell DW, Frank NR, Gaensler EA, Badger TL: Pulmonary function in pregnancy: Serial observations in normal women. Am Rev Tuberc **67**:568, 1953.

Cullen JH, Brum VC, Reid TWH: The respiratory effects of progesterone in severe pulmonary emphysema. Am J Med **27**:551, 1959.

De Groot R, Smith AL: Antibiotic pharmacokinetics in cystic fibrosis: Differences and clinical significance. Clin Pharmacokinet **13**:228, 1987.

Den Heijer M, Koster T, Blom HJ, et al: Hyperhomocysteinemia as a risk factor for deep-vein thrombosis. N Engl J Med **334**:759, 1996.

Dinsmoor MJ: HIV infection and pregnancy. Med Clin North Am **73**:701, 1989.

Diwan VK, Thorson A: Sex, gender and tuberculosis. Lancet **353**:1000, 1999.

Dombrowski MP: Should the definitions of asthma severity be modified during pregnancy? Am J Obstet Gynecol **182**:S167, 2000.

Dombrowski MP: Randomized trial of inhaled beclomethasone versus theophylline for asthma during pregnancy. Am J Obstet Gynecol **184**:S2, 2001.

Dombrowski MP, Bottoms SF, Boike GM, et al: Incidence of preeclampsia among asthmatic patients lower with theophylline. Am J Obstet Gynecol **155**:265,1986.

Dombrowski MP, Brown CL, Berry SM: Preliminary experience with triamcinolone acetonide during pregnancy. J Matern Fetal Med **5**:310, 1996.

Doull IJM, Freezer JN, Holgate ST: Growth of prepubertal children with mild asthma treated with inhaled beclomethasone dipropionate. Am J Respir Crit Care Med **151**:1715, 1995.

Dowsett J: An overview of nutritional issues for the adult with cystic fibrosis. Nutrition **16**:566, 2000.

Dutoit JI, Salome CM, Woolcock AJ: Inhaled corticosteroids reduce the severity of bronchial hyper-responsiveness in asthma but oral theophylline does not. Am Rev Respir Dis **136**:1174, 1987.

Edenborough FP, Mackenzie WE, Stableforth DE: The outcome of 72 pregnancies in 55 women with cystic fibrosis in the United Kingdom 1977–1996. Br J Obstet Gynaecol **107**:254, 2000.

Edenborough FP, Stableforth DE, Webb AK, et al: Outcome of pregnancy in women with cystic fibrosis. Thorax **50**:170, 1995.

Eng M, Butler J, Bonich JJ: Respiratory function in pregnant obese women. Am J Obstet Gynecol **123**:241, 1975.

Ernst P, Spetzer WO, Suissa S, et al: Risk of fatal and near-fatal asthma in relation to inhaled corticosteroid use. JAMA **268**:3462, 1992.

Esmonde TG, Herdman G, Anderson G: Chickenpox pneumonia: An association with pregnancy. Thorax **44**:812, 1989.

Evans DJ, Taylor DA, Zetterstrom O, et al: A comparison of low-dose inhaled budesonide plus theophylline and high-dose inhaled budesonide for moderate asthma. N Engl J Med **337**:1412, 1997.

Ezri T, Szmuk P, Stein A, et al: Peripartum general anesthesia without tracheal intubation: Incidence of aspiration pneumonia. Anaesthesia **55**:421, 2000.

Finland M, Dublin TD: Pneumococcic pneumonias complicating pregnancy and the puerperium. JAMA **112**:1027, 1939.

Fitzsimmons R, Greenberger PA, Patterson R: Outcome of pregnancy in women requiring corticosteroids for severe asthma. J Allergy Clin Immunol **78**:349, 1986.

Fox CW, George RB: Current concepts in the management and prevention of tuberculosis in adults. J La State Med Soc **144**:363, 1992.

Freeman DW, Barno A: Deaths from Asian influenza associated with pregnancy. Am J Obstet Gynecol **78**:1172, 1959.

Frieden TR, Sterling T, Pablos-Mendez A, et al: The emergence of drug-resistant tuberculosis in New York City. N Engl J Med **328**:521, 1993.

Fung DL: Emergency anesthesia for asthma patients. Clin Rev Allergy **3**:127, 1985.

Galant SP, Lawrence M, Meltzer EO, et al: Fluticasone propionate compared with theophylline for mild-to-moderate asthma. Ann Allery Asthma Immunol **77**:112, 1996.

Gazioglu K, Kaltreider NL, Rosen M, et al: Pulmonary function during pregnancy in normal women and in patients with cardiopulmonary disease. Thorax **25**:445, 1970.

Gemzell CA, Robbe H, Strom G, et al: Observations on circulatory changes and muscular work in normal labor. Acta Obstet Gynaecol Scand **36**:75, 1957.

Gilljam M, Antoniou M, Shin J, et al:. Pregnancy in cystic fibrosis. Chest **118**:85, 2000.

Gleicher N, Midwall J, Hochberger D, et al: Eisenmenger's syndrome and pregnancy. Obstet Gynecol Surv **34**:721, 1979.

Good JT, Iseman MD, Davidson PT, et al: Tuberculosis in association with pregnancy. Am J Obstet Gynecol **140**:492, 1981.

Goodland RL, Pommerenke WT: Cyclic fluctuations of the alveolar carbon dioxide tension during the normal menstrual cycle. Fertil Steril **3**:394, 1952.

Grand RJ, Talamo RC, di Sant' Agnese PA, et al: Pregnancy in cystic fibrosis of the pancreas. JAMA **195**:993, 1966.

Greenberger PA, Patterson R: Beclomethasone dipropionate for severe asthma during pregnancy. Ann Intern Med **98**:478, 1983.

Greenberger PA, Patterson R: The outcome of pregnancy complicated by severe asthma. Allergy Proc **9**:539, 1988.

Griffith DE: Mycobacteria as pathogens of respiratory infection. Infect Dis Clin North Am **12**:593, 1998.

Groot CAR, Lammers J-WJ, Molema J, et al: Effect of inhaled beclomethasone and nedocromil sodium on bronchial hyper responsiveness to histamine and distilled water. Eur Respir J **5**:1075, 1992.

Haahtela T, Jarvinen M, Kava T, et al: Comparison of β2-agonist, terbutaline, with an inhaled corticosteroid, budesonide, in newly detected asthma. N Engl J Med **325**:338, 1991.

Haake DA, Zakowski PC, Haake DL, et al: Early treatment with acyclovir for varicella pneumonia in otherwise healthy adults: Retrospective controlled study and review. Rev Infect Dis **12**:788, 1990.

Hägerdal M, Morgan CW, Sumner AE, et al: Minute ventilation and oxygen consumption during labor with epidural analgesia. Anesthesiology **59**:425, 1983.

Hamadeh MA, Glassroth J: Tuberculosis and pregnancy. Chest **101**:1114, 1992.

Harger JH, Ernest JM, Thurnau GR, et al: Risk factors and outcome of varicella-zoster virus pneumonia in pregnant women. J Infect Dis **185**:422, 2002.

Harris JW: Influenza occurring in pregnant women. JAMA **72**:978, 1919.

Harris RE, Rhades ER: Varicella pneumonia complicating pregnancy: Report of a case and review of literature. Obstet Gynecol **25**:734, 1965.

Haynes de Regt R: Sarcoidosis and pregnancy. Obstet Gynecol **70**:369, 1987.

Heidenreich J, Kafarnik D, Westenburger U, et al: Statische und Dynamische Ventilationsgrossen in der Schwangerschaft und im Wochenbett. Arch Gynakol **210**:208, 1971.

Heikkila A, Erkkola R: Review of β-lactam antibiotics in pregnancy: The need for adjustment of dosage schedules. Clin Pharmacokinet **27**:49, 1994.

Hendeles L, Jenkins J, Temple R: Revised FDA labeling guideline for theophylline oral dosage forms. Pharmacotherapy **15**:409, 1995.

Hicks ML, Nolan GH, Maxwell SL, et al: Acquired immuno-deficiency syndrome and *Pneumocystis carinii* infection in a pregnant woman. Obstet Gynecol **76**:480, 1990.

Hilman BC, Aitken ML, Constantinescu M: Pregnancy in patients with cystic fibrosis. Clin Obstet Gynecol **39**:70, 1996.

Hollingsworth HM, Pratter MR, Irwin RS: Acute respiratory failure in pregnancy. J Intens Care Med **4**:11, 1989.

Holmes CB, Hausler H, Numm P: A review of sex differences in the epidemiology of tuberculosis. Int F Tuberc Lung Dis **2**:96, 1998.

Hopwood HG: Pneumonia in pregnancy. Obstet Gynecol **25**:875, 1965.

Hussain A, Mehta NJ, Manikal VM, et al: *Pneumocystis carinii*—Pneumonia in pregnancy. Chest **120**:666, 2001.

Jana N, Vasishta K, Saha SC, et al: Obstetrical outcomes among women with extrapulmonary tuberculosis. N Engl J Med **341**:645, 1999.

Jensen LP, O'Sullivan MJ, Gomez-del-Rio M, et al: Acquired immunodeficiency (AIDS) in pregnancy. Am J Obstet Gynecol **148**:1145, 1984.

Joad JP, Ahrens RC, Lindgren SD, et al: Relative efficacy of maintenance therapy with theophylline, inhaled albuterol, and the combination for chronic asthma. J Allergy Clin Immunol **79**:78, 1987.

Juergens UR, Degenhardt V, Stober M, et al: New insights in the bronchodilatory and anti-inflammatory mechanisms of action of theophylline. Arzneimittelforschung **49**:694, 1999.

Jusko WJ, Mosovich LL, Gerbracht LM, et al: Enhanced renal excretion of dicloxacillin in patients with cystic fibrosis. Pediatrics **56**:1038, 1975.

Kallen B, Fydhstroem H, Aberg A: Congenital malformations after use of inhaled budesonide in early pregnancy. Obstet Gynecol **93**:392, 1999.

Kaunitz AM, Hughes JM, Grimes DA, et al: Causes of maternal mortality in the United States. Obstet Gynecol **65**:605, 1985.

Kell PD, Barton SE, Smith DE, et al: A maternal death caused by AIDS. Case report. Br J Obstet Gynaecol **98**:725, 1991.

Kent NE, Farquharson DF: Cystic fibrosis in pregnancy. Can Med Assoc J **149**:809, 1993.

Kerem B, Rommens JM, Buchanan JA, et al: Identification of the cystic fibrosis gene: Genetic analysis. Science **245**:1073, 1989.

King TE Jr. Restrictive lung disease in pregnancy. Clin Chest Med **13**:607, 1992.

Kirshon B, Faro S, Zurawin RK, et al: Favorable outcome after treatment with amantadine and ribavirin in a pregnancy complicated by influenza pneumonia: A case report. J Reprod Med **33**:399, 1988.

Klaften E, Palugyay J: Zr Physiologie der Atmung in der Schwangerschaft. Arch Gyn **129**:414, 1926.

Klaften E, Palugyay J: Verleichende Untersuchungen über Lage und Ausdehnung von Herz und Lunge in der Schwangerschaft und im Wochenbett. Arch Gyn **131**:347, 1927.

Knorr B, Matz J, Bernstein JA, et al: Montelukast for chronic asthma in 6 to 14 year old children. JAMA **279**:1181, 1998.

Knuttgen HG, Emerson K: Physiological response to pregnancy at rest and during exercise. J Appl Physiol **36**:549, 1974.

Koonin LM, Ellerbrock TV, Atrash HK, et al: Pregnancy-associated deaths due to AIDS in the United States. JAMA **261**:1306, 1989.

Kopito LE, Kosasky HJ, Shwachman H: Water and electrolytes in cervical mucus from patients with cystic fibrosis. Fertil Steril **24**:512, 1973.

Kort BA, Cefalo RC, Baker VV: Fatal influenza A pneumonia in pregnancy. Am J Perinatol **3**:179, 1986.

Kotloff RM, FitzSimmons SC, Fiel SB: Fertility and pregnancy in patients with cystic fibrosis. Clin Chest Med **13**:623, 1992.

Kraan J, Koeter GH, Van Der Mark THW, et al: Dosage and time effects of inhaled budesonide on bronchial hyperactivity. Am Rev Respir Dis **137**:44, 1988.

Krantz ML, Edwards WL: The incidence of nonfatal aspiration in obstetric patients. Anesthesiology **30**:84, 1973.

Lehmann V, Fabel H: Lungenfunktionsuntersuchungen an Schwangeren. I. Lungenvolumina. Z Geburtshilfe Perinatol **177**:387, 1973a.

Lehmann V, Fabel H: Lungenfunktionsuntersuchungen an Schwangeren. II. Ventilation, Atemmechanik und Diffusionkapazitt. Z Geburtshilfe Perinatol **177**:397, 1973b.

Lemna WK, Feldman GL, Kerem B, et al: Mutation analysis for heterozygote detection and the prenatal diagnosis of cystic fibrosis. N Engl J Med **322**:291, 1990.

Lipworth BJ: Airway and systemic effects of inhaled corticosteroids in asthma: Dose response relationship. Pulm Pharmacol **9**:19, 1996.

Lowhagen O, Rak S: Modification of bronchial hyper-reactivity after treatment with sodium cromoglycate during pollen season. J Allergy Clin Immunol **75**:460, 1985.

Lyons HA, Antonio R: The sensitivity of the respiratory center in pregnancy and the administration of progesterone. Trans Assoc Am Physicians **72**:173, 1959.

Lyons HA, Huang CT: Therapeutic use of progesterone in alveolar hypoventilation associated with obesity. Am J Med **44**:881, 1968.

Mabie WC, Barton JR, Wasserstrum N, et al: Clinical observations and asthma in pregnancy. J Matern Fetal Med **1**:45, 1992.

MacDonald NE, Anas NG, Peterson RG, et al: Renal clearance of gentamicin in cystic fibrosis. J Pediatr **103**:985, 1983.

Machida GL: Influence of progesterone on arterial blood and CSF acid-base balance in women. J Appl Physiol **51**:1433, 1981.

Madinger NE, Greenspoon JS, Gray-Ellrodt A: Pneumonia during pregnancy: Has modern technology improved maternal and fetal outcome? Am J Obstet Gynecol **161**:657, 1989.

Margono F, Mroveh J, Garely A, et al: Resurgence of active tuberculosis among pregnant women. Obstet Gynecol **83**:911, 1994.

Maycock RL, Sullivan RD, Greening RR, et al: Sarcoidosis and pregnancy. JAMA **164**:158, 1957.

McAnulty JH, Metcalfe J, Ueland K: Cardiovascular disease. In Burrow GN, Ferris TF (eds): Medical Complications During Pregnancy, 3rd ed, Philadelphia, Saunders, 1988.

McGinty AP: The comparative effect of pregnancy and phrenic nerve interruption on the diaphragm and their relation to pulmonary tuberculosis. Am J Obstet Gynecol **35**:237, 1938.

McKinney WP, Volkert P, Kaufman J: Fatal swine influenza pneumonia during late pregnancy. Arch Intern Med **150**:213, 1990.

Mendelson CL: The aspiration of stomach contents into the lungs during obstetric anesthesia. Am J Obstet Gynecol **52**:191, 1946.

Milne JA: The respiratory response to pregnancy. Postgrad Med J **55**:318; 1979.

Minkoff H, deRegt R, Landesman S, Schwarz R: *Pneumocystis carinii* associated with acquired immunodeficiency syndrome in pregnancy: A report of three maternal deaths. Obstet Gynecol **67**:284, 1986.

MMWR: Initial therapy for tuberculosis in the era of multidrug resistance—recommendations of the advisory council for the elimination of tuberculosis. MMWR Morb Mortal Wkly Rep **42**:536, 1993.

Mobius WV: Abrung und Schwangerschaft. Munch Med Woschenschr **103**:1389, 1961.

Mullooly JP, Barker WH, Nolan TF Jr: Risk of acute respiratory disease among pregnant women during influenza A epidemics. Public Health Rep **101**:205, 1986.

National Asthma Education Program (NAEP): Guidelines for the Diagnosis and Management of Asthma, Expert Panel Report, August 1991. NIH Publication No. 91–3042.

National Asthma Education Program (NAEP): Management of Asthma During Pregnancy, Report of the Working Group on Asthma and Pregnancy, September 1993. NIH Publications No. 93–3279.

National Center for Health Statistics: National hospital discharge survey: Annual summary 1990. Vital Health Stat **13**:1, 1992.

National Council on Radiation Protection and Measurements: Medical Radiation Exposure of Pregnant and Potentially Pregnant Women. Washington, DC, 1977.

Nelson HS, Spector SL, Whitsett TL, et al: The bronchodilator response to inhalation of increasing doses of aerosolized albuterol. J Allergy Clin Immunol **72**:371, 1983.

Nitta AT, Milligan D: Management of four pregnant women with multidrug-resistant tuberculosis. Clin Infect Dis **28**:1298, 1999.

Nolten W, Rueckert P: Elevated free cortisol index in pregnancy: Possible regulatory mechanisms. Am J Obstet Gynecol **139**:492, 1981.

Novy MJ, Tyler JM, Shwachman H, et al: Cystic fibrosis and pregnancy. Report of a case with a study of pulmonary function and arterial blood gases. Obstet Gynecol **30**:530, 1967.

Olson GL: Cystic fibrosis in pregnancy. Sem Perinatol **21**:307, 1997.

Oxhorn H: The changing aspects of pneumonia complicating pregnancy. Am J Obstet Gynecol **70**:1057, 1955.

Paciorek J, Spencer N: An association between plasma progesterone and erythrocyte carbonic anhydrase I concentration in women. Clin Sci **58**:161, 1980.

Palmer J, Dillon-Baker C, Tecklin JS, et al: Pregnancy in patients with cystic fibrosis. Ann Intern Med **99**:596, 1983.

Pauwels R, Van Renterghem D, Van Der Straeten M, et al: The effect of theophylline and enprofylline on allergen-induced bronchoconstriction. J Allergy Clin Immunol **76**:583, 1985.

Perlow JH, Montgomery D, Morgan MA, et al: Severity of asthma and perinatal outcome. Am J Obstet Gynecol **167**:963, 1992.

Pernoll ML, Metcalfe J, Kovach PA, et al: Ventilation during rest and exercise in pregnancy and postpartum. Respir Physiol **25**:295, 1975.

Perutz MF: Hemoglobin structure and respiratory transport. Sci Am **239**:92, 1978.

Pickard RE: Varicella pneumonia in pregnancy. Am J Obstet Gynecol **101**:504, 1968.

Poort SR, Rosendaal FR, Reitsma PH, et al: A common genetic variation in the 3'-untranslated region of the prothrombin gene is associated with elevated plasma prothrombin levels and an increase in venous thrombosis. Blood **88**:3698, 1996.

Prowse CM, Gaensler EAL: Respiratory and acid base changes during pregnancy. Anesthesiology **26**:31, 1965.

Puranik BM, Kaore SB, Kurhade GA, et al: A longitudinal study of pulmonary function tests during pregnancy. Indian J Physiol Pharmacol **38**:129, 1994.

Rackow EC, Astiz M: Pathophysiology and treatment of septic shock. JAMA **266**:548, 1991.

Reisfield DR: Boeck's sarcoid and pregnancy. Am J Obstet Gynecol **75**:795, 1958.

Rendig EK Jr: The place of BCG vaccine in the management of infants born to tuberculosis mothers. N Engl J Med **281**:520, 1969.

Riley L: Pneumonia and tuberculosis in pregnancy. Infect Dis Clin North Am **11**:119, 1997.

Riordan JR, Rommens JM, Kerem B, et al: Identification of the cystic fibrosis gene: Cloning and characterization of complementary DNA. Science **245**:1066, 1989.

Robinson CA, Rose NC: Tuberculosis: Current implications and management in obstetrics. Obstet Gynecol Surv **51**:115, 1999.

Robinson GC, Cambion K: Hearing loss in infants of tuberculosis mothers treated with streptomycin during pregnancy. N Engl J Med 271:949, 1964.

Rodrigues J, Niederman MS: Pneumonia complicating pregnancy. Clin Chest Med 13:679, 1992.

Rommens JM, Iannuzzi MC, Kerem B, et al: Identification of the cystic fibrosis gene: Chromosome walking and jumping. Science 245:1059, 1989.

Rush D, Johnstone FD, King JC: Nutrition and pregnancy. In Burrows GN, Ferris TF (eds): Medical Complications During Pregnancy, 3rd ed, Philadelphia, Saunders, 1988.

Scadding JG: Sarcoidosis. London, Eyre and Spottiswoode, 1967.

Schatz M, Zeiger RS, Harden KM, et al: The safety of inhaled β-agonist bronchodilators during pregnancy. J Allergy Clin Immunol 82:686, 1988.

Schatz M, Zeiger RS, Hoffman C: Intrauterine growth is related to gestational pulmonary function in pregnant asthmatic women. Kaiser-Permanente Asthma and Pregnancy Study Group. Chest 98:389, 1990.

Schatz M, Zeiger R, Hoffman C, et al: Perinatal outcomes in the pregnancies of asthmatic women: A prospective controlled analysis. Am J Respir Crit Care Med 151:1170, 1995.

Schenker JG, Ben-Yoseph Y, Shapira E: Erythrocyte carbonic anhydrase B levels during pregnancy and use of oral contraceptives. Obstet Gynecol 39:237, 1972.

Schulman S, Rhedin AS, Lindmarker P, et al: A comparison of six weeks with six months of oral anticoagulant therapy after a first episode of venous thromboembolism. N Engl J Med 332:1661, 1995.

Sears MR, Taylor DR. Print CG, et al: Regular inhaled β-agonist treatment in bronchial asthma. Lancet 336:1391, 1990.

Shibutani K, Komatsu T, Kubal K, et al: Critical level of oxygen delivery in anesthetized man. Crit Care Med 11:640, 1983.

Shoemaker WC, Ayres S, Grenvik A, et al: Textbook of Critical Care, 2nd ed. Philadelphia, Saunders, 1989.

Siegel B, Siegel S: Pregnancy and delivery in a patient with CF of the pancreas: Report of a case. Obstet Gynecol 16:439, 1960.

Sims CD, Chamberlain GVP, de Swiet M: Lung function tests in bronchial asthma during and after pregnancy. Br J Obstet Gynaecol 88:434, 1976.

Skatrud JB, Dempsey JA, Kaiser DG: Ventilatory response to medroxyprogesterone acetate in normal subjects: Time course and mechanism. J Appl Physiol 44:939, 1978.

Smego RA, Asperilla MO: Use of acyclovir for varicella pneumonia during pregnancy. Obstet Gynecol 78:1112, 1991.

Soreide E, Bjornestad E, Steen PA: An audit of perioperative aspiration pneumonitis in gynaecological and obstetric patients. Acta Anaesth Scand 40:14, 1996.

Spino M, Chai RP, Isles AF, et al: Cloxacillin absorption and disposition in cystic fibrosis. J Pediatr 105:829, 1984.

Spitzer WO, Suissa S, Ernst P, et al: The use of β-agonists and the risk of death and near death from asthma. N Engl J Med 326:501, 1992.

Stenius-Aarniala BSM, Hedman J, Teramo KA: Acute asthma during pregnancy. Thorax 51:411, 1996.

Stratton P, Mofenson LM, Willoughby AD: Human immunodeficiency virus infection in pregnant women under care at AIDS clinical trials in the United States. Obstet Gynecol 79:364, 1992.

Sturridge F, deSwiet M, Letsky E: The use of low molecular weight heparin for thromboprophylaxis in pregnancy. Br J Obstet Gynaecol 101:69, 1994.

Sutton FD, Zwillich CW, Creagh CE, et al: Progesterone for outpatient treatment of Pickwickian syndrome. Ann Intern Med 83:476, 1975.

Svendsen UG, Frolund L, Madsen F, et al: A comparison of the effects of sodium cromoglycate and beclomethasone dipropionate on pulmonary function and bronchial hyper-reactivity in subjects with asthma. J Allergy Clin Immunol 80:68, 1987.

Tabachnik E, Zadik Z: Clinical and laboratory observations: Diurnal cortisol secretion during therapy with inhaled beclomethasone dipropionate in children with asthma. J Pediatr 118:294, 1991.

Tanser SJ, Hodson ME, Geddes DM: Case reports of death during pregnancy in patients with cystic fibrosis—Three out of four patients were colonized with Burkholderia cepacia. Respir Med 94:1004, 2000.

Templeton AA, Kelman GR: Maternal blood-gases. (Pao₂-PaO₂) physiological shunt and VD/VT in normal pregnancy. Br J Anaesth 48:1001, 1976.

Thomas BC, Stanhope R, Grant DB: Impaired growth in children with asthma during treatment with conventional doses of inhaled corticosteroids. Acta Paediatr 83:196, 1994.

Thomson KJ, Cohen ME: Studies on the circulation in normal pregnancy. II. Vital capacity observations in normal pregnant women. Surg Gynecol Obstet 66:591, 1938.

Tinkelman DG, Reed CE, Nelson HS, et al: Aerosol beclomethasone dipropionate compared with theophylline as primary treatment of chronic, mild to moderately severe asthma in children. Pediatrics 92:64, 1993.

Tomlinson MW, Caruthers TJ, Whitty JE, et al: Does delivery improve maternal condition in the respiratory-compromised gravida? Obstet Gynecol 91:108, 1998.

Twentyman OP, Finnerty JP, Holgate ST: The inhibitory effect of nebulized albuterol on the early and late asthmatic reactions and increase in airway responsiveness provoked by inhaled allergen in asthma. Am Rev Respir Dis 144:782, 1991.

Ueland K, Hansen JM: Maternal cardiovascular hemodynamics. II. Posture and uterine contractions. Am J Obstet Gynecol 103:1, 1969.

Uszynski M, Abildgaard U: Separation and characterization of two fibrinolytic inhibitors from human placenta. Thromb Diath Haemorr 25:580, 1971.

Vallejo JC, Starke JR: Tuberculosis and pregnancy. Clin Chest Med 13:693, 1992.

Van Rie A, Warren R, Richardson M, et al: Classification of drug-resistant tuberculosis in an epidemic era. Lancet 356:22, 2000.

Weinberger SE, Weiss ST, Cohen WR, et al: Pregnancy and the lung. Am Rev Respir Dis 121:559, 1980.

Wendel PJ, Ramin SM, Barnett-Hamm C, et al: Asthma treatment in pregnancy: A randomized controlled study. Am J Obstet Gynecol 175:150, 1996.

Wenzel SE: New approaches to anti-inflammatory therapy for asthma. Am J Med 104:287, 1998.

West JB: Pulmonary pathophysiology. Baltimore, Williams & Wilkins, 1978, p. 92.

Wilbrand U, Porath CH, Matthaes P, et al: Der einfluss der Ovarial-steroide auf die Funktion des Atemzentrums. Arch Gynäkol 191:507, 1959.

Yaffe SJ, Gerbracht LM, Mosovich LL, et al: Pharmacokinetics of methicillin in patients with cystic fibrosis. J Infect Dis 135:828, 1977.

Zaborny BA, Lukacsko P, Barinov-Colligaon I, et al: Inhaled corticosteroids in asthma: A dose-proportionality study with triamcinolone acetonide aerosol. J Clin Pharmacol 32:463, 1992.

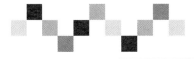

Chapter 47

MATERNAL HEMATOLOGIC DISORDERS

Sarah J. Kilpatrick, MD, PhD, and Russell K. Laros Jr., MD, MSc

ABNORMALITIES OF THE RED AND WHITE BLOOD CELLS

Anemia

Anemia is usually defined as a "hemoglobin (Hgb) value below the lower limits of normal not explained by the state of hydration." The normal Hgb level for the adult female is 14.0 ± 2.0 g/dL (Laros, 1986). This definition has physiologic validity, in that it is the amount of hemoglobin per unit volume of blood that determines the oxygen-carrying capacity of blood. Based on the aforementioned normal value, 20% to 60% of prenatal patients will be found to be anemic at some time during their pregnancy. The CDC defines anemia in pregnancy as an Hgb level below 11 g/dL in the first and third trimesters, and below 10.5 g/dL in the second trimester (Alper et al., 2000). Although this practice will decrease the number of gravidas found to be anemic, it does so by calling some mildly anemic patients normal and thus delaying additional hematologic evaluation. Such a decision is practical and appropriate, as long as the practitioner remembers to obtain a follow-up hemogram to be sure that the anemia has not progressed.

Clinical Presentation

Symptoms caused by anemia are those resulting from tissue hypoxia, the cardiovascular system's attempts to compensate for the anemia, or an underlying disease. Tissue hypoxia produces fatigue, lightheadedness, weakness, and exertional dyspnea. Cardiovascular compensation leads to a hyperdynamic circulation, with the attendant symptoms of palpitations and tachycardia. Clinical conditions commonly associated with anemia include multiple pregnancy, trophoblastic disease, chronic renal disease, arthritis, chronic liver disease, and chronic infection. In obstetric patients, however, anemia is most commonly discovered not because of symptoms but because a complete blood count (CBC) is obtained as part of routine laboratory evaluation either at the initial prenatal visit or at repeat screening at 24 to 28 weeks' gestation.

Additional information of value is the use of "tonics," a family history of anemia or splenectomy, and a history of gastrointestinal bleeding and melena, genitourinary bleeding, or, in individuals at risk for glucose-6-phosphate dehydrogenase (G6PD) deficiency, exposure to oxidant agents. Such agents include antimalarials, sulfonamides, sulfones, nitrofurans, various analgesics, fava beans, moth balls, para-aminosalicylic acid, probenecid, and isoniazid.

Use of the Complete Blood Count

Anemia is not a diagnosis but, like fever or edema, a sign. The key issue in the evaluation of anemia is to define the mechanism or disease process. Although a mild anemia caused by iron deficiency during pregnancy is of little consequence to either the mother or the fetus, a similarly mild anemia caused by carcinoma of the colon has grave implications. One must also keep in mind the genetic implications of many anemias such as the hemoglobinopathies and hereditary spherocytosis.

Table 47-1 presents a classification of anemia based on the pathophysiologic mechanism involved. Although a mechanistic classification of anemia provides an exhaustive catalog of diagnoses, it does not lend itself to a systematic investigation of an individual patient (Horowitz and Laros, 1979). Rather, when the patient is anemic one wants to know the following:

1. What is the morphology of the anemia?
2. What is the reticulocyte count?

Determining the answers to these questions allows one to make a first approximation of a specific diagnosis and to answer the following questions:

4. What is the mechanism of the anemia?
5. Is there an underlying disease?
6. What is appropriate treatment?

The CBC and the reticulocyte count provide the answers to the first three questions. These data allow a morphologic classification of the anemia and indicate whether the marrow is hyper- or hypoproliferative. Table 47-2 presents normal values for women. The Hgb is determined by converting the pigment to cyanmethemoglobin and quantitating the amount spectrophotometrically. The remainder of the values are obtained by flow cytometry with an electronic cell counter.

Based on the size of the red blood cells (RBCs), anemia can be classified as microcytic, normocytic, or macrocytic. The appearance of the RBCs may also provide a clue to the mechanism of the anemia. For example, hypochromic microcytic cells associated with a low reticulocyte count suggest iron deficiency, thalassemia trait, sideroblastic anemia, or lead poisoning. Oval macrocytes combined with a low reticulocyte count and hypersegmented polymorphonuclear leukocytes suggest megaloblastic

TABLE 47-1. ANEMIA CLASSIFIED BY PATHOPHYSIOLOGIC MECHANISM

I. Dilutional (expansion of the plasma volume)
  A. Pregnancy
  B. Hyperglobulinemia
  C. Massive splenomegaly
II. Decreased RBC production
  A. Bone marrow failure
    1. Decreased building blocks or stimulation
      a. Iron, protein
      b. Chronic infection, chronic renal disease
    2. Decreased erythron
      a. Hypoplasia (hereditary, drugs, radiation, toxins)
      b. Marrow replacement (tumor, fibrosis, infection)
  B. Ineffective production
    1. Megaloblastic (vitamin B_{12} and folate deficiency, myelodysplasia, erythroleukemia)
    2. Normoblastic (refractory anemia, thalassemia)
III. Increased RBC loss
  A. Acute hemorrhage
  B. Hemolysis
    1. Intrinsic RBC disorders
      a. Hereditary
        (1) Hemoglobinopathies
        (2) RBC enzyme deficiency
        (3) Membrane defects
        (4) Porphyrias
      b. Acquired
        (1) Paroxysmal nocturnal hemoglobinuria
        (2) Lead poisoning
    2. Extrinsic RBC disorders
      a. Immune
      b. Mechanical
      c. Infection
      d. Chemical agents
      e. Burns
      f. Hypersplenism
      g. Liver disease

RBC, red blood cell.

anemia (vitamin B_{12} or folate deficiency). Oval microcytes and an elevated reticulocyte count are characteristic of hereditary spherocytosis. Various poikilocytes, such as sickle cells, acanthocytes, target cells, and schistocytes, suggest sickle cell disease, acanthocytosis, hemoglobin C disease, and mechanical RBC destruction, respectively.

The peripheral blood smear also allows evaluation of the white blood cells (WBCs). In most cases of leukemia, abnormal granulocytes or lymphocytes appear. The presence of nucleated RBCs in association with marked poikilocytosis suggests erythroleukemia, myeloid metaplasia, or marrow infiltration with solid tumor or granulomatous infection.

Additional Laboratory Studies

Although the CBC is an excellent first step in the approximate diagnosis of anemia, additional studies are usually necessary to confirm the diagnosis. Table 47-3 lists laboratory studies frequently used in the evaluation of an anemic patient.

Serum Hgb and serum haptoglobin levels are useful in defining intravascular hemolysis. When serum haptoglobin is absent or at a low level in conjunction with elevated serum Hgb,

the presence of intravascular hemolysis is established. Further studies are necessary to rule in or rule out specific causes of intravascular hemolysis, such as severe autoimmune hemolytic anemia (direct Coombs test), paroxysmal nocturnal hemoglobinuria (osmotic fragility), and hemoglobinopathies such as sickle cell disease and thalassemia major (Hgb electrophoresis).

The total bilirubin is elevated modestly in hemolytic anemia (rarely in excess of 4 mg/dL). The increase is due predominantly to an increase in the indirect fraction. However, significant hemolysis can occur without an elevation in the bilirubin. Thus, the bilirubin level is helpful only when it is elevated.

The direct Coombs test uses antihuman globulin to detect globulins attached to the surface of RBCs. A positive test indicates an immune cause for a hemolytic anemia. In such cases, it is important to search for underlying causes for autoimmunity, such as connective tissue disease, lymphoma, carcinoma, and sarcoidosis. The diagnosis and management of G6PD and of the various hemoglobinopathies are discussed later in this chapter (see under Enzymopathies: G6PD Deficiency and Others, and under Hemoglobinopathies).

The free erythrocyte protoporphyrin (FEP) (Schifman et al., 1987), plasma iron, plasma total iron-binding capacity (Ho et al., 1987), and serum ferritin level (Puolakka et al., 1980; Haram et al., 2001) are useful in establishing a diagnosis of iron deficiency. Serum ferritin correlates closely with body iron stores, and many investigators support the utilization of serum ferritin as the best single test in patients with anemia to make a diagnosis of iron deficiency anemia (Alper et al., 2000; Haram et al., 2001). A ferritin level of 12 ng/dL or lower is consistent with iron deficiency anemia. Plasma iron and serum ferritin levels are both increased following the ingestion of iron (Taylor et al., 1982; Seligman et al., 1983). Thus, iron therapy must be discontinued for 24 to 48 hours before these studies are carried out. In iron deficiency, the FEP increases approximately fivefold. Iron is transported in the plasma bound to transferrin. In the iron-deficient state, the plasma iron decreases, the iron-binding capacity increases, and the percent saturation decreases. In contrast, with chronic infection, both the plasma iron and the iron-binding capacity are decreased while the percent saturation remains normal. It is still debatable which

TABLE 47-2. NORMAL VALUES FOR RED BLOOD CELLS

Erythroid values	
Hemoglobin (Hgb)	12–16 g/dL
Hematocrit (Hct)	36–41 ml/dL
Red blood cell (RBC) count	$4.0–5.2 \times 10^{12}$/liter
Erythroid indices	
Mean corpuscular volume (MCV)	80–100 μm^3
Mean corpuscular hemoglobin concentration (MCHC)	31–36 g/dL
Red blood cell morphology	
Anisocytosis	Variation in cell size
Poikilocytosis	Variation in cell shape
Polychromatophilia	Amount of "blueness"
Hypochromia	Amount of central pallor
Platelet estimate	5–10 platelets per oil immersion field
Reticulocyte count	$48–152 \times 10^9$/liter
White blood cell (WBC) count	$5–14 \times 10^9$/liter

<table>
<tr><td colspan="2">■ **TABLE 47-3.** LABORATORY STUDIES USEFUL IN EVALUATION OF ANEMIA</td></tr>
</table>

Study	Normal Value
Serum hemoglobin (Hgb)	<1.0 mg/dL
Serum haptoglobin	30–200 mg/dL
Total bilirubin	0.1–1.2 mg/dL
Direct Coombs test	Negative
G6PD	
Electrophoresis	B+
	(A+, A–, B–, 150 others are abnormal)
Quantitative study	4–8 units/g of Hgb
Hemoglobin electrophoresis	>98% A
	<3.5% A_2
	<2% F
RBC enzymes	Multiple types; pyruvate kinase most common
Osmotic fragility	Preincubation: 0.40%–0.46% NaCl
	Postincubation: 0.48%–0.60% NaCl
Serum ferritin	>10 μg/liter
Free erythrocyte protoporphyrin (FEP)	<3.0 μg/g
Plasma iron	40–175 μg/dL
Plasma total iron-binding capacity	216–400 μg/dL
Transferrin saturation	16–60%
Stool guaiac	Negative
Folate level	
Serum	6–12 μg/liter
RBC	165–760 ng/liter
Serum B_{12}	190–950 ng/liter
Anti-intrinsic factor antibody (AIF)	Negative
Bone marrow	Normal distribution of erythroid and myeloid precursors

RBC, red blood cell.

of the aforementioned studies is the most sensitive and specific for making the diagnosis of iron deficiency.

Serum folate, RBC folate, and serum vitamin B_{12} levels are useful in defining the cause of macrocytic anemia. Because the RBC folate more accurately reflects the body's folate stores, many laboratories no longer offer the serum folate determination. The presence of serum intrinsic factor antibodies is specific for pernicious anemia. However, since they are absent in approximately 40% of cases, the absence of these antibodies does not rule out a diagnosis of pernicious anemia.

Examination of the bone marrow by aspiration or biopsy can add much useful information. In addition to providing a ratio of myeloid to erythroid production (normally, approximately 3:1), it provides a measure of iron stores, allows a differential count of myeloid and erythroid precursors, provides evidence of infiltration with neoplasm, and allows histologic and bacteriologic confirmation of infection.

Normal Hematologic Events Associated with Pregnancy

Blood Volume Changes

During pregnancy, there is normally a 36% increase in the blood volume, the maximum being reached at 34 weeks' gestation (Peck and Arias, 1979). The plasma volume increases by 47%, whereas the RBC mass increases only by 17%. The latter reaches its maximum at term. As shown in Figure 47-1, there is relative hemodilution throughout pregnancy, and this reaches its maximum between 28 and 34 weeks. Although this dilutional effect lowers the Hgb, hematocrit (Hct), and RBC count, it causes no change in the mean corpuscular volume or in the mean corpuscular Hgb concentration. Thus, serial evaluation of these two indices is useful in differentiating dilutional anemia from progressive iron-deficiency anemia during pregnancy. In the former, the indices do not change; in the latter, they decrease progressively.

Iron Kinetics

The classic study by Scott and Pritchard (1967) shows that iron stores in healthy women are marginal at best. These authors evaluated iron stores found in the bone marrow of healthy white college students who had never been pregnant and had never donated blood. Approximately two thirds had minimal iron stores. In another study, Pritchard and colleagues (1969) demonstrated that almost 50% of healthy primigravidas had minimal iron stores in the marrow during the first trimester.

The major reason for poor iron stores is thought to be menstrual loss. Monsen and colleagues' data (1967) indicate that the usual menstrual loss is 25 to 30 mL of whole blood. This is equivalent to 12 to 15 mg of elemental iron, since each milliliter of blood contains 0.5 mg of iron. To meet the iron loss for menses

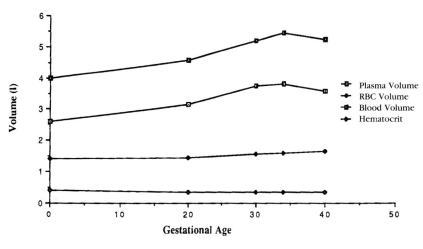

FIGURE 47-1 ■ Hematologic changes during pregnancy. RBC, red blood cell. (Redrawn from Peck TM, Arias F: Hematologic changes associated with pregnancy. Clin Obstet **22**:785, 1979.)

alone, a woman must absorb 1.5 to 2.0 mg of elemental iron from her diet each day. Because only 10% of dietary iron is usually absorbed, and the average diet contains only 6 mg/1000 kilocalories, a woman's iron balance is precarious at best.

Pregnancy presents substantial demands on iron balance above and beyond what is saved by 9 months of amenorrhea (Pritchard et al., 1969). Table 47-4 lists the iron requirements for pregnancy. If available iron stores are insufficient to meet the demands of pregnancy, iron-deficient erythropoiesis results. Fenton and colleagues (1977) used serum ferritin level to evaluate iron stores in pregnant women and found significantly higher ferritin levels in those who were receiving iron supplementation than in those who were not.

Thus, most young women enter their first pregnancy with marginal iron stores. Pregnancy places a large demand on iron balance that cannot be met with the usual diet. In the absence of supplementation, iron deficiency develops. Supplementation with 60 mg of elemental iron per day during the second and third trimesters meets the daily requirement. The Institute of Medicine (1993) has recommended that supplementation be offered only to women whose serum ferritin level is less than 20 μg/liter. Although this is a valid recommendation scientifically, the high cost of the screening study limits its applicability. The usual sequence of events in regard to iron deficiency is an absence of iron in the marrow followed by the development of abnormal plasma iron studies (transferrin, ferritin, or free RBC protoporphyrin). The RBCs first become microcytic, then hypochromic. Finally, anemia develops.

Folate

Folic acid, a water-soluble vitamin, is generally widely available in the diet. Dietary folates are, in fact, a family of compounds and appear as polyglutamates. In humans, the only source of folate is the diet, and absorption occurs primarily in the proximal jejunum. Before folate can be absorbed, it must be reduced to the monoglutamate form (Herbert et al., 1975). Pancreatic conjugases within the intestine are responsible for this process. The activity of conjugase is decreased by anticonvulsants, oral contraceptives, alcohol, and sulfa drugs (Shojania and Hornady, 1973). Thus, in addition to an absolute diminution in the dietary intake, the combination of increased need (as in multiple pregnancy and hemolytic anemia) and decreased absorption can lead to folate deficiency (Pritchard et al., 1970; Iyengar, 1975; Johan and Magnus, 1981).

TABLE 47-4. IRON REQUIREMENTS FOR PREGNANCY

Required for	Average (mg)	Range (mg)
External iron loss	170	150–200
Expansion of red blood cell mass	450	200–600
Fetal iron	270	200–370
Iron in placenta and cord	90	30–170
Blood loss at delivery	150	90–310
Total requirement	980	580–1340
Requirement less red blood cell expansion	840	440–1050

The folate requirement of 50 μg per day for a nonpregnant woman increases to 300 to 500 μg per day during pregnancy (Kitay, 1969; Pritchard et al., 1969). Because adequate folate intake before and during the first weeks of pregnancy reduces the occurrence of neural tube defects, all women considering becoming pregnant should consume 400 μg of folate per day (Centers for Disease Control [CDC], 1991). A recent study estimated that a daily supplement of 400 μg per day would reduce the risk of neural tube defects by 36%, and that a daily supplement of 5 mg would reduce the risk by 85% (Wald and colleagues, 2001). If a previous pregnancy has been complicated by a neural tube defect, the mother's intake of folate should be 4 mg per day in the next pregnancy, starting at least 4 weeks before conception and continuing through the first 3 months of pregnancy (CDC, 1991; American College of Obstetricians and Gynecologists, 1993). When folate depletion occurs, the usual sequence of events is a decreased serum folate, hypersegmentation of polymorphonuclear leukocytes, a decrease in RBC folate, the appearance of ovalocytes in the blood, development of an abnormal marrow, and finally anemia (Herbert et al., 1975).

Vitamin B$_{12}$

Vitamin B$_{12}$, also abundantly available in the diet, is bound to animal protein. Absorption requires hydrochloric acid and pepsin to free the cobalamin molecule from protein. Intrinsic factor is also essential for absorption. Following absorption, transport occurs by binding to transcobalamin II. Most of the vitamin B$_{12}$ is stored in the liver, and individuals generally have a 2- to 3-year store available (Ho et al., 1987).

Morphologic Classification of Anemia

As discussed, a CBC allows placement of a given case of anemia into one of three major groups based on size and Hgb content of the RBCs. The classification is augmented by the reticulocyte count, which adds information about bone marrow activity.

Microcytic Anemia

The microcytic anemias are characterized by abnormal Hgb synthesis with normal RBC production. A logical progression of diagnostic steps requires first that iron-deficiency anemia be ruled out. When iron-deficiency anemia is diagnosed rather than ruled out, however, it is then essential to rule out gastrointestinal bleeding as the cause for the iron deficit. This is accomplished by testing the stool for the presence of occult blood with guaiac or some other equally sensitive reagent. When a microcytic anemia is not due to iron deficiency, one must then seek another cause, such as hemoglobinopathy, chronic infection, or the various sideroblastic anemias. For this purpose, the following tests are indicated:

Hgb electrophoresis
Plasma iron and total plasma iron-binding capacity
FEP
Deoxyribonucleic acid (DNA) probing for a-genes
Bone marrow examination

Anemia of chronic disorders is associated with decreased plasma iron and total plasma iron-binding capacity or elevated

FEP. If the plasma iron and total plasma iron-binding capacity are normal or increased and FEP is normal, one usually is dealing with thalassemia or a sideroblastic anemia. Hemoglobin electrophoresis and DNA probes are used to define the thalassemias, and ring sideroblasts are present in the bone marrow of individuals with hereditary or acquired sideroblastic anemia.

Normocytic Anemia

Evaluation of normocytic anemia is the most difficult because of the diverse nature of this type of anemia. The reticulocyte count varies according to whether RBC production is increased, normal, or decreased. If erythropoiesis is increased, one must then differentiate between hemorrhage and an increased rate of destruction. The blood smear may reveal a type of RBC that is virtually diagnostic. Fragmented cells are seen in microangiopathic hemolysis, as in *HELLP syndrome* [hemolysis, elevated liver enzymes, low platelets] and thrombotic thrombocytopenic purpura; and in association with prosthetic heart valves. Other types of poikilocytes identified include sickle cells, target cells, stomatocytes, ovalocytes, spherocytes, elliptocytes, and acanthocytes.

The Coombs test differentiates *immune* from *nonimmune* causes of hemolysis. Immune hemolysis is related to alloantibodies, drug-induced antibodies, and autoantibodies. Nonimmune causes of hemolysis include various hemoglobinopathies, hereditary disorders of the RBC membrane (spherocytosis and elliptocytosis), hereditary deficiency of an RBC enzyme, and the porphyrias. Acquired, nonimmune hemolysis is due either to paroxysmal nocturnal hemoglobinuria or to lead poisoning.

Bone marrow examination is essential for the evaluation of patients with hypoproliferative anemias with normal iron studies. If erythropoiesis is megaloblastic, folate or vitamin B_{12} deficiency is a likely cause. If it is sideroblastic, both acquired and hereditary forms of sideroblastic anemia must be considered.

Finally, if erythropoiesis is normoblastic, etiologic mechanisms fall into two major categories. The first category has myeloid to erythroid production ratios greater than 4:1 and includes aplasia, infiltration, effects of chronic diseases, and endocrine disorders, such as hypothyroidism and hypopituitarism. In the second category, there is ineffective erythropoiesis, usually associated with a myeloid to erythroid production ratio less than 2:1.

Macrocytic Anemia

Macrocytic anemia is associated with either (1) an increased rate of RBC production and release of less than fully mature RBCs or (2) disorders of impaired DNA synthesis. Early use of a bone marrow examination is helpful in pointing the investigation in the correct direction. When maturation is megaloblastic, abnormal serum vitamin B_{12} and RBC folate levels allow a diagnosis of vitamin B_{12} or folate deficiency. If a diagnosis of folate deficiency is confirmed, the various causes of decreased deconjugation of the polyglutamate and malabsorption must be considered. If anti–intrinsic factor antibodies are present, a diagnosis of *pernicious anemia* is ensured. If anti–intrinsic factor antibodies are absent, a Schilling test is required to differentiate between pernicious anemia and a small bowel malabsorption syndrome.

Anemia and Perinatal Morbidity and Mortality

Effects of Anemia

Although it has been traditionally taught that significant maternal anemia is associated with suboptimal fetal outcome, data supporting this concept are scarce. Most recent studies, including a meta-analysis, reported a significant relationship between women with anemia early in pregnancy and preterm delivery but no significant association with neonates small for gestational age (Scanlon et al., 2000; Xiong et al., 2000; Bondevik et al., 2001). Earlier studies reporting maternal anemia and poor fetal outcome produced conflicting data (Klebanoff et al., 1991; Lu et al., 1991; Scholl et al., 1992; Goldenberg et al., 1996). Elevated Hgb early in pregnancy has also been associated with poor perinatal outcome including stillbirth and neonates small for gestational age (Sagen, 1984; Stephansson et al., 2000). In a case-control study, women with stillbirths had a significantly higher incidence of Hgb above 14.5 than did control women with no stillbirth (Stephansson et al., 2000). Although the mechanism for this association is unknown, the authors hypothesized that high Hgb may be a marker for lack of plasma-volume expansion and hence reduced blood flow to the intervillous space, since high Hgb has also been associated with low-birth-weight neonates. An alternate hypothesis was offered by Sagen (1984), who believed that these data were evidence of chronic hypoxia. Studies in sheep show that fetal oxygen consumption is maintained until the maternal Hct concentration is reduced by more than 50% (Paulone et al., 1987). Furthermore, there are several anecdotal reports in which fetal distress, noted in a fetal heart-rate tracing, was completely relieved by correction of maternal anemia. Thus, although profound maternal anemia can have adverse effects on the fetus, the margin of safety appears to be large. In Africa, Asia, and Latin America, the relative risk of maternal mortality with severe anemia (hemoglobin below 4.7 mg/liter) was significantly elevated at 3.5 (Brabin et al., 2001). It may be that in industrial countries the prevalence of severe anemia is too low to see consistent associations with poor fetal or maternal outcomes.

Effects of Specific Nutritional Defects

Fortunately, the fetal compartment preferentially obtains iron (Galbraith et al., 1980; Okuyama et al., 1985), folate, and vitamin B_{12} (Johan and Magnus, 1981) from and at the expense of the mother. In several studies, the umbilical cord blood ferritin levels of infants whose mothers were iron-deficient were reduced below those of infants whose mothers were not iron-deficient (Fenton et al., 1977; Singla et al., 1996). Yet infants whose ferritin levels were low were not anemic and had normal iron kinetics, and their serum ferritin values were not in the iron-deficient range. In a study of newborns of women with severe folate deficiency, Pritchard and colleagues (1969) found normal neonatal levels of folate.

Genetic Implications

Many of the hemolytic anemias are inherited as either autosomal-dominant or -recessive traits. Thus, once the correct diagnosis has been made, the genetic implications should be thoroughly discussed with the patient and her partner. When appropriate, the discussion should include antenatal diagnosis.

Specific Anemias

Space does not allow a detailed discussion of the diagnosis and treatment of literally hundreds of different anemias. Instead, we present a scheme of diagnostic studies useful in evaluating any anemia and limit discussion of specific anemias to a few that are commonly seen during the course of pregnancy.

Iron-Deficiency Anemia

Iron deficiency is among the most common causes of anemia in pregnant women and may be as prevalent as 47% (Swensen et al., 2001; Jaime-Perez and Gomez-Almaguer, 2002). Clinical symptoms include easy fatigue, lethargy, and headache. *Pica*, which may involve the ingestion of clay, dirt, ice, or starch, is a classic manifestation of iron deficiency and was significantly associated in one study with lower maternal hemoglobin but not with adverse pregnancy outcomes (Rainville, 2001). Clinical findings include pallor, glossitis, and cheilitis. *Koilonychia* has been associated with iron-deficiency anemia but is a rare finding.

The laboratory characteristics of iron-deficiency anemia are a microcytic, hypochromic anemia with evidence of depleted iron stores, low plasma iron, high total iron-binding capacity, low serum ferritin, and/or elevated FEP. If a bone marrow examination is done, stainable iron is markedly depleted or absent.

Although it is difficult to show a consistent association between poor perinatal outcome and maternal anemia in the United States; and iron supplementation has not been shown to alter perinatal outcome, the CDC strongly recommends screening and treatment of iron-deficiency anemia in pregnancy (CDC, 1998; Haram et al., 2001; Sloan et al., 2002). The rationale is that treatment maintains maternal iron stores and may be beneficial for neonatal iron stores (Haram et al., 2001). Iron supplementation is probably indicated only in women with anemia, since a randomized trial of routine versus indicated (hemoglobin below 10 mg/liter) treatment with iron revealed no difference in perinatal outcome or long-term outcome, including subsequent pregnancies (Hemminki and Merilainen, 1995).

The specific treatment is oral iron, most commonly ferrous sulfate, 320 mg one to three times daily. Other iron preparations are more expensive and do not offer any advantage over ferrous sulfate if equal amounts of elemental iron are given. Reticulocytosis should be observed after 7 to 10 days of therapy, and the Hgb can rise by as much as 1 g per week in severely anemic individuals. Absorption from the gastrointestinal tract can be enhanced by administration of 500 mg of ascorbic acid with each dose of iron. Gastrointestinal symptoms associated with iron therapy include nausea, vomiting, abdominal cramps, diarrhea, and constipation. These symptoms correspond to the dose of elemental iron ingested; if symptoms are troublesome, the dose of iron should be reduced. Ferrous sulfate syrup is an effective way of tailoring the dose to the patient's tolerance.

Once the anemia has resolved, the patient should continue to receive iron therapy for an additional 6 months to replace iron stores. Parenteral administration of iron dextran is rarely indicated and should be reserved for patients with a malabsorption syndrome or those who absolutely will not take oral iron and are significantly anemic (Hgb below 8.5 g/dL) (Hamstra et al., 1980). In a recent study, oral iron was compared to intravenous iron sucrose in a randomized trial of pregnant women with hemoglobin of 8 to 10 g/dL (Bayoumeu et al., 2002). The increase in hemoglobin of 2 g/dL was the same in both groups at day 30. Because severe anaphylaxis can occur, a test dose should be administered first. In the absence of any reaction, the full dose can be administered at a maximum rate of 1 mL per minute. The required dose of iron dextran to correct anemia and replenish stores can be calculated as

$$\text{iron dextran (mL)} = (14 - \text{patient's Hgb})$$

$$\times \ (\text{wt in kg}) \times (0.0476) \ + \ \frac{\text{wt in kg}}{5} \ \text{[maximum 14]}$$

Subcutaneous erythropoietin with or without oral iron therapy or intravenous iron sucrose has been used successfully to treat severe iron-deficiency anemia in pregnancy with no significant risks to the mother (Vora and Gruslin, 1998; Breymann et al., 2001; Sifakis et al., 2001). In one study in women who had failed oral iron therapy and had hemoglobin below 8.5 g/dL, the addition of erythropoietin to oral iron was associated with normalization of hemoglobin in 2 weeks in 73% of the women (Sifakis et al, 2001).

Megaloblastic Anemia

Megaloblastic anemia is the second most common nutritional anemia seen during pregnancy. Most commonly, folate deficiency is the cause, but a deficiency in vitamin B_{12} must also be considered. Patients with folate deficiency present with the typical symptoms of anemia plus roughness of the skin and glossitis. The CBC reveals a macrocytic, normochromic (or normocytic, normochromic) anemia with hypersegmentation of the polymorphonuclear leukocytes. The reticulocyte count is normal or low, and the WBC and platelet counts are frequently decreased. Bone marrow examination is not usually necessary for diagnosis, but if it is done, megaloblastic erythropoiesis is noted. The RBC folate level is decreased to below 165 µg/dL (serum folate below 6 mg/L), and the vitamin B_{12} level is normal.

Treatment consists of oral folic acid administered in a dose of 1 mg daily. Parenteral folic acid may be indicated in individuals with malabsorption. A reticulocyte response should be seen in 48 to 72 hours, and the platelet count normalizes within a few days. The neutrophils normalize after 1 to 2 weeks.

In addition to anemia, individuals with vitamin B_{12} deficiency may also manifest neurologic defects relating to damage to the posterior columns of the spinal cord. It is critical that individuals with vitamin B_{12} deficiency not be treated with folic acid alone. Such treatment may well improve the anemia but has absolutely no salutary effect on the neuropathy and, in fact, may make it worse. As with folate deficiency, vitamin B_{12} deficiency is associated with dietary deficiency, an increased requirement, or both. Except in strict vegetarians who avoid all animal products, dietary deficiency is rare.

The most common causes of vitamin B_{12} deficiency are inadequate production of intrinsic factor (pernicious anemia), inadequate production of intrinsic factor after gastrectomy, and the presence of a malabsorption syndrome. The morphologic features of B$_{12}$ deficiency are similar to those of folate deficiency. In this instance, the serum vitamin B$_{12}$ level is low and the folate level is normal. Because ineffective erythropoiesis is a prominent feature, evidence of low-grade hemolysis may be present (increased bilirubin and decreased haptoglobin). The measurement of anti–intrinsic factor antibodies are useful.

Treatment consists of 100 μg of B$_{12}$ per day for the 1st week. The dose can then be decreased to reach a total of 2000 μg by 6 weeks, followed by monthly administration for life in cases of pernicious anemia. Again, a prompt reticulocyte response is anticipated after 3 to 5 days of therapy.

Hereditary Spherocytosis and Elliptocytosis

Spherocytosis is the most common form of inherited hemolytic anemia. The inheritance is as an autosomal-dominant trait with variable penetrance. The exact defect in the RBC leading to the anemia is unknown but is most likely a structural defect in the cell wall. The classic characteristic is an increased RBC osmotic fragility. The prevalence of the gene is 2.2×10^{-4}, which should account for more than 650 pregnancies annually in women with spherocytosis. A hemolytic crisis can be precipitated by many conditions, such as infection, trauma, and pregnancy itself (Moore et al., 1976). A relationship between increased hemolysis and increased maternal blood volume and splenic blood flow has been proposed. An alternative suggestion is an increased osmotic fragility during the third trimester of pregnancy (Magid et al., 1982).

The diagnosis is suspected on the basis of family history and findings in the CBC and reticulocyte count that suggest a hyperproliferative anemia. Confirmation is obtained with the *osmotic fragility test*. Prenatal care of women with hereditary spherocytosis who have not had a splenectomy requires vigilance for hemolytic crisis and folate supplementation to ensure adequate marrow function (Maberry et al., 1992). A hemolytic crisis can be treated conservatively with replacement transfusions or with splenectomy. Because splenectomy is mechanically difficult to accomplish during the third trimester of pregnancy, it is sometimes preceded by delivery. In the absence of severe, untreated anemia, spherocytosis does not contribute to perinatal morbidity or mortality.

Hereditary elliptocytosis, also inherited as an autosomal-dominant trait, is a milder hemolytic state also caused by a structural defect in the RBC wall. The signs and symptoms are similar to those of spherocytosis but are not as severe. Most cases detected during pregnancy have been successfully treated with supportive therapy alone (Breckenridge and Riggs, 1968).

Autoimmune Hemolytic Anemia

There are two major types of antibodies responsible for autoimmune hemolytic anemia: *warm-reactive* and *cold-reactive*. Most warm-reactive antibodies are of the immunoglobulin G (IgG) class and are directed against some component of the Rh system on the surface of the RBC. In contrast, most cold-reactive antibodies are IgM; they are usually specific for anti-I or anti-i. Autoimmune hemolytic anemia with warm-reactive antibodies is frequently seen in association with various hematologic malignancies (chronic lymphocytic leukemia, lymphoma), lupus erythematosus, viral infections, and drug ingestion. Penicillin, stibophen, and α-methyldopa have all been reported to cause autoimmune hemolytic anemia. Cold-reacting antibodies can be seen in association with mycoplasmal infections, infectious mononucleosis, and lymphoreticular neoplasms.

Unfortunately, in a large number of cases, no specific inciting event can be identified (Sacks et al., 1981). Diagnosis is suspected when a hyperproliferative, macrocytic anemia is identified. The stained smear of the peripheral blood often reveals microcytes, polychromatophilia, poikilocytosis, and the presence of normoblasts. Leukocytosis is frequently seen and is a result of marrow hyperactivity. The critical study to confirm the diagnosis is a positive direct Coombs test.

Treatment of autoimmune hemolytic anemia is directed toward both the hemolytic process and the underlying disease. Blood transfusion, corticosteroid therapy, immunosuppression, and splenectomy are the most frequently used measures. In cases with warm-reactive antibodies, corticosteroid should be tried initially, because approximately 80% of patients will respond dramatically. Splenectomy is an effective form of treatment in approximately 60% of patients with warm-reactive antibodies. If the patient is refractory to both corticosteroid therapy and splenectomy, a trial of immunosuppression is warranted. The treatment of cold-reactive antibodies depends on the severity of the hemolytic process. In patients with mild anemia, avoidance of cold temperatures is all that is required. Corticosteroid therapy and splenectomy are usually not effective if the majority of RBC breakdown occurs intravascularly. In patients with severe anemia, a trial of immunosuppression or plasmapheresis should be considered.

Enzymopathies: G6PD Deficiency and Others

More than 20 different hereditary RBC enzyme defects have been described, most with an associated hemolytic anemia. Of these, only G6PD deficiency occurs with more than occasional frequency. The genetic locus controlling G6PD synthesis is on the X chromosome, and males with an abnormal gene may suffer hemolysis, especially if they are exposed to oxidant drugs that stress the pentose phosphate pathway of the erythrocyte. Female heterozygotes are generally clinically unaffected by similar exposure. The G6PD activity of the RBCs in heterozygous females is usually intermediate between activity in hemizygous males and that in normal subjects. Some female carriers, however, have normal G6PD activity, whereas others have activity that falls within the range in affected males. It has been proposed that this is consistent with the *Lyon hypothesis*—that is, one of the two X chromosomes of every female cell is randomly inactivated in early embryonic life and continues to be inactive throughout all cell divisions (Beutler, 1991). Thus, a few heterozygous women may be severely deficient in G6PD activity, but most will have sufficient activity to withstand added stress on this critical metabolic pathway in erythrocytes.

The ethnic groups in which variants of the deficiency occur with greatest frequency are blacks, Mediterranean peoples, Sephardic and Asiatic Jews, and selected Asian populations. Of African American males in the United States, 12% are reported to be deficient in G6PD activity. Most affected individuals are hematologically normal unless they have been exposed to certain drugs or chemicals or have experienced metabolic disturbances or infections that precipitate an acute hemolytic episode. Most affected African Americans carry a variant with these properties. Their hemolytic episodes are relatively mild. Greeks, Sardinians, and Sephardic Jews are more likely to carry G6PD Mediterranean, in which hemolysis is characteristically more severe, and favism (hemolysis induced by ingestion of fava beans) occurs. G6PD-deficient African American populations have not been reported to experience favism.

It is relatively unusual for a pregnant woman to experience severe difficulty because of G6PD deficiency. However, Silverstein and associates (1974) reported Hct levels below 30% in 62% of 180 G6PD-deficient women. Prudence would argue against exposure of a known carrier to precipitants of hemolysis. Sulfonamides, sulfones, some antimalarials, nitrofurans, naphthalene, probenecid, para-aminosalicylic acid–isoniazid, and nalidixic acid are among the medications and commonly occurring environmental chemicals known to precipitate RBC destruction.

One report suggested an increased incidence of low-birthweight infants born to G6PD-deficient mothers, but no correction for the effects of anemia or urinary tract infection was made (Perkins, 1976). Affected male infants born of carrier females have a higher incidence of neonatal hyperbilirubinemia—sometimes severe—than do normal infants, and careful observation of those at risk is strongly advised. The incidence of severe jaundice in G6PD-deficient newborn males is approximately 5%, rising to 50% if there is a history of an icteric sibling. Occasionally, hemolysis has been reported in breast-fed infants whose mothers have eaten fava beans or have been exposed to an oxidant. The neonatal manifestations of G6PD deficiency and other enzymopathies have been reviewed by Matthay and Mentzer (1981).

If a hemolytic episode occurs during pregnancy because of G6PD deficiency in a female heterozygote (or the very rare homozygote), management should include prompt discontinuation of any medication or other agent that may be responsible, treatment of any intercurrent illness, and if clinically indicated, transfusion support. In patients with the variant common in African Americans, the G6PD activity of young RBCs is, even in the male hemizygote, much higher than in RBCs that have circulated for weeks and months. Old cells may be totally devoid of activity. Hence, the hemolytic episode recognized early is generally relatively mild and can be limited to the oldest population of circulating RBCs if the inciting agent is eliminated.

Aplastic and Hypoplastic Anemia

Aplastic anemia is characterized by a reduction in the number of circulating RBCs, neutrophils, and platelets and by the presence of a hypocellular bone marrow. Three mechanisms have been postulated to explain the development of aplastic anemia: (1) insufficient stem cells resulting from an intrinsic defect or a reduction in number after exposure to a noxious agent, (2) presence of a suppressor substance that inhibits the maturation of the myeloid precursors, and (3) development of an autoimmune reaction that causes death of the stem cells.

Agents such as benzene, ionizing radiation, nitrogen mustard, antimetabolites, antimitotic agents, certain antibi-

otics, and toxic chemicals predictably lead to marrow aplasia. In another category are agents such as chloramphenicol, anticonvulsants, analgesics, and gold salts, which induce aplasia only occasionally. Finally, hundreds of agents of various types have been implicated in several cases as causes of aplastic anemia. Unfortunately, in about 50% of the cases, careful search does not reveal any causative agent.

Holly (1953) described eight patients with hypoplastic anemia detected during pregnancy that remitted spontaneously after delivery. The bone marrow was described as hypocellular with an increase in megakaryocytes. To date, over 80 cases have been reported (Fleming, 1973; Snyder et al., 1991; Ascarelli et al., 1998; Ohba et al., 1999). These cases present a spectrum of clinical and bone marrow findings that make it difficult to substantiate the existence of a hypoplastic anemia specifically related to pregnancy. Support for such a hypothesis is found only when recovery occurs after delivery, an entirely normal marrow is documented between pregnancies, and relapse occurs with a subsequent pregnancy.

Patients with aplastic anemia seek medical attention because of symptoms relating to profound anemia, bleeding, or infection. The CBC reveals pancytopenia with a hypoproliferative reticulocyte count. Examination of the bone marrow reveals hypoplasia with normoblastic erythropoiesis. Severe aplastic anemia is fatal for more than 50% of affected patients (Lynch et al., 1975).

Bone marrow transplantation is now the treatment of choice, and long-term survival of 50% to 70% can be expected. Alternatives include antithymocyte globulin, immunosuppressive therapy, and other supportive therapy listed below (Kojima et al., 2000). Survivors have had successful pregnancies following transplantation (Deeg et al., 1983; Doney et al., 1985; Schmidt et al., 1987; Sanders et al., 1996). The largest series examines pregnancy outcomes in 146 pregnancies occurring after treatment for aplastic anemia in 41 women (Sanders et al., 1996). The outcomes in cases treated with total-body irradiation and bone marrow transplantation were compared with those in cases treated with high-dose chemotherapy and bone marrow transplantation. These data demonstrate no increase in the incidence of congenital anomalies in infants. However, total-body irradiation was associated with an increased risk of spontaneous abortion. Twenty-five percent of the pregnancies ended with a preterm delivery or delivery of a low-birthweight infant.

During pregnancy, supportive therapy remains the major objective, since bone marrow transplantation is still relatively contraindicated in pregnancy. In recent years, with modern supportive therapy, the maternal mortality rate has been only 15%, and more than 90% of patients survive in remission. Treatment consists of maintenance of Hgb levels by periodic transfusion, prevention and treatment of infection, stimulation of hematopoiesis with androgens, splenectomy, therapeutic abortion and premature delivery, intravenous gamma globulin, and intravenous steroids (McGuire et al., 1987). Two recent case reports described successful pregnancies with a combination of RBC and platelet transfusions, cyclosporine, human granulocyte-colony–stimulating factor, high-dose intravenous prednisone, and intravenous immunoglobulin (Ascarelli et al., 1998; Ohba et al., 1999). Androgen therapy can be effective at stimulating erythropoiesis. However, androgens are contraindicated during pregnancy unless the fetus is demonstrated to be male. Agents commonly used include fluoxymesterone (0.25 mg/kg/day), oxymetholone (3 to 5 mg/kg/day), nandrolone decanoate (3 to 4 mg/kg/week), or testosterone enanthate (1 to 3 mg/kg/week). Adrenocorticosteroids have also been widely used with some benefit. Unfortunately, the remission rate with steroids is only 12%.

Because of the anecdotal reports of complete remission following pregnancy termination, it is tempting to consider therapeutic abortion. However, thorough examination of the available literature indicates that abortion or premature termination of pregnancy is not associated with a more favorable outcome. The only reason to terminate pregnancy prematurely is the inability to treat the patient satisfactorily during pregnancy with transfusion alone and thus the need to proceed to marrow transplantation.

Paroxysmal nocturnal hemoglobinuria (PNH) hemolysis occurs as a result of an unexplained structural defect in the RBC. There are distinct cohorts of long-lived and short-lived cells. The inherent defect makes the RBCs unusually susceptible to lysis by complement. PNH usually begins insidiously; there is no familial tendency. Considerable variability exists in severity of the disease, and the classic presentation of hemoglobinuria is seen in only 25% of patients. Exacerbations of the hemolytic process are precipitated by infection, menstruation, transfusion, surgery, and ingestion of iron.

The most serious complications are marrow aplasia, thrombosis, and infection. Thrombosis accounts for 50% of deaths and is of particular concern during pregnancy. Although anemia is the most prominent hematologic feature of PNH, leukopenia and thrombocytopenia also occur frequently. The diagnosis is based on a series of special tests that demonstrate the sensitivity of the patient's RBCs to complement.

The ideal treatment of PNH is replacement of the abnormal stem cell with cells capable of producing the normal cellular components. This has been accomplished by bone marrow transplantation. The major therapeutic modalities during pregnancy are iron therapy, androgen treatment (if the fetus is male), corticosteroids, and transfusions (Frakes et al., 1976; Hurd et al., 1982; Solal-Celigny et al., 1988). Iron can be administered orally to replace the considerable amount lost in the urine. Unfortunately, in patients with significant iron deficiency, such treatment may lead to a burst of erythropoiesis, with delivery of a cohort of cells susceptible to the lytic action of complement. If a hemolytic episode follows iron therapy, it should be treated with either suppression of erythropoiesis by transfusion or suppression of hemolysis with corticosteroids. Prednisone in a dose of 1 mg/kg/day is an effective regimen.

When acute hemolytic episodes occur, treatment is aimed at diminishing hemolysis and preventing complications. Patients with PNH have frequent episodes of venous thrombosis, which must be watched for carefully. In cases of acute deep venous thromboses, anticoagulation therapy should be begun. Care must be taken in the use of heparin because hemolytic episodes clearly can be related to its use. During pregnancy, heparin is the anticoagulant of choice; however, during the puerperium or nonpregnant state, warfarin is preferred. Only a few pregnancies have been reported in women with PNH, and both spontaneous abortion and thrombotic events appear to be increased in frequency.

Hemoglobinopathies

Our understanding of the molecular genetics of the hemoglobinopathies and our ability to make specific diagnoses have evolved rapidly over the past three decades (Weatherall and Clegg, 1981; Steinberg and Adams, 1982; Bunn and Forget, 1986). The hemoglobinopathies can be broadly divided into two general types. In the thalassemia syndromes, normal Hgb is synthesized at an abnormally slow rate. In contrast, the structural hemoglobinopathies occur because of a specific change in the amino acid content of Hgb. These structural changes may have either no effect or profound effects on the function of Hgb, including instability of the molecule, reduced solubility, methemoglobinemia, and increased or decreased oxygen affinity.

Thalassemia Syndromes

The thalassemia syndromes are named and classified by the type of chain that is inadequately produced. The two most common are δ-thalassemia and β-thalassemia, both of which affect the synthesis of hemoglobin A. Reduced synthesis of γ or δ chains and combinations in which two or more globin chains are affected are relatively rare. In each instance, the thalassemia is a quantitative disorder of globin synthesis.

α-THALASSEMIA

In patients with α-thalassemia, one or more structural genes are physically absent from the genome. The various α-thalassemia genotypes are summarized in Figure 47-2. In blacks, the most common two-gene deletion state consists of one gene missing on each chromosome. In Asians, most often both genes are missing from the same chromosome. In the homozygous stage, all four genes are deleted and no chains are produced. Thus, the fetus is unable to synthesize normal Hgb F or any adult hemoglobins. This deficiency results in high-output cardiac failure, hydrops fetalis, and stillbirth (Higgs et al., 1989).

The most severe form of α-thalassemia compatible with extrauterine life is hemoglobin H disease, which results from deletion of three α genes. In these patients, abnormally high quantities of both Hgb H (β_4) and Hgb Barts (γ_4) accumulate. Because Hgb H precipitates within the RBC, the cell is removed by the reticuloendothelial system, leading to a moderately severe hemolytic anemia. In α-thalassemia minor (α-thalassemia 1) two genes are deleted, resulting in a mild hypochromic, microcytic anemia that must be differentiated from iron deficiency. A single gene deletion (α-thalassemia 2) is clinically undetectable and is called the "silent carrier" state. Thus, the α-thalassemia trait presents in the adult as mild hypochromic, microcytic anemia.

The diagnosis is presumptive by exclusion of iron deficiency and α-thalassemia. Although α-thalassemia trait does not present a hazard to the adult, there are serious genetic implications when a mating of two individuals with the trait occurs. Under these circumstances, one must make a specific diagnosis by using restriction endonuclease techniques or a DNA probe before undertaking antenatal diagnosis (Kan et al., 1976; Miller, 1982).

β-THALASSEMIA

β-Thalassemia is autosomal recessive and is more common in people of Mediterranean, Middle Eastern, and Asian descent. The underproduction of β-globulin chains is caused

GENOTYPE

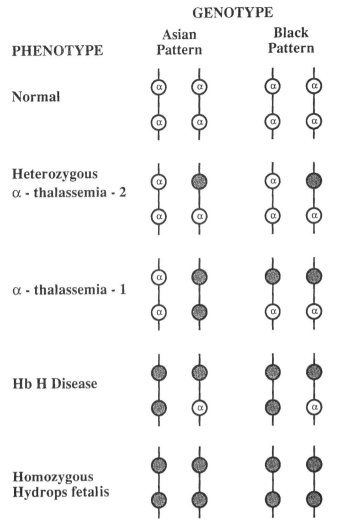

FIGURE 47-2 ■ Genotypes of the various α-thalassemia syndromes. Hgb, hemoglobin.

by point mutations with single nucleotide substitution or oligonucleotide addition or deletion (Cao et al., 1997). The β-globin genes are on chromosome 11. In homozygous β-thalassemia, α-chain production is unimpeded, and these highly unstable chains accumulate and eventually precipitate. Markedly ineffective erythropoiesis and severe hemolysis result in a condition known as *thalassemia major* or *Cooley anemia*. The fetus is protected from severe disease by α-chain production. However, this protection disappears rapidly after birth, with the affected infant becoming anemic by 3 to 6 months of age. The infant has splenomegaly and requires blood transfusions every 3 to 4 weeks. Death generally occurs by the third decade of life and is usually secondary to myocardial hemochromatosis. Female infants surviving until puberty are usually amenorrheic and have severely impaired fertility (Kazazian and Boehm, 1988; Fosburg and Nathan, 1990).

β-Thalassemia minor results in a variable degree of illness, depending on the rate of β-chain production. The characteristic findings include a relatively high RBC, moderate to marked microcytosis, and a peripheral smear resembling iron deficiency. Hgb electrophoresis characteristically shows an elevation of Hgb A_2. β-Thalassemia trait does not impair fertility, and the incidence of prematurity, low-birth-weight

infants, and infants of abnormal size for gestational age is identical to that in normal women (Fleming and Lynch, 1967; Alger et al., 1979). Nineteen women with β–thalassemia major or intermedia were followed through 22 pregnancies; 21 viable infants were delivered (Aessopos et al., 1999). These patients all had intensive treatment including transfusions and iron-chelating agents, if necessary, prior to pregnancy, or their Hgb was above 7 g/dL. In addition, all women had a prepregnancy cardiac echo with left ventricular ejection fraction greater than 55%. These results suggest that women with well-managed, stable β-thalassemia can do very well during pregnancy (Aessopos et al., 1999). The clinical characteristics and hematologic findings of the various thalassemias are summarized in Table 47-5.

Because of increased Asian immigration, the number of β-thalassemia cases has risen, so maternal screening of appropriate women is important (Lorey and Cunningham, 1998). In California, cases of β-thalassemia major, Hgb E/β-thalassemia, and other combined structural Hgb abnormalities are more common than phenylketonuria or galactosemia (Lorey and Cunningham, 1998). A suggestion for easy antenatal maternal screening for β- and α-thalassemia is shown in Figure 47-3 (Alger et al., 1979; Kilpatrick and Laros, 1995). Prenatal diagnosis is now available for β-thalassemia by polymerase chain reaction techniques of mutation detection on fetal blood or DNA (Cao et al., 1997; De Rycke et al., 2001).

Structural Hemoglobinopathies

To date, several hundred variants of α, β, γ, and δ chains have been identified. Most differ from normal chains by only one amino acid. The nomenclature and frequency of the most common hemoglobinopathies in African Americans are depicted in Table 47-6 (Motulsky, 1973). Confirmation of a diagnosis of a specific hemoglobinopathy requires identification of the abnormal Hgb by means of Hgb electrophoresis.

Sickle Cell Trait

In general, women with sickle cell trait do well during pregnancy and labor. Because there is a twofold increase in the rate of urinary tract infection, prenatal patients should be screened for asymptomatic bacteriuria (Whalley et al., 1963, 1964; Blattner et al., 1977). A recent study suggested that the risk of preeclampsia was increased to 25%, compared to 10% in a sickle-negative control group (Larrabee and Monga, 1997). These patients may become iron deficient, and iron supplementation during pregnancy is indicated.

Sickle Cell Anemia

Patients with sickle cell anemia (SCA) suffer from lifelong complications, in part a result of the markedly shortened life span of their RBCs. Most observers believe that the pre-pregnancy course of a woman is a good index of how she will fare during pregnancy. Although fetal outcomes are generally good in pregnancies complicated by SCA, there continues to be an increased risk of prematurity and intrauterine growth restriction (Morrison and Wiser, 1976; Cunningham et al., 1983; Smith et al., 1996; Sun et al., 2001). The most recent series showed an incidence of intrauterine growth restriction and

TABLE 47-5. HEMATOLOGIC AND CLINICAL ASPECTS OF THE THALASSEMIA SYNDROMES

Condition	Hemoglobin (Hb) Pattern*				Clinical Severity
	Hb Level	Hb A₂	Hb F	Other Hb	
Homozygotes					
α-thalassemia	↓↓↓↓	0	0	80% Hb Barts, remainder Hb H and Hb Portland Some Hb A	Hydrops fetalis
β⁺-thalassemia	↓↓↓	Variable	↑↑	Some Hb A	Moderately severe Cooley anemia
β⁰-thalassemia	↓↓↓↓	Variable	↑↑↑	No Hb A	Severe Cooley anemia
δβ⁰-thalassemia	↓↓	0	100%	No Hb A	Thalassemia intermedia
Heterozygotes					
α-thalassemia silent carrier	N	N	N	1%–2% Hb Barts in cord blood at birth	N
α-thalassemia trait	↓	N	N	5% Hb Barts in cord blood at birth	Very mild
Hb H disease	↓↓	N	N	4%–30% Hb H in adults; 25% Hb Barts in cord blood	Thalassemia intermedia
β⁺-thalassemia	↓ to ↓↓	↑	↑	None	Mild
β⁰-thalassemia	↓ to ↓↓	↓	↑↑↑	None	Mild

* ↑, increased; ↓, decreased; number of arrows indicates relative intensity.
N, normal.

preterm delivery of 45% each; both were significantly more common in women with SCA than in the control group without SCA (Sun et al., 2001).

Virtually all signs and symptoms of SCA are secondary to hemolysis, vaso-occlusive disease, or an increased susceptibility to infection (Table 47-7). Clinical manifestations may affect growth and development, with growth restriction and skeletal changes secondary to expansion of the marrow cavity. Painful crises may occur in the long bones, abdomen, chest, or back. The cardiovascular manifestations are those of a hyperdynamic circulation, and pulmonary signs may be secondary to either infection or vaso-occlusion. In addition to painful vaso-occlusive episodes, patients may exhibit hepatomegaly, signs and symptoms of hepatitis, cholecystitis, and painful splenic infarcts. Genitourinary signs include hyposthenuria, hematuria, and pyelonephritis.

Whether or not pregnancy in women with SCA is associated with more complications is controversial. A comparison of pregnancy outcomes between women with SCA and those without it revealed no significant differences (Smith et al., 1996). Rates of maternal morbidity from SCA were the same during pregnancy as in the nonpregnant state. However, another study showed a significant increase in antepartum admissions, preterm labor or preterm premature rupture of membranes, and postpartum infection in women with SCA compared to women without SCA (Sun et al., 2001).

Treatment has been largely symptomatic, with the major objectives being to end a painful crisis and to combat infection. Urinary tract and pulmonary infections should be diagnosed promptly and treated vigorously with appropriate antibiotics. Appropriate ultrasounds should be done throughout the pregnancy to ensure normal fetal growth. There are no prospective studies on the use of antepartum fetal testing in women with sickle cell disease, so this should be instituted at the discretion of the physician.

Transfusion therapy has been used widely for years in the treatment of symptomatic patients. More recently, partial exchange transfusions or prophylactic transfusions have been advocated (Cunningham et al., 1979; Francis and Johnson, 1991). The goal of partial exchange transfusions is to keep the Hgb A above 50% and Hct above 25% (Rust and Perry, 1995). A prospective, randomized study of 72 patients with SCA showed no significant difference in perinatal outcome between women treated with prophylactic transfusion and those receiving transfusion only if Hgb fell below 6 g/dL or Hct fell below 18% (Koshy et al., 1988). However, this study did report a significant decrease in crises during pregnancy in the group receiving prophylactic transfusions. Sixty-six patients with sickle cell–Hgb C disease and 23 with sickle cell–β-thalassemia received transfusions for hematologic reasons only and experienced similar perinatal outcomes. However, the benefits attained must be balanced against a 25% incidence of alloimmunization and 20% delayed transfusion reaction. The use of prophylactic transfusions should be individualized. A recent excellent review of SCA in nonpregnant individuals suggested that transfusion is indicated for symptomatic acute anemia, severe symptomatic chronic anemia, acute chest syndrome with hypoxia, and surgery with general anesthesia and may be useful for severe protracted pain episodes (Steinberg, 1999). In addition, preimplantation genetic diagnosis with polymerase chain reaction assays are available for SCA (De Rycke et al., 2001).

During labor and delivery, the patient must remain well oxygenated and hydrated. In an untransfused patient, regional anesthesia should be administered with great caution (Maduska et al., 1975; Finer et al., 1988). Careful fetal monitoring should be carried out throughout labor. However, if an exchange transfusion protocol has been used and the Hgb A level is above 40%, painful crises are distinctly unusual (Morrison et al., 1978).

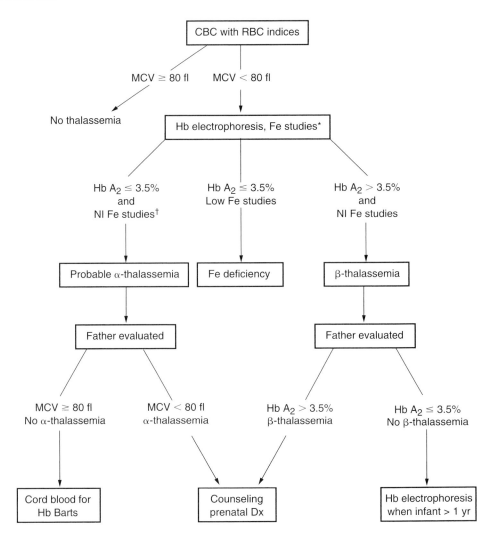

FIGURE 47-3 ■ Maternal screening for α- and β-thalassemia. CBC, complete blood count; Dx, diagnosis; MCV, mean corpuscular volume; RBC, red blood cell.

* May be serum Fe, total Fe binding capacity.
† Percent saturation > 15 or ferritin > 12 ng/mL.

Hemoglobin Sickle Cell Disease

Women who are doubly heterozygous for both the Hgb S and the Hgb C genes are said to have hemoglobin SC disease (Hgb SCD). Hemoglobin electrophoresis reveals approximately 60% Hgb C and 40% Hgb S. Patients with Hgb SCD generally have a normal habitus, a healthy childhood, and a normal life span. If a systematic screening program has not been used, the condition may first be detected in many women during the latter part of pregnancy, when a complication occurs. At the beginning of pregnancy, most women are mildly anemic and splenomegaly is present. Examination of a peripheral blood smear shows numerous target cells. Hemoglobin electrophoresis ensures the correct diagnosis (Laros, 1967; Maberry et al., 1990).

During pregnancy, 40% to 60% of patients with Hgb SCD present as if they had SCA. In contrast to patients with SCA, those with Hgb SCD frequently experience rapid and severe anemic crises resulting from splenic sequestration. These patients also have a greater tendency to experience bone marrow necrosis with the release of fat-forming marrow emboli.

The clinical manifestations of Hgb SCD are otherwise similar to those of SCA but milder, and the general management of symptomatic patients is identical. Considerations for the management of labor are the same as with SCA. In a recent report, women with Hgb SCD had a significantly increased risk of antepartum admission, intrauterine growth

TABLE 47-6. NOMENCLATURE AND FREQUENCY OF THE MOST COMMON HEMOGLOBINOPATHIES IN ADULT AFRICAN AMERICANS

Hemoglobinopathy	Abbreviated Name	Frequency
Sickle cell trait	Hb SA	1:122
Sickle cell anemia	Hb SS	1:708
Sickle cell–hemoglobin C disease	Hb SC	1:757
Hemoglobin C disease	Hb CC	1:4790
Hemoglobin C trait	Hb CA	1:41
Hemoglobin S–β-thalassemia	Hb S–β-thal	1:1672
Hemoglobin S–high F	Hb S–HPFH	1:3412

TABLE 47-7. CLINICAL MANIFESTATIONS OF SICKLE CELL ANEMIA

I. **Growth and development**
   A. Retarded growth
   B. Skeletal changes
   C. Decreased life span
II. **Sickle cell crisis**
   A. Painful vaso-occlusive episodes: bones, abdomen, chest, and back
III. **Cardiovascular manifestations of hyperdynamic circulation**
   A. Cardiomegaly
   B. Systolic murmurs
   C. Failure
IV. **Pulmonary signs**
   A. Infection—pneumococcus, mycoplasma, hemophilus, salmonella
   B. Vascular occlusion
V. **Abdominal involvement**
   A. Painful vaso-occlusive episodes
   B. Hepatomegaly
   C. Hepatitis
   D. Cholecystitis
   E. Splenic infarction
VI. **Bone and joint changes**
   A. Bone marrow infarction
   B. Osteomyelitis—salmonella
   C. Arthritis
VII. **Genitourinary signs**
   A. Hyposthenuria
   B. Hematuria
   C. Pyelonephritis
VIII. **Neurologic manifestations**
   A. Vascular occlusion
   B. Convulsions
   C. Hemorrhage
   D. Visual disturbances
IX. **Ocular manifestations**
   A. Conjunctival vessel changes
   B. Vitreous hemorrhage

restriction, and postpartum infection compared to women without sickle disease, but these risks were half those of the women with SCA (Sun et al., 2001).

Hemoglobin S-β-Thalassemia

Patients with Hgb S-β-thalassemia are heterozygous for the sickle cell and the β-thalassemia genes. In addition to decreased β-chain production, there is a variably increased production of Hgb F and Hgb A_2. Because of this variable production rate, Hgb electrophoresis reveals a spectrum of Hgb concentrations. Hgb S may account for 70% to 95% of the Hgb present, with Hgb F rarely exceeding 20% (Laros and Kalstone, 1971). Because of the thalassemia influence, Hgb S concentration exceeds Hgb A concentration. This is in sharp contrast to patients with sickle cell trait, in whom Hgb A levels exceed the concentration of Hgb S.

The diagnosis is made in an anemic patient by demonstrating increased Hgb A_2 and Hgb F levels in association with a level of Hgb S exceeding that of Hgb A. The peripheral smear reveals hypochromia and microcytosis with anisocytosis, poikilocytosis, basophilic stippling, and target cells. The clinical

manifestations of this disorder parallel those of SCA but are generally milder. Painful crises may occur; however, these patients have a normal body habitus and frequently enjoy an uncompromised life span. We believe that the role of exchange transfusion should be similar to that in patients with Hgb SCD; that is, exchange transfusion should be reserved for the woman who experiences painful crises or whose anemia leads to an Hct below 25%.

Hemoglobin C Trait and Disease

Hemoglobin C trait is an asymptomatic trait without reproductive consequences. Target cells are found in the peripheral smear, but anemia is not present. Hemoglobin C disease is the homozygous state and is a mild disorder usually discovered during a medical evaluation. Mild hemolytic anemia with an Hct in the range of 25% to 35% is characteristic. The RBCs show microspherocytes and characteristic targeting. No increased morbidity or mortality is associated with pregnancy, and no specific therapy is indicated.

Hemoglobin E Disease

The recent resettlement of Southeast Asians in the United States has resulted in an increase in the number of individuals with hemoglobin E trait and disease. The clinical and laboratory manifestations of the various Hgb E syndromes are outlined in Table 47-8 (Wong and Ali, 1982; Ferguson and O'Reilly, 1985). Most individuals have a mild microcytic anemia that is of no clinical significance, and no treatment is necessary. However, patients homozygous for Hgb E have a greater degree of microcytosis and are frequently anemic. Target cells are prominent. As with Hgb C trait and disease, no specific therapy is required and reproductive outcome is normal.

Anemias Associated with Systemic Disease

The normal bone marrow has the capacity to increase its RBC production six- to eightfold in response to anemia. This compensatory mechanism, responsible also for the increase in RBC mass in normal pregnancy, is triggered by tissue hypoxia and mediated by erythropoietin. The response may be absent or blunted in some circumstances, most commonly in chronic disorders. Chronic infections, rheumatoid arthritis, and other inflammatory states are characterized by a mild normocytic, normochromic (or sometimes hypochromic, microcytic) anemia with low serum iron concentration, low transferrin level, inappropriately low reticulocyte count, and generous but poorly utilized stores of reticuloendothelial iron. Although the bone marrow is normally cellular, it does not respond appropriately to the mildly accelerated RBC destruction typical of chronic inflammation. Studies thus far have not determined whether the defect in erythropoiesis can be attributed to inadequate erythropoietin secretion. In the absence of pregnancy, the Hgb is, in these chronic states, frequently 9 to 10 g/dL, and the Hct concentration is about 30%. The hydremia of pregnancy may lower these values somewhat.

A similar but frequently more complicated anemia accompanies renal failure. Here, more often perhaps than in chronic inflammatory states, blood loss and hemolysis are contributory factors, and the serum iron and transferrin changes noted

TABLE 47-8. VARIOUS GENOTYPES OF HEMOGLOBIN E AND THEIR PHENOTYPIC EXPRESSION

Genotype	Degree of Anemia*	MCV†	Electrophoresis (%)				Phenotype Expression
			A + A₂	E	F	S	
A/E	0	↓	68	30	<2	0	None
E/E	0 to +	↓↓	<4	94	<2	0	None
E/α-thal	+ to + +	↓	50	15	35	0	None
S/E	+ +	↓	0	40	0	60	None
E/β⁺-thal	+ +	↓↓	10	60	30	0	Splenomegaly
E/β⁰-thal	+ + +	↓↓	0	60	40	0	Splenomegaly

* Number of + symbols indicates relative severity.
† Number of arrows indicates relative amount of decrease.
MCV, mean corpuscular volume.

above are less regular. In many of these situations, diminished erythropoietin is important in the pathogenesis.

Renal failure and chronic inflammation are rare in pregnancy, so management of the associated anemias is seldom a clinical problem in obstetric patients. Occasionally, however, it is the anemia that calls attention to the underlying disease. These anemias do not respond to hematinic agents or steroid hormones (unless the adrenal steroids play some role in controlling the underlying disease, as in rheumatoid arthritis or lupus). Erythropoietin is useful in treating patients with chronic renal disease and can often obviate repeated RBC transfusion (Erslev, 1991).

Neutropenia and Agranulocytosis

White Blood Cells

Pregnancy is associated with an increase in the neutrophilia count beginning during the 2nd month. The total WBC count increases because of this increase in neutrophils. The neutrophilia begins in the first trimester and reaches a plateau in the second or third trimester, when total counts usually range between 9 and 15 x 10⁹ cells per liter. Kuvin and Brecher (1962) reported that 20% of their group of 88 normal pregnant women had total counts greater than 10.0 x 10⁹ cells per liter. Among subjects with higher counts, 21% had occasional myelocytes and metamyelocytes on peripheral blood smears. A similar proportion of those with total counts less than 10.0 x 10⁹ cells per liter also had these immature forms in the peripheral blood. The authors concluded that this left shift is a common occurrence in normal pregnancy. If the normal pregnant woman should experience any complicating illness usually associated with a polymorphonuclear leukocytosis (i.e., a bacterial infection), a substantial rise in the WBC count is noted. In the absence of complications, the total WBC count falls to within the normal range for nonpregnant women by the 6th postpartum day.

Döhle bodies, blue-staining cytoplasmic inclusions seen in granulocytes stained with Romanovsky dyes (Wright stain, Giemsa stain) and initially identified in individuals with bacteremia, are found on nearly all peripheral smears from pregnant women. By means of electron microscopy, they have been identified as aggregates of rough endoplasmic reticulum. Minor increases in eosinophils have been reported during pregnancy, and basophils decrease slightly. No systematic changes in monocytes have been observed. Neither the absolute lymphocyte count nor the relative numbers of T and B cells are

changed by pregnancy, but cell-mediated immunity is depressed. The mechanisms responsible are poorly understood; however, the process is certainly in part directed by the physiologic hormonal changes accompanying normal pregnancy.

Neutropenia

Isolated neutropenia is uncommon in pregnant women. It has become standard practice among physicians experienced in the chemotherapy of leukemias and other neoplastic diseases to regard 1 x 10⁹/liter as a "safe" number, sufficient to cope with most infections against which neutrophils would provide defense. Although translation of this lower limit of acceptability into other clinical situations has not been established, a count above 1 x 10⁹/liter is probably "safe" in most situations.

Because most cases of neutropenia among pregnant women are caused by drugs or other environmental agents, the importance of recognizing a low WBC count is in alerting the physician to the possible presence of a dangerous drug or chemical or a complicating disorder. Neutropenia may occasionally herald the appearance of lupus erythematosus, acute leukemia, neoplasia involving the marrow, human immunodeficiency virus, or other serious intercurrent disease. Megaloblastic anemia is often accompanied by neutropenia. When an isolated low WBC count is observed, a careful history of medication and other exposure should be taken. Clues suggesting systemic disorders should be sought, and if these efforts are unrewarding, the bone marrow should be examined.

Management is supportive. Complicating illness should be treated, and potentially myelosuppressive substances should be excluded from the patient's medications and environment. A partial list of drugs reported to cause neutropenia is given in Table 47-9. Deficiencies should be corrected, and supportive care, with prompt evaluation and treatment of infection, should be instituted. Transfusions of WBCs have been of limited value.

Hematologic Neoplasia and Pregnancy

Advances over the past 30 years in the management of some leukemias, Hodgkin's disease, and the non-Hodgkin's lymphomas have substantially improved the prognosis for most patients with these malignancies. The former high mortality rates and poor reproductive potential for children and young adults with hematologic neoplastic disease no longer apply in

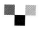

TABLE 47-9. SOME COMMON AGENTS OCCASIONALLY REPORTED TO CAUSE NEUTROPENIA

Analgesics and Anti-inflammatory Agents

Aminopyrine
Phenylbutazone

Anticonvulsants

Diphenylhydantoin sodium
Trimethyloxazolidine

Tranquilizers

Phenothiazines
Meprobamate
Haloperidol

Antimicrobials

Chloramphenicol
Metronidazole
Isonicotinic acid hydrazide
Sulfonamides

Diuretics

Oral Hypoglycemics

Antithyroid Drugs

Propylthiouracil
Methimazole

Miscellaneous

Penicillamine
Cimetidine
Quinine
Gold salts

all cases, and an increasing number of these patients now achieve complete, durable remissions and even cure. This improved prognosis has raised new questions concerning both the possibility and the outcome of pregnancy.

Acute Leukemia

The classification of the acute leukemias by cell type has become increasingly important in evaluation of studies designed to identify the therapeutic regimens most likely to succeed in a given case. Identification of cell-surface markers, histochemical staining, and careful study of the neoplastic cells in peripheral blood and bone marrow stained by conventional methods have allowed more precise classification and sub-classification, and these carry reasonably accurate therapeutic and prognostic implications. For purposes of this discussion, the terms *acute lymphoblastic leukemia* (ALL) and *acute nonlymphoblastic leukemia* (ANLL) are used.

ALL, the most common acute leukemia of childhood, is the disorder in which prolonged remissions and even cures have most often been achieved. In general, the probability of a favorable outcome of therapy is usually inversely related to age, with young children being more likely to do well. The disorder occurs occasionally in young adults, with a less favorable prognosis.

ANLL may occur at any age but is rare in childhood. Its many variants are the common acute leukemias of adults, and although hematologic remissions are being achieved in an increasing proportion of cases, ultimate relapse and resistance to further therapy remain the rule. Newer techniques,

including bone marrow transplantation, show some promise for improving the survival in these cases, but these therapeutic modalities continue to have many biological and practical limitations.

Prepubertal girls who are successfully treated for ALL with chemotherapy and irradiation usually experience normal sexual development (Siris et al., 1976). Catanzarite and Ferguson (1984) were able to identify 10 mothers cured of childhood ALL who bore a total of 13 children, all carried to term and all apparently normal at birth. Dara and coworkers (1981) have reported a successful outcome in a pregnancy that began while the mother was receiving 6-mercaptopurine and methotrexate maintenance therapy for ALL in remission. Relapse occurred in the 4th month, but additional chemotherapy induced a second hematologic remission. The infant appeared normal at birth and showed normal growth and development during the first 6 months.

Pregnancy in women with ANLL is a rare event, and ANLL complicating an established pregnancy is equally uncommon. In a published review in 1977, Lilleyman and associates determined that if ANLL was detected during the first half of pregnancy, a live healthy baby was produced in fewer than 50% of the cases. Abortion, stillbirth, or maternal death accounted for the fetal wastage. In only 1 of the 32 cases included in the report was a fetal abnormality (trisomy C) identified, although nearly two thirds of the mothers received cytotoxic drugs.

Acute promyelocytic leukemia, a form of *acute myeloblastic leukemia*, is commonly associated with disseminated intravascular coagulation (DIC), which has been reported in pregnancy (Roy et al., 1989; Hoffman et al., 1995). A review of 23 pregnant women with acute promyelocytic leukemia noted an 83% live birth rate, with the majority of women receiving chemotherapy during pregnancy (Hoffman et al., 1995). Further, acute promyelocytic leukemia has been treated successfully after the first trimester of pregnancy with all-*trans*-retinoic acid without reported fetal or neonatal morbidity (Hoffman et al., 1995; Giagounidis et al., 2000).

Careful analysis of the reported cases of acute leukemia in pregnancy strongly suggests that the course of the leukemia is not directly influenced by the pregnancy. Some women (and their physicians), however, may be reluctant to expose the fetus to possibly teratogenic or mutagenic drugs. There is no question that acute leukemia that remains untreated or that recurs exerts a potentially devastating effect on both the fetus and the mother (Greenlund et al., 2001). The natural history of both ALL and ANLL managed without cytotoxic drugs is one of death from bleeding or infection in a few months at most. Measures to avoid conception are strongly advocated for young women with acute leukemia requiring chemotherapy, and a solid case for interruption of pregnancy in this same group of patients can be made. However, this advice is not acceptable to all patients.

The frequency and severity of the teratogenic effects of the drugs employed in the treatment of acute leukemia are not known with certainty, because the collected series are small (Pizzuto et al., 1980; Schafer, 1981; Plows, 1982; Sanz and Rafecas, 1982). The occurrence of leukemia in a newborn of a leukemic mother is exceedingly rare, however. Even less is known about the late effects of antileukemic therapy on the surviving offspring of women exposed to these agents during pregnancy. A recent report is very encouraging. Aviles and Neri (2001) performed long-term follow-up of 84 children who were exposed *in utero* to maternal chemotherapy for hematologic malignancies. Over a median of 18 years of follow-up, the authors found no cancers including leukemia, and no congenital, neurological, or psychological abnormalities. Information is also available about the children of individuals themselves treated in childhood for a variety of neoplasms (Li et al., 1979; Green et al., 1991). In 286 completed pregnancies in which one or the other parent had been treated for childhood cancer, there was no excess of congenital anomalies in comparison with published figures for the general population (Li et al., 1979). However, pre-pregnancy parental treatment with dactinomycin may be associated with an increase in congenital cardiac anomalies (Green et al., 1991). Additional information is recorded about the obstetric experience of women treated with chemotherapy for trophoblastic neoplasms (Walden and Bagshawe, 1979). In successfully treated patients, there was no increase in the rate of abnormal pregnancies or fetal abnormalities.

It is therefore evident that live, healthy infants can be born to some pregnant women who develop acute leukemia and to some women with leukemia who become pregnant. Chemotherapy is not invariably teratogenic, but the precise risk of a congenital abnormality is not known. The risk of fetal abnormality may be greater if treatment is started in the early weeks of pregnancy rather than in the latter half, but this hazard must be balanced against the real threat of maternal death inherent in untreated leukemia. As more cases appear with few poor neonatal outcomes, the advantage of maternal life expectancy will begin to outweigh the risk of neonatal exposure to chemotherapeutic agents (Giagounidis et al., 2000; Aviles and Neri, 2001; Hansen et al., 2001). Nonetheless, the patient still has a difficult decision, and it should be made with all available information. Because of the complexities inherent in caring for these women, they should be managed by a multidisciplinary group including a perinatologist and a hematologic oncologist.

Chronic Leukemia

Chronic myelogenous leukemia (CML), sometimes called *chronic granulocytic leukemia*, occurs most often in those over 40 years of age but also occasionally in women in the reproductive years. In most cases, significant elevation of the WBC count (in the absence of infection), with a marked left shift, including variable numbers of myelocytes and myeloblasts, calls attention to the possibility of a blood dyscrasia. In early cases, anemia is usually absent or mild, and the platelet count is often increased.

About 75% of the patients have splenomegaly. Many patients are treated with busulfan, an agent often responsible for amenorrhea and ovarian failure; on this account, pregnancy in a patient with established and treated CML is very rare. However, a number of women have been discovered to have CML after pregnancy has begun. Because the life-threatening complications common in acute leukemia (hemorrhage secondary to thrombocytopenia and infection) are rarely encountered in the early months in patients with CML, the pregnancy can usually be carried to term without the use of chemotherapy or other modalities except, in some cases, transfusion for significant anemia. In this way, the risks to the fetus of potentially mutagenic or teratogenic interventions can be avoided. However, a small number of women with CML have been

treated with interferon-α during pregnancy, with normal pediatric follow-up for as long as 30 months (Mubarak et al., 2002). In addition, hydroxyurea has treated CML successfully in pregnancy (Fadilah et al., 2002).

Splenomegaly can be a problem of clinical importance. A large spleen may be uncomfortable, may be the site of recurrent infarction with perisplenitis, or may compete for space in an abdomen already attempting to accommodate an enlarging uterus. Richards and Spiers (1975), employing localized radiation therapy, have reported successful reduction in spleen size with no obstetric or detectable fetal complications.

The overall average duration of survival from time of diagnosis in CML is between 3 and 4 years. Young women frequently experience a more prolonged survival. Although cures are virtually nonexistent, most patients treated with oral agents enjoy a lengthy clinical remission. Ultimately, the disease becomes refractory to therapy or assumes an accelerated phase that resembles acute leukemia morphologically but is generally resistant to treatment. Successful bone marrow transplantation for chronic-phase CML has been increasingly reported, but good outcomes have usually been limited to young patients whose donors were human leukocyte antigen–identical siblings (Champlin et al., 1988). The other forms of chronic leukemia occur so infrequently in patients under 50 years of age that they are not discussed here.

Hodgkin's Disease

Several factors have combined to make Hodgkin's disease a hematologic neoplasm of increasing importance in obstetric practice. First, there is a peculiar predilection for young adults of both sexes. Second, long-term cures in selected cases following adequate and appropriate radiation therapy are well known. Third, more commonly than for any other tumor (except childhood acute leukemia), durable remissions and cures occur in patients with advanced or extensive disease treated with both combination chemotherapy and high-dose radiation.

An increasing number of young women who have been treated successfully for Hodgkin's disease wish to and do become pregnant. In addition, the management decisions necessary (for both patient and physician) when the disorder first manifests during pregnancy have become increasingly complex. Data are being accumulated that can assist physicians as they advise patients in each of these two situations about the effect of Hodgkin's disease and its treatment on fertility, pregnancy, and the fetus. It is now well established that pregnancy *per se* does not affect Hodgkin's disease, although treatment plans may have to be modified if the fetus is to be protected (Anselmo et al., 1999; Pohlman and Macklis, 2000).

Young women who have been successfully treated for Hodgkin's disease with total lymphoid irradiation, combination chemotherapy, or combined radiation and chemotherapy frequently experience amenorrhea (Horning et al., 1981; Schilsky et al., 1981). Absence of menses may occur even in patients who had undergone midline oophoropexy in an attempt to provide increased protection for the ovaries during radiation therapy. For some, the amenorrhea is temporary. Persistent amenorrhea occurs more often in those receiving combination therapy (radiation and cytotoxic drugs) and in those who are 25 years of age or older at the initiation of treatment.

In a series reported by Horning and colleagues (1981), pregnancy occurred after treatment for Hodgkin's disease in 28 women. Twenty of these resulted in 21 normal live births, including a set of twins; there were two premature infants, one low-birth-weight infant, and five elective therapeutic abortions. Schilsky et al. (1981) reported a total of 15 pregnancies in 27 treated women. Two elective abortions were performed, but the remaining 13 pregnancies were uneventful, and the infants appeared normal. Holmes and Holmes (1978) reported an excess of unfavorable outcomes in pregnancies among women given combination therapy. The treatment programs employed in their study, which covered patients treated between 1944 and 1975, were variable and probably cannot be fairly compared with those in the more recently reported series.

One can conclude, therefore, that women successfully treated with irradiation alone, combination chemotherapy alone, or irradiation and chemotherapy may experience premature ovarian failure; however, this occurrence is not universal, and successful pregnancies without obvious neonatal malformations can occur. Some of the late effects of intensive radiation and chemotherapy, especially the appearance of second neoplasms in some individuals cured of Hodgkin's disease, are well-recognized risks of modern treatment with curative intent. Only careful follow-up of patients with Hodgkin's disease and their progeny will provide meaningful and more precise information concerning the frequency of these late complications. It is too early to suggest that delayed complications or toxic effects may appear in the offspring.

The special problems surrounding pregnancy and Hodgkin's disease involve the limitations that pregnancy imposes on both evaluation of the extent of the disease (staging) and treatment. It is well established that the chances for successful treatment and cure are greatly enhanced if the full extent of disease can be determined and therapy can be planned to eradicate present or suspected tumor. Optimal staging often includes numerous radiographic and scanning procedures and possibly even exploratory laparotomy and splenectomy, procedures that are generally contraindicated in pregnancy. Similarly, exposure of the fetus to potentially mutagenic and teratogenic drugs or to therapeutic radiation, especially in the first trimester, is undesirable. Most experienced authorities recommend interruption of pregnancy if Hodgkin's disease is discovered early or if the patient has received radiation or cytotoxic drugs during the first trimester. If the diagnosis is made later in pregnancy, or relapse of previously known disease occurs at that time, thorough staging evaluations and treatment can sometimes be deferred until after delivery, especially if early delivery is feasible. Carefully planned supradiaphragmatic radiation has occasionally been necessary during pregnancy, and rare patients with progressive, symptomatic disease have been given systemic chemotherapy during late pregnancy without apparent untoward effects on the neonate (Thomas and Peckham, 1976; Anselmo et al., 1999; Fenig et al., 2001).

Management of the patient with Hodgkin's disease during pregnancy must be tailored individually. Young women about to be treated for the disease should undergo tests for pregnancy before therapy is initiated. Effective measures to avoid conception should be stressed as treatment is undertaken. If pregnancy occurs, interruption should be recommended during the first trimester. The management of the patient with Hodgkin's disease who wishes to continue a pregnancy or who has suf-

fered relapse during pregnancy will require the advice of physicians who are experienced in the use of modern radiation and chemotherapeutic modalities and who are familiar with the behavior of the many subtypes of this neoplasm.

Non-Hodgkin's Lymphoma

The non-Hodgkin's lymphomas, the collective term currently employed for malignant disorders (other than Hodgkin's disease and the lymphoid leukemias) primarily affecting lymphoid tissues, are extremely rare in pregnancy. Falkson and co-workers (1980), in a review of the literature, found 13 cases to which they added 1 of their own. Of the 14 women, only 2 were successfully treated during pregnancy; both women received combination chemotherapy and delivered apparently normal infants. A more recent review summarizing more than 57 reported cases suggested that although non-Hodgkin's lymphomas in pregnancy are aggressive tumors, pregnancy does not affect outcome and the best maternal outcome is associated with aggressive chemotherapy (Lishner et al., 1994).

Management of non-hematologic malignancies coincidental with pregnancy are addressed in Chapter 58.

ABNORMALITIES OF COAGULATION

The Coagulation Mechanism

The initial coagulation mechanism for thrombus formation *in vivo* is adhesion of platelets to the injured vessel walls (Shattil and Bennett, 1981). Exposed subendothelium of the injured tissue initiates adhesion, which is promptly followed by a change in shape of the platelet:

$$\text{injury} + \text{platelets} \xrightarrow[\text{aggregation}]{\text{adhesion}} \text{platelet factors} + \text{ADP}$$

Both the platelet membrane and release of the contents of δ-, α-, and γ-granules are involved in platelet adhesion and aggregation as well as in the initiation of the plasma phase of coagulation. The adenosine diphosphate released from platelets attracts more platelets to the area, resulting in *platelet aggregation*. The aggregation phenomenon tends to perpetuate itself, because newly attracted platelets in turn release adenosine diphosphate and attract additional platelets. Increasingly large amounts of platelet factors become available for initiation of the plasma phase of coagulation.

Table 47-10 presents some of the properties of the coagulation factors (Colman et al., 1987). With the exceptions of fibrinogen, prothrombin, and calcium, the coagulation factors are trace proteins. Factor III is not listed in the table and is, in fact, the tissue factor thromboplastin. The preferred descriptive name and several common synonyms for the coagulation factors are as follows:

V (proaccelerin, labile factor)
Factor VII (proconvertin, serum prothrombin conversion accelerator)
Factor VIII (antihemophilic factor, antihemophilic globulin)
Factor IX (plasma thromboplastin component, Christmas factor)
Factor X (Stuart factor, Prower factor)
Factor XI (plasma thromboplastin antecedent)

TABLE 47-10. SOME PROPERTIES OF COAGULATION FACTORS

Factor	Biochemistry	Site of Biosynthesis	Biological Half-Life (hr)	Function
Fibrinogen (I)	Glycoprotein; MW 340,000; 3 globular subunits	Liver	72–120	Common pathway; fibrin precursor
Prothrombin (II)	Monomeric glycoprotein; MW 69,000	Liver; vitamin K*	67–106	Common pathway; proenzyme precursor of thrombin
Calcium (IV)	Ionic calcium	—		Extrinsic, intrinsic, and common pathways
Factor V	Multimeric; MW 200,000–400,000	Liver	12–36	Common pathway
Factor VII	Monomeric glycoprotein; MW 63,000	Liver; vitamin K	4–6	Extrinsic pathway; proenzyme
Factor VIII	Multimeric glycoprotein; MW 330,000; circulates bound to multimeric von Willebrand factor	Probably by liver	10–14	Intrinsic pathway
Factor IX	Monomeric glycoprotein; MW 62,000	Liver; vitamin K	24	Intrinsic pathway; coenzyme
Factor X	Two-chain glycoprotein; MW 59,000	Liver; vitamin K	24–60	Common pathway; proenzyme
Factor XI	Two-chain glycoprotein; MW 200,000	Liver	48–84	Intrinsic pathway; proenzyme
Factor XII	Monomeric glycoprotein; MW 80,000	Unknown	52–60	Intrinsic pathway; proenzyme
Factor XIII	Multimeric glycoprotein; MW 320,000; 4 subunits	Liver; megakaryocytes	72–168	Common pathway; proenzyme; transglutaminase
von Willebrand	Series of macromolecules; MW 1–15×10^6	Endothelial cells and megakaryocytes	12–36	Intrinsic pathway; forms a stable complex with factor VIII

* Vitamin K required for synthesis.
MW, molecular weight.

Factor XII (Hageman factor, glass factor, contact factor)
Factor XIII (fibrin-stabilizing factor)

The third column in the table indicates the site of biosynthesis for each factor. It is noteworthy that prothrombin, factor VII, factor IX, and factor X are dependent on vitamin K for their synthesis and thus are the factors depleted when a patient is receiving a vitamin K antagonist, such as sodium warfarin. The biological half-life is also listed for each factor and can be used to calculate a rough estimate of the frequency of replacement therapy needed during an acute bleeding problem.

The remainder of the coagulation process can be broadly divided into three phases: the extrinsic pathway, intrinsic pathway, and common pathway. The pathway of function for each of the plasma factors is also noted in Table 47-11. The remainder of the coagulation scheme can be summarized by the following six schematized formulas (PF3 = platelet factor 3):

$$(1) \quad \text{tissue thromboplastin} + \text{VII} \xrightarrow[\text{Ca}^{++}]{\text{Ca}^{++}} \text{extrinsic activator}$$

$$(2) \quad \text{XII} + \text{XI} + \text{IX} + \text{PF3} + \text{VIII} \longrightarrow \text{intrinsic activator}$$

$$(3) \quad \text{X} + \text{V} + \text{PF3} + \text{Ca} \xrightarrow[\text{intrinsic activator}]{\text{extrinsic activator}} \text{common activator}$$

$$(4) \quad \text{prothrombin} \xrightarrow[\text{Ca}^{++}]{\text{common activator}} \text{thrombin}$$

$$(5) \quad \text{fibrinogen} \xrightarrow{\text{thrombin}} \text{fibrin polymer}$$

$$(6) \quad \text{fibrin polymer} + \text{VIII} \xrightarrow{\text{Ca}^{++}} \text{stabilized fibrin}$$

The basic feature of coagulation is the conversion of circulating fibrinogen into a stabilized fibrin clot; it occurs in two steps. First, fibrinogen is enzymatically converted to fibrin monomer by the action of thrombin, and the fibrin monomeric units polymerize (formula 5). Second, the resulting fibrin clot is strengthened and further rendered insoluble by the action of factor XIII (formula 6).

For fibrinogen to be converted to fibrin, thrombin must be generated from its precursor prothrombin. This reaction is catalyzed by a complex, common activator, which consists of the activated form of factor X, factor V, calcium, and platelet factors (formula 4). The production of the common activator can occur as a result of two different pathways, the intrinsic and extrinsic (formula 3). The intrinsic is so named because all of its components are present in the circulating plasma (formula 2). This pathway is probably triggered by both endothelial damage and platelet factors. The extrinsic pathway is so named because it is triggered by tissue thromboplastin (formula 1).

Finally, the fibrinolytic system must be briefly considered. Fibrinolysis is the major physiologic means for disposal of fibrin after its hemostatic function has been fulfilled. The mechanism of fibrinolysis is schematically summarized by formulas 7 and 8:

$$(7) \quad \begin{array}{l} \text{plasminogen} \\ \text{fibrin} \\ \text{fibrinogen} \end{array} \xrightarrow{\text{activators}} \text{plasmin}$$

$$(8) \quad \begin{array}{l} \text{complement} \\ \text{factor VIII} \end{array} \xrightarrow{\text{plasmin}} \text{degradation products}$$

Plasminogen is a β-globulin with a molecular mass of 81 kD. It circulates in the plasma in concentrations of 10 to 20 mg/dL. It is activated by a heterogeneous group of substances termed "plasminogen activators" (formula 7). Activators reside within the lysozyme of most cells, and urokinase and streptokinase are examples of specifically identified activators. The activated

TABLE 47-11. SCREENING COAGULATION TESTS

Study	Measures	Normal Values
Bleeding time	Platelets and vascular integrity	1–5 minutes (Ivy)
Platelet count	Number of platelets	$140–440 \times 10^3/mm^3$
Partial thromboplastin time	II, V, VIII, IX, X, XI	24–36 seconds
Prothrombin time	II, V, VII, X	11–12 seconds
Thrombin time	I, II, circulating split products, heparin	16–20 seconds
Plasma fibrinogen	II (fibrinogen)	175–433 mg/dL
Fibrin D-dimer	Fibrin degradation	<0.05 μg/mL

form of plasminogen, plasmin, is a proteolytic enzyme with a wide spectrum of activity. It cleaves arginyl-lysine bonds in a large variety of substrates, including fibrinogen, fibrin, factor VIII, and various components of complement (formula 8). It has a very short life in plasma owing to its inactivation by humoral antiplasmins.

A number of plasma proteases also function as inhibitors of coagulation and fibrinolysis. They serve to control both the speed and extent of coagulation and fibrinolysis. The major inhibitor of the extrinsic phase is C1 inhibitor, which inactivates factor VIIa and kallikrein. The major inhibitor of the intrinsic phase is antithrombin III, which inhibits factor IXa, factor Xa, and thrombin. Other inhibitors are α_1-antitrypsin, α_2-macroglobulin, and α_2-antiplasmin. Protein C is also a potent inhibitor of coagulation. Activated protein C (with its cofactor, protein S) reacts with factors V and VIII to destroy their coagulation property.

Laboratory Methods for Study of Blood Coagulation

No single test is suitable as an overall laboratory screening study of hemostasis and blood coagulation. Commonly, the combination of bleeding time, platelet count, activated partial thromboplastin time (aPTT), prothrombin time (PT) or international normalized ratio, and thrombin time is used as a screening battery. Table 47-11 indicates which factors are measured by each study and shows the normal value for the study in question. A large number of additional studies define specific abnormalities of platelet function or allow measurement of a specific plasma clotting factor. The Rumpel-Leede test, platelet adhesiveness, platelet aggregation, whole blood prothrombin activation rate, and clot retraction are all examples of studies that further define abnormalities of platelet function.

Precise levels of each circulating plasma factor can be determined by either the thromboplastin generation test or cross-correction studies with normal plasma and plasma known to be deficient in the factor being assayed. A specific assay for factor XIII is also available. Several accurate methods are available for the quantitative assay of plasma fibrinogen. Normal values range from 175 to 430 mg/dL. Values are abnormal in acquired hypofibrinogenemia secondary to DIC and in the hereditary afibrinogenemias and dysfibrinogenemias.

Studies used in the evaluation of fibrinolysis include the euglobulin clot lysis time and the demonstration of fibrin-fibrinogen degradation products by a variety of techniques. The *D-dimer study* is specific for identifying fibrinolysis in contrast to fibrinogenolysis. It is important to remember that the screening coagulation studies do not provide a specific etiologic diagnosis. Such a diagnosis is important in that it is necessary for optimal treatment of excessive bleeding, should it occur during surgery. Furthermore, the presence of an adequate coagulation screen in a patient suspected of having a coagulation abnormality does not diminish the necessity of pursuing a specific diagnosis and making available specific therapy, if it is needed.

Several extensive reviews indicate that the utility of the bleeding time has not been enhanced by standardization of the method, that there is no clinically useful correlation between the bleeding time and platelet count in thrombocytopenic individuals, and that no evidence exists that the bleeding time is a predictor of the risk of either spontaneous or surgically induced hemorrhage (Rodgers and Levin, 1990; Lind, 1991). Therefore, bleeding time is no longer commonly used.

Diagnosis and Treatment of Specific Coagulation Disorders

Acquired disorders of coagulation are far more common than congenital ones, and those seen most frequently include idiopathic thrombocytopenic purpura (ITP), DIC, liver disease, and anticoagulant therapy. The congenital disorders seen most frequently are von Willebrand's disease and factor XI deficiency.

Platelet Disorders

Thrombocytopenia, the most common platelet disorder, is due to either diminished production or increased destruction of platelets. The severity of bleeding is roughly proportional to the degree to which the platelet count has been lowered. A specific diagnosis is obviously essential for the proper total management of a patient with thrombocytopenia. However, when hemorrhage is due to thrombocytopenia, platelet transfusions are frequently of value (Cash, 1972). The success of platelet transfusion therapy depends on the functional integrity of the transfused platelets, the underlying cause of the platelet defect in the recipient, and the presence and level of antiplatelet antibodies. Platelet transfusions are available both as platelet-rich plasma and as platelet concentrates. When platelet concentrates are used, a relatively large number of platelets remain in the bag and can be harvested by adding a small amount of normal saline solution after evacuation of each bag to resuspend platelets remaining in the bag. One can expect an increase in platelet count of 5 to 10×10^9 per liter per unit of platelets transfused. The exact incremental rise and the length of platelet survival depend on both the underlying disease process and the freshness of the platelets.

The complications of platelet transfusion are less common and less serious than are those accompanying transfusion of whole blood. They include bacterial contamination, infectious hepatitis, febrile transfusion reaction, and posttransfusion purpura. However, platelets are usually transfused as random donor components; thus multiple donors are utilized with each set of platelets.

GESTATIONAL THROMBOCYTOPENIA

Approximately 7% of women at delivery have thrombocytopenia, defined as a platelet count below 150,000/mm³ (Burrows and Kelton, 1993). In a study by these authors, the most common cause of maternal thrombocytopenia was incidental or gestational thrombocytopenia, accounting for 74% of thrombocytopenic patients. Hypertensive disorders of pregnancy were associated with 21%, and immune disorders, including ITP, accounted for only 3% of the thrombocytopenic patients (Burrows and Kelton, 1993). Gestational thrombocytopenia was defined as thrombocytopenia unassociated with underlying medical disorders, not known to precede pregnancy, and resolved postpartum. Only one infant born to the women with gestational thrombocytopenia had thrombocytopenia, and that infant also had Down syndrome and congenital marrow dysfunction.

The diagnosis of gestational thrombocytopenia is made by ruling out preeclampsia and underlying medical disease and making sure that the patient is not taking any medications associated with thrombocytopenia. Resolution postpartum confirms the diagnosis. Platelet-associated IgG is not specific enough to confirm or refute a diagnosis of gestational thrombocytopenia. Women with gestational thrombocytopenia can have platelet antibodies, and women with ITP may not have platelet antibodies (Lescale, 1996; Clark and Gall, 1997). Because gestational thrombocytopenia is not associated with maternal or neonatal morbidity, these women should receive routine prenatal care and delivery (Burrows and Kelton, 1993; Sullivan and Martin, 1995). Boehlen and colleagues (2000) reported that 97%, 90%, and 47% of thrombocytopenic women with platelets above 115,000, between 75,000 and 115,000, and below 75,000, respectively, had gestational thrombocytopenia. They recommended that if the platelets were above 115,000, and the woman had no significant history and no preeclampsia, no other workup was necessary.

IDIOPATHIC THROMBOCYTOPENIC PURPURA

Also called *isoimmune thrombocytopenic purpura*, ITP is an autoimmune disorder in which platelet destruction is caused by an antiplatelet antibody of the reticuloendothelial system. The antibody is usually of the IgG class and is directed against a platelet-associated antigen. Although the spleen is usually the major site of antibody production, bone marrow cells also synthesize antiplatelet IgG (Cines and Blanchette, 2002).

In most patients with ITP, the level of platelet-associated IgG is increased, and an inverse relationship exists between platelet-associated-IgG level and platelet count. Another group of patients has activated complement C3, causing elevated levels of both C3 and platelet-associated IgG. A third group of patients, constituting 10% to 30% of cases of ITP, has normal levels of platelet-associated IgG but elevated levels of platelet-associated C3.

Both direct and indirect techniques are available for measuring antiplatelet antibodies (Cines et al., 1982). In the *direct* technique, the patient's platelets are incubated with ^{125}I-labeled anti-IgG, and the platelet-associated radioactivity is measured after washing. This test is equivalent to the direct Coombs test for detecting RBC antigen-antibody complexes. In the *indirect* test, normal platelets are incubated with the patient's plasma and washed, and the radioactivity is then measured as in the direct technique. This study is analogous to the indirect Coombs test. Samuels and associates (1990) have reported a correlation between the level of indirect antibody and the fetal platelet count.

The diagnosis is one of exclusion and is made according to established criteria (Cines and Blanchette, 2002) that include the following:

- Normal blood count, except for thrombocytopenia
- Bone marrow with increased size and number of megalokaryocytes
- A blood smear showing an increased percentage of large platelets
- Normal coagulation studies
- No other obvious cause of thrombocytopenia

The incidence of ITP in pregnancy is less than 1% (Burrows and Kelton, 1993). The goal of treatment for patients with ITP is remission, not cure, and the overall management of pregnant women with this disorder should be similar to that of nonpregnant patients. Thus, therapy is stepwise: corticosteroids, then splenectomy, and then consideration of immunosuppressive therapy or plasmapheresis. Each step is determined by the severity of the clinical situation. The starting dose of prednisone is 1 mg/kg, and the usual goal is to keep the platelet count above 30,000 (Cines and Blanchette, 2002). If an adequate response to corticosteroids is not achieved, splenectomy is indicated and should be performed, if possible, during the middle trimester. Corticosteroids have been used for the last 30 years and owe their effectiveness to both an immunosuppressive effect and a slowing in the rate of platelet destruction by the reticuloendothelial system. By themselves, corticosteroids produce a transient remission in 75% of cases in adults but a sustained remission in only 14% to 33% of cases. More recently, immunosuppression with high-dose serum immune globulin has been found to be useful, and this option now is often used during pregnancy before splenectomy is considered (Clark and Gall, 1997). Other agents include danazol, cyclophosphamide, azathioprine, vincristine, and vinblastine, all of which are relatively contraindicated in pregnancy (Brunskill, 1992; Cines and Blanchette, 2002).

The historical controversy about the route of delivery for fetuses of mothers with ITP was based on faulty assumptions that the likelihood of severe neonatal thrombocytopenia was high, the likelihood of neonatal bleeding with thrombocytopenia was high, and cesarean section prevented neonatal bleeding. These beliefs led to recommendation of multiple interventions to prevent neonatal hemorrhage, including cesarean section for all women with ITP and fetal scalp samples or cordocentesis for fetal platelet counts. Several reports have indicated that there is little morbidity related to neonatal thrombocytopenia associated with maternal ITP (Kagan and Laros, 1983; Burrows and Kelton, 1990, 1993; Payne et al.,

1997). Burrows and Kelton (1990, 1993) reported that only 6% of neonates born to mothers with ITP had a platelet count below 50,000, and none of these infants had significant morbidity related to thrombocytopenia. One paper estimated the rate of ITP attributable neonatal intracranial hemorrhage to be 2 per 100,000 births (Rouse et al., 1998). Further, maternal platelet count, presence of platelet-associated IgG, and maternal treatment for thrombocytopenia did not predict neonatal platelet count (Kelton et al., 1982; Burrows and Kelton, 1990; Samuels et al., 1990; Payne et al., 1997).

In addition, there is no evidence that cesarean section offers benefits to a thrombocytopenic infant (Kagan and Laros, 1983; Cook et al., 1991; Silver et al., 1995). Of 134 infants delivered vaginally, 28 (21%) had counts below 30 x 10^9/liter, but only 1 had intracerebral bleeding (Kagan and Laros, 1983). By contrast, of the 31 infants born by cesarean section, 9 (29%) had platelets below 30 x 10^9/liter. Three serious hemorrhages occurred, including one intracranial hemorrhage at 3 days of age. These data do not support the premise that delivery by cesarean section is beneficial for thrombocytopenic infants of women with ITP. Finally, fetal platelet count by fetal scalp sample does not correlate well with actual fetal platelet count. There was only a 50% positive predictive value for fetal platelet count less than 50,000 by fetal scalp sample—equivalent to flipping a coin (Payne et al., 1997).

These data suggesting that neonatal thrombocytopenia resulting from maternal ITP is not associated with significant neonatal morbidity, that there are no reliable predictors of neonatal platelet count, and that cesarean delivery is of no proven benefit in preventing neonatal bleeding form the basis on which two studies recommended discontinuing invasive procedures, namely, cordocentesis, fetal scalp sampling, and prophylactic cesarean delivery, in the management of maternal ITP (Silver et al., 1995; Payne et al., 1997).

There are multiple reports of epidural anesthetic use in patients with platelets below 100 x 10^9/liter without any neurologic sequelae (Rolbin et al., 1988; Hew-Wing et al., 1989; Beilin et al., 1997). However, there is ongoing controversy concerning the lowest safe platelet count for epidural use. It is likely somewhere between 50,000 and 100,000 per cubic millimeter (Hew-Wing et al., 1989; Beilin et al., 1997). One source concluded that "the current belief, that epidural anesthesia is contraindicated in patients whose platelet counts are below 100 x 10^9 per liter, has no supporting data" (Hew-Wing et al., 1989). Certainly, an epidural should only be considered in women with thrombocytopenia if the platelet count is stable, the PT and PTT (partial thromboplastin time) and fibrinogen are normal, and there are no signs of abnormal bleeding.

NEONATAL ALLOIMMUNE THROMBOCYTOPENIA

Unlike ITP-associated thrombocytopenia, neonatal alloimmune thrombocytopenia carries significant morbidity, including intracranial hemorrhage. This is a disorder of the fetus, not of the mother. It is the platelet analog of Rh disease of the newborn; the mother mounts an immune response to platelet antigens present in the fetus, and the antibody crosses the placenta and attacks fetal platelets. Although fetomaternal incompatibility with ABO, human leukocyte antigen class I, and platelet-specific antigens on the platelet surface is possible, most cases are the result of antibodies directed against the platelet-specific antigens Zw (Pl^A), Pl^E, Bak, Yuk, Br, and DUZO.

The frequency of the disorder is only 1 or 2 per 10,000 births, and it is virtually never anticipated until a mother has an affected infant (Taaning and Skibsted, 1990). In more than 50% of cases, neonatal alloimmune thrombocytopenia occurs in a first pregnancy; recurrence risk is above 80% (Muller, 1988). Unfortunately, antepartum serum studies do not predict severity, but in subsequent affected children the disorder can be as severe as or more severe than the index case. The major threat to the fetus is from intracranial hemorrhage, which can occur before, during, or after labor and delivery.

The diagnosis is made by demonstrating maternal-paternal platelet antigen incompatibility, the presence of antiplatelet antibody in maternal serum, and platelet-bound antibody on the platelets of the fetus or newborn. Fetal antigen type and platelet count can be obtained by fetal cordocentesis as early as 20 weeks' gestation. If significant thrombocytopenia exists, transfusion with irradiated maternal platelets is performed (Daffos et al., 1984). However, there is significant risk of fetal exsanguination with cordocentesis in fetuses with alloimmune thrombocytopenia, suggesting that these procedures be performed only when platelets are available and by those with experience with this technique and disorder (Paidas et al., 1995).

Intravenous γ-globulin with and without steroids has been advocated for antepartum management to increase fetal platelet count and decrease the risk of severe fetal hemorrhage (Bussel et al., 1988, 1996). A randomized trial of women with alloimmune thrombocytopenia and documented fetal thrombocytopenia comparing intravenous γ-globulin alone to intravenous γ-globulin with dexamethasone found no benefit of dexamethasone (Bussel et al., 1996). There were no intracranial hemorrhages in either group, and 74% responded with increased fetal platelet counts. Cesarean section was performed unless the fetal platelet count was 50,000 x 10^9 per liter shortly before delivery (Bussel et al., 1996). After birth, either platelet or exchange transfusion with maternal blood is effective treatment (McIntosh et al., 1973). The fetal platelet count should be sampled by percutaneous fetal blood sampling before either vaginal or cesarean delivery. Sia and associates (1985) reported two cases of intracranial hemorrhage despite delivery by cesarean section.

TRANSFUSION-INDUCED THROMBOCYTOPENIA

Thrombocytopenia may be induced by blood transfusion by one of two mechanisms. The first is simply dilutional and may occur in any patient who rapidly receives large volumes of RBCs or stored whole blood (6 units or more) for replacement in a major hemorrhage. Addition of platelet concentrates to the replacement fluids is the treatment of choice if correction must be made promptly. Megakaryocytic hyperplasia and the appearance of newly produced endogenous platelets follow the acute thrombocytopenia if the marrow reacts normally.

A second rare type of transfusion-related thrombocytopenia may occur in women who were previously sensitized by transfusion or pregnancy to naturally occurring platelet antigens. After this sensitization, the patients demonstrate abrupt onset of severe thrombocytopenia and purpura about 10 days after receiving subsequent transfusion of even a single unit of RBCs, whole blood, or plasma. Exchange transfusion has been dramatically effective in two reported cases (Shulman et al., 1961; Cimo and Aster, 1972).

FUNCTIONAL PLATELET DEFECTS

Functional platelet defects are far less common than quantitative disorders. Primary hemostasis is normally accomplished by the interaction of vasoconstriction, endothelial cell reaction to injury, and a series of biochemical events involving platelets that promote adhesion and aggregation, with the formation of the initial hemostatic platelet plug. Normal platelets also contribute significantly to the initiation of blood coagulation and thus the formation of fibrin, and they are necessary for clot retraction. Platelet prostaglandin cyclooxygenase plays a key role in the generation of the intermediate cyclic endoperoxides, which are converted into the active thromboxanes and prostaglandins important in the initiation and modulation of the platelet-release reaction, the process by which a variety of biologically active substances stored in platelet granules and dense bodies are extruded from the platelet to participate in the ongoing hemostatic and coagulation process.

Bleeding may occur because of acquired or congenital abnormalities of platelet function. Except for the platelet defect seen in von Willebrand's disease, the recognized hereditary disorders are rare and beyond the scope of this text; Weiss (1980) has provided a comprehensive review. On the other hand, acquired platelet dysfunction is a common occurrence because it can be produced by a great many biologically active compounds and may accompany a wide variety of disorders. Such disorders, which include uremia, myeloproliferative syndromes, and cyanotic congenital heart disease, are themselves unusual in pregnancy, but drug-induced platelet abnormalities may be responsible for mild bleeding manifestations in many pregnant women and may create more serious problems in those whose hemostatic and clotting mechanisms are already compromised by thrombocytopenia, the use of anticoagulants, or the presence of some other coagulation defect.

Of the drugs in common use that have a significant effect on platelet function, aspirin is the most important because of its ubiquity and the duration of its effect. Aspirin inhibits the platelet-release reaction by acetylating platelet cyclooxygenase; this effect persists in the platelet for the remainder of its life span and results in prolongation of bleeding time and deficient platelet aggregation in the presence of collagen. Patients taking aspirin may note increased bruisability and minor bleeding symptoms, manifestations that persist for several days following a single dose. Ordinarily, these symptoms are inconsequential; during pregnancy and especially at term, however, hemorrhagic complications can be of more than trivial importance. Normal pregnant women given usual doses of aspirin within 10 days of delivery undergo increased intrapartum or postpartum blood loss, and their infants sustain a higher incidence of hemostatic abnormalities than do control maternal-neonatal pairs (Stuart et al., 1982). Low doses of aspirin (60 to 80 mg) in studies to prevent preeclampsia have not appeared to cause hemostatic problems, and large studies of this issue are under way.

Most other nonsteroidal anti-inflammatory agents inhibit prostaglandin synthesis and have been shown to affect platelet function. In general, they are less powerful and shorter-acting antagonists than aspirin, but they should be avoided in pregnancy except for extraordinary indications. Acetaminophen is a safe antipyretic from the standpoint of platelet function; the choice of an analgesic that is safe in pregnancy must be made on an individual basis.

Several antimicrobial agents impair platelet aggregation and the release reaction. In general, these effects have been of no clinical significance, but carbenicillin has been reported to be responsible for serious hemorrhage. Numerous other classes of drugs, when tested, have demonstrated at least in vitro effects on platelet activity. One of importance, because it is commonly included in over-the-counter cough and cold remedies, is glyceryl guaiacolate. Pregnant women should be warned to avoid preparations containing this compound.

The diagnostic hallmark of platelet dysfunction is a significantly prolonged template bleeding time. Devices for performing the Ivy bleeding time test by the template technique are readily available commercially and provide reasonably reproducible results in the hands of experienced operators. Prolonged bleeding times may be seen in thrombocytopenic states (platelet counts below 100×10^9/liter) and most cases of von Willebrand's disease. The differential diagnosis among these three entities is generally readily accomplished.

Drug-induced disorders of platelet function are best managed prophylactically; medications influencing platelet activity should be used with great care in pregnancy and only for compelling reasons. If they are employed and serious bleeding ensues, however, platelet transfusion is generally beneficial in controlling the hemorrhage. Heparin and quinidine are examples of drugs known to be occasionally associated with thrombocytopenia.

Acquired and Congenital Plasma Factor Disorders

VON WILLEBRAND'S DISEASE

Von Willebrand's disease, inherited as an autosomal-dominant trait, is characterized by abnormal bleeding of varying severity. The disease has multiple subtypes, all of which involve a reduction, a qualitative abnormality, or both, of von Willebrand factor vWF. vWF is necessary for platelet adhesion and platelet aggregation, so an abnormal quantity or quality of vWF causes bleeding by impairing blood clotting or platelet adhesion (Batlle et al., 1997). There are three general types of the disease: type 1 is a partial quantitative deficiency; type 2 is a qualitative deficiency, and type 3 is a complete deficiency of vWF. The pathophysiologic basis for the disease is a marked decrease or absence of both clottable and antigenic factor VIII. Criteria for laboratory diagnosis are complex, and the reader is referred to an excellent review (Batlle et al., 1997). Von Willebrand's disease type 1 is difficult to diagnosis definitively, whereas types 2 and 3 are easier to diagnose. Type 1 is the most common and usually involves similar decreases in vWF antigen, ristocetin cofactor, and factor VIII; vWF monomers are present. Type 2 has multiple subtypes, all of which involve prolonged bleeding time, decreased ristocetin cofactor, absence of large functional multimers of vWF, and normal to slightly decreased VIII:C and VIII antigen. Type 3 is autosomal recessive and features absence of factor VIII:C, factor VIII antigen, and ristocetin cofactor activity. Factor VIII coagulant activity to factor VIII antigen will have a ratio of 1:1. (The factor VIII level should be checked periodically during the antenatal course, with pretreatment reserved for patients with levels below 25% of normal.)

DDAVP (1-deamino-8-D-argenine-vasopressin) should be used instead of cryoprecipitate for cases known to be responsive (type I and some IIa). Treatment is begun when the patient presents in labor. The dose is 0.3 µg/kg of DDAVP given over 30 minutes, with the total dose not to exceed 25 µg. Treatment is repeated every 12 hours with infusions being progressively less effective.

The specific treatment of serious hemorrhagic manifestations in patients who are not responsive to DDAVP is cryoprecipitate or fresh frozen plasma. Serious bleeding (and thus treatment) is rare if the factor VIII level is higher than 25% of normal or the bleeding time is under 15 minutes. If cesarean delivery is required for obstetric reasons, treatment is indicated if the level is below 40%. Cryoprecipitate is given in an initial dose of 24 to 36 units/kg (0.24 to 0.39 bags/kg), followed by half of this amount every 12 hours for 3 to 8 days. If possible, treatment should be started 24 hours preoperatively to allow new factor VIII synthesis in addition to the elevation obtained from the therapeutic material.

When unanticipated acute bleeding is encountered or immediate cesarean section planned, the initial therapeutic dose should be increased by approximately 50%, and a second dose should be given approximately 12 hours later (Shulman, 1967). Levels should be checked daily after vaginal delivery or cesarean section, with therapy given if the level falls below 25% or bleeding occurs (Noller et al., 1973; Krishanamurth and Miotti, 1977; Lipton et al., 1982; Cohen and Goldiner, 1989). The various glycine-precipitated antihemophilic factors available for treatment of classic hemophilia should not be used. Although they are effective in raising factor VIII levels, they do not correct the bleeding time, the ristocetin platelet aggregation defect, or, in fact, the clinical bleeding.

Pregnancies in women with von Willebrand's disease should be managed normally and the delivery route determined by the usual obstetric indications. Burlingame and colleagues (2001) reported six pregnancies in two women with von Willebrand's disease type 2 managed with cryoprecipitate, alphanate and/or platelet transfusions. All delivered vaginally without maternal or neonatal complications.

HEMOPHILIA A (FACTOR VIII DEFICIENCY) AND HEMOPHILIA B (FACTOR IX DEFICIENCY)

Hemophilia A and B are transmitted as sex-linked recessive traits. Therefore, severe genetically determined disease is unlikely to occur in pregnant women. The heterozygous carrier of factor VIII or IX deficiency is usually free of bleeding manifestations. Occasionally, carriers whose normal X chromosome has been inactivated in early fetal life may have unusually low levels of factor VIII or IX (Lusher and McMillan, 1978). They may be troubled with menorrhagia (usually responsive to oral contraceptives) and even hemarthroses, but pregnancy and delivery are usually free of serious hemorrhage. Successful treatment for bleeding in the factor VIII–deficient woman has been accomplished with the administration of cryoprecipitate or factor VIII concentrate. Individuals with factor IX deficiency have received fresh frozen plasma or factor IX concentrate for bleeding or surgery.

Sons born to hemophilia A or B carriers have a 50% chance of being affected with the disease. Carrier detection in hemophilia A, employing the techniques of procoagulant and antigenic assay for factor VIII and pedigree analysis, is reliable even during pregnancy (Hoyer, 1994). Prenatal diagnosis of hemophilia can be accomplished by DNA analysis from either chorionic villus sampling or amniocytes (Hoyer, 1994). Intrauterine detection of hemophilia is being accomplished in a few laboratories (Alter, 1984; Weatherall, 1985; White and Shoemaker, 1989), either using a specific DNA probe or taking advantage of restriction-fragment length polymorphism linked to the factor VIII gene. Affected sons born to carriers experience remarkably little bleeding during vaginal delivery, but there are anecdotal reports of massive cephalohematomas in such infants subjected to fetal scalp monitoring during labor. The presence or absence of the disease in newborn males can generally be established by simultaneous assays of maternal and cord blood. Factors VIII and IX do not cross the placenta.

Most female carriers for hemophilia B have no clinical manifestations, but carriers with levels as low as 10% have been reported (Lusher and McMillan, 1978). Women with low levels are at risk for intrapartum and postpartum bleeding and should be given factor IX concentrate if their factor IX level is less than 25% at term (Rust et al., 1975). The appropriate dose of factor IX is 50 units/kg, which usually calculates to 2500 to 3000 units as an initial dose, followed by 1500 units every 12 to 24 hours. The half-life of factor IX varies in individual patients, and the dosage schedule should be modified based on analysis of each patient's factor IX level after transfusion.

Carrier detection for factor IX relies on coagulation assay for factor IX, and carriers have a broad overlap with the normal range. Prenatal diagnosis of fetuses at risk is difficult. Direct fetal blood sampling may be contaminated by factor IX activity in amniotic fluid, and most families do not have a revealing polymorphism (Miller and Hoyer, 1986).

ANTIBODIES TO FACTOR VIII

Antibodies to factor VIII produce hemorrhagic disease. The onset is usually in the postpartum period and can be very dramatic, as illustrated by a recent case report (Shobeiri et al., 2000). In this case the patient was eventually treated with activated prothrombin complex concentrate after hysterectomy, over 50 units of blood products, hypogastric artery ligation, several additional surgeries, and iliac artery embolization, all over a 55-day stay in the hospital. The disorder is caused by the spontaneous development of an inhibitor to factor VIII. The pathogenesis of the disorder is unknown. The inhibitor is an immunoglobulin, usually an IgG but occasionally an IgM. Polyclonal inhibitors have been described.

The clinical manifestations mimic those seen in hemophilia A, with soft-tissue bleeding and even hemarthroses after minimal trauma. A prolonged aPTT that is not corrected by addition of normal plasma after incubation of the mixture is characteristic. All other screening coagulation studies are normal, but the level of factor VIII is low when specific assays are carried out. The natural history of the illness is one of gradual disappearance of the inhibitor over time. The clinical course in patients with spontaneously occurring factor VIII inhibitors can often be modified by the use of prednisone. The infant of an affected mother is rarely affected, and subsequent pregnancies (when they have occurred) have usually not been marred by recurrence of the inhibitor (Coller et al., 1981).

FACTOR X DEFICIENCY

Factor X deficiency is a rare autosomal-recessive bleeding disorder recently described in pregnancy (Konje et al., 1994; Bofill et al., 1996). Factor X levels increase in pregnancy, and the two patients described were managed with fresh frozen plasma and/or factor IXA transfusions for bleeding episodes and prophylactically for delivery. One patient had a vaginal delivery, and one underwent cesarean delivery.

FACTOR XI DEFICIENCY

Also called *plasma thromboplastin antecedent deficiency*, this hereditary disorder is transmitted as an incompletely recessive-autosomal trait manifested either as a major defect in homozygous individuals, with factor XI levels below 20%, or as a minor defect in heterozygous individuals, with levels ranging from 30% to 65% of normal (Leiba et al., 1965). However, severity of bleeding does not always correlate with the level of factor XI (Purcell and Nossel, 1970; Rimon et al., 1976). The aPTT is usually prolonged in individuals with factor XI deficiency, and the specific diagnosis is confirmed when the factor XI level is shown to be below 65% of normal.

Even though factor XI levels normally decrease during pregnancy (Phillips et al., 1973), most gravidas do not encounter bleeding problems. In one series, nine women went through 17 pregnancies without a major hemorrhage (Rapaport et al., 1961). Therapy is based on maintaining the factor XI level above 40% for minor procedures (including delivery) and above 50% for major procedures. Treatment consists of fresh frozen plasma in a loading dose of 10 mL/kg, followed by a maintenance dose of 5 mL/kg/day.

FACTOR XIII DEFICIENCY

Probably transmitted as an autosomal-recessive trait, factor XIII deficiency is extremely rare. It is included in this discussion primarily because two manifestations of the disorder are especially pertinent to any consideration of hematologic problems in obstetrics (Kitchens and Newcomb, 1979; Lorand et al., 1980), First, persistent, even fatal, bleeding from the umbilical stump has been reported as a common event in infants affected by the disorder. Second, affected women experience a very high incidence of spontaneous abortion.

Other clinical manifestations include intracranial bleeding after trivial trauma (an incidence of 30% is reported in some series—much higher than that observed in most coagulation defects) and defective wound healing. The diagnosis is established by demonstrated dissolution of the clot in 5 molar urea; results of all other commonly employed coagulation tests are normal.

Successful results of replacement therapy with fresh and stored plasma, whole blood, and cryoprecipitate have all been reported. Levels adequate for normal hemostasis are low, and transfusion of small amounts of normal plasma given infrequently has served as adequate therapy or prophylaxis. Fisher and colleagues (1966) reported a successful outcome for one woman who received 300 ml of plasma every 10 days during her pregnancy.

LIVER DISEASE

Virtually every hemostatic function may be impaired in liver disease. Deficiencies of prothrombin and of factors VII, IX, and X generally result from decreased synthesis by the damaged liver. Factor V and fibrinogen are also synthesized by the liver; however, their levels are usually not as severely depressed. The diversity of the coagulation abnormality is reflected in the laboratory studies by abnormalities in the aPTT, PT, and fibrinogen levels and by abnormal fibrinolysis. The international normalized ratio, another common test, is similar to the PT but is a calculated index of degree of anticoagulation utilizing the patient's PT and the mean value of a normal control. A value of 1 is normal.

Treatment consists of both vitamin K and procoagulant replacement therapy. Vitamin K can be administered as vitamin K_1 in a dose of 50 mg intramuscularly; the vitamin produces improvement in approximately 30% of patients with liver disease. Replacement therapy is accomplished with fresh frozen plasma in a dose of 10 to 20 mL/kg (Spector and Corn, 1967).

DISSEMINATED INTRAVASCULAR COAGULATION

DIC is a syndrome produced as part of an underlying disease that in some way leads to initiation of the clotting mechanisms (Laros, 1986). In the area of obstetrics and gynecology, DIC is seen in association with placental abruption (Colman et al., 1987), dead fetus syndrome (Sutton et al., 1971), amniotic fluid embolism (Phillips et al., 1964), gram-negative sepsis (Phillips and Davidson, 1972), saline abortions (Phillips et al., 1967; Laros and Penner, 1976), and severe preeclampsia-eclampsia (Pritchard et al., 1976; Bick, 2000).

The first effect of DIC is a disturbance of the coagulation mechanism. This results from the consumption of plasma factors and from the production of anticoagulants by the fibrinolytic system. The coagulation factors consumed are platelets, fibrinogen, prothrombin, factor V, and factor VIII. The body has a limited capacity to produce circulating plasma factors and platelets necessary for clot formation. When the available plasma factors are consumed by intravascular coagulation, the circulating blood becomes deficient in clotting factors. Without sufficient clotting factors, a severe bleeding diathesis may result. Activation of the fibrinolytic system produces fibrin degradation products. These split products serve to interfere further with the coagulation mechanism. The pathophysiology of DIC is summarized in Figure 47-4.

The second major result of DIC is the presence of small clots in the microcirculation. These clots can cause plugging of small vessels and ischemia of various organs. DIC occurs when the coagulation mechanism is inappropriately triggered by any of several underlying disease processes that have in common the ability to disrupt the normal coagulation mechanism.

Disease entities associated with DIC are classified into three major groups according to the mechanisms by which the

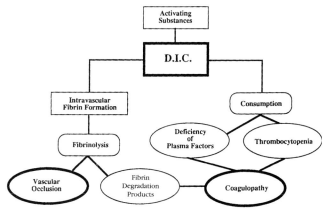

FIGURE 47-4 ■ Pathophysiology of disseminated intravascular coagulation (DIC).

primary disease initiates intravascular clotting. In the first group, the underlying mechanism is the intravascular infusion of thromboplastic substances, tissue thromboplastins that activate the extrinsic coagulation system. Placental abruption and the dead fetus syndrome fall into this category. With abruption, consumption is rapid and fulminant; with the dead fetus syndrome, consumption takes place slowly, occurring over a period of weeks.

The second group of pathologic conditions causing DIC includes conditions associated with endothelial damage. Both the extrinsic and the intrinsic coagulation systems are activated by endothelial damage. Eclampsia-preeclampsia is thought to fall into this category. Several prospective studies have documented subclinical changes including HELLP syndrome in the coagulation system of patients with eclampsia-preeclampsia. However, the specific changes noted and the frequency of the changes have varied widely (Kitzmiller et al., 1974; Pritchard et al., 1976; Weiner and Brandt, 1982; Stubbs et al., 1984; Weenink et al., 1984; Kelton et al., 1985; Socol et al., 1985; Weinstein, 1985). Table 47-12 compares findings in the various syndromes having thrombocytopenia and RBC fragmentation in common.

The third group of conditions associated with DIC encompasses nonspecific or indirect effects of certain diseases. This group includes amniotic fluid embolism, gram-negative sepsis, and saline abortions.

Signs and symptoms are basically those of the underlying disease. The clinical presentation may be hemorrhagic, thrombotic, or both. With acute presentation, hemorrhagic problems predominate, whereas in more indolent presentations, thrombotic problems predominate. Hemorrhagic presentations of DIC involving the skin or mucous membranes include ecchymoses, petechiae, epistaxis, gingival bleeding, hematuria, gastrointestinal bleeding, and venipuncture oozing. Intracranial or intracerebral bleeding is another possible hemorrhagic manifestation. Thrombotic presentations of DIC may be neurologic—as seen in multifocal lesions, delirium, and coma—or dermatologic, with focal ischemia and superficial gangrene. Renal examples of thrombotic presentation are cortical necrosis and uremia. Acute ulceration with bleeding is an example of a gastrointestinal thrombotic presentation. Infarcts and emboli represent pulmonary vascular obstruction, whereas phlebitis and peripheral gangrene are results of thrombotic effects within peripheral veins and arteries.

The laboratory diagnosis of DIC can be relatively easy. All the routine screening tests of coagulation yield grossly abnormal results. The platelet count is almost always decreased or falls progressively, fibrinogen is low (usually below 200 in pregnancy), and circulating fibrin degradation products are increased. The PT and aPTT may be normal, prolonged, or shortened. The shortening occurs early in the progression of the syndrome, when excess amounts of activated factor V and X are in circulation, but before much consumption of these factors has occurred and before the level of fibrin degradation products with their antithrombin properties has increased, leading to prolongation of the PT and aPTT. Indirect evidence of an obstructed microcirculation can be found by examining a peripheral blood smear. As normal RBCs are forced through the obstructed capillary beds, they tend to fragment. Bizarre cell forms called *schistocytes* and *helmet cells* are formed and can readily be identified. If the rate of RBC destruction is brisk, the patient may show evidence of intravascular hemolysis by the appearance of an elevated plasma Hgb level and hemoglobinuria.

The most important step in treating DIC is recognition and treatment of the underlying disease process. Bleeding poses the greatest threat to the patient with DIC, and administration of procoagulants is essential. Platelets are administered as platelet concentrates. The clotting factors may be replaced with fresh frozen plasma. Factor VIII and fibrinogen may be replaced with cryoprecipitate. Appropriate doses are 10 to 20 mL/kg of fresh frozen plasma or 0.1 to 0.2 bags/kg.

Heparin is rarely required in the treatment of DIC but should be considered when there is evidence of progressive renal dysfunction, gangrene of the digits, or other special circumstances. Heparin is administered in a dose of 500 to 1000 units per hour intravenously following a loading dose of 5000 units. Laboratory control of heparin therapy may be difficult; however, unless the fibrinogen level is very low, an adequate end point (thrombin time or aPTT increased to approximately 1.5 times the control value) can usually be attained. Platelet transfusions are particularly important if heparin is to be administered in the face of significant thrombocytopenia (below 30 x 10⁹/liter). Other authors prefer subcutaneous low-dose heparin (Bick, 2000) or antithrombin therapy instead of heparin therapy (Kobayashi et al., 2001). In most instances, if therapy other than delivery, control of bleeding, and product replacement is needed, a hematologist should be consulted.

Fortunately, in obstetric practice the diseases associated with DIC are usually cured by delivery. Therefore, specific treatment for the coagulopathy produced by DIC is also limited in scope. After delivery, the DIC is ameliorated and the coagulation abnormalities resolve. Because of the liver's immense capacity for protein synthesis, the plasma factors return to normal within 24 hours of cessation of DIC. The return of the platelet count to normal takes place slowly (5 to 7 days) because of the time required for generation, maturation, and release by the bone marrow.

THROMBOTIC THROMBOCYTOPENIC PURPURA

Thrombotic thrombocytopenic purpura (TTP) and hemolytic uremic syndrome (HUS) are both thrombotic microangiopathic diseases characterized by intravascular platelet

TABLE 47-12. SYNDROMES ASSOCIATED WITH THROMBOCYTOPENIA AND RED BLOOD CELL FRAGMENTATION

	Disease			
Findings	**PE/E***	**DIC***	**HUS***	**TTP***
Neurologic findings	±	±	±	+
Fever	−	±	±	+
Hypertension	+	±	+	±
Renal dysfunction	+	±	+	±
Thrombocytopenia	±	+	+	+
Hemolytic anemia	±	±	+	+
Elevated FDPs	±	+	±	±
Low fibrinogen	±	+	−	−

* +, usually present; ±, variably present; −, absent.

DIC, disseminated intravascular coagulation; FDP, fibrin degradation product; HUS, hemolytic uremic syndrome; PE/E, preeclampsia/eclampsia; TTP, thrombotic thrombocytopenic purpura.

aggregation causing transient ischemia (Esplin and Branch, 1999). Both involve thrombocytopenia and hemolytic anemia and can progress to multisystem organ failure. Clinically distinguishing them from each other can be difficult but may not be critical, since treatment is similar (Esplin and Branch, 1999). However, the two entities will be described below.

TTP usually presents with a pentad of clinical and laboratory manifestations: hemolytic anemia, thrombocytopenia, neurologic symptoms, renal abnormalities, and fever. It occurs in either sex and at any age but is most common in women in their 20s and 30s. Numerous variants have been described (acute, chronic, familial), and in some instances the clinical manifestations have appeared in association with other conditions (including neoplasia, connective tissue disorders, infection, pregnancy and the puerperium), but many cases remain idiopathic. The etiology of TTP is unknown. Several excellent comprehensive reviews are available (Bukowski, 1982; Esplin and Branch, 1999).

Presenting symptoms of TTP include abnormal bleeding (usually into skin and from mucous membranes; vaginal bleeding is also common); jaundice; neurologic symptoms (including cranial nerve palsies, headache, alterations of consciousness, paresis, organic brain syndromes, syncope, seizures, visual disturbance) that typically fluctuate in severity and may be transient; and fever. Classically, the neurologic symptoms are more common in TTP than in HUS. Noteworthy physical findings are pallor, jaundice, purpura, and neurologic abnormalities; splenic enlargement is unusual.

The peripheral blood is characteristic: moderate to severe thrombocytopenia, moderate to severe anemia with numerous fragmented erythrocytes, polychromatophilia (indicating a brisk reticulocytosis), and numerous nucleated RBCs are found together with a moderate polymorphonuclear leukocytosis. Half of the patients will have a platelet count below 20,000 (Esplin and Branch, 1999). The bone marrow shows intense normoblastic erythroid hyperplasia and an adequate-to-increased number of megakaryocytes. This hematologic appearance has been termed *microangiopathic hemolysis*, in reference to the fragmentation of RBCs within the microcirculation. The indirect serum bilirubin and the lactate dehydrogenase levels are elevated, and hematuria is commonly found. Elevations of blood urea nitrogen and creatinine, sometimes not found at first presentation, usually develop but seldom go beyond 100 mg/dL and 3 mg/dL, respectively. The Coombs antiglobulin reaction is almost invariably negative. The natural history of the disease is nearly always one of progressive deterioration, and survival beyond 3 months from onset is unusual unless therapy is successful.

At presentation, diagnostic considerations include lupus erythematosus, Evans syndrome, and sepsis (particularly *Clostridium perfringens* endometritis in young women with vaginal bleeding) together with DIC, but these conditions can usually be promptly excluded on clinical, immunologic, and bacteriologic grounds. As noted above, HUS presents a more difficult problem in differential diagnosis because microangiopathic hemolysis, thrombocytopenia, and renal failure are the hallmarks of this condition.

HEMOLYTIC UREMIC SYNDROME

Although HUS shares many of the clinical and laboratory features of TTP, it occurs primarily in children and produces a paucity of neurologic symptoms and a far greater degree of renal dysfunction. In nonpregnant adults, HUS is now often treated with plasma exchange, because the more benign course seen in young children and successfully treated with careful supportive measures (sometimes including dialysis) is less commonly observed in older patients. Studies without controls suggest that plasma exchange is often the key to beginning improvement in renal function and hematologic status. With the present state of our knowledge, acceptance of these reports makes diagnostic certainty between TTP and HUS less important. It is not known whether plasma exchange influences the course of HUS in postpartum patients. The three patients reviewed by Egerman and associates (1996) all received multiple units of fresh frozen plasma, and only one underwent plasmapheresis. Two of these women suffered from chronic renal disease requiring dialysis.

Features that help to distinguish the two disorders clinically are as follows:

- History of a viral or bacterial gastrointestinal illness, especially with diarrhea, is common in HUS but rare in TTP.
- Early, severe renal failure with oliguria, anuria, and hypertension is typical of HUS but is less common and less severe and appears later in TTP.
- HUS is predominantly a disease of childhood, although *bona fide* cases have been reported in adults of all ages as well as during pregnancy and the postpartum period (Segonds et al., 1979; Lazebnik et al., 1985).
- Bleeding and thrombocytopenia are generally more severe in TTP.
- Neurologic manifestations (except for alterations of consciousness and even seizures consistent with profound renal failure and hypertensive encephalopathy) are unusual in HUS.

None of these differential points can be considered absolute, but taken together they are helpful in making the distinction between the two conditions. Although the treatment of choice for both TTP and HUS today is plasmapheresis, the prognosis remains worse for HUS, which may be an important reason to attempt to distinguish between the two syndromes (Esplin and Branch, 1999).

Further compounding the diagnostic difficulties when microangiopathic hemolysis is recognized in pregnancy and the postpartum period is the observation that some women with severe toxemia or eclampsia are noted to have fragmentation hemolytic anemia, thrombocytopenia, and renal failure. In 1978, Schwartz and Brenner reviewed the reported cases of TTP in pregnancy. They concluded that in most instances, the diagnosis of TTP was in error and treatment for eclampsia should take precedence over that for TTP unless there is positive evidence that TTP either preceded pregnancy or occurred without evidence of toxemia. This review cites several eclamptic patients with microangiopathy who were successfully managed with the measures directed toward control of eclampsia. Treatments directed at control of TTP (with heparin, antiplatelet agents, dextrose, steroids, dialysis, and splenectomy, in various combinations) in many cases had disastrous results.

Case reports and reviews including case reports of 25 women with TTP or HUS during pregnancy suggested that for the best outcome, aggressive treatment with plasmapheresis is warranted (Egerman et al., 1996; Ezra et al., 1996; Dashe et al., 1998; Brostrom and Bergmann, 2000). However, despite aggressive treatment, there were four maternal deaths and at least two cases of chronic renal disease, underscoring the severity of TTP. Fetal and neonatal outcome was similarly poor, with a 38% perinatal mortality rate. Interestingly, Ezra and coworkers (1996) observed 16 pregnancies in 5 women with TTP and concluded that TTP tended to be recurrent; whether pregnancy affected outcome or recurrence rate was unclear. In another study, 50% of the women with TTP or HUS first diagnosed in pregnancy had a recurrence within 8 years of follow-up (Dashe et al, 1998). Although pregnancy is the most common condition associated with TTP, it is not clear whether pregnancy initiates or aggravates TTP, and thus it is not clear whether termination is useful in managing the condition (Elliot and Nichols, 2001).

Without treatment, TTP is fatal in nearly 90% of cases. Current treatment of TTP with or without pregnancy is plasmapheresis (Rock et al., 2000). It is proposed that the patient's plasma contains some substance favoring platelet aggregation or lacks some material that protects endothelial cells from platelet adhesion. Plasmapheresis has been associated with a fall in mortality from 80% to 10% and should be considered the standard of care for management of TTP in pregnancy (Watson et al., 1990; Esplin and Branch, 1999). Some authors also advocate using glucocorticoids for additional treatment, and if these treatments fail, immunotherapy such as vincristine should be considered (Bell et al., 1991; Esplin and Branch, 1999).

The antiphospholipid antibody syndrome and thrombophilias are discussed in Chapter 48.

REFERENCES

Aessopos A, Karabatsos F, Farmakis D, et al: Pregnancy in patients with well-treated β-thalassemia: Outcome for mothers and newborn infants. Am J Obstet Gynecol **180**:360, 1999.

Alger LS, Golbus MS, Laros RK Jr: Thalassemia and pregnancy. Am J Obstet Gynecol **134**:662, 1979.

Alper BS, Kimber R, Reddy AK: Using ferritin levels to determine iron-deficiency anemia in pregnancy. J Fam Practice **49**:829, 2000.

Alter BP: Advances in prenatal diagnosis of hematologic disease. Blood **64**:329, 1984.

American College of Obstetricians and Gynecologists: Folic acid for the prevention of recurrent neural tube defects. ACOG Committee Opinion 120. Washington, DC: ACOG, 1993.

Anselmo AP, Cavalieri E, Enrici RM, et al: Hodgkin's disease during pregnancy: Diagnostic and therapeutic management. Fetal Diag Therapy **14**:102, 1999.

Ascarelli MH, Emerson ES, Bigelow CL, et al: Aplastic anemia and immune-mediated thrombocytopenia: Concurrent complications encountered in the third trimester of pregnancy. Obstet Gynecol **91**:803, 1998.

Aviles A, Neri N: Hematological malignancies and pregnancy: A final report of 84 children who received chemotherapy in utero. Clin Lymphoma **2**:173, 2001.

Batlle J, Torea J, Rendal E, et al: The problem of diagnosing von Willebrand's disease. J Intern Med **242**:121, 1997.

Bayoumeu F, Subiran-Buisset C, Baka NE, et al: Iron therapy in iron deficiency anemia in pregnancy: Intravenous route versus oral route. Am J Obstet Gynecol **186**:518, 2002.

Beilin Y, Zahn J, Comerford M: Safe epidural analgesia in 30 parturients with platelet counts 69,000 to 98,000. Anesth Analg **85**:385, 1997.

Bell WR, Braine HG, Ness PM, et al: Improved survival in thrombotic thrombocytopenic purpura–hemolytic uremic syndrome. N Engl J Med **325**:398, 1991.

Beutler E: Glucose-6-phosphate dehydrogenase deficiency. N Engl J Med **324**:169, 1991.

Bick RL: Syndromes of disseminated intravascular coagulation in obstetrics, pregnancy, and gynecology. Hematol Oncol Clin N Am **14**:999, 2000.

Blattner P, Dar H, Nitowski HM: Pregnancy outcome in women with sickle cell trait. JAMA **238**:1392, 1977.

Boehlen F, Hohlfeld P, Extermann P, et al: Platelet count at term pregnancy: A reappraisal of the threshold. Obstet Gynecol **95**:29, 2000.

Bofill JA, Young RA, Perry KG: Successful pregnancy in a woman with severe factor X deficiency. Obstet Gynecol **88**:723, 1996.

Bondevik GT, Lie RT, Ulstein M, et al: Maternal hematological status and risk of low birth weight and preterm delivery in Nepal. Acta Obstet Gynecol Scand **80**:402, 2001.

Brabin BJ, Hakimi M, Pelletier D: An analysis of anemia and pregnancy-related maternal mortality. J Nutrition **131**:604S, 2001.

Breckenridge RL, Riggs JA: Hereditary elliptocytosis with hemolytic anemia complicating pregnancy. Am J Obstet Gynecol **101**:861, 1968.

Breymann C, Visca E, Huch R, et al: Efficacy and safety of intravenously administered iron sucrose with and without adjuvant recombinant human erythropoietin for the treatment of resistant iron-deficiency anemia during pregnancy. Am J Obstet Gynecol **184**:662, 2001.

Brostrom S, Bergmann OJ: Thrombotic thrombocytopenic purpura: A difficult differential diagnosis in pregnancy. Acta Obstet Gynecol Scand **79**:84, 2000.

Brunskill PJ: The effects of fetal exposure to danazol. Br J Obstet Gynaecol **99**:212, 1992.

Bukowski RM: Thrombotic thrombocytopenic purpura: A review. Prog Hemost Thromb **6**:287, 1982.

Bunn HF, Forget BJ: Human Hemoglobins. Philadelphia, WB Saunders, 1986.

Burlingame J, McGaraghan A, Kilpatrick S, et al: Maternal and fetal outcomes in pregnancies affected by von Willebrand disease type 2. Am J Obstet Gynecol **184**:229, 2001.

Burrows RF, Kelton JG: Low fetal risks in pregnancies associated with idiopathic thrombocytopenic purpura. Am J Obstet Gynecol **163**:1147, 1990.

Burrows RF, Kelton JG: Fetal thrombocytopenia and its relation to maternal thrombocytopenia. N Eng J Med **329**:1463, 1993.

Bussel JB, Berkowitz RL, Lynch L, et al: Antenatal management of alloimmune thrombocytopenia with intravenous gamma-globulin: A randomized trial of the addition of low-dose steroid to intravenous gamma-globulin. Am J Obstet Gynecol **174**:1414, 1996.

Bussel JB, Berkowitz RL, McFarland JG, et al: Antenatal treatment of neonatal alloimmune thrombocytopenia. N Engl J Med **319**:1374, 1988.

Cao A, Saba L, Galanello R, et al: Molecular diagnosis and carrier screening for β thalassemia. JAMA **178**:1273, 1997.

Cash JD: Platelet transfusion therapy. Clin Hematol **1**:395, 1972.

Catanzarite VA, Ferguson JE II: Acute leukemia and pregnancy: A review of management and outcome, 1972–1982. Obstet Gynecol Surv **39**:663, 1984.

Centers for Disease Control (CDC): Use of folic acid for prevention of spina bifida and other neural tube defects—1983–1991. MMWR Morb Mortal Wkly Rep **40**:513, 1991.

Centers for Disease Control and Prevention (CDC): Recommendations to prevent and control iron deficiency anemia in the United States. MMWR Morb Mortal Wkly Rep **47**:1, 1998.

Champlin RE, Goldman JM, Gale RP: Bone marrow transplantation in chronic myelogenous leukemia. Semin Hematol **25**:74, 1988.

Cimo PL, Aster RH: Post-transfusion purpura: Successful treatment with exchange transfusion. N Engl J Med **287**:290, 1972.

Cines D, Dussk B, Tomaski A, et al: Immune thrombocytopenic purpura and pregnancy. N Engl J Med **306**:106, 1982.

Cines DB, Blanchette VS: Immune thrombocytopenic purpura. N Engl J Med **346**:995, 2002.

Clark AL, Gall SA: Clinical uses of intravenous immunoglobulin in pregnancy. Am J Obstet Gynecol **176**:241, 1997.

Cohen S, Goldiner PL: Epidural analgesia for labor and delivery in a patient with von Willebrand's disease. Regional Anesth **14**:95, 1989.

Coller BS, Hultin MB, Hoyer LW, et al: Normal pregnancy in a patient with a prior postpartum factor VIII inhibitor: With observations on pathogenesis and prognosis. Blood **58**:619, 1981.

Colman RW, Hirsh J, Marder VJ, et al: Hemostasis and Thrombosis. Philadelphia, Lippincott, 1987.

Cook RL, Miller RC, Katz VL, et al: Immune thrombocytopenic purpura in pregnancy: A reappraisal of management. Obstet Gynecol **78**:578, 1991.

Cunningham FG, Pritchard JA, Mason RA: Pregnancy and sickle cell hemoglobinopathies. Obstet Gynecol **62**:419, 1983.

Cunningham FG, Pritchard JA, Mason RA, et al: Prophylactic transfusion of normal red blood cells during pregnancy complicated by sickle cell hemoglobinopathies. Am J Obstet Gynecol **135**:994, 1979.

Daffos F, Forestier F, Muller JY, et al: Prenatal treatment of alloimmune thrombocytopenia. Lancet **2**:632, 1984.

Dara P, Slater LM, Armentrout SA: Successful pregnancy during chemotherapy for acute leukemia. Cancer **47:**845, 1981.

Dashe JS, Ramin SM, Cunningham FG: The long term consequences of thrombotic microangiopathy (thrombotic thrombocytopenic purpura and hemolytic uremic syndrome) in pregnancy. Obstet Gynecol **91:**662, 1998.

De Rycke M, Van de Velde H, Sermon K, et al: Preimplantation genetic diagnosis for sickle-cell anemia and for beta-thalassemia. Prenat Diagn **21:**214, 2001.

Deeg HJ, Kennedy MS, Sanders JR, et al: Successful pregnancy after marrow transplantation for severe aplastic anemia and immunosuppression with cyclosporine. JAMA **250:**647, 1983.

Doney K, Storb R, Buckner CD, et al: Marrow transplantation for treatment of pregnancy-associated aplastic anemia. Exp Hematol **13:**1080, 1985.

Egerman RS, Witlin AG, Friedman SA, et al: Thrombotic thrombocytopenic purpura and hemolytic uremic syndrome in pregnancy: Review of 11 cases. Am J Obstet Gynecol **175:**950, 1996.

Elliot MA, Nichols WL: Thrombotic thrombocytopenic purpura and hemolytic uremic syndrome. Mayo Clin Proc **76:**1154, 2001.

Erslev AJ: Erythropoietin. N Engl J Med **324:**1339, 1991.

Esplin MS, Branch DW: Diagnosis and management of thrombotic microangiopathies during pregnancy. Clin Obstet Gynecol **42:**360, 1999.

Ezra Y, Rose M, Eldor A: Therapy and prevention of thrombotic thrombocytopenic purpura during pregnancy: A clinical study of 16 pregnancies. Am J Hematol **51:**1, 1996.

Fadilah SA, Ahmad-Zailani H, Soon-Keng C, et al: Successful treatment of chronic myeloid leukemia during pregnancy with hydroxyurea. Leukemia **16:**1202, 2002.

Falkson HC, Simson IW, Falkson G: Non-Hodgkin's lymphoma in pregnancy. Cancer **45:**1679, 1980.

Fenig E, Mishaeli M, Kalish Y, et al: Pregnancy and radiation. Cancer Treat Rev **27:**1, 2001.

Fenton V, Cavill J, Fisher J: Iron stores in pregnancy. Br J Haematol **37:**145, 1977.

Ferguson JE, O'Reilly RA: Hemoglobin E and pregnancy. Obstet Gynecol **66:**136, 1985.

Finer P, Blair J, Rowe P: Epidural analgesia in the management of labor pain and sickle cell crisis: A case report. Anesthesiology **68:**799, 1988.

Fisher S, Rikover M, Naor S: Factor XIII deficiency with severe hemorrhagic diathesis. Blood **28:**34, 1966.

Fleming AF: Hypoplastic anaemia in pregnancy. Clin Haematol **2:**477, 1973.

Fleming AF, Lynch W: Beta-thalassemia minor during pregnancy with particular reference to iron status. J Obstet Gynaecol Br Comm **76:**451, 1967.

Fosburg MT, Nathan DG: Treatment of Cooley's anemia. Blood **76:**435, 1990.

Frakes JT, Burmeister RE, Giliberti JJ: Pregnancy in a patient with paroxysmal nocturnal hemoglobinuria. Obstet Gynecol **47:**22S, 1976.

Francis RB, Johnson CS: Vascular occlusion in sickle cell disease: Current concepts and unanswered questions. Blood **77:**1405, 1991.

Galbraith GMP, Galbraith RM, Temple A, et al: Demonstration of transferrin receptors on human placental trophoblast. Blood **55:**240, 1980.

Giagounidis AA, Beckmann MW, Giagounidis AS, et al: Acute promyelocytic leukemia and pregnancy. Eur J Haematol **64:**267, 2000.

Goldenberg RL, Tamura T, DuBard M, et al: Plasma ferritin and pregnancy outcome. Am J Obstet Gynecol **175:**1356, 1996.

Green DM, Zevon MA, Lowrie G, et al: Congenital anomalies in children of patients who received chemotherapy for cancer in childhood and adolescence. N Engl J Med **325:**141, 1991.

Greenlund LJ, Letendre L, Tefferi A: Acute leukemia during pregnancy: A single institutional experience with 17 cases. Leuk Lymphoma **41:**571, 2001.

Hamstra RD, Block MH, Schocket AL: Intravenous iron dextran. JAMA **233:**1726, 1980.

Hansen WF, Fretz P, Hunter SK, et al: Leukemia in pregnancy and fetal response to multiagent chemotherapy. Obstet Gynecol **97:**809, 2001.

Haram K, Nilsen ST, Ulvik RJ: Iron supplementation in pregnancy—evidence and controversies. Acta Obstet Gynecol Scand **80:**683, 2001.

Hemminki E, Merilainen J: Long term follow-up of mothers and their infants in a randomized trial on iron prophylaxis during pregnancy. Am J Obstet Gynecol **173:**205, 1995.

Herbert V, Colman N, Spivack M: Folic acid deficiency in the United States: Folate assays in a prenatal clinic. Am J Obstet Gynecol **123:**175, 1975.

Hew-Wing R, Rolbin SH, Hew E, et al: Epidural anesthesia and thrombocytopenia. Anaesthesia **44:**775, 1989.

Higgs DR, Vickers MA, Wilkie AOM, et al: A review of the molecular genetics of the human a-globin gene cluster. Blood **73:**1081, 1989.

Ho CH, Yuan CC, Yeh SH: Serum ferritin, folate and cobalamin levels and their correlation with anemia in normal full-term pregnant women. Eur J Obstet Gynecol Reprod Biol **26:**7, 1987.

Hoffman MA, Wiernik PH, Kleiner GJ: Acute promyelocytic leukemia and pregnancy. Cancer **76:**2237, 1995.

Holly RG: Hypoplastic anemia in pregnancy. Obstet Gynecol **1:**533, 1953.

Holmes GE, Holmes FF: Pregnancy outcome of patients treated for Hodgkin's disease: A controlled study. Cancer **41:**1317, 1978.

Horning SJ, Hopp RT, Kaplan HS, Rosenberg SA: Female reproductive potential after treatment for Hodgkin's disease. N Engl J Med **304:**1377, 1981.

Horowitz JJ, Laros RK Jr: Anemia and pregnancy: A review of the pathophysiology, diagnosis and treatment. J Cont Ed Obstet Gynecol **1:**9, 1979.

Hoyer LW: Hemophilia A. N Engl J Med **330:**38, 1994.

Hurd WW, Miodovnik M, Stys SJ: Pregnancy associated with paroxysmal nocturnal hemoglobinuria. Obstet Gynecol **60:**742, 1982.

Institute of Medicine: Iron deficiency anemia: Recommended guidelines for prevention, detection and management among U.S. children and women of childbearing age. Washington, DC, National Academy Press, 1993.

Iyengar L: Folic acid absorption in pregnancy. Br J Obstet Gynaecol **82:**20, 1975.

Jaime-Perez JC, Gomez-Almaguer D: Iron stores in low-income pregnant Mexican women at term. Arch Med Res **33:**81, 2002.

Johan E, Magnus EM: Plasma and red blood cell folate during normal pregnancy. Acta Obstet Gynaecol Scand **60:**247, 1981.

Kagan R, Laros RK Jr: Immune thrombocytopenia. Clin Obstet Gynecol **26:**537, 1983.

Kan YW, Golbus MS, Dozy AM: Prenatal diagnosis of alpha-thalassemia. N Engl J Med **295:**1165, 1976.

Kazazian HH, Boehm CD: Molecular basis and prenatal diagnosis of β-thalassemia. Blood **72:**1107, 1988.

Kelton JG, Hunter DJS, Neame PB: A platelet function defect in preeclampsia. Obstet Gynecol **65:**107, 1985.

Kelton JG, Inwood MJ, Barr RM, et al: The prenatal prediction of thrombocytopenia in infants of mothers with clinically diagnosed immune thrombocytopenia. Am J Obstet Gynecol **144:**449, 1982.

Kilpatrick SJ, Laros RK: Thalassemia in pregnancy. Clin Obstet Gynecol **38:**485, 1995.

Kitay DZ: Folic acid deficiency in pregnancy. Am J Obstet Gynecol **104:**1067, 1969.

Kitchens CS, Newcomb TF: Factor XIII. Medicine (Baltimore) **58:**413, 1979.

Kitzmiller JL, Lang JE, Yelenosky PF, et al: Hematologic assays in preeclampsia. Am J Obstet Gynecol **118:**362, 1974.

Klebanoff MA, Shiono PH, Shelby JV, et al: Anemia and spontaneous preterm birth. Am J Obstet Gynecol **59:**164, 1991.

Kobayashi T, Terao T, Maki M, et al: Diagnosis and management of acute obstetrical DIC. Semin Thromb Hemost **27:**161, 2001.

Kojima S, Nakao S, Tomonaga M, et al: Consensus conference on the treatment of aplastic anemia. Int J Hematol **72:**118, 2000.

Konje JC, Murphy P, de Chazal R, et al: Severe factor X deficiency and successful pregnancy. Br J Obstet Gynaecol **101:**910, 1994.

Koshy M, Burd L, Wallace D, et al: Prophylactic red-cell transfusion in pregnant patients with sickle cell disease. N Engl J Med **319:**1447, 1988.

Krishanamurth M, Miotti AB: Von Willebrand's disease and pregnancy. Obstet Gynecol **49:**244, 1977.

Kuvin SF, Brecher G: Differential neutrophil counts in pregnancy. N Engl J Med **266:**877, 1962.

Laros RK Jr: Sickle cell hemoglobin C disease in pregnancy. Pa Med **70:**73, 1967.

Laros RK Jr (ed): Blood Disorders in Pregnancy. Philadelphia, Lea & Febiger, 1986.

Laros RK Jr, Kalstone C: Sickle cell beta-thalassemia and pregnancy. Obstet Gynecol **37:**67, 1971.

Laros RK Jr, Penner JA: Pathophysiology of disseminated intravascular coagulation in saline-induced abortion. Obstet Gynecol **48:**353, 1976.

Larrabee KD, Monga M: Women with sickle cell trait are at increased risk for preeclampsia. Am J Obstet Gynecol **177:**425, 1997.

Lazebnik N, Jaffa AJ, Peyeser R: Hemolytic-uremic syndrome in pregnancy: Review of the literature and report of a case. Obstet Gynecol Surv **40:**618, 1985.

Leiba H, Ramot B, Many A: Heredity and coagulation studies in ten families with factor XI deficiency. Br J Haematol **11:**654, 1965.

Lescale KB, Eddleman KA, Cines DB, et al: Antiplatelet antibody testing in thrombocytopenic pregnant women. Am J Obstet Gynecol **174:**1014, 1996.

Li FP, Fine W, Jaffe N, et al: Offspring of patients treated for cancer in childhood. J Natl Cancer Inst **62:**1193, 1979.

Lilleyman JS, Hill AS, Anderton KJ: Consequences of acute myelogenous leukemia in early pregnancy. Cancer **40**:1300, 1977.

Lind SE: The bleeding time does not predict surgical bleeding. Blood **77**:2547, 1991.

Lipton RA, Ayromlooi J, Coller BS: Severe von Willebrand's disease during labor and delivery. JAMA **248**:1355, 1982.

Lishner M, Zemlickis D, Sutcliffe SB, et al: Non-Hodgkin's lymphoma and pregnancy. Leuk Lymphoma **14**:411, 1994.

Lorand L, Losowsky MS, Miloszewski KJM: Human factor XIII: Fibrin-stabilizing factor. Prog Hemost Thromb **5**:245, 1980.

Lorey F, Cunningham G: Impact of Asian immigration on thalassemia in California. Ann N Y Acad Sci **859**:442, 1998.

Lu ZM, Goldenberg RL, Cliver SP, et al: The relationship between maternal hematocrit and pregnancy outcome. Obstet Gynecol **77**:190, 1991.

Lusher JM, McMillan CW: Severe factor VIII and factor IX deficiency in females. Am J Med **65**:637, 1978.

Lynch RE, Williams DM, Reading JC, et al: The prognosis in aplastic anemia. Blood **45**:517, 1975.

Maberry MC, Mason RA, Cunningham FG, et al: Pregnancy complicated by hemoglobin CC and C-β-thalassemia disease. Obstet Gynecol **76**:324, 1990.

Maberry MC, Mason RA, Cunningham FG, et al: Pregnancy complicated by hereditary spherocytosis. Obstet Gynecol **79**:735, 1992.

Maduska AL, Guinee WS, Heaton AJ, et al: Sickling dynamics of red blood cells and other physiologic studies during anesthesia. Anesth Analg **54**:361, 1975.

Magid MS, Perkins M, Gottfried EL: Increased erythrocyte osmotic fragility in pregnancy. Am J Obstet Gynecol **144**:910, 1982.

Matthay KK, Mentzer WC: Erythrocyte enzymes in the newborn. Clin Haematol **10**:31, 1981.

McGuire WA, Yang HH, Bruno E, et al: Treatment of antibody-mediated pure red-cell aplasia with high-dose intravenous gamma globulin. N Engl J Med **317**:1004, 1987.

McIntosh S, O'Brien RT, Schwartz AD, et al.: Neonatal isoimmune purpura: Response to platelet infusions. J Pediatr **82**:1020, 1973.

Miller CH, Hoyer LW: Prenatal diagnosis of two sporadic cases of hemophilia. N Engl J Med **314**:584, 1986.

Miller JM: Alpha thalassemia minor in pregnancy. J Reprod Med **27**:207, 1982.

Monsen ER, Kuhn JH, Finch CA: Iron status of menstruating females. Am J Clin Nutr **20**:842, 1967.

Moore A, Sherman MM, Strongin MJ: Hereditary spherocytosis with hemolytic crisis during pregnancy. Obstet Gynecol **47**:19S, 1976.

Morrison JC, Whybrew WD, Bucovary ET: Use of partial exchange transfusion preoperatively in patients with sickle cell hemoglobinopathies. Am J Obstet Gynecol **132**:59, 1978.

Morrison JC, Wiser WL: The use of prophylactic partial exchange transfusion in pregnancies associated with sickle cell hemoglobinopathies. Obstet Gynecol **48**:510, 1976.

Motulsky AG: Frequency of sickling disorders in U.S. blacks. N Engl J Med **288**:31, 1973.

Muller JY: Alloimmune thrombocytopenia in the newborn. Curr Stud Hematol Blood Transfus **55**:94, 1988.

Mubarak AA, Kakil IR, Awide A, et al: Normal outcome of pregnancy in chronic myeloid leukemia treated with interferon-alpha in first trimester: report of 3 cases and review of the literature. Am J Hematol **69**:115, 2002.

Noller KL, Bowie EJW, Kempers RD, et al: Von Willebrand's disease in pregnancy. Obstet Gynecol **41**:865, 1973.

Ohba T, Yoshimura T, Araki M, et al: Aplastic anemia in pregnancy: Treatment with cyclosporine and granulocyte-colony stimulating factor. Acta Obstet Gynecol **78**:458, 1999.

Okuyama T, Tawada T, Furuya H, et al: The role of transferrin and ferritin in the fetal-maternal-placental unit. Am J Obstet Gynecol **152**:344, 1985.

Paidas MJ, Berkowitz RL, Lynch L, et al: Alloimmune thrombocytopenia: Fetal and neonatal losses related to cordocentesis. Am J Obstet Gynecol **172**:475, 1995.

Paulone ME, Edelstone DI, Shedd A: Effects of maternal anemia on uteroplacental and fetal oxidative metabolism in sheep. Am J Obstet Gynecol **156**:230, 1987.

Payne SD, Resnik R, Moore TR, et al: Maternal characteristics, risk of severe neonatal thrombocytopenia and intracranial hemorrhage in pregnancies complicated by autoimmune thrombocytopenia. Am J Obstet Gynecol **177**:149, 1997.

Peck TM, Arias F: Hematologic changes associated with pregnancy. Clin Obstet **22**:785, 1979.

Perkins RP: The significance of glucose-6-phosphate dehydrogenase deficiency in pregnancy. Am J Obstet Gynecol **125**:215, 1976.

Phillips LL, Davidson EC: Procoagulant properties of amniotic fluid. Am J Obstet Gynecol **113**:911, 1972.

Phillips LL, Rosano L, Skrodelis V: Changes in factor XI levels during pregnancy. Am J Obstet Gynecol **116**:1114, 1973.

Phillips LL, Skrodelis V, Kers TA: Hypofibrinogenemia and intrauterine fetal death. Am J Obstet Gynecol **89**:903, 1964.

Phillips LL, Skrodelis V, Quigley HJ: Intravascular coagulation in septic abortion. Obstet Gynecol **30**:350, 1967.

Pizzuto J, Aviles A, Noriega L, et al: Treatment of acute leukemia during pregnancy: Presentation of nine cases. Cancer Treat Rep **64**:679, 1980.

Plows CW: Acute myelomonocytic leukemia in pregnancy: Report of a case. Am J Obstet Gynecol **143**:41, 1982.

Pohlman B, Macklis RM: Lymphoma and pregnancy. Semin Oncol **27**:657, 2000.

Pritchard JA, Cunningham FG, Mason RA: Coagulation changes in eclampsia. Am J Obstet Gynecol **124**:855, 1976.

Pritchard JA, Whalley PJ, Scott DE: The influence of maternal folate and iron deficiency on intrauterine life. Am J Obstet Gynecol **104**:388, 1969.

Pritchard JA, Whalley PJ, Scott DE: Infants of mothers with megaloblastic anemia due to folate deficiency. JAMA **211**:1982, 1970.

Puolakka A, Janne O, Pararinen A, et al: Serum ferritin in the diagnosis of anemia during pregnancy. Acta Obstet Gynaecol Scand **95**(Suppl):57, 1980.

Purcell G, Nossel HL: Factor XI (PTA) deficiency. Obstet Gynecol **35**:69, 1970.

Rainville AJ: Pica practices of pregnant women are associated with lower maternal hemoglobin level at delivery. J Am Diet Assoc **101**:318, 2001.

Rapaport SI, Proctor RR, Patch MJ, et al: The mode of inheritance of PTA disease. Blood **18**:149, 1961.

Richards HGH, Spiers ASD: Chronic granulocytic leukemia in pregnancy. Br J Radiol **48**:261, 1975.

Rimon A, Schiffman S, Feinstein D, et al: Factor XI activity and factor XI antigen in homozygous and heterozygous factor XI deficiency. Blood **48**:165, 1976.

Rock G, Porta C, Bobbio-Pallavicini E: Thrombotic thrombocytopenic purpura treatment in year 2000. Haematologica **85**:410, 2000.

Rodgers RPC, Levin J: A critical reappraisal of the bleeding time. Semin Thromb Hemost **16**:1, 1990.

Rolbin SH, Abbott D, Musclow E, et al: Epidural anesthesia in pregnant patients with low platelet counts. Obstet Gynecol **71**:918, 1988.

Rouse DJ, Owen J, Goldenberg RL: Routine maternal platelet count: An assessment of a technicologically driven screening tool. Am J Obstet Gynecol **179**:573, 1998.

Roy V, Gutteridge CN, Nysenbaum A, et al: Combination chemotherapy with conservative obstetric management in the treatment of pregnant patients with acute myeloblastic leukaemia. Clin Lab Haematol **11**:171, 1989.

Rust LA, Goodnight SH, Freeman RK, et al: Pregnancy and delivery of a woman with hemophilia B. Obstet Gynecol **46**:483, 1975.

Rust OA, Perry KG: Pregnancy complicated by sickle hemoglinopathy. Clin Obstet Gynecol **38**:472, 1995.

Sacks DA, Platt L, Johnson CS: Autoimmune hemolytic anemia during pregnancy. Am J Obstet Gynecol **140**:942, 1981.

Sagen N, Nilsen ST, Kim HC, et al: Maternal hemoglobin concentration is closely related to birth weight in normal pregnancies. Acta Obstet Gynecol **63**:245, 1984.

Samuels P, Bussel JB, Braitman LE, et al: Estimation of the risk of thrombocytopenia in the offspring of pregnant women with presumed immune thrombocytopenic purpura. N Engl J Med **323**:229, 1990.

Sanders JE, Hawley J, Levy W, et al: Pregnancies following high-dose cyclophosphamide with or without high-dose busulfan or total-body irradiation and bone marrow transplantation. Blood **87**:3045, 1996.

Sanz MA, Rafecas FJ: Successful pregnancy during chemotherapy for acute promyelocytic leukemia. N Engl J Med **306**:939, 1982.

Scanlon KS, Yip R, Schieve LA, Cogswell ME: High and low hemoglobin levels during pregnancy: Differential risks for preterm birth and small for gestational age. Obstet Gynecol **96**:741, 2000.

Schafer AI: Teratogenic effects of antileukemia chemotherapy. Arch Intern Med **141**:514, 1981.

Schifman RB, Thomasson JE, Evers JM: Red blood cell zinc protoporphyrin testing in iron-deficiency anemia in pregnancy. Am J Obstet Gynecol **157**:304, 1987.

Schilsky R, Sherins R, Hubbard S, et al: Long term follow-up of ovarian function in women treated with MOPP chemotherapy for Hodgkin's disease. Am J Med **71**:552, 1981.

Schmidt H, Ehninger G, Dopfer R, et al: Pregnancy after bone marrow transplantation for severe aplastic anemia. Bone Marrow Transplant **2**:329, 1987.

Scholl TO, Hediger ML, Fischer RL, et al: Anemia vs. iron deficiency: Increased risk of preterm delivery in a prospective study. Am J Clin Nutr **55**:985, 1992.

Schwartz ML, Brenner WE: The obfuscation of eclampsia by thrombotic thrombocytopenic purpura. Am J Obstet Gynecol **131**:18, 1978.

Scott DE, Pritchard JA: Iron deficiency in healthy young college women. JAMA **199**:147, 1967.

Segonds A, Louradour N, Suc JM, et al: Postpartum hemolytic uremic syndrome: A study of three cases with a review of the literature. Clin Nephrol **12**:229, 1979.

Seligman PA, Caskey JH, Frazier JI, et al: Measurements of iron absorption from prenatal multivitamin-mineral supplements. Obstet Gynecol **61**:356, 1983.

Shattil SJ, Bennett JS: Platelets and their membranes in hemostasis: Physiology and pathophysiology. Ann Intern Med **94**:108, 1981.

Shobeiri SA, West EC, Kahn MJ, et al: Postpartum acquired hemophilia (factor VIII inhibitors): A case report and review of the literature. Obstet Gynecol Surv **55**:729, 2000.

Shojania AM, Hornady GJ: Oral contraceptives and folate absorption. J Lab Clin Med **82**:869, 1973.

Shulman NR: The physiologic basis for therapy of classic hemophilia and related disorders. Ann Intern Med **67**:856, 1967.

Shulman NR, Aster RH, Leitner A, et al: Immunoreactions involving platelets: V. Posttransfusion purpura due to a complement-fixing antibody against a genetically-controlled platelet antigen: A proposed mechanism for thrombocytopenia and its relevance in autoimmunity. J Clin Invest **40**:1597, 1961.

Sia CG, Amigo NC, Harper RG, et al: Failure of cesarean section to prevent intracranial hemorrhage in siblings with isoimmune neonatal thrombocytopenia. Am J Obstet Gynecol **153**:79, 1985.

Sifakis S, Angelakis E, Vardaki E, et al: Erythropoietin in the treatment of iron deficiency anemia during pregnancy. Gynecol Obstet Invest **51**:150, 2001.

Silver RM, Branch DW, Scott JR: Maternal thrombocytopenia in pregnancy: Time for a reassessment. Am J Obstet Gynecol **173**:479, 1995.

Silverstein E, Roadman C, Byers RH, et al: Hematologic problems in pregnancy: III. Glucose-6-phosphate dehydrogenase deficiency. J Reprod Med **12**:153, 1974.

Singla PN, Tyagi M, Shankar R, et al: Fetal iron status in maternal anemia. Acta Paediatr **85**:1327, 1996.

Siris ES, Leventhal BG, Vaitukaitis JL: Effects of childhood leukemia and chemotherapy on puberty and reproductive function in girls. N Engl J Med **294**:1143, 1976.

Sloan NL, Jordan E, Winkoff B: Effects of iron supplementation on maternal hematologic status in pregnancy. Am J Public Health **92**:288, 2002.

Smith JA, Espeland M, Bellevue R, et al: Pregnancy in sickle cell disease: Experience of the Cooperative Study of Sickle Cell Disease. Obstet Gynecol **87**:199, 1996.

Snyder TE, Lee LP, Lynch S: Pregnancy-associated hypoplastic anemia: A review. Obstet Gynecol Surv **46**:264, 1991.

Socol ML, Weiner CP, Louis G, et al: Platelet activation in preeclampsia. Am J Obstet Gynecol **151**:494, 1985.

Solal-Celigny P, Tertian G, Fernandez H, et al: Pregnancy and paroxysmal nocturnal hemoglobinuria. Arch Intern Med **148**:593, 1988.

Spector I, Corn M: Laboratory tests of hemostasis: The relation to hemorrhage in liver disease. Arch Intern Med **119**:577, 1967.

Steinberg MH: Management of sickle cell disease. New Eng J Med **340**:1021, 1999.

Steinberg MH, Adams JG: Thalassemia: Recent insights into molecular mechanisms. Am J Hematol **12**:81, 1982.

Stephansson O, Dickman PW, Johansson A, et al: Maternal hemoglobin concentration during pregnancy and risk of stillbirth. JAMA **284**:2611, 2000.

Stuart MJ, Gross SJ, Elred H, et al: Effects of acetylsalicylic acid ingestion on maternal and neonatal hemostasis. N Engl J Med **307**:909, 1982.

Stubbs TM, Lazarchick J, Horger EO: Plasma fibronectin levels in preeclampsia: A possible biochemical marker for vascular endothelial damage. Am J Obstet Gynecol **150**:885, 1984.

Sullivan CA, Martin JN: Management of the obstetric patient with thrombocytopenia. Clin Obstet Gynecol **38**:521, 1995.

Sun PM, Wilburn W, Raynor D, et al: Sickle cell disease in pregnancy: Twenty years of experience at Grady Memorial Hospital, Atlanta, Georgia. Am J Obstet Gynecol **184**:1127, 2001.

Sutton DMC, Hauser R, Kulaping S, et al: Intravascular coagulation in abruptio placentae. Am J Obstet Gynecol **109**:604, 1971.

Swensen AR, Harnack LJ, Ross JA: Nutritional assessment of pregnant women enrolled in the Special Supplemental Program for Women, Infants, and Children (WIC). J Am Diet Assoc **101**:903, 2001.

Taaning E, Skibsted L: The frequency of platelet alloantibodies in pregnant women and the occurrence and management of neonatal alloimmune thrombocytopenic purpura. Obstet Gynecol Surv **45**:521, 1990.

Taylor DJ, Mallen C, McDougall N, et al: Effect of iron supplement on serum ferritin levels during and after pregnancy. Br J Obstet Gynaecol **89**:1011, 1982.

Thomas PRM, Peckham MJ: The investigation and management of Hodgkin's disease in the pregnant patient. Cancer **38**:1443, 1976.

Vora M, Gruslin A: Erythropoietin in obstetrics. Obstet Gynecol Surv **53**:500, 1998.

Wald NJ, Law MR, Morris JK, et al: Quantifying the effect of folic acid. Lancet **358**:2069, 2001.

Walden PAM, Bagshawe KD: Pregnancies after chemotherapy for gestational trophoblastic tumours. Lancet **2**:1241, 1979.

Watson WJ, Katz VL, Bowes WA: Plasmapheresis during pregnancy. Obstet Gynecol **76**:451, 1990.

Weatherall DJ: The New Genetics and Clinical Practice. New York, Oxford University Press, 1985.

Weatherall DJ, Clegg JB: The Thalassemia Syndromes, 2nd ed. Oxford, Blackwell Scientific, 1981.

Weenink GH, Treffers PE, Vijn P, et al: Antithrombin III levels in preeclampsia correlate with maternal and fetal morbidity. Am J Obstet Gynecol **148**:1092, 1984.

Weiner CP, Brandt J: Plasma antithrombin III: An aid in the diagnosis of preeclampsia-eclampsia. Am J Obstet Gynecol **142**:275, 1982.

Weinstein L: Preeclampsia/eclampsia with hemolysis, elevated liver enzymes, and thrombocytopenia. Obstet Gynecol **66**:657, 1985.

Weiss HJ: Congenital disorders of platelet function. Semin Hematol **17**:228, 1980.

Whalley PJ, Martin FG, Pritchard JA: Sickle cell trait and urinary tract infections during pregnancy. JAMA **189**:903, 1964.

Whalley PJ, Pritchard JA, Richards JR: Sickle cell trait and pregnancy. JAMA **186**:1132, 1963.

White GC, Shoemaker CB: Factor VIII gene and hemophilia A. Blood **73**:1, 1989.

Wong SC, Ali MAM: Hemoglobin E disease. Am J Hematol **13**:15, 1982.

Xiong X, Buekens P, Alexander S, et al: Anemia during pregnancy and birth outcome: a meta-analysis. Am J Perinatol **17**:137, 2000.

Chapter 48
THROMBOPHILIAS IN PREGNANCY

Charles J. Lockwood, MD, and Robert Silver, MD

Venous thromboembolism (VTE) of the systemic and pulmonary circulation is a leading cause of maternal mortality in the United States. Second and third trimester fetal loss, intrauterine fetal growth restriction (IUGR), abruption, and severe, early-onset, preeclampsia are associated with thrombosis of the uteroplacental circulation and are leading causes of perinatal morbidity and mortality. Inherited and acquired thrombophilias have recently been linked to many cases of maternal VTE as well as these adverse obstetrical outcomes (Lockwood and Rand, 1994; Girling and de Swiet, 1998; Guideline, 2001; Lockwood, 2001). Identification of these thrombophilic states can provide a unique opportunity to identify patients at risk and prevent untoward maternal and fetal outcomes.

The inherited thrombophilias vary in terms of prevalence and thrombogenic potential. The rarest and most thrombogenic of these conditions are homozygosity or compound heterozygosity for the factor V Leiden and prothrombin G20210A mutations and autosomal dominant antithrombin deficiency. Conversely, the most common (though least thrombogenic) of the inherited thrombophilias are homozygosity for the 4G/4G mutation in the type-1 plasminogen activator inhibitor (PAI-1) gene and the thermolabile variant of methylenetetrahydrofolate reductase (C677T MTHFR) gene. The latter is the most common cause of hyperhomocysteinemia. Inherited thrombophilias that are both relatively common and relatively thrombogenic are heterozygosity for the factor V Leiden and prothrombin G20210A mutation and autosomal dominant deficiencies of protein C and protein S. Taken together, these conditions are present in 15%–20% of ethnic European populations (Guideline, 2001).

The most common acquired thrombophilic condition is the antiphospholipid antibody syndrome present in 0.2%–2% of obstetrical patients (Lockwood and Rand, 1994). These antibodies result from perturbations in endothelial and platelet cell membranes, which cause conformation changes in negatively charged phospholipid-binding proteins such as prothrombin and β-2-glycoprotein-1. This conformational change renders them antigenic, and the resultant antibodies promote thrombosis.

Taken together, the inherited and acquired thrombophilias cause more than half of all maternal VTE and have been linked to a two- to fivefold increased risk of fetal loss, IUGR, abruption and early-onset, severe preeclampsia (Preston et al., 1996; Girling and de Swiet, 1998; Kupferminc et al., 1999; Gris et al., 1999; Lockwood, 2001; Rey et al., 2003). This chapter will review the physiological initiation and regulation of clotting, the effects of pregnancy on hemostasis, and the etiology, patho-genesis, diagnosis, and management of the inherited and acquired thrombophilias.

PHYSIOLOGICAL REGULATION OF HEMOSTASIS

Initiation and Maintenance of Hemostasis

Tissue factor (TF), a cell membrane-bound glycoprotein, is the primary initiator of hemostasis. It is expressed by perivascular cells throughout the body, but not by endothelial cells (Fig. 48-1) (Lockwood, 2001). In the reproductive tract, uterine decidual cells synthesize tissue factor in high abundance (Lockwood et al., 1993, Lockwood et al., 1994; Runic et al., 1997); there, its presence appears vital to the prevention of lethal postpartum hemorrhage (Parry et al., 1998). Indeed, complete deficiency in tissue factor expression is lethal in the transgenic mouse embryo. Following blood vessel damage, cell membrane-bound TF complexes with plasma-derived factor VII. The complex of TF and factor VII directly converts factor X to Xa (formerly termed the *extrinsic pathway*). Factor VIIa is the only clotting factor zymogen to display innate enzymatic activity (Nemerson, 1988). Activation of factor VII by thrombin or factor Xa, however, results in a 100-fold increase in activity.

The TF/VIIa complex can also indirectly generate Xa by converting factor IX to IXa, which, in turn, complexes with its cofactor, factor VIIIa, to convert X to Xa (formerly termed the *intrinsic pathway*). The TF pathway inhibitor (TFPI), which binds to the TF/VIIa/Xa complex, rapidly inhibits this initial clotting activity. The clotting cascade, however, is maintained via thrombin and factor XIIa-activated factor XIa, which serves as an alternative activator of factor IX on the surface of newly aggregated platelets embedded in the nascent fibrin clot. Regardless of how it is generated, factor Xa then complexes with its cofactor, Va, to convert prothrombin (factor II) to thrombin (IIa). Thrombin cleaves fibrinogen to generate fibrin monomers, which spontaneously polymerize and are cross-linked by thrombin-activated factor XIIIa to form the stable clot (see Fig. 48-1).

Physiological Inhibition of Hemostasis

Hemostasis is inhibited by a series of potent antiproteases (Fig. 48-2). These include the TFPI, activated Protein C complexed with Protein S (APC/S), and the potent antithrombin/

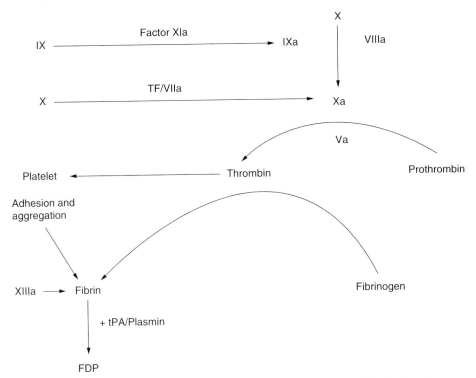

FIGURE 48-1 ■ The hemostatic system showing the coagulation and fibrinolytic pathways.

factor Xa agents, antithrombin, heparin cofactor II, and α-2-macroglobulin. Fibrinolysis is mediated by tissue-type plasminogen activator (tPA) and is primarly inhibited by plasminogen activator inhibitor-1 (PAI-1). The latter also exerts antithrombin effects.

The tissue factor (a.k.a. the extrinsic pathway) inhibitor (TFPI) is the initial inhibitor of TF/VIIa mediated clotting (Lockwood, 1999). The TFPI molecule contains two Kunitz-type inhibitory domains; the first binds to factor Xa, while the second binds to the TF/VIIa complex (Girard et al., 1989). The resultant quaternary inhibitory complex blunts TF-VII generated clotting (see Fig. 48-2). Endothelial cells synthesize and sequester TFPI, with 80% of the circulating moiety bound to lipoproteins. Heparin promotes release of endothelial TFPI and enhances its activity (Bombell et al., 1997). Plasma levels of TFPI also increase in the third trimester and in labor (Girard et al., 1989; Warr et al., 1989; Novotny et al., 1991; Bombell et al., 1997; Lockwood, 1999).

Thrombin binds to endothelial cell membrane-bound thrombomodulin in the presence of ionized calcium, and the resultant complex induces a conformational change in thrombin resulting in its ability to activate protein C (PC) (Esmon, 1993; Bombell et al., 1997) (Fig. 48-3). Activated PC attaches to negatively charged (anionic) endothelial cell membrane phospholipids or binds to the Endothelial Cell Protein C Receptor (EPCR) to inactivate procoagulant factors Va and VIIIa. Activated PC's (APC) inactivation of factor Va and VIIIa is enhanced twofold and 6.4-fold, respectively, by binding to its cofactor, protein S (PS). This process can occur on both endothelial and activated platelet membranes and is a crucial damper of the clotting cascade. Protein S also can act as a direct anticoagulant protein by binding exposed, prothrombotic, anionic phospholipids. Protein C and PS have

short half-lives in the circulation—8 and 42 hours, respectively. Circulating PS exists in both free (40%) and bound (60%) forms. The complement 4b-binding protein (C4b-BP) serves as a carrier protein for PS. Pregnancy, inflammation, and surgery increase C4b-BP levels and reduce PS activity (Delorme et al., 1992). Levels of total and free protein S decline about 40% during pregnancy (Delorme et al., 1992).

Thrombin plays the pivotal role in hemostasis, yet overproduction of thrombin can lead to fatal thrombotic diseases (Seiler, 1996). It is not surprising that a large number of potent serine protease inhibitors (SERPINs), including heparin cofactor II, α-2 macroglobulin, and antithrombin, can serve to inactivate both thrombin and factor Xa (see Fig. 48-2). After either thrombin or factor Xa complexes to one of these inhibitors, the resultant complex binds to vitronectin (Vn), a large plasma and extracellular matrix glycoprotein (Preissner et al., 1996). This three-molecule (ternary) complex then binds heparin or other glycosaminoglycans, a step which greatly augments the rate of thrombin or factor Xa inactivation (Ill and Rouslahti, 1985; Preissner et al., 1987; Delorme et al., 1992; de Boer et al., 1993; Esmon, 1993; Seiler, 1996; Preissner et al., 1996). The most physiologically active anti-thrombin/factor Xa compound is the aptly named antithrombin (AT). Levels of the thrombin-AT complex increase during pregnancy, indicating that pregnancy is associated with increased thrombin generation, but absolute AT levels remain unchanged in pregnancy (Delorme et al., 1992).

A last level of inhibition of fibrin clot propagation is the fibrinolytic system. Tissue-type plasminogen activator (tPA) binds to the fibrin clot to generate plasmin (see Fig. 48-2). Plasmin cleaves fibrin to generate fibrin degradation products (FDPs). Type-1 plasminogen activator inhibitor (PAI-1) is the 50,000 MW fast inactivator of the plasminogen activators.

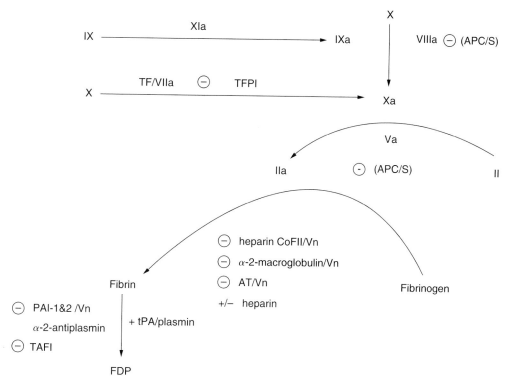

FIGURE 48-2 ■ The hemostatic system showing the coagulation, anticoagulation, fibrinolytic, and antifibrinolytic pathways. Circulating or endothelial-bound TF pathway inhibitor (TFPI) binds to the TF/VIIa/Xa complex to quickly stop TF-mediated clotting. Thrombin-activated factor XI maintains clotting, however, by serving as an alternative activator of factor IX. Thus, dampening of the clotting cascade requires activated protein C complexed with protein S (APC/S) inactivation of the factor IXa and Xa cofactors, VIIIa and Va, respectively. The most crucial endogenous anticoagulants directly inactivate thrombin and Xa and include alpha-2-macroglobulin, heparin cofactor II and, most important, antithrombin (AT). These antiproteases bind to heparin and vitronectin (Vn) as well as thrombin or Xa to shut down the clotting cascade. Finally, fibrinolysis breaks down the fibrin clot. Fibrinolysis is mediated by tissue-type plasminogen activator (tPA), which binds to fibrin, where it activates plasmin. Plasmin, in turn, degrades fibrin but can be inactivated by alpha-2-antiplasmin embedded in the fibrin clot. Fibrinolysis is primarily inhibited by type-1 plasminogen activator inhibitor (PAI-1), the fast inactivator of tPA, and in pregnancy, placental-derived PAI-2, which exists in its active form bound to Vn. TAFI acts as a third potent antifibrinolytic.

Another member of the SERPIN family of antiproteases, PAI-1 acts as the primary inhibitor of fibrinolysis (see Fig. 48-2). The principal source of PAI-1 is the endothelium. In pregnancy, the uterine decidua is an alternative rich source of PAI-1 synthesis (Schatz and Lockwood, 1993), while the placenta produces PAI-2 (Estelles et al., 1989). The PAIs are also maintained in their active forms in plasma as a result of tight binding to Vn (van Meijer et al., 1994). Levels of a third antifibrinolytic protein, thrombin-activatable fibrinolysis inhibitor (TAFI), also increase in pregnancy (Chabloz et al., 2001).

Plasmin is directly inhibited by the action of α-2-antiplasmin, which is embedded in the fibrin clot (Lijnen, 2001).

Pregnancy-Associated Changes in Hemostasis and Fibrinolysis

Pregnancy is associated with up to a 200% increase in levels of fibrinogen and factors II, VII, X, VIII, and XII and PAI-1 (Lockwood, 2001). As noted previously, pregnancy causes significant reductions in PS and significant increases in PAI-1 and PAI-2. The net effect of these pregnancy-induced changes is to exacerbate the clinical effects of the inherited thrombophilias (Lockwood, 2001).

PATHOPHYSIOLOGY OF THE INHERITED AND ACQUIRED THROMBOPHILIAS

Inherited Thrombophilias

Factor V Leiden Mutation

The factor V Leiden (FVL) mutation is the most common clinically significant thrombophilia in ethnic European populations, with a prevalence varying from 5% to 15% (Guideline, 2001; Lockwood, 2001). It is rarely found in persons of Asian or African descent (Guideline, 2001; Lockwood, 2001). A (G→A) mutation in nucleotide 1691 of the factor V gene results in the substitution of a glutamine for an arginine at position 506 in the factor V polypeptide (FV Q506). Because amino acid 506 is the site of APC/S's inactivation, the FVL mutation confers resistance to APC. Indeed, the FVL mutation is the most common cause of APC

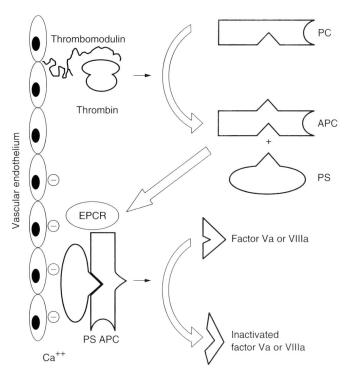

FIGURE 48-3 ■ Thrombin binds to thrombomodulin to activate protein C (APC). The latter either attaches directly to endothelial cell negatively charged phospholipids or binds to the endothelial protein C receptor (EPCR) and inactivates procoagulant factors VIIIa and Va. Activated PC's inactivation of factor Va and VIIIa is enhanced by binding to its cofactor, protein S (PS). (Reprinted with permission from Lockwood CJ: Heritable coagulopathies in pregnancy. Obstet Gynecol Surv **54**:754, 1999.)

resistance. Heterozygosity for the FVL mutation is present in 20%–40% of nonpregnant patients with VTE. Homozygosity for the FVL mutation confers a far greater (more than 100-fold) risk of VTE (Lockwood, 2001).

Pregnancy-induced reductions in protein S and concomitant increases in factor VIII enhance FVL's prothrombotic effects. The mutation is present in 40% of pregnant women with VTEs (Girling and de Swiet, 1998; Gerhardt et al., 2000; Lockwood, 2001). But despite this high attributable risk, given the low prevalence of thromboembolism in pregnancy, the actual risk of VTE in asymptomatic FVL carriers is only 0.2% (Gerhardt et al., 2000). In contrast, homozygosity for the mutation, although rare, is associated with a 15.8% (95% CI, 3.4–39.6) prevalence of venous thrombosis and confers a relative risk of pregnancy-related VTE of 41.3 (4.1–419.7) (Martinelli et al., 2001). Compound heterozygotes (i.e., carriers of one allele each) for the FVL and prothrombin gene mutations have a lower, 4.6%, risk of pregnancy-related VTE (Martinelli et al., 2001).

The FVL mutation appears to be associated with second- and third-trimester fetal loss, severe IUGR, abruption, severe, early-onset preeclampsia, and preterm delivery (Preston et al., 1996; Brenner et al., 1997; Gris et al., 1999; Kupferminc et al., 1999; Erhardt et al., 2000; Gerhardt et al., 2000; Glueck et al., 2000; Guideline, 2001; Lockwood, 2001; Rey et al., 2003). Consistent with the generation of uteroplacental thrombosis and vascular insufficiency, when compared with non-carriers, FVL carriers demonstrate an increased proportion of pathological Doppler measurements, including bilateral uterine artery notches (8.1% versus 21.2%; relative risk of 3.1 [95% CI: 1.2–8.1]) (Lindqvist et al., 2001).

In contrast, with the increased occurrence of later adverse pregnancy outcomes, the association between FVL heterozygosity and recurrent first-trimester loss remains controversial, with a number of authors finding no association (Preston et al., 1996; Pihusch et al., 2001; Rai et al., 2001; Ozcan et al., 2001; Rey et al., 2003) while others have demonstrated a weak association (Kupferminc et al., 1999; Souza et al., 1999; Foka et al., 2000; Rey et al., 2003). However, these later studies failed to discriminate between early (<10 weeks) and later (10–14 weeks) spontaneous abortion. Roque and colleagues noted a "protective" effect of FVL and other maternal thrombophilias on losses prior to 10 weeks' gestation but not on later (10–14 weeks) pregnancy loss (Roque et al., 2001). Consistent with this protective effect is the observation that *in vitro* fertilization (IVF) success rates were substantially higher among FVL carriers than among noncarriers (90% [9/10] versus 49% [45/92] [$P = 0.02$]) (Gopel et al., 2001).

The paradoxical observation that FVL and the other maternal thrombophilias are protective of early pregnancy loss suggests that maintenance of a low-oxygen environment prior to 10 weeks of gestation could be crucial to early pregnancy survival. Early pregnancy can be characterized as a relatively hypoxic state. Rodesch and associates noted an endometrial/intervillous oxygen pressure of 17 ± 6.9 mm Hg at 8–10 weeks of gestation that increased to 60.7 ± 8.5 mm Hg by 13 weeks' gestation (Rodesch et al., 1992). Jaffe and associates reported the presence of trophoblast plugging of the intervillous space in placental histology sections obtained prior to 10 weeks' gestation and observed only low-flow Doppler velocimetry of the intervillous space prior to that stage (Jaffe, 1993). That oxygen could be harmful during the embryonic period is suggested by the undetectable levels of superoxide dismutase, an enzyme responsible for the conversion of the superoxide anions, in embryos prior to 10 weeks' gestation (Watson et al., 1998). Conversely, following establishment of the uteroplacental circulation, uteroplacental thrombosis would convey progressively more harmful effects, accounting for the link between FVL and the other maternal thrombophilias and later adverse pregnancy outcomes.

Prothrombin Gene (G20210A) Mutation

A mutation in the promoter region of the prothrombin gene (G20210A) is present in 2%–3% of ethnic European populations (Guideline, 2001; Lockwood, 2001). It enhances circulating levels of prothrombin (150%–200%), increasing the risk of VTE (Gerhardt et al., 2000; Lockwood, 2001). Although the mutation accounts for 17% of VTE in pregnancy (Gerhardt et al., 2000), given the low prevalence of VTE in pregnancy, the actual risk of thrombosis in an asymptomatic pregnant carrier of the prothrombin G20210A mutation is only 0.5% (Gerhardt et al., 2000). As with the FVL mutation, the prothrombin mutation has also been associated with an increased risk of fetal loss, abruption, severe preeclampsia, and IUGR (Kupferminc et al., 1999; Foka et al., 2000; Martinelli et al., 2000; Guideline, 2001; Lockwood, 2001). Again, as with the FVL mutation, there appears to be at best a weak association between the prothrombin mutation and recurrent first-trimester loss (Pickering et al., 2001; Roque et al., 2001; Rey et al., 2003). Homozygosity for the prothrombin mutation confers a high risk of VTE, equivalent to AT deficiency or FVL homozygosity (Lockwood, 2001).

Protein C and S Deficiencies

Deficiencies of PC are generally autosomal dominant and can result from protean mutations producing two primary phenotypes: Type I, in which both immunoreactive protein levels and PC activity are reduced; and Type II, in which immunoreactive levels are normal but activity is reduced (Lockwood, 2001). Protein S deficiency has three subtypes: Type I, characterized by reduced total and free immunoreactive protein levels and activity; Type II, characterized by normal total and free immunoreactive PS levels but reduced activity; and Type III, in which there are normal total immunoreactive levels but reduced free immunoreactive levels and activity because of increased binding to the C4b-BP carrier protein. The prevalence of primary PC and PS deficiencies is 0.5% and 0.08%, respectively; however, acquired PS deficiency may be present in up to 8% of patients as a result of transient elevations in C4b-BP levels due to inflammation and other stressors (Girling and de Swiet, 1998; Guideline, 2001; Lockwood, 2001).

The reported risks of VTE during pregnancy or the postpartum period with either PC or PS deficiency (<5%) appear to be more comparable to the risk incurred by the FVL and prothrombin mutations than the risk associated with AT deficiency (Walker, 1991). Because of their relative rarity, there is a paucity of reports on the effects of isolated PC and PS deficiencies on pregnancy outcome. There appears, however, to be an increased risk of stillbirth with both PC and PS deficiencies with significant adjusted odds ratios (95% CI) of 2.3 (0.6–8.3) and 3.3 (1.0–11.3), respectively, but not an increased risk of spontaneous abortion with nonsignificant adjusted odds ratios of 1.4 (0.9–2.2) and 1.2 (0.7–1.9), respectively (Preston et al., 1996). Sanson and colleagues also found the relative risk of fetal loss among protein C-, S-, or AT-deficient women to be 2.0 (1.2–3.3) (Sanson et al., 1996); while Rey and colleagues noted in a meta-analysis that PS was associated with recurrent fetal loss (OR, 14.72 [0.99–218]) while PC and AT deficiencies were not associated with such losses (Rey et al., 2003). In addition, rates of severe preeclampsia, abruption, and IUGR appear increased in affected patients (Dekker et al., 1995; Kupferminc et al., 1999; Kupferminc et al., 2000; Lockwood, 2001). Homozygotes for PC and PS deficiency present with neonatal purpura fulminans and are rarely encountered clinically.

Antithrombin Deficiency

The rarest and most thrombogenic of the inherited thrombophilias, AT deficiency can result from a myriad of possible mutations, usually inherited in an autosomal dominant fashion (Eriksson et al., 1995; Gris et al., 1999; Lockwood, 2001). The disorder has two principal forms: Type I, characterized by reductions in both circulating immunoreactive protein levels and activity; and Type II, characterized by normal immunoreactive protein levels but decreased activity (Lane et al., 1997). Although the risk of thrombosis among affected patients is up to 60% during pregnancy and 33% during the puerperium, its prevalence is low (1/1000 to 1/5000), and it accounts for 1% to 20% of maternal VTE (Girling and de Swiet, 1998; Conrad et al., 1990). The risk of early fetal loss and stillbirth are both increased with AT deficiency with odd ratios (95% CI) of 1.7 (1.0–2.8) and 5.2 (1.5–18.1), respectively (Preston et al., 1996). AT deficiency is rarely a cause of stillbirth, severe preeclampsia, IUGR or abruption, however, because of its low prevalence (Kupferminc et al., 1999; Lockwood, 2001).

4G/4G Type-1 Plasminogen Activator Inhibitor Mutation (PAI-1)

The promoter region of the PAI-1 gene contains at least two alternate alleles producing either a four or five guanine (G) base-pair region. While the larger 5G allele permits the binding of transcription factor inhibitors, the smaller 4G allele does not permit the binding of gene repressors. Thus, homozygotes for the 4G/4G allele have a three- to fivefold higher level of circulating PAI-1 compared with those having the 5G/5G alleles (Kohler and Grant, 2000). Homozygosity for the 4G/4G allele could be present in up to a quarter of the population (Eriksson et al., 1995) and causes a modestly increased risk of thromboembolism, fetal loss, IUGR, preeclampsia, and preterm delivery (Glueck et al., 2000; Yamada et al., 2000).

Hyperhomocysteinemia

Homocysteine, generated from the metabolism of the amino acid methionine (Fig. 48-4), normally circulates in the plasma at concentrations of 5–12 μmol/L (Lockwood, 2001).

HOMOCYSTEINE METABOLISM

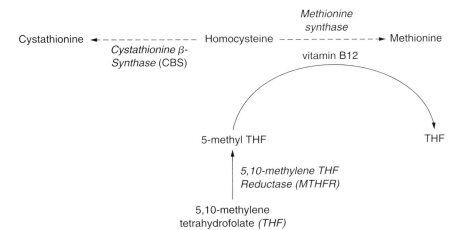

FIGURE 48-4 ■ Mutations in the genes for methionine synthase, cystathionine synthase, or methylene THF reductase with low folate or vitamin B$_{12}$ levels cause elevated homocysteine levels.

Hyperhomocysteinemia can be caused by a number of mutated genes for enzymes in the methionine metabolic pathway and is exacerbated by deficiencies in vitamin B_{12} and folic acid. Hyperhomocysteinemia can be diagnosed by measuring fasting homocysteine levels through gas-chromatography mass spectrometry. The disorder is classified by the fasting homocysteine level:

1. Severe (greater than 100 μmol/L)
2. Moderate (25–100 μmol/L)
3. Mild (16–24 μmol/L).

The severe form results from extremely rare (less than 1/200,000) homozygous deficiencies in either cystathionine β-synthase (CBS) or methylenetetrahydrofolate reductase (MTHFR) enzymes (Lockwood, 2001). Severe hyperhomocysteinemia presents with neurological abnormalities, premature atherosclerosis, and recurrent VTE.

Homozygosity for the 667C-T MTHFR thermolabile mutant is present in up to 11% of ethnic European populations and is the leading cause of mild and moderate hyperhomocysteinemia (Lockwood, 2001). Mild and moderate hyperhomocysteinemia patients are also at risk for fetal neural tube defects (Lockwood, 2001). Eskes (2001) noted that hyperhomocysteinemia resulted in an odds ratio of 4.7 (1.6–14.0) for abruption, while homozygosity for the C677T mutation produced an odds ratio of 2.5 (1.0–6.0). Hyperhomocysteinemia has also been linked with severe preeclampsia, stillbirths, and IUGR (Dekker et al., 1995; de Vries et al., 1997; Kupferminc et al., 1999; Lockwood, 2001). There is no consistent association between hyperhomocysteinemia and recurrent spontaneous abortions (Foka et al., 2000; Murphy et al., 2000; Nelen et al., 2000; Roque et al., 2001; Lachmeijer et al., 2001; Lockwood, 2001).

Acquired Thrombophilias

Antiphospholipid Syndrome

Antiphospholipid syndrome (APS) is an autoimmune disorder defined by the presence of characteristic clinical features and specified levels of circulating antiphospholipid antibodies (APLAs) (Table 48-1). Although several APLAs have been described, the lupus anticoagulant (LA) and anticardiolipin antibodies (aCL) antibodies are most widely accepted for clinical use. These antibodies have been associated with a variety of medical problems, including arterial and venous thromboses, autoimmune thrombocytopenia, and fetal loss (Harris et al., 1986; Harris, 1987; Asherson et al., 1989; Alarcon-Segovia et al., 1992; Viard et al., 1992; Levine et al., 2002). In addition to fetal loss, several obstetric disorders have been associated with APLAs. Pregnancies resulting in surviving infants are frequently complicated by preeclampsia, fetal growth restriction, placental insufficiency, and preterm delivery (Branch et al., 1992; Lima et al., 1996). Other autoimmune conditions, especially systemic lupus erythematosus (SLE), often coexist with APS. Individuals meeting criteria for APS who have another underlying autoimmune disease are considered to have *secondary* APS (Harris, 1987; Alarcon-Segovia et al., 1992). *Primary* APS refers to patients with APS but no other recognized autoimmune disorders (Harris, 1987; Asherson et al., 1989; Wilson et al., 1999). Approximately 70% of individuals with APS are female (Lockshin, 1997).

Antiphospholipid Antibodies

Laboratory testing for APLAs has been extremely confusing for practicing clinicians. Because this is a new and evolving science, controversy and uncertainty exist among experts about the exact nature and specificity of clinically relevant APLAs. Additional problems with APLA testing have included non-

---

TABLE 48-1. INTERNATIONAL CONSENSUS STATEMENT ON PRELIMINARY CRITERIA FOR THE CLASSIFICATION OF THE ANTIPHOSPHOLIPID SYNDROME*

Clinical Criteria

Vascular thrombosis

One or more clinical episodes of arterial, venous, or small-vessel thrombosis, occurring within any tissue or organ

Complications of pregnancy

One or more unexplained deaths of morphologically normal fetuses at or after the 10th week of gestation; or
One or more premature births of morphologically normal neonates at or before the 34th week of gestation; or
Three or more unexplained consecutive spontaneous abortions before the 10th week of gestation

Laboratory Criteria

Anticardiolipin antibodies

Anticardiolipin IgG or IgM antibodies present at moderate or high levels in the blood on two or more occasions
    at least six weeks apart

Lupus anticoagulant antibodies

Lupus anticoagulant antibodies detected in the blood on two or more occasions at least six weeks apart,
    according to the guidelines of the International Society on Thrombosis and Hemostasis

---

* A diagnosis of definite antiphospholipid syndrome requires the presence of at least one of the clinical criteria and at least one of the laboratory criteria. No limits are placed on the interval between the clinical event and the positive laboratory findings.

From Wilson WA, Gharavi AE, Koike T, et al.: International consensus statement on preliminary classification criteria for definite antiphospholipid syndrome: Report of an international workshop. Arthritis Rheum **42:**1309, 1999.

standardized assays, unacceptable interlaboratory variation, and inadequate quality control (Coulam et al., 1990; Peaceman et al., 1992). These issues are further compounded by the introduction and widespread availability of new assays with unproven clinical utility. Many of these issues are being resolved through international workshops. Meanwhile, clinicians should recognize the limitations of available assays and attempt to use a reliable laboratory with expertise in APLA testing.

The two APLAs that are best characterized and most useful clinically are LA and aCL. Many women with LA also have aCL and vice versa, but the correlation is imperfect (Triplett et al., 1988; Lockshin, 1997). Some investigators believe that they are related but different immunoglobulins because LA and aCL can be separated in the laboratory (Chamley et al., 1991). Others suggest that LA and aCL are the same antibody detected by different methods (Pierangeli et al., 1993). Regardless, LA and aCL are both independently associated with the clinical feature of APS. Because some individuals with APS have either LA or aCL, but not both, testing for both antibodies is recommended.

Lupus Anticoagulant

Lupus anticoagulant is an unusual name for an antibody and a double misnomer as well. LA is present in many individuals without SLE and is associated with thrombosis, not anticoagulation. It can be detected in plasma by any one of several phospholipid-dependent clotting assays. Examples include the activated partial thromboplastin time (aPTT), kaolin clotting time (KCT), dilute Russell viper venom time (dRVVT), and plasma clotting time. In these assays, phospholipids serve as a template on which enzymes and cofactors of the clotting cascade interact. If LA is present, it can bind to phospholipids, proteins, or epitopes created by phospholipid-protein interactions, interfering with the interaction of the clotting factors and prolonging the time to clot formation. The sensitivity and specificity of each test for LA are greatly affected by the reagents used and vary among laboratories. Thus, studies that compare the merit of each assay may not be applicable to every institution, and the "best" test for LA could differ from laboratory to laboratory.

Prolonged clotting times in these assays can be due to factors other than LA, such as improperly processed specimens, anticoagulant medications, clotting factor deficiencies, and factor-specific inhibitors. Thus, plasma suspected of containing LA based on a prolonged clotting time should be subjected to confirmatory testing (Fig. 48-5). First, a mixing study is done wherein the patient's plasma is mixed with normal plasma. If the prolonged clotting time is due to a factor deficiency, the addition of normal plasma (containing the missing factor) allows a normal clotting time on repeat testing. In contrast, if an inhibitor such as LA is present, the clotting time remains prolonged.

Some authorities recommend a second confirmatory test involving the addition or removal of phospholipid from the assay. For example, if LA is present, preincubation of plasma with phospholipid removes LA and normalizes clotting time. The platelet neutralization test is frequently used as a second confirmatory assay.

The sequence of assays used to detect LA is complex, and results can be confusing. Fortunately, clinicians need only order a test for LA, which includes some combination of phospholipid-dependent clotting assays and confirmatory tests.

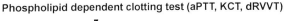
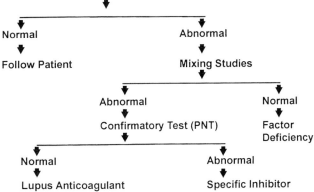

FIGURE 48-5 ■ Detection of lupus anticoagulant. aPTT, activated partial thromboplastin time; dRVVT, dilute Russell viper venon time; KCT, kaolin clotting time; PNT, platelet neutralization test. (From Silver RM, Branch DW: Recurrent miscarriage: Autoimmune considerations. Clin Obstet Gynecol **37**:745, 1994.)

Regardless of the assays used, LA cannot be quantified and is reported as present or absent.

Anticardiolipin Antibodies

Anticardiolipin antibodies (ACA) are detected by conventional immunoassays using purified cardiolipin to bind target proteins. Interlaboratory variation in this assay (Coulam et al., 1990; Peaceman et al., 1992) prompted the development of standard sera, available from the Antiphospholipid Standardization Laboratory in Atlanta, Georgia (Harris and Spinnato, 1991). Assays using these standard positive serum calibrators are quite reliable and allow for the semiquantification of antibody levels. Standard sera have been assigned numeric values termed GPL (immunoglobulin G [IgG] aCL), MPL (IgM aCL), and APL (IgA aCL) units and are reported as negative or as low, medium, or high positive (GPL = IgG binding units; MPL = IgM binding units; APL = IgA binding units).

Low positive aCL and isolated IgM aCL are of questionable clinical significance and should not be considered diagnostic of APS (Silver et al., 1996). The relevance of positive tests for IgA aCL is also uncertain. Low levels of IgG aCL and IgM aCL are sometimes found in healthy individuals (Harris and Spinnato, 1991) and can result from infections (Vaarala et al., 1986) and nonspecific binding. In contrast, several studies have shown a correlation between increasing titers of aCL and APLA-related disorders (Harris et al., 1986; Lockshin et al., 1989; Silver et al., 1996). Thus, only medium-high levels of IgG or IgM aCL, LA, or both are considered sufficient laboratory criteria for the definitive diagnosis of APS (Harris, 1987; Alarcon-Segovia et al., 1992). Positive tests for APLA can be transient and should be confirmed on two occasions at least several weeks apart (Harris, 1987; Rai, Regan, et al., 1995).

Other Antibodies Associated with APS

The antibody responsible for the biologically false-positive serologic test for syphilis (BF-STS) is also an APLA and is often present in patients having LA or aCL. Compared with LA and aCL, the BF-STS correlates poorly with the development of medical problems associated with APLA. Thus, the STS is not recommended in the routine evaluation of APS.

Several other APLAs can be identified with immunoassays using antibodies to phospholipid antigens other than cardiolipin, such as phosphatidylserine, phosphatidylethanolamine, phosphatidylinositol, phosphatidylglycerol, phosphatidylcholine, and phosphatidic acid. APLAs other than LA or aCL, especially antiphosphatidylserine antibodies, are sometimes found in patients with clinical problems associated with APLA (Yetman and Kutteh, 1996; Branch et al., 1997). Most individuals with positive tests for other APLAs, however, also have IgG aCL and LA (Branch et al., 1997). In addition, these assays have not been subjected to quality control or standardization. Tests for APLA other than LA and aCL could prove useful, but they cannot be recommended for routine clinical use.

Instead of directly binding phospholipids, APLAs likely bind either phospholipid-associated proteins or a phospholipid-protein complex. In 1990, three groups conclusively demonstrated that the abundant plasma glycoprotein, β_2-glycoprotein-I (β_2-GP-I), greatly enhances the binding of APLA to phospholipid (Galli et al., 1990; Matsuura et al., 1990; McNeil et al., 1990). Thus, β_2-GP-I was considered a critical cofactor for APLA binding. aCL can be separated into β_2-GP-I–dependent and β_2-GP-I–independent antibodies (Matsuura et al., 1990; Hunt et al., 1992; Aoki et al., 1995). Furthermore, β_2-GP-I–dependent aCL has been reported to correlate better with APS than β_2-GP-I–independent aCL (Hunt et al., 1992; Aoki et al., 1995). The standard assay for aCL uses sera containing β_2-GP-I and consequently identifies β_2-GP-I–dependent aCL.

Many investigators now believe that β_2-GP-I may actually be the true antigen recognized by APLA (Koike and Matsuura, 1991; Roubey, 1994). Antibodies recognizing β_2-GP-I in the absence of phospholipid can be measured and have been associated with the same clinical problems as APLA (Viard et al., 1992; Cabiedes et al., 1995; McNally et al., 1995). In fact, some investigators have suggested that anti–β_2-GP-I may correlate better with APS than does APLA (Cabiedes et al., 1995). Also, some patients with APS may test negative for LA and aCL but positive for anti–β_2-GP-I (Cabral et al., 1996). Anti–β_2-GP-I, however, strongly correlates with aCL, and testing for both antibodies was not found to be superior to aCL testing alone in a cohort of women with recurrent pregnancy loss (Lee et al., 1999). Thus, the clinical utility and cost effectiveness of anti–β_2-GP-I testing in women with obstetric features of APS remain to be determined. It is noteworthy that anti–β_2-GP-I are not currently included in the diagnostic criteria for the APS, but this could change as more data become available.

Several other APLAs or antibodies against phospholipid binding proteins other than cardiolipin-bound β_2 glycoprotein-I have been described. Examples include antibodies against annexin V, prothrombin, protein C, and protein S. As with anti–β_2-GP-I, the clinical utility of testing for these antibodies is uncertain.

Medical Complications

Arguably, the most worrisome complication associated with APLAs is thrombosis (Harris et al., 1986; Hughes et al., 1986; Harris, 1987). Most thrombotic events (65%–70%) are venous, but arterial thromboses and stroke are common (Rosove and Brewer, 1992; Khamashta et al., 1995). The most frequent site of venous thrombosis is the lower extremity, and up to one-half of patients suffer at least one pulmonary embolus. Thrombosis can occur in almost any blood vessel in the body, and occlusions

in unusual locations should prompt clinicians to consider the diagnosis of APS. APLAs account for 2% of VTE (Malm et al., 1992). Thus, unexplained thrombosis in otherwise healthy patients is an indication for APLA testing.

APLAs are also associated with arterial thrombosis, which can occur in atypical sites such as retinal, subclavian, digital, or brachial arteries. Stroke is the most common arterial event, and the most frequently involved vessel is the middle cerebral artery. Transient ischemic attacks (TIAs) and amaurosis fugax are also associated with APLAs (Silver, Draper, Scott, et al., 1994; Silver et al., 1996). Among otherwise healthy individuals with stroke who are younger than 50 years of age, 4%–6% have positive tests for APLAs (Brey et al., 1990; Ferro et al., 1993). Coronary occlusions are also common (Asherson et al., 1989). Individuals with unexplained arterial thrombosis, stroke, amaurosis fugax, or transient ischemic attacks should undergo testing for APLAs.

Pregnancy and the use of estrogen-containing oral contraceptives appear to increase the risk for thrombosis in women with APS. In retrospective analyses of women with APS, most thromboses occurred in association with pregnancy or oral contraceptive use (Branch et al., 1992; Silver, Draper, Scott, et al., 1994). Similarly, 25% of VTE events occurred during pregnancy or the postpartum period in a large cohort study (Silver, Draper, Scott, et al., 1994). These findings were confirmed in prospective studies indicating a 5%–12% risk of thrombosis during pregnancy or the puerperium in women with APS (Branch et al., 1992; Lima et al., 1996). These data provide the rationale for the avoidance of estrogen-containing oral contraceptives and the use of thromboprophylaxis during pregnancy in women with well-characterized APS.

Individuals with APS and previous thrombosis are at substantial risk for recurrent thrombosis. One large cohort study found a recurrence rate of 25% per year in untreated patients with APS and prior thrombosis (Khamashta et al., 1995). More than 69% of these individuals experienced at least one recurrent event during a relatively short follow-up interval. Fortunately, anticoagulation with coumarin to achieve an International Normalized Ratio (INR) of 3 decreases the risk for recurrent thrombosis (Khamashta et al., 1995). It is noteworthy that discontinuation of coumarin is associated with an increased risk of thrombosis.

Autoimmune thrombocytopenia has also been strongly associated with APLA, occurring in 40%–50% of individuals with primary APS (Harris et al., 1985; Asherson et al., 1989; Alarcon-Segovia et al., 1992). Thrombocytopenia associated with APLA is extremely difficult to distinguish from idiopathic thrombocytopenic purpura (ITP). Although the pertinent platelet antigens appear to differ in APS and ITP, no tests distinguish the two disorders reliably. Fortunately, cases of thrombocytopenia caused by ITP and APS are treated identically.

A variety of other medical conditions have been associated with APLAs, including autoimmune hemolytic anemia, livedo reticularis, cutaneous ulcers, chorea gravidarum, multi-infarct dementia, and transverse myelitis (Asherson et al., 1989; Alarcon-Segovia et al., 1992). Occasionally, patients with APS suffer fulminant, life-threatening manifestations of the disease. Some individuals incur progressive thromboses and multiorgan failure, termed *catastrophic antiphospholipid syndrome* (Asherson et al., 1998). Others have a severe illness postpartum consisting primarily of cardiopulmonary failure and fever as well as renal insufficiency and multiple thromboses (Kochenour et al., 1987; Hochfeld et al., 1994; Kupferminc et al., 1994). Both conditions can be fatal.

Obstetric Complications

Numerous retrospective studies have established a strong relationship between the presence of circulating LA and aCL and pregnancy loss (Beaumont, 1954; Reece et al., 1984; Branch et al., 1985; Lockshin et al., 1985; Harris et al., 1986). In fact, the rate of fetal loss in untreated women with LA and previous pregnancy failure could be greater than 80% (Branch and Scott, 1991; Branch et al., 1992; Rai, Clifford, et al., 1995). These data have been confirmed by cohort studies in unselected populations (Lockwood et al., 1989; Pattison et al., 1993; Lynch et al., 1994; Yasuda et al., 1995) and in women with APS (Branch et al., 1992; Cowchock et al., 1992; Out et al., 1992; Rai, Clifford, et al., 1995), demonstrating APLA to be a prospective risk factor for pregnancy loss.

A remarkably large proportion of APLA-related pregnancy losses are second- or third-trimester fetal deaths. Although fetal deaths account for only a few percent of all pregnancy losses in the general population (Goldstein, 1994), 50% of losses in a cohort of 76 women (333 pregnancies) with APS at the University of Utah were fetal deaths (Oshiro et al., 1996). Of these women, 80% had suffered at least one fetal death.

APLAs have been inconsistently associated with recurrent early pregnancy loss. Cohort and case-control studies have not consistently documented positive tests for ACA in a higher proportion of women with recurrent spontaneous abortion than in controls (Petri et al., 1987; Barbui et al., 1988; Out, Bruinse, Christaens, et al., 1991; Parazzini et al., 1991; Parke et al., 1991; MacLean et al., 1994; Rai, Regan, et al., 1995; Balasch et al., 1996; Yetman and Kutteh, 1996). Most investigators report positive tests for APLA in 5%–20% of women with recurrent pregnancy loss (Table 48-2). Many positive results, however, are low-titer or IgM isotype only. Although low levels of APLA could prove relevant to obstetric outcome, as stated earlier, they identify a distinct population at lower risk for APLA-related disorders than patients with APS (Silver et al., 1996). The group at the University of Utah has detected high-titer APLA (LA or medium-high positive IgG aCL) in 4%–5% of a referral population with recurrent spontaneous abortion; however, this study did not distinguish early from late spontaneous abortion (Branch and Scott, 1991).

In contrast to recurrent pregnancy loss, APLAs are not associated with sporadic preembryonic or embryonic pregnancy loss (Infante-Rivard et al., 1991). This is an expected observation given the myriad causes of individual pregnancy loss, the infrequency of APS, and the aforementioned minimal uteroplacental blood flow presents prior to 10 weeks' gestation. Thus, testing for APLA in women with isolated preembryonic or embryonic pregnancy loss is neither clinically useful nor recommended. It is uncertain whether APLAs are related to sporadic fetal death. Some (Bocciolone et al., 1994; Ahlenius et al., 1995) but not all (Haddow et al., 1991) studies have detected increased rates of APLA in unselected women with fetal deaths.

In addition to pregnancy loss, several obstetric disorders have been associated with APLAs. Successful pregnancies in women with APS are frequently complicated by preeclampsia, fetal growth impairment, abnormal fetal heart rate tracings, and preterm birth. These disorders are all characterized by uteroplacental insufficiency and can result in fetal death without obstetric intervention.

Preeclampsia is very common in women with well-characterized APS (Branch et al., 1992; Lima et al., 1996). At the University of Utah, 50% of women with APS had preeclampsia and 25% had severe preeclampsia (Branch et al., 1992). APLAs have been a prospective risk factor for the development of preeclampsia in some (Pattison et al., 1993; Yasuda et al., 1995), but not all, selected populations (Lynch et al., 1994).

APLAs are also present in some women with preeclampsia, especially severe preeclampsia requiring delivery prior to 34 weeks' gestation. An 11%–17% rate of positive tests for APLA has been reported in women with preeclampsia (Branch et al., 1989; Milliez et al., 1991; Sletnes et al., 1992; Moodley et al., 1995). Conversely, routine term preeclampsia is not associated with increased levels of APLAs (Scott, 1987). Thus, the association is strongest in women with severe, early-onset (prior to 34 weeks' gestation) preeclampsia. Prospective testing for APLAs in women at risk for preeclampsia is of little prognostic value and is not recommended (Branch et al., 2001).

Intrauterine growth restriction (IUGR) is also common in APS pregnancies, occurring in 15%–30% in most series (Branch et al., 1992; Caruso et al., 1993; Kutteh, 1996; Lima et al., 1996). Positive tests for APLA occur in 25% of women delivering IUGR fetuses (Polzin et al., 1991), and APLAs have been associated with IUGR in pregnancies complicated

TABLE 48-2. POSITIVE TESTS FOR ANTIPHOSPHOLIPID ANTIBODIES IN WOMEN WITH RECURRENT PREGNANCY LOSS (RPL) AND CONTROLS

Author	Lupus Anticoagulant		IgG Anticardiolipin		Total Positive	
	RPL (%)	Controls (%)	RPL (%)	Controls (%)	RPL (%)	Controls (%)
Petri et al., 1987	4/44 (9)	0/40 (0)	5/44 (11)	1/40 (2)	7/44 (16)	1/40 (2)
Barbui et al., 1988	7/49 (14)	0/141 (0)	4/49 (8)	0/141 (0)	7/49 (14)	0/141 (0)
Parazzini et al., 1991	16/220 (7)	0/193 (0)	11/99 (11)	4/157 (3)	10/99 (10)	4/157 (3)
Parke et al., 1991	4/81 (5)	4/88 (5)	6/81 (7)	0/88 (0)	8/81 (10)	4/88 (5)
Out et al., 1991	5/102 (5)	NA	8/102 (8)	2/102 (8)	11/102 (11)	NA
Yetman and Kutteh, 1996	NA	NA	135/866 (16)	12/288 (4)	NA	NA
MacLean et al., 1994	16/243 (7)	NA	20 (8)	NA	41/243 (17)	NA
Rai et al., 1995	46/500 (9)	NA	15/500 (3)	NA	61/500 (12)	NA
Balasch et al., 1996	17/199 (8)	0/125 (0)	14/199 (7)	0/125 (0)	24/199 (12)	0/125 (0)
MEDIAN	8%	0%	8%	2%	12%	2%

Ig, immunoglobulin; NA, not available.

From Silver RM, Branch DW: Autoimmune disease in pregnancy: Systemic lupus erythematosus and anti-phospholipid syndrome. Clin Perinatol **24:**291, 1997.

by preeclampsia (Sletnes et al., 1992). Other studies have not found a correlation between APLA and IUGR (Pattison et al., 1993; Lynch et al., 1994). This discrepancy could be due to the inclusion of some women with low positive tests for APLA, because the risk of IUGR increases with increasing titers of APLA (Lockshin et al., 1989; Kutteh, 1996; Lima et al., 1996).

Uteroplacental insufficiency, as indicated by abnormal fetal heart rate tracings, occurs in up to 50% of pregnancies with APS (Branch et al., 1992; Lima et al., 1996). It is noteworthy that placental insufficiency can be evident in the second trimester. Druzin and coworkers (1987) noted spontaneous decelerations of the fetal heart rate (FHR) during the second trimester in several fetuses who subsequently died in utero. Uteroplacental insufficiency, preeclampsia, and IUGR all increase the risk of iatrogenic preterm birth in women with APS. Although variably defined, preterm birth has been reported in 12%–35% of individuals with APLA (Branch et al., 1992; Yasuda et al., 1995; Kutteh, 1996; Lima et al., 1996). The risk is greatest in women with high titers of APLA who meet strict criteria for APS. Branch and colleagues (1992) have reported that approximately a third of APS pregnancies resulting in live births deliver prior to 34 weeks' gestation.

Indications for APLA Testing

Generally accepted indications for APLA testing are listed in Table 48-3. Although most are straightforward, the obstetric indications are a matter of some controversy. In part, this is due to poorly characterized obstetric details in available studies as well as a need for additional information.

APLAs, especially low levels of IgM aCL, are present in a few healthy people (Lockwood et al., 1989; Harris and Spinnato, 1991) and are probably meaningless. Clinicians who test for APLAs in women without clinical features of APS may be left with an uninterpretable positive test and a management dilemma. It is best to avoid such problems by testing only patients with disorders clearly related to APLA.

Pathogenesis of Antiphospholipid Syndrome

Because APS is characterized by thrombosis and uteroplacental insufficiency, investigators proposed that thrombosis within the uteroplacental circulation leads to placental infarction and eventual fetal death. This hypothesis has been supported by numerous case reports and case series of extensive thrombosis, infarction, and necrosis in the placentas of women with APS and fetal death (Fig. 48-6) (DeWolf et al., 1982; Branch et al., 1985; Silver, Draper, Byrne, et al., 1994; Nayar and Lage, 1996). In addition to thrombosis and infarction, a decidual vasculopathy characterized by atherosis, intimal thickening, fibrinoid necrosis, and a lack of "normal physiologic changes" in the spiral arteries has been reported in the placentas of APS pregnancies (DeWolf et al., 1982; Nayar and Lage, 1996). This spiral arterial vasculopathy has also been associated with preeclampsia and IUGR (Khong et al., 1986). These findings have been confirmed in a large, case-controlled, histologic evaluation of placentas in women with APLAs and fetal loss (Out, Kooijman, et al., 1991).

Unfortunately, the histologic abnormalities described in these studies are nonspecific (Khong et al., 1986) and are not consistent findings in all pregnancies complicated by APS (Lockshin et al., 1985; Salafia and Parke, 1997). A lack of cor-

TABLE 48-3. INDICATIONS FOR ANTIPHOSPHOLIPID ANTIBODY TESTING

Recurrent spontaneous abortion*
Unexplained second or third trimester fetal death
Severe preeclampsia prior to 34 weeks' gestation
Unexplained venous thrombosis
Unexplained arterial thrombosis
Unexplained stroke
Unexplained transient ischemic attack or amaurosis fugax
Systemic lupus erythematosus or other connective tissue disease
Autoimmune thrombocytopenia
Autoimmune hemolytic anemia
Livedo reticularis
Chorea gravidarum
False-positive serologic test for syphilis
Unexplained prolongation in clotting assay
Unexplained severe intrauterine growth restriction

* Three or more spontaneous abortions with no more than one live birth.

relation between placental findings and fetal outcome has also been noted. It is likely that factors other than placental thrombosis contribute to APLA-related pregnancy loss.

Several possible mechanisms for the decidual vasculopathy and associated thrombosis have been suggested (Fig. 48-7). An attractive and popular hypothesis among obstetricians is that APLAs lead to an increase in the thromboxane:prostacyclin ratio in gestational tissues. Similar pathophysiology has been associated with preeclampsia and IUGR (Walsh, 1985), conditions which similarly are linked to APLA. APLAs can increase the in vitro production of thromboxane by placental explants without altering prostacyclin formation (Peaceman and Rehnberg, 1992, 1993). APLA-induced thromboxane production can be inhibited by aspirin (Peaceman and Rehnberg, 1995), providing a rationale for the clinical use of low-dose aspirin in pregnancies complicated by APS. In addition, fetal loss can be reduced in a murine model of APS by thromboxane inhibition in vivo (Shoenfeld and Blank, 1994). Other investigators, however, have found that APLAs do not alter prostaglandin production (Walker et al., 1988; Dudley et al., 1990). Although intriguing, the roles of thromboxane and

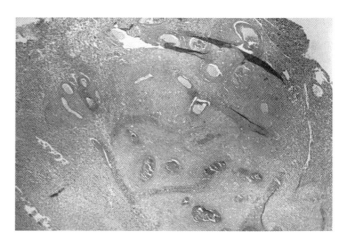

FIGURE 48-6 ■ Placenta demonstrating extensive infarction and vascular thrombosis, taken from a pregnancy resulting in second trimester fetal death in a patient with antiphospholipid syndrome (APS). (From Silver RM, Branch DW: Autoimmune disease in pregnancy: Systemic lupus erythematosus and anti-phospholipid syndrome. Clin Perinatol **24**:291, 320, 1997.)

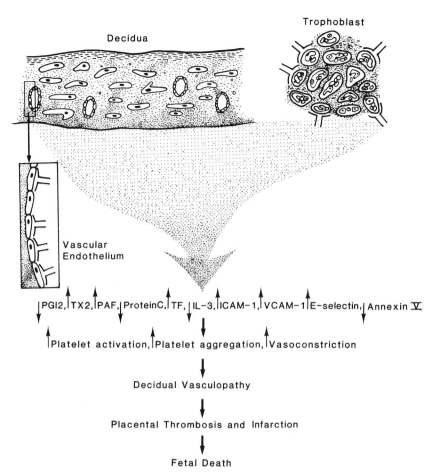

Decidua

Trophoblast

Vascular
Endothelium

| PGI2,|TX2,|PAF,|ProteinC,|TF,|IL-3,|ICAM-1,|VCAM-1|E-selectin,|Annexin Ⅴ|

↑Platelet activation,|Platelet aggregation,|Vasoconstriction

Decidual Vasculopathy

Placental Thrombosis and Infarction

Fetal Death

FIGURE 48-7. ■ Proposed mechanisms of fetal loss associated with antiphospholipid antibodies. (Modified from Silver RM, Branch DW: Recurrent miscarriage: Autoimmune considerations. Clin Obstet Gynecol **37**:745, 1994.)

prostacyclin in human pregnancy loss associated with APLAs remain uncertain.

Numerous other mechanisms have been proposed to explain the episodic vascular thromboses and placental pathology associated with APLAs. Most investigators have focused on the ability of APLAs (or anti–β_2-GP-I) to initiate a prothrombotic cascade of events after binding to either native or damaged gestational tissues, platelets, or endothelium. Thrombogenic mediators induced by APLAs *in vitro* include tissue factor (Tannenbaum et al., 1986; Branch and Rogers, 1993), platelet-activating factor (Silver et al., 1991), thrombin (Ginsberg et al., 1993), E-selectin, and vascular cell adhesion molecule 1 (VCAM-1) (Simantov et al., 1995). APLAs also can promote thrombosis via platelet activation and aggregation (Khamashta et al., 1988; Campbell et al., 1995) and the inhibition of protein C, protein S, and thrombomodulin (Cariou et al., 1988; Lockshin, 1997). Of particular interest to obstetricians is the discovery that APLAs can inhibit the function of placental anticoagulant protein I, also known as annexin V (Sammaritano et al., 1992; Rand et al., 1997). APLAs could promote intervillous thrombosis by displacing this endogenous anticoagulant protein on the surface of trophoblast (Rand et al., 1997). Another potential mechanism for APLA-induced fetal loss is complement activation. Holers and colleagues (2002) demonstrated that complement C3 activation is required for fetal loss in a murine model of APS. All of these theories are promising, but none adequately explains the heterogeneous clinical features associated with APLA.

An important and unresolved issue is whether APLAs are directly pathogenic. Passive immunization with either purified APLAs or APLA-containing IgG fraction can result in murine fetal loss and the facilitation of thrombosis in animal models (Branch et al., 1992; Shoenfeld and Blank, 1994; Pierangeli et al., 1994). These data strongly implicate APLA as an effector of thrombosis and pregnancy loss. Conversely, many APLAs do not cause harm in animal models (Silver et al., 1995; Silver et al., 1997), antibody titer does not always correlate with disease severity, and several individuals have been shown to develop APLA only after the onset of clinically apparent APS (Silver et al., 1996). Thus, APLAs could be a marker for, rather than a cause of, disease.

MANAGEMENT OF THROMBOPHILIAS

Inherited Thrombophilias

The inherited thrombophilias increase the risk of maternal VTE as well as fetal loss after 10 weeks' gestation, abruptions, IUGR, and severe, early-onset preeclampsia up to fivefold. There are no randomized clinical trials, however, to judge the efficacy of anticoagulation therapy in preventing adverse maternal or fetal outcomes. Management paradigms can logically be divided between the extremely rare, highly thrombogenic and the common (but less thrombogenic) inherited thrombophilias.

Management of the highly thrombogenic thrombophilias is quite straightforward. Regardless of prior medical or obstetrical histories, any pregnant patient with AT deficiency or those who are found to be homozygotes for the FVL or prothrombin G20210A mutations are at very high risk for maternal VTE and later adverse pregnancy outcomes. For this reason, they require therapeutic unfractionated or therapeutic low-molecular-weight heparin therapy throughout pregnancy (Lockwood, 2001). This therapy should be continued throughout the antepartum period until the onset of labor. Because low-molecular-weight heparin use has been associated with epidural hematoma formation because of its longer half-life compared with unfractionated heparin, spinal or epidural anesthesia should not be used within 18–24 hours of the last dose. Alternatively, one can replace low-molecular-weight heparin with unfractionated heparin at 36–37 weeks to facilitate the use of epidural anesthesia in labor. Among patients with AT deficiency, antithrombin concentrates can be used during labor and delivery in lieu of heparin to minimize both hemorrhagic and thrombotic risks (Lockwood, 2001). Around 6–12 hours after delivery, heparin therapy should be resumed and coumadin therapy initiated. Heparin must be continued for at least four days after starting coumadin and not discontinued until the INR has been in the therapeutic range (2–2.5) for two consecutive days. Although controversial in pregnancy, premature cessation of heparin may cause a paradoxical thrombosis because coumadin lowers protein C and S levels prior to that of the vitamin K-dependent clotting factors. Coumadin should be continued for at least six weeks, and longer (three to six months) if there has been a prior VTE.

Management of the less thrombogenic thrombophilias is more complex. Antenatal heparin treatment does not appear to be required in asymptomatic patients incidentally found to have a less thrombogenic inherited thrombophilia who are without a history of prior VTE or characteristic adverse pregnancy outcome. Their risks of either VTE and/or characteristic adverse pregnancy outcomes are likely less than 1% (Gerhardt et al., 2000; Lockwood, 2001). Postpartum prophylaxis may be appropriate for patients with affected first-degree relatives or other risk factors for thrombosis and should be given to those who have undergone a cesarean delivery. In contrast, patients with the less thrombogenic thrombophilias as well as compound heterozygotes for the FVL and prothrombin G20210A mutations and a prior VTE should receive prophylactic heparin therapy in the antepartum period. Coumadin can be begun in the immediate postpartum period, with the heparin continued for at least four days and until the INR has been therapeutic for 48 hours. Coumadin is continued for four to six weeks. The broad issue of VTE is discussed in detail in Chapter 42.

Women with a history of recurrent characteristic adverse pregnancy outcomes subsequently found to have an inherited thrombophilia may benefit from antepartum heparin therapy. Observational studies of low-dose aspirin and low-molecular-weight heparin have reported improvement in birth weight compared to untreated pregnancies (Kupferminc et al., 2001; Riyazi et al., 1998). Such patients may benefit from postpartum anticoagulation prophylaxis if they have an affected first-degree relative or other thrombotic risk and should receive such therapy if they have undergone a cesarean delivery.

If patients have characteristic adverse pregnancy outcomes and hyperhomocysteinemia is the sole defect detected, treatment with vitamin B_6, B_{12}, and folic acid (4 mg p.o., q.d.) supplementation appears justified prior to and throughout the pregnancy. Although there are no randomized clinical trials, observational studies support such an approach (Leeda et al., 1998), the toxicity of this therapy is minimal, and folic acid has proven of value in reducing the occurrence of fetal neural tube defects. Prophylactic heparin should be considered among hyperhomocysteinemic patients with a history of VTE or characteristic adverse pregnancy outcomes whose elevated homocysteine levels are unresponsive to such vitamin therapy.

Antiphospholipid Syndrome

Obstetric Management of Antiphospholipid Syndrome

MEDICAL THERAPY. Prompted by poor obstetric outcome in untreated pregnancies, clinicians have used a variety of medications in an attempt to improve fetal survival in women with APS. Medical therapies are based on proposed mechanisms of APLA-related pregnancy loss. Treatments are intended to suppress the immune system (steroids and intravenous immune globulin [IVIG]), to prevent thrombosis in the uteroplacental circulation (heparin and aspirin), and to improve placental blood flow by decreasing the thromboxane:prostacyclin ratio (low-dose aspirin [LDA]).

Lubbe and colleagues (1982) first suggested the use of high-dose prednisone (40–60 mg/day) and low-dose aspirin (60–85 mg/day) to treat women with LA and recurrent pregnancy loss. Since that time, investigators have reported markedly improved pregnancy outcomes using this regimen compared with previous pregnancies in the same women. Indeed, most case series have reported a 60%–70% rate of successful APS pregnancies with prednisone and low-dose aspirin. On the other hand, one group using lower doses of prednisone found no benefit (Lockshin et al., 1989). In addition, a meta-analysis of therapeutic trials showed no reduction in pregnancy loss in women treated with prednisone and low-dose aspirin (Empson et al., 2002). Direct comparison of studies is difficult because subjects had different clinical and laboratory features, dosing regimens varied, and many trials were unrandomized and poorly controlled. Thus, the efficacy of prednisone in pregnancies complicated by APS remains uncertain.

Heparin was first reported as a treatment for APS in 1984 (Garlund, 1984). Over the past two decades, several case series have documented successful pregnancies in approximately 70% of patients treated with heparin and low-dose aspirin (Rosove et al., 1990; Branch et al., 1992; Cowchock et al., 1992). Although full anticoagulation (mean daily dose, 24,700 units of unfractionated heparin) was achieved in one study (Rosove et al., 1990), pregnancy outcomes are similar using lower or "prophylactic" doses (15,000–20,000 units/day in divided doses) (Branch et al., 1992; Cowchock et al., 1992). These findings have been confirmed in two prospective randomized trials comparing prophylactic doses of heparin and low-dose aspirin to low-dose aspirin alone in women with recurrent pregnancy loss and positive tests for APLA (Kutteh, 1996; Rai et al., 1997). Both studies demonstrated significantly improved pregnancy outcomes in patients treated with heparin. The reduction in risk for pregnancy loss was 0.46 (95% CI, 0.29, 0.71) (Empson et al., 2002).

A small randomized trial showed that heparin and low-dose aspirin are as efficacious as prednisone and low-dose aspirin in achieving a successful pregnancy outcome (Cowchock et al., 1992). Women treated with prednisone, however, had an increased rate of preterm premature rupture of membranes (PROM), preterm delivery, and preeclampsia. Another randomized trial using prednisone in women with APLA confirmed the association of prednisone with these obstetric complications (Silver et al., 1993), and the meta-analysis reported an increase in prematurity in pregnancies treated with prednisone (RR, 4.83; 95% CI, 2.85, 8.21) (Empson et al., 2002). Because heparin has fewer side effects than prednisone and provides prophylaxis against thrombosis, heparin and low-dose aspirin are now recommended as primary therapy in women with APS.

Heparin use also has the potential for adverse effects including bleeding, thrombocytopenia, and osteoporosis with fracture. Because the risks of osteoporosis and bleeding increase with increasing doses of heparin, and anticoagulant doses are not better than prophylactic doses in improving fetal survival, prophylactic doses should be used in the absence of another indication for anticoagulation (such as prior thrombosis with APS, prior loss on prophylactic doses, and, perphas, very high ACA levels [e.g., >50 GPL or MPL units]). Axial skeleton weight-bearing exercise and calcium and vitamin D supplementation should be encouraged with the aim of lessening the risk of osteoporosis. If possible, heparin and prednisone should not be used simultaneously. Both predispose women to osteopenic fractures, and fetal outcome is no better with combination therapy than with either drug alone (Branch et al., 1992).

The optimal time to initiate heparin therapy is somewhat controversial. There are theoretical benefits to initiating treatment prior to conception. The side effects of prolonged therapy, however, likely offset these unproven advantages, and it seems reasonable to start heparin after the confirmation of a live, intrauterine embryo. Thromboprophylaxis should be continued through 6 weeks postpartum to minimize the risk of maternal thromboembolism. After delivery, this can be accomplished safely with coumarin. Low-molecular-weight heparin has been used safely in pregnancy (Pauzner et al., 2001) and may be substituted for unfractionated heparin in the treatment of APS.

It is uncertain whether low-dose aspirin improves outcome compared with heparin alone. Three trials comparing aspirin alone versus placebo showed no difference in pregnancy loss in women with positive tests for APLAs (Pattison et al., 2000; Empson et al., 2002). Thus, heparin appears to be more important than aspirin for the treatment of APS during pregnancy.

Despite increased rates of live births, pregnant women treated with heparin or prednisone are frequently plagued by obstetric complications. Of 31 pregnancies in women with APS who were treated with heparin at the University of Utah, two-thirds suffered preeclampsia, more than 40% had IUGR, and 25% delivered prior to 32 weeks' gestation (Branch et al., 1992). These complications, as well as pregnancy losses in patients treated with heparin or prednisone, have prompted a search for better therapies.

Treatment with IVIG has been promising in a small number of cases refractory to heparin or prednisone (Carreras et al., 1988; Scott et al., 1988; Spinnato et al., 1994). Obstetric complications also have been rare in patients treated with IVIG (Spinnato et al., 1994). Most of these women, however, were also treated with heparin or prednisone and low-dose aspirin. A recent, small, randomized, controlled study demonstrated no benefit to IVIG (plus heparin and aspirin) compared with heparin and aspirin alone (Branch et al., 2000). Because the efficacy of IVIG has not been proven in appropriately designed studies and the drug is extremely expensive, it is not recommended as primary therapy.

It is unclear whether women with low levels of APLA or isolated IgM APLA need treatment during pregnancy. Conclusions from studies of women with APS cannot be applied to patients with low levels of APLA because these populations have very different risks for the development of APLA-related disorders (Silver et al., 1996). Three prospective, randomized clinical trials included some patients with recurrent pregnancy loss and low-titer APLA who did not meet other criteria for APS. One study excluded women with SLE or previous thromboembolism (Rai et al., 1997), and the other two included very few women with these conditions (Silver et al., 1993; Kutteh, 1996). Thus, the subjects in these studies appeared to form a different population than studies including women with medical disorders associated with aPL (Branch et al., 1992; Lima et al., 1996). One trial showed that prednisone and low-dose aspirin did not improve fetal outcome compared with low-dose aspirin alone (Silver et al., 1993); however, the other two studies noted increased fetal survival in subjects treated with heparin and low-dose aspirin compared with low-dose aspirin alone (Kutteh, 1996; Rai et al., 1997).

CLINICAL MANAGEMENT. Women with APS should receive preconception counseling regarding their risk for pregnancy loss, preeclampsia, IUGR, preterm birth, cesarean delivery, and thrombosis. If the diagnosis of APS is uncertain, relevant levels of LA and IgG aCL should be confirmed. Although advocated by some, the benefits of serial antibody testing during pregnancy or in titrating medical therapy to suppress antibody levels have not been confirmed. There is no value in serial APLA testing once the diagnosis of APS is certain. Intensive surveillance (e.g., weekly clinic visits and twice weekly non-stress testing) for preeclampsia, IUGR, and placental insufficiency should be instituted at 30–32 weeks' gestation. Fetal monitoring earlier in gestation (24–25 weeks) and serial sonograms could be beneficial in selected cases, such as women with preeclampsia, IUGR, and prior midtrimester fetal death. Some authors (Druzin et al., 1987) have noted spontaneous decelerations during the second trimester in pregnancies complicated by APS. Iatrogenic preterm delivery may improve outcome in severe cases. Finally, women with associated disorders such as SLE, autoimmune thrombocytopenia, and renal disease may require additional specialized care.

After delivery, patients with APS should be advised of their risk for development of nonobstetric disorders associated with APLA (Silver, Draper, Scott, et al., 1994). Some authorities advise that women with previous thrombotic episodes should receive anticoagulation with coumadin to achieve an INR of 2.5–3 throughout their lifetime (Rosove and Brewer, 1992; Khamashta et al., 1995). Intermediate-intensity coumadin (INR 2.0–2.9) may be equally effective with fewer side effects, but proof is lacking. Aspirin alone, however, was not protective against recurrent thrombosis. Acute thromboembolism is treated in the usual fashion with heparin or low-molecular-weight heparin to achieve antifactor Xa levels of 0.6 to 1.2 μ/mL 4 hours after injection or a thrombin time (TT) greater than 100 seconds. Assays such as the aPTT are unreliable for the management of anticoagulation in patients with LA. It is unclear whether patients with APS and no previous thromboses require thromboprophylaxis. Aspirin (325 mg/day) may reduce the risk of thrombosis in nonpregnant women with APS and previous pregnancy loss (but no prior thrombosis) (Erkan et al., 2001). Finally, women with APS should not take estrogen-containing oral contraceptives.

REFERENCES

Ahlenius I, Floberg J, Thomassen P: Sixty-six cases of intrauterine fetal death: A prospective study with an extensive test protocol. Acta Obstet Gynecol Scand **74**:109, 1995.

Alarcon-Segovia D, Perez-Vasquez ME, Villa AR, et al: Preliminary classification criteria for the antiphospholipid syndrome within systemic lupus erythematosus. Semin Arthritis Rheum **21**:275, 1992.

Aoki K, Dudkiewicz AB, Matsuura E, et al: Clinical significance of β_2-glycoprotein I-dependent anticardiolipin antibodies in the reproductive autoimmune failure syndrome: Correlation with conventional antiphospholipid antibody detection systems. Am J Obstet Gynecol **172**:926, 1995.

Asherson RA, Cervera R, Piette J-C, et al. Catastrophic antiphospholipid syndrome: Clinical and laboratory features of 50 patients. Medicine **77**:195, 1998.

Asherson RA, Khamashta MA, Ordi-Ros J, et al: The "primary" antiphospholipid syndrome: Major clinical and serologic features. Medicine **68**:366, 1989.

Balasch J, Creus M, Fabregues F, et al: Antiphospholipid antibodies and human reproductive failure. Hum Reprod **11**:2310, 1996.

Barbui T, Cortelazzo S, Galli M, et al: Antiphospholipid antibodies in early repeated abortions: A case controlled study. Fertil Steril **50**:589, 1988.

Beaumont JL: Syndrome hemorrhagique acquis du a un anticoagulant circulant. Sangre **25**:1, 1954.

Bocciolone L, Meroni P, Parazzini F, et al: Antiphospholipid antibodies and risk of intrauterine late fetal death. Acta Obstet Gynecol Scand **73**:389, 1994.

Bombell T, Mueller M, Haeberli A: Anticoagulant properties of the vascular endothelium. Thromb Haemost **77**:408, 1997.

Branch DW, Andres R, Digre KB, et al: The association of antiphospholipid antibodies with severe preeclampsia. Obstet Gynecol **73**:541, 1989.

Branch DW, Peaceman AM, Druzin M, et al. A multicenter, placebo-controlled pilot study of intravenous immune globulin treatment of antiphospholipid syndrome during pregnancy. Am J Obstet Gynecol **182**:122, 2000.

Branch DW, Porter TF, Rittenhouse L, et al. Antiphospholipid antibodies in women at risk for preeclampsia. Am J Obstet Gynecol **184**:825, 2001.

Branch DW, Rodgers GM: Induction of endothelial cell tissue factor activity by sera from patients with antiphospholipid syndrome: A possible mechanism of thrombosis. Am J Obstet Gynecol **168**:206, 1993.

Branch DW, Scott JR: Clinical implications of antiphospholipid antibodies: The Utah experience. In Harris EN, Exner T, Hughes GRV, Asherson RA (eds): Phospholipid Binding Antibodies. Boca Raton, Fla, CRC Press, 1991, p. 335.

Branch DW, Scott JR, Kochenour NK, et al: Obstetric complications associated with the lupus anticoagulant. N Engl J Med **313**:1322, 1985.

Branch DW, Silver RM, Blackwell JL, et al: Outcome of treated pregnancies in women with antiphospholipid syndrome: An update of the Utah experience. Obstet Gynecol **80**:614, 1992.

Branch DW, Silver RM, Pierangeli SS, et al: Antiphospholipid antibodies in women with recurrent pregnancy loss, fertile controls, and antiphospholipid syndrome. Obstet Gynecol **89**:549, 1997.

Brenner B, Mandel H, Lanir N, et al: Activated protein C resistance can be associated with recurrent fetal loss. Br J Haematol **97**:551, 1997.

Brey RL, Hart RG, Sherman DG, et al: Antiphospholipid antibodies and cerebral ischemia in young people. Neurology **40**:1190, 1990.

Cabiedes J, Cabral AR, Alarcon-Segovia D: Clinical manifestations of the antiphospholipid syndrome in patients with systemic lupus erythematosus associate more strongly with anti-β_2-glycoprotein-I than with antiphospholipid antibodies. J Rheumatol **22**:1899, 1995.

Cabral AR, Amigo MC, Cabiedes J, et al: The antiphospholipid/cofactor syndromes: A primary variant with antibodies to beta$_2$-glycoprotein-I but no antibodies detectable in standard antiphospholipid assays. Am J Med **101**:472, 1996.

Campbell AL, Pierangeli SS, Wellhausen S, et al: Comparison of the effects of anti-cardiolipin antibodies from patients with the antiphospholipid syndrome and with syphilis on platelet activation and aggregation. Thromb Haemost **73**:529, 1995.

Cariou R, Tobelem G, Bellucci S, et al: Effect of lupus anticoagulant on antithrombogenic properties of endothelial cells: Inhibition of thrombomodulin dependent protein C activation. Thromb Haemost **60**:54, 1988.

Carreras LO, Perez GN, Vega HR, et al: Lupus anticoagulant and recurrent fetal loss: Successful treatment with gammaglobulin. Lancet **ii**:393, 1988.

Caruso A, DeCarolis S, Ferrazzani S, et al: Pregnancy outcome in relation to uterine artery flow velocimetry waveforms and clinical characteristics in women with antiphospholipid syndrome. Obstet Gynecol **82**:970, 1993.

Chabloz P, Reber G, Boehlen F, et al: TAFI antigen and D-dimer levels during normal pregnancy and at delivery. Br J Haematol **115**:150, 2001.

Chamley LW, Pattison NS, McKay EJ: Separation of lupus anticoagulant from anticardiolipin antibodies by ion-exchange and gel filtration chromatography. Haemostasis **21**:25, 1991.

Conrad J, Horellou MH, Dreden P, et al: Thrombosis and pregnancy in congenital deficiencies of AT III, protein C, or protein S: Study of 78 women. Thromb Haemost **63**:319, 1990.

Coulam CB, McIntyre JA, Wagenknecht D, et al: Interlaboratory inconsistencies in detection of anticardiolipin antibodies. Lancet **335**:865, 1990.

Cowchock FS, Reece EA, Balaban D, et al: Repeated fetal losses associated with antiphospholipid antibodies: A collaborative randomized trial comparing prednisone to low-dose heparin treatment. Am J Obstet Gynecol **166**:1318, 1992.

Cowchock FS, Smith JB, Gocial B: Antibodies to phospholipids and nuclear antigens in patients with repeated abortions. Am J Obstet Gynecol **155**:1002, 1986.

de Boer HC, de Groot PG, Bouma BN, et al: Ternary vitronectin-thrombin-antithrombin III complexes in human plasma: Detection and mode of association. J Biol Chem **257**:3243, 1993.

de Vries JI, Dekker GA, Huijgens PC, et al: Hyperhomocysteinaemia and protein S deficiency in complicated pregnancies. Br J Obstet Gynaecol **104**:1248, 1997.

Dekker GA, de Vries JI, Doelitzsch PM, et al: Underlying disorders associated with severe early-onset preeclampsia. Am J Obstet Gynecol **173**:1042, 1995.

Delorme MA, Burrows RF, Ofosu FA, et al: Thrombin regulation in mother and fetus during pregnancy. Semin Thromb Hemost **18**:81, 1992.

DeWolf F, Carreras LO, Moerman P, et al: Decidual vasculopathy and extensive placental infarction in a patient with repeated thromboembolic accidents, recurrent fetal loss, and a lupus anticoagulant. Am J Obstet Gynecol **142**:829, 1982.

Druzin ML, Lockshin M, Edersheim TG, et al: Second trimester fetal monitoring and preterm delivery in pregnancies with systemic lupus erythematosus and/or circulating anticoagulant. Am J Obstet Gynecol **157**:1503, 1987.

Dudley DJ, Mitchell MD, Branch DW: Pathophysiology of antiphospholipid antibodies: Absence of prostaglandin-mediated effects on cultured endothelium. Am J Obstet Gynecol **162**:953, 1990.

Empson M, Lassere M, Craig JC, et al: Recurrent pregnancy loss with antiphospholipid antibody: A systematic review of therapeutic trials. Obstet Gynecol **99**:135, 2002.

Erhardt E, Stankovics J, Molnar D, et al: High prevalence of factor V Leiden mutation in mothers of premature neonates. Biol Neonate **78**:145, 2000.

Eriksson P, Kallin B, van 't Hooft FM, et al: Allele-specific increase in basal transcription of the plasminogen-activator inhibitor 1 gene is associated with myocardial infarction. Proc Natl Acad Sci U S A **92**:1851, 1995.

Erkan D, Merrill JT, Yazici Y, et al: High thrombosis rate after fetal loss in antiphospholipid syndrome: Effective prophylaxis with aspirin. Arthritis Rheum **44**:1466, 2001.

Eskes TK: Clotting disorders and placental abruption: Homocysteine—a new risk factor. Eur J Obstet Gynecol Reprod Biol **95**:206, 2001.

Esmon CT: Molecular events that control the protein C anti-coagulant pathway. Thromb Haemostas **70**:29, 1993.

Estelles A, Gilabert J, Anar J, et al: Changes in plasma levels of type 1 and type 2 plasminogen activator inhibitors in normal pregnancy and in patients with severe preeclampsia. Blood **74**:1332, 1989.

Ferro D, Quintarelli C, Rasura M, et al: Lupus anticoagulant and the fibrinolytic system in young patients with stroke. Stroke **24**:368, 1993.

Foka ZJ, Lambropoulos AF, Saravelos H, et al: Factor V leiden and prothrombin G20210A mutations, but not methylenetetrahydrofolate reductase C677T, are associated with recurrent miscarriages. Hum Reprod **15**:458, 2000.

Galli M, Comfurius P, Maassen C, et al: Anticardiolipin antibodies (ACA) directed not to cardiolipin but to a plasma protein cofactor. Lancet **335**:1544, 1990.

Garlund B: The lupus inhibitors in thromboembolic disease and intrauterine fetal death in the absence of systemic lupus. Acta Med Scand **5**:293, 1984.

Gatenby PA, Cameron K, Shearman RP: Pregnancy loss with phospholipid antibodies: Improved outcome with aspirin containing treatment. Aust N Z J Obstet Gynaecol **29**:294, 1989.

Gerhardt A, Scharf RE, Beckman MW, et al: Prothrombin and factor V mutations in women with a history of thrombosis during pregnancy and the puerperium. N Engl J Med **342**:374, 2000.

Ginsberg JS, Demers C, Brill-Edwards P, et al: Increased thrombin generation and activity in patients with systemic lupus erythematosus and anticardiolipin antibodies: Evidence for a prothrombotic state. Blood **81**:2958, 1993.

Girard TJ, Warren LA, Novotny WF, et al: Functional significance of the Kunitz-type inhibitory domains of lipoprotein-associated coagulation inhibitor. Nature **338**:518, 1989.

Girling J, de Swiet M: Inherited thrombophilia and pregnancy. Curr Opin Obstet Gynecol **10**:135, 1998.

Glueck CJ, Phillips H, Cameron D, et al: The 4G/4G polymorphism of the hypofibrinolytic plasminogen activator inhibitor type 1 gene: An independent risk factor for serious pregnancy complications. Metabolism **49**:845, 2000.

Goldstein SR: Embryonic death in early pregnancy: A new look at the first trimester. Obstet Gynecol **84**:294, 1994.

Gopel W, Ludwig M, Junge AK, et al: Selection pressure for the factor-V-Leiden mutation and embryo implantation. Lancet **358**:1238, 2001.

Gris JC, Quere I, Monpeyroux F, et al: Case-control study of the frequency of thrombophilic disorders in couples with late foetal loss and no thrombotic antecedent. The Nimes Obstetricians and Haematologists Study (NOHA). Thromb Haemost **81**:891, 1999.

Guideline: Investigation and management of heritable thrombophilia. Br J Haematol **114**:512, 2001.

Haddow JE, Rote NS, Dostal-Johnson D, et al: Lack of an association between late fetal death and antiphospholipid antibody measurements in the second trimester. Am J Obstet Gynecol **165**:1308, 1991.

Harger JH, Laifer SA, Bontempo FA, et al: Low-dose aspirin and prednisone treatment of pregnancy loss caused by lupus anticoagulants. J Perinatol **15**:463, 1995.

Harris EN: Syndrome of the black swan. Br J Rheumatol **26**:324, 1987.

Harris EN: The Second International Anti-Cardiolipin Standardization Workshop: The Kingston Anti-Phospholipid Antibody Study (KAPS) group. Am J Clin Pathol **94**:476, 1990.

Harris EN, Asherson RA, Gharavi AE, et al: Thrombocytopenia in SLE and related autoimmune disorders: Association with anticardiolipin antibody. Br J Haematol **59**:227, 1985.

Harris EN, Chan JK, Asherson RA, et al: Thrombosis, recurrent fetal loss and thrombocytopenia: Predictive value of the anticardiolipin antibody test. Arch Intern Med **146**:2153, 1986.

Harris EN, Spinnato JA: Should anticardiolipin tests be performed in otherwise healthy pregnant women? Am J Obstet Gynecol **165**:1272, 1991.

Hochfeld M, Druzin ML, Maia D, et al: Maternal-fetal catastrophe: Fulminant and fatal thrombosis in pregnancy complicated by primary antiphospholipid syndrome. Obstet Gynecol **83**:804, 1994.

Holers VM, Girardi G, Mo L, et al: Complement C3 activation is required for antiphospholipid antibody-induced fetal loss. J Exp Med **195**:211, 2002

Hughes GRV, Harris EN, Gharavi AE: The anticardiolipin syndrome. J Rheumatol **13**:486, 1986.

Hunt JE, Adelstein S, Krilis SA: A phospholipid-β_2-glycoprotein I complex is an antigen for anticardiolipin antibodies occurring in autoimmune disease but not with infection. Lupus **1**:83, 1992.

Ill CR, Rouslahti E: Association of thrombin-antithrombin III complex with vitronectin in serum. J Biol Chem **260**:15610, 1985.

Infante-Rivard C, David M, Gauthier R, et al: Lupus anticoagulants, anticardiolipin antibodies, and fetal loss: A case-control study. N Engl J Med **325**:1063, 1991.

Jaffe R: Investigation of abnormal first-trimester gestations by color Doppler imaging. J Clin Ultrasound **21**:521, 1993.

Khamashta MA, Cuadrado MJ, Mujic F, et al: The management of thrombosis in the antiphospholipid-antibody syndrome. N Engl J Med **332**:993, 1995.

Khamashta MA, Harris EN, Gharavi AE, et al: Immune mediated mechanism for thrombosis: Antiphospholipid antibody binding to platelet membranes. Ann Rheum Dis **47**:849, 1988.

Khong TY, DeWolf F, Robertson WB, et al: Inadequate maternal vascular response to placentation in pregnancies complicated by preeclampsia and by small for gestational age infants. Br J Obstet Gynaecol **93**:1049, 1986.

Kochenour NK, Branch DW, Rote NS, et al: A new postpartum syndrome associated with antiphospholipid antibodies. Obstet Gynecol **69**:460, 1987.

Kohler HP, Grant PJ: Plasminogen-activator inhibitor type-1 and coronary artery disease. New Engl J Med. **342**:1792, 2000.

Koike T, Matsuura E: What is the "true" antigen for anticardiolipin antibodies? Lancet **337**:671, 1991.

Kupferminc MJ, Eldor A, Steinman N, et al: Increased frequency of genetic thrombophilia in women with complications of pregnancy. N Engl J Med **340**:9, 1999.

Kupferminc MJ, Fait G, Many A, et al: Severe preeclampsia and high frequency of genetic thrombophilic mutations. Obstet Gynecol **96**:45, 2000.

Kupferminc MJ, Fait G, Many A, et al: Low-molecular-weight heparin for the prevention of obstetric complications in women with thrombophilias. Hypertens Pregnancy **20**:35, 2001.

Kupferminc MJ, Lee MJ, Green D, et al: Severe postpartum pulmonary, cardiac, and renal syndrome associated with antiphospholipid antibodies. Obstet Gynecol **83**:806, 1994.

Kutteh WH: Antiphospholipid antibody associated recurrent pregnancy loss: Treatment with heparin and low-dose aspirin is superior to low dose aspirin alone. Am J Obstet Gynecol **174**:1584, 1996.

Lachmeijer AM, Arngrimsson R, Bastiaans EJ, et al: Mutations in the gene for methylenetetrahydrofolate reductase, homocysteine levels, and vitamin status in women with a history of preeclampsia. Am J Obstet Gynecol **184**:394, 2001.

Lane DA, Bayston T, Olds RJ, et al: Antithrombin mutation database: 2nd (1997) update. For the Plasma Coagulation Inhibitors Subcommittee of the Scientific and Standardization Committee of the International Society on Thrombosis and Haemostasis. Thromb Haemost **77**:197, 1997.

Lee RM, Emlen W, Branch DW, et al: Anti-beta-2 glycoprotein I antibodies in women with recurrent spontaneous abortion, unexplained fetal death, and antiphospholipid syndrome. Am J Obstet Gynecol **181**:642, 1999.

Leeda M, Riyazi N, de Vries JI, et al: Effects of folic acid and vitamin B_6 supplementation on women with hyperhomocysteinemia and a history of preeclampsia or fetal growth restriction. Am J Obstet Gynecol **179**:135, 1998.

Levine JS, Branch DW, Rauch J: The antiphospholipid syndrome. N Engl J Med **346**:752, 2002.

Lijnen HR: Elements of the fibrinolytic system. Ann N Y Acad Sci. **936**:226, 2001.

Lima F, Khamashta MA, Buchanan NMM, et al: A study of sixty pregnancies in patients with the antiphospholipid syndrome. Clin Exp Rheumatol **14**:131, 1996.

Lindqvist PG, Gudmundsson S: Maternal carriership of factor V Leiden associated with pathological uterine artery Doppler measurements during pregnancy. BJOG **108**:1103, 2001.

Lockshin MD: Antiphospholipid antibody: Babies, blood clots, biology. JAMA **277**:1549, 1997.

Lockshin MD, Druzin ML, Goei S, et al: Antibody to cardiolipin as a predictor of fetal distress or death in pregnant patients with systemic lupus erythematosus. N Engl J Med **313**:152, 1985.

Lockshin MD, Druzin ML, Qamar T: Prednisone does not prevent recurrent fetal death in women with antiphospholipid antibody. Am J Obstet Gynecol **160**:439, 1989.

Lockwood CJ: Heritable coagulopathies in pregnancy. Obstet Gynecol Surv **54**:754, 1999.

Lockwood CJ: Inherited thrombophilias in pregnant patients. Prenat Neonat Med **6**:3, 2001.

Lockwood CJ, Krikun G, Papp C, et al: Biological mechanisms underlying RU 486 clinical effects: Inhibition of endometrial stromal cell tissue factor content. J Clin Endocrinol Metab **79**:786, 1994.

Lockwood CJ, Nemerson Y, Guller S, et al: Progestational regulation of human endometrial stromal cell tissue factor expression during decidualization. J Clin Endocrinol Metab **76**:231, 1993.

Lockwood CJ, Rand J: The immunobiology and obstetrical consequences of antiphospholipid antibodies. Obstet Gynecol Surv **49**:432, 1994.

Lockwood CJ, Romero R, Feinberg RF, et al: The prevalence and biologic significance of lupus anticoagulant and anticardiolipin antibodies in a general obstetric population. Am J Obstet Gynecol **161**:369, 1989.

Lubbe WF, Palmer SJ, Butler WS, et al: Fetal survival after prednisone suppression of maternal lupus anticoagulant. Lancet **i**:1361, 1983.

Lubbe WF, Walkom P, Alexander CJ: Hepatic and splenic hemorrhage in a patient with circulating lupus anticoagulant. N Z Med J **95**:842, 1982.

Lynch A, Marlar R, Murphy J, et al: Antiphospholipid antibodies in predicting adverse pregnancy outcome. Ann Intern Med **120**:470, 1994.

MacLean MA, Cumming GP, McCall F, et al: The prevalence of lupus anticoagulant and anticardiolipin antibodies in women with a history of first trimester miscarriages. Br J Obstet Gynaecol **101**:103, 1994.

Malm J, Laurell M, Nilsson IM, et al: Thromboembolic disease: Critical evaluation of laboratory investigation. Thromb Haemost **68**:7, 1992.

Martinelli I, Legnani C, Bucciarelli P, et al: Risk of pregnancy-related venous thrombosis in carriers of severe inherited thrombophilia. Thromb Haemost **86**:800, 2001.

Martinelli I, Taioli E, Cetin I, et al: Mutations in coagulation factors in women with unexplained late fetal loss. N Engl J Med **343**:1015, 2000.

Matsuura E, Igarashi Y, Fujimoto M: Anticardiolipin cofactor(s) and differential diagnosis of autoimmune disease. Lancet **336**:177, 1990.

McNally T, Purdy G, Mackie IJ, et al: The use of an anti-β_2-glycoprotein-I assay for discrimination between anticardiolipin antibodies associated with infection and increased risk of thrombosis. Br J Haematol **91**:471, 1995.

McNeil HP, Simpson RJ, Chesterman CN, et al: Antiphospholipid antibodies are directed against a complex antigen that includes a lipid binding inhibitor of aggregation: β_2 glycoprotein I (apolipoprotein H). Proc Natl Acad Sci USA **87**:4120, 1990.

Milliez J, Lelong F, Bayani N, et al: The prevalence of autoantibodies during third trimester pregnancy complicated by hypertension or idiopathic fetal growth retardation. Am J Obstet Gynecol **165**:51, 1991.

Moodley J, Bhoola V, Duursma J, et al: The association of antiphospholipid antibodies with severe early onset preeclampsia. S Afr Med J **85**:105, 1995.

Murphy RP, Donoghue C, Nallen RJ, et al: Prospective evaluation of the risk conferred by factor V Leiden and thermolabile methylenetetrahydrofolate reductase polymorphisms in pregnancy. Arterioscler Thromb Vasc Biol **20**:266, 2000.

Nayar R, Lage JM: Placental changes in a first trimester missed abortion in maternal systemic lupus erythematosus with antiphospholipid syndrome: A case report and review of the literature. Hum Pathol **27**:201, 1996.

Nelen WL, Blom HJ, Steegers EA, et al: Hyperhomocysteinemia and recurrent early pregnancy loss: A meta-analysis. Fertil Steril **74**:1196, 2000.

Nemerson Y: Tissue factor and hemostasis. Blood **71**:1, 1988.

Novotny WF, Brown SG, Miletich JP, et al: Plasma antigen levels of the lipoprotein-associated coagulation inhibitor in patient samples. Blood **78**:387, 1991.

Ordi J, Barquinero J, Vilardelli M, et al: Fetal loss treatment in patients with antiphospholipid antibodies. Ann Rheum Dis **48**:798, 1989.

Oshiro BT, Silver RM, Scott JR, et al: Antiphospholipid antibodies and fetal death. Obstet Gynecol **87**:489, 1996.

Out HJ, Bruinse HW, Christaens GC, et al: Prevalence of antiphospholipid antibodies in patients with fetal loss. Ann Rheum Dis **50**:553, 1991.

Out HJ, Bruinse HW, Derksen RHWM: Antiphospholipid antibodies and pregnancy loss. Hum Reprod **6**:889, 1991.

Out HJ, Bruinse HW, Godlieve CML, et al: A prospective, controlled multicenter study on the obstetric risks of pregnant women with antiphospholipid antibodies. Am J Obstet Gynecol **167**:26, 1992.

Out HJ, Kooijman CD, Bruinse HW, et al: Histopathological findings from patients with intrauterine fetal death and antiphospholipid antibodies. Eur J Obstet Gynaecol **41**:179, 1991.

Ozcan T, Rinder HM, Murphy J, et al: Genetic thrombophilia mutations are not increased in patients with recurrent losses. Obstet Gynecol **97**:S31, 2001.

Parazzini F, Acaia B, Faden D, et al: Antiphospholipid antibodies and recurrent abortion. Obstet Gynecol **77**:854, 1991.

Parke AL, Wilson D, Maier D: The prevalence of antiphospholipid antibodies in women with recurrent spontaneous abortion, women with successful pregnancies, and women who have never been pregnant. Arthritis Rheum **34**:1231, 1991.

Parry GC, Erlich JH, Carmeliet P, et al: Low levels of tissue factor are compatible with development and hemostasis in mice. J Clin Invest. **101**:560, 1998.

Pattison NS, Chamley LW, Birdsall M, et al: Am J Obstet Gynecol **183**:1008, 2000.

Pattison NS, Chamley LW, McKay EJ, et al: Antiphospholipid antibodies in pregnancy: Prevalence and clinical associations. Br J Obstet Gynaecol **100**:909, 1993.

Pauzner R, Dulitki M, Langevitz P, et al: Low molecular weight heparin and warfarin in the treatment of patients with antiphospholipid syndrome during pregnancy. Thromb Haemost **86**:1379, 2001.

Peaceman AM, Rehnberg K: The immunoglobulin G fraction from plasma containing antiphospholipid antibodies causes increased placental thromboxane production. Am J Obstet Gynecol **167**:1543, 1992.

Peaceman AM, Rehnberg KA: The effect of immunoglobulin G fractions from patients with lupus anticoagulant on placental prostacyclin and thromboxane production. Am J Obstet Gynecol **169**:1403, 1993.

Peaceman AM, Rehnberg KA: The effect of aspirin and indomethacin on prostacyclin and thromboxane production by placental tissue incubated with immunoglobulin G fractions from patients with lupus anticoagulant. Am J Obstet Gynecol **173**:1391, 1995.

Peaceman AM, Silver RK, MacGregor SN, et al: Interlaboratory variation in antiphospholipid antibody testing. Am J Obstet Gynecol **166**:1780, 1992.

Petri M, Golbus M, Anderson R, et al: Antinuclear antibody, lupus anticoagulant, and anticardiolipin antibody in women with idiopathic habitual abortion. A controlled, prospective study of forty-four women. Arthiris Rheum **30**:601, 1987.

Pickering W, Marriott K, Regan L: G20210A prothrombin gene mutation: Prevalence in a recurrent miscarriage population. Clin Appl Thromb Hemost **7**:25, 2001.

Pierangeli SS, Barker JH, Stikovac D, et al: Effect of human IgG antiphospholipid antibodies on an in vivo thrombosis model in mice. Thromb Haemost **71**:670, 1994.

Pierangeli SS, Harris EN, Gharavi AE, et al: Are immunoglobulins with lupus anticoagulant activity specific for phospholipids? Br J Haematol **85**:124, 1993.

Pihusch R, Buchholz T, Lohse P, et al: Thrombophilic gene mutations and recurrent spontaneous abortion: prothrombin mutation increases the risk in the first trimester. Am J Reprod Immunol **46**:124, 2001.

Polzin WJ, Kopelman JN, Robinson RD, et al: The association of antiphospholipid antibodies with pregnancy complicated by fetal growth restriction. Obstet Gynecol **78**:1108, 1991.

Preissner KT, De Boer H, Pannekoek H, et al: Thrombin regulation by physiological inhibitors: The role of vitronectin. Semin Thromb Hemost **22**:165, 1996.

Preissner KT, Zwicker L, Muller-Berghaus G: Formation, characterization and detection of a ternary complex between S protein, thrombin and antithrombin III in serum. Biochem J **243**:105, 1987.

Preston FE, Rosendaal FR, Walker ID, et al: Increased fetal loss in women with heritable thrombophilia. Lancet **348**:913, 1996.

Rai RS, Clifford K, Cohen H, et al: High prospective fetal loss rate in untreated pregnancies of women with recurrent miscarriage and antiphospholipid antibodies. Hum Reprod **10**:3301, 1995.

Rai R, Cohen H, Dave M, et al: Randomized controlled trial of aspirin plus aspirin and heparin in pregnant women with recurrent miscarriage associated with phospholipid antibodies (or antiphospholipid antibodies). BMJ **314**:253, 1997.

Rai RS, Regan L, Clifford K, et al: Antiphospholipid antibodies and β_2-glycoprotein-I in 500 women with recurrent miscarriage: Results of a comprehensive screening approach. Hum Reprod **10**:2001, 1995.

Rai R, Shlebak A, Cohen H, et al: Factor V Leiden and acquired activated protein C resistance among 1000 women with recurrent miscarriage. Hum Reprod **16**:961, 2001.

Rand JH, Wu X-X, Andree HAM, et al: Pregnancy loss in the antiphospholipid-antibody syndrome: A possible thrombogenic mechanism. N Engl J Med **337**:154, 1997.

Reece EA, Gabrielli S, Cullen MT, et al: Recurrent adverse pregnancy outcome and antiphospholipid antibodies. Am J Obstet Gynecol **163**:162, 1990.

Reece EA, Romero R, Clyne LP, et al: Lupus-like anticoagulant in pregnancy. Lancet **1**:344, 1984.

Rey E, Kahn SR, David M, et al: Thrombophilic disorders and fetal loss: A meta-analysis. Lancet **361**:901, 2003.

Riyazi N, Leeda M, de Vries JL, et al: Low-molecular-weight heparin combined with aspirin in pregnant women with thrombophilia and a history of preeclampsia or fetal growth restriction: a preliminary study. Eur J Obstet Gynecol Reprod Biol **80**:49, 1998.

Rodesch F, Simon P, Donner C, et al: Oxygen measurements in endometrial and trophoblastic tissues during early pregnancy. Obstet Gynecol **80**:283, 1992.

Roque H, Paidas M, Rebarber A, et al: There is no association between maternal thrombophilia and recurrent first-trimester loss. Am J Obstet Gynecol **184**:S15, 2001.

Rosove MH, Brewer PMC: Antiphospholipid thrombosis: Clinical course after the first thrombotic event in 70 patients. Ann Intern Med **117**:303, 1992.

Rosove MH, Tabsh K, Wasserstrum N, et al: Heparin therapy for pregnant women with lupus anticoagulant or anticardiolipin antibodies. Obstet Gynecol **75**:630, 1990.

Roubey RAS: Autoantibodies to phospholipid-binding plasma proteins: A new view of lupus anticoagulants and other "antiphospholipid" autoantibodies. Blood **84**:2854, 1994.

Runic R, Schatz F, Krey L, et al: Alterations in endometrial stromal cell tissue factor protein and mRNA expression in patients experiencing abnormal uterine bleeding while using Norplant-2 contraception. J Clin Endocrinol Metab **82**:83, 1997.

Salafia CS, Parke AL: Placental pathology in systemic lupus erythematosus and phospholipid antibody syndrome. Rheum Dis Clin North Am **23**:85, 1997.

Sammaritano LR, Gharavi AE, Soverano C, et al: Phospholipid binding antiphospholipid antibodies and placental anticoagulant protein. J Clin Immunol **12**:27, 1992.

Sanson BJ, Friederich PW, Simioni P, et al: The risk of abortion and stillbirth in antithrombin-, protein C-, and protein S-deficient women. Thromb Haemost **75**:387, 1996.

Schatz F, Lockwood CJ: Progestin regulation of plasminogen activator inhibitor type-1 in primary cultures of endometrial stromal and decidual cells. J Clin Endocrinol Metab **77**:621, 1993.

Scott JR, Branch DW, Kochenour NK, et al: Intravenous immunoglobulin treatment of pregnant patients with recurrent pregnancy loss caused by antiphospholipid antibodies and Rh immunization. Am J Obstet Gynecol **159**:1055, 1988.

Scott RAH: Anticardiolipin antibodies and preeclampsia. Br J Obstet Gynaecol **94**:604, 1987.

Seiler SM: Thrombin receptor antagonists. Semin Thromb Hemost **22**:223, 1996.

Shoenfeld Y, Blank M: Effect of long-acting thromboxane receptor antagonist (BMS 180, 291) on experimental antiphospholipid syndrome. Lupus **3**:397, 1994.

Silveira LH, Hubble CL, Jara LJ, et al: Prevention of anticardiolipin antibody related pregnancy losses with prednisone and aspirin. Am J Med **93**:403, 1992.

Silver RK, Adler L, Hickman AR, et al: Anticardiolipin antibody positive serum enhances endothelial cell platelet activating factor production. Am J Obstet Gynecol **165**:1748, 1991.

Silver RK, MacGregor SN, Sholl JS, et al: Comparative trial of prednisone plus aspirin versus aspirin alone in the treatment of anticardiolipin antibody-positive obstetric patients. Am J Obstet Gynecol **169**:1411, 1993.

Silver RM, Draper ML, Byrne JLB, et al: Unexplained elevations of maternal serum alpha-fetoprotein in women with antiphospholipid antibodies: A harbinger of fetal death. Obstet Gynecol **83**:150, 1994.

Silver RM, Draper ML, Scott JR, et al: Clinical consequences of antiphospholipid antibodies: An historic cohort study. Obstet Gynecol **83**:372, 1994.

Silver RM, Pierangeli SS, Gharavi AE, et al: Induction of high levels of anticardiolipin antibodies in mice by immunization with beta-2 glycoprotein I does not cause fetal death. Am J Obstet Gynecol **173**:1410, 1995.

Silver RM, Porter TF, van Leeuwen I, et al: Anticardiolipin antibodies: Clinical consequences of "low titers." Obstet Gynecol **87**:494, 1996.

Silver RM, Smith LA, Edwin SS, et al: Variable effects on murine pregnancy of immunoglobulin G fractions from women with antiphospholipid antibodies. Am J Obstet Gynecol **177**:229, 1997.

Simantov R, Lo SK, Gharavi A, et al: Activation of cultured vascular endothelial cells by antiphospholipid antibodies. J Clin Invest **96**:2211, 1995.

Sletnes KE, Wislof F, Moe N, et al: Antiphospholipid antibodies in preeclamptic women: Relation to growth retardation and neonatal outcome. Acta Obstet Gynecol Scand **71**:112, 1992.

Souza SS, Ferriani RA, Pontes AG, et al: Factor V leiden and factor II G20210A mutations in patients with recurrent abortion. Hum Reprod **14**:2448, 1999.

Spinnato JA, Clark AL, Pierangeli SS, et al: The antiphospholipid syndrome in pregnancy: Immunoglobulin therapy. Am J Obstet Gynecol **170**:334, 1994.

Tannenbaum SH, Finko R, Cines DB: Antibody and immune complexes induce tissue factor production by endothelial cells. J Immunol **137**:1532, 1986.

Triplett DA, Brandt JT, Musgrave MT, et al: The relationship between lupus anticoagulants and antibodies to phospholipid. JAMA **259**:550, 1988.

Vaarala O, Palusuo T, Kleemola M, et al: Anticardiolipin response in acute infections. Clin Immunol Immunopathol **41**:8, 1986.

van Meijer, Gebbink RK, Preissner KT, et al: Determination of the vitronectin binding site on plasminogen activator inhibitor 1 (PAI-1). FEBS Letters **352**:342, 1994.

Viard JP, Amoura Z, Bach JF: Association of anti-beta-2 glycoprotein I antibodies with lupus-type circulating anticoagulants and thrombosis in systemic lupus erythematosus. Am J Med **93**:181, 1992.

Walker ID. Management of thrombophilia in pregnancy. Blood Rev **5**:227, 1991.

Walker TS, Triplett DA, Javed N, et al: Evaluation of lupus anticoagulants: Antiphospholipid antibodies, endothelial cell immunoglobulin, endothelial prostacyclin secretion, and antigenic protein S levels. Thromb Res **51**:267, 1988.

Walsh SW: Preeclampsia: An imbalance in placental prostacyclin and thromboxane production. Am J Obstet Gynecol **152**:335, 1985.

Warr TA, Warn-Cramer BJ, Rao LV, et al: Human plasma extrinsic pathway inhibitor activity: I. Standardization of assay and evaluation of physiologic variables. Blood **74**:201, 1989.

Watson AL, Skepper JN, Jauniaux E, et al: Susceptibility of human placental syncytiotrophoblastic mitochondria to oxygen-mediated damage in relation to gestational age. J Clin Endocrinol Metab **83**:1697, 1998.

Wilson WA, Gharavi AE, et al: International consensus statement on preliminary classification criteria for definite antiphospholipid syndrome: report of an international workshop. Arthritis Rheum **42**:1309, 1999.

Yamada N, Arinami T, Yamakawa-Kobayashi K, et al: The 4G/5G polymorphism of the plasminogen activator inhibitor-1 gene is associated with severe preeclampsia. J Hum Genet **45**:138, 2000.

Yasuda M, Takakuwa K, Tokunaga A, et al: Prospective studies of the association between anticardiolipin antibody and outcome of pregnancy. Obstet Gynecol **86**:555, 1995.

Yetman DL, Kutteh WH: Antiphospholipid antibody panels and recurrent pregnancy loss: Prevalence of anticardiolipin antibodies compared with other antiphospholipid antibodies. Fertil Steril **66**:540, 1996.

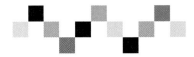

Chapter 49

DIABETES IN PREGNANCY

Thomas R. Moore, MD

In the United States today, 17 million people (6.2% of the population) have been diagnosed with some form of diabetes. Another 6 million with diabetes are undiagnosed. Clinic-based reports and regional studies indicate that type 2 diabetes is increasingly common among American Indian, African American, and Hispanic children and adolescents (National Institute of Diabetes and Digestive and Kidney Diseases, 2002). Higher-than-expected rates of pregestational diabetes in women of childbearing age have already been reported among many immigrant populations undergoing lifestyle changes (e.g., changes in physical activity and diet). In 1995, the rate of diabetes during pregnancy was 25.3 per 1000 women, but the prevalence rates by maternal race/ethnicity ranged from 56.1 for Asian Indian women to 19.3 for Korean women. Diabetes rates increased progressively with age—from 8.3 per 1000 women under 20 years old to 65.6 for women aged 40 to 45 years (Centers for Disease Control and Prevention, 1998) (Fig. 49-1).

Recent studies suggest that the prevalence of diabetes among women of childbearing age is increasing in the United States (Harris et al., 1998). Continued immigration among populations with high rates of type 2 diabetes and the impact of changes in diet (increased calories and fat content) and lifestyle (sedentary) portend marked increases in the percentage of patients with preexisting diabetes who will become pregnant in the future. A virtual epidemic of childhood obesity is occurring presently in the United States, bringing with it a sharp rise in childhood and adolescent diabetes. This trend will have a profound impact on obstetrics and pediatrics in the next two decades and beyond (American Diabetes Association, 2000). Increased outreach efforts to provide care to the populations experiencing rising rates of pregestational diabetes will be necessary if a significant increase in maternal and newborn morbidity is to be avoided (Persson and Hanson, 1998). In infants of diabetic mothers (IDMs), compared with weight-matched controls, the risk of serious birth injury is doubled, the likelihood of cesarean section is tripled, and the incidence of newborn intensive care unit admission is quadrupled (Berkus et al., 1999).

Although pregnancy in the diabetic woman during the 19th century portended death of mother, fetus, or both, today centers providing meticulous metabolic and obstetrical surveillance report perinatal loss rates approaching those seen in the nondiabetic population (McElvy et al., 2000; Wylie et al., 2002). Nevertheless, major problems with both fetal and maternal management persist. Stillbirth rates have fallen dramatically, but congenital fetal anomalies, many of them

life-threatening and debilitating, remain three to four times as frequent in diabetic as in nondiabetic pregnancy. Macrosomia and birth injury occur 10 times as frequently in diabetic fetuses. Recent studies indicate that the magnitude of such risks is proportional to the degree of maternal hyperglycemia (Rudge et al., 2000; Kjos et al., 2001). To a great extent, the excessive fetal and neonatal morbidity of diabetes in pregnancy is preventable or at least reducible by meticulous prenatal and intrapartum care. This chapter reviews the pathophysiology of this complex group of disorders and identifies the obstetric interventions that can potentially improve outcome.

CLASSIFICATION AND PATHOBIOLOGY OF DIABETES MELLITUS

A classification scheme based on the etiopathology of hyperglycemia was developed by the National Diabetes Data Group of the National Institutes of Health in 1979 and has been adopted by the American Diabetes Association (2002e). The types are summarized in Table 49-1. This nomenclature is a useful guide because it categorizes patients by their underlying pathogenesis (insulin-deficient—type 1, and insulin-resistant—type 2, and gestational). The terms insulin-dependent diabetes mellitus (IDDM) and non–insulin-dependent diabetes mellitus (NIDDM) are no longer favored because they have frequently resulted in classifying the patient based on treatment rather than etiology.

An alternative classification in common use (Table 49-2), first proposed by Priscilla White, MD, at the Joslin Clinic in 1932, categorizes patients on the basis of the duration of their disease and the secondary vascular and other end-organ complications evident (Table 49-3). Although the White classification is somewhat descriptive of risk and health status, it does not differentiate by underlying pathophysiology. For this reason, the National Diabetes Data Group scheme is currently favored. The key clinical features differentiating type 1 from type 2 diabetes are listed in Table 49-4. Etiologic differences in these categories are discussed subsequently.

Type 1 Diabetes

Type 1 diabetes is a chronic autoimmune disease that results from a complex interaction of genetic and environmental factors. The natural history of this disorder can be subdivided into three stages (Atkinson and Maclaren, 1994):

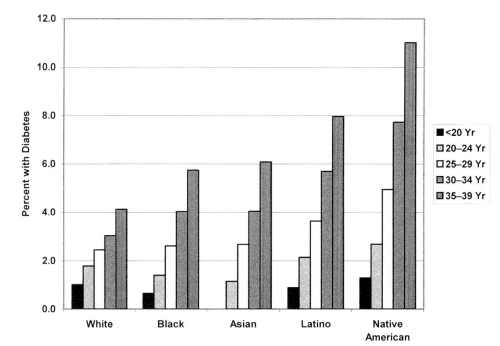

FIGURE 49-1 ■ Prevalence of diabetes during pregnancy by ethnicity and maternal age. (From Centers for Disease Control and Prevention: Diabetes during pregnancy: United States, 1993–1995. MMWR Morb Mortal Wkly Rep **47**:408, 1998.)

- The *pancreatic beta-cell injury stage*, mediated by both humoral and cellular autoimmune activity
- The *pre-diabetic stage*, during which progressive islet cell destruction leads to loss of the first-phase insulin response to glucose challenge
- The *overt diabetes stage*, in which inadequate insulin production by the islet cell–depleted pancreas leads to severe metabolic consequences

One or more autoantibodies, including islet cell autoantibodies, insulin autoantibodies, and autoantibodies to glutamic acid decarboxylase, can be detected in the serum of over 80% of patients during the autoimmune destruction process. A great deal of current research is focused on understanding and, ultimately, preventing the progressive autoimmune process that relentlessly destroys pancreatic tissue and finally leads to type 1 diabetes.

There is a strong genetic susceptibility component to the epidemiology of type 1 diabetes. Convincing evidence indicates the linkage of at least two chromosome regions, including the HLA region on chromosome 6p21 and the insulin gene region on 11p15. Approximately 40% of type 1 and 10% of type 2 diabetes have one or both of these regions involved (Pietropaolo and Le Roith, 2001). Environmental triggers play an additional role in the pathogenesis of diabetes. Even in genetically susceptible subjects, an environmental agent such as a virus is probably necessary to set in motion the intense and progressive autoimmune destruction of the pancreatic islet cells that ultimately ensues.

Type 2 Diabetes

Type 2 diabetes is a disease arising from progressive tissue insulin resistance, hyperglycemia, and hyperlipidemia, mediated by obesity and sedentary lifestyle. Autoimmune destruction of β-cells does not occur in type 2 diabetes, and ketoacidosis seldom occurs except during severe illness. The natural history of this disorder can be subdivided into the following stages:

- *Tissue insulin-resistance stage.* During this stage, factors that promote insulin resistance in muscle and adipose tissue lead to altered tissue glucose uptake and asymptomatic hyperglycemia. Among the factors known to promote insulin resistance are obesity, sedentary lifestyle, family history/genetics, and pregnancy. During this silent stage, lifestyle interventions such as exercise and weight loss can improve insulin sensitivity, reduce hyperglycemia, and arrest or slow the progression of the disease.
- *Glucotoxicity stage.* Hyperglycemia directly inhibits glucose uptake into target cells, acting by down-regulating the glucose transporter system GLUT4. Toxicity of hyperglycemia leads to inadequate insulin

TABLE 49-1. CLASSIFICATION OF GLUCOSE INTOLERANCE IN PREGNANCY

Nomenclature	Old Names	Clinical Features
Type I Insulin-dependent diabetes mellitus (IDDM)	Juvenile-onset diabetes	Ketosis-prone, insulin-deficient
Type II Non-insulin-dependent diabetes (NIDDM)	Adult-onset diabetes	Ketosis-resistant, insulin-resistant; obesity, family history, and age are common factors
Type III Gestational diabetes (GDM)	Gestational diabetes	Occurs only during pregnancy; established by glucose tolerance testing; obesity and age are common risk factors

TABLE 49-2. WHITE'S CLASSIFICATION OF DIABETES IN PREGNANCY

White's Class	Age at Onset (Years)	Duration (Years)	Complications
A	Any	Any	Diagnosed prior to pregnancy; no vascular disease
B	≥20 or	<10	No vascular disease
C	10–19 or	10–19	No vascular disease
D	<10 or	≥20	Background retinopathy only or hypertension
E			Calcification of pelvic arteries (no longer used)
F			Nephropathy (>500 mg/day proteinuria)
H			Arteriosclerotic heart disease
R			Proliferative retinopathy or vitreous hemorrhage
T			After renal transplantation

Adapted from Hare JW, White P: Gestational diabetes and the White classification. Diabetes Care **3**:394, 1980. Copyright © 1980 by American Diabetes Association, Inc.

response, with subsequent heightened early hyperglycemia. Early on, there is a marked disruption in pulsatile insulin delivery, which contributes to further insulin resistance. Later, after glucose intolerance has become overt, several other secretory abnormalities develop coincident with loss of beta-cell glucorecognition. The net result is further deterioration in timing of insulin delivery and postprandial hyperglycemia.

- *Lipotoxicity stage.* Tissue insulin resistance leads to enhanced lipolysis in the visceral fat depot. As obesity increases, the increasing insulin resistance enhances the rate of lipolysis. Chronically elevated free fatty acid levels inhibit glucose-mediated insulin release from the pancreas and worsen insulin resistance at the tissue level (liver and muscle). During the preclinical stages of type 2 diabetes, beta-cell response is abnormal even though normoglycemia is maintained. Lipotoxicity mediates oxidative damage to key organs including the heart and kidneys.
- *Impaired glucose tolerance stage.* In this pre-diabetic stage, by definition, fasting hyperglycemia is present, glucotoxicity and lipotoxicity are ongoing, and progressive tissue damage occurs (see below).
- *Overt diabetes stage.* In this stage, the patient's blood glucose levels are elevated in the fasting and postprandial state and meet criteria set forth by the American Diabetes Association.

The risk of developing type 2 diabetes is affected by age, obesity, and lack of physical activity (Harris et al., 1995), and the condition occurs more frequently in women with prior gestational diabetes mellitus (GDM) and in individuals with hypertension or dyslipidemia. It is often associated with a strong genetic predisposition, more so than is the autoimmune

form of type 1 diabetes, but the genetics of this form of diabetes are complex and not clearly defined as in type 1.

Impaired Glucose Tolerance and Impaired Fasting Glucose

The terms *impaired glucose tolerance* (IGT) and *impaired fasting glucose* (IFG) refer to an intermediate stage between normal glucose homeostasis and diabetes. IFG and IGT are not clinical entities in their own right but rather are intermediate stages to the destination of type 2 diabetes. This stage involves fasting glucose levels above 110 mg/dL (6.1 mmol/liter) but below 126 mg/dL (7 mmol/liter). Note that many individuals with IGT are euglycemic in their daily lives and usually have normal glycohemoglobin levels. All women with a prior diagnosis of IGT should be tested early in pregnancy for the presence of gestational diabetes.

Gestational Diabetes Mellitus

GDM is defined as glucose intolerance that begins or is first recognized during pregnancy (American Diabetes Association, 2002c). Almost uniformly, GDM arises from significant maternal insulin resistance, a state similar to type 2 diabetes. Indeed, in many cases GDM is simply preclinical type 2 diabetes unmasked by the hormonal stress imposed by the pregnancy. Since type 2 diabetes may be first diagnosed as GDM, postpartum testing 6 weeks or more after the pregnancy ends is necessary. Although nationally GDM complicates no more than 2.5% of pregnancies (which translates to more than 135,000 cases annually) (Engelgau et al., 1995), the prevalence of GDM in specific populations varies from 1% to 14% (American Diabetes Association, 2002c). Clinical recognition of GDM is

TABLE 49-3. MATERNAL MORBIDITY ASSOCIATED WITH DIABETIC PREGNANCY BY WHITE'S CLASSIFICATION

Complication	GDM or A (%)	B, C (%)	D, F, R (%)	Total (%)
Preeclampsia	10	8	16	12
Chronic hypertension	10	8	17	10
All hypertension	15	15	31	18
Ketoacidosis	8	7	9	
Hydramnios	5		18	18
Preterm labor	8	5	10	
Cesarean section	12	44	57	—

GDM, gestational diabetes mellitus.

Adapted from Cousins L. Pregnancy complications among diabetic women: Review. Obstet Gynecol Surv **42**:140, 1987.

TABLE 49-4. DIFFERENTIATING FEATURES OF TYPE I AND TYPE II DIABETES*

Clinical Features	IDDM (Type I)	NIDDM (Type II)
Obesity at onset	Uncommon	Common; often of central or masculine type
Metabolic ketoacidosis	Prone to ketosis	Ketosis less likely
Age at onset	Predominantly young (<30 yr)	Predominantly older (>30 yr)
Seasonal trend	Fall and winter	None
Insulin levels	Low to absent	Variable
Appearance of symptoms	Acute or subacute	Variable, usually slow
Inflammatory cells in islets	Present initially	Absent
Treatment	Insulin is required for life	Diet control or oral hypoglycemics may be sufficient, although insulin may be required to control hyperglycemia
Family history of diabetes	Uncommon, but increased prevalence of IDDM	Common with increased prevalence of NIDDM
Twin studies	20%–50% concordance in monozygotic twins	Close to 100% concordance in monozygotic twins
Association with other autoimmune endocrine diseases and antibodies	Yes	No
Islet cell antibodies	Yes	No
HLA associations	Yes	No
Further subtypes	DR3, DR4 associated	MODY, mutant insulins

* Both types may present initially during pregnancy as gestational carbohydrate intolerance.
HLA, human leukocyte antigen; IDDM, insulin-dependent diabetes mellitus; MODY, maturity-onset diabetes of the young; NIDDM, non–insulin-dependent diabetes mellitus.

important because therapy, including medical nutrition therapy, insulin when necessary, and antepartum fetal surveillance, can reduce GDM-associated perinatal morbidity and mortality.

MATERNAL-FETAL METABOLISM IN NORMAL AND DIABETIC PREGNANCY

Normal Maternal Glucose Regulation

With each feeding episode, a complex combination of maternal metabolic interactions—a rise in blood glucose as nutrients are absorbed from the gut, and the secondary secretion of pancreatic insulin, glucagon, somatomedins, and adrenal catecholamines—ensures an ample but not excessive supply of glucose to mother and fetus during pregnancy. The key features of maternal-fetal metabolic regulation during pregnancy are shown in Figure 49-2 and include the following:

- A maternal tendency to develop hypoglycemia between meals and at night while fasting occurs because the fetus continues to draw glucose from the maternal bloodstream across the placenta, even during periods of fasting. Interprandial hypoglycemia becomes increasingly marked as pregnancy progresses and fetal glucose demand grows.
- Levels of the diabetogenic placental steroid and peptide hormones—estrogens, progesterone, and chorionic

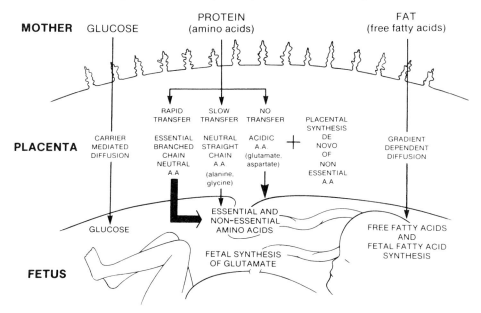

FIGURE 49-2 ■ Transport of maternal fuels to the placental and fetal compartments. The placenta serves as a modulator for the total parenteral alimentation of the fetus. (From Hollingsworth DR: Alterations of maternal metabolism in normal and diabetic pregnancies in insulin-dependent, non–insulin-dependent, and gestational diabetes. Am J Obstet Gynecol **146**:417, 1983.)

somatomammotropin—rise linearly throughout the second and third trimesters, resulting in a progressively increasing tissue resistance to maternal insulin action.

- Progressive maternal insulin resistance requires augmentation in pancreatic insulin production to more than twice nonpregnant levels during feeding to maintain euglycemia. Twenty-four-hour mean insulin levels are 30% higher in the third trimester than in the nonpregnant state.
- Failure to augment pancreatic insulin output (or exogenous insulin supplementation) adequately results in maternal, then fetal, hyperglycemia. The degree of hyperglycemia, and its timing, are important factors contributing to glucose-intolerance–associated morbidity in pregnancy.

When postprandial maternal glucose levels surge excessively, the consequent fetal hyperglycemia is accompanied by episodic fetal hyperinsulinemia. Fetal hyperinsulinemia, lasting only for 1 to 2 hours, has detrimental consequences to fetal growth and well-being. It promotes storage of excess nutrients, resulting in macrosomia, and drives catabolism of the oversupply of fuel, using energy and depleting fetal oxygen stores. Episodic fetal hypoxia stimulated by episodic maternal hyperglycemia leads to an outpouring of adrenal catecholamines, which in turn causes hypertension, cardiac remodeling, and hypertrophy, as well as stimulation of erythropoietin, red blood cell hyperplasia, and increased hematocrit level. High hematocrits, in turn, lead to poor circulation and postnatal hyperbilirubinemia.

These principles are illustrated in Figure 49-3. As seen in studies of normoglycemic women receiving three test meals in a supervised clinical research center, mean fasting blood glucose levels in normal women decline into the third trimester to a remarkably low value of 74 ± 2.7 mg/dL (Cousins et al., 1980). On the other hand, peak postprandial blood glucose values rarely exceed 120 mg/dL at any point in pregnancy. To maintain this strict control of glucose availability in the maternal bloodstream, the output of pancreatic insulin in response to feeding must nearly double. The task of metabolic management in diabetic pregnancy is to mimic (as much as possible) the profiles shown in this figure.

COMPLICATIONS OF DIABETES DURING PREGNANCY

Maternal Morbidity

Women with diabetes prior to pregnancy are at risk for a number of obstetric and medical complications. The relative risk of these problems is proportional to the duration and severity of disease.

Retinopathy

Diabetic retinopathy is the leading cause of blindness between the ages of 24 and 64 years (Elman et al., 1990). Some form of retinopathy is present in virtually 100% of women who have had type 1 diabetes for 25 years or more; approximately 20% of these women are legally blind. The topic of diabetic retinopathy has recently been reviewed (Aiello et al., 1998).

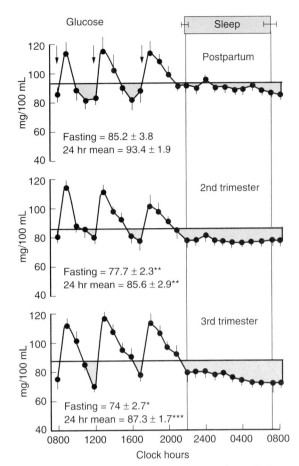

FIGURE 49-3 ■ Profile of blood glucose over 24 hours in the second and third trimesters of pregnancy, with postpartum observations used as a control. Error bars represent standard error. (From Cousins L, Rigg L, Hollingsworth D, et al: The 24-hour excursion and diurnal rhythm of glucose, insulin and C peptide in normal pregnancy. Am J Obstet Gynecol **136**:483, 1980.)

The progression of diabetic retinopathy is predictable, going from mild nonproliferative abnormalities, associated with increased vascular permeability, to moderate and severe nonproliferative diabetic retinopathy, characterized by vascular closure, to proliferative diabetic retinopathy, characterized by the growth of new blood vessels on the retina and posterior surface of the vitreous. Pregnancy has been documented to accelerate these changes, although the precise mechanism is controversial (Schocket et al., 1999). Vision loss resulting from diabetic retinopathy results from several mechanisms. First, central vision may be impaired by macular edema or capillary nonperfusion. Second, the new blood vessels of proliferative diabetic retinopathy and contraction of the accompanying fibrous tissue can distort the retina and lead to tractional retinal detachment, producing severe and often irreversible vision loss. Third, the new blood vessels may bleed, adding the further complication of preretinal or vitreous hemorrhage.

FACTORS AFFECTING PROGRESSION OF RETINOPATHY DURING PREGNANCY

Several studies have suggested that rapid induction of glycemic control in early pregnancy stimulates retinal vascular proliferation (Kroc Collaborative Study Group, 1988; Hopp et al., 1995). However, more recent investigations indicate that the severity and duration of diabetes prior to pregnancy have a greater effect. Temple and colleagues (2001) studied 179 women with pregestational type 1 diabetes, performing dilated fundal examination at the first prenatal visit, 24 weeks, and 34 weeks. Progression to proliferative diabetic retinopathy was noted in only 2.2%, and moderate progression in 2.8%. However, progression was significantly greater in women who had had diabetes for more than 10 years (10% versus 0%; $P = 0.007$) and in women with moderate to severe background retinopathy before pregnancy (30% versus 3.7%; $P = 0.01$). Similar findings were reported by Lauszus and colleagues (2000), who noted that there was an association between grade of retinopathy and hemoglobin (Hb) A_{1c} before and after pregnancy ($P < 0.02$). However, no such correlation was evident when glycemic control was kept tight. Women whose retinopathy progressed during or after pregnancy were significantly younger at diagnosis of diabetes mellitus (14 ± 8 years) than were those showing improvement or no progression of retinopathy (19 ± 8 years; $P < 0.04$). There was no association between retinopathy progression and HbA_{1c}, blood pressure, adverse perinatal outcome, or any of the other variables studied. Serup's (1986) prospective study showed that although half of patients with preexisting retinopathy experienced deterioration during pregnancy, all had partial regression following delivery, and all returned to normal by 6 months after delivery.

OPHTHALMOLOGIC MANAGEMENT DURING PREGNANCY

Screening for retinopathy by a qualified ophthalmologist is recommended prior to pregnancy and again during the first trimester for patients with pregestational diabetes, because of demonstrated effectiveness of laser photocoagulation therapy in arresting progression. Patients with minimal disease should be reexamined once or twice during the pregnancy and at 3 and 6 months after delivery. Those with significant retinal pathology may require monthly follow-up (American Diabetes Association, 2002b).

Nephropathy

Diabetes has become the most common single cause of end-stage renal disease in the U.S. and Europe. In the United States, diabetic nephropathy accounts for about 40% of new cases of this condition, and in 1997, the cost for treatment of diabetic patients with end-stage renal disease was in excess of $15.6 billion. About 20% to 30% of patients with type 1 or type 2 diabetes develop evidence of nephropathy over time, but the rate and extent of progression are highly individual (American Diabetes Association, 2002a).

The pathophysiology of diabetic renal disease is incompletely understood, and the relative roles of genetic susceptibility, control of hyperglycemia, and hypertension are not entirely clear. Additional insults, such as repeated urinary tract infections, excessive glycogen deposition, and papillary necrosis, all hasten deterioration of renal function. The kidney is normal at the onset of diabetes, but within a few years glomerular basement membrane thickening can be appreciated. By 5 years, there is expansion of the glomerular mesangium, resulting in diffuse diabetic glomerulosclerosis. All patients with marked mesangial expansion experience more than 400 mg of urinary protein excretion in 24 hours. The peak incidence of nephropathy occurs after about 16 years of diabetes.

DEFINITIONS

Categories of diabetic nephropathy are distinguished by the level of urinary protein excretion. Table 49-5 shows normal values and the current clinical criteria microalbuminuria, and nephropathy. Screening for microalbuminuria can be performed by three methods: (1) measurement of the albumin-to-creatinine ratio in a random spot collection; (2) 24-hour collection with creatinine, allowing the simultaneous measurement of creatinine clearance; and (3) timed (e.g., 4-hour or overnight) collection. The first method is often found to be the easiest to carry out in an office setting and generally provides accurate information; first-void or other morning collections are preferred because of the known diurnal variation in albumin excretion. Specific assays are needed to detect microalbuminuria because standard hospital laboratory assays for urinary protein are not sufficiently sensitive to measure such levels.

THE EFFECT OF PREGNANCY ON PROGRESSION OF NEPHROPATHY

Some nephrologists discourage pregnancy in women with diabetic renal disease, especially if there is coexisting hypertension, because of concerns of permanent renal deterioration as a result of the pregnancy. However, more recent data indicate that pregnancy does not measurably alter the time course of diabetic renal disease. A study of renal function for 4 years before and 4 years after pregnancy in 11 patients with diabetic nephropathy (Reece, Winn, Hayslett, et al., 1990) showed that the gradual rise in serum creatinine over that period was unaffected by the intervening pregnancy.

As in other complications of diabetes, the progression of renal disease appears to be related to duration of diabetes and degree of glycemic control. Feldt-Rasmussen and associates (1986a,b) reported the effect of 2 years of strict metabolic control on progression of nephropathy in 36 patients randomized to conventional treatment or insulin pump therapy. None

■◾ **TABLE 49–5.** CATEGORIES OF DIABETIC RENAL DISEASE*

Category	24-hr Collection (Mg/24 Hr)	Timed Collection (µg/Min)	Spot Collection (µg/Min)
Normal	<30	<20	<30
Microalbuminuria	30–299	20–199	30–299
Nephropathy	≥300	≥200	≥300

* Two of three collections should be abnormal for a diagnosis of microalbuminuria or nephropathy.

American Diabetes Association: Standards of medical care for patients with diabetes mellitus. Diabetes Care **25**(Suppl 1):S33, 2002.

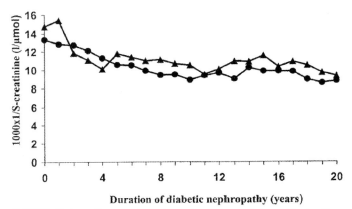

FIGURE 49-4 ■ Changes in reciprocal-serum creatinine with duration of diabetes: a comparison of ever-pregnant (*triangles*) and never-pregnant (*circles*) groups. (Adapted from Rossing K, Jacobsen P, Hommel E, et al: Pregnancy and progression of diabetic nephropathy. Diabetologia **45**(1):36, 2002.)

of the patients managed on the insulin pump experienced progression to clinical nephropathy, whereas five in the conventional treatment group did.

Rossing and colleagues (2002) evaluated the effect of pregnancy on deterioration of renal function in 93 women over 20 years. Groups of never-pregnant and ever-pregnant women, receiving similar medical therapy and with similar renal function at the start of the study, were compared. The results are shown in Figures 49-4 and 49-5. Based on this excellent prospective study, it is evident that pregnancy neither alters the time course of renal disease nor increases the likelihood of transition to end-stage renal disease.

COURSE OF DIABETIC NEPHROPATHY DURING PREGNANCY

In general, patients with underlying renal disease prior to pregnancy can be expected to experience varying degrees of deterioration during pregnancy. The physiologic changes associated with normal pregnancy increase renal blood flow and glomerular filtration by 30% to 50%. Most women with preexisting diabetic nephropathy experience this improvement in renal function, especially during the second trimester (Jovanovic and Jovanovic, 1984). During the third trimester, however, when mean arterial pressure and peripheral vascular resistance typically rise, women with diabetic microvascular disease may experience marked diminution of renal function, an exacerbation in hypertension, and in many cases, preeclampsia. Rising maternal blood pressure and a rapid fall in creatinine clearance are among the most common precipitating events leading to preterm delivery in diabetic women in this time frame. Although delivering the fetus to interrupt the precipitous rise in blood pressure may result in premature birth, this is usually preferable to the risk of renal failure or stroke in the mother (see Pregnancy Outcomes, below).

Reece, Leguizamon, and colleagues (1998) reviewed the outcomes of 315 patients with diabetic nephropathy from the world's literature in 1998. Of these women, 17% ultimately developed end-stage renal disease, and 5% died as a result of renal insufficiency. During pregnancy, proteinuria and mean arterial pressure significantly increased from the first to the third trimester (P <0.05). A smaller study reported by Purdy and coworkers (1996) demonstrated a rise in mean serum

creatinine from 159 μmol/liter (1.8 mg/dL) before pregnancy to 221 μmol/liter (2.5 mg/dL) in the third trimester. Renal function was stable in 27%, showed transient worsening in pregnancy in 27%, and demonstrated a permanent decline in 45%. Proteinuria increased in pregnancy in 79%. Exacerbation of hypertension or preeclampsia occurred in 73%.

PREGNANCY OUTCOMES IN WOMEN WITH DIABETIC NEPHROPATHY

Ekbom and colleagues (2001) compared the outcomes of patients with microalbuminuria or overt nephropathy and those without. Their results, illustrated in Figure 49-6, indicate that the likelihood of preterm delivery is considerably increased in women with microalbuminuria, mainly because of preeclampsia. Classification according to urinary albumin excretion and metabolic control around the time of conception are superior to the White classification in predicting preterm delivery in women with type 1 diabetes.

RENAL DIALYSIS IN DIABETIC PREGNANT WOMEN

Although women receiving maintenance dialysis for end-stage renal failure are often amenorrheic or at least anovulatory, pregnancies are now not uncommon (Wing et al., 1980). Nevertheless, the prognosis for successful pregnancy in diabetic patients with end-stage renal disease is exceedingly poor. Fetal loss in the second trimester and third trimester and neonatal death are frequent. About 60% of births are premature, often because of uncontrollable hypertension, renal failure, or fetal growth failure (Romao et al., 1998). Of the 20% or 25% of pregnancies ending in live births, 40% of babies are severely growth-restricted.

Neither chronic hemodialysis nor chronic peritoneal dialysis corrects uremia. Instead, these modes of therapy limit uremia to a level that allows a tolerable degree of health and rehabilitation (Ward, 1988). A major practical problem with achieving successful pregnancy outcome while on hemodialysis is proper maintenance of maternal vascular volume. Dialysis teams are accustomed to taking off fluid at each session. The pregnant patient requires a progressive increase in vascular volume of at least 20% to 30% above nonpregnant values from 8 to 30 weeks' gestation, however. This volume augmentation

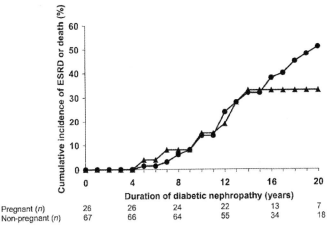

Pregnant (*n*)	26	26	24	22	13	7
Non-pregnant (*n*)	67	66	64	55	34	18

FIGURE 49-5 ■ Cumulative incidence of end-stage renal disease (ESRD) in ever-pregnant (*triangles*) and never-pregnant (*circles*) groups. (From Rossing K, Jacobsen P, Hommel E, et al: Pregnancy and progression of diabetic nephropathy. Diabetologia **45**(1):36, 2002.)

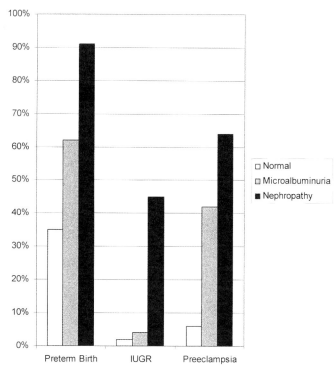

FIGURE 49-6 ■ Pregnancy outcomes in diabetic women with underlying renal disease. IUGR, intrauterine growth restriction. (Adapted from Ekbom P, Damm P, Feldt-Rasmussen U, et al: Pregnancy outcome in type 1 diabetic women with microalbuminuria. Diabetes Care **24**(10):1739, 2001. Copyright © American Diabetes Association. Reprinted with permission from The American Diabetes Association.)

appears to be necessary to maintain uteroplacental perfusion. Pregnancies in which vascular volume does not increase have a high incidence of fetal growth restriction and stillbirth. Difficulties with vascular underfill (hypertension, poor fetal growth, asphyxia) and overfill (hypertension) are common in pregnant patients on hemodialysis and often difficult to rectify (Hou and Firanek, 1998).

The poor prognosis associated with hemodialysis, together with other considerations, has prompted increased interest in continuous ambulatory peritoneal dialysis. Several successful pregnancy series have been reported (Davison, 1987; Romao et al., 1998). Although fluid and chemical balance is constant and heparinization is not necessary, intrauterine deaths, abruption, prematurity, hypertension, and fetal distress still occur. At present, the best strategy for most diabetic women on dialysis desiring pregnancy is to undergo kidney transplantation.

RENAL TRANSPLANTATION

Successful pregnancy with a renal transplant is now a reality. Davison (1987) reviewed data from 1569 pregnancies in 1009 women. Of the 60% of pregnancies that extended beyond the first trimester, 92% resulted in a viable infant. Preeclampsia occurred in 30%, preterm delivery in about 50%, and intrauterine growth restriction (IUGR) in 20%. Patients with the worst renal function had the poorest pregnancy outcomes. Similar results were reported by Armenti and colleagues (1994). Pre-pregnancy factors that increase perinatal risk include the need for antihypertensive therapy and serum creatinine greater than or equal to 1.5 mg/dL.

Sgro and colleagues (2002) reported their experience with 44 pregnancies after renal transplantation, of which 77% resulted in live-born infants. The mean gestational age at delivery was 36.5 ± 2.7 weeks compared to 40.2 ± 1.6 weeks in controls with normal renal function (P <0.001). The mean birthweight in the study group was 2.54 ± 0.67 kg, compared to 3.59 ± 0.53 kg in the control group (P <0.0001). The authors concluded that although patients with a renal transplant have significantly more stillbirths, preterm deliveries, and infants of low birth weight, most pregnancies in the study group went well.

Based on these findings, perinatal outcomes are better in patients who have undergone renal transplantation than in those with end-stage renal disease. Unfortunately, most patients with advanced nephropathy are unwilling to delay pregnancy until after stabilization of renal function following transplantation. This issue is addressed in Chapter 44.

Cardiovascular Complications

Cardiovascular complications experienced by pregnant women with diabetes include chronic hypertension, pregnancy-induced hypertension, and (rarely) atherosclerotic heart disease. In composite studies of all types of diabetic pregnancies, the incidence of hypertensive disorders during pregnancy varies from 15% to 30% (Gabbe et al., 1977a,b; Tevaarwerk et al., 1981).

CHRONIC HYPERTENSION

Chronic hypertension (defined as blood pressure at or above 140/90 mm Hg before the 20th week of gestation) complicates 10% to 20% of pregnancies in diabetic women and up to 40% of those in diabetic women with preexisting renal or retinal vascular disease (Sibai, 2000; Cundy et al., 2002). The perinatal problems encountered with chronic hypertension include IUGR, maternal stroke, preeclampsia, and abruptio placentae (American Diabetes Association, 2002f). In type 1 diabetes, the prevalence of chronic hypertension increases with duration of diabetes and is closely associated with nephropathy (Leguizamon and Reece, 2000).

The Diabetes in Early Pregnancy (DIEP) study reported that women with type 1 diabetes have higher mean blood pressures throughout pregnancy than do normal controls (Peterson et al., 1992). In a significant proportion of patients, this difference is probably evidence of underlying renal compromise. Preexisting chronic hypertension should be suspected when the diabetic patient's systolic blood pressure exceeds 130/80 mm Hg before the third trimester. The diagnosis is strengthened by finding (1) a failure of mean blood pressure to decline normally in the late second trimester, (2) elevation in blood urea nitrogen above 10 mg/dL, (3) serum creatinine above 1 mg/dL, (4) creatinine clearance less than 100 mL/minute, or a combination thereof.

PREECLAMPSIA

Preeclampsia is more frequent among women with diabetes, occurring two to three times as frequently in women with pregestational diabetes as in those without diabetes (Sibai et al., 2000). However, the risk of developing preeclampsia is proportional to the duration of diabetes prior to pregnancy and the existence of nephropathy and hypertension; more than one third of pregnant women who have had diabetes for over

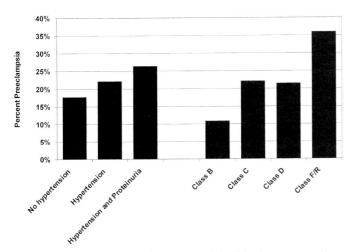

FIGURE 49-7 ■ Likelihood of preeclampsia in diabetic pregnancy by White's class and preexisting hypertension. (From Sibai BM, Caritis S, Hauth J, et al: Risks of preeclampsia and adverse neonatal outcomes among women with pregestational diabetes mellitus. National Institute of Child Health and Human Development Network of Maternal-Fetal Medicine Units. Am J Obstet Gynecol **182**(2):364, 2000.)

20 years develop this condition (Sibai et al., 2000). As is shown in Figure 49-7, patients with White's class B diabetes have a risk profile similar to that of nondiabetic patients, but women with evidence of renal or retinal vasculopathy (classes D, F, or R) have a 50% excess risk of hypertensive complications over the rate observed in those with no hypertension. Similar rates of preeclampsia are experienced by women with diabetic nephropathy.

Renal function assessments should be performed in each trimester in women with overt diabetic vascular disease and in those who have had diabetes for more than 10 years. Significant proteinuria, plasma uric acid levels above 6 mg/dL, or evidence of HELLP syndrome (*h*emolysis, *e*levated *l*iver enzymes, and *l*ow *p*latelets) should prompt a workup for preeclampsia.

HEART DISEASE

Although coronary heart disease is rarely encountered in pregnant women with diabetes, studies by Airaksinen and colleagues (1986) suggest that such women may have preclinical cardiomyopathy and autonomic neuropathy. Diabetic women studied had less than the normal increase in left ventricular size and stroke volume, lower heart-rate increases, and smaller increments in cardiac output.

Although uncommon, atherosclerotic heart disease (White's class H) may afflict diabetic patients in the later reproductive years. Patients with this complication have a mean age of 34 years and exhibit other evidence of diabetic vascular involvement (White's class D or R) (Silfen et al., 1980). For diabetic women with cardiac involvement, pregnancy outcome is dismal, with maternal mortality 50% or higher and perinatal loss rates approaching 30% (Gordon et al., 1996). Recognition of cardiac compromise in the pregnant women with diabetes may be difficult because of the decrease in exercise tolerance that occurs in normal pregnancy. Compromised cardiac function may also be difficult to detect in patients restricted to bed rest for hypertension or poor fetal growth. Thus, it is prudent to obtain a detailed cardiovascular history in all diabetic patients and to consider electrocardi-ography and more extensive cardiology evaluation (e.g., an echocardiogram) in patients who have type 1 diabetes and are over the age of 30 or in patients who have had diabetes for 10 years or more. With intensive monitoring, successful pregnancy is possible albeit hazardous for women with significant cardiac disease (Reece et al., 1986).

Diabetic Ketoacidosis

Diabetic ketoacidosis (DKA) during pregnancy is a medical emergency for both mother and fetus. Pregnant women with type 1 diabetes are at increased risk for DKA (Montoro et al., 1993) although the incidence and morbidity of this complication have decreased from 20% or more in the older literature to approximately 2% in recent years (Chauhan et al., 1996; Cullen et al., 1996). Intrauterine fetal death, formerly as high as 35% with DKA during pregnancy, has dropped to 10% or less.

Precipitating factors include pulmonary, urinary, or soft tissue infections; poor compliance; and very importantly, unrecognized new onset of diabetes. Because severe DKA is life-threatening to mother and fetus, prompt treatment is essential. Fetal well-being in particular is in jeopardy until maternal metabolic homeostasis is reestablished. High levels of plasma glucose and ketones are readily transported to the fetus, which may be unable to secrete sufficient quantities of insulin to prevent DKA *in utero*.

DKA evolves from inadequate insulin action and functional hypoglycemia at the target tissue level. This leads to increased hepatic glucose release but decreased or absent tissue disposal of glucose. Glucose-lacking tissues release ketone bodies, while vascular hyperglycemia promotes osmotic diuresis. Over time, this diuresis causes profound vascular volume depletion and loss of electrolytes. The release of stress hormones (catecholamines, glucagon, growth hormone, and cortisol) further impairs insulin action and contributes to insulin resistance. Left unchecked, this cycle of dehydration, tissue hypoglycemia, and electrolyte depletion will lead to multisystem collapse, coma, and death.

Early in the illness, hyperglycemia and ketosis are moderate. If hyperglycemia is not corrected, diuresis, dehydration, and hyperosmolality follow. Pregnant women in the early stages of ketoacidosis respond quickly to appropriate treatment of the initiating cause (broad-spectrum antibiotics), additional doses of regular insulin, and volume replacement.

Patients with advanced DKA usually present with typical findings, including hyperventilation, normal or obtunded mental state (depending on severity of the acidosis), dehydration, hypotension, and a fruity odor to the breath. Abdominal pain and vomiting may be prominent symptoms. The diagnosis of DKA is confirmed by the presence of hyperglycemia (glucose >200 mg/100 mL) with positive serum ketones at a level of 1:4 or greater.

It is important to recognize that as many as one third of patients may, in early or very late stages of DKA, have initial blood glucose levels less than 200 mg/dL (Cullen et al., 1996). A pregnant diabetic patient with a history of poor food intake or vomiting for more than 12 to 16 hours should be thoroughly worked up for DKA, including a complete blood count and electrolytes. A serum bicarbonate level below 18 mg/dL should prompt performance of an arterial blood gas analysis. In all cases of DKA, the diagnosis is confirmed by arterial blood gases demonstrating a metabolic acidemia (base excess –4 or lower).

TABLE 49–6. TREATMENT PROTOCOL FOR DIABETIC KETOACIDOSIS*

	Initial Phase	Recovery Phase
Insulin	10–20 U insulin IV bolus plus 5–10 U/hr IV (infusion), IM, or SC. IV route should be used in any hypotensive patient[†] Increase hourly dose if serum glucose does not fall despite adequate fluid therapy	As acidosis is reversed, decrease to 5–10 every 2–4 hr When patient is eating, begin long-acting insulin
Fluids	0.9% NaCl at 1000 mL/hr Replace sodium deficit in 4–6 hr (average 500 mEq)	When blood pressure is stable, urine output brisk, and serum glucose falling, decrease to 0.45% NaCl at 250–500 mL/hr When serum glucose <250 mg/dL, add 5% glucose to IV fluids Replace water deficit over 12–24 hr (average 5–10 liters)
Potassium	If serum K+ high, begin KCl at 20 mEq/hr after urine output is established If serum K+ low or normal, begin KCl at 20 mEq/hr immediately; reduce rate by 50% if patient is oliguric Monitor ECG; measure serum K+ every 2–4 hr	Adjust dose of KCl according to serum K+ measurements Continue oral KCl replacement for 1 wk to correct total deficit
Bicarbonate	If pH <7.0, give as needed to raise pH to 7.0 If pH 7.0–7.2, ± small amounts (≤88 mEq) If pH >7.2, give no bicarbonate	Give no bicarbonate
Phosphorus	If patient not oliguric, potassium phosphate may be given at 10 mEq/hr (decrease dosage of KCl accordingly) Measure serum phosphorus and calcium frequently	Give no phosphorus
General measures	If patient is comatose, establish nasogastric tube and bladder catheter Identify and treat any precipitating illness Consider low-dosage heparin	Remove catheter as soon as possible Continue to observe for signs of precipitating or complicating illness

* These are general guidelines. Because there may be wide variation in individual patient needs, there is no substitute for careful monitoring of each patient, particularly in the initial phase of therapy.

† In pregnant women, constant intravenous insulin infusion with an IVAC is preferable.

ECG, electrocardiogram; IM, intramuscular; IV, intravenous; KCl, potassium chloride; NaCl, sodium chloride; SC, subcutaneous.

Adapted from Porte D Jr, Halter JB: The endocrine pancreas and diabetes mellitus. *In* Williams RH (ed): Textbook of Endocrinology. 6th ed. Philadelphia, WB Saunders, 1981.

Table 49-6 contains a protocol for treatment of DKA. The important steps in management should include the following:

- Search for and treat the precipitating cause. These include pyelonephritis and pulmonary or gastrointestinal viral infections.
- Perform vigorous and sustained volume resuscitation. The patient will continue to generate vascular volume deficits until her metabolic abnormalities are largely resolved. A physiologic fluid such as 0.9% NaCl with 20 mEq/liter potassium should be used and continued until the acidosis is substantially corrected (base excess –2 or less). This typically requires an infusion at 1 to 2 liters per hour for the first 1 to 2 hours, then reduced rates (150 to 200 mL/hour) until the base deficit nears normal.
- Place a Foley catheter to monitor urine output.
- Use insulin to correct hyperglycemia, either as a continuous infusion or by intermittent injections of regular insulin. When giving insulin as a continuous infusion, 1 to 2 units/hour will gradually correct the patient's glucose abnormality over 4 to 8 hours. Attempts to normalize plasma glucose levels rapidly (in less than 2 to 3 hours) may result in hypoglycemia and further physiologic counterregulatory responses.
- Follow serum bicarbonate levels and base deficits reported from arterial blood gas analysis to guide

management. Even when blood glucose level is normalized, ongoing acidemia may be present, as evidenced by continuing abnormalities in the patient's electrolytes. Unless volume therapy is continued until electrolytes have substantially returned to normal, DKA may reappear, and the cycle of metabolic derangement will be renewed.

When DKA occurs after 24 weeks' gestation, fetal status should be continuously monitored via fetal heart rate monitoring, biophysical profile, or both. However, even when fetal status is questionable during the phase of volume and plasma-glucose correction, the temptation to perform emergency cesarean section should be avoided. Usually, correction of the maternal metabolic disorder is remarkably effective in normalizing fetal status (Hughes, 1987). Nevertheless, if a reasonable effort has been expended in correcting the maternal metabolic disorder and fetal status is of concern, delivery should not be delayed.

Fetal Morbidity and Mortality

Perinatal mortality in diabetic pregnancy has decreased 30-fold since the discovery of insulin in 1922 and the institution of intensive obstetric and infant care in the 1970s. Improved techniques of maintaining maternal euglycemia

TABLE 49–7. PERINATAL MORTALITY RATES IN DIABETIC PREGNANCY*

	Gestational	Overt	Normals[†]
Fetal mortality (%)	4.7	10.4	5.7
Neonatal mortality (%)	3.3	12.2	4.7
Perinatal mortality (%)	8.0	22.6	10.4

* Mortality rates = deaths per 1000 live births.
[†] Normal = California data from 1986; birth weight, sex, and race corrected.

have led to later timing of delivery and reduced iatrogenic respiratory distress syndrome. Nevertheless, the perinatal mortality rates currently reported for diabetic women remain approximately twice those observed in the nondiabetic population (Table 49-7). Congenital malformations, respiratory distress syndrome, and extreme prematurity account for most perinatal deaths in diabetic pregnancy today.

Miscarriage

Current data indicate that miscarriage rates among women with diabetes, especially those with poor glucose control, are excessive and proportional to degree of maternal hyperglycemia during the periconceptional period. Given the well-documented associations between congenital anomalies and both diabetes and miscarriage, such a finding is not surprising. A retrospective study by Sutherland and Pritchard (1986) of 164 diabetic pregnancies managed with relaxed glycemic control demonstrated a spontaneous abortion rate of almost double the expected rate. Key and associates (1987) reported that glycosylated hemoglobin levels in early pregnancy were significantly higher in women who aborted than in those who delivered successfully (12.8% versus 11.2%). Miodovnik and coworkers (1984) studied spontaneous abortion in diabetic pregnancy prospectively and found an increasing rate among patients with more advanced classes of diabetes. (Rates for classes C, D, and F were 25%, 44%, and 22%, respectively.) In one study, patients with preconceptional metabolic care had a miscarriage frequency one third that of patients who began care later during pregnancy (Rosenn et al., 1991). More recent studies from populations with better glycemic control report miscarriage rates similar to those in the nondiabetic population (Nordstrom et al., 1998; Platt et al., 2002), suggesting that diabetic women with excellent glycemic control have a risk of miscarriage equivalent to that of the nondiabetic patient.

These studies can be used to encourage patients who have not yet conceived to achieve excellent glycemic control. Patients presenting in early pregnancy with normal glycohemoglobin values can be reassured that the overall elevation in risk of miscarriage is modest. However, in patients with glycohemoglobin values 2 to 3 standard deviations above the norm, intense early pregnancy surveillance is indicated.

Congenital Anomalies

A major threat to the infant of a diabetic mother is the possibility of a life-threatening structural anomaly. Among the general population, the risk in pregnancy of a major birth defect is 1% to 2%. Among women with overt diabetes prior to conception, the risk of a structural anomaly in the fetus is

increased four- to eightfold (Reece, Sivan, et al., 1998). The typical defects and their frequency of occurrence according to a prospective study of infants with major malformations are noted in Table 49-8. The majority of lesions involve the central nervous system and the cardiovascular system, although other series have reported an excess of genitourinary and limb defects as well.

There is no increase in birth defects among offspring of diabetic fathers, normoglycemic women, and women who develop gestational diabetes after the first trimester, suggesting that glycemic control during embryogenesis is the main factor in the genesis of diabetes-associated birth defects. A classic report by Miller and co-authors (1981) compared the frequency of congenital anomalies in patients with normal or high first-trimester maternal glycohemoglobin and found only a 3.4% rate of anomalies with HbA_{1c} less than 8.5%, whereas the rate of malformations in patients with poorer glycemic control in the periconceptional period (HbA_{1c} above 8.5) was 22.4%. Lucas and coworkers (1989) reported an overall malformation rate of 13.3% in 105 diabetic patients. However, the risk of delivering a malformed infant was nil with HbA_1 less than 7%, 14% with HbA_1 between 7.2% and 9.1%, 23% with HbA_1 between 9.2% and 11.1%, and 25% with HbA_1 greater than 11.2%.

PATHOGENESIS

The mechanism by which hyperglycemia disturbs embryonic development is multifactorial. The potential teratologic role of disturbances in the metabolism of inositol, prostaglandins, and reactive oxygen species has been established (Eriksson et al., 2000). Embryonic hyperglycemia may promote excessive formation of oxygen radicals in susceptible fetal tissues, which are inhibitors of prostacyclin (Warso and Lands, 1983). The resulting overabundance of thromboxanes and other prostaglandins may then disrupt the vascularization of developing tissues. In support of this theory, addition of prostaglandin inhibitors to mouse embryos in culture medium prevented glucose-induced embryopathy (Pinter et al., 1986). The pathogenic role of free-radical species in teratogenesis with diabetes has been underscored through demonstrating the effect of dietary antioxidants experimentally: High doses of vitamins C and E decreased fetal dysmorphogenesis to nondiabetic levels in rat pregnancy and rat embryo culture (Cederberg et al., 2001; Zaken et al., 2001).

TABLE 49–8. CONGENITAL MALFORMATIONS IN INFANTS OF INSULIN-DEPENDENT DIABETIC MOTHERS

Anomaly	Approximate Risk Ratio	Percent Risk (%)
All cardiac defects	18×	8.5
All CNS anomalies	16×	5.3
Anencephaly	13×	
Spina bifida	20×	
All congenital anomalies	8×	18.4

CNS, central nervous system.

Adapted from Becerra JE, Khoury MJ, Cordero JF, et al: Diabetes mellitus during pregnancy and the risks for specific birth defects: A population based case-control study. Pediatrics **85**:1, 1990.

PREVENTION

Because the critical time for teratogenesis is during the period 3 to 6 weeks after conception, nutritional and metabolic intervention must be instituted preconceptionally to be effective. Several clinical trials of preconceptional metabolic care have demonstrated that malformation rates equivalent to those in the general population can be achieved with meticulous glycemic control (Fuhrmann et al., 1983). Although studies of dietary folate supplementation have demonstrated success in reducing the incidence of neural tube defects in nondiabetic populations, the efficacy of a high-antioxidant diet in preventing renal and cardiac anomalies more frequent in diabetes has not been adequately explored. Preconceptional management of pregestational diabetics is discussed fully below.

Intrauterine Growth Restriction

Although the weights of IDMs are generally skewed into the upper range, IUGR occurs with significant frequency in diabetic pregnancy, especially in women with underlying vascular disease. Additional factors that increase the risk of IUGR in diabetic pregnancy include the higher incidence of structural anomalies and maternal hypertension (see also Chapters 28 and 43).

As noted above, asymmetric IUGR is encountered most frequently in patients with vasculopathy (retinal, renal, or chronic hypertension) (Reece, Sivan, et al., 1998). This association suggests that uteroplacental vasculopathy may result in restricted fetal growth in these patients (Van Assche et al., 2001). Patients with brittle control and frequent episodes of ketosis and hypoglycemia are also prone to preeclampsia and poor fetal growth. Whether fetal growth restriction results from poor maternal-placental blood flow or intrinsically poor placental function is unresolved (Padmanabhan and Shafiullah, 2001).

Fetal Obesity

Fetal obesity is increased threefold in diabetic pregnancies as compared to normoglycemic controls (Combs et al., 1992) and is associated with much of the morbidity experienced by the infant of the diabetic mother (Van Assche et al., 2001). Although controversy exists concerning the optimal criterion to define fetal macrosomia (birthweight or estimated fetal weight above the 90th percentile for gestational age, above 4000 g, above 4250 g, or above 4500 g), the prevalence of oversized infants is markedly increased at each gestational age of diabetic pregnancy compared to normals (Sacks, 1993).

The characteristics of the growth dynamics seen in these infants are unique, in that skeletal growth is largely unaffected, while adipose accumulation, particularly in the third trimester, is excessive and distributed predominantly into the truncal regions. McFarland and colleagues (1998) calculated lean and fat body mass in normal and IDMs and demonstrated that macrosomic infants of diabetic mothers were characterized by larger shoulder and extremity circumferences, a decreased head-to-shoulder ratio, significantly higher body fat, and thicker upper-extremity skinfolds than were with nondiabetic control infants of similar birth weight and birth length.

GROWTH DYNAMICS

During the first and second trimesters, differentiation of diabetic from nondiabetic fetuses is difficult using ultrasound measurements, suggesting that the period of fetal fat deposition (28 weeks and onward) is when most abnormal fetal growth occurs. Ogata and coworkers (1980) used serial ultrasound examinations of fetuses of diabetic women to demonstrate that the rate of abdominal circumference growth typically begins to rise significantly above normal after 24 weeks. Reece, Winn, Smikle, and associates (1990) showed that fetuses of diabetic women have normal head growth and skeletal growth, even when hyperglycemia and fetal abdominal obesity are markedly advanced. Landon and colleagues (1989) confirmed these observations, noting that although head and femur growth in fetuses of diabetic mothers was similar to such growth in normals, abdominal circumference growth exceeded that of controls beginning at 32 weeks.

THE PATHOPHYSIOLOGY OF FETAL OVERGROWTH

The process of excessive fetal fat accumulation in the second half of pregnancy reflects the delivery of an abnormal nutrient mixture from the maternal bloodstream to the fetoplacental unit. In 1952, Pedersen hypothesized that maternal hyperglycemia stimulates fetal hyperinsulinemia, which in turn mediates accelerated fuel use and growth.

MATERNAL GLUCOSE LEVELS. Excessive maternal blood glucose levels are an important, if not the only, element promoting fetal macrosomia (Jovanovic-Peterson, 1991). Findings from the DIEP project indicate that fetal birth weight correlates best with second- and third-trimester postprandial blood glucose levels, not fasting or mean glucose levels. When 2-hour postprandial blood glucose values averaged 120 mg/dL or less, approximately 20% of infants were macrosomic; when postprandial levels ranged up to 160 mg/dL, macrosomia rates reached 35%. Similar findings were reported by Persson and Hanson (1998), who showed that the fasting glucose level contributes only 12% of the birth-weight variance in diabetic pregnancy, and Combs and colleagues (1992), who found that higher postprandial glucose levels up to 32 weeks correlated with the risk of infant macrosomia.

FETAL INSULIN LEVELS. Pedersen's hypothesis highlighting the central role of excessive fetal insulin levels in mediating excessive fetal growth in diabetic pregnancy has been confirmed by multiple studies (Akinbi and Gerdes, 1995). The central role of insulin in mediating intrauterine growth is illustrated by the severe growth restriction observed in infants with congenital glucokinase mutation resulting in markedly reduced fetal insulin production *in utero* (Spyer et al., 2001). When Simmons and colleagues (1995) compared umbilical cord sera in newborn IDMs and normals, they found that the heavier, fatter babies from diabetic pregnancies were also hyperinsulinemic (130.6 versus 90.4 pmol/liter, respectively; $P < 0.01$). Schwartz and coauthors (1994) found that umbilical cord insulin levels at delivery correlated with the degree of macrosomia. Cordocentesis at 36 to 39 weeks' gestation in diabetic pregnancies showed that the fetal plasma insulin-to-glucose ratio and the degree of macrosomia were strongly related ($r = 0.76$; $P < 0.0001$) (Salvesen et al., 1993).

Insulin concentrations in the amniotic fluid have been correlated with fetal plasma insulin levels, birthweight, and the risk of neonatal hypoglycemia (Fraser and Bruce, 1999). Indeed, elevated amniotic fluid insulin levels obtained from nondiabetic patients during amniocentesis at 14 to 20 weeks' gestation (range, 1.4 to 44.5 pmol/liter), adjusted for maternal age and weight, correlated with the likelihood of subsequently diagnosed GDM (odds ratio [OR] = 1.9; 95% confidence interval [CI] = 1.3 to 2.4; P = 0.029). Each unit increase in amniotic fluid insulin multiple of median was associated with a threefold increase in fetal macrosomia incidence (Carpenter et al., 2001).

Krew and colleagues (1994) observed that amniotic fluid C-peptide levels, measured 1 week before delivery, correlated strongly with neonatal fat mass (P = 0.008). Lean body mass did not correlate with C-peptide levels. Weerasiri and co-workers (1993) noted highly significant associations between elevated amniotic fluid insulin values and macrosomia (P <0.0045), birth weight (P <0.00004), and neonatal blood glucose levels (P = 0.042) in gestational diabetic pregnancies.

These studies, which consistently identify a powerful relationship between fetal plasma insulin concentrations and fetal fat percentages, provide strong support for Pedersen's assertion that fetal insulin response to maternal hyperglycemia is a central factor underlying diabetic fetopathy (Fraser and Bruce, 1999).

GROWTH FACTORS. There has been considerable interest in the role of insulinlike growth factors (IGFs) in fetal growth. D'Ercole (1999) has reviewed the current understanding of IGFs and fetal growth, noting that studies of knockout mice have demonstrated the essential roles of the IGFs (IGF-I and -II), insulin, and their receptors in embryonic and fetal growth, providing compelling evidence that increased IGF-II gene expression and/or abundance can stimulate excessive fetal somatic growth. Lauszus and colleagues (2001) observed that maternal levels of IGF-I and -II were proportional to newborn birthweight centile (P <0.01). Jaksic et al (2001) compared IGF-I values in umbilical sera of macrosomic and nonmacrosomic offspring of nondiabetic women, finding the macrosomic infants had significantly higher values of insulin and IGF-I. Roth and co-authors (1996) reported that levels of cord serum IGF-I in macrosomic neonates of mothers with diabetes (83 ± 4.2 ng/mL) were severalfold higher than those in nonmacrosomic infants of nondiabetic (38 ± 1.9 ng/mL) or diabetic mothers (13 ± 3.5 ng/mL). IGF-II cord serum levels were also elevated in the pregnancies of diabetic women compared with those of nondiabetic women. There was a direct linear correlation between cord serum IGF-I and infant birth weight, independent of diabetes (P <0.01).

MATERNAL OBESITY. Because adult-onset diabetes and obesity frequently coexist, the effect of maternal body fat on fetal growth should not be overlooked (Michlin et al., 2000). Several studies suggest that maternal obesity before pregnancy has an independent effect on fetal macrosomia (Essel and Opai-Tetteh, 1995; Nasrat et al., 1996). Vohr and associates (1995) analyzed various risk factors for neonatal macrosomia in women with overt and gestational diabetes compared with obese and normal-weight controls. Multiple-regression analyses revealed that pre-pregnancy weight and weight gain were significant predictors for both infants of gestational diabetic mothers and control infants. Cundy and associates (1993) reported that birth weight was largely determined by maternal factors other than hyperglycemia, with the most significant influencing variables being gestational age at delivery, pre-pregnancy body mass index, maternal height, pregnancy weight gain, the presence of hypertension, and cigarette smoking. When Kumari (2001) assessed the pregnancy outcomes of women with body mass index (BMI) greater than 40 to those of normal-weight women, the incidence of macrosomic infants was tripled, even when women with diabetes were excluded. Perlow and col-

leagues (1992) reported a doubling of macrosomia in non-diabetic, very obese women (weight above 300 pounds). Compared with normal-weight women, massively obese women had more than twice the prevalence of macrosomia, suggesting that maternal obesity has a strong, diabetes-independent influence on fetal growth. This may explain the failure of glycemic control alone to prevent fetal macrosomia in several series (Moore et al., 1987).

OTHER FUELS. As noted by Freinkel and Metzger (1979), other fuels including amino acids, lipids, and growth factors may be supplied to the fetus in abnormal proportions in diabetic pregnancy. Hod and Lapidot (1996) noted that transplacental fluxes of glycine were significantly higher in the overt, preexisting diabetic pregnant patient than in patients with normal pregnancy. A study by Knopp and coworkers (1992) demonstrated that mid-trimester triglyceride levels were a better predictor of a subsequent macrosomic fetus than the glucose tolerance test.

Kitajima et al (2001) examined lipid profiles in women with abnormal glucose challenge tests during pregnancy and found that triglyceride levels correlated with birth weight (r = 0.22; P = 0.009), an association that remained significant after adjusting for pre-pregnant BMI, maternal weight gain, fasting plasma glucose levels, fetal gender, and gestational age at birth (P = 0.01). Fasting maternal hypertriglyceridemia (over 259 mg/dL) was the significant predictor of infants born large for gestational age, independent of pre-pregnant BMI, maternal weight gain, and maternal plasma glucose levels (OR = 11.6; 95% CI = 1.1, 122; P = 0.04).

Birth Injury

Birth injury, including shoulder dystocia (Nesbitt et al., 1998) and brachial plexus trauma, is more common among IDMs, and macrosomic fetuses are at the highest risk (Gilbert et al., 1999). The most common birth injuries associated with diabetes are brachial plexus, facial nerve injury, and cephalhematoma. Interestingly, the current assessments of birth injury among IDMs managed with strict glycemic control show a rate only slightly higher than that among appropriately selected controls (3.2% versus 2.5%) (Mimouni et al., 1992).

Most of the birth injuries occurring to IDMs are associated with difficult vaginal delivery and shoulder dystocia. Although shoulder dystocia occurs in 0.3% to 0.5% of vaginal deliveries among normal pregnant women, the incidence is two- to fourfold higher in women with diabetes, probably because the hyperglycemia of diabetic pregnancy causes the fetal shoulder and abdominal widths to become massive (McFarland et al., 1998; Cohen et al., 1999). Although half of shoulder dystocias occur in infants of normal birth weight (2500 to 4000 g), the incidence of shoulder dystocia rises 10-fold to 5% to 7% among infants weighing 4000 g or more. However, if maternal diabetes is present, the risk at each birth-weight class is increased fivefold (Langer et al., 1991). These risks are further magnified if forceps or vacuum delivery is performed (Keller et al., 1991; Nesbitt et al., 1998) (Fig. 49-8). Although it would be desirable to predict shoulder dystocia on the basis of warning signs during labor such as labor protraction, suspected macrosomic infant, or need for midpelvic forceps delivery, fewer than 30% of these events can be predicted from such clinical factors (Sandmire and O'Halloin, 1988).

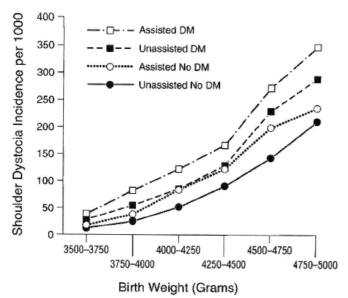

FIGURE 49-8 ■ Risk of shoulder dystocia by diabetes status and instrumental delivery. DM, diabetes mellitus. (From Nesbitt TS, Gilbert WM, Herrchen B: Shoulder dystocia and associated risk factors with macrosomic infants born in California. Am J Obstet Gynecol **179**(2):476, 1998.)

Neonatal Morbidity and Mortality

Polycythemia and Hyperviscosity

Polycythemia (central venous hemoglobin concentration >20 g/dL or hematocrit >65%) occurs in 5% to 10% of IDMs and is apparently related to glycemic control. Hyperglycemia is a powerful stimulus to fetal erythropoietin production, probably mediated by decreased fetal oxygen tension (Widness et al., 1990). Untreated, neonatal polycythemia may promote vascular sludging, ischemia, and infarction of vital tissues, including the kidneys and central nervous system.

Neonatal Hypoglycemia

Hyperinsulinemic IDMs, especially those from pregnancies with poor glycemic control, are at increased risk for low plasma glucose levels after birth (Simmons et al., 2000). This complication is usually much milder and less common in infants of mothers who are euglycemic during labor and delivery and whose diabetes mellitus is well controlled throughout the *entire* pregnancy. A detailed study by Taylor and associates (2002) found no correlation between the likelihood of neonatal hypoglycemia and HbA_{1c}, whereas mean maternal glucose levels during labor were strongly predictive. Unrecognized postnatal hypoglycemia may lead to neonatal seizures, coma, and brain damage. Thus it is imperative that the nursery receiving the IDM have a protocol for frequent monitoring of the infant's blood glucoses until metabolic stability is ensured.

Neonatal Hypocalcemia and Hyperbilirubinemia

Low levels of serum calcium (<7 mg/100 mL) have been reported in up to 50% of IDMs during the first 3 days of life, although more recent series record an incidence of 5% or less with better-managed pregnancies (Cordero et al., 1998). Tsang

and coworkers (1979) have studied this problem extensively. They have reported normal levels of parathyroid hormone in cord blood of IDMs, indicating normal fetal parathyroid function. Decreased parathyroid function in such infants was associated with decreased serum calcium levels and increased serum phosphorus values. These changes in infants of insulin-dependent diabetics did not evoke an increase in serum parathyroid hormone. The resulting functional hypoparathyroidism was judged to be related to prematurity, birth asphyxia, or suppressed parathyroid function secondary to hypercalcemia *in utero*. A fourth possibility, hypersecretion of calcitonin, has also been suggested, but serum calcitonin levels in IDMs are not different from those in normal term infants (Cruikshank et al., 1980).

Neonatal hyperbilirubinemia occurs in approximately 25% of IDMs, a rate approximately double that in normal infants (Cordero et al., 1998). There are multiple causes of hyperbilirubinemia in IDMs, but prematurity and polycythemia are the primary contributing factors. Increased destruction of red blood cells contributes to the risk of jaundice and kernicterus. Close monitoring of the newborn and prompt treatment is necessary to avoid the further morbidity of kernicterus, seizures, and neurological damage.

Hypertrophic and Congestive Cardiomyopathy

In some macrosomic, plethoric infants of mothers with poorly controlled diabetes, a thickened myocardium and significant asymmetric septal hypertrophy has been described (Halliday, 1981). The prevalence of clinical and subclinical asymmetric septal hypertrophy in IDMs has been estimated to be as high as 30% at birth, with resolution by 1 year of age (Mace et al., 1979). As noted in the report by Kjos and colleagues (1990), cardiac dysfunction associated with this entity often leads to respiratory distress, which may be mistaken for hyaline membrane disease.

IDMs who manifest cardiac dysfunction in the neonatal period may have either congestive or hypertrophic cardiomyopathy. This condition is often asymptomatic and unrecognized. Echocardiograms show a hypercontractile, thickened myocardium, often with septal hypertrophy disproportionate to the ventricular free walls (Jaeggi et al., 2001). The ventricular chambers are often smaller than normal, and there may be anterior systolic motion of the mitral valve, producing left ventricular–outflow tract obstruction.

The pathogenesis of hypertrophic cardiomyopathy in IDMs is unclear, although it is recognized to be associated with poor maternal metabolic control. There is evidence that the fetal myocardium is particularly sensitive to insulin during gestation, and Susa and associates (1979) reported a 100% increase in cardiac mass in fetal hyperinsulinemic rhesus monkeys. The myocardium is known to be richly endowed with insulin receptors (Steven and Whitset, 1979).

Cooper and coworkers (1995) performed serial echocardiography on the fetuses of 61 pregnant diabetic women and correlated the ultrasound findings with indices of glycemic control. Although there was a persistent antenatal trend toward excessive ventricular septal thickness in the fetuses with postnatally diagnosed asymmetric septal hypertrophy (n = 19, 46%), this became statistically significant only after 31 weeks. When the newborns with asymmetric septal hypertrophy were compared with normal infants, birth weights (4009 g versus 3457 g; $P < 0.01$) and maternal glycosylated hemoglobin levels (6.7% versus 5.7%) were higher in infants with cardiomyopathy. This study demonstrates the association of fetal septal hypertrophy and poor maternal glycemic control.

IDMs may also have *congestive* cardiomyopathy without hypertrophy. On echocardiogram, the myocardium is overstretched and poorly contractile. This condition is often rapidly reversible with correction of neonatal hypoglycemia, hypocalcemia, and polycythemia; it responds to digoxin, diuretics, or both. In contrast, treatment of hypertrophic cardiomyopathy with an inotropic or diuretic agent tends to decrease the size of the ventricular chambers further and leads to obstruction of blood flow (Cooper et al., 1995).

Respiratory Distress Syndrome

Until recently, respiratory distress syndrome was the most common and most serious disease in IDMs. In the 1970s, improved prenatal maternal management for diabetes and new techniques in obstetrics for timing and mode of delivery resulted in a dramatic decline in its incidence, from 31% to 3% (Frantz and Epstein, 1979). However, even when matched by gestational week of pregnancy, IDMs are more than 20 times as likely as an infant from a normal pregnancy to develop respiratory distress syndrome (Robert et al., 1976).

The increased susceptibility to respiratory distress may be due to altered production of alveolar surfactant or abnormal pulmonary function. Kulovich and Gluck (1979) reported delayed timing of phospholipid production in diabetic pregnancy, as indicated by a delay in the appearance of phosphatidylglycerol in the amniotic fluid. In their study, maturational delay occurred only in gestational diabetes (White's class A patients); fetuses of women with other forms of diabetes showed normal or accelerated maturation of pulmonary phospholipid profiles.

Although some investigators have failed to demonstrate a delay in lung maturation in diabetic pregnancy (Tabsh et al., 1982; Ojomo and Coustan, 1990), the majority of the literature indicates a significant biochemical and physiological delay in IDMs. Tyden and colleagues (1984) and Landon and coworkers (1987) reported that fetal lung maturity occurred later in pregnancies with poor glycemic control (mean plasma glucose level >110 mg/dL) regardless of class of diabetes when these infants were stratified by maternal plasma glucose levels. These findings were recently elucidated in greater detail by Moore (2002), who demonstrated that the linear increase in the amniotic fluid lecithin/sphyngomyelin (L/S) ratio in the third trimester appears unaffected by maternal diabetes (type of diabetes or degree of glucose control), but that amniotic fluid phosphatidyl glycerol was delayed by 1 to 1.5 weeks among women with diabetes (either pregestational or GDM) when compared to controls (Fig. 49-9). This delay in phosphatidyl glycerol was associated with an earlier and higher peak in phosphatidyl inositol in the diabetic cases, suggesting that elevated maternal plasma levels of myoinositol in diabetic women may inhibit or delay the production of phosphatidyl-glycerol in the fetus (Bourbon and Farrell, 1985).

It is possible that poor neonatal respiratory performance in the IDM may have a histologic basis in addition to a biochemical etiology. Studies of fetal lung ion transport in the diabetic rat by Pinter and colleagues (1991) demonstrated decreased

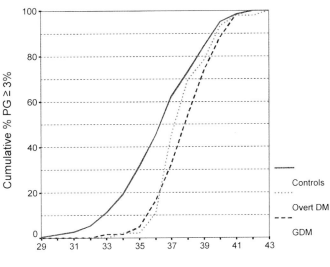

FIGURE 49-9 ■ Delay in fetal pulmonary phosphatidyl glycerol associated with a sustained peak in phosphatidyl inositol in diabetic pregnancy. DM, diabetes mellitus; GDM, gestational diabetes mellitus; PG, phosphatidyl glycerol. (From Moore TR: A comparison of amniotic fluid fetal pulmonary phospholipids in normal and diabetic pregnancy. Am J Obstet Gynecol **186**(4):641, 2002.)

fluid clearance and lack of thinning of the lung's connective tissue compared with controls. Bhavnani and coworkers (1988) reported higher lung glycogen levels and reduced pulmonary compliance in offspring of diabetic rabbits compared with controls. In humans, Kjos and co-authors (1990) noted respiratory distress in 18 of 526 infants delivered of diabetic gestations (3.4%). Surfactant-deficient airway disease accounted for less than one third of cases, however, with transient tachypnea, hypertrophic cardiomyopathy, and pneumonia responsible for the majority.

Thus, the near-term infant of a mother with poorly controlled diabetes is more likely to have neonatal respiratory distress syndrome than is the baby of a nondiabetic mother. This unfortunate circumstance further compounds the IDM's metabolic and cardiovascular difficulties after birth. The observations of Moore (2002) indicate that the nondiabetic fetus achieves pulmonary maturity at a mean gestational age of 34 to 35 weeks, with more than 99% of normal newborns having a mature phospholipid profile by 37 weeks. In diabetic pregnancy, however, it cannot be assumed that lung maturity is assured until after 38.5 gestational weeks have been completed. Any delivery contemplated before 38.5 weeks of gestation for other than the most urgent fetal and maternal indications should be preceded by documentation of pulmonary maturity by amniocentesis. The numerous neonatal complications of the IDM are also summarized in Chapter 60.

Childhood Obesity and Glucose Intolerance

Fetal overgrowth is arguably the most significant problem in pregnancies complicated by diabetes (Table 49-9). Typically defined as birth weight above the 90th percentile for gestational age or greater than 4000 g, macrosomia occurs in 15% to 50% of diabetic pregnancies, compared to 10% to 14% of normal pregnancies (Delgado Del Rey et al., 2001; Lepercq

TABLE 49-9. INCIDENCE OF GROWTH ABNORMALITIES IN DIABETIC PREGNANCY BY WHITE'S CLASS

	Gestational (%)	Class A, B, C (%)	Class D, F, R (%)	Total (%)
Macrosomic (>90th percentile)	22	31	22	24
Small for dates (<10th percentile)	4	5	5	4

Adapted from California Department of Health Services, Maternal and Child Health Branch: Status Report of the Sweet Success California Diabetes and Pregnancy Program 1986–1989, Sacramento, March 31, 1991.

et al., 2001). A 20-year study by Shelley-Jones and associates (1992) indicated that 21% of infants with birth weight greater than or equal to 4540 g were born to glucose-intolerant mothers, a rate clearly disproportionate to the 2% to 8% of gravidas with some form of diabetes.

Obese newborns of diabetic mothers experience excessive morbidity in the neonatal period, as illustrated by a study by Hunter and colleagues (1993). When 230 infants of women with IDDM were compared to 460 infants of euglycemic women, the infants of women with IDDM had significantly higher rates of severe hypoglycemia (OR = 5.38), macrosomia (OR = 4.15), and neonatal jaundice (OR = 1.94). The risk of hyperbilirubinemia ($P = 0.02$), hypoglycemia ($P = 0.01$), and neonatal acidosis ($P = 0.01$) was highest in infants with macrosomia.

Excessive body fat stores, begun in utero and stimulated by excessive glucose delivery during diabetic pregnancy, may extend into childhood and adult life. Vohr and McGarvey (1997) compared infant size at 1 year among those born large for gestational age and those born appropriate for gestational age in gravidas with and without diabetes. Large-for-gestational-age infants of diabetic mothers had a greater BMI, waist circumference, and abdominal skinfold at age 1 year compared with infants in all other study groups. Among all infants of diabetic mothers, the 1-year waist circumference ($r = 0.28$; $P < 0.04$) and subscapular skinfold ($r = 0.37$; $P < 0.007$) correlated with the mean 2-hour postprandial glucose value for the second and third trimester. These investigators concluded that macrosomic infants of mothers with GDM have unique patterns of adiposity that are present at birth and persist at age 1 year.

The downstream effects of deranged maternal metabolism on the offspring has been documented well into puberty. Silverman and co-authors (1995) performed yearly metabolic follow-up of macrosomic offspring of diabetic mothers (ODM) through 14 years of age. When the 88 ODM (12.3 ± 1.7 years) were compared with 80 control subjects of the same age and pubertal stage, ODM had higher 2-hour glucose (6.8 ± 1.4 versus 5.7 ± 0.9 mmol/liter; $P < 0.001$) and insulin (660 ± 720 versus 455 ± 285 pmol/liter; $P < 0.03$) concentrations. In ODM, the prevalence of IGT (2-hour glucose concentration >7.8 mmol/liter) was 1.2% at <5 years, 5.4% at 5 to 9 years, and 19.3% at 10 to 16 years. IGT was not associated with the etiology of the mother's diabetes (gestational versus pregestational).

In a further report by the same group (Silverman et al. 1998), the macrosomia observed at birth in ODM resolved by 1 year of age, but significant obesity recurred in childhood; by 14 to 17 years, the mean BMI was 24.6 ± 5.8 kg/m² in ODM versus 20.9 ± 3.4 kg/m² in control subjects. IGT was found in 36% of ODM. These differences correlated with elevated amniotic fluid insulin values obtained from each individual in the third trimester in utero.

These data provide strong evidence of the adverse influence of fetal obesity associated with excessive nutrient delivery during diabetic pregnancy on long-term adult health. Efforts to reduce fetal overgrowth during pregnancy are likely to have benefits beyond the perinatal period.

Childhood Neurological Abnormalities

Several recent reports have suggested childhood neurodevelopmental abnormalities in ODM. Rizzo and colleagues (1997) compared the offspring of 201 mothers with diabetes with 83 children of normal mothers and correlated subsequent childhood obesity in the ODM with internalizing behavior problems, somatic complaints, anxiety/depression, and social problems. Ornoy and associates (2001) assessed IQ scores on the WISC-R and Bender tests of the children born to diabetic mothers. No differences were found between the study groups in various sensorimotor functions in comparison to controls, but the children of diabetic mothers performed less well than controls in fine and gross motor functions and also performed worse on the Pollack taper test, which is designed to detect inattention and hyperactivity. These investigators also found a negative correlation between the severity of maternal hyperglycemia, as assessed by blood glycosylated hemoglobin levels, and the performance on various neurodevelopmental and behavioral tests by children born to mothers with pregestational diabetes.

These studies, taken together, strongly suggest that childhood and adult body habitus and insulin resistance can be programmed during life in utero, which is strongly influenced by maternal glycemic control. Although it is difficult to assign specific pregnancy-related causation to neurodevelopmental disturbances later in childhood, accumulating evidence indicates that suboptimal maternal glycemic control may have consequences far beyond the neonatal period.

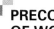 **PRECONCEPTIONAL MANAGEMENT OF WOMEN WITH PREGESTATIONAL DIABETES**

Despite widespread underutilization, preconceptional care programs have consistently been associated with decreased morbidity and mortality (Diabetes Control and Complications Trial Research Group, 1996). Patients who enroll in a preconceptional diabetes-management program obtain earlier prenatal care and have lower HbA$_{1c}$ values in the first trimester (Dunne et al., 1999). A comparison of outcomes among women participating in a preconceptional intensive metabolic program over a span of 15 years to outcomes among women receiving

TABLE 49-10. PRECONCEPTIONAL EVALUATION OF THE DIABETIC PATIENT

Procedure	Tests	Recommendations
Medical history, family history, review of symptoms	Selected patients: fasting and postprandial C-peptide determinations to clarify type of diabetes	Avoid pregnancy until HbA$_{1c}$ is in the normal, nonpregnant range
Physical examination		
Positive findings:		
Hypertension	ECG, cardiac, renal evaluation	Antihypertensive medications
Retinopathy	Retinal evaluation	Ophthalmology consultation
Goiter	T$_4$, thyroid-stimulating hormones, antibodies	
Neuropathy		Vascular, podiatric evaluation
Obesity		Exercise, weight loss
Proteinuria	24-hr urine for protein, creatinine	Nephrology consultation if renal function abnormal
Diabetes assessment	HbA$_{1c}$	
Glycemic control	Home glucose monitoring	
	Stable glycemic profile	
Nutrition		Dietitian consultation
Occupational and family life assessment		Help prepare patient for lifestyle commitments necessary for tight glycemic control

ECG, electrocardiogram; Hb, hemoglobin.

standard treatment demonstrated lowered perinatal mortality (0% versus 7%) and reduced rate of congenital anomalies (2% versus 14%). Unfortunately, when that preconceptional program was discontinued because of lack of funds, the congenital anomaly rate increased by over 50% (McElvy et al., 2000).

The goals of preconceptional counseling and management are to provide prognostic information to the patient and her family, taking into consideration her glycemic, cardiovascular, renal, and ophthalmologic status, to provide advice regarding risks and alternatives to the medications she may be taking, and to provide direct management or referral in normalizing her preconceptional glucose levels (Kitzmiller et al., 1996)

Risk Assessment

Factors to consider in preconceptional diabetes risk assessment (summarized in Table 49-10) are as follows:

- Glycemic control *should be assessed.*
- For patients who have had diabetes for 10 years or more, an electrocardiogram, an echocardiogram, and 24-hour protein and creatinine studies should be performed. The patient who requires antihypertensive agents deserves special attention. Particular attention should be paid to the level of proteinuria: urinary protein exceeding 190 mg per 24 hours prior to pregnancy is associated with a tripled risk of hypertensive disorders in the second half of pregnancy.
- Since retinopathy can progress during pregnancy, the patient should establish a relationship with a qualified ophthalmologist. A baseline retinal evaluation should be completed within the year prior to conception, with laser photocoagulation performed if needed. Previous laser treatment is not a contraindication to pregnancy and may avoid significant hemorrhage during pregnancy.
- Thyroid function (thyroid-stimulating hormone and free thyroxine) should be evaluated and corrected as necessary in all patients with pregestational diabetes

because of the frequent coincidence of autoimmune thyroid disease and diabetes.

- A daily prenatal vitamin that provides 1 mg of folic acid should be prescribed for a minimum of 3 months prior to conception, because folate supplementation significantly reduces the risk of congenital neural tube defects.
- The patient's occupational, financial, and personal situation should be reviewed, since job and family pressures can become barriers to achieving and maintaining excellent glycemic control. In patients with pre-pregnancy hypertension or proteinuria, particular emphasis should be given to defining support systems that permit extended bed rest in the third trimester, should it become necessary.

Metabolic Management

A regimen of frequent and regular monitoring of both pre- and postprandial capillary glucose levels should be instituted. Although there are no data indicating that post-meal glucose monitoring is required prior to pregnancy to achieve adequate control, monitoring these levels increases the preconceptional woman's awareness of the interaction of dietary content and quality with postprandial glycemic excursions. The insulin regimen should result in a smooth glucose profile throughout the day, with no hypoglycemic reactions between meals or at night.

The intensified insulin regimen should be initiated long enough before pregnancy that the glycohemoglobin level is lowered into the normal range for at least 3 months prior to conception. The patient should be skilled in managing her glucose levels in a narrow band well before pregnancy begins, so that the inevitable insulin adjustments necessitated by the appetite, metabolic, and activity changes of early pregnancy can be accomplished smoothly.

Target glucose levels recommended by the American Diabetes Association (2002d) for preconceptional programs are as follows:

Before meals: capillary *whole-blood* glucose 70 to 100 mg/dL (3.9 to 5.6 mmol/liter), or capillary *plasma* glucose 80 to 110 mg/dL (4.4 to 6.1 mmol/liter)

1 to 2 hours after meals: capillary *whole-blood* glucose less than 140 mg/dL (7.8 mmol/liter), or capillary *plasma* glucose less than 155 mg/dL (8.6 mmol/liter)

Oral Hypoglycemic Agents

A recent longitudinal trial in the United Kingdom of intensified metabolic therapy in nonpregnant women with type 2 diabetes (UK Prospective Diabetes Study Group, 1998) demonstrated that oral agents were more effective than insulin in lowering HbA_{1c} levels. This effect was attributed to improved compliance and fewer hypoglycemic reactions. For this and other reasons, most women with type 2 diabetes utilize one or more oral agents for glycemic control—typically metformin and a sulfonylurea or thiazolidinediones. Details of the mechanism of action and pharmacology of these oral hypoglycemic agents are discussed below. Despite the absence of evidence of teratogenicity for most of these compounds, none are recommended for use in pregnancy. Accordingly, standard practice is to transition these patients to insulin management preconceptionally.

A possible exception is the use of metformin in infertile patients with polycystic ovary syndrome who are otherwise oligo-ovulatory. These patients have higher conception and lower miscarriage rates with metformin treatment (Batukan and Baysal, 2001; Jakubowicz et al., 2002). Although two small series documenting the apparent safety of continuing metformin during pregnancy have been published (Glueck et al., 2001, 2002), discontinuing metformin after pregnancy is established is recommended (American Diabetes Association, 2002).

Antihypertensive Medications

Hypertension is a common comorbidity of diabetes, being found in 20% to 30% of women who have had diabetes for longer than 10 years. Although treatment of modest degrees of hypertension (<160 mm Hg systolic) during pregnancy has not been shown to be beneficial in improving perinatal outcome (Sibai, 2000), treatment in non-pregnant diabetic women is recommended when blood pressure is consistently higher than 130/80 mm Hg (American Diabetes Association, 2002d). The UK Prospective Diabetes Study and the Hypertension Optimal Treatment trial both demonstrated improved outcomes, especially in preventing stroke, in patients assigned to lower blood pressure targets. Thus patients will frequently enter the preconceptional period taking one or more antihypertensive medications (Arauz-Pacheco and Raskin, 2002d).

Current evidence indicates that none of the commonly used antihypertensive medications (calcium channel blockers, beta-blockers, methyldopa) are teratogenic. However, prudence and lack of efficacy in improving pregnancy outcomes suggest that these should be discontinued unless pressing indications (overt nephropathy) exist to continue them.

Angiotensin-converting–enzyme inhibitors deserve special mention. They have been shown to ameliorate proteinuria and delay progression to end-stage renal disease in patients with diabetic nephropathy. These medications are therefore considered first-line agents for diabetic women with significant proteinuria (UK Prospective Diabetes Study Group, 1998).

Many women with type 1 diabetes will present for consultation preconceptionally or even in early pregnancy while taking these medications. It is not clear that these medications have teratogenic effects when used in the first trimester, but usage in the second trimester and beyond has been shown to cause a marked reduction in fetal renal blood flow, resulting in oligo-hydramnios and even frank fetal renal failure (Buttar, 1997). For this reason, these medications should not be used during pregnancy, especially after the first trimester. Similar concerns exist for other agents in this family (angiotensin receptor blockers and receptor antagonists) (Briggs and Nageotte, 2001) (see also Chapters 41, 43, and 44).

DIAGNOSING DIABETES

Overt Diabetes

Patients with type 1 diabetes are typically diagnosed in childhood or adolescence during an episode of hyperglycemia, ketosis, and dehydration. Type 1 diabetes is only rarely diagnosed during pregnancy and is most often accompanied by unexpected coma, because early pregnancy may provoke instability of diet and glycemic control in patients with occult diabetes. Thus, a pregnancy test should be ordered in all reproductive-aged women admitted to the hospital for blood glucose management.

The diagnosis of type 2, or insulin-resistant, diabetes cannot be accomplished during pregnancy because severe, early forms of gestational diabetes and preexisting, occult adult-onset diabetes have similar clinical characteristics. Although the finding of elevated HbA_{1c} in early pregnancy may be suggestive, definitive diagnosis of type 2 diabetes must be made after pregnancy. The diagnostic criteria recommended by the American Diabetes Association) for diabetes are listed in Table 49-11.

Hyperglycemia not sufficient to meet the diagnostic criteria for diabetes is categorized as either IFG or IGT, depending on whether it is identified through a random fasting plasma glucose or a 75-gram, 2-hour oral glucose tolerance test (OGTT) (American Diabetes Association, 2002e):

IFG: fasting plasma glucose 110 mg/dL to 126 mg/dL (6.1 mmol/liter to 7 mmol/liter)

IGT: 2-hour plasma glucose 140 mg/dL to 199 mg/dL (7.8 mmol/liter to 11 mmol/liter)

Patients with either IFG or IGT prior to pregnancy should be considered at extremely high risk of developing GDM during pregnancy. GDM patients whose postpartum testing results in the diagnosis of IFG or IGT are at significant risk for evolving into frank diabetes in the near future (5 to 10 years). Recent studies have shown that lifestyle interventions can reduce the rate of progression to type 2 diabetes in these individuals (Tuomilehto et al., 2001).

Gestational Diabetes

Universal versus Targeted Screening

Previously, screening of all pregnant women for GDM was recommended by the American Diabetes Association (Metzger, 1991). However, the recommendations for universal

TABLE 49-11. DIAGNOSTIC CRITERIA FOR DIABETES MELLITUS*†

Symptoms of diabetes and a casual plasma glucose >200 mg/dL (11.1 mmol/liter). "Casual" is defined as any time of day, without regard to time since last meal. The classic symptoms of diabetes include polyuria, polydipsia, and unexplained weight loss.

or

Fasting plasma glucose >126 mg/dL (7.0 mmol/liter). "Fasting" is defined as no caloric intake for at least 8 hr.

or

2-hr plasma glucose >200 mg/dL (11.1 mmol/liter) during a 75-g, 2-hr oral glucose tolerance test.

* In the absence of unequivocal hyperglycemia with acute metabolic decompensation, the diagnosis should be confirmed by repeat testing on a different day.
† The oral glucose tolerance test is not recommended for routine clinical use in nonpregnant subjects but may be required in the evaluation of patients with impaired fasting glucose (see text) or when diabetes is suspected despite a normal fasting plasma glucose.

American Diabetes Association: Standards of medical care for patients with diabetic mellitis. Diabetes Care 25(Suppl 1):S, 2002.

screening have been modified by the Fourth International Workshop-Conference on Gestational Diabetes and the American College of Obstetricians and Gynecologists (Metzger and Coustan, 1998; American College of Obstetricians and Gynecologists, 2001), based on certain factors that have been shown to place women at lower risk for the development of GDM. In patients meeting all of the criteria listed in Table 49-12, it may be cost effective to avoid screening. This recommendation is based on the findings of Naylor and colleagues (1997), who reported the results of screening 4274 Canadian women at 26 weeks' gestation, all of whom received the 3-hour, 100-g glucose tolerance test. From this extensive database, they identified several risk factors that significantly increased the likelihood of GDM (maternal age = 35 years, BMI >22, and Asian or "other" ethnicity). Women with one or no risk factors had a 0.9% risk of GDM, whereas 4% to 7% of those with two to five factors were diagnosed with GDM. By limiting screening to gravidas with more than one risk factor, these investigators were able to reduce testing by 34% while retaining a sensitivity of approximately 80% with a false-positive rate of 13%.

Notwithstanding the findings of Naylor and colleagues (1997), multiple studies have affirmed the inadequacy of screening based on risk factors alone, especially in the heterogeneous populations typically encountered in U.S. urban practices. Lavin and coworkers (1981) noted that the number of cases of GDM detected was similar in women who had clinical risk factors (1.5%) and those who did not (1.4%). A more recent study (Weeks et al., 1995) that assessed the impact of screening only patients with risk factors reported that selective screening would have failed to detect 43% of GDM cases. Moreover, 28% of the women with undiagnosed GDM would have required insulin, and they had a several-fold increased risk of cesarean section because of macrosomia. Similar findings were reported by Danilenko-Dixon and colleagues (1999), who studied predominantly white women in Rochester, Minnesota. They noted that exempting patients who were white and less than 25 years old, with a BMI below 25 and a negative family history would decrease the number of screening tests by only 10% while adding significant complexity to the screening process.

According to current guidelines, therefore, universal screening should be performed in ethnic groups recognized to be at higher risk for glucose intolerance during pregnancy—namely women of Hispanic, African, Native American, South or East Asian, Pacific Island, or Indigenous Australian ancestry. For simplicity of administration of a clinical GDM screening program, universal screening, with the possible

exception of the very lowest risk category, is probably the most reliable policy.

One- or Two-Step Screening

The diagnosis of GDM is based on a positive OGTT. Guidelines issued by the Fourth International Workshop-Conference on Gestational Diabetes Mellitus (Metzer and Coustan, 1998), the American Diabetes Association (American Diabetes Association, 2002c), and American College of Obstetricians and Gynecologists (2001) currently recommend the use of the Carpenter and Coustan diagnostic criteria for the 3-hour, 100-g glucose OGTT (Table 49-13). However, these expert bodies now also acknowledge the alternative use of a single-step, 2-hour, 75-g glucose OGTT in certain high-prevalence populations. Use of these two modalities is discussed below.

ONE-STEP APPROACH

The one-step, 75-g glucose, 2-hour OGTT, commonly used as the preferred test outside the United States, is performed without prior plasma or serum glucose screening. The threshold plasma glucose values defining a positive 2-hour OGTT are identical to the criteria for the 3-hour, 100-g glucose OGTT, and two or more values must be met or exceeded for the diagnosis of GDM. Sacks and colleagues (1995) reported experience with the 75-g, 2-hour OGTT in 3505 pregnant women in a California population. Although a positive association was found between the glucose values on the 75-g glucose, 2-hour OGTT and birth-weight percentiles, no statistically meaningful glucose threshold values relative to birth weight or macrosomia were seen. Similarly, Brustman and colleagues (1995)

TABLE 49-12. "LOW RISK" CRITERIA FOR GESTATIONAL DIABETES*

- Age <25 years
- Normal pre-pregnancy body weight
- No first-degree relatives with diabetes
- Not a member of an ethnic group at high risk for GDM
- No history of GDM in prior pregnancy
- No history of adverse pregnancy outcome

* ALL criteria must be met to omit screening for GDM.
GDM, gestational diabetes mellitus.

From Metzger BE, Coustan DR, Committee To: Summary and recommendations of the Fourth International Workshop-Conference on Gestational Diabetes Mellitus. Diabetes Care 21(Suppl 2), 1998.

TABLE 49-13. ORAL GLUCOSE TOLERANCE TEST
FOR GESTATIONAL DIABETES

Test Prerequisites

- 1-hr, 50-g glucose challenge result ≥ 135 mg/dL
- Overnight fast of 8–14 hr
- Carbohydrate loading 3 d including ≥ 150 g carbohydrate
- Seated, not smoking during the test
- Two or more values must be met or exceeded
- Either a 2-hr (75-g glucose) or 3-hr (100-g glucose) can be performed

Plasma Glucose Criteria for Gestational Diabetes	100-g Glucose Load mg/dL (mmol/liter)	75-g Glucose Load mg/dL (mmol/liter)
Fasting	95 (5.3)	95 (5.3)
1-hr	180 (10.0)	180 (10.0)
2-hr	155 (8.6)	155 (8.6)
3-hr	140 (7.8)	

tested 32 pregnant women with both the 75-g, 2-hour and the 100-g, 3-hour OGTT. Despite a strong positive correlation between the results of the two tests, the glucose values of the 100-g OGTT were significantly higher than those of the 75-g OGTT, and the 100-g OGTT diagnosed 50% of the women with GDM, whereas the 75-g OGTT diagnosed only 38%.

Because the data correlating the one-step, 75-g OGTT and outcome are less well established than those with the 3-hour OGTT, the one-step, 2-hour test should be reserved for high-prevalence populations (e.g., Native Americans). It may also be useful in patients with a pre-pregnancy diagnosis of IGT or those with multiple risk factors for GDM.

TWO-STEP APPROACH

In the two-step approach, a screening or glucose challenge test (GCT) is performed using 50 g of glucose in the fasting or nonfasting state. For those whose plasma glucose value obtained after 1 hour exceeds a critical threshold value, a 100-g, 3-hour OGTT is administered.

THRESHOLD VALUE FOR THE GLUCOSE CHALLENGE TEST

The sensitivity of the GDM testing regimen depends on the threshold value used for the 50-g glucose challenge. Current recommendations from the American Diabetes Association and American College of Obstetricians and Gynecologists (2002c) do not specify the ideal threshold for glucose challenge testing. The commonly utilized value of 140 mg/dL results in approximately 10% to 15% of patients requiring the 3-hour OGTT, depending on the population studied. Of these, 20% to 40% (2% to 7% of the total patients tested) will be found to have GDM. Studies in which all patients undergo a 3-hour OGTT after a GCT indicate that the 140-mg/dL threshold results in 80% sensitivity. This leaves one fifth of patients with GDM undiagnosed and at risk for potentially avoidable perinatal morbidity.

A number of investigators have advocated lowering the GCT threshold value to improve the diagnostic sensitivity. Values of 130 mg/dL and 135 mg/dL have been proposed (Coustan, 1994). A potential disadvantage of using a lower value is an increase in the number of OGTTs performed, resulting in an increase in net program cost that would have to be offset by savings associated with decreased perinatal mor-

bidity. Studies by Ray and associates (1996) found that lowering the GCT threshold to 135 mg/dL increased the number of 3-hour OGTTs performed by 42% while increasing the detection frequency of GDM to 99%.

The Canadian study previously mentioned (Naylor et al., 1997) examined screening thresholds with a view to reduce overall program cost. They calculated, based on receiver-operator curve analysis, that diagnostic efficiency was optimized when a GCT threshold of 130 mg/dL was utilized for intermediate-risk women (two to four risk factors) and 128 mg/dL for higher-risk women.

Although the Canadian testing scheme improved cost-efficiency and detection sensitivity, it is somewhat complicated, suggesting that compliance might be suboptimal when the program is applied elsewhere. The importance of clear and simple screening guidelines was underscored by a study of screening program compliance by Moses and Colagiuri (1997), which found that only 50% of patients eligible to be screened actually underwent the test. These issues are summarized in Table 49-14.

At present, a threshold plasma glucose value of 135 mg/dL or higher is used in most centers because it provides excellent test sensitivity for GDM (>90%) with acceptable cost. Definitive studies regarding cost effectiveness with respect to perinatal outcomes and neonatal costs have not yet been performed, although one such multicenter trial is under way.

MAXIMUM VALUE FOR THE GLUCOSE CHALLENGE TEST

The risk of GDM is approximately proportional to the result of the 1-hour glucose challenge. Dooley and coworkers (1991) found that among nonwhite women, the risk of GDM with a 1-hour glucose value of 200 mg/dL or more is greater than 90%. The value in whites is approximately 66%. For this reason, Coustan (1994) has recommended that no further testing be ordered for women in whom 1-hour challenge responses are above 200 mg/dL. Bobrowski and co-authors (1996) reported that all patients with a screening result above 216 mg/dL yielded a positive 3-hour OGTT result. The data of Dooley and associates noted earlier indicate that many women, especially white women, should undergo definitive testing (100-g, 3-hour GTT) before the diagnosis of GDM is confirmed in order to avoid incorrect designation of

TABLE 49-14. SENSITIVITY AND COST ASSOCIATED WITH UNIVERSAL AND SELECTIVE SCREENING WITH VARIOUS GLUCOSE CHALLENGE THRESHOLDS

	Threshold Value for 1-hr, 50-g Glucose Challenge		
	130 mg/dL	135 mg/dL	140 mg/dL
Sensitivity (%)	100	98	79
% of Population Requiring OGTT	22	20	13

	Threshold Value (mg/dL)	Cost per GDM Case ($)	Sensitivity (%)
Universal	140	222	90
	130	249	100
Risk Factors + Age	140	192	85
≥ 25 yr	130	215	95

GDM, gestational diabetes mellitus; OGTT, oral glucose tolerance test.

Adapted from Coustan DR, Nelson C, Carpenter MW, et al: Maternal age and screening for gestational diabetes: A population based study. Obstet Gynecol **73**:557, 1989.

euglycemic patients as having GDM, as occurs in 10% to 20% of cases. Most experts omit the 3-hour GTT in patients with GCT results of 200 mg/dL or greater and manage the patient as a gestational diabetic.

DIAGNOSTIC VALUES FOR THE 100-G, 3-HOUR OGTT

The cutoff values for the 100-g OGTT originally offered by O'Sullivan and Mahan (1964) (fasting, >105 mg/dL; 1 hour, >190 mg/dL; 2 hour, >165 mg/dL; 3 hour, >145 mg/dL) had been the definitive standard for diagnosing GDM in the United States for two decades. However, these have now been abandoned in favor of lower thresholds proposed by Carpenter and Coustan (1982). The Carpenter and Coustan values were derived to reflect the contemporary practice in most laboratories of measuring plasma, rather than whole blood glucose concentrations. (Plasma glucose levels are typically 10% to 15% lower than whole blood values.) Two or more of the venous plasma concentrations must be met or exceeded for a positive diagnosis. The test should be done in the morning after an overnight fast of between 8 and 14 hours and after at least 3 days of unrestricted diet (>150 g carbohydrate per day) and unlimited physical activity. The subject should remain seated and should not smoke throughout the test.

Naylor and coworkers (1996) assessed the effect of lowering the thresholds for the 3-hour OGTT by evaluating the outcomes of a group of patients considered nondiabetic by the older O'Sullivan and Mahan criteria but defined as GDM by the Carpenter and Coustan criteria. Compared to normal controls, the Carpenter and Coustan group had increased rates of macrosomia (28.7% versus 13.7%; P <0.001) and cesarean delivery (29.6% versus 20.2%; P = 0.02). These findings validate the importance of using the lower values of Carpenter and Coustan if adequate diagnostic accuracy for GDM is to be maintained.

SINGLE ABNORMAL VALUE ON THE 3-HOUR OGTT

A fasting plasma glucose level exceeding 126 mg/dL should be considered highly suspicious for diabetes at any time, whether or not the patient is pregnant. Individuals with fasting plasma glucose above 126 mg/dL should have another fasting test; if the second test is high, gestational diabetes is confirmed.

Patients with a single abnormal OGTT value have increased risk for macrosomia and neonatal morbidity. Berkus and colleagues (1993) followed 764 patients with GDM, stratified by the number of abnormal values on their OGTT. Patients with one or more abnormal GTT values had double the incidence of macrosomic infants (23% to 27% versus 13%; P <0.01). When Langer and coworkers (1987) compared perinatal outcomes in patients with a single abnormal OGTT value with normals and with aggressively managed GDM patients, they found the incidence of macrosomia to be more than threefold higher in the single abnormal value group than in the normal (34% versus 9%) and GDM (34% versus 12%) groups. Neonatal morbidity was fivefold higher in the single abnormal OGTT value group (15%) when compared with the control and GDM groups (3%). It is reasonable to conclude that, if left untreated, one abnormal value on an oral glucose tolerance test is strongly associated with adverse perinatal outcome.

These results underscore the problems associated with current methodologies to identify patients with GDM. The relationship among carbohydrate metabolism, macrosomia, and neonatal morbidity is a continuum that defies a single, clear-cut criterion for diagnosis in all populations. The currently recommended schemes identify at most 90% of pregnancies susceptible to hyperglycemia and fetal macrosomia. The astute clinician should approach women with several GDM risk factors and a single abnormal OGTT value with suspicion. When in doubt, a trial of capillary glucose testing may help to clarify the patient's metabolic status.

Other Tests for Gestational Diabetes

A number of investigators have searched for a single, non-glucose blood test that would accurately predict the results of the OGTT. Because of the proportional relationship of glycated proteins and long-term plasma glucose concentrations, both fructosamine and HbA_{1c} screening have been proposed. Roberts and colleagues (1983) suggested that fructosamine screening for GDM could produce a sensitivity of 85% with a specificity of 95%. A positive relationship between fructosamine levels and macrosomia was demonstrated (Roberts and Baker, 1987; Page et al., 1996). However, subsequent studies have reported significantly lower sensitivities (Nasrat et al., 1988; Huter et al., 1992).

Similarly inferior sensitivity and predictive values have been reported for glycohemoglobin measurements (i.e., HbA_1 and HbA_{1c}) by Shah and colleagues (1982), Baxi and colleagues (1984) and Artal and coworkers (1984) (22%, 63%, and 74%, respectively). A more recent study by Agarwal and associates (2001) assessed the use of lower cutoffs for fructosamine and HbA_{1c} to exclude subjects from further GDM screening and higher cutoffs for one-step diagnosis. The lower cutoffs achieved sensitivities of 90% with negative predictive values of over 85%. However, the upper cutoff values did not achieve acceptable positive predictive values to be useful for diagnosing GDM. Thus the role of these tests would be to identify patients rather than to screen for GDM, but utilizing them would impose an additional step and cost into the diagnostic regimen.

Although screening with glycosylated proteins could theoretically reduce the number of two-step diagnostic procedures, their lack of sensitivity in diagnosis and additional time and cost have left these studies currently of limited use in screening for GDM.

Timing of Gestational Diabetes Screening

FIRST-TRIMESTER SCREENING

The timing of glucose tolerance testing during pregnancy is critical, since delayed diagnosis increases the duration of deranged maternal metabolism and accelerated fetal growth. A surprising percentage of patients (6% to 20%) with GDM can be diagnosed in the first trimester. A majority of these have significant risk factors for glucose intolerance. Moses and associates (1995) assessed the prevalence of GDM in patients with various risk factors: GDM was present in 6.7% overall, in 8.5% of women 30 years old or older, in 12.3% of women with a BMI of 30 or more, and in 11.6% of women with a family history of diabetes. A combination of risk factors predicted GDM in 61% of cases compared with 4.8% of those without risk factors. The additional effect of ethnicity on the prevalence of GDM is summarized in Table 49-15.

Risk factor assessment for GDM (maternal age, ethnicity, obstetric and family history, body habitus, prior GDM, prior IGT, prior macrosomic infant or unexplained stillbirth) should be performed at the first prenatal visit in all pregnant women. Patients with any of these risk factors (Table 49-16) should undergo two-step screening as soon as feasible.

THIRD-TRIMESTER SCREENING

Because the insulin resistance that causes hyperglycemia becomes increasingly evident as the third trimester progresses, early testing may miss some patients who later become glucose-intolerant. Performing the test too late in the third trimester limits the time in which metabolic intervention can take place. For this reason, it is recommended that glucose tolerance testing be performed in all patients at 24 to 28 weeks' gestation (American College of Obstetricians and Gynecologists. 2001).

Whether administered at 12 or 26 weeks, the GCT can be performed without regard to recent food intake (i.e., nonfasting state). Indeed, Coustan and coworkers (1986) have shown that tests performed in fasting subjects are more likely to yield falsely elevated results than are tests conducted between meals. This finding was confirmed by Sermer et al (1994).

TABLE 49-15. PREVALENCE OF GESTATIONAL DIABETES IN VARIOUS NATIONAL AND ETHNIC GROUPS

Reference	Population	Prevalence (%)
Harris et al., 1997	Native American (Cree)	8.3
Henry et al., 1993	Australian	7.8
	Vietnamese	4.3
Nahum et al., 1993	African American	7.5
	White	4.7
	Asian	4.2
Lopez-de la Pena et al., 1997	Mexican	6.9
Yalcin et al., 1996	Turkish	6.6
Rith-Najarian et al., 1996	Native American (Chippewa)	5.8
Fraser et al., 1994	Israeli	5.7
	Bedouin	2.4
Rizvi et al., 1992	Pakistani	3.5
Miselli et al., 1994	Italian	2.3
Serirat et al., 1992	Thai	2.2
Jang et al., 1995	Korean	2.2
Mazze et al., 1992	Minnesota White	1.5

METABOLIC MANAGEMENT OF WOMEN WITH PREGESTATIONAL DIABETES

The goal of metabolic management (glycemic monitoring, dietary regulation, and insulin therapy) in diabetic pregnancy is to prevent or minimize the postnatal sequelae of diabetes—macrosomia, shoulder dystocia, birth injury, and postnatal metabolic instability—in the newborn. If this goal is to be achieved, glycemic control must be instituted early and aggressively.

Principles of Medical Nutritional Therapy

There is a surprising lack of well-controlled research on the optimal diet for lean or obese women with diabetes. Thus, most recommendations regarding dietary therapy are based on common sense and experience. Because women with all types of diabetes experience inadequate insulin action after feeding, the goal of medical nutritional therapy is to avoid single, large meals containing foods with a high percentage of simple carbohydrates that release glucose rapidly from the maternal gut. Three major meals and three snacks are preferred, since this multiple-feeding regimen limits the amount of calories presented to the bloodstream during any given interval. The use of nonglycemic foods that release calories from the gut slowly also improves metabolic control. Examples include foods with complex carbohydrates and cellulose, such as whole-grain breads and legumes. Carbohydrates should account for no more than 50% of the diet, with protein and fats equally accounting for the remainder (American Diabetes Association, 2002c).

Medical nutritional therapy should be supervised by a trained professional—ideally, a registered dietitian. In many programs, dietary counseling is capably provided by a certified diabetes educator. In any case, formal dietary assessment and

TABLE 49-16. RISK FACTORS
FOR GESTATIONAL DIABETES

*Patients with any of these factors should be screened for GDM at the
first prenatal visit:*
1. Maternal age >25 yr
2. Previous macrosomic infant
3. Previous unexplained fetal demise
4. Previous pregnancy with GDM
5. Strong immediate family history of NIDDM or GDM
6. Obesity (>90 kg)
7. Fasting glucose >140 mg/dL (7.8 mM) or random glucose
   >200 mg/dL (11.1 mM)

GDM, gestational diabetes mellitus; NIDDM, non–insulin-dependent diabetes
mellitus.

counseling should be provided at several points during the
pregnancy in order to design a dietary prescription that will
provide adequate quantity and distribution of calories and
nutrients to meet the needs of the pregnancy and support
achieving the plasma glucose targets that have been established. For obese women (BMI >30 kg/m²), a 30% to 33%
calorie restriction (to 25 kcal/kg actual weight per day or less)
has been shown to reduce hyperglycemia and plasma triglycerides with no increase in ketonuria.

Moderate restriction of dietary carbohydrates to 35% to 40%
of calories has been shown to decrease maternal glucose levels
and improve maternal and fetal outcomes (Major et al., 1998).
In a nonrandomized study, subjects with low-carbohydrate
intake (<42%) frequently required the addition of insulin for
glucose control (relative risk [RR] = 0.14; P <0.05), had a
significantly lower rate of macrosomia (RR = 0.22; P <0.04),
and had a lower rate of cesarean deliveries for cephalopelvic
disproportion and macrosomia (RR = 0.15; P <0.04).

Low-Glycemic Foods

Manipulation of the type of carbohydrate in the diet can
provide additional benefits in glycemic control. Crapo and coauthors (1981) compared the blood glucose excursions
induced by the ingestion of 50 g of carbohydrate from dextrose,
rice, potatoes, corn, and bread. They observed that the highest
glucose response occurred with dextrose and potatoes, with
much lower peaks after intake of corn and rice. This has led to
the concept of classifying foods by their glycemic index related
to their tendency to induce hyperglycemia. In general, low-
glycemic foods, such as complex (rather than simple) carbohydrates and those with higher soluble fiber content, are
associated with a more gradual release of glucose into the
bloodstream.

Formal dietary consultation at periodic intervals during the
pregnancy improves metabolic control. Timing and content of
meals should be reviewed at each visit together with the
patient's individual food preferences. In all pregnant women,
the continuing fetal consumption of glucose from the maternal
bloodstream results in a steady downward drift in maternal
glucose levels unless feeding occurs. In patients taking insulin
or oral hypoglycemics, prolonged periods (>4 hours) without
food intake increase the risk of hypoglycemic episodes. In these
patients, a rather rigid schedule of three meals plus snacks at
mid-morning, mid-afternoon, and bedtime is often necessary to

achieve smooth control. Because insulin resistance changes
dynamically during pregnancy, the dietary prescription must be
continually adjusted according to the patient's weight gain,
insulin requirement, and pattern of exercise.

Avoiding Nocturnal Hypoglycemia

Unopposed intermediate-acting insulin action during the
hours of sleep frequently results in severe nocturnal hypoglycemia at 3 to 4 AM in individuals with type 1 diabetes.
Reducing the insulin dose to avoid this complication typically leads to unacceptably high glucose levels on rising at
6 to 7 AM, whereas adding a bedtime snack helps to moderate
the effect of bedtime insulin and to sustain glucose levels
during the night. The snack should contain a minimum of
25 g of complex carbohydrate, together with enough protein
or fat to help prolong release from the gut during the hours
of sleep.

Avoiding Ketosis

The issue of maternal ketosis and its potential effect on
childhood mental performance is a source of continuing controversy. Churchill and associates (1969) reported that
ketonuria during pregnancy is associated with impairment of
neuropsychological development of offspring. This report has
resulted in admonitions to avoid caloric reduction in any pregnant woman. The methodology in Churchill and associates'
study has been criticized, however, because the ketonuria data
were obtained from many different hospitals by having a nurse
obtain a single urine sample for ketones on the day of delivery.

Coetzee and colleagues (1980), however, found morning
ketonuria in 19% of women with insulin-independent diabetes
on a 1000-calorie diet, 14% of those on a 1400- to 1800-calorie
diet, and 7% of normal pregnant women on a free diet. There
were no untoward neonatal events in infants of any of the
ketonuric mothers. Rizzo and coworkers (1991) studied 223
pregnant women with diabetes and their offspring and 35 with
normal glucose tolerance and found no relationship between
maternal hypoglycemia and intellectual function of offspring.

Thus, there may be a difference between starvation ketosis
and the ketosis that develops with poorly controlled diabetes.
Ketonuria develops in 10% to 20% of normal pregnancies after
an overnight fast and may in fact protect the fetus from starvation in the nondiabetic mother. In the final analysis,
significant maternal ketonemia resulting in maternal acidemia
is probably unfavorable for mother and fetus. The small
degrees of ketosis noted in many pregnant women, including
those with diabetes, are unlikely to lead to measurable deficits
in the newborn, however.

Principles of Glucose Monitoring

Glycohemoglobin

Measurements of glycosylated hemoglobin have proved to
be a useful index of glycemic control over the long term (4 to
6 weeks), providing a numeric index of the patient's overall
compliance (Parfitt et al., 1993). Although assessing HbA_{1c}
levels every 4 to 6 weeks during pregnancy rarely alters management significantly, it provides the patient with a score by
which she can rate the success of her hourly efforts to keep her

TABLE 49-17. TIMING OF HOME CAPILLARY GLUCOSE MONITORING

Capillary Glucose Assessment	Advantage	Disadvantage
Preprandial	Permits prospective adjustment of food intake, supplementation of preprandial insulin	Preprandial or fasting glucose levels correlate poorly with fetal morbidity; significant postprandial hyperglycemia may go undetected
Postprandial	Permits supplementation of insulin to reduce postprandial glucose overshoots; improved postprandial control correlates with improved fetal/neonatal outcome	Results are obtained after food intake
Bedtime	Permits adjustment of calories at bedtime snack, adjustment of bedtime insulin	
3–4 AM	Permits detection of nocturnal hypoglycemia	Interrupts sleep, may increase stress

blood glucoses within a narrow band. Glycohemoglobin levels are too crude to guide the adjustments to insulin, however.

Self-Monitoring of Blood Glucose

The availability of capillary glucose chemical test strips has revolutionized the management of diabetes, and they should now be considered the standard of care for pregnancy monitoring. The discipline of measuring and recording blood glucose levels prior to and after meals clearly has a positive effect on improving glycemic control (Goldberg et al., 1986).

TIMING OF CAPILLARY GLUCOSE MONITORING

The frequency and timing of home glucose monitoring should be individualized (Table 49-17), but *postprandial* values must be assessed because they have the strongest correlation with fetal growth. The DIEP study reported that when postprandial glucose values averaged 120 mg/dL, approximately 20% of infants were macrosomic, whereas a modest 30% rise in postprandial glucose levels to a mean of 160 mg/dL resulted in a 35% macrosomia rate (Jovanovic-Peterson et al., 1991). Similar results emphasizing postprandial blood glucose monitoring were reported by de Veciana and associates (1995), who randomized diabetic women to use of preprandial or postprandial blood glucose levels for dietary and insulin management. The women managed using postprandial levels had markedly better results than did those managed using preprandial levels. In the postprandial group, with the mean (± standard deviation) change in the glycosylated hemoglobin value greater ($-3 \pm 2.2\%$ versus $0.6 \pm 1.6\%$; $P < 0.001$), the birth weights were lower (3469 ± 668 g versus 3848 ± 434 g; $P = 0.01$) and the rates of neonatal hypoglycemia (3% versus 21%; $P = 0.05$) and macrosomia (12% versus 42%; $P = 0.01$) were lower.

With these facts in mind, a typical glucose monitoring schedule involves capillary glucose checks on rising in the morning, 1 or 2 hours after breakfast, before and after lunch, before dinner, and at bedtime. For patients taking intermediate- or long-acting insulin at bedtime, obtaining a capillary glucose level between 3 and 4 AM two to three times per week is helpful in interpreting the glucose values in the morning.

It is important for the clinician to be aware of the specific type of capillary glucose reflectance meter being utilized by the patient, since plasma glucose values are 10% to 15% less than those measured in whole blood from the same sample. Most of the newer reflectance meters are calibrated for plasma glucose readings. Clearly the target glucose values utilized in management will be different, depending on the type of meter in use.

TARGET CAPILLARY GLUCOSE LEVELS

Controversy exists as to whether the target glucose levels to be maintained during diabetic pregnancy should be designed to limit macrosomia or to closely mimic non-diabetic pregnancy profiles. The American Diabetes Association (2002c) currently recommends the following, based on evidence from the DIEP (Jovanovic-Peterson et al., 1991):

Fasting *whole blood* glucose <95 mg/dL (5.3 mmol/liter)
Fasting *plasma* glucose <105 mg/dL (5.8 mmol/liter)
and
1-hour postprandial *whole blood* glucose <140 mg/dL (7.8 mmol/liter)
1-hour postprandial *plasma* glucose <155 mg/dL (8.6 mmol/liter)
or
2-hour postprandial *whole blood* glucose <120 mg/dL (6.7 mmol/liter)
2-hour postprandial *plasma* glucose <130 mg/dL (7.2 mmol/liter)

Surprisingly, only limited data exist that can be utilized to define normal glucose variations during pregnancy in normoglycemic gravidas. The profiles from Cousins and colleagues (1980), depicted in Figure 49-3, are derived from highly controlled studies in which volunteer subjects were fed test meals with specific caloric content on a rigid schedule. More recently, Parretti and coworkers (2001) have profiled normal pregnant women twice monthly pre- and postprandially during the third trimester. Testing was with capillary glucose meters, and the women ate a spontaneous diet. The results of the 95th percentile of the plasma glucose excursions are shown in Figure 49-10. It can be seen that fasting and pre-meal plasma glucose levels are usually below 80 mg/dL and often below 70 mg/dL. Peak postprandial plasma glucose values rarely exceed 110 mg/dL.

In consideration of these facts, the target plasma glucose values to be utilized during pregnancy management of women with diabetes should range from 65 to 95 mg/dL preprandially and never exceed 130 to 140 mg/dL postprandially at 1 hour. Superb glycemic control requires attention to both preprandial and postprandial glucose levels. Langer and colleagues (1994)

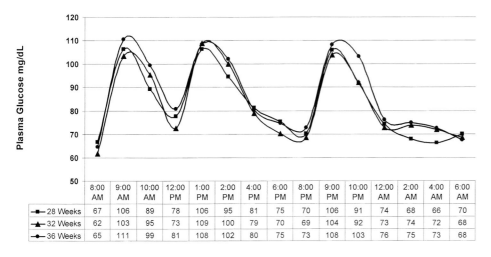

	8:00 AM	9:00 AM	10:00 AM	12:00 PM	1:00 PM	2:00 PM	4:00 PM	6:00 PM	8:00 PM	9:00 PM	10:00 PM	12:00 AM	2:00 AM	4:00 AM	6:00 AM
28 Weeks	67	106	89	78	106	95	81	75	70	106	91	74	68	66	70
32 Weeks	62	103	95	73	109	100	79	70	69	104	92	73	74	72	68
36 Weeks	65	111	99	81	108	102	80	75	73	108	103	76	75	73	68

FIGURE 49-10 ■ Diurnal plasma glucose profile in normoglycemic third-trimester gravidas. Numbers represent the 95th percentile values. (Adapted from Parretti E, Mecacci F, Papini M, et al: Third-trimester maternal glucose levels from diurnal profiles in nondiabetic pregnancies: Correlation with sonographic parameters of fetal growth. Diabetes Care **24**(8):1317, 2001. Copyright © American Diabetes Association. Reprinted with permission from The American Diabetes Association.)

assessed the effectiveness of a program of intensified self-monitoring of blood glucose using glucose guidelines similar to these. Women in the intensified management group had lower rates of macrosomia, cesarean section, metabolic complications, shoulder dystocia, stillbirth, and respiratory complications and fewer neonatal intensive care unit days than did those in the conventional management group and were comparable in these parameters to the nondiabetic controls.

Principles of Insulin Therapy

Despite the fact that no available insulin delivery method approaches the precise secretion of the hormone from the human pancreas, the judicious use of modern insulins can mimic these patterns remarkably well. The goal of exogenous insulin therapy during pregnancy must be to achieve diurnal glucose excursions similar to those of nondiabetic pregnant women. Given that in normal pregnant women, postprandial blood glucose excursions are maintained within a relatively narrow range (70 to 120 mg/dL), the task of reproducing this profile is daunting and requires meticulous daily attention by both patient and physician.

As pregnancy progresses, the increasing fetal demand for glucose results in lower fasting and between-meal blood glucose levels, increasing the risk of symptomatic hypoglycemia. Upward adjustment of short-acting insulins to control postprandial glucose surges within the target band only exacerbates the tendency to interprandial hypoglycemia. Thus, any insulin regimen for pregnant women requires combinations and timing of insulin injections different from those that would be effective in the nonpregnant state. In addition, the regimens must be modified continually as the patient progresses from the first to the third trimester and as insulin resistance rises. The regimen should always be matched to the patient's unique physiology, work, rest, and food intake schedule.

Types of Insulin

The types of insulin frequently used in diabetes control are listed in Table 49-18. Several newer insulins are available for use, but most have not been extensively evaluated in pregnancy. These include an additional short-acting insulin similar to lispro (Humalog), called insulin aspart (Novolog), which has kinetics similar to lispro, and a new, very-long-acting molecularly modified insulin glargine (Lantus). The activity profile of the intermediate and long-acting insulins is shown graphically in Figure 49-11 (Lepore et al., 2000).

TABLE 49–18. INSULIN PREPARATIONS AND PHARMACOKINETICS*

Insulin Preparation	Time to Peak Action (hr)	Total Duration of Action (hr)	Comment
Humalog Insulin lispro Insulin aspart	1	2	Onset within 10 min of injection. No need to delay meal onset after injection.
Regular insulin	2	4	Good coverage of individual meals if injected 20 min prior to eating. Increased risk of postprandial hypoglycemia with unopposed action 2–3 h after eating.
NPH insulin Lente insulin	4	8	Provides intermediate-acting control. Give on rising and at bedtime. Risk of 3 AM hypoglycemia.
Ultralente	8	20	Provides long-acting basal insulin action. High risk of nocturnal hypoglycemia. Does not cover a full 24 h in pregnancy.
Insulin glargine Lantus	5	<24	Prolonged flat action profile. Limited pregnancy experience. Increased risk of nocturnal hypoglycemia or undertreatment during the day.

* Times are approximate in typical pregnant women with diabetes.

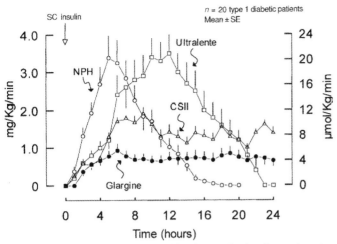

FIGURE 49-11 ■ Kinetics of NPH, Ultralente, glargine (Lantus), and continuous subcutaneous insulin infusion with lispro insulin. Curves show the glucose infusion rate necessary to maintain plasma glucose at 130 mg/dL. CSII, continuous subcutaneous insulin infusion; SC, subcutaneous; SE, standard error. (From Lepore M, Pampanelli S, Fanelli C, et al: Pharmacokinetics and pharmacodynamics of subcutaneous injection of long-acting human insulin analog glargine, NPH insulin, and Ultralente human insulin and continuous subcutaneous infusion of insulin lispro. Diabetes **49**:2142, 2000. Copyright © American Diabetes Association. Reprinted with permission from The American Diabetes Association.)

Typical Insulin Regimens

Flexibility is important in dosing and adjusting insulin during pregnancy. Although most patients find it necessary to organize their mealtimes and physical activity around their insulin regimen, changing timing of insulin injections and types of insulin is frequently necessary to match lifestyle and occupation needs and optimize glycemic control. The following guidelines and examples may help in managing and adjusting insulin during pregnancy:

1. *In the first trimester, reduce insulin dose by 10% to 25% to avoid hypoglycemia.* Reduced physical activity and caloric intake associated with the appetite changes and fatigue of early pregnancy lead to increased insulin effectiveness and interprandial hypoglycemia. It is typical to reduce insulin progressively from the 6th to the 14th week, then to begin restoring it as the insulin resistance mediated by rising placental hormones returns in the second trimester. Jovanovic and colleagues (2001) reported from the DIEP that a significant 18% increase in mean weekly dosage was observed between weeks 3 and 7 (P <0.0001), followed by a significant 9% decline from week 7 through week 15 (P <0.0001). In women with pregestational diabetes, continual downward adjustment in insulin is typically required from the first prenatal visit until approximately 14 to 16 weeks, whereupon requirements begin to rise steadily.

2. *A typical total insulin dose is 0.7 units/kg in the first trimester, but this must be increased progressively with pregnancy duration.* In women with type 1 diabetes, insulin increases are usually 10% to 20% over nonpregnant baseline by the end of pregnancy (Fig. 49-12) (Langer, 1998). In insulin-resistant type 2 patients, 30% to 90% increases are not unusual. Insulin requirements normally plateau after 35 weeks' gestation and may drop significantly after 38 weeks.

3. *A combination of short- and intermediate-acting insulins is necessary to maintain glucose levels in an acceptable range.* A typical regimen involves intermediate-acting insulin (NPH or Lente) prior to breakfast and at bedtime, with injections of regular or short-acting insulin before breakfast and before dinner. Two thirds of insulin is given in the morning and one third in the afternoon and at bedtime.

   Example: 20 units of NPH and 10 units of regular insulin in the morning, 8 units of regular insulin with dinner, 8 units of NPH at bedtime. NPH covers the pre- and post-lunch periods. *Avoid NPH or Lente injections at dinner time because the peak occurs at 2 to 3 AM, creating symptomatic hypoglycemia.* Bedtime dosing with NPH (after 10 PM) is preferable because it peaks at approximately 6 AM, which coincides with the early morning spontaneous rise in maternal glucose (the dawn effect).

4. *Preprandial doses of regular insulin sufficient to keep 1-hour postprandial plasma glucose below 130 mg/dL may result in hypoglycemia 3 to 4 hours later* (e.g., regular insulin before breakfast often causes hypoglycemia at 11 AM). When regular insulin is used to cover the major meals, snacks are essential in the late morning, the late afternoon, and prior to bedtime to avoid interprandial hypoglycemia. This interprandial hypoglycemia effect is intensified if the regular insulin injection is not given at least 20 to 30 minutes prior to the meal. This precaution is particularly relevant for hospitalized patients (since meals do not always arrive on schedule) and when taking meals in restaurants.

5. *The new, short-acting insulins lispro (Humalog) and aspart (Novolog) can reduce interprandial hypoglycemia.* Lispro is manufactured by inverting a short amino acid sequence within the insulin molecule, resulting in a significantly faster onset of action. Lispro injections immediately before meals reduce the risk of hangover hypoglycemia because of the short duration of action. Compared with values for regular human insulin, the peak serum insulin concentration of insulin lispro is three times as high, time to peak is 4.2 times as fast, the absorption rate constant is double, and the duration of action is half as long (Lepore et al., 2000).

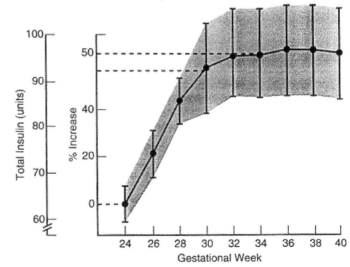

FIGURE 49-12 ■ Change in insulin requirement in women with gestational diabetes. (From Langer O: Maternal glycemic criteria for insulin therapy in gestational diabetes mellitus. Diabetes Care **21**(Suppl 2):B91, 1998.)

These kinetics allow the patient to inject insulin just prior to eating, rather than having to delay 20 to 30 minutes to allow regular insulin to begin its effect. When lispro was compared with regular insulin, lispro reduced postprandial hyperglycemia and decreased the rate of mild hypoglycemic episodes; it was also associated with lower predelivery HbA$_{1c}$ and received higher patient satisfaction scores (Bhattacharyya et al., 2001). Similar findings have been reported when insulin aspart was compared to regular insulin (Hermansen et al., 2002). In summary, lispro or aspart insulin can be substituted 1:1 for regular insulin and is highly effective when given before meals in reducing postprandial glycemia while avoiding insulin hangover, which increases patient compliance. Short-acting insulins have been shown to be effective when used in the insulin pump (see later) (Bode et al., 2002).

6. *Ultralente or glargine (Lantus) insulin can be used to provide a long-acting basal rate of insulin action but risks nocturnal hypoglycemia.* Ultralente is a long-acting insulin preparation with an effective duration of 24 to 30 hours in nonpregnant subjects and approximately 16 to 20 hours during pregnancy. These more rapid kinetics are probably associated with increased renal clearance of insulin during pregnancy. Ultralente can be used effectively to provide a steady and continuous insulin effect with less peak/burn-off effect with associated hypoglycemia/hyperglycemia transients. Ultralente is particularly useful in patients with significant insulin resistance who require high doses of intermediate-acting insulin (e.g., those with type 2 diabetes).

Example: 14 units of Ultralente and 10 units of lispro in the morning, 4 units of lispro prior to lunch, 14 units of Ultralente and 6 units of lispro prior to dinner. A typical dose of Ultralente is 0.1 to 0.2 units/kg (10 to 15 U) given at dinnertime, which results in peak action in the early morning hours (5 to 7 AM). A second dose of Ultralente is often required in the morning to provide basal coverage in afternoon and evening. Because Ultralente does not peak until 10 to 12 hours after injection, the morning dose does not cover the midday meal adequately, typically necessitating a preprandial injection of a short-acting insulin.

Riccio and coworkers (1994) compared use of NPH and Ultralente insulin in nonpregnant women. They found that Ultralente at suppertime was associated with a significantly greater decline in the fasting and average daily plasma glucose concentrations and with lower glucose area under the curve than was NPH insulin. In pregnant patients, especially those with brittle diabetes, the practitioner must use Ultralente with caution, because of the greater risk of hypoglycemia. Ultralente can be substituted for the bedtime dose of NPH insulin, but the morning NPH dose is often still necessary to avoid mid-day hyperglycemia.

Similar concerns exist regarding the use of insulin glargine (Lantus) during pregnancy. In three large comparative trials of nonpregnant subjects, insulin glargine decreased glycosylated hemoglobin and/or fasting blood glucose levels to an extent similar to that seen with NPH insulin. A lower incidence of hypoglycemia, especially at night, was reported in most trials with insulin glargine as compared with NPH insulin (Gillies et al., 2000). However, experience is presently minimal with pregnancy. Although the relatively flat activity profile of glargine is attractive, the dose must be regulated to keep basal insulin action during the night from causing hypoglycemia. During the day, when insulin resistance and insulin requirements are higher, the nocturnal basal rate is usually inadequate. Great care must be exercised in using insulin glargine to avoid severe nocturnal hypoglycemia. At present, glargine appears to be safe for use during embryogenesis if glucose control is adequate (Hofmann et al., 2002).

Adjusting Insulin Dosage Using Carbohydrate Counting, Preprandial Glucose Levels, and Insulin Corrections

Intermediate- and long-acting insulins should be adjusted no more frequently than weekly or biweekly to keep preprandial plasma glucose levels in the target range (70 to 105 mg/dL). However, with short-acting insulins, glycemic control is better when the patient is able to vary, within a reasonable range, the insulin dose she uses to cover a meal, depending on its calorie content (grams of carbohydrate) and the plasma glucose level existing at the time she begins eating. This often means varying short-acting insulin dosage with every injection.

CARBOHYDRATE COUNTING

Patients with pregestational diabetes are usually taught to count the grams of carbohydrate in their meals and adjust the short-acting insulin dosage accordingly. A typical meal containing 60 grams of carbohydrate may require 4 to 6 units of lispro (ratio of carbohydrate to insulin 15:1) in the nonpregnant individual. In the first trimester, typical ratios are 15:1 to 12:1. However, by the second trimester, more insulin is required (12:1 to 10:1) and in the third trimester, especially in patients with some degree of insulin resistance, ratios fall to the 10:1 or even 8:1 levels. The clinician should anticipate these increases in insulin as pregnancy progresses, since the patient often interprets these changes as errors or failure.

However, it should be noted that carbohydrate counting has limits in accuracy (miscalculation of carbohydrate content, individual differences in glucose uptake dynamics), which may result in erratic control. During pregnancy, patients who relatively strictly regiment their food quantity, content, and timing, so that carbohydrate calculations are within a reasonably narrow range, have better control.

PREPRANDIAL GLUCOSE LEVELS

Given the same calorie content of a given meal, achieving target postprandial plasma glucose levels will require more insulin if the preprandial glucose level is higher. Allowing patients to add 2 U lispro when the preprandial glucose level exceeds 120 mg/dL, and to reduce lispro dosage by 2 units when preprandial glucose is below 80 mg/dL, provides smoother control and avoids undesired postprandial glycemic excursions when the preprandial glucose is outside of target range.

INSULIN CORRECTIONS

Women with pregestational diabetes are frequently taught how to perform pre- and postprandial insulin corrections. A typical regime is to add 1 to 2 units of lispro for every 50 mg/dL that the glucose level is out of target range. Thus a preprandial glucose level of 130 mg/dL would require 1 unit of lispro over the prescribed dose for that meal. As pregnancy progresses, corrections increase from 1 per 50 to 1 per 20 mg/dL. However, the patient must be instructed not to take more than 4 to 6 correction units in a single bolus during pregnancy but rather to retest glucose in 1 to 2 hours and apply an additional correction at that time.

Use of the Insulin Pump

Most of the principles mentioned above to enhance and smooth glycemic control by manipulating timing, quantity, and type of insulin can be utilized with greater facility with a continuous subcutaneous insulin infusion via programmable pump. These devices, which infuse insulin by means of a convenient catheter placed into the subcutaneous tissue near the abdomen, can be programmed to provide varying basal and bolus levels of insulin, which change smoothly even while the patient sleeps or exercises.

Several investigators have reported successful outcomes with use of continuous subcutaneous insulin infusion in pregnancy (Gabbe et al., 2000; Simmons et al., 2001; Bode et al., 2002). Caruso and co-authors (1987) compared continuous subcutaneous insulin infusion with intensive mixed subcutaneous injections in 12 pregnant patients with poorly controlled diabetes. Patients with good control with intermittent insulin therapy experienced a reduction in the variation of glucose excursions and a reduction in the total daily insulin requirement when switched to the insulin pump. Jennings and associates (1991) noted that subjects using continuous subcutaneous insulin infusion had lower HbA$_{1c}$ levels and better overall control than did those using conventional therapy.

When Allouche and colleagues (1994) compared insulin pump therapy to intensive intermittent treatment, however, no difference in mean glucose or incidence of fetal macrosomia occurred. Moreover, Mecklenburg and coworkers (1984) reported that although diabetes control improved significantly with insulin pump therapy, 42% of patients experienced at least one major complication, including DKA, infection, or hypoglycemic coma. Significantly, episodes of DKA increased markedly after institution of pump therapy when compared with the patients' own control period.

These findings suggest that continuous, programmable insulin infusion has many advantages over conventional treatment, including the convenience of changing basal rates automatically when the patient is asleep or otherwise occupied and providing programmable but adjustable boluses discreetly from a pump worn under the clothing without the need for needle, syringe, and medication vials. Because pump malfunctions, precipitation of insulin inside the pump mechanism, abscess formation, and poor uptake from the infusion site can occur

unexpectedly, successful insulin pump use requires a meticulous patient, a knowledgeable diabetologist or perinatologist, and prompt availability of emergency counseling and assistance on a 24-hour basis (Caruso et al., 1987).

A properly designed insulin pump infusion scheme allows convenient tailoring of the insulin administration profile to the patient's individual metabolic and lifestyle rhythms. An example regimen is shown in Table 49-19. Note that the lowest infusion rate of the day is between 11 PM and 4 AM, set at about 80% of the mean rate needed during the day. The basal rate must be increased to 1.3 to 1.5 times the mean daily rate between 4 AM and 10 AM to provide extra insulin coverage for the high insulin-resistance period as the day begins (dawn effect). For the remainder of the day (10 AM to 11 PM), a steady mean infusion rate is usually sufficient. Insulin boluses, programmed to limit the postprandial excursion to less than or equal to 130 mg/dL at 1 hour, are given as often as needed. The enhanced ability for the patient to administer extra insulin doses without syringes and insulin vials is of great value in improving the smoothness of glycemic control.

Starting Insulin with Gestational Diabetes

Clinicians and patients are reluctant to start insulin in patients with gestational diabetes, but this intervention may be essential if macrosomia is to be reduced or avoided. Because the period of maximum fetal growth velocity (200 g/week) and fat accretion occurs from 28 to 33 weeks' gestation, delaying definitive therapy with repeated attempts to correct a suboptimal glucose profile with dietary adjustments may, by 33 to 34 weeks, have missed the time when glycemic intervention is effective in modulating fetal growth. It is reasonable to allow a 1- to 2-week trial of dietary management before resorting to other measures, but waiting longer does not significantly increase the likelihood of good control. McFarland and colleagues (1999) have shown that, in the first 2 weeks of dietary therapy, approximately 50% of patients will have achieved good glycemic control, but by the 4th week only an additional 10% will have attained acceptable blood glucose levels.

The effects of prompt and aggressive insulin administration were assessed by Jovanovic-Peterson and colleagues (1997), who reported a protocol in which GDM patients were treated with insulin if any fasting glucose exceeded 90 mg/dL or postprandial glucose exceeded 120 mg/dL. Over a period of 6 years, this protocol resulted in a decrease in macrosomic infants from 18% to 7% and a drop in the cesarean rate from 30% to 20%. Buchanan and associates (1994) utilized ultrasound screening of fetal abdominal circumference in 303 diet-controlled GDM

TABLE 49–19. A TYPICAL ADMINISTRATION PROFILE USING CONTINUOUS SUBCUTANEOUS INSULIN INFUSION PUMP

Time	Basal Rate	Bolus (U)	Comment
12 midnight	0.6 U/hr		Lower basal rate for sleep
4 AM	1.3 U/hr		Higher basal rate opposes the "dawn effect" of rising serum glucose from 4 to 6 AM
7 AM		8	Pre-breakfast bolus
10 AM	1.0 U/hr		Lower basal rate to match increased physical activity, decreased insulin needs
12 noon		4	Pre-lunch bolus
6 PM		4	Pre-dinner bolus
10 PM	0.6 U/hr		Lower basal rate for sleep

patients at 28 weeks to identify early macrosomia that might benefit from insulin treatment. When pregnancies with a fetal abdominal circumference above the 75th percentile were randomized to continued diet or twice-daily insulin therapy, birth weights and percentage of macrosomic infants were reduced in the insulin group (3647 ± 67 g versus 3878 ± 84 g, P <0.02, and 13% versus 45%, P <0.02, respectively). Neonatal obesity, as reflected by skinfold measurements at three sites (P <0.005) was lower as well.

The same group subsequently randomized GDM patients with fasting glucose levels between 105 mg/DL and 120 mg/dL to insulin therapy or monthly ultrasound fetal abdominal circumference screening (Kjos et al., 2001). Insulin therapy was withheld if the fetal abdominal circumference was below the 70th percentile and all fasting glucose measurements were below 120 mg/dL. Although birth weights and incidence of macrosomia were similar in the two groups, insulin therapy was avoided in 38% of the ultrasound group.

The insulin regimen should be designed to address the patient's individual glucose profile. Typically, one to several postprandial glucose levels become consistently above target as the patient's ability to compensate for rising insulin resistance becomes inadequate with diet alone. In such cases, giving lispro or regular insulin injections (4 to 8 U to start) before meals is helpful. If more than 10 units of regular insulin are needed before meals, adding a 6- to 8-unit dose of NPH prior to breakfast helps to achieve smoother control. Should the fasting glucose levels rise above 95 mg/dL, 4 to 6 units of NPH insulin should be administered at bedtime. The doses are scaled up as necessary, once or twice weekly, to keep glucose levels within the target range.

Use of Oral Agents

Maintaining glucose levels within the target range requires meticulous attention to diet and physical activity. For many patients, monitoring capillary glucose several times daily and injecting insulin frequently is impossible. For this reason, there are many current initiatives to augment glucose control with oral agents, particularly in patients with insulin-resistant type 2 diabetes. An ideal treatment would reduce insulin resistance, improve insulin secretion or action, and delay the uptake of glucose from the gut. Current strategies are aimed at augmentation of insulin supply (sulfonylurea and insulin therapy), amelioration of insulin resistance (exercise, weight loss, metformin and troglitazone therapy), and limitation of postprandial hyperglycemia (acarbose therapy).

Pharmacology and Safety

Sulfonylurea compounds, commonly prescribed in the past for patients with type 2 diabetes, have been considered contraindicated during pregnancy because of a high degree of transplacental penetration of most of these agents and the clinical reports of drug concentrations in the neonate higher than maternal levels associated with prolonged and severe neonatal hypoglycemia (Zucker and Simon, 1968). However, rigorously designed trials have not been performed to assess these agents during pregnancy. Reports of fetal anomalies have been largely anecdotal: an increased rate of congenital malformations, particularly ear anomalies, has been reported from a small case-control study (Piacquadio et al., 1991). When

Towner and coworkers (1995) evaluated the frequency of birth defect in fetuses of patients who took oral hypoglycemics during the periconceptional period, they noted that first-trimester glycohemoglobin level and duration of diabetes were strongly associated with fetal congenital anomalies, but use of oral hypoglycemic medications was not.

Interest in glyburide, a second-generation oral sulfonylurea available in the United States since 1984, has recently been rekindled. When glyburide was compared with first-generation sulfonylureas, it was equally effective, had a lower incidence of side effects, and reduced fasting blood glucose and glycohemoglobin levels, without the inconvenience of the additional training required to administer insulin. Because of its ability to enhance target tissue insulin sensitivity, glyburide has been shown to improve glycemic control in many type 2 diabetic patients who have previously failed therapy. As adjunctive therapy, glyburide can reduce the daily dosage for those who require large amounts of insulin (Kolterman, 1992).

Glyburide in Pregnancy

A unique characteristic of glyburide that allows its use in pregnancy is its minimal transport across the human placenta (Koren, 2001). A study by Elliott and colleagues (1991) evaluated glyburide transport in 10 term human placentas with the single-cotyledon placental model, finding virtually no transfer of glyburide even at concentrations 100 times the typical therapeutic levels. This surprisingly low placental transfer may be due to the very high plasma-protein binding of glyburide coupled with a short elimination half-life (4 to 8 hours) (Elliott et al., 1994; Koren, 2001).

Based on findings consistently showing minimal transfer of glyburide across the placenta, Langer and colleagues (2000) designed a randomized trial to compare this oral agent with insulin in patients with gestational diabetes. They randomized 404 women with second- and third-trimester singleton pregnancies who had gestational diabetes requiring treatment to receive glyburide or insulin in an intensified treatment protocol. At the conclusion of the trial, there was no difference between the groups in mean maternal blood glucose, percentage of infants who were large for gestational age (12% and 13%, respectively), birth weight at or above 4000 g (7% and 4%), or neonatal complications (pulmonary, 8% and 6%; hypoglycemia, 9% and 6%; admission to neonatal intensive care unit, 6% and 7%; fetal anomalies, 2% and 2%). Only 4% of the glyburide group required insulin therapy. Glyburide was not detected in the cord serum of any infant in the glyburide group.

Beyond this single encouraging study, experience with glyburide during pregnancy is limited (Coetzee and Jackson, 1985; Lim et al., 1997). Chmait et al (2002), reporting experience with 69 patients with gestational diabetes managed on glyburide, found a failure rate of 19% (>10% glucose values above target). Failure rate was higher in women diagnosed earlier in pregnancy (20 versus 27 weeks; P <0.003) and whose average fasting glucose in the week prior to starting glyburide was higher (126 versus 101 mg/dL). No cases of neonatal hypoglycemia occurred in the glyburide group. Until more studies of glyburide in pregnancy have been reported, the American College of Obstetricians and Gynecologists (2001) considers this agent to be experimental.

Glyburide dosing during pregnancy is similar to using a 70:30 mixture of NPH and regular insulin (effective duration

4 to 8 hours). Glyburide should be taken at least 30 minutes, and preferably 60 minutes, prior to meals so that the peak action covers the postprandial glucose surge. A 2.5-mg tablet at bedtime (after 10 PM) is effective in lowering fasting plasma glucose in the morning. Significant interprandial hypoglycemia can occur with glyburide, and patients should carry glucose tablets with them at all times as a precaution. The maximum dose is 20 mg per day, and no more than 7.5 mg should be taken at a single time.

Other Agents

Metformin is frequently employed in patients with polycystic ovary syndrome and type 2 diabetes to improve insulin resistance and fertility (Diamanti-Kandarakis et al., 1998). Although it has been clearly documented that metformin therapy improves success of ovulation induction (Vandermolen et al., 2001) and reduces first-trimester pregnancy loss in women with polycystic ovary syndrome (Jakubowicz et al., 2002), the effects of continuing metformin during pregnancy are not so clear. Coetzee and Jackson (1979) treated pregestational and gestational diabetics with metformin, but the treatment failed in 54% and 29%, respectively. The perinatal mortality rate in the metformin patients was 61 per 1000, and neonatal jaundice was increased. Hellmuth and colleagues (2000) reported a series of women with gestational diabetes treated with metformin or tolbutamide before 1984. Women treated with metformin had a fourfold increase in preeclampsia and a higher perinatal mortality rate compared with those who were receiving tolbutamide. However, metformin-treated women were older, more obese, and treated later in pregnancy. Glueck and coworkers (2002) compared nondiabetic women with polycystic ovary syndrome (n = 28) who conceived while taking metformin and continued the agent through delivery to matched women without metformin therapy (n = 39). Gestational diabetes developed in 31% of women who did not take metformin versus 3% of those who did (OR = 0.115; 95% CI = 0.014 to 0.938).

Because of the beneficial effect of metformin on first-trimester miscarriage, many patients with polycystic ovary syndrome will enter prenatal care taking this medication. However, none of the existing studies of metformin have adequately addressed the issues of teratogenesis and neonatal hypoglycemia. Given that metformin crosses the placenta, greater experience with this agent is necessary before it can be recommended for use throughout pregnancy.

Alpha-glucosidase inhibitors, another class of oral agents, reversibly inhibit pancreatic amylase and alpha-glucosidase enzymes in the small intestine, delaying cleavage of complex sugars to monosaccharides and thus reducing the rise of blood glucose after a meal. Although these agents offer particular promise in pregnant women because of limited uptake from the gut, few studies in pregnancy are available to assess efficacy. One study (Zarate et al., 2000) of six pregnant women with moderately elevated fasting and postprandial glucose levels who were treated with acarbose three times daily before meals had normalization of glucose control and delivered infants who were considered normal. Acarbose was associated with intestinal discomfort (flatulence and bloating), which persisted for the duration of treatment (de Veciana et al., 2002) reported in abstract a prospective randomized trial of acarbose versus insulin in 91 patients with GDM. Glycemic control was con-

sidered equivalent in the two groups, although 6% of the acarbose group required insulin therapy because of gastrointestinal side effects. No significant adverse reactions or fetal anomalies occurred. Acarbose is given prior to meals, initially 25 mg orally three times daily, to a maximum of 100 mg orally three times daily.

PREGNANCY MANAGEMENT OF THE DIABETIC PATIENT AND FETUS

Fetal Surveillance

The goals of third-trimester management of diabetic pregnancy are to prevent stillbirth and asphyxia while optimizing the opportunity for a safe vaginal delivery. This involves monitoring fetal growth to determine the proper timing and route of delivery and testing for fetal well-being at frequent intervals.

A regimen for fetal surveillance throughout the entire pregnancy is presented in Table 49-20. The principle is to verify fetal viability in the first trimester, validate fetal structural integrity in the second trimester, monitor fetal growth during most of the third trimester, and ensure fetal well-being in the late third trimester.

A variety of fetal biophysical tests are available, including fetal heart rate testing, fetal movement counting, ultrasound biophysical scoring, and fetal Doppler studies. These tests, described in detail in Chapter 21, are summarized in Table 49-21.

Testing should be initiated early enough to avoid the risk of stillbirth but not so early that a high rate of false-positive results is encountered. Since the risk of fetal death is roughly proportional to the degree of hyperglycemia, testing should

TABLE 49–20. FETAL SURVEILLANCE IN TYPE I AND II DIABETIC PREGNANCIES

Time	Test
Preconception	Maternal glycemic control
8–10 wk	Sonographic crown-rump measurement
16 wk	Maternal serum α-fetoproten level
20–22 wk	High-resolution sonography, fetal cardiac echography in women in suboptimal diabetic control (abnormal HbA$_{1c}$) at first prenatal visit
24 wk	Baseline sonographic growth assessment of the fetus
28 wk	Daily fetal movement counting by the mother
32 wk	Repeat sonography for fetal growth
34 wk	Biophysical testing: 2× weekly NST or weekly CST or weekly biophysical profile
36 wk	Estimation of fetal weight by sonography
37–38.5 wk	Amniocentesis and delivery for patients in poor control (persistent daily hyperglycemia)
38.5–40 wk	Delivery without amniocentesis for patients in good control who have excellent dating criteria*

* See test for description.

CST, contraction stress test; NST, non-stress test.

■ **TABLE 49–21.** TESTS OF FETAL WELL-BEING

Test	Frequency	Reassuring Result	Comment
Fetal movement counting	Every night from 28 wk	10 movements in < 60 min	Performed in all patients
Non-stress test	Twice weekly	2 heart-rate accelerations in 20 min	Begin at 28–34 wk with insulin-dependent diabetes; start at 36 wk in diet-controlled gestational diabetes
Contraction stress test	Weekly	No heart-rate decelerations in response to ≥3 contractions in 10 min	Same as for non-stress test
Ultrasound biophysical profile	Weekly	Score of 8 in 30 min	3 movements = 2 1 flexion = 2 30 sec breathing = 2 2 cm amniotic fluid = 2

begin as early as 28 weeks of gestation in patients with poor glycemic control or significant hypertension. In lower-risk patients, testing should begin by 34 weeks. Fetal movement counting is performed in all pregnancies from 28 weeks onward. A Fetal Movement Card for monitoring fetal movement is shown in Figure 49-13.

Timing and Route of Delivery

Assessing Fetal Size

Monitoring of fetal growth and prediction of birthweight continues to be a challenging and highly inexact process. The purpose of such monitoring is to identify the obese fetus and, if possible, avoid birth injury. Newborns weighing more than 4000 g are responsible for 42% to 74% of shoulder dystocias and 56% to 76% of all brachial plexus injuries, even though they account for only 6% of births (Sacks and Chen, 2000). To identify the highest-risk fetuses, use of third trimester ultrasound has been proposed, including serial plotting of biometric parameters, using a cutoff value for estimated fetal weight, and applying a cutoff to a specific parameter (e.g., abdominal circumference) (Chauhan et al., 2000).

Since the risk of birth injury is proportional to birthweight (Nesbitt et al., 1998), much effort has been focused on sonographic estimation of fetal weight (EFW). A number of polynomial formulas using combinations of head, abdomen, and limb measurements have been developed (O'Reilly-Green and Divon, 2000; Sokol et al., 2000). Unfortunately in such formulas, even small errors in measurements of the head, abdomen, and femur are multiplied together, resulting in accuracies of no better than ±15%. In the obese fetus, the inaccuracies are further magnified. Perhaps this is why no single formula has proved to be adequate for identifying the macrosomic fetus (Landon, 2000). In the study by Combs and colleagues (2000), an EFW of ≥ 4000 g had a sensitivity of 45% and a positive predictive value of 81%. To achieve 90% sensitivity would have required using an EFW cutoff of 3535 g, which would have included 46% of the population and produced a 42% false-positive rate. Indeed, Diase and Monga (2002) demonstrated that the mean absolute error of EFW prediction was similar among physicians' clinical estimates (11%), ultrasound estimates (8%), and estimates by the diabetic mothers themselves (8%).

Considering the inaccuracy of weight prediction from a single set of sonographic measurements, serial analysis of parameters every 1.5 to 3 weeks is commonly utilized. However, trended serial EFW calculations compared to a single measurement appear to be no better than a single estimate performed near term. Predictions based on the average of serial EFWs, linear extrapolation from two estimates, or extrapolation by second-order equations fitted to four estimates were no better than the prediction from the last estimate before delivery (Hedriana and Moore, 1994).

Several investigators have assessed the utility of using only the abdominal circumference to discriminate the large fetus (Holcomb et al., 2000). Al-Inany and coworkers (2001) applied an abdominal circumference cutoff of 37 cm to define macrosomia (weight >4000 g), but the moderately high sensitivity (77%) carried a very high false-positive rate (25%). Gilby and colleagues (2000) found that 99% of infants weighing more than 4500 g had an abdominal circumference of 35 cm or more, but the false positive rate was over 30%. An abdominal circumference cutoff of 38 cm or more improved the false-positive rate but lowered the sensitivity unacceptably, to 54%. Ultrasonographic studies of fetal fat thickness on various body parts have been similarly disappointing (Rotmensch et al., 1999).

In view of the presently inadequate methods to diagnose macrosomia antenatally, the widespread practice of estimating fetal weight using ultrasound near term in diabetic pregnancy must be questioned. Parry and colleagues (2000) compared the cesarean rate in neonates falsely diagnosed on ultrasound as macrosomic (false-positives) with the rate in those correctly diagnosed as nonmacrosomic (true negatives). They found that the cesarean rate was significantly higher among the false-positive macrosomics than among the true negatives (42.3% versus 24.3%; RR = 1.74; P <0.05). Thus even with nonmacrosomic fetuses, the availability to the clinician of a sonographic estimate of fetal weight significantly increases the risk of cesarean delivery.

Predicting Shoulder Dystocia

In an effort to minimize the incidence of shoulder dystocia and associated birth injury associated with suspected macrosomia, a number of management schemes have been proposed. Weeks and colleagues (1995) assessed the management of 500 pregnancies with suspected macrosomia and found a high bias toward cesarean section and failed induction. Patients

FETAL MOVEMENT RECORD

Name:_____

Due Date:_____

Start Date	Number of weeks pregnant

INSTRUCTIONS

1. Count the baby's movements **EVERY NIGHT**.

2. A movement may be a kick, swish or roll. Do not count hiccups or small flutters.

3. You can start counting any time in the evening when the baby is active. BUT: **COUNT EVERY NIGHT**.

4. Count baby's movements while lying down, preferably on your left side.

5. Mark down the <u>time</u> you feel the baby move for the first time.

6. Mark down the <u>time</u> you feel the 10th fetal movement.

7. You should feel at least 10 fetal movements within one hour. Call Labor and Delivery **immediately** if

   a) you do not feel 10 movements within 1 hour.

   b) it takes longer and longer for your baby to move 10 times.

   c) you have not felt the baby move all day.

DO NOT WAIT UNTIL TOMORROW.

Date	Time First Movement Felt	Time 10th Movement Felt	Total Time
EXAMPLE 11/4/91	6:50 p.m.	7:28 p.m.	38 minutes

FIGURE 49-13 ■ A Fetal Movement Card. The patient is instructed to note the time at which she begins monitoring fetal movements, then to note the time at which the 10th movement is felt. If she has not recorded 10 movements in 1 hour, she is to call her physician.

with a sonographic EFW greater than 4200 g underwent induction more often (42.5% versus 26.6%), failed to achieve active labor more frequently (49% versus 16.5%), and underwent cesarean section more frequently (52% versus 30%), regardless of actual birthweight. Despite these changes in labor management, the incidence of shoulder dystocia in the predicted and nonpredicted groups was the same (11.8% and 11.7%, respectively).

Thus, there is presently no clinical method of reliably identifying the fetus likely to experience shoulder dystocia and injury during birth without an unacceptably high false-positive rate. Given that 8% to 20% of fetuses from diabetic pregnancy weighing 4500 g or more will experience shoulder dystocia, that 15% to 30% of these will have recognizable brachial plexus injury, and that 5% to 15% of these injuries will result in permanent deficit, approximately 443 to 489 cesarean sections would have to be performed for suspected macrosomia to prevent one case of permanent injury from shoulder dystocia (Rouse and Owen, 1999).

Delivery Timing

Timing of delivery should minimize neonatal morbidity and mortality while maximizing the likelihood of vaginal delivery. Delaying delivery to as near the estimated due date as possible increases cervical ripeness and improves the chances of vaginal birth. Yet the risks of fetal macrosomia, birth injury, and fetal death increase as the due date approaches. Earlier delivery may reduce the risk of shoulder dystocia, but the increase in failed labor inductions and neonatal respiratory distress is appreciable. When all these factors are considered, the optimal time for delivery of most diabetic pregnancies is between 38.5 and 40 weeks. Indications for delivery of the diabetic pregnancy are

summarized in Table 49-22. Because of the apparent delay in fetal lung maturity in these pregnancies, delivery before 38.5 weeks' gestation should be performed only for compelling maternal or fetal reasons.

It may be tempting to consider early delivery in a diabetic pregnancy with evolving macrosomia on ultrasonography. Since fetal growth between 37 and 40 weeks of gestation in a 90th-percentile fetus is approximately 100 to 150 g per week, inducing labor 2 weeks early may reduce the risk of shoulder dystocia in some cases. Kjos and co-authors (1993) compared the outcomes associated with labor induction at 38 weeks versus expectant management in women with gestational diabetes. They found that expectant management increased the gestational age at delivery by 1 week, but the cesarean delivery rate was not significantly different. Macrosomia was

TABLE 49–22. INDICATIONS FOR DELIVERY IN DIABETIC PREGNANCY

Fetal	Nonreactive, positive CST
	Reactive positive CST, mature fetus
	Sonographic evidence of fetal growth arrest
	Decline in fetal growth rate with decreased amniotic fluid
	40–41 weeks' gestation
Maternal	Severe preeclampsia
	Mild preeclampsia, mature fetus
	Markedly falling renal function (creatinine clearance <40 mL/min)
Obstetric	Preterm labor with failure of tocolysis
	Mature fetus, inducible cervix

CST, contraction stress test.

TABLE 49–23. CONFIRMATION OF FETAL MATURITY BEFORE INDUCTION OF LABOR OR PLANNED CESAREAN DELIVERY IN DIABETIC PREGNANCY

1. Phosphatidylglycerol >3% in amniotic fluid collected from vaginal pool or by amniocentesis
2. Completion of 38.5 weeks' gestation
3. Normal last menstrual period
4. First pelvic examination before 12 wk confirms dates
5. Sonogram before 24 wk confirms dates
6. Documentation of more than 18 wk of unamplified (fetoscope) fetal heart tones

present in 23% of the expectantly managed group versus 10% in those induced at 38 weeks.

Fetal lung maturity should be verified in all patients delivered prior to 38.5 weeks by the presence of greater than 3% phosphatidylglycerol or the equivalent on an amniocentesis specimen (Table 49-23). If obstetrical dating is suboptimal, amniocentesis should be performed. Since an unripe cervix, prolonged labor, and increased likelihood of cesarean section frequently complicate labor induction at 37 to 38 weeks, delivery is best timed at 39 to 40 weeks for optimal neonatal outcome. In patients with GDM and superb glycemic control, continued fetal testing and expectant management can be considered until 41 weeks (Lurie et al., 1992). After 40+ weeks, the benefits of continued conservative management are less than the danger of fetal compromise. Induction of labor before 42 weeks in diabetic pregnancy—regardless of the readiness of the cervix—is prudent.

Labor or Primary Cesarean

The American College of Obstetricians and Gynecologists (2000) has recommended that primary cesarean delivery be discussed with diabetic gravidas with an EFW greater than 4500 g. This may reduce the risk of shoulder dystocia to some degree for an individual patient, but the effect on the larger obstetrical population is less clear.

Gonen and associates (2000) retrospectively assessed the impact of a policy of elective cesarean in cases with EFW above 4500 g. During the 4 years of the study with over 16,000 deliveries, macrosomia was correctly predicted in only 18% of cases. Of the 115 undiagnosed macrosomic cases, 13 infants were delivered by emergency cesarean, and 99 were delivered vaginally. Three infants with macrosomia (3%) and 14 infants without macrosomia (0.1%) sustained brachial plexus injury. The policy of preemptive cesarean for EFW greater than 4500 g prevented at most a single case of brachial palsy.

Conway and Langer (1998) performed a prospective trial in diabetic women in which those with EFW of 4250 g or more underwent elective cesarean section. Ultrasonography correctly identified the presence or absence of macrosomia in 87% of patients. The cesarean section rate increased slightly after the protocol was initiated (22% versus 25%), but overall, shoulder dystocia was less frequent (2.4% versus 1.1%).

Given these data, the decision to attempt vaginal delivery or perform a cesarean is inevitably based on very limited data. The patient's past obstetric history, the best EFW, a fetal

adipose profile (abdomen larger than head), and clinical pelvimetry should all be considered. Midpelvic operative deliveries should be avoided when macrosomia is suspected, and low pelvic or even outlet operative deliveries must be approached with extreme caution if labor is protracted. With an EFW greater than 4500 g, a prolonged second stage of labor or arrest of descent in the second stage is an indication for cesarean delivery (American College of Obstetricians and Gynecologists, 2000). Most large series of diabetic pregnancies report a cesarean section rate of 30% to 50%. The best means by which this rate can be lowered is by early and strict glycemic control in pregnancy. Conducting long labor inductions in patients with a large fetus and a marginal pelvis may increase, rather than lower, morbidity and costs.

Intrapartum Glycemic Management

Perinatal asphyxia and neonatal hypoglycemia correlate with maternal hyperglycemia during labor (Mimouni and Tsang, 1988). Unfortunately, strict maternal euglycemia during labor does not guarantee newborn metabolic stability in infants with macrosomia and islet cell hypertrophy. The use of a combined insulin and glucose infusion during labor maintains maternal plasma glucose in a narrow range (80 to 110 mg/dL) and reduces the incidence of neonatal hypoglycemia (Balsells et al., 2000). A protocol for administration of a continuous insulin infusion in labor is outlined in Table 49-24. Typical infusion rates are 5% dextrose in Ringer's lactate at 100 mL per hour and regular or lispro insulin at 0.5 to 1 units per hour. Capillary blood glucose is monitored hourly in such patients. For patients with diet-controlled

TABLE 49–24. INTRAPARTUM MATERNAL GLYCEMIC CONTROL

1. *Insulin Infusion Method*
   a. Withhold AM insulin injection.
   b. Begin and continue glucose infusion (5% dextrose in water) at 100 mL/hr throughout labor.
   c. Begin infusion of regular insulin at 0.5 U/hr.
   d. Begin oxytocin as needed.
   e. Monitor maternal glucose levels hourly using capillary reflectance meter at bedside and/or laboratory determinations.
   f. Adjust insulin infusion.

Plasma/Capillary Glucose (mg/dL)	Infusion Rate (U/hr)
<80	Insulin off
80–100	0.5*
101–140	1.0
141–180	1.5
181–220	2.0*
>220	2.5*

2. *Intermittent Subcutaneous Injection Method*
   a. Give one half the usual insulin dose in AM
   b. Begin and continue glucose infusion (5% dextrose in water) at 100 mL/hr throughout labor.
   c. Begin oxytocin as needed.
   d. Monitor maternal glucose levels hourly using capillary reflectance meter at bedside and/or laboratory determinations.
   e. Administer regular insulin in small (2–5 U) doses to maintain glucose 80–120 mg/dL.

* Bolus 2–5 units intravenously when rate increased.

GDM or mild type 2 diabetes, avoiding dextrose in all intravenous fluids during labor usually maintains excellent glucose control. After 1 to 2 hours, no further assessments of capillary blood glucose are typically necessary.

When cesarean section is planned in diabetic pregnancy, the procedure should be performed early in the day to avoid prolonged periods of fasting. On the night before surgery, insulin-requiring patients should be instructed to take their full dose of NPH, and only half the usual dose of Ultralente. No morning insulin should be taken. A glucose-containing intravenous line should be established promptly on arrival at the hospital, with insulin given as intravenous boluses on a sliding scale as needed every 1 to 4 hours to maintain maternal plasma glucose in the 80- to 160-mg/dL range.

Postpartum Metabolic Management

In the recovery room and postpartum, insulin can be given subcutaneously to women with type 2 diabetes, utilizing a sliding scale until regular diet is established. The insulin doses required postpartum are typically 40% to 50% of the preprandial doses required during pregnancy just prior to delivery. Type 1 patients require more intensive glucose monitoring postpartum, because many experience a honeymoon phase, in which insulin requirements fall dramatically. Use of a continuous glucose-insulin intravenous infusion in type 1 patients, especially those who have had a cesarean delivery, for 2 to 3 days until diet has normalized reduces the risk of severe hypoglycemia.

◼ MANAGEMENT OF THE NEONATE

Neonatal Transitional Management

Unmonitored and uncorrected neonatal hypoglycemia can lead to neonatal seizures, brain damage, and death. The degree of hypoglycemia correlates roughly with the degree of maternal glycemic control over the 6 weeks prior to birth. Pancreatic hypertrophy and chronic fetal hyperinsulinemia—holdovers from the chronically glucose-rich intrauterine environment—can lead to significant hypoglycemia once the umbilical supply of nutrients is interrupted by delivery. Infants of diabetic mothers also appear to have disorders of both catecholamine and glucagon metabolism and have diminished capability to mount normal compensatory responses to hypoglycemia. Thus, current recommendations specify frequent blood glucose checks and early oral feeding when possible (ideally from the breast), with infusion of intravenous glucose if oral measures prove insufficient.

Ordinarily, blood glucose levels can be controlled satisfactorily with an infusion of 10% glucose. If greater amounts of glucose are required, bolus administration of 5 mL/kg of 10% glucose is recommended, with gradually increasing concentrations of glucose administered every 30 to 60 minutes, if necessary.

Breast-Feeding

Considering the number of perinatal complications experienced by many women with diabetes—preeclampsia, macrosomia-induced cesarean section, neonatal hypoglycemia—

achieving a high rate of breast-feeding may seem to be a superfluous goal. However, mounting evidence indicates that breast-fed infants have a much lower risk of developing diabetes than do those exposed to the proteins in cow's milk (McKinney et al., 1999; Schrezenmeir and Jagla, 2000). Pettitt and associates (1997) found that children who were exclusively breast-fed had significantly lower rates of NIDDM than did those who were exclusively bottle-fed in all age groups. The odds ratio for NIDDM in exclusively breast-fed persons, compared with exclusively bottle-fed individuals, was 0.41 (95% CI = 0.18 to 0.93), adjusted for age, sex, birth date, parental diabetes, and birth weight. A study by Gimeno and de Souza (1997) found that a shorter duration of exclusive breast-feeding was a risk factor for childhood diabetes (OR = 2.13; 95% CI = 1.8 to 3.55) and that the introduction to cow's milk products before age 8 days was an important risk factor for the disease. Given the increased risk of diabetes in offspring of women with diabetes, these data underscore the importance of encouraging breast-feeding in all postpartum women with diabetes.

Most neonatologists maintain strict monitoring of glucose levels in newborn IDMs for at least 4 to 6 hours (frequently 24 hours), often necessitating admission to a newborn special care unit. This early separation of mother and neonate impedes breast-feeding and infant attachment and may delay the onset of lactogenesis in the diabetic mother. Neubauer and colleagues (1993) observed that milk of women with IDDM came in later than it did in controls and had significantly lower lactose and higher total nitrogen at 2 to 3 days after delivery. The infants of these diabetic mothers had significantly less milk intake 7 to 14 days after delivery than did those of the control women. Delayed lactogenesis in the women with IDDM was most likely in those with poor metabolic control, however. A study by van Beusekom and co-authors (1993) reported concentrations of micro- and macronutrients in milk and capillary blood and that tight glycemic control was associated with normal proportions of milk nutrients as compared with the multitude of milk abnormalities seen with moderate and poor control.

Thus, current evidence indicates that, with proper encouragement, sustained breast-feeding is possible for a significant proportion of patients with overt diabetes. Webster and co-workers (1995) longitudinally compared breast-feeding habits between women with diabetes and normals. At discharge, 63% of mothers with IDDM and 78% of mothers without IDDM were breast-feeding. At 8 weeks, the proportions of each were nearly identical (58% and 56%, respectively), and at 3 months of age, 47% of mothers with IDDM and 33% of women without IDDM continued to breast-feed. Most important, the study showed that infants of diabetic mothers delivered atraumatically, and infants who are well oxygenated, with mature lungs and excellent antecedent glucose control, can be kept with their mothers under close glycemic monitoring for the first 1 to 2 hours of life. This permits early breast-feeding, which may reduce the need for intravenous glucose therapy.

The actual techniques of infant nursing require some modification in women with overt diabetes, especially insulinopenic type 1 patients. Increased maternal calorie and fluid intake is necessary to maintain milk supply in all women. The calorie expenditure during nursing and for the 30 to 45 minutes thereafter (probably during post-nursing lactogenesis) may precipitate severe hypoglycemia if compensatory calories are not ingested, however. This is especially common during nursing late at night. Thus, breast-feeding women with type 1 diabetes should be encouraged to take in fluids and food (100 to 300 calories per feeding episode) while nursing to avoid reactive hypoglycemia.

Fortunately, studies of breast-feeding women with diabetes indicate that lactation, even for a short duration, has a beneficial effect on overall maternal glucose and lipid metabolism. For postpartum women who have GDM during their pregnancies, breast-feeding may offer a practical, low-cost intervention that helps to reduce or delay the risk of subsequent diabetes.

REFERENCES

Agarwal MM, Hughes PF, Punnose J, et al: Gestational diabetes screening of a multiethnic, high-risk population using glycated proteins. Diabetes Res Clin Pract **51**:67, 2001.

Aiello LP, King GT, Blankenship GL, et al: Diabetic retinopathy. Diabetes Care **21**:156, 1998.

Airaksinen KEJ, Ikaheimo MJ, Salmela PI, et al: Impaired cardiac adjustment to pregnancy in type 1 diabetes. Diabetes Care **9**:376, 1986.

Akinbi HT, Gerdes JS: Macrosomic infants of nondiabetic mothers and elevated C-peptide levels in cord blood. J Pediatr **127**:481, 1995.

Al-Inany H, Alaa N, Momtaz M, et al: Intrapartum prediction of macrosomia: Accuracy of abdominal circumference estimation. Gynecol Obstet Invest **51**:116, 2001.

Allouche C, Barjot P, Six T, et al: [Insulin dependent diabetes and pregnancy: Evaluation of the insulin pump.] J Gynecol Obstet Biol Reprod (Paris) **23**:706, 1994.

American College of Obstetricians and Gynecologists: Fetal macrosomia. ACOG Practice Bulletin no 22, 2000.

American College of Obstetricians and Gynecologists: Gestational diabetes. ACOG Practice Bulletin no 30. Obstet Gynecol **98**:525, 2001.

American Diabetes Association: ADA consensus statement: Type 2 diabetes in children and adolescents. Diabetes Care **12**:381, 2000.

American Diabetes Association: Diabetic nephropathy. Diabetes Care **25**(Suppl 1):S85, 2002a.

American Diabetes Association: Diabetic retinopathy. Diabetes Care **25**(Suppl 1):S90, 2002b.

American Diabetes Association: Gestational diabetes mellitus position statement. Diabetes Care **25**(Suppl 1):S94, 2002c.

American Diabetes Association: Preconception care of women with diabetes (position statement). Diabetes Care **25**(Suppl 1):S82, 2002d.

American Diabetes Association: Report of the Expert Committee on the Diagnosis and Classification of Diabetes Mellitus. Diabetes Care **25** (Suppl 1):S5, 2002e.

American Diabetes Association: Treatment of hypertension in adults with diabetes. Diabetes Care **25**(Suppl 1):S71, 2002f.

Arauz-Pacheco C, Raskin PM: The treatment of hypertension in adult patients with diabetes. Diabetes Care **25**:134, 2002.

Armenti VT, Ahlswede KM, Ahlswede BA, et al: National Transplantation Pregnancy Registry—outcomes of 154 pregnancies in cyclosporine-treated female kidney transplant recipients. Transplantation **57**(4):502, 1994.

Artal R, Mosley GM, Dorey FJ: Glycohemoglobin as a screening test for gestational diabetes. Am J Obstet Gynecol **148**:412, 1984.

Atkinson MA, Maclaren NK: The pathogenesis of insulin dependent diabetes. N Engl J Med **131**:1428, 1994.

Balsells M, Corcoy R, Adelantado JM, et al: Gestational diabetes mellitus: Metabolic control during labour. Diabetes Nutr Metab **13**:257, 2000.

Batukan C, Baysal B: Metformin improves ovulation and pregnancy rates in patients with polycystic ovary syndrome. Arch Gynecol Obstet **265**:124, 2001.

Baxi L, Barad D, Reece EA, et al: Use of glycosylated hemoglobin as a screen for macrosomia in gestational diabetes. Obstet Gynecol **64**:347, 1984.

Becerra JE, Khoury MJ, Cordero JF, et al: Diabetes mellitus during pregnancy and the risks for specific birth defects: A population based case-control study. Pediatrics **85**:1, 1990.

Berkus MD, Conway D, Langer O: The large fetus. Clin Obstet Gynecol **42**:766, 1999.

Berkus MD, Langer O: Glucose tolerance test: Degree of glucose abnormality correlates with neonatal outcome. Obstet Gynecol **81**:344, 1993.

Bhattacharyya A, Brown S, Hughes S, et al: Insulin lispro and regular insulin in pregnancy. QJM **94**:255, 2001.

Bhavnani BR, Enhorning G, Ekelund L, et al: Maternal diabetes and its effect on biochemical and functional development of rabbit fetal lung. Biochem Cell Biol **66**:396, 1988.

Bobrowski RA, Bottoms SF, Micallef JA, et al: Is the 50-gram glucose screening test ever diagnostic? J Matern Fetal Med **5**:317, 1996.

Bode B, Weinstein R, Bell D, et al: Comparison of insulin aspart with buffered regular insulin and insulin lispro in continuous subcutaneous insulin infusion: A randomized study in type 1 diabetes. Diabetes Care **25**:439, 2002.

Bourbon JR, Farrell PM: Fetal lung development in the diabetic pregnancy. Pediatr Res **19**:253, 1985.

Briggs GG, Nageotte MP: Fatal fetal outcome with the combined use of valsartan and atenolol. Ann Pharmacother **35**:859, 2001.

Brustman LE, Gela BD, Moore M, et al: Variations in oral glucose tolerance tests: The 100- versus 75-g controversy. J Assoc Acad Minor Phys **6**:70, 1995.

Buchanan TA, Kjos SL, Montoro MN, et al: Use of fetal ultrasound to select metabolic therapy for pregnancies complicated by mild gestational diabetes. Diabetes Care **17**:275, 1994.

Buttar HS: An overview of the influence of ACE inhibitors on fetal-placental circulation and perinatal development. Mol Cell Biochem **176**:61, 1997.

California Department of Health Services: Status report of the Sweet Success California Diabetes and Pregnancy Program 1986–1989. Sacramento, Calif, Maternal and Child Health Branch, 1991.

Carpenter MW, Canick JA, Hogan JW, et al: Amniotic fluid insulin at 14–20 weeks' gestation: Association with later maternal glucose intolerance and birth macrosomia. Diabetes Care **24**:1259, 2001.

Carpenter MW, Coustan DR: Criteria for screening tests for gestational diabetes. Am J Obstet Gynecol **144**:763, 1982.

Caruso A, Lanzone A, Bianchi V, et al: Continuous subcutaneous insulin infusion (CSII) in pregnant diabetic patients. Prenat Diagn **7**:41, 1987.

Cederberg J, Siman CM, Eriksson UJ: Combined treatment with vitamin E and vitamin C decreases oxidative stress and improves fetal outcome in experimental diabetic pregnancy. Pediatr Res **49**:755, 2001.

Centers for Disease Control and Prevention: Diabetes during pregnancy—United States, 1993–1995. MMWR Morb Mortal Wkly Rep **47**:408, 1998.

Chauhan SP, Perry KG Jr, McLaughlin BN, et al: Diabetic ketoacidosis complicating pregnancy. J Perinatol **16**:173, 1996.

Chauhan SP, West DJ, Scardo JA, et al: Antepartum detection of macrosomic fetus: Clinical versus sonographic, including soft-tissue measurements. Obstet Gynecol **95**:639, 2000.

Chmait R, Dinise T, Daneshmand S, et al: Prospective cohort study to establish predictors of glyburide success in gestational diabetes mellitus. Am J Obstet Gynecol **185**:S197, 2002.

Churchill JA, Berrendes H, Nemore W, et al: Neuropsychological deficits in children of diabetic mothers: A report from the Collaborative Study of Cerebral Palsy. Am J Obstet Gynecol **105**:257, 1969.

Coetzee EJ, Jackson WP: Metformin in management of pregnant insulin-independent diabetics. Diabetologia **16**:241, 1979.

Coetzee EJ, Jackson WP: The management of non–insulin-dependent diabetes during pregnancy. Diabetes Res Clin Pract **1**:281, 1985.

Coetzee EJ, Jackson WPU, Berman PA: Ketonuria in pregnancy—with special reference to calorie-restricted food intake in obese diabetics. Diabetes **29**:177, 1980.

Cohen BF, Penning S, Ansley D, et al: The incidence and severity of shoulder dystocia correlates with a sonographic measurement of asymmetry in patients with diabetes. Am J Perinatol **16**:197, 1999.

Combs CA, Gunderson E, Kitzmiller J, et al: Relationship of fetal macrosomia to maternal postprandial glucose control during pregnancy. Diabetes Care **15**:1251, 1992.

Combs CA, Rosenn B, Miodovnik M, et al: Sonographic EFW and macrosomia: Is there an optimum formula to predict diabetic fetal macrosomia? J Matern Fetal Med **9**:55, 2000.

Conway DL, Langer O: Elective delivery of infants with macrosomia in diabetic women: Reduced shoulder dystocia versus increased cesarean deliveries. Am J Obstet Gynecol **178**:922, 1998.

Cooper MJ, Enderlein MA, Dyson DC, et al: Fetal echocardiography: Retrospective review of clinical experience and an evaluation of indications. Obstet Gynecol **86**:577, 1995.

Cordero L, Treuer SH, Landon MB, et al: Management of infants of diabetic mothers. Arch Pediatr Adolesc Med **152**:249, 1998.

Cousins L: Pregnancy complications among diabetic women: Review. Obstet Gynecol Surv **42**:140, 1987.

Cousins L, Rigg L, Hollingsworth DR, et al: The 24-hour excursion and diurnal rhythm of glucose, insulin and C peptide in normal pregnancy. Am J Obstet Gynecol **136**:483, 1980.

Coustan DR: Screening and diagnosis of gestational diabetes. Semin Perinatol 18:407, 1994.

Coustan DR, Nelson C, Carpenter MW, et al: Maternal age and screening for gestational diabetes: A population based study. Obstet Gynecol 73:557, 1989.

Coustan DR, Widness JA, Carpenter MW, et al: Should the fifty-gram, one-hour plasma glucose screening test for gestational diabetes be administered in the fasting or fed state? Am J Obstet Gynecol 154:1031, 1986.

Crapo PA, Insel J, Sperling MA, et al: Comparison of serum glucose, insulin and glucagon responses to different types of complex carbohydrate in non–insulin-dependent diabetic patients. Am J Clin Nutr 34:184, 1981.

Cruikshank DP, Pitkin RM, Reynolds WA, et al: Altered maternal calcium homeostasis in diabetic pregnancy. J Clin Endocrinol Metab 50:264, 1980.

Cullen MT, Reece EA, Homko CJ, et al: The changing presentations of diabetic ketoacidosis during pregnancy. Am J Perinatol 13:449, 1996.

Cundy T, Gamble G, Manuel A, et al: Determinants of birth-weight in women with established and gestational diabetes. Aust N Z J Obstet Gynaecol 33:249, 1993.

Cundy T, Slee F, Gamble G, et al: Hypertensive disorders of pregnancy in women with type 1 and type 2 diabetes. Diabet Med 19:482, 2002.

Danilenko-Dixon DR, Van Winter JT, Nelson RL, et al: Universal versus selective gestational diabetes screening: Application of 1997 American Diabetes Association recommendations. Am J Obstet Gynecol 181:79, 1999.

Davison JM: Renal transplatation in pregnancy. Am J Kidney Dis 9:374, 1987.

de Veciana M, Major CA, Morgan MA, et al: Postprandial versus preprandial blood glucose monitoring in women with gestational diabetes mellitus requiring insulin therapy. N Engl J Med 333:1237, 1995.

de Veciana M, Trail PA, Evans AT, et al: A comparison of oral acarbose and insulin in women with gestational diabetes mellitus. Am J Obstet Gynecol 99(4, Suppl):S5, 2002.

Delgado Del Rey M, Herranz L, Martin Vaquero P, et al: [Effect of preconceptional metabolic control on the course of pregnancy in diabetic patients.] Med Clin (Barc) 117:45, 2001.

D'Ercole AJ: Mechanisms of in utero overgrowth. Acta Paediatr Suppl 88(428):31, 1999.

Diabetes Control and Complications Trial Research Group: Pregnancy outcomes in the Diabetes Control and Complications Trial. Am J Obstet Gynecol 174:1343, 1996.

Diamanti-Kandarakis E, Kouli C, Tsianateli T, et al: Therapeutic effects of metformin on insulin resistance and hyperandrogenism in polycystic ovary syndrome. Eur J Endocrinol 138:269, 1998.

Diase K, Monga M: Maternal estimates of neonatal birth weight in diabetic patients. South Med J 95:92, 2002.

Dooley SL, Metzger BE, Cho NH, et al: The influence of demographic and phenotypic heterogeneity on the prevalence of gestational diabetes mellitus. Int J Gynaecol Obstet 35:13, 1991.

Dunne FP, Brydon P, Smith T, et al: Pre-conception diabetes care in insulin-dependent diabetes mellitus. QJM 92:175, 1999.

Ekbom P, Damm P, Feldt-Rasmussen B, et al: Pregnancy outcome in type 1 diabetic women with microalbuminuria. Diabetes Care 24:1739, 2001.

Elliott BD, Langer O, Schenker S, et al: Insignificant transfer of glyburide occurs across the human placenta. Am J Obstet Gynecol 165:807, 1991.

Elliott BD, Schenker S, Langer O, et al: Comparative placental transport of oral hypoglycemic agents in humans: A model of human placental drug transfer. Am J Obstet Gynecol 171:653, 1994.

Elman KD, Welch RA, Frank RN, et al: Diabetic retinopathy in pregnancy: A review. Obstet Gynecol 75:119, 1990.

Engelgau MM, Herman WH, Smith PJ, et al: The epidemiology of diabetes and pregnancy in the US, 1988. Diabetes Care 18:1029, 1995.

Eriksson UJ, Borg LA, Cederberg J, et al: Pathogenesis of diabetes-induced congenital malformations. Ups J Med Sci 105:53, 2000.

Essel JK, Opai-Tetteh ET: Macrosomia—maternal and fetal risk factors. S Afr Med J 85:43, 1995.

Feldt-Rasmussen B, Mathiesen ER, Deckert T: Effect of two years of strict metabolic control on progression of incipient nephropathy in insulin-dependent diabetes. Lancet 2:1300, 1986a.

Feldt-Rasmussen B, Mathiesen ER, Hegedus L, et al: Kidney function during 12 months of strict metabolic control in insulin-dependent diabetic patients with incipient nephropathy. N Engl J Med 314:665, 1986b.

Frantz ID III, Epstein MF: Fetal lung development in pregnancies complicated by diabetes. In Merkatz IR, Adam PAJ (eds): The Diabetic Pregnancy: A Perinatal Perspective. New York, Grune & Stratton, 1979.

Fraser RB, Bruce C: Amniotic fluid insulin levels identify the fetus at risk of neonatal hypoglycaemia. Diabet Med 16:568, 1999.

Fraser D, Weitzman S, Leiberman JR, et al: Gestational diabetes among Bedouins in southern Israel: Comparison of prevalence and neonatal outcomes with the Jewish population. Acta Diabetol 31(2):78, 1994.

Freinkel N, Metzger BE: Pregnancy as a tissue culture experience: The critical implications of maternal metabolism for fetal development. In Freinkel N (ed): Pregnancy Metabolism, Diabetes and the Fetus: CIBA Foundation Symposium 63 (new series). Amsterdam, Excerpta Medica, 1979.

Fuhrmann K, Reiher H, Semmler K, et al: Prevention of congenital malformations in infants of insulin-dependent diabetic mothers. Diabetes Care 6:219, 1983.

Gabbe SG, Holing E, Temple P, et al: Benefits, risks, costs, and patient satisfaction associated with insulin pump therapy for the pregnancy complicated by type 1 diabetes mellitus. Am J Obstet Gynecol 182:1283, 2000.

Gabbe SG, Mestman JH, Freeman RK, et al: Management and outcome of diabetes mellitus. Am J Obstet Gynecol 127:465, 1977a.

Gabbe SG, Mestman JH, Freeman RK, et al: Management and outcome of diabetes mellitus, classes B to R. Am J Obstet Gynecol 129:723, 1977b.

Gilbert WM, Nesbitt TS, Danielsen B: Associated factors in 1611 cases of brachial plexus injury. Obstet Gynecol 93:536, 1999.

Gilby JR, Williams MC, Spellacy WN: Fetal abdominal circumference measurements of 35 and 38 cm as predictors of macrosomia: A risk factor for shoulder dystocia. J Reprod Med 45:936, 2000.

Gillies PS, Figgitt DP, Lamb HM: Insulin glargine. Drugs 59:253, 2000.

Gimeno SG, de Souza JM: IDDM and milk consumption: A case-control study in Sao Paulo, Brazil. Diabetes Care 20:1256, 1997.

Glueck CJ, Phillips H, Cameron D, et al: Continuing metformin throughout pregnancy in women with polycystic ovary syndrome appears to safely reduce first-trimester spontaneous abortion: A pilot study. Fertil Steril 75:46, 2001.

Glueck CJ, Wang P, Kobayashi S, et al: Metformin therapy throughout pregnancy reduces the development of gestational diabetes in women with polycystic ovary syndrome. Fertil Steril 77:520, 2002.

Goldberg JD, Franklin B, Lasser D, et al: Gestational diabetes: Impact of home glucose monitoring on neonatal birth weight. Am J Obstet Gynecol 154:546, 1986.

Gonen R, Bader D, Ajami M: Effects of a policy of elective cesarean delivery in cases of suspected fetal macrosomia on the incidence of brachial plexus injury and the rate of cesarean delivery. Am J Obstet Gynecol 183:1296, 2000.

Gordon MC, Landon MB, Boyle J, et al: Coronary artery disease in insulin-dependent diabetes mellitus of pregnancy (class H): A review of the literature. Obstet Gynecol Surv 51:437, 1996.

Halliday HL: Hypertrophic cardiomyopathy in infants of poorly-controlled diabetic mothers. Arch Dis Child 56:258, 1981.

Hare JW, White P: Gestational diabetes and the White classification. Diabetes Care 3:394, 1980.

Harris SB, Caulfield LE, Sugamori ME, et al: The epidemiology of diabetes in pregnant Native Canadians: A risk profile. Diabetes Care 20(9):1422, 1997.

Harris MI, Couric CC, Reiber G, et al (eds): Diabetes in America. Washington, DC, US Government Printing Office, 1995.

Harris MI, Flegal KM, Cowie CC: Prevalence of diabetes, impaired fasting glucose and impaired glucose tolerance in US adults. Diabetes Care 21:518, 1998.

Hedriana H, Moore TR: Comparison of single vs multiple growth sonography in predicting birthweight. Am J Obstet Gynecol 170:1600, 1994.

Hellmuth E, Damm P, Molsted-Pedersen L: Oral hypoglycaemic agents in 118 diabetic pregnancies. Diabet Med 17:507, 2000.

Henry OA, Beischer NA, Sheedy MT, Walstab JE: Gestational diabetes and follow-up among immigrant Vietnam-born women. Aust N Z J Obstet Gynaecol 33(2):109, 1993.

Hermansen K, Vaaler S, Madsbad S, et al.: Postprandial glycemic control with biphasic insulin aspart in patients with type 1 diabetes. Metabolism 51:896, 2002.

Hod M, Lapidot A: Dynamic parameters of maternal amino acid metabolism and fetal growth. Isr J Med Sci 32:530, 1996.

Hofmann T, Horstmann G, Stammberger I: Evaluation of the reproductive toxicity and embryotoxicity of insulin glargine (Lantus) in rats and rabbits. Int J Toxicol 21:181, 2002.

Holcomb WL Jr, Mostello DJ, Gray DL: Abdominal circumference vs estimated weight to predict large for gestational age birth weight in diabetic pregnancy. Clin Imaging 24:1, 2000.

Hopp H, Vollert W, Ebert A, et al: [Diabetic retinopathy and nephropathy—complications in pregnancy and labor]. Geburtshilfe Frauenheikunde, 55(5):275, 1995.

Hou S, Firanek C: Management of the pregnant dialysis patient. Adv Ren Replace Ther 5:24, 1998.

Hughes AB: Fetal heart rate changes during diabetic ketosis. Acta Obstet Gynecol Scand 66:71, 1987.

Hunter DJ, Burrows RF, Mohide PT, et al: Influence of maternal insulin-dependent diabetes mellitus on neonatal morbidity. Can Med Assoc J 149(1):47, 1993.

Huter O, Brezinka C, Solder E, et al: [Postpartum diabetes screening: value of fructosamine determination.] Zentralbl Gynakol 114:18, 1992.

Jaeggi ET, Fouron JC, Proulx F: Fetal cardiac performance in uncomplicated and well-controlled maternal type I diabetes. Ultrasound Obstet Gynecol 17:311, 2001.

Jaksic J, Mikulandra F, Perisa M, et al: Effect of insulin and insulin-like growth factor I on fetal macrosomia in healthy women. Coll Antropol 25:535, 2001.

Jakubowicz DJ, Iuorno MJ, Jakubowicz S, et al: Effects of metformin on early pregnancy loss in the polycystic ovary syndrome. J Clin Endocrinol Metab 87:524, 2002.

Jang HC, Cho NH, Jung KB, et al: Screening for gestational diabetes mellitus in Korea. Int J Gynaecol Obstet 51(2):115, 1995.

Jennings AM, Lewis KS, Murdoch S, et al: Randomized trial comparing continuous subcutaneous insulin infusion and conventional insulin therapy in type II diabetic patients poorly controlled with sulfonylureas. Diabetes Care 14:738, 1991.

Jovanovic R, Jovanovic L: Obstetric management when normoglycemia is maintained in diabetic pregnant women with vascular compromise. Am J Obstet Gynecol 149:617, 1984.

Jovanovic L, Knopp RH, Brown Z, et al: Declining insulin requirement in the late first trimester of diabetic pregnancy. Diabetes Care 24:1130, 2001.

Jovanovic-Peterson L: What is so bad about a prolonged pregnancy? J Am Coll Nutr 10:1, 1991.

Jovanovic-Peterson L, Bevier W, Peterson CM: The Santa Barbara County Health Care Services Program: Birth weight change concomitant with screening for and treatment of glucose-intolerance of pregnancy: A potential cost-effective intervention? Am J Perinatol 14:221, 1997.

Jovanovic-Peterson L, Peterson CM, Reed GF, et al: Maternal postprandial glucose levels and infant birth weight: The Diabetes in Early Pregnancy Study. Am J Obstet Gynecol 164:103, 1991.

Keller JD, Lopez-Zeno JA, Dooley SL, et al: Shoulder dystocia and birth trauma in gestational diabetes: A five-year experience. Am J Obstet Gynecol 165:928, 1991.

Key TC, Giuffrida R, Moore TR: Predictive value of early pregnancy glyco-hemoglobin in the insulin-treated diabetic patient. Am J Obstet Gynecol 156:1096, 1987.

Kitajima M, Oka S, Yasuhi I, et al: Maternal serum triglyceride at 24–32 weeks' gestation and newborn weight in nondiabetic women with positive diabetic screens. Obstet Gynecol 97:776, 2001.

Kitzmiller JL, Buchanan TA, Kjos S, et al: Pre-conception care of diabetes, congenital malformations, and spontaneous abortions. Diabetes Care 19:514, 1996.

Kjos SL, Henry OA, Montoro M, et al: Insulin-requiring diabetes in pregnancy: A randomized trial of active induction of labor and expectant management. Am J Obstet Gynecol 169(3):611, 1993.

Kjos SL, Schaefer-Graf U, Sardesi S, et al: A randomized controlled trial using glycemic plus fetal ultrasound parameters versus glycemic parameters to determine insulin therapy in gestational diabetes with fasting hyperglycemia. Diabetes Care 24:1904, 2001.

Kjos SL, Walther FJ, Montoro M, et al: Prevalence and etiology of respiratory distress in infants of diabetic mothers: Predictive value of fetal lung maturation tests. Am J Obstet Gynecol 163:898, 1990.

Knopp R., Magee MS, Walden CE, et al: Prediction of infant birth weight by GDM screening tests: Importance of plasma triglyceride. Diabetes Care 15:1605, 1992.

Kolterman OG: Glyburide in non–insulin-dependent diabetes: An update. Clin Ther 14:196, 1992.

Koren G: Glyburide and fetal safety; transplacental pharmacokinetic considerations. Reprod Toxicol 15:227, 2001.

Krew MA, Kehl RJ, Thomas A: Relation of amniotic fluid C-peptide levels to neonatal body composition. Obstet Gynecol 84:96, 1994.

Kroc Collaborative Study Group: Diabetic retinopathy after two years of intensified insulin treatment: Followup of the Kroc Collaborative Study. JAMA 260:37, 1988.

Kulovich MV, Gluck L: The lung profile. II. Complicated pregnancy. Am J Obstet Gynecol 135:64, 1979.

Kumari AS: Pregnancy outcome in women with morbid obesity. Int J Gynaecol Obstet 73:101, 2001.

Landon MB: Prenatal diagnosis of macrosomia in pregnancy complicated by diabetes mellitus. J Matern Fetal Med 9:52, 2000.

Landon MB, Gabbe SG, Piana R, et al: Neonatal morbidity in pregnancy complicated by diabetes mellitus: Predictive value of maternal glycemic profiles. Am J Obstet Gynecol 156:1089, 1987.

Landon MB, Mintz M, Gabbe SG: Sonographic evaluation of fetal abdominal growth: Predictor of the large-for-gestational-age infant in pregnancies complicated by diabetes mellitus. Am J Obstet Gynecol 160:115, 1989.

Langer O: Maternal glycemic criteria for insulin therapy in gestational diabetes mellitus. Diabetes Care 21(Suppl 2):B91, 1998.

Langer O, Berkus MD, Huff RW, et al: Shoulder dystocia: Should the fetus weighing greater than or equal to 4000 grams be delivered by cesarean section? Am J Obstet Gynecol 165:831, 1991.

Langer O, Brustman L, Anyaegbunam A, et al: The significance of one abnormal glucose tolerance test value on adverse outcome in pregnancy. Am J Obstet Gynecol 157:758, 1987.

Langer O, Conway DL, Berkus MD, et al: A comparison of glyburide and insulin in women with gestational diabetes mellitus. N Engl J Med 343:1134, 2000.

Langer O, Rodriguez DA, Xenakis EM, et al: Intensified versus conventional management of gestational diabetes. Am J Obstet Gynecol 170:1036, 1994.

Lauszus F, Klebe JG, Bek T: Diabetic retinopathy in pregnancy during tight metabolic control. Acta Obstet Gynecol Scand 79:367, 2000.

Lauszus FF, Klebe JG, Flyvbjerg A: Macrosomia associated with maternal serum insulin-like growth factor–I and –II in diabetic pregnancy. Obstet Gynecol 97:734, 2001.

Lavin JP Jr, Barden TP, Miodovnik M: Clinical experience with a screening program for gestational diabetes. Am J Obstet Gynecol 141:491, 1981.

Leguizamon G, Reece EA: Effect of medical therapy on progressive nephropathy: Influence of pregnancy, diabetes and hypertension. J Matern Fetal Med 9:70, 2000.

Lepercq J, Taupin P, Dubois-Laforgue D, et al: Heterogeneity of fetal growth in type 1 diabetic pregnancy. Diabetes Metab 27:339, 2001.

Lepore M, Pampanelli S, Fanelli C, et al: Pharmacokinetics and pharmacodynamics of subcutaneous injection of long-acting human insulin analog glargine, NPH insulin, and Ultralente human insulin and continuous subcutaneous infusion of insulin lispro. Diabetes 49:2142, 2000.

Lim JM, Tayob Y, O'Brien PM, et al: A comparison between the pregnancy outcome of women with gestation diabetes treated with glibenclamide and those treated with insulin. Med J Malaysia 52:377, 1997.

Lopez-de la Pena XA, Cajero Avelar JJ, De Leon Romo LF: Prevalence of gestational diabetes in a group of women receiving treatment at the Mexican Institute of Social Security in Aguascalientes, Mexico. Ach Med Res 28(2):281, 1997.

Lucas MJ, Leveno KJ, Williams ML, et al: Early pregnancy glycosylated hemoglobin, severity of diabetes, and fetal malformations. Am J Obstet Gynecol 161:426, 1989.

Lurie S, Matzkel A, Weissman A, et al: Outcome of pregnancy in class A1 and A2 gestational diabetic patients delivered beyond 4 weeks' gestation. Am J Perinatol 9(5–6):484, 1992.

Mace S, Hirschfeld SS, Riggs T, et al: Echocardiographic abnormalities in infants of diabetic mothers. J Pediatr 95:1013, 1979.

Major CA, Henry MJ, De Veciana M, et al:. The effects of carbohydrate restriction in patients with diet-controlled gestational diabetes. Obstet Gynecol 91:600, 1998.

Mazze RS, Krogh CL: Gestational diabetes mellitus: Now is the time for detection and treatment. Mayo Clin Proc 67(10):995, 1992.

McElvy SS, Miodovnik M, Rosenn B, et al: A focused preconceptional and early pregnancy program in women with type 1 diabetes reduces perinatal mortality and malformation rates to general population levels. J Matern Fetal Med 9:14, 2000.

McFarland MB, Langer O, Conway DL, et al: Dietary therapy for gestational diabetes: How long is long enough? Obstet Gynecol 93:978, 1999.

McFarland MB, Trylovich CG, Lange O: Anthropometric differences in macrosomic infants of diabetic and nondiabetic mothers. J Matern Fetal Med 7:292, 1998.

McKinney PA, Parslow R, Gurney KA, et al: Perinatal and neonatal determinants of childhood type 1 diabetes: A case-control study in Yorkshire, UK. Diabetes Care 22:928, 1999.

Mecklenburg RS, Benson EA, Benson JW Jr, et al: Acute complications associated with insulin infusion pump therapy: Report of experience with 161 patients. JAMA 252:3265, 1984.

Metzger BE: Summary and recommendations of the Third International Workshop-Conference on Gestational Diabetes Mellitus. Diabetes 40(Suppl 2):197, 1991.

Metzger BE, Coustan DR: Summary and recommendations of the Fourth International Workshop-Conference on Gestational Diabetes Mellitus. Diabetes Care **21**(Suppl 2), 1998.

Michlin R, Oettinger M, Odeh M, et al: Maternal obesity and pregnancy outcome. Isr Med Assoc J **2**:10, 2000.

Miller E, Hare JW, Cloherty JP, et al: Elevated maternal hemoglobin A1c in early pregnancy and major congenital anomalies in infants of diabetic mothers. N Engl J Med **304**:1331, 1981.

Mimouni F, Miodovnik M, Rosenn B, et al: Birth trauma in insulin-dependent diabetic pregnancies . Am J Perinatol **9**(3):205, 1992.

Mimouni F, Tsang RC: Pregnancy outcome in insulin-dependent diabetes: Temporal relationships with metabolic control during specific pregnancy periods. Am J Perinatol **5**:334, 1988.

Miodovnik M, Lavin JP, Knowles HC, et al: Spontaneous abortion among insulin-dependent diabetic women. Am J Obstet Gynecol **150**:372, 1984.

Miselli V, Pagliani U, Bisi S, et al: [Epidemiology of gestational diabetes in Scandiano health district 12 (USL 12)]. Minerva Endocrinol **19**(2):63, 1994.

Montoro MN, Myers VP, Mestman JH, et al: Outcome of pregnancy in diabetic ketoacidosis. Am J Perinatol **10**(1):17, 1993.

Moore TR: A comparison of amniotic fluid fetal pulmonary phospholipids in normal and diabetic pregnancy. Am J Obstet Gynecol **186**:641, 2002.

Moore TR, Hollingsworth DR, Kolterman O: Continuous subcutaneous insulin infusion in an obese insulin-resistant pregnant woman with type II diabetes: Accelerated fetal growth and neonatal complications. Obstet Gynecol **70**:480, 1987.

Moses R, Griffiths RD, Davis W: Gestational diabetes: Do all women need to be tested? Aust N Z J Obstet Gynaecol **35**:387, 1995.

Moses RG, Colagiuri S: The extent of undiagnosed gestational diabetes mellitus in New South Wales. Med J Aust **167**:14, 1997.

Nahum GG, Huffaker BJ: Racial differences in oral glucose screening test results: Establishing race-specific criteria for abnormality in pregnancy. Obstet Gynecol **81**(4):517, 1993.

Nasrat AA, Johnstone FD, Hasan SAM: Is random plasma glucose an efficient screening test for abnormal glucose tolerance in pregnancy? Br J Obstet Gynaecol **95**:855, 1988.

Nasrat, H, Fageeh W, Abalkhail B, et al: Determinants of pregnancy outcome in patients with gestational diabetes. Int J Gynaecol Obstet **53**:117, 1996.

National Institute of Diabetes and Digestive and Kidney Diseases: Epidemiology of diabetes in the United States. Available at www.niddk.nih.gov/health/diabetes/pubs/dmstats.htm. Accessed May 16, 2002.

Naylor CD, Sermer M, Chen E, et al: Cesarean delivery in relation to birth weight and gestational glucose tolerance: Pathophysiology or practice style? JAMA **275**:1165, 1996.

Naylor CD, Sermer M, Chen E, et al: Selective screening for gestational diabetes mellitus. N Engl J Med **337**:1591, 1997.

Nesbitt TS, Gilbert WM, Herrchen B: Shoulder dystocia and associated risk factors with macrosomic infants born in California. Am J Obstet Gynecol **179**:476, 1998.

Neubauer SH, Ferris AM, Chase CG, et al: Delayed lactogenesis in women with insulin-dependent diabetes mellitus. Am J Clin Nutr **58**:54, 1993.

Nordstrom L, Spetz E, Wallstrom K, et al:. Metabolic control and pregnancy outcome among women with insulin-dependent diabetes mellitus: A twelve-year follow-up in the country of Jamtland, Sweden. Acta Obstet Gynecol Scand **77**:284, 1998.

Ogata ES, Sabbagha R, Metzger BE, et al: Serial ultrasonography to assess evolving fetal macrosomia: Studies in 23 pregnant diabetic women. JAMA **243**:2405, 1980.

Ojomo EO, Coustan DR: Absence of evidence of pulmonary maturity at amniocentesis in term infants of diabetic mothers. Am J Obstet Gynecol **163**:954, 1990.

O'Reilly-Green C, Divon M: Sonographic and clinical methods in the diagnosis of macrosomia. Clin Obstet Gynecol **43**:309, 2000.

Ornoy A, Ratzon N, Greenbaum C, et al: School-age children born to diabetic mothers and to mothers with gestational diabetes exhibit a high rate of inattention and fine and gross motor impairment. J Pediatr Endocrinol Metab **14**(Suppl 1):681, 2001.

O'Sullivan JB, Mahan CM: Criteria for the glucose tolerance test in pregnancy. Diabetes **13**:278, 1964.

Padmanabhan R, Shafiullah M: Intrauterine growth retardation in experimental diabetes: Possible role of the placenta. Arch Physiol Biochem **109**:260, 2001.

Page RC, Kirk BA, Fay T, et al: Is macrosomia associated with poor glycaemic control in insulin-dependent diabetic pregnancy? Diabet Med **13**:170, 1996.

Parfitt VJ, Clark JD, Turner GM, et al: Use of fructosamine and glycated haemoglobin to verify self blood glucose monitoring data in diabetic pregnancy. Diabetic Med **10**(2):162, 1993.

Parretti E, Mecacci F, Papini M, et al: Third-trimester maternal glucose levels from diurnal profiles in nondiabetic pregnancies: Correlation with sonographic parameters of fetal growth. Diabetes Care **24**:1317, 2001.

Parry S, Severs CP, Sehdev HM, et al: Ultrasonographic prediction of fetal macrosomia: Association with cesarean delivery. J Reprod Med **45**:17, 2000.

Pedersen J: Diabetes and Pregnancy: Blood Glucose of Newborn Infants. Copenhagen, Danish Science, 1952.

Perlow JH, Morgan MA, Montgomery D, et al: Perinatal outcome in pregnancy complicated by massive obesity. Am J Obstet Gynecol **167**:958, 1992.

Persson B, Hanson U: Neonatal morbidities in gestational diabetes mellitus. Diabetes Care **21**(Suppl 2):B79, 1998.

Peterson CM, Jovanovic-Peterson L, Mills JL, et al: The Diabetes in Early Pregnancy Study: Changes in cholesterol, triglycerides, body weight, and blood pressure: The National Institute of Child Health and Human Development—the Diabetes in Early Pregnancy Study. Am J Obstet Gynecol **166**:513, 1992.

Pettitt DJ, Forman MR, Hanson RL: Breastfeeding and incidence of non–insulin-dependent diabetes mellitus in Pima Indians. Lancet **350**:166, 1997.

Piacquadio K, Hollingsworth DR, Murphy H: Effects of in-utero exposure to oral hypoglycaemic drugs. Lancet **338**:866, 1991.

Pietropaolo M, Le Roith D: Pathogenesis of diabetes: Our current understanding. Clin Cornerstone **4**:1, 2001.

Pinter E, Peyman JA, Snow K, et al: Effetcs of maternal diabetes on fetal rat lung ion transport: Contribution of alveolar and bronchiolar epithelial cells to Na, K() ATPase expression. J Clin Invest **87**:821, 1991.

Pinter E, Reece EA, Leranth CZ, et al: Arachidonic acid prevents hyperglycemia-associated yolk sac damage and embryopathy. Am J Obstet Gynecol **155**:691, 1986.

Platt MJ, Stanisstreet M, Casson IF, et al: St Vincent's declaration 10 years on: Outcomes of diabetic pregnancies. Diabet Med **19**:216, 2002.

Purdy LP, Hantsch CE, Molitch ME, et al: Effect of pregnancy on renal function in patients with moderate-to-severe diabetic renal insufficiency. Diabetes Care **19**:1067, 1996.

Ray R, Heng BH, Lim C, et al: Gestational diabetes in Singaporean women: Use of the glucose challenge test as a screening test and identification of high risk factors. Ann Acad Med Singapore **25**:504, 1996.

Reece EA, Egan JFX, Coustan DR, et al: Coronary artery disease in diabetic pregnancies. Am J Obstet Gynecol **154**:150, 1986.

Reece EA, Leguizamon G, Homko C: Pregnancy performance and outcomes associated with diabetic nephropathy. Am J Perinatol **15**:413, 1998.

Reece EA, Sivan E, Francis G, et al: Pregnancy outcomes among women with and without diabetic microvascular disease (White's classes B to FR) versus non-diabetic controls. Am J Perinatol **15**:549, 1998.

Reece EA, Winn HN, Hayslett JP, et al: Does pregnancy alter the rate of progression of diabetic nephropathy? Am J Perinatol **7**:193, 1990.

Reece EA, Winn HN, Smikle C, et al: Sonographic assessment of growth of the fetal head in diabetic pregnancies compared with normal gestations. Am J Perinatol **7**:18, 1990.

Riccio A, Avogaro A, Valerio A, et al: Improvement of basal hepatic glucose production and fasting hyperglycemia of type 1 diabetic patients treated with human recombinant Ultralente insulin. Diabetes Care **17**:535, 1994.

Rith-Najarian SJ, Ness FK, Faulhaber T, et al: Screening and diagnosis for gestational diabetes mellitus among Chippewa women in northern Minnesota. Minn Med **79**(5):21, 1996.

Rizvi JH, Rasul S, Malik S, et al: Experience with screening for abnormal glucose tolerance in pregnancy: Maternal and perinatal outcome. Asia-Oceania J Obstet Gynaecol **18**(2):99, 1992.

Rizzo TA, Metzger BE, Burns WJ, et al: Correlations between antepartum maternal metabolism and intelligence of offspring. N Engl J Med **325**:911, 1991.

Rizzo TA, Silverman BL, Metzger BE, et al: Behavioral adjustment in children of diabetic mothers. Acta Paediatr **86**:969, 1997.

Robert MF, Neff RK, Hubbell JP, et al: Association between maternal diabetes and the respiratory distress syndrome. N Engl J Med **12**:357, 1976.

Roberts AB, Baker JR: Relationship between fetal growth and maternal fructosamine in diabetic pregnancy. Obstet Gynecol **70**:242, 1987.

Roberts AB, Court DJ, Henley P, et al: Fructosamine in diabetic pregnancy. Lancet **2**:998, 1983.

Romao JE Jr, Luders C, Kahhale S, et al: Pregnancy in women on chronic dialysis: A single-center experience with 17 cases. Nephron **78**:416, 1998.

Rosenn B, Miodovnik M, Combs CA, et al: Pre-conception management of insulin-dependent diabetes: Improvement of pregnancy outcome. Obstet Gynecol **77**:846, 1991.

Rossing K, Jacobsen P, Hommel E, et al: Pregnancy and progression of diabetic nephropathy. Diabetologia **45**:36, 2002.

Roth S, Abernathy MP, Lee WH, et al: Insulin-like growth factors I and II peptide and messenger RNA levels in macrosomic infants of diabetic pregnancies. J Soc Gynecol Investig 3:78, 1996.

Rotmensch S, Celentano C, Liberati M, et al: Screening efficacy of the subcutaneous tissue width/femur length ratio for fetal macrosomia in the nondiabetic pregnancy. Ultrasound Obstet Gynecol 13:340, 1999.

Rouse DJ, Owen J: Prophylactic cesarean delivery for fetal macrosomia diagnosed by means of ultrasonograph—a Faustian bargain? Am J Obstet Gynecol 181:332, 1999.

Rudge MV, Calderon IM, Ramos MD, et al: Perinatal outcome of pregnancies complicated by diabetes and by maternal daily hyperglycemia not related to diabetes: A retrospective 10-year analysis. Gynecol Obstet Invest 50:108, 2000.

Sacks DA: Fetal macrosomia and gestational diabetes: What's the problem? Obstet Gynecol 81:775, 1993.

Sacks DA, Chen W: Estimating fetal weight in the management of macrosomia. Obstet Gynecol Surv 55:229, 2000.

Sacks DA, Greenspoon JS, Abu-Fadil S, et al: Toward universal criteria for gestational diabetes: The 75-gram glucose tolerance test in pregnancy. Am J Obstet Gynecol 172:607, 1995.

Salvesen DR, Brudenell JM, Proudler AJ, et al: Fetal pancreatic beta-cell function in pregnancies complicated by maternal diabetes mellitus: Relationship to fetal acidemia and macrosomia. Am J Obstet Gynecol 168:1363, 1993.

Sandmire HF, O'Halloin TJ: Shoulder dystocia: Its incidence and associated risk factors. Int J Gynaecol Obstet 26:65, 1988.

Schocket LS, Grunwald JE, Tsang AF: The effect of pregnancy on retinal hemodynamics in diabetic versus nondiabetic mothers. Am J Ophthalmol 128:477, 1999.

Schrezenmeir J, Jagla A: Milk and diabetes. J Am Coll Nutr 19 (2, Suppl):176S, 2000.

Schwartz R, Gruppuso PA, Petzold K, et al: Hyperinsulinemia and macrosomia in the fetus of the diabetic mother. Diabetes Care 17:640, 1994.

Serirat S, Deerochanawong C, Sunthornthepvarakul T, et al: Gestational diabetes mellitus. J Med Assoc Thailand 75(6):315, 1992.

Sermer M, Naylor CD, Gare D, et al: Impact of time since last meal on the gestational glucose challenge test. Am J Obstet Gynecol 171:607, 1994.

Serup L: Influence of pregnancy on diabetic retinopathy. Acta Endocrinol 112(Suppl 227):122, 1986.

Sgro MD, Barozzino T, Mirghani HM, et al: Pregnancy outcome postrenal transplantation. Teratology 65:5, 2002.

Shah BD, Cohen AW, May C: Comparison of glycohemoglobin determination and the one-hour oral glucose screen in the identification of gestational diabetes. Am J Obstet Gynecol 144:774, 1982.

Shelley-Jones DC, Beischer NA, Sheedy MT, et al: Excessive birth weight and maternal glucose tolerance—a 19-year review. Aust N Z J Obstet Gynaecol 32:318, 1992.

Sibai BM: Risk factors, pregnancy complications, and prevention of hypertensive disorders in women with pregravid diabetes mellitus. J Matern Fetal Med 9:62, 2000.

Sibai BM, Caritis S, Hauth J, et al: Risks of preeclampsia and adverse neonatal outcomes among women with pregestational diabetes mellitus. Am J Obstet Gynecol 182:364, 2000.

Silfen SL, Wapner RL, Gabbe SG: Maternal outcome in class H diabetes mellitus. Obstet Gynecol 56:749, 1980.

Silverman BL, Metzger BE, Cho NH: Impaired glucose tolerance in adolescent offspring of diabetic mothers: Relationship to fetal hyperinsulinism. Diabetes Care 18:611, 1995.

Silverman BL, Rizzo TA, Cho NH: Long-term effects of the intrauterine environment. Diabetes Care 21(Suppl 2):B142, 1998.

Simmons D: Interrelation between umbilical cord serum sex hormones, sex hormone–binding globulin, insulin-like growth factor I, and insulin in neonates from normal pregnancies and pregnancies complicated by diabetes. J Clin Endocrinol Metab 80:2217, 1995.

Simmons D, Thompson CF, Conroy C: Incidence and risk factors for neonatal hypoglycaemia among women with gestational diabetes mellitus in South Auckland. Diabet Med 17:830, 2000.

Simmons D, Thompson CF, Conroy C, et al: Use of insulin pumps in pregnancies complicated by type 2 diabetes and gestational diabetes in a multiethnic community. Diabetes Care 24:2078, 2001.

Sokol RJ, Chik L, Dombrowski MP, et al: Correctly identifying the macrosomic fetus: Improving ultrasonography-based prediction. Am J Obstet Gynecol 182:1489, 2000.

Spyer G, Hattersley AT, Sykes JE, et al: Influence of maternal and fetal glucokinase mutations in gestational diabetes. Am J Obstet Gynecol 185:240, 2001.

Susa JB, McCormick KL, Widness JA, et al: Chronic hyperinsulinemia in the fetal rhesus monkey: Effects of fetal growth and composition. Diabetes 25:1058, 1979.

Sutherland HW, Pritchard CW: Increased incidence of spontaneous abortion in pregnancies complicated by maternal diabetes mellitus. Am J Obstet Gynecol 155:135, 1986.

Tabsh KM, Brinkman CR III, Bashore RA: Lecithin:sphingomyelin ratio in pregnancies complicated by insulin-dependent diabetes mellitus. Obstet Gynecol 59:353, 1982.

Taylor R, Lee C, Kyne-Grzebalski D, et al: Clinical outcomes of pregnancy in women with type 1 diabetes (1). Obstet Gynecol 99:537, 2002.

Temple RC, Aldridge VA, Sampson MJ, et al: Impact of pregnancy on the progression of diabetic retinopathy in type 1 diabetes. Diabet Med 18:573, 2001.

Tevaarwerk GJM, Harding PGR, Milne KJ, et al: Pregnancy in diabetic women: Outcome with a program aimed at normoglycemia before meals. Can Med Assoc J 125:435, 1981.

Towner D, Kjos SL, Leung B, et al: Congenital malformations in pregnancies complicated by NIDDM. Diabetes Care 18(11):1446, 1995.

Tsang RC, Brown DR, Steicher JJ: Diabetes and calcium: Calcium disturbances in infants of diabetic mothers. In Merkatz SR, Adam PAJ (eds): The Diabetic Pregnancy: A Perinatal Perspective. New York, Grune & Stratton, 1979.

Tuomilehto J, Lindstrom J, Eriksson JG, et al: Prevention of type 2 diabetes mellitus by changes in lifestyle among subjects with impaired glucose tolerance. N Engl J Med 344:1343, 2001.

Tyden O, Berne C, Eriksson UJ, et al: Fetal maturation in strictly controlled diabetic pregnancy. Diabetes Res 1:131, 1984.

UK Prospective Diabetes Study Group: Tight blood pressure control and risk of macrovascular and microvascular complications in type 2 diabetes. BMJ 317:703, 1998.

Van Assche FA, Holemans K, Aerts L: Long-term consequences for offspring of diabetes during pregnancy. Br Med Bull 60:173, 2001.

van Beusekom CM, Zeegers TA, Martini IA, et al: Milk of patients with tightly controlled insulin-dependent diabetes mellitus has normal macronutrient and fatty acid composition. Am J Clin Nutr 57:938, 1993.

Vandermolen DT, Ratts VS, Evans WS, et al: Metformin increases the ovulatory rate and pregnancy rate from clomiphene citrate in patients with polycystic ovary syndrome who are resistant to clomiphene citrate alone. Fertil Steril 75:310, 2001.

Vohr BR, McGarvey ST: Growth patterns of large-for-gestational-age and appropriate-for-gestational-age infants of gestational diabetic mothers and control mothers at age 1 year. Diabetes Care 20:1066, 1997.

Vohr BR, McGarvey ST, Coll CG: Effects of maternal gestational diabetes and adiposity on neonatal adiposity and blood pressure. Diabetes Care 18:467, 1995.

Ward DM: Hypertension, renal diseases and kidney transplantation. In Hollingsworth DR, Resnik R (eds): Medical Counseling Before Pregnancy. New York, Churchill Livingstone, 1988.

Warso MA, Lands WEM: Lipid peroxidation in relation to prostacyclin and thromboxane physiology and pathophysiology. Br Med Bull 39:277, 1983.

Webster J, Moore K, McMullan A: Breastfeeding outcomes for women with insulin dependent diabetes. J Hum Lactation 11:195, 1995.

Weeks JW, Pitman T, Spinnato JA: Fetal macrosomia: Does antenatal prediction affect delivery route and birth outcome? Am J Obstet Gynecol 173:1215, 1995.

Weerasiri T, Riley SF, Sheedy MT, et al: Amniotic fluid insulin values in women with gestational diabetes as a predictor of emerging diabetes mellitus. Aust N Z J Obstet Gynaecol 33:358, 1993.

Widness JA, Teramo KA, Clemons GK, et al: Direct relationship of antepartum glucose control and fetal erythropoietin in human type 1 (insulin dependent) diabetic pregnancy. Diabetologia 33(6):378, 1990.

Wing AJ, Brunner FP, Brynger H, et al: Successful pregnancies in women treated by dialysis and kidney transplantation. Br J Obstet Gynaecol 87:839, 1980.

Wylie BR, Kong J, Kozak SE, et al: Normal perinatal mortality in type 1 diabetes mellitus in a series of 300 consecutive pregnancy outcomes. Am J Perinatol 19:169, 2002.

Yalcin HR, Zorlu CG: Threshold value of glucose screening tests in pregnancy: Could it be standardized for every population? Am J Perinatol 13(5):317, 1996.

Zaken V, Kohen R, Ornoy A: Vitamins C and E improve rat embryonic antioxidant defense mechanism in diabetic culture medium. Teratology 64:33, 2001.

Zarate A, Ochoa R, Hernandez M: [Effectiveness of acarbose in the control of glucose tolerance worsening in pregnancy.] Ginecol Obstet Mex 68:42, 2000.

Zucker P, Simon G: Prolonged symptomatic neonatal hypoglycemia associated with maternal chlorpropamide therapy. Pediatrics 42:824, 1968.

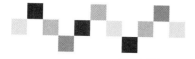

Chapter 50
THYROID DISEASE AND PREGNANCY

Shahla Nader, MD

Thyroid disorders are among the most common endocrinopathies in young women of childbearing age. In large areas of the world, iodine deficiency is the predominant etiology of these disorders. In the western hemisphere, however, these disorders are most often related to altered immunity. The hormonal and immunologic perturbations of pregnancy and the postpartum period, as well as the dependence of the fetus on maternal iodine and thyroid hormone, have profound influences on maternal thyroid function and consequently on fetal well being. Appropriate antepartum and postpartum care requires a basic knowledge of thyroid function, its alteration in pregnancy, and the more common thyroid diseases afflicting women in the setting of pregnancy, all of which are summarized in this chapter.

MATERNAL-FETAL THYROID PHYSIOLOGY

Normal Thyroid Physiology

The thyroid gland is located in the anterior neck below the hyoid bone and above the sternal notch. Consisting of two lobes and connected by the isthmus, it weighs approximately 20–25 grams. Each lobe is divided into lobules, which contain 20–40 follicles apiece. The follicle consists of follicular cells, which surround a glycoprotein material named colloid. The hypothalamic pituitary axis governs the production of thyroid hormone by the follicular cells. Tonic stimulation of thyrotropin releasing hormone (TRH) is required to maintain normal thyroid function, and hypothalamic injury or disruption of the stalk results in hypothyroidism. TRH, a tripeptide, is produced in the paraventricular nucleus of the hypothalamus, and its local production as determined by mRNA is inversely related to concentrations of circulating thyroid hormones. Traversing the pituitary stalk, TRH is delivered to the pituitary thyrotroph via the pituitary portal circulation and affects the production and release of thyrotropin (TSH). A glycoprotein, TSH is composed of α and β subunits, the β subunit conferring specificity. Control of TSH secretion is via negative feedback (from circulating thyroid hormone, somatostatin, dopamine) or via stimulation by TRH.

Thyroid gland production of thyroxine (T_4) and tri-iodothyronine (T_3) is regulated by TSH. Upon binding to its receptor, TSH induces thyroid growth, differentiation, and all phases of iodine metabolism from uptake of iodine to secretion of the two thyroid hormones. In the nonpregnant state, 80–100 micrograms of iodine are taken up by the gland daily.

Dietary iodine is reduced to iodide, absorbed and cleared by the kidney (80%) and thyroid (20%). Iodide is actively trapped by the thyroid and is the rate-limiting step in hormone biosynthesis. The iodide is converted back to iodine and organified by binding to tyrosyl residues, which are part of a glycoprotein called thyroglobulin. This process requires the enzyme thyroid peroxidase. Iodination can give rise to monoidotyrosine (MIT) or di-iodotyrosine (DIT), the ratio depending on prevailing iodine availability. Coupling of two DITs form T_4 and a DIT and MIT form T_3. Thyroglobulin is extruded into the colloid space at the center of the follicle, and hence thyroid hormone is stored as colloid. Hormone secretion by thyroid cells, which is also under TSH control, involves digestion of thyroglobulin and extrusion of T_4 and T_3 into the capillaries. Daily secretion rates approximate 90 mcg of T_4 and 30 mcg of T_3. Both circulate highly bound to protein (mainly thyroxine-binding globulin), with less than 1% in free form (0.3% of T_3, 0.03% for T_4). Other binding proteins include thyroxine-binding prealbumin and albumin. It is the free hormone that enters cells and is active.

Whereas T_4 is completely thyroidal in origin, only approximately 20% of T_3 comes directly from the thyroid. Thyroxine is metabolized in most tissues (particularly in the liver and kidneys) to T_3 by deiodination. It is also metabolized to reverse T_3, a metabolically inactive hormone. Removal of an iodine by $5'$ monodeiodination from the outer ring of T_4 results in T_3, which is metabolically active. When iodine is removed from the inner ring, reverse T_3 is produced (Fig. 50-1). Monodeiodinase type I and type II catalyze the formation of T_3, whereas reverse T_3 is catalyzed by monodeiodinase type III. Normally, approximately 35% of T_4 is converted to T_3, and 40% is converted to reverse T_3, but this balance is shifted in favor of the metabolically inert reverse T_3 in illness, starvation, or other catabolic states (Brennan and Bahn, 1998; DeGroot, 1999). Some 80% of circulating T_3 is derived from peripheral conversion. The half-life of T_4 is one week; five to six weeks are necessary before a change in dose of T_4 therapy is reflected in steady-state T_4 values. The half-life of T_3 is one day.

Free thyroid hormone enters the cell and binds to nuclear receptors and in this way signals its cellular responses (Dillman 1985; Brent, 1994). The affinity of T_3 for nuclear receptors is tenfold that of T_4, which helps to explain the greater biological activity of T_3. Thyroid hormone receptors belong to a large superfamily of nuclear-hormone receptors that include the steroid hormone, vitamin D, and retinoic acid receptors. Thyroid hormones have diverse effects on cellular growth, development, and metabolism. The major effects of thyroid

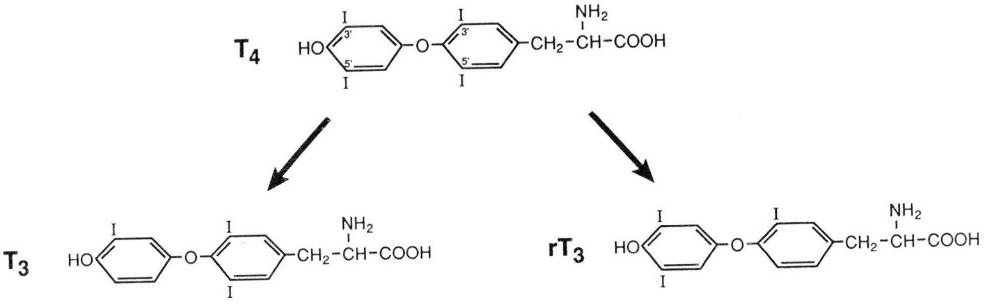

$$T_4 \quad HO - \bigcirc - O - \bigcirc - CH_2 - CH(NH_2) - COOH$$

FIGURE 50-1 ■ Removal of an iodine by 5'-monodeiodination from the outer ring of thyroxine (T_4) results in formation of metabolically active triiodothyronine (T_3). Removal of an iodine from the inner ring results in formation of the metabolically inactive reverse triiodothyronine (rT_3).

hormones are genomic, stimulating transcription and translation of new proteins in a concentration- and time-dependent manner.

Maternal Thyroid Physiology

Not only does pregnancy alter thyroidal economy but the hormone changes of pregnancy also result in profound alterations in the biochemical parameters of thyroid function. This section reviews maternal thyroid physiology, the role of maternal hormones in fetal growth and development, and the development of the fetal hypothalamic-pituitary-thyroid axis. This topic was recently reviewed by Glinoer (1999).

Three series of events occur at different time points of gestation:

1. Starting in the first half of gestation and continuing until term, there is an increase in thyroxine-binding globulin (TBG), a direct effect of increasing circulating estrogen concentrations. Basal levels increase two- to threefold. This increase is accompanied by a trend toward lower free hormone concentrations (T_4 and T_3), which results in stimulation of the hypothalamic-pituitary-thyroid axis. Under conditions of iodine sufficiency, the decrease in free hormone levels is marginal (10%–15% on average). When the supply of iodine is insufficient, more pronounced effects occur, and these are covered in the section Iodine Deficiency, Hypothyroidism, and Pregnancy. For this reason, there is usually a trend toward a slight increase in TSH between the first trimester and term.
2. The second event takes place transiently during the first trimester and is a consequence of thyroid stimulation by increasing concentrations of human chorionic gonadotropin (hCG). As hCG peaks late in the first trimester, there is partial inhibition of the pituitary and transient lowering of TSH between weeks 8 and 14 of gestation (Fig. 50-2). In about 20% of women, TSH falls below the lower limit of normal, and these women often have significantly higher hCG concentrations (Glinoer et al., 1993). The stimulatory action of hCG has been broadly quantified; a 10,000 IU/L increment is associated with a lowering of basal TSH of 0.1 mU/liter. In most normal pregnancies, this is of minor consequence (Grün et al., 1997).
3. Alterations in the peripheral metabolism of thyroid hormone occur throughout pregnancy but are more prominent in the second half. Three enzymes deiodinate thyroid hormones; these are named types I, II, and III deiodinases. Type I is not significantly modified. Type II, which is expressed in the placenta, can maintain T_3 production locally, which could be critical when maternal T_4 concen-

trations are reduced. Type III is also found abundantly in the placenta, catalyses the conversion of T_4 to reverse T_3 and of T_3 to T_2, and this abundance may explain the low T_3 and high reverse T_3 concentrations characteristic of fetal thyroid hormone metabolism (Burrow et al., 1994).

These physiological adaptations to pregnancy, depicted in Figure 50-3 (Color Plate 20), are attained without difficulty by the normal thyroid gland in a state of iodine sufficiency. This does not apply when thyroid function is compromised and/or iodine supply insufficient.

Iodine Deficiency and Goiter

Increased vascularity and some glandular hyperplasia can result in mild thyroid enlargement, but frank goiter occurs because of iodine deficiency or other thyroidal disease. Although iodine deficiency is usually not a problem in the United States, Japan, and parts of Europe, 1–1.5 billion people in the world are at risk, with 500 million living in areas of overt iodine deficiency. The World Health Organization recommends 150 mcg iodine per day for adults and 200 mcg for pregnant women. This is because there is increased renal iodine clearance during pregnancy, and in the latter part of gestation a significant amount of iodine is diverted toward the fetoplacental unit to allow the fetal thyroid to produce its own thyroid hormones. This physiologic adaptation occurs easily with minimal hypothyroxinemia and no goiter formation in areas of iodine sufficiency. Through hypothalamic-pituitary feedback, however, borderline iodine intake chronically enhances thyroid stimulation. The iodine deficiency manifests as greater hypothyroxinemia and subsequently increased TSH, thyroglobulin, and thyroid hypertrophy (Fig. 50-4).

In a study of otherwise healthy pregnant women living under conditions of relative iodine restriction, thyroid volume, as assessed by ultrasonography, increased an average of 30% during pregnancy (Glinoer et al., 1994). In a selected group of these women with goitrogenesis, follow-up a year after delivery did not show a return of thyroid volumes to those found in early pregnancy. Thus, iodine intake should also be increased postpartum, especially in breast-feeding women. Ultrasonography of neonates revealed that thyroid volume was 38% larger in neonates of untreated mothers versus neonates of mothers treated with iodine supplementation (Glinoer, 1997).

Other than iodine deficiency, goiter in pregnancy can be related to the following:

- Graves disease
- Hashimoto's thyroiditis
- Excessive iodine intake

Mother

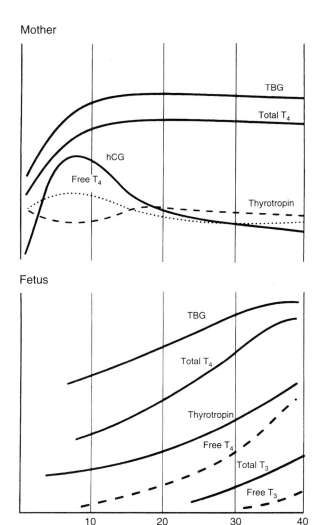

Fetus

Week of Pregnancy

FIGURE 50-2 ■ Relative changes in maternal and fetal thyroid function during pregnancy. The effects of pregnancy on the mother include a marked and early increase in hepatic production of thyroxine-binding globulin (TBG) and placental production of human chorionic gonadotropin (hCG). The increase in serum TBG, in turn, increases total serum thyroxine (T_4) concentrations; hCG has thyrotropin–like activity and stimulates maternal T_4 secretion. The transient hCG-induced increase in serum free T_4 inhibits maternal secretion of thyrotropin. (Reprinted by permission from Burrow GN, Fisher DA, Larsen PR: Maternal and fetal thyroid function. N Engl J Med **331**:1072, 1994).

- Lymphocytic thyroiditis
- Thyroid cancer
- Lymphoma
- Therapy with lithium or thionamides

In the United States, clinical studies of pregnant women and nonpregnant controls have not revealed an increase in goiter in pregnancy (Levy et al., 1980), and ultrasound studies from other areas replete in iodine have confirmed these findings (Nelson et al., 1987; Brander and Kivisaari, 1989).

Iodine Metabolism in Pregnancy

Although radioactive iodine is now absolutely contraindicated in pregnancy, early studies using I^{132} showed a threefold increase in thyroidal iodine clearance in pregnant women.

Another set of studies in 25 pregnant women also revealed increased radioactive iodine uptake during pregnancy compared with the nonpregnant or postpartum state (Halnan, 1958; Abdoul-Khair et al., 1964). The mean renal iodine clearance almost doubles, secondary to increased renal blood flow and a rise in glomerular filtration rate of as much as 50% (Ferris, 1988). If iodine excretion is greater than 100 mcg in a 24-hour period, the patient's iodine intake is assumed to be sufficient (Beckers, 1992).

■ PLACENTAL-FETAL THYROID PHYSIOLOGY

The thyroid gland forms as a midline outpouching of the anterior pharyngeal floor, migrates caudally, and reaches its final position by 7 weeks' gestation. Laternal contributions from the fourth and fifth pharyngeal pouches give it its bilateral shape by weeks 8–9 of gestation. Active trapping of iodide is detectable by week 12, and the first indication of T_4 production is detectable by week 14. Hypothalamic TRH is detectable at weeks 8–9, and the pituitary portal circulation is functional by weeks 10–12. Until midgestation, fetal TSH and

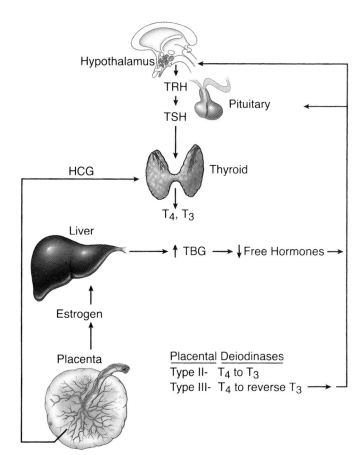

FIGURE 50-3 ■ Schematic representation of the physiologic adaptation to pregnancy showing increased thyroxine-binding globulin concentrations (TBG), increased human chorionic gonadotropin (hCG) with its thyrotropin-like activity, and alterations in peripheral metabolism of thyroid hormones in the placenta. TRH, thyrotropin releasing hormone; TSH, thyroid stimulating hormone. See Color Plate 20. (Adapted from Glinoer D: What happens to the normal thyroid during pregnancy? Thyroid **9**:631, 1999.)

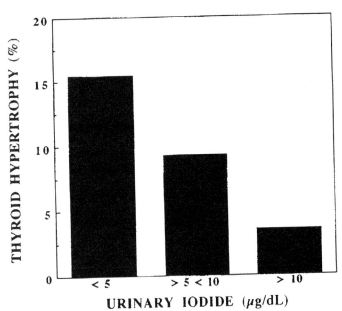

FIGURE 50-4 ■ Percentage of maternal thyroid hypertrophy (thyroid volume >18 mL) in relation to urinary iodine concentration measured during the first trimester of pregnancy. (Reprinted by permission from Caron P, Hoff M, Bassi S, et al: Urinary iodine excretion during normal pregnancy in healthy women living in the southwest of France: Correlation with maternal thyroid parameters. Thyroid **7**:749, 1997.)

T_4 concentrations remain low. At 18–20 weeks' gestation, both the fetal thyroid gland iodine uptake and serum T_4 concentrations begin to increase (Glinoer and Delange, 2000). Concentrations of T_4 increase from 2 mcg/dL at 20 weeks to 10 mcg/dL at term, with increasing TBG concentrations contributing to this rise. Similarly, free fetal T_4 concentrations increase from 0.1 ng/dL at 12 weeks' gestation to 1.5 ng/dL near term. Increases in T_3 and free T_3 are smaller, presumably because of the availability of placental type III deiodinase, which converts T_4 rapidly to reverse T_3. Fetal serum T_3 rises from 6 ng/dL at 12 weeks' gestation to 45 ng/dL near term. Fetal serum TSH increases from 4 to 8 mU/L between weeks 12 and term (Radunovic et al., 1991; LaFranchi, 1999). In summary, most fetal T_4 is inactivated to reverse T_3. Tri-iodothyronine (from T_4 conversion or direct fetal thyroid secretion) is limited in availability. Fetal tissues that depend on T_3 for development (such as the brain structures) are supplied by local T_4 to T_3 conversion via deiodinase type II (Fisher, 1999).

Placental Transfer of Thyroid Hormones

While earlier studies suggested only limited T_4 and T_3 transfer through the placenta, more recent studies have shown that T_4 can be found in first-trimester celomic fluid by 6 weeks' gestation. In addition, nuclear T_3 receptors can be identified in the brain of 10-week-old fetuses and increase tenfold by 16 weeks' gestation before the fetal thyroid becomes fully functional (Bernall and Pekonen, 1984). These studies suggest that maternal T_4 transfer occurs early in gestation and that low levels of T_4 are sustained in the fetus at this time (Santini et al., 1999). Finally, Vulsma and colleagues (1989) have reported that cord serum T_4 levels in hypothyroid neonates with glandular agenesis represented as much as 30% of normal circulating values, a strong indication of maternal

T_4 transfer, although this has not been a uniform finding (DeLange et al., 1989).

It would thus appear that the first phase of maximum-growth velocity of developing brain structures—namely, neuronal multiplication and organization occurring during the second trimester—corresponds to a phase during which the supply of thyroid hormones to the fetus is almost exclusively of maternal origin (Glinoer and DeLange, 2000). In the second phase of maximum fetal brain growth velocity, occurring from the third trimester to 2–3 years postnatally, the supply of thyroid hormone is of fetal and neonatal origin. Hence, low maternal thyroxine concentrations in the second trimester can result in irreversible neurologic deficit in the offspring. When it occurs later, the damage to the fetal brain is less, and partially reversible.

Concentrations of TSH, T_4, T_3, and reverse T_3 are measurable in the amniotic fluid and correlate with the fetal rather than maternal serum.

Neonatal Thyroid Function

Immediately following birth, there is a surge of TRH and TSH followed by a rise in T_3 (from increased T_4 to T_3 conversion) and more moderately, in T_4 (Burrow, 1994). Within a few days, the increased TSH falls to adult levels through T_4 and T_3 negative feedback inhibition. Neonatal T_4 and T_3 concentrations return to normal adult levels within 4–6 weeks (Fisher and Polk, 1989). The transient hyperthyroxinemia can be triggered by neonatal cooling and may represent an adaptation of thermogenesis to extrauterine life (Fisher et al., 1977; Polk, 1988).

In premature neonates, free T_4 levels are low, TSH levels are normal (adult) and T_4 levels relate to gestational age. The clinical consequence of this transient hypothalamic hypothyroidism is unknown; it may cause impaired neurologic and mental development (Fisher and Klein, 1981; Fisher and Foley 1989; Reuss et al., 1996; Vulsma and Kok, 1996).

Placental Transfer of Drugs Affecting Thyroid Function

The potential influence of the placenta on fetal thyroid and neurological development is evident by the ready transfer of several agents that affect thyroid function (Burrow et al., 1977; Fisher, 1977; Roti et al., 1983). These agents include the following:

- Iodine
- Thionamides
- Beta-adrenergic receptor blockers
- Somatostatin
- Exogenous TRH
- Dopamine agonists and antagonists
- Thyroid-stimulating immunoglobulins and other antibodies

TSH does not cross the placenta. TRH and corticosteroid administered antenatally before 32 weeks of gestation stimulates T_4 release and decreases the frequency of chronic lung disease in the neonate (Ballard et al., 1992). Also, intraamniotic administration of T4 in the preterm setting increases fetal maturation as reflected by an increase in the lecithin/sphingomyelin ratio and a decrease in respiratory distress syndrome of the newborn (Romaguera et al., 1993).

PREGNANCY, THE IMMUNE SYSTEM AND THYROID DISEASE

The reader is referred to Chapter 7 for a detailed review of pregnancy immunology. The fetus, with its complete set of paternal antigens, survives because of adjustments in the maternal-placental-fetal immune systems. This immunological compromise of pregnancy is orchestrated primarily by the placental tissues and passaged fetal cells that are able to modulate the local and systemic maternal immune responses (Davies, 1999; Weetman et al., 1999). Hence, autoimmune responses are usually reduced in pregnancy, as evidenced by amelioration of Graves disease, rheumatoid arthritis, and multiple sclerosis (Nelson et al., 1993; Buyon et al., 1996; Confavreuz et al., 1998). Although there is a shift from proinflammatory Th1 cytokines to Th2 cytokines driven, perhaps, by progesterone (Piccinini al., 1995), it is occurring on a background of reduced B-cell reactivity. The reduced B-cell responses are thought to be secondary to placental sex steroids, which are powerful negative regulators of B-cell activity. Whereas most of the immune changes in pregnancy return to normal by 12 months postpartum, there is a marked increase after most pregnancies in many different types of autoantibody secretion and an exacerbation of autoimmune disease. In most studies, total immunoglobulin G as well as autoantibody levels rise above prepregnancy levels during the first 6 months postpartum, suggesting continuing nonspecific immune stimulation (Davies, 1999).

LABORATORY EVALUATION OF THYROID FUNCTION DURING PREGNANCY

Thyrotropin (TSH) and Thyroid Hormones

Table 50-1 outlines values of maternal TSH as well as total and free T_4, T_3, and TBG concentrations during the three trimesters of a normal pregnancy. It is important to remember that total T_4 and total T_3 are elevated because of increased TBG production and reduced clearance induced by the hyperestrogenic state of pregnancy (Ain et al., 1987). The T_3 resin

uptake (an indirect laboratory measure of available TBG binding sites) is reduced in pregnancy because increased TBG binding sites take up more of the added T_3, leaving less to bind to resin. Thus, the free thyroxine Index, which is a product of the total T_4 and T_3 resin uptake, usually falls within the normal range in pregnancy. Because free T_4 can be determined, however, a third-generation TSH and free T_4 are the best ways to evaluate thyroid function in pregnancy. If the TSH is suppressed, suggesting overproduction of thyroid hormones, free T_3 can also be determined. The third-generation TSH assays also allow distinction between profound and marginal suppression. As outlined in an earlier section, free T_3 and T_4 concentrations can be in the high-normal range and TSH can be low early in pregnancy because of the stimulatory effects of hCG. Free hormone levels then fall through the rest of the pregnancy but usually not below the lower limit of normal (Glinoer et al., 1991). Free hormone may be determined by either equilibrium dialysis (usually used for research purposes) or radioimmunoassys (Sturgess et al., 1987). Total T_4 levels in excess of 15 mg/dL and total T_3 concentrations greater than 250 ng/dL are rare in a normal pregnancy (Burrow, 1985; Glinoer et al., 1990). Table 50-2 outlines factors that influence TBG and hence total hormone concentrations.

Resistance to thyroid hormone is a rare condition encompassing a number of different defects. The pituitary and/or other peripheral tissues can manifest this resistance. These patients present with an increased free T_4 concentration along with an inappropriately elevated or nonsuppressed TSH and, clinically, may manifest goiter. Whereas patients with thyroid hormone resistance have normal alpha-subunit concentrations, patients with TSH-secreting tumors (the differential diagnosis of thyroid hormone resistance) often have elevated serum alpha-subunit levels (Weintraub, 1981). In a case reported by Anselmo and colleagues (2001), transient thyrotoxicosis occurred during pregnancy in a subject with resistance to thyroid hormone caused by a mutation in the thyroid receptor beta gene. This thyrotoxicosis manifested clinically by hypermetabolic features and paralleled the rise and peak of hCG concentrations. Symptoms ameliorated and thyroid hormone concentrations declined as pregnancy progressed and hCG concentrations fell.

TABLE 50-1. BIOCHEMICAL PARAMETERS OF MATERNAL THYROID FUNCTION DURING GESTATION

	Trimester		
	First	**Second**	**Third**
Total T_4 (3.9–11.6 µg/dL)	10.7 ± 0.20	$11.5 \pm 0.20^*$	$11.5 \pm 0.20^\dagger$
Total T_3 (90.9–208 ng/dL)	205 ± 2.00	$231 \pm 3.00^*$	$233 \pm 2.00^\dagger$
Molar T_3/T_4 (10–23×10^3)	23.1 ± 0.30	$24.3 \pm 0.30^\ddagger$	$24.8 \pm 0.30^\dagger$
Thyroxine-binding globulin (11–21 mg/liter)	21.2 ± 0.30	$28.5 \pm 0.40^*$	$31.5 \pm 0.30^*$
TBG saturation (28–60%)	39.3 ± 0.60	$30.9 \pm 0.40^*$	$27.9 \pm 0.30^*$
Free T_4 (0.8–2.0 ng/dL)	1.4 ± 0.02	$1.1 \pm 0.01^*$	$1.0 \pm 0.01^*$
Free T_3 (190–710 pg/dL)	330 ± 0.06	$270 \pm 0.06^*$	$250 \pm 0.06^*$
TSH (0.2–4.0 mU/liter)	0.75 ± 0.04	$1.1 \pm 0.04^*$	$1.29 \pm 0.04^*$
hCG (IU/liter $\times 10^3$)	38.5 ± 1.50	$16.4 \pm 0.90^*$	$13.0 \pm 1.50^\dagger$

* $P < .001$.
† $P = $ NS.
‡ $P < .005$.

hCG, human chorionic gonadotropin; TBG, thyroxine-binding globulin; TSH, thyroid-stimulating hormone; T_3, L-triiodothyronine; T_4, L-thyroxine.

TABLE 50-2. FACTORS AFFECTING THYROXINE-BINDING GLOBULIN

Increase	Decrease
Oral contraceptives	Testosterone
Pregnancy	Nephrotic syndrome
Estrogen	Cirrhosis
Hepatitis	Glucocorticoids
Acute intermittent porphyria	Severe illness
Inherited	Inherited

Thyrotropin Receptor Antibodies

Several functional types of TSH receptor antibodies are now recognized to exist. Some antibodies promote gland function (thyroid stimulating immunoglobulins or TSI), some inhibit binding of TSH to its receptor (thyroid-binding inhibitory immunoglobulins or TBII), and some enhance or inhibit thyroid growth. These antibodies can be measured by a variety of bioassays and receptor assays. For example, maternal production of TSI causes maternal Graves, is transferred across the placenta, and can lead to neonatal Graves disease. Excess TBII can cause both maternal and neonatal hypothyroidism.

Antithyroid Antibodies

Patients with autoimmune thyroid disease commonly develop antibodies to thyroid antigens. The two most commonly determined antibodies are those to thyroglobulin and to thyroid peroxidase (anti-TPO) (Mariotti et al., 1989). Among nonpregnant women, the incidence of anti-TPO antibodies is about 3%, the incidence ranging from 5%–15% in pregnant women. A substantial proportion of women with positive anti-TPO antibodies in early pregnancy develop postpartum thyroiditis (Learoyd et al., 1992; Weetman and McGregor, 1994).

Drugs and Thyroid Function

Table 50-3 outlines drug effects on thyroid function and metabolism, absorption of thyroid hormones, and interpretation of thyroid function tests. Iodine and lithium inhibit thyroid function. Propranolol and iopadate block T_4 to T_3 conversion, as do glucocorticoids; however, glucocorticoids also reduce release of TSH from the pituitary, as do dopamine, dopamine agonists, and somatostatin. The antiseizure medication phenytoin results in a reduced total T_4 (by up to 30%) by inhibiting the binding of thyroid hormones to binding proteins and increasing T_4 clearance. Ferrous sulfate, aluminum hydroxide, and sucrafate may inhibit thyroid hormone absorption substantially—an important interaction to note in pregnant women who are taking both iron and thyroid hormones.

Amiodarone, an iodine-rich drug, has been used in pregnancy for maternal or fetal tachyarrhythmias. Amiodarone and the iodine are transferred across the placenta, exposing the fetus to the drug and iodine overload. This iodine overload could cause fetal/neonatal hypothyroidism and goiter, because the fetus acquires the capacity to escape from the acute Wolff-Chaikoff effect (decrease in peroxidase activity and organification that follow iodine excess) only late in gestation. Among 64 pregnancies in which amiodarone was given to the mother, 17% of progeny developed hypothyroidism (both goitrous and nongoitrous). Hypothyroidism was transient, though a few of the infants were treated short-term with thyroid hormones. Only two newborns had transient hyperthyroxinemia. Although breast-feeding resulted in substantial infant amiodarone ingestion, it did not cause major changes in neonatal thyroid function. The authors concluded that amiodarone should be used only when tachyarrhythmias are unresponsive to other drugs and life threatening, and hypothyroid neonates (and perhaps the fetus *in utero*) should be treated. It would also be prudent to monitor the infants of breast-feeding mothers who continue to use the medication (Bartalena et al., 2001).

Nonthyroidal Illness and Thyroid Function

This has been the topic of various reviews and commentaries (Wartofsky and Burman, 1982; Brennan and Bahn, 1998; DeGroot, 1999). Severely ill patients can manifest thyroid function test abnormalities that could relate to functional inhibition of the hypothalamic-pituitary-thyroid axis, impaired T_4 to T_3 conversion (a constant accompaniment of nonthyroidal illness), and abnormalities in binding and clearance of thyroid hormone. Reverse T_3 levels are substantially elevated because of increased T_4 to reverse T_3 conversion and impaired metabolic clearance of reverse T_3. TSH concentrations can be low, normal, or elevated, though seldom higher than 20 mU/L (Wartofsky and Burman, 1982). The more severe the illness, the lower the T_4 values, and this has been used as a prognostic indicator, as a high correlation has been found between a low T_4 and a fatal outcome (Brent and Hershman, 1986). The best test for assessing thyroid function

TABLE 50-3. EFFECTS OF DRUGS ON THYROID HORMONES AND FUNCTION TESTS

1. Inhibit thyroid function
   a. Iodine
   b. Lithium
2. Inhibit T_4 to T_3 conversion
   a. Glucocorticoid
   b. Ipodate
   c. Propranolol
   d. Amiodarone
   e. Propylthiouracil
3. Increase TSH
   a. Iodine
   b. Lithium
   c. Dopamine antagonists
4. Decrease TSH
   a. Glucocorticoids
   b. Dopamine agonists
   c. Somatostatin
5. Inhibit T_4 and T_3 binding to binding proteins
   a. Phenytoin
   b. Salicylates
   c. Sulphonylureas
6. Inhibit gastrointestinal absorption of thyroid hormone
   a. Ferrous sulfate
   b. Sucrafate
   c. Cholestyramine
   d. Aluminum hydroxide

TSH, thyroid-stimulating hormone; T_3, L-triiodothyronine; T_4, L-thyroxine.

in severely or chronically ill patients is the free T_4 concentration. Despite the low T_3 and total T_4 state, it is felt that this situation does not represent true hypothyroidism but rather an adaptation to stress, and that it should not be treated.

THYROID DYSFUNCTION AND REPRODUCTIVE DISORDERS

Thyroid hormones are important for normal reproductive function. Deficiency of thyroid hormone can result in delayed sexual development. As reviewed by Winters and Berga (1997) and Krassas (2000), all women with infertility and menstrual disturbances should have thyroid function tests, usually T_4, T_3, and TSH. Also, women with type I diabetes, who have a relatively high incidence of hypothyroidism, should probably undergo screening prior to conception.

Hyperthyroidism

Hyperthyroidism has been linked to oligomenorrhea, hypomenorrhea, amenorrhea, and infertility, although many thyrotoxic women remain ovulatory. In a more recent survey only 21.5% of 214 thyrotoxic patients had menstrual disturbances compared with 50%–60% in older series (Krassas et al., 1994). Thyroxine upregulates the production of sex hormone binding globulin. Elevated circulating testosterone and estrogen may be observed, and the clearance of testosterone is reduced. Gonadotropin concentrations can be tonically elevated (Akande and Hockaday, 1972; Tanaka et al., 1981). The substantial weight loss seen in some hyperthyroid patients can affect the hypothalamic-pituitary-gonadal axis and also can contribute to the infertility of severe hyperthyroidism.

Hypothyroidism

Hypothyroidism in fetal life does not affect the development of the reproductive tract; during childhood, however, it leads to sexual immaturity and usually a delay in puberty, followed by anovulatory cycles. Almost 25% of women with untreated hypothyroidism have menstrual irregularities. Menorrhagia occurs frequently and can reflect interference with the endometrial maturational process and response to ovarian steroids; it generally responds to thyroxine treatment (Wilansky and Greisman, 1989). The increased miscarriage rate seen in hypothyroid patients may possibly be reflective of disrupted endometrial maturation. Hypothyroidism, through increased thyrotropin-releasing hormone, also can be associated with hyperprolactinemia, which itself can disrupt reproductive function and menstrual cyclicity (del Pozo et al., 1979), leading to oligomenorrhea or amenorrhea. Galactorrhea can sometimes be seen in this setting, as can elevated LH, possibly through diminished dopamine secretion (Thomas and Reid, 1987). Women with hypothyroidism have diminished rates of metabolic clearance of androstenedione and estrone and an increase in peripheral aromatization. Whereas plasma concentrations of testosterone and estradiol are decreased because of diminished binding activity, their unbound fractions are actually increased. Several studies have suggested increased risk of miscarriage in the presence of thyroid antibodies, even in the face of a euthyroid status. There is no documented benefit, however, in using T_4 to treat euthyroid women with recurrent spontaneous abortions (Glinoer et al., 1994; Bussen and Steck, 1995; Wasserstrum and Anania, 1997; Montoro, 1997).

Radioiodine and Gonadal Function

The prevalence of infertility, premature births, miscarriage, and genetic damage in the offspring of women treated with radioactive iodine for thyrotoxicosis does not seem to be increased (Greig, 1973; Safa et al., 1975). Even thyroid cancer doses of I_{131} produce little reproductive toxicity in women, and exposure to radioiodine does not appear to reduce fecundity (Krassas, 2000). In a study of 32 women who conceived following I_{131} treatment for thyroid cancer (resulting in 60 term deliveries), two children conceived within a year of I_{131} had birth defects, but no anomalies were seen in the remaining 58 (Smith et al., 1994). Thus, contraception has been generally recommended for one year following I_{131} treatment. In a large study, Schlumberger and associates (1996) obtained data on 2113 pregnancies conceived after exposure to 30–100 mCi of radioiodine given for thyroid cancer. The incidences of stillbirths, preterm labor, low birth weight, congenital malformations, and death during the first year of life were not significantly different between pregnancies conceived before or after radioiodine therapy. Miscarriages were more frequent in the women treated with I_{131} in the year preceding conception (40%). All women need pregnancy tests prior to I_{131} treatment; such treatment late in the first trimester and in the second trimester could result in irreversible hypothyroidism in the fetus. Lactating mothers who have received diagnostic or therapeutic doses of I_{131} should not breast-feed their infants. These topics are reviewed by Gorman (1999) and Berlin (2001).

HYPERTHYROIDISM AND PREGNANCY

Signs and Symptoms

The prevalence of hyperthyroidism in pregnant women has been reported to range from 0.05% to 0.2% (Fernandez-Soto et al., 1998). The signs and symptoms of mild to moderate hyperthyroidism—namely, heat intolerance, diaphoresis, fatigue, anxiety, emotional lability, tachycardia, and a wide pulse pressure—could be mimicked by the hypermetabolic state of normal pregnancy. On the other hand, weight loss, tachycardia greater than 100 beats/minute, and diffuse goiter are features that may suggest hyperthyroidism. Graves ophthalmopathy can also be helpful but does not necessarily indicate active thyrotoxicosis (Seely and Burrow, 1991). Gastrointestinal symptoms such as severe nausea and excessive vomiting can accompany thyrotoxicosis in pregnancy, as can diarrhea, myopathy, lymphadenopathy, and congestive heart failure.

Diagnosis

Biochemical confirmation of the hyperthyroid state can be obtained through laboratory measurement of free T_4, free T_3, and TSH. Typically, elevated free T_4 and T_3 and greatly suppressed TSH are found, but normal free T_4 can be seen in "T_3 toxicosis." Other laboratory features include normochromic, normocytic anemia, mild neutropenia, elevated liver enzymes and alkaline phosphatase, and mild hypercalcemia. Antithyroid antibodies, namely antithyroglobulin and antithyroid peroxidase, may be positive but are not specific to Graves disease. Thyroid stimulating immunoglobulins (TSI) are considered to be the antibodies specific to Graves disease and can be measured by bioassays or receptor assays (Costagliola et al., 1999).

Differential Diagnosis

Causes of hyperthyroidism are outlined in Table 50-4. Approximately 90%–95% of hyperthyroid pregnant women have Graves disease, and this can be diagnosed with certainty in a thyrotoxic pregnant woman who has diffuse thyromegaly with a bruit and ophthalmopathy. Whereas excess circulating thyroid hormones cause lid retraction and lid lag, proptosis and external ocular muscle palsies reflect infiltrative ophthalmopathy of Graves disease. Graves disease is an autoimmune disease mediated by antibodies (TSI) that activate the TSH receptor and stimulate the thyroid follicular cell. It is an extremely common disease in young women, affecting 3% of women of reproductive age (Varner, 1991). The treatment and course of Graves disease will be outlined first, followed by a discussion of other causes of hyperthyroidism in pregnancy.

Treatment

The outcome of treatment before pregnancy is better than that of treatment in pregnancy (Davis et al., 1989), and thus hyperthyroidism is best treated prior to conception. If untreated or treated inadequately, women may have more complications during pregnancy and delivery. Very mild cases of hyperthyroidism, with adequate weight gain and appropriate obstetric progress, may be followed carefully, but moderate or severe cases must be treated. In a retrospective study of 60 thyrotoxic pregnant women, preterm delivery, perinatal mortality, and maternal heart failure were significantly increased in women who remained thyrotoxic. Also, thyroid hormone status at delivery correlated directly with pregnancy outcome (Davis et al., 1989). In another study by Momotani and Ito (1991), hyperthyroidism at conception was associated with 25% abortion and 15% premature delivery versus 14% and 10%, respectively, in euthyroid patients.

Thionamide Therapy

This topic is reviewed by Mandel and Cooper (2001). The thionamides inhibit the iodination of thyroglobulin and thyroglobulin synthesis by competing with iodine for the enzyme

peroxidase. Propylthiouracil (PTU) is more frequently prescribed in the United States. Carbimazole (a drug metabolized to methimazole) and methimazole itself are used often in Europe and Canada. PTU (but not methimazole) also inhibits the conversion of T_4 to T_3. The goal of therapy is to control the hyperthyroidism without fetal or neonatal hypothyroidism (Momotani et al., 1986). Maternal free T_4 should be maintained in the high-normal range. PTU is given every 8 hours at doses of 100–150 mg (300–450 mg total daily dosage) according to thyrotoxicosis severity. The occasional patient may require higher doses such as 600 mg or more because the risk of uncontrolled maternal hyperthyroidism is greater than that of high-dose PTU (Davis et al., 1989). It could take 6–8 weeks for major clinical effects to manifest. Once the patient is euthyroid (as reflected by monthly free T_4 and free T_3), the dose of PTU should be tapered (for example, halved), with further reduction as the pregnancy progresses. In many patients, PTU can be discontinued by 32–36 weeks' gestation.

Maternal side effects of PTU treatment include rash (approximately 5%), pruritus, drug fever, hepatitis, a lupus-like syndrome, or bronchospasm. An alternative thionamide can be used, although cross-sensitivity occurs in 50%. Agranulocytosis, clearly the most serious side effect, develops in only 0.1%, especially occurring in older women and those receiving higher doses (Cooper, 1983). All patients experiencing fever or unexpected sore throat on therapy should discontinue the drug and have white blood count monitoring. Agranulocytosis is a contraindication to further thionamide therapy; the blood count gradually improves over days or weeks.

Methimazole is not used in the United States because of possible increased transplacental passage (though this is not supported by *in vitro* data [Mortimer et al., 1997]) and because of the risk of cutis aplasia, a scalp deformity (Milham and Elledge, 1972; Van Djike et al., 1987; Martinez-Frias et al., 1992). Although rare, there are also some reports of methimazole embryopathy, with choanal atresia, tracheoesophageal fistula, and facial anomalies (Johnsson et al., 1997; Clementi et al., 1999; Di Gianantonio et al., 2001).

In relation to the risk of antithyroid medications, the risks of untreated hyperthyroidism need to be considered. They appear to relate directly to the control and severity of the hyperthyroidism. In a study of hyperthyroid pregnant women, the odds ratio for low birth weight was 2.4 for those treated during pregnancy and 9.2 for those uncontrolled during pregnancy compared with a group who was euthyroid and remained so. Similarly, prematurity was more common in the hyperthyroid group, the odds ratio being 2.8 in the controlled group and 16.5 in the uncontrolled. Similar findings related to preeclampsia, with an odds ratio of 4.7 in the controlled group (Millar et al., 1994). This was confirmed by a more recent study (Phoojaroenchanachai et al., 2001). In other reports, a higher frequency of small-for-gestational age births, congestive heart failure, and stillbirths have been found (Davis et al., 1989; Mitsude et al., 1992). It is uncertain whether untreated Graves disease is associated with a higher frequency of congenital malformation (Momotani et al., 1984; Wing et al., 1994).

Infants of mothers receiving thionamides should be evaluated ultrasonographically for signs of hypothyroidism such as goiter, bradycardia, and intrauterine growth restriction. If needed, cordocentesis may be performed and fetal thyroid function determined; reference ranges have been reported (Thorpe-Beeston et al., 1991).

TABLE 50-4. ETIOLOGY OF HYPERTHYROIDISM IN PREGNANCY

1. Graves disease
2. Toxic adenoma
3. Toxic multinodular goiter
4. Hyperemesis gravidarum
5. Gestational trophoblastic disease
6. TSH-producing pituitary tumor
7. Metastatic follicular cell carcinoma
8. Exogenous T_4 and T_3
9. De Quervain (subacute) thyroiditis
10. Painless lymphocytic thyroiditis
11. Struma ovarii

TSH, Thyroid-stimulating hormone; T_3, L-triiodothyronine; T_4, L-thyroxine.

PLATE 20

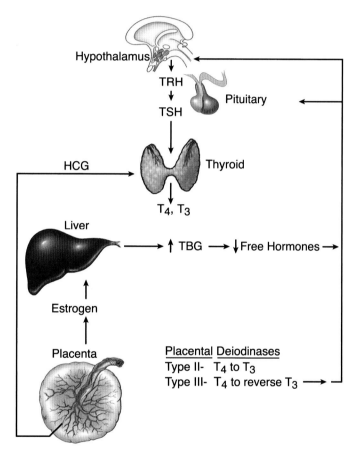

FIGURE 50-3 ■ Schematic representation of the physiologic adaptation to pregnancy showing increased thyroxine-binding globulin concentrations (TBG), increased human chorionic gonadotropin (hCG) with its thyrotropin-like activity, and alterations in peripheral metabolism of thyroid hormones in the placenta. TRH, thyrotropin releasing hormone; TSH, thyroid stimulating hormone. (Adapted from Glinoer D: What happens to the normal thyroid during pregnancy? Thyroid **9:**631, 1999.)

As regards lactation, PTU is not significantly concentrated in breast milk (10% of serum) and does not appear to affect the infant's thyroid hormone levels in any major way. Methimazole also does not appear to affect the child's subsequent somatic or intellectual growth in children exposed to it during lactation (Kampmann et al., 1980; Momotani et al., 1986; Azzizi, 1996). Antithyroid medication should be taken just after breast-feeding, allowing a 3- to 4-hour interval before she lactates again.

Beta-Blockers

These agents are useful for the control of adrenergic symptoms, and in particular maternal heart rate. Propranolol is commonly used in doses of 20–40 mg two or three times daily and also inhibits T_4 to T_3 conversion. Alternately, atenolol, 50–100 mg daily, may be used, and in an emergency esmolol, an ultra short-acting cardioselective intravenous beta-blocker, has been used successfully (Isley et al., 1990). Prolonged therapy with beta-blockers can potentially be associated with intrauterine growth restriction, fetal bradycardia, and hypoglycemia.

Iodides

Iodides decrease circulating T_4 and T_3 by up to 50% within 10 days by acutely inhibiting the release of stored hormone. Their use is appropriate in combination with thionamides (which should be started prior to the iodide) and beta-blockers in severe thyrotoxicosis or thyroid storm. Potassium iodide (SSKI), 5–10 drops twice daily, is given. Sodium ipodate, a radiographic contrast agent, is an alternative and has the added benefit of inhibiting T_4 to T_3 conversion; its safety in pregnancy has not been documented.

Because iodides cross the placenta readily, their use should be short-term (no longer than two weeks), or fetal goiter could result. Inadvertent use of iodides also follows use of betadine cleansing solutions, iodine-containing bronchodilators, and use of the drug amiodarone.

I_{131} thyroid ablation is of course contraindicated in pregnancy: The radioactive iodine is concentrated in the fetal thyroid after 10–12 weeks' gestation. Should a woman inadvertently receive I_{131} in pregnancy, SSKI should be given immediately, along with PTU, to block organification and reduce radiation exposure to the fetal thyroid by a factor of 100 and to the fetal whole body by a factor of 10. To be of benefit, SSKI and PTU treatment must be given within 7–10 days of exposure (Gorman, 1999).

Surgery

In select cases of thyrotoxicosis with severe complications or noncompliance, surgery can be performed in the pregnant patient. Two weeks of iodine therapy preoperatively will reduce gland vascularity. Surgery is best performed in the second trimester, although, if necessary, it can be done in the first or third trimester (Burrow, 1985). As usual, the risks are those of anesthesia, hypoparathyroidism, and recurrent laryngeal nerve paralysis.

Thyroid Storm

When labor and delivery, caesarean section, infection, or preeclampsia threaten to precipitate thyroid storm, combination therapy is indicated. This is achieved with PTU (given before iodide), beta-blockers, and SSKI, with attentive fluid management, nutritional support, and control of fever.

■ FETAL AND NEONATAL HYPERTHYROIDISM

This topic was recently reviewed by Zimmerman (1999). Fetal and neonatal hyperthyroidism are usually produced by transplacental passage of thyroid stimulating immunoglobulins (TSI). While commonly a component of active Graves disease, the antibodies can continue to be present in the maternal circulation after surgical (Fig. 50-5) or radioactive iodine ablation or even in Hashimoto's thyroiditis. Fetal hyperthyroidism occurs when TSIs cross the placenta and activate the fetal thyroid; it occurs in 1% of babies born to such women. Maternal TSI levels in excess of 300% of control values are predictive of fetal hyperthyroidism (Mitsuda et al., 1992) and should probably be measured at 28–30 weeks. The assay used should be a functional one, as TSH-receptor antibodies are heterogeneous and can either stimulate or block the TSH receptor (Clavel et al., 1990; Mitsuda et al., 1992). Neonatal syndromes have been described by transplacental passage of both stimulating and blocking antibodies (Zakarija et al., 1986).

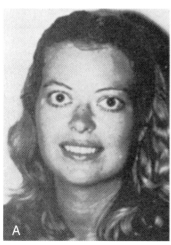
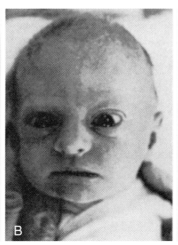
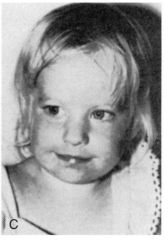

FIGURE 50-5 ■ A, Hypothyroid 21-year-old woman who developed Graves disease at age 7 and was treated by subtotal thyroidectomy. She was given maintenance therapy with thyroid hormone (Synthyroid) 0.15 mg throughout pregnancy. **B,** Her daughter was born at term with severe Graves disease, goiter, and exophthalmos that persisted for 6 months. **C,** The child was normal at age 20 months.

Fetal Thyrotoxicosis

Fetal features include a heart rate greater than 160 beats/minute, growth retardation, advanced bone age, and craniosynostosis, all of which can be detected by ultrasound examination (Becks and Burrow, 1991). Occasionally, nonimmune fetal hydrops and fetal death occur with associated diminished subcutaneous fat and thyroid enlargement. *In utero*, most cases are likely treated by the PTU given to the mother. This problem can arise if the mother is euthyroid but has elevated TSIs (Houck et al., 1988). Cordocentesis can be used for diagnosis and for monitoring therapy. A combination of PTU and T_4 treat the fetal hyperthyroidism while keeping the mother euthyroid.

Neonatal Thyrotoxicosis

Features in the neonate include hyperkinesis, diarrhea, poor weight gain, vomiting, exophthalmos, arrhythmias, cardiac failure, hypertension (both systemic and pulmonary), hepatosplenomegaly, thrombocytopenia, and craniosynostosis. The baby should be examined immediately after birth. Cord blood will reflect the *in utero* environment, and by day two of life, the maternal antithyroid drug effects will have receded. Affected neonates are treated with PTU, beta-blockers, iodine, and, as needed, glucocorticoids and digoxin. Ipodate could be preferable, as it blocks T_4 to T_3 conversion. Remission by 20 weeks is most common and nearly always occurs by 48 weeks; occasionally, there is persistent disease where there is a strong family history of Graves disease.

Other mechanisms of fetal and neonatal hyperthyroidism include activating mutations of the stimulatory G protein in McCune-Albright syndrome and activating mutations of the TSH receptor (Yoshimoto et al., 1991; Kopp et al., 1995).

HYPERTHYROIDISM RELATED TO hCG

When hyperthyroidism is diagnosed during the first trimester, the physician has a challenging differential diagnosis, usually that of Graves disease versus hCG-mediated hyperthyroidism. As indicated in an earlier section, hCG has TSH-like stimulatory activity, which could result in overproduction of thyroid hormone when the concentrations are high or when there is a change in its molecular structure. Molecular variants of hCG with increased thyrotropic potency include basic molecules with reduced sialic acid content, truncated molecules lacking the C-terminal tail, or molecules in which the 47–48 peptide bond in the β-subunit loop is nicked (Hershman, 1999). This relationship is further complicated by differences in hCG clearance rates of different hCG glycoforms (Talbot et al., 2001). The *in vivo* thyrotopic activity is regulated by both the glycoforms and the plasma half-life.

Human chorionic gonadotropin concentrations peak at 6–12 weeks and then decline to a plateau after 18–20 weeks. The stimulation of thyroid hormone production can suppress the TSH to low or suppressed values in up to 20% of normal pregnancies. Twin pregnancies could be associated with biochemical hyperthyroidism (Grün et al., 1997), as may pregnancies complicated by trophoblastic disease. Several clinical scenarios can arise and are briefly described as follows.

Gestational Transient Thyrotoxicosis (GTT)

Gestational transient thyrotoxicosis occurs in the first trimester in women without a personal or family history of autoimmune disease. It results directly from hCG stimulation of the thyroid. Glinoer and colleagues (1993) found an overall prevalence of GTT in 2.4% in a prospective cohort study between the eighth and 14th week of gestation. Symptoms compatible with thyrotoxicosis were often present, and elevated free T_4 concentrations were found. The GTT was transient, paralleled the decline in hCG, and usually did not require treatment. The thyroid gland was not enlarged. Occasionally, beta-blockers were used. GTT was not associated with a less favorable outcome of pregnancy.

Hyperemesis Gravidarum

Hyperemesis gravidarum is a serious pregnancy complication associated with weight loss and severe dehydration, often necessitating hospitalization (Bashiri et al., 1995). Biochemical hyperthyroidism is found in most women with this condition (Goodwin et al., 1992a, 1992b). Whereas the latter authors found that the severity of disease varied directly with the hCG concentration, Wilson and associates (1992) did not find such a correlation. As in the case of GTT, certain hCG fractions could be more important than total hCG as thyroid stimulators (Pekary et al., 1993). The duration of the hyperthyroidism varies widely from 1–10 weeks but is usually self-limited. Vomiting and normalization of T_4 occur by 20 weeks, though TSH may remain suppressed a little longer. Treatment is usually supportive, with correction of dehydration, antiemetics and, occasionally, parenteral nutrition. The vomiting may not be controlled by normalization of thyroid hormones. In patients who require treatment, PTU therapy can be attempted if tolerated; methimazole suppositories can also be used.

Gestational Trophoblastic Disease

Both hydatidiform mole and choriocarcinoma can be associated with hCG levels that are greater than 1000 times normal and thus can cause hyperthyroidism (biochemically seen in approximately 50% of such women). The thyroid is usually not enlarged. Treatment of the hydatidiform mole or choriocarcinoma restores thyroid function to normal. Treatment with antithyroid drugs and beta-blockers is frequently necessary, however, before surgical treatment of the mole (Morgan, 1990).

Recurrent Gestational Hyperthyroidism

Cases of recurrent gestational hyperthyroidism have also been described (Nader and Mastrobattista, 1996; Rodien et al., 1998). In the case described by Rodien and colleages, the hyperthyroidism was caused by a mutant TSH receptor that was hypersensitive to hCG.

Other Causes of Hyperthyroidism

Other much less common causes of hyperthyroidism include thyrotoxicosis factitia (ingestion of exogenous hormone surreptitiously); in such cases serum thyroglobulin, which is produced by the thyroid, is suppressed (Mariotti et al., 1982). Women with large nodular goiters may have hyperthyroidism from autonomously functioning nodules within such goiters. Alternatively, women can have hyperthyroidism from a single toxic adenoma. If either of these entities is diagnosed during pregnancy, the correct treatment is control of hyperthyroidism with antithyroid drugs until definitive treatment (either surgery or radioactive iodine) can be administered postpartum.

Other, even less common, causes of hyperthyroidism in pregnancy are listed in Table 50-4 and include TSH-producing pituitary tumors, metastatic follicular thyroid cancer, viral (de Quervain) thyroiditis, and struma ovarii—an ovarian dermoid tumor in which more than 50% of the neoplasm consists of thyroid tissue.

IODINE DEFICIENCY, HYPOTHYROIDISM, AND PREGNANCY

A schematic representation of the clinical conditions that can affect thyroid function in the mother, fetus, or fetomaternal unit is shown in Figure 50-6.

Iodine Deficiency

Although rare in the United States, iodine deficiency is a common cause of maternal, fetal, and neonatal hypothyroidism in the world, where 1–1.5 billion are at risk and 500 million live in areas of overt iodine deficiency. Worldwide, it is, sadly, the most common cause of mental retardation. In the last few decades, the physiology of maternal and fetal iodine, thyroid hormone metabolism, and fetal brain development, as well as the pathophysiology of iodine deficiency, have

been unraveled. These findings have revealed a fascinating aspect of pregnancy physiology and will be reviewed here briefly, in part because of the lessons we have learned and mainly because it continues to be a worldwide problem worthy of resolution. This topic also has been a subject of numerous reviews (Lazarus, 1999b; Glinoer, 2001; Dunn and Delange, 2001; Delange et al., 2001). Even in the United States, iodine intake has declined, and 15% of women of childbearing age and 7% of pregnant women were recently found to have urinary iodine excretions below 50 μg/L, indicative of moderate iodine deficiency (Hollowell et al., 1998).

Pregnancy is an environmental trigger to the thyroid machinery, inducing changes in certain geographic areas that have iodine deficiency. Four biochemical markers are useful markers of the changes induced:

1. Relative hypothyroxinemia
2. Preferential T_3 secretion as reflected by an elevated T_3/T_4 molar ratio
3. Increased TSH after the first trimester, progressively till term
4. Supranormal thyroglobulin concentrations correlating with gestational goitrogenesis

Goitrogenesis also occurs in the fetus, indicating the exquisite sensitivity of the fetal thyroid gland to the consequences of maternal iodine deficiency. This process can start during the earliest stages of fetal thyroid development. All this occurs on a background of low initial maternal intrathyroidal iodine stores, the increased need for iodine once pregnancy occurs, and the insufficiency of iodine intake throughout the gestation.

It appears that maternal thyroxine, traversing the placenta during the first trimester and subsequently, is necessary for fetal brain development. Even before fetal thyroid hormone synthesis, T_3 receptors are found in fetal brain tissues, and local conversion of T_4 to T_3 can occur. Iodine deficiency perpetuates the process, as the fetus, too, is less able to synthesize thyroid hormones even when the fetal thyroid has developed.

In severe iodine deficiency (intake 20–25 μg/day), a condition known as endemic cretinism (with prevalence up to 15% in severely affected populations) occurs. These infants are characterized by severe mental retardation with a neurological picture including deaf-mutism, squint, and pyramidal and extrapyramidal syndromes. There are few clinical signs of thyroid failure as such. A remarkable exception to this picture has emerged from Africa, where the cretins have less mental retardation and less in the way of neurological deficits. The clinical picture is that of severe thyroid failure with dwarfism, delayed sexual maturation, and myxedema. Thyroid function is grossly impaired.

The present consensus is that the neurologic picture of endemic cretinism results from insults to the developing brain, occurring perhaps during the first trimester (in the case of deafness) and mostly during the second trimester, with the cerebellar abnormalities resulting from postnatal insult. This is supported by the observation that the full picture can only be prevented when the iodine deficiency is corrected before the second trimester and, optimally, even before conception (Pharoah et al., 1971). The pattern found in Africa is explained by the fact that in Africa, iodine deficiency is complicated by selenium deficiency. The deficiency of selenium leads to accumulation of peroxide, and excess peroxide leads to destruction of thyroid cells and hypothyroidism (Vanderpas et al., 1990).

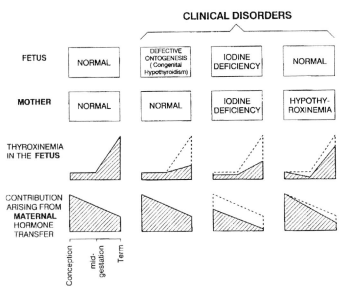

CLINICAL DISORDERS

FIGURE 50-6 ■ Schematic representation of the three sets of clinical conditions that can affect thyroid function in the mother alone, in the fetus alone, or in the fetomaternal unit, showing the relative contributions of an impaired maternal and/or fetal thyroid function that may eventually lead to alterations in fetal thyroxinemia. (Reprinted by permission from Glinoer D, Delange F: The potential repercussions of maternal, fetal and neonatal hypothyroxinemia on the progeny. Thyroid **10**:871, 2000.)

Selenium deficiency also induces monodeiodinase-I (a seleno enzyme) deficiency, resulting in reduced T_4 to T_3 conversion and therefore, in turn, increased availability of maternal T_4 for the fetal brain. Such a protective mechanism may prevent the development of neurologic cretinism, and the combined iodine-selenium deficiency prevalent in Africa could help explain the predominance of the myxedematous type observed in Africa.

Thus, the neurological abnormalities and mental retardation depend ultimately on the timing and severity of the brain insult. Endemic cretinism constitutes only the extreme expression of the spectrum of physical and intellectual abnormalities. In a meta-analysis of 18 studies in areas of iodine deficiency, this appeared to be responsible for an IQ loss of 13.5 points (Bleichrodt and Born, 1994). Even borderline iodine deficiency, as seen in Europe, could be accompanied by impaired school achievements in apparently normal children as reviewed by Glinoer (2001). Actions taken to eradicate iodine deficiency have prevented the occurrence of mental retardation in millions of infants throughout the world. In a study by Xue-Yi and coauthors (1994), in a severely iodine-deficient area of the Xinjiang region of China, iodine was administered to pregnant women. The prevalence of moderate or severe neurologic abnormalities among 120 infants whose mothers received iodine in the first or second trimester was 2% compared to 9% (of 952 infants) when the mothers received iodine in the third trimester ($P = 0.008$). Although treatment in the third trimester did not improve neurologic status, head growth and developmental quotients improved slightly. Finally, the importance of thyroid hormone to fetal and neonatal well being and development was highlighted by a remarkable case of a baby born to a mother with strongly positive TSH receptor-blocking antibodies. The mother was profoundly hypothyroid when tested after delivery. The baby was delivered by cesarean section because of bradycardia. She was also profoundly hypothyroid and required intubation. Her brain size was reduced, and her auditory brain stem response was absent at age 2 months. The audiogram at age 4 revealed sensorineural deafness. At age 6 years, motor development was the same as at age 4 months. She required T_4 for 8 months until the antibody effect had worn off. Her physical growth was normal. Thus the outcome of severe thyroid hormone deficiency *in utero* was fetal distress, permanent auditory deficit, brain atrophy, and severely impaired neuromotor development despite adequate neonatal treatment (Yasuda et al., 1999).

Currently, the Institute of Medicine of the National Academy of Sciences has set iodine requirement as 110 μg for infants 0–6 months, 130 μg for infants 7–12 months, 90 μg for children 1–8 years, 120 μg for those 9–13 years, and 150 μg for those older than 13. The recommended intake for pregnancy and lactation is 200 μg/day.

■ HYPOTHYROIDISM

Signs and Symptoms

Hypothyroidism is said to occur with a frequency of 1 in 1600–2000 deliveries (Montoro, 1997). Population screening studies have revealed a higher incidence, however. In a study in the United States, serum TSH was determined in 2000 women between gestational weeks 15–18; 49 (2.5%) had TSH levels greater than or equal to 6 mU/L, and positive thyroid antibodies were found in 58% of these 49 women compared with 11% of control euthyroid pregnant women (Klein et al., 1991). In a Japanese study, however, only 0.29% had an elevated TSH (Kamijo et al., 1990). In another U.S. study, 1 case out of 1629 deliveries had hypothyroidism (Leung et al., 1993). Women with hypothyroidism have higher pregnancy complication rates. As well as miscarriages, these include preeclampsia, placental abruption, low birth weight, prematurity, and stillbirths (Davis et al., 1988). These outcomes can be improved with early therapy. Gestational hypertension is also more common (Leung et al., 1993).

The symptoms of hypothyroidism are insidious and can be masked by the hypermetabolic state of pregnancy. Symptoms can include modest weight gain, decrease in exercise capacity, lethargy, and intolerance to cold. In moderately symptomatic patients, constipation, hoarseness, hair loss, brittle nails, and dry skin also can occur. Physical signs may include a goiter, a thyroidectomy scar, and delay in the relaxation phase of deep tendon reflexes.

Laboratory confirmation is obtained from an elevated TSH, with or without suppressed free T_4. Positive thyroid autoantibodies may also be found (antithyroglobulin and antithyroid peroxidase). Other laboratory abnormalities can include elevated creatine phosphokinase, cholesterol, carotene, and liver function abnormalities. Macrocytic or normochromic, normocytic anemia can also be seen. Hypothyroidism may occur more frequently in pregnant women with type I diabetes, and T_4 replacement therapy can increase insulin requirements (Jovanovic-Peterson and Peterson, 1988).

Differential Diagnosis

Hashimoto's thyroiditis, also known as chronic lymphocytic thyroiditis, an autoimmune disease, is the most common cause of hypothyroidism and can occur in 8%–10% of women of reproductive age. It is characterized by the presence of antithyroid antibodies, and a goiter can be present. Titers of antithyroglobulin are elevated in 50%–70% of patients, and almost all have antithyroid peroxidase antibodies (Weetman and McGregor, 1984). The goiter is firm and diffusely enlarged and painless, and the gland is infiltrated by lymphocytes and plasma cells. Many patients with Hashimoto's thyroiditis are actually euthyroid but can subsequently develop hypothyroidism. The thyroid gland can also be atrophic and the antibodies negative—so-called idiopathic hypothyroidism. Patients with other autoimmune disease also can develop Hashimoto's thyroiditis.

Other important and common causes of hypothyroidism include post-I_{131} ablation for Graves disease and post-thyroidectomy (for thyroid cancer, for example). Of patients who receive I_{131}, 10%–20% are hypothyroid within the first 6 months, and 2%–4% become hypothyroid each year thereafter (Werner, 1977). Hypothyroidism also can result from subacute viral thyroiditis and, much less commonly, from suppurative thyroiditis.

Drugs known to inhibit the synthesis of thyroid hormones include thionamide therapy, iodides, and lithium. Carbamazepine, phenytoin, and rifampin can increase thyroid clearance. Aluminum hydroxide, cholestyramine, and, most important, ferrous sulfate and sucrafate, can interfere with the intestinal absorption of thyroxine.

Hypothyroidism secondary to hypothalamic or pituitary disease is rare but can occur in the setting of pituitary tumors, secondary to pituitary surgery or irradiation, and in Sheehan's syndrome and lymphocytic hypophysitis, an autoimmune disease with a predilection for women, especially in the setting of pregnancy (see Chapter 51). In secondary hypothyroidism, the TSH could be low or normal, but the free T_4 is low.

Treatment of Hypothyroidism

Hypothyroidism must be treated promptly, and a dose of T_4, 0.1–0.15 mg/day, should be initiated. The dose is adjusted every 4 weeks until the TSH is in the lower end of the normal range. Women who are euthyroid, on T_4, in early pregnancy, need to be rechecked every 8 weeks or so, as the requirements for thyroid hormone increase during pregnancy. In a study of 12 pregnant women with hypothyroidism, 9 required a higher T_4 dose, with a mean dose increase of 45% (Mandel et al., 1990). In a review of 77 pregnancies in 65 hypothyroid women, serum TSH became abnormal in 70% of women with prior I_{131} ablation therapy and in 47% of women with chronic thyroiditis. When data from other studies were pooled, overall, TSH increased above normal in 45%, with a mean daily thyroxine dose of 146 μg (Kaplan, 1992; Kaplan, 1996). It was estimated that the increment in dose could be predicted according to the TSH value at first evaluation. TSH should be redetermined 4–6 weeks after dose adjustment.

The causes of increased T_4 requirements include a real increased demand for T_4 in pregnancy (Mestman, 1999) in patients whose thyroid reserve is compromised, and also, in some cases, iron therapy. Ferrous sulfate interferes with T_4 absorption and should be taken at a different time of day from thyroxine therapy (Brent, 1999). Patients with thyroid cancer whose target TSH is below the normal range will almost uniformly require an increased dose to maintain their suppressed TSH and should be followed closely (Brent, 1999). After delivery, the dose should be reduced to prepregnancy levels, and TSH should be measured 6–8 weeks later.

The topic of thyroid hormone and intellectual development has received widespread publicity and has been the topic of papers and reviews in the past few years (Haddow et al., 1999; Lazarus, 1999b; Klein and Mitchell, 1999). In 1969, Man and Jones studied a cohort of 1349 children and concluded that mild maternal hypothyroidism alone was associated with lower IQ levels in the offspring. In 1990, Matsuura and Konishi documented that fetal brain development is affected adversely when both mother and fetus have hypothyroidism caused by chronic autoimmune thyroiditis. With the background of this information and the association between iodine deficiency, its consequent maternal hypothyroxinemia, and abnormal fetal brain development, Haddow and associates (1999) conducted a study measuring TSH from stored samples in more than 25,000 pregnant women. They located 62 women with high TSH and 124 matched women with normal values. Their 7- to 9-year-old children, none of whom had hypothyroidism as newborns, underwent 15 tests relating to intelligence, attention, language, reading ability, school performance, and visual-motor performance. The full-scale IQ in children of hypothyroid women was 4 points lower ($P = 0.06$); 15% had scores of 85% or less compared with 5% of controls. The IQ of the children of 48 women whose hypothyroidism was not treated averaged 7 points lower than the

124 controls ($P = 0.005$), and 19% had scores of 85 or lower. The researchers concluded that undiagnosed hypothyroidism can affect fetuses adversely and recommended screening for hypothyroidism in pregnancy. Fukushi and coworkers (1999) reported on such screening in Japan and found hypothyroidism in one out of 692 pregnancies. Proposals for screening have emerged (Klein and Mitchell, 1999; Morreale de Escobar et al., 2000), including a position statement from the American Association of Clinical Endocrinologists (Gharib et al., 1999). This statement recommended the following guidelines:

1. Routine TSH measurements before or in early pregnancy are reasonable.
2. TSH should be determined in all pregnant women with goiter, positive thyroid antibodies, personal history of autoimmune disease, and family history of thyroid disease.
3. Thyroxine should be administered promptly even if the TSH elevation is mild.
4. Women on thyroxine therapy should be monitored during pregnancy.

In a study by Pop and colleagues (1995), even the presence of antithyroid peroxidase antibodies in the maternal circulation was shown to have deleterious effects on child development. The pathophysiology of this finding was hard to explain, but in two other similar studies, thyroid antibody-positive women had lower free T_4 levels, and lower scores on psychomotor tests were found in children of mothers whose free T_4 was below the fifth and tenth percentiles as measured at 12 weeks' gestation (Lazarus et al., 1998; Pop et al., 1999).

FETAL AND NEONATAL HYPOTHYROIDISM

The relationship between iodine deficiency and fetal development has already been discussed. Severe neurologic deficits also occur in children with congenital deficiency of thyroid hormone unrelated to iodine deficiency. Neurologic development is impaired if they are untreated before 3 months of postnatal age. Screening of neonates for thyroid hormone deficiency is mandatory in some states, and with early therapy, their development is reasonably normal (Fisher and Polk, 1989). Causes include thyroid agenesis and inborn errors of metabolism, such as peroxidase deficiency. Congenital pituitary and hypothalamic hypothyroidism also occur but are rare. Thyroid hormone deficiency can also result from maternal blocking antibodies that are transferred to the fetus and block TSH action and/or thyroid growth and development (Dussault and Rousseau, 1987; Bogner et al., 1989).

Gruner and associates (2001) reported on a case of fetal goitrous hypothyroidism in which fetal TSH was determined on three occasions by cordocentesis to monitor weekly intra-amniotic administration of T_4. This therapy was initiated to reduce the fetal goiter and polyhydramnios (which it did) and to aid in fetal neurologic development. They also reviewed other reported cases of such therapy and concluded that the optimal dose of T_4 necessary to correct hypothyroidism could more accurately be determined by cordocentesis than by measurement of amniotic fluid hormone concentrations.

THYROID NODULES, MALIGNANT TUMORS, AND NONTOXIC GOITER IN PREGNANCY

Thyroid tumors are the most common endocrine neoplasms. The majority of these nodules are benign hyperplastic (or colloid) nodules, but between 5% and 20% are true neoplasms, either benign follicular adenomas or carcinomas of follicular or parafollicular (C) cell origin. Nodular thyroid disease is common. When a solitary or a dominant nodule is found within the thyroid, biopsy is recommended. Cytopathologic diagnosis of fine needle aspiration biopsy (FNAB) in women aged 15–40 seen at the Mayo Clinic revealed benign findings in 64% and suspicious findings in 12%; FNAB was positive for cancer in 7% and nondiagnostic in 17% (Hay, 1999). The topic of nodular thyroid disease in pregnancy was also reviewed. During a ten-year period, 40 pregnant women were evaluated at the Mayo Clinic, and 39 had FNAB, 95% of which were diagnostic (Tan et al., 1996). The majority (64%) were benign. Three (8%) were positive for papillary thyroid cancer, and nine (23%) were suspicious for papillary cancer or follicular/Hurthle cell neoplasm. Comparable findings were reported by others (Marley and Oertel, 1997). The principles of nodular thyroid disease diagnosis in pregnancy resemble those for nonpregnant women. Serum TSH and free T_4 should be obtained, and an FNAB should be performed on dominant nodules. Radionucleotide scanning is contraindicated, but ultrasound is often performed and could demonstrate other nodules, lymphadenopathy, or abnormal calcification. FNAB is safe in pregnancy and can be performed at any stage. If a nodule is benign, ultrasound can monitor growth of the nodule in pregnancy. If the nodule is suspicious for follicular or Hurthle cell neoplasm, this usually represents a 10%–15% risk of malignancy. It is generally recommended that surgery be performed postpartum, but if a malignancy is diagnosed in early pregnancy, surgery may be performed in the second trimester in the patient needing reassurance. If the FNAB is positive or suspicious for papillary thyroid cancer, the risk is high (50% for suspicious and 100% for positive), and neck exploration should be performed at the soonest safe date. Figure 50-7 outlines the decisionmaking process.

The impact of pregnancy on papillary thyroid cancer was evaluated by Moosa and Mazzaferri (1977). They compared outcomes in pregnant versus nonpregnant women and found no difference in the rates of recurrence, distant spread, or cause-specific mortality. Outcomes were similar when neck surgery was performed during or after pregnancy. A similar conclusion was reached from a study of thyroid cancer cases from the New Mexico Tumor Registry (Herzon et al., 1994). If medullary thyroid cancer is suspected, early surgery is advised.

POSTPARTUM THYROID DISEASE

Autoimmune thyroid disease, which is suppressed during pregnancy, is exacerbated in the postpartum period. New-onset autoimmune thyroid disease occurs in up to 10% of all postpartum women (Davies, 1999). Up to 60% of Graves patients in the reproductive years give a history of postpartum onset (Janssen, 1987). Most of the immune changes of pregnancy gradually return to normal in the 12-month postpartum period.

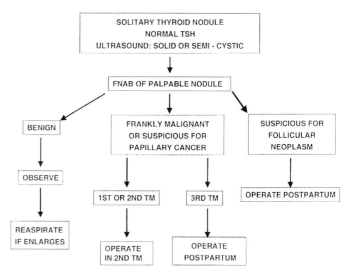

FIGURE 50-7. ■ Evaluation of a solitary thyroid nodule in pregnancy. (Adapted from Tan GH, Gharib H, Goellner JR, et al: Management of thyroid nodules in pregnancy. Arch Intern Med **156**:2317, 1996. *Copyright © 1996, American Medical Association.* All rights reserved.)

As opposed to pregnancy, the major immune changes in T and B cells in the postpartum period are overall T-cell deactivation, enhanced Th_1-type T-cell function, loss of tolerance for fetal alloantigens, enhanced IgG secretion, and autoantibody secretion. Possible mechanisms explaining postpartum autoimmune exacerbation suggested by Davies (1999) include (1) reduced number of fetal cells leading to loss of maternal tolerance to remaining microchimeric cells and (2) loss of placental major histocompatibility complex-peptide complexes, which were inducing T-cell anergy during pregnancy.

Postpartum Graves Disease

The onset of Graves disease postpartum correlates with the development of thyroid stimulating immunoglobulins. Peak antibody production is observed 3–6 months postpartum. Almost all patients with persisting TSI at the end of pregnancy will develop recurrence of Graves if antithyroid drugs are withdrawn. The prevalence of postpartum Graves, which can be either transient or persistent, is estimated at 11% of those with postpartum thyroid dysfunction (Amino et al., 1999).

Postpartum Thyroiditis (PPT)

The topic of postpartum thyroidits (PPT) has been the focus of numerous reviews (Amino et al., 1999; Davies, 1999; Lazarus 1999a; Lucas et al., 2000; Stagnaro-Green, 2000). For the diagnosis of PPT, there must be a documented abnormal TSH (suppressed or elevated) during the first postpartum year in the absence of positive thyroid stimulating immunoglobulins (thus excluding Graves) or a toxic nodule.

Classically, PPT presents with a transient hyperthyroid phase 6 weeks to 6 months postpartum. A hypothyroid phase follows and can last up to one year postpartum. Figure 50-8 schematically demonstrates this and the accompanying changes in serum thyroid antibody concentrations. A review of 11 studies of PPT (Stagnaro-Green, 1993) revealed that only 26% of patients presented in this classic manner. Most patients present with hyperthyroidism alone (38%) or hypothyroidism alone (36%). The incidence of PPT is 6%–9%. It is an auto-

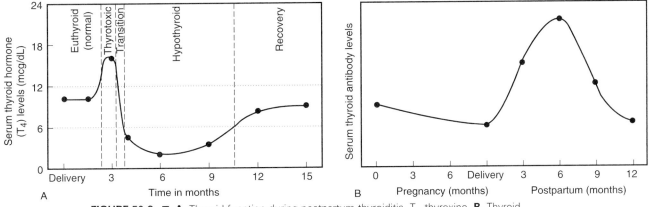

FIGURE 50-8. ■ **A,** Thyroid function during postpartum thyroiditis. T₄, thyroxine. **B,** Thyroid antibody levels during and after pregnancy. (From Smallridge RC, Fein HC, Hayship CC: Postpartum thyroiditis. Bridge **3**:3, 1988. Newsletter of the Thyroid Foundation of America, Inc.)

immune disorder, and, not surprisingly, patients with type I diabetes have an increased incidence, approximately 25% in two North American studies (Gerstein, 1993; Alvarez-Marfany et al., 1994). Women with a history of previous PPT in a prior pregnancy had a 69% recurrence rate in the subsequent pregnancy.

Symptoms of the hyperthyroid phase of PPT include fatigue, palpitations, heat intolerance, and nervousness. This destructive hyperthyroid phase always has a limited duration (a few weeks to a few months). Although beta-blockers may reduce symptoms, antithyroid medications have no role to play.

The hypothyroid phase can be marked by fatigue, hair loss, depression, impairment of concentration, and dry skin. The hypothyroid phase frequently requires treatment, but it is reasonable to wean the patient off therapy 6 months following initiation. Some recommend maintaining T₄ therapy in such patients until the childbearing years are over, and then attempting to wean her off the therapy a year after the last delivery.

The thyroid gland is enlarged in PPT, and thyroid hypoechogenicity appears to be the characteristic ultrasonographic finding (Adams et al., 1992). As indicated previously, PPT is an autoimmune disorder, and there is an association between it and HLA-DR3, HLA-DR4, and HLA-DR5 status. There is lymphocytic infiltration similar to that seen in Hashimoto's thyroiditis. Stagnaro-Green (2000) reported that 33% of women who were antithyroid antibody-positive in the first trimester of pregnancy experienced PPT, in comparison with 3% of women who were antibody-negative.

The laboratory hallmarks of PPT, which is a destructive process, are positive antithyroid antibodies (antithyroglobulin and antithyroid peroxidase), suppressed TSH, and high T₄ (released from destroyed thyroid cells) in the hyperthyroid phase, along with a profoundly suppressed radioactive iodine uptake (contraindicated in a breast-feeding woman). The absence of TSI usually rules out Graves disease, which can also be distinguished by high radioactive iodine uptake.

Depression and Postpartum Thyroiditis

Both depression and postpartum thyroiditis are common postpartum events (Pedersen, 1999). Four large-scale studies have been performed to evaluate their association. Harris and colleagues (1989) evaluated 147 women (65 thyroid antibody-positive, 82 negative) at 6–8 weeks postpartum for thyroid

status and depression. Although there was a positive correlation between postpartum thyroiditis and postpartum depression, there was no association between antibody positivity and depression. Pop and associates (1991) evaluated 293 women during the third trimester and then every 6 weeks up to 34 weeks postpartum. They found that 38% of women with postpartum thyroiditis experienced depression compared with 9.5% of women in a matched control group, and the difference was highly significant. Status of antibodies was not reported. Harris and coauthors (1992) again investigated this association in 232 women (110 thyroid antibody-positive). The women had psychiatric assessment five times during the first 28 weeks postpartum. No association was found between PPT and depression, but an association was found between depression and antibody-positivity. They concluded that 4% of women will experience postpartum depression that has an autoimmune etiology. Pop and colleagues (1993) performed a further analysis of the same 293 women in their earlier study; antibody status was determined during the pregnancy, but only a slight increased association between the presence of antibody and depression was found, and they concluded that antibody status during pregnancy was an important predictor of PPT but not of depression. In a subsequent study, Pop and associates (1998) reported an association between thyroid antibodies and depression in postmenopausal women. In summary, the data suggest some association between PPT, thyroid antibodies, and depression. Of the four clinical trials, two demonstrated an association between PPT and depression, while two demonstrated an association between thyroid antibodies and depression. The role of potential interventions such as T₄ therapy has not been evaluated systematically.

Hypothyroidism

Recovery of thyroid function in women with PPT is not universal, and some women remain permanently hypothyroid. In a study of 44 women with PPT with a mean follow-up of 8.7 years postpartum, Tachi and associates (1988) reported that 77% of the women recovered during the first postpartum year and remained euthyroid. In the other 23%, permanent hypothyroidism developed; half of these never recovered euthyroid function after the initial postpartum insult, while the other half developed hypothyroidism during the years of follow-up. A 23% incidence of permanent hypothyroidism at long-term follow-up (mean 3.5 years) was also reported by Othman and coworkers (1990). It is recommended that women with a history of PPT be evaluated annually for the possible development of hypothyroidism.

Post-abortion Thyroiditis

Several studies have described cases of thyroiditis occurring after an abortion (Stagnaro-Green, 1992; Marqusee et al., 1997). Neither the incidence nor clinical sequelae are known. In the case of Stagnaro-Green (1992), the patient developed transient hypothyroidism following a spontaneous miscarriage. Following a subsequent full-term delivery, the patient became severely hypothyroid, and this condition remained permanent.

Prevention and Screening of Postpartum Thyroiditis

Levothyroxine (0.1 mg daily) or iodide (0.15 mg daily) were administered for 40 weeks postpartum in women who were thyroid antibody-positive during pregnancy. A control group of antibody-negative women received no treatment. The incidence of PPT was similar in all three groups, and the degree of postpartum elevation of thyroid peroxidase antibodies was indistinguishable in the three groups (Kampe et al., 1990).

Whether screening for PPT is worthwhile is a contentious issue. A recent "Therapeutic Controversy" in the Journal of Clinical Endocrinology and Metabolism addressed this topic (Amino et al., 1999). Arguments for and against screening were presented. It was suggested that screening and treatment of symptomatic hypothyroidism would improve the quality of life of the mother, and the importance of recognizing postpartum depression was stressed. Counter-arguments were that the optimal screening strategy was as yet undefined and that no cost-benefit analysis has been performed. It is agreed that women who present with symptoms should have a TSH performed. In addition, high-risk women (women with a history of PPT and women with type I diabetes) should be screened (Alvarez-Marfany et al., 1994; Weetman, 1994).

REFERENCES

Abdoul-Khair SA, Crooks J, Turnbull AC, et al: The physiological changes in thyroid function during pregnancy. Clin Sci 27:195, 1964.

Adams H, Jones MC, Othman S, et al: The sonographic appearances in postpartum thyroiditis. Clin Radiol 145:311, 1992.

Ain KB, Mori Y, Refetoff F: Reduced clearance rate of thyroxine-binding globulin (TBG) with increased sialylation: A mechanism for estrogen induced elevation of serum TBG concentration. J Clin Endocrinol Metab 65:689, 1987.

Akande EO, Hockaday TD: Plasma estrogen and luteinizing hormone concentrations in thyrotoxic menstrual disturbances. Proc R Soc Med 65:789, 1972.

Alvarez-Marfany M, Roman SH, Drexler AJ, et al: Long-term prospective study of postpartum thyroid dysfunction in women with insulin dependent diabetes mellitus. J Clin Endocrinol 79:10, 1994.

Amino N, Tada H, Hidaka Y: Postpartum autoimmune thyroid syndrome: A model of aggravation of autoimmune disease. Thyroid 9:705, 1999.

Anselmo J, Kay T, Dennis K, et al: Resistance to thyroid hormone does not abrogate the transient thyrotoxicosis associated with gestation: Report of a case. J Clin Endocrinol Metab 86:4273, 2001.

Azzizi F: Effect of methimazole treatment of maternal thyrotoxicosis on thyroid function in breast-feeding infants. J Pediatr 128:855, 1996.

Ballard RA, Ballard PL, Creast RK, et al. Respiratory disease in very-low-birthweight infants after prenatal thyrotropin-releasing hormone and glucocorticoid. Lancet 339:510, 1992.

Bartalena L, Bogazzi F, Braverman LE, et al: Effect of amiadarone administration during pregnancy on neonatal thyroid function and subsequent neurodevelopment. J Endocrinol Invest 24:116, 2001.

Bashiri A, Neumann L, Maymon E, et al: Hyperemesis gravidarum: Epidemiologic features, complications and outcome. Eur J Obstet Gynecol Reprod Biol 63:135, 1995.

Bech K, Hoier-Madsen M, Feldt-Rasmussen U, et al: Thyroid function and autoimmune manifestations in insulin-dependent diabetes mellitus during and after pregnancy. Acta Endocrinol (Copenh) 124:324, 1991.

Beckers C: Iodine economy in and around pregnancy. In Beckers C, Reinwein D (eds): The Thyroid and Pregnancy. New York, John Wiley and Sons, 1992.

Becks GP, Burrow G: Thyroid disease and pregnancy. Med Clin North Am 75:121, 1991.

Berlin L: Malpractice issues in radiology. Iodine I_{131} and the pregnant patient. Am J Radiol 176:869, 2001.

Bernal J, Perkonen F: Ontogenesis of the nuclear 3, 5, 3'-triiodothyronine receptor in the human fetal brain. Endocrinology 114:677, 1984.

Bleichrodt N, Born MP: A meta-analysis of research on iodine and its relationship to cognitive development. In Stanbury JB (ed): The Damaged Brain of Iodine Deficiency. New York, Cognizant Communication, 1994, p. 195.

Bogner U, Gruters A, Sigle B, et al: Cytotoxic antibodies in congenital hypothyroidism. J Clin Endocrinol Metab 68:671, 1989.

Brander A, Kivsaari L: Ultrasonography of the thyroid during pregnancy. J Clin Ultrasound 17:403, 1989.

Brennan MD, Bahn RS: Thyroid hormones and illness. Endocr Pract 4:396, 1998.

Brent GA: The molecular basis of thyroid hormone action. N Engl J Med 331:847, 1994.

Brent GA: Maternal hypothyroidism recognition and management. Thyroid 9:661, 1999.

Brent GA, Hershman JM: Thyroxine therapy in patients with severe nonthyroidal illnesses and low serum thyroxine concentration. J Clin Endocrinol Metab 63:1, 1986.

Burrow GN: The management of thyrotoxicosis in pregnancy. N Engl J Med 313:562,1985.

Burrow GN, Fisher DA, Larsen PR: Maternal and fetal thyroid function. N Engl J Med 331:1072, 1994.

Burrow GN, May PB, Spaulding SW, et al: TRH and dopamine interactions affecting pituitary hormone secretion. J Clin Endocrinol Metab 45:65, 1977.

Bussen S, Steck T: Thyroid autoantibodies in euthyroid non-pregnant women with recurrent spontaneous abortions. Hum Reprod 10:2938, 1995.

Buyon JP, Nelson JL, Lockshine MD: The effects of pregnancy on autoimmune thyroid diseases. Clin Immunol Immunopathol 79:99, 1996.

Clavel S, Madec A, Bornet H, et al: Anti TSH-receptor antibodies in pregnant patients with autoimmune thyroid disorder. Br J Obstet Gynaecol 97:1003, 1990.

Clementi M, DiGianantonio E, Pelo E, et al: Methimazole embryopathy: Delineation of the phenotype. Am J Med Genet 83:43, 1999.

Confavreuz C, Hutchinson M, Hours MH, et al: Rate of pregnancy related relapse in multiple sclerosis. New Engl J Med 339:285, 1998.

Cooper DS, Goldminz D, Levin AA, et al: Agranulocytosis associated with antithyroid drugs. Ann Intern Med 98:26, 1983.

Costagliola S, Morgenthaler NG, Hoermann R, et al: Second generation assay for thyrotoxicosis receptor and bodies has superior diagnostic sensitivity for Graves disease. J Clin Endocrinol Metab 84:90, 1999.

Davies TF: The thyroid immunology of the postpartum period. Thyroid 9:675, 1999.

Davis LE, Leveno KJ, Cunningham FG: Hypothyroidism complicating pregnancy. Obstet Gynecol 72:108, 1988.

Davis LE, Lucas MJ, Hankins GDV, et al: Thyrotoxicosis complicating pregnancy. Am J Obstet Gynecol 160:63, 1989.

DeGroot LJ: Dangerous dogmas in medicine: The non-thyroidal illness syndrome. J Clin Endocrinol Metab 84:151, 1999.

Del Pozo E, Wyss H, Tolis G, et al: Prolactin and deficient luteal function. Obstet Gynecol 53:282, 1979.

Delange F, de Benoist B, Pretell E, et al: Iodine deficiency in the world: Where do we stand at the turn of the century? Thyroid 11:437, 2001.

Delange F, de Vilder JJ, Morreale de Escobar G, et al: Significance of early diagnostic data in congenital hypothyroidism: Report of the subcommittee on neonatal hypothyroidism of the European Thyroid Association. In Delange F, Fisher DA, Glinoer D (eds): Research in Congenital Hypothyroidism. New York, Plenum Press, 1989.

Delange F, Lecomte P: Iodine supplementation—Benefits outweigh risks. Drug Safety 22:89, 2000.

Di Gianantonio E, Schaefer C, Mastroiacovo PP, et al: Adverse effects of prenatal methimazole exposure. Teratology 64:262, 2001.

Dillman WH: Mechanism of action of thyroid hormones. Med Clin North Am **69**:849, 1985.

Dunn JT, Delange F: Damaged reproduction: The most important consequence of iodine deficiency. J Clin Endocrinol Metab **86**:2360, 2001.

Dussault JH, Rousseau F: Immunologically-mediated hypothyroidism. Endocrinol Metab Clin North Am **16**:417, 1987.

Fernandez-Soto ML, Jovanovic LG, Gonzalez-Jimenez A, et al: Thyroid function during pregnancy and the postpartum period iodine metabolism and disease status. Endocr Prac **4**:97, 1998.

Ferris TF: Renal disease. *In* Burrow GN, Ferris TF (eds): Medical Complications During Pregnancy. Philadelphia, WB Saunders, 1988, p. 277.

Fisher DA: Hypothyroxinemia in premature infants: Is thyroxine treatment necessary? Thyroid **9**:715, 1999.

Fisher DA, Dussault JH, Sack J, et al: Ontogenesis of hypothalamic-pituitary-thyroid function and metabolism in man, sheep and rat. Recent Progr Horm Res **3**:59, 1977.

Fisher DA, Foley BL: Early treatment of congenital hypothyroidism. Pediatrics **83**:785, 1989.

Fisher DA, Klein AH: Thyroid development and disorders of thyroid function in the newborn. N Engl J Med **304**:702, 1981.

Fisher DA, Polk DH: Development of the thyroid. Baillieres Clin Endocrinol Metab **3**:627, 1989.

Fukushi M, Honma IC, Fujita K: Maternal thyroid deficiency during pregnancy and subsequent neuropsychological development of the child (letter). N Engl J Med **341**:556, 1999.

Gerstein HC: Incidence of postpartum thyroid dysfunction in patients with type I diabetes mellitus. Ann Intern Med **188**:419, 1993.

Gharib H, Cobin RH, Dickey RA: Subclinical hypothyroidism during pregnancy: Position statement from the American Association of Clinical Endocrinologists. Endocrine Pract **5**:367, 1999.

Glinoer D: The regulation of thyroid function in pregnancy: pathways of endocrine adaptation from physiology to pathology. Endocr Rev **18**:404, 1997.

Glinoer D: What happens to the normal thyroid during pregnancy? Thyroid **9**:631, 1999.

Glinoer D: Pregnancy and iodine. Thyroid **11**:471, 2001.

Glinoer D, De Nayer P, Bourdoux P, et al: Regulation of maternal thyroid during pregnancy. J Clin Endocrinol Metab **71**:276, 1990.

Glinoer D, De Nayer P, Delange F, et al: A randomized trial for the treatment of mild iodine deficiency during pregnancy: Maternal and neonatal effects. J Clin Endocrinol Metab **80**:258, 1995.

Glinoer D, De Nayer P, Robyn C, et al: Serum levels of intact human chorionic gonadotropin (hCG) and its free α and β subunits, in relation to maternal thyroid stimulation during normal pregnancy. J Endocrinol Invest **16**:881, 1993.

Glinoer D, Delange F: The potential repercussions of maternal, fetal and neonatal hypothyroxinemia on the progeny. Thyroid **10**:871, 2000.

Glinoer D, Lemore M, Bourdoux P, et al: Partial reversibility during late postpartum of thyroid abnormalities associated with pregnancy. J Clin Endocrinol Metab **74**:453, 1992.

Glinoer D, Riahi M, Grn JP, et al: Risk of subclinical hypothyroidism in pregnant women with asymptomatic autoimmune thyroid disorders. J Clin Endocrinol Metab **79**:197, 1994.

Glinoer D, Soto MF, Bouroux P, et al: Pregnancy in patients with mild thyroid abnormalities: Maternal and neonatal repercussions. J Clin Endocrinol Metab **73**:421, 1991.

Goodwin TM, Montoro M, Mestman JH: The role of chorionic gonadotropin in transient hyperthyroidism of hyperemesis gravidarum. J Clin Endocrinol Metab **75**:1333, 1992a.

Goodwin TM, Montoro M, Mestman JH: Transient hyperthyroidism and hyperemesis gravidarum: Clinical aspects. Am J Obstet Gynecol **167**:648, 1992b.

Gorman CA: Radio iodine and pregnancy. Thyroid **9**:721, 1999.

Greig WR: Radioactive iodine therapy for thyrotoxicosis. Br J Surg **758**:765, 1973.

Grün JP, Meuris S, DeNayer P, et al: The thyrotropic role of human chorionic gonadotropin (hCG) in the early stages of twin (versus single) pregnancy. Clin Endocrinol **46**:719, 1997.

Gruner C, Kollert A, Wildt L, et al: Intrauterine treatment of fetal goitrous hypothyroidism controlled by determination of thyroid-stimulating hormone in fetal serum. A case report and review of the literature. Fetal Diagn Ther **16**:47, 2001.

Haddow JE, Palomaki GE, Alan WC, et al: Maternal thyroid deficiency during pregnancy and subsequent neuropsychological development of the child. N Engl J Med **341**:549, 1999.

Halnan KE: The radioiodine uptake of the human thyroid in pregnancy. Clin Sci **17**:281, 1958.

Harris B, Fung H, Johns S, et al: Transient postpartum thyroid dysfunction and postnatal depression. J Affect Disord **17**:243, 1989.

Harris B, Othman S, Davies JA, et al: Association between postpartum thyroid dysfunction and thyroid antibodies and depression. BMJ **305**:152, 1992.

Hay ID: Nodular thyroid disease diagnosed during pregnancy: How and when to treat. Thyroid **9**:667, 1999.

Hershman JM: Human chorionic gonadotropin and the thyroid: Hyperemesis gravidarum and trophoblastic tumors. Thyroid **9**:653,1999.

Herzon FS, Morris DM, Segal MN, et al: Coexistent thyroid cancer and pregnancy. Arch Otolaryngol Head Neck Surg **120**:1191, 1994.

Hollowell JG, Staehling NW, Hannon WH, et al: Iodine nutrition in the United States. Trends from public health implications: Iodine excretion data from National Health and Nutrition Examination Surveys I and III (1971–1974 and 1988–1994). J Clin Endocrinol Metab **83**:3401, 1998.

Houck JA, Davis RE, Sharma HM: Thyroid-stimulating immunoglobulin as a cause of recurrent intrauterine fetal death. Obstet Gynecol **71**:1018, 1988.

Isley WL, Dahl S, Gibbs H: Use of esmolol in managing a thyrotoxic patient needing emergency surgery. Am J Med **89**:122, 1990.

Janssen R, Dahlberg PA, Winsa B, et al: The postpartum period constitutes an important risk for the development of clinical Graves' disease in young women. Acta Endocrinol **116**:321, 1987.

Johnsson E, Larsson G, Ljunggren M: Severe malformations in infants born to hyperthyroid women on methimazole. Lancet **350**:1520, 1997.

Jovanovic-Peterson L, Peterson CM: De novo clinical hypothyroidism in pregnancies complicated by type I diabetes, subclinical hypothyroidism and proteinuria. Am J Obstet Gynecol **159**:442, 1988.

Kamijo K, Saito T, Saito M, et al: Transient subclinical hypothyroidism in early pregnancy. Endocrinol Jpn **37**:387, 1990.

Kampe O, Jansson R, Karlsson FA: Effects of L-thyroxine and iodide on the development of autoimmune postpartum thyroiditis. J Clin Endocrinol Metab **70**:1014, 1990.

Kampmann JP, Johansen K, Hansen JM, et al: Propylthiouracil in human milk: Revision of a dogma. Lancet **1**:736, 1980.

Kaplan MM: Monitoring thyroxine treatment during pregnancy. Thyroid **2**:147, 1992.

Kaplan MM: Management of thyroxine therapy during pregnancy. Endocr Pract **2**:281, 1996.

Khalil A, Kovacs K, Sima AAF, et al: Pituitary thyrotroph hyperplasia mimicking prolactin-secreting adenoma. J Endocrinol Invest **7**:399, 1984.

Klein RZ, Haddow JE, Faix JD, et al: Prevalence of thyroid deficiency in pregnant women. Clin Endocrinol **35**:41, 1991.

Klein RZ, Mitchell ML: Maternal hypothyroidism and child development. Horm Res **52**:55, 1999.

Kopp P, Van Sande J, Parmer J, et al: Brief report: Congenital hyperthyroidism caused by a mutation in the thyrotropin receptor gene. N Engl J Med **322**:150, 1995.

Krassas GE: Thyroid disease and female reproduction. Fertil Steril **74**:1063, 2000.

Krassas GE, Pontikides N, Kaltsas TH, et al: Menstrual disturbances in thyroidism. Clin Endocrinol **40**:641, 1994.

LaFranchi S: Thyroid function in the preterm infant. Thyroid **9**:71, 1999.

Lazarus JH: Clinical manifestations of postpartum thyroid disease. Thyroid **9**:685, 1999a.

Lazarus JH: Thyroid hormone and intellectual development: A clinician's view. Thyroid **9**:659, 1999b.

Lazarus JH, Aloa A, Parkes AB, et al: The effect of anti–TPO antibodies on thyroid function in early gestation: Implications for screening. American Thyroid Association meeting, Portland, Oregon, 1998.

Learoyd DL, Fund HYM, McGregor AM: Postpartum thyroid dysfunction. Thyroid **2**:73, 1992.

Leung AS, Millar LK, Koonings PP, et al: Perinatal outcome in hypothyroid patients. Obstet Gynecol **81**:349, 1993.

Levy RP, Newman M, Rejah LS, et al: The myth of goiter in pregnancy. Am J Obstet Gynecol **137**:701, 1980.

Lucas A, Pizarro E, Granada ML, et al: Postpartum thyroiditis: Epidemiology and clinical evolution in a non-selected population. Thyroid **10**:71, 2000.

Man EB, Jones WS: Thyroid function in human pregnancy. V. Incidence of maternal serum low butanol-extractable iodines and of normal gestational TBG and TBPA capacities: Retardation of 8-month old infants. Am J Obstet Gynecol **44**: 898, 1969.

Mandel SJ, Cooper DS: The use of antithyroid drugs in pregnancy and lactation. J Clin Endocrinol Metab **86**:2354, 2001.

Mandel SJ, Larsen PR, Seely EW, et al: Increased need for thyroxine during pregnancy in women with primary hypothyroidism. N Engl J Med **323**:91, 1990.

Marley EF, Oertil YC: Fine needle aspiration of thyroid lesions in 57 pregnant and postpartum women. Diagn Cytopathol **16**:122, 1997.

Mariotti S, Chiovato L, Vitti P, et al: Recent advances in the understanding of humoral and cellular mechanisms implicated in thyroid autoimmune disorders. Clin Immunol Immunopathol 50:573, 1989.

Mariotti S, Martino E, Cupini C: Low serum thyroglobulin as a clue to the diagnosis of thyrotoxicosis factitia. N Engl J Med 307:410, 1982.

Marqusee E, Hill JA, Mandel SJ: Thyroiditis after pregnancy loss. J Clin Endocrinol Metab 82:2455, 1997.

Martinez-Frias ML, Cereijo A, Rodriguez-Pinella E, et al: Methimazole in animal feed and congenital aplasia cutis. Lancet 399:742, 1992.

Matsuura N, Konishi J: Transient hypothyroidism in infants born to mothers with chronic thyroiditis—A nationwide study of 23 cases. Endocrinol Jpn 37:767, 1990.

Mestman JH: Thyroid disease in pregnancy other than Graves' and post partum thyroid dysfunction. Endocrinologist 9:294, 1999.

Milham S, Elledge W: Maternal methimazole and congenital defects in children. Teratology 5:525, 1972.

Millar LK, Wing DA, Leung AS, et al: Low birth weight and preeclampsia in pregnancies complicated by hyperthyroidism. Obstet Gynecol 84:946, 1994.

Mitsuda N, Tamaki H, Amino N, et al: Risk factors for development disorders in infants born to women with Graves' disease. Obstet Gynecol 80:359, 1992.

Momotani N, Ito K: Treatment of pregnant patients with Basedow's disease. Exp Clin Endocrinol 97:268, 191.

Momotani N, Noh J, Oyanagi H, et al: Antithyroid drug therapy for Graves' disease during pregnancy. N Engl J Med 315:24, 1986.

Montoro MN: Management of hypothyroidism during pregnancy. Clin Obstet Gynecol 40:65, 1997.

Moosa M, Mazzaferri EL: Outcome of differentiated thyroid cancer diagnosed in pregnant women. J Clin Endocrinol Metab 82:2862, 1997.

Morgan LS: Hormonally active gynecologic tumors. Semin Surg Oncol 6:83, 1990.

Morreale de Escobar G, Obregon MJ, Escobar del Rey F: Is neuropsychological development related to maternal hypothyroidism or to maternal hypothyroxinemia? J Clin Endocrinol Metab 85:3975, 2000.

Mortimer RH, Cannell GR, Addison RS, et al: Methimazole and propylthiouracil equally cover the perfused human term placental lobule. J Clin Endocrinol Metab 82:3099, 1997.

Mujtaba Q, Burrow GN: Treatment of hyperthyroidism in pregnancy with PTU and methimazole. Obstet Gynecol 46:282, 1975.

Nader S, Mastrobattista J: Recurrent hyperthyroidism in consecutive pregnancies characterized by hyperemesis. Thyroid 6:465, 1996.

Nelson JL, Hughes KA, Smith AG, et al: Maternal fetal disparity in HLA class II alloantigens and the pregnancy induced amelioration of rheumatoid arthritis. N Engl J Med 329:466, 1993.

Nelson M, Wickos GG, Caplan RH, et al: Thyroid gland size in pregnancy. J Repro Med 32:888, 1987.

Othman S, Phillips DL, Parkes AB, et al: Long-term follow-up of postpartum thyroiditis. Clin Endocrinol 32:559, 1990.

Pedersen CA: Postpartum mood and anxiety disorders: A guide for the non-psychiatric clinician with an aside on thyroid associations with postpartum mood. Thyroid 9:691, 1999.

Pekary AE, Jackson IM, Goodwin TM, et al: Increased in vitro thyrotropic activity of partially sialated human chorionic gonadotropin extracted from hydatidiform moles of patients with hyperthyroidism. J Clin Endocrinol Metab 76:70, 1993.

Pharoah PQ, Butterfield IH, Hetzel BS: Neurological damage to the fetus resulting from severe iodine deficiency during pregnancy. Lancet 1:308, 1971.

Phoojaroenchanachai M, Sriussadaporn S, Peerapatdir T, et al: Effect of maternal hyperthyroidism during late pregnancy on the risk of neonatal low birth weight. Clin Endocrinol 54:365, 2001.

Piccinini MP, Giudizi MG, Biagiotti R, et al: Progesterone favors the development of human T helper cells producing Th2-type cytokines and promotes both 1L-4 production and membrane CD30 expression in established Th1 cell clones. J Immunol 155:128, 1995.

Polk DH: Thyroid hormone effects on neonatal thermogenesis. Semin Perintal 12:151, 1988.

Pop VJM, de Rooy HAM, Vader HL, et al: Postpartum thyroid dysfunction and depression in an unselected population. N Engl J Med 324:1815, 1991.

Pop VJM, de Rooy HAM, Vader VL, et al: Microsomal antibodies during gestation in relation to postpartum thyroid dysfunction and depression. Acta Endocrinol 129:26, 1993.

Pop VJM, deVries E, van Baar AL, et al: Maternal thyroid peroxidase antibodies during pregnancy: A marker of impaired child development? J Clin Endocrinol Metab 80:3561, 1995.

Pop VJM, Kuijpens JV, van Baar AL, et al: Low maternal FT$_4$ concentrations during early pregnancy associated with impaired psychomotor development in infancy. Clin Endocrinol 50:149, 1999.

Pop VJM, Maarteens LH, Levsink G, et al: Are autoimmune thyroid dysfunction and depression related? J Clin Endocrinol Metab 83:3194, 1998.

Radunovic N, Domez Y, Mandelbrot L, et al: Thyroid function in fetus and mother during the second half of normal pregnancy. Biol Neonate 59:139, 1991.

Reuss ML, Paneth N, Pinto-Martin JA, et al: The relation of transient hypothyroxinemia in preterm infants to neurologic development at two years of age. N Engl J Med 443:821, 1996.

Rodien P, Bremont C, Sanson M-LR, et al: Familial gestational hyperthyroidism caused by a mutant thyrotropic receptor hypersensitive to human chorionic gonadotropin. N Engl J Med 339:1823, 1998.

Romaguera J, Ramirez M, Adamsons K: Intra-amniotic thyroxine to accelerate fetal maturation. Sem Perinatol 17:260, 1993.

Roti E, Gnudi A, Braverman LE: The placental transport, synthesis and metabolism of hormones and drugs, which affect thyroid function. Endocrinol Rev 4:131, 1983.

Safa AM, Schumacher OP, Rodriguez-Antunez A: Long-term follow-up results in children and adolescents treated with radioactive iodine (I$_{131}$) for hyperthyroidism. N Engl J Med 292:167, 1975.

Santini F, Chiovato L, Ghirri P, et al: Serum iodothyronines in the human fetus and the newborn: Endocr for an important role of placenta in fetal thyroid hormone homeostasis. J Clin Endocrinol Metab 84:493, 1999.

Schlumberger M, deVathaire F, Ceccarelli C, et al: Exposure to radioactive iodine I$_{131}$ for scintigraphy or therapy does not preclude pregnancy in thyroid cancer patients. J Nucl Med 37:606, 1996.

Seely BL, Burrow GN: Thyrotoxicosis in pregnancy. Endocrinologist 7:409, 1991.

Smallridge RC: Thyroid function tests. In Beckers KL (ed): Principles and Practice of Endocrinology and Metabolism. Philadelphia, Lippincott Williams and Wilkins, 2001, p. 329.

Smallridge RC, Fein HG, Hayslip CC: Postpartum thyroiditis. Bridge 3:3, 1988.

Smith MB, Xue H, Takahashi H, et al: Iodine I$_{131}$ thyroid ablation in female children and adolescents: Long term risk of infertility and birth defects. Ann Surg Oncol 1:128, 1994.

Stagnaro-Green AS: Post-miscarriage thyroid dysfunction. Obstet Gynecol 803:490, 1992.

Stagnaro-Green AS: Postpartum thyroiditis: Prevalence, etiology, and clinical implications. Thyroid Today 16:1, 1993.

Stagnaro-Green AS: Recognizing, understanding and treating postpartum thyroiditis. Endocrinol Metab Clinics NA 29:417, 2000.

Sturgess ML, Weeks I, Ebans PI, et al: An immunochemiluminometric assay for serum free thyroxine. Clin Endocrinol 27:383, 1987.

Tachi J, Amino N, Tamaski H, et al: Long-term follow-up and HLA association in patients with postpartum hypothyroidism. J Clin Endocrinol Metab 66:480, 1988.

Talbot JA, Lambert A, Anobile LJ, et al: The nature of human chorionic gonadotropin glycoforms in gestational thyrotoxicosis. Clin Endocrinol 55:33, 2001.

Tan GH, Gharib H, Goellner JR, et al: Management of thyroid nodules in pregnancy. Arch Intern Med 156:2317, 1996.

Tanaka T, Tamin H, Kuma K, et al: Gonadotropin response to luteinizing hormone releasing hormone in hyperthyroid patients with menstrual disturbances. Metabolism 30:323, 1981.

Thomas R, Reid RL: Thyroid disease and reproductive dysfunction. Obstet Gynecol 70:789, 1987.

Thorpe-Beeston JG, Nicolaides KH, Felton CV, et al: Maturation of the secretion of thyroid hormone and thyroid-stimulating hormone in the fetus. N Engl J Med 324:532, 1991.

Van Djihe UP, Heydendael RJ, De Kleine MR: Methimazole, carbimazole and congenital skin defects. Ann Intern Med 106:60, 1987.

Vanderpas JB, Contempré B, Dvale NL, et al: Iodine and selenium deficiency associated with cretinism in Northern Zaire. Am J Clinic Nutr 52:1087, 1990.

Varner MW: Autoimmune disorders and pregnancy. Semin Perinatol 15:238, 1991.

Vulsma T, Gons MH, de Vijlder JJ: Maternal-fetal transfer of thyroxine in congenital hypothyroidism due to a total organification defect or thyroid agenesis. N Engl J Med 321:13, 1989.

Vulsma Y, Kok JK: Prematurity-associated neurological and development abnormalities and neonatal thyroid function. N Engl J Med 3343:857, 1996.

Wartofsky L, Burman KD: Alterations in thyroid function in patients with systemic illness: The "euthyroid sick syndrome." Endocrinol Rev 3:164, 1982.

Wasserstrum N, Anania CA: Perinatal consequences of maternal hypothyroidism in early pregnancy and inadequate replacement. Clin Endocrinol 42:343, 1997.

Weetman AP: Editorial: Insulin-dependent diabetes mellitus and postpartum thyroiditis: An important association. J Clin Endocrinol Metab **79**:7, 1994.

Weetman AP: The immunology of pregnancy. Thyroid **9**:643, 1999.

Weetman AP, McGregor AM: Autoimmune thyroid disease: Further developments in our understanding. Endocrinol Rev **15**:788, 1994.

Weintraub BD: Inappropriate secretion of thyroid-stimulating hormone. Ann Intern Med **95**:339, 1981.

Werner S: Modification of the classification of eye changes of Graves' disease: Recommendation of the Ad Hoc Committee of the American Thyroid Association. J Clin Endocrinol Metab **44**:203, 1977.

Wilansky DL, Greisman B: Early hypothyroidism in patients with menorrhagia. Am J Obstet Gynecol **160**:673, 1989.

Wilson R, McKillop JH, MacLean M, et al: Thyroid function tests are rarely abnormal in patients with severe hyperemesis gravidarum. Clin Endocrinol (Oxf.) **37**:331, 1992.

Wing DA, Millar LK, Kooings PP, et al: A comparison of propylthiouracil versus methimazole in the treatment of hyperthyroidism in pregnancy. Am J Obstet Gynecol **170**:90, 1994.

Winters SJ, Berga SL: Gonadal dysfunction in patients with thyroid disease. Endocrinologist **7**:167, 1997.

Xue-Yi C, Xin-Min J, Zhi-Hong D, et al: Time of vulnerability of the brain to iodine deficiency in endemic cretinism. N Engl J Med **331**:1739, 1994.

Yasuda T, Ohnishi H, Wataki K, et al: Outcome of a baby born from a mother with acquired juvenile hypothyroidism having undetectable thyroid hormone concentrations. J Clin Endocrinol Metab **84**:2630, 1999.

Yoshimoto M, Nakayama Itoi, Baba P, et al: A case of neonatal McCune-Albright syndrome with Cushing syndrome and hyperthyroidism. Acta Pediatr Scand **89**:984, 1991.

Zakarija M, McKenzie JM: Pregnancy-associated changes in thyroid-stimulating antibody of Graves' disease and the relationship to neonatal hyperthyroidism. J Clin Endocrinol Metab **57**:1036, 1983.

Zimmerman D: Fetal and neonatal hyperthyroidism. Thyroid **9**:727, 1999.

Chapter 51

OTHER ENDOCRINE DISORDERS OF PREGNANCY

Shahla Nader, MD

The staggering advancements that have been made in endocrinology over the last few decades have permitted precise descriptions and scientific delineation of derangements of normal physiology. In tandem, technologic and pharmaceutical advances have followed that allow correction and management of prevailing problems with a precision that is lacking in many other fields of medicine. When pregnancy is superimposed on abnormal endocrine function in the mother, the consequences for the mother and the fetus can be adverse and sometimes disastrous. Awareness of this danger, combined with the knowledge that accurate diagnostic and therapeutic measures are often available, places a substantial burden on the obstetrician caring for the pregnant patient. This chapter summarizes the normal maternal endocrine adaptation to pregnancy and outlines maternal disorders, some of which are almost specific to pregnancy.

HYPOTHALAMUS AND PITUITARY

The sella turcica of the sphenoid bone, lined by dura mater, is occupied by the pituitary gland. The dura covering the roof, called the *diaphragm sella*, is perforated centrally by the pituitary stalk. Directly above this diaphragm and anterior to the stalk lies the optic chiasm. The gland consists of two lobes, anterior (adenohypophysis) and posterior (neurohypophysis), the former accounting for five-sixths of the volume of the gland. The pituitary stalk not only comprises the direct neural connections between the hypothalamic nuclei and the posterior lobe but also is the vascular link between the hypothalamus and the anterior lobe, thus enabling hypothalamic neurohumoral secretions to influence the activity of the anterior lobe cells. Paired superior hypophyseal arteries, arising from the internal carotids, anastomose around the upper part of the stalk. These terminate within elongated coiled capillary loops into which the hypothalamic hormones are discharged. The capillary bed drains into portal veins that empty into sinusoids of the anterior lobe (Fig. 51-1). Paired inferior hypophyseal arteries supply the posterior lobe. The venous drainage of both lobes is into the cavernous sinuses.

Figure 51-2 is a diagram of the interrelationships and feedback mechanisms of higher brain centers, hypothalamus, pituitary, and target endocrine glands in normal, nonpregnant women (Frohman, 1980). The adenohypophysis produces gonadotropins (luteinizing hormone [LH], follicle-stimulating hormone [FSH]), growth hormone (GH), thyrotropin or thyroid-stimulating hormone (TSH), prolactin, and adrenocorticotropin or adrenocorticotropic hormone (ACTH) and its related peptide β-lipotropin, from which melanocyte-stimulating hormone (β-MSH) is derived.

Since 1947 (when the concept that control of the anterior pituitary is exerted through a neurohumoral mechanism was formulated), several peptides have been isolated from the hypothalamus that indeed function in this capacity. Thus, thyrotropin-releasing hormone (TRH) causes release of TSH (and also of prolactin); growth hormone-releasing factor (GHRF) releases GH; gonadotropin-releasing hormone (GnRH) allows release of LH and FSH; and corticotropin-releasing hormone (CRH) releases ACTH. In addition, substances with an inhibitory rather than a stimulatory influence have been identified: Somatostatin inhibits the release of GH (and many other hormones), while dopamine inhibits the release of prolactin. This inhibition of the lactotroph is clinically important; disturbances of the stalk or vascular dissociation of the hypothalamus from the anterior pituitary results in deficiency of all anterior pituitary hormones with the exception of prolactin. Thus, the lactotroph is normally under predominantly inhibitory control.

Physiologic Changes during Pregnancy

During pregnancy and in the immediate postpartum period, the anterior lobe of the pituitary can double or triple in size because of hyperplasia and hypertrophy of lactotrophs. This is evident at 1 month and continues throughout gestation. At delivery, involution of pregnancy cells occurs for a period of several months but seems to be retarded by lactation (Scheithauer et al., 1990). Magnetic resonance imaging (MRI) studies of normal primigravid patients have confirmed progressively increasing pituitary volumes during gestation (Gonzalez et al., 1988); at the end of pregnancy, there is an overall increase in pituitary gland size of 136% compared with control nulliparous subjects. Similar results have been obtained by Dinc and colleagues (1998), who found changes in pituitary gland volume of 40%, 75%, and a maximum of 120% in the second, third, and immediate postpartum periods, respectively. The major accompanying physiologic change is a progressive increase in serum prolactin concentrations (Tyson et al., 1972), with an approximately tenfold increase during gestation (Fig. 51-3).

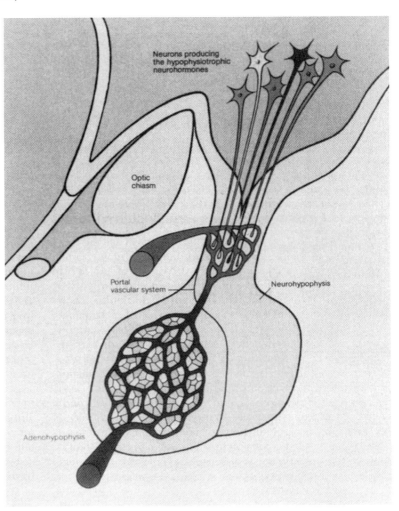

FIGURE 51-1 ■ Schematic illustration of the hypothalamus, pituitary gland, and neurohumoral mechanism controlling the anterior pituitary. (From Halasz B: Introduction to neuroendocrinology. *In* Fluckiger E, Muller EE, Thorner MO: Basic and Clinical Aspects of Neuroscience: The Dopaminergic System. Berlin, Springer-Verlag, 1985, p. 1. Courtesy of Sandoz, East Hanover, NJ.)

Placental estrogens stimulate lactotroph deoxyribonucleic acid (DNA) synthesis, mitotic activity, and prolactin secretion. Prolactin's role is in the preparation of the breasts for initiation and maintenance of lactation. Despite this dramatic increase, the lactotroph maintains its ability to respond to TRH, its releasing hormone (in contradistinction to prolactinomas, in which this response is usually blunted or absent).

Other physiologic changes during pregnancy include the following (Itskovitz and Rosenwaks, 1989):

1. A decline in gonadotropin concentrations with a progressively diminishing response to GnRH
2. A decline of pituitary GH with an increase of a placental variant of GH: This variant has similar somatogenic but less lactogenic bioactivity than pituitary GH, with increases in insulin-like growth factor I (IGF-I or somatomedin-C) commensurate with elevated GH variant. Pituitary GH is the only detectable form during the first trimester. Thereafter, placental GH increases progressively.
3. An increase in CRH (probably of placental origin) during the second and third trimesters
4. A twofold to fourfold increase in ACTH concentrations occurring despite a rise in both bound and free plasma cortisol, suggesting that factors other than cortisol may regulate its release or that an alternative source of ACTH exists

The diurnal variation of cortisol, although blunted, is preserved during pregnancy (see the section of this chapter under Adrenal Glands). Thyrotropin, decreasing slightly in the first trimester, is otherwise essentially unchanged.

The posterior pituitary is a storage terminal for the neurohypophyseal hormones oxytocin and vasopressin. Produced by the supraoptic and paraventricular hypothalamic nuclei along with their respective binding proteins or neurophysins, these hormones are transported as neurosecretory granules along the supraopticohypophyseal tract to the pituitary and from there find their way into the circulation. Vasopressin plays a central role in osmolarity and volume regulation. Osmoreceptors are located in the anterior hypothalamus, and vasopressin release increases when plasma osmolality rises (Fig. 51-4).

Early in pregnancy, plasma osmolality decreases to values 5–10 mOsm/kg below the normal mean of 285 mOsm/kg in nonpregnant women (Davison et al., 1983). Plasma levels of vasopressin and its response to water loading and dehydration, however, are normal in pregnancy, indicating a resetting of the threshold—that is, vasopressin is secreted at a lower plasma osmolality (see Fig. 51-4). Similarly, the plasma osmolality at which thirst is experienced is lower in the pregnant state. Along with these changes, the metabolic clearance of vasopressin increases markedly between gestational week 10 and midpregnancy. This is paralleled by the appearance and increase of circulating vasopressinase (Lindheimer et al., 1991).

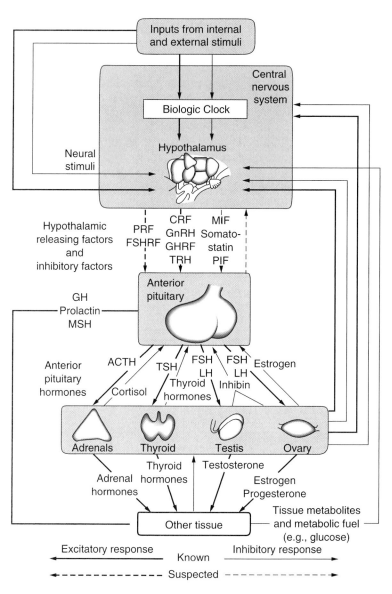

FIGURE 51-2 ■ Schematic drawing of the relationships and feedback mechanism of the neuroendocrine system. The components include the central nervous system, hypothalamus, anterior pituitary gland, and target glands and tissues. *Heavy lines* indicate hormone secretion; *thin lines* indicate inhibitory effect; *dotted lines* indicate suspected pathways. ACTH, adrenocorticoptropin; CRF, corticotropin-releasing factor; FSH, follicle-stimulating hormone; GH, growth hormone; GHRF, growth hormone–releasing factor; GnRH, gonadotropin-releasing hormone; LH, luteinizing hormone; MIF, melanocyte-stimulating hormone-inhibiting factor; MSH, melanocyte-stimulating hormone; PIF, prolactin-inhibiting factor; PRF, prolactin-releasing factor; TRH, thyrotropin-releasing factor; TSH, thyroid-stimulating hormone. (From Frohman LA: Neurotransmitters as regulators of endocrine function. *In* Krieger DR, Hughes JC [eds]: Neuroendocrinology: A Hospital Practice Book. Sunderland Mass, Sinauer Associates, 1980. Illustration by Nancy Kou Gahan and Albert Miller.)

Oxytocin is involved in the process of parturition (Dawood and Khan-Dawood, 1990) and in suckling. Although the role of oxytocin in the initiation of labor is unclear, there is significant preterm increase in plasma concentrations of oxytocin. During nursing, nipple stimulation initiates a neurogenic reflex that is transmitted to the hypothalamus, thus triggering oxytocin release from the posterior pituitary. Oxytocin then induces contraction of the myoepithelial cells and mammary duct smooth muscle, resulting in milk ejection.

Fetal Hypothalamic and Pituitary Development

Figure 51-5 shows the gradual development of the structural and functional aspects of the neuroendocrine system in the fetus. By 10–13 weeks' gestation, fetal pituitary and hypothalamic tissues can respond *in vitro* to stimulatory or inhibitory stimuli. By midgestation, the fetal hypothalamic-pituitary axis is a functional and autonomous unit subject to feedback

control mechanisms. The posterior lobe of the fetal pituitary serves as a storage depot for neuropeptides.

Disorders of the Hypothalamus

Disorders of the hypothalamus can be congenital (Lawrence-Moon-Bardet-Biedl syndrome) or acquired inflammatory (meningitis, encephalitis), space-occupying (tumors, cysts), vascular, or degenerative. In many of these conditions, reproduction is impossible or undesirable. In the autosomal-recessive Lawrence-Moon-Bardet-Biedl syndrome of polydactyly, obesity, retinitis pigmentosa, and mental retardation, 45%–53% of affected females are hypogonadal, but several pregnancies have been reported in such patients (Green et al., 1989). Craniopharyngiomas are derived from vestigial remnants of Rathke's pouch or craniopharyngeal anlage. Manifestations can include headaches, visual disturbances, and hypothalamic dysfunction, including diabetes insipidus. Six craniopharyngiomas have been reported in pregnancy. In two, the tumor recurred, and its enlargement resulted in

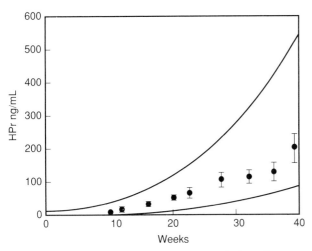

FIGURE 51-3 ■ Basal serum prolactin (HPr) levels throughout normal gestation. Points represent the mean ± standard error of the mean (SEM); *solid lines* represent the range of prolactin levels found in pregnancy. (From Tyson JE, Hwang P, Guyden A, et al: Studies of prolactin secretion in human pregnancy. Am J Obstet Gynecol **113**:14, 1972.)

loss of vision in a subsequent pregnancy (Aydin et al., 1999). Two of the case reports of craniopharyngiomas, previously undiagnosed, presented with diabetes insipidus in pregnancy (Hiett and Barton, 1990). One of these patients also had visual field disturbances and symptoms of raised intracranial pressure. Surgery was performed 3 days after delivery at 34 weeks' gestation because of deteriorating visual acuity. Thus, craniopharyngiomas could potentially require surgery during pregnancy.

Disorders of the Pituitary

Anterior Lobe

Most commonly, tumors, and less commonly, vascular mishaps and inflammatory changes afflict the anterior lobe. In their evaluation, one must consider both anatomic derangements and the effects of excess or deficient hormones that can accompany these disorders. Given the additional physiologic changes in pregnancy outlined previously, the combination of pregnancy and pituitary disorders poses a challenge to the obstetrician and endocrinologist in their endeavors for a safe outcome for both mother and fetus.

PITUITARY TUMORS

The topic of pituitary tumors in pregnancy was reviewed recently by Frohman (2001). Pituitary tumors can be classified into hormonally functioning and functionless lesions. Examples of the former include GH-producing tumors resulting in acromegaly, ACTH-producing tumors giving rise to Cushing's disease, and prolactinomas. Prolactinoma is by far the most common pituitary tumor encountered in pregnancy. Hormonally functionless pituitary tumors are less common (although some of these produce subunits of pituitary hormones, they are, clinically speaking, hormonally functionless). Because they are functionless, these pituitary tumors are relatively asymptomatic in their early stages and tend to be larger at the time of diagnosis. If diagnosed, the patient should undergo appropriate surgical treatment before becoming pregnant. Tumor expansion with visual field defects during pregnancy has been reported (Kupersmith et al., 1994).

PROLACTINOMA

The advent of prolactin radioimmunoassay in the early 1970s permitted the correct diagnosis of prolactinomas in many patients previously thought to have functionless pituitary tumors. Because of the negative impact of excess prolactin on the hypothalamic-pituitary-gonadal axis, the majority of these women, who were also in their childbearing years, presented with amenorrhea and consequently, with infertility. Parallel with the development of the prolactin assay and improved radiologic techniques for diagnosing these tumors came the development and refinement of trans-sphenoidal microsurgical techniques and a powerful new drug, bromocriptine mesylate, which can suppress elevated prolactin concentrations to normal levels. Numerous pregnancies resulted from restoring normal gonadal function in these women, and in the 1980s, information concerning these pregnancies was consolidated. Given the physiologic changes that occur in the pituitary in a normal pregnancy—namely, enlargement of the gland and hyperplasia of the lactotrophs with a tenfold increase in serum prolactin—concerns about women with prolactinomas becoming pregnant were reasonable.

EFFECT OF PROLACTINOMA AND ITS TREATMENT ON PREGNANCY AND THE FETUS: SAFETY OF BROMOCRIPTINE IN PREGNANCY. Bromocriptine mesylate is an ergot derivative with potent dopamine receptor agonist activity. Administered orally, it is a potent inhibitor of prolactin secretion, the effects usually lasting only for the duration of treatment. Numerous accounts of the use and safety of bromocriptine in pregnancy are available, but they are best summed up by Krupp and Monka (1987) from the Drug Monitoring Center, Clinical Research, Sandoz, Basel, Switzerland. They collected data from 2587 pregnancies in 2437 women treated with bromocriptine during some stage of gestation. The results showed that its use was not associated with an increased risk of spontaneous abortion, multiple pregnancy, or congenital malformation in their progeny.

In addition, these authors followed 546 children postnatally up to the age of 9 years and found no adverse effect on postnatal development. In the majority of women treated, bromocriptine was discontinued upon confirmation of pregnancy. These results are important insofar as investigations indicate that bromocriptine crosses the placental barrier and can be found in dose-related concentrations in fetal blood and in the amniotic fluid (del Pozo and Krupp, 1984). A new synthetic dopamine agonist, cabergoline, is now also approved for treatment of prolactinomas. As with bromocriptine, the drug should be discontinued once pregnancy is established. Its twice-weekly administration and reduced side effect profile makes it more palatable for some patients (Colao et al., 1997). The experience with cabergoline use in pregnancy, albeit in fewer patients, appears to be similar to that with bromocriptine (Robert et al, 1996).

EFFECTS OF PREGNANCY ON THE PROLACTINOMA. Prolactinomas are subclassified, according to their size, into microadenomas (less than 10 mm) (Fig. 51-6) and macroadenomas (greater than or equal to 10 mm). In a review of the subject with data collected and combined from many studies, Albrecht and Betz (1986) noted the following. Of 352 pregnant patients with untreated microadenomas, eight

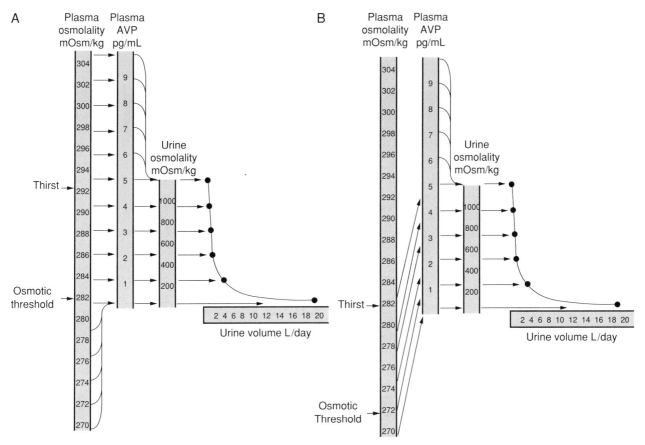

FIGURE 51-4 ■ **A,** Idealized schematic diagram of normal physiologic relationships showing the direct relationship between plasma osmolality and plasma vasopressin and the direct relationship between plasma vasopressin and urine osmolality. The osmotic threshold is illustrated as a floor for plasma osmolality below which the plasma osmolality will not normally fall because of excretion of a high volume of dilute urine. Thirst is illustrated as a physiologic ceiling for plasma osmolality, because above this level thirst will be sensed and water imbibed to avoid further elevation of plasma osmolality. **B,** Idealized schematic diagram of the reset osmostat (as occurs in pregnancy). For the patient to function normally around a lower osmolality, it is necessary that both thirst and the osmotic threshold be lowered and maintain their relative relationship one to the other. Urine osmolality and urine volume follow appropriately for the level of vasopressin in plasma. The subjects experience extreme thirst if the osmolality is raised into the normal range. (From Robinson AG: Disorders of antidiuretic hormone secretion. Clin Endocrinol Metab **14**:55, 1985.)

(2.3%) experienced visual disturbances, 17 (4.8%) experienced headaches, and two (0.6%) had diabetes insipidus. The corresponding figures for 144 pregnant women with macroadenomas were visual disturbances in 22 (15.3%), headaches in 22 (15.3%), and diabetes insipidus in two (1.4%).

In the same review, the outcomes of 318 pregnancies in patients with microadenomas and macroadenomas treated (with surgery, radiation therapy, or both) prior to pregnancy were analyzed. There were visual disturbances in 10 (3.1%), headaches in 12 (3.8%), and diabetes insipidus in one (0.3%). Symptoms related to a pregnancy-induced increase in the size of a pituitary tumor can begin as early as the first trimester, with a mean time for the onset of visual symptoms at 14 weeks' gestation (Magyar and Marshall, 1978). Headaches usually precede visual changes. The time from beginning of pregnancy to onset of symptoms in 91 pregnancies in women with previously untreated tumors is shown in Figure 51-7.

These data can be used to counsel patients with prolactinomas who are planning pregnancy. Definitive treatment of macroadenomas before pregnancy is currently recommended, especially if they are associated with destruction of the sella turcica or with suprasellar extension. Recommendations for management of patients with prolactinomas are outlined in Tables 51-1 and 51-2. Despite prior surgical intervention, complications still can occur during pregnancy (Belchetz et al., 1986). Monthly measurement of serum prolactin is not necessary. Prolactin concentrations measured in a group of patients with surgically untreated microadenomas were found to be elevated early in gestation but did not increase further with advancing gestation (Divers and Yen, 1983), in contrast with normal pregnant controls (Fig. 51-8). A small subset of women appears to experience decrease or normalization of prolactin levels postpartum. Tumor necrosis may have occurred in some. In addition, use of bromocriptine has been associated with tumor fibrosis (Borges et al, 2000).

MANAGEMENT OF PROLACTINOMA COMPLICATIONS DURING PREGNANCY. Before the bromocriptine era and in the early stages of its use, the management of tumor complications in pregnancy was difficult and included surgery, radiotherapy, early delivery, or a combination of these therapies. Fortuitously, it was soon observed that bromocriptine, in addition to its prolactin-lowering effects, can shrink the volume of

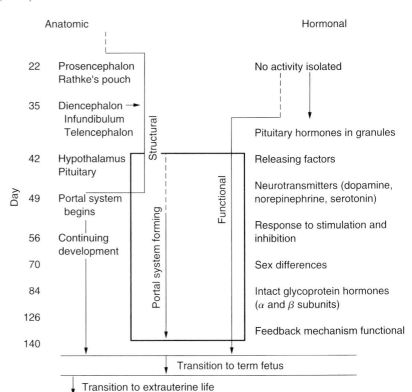

	Anatomic				Hormonal

Day

22 — Prosencephalon / Rathke's pouch — No activity isolated

35 — Diencephalon → / Infundibulum / Telencephalon — Pituitary hormones in granules

42 — Hypothalamus / Pituitary — Releasing factors

49 — Portal system begins — Neurotransmitters (dopamine, norepinephrine, serotonin)

56 — Continuing development — Response to stimulation and inhibition

70 — Sex differences

84 — Intact glycoprotein hormones (α and β subunits)

126 — Feedback mechanism functional

140 — Transition to term fetus

Transition to extrauterine life

FIGURE 51-5 ■ Structural and functional development of neuroendocrine tissue in the human fetus. (From Decherney A, Naftolin F: Hypothalamic and pituitary development in the fetus. Clin Obstet Gynecol **23**:749, 1980.)

pituitary tumors, including large macroadenomas causing visual field defects. Given the lack of known adverse effects of bromocriptine use in pregnancy and the predicament of a pregnant patient with symptomatic tumor enlargement, bromocriptine has been used successfully in the treatment of such complications and is the treatment of choice (Molitch, 1985). It should be administered with food and the dose adjusted according to symptoms (e.g., 2.5–5 mg, two or three times daily). Glucocorticoids may also be given to expedite recovery of visual defects. Surgery is recommended only if there is no response to bromocriptine.

As indicated previously, the majority of patients with microadenomas have uncomplicated pregnancies, whereas a disturbing number of patients with untreated macroadenomas have symptomatic tumor enlargement. Given the tumor-shrinking properties of bromocriptine, it is not surprising that the continuous use of bromocriptine in pregnancy has been advocated and indeed carried out in patients with macroadenomas (Ruiz-Velasco and Tolis, 1984). Until the safety of such therapy on the developing fetus is more fully established, however, such therapy cannot be recommended at present except in special circumstances. Although the rates of abortion and perinatal mortality do not differ in women with pituitary tumors that are untreated or treated before or during pregnancy, there is a significant increase in prematurity in those treated (with surgery, radiotherapy, or both) during pregnancy, compared with those not requiring such treatment or with those treated prior to pregnancy (Magyar and Marshall, 1978). Pituitary apoplexy, itself a rare event, has also been reported in a patient with a macroadenoma in early pregnancy (O'Donovan et al., 1986).

BREAST-FEEDING AND POSTPARTUM CARE. There is no reason to avoid breast-feeding when a patient with prolactinoma wishes to nurse her child. In a small study of 14 women

with microadenomas who breast-fed for 6–14 months, serum prolactin was not significantly higher than it was before pregnancy (Zarate et al., 1979). In another study, the increase in prolactin associated with suckling was absent in women with pathologic hyperprolactinemia. For those wishing to inhibit lactation, bromocriptine is the treatment of choice, a dose of approximately 2.5 mg three times daily with food usually being appropriate.

Although occasional case reports have described seizures or strokes in women who used bromocriptine to inhibit postpar-

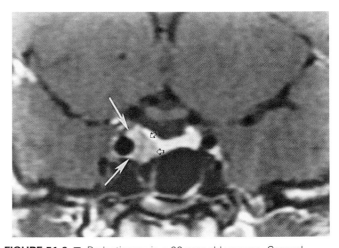

FIGURE 51-6 ■ Prolactinoma in a 26-year-old woman. Coronal magnetic resonance image (SE 600/25) after injection of gadolinium-DTPA reveals a 9 × 8 mm solid mass *(black open arrows)* of intermediate signal intensity, involving the right side of the pituitary gland. The mass is abutting the dura *(white solid arrows)*, which is surrounding the right internal carotid artery. The gadolinium-DTPA has increased the signal intensity of normal pituitary tissue, enhancing the contrast between normal and adenomatous areas.

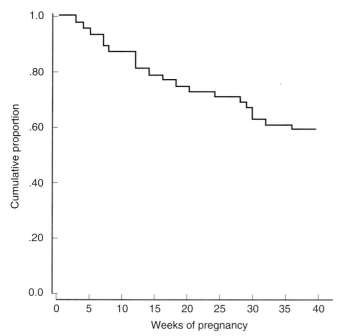

FIGURE 51-7 ■ Time from beginning of pregnancy to onset of symptoms (i.e., headache or visual disturbances) in 91 pregnancies in women with previously untreated pituitary tumors. Sixty-one percent did not experience either headache or visual disturbance during pregnancy. Occurrence of symptoms is fairly evenly distributed throughout pregnancy. (From Magyar DM, Marshall JR: Pituitary tumors and pregnancy. Am J Obstet Gynecol **132**:739, 1978.)

tum lactation—and it should be kept in mind that suppression of lactation is no longer an approved indication for the use of this agent—a recent case-control study failed to link these events to the actual use of bromocriptine (Rothman et al., 1990). Estrogen should not be used to inhibit lactation because the tumor can expand. Ophthalmologic and radiologic evaluation and determination of serum prolactin concentrations are in order 6–8 weeks after delivery. In most instances, the sella returns to its original size and prolactin decreases to previous levels. Further pregnancies are not contraindicated in patients with prolactinomas. Indeed, decreases in prolactin and tumor size have been reported in patients with multiple bromocriptine-induced pregnancies (Ahmed et al., 1992).

ACROMEGALY

Acromegaly is the result of excessive GH secretion in adults, this usually being associated with acidophilic or chromophobic pituitary adenomas. Women with acromegaly slowly develop coarse facial features, prognathism, and spade-like hands and feet. When clinical evidence exists, a glucose tolerance test is performed; lack of suppression of GH below 2 ng/mL during this test is in keeping with a diagnosis of acromegaly in nonpregnant patients. Because the biological effect of GH is mediated through somatomedin-C, elevation of serum concentration of this growth factor not only is considered a useful confirmatory test but also has been used to monitor the progression of the disease. In the context of pregnancy, however, somatomedin-C concentrations should be interpreted with caution because they can be elevated (Furlanetto et al., 1978). In addition, because of the production of a placental variant of GH, special assays using antibodies that recognize specific epitopes on the two hormones are necessary to distinguish normal from placental GH (Frankenne et al., 1988). The placental variant is undetectable within 24 hours after delivery. TRH testing may distinguish pituitary from placental GH: 70% of patients with acromegaly experience a GH response to TRH, whereas the placental variant does not cause a response (Beckers et al., 1990).

Menstrual irregularity or amenorrhea is an extremely frequent finding in acromegalic women. Nonetheless, pregnancy can occur in women with acromegaly and has been reported in 70 patients (Herman-Bonert et al., 1998). It can be accompanied by tumor expansion in approximately 10%, necessitating hypophysectomy. Despite other soft-tissue changes, no major changes occur in the genital tract that would complicate delivery. Definitive treatment before conception is the treatment of choice in acromegalics desiring children. Carbohydrate intolerance occurs in up to 50% and overt diabetes in up to 20% of acromegalics, and the insulin resistance of pregnancy is additive. Hypertension is present in 25%–35% of acromegalics, and cardiac disease is common.

An algorithm for the management of acromegaly in pregnancy has been presented by Herman-Bonert and colleagues (1998). The observation that levodopa (L-dopa) causes a paradoxical decrease in GH in acromegaly led to the use of dopaminergic agonists in the treatment of acromegaly. In two reported cases, pregnancy occurred in acromegalics during bromocriptine therapy. Continuation of treatment during pregnancy did not lead to tumor expansion (Luboshitzky et al., 1980). Tumor expansion resulting in visual field defects, however, has been reported in one of two patients with acromegaly and macroadenomas during pregnancy (Kupersmith et al., 1994).

If acromegaly is diagnosed in a pregnant patient, management depends on the activity of the disease, the tumor size, and the stage of pregnancy. Active disease during pregnancy may respond to bromocriptine until fetal lung maturation is documented. If signs and symptoms related to suprasellar extension do not abate with bromocriptine, transsphenoidal surgery could be necessary.

In a case reported by Yap and associates (1990), acromegaly was diagnosed in the second trimester. Bromocriptine corrected visual field defects and suppressed prolactin secretion but did not reduce fasting GH levels. It was suggested that suppression of physiologic lactotroph hyperplasia by bromocriptine may permit noninvasive management of the

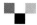

TABLE 51-1. RECOMMENDATIONS FOR TREATMENT OF PATIENTS WITH PROLACTINOMAS WHO DESIRE PREGNANCY

Treatment	Microadenomas	Macroadenomas
Primary	Bromocriptine	Transsphenoidal surgery followed by bromocriptine
Alternative	Transsphenoidal surgery followed by bromocriptine (if necessary)	(i) Radiotherapy plus bromocriptine (ii) Continuous bromocriptine (see text)

TABLE 51-2. MANAGEMENT OF PATIENTS HARBORING PROLACTINOMAS DURING GESTATION

	Microadenomas	Macroadenomas
Asymptomatic patient	**Stop** bromocriptine Routine obstetric care with evaluation for symptoms of tumor expansion Check visual fields each trimester	**Stop** bromocriptine Monthly evaluation for symptoms of tumor expansion Check visual fields each month
Symptomatic patient		Check visual fields Measure serum prolactin concentration Magnetic resonance imaging of pituitary gland Initiate bromocriptine ± dexamethasone for visual complications Trans-sphenoidal surgery if unresponsive to bromocriptine

pituitary adenoma in pregnancy. The somatostatin analogs ocreotide and lanreotide have been used in at least nine patients (de Menis et al., 1999; Neal, 2000). In three patients, the drug was continued throughout pregnancy without reported ill effects on the fetus, despite documented transplacental passage (Caron et al., 1996). While at present, somatostatin analogs should be discontinued in acromegalic patients contemplating pregnancy, they may be considered an alternative to transsphenoidal surgery in pregnancy for an expanding tumor if the patient does nor respond to dopaminergic agonists such as bromocriptine. The maternal-fetal transfer of GH has been said to be negligible, and apart from the effect of glucose intolerance, the fetus is not thought to be affected by acromegaly.

CUSHING'S SYNDROME

Cortisol secretion is controlled by the hypothalamic-pituitary axis (see previous sections and "Adrenal Glands," which follows). Cushing's syndrome is a state of hypercorti-

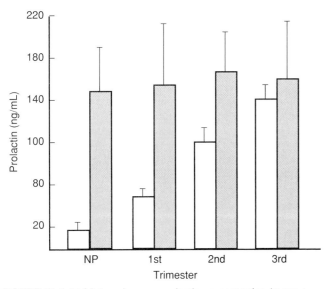

FIGURE 51-8 ■ Maternal serum prolactin concentration (mean ± SEM) in patients with microadenoma (*shaded bars, n* = 237) and controls (*open bars, n* = 215) while nonpregnant (NP) and during each trimester of pregnancy. (From Divers WA, Yen SSC: Prolactin producing microadenomas in pregnancy. Obstet Gynecol **62**:425, 1983. Reprinted with permission of the American College of Obstetricians and Gynecologists.)

solism and can arise from excess ACTH produced by the pituitary or an ectopic ACTH source such as a tumor, both of which can lead to bilateral adrenal hyperplasia. In addition, an adrenal lesion (adenoma or carcinoma) may itself be the direct source of excess cortisol. Pregnancy is uncommon in patients with this syndrome because of its association with a high incidence of menstrual disturbances and anovulation. Pituitary-dependent Cushing's (also called Cushing's disease) gives rise to bilateral adrenal hyperplasia and a state of hypercortisolism. Although pituitary-dependent Cushing's syndrome is the most common etiology in nonpregnant patients, it is relatively less commonly associated with pregnancy, hyperfunctioning adrenal tumors being relatively more common in pregnant patients with this syndrome. A possible explanation for this discrepancy could be a greater degree of ovulatory disturbance in patients with pituitary-dependent Cushing's syndrome (Buescher, 1996).

In a recent series of 67 pregnancies (in 58 patients), incorporating 63 pregnancies from the world literature and four new cases (Aaron et al., 1990), 23 patients had adrenal adenoma (40%), six patients had adrenal cortical carcinoma (10%), and one patient had ectopic ACTH syndrome resulting from an ACTH-secreting pheochromocytoma (2%). In four cases, the cause was not determined (7%), and in the remaining 24 (41%), bilateral adrenal hyperplasia was found, suggestive of pituitary-dependent Cushing's syndrome. Because the placenta can elaborate both CRH and ACTH, however, these hormones could conceivably lead to adrenal stimulation. This phenomenon also explains apparent exacerbation of Cushing's syndrome in pregnancy with amelioration or remission after pregnancy (Pickard et al., 1990; Buescher, 1996).

DIAGNOSIS. The diagnosis of Cushing's syndrome in pregnancy can be rendered more difficult because weight gain, hypertension, striae, edema, and pigmentation may occur in normal pregnancy. More specific signs, such as thinning of the skin, spontaneous bruising, and muscle weakness, should be sought. Furthermore, the laboratory diagnosis is complicated by the changes in adrenal function that occur during normal pregnancy. These include an increase in bound and free serum cortisol, increased urinary free cortisol, and lack of adequate suppression of cortisol following low-dose dexamethasone treatment.

Urinary free cortisol excretion (less than 100 μg/24 hours in the nonpregnant state) is increased during normal pregnancy (averaging 127 μg/24 hours in the third trimester, with values ranging from 68 to 252 μg/24 hours). Bearing these changes in mind—and although urinary free cortisol excretion is still useful as a test of Cushing's syndrome—a low-dose dexamethasone suppression test (2 mg/day), preferably for 8 days (rather than the customary 2 days), is the more appropriate test for diagnosis, and failure of suppression is in keeping with Cushing's syndrome. Even dexamethasone suppressibility of plasma cortisol, however, as judged by standard criteria (less than 6 µg/dL), may be impaired (as occurs in patients receiving estrogen therapy). To be more certain, one should measure both plasma cortisol and 24-hour urinary steroids (free cortisol, 17-ketogenic and 17-ketosteroids) during dexamethasone suppression tests in pregnancy. Loss of diurnal variation in serum cortisol and in the case of pituitary-dependent Cushing's, suggesting an elevated incremental response to CRH, could be quite helpful in the diagnosis of Cushing's in pregnancy, especially as the response to CRH is lost by late third trimester.

To distinguish pituitary-dependent Cushing's from hyperfunctioning adrenal tumors, a high-dose dexamethasone suppression test is recommended (8 mg/day for at least 2 days). Significant (greater than or equal to 50%) suppression of plasma cortisol is the rule in pituitary-dependent Cushing's syndrome, and failure of suppression with high-dose dexamethasone, along with low or undetectable ACTH concentrations, strongly suggests an adrenal source. Because the placenta also produces ACTH, however, this test may not always be reliable. Ectopic ACTH syndrome also causes failure to suppress. The pituitary (and the adrenal) can be evaluated during pregnancy by means of MRI (Schultz et al., 1984; Gonzalez et al., 1988). In the absence of a pituitary tumor, if ACTH is elevated, pituitary disease can be distinguished from ectopic ACTH by inferior petrosal sinus sampling combined with CRH stimulation. There is one report of such testing in pregnancy (Pinette et al., 1994).

MATERNAL-FETAL COMPLICATIONS. Although congenital malformations are not more common in Cushing's syndrome than in normal pregnancy (Pickard et al., 1990), maternal and fetal complications can occur. In the series of Aaron and coworkers (1990), premature birth occurred in 35 of 57 cases (61%) and was associated with morbidity and mortality. There were seven spontaneous abortions (pregnancies terminating before 20 weeks' gestation) and six stillbirths. Intrauterine growth restriction is prevalent, occurring in approximately one half of reported cases (Buescher, 1996). Possible causes include hypertension and cortisol excess itself. Neonatal adrenal insufficiency also has been reported and is presumably due to suppression of the fetal hypothalamic-pituitary-adrenal axis from transplacental transport of excess maternal cortisol (see Fig. 51-5). Maternal complications included hypertension (87%), abnormal carbohydrate metabolism (61%), congestive heart failure, decreased wound healing, and maternal death in three of the 67 cases (Aaron et al., 1990).

THERAPY. Given the poor fetal outcome, therapy aimed at controlling the hypercortisolism has been attempted. Treatment does not appear to influence premature birth, intrauterine growth restriction, or perinatal morbidity, but the incidence of intrauterine fetal demise is decreased (Buescher, 1996). The following recommendations for treatment have been suggested and seem reasonable (Van der Spuy and Jacobs, 1984).

In the first trimester, pituitary surgery for pituitary-dependent Cushing's syndrome and adrenal surgery for tumors of adrenal origin (especially to rule out carcinoma) should be performed. In the third trimester, early delivery of the fetus—preferably vaginal—may be attempted. Metyrapone therapy (to block cortisol secretion) may reduce hypercortisolism until fetal maturity is attained (Close et al., 1993). In the second trimester, treatment should be individualized, the alternatives being definitive surgery versus medical therapy aimed at ameliorating hypercortisolism. Successful transsphenoidal surgery has been reported in the second trimester (Mellor et al, 1998). The risks of treatment with metyrapone, ketoconazole, and aminoglutethimide, all of which block cortisol secretion, are uncertain because transplacental passage occurs and fetal adrenal steroid synthesis may be affected (Gormley et al., 1982). In addition, risk of teratogenicity, virilization of female fetuses (aminoglutethimide), or inadequate masculinization of a male fetus (ketoconazole) discourage the use of these two agents.

NELSON SYNDROME. When a patient with pituitary-dependent Cushing's syndrome undergoes bilateral adrenalectomy as definitive treatment for hypercortisolism and the pituitary lesion is not adequately addressed, a syndrome of hyperpigmentation along with an expanding intrasellar ACTH-producing tumor can result and is called *Nelson syndrome*. The association of this syndrome and pregnancy is rare. In a series involving ten cases, five required postpartum treatment of their pituitary tumors, four were only observed, and one required surgical treatment during the pregnancy, with successful outcome for both mother and child (Surrey and Chang, 1985). A more recent case also documented an uncomplicated pregnancy and normal lactation (Beasley, 1999).

HYPOPITUITARISM

Diminished or decreased production of anterior pituitary hormones results in inadequate activity of target organs, such as thyroid, adrenal, and gonads. The deficiency can be partial—affecting trophic hormones in varying degrees—or it can be complete, resulting in panhypopituitarism. The role of the obstetrician-gynecologist in this context is twofold:

1. To be alert to and aware of the possibility of two disease processes that can affect the pregnant patient, namely Sheehan syndrome and lymphocytic hypophysitis
2. To recognize and treat hypopituitarism in a pregnant patient, thus avoiding undesirable consequences

SHEEHAN SYNDROME

In 1937, Sheehan drew attention to the relationship between postpartum hemorrhage and anterior pituitary necrosis. Because the syndrome is distinctly uncommon with other conditions associated with shock and vascular collapse, it is assumed that the hyperplastic gland in pregnancy is more vulnerable to an inadequate blood supply. In a retrospective survey by Hall (1962), pregnant patients admitted for hemorrhagic collapse were subsequently traced and evaluated for hypopituitarism, the incidence being approximately 3.6%. There is said to be no direct correlation between the severity of the hemorrhage and the occurrence of Sheehan syndrome, but the major part of the pituitary must be destroyed before symptoms become evident (Hall, 1962).

In a series of 25 cases (Drury and Keelan, 1966), 50% of patients had permanent amenorrhea, the remainder experiencing rare and scanty menses. Only one patient menstruated normally, and in most, lactation was poor or absent. There was a surprisingly long interval between the obstetric event and diagnosis (more than 10 years) in more than half the cases.

Although pregnancy in hypopituitary patients is rare, inability to establish the diagnosis and institute proper therapy could have lethal consequences for both mother and fetus. Grimes and Brooks (1980) reviewed pregnancies among patients with Sheehan syndrome. There were 87% live births, 13% abortions, and no stillbirth or maternal death in 15 pregnancies in patients receiving hormonal therapy. In sharp contrast, in 24 pregnancies among 11 women in whom hormone replacement was not provided, there were 58% live births, 42% abortions, a stillbirth, and three maternal deaths.

In nonpregnant patients thought to have Sheehan syndrome, the diagnosis and the extent of pituitary damage can be determined by tests of target organ function (e.g., thyroid function tests, cortisol concentration) as well as tests of pituitary reserve (Lufkin et al., 1983). An ongoing pregnancy does not constitute evidence against the diagnosis of Sheehan syndrome, and it should be considered in all patients with a past history of postpartum hemorrhage, especially if the patient is currently symptomatic. The finding of a low serum thyroxine and low TSH level is in keeping with secondary hypothyroidism; low cortisol concentrations (compared with those of normal pregnant women), along with failure of cortisol and ACTH to increase during times of stress, are in keeping with diminished ACTH reserve. Imaging studies are likely to reveal an empty sella turcica (Scheller and Nader, 1997).

Treatment of pituitary insufficiency during pregnancy does not present special problems. Oral L-thyroxine (0.1–0.2 mg/day) and cortisol (20 mg in the morning, 10 mg in the evening) or prednisone (5 mg in the morning, 2.5 mg in the evening) are administered. There is no need for mineralocorticoids. As in the nonpregnant state, glucocorticoid requirements may increase during episodes of intercurrent illness. During labor, a good state of hydration should be maintained and parenteral glucocorticoids administered. This is most easily achieved by the intravenous infusion of hydrocortisone (cortisol). The dose can be adjusted as appropriate for the patient's state, ranging from 25 to 75 mg every 6 hours. After delivery, parenteral glucocorticoids should be continued, in the smaller doses, for a few days along with intravenous fluids.

PITUITARY NECROSIS

Spontaneous pituitary necrosis and hypopituitarism can occur in pregnant diabetic patients, possibly related to diabetic vascular changes and the general susceptibility of the anterior pituitary to ischemia in pregnancy. It is manifested by severe, midline headaches and vomiting during the third trimester, followed by a decrease in insulin requirements. In three of eight patients reported, the condition was associated with fetal death followed by maternal death (Dorfman et al., 1979)—hence the need for early recognition and prompt management.

LYMPHOCYTIC HYPOPHYSITIS

In 1962, Goudie and Pinkerton described the case of a 22-year-old woman who died of circulatory collapse 8 hours after appendectomy. This occurred 14 months after a normal pregnancy and delivery, but she had developed secondary amenorrhea after delivery. Autopsy revealed lymphocytic infiltration of the pituitary and of the thyroid—the authors postulated an autoimmune mechanism to explain both.

Forty-three of 44 pathologically documented cases reported in the last few decades were in women (Cosman et al., 1989; Bitton et al., 1991; Feigenbaum et al., 1991; Stelmach and O'Day, 1991). In addition, a number of cases have been reported that fit the description just given, but for which pathologic confirmation is not available because surgery was not performed (Nader and Orlander, 1990).

In 32 of the 43 women with pathologically documented lymphocytic hypophysitis, the disease occurred in relation to pregnancy. The features of these 32 patients are outlined in Table 51-3. In 13 patients, the symptoms were noted after delivery; in the other 19, symptoms occurred during the pregnancy and included headache, lethargy, weight loss, and (in one case) collapse and death during labor. Twenty-two of the cases involved varying degrees of hypopituitarism, and 18 involved visual disturbances. Eight cases involved inappropriate hyperprolactinemia, galactorrhea, or both; pituitary stalk disturbance with relative lack of the prolactin inhibitory factor, dopamine, has been suggested as the mechanism likely to explain this phenomenon. In seven cases, the diagnosis was made at autopsy; in the remaining 25, pituitary surgery was performed for suspected tumor.

Seven of the women had evidence of an autoimmune disease. Given this association, antipituitary antibodies have been sought and found in both pregnancy-related and -unrelated cases (Nader and Orlander, 1990). The close temporal association of this disease with pregnancy is most intriguing. Flare-up of autoimmune disease processes in the postpartum period has been well documented, but given the relative immunologic tolerance during pregnancy, the occurrence of lymphocytic hypophysitis during a pregnancy is less well explained. Exacerbation of the disease after delivery, even when it initially presents in pregnancy, has also been described (Meichner et al., 1987).

The association of this disease with pregnancy is also highlighted in an immunohistochemical study performed on pituitary material obtained at autopsy in 69 women who were pregnant or who had undergone delivery; among these were five cases of mild lymphocytic hypophysitis (Scheithauer et al., 1990). In four of these five cases, the patients died at 38–41 weeks' gestation.

The importance of this condition is that it is a potentially life-threatening but treatable disease affecting young women

TABLE 51-3. CHARACTERISTICS OF 32 WOMEN WITH PREGNANCY-RELATED AND PATHOLOGICALLY DOCUMENTED LYMPHOCYTIC HYPOPHYSITIS

Age	Mean 28 years
	Range 18–38 years
History of onset	19 during gestation
	13 postpartum
Hypopituitary*	22 cases
Visual disturbance*	18 cases
Hyperprolactinemia/galactorrhea	8 cases
Associated disorders	
Thyroiditis	4
Thyroiditis and adrenalitis	1
Pernicious anemia	1
Positive smooth muscle antibody	1
Diagnosis	
Autopsy	7
Biopsy (tumor suspected)	25

* Not documented in one of the cases.

during or after pregnancy. Thus, the diagnosis should be considered in women of reproductive age presenting with signs and symptoms of anterior pituitary hormone deficiencies (isolated or in combination) before or after delivery (especially in the absence of significant bleeding during labor). The diagnosis should also be considered in pregnant or postpartum women with visual symptoms and changes. In the absence of a threat to vision, such patients should be treated medically with hormone replacement and their progress observed. MRI should be used to delineate and follow the anatomic defects.

It is also noteworthy that the use of steroids has been associated with amelioration of visual symptoms (Stelmach and O'Day, 1991; Bitton et al., 1991), and the sellar mass has been shown to regress spontaneously. In another reported case (Bitton et al., 1991), partial hypopituitarism resolved after delivery in a biopsy-diagnosed case of lymphocytic hypophysitis. Finally, in a case reported by Brandes and Cerletty (1989) in which the data strongly supported a presumptive diagnosis of lymphocytic hypophysitis, and despite persistent partial hypopituitarism, the patient's menses resumed, she became pregnant, and she had an uncomplicated pregnancy while on thyroid and cortisol replacement. Although considered a disease of the anterior pituitary, lymphocytic hypophysitis can present as diabetes insipidus with thickening and prominence of the pituitary stalk (Ober and Elster, 1994).

Disorders of the Pituitary Gland: Posterior Lobe

Diabetes Insipidus

Vasopressin and oxytocin, produced in the supraoptic and paraventricular nuclei of the hypothalamus, are released into the posterior lobe and from there into the circulation. No disease process with oxytocin deficiency or excess has yet been described. Lack of vasopressin results in diabetes insipidus, however, and this can occur as a primary or idiopathic disorder (approximately 30% of cases) or can be acquired secondary to a variety of pathologic lesions, including cranial injuries (16%), infections, sellar and suprasellar tumors (25%), and vascular lesions. The main symptoms are polyuria, polydipsia, and low urinary specific gravity. The diagnosis is confirmed by water deprivation. During this test, increasing serum osmolality in the face of low urine osmolality, is diagnostic of diabetes insipidus; a return toward normal after vasopressin administration confirms vasopressin deficiency.

EFFECT OF DIABETES INSIPIDUS ON PREGNANCY. Hendricks (1954), in a comprehensive review, concluded that the prior existence of diabetes insipidus in a woman did not appear to alter her fertility, the course of pregnancy, the effectiveness of labor, or lactation. Because oxytocin is also produced in the same hypothalamic nuclei, diabetes insipidus is of particular interest in the pregnant woman because of the possible relationship of decreased oxytocin with decreased uterine contractions during labor. Despite one report of uterine atony (Maranon, 1947), it would appear that labor is normal in most patients with diabetes insipidus.

EFFECT OF PREGNANCY ON DIABETES INSIPIDUS. This topic has been reviewed by Durr and Lindheimer (1996). Diabetes insipidus during pregnancy appears to be characterized by several distinct clinical entities: (1) pregnancy in patients with diabetes insipidus antedating gestation, (2) tran-

sient arginine vasopressin (AVP)–resistant but L-deamino, 8-D-arginine vasopressin (DDAVP)–responsive diabetes insipidus, (3) transient diabetes insipidus during pregnancy in patients with acquired or hereditary latent diabetes insipidus, (4) diabetes insipidus after a complicated delivery, and (5) transient de novo nephrogenic diabetes insipidus, resistant to both AVP and DDAVP.

Pregnancy in patients with diabetes insipidus antedating gestation. The effect of pregnancy on established diabetes insipidus varies. In a review of the subject, Hime and Richardson (1978) found that 58% of patients deteriorated, 20% improved, and 15% remained the same. The metabolic clearance of vasopressin markedly increases between gestational week 10 and midpregnancy and is associated with parallel increases in circulating vasopressinase. Placental inactivation of vasopressin with the production of large quantities of vasopressinase by the placenta may contribute to this increase in clearance rate (Lindheimer et al., 1991). Interestingly, in a few patients in whom preeclampsia developed, the diabetes insipidus improved. The decreased contribution of the placenta to destruction of vasopressin is thought to explain this improvement (Campbell, 1980).

Transient arginine vasopressin (AVP)–resistant but L-deamino, 8-D-arginine vasopressin (DDAVP)–responsive diabetes insipidus. This disorder is attributable to excessively high quantities of circulating vasopressinase (Hamai et al., 1997). It is often associated with liver abnormalities in the mother, such as acute fatty liver or *HELLP syndrome* (hemolysis, elevated liver enzymes, low platelets). Vasopressinase isoenzymes are proteins that are cleared by the liver and, under these circumstances, excessive amounts are made available.

Transient diabetes insipidus during pregnancy in patients with acquired or hereditary latent diabetes insipidus. Patients with limited vasopressin-secreting capacity (latent-central defect) may be unable to sustain the increased production rates necessary during gestation. Clinically, transient diabetes insipidus manifests in the latter part of gestation coinciding with peak vasopressinase levels, and subsequent pregnancies may involve multiple recurrences. A history of prior insult to the area, such as histiocytosis X or Sheehan syndrome, may be obtained. Classic hereditary nephrogenic diabetes insipidus is due to X-linked recessive mutation of the renal vasopressin receptor gene; symptomatic diabetes insipidus in female carriers is thus extremely rare. Some of these carriers, however, do have defects in renal concentrating ability, and it has been hypothesized that nonrandom X-chromosome inactivation in the kidneys could be responsible for the variable expression. Unmasking of a mild defect in vasopressin action (nephrogenic diabetes insipidus) could thus occur: The increased disposal of vasopressin could lead to decompensation. In addition, lowering of the osmotic threshold for thirst, which occurs normally in pregnancy (see Fig. 51-4), causes polydipsia and, hence, unacceptable polyuria in a patient with previously compensated nephrogenic diabetes insipidus (Robinson and Amico, 1991).

Diabetes insipidus after a complicated delivery. This is often associated with severe blood loss leading to various degrees of pituitary apoplexy or Sheehan syndrome.

Transient de novo nephrogenic diabetes insipidus, resistant to both AVP and DDAVP. Ford and Lumpkin (1986) found high prostaglandin E_2 concentrations. Reduced renal sensitivity to vasopressin has been proposed (Nakamura et al., 1991).

TREATMENT. The treatment of choice for central diabetes insipidus is DDAVP or desmopressin acetate, a synthetic analog of vasopressin, administered intranasally. Clinical experience with DDAVP, in a study involving many infants exposed during gestation, has confirmed its safety (Kallen et al., 1995; Ray, 1998). Dosages range from 10–20 μg given once or twice daily. In a study by Burrow and coauthors (1981), the drug was administered and DDAVP concentrations were measured as vasopressin by radioimmunoassay in maternal serum and breast milk. Whereas maternal serum concentrations rose about sevenfold, breast milk concentrations showed little change. This suggests that, given the low levels of DDAVP in milk, these mothers might also breast-feed. It is also noteworthy that DDAVP has little pressor or uterotonic action and is not affected by vasopressinase.

Primary Polydipsia during Gestation

Primary polydipsia has rarely been reported in gestation (Shalev et al., 1980); the pregnancy was merely incidental and had no role in the polydipsia.

ADRENAL GLANDS

The adrenal cortex plays an important and essential metabolic role in humans. Adrenal steroidogenesis leads to the production of three types of steroids. *Mineralocorticoids* are produced by the zona glomerulosa, *glucocorticoids* primarily in the zona fasciculata, and *sex steroids* in the zona reticularis. Figure 51-9 depicts the biosynthetic pathways diagrammatically.

Control of Adrenocortical Hormones

Aldosterone is primarily under the control of the renin-angiotensin system, although ACTH and hyperkalemia also have a stimulatory role. Renin, which is secreted by the juxtaglomerular apparatus of the kidney, converts angiotensinogen (an alpha$_2$-globulin produced by the liver) to angiotensin I, which is itself converted to angiotensin II. Angiotensin II, in addition to its pressor action, stimulates aldosterone secretion.

In turn, although an increase in angiotensin II suppresses renin production, volume and sodium depletion stimulate its release.

Cortisol secretion is controlled by the hypothalamic-pituitary axis. CRH is secreted by the paraventricular nucleus of the hypothalamus. It is a 1-41-NH$_2$ polypeptide that binds to the corticotroph membrane, activating the adenyl cyclase system. ACTH is a 1-39 polypeptide derived from a much larger precursor, pro-opiomelanocortin (POMC). This precursor is processed mainly into ACTH. There is a diurnal rhythm of cortisol secretion, the main secretory phase occurring during the late hours of sleep and early morning. Long- and short-loop negative feedback mechanisms are operating. In the long loop, the adrenal inhibits the anterior pituitary through the plasma cortisol by inhibiting ACTH release and by inhibition of the genome responsible for POMC synthesis. In the short loop, ACTH regulates its own secretion by inhibiting CRH release.

Although control of adrenal androgens is not understood, ACTH has a stimulatory effect on them. The major androgens are androstenedione, dehydroepiandrosterone, and its sulfate. Androstenedione is converted peripherally to testosterone as well as to estrone and estradiol.

Physiologic Changes during Pregnancy

Plasma CRH increases progressively during the second and third trimester, peaking at delivery. The placenta is the likely source (Sasaki et al., 1984). ACTH concentrations also increase during pregnancy and could be of placental origin (Rees et al., 1975); the diurnal variation of both cortisol and ACTH, although blunted, is maintained. Corticosteroid-binding globulin concentrations increase by three times during pregnancy, resulting in an increase in the total plasma cortisol and a fall in its metabolic clearance. The unbound fraction also increases, however, and this is reflected by a rise in urinary free cortisol. These changes are depicted in Figure 51-10. In the third trimester, the 9 A.M. plasma cortisol level ranges between 25 and 46 μg/dL, and the urinary free cortisol excretion ranges between 68 and 252 μg/24 hours. Neither placental ACTH nor CRH are suppressible *in vitro* with exogenous glucocorticoids.

Renin activity increases early, peaking at 12 weeks' gestation, with a decline in the third trimester (Wilson et al., 1980).

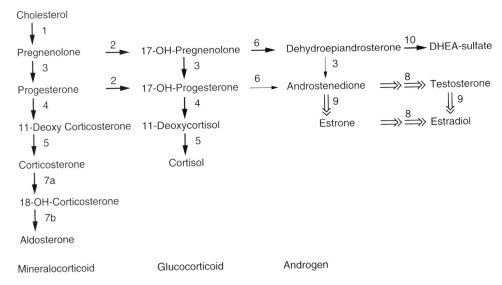

FIGURE 51-9 ■ Adrenal steroidogenic pathways of mineralocorticoid, glucocorticoid, and androgen synthesis. Major pathways are indicated by *thick arrows*, minor ones by *thin arrows*. Extra-adrenal conversion of sex steroids is denoted by *double arrows. Numbers* indicate enzymatic steps as follows: 1, 20α-hydroxylase, 22-hydroxylase, 20-22-desmolase; 2, 17α-hydroxylase; 3, 3β-hydroxysteroid dehydrogenase, 5-4 isomerase; 4, 21-hydroxylase; 5, 11β-hydroxylase; 6, C17-20-lyase; 7a, 18-hydroxylase; 7b, 18-dehydrogenase; 8, 17β-hydroxysteroid dehydrogenase; 9, aromatase; 10, sulfatase.

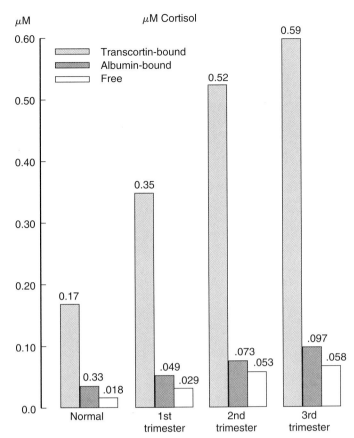

FIGURE 51-10. ■ Absolute distribution of bound and free cortisol in µM/liter pregnancy plasma. (From Rosenthal HE, Slaunwhite WR, Sandberg AA: Transcortin: A corticosteroid-binding protein of plasma: X. Cortisol and progesterone interplay and unbound levels of these steroids in pregnancy. J Clin Endocrinol Metab **29**:352, 1969. Copyright © The Endocrine Society.)

The decline is probably related to the rise in angiotensin II that occurs at this time. Thus, plasma aldosterone concentrations reach values five to eight times that of the nonpregnant state by the third trimester. The activation of the renin-angiotensin-aldosterone axis could be secondary to the fall in blood pressure, which is itself secondary to decreased vascular responsiveness to angiotensin II and decreased vascular resistance. High serum progesterone blocks aldosterone action, preventing kaliuresis.

Total testosterone increases in pregnancy because of an increase in sex hormone–binding globulin with a reduction in the percentage unbound; although the amount of free testosterone is low-normal in the first 28 weeks, it increases thereafter, with values often exceeding the normal range for nonpregnant women (Kerian et al., 1994). Mean levels of androstenedione also increase in the latter part of pregnancy, whereas dehydroepiandrosterone sulfate concentrations fall because of a major rise in the metabolic clearance rate.

Fetal Adrenal Development

This topic was reviewed recently by Keller-Wood and Wood (2001). The fetal adrenal can synthesize cortisol *in vitro* by 8 weeks' gestation. *In vivo*, placental 5-pregnenolone and 4-progesterone are used to synthesize steroids (Peterson, 1977). Two adrenal cortical zones can be identified in the fetus. The

inner, or fetal, zone, which accounts for about 80% of the cortex *in utero*, involutes in the first few months of extrauterine life. The outer zone becomes the adult adrenal cortex. The fetal zone lacks 3β-hydroxysteroid dehydrogenase and is therefore unable to synthesize glucocorticoids or mineralocorticoids. The most abundant product is DHEA, which forms the substrate for placental estrogen synthesis. During most of gestation, the majority of cortisol in the fetal circulation is supplied by the mother through transplacental passage, although fetal cortisol concentrations are lower than maternal because of placental cortisol metabolism.

Disorders of the Adrenal Cortex during Pregnancy

Disrupted reproductive function commonly accompanies significant genetic or acquired abnormalities of adrenal cortical function—thus, these abnormalities are usually diagnosed prior to conception. In patients with previously recognized adrenal disorders, replacement hormone therapy is continued throughout gestation, and the patient is monitored. The pregnancy-associated changes in normal values must be borne in mind.

Primary Adrenocortical Insufficiency (Addison Disease)

Atrophy of the adrenals on an autoimmune basis is the most common cause of adrenal failure, accounting for 75% of the cases. Other causes include hemorrhage (usually associated with sepsis and burns), infections (viral, fungal, or tuberculous), and infiltrative disorders, including metastases, lymphoma, and amyloidosis. With the availability of hormone replacement, pregnancy is no longer contraindicated.

DIAGNOSIS DURING PREGNANCY. In a review of 40 cases, some five decades ago, of Addison disease in pregnancy, 18 died during pregnancy; 12 of 22 who delivered had a crisis in the puerperium, and seven of these died (Brent, 1950). The diagnosis of Addison disease in pregnancy is uncommon and could relate to fetal contribution to maternal steroids. The symptoms include weakness, lassitude, nausea with or without vomiting, pigmentation, weight loss, anorexia, and abdominal pain. Some of these symptoms are also common in normal pregnant women. Thus, the index of suspicion should be raised when a thin pregnant woman complains of prolonged nausea and vomiting, weakness, postural hypotension, and personality changes. A history of polyendocrine autoimmune disorders, type I diabetes, adrenogenital syndrome, tuberculosis, and acquired immunodeficiency syndrome (AIDS) places the pregnant woman at increased risk for adrenocortical insufficiency.

The signs and symptoms and laboratory tests are outlined in Table 51-4. In acutely ill patients, replacement therapy must be initiated immediately and the diagnosis confirmed retrospectively via a pretreatment serum or plasma sample for measuring electrolytes, cortisol, and ACTH. In patients whose illness is less severe, a rapid ACTH stimulation test using synthetic ACTH may be performed; 250 µg is administered intravenously and blood samples are obtained at baseline, 30 minutes, and 60 minutes. Although a cortisol level exceeding 18 µg/dL and an increment exceeding 7 µg/dL is considered normal in the nonpregnant state, the mean increments have

TABLE 51-4. DIAGNOSIS OF PRIMARY ADRENAL INSUFFICIENCY DURING PREGNANCY

Signs and Symptoms

Nausea with or without vomiting, anorexia
Systolic blood pressure <100 mm Hg with postural fall
Increased pigmentation
Abdominal pain
Personality changes
Weakness, fatigue
Muscle and joint pain
Salt craving

Laboratory Findings

Decreased sodium
Increased potassium, BUN, creatinine
Hypoglycemia
Plasma cortisol below normal pregnancy level
Urinary-free cortisol: 24-hour excretion below normal pregnancy level
Increased plasma ACTH
Abnormal cortisol response to rapid ACTH stimulation test

ACTH, adrenocorticotropin or adrenocorticotropic hormone; BUN, blood urea nitrogen.

been reported as 18, 23, and 26 μg/dL in the first, second, and third trimester of pregnancy, respectively (Nolten et al., 1978).

TREATMENT. Replacement regimens are similar to those used in nonpregnant women. This is usually accomplished by hydrocortisone (cortisol), 20 mg in the morning and 10 mg in the evening, along with 9α-fludrocortisone, 0.05–0.1 mg daily. The dose of 9α-fludrocortisone is increased if postural hypotension or hyperkalemia persists and is decreased if hypertension or hypokalemia occurs. The dose of cortisol should be doubled or tripled in any situation associated with stress, including systemic illness or trauma. Breast-feeding has been discouraged because of the potential hazard of corticosteroids passing into the maternal milk, but some investigators disagree (Albert et al., 1989). Labor should be managed with stress doses of 300 mg of hydrocortisone over 24 hours with subsequent tapering.

ACUTE ADRENAL INSUFFICIENCY DURING PREGNANCY, LABOR, DELIVERY, OR THE PUERPERIUM. Addisonian crisis is a rare but life-threatening event in pregnant women (Seaward et al., 1989). The onset could be confused with an abdominal surgical emergency because of the prominence of abdominal pain, nausea, vomiting, and shock. After necessary blood samples are obtained for electrolytes, cortisol, and ACTH determinations, intravenous therapy should be started immediately with 100 mg of hydrocortisone sodium succinate along with an infusion of normal saline and 5% glucose. During the first 24 hours, 300–400 mg of intravenous hydrocortisone sodium succinate should be given continuously, and this can conveniently be added to the replacement fluids administered.

Recovery occurs quickly, and by 24 hours the patient may be able to return to oral feedings and replacement doses of oral hydrocortisone and 9α-fludrocortisone. If not, hydrocortisone may be continued intravenously, usually in diminished dosage. An effort should be made to determine the cause of the adrenal crisis, and the patient should receive careful post-pregnancy supervision. Patients with mild deficiency are especially at risk during labor, delivery, and the immediate postpartum period (Albert et al., 1989).

EFFECT OF MATERNAL ADDISON DISEASE ON THE NEWBORN. Infants born to mothers with Addison disease usually do not have any recognizable defects. Fetal growth, however, could be suboptimal with lower-than-normal birth weights, especially if the diagnosis is confirmed late in pregnancy or during the postpartum period (Drucker et al., 1984). Fetal death has also been reported (Keller-Wood and Wood, 2001). Maternal antibodies to the adrenal cortex do cross the placenta but do not significantly affect neonatal adrenal function.

Cushing's Syndrome

Cushing's syndrome results from an excess of glucocorticoids and is rare during pregnancy. See the previous discussion of hypothalamic and pituitary disorders and a review by Buescher (1996).

Primary Hyperaldosteronism

The autonomous secretion of aldosterone in primary hyperaldosteronism could be due to an adrenal adenoma, bilateral hyperplasia, or—rarely—an adrenocortical carcinoma. In pregnancy, the clinical picture of hyperaldosteronism is similar to that of the nonpregnant patient with hypertension, hypokalemia, and often kaliuresis and elevated serum bicarbonate (Lotgering et al., 1986). The electrolyte disturbances and hypertension could be first apparent in the peripartum period, coinciding with the removal of the protective antialdosterone effect of progesterone. All but one of the pregnancy-related cases of hyperaldosteronism have harbored adenomas (Neerhof et al., 1991; Robar et al., 1998).

DIAGNOSIS. After standardizing the patient for dietary sodium (100–150 mEq daily) and posture (recumbent) and the replacement of plasma potassium, one measures renin activity and aldosterone concentrations. The renin activity is lower and the aldosterone concentration higher than those found in normal pregnancy (Lotgering et al., 1986). Suppression of the aldosterone axis can also be attempted with salt loading (200–300 mEq/day for 3–5 days), the hallmark of primary hyperaldosteronism being lack of suppression of serum aldosterone concentration. If surgery is contemplated, MRI may be used to localize the adenoma. The course of pregnancy is one of difficult-to-treat hypertension. Neonatal morbidity and mortality relate to placental insufficiency.

TREATMENT. Medical treatment with standard antihypertensive drugs should be provided, along with potassium supplements. Surgery in the second trimester could be required if medical treatment fails; surgery has gained wider acceptance since the advent of laparoscopic adrenalectomy. Spironolactone is contraindicated in pregnancy, especially in the first trimester, because of its possible feminizing effects. In the first case report of a pregnant patient with hyperaldosteronism associated with bilateral hyperplasia, documented by Neerhof and colleagues (1991), enalapril maleate, an angiotensin-converting enzyme inhibitor, successfully lowered blood pressures in a patient unresponsive to other medications. The safety of this type of medication in pregnancy is questionable, as there are reports of adverse effects (Kreft-Jais et al., 1988), including fetal skull ossification defects, preterm birth, low birth weight, and oligohydramnios (see Chapter 19).

Congenital Adrenal Hyperplasia

The congenital adrenal hyperplasias (CAHs) involve inherited enzymatic defects of adrenal steroidogenesis. The most severe and life-threatening disorders occur early in the biosynthetic cascade and are usually fatal or incompatible with successful reproduction. Deficiency of 21-hydroxylase is the most common defect (see Fig. 51-7), accounting for 90%–95% of cases with an incidence of about 1 in 14,000, although in some areas, such as Alaska, it is more frequent (Pang et al., 1988). The second most common form is 11-hydroxylase deficiency. CAH in pregnancy and its prenatal treatment was reviewed by New (2001).

GENETICS. All CAHs are autosomal-recessive disorders. Thus, the parents of an affected child have at least one haplotype for the defect, giving each subsequent offspring a 25% chance of having the condition and a 50% chance of being a carrier. An affected individual produces 100% carriers if her partner is nonaffected; if her partner is a carrier, 50% of the offspring are affected and the other 50% are carriers. Siblings or spouses who want to know whether they are heterozygotes for 21-hydroxylase deficiency can be tested by undergoing measurements of adrenal steroids (notably 17-hydroxyprogesterone) before and after ACTH stimulation (White et al., 1987a).

21-HYDROXYLASE DEFICIENCY. 21-Hydroxylase deficiency arises because of genetic mutations of the 21-hydroxylase gene located at a site linked to the human leukocyte antigen (HLA) histocompatibility complex on the short arm of the sixth chromosome. The variation in severity of the deficiency can be accounted for by allelic variation at the gene locus (White and New, 1992). The enzyme block results in inadequate synthesis of 11-deoxycortisol and cortisol; the resulting excess ACTH stimulates adrenal precursors, notably 17-hydroxyprogesterone. Shunting of these excess precursors results in excess androgens, leading to masculinization of genitalia of the female fetus and excess masculinization of the male infant.

If the defect is severe, mineralocorticoid deficiency also occurs with salt wasting. Diagnosis is confirmed by the finding of excess basal 17-hydroxyprogesterone concentrations; in milder forms, ACTH stimulation is necessary and shows an excessive rise in 17-hydroxyprogesterone. Physiologic replacement doses of glucocorticoids (usually cortisol) are used as therapy, dosage being based on surface area. Concentrations of 4-androstenedione, testosterone, and 17-hydroxyprogesterone are used to monitor adequacy of suppression. Fludrocortisone is indicated in salt-losing forms and in non–salt-losing forms with increased plasma renin activity. Virilized females could require surgical reconstruction of the genitalia to provide for normal appearance, intercourse, and pregnancy.

MATERNAL AND FETAL CONSIDERATIONS. Although poor control of CAH results in irregular or absent menses, patients in whom the condition is well controlled may achieve pregnancy, although not so often as one might predict, possibly owing to postnatal intervals of excess androgen exposure. Usually, the same dose of cortisol can be continued through gestation, with additional amounts given during labor, delivery, and the immediate postpartum period. Cesarean section rates are higher because of abnormal maternal external genitalia or a small bony pelvis from premature closure of the epiphyses (Mori and Miyakawa, 1970). Most children of mothers with CAH are normal, although women receiving suboptimal doses of replacement therapy have elevated circulating androgens, which may cross the placenta and virilize the fetus. Free testosterone levels do not change significantly during gestation and can be used as a marker for monitoring therapy. Conversely, excessive glucocorticoid therapy of the mother with CAH could result in suppression of fetal adrenals with resulting transient adrenocortical insufficiency of the neonate.

PRENATAL DIAGNOSIS AND TREATMENT. Prenatal diagnosis of 21-hydroxylase deficiency for offspring of known heterozygotes first became possible with the finding of elevated levels of 17-hydroxyprogesterone in amniotic fluid, obtained by amniocentesis (White et al., 1987b). Since by the time amniocentesis is performed (in the second trimester) it is too late to prevent virilization, dexamethasone is administered in a pregnancy at risk before the end of the seventh week from conception (ninth week gestation). This treatment results in suppression of 17-hydroxyprogesterone and renders it unreliable for diagnosis. When HLA was found to be linked to CAH, diagnoses were made using HLA linkage marker analysis using amniotic cells. To avoid errors resulting from recombination or haplotype sharing, however, direct DNA analysis of the 21-hydroxylase gene (CYP 21) with molecular genetic techniques is currently recommended. Chorionic villus sampling should preferably be used to obtain fetal tissue sooner, at 9–11 weeks' gestation for diagnosis by molecular genetic analysis (New et al., 2001).

Prenatal treatment of the mother with high-dose glucocorticoids has been shown to be effective in preventing virilization of the affected female fetus; the glucocorticoid crosses the placenta and suppresses ACTH secretion from the fetal pituitary (White et al., 1987b). The present-day approach is to treat all such mothers with glucocorticoids. Dexamethasone (20 μg/kg of pre-pregnancy weight) is given orally in divided daily doses once pregnancy has been confirmed. This treatment must be given before the end of the seventh week from conception. Chorionic villus sampling is then performed. If the fetus is male, maternal treatment is discontinued; if female, the treatment is continued until the results of DNA analysis of the 21-hydroxylase gene are available. The glucocorticoids are discontinued only if the female fetus is considered unaffected.

A review of 532 pregnancies prenatally diagnosed using amniocentesis or chorionic villus sampling between 1978 and 2001 was reported by New and associates (2001). Of these 532 pregnancies, 281 were treated prenatally for congenital adrenal hyperplasia because of the risk of 21-hydroxylase deficiency. Of 116 babies affected with CAH, 61 were female, and 49 of them were treated prenatally with dexamethasone. If given in proper dosage, dexamethasone administered at or before week 9 of gestation was effective in reducing virilization. With the exception of striae, weight gain, and edema, there were no other differences in symptoms in treated versus untreated mothers. Prenatally treated newborns had weights that matched untreated and unaffected newborns, and no enduring side-effects were noted. Thus, prenatal diagnosis and treatment of 21-hydroxylase deficiency is both possible and effective. An algorithm showing prenatal management of pregnancies in families at risk for a fetus affected by 21-hydroxylase deficiency is shown in Figure 51-11.

11-HYDROXYLASE DEFICIENCY. 11-Hydroxylase deficiency, an enzyme defect that is not HLA-linked, results in blocked production of cortisol and aldosterone with resulting excess precursors, 11-deoxycortisol and deoxycorticosterone (White et al., 1987b). A shunt toward excess androgens occurs, and

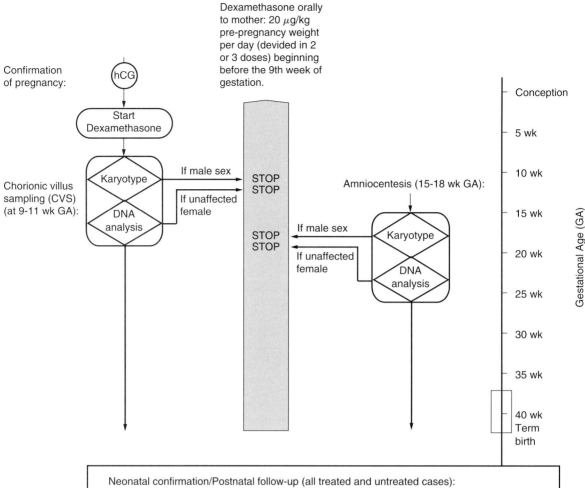

FIGURE 51-11. ■ Algorithm depicting prenatal management of pregnancy in families at risk for a fetus affected with 21-hydroxylase deficiency. (From New MI et al: Extensive personal experience: Prenatal diagnosis for congenital adrenal hyperplasia in 532 pregnancies. J Clin Endocrinol Metab **86**[12]:5651–5657, 2001. Copyright © The Endocrine Society.)

the presentation is that of androgen excess and hypertension. Diagnosis is based on elevated 11-deoxycortisol and deoxycorticosterone concentrations, either basally or after ACTH stimulation. Heterozygotes have no demonstrable biochemical abnormality, even with ACTH stimulation. Treatment is with glucocorticoid replacement. Prenatal diagnosis is confirmed by measuring amniotic fluid 11-deoxycortisol concentrations (Rosler et al., 1979). Prenatal treatment of the mother with dexamethasone, as in 21-hydroxylase deficiency, has been reported, resulting in a female without virilization or ambiguous genitalia, who was genetically affected (Cerame, 1999). Mutations in the 11-hydroxylase gene that could facilitate prenatal diagnosis have also been reported (White et al., 1994).

OTHER CONGENITAL ADRENAL HYPERPLASIA ENZYME DEFICIENCIES. There are a few other rare forms of CAH (see Fig. 51-9). In 17-hydroxylase deficiency, the sex steroid pathway is blocked both in the adrenal cortex and gonad, resulting in a hypogonadal state and primary amenorrhea. Deficiency of 3β-hydroxysteroid dehydrogenase, if severe, presents as lack of pubertal development. Milder forms present pubertally with hyperandrogenism (Rosenfeld et al., 1980).

Long-Term Therapy with Pharmacologic Doses of Steroids

The occurrence of congenital anomalies in animal experiments—cleft palate in particular—raised concerns about pregnant women receiving glucocorticoids during pregnancy. In a review involving 260 pregnancies in which glucocorticoids had been administered to women in pharmacologic doses, however, only two infants had cleft palate (Bongiovanni and McPadden, 1960). Both mothers had received steroids in large doses early in pregnancy. Because closure of the palatal process occurs by the 12th week of gestation, it is possible that the anomaly was related to the medication. While other, smaller studies have not supported this association (Snyder and Snyder, 1978), a prospective cohort study and meta-analysis of epidemiologic studies concluded that prednisone increases the risk of oral clefts by an order of 3.4 fold (Park-Wyllie et al., 2000).

It is also important to remember that the hypothalamic-pituitary-adrenal axis is suppressed with long-term supraphysiologic doses of glucocorticoids, and abrupt withdrawal should be avoided because it could precipitate maternal adrenocortical insufficiency. Glucocorticoids are excreted in breast milk and have the potential to cause growth restriction in the neonate. In addition, neonatal adrenal insufficiency, although rare, can occur in infants born to mothers being treated with exogenous glucocorticoids (Bongiovanni and McPadden, 1960).

Disorders of the Adrenal Medulla during Pregnancy

Pheochromocytoma

Pheochromocytomas are tumors of chromaffin cells. These cells cluster predominantly in the adrenal medulla, and 90% of pheochromocytomas are found in this location. Extra-adrenal tumors range in site from the carotid body to the pelvic floor. They occur either sporadically or as part of the familial multiple endocrine neoplasia, type 2, syndrome. Approximately 12% are malignant, although this percentage is higher in pheochromocytomas occurring in extra-adrenal sites.

SYMPTOMS. Pheochromocytoma is a rare but potentially lethal cause of hypertension in pregnancy. Its possibility should be considered in women with intermittent, labile hypertension or paroxysmal symptoms such as anxiety, diaphoresis, headache, and palpitations. Other symptoms include chest or abdominal pain, unusual reactions to drugs affecting catecholamine release and actions, visual disturbances, convulsions, and collapse. Symptoms tend to be similar in pregnant and nonpregnant women. The occurrence of symptoms during pregnancy only, with recurrence in subsequent pregnancies, has also been described. Increased vascularity of the tumor in pregnancy, as well as the mechanical effect of an enlarging uterus, could explain this phenomenon. In many cases, severe symptoms develop in the peripartum and postpartum periods.

LABORATORY DIAGNOSIS. Laboratory diagnosis involves biochemical demonstration of elevated vanillylmandelic acid, catecholamines, and metanephrines in the 24-hour urine specimen. Plasma catecholamine levels can also be determined. Values in pregnant women are similar to those in nonpregnant subjects. They are elevated for 24 hours after eclamptic

seizures, however. Because methyldopa interferes with catecholamine measurements, it should be discontinued prior to testing. If necessary, the tumor may be localized during pregnancy by means of ultrasonography (Griffin et al., 1984) or MRI (Glazer et al., 1986).

TREATMENT. Treatment of pheochromocytoma in pregnancy is somewhat controversial. Most authors agree that when the diagnosis is confirmed in the second half of pregnancy, alpha-adrenergic blockade with phenoxybenzamine is the treatment of choice. This drug is given orally, starting with 10 mg twice daily, gradually increasing by 10–20 mg daily until hypertension is controlled. When fetal maturity is achieved, cesarean section should be performed, with simultaneous or subsequent excision of the tumor (Fudge et al., 1980; Harper et al., 1989) during adrenergic blockade.

In tumors detected before the 24th week of gestation, surgery during pregnancy has been advocated (Harper et al., 1989) to avoid fetal wasting. A number of such cases have been managed successfully during pregnancy with alpha- and beta-blockade with good fetal outcome, however (Lyons and Colmorgen, 1988; Oliver et al., 1990). The arguments against medical therapy are the unknown effects of alpha- and beta-blockade on the fetus in the long term, the teratogenic potential of phenoxybenzamine, and the risk of a malignant lesion. Beta-blockade alone should not be used without prior alpha-blockade because unopposed alpha-adrenergic activity could lead to generalized vasoconstriction and a steep rise in blood pressure. Anesthetic management of pheochromocytoma resection during pregnancy requires special consideration (Mitchell et al., 1987).

PROGNOSIS. Pheochromocytoma constitutes a life-threatening disease for both the mother and the fetus, although with better management and the availability of alpha- and beta-adrenergic blockade, the prospects for both have improved. Table 51-5 reflects the changes in maternal and fetal mortality rates over the last few decades and indicates the improved prognosis when the diagnosis is made during pregnancy (Schenker and Granat, 1982; Harper et al., 1989). Conversely, in a recent report, a 36-year-old died at 27 weeks' gestation from an autopsy-diagnosed pheochromocytoma (Harrington et al., 1999). Fetal growth restriction could occur secondary to reduced uteroplacental perfusion, and fetal death may occur during acute hypertensive crises.

Four cases of malignant pheochromocytomas in pregnancy were reviewed by Ellison and associates (1988) and another by Devoe and co-workers (1986); alpha-methyl paratyrosine, a dopamine synthesis inhibitor, was used in the latter case. Several cases of pregnancy with pheochromocytoma as part of multiple endocrine neoplasia, type 2, also have been reported (Harper et al., 1989; van der Vaart et al., 1993; Tewari et al., 2001).

TABLE 51-5. CHANGES IN MATERNAL AND FETAL MORTALITIES IN OVER 200 PREGNANCIES COMPLICATED BY PHEOCHROMOCYTOMA, SPANNING SEVERAL DECADES

Time of Diagnosis	Maternal Mortality			Fetal Mortality		
	Before 1969	1969–1979	1980–1987	Before 1969	1969–1979	1980–1987
During pregnancy	18%	4%	0%	50%	42%	15%
Postpartum period	58%	50%	17%	56%	56%	35%

HIRSUTISM AND VIRILIZATION IN PREGNANCY

Hirsutism and virilization in pregnancy was reviewed by McClamrock and Adashi (1992). Women and their female fetuses are protected from the increased concentrations of androgens by the enhanced binding to sex hormone–binding globulin, competition by progestins either for binding to the androgen receptor or for disposition of androgens to more biologically potent compounds, and placental aromatization of androgens. Nevertheless, maternal hirsutism and virilization can occur in pregnancy, nearly always secondary to ovarian disease (or iatrogenic insult). In addition, the female fetus can be affected by elevated circulating maternal androgens. Differentiation of the female external genitalia occurs between the 7th and 12th week of gestation, and exposure to excess androgens could result in partial or complete labial fusion and clitoromegaly. Clitoromegaly may still occur after the 12th week of gestation. The approach to maternal hirsutism and virilization in pregnancy is outlined in Table 51-6.

The two major causes of gestational hyperandrogenism are luteomas and hyperreactio luteinalis (gestational ovarian theca-lutein cysts). Luteomas are benign, solid tumors of the ovary; they are often multinodular and bilateral, and they are usually yellow to tan in color. Regardless of their virilizing effect, luteomas have been associated with elevated circulating maternal androgens.

Not all luteomas cause maternal virilization (overall incidence of virilization = 35%); this could depend on the amount of androgen secreted, the end-organ sensitivity, and the degree of aromatization by the placenta to nonandrogenic steroids. Approximately 80% of female infants born to mothers with virilizing luteomas are virilized, usually exhibiting clitoromegaly. Although luteomas are considered intrapartum lesions that regress after delivery, this concept has been challenged and could account for recurrence of virilization in subsequent pregnancies (Shortle et al., 1987). In contrast with hyperreactio luteinalis, luteomas occur more frequently in black multiparas and are not associated with toxemia, erythroblastosis, or multiple gestation.

Hyperreactio luteinalis is characterized by ovarian enlargement with multiple large-follicle cysts, corpora lutea, or both with marked edema of the stroma. It is generally bilateral,

affecting white primigravidas, and is often associated with conditions resulting in increased human chorionic gonadotropin (hCG), such as molar pregnancies and multiple gestation. Maternal hirsutism or virilization has been documented in approximately 30% of reported cases. There are no reported cases of fetal masculinization, even if the mother is virilized. It has been suggested that the condition could represent an excessive ovarian sensitivity to hCG. The lack of fetal virilization in this condition is intriguing and has been attributed to androgen aromatization in the placenta. As with luteomas, recurrence of hyperreactio luteinalis in consecutive pregnancies has been reported (Bachman et al., 1974).

In a few cases (Sarlis et al, 1999; de Butros and Hatipoglu, 2001; author's personal experience), insulin-resistant polycystic ovary syndrome patients who achieve pregnancy may become extremely androgenized during pregnancy. Metformin was used in one of these cases (Sarlis et al., 1999). Other ovarian lesions that could cause maternal virilization include Sertoli-Leydig cell tumors (arrhenoblastomas), Krukenberg tumors, Brenner tumors, lipoid cell tumors, dermoid cysts, and mucinous and serous cystadenocarcinomas. The majority of Sertoli-Leydig cell tumors coexisting with pregnancy are associated with maternal virilization, and virilization of the female fetus could occur. The malignancy rate for these tumors is high (44%), with substantial maternal (31%) and perinatal (50%) mortality rates. Krukenberg tumors, which are gastrointestinal tumors metastatic to the ovary, are often bilateral and have caused maternal and fetal virilization in all reported cases.

Adrenal tumors, including adrenocortical carcinoma, can cause maternal and fetal virilization (Miyata et al., 1989). Finally, masculinization of the female fetus has been associated with the gestational administration of progestins and androgens and could be unaccompanied by maternal virilization.

PARATHYROID GLANDS AND CALCIUM METABOLISM

Maternal and Fetal Physiology and Lactation

Serum calcium is tightly regulated and maintained within normal limits by parathyroid hormone (PTH) and vitamin D. Vitamin D can be synthesized in the skin under the influence of ultraviolet irradiation or can be absorbed from dietary sources via the gastrointestinal tract. Vitamin D is 25-hydroxylated in the liver and then 1-hydroxylated in the kidney. The physiologically active form of vitamin D is $1,25(OH)_2$ D, which is responsible for increasing intestinal absorption of calcium and for bone resorption. The parathyroid glands, which produce PTH, are stimulated by hypocalcemia and suppressed by high concentrations of calcium, magnesium, and $1,25(OH)_2$ D as well as by hypomagnesemia. PTH influences calcium metabolism, not only by directly resorbing bone, but also by stimulating $1,25(OH)_2$ D formation. There are three major forms of circulating calcium—namely, ionized, protein-bound, and chelated fractions. The ionized fraction is physiologically active and homeostatically regulated.

Calcium homeostasis in pregnancy was reviewed by Hosking (1996). Large amounts of calcium and phosphorus are transferred against a concentration gradient from the mother to the fetus (Pitkin, 1985), the net accumulation of calcium being 25–30 g by term (mostly in the third trimester).

TABLE 51-6. APPROACH TO MATERNAL HIRSUTISM AND VIRILIZATION IN PREGNANCY

History

Acute onset in pregnancy: Investigate as indicated below.
Androgenic drug exposure: Stop drug.

Physical Exam/Ovarian Ultrasound	*Possible Virilization of Female Fetus*
Bilateral cystic: Theca lutein cysts: rule out high hCG states	No
Bilateral solid: Luteoma very likely	Yes
Unilateral solid: Surgery to rule out malignancy	Yes
No ovarian mass: Investigate adrenal glands	Yes

hCG, human chorionic gonadotropin.

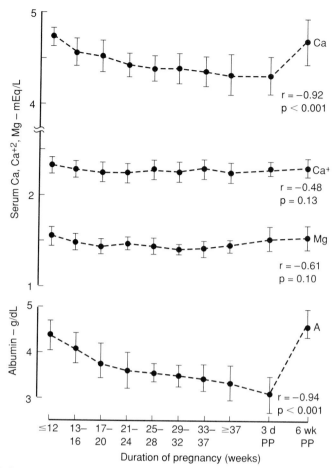

FIGURE 51-12. ■ Mean (± SD) levels of calcium (Ca), ionized calcium (Ca²), magnesium (Mg), and albumin during pregnancy and the puerperium. (From Pitkin RM, Reynolds WA, Williams GA, et al: Calcium metabolism in normal pregnancy: A longitudinal study. Am J Obstet Gynecol **133**:781, 1979.)

Maternal calcium absorption rises during pregnancy to meet these demands. Increased 1,25 $(OH)_2$ D synthesis of placental as well as maternal renal origin leads to the opening of voltage-gated calcium channels in the enterocyte membrane (Steinchen et al., 1980). In the maternal circulation, there is little change in ionized calcium (Pitkin et al., 1979), whereas total serum calcium concentrations fall during gestation, paralleling a decline in serum albumin (Fig. 51-12).

In addition to placental calcium transfer, an expanding extracellular volume and increased urinary calcium losses place further stress on maternal calcium homeostasis. Studies of PTH using traditional radioimmunoassays have supported a concept of physiologic hyperparathyroidism in pregnancy (Pitkin et al., 1979). The advent of new immunoradiometric assays for intact PTH have shown a decline in PTH during pregnancy (Seki et al., 1994). This decline, however, appears to be offset by increased parathyroid-related protein (PTHrp) of fetal origin. This peptide shares considerable homology with PTH as well as a common receptor. It appears that PTHrp is produced both by the fetal parathyroid glands and by the placenta and is the predominant regulator of active placental calcium transport. Transtrophoblastic calcium transfer also depends on an increase in calcium-binding protein, which reaches maximal concentrations in the third trimester when

fetal growth is most rapid. Serum calcitonin concentrations have been variously reported as showing a rise or no consistent change during pregnancy.

Fetal parathyroid tissue has been identified by 6 weeks' gestation, and skeletal mineralization is apparent by the eighth week. Total and ionized calcium concentrations are elevated in the fetus at term and decrease to normal in the newborn period. PTH levels are low in the fetus and increase after birth (Pitkin, 1985). PTHrp is produced by fetal parathyroid glands and is the main regulator of fetal serum calcium. Calcitonin is elevated in the fetus. These events are summarized in Table 51-7. During lactation, the average daily loss of calcium in human milk is 220–340 mg. There is a small drop in serum calcium accompanied by a rise in PTH and 1,25$(OH)_2$ D concentrations.

Disorders of the Parathyroid Glands

Primary Hyperparathyroidism and Hypercalcemia

Hyperparathyroidism is rare in pregnancy. Of 750 cases of parathyroid surgery performed over a 21-year period (Kort et al., 1999), only six occurred in pregnant women (0.8%). The topic of parathyroid disorders in pregnancy was reviewed by Mestman (1998). As in nonpregnant women, the histopathology of hyperparathyroidism in pregnant women involves a single adenoma in the vast majority, although hyperplasia and carcinoma have also been reported (Kristofferson et al., 1985; Gelister et al., 1989). Although many patients are asymptomatic, clinical features of the associated hypercalcemia are summarized in Table 51-8.

In the 102 pregnancies (in 73 women) reported by Kristofferson and coauthors (1985), the clinical history was known in 45. Abdominal symptoms, including nausea, vomiting, pain, and renal colic, were the most frequent, followed by muscular weakness, mental symptoms, and polyuria; 20% were asymptomatic. The diagnosis of hyperparathyroidism during pregnancy is suggested by hypercalcemia. The fall in total serum calcium during pregnancy may mask the diagnosis (or be associated with a postpartum flare-up), and ionized serum calcium should be measured in patients suspected of having primary hyperparathyroidism. One then confirms the diagnosis

TABLE 51-7. MINERALS AND HORMONES INVOLVED IN CALCIUM HOMEOSTASIS

Mineral/Hormone	Mother	Fetus	Newborn
Total calcium*	Low	High	Falls[†]
Ionized calcium*	Low normal	High	Falls
Magnesium*	Low normal	High normal	Falls
Phosphorus*	Low	High	Rises[†]
PTH	Low	Low	Rises
Calcitonin	Normal/High	High	Falls
25(OH) D*	Variable	Variable	Variable
1,25$(OH)_2$ D	High	Low	Rises
PTHrp	High[‡]	High	

* Placental transfer.
[†] Toward nonpregnant adult values.
[‡] Of fetal origin.

PTH, parathyroid hormone; PTHrp, parathyroid-related protein.

TABLE 51-8. MATERNAL FEATURES OF HYPERCALCEMIA

Urinary system	Nephrolithiasis
	Nephrocalcinosis
	Polyuria
Neuromuscular	Weakness
Gastrointestinal	Peptic ulcer disease
	Constipation
	Anorexia
	Nausea/vomiting
Cardiovascular	Hypertension
	Arrhythmias
Skeletal	Osteitis fibrosa cystica
	Osteopenia and fractures
Neuropsychiatric	Depression
	Psychosis
	Obtundation
	Coma
Miscellaneous	Thirst
	Pruritus

by finding inappropriately elevated PTH concentrations as well as an increase in urinary nephrogenic cyclic adenosine monophosphate levels (cAMP).

The differential diagnosis of hypercalcemia includes malignant disease, granulomatous disease, thyrotoxicosis, hypervitaminosis D or A, and immobilization as well as familial hypocalciuric hypercalcemia (FHH), which is an autosomal dominant, inherited form of mild, benign hyperparathyroidism associated with low urinary calcium excretion. Affected neonates of mothers with FHH could manifest symptomatic hypercalcemia; if unaffected, they could develop severe neonatal hypocalcemia because of suppression of fetal parathyroid function. In addition, severe neonatal hypercalcemia could be the homozygous variant of FHH. An altered calcium ion-sensing receptor gene, changing the set-point for PTH secretion, is the underlying defect in FHH. Hypercalcemia associated with increased production of PTHrp has also been described during pregnancy and postpartum (Lepre et al., 1993). In one case, production of PTHrp by hypertrophied breast tissue led to hypercalcemia (Khosla et al., 1990). In another, hypercalcemia developed postpartum in a hypoparathyroid woman on vitamin D (Shomali and Ross, 1999).

During pregnancy, calcium transport across the placenta provides a degree of protection in the mother against hypercalcemia, this protection being greatest in the third trimester. Loss of this protection with delivery can cause acute postpartum maternal hypercalcemia. In many patients, the diagnosis is confirmed after delivery following the occurrence of neonatal tetany. Ten of 15 cases of hyperparathyroidism reported by Gelister and colleagues (1989) presented in this way, the others presenting with hyperemesis, hypertension, and a jaw fracture in a patient who turned out to have a parathyroid carcinoma.

COMPLICATIONS. Complications of hyperparathyroidism affect both mother and infant. Maternal complications include hyperemesis, renal calculi (36%), pancreatitis (13%), hypertension (10%), bone disease (19%), hypercalcemic crises (8%), and psychiatric problems. The overall maternal mortality rate remains low (one out of 73 in the collected series of Kristofferson et al., 1985).

Fetal morbidity and mortality are significant, however. In the 102 pregnancies involving 73 women reviewed by Kristofferson and associates (1985), there were 53 (52%) normal children, 24 (23.5%) cases of neonatal tetany, 10 (9.8%) stillbirths, and a few cases of prematurity and neonatal death. In the series of Gelister and coworkers (1989), 10 of 15 patients presented with neonatal hypocalcemia, and there was one stillbirth.

Although neonatal hypocalcemia with tetany is usually a transient phenomenon related to suppression of fetal parathyroid glands resulting from maternal-fetal hypercalcemia, it can be more prolonged in less mature infants or in infants with birth asphyxia. Hypercalcemic crisis also can occur during pregnancy or after delivery with high serum calcium (greater than 14 mg/dL), generalized weakness, vomiting, and altered mental status. Aggravation of hypercalcemia can occur because of an increase in placental production of 1,25 (OH)$_2$ D by the end of gestation and the removal of the placenta and thus loss of the shunt that transfers calcium from mother to fetus.

TREATMENT. For hyperparathyroidism presenting during pregnancy, standard practice favors surgical treatment. In the collected series of Kristofferson and colleagues (1985), there were 79 pregnancies among 50 women who did not undergo surgery; there were complications in 41 of the pregnancies (52%), and neonatal tetany occurred in 21 (26.6%). This was contrasted with the more favorable outcome in 23 pregnancies involving 23 women who underwent surgical treatment during pregnancy; five had complications (22%), and there were three cases of neonatal tetany (13%). Surgery should be performed in the second trimester, when fetal organs are developed and the uterus is less likely to undergo labor (Nudelman et al., 1984). Conservative treatment of mildly affected, asymptomatic patients has also been suggested (Lowe et al., 1983). In a case reported by Haenel and Mayfield (2000), oral phosphate and parenteral saline were used to tide the patient over during the third trimester.

The treatment of life-threatening hypercalcemia can be problematic and could require hydration, furosemide, phosphates, and even hemodialysis (Monturo et al., 1980; Kleinman et al., 1991; Iqbal et al., 1999). This is summarized in Table 51-9. Calcitonin inhibits bone resorption; its effects are generally short-lived, and it does not cross the placenta. It has been used briefly in pregnancy in the third trimester in one case (Murray et al., 1997). In life-threatening situations, mithramycin (plicamycin) lowers calcium by inhibiting bone resorption. It is an antineoplastic agent and toxic to the fetus. In nonpregnant patients, bisphosphonates (such as pamidronate), given intravenously, are also effective in lowering calcium. There are no data on their use in pregnancy.

PARATHYROID CARCINOMA IN PREGNANCY. Four cases of parathyroid carcinoma during pregnancy were reviewed by Montoro and associates (2000). Severe hypercalcemia, hypertension, and a palpable neck mass were consistent features, whereas palpable masses were found in only 5% and hypertension in 10% of parathyroid adenomas in pregnant patients. Because survival depends on complete initial resection, early surgical intervention is important.

Hypoparathyroidism

This topic was reviewed by Mestman (1998). Hypoparathyroidism in pregnancy usually occurs in patients who have previously undergone neck surgery but can occur in other, less

TABLE 51-9. TREATMENT OF HYPERCALCEMIA

Treatment	Adverse Effects
General	
Hydration	
Discontinue offending drugs	
Restrict calcium	
Increase Renal Calcium Excretion	
0.9% saline 200–500 mL/hr	Volume overload
Furosemide 20–60 mg IV q2–4h	Volume depletion
	Hypokalemia
Dialysis	
Calcium Chelation with Phosphates	
Oral: Neura-phos 500–750 mg q6–8h	Extraskeletal
Rectal: Phosphosoda 5 mL q6–8h	calcification
IV: 50 mM phosphate over 8–12 hours	
Decrease Bone Resorption	
Calcitonin 4–8 IU/kg IM or SC every	Allergic reaction
6–12 hours*	Nausea
Pamidronate (bisphosphonate)	Renal toxicity
30–60 mg IV as single infusion over	
24 hours	
Mithramycin 25 µg/kg IV† every	Low platelets
48–72 hours	Renal toxicity
	Hepatotoxicity

* No reports of congenital defects; does not cross placenta.
† No reports on use in pregnancy; antineoplastic.
IV, intravenously; IM, intramuscularly; SC, subcutaneously.

common circumstances (Table 51-10). The diagnosis is confirmed by the combination of hypocalcemia with low PTH, $1,25(OH)_2$ D, and nephrogenous cAMP concentrations. Other hypocalcemic states that need to be distinguished from hypoparathyroidism include vitamin D deficiency (with a finding of high PTH), excessive chelation (following blood transfusion), pancreatitis, and septic states.

Clinical features include tetany, which may be elicited in latent form via the Chvostek test (tapping of the facial nerve) and Trousseau test (occurrence of tetany within 3 minutes of the induction of ischemia in the upper extremity). Other symptoms include paresthesia, stridor, muscle cramps, and mental changes, including frank psychosis. The electrocardiogram may reveal prolongation of the Q-T interval.

COMPLICATIONS. Neonatal hyperparathyroidism may develop secondary to maternal hypocalcemia. This can cause fetal bone demineralization and growth restriction (Fleischman, 1980). Although this condition is transient, death from complications of skeletal fractures can occur. Loughhead and colleagues (1990) reviewed 16 cases of congenital hyperparathyroidism secondary to maternal hypocalcemia; bone features of hyperparathyroidism were documented in 13 cases. Six of the neonates died within the first 3 months of life. In their conclusion, these authors stated that the presentation varied highly, ranging from clinically and radiologically silent cases to neonates with severe skeletal disease and bone demineralization.

TREATMENT. The maternal serum calcium level should be maintained within normal limits. Vitamin D (50,000–100,000 units/day or more) and calcium salts (1.0 or 1.5 g of elemental calcium per day) are given to maintain normo-

calcemia. More recently, calcitriol ($1,25[OH]_2$ D), which has a more rapid onset of action and a shorter half life, has been used, the usual dose being 0.5–1.0 µg/day (Salle et al., 1981).

The normal replacement dose of vitamin D in a hypoparathyroid woman may need to be increased, possibly because of increased binding of vitamin D to vitamin D–binding protein. In a patient treated with calcitriol, the dose had to be doubled during pregnancy to maintain normocalcemia, similar to the physiologic twofold rise in $1,25(OH)_2$ D during pregnancy (Sadeghi-Nejad et al., 1980). The aim should be serum calcium concentrations in the range of 8–9 mg/dL with avoidance of hypercalciuria (greater than 250 mg/24 hours), which could lead to nephrolithiasis. A prompt decrease to prepregnancy doses of vitamin D is necessary after delivery so that hypercalcemia can be avoided (Caplan and Beguin, 1990). Although lactating women usually require continuation of pregnancy doses of vitamin D, hypercalcemia has been reported (Caplan and Beguin, 1990), and close monitoring would be prudent. This finding could relate to the production of PTHrp by the breasts (Shomali and Ross, 1999; Mather et al., 1999). It could also relate to induction of 1α-hydroxylase by prolactin.

Acute symptomatic hypocalcemia is a medical emergency and should be treated with intravenous calcium (e.g., 10 mL of 10% calcium gluconate over 10 minutes followed by an infusion of 0.5–2.0 mg/kg/hour of elemental calcium, diluted with dextrose to avoid irritation to veins).

Infants receiving breast milk from mothers consuming large doses of vitamin D should undergo periodic calcium determinations, because the breast milk will have higher-than-normal levels of vitamin D (Greer et al., 1984), which could cause hypercalcemia and impaired linear growth in the infant.

Pregnancy-Related Osteoporosis

Osteoporosis is a disorder characterized by loss of bone mass and microarchitectural deterioration, resulting in an increased risk of fracture. Normally, bone formation and resorption are coupled. Bone loss secondary to reduced formation or increased resorption may occur in estrogen-deficiency states, glucocorticoid-excess syndromes, thyrotoxicosis, and other circumstances.

The effect of pregnancy on bone turnover was evaluated by Black and colleagues (2000). In a detailed study using biochemical markers of bone formation and resorption and

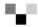

TABLE 51-10. CLASSIFICATION OF HYPO-PARATHYROID DISORDERS

Defect	Etiology
Absence of PTH or insufficiency	Previous thyroid or parathyroid surgery
	Idiopathic hypoparathyroidism (familial or sporadic)
	Di George syndrome
	Iron overload (rare)
	Previous irradiation with [131]I (rare)
Absence of and resistance to PTH	Magnesium depletion
PTH resistance	Pseudohypoparathyroidism

PTH, parathyroid hormone.

dual energy x-ray absorptiometry (DEXA) before, during (forearm), and after pregnancy (hip, spine, and forearm), the authors reported increased markers of bone resorption by 14 weeks' and further by 28 weeks', whereas markers of bone formation did not increase significantly till 28 weeks. Lumbar spine and hip bone mineral density decreased significantly during pregnancy. Thus, it appeared that bone remodeling became uncoupled, with an increase in resorption during the first two trimesters, the increase in formation becoming evident only in the third trimester.

In 1955, Nordin and Roper reported on four young women with backache and vertebral compression fractures diagnosed as idiopathic osteoporosis. Their symptoms developed during or shortly after pregnancy and improved with follow-up. These authors suggested that the association between osteoporosis and pregnancy may not have been fortuitous. Since that time, sporadic cases and small series of patients with osteoporosis in relation to pregnancy and lactation have been reported (Di Gregorio et al., 2000; Honjo and Mizunuma, 2001). Smith and coworkers (1985) suggested that failure of calcium accretion by the maternal skeleton, normally facilitated by increased calcium absorption in response to higher $1,25(OH)_2D$ concentrations, may explain this occurrence; these vitamin concentrations were low in several patients with osteoporosis. In addition, they suggested failure of the calcitonin response to pregnancy as another mechanism; calcitonin has antiresorptive properties and could increase during pregnancy.

In a study of 29 women with idiopathic osteoporosis associated with pregnancy (Dunne et al., 1993), it was observed that pain occurring late in the first full-term pregnancy was the most common presentation and that the natural history was improvement over time. Adult-related fractures occurring at an earlier age were more prevalent in the mothers of these women, suggesting possible genetic factors in the etiology. Low $1,25(OH)_2 D$ concentrations were demonstrated in a case by Khan and colleagues (1995); the abnormality reversed over time. Subsequent pregnancies are not necessarily affected.

During lactation, a substantial part of the calcium demand is mobilized from the maternal skeleton (secondary to low estrogen and high PTHrp from the breasts (Grill et al., 1992). In a study of 18 exclusively breast-feeding women, compared with 18 women in whom lactation was inhibited by bromocriptine, there was a significant decrease in lumbar spine and distal radius and in bone density as well as biochemical evidence of increased bone turnover during breast-feeding, with an incomplete recovery 6 months after breast-feeding cessation (Affinito et al., 1996). In the bromocriptine-treated women, bone-mineral density did not change. Overall, it appears that healthy young women have significant early losses of bone mineral density at the axial spine and hip during six months of lactation (Eisman, 1998). Loss, however, does not continue beyond 6 months despite continuing lactation, and bone mineral density loss is generally restored with the return of normal menses. The calcium demands of late pregnancy and lactation are about 0.3 grams per day. There are limited long-term data on the effects of extended and repeated lactation. Whereas some studies have shown an adverse effect (Lissner et al., 1991), parity and lactation have not been associated with low bone-mineral density or osteoporotic fracture risk in epidemiologic or case-control cohort studies (Tuppurainen et al., 1995).

REFERENCES

Hypothalamus and Pituitary

Aaron D, Schwall AM, Sheeler LR: Cushing's syndrome and pregnancy. Am J Obstet Gynecol **162**:244, 1990.

Ahmed M, Al-Dossary E, Woodhouse NJY: Macroprolactinoma with suprasellar extension: Effect of bromocriptine withdrawal during one or more pregnancies. Fertil Steril **58**:492, 1992.

Albrecht BH, Betz G: Prolactin-secreting pituitary tumors and pregnancy. In Olefsy JM, Robbins RJ (eds): Contemporary Issues in Endocrinology and Metabolism: Prolactinomas. Vol 2. New York, Churchill Livingstone, 1986, p. 195.

Aydin Y, Can SM, Gulkilik A, et al: Rapid enlargement and recurrence of a preexisting intrasellar craniopharyngioma during the course of two pregnancies. J Neurosurg **91**:322, 1999.

Beasley EW: Pregnancy and lactation in Nelson's Syndrome. Endocrinologist **9**:313, 1999.

Beckers A, Stevenaert A, Foidart JM, et al: Placental and pituitary growth hormone secretion during pregnancy in acromegalic women. J Clin Endocrinol Metab **71**:725, 1990.

Belchetz PE, Carty A, Clearkin LG: Failure of prophylactic surgery to avert massive pituitary expansion in pregnancy. Clin Endocrinol **25**:325, 1986.

Bitton RN, Slavin M, Decker RE, et al: The course of lymphocytic hypophysitis. Surg Neurol **36**:40, 1991.

Borges F, Horta C, Mendes P, et al: Factors of cure in hyperprolactinemic women (abstract) Proceedings of the 11th International Congress of Endocrinology, Sydney Australia, 402, 2000.

Brandes JC, Cerletty JM: Pregnancy in lymphocytic hypophysitis. Wis Med J **88**:29, 1989.

Buescher MA: Cushing's syndrome in pregnancy. Endocrinologist **6**:357, 1996.

Burrow GN, Wassenaar W, Robertson GL, et al: DDAVP treatment of diabetes insipidus during pregnancy and the postpartum period. Acta Endocrinol **97**:23, 1981.

Campbell JW: Diabetes insipidus and complicated pregnancy. JAMA **243**:1744, 1980.

Caron P, Gerbeau C, Pradayrol L, et al: Successful pregnancy in an infertile woman with a thyrotropin-secreting macroadenoma treated with somatostatin analog (Oceteotride). J Clin Endocrinol Metab **81**:1164, 1996.

Close CF, Mann MC, Watts JF, et al: ACTH independent Cushing's syndrome in pregnancy with spontaneous resolution after delivery: Control of the hypercortisolism with metyrapone. Clin Endocrinol (Oxf) **39**:375, 1993.

Colao A, Sarno AD, Sarnacchiaro F, et al: Prolactinomas resistant to standard dopamine agonists respond to chronic cabergoline treatment. J Clin Endocrinol Metab **82**:876, 1997.

Cosman F, Post KD, Holub DA, et al: Lymphocytic hypophysitis. Report of 3 cases and review of the literature. Medicine **68**:240, 1989.

Davison JM, Gilmore EA, Durr JS, et al: Altered osmotic thresholds for vasopressin secretion and thirst in human pregnancy. Am J Physiol **246**:105, 1983.

Dawood MY, Khan-Dawood FS: The posterior pituitary pathway. In Droegemveller W, Sciarra J (eds): Gynecology and Obstetrics, Vol 5. Philadelphia, JB Lippincott, 1990.

de Menis E, Billeci D, Marton E, et al: Uneventful pregnancy in an acromegalic patient treated with slow-release lanreotide: A case report. J Clin Endocrinol Metab **84**:1489, 1999.

del Pozo E, Krupp P: Endocrine effects of dopamine receptor stimulation on the feto-maternal unit. In Krauer B, et al (eds): Drugs and Pregnancy. London, Academic Press, 1984, p. 191.

Decherney A, Naftolin F: Hypothalamic and pituitary development in the fetus. Clin Obstet Gynecol **23**:749, 1980.

Dinc H, Esen F, Demirci A, et al: Pituitary dimensions and volume measurements in pregnancy and postpartum. Acta Radiol **39**:64, 1998.

Divers WA, Yen SSC: Prolactin-producing microadenomas in pregnancy. Obstet Gynecol **62**:425, 1983.

Dorfman SG, Dillaplain RP, Gambrell RD: Antepartum pituitary infarction. Obstet Gynecol **53**(Suppl):21S, 1979.

Drury MI, Keelan DM: Sheehan's syndrome. J Obstet Gynaecol Br Commonw **73**:802, 1966.

Durr JA, Lindheimer MD: Diagnosis and management of diabetes insipidus during pregnancy. Endocr Pract **2**:353, 1996.

Feigenbaum S, Martin MC, Wilson CB, et al: Lymphocytic adenohypophysitis: A pituitary mass lesion occurring in pregnancy. Am J Obstet Gynecol **164**:1549, 1991.

Ford SM, Lumpkin HL: Transient vasopressin-resistant diabetes insipidus of pregnancy. Obstet Gynecol **68**:726, 1986.

Frankenne F, Closset J, Gomez F, et al: The physiology of growth hormones in pregnant women and partial characterization of the placental GH variant. J Clin Endocrinol Metab **66**:1171, 1988.

Frohman LA: Neurotransmitters as regulators of endocrine function. *In* Krieger DT, Hughes JC (eds): Neuroendocrinology: A Hospital Practice Book. Sunderland, Mass, Sinauer Associates, 1980.

Frohman LA: Pituitary Tumors in Pregnancy. Endocrinologist **11**:399, 2001.

Furlanetto RW, Underwood LE, Van Wyk JJ, et al: Serum immunoreactive somatomedin-C is elevated late in pregnancy. J Clin Endocrinol Metab **47**:695, 1978.

Gonzalez JF, Elizondo G, Saldivar D, et al: Pituitary gland growth during normal pregnancy: An in vivo study using magnetic resonance imaging. Am J Med **85**:217, 1988.

Gormley MJJ, Hadden DR, Kennedy TL, et al: Cushing's syndrome in pregnancy—Treatment with metyrapone. Clin Endocrinol **16**:283, 1982.

Goudie RB, Pinkerton PH: Anterior hypophysitis and Hashimoto's disease in a young woman. J Pathol Bacteriol **83**:585, 1962.

Green JS, Parfrey PS, Harnett JD, et al: The cardinal manifestations of Bardet-Biedl syndrome, a form of Lawrence-Moon-Biedl syndrome. N Engl J Med **321**:1002, 1989.

Grimes HG, Brooks MH: Pregnancy in Sheehan's syndrome: Report of a case and review. Obstet Gynecol Surv **35**:481, 1980.

Hall MRP: Incidence of anterior pituitary deficiency following post-partum hemorrhage: Cases reviewed from the Oxfordshire and Buckinghamshire area. Proc Soc Med **55**:468, 1962.

Hamai Y, Fujii T, Nishina H, et al: Differential clinical courses of pregnancies complicated by diabetes insipidus, which does or does not predate the pregnancy. Hum Reprod **12**:1816, 1997.

Hendricks CH: The neurohypophysis in pregnancy. Obstet Gynecol Surv **9**:323, 1954.

Hermann-Bonert V, Seliverstov M, Melmed S: Pregnancy in acromegaly: successful therapeutic outcome. J Clin Endocrinol Metab **83**:727, 1998.

Hiett AK, Barton JR: Diabetes insipidus associated with craniopharyngioma in pregnancy. Obstet Gynecol **76**:982, 1990.

Hime MC, Richardson JA: Diabetes insipidus and pregnancy: Case report, incidence and review of literature. Obstet Gynecol Surv **33**:375, 1978.

Itskovitz J, Rosenwaks Z: Pituitary disease in pregnancy. *In* Brody S, Velard K (eds): Endocrine Disorders in Pregnancy. Norwalk, Conn, Appleton and Lange, 1989.

Kallen BAJ, Carlsson SS, Bengtsson BKA: Diabetes insipidus and use of desmopressin during pregnancy. Eur J Endocrinol **132**:144, 1995.

Krupp P, Monka C: Bromocriptine in pregnancy: Safety aspects. Klin Wochenschr **65**:823, 1987.

Kupersmith MJ, Rosenberg C, Kleinberg D: Visual loss in pregnant women with pituitary adenomas. Ann Intern Med **121**:473, 1994.

Lindheimer MD, Barron WM, Davison JM: Osmotic volume control of vasopressin release in pregnancy. Am J Kidney Dis **17**:105, 1991.

Luboshitzky R, Dickstein G, Barzilai D: Bromocriptine induced pregnancy in an acromegalic patient. JAMA **244**:584, 1980.

Lufkin EG, Kao PC, O'Fallon WM, et al: Combined testing of anterior pituitary gland with insulin, thyrotropin-releasing hormone and luteinizing hormone-releasing hormone. Am J Med **75**:471, 1983.

Magyar DM, Marshall JR: Pituitary tumors and pregnancy. Am J Obstet Gynecol **132**:739, 1978.

Maranon G: Diabetes insipidus and uterine atony. Br Med J **2**:769, 1947.

Meichner RH, Riggio S, Manz HJ, et al: Lymphocytic adenohypophysitis causing pituitary mass. Neurology **37**:158, 1987.

Mellor A, Harvey RD, Pobereskin LH, et al: Cushing's disease treated by transsphenoidal selective adenomectomy in mid-pregnancy. Br J Anaesth **80**:850, 1998.

Molitch ME: Pregnancy and the hyperprolactinemic woman. N Engl J Med **312**:1364, 1985.

Nader S, Orlander P: Lymphocytic hypophysitis: A case report and review of the literature. Infertility **13**:145, 1990.

Nakamura Y, Takagi H, Sakurai S, et al: Transient diabetes insipidus during and after pregnancy. N Engl J Med **325**:285, 1991.

Neal JM: Successful pregnancy in a women with acromegaly treated with octreotide. Endocr Pract **6**:148, 2000.

Ober KP, Elster A: Spontaneously resolving lymphocytic hypophysitis as a cause of postpartum diabetes insipidus. Endocrinologist **4**:107, 1994.

O'Donovan PA, O'Donovan PJ, Ritchie EH: Apoplexy into a prolactin secreting macroadenoma during early pregnancy with successful outcome. Br J Obstet Gynaecol **93**:389, 1986.

Pickard J, Jochen AL, Sadur CN, et al: Cushing's syndrome in pregnancy. Obstet Gynecol Surv **45**:87, 1990.

Pinette NG, Pan YQ, Oppenheim D, et al: Bilateral inferior petrosal sinus corticotropin sampling with corticotropin releasing hormone stimulation in a pregnant patient with Cushing's syndrome. Am J Obstet Gynecol **171**:563, 1994.

Ray JG: DDAVP use during pregnancy: An analysis of its safety for mother and child. Obstet Gynecol Surv **53**:450, 1998.

Robert E, Musatti L, Piscitelli G, et al: Pregnancy outcome after treatment with the ergot derivative cabergoline. Repro Toxicol **10**:333, 1996.

Robinson AG: Disorders of antidiuretic hormone secretion. Clin Endocrinol Metab **14**:55, 1985.

Robinson AG, Amico JA: "No-sweet" diabetes of pregnancy. N Engl J Med **324**:556, 1991.

Rothman KJ, Funch DP, Dreyer NA: Bromocriptine and puerperal seizures. Epidemiology **1**:232, 1990.

Ruiz-Velasco V, Tolis G: Pregnancy in hyperprolactinemic women. Fertil Steril **41**:793, 1984.

Scheithauer BW, Sano T, Kovacs KT, et al: The pituitary gland in pregnancy: A clinicopathologic and immunohistochemical study of 69 cases. Mayo Clin Proc **65**:461, 1990.

Scheller TJ, Nader S: Magnetic resonance imaging in Sheehan's syndrome. Case report and literature review of imaging studies. Endocr Pract **3**:82, 1997.

Schultz CL, Haaga JR, Fletcher BD, et al: Magnetic resonance imaging of the adrenal glands: A comparison with computed tomography. AJR **143**:1235, 1984.

Shalev E, Goldstein D, Zuckerman H: Compulsive water drinking in pregnancy. Int J Gynaecol Obstet **18**:465, 1980.

Sheehan HL: Post-partum necrosis of the anterior pituitary. J Pathol Bacteriol **45**:189, 1937.

Stelmach M, O'Day J: Rapid change in visual fields associated with suprasellar lymphocytic hypophysitis. J Clin Neuroophthalmol **11**:19, 1991.

Surrey ES, Chang RJ: Nelson's syndrome in pregnancy. Fertil Steril **44**:548, 1985.

Tyson JE, Hwang P, Guyden A, et al: Studies of prolactin secretion in human pregnancy. Am J Obstet Gynecol **113**:14, 1972.

Van der Spuy ZM, Jacobs HS: Management of endocrine disorders and pregnancy: Part II. Pituitary, ovarian, and adrenal disease. Postgrad Med J **60**:312, 1984.

Yap AS, Clouston WM, Mortimer RH, et al: Acromegaly first diagnosed in pregnancy: The role of bromocriptine therapy. Am J Obstet Gynecol **163**:477, 1990.

Zarate A, Canales ES, Alger M: The effect of pregnancy and lactation on pituitary prolactin secreting tumors. Acta Endocrinol **92**:407, 1979.

Adrenal Glands

Albert E, Dalaker K, Jorde R, et al: Addison's disease and pregnancy. Acta Obstet Gynecol Scand **68**:185, 1989.

Bongiovanni AM, McPadden AJ: Steroids during pregnancy and possible fetal consequences. Fertil Steril **11**:181, 1960.

Brent F: Addison's disease and pregnancy. Am J Surg **79**:645, 1950.

Buescher MA: Cushing's syndrome in pregnancy. Endocrinologist **6**:357, 1996.

Buescher MA, McClamrock HD, Adashi EY: Cushing syndrome in pregnancy. Obstet Gynecol **79**:130, 1992.

Cerame BI, Newfield RS, Pascoe L, et al: Prenatal diagnosis and treatment of 11 β-hydroxylase deficiency congenital adrenal hyperplasia resulting in a normal female genitalia. J Clin Endocrinol Metab **84**:3129, 1999.

Devoe LD, O'Dell BE, Castillo RA, et al: Metastatic pheochromocytoma in pregnancy and fetal biophysical assessment after maternal administration of α-adrenergic, β-adrenergic, and dopamine antagonists. Obstet Gynecol **68**:155, 1986.

Drucker D, Shumak S, Angel A: Schmidt syndrome presenting with intrauterine growth retardation and postpartum Addisonian crises. Am J Obstet Gynecol **149**:229, 1984.

Ellison GT, Mansberger JA, Mansberger AR: Malignant recurrent pheochromocytoma during pregnancy. Case report and review of the literature. Surgery **103**:484, 1988.

Fudge TL, McKinnon WMP, Greary WL: Current surgical management of pheochromocytoma during pregnancy. Arch Surg **115**:1224, 1980.

Garner PR: Management of congenital adrenal hyperplasia during pregnancy. Endocr Pract **2**:397, 1996.

Glazer GM, Woolsey JM, Borrello J, et al: Adrenal tissue characterization using MR imaging. Radiology **158**:73, 1986.

Griffin J, Brooks N, Patricia F, et al: Pheochromocytoma in pregnancy. Diagnosis and collaborative management. South Med J **77**:1325, 1984.

Harper A, Murnaghan GA, Kennedy L, et al: Pheochromocytoma in pregnancy. Five cases and a review of the literature. Br J Obstet Gynecol **96**:594, 1989.

Harrington JL, Farley DR, Van Heerden JA, et al: Adrenal tumors and pregnancy. World J Surg **23**:182, 1999.

Keller-Wood M, Wood CE: Pituitary-adrenal physiology during pregnancy. Endocrinologist **11**:159, 2001.

Kerian V, Nahoul K, LeMartelot MT, et al: Longitudinal study of maternal plasma bioavailable testosterone and androstenediol glucuronide levels during pregnancy. Clin Endocrinol (Oxf) **40**:263, 1994.

Kreft-Jais C, Plovin PF, Tchobrovtsky C, et al: Angiotensin-converting enzyme inhibitors during pregnancy: A survey of 22 patients given captopril and nine given enalapril. Br J Obstet Gynaecol **95**:420, 1988.

Lotgering FK, Derhx FMH, Wallenburg HCS: Primary hypoaldosteronism in pregnancy. Am J Obstet Gynecol **155**:986, 1986.

Lyons CW, Colmorgen GHC: Medical management of pheochromocytoma in pregnancy. Obstet Gynecol **72**:450, 1988.

Mercado AB, Wilson RC, Cheng KC, et al: Prenatal treatment and diagnosis of congenital adrenal hyperplasia owing to steroid 21-hydroxylase deficiency. J Clin Endocrinol Metab **80**:2014, 1995.

Mitchell SZ, Freilich JD, Brant D, et al: Anesthetic management of pheochromocytoma resection during pregnancy. Anesth Analg **66**:478, 1987.

Mori N, Miyakawa I: Congenital adrenogenital syndrome and successful pregnancy. Obstet Gynecol **35**:394, 1970.

Mornet E, Couillin P, Kutten F, et al: Associations between restriction fragment length polymorphisms detected with a probe for human 21-hydroxylase and two clinical forms of 21-hydroxylase deficiency. Hum Genet **74**:402, 1986.

Neerhof MG, Shlossman PA, Ludomirsky A, et al: Idiopathic aldosteronism in pregnancy. Obstet Gynecol **78**:489, 1991.

New MI: Prenatal treatment of congenital adrenal hyperplasia: The United States Experience. Endocrinol Metab Clin North Am **30**:1, 2001.

New MI, Carlson A, Obeid J, et al: Prenatal diagnosis for congenital adrenal hyperplasia in 532 pregnancies. J Clin Endocrinol Metab **86**:5651, 2001.

Nolten WE, Lindheimer MD, Oparil S, et al: Deoxycorticosterone in normal pregnancy. Am J Obstet Gynecol **132**:414, 1978.

Oliver MD, Brownjohn AM, Vinali PS: Medical management of pheochromocytoma in pregnancy. Aust N Z J Obstet Gynaecol **30**:268, 1990.

Pang S, Wallace MA, Hofman L, et al: Worldwide experience in newborn screening for classical congenital adrenal hyperplasia due to 21-hydroxylase deficiency. Pediatrics **81**:866, 1988.

Park-Wyllie L, Mazzotta P, Pastuszak A, et al: Birth defects after maternal exposure to corticosteroids: Prospective cohort study and meta-analysis of epidemiological studies. Teratology **62**:385, 2000.

Peterson RE: Cortisol. In Fuchs F, Klopper A (eds): Endocrinology of Pregnancy, 2nd ed. Hagerstown, Md, Harper and Row, 1977.

Rees LH, Burke CW, Chard T, et al: Possible placental origin of ACTH in normal human pregnancy. Nature **254**:620, 1975.

Robar CA, Pozemba JA, Pelton JJ, et al: Current diagnosis and management of aldosterone producing adenomas during pregnancy. Endocrinologist **8**:403, 1998.

Rosenfeld RL, Rich BL, Wolfsdorf JI, et al: Pubertal presentation of congenital 5-3B-hydroxysteroid dehydrogenase deficiency. J Clin Endocrinol Metab **51**:345, 1980.

Rosenthal HE, Slaunwhite WR, Sandberg AA: Transcortin: A corticosteroid binding protein of plasma: X. Cortisol and progesterone interplay and unbound levels of these steroids in pregnancy. J Clin Endocrinol Metab **29**:352, 1969.

Rosler A, Leiberman E, Rosenmann A, et al: Prenatal diagnosis of 11 beta hydroxylase deficiency congenital adrenal hyperplasia. J Clin Endocrinol Metab **49**:546, 1979.

Sasaki A, Liotta AS, Luckey MM, et al: Immunoreactive corticotropin-releasing factor is present in human maternal plasma during the third trimester of pregnancy. J Clin Endocrinol Metab **59**:812, 1984.

Schenker JG, Granat M: Pheochromocytomas and pregnancy—An updated appraisal. Aust N Z J Obstet Gynaecol **22**:1, 1982.

Seaward PGR, Guidozzi F, Sonnendecker EWW: Addisonian crisis in pregnancy: Case Report. Br J Obstet Gynaecol **96**:1348, 1989.

Snyder RD, Snyder D: Corticosteroids for asthma during pregnancy. Ann Allergy **41**:340, 1978.

Tewari KS, Steiger RM, Lam ML, et al: Bilateral pheochromocytoma in pregnancy, heralding multiple endocrine neoplasia syndrome IIA. J Repro Med **46**:385, 2001.

van der Vaart CH, Heringa MP, Dullaart RPF, et al: Multiple endocrine neoplasia presenting as phaeochromocytoma during pregnancy. Br J Obstet Gynaecol **100**:1144, 1993.

White PC, Curnow KM, Pascoe L: Disorders of steroid 11 beta-hydroxylase isoenzymes. Endocr Rev **15**:421, 1994.

White PC, New MI: Genetic basis of endocrine disease: 2. Congenital adrenal hyperplasia due to 21-hydroxylase deficiency. J Clin Endocrinol Metab **74**:6, 1992.

White PC, New MI, Dupont BO: Congenital adrenal hyperplasia. N Engl J Med **316**:1519, 1987a.

White PC, New MI, Dupont BO: Congenital adrenal hyperplasia. N Engl J Med **316**:1580, 1987b.

Wilson M, Morganti AA, Zervoudakis I, et al: Blood pressure, the renin-aldosterone system and sex steroids throughout normal pregnancy. Am J Med **68**:97, 1980.

Hirsutism and Virilization in Pregnancy

Bachman R, Gennser G, Hakfelt B, et al: Steroid studies in a case of ovarian hyperluteinization with virilism in two consecutive pregnancies. Acta Endocrinol **76**:747, 1974.

de Butros A, Hatipoglu B: Testosterone storm during pregnancy. Endocrinologist **11**:57, 2001.

McClamrock HD, Adashi EY: Gestational hyperandrogenism. Fertil Steril **57**:257, 1992.

Miyata M, Nishihara M, Tokunaka KS, et al: A maternal functioning adrenocortical adenoma causing fetal female pseudohermaphroditism. J Urol **142**:806, 1989.

Sarlis NJ, Weil SJ, Nelson LM: Administration of metformin to a diabetic woman with extreme hyperandrogenemia of non-tumoral origin: Management of infertility and prevention of inadvertent masculinization of a female fetus. J Clin Endocrinol Metab **84**:1510, 1999.

Shortle BE, Warren MP, Tsin D: Recurrent androgenicity in pregnancy: A case report and literature review. Obstet Gynecol **70**:462, 1987.

Parathyroid Glands and Calcium Metabolism

Affinito P, Tommaselli GA, Carlo CD, et al: Changes in bone mineral density and calcium metabolism in breast feeding women. A one year follow-up study. J Clin Endocrinol Metab **81**:2314, 1996.

Black AJ, Topping J, Durham B, et al: A detailed assessment of alterations in bone turnover, calcium homeostasis and bone density in normal pregnancy. J Bone Miner Res **15**:557, 2000.

Caplan RH, Beguin EA: Hypercalcemia in a calcitriol-treated hypoparathyroid woman during lactation. Obstet Gynecol **76**:485, 1990.

Di Gregorio S, Danilowicz K, Rubin Z, et al: Osteoporosis with vertebral fractures associated with pregnancy and lactation; Nutrition **16**:1052, 2000.

Dunne F, Walters B, Marshall T, et al: Pregnancy associated osteoporosis. Clin Endocrinol (Oxf) **39**:487, 1993.

Eisman J: Relevance of pregnancy and lactation to osteoporosis (Commentary). Lancet **352**:504, 1998.

Fleischman AR: Fetal parathyroid gland and calcium homeostasis. Clin Obstet Gynecol **23**:791, 1980.

Gelister JSK, Sanderson JD, Chapple CR, et al: Management of hyperparathyroidism in pregnancy. Br J Surg **76**:1207, 1989.

Greer FR, Hollis BW, Napoli JL: High concentrations of vitamin D_2 in human milk associated with pharmacologic doses of vitamin D_2. J Pediatr **105**:61, 1984.

Grill V, Hillary J, Ho PM, et al: Parathyroid hormone related protein: A possible endocrine function on lactation. Clin Endocrinol (Oxf) **37**:405, 1992.

Haenel LC, Mayfield RK: Primary hyperparathyroidism in a twin pregnancy and review of fetal-maternal calcium homeostasis. Am J Med Sci **319**:191, 2000.

Honjo S, Mizunuma H: Changes in biochemical parameters of bone turnover and bone mineral density in post-pregnancy osteoporosis. Am J Obstet Gynecol **185**:246, 2001.

Hosking DJ: Calcium homeostasis in pregnancy. Clin Endocrinol (Oxf) **45**:1, 1996.

Iqbal N, Aldasouqi S, Peacock M, et al: Life threatening hypercalcemia associated with primary hyperparathyroidism during pregnancy: Case report and review of literature. Endocr Pract **5**:337, 1999.

Khan AA, Ahmed MM, Pritzker KPH: Osteoporosis associated with pregnancy: Case report and review. Endocr Pract **1**:236, 1995.

Khosla S, Van Heerden JA, Gharib H, et al: Parathyroid hormone related protein and hypercalcemia secondary to massive mammary hyperplasia. N Engl J Med **322**:1157, 1990.

Kleinman GE, Rodriguez H, Good MC, et al: Hypercalcemic crisis in pregnancy associated with excessive ingestion of calcium carbonate antacid: Successful treatment with hemodialysis. Obstet Gynecol **78**:496, 1991.

Kort KC, Schiller HJ, Numann PJ: Hyperparathyroidism and pregnancy. Am J Surg **177**:66, 1999.

Kristofferson A, Dahlgren S, Lithner F, et al: Primary hyperparathyroidism and pregnancy. Surgery **97**:326, 1985.

Lepre F, Grill V, Martin TJ: Hypercalcemia in pregnancy and lactation associated with parathyroid hormone related protein. N Engl J Med **328**:666, 1993.

Lissner L, Bengtsson C, Hanson T: Bone mineral content in relation to lactation history in pre and post menopausal women. Calcif Tissue Int **48**:319, 1991.

Loughead JL, Mughal Z, Mimouni F, et al: Spectrum and natural history of congenital hyperparathyroidism secondary to maternal hypocalcemia. Am J Perinatol **7**:350, 1990.

Lowe DK, Orwoll ES, McClung MR, et al: Hyperparathyroidism and pregnancy. Am J Surg **145**:611, 1983.

Mather KJ, Chik CL, Corenblum B: Maintenance of serum calcium by parathyroid hormone related peptide during lactation in a hypoparathyroid patient. J Clin Endocrinol Metab **84**:424, 1999.

Mestman JH: Parathyroid disorders of pregnancy. Semin Perinatol **22**:485, 1998.

Monturo MN, Collea JV, Mestman JH: Management of hyperparathyroidism in pregnancy with oral phosphate therapy. Obstet Gynecol **55**:431, 1980.

Montoro MN, Paler RJ, Goodwin TM, et al: Parathyroid carcinoma during pregnancy. Obstet Gynecol **95**:841, 2000.

Murray JA, Newman WA, Dacus JV: Hyperparathyroidism in pregnancy: Diagnostic Dilemma. Obstet Gynecol Surv **52**:202, 1997.

Nordin BEC, Roper A: Post pregnancy osteoporosis. A syndrome? Lancet **1**:431, 1955.

Nudelman J, Deutsch A, Sternberg A, et al: The treatment of primary hyperparathyroidism during pregnancy. Br J Surg **71**:217, 1984.

Pitkin RM: Calcium metabolism in pregnancy and the perinatal period. A review. Am J Obstet Gynecol **151**:99, 1985.

Pitkin RM, Reynolds WA, Williams GA, et al: Calcium metabolism in normal pregnancy: A longitudinal study. Am J Obstet Gynecol **133**:781, 1979.

Sadeghi-Nejad A, Wolfsdorf JI, Senior B: Hypoparathyroidism and pregnancy: Treatment with calcitriol. JAMA **243**:254, 1980.

Salle BL, Berthezene F, Glorieux FH, et al: Hypoparathyroidism during pregnancy: Treatment with calcitriol. J Clin Endocrinol Metab **52**:810, 1981.

Seki K, Wada S, Nagata N, et al: Parathyroid hormone–related protein during pregnancy and the perinatal period. Gynecol Obstet Invest **37**:83, 1994.

Shomali ME, Ross DS: Hypercalcemia in a woman with hypoparathyroidism associated with increased parathyroid hormone related protein during lactation. Endocr Pract **5**:198, 1999.

Smith R, Stevenson JC, Winearls CG, et al: Osteoporosis of pregnancy. Lancet **1**:1178, 1985.

Steinchen JJ, Tsang RC, Grafton TL, et al: Vitamin D homeostasis in the perinatal period: 1,25-dihydroxyvitamin D in maternal, cord and neonatal blood. N Engl J Med **302**:315, 1980.

Tuppuraineen M, Kroger H, Honkanen R, et al: Risks of perimenopausal fractures—a prospective population–based study. Acta Obstet Gynecol Scand **7**:624, 1995.

Chapter 52

GASTROINTESTINAL DISEASE IN PREGNANCY

Larry D. Scott, MD, MA, and Emad Abu-Hamda, MD

Gastrointestinal function may be altered during pregnancy, resulting in a variety of problems and complaints. Moreover, the unique hormonal and metabolic environments created by pregnancy can alter the course of preexisting gastrointestinal disease with the potential for both favorable and unfavorable effects. On the other hand, gastrointestinal disease itself or its management can alter the course of pregnancy and affect its outcome. The interrelationships among pregnancy and gastrointestinal function, symptoms, and disease on all these levels are the focus of this chapter.

GASTROINTESTINAL SYMPTOMS DURING PREGNANCY

A long-held concept, based on animal studies and clinical experience in humans, is that gastrointestinal motility is inhibited during pregnancy (Baron et al., 1993). Elevated levels of sex steroids, particularly progesterone, are thought to mediate this inhibitory effect, which in turn can give rise to myriad digestive complaints and problems. Although many of these are commonly thought to be pregnancy-related, surveys that actually define and quantify gastrointestinal symptoms that may be unique to pregnancy are few.

In one such study (Table 52-1), 12 symptoms were experienced more frequently by pregnant women during one, two, or all three trimesters than by a group of nonpregnant women from the same population. The study population was composed of respondents to a questionnaire regarding the occurrence and frequency of digestive symptoms. These women were largely from a low socioeconomic group attending a university teaching clinic (Scott et al., 1986).

Several of these 12 symptoms (e.g., heartburn) are consistent with long-held concepts. On the other hand, 22 other digestive symptoms were evenly distributed among the four groups and did not appear to be related to pregnancy (Table 52-2). Contrary to traditional beliefs, this latter list included symptoms usually indicative of constipation (hard or dry stools, straining at defecation, hemorrhoids); furthermore, a need to use laxatives actually was noted more frequently in the nonpregnant women (see Table 52-1). No firm conclusions can be drawn from one survey, and personal experience may well dictate alternative views; nonetheless, the survey does imply that it is not always possible to state unequivocally which symptoms and conditions are causally related to pregnancy.

Although categorical statements regarding gastrointestinal symptoms during pregnancy may not be possible, some symptoms have been evaluated in more detail. One of these is heartburn, the cardinal symptom of gastroesophageal reflux. In the study just discussed, 48.5% of women in the third trimester reported heartburn, a figure similar to the 48% incidence in late pregnancy reported by Nagler and Spiro (1962) more than 40 years ago. The number of women experiencing heartburn daily was more than twice that reported by nonpregnant women. The mechanisms that may underlie increased occurrence of gastroesophageal reflux during pregnancy are discussed in a later section of this chapter.

Increased appetite, although not specifically a gastrointestinal symptom, nonetheless can reflect gastrointestinal function. Teleologically, this finding is consistent with increased nutritional demands during pregnancy. Influences of sex steroids on appetite have been described, with progesterone thought to be an appetite stimulant (Van Thiel and Schade, 1986).

Although nausea and vomiting are clearly pregnancy-related, other symptoms of gastric origin can occur also—for example, early satiety is common in third-trimester pregnancy. This may reflect the mechanical effect of an enlarging uterine fundus but also raises questions about gastric emptying, which may be impaired. Reports on this possibility are conflicting (Hunt and Murray, 1958; Davison et al., 1970; Schade et al., 1984). If delayed gastric emptying does occur during pregnancy, it could be confined to term, possibly related to drugs given during labor (La Salvia and Steffen, 1950); as such, it does not reflect a pregnancy-related phenomenon.

The issue of constipation is an interesting one. In the survey reported here (Scott et al., 1986), it was not, by the definition used, more common during pregnancy. In a study of 1000 Israeli women, half the study population reported no change in bowel movement frequency during pregnancy, with an additional third reporting an increase in frequency (Levy et al., 1971). More recently, constipation, undefined in the study, was reported in 39% of women in the first trimester, but the prevalence had fallen to 20% by 36 weeks; no postpartum data were recorded (Meyer et al., 1994). Although obstetric textbooks describe constipation as common, survey data from these and other studies call into question some traditionally held concepts.

In summary, although the data reported in Table 52-1 include statistically significant differences in frequency, they may not be reproducible in another population. That digestive symptoms can be pregnancy-related is not surprising, and in

TABLE 52-1. SYMPTOMS SHOWING SIGNIFICANT DIFFERENCES IN DISTRIBUTION AMONG THE STUDY POPULATION (*n* = 550)*

Symptom	1st Trimester	2nd Trimester	3rd Trimester	Not Pregnant
	(*n* = 85)	(*n* = 149)	(*n* = 225)	(*n* = 91)
Xerostomia	42.6†	47.5	46.5†	37.5
Regurgitation	53.6†	33.5	49.2†	34.0
Heartburn	29.2†	29.4	48.5†	27.5
Eructation	31.5†	28.2†	34.0†	13.5
Improved appetite	47.8†	52.1†	52.1†	23.6
Early satiety	43.3†	57.0	59.8†	41.3
Epigastric pain	28.7†	20.8	21.9†	19.2
Nocturnal pain	21.7†	21.0	36.6†	24.0
Nausea	65.8†	59.8†	45.8†	35.1
Vomiting	44.2†	32.5	28.4	17.0
Laxative use	22.7†	19.8	21.7	35.9‡
Black stools	13.3†	25.4†	34.6†	12.0
Pruritus	31.5†	44.1†	47.6†	28.3

* Data shown are for symptoms with significant differences in distribution of responses among the four groups; numbers reflect percent of subjects experiencing symptoms regardless of frequency.
† Denotes group within which frequency of occurrence differed significantly from nonpregnant group.
‡ Denotes group within which frequency of occurrence differed significantly from each pregnant group.

specific patients, pregnancy may be the key to symptom production. With the few exceptions just noted, however, generalities could be difficult, if not impossible, to make.

ALTERATIONS IN GASTROINTESTINAL FUNCTION

Table 52-3 summarizes, by organ system, the physiologic alterations that can occur during pregnancy and their clinical implications. Discussion of these alterations follows.

Esophagus

The function of the esophagus is to transport the swallowed bolus from the pharynx to the stomach. At the same time, it must defend itself against reflux of gastric or gastroduodenal contents that may injure the esophageal mucosa or be subject

TABLE 52-2. SYMPTOMS *NOT* SHOWING SIGNIFICANT DIFFERENCES IN DISTRIBUTION AMONG THE STUDY POPULATION (*n* = 550)

Sialorrhea	Antacid use
Bitter taste	Reduced appetite
Water brash	Postprandial bloating
Solid or liquid dysphagia	Epigastric pain after meals
Odynophagia	
Chest pain	Clay-colored stools
	Dark urine
Oily-appearing stools	Jaundice
Hard or dry stools	Abdominal pain radiating to back
Unformed or watery stools	
Antidiarrheal drug usage	
Straining at defecation	
Flatulence	
Hematochezia	
Hemorrhoids	

to aspiration with subsequent pneumonitis, laryngitis, bronchospasm, or other harmful effects. These functions of transport and defense are largely the province of esophageal motility. With normal swallowing, sequential peristaltic contractions propel the bolus caudally through a relaxed lower esophageal sphincter (LES), which then regains tone, serving as a barrier against gastroesophageal reflux. Should reflux occur, a primary (*swallow-induced*) or secondary (*distention-induced*) peristaltic sequence returns the refluxed contents back to the gastric lumen.

There have been limited observations of esophageal motility in pregnancy. In one series, amplitude and duration of contractions were similar in pregnant and nonpregnant women, although the velocity of spread of wave forms in the lower third of the esophageal body was decreased by about a third in pregnancy. The values for both groups, however, were still within normal limits (Ulmsten and Sundstrom, 1978). Another study of heartburn in pregnancy showed no differences in motility in the body of the esophagus between pregnant and nonpregnant women (Nagler and Spiro, 1961). Although observations have been limited, it is probably safe to conclude that peristaltic motility of the esophageal body is unaltered in pregnancy.

Such is not the case with the LES, which traditionally is evaluated by intraluminal measurements of resting (basal) pressure. In animal models, as well as in most observations in human pregnancy, resting pressures are lowered (Ostick et al., 1976; Van Thiel et al., 1977). In a study of early pregnancy, pressures were not affected by pregnancy, but the response of the LES to stimulation by various agonists was reduced (Fisher et al., 1978). Perhaps the most convincing observation was by Van Thiel and associates, who measured LES pressure serially in the same group of women during each trimester of pregnancy and during the postpartum period, showing a stepwise reduction in relation to duration of gestation with recovery following delivery (Van Thiel et al., 1977) (Fig. 52-1). This phenomenon could well be a major variable in the genesis of gastroesophageal reflux and heartburn and will be discussed shortly.

■ TABLE 52-3. IMPLICATIONS OF ALTERATIONS IN GASTROINTESTINAL FUNCTION IN PREGNANCY

Physiologic Alterations	Clinical Implications
Esophagus	
Reduction in resting LES pressure	Gastroesophageal reflux
	Heartburn
Reduction in responsiveness of LES to pharmacologic and physiologic stimulation	Uncertain risk for erosive esophagitis and stricture formation
Questionable changes in wave-form characteristics and spread	
Stomach	
Slow gastric emptying with increased residual volume (term)	Gastroesophageal reflux (?)
	Nausea and vomiting (?)
	Risk of aspiration with general anesthesia for delivery
Equivocal changes in acid + pepsin secretion	Decreased incidence of duodenal ulcer
Small Intestine	
Increased transit time	Stasis and bacterial overgrowth
Changes in propulsive motility	Sequestration of bile acids
Reduced contractile responsiveness of intestinal muscle (*in vitro*)	Pseudo-obstruction syndrome
Increased activity of brush border enzymes, gut hypertrophy, and increased villus height	Enhanced efficiency of absorption of some nutrients
Folate malabsorption (?)	Megaloblastic anemia
	Neural tube defects
Colon	
Increased transit time (?)	Constipation and its attendant symptoms
Contractile responsiveness of colonic smooth muscle reduced	Pseudo-obstruction syndrome
Increased sodium and water absorption	

LES, lower esophageal sphincter.

The explanation for these changes is not certain. The theory most often put forward is that reduced LES pressure is due to high circulating levels of progesterone, which has an inhibitory effect on both gastrointestinal and uterine smooth muscle (Kumar, 1962; Ryan and Pellechia, 1982). This is a plausible theory, but the evidence remains circumstantial; at least in one study, the degree of reduction in LES pressure did not correlate with the concentration of progesterone in the peripheral blood (Ostick et al., 1976).

Stomach

Gastric function is primarily secretory and motor. The secretory function manifests in the production of hydrogen ion by the parietal cell located in fundic mucosa of the gastric body. The production of acid creates a hostile environment for potentially pathogenic microorganisms while also providing the optimal pH for activation of pepsinogen to pepsin, which has proteolytic function. The presence of acid also could facilitate absorption of certain elements, such as ionic iron and ascorbic acid. In practice, however, the importance of this function is limited because patients with achlorhydria do not appear to experience an increased risk from infections and are not jeopardized nutritionally. On the other hand, acid, while serving the physiologic role just discussed, also can serve as a pathogenetic factor in the production of duodenal ulcers, gastric ulcers, and gastroesophageal reflux disease. It is thus reasonable to ask whether acid secretion is altered by pregnancy and, if so, whether there are physiologic or perhaps pathophysiologic consequences.

Most of the studies of gastric physiology have been carried out in experimental animals and to a lesser extent in small groups of pregnant women. As is discussed later, ulcer patients may experience fewer symptoms during pregnancy, which suggests that acid secretion is reduced. At least two studies

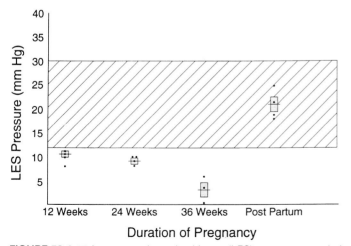

FIGURE 52-1 ■ Lower esophageal sphincter (LES) pressure recorded in four volunteer women during pregnancy and in the postpartum period. The *shaded area* shows the range of values for LES pressure in normal nonpregnant women. The *horizontal bars* and *stippled areas* represent the mean ± SEM for each time period. (From Van Thiel DH, Gavaler J, Joshi SN, et al: Heartburn of pregnancy. Gastroenterology **72**:666, 1977, copyright © by The American Gastroenterological Association.)

addressing acid secretion in pregnancy have concluded that both basal acid secretion and stimulated acid secretion are in fact reduced during pregnancy (Murray et al., 1957; Hunt and Murray, 1958); however, other studies report no change (Waldum et al., 1980) or even an increase in acid production in the third trimester (Gryboski and Spiro, 1956). Clearly, this issue is unsettled. The implications of changes in acid secretion could be more relevant to ulcer symptoms in patients so affected. For the reasons stated previously, it is unlikely that any changes have adverse effects on nutrition or susceptibility to infection.

Motor function of the stomach has received more attention in recent publications, although investigations remain somewhat limited because of methodology (e.g., radioisotope scanning), which is contraindicated in pregnancy. The motor function of the stomach is designed both to receive ingested food or fluids (a process called *receptive relaxation*) and to prepare the gastric contents for digestion and absorption by grinding solid material into very fine particles prior to intermittently emptying small amounts into the duodenum (Minami and McCallum, 1984). This latter function is carried out by peristaltic contractions in the gastric antrum and the variable size of the pyloric lumen at the gastroduodenal junction.

Gastric motility and emptying in pregnancy have been of interest for two reasons. The first is the common occurrence of nausea and vomiting, particularly early in pregnancy, and the possibility of altered gastric motor function, regardless of the cause, which may underlie this complaint. The other is the concern—expressed by anesthesiologists—about gastric contents in a pregnant woman at term who is undergoing sedation or even general anesthesia without adequate preparation, and the attendant risk of aspiration. Various methods used to examine this question have led to the conclusion that pregnancy has no influence on gastric emptying (La Salvia and Steffen, 1950; Schade et al., 1984; Radberg et al., 1989) in first, second, and third trimesters. Slowing of emptying sometimes occurs at term, but this appears to be related to analgesics and sedative agents used during labor (La Salvia and Steffen, 1950; O'Sullivan et al., 1987). In summary, any effects of pregnancy on gastric function, whether secretory or motor, are limited.

Small Intestine

As the site of digestion and absorption of nutrients, the small intestine assumes considerable importance during pregnancy because of the unique nutritional demands of this state. Pancreaticobiliary function is also intrinsic to nutrient digestion and absorption and is discussed in Chapter 53.

One way to measure small intestinal function is to look at the movement of intraluminal contents through the duodenum, jejunum, and ileum. Both animal (Scott and DeFlora, 1983) and human studies (Parry et al., 1970a; Lawson et al., 1985; Braverman et al., 1988) agree that transit time through the small intestine is prolonged during pregnancy (Fig. 52-2). In one animal study, propulsive motility, as reflected in the cycling characteristics of the migrating motor complex, was altered (Scott and DeFlora, 1983). The observations are sufficiently limited to make it difficult to conclude the stage of pregnancy in which this phenomenon is most likely to occur, although in one series, transit time was longest in the third trimester and returned to normal after delivery (Wald et al., 1982).

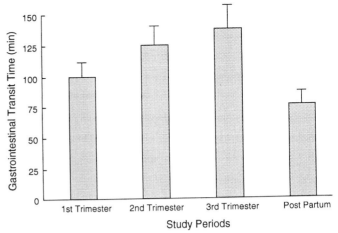

FIGURE 52-2 ■ Orocecal gastrointestinal transit time in women in the first ($n = 8$), second ($n = 12$), and third ($n = 22$) trimesters of pregnancy and postpartum ($n = 17$); data shown are mean values ± SD. Transit time was longest in second-trimester and third-trimester women and was similar in first-trimester and postpartum women. (Adapted from Lawson M, Kern F Jr, Everson GT: Gastrointestinal transit time in human pregnancy: Prolongation in the second and third trimesters followed by postpartum normalization. Gastroenterology **89**:996, 1985, copyright © by The American Gastroenterological Association.)

As *transit time*, a function of intestinal motility, is prolonged, theoretically there can be both beneficial and negative effects; certainly, prolonged contact of nutrients with the mucosal surface could facilitate absorption. Mixing of chyme with digestive enzymes and bile salts—also a function of motility—contributes significantly to digestion and absorption as well, however, and is not measured in these studies. On the other hand, delayed transit conceivably could give rise to unpleasant symptoms such as bloating and distention or, possibly, bacterial overgrowth, which can affect absorption adversely. These absorption questions remain unanswered. Progesterone is again offered as a possible explanation for the prolonged transit time because of its inhibitory effect on gastrointestinal smooth muscle (Wald et al., 1982; Lawson et al., 1985).

Teleologically, it would not be surprising if absorptive function were enhanced during pregnancy, and authors of earlier discussions of this issue have referred to such a possibility (Parry et al., 1970a). Vitamin B_{12} absorption, for example, is increased during pregnancy in laboratory animals (Brown et al., 1977), and transport of certain amino acids is increased (Dugas et al., 1970; Butt and Fleshler, 1971); on the other hand, folic acid deficiency can occur (Rothman, 1970).

Absorptive efficiency or capacity is difficult to measure, and virtually no studies in human pregnancy answer this question. Animal studies have shown an increase in small intestinal weight during pregnancy, much of which is mucosal (Burdett and Reek, 1979). Morphologically, mucosal hypertrophy and increase in villus height have occurred (Cripps and Williams, 1975; Prieto et al., 1994). Activities of some (but not all) brush border enzymes are actually more pronounced during lactation and then resolve following weaning (Cripps and Williams, 1975; Elias and Dowling, 1976). Whether these presumed adaptive changes in animals are a response to increased nutrient intake, hormonal factors, or both is not clear (Dowling, 1982).

Colon

Little is known about colonic function in pregnancy. Normally, the proximal colon is a major site of electrolyte and water absorption, concentrating and desiccating the largely fluid material that enters from the ileum. Colonic motility is responsible for periodic transfer of luminal contents from the proximal colon to the distal colon and rectum with subsequent evacuation of stool, which—although still 60%–85% water in composition—is normally in solid form (Powell, 1991).

As has been suggested for other regions of the gastrointestinal tract, it is generally thought that colonic motility is reduced during pregnancy; this hypothesis has only been measured in animal models of pregnancy, however. Colonic smooth muscle in pregnant guinea pigs is less responsive to stimulation by agonists (Scott and DeFlora, 1989), and transit time is increased in pregnant rats, although not out of proportion to other circumstances in which sex steroid levels are increased (Ryan and Bhojwani, 1986). In pharmacologic experiments, progesterone does exert an inhibitory effect on colonic smooth muscle, a finding which again supports the hypothesis that this steroid mediates the general inhibition of gut motility during pregnancy (Gill et al., 1985). There is also evidence for increased activity of endogenous opioids during pregnancy, and theoretically, this may also inhibit colonic motility (Iwasaki et al., 1991).

In a study of early pregnancy in women scheduled for therapeutic abortion, sodium and water absorption in the proximal colon was increased, possibly because of increased mineralocorticoid activity (Parry et al., 1970b). If these limited observations are valid, it would not be surprising that constipation is often thought to be a problem during pregnancy.

SPECIFIC GASTROINTESTINAL DISORDERS IN PREGNANCY

Nausea and Vomiting

Although obviously not a specific disease, nausea, sometimes accompanied by vomiting, is so common during pregnancy that it is necessarily included in any discussion of gastrointestinal disorders. In the survey of gastrointestinal symptoms noted previously (Scott et al., 1986), 66% of women in their first trimester had some degree of nausea, and 44% complained of vomiting; 18% of the total population surveyed had vomited more than once daily. The onset of nausea and vomiting of pregnancy is typically 4–6 weeks into gestation, with the peak occurrence at 8–12 weeks; resolution is expected by the 20th week. Other reports cite frequencies of 70% or higher (Jarnfelt-Samsioe et al., 1983; Klebanoff et al., 1985; Whitehead et al., 1992; Gadsby et al., 1993).

The disorder spans a spectrum of problems, ranging from troublesome but tolerable "morning sickness," which can be managed with dietary discretion and simple remedies, to severe cases, also called *hyperemesis gravidarum*, in which fluid and electrolyte status and nutritional status could be jeopardized. Liver function test results (alanine aminotransferase [ALT]), aspartate aminotransferase [AST]) can also be mildly elevated in hyperemesis (Abell and Riely, 1992). Fortunately, hyperemesis is unusual; reported frequencies range from 3.3 to 10 cases per 1000 pregnancies. Circumstances in which this condition is more likely include increased body weight, nulli-

parity, and twin gestation (Broussard and Richter, 1998; Van Thiel and Schade, 1986; Abell and Riely, 1992). Although nausea and vomiting in pregnancy are common, they remain perhaps the least understood of the disorders that accompany gestation.

Nausea, particularly when associated with vomiting, implies a specific disorder of the upper gastrointestinal tract. For example, the nausea and vomiting that sometimes complicate diabetes (*gastroparesis diabeticorum*) are thought to be due to a primary disturbance of gastric motility in which propulsive activity is reduced or absent (Janssens et al., 1990). A similar phenomenon can occur after vagotomy or even in the absence of an identifiable underlying disease process (Malagelada, 1982).

As noted previously, however, although gastrointestinal motility can be reduced during pregnancy, studies attempting to document a defect in gastric emptying as a measure of gastric motility have generally been unrevealing. Using a different approach, investigators measured gastric electrical activity (a correlate of motility) in pregnant women and reported abnormalities in patients complaining of nausea (Koch et al., 1990). In this study, surface electrodes placed on the skin of the upper abdomen recorded electrical events in the wall of the stomach, a technique called *electrogastrography*. Abnormalities correlated with a higher nausea score during the test as determined subjectively. In a small subgroup who had nausea, the abnormalities subsequently disappeared following delivery. In a subsequent study, the baseline electrogastrogram did not differ in pregnant women with and without nausea (Riezzo et al., 1992). These findings imply that this problem is not in fact a primary disorder of gastric motility.

Although nausea and vomiting can reflect an intrinsic abnormality of the stomach, these symptoms also can arise via events in the central nervous system. The major participants at this level are the chemoreceptor trigger zone (CTZ), located in the area postrema of the brain stem, and the nearby "vomiting center," which includes the motor nuclei of cranial nerves, among them the dorsal motor nucleus of the vagus (Koch, 1995). The vomiting center receives afferent input not only from peripheral sites but also from the CTZ and coordinates the motor events associated with the act of vomiting. The CTZ can be affected by a number of diverse stimuli; examples include adverse effects of medication (e.g., morphine) or the nausea that accompanies severe pain.

It is possible that during pregnancy, one or more factors create disturbances in gastroduodenal motility through such central effects. Some authors have theorized that such a mechanism involves hormonal factors (human chorionic gonadotropin [hCG], thyroxin, cortisol, other steroid hormones), although there are no clear-cut relationships between increased or decreased circulating levels and women with these complaints (Jarnfelt-Samsioe, 1987; Andrews and Whitehead, 1990). Alternatively, the CTZ could be more sensitive to otherwise normal levels of a particular hormone or metabolite in some individuals (Jarnfelt-Samsioe et al., 1985; Whitehead et al., 1992).

In patients with severe nausea and vomiting of pregnancy (hyperemesis), these various hormonal and metabolic variables have received closer scrutiny. Thyroxin and the various gestational hormones have been the basis for many pathogenetic theories; for example, some women with hyperemesis appear to be hyperthyroid, and this condition could in some way be associated with either higher levels of circulating hCG or hCG with higher biological activity (Kimura et al., 1993; Broussard and Richter, 1998). There also have been a few case reports of hyperparathyroidism secondary to parathyroid adenomas that were associated with hyperemesis gravidarum (Abell and Riely, 1992).

Psychological and social factors have also been thought to be important (Deuchar, 1995). Support for these variables has been derived from observations that the problem is more common in overcrowding or unfamiliar circumstances. Hyperemesis may be more common in unwanted or unplanned pregnancies. Although social and psychological or emotional factors are not likely a primary cause of hyperemesis, it is certainly possible that such issues adversely affect its clinical expression (Broussard and Richter, 1998).

Having considered the potential importance of central mechanisms in hyperemesis gravidarum, were turn to consideration of a gastric role, which recently has been suggested. There are now several reports of a higher prevalence of *Helicobacter pylori* (*H. pylori*) seropositivity in hyperemesis patients when compared with asymptomatic pregnant controls (Frigo et al., 1998; Erdem et al., 2002). There also has been a case report showing a response to *H. pylori* eradication therapy in three patients with hyperemesis gravidarum who had failed conventional therapy (Jacoby and Porter, 1999). Although these reports speculate about a potential role of *H. pylori* gastritis in patients with hyperemesis gravidarum, a positive serologic test does not necessarily indicate active infection. Any suggestion of a role for this bacterium in this disorder is thus premature. Additional consideration of *H. pylori* in peptic ulcer disease appears later in this chapter.

Management options are few, although fortunately, as noted earlier, the problem often lessens spontaneously as the pregnancy progresses. One must be sure that the symptom does not represent the development of other disorders in which nausea may sometimes occur—for example, biliary disease, pancreatitis, and peptic ulcer disease (PUD) should be considered, although distinguishing features usually aid differential diagnosis.

Symptomatic management with attention to fluid balance is the mainstay of management; small meals with avoidance of potential irritants are often recommended. Pharmacologic agents can be used; however, as with any situation during pregnancy, they should be used judiciously. In the past, pyridoxine (vitamin B_6) has been advocated; although its efficacy may not be predictable, it is probably innocuous and is rated category "A" by the U.S. Food and Drug Administration (FDA). Randomized, double-blind, placebo-controlled trials have suggested efficacy in women taking up to 75 mg of pyridoxine daily (Vutyavanich et al., 1995; Mazzotta and Magee, 2000).

Metoclopramide (Reglan) has been used more often in recent years, although there have been no randomized, controlled trials that have been published demonstrating its efficacy in the treatment of nausea and vomiting of pregnancy (Mazzotta and Magee, 2000; Magee et al., 2002). Placental transfer does occur, but the experience has been favorable and it appears to be safe, justifying a "B" rating (no evidence of risk in humans) by the FDA. Meclizine (Antivert) has received a similar rating and has been shown to be effective (Broussard and Richter, 1998). Phenothiazines (promethazine, prochlorperazine, and others) are also probably safe and effective (Mazzotta and Magee, 2000). There has been limited reported experience with ondansetron. Although this agent is very effective in the treatment of chemotherapy-induced nausea and vomiting, it may be no more effective than promethazine in nausea and vomiting of pregnancy (Magee et al., 2002).

Finally, although there are no controlled studies, supportive psychotherapy (encouragement, explanation, reassurance, opportunity to ventilate emotions) and, if indicated, focal psychotherapy targeting a specific conflict have been advocated as essential to a comprehensive management plan (Deuchar, 1995; Murphy, 1998).

In severe cases of hyperemesis, more aggressive support could be required, including both fluid and nutritional resuscitation (Levine and Esser, 1988). Home infusion therapy can be administered safely to selected patients (Naef et al., 1995). Maternal ketosis should be avoided because of concern about the adverse effects of maternal ketones, which are readily transported across the placenta, on fetal development (Hod et al., 1994). Ketones can be used in fetal metabolism, however, and theoretically, they have a beneficial effect in the setting of maternal starvation.

Interestingly, nausea and vomiting of pregnancy have been associated with a decreased risk of spontaneous abortion in the first half of pregnancy. This "protective" characteristic has also been noted with hyperemesis (Abell and Riely, 1992; Bashiri et al., 1995). Although some reports on outcome have suggested an increased risk for intrauterine growth retardation and low-birth-weight neonates in patients with hyperemesis, this remains controversial, and there does not seem to be any difference in the likelihood of congenital defects (Abell and Riely, 1992; Deuchar, 1995). Because this condition is a first-trimester problem, another potentially important variable in outcome is how the problem is managed, in particular the pharmacologic agent chosen (Klebanoff and Mills, 1986).

Gastroesophageal Reflux Disease

Gastroesophageal reflux disease (GERD), defined as the abnormal reflux of acidic gastric content into the esophagus, is a common disorder in the general population (Nebel et al., 1976; Talley et al., 1992). The cardinal symptom, heartburn, is one experienced by many people, although only a minority actually have a problem severe enough to cause them to seek medical attention. Symptoms, however, do not always mean esophagitis with mucosal injury and inflammation. In fact, although some patients with heartburn have esophagitis, most patients with these complaints actually have normal esophageal mucosa. There is yet a third group of patients with reflux and esophageal injury but with few or no symptoms. These patients are at highest risk for complications, primarily stricture, because the disease is not recognized until these late problems develop.

During pregnancy, conditions can develop that favor the occurrence of gastroesophageal reflux; however, virtually all of these patients fall into the group of symptomatic patients without overt esophagitis, possibly in part because the duration of the problem is limited. Endoscopically determined esophagitis and stricture have been reported during pregnancy, but in this case, it was a sequela of protracted vomiting in a patient with hyperemesis gravidarum (Swinhoe et al., 1981). For the most part, therefore, the problem is one of symptoms—often severe, but with esophageal injury unlikely.

Four major variables can affect gastroesophageal reflux (Dodds et al., 1981). The first and the one most often cited is the strength of the antireflux barrier. Contributing to this barrier is the closure tension, also known as *resting* or *basal pressure*, of the LES, a zone of high pressure associated with specialized circular muscle located anatomically at the gastroesophageal junction. Although reflux may predictably occur when basal sphincter pressure is reduced or in some cases absent, it may also occur during a phenomenon called *transient LES relaxation*. Sometimes called *inappropriate relaxations* because they occur spontaneously, unassociated with swallowing, they explain the sometimes paradoxical occurrence of reflux in patients with normal LES basal pressures (Pope, 1994).

Mechanical factors also serve a barrier function. These are defined by the anatomic configuration of the esophagogastric junction, the diaphragm, and associated supporting structures. The other variables include the potency and volume of refluxed fluid, a function of both acid secretion and gastric emptying; esophageal clearance, a function of propulsive motility in the esophageal body; and tissue resistance, which is poorly understood but probably influenced by nutritional factors and blood flow.

Although a large body of information has been generated regarding these variables in healthy people and patients with reflux, little is known about them during pregnancy. As noted earlier, however, LES resting pressure appears to be reduced during pregnancy, although there is no information regarding transient LES relaxation. If basal pressure is reduced, the barrier against reflux could be jeopardized. Moreover, in addition to the possible changes in the antireflux barrier, the abdominothoracic pressure gradient could be increased by the enlarging uterine fundus and could contribute to the tendency for reflux to occur, although this concept is not universally accepted (Van Thiel and Wald, 1981).

Observations of esophageal motility are sufficiently limited that no conclusions are possible, although the single report of reduced contractile amplitude and wave-form velocity (Ulmsten and Sundstrom, 1978) implies a possible defect in esophageal clearance of refluxed acid (Marrero et al., 1992). Based on information cited previously, alterations in gastric function are not likely to play a role in pregnancy-related reflux. In the absence of observations of intraesophageal pH in ambulatory patients over time—24 hours or longer—conclusions about the magnitude and pathogenesis of the problem remain speculative (Mattox and Richter, 1990; Hewson et al., 1991).

As noted earlier, heartburn of pregnancy occurs in about 50% of women in the third trimester; by other estimates, it can occur in as many as 80% of patients (Olans and Wolf, 1994). Management of the reflux problem involves some degree of lifestyle modification and, if needed, pharmacologic intervention. Many physicians have a nihilistic view of reflux therapy during pregnancy, primarily because it is a self-limited problem with resolution during the postpartum period. Standard antireflux measures, including head-of-bed elevation during sleep, small meals, a reduced-fat diet, and smoking cessation, are of some value. Attempts to decrease intra-abdominal pressure (e.g., avoidance of tight clothing) are of little value during pregnancy.

Antacids can be useful for symptoms and are generally safe if not taken in excess. Adverse reactions associated with excessive use of antacids include diarrhea and metabolic and electrolyte alterations such as hypercalcemia, hypermagnesemia, and hypophosphatemia. Moreover, magnesium-containing antacids should be avoided in the late stages of pregnancy, because of the theoretical potential for magnesium to alter labor (Katz and Castell, 1998).

The mainstay of symptomatic management for reflux, however, has been the inhibition of acid secretion using H_2 receptor antagonists, which currently are available over the counter. Although use of these agents during pregnancy cannot be encouraged, selected patients who remain symptomatic despite antacid therapy may benefit. As a group of drugs, they are among the safest available, and their use during pregnancy, although not sanctioned by the FDA, appears to be safe despite transfer of the drug across the placenta (Dicke et al., 1988) (Table 52-4). Cimetidine, ranitidine, famotidine, and nizatidine are all rated category B drugs for use during pregnancy (Physicians' Desk Reference, 2002).

Both clinical and published experience attest to the safety and efficacy of these drugs during pregnancy when used in patients with persistent symptoms that do not respond to antacids (Magee et al., 1996; Larson et al., 1997; Kallen, 1998; Rayburn et al., 1999). Although fetal abnormalities and spontaneous abortions have been reported in case reports, their relationship to the drug given was equivocal (Cipriani et al., 1983; Colin-Jones et al., 1985; Koren and Zemlickis, 1991). The literature on limited use of these drugs in obstetric anesthesia to reduce the risk of acid aspiration pneumonitis is extensive (Hodgkinson et al., 1983; Sacco et al., 1986; Colman et al., 1988), with no unfavorable outcomes noted. Although H_2 receptors are present in myometrium, no changes in contractility, fetal heart rate, or course of labor have been noted in women taking H_2 antagonists (Smallwood et al., 1995).

The newest group of drugs in the therapeutic armamentarium to treat gastroesophageal reflux disease are the proton pump inhibitors (omeprazole, lansoprazole, rabeprazole, pantoprazole,

TABLE 52-4. MAJOR GASTROINTESTINAL DRUGS USED IN PREGNANCY

Drug	Potential Use	FDA Category*
Metoclopramide	Nausea/GERD	B
Cimetidine	GERD/PUD	B
Ranitidine	GERD/PUD	B
Famotidine	GERD/PUD	B
Nizatidine	GERD/PUD	B
Sucralfate	PUD	B
Omeprazole	GERD/PUD	C
Lansoprazole	GERD/PUD	B
Rabeprazole	GERD/PUD	B
Pantoprazole	GERD/PUD	B
Esomeprazole	GERD/PUD	B
Sulfasalazine	IBD	B
Olsalazine	IBD	C
Mesalamine	IBD	B
Balsalazide	IBD	C
Prednisone	IBD	B
Budesonide	IBD	C

* B = no evidence of risk in humans; C = risk cannot be ruled out.

FDA, Food and Drug Administration; GERD, gastroesophageal reflux disease; IBD, inflammatory bowel disease; PUD, peptic ulcer disease.

and esomeprazole). These drugs block the hydrogen-potassium ATPase located on the apical membrane of the parietal cell in the gastric secretory epithelium. This is the final common pathway in acid secretion and, not surprisingly, these agents are extremely potent. They are currently the mainstay of therapy in reflux esophagitis outside of pregnancy. They are all classified as category B except for omeprazole, which is classified as category C by the FDA (Physicians' Desk Reference, 2002). Omeprazole does cross the placenta to a limited extent, and there is a potential for fetal toxicity (Ching et al., 1986). As with H$_2$ receptor antagonists, however, published reports of the use of proton pump inhibitors in pregnancy have documented safety. Therefore, selective use in pregnancy could be considered in refractory cases (Kallen, 2001; Ruigomez et al., 1999; Lalkin et al., 1998). The safety and efficacy of proton pump inhibitors to decrease the risk of aspiration pneumonitis in obstetric anesthesia in women undergoing emergency cesarean section has also been well documented (Orr et al., 1993; Rocke et al., 1994).

Yet another group of agents has found a role in the management of gastroesophageal reflux; these are collectively known as *prokinetic* or *promotility drugs* because they accelerate gastric emptying and can increase both basal pressure in the LES and propulsive esophageal motility. Metoclopramide (Reglan) is the only agent of this type currently available in the United States, but because of questionable efficacy in this setting and problematic adverse effects, its use in pregnancy has been confined to obstetric anesthesia (Orr et al., 1993). It is unlikely that prokinetic drugs would be needed to manage heartburn of pregnancy. The major treatment focus, generally successful, has been on lifestyle modifications and acid neutralization or suppression, as discussed previously.

Peptic Ulcer Disease

Views are conflicting regarding any significant change in motor or secretory gastric function during pregnancy; based on those observations, one might not expect any alteration in the clinical expression of peptic ulcer disease during pregnancy. In addition, ulcer is a greater problem among males than among females. For several years, the general consensus has been that pregnancy has a salutary effect on the course of ulcer in women who already carry that diagnosis, and new-onset ulcer during pregnancy is rare. In the largest series reported, covering 313 pregnancies that took place following the diagnosis of ulcer, 45% of patients had no symptoms, 44% improved, and only 12% experienced no improvement (Clark, 1953). These findings may be explained partly by the avoidance of nonsteroidal anti-inflammatory drugs (NSAIDs) and smoking during pregnancy, both of which are known risk factors for ulcerogenesis (Michaletz-Onody, 1992). Other theories include the potential for estrogen to exert a protective effect on the gastric and duodenal mucosa (Doll et al., 1965) and immunological tolerance that occurs during pregnancy, which may permit H. *pylori* to exist in the gastric mucosa with little inflammatory response and risk for ulcer (Cappell and Garcia, 1998). On the other hand, although the pathogenetic role of gastritis caused by the bacterium H. *pylori* in most patients with duodenal and gastric ulcer not related to nonsteroidal anti-inflammatory agents (NSAIDs) is now accepted, it has not been investigated in the context of pregnancy (Peura, 1996).

Despite what appears to be a reduced occurrence of ulcer, complications—primarily perforation—have been reported during pregnancy (Baird, 1966; Paul et al., 1976). As with many conditions that present during pregnancy, symptoms may not be classic, with the result that diagnosis could be delayed. Although bleeding as a complication of ulcer is more common than perforation in the general population, the reverse could be true in pregnancy. In one series of 12 pregnant women with upper gastrointestinal bleeding, no cases were due to peptic ulcer disease (Palmer, 1961), in contrast with a nearly 50% expectancy rate in the nonpregnant population presenting with this problem (Laine, 1993). Although uncommon, hemorrhage from ulcer is more likely late in pregnancy or in the early postpartum period (Aston et al., 1991). Gastric outlet obstruction resulting from ulcer has been rarely reported in pregnancy (Goh et al., 1993).

In the general population, the diagnosis of uncomplicated ulcer in an otherwise healthy patient can often be based on presenting symptoms (e.g., epigastric burning pain, worse pain on an empty stomach, often awakening the patient in the early morning hours, and relieved with food or antacids). Empirical therapy in this setting includes a therapeutic dosing regimen of an H$_2$-receptor antagonist or a proton pump inhibitor; if the patient responds, 6 to 8 weeks of therapy should be completed. If there is no response within 10–14 days, a diagnostic study (usually upper gastrointestinal endoscopy) is indicated.

As in the nonpregnant state, diagnosis of uncomplicated ulcer in pregnancy, although infrequent, should also be clinically based, and treatment likewise can be initiated empirically (Kahn and Greenfield, 1985; Cappell and Garcia, 1998). One might have concern, however, using drugs that are placentally transferred, and management—in contrast with that of the nonpregnant patient—may not initially include H$_2$ antagonists or proton pump inhibitors. One would be left with attention to diet with regular meals, avoidance of symptom-producing foods, judicious use of antacids, and avoidance of potentially adverse factors such as smoking, coffee and caffeine-containing foods, alcohol, and aspirin and other NSAIDs. Sucralfate, as a nonabsorbed agent that accelerates healing of ulcer by improving mucosal defense at the ulcer site, is an attractive alternative. Practically speaking, however, the safety profile of many of the H$_2$ antagonists is so favorable, as already noted, that one need not hesitate to use such agents if justified by the clinical circumstances (Magee et al., 1996). A similar argument can be made for empirical use of proton pump inhibitors. The use of endoscopy during pregnancy is discussed later in this chapter.

Because of the association of many ulcers with H. *pylori* infection in the stomach, the standard of practice in the general population has now evolved to testing for the presence of this bacterium in all patients with active ulcer. Both endoscopic and noninvasive testing are available, which provide a high degree of sensitivity and specificity (National Institutes of Health, 1994). If test results are positive, patients should receive eradication therapy, usually a combination of two antibiotics, often given with bismuth and a proton pump inhibitor.

There are no guidelines for such a program during pregnancy. Because of the relative ease with which active ulcer disease can be managed with acid reduction therapy and the safety of available agents for this purpose, however, there would be no urgency to resolve an H. *pylori* question in a patient with active ulcer during pregnancy. Active maternal infection does not pose an increased risk to infants during the first year of life (Blecker et al., 1994; Ashorn et al., 1996). Further, eradication regimens that involve multiple agents pose additional hazards in this setting, and diagnosis and treatment of infection can be deferred to the postpartum period.

A rare cause of peptic ulcer disease is the *Zollinger-Ellison syndrome*, in which pathologic hypersecretion of gastric acid results from a gastrin-producing endocrine tumor. Women with this syndrome may become pregnant, and successful management of both the ulcer diathesis and the pregnancy have now been documented using high doses of H_2 antagonists and proton pump inhibitors without fetal toxicity (Harper et al., 1995; Stewart et al., 1997).

Inflammatory Bowel Disease

Inflammatory bowel disease (IBD), comprising both ulcerative colitis and Crohn disease, is the one gastrointestinal disorder whose relationship with pregnancy generates the most controversy. Several studies examining similar issues often have drawn conflicting conclusions. Further, there may well be differences between these disorders in how they impact pregnancy and vice versa.

Ulcerative colitis is primarily a mucosal disease, always involving the rectum and extending proximally in a continuous fashion. The extent of involvement varies, but in some patients it affects the entire colon. Other regions of the gastrointestinal tract are spared. Symptoms are primarily diarrhea, often with bleeding, and some degree of abdominal pain. *Crohn disease*, on the other hand, is a transmural granulomatous inflammatory process that involves the rectum only about 50% of the time. It may involve any region of the gastrointestinal tract but is most common in the colon and terminal ileum. Although diarrhea and bleeding may occur, these symptoms are less predictable, particularly in the absence of significant colonic disease, and the diagnosis can be elusive. Abdominal pain is almost always a problem, and nutritional deficiencies occur more often in Crohn disease than in ulcerative colitis. Fistulous complications, including rectovaginal fistula, can be particularly troublesome.

In the past, fertility was thought to be jeopardized in patients with IBD of either type (DeDombal et al., 1965); today, that seems to be less likely. In the most often quoted study, women with ulcerative colitis had a fertility rate of 81% and an incidence of involuntary infertility of 7%. If one looked at the number of children per family as an index of fertility, the numbers among women with IBD were similar to those among the general population (Willoughby and Truelove, 1980). Other reviews of this topic also conclude that, at least in ulcerative colitis, fertility rate is unaffected (Singer and Brandt, 1991; Hanan, 1998; Jospe and Peppercorn, 1999; Moum, 2000; Alstead, 2002). The only exception may be ulcerative colitis patients who have undergone proctocolectomy with ileoanal anastamosis with J-pouch (Olsen et al, 2002). In this study, these patients had a significantly prolonged time to pregnancy compared with women in the reference population, possibly because of impaired fertility from surgery-related pelvic adhesions. The effect of Crohn disease on fertility is less clear-cut; one might predict that, at least in some patients who have small bowel disease with extensive perienteric inflammation—often with fistulous tracts—pelvic inflammation with infertility could easily occur. Indeed, many recent reviews conclude that fertility is slightly lower among patients with Crohn disease when compared with healthy women (Hanan, 1998; Jospe and Peppercorn, 1999; Moum, 2000; Alstead, 2002). Again, studies present conflicting results, but the critical variable is probably the degree of disease activity (Hudson et al., 1997). Fertility is highest among women in remission or

following surgical resection of active disease (DeDombal et al., 1972; Donaldson, 1985). Much of the controversy surrounding this issue reflects the lack of a consistent definition of infertility. Infertility could result from anatomic causes, but in large population surveys, other variables, such as physician advice, impaired sexuality caused by psychological and physical components of the illness, and even male infertility, are not usually considered.

The general consensus from early studies is that ulcerative colitis does not have an adverse effect on pregnancy outcome as measured by the occurrence of spontaneous abortion, stillbirth, congenital abnormality, or premature delivery (DeDombal et al., 1972; Mogadam, Korelitz, et al., 1981; Nielson et al., 1983; Porter and Stirrat, 1986). This statement should be qualified, however, by the fact that most studies report that women with inactive disease have the most favorable course (Willoughby and Truelove, 1980; Korelitz, 1992). Other evidence suggests that there could be an increased risk of pregnancy complications; however, disease activity is not always assessed in these surveys, yet this may be the important determinant in outcome (Fedarkow et al., 1989; Baird et al., 1990; Kornfeld et al., 1997; Alstead, 2002). Similar conclusions can be drawn for women with Crohn disease. In particular, among those with emergence of disease activity either at the outset of gestation or during its course, an increased risk of preterm birth, low birth weight, and small-for-gestational-age infants can result (Mogadam, Dobbins, et al., 1981; Nielson et al., 1984; Fedarkow et al., 1989; Baird et al., 1990, Kornfeld et al., 1997; Fonager et al., 1998; Alstead, 2002).

The need for any surgical intervention to treat complications of ulcerative colitis, such as hemorrhage or toxic megacolon, imposes a great risk for fetal survival (Korelitz, 1985; Fedorkow et al., 1989). Although surgery for Crohn disease during pregnancy has traditionally been associated with significant maternal and fetal mortality, favorable outcomes sometimes are achieved (Hill et al., 1997).

In general, the rate of cesarean section at term does not appear to be affected by an underlying diagnosis of IBD (Crohn et al., 1956; Nielson et al., 1984; Porter and Stirrat, 1986). A more recent study, however, showed a slightly increased rate of cesarean sections in patients with inflammatory bowel disease (Kornfeld et al., 1997). Cesarean section may be the preferred mode of delivery in patients with active or inactive perirectal, perianal, or rectovaginal fistulas because it avoids the potential for poor healing of the episiotomy site (Moum, 2000). These are not issues for women who have undergone ileoanal anastomosis with J-pouch after total proctocolectomy for ulcerative colitis. Successful pregnancies without undue complications have occurred. Vaginal delivery is safe for these patients, and the decision regarding mode of delivery in women with ulcerative colitis can be based solely on obstetrical issues (Scott et al., 1996).

Does pregnancy pose a risk for the patient with IBD? In most patients, the answer is probably no, although the key variable again appears to be the degree of activity of IBD at the time of conception. If activity is quiescent, the odds are favorable that it will remain so for the duration of the pregnancy, whereas active disease at conception tends to persist and may worsen (Willoughby and Truelove, 1980; Nielson et al., 1983; Rogers and Katz, 1995; Hanan, 1998; Jospe and Peppercorn, 1999; Moum, 2000; Alstead, 2002).

Relapses do occur but apparently no more often than in the nonpregnant population (Nielson et al., 1983; Hanan, 1998;

Jospe and Peppercorn, 1999; Moum, 2000; Alstead, 2002). IBD can also present initially during pregnancy, possibly more often in ulcerative colitis than in Crohn disease (Hanan and Kirsner, 1986; Hanan, 1998). Along with exacerbations of already established IBD, such initial presentations are more likely early in gestation, primarily during the first trimester (Nielson et al., 1983; Korelitz, 1985). Contrary to prior reports (Banks et al., 1957), IBD initially presenting during pregnancy does not seem to run a more severe course than disease presenting at any other time (Subhani and Hamilton, 1998).

The postpartum period at one time was thought to be a particularly high-risk time for exacerbation of previously quiescent IBD or for onset of new disease; this does not now appear to be the case (Willoughby and Truelove, 1980; Mogadam, Korelitz, et al., 1981; Korelitz, 1982; Jospe and Peppercorn, 1999). The degree of activity at term is probably what would be expected during the postpartum period. The anatomic distribution of Crohn disease has been speculated to be important, with small bowel disease patients more likely to do well than patients with colitis, but this remains controversial (Fagan, 1989).

Whereas pregnancy may or may not affect IBD or vice versa, it does seem clear that active IBD and pregnancy together, although not a common occurrence, can be problematic from an evaluation as well as from a management standpoint. Complaints of diarrhea (particularly with bleeding) and abdominal pain should at least alert one to the possibility of IBD. Constitutional symptoms of fever, anorexia, and anemia also can occur. Pregnancy per se, particularly in the first trimester, may be accompanied by some of these complaints, and suspicion of underlying IBD would not be as great as it might be in other clinical situations.

As a process involving primarily mucosa and always involving at least the distal colon (if not the more proximal large bowel), ulcerative colitis can more quickly be recognized and diagnosis can more easily be attained via proctoscopy. At least some rectal bleeding almost always occurs, and the change in bowel habit toward diarrhea varies with the extent of colonic involvement. Because it spares the rectum in many patients and may involve the small as well as the large intestine, Crohn disease may be more difficult to diagnose. As noted earlier, *de novo* occurrence of these disorders during pregnancy is not common, so this dilemma is unusual (Singer and Brandt, 1991; Hanan, 1998). In the patient with known disease, one's index of suspicion is necessarily heightened already. The feasibility of various diagnostic modalities, which can certainly come into play with these disorders, is discussed later in this chapter.

Pharmacologic management of IBD is a topic that in the past has been controversial; more recent experience and published reports suggest the more uniform conclusion that most drugs useful in managing IBD in nonpregnant women are also useful and, more importantly, safe in pregnant women, although there are exceptions (Hanan and Kirsner, 1986; Singer and Brandt, 1991; Connell, 1996). Generally, drug administration has already been initiated, and the decision required is not so much whether to start medication as whether to discontinue the drug or alter the dosage. As noted previously, disease that is quiescent in women who become pregnant more often than not remains quiescent, but in many cases, particularly with ulcerative colitis, this quiescence or remission is medication-dependent. In the unusual situation in which IBD begins during pregnancy, one must be confident in the ability of early use of these agents to control the disease.

Over time, the major agents in the management of IBD have been corticosteroids (particularly prednisone) and sulfasalazine (see Table 52-4). The latter is a particularly interesting agent in that the active moiety, 5-amino salicylate (5-ASA, mesalamine), works locally within the colonic lumen, but only because its absorption in the small intestine following oral ingestion is largely prevented by its coupling with sulfapyridine. It is the colonic bacteria that break the bond, releasing the salicylate, which exerts an anti-inflammatory effect through inhibition of both the cyclooxygenase and lipoxygenase pathways of arachidonic acid metabolism (Stenson, 1995).

Sulfapyridine has no active role in treating IBD, serving only as a vehicle for transport of 5-ASA; it is, however, absorbed in the colon and is responsible for both the orange color of the urine noted by many patients and the adverse reactions—notably headache and hypersensitivity—that can occur during sulfasalazine therapy. Sulfapyridine can also cross the placenta and appears in breast milk in small concentrations, raising concern about the potential to displace unconjugated bilirubin from albumin and cause kernicterus in the breast-fed newborn. Outcome studies, however, have shown no increase in neonatal jaundice in women taking sulfasalazine (Willoughby and Truelove, 1980; Mogadam, Dobbins, et al., 1981; Nielson et al., 1983; Nielson et al., 1984). Moreover, the drug is safe during pregnancy, with no evidence of adverse effect on mother or fetus (Willoughby and Truelove, 1980; Mogadam, Dobbins, et al., 1981; Nielson et al., 1983). There should be no hesitation, therefore, in using sulfasalazine during pregnancy.

Folic acid supplements, a mainstay of nutritional management of pregnancy, are of particular importance for pregnant women who are taking sulfasalazine, which can inhibit absorption and metabolism of folate; such supplements should be prescribed for these patients. An increase in neural tube defects as well as other congenital defects can occur with the use of folate antagonists. There has been no evidence directly linking sulfasalazine to these congenital defects, but in view of this study, folate supplementation should be prescribed and emphasized (Hernandez-Diaz et al., 2000; Alstead, 2002).

In the 1990s, newer formulations of 5-ASA were developed that lack the sulfapyridine moiety, with a hoped-for reduction in adverse reactions. With these agents, delivery of 5-ASA to the distal small intestine and colon is accomplished through either a pH-dependent or a diffusion-dependent release system. Another agent (olsalazine) uses a 5-ASA dimer with an azo bond that can be cleaved only by bacterial enzymes in the colon. The newest 5-ASA is balsalazide, a prodrug that is also converted to its active form by colonic bacteria. Small amounts of 5-ASA are absorbed systemically through both placental transfer and excretion in breast milk. Although published experience to date has been limited, the use of these newer agents during pregnancy does not appear to be associated with adverse effects (Habal et al., 1993; Christensen et al., 1994; Diav-Citrin et al., 1998; Alstead, 2002). This is expected, given the favorable experience with sulfasalazine, and in conventional doses, it appears likely that these agents can be used safely during pregnancy. It must be noted, however, that the majority of patients in these studies were on low-dose 5-ASA (less than 2.4 gm mesalamine). There have been reports of interstitial nephritis in newborns of mothers on high-dose mesalamine; therefore, in scenarios where higher doses are required, caution should be exercised, or it may be more appropriate to use steroids in those situations (Diav-Citrin et al., 1998; Alstead, 2002).

Similar conclusions have been drawn regarding the use of prednisone, which is rapidly metabolized to prednisolone in the maternal liver and does not cross the placenta in significant amounts (Singer and Brandt, 1991). The experience with prednisone is greater than that with sulfasalazine because of its use in other disorders besides IBD. Comparative studies of women taking and not taking prednisone have not shown any detrimental effect on either maternal or fetal outcome (DeDombal et al., 1972; Mogadam, Dobbins, et al., 1981; Khosla et al., 1984). Supplemental corticosteroids are advisable during labor and delivery, however, and the neonate should be observed for signs of adrenal insufficiency even though this is unlikely (Connell, 1996; Subhani and Hamilton, 1998; Jospe and Peppercorn, 1999).

Budesonide is a new glucocorticoid that is used in the induction of remission in Crohn disease involving the terminal ileum and right colon. It is delivered in a time-release formulation and exerts its anti-inflammatory effect topically. Although well absorbed, it has low systemic activity because of extensive first-pass metabolism in the liver, with fewer side effects compared to conventional steroids. While theoretically safe, data relevant to use during pregnancy are lacking.

Immunosuppressive therapy with azathioprine or 6-mercaptopurine, sometimes useful in IBD, has been reported to be safe when used during pregnancy (Miller, 1986; Alstead et al., 1990; Connell, 1996; Hanan, 1998; Alstead, 2002) despite theoretical concerns with agents of this type. Experience is limited, however, and largely derived from reports in renal transplant patients. There can be an increased frequency of intrauterine growth retardation and prematurity; fetal risk, however, is low. If the immunosuppressive agent has been used effectively to keep the disease in remission in a given patient, there appears to be justification for continuing it throughout the pregnancy (Connell, 1996). Clearly, this is a situation in which the patient should participate in the decisionmaking process, weighing the possible risks of drug toxicity to the fetus against the risks of a flare-up of the disease process and its inherit risks to the fetus. Mothers on immunosuppressive agents should be advised not to breast feed because of the unknown effects on the newborn (Jospe and Peppercorn, 1999; Moum, 2000).

Other agents used occasionally—such as metronidazole and, more recently, novel therapy with methotrexate or cyclosporine—should probably not be used in the absence of well-documented safety and indications (Peppercorn, 1990; Connell, 1996). Cyclosporine, a potent immunosuppressive in managing organ transplantation, has recently become another effective treatment option in managing severe colitis (Lichtiger et al., 1994). Its use in pregnancy is still controversial because of its side-effect profile; however, it has not been associated with adverse risks to the fetus (Radomski et al., 1995; Bermas et al., 1995). Currently, its use should be limited to those patients with fulminant colitis not responding to steroids, in order to avoid a colectomy that would pose an overwhelming risk to the fetus. Methotrexate is used occasionally in patients with Crohn disease; however, its use in pregnancy is contraindicated because of its documented teratogenicity (Donnenfield et al., 1994). Total parenteral nutrition, although not primary therapy for IBD, is nonetheless a potentially useful adjunct in some patients, particularly those with Crohn disease and associated nutritional deficiencies. Experience is limited, but there are increasing numbers of reports of successful use during pregnancy (Lang et al., 1987; Watson et al., 1990; Amato and Quercia, 1991).

Infliximab is a new chimeric mouse human monoclonal antibody directed against tumor necrosis factor alpha, a key proinflammatory cytokine in inflammatory bowel disease. It is used primarily to treat refractory and/or fistulizing Crohn disease. It is not currently used in pregnant patients or those who are breast feeding. The only currently available data on its use in pregnancy is a postmarketing survey, which identified 35 patients exposed to infliximab in whom pregnancy outcome information was available. 74% of these pregnancies ended in live births, 5% in miscarriages, and 4% in therapeutic terminations, suggesting that pregnant women exposed to infliximab had outcomes no different from those of healthy women. Further data, however, is required before a final determination on the role of infliximab during pregnancy can be made (Katz et al., 2001).

Assuming the delivery of a healthy infant in a woman with IBD, the question often remains as to the child's risk for subsequent development of the disease during his or her lifetime. This question is often posed by parents in family planning. The risk is unequivocally increased by virtue of having a parent with IBD but is difficult to quantify because it is the susceptibility to the disease that is likely inherited rather than the disease itself. The best estimates indicate a lifetime risk of less than 10%; Jews are more predisposed than non-Jews (Yang et al., 1993).

Appendicitis

Acute appendicitis is thought to be the most common nonobstetric cause of acute abdominal pain leading to exploratory laparotomy in pregnancy (Al-Mulhim, 1996; Firstenberg and Malangoni, 1998; Mourad et al., 2000; Castro et al., 2001), even though it may be less common in this setting than in the general population (Andersson and Lambe, 2001). The incidence of proven appendicitis approximates one in 1500 deliveries (Mazze and Kallen, 1991; Al-Mulhim, 1996; Firstenberg and Malangoni, 1998; Mourad et al., 2000; Castro et al., 2001) and can occur in any trimester as well as in the postpartum period, with a slight predominance in the second trimester (Al-Mulhim, 1996; Hee and Viktrup, 1999; Andersen and Nielsen, 1999; Mourad et al., 2000).

Maternal and fetal mortality and morbidity are increased when appendicitis is associated with pregnancy, and the risks rise significantly if perforation and peritonitis occur (Cunningham and McCubbin, 1975; Horowitz et al., 1985; Al-Mulhim, 1996; Firstenberg and Malangoni, 1998). Although maternal mortality is extremely rare (Al-Mulhim, 1996; Hee and Viktrup, 1999), fetal loss is between 10% and 20% in most reports and is due mainly to preterm labor or intrauterine demise, particularly if perforation has occurred. Preterm labor associated with acute appendicitis usually occurs within 5 days of surgery (Al-Mulhim, 1996). The preterm labor is thought to be due to the infectious process but could be secondary to the surgical process itself. As Babler (1908) stated almost a century ago, "the mortality of appendicitis is the mortality of delay."

As pregnancy progresses, the diagnosis of appendicitis becomes more difficult and is mainly a clinical one. Cunningham and McCubbin (1975) noted no delays in diagnosis in the first trimester, in contrast to delays occurring in 18% in the second trimester and 75% in the third trimester. This delay in diagnosis is reflected in the increased maternal and fetal mortality with advanced gestation because of a higher incidence of complications, such as perforation with generalized peritonitis

(Firstenberg and Malangoni, 1998; Hoshino et. al., 2000). Pain, frequently vague and diffuse, is usually present on the right side of the abdomen. The cecum and appendix have been reported to be displaced upward and laterally as pregnancy progresses (Baer et al., 1932), but the frequency of this clinical dictum needs to be reevaluated with modern technology. A recent study was unable to validate the long-held belief that patients presenting with appendicitis in the third trimester had right upper quadrant pain resulting from the appendiceal migration upwards from the gravid uterus. In fact, right lower quadrant pain was by far the most common presentation in all three trimesters (Mourad et al., 2000). Other reports have arrived at similar conclusions (Al-Mulhim, 1996; Andersen and Nielsen, 1999). Although the appendix can be found near its usual location, the gravid uterus displaces the anterior peritoneum, and this can lead to vague symptoms of a nonlocalizing nature. Nausea is frequently present but is difficult to evaluate in the first trimester. Anorexia is less common, as are diarrhea and urinary symptoms (Cunningham and McCubbin, 1975).

Vital signs are frequently normal, and fever is usually low-grade or absent. Direct abdominal tenderness is variable as well. Rebound tenderness, along with rectal tenderness, are highly suggestive of appendicitis; these signs become less frequent as pregnancy progresses. Laboratory findings are usually of little help in the diagnosis. The leukocytosis of pregnancy diminishes the value of a white blood cell count, but a left shift in the white cell count differential may be helpful in distinguishing those patients with appendicitis from those with a normal appendix (Al-Mulhim, 1996; Firstenberg and Malangoni, 1998). Pyuria and hematuria, suggestive of urinary tract disease, can occur in as many as one-fourth of patients with appendicitis in pregnancy (Weingold, 1983). Graded-compression ultrasonography, although useful in nonpregnant patients (Puylaert et al., 1987), has been used in only a few pregnant patients with appendicitis (Barloon et al., 1995). Favorable but limited experience with helical computed tomography as a diagnostic aid in pregnant patients with suspected acute appendicitis has been reported (Castro et al., 2001).

The differential diagnosis of acute appendicitis in pregnancy includes pyelonephritis, cholecystitis, renal or ureteral calculi, adnexal torsion, degenerating myoma, extrauterine pregnancy, and placental abruption.

Treatment of appendicitis in pregnancy is appendectomy, with care taken to avoid maternal hypotension and hypoxemia. Most authorities advise that the incision, generally a muscle-splitting type, be made over the point of maximal tenderness. Appendectomy must be done immediately once appendicitis is diagnosed. The only situation in which appendectomy may be delayed is if the patient is in active labor. If labor becomes prolonged or if appendiceal perforation is suspected, then an immediate cesarean section followed by an appendectomy is indicated (Firstenberg and Malangoni, 1998).

The routine use of antibiotics is controversial, but these agents should be administered if a phlegmon, perforation, abscess, or significant peritonitis is found. If antibiotics are given for appendicitis, then a second-generation cephalosporin with anaerobic coverage or broad-spectrum penicillin with anaerobic coverage should be given (Firstenberg and Malangoni, 1998). Postoperatively, the patient should be observed closely for preterm labor. Any benefit from prophylactic use of tocolytic agents is unknown (Hee and Viktrup, 1999).

Laparoscopic surgery, once thought to be contraindicated during pregnancy, has been reported with increasing frequency

in recent years, with no negative impact on fetal or maternal outcome, although special precautions are advised (Lemaire and van Erp, 1997) Cholecystectomy and appendectomy are the most common procedures reported and have the advantage of decreasing hospitalization time, reducing narcotic use, and bringing about a quicker return to the regular diet. There is also the theoretical advantage of decreased uterine manipulation with perhaps a decreased risk of preterm labor. One report suggests a potential benefit of laparoscopy as a diagnostic tool that may enable an earlier diagnosis of appendicitis (Gurbuz and Peetz, 1997). Two recent studies showed the safety of laparoscopic appendectomy in all three trimesters when compared with open appendectomy; there was no increased risk of preterm delivery or adverse outcomes (Affleck et al., 1999; Lyass et al., 2001).

OTHER GASTROINTESTINAL DISORDERS

Constipation

As noted previously, there is no strong information to support the occurrence of constipation as a pregnancy-related problem, and indeed the issue is not a crucial one. Constipation is common in the general population, and it is not surprising that it occurs during pregnancy with some frequency.

Diagnostic studies as to cause are seldom required, and empirical management is appropriate in most cases. As in the nonpregnant patient, attention to adequate dietary fiber along with increasing oral fluid intake is fundamental to management. Although inadequate fiber cannot be implicated as a cause of constipation occurring during pregnancy (Anderson, 1986), fiber supplements have been effective in increasing frequency of bowel movements and producing a softer stool consistency (Anderson and Whichelow, 1985; Jewell and Young, 2001). One source of supplemental fiber takes the form of psyllium preparations; if necessary, judicious use of an osmotic laxative, such as milk of magnesia (magnesium hydroxide), which mobilizes fluid within the gut lumen, may be considered. Experience with senna preparations during pregnancy has been favorable, and intermittent use is probably safe and effective (Biggs and Vesey, 1980). Likewise, lactulose, which exerts its effect in the colonic lumen, is an acceptable alternative (Muller and Jaquenoud, 1995). Castor oil and mineral oil should be avoided during pregnancy because of potential adverse maternal and fetal effects (Lewis and Weingold, 1985).

Colonic Ileus

There have also been reports of more dramatic problems involving the colon during pregnancy or the early postpartum period. One of these is colonic ileus which, in effect, is colonic pseudo-obstruction (Slemmons and Williams, 1938; Charles and Stronge, 1972; Moore et al., 1986). In nonpregnant settings, this condition has also been called *Ogilvie's syndrome* and clinically manifests as an acutely dilated, gas-filled colon in the absence of distal obstruction (Nanni et al., 1982). Although uncommon in association with pregnancy, it is most likely to occur over a 2- to 3-day period following either cesarean section or vaginal delivery (Sharp, 1994; Mayer and Hussain, 1998). Case reports of adynamic colonic ileus occurring during pregnancy have also been published, however (Rieger et al.,

1996; Pecha and Danilewitz, 1996). Abdominal distention can be striking in the already protuberant gravid abdomen, and pain, nausea, vomiting, and obstipation can occur.

A problem of this type adds additional support to the concept that gut motility is inhibited during pregnancy. Although the gestational metabolic and hormonal environment may predispose to ileus, ileus can also occur during pregnancy under other circumstances—for example, it is a recognized complication of tocolytic therapy for premature labor using magnesium sulfate (Hill et al., 1985; Dudley et al., 1989), especially if used in combination with nifedipine (Pecha et al., 1996). Patients should initially be managed conservatively with correction of any contributing factors, such as electrolyte abnormalities. Any anticholinergic or opiate medications should be discontinued if possible. Failure to respond to conservative measures after 48–72 hours, or a cecal diameter greater than 12 cm at any time, is an indication for decompression (Rieger et al., 1996; Luckas and Buckett, 1997). Colonoscopic decompression may be feasible and successful in selected patients with these disorders, however, and it appears to be safe in pregnancy and the postpartum period (Moore et al., 1986) (see the discussion under Gastrointestinal Endoscopy later in this chapter). Any clinical signs of perforation prior to colonoscopy or signs of colonic ischemia during colonoscopy, however, should be an indication for emergent laparotomy. Neostigmine has been used as a parasympathomimetic to decompress acute colonic pseudoobstruction, with excellent immediate results, but experience during pregnancy is lacking (Ponec et al., 1999). A similar clinical presentation could occur with volvulus. Both cecal and sigmoid volvulus have been reported in pregnancy and could require colonoscopy and/or surgery for management (John et al., 1996; Lord et al., 1996; Montes and Wolf, 1999).

Miscellaneous Conditions (Inflammation, Carcinoma, Obstruction, and Infection)

Pancreatitis and biliary disease during pregnancy are discussed in Chapter 53. The pregnant patient is not protected from other gastrointestinal disorders. For example, there are case reports of carcinoma of the stomach (Davis and Chen, 1991; Sommerville et al., 1991), carcinoma of the colon (Nesbitt et al., 1985; Shushan et al., 1992; Shioda et al., 1994), intestinal obstruction (Connolly et al., 1995; Meyerson et al., 1995), celiac sprue (Ogborn, 1975; Molteni et al., 1990), giardiasis (Kreutner et al., 1981), and amebiasis (Wig et al., 1984), which can occur during pregnancy. Undoubtedly, other conditions have been seen as well, and all present unique problems in evaluation and management that must be considered case by case.

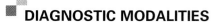

DIAGNOSTIC MODALITIES

Imaging Studies

Experience with imaging techniques—including barium contrast studies and computed tomography (CT)—in the diagnosis and management of gastrointestinal problems in pregnancy is limited, primarily because of the potential adverse effects of ionizing radiation on the fetus (American Academy of Pediatrics, 1978; Brent, 1989). Such studies have undoubtedly been carried out inadvertently in the first trimester, but

their impact is difficult to quantify. Nonetheless, although brief radiation exposure may be harmless in many cases, there is a defined risk, and the decision to use this modality must be made judiciously (Wyte, 1994). In many maternal conditions, the need to use conventional radiographic methods could be small because of (depending on the problem) the response to empirical therapy, the self-limited nature of the problem, and the ease and safety of gastrointestinal endoscopy in diagnosis and treatment of the occasional patient with a difficult clinical dilemma.

In contrast with diagnostic methods that use ionizing radiation, ultrasonography appears to pose no risk to mother or fetus during pregnancy (Wyte, 1994); however, its application to the hollow viscus disorders discussed in this chapter is limited. Ultrasonography has its major use in pancreatic and hepatobiliary disease. The use of magnetic resonance imaging (MRI) during pregnancy is increasing and appears to be safe (Wyte, 1994; Shoenut et al., 1993), although caution is still advisable, especially during the first trimester because of limited experience with MRI during organogenesis.

Gastrointestinal Endoscopy

The major indications for gastrointestinal endoscopy, as outlined by the American Society for Gastrointestinal Endoscopy (2000), are listed in Table 52-5. These indications would also apply to the pregnant woman insofar as timely conduction of the procedure affects the care of the patient. A situation calling for endoscopy is usually one in which empirical management was without benefit or in which the urgency of the situation warrants prompt intervention. An example of the latter is gastrointestinal hemorrhage. On the other hand, elective endoscopy, particularly for issues unrelated to pregnancy (e.g., surveillance for colon cancer in a high-risk patient), usually can be deferred until after delivery.

There are several reasons why endoscopy, as both a diagnostic and a therapeutic tool, could be particularly well suited to and valuable in pregnancy. Radiographic imaging is

TABLE 52-5. MAJOR INDICATIONS FOR GASTROINTESTINAL ENDOSCOPY IN A GENERAL POPULATION

Esophagogastroduodenoscopy (EGD)

Persistent upper abdominal distress or gastroesophageal reflux
Upper abdominal distress associated with symptoms/signs of serious organic disease
Dysphagia or odynophagia
Gastrointestinal bleeding
Unexplained or persistent vomiting
Concomitant disease in which the presence of upper gastrointestinal pathology might have impact on management

Colonoscopy

Gastrointestinal bleeding suggestive of colorectal origin
Unexplained iron deficiency anemia
Surveillance of colorectal neoplasia
Evaluation of suspected or known inflammatory bowel disease
Clinically significant, unexplained diarrhea

Modified and adapted from American Society for Gastrointestinal Endoscopy: Consensus statement: Appropriate use of gastrointestinal endoscopy. Gastrointest Endosc **52**:831, 2000. Copyright © by The American Society for Gastrointestinal Endoscopy.

relatively contraindicated during pregnancy because of fetal radiation exposure. Depending on the agent, prescribing medications without a definitive diagnosis could be problematic if the proposed medication has the potential for fetal harm. Finally, to control active gastrointestinal bleeding, endoscopy offers a relatively safe therapeutic alternative to surgery, which is associated with a high risk of fetal death (Cappell, 1998).

Concerns regarding the safety of gastrointestinal endoscopy are twofold:

1. Effects of medication given during the procedure, as premedication is often used for endoscopic procedures
2. Effects of the manipulation of the endoscope per se, if any

Little information has been published regarding either of these issues (particularly the latter) apart from case reports of unusual gastrointestinal problems that occurred during pregnancy. In many of these reports, gastrointestinal endoscopy was used in the care of the patient, and no ill effects occurred (Moore et al., 1986; Hirabayashi et al., 1987; Davis and Chen, 1991; Sommerville et al., 1991).

A survey of the membership of the American Society for Gastrointestinal Endoscopy resulted in a report of experience in 110 endoscopic procedures (Rustgi et al., 1986). These procedures were distributed among upper gastrointestinal endoscopy (73), flexible sigmoidoscopy and colonoscopy (26), and rigid proctosigmoidoscopy (11). No complications or ill effects were reported. More than 50% of the patients received premedication—usually meperidine, diazepam, or a combination—without apparent difficulty. Fetal outcome was not specifically looked at in the survey, but one spontaneous abortion was noted at 14 weeks' gestation (4 weeks after the procedure), and one premature delivery was noted at 8 months' gestation in a patient who had undergone esophagogastroduodenoscopy at 3 weeks' gestation. The authors concluded that gastrointestinal endoscopy was safe when performed during pregnancy and in some cases may be the procedure of choice given the limitations imposed by radiation risks plus accuracy of diagnosis.

A more recent report of upper gastrointestinal endoscopy in 83 pregnant women reported a similarly favorable experience (Cappell et al., 1996a). Indications were equally divided between acute gastrointestinal bleeding and abdominal pain, vomiting, or both. Diagnostic accuracy was high, particularly in the bleeding patients, in whom the procedure also offered an opportunity for hemostatic therapy. There was no induction of labor, and there were no adverse effects on fetal outcome. The various studies looking at the role of upper gastrointestinal endoscopy during pregnancy suggests that in upper gastrointestinal bleeding, the benefits of the procedure outweigh the risks. Therefore, when patients present with melena or hematemesis with hemodynamic instability or requirement for blood transfusion, upper gastrointestinal endoscopy is generally recommended. On the other hand, for patients presenting with nausea, vomiting, or abdominal pain, the yield of upper gastrointestinal endoscopy is low. In this setting, endoscopy is generally not necessary unless the symptoms are severe and refractory to medical therapy or accompanied by bleeding (Cappell, 1998).

A report from the same institution describing experience with flexible sigmoidoscopy (48 cases) and colonoscopy (8 cases) drew similar conclusions (Cappell et al., 1996b). Because of the lack of sufficient data regarding safety of colonoscopy during pregnancy, however, this procedure should be considered only in uncontrolled colonic bleeding when the only alternative is surgery, and in cases of suspected colon cancer (Cappell, 1998).

Although its primary application is in pancreaticobiliary disease, endoscopic retrograde cholangiopancreatography (ERCP) can be performed safely during pregnancy if special precautions are taken (Baillie et al., 1990; Hoffman and Cunningham, 1992; Jamidar et al., 1995; Cappell, 1998). The most common clinical circumstance, often also requiring endoscopic sphincterotomy, is the patient with choledocholithiasis, with or without associated pancreatitis.

There have been rare case reports describing placement of percutaneous endoscopic gastrostomy (PEG) tubes for nutritional support during pregnancy in patients with severe malnutrition endangering the well being of the mother and fetus. PEG tubes can be considered when enteral support is desired and nasogastric and nasoduodenal tubes are not tolerated; however, efficacy and safety data are too limited to permit conclusions (Shaheen et al., 1997).

Careful and judicious use of endoscopy can have an important role in the management of selected pregnant patients in whom prompt diagnosis is deemed necessary for successful management.

SUMMARY

Pregnancy is a unique metabolic and hormonal state with effects on many body systems, not the least of which is the gastrointestinal tract. Many symptoms and complaints result from these changes. Similarly, patients with chronic gastrointestinal disorders can experience changes in symptoms or may experience problems for which diagnosis and management can be a challenge. Careful selection of diagnostic and therapeutic options can result in successful outcomes for both mother and fetus.

REFERENCES

Abell TL, Riely CA: Hyperemesis gravidarum. Gastroenterol Clin North Am **21**:835, 1992.

Affleck DG, Handrahan DL, Egger MJ, et al: The laparoscopic management of appendicitis and cholelithiasis during pregnancy. Am J Surg **178**:523, 1999.

Al-Mulhim AA: Acute appendicitis in pregnancy. A review of 52 cases. Int Surg **81**:295, 1996.

Alstead EM: Inflammatory bowel disease in pregnancy. Postgrad Med J, **78**:23, 2002.

Alstead EM, Ritchie JK, Lennard-Jones JE, et al: Safety of azathioprine in pregnancy in inflammatory bowel disease. Gastroenterology **99**:443, 1990.

Amato P, Quercia RA: A historical perspective and review of the safety of lipid emulsion in pregnancy. Nutr Clin Pract **6**:189, 1991.

American Academy of Pediatrics Committee on Radiology: Radiation of pregnant women. Pediatrics **61**:117, 1978.

American Society for Gastrointestinal Endoscopy: Consensus statement: Appropriate use of gastrointestinal endoscopy: Gastrointest Endosc **52**:831, 2000.

Anderson AS: Dietary factors in the aetiology and treatment of constipation during pregnancy. Br J Obstet Gynaecol **93**:245, 1986.

Anderson AS, Whichelow MJ: Constipation during pregnancy: Dietary fibre intake and the effect of fibre supplementation. Hum Nutr Appl Nutr **39**:202, 1985.

Andersen B, Nielsen TF: Appendicitis in pregnancy: Diagnosis, management and complications. Acta Obstet Gynecol Scand **78**:758, 1999.

Andersson RE, Lambe M: Incidence of appendicitis during pregnancy. Int J Epidemiol **30**:1281, 2001.

Andrews P, Whitehead S: Pregnancy sickness. NIPS **5**:5, 1990.

Ashorn M, Miettinen A, Ruuska T, et al: Seroepidemiological study of *Helicobacter pylori* infection in infancy. Arch Dis Child Fetal Neonatal Ed **74**:F141, 1996.

Aston NO, Kalaichandran S, Carr JV: Duodenal ulcer hemorrhage in the puerperium. Can J Surg **34**:482, 1991.

Babler EA: Perforative appendicitis complicating pregnancy. JAMA **51**:1310, 1908.

Baer JL, Reis RA, Artens RA: Appendicitis in pregnancy with changes in position and axis of the normal appendix in pregnancy. JAMA **98**:1359, 1932.

Baillie J, Carins SR, Putnam WS, et al: Endoscopic management of choledocholithiasis during pregnancy. Surg Gynecol Obstet **171**:1, 1990.

Baird DD, Narendranathan M, Sandler RS: Increased risk of preterm birth for women with inflammatory bowel disease. Gastroenterology **99**:987, 1990.

Baird RM: Peptic ulcer in pregnancy: Report of a case with perforation. Can Med Assoc J **94**:861, 1966.

Banks BM, Korelitz BI, Zetzel L: The course of nonspecific ulcerative colotis: Review of twenty years' experience and late results. Gastroenterology **32**:983, 1957.

Barloon TJ, Brown BP, Abu-Yousef MM, et al: Sonography of acute appendicitis in pregnancy. Abdom Imaging **20**:149, 1995.

Baron TH, Ramirez B, Richter JE: Gastrointestinal motility disorders during pregnancy. Ann Intern Med **118**:366, 1993.

Bashiri A, Neumann L, Maymon E, et al: Hyperemesis gravidarum: Epidemiologic features, complications and outcome. Eur J Obstet Gynecol Reprod Biol **63**:135, 1995.

Bermas BL, Hill JA: Effects of immunosuppressive drugs during pregnancy. Arthritis Rheum **38**:1722, 1995.

Biggs JSG, Vesey EJ: Treatment of gastrointestinal disorders of pregnancy. Drugs **19**:70, 1980.

Blecker U, Lanciers S, Keppens E, et al: Evolution of *Helicobacter pylori* positivity in infants born from positive mothers. J Pediatr Gastroenterol Nutr **19**:87, 1994.

Braverman DZ, Herbet D, Goldstein R, et al: Postpartum restoration of pregnancy-induced cholecystoparesis and prolonged intestinal transit time. J Clin Gastroenterol **10**:642, 1988.

Brent RL: The effect of embryonic and fetal exposure to x-ray, microwaves, and ultrasound: Counseling the pregnant and nonpregnant patient about these risks. Semin Oncol **16**:347, 1989.

Broussard CN, Richter JE: Nausea and vomiting of pregnancy. Gastroenterol Clin North Am **27**:123, 1998.

Brown J, Robertson J, Gallagher N: Humoral regulation of vitamin B_{12} absorption by pregnant mouse small intestine. Gastroenterology **72**:881, 1977.

Burdett K, Reek C: Adaptation of the small intestine during pregnancy and lactation in the rat. Biochem J **184**:245, 1979.

Butt J, Fleshler B: Increase in maternal gut amino acid transport in late gestation in the guinea pig (abstr). J Lab Clin Med **78**:827, 1971.

Cappell MS: The safety and efficacy of gastrointestinal endoscopy during pregnancy. Gastroenterol Clin North Am **27**:37, 1998.

Cappell MS, Colon VJ, Sidhom OA: A study of eight medical centers of the safety and clinical efficacy of esophagogastroduodenoscopy in 83 pregnant females with follow-up of fetal outcome with comparison control groups. Am J Gastroenterol **91**:348, 1996a.

Cappell MS, Colon VJ, Sidhom OA: A study at 10 medical centers of the safety and efficacy of 48 flexible sigmoidoscopies and 8 colonoscopies during pregnancy with follow-up of fetal outcome and with comparison to control groups. Dig Dis Sci **41**:2353, 1996b.

Cappell MS, Garcia A: Gastric and duodenal ulcers during pregnancy. Gastroenterol Clin North Am **27**:169, 1998.

Castro AM, Shipp TD, Castro EE, et al: The use of helical computed tomography in pregnancy for the diagnosis of acute appendicitis. Am J Obstet Gynecol **184**:954, 2001.

Charles D, Stronge J: Special problems of the colon and rectum in obstetric practice. Clin Obstet Gynecol **15**:522, 1972.

Ching MS, Morgan DJ, Mihaly GW, et al: Placental transfer of omeprazole in maternal and fetal sheep. Dev Pharmacol Ther **9**:323, 1986.

Christensen LA, Rasmussen SN, Hansen SH: Disposition of 5-aminosalicylic acid and N-acetyl-5-aminosalicylic acid in fetal and maternal body fluids during treatment with different 5-aminosalicylic acid preparations. Acta Obstet Gynecol Scand **73**:399, 1994.

Cipriani S, Conti R, Vella G: Ranitidine in pregnancy: Three case reports. Clin Eur **22**:1, 1983.

Clark DH: Peptic ulcer in women. Br Med J **1**:1254, 1953.

Colin-Jones DG, Langman MJS, Lawson DH, et al: Post-marketing surveillance of the safety of cimetidine: 12-month morbidity report. Q J Med **54**:253, 1985.

Colman RD, Frank M, Loughnan BA, et al: Use of intramuscular ranitidine for the prophylaxis of aspiration pneumonitis in obstetrics. Br J Anaesth **61**:720, 1988.

Connell WR: Safety of drug therapy for inflammatory bowel disease in pregnant and nursing women. Inflamm Bowel Dis **2**:33, 1996.

Connolly MM, Unti JA, Nora PF: Bowel obstruction in pregnancy. Surg Clin North Am **75**:101, 1995.

Cripps AW, Williams VJ: The effect of pregnancy and lactation on food intake, gastrointestinal anatomy and the absorptive capacity of the small intestine in the albino rat. Br J Nutr **33**:17, 1975.

Crohn BB, Yarnis H, Korelitz BI: Regional ileitis complicating pregnancy. Gastroenterology **31**:615, 1956.

Cunningham FG, McCubbin JH: Appendicitis complicating pregnancy. Obstet Gynecol **45**:415, 1975.

Davis JL, Chen MD: Gastric carcinoma presenting as an exacerbation of ulcers during pregnancy: A case report. J Reprod Med **36**:450, 1991.

Davison JS, Davison MC, Hay DM: Gastric emptying time in late pregnancy and labour. J Obstet Gynaecol Br Commonw **77**:37, 1970.

DeDombal FT, Burton IL, Goligher JC: Crohn's disease and pregnancy. Br Med J **3**:550, 1972.

DeDombal FT, Watts JM, Watkinson G, et al: Ulcerative colitis in pregnancy. Lancet **2**:599, 1965.

Deuchar N: Nausea and vomiting in pregnancy: A review of the problem with particular regard to psychological and social aspects. Br J Obstet Gynaecol **102**:6, 1995.

Diav-Citrin O, Park YH, Veerasuntharam G, et al: The safety of mesalamine in human pregnancy: A prospective controlled cohort study. Gastroenterology **114**:23, 1998.

Dicke JM, Johnson RF, Henderson GI, et al: A comparative evaluation of the transport of H_2-receptor antagonists by the human and baboon placenta. Am J Med Sci **295**:198, 1988.

Dodds WJ, Hogan WJ, Helm JF, et al: Pathogenesis of reflux esophagitis. Gastroenterology **81**:376, 1981.

Doll R, Hill ID, Hutton CF: The treatment of gastric ulcer with carbenoxolone sodium and estrogens. Gut **6**:10, 1965.

Donaldson RM: Management of medical problems in pregnancy: Inflammatory bowel disease. N Engl J Med **312**:1616, 1985.

Donnenfield AE, Pastuszak A, Noah JS, et al: Methotrexate exposure prior to and during pregnancy. Teratology **49**:79, 1994.

Dowling RH: Small bowel adaptation and its regulation. Scand J Gastroenterol **17**(Suppl 74):53, 1982.

Dudley D, Gagnon D, Varner M: Long-term tocolysis with intravenous magnesium sulfate. Obstet Gynecol **73**:373, 1989.

Dugas MC, Hazlewood RC, Lawrence AL: Influence of pregnancy and/or exercise on intestinal transport of amino acids in rats. Proc Soc Exp Biol Med **135**:127, 1970.

El Younis CM, Abulafia O, Sherer DM: Rapid marked response of sever hyperemesis gravidarum to oral erythromycin. Am J Perinatol **15**:533, 1998.

Elias E, Dowling RH: The mechanism for small bowel adaptation in lactating rats. Clin Sci Mol Med **51**:427, 1976.

Erdem A, Arslan M, Erdem M, et al: Detection of *Helicobacter pylori* seropositivity in hyperemesis gravidarum and correlation with symptoms. Am J Perinatol **19**:87, 2002.

Fagan EA: Disorders of the gastrointestinal tract. In de Swiet M (ed): Medical Disorders in Obstetric Practice. 2nd ed. Oxford, Blackwell Scientific Publications, 1989, p. 521.

Fedarkow DM, Persaud D, Nimrod CA: Inflammatory bowel disease: A controlled study of late pregnancy outcome. Am J Obstet Gynecol **160**:98, 1989.

Firstenberg MS, Malangoni MA: Gastrointestinal surgery during pregnancy. Gastroenterol Clin North Am **27**:73, 1998.

Fisher RS, Roberts GS, Grabowski CJ, et al: Altered lower esophageal sphincter function during early pregnancy. Gastroenterology **74**:1233, 1978.

Fonager K, Sorensen HT, Olsen J, et al: Pregnancy outcome for women with Crohn's disease: A follow-up study based on linkage between national registries. Am J Gastroenterol **93**:2426, 1998.

Francella A, Dayan A, Rubin P, et al: 6-mercaptopurine (6-MP) is safe therapy for child bearing patients with inflammatory bowel disease (IBD): A case controlled study. Gastroenterology **110**:A909, 1996.

Frigo P, Lang C, Reisenberger K, et al: Hyperemesis gravidarum associated with *Helicobacter pylori* seropositivity. Obstet Gynecol **91**:615, 1998.

Gadsby R, Barnie-Adshead AM, Jagger C: A prospective study of nausea and vomiting during pregnancy. Br J Gen Pract **43**:245, 1993.

Gill RC, Bowes KL, Kingma YJ: Effect of progesterone on canine colonic smooth muscle. Gastroenterology **88**:1941, 1985.

Goh JT, Flynn MB, Florin TH: Active chronic peptic ulcer disease complicated by gastric outlet obstruction in pregnancy. Aust N Z J Obstet Gynecol **33**:89, 1993.

Gryboski WA, Spiro HM: The effect of pregnancy on gastric secretion. N Engl J Med **255**:1131, 1956.

Gurbuz AT, Peetz ME: The acute abdomen in the pregnant patient: Is there a role for laparoscopy? Surg Endosc **11**:98, 1997.

Habal FM, Hui G, Greenberg GR: Oral 5-aminosalicylic acid for inflammatory bowel disease in pregnancy: Safety and clinical course. Gastroenterology **105**:1057, 1993.

Hanan IM: Inflammatory bowel disease in the pregnant woman. Compr Ther **24**:409, 1998.

Hanan IM, Kirsner JB: Inflammatory bowel disease in pregnancy. *In* Rustgi VK, Cooper JN (eds): Gastrointestinal and Hepatic Complications in Pregnancy. New York, John Wiley and Sons, 1986, p. 69.

Harper MA, McVeigh JE, Thompson W, et al: Successful pregnancy in association with Zollinger-Ellison syndrome. Am J Obstet Gynecol **173**:863, 1995.

Hee P, Viktrup L: The diagnosis of appendicitis during pregnancy and maternal and fetal outcome after appendectomy. Int J Gynaecol Obstet **65**:129, 1999.

Hernandez-Diaz S, Werler MM, Walker AM, et al: Folic acid antagonists during pregnancy and the risk of birth defects. N Engl J Med **343**:1608, 2000.

Hewson EG, Sinclair JW, Dalton CB, et al: Twenty-four-hour esophageal pH monitoring: The most useful test for evaluating non-cardiac chest pain. Am J Med **90**:576, 1991.

Hill JA, Clark A, Scott NA: Surgical treatment of acute manifestations of Crohn's disease during pregnancy. J R Soc Med **90**:64, 1997.

Hill WC, Gill PJ, Katz M: Maternal paralytic ileus as a complication of magnesium sulfate tocolysis. Am J Perinatol **2**:47, 1985.

Hirabayashi M, Veo H, Okudaira Y, et al: Early gastric cancer and a concomitant pregnancy. Am Surg **53**:730, 1987.

Hod M, Orvieto R, Kaplan B, et al: Hyperemesis gravidarum: A review. J Reprod Med **39**:605, 1994.

Hodgkinson R, Glassenberg R, Joyce TH III, et al: Comparison of cimetidine with antacid for safety and effectiveness in reducing gastric acidity before elective caesarean section. Anesthesiology **59**:86, 1983.

Hoffman BJ, Cunningham JT: Radiation exposure to the pregnant patient during ERCP (abstr). Gastrointest Endosc **38**:253, 1992.

Horowitz MD, Gomez GA, Santiesteban R, et al: Acute appendicitis during pregnancy. Arch Surg **120**:1362, 1985.

Hoshino T, Ihara Y, Suzuki T: Appendicitis during pregnancy. Int J Gynaecol Obstet **69**:271, 2000.

Hudson M, Flett G, Sinclair TS, et al: Fertility and pregnancy in inflammatory bowel disease. Int J Gynaecol Obstet **58**:229, 1997.

Hunt JN, Murray FA: Gastric function in pregnancy. J Obstet Gynaecol Br Commomw **65**:78, 1958.

Iwasaki H, Collins JG, Saito Y, et al: Naloxone-sensitive, pregnancy-induced changes in behavioral responses to colorectal distension: Pregnancy-induced analgesia to visceral stimulation. Anesthesiology **74**:927, 1991.

Jacoby EB, Porter KB: *Helicobacter pylori* infection and persistent hyperemesis gravidarum. Am J Perinatol **16**:85, 1999.

Jamidar PA, Beck GJ, Hoffman BJ, et al: Endoscopic retrograde cholangiopancreatography in pregnancy. Am J Gastroenterol **90**:1263, 1995.

Jarnfelt-Samsioe A: Nausea and vomiting in pregnancy: A review. Obstet Gynecol Surg **42**:422, 1987.

Jarnfelt-Samsioe A, Eriksson B, Waldenstrom J: Some new aspects on emesis gravidarum: Relations to clinical data, serum electrolytes, and creatinine. Gynecol Obstet Invest **19**:174, 1985.

Jarnfelt-Samsioe A, Samsioe G, Velinder G: Nausea and vomiting in pregnancy: A contribution to its epidemiology. Gynecol Obstet Invest **16**:221, 1983.

Janssens J, Peeters TL, Vantrappen G, et al: Improvement in gastric emptying in diabetic gastroparesis by erythromycin: Preliminary studies. N Engl J Med **322**:1028, 1990.

Jewell D, Young G: Interventions for nausea and vomiting in early pregnancy. Cochrane Database Syst Rev **(1)**:CD000145, 2001.

John H, Gyr T, Giudici G, et al: Cecal volvulus in pregnancy: Case report and review of literature. Arch Gynecol Obstet **258**:161, 1996.

Jospe ES, Peppercorn MA: Inflammatory bowel disease and pregnancy: a review. Dig Dis **17**:201, 1999.

Kahn K, Greenfield S (for Health and Public Policy Committee, American College of Physicians): Endoscopy in the evaluation of dyspepsia. Ann Intern Med **102**:266, 1985.

Kallen B: Delivery outcome after the use of acid-suppressing drugs in early pregnancy with special reference to omeprazole. Br J Obstet Gynaecol **105**:877, 1998.

Kallen BA: Use of omeprazole during pregnancy—No hazard demonstrated in 955 infants exposed during pregnancy. Eur J Obstet Gynecol Reprod Biol **96**:63, 2001.

Katz JA, Lichtenstein GR, Keenan GF, et al: Outcome of pregnancy in women receiving REMICADE (infliximab) for the treatment of Crohn's disease or rheumatoid arthritis **120**(S1):A-69, 2001.

Katz PO, Castell DO: Gastroesophageal reflux disease during pregnancy. Gastroenterol Clin North Am **27**:153, 1998.

Khosla R, Willoughby CP, Jewell DP: Crohn's disease and pregnancy. Gut **25**:52, 1984.

Kimura M, Amino N, Tamaki H, et al: Gestational thyrotoxicosis and hyperemesis gravidarum: Possible role of hCG with higher stimulating activity. Clin Endocrinol **38**:345, 1993.

Klebanoff MA, Koslowe PA, Kaslow R, et al: Epidemiology of vomiting in early pregnancy. Obstet Gynecol **66**:612, 1985.

Klebanoff MA, Mills JL: Is vomiting during pregnancy teratogenic? Br Med J (Clin Res Ed) **292**:724, 1986.

Koch KL: Approach to the patient with nausea and vomiting. *In* Yamada T (ed): Textbook of Gastroenterology, 2nd ed. Philadelphia, JB Lippincott, 1995, p. 731.

Koch KL, Stern RM, Vasey M, et al: Gastric dysrhythmias and nausea of pregnancy. Dig Dis Sci **35**:961, 1990.

Korelitz BI: Epidemiological and psychosocial aspects of inflammatory bowel disease with observations on children, families, and pregnancy. Am J Gastroenterol **77**:929, 1982.

Korelitz BI: Pregnancy, fertility and inflammatory bowel disease. Am J Gastroenterol **80**:365, 1985.

Korelitz BI: Inflammatory bowel disease in pregnancy. Gastroenterol Clin North Am **21**:827, 1992.

Koren G, Zemlickis DM: Outcome of pregnancy after first-trimester exposure to H₂ receptor antagonists. Am J Perinatol **8**:37, 1991.

Kornfeld D, Cnattingius S, Ekbom A: Pregnancy outcomes in women with inflammatory bowel disease—A population-based cohort study. Am J Obstet Gynecol **177**:942, 1997.

Kreutner AK, Del Bene VE, Amstey MS: Giardiasis in pregnancy. Am J Obstet Gynecol **140**:895, 1981.

Kumar D: In vitro inhibitory effect of progesterone on extrauterine human smooth muscle. Am J Obstet Gynecol **84**:1300, 1962.

La Salvia LA, Steffen EA: Delayed gastric emptying time during labor. Am J Obstet Gynecol **59**:1075, 1950.

Laine L: Rolling review: Upper gastrointestinal bleeding. Aliment Pharmacol Ther **7**:207, 1993.

Lalkin A, Loebstein R, Addis A, et al: The safety of omeprazole during pregnancy: A multicenter prospective controlled study. Am J Obstet Gynecol **179**:727, 1998.

Lang CE, Johnson DJ, Sax HC, et al: Total parenteral nutrition in pregnancy: A case report. J Pediatr Perinat Nutr **1**:61, 1987.

Larson JD, Patatanian E, Miner PB Jr, et al: Double-blind, placebo-controlled study of ranitidine for gastroesophageal reflux symptoms during pregnancy. Obstet Gynecol **90**:83, 1997.

Lawson M, Kern F Jr, Everson GT: Gastrointestinal transit time in human pregnancy, prolongation in the second and third trimesters followed by postpartum normalization. Gastroenterology **89**:996, 1985.

Lemaire BM, van Erp WF: Laparoscopic surgery during pregnancy. Surg Endosc **11**:15, 1997.

Levine MJ, Esser D: Total parenteral nutrition for the treatment of severe hyperemesis gravidarum: Maternal nutritional effects and fetal outcome. Obstet Gynecol **72**:102, 1988.

Levy N, Lemberg L, Sharf M: Bowel habit in pregnancy. Digestion **4**:216, 1971.

Lewis JH, Weingold AB: The use of gastrointestinal drugs during pregnancy and lactation. Am J Gastroenterol **80**:912, 1985.

Lichtiger S, Present DH, Kornbluth A, et al: Cyclosporine in severe ulcerative colitis refractory to steroid therapy. N Engl J Med **330**:1841, 1994.

Lord SA, Boswell WC, Hungerpiller JC: Sigmoid volvulus in pregnancy. Am Surg **62**:380, 1996.

Luckas M, Buckett W: Acute colonic pseudo-obstruction in the obstetric patient. Br J Hosp Med **57**:378, 1997.

Lyass S, Pikarsky A, Eisenbert VH, et al: Is laparoscopic appendectomy safe in pregnant women? Surg Endosc **15**:377, 2001.

Magee LA, Inocencion G, Kamboj L, et al: Safety of first trimester exposure to histamine H₂ blockers: A prospective cohort study. Dig Dis Sci **41**:1145, 1996.

Magee LA, Mazzotta P, Koren G: Evidence-based view of safety and effectiveness of pharmacologic therapy for nausea and vomiting of pregnancy (NVP). Am J Obstet Gynecol **185**:S256, May 2002.

Malagelada JR: Gastric emptying disorders: Clinical significance and treatment. Drugs **24**:353, 1982.

Marrero JM, Goggin PM, et al: Determinants of pregnancy heartburn. Br J Obstet Gynaecol **99**:731, 1992.

Mattox HE, Richter JE: Prolonged ambulatory esophageal pH monitoring in the evaluation of gastroesophageal reflux disease. Am J Med **89**:345, 1990.

Mayer IE, Hussain H: Abdominal pain during pregnancy. Gastroenterol Clin North Am **27**:1, 1998.

Mazze RI, Kallen B. Appendectomy during pregnancy: A Swedish registry study of 778 cases. Obstet Gynecol **77**:835, 1991.

Mazzotta P, Magee LA: A risk-benefit assessment of pharmacological and non-pharmacological treatments for nausea, vomiting of pregnancy. Drugs **59**:781, 2000.

Meyer LC, Peacock JL, Bland JM, et al: Symptoms and health problems in pregnancy: Their association with social factors, smoking, alcohol, caffeine and attitude to pregnancy. Paediatr Perinat Epidemiol **8**:145, 1994.

Meyerson S, Holtz T, Ehrinpreis M, et al: Small bowel obstruction in pregnancy. Am J Gastroenterol **90**:299, 1995.

Michaletz-Onody PA: Peptic ulcer disease in pregnancy. Gastroenterol Clin North Am **21**:817, 1992.

Miller JP: Inflammatory bowel disease in pregnancy: A review. J R Soc Med **79**:221, 1986.

Minami H, McCallum RW: The physiology and pathophysiology of gastric emptying in humans. Gastroenterology **86**:1592, 1984.

Mogadam M, Dobbins WD, Korelitz BI, et al: Pregnancy in inflammatory bowel disease: Effect of sulfasalazine and corticosteroids on fetal outcome. Gastroenterology **80**:72, 1981.

Mogadam M, Korelitz BI, Ahmed SW, et al: The course of inflammatory bowel disease during pregnancy and postpartum. Am J Gastroenterol **75**:265, 1981.

Molteni N, Bardella MT, Bianchi PA: Obstetrical and gynecological problems in women with untreated celiac sprue. J Clin Gastroenterol **12**:37, 1990.

Montes H, Wolf J: Cecal volvulus in pregnancy. Am J Gastroenterol **94**:2554, 1999.

Moore JG, Gladstone NS, Lucas GW, et al: Successful management of post-caesarean section acute pseudo-obstruction of the colon (Ogilvie's syndrome) with colonoscopic decompression: A case report. J Reprod Med **31**:1001, 1986.

Moum B: Chronic inflammatory bowel disease and pregnancy. Scand J Gastroenterol **35**:673, 2000.

Mourad J, Elliott JP, Erickson L, et al: Appendicitis in pregnancy: New information that contradicts long-held clinical beliefs. Am J Obstet Gynecol **182**:1027, 2000.

Muller M, Jaquenoud E: Treatment of constipation in pregnant women: A multicenter study in a gynecological practice. Schweiz Med Wochenschr **125**:1689, 1995.

Murphy PA: Alternative therapies for nausea and vomiting of pregnancy. Obstet Gynecol **91**:149, 1998.

Murray FA, Erskine JP, Fielding J: Gastric secretion in pregnancy. J Obstet Gynaecol Br Commonw **64**:373, 1957.

Naef RW III, Chauhan SP, Roach H, et al: Treatment for hyperemesis gravidarum in the home: An alternative to hospitalization. J Perinatol **15**:289, 1995.

Nagler R, Spiro HM: Heartburn in late pregnancy: Manometric studies of esophageal motor function. J Clin Invest **40**:954, 1961.

Nagler R, Spiro HM: Heartburn in pregnancy. Am J Dig Dis **7**:648, 1962.

Nanni G, Garbini A, Luchetti P, et al: Ogilvie's syndrome (acute colonic pseudo-obstruction): Review of the literature (October 1948 to March 1980) and report of four additional cases. Dis Colon Rectum **25**:157, 1982.

National Institutes of Health: NIH Consensus Development Panel: *Helicobacter pylori* in peptic ulcer disease. JAMA **272**:65, 1994.

Nebel OT, Fornes MF, Castell DO: Symptomatic gastroesophageal reflux: Incidence and precipitating factors. Dig Dis Sci **21**:953, 1976.

Nesbitt JC, Moise KJ, Sawyers JL: Colorectal carcinoma in pregnancy. Arch Surg **120**:636, 985.

Nielson OH, Andreasson B, Bondesen S, et al: Pregnancy in ulcerative colitis. Scand J Gastroenterol **18**:735, 1983.

Nielson OH, Andreasson B, Bondesen S, et al: Pregnancy in Crohn's disease. Scand J Gastroenterol **19**:724, 1984.

Ogborn ADR: Pregnancy in patients with coeliac disease. Br J Obstet Gynaecol **82**:293, 1975.

Olans LB, Wolf JL: Gastroesophageal reflux in pregnancy. Gastrointest Endosc Clin North Am **4**:699, 1994.

Olsen KO, Juul S, Berndtsson I, et al: Ulcerative colitis: Female fecundity before diagnosis, during disease, and after surgery compared with a population sample. Gastroenterology **122**:15, 2002.

Orr DA, Bill KM, Gillon KR, et al: Effects of omeprazole, with and without metoclopramide, in elective obstetric anaesthesia. Anaesthesia **48**:114, 1993.

Ostick DG, Cowley DJ, Hey VM, et al: A study of gastroesophageal reflux in late pregnancy. *In* Vantrappen G (ed): Proceedings of the Fifth International Symposium on Gastrointestinal Motility. Herentals, Belgium, Typoff Press, 1976, p. 358.

O'Sullivan GM, Sutton AJ, Thompson SA, et al: Noninvasive measurement of gastric emptying in obstetric patients. Anesth Analg **66**:505, 1987.

Palmer ED: Upper gastrointestinal hemorrhage during pregnancy. Am J Med Sci **242**:223, 1961.

Parry E, Shields R, Turnbull AC: Transit time in the small intestine in pregnancy. J Obstet Gynaecol Br Commonw **77**:900, 1970a.

Parry E, Shields R, Turnbull AC: The effect of pregnancy on the colonic absorption of sodium, potassium, and water. J Obstet Gynaecol Br Commonw **77**:616, 1970b.

Paul M, Tew WL, Holliday RL: Perforated peptic ulcer in pregnancy with survival of mother and child: Case report and review of the literature. Can J Surg **19**:427, 1976.

Pecha RE, Danilewitz MD: Acute pseudo-obstruction of the colon (Ogilvie's syndrome) resulting from combination tocolytic therapy. Am J Gastroenterol **91**:1265, 1996.

Peppercorn MA: Advances in drug therapy for inflammatory bowel disease. Ann Intern Med **112**:50, 1990.

Peura DA: *Helicobacter pylori* and ulcerogenesis. Am J Med **100**:19S, 1996.

Physicians' Desk Reference. Montvale, NJ, Medical Economics Co, 2002.

Ponec RJ, Saunders MD, Kimmey MB: Neostigmine for the treatment of acute colonic pseudo-obstruction. N Engl J Med **341**:137, 1999.

Pope CE: Acid-reflux disorders. N Engl J Med **331**:656, 1994.

Porter RJ, Stirrat GM: The effects of inflammatory bowel disease on pregnancy: A case-controlled retrospective analysis. Br J Obstet Gynaecol **93**:1124, 1986.

Powell DW: Approach to the patient with diarrhea. *In* Yamada T (ed): Textbook of Gastroenterology. Philadelphia, JB Lippincott, 1991, p. 732.

Prieto RM, Ferrer M, Fe JM, et al: Morphological adaptive changes of small intestinal tract regions due to pregnancy and lactation in rats. Ann Nutr Metab **38**:295, 1994.

Puylaert JBCM, Rutgers PH, Lalisang RI: A prospective study of ultrasound in the diagnosis of appendicitis. N Engl J Med **317**:666, 1987.

Radberg G, Asztely M, Cautor P, et al: Gastric and gallbladder emptying in relation to the secretion of cholecystokinin after a meal in late pregnancy. Digestion **42**:174, 1989.

Radomski JS, Ahlswede BA, Jarrell BE, et al: Outcomes of 500 pregnancies in 335 female kidney, liver, and heart transplant recipients. Transplant Proc **27**:1089, 1995.

Rayburn W, Liles E, Christensen H, et al: Antacids vs. antacids plus non-prescription ranitidine for heartburn during pregnancy. Int J Gynaecol Obstet **66**:35, 1999.

Rieger NA, Lyon WJ, Bryce RL, et al: A case of acute colonic pseudoobstruction in pregnancy. Aust N Z J Obstet Gynaecol **36**:363, 1996.

Riezzo G, Pezzolla F, Darconza G, et al: Gastric myoelectrical activity in the first trimester of pregnancy: A cutaneous electrogastrographic study. Am J Gastroenterol **87**:702, 1992.

Rocke DA, Rout CC, Gouws E: Intravenous administration of the proton pump inhibitor omeprazole reduces the risk of acid aspiration at emergency cesarean section. Anesth Analg **78**:1093, 1994.

Rogers RG, Katz VL: Course of Crohn's disease during pregnancy and its effect on pregnancy outcome: A retrospective review. Am J Perinatol **12**:262, 1995.

Rothman D: Folic acid in pregnancy. Am J Obstet Gynecol **108**:149, 1970.

Ruigomez A, Garcia Rodriguez LA, Cattaruzzi C, et al: Use of cimetidine, omeprazole, and ranitidine in pregnant women and pregnancy outcomes. Am J Epidemiol **150**:476, 1999.

Rustgi VK, Cooper JN, Colcher H: Endoscopy in the pregnant patient. *In* Rustgi VK, Cooper JN (eds): Gastrointestinal and Hepatic Complications in Pregnancy. New York, John Wiley and Sons, 1986, p. 104.

Ryan JP: Effect of pregnancy on intestinal transit: Comparison of results using radioactive and nonradioactive test meals. Life Sci **31**:2635, 1982.

Ryan JP, Bhojwani A: Colonic transit in rats: Effect of ovariectomy, sex steroid hormones, and pregnancy. Am J Physiol **251**:G46, 1986.

Ryan JP, Pellechia D: Effect of ovarian hormone pretreatment on gallbladder motility in vitro. Life Sci **31**:1445, 1982.

Sacco T, Corinaldesi R, Miglioli M, et al: The prevention of Mendelson's syndrome: Oral and intravenous administration of ranitidine. Clin Trials J **23**:193, 1986.

Schade RR, Pelekanos MJ, Tauxe WN, et al: Gastric emptying during pregnancy (abstr). Gastroenterology **86**:1234, 1984.

Scott HJ, McLeod RS, Blair J, et al: Ileal pouch-anal anastomosis: Pregnancy, delivery and pouch function. Int J Colorectal Dis **11**:84, 1996.

Scott LD, DeFlora E: Intestinal transit in female rats: Effect of pregnancy, estrous cycle and castration (abstr). Gastroenterology **84**:1303, 1983.

Scott LD, DeFlora E: Cholinergic responsiveness of intestinal muscle in the pregnant guinea pig. Life Sci **44**:593, 1989.

Scott LD, Kozinetz C, Gonik B: Gastrointestinal function in pregnancy (abstr). Gastroenterology **90**:1624, 1986.

Scott LD, Lester R, Van Thiel DH, et al: Pregnancy-related changes in small intestinal myoelectric activity in the rat. Gastroenterology **84**:301, 1983.

Shaheen NJ, Crosby MA, Grimm IS, et al: The use of percutaneous endoscopic gastrostomy in pregnancy. Gastrointest Endosc **46:**564, 1997.

Sharp HT: Gastrointestinal surgical conditions during pregnancy. Clin Obstet Gynecol **37:**306, 1994.

Shioda Y, Koizumi S, Furuya S, et al: Intussusception caused by a carcinoma of the cecum during pregnancy: Report of a case and review of the literature. Surg Today **23:**556, 1994.

Shoenut JP, Semelka RC, Silverman R, et al: MIR in the diagnosis of Crohn's disease in two pregnant women. J Clin Gastroenterol **17:**244, 1993.

Shushan A, Stemmer SN, Reubinoff BE, et al: Carcinoma of the colon during pregnancy. Obstet Gynecol Surv **47:**222, 1992.

Singer AJ, Brandt LJ: Pathophysiology of the gastrointestinal tract during pregnancy. Am J Gastroenterol **86:**1695, 1991.

Slemmons JM, Williams NH: Ileus in pregnancy. West J Surg Obstet Gynecol **46:**84, 1938.

Smallwood RA, Berlin RG, Castagnoli N, et al: Safety of acid-suppressing drugs. Dig Dis Sci **40:**63S, 1995.

Sommerville M, Koonings PP, Curtin JP, et al: Gastrointestinal signal ring carcinoma metastatic to the cervix during pregnancy. J Reprod Med **36:**813, 1991.

Stenson WF: Inflammatory bowel disease. *In* Yamada T (ed): Textbook of Gastroenterology, 2nd ed. Philadelphia, JB Lippincott, 1995, p. 1748.

Stewart CA, Termanini B, Sutliff VE, et al: Management of the Zollinger-Ellison syndrome in pregnancy. Am J Obstet Gynecol **176:**224, 1997.

Subhani JM, Hamiliton MI: Review article: The management of inflammatory bowel disease during pregnancy. Aliment Pharmacol Ther. **12:**1039, 1998.

Swinhoe JR, Cochrane GW, Wishart R: Oesophageal stricture due to reflux oesophagitis of pregnancy. Br J Obstet Gynaecol **88:**1249, 1981.

Talley NJ, Zinsmeister AR, Schleck C, et al: Natural history of gastroesophageal reflux: A population-based study (abstr). Gastroenterology **102:**A28, 1992.

Truelove SC: Stilboestrol, phenobarbitone and diet in chronic duodenal ulcer. Br Med J **2:**559, 1960.

Ulmsten V, Sundstrom G: Esophageal manometry in pregnant and nonpregnant women. Am J Obstet Gynecol **132:**260, 1978.

Van Thiel DH, Gavaler J, Joshi SN, et al: Heartburn of pregnancy. Gastroenterology **72:**666, 1977.

Van Thiel DH, Wald A: Evidence refuting a role for increased abdominal pressure in the pathogenesis of the heartburn associated with pregnancy. Am J Obstet Gynecol **140:**420, 1981.

Van Thiel DH, Schade RR: Pregnancy: Its physiologic course, nutrient cost, and effects on gastrointestinal function. *In* Rustgi VK, Cooper JN (eds): Gastrointestinal and Hepatic Complications in Pregnancy. New York, John Wiley and Sons, 1986, p. 1.

Vutyavanich T, Wongtra-ngan S, Ruangsri R: Pyridoxine for nausea and vomiting of pregnancy: A randomized, double-blind, placebo-controlled trial. Am J Obstet Gynecol **173:**881, 1995.

Wald A, Van Thiel DH, Hoechstetter L, et al: Effect of pregnancy on gastrointestinal transit. Dig Dis Sci **27:**1015, 1982.

Waldum HL, Straume BK, Lundgren R: Serum group I pepsinogens during pregnancy. Scand J Gastroenterol **15:**61, 1980.

Watson LA, Bommarito AA, Marshall JF: Total peripheral parenteral nutrition in pregnancy. J Paren Enteral Nutr **14:**485, 1990.

Weingold A: Appendicitis in pregnancy. Clin Obstet Gynecol **26:**80, 1983.

Whitehead SA, Andrews PLR, Chamberlain GVP: Characterisation of nausea and vomiting in early pregnancy: A survey of 1000 women. J Obstet Gynaecol **12:**364, 1992.

Wig JD, Bushnurmath SR, Kaushik SP: Complications of amoebiasis in pregnancy and puerperium. Ind J Gastroenterol **3:**37, 1984.

Willoughby CP, Truelove SC: Ulcerative colitis and pregnancy. Gut **21:**469, 1980.

Wyner J, Cohen SE: Gastric volume in early pregnancy. Anesthesiology **57:**209, 1982.

Wyte CD: Diagnostic modalities in the pregnant patient. Emerg Med Clin North Am **12:**9, 1994.

Yang H, McElree C, Roth M-P, et al: Familial empirical risks for inflammatory bowel disease: Differences between Jews and non-Jews. Gut **34:**517, 1993.

Chapter 53

DISEASES OF THE LIVER, BILIARY SYSTEM, AND PANCREAS

Mark B. Landon, MD

As with any other medical condition, liver disease may antedate pregnancy or develop during pregnancy itself. Also, several liver disorders are unique to or are commonly associated with pregnancy. Many of these diseases are so uncommon that a seasoned clinician or specialist in maternal-fetal medicine may rarely encounter certain liver disorders during a career. Thus, it is important to have some background knowledge concerning the various liver diseases complicating pregnancy and reliable references to aid in diagnosis and management. This chapter reviews both preexisting liver conditions and those that are primarily associated with pregnancy. The reciprocal effects of disease and pregnancy are considered along with the principles of clinical management.

LIVER IN NORMAL PREGNANCY

Whereas liver size may increase in normal pregnancy in experimental animals, there is no evidence that enlargement of the liver occurs during human gestation. Thus, hepatomegaly can be considered a potential pathologic finding, signifying the need to determine whether underlying liver disease exists. There is also little evidence that the liver undergoes any major histologic changes during pregnancy. The liver may be displaced superiorly during normal pregnancy primarily as a result of the expanding uterus and to a lesser extent displacement of the intestines.

Hepatic blood flow remains constant in pregnancy (25% to 33% of cardiac output). Because cardiac output and blood flow increases to other organs and hepatic blood flow is unaltered, it follows that there is a decrease in the proportion of cardiac output to the liver.

DIAGNOSIS OF LIVER DISEASE

As previously mentioned, hepatomegaly is an abnormal physical finding and may signify infiltrative disease (such as acute fatty liver of pregnancy [AFLP]) or an inflammatory condition (such as hepatitis). The liver may also enlarge as a result of passive congestion (right-sided heart failure) or in the Budd-Chiari syndrome. Malignancy is rarely a cause of liver enlargement in a reproduction-aged individual.

Dermatologic findings of both chronic liver disease and acute liver failure such as palmar erythema and spider nevi are often found in normal pregnancy. In contrast, jaundice and scleral icterus are clearly abnormal findings and warrant further evaluation.

Imaging of the liver may be complicated in pregnancy, particularly if radiation is used. Precautions are taken to shield the fetus or to provide dosimetry estimates if significant exposure is likely. Thus, ultrasound remains a primarily imaging tool, yet it is often of limited value in assessing liver architecture. Computed tomography (CT) and endoscopic retrograde cholangiopancreatography can be used during pregnancy, again with care to shield the fetus from radiation. Magnetic resonance imaging has the advantage of no radiation exposure and has an established safety profile in pregnancy.

On rare occasions, histologic diagnosis may be essential to management in a pregnant woman. This is most often an issue when AFLP is being weighed in the differential diagnosis and confirmatory biopsy is likely to influence the decision to proceed with delivery. The procedure remains safe in expert hands provided that coagulation parameters are within normal limits.

LIVER FUNCTION IN NORMAL PREGNANCY

During normal pregnancy, profound changes occur in the serum concentration of plasma proteins (Table 53-1). Serum proteins synthesized by the liver are also affected by the hyperestrogenic state of pregnancy. The alterations in serum concentration may persist for a few months after delivery.

With an expansion in plasma volume, total serum protein concentration diminishes 20% by mid-pregnancy. Most of this reflects a fall in serum albumin because small increases in α and β globulin fractions occur. Maher and colleagues (1993) suggested a reciprocal relationship between rising levels of α-fetoprotein and the fall in serum albumin.

Serum fibrinogen reliably rises in concentration during pregnancy. Fibrinogen biosynthesis and manufacture of other coagulation factors (VII, VIII, IX, and X) are increased in pregnancy and also with estrogen administration. Estrogens increase hepatic rough endoplasmic reticulum and accelerate synthesis of proteins. Increased amounts of progesterone, in turn, lead to proliferation of smooth endoplasmic reticulum and an increase in cytochrome P-450. Other serum proteins such as ceruloplasmin and transferrin also rise with gestation.

TABLE 53-1. LIVER FUNCTION TESTS IN NORMAL PREGNANCY

Prothrombin time	Unchanged
Total bilirubin	Unchanged
Aspartate aminotransferase	Unchanged
Alanine aminotransferase	Unchanged
Liver alkaline phosphatase	Unchanged
γ-Glutamyl-transpeptidase	Unchanged
5'-Nucleotidase	Unchanged
Total alkaline phosphatase (includes placental isoenzyme)	Increased
Binding globulins (thyroxine, cortisol, sex steroid)	Increased
Cholesterol	Increased
Fibrinogen	Increased
Ceruloplasmin	Increased
Transferrin	Increased
Lactate dehydrogenase	Increased
Total protein, albumin	Decreased

Serum binding capacity for thyroxine, vitamin D, cortisol, and testosterone also accompany normal pregnancy and affect the concentration of the bound portion of these hormones.

Liver function tests were studied in a prospective analysis of 103 pregnant women and matched control subjects (Bacq et al., 1997). This study confirmed that bilirubin levels remain normal during pregnancy as do serum aminotransferases (aspartate aminotransferase and alanine aminotransferase). Thus, an elevation in bilirubin suggests either liver disease or hemolysis, whereas a rise in the two serum enzyme levels indicate liver damage.

Total serum alkaline phosphatase is elevated by the third trimester in normal pregnancy. Most of this elevation stems from placental production, with a return to normal levels within a few weeks postpartum. First-trimester placental production is limited, so that this assay is only useful in early gestation. Estrogens may produce injury to canalicular membranes, resulting in bile duct obstruction and intrahepatic cholestasis with a resultant rise in serum alkaline phosphatase. In contrast, levels of γ-glutamyl-transpeptidase are normal or deceased in the third trimester (Bacq et al., 1997). Serum lactate dehydrogenase and ornithine transcarbamylase are increased at term.

LIVER DISORDERS UNIQUE TO PREGNANCY

Intrahepatic Cholestasis of Pregnancy

Intrahepatic cholestasis of pregnancy (IHCP) is the most common liver condition unique to pregnancy, yet it is a rare disease, with a prevalence of 1 in 1000 to 1 in 10,000 deliveries (Reyes and Simon, 1993). The disease usually presents in the third trimester and is characterized by pruritus and mild jaundice. The disease has been reported in highest frequencies in Chile and Scandinavia (Reyes and Simon, 1993). The frequency in singleton pregnancies in Chile was reported as 4.7% compared with 20.9% in twin gestations (Gonzales et al., 1989). In Sweden, between 1.0% and 1.5% of pregnancies may be affected (Berg et al., 1986). Hepatitis C virus infection may predispose to IHCP, as one report found 15.9% of women

affected compared with 0.8% of control subjects (Locatelli et al., 1999).

The etiology of IHCP is unknown, yet familial history and an association with cholestasis while taking oral contraceptives strongly suggest an inherited susceptibility to alterations in steroid and bile acid metabolism (Knox and Olans, 1996). A family history is present in up to 50% of women in association with histocompatibility antigen haplotypes HLA-B8 and HLA-BW16. Specific mutations of the MDR3 gene (also called ABCB4) have been reported (Dixon et al., 2000).

Derangements in the metabolism of bile acids and progesterone in IHCP featuring increased levels of sulfated progesterone metabolites and a reduction in glucuronidated intermediates are features of this disorder (Meng et al., 1997). It has been suggested that a defect in biliary excretion of sulfated steroid metabolites in IHCP results in cholestasis via saturation of hepatic transport systems (Reyes and Sjovall, 2000). Impaired transport of bile acids across the placenta from the fetal to maternal circulation seems to play a key role in the pathogenesis of fetal compromise associated with IHCP (Serrano et al., 1998). Bile acid exchanges apparently exist on both sides of the trophoblast. In vitro studies reveal impairment of efficiency and diffusion of vesicle trophoblastic transplant of bile acids from fetus to mother in IHCP (Serrano et al., 1998). There is also an independent increased flow of maternal bile acids to the fetus in IHCP via an adenosine triphosphate-dependent transporter.

The pruritus of IHCP may be attenuated by opioid antagonists, suggesting a central etiology for this symptom (Jones and Bergasa, 1999). Older teaching stressed that subcutaneous deposit of bile acids were primarily responsible for this phenomenon. However, studies in which sera from affected women were injected into the medullary dorsal horn of monkeys induced scratching, which did not occur when control sera were injected Jones and Bergasa, 1999). Naloxone apparently can alleviate pruritus of IHCP (Jones and Bergasa, 1999); however, its clinical utility is limited because of its short half life.

Clinical Presentation

IHCP presents typically with progressive pruritus during the third trimester. It presents initially in the evening and eventually becomes evident throughout the day. Several weeks later, clinical jaundice may develop in up to 75% of cases (Brites et al., 1998). The symptoms generally resolve within days of delivery. The differential diagnosis typically includes gallbladder disease with cholestasis or hepatitis (Table 53-2). Absence of fever, malaise, abdominal pain, nausea, and vomiting point to IHCP as a strong possibility. The clinical diagnosis is then confirmed by laboratory investigation. There is, however, no uniform criteria for the diagnosis for IHCP. Serum alkaline phosphatase levels are typically increased 5- to 10-fold; however, this enzyme is elevated in normal later pregnancy. Serum and urinary total sulfated progesterone metabolites are increased in IHCP (Meng et al., 2000). Bilirubin is typically mildly elevated, with primarily direct levels rarely exceeding 5 mg/dL. If cholestasis persists for weeks, decreased vitamin K reabsorption and diminished prothrombin synthesis may lead to a prolonged prothrombin time. Elevations in serum transaminases are variable, with reports of normal values ranging to severalfold increases (Knox and Olans, 1996).

TABLE 53-2. DIFFERENTIAL DIAGNOSIS OF LIVER DISEASE IN PREGNANCY

	Incidence	Trimester Affected	Total Bilirubin (mg/dL)	Serum Transamalase Levels (IU/L)	Renal Abnormalities	Distinguishing Features
Intrahepatic cholestatis	1 in 1000– 1 in 10,000	Usually third	<5 primary direct	<300	No	Intense pruritus, elevated bile acids
Acute fatty liver	1/7000– 1/16,000	Usually third	2–10	<1000	May be present	Hypoglycemia, fatty infiltration on liver biopsy overlap with preeclampsia common
HELLP* syndrome, severe preeclampsia	1 in 500	Late second or typically third	<5	50–2000	May be present	Hypertension, thrombocytopenia, proteinuria
Viral hepatitis	1–2/1000	Any	>5 maybe up to 30 with fulminant disease	500–3000	No	Serologic diagnosis

* Hemolysis, elevated liver enzymes, and low platelets.

Serum cholesterol and triglyceride levels are elevated beyond the normal physiologic rises seen in pregnancy.

Serum bile acids (chenodeoxycholic acid, deoxycholic acid, and cholic acid) are elevated in most cases and have been reported to be the most sensitive laboratory abnormality (Palma et al., 1992). The degree of pruritus, however, does not correlate with serum bile acid levels. Fasting levels of bile acids are best obtained to secure a diagnosis, yet others suggest that IHCP can be diagnosed clinically based on the absence of cholestatic gallbladder disease, hepatitis, and any other disorder that might result in pruritus (Rioseco et al., 1994). A review of 100 cases of IHCP documented elevated fasting bile acid levels in only 50% of women (Lopez et al., 1982).

Liver biopsy is rarely necessary in affected individuals. Typical histologic changes include centrilobular dilated bile canaliculi with plugging. Abundant bile pigment is present in hepatocytes (Reyes and Sjovall, 2000).

Clinical Management

MATERNAL THERAPY

The goal of maternal treatment is to reduce pruritus. Antihistamines are of limited value in this regard. For many years, cholestyramine, an anion-binding resin that disrupts the enterohepatic circulation and reabsorption of bile acids, was used as a primary medical therapy in IHCP. This drug, however, comes as a powder and must be mixed, which makes it difficult to take. It also has the disadvantage of a delayed affect (approximately 2 weeks) and, more importantly, may lead to malabsorption of fat-soluble vitamins such as vitamin K. With prolonged therapy, parenteral vitamin K has been suggested along with obtaining prothrombin times. Unlike cholestyramine, phenobarbital induces hepatic microsomal enzymes and thus increases bile salt secretion and bile flow (Laatikinen, 1978). Aside from its unsatisfactory sedative properties, this medication also may require a week or more to be effective.

Dexamethasone suppresses fetal–placental estrogen synthesis and has been shown to alleviate pruritus and improve liver function in IHCP (Hirvioja et al., 1992). Conflicting data

regarding efficacy of dexamethasone have limited its use in IHCP (Kretowica and McIntyre, 1994).

Guar gum, a gel-like fiber that augments fetal elimination of bile acids, has been shown to improve pruritus and stabilize bile levels in two small randomized trials of 96 women (Gylling et al., 1998; Riikonen et al., 2000). The two most promising agents for treatment of IHCP are S-adenyl-methionine and ursodeoxycholic acid (UDCA). S-adenyl-methionine reverses estrogen-induced impairment of bile secretion, whereas UDCA is a naturally occurring hydrophilic bile acid that competes with other more cytotoxic bile acids. Its effects are mediated by amelioration of damage to cell membranes caused by retained toxic bile acids (Kowdley, 2000). UDCA improves maternal pruritus and liver function abnormalities and also acts to reverse abnormalities of bile acid transport across the placenta (Serrano et al., 1998)

A small study of 32 women with IHCP suggested that combination therapy of S-adenyl-methionine and UDCA might be more effective than either drug alone (Nicastri et al., 1998). A randomized, double-blind, placebo-controlled study in which treated women took a gram of UDCA daily for 3 weeks revealed a significant decrease in pruritus and liver function abnormalities (Palma et al., 1997). The recommended dosage of UDCA is 14 to 16 mg/kg/day (Palma et al., 1997; Brites et al., 1998). Serrano and colleagues (1998) demonstrated that UDCA improves the efficiency of bile transport from the fetal to maternal compartment across the trophoblast in a postdelivery placental study using placentas from women with IHCP. These authors noted that treatment with UDCA both improves maternal hepatic bile acid transport and restores trophoblastic transport mechanisms, with a net effect of transfer to the maternal circulation.

FETAL CONCERNS

There is an increased risk of preterm birth and fetal demise in women affected by IHCP (Heinonen and Kirkinen, 1999). In a study of 83 pregnancies complicated by IHCP, meconium occurred in 45%, spontaneous preterm labor in 44%, and intrapartum fetal distress in 22% (Fisk et al., 1988). The overall perinatal mortality has ranged from 3% to 20% (Fisk et al., 1988; Rioseco et al., 1994). The cause of fetal death is unknown, but fetal heart rate abnormalities suggest that elevated serum bile acid levels might impair cardiomyocyte function (Williamson et al., 2001). Secondary bile acids are capable of inducing death, malformation, and growth delay (Zimber and Zussman, 1990). Using a rat model, Williamson and associates (2001) studied the effects of primary bile taurocholate on cardiomyocytes. Addition of taurocholate to a network of synchronously beating cells caused a decrease in the rate of contraction, indicating that raised levels of this bile acid in the fetal serum in IHCP may contribute to fetal dysrhythmia and sudden intrauterine fetal death. This finding is of interest because fetal heart rate testing has been reported as normal until hours before delivery in cases of fetal demise (Palma et al., 1997). Most fetal deaths occur late in pregnancy. For this reason, some have advocated proceeding with early delivery once fetal lung maturity is established (Davies et al., 1995). Before term, non-stress testing has been used, yet sudden fetal death has occurred with various testing regimens (Rioseco et al., 1994). It should be emphasized that various indices of maternal disease such as bile acid levels and liver enzyme abnormalities may not correlate with fetal risk, because stillbirth has occurred in women without biochemical evidence of disease and only pruritus (Reid et al., 1976).

Overlap Syndromes with Liver Dysfunction: Preeclampsia, HELLP Syndrome, Acute Fatty Liver of Pregnancy, and Liver Rupture

These conditions, which generally occur during the third trimester and postpartum, are often characterized by hypertension, elevated liver enzymes, and thrombocytopenia (see Chapter 43). Most often, resolution follows delivery; however, progressive disease and multisystem organ failure may lead to maternal mortality. HELLP syndrome (hemolysis, elevated liver enzymes, and low platelets) is most often a variant of severe preeclampsia because hypertension and proteinuria are generally accompanying features. There is also overlap between AFLP and preeclampsia, which is present in approximately 50% of cases of AFLP. The association with primigravid women, multiple gestation, and amelioration with delivery all support a common underlying etiology with preeclampsia. It is essential for the clinician to differentiate the overlap syndromes from unrelated conditions, which do not improve after delivery. Because of the rare nature of AFLP, for example, a multidisciplinary team approach consisting of maternal-fetal medicine and liver specialists is recommended to guide therapy.

Fatty Acid Oxidation Pathways: Acute Fatty Liver of Pregnancy, Overlap Syndrome and Long-Chain 3-Hydroxyacyl-Coenzyme A Dehydrogenase Deficiency

Over the past dozen years, clinical observations have demonstrated an association between AFLP, HELLP syndrome, and a recessively inherited fatty acid oxygenation disorder, long-chain 3-hydroxyacyl-coenzyme A dehydrogenase (LCHAD) deficiency (Ibdah et al., 2000). This enzyme resides in the mitochondrial trifunctional protein, which also contains the active site of long-chain 2,3-enoly-coenzyme A thiolase. Considerable evidence suggests that LCHAD deficiency,

when present in the homozygous fetus, may cause maternal liver disease of pregnancy in susceptible heterozygous mothers (Schoeman et al., 1991). Hagerfeldt and colleagues (1995) first reported a woman with AFLP whose infant was later discovered to have a B-oxidation defect characterized by 3-hydroxydicarboxylic aciduria and accumulation of 3-hydroxy fatty acid intermediates, indicating LCHAD deficiency. This woman had also developed AFLP in a prior pregnancy, and the infant delivered died at 11 months of age. Schoeman and coworkers (1991) reported cases of recurrent AFLP in two successive pregnancies in which both children had 3-hydroxycarboxylic aciduria. Wilcken and colleagues (1993) later described five women who developed AFLP or HELLP syndrome during six pregnancies in which all offspring were subsequently discovered to have LCHAD deficiency. The specific molecular defects present in families with maternal liver disease of pregnancy and offspring with LCHAD deficiency have been documented (Sims et al., 1995; Issacs et al., 1996).

Ibdah and coworkers (1999) reported their experience in 24 families, 19 with isolated LCHAD deficiency and 5 with complete trifunctional protein deficiency. These authors used DNA amplification and nucleotide sequence analysis to identify mutations in the α subunit of the trifunctional protein. In addition to the isolated defect in 19 infants, children were identified as homozygous for a mutation in which glutamic acid at reside 474 was changed to glutamine. Eleven children were compound heterozygotes, with this mutation in one allele of the α subunit and a different mutation in the other allele. Seventy-nine percent of heterozygous mothers carrying a fetus with the Glu 474 Gln mutation developed AFLP or HELLP syndrome during pregnancy. Of the five children with complete deficiency of the trifunctional protein, none had the Glu 474 Gln mutation and none of their mothers developed liver disease during pregnancy. The Glu 474 Gln mutation appears to be a unique defect in Scandinavian populations (Tyni et al., 1998). Tyni and coworkers (1998) reported on 63 pregnancies in 18 Finnish families with LCHAD deficiency and confirmed that maternal liver disease is more common with affected fetuses compared with those presumed heterozygotes or normal. Affected fetuses also had a higher frequency of prematurity asphyxia and growth retardation when compared with their unaffected siblings.

The mechanism by which LCHAD deficiency in the fetus results in severe liver disease in the heterozygote mother is unknown. The presence of third-trimester disease along with amelioration after delivery suggests that changes in maternal metabolism contribute to this phenomenon. The considerable rise in estrogen in late pregnancy along with reduced fatty acid oxidation and increased ketone, triglyceride, and ULDL production compounded by 3-hydroxy fatty acid metabolites produced by an affected fetus might stress the mitochondrial oxidation pathways of a heterozygous mother. Ibdah and associates (2000) suggested that 15% to 20% of pregnancies complicated by AFLP and less than 2% of pregnancies complicated by HELLP syndrome are associated with fetal LCHAD deficiency. A Dutch study (den Boer et al., 2000) reported the prevalence of the common LCHAD mutation to be 1 in 113 in women with a history of HELLP syndrome. Nonetheless, molecular screening in pregnancies complicated by AFLP and HELLP syndrome may identify a potentially fatal disorder in the offspring. This is recommended for women with a history of AFLP and considered for those with recurrent

HELLP syndrome (Ibdah et al., 2000). Molecular prenatal diagnosis in families with proven LCHAD deficiency can identify an affected fetus and thereby assess the risk for serious maternal liver disease as well (Ibdah et al., 2000).

Acute Fatty Liver of Pregnancy

AFLP remains a rare condition with a prevalence of 1 in 7000 to 16,000 deliveries (Moise and Shah, 1987; Reyes et al., 1994). It is more likely with a male fetus and twin gestation. Older studies reported a nearly 70% mortality rate, yet today maternal survival is likely in the 75% range (Moise and Sha, 1987). Prompt recognition and early diagnosis with delivery has reversed these survival statistics over time (Ebert et al., 1984). Castro and colleagues (1999) reviewed 28 cases of AFLP after 1982 and reported no maternal mortalities and only two perinatal deaths.

Clinical and Laboratory Manifestations

Women with AFLP typically present during the third trimester with nausea and vomiting (Purdie and Walters, 1988; Usta et al., 1994). Abdominal pain, often localized to the right upper quadrant, follows, with the development of hepatic failure if delivery is not promptly undertaken. Despite right upper quadrant discomfort, hepatomegaly is often absent. Progressive jaundice, malaise, and eventual consciousness changes of somnolence and coma may follow. Massive liver dysfunction can produce coagulopathy and spontaneous bleeding. Renal dysfunction manifested by oliguria and azotemia complicates nearly half of all cases (Purdie and Walters, 1988). Diabetes insipidus has also been reported to coexist with AFLP. In severe cases complicated by coagulopathy and renal failure, hypoglycemia and pancreatitis may precede maternal death (Moise and Shah, 1987). Liver rupture has also been reported (Roh, 1986; Minuk et al., 1987).

Differentiating AFLP from other causes of liver disease during pregnancy can be challenging (see Table 53-2). Moreover, AFLP may occur with severe preeclampsia (Amon et al., 1991), chronic active hepatitis (Minton et al., 1993), and cholestasis of pregnancy (Vanjak et al., 1991). Laboratory diagnosis is helpful in distinguishing AFLP from other processes. In AFLP, liver transaminases are elevated but are generally less than 500 IU/L (Ebert et al., 1984). This is a similar range to severe preeclampsia and HELLP but far lower than observed with acute viral hepatitis. Maternal and fetal outcome do not correlate with liver enzyme levels. If coagulopathy is present, prothrombin time is prolonged before partial thromboplastin time, reflecting hepatic-dependent vitamin K biosynthesis of coagulation factors. Elevation of bilirubin is expected in AFLP, with total levels modestly high, in the range of 5 to 10 mg/dL. Liver biopsy reveals microvesicular hepatic steatosis and mitochondrial disruption on electron microscopy (Minakami et al., 1988). This is in contrast to HELLP syndrome, in which histology shows periportal hemorrhage and fibrin deposition, although fatty infiltration may be observed (Minakami et al., 1988). Periportal architecture is preserved in most biopsies of AFLP. Special stains, including oil red O for demonstrating fat, have high sensitivity but are not specific for AFLP. Reyes and colleagues (1994) reported the presence of mega-

mitochondria with paracrystalline inclusions in all women with AFLP. Liver biopsy, however, is generally unnecessary in affected cases. If this procedure is essential to diagnosis, coagulopathy must be corrected before obtaining a histologic specimen. There is continued controversy regarding the utility of CT for establishing the diagnosis of AFLP. Whereas some have reported decreased attenuation consistent with fatty infiltration (Goodacre et al., 1988; Mabie et al., 1988), others have reported limited sensitivity of this technique (Van Le and Podrasky, 1990; Usta et al., 1994). Magnetic resonance imaging may be more helpful by using T2-weighted gradient-echo sequences (Siegelman, 1997).

Management

Delivery is recommended once the diagnosis of AFLP is secured (Bacq et al., 1997). Supportive care is rendered, including correction of any underlying coagulopathy. Intravenous solutions containing glucose are advised because of the threat of hypoglycemia. Whereas vaginal delivery is preferred, cesarean section is advised if induction is likely to be prolonged or if progressive disease warrants prompt intervention. Regional anesthesia is recommended, provided that coagulopathy has been corrected, because it allows the evaluation of consciousness and eliminates the potential noxious effects of inhalation agents, which can be hepatotoxic.

Preeclampsia and HELLP Syndrome

Liver involvement signifies the development of severe preeclampsia. Elevation of liver enzymes may occur as an isolated laboratory abnormality or as a component of HELLP syndrome. Although severe hypertension may be absent in HELLP syndrome, in most instances there is some degree of accompanying hypertension that helps to distinguish these disorders from other diseases. There may be overlap between HELLP syndrome and AFLP, however. Isolated serum transaminase elevations in severe preeclampsia rarely exceed 500 U/L (see Table 53-2). Elevation in serum bilirubin levels is more typical of HELLP syndrome, yet these rarely exceed 2.0 mg/dL. In contrast, bilirubin levels are generally higher in AFLP. Marked elevations of transaminases greater than 1000 U/L and bilirubin levels exceeding 5 mg/dL are more likely a feature of viral hepatitis. Hepatic failure with encephalopathy and coagulopathy are uncommon in preeclampsia and should prompt a differential diagnosis, including fatty liver and other causes of hepatic dysfunction.

Hepatic involvement occurs in approximately 10% of severe preeclampsia cases (Weinstein, 1982). Most of these women have only liver enzyme elevations without epigastric pain. The development of right upper quadrant pain does often signify liver involvement such that liver function tests should be promptly evaluated in this setting. Histologic descriptions of hepatic involvement in preeclampsia include periportal hemorrhage, sinusoidal fibrin deposition, and cellular necrosis (Barton et al., 1992). The pathophysiologic basis of these findings likely includes ischemia, although hepatic blood flow is primarily dependent on the portal venous system.

Women with preeclampsia and liver involvement should generally undergo delivery, although administration of steroids to first promote fetal lung maturity can be undertaken in preterm cases when maternal condition is otherwise stable.

Laboratory abnormalities generally resolve within 48 hours after delivery, although resolution of thrombocytopenia in women with HELLP syndrome may take longer. Because HELLP syndrome may develop during the postpartum period in 20% of cases, liver function testing and potential imaging should be undertaken if abdominal pain or thrombocytopenia is present after delivery in the setting of preeclampsia.

Liver Rupture and Infarction

Rupture of the liver during pregnancy is a rare but often catastrophic event with substantial risk for both fetal and maternal mortality (Smith et al., 1999). Most cases during pregnancy involve severe preeclampsia and HELLP syndrome (Pereira et al., 1997). Subcapsular liver hematoma has been reported in 4 of 442 women with HELLP syndrome (Sibai et al., 1993). Although the pathogenesis of hepatic rupture remains unclear, subcapsular hemorrhage is a common finding at autopsy in cases of maternal preeclampsia. Because significant blood loss may occur in such patients, hypertension may be minimal or absent at the time of presentation. In the previously cited report, the diagnosis was obscured by the presence of disseminated intravascular coagulation, thought to be secondary to abruptio placentae (Sibai et al., 1993).

Spontaneous rupture of the liver is proceeded by the development of subcapsular hemorrhage, which produces stretching of the liver capsule. This stretch or irritation results in significant right upper quadrant pain. Upon rupture of the capsule, hemoperitoneum ensues with the development of peritoneal signs accompanied by hypovolemic shock. If hypertension has not antedated the event, it may only be manifest after vigorous fluid resuscitation.

Laboratory evaluation of women with either subcapsular hematoma or rupture reveals thrombocytopenia, hypofibrinogenemia, or prolonged prothrombin and partial thromboplastin times. Anemia accompanied by hemolysis, with elevation of bilirubin and lactate dehydrogenase, and liver transaminases are present. Thus, the differential diagnosis of unruptured liver hematoma includes AFLP, placental abruption with coagulopathy, thrombotic thrombocytopenic purpura, and cholangitis with sepsis.

In suspected cases, which most often will be in the setting of HELLP syndrome with right upper quadrant pain, diagnostic imaging is required to establish a diagnosis (Barton and Sibai, 1996). Bedside ultrasonography can often demonstrate hemoperitoneum; however, CT or magnetic resonance imaging is the preferred technique for visualizing liver hematomas. Such imaging is critical before consideration of liver biopsy if the diagnosis is unclear. Liver biopsy is contraindicated with suspected subcapsular hemorrhage. To confirm the presence of intraperitoneal bleeding, paracentesis may occasionally be helpful.

Conservative management of an intact hematoma without rupture is recommended, particularly if the patient is hemodynamically stable (Barton and Sibai, 1996). These women should be closely monitored in an intensive care setting with serial imaging studies to define the extent of hemorrhage, progression, and whether leaking has occurred. Excessive palpation of the liver or increases in intra-abdominal pressure from emesis should be avoided. If maternal hemodynamic status deteriorates, rupture is likely and prompt surgical exploration is the treatment of choice. A surgical team skilled in the management of liver trauma is essential. Fluid replacement, transfusion, and correction of coagulopathy are necessary in conjunction with an attempt to control hepatic bleeding. Several approaches have been successfully used, including packing and drainage and control of hemorrhage areas through ligation of bleeding segments. Suturing omentum to exposed areas has also been used along with packing techniques. Radiologic embolization or surgical ligation of the hepatic artery has also been accomplished in selected cases. However, the rare nature of this condition precludes recommending this approach as being superior to others. In a patient who is relatively stable, angiography may be attempted while making preparations for potential laparotomy.

Maternal and fetal mortality may approach 50% in cases of liver rupture. In a series of seven cases, four survivors were reported that were all managed with packing and drainage (Smith et al., 1999). All three women undergoing hepatic lobectomy did not survive. Mortality is often due to massive blood loss and coagulopathy. Patients that survive commonly experience respiratory insufficiency from adult respiratory distress syndrome or pulmonary edema and acute liver failure. Critical care of fluid and respiratory status monitoring (see Chapter 45) is essential, as is follow-up hepatic imaging, to be certain that stabilization has occurred.

Infarction involving multiple areas of liver parenchyma may also be a feature of severe preeclampsia or HELLP syndrome (Krueger et al., 1990). Such individuals experience abdominal pain and often fever. Massive elevations in transaminases accompanied by thrombocytopenia are common features. CT demonstrates clearly demarcated areas of poor vascularization involving multiple liver segments. Biopsy of these areas demonstrates hemorrhage and leukocyte infiltration in areas adjacent to hemorrhage. In the setting of HELLP syndrome, multiple adjacent areas of periportal hemorrhage most likely form these infarcted segments. Although laboratory evidence of liver inflammation is impressive in affected cases, improvement after delivery can be expected.

Maternal Disorders Coincidental to Pregnancy

Viral Hepatitis

Viral hepatitis is the most common cause of jaundice during pregnancy (Dinsmoor, 1997) (see Table 53-2). There are six primary subtypes of hepatitis virus: A, B, C, D, E, and G (Table 53-3). The incubation periods vary, and clinical features of acute infection may overlap. The diagnosis ultimately requires specific serologic markers for acute and chronic infection (see Table 53-3). Importantly, the clinical implications of each virus for maternal and fetal/neonatal health varies considerably.

The maternal management of viral hepatitis is not altered greatly by pregnancy. Supportive therapy is generally sufficient, although occasional cases of certain viral subtypes may lead to progressive liver failure. Hepatitis A and B remain the most common viruses responsible for acute hepatitis in pregnancy in both North America and Europe. Infection during the third trimester is most common. Hepatitis E is rare within the United States. There is some evidence that infection with hepatitis E during pregnancy can be fulminant and is associated with relatively high rates of mortality (Rab et al., 1997). The severity of infection with viruses A through D is, however, not influenced

■ **TABLE 53-3.** COMPARISON OF VARIOUS FORMS OF VIRAL HEPATITIS

Feature	Hepatitis A	Hepatitis B	Hepatitis C	Hepatitis D	Hepatitis E
Viral type	RNA	DNA	RNA	RNA	RNA
Incubation period	12–15 days	30–180 days	30–160 days	30–180 days	14–63 days
Transmission	Fecal–oral	Parenteral	Parenteral	Parenteral	Fecal–oral
Diagnosis	IgM, IgG hepatitis antibody	HBsAg, anti-HBs anti-HBc, HBeAg HBV DNA	Hepatitis C antibody	Delta antigen, IgM specific antibody	IgM anti-HEV
Carrier risk	0	10–15%	50–85%	Up to 80% risk of chronic hepatitis B infection with coinfection of hepatitis D	0
Chronic variety	None	Chronic persistent, chronic acute forms, cirrhosis	Chronic persistent, chronic active forms, cirrhosis	Chronic hepatitis risk as above	None
Vertical fetal transmission risk	No	Yes	Yes	Yes	Yes

anti-HBc, antibody to hepatitis B care antigen; anti-HBs, antibody to hepatitis B surface antigen; anti-HEV, antibody to hepatitis E virus; HBeAg, hepatitis B e antigen; HBsAg, hepatitis B surface antigen.

by gestation. Prematurity and perinatal death are uncommon yet are slightly increased over background rates for the general population. In contrast, miscarriage, fetal growth, retardation, and congenital malformation rates are not increased.

Hepatitis A

Hepatitis A accounts for approximately one third of cases of hepatitis in the United States. The virus is a ubiquitous RNA picornavirus, which is transmitted through fecal–oral contamination, including person-person contact. Poor hygiene and poor sanitation, resulting in contaminated food and water, are the common modes of infection. The disease is endemic to the developing world where inadequately treated sewage may contaminate fruits, vegetables, and shellfish. The disease is more common among immigrants, drug users, and homosexual men (Centers for Disease Control [CDC], 1992).

The incubation period of hepatitis A ranges from 14 to 50 days and is followed by nonspecific symptoms of malaise, headache, fatigue, anorexia, nausea, vomiting, and diarrhea. Cholestasis shortly follows with jaundice, acholic stools, and dark urine. Some patients may experience few symptoms at all. Hepatitis A is a self-limited disease without a chronic process that complicates other viral hepatitis infections.

The diagnostic test most commonly used is an IgM-specific antibody to hepatitis A virus. The presence of IgG antibody to hepatitis A virus indicates postinfection and immunity in developing countries with poor sanitation, childhood infection, or exposure is common. Thus, hepatitis A is uncommon in adult populations in impoverished countries. In the United States, seasonal variation and an increasing frequency in adults has been observed. IgM antibody is detectable 1 month after exposure and may persist for as long as 6 months. IgG antibody to hepatitis A virus appears within 35 to 40 days of exposure and signifies lifelong immunity.

Acute hepatitis A infection rarely requires more than general supportive care. Recovery follows in typical fashion within 4 to 6 weeks. Fulminant hepatitis is observed in less than 1% of cases. These individuals may require intensive care for treatment of coagulopathy and encephalopathy. Hepatitis A virus is excreted in large amounts in stool before the onset of symptoms of jaundice. Affected patients should be advised of their potential risk for transmission. Sexual partners and household contacts are advised to receive immunoprophylaxis consisting of immune globulin (IG). A single intramuscular dose of 0.02 mL/kg may be protective in up to 80% of cases within 2 weeks of exposure. The formalin-inactivated hepatitis A vaccine should also be considered as it appears safe for use in pregnancy (Duff and Duff, 1998). A single intramuscular dose of 0.06 mL is used. Pregnant women embarking on travel to endemic areas should be screened for immunity to hepatitis A and if IgG negative should receive immunoprophylaxis and vaccination.

Perinatal transmission of hepatitis A is rare. In such cases, fecal contamination occurs when maternal incubation coincides with delivery. Infants delivered to a mother manifesting acute hepatitis A should receive IG to prevent horizontal transmission (American College of Obstetricians and Gynecologists, 1993).

Hepatitis B

Hepatitis B accounts for 40% to 45% of all cases of hepatitis in the United States. Acute hepatitis B infection occurs in 1 to 2 per 1000 pregnancies (Dinsmoor, 1997). Over 300,000 new cases of hepatitis B occur annually in the United States, and it is estimated that 1 million individuals are chronic carriers of the hepatitis B virus (HBV). In the United States, each year approximately 20,000 infants are delivered of hepatitis B surface antigen (HBsAg)-seropositive women (CDC, 1996). The frequency of chronic hepatitis B infection in pregnancy is between 5 and 15 per 1000 (Syndman, 1985). Before the introduction of immunoprophylaxis, nearly 3000 infants became chronically infected each year as a result of vertical transmission (CDC, 1996). The high risk of vertical transmission from carrier pregnant women to their offspring and its potential prevention by screening and immunization are areas of special interest to the practicing obstetrician and maternal-fetal specialist. Moreover, there is an increased likelihood of a chronic carrier state in infected newborns compared with adult population of the infected pregnant woman.

ACUTE HEPATITIS B

Hepatitis B is a DNA virus with three major structural antigens: HBsAg, core antigen, and e antigen (HBeAg) (Table 53-4). The intact virus is known as the Dane particle. Transmission occurs principally through parenteral drug use, sexual intercourse, and vertically after perinatal exposure. The peak prevalence of disease is in the reproductive age group, where heterosexual contact for females represents the most common method of infection. Population groups at increased risk include drug addicts, transfusion recipients, dialysis patients, Asians, residents and employees of chronic care facilities, and prisoners.

HBsAg is found in blood 2 to 8 weeks before the development of symptoms or laboratory abnormalities. Serum HBsAg generally remains detectable until the convalescent phase. HBeAg becomes detectable after HBsAg and indicates a high viral inoculum and viral replication. The diagnosis of acute hepatitis B requires the detection of surface antigen and IgM antibody to the core antigen (IgM-anti-HBc). Identification of IgM-anti-HBc is important because certain individuals with fulminant acute hepatitis B may experience a "window" of time when HBsAg is not easily detectable. Clinical recovery is accompanied by clearance of HBV DNA followed by HBeAg and HBsAg antigenemia within 1 to 3 months along with the presence of IgG-anti-HBc and antibody to HBeAg. The presence of antibody to HBsAg indicates recovery and clearance of the virus along with immunity.

CHRONIC CARRIER STATE

After acute hepatitis B infection, 85% to 90% of adults experience complete resolution and develop antibody to HBsAg, which confers immunity. Thus, approximately 10% to 15% of individuals fail to clear the virus and remain HBsAg-seropositive carriers for more than 6 months after acute infection. Of these chronically infected people, 15% to 30% develop chronic acute hepatitis or cirrhosis. A smaller percentage, which includes nearly 800 cases per year of primary liver cancer, follow the chronic infection state. Chronic infection is more likely in those who remain HBeAg positive or become superinfected with hepatitis D (American College of Obstetricians and Gynecologists, 1993). Other factors associated with the chronic carrier state include infection early in life, symptomless infection, immunosuppression, Asian background, and Down syndrome.

Liver damage is related primarily to immunologic events. Cytotoxic T-cell destruction of infected hepatocytes manifesting core antigen results in massive liver injury over time. Exacerbations of inflammatory activity follow viral replication and mirror the load of HBV DNA detectable in serum.

PERINATAL ASPECTS

Acute hepatitis B results in fulminant maternal infection in less than 1% of cases. The principal concern is thus potential transmission of the virus to contacts and during the perinatal period. It has been estimated that vertical transmission accounts for 40% of chronic carrier and more than one million deaths each year from HBV-related hepatic disease. The American College of Obstetricians and Gynecologists (1993) and the CDC (1996) both continue to endorse universal prenatal screening for hepatitis B. Such a strategy has been deemed cost-saving in identifying 20,000 HBsAg-seropositive women and preventing 3000 chronically infected neonates per year in the United States. High-risk status, including individuals of Asian and Eskimo background, admitted intravenous drug users, or prostitutes, may identify no more than 50% of infected women. Screening is performed at the first prenatal visit; however, testing should be repeated later in pregnancy and postpartum in seronegative mothers at high risk (CDC, 1991).

Transmission during labor and birth likely results from the mixing of maternal and fetal blood and contact with infected cervicovaginal secretions and amniotic fluid. Transplacental transmission may occur and explains some failures of immunoprophylaxis (Tang, 1990). Delivery by cesarean and avoidance of breast-feeding do not prevent infection of the newborn.

Without neonatal immunoprophylaxis, perinatal transmission occurs in 10% to 20% of HBsAg-positive women and in nearly 90% of individuals positive for both HBsAg and HBeAg (Sweet, 1990). Over 90% of infants born to HBeAg-seropositive women will continue as chronic carriers of HBV. The presence of HBeAg beyond the second month of life denotes likely chronic carriage. The risk of becoming a chronic carrier is independent of gestational age, birth weight, or viral subtype. A combination of passive and active immunization can effectively prevent most cases of horizontal and vertical transmission of hepatitis B. Individuals who have had household or sexual contact with infected individuals should undergo serologic testing to determine their immune status. If they are found to be seronegative, hepatitis B IG is prescribed at a dose of 0.06 mL/kg by intramuscular injection. Hepatitis B vaccination is also advised (Table 53-5). This sequence is recommended for offspring of seropositive mothers who should receive 0.5 mL intramuscularly hepatitis B IG after birth. The hepatitis B vaccination series is then instituted within 12 hours of birth. This vaccine is composed of inactivated portions of the surface antigen manufactured by recombinant DNA technology. The strategy of neonatal immunoprophylaxis is between 85% and 95% effective in preventing neonatal hepatitis B infection.

TABLE 53-4. SEROLOGIC DIAGNOSIS OF HEPATITIS B

Status	Key Marker	Other Markers
Acute hepatitis B	IgM anti-HBc (high-titer)	HBsAg, HBeAg, HBV DNA
Chronic hepatitis B with high virus replication		HBV DNA, HBeAg
With low virus replication	HBsAg in the absence of high-titer IgM anti-HBc	Anti-HBe and no HBV DNA
With pre-core mutation*		HBeAg seronegative with HBV DNA

* Results in failure of HBeAg production; HBcAg is unaffected.
anti-HBc, antibodies to hepatitis B care antigen; anti-HBe, antibodies to hepatitis B e antigen; HBeAg, hepatitis B e antigen; HBsAg; hepatitis B surface antigen; HBV; hepatitis B virus.

TABLE 53-5. HEPATITIS B VIRUS PERINATAL POSTEXPOSURE RECOMMENDATIONS

HBIG Dose	Timing	Vaccine* Dose[†]	Timing
0.5 mL (250 IU)	Within 12 h	5–10 (μg IM)	Within 12 h

* Fir+-st dose given concurrently with HBIG but at different intramuscular sites. Schedules for basic course: 0, 1, and 6 months or 0, 1, 2, and 12 months.
[†] Dose and schedule depend on manufacturer's recommendations.
HBIG, hepatitis B immune glabulin; IM, intramuscularly.

Adapted from Update on adult immunization. Recommendations of the Immunization Practices Advisory Committee. MMWR Morb Mortal Wkly Rep RR12 **40**:33, 1991.

Women who present in labor with unknown HBsAg status should be considered potentially infectious until serologic testing confirms otherwise. In the absence of known natural serologic status, some institutions have used neonatal combined immunoprophylaxis as a cautionary approach. Despite recommendations for maternal screening and newborn immunoprophylaxis, approximately 10% of neonates of infected mothers fail to receive hepatitis B IG and vaccination after birth (CDC, 1996). Each institution should provide a systematic review of maternal hepatitis B status. Postimmunization testing is also important for high-risk groups likely to have carriers within a household. The CDC has recommended universal hepatitis B vaccination for all infants (CDC, 1991). Testing is recommended at 12 months to ensure presence of antibodies to HBsAg. The detection of IgM-anti-HBc suggests recent infection, whereas maternal IgG-anti-HBc may persist beyond 12 months. Immunization failures are generally believed to result from (1) a genetically predetermined response, (2) in utero infection, (3) immunosuppression such as from intercurrent human immunodeficiency virus (HIV) infection, (4) other diseases, or (5) the emergence of antibody escape variants of HBV (Carmen et al., 1990).

MEDICAL PERSONNEL CONCERNS

Health care workers may acquire hepatitis B infection from patients. Approximately 12,000 American medical and related personnel contract hepatitis B annually as a result of needlesticks or introduction of body fluids into mucous membranes. Of these cases, 1% to 2% develop fulminant hepatitis and die (Jagger et al., 1988). Prevention of such infections is promoted by (1) vaccination of health care workers, (2) vaccination of individuals at high risk for contracting hepatitis B, and (3) following universal precautions as they relate to sharp objects and handling of body fluids. Testing for anti-HBs approximately 1 month after the third vaccine dose is advisable, because poor responders are present in 20% of vaccinated individuals. Levels of anti-HBs fall greatly over time; however, immunocompetence is demonstrated in most individuals by an appropriate rise in antibody to an antigen challenge (immune memory). The minimum level of protective anti-HBs is unknown. Individuals who are poor responders to vaccination should receive hepatitis B IG after an exposure.

Infected health care workers may also pose a risk to patients by transmitting HBV during invasive procedures. If a patient does not have immunity to hepatitis B, an infected health care worker is obligated to inform their patient of the possibility of transmission of the virus if blood to blood exposure should occur. After consent is obtained, great care and caution should be used to prevent any sharp injury.

Hepatitis C

Hepatitis C virus (HCV) infection affects approximately 4 million individuals in the United States and is the primary indication for liver transplantation (Alter and Seef, 2002). The disease follows an indolent course such that only 25% to 30% of infected individuals are diagnosed (CDC, 1997). The prevalence of HCV infection among pregnant women varies from 1% to 5%, with the highest rates of infection present in urban populations (Berger, 1998).

HCV is blood-borne and is thus common in intravenous drug users and individuals having received multiple transfusions. Blood transfusion donors have been routinely tested for HCV since 1990. The disease has a peak incidence in ages 30 to 49 years; however, a large percentage of those affected report no risk factors. Only 24% of infected pregnant women gave a history of receiving blood products, and a similar percentage (27%) deny either transfusion or intravenous drug use (Reinus et al., 1992; Ward et al., 2000).

The incidence of HCV infection has fallen from 150,000 cases in 1994 to approximately 36,000 cases per year (CDC, 1997). Acute hepatitis C is generally a mild disease that is often undiagnosed; however, progression to chronic hepatitis is the norm, with at least 50% developing biochemical evidence of liver dysfunction. Unlike hepatitis B, passive and active immunization interventions do not exist. Whereas 30% to 40% of chronically infected individuals achieve remission after pharmacologic antiviral therapy, most experience a progressive course marked by histologically confirmed chronic hepatitis (Alter and Seef, 2000). Nearly 20% of those individuals eventually develop cirrhosis, and 1% to 6% may develop hepatocellular carcinoma (Alter et al., 1992; Seeff et al., 1992).

Most pregnant women with HCV infection are chronically infected and deny acute illness. Concurrent alcoholism, drug use, and coexisting HIV infection are associated risk factors. Hepatitis C is a 30- to 38-nm single-stranded RNA virus related to the flaviviruses and pestiviruses. The incubation period lasts 5 to 10 weeks. HCV represents a series of closely related quasispecies with six major genotypes having been identified. Genotypes 1 and 2 are most common in the United States. The diagnosis of HCV infection relies on the identification of anti-C antibody. Initial screening generally consists of an enzyme immunoassay. Confirmation is then obtained through a recombinant immunoblot assay against four specific viral antigens. Antibody may not be present until 4 to 5 months after acute infection. Importantly, presence of antibody does not distinguish acute from chronic disease or the extent of viremia present. Branched-chain DNA and reverse transcriptase polymerase chain reaction assays may be used to quantify HCV RNA or viremia loads. This information may have bearing on the risk of vertical transmission to the newborn (Granovsky et al., 1998).

PREGNANCY CONCERNS

There is no evidence that HCV infection affects fertility. The indolent nature of the disease with peek incidence in the childbearing age group make potential HCV infection a primary concern for the obstetrician. There appears to be no increase in miscarriage, prematurity, or obstetric interventions in anti-HCV–positive women compared with control subjects (Jabeen et al., 2000).

Vertical transmission of HCV may occur, although less frequently than HBV infection. Overall, the risk of perinatal transmission is approximately 5% (Resti et al., 1998; Conte et al., 2000). HIV coinfection drug abuse and high HCV viral loads are associated with an increased risk of perinatal transmission (Ohto et al., 1994; Granovsky et al., 1998). Vertical transmission among nonviremic gravidas is rare, yet unfortunately most anti-HCV gravidas are viremic at delivery, because HCV viremia is demonstrated in 55% to 75% of cases. A prospective study of 128 infants of anti-HCV–positive women without demonstrable viral load revealed no cases of perinatal transmission (Resti et al., 1998). Similar results were reported in 100 nonviremic pregnant women (Conte et al., 2000). The few studies revealing occasional vertical transmission in nonviremic women may represent RNA degrading in maternal samples, intermittent viremia, or potentially postnatal infection. Among 275 HCV RNA–positive women, Resti and coworkers (1998) reported a vertical transmission rate of 4.7%. Thirteen infants became infected and 6 were RNA positive at birth, raising the possibility of in utero transmission of HCV. Whereas contamination with maternal blood could explain these results, in utero infection has been reported after midtrimester amniocentesis (Minola et al., 2001). In Resti's report, no statistically significant difference was found between viral loads in mothers transmitting HCV to their offspring versus those not subsequently infected. In contrast, Ohto and associates (1994) found viral loads of mothers of infected newborns to be significantly higher than those of noninfected infants. A review of nine studies of 30 transmitting and 144 nontransmitting HCV-infected mother revealed that viral loads exceeded more than 10^6 copies/mL in 28 of 30 transmitting cases (Thomas et al., 1998).

HCV viremia and transmission appears to be more common in women coinfected with HIV. One report documented an HCV viremia rate of 49% in HIV-negative women compared with 82% in the HIV-positive population (Zanetti et al., 1998). Transmission rates from HIV-negative HCV viremic women averaged 8% in one analysis compared with 21% among HIV coinfected HCV viremic gravidas (Spencer et al., 1997).

PREGNANCY MANAGEMENT

There is no contraindication to pregnancy in HCV-infected women. Clearly, the risk of perinatal infection must be reviewed and the extent of maternal disease considered before making recommendations. Interferon and pegylated interferon alone and in combination with oral ribavirin may ameliorate disease and are being prescribed with increasing frequency to chronically infected individuals (Jaeckel et al., 2001). The potential toxicity of these drugs contraindicates their use in pregnancy at the present time. Their benefit in preventing neonatal infection has yet to be determined.

Whether a benefit exists for cesarean delivery to prevent vertical transmission is unknown. Gibb and colleagues (2000) reported an overall transmission rate of 6.7% with no cases of perinatal transmission in 31 elective cesarean sections. Other studies have shown conflicting results regarding the route of delivery and perinatal HCV transmission. Few studies distinguish between elective and emergency cesarean delivery and HIV coinfectivity. A large study of 275 HCV-positive women (Resti et al., 1998) found no difference in vertical transmission rates (4% vaginal versus 6% cesarean). Viral loads have not

been addressed in such analysis, and the question as to whether vertical transmission may be affected by route of delivery among gravidas with higher viral loads deserves future study. A similar hypothesis exists with respect to breast-feeding, although it has not been contraindicated in anti-HCV–positive women.

There is no current vaccine available for HCV. Whereas passive immunization with immunoglobulin is recommended after percutaneous exposure, immunoprophylaxis of the newborn has not been shown to be beneficial in clinical trials.

Hepatitis D

Hepatitis D is an RNA virus that is dependent on coinfection with hepatitis B for viral replication. It is only found as a simultaneous acute infection acquired with hepatitis B or as a superinfection in an individual who is a chronic hepatitis B carrier. Epidemiologic features of hepatitis D are similar to hepatitis B.

Coinfection with hepatitis B is generally self-limited and carries a similar risk of progression to chronic liver disease as isolated acute hepatitis B infection. However, superinfection with hepatitis D is associated with an 80% progression to chronic hepatitis. Superinfection ultimately occurs in 25% of chronic hepatitis B carriers. Those who develop chronic hepatitis ultimately have a 75% to 80% risk of cirrhosis with potential for liver failure.

The diagnosis of acute coinfection is confirmed by the presence of delta antigen or IgM specific antibody in sera of an individual demonstrating HBsAg and core antigen IgM. Superinfection is marked by specific antigen and IgM to hepatitis D and positive hepatitis B core antigen-IgG, indicating chronic hepatitis B infection.

Women with acute hepatitis D are managed supportively as with acute hepatitis of other etiologies. Those with chronic infection require monitoring of liver function, including coagulation parameters. Perinatal transmission of hepatitis D has been reported (Deinhardt and Gust, 1982); however, neonatal prophylaxis for hepatitis B usually prevents such transmission.

Hepatitis E

The hepatitis E virus is an RNA virus found most frequently in Asia, Africa, and South America. It is similar to hepatitis A in that it is transmitted by the fecal-oral route. The incubation period is 2 to 9 weeks, with an average of 45 days (Chauhan et al., 1992). In developing countries, fulminant maternal infection has been reported with mortality rates from 10% to 20% (Rab et al., 1997). These extreme cases are most common during the third trimester. Cases of hepatitis E in the United States have occurred exclusively in women who traveled to areas of the world where the virus is endemic (CDC, 1993).

Diagnosis of hepatitis E rests on identification of IgM antibody to hepatitis E virus in the sera of infected individuals. A fluorescent antibody assay and Western blot technology have been used to confirm the diagnosis.

Women with hepatitis E infection may require intensive care if liver failure develops. Intrauterine fetal demise may follow profound episodes of hypoglycemia. Although perinatal transmission is uncommon, it has been reported (Khuroo et al., 1995) and is associated with neonatal death. Thus, precaution should be taken when caring for infected women to minimize contact with infected feces and contaminated clothing.

Other Hepatic Viruses

Hepatitis resulting from the herpes viruses is rare during pregnancy, particularly in the immunocompetent woman. In patients receiving immunosuppressive drugs or infected with HIV, hepatitis may result from a variety of infectious causes, including herpes simplex virus and cytomegalovirus (CMV). Mortality rates exceeding 90% have been reported with HSV hepatitis during pregnancy (Young et al., 1996). A high index of suspicion is warranted when disseminated maternal herpes simplex infection is present because typical mucocutaneous lesions and jaundice may be absent in affected cases. Antiviral therapy consisting of acyclovir or vidarabine may be helpful in affected cases (Young et al., 1996).

CMV hepatitis is fairly common in individuals with advanced HIV infection. CMV may also be responsible for mass-like lesions of the hepatobiliary tract, mimicking malignancy or other causes of obstruction. Transplant patients are particularly susceptible to CMV, which may complicate pregnancy and pose a risk for fetal infection (Laifer et al., 1995). Serious CMV infections including hepatitis are treated with intravenous ganciclovir. This drug may induce neutropenia. There are little data regarding the use of this medication during pregnancy, and it is unknown whether maternal treatment prevents fetal infection. Similarly, there are little data regarding the safety of phosphonoformate (foscarnet), another drug used commonly in severe CMV infections. Hepatitis is a common feature of Epstein-Barr virus infection (mononucleosis). Most cases are self-limited, although liver failure may occasionally follow infection.

Human Immunodeficency Virus Infection

Liver diseases is common in late HIV infection and acquired immunodeficiency syndrome (see Chapter 40). Liver abnormalities may follow drug-induced hematoxicity, including the use of the antituberculosis drug isoniazid and trimethoprim-sulfamethoxazole treatment for *Pneumocystis carinii* infection. Acute and chronic hepatitis from common etiologic agents and from herpes viruses may occur as well. Opportunistic and fungal infections may lead to inflammation and obstruction of the biliary tract, cholestasis, and right upper quadrant pain. Potential agents include cryptosporidium, CVM toxoplasmosis, cryptococcus, and histoplasmosis and mycobacterium species. Intrahepatic neoplasms most likely associated with HIV infection include non-Hodgkin lymphoma and Kaposi sarcoma.

The clinical presentation of most liver diseases in women with HIV infection is nonspecific. Fever, hepatomegaly, right upper quadrant pain, and biochemical abnormalities consistent with cholestasis are typical features. Viral loads (RNA levels) are generally high in such cases. Imaging studies are valuable in differentiating HIV-related processes from other causes of cholestatic jaundice. CT, when used, should be accompanied by abdominal shielding. Liver biopsy may be valuable in securing tissue for culture and diagnosis.

■ CHRONIC LIVER DISEASE IN PREGNANCY

Chronic Nonviral Hepatitis

Chronic nonviral hepatitis may result from a variety of autoimmune conditions, alcoholism, and drug- or toxin-induced injury. Most cases of chronic nonviral hepatitis in reproductive-aged women results from autoimmune disease. Autoantibodies to smooth muscle and liver-specific proteins are present, as are antinuclear antibodies in most cases. Whereas amenorrhea and infertility are common in affected women, treatment with immunosuppressive regimens consisting of corticosteroids and azathioprine have stalled progression of disease and also resulted in renewed fertility. If disease activity is well controlled, most women will have a good prognosis for pregnancy. Prematurity, fetal growth retardation, and hypertensive disorders of pregnancy are, however, increased over the general population. Treatment with corticosteroids and azathioprine should be continued during pregnancy. Azathioprine is probably not teratogenic, although neonatal immunosuppression is a possible side effect (Little, 1997).

Cirrhosis

Pregnancy in women with cirrhosis is uncommon because most women experience oligomenorrhea and infertility. Nonetheless, over the years there have been considerable reports of end-stage liver disease coexisting with pregnancy. It is doubtful that any single institution or maternal-fetal specialist has managed a large number of such cases. Most series in the literature are 20 years or older.

Cirrhosis is associated with an increased risk for premature delivery and perinatal mortality. In a series of 95 pregnancies in 78 women with cirrhosis, 10 stillbirths were observed and no significant change in liver function occurred in two thirds of individuals (Huchzermeyer, 1971). Prematurity (20% risk) and need for early termination (18% risk) have also been reported (Schreyer et al., 1982). Maternal complications associated with cirrhosis include anemia, preeclampsia, postpartum hemorrhage, and bleeding from esophageal varices (Schreyer et al., 1982).

Bleeding from esophageal varices remains the most feared complication of cirrhosis and pregnancy. Maternal mortality is clearly a risk secondary to massive esophageal bleeding. Bleeding occurred in 18 of 23 women with known esophageal varices (Cheng, 1977). Portal decompression procedures were used successfully in several cases without adverse maternal-fetal effects. The risk for variceal bleeding increases as pregnancy advances because of increased circulating blood volume, elevation in portal pressure, and vena cava compression resulting in enhanced flow through the azygos venous system. Most bleeds occur during the second and third trimester, with some in the postpartum period. The likelihood of bleeding may be decreased in individuals who have undergone portal caval decompression procedures before pregnancy (Schreyer et al., 1982). It follows that the pregnant woman with cirrhosis must be evaluated endoscopically for varices with appropriate treatment undertaken (see later discussion under Portal Hypertension).

Because most women with cirrhosis will have an uncomplicated pregnancy, careful monitoring should allow progression to term. Nutritional intervention such as limiting protein intake is advised only in advanced cases and after surgical portal decompression. Maneuvers to reduce straining and thus portal pressure are advised if varices have been documented. Vaginal delivery is the preferred route of delivery, with an attempt to shorten the second stage by forceps or vacuum extraction to limit excessive pushing and increases in intra-abdominal pressure. Careful attention to the pharmacokinetics and metabolism of anesthetic agents must be considered. Postpartum bleeding may also be increased such that vitamin K, fresh frozen plasma, and platelets should be readily available.

Treatment for chronic liver disease may be affected by pregnancy. Immunosuppressive therapy for chronic hepatitis should generally be continued during pregnancy, although specific risks associated with therapies must be considered. Combination corticosteroid and azathioprine may be used in select cases. Interferon therapy for chronic active hepatitis B or C infection remains contraindicated in pregnancy largely because of the uncertain effects of this medication on the developing fetus.

Portal Hypertension

Although studies indicate that the pregnant woman with cirrhosis will most often have an uncomplicated pregnancy, the substantial risk of hemorrhage from bleeding varices must be emphasized to the patient and her family. Termination of pregnancy may be recommended if liver disease is deteriorating despite treatment or if significant varices are documented. Thus, any woman with cirrhosis and suspected portal hypertension should undergo esophagogastroduodenoscopy, preferably before or early during gestation. The death rate in pregnant women with cirrhosis ranges from 10% to 18%, with most of these cases complicated by massive gastrointestinal bleeding (Pajor and Lehoczky, 1994). Women at highest risk are those with a history of gastrointestinal bleeding antedating pregnancy.

Management of bleeding varices may be accomplished with sclerotherapy as an alternative to portacaval anastomosis. Some have suggested it is superior to portosystemic shunting to reducing recurrent bleeding episodes. In a study of 11 women with cirrhosis during pregnancy, four of six with documented varices experienced gastrointestinal hemorrhage requiring endoscopic sclerotherapy (Pajor and Lehoczky, 1994). Five of these women had significant coagulation disorders as well. In the entire series, there were six growth-retarded infants, three preterm deliveries, and one neonatal death. In addition to sclerotherapy, portal pressure may be reduced with beta-blocker therapy. Portal decompression surgery has been accomplished during pregnancy; however, it has clearly become a second-line approach to endoscopic sclerotherapy. Another feared complication in association with portal hypertension is the development of splenic artery aneurysm. Pulsed-wave Doppler and CT imaging may be helpful in establishing the diagnosis. Elective laparoscopic surgery with ligation should be strongly considered before pregnancy because rupture carries with it an enormous risk of maternal and fetal death.

Primary Biliary Cirrhosis

Primary biliary cirrhosis is a chronic liver disease of uncertain etiology, which initially presents as cholestasis and progresses eventually to cirrhosis and liver failure. Most patients present initially with pruritus and jaundice. Biochemical evidence of cholestasis is apparent with elevation of alkaline phosphatase and predominantly indirect hyperbilirubinemia. The diagnosis relies on the demonstration of antimitochondrial antibodies and liver histology consistent with cholestasis. Other causes of cholestasis, including mechanical obstruction, must be ruled out. The differential diagnosis includes IHCP, cholelithiasis, sclerosing cholangitis, and disorders of bilirubin metabolism.

Primary biliary cirrhosis rarely complicates pregnancy (Rabinovitz et al., 1995). The outcomes associated with pregnancy are variable and are probably related to disease stage. Nonetheless, fetal surveillance and ultrasonographic monitoring of fetal growth seem prudent. Drug therapy is aimed at relieving symptoms. As with IHCP, UDCA has replaced cholestyramine as primary therapy. Vitamin K supplementation should be considered before delivery.

Wilson Disease

Wilson disease is a rare disorder of copper metabolism characterized by liver failure and neurologic dysfunction. Kayser-Fleischer corneal rings are a hallmark of diagnosis; however, these may be absent in patients with liver disease. Levels of ceruloplasmin are depressed in Wilson disease but may actually increase to normal with advanced liver disease. The diagnosis must be considered in reproductive-aged women presenting with advanced liver disease of unknown etiology.

Treatment of Wilson disease consists primarily of penicillamine or trientine. These chelating agents are well tolerated during pregnancy and should be continued. Deterioration in hepatic function may occur if these medications are abruptly discontinued (Shimono et al., 1991). Several series have reported successful pregnancies in women with treated Wilson disease (Walshe, 1986; Fukuda et al., 1997; Toaff et al., 1977). Pregnancy outcomes do not appear to be affected, yet there is a single report of reversible neonatal cutis laxa in the offspring of a woman treated with 1500 mg penicillamine/day (Little, 1997). The drug clearly crosses the placenta and may result in copper deficiency in the fetus. Toxicity may occur when doses exceed 1500 mg/day. Lower dosing of penicillamine may be accomplished during pregnancy, which might lower the risk of this complication. Successful pregnancy has been reported in women receiving liver transplantation for Wilson disease (Rath et al., 1997).

Budd-Chiari Syndrome

Budd-Chiari syndrome is a rare disorder primarily of women that results from hepatic vein occlusion. This occurrence has been linked to both pregnancy and oral contraceptive use (Khuroo and Datta, 1980). In one series, nearly 15% of cases were associated with pregnancy (Khuroo and Datta, 1980). The disease may present either acutely with obstruction of major hepatic veins or may be chronic, marked by involvement of smaller interlobular veins. The chronic variety is clearly associated with a better prognosis. Both varieties produce congestion and necrosis of centrilobular areas of the liver (Dilawari et al., 1994). Large vein obstruction is often associated with pregnancy and preeclampsia (Gordon et al., 1991). Some have suggested that Budd-Chiari syndrome complicating pregnancy is associated with thrombophilias, including antiphospholipid antibodies and factor V Leiden mutation (Fickert et al., 1996; Segal et al., 1996).

Clinically, this disorder presents with abdominal pain, distention, and ascites. A high protein content of the ascitic fluid is present. Fever, nausea, vomiting, and jaundice may be present in some cases. Laboratory evaluation shows marked elevation of alkaline phosphatase beyond normal pregnancy levels. Liver enzymes are modestly elevated. Histologic examination is nonspecific, demonstrating centrilobular zonal congestion with hemorrhage and necrosis. Diagnosis can be achieved through pulsed-wave Doppler imaging, demonstrating direction and amplitude of flow. Percutaneous hepatic venous catheterization will show elevated hepatic vein pressures, venous occlusion, and collateral circulation. Magnetic resonance imaging may also aid in diagnosis (Gordon et al., 1991).

Women who develop acute major venous obstruction often deteriorate rapidly, with portal hypertension, variceal bleeding, and fulminant hepatic failure. Pregnancy outcome thus is dependent on maternal status. Porta caval shunting may improve portal hypertension and ascites, although many pregnant woman are not surgically stable enough to undergo this procedure. These procedures have been primarily accomplished in postpartum cases. There are reports of successful pregnancies after mesocaval shunting (Huguet et al., 1984). Patients developing Budd-Chiari syndrome should be evaluated for underlying thrombophilias. Even in the absence of such entities, treatment with anticoagulation is advised. Such therapy, however, does not eliminate the risk of recurrent thrombosis.

Sclerosing Cholangitis

Primary sclerosing cholangitis (PSC) is a chronic cholestatic disease of unknown etiology characterized by fibrosis and inflammation of the intra- and extrahepatic bile ducts. The disorder follows a progressive course, leading to biliary cirrhosis, hepatic failure, and ultimately death. Affected individuals are also at risk for the development of cholangiocarcinoma. PSC generally occurs in patients with ulcerative colitis and to a lesser extent Crohn disease. In most cases, the onset of inflammatory bowel disease precedes the development of PSC.

The etiology of PSC remains obscure; however, this disorder may have an immunologic basis. The number and percentage of circulating suppressor T cells are decreased and the T helper to T suppressor ratio is increased in affected patients (Wiesner et al., 1984). The presence of common human leukocyte antigen haplotypes and circulating immune complexes among affected individuals lends support to the theory that PSC is an autoimmune disease of the biliary system (Chapman and Jewell, 1985).

The diagnosis of PSC is based on clinical laboratory and histology findings and includes characteristic cholangiographic appearance of diffuse irregularity and narrowing of the hepatic bile ducts. Pruritus, jaundice, and abdominal pain are typically clinical features. Itching is generally severe enough to require UDCA or other therapies. Favorable pregnancy outcomes have been reported for women with PSC (Landon et al., 1987; Janczewska et al., 1996). In one series of 13 pregnancies including three with onset during gestation, no significant maternal or neonatal morbidity was observed (Janczewska et al., 1996). Individual case reports have detailed variable courses for PSC during pregnancy. In one report, the cholestatic process paradoxically improved with advancing gestation followed by a decline in hepatic function after delivery (Landon et al., 1987). Other reports have described deterioration of liver function (Nolan et al., 1994) and the need for transplantation during pregnancy (Paternoster et al., 1995). Severe elevations in fetal bile acid levels have been documented, including cholylglycine concentrations nearly 20 times greater than normal, indicating placental transfer (Landon et al., 1987). Meconium passage is common, and thus fetal surveillance is recommended with maternal PSC.

Acute Liver Failure*

Acute liver failure is an uncommon medical emergency during pregnancy. Fulminant hepatic failure is defined as the development of hepatic encephalopathy caused by severe liver dysfunction within 8 weeks of onset of symptoms in a patient with a previously normal liver function (Trey and Davidson, 1970). Late-onset hepatic failure (subacute hepatic necrosis) consists of the development of encephalopathy 8 to 26 weeks after the onset of symptoms. Early recognition of acute liver failure is essential because affected individuals should be promptly transferred to a tertiary facility where transplantation is potentially available.

The general management of acute hepatic failure is not altered by pregnancy or the underlying etiology (Lee and Williams, 1997). Assessment includes the likelihood of recovery and suitability for liver transplantation based on clinical indictors. A poor prognosis is associated with renal dysfunction, metabolic acidosis, hypotension, hyponatremia, and thrombocytopenia. Hepatic and portal venous blood flow should be assessed with Doppler ultrasound to document patency and direction of blood flow. Exclusion of HIV infection and previously undiagnosed Wilson disease by appropriate blood testing should be performed. Serial determinations of liver function tests and in particular prothrombin time are key in documenting the degree of liver dysfunction and prognosis.

Survival appears to be influenced by the interval between the onset of symptoms and jaundice and the subsequent development of encephalopathy. A better prognosis is associated with cases in which the interval is less than 7 days, such as occurs with hepatitis A and B infections. Longer intervals are more typical when the etiology of liver failure is indeterminate.

It is imperative to rule out pregnancy-associated diagnoses such as acute fatty liver, HELLP, or preeclampsia because delivery often leads to improvement or resolution of maternal condition. There is no evidence that delivering affects the course of liver failure in cases of viral hepatitis. Most cases of liver failure in North America are of indeterminate etiology; however, no specific data exist regarding the cause found during pregnancy. As mentioned previously, hepatitis E and B may be associated with fulminant liver failure during pregnancy in developing countries. Drug reactions, acetaminophen overdose, and toxin exposures are all potential etiologies. Acetaminophen overdose during pregnancy has been reported on numerous occasions (Riggs et al., 1989). The antidote N-acetylcysteine should be promptly administered in documented cases because the outcome is clearly affected if this is delayed. Maternal and fetal death as a result of maternal hepatotoxicity have been reported (Wang et al., 1997).

Etiology is the most important variable for predicting survival without transplantation. Specific serologic tests are necessary, because clinical features overlap with other causes of acute liver failure (see Table 53-2). Seronegativity for HBsAg is not sufficient to exclude hepatitis B, because this antigen is cleared abnormally rapidly in fulminant hepatitis B. Persistent high-titer HBsAg points to another cause of hepatic failure, especially superinfection of a chronic carrier with other viruses. Multiple viral etiologic mechanisms should also be

---

* This section was adapted from Fagan, EA: Diseases of the Liver, Biliary System, and Pancreas. *In* Creasy RK, Resnik R (eds): Maternal-Fetal Medicine. 4th ed. Philadelphia, WB Saunders, 1999.

considered, especially in intravenous drug users. Acute hepatitis C rarely causes acute liver failure. Hepatitis E is uncommon in the United States and the West but should be considered in travelers returning from high-prevalence countries. Importantly, assays for testing IgM and antibodies to hepatitis E are not sensitive to all serotypes and may be positive only transiently in severe illness, including during pregnancy (Fagan et al., 1994). Hepatitis D antibodies may be negative in the early phase of fulminant hepatitis D and B coinfection. A full panel of serologic markers should be sought repeatedly if negative. These include seroconversion to IgG antibodies for hepatitis A, D, and E and seroconversion to anti-HBs and anti-HBe in fulminant hepatitis B.

The differential diagnosis in pregnancy includes viral hepatitis, AFLP, severe preeclampsia and toxemia of pregnancy, HELLP syndrome, and overlapping conditions such as thrombotic thrombocytopenic purpura and hemolytic-uremic syndrome. Severe hyperemesis gravidarum, Budd-Chiari syndrome, alcohol hepatitis, pancreatitis, septicemias, and infective conditions such as leptospirosis may present with drowsiness, renal impairment, and jaundice. Chronic liver disease, especially Wilson disease and autoimmune chronic active hepatitis, and malignant infiltrations of liver may be clinically indistinguishable (Pereira et al., 1997).

Clinical features of acute liver failure are not diagnostic. Cutaneous stigmata such as spider nevi and palmar erythema can be seen in acute liver failure, chronic liver disease, and healthy pregnancy. Systolic hypertension may indicate cerebral edema. The liver usually is small; a palpable liver in pregnancy may indicate infiltration. Splenomegaly and hemolysis, although uncommon, are found in Wilson disease and other chronic liver disorders.

The polymorphonuclear leukocytosis emphasized in acute fatty liver, hematologic disturbances in disseminated intravascular coagulation, and platelet counts below 100×10^9/liter are common in acute liver failure regardless of etiology (Pereira et al., 1997) because of sepsis, including fungal infection. Low levels of serum transaminase (aspartate aminotransferase or alanine aminotransferase) and platelet count have been reported in acute fatty liver, the toxemias, and HELLP syndrome. However, liver enzymes can rise above 2000 IU/liter with hepatic ischemia, rupture, and infarction. Relatively low levels of bilirubin and serum transaminase indicate extensive hepatocellular necrosis, lack of regeneration of hepatocytes, and a poor prognosis. Histologic documentation of massive hepatocyte necrosis only is of limited practical use.

Administration of fresh frozen plasma without overt bleeding does not alter outcome and obscures results of the prothrombin time. Vaginal delivery is less likely to be associated with excess blood loss compared with cesarean section (Pereira et al., 1997). Parenteral vitamin K_1 and folic acid should be given routinely. Fresh blood and blood products should be available to support any obstetric or surgical intervention. Gastrointestinal bleeding from gastric erosions is decreased by the prophylactic administration of an H_2 antagonist. The stomach should be emptied hourly to prevent aspiration of gastric contents. Early enteral feeding reduces translocation of microbes from the intestinal wall into the circulation and reverses the catabolic state. Elective endotracheal intubation may be required to protect the airway (particularly before transfer and surgical procedures, including delivery) before the development of overt cerebral edema. Intubation must be per-

formed by an experienced anesthetist. All sedation should be withdrawn.

Profound hypoglycemia remains a common cause of fetal and maternal death. Blood glucose levels should be closely monitored and immediate provisions made to administer large quantities of glucose (10% to 50% solutions) via a central venous catheter. The patient should be maintained at 10 to 20 degrees of elevation with minimal turning and stimulation. Early manifestations of cerebral edema include peaks of systolic hypertension and tachycardia and should be treated by mannitol (0.5 to 1.0 g/kg given as a bolus) to induce a diuresis (Lee and Williams, 1997). Mannitol is potentially nephrotoxic and is ineffective in renal failure. Serum osmolalities should be maintained between 290 and 315 mOsm/liter. Ultrafiltration and hemodialysis may be required to remove excess fluid. Levels of blood urea may be misleadingly low. Renal function is best monitored by serial levels of blood creatinine and creatinine clearance. Hyperventilation to reduce the partial pressure of carbon dioxide further reduces the limited brain flow and is no longer recommended. Intracranial pressure monitoring should be considered early on in the patient likely to progress to grade IV coma and in transplant candidates. Seizures seem to be more common than hitherto realized and should be suspected in a deteriorating patient without specific elevations in intracranial pressure. Such patients should be considered for assisted ventilation, especially if they require benzodiazepines and other sedative drugs. Detailed microbiologic cultures and analysis should be performed serially on all body fluids, including blood, urine, and sputum. Infections, including fungal infections, are common in liver failures. Hemoperfusion techniques using columns of charcoal and albumin-coated resin and plasmapheresis have been superseded by broad advances in medical and nursing care in specialized intensive care units (Lee and Williams, 1997).

Health care personnel should handle patients with care and should be provided with protective clothing. Pregnant and nonimmunized (for hepatitis A and B) personnel should not be allowed to nurse patients with suspected hepatitis A, B, or E.

The place of agents that inhibit virus replication, such as nucleoside analogues (lamivudine, famciclovir), protease inhibitors, phosphonoformate trisodium, and interferons, is under study for fulminant hepatitis B. Interferons have been given to three pregnant women with fulminant viral hepatitis, and two survived (Levin et al., 1989). Data on controlled trials in fulminant hepatitis are lacking. In fulminant hepatitis B and D, virus replication is less than in uncomplicated acute infection.

In controlled trials, corticosteroid have been found to be without benefit. The increased risks of microbial infection and known adverse effects on virus replication are sufficient to outweigh any marginal benefits except in the very rare case of drug-induced hypersensitivity with vasculitis.

Liver Transplantation

Liver transplantation has become more common, especially in individuals in the reproductive age group. Such women often are generally fertile after the procedure and thus may represent a challenge during pregnancy (Laifer and Guido, 1995). Aside from the risks associated with the chronic immunosuppressive therapy, there appears to be an increased rate of preeclampsia and prematurity in transplant recipients (Mass et al., 1996). Liver transplant recipients with biopsy-proven acute rejection during pregnancy appear to be at greater risk for both poorer outcomes and recurrent rejection episodes (Armenti et al., 1999). Whereas allograft rejection and graft loss may occur, the prevailing opinion is that pregnancy does not exacerbate or accelerate graft rejection (Laifer et al., 1995). Immunosuppressive therapy commonly used in liver transplant patients such as cyclosporine and tacrolimus do not appear to be teratogenic (Jain et al., 1997). The variation in serum levels of these medications during pregnancy underscores the requirement for cooperative management of these individuals between transplant specialists and maternal-fetal medicine physicians.

A successful outcome for pregnancy can be expected even in women who become pregnant in the first year after transplant (Patapis et al., 1997). Despite this fact, it has been recommended that attempts at conception be deferred for 1 to 2 years after transplant because complications are most likely during this time (Jain et al., 1997). Contraception is a critical issue for such women because oral contraceptives may promote hepatotoxicity of cyclosporine (Deray et al., 1987) and are contraindicated in women with Budd-Chiari syndrome. Regular cervical cytology should be obtained because the incidence of dysplasia is increased in women receiving immunosuppressive therapy (Mass et al., 1996).

For women who do eventually conceive, pregnancy outcome remains favorable. Spontaneous preterm delivery is increased, yet there appears to be no apparent risk for fetal growth restriction. Immunosuppressive drugs do cross the placenta and are concentrated in breast milk. Transient impairment in renal function has been reported in some cases (Laifer et al., 1995). A single case of congenital CMV complicated by hydrops fetalis has also been reported in a transplant patient (Laifer et al., 1995).

Liver transplantation has been undertaken during pregnancy for a variety of conditions, including Budd-Chiari syndrome, viral hepatitis, acute fatty liver, liver rupture, and cirrhosis from chronic hepatitis. Both maternal and fetal mortality are obvious concerns, yet transplantation for acute liver failure that is unlikely to resolve despite delivery of the fetus may become a necessity. In women who survive the transplant operation, increased risks for impaired hemostasis as a result of coagulopathy remain throughout pregnancy and delivery. Infection, renal failure, and adult respiratory distress syndrome are also frequent complications.

■ GALLBLADDER DISEASE

Cholelithiasis is common in the adult population as approximately 15% of women over age 35 have asymptomatic gallstones. Most of these stones contain predominantly cholesterol, and stones are found in 12% of pregnancies (Sung et al., 2000). Biliary sludge increased during pregnancy as a result of delayed gallbladder emptying, and thus pregnancy increases the likelihood of gallstone formation (Bennion and Grundy, 1978). Despite this, the frequency of acute cholecystitis is not increased during gestation (Kammerer, 1979). It has been suggested that the rise in sex steroid hormones during pregnancy inhibits gallbladder contraction with retention of cholesterol crystals, the precursor for stone formation. Gallbladder volume is increased both during fasting and postprandially when compared with nonpregnant women

(Braverman, 1980). Asymptomatic gallstones are frequently visualized when ultrasound is used for other diagnostic purposes during pregnancy (Valdivieso et al., 1993). Surgery is not indicated in such cases. Nonsurgical management of cholelithiasis in the nonpregnant individual has included bile acid therapy, lithotripsy, and dissolution with methyl terbutyl ether; however, none of these approaches is recommended during pregnancy because safety has not been established.

Biliary colic should be distinguished from acute cholecystitis. In the former case, episodes of spasmodic right upper quadrant pain present in a self-limited fashion that often requires no specific treatment. Ultrasonography is used to visualize stones and secure a diagnosis. In contrast, acute cholecystitis is marked by right upper quadrant pain in association with anorexia, nausea, vomiting, fever, and minimal leukocytosis. Obstruction of the cystic duct leads to inflammation and bacterial infection in at least half of cases. In the past, medical management was preferred during pregnancy because many women would respond without serious morbidity and the need for surgery (Landers et al., 1987). Medical management typically involves intravenous hydration, analgesics, nasogastric suction, and antibiotic administration. In a study of 42 women presenting with acute gallbladder disease during pregnancy, 26 responded to conservative therapy alone (Daradkeh et al., 1999). In another study, 15 of 26 women managed medically developed recurrent symptoms during pregnancy (Dixon et al., 1987). In this report, cholecystectomy performed during the second trimester was accompanied by minimal maternal morbidity and reduced hospitalizations. Whereas reported series of such women managed surgically tend to have more advanced disease, it appears that a more aggressive approach may be associated with less prematurity and more favorable outcomes (Lee et al., 2000).

In women who present with ascending cholangitis, common bile duct obstruction, or pancreatitis, cholecystectomy should clearly be performed. Common bile duct stones may be extracted through endoscopic retrograde cholangiopancreatography (Nesbitt et al., 1996). Over the past decade, considerable experience has been gained with laparoscopic cholecystectomy during pregnancy (Affleck et al., 1999; Barone et al., 1999). A laparoscopic approach is apparently feasible during the third trimester as well (Sung et al., 2000). In a report comparing 20 laparoscopies with 26 open cholecystectomies between 1992 and 1996, only one patient undergoing laparoscopy developed preterm labor (Barone et al., 1999). Similar success with favorable outcomes have been documented in a review of over 100 cases of laparoscopic cholecystectomy during pregnancy (Graham et al., 1998). Because nearly 36% of women with symptomatic gallstones initially managed conservatively during pregnancy may eventually require surgery, laparoscopic cholecystectomy should be considered if disease is severe enough to warrant hospitalization (Glasgow et al., 1998).

■ PANCREATITIS

The true incidence of pancreatitis complicating pregnancy is difficult to ascertain. In a series of 500 cases of acute pancreatitis, only seven women developed the disease while pregnant (McKay et al., 1980). The incidence of pancreatitis during pregnancy has ranged from 1 in 1066 to 1 in 3300 pregnancies

(Wilkinson, 1973; Ramin et al., 1995). There appears to be a greater association of gallstones with the development of pancreatitis during gestation. McKay and colleagues (1980) reported 18 of 20 women who developed pancreatitis while pregnant or within 5 months postpartum had cholelithiasis. Block and Kelley (1989) reported that all 21 cases of pancreatitis during pregnancy in their institution were associated with gallstones. In nonpregnant individuals, alcoholism is by far the most common etiologic factor. Other causes for pancreatitis include familial hyperlipidemia, viral infection, hyperparathyroidism, thiazide ingestion, and penetrating duodenal ulcer. The normal hypertriglyceridemia of pregnancy may be exacerbated in patients with familial hyperlipidemia and thereby induce pancreatitis (Achard et al., 1991). These rare cases have been treated successfully with lipoprotein apheresis (Sanderson et al., 1991). Finally, there is an association of AFLP with pancreatitis.

The clinical presentation of pancreatitis is not significantly altered in pregnancy. The disease may occur at any stage in gestation but is more common in the third trimester and the puerperium. Epigastric pain, which may radiate to the flanks or shoulders along with abdominal tenderness, should prompt appropriate laboratory investigation. Occasionally, a patient will present with nausea and vomiting as her only complaints. Mild fever and leukocytosis may be present. Radiologic examination of the abdomen may simply reveal an adynamic ileus. Ultrasound imaging of the pancreas can be difficult. Therefore, if significant pancreatic necrosis is suspected, CT becomes preferable. In most cases, this radiologic study is unnecessary.

In evaluating the pregnant patient with suspected pancreatitis, the differential diagnosis includes most causes of abdominal pain in young women. These are principally peptic ulcer diseases, including perforation, acute cholecystitis, biliary colic, and intestinal obstruction. Specific tests used to corroborate the diagnosis of pancreatitis rely on the measurement of pancreatic enzymes, principally amylase. Elevated values should suggest pancreatitis, although they may be present with other conditions such as cholecystitis, intestinal obstruction, peptic ulcer disease, hepatic trauma, and ruptured ectopic pregnancy. Both serum amylase and lipase levels should be measured in suspected cases. These levels are typically elevated threefold over normal values.

In most cases, acute pancreatitis resolves spontaneously within several days (Ramin et al., 1995). However, in 10% of cases illness is complicated, and such patients are best managed in an intensive care environment. Pancreatic secretory activity should be reduced by not allowing the patient to take anything orally. Nasogastric suction is reserved for those with nausea and vomiting. Meperidine is the drug of choice for analgesia because, unlike morphine, it does not constrict the sphincter of Oddi. Fluid and electrolyte replacement and serial laboratory assays of hemoglobin, white blood cell count, amylase, liver function enzymes, glucose, and calcium are essential. In advanced cases, hypocalcemia may be present, and calcium replacement is necessary. Because there is a high likelihood of associated gallstone disease, endoscopic retrograde cholangiopancreatography may be beneficial if common duct obstruction has occurred. Patients who have been unable to eat for periods of greater than 1 week may also benefit from intravenous alimentation.

Percutaneous aspiration of pancreatic exudate is important in refractory cases. This CT-guided procedure may be necessary to distinguish between sterile and infected pancreatic necrosis. For infected cases, surgical drainage of the pancreatic exudate is necessary. Of course, laparotomy carries with it the added risks of preterm labor and delivery. Patients who relapse may also develop a pseudocyst. This complication required surgical intervention after a period of time in which an adequate drainage procedure can be accomplished.

REFERENCES

Affleck DG, Handrahan DL, Egger MJ, et al: The laparoscopic management of appendicitis and cholelithiasis during pregnancy. Am J Surg **178**:823, 1999.

Alter HJ, Seef LB: Recovery, persistence and sequelae in hepatitis C virus infection: A perspective on long-term outcome. Semin Liver Dis **20**:17, 2000.

Alter MJ, Margolis HS, Krawcsynski K, et al: The natural history of community-acquired hepatitis C in the United State. The Sentinel Counties Chronic non-A, non-B Hepatitis Study Team. N Engl J Med **327**:1899, 1992.

American College of Obstetricians and Gynecologists: Hepatitis in pregnancy. Int J Gynaecol Obstet **42**:189, 1993.

Amon E, Allen SR, Petrie RH, et al: Acute fatty liver of pregnancy associated with preeclampsia: Management of hepatic failure with postpartum liver transplantation. Am J Perinatol **8**:278, 1991.

Archard JM, Westeel PF, Morniere P, et al: Pancreatitis related to severe acute hypertriglyceridemia during pregnancy: Treatment with lipoprotein apheresis. Intensive Care Med **17**:236, 1991.

Armenti VT, Wilson GA, Radomski JS, et al: Report from the National Transplantation Pregnancy Registry (NTPR): Outcomes of pregnancy after transplantation. Clin Transplant **1**:111, 1999.

Bacq Y, Sapey T, Brechot MC, et al: Intrahepatic cholestasis of pregnancy: A French prospective study. Hepatology **26**:358, 1997.

Barone JE, Bears S, Chen S, et al: Outcome study of cholecystectomy during pregnancy. Am J Surv **177**:232, 1999.

Barton JR, Riely CA, Adamec TA, et al: Hepatic histopathologic condition does not correlate with laboratory abnormalities in HELLP syndrome. Am J Obstet Gynecol **167**:1538, 1992.

Barton JR, Sibai BM: Hepatic imaging findings in HELLP syndrome (hemolysis, elevated liver enzymes and low platelet count). Am J Obstet Gynecol **174**:1820, 1996.

Bennion LJ, Grundy SM: Risk factors for the development of cholelithiasis in man. N Engl J Med **299**:1221, 1978.

Berg B, Helm G, Petersohn L, et al: Cholestasis of pregnancy: Clinical and laboratory studies. Acta Obstet Gynaecol Scand **65**:107, 1986.

Berger A: Mother to child transmission of hepatitis C virus: Prospective study of risk factors and timing of infection in children born to women seronegative for HIV-1. Science commentary: Behavior of hepatitis C virus. BMJ **317**:440, 1998.

Block P, Kelley TR: Management of gallstone pancreatitis during pregnancy and the postpartum period. Surg Gynecol Obstet **168**:426, 1989.

Braverman DZ, Johnson ML, Kern F Jr: Effects of pregnancy and contraceptive steroids on gallbladder functions. N Engl J Med **302**:362, 1980.

Brites D, Rodrigues CMP, Oliverira N, et al: Correction of maternal serum bile acid profile during ursodeoxycholic acid therapy in cholestasis of pregnancy. J Hepatol **28**:91, 1998.

Carmen WF, Zanetti AR, Karayiannis P, et al: Vaccine-induced escape mutant of hepatitis B virus. Lancet **336**:325, 1990.

Castro MA, Fassett MJ, Reynolds TB, et al: Reversible peripartum liver failure: A new perspective on the diagnosis, treatment, and cause of acute fatty liver of pregnancy, based on 28 consecutive cases. Am J Obstet Gynecol **181**:289, 1999.

Centers for Disease Control (CDC): Public health service interagency guidelines for screening donors of blood, plasma, organs, tissues, and semen for evidence of hepatitis B and hepatitis C. MMWR Morb Mortal Wkly Rep **40**:1, 1991.

Centers for Disease Control (CDC): Hepatitis A among homosexual men—United States, Canada, and Australia. MMWR Morb Mortal Wkly Rep **4**:155, 1992.

Centers for Disease Control and Prevention (CDC): Hepatitis E among U.S. travelers, 1989–1992. MMWR Morb Mortal Wkly Rep **42**:1, 1993.

Centers for Disease Control and Prevention (CDC): Prevention of perinatal hepatitis B by enhanced case management. MMWR Morb Mortal Wkly Rep **45**:584, 1996.

Centers for Disease Control and Prevention (CDC): Recommendations for prevention and control of hepatitis C virus (HCV) infection and HCV-related disease. MMWR Morb Mortal Wkly Rep 15:1, 1997.

Chapman RWG, Jewell DP: Primary sclerosing cholangitis—an immunologically mediated disease? West J Med 143:193, 1985.

Chauhan A, Jameel S, Chawla YK, et al: Common etiological agent for epidemic and sporadic non-A, non-B hepatitis. Lancet 339:1509, 1992.

Cheng YS: Pregnancy in liver cirrhosis and/or portal hypertension. Am J Obstet Gynecol 128:812, 1977.

Conte D, Fraquelli M, Prati D, et al: Prevalence and clinical course of chronic hepatitis C virus (HVC) infection and rate of HCV vertical transmission in a cohort of 15,250 pregnant women. Hepatology 31:751, 2000.

Daradkeh S, Sumrein I, Paoud F, et al: Management of gallbladder stones during pregnancy: Conservative treatment or cholecystectomy? Hepatogastroenterology 46:3074, 1999.

Davies MH, da Silva RCMA, Jones SR, et al: Fetal mortality associated with cholestasis of pregnancy and the potential benefits of therapy with ursodeoxycholic acid. Gut 37:580, 1995.

Deinhardt F, Gust I: Viral hepatitis. Bull WHO 60:661, 1982.

den Boer ME, Ljlst L, Wijburg FA, et al: Heterozgosity for the common LCHAD mutation (1528 g > C) is not a major cause of HELLP syndrome and the prevalence of the mutation in the Dutch population is low. Pediatr Res 48:151, 2000.

Deray G, le Hoang P, Cacoub P, et al: Oral contraceptives interaction with cyclosporine (letter). Lancet 1:158, 1987.

Dilawari JB, Bambery P, Chawla Y, et al: Hepatic outflow obstruction (Budd-Chiari syndrome): Experience with 177 patients and a review of the literature. Medicine 73:21, 1994

Dinsmoor MJ: Hepatitis in the obstetric patient. Infect Dis North Am 11:77, 1997.

Dixon NF, Faddis DM, Silberman H: Aggressive management of cholecystitis during pregnancy. Am J Surg 154:294, 1987.

Dixon PH, Weerasekera N, Linton KJ, et al: Heterozygous MDR3 missense mutation associated with intrahepatic cholestasis of pregnancy: Evidence for a defect in protein trafficking. Hum Mol Genet 8:1209, 2000.

Ebert EC, Sun EA, Wright SH, et al: Does early diagnosis and delivery in acute fatty liver of pregnancy lead to improvement in maternal and infant survival? Dig Dis Sci 29:453, 1984.

Fagan EA: Intrahepatic cholestasis of pregnancy. Br Med J 309:1243, 1994

Fickert P, Ramschak H, Kenner L, et al: Acute Budd-Chiari syndrome with fulminant hepatic failure in a pregnant woman with factor V Leiden mutation. Gastroenterology 111:1670, 1996.

Fisk NM, Bye WB, Storey GNB: Maternal features of obstetric cholestasis: 20 years experience at King George V Hospital. Aust N Z Obstet Gynaecol 28:172, 1988.

Fukuda K, Ishii A, Matsue Y, et al: Pregnancy and delivery in penicillamine treated patients with Wilson's disease. Tohoku J Exp Med 123:279, 1977.

Glasgow RE, Visser BC, Harris HW, et al: Changing management of gallstone disease during pregnancy. Surg Endosc 12:241, 1998.

Gonzales M, Reyes H, Arrese M, et al: Intrahepatic cholestasis of pregnancy in twin pregnancies. J Hepatol 9:84, 1989.

Goodacre RL, Hunter DJ, Millward S, et al: The diagnosis of acute fatty liver of pregnancy by computed tomography. J Clin Gastroenterol 10:680, 1988.

Gordon S, Polson D, Shirkhoda A: Budd-Chiari syndrome complicating pre-eclampsia: Diagnosis by magnetic resonance imaging. J Clin Gastroenterol 13:460, 1991.

Graham G, Baxi L, Tharakan T: Laparoscopic cholecystectomy during pregnancy: A case series and review of the literature. Obstet Gynecol Surv 53:566, 1998.

Granovsky MO, Minkoff HL, Tess BH, et al: Hepatitis C virus infection in the mothers and infants cohort study. Pediatrics 102:355, 1998.

Gylling H, Riikonen S, Nikkila K, et al: Oral guar gum treatment of intrahepatic cholestasis and pruritus in pregnant women: Effects on serum cholesanol and other non-cholesterol sterols. Eur J Clin Invest 28:359, 1998.

Hagerfeldt N, Venizelos N, Dobeln U: Clinical and biochemical presentation of long chain 3-hydroxyacyl-CoA dehydrogenase deficiency. J Inherit Metab Dis 18:245, 1995.

Heinonen S, Kirkinen P: Pregnancy outcome with intrahepatic cholestasis. Obstet Gynecol 94:189, 1999.

Hirvioja ML, Tuimala R, Vuori J: The treatment of intrahepatic cholestasis of pregnancy by dexamethasone. Br J Obstet Gynaecol 99:109, 1992.

Huchzermeyer H: Pregnancy in patients with liver cirrhosis and chronic hepatitis. Acta Hepatosplenol (Stuttg) 18:294, 1971.

Huguet C, Deliere T, Oliver JM, et al: Budd-Chiari syndrome with thrombosis of the inferior vena cava: Long-term patency of mesocaval and cavoatrial prosthetic bypass. Surgery 95:108, 1984.

Ibdah JA, Yang Z, Bennett MJ: Liver disease in pregnancy and fetal fatty acid oxidation defects. Mol Genet Metab 71:182, 1999.

Ibdah JA, Yang Z, Bennett MJ, et al: Liver disease in pregnancy and fetal fatty acid oxidation defects. Mol Genet Metab 71:182, 2000.

Issacs JD, Sims HF, Powell CK, et al: Maternal acute fatty liver of pregnancy associated with fetal trifunctional protein deficiency: Molecular characterization of a novel maternal mutant allele. Pediatr Res 40:393, 1996.

Jabeen T, Cannon B, Hogan M, et al: Pregnancy and pregnancy outcome in hepatitis C type 1b. Q J Med 93:597, 2000.

Jaeckel E, Cornberg M, Wedemeyer H, et al: Treatment of acute hepatitis C with interferon alpha-2b. N Engl J Med 345:1452, 2001.

Jagger J, Hunt EH, Brand-Elnagger J, et al: Rates of needles-stick injury caused by various devices in a universal hospital. N Engl J Med 319:284, 1988.

Jain A, Venkataramanan R, Fung JJ, et al: Pregnancy after liver transplantation under tacrolimus. Transplantation 64:559, 1997.

Janczewska T, Olsson R, Hultcrantz R, et al: Pregnancy in patients with primary sclerosing cholangitis. Liver 16:326, 1996.

Jones EA, Bergasa NV: The pruritus of cholestasis. Hepatology 29(4):1003, 1999.

Kammerer WS: Nonobstetric surgery during pregnancy. Med Clin North Am 63:1157, 1979.

Khuroo M, Datta D: Budd-Chiari syndrome following pregnancy: Report of 16 cases with roentgenologic hemodynamic and histologic studies of the hepatic outflow tract. Am J Med 8:113, 1980.

Khuroo MS, Kamili S, Jameel S: Vertical transmission of hepatitis E virus. Lancet 345:1025, 1995.

Knox TA, Olans LB: Liver disease in pregnancy. N Engl J Med 335:568, 1996.

Kowdley KV: Ursodeoxycholic acid therapy in hepatobiliary disease. Am J Med 108:690, 2000.

Kretowicz E, McIntyre HD: Intrahepatic cholestasis of pregnancy, worsening after dexamethsone. Aust N Z Obstet Gynaecol 34:211, 1994.

Krueger K, Hoffman B, Lee W: Hepatic infarction associated with eclampsia. Am J Gastroenterol 85:588, 1990.

Laatikinen T: Effect of cholestyramine and phenobarbital on pruritus and serum bile acid levels in cholestasis of pregnancy. Am J Obstet Gynecol 132:501, 1978.

Laifer SA, Ehrlich GD, Huff DS, et al: Congenital cytomegalovirus infection in offspring of liver transplant recipients. Clin Infect Dis 20:52, 1995.

Laifer SA, Guido RS: Reproductive function and outcome of pregnancy after liver transplantation in women. Mayo Clin Proc 70:388, 1995.

Landers D, Carmona R, Crombleholme W, et al: Acute cholecystitis in pregnancy. Obstet Gynecol 69:131, 1987.

Landon MB, Soloway RD, Freeman LJ, et al: Primary sclerosing cholangitis. Obstet Gynecol 69:457, 1987.

Lee S, Bradley JP, Mele MM, et al: Cholelithiasis in pregnancy: Surgical versus medical management. Obstet Gynecol 95:S70, 2000.

Lee WM, Williams R (eds): Acute Liver Failure. Cambridge, England, Cambridge University Press, 1997.

Levin S, Leibowitz E, Torten J, et al: Interferon treatment in acute progressive and fulminant hepatitis. Isr J Med Sci 25:364, 1989.

Little BB: Immunosuppressant therapy during gestation (review). Semin Perinatal 21:143, 1997.

Locatelli A, Roncaglia N, Arreghini A, et al: Hepatitis C virus infection is associated with a higher incidence of cholestasis in pregnancy. Br J Obstet Gynaecol 106:498, 1999.

Lopez J, Glasinovic JC, Marinovic I, et al: Clinical and laboratory characterization in 100 cases of pregnancy cholestasis. Rev Med Chil 47:215, 1982 [In Spanish].

Mabie WC, Dacus JV, Sibai BM, et al: Computed tomography in acute fatty liver of pregnancy, J Reprod Med 35:815, 1988.

Maher J, Goldenberg R, Tamura T, et al: Albumin levels in pregnancy: A hypothesis that decreased levels of albumin are related to increasing levels of alpha-seroprotein. Early Hum Dev 34:209, 1993.

Mass K, Quint EH, Punch MR, et al: Gynecological and reproductive function after liver transplantation. Transplantation 62:476, 1996.

McKay AJ, O'Neill J, Imrie CW: Pancreatitis, pregnancy, and gallstones. Br J Obstet Gynaecol 87:47, 1980.

Meng L-J, Reyes H, Axelson M, et al: Progesterone metabolites and bile acids in serum of patients with intrahepatic cholestasis of pregnancy: Effects of ursodeoxycholic acid therapy. Hepatology 26:1573, 1997.

Meng LJ, Reyes H, Palma J, et al: Profiles of acids and progesterone metabolites in the urine and serum of women with intrahepatic cholestasis or pregnancy. J Hepatol 32:542, 2000.

Minakami H, Oka N, Sato T, et al: Preeclampsia: A microvesicular fat disease of the liver? Am J Obstet Gynecol **159**:1043, 1988

Minola E, Maccabruni A, Pacati I, et al: Amniocentesis as a possible risk factor for mother-to-infant transmission of hepatitis C virus. Hepatology **33**:5, 2001.

Minton D, Yancey MK, Dolson DJ, et al: Acute fatty liver of pregnancy in a patient with chronic active hepatitis and associated hepatocyte alpha 1-antrypsin inclusions. Obstet Gynecol **81**:819, 1993.

Minuk GY, Lui RC, Kelly JK: Rupture of the liver associated with acute fatty liver of pregnancy. Am J Gastroenterol **82**:457, 1987.

Moise JF Jr, Shah DM: Acute fatty liver of pregnancy: Etiology of fetal distress and fetal wastage. Obstet Gynecol **69**:482, 1987.

Nesbitt TH, Kay HH, McCoy MC, et al: Endoscopic management of biliary disease during pregnancy. Obstet Gynecol **87**:806, 1996.

Nicastri PL, Diaferia A, Tartagni M, et al: A randomized placebo-controlled trial of ursodeoxycholic acid and S-adenosylmethionine in the treatment of intrahepatic cholestasis of pregnancy. Br J Obstet Gynaecol **105**:1205, 1998.

Nolan DG, Martin LS, Nataragan S, et al: Fetal complications associated with extreme fetal bile acids and maternal primary sclerosing cholangitis. Obstet Gynecol **84**:695, 1994.

Ohto H, Terazawa S, Sasaki N, et al: Vertical Transmission of Hepatitis C Collaborative Study Group: Transmission of hepatic C virus from mother to infants. N Engl J Med **330**:744, 1994.

Pajor A, Lehoczky D: Pregnancy in liver cirrhosis—assessment of maternal and fetal risks in eleven patients and review of management. Gynecol Obstet Invest **38**:45, 1994.

Palma J, Reyes H, Ribalta J, et al: Effects of ursodeoxycholic acid in patients with intrahepatic cholestasis in pregnancy. Hepatology **15**:1043, 1992.

Palma J, Reyes H, Ribalta, J, et al: Ursodeoxycholic acid in treatment of cholestasis of pregnancy: A randomized, double blinded study controlled with placebo. J Hepatol **27**:1022, 1997.

Patapis P, Trani S, Mirza DF, et al: Outcome of graft function and pregnancy following liver transplantation. Transplant Proc **29**:1563, 1997.

Paternoster DM, Floreani A, Burra P: Liver transplantation and pregnancy. Int J Gynaecol Obstet **50**:199, 1995.

Pereira AP, O'Donohue J, Wendon J, et al: Maternal and perinatal outcome in severe pregnancy-related liver disease. Hepatology **26**:1258, 1997.

Purdie JM, Walters BN: Acute fatty liver of pregnancy: Clinical features and diagnosis. Aust N Z J Obstet Gynaecol **28**:62, 1988.

Rab MA, Bile MD, Mubarik MM, et al: Water-borne hepatitis E virus epidemic in Islamabad, Pakistan. A common source outbreak tracked to the malfunction of a modern water treatment plant. Am J Trop Med **57**:151, 1997.

Rabinovitz M, Appazamy R, Finkelstein S: Primary biliary cirrhosis diagnosed during pregnancy: Does it have a different outcome? Dig Dis Sci **40**:571, 1995.

Ramin KD, Ramin SM, Richey SD, et al: Acute pancreatitis in pregnancy. Am J Obstet Gynecol **173**:187, 1995.

Rath HC, Enger IM, Ruschoff J, et al: Acute hemolytic crisis as the initial manifestation of Wilson's disease. Z Gastroenterol **35**:199, 1997.

Reid R, Ivey KJ, Rencoret RH, et al: Fetal complications of obstetric cholestasis. Br Med J **1**:870, 1976.

Reinus JF, Leikin EL, Alter HJ, et al: Failure to detect vertical transmission of hepatitis C virus. Ann Intern Med **117**:881, 1992.

Resti M, Azzari C, Mannelli F, et al: Tuscany Study Group on Hepatitis C Virus Infection in Children. Mother to child transmission of hepatitis C virus: Prospective study of risk factors and timing of infection in children born to women seronegative for HIV-1. BMJ **317**:437, 1998.

Reyes H, Sandoval L, Wainstein A, et al: Acute fatty liver of pregnancy: A clinical study of 12 episodes in 11 patients. Gut **35**:11, 1994.

Reyes H, Simon F: Intrahepatic cholestasis of pregnancy: An estrogen-related disease. Semin Liver Dis **13**:289, 1993.

Reyes H, Sjovall J: Bile acids and progesterone metabolites in intrahepatic cholestasis of pregnancy. Ann Med **32**:94, 2000.

Riggs BS, Bronstein AC, Kulig K, et al: Acute acetaminophen overdose during pregnancy. Obstet Gynecol **74**:247, 1989.

Riikonen S, Savonius H, Gylling H, et al: Oral guar gum, a gel forming dietary fiber, relieves pruritus in intrahepatic cholestasis of pregnancy. Acta Obstet Gynaecol Scand **79**:260, 2000.

Rioseco AJ, Ivankovic MB, Manzur A, et al: Intrahepatic cholestasis of pregnancy: A retrospective case-control study of perinatal outcome. Am J Obstet Gynecol **170**:890, 1994.

Roh LS: Subcapsular hematoma in fatty liver of pregnancy. J Forensic Sci **31**:1509, 1986.

Sanderson SL, Iverius PH, Wilson DE: Successful hyperlipemic pregnancy. JAMA **265**(14):1858, 1991.

Schoeman MN, Batey RG, Wilcken B: Recurrent acute fatty liver of pregnancy associated with a fatty-acid oxidation defect in the offspring. Gastroenterology **100**:544, 1991.

Schreyer P, Caspi E, El-Hindi J, et al: Cirrhosis—pregnancy and delivery: A review. Obstet Gynecol Surv **37**:304, 1982.

Seeff LB, Buskell-Bales Z, Wright EC, et al: Long-term mortality after transfusion-associated non-A, non-B hepatitis. The National Heart, Lung, and Blood Institute Study Group. N Engl J Med **327**:1906, 1992.

Segal S, Shenhav S, Segal O, et al: Budd-Chiari syndrome complicating severe preeclampsia in a parturient with primary antiphospholipid syndrome. Eur J Obstet Gynaecol Reprod Biol **68**:227, 1996.

Serrano MA, Brites D, Larena MG, et al: Beneficial effects of ursodeoxycholic acid on alterations included by cholestasis of pregnancy in bile acid transport across the human placenta. J Hepatol **28**:829, 1998.

Shimono N, Ishibashi H, Ikematsu H, et al: Fulminant hepatic failure during perinatal period in a pregnant woman with Wilson's disease. Gastroenterol Jpn **26**:69, 1991.

Sibai B, Ramadan M, Usta I, et al: Maternal morbidity and mortality in 442 pregnancies with hemolysis elevated liver enzymes with low platelets (HELLP syndrome). Am J Obstet Gynecol **169**:1000, 1993.

Siegelman ES: MR imaging of diffuse liver disease. Hepatic fat and iron. Magn Reson Imag Clin North Am **5**:347, 1997.

Sims HF, Brackett JC, Powell CK, et al: The molecular basis of pediatric long chain 3-hydroxyacyl-CoA dehydrogenase deficiency associated with maternal acute fatty liver of pregnancy. Proc Natl Acad Sci USA **92**:841, 1995.

Smith LG, Moise KJ Jr, Dildy GA III, et al: Spontaneous rupture of liver during pregnancy: Current therapy. Obstet Gynecol **77**:171, 1999.

Spencer JD, Latt N, Beeby PJ, et al: Transmission of hepatitis C virus to infants of human immunodeficiency virus-negative intravenous drug-using mother: Rate of infection and assessment of risk factors for transmission. J Viral Hep **4**:395, 1997.

Sung H-P, Heinerman PM, Steiner H, et al: Laparoscopic cholecystectomy and interventional endoscopy for gallstone complications during pregnancy. Surg Endosc **14**:267, 2000.

Sweet RL: Hepatitis B infection in pregnancy. Obstet Gynecol Report **2**:128, 1990.

Syndman DR: Hepatitis in pregnancy. N Engl J Med **313**:1398, 1985.

Tang S: Study on the HBV infection and its rate. Chung Hua Lui Using Ping Hsueh Tsa Chih **11**:328, 1990.

Thomas SL, Newell M-L, Peckham CS, et al: A review of hepatitis C virus (HCV) vertical transmission: Risks of transmission to infants born to mother with and without HCV viraemia or human immunodeficiency virus infection. Int J Epidemiol **27**:108, 1998.

Toaff R, Toaff M, Peyser M, et al: Hepatolenticular degeneration (Wilson's disease) and pregnancy. Obstet Gynecol Surv **32**:497, 1977.

Trey C, Davidson CS: The management of fulminant hepatic failure. Progr Liver Dis **3**:282, 1970.

Tyni T, Ekholm E, Pihko H: Pregnancy complications are frequent in long-chain 3-hydroxyacyl-coenzyme A dehydrogenase deficiency. Am J Obstet Gynecol **178**:603, 1998.

Usta IM, Barton JR, Amon EA, et al: Acute fatty liver of pregnancy: An experience in the diagnosis and management of fourteen cases. Am J Obstet Gynecol **171**:1342, 1994.

Valdivieso V, Covarrubias C, Siegel F, et al: Pregnancy and cholelithiasis: Pathogenesis and natural course of gallstones diagnosed in early puerperium. Hepatology **17**:1, 1993.

Vanjak D, Moreau R, Roche-Sicot J, et al: Intrahepatic cholestasis of pregnancy and acute fatty liver of pregnancy: An unusual, but favorable association? Gastroenterology **110**:1123, 1991.

Van Le L, Podrasky A: Computed tomographic and ultrasonographic findings in women with acute fatty liver of pregnancy. J Reprod Med **35**:815, 1990.

Walshe JM: The management of pregnancy in Wilson's disease treated with trientine. Q J Med **58**:81, 1986.

Wang PH, Yang MJ, Lee WL, et al: Acetaminophen poisoning in late pregnancy. A case report. J Reprod Med **42**:367, 1997.

Ward C, Tudor-Williams G, Cotzias T, et al: Prevalence of hepatitis C among pregnant women attending an inner London obstetric department: Uptake and acceptability of named antenatal testing. Gut **27**:277, 2000.

Weinstein L: Syndrome of hemolysis elevated liver enzymes, and low platelet count: A severe consequence of hypertension in pregnancy. Am J Obstet Gynecol **142**:159, 1982.

Wiesner RH, Beaver SJ, Katzmann JA: Alterations of T-cell subsets and β-cells in primary sclerosing cholangitis. Gastroenterology **86:**1346, 1984.

Wilcken B, Leung K-C, Hammond, et al: Pregnancy and fetal long-chain 3-hydroxyacyl coenzyme A hydrogenase deficiency. Lancet **341:**407, 1993.

Williamson C, Gorelik J, Eaton BM, et al: The bile acid taurocholate impairs rate cardiomyocyte function: A proposed mechanism for intra-uterine fetal death in obstetric cholestasis. Clin Sci **4:**363, 2001.

Wilkinson EJ: Acute pancreatitis in pregnancy: A review of 98 cases and a report of 8 new cases. Obstet Gynecol Surg **28:**281, 1973.

Young FJ, Chafizadeh F, Oliveira VL, et al: Disseminated herpes virus infection during pregnancy. Clin Infect Dis **22:**51, 1996.

Zanetti AR, Tanzi E, Romano L, et al: Multicenter trial on mother-to-infant transmission of GBV-C virus. The Lombardy Study Group on Vertical/Perinatal Hepatitis Viruses Transmission. J Med Virol **54:**107, 1998.

Zimber A, Zusman I: Effects of secondary bile acid on the intrauterine development in rats. Teratology **42:**215, 1990.

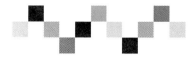

Chapter 54

RHEUMATOLOGIC AND CONNECTIVE TISSUE DISORDERS

Gary D. V. Hankins, MD, and Victor R. Suarez, MD

Connective tissue disorders (CTDs) share a common denominator: persistent, uncontrolled, immunologically mediated tissue damage of various organs (joints, skin, kidney, blood vessels, etc.). These autoimmune diseases arise when the immune system loses its ability to discriminate between self and non-self. Women, particularly during the reproductive years, are disproportionately affected by several of these autoimmune diseases (e.g., systemic lupus erythematosus [SLE], rheumatoid arthritis [RA], scleroderma, and Sjögren syndrome [SS]). These diseases are included within the rheumatologic diseases (CTDs or collagen diseases) because arthralgias and arthritis are very common complaints. Any woman with new-onset arthralgia or arthritis should have a thorough history and physical to rule out autoimmune CTD. Their clinical course is variable; for example, inflammatory polyarthritis can be a self-limiting disease, can develop into RA, or can differentiate into another form of chronic arthritis.

Normal pregnancy is a unique immunologic state where the fetus, despite being non-self (partial allograft), is recognized and tolerated by the maternal immune system while it remains immunocompetent. How the genetically mismatched fetus escapes rejection and how the mother avoids immunosuppression continue to be a biological enigma (see Chapter 7). In addition, why autoimmune diseases predominantly affect women continues to be an unresolved mystery. During pregnancy some of these syndromes improve or worsen, whereas most of the syndromes exacerbate during the postpartum period.

Although relatively rare, autoimmune diseases can be devastating to the patient if not promptly recognized and properly treated. These diseases have not only medical consequences, but also significant financial and social implications associated with treatment costs, lost wages, disability, and increased mortality. This chapter provides a review of the diagnosis and management of autoimmune rheumatic diseases during pregnancy, with detailed attention to the effects of pregnancy on the disease course and the effects of the disease and its treatment on mother and fetus. All pregnancies complicated with autoimmune diseases should be considered high risk and managed jointly between the obstetrician, perinatologist, internist, and the rheumatologist.

RHEUMATOID ARTHRITIS

Definition and Clinical Manifestations

RA is a chronic inflammatory/autoimmune disease characterized by symmetrical polyarthritis of the small joints of the hands and feet. Though polyarthritis is the hallmark of the disease, other organ systems—including the blood vessels, lungs, and cardiopulmonary system—may also be involved (extra-articular manifestations). RA has a prodromal phase that includes malaise, weight loss, arthralgias, or joint stiffness. The onset of the disease itself is usually insidious, with pain and swelling in one or more joints in the upper extremities, with involvement of the metacarpophalangeal and proximal interphalangeal joints. The progression is usually centripetal (from small joints to large joint arthritis); within the first weeks or months the disease tends to settle in the joints symmetrically, with the lower extremities (knees, ankles, toes) becoming also involved. Chronicity and remission are important aspects of the natural history of RA; the progressive erosive synovitis leads to fibrosis, ankylosis, and joint deformation.

Less often, RA starts as an acute process apparently triggered by surgery, trauma, stress, or the puerperium. Although any joint may be affected, involvement of the distal finger joints and lumbar and dorsal spine is rare. The hip joints are not spared, but fortunately their compromise is late and the need for hip abduction during vaginal delivery is not affected. In contrast, involvement of the temporomandibular joint and larynx (arytenoid fixation, nodules, and reflux laryngitis) are quite common in young patients, and this may cause difficulties during intubation for general anesthesia. Subluxation of cervical spine may also be present, although it is usually a late manifestation of RA.

Epidemiology

Although RA is a heterogeneous disease with a diverse spectrum of manifestations and course of illness, some consistent features have been observed across populations. Most RA patients are women (female-to-male ratio ranging from 2:1 to 4:1), its onset is frequently during childbearing age (20 to 40 years), there is an increased familial or immunogenetic risk in early age-onset disease, there is usually a predictable clinical improvement during pregnancy and worsening postpartum, and there is an increased incidence with aging (postmenopause). All the aforementioned suggest that hormonal factors influence the disease (Grossman and Brahn, 1997; Masi et al., 1999). Although RA affects approximately 1% of the general adult population, the exact prevalence during the childbearing years has been difficult to calculate. RA probably complicates pregnancy in 1:1000 to 1:2000 cases.

Despite the beneficial effect of pregnancy on RA, there is controversial epidemiologic data that pregnancy may protect from or at least postpone the development of RA later in life. Hazes and associates (1990) reported that the risk of RA in women who had ever been pregnant compared with women who had never been pregnant was 0.49 (95% confidence interval [CI], 0.27–0.91). They also found that the earlier the first pregnancy, the lower the risk of RA, and yet previable pregnancy had no protective effect. This presumed protective effect of pregnancy was found to be independent of oral contraceptive use, the presence of human leukocyte antigen (HLA)-DR4, or a family history of RA (Hazes et al., 1990).

Previous blood transfusion, smoking, obesity (Ollier et al., 2001), and termination of pregnancy have been associated with a higher risk of developing RA (odds ratio, 3.74; 95% CI, 1.4–9.9) (Carette et al., 2000). Factors associated with poorer prognosis in patients with early RA are female gender, larger number of joints involved, elevated levels of acute phase reactants, presence of rheumatoid factor (RF), and radiologic evidence of joint damage (Bresnihan, 2001).

Etiology

Although the etiology of RA remains unknown, it probably results from the combination of genetic susceptibility and exposure to an appropriate environmental trigger. Monozygotic twins have only a 30% to 50% concordance rate for RA. Genetic associations have been identified, particularly with the major histocompatibility complex class II antigens. Potential RA susceptibility genes include HLA-D, IL-1, aromatase, corticotropin-releasing hormone, and a region on the X chromosome (Ollier et al., 2001). So far, attempts to discover infectious causes have proven unsuccessful. Molecular immunologic studies of RA have identified risk factors for the disease, predictors of disease severity, the molecular mechanisms of inflammatory responses, and mechanisms of tissue destruction. It is known, for example, that inheriting certain genes in the major histocompatibility complex partly dictates susceptibility and severity of RA (Smith and Haynes, 2002).

During pregnancy, clinical improvement in women with RA is frequent. The mechanisms responsible for RA remission during pregnancy are still hypothetical and include theories on temporal changes in the levels of IgG terminal sugars (Alavi et al., 2000), pregnancy-associated β_2-glycoprotein (which has immunosuppressive action) (Unger et al., 1983), changes in the bidirectional communication between the neuroendocrine and the immune system with differences in lymphocyte subpopulations, and interleukin production that affects immune regulation, probably mediated by maternal–fetal disparity in HLA-D alleles (mainly DQ-alpha) (Nelson et al., 1992).

T cells can be categorized according to the cytokines they produce. Type 1 helper T cells (Th1) produce mainly interferon, tumor necrosis factor (TNF), and interleukin (IL)-2, whereas type 2 helper T cells (Th2) produce mainly IL-4 and IL-10. RA is regarded as a T-cell–mediated and Th1 immune response–driven disease. As in most specialized microenvironments, the normal synovial microenvironment represents a state of homeostasis in which Th1 responses are balanced by Th2 immune activation. The fetal–placental unit is a unique microenvironment, in which there is a shift from Th1 to Th2 immune response, increasing the anti-inflammatory cytokines IL-4 and IL-10 in concert with other cytokines, which may contribute to gestational amelioration of RA (Smith and Haynes, 2002). It has been proposed that cell-mediated immunity is suppressed and changed to Th2 by progesterone and prostaglandins.

Diagnosis

Early diagnosis and intervention may provide the greatest hope for reducing the disability associated with RA. Unfortunately, accurate diagnosis is usually delayed in patients with early RA by limited access to a specialist service, slow evolution of the clinical features of disease, and lack of absolute diagnostic criteria until the disease is far advanced. Plain radiographs of the joints are not sensitive (usually normal during the first 6 months of disease), but they are useful as a baseline and in detecting erosion at the end of long bones associated with RA (Davidson and Kaiser, 1997). When juxta-articular osteoporosis, joint erosions, and narrowing of joint spaces are detected in radiographs, they become the most specific of all laboratory tests for RA.

Acute phase reactants, serologic features including presence of RF, and immunohistologic analysis of synovial tissue can provide the basis for differentiating early RA from other forms of arthritis (Bresnihan, 2001). Up to 90% of patients with RA have RF present in blood, although its pathogenic role remains unclear. RF is an autoantibody against an antigenic epitope located on the constant (Fc) portion of IgG and IgM molecules. Despite the extremely strong association of RF with RA, RF clearly does not cause the disease because it occurs with other chronic inflammatory and infectious diseases (see later) and sometimes even in healthy individuals. RF is measured by the antihuman IgG latex agglutination test (Latex test) and anti-rabbit IgG hemagglutination test (RAHA test). One in every five patients with RA also has low titers of antinuclear antibody (ANA). Most autoantibody titers (RF, ANA, extractable nuclear antigen, anti-Jo-1, etc.) do not vary with disease flare-ups and remissions.

Given a compatible history and examination, RF, at titers of 1:160 or higher, is strongly supportive of the diagnosis of RA. RF is usually positive within a year of the onset of disease. Importantly, RF is also found in several chronic inflammatory and infectious diseases such as SLE, sarcoidosis, syphilis, tuberculosis, and endocarditis. The absence of RF will not rule out RA, but its presence confirms it (Davidson and Keiser, 1997).

Effects of Rheumatoid Arthritis on Pregnancy

When RA is already established, there is no indication of any adverse effects on pregnancy outcome (Nelson and Ostensen, 1997). This may reflect minimal or no transplacental passage of maternal pathogenic T cells or their inactivation when traffic does occur. Recently, the Arthritis Research Campaign Epidemiology Unit from the University of Manchester, United Kingdom, reported that infants born to women with arthritis and inflammatory polyarthritis had lower mean birth weight than control subjects (3.3 ± 0.5 kg [± standard deviation] compared with 3.5 ± 0.4 kg; $P = 0.004$), even after adjustment for potential confounding factors (Bowden et al., 2001). Although statistically significant, 200 g at term in appropriate-for-gestational-age weight infants seems of minimal clinical importance. Unfortunately, the authors did not report on the proportion of small-for-gestational-age or intrauterine growth-restricted infants born to RA patients. Pregnancy outcome in women who first developed RA during pregnancy seems un-affected, as well as that of apparently healthy women who later in life developed RA (Siamopoulou-Mavridou et al., 1988; Nelson et al., 1992).

Effects of Pregnancy on Rheumatoid Arthritis

Hormonal and reproductive factors influence RA susceptibility and severity. As mentioned previously, RA is more common in women than men, especially before menopause. Men may be protected by hormonal factors and require a stronger genetic component to develop disease (Ollier et al., 2001). Estrogens have been implicated as enhancers of humoral immunity, and androgens and progesterone are natural immune suppressors. Cutolo (2000) suggested a possible pathogenic role for the decreased levels of the immune-suppressive androgens. Sex hormone concentrations before glucocorticoid therapy have been evaluated in male and female RA patients. Hormonal levels were altered, especially in premenopausal women and male patients, particularly, low levels of gonadal and adrenal androgens (testosterone and dehydrotestosterone, dehydroepiandrosterone and dehydroepiandrosterone sulfate) and a reduced androgen-to-estrogen hormone ratio.

Pregnancy

The ameliorating effect of pregnancy on RA has been well known since 1938 and repeatedly confirmed for 75% of RA pregnancies. Improvement of symptoms usually occurs in the first trimester and increases as pregnancy progresses (Ostensen, 1999). The Epidemiology Unit from Manchester has raised the question that there may be a greater widespread variability in disease response than previously thought. In an attempt to standardize measures of disease activity with uniform assessment of joint symptoms, examination of inflamed joints, and application of the Health Assessment Questionnaire, this study found that only 23 of 140 patients followed prospectively were in complete remission (no joints with active disease and no therapy) during the third trimester (Barrett et al., 1999). The ameliorating effect of pregnancy on RA activity is actually greater than that of some of the newer therapeutic agents (Kanik and Wilder, 2000).

Although the reasons for the ameliorating effect of pregnancy on RA symptoms is not well understood, it is possible that the shift in the balance between Th1-type cytokines and Th2-type cytokines that occurs during pregnancy may play a role.

Puerperium

A relapse (flare) of RA is observed within 6 months after delivery in 90% of women (Ostensen, 1999). Mastorakos and Ilias (2000) proposed that a transient postpartum maternal hypothalamic corticotropin-releasing hormone suppression, together with the steroid withdrawal that follows parturition, might be causally related to mood disorders and the vulnerability to autoimmune diseases such as thyroiditis or RA often observed during this period. Contrarily, pregnancy has been described as a state of relative hypercortisolism. Hypothalamic corticotropin-releasing hormone secretion normalizes within 12 weeks (Mastorakos and Ilias, 2000).

Breast-Feeding

Hyperprolactinemia has been proposed as the explanation for why breast-feeding is associated with higher rates of postpartum RA flares (Barrett et al., 2000). Prolactin enhances inflammatory and antitumor responses (Th1-type cytokine-like effects) *in vitro*. Paradoxically, however, hyperprolactinemia can also be associated with conditions such as pregnancy, where remission of Th1-mediated diseases is known to occur in the context of a Th2-dominated milieu.

Contraception

Minimal supportive evidence exists for the concept that oral contraceptives protect against the development of RA. In fact, Drossaers-Bakker and colleagues (2002) studied the association between hormonal factors and the outcome of RA after a 12-year follow-up. These authors found that oral contraceptive use and pregnancy do not significantly influence outcome in long-term RA. However, they reported a statistical trend for patients with multiple pregnancies and long-term oral contraceptive use to have less radiographic joint damage and a better functional level.

Management

The primary objectives in treating women with RA are reduction of inflammation and pain, preservation of function, and prevention of deformities. Treatment of RA requires both drug and non-drug approaches. Nonpharmacologic measures include systemic and articular rest, appropriate use of heat and cold, assistive devices, and timely physical and occupational therapies.

Current drug therapy for RA consists of combinations of nonsteroidal anti-inflammatory drugs (NSAIDs) and disease-modifying antirheumatic drugs (DMARDs). NSAIDs reduce the pain and inflammation of RA and improve mobility but do not slow the progression of joint damage. DMARDs, which limit potentially irreversible joint damage, may influence the course of disease progression. Methotrexate, hydroxychloroquine, sulfasalazine, and low-dose corticosteroids are usually the mainstays of treatment for younger patients with RA (Bresnihan, 2001).

Analgesics and Anti-Inflammatory Drugs

The frequent prescription of acetaminophen (paracetamol) as the main therapeutic agent in the treatment of RA rather than specific anti-inflammatory agents is not justified. NSAIDs are not teratogenic in humans; thus, their cessation is not necessary periconceptionally. NSAIDs with preferential inhibition of cyclooxygenase II (COX-2) may offer a better safety profile than other NSAIDs. Conventional NSAIDs inhibit both COX isoforms to a similar extent and in an approximately equal dose and concentration range. The two recent clinically available selective COX-2 inhibitors, celecoxib and rofecoxib, are about 100 to 1000 times more selective on the COX-2 than on the COX-1 isoform. COX-2 is mainly an inducible isoform, although also to some extent is present constitutively in the central nervous system, the juxtaglomerular apparatus of the kidney, and in the placenta during late gestation (Everts et al., 2000). The well-known contraindications for NSAIDs, such as late pregnancy, aspirin-induced asthma, congestive heart failure, and renal dysfunction, apply also to the COX-2 inhibitors (Everts et al., 2000).

Although steroids produce a fast anti-inflammatory effect, they may not alter the progression of RA; furthermore, symptoms reappear when the drug is discontinued. At present, steroids are used either for short-term treatment during initiation of therapy, in bursts during acute disease flares, or chronically in low doses. Intra-articular steroid (triamcinolone) injection may be used for symptomatic relief of oligoarthritis, but no more often than four times a year.

Disease-Modifying Antirheumatic Drugs

Methotrexate is contraindicated during pregnancy because of its teratogenic effects. The critical dose for the "aminopterin syndrome" is probably above 10 mg of methotrexate per week, and the critical period is probably between 6 to 8 weeks' gestation (Feldkamp and Carey, 1993). For many rheumatologists, treatment with low-dose methotrexate is the drug of choice for nonpregnant RA patients who fail to respond to NSAIDs. Methotrexate is usually given between 7.5 and 20 mg/wk. Methotrexate is associated with serious side effects in about 5% of cases (hematologic, infectious, or respiratory). Other absolute contraindications include poor compliance and the possibility of mistakes in the timing of the administration, treatment with trimethoprim, hemodialysis, renal insufficiency (clearance no more than 50 mL/min), and alcoholism.

Antimalarials have not been associated with any fetal side effects and can be continued during pregnancy if necessary (Lima et al., 1995). Gold salts are indicated for erosive disease not responding to or not tolerating methotrexate treatment. Although not associated with neonatal malformations, gold salts have been found in the fetus's liver and kidney. Monthly injection of gold salts on the first day of menses ensures that it can be withdrawn as soon as pregnancy is recognized. Sulfasalazine has been used extensively during pregnancy and lactation in patients with inflammatory bowel disease. In such patients, sulfasalazine does not seem to cause an increase in either the incidence of fetal abnormalities or spontaneous abortions (Zeldis, 1989). Immunosuppressive drugs are occasionally used in the treatment of RA. Azathioprine, like methotrexate, is an antimetabolite and is effective for RA patients not responsive to antimalarials or gold. The fetal liver lacks the enzyme that converts azathioprine to its active metabolites; thus, azathioprine does not seem to be teratogenic in humans. Because teratogenicity of penicillamine is

still a debate issue, it seems prudent to discontinue it. Janssen and Genta (2000) published a more extensive review on this topic.

New Drugs

Leflunomide (Arava), a recently approved DMARD, is an isoxazole-based immunomodulator. Leflunomide is contraindicated during pregnancy (Kaplan, 2001). Animal studies have shown an increased rate of malformations and fetal death in various species. Because the drug has a prolonged and unpredictable elimination half-life, it should be stopped as soon as pregnancy is suspected or diagnosed. Ideally, leflunomide must be discontinued for 2 years before attempting conception; this time can be shortened if the patient opts for drug washout with cholestyramine, which enhances elimination (Bresnihan, 2001).

Etanercept (Enbrel) is a TNF blocking agent that has been considered a major advance in the treatment of RA. Etanercept is a fusion protein consisting of the extracellular ligand-binding domain of the 75-kDa receptor for TNF-α and the constant portion (Fc) of human IgG-1. The U.S. Food and Drug Administration approved etanercept for treatment of multidrug-resistant RA in 1998. In patients with active RA (American College of Rheumatologists [ACR] functional classes I to III) who had failed to respond to previous treatment with one or more DMARDs, etanercept, alone or in combination with methotrexate, produced improvements in all components included in the ACR's disease activity measures (Jarvis and Faulds, 1999). Minimal human data exist regarding the impact of anti-TNF-α therapy on human reproductive function. Because TNF-α potentiates collagenolysis and ovulation, there exists a theoretical risk that TNF-α inhibition could exert an undesirable effect on conception. Sills and associates (2001) reported the first case of ovulation induction, intrauterine insemination, normal pregnancy, and singleton delivery of a healthy infant after chronic (more than 1 year) preovulatory TNF-α inhibitor therapy for RA. A recent overview of the use of DMARDs during pregnancy has been published by Chakravarty and associates (2003).

The use of thalidomide during the 1950s resulted in teratogenic effects in thousands of infants. Although thalidomide (Thalomid) is currently approved for the treatment of a complication of leprosy, it is commercially available to treat some rheumatologic diseases through a controlled distribution system. Currently, no definite thalidomide therapeutic effects have been proved for RA patients.

■ SYSTEMIC LUPUS ERYTHEMATOSUS

Definition

SLE is a multisystemic autoimmune rheumatic disease, with protean and often complex manifestations. SLE can follow an unpredictable course and can be either chronic or of a relapsing and remitting form. SLE has serious musculoskeletal, renal, and cardiovascular effects. Most of these adverse consequences are not only secondary to the disease itself but to its associated treatment (corticosteroids) (Petri, 2001).

Pathogenesis

Current evidence suggest that SLE occurs when a patient develops persistent pathogenic autoantibodies (against nuclear antigens) and immune complexes that alter the normal anatomy and function of target tissues and organs (skin, glomeruli, platelets, or erythrocytes, etc.), giving rise to a constellation of symptoms and signs (rash, nephritis, thrombocytopenia, anemia, etc.). Individuals developing SLE are affected by their own genetic susceptibility (HLA and non-HLA genes) to produce a persistent hyperactivation of humoral and cellular autoimmunity with their environment. Ultraviolet B light is a definite environmental factor linked to SLE pathogenesis (Hahn, 2001).

Highly specific autoantibody profiles in the mother (independent of whether she has a clinical disease or not) are associated with fetal demise and neonatal lupus syndromes, the most serious manifestation of which is isolated congenital heart block (CHB). The former is associated with antiphospholipid antibodies and the latter with antibodies directed against SSA/Ro and SSB/La polypeptides.

Arterial or venous thromboses and recurrent fetal loss characterize the antiphospholipid antibody syndrome (APS). It occurs as primary disease but also in the context of SLE. Whereas primary APS induces a thrombotic microangiopathy without significant inflammatory reaction, secondary APS in SLE is usually associated with vasculitis. Patients with SLE frequently have some antiphospholipid antibodies to β_2-glycoprotein-I, prothrombin, protein C, protein S, and annexin V. Thrombotic complications in SLE may depend on the antigenic specificities of these antibodies, alone or in combination. Multivariate analysis has shown that both anti-β_2-glycoprotein-I and anti-prothrombin antibodies are a significant risk factor for arterial thrombosis (odds ratios, 8.8 and 14.5, respectively; 95% CIs, 3.2–25 and 1.8–116, respectively) but not for venous thrombosis. Conversely, the presence of anti-protein S antibodies is a significant risk factor for venous thrombosis (odds ratio, 30.4; 95% CI, 3.3–281) but not for arterial thrombosis. The only significant risk factor for fetal loss was the presence of anti-annexin V antibodies (odds ratio, 5.9; 95% CI, 1.4–14.8) (Nojima et al., 2001). The antiphospholipid syndrome will be considered in more details separately in Chapter 48.

Recent data link sex hormones and prolactin to SLE activity, which may be one of the explanations for the frequency of SLE flares during pregnancy (Khamashta et al., 1997). Additionally, fetal–maternal cell trafficking, or the passage of fetal cells into the maternal circulation and maternal cells into their offspring (maternal microchimerism), has been suggested in the pathogenesis of autoimmune disease, particularly SLE (Lambert et al., 2001).

Diagnosis

Clinical suspicion is the key for SLE diagnosis. SLE is not a single and simple disease entity; it is rather a group of related syndromes with broadly based criteria used for its classification and diagnosis. In 1997 and 1999 the ACR updated the classification criteria for SLE (Table 54-1). The ACR incorporated new immunologic criteria ("positive finding of antiphospholipid antibodies," including IgG or IgM anticardiolipin antibodies and lupus anticoagulant), new neuropsychiatric manifestations of SLE, and deleted the "positive LE cell preparation" criterion (Hochberg, 1997; ACR, 1999). Per consensus, if any 4 or more of the 11 criteria are present, serially or simultaneously during any interval of observation, the definitive diagnosis of SLE is met.

Symptoms and Signs

It is unusual to make the diagnosis *de novo* during pregnancy; however, cases are still encountered. Diagnosis is difficult and often delayed. Most pregnant women with SLE complain of vague symptoms, including fatigue, myalgias, fluctuating low-grade fever (100 to 101°F), and weight loss. The characteristic butterfly rash over the nose and cheeks is absent in most or is subtle and difficult to distinguish from ordinary sunburn or the increased pigmentation of pregnancy. Pleurisy is a common early feature of lupus, but the pain is rarely severe, and sometimes the history emerges only during direct questioning. Vasospastic Raynaud phenomenon may be subtle and is particularly unusual in pregnancy.

Central nervous system manifestations are common and often subtle, occurring in about 50% of the patients and consisting mainly of disorders of thought content and of mood. Central nervous system disease may make the patient inattentive, difficult to communicate with, poorly compliant with therapy, or simply vexing to the physician. These central nervous system manifestations are occasionally heralded by seizures and may be overtly manifested by stroke-like symptoms. Chorea is a rare manifestation of lupus that may be estrogen induced (i.e., in pregnancy or with the combined oral contraceptive) (Donaldson and Espiner, 1971).

Patients' assessment of their own disease is very important. Isenberg (2002) asked 100 consecutive lupus patients about the most troublesome feature of their disease. Surprisingly, it was not fear of facial disfigurement, kidney failure, or death, but rather most patients said that it was fatigue. A useful index to assess this symptom is the Short Form 36. Although not designed specifically for use in lupus patients, it has been studied in numerous other multisystem diseases and normal values are based on approximately 10,000 healthy individuals (available at *www.sf36.com*).

Diagnosis of SLE is also problematic because of the frequent coexistence or later development of at least one other autoimmune disease. In a cohort of more than 200 lupus patients followed long term, 30% of them developed one or more of the following: SS, hyperthyroidism, hypothyroidism, erosive arthritis typical of RA, myasthenia gravis, autoimmune cirrhosis, parathyroidism, or celiac disease (McDonagh and Isenberg, 2000).

Laboratory Testing

Laboratory markers may rule in or rule out the diagnosis. Numerous autoantibodies are associated with SLE. ANAs are highly sensitive but not highly specific and thus are used for screening purposes. Farnam and associates (1984) reported a false-positive rate of 10% for ANA during normal uncomplicated pregnancy compared with only 2% in age-matched nonpregnant control subjects. This screening test collectively detects total ANAs against double-stranded (native) DNA

TABLE 54-1. REVISED CRITERIA FOR CLASSIFICATION OF SYSTEMIC LUPUS ERYTHEMATOSUS*

Criterion	Definition
1. Malar rash	Fixed erythema, flat or raised, over the malar eminences, tending to spare the nasolabial folds
2. Discoid rash	Erythematous raised patches with adherent keratotic scaling and follicular plugging; atrophic scarring may occur in older lesions
3. Photosensitivity	Skin rash as a result of unusual reaction to sunlight, by patient history or physician observation
4. Oral ulcers	Oral or nasopharyngeal ulceration, usually painless, observed by physician
5. Arthritis	Nonerosive arthritis involving 2 or more peripheral joints, characterized by tenderness, swelling, or effusion
6. Serositis	a. Pleuritis—convincing history of pleuritic pain or rubbing heard by a physician or evidence of pleural effusion *OR* b. Pericarditis—documented by ECG or rub or evidence of pericardial effusion
7. Renal disorder	a. Persistent proteinuria greater than 0.5 g/d or greater than 3+ if quantitation not performed *OR* b. Cellular casts—may be red cell, hemoglobin, granular, tubular, or mixed
8. Neurologic disorder	a. Seizures—in the absence of offending drugs or known metabolic derangements; e.g., uremia, ketoacidosis, or electrolyte imbalance *OR* b. Psychosis—in the absence of offending drugs or known metabolic derangements, e.g., uremia, ketoacidosis, or electrolyte imbalance *OR* c. Other central or peripheric neuropsychiatric syndrome[†]
9. Hematologic disorder	a. Hemolytic anemia—with reticulocytosis *OR* b. Leukopenia—less than 4000/mm³ total on 2 or more occasions *OR* c. Lymphopenia—less than 1500/mm³ on 2 or more occasions *OR* d. Thrombocytopenia—less than 100,000/mm³ in the absence of offending drugs

10. Immunologic disorder	a. Anti-DNA: antibody to native DNA in abnormal titer
	OR
	b. Anti-Sm: presence of antibody to Sm nuclear antigen
	OR
	c. Positive finding of antiphospholipid antibodies[‡] based on the following:
	  i. An abnormal serum level of IgG or IgM anticardiolipin antibodies
	    OR
	  ii. A positive test result for lupus anticoagulant using a standard method
	    OR
	  iii. A false-positive serologic test for syphilis known to be positive for at least 6 months and confirmed by *Treponema pallidum* immobilization or fluorescent treponemal antibody absorption test

11. Antinuclear antibody	An abnormal titer of antinuclear antibody by immunofluorescence or an equivalent assay at any point in time and in the absence of drugs known to be associated with "drug-induced lupus" syndrome

* The classification is based on 11 criteria. For the purpose of identifying patients in clinical studies, a person shall be said to have systemic lupus erythematosus if any 4 or more of the 11 criteria are present, serially or simultaneously, during any interval of observation (Tan et al., 1982; Hochberg, 1997).
† The American College of Rheumatology provides case definitions for 19 neuropsychiatric syndromes seen in systemic lupus erythematosus, with reporting standards and recommendations for laboratory and imaging tests (American College of Rheumatology, 1999). Also available at *www.rheumatology.org/ar/1999/aprilappendix.html*.
‡ Standard methods should be used in testing for the presence of antiphospholipid (Harris, 1990; Brandt et al., 1995).

ECG, electrocardiogram.

(anti-dsDNA = anti-nDNA), histones, SSA/Ro, SSB/La, Sm, Sm/RNP, Scl-70, Jo-1, and centromeric antigens. A negative screening result implies that the individual has a high probability of being ANA free, whereas a positive test reflects only the need for further testing. When equivocal ANA results are obtained, the choices are to retest, to test by another method, or to obtain a new sample. Equivocal samples that give positive results when retested should be reported as positive. Equivocal samples that give negative results upon retest should be reported as negative.

Individuals with SLE will, from time to time throughout the course of their disease, have ANA results ranging from very low titers to high titers. A high or low titer does not necessar-ily mean the disease is more or less active, and patients can even have negative results despite being ill. A titer above 1:80 is usually considered positive for lupus. However, perfectly healthy individuals can have a positive ANA, and the laboratory test alone cannot establish the diagnosis of lupus. In relation to the pattern of binding, peripheral pattern is the most specific for SLE.

Further laboratory investigation should be done to confirm the diagnosis of SLE, for example, obtaining anti-dsDNA antibodies. Other second-line autoantibodies are the ones against extractable (soluble) RNA–protein conjugates, also known as extractable nuclear antibodies. These extractable nuclear antigens include anti-Sm, anti-ribonucleoprotein, anti-

SSA/Ro, and anti-SSB/La. Commonly tested antibodies, with a brief comment on their clinical relevance to pregnancy, are listed in Table 54-2. There is currently no evidence that serial serologic (erythrocyte sedimentation rate, complement levels, or autoantibodies titers) determinations during pregnancy are better than timely clinical assessment for the diagnosis of an SLE exacerbation. Certainly, hypocomplementemia and autoantibodies may occur in normal pregnant patients, and its presence does not predict a bad outcome (Adelsberg, 1983; Patton et al., 1987).

Epidemiology

SLE affects predominantly women, and the female-to-male ratio during the reproductive years (ages 15 to 44 years) is 9:1. This ratio before menarche and after menopause is only 3:1. The only other autoimmune disease with such a high female preponderance is Hashimoto thyroiditis (female-to-male ratio of 25 to 50:1).

Investigators from the Mayo Clinic's Rochester Epidemiology Project reported that in 1993 the average incidence rate (age and sex adjusted to the 1970 U.S. white population) was 5.56 per 100,000 (95% CI, 3.93–7.19), compared with an incidence of 1.51 (95% CI, 0.85–2.17) in their 1950 to 1979 cohort (Uramoto et al., 1999). This tripled incidence over the past four decades is likely due to a combination of improved recognition of mild disease and better approaches to therapy. The same group reported that the age- and sex-adjusted prevalence rate as of January 1, 1993 was approximately 1.22 per 1000 (95% CI, 0.97–1.47) (Uramoto et al., 1999). Using a different approach, Hochberg and colleagues (1995) reported that the prevalence of SLE in the United States in 1995 among women aged 18 and above was 124 cases per 100,000 (95% CI, 40–289). This prevalence was obtained from over 4000 telephone-screening interviews and verification of SLE cases by review of medical records.

Minority women (African American, Hispanic, Asian, and Native American) have a risk two to five times that of white women. In African-American women, the prevalence is 1 in 245 (Sacks et al., 2002). Race is a major predictor of clinical manifestations, laboratory and serologic tests, and disease-related morbidity. The effect of race on musculoskeletal morbidity remains even after adjustment for education, insurance status, and smoking (Petri, 1998). Based on 2000 census data, we project that over 250,000 women aged 18 and above have SLE in the United States.

Fertility is not affected except during severe acute disease, in patients with end-stage renal disease, and after cyclophosphamide therapy, which can cause premature ovarian failure (McDermot and Powell, 1996). SLE is therefore relatively common in pregnancy and is the most prevalent CTD during pregnancy. SLE places at risk approximately 1 in 2000 to 3000 deliveries (Yasmeen et al., 2001; Gimovsky et al., 1984).

Morbidity

Cervera and colleagues (1999) prospectively collected 5-year morbidity data on 1000 European SLE patients. Forty percent of these patients had one or more episodes of arthritis, 27% had infections, 26% malar rash, 22% active nephropathy, 14% fever, 14% neurologic involvement, 13% Raynaud phenomenon, 13% serositis, 11% hypertension, 10% thrombocytopenia, 8% osteoporosis, 7% thrombosis, and 6% cytopenia (anemia, leukopenia, thrombocytopenia, bicitopenia, or pancytopenia) resulting from immunosuppressive agents. Of note, 16 patients (1.6%) developed malignancies, with the most frequent primary localizations being the uterus and the breast.

Mortality and Survival

Although many details of pathogenesis of SLE remain unresolved, our understanding has improved and led over the past century to lower morbidity and mortality rates. Cervera and associates (1999) reported a 5-year survival rate of 95%. The most frequent causes of death were active SLE (28.9%), infections (28.9%), and thromboses (26.7%). A lower 5-year survival rate (92%) occurred in patients who had nephropathy at enrollment of the study. In a study from University College in London (Moss et al., 2002), 41 deaths occurred among 300 SLE nonpregnant patients between 1978 and 2000. Overall, malignancy was the most common cause of death (20%). Cause of death varied depending on disease duration. Forty percent of early deaths (less than 5 years after diagnosis of SLE) were due to SLE-related renal disease, whereas 23% of late deaths were due to vascular causes. Death because of

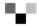

TABLE 54-2. ANTIBODY TESTS HELPFUL IN PERINATAL ASSESSMENT OF LUPUS ERYTHEMATOSUS

Antibody	Clinical Pertinence
Antinuclear antibody	Screening of systemic lupus erythematosus (SLE)
Anti-DNA	Associated with SLE disease activity and nephritis
Anti-Ro (Anti-SSA)	Specific for Sjögren syndrome and SLE; associated with nephritis; highly correlated with neonatal lupus and congenital heart block
Anti-La (Anti-SSB)	Negatively associated with nephritis in anti-Ro–positive patients
Anticentromere	90% in scleroderma's CREST* syndrome
Anticardiolipin	Vascular thromboses, recurrent abortion/miscarriages
Anti-ribonucleoprotein	Mixed connective tissue disease

* Calcinosis cutis, Raynaud phenomenon, esophageal involvement, sclerodactyly, and telangiectasia.

Modified from Hollingsworth DR, Resnik R (eds): Medical Counseling before Pregnancy. New York, Churchill Livingstone, 1988.

infection occurred throughout the follow-up period. The risk of death was reported to be four times higher in the cohort of SLE patients compared with the general population. Multivariate analysis has identified the following prognostic factors for death in SLE patients ($n = 665$) followed prospectively over 20 years: renal damage, thrombocytopenia, lung involvement, SLE disease activity index at least 20 at presentation, and age at least 50 at diagnosis (Abu-Shakra et al., 1995b).

The overall 5-, 10-, 15-, and 20-year survival rates were 93%, 85%, 79%, and 68%, respectively; SLE patients have a fivefold increased risk for death compared with that of the general population (Abu-Shakra et al., 1995a). The Centers for Disease Control and Prevention released a report in May 2002 showing a 60% increase in SLE deaths over a 20-year period (Sacks et al., 2002). The report's most alarming findings were that the death rate among black women aged 45 to 64 years had increased 70% and that more than one third of all deaths resulting from SLE occurred among persons less than 45 years of age. Approximately 80% of new cases of SLE develop among women in their childbearing years, and lupus is up to three times more common among African-American women than among white women (Sacks et al., 2002).

Effects of Pregnancy on Systemic Lupus Erythematosus

Lupus activity during pregnancy continues to be a subject of too much debate and too little research. As is the case with most illnesses that run a fluctuating course, it is difficult to document any unique effect of pregnancy on the course of SLE (Lockshin 1989, 1992a, b). Most studies on this topic are small single-clinic studies in which systematic biases (inclusion and exclusion criteria, control selection, ascertainment, physician behavior) cannot be corrected by meta-analysis. SLE is a syndrome and not a unique disease entity, making it virtually impossible for investigators to stratify patients by not only demographic and obstetric parameters, but by disease activity and damage indices measured immediately before conception and by their particular autoantibody status. A most important step would be to standardize the definition of what constitutes a significant change in disease status, called "flares." Diagnosis of SLE flares can be difficult during pregnancy and must rely on a thorough clinical and laboratory assessment. The so-called flares during pregnancy may not be related to SLE activity but may reflect other pathologic entities, such as preeclampsia. Current measures used to assess disease activity do little to help physicians predict disease flares or complications that may arise. Furthermore, most autoantibodies (ANA, extractable nuclear antigen, RF, anti-Jo-1, etc.) do not vary with disease flare-ups and remissions (Davidson and Keiser, 1997).

Given these limitations, the rates of flare per patients per month in 78 pregnancies in 68 SLE patients attending the lupus pregnancy clinic at St. Thomas's Hospital in England during a 5-year period were compared with a control group of 50 consecutive, nonpregnant, age-matched SLE patients attending the same lupus clinic (Ruiz-Irastorza et al., 1996). Pregnancy and control groups were homogeneous for age, race, disease duration, and distribution of autoantibodies. SLE activity was assessed using the Lupus Activity Index score. An increase of at least 0.26 in the score was considered as a disease flare. Sixty-five percent of the patients flared during pregnancy and/or the puerperium (8 weeks postdelivery), whereas 42% flared in the control group ($P = 0.015$). Less flares occurred during the first trimester compared with the remainder of pregnancy and the puerperium. Flares were not more severe than in nonpregnant patients, and most of them were managed conservatively (nonimmunosuppressive treatment). Forty-three of these pregnant patients continued to be cared for at their regular lupus clinic for the year after puerperium, and their disease course was compared with that which they experienced during pregnancy. They flared more frequently during pregnancy than after ($P = 0.003$) but had no difference in kidney and central nervous system involvement or in terms of frequency of flares, between patients taking and not taking steroids (prednisolone).

Other authors have reported that the rate of SLE exacerbations is similar in pregnant women compared with their matched nonpregnant control subjects (Mintz et al, 1986; Meehan and Dorsey, 1987; Lokshin, 1989). In these studies flare rates during pregnancy ranged between 21% and 60%, and most were mild. When flare rates are stratified based on the patients disease activity at the time of conception, different authors have concluded that the rate of flares and the rate of renal deterioration was lower among pregnancies conceived while on remission (Hayslett and Lynn, 1980; Jungers et al., 1982; Bobrie et al., 1987; Hayslett, 1992; Urowitz, 1993).

In summary, the issue of whether pregnancy predisposes to increased disease SLE flare activity remains unsettled, because individual series vary in the characteristics of patients accepted for study and in definitions of flare. Nevertheless, flares do occur, but their rate is lower if the disease is under good control for at least 6 months before conception. Reported frequencies for flares during pregnancy range between 15% and 60%. SLE may flare during any trimester of pregnancy and in the puerperium. Mild SLE flares usually affecting skin and joints do not confer any adverse prognosis on maternal–fetal outcome, unless it is affecting the kidney. Severe renal flares and permanent impairment of renal function are uncommon (Buyon, 1998; Julkunen, 2001). To date, there is no support that steroids prevent SLE flares during pregnancy, and therefore prophylactic prednisone should not be given routinely (Khamashta et al., 1997). Whether pregnancy per se is a predisposing factor for SLE flares remains an open area of research.

Effect of Systemic Lupus Erythematosus on Pregnancy

A 2-year population-based study using data from the California Health Information for Policy Project, which links records from birth certificates and hospital discharge records of mothers and newborns who delivered in all civilian hospitals in the state of California between 1993 and 1994, showed that SLE was associated with a significant increase in maternal pregnancy complications and in fetal and neonatal morbidity and mortality as compared with the control population. However, this study found significantly fewer adverse outcomes than was previously reported (Yasmeen et al., 2001).

Maternal Outcome

If the lupus patient does not have hypertension, renal impairment, or the antiphospholipid syndrome, her chances of a normal pregnancy are good and may indeed be no worse than those of a normal patient. Specific adverse pregnancy outcomes in SLE as reported by the California Health Information for Policy Project included hypertensive complications, renal disease, preterm delivery, nonelective cesarean section, postpartum hemorrhage, and delivery-related deep vein thrombosis (Yasmeen et al., 2001).

Systemic Lupus Erythematosus Nephritis

Pregnancies in women with lupus nephritis require intense fetal and maternal surveillance. The outlook of pregnancy for women with lupus nephritis is usually favorable if the disease (both renal and nonrenal) has been quiescent for at least 6 months before pregnancy and if, at conception, serum creatinine is no more than 1.5 mg/dL (140 µmol/liter), proteinuria less than 3 g/24 h, and blood pressure controlled (Julkunen, 2001). Proteinuria is the most common presentation of SLE nephritis (75%), followed by hematuria or aseptic pyuria (40%) and presence of urinary casts (33%). The most common and most serious histologic category of SLE nephritis is diffuse proliferative glomerulonephritis. An unpublished meta-analysis of retrospective evaluation of SLE renal disease during pregnancy showed that about one fourth of women experienced renal deterioration and 8.5% of pregnancies were associated with permanent deterioration (Clark et al., 1997). Hayslett and Lynn (1980) noted a 50% fetal loss rate in mothers with a serum creatinine in excess of 1.5 mg/dL. The presence of antiplatelet antibodies is an additional risk factor.

Preeclampsia and Eclampsia

The definitive treatment of preeclampsia is delivery of the fetus. However, the decision to deliver a very preterm infant (less than 32 weeks' gestation) is not that easy. A randomized clinical trial that studied the effects of expectant management of severe preeclampsia remote from term specifically excluded women with CTDs (Sibai et al., 1994), so currently there are no data to support this approach.

Patients with lupus nephritis during pregnancy frequently exhibit increasing proteinuria, hypertension, and deterioration of renal function because of active lupus nephritis, chronic lupus nephritis, and/or superimposed preeclampsia during pregnancy. The clinical features of preeclampsia—which usually run a much more acute course, remits after delivery, and is not associated with other well-known features of SLE such as arthritis—normally distinguish the two conditions. Measurement of ANA, anti-dsDNA, decreased levels of CH50, and active urinary sediment (cellular casts, aseptic leukocyturia, and/or hematuria) may help distinguish an SLE nephritis flare from other renal conditions and preeclampsia. Although histopathology usually will clarify the diagnosis and orient the treatment, there is an understandable reluctance to perform kidney biopsies during pregnancy. Krane and associates (1995) reported four percutaneous renal biopsies in pregnant patients with lupus nephritis. Before the biopsy the mean serum creatinine was 2.9 mg/dL, with a mean creatinine clearance of 66 mL/min and protein excretion of 5.3 g/day. All patients were found to have grade IV lupus nephritis and received pulse methylprednisolone immediately; three received cyclophosphamide as well. All three patients with crescent formation developed end-stage renal disease within 3 years. The fourth patient had normal renal function 3 years after biopsy.

A Taiwanese series of 15 percutaneous renal biopsies performed in pregnant women with idiopathic renal disease presenting before 30 weeks of gestation showed that eight had lupus nephritis (five with diffuse crescenteric changes and three with a mesangial proliferative pattern), three had chronic glomerulonephritis, two had mesangial proliferative glomerulonephritis, and one each had diabetic nephrosclerosis and endocapillary proliferative glomerulonephritis (Chen et al., 2001). Early induction of labor was recommended for the four patients with diabetic nephrosclerosis or glomerulonephritis. The other 11 patients received intravenous pulse methylprednisolone or high-dose oral prednisolone therapy. The responses to steroid therapy in these 11 patients were as follows: 5 achieved complete remission of nephrosclerosis, 3 achieved incomplete remission, and 3 achieved partial remission. Fourteen of the 15 pregnancies resulted in live births; one pregnancy resulted in stillbirth. After 2 years' follow-up, seven mothers achieved complete remission, three had died, three developed chronic renal failure, and two progressed to end-stage renal failure requiring chronic hemodialysis.

In SLE patients, APN nephropathy can occur in SLE in addition to, and independently of, lupus nephritis. Antiphospholipid syndrome nephropathy has particular vaso-occlusive lesions, is associated with lupus anticoagulant but not with anticardiolipin antibodies, and is associated with extrarenal antiphospholipid syndrome, mainly arterial thromboses and fetal loss, but not with the venous thromboses. Additionally, APN nephropathy is an independent risk factor, over and above lupus nephritis, that contributes to an elevated prevalence of hypertension, elevated serum creatinine, and increased interstitial fibrosis. Thus, APN nephropathy may worsen the prognosis in patients with lupus and may also have therapeutic significance in that its recognition should permit a better balance between immunosuppressor and antithrombotic and/or vasoprotective therapy (Daugas et al., 2002).

In summary, histopathologic studies may be useful in counseling regarding continuation or termination of pregnancy, potential maternal and fetal outcome, and recommending specific therapeutic modalities; however, sound clinical judgment is mandatory to decide which patient may benefit from this procedure.

Fetal/Neonatal Outcome

Yasmeen and colleagues (2001) reported that neonatal and fetal outcomes were significantly worse in the SLE group as compared with control subjects. SLE pregnancies had a higher prevalence of fetal growth restriction and neonatal death and longer newborn hospital stays ($P < 0.0001$).

Pregnancy Loss

It has been recognized for decades that SLE is associated with an increased risk for pregnancy loss. Most excess fetal loss in women with SLE occurs in association with antiphospholipid antibodies, which also are associated with pregnancy loss in non-SLE and in healthy women (see Chapter 48). In a Mexican series of 73 pregnancies in 46 severe SLE patients, longer disease duration, ingestion of immunosuppressive drugs during pregnancy, and any related manifestation of APS were correlated with fetal loss (Martinez-Rueda et al., 1996). When SLE is associated with secondary antiphospholipid syndrome and lupus anticoagulant or β_2-glycoprotein antibodies are present, a further increase in the incidence of pregnancy loss is expected (Kiss et al., 2002). In patients diagnosed with SLE, the proportion of pregnancies ending with live birth at term decreased to one third compared with three fourths in those without a diagnosis of SLE, and the incidence of preterm deliveries and spontaneous abortions increased by 6.8 and 4.7 times, respectively (Kiss et al., 2002).

Preterm Labor

SLE increases the risks of preterm delivery as a result of hypertension, renal compromise, and preterm rupture of membranes. Up to a 40% risk of preterm premature rupture of membranes has been reported in SLE patients (Johnson et al., 1995), with the highest incidence between 34 and 37 weeks' gestation. If preterm labor occurs in women with SLE, tocolysis is reasonable unless severe intrauterine growth restriction or maternal disease (active renal flare not responding to steroids or severe preeclampsia) is present.

Growth Restriction

Most investigators have reported higher rates of symmetrical and asymmetrical intrauterine growth restriction in SLE patients. However, disease activity at conception has not been correlated to intrauterine growth restriction or placental size (Fine, 1981; Mintz et al., 1986). In most cases, these children thrive once they are delivered.

Intrauterine Fetal Death

Intrauterine fetal death in the general population is uncommon, usually less than 1% of all births. In one review, stillbirth rates in SLE at at least 20 weeks' gestation vary between 40 and 150 per 1000 births in lupus women (Simpson, 2002). Intrauterine fetal death in SLE patients has been associated with the presence of the APS, history of previous fetal death, and active disease at the time of conception, presence of lupus nephropathy, and chronic hypertension (Bobrie et al., 1987; Jungers et al., 1982).

Neonatal Lupus Syndrome

Neonatal lupus erythematosus (NLE) is a rare disorder described mainly through case reports, characterized by one or more of the following findings: CHB, cardiomyopathy, cutaneous lupus lesions, hepatobiliary disease, and thrombocytopenia. The transplacental transfer of maternal autoantibodies, mainly anti-SSA/Ro, is responsible for the development of the disease. There are some data to suggest that anti-SSB/La and,

rarely, anti-RNP antibodies play an important pathologic role in some cases of NLE. The manifestation of anti-RNP-positive NLE is, however, somewhat atypical. It remains an enigma why all pregnancies are not affected when the putative maternal antibodies are present.

Congenital Heart Block

Anti-SSA/Ro antibody (52 kDa/60 kDa) and anti-SSB/La antibody are associated with CHB. Because the production of anti-Ro and anti-La antibodies is correlated with the presence of HLA-DR3, which is more common in patients with SS, CHB is even more common in patients with SS than in those with lupus (Paredes et al., 1983; Veille et al., 1985). Histologically, antibody-mediated inflammation and subsequent fibrosis of the atrioventricular node causes CHB. In contrast to the atrioventricular node, permanent sinoatrial nodal involvement is not clinically apparent (Askanase et al., 2002). The likelihood of detecting congenital CHB with serial fetal echocardiography (at 18, 24, and 32 weeks' gestation) in pregnant women who are anti-Ro and/or La positive but have no history of previous child with congenital CHB is very low. Gladman and coworkers (2002) found no cases in 102 pregnancies with such characteristics.

Although often initially asymptomatic, mothers tend to develop symptoms of CTDs (Lee, 2001). In a series of 55 children with isolated CHB, all their mothers were positive for antibodies against SSA/Ro alone or to both SSA/Ro and SSB/La. At the time of fetal or neonatal diagnosis, around 40% of the mothers were asymptomatic, 25% had SLE, 15% had SS, and 20% had undifferentiated autoimmune syndrome. The asymptomatic women were followed for a median period of time of 4 years. Almost half developed symptoms of a rheumatic disease. These women, now symptomatic, developed an undifferentiated autoimmune syndrome (55%), SS (18%), and SLE (27%) (Waltuck and Buyon, 1994).

To date, no definite treatment is available prenatally to prevent the occurrence of CHB, but careful maternal screening and serial fetal echocardiograms are warranted. Intrauterine therapeutic options are dexamethasone therapy to suppress maternal and fetal inflammatory reactions and repeated plasmaphereses to reduce autoantibody levels (Zemlin et al., 2002). Buyon and coworkers (1995) reported that CHB was identified between 16 and 24 weeks of gestation in 53% of affected pregnancies, between 25 and 30 weeks in 24%, between 31 and 37 weeks in 11%, and between 38 and 40 weeks in 7%. These authors reported that in 19 pregnancies, women were given fluorinated steroids (betamethasone and dexamethasone) as attempted therapy after the discovery of CHB. Of these, one fetus with second-degree block reverted to sinus rhythm and two with third-degree block exhibited an improvement in the degree of block. In eight fetuses, pleural and/or pericardial effusions resolved.

Eronen and associates (2001) reported that poor fetal outcome in fetuses with CHB diagnosed between 20 and 30 weeks' gestation was associated with low ventricular rate, low left ventricular fractional shortening, and high umbilical artery resistance index. These authors performed echocardiography at 2-week intervals. In relation to the neonatal outcome, one third of the children with autoantibody-associated CHB died in the early neonatal period and, of those who survived, most required pacemakers (Waltuck and Buyon, 1994).

Isolated CHB has an excellent prognosis after pacemaker implantation. Most early deaths result from delayed initiation of pacing therapy or hemodynamic abnormalities associated with congenital heart defects. A multi-institutional case series of 16 infants with CHB who developed late-onset dilated cardiomyopathy despite early institution of cardiac pacing found that these infants required close follow-up not only of their cardiac rate and rhythm, but also ventricular function because of their high risk to develop left ventricular cardiomyopathy (Moak et al., 2001).

The risk of CHB is far greater in association with anti-Ro than with anti-La. Anti-Ro antibodies are quite common in CTDs, so that the risk of CHB in the presence of anti-Ro is only about 1 in 20, although this increases to 1 in 3 if the mother has already had a child with CHB (Olaáh and Gee, 1991). The occurrence of CHB in women known to have CTD with anti-SSA/Ro antibodies has been reported in an Italian series of 100 women (Brucato et al., 2001). Only two of these women had infants who developed CHB *in utero*. The cases were detected at 22 and 20 weeks, respectively. In this series, one of the two mothers had primary SS and the other had mixed or undifferentiated CTD. No case of congenital CHB occurred among the infants of 53 mothers with SLE. No fetal death occurred because of congenital CHB.

In addition, the CHB may be associated with endomyocardial fibrosis (Scott and Esscher, 1979), pericarditis (Fox and Hawkins, 1990), or pericardial effusion (Shenker et al., 1987). Of course, fetuses may have CHB because of a primary cardiac malformation, frequently an atrioventricular canal defect (Shenker et al., 1987). Under these circumstances, there is usually no association with maternal CTD.

The management of the occasional fetus with hydrops and cardiac failure in association with heart block before viability is problematic. Evaluation of the fetus's general condition is difficult, because accurate assessment usually depends on measurement of fetal heart rate, its variability, and its reactivity. Evaluation of biophysical profile and measurement of umbilical blood flow by Doppler ultrasound can be of value. Understandably, many such fetuses are delivered by cesarean section because of inability of fetal heart rate monitoring to evaluate fetal condition.

Neonatal Cutaneous Lupus

NLE skin lesions often appear on the face or the scalp in the second or third month of life, and ultraviolet exposure is thought to be an initiating factor because it can externalize intranuclear autoantigens at the cell surface. Cimaz and coworkers (2002) reported a biopsy-confirmed case of an infant born to an anti-SSA/Ro and anti-SSB/La negative, anti-RNP positive mother, with erythematosus scarring rash in the scalp and face that developed *in utero* and was not associated with sun exposure.

Hematologic, Hepatobiliary, and Neurologic Neonatal Lupus Erythematosus

The hematologic abnormalities are hemolytic anemia, leukopenia, and thrombocytopenia. Because maternal IgG antibodies do not persist in the neonate, hematologic abnormalities are usually transient and are not a major problem (McCauliffe, 1995). Lee and coworkers (2002) reported three clinical variants of hepatobiliary disease: severe liver failure

present during gestation or in the neonatal period, conjugated hyperbilirubinemia with mild or no elevations of aminotransferases, and mild elevations of aminotransferases occurring at approximately 2 to 3 months of life. The prognosis for the children in the last two categories is excellent. A case reported recently included neurologic involvement with spastic paraparesis as the main clinical finding (Besson-Leaud, 2002).

Management of Systemic Lupus Erythematosus in Pregnancy

Obstetricians and perinatologists will be confronted with two types of scenarios: the patient with SLE who is pregnant or desires to become pregnant, and the patient who debuts during pregnancy. "Borderline SLE" or patients with undetermined or mixed CTDs also require proper counseling and medical care.

Preconceptional Counseling

Pregnancy in patients with SLE requires consideration of five major issues:

1. What is the risk to the mother?
2. What is the risk to the fetus?
3. What is the effect and treatment of antiphospholipid antibody?
4. What is the risk of neonatal lupus?
5. What is the stability of the family unit, particularly in the events of maternal disability or death (Lockshin, 1992a)?

Fertility

Wang and colleagues (1995) studied 92 women with SLE treated with oral cyclophosphamide. Menstrual disturbance during cyclophosphamide treatment occurred in 55% of patients: 36% had amenorrhea and 19% had oligomenorrhea. Sustained oligomenorrhea occurred in 12% of patients, and permanent amenorrhea after cessation of oral cyclophosphamide occurred in 27% of women. Hormonal studies in these patients were consistent with ovarian failure. A statistically significant association between amenorrhea and cumulative dose of cyclophosphamide after adjustment for age was found, whereas no such association was linked to the duration of treatment. Fourteen of the 23 women who wished to become pregnant after cessation of treatment conceived, resulting in 20 live births and two abortions. It seems likely that in the next 10 to 15 years we will see major changes in the treatment of patients with lupus. Newer immunosuppressive drugs, such as mycophenolate mofetil acid (Cellsept) and tacrolimus (Progaf) are already used as an alternative to azathioprine or cyclophosphamide in nonpregnant women.

Prenatal Care

SLE patients require increased surveillance and interventions that may lead to more favorable pregnancy outcomes. Cytotoxic drugs and antimetabolites must be discontinued before conception or as soon as pregnancy is recognized. In relation to triple test screening, maternal serum human chorionic gonadotropin levels in SLE patients were 1.48 multiples of the gestation-specific normal medians compared with 0.79 in control subjects. These preliminary findings, reported by Maymon and colleagues (2001), should be further studied to evaluate the implications for Down syndrome screening, detection of SLE cases during pregnancy, and the prediction of adverse outcome in SLE gestations.

Nonpharmacologic Treatment

The primary objectives in treating women with rheumatologic complaints are reduction of inflammation and pain, preservation of function, and prevention of deformities. Nonpharmacologic measures for the treatment of arthralgias and arthritis include systemic and articular rest, appropriate use of heat and cold, and timely physical and occupational therapies. Other general supportive measures include adequate sleep and avoidance of fatiguing activities, because mild exacerbation may resolve within few days of bed rest. Sunscreens (SPF 20 or higher), protective clothing, and direct sun exposure avoidance are needed for patients with photosensitivity. Small isolated skin lesions respond to topical steroids (see later).

Pharmacologic Treatment

The drugs most frequently used for the treatment of mild SLE are simple analgesics, such as acetaminophen and NSAIDs. In more severe cases, antimalarial drugs, corticosteroids, and cytotoxic agents are used. NSAIDs (including the COX-2 inhibitors) are effective treatment for the arthralgias, arthritis, fever, and serositis associated with SLE. Lupus patients are more prone to renal and hepatic toxicities associated with these drugs, and as such they should be avoided if there is active SLE nephritis and during the third trimester. Aspirin in high dosage and other NSAIDs have been associated with neonatal hemorrhage because of platelet inhibition (Stuart et al., 1982). There is the theoretical risk that prostaglandin synthetase inhibitors will cause premature closure of the ductus arteriosus and pulmonary hypertension, especially in late pregnancy.

Antimalarials interfere with normal phagocytic function and antigen processing, inhibit platelet aggregation, and reduce serum lipids, making them important in lupus patients with inflammatory polyarthritis, skin disease, alopecia, severe fatigue, and APS. Antimalarials, in particular hydroxychloroquine, seem to be safe for the fetus. A recent survey among North American and U.K. lupus experts revealed that most continue antimalarials during pregnancy and allow breastfeeding while on antimalarials (Al-Herz et al., 2002). A small randomized clinical trial from Brazil found beneficial effects of hydroxychloroquine (n = 10) compared with placebo (n = 10) during pregnancy (Levyet al., 2001). The patients in the hydroxychloroquine group had no flare-ups, less prednisone dosage changes, lower SLE disease activity index scores at conclusion of the study, and higher gestational age and Apgar scores. Neonatal examination did not reveal congenital anomalies, or abnormalities in neuro-ophthalmological and auditory evaluations at 1.5 to 3 years of age. Thus, these drugs should not be discontinued during pregnancy in a patient with lupus, particularly when the known terminal elimination half-life is 1 to 2 months (Borden and Parke, 2001).

Antimalarials are not effective in the treatment of fever, SLE nephritis, or neurologic or hematologic disease manifestations. Chloroquine may also cause chorioretinitis in adults; however, studies in the United States (Park and Rothfield, 1996) and the United Kingdom (Khamashta et al., 1996) have shown no association with ocular abnormalities in the fetus.

Steroids

Indications for systemic steroids include life-threatening manifestations of SLE (e.g., nephritis, neurologic involvement, thrombocytopenia, and hemolytic anemia). Steroids are also indicated for severe debilitating fatigue or cutaneous manifestations unresponsive to other drugs. Lockshin and Sammaritano (1998) reviewed the pharmacokinetics and pharmacodynamics of steroids in pregnancy. It is accepted that systemic steroids are not teratogenic and that pregnant women receiving steroid therapy suffer the same side effects and benefits as do women who are not pregnant. Clinical experience suggests no abnormalities of children of mothers treated with the usual doses of prednisone and methylprednisolone throughout pregnancy, but premature rupture of amniotic membranes and low-birth-weight infants may occur. The effect on the fetus of bolus doses of methylprednisolone is unknown. Very little of the corticosteroid ingested by the mother enters her breast milk (Lockshin and Sammaritano, 1998). In women with lupus and/or APS receiving heparin throughout pregnancy, corticosteroids must be reduced as much as possible, and calcium plus vitamin D are recommended (Ruiz-Irastorza et al., 2001).

Patients who have life-threatening SLE manifestations may need prednisone 1 to 2 mg/kg orally daily in divided doses for several weeks. After disease is controlled, prednisone should be consolidated to a single daily dose and then tapered slowly, with the dose reduction of no more than 10% every week. Faster tapering schedules result in relapse. Patients who are taking steroids should be regularly checked for gestational diabetes. If a woman has taken regular steroid therapy for more than 1 month in the year before delivery, a parenteral hydrocortisone in stress doses, 100 mg every 8 hours for three doses, should be given to prevent maternal Addisonian collapse during labor and delivery. Intravenous pulse therapy with methylprednisolone is used in rapidly progressive SLE nephritis, severe neurologic disease, and life-threatening thrombocytopenia. Methylprednisolone as a single therapy does not prolong renal survival compared with regimens, including cyclophosphamide (Dooley and Falk, 1998).

Immunosuppresants

Aggressive immunosuppressive therapy should be considered for patients with proliferative lupus nephritis because the risk for progression to end-stage renal disease is high (Dooley and Falk, 1998). Azathioprine may be used during pregnancy but not during lactation. Azathioprine has been used rather widely in pregnancy, chiefly in patients with renal transplants. Azathioprine in combination with steroids may be given to patients with lupus nephritis. For SLE patients without renal involvement, it is given to those who require a maintenance dose of 15 mg or higher of prednisone and for those who experience recurrent flares. It is also effective for patients with skin lesions, pneumonitis, thrombocytopenia, or hemolytic anemia. It has not been shown to increase the risk for the development of malignancies among patients with SLE (Abu-Shakra and Shoenfeld, 2001).

In nonpregnant SLE patients, Euler and coworkers (1994) proposed that treatment-free clinical remission can be achieved by an intensified treatment protocol synchronizing plasmaphereses with subsequent high-dose pulse cyclophosphamide followed by 6 months of oral immunosuppression therapy. Plasmapheresis has been successfully used in pregnancy for maternal severe proximal myopathy induced by steroids (Thomson et al., 1985) and in those with a poor obstetric history (Frampton et al., 1987). Nevertheless, plasmapheresis remains under study and has not shown additional benefit in treatment of severe lupus nephritis (Dooley and Falk, 1998). Cyclophosphamide and methotrexate are contraindicated because of the risk of teratogenesis. The management of APS patients with thromboembolism, arterial or venous, is considered in Chapters 42 and 48.

Thalidomide

Thalidomide (Thalomid, Celgene Corporation, Warren, NJ) has been reapproved for marketing by the U.S. Food and Drug Administration based on its effectiveness in the treatment of cutaneous forms of SLE refractory to other therapies (Karim et al., 2001). This is despite its known teratogenic effects and the frequent recurrence after discontinuation of treatment. Women must use two methods of birth control beginning 4 weeks before starting treatment with thalidomide and continue them for at least 4 weeks after stopping the drug (U.S. Food and Drug Administration, 2002). This unfortunately means that we may again find patients affected by its grave teratogenic and neuropathic effects.

Postpartum Issues

Oral contraceptives containing synthetic estrogens are contraindicated in women with active lupus nephritis, uncontrolled hypertension, history of thromboembolic diseases, or high levels of antiphospholipid antibodies (Julkunen, 2001). During lactation, prednisone and hydroxychloroquine can be used cautiously (Janssen and Genta, 2000).

In summary, acetaminophen is the most frequent analgesic used in pregnancy. Salicylates and NSAIDs are traditionally avoided in the last trimester yet would appear to pose only minor risks. Steroids should be used for life-threatening cases. Because of the risk of dangerous exacerbation of SLE in the puerperium, steroid dosage should be reduced with great care only after delivery. The use of azathioprine should be reserved for life-threatening cases in which steroid therapy has failed or is contraindicated. Supportive care, including rigorous control of hypertension and prevention of osteoporosis, are important clinical goals.

Outcome Measurement in Systemic Lupus Erythematosus

Not all clinical problems reported by a lupus patient are due to the disease; some may be a consequence of therapy and others may be unrelated to lupus. The optimal outcome measures to be used in clinical trials of SLE have yet to be determined. Useful instruments should assess disease outcome in terms of all organ systems involved; distinguish current potentially reversible disease activity, permanent organ damage, and the effect of the disease on the patients' health status; and appraise important issues to the patient. Acticard is a computerized chart that helps monitor disease progression and therapeutic effects in SLE by calculating a summary of five disease activity indices: ECLAM (European Consensus Lupus Activity Measurement), SLAM (Systemic Lupus Activity Measure), SLEDAI (SLE disease activity index), SIS (SLE Index Score), and BILAG (British Isles Lupus Assessment Group). Acticard 2000 is available on the Internet at no cost (www.acticard.org/home.htm). At present there is no drug responder index, which would need to include the above disease activity indices plus measures of drug toxicity and cost.

SCLERODERMA

Progressive systemic sclerosis or scleroderma is a chronic connective tissue disease characterized by localized or diffuse fibrosis of the skin and internal organs (gastrointestinal tract, esophagus, kidneys, and lungs). The cause is unknown, and there is no known cure or disease-modifying therapy. Its pathogenesis has been linked to autoimmunity, fibroblast dysfunction, and exposure to silica. Anticentromere antibody and SCL-70 antibodies unfortunately have low sensitivity and specificity for diagnostic purposes. Patients usually have mild hemolytic anemia, hypergammaglobulinemia, and increased sedimentation rates. Proteinuria and casts are present in patients with renal involvement.

Scleroderma may or may not be associated with systemic disease. In the localized form (morphea or linear scleroderma) the process is limited, usually to the skin of the hands; it is associated with Raynaud phenomenon, and there is no organ involvement. Systemic scleroderma can be either limited (80% of patients) or diffuse (20%). Limited systemic scleroderma is also known as CREST syndrome (calcinosis cutis, Raynaud phenomenon, esophageal involvement, sclerodactyly, and telangiectasia). Although patients with CREST syndrome have a higher prevalence of lung involvement (pulmonary hypertension), overall they have a better prognosis than the patients with diffuse systemic scleroderma. In a series of 91 pregnancies complicated with scleroderma, 10% required cesarean delivery; none had wound infections or complications (Steen, 1999).

Only limited data are available regarding the incidence or outcome for either the mother with scleroderma or her fetus. The prognosis of localized scleroderma is good in general and particularly in pregnancy. The prognosis of systemic scleroderma in pregnancy is far worse than in the localized form. Because many patients deteriorate, often with hypertensive crises (hypertensive renal/uremic syndrome), they have been advised against pregnancy (Black and Stevens, 1989). Renal crisis presents as a hypertensive crisis (urgent or emergency) associated with thrombocytopenia that is very difficult to differentiate from severe preeclampsia. Progressive azotemia (daily increases in serum creatinine) and normal liver function tests may help in the differential diagnosis with preeclampsia. These crises usually occur in scleroderma patients who have had diffuse disease for less than 5 years (Steen, 1999). Despite the association of angiotensin-converting enzyme inhibitors with birth defects and infant kidney dysfunction (Mastrobattista, 1997), angiotensin-converting enzyme inhibitors should be used urgently in the case of hypertensive renal crisis because they are the only drugs that successfully control hypertension in these circumstances (Steen, 1999). Captopril has been advocated as treatment for crisis in patients with scleroderma. Although it is not clear whether pregnancy itself accelerates the inevitable deterioration in these patients, there is no evidence that termination of pregnancy will reverse the renal crisis (Steen, 1999).

Scleroderma patients should have an anesthesiology consult early in pregnancy for airway and skin thickness assessment (difficult intravenous access or epidural regional anesthesia) (Thompson and Conklin, 1983).

SJÖGREN SYNDROME

SS is a rare autoimmune disorder that infiltrates (lymphocyte and plasmocytes) exocrine glands, primarily the lacrimal and salivary glands. Ninety percent of affected individuals are women. The incidence peaks between ages 40 and 60 years. This syndrome can present as an isolated entity but more frequently is associated with other rheumatoid syndromes or diseases (RA, SLE, primary biliary cirrhosis, scleroderma, polymyositis, Hashimoto, etc.). SS is consistent with a normal lifespan when not associated with other rheumatoid disorders.

Characteristic symptoms include dryness of the eyes (keratoconjuctivitis sicca), mouth (xerostomia), and other mucosae. Less specific symptoms like fatigue and myalgias are common. Parotid enlargement develops in one third of patients. Patients with SS have an increased frequency of drug (particularly antibiotics, which may be linked to HLA-DR3) allergy and other allergic manifestations (Fox et al., 1999), distal renal tubular acidosis (type I) (Carminati et al., 2001), Waldenström macroglobulinemia, and lymphomas.

This syndrome is associated with several autoantibodies such as the SS autoantibodies against cytoplasm tic antigens (anti-SSA/Ro, anti-SSB/La), ANAs, and RF. RF can be present in up to 70% of patients. When SS-A autoantibody is present, patients have more systemic manifestations of the syndrome, including dysphagia, pancreatitis, pleuritis, vasculitis, and neuropsychiatric manifestations. The Schirmer test and labial biopsy are useful in diagnosis. The European Cooperative Group has modified the diagnostic criteria for SS to include either a positive minor salivary gland biopsy or a positive autoantibody against SSA/Ro or SSB/La.

Treatment is symptomatic. Artificial tears (Clovis, Murine, Refresh) are safe during pregnancy. They stabilize and thicken the precorneal tear film and prolong tear film breakup time, which occurs with dry eye states. Newly developed topical and oral therapies can ease the oral and ocular dryness. Orally administered agonists of the muscarinic M3 receptor (pilocarpine and cevimeline) are approved by the U.S. Food and Drug Administration to increase salivary secretion. There are no adequate and well-controlled studies in pregnant women (category C) for either pilocarpine (Salagen) or cevimeline (Evoxac). Animal studies using megadoses of cevimeline (five times the maximum recommended) have been associated with a reduction in the mean number of implantations. It is not known whether this drug is secreted in human milk (U.S. Food and Drug Administration, 2002). Topical ocular use of low-dose corticosteroids may decrease conjunctival surface inflammation. Orally administered interferon-α (category C), which improves saliva flow and symptoms, is currently being studied (Fox et al., 1999).

Julkunen and coworkers (1995) analyzed retrospectively the fetal outcome in 55 pregnancies in 21 Finish women with primary SS and compared it with that in 100 pregnancies in 42 patients with SLE and 94 pregnancies in 42 healthy women matched for age, parity, and the onset of the autoimmune disease with respect to pregnancy. These authors found that most pregnancies in women with primary SS occur before the onset of the disease and that these women had an increased risk of fetal loss, which was not associated with elevated levels of anticardiolipin antibody or antibodies against SSA/Ro or SSB/La. The risk of fetal loss in primary SS was similar to that in women with SLE, but fetal growth restriction appears to be more common in SLE than in primary SS (Julkunen et al., 1995). As in SLE, CHB is particularly common in patients with SS because of the presence of anti-Ro (SSA) autoantibody and others, such as La/SSB, U1-RNP antigens, or M1 muscarinic receptor (Borda et al., 1999). Mothers of infants with NLE may be asymptomatic initially or may have SS, SLE, overlap syndrome, or, uncommonly, leukocytoclastic vasculitis (Borrego et al., 1997).

SS should not be confused with Sjögren-Larsson syndrome, which is a triad of spasticity, mental retardation, and congenital ichthyosis in children resulting from microsomal fatty aldehyde dehydrogenase deficiency, because there is available prenatal diagnosis.

ANKYLOSING SPONDYLITIS

Ankylosing spondylitis (AS) is a chronic inflammatory process of the spine, clinically manifested by insidious low backache in young adults (ages 15 to 40 years), progressive stiffening and limitation of back motion, and chest expansion. The ascending spinal involvement starts at the level of the sacroiliac joints to encompass the entire spine, flattening the lumbar curvature and exaggerating the thoracic one. In advanced AS the spine becomes fused by calcification ("bamboo spine" on x-rays) and the sacroiliac joint becomes obliterated and linked by bridges of bone (ankylosis). In AS, clinical manifestations are similar in men and women, whereas radiologic features appear more frequent and severe in males. However, no consistent differences in outcome and mortality between men and women have been disclosed.

Although a role for sex steroids in the pathogenesis of AS is suggested by the male predominance, the peak age at onset in young adults, the increased number of first manifestations and flares after pregnancy, and the fact that sex steroids may modulate immune functions, there is as yet no rationale for the use of medication that modifies sex steroid hormones in the management of AS (Gooren et al., 2000).

Ostensen and Ostensen (1998) published the findings from the AS International Federation questionnaire that included almost a thousand European and North American women with AS. It was found that their mean age at onset of AS was 23 years and that the onset was related to a pregnancy in 21% of them. About half the patients had either peripheral arthritis or acute anterior uveitis. Disease activity worsened in one third of patients and improved in another third. Improvement was associated with a history of peripheral arthritis and carrying a female fetus. Sixty percent of patients had postpartum flares within 6 months after delivery, and this was associated with disease activity at conception. A significant number of patients required cesarean section. General anesthesia may be a problem because of ankylosis of the cervical spine and temporomandibular joints; epidural block may be difficult because of calcification and ankylosis in the vertebral column.

The treatment of AS is similar to that described for RA. Because of possible maternal and fetal side effects, NSAIDs generally are discontinued during the last 8 weeks of pregnancy, but during lactation several NSAIDs can be used. Treatment with sulfasalazine is compatible with pregnancy and lactation (Gran and Ostensen, 1998). Children of AS patients exhibit a slightly increased risk of developing spondyloarthropathies (AS included) later in life (Gran and Ostensen, 1998).

MIXED CONNECTIVE TISSUE DISEASE

Mixed connective tissue disease (undifferentiated connective tissue disease, overlap, or bridge syndrome) should be considered as an important syndrome in any patient who presents with heterogeneous clinical presentation and does not fit into any definite criteria of systemic CTDs. Mixed connective tissue disease is characterized clinically by the overlap of different features of different rheumatologic diseases (most commonly SLE, scleroderma, and polymyositis) and serologically by antibodies to soluble ribonucleoprotein nuclear antigens and by the other ANAs as well. With time many patients will develop more clear features of their underlying disease. Maternal and fetal risks are the same in mixed connective tissue disease as in SLE.

FUTURE STUDIES

It is clear that there is a bidirectional communication between the neuroendocrine and the immune system and that both systems influence each other and interact under physiologic conditions and in response to inflammatory stimuli. The precise role of neuroendocrine, in particular glucocorticoids homeostasis, in pregnancy-induced modification of disease activity in connective tissue diseases still needs to be clarified.

Future studies of maternal–fetal immunology should yield insights not only into the maintenance of normal pregnancy but also into the disproportionate increase of autoimmune diseases in females and the variable course of these diseases during pregnancy. Current research efforts focus on genetic and socioeconomic factors involved in racial differences in expression of connective tissue diseases, hormonal manipulation to preserve gonadal function during cytotoxic therapy, and the potential impact on connective tissue diseases activity of estrogen-containing oral contraceptives or postmenopausal hormone replacement therapy.

REFERENCES

Abu-Shakra M, Shoenfeld Y: Azathioprine therapy for patients with systemic lupus erythematosus. Lupus 10:152, 2001.

Abu-Shakra M, Urowitz MB, Gladman DD, et al: Mortality studies in systemic lupus erythematosus: Results from a single center. I. Causes of death. J Rheumatol 22:1259, 1995a.

Abu-Shakra M, Urowitz MB, Gladman DD, et al: Mortality studies in systemic lupus erythematosus: Results from a single center. II. Predictor variables for mortality. J Rheumatol 22:1265, 1995b.

Adelsberg BR: The complement system in pregnancy. Am J Reprod Immunol 4:38, 1983.

Alavi A, Arden N, Spector TD, et al: Immunoglobulin G glycosylation and clinical outcome in rheumatoid arthritis during pregnancy. J Rheumatol 27:1379, 2000.

Al-Herz A, Schulzer M, Esdaile JM: Survey of antimalarial use in lupus pregnancy and lactation. J Rheumatol 29:700, 2002.

American College of Rheumatology Hoc Committee on Neuropsychiatric Lupus Nomenclature: The American College of Rheumatology nomenclature and case definitions for neuropsychiatric lupus syndromes. Arthritis Rheum 42:599, 1999.

Askanase AD, Friedman DM, Copel J, et al: Spectrum and progression of conduction abnormalities in infants born to mothers with anti-SSA/Ro-SSB/La antibodies. Lupus 11:145, 2002.

Barrett JH, Brennan P, Fiddler M, et al: Does rheumatoid arthritis remit during pregnancy and relapse postpartum? Results from a nationwide study in the United Kingdom performed prospectively from late pregnancy. Arthritis Rheum 42:1219, 1999.

Barrett JH, Brennan P, Fiddler M, et al: Breast-feeding and postpartum relapse in women with rheumatoid and inflammatory arthritis. Arthritis Rheum 43:1010, 2000.

Black CM, Stevens WM: Scleroderma. Rheum Dis Clin North Am 15:193, 1989.

Bobrie G, Liote F, Houillier P, et al: Pregnancy in lupus nephritis and related disorders. Am J Kidney Dis 9:339, 1987.

Borda E, Leiros CP, Bacman S, et al: Sjögren autoantibodies modify neonatal cardiac function via M1 muscarinic acetylcholine receptor activation. Int J Cardiol 70:23, 1999.

Borden MB, Parke AL: Antimalarial drugs in systemic lupus erythematosus: use in pregnancy. Drug Safety 24:1055, 2001.

Borrego L, Rodriguez J, Soler E, et al: Neonatal lupus erythematosus related to maternal leukocytoclastic vasculitis. Pediatr Dermatol 14:221, 1997.

Bowden AP, Barrett JH, Fallow W, et al: Women with inflammatory polyarthritis have babies of lower birth weight. J Rheumatol 28:355, 2001.

Brandt JT, Triplett DA, Alving B, et al: Criteria for the diagnosis of lupus anticoagulants: An update. On behalf of the Subcommittee on Lupus Anticoagulant/Antiphospholipid Antibody of the Scientific and Standardisation Committee of the ISTH. Thromb Haemost 74:1185, 1995.

Bresnihan B: Treating early rheumatoid arthritis in the younger patient. J Rheumatol 62:45, 2001.

Brucato A, Frassi M, Franceschini F, et al: Risk of congenital complete heart block in newborns of mothers with anti-Ro/SSA antibodies detected by counterimmunoelectrophoresis: a prospective study of 100 women. Arthritis Rheum 44:1832, 2001.

Buyon JP: The effects of pregnancy on autoimmune diseases. J Leuk Biol 63:281, 1998.

Buyon JP, Waltuck J, Kleinman C, et al: In utero identification and therapy of congenital heart block. Lupus 4:116, 1995.

Carette S, Surtees PG, Wainwright NW, et al: The role of life events and childhood experiences in the development of rheumatoid arthritis. J Rheumatol 27:2123, 2000.

Carminati G, Chena A, Orlando JM, et al: Distal renal tubular acidosis with rhabdomyolysis as the presenting form in 4 pregnant women. Nefrologia 21:204, 2001.

Cervera R, Khamashta MA, Font J, et al: Morbidity and mortality in systemic lupus erythematosus during a 5-year period. A multicenter prospective study of 1,000 patients. European Working Party on Systemic Lupus Erythematosus. Medicine (Baltimore) 78:167, 1999.

Chakravarty EF, Sanchez-Yamamoto D, Bush TM: The use of disease modifying antirheumatic drugs in women with rheumatoid arthritis of childbearing age: A survey of practice patterns and pregnancy outcomes. J Rheumatol 30:241, 2003.

Chen HH, Lin HC, Yeh JC, et al: Renal biopsy in pregnancy complicated by undetermined renal disease. Acta Obstet Gynecol Scand 80:888, 2001.

Cimaz R, Biggioggero M, Catelli L, et al: Ultraviolet light exposure is not a requirement for the development of cutaneous neonatal lupus. Lupus 11:257, 2002.

Clark SL, Cotton DB, Hankins GDV, et al (eds): Systemic lupus erythematosus. In Critical Care Obstetrics, 3rd ed. Malden, Mass, Blackwell, 1997, p. 485.

Cutolo M: Sex hormone adjuvant therapy in rheumatoid arthritis. Rheum Dis Clin North Am 26:881, 2000.

Daugas E, Nochy D, Huong du LT, et al: Antiphospholipid syndrome nephropathy in systemic lupus erythematosus. J Am Soc Nephrol 13:42, 2002.

Davidson A, Keiser HD: Diagnosing and treating the predominantly female problems of systemic autoimmune diseases. Medscape Womens Health 2:6, 1997.

Davison J: Renal disease. In deSwiet M (ed): Medical Disorders in Obstetric Practice. Oxford, Blackwell, 1989, p. 226.

Donaldson LM, Espiner EA: Disseminated lupus erythematosus presenting as chorea gravidarum. Arch Neurol 25:240, 1971.

Dooley MA, Falk RJ: Immunosuppressive therapy of lupus nephritis. Lupus 7:630, 1998.

Drossaers-Bakker KW, Zwinderman AH, van Zeben D, et al: Pregnancy and oral contraceptive use do not significantly influence outcome in long term rheumatoid arthritis. Ann Rheum Dis **61**:405, 2002.

Eronen M, Heikkila P, Teramo K: Congenital complete heart block in the fetus: Hemodynamic features, antenatal treatment, and outcome in six cases. Pediatr Cardiol **22**:385, 2001.

Euler HH, Schroeder JO, Harten P, et al: Treatment-free remission in severe systemic lupus erythematosus following synchronization of plasmapheresis with subsequent pulse cyclophosphamide. Arthritis Rheum **37**:1784, 1994.

Everts B, Wahrborg P, Hedner T: COX-2-specific inhibitors—The emergence of a new class of analgesic and anti-inflammatory drugs. Clin Rheumatol **19**:331, 2000.

Farnam J, Lavastida MT, Grant JA, et al: Antinuclear antibodies in the serum of normal pregnant women: A prospective study. J Allerg Clin Immunol **73**(5 Pt 1):596, 1984.

FeldKamp M, Carey JC: Clinical teratology counseling and consultation case report: Low dose methotrexate exposure in the early weeks of pregnancy. Teratology **47**:553, 1993.

Fine LG for the UCLA Report on Systemic Lupus Erythematosus in Pregnancy: Systemic lupus erythematosus in pregnancy. Ann Intern Med **94**:667, 1981.

Fox R, Hawkins DF: Fetal-pericardial effusion in association with congenital heart block and maternal systemic lupus erythematosus: Case report. Br J Obstet Gynaecol **97**:638, 1990.

Fox RI, Tornwall J, Michelson P: Current issues in the diagnosis and treatment of Sjögren's syndrome. Curr Opin Rheumatol **11**:364, 1999.

Frampton G, Pameron JA, Thomas M, et al: Successful removal of antiphospholipid antibody during pregnancy using plasma exchange and low-dose prednisolone. Lancet **2**:1023, 1987.

Gimovsky ML, Montoro M, Paul RH: Pregnancy outcome in women with systemic lupus erythematosus. Obstet Gynecol **63**:686, 1984.

Gladman G, Silverman ED, Yuk-Law LL, et al: Fetal echocardiographic screening of pregnancies of mothers with anti-Ro and/or anti-La antibodies. Am J Perinatol **19**:73, 2002.

Gooren LJ, Giltay EJ, van Schaardenburg D, et al: Gonadal and adrenal sex steroids in ankylosing spondylitis. Rheum Dis Clin North Am **26**:969, 2000.

Gran JT, Ostensen M: Spondyloarthritides in females. Baillieres Clin Rheumatol **12**:695, 1998.

Grossman JM, Brahn E: Rheumatoid arthritis: current clinical and research directions. J Women Health **6**:627, 1997.

Hahn BH: Pathogenesis of systemic lupus erythematosus. *In* Ruddy S, Harris ED Jr, Sledge CB (eds): Kelley's Textbook of Rheumatology, 6th ed. Philadelphia, Saunders, 2001.

Harris EN: The second international anticardiolipin standardization workshop: The Kingston Antiphospholipid Antibody Study (KAPS) Group. Am J Clin Pathol **94**:476, 1990.

Hayslett JP: The effect of systemic lupus erythematosus on pregnancy and pregnancy outcome. Am J Reprod Immunol **28**:199, 1992.

Hayslett JP, Lynn RI: Effect of pregnancy in patients with lupus nephropathy. Kidney Int **18**:207, 1980.

Hazes JM, Dijkmans BA, Vandenbroucke JP, et al: Pregnancy and the risk of developing rheumatoid arthritis. Arthritis Rheum **33**:1770, 1990.

Hochberg MC: Updating the American College of Rheumatology revised criteria for the classification of systemic lupus erythematosus. Arthritis Rheum **40**:1725, 1997.

Hochberg MC, Perlmutter DL, Medsger TA, et al: Prevalence of self-reported physician-diagnosed systemic lupus erythematosus in the USA. Lupus **4**:454, 1995.

Isenberg DA: Some thoughts about lupus for the new millennium. Available at *http://www.rheuma21st.com/archives/cutting_edge_lupus.html*. Accessed June 23, 2002.

Janssen NM, Genta MS: The effects of immunosuppressive and anti-inflammatory medications on fertility, pregnancy, and lactation. Arch Intern Med **160**:610, 2000.

Jarvis B, Faulds D: Etanercept: A review of its use in rheumatoid arthritis. Drugs **57**:945, 1999.

Johnson MJ, Petri M, Witter FR, et al: Evolution of preterm delivery in a systemic lupus erythematosus pregnancy clinic. Obstet Gynecol **86**:396, 1995.

Julkunen H: Pregnancy and lupus nephritis. Scand J Urol Nephrol **35**:319, 2001.

Julkunen H, Kaaja R, Kurki P, et al: Fetal outcome in women with primary Sjögren's syndrome. A retrospective case-control study. Clin Exp Rheumatol **13**:65, 1995.

Kanik KS, Wilder RL: Hormonal alterations in rheumatoid arthritis, including the effects of pregnancy. Rheum Dis Clin North Am **26**:805, 2000.

Kaplan MJ: Leflunomide aventis pharma: Current opinion. Invest Drugs **2**:222, 2001.

Karim MY, Ruiz-Irastorza G, Khamashta MA, et al: Update on therapy—Thalidomide in the treatment of lupus. Lupus **10**:188, 2001.

Khamashta MA, Buchanan NMM, et al: The use of hydroxychloroquine in lupus pregnancy: The British experience. Lupus **1**:S65, 1996.

Khamashta MA, Ruiz-Irastorza G, Hughes GR: Systemic lupus erythematosus flares during pregnancy. Rheumatol Dis Clin North Am **23**:15, 1997.

Kiss E, Bhattoa HP, Bettembuk P, et al: Pregnancy in women with systemic lupus erythematosus. Eur J Obstet Gynecol Reprod Biol **101**:129, 2002.

Krane NK, Thallur V, Wood H, et al: Evaluation of lupus nephritis during pregnancy by renal biopsy. Am J Nephrol **15**:186, 1995.

Lambert NC, Stevens AM, Tylee TS, et al: From the simple detection of microchimerism in patients with autoimmune diseases to its implication in pathogenesis. Ann N Y Acad Sci **945**:164, 2001.

Lee LA: Neonatal lupus: Clinical features, therapy, and pathogenesis. Curr Rheumatol Rep **3**:391, 2001.

Lee LA, Sokol RJ, Buyon JP: Hepatobiliary disease in neonatal lupus: Prevalence and clinical characteristics in cases enrolled in a national registry. Pediatrics **109**:E11, 2002.

Levy RA, Vilela VS, Cataldo MJ, et al: Hydroxychloroquine (HCQ) in lupus pregnancy: Double-blind and placebo-controlled study. Lupus **10**:401, 2001.

Lima F, Buchanan NM, Khamashta MA, et al: Obstetric outcome in systemic lupus erythematosus. Semin Arthritis Rheum **25**:184, 1995.

Lockshin MD: Pregnancy does not cause systemic lupus erythematosus to worsen. Arthritis Rheum **32**:665, 1989.

Lockshin MD: Overview of lupus pregnancies. Am J Reprod Immunol **28**:181, 1992a.

Lockshin MD: Treatment of lupus pregnancy: Can we reach consensus? (editorial). Clin Exp Rheumatol **10**:429, 1992b.

Lockshin MD, Sammaritano LR: Corticosteroids during pregnancy. Scand J Rheumatol **107**:136, 1998.

Martinez-Rueda JO, Arce-Salinas CA, Kraus A, et al: Factors associated with fetal losses in severe systemic lupus erythematosus. Lupus **5**:113, 1996.

Masi AT, Chatterton RT, Aldag JC: Perturbations of hypothalamic-pituitary-gonadal axis and adrenal androgen functions in rheumatoid arthritis: An odyssey of hormonal relationships to the disease. Ann N Y Acad Sci **876**:53, 1999.

Mastorakos G, Ilias I: Maternal hypothalamic-pituitary-adrenal axis in pregnancy and the postpartum period. Postpartum-related disorders. Ann N Y Acad Sci **900**:95, 2000.

Mastrobattista JM: Angiotensin converting enzyme inhibitors in pregnancy. Semin Perinatol **21**:124, 1997.

Maymon R, Cuckle H, Sehmi IK, et al: Maternal serum human chorionic gonadotrophin levels in systemic lupus erythematosus and antiphospholipid syndrome. Prenat Diagn **21**:143, 2001.

McCauliffe DP: Neonatal lupus erythematosus: a transplacentally acquired autoimmune disorder. Semin Dermatol **14**:47, 1995.

McDermot EM, Powell RJ: Incidence of ovarian failure in systemic lupus erythematosus after treatment with pulse cyclophosphamide. Ann Rheum Dis **55**:224, 1996.

McDonagh JE, Isenberg DA: Development of additional autoimmune diseases in a population of patients with systemic lupus erythematosus. Ann Rheum Dis **59**:230, 2000.

Meehan RT, Dorsey JK: Pregnancy among patients with systemic lupus erythematosus receiving immunosuppressive therapy. J Rheumatol **14**:252, 1987.

Mintz G, Niz J, Gutierrez G, et al: Prospective study of pregnancy in systemic lupus erythematosus. Results of a multidisciplinary approach. J Rheumatol **13**:732, 1986.

Moak JP, Barron KS, Hougen TJ, et al: Congenital heart block: development of late-onset cardiomyopathy, a previously underappreciated sequela. J Am Coll Cardiol **37**:238, 2001.

Moss KE, Ioannou Y, Sultan SM, et al: Outcome of a cohort of 300 patients with systemic lupus erythematosus attending a dedicated clinic for over two decades. Ann Rheum Dis **61**:409, 2002.

Nelson JL, Hughes KA, Smith AG, et al: Maternal-fetal disparity in HLA class II alloantigens and the pregnancy-induced amelioration of rheumatoid arthritis. N Engl J Med **329**:466, 1993.

Nelson JL, Ostensen M: Pregnancy and rheumatoid arthritis. Rheum Dis Clin North Am 23:195, 1997.

Nelson JL, Voigt LF, Koepsell TD, et al: Pregnancy outcome in women with rheumatoid arthritis before disease onset. J Rheumatol 19:18, 1992.

Nojima J, Kuratsune H, Suehisa E, et al: Association between the prevalence of antibodies to beta (2)-glycoprotein I, prothrombin, protein C, protein S, and annexin V in patients with systemic lupus erythematosus and thrombotic and thrombocytopenic complications. Clin Chem 47:1008, 2001.

Olaáh KS, Gee H: Fetal heart block associated with maternal anti-Ro (SS-A) antibody—Current management: A review. Br J Obstet Gynaecol 98:751, 1991.

Ollier WE, Harrison B, Symmons D: What is the natural history of rheumatoid arthritis? Best Pract Res Clin Rheumatol 15:27, 2001.

Ostensen M: Sex hormones and pregnancy in rheumatoid arthritis and systemic lupus erythematosus. Ann N Y Acad Sci 876:131, 1999.

Ostensen M, Ostensen H: Ankylosing spondylitis—The female aspect. J Rheumatol 25:120, 1998.

Paredes RA, Morgan H, Lachelin GCL: Congenital heart block in a fetus associated with maternal Sjögren's syndrome: Case report. Br J Obstet Gynaecol 90:970, 1983.

Park AL, Rothfield NF: Anti-malarial drugs in pregnancy: The North American experience. Lupus 1:67, 1996.

Patton PE, Coulam CB, Bergstralh E: The prevalence of autoantibodies in pregnant and non-pregnant women. Am J Obstet Gynecol 157:134, 1987.

Petri M: The effect of race on incidence and clinical course in systemic lupus erythematosus: The Hopkins Lupus Cohort. J Am Med Womens Assoc 53:9, 1998.

Petri M: Long-term outcomes in lupus. Am J Managed Care 7 (16 Suppl):S480, 2001.

Ruiz-Irastorza G, Khamashta MA, Nelson-Piercy C, et al: Lupus pregnancy: is heparin a risk factor for osteoporosis? Lupus 10:597, 2001.

Ruiz-Irastorza G, Lima F, Alves J, et al: Increased rate of lupus flare during pregnancy and the puerperium: A prospective study of 78 pregnancies. Br J Rheumatol 35:133, 1996.

Sacks JJ, Helmick CG, Langmaid G, et al for the Division of Adult and Community Health, National Center for Chronic Disease Prevention and Health Promotion, Centers for Disease Control and Prevention: Trends in Deaths from Systemic Lupus Erythematosus—United States, 1979–1998. June 26, 2002.

Scott JS, Esscher E: Congenital heart block and maternal systemic lupus erythematosus. Br Med J 1:1235, 1979.

Shenker L, Reed KL, Anderson CF, et al: Congenital heart block and cardiac anomalies in the absence of maternal connective tissue disease. Am J Obstet Gynecol 157:248, 1987.

Siamopoulou-Mavridou A, Manoussakis MN, Mavridis AK, et al: Outcome of pregnancy in patients with autoimmune rheumatic disease before the disease onset. Ann Rheum Dis 47:982, 1988.

Sibai BM, Mercer BM, Schiff E, et al: Aggressive versus expectant management of severe preeclampsia at 28 to 32 weeks' gestation: a randomized controlled trial. Am J Obstet Gynecol 171:818, 1994.

Sills ES, Perloe M, Tucker MJ, et al: Successful ovulation induction, conception and normal delivery after chronic therapy with etanercept: A recombinant fusion anti-cytokine treatment for rheumatoid arthritis. Am J Reprod Immunol 46:366, 2001.

Simpson LL: Maternal medical disease: Risk of antepartum fetal death. Semin Perinatol 26:42, 2002.

Smith JB, Haynes MK: Rheumatoid arthritis—A molecular understanding. Ann Intern Med 136:908, 2002.

Steen VD: Pregnancy in women with systemic sclerosis. Obstet Gynecol 94:15, 1999.

Stuart MJ, Gross SJ, Elrad H, et al: Effects of acetylsalicylic-acid ingestion on maternal and neonatal hemostasis. N Engl J Med 307:902, 1982.

Tan EM, Cohen AS, Fries JF, et al: The 1982 revised criteria for the classification of systemic lupus erythematosus. Arthritis Rheum 25:1271, 1982.

Thomson BJ, Watson ML, Liston WA, et al: Plasmapheresis in pregnancy complicated by acute systemic lupus erythematosus. Case report. Br J Obstet Gynaecol 92:523, 1985.

Thompson J, Conklin KA: Anesthetic management of a pregnant patient with scleroderma. Anesthesiology 59:69, 1983.

Unger A, Kay A, Griffin AJ, et al: Disease activity and pregnancy associated alpha 2-glycoprotein in rheumatoid arthritis during pregnancy. Br Med J Clin Res Educ 286:750, 1983.

Uramoto KM, Michet CJ, Thumboo J, et al: Trends in the incidence and mortality of systemic lupus erythematosus, 1950–1992. Arthritis Rheum 42:46, 1999.

Urowitz MB, Gladman DD, Farewell VT, et al: Lupus and pregnancy studies. Arthritis Rheum 36:1392, 1993.

U.S. Food and Drug Administration: Center for Drug Evaluation and Research. Frequently asked questions concerning thalidomide. June 28, 2002.

Veille JC, Sunderland C, Bennett RM: Complete heart block in a fetus associated with maternal Sjögren's syndrome. Am J Obstet Gynecol 151:660, 1985.

Waltuck J, Buyon JP: Autoantibody-associated congenital heart block: Outcome in mothers and children. Ann Intern Med 120:544, 1994.

Wang CL, Wang F, Bosco JJ: Ovarian failure in oral cyclophosphamide treatment for systemic lupus erythematosus. Lupus 4:11, 1995.

Yasmeen S, Wilkins EE, Field NT, et al: Pregnancy outcomes in women with systemic lupus erythematosus. J Matern Fetal Med 10:91, 2001.

Zeldis JB: Pregnancy and inflammatory bowel disease. West J Med 151:168, 1989.

Zemlin M, Bauer K, Dorner T, et al: Intrauterine therapy and outcome in four pregnancies of one mother with anti ro-autoantibody positive Sjoegren's syndrome. Zeitschr Geburtsh Neonat 206:22, 2002.

Chapter 55

NEUROLOGIC DISORDERS

Michael J. Aminoff, MD, DSc, FRCP

Women are as susceptible to neurologic disorders during gestation as at other times, and certain disorders may be aggravated or influenced by pregnancy. Moreover, the investigation and management of many neurologic disorders may be complicated by the pregnancy and by concern for the safety of the developing fetus. This chapter does not cover all aspects of neurologic disease (see standard texts) but describes some of the special problems posed by neurologic disorders during pregnancy and, conversely, by pregnancy in patients with neurologic disorders.

EPILEPSY

Women with epilepsy should be advised about possible interactions between anticonvulsant drugs and oral contraceptive agents. Whether oral contraceptives affect seizure frequency or blood levels of antiepileptic drugs is unclear, but certain anticonvulsants (including phenytoin, phenobarbital, primidone, carbamazepine, oxycarbazepine, and topiramate) may interfere with the effectiveness of oral contraceptives, leading to unwanted pregnancy (Janz et al., 1989). Accordingly, the possibility of contraceptive failure must be discussed with women taking these anticonvulsants and documented in the records.

Between 0.3% and 0.6% of pregnant women have epilepsy. Pregnancy may affect the seizure disorder, and the disorder may itself affect the course of the pregnancy and the manner in which it is best managed. Moreover, recurrent seizures and drugs given to the mother in an attempt to control them may affect fetal development. Regular counseling of women with epilepsy is necessary during the reproductive years, because unplanned pregnancy may occur.

Effect of Pregnancy on Seizure Disorders

Pregnancy has an unpredictable and variable influence on epilepsy. In 153 pregnancies in one series of 59 patients with epilepsy, seizure frequency increased in 45%, was reduced in 5%, and remained unchanged in the remainder (Knight and Rhind, 1975). When seizure frequency increased, it most commonly did so in the first trimester and usually reverted to the pregestational pattern at the conclusion of the pregnancy, although a few patients experienced a permanent deterioration in seizure control. In general, control in patients with frequent seizures (more than one a month) before pregnancy was likely to deteriorate during the gestational period, whereas only about 25% of patients with infrequent attacks (less than one every 9 months) experienced an exacerbation during pregnancies.

In a prospective study of 136 pregnancies in 122 epileptic women, seizure frequency increased in 50 pregnancies (37%), often in association with noncompliance with a therapeutic regimen (Schmidt et al., 1983). Among several other series, seizures increased during pregnancy in 23% to 75% of instances (Yerby, 1991). Tanganelli and Regesta (1992) found that seizures were more likely to be exacerbated during pregnancy in women with more frequent seizures before the pregnancy and in those with partial (focal) seizure disorders.

It is usually not possible to predict the outcome in individual cases, regardless of the maternal age, the outcome of previous pregnancies, or any apparent relationship between seizures and the menstrual cycle. None of these provides a guide to the effect that pregnancy will have on the course of epilepsy. Moreover, attacks may occur during pregnancy in patients who have been seizure-free for several years.

Epilepsy may appear for the first time during or immediately after pregnancy. Fewer than 25% of women in this latter group have seizures only in relation to pregnancy and at no other time (i.e., gestational epilepsy) (Montouris et al., 1979). About one third of patients with true gestational epilepsy experience recurrent seizures during pregnancy, and the remainder have only a single convulsion (Knight and Rhind, 1975). Even in this group of patients, however, the occurrence of seizures in one pregnancy is no guide to the course of subsequent gestations.

The seizures that occur during pregnancy do not differ clinically from those occurring in other circumstances, although in women in whom seizures occur for the first time during pregnancy, the attacks and any electroencephalographic abnormalities are often focal (Knight and Rhind, 1975). Improved compliance with an anticonvulsant drug regimen may sometimes account for the reduction in seizure frequency that occasionally occurs during pregnancy in an epileptic.

The increase in seizure frequency that occurs in some epileptic patients during pregnancy may relate to the metabolic, hormonal, or hematologic changes of the gestational period or to fatigue or sleep deprivation. A rapid and excessive gain in weight sometimes occurs before an increase in seizure frequency, providing some support for the belief that fluid retention may occasionally be a factor, perhaps by a dilutional effect on anticonvulsant drug concentration. It is also certainly tempting to relate any change in seizure frequency to hormonal factors because estrogens are epileptogenic in animals and progesterone has both convulsant and anticonvulsant properties. Nausea, vomiting, reduced gastric motility, or use of antacids may also lead to reduced absorption of anticonvulsant drugs.

There is sometimes difficulty in maintaining adequate treatment with anticonvulsant drugs during pregnancy. Serum levels of the older antiepileptic drugs generally decline in pregnancy and rise in the postpartum period. For phenytoin, carbamazepine, and valproate (but not phenobarbital), the decline is less for free levels than total levels. An increase in dosage is frequently required to maintain plasma levels at pre-pregnancy values, but in this regard it is important to appreciate that the free level, rather than the total level, of the drug correlates best with therapeutic efficacy. Several new antiepileptic drugs, such as felbamate, gabapentin, and lamotrigine, have become available, but the effect of pregnancy on their pharmacokinetics is unclear.

The reason for such changes in drug requirements is unknown. Among the various possibilities are the dilutional effect of increasing plasma volume and extracellular fluid volume. Poor compliance with anticonvulsant drug regimen, perhaps relating to nausea and vomiting or to concerns about the effect of medication on the fetus, may also be an important contributory factor, as may decreased plasma protein binding and changes in the absorption and excretion of drugs. The increased metabolic capacity of the maternal liver in pregnancy and possible fetal or placental metabolism of part of the anticonvulsant dose may also bear on the changes in anticonvulsant drug requirements that occur in epileptic women during pregnancy.

Folic acid therapy may lower the plasma phenytoin level, sometimes to below the therapeutic range, and other drugs taken concomitantly with an anticonvulsant medication may also lead to reduced plasma levels of the anticonvulsant. Antacids and antihistamines merit particular mention here because it is not uncommon for them to be taken during pregnancy.

Status epilepticus sometimes complicates pregnancy and may occur without any preceding increase in seizure frequency (Knight and Rhind, 1975), occasionally because of the injudicious discontinuation of anticonvulsant drugs. Fortunately, this is a rare occurrence, but it may lead to a fatal outcome for the mother or fetus. The absence of hypertension, proteinuria, and edema helps in distinguishing this condition from eclamptic convulsions. As in the nonpregnant patient, it is essential to obtain control of the seizures as rapidly as possible, but the former practice of terminating pregnancy is usually unnecessary now.

Status epilepticus is treated with anticonvulsant drug therapy, with the pregnancy being allowed to continue to term. Intravenous diazepam, 10 to 30 mg, or lorazepam, 4 to 8 mg, usually provides temporary control of the seizures, but other anticonvulsant drugs are generally needed as well if seizures are not to recur. Intravenous phenytoin is usually given but is best administered in the form of fosphenytoin sodium, the dose of which is expressed in terms of *phenytoin equivalents.* Fosphenytoin sodium is water soluble, may be infused with dextrose or saline, is better tolerated at the infusion site than phenytoin, and may be infused three times more rapidly than intravenous phenytoin, with the same pharmacologic effects. It is converted in the body to phenytoin, which may be cardiotoxic, so cardiac monitoring is required while the fosphenytoin is given in a loading dose of 15 to 20 mg phenytoin equivalents/kg infused at a rate of up to 150 mg phenytoin equivalents/kg. Other anticonvulsants may also be required, including intravenous phenobarbital or midazolam. It is of paramount importance to maintain control of the airway and of glucose and electrolyte balance.

Effect of Epilepsy on Pregnancy and Lactation

Only a few studies have attempted to document the effect of epilepsy on pregnancy. The results are often difficult to evaluate because of (1) the limited number of cases reported; (2) the lack of comparative data on nonepileptic women attending the same institutions; (3) differences in the severity of the epilepsy and how it has been treated; (4) differences in age, medical background, and socioeconomic status of the patients reported; and (5) the lack of information concerning such relevant social habits as cigarette smoking and alcohol ingestion.

The incidence of vaginal hemorrhage and of toxemia during 371 gestations in epileptic women was found by Bjerkedal and Bahna (1973) to be almost twice that in an unmatched group of 112,530 control pregnancies. Others, however, did not find any meaningful difference in the incidence of toxemia between epileptic and nonepileptic women (Watson and Spellacy, 1971). In a large collaborative study, bleeding occurred during pregnancy in 26% of those with no history of convulsive disorder, in 29.8% of those with such a history, and in 33.7% of those who regularly took phenytoin during early pregnancy (Monson et al., 1973).

Whether preterm labor occurs more commonly in epileptic women, as reported by Bjerkedal and Bahna (1973), is unclear. There is a significantly higher rate of stillbirths in epileptic patients, but there does not seem to be an increased incidence of low-birth-weight infants, at least in some studies (Niswander and Gordon, 1972; Monson et al., 1973; Shapiro et al., 1976). Cesarean section is not indicated simply because of maternal epilepsy except when seizures occur frequently or during labor, when they are precipitated by physical activity, or when patients cannot cooperate during labor because of their neurologic disorder or mental abnormality (Hiilesmaa, 1992). Fetal death can result from maternal seizures, presumably in relation to the accompanying hypoxia and acidosis. The effect on placental blood flow of maternal seizures is not established, but changes in fetal heart rate suggestive of hypoxia have been described (Teramo et al., 1979; Yerby, 1991); they may relate to reduced placental blood flow or to metabolic changes in the mother.

An increased incidence of neonatal death has been reported in the offspring of epileptic mothers (Speidel and Meadow, 1972; Bjerkedal and Bahna, 1973). The increase in perinatal mortality may relate to a number of factors, including congenital malformations, iatrogenic neonatal hemorrhage, seizures per se, socioeconomic factors, and preterm delivery.

Anticonvulsant drugs taken by the mother may be present in breast milk, but their concentration is usually insufficient to have any major effect on the infant. The transmission rate of antiepileptic drugs into breast milk varies with the agent and is about 2% for valproic acid; 30% to 45% for phenytoin, phenobarbital, and carbamazepine; 60% for primidone; and 90% for ethosuximide (Janz et al., 1989). When obvious sedation develops in an infant and is likely to relate to antiepileptic drugs in breast milk, breast-feeding should be discontinued and the infant observed for signs of drug withdrawal. Breast-feeding does not need to be discouraged otherwise, at least not for reasons related to its content of anticonvulsant medication.

Effect of Maternal Epilepsy and Anticonvulsant Drugs on the Fetus and Neonate

The epileptic woman who becomes pregnant usually is concerned that her unborn child might inherit a similar susceptibility to seizures. The risk of epilepsy in the child depends on the nature of the mother's seizure disorder and is higher in idiopathic than acquired maternal epilepsy. Precise quantification of the risk is not possible, but it is probably about 2% to 3%. Although the offspring of women with epilepsy have a significantly higher incidence of epilepsy than the general population, the offspring of affected men do not (Annegers et al., 1976). The cause of this increased risk to the offspring of epileptic mothers is unknown. It may relate to genetic factors, seizures arising during pregnancy, or the metabolic and toxic consequences of seizures or anticonvulsant drugs. In general, pregnancy in epileptic women does not need to be discouraged on these grounds, but reassurance and support are necessary.

A major problem relating to the management of epileptic patients during pregnancy is the possibility that certain anticonvulsant drugs may induce fetal abnormalities, but controversy still exists regarding the potential teratogenicity of these drugs. In reviewing the available data, one must remember that epilepsy has a relatively low prevalence rate, can occur for a multitude of reasons, can vary markedly in severity, can be treated by a variety of drugs either singly or in combination, and can itself be associated with an increased risk of fetal malformations. Moreover, some patients may have a common genetic predisposition to seizures and to fetal malformation. Finally, environmental factors may be important in the genesis of congenital abnormalities, and socioeconomic backgrounds must be matched as far as is possible when comparisons are made of the incidence of malformations in different patient populations.

A number of reports have suggested that anticonvulsant drugs are teratogenic. The most commonly observed malformations in the offspring of mothers taking anticonvulsant drugs are cleft lip, cleft palate, and congenital heart disease. In a detailed study by Annegers and colleagues (1974), the incidence of malformations per 1000 live births was 71 for epileptic mothers taking anticonvulsant drugs and 18 for those not taking such medications. The two groups were similar with regard to the types of seizure experienced, but it was not possible to determine whether there were differences between them in seizure frequency during pregnancy or in the familial occurrence of malformations. The incidence of congenital heart disease in this series was 43 per 1000 live births for epileptic mothers receiving anticonvulsant drugs, zero for epileptic mothers not taking such medication, and 5.7 among the general population subserved by the Mayo Clinic. Corresponding figures for cleft lip or palate were 21, zero, and 1.9, respectively. These figures therefore imply an increase in the incidence of such malformations among the children of epileptic women taking anticonvulsant drugs during pregnancy.

Starreveld-Zimmerman and colleagues (1974) suggested that the frequency of seizures tends to be higher among epileptic mothers with malformed offspring than among those with normal infants. Results of studies in Finland and the United States raise the possibility that fetal damage sometimes attributed to phenytoin and other anticonvulsant drugs may be due to the epilepsy itself (Shapiro et al., 1976). The studies confirmed that treated maternal epilepsy is associated with an increased incidence of malformations, especially cleft anomalies. The malformation rate in children exposed antenatally to phenytoin daily during early pregnancy, however, was similar to that in children born to unexposed epileptic mothers. Moreover, there was no evidence for fetal damage in women taking phenobarbital for indications other than epilepsy.

All the commonly used older antiepileptic drugs are teratogenic to some extent, and malformation rates are higher in the offspring of mothers taking drug combinations. For carbamazepine, the study by Jones and associates (1989) revealed a relatively high incidence of craniofacial defects, fingernail hypoplasia, and developmental delay in children exposed prenatally to this drug. Its use during pregnancy, particularly in combination with other drugs, has also been associated with an increased risk of spina bifida (Rosa, 1991). Valproic acid, however, has an especially high (1% to 2%) rate of neural tube defects (Bjerkedal et al., 1982; Robert and Guibaud, 1982). Trimethadione seems particularly dangerous (Speidel and Meadow, 1972; Feldman et al., 1977) and has been reported to cause fetal malformations and mental retardation in more than 50% of exposed infants. This drug, therefore, should be avoided during pregnancy when possible. Whether newer anticonvulsant drugs, such as felbamate, gabapentin, lamotrigine, tiagabine, topiramate, and vigabatrin, are teratogenic is unknown.

Animal studies lend support to the belief that some anticonvulsants are teratogenic. The mechanism involved is unclear but may relate to folate deficiency or antagonism. Dansky and associates (1992), for example, showed that low blood folate levels before or early in pregnancy are significantly associated with spontaneous abortion and the occurrence of developmental anomalies. It has also been suggested that certain oxidative intermediary metabolites of anticonvulsants may affect cell division and migration.

Although most children born to epileptic mothers are cognitively normal, prenatal antiepileptic drug exposure may also be associated with developmental delay (Dean et al., 2002), particularly when more than one drug has been taken by the mother. The mechanisms involved are unclear, but a genetic predisposition may also be important (Meador, 2002). It is also unclear whether some anticonvulsant drugs pose a greater risk than others.

Maternal use of phenytoin during pregnancy has been associated with a specific syndrome, the so-called *fetal hydantoin syndrome*, characterized by prenatal and postnatal growth deficiency, microcephaly, dysmorphic facies, and mental deficiency. It is alleged that 11% of infants exposed to phenytoin *in utero* have enough clinical features to be classified as having this syndrome and that almost three times as many more show lesser degrees of impairment of performance or morphogenesis (Hanson et al., 1976). Other reports have been unable to confirm the relationship of this syndrome to maternal ingestion of specific anticonvulsants (Shapiro et al., 1976, 1977). The syndrome is not unlike that ascribed to phenobarbital (Seip, 1976) and carbamazepine (Jones et al., 1989), and it resembles the fetal alcohol syndrome. A consistent facial phenotype has also been reported in children exposed to valproic acid or sodium valproate *in utero* (DiLiberti et al., 1984).

Maternal use of barbiturates (60 to 120 mg daily) in late pregnancy may be associated with neonatal withdrawal symptoms beginning a week after birth, including restlessness, constant crying, irritability, tremulousness, difficulty in sleeping, and vasomotor instability but not seizures.

Clinical or subclinical coagulopathy may also occur in the neonate whose mother received anticonvulsants during pregnancy. In a prospective study of neonates born to mothers taking anticonvulsant drugs, 7 of 16 infants had a severe coagulopathy, 1 had a mild defect, and the remainder were normal (Mountain et al., 1970). No evidence of coagulopathy was found in the mothers.

In affected infants, factors II, VII, IX, and X are decreased and factors V and VIII and fibrinogen are normal. The abnormalities are therefore similar to those produced by vitamin K deficiency. Bleeding in affected infants tends to occur within 24 hours of birth, rather than on the 2nd or 3rd day, as in classic hemorrhagic diseases of the newborn, and at relatively unusual sites such as the pleural and abdominal cavities. Prevalence rates average about 10%, but mortality may exceed 30% (Yerby, 1991). Bleeding may also occur in utero, resulting in stillbirth (Speidel and Meadow, 1972).

Maternal ingestion of vitamin K_1 (10 mg daily) during the last month of pregnancy may prevent these hemorrhagic complications in the offspring of treated epileptic mothers (Deblay et al., 1982). Vitamin K_1 administration to the newborn infant usually reverses the bleeding tendency, but the infant may die despite such therapy (Bleyer and Skinner, 1976). It is therefore recommended that prothrombin and partial thromboplastin times of cord blood be measured at delivery if the mother received anticonvulsant drugs. If the value is abnormally low or if there is clinical evidence of a coagulopathy during the neonatal period, treatment with infusion of fresh frozen plasma or concentrates of factors II, VII, IX, and X may have to be considered in addition to the routine administration of vitamin K_1.

General Therapeutic Approaches

It is clearly difficult to make more than general therapeutic recommendations about pregnancy in the epileptic woman. Epilepsy should be treated with the smallest effective dose of an anticonvulsant drug, and monotherapy is preferable to polytherapy. Drug selection is based on seizure type, clinical status, and the maternal and fetal risks (Bruno and Harden, 2002). Folate supplementation (4 mg daily) is generally provided. Prenatal counseling is important. If a nonpregnant epileptic woman asks about pregnancy, it is appropriate to indicate that there is a small risk of her having a malformed child because of either the seizure disorder or the drugs used in its treatment. This risk is probably about double that for the nonepileptic patient (Speidel and Meadow, 1972; Janz, 1975; Smithells, 1976), but there is still a good (more than 90%) chance that she will have a normal child.

Data concerning the relative safety and therapeutic effectiveness of different anticonvulsant drugs in the management of pregnant epileptic patients are insufficient to guide the physician responsible for the care of such patients. It seems clear, however, that trimethadione should not be used, and valproic acid is probably best avoided. If valproic acid must be used, amniocentesis is advisable to detect any increase in α-fetoprotein levels (which is associated with neural tube defects) so that therapeutic abortion can be considered if necessary. Substitution of one anticonvulsant drug for another in

epileptic women who are initially seen after the first trimester is best avoided, because major malformation of the fetus has probably occurred already if it is going to occur at all.

The principles of drug management of a seizure disorder in the pregnant woman are the same as in the nonpregnant woman. Anticonvulsant drugs are as necessary to epileptic patients during pregnancy as at other times. A detailed account of the drugs used in the treatment of epilepsy is unnecessary here, but several points are worthy of comment.

In the first place, a solitary seizure, unrelated to toxemia, should not lead to a diagnosis of epilepsy because there may be no further attacks. Only time will tell whether an individual who has a single seizure is going to have further attacks, thereby justifying a diagnosis of epilepsy and necessitating prophylactic anticonvulsant drug treatment.

Although some physicians start a patient on anticonvulsant medication after one convulsion, others prefer to withhold medication until the patient has had at least two seizures, at least in the nonpregnant state. During pregnancy, however, many physicians initiate anticonvulsant therapy after even a single seizure and arrange for neurologic reevaluation after delivery. This approach merits emphasis because many patients with so-called gestational epilepsy will have only a single convulsion, and continued treatment in such circumstances may therefore be unnecessary. Simple medical and neurologic investigations are indicated in an adult who has an isolated seizure and is otherwise well with no neurologic signs— hematologic and biochemical screening tests, electroencephalogram, and, particularly in the nonpregnant patient, magnetic resonance imaging (MRI) of the head and a chest radiograph. If the findings of such investigations are unremarkable, I discuss the controversial issue of anticonvulsant drug treatment with the patient but generally recommend that treatment be withheld unless a future attack occurs.

Pregnant women experiencing two or more seizures clearly merit prophylactic anticonvulsant drug treatment. In those with a progressive history, abnormal neurologic signs, or a focal electroencephalographic abnormality, it is also necessary to exclude an underlying structural lesion by means of MRI of the head. The management of such a lesion is described later in this chapter.

If prophylactic anticonvulsant drug treatment is necessary, it is generally continued until the patient has been seizure free for at least 2 or 3 years. Treatment is started with a small dose of one of the anticonvulsants, depending on the type of seizure experienced by the patient and the considerations outlined earlier. The dose is increased until seizures are controlled, blood concentrations reach the upper end of the optimal therapeutic range, or side effects limit further increments. If seizures continue despite optimal blood levels of the anticonvulsant drug selected, a second drug should be substituted for the first. Patients often respond preferentially to one or another of the various drugs that are available. Experience during pregnancy with certain newer antiepileptic agents (e.g., felbamate, lamotrigine, gabapentin, and topiramate) is limited, however, and their effect on the developing fetus is uncertain.

Patients must take medication as prescribed, and treatment should be controlled by frequent monitoring of the plasma anticonvulsant drug concentration. Monthly follow-up visits during pregnancy usually permit satisfactory supervision of the patient. At the initial visit, trough values of total and free concentrations of each drug should be measured. Total levels should then be measured each month in patients whose seizures are well controlled; free levels should be monitored monthly in those with poor seizure control, seizures during pregnancy, or a marked (more than 50%) decline in total level. Poor compliance with an anticonvulsant drug regimen can often be improved by encouragement and by explanation of the importance of taking medication regularly. Simplifying the dosage schedule so that medication is taken just once or twice daily may be helpful.

As the pregnancy continues, the dose of the anticonvulsant drug may need to be increased if seizures become more common or the free level of the anticonvulsant drug declines by more than about 30%. In some instances, the required dose may reach a level that would probably cause toxic side effects in a nonpregnant patient. If the anticonvulsant dosage is increased during the pregnancy, reductions will probably be necessary in the puerperium to prevent toxicity, but this change must be based on clinical evaluation and measurement of the plasma concentration of the drug, because the period over which drug requirements decline varies considerably. Because of the poorly defined risks of increased obstetric complications among pregnant epileptic women, close supervision of such patients by the obstetrician is mandatory, and delivery in a hospital is advised.

After delivery, the infant must be inspected for congenital malformations and given an injection of vitamin K_1 (1 mg/kg intramuscularly). Clotting factors should be studied after about 4 hours, and further injections of vitamin K_1 should be given if necessary. If hemorrhage occurs, infusions of fresh frozen plasma or of factors II, VII, IX, and X may also be necessary. Breast-feeding of a healthy infant by an epileptic mother should not be discouraged.

HEADACHE

Headache is a common complaint and may have many causes. Among patients attending headache clinics, symptoms are most frequently attributed to migraine, tension, or depression. Tension headaches are commonly chronic, last all day, are worse in the evening, may have a tight quality to them, may be accompanied by local soreness and concern about lumps or bumps on the head, and are often accompanied by poor concentration and nonspecific symptoms such as dizziness. The pain frequently commences, or is most intense, in the neck and the back of the head. If treatment with mild tranquilizers (such as diazepam) is unsuccessful, a trial of antimigraine preparations may be worthwhile. Depression headaches are somewhat similar but are often worse in the mornings, may be accompanied by other symptoms of depression, and often respond, to a limited extent, to tricyclic antidepressant drugs.

Most patients presenting with headache do not have severe underlying structural disease, but it is important to bear this possibility in mind. About one third of patients with brain tumors present with a primary complaint of headache. The headache in such patients is often an intermittent, dull, nonthrobbing ache that is exacerbated by exercise and may be associated with nausea or vomiting, but these features do not in themselves permit any reliable distinction from migraine. Similarly, the severity of the headache is unhelpful in this regard. Headaches that disturb sleep, however, are more suggestive of an underlying structural lesion, as are exertional headaches and late-onset paroxysmal headaches.

The duration and course of a headache also provide a guide to the underlying cause. A long history of chronic headache without other accompaniments is unlikely to reflect serious disease unless associated with drowsiness, visual disturbances, limb symptoms, seizures, intellectual changes, or other neurologic symptoms. The sudden development of severe headache in a previously well patient is more ominous and may well be due to acute intracranial abnormality (e.g., subarachnoid hemorrhage), glaucoma, or another condition requiring specific treatment.

The evaluation of patients with headaches demands a full general and neurologic examination together with an assessment of mental status. It may be necessary to include examination of the teeth, eyes, paranasal sinuses, and urine, and various investigative procedures may be indicated, depending on the initial clinical impression. If intracranial disease is suspected on the basis of the history or presence of neurologic signs, the need for computed tomography (CT) or MRI of the head, an electroencephalogram, and examination of the cerebrospinal fluid must be decided on an individual basis. Both cranial arteritis and cervical spondylosis are important causes of headache but would not be expected among patients in the childbearing age group.

Post-traumatic headaches generally pose no diagnostic problem because of the relationship to previous injury, and they usually respond to simple analgesics, mild tranquilizers, or antimigraine preparations. Acute sinusitis typically produces a localized throbbing headache accompanied by tenderness; the relationship of symptoms to a respiratory tract infection and the radiologic findings permit the diagnosis to be made with confidence, and treatment is directed at the underlying infection.

Migraine

Among women of childbearing age, migraine is an important cause of headache. In classic migraine, episodic headache is preceded by visual, sensory, or motor symptoms, but in other types there may be no premonitory focal symptoms. Headaches may be lateralized or generalized, generally have a gradual onset, and usually last for less than a day, although they may persist for longer. They may be dull or throbbing; are commonly accompanied by nausea, vomiting, and photophobia; and are often associated with blurring of vision, lightheadedness, and scalp tenderness. Photopsia, fortification spectra, and other focal neurologic symptoms may precede or accompany the headache, and consciousness is sometimes impaired or lost (syncopal attacks or seizures).

About 60% of women with migraine link the periodicity of some of their attacks to the menstrual cycle, with headaches occurring usually just before or during menstruation (Lance, 1973). It is migrainous attacks without aura that are most likely to be related to the menstrual cycle (Silberstein, 2001). Some patients may have headaches that occur only in relationship to the menstrual cycle, although this pattern is much less common. Several studies failed to show any abnormality of hormonal cycles in women with migraine relating to menstruation (Somerville, 1972a; Epstein et al., 1975); however, migraine headache can be postponed by artificial maintenance of elevated plasma estradiol levels, even though menstruation occurs at the expected time (Somerville, 1972a). The manner in which such hormonal factors provoke migraine remains unclear.

Migraine headaches are commonly exacerbated in women using oral contraceptives, but improvement can occur in some patients (Ryan, 1978). Such exacerbation usually becomes apparent within the first few months of oral contraceptive use (Ryan, 1978). Preparations with a relatively higher estrogen content are most likely to influence the headache pattern and are generally not as well tolerated as low-estrogen preparations. Recurrent headache provoked by the use of oral contraceptives may persist despite withdrawal of the offending medications, but whether this is anything more than fortuitous is unclear (Raskin, 1988). Of special concern is evidence suggesting that women with migraine exacerbated by oral contraceptives have an increased risk of cerebral infarction (Collaborative Group, 1975), perhaps caused by intimal hyperplasia of arteries supplying the brain (Irey et al., 1978).

Migraine often improves considerably after the first trimester of pregnancy, but it occasionally worsens or occurs for the first time during pregnancy, most commonly during the first 3 months of gestation (Somerville, 1972b). Lance (1973) found that relief occurred with pregnancy in 64% of those whose attacks were menstrual and in 48% of those with migraine unrelated to the menstrual cycle. A large study by Ratinahirana and colleagues (1990) produced similar findings. The response of migraine to pregnancy does not correlate with sex of the fetus or with differences in plasma progesterone levels, although it may relate to changes in the pattern of circulating estrogens (Somerville, 1972b).

Management of migraine consists of the avoidance of precipitating factors coupled with prophylactic or symptomatic drug treatment, if necessary. In general populations, when simple analgesics do not provide relief, treatment with extracranial vasoconstrictors (e.g., ergotamine or dihydroergotamine), β-adrenergic blockers (propranolol), serotonin agonists (e.g., sumatriptan), tricyclic antidepressants (amitriptyline), or other drugs may be necessary. Menstrual migraine may improve with standard pharmacologic therapy. Hormonal interventions are usually unsuccessful, but bromocriptine (2.5 mg three times daily) is sometimes worthwhile (Hertzog, 1997).

During pregnancy, medication is best avoided if possible. Dietary and other precipitants of headache should be avoided. When drugs are required, simple analgesics should be used. Acetaminophen is preferred over aspirin because aspirin may cause hemorrhagic complications and, in large doses in late pregnancy, may prolong labor and increase the incidence of stillbirth (Niederhoff and Zahrodnik, 1983; Sawle and Ramsay, 1998). Triptans are probably best avoided during pregnancy and breast-feeding, although there is no definite evidence of teratogenicity (Evans and Lipton, 2001). Meperidine suppositories (50 mg) may be prescribed for severe pain (Welch, 1994). A specific effort should be made to avoid ergotamine-containing preparations because of the effect this drug may have on the gravid uterus. Large doses of ergotamine given to animals in early pregnancy caused a number of complications, including fetal death, abortion, cataracts, and various developmental anomalies (Griffith et al., 1978). Ergonovine may induce chromosomal aberrations (Raskin, 1988). Propranolol is also best avoided during pregnancy because it may mildly impair fetal growth (Schoenfeld et al., 1978) and may theoretically lead to β-adrenergic blockade in the fetus or newborn.

Such inhibition of normal β-adrenergic responsiveness to asphyxia or to other stresses may theoretically increase the harmful effects of the latter (Rosen et al., 1979). Other reported potential neonatal complications include prematurity, respiratory depression, hypoglycemia, and hyperbilirubinemia (Ueland et al., 1981; Jackson and Fishbein, 1986).

A comparison of the reproductive histories of 777 women with and 182 women without migraine revealed the incidence of miscarriage, stillbirth, and toxemia of pregnancy to be similar (Wainscott et al., 1978). In addition, the incidence of congenital malformations among offspring of women with migraine was no greater than in the control group or in the general population, but the drug histories of the patients with migraine were incomplete.

Postnatal Headache

About one third of women experience headaches in the week after delivery, and most of them have either a past or family history of migraine (Stein, 1981). The headaches, which are usually mild and bifrontal, generally respond well to simple analgesics and are self-limited.

TUMORS

Any type of intracranial tumor can occasionally appear during the gestational period, and accurate diagnosis may then be delayed because symptoms are erroneously ascribed to toxemia of pregnancy. In addition, although the relationship between the tumor and pregnancy is usually fortuitous, pituitary adenomas, meningiomas, neurofibromas, hemangioblastomas, and vascular malformations occasionally exhibit relapses in relation to pregnancy, with symptoms developing or rapidly worsening during gestation, remitting to some extent after delivery, and recurring in a subsequent pregnancy. Attention here focuses on those aspects of intracranial tumors that relate to pregnancy rather than on a more general account of intracranial neoplasms.

Visual field defects sometimes develop during pregnancy in patients with a pituitary adenoma or a craniopharyngioma, which must be excluded in such circumstances. Meningiomas in the suprasellar or parasellar region or on the medial sphenoidal wing may also produce symptoms, such as diplopia and unilateral scotoma or ptosis, that relapse and remit in relation to pregnancy over several years. Symptoms tend to develop in the last 4 months of gestation and often lead to a mistaken initial diagnosis of multiple sclerosis. Early surgical intervention may help to preserve vision and prevent other neurologic catastrophes.

Symptoms caused by acoustic neuroma may begin or may be aggravated in the latter stages of pregnancy (Allen et al., 1974). Such symptoms in different patients include hearing loss, tinnitus, headaches, vertigo, dysequilibrium, facial weakness, and diplopia. Aggravation of symptoms in one pregnancy does not necessarily indicate that exacerbation will occur in subsequent ones.

In one study, 6 of 12 female patients with cerebellar hemangioblastomas were pregnant at the time of their first symptoms; in each case, however, at least one normal pregnancy had preceded the onset of symptoms (Robinson, 1965). Two patients underwent surgery in early pregnancy; one aborted shortly afterward, and the other carried her child to term. The other four patients went into normal labor and were successfully treated for the tumors later.

How pregnancy may precipitate or exacerbate symptoms caused by intracranial tumors is unclear. The most likely explanation is that pregnancy leads to a slight increase in the size of the tumor. Tumors with symptoms consistently related to pregnancy are usually so placed that only slight enlargement will lead to significant involvement of important neural structures. Thus, symptoms of spinal meningiomas may be exacerbated by pregnancy, but convexity meningiomas, which have room for expansion, are unlikely to show any particular relationship of symptoms to pregnancy.

Several possibilities have been advanced to account for the manner in which pregnancy might influence tumor size. Suggested mechanisms include accelerated growth rate, vascular engorgement, and increased fluid content; supportive evidence for these proposals is lacking. Nevertheless, there is accumulating evidence for sex steroid–binding sites in a number of human tumors, especially meningiomas (Schipper, 2001). The presence of such receptors in tumors suggests that the natural history of these tumors may be modifiable by these hormones or their antagonists.

Patients with intracranial neoplasms may have nonspecific symptoms of cerebral dysfunction, with evidence of raised intracranial pressure or some characteristic combination of symptoms and signs that reflect the location of the lesion. As always, the history and physical findings guide the manner in which such patients are evaluated further. MRI or CT of the head (Figs. 55-1 and 55-2) can now provide an enormous amount of additional information noninvasively. The former is more sensitive for diagnosis of an intracranial tumor and is safe in pregnant women because it does not involve exposure to radiation. When CT or other radiologic investigations are necessary, shielding may help to protect the fetus from excessive radiation.

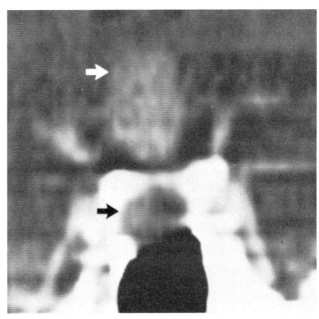

FIGURE 55-2 ■ Coronal reformation of computed tomography of same patient as in Figure 55-1. The intrasellar extent *(black arrow)* and suprasellar extent *(white arrow)* of the pituitary adenoma can be seen.

Each patient must be treated on an individual basis, and essential neurosurgical treatment should not be delayed because of the pregnancy. For pituitary adenomas or other benign tumors encountered in the latter half of pregnancy, operations can sometimes be delayed until a more propitious time if the patient is carefully observed. However, signs of increased intracranial pressure, visual deterioration, an increasing neurologic deficit, or the clinical features of an infratentorial lesion indicate the need for early or immediate intervention. For patients with pituitary adenomas, pharmacologic intervention (e.g., corticosteroids or bromocriptine) may be adequate. In most instances, visual disturbances improve spontaneously after delivery regardless of any pharmacologic measures (Simon, 1988). Cranial irradiation during the first trimester for the treatment of malignant brain tumors is associated with an increased risk of fetal loss or malformation; during later pregnancy, it is associated with an increased risk of childhood leukemia (DeAngelis, 1994).

In general, pregnancy can be allowed to proceed—at least until the fetus is viable and often to term—in patients with intracranial neoplasms; however, therapeutic abortion may be justifiable for some patients with malignant brain tumors and if significant symptoms, such as uncontrollable seizures, occur during pregnancy, particularly when the tumor cannot be removed completely (Kempers and Miller, 1963). Obstetric management must also be determined on an individual basis. Some investigators have proposed that delivery by cesarean section is safer than spontaneous vaginal delivery in women with cerebral tumors because the vaginal delivery may enhance any increase in intracranial pressure caused by the neoplasm. Vaginal delivery with adequate regional anesthesia and judicious shortening of the second stage of labor by use of low forceps (to prevent any increase in intracranial pressure associated with the abdominal pushing efforts of this stage) is often satisfactory, however.

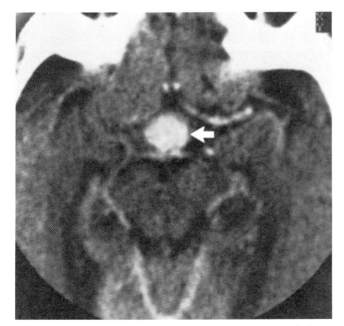

FIGURE 55-1 ■ Computed tomography of a patient with a pituitary adenoma, showing an enhancing lesion *(arrow)* in the suprasellar cistern. More inferior axial scans showed this lesion arising from the sella.

Pregnancy may be followed by the development of choriocarcinoma, which commonly metastasizes to the brain (Weed and Hunter, 1991). Neurologic presentation is typically with symptoms of a space-occupying cerebral lesion or with an acute deficit resulting from hemorrhage into the lesion. Treatment of cerebral metastases may involve chemotherapy, radiation therapy, and, for isolated metastases, surgery (Patchell et al., 1990).

PSEUDOTUMOR CEREBRI

There is a well-recognized association of benign intracranial hypertension with pregnancy and with oral contraceptive preparations. When symptoms do develop during pregnancy, they usually occur in the first trimester or the month after delivery, but they may occur at any time during the gestational period. Symptoms consist of headache and visual disturbances caused by papilledema and possibly diplopia resulting from abducens weakness. The patient looks well despite the grossly abnormal appearance of the optic disks, and neither electroencephalography nor MRI reveals any evidence of a space-occupying lesion. Although lumbar puncture will show increased pressure of the cerebrospinal fluid, the composition of the fluid is unremarkable. The possibility of intracranial venous sinus thrombosis must be kept in mind when the patient is being evaluated.

Although benign intracranial hypertension is self-limiting, remission may not occur until well after delivery, and the disorder sometimes recurs in a subsequent pregnancy. If the condition is left untreated, there is a risk of secondary optic atrophy and subsequent permanent impairment of vision. A number of different therapeutic approaches to lowering intracranial pressure have been reported, including use of high-dose steroids, acetazolamide, furosemide, repeated lumbar punctures, and lumboperitoneal or other shunting procedures. If the response to these measures is unsatisfactory and intracranial pressure remains high enough to endanger vision, optic nerve decompression may be required, as may early delivery of the fetus. There are no specific obstetric complications, and the patient can be expected to give birth to a normal infant.

OCCLUSIVE CEREBROVASCULAR DISEASE

Cerebrovascular disease may develop during an otherwise normal pregnancy as a result of either arterial or venous disease. Pregnancy increases the risk of cerebral infarction to about 13 times the rate expected outside of pregnancy (Wiebers, 1985). The risk seems to be greatest in the few days around the time of delivery (Salonen Ros et al., 2001).

Arterial Occlusive Disease

Arterial disease is not unusual, even in the absence of diabetes or severe hypertension, in women of childbearing age. Major arterial occlusion accounts for approximately two thirds of the cases of nonhemorrhagic hemiplegia that develop during pregnancy or the puerperium (Jennett and Cross, 1967). Numerous cases of occlusion of the middle cerebral artery or one of the other major intracranial arteries have been described during pregnancy, with occlusion generally occurring in the third trimester or the postpartum period. Such a stroke is usually due to the development of a thrombus on a preexisting atheromatous plaque. Predisposing factors may be anemia, hormonal influences, hypertension, increased platelet aggregability, reduced tissue plasminogen activity, changes in blood coagulation factors (especially factors V, VII, VIII, IX, X, and XII and fibrinogen) during late pregnancy, preeclamptic toxemia with hypertension, and puerperal septicemia. Other causes of stroke in young women include a protein C, protein S, and antithrombin III deficiency; hyperhomocysteinemia; arteritis; meningovascular syphilis; sickle cell disease; antiphospholipid antibodies; polycythemia and other hematologic disorders; and cardiomyopathy.

An embolus secondary to rheumatic or ischemic heart disease, subacute bacterial endocarditis, or a cardiac myxoma may occur. Rare instances of arterial occlusion by paradoxical embolization from a pelvic vein via a patent foramen ovale have also been described. Rarely, fat, air, or amniotic fluid embolism may occur in relation to childbirth. Hypotension as a consequence of hemorrhage or related to anesthesia during labor may lead to watershed cerebral infarction.

Transient cerebral ischemic attacks may precede occlusion of one of the major intracranial arteries. The neurologic disorder and the underlying arterial disease must be investigated and treated as in nonpregnant patients. Investigations should include complete blood count, blood smear, erythrocyte sedimentation rate, serum cholesterol and triglyceride levels, prothrombin and partial thromboplastin times, electrocardiogram, echocardiography, and radiologic procedures. CT is an important means of excluding intracranial hemorrhage. Angiography enables the major cerebral vessels to be visualized and may permit recognition of degenerative atherosclerotic disease that is remediable by disobliterative surgery (Fig. 55-3).

When surgically inaccessible disease of the intracranial arteries is present, the possibility that the obstruction is serving as a source of emboli must be borne in mind, and consideration

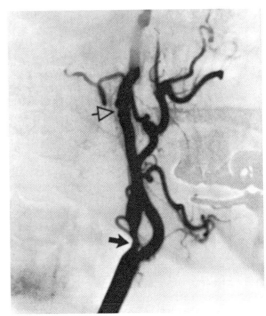

FIGURE 55-3 ■ Common carotid angiogram showing atherosclerotic narrowing of the internal carotid artery *(solid arrow)* at its origin. There is some corrugation of the internal carotid artery more rostrally at the level of C-1 and C-2, reflecting fibromuscular dysplasia *(open arrow).*

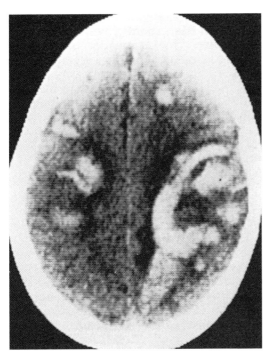

FIGURE 55-4 ■ Patient with superior sagittal sinus thrombosis. Computed tomography shows curvilinear areas of high density representing cortical venous thromboses and adjacent parenchymal venous infarcts.

must therefore be given to treatment with anticoagulants or aspirin. Warfarin is best avoided, if possible, because it crosses the placenta and increases hemorrhagic complications, and especially during the first trimester, because of the risks of teratogenicity and fetal wastage (Wiebers, 1985). Patients requiring anticoagulation during pregnancy are maintained instead on subcutaneously administered heparin, which usually is discontinued when labor begins and resumed about 12 hours after vaginal delivery or 24 hours after cesarean section. With regard to subsequent obstetric management, vaginal delivery, unless specifically contraindicated, is preferable to cesarean section. Other diseases that may be associated with arterial occlusive disease in pregnancy (e.g., eclampsia, thrombotic thrombocytopenic purpura) are discussed in Chapters 43 and 47.

The association of stroke with oral contraceptive use is now widely known. The risk can probably be reduced by lowering other risk factors, such as hypertension. A variety of mechanisms may be involved, including a predisposition to hypercoagulability, but the precise mechanisms have not been defined.

Intracranial Venous Occlusive Disease

Intracranial venous occlusive disease is an uncommon complication of pregnancy and childbirth. When the thrombosis occurs in the first trimester, it usually follows a complication such as spontaneous abortion, therapeutic abortion, or stillbirth, but it may occur in an otherwise normal pregnancy (Fishman et al., 1957; Stevens and Ammerman, 1959; Eckerling et al., 1963). Intracranial venous thrombosis is more likely in the third trimester or in the puerperium and is sometimes related to preeclampsia.

Intracranial venous thrombosis is characterized clinically by headache, paresis, focal or generalized convulsions, drowsiness, and confusion; disturbances of speech, sensation, or vision are not uncommon, and a mild pyrexia may be present. There may be signs of meningeal irritation caused by subarachnoid bleeding secondary to cortical infarction, and fluctuating hypertension is sometimes found (Goldman et al., 1964). Papilledema may be present, particularly if the superior sagittal sinus is involved. The cerebrospinal fluid pressure may be increased, and often the protein or cell content is elevated; occasionally the fluid is frankly bloodstained. The diagnosis may be confirmed by CT and magnetic resonance angiography, which are also necessary to exclude arterial pathology and vascular malformation (Figs. 55-4 and 55-5).

The symptoms and signs of intracranial venous thrombosis are sometimes ascribed mistakenly to eclampsia, but the absence of previous signs of preeclampsia should help in preventing diagnostic confusion.

The prognosis is not encouraging. In about one third of cases, intracranial venous thrombosis has a fatal outcome. Moreover, if patients do survive, thrombosis may recur later in the same pregnancy or the puerperium or in subsequent pregnancies.

The etiologic basis of aseptic intracranial venous thrombosis is uncertain; coagulation abnormalities, changes in the constituents of the peripheral blood, and intimal damage to the dural sinuses have been suggested as causes. Protein C, protein S, and antithrombin III deficiencies are common inherited prothrombotic states. Protein S deficiency, in particular, has been associated with cerebral venous thrombosis (Confavreux et al., 1994). Low levels of protein C and S have been reported during pregnancy (Markus and Hambley, 1998). Activated protein C resistance has been noted in a number of

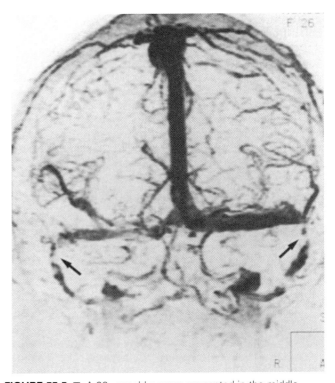

FIGURE 55-5 ■ A 26-year-old woman presented in the middle trimester of pregnancy with headache and had bilateral papilledema. Imaging studies of the brain were normal. This coronal view of her magnetic resonance venogram (obtained using a two-dimensional time-of-flight technique) shows loss of flow-related enhancement in both transverse sinuses *(arrows)* consistent with thrombus formation.

patients with venous thromboembolic events and also with cerebral venous thrombosis. Deschiens and associates (1996) found that 6 of 40 patients with cerebral venous thrombosis had protein C or S deficiency or activated protein C resistance, and 3 of 12 patients were similarly found by Weih and coworkers (1998) to have the factor V Leiden mutation (a common cause of activated protein C resistance).

The treatment of intracranial venous thrombosis is controversial. It may include anticonvulsant drugs if seizures have occurred and antiedemic agents, such as dexamethasone and mannitol, to reduce the intracranial pressure. Anticoagulant drugs have been used in the belief that they may prevent extension of thrombosis, but they may provoke hemorrhagic intracranial complications (Gettelfinger and Kokmen, 1977). The risk of intracranial hemorrhage has probably been exaggerated, and one study suggests that anticoagulation with dose-adjusted intravenous heparin is effective treatment for venous sinus thrombosis (Einhaupl et al., 1991).

Labor can usually be allowed to commence spontaneously, with forceps assistance of delivery, if the thrombosis has occurred early in pregnancy. If thrombosis occurs shortly before or during labor, however, cesarean section may be necessary.

Several other reports have stressed that a strong relationship exists between factor V Leiden mutation and cerebral venous thrombosis (Dulli et al., 1996; Martinelli et al., 1996; Pugliese et al., 1998), particularly in women taking oral contraceptive preparations (Bloemenkamp et al., 1995). Whether all women should be tested for factor V Leiden before receiving oral contraceptive agents is unsettled. It does seem reasonable, however, to test for activated protein C resistance in patients experiencing a stroke during pregnancy or the postpartum period or while receiving oral contraceptives.

Pituitary Infarction

Sheehan syndrome is a well-recognized complication of the peripartum period (see Chapter 51).

INTRACRANIAL (SUBARACHNOID) HEMORRHAGE

Subarachnoid hemorrhage is more common in women than in men. Mhurchu and colleagues (2001) found that menstrual and reproductive history (other than an older age at birth of first child) did not influence the risk of hemorrhage; the risk was not affected by use of oral contraceptive agents. Okamoto and associates (2001), however, noted an increased risk of subarachnoid hemorrhage with an earlier age of menarche and with nulligravity; they found no association with regularity of menstrual cycle, age at pregnancy or first birth, or number of births.

When intracranial hemorrhage occurs during pregnancy, it is usually, at least in part, into the subarachnoid space. Sudden severe headache, sometimes accompanied by nausea and vomiting, is the main symptom. Examination reveals signs of meningeal irritation that may be accompanied by depressed consciousness, cranial nerve abnormalities, and a neurologic deficit in the limbs.

In patients in whom subarachnoid hemorrhage complicates otherwise normal pregnancies, the underlying source is most commonly an aneurysm and less often an angioma or of indeterminate cause. Other less common causes of intracranial hemorrhage include mycotic aneurysms, vasculitides, various hematologic disorders, disseminated intravascular coagulation, eclampsia, and metastatic choriocarcinoma. Treatment is of the underlying cause. Although bleeding may occur at any time during the pregnancy, aneurysms are somewhat more likely to bleed in the latter half of the gestational period.

Cerebral angiomas, which are located supratentorially in at least 70% of patients, may appear at any age. Intracranial or subarachnoid hemorrhage is the most common presentation. The peak age for hemorrhage is between 15 and 20 years, and about 70% of all angiomas that are going to bleed will have done so by the time patients reach age 40 years (Perret and Nishioka, 1966). The mortality rate from an initial hemorrhage is approximately 10% but has varied in different series; survivors are more likely to experience further hemorrhage than patients who have never had one. Other patients with intracranial angiomas may present with focal or generalized seizures, headache, focal neurologic deficits, or nonspecific neurologic symptoms. Robinson and colleagues (1974) reported that pregnancy has a deleterious effect on intracranial angiomas, making them more likely to bleed, but their impression has not been substantiated by others (Parkinson and Bachers, 1980) unless there is a history of earlier bleeds (Horton et al., 1990).

Intracranial saccular aneurysms arise from a developmental arterial defect, and with increasing age they become more common sources of hemorrhage than angiomas. They are generally located at sites of vessel branching, occurring with particular frequency in relation to the anterior or posterior communicating arteries. Although such aneurysms sometimes cause focal symptoms that relate to compression of neighboring structures, patients generally present with hemorrhage that occurs without warning, owing to aneurysmal rupture. Such hemorrhage seems to occur more commonly in the late rather than early stages of pregnancy (Sadasivan et al., 1990), but occurrence during labor and delivery has been reported only rarely. In addition to the signs of subarachnoid hemorrhage, focal or lateralizing neurologic signs may be present and help to localize the source of bleeding.

In the evaluation of patients presenting with symptoms of intracranial hemorrhage, the first diagnostic study now performed is usually a CT of the head, which is a reliable means of detecting recent subarachnoid or intracerebral hemorrhage and may permit the source of bleeding to be localized (Fig. 55-6). In patients with angiomas, nonhomogeneous areas of mixed density with irregular calcifications are typical, and vermiform areas of enhancement are seen after infusion of contrast material. Aneurysms are seen as small, round, dense areas after infusion of contrast material and are sometimes evident even without contrast. If CT findings are normal, the cerebrospinal fluid should be examined and angiography undertaken if the fluid is bloodstained or xanthochromic.

Angiography permits the identity of the lesion to be established with certainty and provides important additional information concerning its anatomic features (Fig. 55-7). Special shielding during this and other radiologic procedures should be provided for pregnant patients. All the major intracranial vessels should be opacified; feeding vessels to angiomas sometimes arise from the contralateral side, and it is not uncommon for aneurysms to be multiple. Angiography does not reveal the malformation in the occasional patient with a suspected

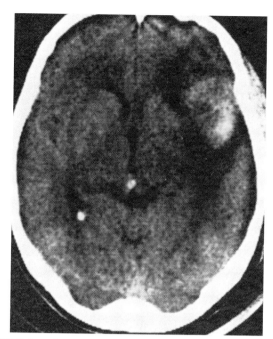

FIGURE 55-6 ■ Computed tomography showing hemorrhage into the sylvian fissure and adjacent parenchyma, with surrounding edema and/or ischemia. The findings are indicative of subarachnoid and intracerebral hemorrhage and localize the source of bleeding to the middle cerebral artery.

angioma, possibly because the lesion was small and destroyed itself when it bled ("cryptic malformation"). Nevertheless, if angiography shows neither an angioma nor an aneurysm in a patient presenting with subarachnoid hemorrhage, the study should be repeated after about 14 days because vascular spasm after a bleed may obscure an aneurysm.

The management of subarachnoid hemorrhage consists of bed rest, with sedation and analgesia as necessary and operative or endovascular treatment of the underlying lesion if feasible. Surgical treatment is aimed at preventing further hemorrhages, but induction of hypotension during the course of the intracranial operation should be avoided unless it is essential because it may be followed by premature labor or fetal death; hypothermia is well tolerated (Robinson et al., 1974).

If the anomalous vessels constituting an angioma are surgically accessible and do not involve a critical vessel or area of the brain, they can often be excised. Such surgery is commonly preceded by embolization of the main vessels feeding the malformation in an attempt to reduce the size of the latter. Other obliterative techniques have been developed (Aminoff, 1983). The optimal time for treatment of an angioma is uncertain, but therapeutic intervention is often delayed until after childbirth (Sadasivan et al., 1990). In the patient with an aneurysm that has bled, the risk of further bleeding is much greater, especially in the weeks after the initial hemorrhage. Accordingly, operative treatment, if indicated by the angiographic findings and the condition of the patient, should not be delayed because of the pregnancy (Stoodley et al., 1998). An endovascular approach may be successful (Piotin et al., 2001) and is being favored increasingly over surgery.

In patients with aneurysms that have been successfully obliterated or that ruptured before the last trimester, pregnancy and delivery can generally be allowed to proceed normally. In patients with incompletely obliterated or unop-

erated aneurysms that ruptured in the last 2 months of pregnancy, cesarean section is probably advisable at 38 weeks' gestation. Some authorities also advocate delivery by elective cesarean section at 38 weeks in patients with arteriovenous malformations and further recommend that concomitant sterilization be considered (Robinson et al., 1974), presumably if the malformation itself is inoperable. However, the need for either procedure in this context is unclear, and arguments for them are without adequate foundation. In patients showing a steady deterioration in neurologic status and for whom a fatal outcome seems likely, preparations should be made so that the fetus, if viable, can be delivered before it dies from anoxia.

VASCULAR ANOMALIES AND THE NERVOUS SYSTEM

The most important vascular anomalies that occur in relation to the nervous system are intracranial aneurysms and cerebral angiomas (see preceding section). However, several other types of vascular anomalies may become manifest during pregnancy and merit brief discussion.

Intracranial Dural Vascular Anomalies

Certain intracranial dural vascular anomalies may become evident for the first time during pregnancy. They consist of abnormal arteriovenous shunts involving meningeal branches of the carotid and vertebral arteries and the dural veins and sinuses. Although some represent a developmental anomaly, others are acquired in adult life, occasionally after trauma, presumably because of the close anatomic relationship of certain meningeal arteries and veins. A detailed account of these anomalies is provided by Aminoff (1983).

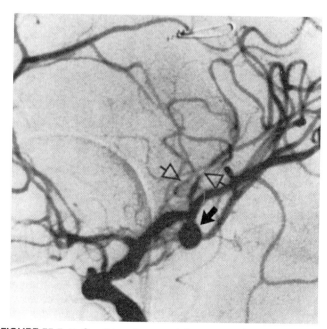

FIGURE 55-7 ■ Carotid angiogram of the same patient as in Figure 55-6. An aneurysm *(solid arrow)* is shown at the trifurcation of the middle cerebral artery. There is some spasm of vessels in the vicinity of the aneurysm *(open arrows)*.

Shunts involving the anterior–inferior group of dural sinuses (cavernous, intercavernous, sphenoparietal, superior and inferior petrosal, and basilar plexus) are characterized clinically by unilateral orbital or head pain, diplopia, a red or protruding eye, and tinnitus. The onset of symptoms sometimes follows abortion or relates to the postpartum period (Newton and Hoyt, 1970; Taniguchi et al., 1971), possibly because of rupture of the thin-walled dural arteries during the straining of labor or because of the circulatory changes that occur in pregnancy.

On examination, there is usually a mild proptosis, distended conjunctival veins, increased intraocular pressure, a transient sixth nerve palsy, or a bruit over the eye. Angiography reveals a low-volume shunt supplied from meningeal branches of the internal or external carotid arteries, sometimes from the contralateral side. Drainage may be directly into the cavernous sinus or into a more distant dural sinus or venous structure that communicates with the cavernous sinus. The fistula may close spontaneously, but if it remains patent, embolization of the feeding vessels may help to relieve intolerable symptoms or failing vision.

Arteriovenous shunts to the superior–posterior group of dural sinuses (superior and inferior sagittal, straight, transverse, sigmoid, and occipital) may also occur, with a female predominance among the reported cases. Symptoms and signs may relate to the shunt itself, to subarachnoid hemorrhage, to increased intracranial pressure, or to cerebral ischemia.

Tinnitus is the most common complaint, but headache, visual deterioration, subarachnoid hemorrhage, seizures, and various neurologic deficits may also occur. A bruit is often present and may be the sole finding on examination; it is best heard over the mastoid region or behind the ear. Papilledema may be present, and other neurologic signs are sometimes encountered. The arterial supply is commonly from branches of the external carotid artery, tentorial branches of the internal carotid artery, and meningeal branches of the vertebral artery. Ligation or embolization of feeding vessels or a direct surgical approach to the lesion may be helpful in patients with disabling symptoms or a history of hemorrhage.

Dural and Intradural Spinal Angiomas

Spinal angiomas are uncommon but are important to recognize because most are readily treated by surgery. Most are arteriovenous malformations, and most of these are dural; if intradural, they are commonly extramedullary, are posterior to the cord, and are fed by one or more arteries that either fail to supply the cord or contribute only to the posterior spinal circulation (Aminoff, 1976).

Spinal arteriovenous malformations may lead to spinal subarachnoid hemorrhage but more commonly give rise to a gradual disturbance in function of cord, nerve roots, or both. Spinal subarachnoid hemorrhage is much more common in patients with a cervical malformation than a more caudal lesion, may sometimes occur from an associated (arterial) aneurysm, and is associated with an overall mortality of at least 15%. It may be the first symptom produced by the lesion. Approximately half of the patients who survive the first hemorrhage have a second, and half of the subsequent survivors have further bleeding episodes unless the underlying malformation is treated. The spinal source of the hemorrhage may not be recognized until the later development of symptoms and signs of cord dysfunction, despite the local occurrence of sudden severe pain at the onset of bleeding, accompanied by signs of meningeal irritation.

Myelopathy or radiculopathy, or both, of gradual or sudden onset, is the more common mode of presentation. By the time of diagnosis, approximately two thirds of patients complain of leg weakness, sensory symptoms, pain, and a sphincter disturbance. In some patients, symptoms, especially pain, are precipitated or aggravated by exercise and relieved by rest, whereas symptoms in other patients may relate to specific postures, such as sitting or bending forward. Symptoms occasionally relate to pregnancy, the menstrual cycle, nonspecific infective illness, a transient increase in body temperature, or trauma. On examination, signs of an upper or lower motor neuron disturbance or a mixed motor deficit are usually found in the legs; sensory deficits are common and are usually extensive, but occasionally they may be restricted to a radicular distribution. There may be a coexisting cutaneous angioma that occasionally relates segmentally to the spinal lesion, and a bruit may be audible over the spine on auscultation.

Numerous case reports illustrating the influence of pregnancy on these lesions have been published. In one case that I encountered, symptoms occurred during each of three pregnancies, with complete clearing after delivery. Their basis was not recognized until the patient later experienced leg weakness and urinary retention that necessitated immediate hospitalization; myelography and spinal angiography then demonstrated an arteriovenous malformation that was treated surgically.

The relationship of symptoms to pregnancy in such cases may be based in part on enhancement of preexisting cord ischemia by hemodilution and anemia. Moreover, pressure on pelvic and abdominal veins by an enlarged uterus may aggravate symptoms of caudally situated malformations by obstructing venous return to the heart, with a consequent reduction in intramedullary arteriovenous pressure gradient and thus in cord blood flow (Aminoff, 1976).

Diagnosis depends on radiologic investigations, which must not be postponed out of concern for the developing fetus, because any delay in establishing the diagnosis may lead to increased, often irreversible, disability in the mother. Spinal MRI may fail to detect the lesion. At myelography, the characteristic abnormality consists of vermiform defects caused by vascular impressions in the column of contrast material, usually without any obstruction in the subarachnoid space. If myelography suggests a vascular malformation, spinal angiography is undertaken to determine the level and extent of the vascular abnormality; the position of the arteriovenous shunt in relation to the cord; the number, origin, and anatomic location of arteries feeding the malformation; and the main supply to the cord in the region of the malformation.

Treatment is indicated in all patients who have progressive symptoms or functional incapacity or have had a hemorrhage. Delay in these cases may lead to irreversible disability or even death. When the angioma is dural or intradural but mainly or completely extramedullary, is posterior to the cord, and is fed by vessels that do not contribute to the anterior spinal circulation, surgical treatment or embolization generally poses no specific problem. Feeding vessels are obliterated, and the fistulous portion of the malformation is removed. Malformations located anterior to or within the cord are more difficult to treat because of their inaccessibility and because they are often supplied by the anterior spinal artery or one of its feeders. Such lesions are often regarded as inoperable, and experience in their treatment remains limited.

INFECTIONS

The central nervous system may be infected by bacterial, viral, fungal, or other organisms through the blood supply, by extension from infected adjacent structures, or by direct inoculation such as may follow trauma. The neural parenchyma may be involved diffusely (as in encephalitis) or focally (as with cerebral abscess), or infection may primarily involve the meninges and parameningeal structures (such as in meningitis or subdural empyema). Although the resulting neurologic disorder may complicate pregnancy or delivery or may necessitate antimicrobial therapy that can harm the developing fetus, the clinical features, diagnosis, and management of such infections during pregnancy are essentially the same as at other times. Accordingly, further discussion is limited to certain infections that either pose some particular problem when they occur during pregnancy or are especially likely to develop in relation to pregnancy.

Poliomyelitis

The development of an effective vaccine has all but eradicated paralytic poliomyelitis in developed countries. Even pregnant women can be included safely in programs of mass vaccination with live oral poliovirus vaccine (Harjulehto-Mervaala et al., 1994). Nevertheless, the disorder still occurs in unprotected persons and remains common in many parts of the world. Moreover, people with residual disability from previous poliomyelitis are still seen fairly regularly in most large medical centers; obstetric management of such patients may be complicated by their neurologic deficits.

Most patients infected with poliovirus either are asymptomatic or have only minor nonspecific respiratory or gastrointestinal symptoms. Nervous system involvement occurs in only a few instances; its clinical manifestations are described in standard neurologic textbooks. Patients with neurologic involvement should be hospitalized, with care taken to provide for any circulatory or respiratory complications that may develop. Simple analgesics can be provided for relief of pain, and physical therapy may be helpful once muscle weakness has stabilized.

Pregnancy increases the susceptibility of women to clinical poliomyelitis (Weinstein et al., 1951). In one large series of patients admitted with poliomyelitis, 34% of the married women and 26% of all the women of reproductive age were pregnant (Hunter and Millikan, 1954). It is unclear, however, whether pregnant women become more susceptible to the initial viral infection or merely become more susceptible to invasion of the nervous system. Pregnancy may also alter the course of the infection. The course is unaffected if poliomyelitis develops early in pregnancy, but an increase in severity or distribution of the muscle weakness may occur if childbirth takes place during the acute phase or shortly thereafter (Weinstein et al., 1951).

In early pregnancy, and especially during the first trimester, spontaneous abortion may occur either in association with a febrile reaction in the acute phase of poliomyelitis or in relation to apparently mild nonparalytic attacks of the disease. Abortion or fetal loss may also occur spontaneously in the second or third trimester but often with maternal illness of such severity that assisted respiration may be necessary.

Even patients with severe poliomyelitis necessitating respirator assistance can usually be managed supportively, and labor can be managed similarly to that in normal women unless there are specific obstetric indications for operative delivery or induction of labor. The uterine muscle is not paralyzed.

Fetal poliomyelitis is exceedingly rare. Normal offspring can generally be anticipated, although Schaeffer and colleagues (1954) reported the presence of the virus in both the fetus and placenta after a spontaneous abortion that occurred 11 days after a clinical attack of poliomyelitis in a 24-year-old woman.

Neonatal cases of poliomyelitis are well recognized. If an infant is affected within the first 5 days of life, the disorder is assumed to be secondary to transplacental transmission of the virus. Such neonatal cases are associated with a mortality rate of at least 50%, but subclinical infection with poliovirus may certainly also occur in newborn infants.

Tetanus

A worldwide disease, tetanus is rarely encountered in developed countries where immunization procedures are freely available. *Clostridium tetani* infection via tetanus spores may follow injury, surgical procedures, childbirth, abortion, and injections. If the spores are converted into vegetative grampositive rods and favorable anaerobic conditions are present, tetanospasmin, a toxin that is responsible for the symptoms of tetanus, is produced.

The incubation period is variable. In generalized tetanus, the most common presenting symptom is trismus and the disorder itself is characterized by frequent spasms of various muscles that can be provoked by minor external stimuli and may occur against a background of continuous tonic muscle contractions. Typically, the trunk is hyperextended, the arms are flexed, and the legs are extended; laryngospasm may lead to respiratory obstruction.

Localized tetanus is more benign and is characterized by persistent rigidity of muscles close to the site of inoculation with the organism. A splanchnic form is described after abdominal and pelvic operations or uterine trauma, with prominent involvement of the muscles of deglutition and respiration.

The morbidity and mortality rates also vary. Respiratory complications are a leading cause of death, as is the autonomic hyperactivity that sometimes complicates tetanus. Treatment is directed at the following:

1. Neutralizing unbound toxin with antitoxin
2. Reducing further toxin production by surgical toilet and antibiotic treatment
3. Controlling tetanic spasms by drugs such as diazepam, chlorpromazine, and barbiturates
4. Assisting respiration mechanically if necessary
5. Undertaking general supportive measures

Tetanus may develop as a complication of childbirth or abortion, especially in underdeveloped countries. It leads to abortion in many instances and has a maternal mortality rate that often exceeds 50%. In addition to the measures just listed, evacuation of products retained in the uterus may be necessary, and hysterectomy is sometimes required (Speroff, 1966; Reid, 1967).

Tetanus is also a common cause of neonatal death in underdeveloped countries. Infection usually results from a lack of hygiene during delivery, with consequent contamination of the umbilical cord. The clinical manifestations differ from those in older children or adults, in that dysphagia and respiratory problems are often more marked, fever is usually higher, and the disease is generally more severe, often fulminating. Most affected infants are 6 to 9 days old when admitted and have a typical history of continuous crying for up to 48 hours, followed by cessation of sucking and then of crying, accompanied by convulsions and often fever.

In regions where neonatal tetanus is common, the mortality rate may approach 10% of births. Improvement of delivery practices and obstetric services may prevent the disorder, as may the active immunization of pregnant women and the substitution of disinfectants for traditional cord-care practices (Axelsson, 2002). Unfortunately, in most areas with a high incidence of tetanus neonatorum, there are no widely available maternity services, and any prophylactic approach that depends on the early identification of pregnant women is impractical. In one series, however, immunization of women with two or three intramuscular injections of tetanus toxoid resulted in complete absence of neonatal tetanus among the offspring of subsequent pregnancies for more than 4 years (Newell et al., 1966).

Miscellaneous Maternal Infections

Clinical or subclinical maternal infection may involve the fetus and may affect the developing nervous system and thus the neonate. The resulting neurologic complications merit brief comment here. Fetal infection may be inconsequential or may result in abortion, stillbirth, growth retardation, congenital disease, or developmental anomalies. Gestational age at the time of infection influences the effects (see Chapter 39).

Infection with *Listeria monocytogenes* is an important cause of habitual abortion and may also lead to a variety of other manifestations in pregnant women. In neonates, infection may take an early-onset predominantly septicemic form, characterized by prematurity, respiratory distress, heart failure, and increased neonatal mortality, or a late-onset predominantly meningitic or meningoencephalitic form. Diagnosis depends on the bacteriologic and serologic findings. Treatment consists of appropriate antibiotic therapy, usually with ampicillin.

Maternal rubella, especially when it occurs in the first 2 months of pregnancy, may cause fetal infection and a congenital syndrome characterized by ocular abnormalities, deafness, mental retardation, seizures, focal neurologic deficits, cardiac anomalies, hepatosplenomegaly, and other abnormalities in a variety of combinations. In rare patients with congenital rubella, pyramidal and extrapyramidal signs, seizures, and dementia occur as part of a progressive panencephalitic illness during the second decade of life; high antibody titers to rubella virus occur in blood and cerebrospinal fluid, and the virus may even be isolated from the brain (Townsend et al., 1975; Weil et al., 1975).

In *congenital toxoplasmosis*, seizures and pyramidal defects may result from meningoencephalitis together with chorioretinitis, obstructive hydrocephalus, and cerebral calcification. There may be respiratory and feeding difficulties. Later mental development may be retarded. For prophylactic purposes, pregnant women should be advised to avoid contact with cat feces and ingestion of raw or undercooked meat.

Fetal infections with *cytomegalovirus* may cause hepatosplenomegaly, jaundice, petechiae, ocular defects, cardiac defects, and other abnormalities. Involvement of the nervous system may lead to cerebral malformation, microcephaly, mental retardation, seizures, obstructive hydrocephalus, cerebral calcification, deafness, or chorioretinitis.

Herpes simplex virus infection in the neonate is characterized primarily by visceral involvement, but the brain may be affected. Seizures, irritability, motor deficits, increased intracranial pressure, and depression of consciousness may all occur, sometimes in the apparent absence of more widespread disease.

Children born to women infected with the *human immunodeficiency virus* are at risk of infection with the virus. The risk varies in different series for uncertain reasons. The virus may infect the fetus *in utero* or the neonate during birth or through breast milk. Infected children may develop acquired immunodeficiency syndrome after an interval ranging from several months to several years. This leads typically to developmental delay and regression as a result of progressive encephalopathy. Calcification of the basal ganglia may occur. Systemic features include failure to thrive, pneumonitis, hepatosplenomegaly, and recurrent bacterial infections. Management of pregnant women with human immunodeficiency virus infection therefore includes minimizing the risk of transmitting the infection to offspring, recognizing neonatal infection early, reducing the risk of opportunistic infection, and managing psychosocial aspects. Antiretroviral therapy of infected women during pregnancy and zidovudine therapy of neonates for 6 weeks (or longer and with combination therapy if necessary) may be helpful. The protective effect of maternal therapy depends on the complexity and duration of treatment, and HAART (highly active antiretroviral therapy) is associated with the lowest transmission rates (Cooper et al., 2002). Compared with no antiretroviral treatment or monotherapy, combination therapy does not seem to be associated with increased risks of prematurity or other adverse outcomes of pregnancy (Tuomala et al., 2002). The use of infant formula to prevent postnatal transmission through breast milk has helped to reduce the incidence of infection in developed countries (Fowler et al., 2000; Mofenson and McIntyre, 2000). Infants may require monitoring for 1 to 2 years with testing for human immunodeficiency virus to exclude infection. For further discussion, see Chapter 40.

The possibility of *syphilitic infection* must be borne in mind during the evaluation of all pregnant women. Effective treatment of maternal syphilis at an early stage of pregnancy generally prevents fetal involvement, and treatment in later pregnancy affects both mother and fetus. Syphilis may severely affect pregnancy, leading to increased chances of abortion and perinatal mortality and to symptomatic congenital syphilis in many of the surviving infants. Infants may also be infected at birth if they come into contact with an infective lesion. The possibility of congenital infection can be confirmed by various serologic tests. The clinical features of congenital neurosyphilis, which may become apparent after the first few weeks of life or may be delayed for several years, are essentially the same as those of neurosyphilis in adults. Infants with clinical or laboratory evidence of infection require treatment to prevent its occurrence, penicillin being the drug of choice.

◼ METABOLIC DISORDERS

A number of metabolic disorders are considered elsewhere in this chapter, including Wilson disease, hepatic porphyria, and the Wernicke-Korsakoff syndrome. In this section, attention is confined to two other disorders that are important to recognize for therapeutic purposes: vitamin B$_{12}$ deficiency and phenylketonuria (PKU).

Vitamin B$_{12}$ Deficiency

Vitamin B$_{12}$ deficiency is a well-known cause of neurologic disease (myelopathy characterized predominantly by pyramidal and posterior column deficits, polyneuropathy, mental changes, optic neuropathy) in adults, in whom it may arise from malabsorption, dietary inadequacy, or other causes. There is often an accompanying megaloblastic anemia, but this may be obscured if folic acid supplements have been taken. Clinical presentation during pregnancy does not differ from that in the nongestational period. Treatment with parenteral vitamin B$_{12}$ prevents further progression and may lead to improvement, at least in part, of the neurologic disorder.

It is not widely recognized that maternal vitamin B$_{12}$ deficiency during pregnancy and the puerperium may lead to a similar deficiency in the fetus and neonate. A reduced content of vitamin B$_{12}$ in maternal milk may then lead to frank deficiency in breast-fed infants. The resulting clinical syndrome among such infants is characterized by megaloblastic anemia, cutaneous pigmentation, apathy, developmental delay or regression, and involuntary movements (Jadhav et al., 1962). The clinical and biochemical abnormalities are rapidly corrected by vitamin supplementation.

Phenylketonuria

An autosomal recessive disorder, PKU is an important cause of mental retardation, which develops in the absence of adequate dietary treatment. Screening programs for neonates with PKU have permitted the identification and treatment of affected infants to prevent intellectual deterioration, but the optimal duration of treatment remains unclear (Scriver and Clow, 1980). Women with PKU have a high rate of spontaneous abortion, and their nonphenylketonuric (heterozygote) offspring have a high incidence of certain abnormalities. Among the offspring of pregnancies during which the maternal PKU is untreated, there are marked increases in the incidence of mental retardation, microcephaly, and congenital heart disease compared with the normal population, and these increases correlate with maternal blood levels of phenylalanine (Lenke and Levy, 1980).

The fetal effects of maternal PKU occur because of the high maternal blood levels of phenylalanine, not because the infant has PKU. Dietary treatment during early pregnancy (i.e., within the first 2 months) may prevent the fetal effects (Koch et al., 2000). Treatment of women known to have PKU is best reinitiated before conception, however, and may need to be in effect at conception for maximal benefit. Even so, a normal child cannot be ensured.

The mother with undiagnosed PKU poses different problems. Antenatal screening for maternal PKU (or testing for PKU at the first antenatal visit of a woman with a family history of the disease, low intelligence of uncertain etiology, or a history of microcephalic offspring) may be justifiable.

The newborn offspring of a mother with PKU will be homozygous or heterozygous for the disorder. The homozygotes definitely require a diet low in phenylalanine, but the proper nutritional management of heterozygotes is less clear. The mother, however, should be advised against breast-feeding because her milk will contain a high concentration of phenylalanine.

Elevation of blood phenylalanine levels is only minimal during pregnancy in mothers who are heterozygous for the disorder, and the incidence of congenital anomalies and brain damage is not excessive in their offspring, except for congenital pyloric stenosis (Scriver and Clow, 1980).

■ MOVEMENT DISORDERS

When *dystonia* develops during pregnancy, it usually presents acutely as a consequence of treatment with antiemetic dopamine antagonists (such as metoclopramide), neuroleptic drugs, or levodopa. In patients with established dystonia, genetic counseling may be prudent if the disorder has a hereditary basis, and the need to continue on pharmacologic treatment should be evaluated before planned pregnancy. *Parkinson disease* shows no consistent change during pregnancy, but little information is available concerning the safety of antiparkinsonian agents when taken during the gestational period.

Chorea Gravidarum

The term "chorea" refers to involuntary rapid muscle jerks that occur unpredictably in different parts of the body. When the disorder is florid, choreic limb movements and facial grimacing are unmistakable and distort any concomitant voluntary activity. In mild cases, there may be no more than a persistent restlessness and clumsiness.

Sydenham chorea is generally regarded as a complication of infection with group A hemolytic streptococci, the underlying pathology possibly being an arteritis. When it occurs during pregnancy, it is referred to as "chorea gravidarum." This disease occurs most commonly in primigravidas, with symptoms tending to occur in the early part of pregnancy and remitting after delivery. A history of chorea and rheumatic fever is obtained in about two thirds of patients, and the other third have clinical signs of rheumatic heart disease. Psychological disturbance may occasionally be conspicuous. Willson and Preece (1932) found that 20% of women with the disorder have a recurrence in later pregnancies. Death, primarily caused by underlying rheumatic heart disease, is rare (Beresford and Graham, 1950).

Symptomatic benefit follows bed rest and sedation, and there is no indication for termination of pregnancy. The prognosis is essentially that of any cardiac complication. No specific obstetric complications are associated with chorea gravidarum, and a normal healthy infant can generally be anticipated.

Although many cases of chorea gravidarum relate to preceding streptococcal infection, in other instances there is no clinical or laboratory evidence of such an association. Instead, clinical impression suggests that pregnancy has, in some way, merely exacerbated some preexisting disturbance that then becomes clinically evident. Similarly, chorea is occasionally induced by oral contraceptives in women with preexisting basal ganglia abnormalities resulting from various causes. The dyskinesia in such cases usually begins within about 3 months of the introduction of contraceptive therapy, evolves subacutely, is often asymmetrical or unilateral, and resolves with discontinuation of the offending substance. The pathophysiologic basis of hormonal contraceptive-induced chorea is uncertain, but a vascular mechanism (Lewis and Harrison, 1969), an immunologic mechanism (Gamboa et al., 1971), and a hormone-dependent alteration in central dopaminergic activity (Nausieda et al., 1979) have tentatively been advanced as the underlying causes.

Barber and colleagues (1976) described a young woman with hemichorea that developed with the use of oral contraceptives, later recurred in early pregnancy, and cleared after therapeutic abortion. Subsequent challenge with a combined estrogen–progestogen pill led to recurrence of chorea, but the patient was then successfully managed with progestogen alone without further symptoms, suggesting that the estrogen component was responsible for the dyskinesia. Estrogens may certainly influence catecholamine turnover rates in parts of the brain (Yen, 1977), and this process may therefore be the mechanism by which both chorea gravidarum and contraceptive-induced chorea occur in patients with previous damage, subclinical or evident, to the basal ganglia. Other observations, summarized by Nausieda and coworkers (1979), imply that a more complex interaction between estrogenic and progestational hormonal levels is involved.

Chorea developing for the first time during pregnancy must not automatically be regarded as a variant of Sydenham chorea, because it may arise for other reasons. The choreic movements of Huntington disease occasionally occur for the first time during pregnancy, but the subsequent course of events and the family history will point to the correct diagnosis. Systemic lupus erythematosus may also cause chorea that sometimes commences during pregnancy, and a thorough search for evidence of this disorder, therefore, should be made in all patients without clear evidence of a rheumatic basis for chorea. Finally, as in nonpregnant patients, chorea may relate to polycythemia vera rubra, thyrotoxicosis, hypocalcemia, Wilson disease, and treatment with phenytoin or a major tranquilizing drug.

Restless Legs Syndrome

Between 10% and 20% of pregnant patients are said to experience unpleasant creeping sensations deep in the legs and occasionally in the arms (Goodman et al., 1988). Symptoms generally occur when patients are relaxed, especially at night, and induce a need to move about. These symptoms usually develop in the latter half of pregnancy, subsiding soon after delivery (Ekbom, 1970). Similar symptoms may also occur without any relation to pregnancy.

No abnormalities are found on neurologic examination. The cause of the disorder is unknown, but symptoms sometimes resolve after correction of any coexisting anemia or iron deficiency. Persistent or intolerable symptoms may respond to treatment with drugs such as diazepam or clonazepam. Other drugs that are sometimes helpful include levodopa, bromocriptine, clonazepam, and opiates, but these are better avoided during pregnancy if possible.

Wilson Disease

An autosomal recessive disorder caused by a gene defect on the long arm of chromosome 13, Wilson disease is characterized by the accumulation of copper in the brain, liver, and other organs. Neurologic and mental symptoms such as intellectual disturbances, abnormal movements of all sorts, dysarthria, dysphagia, and rigidity are common presenting complaints. Once neurologic signs are present, careful examination of the eyes invariably shows the presence of Kayser-Fleischer rings, which are brown deposits of copper along the edge of the cornea in Descemet membrane. Clinical evidence of hepatic involvement may be present but is variable.

The diagnosis is suggested by the family history, low serum copper and ceruloplasmin concentrations, and increased 24-hour urinary excretion of copper. Treatment with a low-copper diet and with penicillamine, a chelating agent that promotes copper excretion, may lead to marked improvement of neurologic and hepatic status.

There is a high miscarriage rate in patients with untreated Wilson disease. Pregnancy generally proceeds normally in patients who have received adequate chelation therapy and carries no particular hazard for the mother or fetus. There is no clinical evidence that penicillamine gives rise to fetal connective tissue abnormalities when its use is continued during pregnancy (Scheinberg and Sternlieb, 1975; Walshe, 1977). It may be prudent to reduce the dose of penicillamine to 250 mg daily about 6 weeks before delivery if cesarean section is planned, however, to avoid impairment of wound healing (Scheinberg and Sternlieb, 1975). An alternative approach is treatment with trientine and zinc (Walshe, 1986), but experience with oral zinc salts taken during pregnancy is limited, and trientine is teratogenic in rats (Hartard and Kunze, 1994). Labor and delivery may be complicated in patients with portal hypertension. Hemorrhage from esophageal varices may occur, especially during the second or third trimesters. Extradural analgesia helps to avoid straining during vaginal delivery; cesarean section is best reserved for obstetric indications (Furman et al., 2001).

■ MULTIPLE SCLEROSIS

Multiple sclerosis is a disorder in which plaques of demyelination develop at different times and in different sites throughout the central nervous system. Its etiology remains uncertain; clinical onset is usually in early adult life. There is considerable variability in the tempo and character of neurologic symptoms and signs. The disorder is classically associated with unpredictable exacerbations during which neurologic deficits develop, followed by remissions during which symptoms and signs may partially or completely resolve. With time, patients become increasingly disabled, although perhaps not for many years after appearance of the initial symptoms. In other patients, the disorder follows a progressive course from its onset.

Several epidemiologic studies have suggested a tendency for remissions during pregnancy and an increased frequency of multiple sclerosis exacerbations in the first 3 to 6 months after childbirth (Korn-Lubetzki et al., 1984; Birk and Rudick, 1986; Abramsky, 1994). Pregnancy itself, or number of pregnancies, however, has no effect on subsequent neurologic disability (Thompson et al., 1986; Weinshenker et al., 1989; Sadovnick et al., 1994). The remission of multiple sclerosis during pregnancy probably relates to a gestational immunosuppressive state that in turn has a multifactorial basis (Abramsky, 1994). Similarly, multiple sclerosis does not influence the natural course of pregnancy or childbirth (Poser and Poser, 1983).

The possibility of a familial incidence of multiple sclerosis is widely known, but this pattern is uncommon and tends to involve siblings rather than different generations. It may merely reflect common exposure to some currently unrecognized etiologic agent rather than genetic predisposition to the disorder. With these points in mind, inquiries by a pregnant woman with multiple sclerosis who is worried that her child may later become affected should be met with firm reassurance. A patient with multiple sclerosis does not need to be discouraged from pregnancy unless she is already so disabled by the disorder that she will clearly be incapable of coping with the responsibilities and physical demands of parenthood. Patients with minimal incapacity who are anxious to have a child will usually do so anyway and do not need to be discouraged as long as they have some understanding of the nature of their disorder and its unpredictable course. In discussions between such patients and physicians, it seems reasonable to provide optimistic assurance that multiple sclerosis does not shorten life and that significant disability may not occur for many years, if at all.

The management of multiple sclerosis during pregnancy is supportive. The treatment of acute exacerbations generally consists of bed rest and prescription of a brief course of steroids, which may hasten recovery without necessarily influencing its extent. Patients with sphincter disturbances or who are paraplegic may experience increased difficulties during pregnancy. The method of delivery should depend solely on obstetric factors.

OPTIC NEURITIS

Any type of optic neuropathy may develop fortuitously during gestation. Thus, optic neuritis may develop during pregnancy or lactation (Retzloff et al., 2001) in patients with established multiple sclerosis or in patients who will later develop other manifestations of that disorder. Optic nerve involvement by tumors or vascular malformations may also appear for the first time in the gestational period, as may the optic neuropathy that sometimes complicates vitamin deficiency. Optic nerve involvement may complicate hyperemesis gravidarum, with rapid onset of marked, usually bilateral, visual loss; the entity is rare, but if vomiting is unresponsive to treatment, it may be necessary to terminate pregnancy.

Leber optic atrophy is a hereditary disorder that usually occurs in early adult life. It commonly has a sex-linked recessive mode of inheritance, so that the male offspring of women carriers of the disorder may be affected. Other modes of inheritance have also been described. The clinical deficit commences abruptly with visual loss and leads ultimately to bilateral central scotoma with optic atrophy. No abnormalities are found in the neonate. Other forms of hereditary optic atrophy have also been described in which the disorder is congenital or develops in infancy or early childhood and may have either a dominant or a recessive mode of transmission. The family pedigree is thus important for diagnostic and counseling purposes in all such instances.

TRAUMATIC PARAPLEGIA

When spinal cord injury resulting in paraplegia occurs during the course of an established pregnancy, it may be followed by spontaneous abortion or stillbirth. If the pregnancy continues, the detailed radiologic investigations that are needed to determine the nature and extent of the spinal injury may be hazardous to the developing fetus, especially if it is still very immature (see Chapter 19). In such circumstances, however, the interests of the mother are of paramount importance.

Many patients with established paraplegia are eager to experience motherhood, and because they are capable of sexual intercourse, they inquire about the possibility and potential hazards of childbirth. Urinary tract infection, a common complication of paraplegia, can be exacerbated by pregnancy but is not a contraindication to pregnancy if there is no gross impairment of renal function. In the management of paraplegics, it is important to reeducate the paralyzed bladder so that only a minimal amount of residual urine remains after micturition. If this is achieved, difficulty with micturition can usually be postponed to the last stages of pregnancy, when catheterization is often necessary.

Pregnancy may increase the likelihood of development of pressure sores in paraplegic women. Patients and their families should be informed about the cause of these sores and the manner in which prolonged pressure can be avoided. Because anemia lowers the resistance of paraplegic patients to infection and pressure, particular care must be taken to prevent its development during pregnancy.

The uterus itself contracts normally in labor despite interruption of its nerve supply. However, patients with complete spinal cord lesions above the tenth thoracic segment cannot appreciate the onset of labor or feel any pain during it because afferent fibers from the uterus enter the cord more caudally. Medical attendants then need to examine the state of the cervix to identify the onset of labor with certainty. Because labor often commences before term in such circumstances, the cervix is often examined at each antenatal visit after 24 to 26 weeks of pregnancy; the patient should be hospitalized if the cervix is found to be dilated (Robertson, 1972).

The occurrence of symptoms such as leg spasms in association with uterine contractions may be helpful in signaling the onset of labor, as may uterine palpation by the patient's spouse. Routine hospitalization after the 32nd week should be considered. In patients with cord lesions below the 10th or 11th thoracic segment, uterine contractions produce normal pain sensations. A patient with spasticity resulting from the cord lesion may develop painful flexor spasms and ankle clonus during uterine contractions.

Pregnant women with complete cord lesions above the fifth or sixth thoracic segment (above the splanchnic outflow) may develop the syndrome of autonomic hyperreflexia with excessive activity of a viscus. This is characterized by throbbing headache, hypertension, reflex bradycardia, sweating, nasal congestion, and cutaneous vasodilatation and piloerection above the level of the lesion. During labor, these symptoms are most conspicuous with uterine contractions and become especially prominent just before delivery. Electrocardiographic monitoring may facilitate recognition of any changes in cardiac rate or rhythm that occur during uterine contractions. Symptoms are due to the sudden release of catecholamines.

Treatment has generally been with reserpine (which depletes catecholamines from sympathetic nerve terminals but also can cause potentially dangerous nasal congestion in the nasal-breathing neonate), atropine, clonidine, glyceryl trinitrate, or hexamethonium (a ganglion blocker). The syndrome can be prevented by spinal or epidural anesthesia extending to the level of the tenth thoracic segment, and early consultation with an anesthesiologist may therefore be helpful.

Cesarean section is not indicated by paraplegia per se, but it may be required because of bony deformity of the spine or pelvis. If the patient has a permanent suprapubic cystostomy, a vertical incision rather than a lower segment transverse incision must be used. Forceps delivery or vacuum extraction is often required because the muscles responsible for the expulsive efforts of the second stage are paralyzed and because severe hypertension sometimes necessitates shortening the second stage (Robertson, 1963).

Absorbable sutures, such as catgut, are poorly absorbed in paraplegics, and sterile abscesses commonly form around buried catgut; thus, nonabsorbable sutures, such as nylon, are preferred for repairing an episiotomy (Robertson, 1963). Paraplegic and quadriplegic patients can successfully breast-feed their infants, and they have a normal letdown (milk ejection) reflex during suckling (Robertson, 1972).

ROOT LESIONS

Prolapsed Intervertebral Disk and Pregnancy

Pregnancy is one etiologic factor in the development of prolapsed lumbar intervertebral disks (O'Connell, 1960). From a review of the case notes of 347 consecutive women with verified disk prolapse, O'Connell (1960) found that low back pain or sciatic pain attributable to the prolapse occurred commonly during or immediately after pregnancy. O'Connell (1944) suggested that the postural and mechanical stresses of pregnancy may well be responsible, particularly if hormonal factors render the lumbar intervertebral disks more vulnerable to stress by inducing changes in them analogous to those occurring in the pelvic joints. Other authors have concluded, however, that acute herniation of a lumbar disk during pregnancy is uncommon (LaBan et al., 1983).

The symptoms and signs of lumbar disk protrusion during pregnancy are similar to those occurring in nonparous women. Radicular and low back pain are usually conspicuous features, and there may be a segmental motor and sensory disturbance in the limbs. When the disk prolapses centrally rather than laterally, symptoms and signs in the legs may be bilateral, and sphincter disturbances occur more commonly.

Lumbar disk protrusion must be distinguished from other causes of leg weakness developing during or soon after pregnancy. Lumbosacral palsy may arise during labor from compressive injury of the plexus, but tenderness and rigidity of the lumbar spine, sciatica, and signs of root tension favor the diagnosis of protruded disk. The distribution of muscular weakness may also be helpful; depending on their location, plexus lesions cause weakness and sensory symptoms in a polyradicular or peripheral nerve distribution in the legs. Moreover, because only the anterior primary rami contribute to the plexus, a proximal radiculopathy can be distinguished from a plexus lesion by electromyographic examination of muscles supplied by the posterior primary rami, namely the paraspinal muscles, involvement of which therefore favors a root lesion.

In patients with lateral protrusion of a lumbar disk, simple analgesics provide symptomatic relief. Imaging studies and surgery can usually be deferred until after childbirth. However, laminectomy and excision of the protruded disk may be necessary during pregnancy, especially if symptoms are bilateral or if there is any disturbance of sphincter function.

Other Lumbosacral Root Lesions

Most disk lesions involve the L-5 or S-1 roots. Although a disk lesion may occasionally affect the L-4 root, involvement of an upper lumbar nerve root suggests other compressive disease. Moreover, in a patient presenting with an L-5 or S-1 radiculopathy, there may be a more rostrally situated lesion if no abnormality, such as a protruded disk, is seen in the L4-5 or L5-S1 region, because the spinal cord ends at the lower border of L-1 and the roots then descend intradurally before exiting through their respective intervertebral foramina. In such circumstances, the possibility of other compressive lesions must be considered. As with nonpregnant patients, each case is best managed on an individual basis (see standard neurologic textbooks for further details).

PLEXUS LESIONS AND PERIPHERAL MONONEUROPATHIES

Certain peripheral entrapment neuropathies are particularly liable to develop in pregnancy and may lead to troublesome symptoms. Recognition of the basis of such symptoms is important because, with reassurance about their benign nature, most patients can tolerate them until they give birth, when the symptoms generally subside spontaneously. A number of other peripheral nerve or plexus lesions may develop during labor or obstetric surgical procedures as a result of compression or stretch of nerves, especially in anesthetized patients.

Disorders of peripheral nerves may be characterized by slowing or blocking of conduction along intact axons or by axonal degeneration. The former carries a much more favorable prognosis for recovery than the latter, in that once axonal degeneration has occurred, recovery can take place only by regeneration, a process that may take many months and may never be complete.

Electrophysiologic Evaluation

In the evaluation of patients with suspected nerve lesions, electrophysiologic techniques have been helpful in several ways (Aminoff, 1998). Electromyography can aid in determining whether weakness is neurogenic; if so, the electromyographically demonstrated pattern of affected muscles may indicate the location of the lesion (i.e., whether root, plexus, or individual peripheral nerve has been affected). The findings may also indicate whether neurogenic weakness is a consequence of impaired conduction along otherwise intact axons or of axonal degeneration, a distinction that is of prognostic importance.

The motor responses to nerve stimulation provide complementary information. If axonal degeneration results from a focal lesion in a peripheral nerve, the motor responses to electrical stimulation either proximal or distal to the lesion become small or absent about a week after injury, depending on the completeness of the lesion. In contrast, in patients with a conductive disturbance caused by an acute focal lesion, the motor responses to stimulation beyond (distal to) the lesion are generally normal, whereas those elicited by more proximal stimulation may be small.

Motor and sensory conduction velocity can be measured in various accessible segments of peripheral nerves, and focal slowing may provide confirmatory evidence of an underlying entrapment or focal neuropathy. Moreover, in patients presenting with a mononeuropathy, nerve conduction studies can be used to exclude the real possibility of an underlying subclinical polyneuropathy.

Lumbosacral Plexus Lesion

The roots of the sciatic nerve may be compressed in the pelvis by the fetal head or obstetric forceps, and the brunt of the resulting motor deficit is then borne by muscles supplied by the common peroneal fibers because of their relationship to the bony pelvis. This type of injury to the maternal lumbosacral plexus is more likely when a short patient with a small pelvis carries a rather large infant, so that labor is complicated by minor disproportion, or when mid-forceps are used during delivery because of malpresentation. The features of the pelvis that predispose to this complication include a straight sacrum, a flat wide posterior pelvis, posterior displacement of the transverse diameter of the inlet, wide sacroiliac notches, and prominent ischial spines.

Symptoms are generally unilateral. They usually develop immediately after delivery but may not be noticed until the patient is allowed out of bed. When the common peroneal fibers are involved, the main complaint is of leg weakness, which is sometimes erroneously attributed to a painful episiotomy. In more severe cases, there is footdrop. Numbness and paresthesias may occur over the dorsum of the foot and lateral aspect of the leg, and cutaneous sensation may be impaired in this distribution.

Unless the injury has been severe, the predominant pathologic change is demyelination of the affected fibers, and this is reflected in the electrophysiologic findings. With mild injuries, the prognosis for recovery is excellent; if Wallerian degeneration has occurred, recovery may take many months and may never be complete.

Physical therapy is all that is needed for the treatment of mild cases, but calipers and night casts may be required in more severe instances to prevent contracture.

Subsequent pregnancies can be allowed to proceed normally if an easy vaginal delivery is anticipated. Low forceps can be used with caution if necessary, but the use of mid-forceps may be hazardous. It would seem sensible to advise cesarean section if the infant is clearly very large or if premonitory symptoms suggesting nerve compression occur with attempted engagement of the fetal head in the pelvic brim during the last 4 weeks of pregnancy in a patient with a history of obstetric lumbosacral plexus palsy.

Acute Familial Brachial Neuritis

Several reports document the rare occurrence of brachial plexus neuropathy on a familial basis. Taylor (1960) reported that 24 of 119 members of a family covering five generations had experienced single or multiple attacks of acute brachial neuropathy. This was characterized by pain, weakness, atrophy, and sensory loss that was usually unilateral but occasionally bilateral and from which gradual recovery generally occurred. Both males and females were affected, but among females there was a striking association of attacks with pregnancy or the puerperium, in contrast to the more common idiopathic disorder, which is rarely associated with pregnancy. In some instances of the familial disease, the lower cranial nerves were involved and isolated mononeuropathies of the other extremities were present. Ungley (1933) described a similar syndrome in a mother and both of her daughters, and other cases have also been described. Treatment with oral steroids may be helpful in relieving pain but does not seem to affect the rate of recovery.

Carpal Tunnel Syndrome

Compression of the median nerve may occur in the carpal tunnel at the wrist, especially when (1) the normal size of the carpal tunnel is reduced, as by degenerative arthritis, or (2) the volume of its contents is increased, as in inflammatory disorders involving the tendons and connective tissues at the wrist. The *carpal tunnel syndrome* is common during pregnancy, perhaps because of excessive fluid retention (Padua et al., 2001). Pain and paresthesias are early symptoms and frequently occur at night, awakening the patient from sleep. The symptoms usually involve the first three digits and the lateral border of the ring finger, but some patients report that all digits are affected. Pain may also occur in the forearm and, occasionally, in the upper arm. With time, weakness of the thenar muscles may develop. On examination, it is often possible to elicit *Tinel's sign* (percussion of the nerve at the wrist causing paresthesias in its distal distribution), and *Phalen's maneuver* (flexion at the wrist for more than a minute) sometimes reproduces or enhances symptoms. There may be mild weakness and wasting of the abductor pollicis brevis and opponens pollicis muscles, impaired cutaneous sensation in a median nerve distribution in the hand, or both motor and sensory signs.

Electrophysiologic testing usually suggests or confirms the diagnosis (Fig. 55-8). In the evaluation of patients, it is important to remember that the carpal tunnel syndrome is commonly bilateral, even though it may be unilaterally symptomatic, and an entrapment neuropathy may be the first manifestation of a subclinical polyneuropathy. These possibilities can be excluded by appropriate electrophysiologic studies.

Symptoms developing or worsening during pregnancy usually respond to the nocturnal use of a wrist splint and generally clear within about 3 months of delivery, although they may recur in subsequent pregnancies. The splint is placed on the dorsal surface so that the wrist can be maintained in a neutral or slightly flexed position. Some patients are helped by injection of steroids into the carpal tunnel and others by treatment with diuretics. Time must be taken to explain to the patient that her symptoms are benign and will generally subside spontaneously after the pregnancy. With such reassurance, most patients accept their symptoms without difficulty (Stolp-Smith et al., 1998).

Surgical division of the anterior carpal ligament may be necessary, however, if symptoms are intolerable or do not clear in the weeks after delivery. Surgical treatment may also be necessary in a patient with clinical or electrophysiologic evidence of increasing nerve dysfunction despite conservative measures, but it can usually be avoided during the pregnancy itself.

FIGURE 55-8 ■ Nerve conduction studies in a patient with left-sided carpal tunnel syndrome. **A,** Responses of the abductor pollicis brevis muscle to supramaximal electrical stimulation of the median nerves at the wrist. The prolonged latency of the response on the left is evident. **B,** The sensory action potentials recorded over the median nerve at the wrist after electrical stimulation of digital sensory fibers in the index fingers. Those on the left are smaller in amplitude and more prolonged in latency than those on the right. Maximal motor conduction velocity in the forearm segments of the median nerves was normal.

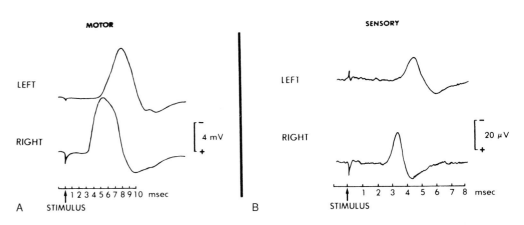

Meralgia Paresthetica

The lateral femoral cutaneous nerve, a purely sensory nerve derived from the L-2 and L-3 roots, is particularly susceptible to compression or stretch injury during pregnancy, especially during the third trimester. Obesity and diabetes mellitus are other predisposing factors. The nerve usually runs under the outer portion of the inguinal ligament to reach the thigh, but the ligament sometimes splits to enclose the nerve. In the latter circumstance, hyperextension of the hip or an increased lumbar lordosis, such as occurs during pregnancy, leads to compression of the nerve by the posterior fascicle of the ligament (Pearson, 1957; Rhodes, 1957). Entrapment of the nerve at any point along its course may lead to similar symptoms, however, and several anatomic variations may predispose the nerve to damage when it is stretched. Pain, paresthesias, and numbness may occur about the outer aspect of the thigh and are sometimes relieved by sitting. Symptoms are unilateral in approximately 80% of cases.

Little may be found on physical examination, but in severe cases cutaneous sensation is disturbed in the affected area. Symptoms, which are usually mild, subside spontaneously in the puerperium or within a few weeks of delivery. Accordingly, patients should be reassured about the benign nature of the disorder. In a few instances, however, pain has been so severe that labor has had to be induced early. Hydrocortisone injections in the region where the nerve lies medial to the anterior superior iliac spine may relieve persistent symptoms for a time, and nerve decompression by transposition may provide more lasting relief (Keegan and Holyoke, 1962) but is required very rarely.

Traumatic Mononeuropathies

The causes and clinical features of traumatic mononeuropathies that are likely to develop in relation to obstetric procedures are listed here.

The *obturator nerve* originates within the psoas muscle from the L-2, L-3, and L-4 nerves; emerges from the medial border of psoas; and enters the pelvis immediately in front of the sacroiliac joint. It sweeps around the lateral pelvic wall and then passes through the obturator foramen, dividing into branches that supply the adductor, gracilis, and external obturator muscles; the skin over part of the medial thigh; and the hip joint. The nerve may be injured during genitourinary operations involving the lithotomy position, owing to angulation as it leaves the obturator foramen or to compression between the fetal head (or a pelvic mass) and the bony pelvic wall. An obturator nerve palsy leads to impaired gait, because of weakness of the adductor muscles, and to a sensory disturbance involving particularly the medial part of the mid-thigh and lower thigh. Pain may also occur and tends to radiate from the groin down the inner side of the thigh.

The *femoral nerve* originates within the psoas muscle from the L-2, L-3, and L-4 nerves and passes beneath the inguinal ligament to enter the thigh. It innervates the iliacus, sartorius, pectineus, and quadriceps femoris muscles, and its cutaneous branches supply anterior and medial portions of the thigh and, through the saphenous nerve, the medial portions of the lower leg. Clinical features of a femoral nerve palsy are weakness and, in severe cases, wasting of the quadriceps muscle, sensory impairment over the anteromedial aspect of the thigh and occasionally of the leg to the medial malleolus, and depression or absence of the knee jerk. Such a palsy can occur as an isolated phenomenon in the patient with diabetes mellitus, a bleeding tendency, or retroperitoneal neoplasm, and may sometimes arise by angulation and pressure from the inguinal ligament when the thighs are markedly flexed and abducted, as in the lithotomy position in anesthetized patients.

The *saphenous nerve*, the branch of the femoral nerve that supplies sensation to the medial aspect of the leg below the knee, may itself be damaged by pressure from leg braces when the patient is improperly suspended in the lithotomy position (Slocum et al., 1948; Britt and Gordon, 1964), leading to numbness and paresthesias that are usually fairly short-lived.

Sciatic or *common peroneal nerve palsies* are easy to confuse with a plexus palsy because, as already indicated, their constituent fibers are susceptible to compressive injury in the sacral plexus during labor. Misplaced deep intramuscular injections are probably still the most common cause of sciatic nerve palsy. The sciatic nerve may also be injured by stretching when a patient is positioned in stirrups on the obstetric table. To avoid this injury, the knee and hip joints should be well flexed, and extreme external rotation of the hip should be avoided (Burkhart and Daly, 1966).

In patients with a sciatic nerve palsy, the resulting weakness and sensory disturbance depend on whether the entire nerve has been affected or certain fibers are selectively involved. In general, the peroneal fibers of the sciatic nerve are much more likely to be damaged than fibers destined for the tibial nerve.

Accordingly, the clinical features of a sciatic nerve lesion may simulate those of a peroneal neuropathy, although electromyographic evidence of involvement of the short head of the biceps femoris muscle favors the former. The common peroneal nerve itself is vulnerable to compression or direct trauma in the region of the head and neck of the fibula and may certainly be injured at this site by pressure from the leg braces of the obstetric table, especially in anesthetized patients. Weakness of dorsiflexion and eversion of the foot are accompanied by numbness or blunted sensation of the anterolateral aspect of the calf and the dorsum of the foot.

Bell's Palsy

Sir Charles Bell first established the motor function of the seventh cranial nerve in the early 19th century. His name soon came to be associated with all forms of facial paralysis, but the designation Bell's palsy is now used for facial paresis of lower motor neuron type when no specific etiologic agent can be found. Some cases have been attributed to viral infection or related to an inflammatory reaction involving the facial nerve near the stylomastoid foramen or in the bony facial canal.

Although a possible association with pregnancy was alluded to by Bell himself, only recently has such an association been substantiated. The incidence of Bell's palsy in nonpregnant women of childbearing age is 17.4 per 100,000 per year, whereas the incidence during pregnancy is 45.1 per 100,000 births (Hilsinger et al., 1975). Per year of exposure, the risk to pregnant women is more than three times that to nonpregnant women of similar age, with approximately 85% of cases appearing in the third trimester or immediate puerperium (Hilsinger et al., 1975). A previously suggested relationship with hypertension or preeclampsia is supported by the study of Shmorgun and coworkers (2002).

The clinical features of Bell's palsy are well known. The facial paresis is generally abrupt in onset, although it may worsen over the following day. Pain around the ear may precede or accompany the weakness in about half the cases but usually lasts for only a few days. The face itself feels stiff and pulled to one side. It may be difficult to close the eye on the affected side, and ipsilateral epiphora may occur. The patient may have difficulty with eating and with fine facial movements (as when applying cosmetics). A disturbance of taste, caused by involvement of chorda tympani fibers, is common, and hyperacusis, caused by involvement of fibers to the stapedius, is occasionally troublesome.

Treatment is controversial. Most patients recover without treatment, and only about 10% of all patients are seriously dissatisfied with the final outcome because of permanent disfigurement or other long-term sequelae. Clearly, treatment is best reserved for patients in whom an unsatisfactory outcome can be predicted soon after onset. To be effective, treatment should commence within the first 5 or 6 days.

The best clinical guide to prognosis at an early stage is the severity of the palsy. Patients who have clinically complete palsy when they are first seen are less likely to recover fully than those with an incomplete palsy. Other clinical indicators for a poor prognosis for recovery include advancing age, hyperacusis, and the presence of severe initial pain.

The only medical treatment that may influence the outcome of Bell's palsy is steroid therapy (Taverner et al., 1966, 1967, 1971; Adour et al., 1972), although rigorously controlled trials have not demonstrated benefit (May et al., 1976; Wolf et al., 1978). Despite, or because of, the uncertainty about their effectiveness, many physicians routinely prescribe steroids to patients who are seen within 5 days of onset. Surgical procedures to decompress the facial nerve have not been beneficial.

POLYNEUROPATHIES

There were several early reports of the occasional occurrence of a polyneuropathy during pregnancy, but there does not appear to be any specific "polyneuritis of pregnancy." Any type of polyneuropathy (such as that caused by diabetes mellitus) may develop during the gestational period. Discussion here is limited to those most likely to become manifest clinically or to pose a management problem during pregnancy.

Nutritional Neuropathies

Nutritional deficiency may be the most probable cause of peripheral nerve involvement in patients who come from underdeveloped countries or have hyperemesis. Signs of peripheral nerve involvement may be found in patients with hyperemesis gravidarum who have Wernicke encephalopathy (Campbell and Biggart, 1939; Barnes, 1962). In the limbs, numbness, paresthesias, and dysesthesias are accompanied by cutaneous sensory loss, depressed tendon reflexes, and distal weakness. Retrobulbar neuropathy may also occur, and tachycardia, postural hypotension, exertional dyspnea, and sphincter disturbances are sometimes conspicuous. The polyneuropathy is accompanied by ophthalmoplegia (horizontal and vertical nystagmus, impaired lateral gaze, conjugate gaze palsies), ataxia of gait, and a confusional state. The features of *Korsakoff psychosis*, which consists of impaired memory and an inability to acquire new information, sometimes accompanied by confabulation, may also be conjoined.

The diagnosis is confirmed by the finding of a marked reduction in blood transketolase activity and a marked thiamine pyrophosphate effect. Treatment is with thiamine, 50 mg, given once intravenously and then intramuscularly for several days until a satisfactory dietary intake is assured.

In other instances, a severe polyneuropathy may develop without an accompanying encephalopathy, presumably in relation to a nutritional deficiency, although the specific factors responsible for the peripheral nerve involvement are not known. Patients may complain of pain, paresthesias, and dysesthesias in the extremities; of limb weakness; or of ataxia. There may be accompanying cardiac involvement, with tachycardia, exertional dyspnea, and heart failure. Treatment consists of a balanced diet and supplements of vitamins, especially those of the B group.

Vitamin B_{12} deficiency may lead to maternal polyneuropathy and other neurologic abnormalities and can affect the fetus and neonate.

Acute Idiopathic Polyneuropathy
Guillain-Barré Syndrome

An acute or subacute polyneuropathy that sometimes follows infective illnesses, inoculations, or surgical procedures but often occurs without any obvious preceding event characterizes acute idiopathic polyneuropathy. In many such instances, the neuropathy follows clinical or subclinical infection with *Campylobacter jejuni*. The disorder may have an immunologic basis, but the precise mechanism is unclear. It can pose an especially difficult management problem when it occurs during pregnancy.

The main complaint is of weakness that varies widely in severity in different patients, is often more marked proximally than distally, and is often symmetrical in distribution. It usually begins in the legs, frequently comes to involve the arms, and often affects one side or both sides of the face. Weakness may progress to total paralysis and may be life-threatening if the muscles of respiration or deglutition are involved. Sensory symptoms are common but are usually less conspicuous than motor symptoms. Autonomic dysfunction may be manifested by tachycardia, cardiac irregularities, hypotension or hypertension, facial flushing, disturbances of sweating, disturbed pulmonary function, and other signs and symptoms.

Examination of the cerebrospinal fluid reveals characteristic changes; the protein content is significantly increased but the cell content is normal. Measurement of motor and sensory conduction velocity in the peripheral nerves may reveal marked slowing, but the chronology of this reduction does not necessarily parallel that of the clinical disorder. In some patients, the conduction velocity remains normal, presumably because disease is restricted to the nerve roots or proximal segments of the nerves. Most patients eventually make a good recovery, but it may take many months and some patients are left with persisting disability.

There is no convincing evidence that the Guillain-Barré syndrome occurs more commonly during gestation than at other times, and the course of the disorder does not seem to be influenced by pregnancy. Improvement in neurologic status may certainly occur before delivery and is not necessarily delayed until the infant is born.

Treatment is symptomatic, with attention directed at the prevention of complications, such as respiratory failure and vascular collapse. Plasmapheresis or treatment with intravenous immunoglobulins is helpful in patients with rapidly advancing or severe disease. Severely affected patients are best managed in intensive care units, where respiratory and circulatory function can be monitored and assisted respiration can be started as soon as is necessary. Ventilatory support may help to avert fetal hypoxia (Gauthier et al., 1990). Ultrasonographic fetal monitoring generally reveals normal fetal movements even when the mother is severely paralyzed (Nelson and McLean, 1985).

Approximately 3% of patients with acute idiopathic polyneuropathy have one or more relapses, sometimes several years after the initial illness. Such relapses, which are clinically similar to the original illness, occasionally occur in relation to pregnancy (Calderon-Gonzalez et al., 1970; Novak and Johnson, 1973; Jones and Berry, 1981).

Porphyric Neuropathy

In the hepatic forms of porphyria, both the central and peripheral nervous systems may be affected. *Acute intermittent porphyria*, inherited as an autosomal recessive trait, is characterized by increased production and urinary excretion of porphobilinogen and δ-aminolevulinic acid. The Watson-Schwartz test, a useful qualitative test for increased urinary porphobilinogen, is of great value in establishing the diagnosis (Tschudy et al., 1975). Colicky abdominal pain is often the most conspicuous symptom, but the usual neurologic manifestation is a polyneuropathy, predominantly motor but sometimes with pronounced autonomic involvement, that may take weeks or months to regress, depending on its severity. Cerebral manifestations may also occur, often preceding the development of a severe polyneuropathy and similarly clearing after a variable time. Clinical indicators of disease activity include tachycardia, fever, and a peripheral leukocytosis. In variegate porphyria, cutaneous sensitivity to sunlight is an additional clinical feature.

Attacks may be precipitated by pharmacologic agents such as barbiturates, sulfonamides, and estrogens. Some women have found that relapses are most likely to occur premenstrually; long-term combination oral contraceptives may prevent attacks in these patients (Perlroth et al., 1965). In other patients, oral contraceptives may precipitate exacerbations, and this form of contraception is probably best avoided in women with a blood relative who has a hepatic type of porphyria (Donaldson, 1978).

Pregnancy may also lead to an acute exacerbation and may even have a fatal outcome, but many patients tolerate attacks without apparent ill effect. When relapses occur, they usually do so in early pregnancy and may lead to spontaneous abortion (Donaldson, 1978). However, exacerbations may occur at any time during pregnancy or postpartum. The implications and uncertain outcome must therefore be explained to patients who are contemplating pregnancy, and close supervision should be provided during the gestational period. Latent cases may be exacerbated by medication used during or after labor, and particular care must be exercised in this regard. In general, if the pregnancy proceeds satisfactorily, a healthy infant can be anticipated.

■ MYASTHENIA GRAVIS

Variable weakness and fatigability of skeletal muscles, resulting from defective neuromuscular transmission, are the clinical hallmarks of myasthenia gravis. The disorder has an autoimmune basis. It is characterized by a reduced number of available acetylcholine receptors at the neuromuscular junctions. Myasthenia gravis is more common in females. In some patients, the external ocular muscles or levator palpebrae are especially affected; in others, the facial and bulbar muscles are selectively involved. In yet others, the limb muscles, especially the proximal ones, are predominantly affected. Weakness may remain localized to a few muscle groups or may become generalized, and it can be life-threatening if the muscles of respiration or deglutition are involved.

Patients are particularly sensitive to even small doses of neuromuscular blocking agents, such as tubocurarine, but improvement results from treatment with acetylcholinesterase inhibitors. Thymectomy often leads to a remission of symptoms, and myasthenia gravis may be associated with thymoma. Repetitive supramaximal electrical stimulation of motor nerves may lead to an abnormal decline in size of the evoked muscle action potentials. This finding is sometimes of diagnostic help, as is the finding of elevated levels of circulating acetylcholine receptor antibodies and the clinical response to edrophonium or neostigmine. In addition to thymectomy in appropriate cases, treatment may involve the use of anticholinesterases, steroids, intravenous immunoglobulins, and plasmapheresis (see general neurologic textbooks for standard medical management of this disease).

Exacerbations of myasthenia gravis sometimes occur shortly before the onset of the menstrual period and tend to improve once menstruation has begun. Such an association may disappear after thymectomy.

Myasthenia gravis may first appear during or shortly after pregnancy, but it is difficult to predict the influence of pregnancy on a patient with the disorder. Moreover, the effect of pregnancy may vary on different occasions, so that the outcome in individual cases cannot be predicted on this basis. Relapses are not uncommon in early pregnancy, with partial or complete remission often occurring at a later stage. Batocchi and associates (1999) found during pregnancy that myasthenia relapsed in 17% of asymptomatic patients who were not on treatment before conception; among patients on therapy, symptoms improved in 39% of pregnancies, were unchanged in 42%, and worsened in 19%. Further, myasthenic symptoms worsened after delivery in 28% of pregnancies. It may be tempting to terminate a pregnancy because of the severity of myasthenic symptoms—death has been reported in pregnancy complicated by myasthenia gravis—and because of the difficulties in their treatment, but termination does not necessarily lead to clinical benefit. Myasthenia gravis, therefore, should be managed in pregnant patients just as in nonpregnant patients.

Myasthenia gravis has little effect on the pregnancy itself. Moreover, there may be a marked contrast during labor between the strength of uterine contractions in the second stage and the skeletal muscle weakness exhibited by the patient. If the expulsive phase of labor is prolonged, instrumental assistance may help to avoid maternal exhaustion. Cesarean section should be reserved for patients in whom it is indicated on obstetric grounds. Regional analgesia is preferable to general anesthesia, and the use of muscle relaxant drugs is avoided if possible. Similarly, the use of magnesium sulfate for eclampsia should be avoided because it may precipitate myasthenic crisis.

Infants born to myasthenic patients should be carefully watched during the week after delivery for signs of neonatal myasthenia. Such signs include a poor cry, respiratory difficulties, weakness in sucking, a weak Moro reflex, and feeble limb movements, usually becoming apparent within the first 72 hours of birth. Symptoms are usually not evident immediately after birth, and this delay has been attributed to protection of the infant by placental transfer of maternal anticholinesterase drugs.

Neonatal myasthenia is a transient disorder that relates to placental transfer of maternal antibody against acetylcholine receptors (Keesey et al., 1977). It occurs in 10% to 15% of infants born to myasthenic mothers and does not seem to be related to the duration or severity of maternal illness, although disease in mothers of myasthenic newborns is usually generalized rather than localized. It can be treated with anticholinesterase drugs, usually subsides within 6 weeks of delivery, but may result in death caused by aspiration or respiratory failure. Facilities should thus be available for the immediate resuscitation of affected infants or those at risk of being

affected. Immunosuppressive therapy is sometimes required. Maternal myasthenia has also been incriminated as a rare cause of congenital arthrogryposis (Polizzi et al., 2000).

The birth of a child with neonatal myasthenia does not necessarily imply that future children will also have the disorder, although they often do.

The transient neonatal disorder that may occur in the offspring of a myasthenic mother must not be confused with congenital myasthenia gravis. The latter is rare, occurs in children born of healthy mothers, and is usually permanent.

DISORDERS OF MUSCLE

Myotonic Dystrophy

Myotonic dystrophy is a slowly progressive dominantly inherited disorder that usually appears in early adult life but may become manifested in childhood. It has been related to an expanded trinucleotide repeat in a gene localized to 19cen-q13.2. Increasing number of triplet repeat expansions governs clinical expression of disease; prenatal detection of the disorder is possible (Redman et al., 1993; Shelbourne et al., 1993). Myotonia is accompanied by weakness of the facial, sternomastoid, and distal limb muscles. There may be a number of associated features, including cataracts, frontal baldness, cardiac and endocrine disturbances, and intellectual changes. During pregnancy, the weakness and myotonia may be aggravated, and the course of the disorder is sometimes accelerated. When deterioration does occur, it often begins at about the 6th or 7th month of pregnancy.

In the antepartum period, the major reported obstetric complications of myotonic dystrophy include threatened, spontaneous, and habitual abortion. Hydramnios, which may also occur, has been attributed to decreased fetal swallowing, as demonstrated radiographically by intra-amniotic injection of radiopaque dye (Dunn and Dierker, 1973), suggesting fetal muscle involvement. Premature onset of labor in patients with myotonic dystrophy has been attributed in some instances to abnormalities of uterine muscle. Labor may also be abnormal in patients with myotonic dystrophy owing to a failure of the uterus to contract normally. Thus, the first stage may be prolonged and retention of the placenta and postpartum hemorrhage may occur. Manual removal of the placenta is sometimes necessary. Skeletal muscle weakness may also lead to poor voluntary assistance in the second stage.

Myotonic dystrophy may become manifest in infancy, occurring congenitally among the offspring of mothers who have the disorder, sometimes only mildly. In such cases, it is often possible to obtain a history of hydramnios or reduced fetal movements during the latter part of pregnancy. Some affected infants die within hours or a few days of birth. The clinical features in affected infants include facial diplegia, hypotonia, neonatal respiratory distress, feeding difficulties, delayed motor development, and mental retardation (Harper, 1989). Myotonia, a cardinal feature of the adult disease, is absent in the congenital form. The neonatal respiratory distress may be due to involvement of the respiratory muscles, pulmonary immaturity, aspiration pneumonia, and impaired neural control of respiration. Talipes is present at birth in about half of all cases and may require surgical correction.

Familial studies have indicated that in almost every case of congenital myotonic dystrophy, transmission has occurred via the mother. Such transmission does not fit with an autosomal dominant pattern of inheritance. Genetic data suggest that the congenital form results from the combination of the gene responsible for the disorder in adults with some additional maternally transmitted factor. The nature of this maternal factor is unclear. Others have suggested that the maternal transmission of the congenital form relates to relative male infertility.

The management of patients requiring anesthesia for obstetric or other reasons merits brief comment. Hook and coworkers (1975) emphasized that depolarizing muscle relaxant drugs should be avoided because they may cause myotonic spasm and that nondepolarizing agents, such as tubocurarine, can be used but should be given in reduced dosage to patients receiving quinine for myotonia. Thiopental sodium (Pentothal) may lead to marked respiratory depression and is best avoided, as are other respiratory depressant drugs, especially if the patient already has impaired respiratory function. Electrocardiographic monitoring permits the early recognition of any cardiac arrhythmias, to which patients with myotonic dystrophy are prone. For these reasons, regional analgesia is the preferred method of management.

Myotonia Congenita

The dominant form of myotonia congenita (*Thomsen disease*) is usually present from birth, although symptoms may not appear until early childhood. Patients complain of muscle stiffness (myotonia) that is enhanced by cold or inactivity and is relieved by exercise; power is full, but the muscles may be diffusely hypertrophied. Pregnancy may aggravate the myotonia, especially in the latter half of the gestational period, with improvement occurring after delivery. Several illustrative case reports have been published (Hakim and Thomlinson, 1969).

Polymyositis

In polymyositis or dermatomyositis, which can occur at any age, there is weakness and wasting, especially of the proximal musculature, as a result of inflammatory infiltration of muscles and destruction of muscle fibers. The muscles are often painful and tender. There may be an association with malignancy or one of the collagen diseases. The erythrocyte sedimentation rate and serum creatine kinase levels are elevated. Histologic examination of a muscle biopsy specimen usually permits the diagnosis to be made with confidence so that treatment with steroids can be instituted. Pregnancy has a variable effect on the muscle weakness, but a high perinatal mortality rate has been reported (Tsai et al., 1973).

■ PSYCHIATRIC DISORDERS

Pregnancy may occur during the course of established psychiatric illness, and conversely, psychiatric disorders may first develop during or shortly after pregnancy, although no specific disorders relate to this period. In the evaluation of patients with psychiatric disorders, it must be borne in mind that pregnancy can have a number of different psychopathologic implications, depending on the patient's social, cultural, educational, emotional, and medical background. The attitude of a patient to pregnancy, especially with regard to whether it was desired, influences her psychological response, and her capacity to cope with pregnancy depends on her acceptance of it. If the pregnancy was planned, the factors that motivated it are also of some relevance because the aim may have been to overcome marital disharmony, to keep up with peers, and so on. These aspects clearly govern the response of an individual patient to pregnancy. See Chapter 56 for a discussion of psychiatric disorders.

REFERENCES

Abramsky O: Pregnancy and multiple sclerosis. Ann Neurol 36(Suppl):38, 1994.

Adour KK, Wingerd J, Bell DN: Prednisone treatment for idiopathic facial paralysis (Bell's palsy). N Engl J Med 287:1268, 1972.

Allen J, Eldridge R, Koerber T: Acoustic neuroma in the last months of pregnancy. Am J Obstet Gynecol 119:516, 1974.

Aminoff MJ: Spinal Angiomas. Oxford, Blackwell, 1976.

Aminoff MJ: Angiomas and fistulae involving the nervous system. In Ross Russell RW (ed): Vascular Disease of the Central Nervous System, 2nd ed. Edinburgh, Churchill Livingstone, 1983.

Aminoff MJ: Electromyography in Clinical Practice, 3rd ed. New York, Churchill Livingstone, 1998.

Annegers JF, Elveback LR, Hauser WA, et al: Do anticonvulsants have a teratogenic effect? Arch Neurol 31:364, 1974.

Annegers JF, Hauser WA, Elveback LR, et al: Seizure disorders in offspring of parents with a history of seizures: A maternal-paternal difference? Epilepsia 17:1, 1976.

Axelsson I: A Cochrane review on the umbilical cord care and prevention of infections. Lakartidningen 99:1563, 2002.

Barber PV, Arnold AG, Evans G: Recurrent hormone dependent chorea: Effects of oestrogens and progestogens. Clin Endocrinol 5:291, 1976.

Barnes J: Obstetrical complications in neurological disorders. Proc R Soc Med 55:575, 1962.

Batocchi AP, Majolini L, Evoli A, et al: Course and treatment of myasthenia gravis during pregnancy. Neurology 52:447, 1999.

Beresford OD, Graham AM: Chorea gravidarum. J Obstet Gynaecol Br Emp 57:617, 1950.

Birk K, Rudick R: Pregnancy and multiple sclerosis. Arch Neurol 43:719, 1986.

Bjerkedal T, Bahna SL: The occurrence and outcome of pregnancy in women with epilepsy. Acta Obstet Gynaecol Scand 52:245, 1973.

Bjerkedal T, Czeizel A, Goujard J, et al: Valproic acid and spina bifida. Lancet 2:1096, 1982.

Bleyer WA, Skinner AL: Fatal neonatal hemorrhage after maternal anticonvulsant therapy. JAMA 235:626, 1976.

Bloemenkamp KW, Rosendaal FR, Helmerhorst FM, et al: Enhancement by factor V Leiden mutation of risk of deep-vein thrombosis associated with oral contraceptives containing a third-generation progestagen. Lancet 346:1593, 1995.

Britt BA, Gordon RA: Peripheral nerve injuries associated with anaesthesia. Can Anaesth Soc J 11:514, 1964.

Bruno MK, Harden CL: Epilepsy in pregnant women. Curr Treat Options Neurol 4:31, 2002.

Burkhart FL, Daly JW: Sciatic and peroneal nerve injury: A complication of vaginal operations. Obstet Gynecol 28:99, 1966.

Calderon-Gonzalez R, Gonzalez-Cantu N, Rizzi-Hernandez H: Recurrent polyneuropathy with pregnancy and oral contraceptives. N Engl J Med 282:1307, 1970.

Campbell ACP, Biggart JH: Wernicke's encephalopathy (polioencephalitis haemorrhagica superior): Its alcoholic and nonalcoholic incidence. J Pathol Bacteriol 48:245, 1939.

Collaborative Group for the Study of Stroke in Young Women: Oral contraceptives and stroke in young women: Associated risk factors. JAMA 231:718, 1975.

Confavreux C, Brunet P, Petiot P, et al: Congenital protein C deficiency and superior sagittal sinus thrombosis causing isolated intracranial hypertension. J Neurol Neurosurg Psychiatry 57:655, 1994.

Cooper ER, Charurat M, Mofenson L, et al: Combination antiretroviral strategies for the treatment of pregnant HIV-1-infected women and prevention of perinatal HIV-1 transmission. J Acquir Immune Defic Syndr 29:484, 2002.

Dansky LV, Rosenblatt DS, Andermann E: Mechanisms of teratogenesis: Folic acid and antiepileptic therapy. Neurology 42(Suppl 5):32, 1992.

Dean JC, Hailey H, Moore SJ, et al: Long term health and neurodevelopment in children exposed to antiepileptic drugs before birth. J Med Genet 39:251, 2002.

DeAngelis LM: Central nervous system neoplasms in pregnancy. In Devinsky O, Feldmann E, Hainline B (eds): Neurological Complications of Pregnancy. New York, Raven Press, 1994, p. 139.

Deblay MF, Vert P, Andreá M, et al: Transplacental vitamin K prevents haemorrhagic disease of infant of epileptic mother (letter). Lancet 1:1247, 1982.

Deschiens MA, Conard J, Horellou MH, et al: Coagulation studies, factor V Leiden, and anticardiolipin antibodies in 40 cases of cerebral venous thrombosis. Stroke 27:1724, 1996.

DiLiberti JH, Farndon PA, Dennis NR, et al: The fetal valproate syndrome. Am J Med Genet 19:473, 1984.

Donaldson JO: Neurology of Pregnancy. Philadelphia, Saunders, 1978.

Dulli DA, Luzzio CC, Williams EC, et al: Cerebral venous thrombosis and activated protein C resistance. Stroke 27:1731, 1996.

Dunn LJ, Dierker LJ: Recurrent hydramnios in association with myotonia dystrophica. Obstet Gynecol 42:104, 1973.

Eadie MJ, Lander CM, Tyrer JH: Plasma drug level monitoring in pregnancy. Clin Pharmacokinet 2:427, 1977.

Eckerling B, Goldman JA, Gans B: Intracranial sinus thrombosis, a rare complication of early pregnancy: Report of three cases. Obstet Gynecol 21:368, 1963.

Einhaupl KM, Villringer A, Meister W, et al: Heparin treatment in sinus venous thrombosis. Lancet 338:597, 1991.

Ekbom KA: Restless legs. In Vinken PJ, Bruyn GW (eds): Handbook of Clinical Neurology, vol 8. Amsterdam, North Holland, 1970.

Epstein MT, Hockaday JM, Hockaday TDR: Migraine and reproductive hormones throughout the menstrual cycle. Lancet 1:543, 1975.

Evans RW, Lipton RB: Topics in migraine management: A survey of headache specialists highlights some controversies. Neurol Clin 19:1, 2001.

Feldman GL, Weaver DD, Lovrien EW: The fetal trimethadione syndrome: Report of an additional family and further delineation of this syndrome. Am J Dis Child 131:1389, 1977.

Fishman RA, Cowen D, Silbermann M: Intracranial venous thrombosis during the first trimester of pregnancy. Neurology 7:217, 1957.

Fowler MG, Simonds RJ, Roongpisuthipong A: Update on perinatal HIV transmission. Pediatr Clin North Am 47:21, 2000.

Furman B, Bashiri A, Wiznitzer A, et al: Wilson's disease in pregnancy: five successful consecutive pregnancies of the same woman. Eur J Obstet Gynaecol Reprod Biol 96:232, 2001.

Gamboa ET, Isaacs G, Harter DH: Chorea associated with oral contraceptive therapy. Arch Neurol 25:112, 1971.

Gauthier PE, Hantson P, Vekemans MC, et al: Intensive care management of Guillain-Barré syndrome during pregnancy. Intensive Care Med 16:460, 1990.

Gettelfinger DM, Kokmen E: Superior sagittal sinus thrombosis. Arch Neurol 34:2, 1977.

Goldman JA, Eckerling B, Gans B: Intracranial venous sinus thrombosis in pregnancy and puerperium: Report of fifteen cases. J Obstet Gynaecol Br Commonw 71:791, 1964.

Goodman JDS, Brodie C, Ayida GA: Restless leg syndrome in pregnancy. Br Med J 297:1101, 1988.

Griffith RW, Grauwiler J, Hodel C, et al: Toxicologic considerations. In Berde B, Schild HO (eds): Ergot Alkaloids and Related Compounds: Handbook of Experimental Pharmacology, vol 49. New York, Springer-Verlag, 1978.

Hakim CA, Thomlinson J: Myotonia congenita in pregnancy. J Obstet Gynaecol Br Commonw 76:561, 1969.

Hanson JW, Myrianthopoulos NC, Harvey MAS, et al: Risks to the offspring of women treated with hydantoin anticonvulsants, with emphasis on the fetal hydantoin syndrome. J Pediatr 89:662, 1976.

Harjulehto-Mervaala T, Aro T, Hiilesmaa VK, et al: Oral polio vaccination during pregnancy: Lack of impact on fetal development and perinatal outcome. Clin Infect Dis 18:414, 1994.

Harper PS: Myotonic Dystrophy, 2nd ed. Philadelphia, Saunders, 1989.

Hartard C, Kunze K: Pregnancy in a patient with Wilson's disease treated with D-penicillamine and zinc sulfate. Eur Neurol 34:337, 1994.

Hertzog AG: Continuous bromocriptine therapy in menstrual migraine. Neurology 48:101, 1997.

Hiilesmaa VK: Pregnancy and birth in women with epilepsy. Neurology 42 (Suppl 5):8, 1992.

Hilsinger RL, Adour KK, Doty HE: Idiopathic facial paralysis, pregnancy, and the menstrual cycle. Ann Otol Rhinol Laryngol 84:433, 1975.

Hook R, Anderson EF, Noto P: Anesthetic management of a parturient with myotonia atrophica. Anesthesiology 43:689, 1975.

Horton JC, Chambers WA, Lyons SL, et al: Pregnancy and the risk of hemorrhage from cerebral arteriovenous malformations. Neurosurgery 27:867, 1990.

Hunter JS, Millikan CH: Poliomyelitis with pregnancy. Obstet Gynecol 4:147, 1954.

Irey NS, McAllister HA, Henry JM: Oral contraceptives and stroke in young women: A clinicopathologic correlation. Neurology 28:1216, 1978.

Jackson CD, Fishbein L: A toxicological review of beta-adrenergic blockers. Fundam Appl Toxicol 6:395, 1986.

Jadhav M, Webb JKG, Vaishnava S, et al: Vitamin-B_{12} deficiency in Indian infants: A clinical syndrome. Lancet 2:903, 1962.

Janz D: The teratogenic risk of antiepileptic drugs. Epilepsia 16:159, 1975.

Janz D, Beck-Mannagetta G, Andermann E, et al: Guidelines for the care of epileptic women of childbearing age. Epilepsia 30:409, 1989.

Jennett WB, Cross JN: Influence of pregnancy and oral contraception on the incidence of strokes in women of childbearing age. Lancet 1:1019, 1967.

Jones KL, Lacro RV, Johnson KA, et al: Pattern of malformations in the children of women treated with carbamazepine during pregnancy. N Engl J Med 320:1661, 1989.

Jones MW, Berry K: Chronic relapsing polyneuritis associated with pregnancy. Ann Neurol 9:413, 1981.

Keegan JJ, Holyoke EA: Meralgia paresthetica: An anatomical and surgical study. J Neurosurg 19:341, 1962.

Keesey J, Lindstrom J, Cokely H, et al: Anti-acetylcholine receptor antibody in neonatal myasthenia gravis. N Engl J Med 296:55, 1977.

Kempers RD, Miller RH: Management of pregnancy associated with brain tumors. Am J Obstet Gynecol 87:858, 1963.

Knight AH, Rhind EG: Epilepsy and pregnancy: A study of 153 pregnancies in 59 patients. Epilepsia 16:99, 1975.

Koch R, Friedman E, Azen C, et al: The International Collaborative Study of Maternal Phenylketonuria: Status report 1998. Eur J Pediatr 159 (Suppl 2):S156, 2000.

Korn-Lubetzki I, Kahana E, Cooper G, et al: Activity of multiple sclerosis during pregnancy and puerperium. Ann Neurol 16:229, 1984.

LaBan MM, Perrin JCS, Latimer FR: Pregnancy and the herniated lumbar disc. Arch Phys Med Rehabil 64:319, 1983.

Lance JW: The Mechanism and Management of Headache, 2nd ed. London, Butterworths, 1973.

Lenke RR, Levy HL: Maternal phenylketonuria and hyperphenylalaninemia: An international survey of the outcome of untreated and treated pregnancies. N Engl J Med 303:1202, 1980.

Lewis PD, Harrison MJG: Involuntary movements in patients taking oral contraceptives. Br Med J 4:404, 1969.

Markus HS, Hambley H: Neurology and the blood: haematological abnormalities in ischaemic stroke. J Neurol Neurosurg Psychiatry 64:150, 1998.

Martinelli I, Landi G, Merati G, et al: Factor V gene mutation is a risk factor for cerebral venous thrombosis. Thromb Haemost 75:393, 1996.

May M, Wette R, Hardin WB, et al: The use of steroids in Bell's palsy: A prospective controlled study. Laryngoscope 86:1111, 1976.

Meador KJ: Neurodevelopmental effects of antiepileptic drugs. Curr Neurol Neurosci Rep 2:373, 2002.

Mhurchu CN, Anderson C, Jamrozik K, et al: Hormonal factors and risk of aneurysmal subarachnoid hemorrhage: an international population-based, case-control study. Stroke 32:606, 2001.

Mofenson LM, McIntyre JA: Advances and research directions in the prevention of mother-to-child HIV-1 transmission. Lancet 355:2237, 2000.

Monson RR, Rosenberg L, Hartz SC, et al: Diphenylhydantoin and selected congenital malformations. N Engl J Med 289:1049, 1973.

Montouris GD, Fenichel GM, McLain LW: The pregnant epileptic: A review and recommendations. Arch Neurol 36:601, 1979.

Mountain KR, Hirsh J, Gallus AS: Neonatal coagulation defect due to anticonvulsant drug treatment in pregnancy. Lancet 1:265, 1970.

Nausieda PA, Koller WC, Weiner WJ, et al: Chorea induced by oral contraceptives. Neurology 29:1605, 1979.

Nelson LH, McLean WT: Management of Landry-Guillain-Barré syndrome in pregnancy. Obstet Gynecol 65 (Suppl):25S, 1985.

Newell KW, Lehmann AD, Leblanc DR, et al: The use of toxoid for the prevention of tetanus neonatorum: Final report of a double-blind controlled field trial. Bull WHO 35:863, 1966.

Newton TH, Hoyt WF: Dural arteriovenous shunts in the region of the cavernous sinus. Neuroradiology 1:71, 1970.

Niederhoff H, Zahrodnik H-P: Analgesics during pregnancy. Am J Med 75 (Suppl):117, 1983.

Niswander KR, Gordon M: The Collaborative Perinatal Study of the National Institute of Neurological Diseases and Stroke: The Women and Their Pregnancies. Washington, DC, Department of Health, Education and Welfare, Publication No. NIH 73-379, 1972.

Novak DJ, Johnson KP: Relapsing idiopathic polyneuritis during pregnancy. Arch Neurol 28:219, 1973.

O'Connell JEA: Maternal obstetrical paralysis. Surg Gynecol Obstet 79:374, 1944.

O'Connell JEA: Lumbar disc protrusions in pregnancy. J Neurol Neurosurg Psychiatry 23:138, 1960.

Okamoto K, Horisawa R, Kawamura T, et al: Menstrual and reproductive factors for subarachnoid hemorrhage risk in women: a case-control study in Nagoya, Japan. Stroke 32:2841, 2001.

Padua L, Aprile I, Caliandro P, et al: Symptoms and neurophysiological picture of carpal tunnel syndrome in pregnancy. Clin Neurophysiol 112:1946, 2001.

Parkinson D, Bachers G: Arteriovenous malformations: Summary of 100 consecutive supratentorial cases. J Neurosurg 53:285, 1980.

Patchell RA, Tibbs PA, Walsh JW, et al: A randomized trial of surgery in the treatment of single metastases to the brain. N Engl J Med 322:494, 1990.

Pearson MG: Meralgia paresthetica with reference to its occurrence in pregnancy. J Obstet Gynaecol Br Emp 64:427, 1957.

Perlroth MG, Marver HS, Tschudy DP: Oral contraceptive agents and the management of acute intermittent porphyria. JAMA 194:1037, 1965.

Perret G, Nishioka H: Report on the cooperative study of intracranial aneurysms and subarachnoid hemorrhage. Section VI. Arteriovenous malformations. J Neurosurg 25:467, 1966.

Piotin M, de Souza Filho CB, Kothimbakam R, et al: Endovascular treatment of acutely ruptured intracranial aneurysms in pregnancy. Am J Obstet Gynecol 185:1261, 2001.

Polizzi A, Huson SM, Vincent A: Teratogen update: maternal myasthenia gravis as a cause of congenital arthrogryposis. Teratology 62:332, 2000.

Poser S, Poser W: Multiple sclerosis and gestation. Neurology 33:1422, 1983.

Pugliese D, Nicoletti G, Andreula C, et al: Combined protein C deficiency and protein C activated resistance as a cause of caval, peripheral, and cerebral venous thrombosis. Angiology 49:399, 1998.

Raskin NH: Headache, 2nd ed. New York, Churchill Livingstone, 1988.

Ratinahirana H, Darbois Y, Bousser MG: Migraine and pregnancy: A prospective study in 703 women after delivery. Neurology 40(Suppl 1):437, 1990.

Redman JB, Fenwick RG, Fu YH, et al: Relationship between parental trinucleotide CGT repeat length and severity of myotonic dystrophy in offspring. JAMA 269:1960, 1993.

Reid DE: Assessment and management of the seriously ill patient following abortion. JAMA 199:805, 1967.

Retzloff MG, Kobylarz EJ, Eaton C: Optic neuritis with transient total blindness during lactation. Obstet Gynecol 98:902, 2001.

Rhodes P: Meralgia paraesthetica in pregnancy. Lancet 2:831, 1957.

Robert E, Guibaud P: Maternal valproic acid and congenital neural tube defects. Lancet 2:937, 1982.

Robertson DNS: The paraplegic patient in pregnancy and labour. Proc R Soc Med 56:381, 1963.

Robertson DNS: Pregnancy and labour in the paraplegic. Paraplegia 10:209, 1972.

Robinson JL, Hall CS, Sedzimir CB: Arteriovenous malformations, aneurysms, and pregnancy. J Neurosurg 41:63, 1974.

Robinson RG: Aspects of the natural history of cerebellar haemangioblastomas. Acta Neurol Scand 41:372, 1965.

Rosa FW: Spina bifida in infants of women treated with carbamazepine during pregnancy. N Engl J Med 324:674, 1991.

Rosen TS, Lin M, Spector S, et al: Maternal, fetal, and neonatal effects of chronic propranolol administration in the rat. J Pharmacol Exp Ther 208:118, 1979.

Ryan RE: A controlled study of the effect of oral contraceptives on migraine. Headache 17:250, 1978.

Sadasivan B, Malik GM, Lee C, et al: Vascular malformations and pregnancy. Surg Neurol 33:305, 1990.

Sadovnick AD, Eisen K, Hashimoto SA, et al: Pregnancy and multiple sclerosis: A prospective study. Arch Neurol 51:1120, 1994.

Salonen Ros H, Lichtenstein P, Bellocco R, et al: Increased risk of circulatory diseases in late pregnancy and puerperium. Epidemiology 12:456, 2001.

Sawle GV, Ramsay MM: The neurology of pregnancy. J Neurol Neurosurg Psychiatry 64:711, 1998.

Schaeffer M, Fox MJ, Li CP: Intrauterine poliomyelitis infection: Report of a case. JAMA 155:248, 1954.

Scheinberg IH, Sternlieb I: Pregnancy in penicillamine-treated patients with Wilson's disease. N Engl J Med 298:1300, 1975.

Schipper HM: Sex hormones and the nervous system. In Aminoff MJ (ed): Neurology and General Medicine, 3rd ed. New York, Churchill Livingstone, 2001, p. 365.

Schmidt D, Canger R, Avanzini G, et al: Change of seizure frequency in pregnant epileptic women. J Neurol Neurosurg Psychiatry 46:751, 1983.

Schoenfeld N, Epstein O, Nemesh L, et al: Effects of propranolol during pregnancy and development of rats. 1. Adverse effects during pregnancy. Pediatr Res 12:747, 1978.

Scriver CR, Clow CL: Phenylketonuria: Epitome of human biochemical genetics. N Engl J Med 303:1336, 1980.

Seip M: Growth retardation, dysmorphic facies and minor malformations following massive exposure to phenobarbitone in utero. Acta Paediatr Scand 65:617, 1976.

Shapiro S, Slone D, Hartz SC, et al: Anticonvulsant and parental epilepsy in the development of birth defects. Lancet 1:272, 1976.

Shapiro S, Slone D, Hartz SC, et al: Are hydantoins (phenytoins) human teratogens? J Pediatr 90:673, 1977.

Shelbourne P, Davies J, Buxton J, et al: Direct diagnosis of myotonic dystrophy with a disease-specific DNA marker. N Engl J Med 328:471, 1993.

Shmorgun D, Chan WS, Ray JG: Association between Bell's palsy in pregnancy and pre-eclampsia. QJM 95:359, 2002.

Silberstein SD: Headache and female hormones: what you need to know. Curr Opin Neurol 14:323, 2001.

Simon RH: Brain tumors in pregnancy. Semin Neurol 8:214, 1988.

Slocum HC, O'Neal KC, Allen CR: Neurovascular complications from malposition on the operating table. Surg Gynecol Obstet 86:729, 1948.

Smithells RW: Environmental teratogens of man. Br Med Bull 32:27, 1976.

Somerville BW: The role of estradiol withdrawal in the etiology of menstrual migraine. Neurology 22:355, 1972a.

Somerville BW: A study of migraine in pregnancy. Neurology 22:824, 1972b.

Speidel BD, Meadow SR: Maternal epilepsy and abnormalities of the fetus and newborn. Lancet 2:839, 1972.

Speroff L: Bacterial shock in obstetrics and gynecology, with emphasis on the surgical management of septic abortion. Am J Obstet Gynecol 95:139, 1966.

Starreveld-Zimmerman AAE, van der Kolk WJ, Elshove J, et al: Teratogenicity of antiepileptic drugs. Clin Neurol Neurosurg 77:81, 1974.

Stein GS: Headaches in the first postpartum week and their relationship to migraine. Headache 21:201, 1981.

Stevens H, Ammerman HH: Intracranial venous thrombosis in early pregnancy. Am J Obstet Gynecol 78:104, 1959.

Stolp-Smith KA, Pascoe MK, Ogburn PL: Carpal tunnel syndrome in pregnancy: Frequency, severity, and prognosis. Arch Phys Med Rehabil 79:1285, 1998.

Stoodley MA, Macdonald RL, Weir BK: Pregnancy and intracranial aneurysms. Neurosurg Clin North Am 9:549, 1998.

Tanganelli P, Regesta G: Epilepsy, pregnancy, and major birth anomalies: An Italian prospective, controlled study. Neurology 42(Suppl 5):89, 1992.

Taniguchi RM, Goree JA, Odom GL: Spontaneous carotid-cavernous shunts presenting diagnostic problems. J Neurosurg 35:384, 1971.

Taverner D, Cohen SB, Hutchinson BC: Comparison of corticotrophin and prednisolone in treatment of idiopathic facial paralysis (Bell's palsy). Br Med J 4:20, 1971.

Taverner D, Fearnley ME, Kemble F, et al: Prevention of denervation in Bell's palsy. Br Med J 1:391, 1966.

Taverner D, Kemble F, Cohen SB: Prognosis and treatment of idiopathic facial (Bell's) palsy. Br Med J 4:581, 1967.

Taylor RA: Heredofamilial mononeuritis multiplex with brachial predilection. Brain 83:113, 1960.

Teramo K, Hiilesmaa V, Bardy A, et al: Fetal heart rate during a maternal grand mal epileptic seizure. J Perinat Med 7:3, 1979.

Thompson DS, Nelson LM, Burns A, et al: The effects of pregnancy in multiple sclerosis: A retrospective study. Neurology 36:1097, 1986.

Townsend JJ, Baringer JR, Wolinsky JS, et al: Progressive rubella panencephalitis: Late onset after congenital rubella. N Engl J Med 292:990, 1975.

Tsai A, Lindheimer MD, Lamberg SI: Dermatomyositis complicating pregnancy. Obstet Gynecol **41**:570, 1973.

Tschudy DP, Valsamis M, Magnussen CR: Acute intermittent porphyria: Clinical and selected research aspects. Ann Intern Med **83**:851, 1975.

Tuomala RE, Shapiro DE, Mofenson LM, et al: Antiretroviral therapy during pregnancy and the risk of an adverse outcome. N Engl J Med **346**:1842, 2002.

Ueland K, McAnulty JH, Ueland FR, et al: Special considerations in the use of cardiovascular drugs. Clin Obstet Gynecol **24**:809, 1981.

Ungley CC: Recurrent polyneuritis in pregnancy and the puerperium affecting three members of a family. J Neurol Psychopathol **14**:15, 1933.

Wainscott G, Sullivan FM, Volans GN, et al: The outcome of pregnancy in women suffering from migraine. Postgrad Med J **54**:98, 1978.

Walshe JM: Pregnancy in Wilson's disease. Q J Med **46**:73, 1977.

Walshe JM: The management of pregnancy in Wilson's disease treated with trientine. Q J Med **58**:81, 1986.

Watson JD, Spellacy WN: Neonatal effects of maternal treatment with the anticonvulsant drug diphenylhydantoin. Obstet Gynecol **37**:881, 1971.

Weed JC, Hunter VJ: Diagnosis and management of brain metastasis from gestational trophoblastic disease. Oncology **5**:48, 1991.

Weih M, Vetter B, Ziemer S, et al: Increased rate of factor V Leiden mutation in patients with cerebral venous thrombosis. J Neurol **245**:149, 1998.

Weil ML, Itabashi HH, Cremer NE, et al: Chronic progressive panencephalitis due to rubella virus simulating subacute sclerosing panencephalitis. N Engl J Med **292**:994, 1975.

Weinshenker BG, Hader W, Carriere W, et al: The influence of pregnancy on disability from multiple sclerosis: A population-based study in Middlesex County, Ontario. Neurology **39**:1438, 1989.

Weinstein L, Aycock WL, Feemster RF: The relation of sex, pregnancy and menstruation to susceptibility in poliomyelitis. N Engl J Med **245**:54, 1951.

Welch KMA: Migraine and pregnancy. In Devinsky O, Feldmann E, Hainline B (eds): Neurological Complications of Pregnancy. New York, Raven Press, 1994, p. 77.

Wiebers DO: Ischemic cerebrovascular complications of pregnancy. Arch Neurol **42**:1106, 1985.

Willson P, Preece AA: Chorea gravidarum. Arch Intern Med **49**:471, 1932.

Wolf SM, Wagner JH, Davidson S, et al: Treatment of Bell palsy with prednisone: A prospective, randomized study. Neurology **28**:158, 1978.

Yen SSC: Neuroendocrine aspects of the regulation of cyclic gonadotropin release in women. In Martini L, Besser GM (eds): Clinical Neuroendocrinology. New York, Academic Press, 1977.

Yerby MS: Pregnancy and epilepsy. Epilepsia **32**(Suppl 6):S51, 1991.

Chapter 56

MANAGEMENT OF DEPRESSION AND PSYCHOSES DURING PREGNANCY AND THE PUERPERIUM

Barbara L. Parry, MD

The recognition and management of depression and psychoses during pregnancy and the puerperium are of critical importance. Particularly in the United States, these disorders often are underrecognized and undertreated, potentially contributing to devastating effects on the child, the mother, the family, and society. With the goal of improving health care in maternal-fetal medicine, this chapter will be devoted to the detection and management of these disorders. As symptoms of depression and psychosis are similar whether they present during pregnancy or postpartum, the clinical phenomenology of these syndromes will be described together first. Treatment, however, differs according to the reproductive state (e.g., effects of pharmacological agents on the fetus during pregnancy are not the same as on the infant during breast-feeding postpartum); therefore, management of symptoms during pregnancy versus the postpartum period will be addressed separately.

CLINICAL PHENOMENOLOGY

SYNDROMES. A range of mood syndromes can occur during pregnancy or postpartum. These include maternity or baby blues, major depression, and psychosis.

Maternity or Baby Blues

SYMPTOMATOLOGY. This subclinical syndrome is characterized by symptoms of crying, irritability, rapid mood shifts, and anxiety.

EPIDEMIOLOGY. The symptoms occur in 50%–80% of women (Stein, 1982). Given their transient nature and the fact that they are not severe enough to consistently affect the woman's ability to function, this syndrome is not considered a clinical disorder.

COURSE. The symptoms usually have their onset three days after delivery and generally resolve by the tenth day postpartum.

RISK FACTORS. Symptoms of premenstrual syndrome experienced prior to pregnancy may predispose a woman to maternity blues.

Major Depression

SYMPTOMATOLOGY. The symptoms in women with postpartum depression are similar to those in women who have major depressive episodes unrelated to childbirth (Wisner et al., 1994). The symptoms of depression in pregnancy are also similar to those occurring outside the puerperium, although the clinician must recognize that many vegetative manifestations of depression—for example, fatigue, sleep disturbance, appetite changes, or weight changes—are normal physical symptoms of pregnancy. In these cases, in addition to eliciting symptoms of depression, dysphoria or anxiety, it is important for the clinician to ask about symptoms of anhedonia (loss of pleasure in usually pleasurable activities), social withdrawal, cognitive disturbances (e.g., the inability to concentrate), guilt, hopelessness, helplessness, sense of worthlessness, or suicidal ideation to establish the diagnosis of a major depressive episode. Major depression is defined by the presence of five of the symptoms listed in Table 56-1, one of which must be either depressed mood or decreased interest or pleasure in activities. The symptoms must be present for most of the day nearly every day for two weeks or longer. The diagnosis of major depression also requires a decline from and substantial impairment of the woman's previous level of functioning.

In the Diagnostic and Statistical Manual of Mental Disorders, fourth edition (DSM-IV) (American Psychiatric Association, 1994), symptoms characterizing postpartum depression are listed under mood disorders, with a postpartum onset specifier. (Depressive symptoms during pregnancy are not addressed.) Postpartum onset is defined as within four weeks of delivery. Most clinicians and investigators, however, use a more inclusive timeline including up to three months after delivery based on the epidemiological studies of Kendell and colleagues (1987). The Marcé Society, an international organization for the study of mental illness related to childbearing, defines onset of a postpartum illness as one that occurs within 12 months of delivery.

An effective screening tool that is easy to administer to establish the diagnosis of postpartum depression, and which also has been validated for use during pregnancy, is the Edinburgh Postnatal Depression Scale (Cox et al., 1987; Green and Murray, 1994). If a woman has a total score on the Edinburgh Postnatal Depression Scale of 10 or higher or

TABLE 56-1. CRITERIA FOR MAJOR DEPRESSIVE EPISODE

A. Five (or more) of the following symptoms have been present during the same 2-week period and represent a change from previous functioning; at least one of the symptoms is either (1) depressed mood or (2) loss of interest or pleasure.*
  1. Depressed mood most of the day, nearly every day, as indicated by either subjective report (e.g., feels sad or empty) or observation made by others (e.g., appears tearful)[†]
  2. Markedly diminished interest or pleasure in all, or almost all, activities most of the day, nearly every day (as indicated by either subjective account or observation by others)
  3. Significant weight loss or weight gain when not dieting (e.g., a change of more than 5% of body weight in a month), or decrease or increase in appetite nearly every day.[‡]
  4. Insomnia or hypersomnia nearly every day
  5. Psychomotor agitation or retardation nearly every day (observable by others, not merely subjective feelings of restlessness or being slowed down)
  6. Fatigue or loss of energy nearly every day
  7. Feelings of worthlessness or excessive or inappropriate guilt (which may be delusional) nearly every day (not merely self-reproach or guilt about being sick)
  8. Diminished ability to think or concentrate, or indecisiveness, nearly every day (either by subjective account or as observed by others)
  9. Recurrent thoughts of death (not just fear of dying), recurrent suicidal ideation without a specific plan, or a suicide attempt or a specific plan for committing suicide
B. The symptoms do not meet criteria for a Mixed Episode.
C. The symptoms cause clinically significant distress or impairment in social, occupational, or other important areas of functioning.
D. The symptoms are not due to the direct physiological effects of a substance (e.g., a drug of abuse, a medication) or a general medical condition (e.g., hypothyroidism).
E. The symptoms are not better accounted for by bereavement, i.e., after the loss of a loved one, the symptoms persist for longer than 2 months or are characterized by marked functional impairment, morbid preoccupation with worthlessness, suicidal ideation, psychotic symptoms, or psychomotor retardation.

* Symptoms that are clearly due to a general medical condition or mood-incongruent delusions or hallucinations are not included.
† Can be irritable mood.
‡ Consider failure to make expected weight gains.

From American Psychiatric Association: Diagnostic and Statistical Manual for Mental Disorders, 4th ed. Washington, DC, American Psychiatric Association, 1994.

indicates that "the thought of harming myself has occurred to me" either "sometimes" (a score of 2) or "quite often" (a score of 3), a brief clinical interview to review symptoms and establish the diagnosis of depression is warranted.

EPIDEMIOLOGY. Postpartum depression, the most common complication of childbearing, occurs in 13% of women (O'Hara and Swain, 1996). Given that there are nearly four million births in the United States annually, half a million women have this disorder every year. Most women with a pregnancy-onset of major depression have a previous history of a mood disorder.

COURSE. Once a woman has had a postpartum depression, the risk for recurrence (defined as a return of symptoms that fulfill the DSM-IV criteria for major depression) is 25% (Wisner et al., 2001). Often, the symptoms of depression can have an insidious onset, not peaking until the third or fourth month postpartum. If left untreated, they may progress into the second postpartum year. Without treatment, the average duration of a postpartum episode of depression is seven months (O'Hara et al., 2000). Fifty to 85% of patients with a single episode of major depression will have at least one more episode of major depression after the discontinuation of medication, and the risk increases with the number of previous episodes (American Psychiatric Association, 2000). A depressive disorder during pregnancy usually extends into the postpartum period.

RISK FACTORS. A personal or family history of a mood disorder (not necessarily related to childbearing) and stressful life events predispose a woman to the development of a depressive disorder during pregnancy or the postpartum period, as they do at other times (O'Hara and Swain, 1996; Swendsen and Mazure, 2000; Wisner and Stowe, 1997). Primiparous women

are at greatest risk, but the occurrence of a depressive episode does not appear to be related to a woman's educational level, the sex of the infant, breast-feeding, the mode of delivery, or whether or not the pregnancy was planned.

Psychosis

SYMPTOMATOLOGY. Psychosis occurring during pregnancy or postpartum is a clinical emergency that requires immediate intervention because of the risk of infanticide or suicide, particularly in teenage mothers (Davidson and Robertson, 1985; Appleby, 1991). It differs from other psychotic episodes in that it can present with symptoms of sleep disturbance (even when the child is sleeping) and depersonalization (feeling removed or distant from people and the surrounding environment) and progresses rapidly to confusion, extreme disorganization of thought, bizarre behavior, delusions, and unusual visual, olfactory, or tactile hallucinations, all of which suggest an organic cause (Brockington and Meakin, 1994). The symptoms could be a manifestation of an underlying bipolar disorder, which has a high frequency of occurrence during the postpartum period (Targum et al., 1979).

EPIDEMIOLOGY. Postpartum psychosis occurs in 1/500–1/1000 primiparous women. With subsequent deliveries, the risk increases to 1/3–1/5 (Kendell et al., 1987). In about 33% of susceptible women, episodes recur outside the postpartum period. Episodes during pregnancy generally are in women with a previous history of mood disorders, particularly that of bipolar illness.

COURSE. The onset of symptoms usually occurs within the first two weeks after delivery. Treatment should be instituted immediately to prevent development into a more refractory illness that may be resistant to treatment, and treatment should be maintained for at least the first 6 weeks postpartum. Often, psychotic episodes, even with treatment, can progress to a depressive illness later in the postpartum period, about 3 to 4 months after delivery. There is a high recurrence rate in the first 6 months postpartum.

RISK FACTORS. A previous episode of a postpartum psychosis predisposes a woman to the development of a psychosis after a subsequent delivery. Primiparous women are at increased risk. Women with a personal or family history of bipolar illness are at three times the risk for the development of a postpartum psychosis compared with women without such histories. Women with a previous history of a mood disorder also are at increased risk for a recurrence during pregnancy.

EVALUATION

If a woman has considered a plan to act on suicidal thoughts or has thoughts about harming her infant, provisions for safety and urgent referral for psychiatric care are recommended. Women who have major functional impairment (as evidenced by the avoidance of family or friends, an inability to attend to hygiene, or an inability to care adequately for the infant) and those with coexisting substance abuse are also candidates for rapid referral. Women who report depressive symptoms without suicidal ideation or major functional impairment (or who register a score between 5 and 9 on the Edinburgh Postnatal Depression Scale) should be evaluated again 2 to 4 weeks later in order to determine whether an episode of depression has evolved or whether symptoms have subsided.

A careful history and physical examination are warranted in all women. Thyroid function should be assessed (see Chapter 50), as both hypothyroidism and hyperthyroidism are frequent during the puerperium and can contribute to mood changes. In women with thyroid disorders, treatment of both thyroid and depressive disorders generally is required.

Any presentation of psychotic symptoms (hallucinations, delusions, bizarre behavior) necessitates immediate psychiatric referral and usually hospitalization because of the imminent risk of infanticide or suicide. Psychotic symptoms often are a manifestation of bipolar disorder that can present with either a psychotic depressive or manic episode. Manic symptoms can be detected by the following questions: "Have you ever had four continuous days when you were feeling so good, high, excited, or 'hyper' that other people thought you were not your normal self or you got into trouble?" and "Have you experienced four continuous days when you were so irritable that you found yourself shouting at people or starting fights or arguments?" With these symptoms, the more rapid the intervention, the better the prognosis.

TREATMENT

General Principles

This section addresses pharmacologic, hormonal, psychotherapeutic, and chronobiologic interventions for major depression and psychosis during pregnancy and for postpartum women who are breast-feeding. Treatment for these disorders requires the clinician to weigh the benefits of treatment against many unknown potential risks. Information is often scarce, as double-blind, placebo-controlled trials of medication during pregnancy or in women who are lactating are not feasible. An increasing database supports replicated observations that untreated depression in the mother can impair neurocognitive development of the child (Dawson et al., 1992; Murray, 1992), observations that also are supported by animal models (Newport et al., 2002). Furthermore, Weissman and colleagues (1987, 1997) reported that children of depressed parents were at higher risk not only for early-onset major depressive disorder but also for anxiety disorders, alcohol abuse, social impairment, and medical problems. Studies to date indicate that most psychotropic medications in dosages commonly used have no major teratogenic effects. Long-term behavioral effects of these medications are unknown, however. Thus, in many instances the risk of psychiatric illness (e.g., major depression or psychosis) is much worse for the brain and the interaction of mother and child than the potential adverse effects of psychotropic medication. Whenever possible, the lowest possible dosage of medication should be used, and alternative nonpharmacologic interventions such as outpatient psychotherapy, hospitalization, or milieu therapy should always be considered as alternative or adjunctive treatments. For example, with maternity blues, treatment with education and reassurance generally is sufficient and does not require routine use of psychotropic medication.

Before a planned pregnancy, psychotropic medication should be evaluated. The hormonal effects of pregnancy and the puerperium may alter the course of the illness. With relatively mild or moderate psychiatric illness, for example, pregnancy could improve symptoms, and thus pre-existing psychotropic medication could be withdrawn or not reinstituted. With more severe or worsening illness, however, maintenance or altered dosing of psychotropic medication may be required to prevent exacerbations of the illness during pregnancy or the postpartum period. As organ formation occurs between the second and sixth week of gestation, this time is the most critical interval in which to avoid the use of medication if possible. It is not necessary, however, to induce unwarranted guilt or to have the woman consider terminating pregnancy if she does become pregnant while on psychotropic medication. The importance of close rapport between the treating physician and the pregnant or breast-feeding patient cannot be overstated and will obviate or decrease reliance on psychotropic medication in many cases. Women with previous episodes of depression or psychoses occurring during pregnancy or the puerperium may develop significant anticipatory anxiety about suffering from the potentially devastating effects of these illnesses again, anxiety that can be mitigated dramatically by the ongoing care and effective management by the health care provider. In the United Kingdom, Australia, and certain European countries, for example, the existence of mother-baby units and home health care providers have a major impact in improving the recognition and management and reducing the adverse consequences of these disorders. Whether treatment interventions are psychosocial or pharmacologic, early intervention with close follow-up and maintenance throughout the puerperium have the best prognosis and prevent the untoward consequences and refractory course that otherwise could develop.

Pharmacologic Interventions

Pregnancy

MAJOR DEPRESSION. For women with a diagnosis of major depression, treatment with antidepressants is appropriate. Surprisingly little information exists on the use of tricyclic and other antidepressants in pregnancy, especially considering the frequency of major depression in women of reproductive age. Depression in the first trimester, if not moderate to severe, should be treated if possible by supportive measures, as pregnancy itself may improve minor depressive symptoms. Cases of suicidality, incapacitating vegetative signs, or psychosis warrant hospitalization. Use of antidepressants, including selective serotonin-reuptake inhibitors (SSRIs), is indicated for vegetative signs that accompany a major depressive episode and do not resolve with supportive intervention. The available data show no evidence for a statistically significant association between fetal exposure and high rates of congenital malformations in fetuses exposed to tricyclic or other antidepressant drugs, although isolated cases of abnormalities have been reported in clinical and animal studies (Altshuler et al., 1996; Wisner et al., 1999). The clinician also needs to inform women about the potential for neonatal toxicity and long-term behavioral teratogenicity. There has been concern about the effects of the use of antidepressant drugs in the second and third trimesters on the neurological development of the fetus, particularly with respect to neurotransmitter systems. In studies of rodents, fluoxetine affects neurotransmitter systems in the brain (Cabrera and Battaglia, 1994), although it is difficult to know how these findings could apply to humans.

If antidepressants are used in the third trimester, the pediatrician should be warned to anticipate the possibility of withdrawal symptoms in the infant, and any marked change in maternal blood pressure is an indication for obstetrical surveillance of uteroplacental sufficiency.

For new onsets of depression, an SSRI may be tried initially because such agents are associated with a low risk of toxic effects in patients taking an overdose, as well as with ease of administration. If the patient has had a previous positive response to a specific drug from any class of antidepressants, however, that agent should be strongly considered. Women may be more likely to have a response to serotonergic agents, such as the SSRIs and venlafaxine, than to nonserotonergic tricyclic antidepressants (TCAs) (Kornstein, 1997). Slow increases in the dose are helpful in managing side effects. Dosages of certain drugs (i.e., TCAs, lithium) may need to be increased in the third trimester (Stewart et al., 1991; Wisner et al., 1993).

TRICYCLIC ANTIDEPRESSANTS

Amitriptyline (Elavil) and trimipramine (Surmontil) have been associated with adverse pregnancy outcomes in rats and rabbits. Trazadone (Desyrel) and amoxapine (Ascendin) also have been associated with poor fetal outcome in lower mammals. In general, therefore, although teratogenicity has not been proven, it is advisable to avoid using tricyclic drugs in the first trimester. In addition, these agents may interfere with normal labor. Isolated case reports have documented a withdrawal syndrome in neonates, including symptoms of cyanosis, difficulty breathing, and feeding difficulties after desipramine (Norpramin); urinary retention following nortriptyline (Pamelor); and dystonic movements and seizures after imipramine (Tofranil). These findings have led some authors to recommend a prelabor withdrawal period for patients on tricyclic drugs. No evidence, however, indicates that intrauterine withdrawal is safer than extrauterine withdrawal. Because fetal hyperactivity and seizures are possible, extrauterine withdrawal may be safer. Like phenothiazines, tricyclic drugs can cause hypotension.

SELECTIVE SEROTONIN REUPTAKE INHIBITORS (SSRIs)

Pastuszak and associates (1993) compared pregnancy outcomes following primarily first-trimester exposure to fluoxetine, TCAs, and agents known not to be teratogenic. Infants born to women treated with either fluoxetine or TCAs had more neonatal complications than the group exposed to nonteratogens, but no increased teratogenic risk. Chambers and coworkers (1996) found that women taking fluoxetine during pregnancy do not have an increased risk of spontaneous pregnancy loss or major fetal anomalies, but infants exposed to fluoxetine in the third trimester are at increased risk for more perinatal complications (premature delivery, admission to special-care nurseries, poor neonatal adaptation including respiratory difficulty, cyanosis on feeding, jitteriness, lower birth weight, and shorter birth length). These investigators recommend that fluoxetine be discontinued if possible before the last trimester. Nulman and colleagues (1997) found that the neurodevelopment of preschool children exposed *in utero* to tricyclic drugs or fluoxetine during pregnancy and followed from birth until 86 months did not differ from that of the control group. There were no significant differences in temperament, mood, arousability, activity level, distractibility, global intelligence quotient (IQ), or language development in children exposed to SSRIs in fetal life. Kulin and associates (1998) reported pregnancy outcomes following maternal use of the SSRIs fluvoxamine, paroxetine, and sertraline and found that outcomes among women who took an SSRI throughout pregnancy did not differ from outcomes among those who took the drug only during the first trimester or among those who were exposed to nonteratogens.

MONOAMINE OXIDASE INHIBITORS

The use of monoamine oxidase inhibitors (MAOIs) is contraindicated in pregnancy for several reasons:

1. Studies found growth retardation in animals receiving doses in excess of the maximum human recommended dose.
2. Pregnancy-induced hypertension is a common complication of pregnancy that often has an insidious onset; further exacerbation of that condition by use of MAOIs could lead to placental hypoperfusion and have serious fetal consequences.
3. If premature labor occurs, tocolysis with betamimetics may be obstetrically indicated but not feasible because of potential interaction with the MAOI.
4. Anesthetic management in labor could be complicated by the relative contraindication of opioids in patients taking MAOIs.

When pregnancy occurs while the woman is taking MAOIs, the drug should be discontinued. Guidelines have been suggested for appropriate obstetrical anesthesia and analgesia for women treated with MAOIs (Pavy et al., 1995; Gracious and Wisner, 1997).

PSYCHOSIS. Psychosis is a medical emergency because of the potential risk for infanticide or suicide. Imminent referral to a psychiatrist, hospitalization, or initiation of antipsychotic medication is indicated. Psychotic illness itself confers the greatest increase in risk of poor fetal outcome.

ANTIPSYCHOTICS

No conclusive evidence indicates that antipsychotics are teratogenic. Unless the patient presents a danger to herself, her unborn child, or others, or hospitalization does not adequately control her psychosis, phenothiazines should be avoided in the first trimester because they could increase the risk of congenital anomalies slightly (0.4%) (Altshuler et al., 1996). Use of these agents in the second and third trimester is unlikely to cause fetal malformation, and in contrast to data in animals, in humans there is no evidence of long-term effects on behavioral functioning or IQ up to 5 years of age (Kris, 1965; Edlund and Craig, 1984). The pediatrician should be alert to the possibility of transient perinatal syndromes (motor restlessness, tremor, hypertonicity, abnormal movements, difficulty with feeding, and possible neonatal jaundice and functional bowel obstruction) that generally resolve within days but can last up to 10 months after birth.

In view of the potential for hypotension with aliphatic phenothiazines and thioridazine (Mellaril) and the possible increased risk of fetal malformations with chlorpromazine (Thorazine), use of high-potency agents appears preferable as first-line management; low-potency agents should be used only if unacceptable adverse effects occur with the use of other agents. The newer atypical antipsychotic medications such as risperidone (Risperdal) or clozapine (Clozaril), perhaps because they are not specific for D_2 receptors linked with puerperal psychosis (Wieck et al., 1991), do not appear to be as effective as the high-potency dopamine blockers such as haloperidol (Haldol) in reducing psychotic symptoms during the puerperium. Medications to treat the extrapyramidal side effects of neuroleptics generally are not needed during pregnancy because of the effect of estrogen on dopamine receptors (Nausieda et al., 1979). Their routine use is not advised, given the association between the use of these drugs, such as benztropine (Cogentin), trihexyphenidyl (Artane), and amantadine (Symmetrel) and malformations (Heinonen et al., 1977).

Maintenance on antipsychotic medication for at least six weeks is warranted, with close monitoring at least at weekly intervals. Following resolution of the psychosis, which if recognized in its early stages and treated aggressively has a good prognosis, nonpsychotic depressive symptoms could present later in the course of the illness. If recognition or treatment of psychosis is delayed, it often develops into a chronic illness that becomes more refractory to intervention.

MANIA. In women with pre-existing illness, there is a high recurrence of mania during pregnancy that can present as psychosis (Kendell et al., 1987); therefore, maintenance on lithium is important to deter the development of adverse sequelae to the mother and infant. The risks of the development of Ebstein's cardiac anomaly in the first trimester with use of lithium is lower than previously thought (Cohen et al., 1994). Lithium crosses the placenta freely, and maternal and fetal plasma concentrations are similar. Reversible goiter from transplacental lithium poisoning can occur. Neonates exposed to lithium *in utero* have exhibited a variety of neurological side effects, including muscle flaccidity, inhibition of normal neonatal reflexes, lethargy, and cyanosis and cardiovascular effects, including atrial flutter, tricuspid regurgitation, and congestive heart failure. Careful monitoring of lithium concentration is required because of the dramatic shifts in fluid volume during pregnancy. A higher glomerular filtration rate, coupled with the increased plasma volume, often leads to a requirement for higher dosages in the gravid woman to achieve serum lithium concentrations comparable to those in the nongravid patient. Dehydration can occur during labor, and there could be a rapid loss of fluid volume after delivery. Thus, when lithium is used in the second and third trimesters, the clinician should monitor lithium levels every 2 weeks and taper lithium slowly to 25%–50% of the usual dosage 2 weeks before the estimated date of confinement, if clinically indicated. The anticonvulsants, carbamazepine (Tegretol) and valproic acid (Depakote), have not proved to be safer than lithium. Although they are effective mood stabilizers, their use has been associated with a 1%–5% incidence of spina bifida or other neural tube defects. The risk is thought to be higher with valproic acid. If mania cannot be controlled with antipsychotics or mood stabilizers, clonazepam (Klonopin) is a reasonable alternative. Benzodiazepines such as diazepam (Valium) cross the placenta throughout gestation; the use of Valium has been associated with cleft lip and palate (Heinonen et al., 1977), although the relationship remains uncertain. It is advisable to use a low-dose neuroleptic for treating the symptoms of mania and attendant anxiety.

Postpartum

DEPRESSION. Maternity blues can be managed by education and reassurance. For major depression, antidepressant medication is indicated. Only one placebo-controlled trial and three open trials that specifically address postpartum depression, however, have been published. Fluoxetine, an SSRI, was compared with psychotherapy, and both treatments were similarly effective. Fluoxetine was significantly more effective than placebo (Appleby et al., 1997). In open trials, sertraline (Stowe et al., 1995), venlafaxine (Cohen et al., 2001), and drugs grouped according to class (SSRIs and TCAs)(Wisner et al., 1999) were effective.

Women who have given birth recently often are sensitive to the side effects of medications (Wisner et al., 1997). Treatment should be initiated at half the recommended starting does (e.g., 25 mg of sertraline per day or 10 mg of paroxetine per day) for four days, and doses should be increased by small increments (e.g., 25 mg of sertraline per week or 10 mg of paroxetine per week) as tolerated until full remission is achieved. If the patient has a response to an initial trial of medication lasting 6–8 weeks, the same dose should be continued for a minimum of six months after a full remission has been achieved, in order to prevent a relapse (American Psychiatric Association, 2000). If there is no improvement after 6 weeks of drug therapy, of if the patient has a response but then has a relapse, referral to a psychiatrist should be considered. Long-term treatment for the prevention of recurrence should be considered for women who have had three or more episodes of severe depression. Because depressive symptoms often present with anxious, agitated features early in the postpartum course, antidepressant treatment for these symptoms is superior to use of the benzodiazepines, given the high excretion of benzodiazepines in breast milk and their propensity to induce respiratory depression.

BREAST-FEEDING

All antidepressants are excreted in breast milk. Therefore, the lowest effective dose of antidepressants should be used in a lactating mother. Observation of the infant's behavior before the mother is treated permits clinicians to avoid misinterpreting typical behavior as potentially drug-related.

TCAs are not typically found in measurable amounts in nursing infants (Wisner et al., 1996). Of the TCAs, nortriptyline and desipramine have few side effects. The only adverse outcomes reported with any TCA—respiratory depression and sedation—occurred in an infant whose mother was taking doxepin (Wisner et al., 1996). Of the drugs in this class, nortriptyline has been studied the most as a treatment for breast-feeding women. Children who were exposed to TCAs through breast milk have been followed through preschool and compared with children who were not exposed to these drugs, and no developmental problems were found (Yoshida et al., 1997). TCAs are not first-line drugs for the treatment of depression, however.

SSRIs

Based on an Expert Consensus Guideline Series (Althsuler et al., 2001) it is recommend that sertraline be used as a first-line treatment for breast-feeding mothers because of its low risk, although sporadic high levels have been observed in some infants (Stowe et al., 1997; Wisner et al., 1998). Epperson and colleagues (2001) observed minimal change in infants who were exposed to small amounts of sertraline through breast milk, assessing platelet serotonin level, which is reflective of central neuronal serotonin transporters. Other investigators have not observed adverse effects in breast-fed infants whose mothers were treated with sertraline, paroxetine, or fluvoxamine (Stowe et al., 2000; Misri et al., 2000; Hendrick et al., 2001). In one report, citalopram, which has a relatively short half-life, was associated with "uneasy sleep" in an infant with a measurable serum level (Jenson et al., 1997). With fluoxetine, breast-fed infants of fluoxetine-treated mothers gain less weight after birth, although unusual behavior was not observed in these infants (Chambers et al., 1999). Colic has been reported in three infants who were breast-fed by mothers taking fluoxetine. The infants had serum levels of fluoxetine and norfluoxetine (the active metabolite) that were in the therapeutic range for adults (Lester et al., 1993; Kristensen et al., 1999). As both fluoxetine and norfluoxetine have long half-lives (84 and 146 hours, respectively), continuous exposure to fluoxetine through breast milk is more likely than exposure to other SSRIs to lead to measurable serum levels (Wisner et al., 1996).

There are no published long-term evaluations of infants exposed to SSRIs through breast milk. As most of the published studies on antidepressant levels in infants exposed through breast milk are in full-term infants, close clinical monitoring and measurement of serum levels are warranted for premature or sick newborns. The full-term neonatal cytochrome P-450 activity is approximately one-half that found in adults (Morseli, 1980). The collective data on serum levels suggest that infants more than 10 weeks of age are at low risk for adverse effects, at least from TCAs. The higher lipid content of hind milk makes it likely that the second half will have a higher concentration of maternal medication than the fore milk. Taking medication immediately after breast-feeding minimizes the amount present in milk and maximizes clearance before the next feeding (Kacew, 1993).

PSYCHOSIS. Given the high risk to the mother and infant during a psychosis, and the minimal side effects of antipsychotic medication during breast-feeding, imminent use of low-dose, high-potency neuroleptics is warranted for this condition. The patient should be left on the medication for at least six weeks following the resolution of the psychosis, as recurrences are common, particularly in the early postpartum period. Only minimal dosages may be required to control symptoms. The milk-to-plasma ratio of chlorpromazine (Thorazine) is 0.3:1, and the ratio for perphenazine (Trilafon) is 1:1. The use of phenothiazines in lactating women has not been associated with serious consequences (Burt et al., 2001), although developmental delays were observed at 12–18 months in three infants exposed to a combination of haloperidol and chlorpromazine in one study, in which only one of the infants had detectable serum levels of neuroleptic (Yoshida et al., 1998). Thus, breast-feeding by mothers taking these medications is not contraindicated, but monotherapy is advised whenever possible. Given the risks of inducing hypotension with phenothiazines, the clinician is wise to use higher-potency neuroleptics (such as haloperidol) in small dosages (1–2 mg) instead. Because clozapine could induce fatal agranulocytosis in adults and there is lack of data on infants exposed to other atypical antipsychotics, it is imprudent to use these medications as a first-line treatment or for women treated with these agents to breast-feed. Because estrogen could modulate dopamine receptors (Ali and Peck, 1985), anti-parkinsonian medication is typically not needed. Furthermore, as described previously, these agents have not been adequately tested and could be associated with significant side effects. Thus, they should not be used routinely and should be administered only to treat intolerable adverse effects associated with the use of antipsychotic medications.

MANIA. Because there is a high incidence of mania in the postpartum period, antipsychotic medication or mood stabilizers could be required in order to control it. Although lithium carbonate is a first-line prophylactic treatment for mania in women who are not childbearing, its excretion through the breast milk in mothers and through the kidneys in infants makes its use problematic during lactation: The mean concentration of lithium in breast milk is approximately half the maternal serum concentration (Sykes et al., 1976), with a range from 25% to 77%. Lithium concentrations in the serum of breast-feeding infants are estimated to be one-tenth to one-half of those in maternal serum. During the first several months of life, the infant's kidney function is not fully developed, and the lithium excretion is slower than that of an older child. Several reports of lithium toxicity in breast-feeding infants exist, including cyanosis, T-wave abnormalities, and decreased muscle tone. Toxicity is especially likely during dehydration, such as during infection. Thus, because of this potential for toxicity, lithium is contraindicated in breast-feeding women. Valproic acid (Depakote) and carbamazepine (Tegretol) also are used as mood stabilizers in the treatment of mania. Because of rapid metabolism, their use in lactating women is safer than lithium in the postpartum patient who cannot be controlled adequately on neuroleptics but who insists upon breast-feeding, provided that the infant is carefully monitored for pediatric clinical status, liver enzymes, and platelets. Because benzodiazepines such as diazepam (Valium) and chlordiaxepoxide (Librium) are excreted in breast milk and could contribute to respiratory depression, nursing mothers should avoid the use of these compounds. If necessary, occasional low doses of shorter-acting compounds are safer.

Hormonal Therapy

Estrogen and progesterone have been used to treat postpartum depression. Gregoire and colleagues (1996) compared 17β-estradiol (200 μg per day) with placebo. The estradiol-treated group had a significant reduction in depression scores during the first month. Half of the women, however, were on antidepressant treatment. Transdermal estradiol may be used with antidepressants for women with postpartum depression without interfering significantly with lactation. Given the lack of controlled randomized trials, use of progesterone as a treatment or as prophylaxis in the management of postpartum mood disorders is not advised (Granger and Underwood, 2001). Prophylactic administration of a progestogen after delivery increased the risk of postpartum depression compared with placebo (Lawrie et al., 1998). To investigate the hormonal basis of postpartum depression, Bloch and associates (2000) simulated the decline in reproductive hormones after delivery in nonpregnant women with the use of the GnRh agonist leuprolide to induce a hypogonadal state. The women then were treated with supraphysiological doses of estradiol and progesterone, and then both steroids were withdrawn under double-blind conditions. Five of eight women with a history of postpartum depression, but none of eight women without previous depression, had mood changes. Thus, women with postpartum depression appear differentially sensitive to the effects of the withdrawal of gonadal steroids on mood.

Psychotherapy

Pregnancy

Spinelli (1997) found that a 16-week pilot trial of interpersonal psychotherapy was effective in significantly reducing depressive ratings in 13 women with antepartum major depression. In a study of 35 economically disadvantaged women, Zlotnick and coauthors (2001) administered a group intervention based on interpersonal psychotherapy during pregnancy, which prevented postpartum depression.

Postpartum

O'Hara and colleagues (2000) studied 120 postpartum women who were given either a 12-session treatment with interpersonal psychotherapy that focuses on changing roles and important relationships or were put on a waiting list for therapy (control condition). The active therapy was effective in relieving depressive symptoms and improving psychosocial functioning. In the study by Appleby and associates (1997), psychotherapy in addition to fluoxetine did not improve outcomes more than fluoxetine alone in women with postpartum depression.

ELECTROCONVULSIVE THERAPY (ECT)

ECT is an effective treatment for pregnancy and postpartum depression and psychosis, although it requires referral to a psychiatrist to implement.

Prophylactic Treatment

If a woman has brittle bipolar illness, she should remain on her psychotropic medication during pregnancy, as the adverse effects of a recurrence of her illness outweigh the risks from medication. Preventive therapy after delivery should be considered for women with any previous history of depression. The drug to which the patient previously responded or an SSRI are reasonable choices. The TCA nortriptyline did not confer protection compared with placebo in a follow-up study (Wisner et al., 2001). Stewart and associates (1991) found that lithium carbonate served as an effective prophylactic agent. An international trial is underway to investigate this work further by testing the efficacy of a neuroleptic medication (Haloperidol) versus lithium carbonate in the prevention of recurrent postpartum psychosis.

Chronobiological Therapy

One theory for depression includes desynchronization of circadian rhythms (Wehr and Wirz-Justice, 1981). Treatment implications are to resynchronize the biological rhythms of sleep and activity with those of other underlying circadian rhythms such as melatonin, cortisol, thyroid-stimulating hormone (TSH), or prolactin. This end may be achieved by administration of bright light (greater than 2500 lux) or wake therapy (sleep deprivation) at critical times of the day. Although still in its experimental stages, the use of bright light or wake therapy in women with pregnancy or postpartum depression has had promising results in pilot studies (Parry et al., 2000; Corral et al., 2000; Oren et al., 2002). Further studies in this area would be worthwhile given the relatively short onset of action of these treatments and the avoidance of risks associated with pharmacological interventions.

■ CONCLUSION

It is critical to recognize the symptoms of depression and psychosis during pregnancy and postpartum. The earlier the symptoms are recognized, the earlier they can be treated; intervention dramatically improves their prognosis and prevents the otherwise potentially devastating effects of these illnesses on the child, mother, family, and society.

R E F E R E N C E S

Ali SF, Peck EJ: Modulation of anterior pituitary dopamine receptors by estradiol 17-β: dose-response relationship. J Neurosci Res **13**:497, 1985.

Altshuler LL, Cohen LS, Moline ML, et al: The Expert Consensus Guideline Series: Treatment of depression in women. Postgrad Med (A Special Report) **107**:1, 2001.

Altshuler LL, Cohen L, Szuba MP, et al: Pharmacologic mangement of psychiatric illness during pregnancy: Dilemmas and guidelines. Am J Psychiatry **153**:592, 1996.

American Psychiatric Association. Guidelines for the treatment of patients with major depressive disorder. Am J Psychiatry **157**:S1, 2000.

Appleby L: Suicide during pregnancy and in the first postnatal year. BMJ **302**:137, 1991.

Appleby L, Warner R, Whitton A, et al: A controlled study of fluoxetine and cognitive-behavioural couselling in the treatment of postnatal depression. BMJ **314**:932, 1997.

Bloch M, Schmidt PJ, Danaceau M, et al: Effects of gonadal steroids in women with a history of postpartum depression. Am J Psychiatry **157**:924, 2000.

Brockington IF, Meakin CJ: Clinical cues to the aetiology of puerperal psychosis. Prog Neuropsychopharmacol Biol Psychiatry **18**:417, 1994.

Burt VK, Suri R, Altshuler L, et al: The use of psychotropic medications during breast-feeding. Am J Psychiatry **158**:1001, 2001.

Cabrera FM, Battaglia G: Delayed decreases in brain 5-HT 2a and 2c receptor density and function in male rat progeny following prenatal fluoxetine. J Pharmacol Exp Ther **269**:637, 1994.

Chambers CD, Anderson PO, Thomas RG, et al: Weight gain in infants breastfed by mothers who take fluoxetine. Pediatrics **104**:1120, 1999.

Chambers CD, Johnson KA, Dick LM, et al: Birth outcomes in pregnant women taking fluoxetine. N Engl J Med **335**:1010, 1996.

Cohen LS, Friedman JM, Jefferson JW, et al: A reevaluation of risk of *in utero* exposure to lithium. JAMA **271**:146, 1994; correction, **271**:1485, 1994.

Cohen LS, Viguera AC, Bouffard SM, et al: Venlafaxine in the treatment of postpartum depression. J Clin Psychiatry **62**:592, 2001.

Corral M, Kuan A, Kostara D: Bright light therapy's effect on postpartum depression (letter). Am J Psychiatry **157**:303, 2000.

Cox JL, Holden JM, Sagovsky R: Detection of postnatal depression: Development of the 10-item Edinburgh Postnatal Depression Scale. Br J Psychiatry **150**:782, 1987.

Davidson J, Robertson E: A follow-up study of post partum illness, 1946–1978. Acta Psychiatr Scand **71**:451, 1985.

Dawson G, Klinger LG, Panagiotides H, et al: Frontal lobe activity and affective behavior of infants of mothers with depressive symptoms. Child Dev **63**:725, 1992.

Desmond MM, Rudolph AJ, Hill RM, et al: Behavior alteration in infants born to mothers on psychoactive medication during pregnancy. *In* Austin F (ed): Congenital Mental Retardation. Austin Tex, University of Texas Press, 1967, p. 235.

The Diagnostic and Statistical Manual of Mental Disorders, 4th ed.: DSM-IV. Washington, DC, American Psychiatric Association, 1994, p. 386.

Edlund MJ, Craig TJ: Antipsychotic drug use and birth defects: An epidemiologic reassessment. Compr Psychiatry **25**:32, 1984.

Epperson N, Czarkowski KA, Ward-O'Brien D, et al: Maternal sertraline treatment and serotonin transport in breast-feeding mother-infant pairs. Am J Psychiatry **158**:1631, 2001.

Gracious BL, Wisner KL: Phenelzine use throughout pregnancy and the puerperium period: Case report, review of the literature and management recommendations. Depress Anxiety **6**:124, 1997.

Granger ACP, Underwood MR: Review of the role of progesterone in the management of postnatal mood disorder. J Psychosom Obstet Gynecol **22**:49, 2001.

Green JM, Murray D: The use of the Edinburgh Postnatal Depression Scale in research to explore the relationship between antenatal and postnatal dysphoria. *In* Cox J, Holden J (eds): Perinatal Psychiatry: Use and Misuse of the Edinburgh Postnatal Depression Scale. London, Royal College of Psychiatrists, 1994, p. 180.

Gregoire AJP, Kumar R, Everitt B, et al: Transdermal oestrogen for treatment of severe postnatal depression. Lancet **347**:930, 1996.

Heinonen OP, Slone D, Shapiro S: Birth Defects and Drugs in Pregnancy. Littleton Mass, Publishing Services Group, 1977, p. 322.

Hendrick V, Fukuchi A, Althsuler L, et al: Use of sertraline, paroxetine and fluvoxamine by nursing women. Br J Psychiatry **179**:163, 2001.

Jenson PN, Olesen OV, Bertelsen A, et al: Citalopram and desmethylcitalopram concentrations in breast milk and in serum of mother and infant. Ther Drug Monit **19**:236, 1997.

Kacew S: Adverse effects of drugs and chemicals in breast milk on the nursing infant. J Clin Pharmacol **33**:213, 1993.

Kendell RE, Chalmers JC, Platz C: Epidemiology of puerperal psychoses. Br J Psychiatry **150**:662, 1987.

Kornstein SG: Gender differences in depression: Implications for treatment. J Clin Psychiatry **58**:S12, 1997.

Kris EB: Children of mothers maintained on pharmacotherapy during pregnancy and postpartum. Curr Ther Res **7**:785, 1965.

Kristensen JH, Ilett KE, Hackeett LP, et al: Distribution and excretion of fluoxetine and norfluoxetine in human milk. Br J Clin Pharmacol **48**:521, 1999.

Kulin NA, Pastuszak A, Sage SR, et al: Pregnancy outcome following maternal use of the new selective serotonin reuptake inhibitors. JAMA **279**:609, 1998.

Lawrie TA, Hofmeyr GJ, De Jager M, et al: A double-blind randomized placebo-controlled trial of postnatal norethisterone enanthate: The effect on postnatal depression and serum hormones. Br J Obstet Gynaecol **105**:1082, 1998.

Lester BM, Cucca J, Andreozzi L, et al: Possible association between fluoxetine hydrochloride and colic in an infant. J Am Acad Chil Adoles Psychiatry **32**:1253, 1993.

Misri S, Kim J, Riggs KW, et al: Paroxetine levels in postpartum depressed women, breast milk, and infant serum. J Clin Psychiatry **61**:828, 2000.

Morseli PL: Clinical pharmacokinetics in newborns and infants. Clin Pharmacokinet **5**:485, 1980.

Murray L: The impact of postnatal depression on infant development. J Child Psychol Psychiatry **33**:343, 1992.

Nausieda PA, Koiller WC, Weiner WJ, et al: Modification of postsynaptic dopaminergic sensitivity by female sex hormones. Life Sci **25**:521, 1979.

Newport JD, Stowe ZN, Nemeroff CB: Parental depression: Animal models of an adverse life event. Am J Psychiatry **159**:1265, 2002.

Nulman I, Rovet J, Stewart DE, et al: Neurodevelopment of children exposed *in utero* to antidepressant drugs. N Engl J Med **336**:258, 1997.

O'Hara MW, Stuart S, Gorman LL, et al: Efficacy of interpersonal psychotherapy for postpartum depression. Arch Gen Psychiatry **57**:1039, 2000.

O'Hara MW, Swain AM: Rates and risk of postpartum depression: A meta analysis. Int Rev Psychiatry **8**:7, 1996.

Oren DA, Wisner KL, Spinelli M, et al: An open trial of morning light therapy for treatment of antepartum depression. Am J Psychiatry **159**:666, 2002.

Parry BL, Curran ML, Stuenkel CA, et al: Can critically timed sleep deprivation be useful in pregnancy and postpartum depressions? J Affective Disorders **60**:201, 2000.

Pastuszak A, Schick-Boschetto B, Zuber C: Pregnancy outcome following first-trimester exposure to fluoxetine (Prosac). JAMA **269**:2246, 1993.

Pavy TJ, Kliffer AP, Douglas MJ: Anesthetic management of labour and delivery in a woman taking long-term MAOI. Can J Aneth **42**:618, 1995.

Spinelli MG: Interpersonal psychotherapy for depressed antepartum women: A pilot study. Am J Psychiatry **154**:1028, 1997.

Stein G: The Maternity Blues. *In* Brockington IF, Kumar R (eds): Motherhood and Mental Illness. London, Academic Press, 1982, p. 119.

Stewart DE, Klompenhouwer JL, Kendell RE, et al: Prophylactic lithium in puerperal psychosis: The experience of three centres. Br J Psychiatry **158**:393, 1991.

Stowe ZN, Casarella J, Landry J, et al: Sertraline in the treatment of women with postpartum major depression. Depression **3**:49, 1995.

Stowe ZN, Cohen LS, Hostetter A, et al: Paroxetine in human breast milk and nursing infants. Am J Psychiatry **157**:185, 2000.

Stowe ZN, Owens MJ, Landry JC, et al: Sertraline and desmethylsertraline in human breast milk and nursing infants. Am J Psychiatry **154**:1255, 1997.

Swendsen JD, Mazure CM: Life stress as a risk for postpartum depression: Current research and methodological issues. Clin Psychol Sci Pract **7**:17, 2000.

Sykes PA, Quarrie J, Alexander FW: Lithium carbonate and breast-feeding. Br Med J **2**:1299, 1976.

Targum SD, Davenport YB, Webster MJ: Postpartum mania in bipolar manic-depressive patients withdrawn from lithium carbonate. J Nerv Ment Dis **167**:572, 1979.

Wehr TA, Wirz-Justice A: Internal coincidence model for sleep deprivation and depression. *In* Koella, WP (ed): Sleep 1980, Fifth European Congress on Sleep Research. Amsterdam, Karger, Basel, Switzerland, 1981, p. 26.

Weissman MM, Gammon D, John K, et al: Children of depressed parents. Arch Gen Psychiatry **44**:847, 1987.

Weissman MM, Warner V, Wickramarate P, et al: Offspring of depressed parents. Arch Gen Psychiatry **54**:932, 1997.

Wieck A, Kumar R, Hirst AD, et al: Increased sensitivity of dopamine receptors and recurrence of affective psychosis after childbirth. Br Med J **303**:613, 1991.

Wisner KL, Gelenberg AJ, Leonard H, et al: Pharmacologic treatment of depression during pregnancy. JAMA **282**:1264, 1999.

Wisner KL, Peindl KS, Gigliotti TV: Tricyclics vs. SSRIs for postpartum depression. Arch Women's Mental Health **1**:189, 1999.

Wisner KL, Peindl KS, Hanusa BH: Symptomatology of affective and psychotic illnesses related to childbearing. J Affect Disord **30**:77, 1994.

Wisner KL, Perel JM, Blumer J: Serum sertraline an N-desmethylsertraline levels in breast-feeding mother-infant pairs. Am J Psychiatry **155**:690, 1998.

Wisner KL, Perel JM, Findling RL: Antidepressant treatment during breast-feeding. Am J Psychiatry **153**:1132, 1996.

Wisner KL, Perel JM, Peindl KS, et al: Effects of the postpartum period on nortriptyline pharmacokinetics. Psychopharmacol Bull **33**:243, 1997.

Wisner KL, Perel JM, Peindl KS, et al: Prevention of recurrent postpartum depression: A randomized clinical trial. J Clin Psychiatry **62**:82, 2001.

Wisner KL, Perel JM, Wheeler SB: Tricyclic dose requirements across pregnancy. Am J Psychiatry **150**:1541, 1993.

Wisner KL, Stowe ZN: Psychobiology of postpartum mood disorders. Semin Reprod Endocrinol **15**:77, 1997.

Yoshida K, Smith B, Craggs M, et al: Neuroleptic drugs in breast-milk: A study of pharmacokinetics and of posssible adverse effcts in breast-fed infants. Psychol Med **28**:81, 1998.

Zlotnick C, Johnson SL, Miller IW, et al: Postpartum depression in women receiving public assistance: Pilot study of an interpersonal-therapy-oriented group intervention. Am J Psychiatry **158**:638, 2001.

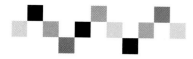

Chapter 57
THE SKIN AND PREGNANCY

Ronald P. Rapini, MD

The physical and hormonal alterations induced by pregnancy, childbirth, and the puerperium are associated with numerous cutaneous changes. Some of these occur so frequently that they are not considered abnormal and vary only in degree. This chapter discusses these physiologic changes as well as the pathologic rashes of pregnancy and the effects of pregnancy on preexisting dermatologic diseases.

COMMON SKIN CHANGES INDUCED BY PREGNANCY

Pigmentary Changes

Hyperpigmentation occurs in almost all pregnant women (Elling and Powell, 1997). Much of this is presumed to be due to the effects of increased levels of melanocyte-stimulating hormone (MSH) (Ances and Pomerantz, 1974) or estrogen and progesterone (Maeda et al., 1996) on the melanocytes in the epidermis (see Chapter 9 for details of endocrine changes in pregnancy). Altmeyer and associates (1989) showed a significant increase in the levels of alpha-MSH, melatonin, adrenocorticotropin or adrenocorticotropic hormone (ACTH), and progesterone from the first to the third trimester. Nearly all pregnant women experience mild generalized hyperpigmentation, with accentuation in the areolae and genital skin. The neck can become hyperpigmented. If the neck becomes velvety or papillomatous, then acanthosis nigricans should be considered. Hyperpigmentation of the linea alba, the longitudinal demarcation line on the midline of the abdomen, is called *linea nigra*. All of these pigmentary changes generally regress following delivery.

Melasma is diffuse macular hyperpigmentation of the face, usually involving the forehead, cheeks, and bridge of the nose (Grimes, 1995). Although the antequated term *chloasma* has often been used as a synonym, it was typically restricted to those cases occurring during pregnancy ("mask of pregnancy"). Melasma occurs in about 70% of pregnant women but also can occur in women who are not pregnant, especially those taking oral contraceptives and other hormones. Increased expression of alpha-MSH has been found in lesional skin (Im et al., 2002). The hyperpigmentation is usually blotchy and poorly demarcated and is bilaterally symmetric. It usually resolves after delivery; however, it persists for months or years in about 30% of patients. An increased incidence of thyroid abnormalities has been reported in patients with melasma (Lutfi et al., 1985), but in many instances this is mild and subclinical.

Avoidance of exposure to sun during pregnancy helps prevent or minimize the formation of melasma. Topical sunscreen lotions with sun protective factor ratings of 15 or greater are important. For troublesome hyperpigmentation that persists after delivery, topical hydroquinone bleaching creams and solutions, such as Claripel, Lustra, Alustra, Melanex, or Solaquin, are sometimes useful. Treatment is frequently prolonged for months. Cosmetics are useful for covering irregular pigmentation. Additional therapeutic options for melasma persisting after pregnancy include daily topical retinoic acid (tretinoin [Retin-A, Avita]) (Kimbrough-Green et al., 1994), salicylic acid (SalAc cleanser), or azelaic acid (Azelex). A combination of topical fluocinolone, hydroquinone, and tretinoin (Tri-Luma cream) has recently been approved. Chemical peels with trichloroacetic acid, phenol, glycolic acid, Jessner's solution, or kojic acid may be effective (Garcia and Fulton, 1996; Lawrence et al., 1997). Although the Q-switched lasers (yttrium-aluminum-garnet, ruby, or alexandrite) have been useful for many other pigmentary problems, they usually are of little help with melasma (Taylor and Anderson, 1994).

Pregnancy has been reported to induce the appearance of *new melanocytic nevi* or enlargement of preexisting nevi, but the incidence of changes in nevi and the formation of melanoma seems to be no greater than in nonpregnant women (Katz et al., 2002). Most melanomas exhibit asymmetry, an irregular border, variegated colors (red or white in addition to black or blue), and a diameter greater than 6 mm. Suspicious lesions should be excised immediately (Gormley, 1990). Local anesthetic agents, such as lidocaine, are generally regarded as safe. The use of epinephrine in low doses along with lidocaine could help to expedite surgery. The subject of malignant melanoma during pregnancy is addressed in Chapter 58.

Vascular Changes

Pregnancy induces dilation and proliferation of blood vessels. Although this is thought to be largely due to estrogen, the mechanism is not completely understood. *Telangiectasias* (persistently dilated blood vessels) that resemble those seen with chronic sunlight or radiation exposure can occur in pregnancy. *Spider angioma* (nevus araneus) is characterized by a central arteriole with radiating vascular "legs" resembling those of a spider and is most prevalent in sun-exposed areas. Multiple spider angiomas also can occur in liver disease (resulting from decreased hepatic estrogen catabolism), with estrogen therapy, and in normal nonpregnant women. These lesions can regress spontaneously. Persistent lesions are best treated with light electrocoagulation or laser ablation.

Palmar erythema occurs in many normal pregnant women and could be associated with liver disease, estrogen therapy, and collagen vascular diseases. These vascular changes require no therapy and usually resolve after delivery.

Pyogenic granuloma is a misnomer for a juicy-red, nodular, often pedunculated, exuberant proliferation of granulation tissue (not really a granuloma, which is a nodular aggregate in which macrophages predominate). These lesions can occur anywhere on the skin but are especially common on the gums, often resulting from gingivitis or trauma. The terms *lobular capillary hemangioma*, *pregnancy tumor*, and *granuloma gravidarum* are synonyms for pyogenic granuloma (Mooney and Janniger, 1995). Therapy consists of surgical excision or electrosurgical destruction (Sills et al., 1996); however, this can often be delayed until after delivery because some lesions regress spontaneously. Immediate biopsy should be performed if the clinical diagnosis is in doubt because occasional neoplasms, such as amelanotic melanomas, can resemble a pyogenic granuloma.

Venous congestion and increased vascular permeability during pregnancy commonly cause edema of the skin and subcutaneous tissue, particularly of the vulva and lower legs. *Severe labial edema* has occasionally been reported during pregnancy (Morris et al., 1990), and sometimes a search for other causes is warranted. *Varicosities* are common on the legs and around the anus (hemorrhoids). These may regress after delivery but usually not completely (Wong and Ellis, 1989).

Connective Tissue Changes

The mechanisms by which collagen and other connective tissue elements are influenced during pregnancy are poorly understood. *Striae* ("stretch marks") represent linear tears in dermal connective tissue and appear as red or purple atrophic bands over the abdomen, breasts, thighs, buttocks, groin, and axillae. Sometimes these lesions are pruritic. Genetic susceptibility may be involved, because no striae form in pregnant women with Ehlers-Danlos syndrome, and they do not develop in some normal women. Striae are more common in younger women with greater total weight gain (Madlon-Kay, 1993).

Despite numerous anecdotal claims of therapeutic efficacy, no topical therapy prevents or affects the course of striae, which ordinarily become less apparent as the red or purple color fades after delivery. There are numerous testimonials regarding the value of olive oil, cocoa butter, vitamin E, tretinoin (Rangel et al., 2001), and nutritional therapy, but none of these has proved valuable in controlled studies (Pribanich et al., 1994). The pulsed dye laser has been reported to be helpful, particularly in obliterating the red color of early lesions, but it is difficult to determine whether the short-term improvement is better than that following long-term observation.

Skin tags (acrochordons or molluscum fibrosum gravidarum) are soft papular or pedunculated growths of fibrous and epithelial tissue that are common in obesity as well as in pregnancy. They are usually skin-colored to brown and usually appear on the neck, axillae, or groin. Skin tags often persist after delivery and can easily be electrocoagulated or snipped off with scissors.

Hair Cycle and Growth Changes

The hair growth cycle is divided into three phases: anagen, catagen, and telogen. The duration of the growing phase (anagen) of each scalp hair follicle persists 3–4 years, with an average daily growth rate of approximately 0.34 mm. Growth activity is followed by a relatively short transitional (catagen) phase, lasting about 2 weeks, followed by a resting phase (telogen), lasting several weeks. When the next hair cycle starts, newly forming hair causes shedding of the older telogen hairs.

The activity of each of about 100,000 follicles on the human scalp cycles randomly and independently from the activity of neighboring follicles. At any given time, approximately 10%–15% of hair follicles are in telogen. If the average duration of growth of each follicle is approximately 1000 days (3 years), it can be calculated that about 100 hairs are shed normally each day.

In late pregnancy, hormones appear to increase the number of anagen hairs and decrease those in telogen (Randall, 1994). Following hormone withdrawal in the postpartum period, telogen hairs can rise to 35% or more of scalp hairs, resulting in a transient hair loss peaking about 3–4 months after parturition (Schiff and Kern, 1963). This diffuse hair loss has been called *telogen effluvium*, whether it occurs after delivery, surgery, illness, crash dieting, or some other stressful event. The severity varies greatly, and it takes a total hair loss of 40%–50% to become noticeable. Telogen effluvium is generally easy to distinguish from other causes of hair loss, and patients should be reassured that regrowth is likely to occur by 9 months after delivery without any treatment.

Hirsutism of the lower facial or sexual skin areas is uncommon but occasionally occurs in the second half of pregnancy and can be accompanied by acne. The cause is presumed to relate to the effects of ovarian and placental androgens on the pilosebaceous unit. The possibility of an underlying androgen-secreting tumor of the ovary, of a luteoma, or of a lutein cyst should be considered, although polycystic ovary disease appears to be the most frequent cause.

Several different *nail changes* have been reported during pregnancy but do not occur regularly. These changes include transverse grooving, increased brittleness, softening, or distal onycholysis (Wong and Ellis, 1989).

■ SKIN CONDITIONS SPECIFIC TO PREGNANCY

Table 57-1 lists the rashes specific to pregnancy. Because of a lack of understanding of the pathogenesis of most of these conditions and the lack of specific diagnostic criteria, the terminology has been confusing (Harahap and Wallach, 1995; Black et al., 2002). Many of these diseases have been described by different authors using different names for the same conditions (Al-Fares et al., 2001). In general, all tend to be pruritic and usually resolve within a few weeks after delivery. They all can recur in subsequent pregnancies except the polymorphic eruption of pregnancy and prurigo gestationis. Three of the diseases have been claimed to be associated with increased fetal mortality. It is important to keep in mind that pregnant women also can experience other dermatoses

TABLE 57-1. RASHES OF PREGNANCY

Disease	Estimated % of All Pregnancies	Lesion Morphology	Most Common Location	Important Laboratory Features	Usual Trimester of Onset	Increased Fetal Mortality
Pruritus gravidarum	1.5–2.0	Pruritus, no rash	Anywhere	Sometimes increased bile salts, LFTs	3	Yes (?)
Pruritic urticarial papules and plaques of pregnancy (PUPPP)	0.6	Papules, plaques, urticaria	Abdomen, thighs, especially in striae	None	3	No
Prurigo gestationis (Besnier)	0.3	Excoriated papules	Extremities	None	2	No
Pemphigoid gestationis (herpes gestationis)	0.002	Papules, vesicles	Anywhere	Direct IF biopsy	2 or 3	Yes (?)
Impetigo herpetiformis	Very rare	Pustules	Intertriginous, trunk	Biopsy subcorneal pustule	1, 2, or 3	Yes
Autoimmune progesterone dermatitis	Very rare	Acneiform, urticarial	Buttocks, extremities	Progesterone intradermal skin test	1	(?)

IF, immunofluorescence; LFTs, liver function tests.

besides those specific to pregnancy. For example, contact dermatitis, eczema, superficial fungal infections, folliculitis (Zoberman and Farmer, 1981), erythema multiforme, urticaria, vasculitis, viral exanthems, scabies, secondary syphilis, and drug eruptions all can occur, and it can be difficult to distinguish these from some of the pregnancy-specific rashes discussed here.

General Treatment

The same treatment principles apply to all of the specific dermatoses of pregnancy. Few drugs have been proved safe during pregnancy, and the risk-benefit ratio must be considered. Milder disease is treated with topical emollients, calamine lotion, cool compresses or baths, and topical corticosteroids. Topical corticosteroids (e.g., hydrocortisone and triamcinolone) are classified as U.S. Food and Drug Administration (FDA) Pregnancy Risk Category C, but they are still widely used during pregnancy when the possible benefits outweigh the risks of minimal percutaneous absorption. Some of the very high-potency topical corticosteroids, such as clobetasol, have potential for significant absorption on large body surface areas.

Many oral antihistamines, including the nonsedating fexofenadine (Allegra) and desloratadine (Clarinex), are labeled as FDA Pregnancy Risk Category C because available data are insufficient. Hydroxyzine (Atarax) is not recommended in the first trimester because it has been associated with a slightly increased rate (5.8%) of congenital malformations, but otherwise it is in Category C (Hale and Pomeranz, 2002). Those oral antihistamines classified as Category B (e.g., cetirizine [Zyrtec], chlorpheniramine, cyproheptadine [Periactin], diphenhydramine [Benadryl], and loratadine [Claritin]) could be worth trying in patients with bothersome pruritus. Cetirizine and loratadine are the relatively nonsedating agents. The favorite antihistamine in pregnancy appears to be diphenhydramine, even though it produces annoying drowsiness. One study associated diphenhydramine with cleft palate, but this has been disputed in other studies (Hale and Pomeranz, 2002). There has been an increased rate of retrolental fibroplasia reported in premature infants whose mothers took antihista-

mines within 2 weeks of delivery. No antihistamines are recommended during lactation by the manufacturers, but the American Academy of Pediatrics considers diphenhydramine to be safe during lactation, as levels in breast milk are low.

Use of systemic corticosteroids (e.g., prednisone, prednisolone) in patients with severe disease appears to be relatively safe in humans (pregnancy Class B). Although cleft palates have occurred in offspring of pregnant rabbits undergoing such therapy, this relationship has not been demonstrated in humans. Infants of mothers treated with systemic corticosteroids should be monitored for evidence of adrenal insufficiency.

Pruritus Gravidarum

Pruritus gravidarum can be defined as generalized itching during pregnancy without the presence of a rash (although excoriations can be present). Up to 14% of pregnant women complain of itching, but pruritus associated with cholestasis occurs in only about 1.5%–2% of pregnant women, with onset usually in the third trimester. Some authorities seem to confuse definitions by reserving the term pruritus gravidarum for patients with cholestasis of pregnancy (Roger et al., 1994). Frank clinical jaundice occurs in only 0.02% of pregnancies. Pruritus limited to the anterior abdominal wall is common and is usually due to skin distention and development of striae rather than cholestasis.

Cholestatic itching correlates better with serum bile acid levels than with other biochemical "liver function tests" such as alkaline phosphatase, aspartate aminotransferase (AST, or SGOT), alanine aminotransferase (ALT, or SGPT), and bilirubin. The mechanism of biliary obstruction in pregnancy is discussed in Chapter 53. It has been stressed that some patients with skin lesions indicative of one of the other pregnancy rashes described in this chapter have coexisting cholestasis of pregnancy, so screening with liver function tests could be reasonable for patients with pregnancy rashes as well as for those experiencing pruritus without rash (Borradori and Saurat, 1994). It is also important to point out that pruritus can precede the findings of abnormal liver function tests or total serum bile acids, so that follow-up testing for obstetric cholestasis may be needed in itchy pregnant patients with initial normal findings (Kenyon et al., 2001).

Pruritus gravidarum appears to be associated with an increased chance of twin pregnancies (Roger et al., 1994). Pruritus usually disappears shortly after delivery but recurs in approximately 50% of subsequent pregnancies. An increased incidence of cholelithiasis has been observed in pregnant women with pruritus and recurrent cholestasis (Furhoff, 1974). Oral contraceptives could precipitate recurrent symptoms in this group. Reported increases in rates of premature delivery and perinatal mortality appear to be restricted to those in whom frank clinical jaundice develops (Friedlander and Osler, 1967). Slightly shortened gestational times, lower birth weights, and increased meconium staining occur in pregnancies without clinical jaundice; their clinical significance awaits further information.

Treatment is symptomatic, and mild cases usually respond to adequate skin lubrication and topical antipruritics (see the general treatment guidelines discussed previously). Oral antihistamines could be of some benefit. Ultraviolet light treatment or judicious sun exposure could also decrease pruritus. In more severe cases, phenobarbital or bile-sequestering agents such as cholestyramine, supplemented with fat-soluble vitamins, could be beneficial (Laatikainen, 1978), although there is no agreement about efficacy (Black et al., 2002). A review of published studies concluded that there is insufficient evidence to recommend guar gum, activated charcoal, S-adenosylmethionine, and ursodeoxycholic acid (Burrows et al, 2001). Other authorities are convinced that ursodeoxycholic acid reduces premature labor, fetal distress, and fetal deaths (Black et al., 2002).

Pruritic Urticarial Papules and Plaques of Pregnancy

Pruritic urticarial papules and plaques of pregnancy (PUPPP) (Lawley et al., 1979) is a poorly defined disorder characterized by erythematous papules, plaques, and urticarial lesions and usually begins in the third trimester. It is probably the most common pregnancy rash. The rash has also been named *polymorphic eruption of pregnancy (PEP)* by Holmes and Black in 1982 (Black et al., 2002), and this term is preferred in Europe. The term PUPPP is most popular in the United States. The eruption has also been called *toxemic rash of pregnancy* (Bourne, 1962) and *late-onset prurigo of pregnancy* (Nurse, 1968) in the past.

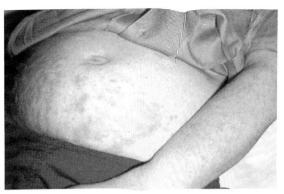

FIGURE 57-2 ■ Pruritic urticarial papules and plaques of pregnancy (PUPPP). Urticarial involvement of striae, with papular eruption on the arms. See Color Plate 21.

PUPPP is almost always pruritic, and itching is severe in 80% of patients. The lesions begin on the abdomen in 80%–90% of cases, often sparing the umbilicus (Fig. 57-1; see Color Plate 21). The striae become involved in 67% of cases, suggesting that abdominal distention may contribute to the inflammation occurring with this rash (Figs. 57-2 and 57-3; see Color Plate 21). In many cases, the eruption spreads to the proximal thighs, buttocks, and proximal arms. The face is nearly always spared. Sometimes erythema multiforme–like target lesions are present.

The rash usually resolves before or within several weeks after delivery. Some patients have had significant reductions in serum cortisol levels (Vaughn Jones et al., 1999). The disease is most prevalent in primigravidas. There appears to be an association with increased maternal weight gain, increased newborn birth weight, and an increased twin pregnancy rate of 10% of cases (Cohen et al., 1989). Unlike most of the other rashes of pregnancy, PUPPP does not tend to recur with subsequent pregnancies (Yancey et al., 1984). There is no increase in the fetal mortality rate.

Routine skin biopsies show nonspecific changes, including variable parakeratosis, spongiosis, acanthosis, dermal edema, and perivascular lymphocytes and eosinophils. Vesicles occur in a minority of cases and can cause confusion with pemphigoid gestationis, but the results of direct immunofluorescence (IF) of skin biopsy specimens are usually negative. A few cases have shown linear immunoglobulin M (IgM) at the dermal-epidermal junction (Vaughan Jones et al., 1996). Treatment depends on the severity of the condition, as mentioned previously for pregnancy rashes in general.

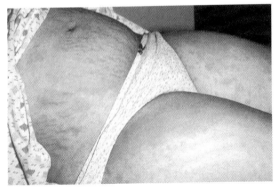

FIGURE 57-1 ■ Pruritic urticarial papules and plaques of pregnancy (PUPPP). Lesions commonly begin in the abdominal striae. Confluent erythematous urticarial papules and plaques are also present on the ˌˌs in this patient. See also Color Plate 21.

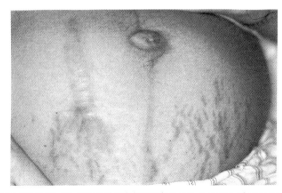

FIGURE 57-3 ■ Pruritic urticarial papules and plaques of pregnancy (PUPPP). The eruption often begins in itchy red striae. Note the linea nigra. See also Color Plate 21.

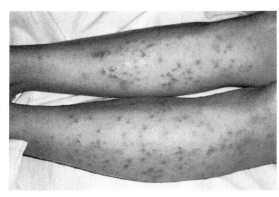

FIGURE 57-4 ■ Prurigo gestationis. The predominant lesions are excoriated papules. See also Color Plate 21.

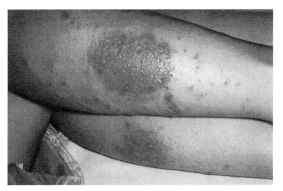

FIGURE 57-6 ■ Prurigo gestationis. Although papules are more common, occasional lesions can coalesce into crusty plaques. See also Color Plate 21.

Prurigo Gestationis

The pathogenesis of prurigo gestationis is unknown. The general term *prurigo* designates an intensely pruritic skin eruption in which excoriation predominates, suggesting a prominent emotional component. Many of these patients have a genetic predisposition toward atopic dermatitis, and many examples of this "disease" may in fact represent patients with eczema or dermatitis (Vaughan Jones et al., 1999). Prurigo gestationis was first described by Besnier in 1904 and is similar to the early prurigo of pregnancy later described by Nurse in 1968 (Vaughan Jones et al., 1999). The lesions consist of excoriated papules or nodules mostly over the extremities, usually beginning in the middle of pregnancy (Figs. 57-4 to 57-6; Color Plate 21). Elevated liver function test results have been reported in some cases, but this probably represents an overlap of patients with pruritus gravidarum. The eruption usually clears by 3 months after delivery, and the recurrence rate in subsequent pregnancies is low. Treatment depends on the severity of the condition, as discussed previously.

Papular dermatitis of pregnancy was separated out as a distinct entity by Spangler and coauthors (1962) on the basis of markedly elevated levels of 24-hour urinary human chorionic gonadotropin (hCG) for that stage of pregnancy and decreased levels of plasma and urinary estriol and plasma cortisol. In addition, the lesions were noted to be more widespread than lesions of the other pregnancy rashes. Whether these criteria are sufficient to determine a separate disease is questionable.

There have been few case reports, and some of the reported cases of papular dermatitis have been questionable because of the lack of appropriate laboratory studies to exclude the other pregnancy rashes discussed in this chapter. Vaughan Jones and coworkers (1999) concluded that papular dermatitis of Spangler is not a separate entity because they were unable to identify any patients with decreased estradiol in a large series of patients with pregnancy rashes.

Pemphigoid Gestationis

Pemphigoid gestationis is a rare, autoimmune, blistering dermatosis of pregnancy and the immediate postpartum period (Lin et al., 2001). It is not related to infection by herpesvirus; the (unfortunately) common synonym *herpes gestationis* refers to the grouped (herpetiform) nature of the blisters (which often are not really herpetiform at all) (Black et al., 2002). It is best to avoid the term *herpes gestationis* because of the risk of misleading patients and misinformed health care workers; not using the term avoids potentially inappropriate treatments for herpesvirus. The onset is usually during the second or third trimester, but cases beginning in the first trimester or the immediate postpartum period have been well documented. A high frequency of human leukocyte antigen (HLA) haplotypes B8 and DR3/DR4 has been reported (Shornick, 1993).

Lesions usually begin on the abdomen, often around the umbilicus (Fig. 57-7; Color Plate 22). Other commonly involved areas include the trunk, buttocks, and extremities. The face and mucous membranes are rarely affected. Vesicles and bullae are the most important clinical lesions (Figs. 57-8 and

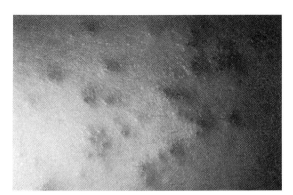

FIGURE 57-5 ■ Prurigo gestationis. Close-up view of excoriated papules (same patient as in Fig. 57-1). See also Color Plate 21.

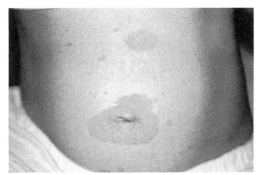

FIGURE 57-7 ■ Pemphigoid gestationis. Characteristic periumbilical urticarial plaque. Blisters may or may not be present. See also Color Plate 22.

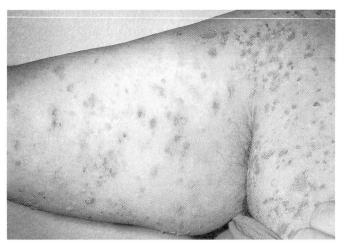

FIGURE 57-8 ■ Pemphigoid gestationis. Crusts and blisters on mother of child seen in Figure 57-10. See also Color Plate 22.

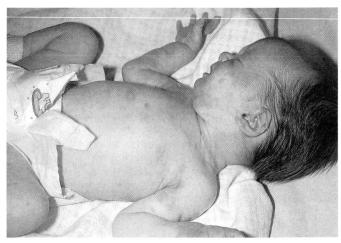

FIGURE 57-10 ■ Pemphigoid gestationis. Newborn child of mother seen in Figure 57-8. Urticarial erythematous patches with rare blisters. See also Color Plate 22.

57-9; Color Plate 22). Erythematous plaques, often annular or urticaria-like, frequently are present, and these could resemble PUPPP. The extent of the disease process and the degree of accompanying pruritus can be mild to severe.

A mortality rate in infants born to affected mothers has been estimated to be as high as 30%, although this figure has been disputed (Shornick and Black, 1992). Increased prematurity has also been reported (Mascaro et al., 1995). With systemic corticosteroid treatment of severe cases, fetal risk appears to be minimal. There is an increase in premature and small-for-gestational-age infants (Shornick and Black, 1992). Most infants do not have skin lesions, although transient urticarial and vesicular lesions thought to be due to transplacental antibody transfer have been noted in less than 5% of infants born of affected mothers (Figs. 57-10 and 57-11; Color Plate 22) (Katz et al., 1977).

Postpartum flares occur in 50%–75% of patients with pemphigoid gestationis. Exacerbation typically begins within 24–48 hours after delivery and can last for several weeks or several months. Skin lesions have been reported to persist for more than a year in women who do not breast-feed compared with those who do (average postpartum duration is 1–6 months) (Black and Stephens, 1992). Flares also can occur with subsequent menses, ovulation, or treatment with estrogen or progesterone. About 20%–50% of patients who have had pemphigoid gestationis experience recurrent skin lesions when treated with oral contraceptives.

Although not diagnostic, the routine histopathologic features are characteristic. Blistering lesions are usually subepidermal but sometimes are intraepidermal as a result of spongiosis. Focal necrosis of basal keratinocytes can occur. There are perivascular lymphocytes in the dermis with a significant number of eosinophils.

Immunopathologically, pemphigoid gestationis and bullous pemphigoid (an autoimmune disease most prevalent in the elderly) are strikingly similar. Heavy linear deposits of C3 are present in the epidermal basement membrane zone (BMZ) of pemphigoid gestationis perilesional skin (Fig. 57-12; Color Plate 22), usually in the absence of IgG deposits when direct IF staining methods are used. BMZ C3 deposits have also been described in some infants born to affected mothers with pemphigoid gestationis. By contrast, direct IF of bullous pemphigoid shows both C3 and IgG.

Unlike the case with bullous pemphigoid, however, circulating anti-BMZ IgG autoantibodies are measurable in the serum by indirect IF in only 10%–20% of cases of pemphigoid gestationis. When antibodies are present, titers are usually low,

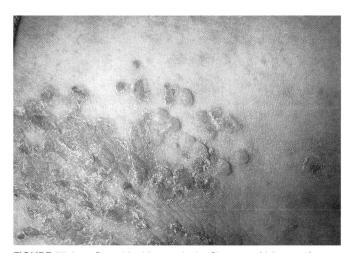

FIGURE 57-9 ■ Pemphigoid gestationis. Close-up of blisters of mother seen in Figure 57-8. See also Color Plate 22.

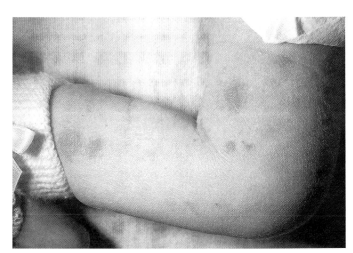

FIGURE 57-11 ■ Pemphigoid gestationis. Close-up of erythematous patches seen in Figure 57-10. See also Color Plate 22.

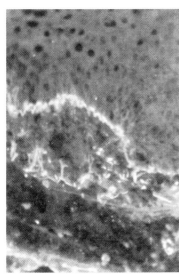

FIGURE 57-12 ■ Pemphigoid gestationis. This skin biopsy specimen, taken for direct immunofluorescence, demonstrates a linear band of C3 at the basement membrane zone. See also Color Plate 22.

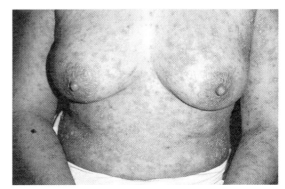

FIGURE 57-13 ■ Impetigo herpetiformis (pustular psoriasis). Extensive sterile pustules. See also Color Plate 23.

again in contrast to bullous pemphigoid. Circulating IgG1 autoantibodies (herpes gestationis factor, also called pemphigoid gestationis factor) avidly fix complement to the BMZ in pemphigoid gestationis. They are present in such low levels, however, that they often escape detection by routine methods. Bullous pemphigoid IgG subclasses are more heterogeneous, with IgG4 predominating over IgG1. Pemphigoid gestationis autoantibodies usually react with a 180-kD protein associated with hemidesmosomes of basal keratinocytes (Matsumura et al., 1996), whereas bullous pemphigoid autoantibodies potentially react with two protein bands, almost always with a 230-kD protein (BPAg1) and sometimes also with the same 180-kD protein that is the main target in pemphigoid gestationis (BPAg2, also called type XVII collagen). Only a small number of patients with pemphigoid gestationis have autoantibodies directed against the BPAg1.

There is an increased incidence of antithyroid antibodies, but clinically apparent thyroid dysfunction is rare (Shornick, 1993). Patients are at an increased risk for Graves' disease, but usually this does not occur simultaneously with pemphigoid gestationis.

Treatment of pemphigoid gestationis should not be designed to suppress the disease process entirely, because the higher doses of therapy needed to suppress disease activity completely could have more serious side effects. Instead, therapy should be directed toward suppressing the appearance of new lesions and relieving the intense pruritus. Potent topical corticosteroids can be attempted in mild to moderate cases. In moderate to severe cases, prednisone, 20–40 mg/day, is often adequate to suppress new blister formation and relieve symptoms. Once new blister formation has been suppressed, the prednisone dose can be tapered to lower doses or to just enough to maintain control and relieve symptoms. Eventually, alternate-day therapy may become more appropriate and should be attempted.

If the disease flares in the immediate postpartum period, treatment with prednisone, 20–40 mg/day, should be reinstituted. Higher doses may be instituted at this time if necessary. Infants of mothers treated with prednisone should be monitored for evidence of adrenal insufficiency. Minocycline and nicotinamide have been used anecdotally as an alternative to prednisone in pregnancy (Loo et al., 2001). Plasmapheresis is used for severe cases (Black et al, 2002). Dapsone is often used for other autoimmune blistering disorders but is contraindicated during pregnancy, as it can cause hemolytic disease of the newborn. Alternative therapies that may be useful in the postpartum period have been reviewed (Shornick, 1993). Other treatment modalities useful for all pregnancy rashes have been discussed previously.

Impetigo Herpetiformis

First described in 1872 by von Hebra, impetigo herpetiformis is a severe, generalized pustular dermatosis associated with pregnancy. The name is unfortunate because it is unrelated to either bacterial infection (impetigo) or herpesvirus infection. The onset of the disease usually is in the third trimester, but well-documented cases have occurred as early as the first trimester. The disease usually subsides between pregnancies but can recur with subsequent pregnancies (and usually earlier in a subsequent pregnancy). Hypoparathyroidism, hypocalcemia, hypophosphatemia, decreased vitamin D levels, elevated erythrocyte sedimentation rate, and leukocytosis can be present (Wolf et al., 1995). The etiology remains unknown, but it could be a reaction to drugs or occult infection in a genetically predisposed patient.

Clinically, the disease is characterized by hundreds of translucent, white, sterile pustules (Figs. 57-13 and 57-14; Color Plate 23) that arise on irregular erythematous bases or

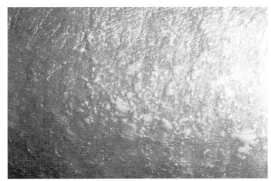

FIGURE 57-14 ■ Impetigo herpetiformis (pustular psoriasis). Close-up view of superficial pustules (just beneath the stratum corneum) with characteristic coalescence into "lakes of pus." See also Color Plate 23.

plaques. These lesions extend peripherally while central pustules rupture owing to their superficial locations, leaving denuded surfaces with crusts as occur in some forms of pemphigus. Common areas of involvement include the axillae, inframammary areas, umbilicus, groin, and gluteal crease. Pustular lesions can also occur on the hands and involve the nails with subsequent nail loss or onycholysis.

Constitutional symptoms are common and include fever, chills, nausea, vomiting, and diarrhea with severe dehydration. Delirium, tetany, and convulsions are rare complications usually associated with hypocalcemia. Death may occur, again in association with these complications and septicemia. Impetigo herpetiformis is now thought to be a form of generalized pustular psoriasis that occurs during pregnancy. The clinical presentation and histopathology of both disease entities are identical. The majority of the pregnant patients do not have a previous history of psoriasis.

Histopathologically, impetigo herpetiformis is characterized by subcorneal pustules containing neutrophils and degenerated keratinocytes. Cultures of pustular lesions are usually negative unless secondarily infected.

Systemic corticosteroid therapy is the treatment of choice for impetigo herpetiformis. Usually, 20–40 mg of prednisone per day is sufficient to control new lesion formation. Systemic antibiotics could help when secondary infection is present. Topical measures, such as wet compresses with or without topical corticosteroid preparations, are also useful as general treatment for itchy pregnancy rashes, as discussed previously. Intravenous fluids and electrolytes are important for patients with diarrhea, vomiting, high fever, and extensive skin pustulation. Cyclosporine has been used successfully in pregnancy for severe cases (Imai et al., 2002). Acitretin (a synthetic vitamin A derivative given orally) and methotrexate, both used commonly for generalized pustular psoriasis, are contraindicated during pregnancy.

Autoimmune Progesterone Dermatitis

This autoimmune dermatosis is a rare, poorly defined, urticarial, papular, vesicular, or pustular eruption thought to be caused by hypersensitivity to progesterone, usually appearing as a recurrent cyclic eruption during the luteal phase of the menstrual cycle (Herzberg et al., 1995; Moody and Schatten, 1997). Less than 50 cases have been reported. Only five cases involved onset or worsening of this condition with pregnancy. Two of these cases were associated with spontaneous abortion. In other cases of autoimmune progesterone dermatitis, the rash improved or cleared during pregnancy. *Estrogen dermatitis* has been described in seven patients, all of whom had severe premenstrual exacerbations of a variety of skin eruptions (Shelley et al., 1995). Skin test results were positive for estrogen in all seven cases.

Autoimmune progesterone dermatitis has been documented by the use of intradermal or intramuscular test injections of progesterone (for methods, see Black et al., 2002). Intradermal tests generally produce an immediate local urticarial reaction or a delayed reaction. Intramuscular challenges have caused exacerbations of the rash or even angioedema. Progesterone antibodies have been demonstrated in four cases by indirect IF. An indirect basophil degranulation test has also been used, in which the patient's serum is mixed with synthetic progesterone and rabbit

basophils. Specific therapy for this condition during pregnancy has not been reported. Nonpregnant patients have responded to estrogens (if the allergen was progesterone), the antiestrogen tamoxifen, the anabolic androgen danazol, or oophorectomy (Vasconcelos et al., 2000). Spontaneous remission can occur after successful treatment (Black et al., 2002).

SKIN DISORDERS AFFECTED BY PREGNANCY

The effect of pregnancy on preexisting skin diseases often varies. Table 57-2 lists some skin diseases that improve or become aggravated by pregnancy, although the course of a disease in a given patient is not always predictable. Cutaneous infections are covered in Chapter 39, whereas connective tissue diseases involving the skin are discussed in Chapter 54. Some infectious, autoimmune, or rheumatic diseases tend to worsen during pregnancy.

Acne Vulgaris

Acne is a disease of the pilosebaceous unit. It is partially influenced by androgens such as testosterone and dehydroepiandrosterone sulfate (DHEA-S), which increase sebaceous gland activity. Estrogen reduces sebaceous gland size and activity, but this is probably a function of negative feedback on androgen production by the ovary. Sebaceous gland activity is actually increased during pregnancy. Montgomery tubercles are small sebaceous glands on the areolae of the breasts, and their papular enlargement is one of the first signs of pregnancy.

TABLE 57-2. EFFECT OF PREGNANCY ON SKIN DISEASES

Improved by Pregnancy (Usually)

Fox-Fordyce disease
Hidradenitis suppurativa

Aggravated by Pregnancy (Usually)

Condylomata acuminata (Lynch, 1985)
Ehlers-Danlos syndrome (Winton, 1989)
Erythema multiforme
Erythema nodosum (Buckshee and Chadha, 1996)
Herpes simplex (Winton, 1989)
Lupus erythematosus
Neurofibromatosis (Swapp and Main, 1973)
Pemphigus (Winton, 1989)
Pityriasis rosea
Porphyrias (Winton, 1989)
Pseudoxanthoma elasticum (Winton, 1989)
Scleroderma (increased renal disease)
Tuberous sclerosis (increased seizures)

Unpredictable Response to Pregnancy

Acne
Acquired immunodeficiency syndrome (Winton, 1989)
Atopic dermatitis (Kemmett and Tidman, 1991)
Dermatomyositis
Malignant melanoma (Winton, 1989)
Psoriasis (Boyd et al., 1996)

Acne consists of erythematous papules, pustules, comedones, and cysts on the face, back, and chest. Some cases reported as "pruritic folliculitis of pregnancy" of widespread locations may actually represent hormonally induced acne (Black, 1989). Pregnancy has a variable effect on acne, probably because many other factors are involved in its pathogenesis besides the hormonal influences discussed.

Acne can be controlled during pregnancy or lactation with topical benzoyl peroxide (Category C), salicylic acid, azalaic acid (Azelex, Category B) or topical antibiotics such as erythromycin (Category B) or clindamycin (Cleocin T, Category B). Topical and oral sulfonamides should be avoided near term. Forms of topical metronidazole (MetroLotion, MetroGel, MetroCream, Noritate cream, all Category B) usually are used if other alternatives have failed. More severe disease can be treated with the apparent oral antibiotic of choice, erythromycin, starting with 1 g daily (FDA Pregnancy Category B), even though its efficacy has been dwindling because of the increasing resistance of bacterial flora. It appears to be safe during lactation as well. Erythromycin estolate has been implicated as a cause of hepatotoxicity in pregnancy after prolonged use, so it should be avoided. Tetracycline should be avoided because of its potential risk of fatty liver of pregnancy and adverse effects on fetal dentition. Vitamin A derivatives (retinoids) such as oral isotretinoin are contraindicated because of teratogenic effects. Topical retinoids such as tretinoin (Retin-A, Avita, Category C) or topical adapalene (Differin, Category C) are not contraindicated, but different topical drugs are probably better during pregnancy. Topical tazarotene is in Category X, but healthy babies have been born to six women.

Atopic Dermatitis

Atopic dermatitis is an allergic skin disease characterized by intensely pruritic eczematous lesions that become lichenified when patients are caught in a scratch-itch cycle. There appears to be an inherited irritability of the skin (the "itch that rashes" instead of the rash that itches), and many patients have a personal or family history of eczema, asthma, hay fever, food allergies, or allergic rhinitis beginning in childhood. This disease can worsen (52%) or improve (24%) during pregnancy (Kemmett and Tidman, 1991). Some studies show that breastfeeding reduces the incidence of atopy in infants because cow's milk has been implicated as a significant aggravating factor. Soya milk is often substituted, but it also can be allergenic (Kramer, 2000). The mother's diet has not been shown to make a significant difference during pregnancy and breastfeeding (Herrmann et al., 1996). An increased incidence of atopy in children has also been associated with a wide variety of confusing factors in various studies, such as increased fetal growth and a larger head circumference (Leadbitter et al., 1999), increased gestational age (Olesen et al., 1997), low parity, febrile infections in pregnancy, the use of contraceptives before pregnancy (Xu et al., 1999), and maternal smoking (Schafer et al., 1997).

Treatment with topical emollients, topical corticosteroids, and oral antihistamines is usually effective. If the skin is extremely dry and scaly, greasy ointments could be more effective than creams. Patients should be instructed to use soap sparingly and should always apply topical emollient lotions or creams after bathing. The newer immunomodulators, topical pimecrolimus (Elidel cream) and tacrolimus (Protopic ointment) are Pregnancy Category C. Exceptional patients may require systemic corticosteroids.

Erythema Nodosum

Erythema nodosum is characterized by tender nodules on the anterior lower legs, usually considered to be a reaction to a drug or an infection somewhere else, such as streptococcal pharyngitis or coccidioidomycosis (Arsura et al., 1998). Sarcoidosis and inflammatory bowel disease are also frequent causes (Brodell and Mehrabi, 2000). Women account for 90% of patients. Erythema nodosum is known to be precipitated by pregnancy as well as by oral contraceptives (Coaccioli et al., 1998), which suggests an estrogen influence on this disease (Buckshee and Chadha, 1996). Treatment begins with specific therapy for the underlying inciting cause. Nonsteroidal anti-inflammatory agents other than acetaminophen are usually not recommended because they can constrict the ductus arteriosus or cause prolonged labor because of prostaglandin synthesis inhibition. Systemic corticosteroids may be used in more severe noninfectious cases.

Fox-Fordyce Disease

Fox-Fordyce disease is a rare entity, often called *apocrine miliaria* because it can be thought of as being similar to the "prickly heat" or "heat rash" involving eccrine glands. Fox-Fordyce disease occurs mainly in women, with onset usually shortly after puberty (Ghislain et al., 2002). Multiple pruritic, dome-shaped, follicular papules develop in the axillae and anogenital region, areas rich in apocrine glands. The disease usually improves during pregnancy or with oral contraceptive therapy, probably because of an estrogen effect. Apocrine activity, unlike eccrine activity, appears to be decreased during pregnancy (Elling and Powell, 1997). Response to topical corticosteroids varies.

Genodermatoses

A long list of inherited severe cutaneous diseases involving the mother or other family members can affect fetal mortality or morbidity. New techniques that make it possible to study the molecular, enzymatic, and ultrastructural basis of these conditions are continually evolving. It is impossible to provide up-to-date information on this rapidly changing field in a textbook. More details of prenatal diagnosis are given in Chapter 18.

Modalities useful for detecting severe fetal skin diseases include chorionic villus sampling, amniocentesis (Akiyama and Holbrook, 1994), and fetal skin biopsy (Elias et al., 1994). Although *ichthyosis* and *epidermolysis bullosa* are the two most important groups of disorders, prenatal diagnosis has been successful in many other skin diseases (Holbrook et al., 1993).

There are many types of ichthyosis, all of which cause extensively thickened, scaly skin resembling the scales of a fish. A variety of ichthyotic syndromes have been described that involve other abnormalities besides the skin. Ichthyosiform erythroderma is subdivided into dominant and recessive forms, and generalized involvement is usually present at birth. The collodion and harlequin fetuses are severe examples of ichthyosis in which an infant with grotesque deformities, often resulting in death, is born encased in a horny sheet.

Genetic defects have been discovered in many forms of ichthyosis (Bichakjian et al., 1998; Di Mario et al., 1998; Bitoun et al., 2002).

The multiple forms of epidermolysis bullosa are characterized by extensive blistering that can contribute to excessive fluid loss or predispose to scarring, deformities, and fatal neonatal infection. Genetic defects have been identified in many types of heritable blistering disorders (Uitto and Pulkkinen, 2001). One can distinguish the dystrophic and letalis forms of the disease from the less severe simplex form by using electron microscopy or immunofluorescent staining of BMZ antigens to determine the level of blistering in the skin (Shimizu et al., 1998).

Psoriasis

Psoriasis is a papulosquamous skin condition found in 1%–3% of the population. It is usually mild but sometimes can become severe, generalized, or associated with psoriatic arthritis. The pustular form of psoriasis was discussed in the section on impetigo herpetiformis. In one study, psoriasis remained unchanged during pregnancy in 43% of patients, improved in 41%, and worsened in 14%. In the postpartum period, it remained unchanged in 37%, improved in 11%, and worsened in 49% (Dunna and Finlay, 1989). Psoriasis in pregnancy is commonly treated with topical corticosteroids (mostly Category C agents). Low-potency hydrocortisone is used commonly on delicate skin areas such as the face and intertriginous areas, while medium-potency triamcinolone is used on most other areas. The topical vitamin D derivative calcipotriene (Dovonex, Category C) has not been evaluated during pregnancy or lactation, and use of large quantities can result in hypercalcemia. The topical retinoid tazarotene is a Category X agent. For severe disease, oral cyclosporine (category C) has been used without an apparent increase in problems. Ultraviolet B light therapy is safe in pregnancy. Oral psoralen combined with ultraviolet A light (PUVA) has a Category C designation. The oral retinoid acitretin and the antimetabolite methotrexate are both Category X agents and should not be used.

REFERENCES

Akiyama M, Holbrook KA: Analysis of skin-derived amniotic fluid cells in the second trimester: Detection of severe genodermatoses expressed in the fetal period. J Invest Dermatol **103**:674, 1994.

Al-Fares SI, Jones SV, Black MM: The specific dermatoses of pregnancy: A re-appraisal (review). J Eur Acad Dermatol Venereol **15**:197, 2001.

Altmeyer P, Bernd A, Holzmann H, et al: Alpha-MSH and pregnancy. Z Hautkr **64**:577, 1989.

Ances JG, Pomerantz SH: Serum concentrations of beta-MSH in human pregnancy. Am J Obstet Gynecol **119**:1062, 1974.

Arsura EL, Kilgore WB, Ratnayake SN: Erythema nodosum in pregnant patients with coccidioidomycosis. Clin Infect Dis **27**:1201, 1998.

Bichakjian CK, Nair RP, Wu WW, et al: Prenatal exclusion of lamellar ichthyosis based on identification of two new mutations in the transglutaminase 1 gene. J Invest Dermatol **110**:179, 1998.

Bitoun E, Bodemer C, Amiel J, et al: Prenatal diagnosis of a lethal form of Netherton syndrome by SPINK5 mutation analysis. Prenat Diagn **22**:121, 2002.

Black MM: Prurigo of pregnancy, papular dermatitis of pregnancy, and pruritic folliculitis of pregnancy. Semin Dermatol **8**:23, 1989.

Black MM, McKay M, Braude PR, et al: Obstetric and Gynecologic Dermatology, 2nd ed. London, Mosby, 2002.

Black MM, Stephens CJM: The specific dermatoses of pregnancy: The British perspective. Adv Dermatol **7**:105, 1992.

Borradori L, Saurat J-H: Specific dermatoses of pregnancy: Toward a comprehensive view. Arch Dermatol **130**:778, 1994.

Bourne G: Toxaemic rash of pregnancy. J R Soc Med **55**:462, 1962.

Boyd AS, Morris LF, Phillips CM, et al: Psoriasis and pregnancy: Hormone and immune system interaction. Int J Dermatol **35**:169, 1996.

Brodell RT, Mehrabi D: Underlying causes of erythema nodosum. Lesions may provide clue to systemic disease. Postgrad Med **108**:147, 2000.

Buckshee K, Chadha S: Post tonsillitic erythema nodosum in pregnancy. Int J Gynaecol Obstet **55**:293, 1996.

Burrows RF, Clavisi O, Burrows E: Interventions for treating cholestasis in pregnancy. Cochrane Database System Review **4**:CD000493, 2001.

Coaccioli S, Donati D, Di Cato L, et al: Onset of erythema nodosum during pregnancy: A case report. Clin Exp Obstet Gynecol **25**:50, 1998.

Cohen LM, Capeless EL, Krusinski PA, et al: Pruritic urticarial papules and plaques of pregnancy and its relationship to maternal-fetal weight gain and twin pregnancy. Arch Dermatol **125**:1534, 1989.

Di Mario M, Ferrari A, Morales V, et al: Antenatal molecular diagnosis of X-linked ichthyosis by maternal serum screening for Down's syndrome. Gynecol Obstet Invest **45**:277, 1998.

Dunna SF, Finlay AY: Psoriasis: improvement during and worsening after pregnancy. Br J Dermatol **120**:584, 1989.

Elias S, Emerson DS, Simpson JL, et al: Ultrasound-guided fetal skin sampling for prenatal diagnosis of genodermatoses. Obstet Gynecol **83**:337, 1994.

Elling SV, Powell FC: Physiologic changes in the skin during pregnancy. Clin Dermatol **15**:35, 1997.

Friedlander P, Osler M: Icterus and pregnancy. Am J Obstet Gynecol **97**:894, 1967.

Furhoff AK: Itching in pregnancy. Acta Med Scand **196**:403, 1974.

Garcia A, Fulton JE: The combination of glycolic acid and hydroquinone or kojic acid for the treatment of melasma and related conditions. Dermatol Surg **22**:443, 1996.

Ghislain PD, van Der Endt JD, Delescluse J: Itchy papules of the axillae. Arch Dermatol **138**:259, 2002.

Gormley DE: Cutaneous surgery and the pregnant patient. J Am Acad Dermatol **23**:269, 1990.

Grimes PE: Melasma: Etiologic and therapeutic considerations. Arch Dermatol **131**:1453, 1995.

Hale EK, Pomeranz MK: Dermatologic agents during pregnancy and lactation: An update and clinical review. Int J Dermatol **41**:197, 2002.

Harahap M, Wallach RC: Skin Changes and Diseases in Pregnancy. New York, Marcel Dekker, 1995.

Herrmann M-E, Dannemann A, Gruters A, et al: Prospective study on the atopy preventive effect of maternal avoidance of milk and eggs during pregnancy and lactation. Eur J Pediatr **155**:770, 1996.

Herzberg AJ, Strohmeyer CR, Cirillo-Hyland VA: Autoimmune progesterone dermatitis. J Am Acad Dermatol **32**:335, 1995.

Holbrook KA, Smith LT, Elias S: Prenatal diagnosis of genetic skin disease using fetal skin biopsy samples. Arch Dermatol **129**:1437, 1993.

Im S, Kim J, On WY, et al: Increased expression of alpha-melanocyte-stimulating hormone in the lesional skin of melasma. Br J Dermatol **146**:165, 2002.

Imai N, Watanabe R, Fujiwara H, et al: Successful treatment of impetigo herpetiformis with oral cyclosporine during pregnancy. Arch Dermatol **138**:128, 2002.

Katz A, Minta JO, Toole JWP, et al: Immunopathologic study of herpes gestationis in mother and infant. Arch Dermatol **113**:1069, 1977.

Katz VL, Farmer RM, Dotters D: Focus on primary care: from nevus to neoplasm: Myths of melanoma in pregnancy. Obstet Gynecol Survey **57**:112, 2002.

Kemmett D, Tidman MJ: The influence of the menstrual cycle and pregnancy on atopic dermatitis. Br J Dermatol **125**:59, 1991.

Kenyon AP, Piercy CN, Girling J, et al: Pruritus may precede abnormal liver function tests in pregnant women with obstetric cholestasis: A longitudinal analysis. BJOG **108**:1190, 2001.

Kimbrough-Green CK, Griffiths CEM, Finkel LJ, et al: Topical retinoic acid (tretinoin) for melasma in black patients. Arch Dermatol **130**:727, 1994.

Kramer MS: Maternal antigen avoidance during lactation for preventing atopic eczema in infants. Cochrane Database System Review **2**:CD000131, 2000.

Laatikainen M: Effect of cholestyramine and phenobarbital on pruritus and serum bile acid levels in cholestasis of pregnancy. Am J Obstet Gynecol **132**:501, 1978.

Lawley TJ, Hertz KC, Wade TR, et al: Pruritic urticarial papules and plaques of pregnancy. JAMA **241**:1696, 1979.

Lawrence N, Cox SE, Brody HJ: Treatment of melasma with Jessner's solution versus glycolic acid. J Am Acad Dermatol **36**:589, 1997.

PLATE 21

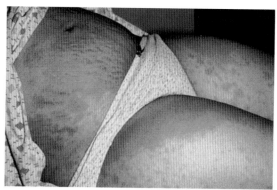

FIGURE 57-1 ■ Pruritic urticarial papules and plaques of pregnancy (PUPPP). Lesions commonly begin in the abdominal striae. Confluent erythematous urticarial papules and plaques are also present on the thighs in this patient.

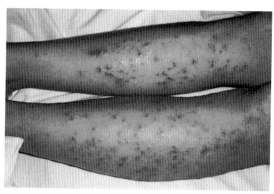

FIGURE 57-4 ■ Prurigo gestationis. The predominant lesions are excoriated papules.

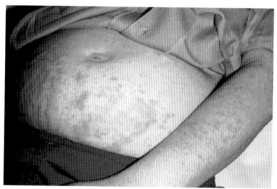

FIGURE 57-2 ■ Pruritic urticarial papules and plaques of pregnancy (PUPPP). Urticarial involvement of striae, with papular eruption on the arms.

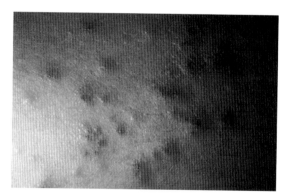

FIGURE 57-5 ■ Prurigo gestationis. Close-up view of excoriated papules (same patient as in Fig. 57-1).

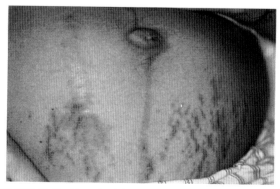

FIGURE 57-3 ■ Pruritic urticarial papules and plaques of pregnancy (PUPPP). The eruption often begins in itchy red striae. Note the linea nigra.

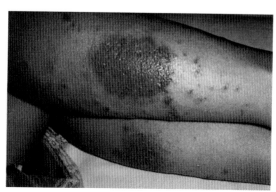

FIGURE 57-6 ■ Prurigo gestationis. Although papules are more common, occasional lesions can coalesce into crusty plaques.

PLATE 22

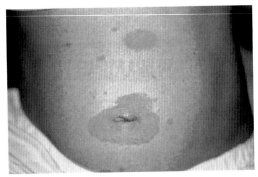

FIGURE 57-7 ■ Pemphigoid gestationis. Characteristic periumbilical urticarial plaque. Blisters may or may not be present.

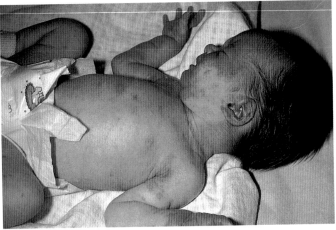

FIGURE 57-10 ■ Pemphigoid gestationis. Newborn child of mother seen in Figure 57-8. Urticarial erythematous patches with rare blisters.

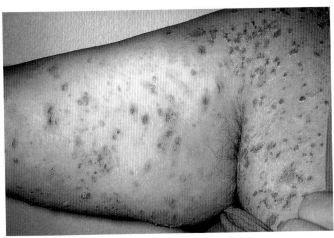

FIGURE 57-8 ■ Pemphigoid gestationis. Crusts and blisters on mother of child seen in Figure 57-10.

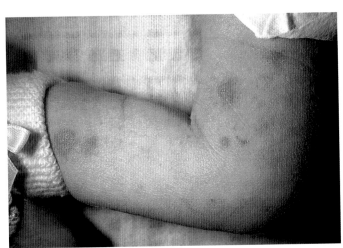

FIGURE 57-11 ■ Pemphigoid gestationis. Close-up of erythematous patches seen in Figure 57-10.

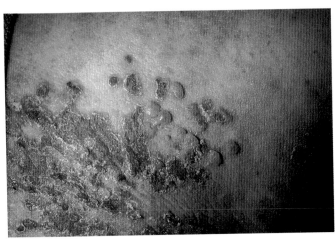

FIGURE 57-9 ■ Pemphigoid gestationis. Close-up of blisters of mother seen in Figure 57-8.

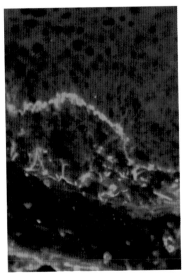

FIGURE 57-12 ■ Pemphigoid gestationis. This skin biopsy specimen, taken for direct immunofluorescence, demonstrates a linear band of C3 at the basement membrane zone.

PLATE 23

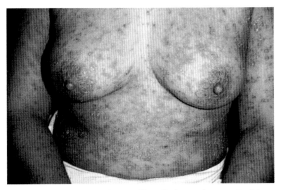

FIGURE 57-13 ■ Impetigo herpetiformis (pustular psoriasis). Extensive sterile pustules.

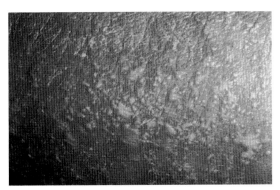

FIGURE 57-14 ■ Impetigo herpetiformis (pustular psoriasis). Close-up view of superficial pustules (just beneath the stratum corneum) with characteristic coalescence into "lakes of pus."

Leadbitter P, Pearce N, Cheng S, et al: Relationship between fetal growth and the development of asthma and atopy in childhood. Thorax 54:905, 1999.

Lin MS, Arteaga LA, Diaz LA: Herpes gestationis (review). Clin Dermatol 19:697, 2001.

Loo WJ, Dean D, Wojnarowska F: A severe persistent case of pemphigoid gestationis successfully treated with minocycline and nicotinamide. Clin Exp Dermatol 26:726, 2001.

Lutfi RJ, Fridmanis M, Misiunas AL, et al: Association of melasma with thyroid autoimmunity and other thyroidal abnormalities and their relationship to the origin of melasma. J Clin Endocrinol Metab 61:28, 1985.

Lynch PJ: Condyloma acuminata (anogenital warts). Clin Obstet Gynecol 28:142, 1985.

Madlon-Kay DJ: Striae gravidarum: Folklore and fact. Arch Fam Med 2:507, 1993.

Maeda K, Naganuma M, Fukuda M, et al: Effect of pituitary and ovarian hormones on human melanocytes in vitro. Pigment Cell Res 9:204, 1996.

Mascaro JM Jr, Lecha M, Mascaro JM: Fetal morbidity in herpes gestationis. Arch Dermatol 131:1209, 1995.

Matsumura K, Amagai M, Nishikawa T, et al: The majority of bullous pemphigoid and herpes gestationis serum samples react with the NC16a domain of the 180-kDa bullous pemphigoid antigen. Arch Dermatol Res 288:507, 1996.

Moody BR, Schatten S: Autoimmune progesterone dermatitis. South Med J 90:845, 1997.

Mooney MA, Janniger CK: Pyogenic granuloma. Cutis 55:133, 1995.

Morris LF, Rapini RP, Hebert AA, et al: Massive labial edema in pregnancy. South Med J 83:846, 1990.

Nurse DS: Prurigo of pregnancy. Australas J Dermatol 9:258, 1968.

Olesen AB, Ellingsen AR, Olesen H, et al: Atopic dermatitis and birth factors: Historical follow up by record linkage. BMJ 314:1003, 1997.

Pribanich S, Simpson FG, Held B, et al: Low-dose tretinoin does not improve striae distensae: A double-blind, placebo controlled study. Cutis 54:121, 1994.

Randall VA: Androgens and human hair growth. Clin Endocrinol 40:439, 1994.

Rangel O, Arias I, Garcia E, et al: Topical tretinoin 0.1% for pregnancy-related abdominal striae: An open-label, multicenter, prospective study. Adv Ther 18:181, 2001.

Roger D, Vaillant L, Fignon A, et al: Specific pruritic diseases of pregnancy: A prospective study of 3192 pregnant women. Arch Dermatol 130:734, 1994.

Schafer T, Dirschedl P, Kunz B, et al: Maternal smoking during pregnancy and lactation increases the risk for atopic eczema in the offspring. J Am Acad Dermatol 36:550, 1997.

Schiff BL, Kern AB: A study of postpartum alopecia. Arch Dermatol 87:609, 1963.

Shelley WB, Shelley ED, Talanin NY, et al: Estrogen dermatitis. J Am Acad Dermatol 32:25, 1995.

Shimizu H, Horiguchi Y, Suzumori K, et al: Successful prenatal exclusion of an unspecified subtype of severe epidermolysis bullosa. Int J Dermatol 37:364, 1998.

Shornick JK: Herpes gestationis. Dermatol Clin 11:527, 1993.

Shornick JK, Black MM: Fetal risks in herpes gestationis. J Am Acad Dermatol 26:63, 1992.

Sills ES, Zegarelli DJ, Hoschander MM, et al: Clinical diagnosis and management of hormonally responsive oral pregnancy tumor (pyogenic granuloma). J Reprod Med 41:467, 1996.

Spangler AS, Reddy W, Bardawil WA, et al: Papular dermatitis of pregnancy: A new clinical entity? JAMA 181:577, 1962.

Swapp GH, Main RA: Neurofibromatosis in pregnancy. Br J Dermatol 88:431, 1973.

Taylor CR, Anderson RR: Ineffective treatment of refractory melasma and postinflammatory hyperpigmentation by Q-switched ruby laser. J Dermatol Surg Oncol 20:592, 1994.

Uitto J, Pulkkinen L: Molecular genetics of heritable blistering disorders (review). Arch Dermatol 137:1458, 2001.

Vasconcelos C, Xavier P, Vieira AP, et al: Autoimmune progesterone urticaria. Gynecol Endocrinol 14:245, 2000.

Vaughan Jones SA, Dunnill MGS, Black MM: Pruritic urticarial papules and plaques of pregnancy (polymorphic eruption of pregnancy): Two unusual cases. Br J Dermatol 135:102, 1996.

Vaughan Jones SA, Hern S, Nelson-Piercy C, et al: A prospective study of 200 women with dermatoses of pregnancy correlating clinical findings with hormonal and immunopathological profiles. Br J Dermatol 141:71, 1999.

Winton GB: Skin diseases aggravated by pregnancy. J Am Acad Dermatol 20:1, 1989.

Wolf Y, Groutz A, Walman I, et al: Impetigo herpetiformis during pregnancy: Case report and review of the literature. Acta Obstet Gynecol Scand 74:229, 1995.

Wong RC, Ellis CN: Physiologic skin changes in pregnancy. Semin Dermatol 8:7, 1989.

Xu B, Jarvelin MR, Pekkanen J: Prenatal factors and occurrence of rhinitis and eczema among offspring. Eur J Allergy Clin Immunol 54:829, 1999.

Yancey KB, Hall RP, Lawley TJ: Pruritic urticarial papules and plaques of pregnancy: Clinical experience in twenty-five patients. J Am Acad Dermatol 10:473, 1984.

Zoberman E, Farmer ER: Pruritic folliculitis of pregnancy. Arch Dermatol 117:20, 1981.

Chapter 58

PELVIC MALIGNANCIES, GESTATIONAL TROPHOBLASTIC NEOPLASIA, AND NONPELVIC MALIGNANCIES

Michael L. Berman, MD, Philip J. Di Saia, MD, and Krishnansu S. Tewari, MD

The frequency of cancer in association with pregnancy is only approximately 1 per 1000 live births; nevertheless, it is difficult to imagine a set of circumstances more stressful for a patient and her physician than the discovery of a malignancy in a pregnant woman. As summarized in Table 58-1, several questions come to mind, including the following:

- Is it necessary to terminate the pregnancy while the fetus is immature?
- Can the tumor metastasize to the fetus?
- Will treatment of the malignancy adversely affect the conceptus?
- Can definitive therapy be deferred safely until the fetus is viable?
- Does pregnancy adversely affect prognosis for the pregnant patient?

Because coexistence of pregnancy with malignant disease is a relatively rare occurrence, and since pregnancy typically occurs at an earlier age than that associated with most cancer diagnoses, clear therapeutic decisions may not be readily at hand when the diagnosis is made. On the other hand, the increasing trend among many women to delay childbearing to the latter portion of the reproductive years will undoubtedly result in an increased frequency of a cancer diagnosis in older parturients.

In 1963, Barber and Brunschwig reviewed 700 cases of cancer in pregnancy (Di Saia and Creasman, 1981). The most common malignancies, in order of frequency, were breast cancer, leukemia and lymphomas as a group, melanoma, gynecologic cancers, and bone tumors. (Leukemia and lymphoma are discussed in Chapter 47.) The relative frequencies of cancers in pregnancy by site appear not to have changed over the past three decades.

In theory, the hormonal, metabolic, hemodynamic, and immunologic changes that occur during pregnancy impose many possible adverse effects in these women. These theoretical concerns are greatest for tumors arising in tissues and organs that are under hormonal control or that respond to hormonal stimulation. Increased vascularity in the breasts and pelvic organs, enhanced lymphatic drainage of many organs, and the state of immunologic tolerance that characterizes pregnancy may contribute to early dissemination of the malignant process. This indirect and hypothetical reasoning, in most instances, has not been substantiated and often has led to erroneous conclusions resulting in a recommendation for therapeutic abortion. Although these hypotheses are intellectually stimulating, much of the material that follows suggests that the validity of such conclusions usually lacks solid supporting clinical data.

PELVIC MALIGNANCIES IN PREGNANCY

Cervical Cancer

Cervical cancer is the most frequently diagnosed invasive neoplasm in pregnancy, occurring in approximately 1 per 2000 to 2500 pregnancies (Shivvers and Miller, 1997). It constitutes approximately 25% of all malignancies in pregnant women. Nearly 3% of all cervical cancers are found during pregnancy, emphasizing the need for careful evaluation of all pregnant women for cervical cancer and its precursor lesions (Hacker et al., 1982).

As part of every first prenatal visit, the physician should obtain a Papanicolaou smear from both the cervix and the endocervical canal. Occult malignancies in the endocervix often are not detected if this area is not evaluated with either a cotton-tipped applicator or an endocervical aspirator. A wire brush sampling device should be avoided in pregnancy because of the small risk of rupturing the fetal membranes. Although the Papanicolaou smear is a sensitive screening tool, one should not rely on it to rule out invasive disease in the presence of a suspected cervical lesion, because up to 30% of invasive cancers can be associated with negative cytologic findings. Thus, office punch biopsy of suspected lesions should be done even in the presence of a normal Papanicolaou smear. The moderate bleeding that ensues can be controlled adequately with Monsel's solution and silver nitrate.

Although cervical cancer is an uncommon cause of bleeding in pregnancy, a high index of suspicion can avoid unnecessary delays in the diagnosis of the occasional case. Thus, a careful speculum examination of the lower genital tract to rule out the existence of a friable exophytic lesion is essential to evaluate this complaint. Other nonobstetric causes of bleeding, such as a cervical polyp or a vaginal laceration, can also be excluded in this manner.

TABLE 58-1. CANCER IN PREGNANCY: ISSUES TO CONSIDER

Oncologic

Timing of therapy
Type of therapy
Maternal effects of therapy
Maternal surveillance

Obstetric

Fetal effects of therapy
Antepartum fetal surveillance
Corticosteroid use
Amniocentesis
Timing of delivery
Route of delivery

Ethical, Religious, Medicolegal, and Socioeconomic

Pregnancy termination
Advocate for fetus
Fetal viability
Maternal risk
Health care costs
Right to autonomy
Mother's overall prognosis (length of time mother will live to spend with the baby)

The methods used for diagnosis and treatment of cervical cancer and its precursors in either pregnant or postpartum patients are the same as those used in nonpregnant patients. Although the Papanicolaou smear is helpful in detecting preclinical disease in the cervix, its accuracy in invasive disease can be compromised by the presence of blood and a marked inflammatory reaction that may obscure the underlying diagnosis. The major diagnostic difficulty lies in the hesitancy of some physicians to take a biopsy specimen of the cervix of a pregnant patient. Such specimens are unquestionably necessary, and in the absence of a visible lesion, the process should be carried out with colposcopic visualization.

The general philosophy for diagnosis and treatment of intraepithelial neoplasia of the cervix detected during pregnancy is one of expectant therapy after careful analysis. The pregnant patient who has an abnormal Papanicolaou smear should undergo colposcopically directed biopsy of "suspicious" areas to rule out invasive disease. Depending on the experience of the colposcopist, areas of abnormality that are clearly not invasive, such as those with minimal white epithelium but no underlying vascular changes, may be observed without biopsy until the postpartum period.

Colposcopic Evaluation of the Pregnant Cervix

Because the glandular epithelium is usually visible on the ectocervix, the pregnant cervix lends itself to colposcopic visualization. When needing to evaluate a patient with an abnormal Papanicolaou smear, it is imperative that the colposcopist be familiar with the physiologic changes of the pregnant cervix, since they may lead to an overestimation of the severity of any given cervical lesion. In pregnancy, the cervix often undergoes softening and cyanosis, and through hypertrophy of the fibromuscular stroma, there is an increase in cervical volume. Endocervical gland hyperplasia increases the number of glands, and the transformation zone typically undergoes eversion. The physiologic metaplasia of pregnancy may be mistaken for acetowhite changes, punctation, or mosaicism. Finally, a decidual reaction coupled with increased vascularity may result in polypoid projections that may suggest cancer. All of these physiologic changes are benign and can be recognized by an experienced colposcopist, who at the same time must not overlook premalignant and malignant lesions (Baldauf et al., 1995).

Patients with intraepithelial neoplasia of the cervix may deliver vaginally, with subsequent reassessment performed postpartum. Interestingly, many of these patients do not demonstrate persistent intraepithelial neoplasia when they are reevaluated 6 weeks after delivery. Although an explanation for these changes is obscure, they probably result from either spontaneous regression or traumatic loss of the epithelium during the birth process.

Conization of the Pregnant Cervix

When invasion is suspected on the basis of clinical or cytologic assessment, a carefully directed incisional biopsy of sufficient depth to permit an accurate diagnosis should be carried out. A diagnosis of microinvasion on biopsy must be followed as soon as possible by a cone biopsy to rule out frankly invasive disease (Table 58-2). This is the only absolute indication for conization during pregnancy. Conization results distinguish patients with microinvasion (whose pregnancy can proceed to term without appreciable maternal risk) from those with frank invasion (in whom consideration must be given to early interruption of the pregnancy).

"Microinvasion," or "early stromal invasion," of the cervix is an invasive cancer that, as defined by the Society of Gynecologic Oncologists (Creasman, 1995), (1) does not penetrate the stroma more than 3 mm below the basement membrane of

TABLE 58-2. RECOMMENDATIONS FOR MANAGEMENT OF THE PREGNANT PATIENT WITH ABNORMAL CYTOLOGIC FINDINGS

Results of Colposcopically Directed Biopsy	Management
CIN I–III (cytology consistent with CIN)	Deter further diagnostic and therapeutic procedures until 6 weeks postpartum
CIN I–III (cytology consistent with invasive cancer)	Cone biopsy*
Microinvasive tumor	Cone biopsy*
Invasive cancer	Radical hysterectomy or radiotherapy

* Proceed to radical hysterectomy or radiotherapy if invasive cancer is present.
CIN, cervical intraepithelial neoplasia.

Adapted from Di Saia PJ, Creasman WT: Clinical Gynecologic Oncology. St. Louis, CV Mosby, 1981.

the epithelium from which the invasive lesion arises, (2) does not manifest vascular or lymphatic invasion, (3) is free of confluent tongues of tumor, and (4) does not extend to the margins of the surgical specimen.

By International Federation of Gynecology and Obstetrics (Benedet et al., 2001) staging criteria, such lesions must be less than 7 mm in diameter to qualify as stage IA_1. When histologic criteria for stage IA_1 disease have been met, the patient is advised that pregnancy may continue safely to term. Cesarean section is not necessary for this group of patients, and the route of delivery should be determined by obstetric indications. A recommendation for postpartum hysterectomy is not essential in these patients if they desire to bear more children.

A second category of microinvasive cancer includes the lesions that invade between 3.1 and 5 mm and are less than 7 mm in diameter (International Federation of Gynecology and Obstetrics stage IA_2). An expectant approach to definitive management may be considered in such patients; however, definitive treatment by modified radical hysterectomy with pelvic lymphadenectomy should be considered following delivery.

The performance of a cone biopsy in the pregnant patient is a formidable undertaking with an increased risk of hemorrhage and spontaneous abortion. Excessive bleeding is reported to occur in approximately 10% of pregnant women undergoing the procedure, and the risk of perinatal death is 3% to 6%.

To reduce the risk of hemorrhage, we recommend using six hemostatic sutures evenly distributed around the portion of the cervix close to the vaginal reflection (Fig. 58-1). These sutures reduce blood flow to the cone bed, evert the squamocolumnar junction, and facilitate performance of a shallow cone biopsy with little interruption of the endocervical canal. The surgical procedure described for pregnancy might be envisioned as excising a "coin" rather than a cone of tissue (Fig. 58-2). The loop electrocautery excision procedure is especially well adapted to excision of a shallow cone of sufficient breadth and depth to permit treatment decisions while a more extensive invasive process is ruled out. In the pregnant patient, such a procedure should be done in the operating room rather than in the office setting.

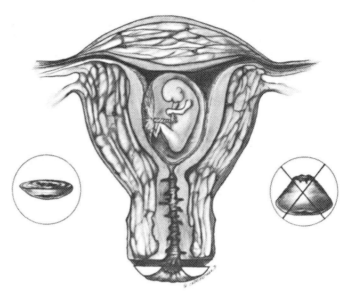

FIGURE 58-2 ■ The shallow "coin biopsy" of the cervix appropriate in pregnancy. (From Creasy RK, Resnik R: Maternal-Fetal Medicine, 4th ed. Philadelphia, WB Saunders, 1999, p. 1130, Fig. 61-2.)

To offset the risk of cervical incompetence, Goldberg and colleagues (1991) performed 17 conization procedures between 12 and 27 weeks' gestation and placed a cerclage through the cervix once the conization specimen was obtained. All of these procedures were complication-free, and all 17 women had uneventful pregnancies, delivering viable infants beyond 35 weeks' gestation. Although these results are interesting, cone-cerclage should be investigated further before it becomes a part of clinical practice.

Presentation

Cervical cancer in pregnancy is most often diagnosed at an early stage, when the likelihood of cure is high. It occurs at a mean age of approximately 35 years in women typically of higher parity (mean, 4.5). Symptoms, when present, include vaginal and postcoital bleeding, vaginal discharge, and pelvic pain. It appears that the distribution of tumor-cell type is similar to that reported in nonpregnant patients, with squamous-cell carcinomas accounting for up to 85%; adenocarcinomas, 10% to 15%; and other cell types (such as neuroendocrine and villoglandular), up to 5% of the cancers.

Cervical cancers are staged clinically rather than surgically because many patients undergo primary radiation therapy rather than surgery for definitive management (Creasman, 1995). Procedures permitted by the International Federation of Gynecology and Obstetrics for use in assigning a stage to a given cervical cancer are comprehensive physical examination, cervical biopsy, chest x-ray, intravenous pyelography, cystoscopy, and sigmoidoscopy. The pelvic examination is crucial and should include visual inspection of the cervix and a bimanual exam to determine if the cancer has spread to the parametria or vaginal wall. Many centers now incorporate magnetic resonance imaging to assess tumor volume and disease extent since this noninvasive modality does not place the fetus at risk of exposure to ionizing radiation.

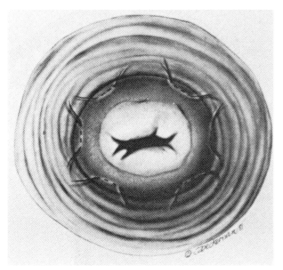

FIGURE 58-1 ■ Location of six hemostatic sutures made in the cervix after cone biopsy. (From Creasy RK, Resnik R: Maternal-Fetal Medicine, 4th ed. Philadelphia, WB Saunders, 1999, p. 1130, Fig. 61-1.)

Therapy

Confusion concerning the course of this disease in pregnancy has been attended by controversy concerning optimal therapy. Support can be found for therapeutic approaches that include radiation therapy, radical surgery, or a combined approach (Method and Brost, 1999; Marana et al., 2001). The dissenting opinions are not resolved easily because most reports contain a limited number of cases from which conclusions can be drawn. As is often true when many therapeutic approaches are advocated for a given disease, in some instances there are clear advantages to one approach over another, whereas in other situations any of several approaches is satisfactory. The therapeutic modalities and their respective roles are discussed in detail later.

Treatment depends not only on the tumor stage and the mother's general health, but also on the gestational age of the fetus and the mother's beliefs regarding pregnancy termination and continuation. A multidisciplinary approach must be undertaken and should include the obstetrician, the mother, and her family, as well as a gynecologic oncologist, a maternal-fetal–medicine specialist, a neonatologist, a pathologist, and an anesthesiologist. A medical social worker and informed labor and delivery nurses may also be considered for inclusion. In difficult situations, especially when the fetus is at the threshold of viability (i.e., 23 to 25 weeks' gestation), it may even be necessary to consult with the risk-management office (or legal counsel) and the hospital chaplain and to convene a medical ethics committee (Tewari , Cappuccini, et al., 1998, 1999).

Microinvasive tumors with less than 3 mm of invasion (stage IA$_1$) and no lymphovascular space involvement may be managed expectantly until the postpartum period. The route of delivery in such cases is determined solely by obstetric indications. Radical surgery or radical radiotherapy is generally advised for stage I tumors with greater than 3 mm of invasion and for stage IIA lesions. Both treatment modalities are equally efficacious for early-stage cervical cancer. Although complications of radical surgery can include excessive blood loss, ureteral injury, prolonged bladder dysfunction, lymphocyst formation, vesicovaginal fistulization, obstipation, and occasionally pulmonary embolism, radiation therapy carries a greater risk for chronic morbidities including vaginal stricture and sexual dysfunction, colonic-, rectal- or vesicovaginal-fistula formation, and bowel stricture. In addition, premenopausal patients will experience premature ovarian failure if the pelvis is irradiated, with an increased risk of cardiovascular disease and osteoporosis. Therefore, radical surgery is the most frequently chosen option for pregnant women, provided they are otherwise in good general health. An outline of recommended treatment for cervical cancer in pregnancy is shown in Table 58-3.

Cesarean/Radical Abdominal Hysterectomy

The surgical procedure of choice is the radical abdominal hysterectomy with bilateral pelvic and aortocaval lymphadenectomy. This is associated with relatively low morbidity and results in the preservation of ovarian function. Although vascular supply to the pelvis is increased, normal tissue planes are very distinct, thereby facilitating pelvic dissection. In this procedure, the cervix and corpus are removed, and the parametrial tissues along the length of the cardinal and uterosacral ligaments, upper vagina, and retroperitoneal lymph nodes are excised as well. Lateral ovarian transposition should also be performed at the time of radical abdominal hysterectomy, with metallic clips placed between the hilum of the ovary and the mesosalpinx. This will permit radiographic identification of the ovaries in case postoperative adjuvant radiation therapy is required because of high-risk pathologic features of the tumor. The radiation fields, when required, can often be designed so that the ovaries can be avoided.

Before 20 weeks' gestation, the entire surgical procedure may be performed with the fetus *in situ*. After 20 weeks, evacuation of the fetus is recommended to obtain improved visualization. A high vertical hysterotomy incision is performed to avoid disturbing the lower uterine segment and the carcinoma. Similarly, if the fetus is viable and a cesarean/radical hysterectomy is elected, a classical uterine incision is required.

Several reports have confirmed that radical hysterectomy can be performed safely during pregnancy. For example, Monk and Montz (1992) reported that intraoperative complications

TABLE 58-3. SUGGESTED THERAPY FOR CERVICAL CANCER IN PREGNANCY

Length of Pregnancy	Stage of Cancer	
	I–IIA	IIB–IIIB

Up to 20 wk	4500 WP:
	    If spontaneous abortion, 6000 B
	    If no abortion, modified radical hysterectomy
	        or
	    Radical hysterectomy with bilateral pelvic
	        lymphadenectomy
		5000 WP:
		    If spontaneous abortion, 5000 B
		    If no spontaneous abortion, type II radical hysterectomy,
		        no lymphadenectomy

Beyond 20 wk	Cesarean section when fetus viable followed by
	    5000 WP and 5000 B
	        or
	    Cesarean radical hysterectomy with bilateral pelvic
	        lymphadenectomy
		Cesarean section when fetus viable followed by
		    5000–6000 WP and 4000–5000 B

B, brachytherapy—vaginal radium in two applications, with number indicating mg/hr; WP, whole-pelvis irradiation, with number indicating cGy.

Modified from Di Saia PJ, Creasman WT: Clinical Gynecologic Oncology. St. Louis, CV Mosby, 1981.

and postoperative morbidity were minimal in 13 patients so managed. The average blood loss was greater when a radical hysterectomy was performed during pregnancy (1493 versus 1065, $P < 0.05$) compared to nonpregnant matched controls; however, there were no differences in the number of blood transfusions or mean hospital stays between pregnant and nonpregnant patients.

Radical Radiotherapy

If spontaneous abortion does not occur by completion of the external beam therapy, a modified radical hysterectomy without pelvic lymphadenectomy should be performed to excise the remaining central neoplasm. This strategy delivers potentially curative doses of radiation to the pelvic lymph nodes, followed by surgical resection of the remaining central tumor. This approach is preferable to completion of therapy with brachytherapy because the gravid uterus is not suitable for intracavitary radium or cesium. Although some institutions prefer an extended extrafascial hysterectomy following 5000 cGy of whole-pelvis irradiation in patients with early lesions, we prefer the more extensive modified radical hysterectomy. This approach accomplishes adequate excision of the cervix, the medial parametria, and the upper vagina, thereby including all the tissues that would have been effectively irradiated by the pear-shaped isodose distribution of a tandem and ovoid application of brachytherapy. Those who advocate an extrafascial hysterectomy often advise further vaginal vault irradiation following the surgical procedure in order to treat the upper vagina and medial parametria more completely. An alternative approach in the patient who has not aborted is to evacuate the uterus by means of a hysterotomy, followed by conventional intracavitary irradiation delivered within 1 to 2 weeks (Sood et al., 1997).

Patients who are at least 20 weeks pregnant may delay radiotherapy until fetal viability is reached unless hemorrhage necessitates earlier intervention. The timing of cesarean delivery is determined by the status of fetal lung maturity, as described previously. The basic radiotherapeutic plan employed for cancer of the cervix in the nonpregnant patient can generally be used after uterine involution is completed for patients in whom only cesarean section has been performed. Whole-pelvis irradiation commences immediately after the abdominal incision has healed, typically within 3 weeks after surgery. Intracavitary radiation can follow completion of uterine involution and treatment to the whole pelvis.

Deliberate Delay in Therapy

At times a delay in definitive therapy must be considered to permit a fetus to reach a stage where viability is likely. Factors that must be taken into account include the mother's feelings regarding pregnancy termination, fetal viability, and maternal risk. Traditionally, women who present before 20 weeks' gestation have been advised to undergo immediate treatment with sacrifice of the pregnancy, while those presenting at or beyond 20 weeks have been offered deliberate delays, provided their tumor had not progressed beyond the cervix (Sorosky et al., 1995). However, fetal viability is a complex issue, and through the use of corticosteroids, recombinant surfactant, and improved neonatal intensive care units, the threshold of survivability has been lowered to earlier gestations. Still, it is not possible to recommend a specific minimum gestational age at which a planned delay in therapy is safe.

Duggan and colleagues (1993) reported a mean delay of 144 days among eight patients with stage I disease who wanted to maximize their chances for a good fetal outcome. All eight babies were viable at delivery, and at a follow-up of 3 to 124 months, there have been no recurrences among these eight women. The investigators suggested that a deliberate delay in therapy is a reasonable alternative for informed pregnant women with stage I cervical disease.

If a woman in early pregnancy with stage I disease opts to delay therapy for fetal well-being, then accurately dating the pregnancy using ultrasonography is imperative. This is crucial in order to effect delivery and institute definitive therapy as soon as fetal pulmonary maturity can be demonstrated, usually by 32 to 34 weeks' gestation. Thus, amniocentesis for fetal maturity testing will be necessary, as will administration of antepartum steroids. Implicit in this concept is the need for a neonatal intensive care unit for care of the preterm newborn.

In summary, delays in definitive treatment of an early-stage cervical cancer of 4 to 14 weeks are usually appropriate when required to assure fetal viability. Cesarean radical hysterectomy at 34 weeks' gestation usually ensures fetal viability while delaying definitive therapy by a maximum of 14 weeks for patients whose diagnosis is confirmed during the second half of pregnancy. The former beliefs that pregnancy may accelerate tumor growth and that parturition may squeeze viable cells into the vascular system and increase the incidence of metastatic spread have not been substantiated either by hormone receptor data or by clinical observation. Even cervical adenocarcinomas have low or absent sex steroid hormone receptors, with supporting data showing that, stage for stage, the outcome for pregnant patients with cervical cancer is approximately the same as for young nonpregnant patients. It should be emphasized that this discussion regarding treatment delays should apply only to squamous cell carcinomas and that these issues are not as clear for adenocarcinomas. All treatment delays are contraindicated for some of the rarer cell types, such as the neuroendocrine small-cell carcinoma of the cervix, which may be extraordinarily virulent (Balderston, 1998).

Prognosis

Although many early reports suggested that pregnancy may accelerate the growth of carcinoma of the cervix, most recent studies show that pregnancy has little effect on tumor growth. There are conflicting reports whether the prognosis in cancer patients under age 35 years tends to differ from that in women in whom disease is detected after this age. The perception of a worse prognosis is probably related to aggressive histologic subtypes of cancer in younger patients. Because cervical cancer in pregnancy usually occurs in the younger patients, survival statistics for these women must be compared with that in a group of nonpregnant cervical cancer patients whose age distribution is similar to that of the group of pregnant patients. When such comparisons are made, pregnancy is found to have little adverse effect on the overall survival for this disease (Hopkins and Morley, 1992; Sivanesaratnam et al., 1992; van der Vange, 1995). In addition, patients with diethylstilbestrol-associated clear cell carcinoma of the cervix (and vagina) diagnosed during pregnancy have 5- and 10-year survival rates that are not significantly different from those reported for nonpregnant women with this diagnosis.

Thus, as would be expected for nonpregnant patients, the prognosis for this disease in pregnancy is a function of stage and tumor volume (Zemlickis et al., 1991). When primary surgery or a staging laparotomy is done, the survival probability can be refined further based on the status of lymph nodes in the pelvis and along the abdominal aorta and inferior vena cava.

Because women with more advanced disease may have difficulty in attaining pregnancy, there have been too few reports of such women to draw conclusions regarding maternal outcome. Cervical cancer by itself does not adversely affect the fetus. There have been no reports of cervical cancer metastasis to the placenta or the fetus.

Ovarian Cancer

Among malignancies arising in the pelvic region, ovarian cancers are second in frequency to cervical cancer, but they are exceedingly rare during pregnancy, occurring in only 1 in 20,000 to 30,000 pregnancies (Jubb, 1963). The differential diagnosis of ovarian masses during pregnancy is complicated by (1) their location outside the pelvis during the second half of pregnancy and (2) the difficulty in distinguishing between the consistency of a gravid uterus and that of an ovarian neoplasm. Despite this diagnostic dilemma, the routine use of ultrasonography to assess fetal development and investigate potential fetal anomalies increases the likelihood of finding unexpected ovarian masses. The routine use of ultrasound technology, however, also creates the clinical dilemma of identifying subclinical masses, which rarely prove to be malignant but which may necessitate some type of diagnostic intervention.

Adnexal Masses in Pregnancy

The finding of an ovarian mass presents challenging problems in diagnosis and management. Eastman and Hellman (1966) reported finding ovarian cysts in 1 of 81 pregnancies, and Grimes and coworkers (1954) reported a cyst "large enough to be hazardous" in 0.3% of pregnancies. Management of ovarian cysts can be complicated by pelvic impaction, obstructed labor, torsion, hemorrhage into the tumor, rupture of the cyst, infection, and rarely, malignancy (Hess et al., 1988). Although malignancy is relatively uncommon and is the least acute complication in pregnancy, it should always be foremost in the clinician's mind.

Torsion of an ovarian neoplasm is particularly common in pregnancy, with a reported incidence of 10% to 15%. Most cases of ovarian torsion occur either when the uterus is growing at a rapid rate between the 8th and 16th weeks of gestation or when the uterus is involuting rapidly during the puerperium. About 60% of the cases occur during the first half of pregnancy, and most of the remaining cases occur in the puerperium. The usual sequence of events is sudden lower abdominal pain, nausea with vomiting, and in some instances, a shocklike syndrome. The abdomen is often tense and tender, and there may be rebound tenderness with guarding.

Most ovarian masses found in pregnancy are corpus luteum cysts, which are usually no more than 5 cm in diameter. Their management in early pregnancy should be expectant, because more than 90% of these functional cysts disappear as pregnancy progresses and are undetectable by the 14th week of gestation. As the uterus begins to rise out of the pelvis at the end of the first trimester, ovarian enlargement is best evaluated by pelvic and abdominal ultrasound study because the ovaries often are not easily palpated.

It is especially difficult to distinguish an ovarian tumor in pregnancy from other pelvic structures on the basis of a pelvic examination alone because of the size and cystic consistency of the gravid uterus. When a tumor is palpable within the pelvis, it must be differentiated from a retroverted pregnant uterus, a pedunculated uterine leiomyoma, carcinoma of the rectosigmoid colon, a pelvic kidney, a retroperitoneal mass, or a uterine congenital anomaly such as an accessory uterine horn. In the patient with a mass that is suggestive of malignancy, diagnostic studies should include ultrasound of the abdomen and pelvis to detect ascites when present and to be certain that the mass is extrauterine. Additional studies can include an intravenous pyelogram to rule out a pelvic kidney and possible ureteral obstruction, as well as a limited barium enema to be certain that colon cancer is not present. These radiologic studies should be avoided, if possible, during the first trimester to prevent the potential mutagenic effects of ionizing radiation to the developing fetus during organogenesis. In the latter half of pregnancy, ovarian tumors are particularly difficult to detect because the adnexa are located in the abdomen, beyond the reach of examining fingers in the vaginal area. Abdominal examination, the chief method of diagnosis in the second half of pregnancy, is unreliable because of the large uterus, even when ascites is present.

When an ovarian tumor is not detected during the first half of pregnancy, often the diagnosis cannot be made until labor or delivery. If the ovarian mass obstructs the birth canal during labor, exploratory laparotomy is indicated for both delivery of the infant and management of the ovarian neoplasm. Allowing a labor to proceed while an ovarian neoplasm obstructs the birth canal can result in rupture of the ovarian mass, followed by hemorrhage, peritonitis, tumor dissemination, or shock. Even if an ovarian cyst does not rupture, the trauma of labor can cause hemorrhage into the tumor, followed by necrosis and suppuration. Yet Brodsky and coworkers (1980) reported up to a fivefold increase in second-trimester pregnancy loss associated with operative intervention for a pelvic mass. Despite this adverse effect of operative intervention, we believe that the benefits of earlier cancer diagnosis and prevention of subsequent complications outweigh the risks of avoiding operative intervention during the second trimester.

Management of the Adnexal Mass in Pregnancy

The gestational age of the pregnancy, the mother's symptoms, and the size and characteristics of the mass are considered when formulating a management strategy for the adnexal mass in pregnancy. Unilateral, unilocular, mobile masses less than 6 cm in maximal diameter that are discovered early in pregnancy may be observed, since most will be functional cysts and cancer is not a realistic concern. Solid masses, as well as those that are bilateral, greater than 6 cm in maximal diameter, and/or persist into the second trimester, are best managed by laparotomy. Elective resection during the 16th to 18th week of gestation is associated with pregnancy interruption less often than is emergent surgery for ovarian torsion or hemorrhage. Table 58-4 lists the ovarian neoplasms most commonly encountered during pregnancy.

TABLE 58-4. ADNEXAL MASSES REMOVED DURING PREGNANCY

Mass	%
Mucinous or serous cystadenoma	34
Mature teratoma	27
Luteal cyst	18
Other, nonmalignant	16–19
Other, malignant*	2–5

*Dysgerminoma is the most common of the malignant ovarian tumors in pregnancy; other malignant germ cell tumors, tumors of low malignant potential (i.e., borderline), frankly invasive epithelial cancers, granulose cell tumors, and Sertoli-Leydig tumors have also been discovered in pregnancy.

Of course, any clinical scenario consistent with torsion, hemorrhage, or ovarian rupture necessitates immediate celiotomy. During the first trimester, this most often occurs as a torsed corpus luteum. Excision of an infarcted adnexa in this setting should be accompanied by prophylactic administration of progestational agents until the placenta matures (56 to 70 days of gestation).

Elective surgery deferred to the 16th to 18th week provides a reduced risk of spontaneous abortion and assures hormonal independence from the corpus luteum. A vertical midline or paramedian incision should be employed because it requires minimal uterine manipulation. Because the ovarian pedicle is usually long, the gravid uterus does not require handling while the ovaries are mobilized into the incision. Careful inspection of the contralateral ovary is imperative, whether the primary neoplasm is benign or malignant. Because a benign neoplasm will be encountered in most instances, ovariectomy can usually be avoided. Following ovarian cystectomy, the neoplasm should be opened in the operating room, and if the diagnosis is uncertain, a frozen section should be examined prior to closure of the abdominal incision.

Epithelial Ovarian Cancer in Pregnancy

Epithelial tumors, which include serous, mucinous, endometrioid, and clear cell cancers, account for nearly 50% of malignant ovarian neoplasms found in pregnancy (Boulay and Podczaski, 1998). The diagnosis is usually fortuitous; the tumor is found at exploratory laparotomy for an adnexal mass or at cesarean section. Characteristically, these tumors are of early stage and low grade; indeed, many epithelial cancers of the ovary during pregnancy prove to be tumors of low malignant potential (Mooney et al., 1997).

Should the surgeon find a frankly invasive ovarian malignancy during pregnancy, the first obligation is to stage the disease properly (Table 58-5) while providing operative intervention. Treatment should be appropriate for the stage of the disease, regardless of the pregnancy. It is appropriate to treat stage IA lesions conservatively with a unilateral salpingo-oophorectomy, provided that a thorough exploration of the abdominal cavity has been carried out, inclusive of surgical staging. The exploration should be performed through a midline or paramedian incision extending above the umbilicus. The operative procedure should include collection of peritoneal fluid or washings for cytologic evaluation, visualization of the liver and diaphragm, biopsy of the omentum and peritoneum in the pelvis and pericolic areas, and careful evaluation of the pelvic and periaortic lymph nodes. From prospective data in nonpregnant women, up to 30% of women with clinical stage I disease will be upstaged by virtue of microscopic metastases in the omentum, peritoneal surfaces, and/or retroperitoneal lymph nodes. More advanced lesions should not be treated conservatively unless they are tumors of low malignant potential, in which case definitive surgical therapy can be deferred until fetal viability is achieved. Of course, the decision regarding the degree of surgical radicality in the setting of advanced disease (which may include hysterectomy while the fetus is still immature) ultimately rests with the

TABLE 58-5. FIGO STAGE GROUPING FOR PRIMARY CARCINOMA OF THE OVARY (1985)*

Stage I. Growth limited to the ovaries
  A. Growth limited to one ovary; no ascites. No tumor on the external surface; capsule intact
  B. Growth limited to both ovaries; no ascites. No tumor on the external surfaces; capsules intact
  C.† Tumor either stage IA or IB but with tumor on the surface of one or both ovaries; or with capsule(s) ruptured; or with ascites present containing malignant cells or with positive peritoneal washings

Stage II. Growth involving one or both ovaries with pelvic extension
  A. Extension and/or metastases to the uterus and/or tubes
  B. Extension to other pelvic tissues
  C.† Tumor either stage IIA or IIB but with tumor on the surface of one or both ovaries; or with capsule(s) ruptured; or with ascites present containing malignant cells or with positive peritoneal washings

Stage III. Tumor involving one or both ovaries with peritoneal implants outside the pelvis and/or positive retroperitoneal or inguinal nodes. Superficial liver metastasis equals stage III. Tumor is limited to the true pelvis but with histologically verified malignant extension to small bowel or omentum
  A. Tumor grossly limited to the true pelvis with negative nodes but with histologically confirmed microscopic seeding of abdominal peritoneal surfaces
  B. Tumor of one or both ovaries with histologically confirmed implants of abdominal peritoneal surfaces, none exceeding 2 cm in diameter; nodes negative
  C. Abdominal implants >2 cm in diameter and/or positive retroperitoneal or inguinal nodes

Stage IV. Growth involving one or both ovaries with distant metastasis. If pleural effusion is present, there must be positive cytologic test results to allot a case to stage IV; parenchymal liver metastasis equals stage IV

* These categories are based on findings at clinical examination and/or surgical exploration. The histologic characteristics are to be considered in the staging, as are results of cytologic testing as far as effusions are concerned. It is desirable that a biopsy be performed on suspicious areas outside the pelvis.
† In order to evaluate the impact on prognosis of the different criteria for allotting cases to stage IC or IIC, it would be of value to know if rupture of the capsule was (1) spontaneous or (2) iatrogenic, and if the source of malignant cells detected was (1) peritoneal washings or (2) ascites.
FIGO, International Federation of Gynecology and Obstetrics.

From Creasy RK, Resnik R: Maternal-Fetal Medicine, 4th ed. Philadelphia, WB Saunders, 1999, p. 1133.

patient and her desire to continue the pregnancy. Accordingly, preoperative counseling of the patient concerning all of the possible findings and the treatment options is most important.

Malignant Germ Cell Tumors of the Ovary in Pregnancy

Germ cell tumors are the most common ovarian neoplasms in pregnancy. The most frequently encountered germ cell tumor to complicate pregnancy is the mature teratoma. When a mature teratoma is discovered at surgery, the uninvolved ovarian tissue can usually be preserved because these neoplasms are well encapsulated and can easily be dissected away from the remainder of the ovary.

The malignant germ cell tumors include dysgerminomas, embryonal carcinomas, immature teratomas, and yolk sac tumors (previously called endodermal sinus tumors). Sometimes a mixture of these various elements is present within the same malignancy; this is termed a *mixed germ cell tumor* (Horbelt et al., 1984). Of the malignant germ cell tumors, dysgerminomas are the most commonly reported.

Ovarian dysgerminomas are unique among the malignant germ cell tumors because of their overall good prognosis in stage I, when treated by surgery alone, and their exquisite sensitivity to radiation therapy in addition to chemotherapy. In this latter regard, they behave in a fashion that is identical to the seminoma of the testis, which shares the same histologic and biological features. Dysgerminomas in stage IA may be managed with a unilateral adnexectomy and continuation of the pregnancy without additional therapy. As stated earlier, optimal staging is mandatory and should include a lesion-directed unilateral pelvic lymphadenectomy and bilateral aortocaval lymph node sampling, because dysgerminomas metastasize primarily via the lymphatic system to the ipsilateral pelvic and bilateral aortocaval lymph nodes. Peritoneal metastases are often seen in this germ cell malignancy. Careful surgical staging is essential because lymphangiography and computed tomography (CT), which are recommended in the evaluation of the nonpregnant patient, are contraindicated when the pregnancy is to be continued.

Emergency surgical intervention and obstetric complications are commonly reported in patients with dysgerminomas. Karlen and associates (1979) reviewed 27 cases of dysgerminoma associated with pregnancy. Torsion and incarceration were commonly found in this group of patients, whose rapidly enlarging neoplasms averaged 25 cm in diameter. Obstetric complications occurred in nearly one half of patients and fetal demise in one fourth. Surprisingly, recurrences were seen in 30% of 23 stage IA tumors treated by unilateral oophorectomy, therefore casting doubt on the philosophy of treating these patients conservatively. The extent to which these patients underwent surgical exploration was not known in most cases, however, and therefore accuracy of staging cannot be assessed.

Dysgerminomas confined to one ovary carry approximately a 10% recurrence rate, usually during the first 2 years after surgery. These patients can continue pregnancy safely once appropriate surgical staging has been performed. Because chemotherapy or radiation therapy is successful in curing more than 75% of patients even with metastatic or recurrent dysgerminoma, and because there is a low incidence of recurrence in carefully staged patients with stage IA disease, a conservative approach to these tumors is recommended when the diagnosis is made during pregnancy.

Chemotherapy for Malignant Germ Cell Tumors in Pregnancy

Chemotherapy is required for all malignant germ cell tumors of the ovary during pregnancy except stage I dysgerminoma or a stage IA grade I immature teratoma (Buller et al., 1992; Tewari Rose, et al., 1998). Accordingly, recommendations for treatment with all other malignant germ cell tumors during the first trimester include pregnancy termination via uterine evacuation because of the potential for teratogenicity when chemotherapy is administered during the period of fetal organogenesis. Beyond embryogenesis, combination chemotherapy can be safely administered during the second and third trimesters. The most common regimen deployed in treating germ cell malignancies are bleomycin, etoposide, and cisplatin in combination.

Unusual Malignant Ovarian Tumors in Pregnancy

The luteoma of pregnancy, hyperreactio lutinalis, the large solitary luteinized follicle cyst of pregnancy and puerperium, granulose cell proliferations, hilus cell hyperplasia, and the ectopic deciduas are non-neoplastic ovarian lesions associated with pregnancy or the postpartum period that can be confused with true sex cord-stromal tumors. Although these alterations can simulate a neoplastic process on clinical, gross, or microscopic examination, they involute spontaneously after the termination of pregnancy.

True sex cord–stromal ovarian tumors have been observed to complicate pregnancy (Young et al., 1984; Kalir and Friedman, 1998). Young and colleagues (1984) reported 17 granulosa cell tumors in pregnancy and 13 Sertoli-Leydig cell tumors. Twenty-seven patients presented with abdominal pain, shock, vaginal bleeding, and/or virilization, and three were asymptomatic. All but one were treated conservatively with unilateral adnexectomy, and the authors noted that the biological behavior of these tumors diagnosed during gestation was similar to that of sex cord–stromal cancers unassociated with pregnancy. Typically, they present at stage I and have a high cure rate when managed by surgery alone.

Perhaps the most aggressive primary ovarian malignancy is the small cell ovarian cancer, for which survival rates beyond 6 months following diagnosis are uncommon. The only 5-year survivor of an advanced stage, small cell ovarian cancer in pregnancy occurred after treatment with a six-drug chemotherapy regimen (Tewari, Brewer, et al., 1997).

Finally, metastatic cancers to the ovary have been described in pregnancy, most commonly, the Krukenberg tumor arising from the pylorus of the stomach; these tumors may have a predilection for bilaterality and contain neoplastic signet ring cells that exhibit intracellular mucin production (Sandmeier et al., 2000). Carcinomas from the large intestine, appendix, and breast have also metastasized to the ovary during pregnancy (Sebire et al., 2000).

Summary of Ovarian Cancer in Pregnancy

The pregnant state does not appear to have a direct adverse effect on the prognosis of the patient with an ovarian malignancy, although its continuation can compromise both the initial operation and the initiation of postoperative therapy. Ovarian cancers are not sensitive to either exogenous or endogenous sources of sex steroids; therefore, the prognosis is unaffected by the pregnancy. Similarly, there is no adverse consequence of hormone-replacement therapy following removal of the ovaries for a cancer diagnosis.

In summary, diagnosis and treatment of the pregnant woman with an ovarian tumor is a complex matter for the clinician, the solution of which is often not clear-cut. One must have a high index of suspicion and must endeavor to diagnose early and treat promptly, preferably early in the second trimester. The difficulty arises when both patient and physician resist an abdominal exploration during pregnancy because of the fear of precipitating fetal loss. However, the potential danger to the mother of a delay in diagnosis exceeds the risk to the fetus. Most of the dangers seen with ovarian tumors are those created by acts of omission rather than of commission. The possibility of an ovarian cancer must be kept foremost in the minds of physicians caring for pregnant patients, and any adnexal mass in pregnancy persisting after the 14th week of gestation, excluding thin-walled unilocular cysts, should be surgically removed.

Other Pelvic Malignancies

Colorectal Cancer

Three percent of colorectal cancer patients are younger than 40 years. The incidence of this neoplasm in pregnancy is estimated to be 1 in 50,000 to 100,000 pregnancies (Bernstein et al., 1993). Interestingly, the majority (up to 65%) of colorectal cancers diagnosed during gestation are rectal carcinomas. To date, only 32 cases of colonic cancer arising above the peritoneal reflection during pregnancy have been reported in the literature (Woods et al., 1992). Ochshorn and colleagues (2000) has noted that this distribution is opposite to that observed in the general population, where cancers occur predominantly above the rectum. This further emphasizes the importance and value of digital rectal examination for pregnant women.

The diagnosis is often delayed because the most common complaint, rectal bleeding during pregnancy, is often attributed to hemorrhoids. Although stage for stage, survival is not different from that for the general population, colorectal carcinoma during pregnancy is associated with a poor prognosis, mostly as a consequence of delay in diagnosis resulting in advanced stage of disease. Locally advanced disease may prompt premature labor or necessitate early therapy, resulting in intrauterine death; only 78% of pregnancies associated with colorectal cancer produce live-born infants. Although the tumor has never been reported to metastasize to the fetus, Rothman and colleagues (1973) identified one case with placental implants.

Management of a rectal cancer can vary based on gestational age (Balloni et al., 2000; Caforio et al., 2000). Prior to 10 weeks' gestation, an abdominal perineal resection can be done without removing the uterus. Between 10 and 20 weeks' gestation, Barber and Brunschwig (1968) advocated routine hysterectomy to gain access to the rectum and to ensure adequate margins in resection. Occasionally, there will be tumor fixation to the uterus, fallopian tubes, or ovaries. Oophorectomy is recommended for all low-lying colonic tumors because of the high incidence of metastatic disease to the ovaries; at times, occult metastases are found even in the normal-appearing ovary. Alternatively, pregnancy termination

followed by neoadjuvant radiotherapy or chemotherapy can be conducted with subsequent surgical extirpation of the tumor.

When the diagnosis is made between 20 and 32 weeks' gestational age, definitive therapy may be postponed until fetal maturation occurs, preferably by 34 weeks' gestational age. The mode of delivery remains a controversial issue. Some investigators favor cesarean delivery to avoid pressure and trauma to the tumor with a vaginal delivery, thereby theoretically decreasing the risk of bleeding and metastases. Furthermore, rectal surgery may be performed with cesarean section. Vaginal delivery, on the other hand, permits regression of the gravid uterus and pelvic vascularity following delivery, which may improve accessibility to the cancer while reducing the risk of bleeding and thromboembolic complications. Additionally, surgery is not always the preferred initial treatment, especially in cases of large tumors, for which neoadjuvant radio-chemotherapy has become a well-established primary treatment modality for rectal carcinoma. Thus treatment typically is determined by the extent of disease, the duration of gestation, and physician and patient preference.

Retroperitoneal Sarcomas

Retroperitoneal sarcomas also can occur during pregnancy and often present great technical difficulties at surgical removal. Most of the lesions are neurofibrosarcomas or sarcomas of similar histologic nature, and their course depends greatly on their grade. Therapy for low-grade sarcomas can be deferred until the postpartum period, when resection should be technically much easier; however, if such a tumor extends into the pelvis, cesarean delivery is often required. High-grade lesions are associated with a poor prognosis, and therapy must be individualized according to the length of gestation and preference of the patient.

GESTATIONAL TROPHOBLASTIC NEOPLASIA

Gestational trophoblastic neoplasia (GTN) is a clinical diagnosis that includes the histologic diagnoses of hydatidiform mole, locally invasive mole, metastatic mole, and choriocarcinoma. GTN describes this spectrum of disease because in most instances the histologic diagnosis is unknown when treatment is initiated.

Prior to the revolutionary developments in detection and treatment in the 1950s, the prognosis for women with this group of diseases, when metastatic, was quite dismal. In 1956, Li and associates reported the first complete and sustained remissions in patients with metastatic choriocarcinoma after methotrexate therapy. Since that time, the treatment has evolved to a point where GTN is the most curable gynecologic malignancy and, indeed, the most curable cancer known to medicine.

Several distinct features of these tumors account for the dramatic change in prognosis. First, a sensitive marker, human chorionic gonadotropin (hCG), is secreted by the tumor, and the amount of this hormone measured in serum is directly related to the number of viable tumor cells. Second, these malignancies are exquisitely sensitive to various chemotherapeutic agents. Third, subgroups of affected patients with various high-risk factors have been identified, permitting individualization of treatment. Fourth, the neoplastic cells are highly antigenic and represent a true allograft.

Hydatidiform Mole

Hydatidiform mole occurs in 1 of every 1200 pregnancies in the United States but much more frequently in other areas of the world. In the Far East and the tropics, it is reported in 1 of every 120 pregnancies. Its frequency increased dramatically in the Philippines during World War II, suggesting a relationship to stress and diet. Molar pregnancies occur relatively more frequently at both ends of the reproductive spectrum, with patients at greatest risk in the early teens and peri-menopausally. Age, parity, and gestational age at the time of diagnosis do not appear to affect the risk of malignant sequelae.

Several clinical presentations, including hyperemesis, preeclampsia, uterine size inconsistent with gestational age, and hyperthyroidism, are often associated with hydatidiform mole and can suggest the diagnosis. Essentially all patients with hydatidiform mole have amenorrhea and can experience characteristic or often exaggerated signs and symptoms of pregnancy.

Vaginal bleeding is the most common presenting symptom, typically occurring during the first trimester. This manifestation ranges from a dark brown discharge to brisk hemorrhage sometimes requiring blood transfusions. Excessive nausea and vomiting are reported to occur in almost one third of patients with hydatidiform mole, although Curry and associates (1975) noted only a 14% incidence in 347 patients studied. Preeclampsia diagnosed in the first trimester of pregnancy is almost pathognomonic of a hydatidiform mole, although only 12% of patients studied by Curry's group (1975) had this complication.

Hyperthyroidism occurs rarely but, when present, can precipitate a clinical emergency. As many as 10% of patients manifest laboratory evidence of hyperthyroidism, although fewer than 1% of the patients studied by Curry and coworkers (1975) had clinical evidence of this disease. The clinical manifestations of hyperthyroidism disappear once the molar pregnancy is evacuated; thyroid suppression can be indicated in the symptomatic patient with discontinuation of therapy after uterine evacuation. Hyperthyroidism in molar pregnancy results from the production of thyrotropin by molar tissue.

In women with hydatidiform moles, there is often a discrepancy between uterine size and duration of pregnancy. Uterine size is excessive for gestational age in about 50% of patients; in approximately one third of the patients, however, the uterus is smaller than expected. Theca-lutein cysts of the ovary, resulting from hyperstimulation of the ovaries from excessive hCG production by the molar pregnancy, can be quite large. About 50% of patients with molar pregnancy have palpable theca-lutein cysts. A patient with either a uterus that is large for date or a theca-lutein cyst appears to have a greater likelihood of malignant sequelae than does a patient with normal ovaries and a uterus that is normal or small for date. More than 50% of the women with both enlarged cystic ovaries and excessive uterine enlargement require therapy for malignant sequelae.

The first clinical evidence to suggest the diagnosis of hydatidiform mole often is the spontaneous passage of vesicles from the uterus. Histologically, the tissue is characterized by the presence of avascular edematous villi with varying degrees of trophoblastic hyperplasia. Cytogenetic studies have shown these tissues to be diploid, XX, with the entire genetic composition to be paternally derived. An unusually elevated hCG level occurring together with an enlarged uterus and vaginal bleeding strongly suggest the diagnosis of hydatidiform mole; however, a single hCG determination cannot be diagnostic. Occasionally, a markedly elevated hCG titer may be seen with a normal single or multiple gestation or a pathologic condition such as erythroblastosis fetalis. Conversely, an hCG titer that is appropriate for the gestational age can be seen with a mole.

A definitive diagnosis prior to spontaneous passage of vesicles can be made by ultrasonography. Indeed, ultrasonography is specific in differentiating between a normal pregnancy and a hydatidiform mole. In a normal pregnancy, a gestational sac is seen early and a fetal pole with cardiac motion is seen at approximately 6 to 7 weeks' gestation. In a molar pregnancy, the characteristic ultrasonogram reveals multiple echoes, which are formed by the interface between the molar villi and the surrounding tissue, in the absence of a gestational sac or fetus. With the new and more refined ultrasound techniques, the presumptive diagnosis of a molar pregnancy can be substantiated in almost all cases.

Rarely, a fetus coexists with a molar gestation, thereby resulting in confusion of the typical ultrasonographic findings. In addition, there is the possibility of a partial or "transitional" mole, in which a fetus can coexist with hydropic villi having lesser degrees of trophoblastic hyperplasia. This clinical entity also can provide an ambiguous picture on ultrasonography. Excessive uterine size, toxemia, and hyperthyroidism are rare with this diagnosis. Cytogenetic studies show these tissues to be triploid, usually with two thirds of the genetic material derived from the father and one third from the mother, unlike the case with the "classic" mole. In some series, 35% of molar pregnancies were partial moles, with approximately one third of the partial moles demonstrating fetal parts. Fewer than 10% of patients with partial moles require chemotherapy for nonmetastatic gestational trophoblastic disease. Prompt response to chemotherapy and failure to metastasize have been characteristic of this diagnosis.

Techniques used to evacuate a molar pregnancy in the past have included dilatation and curettage, hysterotomy, hysterectomy, and various chemical and mechanical induction techniques. Before the use of suction curettage, hysterectomy was frequently used for uteri greater than 12 to 14 weeks in size because of the excessive risk of hemorrhage when evacuation was attempted by sharp curettage. Suction curettage is now the method of choice for evacuating a mole, and hysterectomy is limited to older patients who have finished childbearing, in whom the risk of malignant sequelae can be reduced by this means, and to the occasional younger patient with major hemorrhage.

Suction curettage can be carried out even when the uterus is the size of that in a term pregnancy. It is recommended that all patients with molar pregnancy who desire to maintain fertility undergo suction curettage, with a laparotomy set-up available in case evacuation is not successful. After a moderate amount of tissue has been removed, intravenous oxytocin is usually begun. It is important to avoid uterine stimulation with oxytocin prior to evacuation. Uterine contractions can cause trophoblastic tissue to be engulfed by the large venous sinusoids in the uterus, resulting in embolization of trophoblastic tissue (deportation) to the lungs. When deportation is excessive, severe respiratory embarrassment can occur. A sharp curettage is recommended after suction curettage has been completed and involution has begun.

If a primary hysterectomy is selected for initial therapy, the ovaries can be left undisturbed even when theca-lutein cysts are encountered. These functional cysts will regress completely when hCG is no longer present in the serum. If there is concern for torsion or rupture of the adnexa because of their overall dimension, they can be aspirated to reduce their volume. Even when hysterectomy is used for therapy, the patient must be followed up with serial hCG determinations, as if the uterus had not been removed (Table 58-6).

After uterine evacuation, serial serum quantitative beta-hCG levels should be assessed every 1 to 2 weeks until hCG is undetectable on two consecutive determinations. Two negative readings indicate spontaneous remission and occur in 80% to 85% of patients. The hCG titer should then be repeated every 1 to 2 months for at least a year. It is imperative that the patient use some type of contraceptive during this interval, because a subsequent pregnancy will cause secretion of hCG, suggesting recurrence of GTN. Unless otherwise contraindicated, oral contraceptives should be used, although one report suggests that their administration should be delayed until hCG titer approaches undetectable levels (Bagshawe, 1976). The Gynecologic Oncology Group (Curry et al., 1989) was unable to prove an association between oral contraceptive use and malignant sequelae of GTN. Others have reported a negative association between oral contraceptive use and gestational trophoblastic tumor ($P < 0.001$) (Deicas et al., 1991). Regular pelvic examinations should be performed at 4-week intervals until the hCG titer is undetectable. Additional examinations should be performed at 3-month intervals during the 1st year. After 1 year of negative hCG titers, contraception can be discontinued and further pregnancies may be attempted.

Another molar pregnancy occurs in only 1% of subsequent pregnancies; however, this small subset of patients has a low likelihood of future viable pregnancies. Most patients with a history of molar pregnancy who have desired future childbearing have subsequently had a normal gestation without difficulty, although there may be a slightly increased risk of spontaneous abortion.

The hCG titer will plateau or rise during the observation period in up to 25% of patients, indicating persistent GTN. Interestingly, this risk of malignant sequelae varies among different trophoblastic disease centers, with some reporting the use of chemotherapy in as few as 6% to 8% of patients. The variation in part probably reflects different patient populations and variable criteria used in treatment centers in decisions as to when chemotherapy should be administered. Some authors have suggested starting chemotherapy if hCG titers are still measurable 60 days after uterine evacuation, because persistent GTN will be manifested in at least 50% of such patients. Patients in whom hCG titers are still falling at 60 days can be observed as long as the titer does not plateau or rise and until there is no evidence of metastasis. Although most patients who have not demonstrated a normal regression curve characterized by a weekly 50% or greater drop in hCG levels probably will require chemotherapy, in many such patients the hCG titer will become normal spontaneously. Thus, careful continued observation of hCG titers should minimize the number of patients given chemotherapy.

Considerable controversy also remains concerning the factors that place a patient with a hydatidiform mole at high risk for malignant sequelae; nevertheless, it is agreed that titers plateauing for 3 to 6 consecutive weeks or rising more than 50% necessitate evaluation for metastatic disease followed by prompt chemotherapy.

Coexisting Mole and Normal Fetus

During the preceding decade, several centers reported the rare coexistence of a normal intrauterine pregnancy with a complete mole. These so-called "twin pregnancies" may occur spontaneously or as a consequence of assisted reproductive technology and are estimated to complicate 1 in 100,000 pregnancies. To date, there have been approximately 130 published cases, including higher order gestations, associated with a molar pregnancy.

As expected, the outlook for the normal fetus is compromised in such situations. Bristow and colleagues (1996) reported 25 cases from the literature and one of their own, in which 19 were evacuated before fetal viability and only 7 resulted in a live-born infant. Although there were no differences between the viable and nonviable groups with respect to mean age, gravidity, parity, uterine size, presence of preeclampsia, or presence of theca-lutein cysts, persistent GTN developed in 68.4% of the pre-viable group of patients (who required molar evacuation), but in only 28.6% of those in the viable group. Clinical factors that required termination of the pregnancy might have been surrogates for aggressive trophoblastic growth, and therefore persistent disease and the subsequent need for adjuvant systemic therapy.

Steller's group (1994) from the New England Trophoblastic Disease Center discovered eight well-documented cases of twin pregnancy with complete hydatidiform mole and coexisting fetus. They compared the clinical features of these 8 patients to those of 71 women with singleton complete hydatidiform mole. Although the presenting symptoms were similar in both groups, a twin pregnancy with complete mole and coexisting fetus was diagnosed at a later gestational age, had higher preevacuation beta-hCG levels, and had a greater propensity to develop persistent gestational trophoblastic tumor.

The major obstacles to carrying the normal fetus is the development of a paraneoplastic medical complication, catastrophic vaginal hemorrhage, and formation of metastatic foci. Patients must be counseled regarding these risks, especially if they wish to carry the normal baby to viability or even term gestation. In the exceedingly rare situation in which metastatic GTN coexists with a normal gestation (Nabers et al., 1990;

TABLE 58-6. POSTEVACUATION AND POSTHYSTERECTOMY MANAGEMENT OF HYDATIDIFORM MOLE

1. hCG determination (radioimmunoassay) every wk until negative two times, then monthly for 1 yr
2. Physical examination including pelvis every 4 wk until remission; then every 3 mo for 1 yr
3. Chest film as a baseline study and again should chemotherapy be required
4. Chemotherapy started immediately if hCG titer rises or plateaus during follow-up *or* metastases are detected at any time

hCG, human chorionic gonadotropin.

Modified from Di Saia PJ, Creasman WT: Clinical Gynecologic Oncology. St. Louis, CV Mosby, 1981.

Steigrad et al., 1999), intravenous systemic chemotherapy is necessary during pregnancy, unless the disease is discovered when the baby is of advanced gestational age, in which case, delivery followed by immediate systemic therapy may rarely be an option.

In studies by Goldstein and colleagues (1967, 1970, 1978), methotrexate, administered prophylactically at the time of uterine evacuation, decreased the likelihood of malignant sequelae. This approach has not been accepted widely because the 80% of patients who would have a spontaneous remission would be treated unnecessarily and because overall survival remains close to 100% even if treatment is delayed until hCG titers and clinical evaluations suggest persistent disease. For these reasons, prophylactic chemotherapy should no longer be considered appropriate for patients with hydatidiform mole; however, this therapeutic approach may be considered for the occasional patient who is likely to be lost to follow-up.

Data from the era prior to effective chemotherapy for these diseases in which a tissue diagnosis usually was known showed that approximately 50% of the patients with choriocarcinoma had an antecedent molar gestation; the remainder of cases were approximately evenly divided between term gestation and abortion. Because most patients requiring chemotherapy have an invasive mole, which is always preceded by hydatidiform mole, most patients undergoing therapy for GTN will have had a documented molar gestation.

Delays in diagnosis and inappropriate treatment are seen commonly in patients with GTN, especially when the initial manifestation of the malignancy results from sequelae associated with extrauterine disease. These unfortunate events often occur because of errors in interpreting biopsy findings and a low level of suspicion for this disease process by the clinician. Patients with apparent metastatic tumor sometimes undergo biopsy procedures and extensive operations when serum hCG determinations by the alert clinician with a high index of suspicion would provide the diagnosis. Metastatic tumors have been resected from the lower genital tract, the gastrointestinal tract, the liver, the lung, the brain, and other sites. Unfortunately, many of these lesions have been reported as "anaplastic tumor," compounding the problem of inappropriate surgery with further delays in diagnosis. It should be apparent that any patient of reproductive age presenting with symptoms of metastatic malignancy should have a quantitative hCG determination to rule out GTN. This approach should obviate biopsy and other surgical evaluations and permit immediate treatment.

Although the performance of a diagnostic uterine curettage has been a common practice in patients who may have persistent GTN following evaluation of a molar pregnancy, this procedure is unnecessary, is rarely helpful, and can occasionally result in uterine perforation, massive hemorrhage, and the need for a hysterectomy. It is true that if malignant trophoblastic disease is identified pathologically, the diagnosis and need for chemotherapy are confirmed, but GTN is often deep in the myometrium and unobtainable by curettage. Thus, the need for chemotherapy is not altered by either the presence or the absence of molar tissue or choriocarcinoma on subsequent uterine curettage. In many instances, patients with GTN have metastases in the absence of disease within the uterus.

Proper diagnostic evaluation of women with GTN is essential. The work-up for a diagnosis of persistent GTN should consist of the following:

History and physical examination
Chest x-ray and CT scan of lungs
Liver and brain CT scans
Liver function tests
Hematologic survey
Pretreatment hCG titer

Initial studies should include CT of the liver and brain to evaluate for metastases in these sites. We recommend a CT scan of the lungs in addition to the chest radiograph because the lungs are the most common sites of metastases in GTN, and occasionally these studies document metastases in the presence of normal chest findings. Pretreatment blood studies help to exclude factors that may influence the choice of chemotherapeutic agents. For example, patients with abnormal liver function should not be treated with methotrexate because of its potential hepatotoxicity. In addition, normal renal function is necessary when methotrexate is used, since this agent is excreted by the kidneys. A careful pelvic examination will rule out metastases to the cervix, vagina, and vulva. Once the tests have been obtained, disease can be classified and specific therapy initiated.

Nonmetastatic Trophoblastic Disease

Nonmetastatic trophoblastic disease is the most common diagnosis within the spectrum of GTN and, as expected, carries the best prognosis, with 100% of patients expected to achieve complete sustained remission. This designation is applied when the results of evaluation for metastases are negative, implying that disease is limited to the uterus.

Patients are treated with single-agent chemotherapy (Table 58-7). Both methotrexate and actinomycin D have been used successfully as single agents, with a variety of dosage schemes. Higher doses of methotrexate with folinic acid have been advocated over lower doses of methotrexate without folinic acid or actinomycin D because of the lower toxicity and comparable effectiveness. Single-agent therapy should be repeated as soon as possible, with 7 to 10 days allowed between courses. Toxicity should be monitored carefully (Table 58-8), with longer intervals between courses indicated if stomatitis or bone marrow suppression is present when the subsequent course of chemotherapy is due. The therapy should be continued until three negative weekly hCG titers are obtained.

Employing the methotrexate–folinic acid regimen, Berkowitz and colleagues (1986) reported complete remissions in 90% of 163 patients treated in this way. The remaining patients achieved complete, sustained remissions using sub-

TABLE 58-7. SINGLE-AGENT CHEMOTHERAPY FOR GESTATIONAL TROPHOBLASTIC NEOPLASIA

Agent	Dosage*
Methotrexate	20–25 mg/d IM for 5 d
Actinomycin D	10–12 µg/kg/d IV for 5 d
Methotrexate with folinic acid	1 mg/kg IM on d 1, 3, 5, and 7
	0.1 mg/kg IM on d 2, 4, 6, and 8

* Intervals of 7 to 10 days between courses, if possible, for all three modalities.
IM, intramuscularly; IV, intravenously.

From Creasy RK, Resnik R: Maternal-Fetal Medicine, 4th ed. Philadelphia, WB Saunders, 1999, p. 1138.

TABLE 58-8. MANAGEMENT OF SINGLE-AGENT CHEMOTHERAPY FOR GESTATIONAL TROPHOBLASTIC NEOPLASIA

1. Agent and dosage as listed in Table 58-7; course repeated every 7 to 10 d, depending on toxicity, until hCG titer is normal
2. Contraception begun
3. Chemotherapy postponed in presence of:
   a. Severe oral or gastrointestinal ulceration
   b. Febrile course associated with leukopenia
4. Chemotherapy repeated when:
   a. WBC count > 3000 cells/mm³
   b. Polymorphonuclear leukocyte count > 1500 cells/mm³
   c. Platelet count > 100,000 cells/mm³
   d. BUN, AST, ALT essentially normal
5. Chemotherapeutic agent changed if:
   a. hCG titer rises (twofold or more) or plateaus
   b. Evidence of new metastasis appears
6. Remission defined as three consecutive weekly titers with undetectable levels of hCG

ALT, alanine aminotransferase; AST, aspartate transaminase; BUN, blood urea nitrogen; hCG, human chorionic gonadotropin; WBC, white blood cell.

sequent treatment with actinomycin D or multiagent chemotherapy regimens.

If the hCG titer rises or plateaus after two or more courses of chemotherapy, alternative drugs should be instituted. In general, failure of either actinomycin D or methotrexate warrants switching to the other of these two drugs. If therapy with the second drug fails, the patient can still be treated successfully with intra-arterial infusion of the drug into the uterus, multiagent chemotherapy (as described later for metastatic trophoblastic neoplasia), or hysterectomy. When either hysterectomy or intra-arterial chemotherapy is contemplated, a pelvic arteriogram should be done to verify a resistant focus of tumor within the uterus. Evidence of new metastasis while the patient is being treated is also an indication for changing the chemotherapy.

Once the hCG value has returned to normal levels, appropriate follow-up with monthly hCG titers for 1 year is mandatory (Table 58-9). An effective contraceptive method must be used during this time. A patient who has remained in remission for 1 year and desires more children should be advised that childbearing may be resumed.

Low-Risk Metastatic Trophoblastic Neoplasia

Several staging systems have been proposed to classify patients with metastatic gestational neoplasm. The two most commonly used are the clinical classification of malignant

TABLE 58-9. FOLLOW-UP PROTOCOL FOR GESTATIONAL TROPHOBLASTIC NEOPLASIA AFTER SPONTANEOUS OR CHEMOTHERAPY-INDUCED REMISSION

Three consecutive normal weekly hCG assays
hCG titer determinations monthly for 12 mo; then every 6 mo
Contraception for 1 yr

hCG, human chorionic gonadotropin.

From Creasy RK, Resnik R: Maternal-Fetal Medicine, 4th ed. Philadelphia, WB Saunders, 1999, p. 1139.

gestational trophoblastic disease (Table 58-10) and the staging system proposed by the World Health Organization (Table 58-11). The World Health Organization system is more widely used and effectively categorizes patients as having high, intermediate, or low risk. The variables analyzed in this staging system are age; type of antecedent pregnancy; interval since the antecedent pregnancy; ABO grouping; history of cytotoxic therapy; and sites, number, and size of metastatic lesions. A score of 4 or lower is designated low risk.

Single-agent therapy, employing either methotrexate or actinomycin D (as described for nonmetastatic trophoblastic disease), is the treatment choice. Once a normal hCG value has been achieved, one additional course beyond the first negative reading is required. Should resistance to the initial choice of chemotherapy occur, manifested either by rising or plateauing titers or by the development of new metastasis, multiagent therapy (as described later) should be instituted.

The Southeastern Trophoblastic Center reported 55 patients with "good prognosis" metastatic GTN (Hammond et al., 1980). Thirty-five of 40 patients treated with chemotherapy alone experienced complete remission, and the remaining five, all of whom had resistant foci of disease in the uterus despite complete resolution of the metastatic disease, had a hysterectomy after drug therapy failed, with complete remissions in all cases. The other 15 patients, all of whom achieved remission, underwent chemotherapy and hysterectomy performed primarily. Thus, complete, sustained remission was achieved in all 55 patients. Many other centers have reported similar results in large numbers of patients, most of whom had presented with lung or pelvic metastases, emphasizing the appropriateness of the term "low-risk GTN."

Intermediate-Risk Metastatic Trophoblastic Neoplasia

A World Health Organization system score of 5 to 8 places the patient in the intermediate-risk treatment category. The chemotherapeutic recommendations are treatment with methotrexate, 0.3 mg/kg intramuscularly/intravenously; actinomycin D, 8 µg/kg intravenously, and either cyclophosphamide, 3 mg/kg intravenously, or chlorambucil, 0.15 mg/kg

TABLE 58-10. CLASSIFICATION OF GESTATIONAL TROPHOBLASTIC NEOPLASIA

I. **Nonmetastatic disease:** No evidence of disease outside uterus
II. **Metastatic disease:** Any disease outside uterus
   A. *Good-prognosis* metastatic disease
      1. Short duration (last pregnancy < 4 mo prior)
      2. Low pretreatment hCG titer (<100,000 IU/24-hr urine specimen or < 40,000 mIU/mL of serum)
      3. No metastasis to brain or liver
      4. No prior chemotherapy failure
   B. *Poor-prognosis* metastatic disease (Any one of the following):
      1. Long duration (last pregnancy > 4 mo previously)
      2. High pretreatment hCG titer (>100,000 IU/24-hr urine specimen or > 40,000 mIU/mL of serum)
      3. Brain or liver metastasis
      4. Failed prior chemotherapy

hCG, human chorionic gonadotropin.

Modified from Di Saia PJ, Creasman WT: Clinical Gynecologic Oncology. St. Louis, CV Mosby, 1981.

TABLE 58-11. WORLD HEALTH ORGANIZATION PROGNOSTIC INDEX SCORE FOR GESTATIONAL TROPHOBLASTIC NEOPLASIA

Prognostic Factors	0	1	2	4
Age (yr)	≤35	>35		
Antecedent pregnancy	Hydatidiform mole	Abortion term		
Interval (mo)	<4	4–6	7–12	>12
hCG (IU/liter)	<10^3	10^3–10^4	10^4–10^5	>10^5
ABO blood group type (female × male)		O × A	B	
Largest tumor (cm)		3–5	>5	
Metastatic site		Spleen, kidney	GI tract, liver	Brain
Number of metastases		1–4	4–8	>8
Previous chemotherapy			Single drug	Two or more drugs

B, blood group; GI, gastrointestinal; hCG, human chorionic gonadotropin.

Modified from Hoskins WJ, Perez CA, Young RC: Principles and Practice of Gynecologic Oncology. Philadelphia, Lippincott-Raven, 1996, p. 1056.

orally. Each agent is administered as a 5-day course every 12 to 14 days, or as bone marrow toxicity permits (Table 58-12). This regimen is administered until negative hCG titers are obtained for at least four cycles.

High-Risk Metastatic Trophoblastic Neoplasia

Disease that has been characterized as carrying a poor prognosis presents a serious challenge to the physician and medical team. Many of the patients have been treated with chemotherapy and have developed resistance to that treatment while bone marrow reserves have been depleted. Multiagent chemotherapy is recommended in this case, and a multimodality approach is essential for many patients. Patients should be treated in centers where there are teams of physicians with special interest and expertise in this problem. A health care team of physicians often includes a gynecologic oncologist (who should direct therapy), a radiation therapist, a neurologist, a neurosurgeon, a psychiatrist, a physiatrist, and others. Essential support personnel include a well-trained team of nurse oncologists and specialists in social service, physical therapy, respiratory therapy, occupational therapy, and speech therapy to deal with some of the many problems that may confront patients with this disease.

Some patients will require hospitalization for several months. Life-threatening toxicity from therapy may ensue, and in some instances patients may require specialized care, such as total parenteral nutrition, isolation, mechanical ventilation, and other life-support measures during long periods when their host defense mechanisms are depleted and their medical condition requires continued monitoring and care. The risk posed by such therapy can be markedly reduced by the administration of granulocyte colony–stimulating factors following each course of therapy.

Beginning in 1969 in several centers nationwide, patients with high-risk metastatic GTN were started on multiagent chemotherapy for primary treatment because the experience had been that high-risk patients treated initially with single-agent chemotherapy and later with multiple agents were rarely salvaged. Cerebral or hepatic metastases were treated concurrently with 2000 to 3000 cGy in 10 to 15 days to the whole brain or liver. Since 1979, with the recognition of the exceptional clinical activity of etoposide in GTN, Bagshawe's group has employed a five-drug regimen of etoposide, methotrexate, and actinomycin D (EMA) plus vincristine and cyclophosphamide (CO), alternating the two-drug and three-drug regimens weekly in the treatment of high-risk metastatic patients. Available data for this EMA/CO regimen have suggested its superiority over other regimens previously employed for these patients. Bagshawe's group has reported an 84% overall survival rate, including patients in whom prior chemotherapy had failed, and a 94% survival rate in those who had not received any previous chemotherapy (Newlands et al., 1986).

In treatment of patients with high-risk metastatic GTN, adjunctive modalities, including radiation therapy and surgery, must be considered at all times. These modalities can include hysterectomy, resection of metastatic lesions in the lungs, brain, or elsewhere, and/or irradiation of unresectable lesions.

In nonmetastatic and low-risk metastatic GTN, complete remission is considered only after three consecutive normal weekly hCG titers; however, individuals with high-risk metastatic GTN require at least four courses of chemotherapy after the first negative hCG titer. Follow-up evaluations for high-risk metastatic GTN after complete remission are the same as for nonmetastatic and low-risk metastatic GTN. Patients with liver metastases have the poorest prognosis—a success rate below 50% for metastases at this site.

TABLE 58-12. TREATMENT OF INTERMEDIATE-RISK METASTATIC GESTATIONAL TROPHOBLASTIC NEOPLASIA

Modality or Agent	Dosage
Methotrexate	20–25 mg/d IM for 5 d
Actinomycin D	10–12 μg/kg/d IV for 5 d
Chlorambucil	10 mg/day PO for 5 d
Brain or liver radiation therapy	2000–3000 cGy in 10–15 d

IM, intramuscularly; IV, intravenously; PO, orally.

From Creasy RK, Resnik R: Maternal-Fetal Medicine, 4th ed. Philadelphia, WB Saunders, 1999, p. 1140.

Adverse Effects of Chemotherapy

Most patients with GTN have been cured with chemotherapy, and many have desired future childbearing. Major concerns in this regard have included the potential for chemotherapy-induced sterility or congenital malformations in their offspring.

Rustin and associates (1984) studied these issues in 445 long-term survivors treated with chemotherapy at the Charing Cross Hospital, London. Ninety-seven percent of women who wished to conceive did so, and 86% achieved at least one live birth. In a report of 272 women from the same institution 13 years later, only 56% of such women who attempted to become pregnant were successful (Bower et al., 1997). Women who had received combination chemotherapy were less likely to have a live birth than were those treated with methotrexate alone. In addition, congenital malformations did not occur at an elevated rate in the offspring of these women compared with that expected for women of comparable age who had never received chemotherapy. The risk of second malignancies following chemotherapy in these patients is less certain. Earlier studies largely excluded this potential adverse effect from analysis. More-recent reports have suggested an increase in the incidence of second malignancies following EMA/CO used to treat high-risk metastatic GTN when compared with other chemotherapy regimens.

Bower's group (1997) reported the experience of 272 women at Charing Cross Hospital treated with the EMA/CO regimen. When these women were compared with 1394 women treated with multiagent chemotherapy, the incidence of second malignancies—specifically, myeloid leukemia, melanoma, and colon and breast cancers—was statistically higher ($P = 0.01$).

CANCER THERAPY IN PREGNANCY

Chemotherapy

Theoretically, most cytotoxic agents useful in treating malignant neoplasms are both teratogenic and mutagenic in human fetuses when administered early in pregnancy. Their use evokes complex moral and philosophical questions as well as difficult medical decisions. Both mother and fetus are at risk—the mother from the cancer and the fetus from its treatment. The use of cytotoxic drugs can result in abortion, fetal death, malformations, or growth retardation.

The long-term effect on the viable infant is unknown but requires careful study. The need for long-term observation has been emphasized dramatically with the recognition of diethylstilbestrol-related adenocarcinomas of the vagina and cervix and other congenital effects on reproductive organs that can affect subsequent fertility decades later in young women exposed in utero to this drug during the first trimester. A similarly devastating long-term effect may be found in the offspring of women treated with chemotherapeutic agents during pregnancy. The theoretical dangers to the fetus must be weighed against the possible detrimental effect of withholding these agents from the mother.

The oncologist treating pregnant women with cytotoxic agents should be aware of the many physiologic changes during pregnancy that can affect drug absorption, distribution, and excretion. The effect of pregnancy on gastrointestinal motility can markedly alter the absorption of agents taken orally. Similarly, expanded blood volume and total body water have a marked effect on drug distribution, and the increase in renal blood flow accelerates the excretion of agents eliminated by the kidneys. The complex interaction of these various physiologic changes, coupled with the infrequency of cytotoxic drug administration in pregnancy, has precluded well-conducted pharmacokinetic studies to determine appropriate dosing strategies during pregnancy. In the absence of such data, conventional treatment approaches used in nonpregnant patients are employed when these agents are administering during pregnancy.

Most available data suggesting a teratogenic and mutagenic effect of chemotherapeutic agents have been derived from experiments on gravid laboratory animals. Extrapolation of data from these experiments provides the basis for much of the concern about the potential danger to the human fetus. In addition, because all cytotoxic agents profoundly affect rapidly growing tissues and because a high rate of cell division is characteristic of fetal tissues, one would expect a high likelihood of fetal damage from these drugs. There is surprisingly little information on humans, but what does exist suggests a favorable pregnancy outcome in most instances, belying both the findings in laboratory animals and the theoretical concerns (Doll et al., 1989; Sood et al., 2001).

Unquestionably, the first trimester of pregnancy, in which organogenesis is established, is the period in which the fetus is most vulnerable to anticancer agents. Potential injury can result in either the death of the fetus or induction of abnormalities inadequate to cause fetal demise. During the second and third trimesters, organogenesis is completed but neuronal growth in the brain continues. In general, adverse effects of these drugs have not been reported when therapy has been initiated after the first trimester. Nevertheless, the potential adverse effects, especially as they relate to cortical brain function, warrant careful longitudinal investigation of these children.

Several publications that address the reported adverse effects of cytotoxic chemotherapy emphasize the risk of such therapy in the first trimester but also demonstrate that these effects are not inevitable. Sokal and Lessman (1960) reviewed 50 reports of pregnant women receiving anticancer chemotherapy. They found 8 instances of fetal abnormalities, 16 spontaneous abortions, and 7 therapeutic abortions. Although serious congenital anomalies and spontaneous abortions did occur in some patients receiving chemotherapy in the first trimester, such complications were not inevitable. No obvious fetal malformations were observed in the infants of the women who received chemotherapy after the first trimester.

Similarly, Nicholson (1968) collected 185 reports of human pregnancies during which anticancer chemotherapy was administered. Of 110 women treated during the first trimester, fetal or infant status was recorded in only 68 cases, in which there were 15 instances of fetal abnormalities. Ten of the 15 women received folic acid antagonists, 2 had taken busulfan, and 1 each had been treated with 6-mercaptopurine, chlorambucil, and cyclophosphamide. No malformations were reported in the offspring of 75 women who received chemotherapy during the second and third trimesters, although infant status was recorded in only 73 cases.

In a review of this subject by Schapira and Chudley (1984), the incidence of teratogenicity of chemotherapeutic agents given to women during the first trimester was 12.7%, representing a fivefold increase over that of the offspring of noncancer patients. These data are consistent with findings from a more recent review by Doll and coworkers (1989), in which first-trimester drug exposure in 139 reported cases resulted in 24 infants with malformations (17%). The frequency of malformations was slightly higher in fetuses exposed to antimetabolites (15 of 77 cases, or 19%, including all 3 reported cases of exposure to methotrexate) than in those exposed to alkylating agents (6 of 44 cases, or 14%). Surprisingly, exposure to combinations of cytotoxic agents did not increase the frequency of malformations in the cases reviewed in this report (7 of 45 affected newborns, or 16%).

Avileás and co-authors (1991) reported observations from 43 infants exposed *in utero* to cytotoxic agents. Nineteen were exposed to chemotherapeutic agents during the first trimester, including 6 who were exposed to doses of methotrexate lower than those typically associated with fetal malformations (120 to 250 mg total dose). The children exposed to the chemotherapeutic agents *in utero* have been observed for 3 to 19 years. No congenital or developmental anomalies have been identified when these children was compared to others of the same social and economic background.

Although the greatest effect of cytotoxic therapy in pregnancy is during the first trimester, attention must be given to the possible effects of drug administration late in pregnancy as well. Although commonly employed agents cross the placenta to the fetus, drug elimination by the fetus is accomplished through metabolism by the fetal liver, excretion by the fetal kidneys, and transplacental passage back to the mother. The role of placental excretion has not been defined, but its absence following delivery, coupled with an underdeveloped ability to metabolize or excrete the drug by the neonate, can lead to leukopenia and subsequent neutropenic sepsis as well as thrombocytopenia and risk of hemorrhage.

Reynoso and colleagues (1987), basing their work on the experience of the Toronto Leukemia Study Group, estimated that one third of fetuses exposed to chemotherapy near term will experience pancytopenia. To avoid this potential risk, the physician should withhold such agents, if possible, during the last month of pregnancy. A complete blood count should be done on the newborn, and breast-feeding is contraindicated because all of these agents can be secreted in breast milk.

Of the drugs used to treat cancers, the group most commonly associated with teratogenic effects are the folic acid antagonists. The two drugs in this group, aminopterin and methotrexate, when delivered in sufficient doses in the first trimester of pregnancy, almost invariably result in either spontaneous abortion or an abnormal fetus. The most frequent effects of exposure to these agents include delayed ossification of the bones of the calvarium (cranial dysostosis), hypertelorism, micrognathia, limb deformities, and cerebral anomalies. Speech and intelligence can be severely affected. Therefore, these drugs should not be administered during the first trimester of pregnancy unless there is an immediately life-threatening disease for which no other drugs are established to be effective. If the antifolic agent is used and the mother does not abort spontaneously, therapeutic abortion should be offered. If a therapeutic abortion is declined, fetal effects can be monitored *in utero* with serial ultrasound studies. Minimal data on the use of these drugs later in pregnancy indicate that they do not harm the fetus after the first trimester.

Although most other antitumor drugs (including 6-mercaptopurine, azathioprine, 5-fluorouracil, the alkylating agents, vinca alkaloids, and procarbazine) are teratogenic in laboratory animals, there have been few case reports of fetal abnormalities associated with the use of these agents in the first trimester of human pregnancy. The explanation for this apparent discrepancy is unclear, but the differences may result from variations in placental function between laboratory animals and humans, placental transfer of drugs, and different dosage regimens in experimental animals compared to humans. On the other hand, there have been isolated reports of fetal abnormalities with most drugs, emphasizing the importance of avoiding their use, especially in the first trimester. These findings also emphasize the importance of effective contraception to prevent pregnancy and potential fetal abnormalities in any woman of childbearing age receiving chemotherapy.

Reports of adverse effects of commonly used cytotoxic agents in the treatment of gynecologic malignancies other than GTN are limited. Thus, the effects of agents such as paclitaxel, cisplatin, carboplatin, doxorubicin, altretamine, and the topoisomerase inhibitors on the developing fetus are unknown.

The lack of observations of the long-term status of the offspring of patients treated during pregnancy prevents definite conclusions regarding the relative safety or danger of anticancer chemotherapy to viable offspring who appear normal at birth. Long-term observation is necessary to establish normality, because many defects may not be obvious on inspection and may emerge as impairments of growth, development, learning abilities, or reproductive function, carcinogenesis, or even a teratogenic effect, which may be delayed until the next generation.

A common concern to patients of reproductive age who are taking cytotoxic agents is the potential effect on subsequent reproductive capacity. Indirect evidence of the possible gonadal effects of these drugs can be found in the studies of reproduction following renal transplantation. Recipients are maintained on a regimen of immunosuppressive therapy, typically with azathioprine and prednisone, drugs with immunologic effects similar to those of many anticancer agents. The literature concerning the effects of this therapy on reproductive capacity and fetal outcome is quite optimistic. Women who become pregnant while in an immunosuppressed state appear to deliver healthy babies, barring prematurity and other obstetric problems.

Penn and coworkers (1971) reported on 19 men on immunosuppressive therapy who fathered 23 pregnancies that resulted in 1 spontaneous abortion and 19 live births, including 1 infant with a meningomyelocele. Three pregnancies had not been completed at the time of the report. Much comparable information for women receiving cytotoxic drug therapy concerns those women with a history of GTN treated with methotrexate or actinomycin D, as reported earlier.

Studies of 596 women reported by Rustin (1984), Goldstein (1984), and Bower (1997) and their colleagues show no excess of fetal malformations in the offspring of women treated previously with chemotherapy for GTN. It is unknown whether this favorable experience, found for patients treated mainly by methotrexate or actinomycin D, will carry over to those treated successfully with other agents for other types of malignancies seen in younger women, including breast and hematologic malignancies.

Effect of Chemotherapy on Ovarian Function

The effect of chemotherapy on subsequent fertility has been addressed by Byrne and co-authors (1987). These effects are usually directed against follicular growth and maturation, and patients with a depleted number of follicles are particularly susceptible to cytotoxic agents. In Byrne's review of a retrospective cohort of 2283 survivors of childhood and adolescent cancer, there was no decrease in fertility in either sex following chemotherapy with regimens that excluded alkylating agents. Therapy with alkylating agents reduced fertility in men by nearly 60% but did not affect fertility in a consistent fashion in women. The adverse effect in males results from a loss of spermatogenic function, which relates to both dose and duration of therapy. Alkylating agents in general, and especially cyclophosphamide when employed for more than 6 months in women older than 35 years of age, can also produce amenorrhea and hormonal evidence of ovarian failure. When ovarian biopsies of such women are performed, extensive fibrosis is evident; usually only a small number of ova are present, and these are inactive. This phenomenon is rarely seen in younger women or in those treated for a shorter duration.

In women with breast cancer treated with cytotoxic therapy, amenorrhea has been reported in as many as 53% who receive cyclophosphamide/methotrexate/5-fluorouracil before age 35 years, in 84% of those age 35 to 44 years, and in 94% of those older than 44 years. When ovarian failure occurs in this setting, it is permanent in 86% of women younger than 40 years and in 96% of those older than 40 years (Mehta et al., 1991). Because the prepubescent ovary is resistant to the injurious effects of chemotherapy, several investigators have tried to preserve ovarian function by pharmacologically terminating ovarian function during chemotherapy. Recent studies suggest that the combination of a gonadotropin-releasing hormone agonist given concurrently with chemotherapy may prevent chemotherapy-induced ovarian damage (Blumenfeld et al., 1996). More reports of success with this intervention are needed before definitive recommendations can be made.

Radiation Therapy

Effects on the Fetus

The primary concerns associated with radiation therapy administered during pregnancy include the effect on the fetus (risk of abortion, malformations, impaired reproductive capacity) and the effect on the maternal gonads that may contribute to reproductive difficulties in the future. Thus, the concerns about and potential adverse effects of radiation are identical to those for chemotherapy. Yet, unlike the adverse effect of chemotherapy, these occur with alarming and predictable frequency in patients undergoing radiation therapy. The embryo represents the most radiosensitive stage in human life, and radiation injury to the embryo results in marked developmental and structural anomalies. These exaggerated effects result from a combination of factors: (1) Many cells in the embryo are differentiating and are therefore highly sensitive to ionizing radiation; (2) there is a high rate of mitotic activity in the cells of the embryo, and mitosis is the most radiosensitive period in the cell cycle; and (3) if the embryonic cell is genetically altered or killed during its development, the adult form either will be functionally or structurally altered or will not survive.

The sensitivity to ionizing radiation of different tissues within the human embryo varies markedly. In addition, the adverse effects vary with both duration of gestation and dose of radiation. Of the abnormalities attributed to radiation of the embryo, microcephaly and associated central nervous system conditions have been reported most frequently. Other abnormalities most frequently encountered in surviving children include microphthalmos, cataracts, pigmentary degeneration of the retina, and skeletal and genital tract anomalies. Mental retardation and stunted growth are also frequent sequelae. Experimental studies confirm that fetal anomalies consistently result from a dose of 200 to 300 cGy delivered during the first trimester of pregnancy. An accurate prediction of the incidence of specific anomalies for a given dose of radiation has not been possible.

The fetus is most sensitive to ionizing radiation between days 11 and 56 (Rugh, 1971; Hicks and D'Amato, 1996); after day 56, however, primary organ systems have developed and much larger doses of x-rays or gamma rays are necessary to produce serious abnormalities (United Nations Scientific Committee on the Effects of Atomic Radiation, 1986; International Commission on Radiological Protection, 1990). Therefore, there are three periods of embryogenesis during which similar amounts of radiation can have markedly different radiobiological effects:

1. *Preimplantation and early implantation (days 0 to 10):* In this phase, radiation produces an all-or-none effect, in that it either destroys the embryo or has no apparent adverse effect.
2. *Organ system formation (days 11 to 56):* During this period, radiation exposure often causes visceral organ or somatic damage (Brent, 1977; Donagi and Lesser, 1977). Microcephaly, anencephaly, eye damage, growth retardation, spina bifida, and foot damage have been reported with exposure to 4 cGy or less, doses of ionizing radiation often delivered by a barium enema or intravenous pyelogram. Although cause and effect have not been proved with these lower doses, it is believed that doses as low as 10 cGy can result in a measurable increase in fetal anomalies and that doses of 100 cGy or more during this crucial phase of fetal development result in anomalies in all surviving children, according to observations in survivors of the atomic bombs in Hiroshima and Nagasaki (Jablon and Kato, 1970; Miller and Mulvihill, 1976).
3. *After day 56:* After organ system formation is complete, larger doses are required to produce external malformations. At this time, the nervous system is especially vulnerable to injury, and doses above 50 cGy can produce mental retardation and microcephaly, even in the second trimester. These effects have been reported as late as 20 weeks of gestation; after this time, however, a surviving child is not likely to exhibit overt abnormalities. Some infants exposed late in pregnancy do exhibit skin erythema, abnormal pigmentation, epilation, or hematologic deficiencies.

Radiography

Because the developing fetus can be exquisitely sensitive to ionizing radiation and because there is no threshold dose of radiation below which the fetus cannot be harmed, diagnostic radiologic procedures should be avoided during the first and second trimesters of pregnancy (Stewart and Webb, 1956; Bureau of Radiological Health, 1973; National Council on Radiation Protection, 1977b; Baker and Vandergrift, 1979). The exposure to the fetus and maternal gonads varies with the procedure performed and the precautions taken. A chest x-ray results in an exposure of 0.5 mrem per plate to the chest and a much lower exposure to the pelvic structures. The pelvic dose can be negligible if the patient wears a lead apron. On the other hand, procedures in which multiple x-rays of the pelvis are taken during pregnancy, such as a barium enema, intravenous pyelogram, or x-ray pelvimetry, are of special concern because there is evidence that an exposure of only 3 to 5 cGy may result in an increase in benign or malignant tumors in the child. For example, pelvimetry at term has been associated with an increased risk of childhood leukemia in exposed offspring.

As can be seen in Table 58-13, the dose to the fetus is almost always lower than 1 cGy for radiological examinations outside the abdominal region, and the risk of damage at such low levels is negligible. For pelvic and lower abdominal x-rays, the dose to the fetus is rarely above 5 cGy. Fenig and colleagues (2001) emphasize that only very rarely, if at all, will the level of fetal irradiation in diagnostic radiology justify the termination of pregnancy. It will be necessary to calculate or measure the level of radiation only when women have undergone multiple x-ray examinations in which the fetus is directly exposed to radiation, or when both radiographic and fluoroscopic examinations have been performed (Feige and Kahan, 1976). If the level is found to be greater than 5 to 10 cGy, abortion should be considered (Hamer-Jacobsen, 1959; National Council on Radiation Protection, 1977a).

A very important part of staging in cervical cancer involves determining whether hydronephrosis exists. This is due to ureteral obstruction by the tumor and can be studied using "one shot" intravenous pyelography or a limited computed axial tomography study with contrast material. Each of these procedures places the fetus at minimal risk of exposure to ionizing radiation. Many centers use ultrasonography in pregnant women to rule out hydronephrosis, avoiding all radiation exposure; this modality or magnetic resonance imaging may be substituted for an intravenous pyelography or CT scan.

Radionuclides

Radiation may reach the fetus in pregnant women undergoing radionuclide examinations (e.g., bone scans, ventilation-perfusion studies) via penetrating gamma rays emitted by the radionuclide concentrated in the maternal organs or in the placenta. Additionally, the fetus may take up radionuclides once they have crossed the placenta. The amount of time radioactive atoms remain in the body depends upon the physical half-life of the isotope, its rate of excretion, and its biological half-life. Most nuclear diagnostic examinations will result in a fetal dose of less than 1 cGy.

An important isotope to consider is iodine-131, which may be administered in therapeutic doses to pregnant women with medullary carcinoma of the thyroid, Graves disease, or other forms of thyrotoxicosis. The level of fetal thyroid irradiation in these cases will be a function of the amount of radioactive material crossing the placenta, the degree of uptake by the fetal thyroid itself, and the period when the radioactive iodine is given, keeping in mind that the normal period for the onset of thyroid function is between 10 weeks' and 12 weeks' gestational age. To date, there has been one reported case of cretinism in an infant exposed to iodine-131 in utero.

The use of radiation in pregnancy-associated breast and cervical cancer is described elsewhere in this chapter, and although leukemia and lymphoma are discussed in Chapter 47, we will use Hodgkin's disease in this section to illustrate the use of therapeutic radiation in pregnancy (Becker and Hyman, 1965; Becker, 1968; Thomas and Peckham, 1976; Conley and Jacobson et al., 1977; Jacobs, 1982; Tawil et al., 1983; Nisce et al., 1986). It should be emphasized that the incidence of Hodgkin's disease peaks during the reproductive years, and the condition can be found associated with pregnancy once in every 1000 to 6000 deliveries. Because the disease often presents with supradiaphragmatic lymphadenopathy, radiotherapy is often clinically indicated, and its use during pregnancy has been extensively investigated (Wong et al., 1985). For example, in a presentation of 16 pregnant women (6 to 32 weeks' gestation) with supradiaphragmatic Hodgkin's disease, Woo and colleagues (1992) noted that definitive radiotherapy was employed using the mantle field technique and a lead shield over the uterus. The estimated dose to the mid-fetus ranged from 1.4 cGy to 5.5 cGy with 6 MV photons and 10 cGy to 13.6 cGy for cobalt-60. All 16 babies were delivered at term, without gross malformations or growth restriction; subsequent follow-up disclosed no developmental delays or childhood malignancies.

There has been a recent trend toward using combination chemotherapy with lower-dose, lower-volume radiation fields to treat the early stages of Hodgkin's disease. Such an approach in pregnant women will also reduce the dose absorbed by the fetus.

TABLE 58-13. ESTIMATED AVERAGE DOSE TO FETUS PER RADIOGRAPHIC EXAMINATION

Radiographic Examination	cGy*
Dental	0.00006
Head	<0.0005
Cervical spine	<0.0005
Extremities	<0.0005
Shoulder	0.0005
Thoracic spine	0.0110
Chest	0.0005
Mammography	<0.010
Upper gastrointestinal series	0.170
Femur (distal)	0.001
Lumbar spine	0.720
Pelvis	0.210
Hip and femur (proximal)	0.120
Intravenous pyelography	0.590
Cystography	1.500
Barium enema	0.900
Abdomen	0.220
Pelvimetry	1.270

* For purposes of this discussion, 1 rad = 1 rem = 1000 millirem = 1 cGy. (Note: The rem is the old unit of dose equivalent and is the product of the absorbed dose in rads and modifying factors; the rem is being replaced by the sievert (Sv) in the SI system.)

Modified from Fenig E, Mishaeli M, Kalish Y, et al: Pregnancy and radiation. Cancer Treat Rev **27**:1, 2001.

Effects on Ovarian Function

The adverse effects of radiation on the human gonads include both genetic damage, which can be transmitted from generation to generation, and sterility (Sharma et al., 1981; Byrne et al., 1987; Hall, 1994). As additional clinical and theoretical data are accumulated, frequent changes are made in what is considered the permissible cumulative body dose of radiation. Current maximal dose recommendations range from 10 cGy to 14 cGy during the first 30 years of life. This includes ionizing radiation from both medical and background sources. The tolerance of normal organs to radiation is often described by the dose at which 5% of patients will experience organ-specific toxicity 5 years after exposure (Table 58-14).

The ovaries are exquisitely sensitive to the effects of radiotherapy. The initial targets of ionizing radiation are the dividing granulosa cells that line the developing follicles. With the destruction of these cells, oocytes lose viability and the follicles become atrophic. The dose of radiation to the ovaries required to produce complete and permanent sterility varies with age at the time of radiotherapy or, more precisely, with the number of remaining oocytes. The range of doses fits nicely with the "target theory" of radiation effect, which postulates that the dose that produces total cell kill in any population is proportional to the total number of cells that must be destroyed.

The threshold values for permanent and temporary sterility have not been defined clearly. In women 40 years of age and older, 600 cGy can induce menopause. Adolescent girls treated with 2000 cGy fractionated over 5 to 6 weeks have a 95% likelihood of permanent sterility. With conventional therapeutic doses of radiation, any field that includes the ovaries will cause sterility. This is the case with the standard inverted Y field used in the treatment of Hodgkin's disease. In an effort to prevent this effect in young women with Hodgkin's disease who may desire subsequent childbearing, oophoropexy or surgical movement of the ovaries out of the treatment field is performed at the time of staging laparotomy. During this procedure, the ovaries can be displaced either laterally beyond the planned radiation field or medially behind the uterus, where they are shielded during treatment.

When the ovaries are transposed laterally, the ovarian exposure to radiation is typically 4% to 5% of the total pelvic dose. Feeney and co-workers (1995) reported the Indiana

University Medical Center experience of 132 cervical cancer patients who underwent lateral ovarian transposition. Among the patients who received no adjuvant therapy, 3% had menopausal complaints within 4 years of surgery. Levels of follicle-stimulating hormone in these patients did not consistently corroborate their subjective complaints. Of women who received adjuvant radiotherapy, 50% experienced menopausal symptoms associated with elevated levels of follicle-stimulating hormone during treatment or within 2 years of radiotherapy.

The experience reported by Anderson and colleagues (1993) was even more marked than that of the Feeney study. This group reported that only 33% of patients with transposed ovaries who received radiation therapy retained ovarian function. Only 67% of the women with transposed ovaries who did not receive radiation retained ovarian function at a median follow-up of 75 months. In contrast, extrapelvic irradiation does not contribute to ovarian failure, as the radiation exposure to the ovaries is typically quite low.

Radiation-Induced Carcinogenesis

As described above, the gonads are among the most radiosensitive organs in the human body. For this reason, subfertility and infertility become important issues in women and are age- and dose-dependent and a function of the radiation fields employed. Even if fertility is preserved, however, there is concern regarding the induction of germ-line mutations and chromosomal aberrations that could result not only in birth defects but also in neoplasms in the offspring (Monson and MacMahon, 1984).

Based on animal experiments, the estimated dose of gonadal radiation required to produce a mutation rate equal to the baseline spontaneous lifetime rate in humans is between 100 cGy and 150 cGy. It is estimated that 1 cGy produces five mutations for every 1 million genes exposed. Fortunately, most mutants are recessive, and many are not harmful. Mutant effects are not seen in the first generation and may not be visible for many generations, until two people with the same mutation mate. Most estimates of genetic damage are empirical, but approximately 25 cGy to 150 cGy must be given from birth to the end of reproductive age to double the rate of spontaneous gene mutations.

Fenig and colleagues (2001) illustrated the importance of gaining a proper perspective on the issue, since natural radiation must also be taken into consideration. Humans are exposed to cosmic radiation throughout the world. For example, the natural uranium content of the soil is very high in the Rocky Mountain areas of Colorado, New Mexico, and Utah. In addition, the attenuation of cosmic radiation by the atmosphere is diminished by the high altitudes, and as a result, the annual level of radiation exposure per person exceeds that in other areas of the United States by 100 mrem. A fetus whose mother lives in Colorado will receive a surplus of 85 mrem during the 9 months of pregnancy, equivalent to 150 chest x-rays or 1250 dental radiographs! Interestingly, the incidence of cancer in Colorado is actually about 35% below the national average. This observation is replicated in some regions of India and China, where background radiation is up to 2000 mrem per year, but no increase in radiation-induced morbidity has been documented.

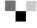

TABLE 58-14. NORMAL ORGAN TOLERANCE TO RADIOTHERAPY

Organ	TD$_{5/5}$* (cGy)
Uterine corpus/cervix	20,000–30,000
Upper vagina	20,000
Lower vagina	20,000
Ovary	Single dose: 650–800
	Fractionated: 1500–2000
Bladder	7000
Ureter	7500
Rectosigmoid colon	6000
Rectovaginal septum	6000
Brain	5000
Stomach	4500
Spinal cord	4500
Small intestine	4000
Liver	2500
Kidney	2000
Lung	2500
Bone marrow	2550
Fetus	200

* Dose that yields 5% radiotoxicity at 5 years.

NONPELVIC MALIGNANCIES IN PREGNANCY

Malignant Melanoma in Pregnancy

As the eighth most common cancer, malignant melanoma is responsible for nearly 1 of every 50 cancer deaths in the United States. There are many myths that have developed regarding the interrelationship of melanoma with pregnancy (Katz et al., 2002), including (1) pregnancy increases the risk of developing melanoma; (2) pregnancy worsens the prognosis; (3) future pregnancies have an adverse effect both on prognosis and on recurrence; and (4) women who have had melanoma should not take oral contraceptives or hormone-replacement therapy because of the theoretical effect of hormones on melanocytes. It is noteworthy that the medical literature does not support these beliefs.

Background on Nevi and Melanoma

All melanomas masquerade as nevi prior to their diagnosis, indicating a possible role for their prophylactic removal in childhood. Unfortunately, about 15 to 20 nevi are present on each individual, and removal of each lesion is thus impractical. Nevertheless, nevi at greatest risk for malignant degeneration, including those on the feet, palms, genitals, and areas of persistent irritation from clothing, should be removed when discovered. Pigmented lesions with irregular borders or surface contour and those that have undergone enlargement or a color change must be excised to rule out the presence of a melanoma. Variations in the color of a lesion should lead the clinician to suspect melanoma. Shades of red or pink suggest inflammation, whereas a bluish hue may result from pigmented cells within the dermis; both conditions suggest a malignant diagnosis. A policy of waiting and watching a suspected pigmented lesion may be detrimental, since early excision of a melanoma often is life-saving.

There are five main types of malignant melanoma. The most common is the superficial spreading melanoma, which accounts for 70% to 75% and tends toward horizontal growth prior to becoming invasive. Approximately 15% of melanomas are nodular and become invasive early. In sun-damaged areas, a lentigo maligna may develop, and in darker-skinned persons, the acral-lentiginous melanoma can be found on palms and soles. Finally, the least common are the amelanotic melanomas, which are difficult to diagnose.

Treatment of melanomas is related to depth and stage (Table 58-15). Lesions less than 1 mm in thickness usually require a 1-cm margin of excision, whereas those between 1 mm and 4 mm need a 2-cm margin. Sentinel lymph node identification and evaluation is indicated for lesions penetrating beyond 1 mm. A wide excision is curative for stage I lesions. The role of alpha interferon for stage II and stage III disease is currently under investigation.

Malignant Melanoma in Pregnancy

Levels of melanocyte-stimulating hormone, produced by the pituitary gland, increase after the 2nd month of pregnancy, suggesting that hormonal secretions during pregnancy may indirectly stimulate the growth of these tumors. Pregnancy is also associated with increased production of adrenocorticotropic hormone, resulting in heightened intrinsic melanocyte-stimulating hormone activity. Thus, increased pigmentation is characteristic of pregnancy, occurring in the nipple, vulva, linea nigra, and on occasion, preexisting nevi. In addition, estrogens, which are produced in enormous quantities during pregnancy, have been shown to control melanocyte activity in the guinea pig. Despite these observations and theoretical concerns, no studies have demonstrated a therapeutic benefit of abortion, delivery, or oophorectomy.

Approximately one third of women with melanomas are of childbearing age, and melanomas account for 8% of cancers in pregnancy. A number of studies have addressed the impact of pregnancy on prognosis of malignant melanoma (Pack and Scharnagel, 1951). In 1960, George and colleagues reported on 115 pregnant patients and compared them to 330 nonpregnant controls. Although no differences were found in 5- or 10-year survival rate, the two groups of patients were not controlled for level or stage of disease. White and colleagues (1961) reported a study of 71 women between 15 and 30 years of age with melanomas; 30 of the women were pregnant. The 5-year survival rate in the pregnant patients was 73%, but the rate in the nonpregnant patients was 53%. The authors concluded that differences in survival between the two groups were not significant. In 1985, Reintgen and coworkers reported the first case-control study; 58 pregnant women were matched with 585 nonpregnant women at the same stage of disease. There was no difference in survival between the two groups. Separate investigations by McNanamny and colleagues (1989), Wong and colleagues (1989), and Slingluff and coworkers (1990) used comparison groups that controlled for

TABLE 58-15. MALIGNANT MELANOMA: THE CLARK, BRESLOW, AND CHUNG MICROSTAGING CLASSIFICATION SYSTEMS

Microstaging Level	Clark et al., 1969	Breslow et al., 1970	Chung et al., 1975
Level I	All tumor cells above basement membrane (*in situ*)	<0.75 mm depth of invasion	Intraepithelial
Level II	Tumor extends to papillary dermis	0.76–1.5 mm depth of invasion	<1 mm invasion into dermis or lamina propria
Level III	Tumor extends to interface between papillary and reticular dermis	1.51–2.25 mm depth of invasion	1 to 2 mm invasion into subepithelial tissue
Level IV	Tumor extends between bundles of collagen of reticular dermis	2.26–3.0 mm depth of invasion	>2 mm invasion into fibrous or fibromuscular tissue
Level V	Tumor invasion of subcutaneous tissue	>3 mm depth of invasion	Extension into subcutaneous fat

tumor thickness, differentiation, and stage and found no difference in survival or disease-free intervals based on pregnancy status.

Grin and co-authors (1996) reviewed five well-controlled case studies involving a total of 427 women with a diagnosis of malignant melanoma, the majority of whom had stage I disease. No adverse effects of pregnancy on overall survival were seen in any of these studies; however, among women whose melanoma recurred, there was a reduced disease-free survival in the pregnant women reported in three of the studies.

The cumulative retrospective case-controlled studies have involved over 450 pregnant women with malignant melanoma. The anatomic location of the primary tumor does not differ between pregnant and nonpregnant women, and no analysis has identified any differences in survival between the two groups. Multivariate analyses have been performed and have revealed that the stage of disease at diagnosis, not the pregnancy, is the only consistent finding that influences prognosis (Borden, 2000). Thus, we conclude that pregnancy does not confer a worse prognosis for this diagnosis when patients are matched for stage of disease.

Epidemiologic evidence has never substantiated the claim that recurrence of melanoma is hastened in patients who become pregnant. The frequent recommendation that women delay conception for 2 years after treatment for malignant melanoma is based mainly on the time during which recurrences are most likely to be identified. Only two case-control studies have examined this potential adverse interaction (Reintgen et al., 1985; MacKie et al., 1991). These authors were unable to identify any difference in disease-free survival or overall survival in the women with stage I melanoma who became pregnant within 5 years of diagnosis of this malignancy.

Finally, melanomas do not have estrogen receptors. A large Danish case-control trial showed, as might therefore be expected, that melanomas are unaffected by the use of hormones, either in birth control pills or in estrogen-replacement therapy (Osterlind et al., 1988).

Some reports in the literature suggest that malignant melanomas are thicker in pregnant than in nonpregnant women, a finding that itself confers a poor prognosis (Travers et al., 1995). This finding might be explained by longer delays in diagnosis of malignant melanoma during pregnancy because of the hyperpigmentation commonly associated with pregnancy. It is essential that all physicians and midwives conduct a full examination of the skin of their patients. A changing skin lesion should be subjected to an excisional biopsy. Early diagnosis of stage I disease will often lead to curative therapy.

The reported low incidence of tumor metastases to the products of conception is probably due to a number of factors, including the unexplained resistance of the placenta to invasion of maternal cancer that has been demonstrated in many animal studies. Metastasis of maternal cancer to the products of conception is rare despite the sizable number of pregnancies at risk. In a comprehensive review of the subject by Dildy and co-authors (1989), only 53 cases of malignancy metastatic to the products of conception, including 12 that metastasized to the fetus, were reported between 1866 and 1987. Although melanoma accounts for only 8% of cancers associated with pregnancy, 30% of all tumors metastasizing to the placenta and more than half metastasizing to the fetus are melanomas. In contrast, breast and cervix combined accounted for more than 50% of the cases in pregnant women; however, only eight cases

have been reported involving spread to the products of conception; none of them involved the fetus.

Breast Cancer

Pregnancy-associated breast cancer (PABC) is generally defined as cancer diagnosed during pregnancy, up to 1 year following delivery, or at any time while the mother is lactating. Breast cancer is uncommon in women under 35 years of age. However, because of the increasing numbers of women delaying childbearing until later in their reproductive years, when breast cancer is found more frequently, breast cancer has become one of the more common malignancies to complicate pregnancy, with an incidence of approximately 1 case per 3000 pregnancies (National Cancer Institute, 2002). Importantly, the first-birth rate for women aged 30 to 34 years has increased from 53.4 per 1000 in 1975 to 92.1 per 1000 in 1997. Furthermore, the first-birth rate for women in the United States aged 35 to 39 years increased from 36.1 per 1000 in 1990 to 44.5 per 1000 in 1997 (Smith et al., 2001). Finally, since 1984, the first-birth rate for women in their 40s has continued to rise (Sondik et al., 2002). The average age of patients with PABC is between 32 and 38 years.

The risk is increased in certain families, with the overall risk doubling in women whose mothers or sisters have had the disease. Risk factors appear to be cumulative; women with multiple risk factors (early menarche, previous benign or premalignant breast disease, and either nulliparity or initial pregnancy after age 34) are more likely to be affected by breast cancer than are those without these factors. For example, the risk in daughters of women who had bilateral breast cancer premenopausally is increased ninefold over women without such a family history. The greatest risk in these offspring occurs during the premenopausal period. These data have led some investigators to advocate prophylactic subcutaneous mastectomy in women at greatest risk for this disease.

BRCA1/BRCA2

Epidemiologic data suggest that having a first pregnancy at a young age decreases a woman's risk of breast cancer; however, women who are carriers of BRCA1 or BRCA2 mutations may not be so protected. Surprisingly, Jernstrom and colleagues (1999) found that parous women with BRCA1 or BRCA2 mutations were significantly more likely to develop breast cancer by age 40 than were nulliparous mutation carriers. In evaluating the relative risk of breast cancer among BRCA carriers, Johannsson and coworkers (1999) noted that the incidence of PABC was higher in women with BRCA1 mutations than in those with BRCA2 mutations. Because these data come from limited population–specific analyses, firm conclusions regarding the risk of PABC among carriers of BRCA1 or BRCA2 mutations cannot be made.

Hormonal Issues

The massive endogenous hormonal production in pregnancy has often been assumed to influence the course of breast cancer adversely. The striking rise in estrogen production during pregnancy has been of sufficient concern that many physicians have considered termination of pregnancy to be an important therapeutic objective, and avoidance of further pregnancies a principle of continuing care. It is still unknown whether the stimulatory effect of increased estrogen production has an adverse effect on prognosis or whether the disproportionate rise of estriol, a relatively weak estrogen, confers some measure of protection.

In many instances, hormonal dependence of these tumors cannot be demonstrated (Clavel-Chapelon, 2002; Mogren et al., 2002). Indeed, some studies have reported estrogen receptor positivity in fewer than 25% of breast cancers associated with pregnancy. Two theories have been advanced to account for these observations: saturation of estrogen receptors as a consequence of high levels of circulating estrogen during pregnancy, and downregulation of estrogen receptors and progesterone receptors at the tumor level secondary to the high levels of circulating estrogens. Because the steroid hormones would then occupy cytoplasmic receptors, none would be available for ligand-binding assays, thus producing a false-negative result.

Accurate determination of hormone receptor status is essential for successful therapy, because, as in breast cancer not associated with pregnancy, the estrogen receptor status and the progesterone receptor status of the primary tumor determines whether antiestrogen therapy is warranted. Although there are no reported trials of tamoxifen or aromatase inhibitors in pregnant women, it is acknowledged that tamoxifen is an antiestrogen and can cause vaginal bleeding, spontaneous abortions, birth defects, and fetal death. In fact, we reported the teratogenic effects of tamoxifen use during pregnancy for an inflammatory breast carcinoma; the 46 XX child was born with labial fusion and clitoromegaly (Tewari, Bonebrake, et al., 1997). Treatment with tamoxifen or aromatase inhibitors should be delayed until the completion of pregnancy to avoid the potential adverse fetal effects.

Additional hormonal substances secreted in increased quantities during pregnancy that may influence neoplastic growths in the breast include the glucocorticoids and prolactin. Because glucocorticoids can reduce cellular immunity and perhaps promote the implantation and growth of malignant neoplasms, their increased production has grave clinical implications for the patient with breast cancer. Similarly, elevated quantities of prolactin produced by the hypophysis, and of human placental lactogen, by the placenta, late in pregnancy and during milk production, may affect breast cancer adversely. Although prolactin promotes the growth of dimethyleneanthracene-induced mammary tumors in mice, its role in humans is unknown and is currently being studied. Prolactin suppression with either ergot compounds or L-dopa has not proved to be of therapeutic value, yet the observation that women with bone pain from metastatic breast cancer sometimes obtain relief from prolactin suppression implicates prolactin as a possible promoter of breast cancer in humans.

Diagnosis

Pregnant women tend to present with a larger primary tumor and a higher incidence of positive lymph nodes than do nonpregnant patients. The prognosis is poorer in pregnant women because regional lymph node metastases are typically present and are frequently associated with occult distant metastases (White, 1954; Guinee et al., 1994; Merkel, 1996; Shousha, 2000). Conversely, patients with negative nodes in pregnancy have a prognosis similar to that for nonpregnant patients with early-stage disease.

The more advanced stage of disease in most pregnant patients has been attributed to multiple factors. First and foremost, the breast engorgement that occurs in pregnancy can delay the diagnosis by obscuring a mass for many months. Second, breast cancer is more difficult to palpate or visualize radiographically in the young premenopausal patient than in the postmenopausal woman in whom normal breast tissue has been largely replaced by fatty tissue. In addition, the increased vascularity and lymphatic drainage from the breast in pregnancy theoretically may assist the metastatic process. Rarely, a pregnant woman may present with metastatic carcinoma in the absence of a known primary lesion. In such instances, breast cancer should be suspected because it is the most common tumor presenting in this fashion during pregnancy.

The obstetrician, more than any other physician, has the opportunity to detect breast cancer early in pregnancy through regular examinations and indirectly by educating patients in self-examination. Needle aspiration of masses or ultrasound can distinguish a cyst or galactocele from a solid tumor; if bloody fluid is obtained, it should be examined cytologically, with core needle or excision biopsy indicated to make a definitive diagnosis. Fine needle–aspiration cytology of solid masses, with a reported sensitivity and specificity approaching 95% in some studies, also can be considered (Bottles and Taylor, 1985). Other investigators report similar specificities but with sensitivities as low as 50% to 66% for fine needle aspiration in pregnancy. Core needle biopsy with stereotactic guidance or excision biopsy should be done in masses from which fluid cannot be aspirated and from suspected masses in which fine needle–aspiration cytology is nondiagnostic. The risk of a breast biopsy to the mother and the fetus is small. Unfortunately, mammography is seldom useful during pregnancy because of the great radiographic density of the breast. Even in nonpregnant women under age 35 years with a palpable malignant breast mass, mammography findings are negative in most instances.

The histopathology of breast cancers in pregnant women is similar to that reported in age-matched nonpregnant controls. Even inflammatory carcinoma, once thought to occur more frequently in pregnancy, occurs with equal frequency in these two patient populations—approximately 1.5% to 4% of cases.

Staging of breast cancer currently conforms to a complicated system recommended jointly by the International Union Against Cancer and the American Joint Committee on Cancer Staging. The Haagensen clinical staging classification for breast cancer is more descriptive, however, because it accounts for the clinical prognostic indicators in this disease process (Table 58-16).

Role of Pregnancy Termination in Management

Although many clinicians believe that localized breast cancer in the first trimester is a valid reason to recommend pregnancy termination, the presence of a fetus does not compromise proper surgical management. More importantly, the belief that abortion improves survival have been refuted by a number of published case series that do not support this hypothesis. Interestingly, Gwyn and Theriault (2001) have published data suggesting that pregnant women who terminate their pregnancies may actually have decreased survival. Thus, pregnancy termination is not an essential component of effective treatment of early disease, despite the theoretical advantage of removing the source of massive estrogen production.

TABLE 58-16. HAAGENSEN CLINICAL CLASSIFICATION FOR STAGING OF BREAST CARCINOMA

Stage A	1.	No clinically involved axillary nodes
	2.	No edema or ulceration of skin, tumor not solidly fixed to chest wall
Stage B	1.	Clinically involved movable axillary nodes <2.5 cm in transverse diameter
	2.	No edema or ulceration of skin, tumor not solidly fixed to chest wall
Stage C		Any one of five grave signs of advanced breast carcinoma
	1.	Edema of skin of limited extent involving less than one third of the skin over the breast
	2.	Ulceration of skin
	3.	Solid fixation of tumor to chest wall
	4.	Axillary lymph nodes ≥ 2.5 cm in transverse diameter
	5.	Fixation of axillary nodes to overlying skin or deeper structures of axilla
Stage D		All other patients with more advanced breast carcinoma, including:
	1.	A combination of any two or more of the five grave signs listed under Stage C
	2.	Extensive edema of skin (involving more than one third of the skin over the breast)
	3.	Satellite skin nodules
	4.	The inflammatory type of carcinoma
	5.	Clinically involved supraclavicular lymph nodes
	6.	Internal mammary metastases as evidenced by a parasternal tumor
	7.	Edema of the arm
	8.	Distant metastases

From Haagensen CD, Bodian C, Haagensen DE Jr: Breast Carcinoma: Risk and Detection. Philadelphia, WB Saunders, 1981.

The relatively infrequent responsiveness to oophorectomy in patients who develop cancers while pregnant suggests that these tumors are frequently receptor-negative. In this situation, the pregnant patient with advanced disease may elect to undergo primary chemotherapy without hormonal ablation by abortion plus castration. As will be discussed later, after the first trimester, the apparent risks of chemotherapy to the fetus are small, and pregnancy can be allowed to proceed.

In contrast, in advanced breast cancer when tumor tissue is estrogen receptor–positive, pregnancy termination is usually necessary for effective palliation. Surgical castration is the usual step in managing women with disseminated mammary cancer, and castration would be useless unless accompanied by pregnancy termination to remove the placental source of hormones. When the pregnancy enters the third trimester, the decision for premature delivery depends heavily on the patient's wishes and the urgency of treatment. A short wait until the fetus is viable may not be accompanied by significant progress of the neoplasm. Continued gestation represents no threat to the fetus, because the risk that cancer will traverse the placenta and metastasize to the fetus is negligible.

Surgical Management

Of patients with breast cancer, 1% to 2% are pregnant when the diagnosis is made; this finding constitutes a difficult challenge to the physician in counseling and treating the patient. The best evidence indicates that pregnancy does not augment the rate of growth or spread of breast cancer and that abortion does not improve the prognosis. If the pregnancy is to be allowed to continue, initial treatment is usually surgical and can consist of radical, modified radical, or simple mastectomy, depending on the extent of disease and the histologic type of tumor. Lumpectomy and quadrantectomy are rarely employed, because the lesions are typically large and with less well-defined clinical margins than in nonpregnant patients. The more extensive operations are tolerated well during pregnancy, and the results of treatment are much the same, stage for stage, as in the nonpregnant state. If a cancer is detected early, is smaller than 2 cm in diameter, is well differentiated, and has not metastasized to regional lymph nodes, the chance of survival is similar to that seen in the nonpregnant patient—between 70% and 80%. Unfortunately, such a presentation in pregnancy is unusual for reasons stated previously. If, however, there is involvement of the subareolar region, inflammatory carcinoma, edema or ulceration of the skin, fixation of the tumor to the chest wall, or involvement of axillary, supraclavicular, or internal mammary lymph nodes, the prognosis is poor.

Optimal treatment of breast cancer during pregnancy is confusing because of a lack of controlled studies evaluating survival of comparable patients in different treatment groups (Keleher et al., 2002). Most studies report small numbers of patients undergoing varying treatment plans in a nonrandomized fashion. Most authorities recommend a radical or modified radical mastectomy without delay in patients with stage I or stage II and some stage III disease. The extent of surgery in treating advanced breast cancer remains a subject of extensive debate throughout the world (Kuerer et al., 1998, 2002).

The timing of surgery for breast cancer diagnosed late in pregnancy is also controversial (Nettleton et al., 1996). Some reports suggest that patients treated after delivery have better cure rates than do those treated in the second and third trimesters. This observation suggests that postponement of therapy for patients near term may be of benefit; however, selection bias probably accounts for survival differences among these retrospective reports. Delays in definitive therapy may have occurred more often for the women with a better prognosis, with immediate treatment carried out more frequently in patients with more extensive disease and a less favorable prognosis. If such treatment bias exists, prompt treatment would not be expected to correlate with good results, and treatment after delivery would appear to be better, owing to a preponderance of favorable cases in the second group.

Pregnancy Following Breast Conservation Therapy

The modified radical mastectomy avoids the inherent risk of radiation exposure to the fetus required for women treated with breast conservation therapy. Reconstruction should be delayed until after delivery, because significant distortion of autologous flaps may result from the enlarging uterus (Parodi et al., 2001).

Breast conservation therapy consists of a lumpectomy and axillary lymph node dissection followed by a 6-week course of radiotherapy to the chest wall. Because of the risk to the fetus, this method is contraindicated, especially when the diagnosis is made in the first or early second trimester.

Sentinel Node Identification

Sentinel lymph node biopsy is replacing axillary lymphadenectomy for women with breast cancer in many centers but has not yet been incorporated into the management of pregnant women with breast cancer (Giuliano et al., 1994). The methods employed to assist in the identification of the sentinel node include the radioisotope technetium-99m and the dye isosulfan blue. Fetal exposure to radiation, if employed during pregnancy, would be very low, because the dose to the breast with technetium-99m is only 500 to 1000 uCi. Lymphazurine is a category C drug and has not been tested in pregnant animals or humans.

Radiotherapy

Despite the trend toward limited surgery combined with radiotherapy for breast conservation, this approach should not be employed in pregnancy, because the dose to the fetus from radiation scatter would be unacceptably high. Embryos in the first 8 weeks of organogenesis are most susceptible to the teratogenic effects of radiation. It has been estimated that the dose of radiation to the true pelvis may amount to 0.1% to 0.3% of the total dose administered to the maternal breast or chest wall, approximately 5 to 15 cGy for a typical breast treatment course of 5000 cGy. The internal scatter of radiation is a function of the distance of the fetus from the central beam (Ngu et al., 1992; Van der Giessen, 1997; Antypas et al., 1998; Kouvaris et al, 2000). Toward the end of pregnancy, the larger fetus could receive up to 200 cGy as the fundus of the uterus extends into the upper abdomen. Although congenital anomalies are rare with advancing gestation, mental retardation and an enhanced lifetime risk of radiation-induced cancer cannot be ignored. Women with early cancers who insist on breast conservation may be considered for management by tumor excision and axillary node dissection followed by full breast irradiation following delivery.

Chemotherapy

A variety of case reports and small series have confirmed the safety of chemotherapy administered to pregnant women with advanced breast cancers (Berry et al., 1999; Giacalone et al., 1999; De Santis et al., 2000; Meyer-Wittkopf et al., 2001; Kuerer, 2002). Occasional transient episodes of leucopenia have been reported in the fetus, in addition to one unexplained neonatal demise. The drugs employed have included doxorubicin, cyclophosphamide, 5-fluorouracil, and docetaxel, all agents commonly used to treat patients with this disease.

Breast-Feeding

There is no uniform agreement about the role of breast-feeding in the postpartum patient with breast cancer. Because many data implicate a viral etiology for breast cancer in laboratory animals, there is concern that a virus may cause human breast cancer as well. Therefore, the possibility exists that the contralateral breast is contaminated with the etiologic agent, which may even be passed on to the fetus. This theory has never been borne out in fact, but most surgeons recommend artificial feeding in such cases to avoid vascular enrichment in the opposite breast, which may also contain a neoplasm. This approach is especially important if systemic cytotoxic therapy is planned, because antineoplastic agents are detectable in breast milk and may cause neonatal bone marrow suppression. There are, however, no convincing data that nursing adversely affects the prognosis of breast cancer patients.

For women who want to breast-feed, a specific issue concerns the effects of breast lumpectomy and irradiation on lactation. Tralins (1995) conducted a national survey of 2582 members of the American Society of Therapeutic Radiology and Oncology and documented that one in four women had achieved successful bilateral lactation following lumpectomy and radiotherapy.

Survival Figures

The reported overall survival rate for women with a diagnosis of breast cancer during pregnancy is poor, reflecting advanced stage of disease at diagnosis in most (King et al., 1985; Ezzat et al., 1996; Bonnier et al., 1997; Kuerer et al., 1997; Ibrahim et al., 2000). Zemlickis and colleagues (1992) compared 188 women with PABC to 269 nonpregnant controls and found that women with PABC were 2.5 times as likely to present with metastatic disease and had a significantly lower chance of presenting with stage I disease.

Holleb and Farrow (1962) reported a series of 283 patients with breast carcinoma in pregnancy; 73 had inoperable disease, and 210 received surgery with or without postoperative radiation. Ninety-three percent of patients with inoperable disease died within 2 years of the diagnosis, including all 7 who had undergone interruption of pregnancy. The majority of the remaining 210 patients underwent radical mastectomy and received postoperative radiation therapy. Seven of 28 patients whose disease was diagnosed in the first trimester survived for 5 years. Half of these 28 patients delivered at or near term, and the other half underwent termination of pregnancy. Continuation of pregnancy did not seem to affect survival adversely, with 33% 5-year survival in the group who carried to term versus 17% in those who underwent abortion. For the small subgroups of patients, these survival differences were not significant. This and other series are shown in Table 58-17.

Peters and Meakin (1965) reported on 70 patients with breast cancer in pregnancy, all of whom were treated with preoperative or postoperative radiotherapy in conjunction with radical mastectomy. The overall survival rate in this series was 32.9% at 5 years and 19.5% at 10 years. Three of 12 patients treated during the first and second trimesters survived 5 years. Only one of the nine patients treated during the third trimester survived 5 years, and she had active disease at the time of the report. The remaining 49 patients who were treated postpartum had a 39% 5-year survival, prompting the authors to suggest that a delay in the treatment of breast carcinoma until after delivery should be considered.

Anderson and co-investigators (1996) reported the experience at Memorial Sloan-Kettering Cancer Center with breast cancer in women younger than 30 years of age. Two hundred and twenty-seven cases were identified, of whom 22 had PABC. The authors confirmed that tumors in women with PABC were usually larger and at more advanced stages at diagnosis than were those in young women who were not pregnant. It is notable, though, that the survival probability for women with early-stage disease was independent of pregnancy status.

TABLE 58-17. FIVE-YEAR SURVIVAL RATES BY NODAL STATUS IN PATIENTS WITH PREGNANCY-ASSOCIATED BREAST CANCER

Year	Author	Institution	N	LN negative (%)	LN positive (%)
1943	Haagensen and Stout	Columbia-Presbyterian	20	0	0
1954	White	University of Washington	40	72	6
1962	Holleb and Farrow	Memorial Sloan-Kettering	45	58	21
1973	Applewhite et al.	Louisiana State University	48	56	18
1985	King et al.	Mayo Clinic	63	75	33
1991	Petrek et al.	Memorial Sloan-Kettering	56	82	47
1997	Kuerer et al.	Mount Sinai	26	60	45
1997	Bonnier et al.	Multicenter French Study	154	63	31

LN negative (%), 5-year survivorship among lymph node–negative patients; LN positive (%), 5-year survivorship among lymph node–positive patients.

From Keleher AJ, Theriault RL, Gwyn KM, et al. Multidisciplinary management of breast cancer concurrent with pregnancy. J Am Coll Surg;**194:**54, 2002.

Pregnancy Following Breast Cancer

Prophylactic oophorectomy in early-stage breast cancer has been advocated by some clinicians to prevent further pregnancy, which may cause recrudescence of the disease through hormonal stimulation. This procedure has also been advocated if the tumor is receptor-positive to eliminate the ovarian source of estrogen production in the hope of preventing or delaying subsequent recurrence.

Neither argument to support this approach is substantiated by the literature. For example, using the International Breast Cancer Study Group database, Gerber and colleagues (2001) retrospectively reviewed the survival outcomes of women who became pregnant after treatment for early-stage breast cancer with those of matched controls (i.e., breast cancer patients who did not subsequently conceive): the overall 5- and 10-year survival rates were 92% and 86%, respectively, for the pregnancy group, compared with 85% and 74% for women who did not become pregnant. Thus, pregnancy following mastectomy does not influence the prognosis, and a few reports have even suggested that future pregnancies may be protective.

The rationale for eliminating the ovarian source of estrogens in the primary treatment of early disease is based on the observation that castration in the presence of observable recurrence results in partial or complete temporary tumor regression in approximately one third of cases. This argument is refuted, however, by two large clinical trials conducted in the United States that did not demonstrate a significant benefit from castration as adjuvant therapy. In one trial, the National Surgical Adjuvant Breast Project, 199 premenopausal breast cancer patients were randomized, with 129 undergoing surgical castration and 70 serving as controls without hormonal ablation (Fisher, 1971). After observation for up to 60 months, there was no evidence that those who were castrated derived any benefit from the procedure.

Although it may be presumptuous to conclude on the basis of retrospective studies that pregnancy protects against recurrence after mastectomy, it is reasonably safe to conclude that it does not increase the risk of recurrence. Consequently, if a pregnancy occurs, there appears to be no justification for recommending its termination in patients without evidence of recurrence (Averette et al., 1999; Velentgas et al., 1999). Finally, patients must be cautioned that an uneventful pregnancy following a cancer diagnosis in no way guarantees against subsequent recurrence. Indeed, there are cases on record in which multiple pregnancies have eventually been followed by recurrence. It is reasonable to recommend that women with favorable tumors without regional or distant spread wait at least 3 years before attempting pregnancy. All such patients should undergo extensive evaluation before conception, including bone and liver scans, chest x-rays, and mammography of the opposite breast, and they all must be observed closely during pregnancy.

Bone Tumors

Both benign and primary or metastatic malignant bone tumors can be found in pregnant women and can pose problems in diagnosis and treatment. Frequently, the diagnosis can be suspected from the characteristic radiographic findings in a patient with bony asymmetry or pain. When the diagnosis is uncertain and malignancy is suspected, a biopsy must be done.

Benign bone tumors are rarely a problem in pregnancy; however, two benign tumors that can affect pregnancy and delivery are endochondromas and benign exostosis, both of which can develop at the pelvic brim. These neoplasms may interfere with progression of labor and engagement of the fetal head by causing mechanical obstruction at the pelvic inlet, necessitating cesarean section.

Primary malignant bone tumors are rarely associated with pregnancy. The most common primary malignant tumors seen in the childbearing years are Ewing's sarcoma, osteogenic sarcoma, and osteocystoma. These tumors usually involve the clavicle, sternum, spine, humerus, or femur and are associated with local pain, mass, and disability. Signs and symptoms of myelitis with radiating pain, paresthesias, and weakness can be produced by primary sarcoma of the spine.

Primary bone cancer is aggressive, frequently having metastasized by the hematogenous route at the time of diagnosis. It is treated initially with surgical excision, usually without regard for the pregnancy. In the past, x-ray therapy and chemotherapy were delayed until delivery if the tumor had not metastasized at the time of diagnosis in the pregnant patient. Because pregnancy does not affect the growth of bone cancers and because these tumors do not affect the pregnancy, indications for pregnancy termination did not exist. Unfortunately, survival in the group of patients for whom chemotherapy was delayed was uniformly poor, with most patients dying of disseminated cancer within 24 months.

Within the past 20 years, the treatment of osteogenic sarcomas has become much more successful, often combining adjuvant chemotherapy with more limited surgery than was previously advocated. Aggressive chemotherapy administered soon after amputation or resection is crucial to prevent the development of clinically detectable metastases in patients with these tumors. Therefore, it is appropriate to recommend early termination of pregnancy for patients whose cancers are discovered in the first or early second trimester. If the diagnosis is made later in pregnancy, early delivery of the infant should take place, and intensive multiagent chemotherapy with doxorubicin, methotrexate, and cisplatin should be instituted.

Alternatively, because the risk of fetal malformations induced by chemotherapy during the second half of the pregnancy is low, continuation of pregnancy can be considered despite administration of a methotrexate-containing multiple-drug regimen. The rarity of these tumors in pregnancy precludes concrete treatment recommendations based on extensive clinical experience. Because most recurrences from bone malignancy appear within the first 3 years after initial therapy, recommendations for future pregnancies should be deferred until that interval has passed.

In women of childbearing age, the most common malignancies that metastasize to bone are those of the breast, cervix, thyroid, and kidney. Metastases occur most frequently in the skull, ribs, spine, and long bones, except for those from the cervix, which can extend directly to involve the pelvis. Patients can present with pain, a pathologic fracture, or paralysis, but lesions in some asymptomatic patients are identified by routine chest x-ray during pregnancy. This finding necessitates careful evaluation for a primary site, with definitive therapy dictated by the source of tumor and the duration of pregnancy at the time of diagnosis.

Thyroid Cancer

Both benign diseases and cancers of the thyroid gland occur more commonly in women than in men. Approximately 65% of all patients with carcinoma of the thyroid are women. Although the majority of patients with thyroid carcinoma are in their 50s and 60s, about 15% are below age 30 years. Some younger patients with thyroid cancer have an antecedent history of thymic radiation during infancy or facial skin radiation in the treatment of adolescent acne.

The identification of a thyroid nodule is usually by physical examination. Physical examination is not sufficient to ensure that the palpated mass is solitary. Thyroid nodules can be present in approximately 1% of women of childbearing age. Seventy-five percent of thyroid nodules discovered and evaluated during pregnancy are benign colloid nodules (Tan et al., 1996). Because approximately 15% of solitary thyroid nodules are malignant, prompt investigation of these nodules is warranted. Since thyroid scanning in pregnancy is contraindicated, evaluation should consist of serum-free thyroxine and triiodothyronine determinations to rule out a benign toxic adenoma and ultrasonography to rule out a cystic mass, which is rarely malignant (<2% of cases). The approach to the evaluation of thyroid nodules in pregnant women should be similar to that for nonpregnant patients. If a solitary solid cold nodule is found, fine needle aspiration or percutaneous needle biopsy is warranted. Pregnancy does not affect the reliability of this procedure.

The diagnosis of carcinoma of the thyroid during pregnancy is not an absolute indication to terminate the pregnancy; neither is pregnancy a contraindication to necessary surgery. Thyroidectomy should be performed for malignant lesions of the papillary type, even during pregnancy, because they tend to be quite aggressive. Definitive treatment of follicular masses can be delayed until the postpartum period because they are much more indolent than papillary tumors. Radioactive iodine therapy, when indicated, must be withheld until after delivery. The recurrence rate is not influenced by subsequent pregnancies but is related to many other factors. The prognosis for younger patients with thyroid cancer appears to be better than that for older patients. Additional prognostic factors include tumor size, histologic type, and grade. Furthermore, anaplastic cancers are associated with a dismal outlook.

METASTASES TO THE PLACENTA AND FETUS

Although cancer during pregnancy is not uncommon, metastases to the placental tissue or the fetus are rare. Most malignancies, when matched stage for stage, portend the same prognosis for the woman whether she is pregnant or not. Exceptions include hepatocellular cancer, lymphoma, thyroid, colon, and nasopharyngeal cancers. In addition to these primary cancer sites, metastatic disease to the products of conception predicts an ominous course for the mother.

The first report of metastases to the placenta and fetus appeared in 1866. In this case, Friedreich observed a mother with disseminated "hepatic" carcinoma that spread to and killed the fetus. There have been no other reports of "hepatic" metastases to the products of conception, and we suspect that Friedreich's patient had a malignant melanoma, which is the most likely to behave in this clinical manner. Indeed, malignant melanoma is the most common cancer to metastasize to the placenta and fetus. Since Friedreich's initial report, there have been fewer than 65 published cases of maternal malignancy metastatic to the gestation. These have been summarized by Ackerman and Gilbert-Barness (1997). Because of its generous blood flow, large surface area, and favorable biological environment for growth, one would consider the placenta to be an ideal site for metastases, and therefore the relative paucity of such events remains unclear. Perhaps immunologic rejection of tumor cells, utero-placental circulatory mechanisms, or even a protective role of the trophoblast limit the establishment of metastatic foci.

Cancers that have been reported to metastasize to the intervillous space or to the placenta proper include sarcomas, carcinomas, lymphomas, leukemias, and melanomas (Aronsson, 1963; Cavell, 1963; Brossard et al., 1994). Importantly, 30% of the cases are melanomas, followed by breast cancer (18%), and then the hematopoietic malignancies (13%).

Nearly half of the reports contain cases of known malignancy diagnosed prior to the onset of pregnancy. Gestational reactivation of malignancy has been reported in women who had been disease free for 5 years prior to becoming pregnant. Unfortunately, 93% of such women died of their disease, sometimes within hours of delivery.

In direct contradistinction to the unfavorable prognosis for women with placental metastases, the prognosis for the infant has been excellent, with 53 of the 63 reported cases revealing no evidence of disease in the baby. In addition, since 1966, there have been no reports of an infant succumbing to metastatic disease, although several reports have described fetal demises as a consequence of complications of prematurity.

One other unusual scenario is that of GTN metastatic to the fetus, with 15 to 20 cases reported to date (Chandra et al., 1990). Interestingly, widely metastatic disease in the delivered neonate can occur in the absence of metastatic GTN in the mother.

TUMOR MARKERS IN PREGNANCY

Serum CA 125 levels are elevated in many women with ovarian cancers, as well as many with a wide variety of noncancerous conditions including pregnancy (Jacobs and Bast, 1989). In pregnant women the CA 125 values are highest during the first trimester, with levels as high as 1250 units reported (Kobayashi et al., 1989). The values typically decrease during the late first trimester and should remain below 35 units per mL of serum until delivery. In some instances the maternal serum CA 125 remains within normal limits throughout uncomplicated pregnancies.

The maternal serum α-fetoprotein is a useful marker for women harboring a malignant germ cell tumor containing an endodermal sinus tumor, immature teratoma, or embryonal component (Horbelt et al., 1984; Montz et al., 1989; Young and Gee, 1990; Frederiksen et al., 1991). Produced initially by the yolk sac, and later by the fetal liver and gastrointestinal tract, α-fetoprotein is readily measured in the mother during fetal development. Accordingly, the use of α-fetoprotein levels to monitor women with a history of endodermal sinus tumor who subsequently become pregnant poses a distinct clinical dilemma.

The use of hCG levels to monitor pregnant women in remission following treatment for gestational trophoblastic disease presents a similar problem. The hCG steadily increases during the first trimester of pregnancy and may reach levels beyond 100,000 units at 10 weeks' gestation. Accordingly, women with a history of trophoblastic neoplasia must undergo transvaginal ultrasonography to document intrauterine pregnancy, and a metastatic work-up should be conducted if the hCG remains markedly elevated during pregnancy or if focal symptoms manifest.

The glycolytic enzyme, lactate dehydrogenase, is a marker for gonadal and extragonadal dysgerminomas (Schwartz and Morris, 1988). Because the enzyme is ubiquitous, the heterogeneity afforded its multiple molecular forms permits electrophoretic separation into five isoenzymes. Isoenzyme fractions 1 and 2 are specifically elevated in women with dysgerminomas. During pregnancy and the puerperium, lactate dehydrogenase values fluctuate very little unless the patient is preeclamptic.

Finally, inhibin is a glycoprotein hormone produced by normal ovarian granulosa cells and testicular Sertoli cells. In the ovary, it inhibits the secretion of follicle-stimulating hormone. Patients with granulosa cell tumors have elevated serum levels of inhibin, and this finding has been used to detect recurrent tumor (Rishi et al., 1997). In pregnancy, serum levels of inhibin do not rise significantly unless the patient has preeclampsia or gestational hypertension (Silver et al., 1999). The use of an inhibin monoclonal antibody can preferentially mark inhibin secreted from granulosa cell tumors and Sertoli-Leydig cell tumors.

REFERENCES

Ackerman J, Gilbert-Barness E: Malignancy metastatic to the products of conception: A case report with literature review. Pediatr Pathol Lab Med 17:577, 1997.

Anderson B, LaPolla J, Turner D, et al: Ovarian transposition in cervical cancer. Gynecol Oncol 49:206, 1993.

Anderson BO, Petrek JA, Byrd DR, et al: Pregnancy influences breast cancer stage at diagnosis in women 30 years of age and younger. Ann Surg Oncol 3:204, 1996.

Antypas C, Sandilos P, Kauvaris J, et al: Fetal dose evaluation during breast cancer radiotherapy. Int J Radiat Oncol Biol Phys 40:995, 1998.

Applewhite RR, Smith LR, DeVicente F: Carcinoma of the breast associated with pregnancy and lactation. Am J Surg 39:101, 1973.

Aronsson S: A case of transplacental tumor metastasis. Acta Paediatr Scand 52:123, 1963.

Averette HE, Mirhashemi R, Moffat FL: Pregnancy after breast carcinoma: The ultimate medical challenge. Cancer 85:2301, 1999.

Avileás A, Diaz-Maques J, Talavera A, et al: Growth and development of children of mothers treated with chemotherapy during pregnancy: Current status of 43 children. Am J Hematol 36:243, 1991.

Bagshawe KD: Risk and prognostic factors in trophoblastic neoplasia. Cancer 38:1373, 1976.

Baker ML, Vandergrift A, Dalrymple GV: Fetal exposure in diagnostic radiology. Health Phys 37:237, 1979.

Baldauf JJ, Dreyfus M, Ritter J, et al: Colposcopy and directed biopsy reliability during pregnancy: A cohort study. Eur J Obstet Gynecol Reprod Biol 62:31, 1995.

Balderston KD, Tewari K, Gregory WT, et al: Neuroendocrine small cell carcinoma of the uterine cervix in pregnancy: Long-term survival following combined therapy. Gynecol Oncol 71:128, 1998.

Balloni L, Pugliese P, Ferrari S, et al: Colon cancer in pregnancy: Report of a case and review of the literature. Tumori 86:95, 2000.

Barber HRK, Brunschwig A: Carcinoma of the bowel: Radiation and surgical management and pregnancy. Am J Obstet Gynecol 100:926, 1968.

Becker MH, Hyman GA: Management of Hodgkin's disease coexistent with pregnancy. Radiology 85:725, 1965.

Becker MH: Hodgkin's disease and pregnancy. Radiol Clin N Am; 6:111, 1968.

Benedet JL, Odicino F, Maisonneuve P, et al: Carcinoma of the cervix uteri. J Epidemiol Biostat 6(1):7, 2001.

Berkowitz RS, Goldstein DP, Bernstein MR: Ten years' experience with methotrexate and folinic acid as primary therapy for gestational trophoblastic disease. Gynecol Oncol 23:111, 1986.

Bernstein MA, Madoff RD, Caushaj PJ: Colon and rectal cancer in pregnancy. Dis Colon Rectum 36:172, 1993.

Berry DL, Theriault RL, Holmes FA, et al: Management of breast cancer during pregnancy using a standardized protocol. J Clin Oncol 17:855, 1999.

Blumenfeld Z, Avivi I, Linn S, et al: Prevention of irreversible chemotherapy-induced ovarian damage in young women with lymphoma by a gonadotropin-releasing hormone agonist in parallel to chemotherapy. Hum Reprod 11:1620, 1996.

Bonnier P, Roman S, Dilhuydy JM, et al: Influence of pregnancy on the outcome of breast cancer: A case-control study. Int J Cancer 72:720, 1997.

Borden EC: Melanoma in pregnancy. Semin Oncol 27:654, 2000.

Bottles K, Taylor R: Diagnosis of breast masses in pregnant and lactating women by aspiration cytology. Obstet Gynecol 66:765, 1985.

Boulay R, Podczaski E: Ovarian cancer complicating pregnancy. Obstet Gynecol Clin N Am 25:385, 1998.

Bower M, Newlands ES, Holden L, et al: EMA/CO for high risk gestational trophoblastic tumors: Results from a cohort of 272 patients. J Clin Oncol 15:2636, 1997.

Brent RI: Radiation and other medical agents. In Wilson LG, Fraser FC (eds): Handbook of Teratology, vol 1. New York, Plenum Press, 1977, p. 60.

Breslow A: Thickness, cross-sectional areas, and depth of invasion in the prognosis of cutaneous melanoma. Ann Surg 172:902, 1970.

Bristow RE, Shumway JB, Khouzami AN, et al: Complete hydatidiform mole and surviving coexistent twin. Obstet Gynecol Surv 51:705, 1996.

Brodsky JB, Cohen EN, Brown BW, et al: Surgery during pregnancy and fetal outcome. Am J Obstet Gynecol 138:1165, 1980.

Brossard J, Abish S, Bernstein ML, et al: Maternal malignancy involving the products of conception: A report of malignant melanoma and medulloblastoma Am J Pediatr Hematol Oncol 16:380, 1994.

Buller RE, Darrow V, Manetta A, et al: Conservative surgical management of dysgerminoma concomitant with pregnancy. Obstet Gynecol 79:887, 1992.

Bureau of Radiological Health: Population exposure to x-rays. DHEW Publication (FD) 73-8047. Washington, DC, US Government Printing Office, 1973.

Byrne J, Mulvihill JJ, Myers MH, et al: Effects of treatment on fertility in long-term survivors of childhood or adolescent cancer. N Engl J Med 317:1315, 1987.

Caforio L, Draisci G, Ciampelli M, et al: Rectal cancer in pregnancy: A new management based on blended anesthesia and monitoring of fetal well being. Eur J Obstet Gynecol Reprod Biol 88:71, 2000.

Cavell B: Transplacental metastasis of malignant melanoma. Acta Paediatr Suppl 146:37, 1963.

Chandra SA, Gilbert EF, Viseskul C, et al: Neonatal intracranial choriocarcinoma. Arch Pathol Lab Med 114:1079, 1990.

Chung Af, Woodruff JM, Lewis JL: Malignant melanoma of the vulva. Obstet Gynecol 45:638, 1975.

Clark WH, From L, Bernardina EA, et al: The histogenesis and biologic behavior of primary human malignant melanomas of the skin. Cancer Res 29:705, 1969.

Clavel-Chapelon F: Differential effects of reproductive factors on the risk of pre- and postmenopausal breast cancer: Results from a large cohort of French women. Br J Cancer 86:723, 2002.

Conley JG, Jacobson A: Modified radiation therapy regimen for Hodgkin's disease in the third trimester of pregnancy. Am J Roentgenol 128:666, 1977.

Creasman WT: New gynecologic cancer staging. Gynecol Oncol 58:157, 1995.

Curry SL, Hammond CB, Tyrey L, et al: Hydatidiform mole: Diagnosis, management and long-term follow-up of 347 patients. Obstet Gynecol 45:1, 1975.

Curry SL, Schlaerth JB, Kohorn EI, et al: Hormonal contraception and trophoblastic sequelae after hydatidiform mole. Am J Obstet Gynecol 1989; 160:805, 1989.

Deicas RE, Miller DS, Rademaker AW, et al: The role of contraception in the development of postmolar gestational trophoblastic tumor. Obstet Gynecol 78:221, 1991.

De Santis M, Lucchese A, De Carolis: Metastatic breast cancer in pregnancy: First case of chemotherapy with docetaxel. Eur J Cancer Care (Engl) 9:235, 2000.

Di Saia PJ, Creasman WT: Clinical Gynecologic Oncology. St Louis, CV Mosby, 1981.

Dildy GA, Moise KJ, Carpenter RJ, et al: Maternal malignancy metastatic to the products of conception: A review. Obstet Gynecol Surv 44:535, 1989.

Doll DC, Ringenberg QS, Yarbro JW: Antineoplastic agents and pregnancy. Semin Oncol 16:337, 1989.

Donagi A, Lesser Y: National evaluation of trends in x-ray exposure of medical patients in Israel. Presented at the 4th Congress of the International Radiation Protection Association, April 1977, Paris.

Duggan B, Muderspach LI, Roman LD, et al: Cervical cancer in pregnancy: Reporting on planned delay in therapy. Obstet Gynecol 82:598, 1993.

Eastman NJ, Hellman LM: Ovarian tumors in pregnancy. In Eastman NJ, Hellman LM (eds): Williams' Obstetrics, 13th ed. New York, Appleton-Century-Crofts, 1966, p. 737.

Ezzat A, Raja MA, Berry J, et al: Impact of pregnancy on non-metastatic breast cancer: A case control study. Clin Oncol (R Coll Radiol) 8:367, 1996.

Feeney DD, Moore DH, Look KY, et al: The fate of the ovaries after radical hysterectomy and ovarian transposition. Gynecol Oncol 56:3, 1995.

Feige Y, Kahan RS: Practical implications of new approaches in evaluating risks from ionizing radiation. Trans Nucl Soc Israel 71, 1976.

Fenig E, Mishaeli M, Kalish Y, et al: Pregnancy and radiation. Cancer Treat Rev 27:1, 2001.

Fisher B: Status of adjuvant therapy: Results of The National Surgical Adjuvant Breast Project studies on oophorectomy, postoperative radiation therapy, and chemotherapy. Other comments concerning clinical trials. Cancer 28(6):1654, 1971.

Frederiksen MC, Casanova L, Schink JC: An elevated maternal serum α-fetoprotein leading to the diagnosis of an immature teratoma, Int J Gynecol Obstet 35:343, 1991.

Friedreich N: Beitrage zur pathologie des Krebses. Virchows Arch (Pathol Anat) 36:30, 1866.

George PA, Fortner JG, Pack GT: Melanoma with pregnancy. Cancer 13:854, 1960.

Gerber S, Coates AS, Goldhirsch A, et al: Effect of pregnancy on overall survival after the diagnosis of early stage breast cancer. J Clin Oncol 19:1671, 2001.

Giacalone PL, Laffargue F, Benos P: Chemotherapy for breast carcinoma during pregnancy: A French national survey. Cancer 86:2266, 1999.

Giuliano AE, Kirgan DM, Guenther JM, et al: Lymphatic mapping and sentinel lymphadenectomy for breast carcinoma. Ann Surg 220:391, 1994.

Goldberg GL, Altaras MM, Bloch B: Cone cerclage in pregnancy. Obstet Gynecol 77:315, 1991.

Goldstein DP: Five years' experience with the prevention of trophoblastic tumors by the prophylactic use of chemotherapy in patients with molar pregnancy. Clin Obstet Gynecol 13:945, 1970.

Goldstein DP, Berkowitz RS, Bernstein MR: Reproductive performance after molar pregnancy and gestational trophoblastic tumors. Clin Obstet Gynecol 27:221, 1984.

Goldstein DP, Reid D: Recent developments in management of molar pregnancy. Clin Obstet Gynecol 10:313, 1967.

Goldstein DP, Saracco P, Osathanondh R, et al: Methotrexate with citrovorum factor rescue for gestational trophoblastic neoplasms. Obstet Gynecol 53:93, 1978.

Grimes WH, Bartholomew RA, Calvin ED: Ovarian cysts in pregnancy. Am J Obstet Gynecol 68:594, 1954.

Grin CM, Driscoll MS, Grant-Kels JM: Pregnancy and prognosis of malignant melanoma. Semin Oncol 23:734, 1996.

Guinee VF, Olsson H, Torgil M, et al: Effect of pregnancy on prognosis for young women with breast cancer. Lancet 343:1587, 1994.

Gwyn K, Theriault R: Breast cancer during pregnancy. Oncology 15:39, 2001.

Haagensen CD, Bodian C, Haagensen DE Jr: Breast Carcinoma: Risk and Detection. Philadelphia: WB Saunders, 1981.

Haagensen CD, Stout AP: Carcinoma of the breast: Criteria of operability. Ann Surg 118:859, 1943.

Hacker NF, Berek JS, Lagasse LD, et al: Carcinoma of the cervix associated with pregnancy. Obstet Gynecol 59:735, 1982.

Hall EJ: Hereditary effects of radiation In Hall EJ (ed): Radiobiology for the Radiologist, 4th ed. Philadelphia, JB Lippincott, 1994, p. 351.

Hamer-Jacobsen E: Therapeutic abortion on account of x-ray. Denver Med Bull 6:113, 1959.

Hammond CB, Weed JC Jr, Currie JL: The role of operation in the current therapy of gestational trophoblastic disease. Am J Obstet Gynecol 136:844, 1980.

Hess LW, Peaceman A, O'Brien WF, et al: Adnexal mass occurring with intrauterine pregnancy: Report of fifty-four patients requiring laparotomy for definitive management. Am J Obstet Gynecol 158:1029, 1988.

Hicks SP, D'Amato CJ: Effects of ionizing radiation on mammalian development. Adv Teratol 1:195, 1966.

Holleb AI, Farrow JH: The relation of carcinoma of the breast and pregnancy in 283 patients. Surg Gynecol Obstet 115:65, 1962.

Hopkins MP, Morley GW: The prognosis and management of cervical cancer associated with pregnancy. Obstet Gynecol 80:9, 1992.

Horbelt D, Delmore J, Meisels R, et al: Mixed germ cell malignancy of the ovary concurrent with pregnancy. Obstet Gynecol 84:662, 1984.

Hoskins WJ, Perez CA, Young RC: Principles and Practice of Gynecologic Oncology. Philadelphia, Lippincott-Raven, 1996.

Ibrahim EM, Ezzat AA, Baloush A, et al: Pregnancy-associated breast cancer: A case-control study in a young population with a high fertility rate. Med Oncol 17:293, 2000.

International Commission on Radiological Protection: ICRP Publication 60. Oxford: Pergamon Press, 1990.

Jablon S, Kato H: Childhood cancer in relation to prenatal exposure to atomic bomb radiation. Lancet 2:1000, 1970.

Jacobs C, Donaldson SS, Rosenberg SA, et al: Management of the pregnant patient with Hodgkin's disease. Ann Intern Med 95:669, 1982.

Jacobs I, Bast RC: The CA 125 tumor–associated antigen: A review of the literature. Hum Reprod 4:1, 1989.

Jernstrom H, Lerman D, Ghadirian P, et al: Pregnancy and risk of early breast cancer in carriers of BRCA1 and BRCA2. Lancet 354:1846, 1999.

Johannsson O, Loman N, Borg A, et al: Pregnancy-associated breast cancer in BRCA1 and BRCA2. Lancet 352:1359, 1999.

Jubb ED: Primary ovarian carcinoma in pregnancy. Am J Obstet Gynecol 85:345, 1963.

Kalir T, Friedman F Jr: Gynandroblastoma in pregnancy: Case report and review of literature. Mt Sinai J Med 65:292, 1998.

Karlen JR, Akbari A, Cook WA: Dysgerminoma associated with pregnancy. Obstet Gynecol 53:330, 1979.

Katz VL, Farmer RM, Dotters D: Focus on primary care: From nevus to neoplasm: Myths of melanoma in pregnancy. Obstet Gynecol Surv 57:112, 2002.

Keleher AJ, Theriault RL, Gwyn KM, et al: Multidisciplinary management of breast cancer concurrent with pregnancy. J Am Coll Surg 194:54, 2002.

King RM, Welch JS, Martin JK Jr, et al: Carcinoma of the breast associated with pregnancy. Surg Gynecol Obstet 160:228, 1985.

Kobayashi F, Sagawa N, Nakamura K, et al: Mechanism and clinical significance of elevated CA125 levels in the sera of pregnant women. Am J Obstet Gynecol **160**:563, 1989.

Kouvaris JR, Antypas CE, Sandilos PH, et al: Postoperative tailored radiotherapy for locally advanced breast carcinoma during pregnancy: A therapeutic dilemma. Am J Obstet Gynecol **183**:498, 2000.

Kuerer HM, Cunningham JD, Bleiweiss IJ, et al: Conservative surgery for breast carcinoma associated with pregnancy. Breast J **4**:171, 1998.

Kuerer HM, Cunningham JD, Brower ST, et al: Breast carcinoma associated with pregnancy and lactation. Surg Oncol **6**:93, 1997.

Kuerer HM, Gwyn K, Ames FC, et al: Conservative surgery and chemotherapy during pregnancy for breast carcinoma. Surgery **131**:108, 2002.

Li M, Hertz R, Spencer DB: Effects of methotrexate therapy upon choriocarcinoma and chorioadenoma. Proc Soc Exp Biol Med **93**:361, 1956.

MacKie RM, Bufalino R, Morabito A: Lack of effect of pregnancy on outcome of melanoma. Lancet **337**:653, 1991.

Marana HRC, de Andrade JM, da Silva Mathes AC, et al: Chemotherapy in the treatment of locally advanced cervical cancer and pregnancy. Gynecol Oncol **80**:272, 2001.

McNanamny DS, Moss ALH, Pocock PV: Melanoma and pregnancy: A long-term follow-up. Br J Obstet Gynecol **96**:1419, 1989.

Mehta RR, Beattie CW, Das Gupta T: Endocrine profile in breast cancer patients receiving chemotherapy. Breast Cancer Res Treat **20**:125, 1991.

Merkel DE: Pregnancy and breast cancer. Semin Surg Oncol **12**:370, 1996.

Method MW, Brost BC: Management of cervical cancer in pregnancy. Semin Surg Oncol **16**:251, 1999.

Meyer-Wittkopf M, Barth H, Emons G, et al: Fetal cardiac effects of doxorubicin therapy for carcinoma of the breast during pregnancy: Case report and review of the literature. Ultrasound Obstet Gynecol **18**:62, 2001.

Miller RW, Mulvihill JJ: Small head size after atomic irradiation. Teratology **14**:355, 1976.

Mogren I, Stenlund H, Hogbert U: Long-term impact of reproductive factors on the risk of cervical, endometrial, ovarian and breast cancer. Acta Oncol **40**:849, 2002.

Monk BJ, Montz FJ: Invasive cervical cancer complicating intrauterine pregnancy: Treatment with radical hysterectomy. Obstet Gynecol **80**:199, 1992.

Monson RR, MacMahon B: Prenatal x-ray exposure and cancer in children. In Boice JD Jr, Fraumeni JF Jr (eds): Radiation Carcinogenesis: Epidemiology and Biological Significance. New York, Raven Press, 1984, p. 187.

Montz FJ, Horenstein J, Platt LD, et al: The diagnosis of immature teratoma by maternal serum alpha-fetoprotein screening. Obstet Gynecol **73**:522, 1989.

Mooney J, Silva E, Tornos C, Gershenson D: Unusual features of serous neoplasms of low malignant potential during pregnancy. Gynecol Oncol **65**:30, 1997.

Nabers J, Splinter TA, Wallenburg HC, et al: Choriocarcinoma with lung metastases during pregnancy with successful delivery and outcome after chemotherapy. Thorax **45**:416, 1990.

National Cancer Institute: Breast cancer in pregnancy. Cancer-Net. Available at *www.cancernet.nci.nih.gov/cgi-bin/srchcgi.exe*. Accessed April 24, 2002.

National Council on Radiation Protection: Review of NCRP radiation dose limit for embryo and fetus in occupationally exposed women. NCRP Report No. 53, Washington, DC, 1977a, p. 25.

National Council of Radiation Protection: Medical radiation exposure of pregnant and potentially pregnant women. NCRP Report No. 54, Washington, DC, 1977b, p. 7.

Nettleton J, Long J, Kuban D, et al: Breast cancer during pregnancy: Quantifying the risk of treatment delay. Ostet Gynecol **87**:414, 1996.

Newlands ES, Bagshawe KD, Begent RH, et al: Developments in chemotherapy for medium- and high-risk patients with gestational trophoblastic tumours. Br J Obstet Gynecol **93**:63, 1986.

Ngu SL, Duval P, Collins C: Foetal radiation dose in radiotherapy for breast cancer. Austral Radiol **36**:321, 1992.

Nicholson HO: Cytotoxic drugs in pregnancy. J Obstet Gynaecol Br Commonw **75**:307, 1968.

Nisce LA, Tome MA, He S, et al: Management of coexisting Hodgkin's disease and pregnancy. Am J Clin Oncol **9**:146, 1986.

Ochshorn Y, Kupferminc MJ, Lessing JB, et al: Rectal carcinoma during pregnancy. A reminder and updated treatment protocols. Eur J Obstet Gynecol Reprod Biol **91**:201, 2000.

Osterlind A, Tucker MA, Stone BJ, et al: The Danish study of cutaneous malignant melanoma: Hormonal and reproductive factors in women. Int J Cancer **42**:821, 1988.

Pack GT, Scharnagel IM: Prognosis for malignant melanoma in the pregnant woman. Cancer **4**:324, 1951.

Parodi PC, Osti M, Longhi P, et al: Pregnancy and tram-flap reconstruction after mastectomy: A case report. Scand J Plast Reconstr Surg Hand Surg **35**:211, 2001.

Penn I, Makowski E, Droegemueller W, et al: Parenthood in renal homograft recipients. JAMA **216**:1755, 1971.

Peters MV, Meakin JW: The influence of pregnancy in carcinoma of the breast. Prog Clin Cancer **1**:471, 1965.

Petrek JA, Dukoff R, Rogatko A: Prognosis of pregnancy associated breast cancer. Cancer **67**:699, 1991.

Reintgen DS, McCarty KS, Vollmer R, et al: Malignant melanoma. Cancer **55**:1340, 1985.

Reynoso EE, Shepherd FA, Messner HA, et al: Acute leukemia during pregnancy: The Toronto Leukemia Study Group experience with long-term follow-up of children exposed in utero to chemotherapeutic agents. J Clin Oncol **5**:1098, 1987.

Rishi M, Howard LN, Bratthauer, GL, et al: Use of monoclonal antibody against human inhibin as a marker for sex cord-stromal tumors of the ovary. Am J Surg Pathol **21**:583, 1997.

Rothman AL, Cohen AJ, Astarloa J: Placental and fetal involvement by maternal malignancy: A report of rectal carcinoma and review of the literature. Am J Obstet Gynecol **116**:1023, 1973.

Rugh R: X-ray induced teratogenesis in the mouse and its possible significance to man. Radiology **99**:433, 1971.

Rustin GJ, Booth M, Dent J, et al: Pregnancy after cytotoxic chemotherapy for gestational trophoblastic tumours. BMJ (Clin Res) **14**:288, 1984.

Sandmeier D, Lobrinus JA, Vial Y, et al: Bilateral Krukenberg tumor of the ovary during pregnancy. Eur J Gynaecol Oncol **21**:58, 2000.

Schapira DV, Chudley AE: Successful pregnancy following continuous treatment with combination chemotherapy before contraception and throughout pregnancy. Cancer **54**:800, 1984.

Schwartz PE, Morris JM: Serum lactic dehydrogenase: A tumor marker for dysgerminoma. Obstet Gynecol **72**:511, 1988.

Sebire NJ, Osborn M, Darzi A, et al: Appendiceal adenocarcinoma with ovarian metastases in the third trimester of pregnancy. J R Soc Med **93**:192, 2000.

Sharma SC, Williamson JF, Khan FM, et al: Measurement and calculation of ovary and fetus dose in extended field radiotherapy for 10 MV x-rays. Int J Radiat Oncol Biol Phys **7**:843, 1981.

Shivvers SA, Miller DS: Preinvasive and invasive breast and cervical cancer prior to or during pregnancy Clin Perinatol **24**:369, 1997.

Shousha S: Breast carcinoma presenting during or shortly after pregnancy and lactation. Arch Pathol Lab Med **124**:1053, 2000.

Silver HM, Lambert-Messerlian GM, Star JA, et al: Comparison of maternal serum total activin A and inhibin A in normal, preeclamptic, and nonproteinuric gestationally hypertensive pregnancies. Am J Obstet Gynecol **180**:1131, 1999.

Sivanesaratnam V, Jayalaksmi P, Loo C: Surgical management of early invasive cancer of the cervix associated with pregnancy. Gynecol Oncol **48**:68, 1992.

Slinguff CL Jr, Reintgen DS, Vollmer RT: Malignant melanoma arising during pregnancy: A study of 100 patients. Ann Surg **211**:5529, 1990.

Smith LH, Dalrymple JL, Leiserowitz GS, et al: Obstetrical deliveries associated with maternal malignancy in California, 1992 through 1997. Am J Obstet Gynecol **184**:1504, 2001.

Sokal JE, Lessman EM: The effects of cancer chemotherapeutic agents on the human fetus. JAMA **172**:1765, 1960.

Sondik EJ, Anderson JR, Curtin LR, et al: Trends in pregnancies and pregnancy rates by outcome: Estimates for the United States, 1976–96. Vital and Health Statistics from the Centers for Disease Control and Prevention Series **21**:56, 2002.

Sood AK, Shahin MS, Sorosky JI: Paclitaxel and platinum chemotherapy for ovarian carcinoma during pregnancy. Gynecol Oncol **83**:599, 2001.

Sood AK, Sorosky JI, Mayr N, et al: Radiotherapeutic management of cervical cancer complicating pregnancy. Cancer **80**:1073, 1997.

Sorosky JI, Squatrito R, Ndubisi BU, et al: Stage I squamous cell cervical carcinoma in pregnancy: Planned delay in therapy awaiting fetal maturity. Gynecol Oncol **59**:207, 1995.

Steigrad SJ, Cheung AP, Osborn RA: Choriocarcinoma co-existent with an intact pregnancy: Case report and review of the literature. J Obstet Gynaecol Res **25**:108, 1999.

Steller MA, Genest DR, Bernstein MR, et al: Natural history of twin pregnancy with complete hydatidiform mole and coexisting fetus. Obstet Gynecol **83**:35, 1994.

Stewart A, Webb J: Malignant disease in childhood and diagnostic irradiation in utero. Lancet **2**:447, 1956.

Tan GH, Gharib H, Goellner JR, et al: Management of thyroid nodules in pregnancy. Arch Intern Med **156**:2317, 1996.

Tawil E, Mercier JP, Dandavino A: Hodgkin's disease complicating pregnancy. J Can Assoc Radiol **36:**133, 1983.

Tewari K, Brewer C, Cappuccini F, et al: Advanced stage small cell carcinoma of the ovary in pregnancy: Long-term survival after surgical debulking and multi-agent chemotherapy. Gynecol Oncol **66:**531, 1997.

Tewari K, Bonebrake RG, Asrat T, et al: Ambiguous genitalia in infant exposed to tamoxifen in utero. Lancet **350:**183, 1997.

Tewari K, Cappuccini F, Balderston KD, et al: Pregnancy in a Jehovah's Witness with cervical cancer and anemia. Gynecol Oncol **71:**330, 1998.

Tewari K, Cappuccini F, Freeman RK, et al: Managing cervical cancer in pregnancy. Contemp OB/Gyn **44:**134, 1999.

Tewari K, Rose GS, Balderston KD, et al: Fertility drugs and malignant germ cell tumour of the ovary in pregnancy. Lancet **351:**957, 1998.

Thomas PRM, Peckham MJ: The investigation and management of Hodgkin's disease in the pregnant patient. Cancer **38:**1443, 1976.

Tralins AH: Lactation after conservative breast surgery combined with radiation therapy. Am J Clin Oncol **18:**40, 1995.

Travers RL, Sover AJ, Berwisk M: Increased thickness of pregnancy-associated melanoma. Br J Dermatol **132:**876, 1995.

United Nations Scientific Committee on the Effects of Atomic Radiation: Genetic and somatic effects of ionizing radiation. New York, United Nations, 1986, p. 16.

Van Der Giessen PH: Measurement of the peripheral dose for the tangential breast treatment technique with co-60 gamma radiation and high energy x-rays. Radiother Oncol **42:**257, 1997.

van der Vange N, Weverling GJ, Ketting BW, et al: The prognosis of cervical cancer associated with pregnancy: A matched cohort study. Obstet Gynecol **85:**1022, 1995.

Velentgas P, Daling JR, Malone KE, et al: Pregnancy after breast carcinoma: Outcomes and influence on mortality. Cancer **85:**2424, 1999.

White LP, Linden G, Breslow L, et al: Studies on melanoma: The effect of pregnancy on survival in human melanoma. JAMA **117:**235, 1961.

White TT: Carcinoma of the breast and pregnancy. Ann Surg **139:**9, 1954.

Wong JH, Sterns EE, Kopald HK: Prognostic significance of pregnancy in stage 1 melanoma. Arch Surg **124:**1227, 1989.

Wong PS, Rosemark PJ, Wexler MC, et al: Doses to organs at risk from mantle field radiation therapy using 10 MV x-rays. Mt Sinai J Med **52:**216, 1985.

Woo SY, Fuller LM, Cundiff JH, et al: Radiotherapy during pregnancy for clinical stages IA-IIA Hodgkin's disease. Int J Radiat Oncol Biol Phys **23:**407, 1992.

Woods JB, Martin JN Jr, Ingram FH, et al: Pregnancy complicated by carcinoma above the rectum. Am J Perinatol **9:**102, 1992.

Young A, Gee H: Raised maternal serum alpha-fetoprotein levels during pregnancy following treatment of an endodermal sinus tumor: Case Report. Br J Obstet Gynaecol **97:**267, 1990.

Young RH, Dudley AG, Scully RE: Granulosa cell, Sertoli-Leydig cell, and unclassified sex-cord stromal tumors associated with pregnancy: A clinicopathological analysis of thirty-six cases. Gynecol Oncol **18:**181, 1984.

Zemlickis D, Lishner M, Degendorfer P, et al: Maternal and fetal outcome after invasive cervical cancer in pregnancy. J Clin Oncol **9:**1956, 1991.

Zemlickis D, Lishner M, Degendorfen P, et al: Maternal and fetal outcome after breast cancer in pregnancy. Am J Obstet Gynecol **166:**781, 1992.

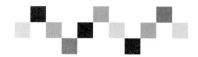

Chapter 59

ANESTHETIC CONSIDERATIONS FOR COMPLICATED PREGNANCIES

Laurence S. Reisner, MD, and Krzysztof M. Kuczkowski, MD

The physiologic changes that occur during normal pregnancy must be considered by the anesthesiologist to facilitate selecting the most appropriate and safest anesthetic drugs and techniques. When pregnancy is complicated by a significant medical disorder, the anesthetic considerations are even more challenging. This chapter reviews the special concerns posed by the more common and complex medical disorders superimposed on pregnancy as well as the most prudent technical solutions to the specific problems. Epidural and combined spinal-epidural analgesia or anesthesia are frequently recommended for the parturient with medical or obstetric complications because of the great flexibility and usefulness of these techniques for virtually any obstetric procedure.

PREECLAMPSIA

The patient with preeclampsia has multiple organ system alterations that affect the selection of analgesia and anesthesia for labor and delivery. The patient with mild preeclampsia rarely poses a major problem regarding anesthesia. Consequently, the focus here is on the patient with severe preeclampsia and eclampsia. Throughout this chapter, intensive care monitoring and the use of pulmonary artery occlusion pressure monitoring are emphasized (see also Chapter 45).

Intravascular Volume Depletion

Intravascular volume depletion is a well-recognized occurrence with severe preeclampsia (Hays et al., 1985). The anesthesiologist is concerned about inducing epidural or spinal anesthesia in the presence of a relative hypovolemia because the ensuing sympathetic blockade could lead to precipitous declines in blood pressure, which can seriously impair critical organ and uteroplacental blood flow. Preanesthetic volume expansion is used with caution to prevent this undesired effect. Such replacement often requires the use of central venous pressure or pulmonary artery pressure monitoring (Cotton et al., 1985). Because many patients with preeclampsia have low central filling pressures, they often require large volumes of fluid to bring the pressures into the middle of the normal range. This measure, however, can result in pulmonary edema in the postpartum period, when colloid osmotic pressure reaches its nadir (Benedetti et al., 1985). More judicious fluid management with slow advancement of an epidural block, particularly

for those undergoing cesarean delivery, is proving effective at maintaining maternal blood pressure while minimizing the risk of fluid overload.

The choice of fluid—crystalloid or colloid—remains controversial. Studies have demonstrated the beneficial effects of albumin administration for these patients (Kirshon et al., 1988). Its use is justified in part by the fact that preeclamptic subjects tend to demonstrate significant reductions in plasma protein levels and colloid osmotic pressure as a result of protein loss through the kidney. Arguments against the routine use of albumin emphasize that the functional changes in membranes that allow edema to occur also allow protein to leak into the tissues, thus making removal of interstitial fluid more difficult. To avoid volume overload, the judicious administration of crystalloid solution (up to 2000 mL) is guided by central venous or pulmonary artery occlusion pressure monitoring. This is accomplished with simultaneous advancement of the regional block, thereby titrating the effects of one against the other. If the patient has marked edema or low colloid osmotic pressure or has not responded to crystalloid infusion, 25% salt-poor albumin is administered to maintain intravascular volume. The objective is to provide sufficient volume to allow the patient to undergo anesthesia and maintain an adequate urine flow rather than totally correct an estimated volume deficit.

Vascular Reactivity

Vascular reactivity is enhanced in preeclampsia, and the increased sensitivity to vasopressor agents such as angiotensin II and catecholamines is well documented (Gant et al., 1973; Zuspan, 1977). Systemic vascular resistance can be increased, and uteroplacental crucial organ blood flow can be compromised. The anesthesiologist must consider the possibility that the administration of regional anesthesia and its attendant sympathetic blockade to a patient who is already experiencing volume depletion and vasoconstriction could result in sudden hypotension. The initiation of epidural blockade with maintenance of an acceptable maternal blood pressure, however, results in increases in uteroplacental blood flow (Joupilla et al., 1979). An acceptable maternal blood pressure is defined as no more than a 25% reduction in systolic blood pressure.

The vasoreactivity also alerts the anesthesiologist to use lower doses of vasopressors to correct maternal hypotension. An arterial catheter can be helpful in monitoring beat-to-beat blood pressure responses in patients requiring aggressive therapy. Patients who undergo general anesthesia for cesarean delivery are at risk for hypertensive crisis at the time of laryngoscopy and intubation as a result of the associated increase in sympathetic tone. This can lead to intracranial hemorrhage or pulmonary edema, and measures should be taken to block this response when general anesthesia is required (Fox et al., 1977).

Coagulation

Coagulation system changes are frequently observed in patients with severe preeclampsia. The most common alteration is a decrease in platelet count. This is usually not a concern unless it falls below 100,000/mm³. Many anesthesiologists are reluctant to administer regional anesthesia when the platelet count is at or below this level for fear that an epidural hematoma may occur. A possible platelet functional defect has also been identified in these patients (Kelton et al., 1985). This results in a prolonged Ivy bleeding time in spite of a normal platelet count. The absolute limit beyond which it is thought unwise to perform regional anesthesia is arbitrary and variable, as there are no documented reports of an epidural hematoma occurring in association with epidural anesthesia in preeclamptic patients with either lowered platelet counts or a prolonged Ivy bleeding time, and some have questioned the diagnostic and predictive ability of the bleeding time (Channing-Rogers et al., 1990).

There is retrospective evidence to suggest that many epidural agents have been placed in such patients without incident (Rolbin et al., 1988). Nevertheless, the potential complication is so serious that the arbitrary limit generally used is as follows: If the bleeding time is less than 12 minutes or if another test of primary hemostasis indicates good platelet function, it is probably safe to use regional anesthesia even if the platelet count is below 100,000/mm³. Other tests of whole-blood clotting (e.g., thromboelastogram, Sonoclot, Platelet Function Analyzer -100) are being evaluated in preeclamptic and healthy parturients, but their usefulness as predictors of surgical or epidural bleeding remains to be defined. Disseminated intravascular coagulation (DIC) is an infrequent occurrence in preeclamptic patients but significantly alters other tests of coagulation.

Edema

Edema is a frequent finding in patients with preeclampsia. Limb edema can make vascular access difficult. Edema in the neck can obscure landmarks for performing internal jugular vein cannulation for central line insertion. The most worrisome edema for the anesthesiologist is that which can occur in the pharynx and larynx. Indeed, difficult or impossible intubation has been encountered with severe maternal consequences. General anesthesia for markedly edematous preeclamptic patients should be avoided, and when absolutely necessary, preparation for alternative methods of securing the airway must be made. Postextubation airway obstruction resulting from edema at the level of the glottis is a serious complication and occurs frequently in these patients.

Pulmonary edema is another complication of preeclampsia. Most of these patients have normal cardiac function with imbalances in pulmonary artery pressure and colloid osmotic pressure.

The observed reduction of colloid osmotic pressure in normal pregnancy is further decreased in preeclampsia. This is due to the loss of albumin, which is the major contributor to colloid osmotic pressure. Modest elevations in pulmonary artery occlusion pressure from exogenous fluid administration and mobilization of endogenous fluid will alter the gradient between colloid osmotic pressure and pulmonary artery pressure so that transudation of fluid into the interstitium is likely.

Drugs

Pharmacologic agents are often required to treat patients with preeclampsia. These drugs can interact with anesthetic agents to produce an undesired effect, and both obstetrician and anesthesiologist should be aware of the pharmacology of the drugs employed, their dosages, and the time of administration.

Magnesium sulfate is the most commonly administered agent in the management of preeclampsia. Adverse effects are few when it is administered appropriately, and overdosage is treated easily with intravenous calcium. Magnesium exerts several important effects at the neuromuscular junction. It inhibits the release of acetylcholine from the presynaptic nerve terminal, depresses the postjunctional membrane response, and depresses the response of the underlying myofibrils (Foldes, 1959). These effects are responsible for the muscle weakness and respiratory depression observed with overdosage. Neuromuscular blocking agents are used to facilitate endotracheal intubation and to maintain a relaxed surgical field when general anesthesia is provided for cesarean delivery (Reisner and Lin, 1999). Magnesium potentiates and prolongs the action of depolarizing agents (e.g., succinylcholine) as well as nondepolarizing agents (e.g., D-tubocurarine, rocuronium, vecuronium, atracurium, pancuronium) (Ghoneim and Long, 1970). Therefore, lower doses of these drugs will be necessary, and electronic monitoring of the neuromuscular junction is helpful.

It is essential that the patient be evaluated carefully at the end of the procedure to ensure that she has regained sufficient muscle strength to maintain and protect her airway and to sustain adequate ventilation. Because drugs used to provide anesthesia are anticonvulsant in nature, it is prudent to discontinue magnesium sulfate therapy in the operating room when general anesthesia is used and to reinitiate use after the patient has regained full neuromuscular function.

The anesthetic options for a patient with severe preeclampsia depend on the mode of delivery. Analgesia for the first stage of labor reduces maternal catecholamine output and perhaps maintains or improves uteroplacental blood flow. Systemic analgesia with narcotics is acceptable, although continuous lumbar epidural analgesia provides the best pain relief with minimal, if any, sedation. The use of segmental epidural analgesia avoids extensive sympathetic blockade. Opioids may be added to the local anesthetic solution to enhance the quality of pain relief without additional sympathetic or motor blockade. If sympathetic blockade must be totally avoided, the use of intrathecal narcotics (e.g., morphine, fentanyl, sufentanil, or meperidine) could be preferable by either single injection or continuous technique. Anesthesia for vaginal delivery may be provided by pudendal nerve block, low spinal anesthesia, or lumbar or caudal epidural anesthesia. Although the choice of anesthetic in the patient who is to undergo cesarean delivery has been controversial, the careful use of epidural anesthesia, with meticulous attention to left uterine displacement and fluid management, is associated with good maternal and fetal outcome and is the preferred approach (Moore et al., 1985).

When general anesthesia is required, measures must be taken to avoid the hypertensive response to laryngoscopy and intubation as well as to extubation. Labetalol administered just before induction, in doses up to 1 mg/kg, have proved effective in reducing this response. Alternative or adjunctive drugs, such as sodium nitroprusside and nitroglycerin, may also be utilized. Sodium nitroprusside, because of its short half-life, provides the advantage of allowing for minute-to-minute blood pressure control.

Inability to intubate the trachea is the leading cause of maternal death associated with general anesthesia. Therefore, alternative means of providing oxygenation and ventilation (e.g., laryngeal mask airway, the Combitube, transtracheal jet ventilation) must be readily available (Reisner, Benumof, et al., 1999). Transtracheal jet ventilation provides adequate oxygenation and ventilation to pregnant patients (Benumof and Scheller, 1989). If airway difficulty is anticipated, an awake intubation, perhaps aided by a fiberoptic bronchoscope, may be necessary.

Spinal anesthesia is usually avoided for cesarean delivery of patients with severe preeclampsia because of concern about rapid onset of profound sympathetic blockade. With the use of a continuous catheter, however, the block may be titrated in a fashion similar to that for epidural anesthesia. On occasion, some patients technically meet the criteria for severe preeclampsia but do not have evidence of significant volume contraction or vasospasm and may be suitable candidates for spinal anesthesia.

■ NEUROLOGIC DISORDERS

Multiple Sclerosis

Multiple sclerosis is a disease of young adults that can occur in young pregnant women. Although there have been many attempts to associate anesthesia and surgery with relapses of symptoms, no controlled studies have directly linked any form of anesthesia to exacerbation (Kytta and Rosenberg, 1984). Routine use of anticholinergic agents is not recommended because they could induce an elevation in temperature, known to be associated with exacerbations.

There has been concern that local anesthetics may be more histotoxic to nervous tissue already damaged by multiple sclerosis. All local anesthetic agents are neurotoxic in concentrations well above those used clinically. Enhanced neurotoxicity from local anesthetic drugs has not been demonstrated in patients with multiple sclerosis, and epidural analgesia and anesthesia have been successfully used for labor and delivery (Crawford et al., 1981; Bader et al., 1988).

The lowest concentration of local anesthesia capable of producing the desired effect should be selected. Epidural and intrathecal narcotics have also been administered without apparent adverse effects.

Paraplegia

The paraplegic patient is able to maintain a far better state of health than in the past, and many do elect to become pregnant. The level and extent of the lesion determine the patient's response to labor. If the spinal cord lesion is below the tenth thoracic dermatome, the patient will have the sensation of labor. If it is above this level, she will have minimal, if any, awareness of contractions. Paraplegic parturients tend to have a normal course of labor but a higher percentage of forceps-assisted deliveries because of weakness of the abdominal muscles and consequent impairment of the ability to bear down effectively in the second stage. The major anesthetic issues are the management of analgesia and anesthesia for labor and delivery, the possibility of autonomic hyperreflexia, and hyperkalemia with the administration of succinylcholine.

The phenomenon of *autonomic hyperreflexia* occurs in patients whose spinal cord lesion is at the seventh thoracic dermatome or higher. This condition is characterized by severe hypertension, bradycardia, headache, premature ventricular contractions, flushing, sweating, and pilomotor erection. The hypertension can be severe and, if uncontrolled, can lead to central nervous system hemorrhage, cardiac decompensation, or death. It is triggered by stimulation below the level of the spinal cord lesion. Common initiating events include bladder or rectal distention, rubbing of the skin, genital stimulation, and contraction of any hollow viscus, including the uterus. The triggering impulse is conducted to the spinal cord, where a reflex response occurs that cannot be modulated or inhibited by higher centers, owing to the isolation invoked by the cord lesion. This results in an uncontrolled adrenergic discharge with norepinephrine release from the peripheral sympathetic nerve endings (Schonwald et al., 1981). The release of adrenal catecholamines may also be involved.

Although a large percentage of patients at risk do exhibit this reflex, some do not. A careful history should reveal those who exhibit such a response. Because preterm labor could be unrecognized by these patients, the sudden onset of paroxysmal hypertension should prompt a search for uterine contractions before the diagnosis of pregnancy-induced hypertension is considered.

During labor, adequate blockade of the afferent impulses can be provided by regional anesthesia, even if no pain is perceived by the patient. Continuous epidural anesthesia with both local anesthetic and narcotic agents has been employed successfully to treat autonomic hyperreflexia during labor and delivery (Baraka, 1985). Spinal anesthesia, both single-injection and continuous, has also been used to control blood pressure (Lambert et al., 1982). With regional anesthesia, it is difficult to determine whether an adequate block is present, as the usual sensory tests are useless below the level of the lesion. The anesthetic block must therefore be titrated to just above the existing sensory level. Autonomic hyperreflexia can also be controlled by a variety of antihypertensive agents, such as phentolamine and sodium nitroprusside.

Finally, general anesthesia can effectively inhibit the hyperreflexia response (Wanner et al., 1987). If general anesthesia is required for a complex vaginal or cesarean delivery, however, the anesthesiologist must determine when the spinal cord injury initially occurred; this is because there is a significant release of potassium from the denervated muscle following use of succinylcholine for endotracheal intubation if it is administered 6 months to 1 year after the injury (Gronert and Theye, 1975). The elevation in serum potassium can reach life-threatening levels.

Ordinarily, although a general anesthetic agent may be utilized safely, an epidural anesthetic agent is preferred. Regional anesthesia has the advantage of blocking afferent input, thereby avoiding autonomic hyperreflexia. In addition, if the lesion is in the upper thoracic region, the patient will have weak abdominal and thoracic musculature. The use of epidural anesthesia is preferable to spinal anesthesia because the degree of motor impairment is less and profound muscle relaxation is not required. The block can be advanced gradually, thus avoiding sudden hypotension from a rapid extensive sympathetic blockade.

Subarachnoid Hemorrhage

Subarachnoid hemorrhage from an intracranial vascular lesion is an infrequent but extremely serious complication of pregnancy (Dias and Sekkar, 1990; Horton et al., 1990). It is possible that the stress induced by the increased cardiac output and blood volume, combined with the softening of vascular connective tissue by the hormonal changes of pregnancy, may predispose a patient to such an event. The diagnosis could be obscured initially because nausea and vomiting are common findings during pregnancy.

Treatment is usually surgical if the lesion is an aneurysm because this significantly improves maternal chances of survival. The decision to treat surgically should be influenced not by the pregnancy but by the site and type of lesion, the clinical condition of the patient, and the presence or absence of vasospasm. Medical management appears to be as effective as surgical management for arteriovenous malformations during pregnancy. Once a patient has undergone surgical correction of an aneurysm, there are no special considerations for anesthetic management of labor and delivery.

The anesthetic concerns regarding the patient without surgical correction are focused on two different clinical situations. The first relates to the patient undergoing neurosurgery for a ruptured aneurysm; the second is anesthetic management of labor and delivery for a patient who has not undergone surgical repair. Anesthesia for the patient having a neurosurgical procedure has the same primary goals as for all patients having surgery during pregnancy, namely, maintaining uteroplacental blood flow and fetal oxygenation and preventing preterm delivery (Leicht, 1990).

The usual neurosurgical anesthetic approach to patients with these types of lesions includes the following:

1. Deliberate hypotension to reduce the risk of cerebral hemorrhage
2. Hypothermia to reduce cerebral metabolism
3. Hyperventilation to reduce cerebral blood flow and brain size
4. Diuresis to promote shrinkage of the brain

Deliberate hypotension can be produced with a volatile anesthetic, sodium nitroprusside, nitroglycerin, or trimethaphan. Each agent carries its own potential hazards in addition to reduction in uteroplacental blood flow. It is generally acknowledged that a reduction in systolic blood pressure of 25%–30% or a mean arterial blood pressure of less than 70 mm Hg will lead to reductions in uteroplacental blood flow. The hypotensive agents also cross the placenta and can induce hypotension in the fetus. Further, nitroprusside is converted to cyanide, and cyanide accumulation and toxicity in the fetus pose at least a theoretical risk in the human. If this agent is used, it should be for only a short time. It should be discontinued if the required infusion rate exceeds 0.5 mg/kg/hour, if maternal metabolic acidosis ensues, or if resistance to the agent is apparent.

Nitroglycerin has yet to be associated with adverse fetal effects. It is metabolized to nitrites, which, experimentally at least, have produced methemoglobinemia. This agent, however, is less predictable in its hypotensive effect than sodium nitroprusside. Trimethaphan often leads to tachyphylaxis, and it interacts with neuromuscular blocking agents. It is a ganglionic blocker, thus intensifying the effects of some of the nondepolarizing muscle relaxants. Fetal heart rate monitoring should be employed, and hypotension should be limited to the shortest period of time possible. Although it is preferable to avoid or limit the period of hypotension in the pregnant patient, successful neonatal outcome after induced hypotension with careful control has been observed (Donchin et al., 1978; Minielly et al., 1979).

Hypothermia is used occasionally to decrease cerebral metabolic requirements and blood flow. The usual goal is to achieve a temperature of approximately 30°C. This measure induces similar temperature changes in the fetus, and fetal bradycardia occurs. The heart rate will increase again with rewarming (Stange and Halldin, 1983). Hyperventilation is commonly used during neuroanesthesia, as the decrease in PCO_2 reduces cerebral blood flow. The goal is to reach a $PaCO_2$ of approximately 20–25 mm Hg. This degree of respiratory alkalosis should not be a problem for the healthy fetus, as a $PaCO_2$ of 32 mm Hg is the norm for pregnant women. Fetal heart rate monitoring should alert the anesthesiologist to compromises in fetal oxygenation, and adjustments may be made accordingly.

Diuresis is often accomplished with osmotic agents or loop diuretics to shrink the brain both intraoperatively and postoperatively. These agents can cause significant negative fluid shifts for the fetus. Obviously, diuretic agents should be given only as necessary and not strictly by protocol for the pregnant patient.

The objectives in managing a patient for labor and delivery who has not undergone surgical repair are to avoid hypertension and to avoid elevations in intracranial pressure. The Valsalva maneuver should be avoided, because the sudden pressure changes at the end of the maneuver can produce a gradient that favors rupture of the lesion. Epidural analgesia and anesthesia can most effectively provide conditions to meet these goals. It could be relatively contraindicated for patients who already have marked increases in intracranial pressure, inasmuch as an unintentional dural puncture can lead to herniation of the cerebellum. There is also a theoretical risk of further increasing intracranial pressure from the volume of fluid placed in the epidural space. This pressure rise is minimal and transient in the normal parturient, however, when the volume administered is kept relatively small and the rate of injection slow.

Other commonly used forms of analgesia may be employed as long as maternal respiratory depression is avoided. Cesarean delivery anesthesia is best provided by the continuous epidural technique. Spinal anesthesia may be used if intracranial hypertension does not exist. If general anesthesia is required, the steps outlined previously for preventing the hypertensive response to laryngoscopy and intubation will be necessary. For more information about these neurologic complications, see Chapter 55.

■ RESPIRATORY DISORDERS

In order to understand the implications of anesthesia superimposed on a pregnant woman with respiratory disease, one should have a knowledge of the physiologic alterations in the respiratory tract during pregnancy. These changes and the various disorders in pregnancy are reviewed in Chapter 46.

Asthma

Asthma is the most common respiratory problem encountered in the population of childbearing age. The disease is characterized by bronchial constriction, bronchial secretions, and bronchial edema. Therapy commonly includes theophylline preparations, inhaled beta-adrenoceptor agonists, anticholinergic agents, corticosteroids, and occasionally, cromolyn sodium. Magnesium sulfate has also been effective in alleviating acute symptoms (Lindeman et al., 1989). The effect of pregnancy on the condition of the asthmatic has been controversial, but it does appear that with proper management and prompt attention to acute episodes, most patients do well (Greenberger, 1990). Maintenance of the patient's medications and hydration are of major importance during labor and delivery.

Analgesia and anesthesia for labor and delivery of the asthmatic patient serve to alleviate anxiety and hyperventilation. Hyperventilation can precipitate an attack and lead to increased fluid losses and dehydration. Narcotic analgesia administered in a judicious fashion may be utilized, but narcotics are bronchoconstrictors and should be avoided if the patient is actively wheezing or in respiratory distress. Epidural analgesia with local anesthetics, opioids, or both is extremely beneficial because pain can be relieved while respiratory depression is avoided (Younker et al., 1987). If the patient is severely asthmatic, it is essential to avoid a high and dense level of anesthesia because accessory muscles of respiration could be impaired. A high thoracic level could completely block sympathetic pathways, and the unopposed parasympathetic tone could lead to bronchoconstriction. Either low spinal anesthesia or a pudendal block is a reasonable choice for vaginal delivery if epidural analgesia is not used.

Regional anesthesia is preferred because the insertion of an endotracheal tube at the light levels of anesthesia traditionally favored for obstetrics frequently results in bronchospasm (Benatar, 1981). Even though pulmonary mechanics are reasonably well maintained under spinal or epidural anesthesia to the fourth thoracic dermatome, the patient should receive an inhaled beta agonist prior to the procedure and bring her inhaler with her to the operating room, as bronchospasm could occur (McGough and Cohen, 1990). Appropriate attention to hydration and maintenance of blood pressure are required, and supplemental oxygen is recommended.

General anesthesia for cesarean delivery in the asthmatic patient poses additional risk. Careful attention to detail is necessary to avoid life-threatening bronchospasm, and general anesthesia should be used only if regional anesthesia is contraindicated. Preoperative preparation should include adequate hydration, intravenous aminophylline, treatment with a beta$_2$ agonist inhaler, antacid therapy, and sufficient time for preoxygenation (a minimum of 3 minutes). A rapid-sequence induction may then be undertaken. The induction agent of choice is ketamine because it is a bronchodilator and does not release histamine (Corssen et al., 1972). Propofol decreases the response to airway manipulation and could prove to be a reasonable alternative. Thiopental administered in the commonly used doses for cesarean delivery produces a plane of anesthesia that is too light to prevent bronchospasm. Larger doses are an alternative to ketamine and may be employed with the small risk that the newborn will be depressed from the anesthetic in the immediate postdelivery period.

The patient with active wheezing requiring a general anesthetic for cesarean delivery could require a slower induction. Anesthesia is induced intravenously, a muscle relaxant is administered, cricoid pressure is applied and maintained, and the patient is ventilated by mask with a volatile anesthetic agent to promote bronchodilation. When a deep plane of anesthesia is reached, the patient is intubated. This technique exposes the patient to a greater risk of regurgitation and aspiration of gastric contents and should be employed only when there are no other reasonable options.

Once anesthesia is induced and the patient has been intubated successfully, maintenance includes the administration of a volatile agent in a humidified gas mixture because all gases in current use (halothane, enflurane, isoflurane, sevoflurane) produce direct bronchial muscle relaxation (Hirshman et al., 1982). If intraoperative wheezing should occur, a beta$_2$ agonist may be aerosolized via the endotracheal tube. Although the effect is synergistic with the halogenated agents, two potential problems must be considered. First, halothane administration in the presence of therapeutic or higher levels of aminophylline has been associated with serious ventricular arrhythmias and cardiac arrest (Richards et al., 1988). Isoflurane, enflurane, or sevoflurane is an acceptable alternative. Second, the volatile agents tend to relax uterine musculature at concentrations that are effective as bronchodilators, and the possibility of enhanced uterine bleeding exists. This effect can usually be counteracted by the administration of oxytocin. The use of prostaglandins to control hemorrhage is not recommended because prostaglandin F$_{2alpha}$ is a bronchoconstrictor. Once the infant has been delivered, ventilation with bag and mask oxygen eliminates most of the volatile agent from the infant in a few minutes.

Muscle relaxation can be maintained with a succinylcholine infusion or with a nondepolarizing agent. Curare, metocurine, and atracurium are associated with histamine release in large doses, whereas pancuronium, vecuronium, rocuronium, and cis-atracurium are not. When a nondepolarizing agent is used, it usually must be reversed at the end of the procedure with an anticholinesterase drug such as neostigmine or edrophonium. This group of nondepolarizing drugs can produce bronchoconstriction and increased production of secretions. Consequently, a sufficient dose of an anticholinergic agent such as atropine or glycopyrrolate must be administered prior to use. The nonpregnant asthmatic patient is usually extubated in a deep plane of anesthesia to avoid the stimulus of the endotracheal tube, but the pregnant patient should be extubated while awake because of the risks of vomiting and aspiration. Intravenous lidocaine can prevent coughing and bronchoconstriction upon emergence.

Postoperative care should include humidified oxygen, incentive spirometry, and the required pharmacologic agents. Epidural and intrathecal narcotics provide excellent postoperative analgesia with minimal sedation.

Cystic Fibrosis

The meticulous use of pulmonary toilet and aggressive antibiotic therapy has made it possible for many women with cystic fibrosis to survive well into their childbearing years (Canny et al., 1991). The pulmonary complications of patients with cystic fibrosis provide significant anesthetic challenges. Thick, excessive mucus production results in obstruction of the small and medium-sized airways with subsequent bronchitis and bronchiectasis. Pneumothorax, atelectasis, progressive hypoxemia, and cor pulmonale are all seen commonly with the disease.

Therapy consists of postural drainage and chest percussion (often on a daily basis), antibiotics for symptoms of infection, bronchodilators for wheezing, intermittent mucolytic therapy (N-acetylcysteine), vitamins, and pancreatic enzyme replacement. Preoperative evaluation should include pulmonary function studies, cardiac evaluation, and measurement of arterial blood gases. Successful completion of gestation with careful attention to medical management is now well documented (Valenzuela et al., 1988; Canny et al., 1991).

Optimal analgesia during the first stage of labor is provided by continuous lumbar epidural anesthesia. Intrathecal opioids should be avoided because they have, on occasion, been associated with severe respiratory depression, particularly if parenteral opioids have been administered as well (Jaffee et al., 1997). Management concerns are similar to those of the severe asthmatic patient. The state of hydration needs to be maintained because these patients often lose a great deal of fluid through sweating. Narcotics should be used in very small amounts because they suppress the cough reflex and produce respiratory depression. Nitrous oxide should probably be avoided because of the frequency of pneumothorax from ruptured bullae. Anesthesia for vaginal delivery may be provided with low spinal, epidural, or pudendal nerve block.

Anesthesia for cesarean delivery also carries with it the same management concerns as for the patient with severe asthma, and carefully titrated continuous epidural anesthesia is recommended. Although general anesthesia can be used safely for patients with cystic fibrosis, the risk of maternal hypoxemia during induction is greater than for asthmatic patients, and the possibility of pneumothorax exists during positive-pressure ventilation. Anticholinergics (drying agents) and narcotics are usually excluded from the regimen, and gases should be humidified. Patients with very advanced disease could require postoperative mechanical ventilation until they regain their full preoperative capabilities.

Morbid Obesity

Morbid obesity is defined as an accumulation of adipose tissue that causes the body mass index (BMI) to increase by 30% or more, as shown by the following equation:

$$BMI = \frac{weight\ (kg)}{[height\ (m)]^2}$$

where weight is in kilograms and height is in meters.

Substantial change takes place over time in the respiratory system. A restrictive lung disease pattern develops, and pulmonary function testing reveals a decrease in expiratory reserve volume, vital capacity, inspiratory capacity, and total lung capacity. Compliance decreases, and the work of breathing increases. There is also a ventilation-perfusion imbalance, leading to hypoxemia, particularly in the supine or Trendelenburg position.

Pregnancy imposes changes in lung volumes similar to those resulting from obesity. Although it would be presumed that these effects are additive, this is not the case. A study evaluat-

ing 12 obese pregnant women revealed that the usual pulmonary changes of pregnancy occurred, but they were not accentuated by the obesity. Hypoxemia existed but was not worsened by pregnancy (Eng et al., 1975).

Labor should be conducted in the sitting or semirecumbent position with left uterine displacement. Supplemental oxygen administration and pulse oximeter monitoring are advised. Epidural or combined spinal-epidural analgesia is recommended but could be technically difficult or impossible to perform because of obscured landmarks, difficult positioning, and excessive layers of adipose tissue. Other forms of analgesia, including intrathecal narcotics, intravenous narcotics, and inhalation of nitrous oxide/oxygen, are all suitable. The anesthetic for vaginal delivery may be any of the commonly used forms; the patient should remain in a semisitting position, if possible, to prevent small airway closure.

Cesarean delivery anesthesia may be provided by either the spinal, epidural, or combined spinal-epidural route (Kuczkowski and Benumof, 2002b). Again, technical difficulties can be encountered, and the dosage of drug needs to be reduced because spread in both the subarachnoid and epidural space is enhanced with morbid obesity (Hodgkinson and Husain, 1980). The physician must take care to avoid a significant motor block, which could compromise ventilation and result in hypoxemia. The Trendelenburg position should be avoided because it shifts the weight of the abdominal viscera and the panniculus toward the chest and diaphragm, further compromising respiration.

Technically, general anesthesia poses several challenges. First, the airway must be secured. Endotracheal intubation can be extremely difficult as a result of excessive tissue and edema. Exceedingly large breasts can interfere with the insertion of a conventional laryngoscope. A careful assessment of the airway must be made; if this assessment appears difficult, a fiberoptic intubation is recommended with the patient awake. If a rapid sequence induction is attempted and the airway cannot be conventionally secured, an alternative means, such as a laryngeal mask airway, Combitube, or transtracheal jet ventilation must be at hand, as hypoxia and acidosis can develop at an extremely rapid rate.

After the airway is secured, mechanical ventilation will be required, and the pressures generated need to be high to move the large body mass. Large tidal volumes help to prevent airway closure. Extubation should be performed only when the patient is fully awake and has regained her full strength. Postoperative analgesia, preferably by the epidural route, is extremely helpful in allowing for deep breathing exercises to avoid atelectasis and pneumonia.

CARDIAC DISEASE

The pregnant patient with heart disease represents a unique challenge for the anesthesiologist. Determination of the appropriate analgesic and anesthetic modalities requires a thorough understanding of the parturient's pathophysiology as well as pharmacologic therapy and how these interact with anesthetic care. Chapter 41 presents an in-depth discussion of the various cardiac disorders in pregnancy.

Over the past two decades, greater awareness of the physiologic burden that pregnancy places on an already compromised cardiovascular system in this subset of pregnant women has led to more accurate counseling before conception and major advances in treatment. Formerly, rheumatic heart disease was the most common cardiac disorder in pregnancy, with mitral stenosis the single most prevalent resulting lesion. In general, the incidence of rheumatic heart disease has decreased, but in some locales it has risen again with the recent influx of immigrants from Asia. Also, many more women with congenital heart defects are reaching childbearing age, a consequence of surgical correction (Spielman, 1986). As more women delay childbearing until later reproductive years, ischemic cardiac disease can be expected to become increasingly prevalent (Roberts and Chestnut, 1987).

General Considerations

Pregnancy normally results in dramatic changes in the cardiovascular system, and these changes as well as cardiac disorders in pregnancy are reviewed extensively in Chapters 8 and 41. Four principal changes that present unique problems to the patient with cardiac disease have been well delineated (Clark, 1991) and have special anesthetic implications.

First, there is a 50% increase in intravascular volume that generally peaks by the early-to-middle third trimester. This relative volume overload could be poorly tolerated in patients whose cardiac output is limited by myocardial dysfunction from ischemia or intrinsic or valvular lesions.

Second, there is a progressive decrease in systemic vascular resistance (SVR) throughout pregnancy, so that mean arterial pressure (MAP) is preserved at normal values despite a 30%–40% increase in cardiac output. This could be of importance in those patients at risk for right-to-left shunting as well as for patients with some types of valvular disease (e.g., aortic stenosis).

Third, the compromised cardiovascular system is further stressed by the marked fluctuations in cardiac output observed during labor. Pain and apprehension can precipitate an increase in cardiac output to as much as 45%–50% over those levels seen in the late second stage of labor (Ueland and Hansen, 1969a). Further, each uterine contraction serves, in effect, as an autotransfusion to the central blood volume, resulting in an increase in cardiac output of 10%–25% (Ueland and Hansen, 1969b). The Valsalva maneuver results in wide swings in both venous and arterial pressures, which have been associated with acute cardiac decompensation. The increases in cardiac output reach a maximum of 80% higher than antepartum levels immediately following delivery secondary to relief of inferior vena cava obstruction and a final autotransfusion of approximately 500 mL from uterine contraction.

The fourth consideration is the hypercoagulability associated with pregnancy and the possible need for appropriate anticoagulation, especially in those patients at increased risk for arterial thrombosis and embolization (prosthetic heart valve or chronic atrial fibrillation). Therapeutic anticoagulation affects the options for anesthetic management—perhaps the location of invasive monitors—and increases the risk of postpartum hemorrhage.

Optimal anesthetic management requires a thorough assessment of the anatomic and functional capacity of the diseased heart along with an analysis of how the described major physiologic changes are likely to affect the specific limitations imposed by the intrinsic disease. Specifically, to determine the most appropriate anesthetic regimen, the anesthesiologist must consider the following:

1. Patient's tolerance to pain during labor or surgery
2. Impact of uterine contraction–induced autotransfusion
3. Postpartum changes induced by relief of vena caval obstruction
4. Potential for postpartum hemorrhage
5. Use of uterine oxytocic agents

The most basic principles of obstetric anesthesia management must always apply (Malinow and Ostheimer, 1987):

1. Provisions for maintenance of uteroplacental perfusion by avoidance of aortocaval compression
2. Minimizing sympathetic blockade coupled with intravascular volume maintenance
3. Standard-of-care monitoring of parturient and fetus
4. Provision for aspiration prophylaxis

Analgesia during the first stage of labor is focused on reducing the pain-related rises in catecholamine levels and avoiding aortocaval compression. Intravenous fluid management should be carefully monitored to avoid both a lack of and an excess of fluids. Arterial, central venous, and/or pulmonary artery monitoring may be required to manage the patient optimally. Although such lines are generally reserved for symptomatic women, patients who have "tight" aortic stenosis, coarctation of the aorta, aortic aneurysm, right-to-left shunts, or primary pulmonary hypertension may benefit from invasive monitoring even with minimal symptoms. See Chapters 41 and 45 for more detailed information.

Appropriate analgesia should be supplied. All of the available modalities have application for some patients. Continuous lumbar epidural analgesia with local anesthetics, narcotics, or both is frequently optimal. Limited sympathetic blockade could prove helpful with mitral valve lesions because of the effect on both preload and afterload. For a patient whose condition is so compromised that even the modest changes induced by segmental epidural analgesia are worrisome, the use of intrathecal narcotic analgesia by single injection or continuous catheter may be beneficial because all of the hemodynamic alterations of sympathetic blockade are avoided.

Once the patient with significant cardiac disease has entered the second stage of labor, it is prudent for her to avoid pushing. The lithotomy position may need to be avoided for patients with lesions such as mitral stenosis, inasmuch as this position results in an acute increase in central blood volume.

For second-stage management, analgesia for uterine contractions and anesthesia of the perineum are the objectives. Uterine contractions spontaneously bring the infant's head to a deliverable position, and delivery can then be assisted by the application of the vacuum extractor or forceps. Again, a regional technique is optimal. Epidural analgesia or anesthesia may be continued. Attention must be paid to extension of the sympathetic blockade. If an epidural block is not used, a low spinal anesthetic may be appropriate. Pudendal nerve block, although it does not provide as complete an analgesia as an epidural, can be employed satisfactorily as an adjunct to regional anesthesia or can be used alone.

It is generally thought that cesarean delivery should be reserved for obstetric indications only and that the presence of heart disease should not influence that decision. The overall stresses of labor and vaginal delivery, as measured by alterations in cardiac output, are approximately the same as with cesarean delivery. Some circumstances, however, may lead to the decision to perform an elective cesarean delivery. The choice of anesthesia depends on the lesion and its severity. Epidural anesthesia provides the least amount of alteration in hemodynamics during cesarean delivery, although general anesthesia can be equally as safe when the abrupt changes associated with laryngoscopy and intubation, as well as suction and extubation, are blunted by the appropriate choice of pharmacologic agents and anesthetic technique.

Anesthetic for Cardiac Surgery during Pregnancy

Surgery of any type is usually avoided during pregnancy because of potential compromise to the unborn infant. The developing fetus may experience teratogenic effects from drugs administered during the course of anesthesia. This has been demonstrated in animals with a multitude of anesthetic adjuvants but has never been clearly documented in humans (Pedersen and Finster, 1979; Levinson and Shnider, 1987; Reisner, 1998). Teratogenic changes could also be induced by hypoxia during the procedure or by decreased uteroplacental perfusion. Premature labor is often associated with surgery during pregnancy, particularly abdominal procedures (Levine and Diamond, 1961). Thus, if surgery is indicated during the course of pregnancy, it is usually performed during the second trimester whenever possible. This strategy avoids the period of organogenesis, and premature labor is said to be less likely. Many centers utilize tocolytic therapy as part of their routine for the surgical patient who is pregnant. Although this can be useful for patients without cardiovascular disease, most of these drugs have potent cardiovascular side effects and would prove less desirable for the patient with heart disease (Ravindran et al., 1980).

The pregnant patient with heart disease is often managed with medical therapy, which can include long periods of bed rest if necessary. If a surgical lesion is present, every attempt is made to delay the definitive procedure until after delivery of the infant. There are patients who decompensate so severely from the cardiovascular stress imposed by pregnancy, however, that their chance of survival is very small unless surgical correction is attempted. These patients usually suffer from rheumatic valvular disease, most often mitral stenosis.

The first cardiac operations performed during pregnancy were closed mitral commissurotomies for severe congestive heart failure caused by mitral stenosis in 1952. A review of 514 cases by Ueland (1975) revealed a maternal mortality of 1.75% and a fetal loss of 8.6%. This was quite favorable when compared with a maternal mortality of 4.2%–18.7% in pregnant patients with NYSHA Class III and IV cardiac disease managed with medical therapy; the fetal loss in that group of patients was approximately 50%. The extremely good surgical survival figures in the cardiac surgery group are probably due to the fact that these patients are young with relatively healthy hearts that were overburdened by the circulatory changes of pregnancy and that the operations did not involve cardiopulmonary bypass. The use of cardiopulmonary bypass for open heart procedures in the pregnant patient soon followed. The risk for both mother and fetus increases with this more complex procedure. A multi-institutional study of cardiopulmonary bypass in this subset of patients by Zitnik and colleagues (1969) revealed a 5% maternal mortality and a fetal loss of 33%. More current data indicate a maternal mortality of 0%–2.9% and a fetal loss of 20% (Pomini et al., 1996). The high fetal loss has been attributed to several factors that could affect fetal oxygen delivery during cardiopulmonary bypass. These include nonpulsatile perfusion, inadequate perfusion pressure, embolic events to the uteroplacental circulation, disturbance of uteroplacental blood flow by cannulae, release of catecholamines and renin, and hypothermia (Parry and Westaby, 1996). Some of these potential hazards can be avoided by the use of fetal monitoring during the operation.

Several reports of the benefit of fetal monitoring during cardiopulmonary bypass have appeared in the literature (Koh et al., 1975; Eilen et al., 1981). In one instance, a fetal heart rate of 60 was restored to 100 by an increase in pump flow from 3100 to 3600 mL/minute (Koh et al., 1975). In addition to identifying potentially threatening events, all authors have reported a sustained fetal bradycardia between 80 and 100 beats per minute during hypothermic cardiopulmonary bypass, which resolves with the restoration of maternal temperature and normal circulation. One meta-analysis revealed that fetal mortality was reduced to 0% when normothermic cardiopulmonary bypass was utilized (Pomini et al., 1996).

Based on the available knowledge of the physiologic changes of pregnancy, the pharmacology of drugs employed during cardiopulmonary bypass, the physiology of extracorporeal circulation, and experiences reported, the following recommendations for cardiopulmonary bypass during pregnancy can be made. Although it would be desirable to avoid such surgery until after pregnancy, no pregnant patient should be denied a definitive operation because of gestation. Whenever possible, the period of organogenesis should be avoided and the second trimester favored. If cardiopulmonary bypass is required after 28 weeks' gestation, it has been suggested that cesarean delivery immediately prior to the cardiac surgery is a reasonable and safe procedure (Parry and Westaby, 1996). We believe that hemostasis must be meticulous in such cases, as full anticoagulation is necessary.

Every effort to ensure adequate fetal oxygenation and perfusion during the procedure should be exercised. Maternal inspired oxygen concentration should be maintained as high as possible, and arterial blood gases should be checked frequently. Maternal ventilation should be adjusted to avoid respiratory alkalosis, as this causes a shift in the oxyhemoglobin dissociation curve to the left, thus potentially decreasing oxygen transport to the fetus. Aortocaval compression must be minimized by utilizing a wedge to provide left uterine displacement if the patient is at 20 weeks of gestation or greater. Calculation of pump flows should include a 30%–50% increase above normal to compensate for the increase in cardiac output that occurs with pregnancy. Pomini and colleagues (1996) recommend maintaining flows at 2.7 L/m²/min or greater. Perfusion pressures of 60 mm Hg or greater appear optimal for maintaining uteroplacental perfusion. Perfusion times should be kept to a minimum, and normothermic bypass should be utilized whenever possible. Electrolyte balance should be maintained, and the impact of vasopressors on the uteroplacental circulation should be considered before they are instituted. Electronic fetal monitoring should be used, with a member of the health care team experienced in its interpretation available.

Monitoring of uterine activity can also be desirable, as increased uterine activity has been associated with cardiopulmonary bypass (Parry and Westaby, 1996).

Valvular Heart Disease

Rheumatic fever continues to be the predominant etiology of valvular heart disease in pregnancy. Complications during pregnancy include univentricular or biventricular failure, atrial dysrhythmias, systemic or pulmonary embolism, and infective endocarditis, with an overall incidence of complications estimated at 15% of all patients with valvular disease. In general, regurgitant lesions are well tolerated during pregnancy because the increased plasma volume and lowered systemic vascular resistance result in increased cardiac output. In contrast, stenotic valvular disease is poorly tolerated with advancing pregnancy, owing to the inability to increase cardiac output sufficient to accommodate the augmented plasma volume; this situation leads to pulmonary venous congestion and, possibly, frank pulmonary edema.

Mitral Stenosis

Mitral stenosis can occur as an isolated lesion or in conjunction with right-sided or aortic valvular disease. It accounts for nearly 90% of rheumatic heart disease in pregnancy, with 25% of patients first experiencing symptoms during pregnancy (Sugrue et al., 1981). The principal pathophysiologic derangement is a decrease in mitral valve orifice, resulting in obstruction to left ventricular filling. This hemodynamic aberration leads to a relatively fixed cardiac output. Although initially, the left atrium may overcome this obstruction, with progression of disease left atrial volume and pressure ultimately increase and lead to a progressive and chronic rise in pulmonary capillary wedge pressure and pulmonary venous pressure; pulmonary hypertension and right ventricular hypertrophy and failure can ensue. An anatomically moderate lesion can become functionally severe with the marked increase in cardiac output that accompanies normal pregnancy, labor, and delivery.

Anesthetic management is oriented toward the avoidance of tachycardia, as the time required for left ventricular diastolic filling is prolonged. Patients who are asymptomatic at term generally require increased vigilance but should not require invasive monitoring. Patients with marked symptoms are at significant risk in the peripartum period and should receive arterial and pulmonary artery catheter monitoring continuing through a minimum of 24 hours postpartum (Clark et al., 1985). An increase in central circulating blood volume can occur suddenly in the immediate postpartum period, and tolerance of this intravascular load may be poor, especially for patients with a fixed cardiac output (Ueland, 1988; Ducey and Ellsworth, 1989).

Anesthesia for labor and vaginal delivery can best be accomplished with segmental lumbar epidural anesthesia to avoid changes in monitored hemodynamic parameters. A sudden decrease in systemic vascular resistance may be poorly tolerated following the development of reflex tachycardia. Although other analgesic modalities may be employed, segmental epidural analgesia allows for careful titration to the desired result while minimizing undesirable changes. The addition of opioids, such as fentanyl, to the dilute local anesthetic mixture enhances the quality of analgesia yet does not add to the sympathetic block-

ade. Opioids alone may be administered by the epidural or intrathecal route for the critically ill patient. Adequate segmental and perineal anesthesia reduces catecholamine-induced increases in heart rate as well as the urge to push, allowing fetal descent to be accomplished by uterine contractions and avoiding the deleterious effects of the Valsalva maneuver during the second stage of labor. When epidural anesthesia has not been used, a low spinal anesthetic may be administered to allow for a controlled second stage and delivery.

Caudal anesthesia is another reasonable option. Pudendal nerve block can provide adequate, although not ideal, pain relief for some patients.

Anesthetic options for cesarean delivery must take into account the additional potential hazards of marked fluid shifts secondary to anesthetic technique, operative blood loss, and the mobilization of fluid in the postpartum period. Either regional or general anesthesia may be used. Epidural anesthesia is preferred over spinal anesthesia because the former results in slower onset of blockade and thus more controllable hemodynamic alterations. Prophylactic ephedrine and arbitrary intravascular volume loading are best avoided; instead, a careful titration of anesthetic level allows judicious and appropriate intravenous fluid administration, which should be guided by hemodynamic monitoring in the symptomatic patient. These patients could be prone to hypotension with epidural anesthesia, secondary to a combination of venous pooling and prior beta-adrenergic blockade and diuretic therapy (Ziskind et al., 1990). The usual vasopressor choice of ephedrine should be avoided, as it could result in tachycardia. Instead, judicious use of metaraminol or low-dose (20–40 µg) phenylephrine assists in restoration of maternal blood pressure with little or no unwanted effect on uteroplacental perfusion.

General anesthesia also can provide a very stable hemodynamic course if the sympathetic stimulation associated with laryngoscopy and intubation as well as with suction and extubation is minimized. This can be accomplished with anesthetic agents and/or beta-adrenergic blockade. Induction of general anesthesia should be accomplished carefully, without drugs that commonly produce tachycardia. Depending on the severity of the disease, the need to blunt the hemodynamic response to endotracheal intubation may necessitate the use of a high-dose narcotic-based technique. Such a strategy also serves to avoid myocardial depression and the decreases in SVR that can occur with commonly employed short-acting barbiturates. Anesthesia is maintained with narcotics, muscle relaxants, nitrous oxide, and oxygen. Emergence must be controlled carefully to ensure return of protective reflexes and avoidance of tachycardia.

Aortic Stenosis

Aortic stenosis is a rare complication of pregnancy, primarily because the natural history of this lesion, which occurs secondary to rheumatic heart disease, typically requires three to four decades to yield severity adequate to produce symptoms. Women with congenitally bicuspid aortic valves and patients with a history of bacterial endocarditis, however, can present in pregnancy with severe aortic stenosis. Unlike mitral stenosis, with aortic stenosis, symptoms of congestive heart failure, angina, and syncope develop relatively late in the course of the disease. The pathophysiology of severe aortic stenosis entails narrowing of the valve orifice to less than 1 cm^2, associated with a transvalvular gradient of 50 mm Hg, which results in significant increases in afterload to left ventricular ejection. The left ventricle appropriately and concentrically hypertrophies and becomes markedly less compliant, although contractility is usually well preserved. The transvalvular gradient increases progressively throughout pregnancy as a result of increasing blood volume and decreasing SVR (Raymond et al., 1987).

Anesthetic management encompasses the following goals:

1. Avoiding both tachycardia and bradycardia
2. Maintaining adequate preload in order that the left ventricle may generate an adequate cardiac output across the stenotic valve
3. Maintaining hemodynamic parameters within a narrow therapeutic window

Patients with transvalvular gradients greater than 50 mm Hg and patients with symptomatic aortic stenosis warrant invasive monitoring with arterial and pulmonary artery catheters in the peripartum period (Easterling et al., 1988).

Provision of labor analgesia with segmental epidural anesthesia remains a controversial issue because these patients may not be able to tolerate the decreases in preload and afterload that can attend epidural analgesia and its associated sympathetic blockade (Sugrue et al., 1981). Easterling and associates (1988) described a series of four patients with moderate to severe aortic stenosis who were managed successfully with epidural anesthesia without untoward sequelae; adequate time was allowed to titrate the level of block carefully and initiate appropriate compensatory actions to correct hemodynamic alterations associated with the anesthetic agent. Intrathecal or epidural opioids, whether alone or in combination with an epidural segmental anesthetic, are other appropriate choices. Spinal opioids have no cardiovascular effects. In particular, myocardial contractility is unaltered, preload is preserved, and, most importantly, SVR is not diminished by this technique (Forster and Joyce, 1989). Local anesthetics and opioids are believed to act synergistically, allowing for a decrease in concentration of both drugs when they are used together. Effective analgesia can prevent the tachycardia associated with labor pain.

For cesarean delivery, either judiciously titrated epidural anesthesia or general endotracheal anesthesia may be used. General anesthesia can be accomplished with the same caution that applies for parturients with mitral stenosis; myocardial depression associated with halogenated volatile anesthetics should be avoided.

Mitral Insufficiency

Mitral valve insufficiency and regurgitation is the second most prevalent valvular lesion in pregnancy. Chronic left ventricular volume overload and work are usually well tolerated, with symptoms developing relatively late in life after childbearing age; thus, most patients with mitral regurgitation tolerate pregnancy well. Complications include an increased risk of atrial fibrillation during pregnancy, bacterial endocarditis requiring antibiotic prophylaxis, systemic embolization, and pulmonary congestion during pregnancy.

In one review of maternal deaths associated with rheumatic valvular lesions, no patient died from complications of mitral regurgitation without the presence of coexisting mitral stenosis (Hibbard, 1975). Congenital mitral valve prolapse is much more common during pregnancy than mitral regurgitation and can be present in 10%–17% of pregnancies. It is a well-tolerated and generally benign form of mitral regurgitation, and therapeutic interventions are thus rarely necessary (Rayburn and Fontana, 1981; Gianopoulos, 1989).

The pathophysiology of regurgitation through an incompetent mitral valve results in chronic volume overload of the left ventricle and dilatation. If left ventricular compromise is sufficiently long-standing and severe, the increase in plasma volume with pregnancy progression can result in pulmonary venous congestion. By contrast, the decreasing SVR associated with pregnancy may serve to improve forward flow across the aortic valve at the expense of regurgitant flow. Increases in SVR, which occur with labor pain, uterine contractions, or surgical stimulation, could result in a rise in the proportion of regurgitant blood flow, perhaps leading to acute left ventricular failure.

Anesthetic management of labor and delivery can be provided safely via any of the available techniques, including segmental lumbar epidural anesthesia. Adequate analgesia and anesthesia minimize the peripheral vasoconstriction, attenuating the increase in left ventricular afterload associated with labor pain and thereby augmenting the forward flow of blood. Sympathetic blockade also serves to decrease SVR and is beneficial in this regard; the caveat here is that venous capacitance will increase, and one must be prepared to augment preload cautiously with intravenous fluid infusion to maintain left ventricular filling volume.

Asymptomatic patients at term are unlikely to require invasive monitoring. Continuous electrocardiographic (ECG) monitoring is a reasonable addition to basic standards of peripartum monitoring. In symptomatic patients, invasive monitoring with arterial and pulmonary arterial catheter should be used.

Aortic Insufficiency

Aortic insufficiency can be congenital or acquired. If congenital, it is commonly associated with other lesions; if acquired, it could be secondary to rheumatic heart disease or endocarditis in association with aortic root dissection. Symptoms following rheumatic fever usually develop during the fourth or fifth decade of life; thus, most women in whom this is the dominant lesion have uneventful pregnancies.

The basic pathophysiology is of chronic volume overloading of the left ventricle resulting in hypertrophy and dilation associated with increased compliance. Because of hypertrophy, myocardial oxygen requirements are higher than normal, yet perfusion pressure (and oxygen supply) can be decreased by a reduction in diastolic pressure and an increased left ventricular end-diastolic pressure.

Anesthetic considerations thus center on the following points:

1. Minimizing pain and, therefore, catecholamine-induced increases in SVR
2. Avoiding bradycardia, which serves to increase time for regurgitant flow
3. Avoiding myocardial depressants, which can exacerbate failure

Because the anesthetic concerns are similar to those for patients with mitral regurgitation, epidural anesthesia for labor and delivery is desirable in order to prevent increases in peripheral vasoconstriction. Epidural anesthesia is also appropriate as a surgical anesthetic agent, as is general anesthesia with judicious avoidance of direct myocardial depressants. Invasive monitoring is a requirement in any patient with symptoms of congestive heart failure.

The parturient who has undergone mitral or aortic valve replacement faces several potential problems, such as thromboembolism, valvular outflow obstruction, endocarditis, and hemolysis. These patients have received anticoagulation, usually with coumarin derivatives, to prevent the thrombotic problems mentioned. Heparin is usually substituted for coumarin anticoagulants during pregnancy to avoid potential congenital anomalies (Shaul and Hall, 1977). Full anticoagulation is a direct contraindication to the use of regional anesthesia because of the risk of causing epidural or spinal hematoma. The use of low-molecular-weight heparin (enoxaparin) has been associated with spinal epidural hematoma when regional anesthesia was used or attempted in Europe and, more recently, in the United States (Porterfield and Wu, 1997). This is probably due to its having a longer half-life than unfractionated heparin. It is therefore recommended that regional anesthesia not be administered unless the drug has been discontinued for at least 12–24 hours, depending upon the dosage. One alternative is to continue heparinization throughout labor and delivery and use systemic analgesia for labor and general anesthesia for delivery. Another option with unfractionated heparin is to discontinue heparin therapy just prior to labor and delivery, normalize the coagulation results, use regional anesthesia, and restart heparin 12 hours later. This may not be practical in an obstetric setting. The choice of strategies depends on the severity of the patient's hemodynamic derangement and the optimal analgesic management.

Congenital Heart Disease

Congenital heart disease is becoming the most common cardiac problem encountered in the pregnant patient (Gianopoulos, 1989). Patients are increasingly likely to survive to childbearing age with the advent of palliative surgery or total correction of their defects. Many of these patients can be expected to have uneventful pregnancies and deliveries.

Left-to-Right Shunts

VENTRICULAR SEPTAL DEFECT. Ventricular septal defect (VSD) occurs in 7% of adults with congenital heart disease. Patients with uncorrected lesions in the absence of pulmonary hypertension do well during pregnancy. In the small percentage of patients with large VSDs and coexisting pulmonary hypertension, maternal mortality ranges from 7% to 40%. Severe right ventricular failure with shunt reversal (*Eisenmenger's syndrome*) is the major ensuing complication. During pregnancy, elevation of plasma volume, cardiac output, and heart rate can increase left-to-right shunt and can further worsen the degree of pulmonary hypertension.

The major goals in peripartum management include awareness that marked increases in peripheral vascular resistance and heart rate could be poorly tolerated, with ventricular failure a distinct possibility. Conversely, acute increases in pulmonary vascular resistance (PVR) and right ventricular compromise can lead to shunt reversal and hypoxia.

Optimal anesthesia for labor and vaginal delivery is achieved with segmental epidural anesthesia consisting of local anesthetics, opioids, or their combination to permit control of painful stimuli, thus minimizing changes in heart rate and

SVR. Anesthesia for cesarean delivery can be accomplished either with slow titration of an epidural anesthetic agent to allow time for correction of pressure changes or with a general anesthetic agent that combines opioid and inhalation technique to depress the adrenergic response to endotracheal intubation and minimize myocardial depression.

ATRIAL SEPTAL DEFECT. Atrial septal defect is one of the most common congenital cardiac lesions in women of childbearing age, and pregnancy is generally well tolerated even when pulmonary blood flow is increased. The risk of left ventricular failure is increased during pregnancy, however. Increases in atrial volume result in biatrial enlargement, and thus supraventricular dysrhythmias are likely.

Pregnancy-associated increases in plasma volume and cardiac output serve to accentuate the left-to-right shunt, right ventricular volume work, and pulmonary blood flow, with the possible development of pulmonary hypertension and left and right ventricular failure. Peripartum management centers on avoiding vascular resistance changes that could increase the degree of shunt. Increases in SVR or decreases in PVR may not be well tolerated.

Although all of the common methods of providing labor analgesia are useful, lumbar epidural analgesia for labor, vaginal delivery, or cesarean delivery attenuates the hazards of increased SVR. General anesthesia for cesarean delivery is also well tolerated, provided that increases in SVR are avoided and sinus rhythm is maintained.

PATENT DUCTUS ARTERIOSUS. Patent ductus arteriosus (PDA) accounts for 15% of all cases of congenital heart disease; today most patients with a large PDA (greater than 1 cm) receive early surgical intervention. Patients with a small PDA typically have normal pregnancies, but in those pregnant women with superimposed pulmonary hypertension, maternal mortality can reach 5%–6% from ventricular failure. The progressive decrease in SVR development throughout pregnancy can be associated with shunt reversal and peripheral cyanosis.

Anesthetic considerations include avoidance of increases in SVR and hypervolemia. Conversely, acute decreases in SVR may result in reversal of shunt in patients with preexisting pulmonary hypertension and right ventricular compromise. Again, all modalities may be used, depending on the severity of the disease. Continuous lumbar epidural analgesia for labor and delivery diminishes the increase in SVR associated with pain. Epidural or general anesthesia is appropriate for cesarean delivery if increases in SVR associated with endotracheal intubation and surgical stimulation are addressed adequately.

Right-to-Left Shunts

Eisenmenger's syndrome consists of pulmonary hypertension, a right-to-left intracardiac shunt resulting from pulmonary hypertension superimposed on a previously left-to-right shunt, and arterial hypoxemia. Pregnancy is not well tolerated by patients in this condition. The maternal mortality rate is estimated at 30%–50%. This entity is responsible for approximately 50% of the maternal mortality in parturients with congenital heart disease (Spielman, 1986).

Anesthetic considerations center on avoidance of any decrease in SVR and, therefore, on avoidance of hypotension or myocardial depression. Hypotension from any cause, including conduction block or hemorrhage, can progress to insufficient right ventricular pressures to perfuse the hypertensive pulmonary arterial bed and can result in sudden death.

Analgesia for vaginal delivery can be accomplished with systemic narcotics, intrathecal narcotics, or cautious application of a segmental epidural if SVR is maintained. During the first stage of labor, epidural or intrathecal opioid administration would be a useful adjunct, and its sole administration has been recommended as the safest approach (Abboud et al., 1983). If an epidural block is employed, epinephrine should be omitted from the test dose because peripheral beta-adrenergic effects could cause a decrease in SVR.

For second-stage analgesia and anesthesia, a caudal epidural block could be preferable to the lumbar route because dense perineal analgesia can be provided without extensive sympathetic blockade. Delivery by cesarean delivery is most safely accomplished via general anesthesia, although regional anesthesia for elective cesarean delivery has been reported (Spinnato et al., 1981; Hytens and Alexander, 1986).

Regardless of the anesthetic technique employed, the postpartum period is probably the most likely time for life-threatening complications of hypoxemia, cardiac dysrhythmias, and thromboembolic events to occur (Gilman, 1991); most maternal deaths, in fact, occur in the first postpartum week (Cobb et al., 1982). The use of invasive monitoring is highly recommended in management of these patients in the peripartum period; pulmonary artery catheters and serial arterial blood gas determinations allow early detection of changes in cardiac output, pulmonary artery pressures, and shunt fraction. Serial measurements of cardiac output and especially SVR are useful in this regard. It should be recognized that technical difficulty in passage of a pulmonary artery catheter and obtaining wedge pressures is well documented, and a central venous catheter may have to suffice (Pollack et al., 1990; Schwalbe et al., 1990).

TETRALOGY OF FALLOT. Tetralogy of Fallot comprises 15% of all congenital heart disease and is the most common etiologic factor in right-to-left shunt in women of childbearing age. Particularly poor prognostic signs include a history of syncope, polycythemia (hematocrit greater than 60), decreased arterial oxygen saturation (less than 80%), right ventricular hypertension, and congestive heart failure. Increased right-to-left shunt can accompany pregnancy-induced decreases in SVR. The stress of labor can increase PVR and thus increase the degree of shunt. Most complications occur in the postpartum period when SVR is lowest, thus exacerbating the right-to-left shunting of blood and worsening the degree of arterial hypoxemia.

Anesthetic considerations must focus on minimizing the hemodynamic changes that would exacerbate the degree of shunt. Strict avoidance of decreased SVR, decreased venous return, and myocardial depression are of paramount importance. Analgesia for labor and vaginal delivery in these patients is most safely provided by systemic medication, inhalational nitrous oxide analgesia, or pudendal block. Intrathecal opioids can prove optimal in some circumstances. Regional anesthetic techniques should be used with extreme caution because the decrease in SVR could result in increased shunt. Low-dose ketamine may prove a reasonable option for forceps-assisted deliveries. Anesthesia for cesarean delivery should be provided by general anesthesia.

Invasive monitoring with arterial and pulmonary artery catheters to evaluate cardiac filling pressures and SVR is warranted in those patients with uncorrected tetralogy or only palliative correction.

PRIMARY PULMONARY HYPERTENSION. Primary pulmonary hypertension predominantly affects women of childbearing age and is associated with a high maternal mortality (greater than 50%). Most deaths occur during labor and the puerperium (Slomka et al., 1988; Roberts and Keast, 1990; Mangano, 1993). Signs and symptoms depend on severity of the disease and are caused by a fixed low cardiac output, the degree of pulmonary hypertension, and the degree of right ventricular compromise.

Anesthetic considerations are focused on the following points:

1. Evaluating the severity of the disease and its responsiveness to therapy
2. Maintaining hemodynamic stability
3. Administering the appropriate analgesia and anesthesia for labor and delivery

In selecting an analgesic or anesthetic regimen, the physician must consider primarily the prevention of increases in PVR from underventilation, pharmacologic agents, pulmonary hyperinflation, and stress. Furthermore, decreases in right ventricular volume from intravascular volume depletion, venodilation, or aortocaval compression are poorly tolerated. Significant decreases in SVR from sympathetic blockade from regional anesthesia or volatile anesthetic agents could produce severe decompensation because the cardiovascular system may be unable to compensate for the decline in afterload (Slomka et al., 1988). Finally, right ventricular contractility could be marginal, and the addition of negative inotropic anesthetic agents could lead to marked depression in cardiac function. The parturient should be monitored with an ECG, pulse oximetry, radial artery catheter, and a pulmonary artery catheter throughout labor and the postpartum period. The use of a pulmonary artery catheter allows early detection of changes in PVR or right ventricular function and serves as a guide to fluid and pharmacologic therapy.

Labor and vaginal delivery can best be managed by the judicious use of systemic narcotic analgesics and pudendal nerve block. Epidural analgesia with local anesthesia may be provided only if the block is slowly titrated in a limited dermatomal fashion from T10 to L1 to avoid extensive sympathetic blockade. Intrathecal or epidural opioids also provide effective first-stage analgesia. Vaginal delivery can be managed by the addition of a caudal catheter or pudendal block.

Regional anesthesia is best avoided for cesarean delivery, and a slow induction with either high-dose narcotics or an inhalation agent is recommended. This practice is necessary to avoid marked increases in PVR with laryngoscopy. Cricoid pressure must be maintained throughout the induction to prevent the aspiration of gastric contents. Ventilation must be adequate, but pulmonary hyperinflation must be avoided. Uterine stimulants should be omitted because they can be associated with significant elevations in PVR.

Coronary Artery Disease

Coronary artery disease is uncommon in women of childbearing age, with a reported incidence of 1 in 10,000 pregnancies. In one review, it was determined that only 13% of gravidas who had a myocardial infarction (MI) had a known history of coronary artery disease; overall maternal mortality was 37%, increasing to 45% if the infarction occurred in the third trimester (Hankins et al., 1985; Burlew, 1990).

The pathophysiology and clinical manifestations are identical to those in the nonpregnant patient. It should be noted that the hemodynamic demands that pregnancy places on the myocardium represent a stress to the coronary circulation. General management guidelines currently include efforts to reduce the cardiac workload with measures such as bed rest, nitrate therapy for preload reduction, and conduction anesthesia during delivery. Cardiac medications, such as beta blockers and nitrates, should be continued throughout the pregnancy, labor, delivery, and puerperium. Effort must be directed toward optimizing myocardial oxygen supply; supplemental oxygen should be provided, anemia treated, and respiratory depression secondary to sedation meticulously avoided.

Although reasonable pain relief can be achieved with systemic narcotic analgesia, the early institution of continuous regional anesthesia for labor and delivery is recommended to minimize the pain and stress that have the potential to precipitate ischemia and angina (Rosenlund and Marx, 1988). Beneficial effects associated with regional anesthesia may also include decreased preload and afterload so that myocardial work is diminished. Marked and sudden decreases in afterload must be avoided because coronary artery perfusion is dependent on diastolic pressure. Also, significant decreases in SVR can precipitate reflex tachycardia, which may increase cardiac workload sufficiently to produce ischemia. Epidural anesthesia effectively attenuates the progressive rise in central venous pressure and cardiac output that occurs during labor in the unanesthetized parturient. Multiple-lead ECG monitoring should be instituted early in labor so that ischemia can be detected and treated promptly.

When one is establishing epidural blockade, it is recommended that epinephrine be omitted from the test dose to avoid potential tachycardia and that the block be established by administration of slower-onset local anesthetic agents, such as bupivacaine or ropivacaine. Additionally, supplementation of a dilute local anesthetic solution with an epidural opioid has been advocated (Hands et al., 1990). Fetal descent during the second stage of labor should be by force of uterine contraction, with avoidance of the Valsalva maneuver, according to the patient's baseline ejection fraction and analysis of the hemodynamic response to contractions. When epidural analgesia for first-stage labor is not employed, a low spinal anesthetic (saddle block) provides excellent conditions for an assisted delivery with minimal hemodynamic trespass.

Elective cesarean delivery can be performed safely with a slowly titrated level of epidural anesthesia, allowing judicious intravenous fluid infusion to maintain pulmonary capillary wedge pressure and blood pressure (Aglio and Johnson, 1990). Spinal anesthesia is much less desirable, given the rapid onset of sympathetic block with great potential for hypotension and reflex tachycardia. When administering general anesthesia for cesarean delivery, the anesthesiologist must take into consideration the importance of minimizing the cardiovascular response to the stress of endotracheal intubation and surgery. In the absence of congestive heart failure, an inhalation technique is recommended.

A history of recent (especially third-trimester) myocardial infarction less than 6 weeks previously, congestive heart failure, or unstable or crescendo angina warrants invasive monitoring with arterial and pulmonary artery catheters (Frenkel et al., 1991). Monitoring should be continued for a minimum of 24 hours into the postpartum period to assess increases in pulmonary capillary wedge pressure as intravascular volume increases following delivery and as anesthesia subsides.

Asymmetric Septal Hypertrophy (Idiopathic Hypertrophic Subaortic Stenosis)

Asymmetric septal hypertrophy (ASH) or idiopathic hypertrophic subaortic stenosis (IHSS) is a disease without a defined etiology, but at least one third of the subjects have a familial history, and it appears to be inherited as an autosomal dominant trait. The primary features of this cardiomyopathy include marked hypertrophy of the left ventricle and interventricular septum and obstruction of the left ventricular outflow tract during systole by the hypertrophied muscle. The anterior leaflet of the mitral valve could be displaced by the hypertrophied muscle and thus contribute to the obstruction in some patients.

The disease commonly presents during the second to fourth decades of life. Common symptoms include angina pectoris, dizziness, and exertional dyspnea. Physical findings include signs of left ventricular hypertrophy, a systolic ejection murmur, and a third heart sound. The ECG indicates left ventricular hypertrophy and, in many cases, evidence of Wolff-Parkinson-White syndrome and evidence of abnormal Q waves. There is wide variability in both the findings and the symptoms of the disease.

The hemodynamic limitations of ASH are produced as the ventricle contracts. The hypertrophied walls narrow the outflow region during systole. The determinants of the degree of obstruction are the volume of the left ventricle at systole, the force of left ventricular contraction, and the degree of left ventricular distention during systolic contraction. The patient therefore requires a high preload in order to maintain a full left ventricle, a reduced contractile force in order to minimize outflow tract narrowing, and a high systemic vascular resistance to maintain distention of the left ventricle during systole.

Therapy is primarily focused on the administration of beta-adrenergic blocking agents to reduce myocardial contractility and heart rate. Some patients can receive calcium channel–blocking drugs as well. Patients with ASH do not tolerate hypovolemia, decreased SVR, or increases in myocardial contractility very well. The cardiovascular and hemodynamic changes of pregnancy have a variable effect on patients with ASH, depending on both the severity and the nature of the disorder. The increase in blood volume associated with pregnancy should yield a beneficial effect, as it increases preload. The usually observed increase in heart rate and stroke volume during pregnancy can have a negative effect, and the decrease in SVR, which begins during the second trimester, may also have a negative impact on cardiac performance. Although the potential for left ventricular failure and cardiac arrhythmias during pregnancy exists, the outcome of patients with ASH has been reasonably good (Oakley et al., 1979).

The therapeutic objectives during parturition should be as follows:

1. Minimizing pain-associated increases in catecholamine levels
2. Maintaining preload by adequate intravenous fluid administration
3. Avoiding the Valsalva maneuver, which decreases preload abruptly

Invasive monitoring with both an arterial line and a pulmonary artery catheter will yield the information necessary to provide precise management. Recommendations for analgesia during the first stage of labor have been to employ systemic narcotics, inhaled analgesics, or paracervical block. Regional analgesia has been considered a substantial risk because of the potential for both venodilation (decreased preload) and arterial dilation resulting in decreased SVR (Oakley et al., 1979). Decreased SVR can possibly be avoided, however, if careful incremental titration of continuous lumbar epidural analgesia is carried out. A limited segmental level of analgesia from T10 to L2 provides adequate analgesia with minimal sympathetic blockade, thus preserving preload. Dilute solutions of a local anesthetic agent with the addition of a narcotic, such as fentanyl, provides optimal analgesia (Minnich et al., 1987). Intrathecal narcotics may also be used, thereby eliminating the risk of sympathetic blockade but adding the potential side effects of respiratory depression, pruritus, and nausea, all of which are easy to treat.

A combined spinal and epidural analgesic approach has been used successfully for a patient with IHSS (Ho et al., 1997). Vaginal delivery can be accomplished with pudendal block, carefully extended epidural analgesia, or low spinal anesthesia (saddle block). The saddle block involves the spinal segments from L2 to S5 and thus avoids the majority of sympathetic nerve elements. Regional anesthesia is effective at blocking the uncontrollable urge to bear down. If hypotension necessitating a vasopressor does occur, the use of ephedrine is relatively contraindicated because it causes tachycardia and increased myocardial contractility. Metaraminol or a pure vasoconstricting drug, such as phenylephrine (20–40 µg), should be employed in the lowest effective doses to minimize its effect on the uterine arteries.

Anesthesia for cesarean delivery offers additional challenges. Left uterine displacement must be maintained and volume requirements carefully assessed in view of the increased blood loss. Invasive monitoring will be needed. Regional anesthesia is usually avoided for the aforementioned reasons, and clearly the level of anesthesia required is likely to produce extensive sympathetic blockade with undesirable consequences (Oakley et al., 1979; Loubser et al., 1984). Nonetheless, a carefully titrated epidural anesthetic with ongoing compensation for the induced hemodynamic changes could prove acceptable. General anesthesia is preferred by many, although the ideal technique is yet to be established and experience is limited (Boccio et al., 1986). Although the use of volatile anesthetic agents is advantageous because they reduce myocardial contractility, they also decrease uterine contractility and SVR. Modest doses should have a minimal effect on both.

As with the preeclamptic patient, the stimulating effects of laryngoscopy and intubation on patients with AHS and IHSS need to be blunted pharmacologically. Oxytocin must be administered cautiously because it tends to decrease SVR and results in tachycardia when administered rapidly. The parturient with ASH requires careful attention by means of appropriate monitoring and immediate availability of the necessary vasopressors, beta blockers, and intravenous volume expanders.

Marfan Syndrome

Marfan syndrome is an autosomal dominant disorder characterized by connective tissue abnormalities of the cardiovascular, skeletal, and ocular systems. The principal cardiovascular involvement is weakness of the aortic media,

which can result in progressive aortic dilatation or acute dissection. This dilatation can begin as early as the first year of life and typically occurs first in the coronary sinuses. Profound aortic regurgitation can predate clinical evidence of aortic dissection, and dissection may not be heralded by the classic chest pain with radiation to the back that usually accompanies aortic dissection from other causes. These patients also can experience coronary artery involvement, pulmonary artery dilatation, redundant chordae tendineae, or an increased incidence of aortic coarctation.

Anesthetic management options for labor and delivery or cesarean delivery has been only rarely reported. In one case report of two patients with Marfan syndrome and evidence of aortic dissection, epidural anesthesia was provided successfully for cesarean delivery with invasive monitoring via pulmonary artery catheter and arterial line (Mor-Yosef et al., 1988). In the asymptomatic patient without cardiovascular manifestations and a normal echocardiographic examination, segmental epidural anesthesia for labor and vaginal delivery without invasive hemodynamic monitoring are appropriate and inherently safe if the severity of associated scoliosis does not preclude the success of this technique. It is apparent that adequate analgesia, as provided by an epidural block, is distinctly advantageous in decreasing pain and catecholamine output, thus diminishing the stress on the aortic wall. Anesthesia for cesarean delivery may be provided by either regional or general technique.

General anesthesia for cesarean delivery in the presence of cardiovascular complications must be tailored to minimize the hemodynamic response to endotracheal intubation and surgical stimuli. Both prophylactic beta-adrenergic blockade and inhalational agents that produce decreased myocardial contractility and slow the force of cardiac ejection have been advocated (Wells, 1987). Control of blood pressure alone with vasodilators may only serve to increase left ventricular ejection velocity and, unless combined with beta-adrenergic blockade, may not prevent dissection. The potential for temporal-mandibular joint laxity and dislocation on endotracheal intubation also exists, although difficult intubation has not been reported.

■ EHLERS-DANLOS SYNDROME

Ehlers-Danlos syndrome (EDS) is a rare, genetically transmitted connective tissue disorder, nonspecific to pregnancy. Because of the multiorgan involvement and varied presentations of this disease, no uniform or routine anesthetic recommendations can be made (Kuczkowski and Benumof, 2002a). The features of EDS that have the greatest impact on the management of anesthesia include fragile, poorly healing skin, excessive bleeding, spontaneous pneumothorax, easy joint dislocation, valvular prolapse, and spontaneous dissections or ruptures of major vessels.

Some of the problems in EDS could have implications for the administration of regional anesthesia. Although bruising, bleeding, and hematomas are common, no consistent coagulation disorder has been identified in association with EDS. Nevertheless, bleeding can complicate arterial, peripheral, or central line and neuraxial needle placement. If general anesthesia is selected for these parturients, the airway must be managed gently in view of the possible presence of spine involvement, periodontal disease, propensity for gingival bleeding, and oropharyngeal tissue fragility (Garahan and

Licata, 1998). Cardiac function must be evaluated preoperatively, and anesthetic implications must be considered. Intraoperatively, low airway pressures are needed because of the increased risk of pneumothorax. If possible, spontaneous ventilation is recommended. Elaborate padding of pressure points is indicated.

■ SPINAL ABNORMALITIES

Kyphoscoliosis occurs in approximately 0.4%–1% of the population in the United States and is associated with both obstetric and anesthetic concerns during pregnancy and delivery (Kafer, 1980). Specific obstetric concerns relate to concomitant disease as well as to the risk of dystocia in labor. Lesions involving the upper spine are commonly associated with disordered cardiorespiratory function. The natural history of an untreated severe curve is progression of deformity over time, resulting in early death from cardiorespiratory failure.

Anesthetic management for labor and vaginal delivery must be designed to minimize respiratory depression from systemic opioids or respiratory embarrassment from excessive intercostal muscle paralysis during high levels of regional anesthesia in patients with preexisting pulmonary dysfunction (Daley et al., 1990a). It is equally important to emphasize the need for adequate analgesia in order to minimize catecholamine-induced increases in cardiac output that can precipitate high-output, right-sided heart failure. A closely monitored segmental epidural analgesic technique would serve all of these purposes and avoid systemic opioid-induced respiratory depression.

Although an epidural analgesic is optimal for the aforementioned reasons, it could be difficult to achieve in the kyphoscoliotic obstetric patient. Distortion of the spinal column and of the epidural space could prevent either proper placement of an epidural catheter or uniform distribution of the local anesthetic solution, resulting in incomplete block. Subarachnoid catheter placement and segmental block have been reported for use in labor and vaginal delivery when epidural anesthesia had been unsuccessful (Elam, 1970).

Both continuous epidural and subarachnoid approaches have been employed to provide surgical anesthesia for cesarean delivery. Both techniques offer the distinct advantage of slow titration of anesthetic level, which allows time for assessment of adequacy of respiratory function and for compensatory hemodynamic mechanisms to become operative. Another significant factor favoring regional anesthesia is that it provides superior analgesia after cesarean delivery in the patient with scoliosis and respiratory impairment. Some investigators have noted attenuation of the decrease in vital capacity following abdominal surgery when epidural anesthesia has been continued postoperatively (Bromage, 1967). Others note that patients undergoing a variety of regional anesthetic and spinal opioid techniques invariably have better pulmonary function than patients receiving systemic opioids (Bromage et al., 1980; Shulman et al., 1984).

General anesthesia for cesarean delivery is indicated when severe scoliosis and cardiorespiratory impairment (cor pulmonale) are apparent at presentation, as respiratory embarrassment is likely to develop in these patients if a high regional anesthetic block is administered. These patients also warrant invasive monitoring of central venous pressure and serial arterial blood gas measurements.

Previous Spinal Surgery

Previous spinal surgery has been thought by some to represent a relative contraindication to regional anesthesia. A potential problem is obliteration of the epidural space from adhesions, which can limit spread of local anesthetics as well as increase the risk of dural puncture. Insertion of an epidural needle in the fused area could be relatively contraindicated or impossible to perform because of the presence of bone graft material and scar tissue, degenerative changes that occur in the spine after fusion, persistent back pain, and the risk of introducing infection in the area of foreign bodies (Daley et al., 1990b). Finally, these patients may express considerable anxiety and reluctance regarding catheter insertion in their backs.

A number of complications are related to epidural anesthesia for these patients. Generally, these include failure to place an epidural catheter, inadequate or patchy anesthesia, and increased risk of dural or vascular puncture. There is an increased risk of failure if the fusion extends to the L5-S1 interspace; significantly higher success rates are noted when the inferior limit of surgery is at L3 (Crosby and Halpern, 1989). Patients who have undergone earlier spinal surgery should be seen in antepartum consultation by the anesthesiologist, and the options for analgesia and anesthesia for labor and delivery should be discussed in detail (Hubbert, 1985). Epidural anesthesia may be offered if the patient accepts the higher incidence of complications and failure rate. Alterations in dosage with larger-than-usual doses of local anesthesia required have been described, and with adjustments and vigilance this technique has been used successfully (Daley et al., 1990a).

Achondroplastic Dwarfism

Although achondroplastic dwarfism is a rare complication of pregnancy, the patient could have a number of anatomic and physiologic abnormalities that contribute to problems with the administration of anesthesia. The airway in patients with achondroplasia typically has narrowed nasal passages and pharyngeal and maxillary hypoplasia. The base of the skull is shortened (because of early fusion of constituent bones) and angulated, yielding limited extension and making endotracheal intubation potentially difficult. Easy-mask general anesthetic ventilation has been described, however (Mayhew et al., 1986). Kyphoscoliosis is a common associated clinical finding in dwarfs, and for this reason respiratory problems caused by decreased functional residual capacity secondary to scoliosis and advancing enlargement of the uterus throughout pregnancy could be encountered (Kalla et al., 1986). Obstructive sleep apnea has become recognized as an insidious cause of morbidity in achondroplasia and is more common than central apnea because of cervicomedullary cord compromise (Reid et al., 1987). Acquired pulmonary hypertension leading to cor pulmonale can occur in achondroplasia, with contributions by restrictive lung disease associated with scoliosis, chronic upper airway obstruction, and sleep apnea.

Abnormalities of the spinal cord can result from severe kyphosis and scoliosis or from odontoid hypoplasia with cervical instability, leading to spinal cord and nerve root compression. The vertebral bodies are abnormally shallow, with underdeveloped vertebral arches yielding narrowing of the subarachnoid and epidural space. Additionally, adults with the condition have hypoplastic intervertebral discs that can prolapse easily into a congenitally stenotic canal and produce neural compression. All of the foregoing could make regional anesthesia difficult or impossible to achieve, with unpredictable spread of local anesthetic solutions and increased risk of unintentional dural puncture.

Cesarean delivery is inevitable for these women because the maternal pelvis is invariably small and contracted, resulting in cephalopelvic disproportion. In this setting, the anesthesiologist must fully understand the aforementioned problems in order to facilitate the safe delivery of anesthesia as well as methods of minimizing the risk of maternal aspiration and avoiding fetal depression.

Pregnancy in achondroplasia compounds many of the outlined problems and presents a unique challenge to the obstetrician and anesthesiologist. General endotracheal anesthesia has traditionally been considered the technique of choice in achondroplasia, even though case reports have detailed difficult endotracheal intubation (Walts et al., 1975). In those instances, extension of the neck was difficult or impossible. These patients warrant early discussion of the probability of intubation while awake after a thorough examination of the airway and review of any available cervical radiographs.

Technically challenging problems are also associated with regional anesthesia owing to the skeletal abnormalities encountered. Epidural anesthesia has been administered successfully (Cohen, 1980; Wardall and Frame, 1990). A relative contraindication to regional anesthesia has been a concern that neurologic sequelae can be attributed to the anesthetic agent. Those patients who have received successful epidural anesthesia have not experienced preoperative or postoperative neurologic dysfunction. Epidural anesthesia is theoretically preferable to spinal anesthesia because it lends itself to titration of the level of block. A smaller dose of anesthesia than usual could be required owing to maternal short stature and kyphoscoliosis. The dangers of intraoperative hypotension and high or total spinal block are greater for spinal than for epidural anesthesia.

SUBSTANCE ABUSE

By definition, substance abuse is described as "self-administration of various drugs that deviates from medically or socially accepted use, which if prolonged can lead to the development of physical and psychological dependence" (Stoelting and Dierdorf, 1993). Most often, abuse of an illicit substance is first suspected or diagnosed during medical management of another condition such as hepatitis, human immunodeficiency syndrome (HIV), or pregnancy. Illicit substances most commonly abused in pregnancy include cocaine, amphetamines, opioids, ethanol, tobacco, marijuana, caffeine, and toluene-based solvents. Polysubstance abuse is very common (Kuczkowski, 2001). Regardless of the drug(s) ingested and the clinical manifestations, it is always difficult to predict the exact anesthetic implications in chemically dependent patients. Most patients with a history of drug abuse deny it when interviewed preoperatively by anesthesiologists or obstetricians (Birnbach, 1999).

Anesthesiologists become involved in the care of drug-abusing patients either in emergency situations—fetal distress,

placental abruption, or uterine rupture—or in more controlled situations, such as a request for labor analgesia. Of the drugs abused, cocaine has the most profound implications for the obstetric anesthesiologist. Both regional and general anesthesia in the cocaine-abusing parturient can be associated with serious complications (Kuczkowski et al., 2000). When regional anesthesia is selected, combative behavior, altered pain perception, cocaine-induced thrombocytopenia, and ephedrine-resistant hypotension could be encountered. Low doses of phenylephrine titrated to the effect usually restore blood pressure to normal. Pronounced abnormalities in endorphin levels and changes in both mu and kappa opioid receptor densities resulting from cocaine addiction could result in perception of pain despite adequate spinal/epidural anesthesia sensory levels.

Hypertension, cardiac arrhythmias, and myocardial ischemia could be encountered under general anesthesia. Propranolol is contraindicated in cocaine-intoxicated patients because of the potential for unopposed alpha-adrenergic stimulation following beta blockade (Lange and Hillis, 2001). Although esmolol may provide effective control of tachycardia and hypertension, beta blockade has also been shown to enhance cocaine-induced coronary vasoconstriction. The short elimination half-life of esmolol could offer some advantages if the drug administration is deemed necessary.

The administration of hydralazine has recently become a standard drug therapy for the treatment of hypertension in cocaine-addicted parturients. The mechanism of this drug action includes vasodilation and decrease in systemic vascular resistance, leading to reflex tachycardia, which may not always be desirable in the patient who is already tachycardic from cocaine intake. Labetalol, a combined nonselectve beta- and alpha-adrenergic blocker, rapidly restores blood pressure without affecting heart rate or uterine blood flow and has been recommended by many in cocaine toxicity. Some have suggested, however, that labetalol should not be used to treat cocaine-induced hypertension because labetalol's antagonism of beta-adrenergic receptors is greater than its effect on alpha-adrenergic receptors (Birnbach, 1999). The use of calcium channel blockers in drug-abusing parturients remains unclear. Many other drugs, such as nitroglycerin and nitroprusside, have been recommended, although the best drug intervention still remains to be established.

All potent volatile anesthetic agents can produce cardiac arrhythmias and increased systemic vascular resistance in cocaine-intoxicated parturients. Halothane has been found to sensitize the myocardium to the effects of catecholamines and therefore should be avoided. When ketamine is used in cocaine-abusing patients, caution is indicated, as ketamine can stimulate the central nervous system and potentiate the cardiac effects of cocaine by further increasing catecholamine levels (Kuczkowski, 2001). Nitroglycerin is safe and effective in the treatment of anginal chest pain secondary to acute cocaine ingestion.

REFERENCES

Abboud JK, Raya J, Noueihed R, et al: Intrathecal morphine for relief of labor pain in a parturient with severe pulmonary hypertension. Anesthesiology **59**:477, 1983.

Aglio LS, Johnson MD: Anesthetic management of myocardial infarction in a parturient. Br J Anaesth **65**:258, 1990.

Bader AM, Hunt CO, Datta S, et al: Anesthesia for the pregnant patient with multiple sclerosis. J Clin Anesth **1**:21, 1988.

Baraka A: Epidural meperidine for control of autonomic hyperreflexia in a paraplegic parturient. Anesthesiology **62**:688, 1985.

Benatar SR: Anaesthesia for the asthmatic. S Afr Med J **59**:409, 1981.

Benedetti TJ, Cotton DB, Williams V: Hemodynamic observations in severe preeclampsia complicated by pulmonary edema. Am J Obstet Gynecol **152**:330, 1985.

Benumof JL, Scheller MS: The importance of transtracheal jet ventilation in the management of the difficult airway. Anesthesiology **71**:769, 1989.

Birnbach DJ: Substance Abuse. In Chestnut DH (ed): Obstetric Anesthesia—Principles and Practice. St. Louis, Mosby, 1999, p. 1027.

Boccio RV, Chung JH, Harrison DM: Anesthetic management of cesarean section in a patient with idiopathic hypertrophic subaortic stenosis. Anesthesiology **65**:663, 1986.

Bromage PR: Extradural analgesia for pain relief. Br J Anaesth **39**:721, 1967.

Bromage PR, Comporesi EM, Chestnut D: Epidural narcotics for postoperative analgesia. Anesth Analg **59**:474, 1980.

Burlew BS: Managing the pregnant patient with heart disease. Clin Cardiol **13**:757, 1990.

Canny GJ, Corey M, Livingstone RA, et al: Pregnancy and cystic fibrosis. Obstet Gynecol **77**:850, 1991.

Channing-Rogers RP, Levin J: A critical reappraisal of the bleeding time. Semin Thromb Hemost **16**:1, 1990.

Clark SL: Cardiac disease in pregnancy. Crit Care Obstet **18**:237, 1991.

Clark SL, Phelan JP, Greenspoon J, et al: Labor and delivery in the presence of mitral stenosis: Central hemodynamic observations. Am J Obstet Gynecol **152**:984, 1985.

Cobb T, Gleicher N, Elkayam V: Congenital heart disease and pregnancy. In Elkayam V, Gleicher N (eds): Cardiac Problems in Pregnancy. New York, Alan R. Liss, 1982, p. 61.

Cohen SE: Anesthesia for cesarean section in achondroplastic dwarfs. Anesthesiology **52**:264, 1980.

Corssen G, Gutierrez J, Reves JG, et al: Ketamine in the anesthetic management of asthmatic patients. Anesth Analg **51**:588, 1972.

Cotton DB, Gonik B, Dorman K, et al: Cardiovascular alterations in severe pregnancy induced hypertension: Relationship of central venous pressure to pulmonary capillary wedge pressure. Am J Obstet Gynecol **151**:762, 1985.

Crawford JS, James FM, Nolte H, et al: Regional analgesia for patients with chronic neurological disease and similar conditions. Anaesthesia **36**:821, 1981.

Crosby ET, Halpern SH: Obstetric epidural anaesthesia in patients with Harrington instrumentation. Can J Anaesth **36**:693, 1989.

Daley MD, Rolbin S, Hew E, et al: Continuous epidural anaesthesia for obstetrics after major spinal surgery. Can J Anaesth **37**:S112, 1990a.

Daley MD, Rolbin SH, Hew EM, et al: Epidural anaesthesia for obstetrics after spinal surgery. Reg Anesth **15**:280, 1990b.

Dias MS, Sekhar LM: Intracranial hemorrhage from aneurysms and arteriovenous malformations during pregnancy and the puerperium. Neurosurgery **25**:855, 1990.

Donchin Y, Amirav B, Sahar A, et al: Sodium nitroprusside for aneurysm surgery in pregnancy. Br J Anaesth **50**:849, 1978.

Ducey JP, Ellsworth SM: The hemodynamic effects of severe mitral stenosis and pulmonary hypertension during labor and delivery. Intensive Care Med **15**:192, 1989.

Easterling TR, Chadwick HS, Otto CM, et al: Aortic stenosis in pregnancy. Obstet Gynecol **72**:113, 1988.

Eilen B, Kaiser IH, Becker RM, et al: Aortic valve replacement in the third trimester of pregnancy: Case report and review of the literature. Obstet Gynecol **57**:119, 1981.

Elam JO: Catheter subarachnoid block for labor and delivery: A differential segmental technique employing hyperbaric lidocaine. Anesth Analg **49**:1007, 1970.

Eng M, Butler J, Bonica JJ: Respiratory function in pregnant obese women. Am J Obstet Gynecol **123**:241, 1975.

Foldes FF: Factors which alter the effects of muscle relaxants. Anesthesiology **20**:464, 1959.

Forster R, Joyce T: Spinal opioids and the treatment of the obstetric patient with cardiac disease. Clin Perinatol **16**:955, 1989.

Fox EJ, Sklar GS, Hiu CH, et al: Complications related to the pressor response to endotracheal intubation. Anesthesiology **47**:524, 1977.

Frenkel Y, Etchin A, Barkai G, et al: Myocardial infarction during pregnancy: A case report. Cardiology **78**:363, 1991.

Gant NF, Daley GL, Chand S, et al: A study of angiotensin II pressor response throughout primigravid pregnancy. J Clin Invest **52**:2682, 1973.

Garahan MB, Licata A: Dermatoses. In Gambling DR, Douglas MJ (eds): Obstetric Anesthesia and Uncommon Disorders. Philadelphia, WB Saunders, 1998, p. 353.

Ghoneim MM, Long IP: Interaction between magnesium and other neuromuscular blocking agents. Anesthesiology **32**:23, 1970.

Gianopoulos JG: Cardiac disease in pregnancy. Med Clin North Am **73**:639, 1989.

Gilman DH: Caesarean section in undiagnosed Eisenmenger's syndrome: Report of a patient with a fatal outcome. Anaesthesia **46**:371, 1991.

Greenberger PA: Asthma during pregnancy. J Asthma **27**:341, 1990.

Gronert GA, Theye RA: Pathophysiology of hyperkalemia induced by succinylcholine. Anesthesiology **43**:89, 1975.

Hands ME, Johnson MD, Saltzman DH, et al: The cardiac, obstetric, and anesthetic management of pregnancy complicated by acute myocardial infarction. J Clin Anesth **2**:258, 1990.

Hankins GD, Wendel GD Jr, Leveno KJ, et al: Myocardial infarction during pregnancy: A review. Obstet Gynecol **65**:139, 1985.

Hays PM, Cruikshank DP, Dunn LJ: Plasma volume determination in normal and preeclamptic pregnancies. Am J Obstet Gynecol **151**:958, 1985.

Hibbard LT: Maternal mortality due to cardiac disease. Clin Obstet Gynecol **18**:27, 1975.

Hirshman CA, Edelstein G, Peetz S, et al: Mechanisms of action of inhalational anesthesia on airways. Anesthesiology **56**:107, 1982.

Ho KW, Kee WDN, Poon MCM: Combined spinal and epidural anesthesia in a parturient with idiopathic hypertrophic subaortic stenosis. Anesthesiology **87**:168, 1997.

Hodgkinson R, Husain J: Obesity and the cephalad spread of analgesia following epidural administration of bupivacaine for cesarean section. Anesth Analg **59**:89, 1980.

Horton JC, Chambers WA, Lyons SL, et al: Pregnancy and the risk of hemorrhage from cerebral arteriovenous malformations. Neurosurgery **27**:867, 1990.

Hubbert CH: Epidural anesthesia in patients with spinal fusion. Anesth Analg **64**:843, 1985.

Hytens L, Alexander JP: Maternal and neonatal death associated with Eisenmenger's syndrome. Acta Anaesth Belg **37**:45, 1986.

Jaffee JB, Drease GE, Kelly T, et al: Severe respiratory depression in the obstetric patient after intrathecal meperidine or sufentanil. Int J Obstet Anesth **6**:182, 1997.

Joupilla R, Joupilla P, Hollmen A, et al: Epidural analgesia and placental blood flow during labor in pregnancies complicated by hypertension. Br J Obstet Gynaecol **86**:969, 1979.

Kafer ER: Respiratory and cardiovascular function in scoliosis and the principle of anesthetic management. Anesthesiology **52**:339, 1990.

Kalla GN, Fening E, Obiaya MO: Anaesthetic management of achondroplasia. Br J Anaesth **58**:117, 1986.

Kelton JG, Hunter DJ, Neame PB: A platelet function defect in preeclampsia. Obstet Gynecol **65**:107, 1985.

Kirshon B, Moise KJ Jr, Cotton DB, et al: Role of volume expansion in severe preeclampsia. Surg Gynecol Obstet **167**:367, 1988.

Koh KS, Friesen RM, Livingstone RA, et al: Fetal monitoring during maternal cardiac surgery with cardiopulmonary bypass. Can Med Assoc J **112**:1102, 1975.

Kuczkowski KM: Drug Abuse in Pregnancy—Anesthetic Implications. Progress Anesthesiol **25**:355, 2001.

Kuczkowski KM, Benumof JL: Cesarean section and Ehlers-Danlos syndrome: Choice of anesthesia. Intl J Obstet Anesth **11**:222, 2002a.

Kuczkowski KM, Benumof JL: Repeat cesarean section in a morbidly obese parturient: A new anesthetic option. Acta Anaesthesiol Scand **46**:753, 2002b.

Kuczkowski KM, Birnabach DJ, van Zundert A: Drug abuse in the parturient. Sem Anestesiol Periop Med Pain **19**:216, 2000.

Kytta J, Rosenberg P: Anaesthesia for patients with multiple sclerosis. Ann Chir Gynaecol **73**:299, 1984.

Lambert DH, Deane RS, Mazuzan JE: Anesthesia and the control of blood pressure in patients with spinal cord injury. Anesth Analg **61**:344, 1982.

Lange RA, Hillis LD: Cardiovascular complications of cocaine use. N Engl J Med **345**:351, 2001.

Leicht CH: Anesthesia for the pregnant patient undergoing nonobstetric surgery. Anesth Clin North Am **8**:131, 1990.

Levine W, Diamond B: Surgical procedures during pregnancy. Am J Obstet Gynecol **81**:1046, 1961.

Levinson G, Shnider SM: Anesthesia for surgery during pregnancy. In Shnider SM, Levinson G (eds): Anesthesia for Obstetrics. Baltimore, Williams and Wilkins, 1987, p. 188.

Lindeman KS, Hirshman CA, Freed AN: Effect of magnesium sulfate on bronchoconstriction in the lung periphery. J Appl Physiol **66**:2527, 1989.

Loubser P, Suh K, Cohen S: Adverse effects of spinal anesthesia in a patient with idiopathic hypertrophic subaortic stenosis. Anesthesiology **60**:228, 1984.

Malinow AM, Ostheimer GW: Anesthesia for the high-risk parturient. Obstet Gynecol **69:**951, 1987.

Mangano DT: Anesthesia for the pregnant cardiac patient. In Shnider SM, Levinson G (eds): Anesthesia for Obstetrics, 2nd ed. Baltimore, Williams and Wilkins, 1993, p. 485.

Mayhew JF, Katz J, Miner M, et al: Anaesthesia for the achondroplastic dwarf. Can J Anaesth **33:**216, 1986.

McGough EK, Cohen JA: Unexpected bronchospasm during spinal anesthesia. J Clin Anesth **2:**35, 1990.

Minielly R, Yupze AA, Drake CG: Subarachnoid hemorrhage secondary to ruptured cerebral aneurysm during pregnancy. Obstet Gynecol **53:**64, 1979.

Minnich ME, Quirk JG, Clark RB: Epidural anesthesia for vaginal delivery in a patient with idiopathic hypertrophic subaortic stenosis. Anesthesiology **67:**590, 1987.

Moore TR, Key TC, Reisner LS, et al: Evaluation of the use of continuous lumbar epidural anesthesia for hypertensive pregnant women in labor. Am J Obstet Gynecol **152:**404, 1985.

Mor-Yosef S, Younis J, Granat M, et al: Marfan's syndrome in pregnancy. Obstet Gynecol Surv **43:**382, 1988.

Oakley GDG, McGarry K, Limb DG, et al: Management of pregnancy in patient with hypertrophic cardiomyopathy. Br Med J **1:**1749, 1979.

Parry AJ, Westaby S: Cardiopulmonary bypass during pregnancy. Ann Thorac Surg **61:**1865, 1996.

Pedersen H, Finster M: Anesthetic risk in the pregnant surgical patient. Anesthesiology **51:**439, 1979.

Pollack KL, Chestnut DH, Wenstrom KD: Anesthetic management of a parturient with Eisenmenger's syndrome. Anesth Analg **70:**212, 1990.

Pomini F, Mercogliano D, Cavalletti C, et al: Cardiopulmonary bypass in pregnancy. Ann Thorac Surg **61:**259, 1996.

Porterfield WR, Wu CL: Epidural hematoma in an ambulatory surgical patient. J Clin Anesth **9:**74, 1997.

Ravindran R, Viegas OJ, Padilla LM, et al: Anesthetic considerations in pregnant patients receiving terbutaline therapy. Anesth Analg **59:**391, 1980.

Rayburn WF, Fontana ME: Mitral valve prolapse and pregnancy. Am J Obstet Gynecol **141:**9, 1981.

Raymond R, Underwood DA, Moodie DS: Cardiovascular problems in pregnancy. Cleveland Clin J Med **54:**95, 1987.

Reid CS, Pyeritz RE, Kopits SE, et al: Cervicomedullary compression in young patients with achondroplasia: Value of comprehensive neurologic and respiratory evaluation. J Pediatr **110:**522, 1987.

Reisner LS: The pregnant patient and the disorders of pregnancy. In Benumof J (ed): Anesthesia and Uncommon Diseases. Philadelphia, WB Saunders, 1998, p. 459.

Reisner LS, Benumof LJ, Cooper SD: The difficult airway: Risk, prophylaxis and management. In Chestnut DH (ed): Obstetric Anesthesia: Principles and Practice. St. Louis, Mosby, 1999, p. 590.

Reisner LS, Lin D: Anesthesia for cesarean section. In Chestnut DH (ed): Obstetric Anesthesia—Principles and Practice. St. Louis, Mosby, 1999, p. 465.

Richards W, Thompson J, Lewis G, et al: Cardiac arrest associated with halothane anesthesia in a patient receiving theophylline. Ann Allergy **61:**83, 1988.

Roberts NV, Keast PJ: Pulmonary hypertension and pregnancy—A lethal combination. Anaesth Intens Care **18:**366, 1990.

Roberts SL, Chestnut DH: Anesthesia for the obstetric patient with cardiac disease. Clin Obstet Gynecol **30:**601, 1987.

Rolbin SH, Abbott D, Musclow E, et al: Epidural anesthesia in pregnant patients with low platelet counts. Obstet Gynecol **71:**918, 1988.

Rosenlund RC, Marx GF: Anesthetic management of a parturient with prior myocardial infarction and coronary artery bypass graft. Can J Anaesth **35:**515, 1988.

Schonwald G, Fish KJ, Perkash I: Cardiovascular complications during anesthesia in chronic spinal cord injured patients. Anesthesiology **55:**550, 1981.

Schwalbe SS, Deshmuk SM, Marx GF: Use of pulmonary artery catheterization in parturients with Eisenmenger's syndrome. Anesth Analg **71:**442, 1990.

Shaul WL, Hall JG: Multiple congenital anomalies associated with oral anticoagulants. Am J Obstet Gynecol **127:**191, 1977.

Shulman M, Sandler AN, Bradley JW, et al: Post-thoracotomy pain and pulmonary function following epidural and systemic morphine. Anesthesiology **61:**569, 1984.

Slomka F, Salmeron S, Zetlaoui P, et al: Primary pulmonary hypertension and pregnancy: Anesthetic management for delivery. Anesthesiology **69:**959, 1988.

Spielman FJ: Anaesthetic management of the obstetric patient with cardiac disease. Clin Anaesth **4:**247, 1986.

Spinnato JA, Kraynack BJ, Cooper MW: Eisenmenger's syndrome in pregnancy: Epidural anesthesia for elective cesarean section. N Engl J Med **304:**1215, 1981.

Stange K, Halldin M: Hypothermia in pregnancy. Anesthesiology **58:**460, 1983.

Stoelting RK, Dierdorf SF: Psychiatric Illness and Substance Abuse. In Stoelting RK, Dierdorf SF (eds): Anesthesia and Co-Existing Disease. New York, Churchill Livingstone, 1993, p. 517.

Sugrue D, Blake S, MacDonald D: Pregnancy complicated by maternal heart disease at the National Maternity Hospital, Dublin, Ireland: 1969 to 1978. Am J Obstet Gynecol **139:**1, 1981.

Ueland K: Cardiac surgery and pregnancy. Am J Obstet Gynecol **92:**148, 1975.

Ueland K: Intrapartum management of the cardiac patient. Clin Perinatol **8:**155, 1988.

Ueland K, Hansen J: Maternal cardiovascular dynamics: II. Posture and uterine contractions. Am J Obstet Gynecol **103:**1, 1969a.

Ueland K, Hansen J: Maternal cardiovascular dynamics: III. Labor and delivery under local and caudal analgesia. Am J Obstet Gynecol **103:**8, 1969b.

Valenzuela GJ, Comunale FL, Davidson BH, et al: Clinical management of patients with cystic fibrosis and pulmonary insufficiency. Am J Obstet Gynecol **159:**1181, 1988.

Walts LF, Finerman G, Wyatt GM: Anaesthesia for dwarfs and other patients of pathological small stature. Can J Anaesth **22:**703, 1975.

Wanner MB, Rageth CJ, Zach GA: Pregnancy and autonomic hyperreflexia in patients with spinal cord lesions. Paraplegia **25:**482, 1987.

Wardall GJ, Frame WT: Extradural anaesthesia for caesarean section in achondroplasia. Br J Anaesth **64:**367, 1990.

Wells DG: Anaesthesia and Marfan's syndrome: Case report. Can J Anaesth **34:**311, 1987.

Younker D, Clark R, Tessem J, et al: Bupivacaine-fentanyl epidural analgesia for a parturient in status asthmaticus. Can J Anaesth **34:**609, 1987.

Ziskind S, Etchin A, Frenkel Y, et al: Epidural anesthesia with the Trendelenburg position for cesarean section with or without a cardiac surgical procedure in patients with severe mitral stenosis: A hemodynamic study. J Cardiothorac Anesth **3:**354, 1990.

Zitnik RS, Brandenberg RO, Sheldon R, et al: Pregnancy and open heart surgery. Circulation **39**(SI):1257, 1969.

Zuspan FP: Pregnancy-induced hypertension: I. Role of the sympathetic nervous system and adrenal gland. Acta Obstet Gynecol Scand **56:**283, 1977.

Part IV
THE NEONATE

Chapter 60

IDENTIFICATION AND MANAGEMENT OF PROBLEMS IN THE HIGH-RISK NEONATE

Avroy A. Fanaroff, MB, BCh(RAND), FRCP(E), FRCPCN, Richard J. Martin, MBBS, FRACP, and Ricardo J. Rodriguez, MD, FAAP

Regionalization of perinatal care is a cost-effective strategy. The risk-adjusted neonatal mortality rate is significantly lower for births within hospitals that have level III neonatal intensive care (subspecialty) units (NICUs) with an average daily census of 15 patients per day, compared with the smaller level III NICUs or the level II NICUs called *specialty units* (Phibbs et al., 1996). Furthermore, the costs of the births of infants at the subspecialty centers was not different from that of infants born at other hospitals. Hence, to keep infant morbidity as low as possible without increasing costs, high-risk deliveries in urban areas should be concentrated in a smaller number of designated subspecialty units.

■ MANAGEMENT OF THE INFANT

In the Delivery Room

A team approach with input from a perinatologist or obstetrician (or both), a neonatologist, and a skilled nursing and respiratory therapy staff is optimal. The combined expertise of this team greatly improves preparedness for obstetric emergencies. When a high-risk delivery is identified, referral to a tertiary center that is expert in high-risk obstetric and neonatal care can reduce morbidity and mortality for both the mother and her child. The cost of providing such care continues to increase, but this cost is balanced by improvement in infant outcome. The ability to sustain this momentum rests on continuing research into the transitional physiology of the infant as well as on scrupulous training of all personnel in the most advanced techniques of neonatal resuscitation.

The neonatal resuscitation curriculum developed by the American Academy of Pediatrics unifies the principles of neonatal resuscitation developed over decades of clinical experience and the evidence-based practice of neonatology. The following discussion reviews the physiology of normal and abnormal postnatal adaptation as well as specific current recommendations for delivery-room management of the infant.

Pulmonary and Circulatory Adaptations at Birth

Following delivery, a remarkable series of physiologic adaptations allows the infant to make a smooth transition from intrauterine to extrauterine life. After birth, the expanding lungs must replace the placenta as the site of gas exchange. The first few breaths clear lung fluid from the airway and alveolar space and establish a functional residual capacity. Clearance of lung fluid is also aided by chest compression as the infant passes through the vaginal canal. Furthermore, expansion of the lungs stimulates surfactant release, which reduces surface tension and stabilizes the infant's functional residual capacity. Expansion of the lungs also lowers pulmonary vascular resistance and increases pulmonary blood flow. Through these processes, the newly expanded lungs develop sufficient exchange surface area and blood flow to permit oxygen uptake and carbon dioxide (CO_2) removal.

Important circulatory changes also accompany occlusion of the umbilical cord. At this point, the low-resistance placental circulation is cut off, and the infant's systemic blood pressure rises. These effects combine to decrease right-to-left shunting of blood at the ductus arteriosus and at the foramen ovale. Furthermore, the increase in PaO_2 that occurs as the infant breathes stimulates physiologic closure of the ductus arteriosus. These important circulatory events reroute blood from the right side of the heart to the infant's lungs and result in an adult-type circulatory pattern in the healthy newborn within the first few hours of life.

Initial Steps in Resuscitation

The ABCs of Resuscitation

A healthy infant's transition to extrauterine life can be assisted by a few simple steps: thermal management, respiratory evaluation, and Apgar score assessment.

THERMAL MANAGEMENT

Immediately after birth, the newborn infant should be placed on a preheated radiant warmer and thoroughly dried, and any wet blankets should be removed promptly. These initial steps are important to minimize heat loss, particularly in premature infants (Fig. 60-1). In these patients, heat loss through evaporation, convection, conduction, and radiation is exaggerated by a lack of subcutaneous fat as well as by the increased ratio of surface area to weight. Moreover, the preterm infant is poorly equipped to generate additional heat because of reduced stores of brown fat and glycogen. Hypothermia can precipitate a cascade of adverse physiologic changes, including hypoglycemia, metabolic acidosis, and reversion to the fetal circulatory pattern, in

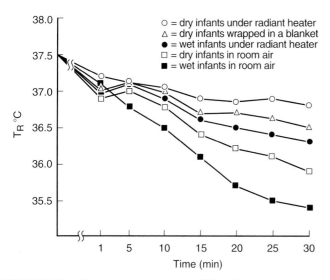

FIGURE 60-1 ■ Mean core temperatures (T_R) in infants showing the effect of drying and thermal protection immediately after birth. (From Dahm LS, James LS: Newborn temperature and calculated heat loss in the delivery room. Pediatrics **49**:504, 1972.)

which circulation bypasses the lungs. To avoid these complications, the infant should be kept in a neutral thermal environment in which oxygen consumption is minimal. This can be achieved by caring for the newborn on a servo-controlled radiant warmer, with the goal of maintaining a normal temperature between 36.5°C and 37.5°C. A knitted cap placed on the infant's head in the delivery room is also important in decreasing evaporative heat loss.

RESPIRATORY EVALUATION

The next step in initial care should be to ensure an open airway. This can be accomplished easily by using a bulb syringe to gently suction first the infant's mouth, then the nose. The special management needed for infants with meconium-stained amniotic fluid is discussed later in this chapter. Once the airway is cleared, the infant's respirations, heart rate, and color should be evaluated. The mildly depressed infant could experience primary apnea at birth. This type of apnea may be due to mild depression of the brain stem respiratory output caused by hypoxia and can be compounded by vagal reflex inhibition caused by suctioning of the pharynx. Within seconds, primary apnea responds easily to tactile stimulation and inhalation of 100% oxygen.

CARDIOVASCULAR ASSESSMENT

The next step in initial management of an infant is evaluation of the heart rate. The normal heart rate of a term infant averages 120 to 140 beats/minute after the initial physiologic

reaction to delivery has subsided. If the heart rate is below 100 beats/minute, initiation of positive-pressure ventilation could be required to provide adequate oxygenation to the heart and brain. In most mildly depressed infants, positive-pressure ventilation promptly restores a heart rate that is above 100 beats/minute, adequate to sustain normal cardiac output.

If the infant is breathing and the heart rate is over 100, the infant's color should be assessed. If peripheral cyanosis is present, supplemental oxygen is not required, but the infant should be evaluated to determine whether core temperature is low and warming is necessary. If central cyanosis is present, free-flow 100% oxygen should be provided by mask. Oxygen acts as a pulmonary vasodilator and restores normal neural and cardiac function through the systemic circulation. If central cyanosis persists despite adequate respiratory effort and inhalation of 100% oxygen, further evaluation of the cause of cyanosis must be promptly undertaken.

These simple steps—the ABCs of newborn resuscitation—often can be completed before the end of the first minute of life and are sufficient for initial delivery-room care of the majority of healthy infants.

APGAR SCORE ASSESSMENT

The next step in an infant's evaluation is assessment of the Apgar score. This scoring system provides a qualitative measure of the infant's success in adapting to the extrauterine environment (Table 60-1). The score consists of two vital signs (respiratory effort and heart rate), color, and two neurologic responses (response to stimulation and general tone). Each of these components is given a score of 0, 1, or 2, with 2 being the best, and 0 indicating no response. Each component is evaluated at 1 and 5 minutes following delivery, and a total score is calculated. When the Apgar score is less than 6 at 5 minutes, a 10- and 15-minute score should be calculated. This scoring system was developed for infants at term. In premature infants (less than or equal to 32 weeks' gestation or less than 1500 g at birth), care must be used in interpretation of a low Apgar score, which can occur in the absence of asphyxia (Tooley et al., 1977).

The neurologic outcome of asphyxiated infants is of the utmost concern to both caregivers and parents. The prognosis for recovery is difficult to determine. Although the Apgar score is a quick method to assess the infant's neurologic status, the scores at 1 and 5 minutes do not correlate with infant outcome. Despite a low initial Apgar score, an infant may well make a full recovery. For example, an Apgar score of 0 to 3 at 5 minutes is associated with only a 1% risk of cerebral palsy. If the infant demonstrates a persistently low Apgar score (0 to 3) at 10, 15, and 20 minutes of life, the correlation with future neurologic outcome is higher, but this still does not indicate the cause of future disability. Much still remains to be learned about the

TABLE 60-1. COMPONENTS OF THE APGAR SCORE

Sign	Score		
	0	1	2
Heart rate	Absent	<100 beats/minute	>100 beats/minute
Respiratory effort	Absent	Slow, irregular	Good cry
Color	Cyanotic, pallid	Acrocyanotic	Pink
Muscle tone	Limp	Minimal	Active
Reflex response	Absent	Minimal	Active

human infant's response to perinatal hypoxia and ischemia as well as about the reliability of physiologic indicators of long-term outcome. The reader is referred to Chapter 61 for a detailed discussion of the pathogenesis of neonatal brain disease.

CARE OF THE DEPRESSED NEWBORN INFANT

Even with the best antenatal management, infants can be born who have suffered a degree of hypoxia or hypoperfusion *in utero*. For such infants, advanced skill in resuscitation is required, with each step designed to reverse the effects of asphyxia as much as possible.

The term *asphyxia*, as used in clinical practice, should be reserved to describe a specific combination of acidemia, hypoxia, and metabolic acidosis. An infant who exhibits acute neurologic injury proximate to asphyxia should show all of the following:

1. Profound metabolic or mixed acidemia (pH < 7) on an umbilical cord arterial blood sample if obtained
2. An Apgar score of 0–3 for longer than 5 minutes
3. Neonatal neurologic manifestations (e.g., seizures, coma, or hypotonia)
4. Multisystem organ dysfunction (e.g., cardiovascular, gastrointestinal, hematologic, pulmonary, or renal abnormalities)

The more profound the asphyxia, the harder it is to establish spontaneous respiration, normal heart rate, and oxygenation. Hypoxic-ischemic injury *in utero* can lead to a form of severe central depression of respiration that is called *secondary apnea*. An infant with this form of apnea is unresponsive to tactile stimulation, and artificial ventilation with oxygen must be initiated at once if the infant fails to respond to the initial ABCs of resuscitation. When effective ventilation is provided, oxygenated blood can begin to perfuse the brain, and the infant's own respiratory drive resumes. Prolonged asphyxia also can result in a depression of heart rate and cardiac contractility, both of which also improve when the infant is ventilated successfully.

If the infant fails to respond to bag-and-mask positive-pressure ventilation and the heart rate remains below 60 beats/minute, intubation and chest compressions should be performed as quickly as possible. Intubating a newborn infant takes practice and skill, and the procedure should be undertaken by health care professionals who are trained and experienced in neonatal resuscitation. Even in the moderately depressed infant, restoration of circulation and artificial ventilation usually dramatically improves color and perfusion before 5 minutes of life, and prolonged cardiorespiratory support may not be necessary.

PERINATAL CARE AT THE THRESHOLD OF VIABILITY

A major challenge is the optimal management of the mother and infant when delivery takes place at the threshold of viability (MacDonald 2002; ACOG, 2002). This complex problem involves medical, social, ethical, religious, and economic issues. These relatively few deliveries tax the resources of any institution and require coordinated effort, skilled professionals, and excellent communication to meet the needs of all the parties involved. Although infants with a birth weight below 1 kg account for approximately 0.4% and those below 750 g account for 0.2% of all deliveries, they are responsible for the bulk of the mortality and contribute disproportionately to the morbidity. Resource utilization is excessive for these infants, with prolonged, technology-dependent intensive care after extensive periods of hospitalization.

Improved survival of extremely immature and low-birth-weight infants has blurred the definition of viability. Furthermore, there will continue to be changes so that specific birth weight, and gestational-age numbers should be used only as a guide for decisionmaking. The available data are for groups, but decisions must be made for individuals. Survival for the lowest gestational ages (23 to 24 weeks) is complicated by very high rates of short- and long-term morbidity (Figs. 60-2, 60-3, and 60-4). These infants are at greater risk for cerebral palsy, mental retardation, deafness, and blindness. The perinatal team must coordinate all the perinatal information, present the available options to the family, be aware of their wishes with regard to active resuscitation and intervention, and communicate the action plan to all persons who might attend the delivery. The prospective parents must be fully informed of the local outcome data and the risks and benefits of various interventions, the complexities of care required for an extremely premature infant, and the potential short- and long-term adverse outcomes. The risks and outlook could change frequently after the birth. Plans for neonatal management made prior to delivery often need to be modified by information that becomes available only after birth, e.g., the infant's condition, weight, presence of anomalies, and responses to simple or invasive resuscitative measures. Repeated discussions with the families and consistency from the health care providers can facilitate a difficult task. Counseling should be sensitive to cultural and ethnic diversity, and a skilled translator should be available for parents whose primary language differs from the language of the care providers.

There is considerable debate as to the appropriate management of babies born at the limits of viability. Reports on the outcomes of these pregnancies relate either to gestational age or birth weight. There are important differences in mortality and morbidity data according to whether they are derived from obstetrical (gestational age-based) or neonatal (birth weight-based) datasets. First, the denominator used to calculate mortality and morbidity from obstetrical datasets use the number of fetuses alive at the onset of labor or alive at birth, and thus include stillborn infants and live-born infants who died in the delivery room. The denominator for neonatal data is the number of admissions to the nursery. This difference results in higher survival rates for neonatal data. In a report from a single center on 278 deliveries between 22 and 25 weeks' gestation from 1993 and 1997, the fetal death rate was 24%. Survival to discharge rates by gestational age with and without fetal deaths were 1.8% and 4.6% at 22 weeks', 34% and 46% at 23 weeks', 49% and 59% at 24 weeks', and 76% and 82% at 25 weeks' gestation (El-Metwally et al., 2000). Second, gestational age as determined by the "best obstetrical estimate" (a combination of menstrual, clinical, and ultrasound data), is a stronger predictor of outcome before delivery than ultrasound estimates of fetal weight (Bottoms et al., 1999). Actual birth weight is superior to both gestational age and estimated fetal weight but is not available until after delivery. Third, despite the sensitivity of antenatal ultrasound to detect anomalies, abnormalities

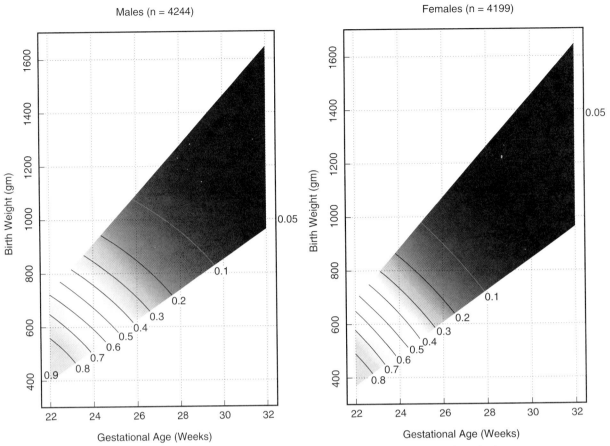

FIGURE 60-2 ■ Estimated mortality risk by birth weight and gestational age based on singleton infants born in NICHD Neonatal Research Network Centers between January 1, 1997, and December 31, 2000. (From Ehrenkranz RE, Wright LL: NICHD Neonatal Research Network: Contributions and future challenges. Sem Perinatol **27** [in press, 2003].)

of development may not be evident until after birth. Parents should be advised that decisions made before delivery necessarily rest upon incomplete data and that a reassessment of the baby's prognosis will be made in the nursery. It is essential that obstetrical and neonatal care providers communicate clearly with one another and especially with the parents about these subtle but important aspects of perinatal care.

Both gestational age and birth weight influence survival and morbidity. The outlook for an infant delivered at 24 1/7 weeks who weighs 550 g is different from an infant at 24 6/7 weeks who weighs 900 g. Other factors that affect

outcome include gender, intrauterine growth pattern (see Fig. 60-2), race, and treatment with antenatal corticosteroids (Tyson et al., 1996). At all weights and gestational ages, females have a better chance of surviving than males. Decisions regarding active resuscitation and viability should thus take into consideration the combination of projected birth weight, gestational age, gender, growth restriction, and maternal history. Unfortunately, the perinatal team often encounters a woman who will deliver imminently with uncertain dates and who has received no prenatal care. In this setting, antenatal ultrasound measurements may be

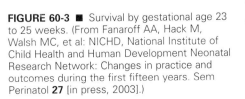

FIGURE 60-3 ■ Survival by gestational age 23 to 25 weeks. (From Fanaroff AA, Hack M, Walsh MC, et al: NICHD, National Institute of Child Health and Human Development Neonatal Research Network: Changes in practice and outcomes during the first fifteen years. Sem Perinatol **27** [in press, 2003].)

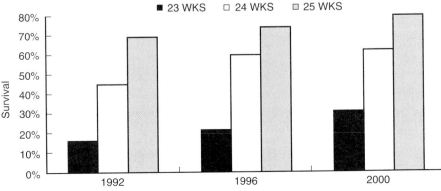

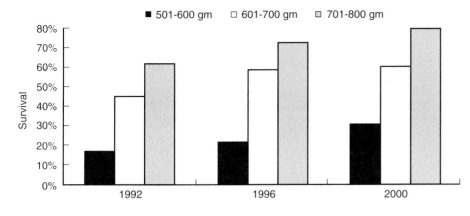

FIGURE 60-4 ■ Survival by birth weight 501 g to 800 g. (From Fanaroff AA, Hack M, Walsh MC, et al: National Institute of Child Health and Human Development Neonatal Research Network: Changes in practice and outcomes during the first fifteen years. Sem Perinatol **27** [in press, 2003].)

the only data available. Although there are no ultrasound criteria to predict neonatal mortality or morbidity, threshold values for biparietal diameter (50 mm) and femur length (37 mm) below which survival is unlikely have been published (Bottoms et al., 1999).

There has been considerable improvement over the past few years for babies with a birth weight above 600 g and a gestational age of 25 weeks or greater. Despite the widespread publicity they receive, survivors with a birth weight below 500 g are few. The majority of these are moderately small-for-gestational-age, female infants. The few survivors mean that follow-up data available for appropriate counseling are minimal.

Neonatal surfactant and antenatal steroid therapies have been credited with improving the survival rates for infants with birth weights below 1500 g. The impact of these treatments for the lowest birth weight (less than 750 g) and gestational age (fewer than 25 weeks) groups when they reach school age remains to be determined. Although survival at 24 weeks' gestation now is around 60%, there is considerable neurodevelopmental disability (40%); the chance of a neurologically intact infant is only 36%. In addition to neurodevelopmental handicap, there are high rates of debilitating lung and eye morbidity at the lower gestations.

There are no clear-cut guidelines regarding the obstetric management of the extremely low-birth-weight infant. A cesarean section often necessitates a vertical uterine incision with increased risk of maternal morbidity. Furthermore, there is no overwhelming evidence of improved outcome with cesarean delivery for extremely premature infants. Management of the infant should be humane and compassionate with provision of warmth and comfort. The Fetus and Newborn Committee, Canadian Pediatric Society, Maternal-Fetal Medicine Committee, and Society of Obstetricians and Gynecologists of Canada have specific guidelines with regard to management of women with threatened birth of an infant of extremely low gestational age:

Fetuses with a gestational age of less than 22 weeks are not viable, and those with an age of 22 weeks are rarely viable. In well-dated pregnancies, their mothers are not candidates for cesarean section, and the newborns should be provided with compassionate care rather than active treatment. The outcomes for infants with gestational ages of 23 and 24 weeks vary greatly. Careful consideration should be given to the limited benefits for

the infants and potential harms of cesarean section, as well as the expected results of resuscitation at birth. Cesarean section, when indicated, and any required neonatal treatment are recommended for infants with gestational ages of 25 and 26 completed weeks; most infants of this age will survive, and most survivors will not be severely disabled. Treatment of all infants with a gestational age of 22–26 weeks should be tailored to the infant and family and should involve fully informed parents.

Recent publications from the American Academy of Pediatrics (MacDonald et al., 2002) and the American College of Obstetricians and Gynecologists (ACOG, 2002) follow similar guidelines, with emphasis on communication with the family.

When resuscitation is not performed because of extreme immaturity or other considerations, the family must be supported carefully. They must be allowed access to support personnel including the hospital staff, clergy, relatives, and close friends. They should be encouraged and permitted to hold, touch, and interact with the fetus. The infant should be weighed and measured and this information provided to the mother. The infant should be gently handled and kept warm and comfortable. Ongoing support following the infant's demise is essential. In summary, the obstetric and pediatric team supported by nursing specialists, social workers, and bioethicists should confer and then counsel the family.

Counseling for future pregnancies is mandatory. Realistic outcomes must be presented, including the risks for moderate or severe disability, mental retardation, cerebral palsy, visual impairment including blindness, hearing loss, and the need for special education. The team must realize that there is no ethical distinction between withholding and withdrawing life-sustaining treatments. Humane care must be provided to all infants, including those from whom life-sustaining interventions have either been withheld or withdrawn. Parents should be encouraged to actively participate in the decision-making process concerning the treatment of their infant. Families should, at all times, be treated with dignity and compassion. In this manner, a course of action for the delivery and immediate management of the fetus can be arrived at. Continuation of care is based on the condition of the infant, with the family fully informed of the condition and plans at all times. The limits of viability remain a moving target as long as viability means the ability to survive so that life would be considered worthwhile to the infant or the parents.

Advanced Resuscitation and the Specific Problems of the Severely Asphyxiated Newborn

The use of medications to support circulation may be required in those rare infants who have a heart rate below 60 beats/minute despite adequate ventilation and chest compressions for a minimum of 30 seconds or who have an undetectable heart rate (Table 60-2). Epinephrine, volume expanders, and sodium bicarbonate are medications for advanced newborn resuscitation that should be available in all delivery rooms.

Two routes are used for emergency administration of such medications to a newborn. Epinephrine may be given intratracheally, from which site rapid absorption into the circulation occurs. Placement of an umbilical venous line provides prompt and convenient access for administration of volume expanders or bicarbonate.

Epinephrine is the first drug to be considered during advanced resuscitation. Epinephrine increases the strength and rate of cardiac contractions and may be given at a dose of 0.1 to 0.3 mL/kg (concentration 1:10,000) by the intravenous or intratracheal route and repeated every 5 minutes if required. Within 15–30 seconds, heart rate and perfusion usually improve.

The severely depressed infant can present with circulatory shock at birth, owing to such problems as asphyxia, hemorrhage, sepsis, pulmonary insufficiency, or structural heart disease. The antenatal history may give valuable clues allowing anticipation of shock in the infant (e.g., if abruptio placentae has occurred or if severe fetal heart rate depression has been diagnosed prior to delivery). Clinical signs of hypovolemia in the infant include pallor, weak pulses, cold extremities, poor capillary refill, poor response to resuscitation, or low blood pressure. Tachypnea, poor urine output, metabolic acidosis, and central nervous system depression may also accompany the picture of shock. The management of shock depends on the underlying mechanism. Three mechanisms that can contribute to shock are decreased blood volume (usually resulting from perinatal blood loss or twin-twin transfusion), decreased cardiac contractility (asphyxia, congenital heart disease, arrhythmias), and decreased peripheral vascular resistance (sepsis).

Volume expansion is the first line of treatment of the clinical picture of shock. This is effective for infants with reduced volume because of blood loss as well as for septic infants in whom vasodilation results in effective reduction of blood volume. The most commonly used volume expanders are normal saline, whole blood (cross-matched with the mother), and Ringer's lactate solution, given intravenously at a dose of 10 mL/kg over 5 to 10 minutes. Care should be taken, however, not to administer excessive fluids to the infant with asphyxia and myocardial dysfunction. In such infants, a combination of fluid administration at the dose just indicated and use of inotropic agents such as dopamine may yield the best outcome. Within minutes of restoration of peripheral circulation, blood pressure, color, perfusion, and neurologic state may improve remarkably and rapidly.

During prolonged asphyxia, diminished oxygen delivery to the tissues can result in a buildup of lactic acid, with resultant metabolic acidosis. When ventilation has been established and metabolic acidosis is documented or strongly suspected on clinical grounds, sodium bicarbonate may be administered intravenously at a dose of 2 mEq/kg of a 0.5 mEq/mL (4.2%) solution. Resolution of the metabolic acidosis reverses pulmonary vasoconstriction and aids in establishment of normal aerobic metabolism. Hypoglycemia may accompany profound asphyxia as well. The provision of intravenous glucose is invaluable for the recovery of all tissues of the asphyxiated infant.

Apparently stillborn infants (Apgar score of 0 at 1 minute) who respond to resuscitative efforts represent a class of children at a very high risk for poor outcome. In a study by Jain and associates (1991), 39% of apparently stillborn infants who were resuscitated survived beyond the neonatal period. Of those who survived, 39% exhibited abnormal development. It should be noted that if an infant exhibited no response to 10 minutes of resuscitation, the survival rate was only 2%. These sobering data should be kept in mind when decisions must be made in the delivery room concerning the extent and duration of neonatal resuscitation.

Extremely-low-birth-weight (ELBW) infants (less than 1 kg at birth) present a particular challenge in the immediate postnatal period. Such infants are prone to hypothermia, with the attendant cascade of adverse effects, including hypoglycemia, reversion to fetal circulatory patterns, acidosis, and hypoxia. Thus, special consideration must be given to provision of a dry and warm space in the delivery room, preferably a preheated radiant warmer. The degree of respiratory insufficiency shown by such babies is in direct proportion to their immaturity; personnel experienced in intubation and stabilization of such infants should be available at the delivery. The process of delivery itself could be stressful to ELBW infants, and complications ranging from bruising of the head, thorax, and extremities to severe asphyxia may be present. Furthermore, if chorioamnionitis has developed prior to delivery, neonatal

■ **TABLE 60-2.** MEDICATIONS USED DURING RESUSCITATION

Drug	Concentration	Dosage	Route
Epinephrine	1:10,000	0.1–0.3 mL/kg	IV or ET
Volume expanders	Whole blood Normal saline Ringer's lactate solution	10 mL/kg	IV
Sodium bicarbonate	0.5 mEq/mL (4.2% solution)	2 mEq/kg	IV; give slowly over at least 2 minutes; give only if infant being effectively ventilated
Naloxone	0.4 mg/mL or 1.0 mg/mL	0.1 mg/kg	IV, ET, preferred; IM, SC acceptable

ET, endotracheal; IM, intramuscular; IV, intravenous; SC, subcutaneous.

infection may have occurred and could compromise the infant further. Thus, delivery of such infants at a tertiary care facility optimizes the chance for a normal outcome.

Prospective parents of ELBW infants often wish to be fully informed of the hazards of immaturity so that they can participate in decisions as to the advisability of aggressive antenatal or postnatal care. Many perinatal and postnatal factors are continuing to increase the rate of survival for small infants at the threshold of viability using strategies that include maternal corticosteroid administration and postnatal surfactant therapy. Survival rates now range from 20% to 35% at 500 to 599 g, 41% to 57% at 600 to 699 g, and 65% to 88% at 700 to 799 g birth weight. Despite advances in care for these infants, however, there has been no change in early childhood neurodevelopmental outcome of recent survivors who weighed 600 to 750 g at birth. For example, mild to severe neurodevelopmental impairment can occur in 20% to 35%, and blindness in 2% to 10% of survivors at this weight range. Because regional differences in outcome can occur, the perinatologists and neonatologists involved in the care of all premature infants need to be informed of the changing patterns of outcome for their own hospital centers so as to best advise these families.

Meconium Aspiration

Meconium staining of the amniotic fluid or fetus (see also Chapter 24) occurs *in utero* in 8% to 20% of all infants and often can be a normal process accompanying delivery. Passage of meconium could indicate fetal distress, however—for example, in infants who are small for gestational age or very postmature, in those with cord complications, or in those in whom other factors are compromising oxygen delivery.

Meconium passage is characteristic of term infants and is almost never observed in the amniotic fluid before 34 weeks' gestation. The presence of meconium in the amniotic fluid should alert the delivery room team to the possibility of a depressed fetus, and a professional skilled in the technique of infant intubation and resuscitation should be present at delivery.

Meconium that remains in the amniotic fluid for a prolonged period can stain the umbilical cord, placenta, and fetus. Normally, the infant exhibits phasic respirations *in utero*, which can increase markedly in depth if asphyxia occurs. Meconium inhaled in this manner can penetrate the infant's airways and, if the consistency of the meconium is pea-soup or particulate, the material can cause obstruction of airways and result in atelectasis. In such infants, pneumothorax can develop after birth and can compromise the infant's cardiorespiratory status.

In the delivery room, management of this problem begins with the obstetrician, who should facilitate clearing of the upper airway by suctioning the pharynx and nares, preferably with wall suction after the head has been delivered. In approximately 10% of infants who have passed meconium *in utero*, residual meconium is left in the trachea below the vocal cords. In cases of meconium-stained amniotic fluid and neonatal depression, endotracheal intubation of the infant is recommended in order to clear the airway of residual meconium. If the meconium is light and the infant is not depressed at birth, intubation is usually not required (Wiswell et al., 2000).

Drug Depression in Infants at Birth

When narcotic analgesics such as meperidine (Demerol) are given intramuscularly to the mother within 1½ to 2 hours before delivery, the drug concentration is at its maximum in the serum of the mother and fetus at the time of birth. Narcotic depression of the infant could present as apnea and hypotonia. These effects on the infant can be reversed by administration of naloxone, 0.1 mg/kg, given either intramuscularly, intravenously, or intratracheally. Typically, the infant's tone and respiratory effort improve dramatically. Naloxone, however, may create acute drug withdrawal in infants whose mothers are addicted to narcotics or are on methadone therapy. In such cases, naloxone administration is contraindicated.

Congenital Malformations

About 2% of newborn infants have a serious malformation that has surgical or cosmetic implications. The majority of defects are of multifactorial inheritance. This pattern of inheritance is exemplified by congenital heart disease, neural tube defects, cleft lip or palate, and clubfoot.

Approximately 20% of all serious malformations are inherited in a mendelian manner, usually autosomal dominant, with a minority autosomal recessive or x-linked recessive. Limb anomalies, including polydactyly and syndactyly, are the most common autosomal dominant anomalies.

The most prevalent syndrome attributed to an abnormal chromosome is Down syndrome, or trisomy 21, which occurs in about one in 1000 births. Other trisomies, such as trisomy 18 and 13, occur at a lesser frequency of one in 10,000 live births. The rate of occurrence of all three trisomies increases with advanced maternal age.

Recently, development of DNA probes for specific mutant genes has allowed prenatal diagnosis of single gene disorders. For example, hemophilia A and B can be detected via fetal DNA from the amniotic fluid. This powerful technology will play an increasing role in prenatal genetic screening of high-risk pregnancies (see Chapters 1 and 18).

Congenital Diaphragmatic Hernia

Congenital diaphragmatic hernia (CDH) results from failure of closure of the posterolateral pleuroperitoneal folds during the eighth to ninth week of gestation, which results in herniation of intestine (90% of cases) and liver (50%) into the thoracic cavity. Most commonly, hernias involve the left hemidiaphragm. In these infants, breath sounds are absent over the left lung, and the cardiac sounds shift to the right. Respiratory distress, persistent cyanosis, and a scaphoid abdomen should make one suspicious of this diagnosis. A left-sided pneumothorax can yield similar auscultatory findings but is usually associated with abdominal distention rather than with a scaphoid abdomen. Because of advances in antenatal ultrasound technique, the prenatal diagnosis of diaphragmatic hernia is possible as early as 26 weeks' gestation, which allows for planning of delivery at a tertiary care center. Delayed operation could improve stability of the infant and decrease reactive pulmonary hypertension. The use and timing of extracorporeal membrane oxygenation (ECMO) in this disorder remains controversial, and the overall mortality rate still ranges from 20% to 60%.

Although most hernias are detected by antenatal ultrasonography, the occasional case still can be diagnosed from a chest radiograph in an infant who fails to respond adequately to cardiopulmonary resuscitation in the delivery room. When a diaphragmatic hernia is discovered, the infant should be intubated, and a nasogastric tube should be placed to decompress the gastrointestinal tract and prevent cardiac tamponade by the overdistended bowel. Successful initial management of the infant with CDH depends on early recognition of the defect, stabilization of acid-base balance, and adequate ventilatory support.

BIRTH TRAUMA/BIRTH INJURIES

The incidence of birth injuries has declined over the last fifty years. Birth injuries reportedly occur in two to seven per 1000 live births. They are not entirely avoidable and can be noted even after the most skilled and careful obstetric care. The fetus can be injured by antenatal or intrapartum interventions as well as by delivery itself. Amniocentesis, cordocentesis, fetal surgical manipulations, intrauterine transfusions, and even fetal heart rate monitoring via the scalp electrode all present some degree of risk for the fetus. The physical process of labor and delivery itself, however, accounts for the vast majority of birth injuries. The most vulnerable infants are those who are macrosomic or premature or who present abnormally. Prolonged labor, dystocia, and cephalopelvic disproportion predispose to injury, as does instrumental intervention with forceps or vacuum extractor. Delivery by cesarean section does not ensure freedom from birth trauma. Furthermore, the neonate can experience trauma during resuscitation.

CEPHALOHEMATOMA. Cephalohematomas are due to subperiosteal hemorrhage that occurs in the parieto-occipital area of the infant's head. Hemorrhage in this location is confined by the sutures and can be associated with hairline fractures of the skull, most frequently over the parietal bones. A cephalohematoma presents as a fluctuant swelling on the second day of life and, if large enough, can result in anemia and subsequent jaundice. Bilateral cephalohematomas also occasionally occur. Cephalohematomas should be differentiated from caput succedaneum, which has overlying bruising and less well-defined margins because the caput is not confined by the suture lines. Compared with a cephalohematoma, a caput resolves quickly over the first few days of life. No therapy is needed for a cephalohematoma, and the fluid should never be aspirated unless infection is suspected. Blood transfusion rarely is required.

SUBGALEAL HEMORRHAGE. Subgaleal hemorrhge (SGH) is a rare but serious condition. Its incidence is estimated at around four per 10,000 deliveries; however, there is a significant increase after instrumental deliveries—for example, up to 64 per 10,000 after vacuum extractions. Skull fractures with injuries to intracranial veins or sinuses also can lead to SGH. Blood collects in the space between the galea aponeurotica and the periosteum of the skull, and because of the loose connective tissue in this area, large amounts of blood can accumulate rapidly, leading to severe hypovolemia and shock. Infants present with pallor and swelling of the scalp. The presence of a fluctuating mass crossing sutures, fontanelles, or both is very suggestive of SGH. A posterior spread of the hemorrhage is usually accompanied by forward protrusion of the ears. Late clinical signs include hypotension, a dropping hematocrit,

and hypovolemic shock. Seizures and disseminated intravascular coagulation (DIC) are also common. The treatment consists of aggressive replacement of blood and blood products to restore intravascular volume and correct DIC. Surgical treatment may be considered in some cases. Mortality is up to 25%.

FACIAL NERVE PALSY. Facial nerve palsy may result from compression of the facial nerve by forceps or from spontaneous compression against the sacral promontory. The paralyzed side of the face appears smooth and full, with obliteration of the nasolabial fold; the eye may remain persistently open, and the corner of the mouth droops. With crying, the mouth is drawn to the side that is not paralyzed. Facial asymmetry needs to be differentiated from congenital hypoplasia or absence of the depressor anguli oris muscle (depressor of the angle of the mouth). If the eye remains open, a pad and methylcellulose drops may be used to prevent corneal injury. Spontaneous resolution of these lesions usually occurs; however, neurologic evaluation and follow-up are warranted if the paralysis does not improve.

FRACTURE OF THE CLAVICLE. Fracture of the clavicle can occur, most notably following shoulder dystocia or a difficult breech delivery. The clavicle is the most frequently fractured bone, and a cracking sound could be audible at the time of delivery. Fractures at this site may be asymptomatic or can be confirmed radiologically after detection of swelling, discoloration, tenderness, or an asymmetric Moro reflex. The affected arm and shoulder are immobilized for 7 to 10 days, by which time pain usually has subsided and callus formation has occurred.

FRACTURES OF THE LONG BONES. Fractures of the long bones are usually in the midshaft region and are sustained most commonly during manipulation of the arms or legs in a breech delivery. The diagnosis is usually made when swelling, pain, deformity, shortening, and lack of movement are observed in the affected limb. Treatment is directed at immobilization by casting, with little concern for careful alignment because of the great capacity for remodeling of bone in the newborn. Complete union is anticipated within 3 to 4 weeks.

BRACHIAL PLEXUS INJURY. Brachial plexus injuries are due to traction on or avulsion of the cranial nerve roots. These injuries are classified according to the site of the lesion. The most common is Erb's palsy, which involves the roots of C5 and C6. Infants with Erb's palsy hold the arm limply alongside the body with the forearm pronated. There is loss of movement and reflexes in the affected limb, including loss of the Moro response. The grasp reflex remains intact. Klumpke's palsy refers to lesions of the lower brachial plexus nerve roots C8–T1. In Klumpke's paralysis, the hand is paralyzed, there are no voluntary movements of the wrist, and the grasp reflex is absent. A claw hand can result from this type of injury. When the first sympathetic root (T1) is affected, Horner's syndrome (dilated pupil, ptosis, and absence of sweating) is observed. Rarely, the whole brachial plexus is involved, with a global palsy of the arm. Lesions of nerves C3, C4, and C5 can result in phrenic nerve paralysis, diaphragmatic paralysis, and respiratory compromise.

Most cases of brachial palsy follow prolonged labor and difficult deliveries in which traction is exerted on the neck (Allen et al., 1991). During a breech presentation, the plexus can be injured as a result of traction on the shoulder when delivery of the head is attempted. In considering the etiology of these injuries, one should remember that a significant number of cases of brachial palsy (often bilateral and in association with other nerve palsies) occur *in utero* and in the absence of birth trauma.

In infants with brachial plexus injuries, radiographs are indicated to exclude fractures of the spine, clavicle, and long bones of the arm. Treatment is expectant, with splinting to avoid contractures and physiotherapy once the initial postinjury period has passed. Because most injuries are mild, recovery can be anticipated by 4 months in 88% and by 2 years in 93% of cases. Residual long-term defects rarely occur but can include muscle atrophy, joint contractures, impaired growth of the limb, and general weakness of the shoulder girdle; therefore, close pediatric and neurologic follow-up of these patients is appropriate.

RESPIRATORY DISORDERS

Respiratory Distress Syndrome

Clinical Features

Respiratory distress syndrome (RDS) is one of the major causes of morbidity in newborn babies, although lack of a precise clinical definition in very-low-birth-weight infants necessitates cautious interpretation of statistics regarding incidence, mortality, and outcome. The diagnosis can be established biochemically by documentation of surfactant deficiency in amniotic fluid or in tracheal or gastric aspirate, although such data are usually unavailable. The greatest risk factor appears to be low gestational age and low birth weight (McIntire et al., 1999); other risk factors include maternal diabetes, hydrops fetalis, and perinatal asphyxia, which could be secondary to placental abruption. The incidence of RDS probably exceeds 80% at a gestation of less than 27 weeks, although severity varies widely. With improved survival, sequelae have increased dramatically—especially bronchopulmonary dysplasia (BPD)—because of the disease process as well as modes of treatment (Bancalari, 2002).

Impaired or delayed surfactant synthesis superimposed on a structurally immature lung appears to be key to the pathogenesis of RDS (Fig. 60-5). The resultant decrease in lung compliance leads to alveolar hypoventilation and ventilation-perfusion imbalance. The resultant hypoxemia can cause metabolic acidosis, and both can contribute to pulmonary vasoconstriction and aggravate hypoxemia. Meanwhile, high inspired oxygen and baro/volu-trauma from assisted ventilation initiate an inflammatory process in the immature lung that paves the way for development of chronic neonatal lung disease or BPD.

Infants with RDS typically present a combination of tachypnea, nasal flaring, subcostal and intercostal retractions, cyanosis, and expiratory grunting. Retractions are prominent and are the result of the very compliant rib cage being drawn in on inspiration as the infant generates high intrathoracic pressures to expand the poorly compliant lungs. The typical expiratory grunt is thought to result from partial closure of the glottis during expiration and in this way, it acts as a means of trapping alveolar air and maintaining an adequate end-expiratory lung volume (or functional residual capacity [FRC]). Although these signs are characteristic for neonatal respiratory disease, they can result from a wide variety of nonpulmonary causes, such as hypothermia, hypoglycemia, anemia, polycythemia, or metabolic acidosis. Furthermore, such nonpulmonary conditions can complicate the clinical course of RDS.

A constant feature of RDS is the early onset of clinical signs of the disease, typically within 1 to 2 hours of delivery. The uncomplicated natural course of clinical disease is characterized by a progressive worsening of symptoms, with a peak severity by days 2 to 3 and onset of recovery by 72 hours. This is now rare because all but the mildest cases of RDS are treated with exogenous surfactant, as discussed later in this chapter. When the disease process requires assisted ventilation and is complicated by the development of air leaks, significant shunting through a patent ductus arteriosus, or BPD, the infant's recovery could be delayed for days to months.

The typical radiographic features consist of a diffuse reticulogranular pattern in both lung fields with superimposed air bronchograms. These findings cannot be differentiated reliably from those of neonatal pneumonia, most commonly caused by group B streptococci. This problem has been the major reason for the widespread use of antibiotics in the initial management of infants with RDS. The increased use of various means of ventilatory support and the enhanced survival of infants with more severe pulmonary disease have resulted in the more frequent diagnosis of BPD at an early postnatal age.

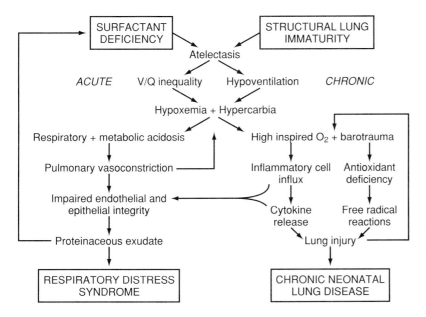

FIGURE 60-5 ■ The acute and chronic events that may lead to neonatal respiratory distress syndrome and accompanying lung injury. (Redrawn from Rodriguez RJ, Martin RJ, Fanaroff AA: Respiratory distress syndrome and its management. *In* Fanaroff AA, Martin RJ (eds): Neonatal-Perinatal Medicine, 7th ed. St. Louis, Mosby-Year Book, 2002, p. 1003.)

Management

When an infant (especially a preterm infant) presents with respiratory symptoms, there is a tendency to conclude that underlying pulmonary parenchymal disease is present; however, the differential diagnosis is extensive and includes nonpulmonary problems. Disorders of the upper airway (e.g., choanal atresia, micrognathia), larynx, trachea, intrathoracic airway, chest wall, central nervous system, cardiovascular system, and musculoskeletal system—together with hematologic and metabolic problems or sepsis—easily may be confused with lung disorders. To avoid serious diagnostic and therapeutic errors, historical information related to pregnancy, delivery, and the neonatal transition must be reviewed thoroughly. Meticulous observation and careful physical examination of the infant must follow. Analysis of simple laboratory data includes blood gases, complete blood cell count with differential, blood glucose and blood culture, together with appropriate radiographic studies. Therapy for RDS comprises the careful application of general supportive measures, exogenous surfactant therapy, and specific measures for controlling or assisting ventilation.

GENERAL MEASURES

Infants with respiratory difficulty require an optimal thermal environment to minimize oxygen consumption and oxygen requirements. The ability to supply an adequate caloric intake to the critically ill infant receiving respiratory assistance is facilitated by intravenous hyperalimentation that includes lipid solutions. The role of nutritional support for these infants cannot be overemphasized. Therefore, hyperalimentation is started on the first day of life, especially for infants weighing less than 1000 g. Once the patient is considered stable, usually within 72 hours after birth, small gavage feeds of formula or breast milk should be started. Fluid and electrolyte balance must be individualized and closely monitored because overenthusiastic attention to calories could result in fluid overload, patent ductus arteriosus, and congestive heart failure. The resultant increase in ventilatory support could contribute to the development of BPD (Costarino et al., 1992). Spontaneous diuresis often precedes improvement in lung function and recovery from RDS, although there is no evidence that diuretic therapy improves the early clinical course.

Metabolic acidosis is most often encountered when the infant has been depressed at birth and required resuscitation. A subsequent metabolic acidosis out of proportion to the degree of respiratory distress could signify hypoperfusion, sepsis, or an intraventricular hemorrhage. It is not necessary to correct metabolic or respiratory acidosis if the pH is greater than 7.25, whereas a pH of less than 7.20 typically requires intervention. In the case of respiratory acidosis, alkali therapy is not indicated until some form of assisted ventilation has been initiated.

It is customary to maintain a venous hematocrit of at least 40% during the acute phase of RDS to support an adequate oxygen-carrying capacity. Arterial oxygen tension (PaO_2) is maintained between 50 and 80 mm Hg. Although umbilical arterial catheters still form the basic means of arterial sampling in infants with RDS, the list of catheter-related thrombotic, embolic, and ischemic complications is formidable. For infants with mild or resolving respiratory distress, noninvasive measurement of PO_2 and PCO_2 via transcutaneous electrodes could make it unnecessary to insert an arterial catheter. Because poor perfusion, hyperoxemia, and advancing postnatal age make transcutaneous PO_2 ($TcPO_2$) somewhat unreliable as a measure of PaO_2, its use has declined, whereas the technique of continuous noninvasive measurement of oxygen saturation via pulse oximetry has gained widespread acceptance.

As hyperoxic levels of PaO_2 are approached, however, saturation becomes less sensitive, with flattening of the hemoglobin dissociation curve, and large changes in PaO_2 cause only minor alterations in saturation. Thus, in the absence of arterial sampling, both oxygen saturation and $TcPO_2$ must be interpreted with caution.

SURFACTANT THERAPY

The discovery that surfactant deficiency (see also Chapters 16 and 25) was key in the pathophysiology of RDS led early investigators to administer artificial aerosolized phospholipids to infants, with only limited therapeutic success. In their landmark study, Fujiwara and associates (1980) developed a mixture of both natural (animal-derived) and synthetic surface active lipids for use in humans. When administered to an initial group of 10 preterm infants with severe RDS who were not improving despite artificial ventilation, a single dose of surfactant instilled into the endotracheal tubes resulted in a dramatic decrease in inspired oxygen and ventilator pressures. None of the infants in this uncontrolled series subsequently succumbed from RDS.

Various other forms of largely natural surfactant subsequently also led to impressive results in preterm infants with RDS. There followed a series of collaborative multicenter trials in which purely synthetic and mixed natural/synthetic preparations were primarily employed. The former studies used protein-free synthetic phospholipid products (such as Exosurf), which contain alcohol to act as a spreading agent for dipalmitoyl phosphatidylcholine at the air/fluid alveolar interface. The latter investigations employed the Fujiwara preparation, a protein-containing extract of minced calf lung supplemented with dipalmitoyl phosphatidylcholine, tripalmitin, and palmitic acid and marketed as Survanta. Since then, a number of natural surfactants, derived primarily from bovine and porcine lungs, have been tested and become available for clinical use. These preparations have performed comparably in clinical trials. A multitude of studies have now employed various combinations of prevention (delivery-room administration) and rescue (administration for established RDS) protocols in North America, Europe, and Japan. A systematic review of comparison trials between synthetic and natural preparations demonstrated a significant decrease in mortality and frequency of pneumothorax. In addition to these benefits, a more rapid physiologic response after the administration of natural (protein-containing) preparations has been shown as manifested by the ability to reduce inspired oxygen and ventilator pressures (Vermont-Oxford Neonatal Network, 1996; Stevens et al., 2002).

Exogenous surfactant therapy requires the presence of an endotracheal tube. There is now clear evidence arising from meta-analysis of several randomized trials that preventive treatment—surfactant administered endotracheally during the first 15 minutes of life—is associated with better outcomes when compared with treatment of established RDS. Specifically, a significant decrease in mortality (in the combined outcome BPD and death) and a significant reduction in pneumothorax are

TABLE 60-3. SURFACTANT THERAPY FOR RESPIRATORY DISTRESS SYNDROME (RDS)

- Decrease in neonatal mortality of preterm infants
- Increase in survival without bronchopulmonary dysplasia (BPD), although incidence of BPD unchanged
- Decrease in incidence of air leaks
- Improvement in arterial oxygenation
- Optimal benefit with antenatal corticosteroids and surfactant retreatment
- Decreased mortality with prophylactic versus rescue therapy in ELBW <29 weeks' gestation
- Unresolved issues include risk factors for pulmonary hemorrhage and role of ventilator strategy (e.g., high frequency) in optimizing surfactant therapy

observed (Soll, 2001). Regardless of the timing of initial surfactant therapy, subsequent retreatments over the first 48 hours of life are often needed for optimal therapeutic effect (Table 60-3). All regimens of surfactant therapy appear to decrease the incidence of air leaks and improve oxygenation of ventilated preterm infants. More strikingly, mortality from RDS and even overall mortality of preterm infants are significantly reduced, especially when multiple-dose surfactant therapy is used for these infants. In contrast with the impressive improvement in mortality, the incidence of BPD, intraventricular hemorrhage (IVH), sepsis, and symptomatic patent ductus arteriosus appears unaltered in most studies (Jobe, 1993).

The overall incidence of BPD has not been reduced by the use of surfactant therapy. This could be a consequence of enhanced survival, and there is evidence that surfactant has increased the rate of survival without BPD (see Table 60-3). The incidence of BPD is significantly reduced in survivors of RDS who have a birth weight of at least 1250 g (Liechty et al., 1991).

Presumably, BPD is more likely to be a direct consequence of barotrauma in the preterm survivors of neonatal intensive care who have a more advanced gestational age, and such diverse factors as impaired respiratory drive, nutritional compromise, intercurrent infection, and congestive heart failure are less of a problem than in the smallest survivors of assisted ventilation (Table 60-4).

Pulmonary hemorrhage has been reported in up to 6% of preterm infants treated with exogenous surfactant and typically occurs in the first 72 hours of life. In surfactant-treated infants, there tends to be extensive intra-alveolar hemorrhage, in contrast with pulmonary hemorrhage in infants not exposed to surfactant in whom such bleeds present as interstitial hemorrhage and localized hematomas (Pappin et al., 1994). Garland and coworkers (1994) reported a significant relationship between pulmonary hemorrhage and a clinically detectable patent ductus arteriosus in surfactant-treated infants. In contrast, Braun and colleagues (1999) did not find such an association in a case-control study of pulmonary hemorrhage either before or after the clinical introduction of surfactant replacement therapy. It remains to be determined whether prophylactic ductal closure would reduce the risk of pulmonary hemorrhage.

Dramatic improvement in oxygenation after surfactant therapy does correlate with an increase in lung volume and resultant stabilization of FRC. This occurs despite the failure of lung compliance to increase rapidly and suggests that surfactant therapy could induce regional over-distention of alveoli.

If lung compliance is compared on spontaneous rather than ventilator breaths, however, or if ventilator pressures are promptly lowered in response to the increase in PaO_2 induced by surfactant therapy, an increase in compliance in response to surfactant occurs (Davis et al., 1988; Kelly et al., 1993).

Some infants do not exhibit the anticipated favorable response to surfactant therapy. Some poor responders appear to develop systemic hypotension during surfactant therapy, and this could enhance right-to-left shunting and prevent oxygenation from improving. When protein-rich pulmonary edema fluid is a prominent component of RDS, this would be expected to inhibit or decrease the surface tension-lowering capacity of surfactant, as noted in Figure 60-5.

The genes that code for the various surfactant proteins A, B, C, and D have been characterized. The application of DNA recombinant technology has led to the development of new synthetic preparations (e.g., human recombinant SPC-based surfactant), which currently are undergoing clinical evaluation. The precise role of surfactant proteins in prevention of RDS is under intensive study. Surfactant protein A–deficient mice have essentially normal metabolism of saturated phosphatidylcholine, which is a critical component of surfactant function (Ikegami et al., 1997). This is consistent with the fact that clinically available surfactants do not contain surfactant protein A despite their well-documented efficacy. Interestingly, these animals could be more prone to bacterial, viral, and fungal infections; thus, SPA may play a significant role in the modulation of the innate immune response of the lung. In contrast, term infants who are genetically deficient in surfactant protein B lack functional pulmonary surfactant and develop irreversible respiratory failure as neonates. Several mutations of this deficiency have been characterized, and only lung transplantation has been successful as therapy for surfactant protein B deficiency (Hamvas et al., 1997). In recent years, mutations of the SPC gene have been described in families with a history of chronic interstitial lung disease in infancy and adulthood. The role of SPC deficiency in neonatal RDS, if any, is still unclear (Amin et al., 2001; Nogee et al., 2001).

No adverse immunologic consequences of foreign tissue protein administration have yet been reported in the recipients of natural surfactant therapy. Currently available data from large numbers of infants in the United States and Europe also indicate no adverse effects on physical growth, respiratory symptoms, or neurodevelopmental outcome. Finally, the improvement in mortality and morbidity induced by surfactant therapy is accompanied by significant cost savings (Schwartz et al., 1994).

TABLE 60-4. MAJOR CAUSES OF INABILITY TO WEAN MECHANICAL VENTILATION IN VERY-LOW-BIRTH-WEIGHT INFANTS

Respiratory	Nonrespiratory
Impaired respiratory drive	Nutritional compromise
Respiratory muscle failure	Neurologic problems
Abnormal pulmonary mechanics	Excessive sedation
	Intercurrent infection (sepsis, NEC)
Localized atelectasis	Congestive heart failure—PDA
Uncontrolled air leaks	

From Fanaroff AA, Martin RJ (eds): Neonatal-Perinatal Medicine. 6th ed. St. Louis, Mosby-Year Book, 1997, p. 1036.

NEONATAL ASSISTED VENTILATION

Assisted ventilation has contributed substantially to improving the outcome of infants with respiratory distress. It is important to consider the mechanical characteristics of the respiratory system to understand the physiologic rationale of the blood gas responses that occur after ventilator setting changes, especially in neonates with RDS whose disease is characterized by rapidly changing pulmonary mechanics. Carbon dioxide elimination is a function of alveolar ventilation and is determined by both the pressure gradient between expiration and inspiration and ventilator frequency. Oxygen uptake is affected not only by ventilation but also largely by the matching of perfusion with ventilation. During assisted ventilation, oxygenation is largely determined by the mean airway pressure, which is a measure of the average pressure to which the lungs are exposed during the respiratory cycle. Changes in inspired oxygen concentration also alter alveolar oxygen tension and thus oxygenation (Carlo et al., 2002).

There is tremendous interest in introducing newer modes of assisted ventilation in order to minimize the risks of ventilator-induced lung injury (VILI) and high supplemental oxygen on an immature respiratory system, all of which are thought to contribute to the pathogenesis of BPD. Various modes of patient-triggered ventilation are being investigated for their ability to synchronize spontaneous and ventilator-triggered breaths, and in particular, to enhance weaning of assisted ventilation. Initial randomized controlled trials have shown a decreased need for sedation and a trend to a decrease in days on mechanical ventilation. Unfortunately, these trials were not powered to demonstrate a significant reduction in BPD.

High-frequency ventilation is being employed widely for infants with severe lung disease in an attempt to minimize VILI, although many issues remain unresolved (Table 60-5). All techniques of high-frequency ventilation have in common the use of high frequencies and small volumes, and currently high-frequency oscillatory ventilation (HFOV) holds the greatest promise. High-frequency oscillatory ventilation delivers extremely small volumes (even less than dead space) at very high frequencies (usually 600–900/minute) with the use of a piston or diaphragm pump. The ventilator strategy most widely employed is designed to optimize lung inflation by initially using relatively high mean airway pressures on which very-low-volume oscillations are superimposed. In an initial large multicenter trial, neither the incidence and severity of BPD nor mortality was improved by high-frequency oscillatory ventilation (HIFI Study Group, 1989). The most disconcerting observations were that high-frequency oscillatory ventilation was associated with a significantly increased incidence of grades III and IV intracranial hemorrhage and periventricular leukomalacia

TABLE 60-5. HIGH-FREQUENCY VENTILATION: UNRESOLVED ISSUES

1. Optimal ventilatory strategy in relation to underlying disease and mode of high-frequency ventilation (jet, oscillator, flow interrupter)
2. Role as primary mode of ventilation versus rescue therapy
3. Ability to decrease rate of bronchopulmonary dysplasia
4. Ability to decrease need for extracorporeal membrane oxygenation
5. Ability to enhance surfactant delivery

(see Table 60-5), although this remains controversial (Clark et al., 1996). A large multicenter, randomized trial in the UK demonstrated no differences in the incidence of BPD between infants randomized to HFOV versus conventional ventilation, while a similar study in the US showed a small but significant benefit when HFOV was used (Courtney et al., 2002). Neither of these trials showed differences in the incidence of periventricular leukomalacia or intraventricular hemorrhage between HFOV versus conventional ventilation (Johnson et al., 2002). HFOV reduced the need for ECMO in neonates with pulmonary hypertension (Clark et al., 1996) and reduced the development of air leaks in premature infants with RDS (HIFI Study Group, 1989). HFOV seems to be most beneficial in selected infants with the most severe derangement of lung function or gas exchange. The lack of consistent results could be due to differences in study design and, more important, could be influenced by wide variations in experience among centers.

Liquid ventilation is a creative research tool that could reduce barotrauma from assisted ventilation applied to the most structurally immature lungs. This approach involves inert perfluorochemical liquids that have high solubility for respiratory gases. The infused liquid is evenly distributed throughout the lungs and essentially eliminates surface tension–related forces (Wolfson et al., 1992). With the liquid ventilation approach, it is possible to maintain cardiopulmonary stability in preterm lambs and accomplish gas exchange in very immature neonates for brief periods. Although it is a highly successful technique in the laboratory setting, liquid ventilation has not yet found a place in the management of newborns with respiratory failure. Potentially, this technique may also develop into an alternative route for drug delivery (e.g., antibiotics, chemotherapeutic agents) to the alveolar surface.

Transient Tachypnea

Transient tachypnea typically presents as respiratory distress in term infants or preterm infants who are close to term. The clinical features comprise various combinations of mild cyanosis, grunting, flaring, retracting, and tachypnea in the first few hours after birth, associated with a modest requirement for supplemental oxygen. The chest radiograph shows prominent perihilar streaking that could represent engorgement of the periarterial lymphatics that participate in the clearance of alveolar fluid. The radiographic appearance usually can be readily distinguished from the diffuse reticulogranular pattern with air bronchograms that is characteristic of RDS. The presence of fluid in the minor fissure is a common but nonspecific finding.

Patchy infiltrates that clear within 48 hours and are associated with perihilar streaking are probably also manifestations of transient tachypnea. Differentiation from neonatal pneumonia or meconium aspiration can be extremely difficult, especially if the antenatal or postnatal history includes risk factors for these disorders. Evaluation, monitoring, and basic supportive care must cover all the various diagnostic contingencies. A course of antibiotic therapy may be begun, depending on the history and clinical status of the infant, and may be terminated at 48 hours if cultures are negative. Transient tachypnea of the newborn by definition is self-limiting with no risk of recurrence or residual pulmonary dysfunction.

Pneumothorax

Pulmonary air leaks comprise a spectrum of disease that includes pneumothorax, pneumomediastinum, pneumopericardium, and pulmonary interstitial emphysema (Madansky et al., 1979). The likelihood of a pneumothorax being symptomatic in an infant without underlying lung disease is small, and many of these cases go undetected. Several interventions and disease states markedly increase the risk of pulmonary air leaks. These include vigorous resuscitation at birth, RDS, meconium aspiration syndrome, and pulmonary hypoplasia. Treatment with assisted ventilation results in an increase in the incidence of pneumothorax and other air leaks in most series, with some variability according to the ventilatory technique employed (Primhak, 1983). There has been a decline in the incidence of air leaks with the use of more cautious ventilatory management and surfactant therapy.

Transillumination of the chest is a useful technique for immediate diagnosis of pneumothorax and invariably yields positive results if the pneumothorax is large. When there are lesser or questionable areas of abnormal transillumination and the infant's condition is stable, radiographic confirmation is indicated before therapeutic intervention is undertaken. This allows precise localization of the pneumothorax and differentiation from a pneumomediastinum. The presence of an isolated pneumomediastinum (or other air leak) requires close observation of vital signs and frequent clinical assessment. In infants with lung disease, the presence of a pneumothorax accentuates the respiratory difficulty and often requires prompt intervention. This consists of the placement of a large-bore, multiple-holed chest tube into the pleural space, preferably anterior to the lung. In cases where rapid hemodynamic deterioration occurs because of a tension pneumothorax, needle aspiration by a skilled caregiver may be life-saving. In an infant who has no underlying pulmonary disease, no specific management is necessary for an asymptomatic (or mildly symptomatic) pneumothorax.

Neonatal Pneumonia and Meconium Aspiration Syndrome

The lungs are a common site for the establishment of sepsis in the neonate. Such infection, be it bacterial or viral in origin, can be acquired before or at the time of birth or in the early postnatal period. Because bacterial pneumonia carries a substantial risk of mortality in the neonate, an extremely high index of suspicion must be maintained for all infants, preterm and term alike, in whom signs of respiratory distress are observed.

Bacterial pneumonia can be acquired by the fetus via transplacental passage of organisms, although ascending infection from the genital tract before or during labor appears to predominate. Prolonged rupture of membranes is a major predisposing factor, although it is possible that bacteria may gain access to the fetus by ascent through intact membranes. Because bacterial colonization of the infant always occurs during vaginal delivery, neonatal pneumonia can develop in the absence of prolonged rupture of membranes or any maternal symptoms.

Group B streptococci (GBS) are the major pathogens producing neonatal pneumonia. The organism is characteristically acquired from the maternal genital tract during labor or delivery, and overt group B streptococcal sepsis develops in approximately 1% of infants colonized in this way. Historically, the incidence of neonatal GBS infection was around 1 to 4 per 1000 live births. With the introduction of universal maternal screening and of intrapartum antibiotic prophylaxis for the prevention of neonatal GBS, the infection rate has fallen substantially, to less than 0.75 cases per 1000 live births. Approximately one third of the infants with group B streptococcal bacteremia are preterm, and the mortality rate is considerably higher in these infants (Weisman et al., 1992). Other bacteria that should be considered when pneumonia is acquired *in utero* or in the immediate perinatal period include *Escherichia coli*, *Klebsiella* organisms, group D streptococci, *Listeria* organisms, and pneumococci, acquired via transmission from the mother. Interestingly, the widespread use of intrapartum antibiotics has resulted in the reemergence of ampicillin-resistant organisms as important pathogens in early neonatal sepsis (Stoll et al., 2002b).

The nonspecific nature of the clinical signs that characterize neonatal sepsis make a high index of suspicion the key to early diagnosis. In some cases of severe pneumonia, the infants totally lack pulmonary symptoms and present only mild or severe neurologic depression. Other alerting features include thermal instability or apneic spells. Chest radiography could reveal streaky densities, confluent opacities, or diffuse granularity, as in RDS. Appropriate antibiotic therapy is almost always begun before antibiotic sensitivities are available. The most effective drug regimen should be continued for at least 10 days.

As with meconium staining of the amniotic fluid, meconium aspiration syndrome occurs predominately in small-for-gestational-age and postmature infants and is thought to occur in about 4% of deliveries complicated by meconium-stained fluid (Wiswell and Bent, 1993). With appropriate preventive management of the airway, the incidence of clinically significant meconium aspiration syndrome can be reduced substantially. Thick meconium, fetal tachycardia, or absence of fetal cardiac accelerations on intrapartum monitoring appear to identify the infant at high risk for meconium aspiration syndrome (Rossi et al., 1989).

Pathophysiologically, the pulmonary problems are due to airway obstruction and a ball-valve phenomenon created by the presence of meconium within the airways. Areas of atelectasis develop within the lung, resulting from total small airway obstruction, adjacent to areas of overexpansion from gas trapping in regions with partial obstruction (Fig. 60-6). Air leaks, including pneumomediastinum and pneumothorax, are more likely to occur after aspiration of meconium and cellular debris. Chemical inflammation secondary to aspirated meconium presumably leads to pneumonitis. In addition, *in vitro* data have shown a concentration-dependent inhibition of surfactant by meconium, all of which could aggravate atelectasis, hypoventilation, and intrapulmonary shunting (Moses et al., 1991).

Preventive management for the infant born with meconium-stained fluid must include thorough suctioning of the oropharynx and nasopharynx at the perineum prior to delivery. Whereas it is widely accepted that subsequent intubation and tracheal suctioning are needed for the depressed infant in the presence of thick meconium, current data do not support a policy of indiscriminate intubation in vigorous infants with light meconium-stained fluid (Wiswell et al., 2000). The subsequent management of meconium aspiration

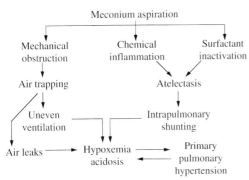

FIGURE 60-6 ■ Pathophysiology of meconium aspiration syndrome. (From Miller MJ, Fanaroff AA, Martin RJ: Respiratory disorders in preterm and term infants. *In* Fanaroff AA, Martin RJ (eds): Neonatal-Perinatal Medicine, 7th ed. St. Louis, Mosby-Year Book, 2002, p. 1026.)

syndrome (or bacterial pneumonia) consists of supportive therapy. Bacterial sepsis may have precipitated the passage and subsequent aspiration of meconium; therefore, management may include the use of antibiotics. Primary pulmonary hypertension of the newborn (PPHN) or persistent fetal circulation can complicate the clinical course of neonatal pneumonia associated with sepsis or meconium aspiration. Several randomized controlled trials have shown that surfactant replacement therapy significantly reduces the need for ECMO in babies with meconium aspiration syndrome. Moreover, the beneficial effects are more pronounced when therapy is instituted early in the course of the disease (Lotze et al., 1998). The optimal method for surfactant administration, however—as a bolus or through bronchoalveolar lavage with dilute surfactant—remains unresolved (Wiswell et al., 2002).

Pulmonary Hypoplasia

Pulmonary hypoplasia represents a broad spectrum of anatomic malformations ranging from bronchial and pulmonary agenesis to mild pulmonary parenchymal hypoplasia. Pulmonary hypoplasia can be unilateral or bilateral and can occur as an isolated entity or secondary to lesions restricting lung growth.

Secondary pulmonary hypoplasia is most commonly encountered in one of two conditions: oligohydramnios or congenital diaphragmatic hernia. The degree of hypoplasia in these conditions, and thus the probability of survival of the infant, depends on the degree to which the lung growth is restricted. Unilateral diaphragmatic hernia, associated with displacement of abdominal viscera into the thoracic cavity, occurs as often as one in 2200 births. Eighty percent of defects involve the left hemidiaphragm. The severity of respiratory insufficiency after birth can be mild or can be so severe as to be incompatible with life, depending on the degree of compression of the lung by the herniated viscus. Accompanying morphologic changes result in restriction to pulmonary blood flow and resultant primary pulmonary hypertension, which is often the dominant clinical problem in the immediate postnatal period.

Infants born with diaphragmatic hernia continue to experience a high mortality rate—approximately 50% for those who are diagnosed in the first 24 hours of life. Early prenatal diagnosis has permitted referral of these high-risk deliveries to tertiary centers so that optimal ventilatory care and surgical expertise are available. Because of the heterogeneity of clinical severity, a number of schema and criteria have been proposed (with varying degrees of success) to grade the degree of physiologic derangement and predict the survival of the infant. The presence of polyhydramnios and prenatal detection early in gestation are negative prognostic indicators. Adequate ventilation of the infant after birth has also permitted estimation of the adequacy of pulmonary function. ECMO has been used perioperatively for infants in whom congenital diaphragmatic hernia is associated with poor pulmonary function and primary pulmonary hypertension. The timing of ECMO and its therapeutic benefit in this disorder remain controversial (Newman et al., 1990). Nitric oxide therapy has also failed to improve outcome.

Bilateral pulmonary hypoplasia commonly occurs in association with oligohydramnios caused either by renal disease in the fetus or chronic leakage of amniotic fluid. The presence of pulmonary hypoplasia in infants with bilateral *renal agenesis* was first recognized by Potter in 1946. A similar picture of lethal pulmonary hypoplasia is visible in conjunction with bilaterally dysplastic kidneys with or without cyst formation and in infants with congenital obstructive uropathy. Characteristic features include premature birth in the breech position, a typical facial appearance (called *Potter facies*), limb malformations, and severe respiratory insufficiency often complicated by pneumothoraces and resulting in a fatal outcome in the vast majority of infants.

Prenatal ultrasound diagnosis of congenital cystic disease of the kidney, renal agenesis, or obstructive uropathy has made early termination of such pregnancies possible in selected cases. Despite attempts at *in utero* decompression of the urinary system, fetal surgery in this disease has met with limited success (see Chapter 27).

Infants subject to oligohydramnios resulting from chronic leakage of amniotic fluid over the course of many weeks can exhibit a varying degree of pulmonary hypoplasia. Oligohydramnios can act by compressing the fetal thorax or by altering the dynamics of lung fluid so that full expansion of the lungs cannot be maintained. The severity of the pulmonary hypoplasia is directly proportional to rupture of membranes early in gestation, longer duration of rupture, and the presence of oligohydramnios during the period of rupture (Vergani et al., 1994). Postnatal management of those infants has improved with the advent of high-frequency ventilation, but eventual survival is still limited by the underlying degree of pulmonary hypoplasia.

Other Respiratory Disorders

Neonatal respiratory distress can be the end result of a diversity of pulmonary and nonpulmonary disorders, as indicated previously. Structural problems in the upper or lower airway and a variety of intrathoracic tumors and malformations can present in this way (Table 60-6). Neuromuscular disease can involve the respiratory system, prevent adequate chest wall expansion, or result in respiratory muscle failure.

Neonatal apnea is a clinical problem in the majority of preterm infants with a birth weight of 1 kg or less. Apnea can be associated with a specific precipitating factor or pathophysiologic disorder other than prematurity, many of which are summarized in Figure 60-7. It appears that the respiratory centers

TABLE 60-6. MAJOR EXTRAPULMONARY CAUSES OF NEONATAL RESPIRATORY DISTRESS

Condition	Causes
Upper airway obstruction	Choanal atresia
	Nasal congestion (infection, trauma)
	Micrognathia
	Enlarged tongue
	Laryngomalacia, webs
	Tumors, hemangiomas
	Vocal cord paralysis
	Tracheal stenosis
Lower airway obstruction	Tracheomalacia
	Bronchomalacia
	Lobar emphysema
Extrinsic mass	Goiter
	Cystic hygroma
	Vascular ring
	Mediastinal mass (cyst, teratoma)
	Tracheoesophageal fistula
	Bronchogenic cyst
	Pleural effusions
Chest wall abnormalities	Dwarfism (e.g., thanatophoric)
	Skeletal dysplasias
	Asphyxiating thoracic dystrophy
Diaphragm disorders	Eventration, congenital diaphragmatic hernia
	Phrenic nerve injury
Neuromuscular disease	Spinal cord injury
	Werdnig-Hoffmann disease
	Myasthenia syndromes
	Muscular dystrophies
Cardiac disease	Total anomalous pulmonary venous drainage
	Congestive heart failure, AV malformations
	Arrhythmias
Metabolic disorder	Metabolic acidosis
Hematologic disorders	Anemia
	Polycythemia

responsible for generation of breathing patterns in preterm infants are sensitive to a bewildering array of peripheral stimuli that can trigger apnea, bradycardia, and desaturation.

In preterm infants, a majority of apneic episodes are accompanied by airway obstruction at the level of the pharynx. The most common type of apnea observed in premature infants is mixed apnea, in which a central respiratory pause is preceded or followed by obstructed breaths. Negative pharyngeal pressure generated during inspiration can produce pharyngeal collapse, particularly if upper-airway dilator muscle activity is decreased.

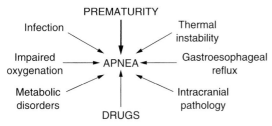

FIGURE 60-7 ■ Specific contributory causes of neonatal apnea. (From Martin RJ, Miller MJ, Carlo WA: Pathogenesis of apnea in preterm infants. J Pediatr **109**:733, 1986.)

Diaphragmatic activity can then continue, although no net airflow results. During apnea with an obstructive component, clinical cardiorespiratory monitoring may demonstrate only bradycardia and desaturation as respiratory movements continue during the period of obstruction.

The first step in evaluating apnea is to rule out treatable causes. When this has been accomplished, the apnea can be considered idiopathic. Methylxanthine (theophylline or caffeine) therapy has become the mainstay of pharmacologic therapy in apnea of premature infants, whether such episodes are central, mixed, or obstructive. In infants with persistent apnea on theophylline therapy requiring intervention, nasal continuous positive airway pressure (CPAP) at 3–5 cm H_2O has proved effective in infants by splinting the upper airway with positive pressure, with the aims of preventing obstruction and stabilizing resting lung volume and resultant gas exchange (Miller et al., 1990).

At the time of discharge, many preterm infants still exhibit apneic episodes of at least 12 seconds' duration, although their clinical significance is unclear (Barrington et al., 1996). The various causes of neonatal apnea are summarized in Figure 60-7.

CARDIOVASCULAR PROBLEMS

Evaluation of Cyanosis

The appearance of persistent central cyanosis in the neonatal period raises the possibility of cyanotic congenital heart disease. This is typically resolved by performing a hyperoxia test in which the infant is exposed to 100% oxygen for 5 to 10 minutes, after which PaO_2 is sampled (or oxygenation is measured noninvasively). Persistent hypoxia after 100% oxygen exposure suggests the presence of fixed right-to-left shunting. The test aids in differentiation between primary lung disease and congenital heart disease with right-to-left shunting. A modification of the hyperoxia test that combines hyperoxia with hyperventilation can be used to distinguish between structural congenital heart disease and primary (or persistent) pulmonary hypertension of the newborn (see later), both of which have right-to-left shunting. In response to 100% oxygen with or without hyperventilation, infants with PPHN usually exhibit PaO_2 levels higher than 100 mm Hg. In contrast, patients with anatomically fixed right-to-left shunting rarely generate a PaO_2 above 40 to 50 mm Hg, even with hyperventilation.

Generally, serious structural heart disease is compatible with a relatively normal intrauterine existence. It is the transition to extrauterine life that makes the cardiac lesion hemodynamically significant. In many infants (e.g., those with lesions dependent on a patent ductus arteriosus to supply the pulmonary or systemic blood flow), a goal of management is to prevent ductal closure and return to an *in utero* circulation until diagnosis is complete and therapy initiated. Apart from cyanosis, respiratory distress should be noted because its presence could indicate cardiac disease associated with poor systemic output or increased pulmonary blood flow. Auscultation of a cardiac murmur rarely provides specific diagnostic information, and the loudest murmur can signify a relatively benign lesion. The presence of systolic ejection clicks can help in the diagnosis of pulmonic or aortic valve stenosis. A careful assessment and comparison of peripheral pulses and perfusion are essential to diagnosing aortic coarctation and conditions associated with poor systemic flow (such as hypoplastic left side of the heart), which may not exhibit any cyanosis (Zahka and Lane, 2002). Although radiography and electrocardiography remain useful diagnostic tools, cardiac ultrasonography is the definitive diagnostic method in evaluation of suspected neonatal cardiac disease.

Primary (Persistent) Pulmonary Hypertension

The normal transition to extrauterine life involves a dramatic decrease in pulmonary vascular resistance. The mediators of neonatal pulmonary vasodilation include mechanical factors related to lung expansion, oxygenation, and the balance of vascular endothelial factors, including endothelin and nitric oxide. Delayed relaxation of the pulmonary vascular bed is a feature of many neonatal pulmonary problems, including lung hypoplasia caused by mechanical compression (e.g., congenital diaphragmatic hernia), meconium aspiration pneumonia, perinatal asphyxia, bacterial pneumonia, and sepsis. It also can occur in the absence of obvious triggering diseases, presumably because of abnormal muscularization of pulmonary arterioles or transient defects in endothelial function. The high degree of pulmonary vascular resistance causes pulmonary and right-sided ventricular hypertension, and the presence of the ductus arteriosus and foramen ovale provides sites of extracardiac and intracardiac shunting that affect the disease dramatically, causing systemic arterial desaturation. Myocardial dysfunction (commonly associated with asphyxia) or decreased systemic vascular resistance associated with infection can further compromise the tenuous balance between the systemic and pulmonary circulation and worsen the hypoxemia.

The primary goal of therapy is to reduce pulmonary vascular resistance selectively (Kinsella and Abman, 2000). A number of effective strategies are employed with variable degrees of success, as summarized in Table 60-7. Discovery of nitric oxide as the endothelium-derived relaxing factor (EDRF) and its role in cardiovascular adaptation to extrauterine life has clearly improved our understanding of the pathophysiologic mechanism involved in PPHN and changed the therapeutic approach to this problem. Results from animal experiments and a number of clinical trials indicated that inhaled NO improved oxygenation in patients with persistent pulmonary hypertension by promoting pulmonary vasodilation selectively. Prompted by these encouraging results, a number of prospective randomized clinical trials followed. Two large, multicenter, randomized controlled trials of inhaled nitric oxide for hypoxic respiratory failure in term and near-term newborn, sponsored by the NICHD Neonatal Network (NINOS Study Group, 1997b) and the Clinical Inhaled Nitric Oxide Research Group, demonstrated a significant reduction in the need for extracorporeal membrane oxygenation. There was no significant difference in mortality rate between the ECMO and the inhaled nitric oxide groups (NINOS, 1997b; Clark et al., 2000). These results led to FDA approval of inhaled NO for use in full-term newborns with hypoxic respiratory failure. Although there seems to be no evidence of acute toxicity of nitric oxide when used appropriately; doses of 80 ppm cause significant methemoglobinemia. Data from long-term follow-up studies of newborn babies treated with inhaled NO suggest similar neurodevelopmental, behavioral, and medical outcomes compared with ECMO-treated patients (NINOS Study Group, 2000).

■ TABLE 60-7. TREATMENT STRATEGIES FOR PERSISTENT PULMONARY HYPERTENSION

Respiratory Management

Supplemental oxygen
Gentle ventilation
High-frequency ventilation
Surfactant replacement for RDS, MAS
Inhaled nitric oxide

Pharmacologic Management

Correct metabolic acidosis
  Sodium bicarbonate
Vasodilators
  Phosphodiesterase inhibitors, e.g., milrinone
  Prostacyclin

Cardiovascular Support

Optimize cardiac output, systemic resistance
  Dopamine
  Maintain adequate intravascular volume
  Normalization of ionized calcium

Environmental Modifications

Sedation
  Fentanyl
  Morphine
Avoidance of noise and light stress
Minimal handling

Extracorporeal Membrane Oxygenation

From Zahka KG, Patel CR: Cardiovascular problems of the neonate. *In* Fanaroff AA, Martin RJ (eds): Neonatal-Perinatal Medicine, 6th ed. St. Louis, Mosby–Year Book, 1997, p. 1163.

Patent Ductus Arteriosus

The ductus arteriosus, which connects the pulmonary artery and the aorta, is an essential structure during fetal life. Because fetal pulmonary vascular resistance is high, nearly 90% of the blood ejected by the fetal right ventricle flows through the ductus arteriosus to the descending aorta. The ductus arteriosus closes in the first few days after birth, and the entire right ventricular output is ejected into the pulmonary arterial bed. If the ductus arteriosus remains patent postnatally and pulmonary vascular resistance falls, blood flow through the ductus is left to right from the aorta to the pulmonary artery. Furthermore, because the connection is open during both systole and diastole and pulmonary artery pressure is lower than the respective aortic pressure, blood flows across the patent ductus arteriosus continuously throughout the cardiac cycle.

The mechanisms responsible for constriction of the ductus arteriosus at birth are not fully understood. The ductus is highly sensitive to changes in oxygen tension; the increase in arterial oxygen tension that normally occurs after birth probably serves as the stimulus for ductal closure. How this response is mediated is less certain; it is likely attributable to a complex interaction between autonomic chemical mediators, nerves, prostaglandin, and the ductal musculature. The ductus arteriosus functionally closes in most full-term infants during the first day of life, but anatomic obliteration of the ductus does not occur until after the first week of life. A persistently patent ductus arteriosus is uncommon in otherwise normal children. In contrast, 10% to 20% of premature babies with RDS and 30% of infants who weighed less than 1.5 kg at birth have a patent ductus arteriosus, possibly as a result of hypoxia and immaturity of the ductal closure mechanisms (Reller et al., 1993).

In the premature infant, failure of spontaneous closure may cause congestive heart failure, and accompanying respiratory distress may require therapy to close the ductus arteriosus. A rapid or progressive increase in ventilator settings and inspired oxygen could be manifestations of congestive heart failure caused by a patent ductus arteriosus in such patients. Persistence of a patent ductus arteriosus has been associated with an increased incidence of BPD and necrotizing enterocolitis. Medical management with fluid restriction and diuretics is occasionally effective. Indomethacin, a prostaglandin synthetase inhibitor, has been shown to close the ductus arteriosus in a large proportion of premature infants up to 14 days of age and occasionally as late as 1 month of age. Contraindications to indomethacin therapy are progressive intracranial hemorrhage, renal failure, or significant hyperbilirubinemia or thrombocytopenia. Failure of indomethacin therapy has been related to extreme immaturity and to greater postnatal age at initiation of therapy (Weiss et al., 1995). Prophylactic use of indomethacin for ductal closure has. its advocates. The NICHD-sponsored study of prophylactic indomethacin for the prevention of intraventricular hemorrhage (TIPPS) demonstrated not only a significant reduction in the incidence of grade III and IV bleeds but also a 26% absolute reduction in the incidence of PDA (Schmidt et al., 2001). Because of the potential side effects of indomethacin on cerebral and renal circulation (vasoconstriction), the use of an alternative drug (e.g., ibuprofen) is currently being evaluated. Preliminary data indicate a similar therapeutic effect with no adverse effects on cerebral or renal perfusion; however, an ongoing randomized controlled trial of ibuprofen prophylaxis for the prevention of PDA was halted because of concerns over severe hypoxemia in three preterm infants after receiving the drug (Courtney et al., 2002). More data are necessary before ibuprofen can be recommended as an alternative treatment for PDA. Surgical ligation of the ductus arteriosus carries minimal risk, even in the smallest infants. Surgery is indicated if the ductus remains hemodynamically significant by clinical or echocardiographic criteria after medical therapy or if indomethacin is contraindicated.

Neonatal Hypertension

Systemic arterial hypertension can be detected in 2% of infants admitted to intensive care units (Leder et al., 1986). In defining hypertension in the neonate, it is essential to take into consideration birth weight, gestational age, and postnatal age as well as the clinical history of the infant. In a prospective study of blood pressure during the first month of life, Stork and coworkers (1984) noted that blood pressure rises acutely during the first 5 days of life and more gradually thereafter. The blood pressure relates to birth weight and remains higher in infants with greater birth weights. No diurnal variation of blood pressure has been found in newborn infants.

Hypertension in the otherwise healthy newborn is usually secondary to renal disease and is most commonly due to renovascular hypertension (Table 60-8). Hypertension is also noted in association with raised intracranial pressure, coarctation of

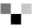

TABLE 60-8. ETIOLOGY OF SYSTEMIC HYPERTENSION IN NEWBORN INFANTS

Renovascular and Renal Parenchymal Disease

Renal vein or artery thrombosis
Abdominal aortic thrombosis
Renal artery stenosis
Autosomal recessive polycystic kidney disease (ARPKD)
Autosomal dominant polycystic kidney disease (ADPKD)
Renal malformations
Acute and chronic renal failure

Cardiac

Coarctation of the aorta
Post ECMO

Pulmonary

Bronchopulmonary dysplasia

Endocrine

Congenital adrenal hyperplasia

Tumors

Congenital mesoblastic nephroma
Pheochromocytoma
Neuroblastoma

Medications

Vasopressors
Corticosteroids
Drug withdrawal syndrome

the aorta, endocrine disorders (including hyperthyroidism, congenital adrenal hyperplasia, or, rarely, pheochromocytoma), and drugs such as phenylephrine, epinephrine, dopamine, and pancuronium. Hypertension also can occur because of intra-aortic thrombosis caused by an indwelling umbilical artery line. Stork and coauthors (1984) found that hypertension occurred with equal frequency when arterial lines were placed in the thoracic or abdominal aorta. Although most infants are asymptomatic, symptoms associated with hypertension include tachypnea, respiratory distress, mottling of the skin, and even congestive heart failure. Retinopathy can occur soon after onset of hypertension and appears to have features similar to those observed in adults.

Clinical investigation of the infant with hypertension should include ultrasonogram of the kidneys with doppler examination of the renal vessels and abdominal aorta. Echocardiography and other laboratory tests (e.g., 17 OH progesterone) are also often required to rule out other specific etiologies.

The onset of hypertension in a neonate is a significant finding, usually indicative of a potentially life-threatening disorder. Therapy should be directed at control of the hypertension, which commonly responds well to hydralazine therapy. In the presence of hemodynamic compromise or malignant hypertension, the use of intravenous, short acting vasodilators (e.g., sodium nitroprusside, beta blockers) is indicated. Depending on the etiology, the management of these patients often requires a multidisciplinary approach. It has been reassuring to note that upon follow-up, the hypertension resolves spontaneously in many infants and there is no evidence of permanent renal impairment.

◼ INTRAUTERINE GROWTH RESTRICTION

Although different rates and patterns of intrauterine growth have been observed for many years, it was not until some 50 years ago that the clinical significance of these patterns was recognized. Technologic advances, as outlined throughout this book, have permitted close monitoring of fetal anatomy, growth, well being, and maturity. Furthermore, the majority of infants with intrauterine growth problems (see also Chapter 28) are now identified prior to delivery, permitting better planning of the delivery and preparation for resuscitation of the neonate. This represents a quantum leap from 20 years ago, when less than a third of such problems with these infants were anticipated prior to labor and delivery, times of great stress and danger for the growth-restricted fetus.

Classification of infants, according to tables relating birth weight to gestational age, are used to determine whether growth has occurred at a normal, accelerated, or diminished rate *in utero*. At any gestational age, both mortality and morbidity are strongly related to the quality of intrauterine growth as reflected by birth weight percentiles. McIntire and colleagues (1999) found strong relationships between mortality and morbidity— for example, the occurrence of respiratory distress (Fig. 60-8) and birth weight percentiles. From a statistical standpoint, only infants born with a birth weight greater than two standard deviations below the mean for any gestational age are truly small for gestational age (SGA). Because they share common clinical problems, however, all infants with birth weights below the 10th percentile for gestational age are regarded as SGA. Furthermore, many infants, particularly those born beyond term, have birth weights above the 10th percentile but demonstrate evidence of weight loss and should be considered within the spectrum of the growth-restricted infant.

Low birth weight (below 2500 g) accounts for 75% of poor perinatal outcomes. Strategies to improve the outcome in these infants have focused on antenatal prevention of conditions associated with low birth weight together with intensive education, extensive intrapartum evaluation and monitoring, and sophisticated and aggressive care of the low-birth-weight fetus and infant. Simple measures in antenatal care, such as elimination of cigarette smoking, improved nutrition, eradication of genitourinary tract infection, and increased awareness of the hazards of preterm birth, have led to lower rates of prematurity in some centers. Recognition and treatment of vaginosis could further reduce premature birth.

Many conditions result in abnormal growth *in utero*. The etiology, together with the timing, duration, and severity of the insult, modify the patterns of growth and hence the problems observed in the fetus and newborn. During the first trimester, global insults, including perinatal infections (*toxoplasmosis, rubella, cytomegalovirus, and herpes simplex—TORCH*), ingested teratogens (e.g., anticonvulsants, alcohol, anticoagulants), chromosomal abnormalities (trisomy 21, 18, and 13 and Turner's syndrome), and aerosol and narcotic drug abuse initiate profound failure of growth of the fetus, resulting in a short infant of low birth weight and often reduced head circumference and hence brain capacity. These infants with reduction of all growth parameters are considered to have *symmetric growth restriction*.

Later onset of fetal growth failure results from disorders of the fetus or placenta or from maternal problems. Delivery of oxygen and nutrients is impeded by maternal or placental factors in what is called *placental insufficiency*. A dramatic effect of how oxygen administration can enhance growth and correct metabolic acidosis in a small group of growth-restricted infants was reported by Nicolaides and coworkers (1987). These factors can become operative at variable times during pregnancy, resulting in less predictable effects on fetal growth. Examples of these factors include, among others, maternal hypertension (preeclampsia and essential hypertension), smoking, malnutrition (undernutrition), and varied forms of maternal vascular and renal diseases. They result in *asymmetric growth restriction*, which is characterized by weight at or below the 10th percentile with length and head circumference above the 10th percentile. These infants have the potential for normal growth and development, yet they are extremely vulnerable to perinatal asphyxia, which must be assiduously avoided. Perhaps equally vulnerable and often overlooked are the group of infants, frequently postterm, with birth weight above the 10th percentile but with evidence of recent weight loss as indicated by loose folds of skin, the result of loss of subcutaneous tissue. Long-standing substrate deprivation can ultimately affect length and head circumference, thus demonstrating the clinical picture of symmetric intrauterine growth restriction (IUGR).

Follow-up data (Hack and Fanaroff, 1984) suggest that IUGR as a consequence of malnutrition secondary to either maternal malnutrition or impaired uteroplacental transfer of nutrients is accompanied by a favorable outcome for the infant. This prompted Warshaw (1985) to question, in a provocative editorial, whether "IUGR resulting from restricted nutrient supply really represents pathology or is it a favorable adaptation of the fetus to maximize the prospects of good outcome? A strong case can be made for the latter." He further emphasizes that decreased fetal size with sparing of brain growth, acceleration of pulmonary maturation, and mild polycythemia—common features in the growth-restricted fetus—initially represent important adaptive strategies that become pathologic when deprivation becomes extreme and fetal distress supervenes. In the typical newborn

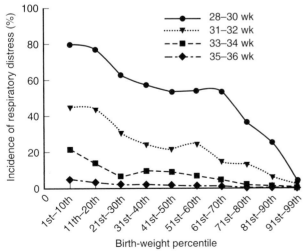

FIGURE 60-8 ◼ Incidence of respiratory distress among 12,317 preterm infants, according to birth-weight percentile after stratification according to gestational age (28 through 30 weeks, 31 or 32 weeks, 33 or 34 weeks, and 35 or 36 weeks). (From McIntire DD, Bloom SL, Casey BM, et al: Birth weight in relation to morbidity and mortality among newborn infants. N Engl J Med **340**:1234, 1999, Fig. 2.)

with nutritionally induced IUGR, body proportions are asymmetric at birth, with brain growth and head circumference spared at the expense of both weight and linear growth. It is postulated that redistribution of the blood flow favors brain growth at the expense of the viscera and skeletal muscles.

Another group of infants with disordered intrauterine growth includes those infants in whom specific genetic, inherited metabolic, or chromosomal anomalies severely restrict the growth potential. The products of multiple gestation and those with other specific syndromes and congenital malformations can also be SGA. In many infants, no cause is identified for their diminished growth. Exposure to tobacco could be significant in this latter group. The variable etiologies and timing of the onset of the insults results in less predictability of growth, with both symmetric and asymmetric patterns observed. Nonetheless, more precise antenatal evaluation of fetal growth is permitting a more rational approach to the perinatal management of these complex problems and has resulted in a significant reduction in the incidence of stillbirths. Uniparental dysomy can be added to the causes of intrauterine growth restriction.

In pregnancies with compromised fetal growth, every effort must be made to avoid asphyxia and ensure an atraumatic delivery. The fetus is monitored closely during labor and delivery, which is accomplished surgically if distress supervenes. When fetal compromise is established before labor, elective cesarean section may be performed. Personnel skilled and experienced in neonatal resuscitation should be present at the delivery. A depressed infant with low Apgar scores should be anticipated. Resuscitative efforts designed to clear the airway, establish ventilation, support the circulation, and correct any metabolic acidosis as already detailed, are initiated promptly. The thermal environment should result in minimal oxygen consumption. If the amniotic fluid contains meconium, the airway is first cleared prior to delivery of the body, and subsequently, the trachea may need to be intubated and aspirated.

Assessment of Gestational Age

Once the initial transfer to extrauterine existence has been accomplished, the first order of business is to establish the birth weight/gestational age relationship.

The clinical course and strategy for management depend on early identification of SGA infants. Thus, it is essential to classify all infants promptly as small, appropriate, or large for gestational age. Historically, the gestational age is determined from a combination of the mother's dates and antenatal parameters, including ultrasonographic examination when available, quickening, and detection of fetal heartbeat. When antenatal dating is not reliable, the neonatal assessment of gestational age is obtained from a combination of assessment of physical and neurologic characteristics according to the method of Dubowitz and associates (1970).

Ballard and colleagues (1979) have produced an abbreviated version of gestational age assessment that has become extremely popular and has been validated statistically. The Ballard maturational score has been refined and expanded (Ballard et al., 1991) to be more accurate and to include extremely premature infants. This new Ballard score has been validated in 578 neonates following accurately dated pregnancies; it has been found to be an accurate gestational assessment tool for extremely premature infants and remains valid for the entire newborn population. For infants born prior to 26 weeks'

gestation, the assessment should be made before age 12 hours. The weight, length, and head circumference should be compared with normal standards to determine first whether growth has been restricted and, if so, whether there is symmetric or asymmetric growth restriction. The Babson charts (birth to 1 year) (Babson and Benda, 1976) are extremely useful for this purpose (Alexander et al., 1996) (Fig. 60-9). If the infant plots out to be SGA, the etiology of the growth retardation must be sought and a management plan enacted that anticipates, prevents, and treats those conditions most prominent in these infants and outlined in Table 60-9.

After the infant's condition has been stabilized in the delivery room, a careful physical examination and additional measurements are necessary to determine whether the infant is SGA. For example, the ponderal index, which relates length to weight, is useful in order to further subclassify symmetric or asymmetric growth restriction and identify wasted infants. Physical and laboratory data are used to distinguish those infants with congenital malformations or congenital infections from those undergrown as a consequence of placental insufficiency.

Growth-restricted infants have relatively large heads for their wasted trunks and extremities, although approximately 50% of SGA very-low-birth-weight infants have head circumferences below the third percentile at birth. There is reduced subcutaneous tissue, as evidenced by skin-fold thickness determinations, and because of a lack of vernix, the skin is often desquamating and stained with meconium. Physical indicators of gestational age, including sole creases, breast dimensions, and external appearance of the genitalia, can be misleading because of variable effects of malnutrition, and the neurologic examination is usually more reliable and indicative of true gestational age. The neurologic examination can show accelerated maturation as a result of intrauterine stress and is obviously not reliable in infants who have been severely asphyxiated.

Many postmature infants demonstrate evidence of late IUGR. Characteristically, their length is of a higher percentile than their birth weight, and they have an anxious, alert appearance. The skin is dry, cracked, and wrinkled from loss of subcutaneous tissue; lacks vernix; and is often stained brownish green or yellow. The nails are long, and the skull is excessively firm. As with SGA infants, perinatal complications include asphyxia, meconium aspiration syndrome, and hypoglycemia.

The clinical problems and the underlying physiologic mechanisms resulting in these problems in SGA infants are outlined in Table 60-10. Combinations of problems frequently occur in the same infant. Furthermore, the reserves of these SGA infants could have been depleted by the labor and delivery process. This renders them extremely vulnerable to physiologic deviations that are readily compensated for by their appropriately grown counterparts. The most common problems include asphyxia neonatorum, hypoglycemia, polycythemia and hyperviscosity, congenital malformations, and congenital infections. Jones and Robertsen (1986) reviewed the hospital course and outcome of 164 infants whose gestation-specific birth weight was less than the 5th percentile and who were greater than or equal to 37 weeks' gestation. Finding a very low incidence of malformations (4%), congenital infections, and significant complications, they concluded that SGA infants of 37 weeks' gestation or more have few neonatal problems and do not require admission to the intensive care unit. They nonetheless still require close

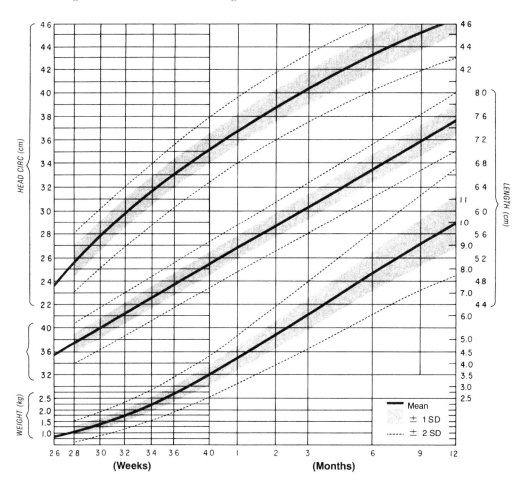

FIGURE 60-9 ■ Infant growth chart. (Adapted from Babson SG, Benda GI: Growth graphs for the clinical assessment of infants of varying gestational age. J Pediatr **89**:814, 1976.)

TABLE 60-9. COMPARISON OF PROBLEMS OF SMALL-FOR-GESTATIONAL-AGE (SGA) AND IMMATURE NEWBORN INFANTS

Problem	Immature AGA	Immature SGA	Mature SGA (Symmetric)	Mature SGA (Asymmetric)
Early weight change	5%–10% loss, then slow gain	5%–10% loss, then slow gain	5%–10% loss, then slow gain	≤5% loss, then rapid gain
Congenital infection	+	+ +	+ +	±
Respiratory problems	Hyaline membrane disease	Hyaline membrane disease	Unusual	Aspiration syndrome Pneumomediastinum Pneumothorax
Persistent fetal circulation	+	+	0	+ +
Apneic spells	+ + + +	+ + + +	0	0
Polycythemia	0	0	±	+ +
Hyperbilirubinemia	+ + + +	+ + + +	+	+ +
Hypoglycemia	+	+	+	+ + +
Hypocalcemia	+	+	±	+
Congenital malformation	±	+	+ +	±
Intracranial hemorrhage	+++	+++	±	+
Asphyxia	++	++	±	++
Growth (linear)	Normal	Subnormal (rare catch-up)	Subnormal (rare catch-up)	Normal
Neurobehavioral residual	+ + (most in very-low-birth-weight infants)	+++	+++	+ (more if asphyxia is severe)

AGA, appropriate for gestational age.

From Klaus MH, Fanaroff AA (eds): Care of the High Risk Neonate, 4th ed. Philadelphia, WB Saunders, 1993.

TABLE 60-10. PERINATAL ADAPTIVE PROBLEMS

Problem	Pathogenesis	Prevention
Perinatal asphyxia	↓ Placental reserve (insufficiency) ↓ Cardiac glycogen stores	Antepartum, intrapartum fetal heart rate monitoring
Meconium aspiration	Hypoxia/stress phenomenon	Oral/pharyngeal/tracheal suction
Fasting hypoglycemia	↓ Hepatic glycogen ↓ Gluconeogenesis	Early alimentation
Alimented hyperglycemia	"Starvation diabetes"	Avoid excessive carbohydrate loads
Polycythemia/hyperviscosity	Fetal hypoxia; ↑ erythropoietin Placental transfusion	Neonatal partial exchange transfusion
Temperature instability	↓ Adipose tissue ↑ Heat loss	Ensure neutral thermal environment
Pulmonary hemorrhage (rare)	Hypothermia, hypoxemia, DIC	Avoid cold stress, hypoxia
Immunodeficiency	"Malnutrition" effect	Unknown

DIC, disseminated intravascular coagulation.

Modified from Gregory GA: Pediatric Anesthesiology. New York, Churchill Livingstone, 1989.

observation in well-baby nurseries. Nine infants (5%) did become hypoglycemic, but only one with associated respiratory distress required intravenous glucose.

The long-term prognosis for SGA infants has emerged slowly. In view of the many variables affecting growth and development and the heterogeneous group of infants covered by the definition of SGA, it is not surprising that reports of outcome range from extremely optimistic to depressingly pessimistic. The ultimate picture depends on the etiology of the aberrant growth, including the presence of congenital infections or malformations, the timing and duration of the insult, the severity of growth retardation, the degree of intrauterine or postnatal asphyxia, the postnatal course, and above all, on the socioeconomic status of the family. Recent reports identify and attempt to control for these variables, facilitating interpretation of the results.

Few preterm infants who are SGA at birth catch up in growth during the neonatal period. Superimposed on their intrauterine causes of growth failure are a variety of postnatal problems that further affect their growth. In our experience, 91% of SGA infants will still be two standard deviations below the norms at 40 weeks' corrected age. Varying patterns of growth are observed during the first year of life, with the most rapid catch-up occurring during this period. Some infants who failed to grow during the neonatal period demonstrate an accelerated growth velocity and catch-up; others demonstrate a normal growth velocity but remain small and never catch up. A few have a decreased growth velocity and frankly "fail to thrive."

Growth during infancy is influenced by many factors, including the persistence of perinatal problems such as bronchopulmonary dysplasia, necrotizing enterocolitis, cholestasis, and malabsorption. Additional factors influencing growth include the need for rehospitalization and the presence of care-taking disorders and feeding problems in children with neurologic impairment. SGA infants rarely catch up in weight after the first year, and at 3 years some 50% of SGA infants still have subnormal weight. Little evidence in the literature supports the concept that they will catch up later in life. Caretakers must, therefore, make every effort during the first year of life to ensure maximal nutritional support and to use nutritional and non-nutritive techniques to optimize caloric utilization.

The growth of the head correlates well with intellectual development as an indirect marker of brain size. It is noteworthy that the SGA infant with small head size at birth may still turn out to be developmentally normal. Some 50% of SGA infants have a small head circumference at birth; catch-up indicates a good outlook. At times it is difficult to distinguish catch-up head growth from hydrocephalus. Ultrasonography should be used to detect, among other things, congenital or acquired anatomic abnormalities, evidence of bleeding, and ventricular size. Computed tomography (CT) is used to clarify suspicious lesions.

The timing, duration, and etiology of the IUGR together with the degree of catch-up growth determine the outcome of both term and preterm growth-restricted infants. The outcome reports of SGA term infants have varied. Normal IQ predominates; however, language delay, behavioral problems, and potential school difficulties despite a normal IQ are emerging as significant problems. As already indicated, early reports on SGA preterm infants were devastating and depressing. Recent reports that exclude infants with congenital infections and major malformations have not found significant differences between SGA and AGA preterm infants. This finding has been attributed to many factors, including earlier recognition, more precise intrauterine monitoring, appropriate delivery with avoidance of asphyxia and trauma, avoidance of hypoglycemia, and improved postnatal nutrition. SGA infants nonetheless appear to exhibit more minor neurologic abnormalities than their AGA counterparts. Infants at greatest risk for poor neurodevelopmental outcome include those weighing less than 1 kg at birth, those with asphyxia and seizures in the neonatal period, those with congenital infections and major malformations, and those who do not catch up in any of the growth parameters.

The follow-up of the SGA infant presents a continuing challenge. All infants should be considered at risk, and every effort should be made by the caretakers to ensure that all the available resources at the medical center are used so that these infants can achieve their maximal potential.

Head circumference correlates with brain volume, brain weight, and cellularity during infancy and childhood. It is an excellent predictor of outcome. Infants with perinatal growth failure as reflected by subnormal head circumference persisting through the first 8 months of life demonstrate the poorest cognitive function, academic achievement, and behavior at age 8 years (Hack et al., 1991).

INFANTS OF DIABETIC MOTHERS

The metabolic derangements are the major abnormality affecting persons with diabetes mellitus. Pregnant women with diabetes should be managed by suitably trained personnel and teams who monitor mother and fetus comprehensively throughout pregnancy. Optimal care of women with diabetes must begin prior to conception because careful preconception control of diabetes demonstrably reduces the incidence of major anomalies. All pregnancies should be screened so that women with gestational diabetes can be identified and managed appropriately. Prevention of ketoacidosis and recognition and treatment of pregnancy-induced hypertension or pyelonephritis are important.

The pathophysiologic alterations induced by pregnancy and the management of the diabetic mother are discussed in Chapter 49. Many potential problems in the offspring can be anticipated. The major problems include macrosomia, birth asphyxia, hypoglycemia, cardiorespiratory disorders, and congenital malformations. The improved ability to monitor fetal growth, maturity, and well-being antenatally and during labor has significantly reduced the incidence of stillbirth, severe birth asphyxia, and RDS. Despite tight control of maternal glucose homeostasis, macrosomia remains a significant problem in approximately one third of diabetic pregnancies. Cesarean section could be indicated for cephalopelvic disproportion; shoulder dystocia is a constant concern for the perinatal team because it can result in a traumatic delivery with an asphyxiated, depressed infant.

A complete physical examination detects the presence of malformations and whether birth trauma or injury has occurred. Brachial plexus injury is the most common nerve injury of the newborn. Brachial plexus stretching—the result of traction of the head and neck in a vertex delivery—results in Erb's palsy (C5, C6), characterized by an adducted shoulder and internally rotated arm with the elbow extended, forearm pronated, and wrist flexed. Diaphragmatic paralysis may occur on the same side (see earlier).

Congenital malformations are observed two to six times more frequently in offspring of diabetics. Whereas any organ system may be involved, anomalies of the cardiovascular system and skeleton predominate. Maternal HbA_{1c} is associated with malformations, with fewer malformations noted in those pregnancies in which the HbA_{1c} remains in the normal range. There is, therefore, a major thrust to control maternal blood glucose rigidly before conception and during the first trimester to reduce the malformation rate. Animal studies demonstrate that this concept is valid. The rationale of the preconception program for a diabetic woman is to optimize the pregnancy outcome for herself and her offspring. Strict glucose control at this time reduces the frequency of congenital malformations and can diminish other perinatal complications, including intrauterine death, macrosomia, and neonatal disorders. Although this concept has been well accepted, not all prospective studies have documented a clear reduction in the incidence of malformations (Mills et al., 1988).

Hypoglycemia remains a prevalent problem in the offspring of women with type I and type II diabetes. Because the clinical manifestations of hypoglycemia can be subtle and the neurologic sequelae of sustained hypoglycemia devastating, all infants at risk should be screened to identify them early and correct hypoglycemia. Screening is accomplished by means of a glucose oxidase-peroxidase chromogen test strip, usually with a reflectance colorimeter. If the screen value is below 45 mg%, a quantitative blood sugar specimen is recommended. In term infants, hypoglycemia is defined as a plasma glucose level below 35 mg/100 mL 2 hours after birth. Most clinicians attempt to maintain the blood glucose above 40 mg% on the basis of the data from Srinivasan and colleagues (1986), which reveal that blood glucose in the normal neonate does not decline below 40 mg% after the first 2 hours of life. There is continuing debate over the definition of hypoglycemia. The debate revolves around broad principles, including whether the definition is statistical or functional. Because hypoglycemia can have far-reaching consequences, it appears wiser to be conservative and maintain the blood glucose above 40 mg%.

Hypoglycemia can manifest dramatically with seizures, but an insidious onset that may be overlooked is more likely. A wide range of symptoms have been attributed to hypoglycemia. These include apathy, poor feeding, apnea, high-pitched or weak cry, hypotonia, and eye rolling. Many of these are nonspecific symptoms frequently observed in normoglycemic infants. In all diabetic offspring, hypoglycemia should be anticipated and the blood glucose monitored hourly initially and then every 2 to 4 hours until it has stabilized in the normal range. Efforts are made to establish early oral feeds and the environment optimized to minimize energy demands. Intravenous infusions are used liberally, with glucose infused by pump at rates of 4 to 9 mg/kg/minute or greater if necessary. If the infant is symptomatic with hypoglycemia, 2 mL/kg of 10% dextrose is infused rapidly followed by an infusion rate of 8 mg/kg/minute, increasing with 2-mg/kg/minute increments to achieve normoglycemia. Diazoxide and then glucocorticoids are added when the rate of glucose infusion exceeds 14 mg/kg/minute. Neurologic sequelae can be noted in 30% to 50% of symptomatic hypoglycemic neonates.

In 1973, Pildes reported that problems of neonatal adaptation could be anticipated in 50% of offspring of insulin-dependent diabetics and in 10% to 20% of offspring of gestational diabetics. Since then, the enhanced ability to evaluate and monitor fetal maturity and well-being has resulted in a marked reduction in respiratory disorders. Functional and anatomic cardiovascular abnormalities have therefore assumed a more significant role. Technologic advances, including Doppler ultrasonography and two-dimensional echocardiography, permit precise definition of the cardiac problems. The unique cardiomyopathy that complicates diabetic pregnancies is only part of the spectrum of heart disease, which includes a fourfold increase in the incidence of congenital heart disease, arrhythmias, persistence of the fetal circulation, disorders of blood pressure, and effects of asphyxia on myocardial function. Gladman and colleagues (1997) prospectively evaluated all pregnant women with type I or type II diabetes by means of fetal echocardiography. Cardiac defects were detected in 7 of 328 pregnancies assessed, for an incidence of 2.1%. Diabetic cardiomyopathy is characterized by cardiomegaly with interventricular septal hypertrophy resulting in functional obstruction akin to the hypertrophic cardiomyopathy observed in adults. Septal hypertrophy can be observed in the fetus and appears to correlate with maternal control as evidenced by HbA_{1c}.

A wide spectrum of clinical presentation is observed in infants with cardiomyopathy. Congestive or hypertrophic symptoms may predominate, and cyanosis, mottling, tachypnea, tachycardia, and features of congestive heart failure could be apparent. The heart is enlarged on radiographs, and the disorder is confirmed echocardiographically. Treatment is symptomatic with careful management of fluids, correction of polycythemia, maintenance of normoglycemia, and close monitoring and correction of electrolyte disorders or hypocalcemia. Although diuretics are used if there is clear evidence of fluid overload, digitalis and inotropic agents are avoided unless poor myocardial contractility is documented. In symptomatic infants with cardiomyopathy, beta blockers, such as propranolol, may be useful.

The disease is self-limited and, in general, symptoms and clinical features resolve within a few weeks, although the septal and wall hypertrophy may take months to resolve.

NUTRITION

Meeting the nutritional and metabolic needs of the increasing number of extremely immature, small, and sick infants who now survive presents a major challenge to the neonatologist. Although ideal growth rates have yet to be defined, we attempt to achieve them. Immaturity of the gastrointestinal tract, together with altered metabolic rates induced by illness, compound the problem. Many infants fail to thrive during their nursery sojourn, as evidenced by declining growth percentiles. Follow-up data indicate that relatively brief periods of failure to thrive are well tolerated, and provided catch-up growth has been achieved by 8 months of corrected age, normal neurodevelopment can be anticipated.

A better understanding of the physiology and development of the gastrointestinal tract is emerging. This should permit a more rational approach to this most important aspect of care. The full-term infant is better equipped to tolerate periods of starvation than the preterm infant, who has extremely low reserves, particularly of fat and glycogen. In all infants, every effort is made to avoid even brief periods of starvation, and energy is supplied intravenously commencing on the first day of life. With a combination of intravenous and oral alimentation, the immature and diseased gastrointestinal tract is not overburdened, and sufficient calories, fluid, minerals and essential amino acids, fatty acids, and glucose can be administered while maturation or recovery occurs. Immaturity, ileus, cardiorespiratory failure, and gastrointestinal or other associated anomalies all can result in an infant too sick to absorb nutrients from the gastrointestinal tract. The provision of 60 calories/kg/day intravenously, provided 10% of these are in the form of protein, prevents tissue catabolism.

Extrauterine adaptation should be normal before oral alimentation is begun. The technique of feeding is determined by weight, gestational age, and condition of the infant. Oral feeding is commenced only when there is clear-cut evidence of a gag reflex (usually at 34 weeks' gestation). Whereas formerly infants with arterial catheters receiving assisted ventilation received nothing by mouth, the tendency is to commence feeding sooner because even small amounts of food placed in the stomach accelerate the maturation of gastrointestinal function.

Basic problems in feeding the preterm infant include lack of coordination between suck and swallow until 34 weeks' gestation, diminished gastric capacity, gastroesophageal reflux (poor sphincter development), diminished gastrointestinal motility,

and malabsorption. Alterations in motility and propulsion are accentuated in asphyxiated infants. During the first weeks of life, nutritional needs are met primarily with intravenous alimentation, and oral feedings are introduced gradually. In order to ensure adequate growth (15 to 30 g/day), it is necessary to provide approximately 120 calories/kg/day.

Breast milk or specially modified humanized formula may be used. There has been a hot debate concerning the adequacy of breast milk for the preterm infant. Although the protein, calcium, and iron content, for example, are theoretically inadequate to meet the growth needs of the premature infant, the unique physical and immunologic properties of human milk make it highly desirable. This translates into reducing the incidence of necrotizing enterocolitis (see later).

Lucas and Cole (1990) were able to document that preterm infants who received either complete or partial enteral alimentation with breast milk had a reduced rate of necrotizing enterocolitis. The milk can be supplemented or fortified. Formula has been modified to resemble human milk and may be offered as 20–24 calories/ounce. Because of low-birthweight infants' limited gastric capacity and delicate fluid balance with a tendency to fluid overload, 24-calorie preparations are popular for them.

Various feeding strategies have been attempted, and there are proponents and opponents of the various regimens. The daily water requirements depend on the thermal environment, maturity, physical environment (i.e., radiant warmers and phototherapy), rate of growth, and intercurrent conditions. Immature infants with high evaporative water losses require large fluid intakes when compared with adults or term infants. Renal immaturity and limited endocrine control further strain the system, diminishing the margins for error. Excess fluid administration has been implicated in the incidence of patent ductus arteriosus, necrotizing enterocolitis, and bronchopulmonary dysplasia. Fluid balance is monitored by closely determining intake/output, body weight, serum and urine osmolarity, urine specific gravity, and urine and serum electrolytes.

Total parenteral nutrition remains an integral part of the feeding program of premature infants and the mainstay of nutritional support for infants with major gastrointestinal anomalies or short bowel following surgical resection. Protein, carbohydrates, fat, electrolytes, trace minerals, vitamins, and water are all provided intravenously. Because of the high complication rate associated with central lines, every effort is made to administer the parenteral nutrition via peripheral veins. This is not always possible, particularly for extremely immature infants and those with short bowel who require prolonged parenteral nutrition. The metabolic, mechanical, and infectious complications of parenteral nutrition are summarized in Tables 60-11 and 60-12.

Fluid Requirements

In *utero*, the fetus participates in an exchange of water involving the mother, fetus, and amniotic fluid. Remarkably large volumes of water are exchanged between the mother and the fetus—approximately 3500 mL/hour at term—with the net flux being in the maternofetal direction. Ultrasonographic studies reveal that fetal swallowing of amniotic fluid amounts to about 20 mL/hour at term and that micturition adds approximately 28 mL/hour at term. Together, swallowing and micturition contribute only about 10% of the hourly water

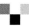

TABLE 60-11. METABOLIC COMPLICATIONS OF TOTAL PARENTERAL NUTRITION AND THEIR PROBABLE CAUSE

Complication	Probable Etiology
Disorders Related to Infusate Components	
Metabolic acidosis	Use of hydrochloride salts of cationic amino acids
Hyperammonemia	Inadequate arginine intake
Abnormal plasma aminograms	Amino acid pattern of nitrogen source
Hepatic disorders	Unknown; suggested causes include prematurity, malnutrition, sepsis, inadequate stimulation of bile flow, toxic effects of amino acids, specific amino acid deficiency, excessive amino acid and/or carbohydrate intake, nonspecific response to lack of feeding
Disorders Related to Metabolic Capacity of Patient	
Hyperglycemia	Excessive intake (either excessive concentration or infusion rate); change in metabolic state (e.g., stress, sepsis)
Hypoglycemia	Sudden cessation of infusion
Azotemia	Excessive nitrogen intake
Electrolyte disorders	Excessive or inadequate intake
Mineral disorders	Excessive or inadequate intake
Vitamin disorders	Excessive or inadequate intake
Essential fatty acid deficiency	Failure to provide essential fatty acids

exchange between the fetus and amniotic fluid. The large fetal renal output is noteworthy; clearly, water conservation is not a priority of the fetal kidney.

The total body water content of the fetus is high and diminishes with advancing gestational age. Total body water accounts for about 90% of fetal weight at 13 weeks, 86% at 26 weeks, and 70% at term. In addition, as maturation proceeds, intracellular water forms a greater percentage of total body water as extracellular water decreases.

Both full-term and preterm infants show appreciable weight loss during the first week of life. This appears to be accounted for by loss of extracellular fluid. *Insensible water loss* is a major source of water loss following delivery. There is an inverse relationship between birth weight, gestational age, and insensible water loss. Hence, immature, low-birth-weight infants have

the largest losses, in some infants exceeding 100 mL/kg/day. Mechanisms accounting for this excess water loss include the relatively large surface-area-to-body-weight ratio, the minimal amount of subcutaneous tissue, and the highly vascularized, permeable, very thin epidermis. Insensible water loss correlates with metabolic rate, and hence water losses increase with cold stress, crying, and activity. Metabolic rate increases with advancing postnatal age in all weight groups and gestational ages. The excessive losses in immature, low-birth-weight infants occur independently of their metabolic rates. One investigator noted that evaporative heat losses account for 65% of heat loss in the first week of life and 43% in the second week in healthy preterm infants. Additional factors increasing evaporative water losses up to two- to threefold include radiant warmers and phototherapy.

TABLE 60-12. COMPLICATIONS OF PARENTERAL NUTRITION

Mechanical Complications		Septic Complications
Catheter Insertion	**Catheter Use**	**Catheter Use**
Pneumothorax	Venous thrombosis	Contamination and infection at catheter site due to improper catheter care
Hemothorax	Superior vena cava syndrome	
Hydromediastinum	Pulmonary embolus	
Subclavian artery injury	Catheter dislodgement	Catheter "seeding" from distant site of infection
Subclavian hematoma	Perforation and/or infusion leaks	
Subclavian vein laceration	(pericardial, pleural, mediastinal)	
Arteriovenous fistula		
Air embolism		
Catheter embolism		
Catheter malposition		
Thoracic duct laceration		
Cardiac perforation and tamponade		
Brachial plexus injury		
Horner syndrome		
Phrenic nerve paralysis		
Carotid artery injury		

Insensible water loss can be reduced by the interposition of a heat shield in an isolette or by the use of double-walled isolettes, thermal blankets, or even plastic wrap when the infants are nursed under a radiant warmer. Topical application of petrolatum also reduces evaporative water losses, which can influence fluid balance significantly. Although control reports suggested decreased colonization when infants were switched to a petrolatum-based product, increased sepsis caused by coagulase-negative *staphylococcus* was documented. The condition of the skin was improved.

It becomes apparent that water requirements vary enormously with the weight and gestational age of the infant as well as with the environmental conditions. The state of the infant is also of vital importance in determining fluid management. For example, infants on ventilators generally experience no respiratory water losses and may even gain water via the respiratory tract. Fluid management is thus determined by frequent assessment of the infant, taking into account clinical status, vital signs, perfusion, weight, urine output, urine specific gravity and osmolality, hematocrit, blood urea nitrogen (BUN), electrolytes, and creatinine levels. Guidelines for fluid management are to commence with 50–60 mL/kg/day on the first day and then adjust upward thereafter on the basis of the aforementioned determinations and observations. Indications for increasing the daily fluid intake include a failing urine output accompanied by rising specific gravity or osmolality, excessive weight loss (more than 2% to 3%/day), and rising BUN and hematocrit. Increased fluid administration is also necessary in infants with third-space losses, as in peritonitis.

Administration of too little fluid can cause dehydration. However, weight loss up to 15% is tolerated in the first week of life provided that hypoglycemia is prevented. Very-low-birth-weight infants who do not lose weight are more likely to develop a PDA and bronchopulmonary dysplasia. Excess fluid administration (generally greater than 140 mL/kg/day) has been associated with clinical patent ductus arteriosus, pulmonary edema, necrotizing enterocolitis, and bronchopulmonary dysplasia.

In summary, total body water is greater in less mature infants. All infants lose weight and water during the first week of extrauterine life. Large insensible water losses should be anticipated in low-birth-weight infants. Daily fluid management is based on clinical observations and measurements together with biochemical monitoring. Excessive fluid administration is possibly more harmful than too little.

Hypocalcemia and Bone Mineralization

Calcium is transferred across the placenta against an uphill maternal-fetal calcium gradient. Fetal levels are about 1 mg/100 mL above maternal levels. Maternal parathyroid hormone and 1,25-dihydroxyvitamin D_3 concentrations are elevated during pregnancy, the latter accounting for increased gastrointestinal calcium absorption. In contrast, fetal levels of 1,25-dihydroxyvitamin D_3 are low as a consequence of minimal placental transfer and decreased fetal production. Bone mineralization *in utero* depends on an adequate supply of calcium (130 to 150 mg/kg/day), phosphate, magnesium, and the appropriate balance between parathyroid hormone, calcitonin, and vitamin D. From 28 weeks until term as fetal weight triples, the calcium content increases fourfold, and bone mineral density increases progressively.

At birth, the constant infusion of calcium from the mother stops abruptly, and serum calcium starts to fall, stimulating parathyroid hormone. 1,25-Dihydroxyvitamin D_3 levels increase to adult levels by 24 hours of life as the neonate prepares to defend the serum calcium and enhance gastrointestinal calcium absorption. With a net absorption of only 20% to 25% of the enteral calcium, however, neither breast milk nor humanized proprietary formulas deliver the same calcium supply to the neonate as that provided to the fetus. Consequently, under usual circumstances, bone mineralization in the preterm infant nurtured in the nursery lags behind that achieved *in utero*. Manipulation of parenteral nutrition and the formula to provide additional calcium and phosphate can correct this process.

Despite the physiologic hormonal adaptive process, there is normally a fall in serum calcium in the first 24 to 48 hours before stabilization. Early neonatal hypocalcemia represents an exaggerated physiologic fall in serum calcium during this time and is noted in 30% to 40% of low-birth-weight infants. Other infants at risk include asphyxiated term infants, infants of diabetic mothers, and those with respiratory disorders, sepsis, and hypoglycemia. Serum calcium should be monitored in infants identified at risk, and calcium infusions should be given to symptomatic infants.

Symptoms of hypocalcemia cover a wide spectrum from normal behavior through jitteriness, twitching, and even convulsions. Nonspecific features, including vomiting, poor feeding, cyanosis, and high-pitched cry, can occur. Chvostek's sign is unreliable, and the diagnosis is confirmed by serum calcium determinations.

Classic neonatal tetany observed on days 5 to 7 of life is associated with hyperphosphatemia. This is secondary to increased phosphate intake. Lactoengineering resulting in better balance between calcium and phosphorus in formulas has made this entity much less common. Hypocalcemia also occurs after exchange transfusions, in neonates with uremia, and as a consequence of chronic diuretic therapy, which may produce hypercalciuria and renal stones.

Treatment of hypocalcemia is to provide 24–35 mg/kg/day of calcium. Calcium gluconate (USP), providing 9 mg calcium/mL, and calcium gluceptate injection (Lilly), which contains 18 mg calcium/mL, are most frequently used. Infusion is given extremely slowly by pump because calcium can cause severe bradycardia or even cardiac arrest if administered too rapidly. In acute situations, such as an infant who is having seizures, a push of calcium gluconate using a dose up to 3 mg/kg may be administered. Heart rate must be monitored closely, and only a secure intravenous line is used because calcium is extremely irritating to tissue and has produced extensive tissue necrosis when solutions containing calcium infiltrate the tissues.

HEMATOLOGIC PROBLEMS

Anemia

There are many causes of anemia in the neonatal period. Anemia can result from any of three causes: hemorrhage, hemolysis, and failure of red blood cell production. The presence of severe anemia at the time of delivery or on the first day of life is usually the result of hemorrhage or hemolysis resulting from isoimmunization. When the anemia is secondary to acute blood loss at the time of birth, there can be evidence of circulatory insufficiency.

Oski and Naiman (1982) classify hemorrhage leading to anemia at birth or early in the neonatal period broadly into five categories:

1. Obstetric accidents and malformations of the placenta and cord
2. Occult hemorrhage prior to birth
3. Internal hemorrhage
4. Iatrogenic blood loss
5. Hemolytic anemias

Obstetric Accidents and Malformations of the Placenta and Cord

This subgroup includes rupture of a normal or abnormal umbilical cord. Rupture of the normal umbilical cord is rare and may result from an unattended precipitous delivery. Severe fetal hemorrhage can accompany placenta previa, abruptio placentae, or accidental incision of the placenta or umbilical cord during cesarean section. Failure of the infant to receive the usual placental transfusion during the cesarean section and clamping the cord with the infant above the placenta aggravates the situation, because fetoplacental hemorrhage will occur. Infants delivered with tight nuchal cords are also at risk for fetoplacental hemorrhage and should be evaluated for signs and symptoms of acute blood loss, including pallor, tachycardia, tachypnea or gasping respiration, hypotension, and evidence of poor perfusion with slow capillary refill. The hemoglobin content may initially be normal but drops precipitously as circulating volume is restored. Anemia is defined as a hemoglobin level less than 12 g/100 mL in the first week of life. The hemoglobin and hematocrit levels both rise 2 to 3 g/100 mL and 3% to 6%, respectively, to peak at 3 to 12 hours of age. The capillary values for both hemoglobin and hematocrit are consistently higher than venous or arterial measurements.

It can be extremely difficult to distinguish the infant with hypovolemic shock from the severely asphyxiated newborn; both can be extremely pale with evidence of poor perfusion and circulatory insufficiency. Both conditions can be present in the same patient. Hypotension is noted when circulating volume has been reduced by 25%. When a depressed, pale infant is to be treated, the resuscitative plan outlined early in this chapter should be followed. Blood pressure and a venous hematocrit are quickly ascertained. Attempts are made to oxygenate and ventilate the patient, to restore cardiac output and circulating volume, to correct metabolic acidosis, and then to correct the anemia with transfusion. Anemia as a result of obstetric accidents or malformations of the placenta and cord is usually diagnosed from historical information and close inspection of the placenta, cord, and membranes.

Occult Hemorrhage Prior to Birth

Although some degree of hemorrhage from the fetus into the maternal circulation occurs during 50% of pregnancies, in only 1% will the amount of fetal loss exceed 40 mL and cause anemia in the newborn. Massive fetomaternal hemorrhage, defined as more than 150 mL of fetal blood in the maternal circulation, is said to account for 3% of perinatal mortality and occurs in approximately 1 in 800 deliveries. Some of the causes of fetomaternal hemorrhage include amniocentesis, external version, fundal pressure during the second stage of labor, the use of intravenous oxytoxics, trauma, placenta previa, and abruptio placentae (Nathan and Orkin, 1998).

The clinical manifestations of fetomaternal hemorrhage depend on the timing and acuity. Chronic bleeding results in a very pale infant, not necessarily in distress or manifesting any features of shock but with enlargement of the liver and spleen. The blood smear is typically microcytic and hypochromic, and there is no evidence of hemolysis. Fetal cells can be demonstrated in the maternal circulation, usually by means of the acid elution technique of Kleihauer and Betke. If fetomaternal hemorrhage of significant proportions has occurred acutely, the clinical features of shock and hypoperfusion (as already described) predominate. The red blood cell morphology is normocytic and normochromic, and no hepatosplenomegaly is present. In contrast with the infants with chronic loss who require only iron supplementation, these latter infants are in dire need of serial infusions to restore intravascular volume, and then blood transfusion.

Occult hemorrhage may also be noted with intrauterine twin-to-twin transfusions. The donor twin is pale and usually smaller than the plethoric recipient. Both twins are at risk and need close observation and appropriate intervention.

Internal Hemorrhage

There are many potential sites for blood loss in the newborn. The detection of anemia during the first days of life should initiate a careful evaluation to determine the source of blood loss. The finding of a large cephalohematoma or extensive swelling of the scalp associated with a subaponeurotic collection of blood is one common site of blood loss. Infants delivered in the breech position can have significant blood loss into the muscles and manifest bruising but not necessarily swelling. The advent of ultrasonography and CT has facilitated the search for intracranial and intra-abdominal sites of blood loss.

Adrenal hemorrhage, rupture of the liver, and rupture of the spleen traditionally all accompany difficult and traumatic deliveries of both macrosomic and premature infants and are more likely to be noted with breech presentation. The usual clinical manifestations of shock are accompanied by specific abdominal findings, which include periumbilical discoloration. Adrenal hemorrhage sometimes is confirmed only by the incidental finding of adrenal calcification. Rupture of the liver is usually contained by the capsule, and the infant experiences decompensation only after about 48 hours.

Iatrogenic Blood Loss

Iatrogenic blood loss is associated with excessive blood withdrawal, bleeding from inadequate clamping of the umbilical cord, bleeding associated with improper management of the umbilical arterial catheters, or excessive bleeding following procedures such as circumcision. The volume of blood withdrawn from sick neonates should be monitored to draw the minimal volume of blood necessary and to restrict the number of laboratory investigations. Strict adherence to protocols regarding care of catheters diminishes the risks of hemorrhage from this source. Close attention to blood withdrawal from premature infants has reduced the donor exposure and diminished the number of blood transfusions in these vulnerable babies.

Hemolytic Anemias

There are many causes of hemolytic disease in the newborn. The presence of jaundice distinguishes the hemolytic from those characterized by blood loss. Major categories of hemolysis of significance in the neonatal period are as follows:

- Isoimmunization
- Congenital defects of the red blood cell
- Acquired defects of the red blood cell

The problem of isoimmunization is dealt with in Chapter 30. Congenital defects of the red blood cell, which include the enzymatic defects, are characterized by specific morphology of the red blood cell or by the presence of abnormal hemoglobin. Among the causes of acquired defects of the red blood cell are a variety of bacterial and viral infections and a multitude of drugs and toxins.

In summary, hemorrhage is the most common cause of early anemia. The cause is usually apparent from the history. The initial evaluation requires a complete blood count with smear and reticulocyte count, total and direct bilirubin, blood type and Coombs' test, and the Kleihauer-Betke test on maternal blood. TORCH titers, a full coagulation profile, red blood cell enzymes, and hemoglobin electrophoresis are analyzed as indicated by the history and physical examination.

If significant hemorrhage has occurred and the neonate manifests shock with a reduced blood pressure and metabolic acidosis, arrangements are made for immediate blood transfusion. In the meantime, circulation is supported with expansion of the intravascular volume, and mechanical ventilation optimizes oxygenation.

Polycythemia

Polycythemia is defined by a venous hematocrit above 65%. In appropriately grown newborns, the incidence is approximately 4%, rising to 18% to 45% in SGA infants. The high hematocrit is thought to be the result of intrauterine hypoxia stimulating erythropoietin but could also be secondary to a twin-to-twin transfusion. Infants with high hematocrits can have hyperviscosity as well as reduced red blood cell deformability. They are susceptible to thrombotic complications. Symptoms attributable to polycythemia include respiratory distress, lethargy, jitteriness, edema, and priapism. Polycythemic infants are also more prone to hypoglycemia and jaundice.

The tendency has been to empirically reduce the hematocrit by means of partial exchange transfusion if the hematocrit is greater than 70% (or greater than 65% if the infant is symptomatic). Partial isovolemic transfusion most effectively lowers the viscosity if normal saline is used. The volume necessary to exchange in order to achieve the desired reduction of hematocrit to approximately 55% is calculated as follows:

$$\text{volume (mL)} = \frac{\text{blood volume} \times (\text{hct 1} - \text{hct 2})}{\text{hct 1}}$$

where hct 1 = initial hematocrit and hct 2 = desired hematocrit.

Currently, indications for intervention in polycythemic neonates remain largely empirical extrapolations from studies of blood viscosity. Some recent studies indicate that the whole-blood viscosity is lower in neonates than in adults at every level of hematocrit and that this results from a lower plasma viscosity. Intervention is not undertaken lightly. The major risk of partial exchange transfusion is an increased incidence of bowel necrosis and necrotizing enterocolitis.

Drew and coworkers (1997) reported that 7-year-old children with cord blood hyperviscosity had a threefold greater chance of neurologic disability than those with normal viscosity. Partial exchange transfusion used to lower hematocrit decreases viscosity, reverses many of the physiologic abnormalities, and ameliorates most symptoms, but it has not been shown to affect the long-term outcomes of these children significantly. Partial exchange with normal saline or even Ringer's solution is as effective and safe as plasma in symptomatic polycythemic newborns. These solutions produce hemodilution comparable to partial exchange with serum and a correction of hypervolemia without subjecting the infants to the risks of blood products (Deorari et al., 1995; Roithmaier et al., 1995).

Jaundice

Hyperbilirubinemia is the most common problem encountered in the full-term neonate. Hyperbilirubinemia is clinically relevant in the neonate because it is associated with kernicterus (yellow staining of the basal ganglia and hippocampus). Bilirubin appears to be responsible for the central nervous system damage, although the precise mechanism and predisposing conditions remain elusive. The interrelationships between total bilirubin, total albumin, and bilirubin-binding capacity, the integrity of the blood-brain barrier, and the factors determining the uptake of bilirubin into the cell remain under close scrutiny. Most reports indicate that in term infants without evidence of hemolysis, kernicterus is unlikely to occur if the serum bilirubin is maintained below 25 mg%, although kernicterus has been reported at autopsy in low-birth-weight infants when the serum bilirubin never exceeded 10 mg%. There has been a resurgence of kernicterus in term and near-term infants attributable to early discharge, poorly supervised breast-feeding, and inadequate follow-up.

Clinical manifestations of kernicterus in the full-term infant include temperature instability, lethargy, poor feeding, high-pitched cry, vomiting, and hypotonia. Subsequently, irritability, opisthotonus, sun-setting appearance of the eyes, and seizures can occur. "Wind-milling" movements of the extremities have been reported. Pulmonary or gastric hemorrhage can occur as a terminal event. Long-term sequelae include the spastic or athetoid form of cerebral palsy, hearing loss (especially high-tone), paralysis of upward gaze, and enamel hypoplasia. Many reports, however, suggest that bilirubin encephalopathy can be asymptomatic in the newborn and subsequently produce neurodevelopmental abnormalities. In the preterm infant, fisting, apnea, and increased tone may be the only acute manifestations. The search continues for a method of identifying infants at greatest risk to determine if and when encephalopathy is imminent.

Bilirubin is produced from breakdown of hemoglobin, myoglobin cytochromes, and other heme-containing compounds mainly in the liver, spleen, and bone marrow. The indirect bilirubin so formed is water-insoluble but fat-soluble, and hence potentially toxic to the central nervous system. Bilirubin is transported in the blood bound to albumin and accepted into the hepatic cells by a receptor ligandin. Under the influence of the enzyme glucuronosyl transferase, the bilirubin is conjugated to form bilirubin diglucuronide, which is water-soluble and excreted in the bile. Bilirubin diglucuronide is deconjugated in the gut by a glucuronidase, reabsorbed, and recirculated to the liver—the so-called enterohepatic circulation of bilirubin. Prior to delivery, the indirect bilirubin is transported across the placenta.

Jaundice usually occurs in term infants on the third day of life and progresses from the head and neck to the trunk and limbs. It disappears in the reverse direction. The onset of jaundice within the first 36 hours of life, persistence beyond the first week of life, a serum bilirubin exceeding 13 mg/dL, elevation of the direct bilirubin, or a combination thereof is an indication for investigation of the jaundice. The level of 13 mg/dL has been selected as the upper limit for "physiologic jaundice" from multiple studies. These revealed that the serum bilirubin ranges between 6 and 7 mg/dL between days 2 and 4. Two standard deviations (SDs) above this is 13%. In a sample of 2421 infants admitted to their nursery, Maisels and Gifford (1986) noted that the mean serum bilirubin on the 2nd to 3rd day of life was 6.2 ± 3.7 mg%. The incidence of infants with bilirubin levels above 12.9 mg/dL was 6.1%— virtually identical to the rate in Caucasian infants in the collaborative study completed in the early 1960s (99% of the Hershey, Pennsylvania, population was Caucasian). The distinction between physiologic and pathologic jaundice at a specific level has been replaced by the introduction of the liver-specific bilirubin. Infants with bilirubin levels above the 90th percentile for their age (in hours) require investigation and treatment.

The major causes of neonatal hyperbilirubinemia are listed in Table 60-13. Important historical data include the blood types of the parents and the isoimmune status, ethnic origin of parents, maternal drug history, gestation history, mode of delivery, past history with regard to jaundiced neonates, stooling pattern, and method of feeding. Jaundice associated with breast-feeding is the most common cause of hyperbilirubinemia in the otherwise healthy full-term infant.

TABLE 60-13. CAUSES OF NEONATAL HYPERBILIRUBINEMIA

Overproduction	Undersecretion	Mixed
A. Hemolytic disorders	**E. Decreased hepatic uptake of bilirubin**	**I. Prenatal infection**
1. Fetomaternal blood group incompatibility ABO, Rh, others	1. Persistent ductus venosus shunt	1. Toxoplasmosis
2. Genetic causes of hemolysis	2. Cytosol receptor protein (y) blocked by:	2. Rubella
a. Hereditary spherocytosis	a. Drugs	3. Cytomegalovirus (CMV)
b. Enzyme defects: G6PD, pyruvate kinase, others	b. Abnormal human milk inhibitor (? NEFA, ? may belong in D. or F.)	4. *Herpesvirus hominis*
c. Hemoglobinopathies: α-thalassemia, β-γ-thalassemia, others		5. Syphilis
3. Drug-induced hemolysis—vitamin K	**F. Decreased bilirubin conjugation**	6. Hepatitis
		7. Others
B. Extravascular blood: petechiae, hematoma, pulmonary and cerebral hemorrhage, swallowed blood	1. Congenital reduction in glucuronyl transferase activity	
C. Polycythemia	a. Familial nonhemolytic jaundice (types I and II)	**J. Postnatal infections (sepsis)**
1. Chronic fetal hypoxia	b. Gilbert's syndrome*	**K. Multisystem disorders**
2. Maternal-fetal or fetofetal transfusion	2. Enzyme inhibitor	1. Prematurity ± respiratory distress syndrome
3. Placental transfusion (cord stripping)	a. Drugs and hormones: novobiocin, ? pregnanediol	2. Infants of diabetic mothers
	b. Galactosemia (early)	3. Severe erythroblastosis
D. Exaggerated enterohepatic circulation	c. Lucey-Driscoll syndrome	
	d. Abnormal human milk	
1. Mechanical obstruction	**G. Impaired transport of conjugated bilirubin out of hepatocyte**	
a. Atresia and stenosis	1. Congenital transport defect: Dubin-Johnson and Rotor's syndromes	
b. Hirschsprung disease	2. Hepatocellular damage secondary to metabolic disorders	
c. Meconium plug syndrome	a. Galactosemia (late)	
2. Reduced peristalsis	b. Alpha$_1$-antitrypsin deficiency*	
a. Fasting or underfeeding	c. Tyrosinemia	
b. Drugs (hexamethoniums, atropine)	d. Hypermethioninemia	
c. Pyloric stenosis	e. Hereditary fructose intolerance*	
	3. Toxic obstruction (IV alimentation)	
	H. Obstruction to bile flow	
	1. Biliary atresia	
	2. Choledochal cyst*	
	3. Cystic fibrosis*	
	4. Extrinsic obstruction (tumor or band)	

* Not seen early in the neonatal period.

IV, intravenous; NEFA, nonesterified fatty acids.

From Poland RL, Ostrea EM Jr: Neonatal hyperbilirubinemia. *In* Klaus MH, Fanaroff AA (eds): Care of the High Risk Neonate, 4th ed. Philadelphia, WB Saunders, 1993.

TABLE 60-14. CONJUGATED HYPERBILIRUBINEMIA OF EARLY INFANCY

Suggested work-up

1. History and physical examination*
2. Complete blood cell count and reticulocyte count
3. Coombs' test
4. Urinalysis, including reducing substances
5. Serum bilirubin concentration, total and direct-reacting
6. Total serum protein and protein electrophoresis
7. Serum transaminases
8. Alpha$_1$-antitrypsin concentration
9. Hepatitis-associated antigen and titers
10. Sweat chloride concentration
11. Serologic titers for rubella, cytomegalovirus, etc.
12. Clotting factors, platelet count
13. Liver biopsy

* May lead one to order other diagnostic tests not listed.

Modified from Poland RL, Ostrea EM Jr: Neonatal hyperbilirubinemia. *In* Klaus MH, Fanaroff AA (eds): Care of the High Risk Neonate, 4th ed. Philadelphia, WB Saunders, 1993, p. 276.

The presence of plethora, bruising, and cephalohematoma should be sought. Hepatosplenomegaly accompanied by pallor, purpura, and rashes could indicate congenital infection or hemolytic disease. The initial evaluation should always include a complete blood count with smear and reticulocyte count, blood type of mother and infant, direct antibody test (DAT), total and direct bilirubin level, and urinalysis to rule out infection and galactosemia. If the infant is sick with jaundice, a blood culture, spinal tap, and chest radiograph are also indicated. If the direct bilirubin exceeds 10% of the total, this indicates either biliary obstruction or hepatocellular damage. Therefore, in addition to the aforementioned studies, serum protein and protein electrophoresis, serum transaminases, alpha$_1$-antitrypsin concentration, hepatitis-associated antigens and titers, TORCH titers, sweat chloride, and clotting profile may be indicated (Table 60-14). An abdominal ultrasound examination may prove extremely productive, as may a CT scan of the liver. A liver biopsy could be indicated.

Persistent elevation of the indirect bilirubin occurs predominantly with hemolytic disease, hypothyroidism, or breast milk jaundice. The latter has been attributed at various times to hormones in the breast milk, to nonesterified fatty acids in the breast milk that inhibit glucuronyl transferase, and to the presence of β-glucuronidase in human milk, which enhances the enterohepatic circulation of bilirubin. ABO incompatibility is the most common cause of hemolytic disease in the newborn. A very high anti-A or anti-B antibody titer can be found in the maternal serum; the infant's blood smear reveals abundant spherocytes, and the reticulocyte count could be elevated. Hemolytic disease of the newborn, secondary to Rh incompatibility, has become extremely rare with the widespread screening and use of Rh immune globulin.

Treatment of Jaundice

No treatment should be instituted without an investigation of the cause of the jaundice. Adequate hydration of jaundiced neonates is important. This has generated considerable controversy because proponents of breast-feeding are convinced that supplementation with formula or water decreases the success of breast-feeding. Evidence is strongly mounting to indicate that a reduced calorie or fluid intake is responsible for the early elevated bilirubin levels noted among breast-fed infants. Breast-feeding should not be discontinued during the first days of life.

Phototherapy has been used extensively for the treatment of jaundice. Light reduces bilirubin levels predominantly by photoisomerization and, to a lesser extent, photo oxidation. Essentially, during photoisomerization, bilirubin is converted rapidly from a relatively insoluble state to water-soluble photoisomers. When bilirubin is exposed to light (Fig. 60-10), native bilirubin is converted to photobilirubin and the structural isomer lumirubin. Lumirubin appears to be the principal route of pigment elimination during phototherapy. Before phototherapy is ordered, the cause of the hyperbilirubinemia should be investigated. Most recent studies on the natural history of jaundice reveal that the early use of phototherapy offers no advantage, and prophylactic phototherapy, even in tiny immature infants, has not proved to be necessary.

Guidelines for the use of phototherapy and exchange transfusions are outlined in Table 60-15. It is important to recognize that these are only guidelines. Therapy should always be dictated by the clinical condition and clinical evaluation, not

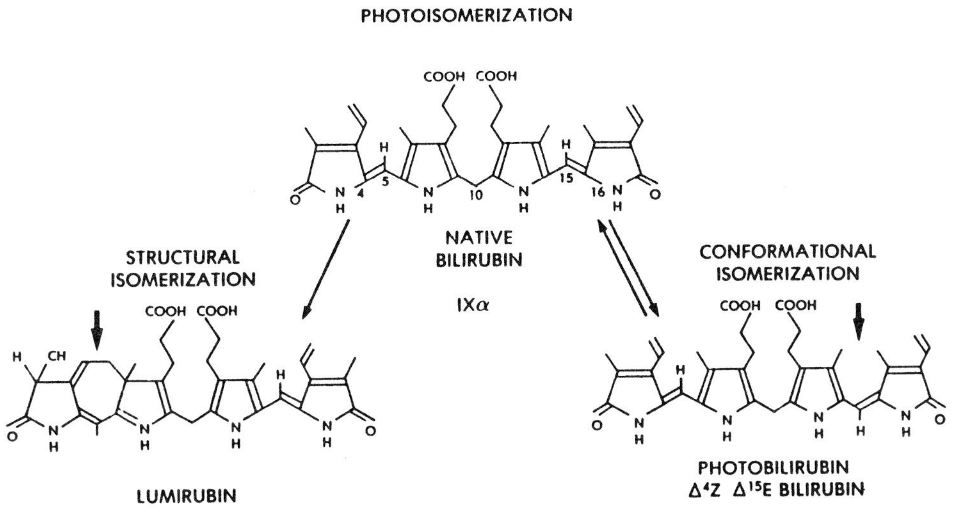

PHOTOISOMERIZATION

FIGURE 60-10 ■ The photoisomerized conversion of bilirubin IX-a (Z,Z) to water-soluble bilirubin IX-a (Z,E) and lumirubin. (From Poland RL, Ostrea EM Jr: Neonatal hyperbilirubinemia. *In* Klaus MH, Fanaroff AA (eds): Care of the High Risk Neonate, 4th ed. Philadelphia, WB Saunders, 1993.)

TABLE 60-15. MANAGEMENT OF HYPERBILIRUBINEMIA IN THE HEALTHY TERM NEWBORN

Age, Hours	Total Serum Bilirubin Level, mg/dL (µmol/L)			
	Consider Phototherapy*	Phototherapy	Exchange Transfusion If Intensive Phototherapy Fails†	Exchange Transfusion and Intensive Phototherapy
≤24‡	—	—	—	—
25–48	≥12 (170)	≥15 (260)	≥20 (340)	≥25 (430)
49–72	≥15 (260)	≥18 (310)	≥25 (430)	≥30 (510)
>72‡	≥17 (290)	≥20 (340)	≥25 (430)	≥30 (510)

* Phototherapy at these total serum bilirubin (TSB) levels is a clinical option, meaning that the intervention is available and may be used on the basis of individual clinical judgment.

† Intensive phototherapy should produce a decline of TSB of 1 to 2 mg/dL within 4–6 hours and the TSB level should continue to fall and remain below the threshold level for exchange transfusion. If this does not occur, it is considered a failure of phototherapy.

‡ Term infants who are clinically jaundiced at 24 hours old or less are not considered healthy and require further evaluation (see text).

merely by laboratory tests. In bruised, asphyxiated, acidotic, or potentially septic infants, more liberal indications for treatment are often used. Since the advent of Rh immune globulin, the number of exchange transfusions has diminished markedly.

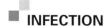
INFECTION

Infection (see also Chapter 39) remains a significant cause of neonatal morbidity and mortality (Stoll et al., 2002a, b). The incidence of neonatal septicemia is inversely related to gestational age; 1 in 250 premature infants and 1 in 1500 term infants experience a systemic bacterial infection in the first month of life. Approximately one third of infants with a birth weight between 501 g and 750 g develop late-onset sepsis. Although the spectrum of organisms involved has changed, the overall incidence of infections has decreased little since the 1980s. On the positive side, mortality rates have continued to decline as a result of earlier detection and better supportive care, combined with specific antibiotic therapy.

Immune Response

Because the immune system of the newborn is defective in many respects, infants are predisposed to a higher risk of infection. The abnormalities in immune defense mechanisms that have been described include abnormal chemotaxis, phagocytosis and bactericidal activity, abnormal opsonic activity, and defects in the complement pathway. In addition, the infant's host defense mechanisms are not intact at birth, and the immunoglobulin M (IgM) and IgG responses to infection are depressed compared with those of the adult. The preterm infant is particularly deficient in circulating immunoglobulin because the serum IgG is acquired transplacentally after the 17th week of gestation. Therefore, the infant's IgG level tends to be less than the maternal level and is directly related to gestational age. The extremely immature infant starts with low levels of IgG that decline to severely hypogammaglobulinemic levels (less than 200 mg/dL). IgM is, in fact, the principal antibody synthesized by the neonate in response to infection *in utero*.

Environmental Risk Factors

The infant *in utero* is surrounded by sterile amniotic fluid that inhibits the growth of most microorganisms. The infant's protected status can be breached by microorganisms via two routes: by hematogenous spread from the maternal circulation and, more commonly, by ascending infection when normal vaginal flora gain access to the uterine cavity. Colonization and infection of the infant by the latter route are more common following rupture of fetal membranes for more than 24 hours. During vaginal delivery, the infant also can become contaminated by an assortment of vaginal flora. Serious infection via this route is more common the heavier the degree of colonization of the infant's skin (e.g., with the group B streptococcal organism).

Evaluation of the Newborn

The signs of sepsis in the newborn are nonspecific and can include poor feeding, apnea, weak suck, lethargy, hypoglycemia, and tachypnea, as well as temperature instability. These signs, when combined with an abnormal complete blood cell count (increased total leukocytes, increased band count) or spinal fluid leukocytosis, could warrant initiation of antibiotic therapy prior to definitive isolation of the infecting organism. Ampicillin (100 to 200 mg/kg/day) and gentamicin (5 mg/kg/day) are commenced for suspected early-onset sepsis, but because coagulase-negative *Staphylococcus* is the predominant cause of nosocomial sepsis, this must be taken into consideration for the therapy of late-onset sepsis.

Group B Streptococcus

Group B streptococcus (GBS) is the principal gram-positive organism responsible for early-onset neonatal septicemia and meningitis. This bacterial pathogen can be acquired from the colonized vaginal tract of the mother, with maternal colonization rates varying between 4% and 30%. The attack rate for colonized infants is low, however (less than 1%), possibly because of passive immunization of the newborn by transplacental protective antibody. Early-onset streptococcal infection presents as a multisystem disease with such symptoms as apnea, respiratory distress, and hypotension. Unless the illness is detected and treated promptly, the infant can develop a shock-like picture rapidly. Fortunately, with early treatment of the septicemic infant, a full recovery is expected. There has been a major thrust to prevent group B streptococcal disease. Detection of maternal colonization through screening at 35 to 37 weeks' gestation, coupled with intrapartum antibiotic therapy commencing at least 4 hours prior to delivery for all colonized and at-risk women, is the recommended strategy

(Schrag et al., 2002). The rates of early-onset GBS have decreased from one to two cases per 1000 to less than 0.5 case per 1000 deliveries.

Congenital Viral Infection

Maternal viral infection that occurs during pregnancy can be relatively asymptomatic. Cytomegalovirus infection is most commonly encountered (Goldenberg and Rouse, 1997) (Table 60-16). In some specific types of infection, however, the viremia can spread to the newborn, resulting in intrauterine infection with potential long-term sequelae. In many cases, antenatal diagnosis of the infection has not occurred, and the complications of infection are apparent only at delivery. Treatment at this stage is either incompletely effective or not available.

There has been an increase in HIV infections in children. More than 90% of infected children in the United States acquire their infection from their mother. The risk of infection for an infant born to an HIV-seropositive mother who did not receive antiviral therapy during pregnancy is somewhere between 13% and 39%. Most infections occur close to or during delivery or after delivery through breast-feeding. Zidovudine therapy during pregnancy has been effective in reducing transmission (AIDS Clinical Trials Group Protocol, 1994). Immediate and aggressive care of the neonate is recommended, with the drug regimen determined by the status of the infant.

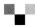

TABLE 60-16. DIAGNOSTIC AIDS FOR CONGENITAL AND PERINATAL INFECTIONS

Infection	Diagnostic Aid
Cytomegalovirus	Isolation of virus from urine within 2 weeks of age
Rubella	Isolation of virus from throat (and stools, conjunctiva, or urine) within 1 month of age; serial determination of antibody between 3 and 9 months of age
Syphilis	Dark-field examination of lesions if present; antibody determination with both reagin (VDRL) and fluorescent antibody test
Toxoplasma	Isolation of *T. gondii* from placenta, CSF, or blood; serial determination of IgG antibody (FA) between 1 and 6 months of age; determination of IgM antibody in cord serum
Enteroviruses	Isolation of virus from feces, CSF, throat, nasopharynx
Hepatitis B	Serial determination of hepatitis B surface antigen, antibody to the surface antigen, and antibody to the hepatitis core antigen
Herpes simplex	Isolation of virus from skin vesicles, conjunctiva, throat, CSF, and stools
Varicella	Isolation of virus from skin lesions
Chlamydia	Isolation or direct staining of organism from conjunctiva and nasopharynx
Epstein-Barr	Serial determination of antibodies; culture of cord lymphocytes
HIV	Serial determination of antibodies; culture of blood

CSF, cerebrospinal fluid; FA, fluorescent antibody: HIV, human immunodeficiency virus; VDRL, Venereal Disease Research Laboratory.

Modified from Stagno S: Diagnosis of viral infections of the newborn infant. Clin Perinatol **8**:579, 1981.

Ophthalmia Neonatorum

The increased incidence of sexually transmitted diseases since the 1980s carries with it a risk for an increase in occurrence of ophthalmia neonatorum caused by *Neisseria gonorrhoeae* and *Chlamydia trachomatis*. In developing countries, the gonococcus remains a common pathogen responsible for ophthalmia. Prevention of gonococcal ophthalmia is best achieved by recognition and treatment of the infection in the mother prior to delivery so as to avoid exposure of the neonate. Cultures of the mother for *N. gonorrhoeae* are recommended in both the first and third trimesters because 30% of women with gonococcal cervicitis in the first trimester experience a recurrence during the third trimester. Similarly, treatment of the mother with *C. trachomatis* infection reduces the risk of infection of the infant. All infants now receive eye prophylaxis against these infections immediately after delivery. Erythromycin ointment (0.5%) has emerged as the agent of choice. In addition to being an effective agent against the common pathogens, erythromycin is better tolerated and causes less chemical conjunctivitis than silver nitrate. Ophthalmic povidone-iodine (2.5%) may offer more effective prophylaxis against ophthalmia neonatorum. A single vial can be used for many infants. The staining of the conjunctivae ensures correct application, and the agent is less toxic and less expensive than agents currently in use.

Clinical features of conjunctivitis in the infant include purulent discharge, erythema, and swelling of the eyelids, with intense congestion of the conjunctivae. Conjunctival exudates and transudates forming pseudomembranes often occur with ophthalmia secondary to *Chlamydia*, and the palpebral conjunctivae may bleed when touched with a cotton swab. The presence of keratitis suggests serious infection with herpes simplex virus. The onset of clinical symptoms usually occurs on the second day and rarely occurs beyond the 10th day of life; bilateral involvement is common.

Laboratory investigation of the affected infant must include a conjunctival smear, bacterial culture for gonococci or staphylococci, and specific rapid antigen detection tests for *Chlamydia*. Chlamydial conjunctivitis in young infants is treated with oral erythromycin (50 mg/kg/day) for 14 days. Infants with evidence of gonococcal ophthalmia must be hospitalized. Susceptibility testing of the strain of *Gonococcus* is recommended because multiple forms of resistance have been reported. Recommended antimicrobial therapy for gonococcal ophthalmia is ceftriaxone, 25–50 mg/kg/day intravenously or intramuscularly for 7 days. Topical therapy cannot eradicate neonatal ophthalmia caused by gonococcus or *Chlamydia*.

If the mother or her sexual partner are infected with either *N. gonorrhoeae* or *C. trachomatis* at the time of delivery, both should be treated, and eye prophylaxis of the infant should be instituted. The infant's eyes should be checked daily during the hospital stay or, with early discharge, the eye condition should be followed closely by the visiting nurse (American Academy of Pediatrics Committee on Infectious Diseases, 2000).

Infections of the Premature Infant

The premature infant, as discussed previously, has a poorly developed immune system with which to resist infection. In addition, the essential barrier of skin integrity can be breached many times in the hospitalized infant, allowing a portal of entry for microorganisms. These factors predispose the premature baby to several unusual types of infection that do not occur in the term newborn.

Coagulase-Negative Staphylococci

These organisms are part of the normal human skin flora and, in the adult or term infant, do not cause systemic illness. Recently, these microorganisms have been recognized as an increasing source of morbidity and mortality in the most premature infants. Infected infants often present after the first week of in-hospital life with recurrent apnea, worsening respiratory distress or increased ventilatory requirements, bradycardia, feeding intolerance, abdominal distention, guaiac-positive stools, and temperature instability. The major risk factors include low birth weight, immaturity, male gender, low immunoglobulin levels, prolonged use of central lines, intralipid infusions, and the use of corticosteroids. Both septicemia and meningitis resulting from staphylococci have been reported, although meningitis is uncommon. Parenteral therapy with vancomycin usually results in an effective cure and full recovery. Handwashing remains a potent measure for prevention of nosocomial infection.

Fungal Infections

Colonization of the newborn skin with C. *albicans* is common, and superficial infection usually presents with oral thrush or a diaper dermatitis. The premature infant is subject to invasive disease from this yeast-like organism, however, which can cause both septicemia and meningitis. The portal of entry for infection, as in the case of *Staphylococcus epidermidis*, could be via indwelling catheters. Deep spread from contagious surface infection can occur, however. When promptly recognized through blood, cerebrospinal fluid, and urine culture, this infection can be treated successfully with intravenous amphotericin B, although the treatment course could require several weeks of therapy. Congenital candidiasis can present with a severe skin eruption; the skin appears boiled and desquamated, and there is often profound leukocytosis. Many species are responsible for infections in the newborn.

Necrotizing Enterocolitis

Premature infants are subject to an unusual and potentially fatal disorder of the gastrointestinal tract called *necrotizing enterocolitis*. This disorder can present in several different ways, ranging from mild abdominal distention with gastric aspirates to fulminant peritonitis, shock, and disseminated intravascular coagulation (Table 60-17). A hallmark feature is the documentation of pneumatosis intestinalis or portal venous gas on abdominal radiograph, both of which could precede intestinal perforation. The injury to the bowel resembles ischemic necrosis, most commonly of the small intestine, although the entire gastrointestinal tract below the esophagus can be involved. The cause of this disorder is unknown. One hypothesis implicates early feeding of a premature infant in colonization of the bowel with pathogenic organisms that then become invasive (Fig. 60-11). In some series of affected infants, bacteremia with gram-negative or gram-positive organisms has been reported; however, this is true in only about 25% of cases.

Treatment usually consists of bowel rest, supportive fluid therapy, and broad-spectrum antibiotic coverage. Surgical con-

TABLE 60-17. SIGNS AND SYMPTOMS ASSOCIATED WITH NECROTIZING ENTEROCOLITIS

Gastrointestinal	Systemic
Abdominal distention	Lethargy
Abdominal tenderness	Apnea/respiratory distress
Feeding intolerance	Temperature instability
Delayed gastric emptying	"Not right"
Vomiting	Acidosis (metabolic and/or
Occult/gross blood in stool	respiratory)
Change in stool pattern/diarrhea	Glucose instability
Abdominal mass	Poor perfusion/shock
Erythema of abdominal wall	Disseminated intravascular
	coagulopathy
	Positive results of blood cultures

sultation and resection of necrotic bowel sometimes is required. More recently, perforations of the bowel have been treated with simple drains in the extremely-low-birth-weight infant. The prognosis for full recovery is best if the segment of the bowel involved is small and surgery is not required. Spontaneous isolated bowel perforations have been recognized in preterm infants. These are often associated with corticosteroid therapy.

NEONATAL SEIZURES

Seizures are the most common and distinctive signal of neurologic disturbance in the first month of life (Volpe, 1999). Convulsions have been noted in 1.5 to 3 per 1000 births. The true incidence could be obscure because the manifestations are extremely subtle and may not be recognized. Newborn infants have less well-organized seizure patterns than those observed in adults. Subtle or fragmentary seizures are the most frequently observed clinical category. Indeed, any abnormal repetitive and stereotypic event could be a clinical seizure. Considerable debate surrounds the mechanism and clinical manifestations of neonatal seizures. Technologic developments permitting continuous monitoring of electrical brain activity together with videotape recordings of neonatal activity could result in reclassification of neonatal seizure disorders (Mizrahi and Kellaway, 1984; Mizrahi, 1986; Scher, 1997).

The etiology of neonatal seizures has been more clearly established as a result of ultrasonography, CT, and magnetic resonance imaging (MRI). Whereas in 1977 the etiology could not be determined in 30% of neonatal seizure disorders, a similar survey in 1986 showed no established etiology in only 2%. Hypoxic-ischemic events are the major cause of neonatal seizures (Table 60-18). Metabolic disorders, including hypoglycemia and hypocalcemia, brain anomalies, cerebrovascular lesions with and without trauma, infections, drug withdrawal, or toxins, in addition to selected genetic syndromes, may all account for the seizure activity.

Types of Convulsive Patterns

Five patterns of seizure activity are recognized in the newborn (Volpe, 1999). This includes the most common variety, designated as *subtle*, wherein sucking, chewing, bicycling, or swimming movements are combined with drooling,

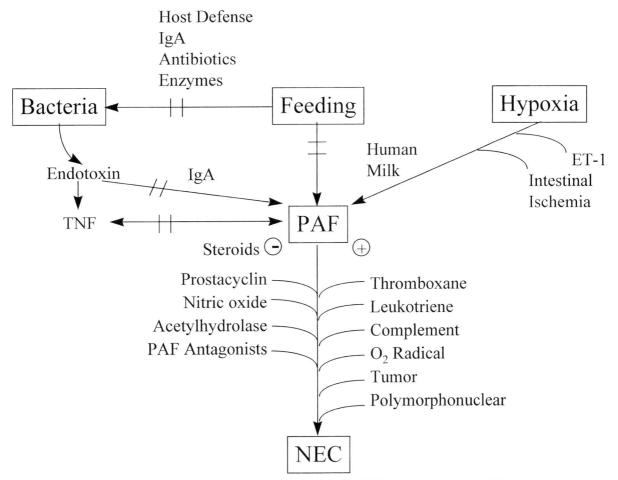

FIGURE 60-11 ■ Pathogenesis of necrotizing enterocolitis (NEC). Ig, immunoglobulin; PAF, platelet-activating factor; TNF, tumor necrosis factor. (From Caplan MS, MacKendrick W: Inflammatory mediators and intestinal injury. Clin Perinatol **21**:235, 1994.)

apnea, tonic deviation of the eyes, and fluttering of the eyelids. *Multifocal clonic seizures* are manifested by migratory movements commencing in one or two limbs and moving in a nonorderly fashion to other parts of the body. *Focal seizures* are well-localized and not usually accompanied by unconsciousness. They begin in a single limb and spread to other body parts on the same side. *Tonic seizures* could resemble the decerebrate or decorticate posturing that occurs in older patients, with tonic extension of all limbs or flexion of upper limbs with extension of the lower limbs. *Myoclonic seizures* are characterized by single or multiple jerks with flexion of upper or lower limbs. They are rare in the newborn period.

 TABLE 60-18. ETIOLOGY OF NEONATAL SEIZURES

Cause	1977	1986
Hypoxic-ischemic encephalopathy	36%	46%
Intracranial hemorrhage	—	15%
Cerebral infarction	—	6%
Hypoglycemia	4%	5%
Hypocalcemia	12%	0%
Intracranial infection	12%	17%
Developmental defects	5%	8%
Drug withdrawal	0%	0%
Unknown	30%	2%

Seizures are distinct from *jitteriness*, a stimulus-sensitive series of synchronous movements not accompanied by other signs, which can be diminished or terminated with passive flexion. There are no abnormalities of gaze or other eye movements in jittery neonates. The infants are generally alert. The onset, nature, and duration of seizures are all important considerations regarding the prognosis for neonatal seizures. If the seizures are controlled easily and the electroencephalogram returns to normal, the outcome is usually good. Persistence of clinical and electrical seizure activity is ominous.

Anticonvulsant Therapy

It is important to recognize and treat the many metabolic disturbances that can result in neonatal seizures. Included among these are hypoglycemia, hypocalcemia, urea cycle disorders, pyridoxine deficiency, ketotic and nonketotic hyperglycinemia, and other inborn errors of metabolism. Withdrawal from drugs rarely causes seizures.

Phenobarbital is the mainstay of anticonvulsant therapy. It limits the spread of seizure activity and could elevate the seizure threshold by increasing the activity of the inhibitory neurotransmitters. Phenobarbital is readily absorbed orally, and cerebrospinal fluid and brain tissue levels are equal to serum levels. The majority of the phenobarbital is metabolized in the liver; the rest is excreted directly via the kidney.

A loading dose of 20 mg/kg is given intravenously and may be followed with 5 mg/kg every 5 minutes up to a total loading dose of 40 mg/kg in order to control status epilepticus. A maintenance dose of 3 to 4 mg/kg/day is recommended, and a serum level of 30 μg/mL is desirable for seizure control (Volpe, 1999). Phenytoin may be used in combination with phenobarbital. It is not absorbed orally, but its activity is similar to that of phenobarbital. The loading dose for phenytoin is 15 to 20 mg/kg. Intravenous benzodiazepines—mainly diazepam—are occasionally used to control seizures.

The duration of anticonvulsant therapy is determined by the clinical course. Medication may be discontinued during the first month of life if clinical recovery appears to be complete as evidenced by a normal neurologic examination together with absence of seizures electrically and clinically (Bergman et al., 1983; Goldberg et al., 1986; Scher et al., 1993).

Legido and associates (1991) used electroencephalography (EEG) to relate neonatal seizures to the neurologic outcome in 40 infants with seizures of varying cause. The outcome was unfavorable in 70%, with the development of epilepsy in 56%, cerebral palsy in 63%, and developmental delay in 67%. The onset of seizures on the first day of life, seizure frequency (more than two per hour), and an abnormal EEG background predicted a poor outcome.

CONGENITAL MALFORMATIONS

As a result of advances in the care of immature low-birth-weight infants, congenital malformations and genetic disorders (see also Chapters 1, 18, and 19) have assumed an important role as causes of morbidity and mortality during the first month of life. Not all malformations are detected at birth. Thus, surveys could underestimate the true incidence. Nonetheless, as noted in a study of 18,155 newborns, Holmes (1976) documented that 2% of newborns have a serious malformation that has surgical or cosmetic importance. Furthermore, the National Foundation of March of Dimes estimates that genetic errors afflict more than 15 million persons in the United States with mental retardation, diabetes, complete or partial blindness, impaired hearing, defects in specific organ systems, and congenital bone, muscle, or joint disease.

There are multiple causes of birth defects or genetic disorders, including chromosomal abnormalities, single gene disorders, environmental agents, multifactorial disorders, and many still classified as unknown. The etiology of many syndromes has been elucidated with the recent advances in genetics and the ability to identify single gene defects as well as microdeletions and other structural changes on the chromosomes. A comprehensive evaluation should be offered to the infants and families when birth defects are noted. This includes a careful history noting family pedigree and history of pregnancy, physical and laboratory studies of both the infant and family members if indicated, genetic counseling, and provision of psychosocial support for the family. The types and etiologies of major malformations are shown in Table 60-19.

As noted in Chapters 18, 19 and 20, birth defects have been recognized with increasing frequency antenatally. Some of the factors that could raise the index of suspicion, prompting a careful anatomic survey of the fetus, include a positive family history, advanced maternal age, exposure during the pregnancy

TABLE 60-19. TYPE AND ETIOLOGY OF MAJOR MALFORMATIONS IN 18,155 NEWBORNS

Malformation		Number
Multifactorial Inheritance		128 (0.7%)
Anencephaly-myelomeningocele-encephalocele	25	
Cardiac anomalies	45	
Cleft lip and/or palate	14	
Clubfoot	21	
Congenital hip dislocation	12	
Hypospadias	8	
Omphalocele	2	
Bilateral renal agenesis	1	
Mendelian Inheritance		67 (0.4%)
Autosomal dominant disorders [excluding polydactyly]	57	
Autosomal recessive disorders	9	
X-linked recessive disorders	1	
Chromosome Abnormalities		27 (0.2%)
Down syndrome	21	
Trisomy 13	3	
Other	3	
Teratogenic Conditions		15 (0.1%)
Infants of diabetic mothers	14	
Effects of warfarin	1	
Unknown		107 (0.6%)
Total number affected		344 (2%)

From Kurezynski TW: Congenital malformations. *In* Fanaroff AA, Martin RJ (eds): Neonatal-Perinatal Medicine. 5th ed. St. Louis. Mosby-Year Book, 1992, p. 372.

to teratogens including drugs (e.g., anticonvulsants), or the antenatal detection of abnormalities in the volume of amniotic fluid, elevated alpha-fetoprotein, or fetal growth restriction. After delivery, all infants are carefully examined for birth defects and should be more closely observed and followed if they are undergrown or have abnormal facial features, multiple minor malformations, a single umbilical artery, or a single palmar crease. Clinical examination may be complemented by ultrasonographic, radiographic, hematologic, biochemical, and chromosomal studies.

Esophageal Atresia and Tracheoesophageal Fistula

Normal division of the foregut into trachea and esophagus occurs during the fourth week of gestation. Any interruption in embryonic septation results in esophageal atresia (EA) and tracheoesophageal fistula (TEF). These abnormalities commonly occur together but occasionally appear separately. The most common form of malformation is EA with distal TEF (87%). Isolated esophageal atresia and isolated tracheoesophageal fistula occur 8% and 4% of the time, respectively (Ashcraft and Holder, 1976). The overall incidence is 1 in 3000 births. The diagnosis should be suspected when there is a history of prematurity (35%) and polyhydramnios. The latter is present in 32% of infants with EA and distal TEF and in 85% of infants with isolated EA.

The presence of excess mucus ("juicy baby") within the first few hours after birth suggests EA with or without TEF.

There could be associated respiratory distress marked by tachypnea and cyanosis. Early diagnosis is important to avoid complications of aspiration and chemical pneumonitis. Resistance to a nasogastric tube 9 to 13 cm from the nares suggests EA. A radiograph of the chest and abdomen shows the radiopaque catheter lying in a blind esophageal pouch. Associated abnormalities are found in 50% of infants with EA and TEF. Air in the gastrointestinal tract indicates patency of the fistula. Cardiac and vertebral anomalies may be seen as part of the VATER (vertebral defects, imperforate anus, tracheoesophageal fistula, and renal and radial dysplasia) association.

Early management requires gastrostomy and continuous suction of the blind upper pouch. Definitive surgical repair usually is undertaken later, when the infant's condition is stable. Primary repairs depend on how closely the esophageal ends are juxtaposed. Postoperative complications are the result of leakage of fluid from the esophageal anastomosis and of poor distal esophageal peristalsis. Outlook is good in infants with isolated EA or TEF.

Abdominal Wall Defects

Defects in the abdominal wall can result from obstruction of the omphalomesenteric vessel resulting in gastroschisis, or from failure of normal embryonic regression of intestine from umbilical stalk into the abdominal coelom during the 10th gestational week, resulting in the development of an omphalocele. Both these lesions can be detected in utero. Understanding this basic embryology allows the clinician to differentiate these.

Initial treatment should be directed at maintaining body temperature and fluid balance and preventing infection. A nasogastric catheter should be placed. Exposed viscera should be covered with warm saline dressings. A plastic bag is recommended to keep the viscera moist, sterile, and to avoid excessive fluid leaks. Frequently, a staged operative closure with the use of a Silastic (silicone) "chimney" is performed. Postoperative complications consist of respiratory embarrassment and pulmonary hypertension, small bowel perforation, and intestinal obstruction. Malrotation of the bowel is present in both conditions.

The mortality rate in infants with gastroschisis used to be as high as 60%, but improved survival has been noted with the introduction of total parenteral nutrition, better anesthesia, and highly trained surgeons—a mortality rate of less than 5% can be anticipated (Grosfeld et al., 1981; Novotny et al., 1993). The outlook for infants with omphalocele relates directly to the presence of associated anomalies.

Neural Tube Defects (Meningomyelocele)

Meningomyelocele results from failure of neural tube closure during the third to fourth week of gestation. The incidence is 1 to 3 per 1000 births, 2% to 3% in a second child with one previous affected sibling, and 5% in a third child with two previous affected siblings. Most cases can be prevented with preconceptual and periconceptual folic acid ingestion (see Chapter 18).

Physical examination demonstrates a thin membrane covering the defect. Leakage of spinal fluid is not uncommon and predisposes the infant to infection. Prognosis for ambulation is determined by identifying the level of sensory and motor func-

tion. Hydrocephalus occurs in 60% to 85% of low lumbar and sacral defects and in 96% of high lumbar and thoracic lesions. Outcome is poor with high lumbar or thoracic defects, severe hydrocephalus (less than 1 cm of frontal cerebral mantle), or other brain malformations and associated anomalies. Immediate closure of the defect confers a 90% chance of survival. Once the defect is closed, a multidisciplinary approach, involving a neurosurgeon, orthopedist, urologist, pediatrician, social worker, physical therapist, and psychologist, is required.

Prenatal detection of neural tube defects has led to ongoing research efforts to repair the defects in utero, but there are currently insufficient data to judge the benefits and risks of this approach (Walsh et al., 2001).

NEONATAL SCREENING FOR METABOLIC DISEASES

The American Academy of Pediatrics has recommended metabolic screening of the infant's blood as a preventive public health measure that should be performed on all neonates prior to discharge from the nursery. All states in the United States currently screen for the disorders phenylketonuria and congenital hypothyroidism. Screening for sickle-cell disease has been recommended by a National Institutes of Health Consensus Conference, and many states also screen for galactosemia and homocystinuria. These disorders have been selected for early screening because detection and prompt treatment in infancy can prevent mental retardation or severe, life-threatening illness.

The most common disorder detected by screening is sickle-cell disease, with an incidence as high as 1 in 400 births. Early identification allows prevention of infection in childhood, as well as prompt medical intervention if sickle-cell crisis develops. Hypothyroidism occurs in 1 in 5000 deliveries and can result in permanent mental retardation unless detected and treated with thyroid hormone replacement. Phenylketonuria is a rare defect in phenylalanine metabolism (1 in 14,000 deliveries) in which severe mental retardation can develop if the infant is not provided with a special formula low in phenylalanine. Galactosemia is also a rare metabolic defect (1 in 50,000 births) in which life-threatening toxic effects of elevated blood galactose can occur in the affected infant after feeding. A special galactose-free diet is essential for survival and normal development of these infants. Homocystinuria is a disorder of methionine metabolism, which may result in mental retardation and severe disability unless detected in infancy and treated with dietary management.

Blood specimens for these disorders are obtained from every neonate before the baby is discharged from the nursery. The specimens are forwarded to the responsible laboratory, and results of the tests are returned to the physician ordering them. Infants with abnormal screening results are then referred for definitive medical evaluation. Earlier discharge of the mother-infant dyad has prompted reorganization of the testing procedure, with home screening when necessary. Phenylketonuria and other disorders may be detected only after the initiation of feeding, when metabolites will accumulate. Hence, if the initial specimen is obtained before 24 hours of age, a second specimen should be obtained at 1 to 2 weeks of age to decrease the probability of missing these disorders. The positive cost/benefit ratio of newborn metabolic screening continues to justify the personnel and financial commitment to these disorders.

NEURODEVELOPMENTAL OUTCOME

Advances in perinatal and neonatal care have largely been responsible for improved survival in high-risk neonates. Following the introduction of modern neonatal intensive care in the 1960s, there was a decrease in adverse neurodevelopmental sequelae compared with the preceding era. During the 1970s and 1980s, mortality continued to decrease so that the absolute number of both healthy and neurologically impaired very-low-birth-weight survivors has actually increased. However, conditions of presumed genetic and prenatal origin account for more children with neurodevelopmental disorders than problems arising out of the perinatal period. Also, because more infants are born full-term, more term children have cerebral palsy than preterm infants. Infants who are at risk for later neurodevelopmental problems include those who had severe asphyxia, extensive intraventricular hemorrhage, periventricular leukomalacia, meningitis, or seizures, as well as infants with multisystem congenital malformations and those of very low birth weight.

Comparisons are inevitably made between results of neurodevelopmental follow-up from various tertiary perinatal centers (Hack, Klein, et al., 1995; Hack and Fanaroff, 2000). Weight-selected samples from different units may not be comparable, however, because outcome is heavily influenced by the following factors:

- Socioeconomic status of the parents
- Incidence of extreme prematurity
- Admission policies
- Proportion of inborn patients at any center

Although regional results do reflect a more accurate picture of outcome because they include all infants born in an area, such expensive and time-consuming studies are rarely available.

General Problems

Neonatal intensive care has resulted in increased morbidity resulting from various medical complications, including chronic neonatal lung disease, increased susceptibility to respiratory infection, sequelae of necrotizing enterocolitis, and cholestatic jaundice. These, in turn, could contribute to multiple rehospitalizations, poor physical growth, and an increase in postneonatal deaths. Up to 33% of infants with birth weight less than 1.5 kg are rehospitalized during the first year of life, and up to 10% are hospitalized during the second and third years of life (Hack, Wright, et al., 1995). Children with neurologic sequelae such as cerebral palsy and hydrocephalus have an even higher rate of rehospitalization for such reasons as shunt complications, orthopedic correction of spasticity, and eye surgery. Bjerager and colleagues (1995) noted that young adults (aged 20 years) born with very low birth weight appeared to have the same quality of life as their normal-birth-weight peers, provided they were free of handicap.

Intracranial Hemorrhage

Intracerebral hemorrhage occurs in up to 50% of very-low-birth-weight infants and is thought to be a substantial cause of morbidity and mortality in these patients. Bleeding occurs in the subependymal germinal matrix and may extend to the lateral ventricles and brain parenchyma. Potential etiologic factors include the following:

1. Capillary fragility
2. Abnormal regulation of cerebral blood flow
3. Coagulation abnormalities
4. Systemic hypertension or hypotension
5. Air leaks
6. Blood gas derangements

The rise of maternal chorioamnionitis and inflammation in the etiology of periventricular hemorrhage and periventricular leukomalacia is also being elucidated (Volpe, 2001).

Follow-up studies demonstrate that only *grade IV* intraventricular hemorrhages (which demonstrate intraparenchymal extension) carry a poor prognosis for neurologic outcome. *Grade I* (subependymal) and *grade II* (subependymal plus intraventricular) hemorrhages are not thought to impair the chances for a normal neurodevelopmental prognosis. *Grade III* hemorrhage is associated with ventricular dilation; the prognosis depends, in part, on the extent of the resultant hydrocephalus. Studies indicate that leukomalacia or intraparenchymal lesions that demonstrate echodensity on ultrasound examination may occur independently of intraventricular hemorrhage, are the result of necrosis secondary to ischemia, and carry a poor prognosis for subsequent normal development (Volpe, 2001).

In premature infants, there are two principal lesions that underlie brain injury: periventricular hemorrhagic infarction and periventricular leukomalacia. These lesions potentially are preventable: Periventricular hemorrhagic infarction can be avoided by preventing germinal-matrix intraventricular hemorrhage, while periventricular leukomalacia can be prevented by identifying and correcting alterations in cerebral blood flow and interrupting the cascade to oligodendroglial cell death by such agents as free-radical scavengers (Volpe, 1997). Antenatal steroid administration between 24 and 34 weeks' gestation reduces the incidence of grades III and IV intraventricular hemorrhage.

Severe intracranial hemorrhage can be prevented by the administration of indomethacin shortly after delivery. Follow-up data reveal no adverse effect of indomethacin on neurodevelopmental outcome in treated infants but no advantage either; cerebral palsy occurred in 7% of both indomethacin-treated and placebo-treated infants at 4.5 years of age (Ment et al., 1996; Ment et al., 2000; Schmidt et al., 2001; Schmidt et al., 2002).

Cranial ultrasound abnormalities are strong predictors of disabling cerebral palsy in low-birth-weight infants. Parenchymal echodensities/lucencies, or ventricular enlargement, are the most powerful predictors. Germinal matrix hemorrhage/intraventricular hemorrhage contribute independently to the risk of disabling cerebral palsy.

Growth Delay

Intrauterine or neonatal growth retardation occurs in up to 95% of very-low-birth-weight infants (Lemons et al., 2001). The poor neonatal growth is related to inadequate nutrition during the acute phase of neonatal disease and to chronic medical sequelae that result in increased caloric requirements.

These include chronic lung disease and malabsorption secondary to necrotizing enterocolitis or cholestatic liver disease. Poor feeding in neurologically impaired children and the lack of an optimal nurturing environment in the nursery could affect neonatal growth as well. As these conditions gradually resolve and an optimal home environment is provided, catch-up body growth could occur during the first 2 to 3 years of life.

Growth after discharge is a good measure of physical, neurologic, and environmental well-being. To promote optimal catch-up growth of high-risk infants, one must maximize neonatal nutrition and provide sufficient calories during the recovery phase. This is especially important because catch-up of head circumference in both appropriate and SGA children occurs only during the first 6 to 12 months after term. As noted earlier, measurement of head growth is a simple means of predicting neurodevelopmental outcome. If head growth, a surrogate for brain growth, does not catch up, the outlook is dismal. Catch-up of height and weight to above the third percentile can occur up to 8 years of age. Very-low-birth-weight infants continue to be smaller than the children delivered at term, however (Hack, Weissman, et al., 1996).

Neurodevelopmental Disorders

A very high incidence of *transient* neurologic abnormalities occurs in high-risk infants. These include abnormalities of muscle tone, such as hypotonia and hypertonia. Some degree of physiologic hypertonia normally exists during the first 3 months, and so it may be difficult to diagnose early spasticity related to cerebral palsy. Children who will develop cerebral palsy have hypotonia initially (poor head control and back support); spasticity of the extremities develops only later. Spasticity during the first 3 to 4 months is a poor prognostic sign. Persistence of primitive reflexes may also be a sign of early cerebral palsy. Although mild hypertonia or hypotonia persisting at 8 months usually resolves by the second year, it may indicate later subtle neurologic dysfunction (Georgieff et al., 1986). In normal awake infants, fidgety movements are seen from the age of 6 weeks to 20 weeks. These writhing movements can involve the whole body and last from seconds to minutes. There is a variable sequence of arm, leg, neck, and trunk movements that wax in intensity, force, and speed. The majority of sequences of flexion and extension movements of the arms and legs is complex, with superimposed rotations and slight changes in direction. Prechtl and colleagues (1997) tested the predictive value of absent or abnormal spontaneous movements for the later development of neurologic deficits. Normal neurologic outcome was found in 67 (90%) of 70 infants with normal fidgety movements. Abnormal quality or total absence of fidgety movements was followed by neurologic abnormalities in 57 (95%) of 60 infants, including cerebral palsy in 49. The specificity and sensitivity of fidgety movements (96% and 95%, respectively) were higher than by ultrasound imaging of the brain (83% and 80%, respectively). The movements are analyzed on videotape, but the technique is simple and nonintrusive. It will be added to the assessment of at-risk infants.

Major neurologic sequelae can usually be detected during the latter part of the first year of life in up to 10% of high-risk newborns or even earlier if signs are severe. Major neurologic handicap is usually classified as one of the following:

- Cerebral palsy (spastic diplegia, spastic quadriplegia, spastic hemiplegia, or paresis)
- Hydrocephalus (with or without accompanying cerebral palsy or sensory deficits)
- Blindness (usually caused by retinopathy of prematurity)
- Seizures
- Deafness

The intellectual outcome of these children can differ greatly according to the neurologic diagnosis. For example, children with spastic quadriplegia usually have severe mental retardation, whereas children with spastic diplegia or hemiplegia can have intact mental functioning. This is not always measurable until after 2 or 3 years of age.

Most neurologic or physical problems either resolve or become permanent during the first year of life. There is a close relationship between abnormal neurologic findings at 1 year in very-low-birth-weight infants and school performance at as late as 7 years (Vohr and Garcia Coll, 1985). During the second year of life, the environmental effects of maternal education and social class begin to play a major role in the various cognitive outcome measures. Further problems can emerge, such as subtle motor, visual, and behavioral difficulties. These are best diagnosed and treated in a psychological and educational rather than in a medical follow-up setting. A disturbing feature in recent years has been the high rates of learning problems and school failure among the low-birth-weight graduates from NICUs, even those with no apparent neurologic impairment and normal IQs. Educators must be alerted to this problem so that they can provide timely support (McCormick, 1997; Hack et al., 2002).

A number of reports have linked long-term poor school performance and neurologic problems with lower neonatal thyroxine concentrations. The risk of cerebral palsy is increased 11-fold, even after adjusting for multiple perinatal variables, including birth weight, gestational age, and prenatal, perinatal, and neonatal variables. Whether this association is causal remains unclear, however. Substitution therapy has not proved helpful in preventing neurologic and learning deficits (den Ouden et al., 1996; Lucas et al., 1996; Vulsma and Kock, 1996).

REFERENCES

AIDS Clinical Trials Group Protocol (Centers for Disease Control and Prevention): Recommendations for the use of zidovudine to reduce perinatal transmission of human immunodeficiency virus. MMWR **43** (No. RR-11):1, 1994.

Alexander GR, Himes JH, Kaufman RB, et al: A United States national reference for fetal growth. Obstet Gynecol **87**:163, 1996.

Allen R, Sorab J, Gonik B: Risk factors for shoulder dystocia: An engineering study of physician applied forces. Obstet Gyneol **77**:352, 1991.

American Academy of Pediatrics Committee on Infectious Diseases: Red Book 2000, 25th ed. Elk Grove Village, Ill, American Academy of Pediatrics Committee on Infectious Diseases, 2000.

American College of Obstetricians and Gynecologists Committee on Obstetrics: Perinatal care at the threshold of viability. ACOG Practice Bulletin No. 38, 2002.

Amin RS, Wert SE, Baughman RP, et al: Surfactant protein deficiency in familial interstitial lung disease. J Pediatr **139**:85, 2001.

Ashcraft KW, Holder TM: Esophageal atresia and tracheoesophageal fistula malformations. Surg Clin North Am **56**:299, 1976.

Babson SG, Benda GI: Growth graphs for the clinical assessment of infants of varying gestational age. J Pediatr **89**:814, 1976.

Ballard JL, Khoury JC, Wedig K, et al: New Ballard score, expanded to include extremely premature infants. J Pediatr **119**:417, 1991.

Ballard JL, Novak KK, Driver M: A simplified score for assessment of fetal maturation of newly born infants. J Pediatr **95**:769, 1979.

Bancalari E: Neonatal chronic lung disease. In Fanaroff AA, Martin RJ (eds): Neonatal-Perinatal Medicine, 7th ed. St. Louis, Mosby-Year Book, 2002, p. 1057.

Barrington KJ, Finer N, Li D: Predischarge respiratory recordings in very low birth weight newborn infants. J Pediatr **129**:6, 1996.

Bergman I, Painter MJ, Hirsch RP, et al: Outcome in neonates with convulsions treated in an intensive care unit. Ann Neurol **1**:219, 1983.

Bjerager M, Steensberg J, Greisen G: Quality of life among young adults born with very low birthweights. Acta Paediatr **84**:1339, 1995.

Bottoms SF, Paul RH, Mercer BM, et al: Obstetric determinants of neonatal survival: Antenatal predictors of neonatal survival and morbidity in extremely low birth weight infants. The NICHD Maternal Fetal Medicine Units Network. Am J Obstet Gynecol **180**:665, 1999.

Braun KR, Davidson KM, Henry M, et al: Severe pulmonary hemorrhage in the premature newborn infant: Analysis of presurfactant and surfactant eras. Biol Neonate **75**:18, 1999.

Caplan MS, MacKendrick W: Inflammatory mediators and intestinal injury. Clin Perinatol **21**:235, 1994.

Carlo WA, Martin RJ, Fanaroff AA: Assisted ventilation and complications of respiratory distress. In Fanaroff AA, Martin RJ (eds): Neonatal-Perinatal Medicine, 7th ed. St. Louis, Mosby-Year Book, 2002, p. 1011.

Clark RH, Dykes FD, Bachman TE: Intraventricular hemorrhage and high-frequency ventilation: A meta-analysis of prospective clinical trials. Pediatrics **98**:6, 1996.

Clark R, Kuese TJ, Walker MW, et al: Low-dose nitric oxide therapy for persistent pulmonary hypertension of the newborn. N Engl J Med **342**:469, 2000.

Costarino AT, Gruskay JA, Corcoran L, et al: Sodium restriction versus daily maintenance replacement in very-low-birth-weight premature infants. J Pediatr **120**:99, 1992.

Courtney S, Durand DJ, Asselin JM, et al. High frequency oscillatory ventilation versus conventional mechanical ventilation for very low birth weight infants. N Engl J Med **347**:643, 2002.

Dahm LS, James LS: Newborn temperature and calculated heat loss in the delivery room. Pediatrics **49**:504, 1972.

Davis JM, Veness-Meehan K, Notter RH, et al: Changes in pulmonary mechanics after the administration of surfactant to infants with respiratory distress syndrome. N Engl J Med **319**:476, 1988.

den Ouden AL, Kok JH, Verkerk PH, et al: The relation between neonatal thyroxine levels and neurodevelopmental outcome at age 5 and 9 years in a national cohort of very preterm and/or very low birth weight infants. Pediatr Res **39**:142, 1996.

Deorari AK, Paul VK, Shreshta L, et al: Symptomatic neonatal polycythemia: Comparison of partial exchange transfusion with saline versus plasma. Indian Pediatr **32**:1167, 1995.

Drew JH, Guaran RL, Cichello M, et al: Neonatal whole blood hyperviscosity: The important factor influencing later neurologic function is the viscosity and not the polycythemia. Clin Hemorheol Microcirc **17**:67, 1997.

Dubowitz L, Dubowitz V, Goldberg C: Clinical assessment of gestational age in the newborn infant. J Pediatr **77**:1, 1970.

El-Metwally D, Vohr B, Tucker R: Survival and neonatal morbidity at the limits of viability in the mid 1990's: 22 to 25 weeks. J Pediatr **137**:616, 2000.

Fujiwara T, Macta H, Chida S, et al: Artificial surfactant therapy in hyaline membrane disease. Lancet **1**:55, 1980.

Garland J, Buck R, Weinberg M: Pulmonary hemorrhage risk in infants with a clinically diagnosed patent ductus arteriosus: A retrospective cohort study. Pediatrics **94**:719, 1994.

Georgieff MK, Bernbaum JC, Hoffman-Williamson M, et al: Abnormal truncal muscle tone as a useful early method for developmental delay in low birth weight infants. Pediatrics **77**:659, 1986.

Gladman G, McCrindle BW, Boutin C, et al: Fetal echocardiographic screening of diabetic pregnancies for congenital heart disease. Am J Perinatol **14**:59, 1997.

Goldberg RN, Moscosco P, Bauer GR, et al: Use of barbiturate therapy in severe perinatal asphyxia: A randomized controlled trial. J Pediatr **109**:851, 1986.

Goldenberg RL, Rouse DJ: Preterm birth, cerebral palsy and magnesium. Nat Med **3**:146, 1997.

Gregory GA: Pediatric Anesthesiology. New York, Churchill Livingstone, 1989.

Grosfeld JL, Dawes L, Weber TR: Congenital abdominal wall defects: Current management and survival. Surg Clin North Am **61**:1037, 1981.

Hack M, Breslau N, Weissman B, et al: Effects of very low birth weight and subnormal head size on cognitive abilities at school age. N Engl J Med **325**:231, 1991.

Hack M, Fanaroff AA: Outcome of growth failure associated with preterm birth. Clin Obstet Gynecol **27**:647, 1984.

Hack M, Fanaroff AA: Outcomes of children of extremely low birth weight and gestational age in the 1990s. Semin Neonatol **5**:89; 2000.

Hack M, Flannery DJ, Schluchter M, et al: Outcomes in young adulthood for very-low-birth-weight infants. N Engl J Med **346**:149, 2002.

Hack M, Klein NK, Taylor HG: Long-term developmental outcomes of low birth weight infants. Future Children **5**:176, 1995.

Hack M, Weissman B, Borawski-Clark E: Catch-up growth during childhood among very low-birth-weight children. Arch Pediatr Adolesc Med **150**:1122, 1996.

Hack M, Wright L, Shankaran S, et al: Very low birth weight outcomes of the National Institutes of Child Health and Human Development Neonatal Network, November 1989 to October 1990. Am J Obstet Gynecol **172**:457, 1995.

Hamvas A, Nogee LM, Mallory GB Jr, et al: Lung transplantation for treatment of infants with surfactant protein B deficiency. J Pediatr **130**:231, 1997.

HIFI Study Group: High frequency oscillatory ventilation compared with conventional mechanical ventilation in the treatment of respiratory failure in preterm infants. N Engl J Med **320**:88, 1989.

Holmes LB: Type and etiology of major malformations in 18,155 newborns. N Engl J Med **195**:204, 1976.

Ikegami M, Korfhagen TR, Bruno MD, et al: Surfactant metabolism in surfactant protein A–deficient mice. Am J Physiol (Lung Cell Mol Physiol) **272**:L479, 1997.

Jain L, Ferre C, Vidyasagar D, et al: Cardiopulmonary resuscitation of apparently stillborn infants: survival and long-term outcome. J Pediatr **118**:778, 1991.

Jobe AH: Pulmonary surfactant therapy. N Engl J Med **328**:861, 1993.

Johnson AH, Peacock JL, Greenough A, et al: High frequency oscillatory ventilation for the prevention of chronic lung disease of prematurity. N Engl J Med **347**:633, 2002.

Jones RAK, Robertsen NRC: Small for dates babies: Are they really a problem? Arch Dis Child **61**:877, 1986.

Kelly E, Bryan H, Possmayer F, et al: Compliance of the respiratory system in newborn infants pre- and postsurfactant replacement therapy. Pediatr Pulmonol **15**:225, 1993.

Kinsella J, Abman S: Clinical approach to inhaled nitric oxide therapy in the newborn with hypoxemia. J Pediatr **136**:6, 2000.

Klaus MH, Fanaroff AA (eds): Care of the High-Risk Neonate, 4th ed. Philadelphia, WB Saunders, 1993.

Kurczynski TW: Congenital malformations. In Fanaroff AA, Martin RJ (eds): Neonatal-Perinatal Medicine, 5th ed. St. Louis, Mosby-Year Book, 1992, p. 372.

Leder ME, Kliegman RM, Fanaroff AA: Epidemiology and management of severe symptomatic neonatal hypertension. Am J Perinatol **3**:235, 1986.

Legido A, Clancy RR, Berman PH: Neurologic outcome after electroencephalographically proven neonatal seizures. Pediatrics **88**:583, 1991.

Lemons JA, Bauer CR, Oh W, et al: Very low birth weight outcomes of the National Institute of Child Health and Human Development Neonatal Research Network, January 1995 through December 1996. NICHD Neonatal Research Network. Pediatrics **107**(1):E1, 2001.

Liechty EA, Donovan E, Purohit D, et al: Reduction of neonatal mortality after multiple doses of bovine surfactant in low birth weight neonates with respiratory distress syndrome. Pediatrics **88**:19, 1991.

Lotze A, Mitchell BR, Bulas DI, et al: Multicenter study of surfactant (beractant) use in the treatment of term infants with severe respiratory failure. Survanta in Term Infants Study Group. J Pediatr **132**:40, 1998.

Lucas A, Cole TJ: Breast milk and neonatal necrotising enterocolitis. Lancet **336**:1519, 1990.

Lucas A, Morley R, Fewtrell MS: Low triiodothyronine concentration in preterm infants and subsequent intelligence quotient (IQ) at 8 year follow up. BMJ **312**:1132, 1996.

MacDonald H. and the Committee on Fetus and Newborn. American Academy of Pediatrics. Perinatal Care at the Threshold of Viability. Pediatrics **110**(5):1024, 2002.

Madansky DL, Lawson EE, Chernick V, et al: Pneumothorax and other forms of pulmonary air leaks in newborns. Am Rev Respir Dis **120**:729, 1979.

Maisels MJ, Gifford K: Normal serum bilirubin levels in the newborn and the effect of breast-feeding. Pediatrics **78**:837, 1986.

Martin RJ, Miller MM, Carlo WA: Pathogenesis of apnea in preterm infants. J Pediatr **109**:733, 1986.

McCormick MC: The outcomes of very low birth weight infants: Are we asking the right questions? (Commentary). Pediatrics **99**:869, 1997.

McIntire DD, Bloom SL, Casey BM, et al: Birth weight in relation to morbidity and mortality among newborn infants. N Engl J Med **340**:1234, 1999.

Ment LR, Vohr B, Allan W, et al: Outcome of children in the indomethacin intraventricular hemorrhage prevention trial. Pediatrics **105**:485, 2000.

Ment LR, Vohr B, Oh W, et al: Neurodevelopmental outcome at 36 months corrected age of preterm infants in the multicenter indomethacin intraventricular hemorrhage prevention trial. Pediatrics **98**:714, 1996.

Miller MJ, DiFiore JM, Strohl KP, et al: Effect of nasal CPAP on supraglottic and total pulmonary resistance in preterm infants. J Appl Physiol **6**:141, 1990.

Miller MJ, Fanaroff AA, Martin RJ: Respiratory disorders in preterm and term infants. *In* Fanaroff AA, Martin RJ (eds): Neonatal-Perinatal Medicine, 7th ed. St. Louis, Mosby, 2002, p. 1025.

Mills JL, Knapp RH, Simpson JL, et al: Lack of relation of increased malformation rates in infants of diabetic mothers to glycemic control during organogenesis. N Engl J Med **318**:671, 1988.

Mizrahi EM: Neonatal electroencephalography: Clinical features of the newborn, techniques of recording, and characteristics of the normal EEG. Am J EEG Technol **26**:81, 1986.

Mizrahi EM, Kellaway P: Seizures of neonates and young infants with and without accompanying EEG epileptiform activity: An EEG/polygraph/video monitoring study. Epilepsia **25**:668, 1984.

Moses D, Holme BA, Spitale P, et al: Inhibition of pulmonary surfactant function by meconium. Am J Obstet Gynecol **164**:477, 1991.

Nathan D, Orkin S: *In* Nathan D, Oski F: Hematology of Infancy and Childhood, 5th edition. Philadelphia, WB Saunders, 1998.

Newman KD, Anderson KD, VanMeurs K, et al: Extracorporeal membrane oxygenation and congenital diaphragmatic hernia: Should any infant be excluded? J Pediatr Surg **25**:1048, 1990.

Nicolaides KH, Bradley RJ, Soothill PW, et al: Maternal oxygen therapy for intrauterine growth retardation. Lancet **i**:942, 1987.

NINOS Study Group: Inhaled nitric oxide and hypoxic respiratory failure in infants with congenital diaphragmatic hernia. Pediatrics **99**:838, 1997a.

NINOS Study Group: Inhaled nitric oxide in full term and nearly full term infants with hypoxic respiratory failure. N Engl J Med **336**:597, 1997b.

NINOS Study Group: Inhaled nitric oxide in term and near term infants: Neurodevelopmental follow-up of The Neonatal Inhaled Nitric Oxide Study Group (NINOS) J Pediatr **136**:611, 2000.

Nogee LM, Dunbar AE, Wert SE, et al: A mutation in the surfactant protein C gene associated with familial interstitial lung disease. N Engl J Med **344**:573, 2001.

Novotny DA, Klein RL, Boeckman CR: Gastroschisis: An 18 year review. J Pediatr Surg **28**:650, 1993.

Oski FA, Naiman JL: Hematologic problems in the newborn. *In* Problems in Clinical Pediatrics. Philadelphia, WB Saunders, 1982.

Pappin A, Shenker N, Hack M, et al: Extensive intraalveolar pulmonary hemorrhage in infants dying after surfactant therapy. J Pediatr **124**:621, 1994.

Phibbs CS, Bronstein JM, Buxton E, et al: The effects of patient volume and level of care at the hospital of birth on neonatal mortality. JAMA **276**:1054, 1996.

Pildes R: Infants of diabetic mothers. N Engl J Med **289**:902, 1973.

Poland RL, Ostrea EM Jr: Neonatal hyperbilirubinemia. *In* Klaus M, Fanaroff AA (eds): Care of the High-Risk Neonate, 4th ed. Philadelphia, WB Saunders, 1993.

Prechtl HFR, Einspeiter C, Cioni G, et al: An early marker for neurological deficits after perinatal brain lesions. Lancet **349**:1361, 1997.

Primhak RA: Factors associated with pulmonary air leak in premature infants receiving mechanical ventilation. J Pediatr **102**:764, 1983.

Reller MD, Rice MJ, McDonald RW: Review of studies evaluating ductal patency in the premature. J Pediatr **122**:S59, 1993.

Rodriguez RJ, Martin RJ, Fanaroff AA: Respiratory distress syndrome and its management. *In* Fanaroff AA, Martin RJ (eds): Neonatal-Perinatal Medicine, 7th ed. St. Louis, Mosby, 2002, p. 1001.

Roithmaier A, Arlettaz R, Bauer K, et al: Randomized controlled trial of Ringer solution versus serum for partial exchange transfusion in neonatal polycythaemia. Eur J Pediatr **154**(1):53–56, 1995.

Rossi EM, Philipson EH, Williams TG: Meconium aspiration syndrome: Intrapartum and neonatal attributes. Am J Obstet Gynecol **161**:1106, 1989.

Scher M: Seizures in the newborn infant: Diagnosis, treatment and outcome. Clin Perinatol **24**:735, 1997.

Scher MS, Aso K, Beggarly ME, et al: Electrographic seizures in preterm and full term neonates: Clinical correlates, associated brain lesions, and risk for neurological sequelae. Pediatrics **91**:128, 1993.

Schmidt B, Davis P, Moddemann D, et al: Long-term effects of indomethacin prophylaxis in extremely-low-birth-weight infants. N Engl J Med **344**:1966; 2001.

Schmidt B, Wright LL, Davis P, et al: Ibuprofen prophylaxis in preterm neonates. Lancet **60**:492, 2002.

Schrag S, Gorwitz R, Fultz-Butts K, et al: Prevention of perinatal group B streptococcal disease. Revised guidelines from CDC. MMWR Recomm Rep **51**(RR-11):1, 2002.

Schwartz RM, Luby AM, Scanlon JW, et al: Effect of surfactant on morbidity, mortality, and resource use in newborn infants weighing 500 to 1500 g. N Engl J Med **330**:1476, 1994.

Soll RF: Multiple versus single-dose natural surfactant extract for severe neonatal respiratory distress syndrome (Cochrane Review). In the Cochrane Library, Issue 2, CD000141, 2001.

Srinivasan G, Pildes RS, Cattamanchi G, et al: Plasma glucose values in normal neonates: A new look. J Pediatr **109**:114, 1986.

Stagno S: Diagnosis of viral infections of the newborn infant. Clin Perinatol **8**:579, 1981.

Stoll BJ, Hansen N, Fanaroff AA: Late-onset sepsis in very low birth weight neonates: the experience of the NICHD Neonatal Research Network. Pediatrics **110**:285; 2002a.

Stevens TP, Blennow M, Soll RF: Early surfactant administration with brief ventilation vs selective surfactant and continued mechanical ventilation for preterm infants with or at risk for RDS. Cochrane Database Syst Rev, CD003063, 2002.

Stoll BJ, Hansen N, Fanaroff AA: Changes in pathogens causing early-onset sepsis in very-low-birth-weight infants. N Engl J Med **347**:240, 2002b.

Stork EK, Carlo WA, Kliegman R, et al: Hypertension redefined for critically ill neonates. Pediatr Res **18**:321A, 1984.

Tooley WH, Phibbs RH, Sohleuter MA: Intrauterine Asphyxia and the Developing Fetal Brain. Chicago, Year Book Medical Publishers, 1977.

Tyson JE, Younes N, Verter J, et al: Viability, morbidity and resource use among newborns of 501–800 g birth weight. JAMA **276**:1645, 1996.

Vergani P, Ghidini A, Locatelli A, et al: Risk factors for pulmonary hypoplasia in second trimester premature rupture of membranes. Am J Obstet Gynecol **170**:273, 1994.

Vermont-Oxford Neonatal Network: A multicenter randomized trial comparing synthetic surfactant with modified bovine surfactant extract in the treatment of neonatal respiratory distress syndrome. Pediatrics **97**:1, 1996.

Vohr BR, Garcia Coll CT: Neurodevelopmental and school performance of very low birth weight infants: A seven-year longitudinal study. Pediatrics **76**:345, 1985.

Volpe JJ: Brain injury in the premature infant: Neuropathology, clinical aspects, pathogenesis, and prevention. Clin Perinatol **24**:567, 1997.

Volpe JJ: Neurology of the Newborn, 4th ed. Philadelphia, WB Saunders, 1999.

Volpe JJ: Neurobiology of periventricular leukomalacia in the premature infant. Pediatr Res **50**:553, 2001.

Vulsma T, Kok JH: Prematurity-associated neurologic and developmental abnormalities and neonatal thyroid function (editorial; comment). N Engl J Med **334**:857, 1996.

Walsh DS, Adzick NS, Sutton LN, et al: The rationale for in utero repair of myelomeningocele. Fetal Diagn Ther **16**:312, 2001.

Warshaw JB: Intrauterine growth retardation: Adaptation or pathology? Commentary. Pediatrics **76**:998, 1985.

Weisman LE, Stoll BJ, Creuss DF, et al: Early onset Group B streptococcal sepsis: A current reassessment. Pediatrics **121**:428, 1992.

Weiss H, Cooper B, Brook M, et al: Factors determining reopening of the ductus arteriosus after successful clinical closure with indomethacin. J Pediatr **127**:466, 1995.

Wiswell TE, Bent RC: Meconium staining and the meconium aspiration syndrome. Pediatr Clin North Am **40**:995, 1993.

Wiswell TE, Gannon CM, Jacob J, et al. Delivery room management of the apparently vigorous meconium stained neonate: Results of the Multicenter, International, Collaborative Trial. Pediatrics **105**:1, 2000.

Wiswell TE, Knight GR, Finer NN, et al: A multicenter, randomized, controlled trial comparing Surfaxin (Lucinactant) lavage with standard care for treatment of meconium aspiration syndrome. Pediatrics **109**:1081, 2002.

Wolfson MR, Greenspan JS, Deoras KS, et al: Comparison of gas and liquid ventilation: Clinical, physiological and histological correlates. J Appl Physiol **723**:1024, 1992.

Zahka KA, Lane JR: Approach to the neonate with cardiovascular disease. *In* Fanaroff AA, Martin RJ (eds): Neonatal-Perinatal Medicine, 7th ed. St. Louis, Mosby-Year Book, 2002, p. 1112.

Chapter 61

CEREBRAL PALSY

Robert L. Goldenberg, MD

In 1862, a London orthopedic surgeon, William John Little, described a group of children with motor abnormalities, or "spastic rigidity," and related this condition to pregnancy complications and preterm birth (Little, 1862). Others soon began studying and attempting to classify the childhood motor disorders, including Sarah McNutt, who reportedly toured widely, lecturing on the relationships among complications of labor, difficult deliveries, the errors of obstetricians, and spastic rigidity (Ingram, 1984).

During the subsequent decades, there was a great deal of activity related to the "birth palsies," and many physicians, including Freud, wrote extensively on this subject. In fact, Freud (1897) described a classification scheme based on the muscles that were affected, which constitutes the foundation of many of the classification schemes used today. Disagreements over the definition of and the most appropriate classification schemes for cerebral palsy, however, have been common since then, and to date, no consensus on the best classification scheme has emerged (Bax, 1964; Ingram, 1984). Nevertheless, there is a relatively wide consensus on the overall definition of cerebral palsy. Perhaps the most commonly used is that of Nelson and Ellenberg (1978), who defined cerebral palsy as "a chronic disability characterized by aberrant control of movement or posture appearing early in life and not the result of recognized progressive disease."

Voluntary and involuntary motor performance are coordinated through a network of central nervous system (CNS) structures, including the cerebral cortex, pyramidal tracts, thalamus, cerebellum, basal ganglia, brain stem, and spinal cord (Fig. 61-1). In making a diagnosis of cerebral palsy, one must differentiate between injury to lower motor neurons and injury to upper motor neurons. Injury to lower motor neurons (i.e., spinal cord or nerve damage) often results in fasciculation, atrophy, flaccidity, hypotonia, and loss of tendon reflexes. In contrast, cerebral palsy, which is associated with upper motor neuron injuries, manifests as excessive muscular tonus, spasticity with increased stretch reflexes, and hyperactive tendon reflexes. Cerebral palsy, therefore, is associated with damage to the upper motor neurons within the brain, not to the spinal cord.

Cerebral palsy is a neuromuscular condition only and does not imply alterations in cognitive function. Although children who have cerebral palsy are statistically more likely to have low intelligence quotients (IQs), mental retardation, or various types of seizure disorders, many children with cerebral palsy have normal intelligence and are free of other types of neurologic disability (Nelson and Ellenberg, 1988).

Despite the absence of a single specific classification system, most systems contain similar components (Ingram, 1984). For example, nearly all systems classify the motor dysfunction by the predominant characteristic, such as spasticity, flaccidity, dyskinesis, or ataxia. Of these types, *spastic cerebral palsy* is by far the most common. Children with spastic cerebral palsy generally present with persistent hypertonia and rigidity (often described as having a "clasp-knife" quality) and often experience contractures and abnormal curvatures of the spine. Spastic cerebral palsy occurs predominantly because of cerebral cortex and pyramidal tract injury. Because of the distribution of the nerve fibers related to specific muscle groups within the pyramidal tracts, periventricular injury is more likely to affect the lower extremities (Fig. 61-2). More diffuse damage to the cortex and pyramidal tracts tends to result in spastic quadriplegia. In this condition's severest form, muscles of the face, chest, and abdomen are affected as well.

Dyskinetic cerebral palsy is thought to involve the basal ganglia and the extrapyramidal tracts. The child is marked by impaired voluntary muscle control that often involves incomplete and fragmented movements. Motor movements can be characterized as bizarre, twisting motions with exaggerated posturing that is more obvious in the distal extremities. This form of cerebral palsy is classified by the type of movement and not by specific muscle groups, because all four extremities are affected. Upper extremities tend to be more involved than lower extremities, however, and facial muscles are often involved as well. Dyskinesis is often associated with increased muscle tone but is often described as "lead pipe" in contrast with the clasp-knife quality. In the past, terms such as *athetoid*, *choreoathetoid*, or *dystonic* were used to describe the varied movements. Dyskinetic cerebral palsy is less common now than in the past, probably because many cases were associated with kernicterus.

Finally, *ataxic cerebral palsy* is marked by poor muscle coordination and lack of balance and position sense. Much of the neurologic damage is believed to occur in the cerebellum because cerebellar injury characteristically results in abnormal muscle coordination, lack of balance, and lack of position sense. The infant is often floppy at birth, but later the hypotonia is replaced by a gradual increase in tone and stiffness. The later years are marked by gait disturbances and muscle instability. In some of these cases, however, the generalized hypotonia persists; this condition is labeled *atonic cerebral palsy*.

Included in nearly all classification schemes are the patterns of motor involvement. Although any muscle group can be affected, several patterns predominate:

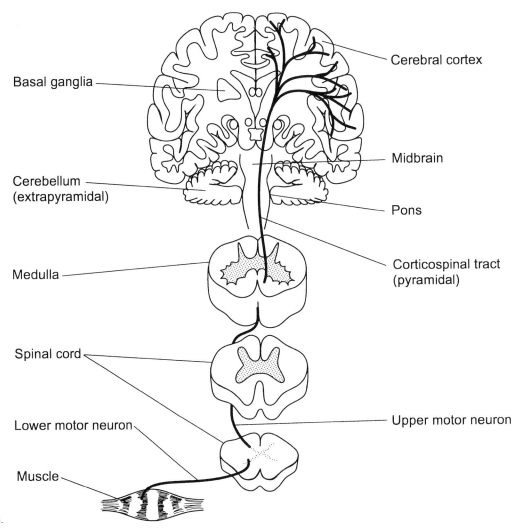

FIGURE 61-1 ■ Motor pathways.

- If all four limbs have major involvement, the cerebral palsy is defined as *quadriplegia*.
- When the lower extremities are predominantly involved, the cerebral palsy is classified as *diplegia*.
- If one side of the body is involved, the cerebral palsy is classified as *right or left hemiplegia*.

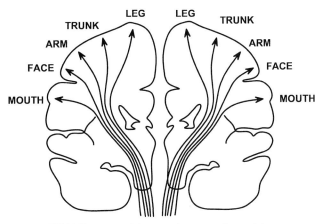

FIGURE 61-2 ■ Motor pathways and ventricles.

- Single-limb involvement, which is rare, is called *monoplegia*.

Most classification schemes emphasize the extremities, but it is clear that many children with cerebral palsy, especially the most severely affected, have motor problems that affect the face and mouth. Therefore, for some children with cerebral palsy, feeding can be problematic because of difficulty with chewing, swallowing, and sucking. These difficulties can be associated with the additional problems of gagging, drooling, and even aspiration. Affected children could also have respiratory difficulties because of an inability to expand the chest and the inability to clear mucus secretions.

With the availability of magnetic resonance imaging (MRI) and other imaging techniques, some authors are now classifying cerebral palsy by the location of brain lesions either in the neonatal period or at the time of diagnosis during childhood. MRI reveals specific brain lesions in 70%–90% of children with cerebral palsy (Yin et al., 2000). At least some authors classify these into pyramidal tract lesions (found mostly in the periventricular area) and extrapyramidal lesions in sites such as the basal ganglia and thalamus. Pyramidal tract lesions are more commonly associated with spastic diplegia and are frequent in children born before term, whereas extrapyramidal lesions are more common in term infants with quadriplegia, often of the dyskinetic variety (Truwit et al., 1992; Candy et al., 1993; Capute and Accardo, 1996).

When the time of origin is known, the cerebral palsy may be classified by time of onset (i.e., prenatal, perinatal, or postnatal). Similarly, when there is a clear etiology such as asphyxia, preterm birth, or viral infection, the cerebral palsy may be classified by its etiology. Usually, some measure of the degree of disability is included in the classification scheme. Mild cerebral palsy, for example, has been defined as cerebral palsy that does not interfere substantially with activities of daily living. Moderate cerebral palsy is marked by substantial disability with a need for wheelchair, bracing, or other assistance. Severe cerebral palsy is marked by the inability to function independently in activities of daily living.

More recently, cerebral palsy has been classified by more complex levels of functioning, including measurements of mobility, physical dependency, pain and suffering, difficulty with schooling, and social, economic, and service burden (Jarvis and Hey, 1984). Children with cerebral palsy often have other associated neurologic impairments. Mental retardation—usually defined as an IQ of less than 70 or 75—is present in about half of cases of cerebral palsy, and one-third to one half of children with cerebral palsy also have a seizure disorder. Even when the disability is severe, however, children with cerebral palsy can have entirely normal intellectual functioning. Other problems, such as strabismus, amblyopia, cortical blindness, and hearing loss, are all more common in children with cerebral palsy than in nonaffected children.

These classification schemes are useful for at least two major purposes. First, understanding the association of various types of cerebral palsy with specific risk factors has been helpful for defining the predictors of this condition. Second, knowledge about the frequency and level of various disabilities has been necessary for predicting the overall need for services in affected children.

ETIOLOGY

Later in this chapter, the many potential causes of cerebral palsy, ranging from preterm birth to asphyxia to various infections and metabolic disorders, are addressed (Table 61-1). At this point, we stress that cerebral palsy is the end result of injury to the brain's motor pathways, and that the term *injury* is basically synonymous with *cell death*. As described previously, the motor pathways can be divided conceptually into pyramidal and extrapyramidal areas.

A number of authors state that particular brain regions are especially vulnerable to injury in certain time periods, a phenomenon known as *selective vulnerability* (Hoon et al., 1997). Johnston and associates (1995) emphasize that because myelinization is in its initial phases in the late second trimester, cerebral white matter is most susceptible to injury at that time. In contrast, the basal ganglia and other nonpyramidal motor areas appear to become most vulnerable to injury later in the pregnancy.

Regardless of the timing or the event leading to injury, it is likely that the cell death follows a similar final pathway that could include increased production of cytokines and nitric oxide, activation of N-methyl-D-aspartate (NMDA) receptors, and finally, calcium influx. If the injury occurs in the late second or early third trimester and is in the periventricular

TABLE 61-1. PUTATIVE ETIOLOGIC MECHANISMS IN CEREBRAL PALSY

Prenatal	Perinatal	Postnatal
Congenital CNS malformation	Abnormal fetal presentation	CNS infections
Fetal infection	Cerebral hemorrhage	Hypoxia Suffocation Drowning
Genetic syndromes Metabolic syndromes Familial ataxia Chromosome abnormalities	CNS infection	Kernicterus
Hypothyroidism	Hypoxia	Trauma
Hypoxia	Intrauterine infection	Vaccination reaction
Radiation exposure	Prematurity	Vascular thrombosis and other cerebrovascular conditions
Toxins (i.e., mercury, alcohol)	Trauma	

CNS, central nervous system.

area, death of oligodendrocytes in the pyramidal tract more likely results in spasticity of the lower extremities. Later in the pregnancy, more diffuse injuries, including injury to the basal ganglia, more likely result in quadriplegia.

PREVALENCE

Because cerebral palsy is a nonprogressive disorder present from infancy, it is probably inappropriate to study its "incidence," or the appearance of new cases over time. Therefore, prevalence, defined as the number of cases of the disease present during a specific time period, is the appropriate statistic to use. The population denominator has varied from study to study. For example, the denominator may include all live births, only neonatal survivors, or only children living in a specific geographic area (Paneth and Kiely, 1984).

Determining which infants to include in the numerator is also important. For example, Nelson and Ellenberg (1978) noted that children with cerebral palsy are more likely to die than children without this condition (10% by age 7 years), and these children could be lost from the numerator over time. In a study from Western Australia, Stanley and Watson (1992), who examined 74 children with an initial diagnosis of spastic diplegia, noted that 16 had already died by the time of the subsequent study. In addition, 15 of the remaining children no longer fulfilled the criteria for the diagnosis of spastic quadriplegia. Therefore, some children with apparent cerebral palsy experience a reduction in motor symptoms, so that at some point they may no longer be classified as having this condition. As another example, Nelson and Ellenberg (1982) reported that as many as 50% of children with a diagnosis of cerebral palsy by 1 year of age were free of any motor handicap at age 7 years, although many had evidence of other neurodevelopmental problems.

Adding to the difficulty in understanding its prevalence, cerebral palsy is not always clearly evident in the first year or two of life, and many series show additional case identifications (especially mildly affected children) through school age. Distinct from age of the child, spasticity or tightness of the lower extremities can variably be classified as cerebral palsy in a number of children. This occurs because abnormalities of motor function include cerebral palsy as well as various categories of decreased fine and gross motor skills and clumsiness. Differentiating these characteristics from cerebral palsy is not always easy. Therefore, the methods of case ascertainment, the rigor of the diagnosis, and the age of the child are all important considerations in defining the prevalence of this condition, and defining the prevalence of cerebral palsy for a particular birth population is particularly problematic. Also, because cerebral palsy is a relatively rare condition, biases resulting in the loss of just a few children or the overdiagnosis of several others can result in apparently dramatic changes in prevalence.

Alberman and Stanley (1984) from Australia emphasized the difficulties involved in studying cerebral palsy. These pitfalls included the following:

1. Cerebral palsy is not a single condition but rather a group of clinical syndromes.
2. It is difficult to classify the individual cerebral palsy syndromes.
3. Syndromes that appear identical may have different causes.
4. Timing of insults can occur anywhere in the prenatal, perinatal, and postpartum periods.
5. Anatomic studies have been few and often far removed from the time of the insult.
6. Cerebral palsy has a low prevalence, and large prospective studies are difficult to undertake, expensive, and time consuming.
7. The diagnosis can occur at least months and often years after birth.
8. The expression of the biological or anatomic damage is affected by a number of other factors (such as the child's environment) that could mitigate the impact of the anatomic damage.
9. In some children with cerebral palsy, the diagnostic classifications change over time; this could mean a change from one diagnostic category to another or a change away from cerebral palsy altogether.

These authors emphasize that many studies of cerebral palsy are flawed because of problems with selection and the confounding effect of interrelated variables. Compared with a pregnancy outcome such as death, the prevalence of cerebral palsy is much harder to define. Although there are death certificates, there are no certificates given or collected for cerebral palsy.

Despite all of these definitional and ascertainment problems, the prevalences of cerebral palsy found across studies have been remarkably consistent (Paneth and Kiely, 1984; Cans, 2000). Using a definition of prevalence as the number of affected living children per thousand live births, virtually all investigators reported a prevalence of cerebral palsy between 1.5 and 2.5 per thousand live births. Nearly all studies of cerebral palsy have been performed in developed countries, however, with most coming from Scandinavia, the United States, Great Britain, and Australia; little information exists about the prevalence of cerebral palsy in less developed areas. Within developed countries, little evidence suggests that the prevalence of cerebral palsy is higher in one location than in

another. Similarly, and although somewhat more controversial, there has been little evidence since about 1950 that the overall prevalence of cerebral palsy is changing; however, some areas report increases in prevalence, while others report decreases (Colver et al., 2000; Grether and Nelson, 2000; Hagberg et al., 2001).

In spite of the lack of evidence of changes in the overall prevalence of cerebral palsy, there is evidence that the prevalence of various subtypes has changed (Riikonen et al., 1989; Stanley and Watson, 1992). For example, since the 1970s, substantial evidence has been accumulating that the prevalence of choreoathetosis usually associated with kernicterus from hemolytic disease of the newborn is decreasing (Stanley, 1984). Among the many reasons for this decrease are the following:

1. Use of anti-D immunoglobulin in Rh-negative women
2. A marked reduction in the number of Rh-sensitized women
3. An overall decrease in parity, resulting in lower numbers of women who are Rh-sensitized in subsequent pregnancies
4. Intrauterine diagnosis and treatment in affected fetuses
5. Vigorous early diagnosis and treatment of neonatal jaundice by means of phototherapy and exchange transfusion

On the other hand, the prevalence of spastic diplegia, which is more common in surviving very-early-gestational-age preterm newborns, appears to be increasing (Colver et al., 2000; Wood et al., 2000).

In Turkey, Ozmen and coworkers (1993) described 1873 cases of cerebral palsy evaluated between 1982 and 1989. They make several important points about the prevalence of cerebral palsy in a country in which very-low-birth-weight infants rarely survive. Most of the cerebral palsy occurred in term infants, and the most common type of cerebral palsy was spastic quadriplegia; spastic diplegia was less common. Perinatal risk factors were often present in these cases. The pattern of cerebral palsy in Turkey versus that in more developed countries suggests that when survival of very-low-birth-weight infants is rare, spastic diplegia is less common, whereas spastic quadriplegia, often associated with asphyxic obstetric events, is more common and will be found predominantly in term infants.

These data and others presented later in the chapter argue strongly that certain types of cerebral palsy tend to be associated with specific causes. For example, spastic diplegia tends to be more common in very preterm infants because of frequent periventricular hemorrhage and leukomalacia. Spastic quadriplegia, which suggests diffuse brain damage, has frequently been associated with prolonged hypoxia-asphyxia. Bilirubin deposition has been associated with choreoathetoid cerebral palsy. Hemiplegias appear to result from brain injury to one cerebral hemisphere and not usually from diffuse brain damage, and they could represent the results of a localized hemorrhage or infarction.

DEMOGRAPHIC, SOCIAL, AND BIOLOGICAL RISK FACTORS

Both maternal age and parity are related to cerebral palsy, with a number of studies showing a U-shaped pattern in which infants of mothers who are younger than 20 and older than 34 years of age are at increased risk (Stanley, 1984). Both maternal age and parity are associated with a number of confounders, however, and it is not at all clear whether either is an independent predictor of cerebral palsy. For example, women of low or high maternal age and women of high parity are more likely to be at risk for prematurity and growth restriction, both of which are independent risk factors for cerebral palsy. As another example, women of high parity may have a greater number of pregnancies because of previous reproductive failures. It is therefore likely that the high parity is not in any way causal but is a surrogate measure for previous reproductive failure. Nevertheless, the decrease in the numbers of women with many pregnancies could be contributing to a small reduction in some types of cerebral palsy, especially that portion of cerebral palsy associated with Rh sensitization and kernicterus.

Low social class is associated with increased rates of low birth weight and preterm birth, and many authors have assumed that cerebral palsy also falls into the group of reproductive failures associated with lower social class. Most of the studies reveal little or no relationship between social class and the prevalence of cerebral palsy, however. In fact, regardless of whether social class has been categorized by income level, by father's occupation, or whether the studies were performed in the United States, Great Britain, or Australia, there is no clear relationship between social class and cerebral palsy. For example, in the U.S. Collaborative Perinatal Study (Nelson and Ellenberg, 1978), when social class was defined by combined scores for occupation, head of household, education, and total household income, social class was not significantly associated with cerebral palsy.

As with socioeconomic class, there is little evidence that differences in race are associated with the prevalence of cerebral palsy (Nelson and Ellenberg, 1978). If anything, in the United States, Caucasian children show slightly higher rates of cerebral palsy than African-American children, and Aboriginal children in Australia do not have higher rates of cerebral palsy than Australian Caucasian children (Stanley, 1984). The similarities in overall rates of cerebral palsy in various racial groups, despite large differences in rates of low birth weight, suggest that factors responsible for one condition may not necessarily be responsible for the other. Stanley (1984) points out, however, that although overall cerebral palsy is not more common in populations of low socioeconomic status, among black children in the United States and Aboriginal infants in Australia, an excess of postnatally acquired cerebral palsy occurs among the minority and presumably less privileged groups. Because postnatal cerebral palsy accounts for only about 10% of the total burden of cerebral palsy, an increase in this small etiologic fraction is not usually obvious in the overall prevalence of cerebral palsy.

Cerebral palsy is more likely to develop in boys than girls. This relationship has been reported in most studies, although one study from western Australia suggests that this observation may not be universal in all geographic areas or time periods (Stanley, 1984). Although an excess of males has been reported in association with a number of pregnancy-related complications, including preeclampsia, placental abruption, death, and other neurologic syndromes, the reasons for any of these differences, including cerebral palsy, are not apparent. The familial form of sex-related or X-linked spastic paraplegia is rare and does not appear to account for the difference in rates of cerebral palsy between male and female children.

MULTIPLE BIRTHS AND CEREBRAL PALSY

The risk for development of cerebral palsy in a twin infant is five or six times greater than that for a singleton, whereas triplets have another fivefold to sixfold increased risk over that in twins (Stanley, 1984; Scheller and Nelson, 1992; Cincotta et al., 2000). In a California study by Grether and coauthors (1992), twins constituted approximately 2% of the population but 10% of the population with cerebral palsy. Therefore, there is little question that cerebral palsy is more common in multiple births.

Twins and triplets are born preterm much more frequently than singleton infants, however, and the major question is whether or not multiple birth contributes to excess cerebral palsy over and above the association with preterm birth. The answer is provided in studies from Australia and California that have made it reasonably clear that at a given low birth weight or gestational age, the risk of cerebral palsy is not substantially greater in twins than in singletons. The higher rate of cerebral palsy in multiple births is largely explained by their tendency to be preterm. Several studies also have indicated that as the infants approach term or as the birth weight approaches 2500 g or more, twin infants have a twofold greater risk of cerebral palsy than their equivalently weighted or aged singleton counterparts. Whether this increased risk is associated with increased asphyxial episodes or the associated increase in fetal growth restriction or is an inherent problem of multiple births is unknown.

The rate of cerebral palsy in twins or triplets, however, is substantially increased if one of the fetuses dies in utero (Melnick, 1977). For example, in a study by Petterson and associates (1993), if one of the twins suffered a death in utero, the prevalence of cerebral palsy in the cotwin was tenfold to 15-fold higher than when both twins were liveborn and 60-fold higher than the prevalence of cerebral palsy in liveborn singletons. This finding is due largely to monochorionic placentation, in which the risk for development of periventricular leukomalacia (PVL) in the surviving cotwin is 30% (Bejar et al., 1990; Glinianaia et al., 2002). For triplets with one fetal death, the prevalence of cerebral palsy in the surviving infants was 15%; when all triplets were born alive, the rate was 3%. Therefore, the risk of cerebral palsy was substantially increased in older twins compared with singletons and in multiple births with a fetal death compared with multiple births without fetal death. These increased risks, plus the substantial increase in multiple births since the late 1970s associated with various ovulation induction and in vitro fertilization techniques, suggest that the contribution of multiple births to the overall cerebral palsy rate is substantial and very likely to be increasing.

PREMATURITY AND GROWTH RESTRICTION

It has been well known for nearly 150 years that low-birth-weight infants are at greater risk for cerebral palsy than full-sized infants. Only since the late 1960s, however, has a relatively clear distinction been made between babies born before term and growth-retarded or small-for-gestational-age (SGA) babies, and only recently has it become clear that cerebral palsy is much more common in preterm infants than in growth-retarded infants. In fact, questions remain about the importance of growth restriction as a predictor of cerebral palsy (Chard et al., 1993).

Prematurity

Although the relative importance of being preterm and the overall contribution of preterm birth to the prevalence of cerebral palsy has been debated over the years, there seems little question that infants born at the lowest extremes of birth weight or gestational age are at extremely high risk for cerebral palsy compared with term infants (Fig. 61-3). Data from several institutions suggest that in infants born at 23–25 weeks' gestation and at 500–600 g who survive, the diagnosis of cerebral palsy is made in about 25% (Finnstrom et al., 1998; Wilson-Costello et al., 1998; O'Shea and Dammann, 2000). When all infants weighing less than 1000 g are considered, approximately 5%–10% have cerebral palsy; however, infants born at 27 or 28 weeks' gestation and weighing about 1000 g have about a 3% likelihood of cerebral palsy. Infants of 36 weeks' gestation have a risk of cerebral palsy of about 5 per 1000, and only 1 per 1000 infants born at 40 weeks' gestation have cerebral palsy. The risk, therefore, decreases steadily as birth weight or gestational age increases (Ellenberg and Nelson, 1979; Hack et al., 1989, 1996; Cooke, 1990; Pharoah et al., 1990; Paneth, 1993).

To illustrate the relationship between preterm birth and cerebral palsy, Hagberg and Hagberg (1984) described a population of 681 children with cerebral palsy. Approximately one third of all the infants with cerebral palsy were born before term, compared with only 6% of the total population being preterm. When the various subclassifications of cerebral palsy were examined, more than 50% of the cases of spastic diplegia were associated with preterm birth. In contrast, only 7% of the cases of spastic quadriplegia were associated with preterm birth.

As the number of very-low-birth-weight (less than 1500 g) infants surviving has increased, the rate of cerebral palsy per 1000 liveborn infants within that birth-weight range has increased dramatically. For example, in Western Australia, cerebral palsy in liveborn infants weighing less than 1500 g rose from 15 per 1000 live births in 1967–1970 to more than 60 per 1000 live births in the period 1983–1985 (Stanley and Watson, 1992). The rate of cerebral palsy in surviving infants did not appear to change dramatically, however. Because there have been such dramatic increases in survival, especially in the infants weighing less than 1000 g, it is crucial to indicate whether the denominator for this group is per 1000 live births or per 1000 neonatal survivors.

As more very-low-birth-weight infants survive, the proportion of infants with cerebral palsy attributable to having very low birth weight increases. For example, the U.S. Collaborative Perinatal Project studied infants born between 1959 and 1966. In that study, only 9% of the cases of cerebral palsy were attributed to infants surviving with a birth weight of less than 1500 g (Nelson and Ellenberg, 1986). Later studies in the United States, however, showed that more than 30%, and perhaps as many as 50% (Doyle et al., 2000; O'Shea and Dammann, 2000) of children with cerebral palsy had birth weights less than 1500 g.

Similar increases have been reported from a number of other countries. In Sweden, from 1975–1982, the proportion of cerebral palsy cases with birth weight less than 1500 g increased from 9% to 18% and over time increased from 6% to 13% in Australia and from 5% to 21% in the United Kingdom (Hagberg et al., 1989). Therefore, as later birth cohorts are considered, a greater percentage of the cases of cerebral palsy

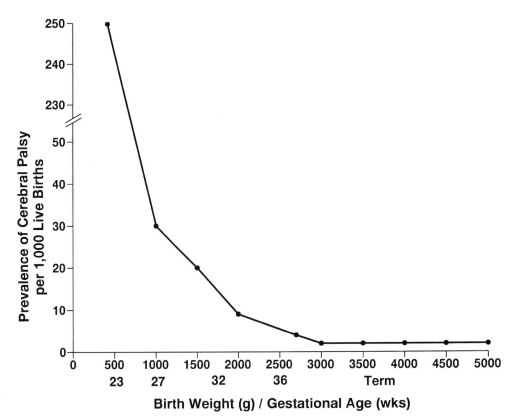

FIGURE 61-3 ■ Prevalence of cerebral palsy by birth weight and gestational age.

are found in the very-low-birth-weight group. When birth weights of less than 2500 g are considered, the contribution of low birth weight to cerebral palsy rose from 10% in the 1960s to 35%–40% in the 1980s and probably to 50% or more in the 1990s (O'Shea and Dammann, 2000; Doyle et al, 2000). Therefore, the rise in survival of very-low-birth-weight infants could be associated with an increase in the prevalence of school-aged children with cerebral palsy. Paneth (1993) notes that population-based registries in Western Australia, Finland, Southern Sweden, the United Kingdom, and Japan all have documented rises in school-aged children with cerebral palsy associated with very-low-birth-weight infants.

Attempting to explain this phenomenon, Paneth (1993) emphasized that in 1960, the mortality rate for Caucasian singletons weighing less than 1000 g in the United States was more than 99%; therefore, among the approximately 10,000 infants born at that weight, only 67 survived to 1 month. In 1983, among the 8500 Caucasian singleton infants born weighing less than 1000 g, nearly 4000 survived to 1 month of age. Thus, in 1983 there were 59 times as many Caucasian singleton survivors weighing less than 1000 g at birth than in 1960. Updating these numbers to 2002, we find that more than 80% of infants weighing less than 1000 g at birth are surviving. This suggests that there will be about 7000 Caucasian survivors of less than 1000 g birth weight, a 100-fold increase since 1960 in the population born weighing less than 1000 g, all of whom are at risk for cerebral palsy. Assuming a constant risk of cerebral palsy in these infants over time of about 10%, the absolute number of Caucasian infants in the United States with birth weights of less than 1000 g who survive with cerebral palsy has increased from about 7 in 1960 to more than 700 in the 1990s.

These types of epidemiologic associations, although clear, do not answer the question as to why preterm births are associated with cerebral palsy. Specifically, is it the gestational age itself or other factors associated with being born before term that predispose these infants to cerebral palsy? These issues are explored later in this chapter.

Growth Restriction

In this discussion, the terms *growth restriction* and *small for gestational age* are used synonymously. Understanding the controversy as to whether being SGA at birth is related to cerebral palsy helps one in the overall picture of ascribing an etiology to cases of cerebral palsy (Chard et al., 1993).

Many study designs have been used to evaluate neurodevelopmental outcome in SGA infants (Allen, 1984; Aylward et al., 1989). One of the most common is a cohort study in which the entire birth population is evaluated prospectively and the outcome associated with being in the lower 10th percentile of birth weight for gestational age is compared with either the entire non-SGA population or a representative sample. This type of study is labor-intensive in that only 10% of the children evaluated are SGA and the outcomes of interest, such as cerebral palsy, occur only occasionally. Therefore, these prospective cohort studies generally are not powerful enough to define significant relationships between SGA and major but rare outcomes, such as cerebral palsy, which are dichotomous. Instead, many of these cohort studies tend to consider continuous neurodevelopmental outcomes, such as the mean IQ score.

A retrospective case-control study is another type of study used to determine adverse outcomes associated with SGA status. In these studies, children with the outcome of interest, such as cerebral palsy, are first identified; then the rate of SGA status in the cases is compared with the rate of SGA status in the control group; and the relative risk of the association between SGA and cerebral palsy is determined. This type of study provides much of the evidence for the relationship between cerebral palsy and SGA.

Before the specific outcomes associated with SGA can be evaluated, it is important to emphasize that many of the factors associated with or that cause SGA could have a direct effect on neurologic development, independent of their effect on fetal growth. For example, many babies with chromosomal abnormalities are SGA. These infants also have several different types of neurodevelopmental handicaps, but it seems inappropriate to consider the SGA to have caused the neurodevelopmental handicaps. Instead, the chromosome anomaly itself is likely responsible for both the SGA and the neurodevelopmental handicap. Several other risk factors, such as congenital infection, various types of structural abnormalities, drug use, alcohol use, and smoking, all can cause growth restriction and may cause neurodevelopmental problems, but the growth restriction itself may not fall in the causative pathway for the neurologic dysfunction.

One of the difficult issues in dealing with adverse neurologic outcome in SGA infants is the relationship among SGA, hypoxia, and the adverse outcome. For example, it is often not clear whether any specific poor neurologic outcome is related to SGA status or to an associated hypoxic episode. Conceptually, poor placental function, a chronic condition, is a cause of at least a portion of the SGA status. If the SGA status is caused by poor transport of essential nutrients and oxygen across the placenta, one can easily imagine that poor fetal oxygenation, especially during labor, is a likely concurrent phenomenon. What is known is that poor oxygenation and the resultant acidemia are more common in SGA infants than in other infants (Low et al., 1982). As discussed later, however, there are no universal definitions for hypoxia, asphyxia, or acidemia. The nature of the association between these conditions and cerebral palsy, as well as other neurologic outcomes, is therefore debatable.

The question naturally arises: Are SGA infants who are not subject to decreased oxygenation in the perinatal period at risk for poor neurologic performance? In a study that addressed this issue, Berg (1989), using data from the Collaborative Perinatal Project, found that in the absence of hypoxia-related factors, neither children with symmetric intrauterine growth restriction (IUGR) nor children with asymmetric IUGR at age 7 years were at higher risk for neurologic morbidity, including cerebral palsy, than non-IUGR children. In the presence of perinatal hypoxia-related factors, however, children with IUGR were more likely to be neurologically abnormal than children without IUGR.

Similar conclusions have been reached by a number of other authors, including Uvebrant and Hagberg (1992), who agreed that at least part of the increase in cerebral palsy in term SGA infants was associated with asphyxia. Other authors have confirmed that low-ponderal-index SGA infants generally had normal outcomes unless they were asphyxiated at birth. Gilles and colleagues (1983) and Sims (1985) both provide data that suggest a mechanism for the increased risk of cerebral palsy associated with growth restriction. They note that an increased frequency of growth restriction and oligohydramnios was associated with perinatal white matter damage. The authors speculated that chronic hypoxia in the fetus that results in growth restriction and oligohydramnios could also be associated with the fetal cerebral ischemia leading to the white matter lesions.

A related issue is whether SGA status that is solely due to acute maternal nutritional deprivation is associated with long-term neurologic deficiencies. One of the few natural experiments in which this issue can be evaluated, the Dutch famine during World War II, showed no increase in cerebral palsy with nutritional deprivation alone (Susser and Stein, 1977). These data suggest that most of the adverse neurologic outcomes associated with SGA in otherwise healthy populations do not have a nutritional etiology but instead are due to nonnutritional causes.

Despite these considerations, review of the available data regarding the relationship between SGA and cerebral palsy allows some conclusions to be drawn. For example, babies born at term who later have cerebral palsy tend to be lighter at birth than those in whom cerebral palsy is not present. Nevertheless, most small babies, even if they are very SGA, do not eventually have cerebral palsy. In fact, most children with cerebral palsy are of normal birth weight. Translated into a measure of risk, being SGA at term appears to double or triple the risk of cerebral palsy (i.e., from 1 or 2 per 1000 live births to 2–6 per 1000 live births). Factors that appear to be associated with increased risk are the severity of the SGA, male sex, and whether asphyxia or other risk factors for cerebral palsy are present.

In many studies of preterm infants and cerebral palsy, preterm SGA infants appear to have less cerebral palsy than appropriate-for-gestational-age (AGA) preterm infants. These SGA preterm infants are frequently born in conjunction with maternal preeclampsia, and most studies suggest a protective effect of preeclampsia against cerebral palsy in preterm SGA infants (Murphy et al., 1995). Even this conclusion is not unanimous, however.

Robertson and coworkers (1990), for example, studying infants who weighed less than 1500 g and were in lower than the 10th percentile for weight, found that preterm SGA infants were not at greater risk for cerebral palsy than were AGA birth weight– or gestational age–matched controls, but all were at substantially greater risk than a term AGA comparison group. On the other hand, Hack and coauthors (1989), studying infants weighing less than 1500 g, observed an 8% rate of cerebral palsy in the AGA group but only a 3% rate ($P < 0.01$) in the SGA group. Veelken and associates (1992) also showed that SGA infants weighing less than 1500 g had less cerebral palsy than preterm AGA infants weighing less than 1500 g.

These data indicate that in cohorts defined by birth weight, SGA infants have less cerebral palsy. In cohorts defined by gestational age, however, SGA infants had similar or higher rates of cerebral palsy.

In summary, previous reviews suggest that SGA is a heterogeneous condition occasionally, but not usually, associated with various types of neurodevelopmental dysfunction including cerebral palsy (Goldenberg et al., 1998). No studies show that improvements in cerebral palsy or other neurologic outcomes can be achieved by any particular course of action in women with an SGA fetus. Logically, however, preventing asphyxia in SGA infants should reduce the prevalence of cerebral palsy, particularly among those who are asymmetric and associated with maternal hypertension. It is less clear whether

interventions directed at the more symmetric or uniformly undergrown infants will improve outcome in the relatively small percentage of these children who have major developmental problems (including cerebral palsy) associated with being SGA.

NONASPHYXIC CAUSES OF CEREBRAL PALSY

One investigative group in Western Australia has energetically studied risk factors for potential pathways leading toward the development of cerebral palsy (Stanley, 1984; Blair and Stanley, 1988, 1990). In one study using a time-ordered multivariate approach to distinguish confounders and their consequences from possible causes, the authors identified 18 factors as having an association with spasticity (Stanley et al., 1993). Only half of the cases of cerebral palsy (versus 14% of control cases) had one or more of these factors, however. No factor was present in more than 11% of cases, and most were present in less than 5% of cases. The authors concluded that many pathways led to the development of cerebral palsy, with each contributing only a small proportion. The authors also divided risk factors by time of onset and found that factors identified as occurring before labor started were present in 35% of all cases, whereas intrapartum initiation of the etiologic pathway was relatively unimportant, being present in only 9% of cases. Postpartum events explained only 10% of cases.

Murphy and associates (1995) found that the frequency of cerebral palsy increased with decreasing gestational age and birth weight. The factors associated with an increased risk of cerebral palsy after adjustment for gestational age included chorioamnionitis (odds ratio [OR] = 4.2), prolonged rupture of membranes (OR = 2.3), and other maternal infection (OR = 2.3). Interestingly, preeclampsia was associated with a reduced risk of cerebral palsy (OR = 0.4), as was delivery without labor (OR = 0.3). Growth restriction was not associated with an increased risk of cerebral palsy.

In a study by Torfs and colleagues (1990), significant predictors of cerebral palsy included unusually long or short interpregnancy intervals, the presence of a birth defect, low birth weight, low placenta weight, abnormal fetal position, and abruptio placentae. Of the children in this study with cerebral palsy, 78% had no evidence of birth asphyxia, whereas the 22% who did have evidence of asphyxia also had other prenatal risk factors.

Nelson and Ellenberg (1986) agreed that most of the predictors of cerebral palsy were present in only a small proportion of the mothers of children with cerebral palsy and accounted for only a small portion of the outcome. Additionally, most mothers with the identified risk factors did not produce infants with cerebral palsy. Because the cause of most cases of cerebral palsy is unknown and no single cause contributes to much of the outcome, no foreseeable specific intervention is likely to prevent a large proportion of cases of cerebral palsy. Specifically, of the maternal-infant pairs in the highest 5% risk for cerebral palsy, only 2.8% produced a child with cerebral palsy; the false-positive rate was therefore 97%. Epidemiologic studies published since then have not provided a reason to change the impression that our ability to identify modifiable causes of cerebral palsy is limited (Kuban and Leviton, 1994). Nevertheless, a discussion of some of these potential risk factors follows.

In a report from Western Australia, Palmer and colleagues (1995) noted that antepartum hemorrhage was a significant risk factor for the development of subsequent cerebral palsy; however, this risk was mediated entirely through the increased premature birth rate associated with antepartum hemorrhage. Neither preeclampsia nor urinary tract infection was significantly associated with cerebral palsy in this study. Blair and Stanley (1993) agreed, estimating that severe midtrimester hemorrhage was associated with a nearly fivefold increased risk of spasticity.

Maternal bleeding in women delivering at term is also associated with increased risk of cerebral palsy, but this increased risk is almost certainly mediated through a pathway that includes placental abruption and fetal asphyxia. Maternal bleeding is probably not an independent risk factor for cerebral palsy but, instead, is likely a surrogate measure for preterm birth, asphyxia, or both. Similarly, in a number of studies, an abnormal lie or a breech presentation was a risk factor for subsequent development of cerebral palsy. Because many infants with an abnormal lie are preterm, the relationship between abnormal lie and preterm birth is mediated at least in part by an increased risk of cerebral palsy in preterm infants.

Yet, the incidence of cerebral palsy is probably increased in term breech infants. Whether this relationship is the result of an increased risk of hypoxic events, more cerebral trauma, or fetal brain abnormalities present prior to labor that result in an inability of the fetus to maneuver into the vertex position is unknown. The increased risk of various congenital anomalies in breech infants, however, suggests that at least part of the statistical association sometimes described between term breech infants and cerebral palsy could be due to various types of congenital or developmental brain anomalies or injuries.

Data from various studies confirm that 20%–25% of cases of severe or moderate cerebral palsy are associated with a congenital malformation. These observations suggest that early-onset developmental abnormalities play a significant role in the etiology of cerebral palsy. Neonatal cretinism, associated with congenital iodine deficiency, presents a characteristic syndrome encompassing mental deficiency, deaf mutism, and spastic rigidity (Pharoah et al., 1971; Halpern et al., 1991). The motor disability is characteristic and differs from the usual forms of cerebral palsy in being primarily proximal, involving the pelvic and shoulder girdles, and tending to spare the feet and, particularly, the hands (McCarrison, 1988). Notable in infants with cretinism is the absence of ataxia and seizures. Lesch-Nyhan syndrome, associated with a deficiency of urea cycle enzyme, has among its characteristics a form of spastic rigidity typical of cerebral palsy. Children with a large number of other genetic metabolic enzyme deficiencies also have the motor characteristics of cerebral palsy (Hoon et al., 1997).

As discussed previously, kernicterus, secondary to bilirubin deposition in the basal ganglia, is one of the best known causal factors for the development of cerebral palsy. Because the bilirubin is cleared effectively by the placenta prior to birth, it is only in the neonatal period that the infant is left to his or her own devices to clear excessive bilirubin. Kernicterus occurs only if bilirubin cannot be cleared. In addition to kernicterus, other postpartum risk factors (e.g., neonatal hypoglycemia) have been associated with the development of cerebral palsy. It is difficult, however, to separate the responsibility of neonatal hypoglycemia from its associated growth restriction and asphyxia. Therefore, it is not clear whether

neonatal hypoglycemia is associated with cerebral palsy (Koivisto et al., 1972).

Many bacterial and viral infections of the fetus, infant, and young child have been associated with cerebral palsy, although quantification is difficult (Fowler et al., 1992). For example, Stanley (1984) notes that a fairly large number of cases of cerebral palsy associated with congenital rubella syndrome were described before the initiation of the rubella vaccination program, but this relationship rarely occurs in the United States today.

Congenital infection with *Toxoplasma gondii* and cytomegalovirus also can cause cerebral palsy. Older literature suggests that infection of the infant or young child with measles, mumps, varicella, and rubella was once reported as a common cause of CNS injury leading to cerebral palsy. Since the development of vaccines for many of the common childhood diseases, however, it appears that a viral etiology for postpartum acquired cerebral palsy is rare. Nelson (1995) agrees, stating that although numeric documentation is lacking, judging from medical writing in the 19th century when infectious diseases were more frequent and less effectively treated, postnatally acquired cerebral palsy was more common than it is now in developed countries.

Because of these reductions, it appears that cytomegalovirus infections have become the most common viral infection associated with a cerebral palsy–like syndrome (Fowler et al., 1992). In addition to the infections described, herpesvirus infection as well as meningococcal, pneumococcal, and group B streptococcal infections of the neonate also can manifest later in life as a cerebral palsy–like syndrome. Finally, about 20% of cases of postpartum cerebral palsy are due to injury, including motor vehicle accidents, near-drownings, and physical abuse. Although the postnatal causes of cerebral palsy contribute to only a small percentage of cases of cerebral palsy, they could lead to the most preventable cases.

Alloimmune thrombocytopenia of the newborn has been reported to cause fetal and neonatal death associated with intracranial hemorrhage but has also been associated with serious neurodevelopmental sequelae, including cerebral palsy. The overall contribution of thrombocytopenia to the prevalence of cerebral palsy is probably very low, however (Bonacossa and Jocelyn, 1996). Chemical teratogenesis has also been shown to result in cerebral palsy (Murakami, 1972; Takeshita et al., 1989). For example, methylmercury, which reached the mother via fish in Minemata, Japan and via contaminated flour in Iraq, resulted in severe spastic quadriplegia with mental retardation in the infant (Gilbert and Grant-Webster, 1995). Severe prenatal alcohol abuse has also been associated with cerebral palsy (Marcus, 1987).

■ BIRTH ASPHYXIA AND CEREBRAL PALSY

In general, we have tended to be quite careless in our use of the terms fetal-neonatal hypoxia, asphyxia, and ischemia and tend to use the terms interchangeably (Paneth, 1992, 1993; MacLennan, 1999; Amato and Donati, 2000). Hypoxia, however, literally means "low oxygen." Reduced oxygen causes a series of metabolic events, including acidosis (a low pH), changes in energy use, and changes in tissue perfusion, which vary with the time and duration of the hypoxic episode. The same chain of events can be initiated by lowered tissue perfusion (ischemia) that results in tissue hypoxia. The ability to measure birth asphyxia (insufficient oxygenation to maintain organ function) is limited because most fetal or newborn measures, including abnormal fetal heart rates, presence of meconium, low Apgar scores, low cord blood pH, and delay in spontaneous breathing, are associated with a variety of conditions besides asphyxia. Furthermore, none of these characteristics measures fetal cerebral oxygen deprivation; nor do they correlate well with each other, and the presence of these markers often does not identify the same infants. Therefore, the lack of clinically reliable indicators for impaired fetal placental gas exchange limits our ability to determine whether birth asphyxia plays a causal role in cerebral palsy, and if it does, how frequently this relationship exists.

Paneth (1993) has stated that the entity called *hypoxic-ischemic encephalopathy*, characterized by seizures, hypotonia, and absent suck and respiratory effort, occurs not only in infants with clear evidence of a hypoxic episode but also in infants with various urea cycle and amino acid disorders, myotonic dystrophy, Down's syndrome, and many other conditions. A number of studies have found that many infants with the clinical findings of hypoxic-ischemic encephalopathy had normal vaginal deliveries with no evidence of fetal distress or birth depression. Nelson and Ellenberg (1984) have emphasized that if a baby shows no neurologic signs after birth, it is unlikely that any subsequent neurologic problems are related to the birth. It is only in the presence of signs of newborn encephalopathy that obstetric factors are likely to have a relationship to cerebral palsy.

The relationship of Apgar scores and umbilical cord gases to the later development of cerebral palsy requires extra mention. The Apgar score was first described in 1953 to help define which newborns required extra attention and was not meant to be used as a predictor of future neurologic status (Apgar, 1953). Further, the Apgar score measures many characteristics other than the infant's oxygen or acid-base status; these include drug use, trauma, hypovolemia, infections, anomalies, and neuromuscular maturity.

As a rule, the earlier the gestational age, the lower the Apgar scores, even in the presence of normal umbilical cord gases (Goldenberg et al., 1984). The presumed relationship between moderately low Apgar scores and cerebral palsy likely originated from a time before it was appreciated that, especially in preterm infants, Apgar scores are a better reflection of gestational age than they are of acid-base status. In preterm infants, at least part of the increased risk of cerebral palsy associated with low Apgar scores probably reflects early-gestational-age susceptibility to intracerebral hemorrhage (ICH) and white matter damage—not asphyxia.

Nevertheless, in the U.S. Collaborative Perinatal Project (Freeman and Nelson, 1988) and other studies (Grant, 1988; Fee et al., 1990), cerebral palsy had a significant association with very low Apgar scores persisting for long periods of time (Fig. 61-4). Subsequent studies show that at the extreme, low Apgar scores correlated with increased risk of cerebral palsy. For example, the correlation of cerebral palsy with 1-minute Apgar scores generally is poor, and even when the 5-minute scores are 3 or below, cerebral palsy develops in only 5% of infants.

Most term infants with very low Apgar scores do not suffer from cerebral palsy. In term infants, only when Apgar scores below 3 persisted for 20 minutes or more was the risk of cerebral palsy greater than 50%. Therefore, the very low late Apgar score in term infants is an extremely powerful predictor of which infants will experience cerebral palsy. In this study of 390 infants with Apgar scores of 0–3 at 10 minutes or later, however, 270 died before 1 year of age. Of the 99 survivors who were evaluated, only 12% had cerebral palsy. Three quarters of these apparently severely asphyxiated newborns were neurologically healthy by school age. Similar findings exist in relationship to umbilical cord gases. Although some authors define a pH of less than 7.2 as "low," it seems relatively clear that only among infants with pH values of less than 7 is there a significantly increased risk of encephalopathy and ultimately cerebral palsy (Winkler et al., 1991). Below this cutoff, however, it appears that the lower the pH, the greater the risk of neonatal brain damage.

Gaffney and coauthors (1995) showed that mothers of infants with neonatal encephalopathy were more likely to be primigravidas, to undergo a pregnancy of greater than 41 weeks'

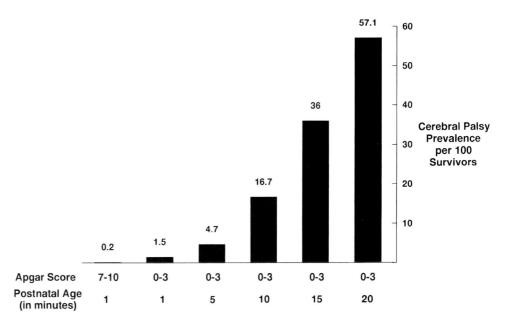

FIGURE 61-4 ■ Cerebral palsy prevalence per 100 survivors by Apgar score and age. (From Freeman JM, Nelson KB: Intrapartum asphyxia and cerebral palsy. Pediatrics **82:**240, 1988. Reproduced with permission.)

| Apgar Score | 7-10 | 0-3 | 0-3 | 0-3 | 0-3 | 0-3 |
| Postnatal Age (in minutes) | 1 | 1 | 5 | 10 | 15 | 20 |

gestation, to have meconium-stained amniotic fluid, and to have an abnormal fetal heart rate tracing. In general, these were the infants at 5 years of age who were more likely to have spastic quadriplegia; however, this group represented only one of 10 cases of all cerebral palsy.

Nelson and Grether (1998) examined obstetric complications capable of limiting fetal oxygen supply and investigated their association with spastic cerebral palsy. These potentially asphyxiating conditions included abruptio placentae, placental previa, prolapsed cord, cord compression, maternal shock, true-cord knot, and tight nuchal cord. Of these, only a tight nuchal cord was statistically associated with an increased risk of cerebral palsy. Because the delivering physician had an opportunity to be aware of the condition of the baby at birth prior to reporting whether a tight nuchal cord was present, however, even the recording of the tight nuchal cord at birth by the physician may simply be a surrogate measure of an infant in trouble in the delivery room. Similarly, in reports of meconium being related to subsequent cerebral palsy, the presence of meconium may be more likely to be recorded in the delivery room if the infant appears to be in distress.

Richmond and associates (1994), examining the relationship between the obstetric management of fetal distress and the development of cerebral palsy, concluded that even if fetal distress were completely eliminated, the prevalence of cerebral

palsy might be reduced by only 16%. Because not all asphyxic episodes are preventable, perfect obstetric management of fetal distress may reduce the prevalence of cerebral palsy by 9% in term infants and 6% overall (MacLennan, 1999; Nelson and Grether, 1999).

Susser and Stein (1988) pointed out that there is no good contemporary evidence for a causal role of obstetric practice in the development of cerebral palsy. This lack of relationship was further confirmed by an earlier study of Niswander and associates (1984).

Gaffney and colleagues (1995) described a flow chart using a series of six questions that help to define both potential causes of cerebral palsy and the proportion of cerebral palsy that may be preventable by improving intrapartum care. In their study of 237 infants, only 26, or about 10%, were classified as showing evidence of suboptimal intrapartum care, suggesting that their cases were potentially preventable (Fig. 61-5). In 1999, an International Cerebral Palsy Task Force evaluated the relationship between birth asphyxia and cerebral palsy (MacLennan, 1999). The group first defined the criteria necessary to implicate an acute intrapartum hypoxic event (Table 61-2). They then went on to name a group of factors that suggest a cause of cerebral palsy other than acute intrapartum hypoxia (Table 61-3) and then listed a series of questions pertinent to assessing the preventability of the cases of cerebral palsy presumed to be due

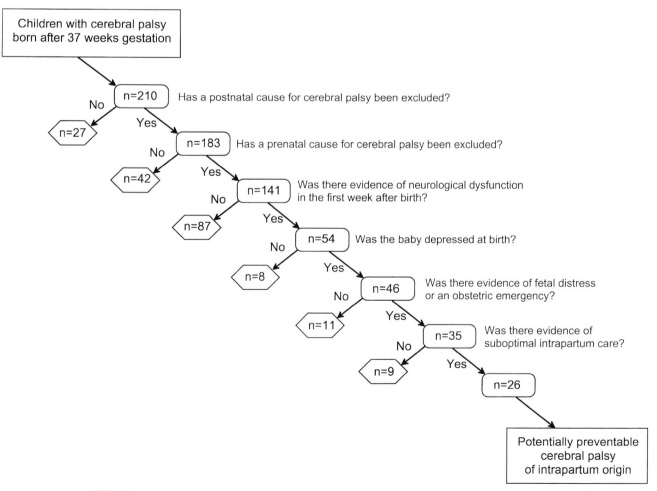

FIGURE 61-5 ■ Potentially preventable cerebral palsy of intrapartum origin. (From Gaffney G, Flavell V, Johnson A, et al: Model to identify potentially preventable cerebral palsy of intrapartum origin. Arch Dis Child **73**:F106, 1995.)

TABLE 61-2. CRITERIA TO DEFINE AN ACUTE INTRAPARTUM HYPOXIC EVENT

Essential Criteria

1. Evidence of a metabolic acidosis in intrapartum fetal umbilical arterial cord, or very early neonatal blood samples (pH <7.00 and base deficit ≥12 mmol/L)
2. Early onset of severe or moderate neonatal encephalopathy in infants of ≥34 weeks' gestation
3. Cerebral palsy of the spastic quadriplegic or dyskinetic type

Criteria That Together Suggest an Intrapartum Timing but by Themselves Are Nonspecific

4. A sentinel (signal) hypoxic event occurring immediately before or during labor
5. A sudden, rapid, and sustained deterioration of the fetal heart rate pattern, usually after the hypoxic sentinel event, where the pattern was previously normal
6. Apgar scores of 0–6 for longer than 5 minutes
7. Early evidence of multisystem involvement
8. Early imaging evidence of acute cerebral abnormality

---

to an intrapartum event (Table 61-4). More recently, the American College of Obstetricians and Gynecologists and the American Academy of Pediatrics convened a task force to review the most current evidence-based publications regarding the mechanisms and timing of possible etiologic events that can lead to neonatal encephalopathy. (Neotatal Encephalopathy and Cerebral Palsy, 2003). With very few differences, the American Task Force came to similar conclusions as those drawn by the International group.

In summary, there is little question that fetal asphyxia is associated with cerebral palsy, usually spastic quadriplegia. This asphyxia appears to account for no more than 15% of all cases of cerebral palsy, however, and of these, only about half can be eliminated by excellent medical care.

INTRACRANIAL HEMORRHAGE AND PERIVENTRICULAR LEUKOMALACIA AS PREDICTORS OF CEREBRAL PALSY

Prior to the use of ultrasonography for the diagnosis of neonatal brain damage, a number of studies examined neonatal white matter lesions based on necropsy. For example, analy-

sis of autopsy data from the Collaborative Perinatal Project (Leviton and Paneth, 1990) showed that periventricular white matter lesions (leukomalacia) were most common in infants born at 28–31 weeks' gestation (Table 61-5) and then decreased as the gestational age at birth increased. Also, the greater the age of the infant at death, the greater the risk that PVL develops before death. Perhaps most interesting, babies with documented bacteremia were nine times more likely to have white matter necrosis. Otherwise, most measures of perinatal distress were not associated with white matter necrosis.

Leviton and Paneth, among others, have produced a prodigious amount of work describing the relationship between neonatal brain damage and cerebral palsy, especially in preterm infants (Papile et al., 1983; Guzetta et al., 1986; Fawer et al., 1987; Leviton and Paneth, 1990; Paneth et al., 1990; Pidcock et al., 1990; Roth et al., 1993; Gaffney, Squier, et al., 1994; Pinto-Martin et al., 1995). They emphasize that many structural abnormalities of cerebral white matter that predict later handicap can now be identified by ultrasound imaging performed in the neonatal intensive care unit. As a result, these images have become the focus of epidemiologic attention. These authors emphasize that because cerebral palsy is relatively rare and cannot be diagnosed near birth, many current

---

TABLE 61-3. FACTORS THAT SUGGEST A CAUSE OF CEREBRAL PALSY OTHER THAN ACUTE INTRAPARTUM HYPOXIA

- Umbilical arterial base deficit less than 12 mmol/L or pH greater than 7.00
- Infants with major or multiple congenital or metabolic abnormalities
- Central nervous system or systemic infection
- Early imaging evidence of long-standing neurological abnormalities—for example, ventriculomegaly, porencephaly, multicystic encephalomalacia
- Infants with signs of intrauterine growth restriction
- Reduced fetal heart rate variability from the onset of labor
- Microcephaly at birth (head circumference less than one third of the centile)
- Major antenatal placental abruption
- Extensive chorioamnionitis
- Congenital coagulation disorders in the child
- Presence of other major antenatal risk factors for cerebral palsy—for example, preterm birth at less than 34 weeks' gestation, multiple pregnancy, or autoimmune disease
- Presence of major postnatal risk factors for cerebral palsy—for example, postnatal encephalitis, prolonged hypotension, or hypoxia resulting from severe respiratory disease
- A sibling with cerebral palsy, especially of the same type.

TABLE 61-4. QUESTIONS PERTINENT TO ASSESSING THE PREVENTABILITY OF CEREBRAL PALSY ASSUMED TO BE DUE TO AN ACUTE INTRAPARTUM EVENT

- Were there risk factors for an antenatal cause of cerebral palsy?
- Was there a sentinel hypoxic event?
- Was an intervention proved to reduce the rate of cerebral palsy available?
- Have the criteria for defining an acute intrapartum hypoxic event been met?
- Could the signs of fetal compromise reasonably have been detected?
- Was there an avoidable major delay in expediting delivery?
- Would quicker delivery of the baby have compromised the mother's health or life?
- Would an earlier delivery, if practical, have prevented or ameliorated the outcome?

MacLennan A, for the International Cerebral Palsy Task Force: A template for defining a causal relation between acute intrapartum events and cerebral palsy: International consensus statement. BMJ **319**(16):1054, 1999.

studies are using surrogate ultrasound measures of brain damage on the temporal pathway to cerebral palsy.

Two conditions—intracranial hemorrhage (ICH), seen on ultrasonography as periventricular echodensities, and echolucencies in the cerebral white matter, often called periventricular leukomalacia (PVL)—are the two best neonatal predictors of cerebral palsy. Because ICH and PVL are relatively easily diagnosed by cranial ultrasonography in the weeks following birth while the preterm infants are still in the hospital, and because cranial ultrasound images have become part of routine care for very preterm infants, collecting this type of data is relatively easy and generally not omitted or lost. Also, because it is collected routinely, from a research perspective, it is not expensive to obtain. Furthermore, because ultrasound scans can be obtained repeatedly and are likely without risk, changes in cerebral white matter can be observed sequentially.

It should be emphasized that several authors caution that despite the frequency with which echodensities and echolucencies are reported as intracranial hemorrhage and PVL, there is still no clear consensus on how to correlate ultrasound observations, including echodensities and echolucencies, with pathologic findings. Nevertheless, many reports assume 100% correlation between various neonatal cranial ultrasound findings and specific pathologic diagnoses such as ICH or PVL.

Despite the reservations expressed by Leviton and others about the translation of various ultrasound observations to specific pathologic diagnoses, much of the ultrasound literature uses these specific anatomic terms.

Leviton and Paneth (1990) reviewed the long-term outcome of children with ultrasound-determined echodense lesions (equivalent to grade IV ICH) in the neonatal period. In these children, the range of prevalence of cerebral palsy was 40%–100% (Table 61-6). Many other studies have confirmed that approximately two thirds of infants with apparent grade IV hemorrhage subsequently suffer from cerebral palsy. Similarly, cystic white matter disorders, characterized by single or multiple echolucent regions, correlate well with subsequent adverse neurologic outcomes. Specifically, cerebral palsy develops in infants with cystic periventricular abnormalities in 62%–100% (Table 61-7) of cases, with a mean of 80%. The presence of cysts larger than 3 cm in diameter has been associated with a 90%–100% risk of subsequent cerebral palsy. In general, the more extensive the hemorrhage and the more severe the leukomalacia, the greater the risk of cerebral palsy (Fawer et al., 1987; Aziz et al., 1995; Dammann and Leviton, 1997).

Data from the National Institute of Child Health and Development (NICHD) Neonatal Network help us understand some of the potential factors that influence the risk of grade III or grade IV ICH in neonates who weigh less than 1500 g. Shankaran and coworkers (1996) and others (Philip et al., 1989; Strand et al., 1990) note that the incidence of severe intracranial hemorrhage has been decreasing in newborns weighing less than 1500 g since the early 1980s. The factors potentially related to the development of ICH considered included birth weight, gestational age, growth restriction, types of presentation, method of delivery, antepartum hemorrhage, antenatal steroid use, maternal age, prenatal care, diabetes, hypertension or preeclampsia, race, and infant gender. In this study, both low gestational age and low birth weight were associated with an increased risk of hemorrhage. African-American race, female infant gender, antenatal steroid use, and hypertension or preeclampsia were associated with a decreased incidence of intracranial hemorrhage.

As stated previously, various areas of the fetal brain develop at different times and therefore have distinct vulnerabilities that depend on the gestational age. For example, the basal ganglia and the motor cortex could be especially vulnerable to injury during the third trimester. Injury at this time tends to be due to asphyxia but may also be associated with kernicterus,

TABLE 61-5. INCIDENCE OF CYSTIC PERIVENTRICULAR LEUKOMALACIA (PVL) ACCORDING TO GESTATIONAL AGE

Gestational Age (Wk)	No.	PVL	Incidence of PVL* (%)
<27	89	5	7.2
<27	75	9	12.9
<28	99	14	15.7
<29	110	11	10.5
<30	128	15	12.4
<31	115	7	6.5
<32	186	8	4.3
TOTAL	802	69	9.2

* Calculated for infants surviving at least 7 days.

From Zupan V, Gonzalez P, Lacaze-Masmonteil T, et al: Periventricular leukomalacia: Risk factors revisited. Dev Med Child Neurol **38**:1061, 1996.

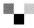

TABLE 61-6. ECHODENSE PARENCHYMAL LESIONS AND THE RISK OF SUBSEQUENT CEREBRAL PALSY

Study	No.	Lesion Description	Survivors with Cerebral Palsy (%)
Papile, 1983	17	Grade IV cerebral ICH	86
Pape, 1985	20	Grade IV ICH	40
Catto-Smith, 1985	3	ICH	67
Guzetta, 1986	22	Periventricular intraparenchymal echolucency	86
Graham, 1987	3	Parenchymal hemorrhage	100
Cooke, 1987	32	Parenchymal hemorrhage or extension	63
TOTAL	97		67

ICH, intracerebral hemorrhage.

Adapted from Leviton A, Paneth N: White matter damage in preterm newborns—an epidemiologic perspective. Early Hum Dev **24:**1, 1990.

infection, or other types of injury such as those associated with metabolic disorders. In the third trimester, white-matter injury is relatively uncommon. According to general consensus, however, because the developmental sequence from the oligodendrocyte precursors to a mature cell capable of synthesizing myelin occurs during the last part of the second trimester, the fetus is more prone to develop white-matter damage toward the end of the second trimester than at any other time. During this period, infants have little stainable myelin in their cerebral hemispheres but do have premyelin glial cells. As these cells begin the process of myelinogenesis at about 26–28 weeks' gestational age, they appear to be particularly vulnerable to injury. Other cells beside the oligodendrocyte that could be particularly susceptible to damage in the last half of the second trimester are the endothelial cells of blood vessels, especially those in the supracaudate germinal matrix.

Johnston and coauthors (1995) also emphasize that the brains of preterm fetuses have more excitatory NMDA receptors than brains of more mature infants. When stimulated, these receptors appear to be more vulnerable to injury. Overstimulation apparently leads to calcium toxicity and cell death. They describe converging mechanisms of injury related to cerebral palsy. In term infants, the likely pathway is as follows: from ischemia to the increased production of gluta-

mate, to the stimulation of the NMDA receptors, to increased calcium entry into cells, to increased nitric oxide synthetase, to an increased production of nitric oxide radicals, and ultimately to cell death (Lipton and Rosenberg, 1994). The cells most likely to die are in the cerebral cortex. At less than 32 weeks' gestation, however, the predominant pathway appears to be related to infection, endotoxins, and cytokines that also can stimulate increased nitric oxide synthesis and increased production of nitric oxide radicals, which again lead to cell death. The cells that are most vulnerable at this time appear to be the oligodendrocytes, which in the next several weeks would start the production of myelin.

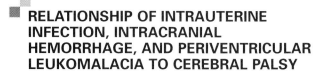

RELATIONSHIP OF INTRAUTERINE INFECTION, INTRACRANIAL HEMORRHAGE, AND PERIVENTRICULAR LEUKOMALACIA TO CEREBRAL PALSY

A number of studies now link chorioamnionitis to the development of cerebral palsy (Dammann, 2000; Yoon, 2000; Wu, 2000). Nelson and Ellenberg (1978), using data from the Collaborative Perinatal Project, showed that in low-birth-weight infants, chorioamnionitis was associated with a tripling

TABLE 61-7. PERCENT OF CHILDREN WITH ECHOLUCENT PARENCHYMAL LESIONS WHO LATER HAVE CEREBRAL PALSY

Study	No.	Lesion Description	Survivors with Cerebral Palsy (%)
DeVries, 1985	10	Extensive or subcortical PVL	100
Graziani, 1985	15	Large periventricular cysts or porencephaly	80
Boyzynski, 1985	4	PVL	100
Weindling, 1985	8	Periventricular cysts	100
Smith, 1986	16	PVL	88
Graham, 1987	13	Cystic PVL	62
	8	Multiple cysts	88
Fawer, 1987	11	Extensive PVL	73
Stewart, 1987	10	Cysts	80
Cooke, 1987	32	Porencephalic cysts	69
Total	127		80

PVL, periventricular leukomalacia.

Adapted from Leviton A, Paneth N: White matter damage in preterm newborns: An epidemiologic perspective. Early Hum Dev **24:**1, 1990.

of the risk of cerebral palsy from 12 per 1000 to 39 per 1000 live births. Among term infants in that study, chorioamnionitis increased the risk of cerebral palsy from 3 per 1000 to 8 per 1000 live births. In a more recent study, Grether and associates (1996) examined prenatal and perinatal factors related to cerebral palsy in very-low-birth-weight California infants. In this study, chorioamnionitis was associated with a fourfold increased risk of cerebral palsy. Even more recently, term infants with evidence of chorioamnionitis had a significantly greater risk of cerebral palsy (Grether and Nelson, 1997). Murphy and colleagues (1995), investigating the relationship of various antenatal and intrapartum risk factors to cerebral palsy in infants born at less than 32 weeks' gestational age, showed that in such infants, chorioamnionitis increased the risk of cerebral palsy from 3% in controls to 17% in infected infants.

In a number of other studies, intrauterine infection has preceded neonatal ICH, a precursor of cerebral palsy. For example, Groome and coworkers (1992), using data from the March of Dimes multicenter study, showed that clinical chorioamnionitis was associated with a two- to threefold increased risk of ICH. Leviton's group also has explored the relationship between maternal intrauterine infection and evidence of brain damage in the preterm newborn (Dammann and Leviton, 1996, 1997). They revealed an association between intrauterine infection in the mother and both ICH and white-matter damage in the newborn. In a study of more than 1000 preterm infants, intrauterine infection was associated with a doubling of the infant's risk for having ICH, PVL, and ventriculomegaly.

Leviton's group also note an increased risk of ICH in the group of infants with infection born after a short duration of ruptured membranes and suggested that infection of the mother prior to delivery could be more important in predicting ICH than the perinatal infections that develop after rupture of the fetal membranes (Dammann and Leviton, 1997). Even after adjusting for gestational age, type of labor, and type of delivery, the relationship between intrauterine infection and ICH persisted. Additional data from the NICHD Neonatal Network (Stoll et al., 1995, 1996) confirm that both early-onset and late-onset sepsis in very-low-birth-weight newborns is associated with an increased incidence of intracerebral hemorrhage.

Bejar and co-authors (1988) found that chorioamnionitis was present in more than half of the preterm infants who developed white-matter echolucencies within 3 days after birth. Leviton (1993) notes that the histologic abnormalities of white matter have been associated with sepsis in the baby and with gynecologic and urinary tract infection in the mother. They also note that increased risks of PVL in newborn infants with sepsis and necrotizing enterocolitis support the hypothesis that a bacterial toxin contributes to the occurrence of PVL in some babies. Mays and colleagues (1995) report that acute appendicitis is associated with ICH and PVL even when the gestational age at birth is controlled for. Therefore, even extrauterine intra-abdominal infections appear to be able to initiate the cascade of events linking infection, labor, and neonatal brain injury (Dammann and Leviton, 1998).

Hansen and associates (2000) studied the correlation between placental pathology and ICH in preterm infants. They observed that ICH was reduced with placental findings suggestive of old and recent infarcts, including histologic features such as increased syncytial knots and villous fibrosis. Placental characteristics of inflammation, including umbilical vasculitis, chorionic vasculitis, and inflammation of the subchorion, chorion, and amnion, were associated with an increased risk of ICH, however. Grafe (1994), Salafia and associates (1995), and others confirmed the relationship between periventricular hemorrhage and leukomalacia and between cerebral palsy and placental membrane and umbilical cord evidence of inflammation and associated thrombosis (Kraus, 1997; Redline and O'Riordan, 2000).

In a further attempt to understand this phenomenon, Kuban and coworkers (1999) studied echolucent images in periventricular white matter in relationship to maternal uterine infection. The odds ratio for development of an echolucency was highest for infants whose placentas had vasculitis of the chorionic plate or umbilical cord (OR = 9.8). Among infants born 1 or more hours after membrane rupture, however, placental vasculitis did not predict the development of echolucencies. These observations suggest that in very-low-birth-weight infants, uterine infections predating membrane rupture contribute to the risk of cerebral white matter damage and perhaps later cerebral palsy. They believe that their data argues against the hypothesis that ascending uterine infection after membrane rupture contributes appreciably to the risk of white matter damage that predicts cerebral palsy.

Zupan and coauthors (1996), in a study of risk factors for PVL, found a strong link between intrauterine infection and the development of PVL and that this relationship was increased in the face of premature rupture of membranes and infection (Fig. 61-6). They also think that most of the PVL originates before birth and that susceptibility to the condition depends closely on the developmental age. They note that factors related to preeclampsia are rarely associated with PVL, and they strongly suggest that the major etiologic components of white-matter lesions in infants born late in the second trimester relate to the presence of an intrauterine infection.

Perlman and colleagues (1996) noted that cystic PVL, which occurred in 3% of infants weighing less than 1500 g, was associated with two clinical indicators: prolonged rupture of membranes and chorioamnionitis. The odds ratio for cerebral palsy after prolonged rupture of membranes was 6.6, and the odds ratio for cerebral palsy with chorioamnionitis was 6.8.

From these data, there seems little question that intrauterine infection, a clear predictor of preterm delivery (Gibbs et al., 1992; Andrews et al., 1995), is also a predictor of white-matter lesions, ICH, and ultimately, cerebral palsy. If, as has been proposed (Goldenberg and Andrews, 1996), 70%–80% of very-low-birth-weight births are associated with an intrauterine infection, the high rate of cerebral palsy in these infants could well be related to the infection. The apparent reduction in cerebral palsy associated with preeclampsia could be a more "normal" baseline level (Blair et al., 1996), and the higher rates of cerebral palsy in babies born following spontaneous labor or preterm premature rupture of membranes may well be due to intrauterine infection. Figure 61-7, based on the work of Leviton, Romero, and others, shows a possible pathway leading from infection to cerebral palsy.

CYTOKINES AND BRAIN DAMAGE

In recent years, much evidence has emerged suggesting that various cytokines mediate the relationship between cerebral palsy and intrauterine infection, ICH, and PVL. Certainly,

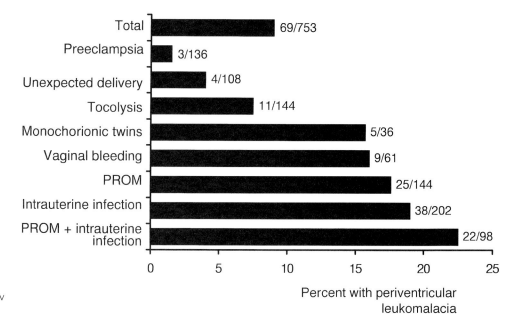

FIGURE 61-6 ■ Risk factors for periventricular leukomalacia. PROM, premature rupture of membranes. (From Zupan V, Gonzalez P, Lacaze-Masmonteil T, et al: Periventricular leukomalacia: Risk factors revisited. Dev Med Child Neurol **38**:1061, 1996.)

various cytokines, such as interleukin-6 (IL-6), IL-1, tumor necrosis factor (TNF), and others, are elevated in the amniotic fluid of pregnant women with chorioamnionitis. Andrews and associates (1995) have emphasized that amniotic fluid cytokines are elevated even with infection confined to the amniotic membranes. Adinolfi (1993) was among the first to propose that cytokines produced in relationship to maternal infection were harmful to the developing brain of the unborn infants. Figueroa and coworkers (1996) showed that elevated amniotic fluid IL-6 predicted neonatal PVL and ICH. Yoon and coauthors (1996b), Kashlan and colleagues (1997), and others showed that elevated IL-6 levels in the umbilical cord were also related to the subsequent development of periventricular echodensities and echolucencies. Recent papers document the association between elevated umbilical cord blood cytokine levels and cerebral palsy (Yoon et al., 2000; Duggan et al., 2001).

Although the exact mechanisms are unclear, the association between high levels of cytokines in the brain secondary to various types of perinatal infections and subsequent brain damage may explain the relationship between intrauterine infection and cerebral palsy. There is also evidence that the elevated TNF-α and other cytokines are associated with an increased risk of PVL (Selmaj et al., 1988; Dammann and Leviton, 1996; Deguchi et al., 1996; Figueroa et al., 1996; Yoon et al., 1996a, 1997; Kashlan et al., 1997). Cytokines appear to induce astrogliosis, cystic necrosis, and deposits of debris in the white matter. In addition, microglial expression of TNF-α was more common in the white matter of infants with PVL than in infants without this condition.

Leviton believes that cytokines may damage cerebral white matter by at least three mechanisms:

1. Hypotension and ischemia
2. Blood vessel obstruction following intravascular coagulation
3. Toxic effects on the oligodendrocytes and myelin

Another possible mechanism by which various cytokines could mediate white matter damage is the stimulation of microglia to produce nitric oxide and related free radicals. Therefore, TNF and other cytokines could be associated with newborn brain damage via oxidant stress. Thus, the cytokines that are stimulated by intrauterine infections and that are, at least in part, responsible for the initiation of the preterm labor are also probably responsible for one sequence of events leading to neonatal brain damage.

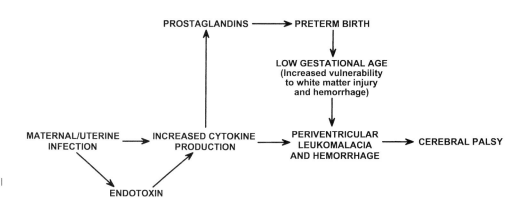

FIGURE 61-7 ■ Pathway to cerebral palsy in preterm infants.

INTERVENTIONS TO REDUCE CEREBRAL PALSY

The two most common potentially preventable causes of cerebral palsy are asphyxia and preterm birth. Because about 10%–15% of cerebral palsy appears to occur in relationship to an apparent hypoxic episode, fetal heart rate monitoring for hypoxic distress and appropriate interventions, including maternal oxygen administration, repositioning, decreased use of oxytocin, and expedited delivery when appropriate, originally were thought to show great promise in reducing cerebral palsy. To date, however, there is little evidence that these interventions are associated with a reduction in cerebral palsy, and it is suggested that cerebral palsy may be increased in the presence of fetal heart rate monitoring (Shy et al., 1990).

Nelson (1995), for example, argues that fetal monitoring may actually increase the risk of cerebral palsy. First, the scalp electrode site itself could provide a portal of entry for herpes and other viruses and bacteria. Second, and probably more important, internal fetal monitoring has been associated with an increased risk of chorioamnionitis, which appears to be a potent risk factor for cerebral palsy. Therefore, the benefit that may be achieved by the use of fetal heart rate monitoring and subsequent interventions (including early delivery) in reducing the asphyxic etiologic components of cerebral palsy may be counterbalanced by an increasing risk of the infectious etiologic components of cerebral palsy. Regardless, the widespread introduction of fetal heart rate monitoring in the 1970s was not associated with any apparent reduction in the prevalence of cerebral palsy (Chalmers, 1979; MacDonald et al., 1985; Grant et al., 1989; Colditz and Henderson-Smart, 1990; Freeman, 1990; MacDonald, 1996; Nelson et al., 1996). These issues are discussed in greater depth in Chapter 22.

Prior to the more frequent use of cesarean section for cephalopelvic disproportion and breech delivery, intracranial trauma and hemorrhage, which at least sometimes was associated with the development of subsequent cerebral palsy, was more common than it is now. Nelson (1995) also thinks that there has been a reduction in cerebral palsy associated with obstetric trauma, partly basing this idea on the observation that in recent years compared with previous time periods, infants born weighing more than 4000 g have the lowest rate of cerebral palsy of any birth weight group. Although there is no way to conclusively prove that reduced trauma was associated with this improvement, this argument appears reasonable (Freeman, 1985). Taking steps to avoid intracranial birth trauma and the associated asphyxia if at all possible makes sense as a strategy to reduce unnecessary mortality and long-term neurologic morbidity, which can include cerebral palsy.

Preterm birth, which occurs in 10% of all pregnancies, is a major problem in modern obstetrics, accounting for the majority of infant mortality and much long-term neurologic morbidity, including cerebral palsy. Adverse outcomes are concentrated in the most preterm infants, those with birth weights of less than 1500 g (2% of all infants) and especially less than 1000 g (~1% of all infants). Evidence suggests that as many as 70% of very preterm births follow intrauterine infection in which increased inflammatory cytokine production precipitates the labor (Gibbs et al., 1992; Andrews et al., 1995). Reducing the rate of preterm birth is therefore crucial to achieving a substantial reduction in cerebral palsy. Because there has been no progress in reducing the preterm birth rate, however, and because most very preterm infants now survive, reducing the long-term neurologic morbidity associated with extreme prematurity is of paramount importance.

Without question, corticosteroids given to the mother prior to birth of certain preterm infants are associated with a reduction in the major precursors of cerebral palsy, intracranial hemorrhage, and PVL. The relationship between corticosteroid use and a reduction in intracranial hemorrhage in preterm infants was first noted by Liggins and Howie in 1972. Since then, this relationship has been confirmed in a number of randomized trials, most recently by Garite and associates (1992) in infants of 24–28 weeks' gestational age and in Finland by Kari and colleagues (1994) in infants of less than 32 weeks' gestational age. In the latter study, both intracranial hemorrhage and PVL were reduced in association with corticosteroid use.

Crowley (1995), using meta-analytical techniques, has concluded that the use of corticosteroids is associated with about a 50% reduction in periventricular hemorrhage. These results are confirmed by reports from the NICHD Neonatal Network (Shankaran et al., 1996) as well as by reports associated with several surfactant trials. Evidence associating corticosteroid use with reduced rates of cerebral palsy itself is less common, but data from Kitchen and colleagues (1985, 1987) in Australia suggest that long-term neurologic disability (including cerebral palsy) is reduced by about 50% in infants exposed to corticosteroids.

Corticosteroids may have beneficial effects on the brain, not only through a mechanism of decreased intracranial hemorrhage but also via enhanced maturation of oligodendrocytes and enhanced antioxidant synthesis, resulting in less white-matter damage. Corticosteroids could reduce the risk of subsequent cerebral palsy via a number of other mechanisms as well. These include reducing the risk of respiratory distress syndrome and chronic lung disease, both of which could be associated with an increased risk of cerebral palsy. Also, because corticosteroids have been noted to stabilize cranial blood flow in the newborn, their use may reduce the risk of both ICH and the development of PVL by improving blood supply and reducing cerebral ischemia. Antenatal steroids, therefore, can be viewed as maturing the fetus, perhaps past the window of vulnerability for brain damage. The specific conditions for corticosteroid use were originally reviewed by the Consensus Conference and the American College of Obstetrics and Gynecology (ACOG, 1994; NIH Consensus Development Panel, 1995). Interestingly, following these reports, not only did the use of single courses of corticosteroids increase, but so did the use of repeated weekly courses. Because of several reports relating repeated courses of corticosteroids to decreased head growth and other potential side effects, a subsequent NICHD Consensus strongly advised against this practice (Baud et al., 1999; Goldenberg and Wright, 2001; NIH Consensus Development Panel, 2001). More recently, there have been several studies that strongly suggest that the use of postnatal corticosteroids, given to the preterm newborn to reduce the risk of chronic lung disease, substantially increases the risk of cerebral palsy (Yeh et al., 1998; O'Shea et al., 1999; Shinwell et al., 2000).

MAGNESIUM SULFATE AND CEREBRAL PALSY

The magnesium ion plays an important role in many biological functions. Magnesium catalyzes or activates more than 300 different enzymes, decreases membrane excitability, and regulates vascular tone (Nelson, 1996). Magnesium sulfate has been used therapeutically in obstetrics for many years, originally to prevent eclamptic convulsions and more recently as a tocolytic to inhibit uterine contractions so as to forestall preterm birth. Given intravenously, magnesium crosses the placenta rapidly, and after 3 hours of administration, fetal levels are comparable to maternal levels.

For a number of years, it has been believed that infants born to preeclamptic mothers experience less cerebral palsy than do other infants born at similar gestational ages. On the strength of this observation and animal research indicating a protective effect of magnesium on brain injury, Nelson and Grether (1995) undertook a retrospective case-controlled analysis of cerebral palsy in infants with birth weights below 1500 g. Three of the 42 infants with cerebral palsy had been exposed to magnesium, whereas 27 of 75 controls had not. This finding was statistically significant, with an odds ratio of 0.14. Multivariate analysis adjusting for many potential confounders confirmed the results.

Schendel and colleagues (1996), in a larger population-based cohort study, evaluated the relationship between maternal magnesium sulfate exposure, cerebral palsy, and mental retardation in children with birth weights of less than 1500 g born from 1986 through 1988. Of the 519 infants who survived infancy, 17% were identified as magnesium-exposed. In the univariate analyses, magnesium use was associated with a significant reduction (OR = 0.11) in cerebral palsy. Adjusting for a number of confounders did not change these results. Subsequent reports have shown conflicting results (Grether et al., 2000; Boyle et al., 2000; Matsuda et al., 2000).

What might predelivery maternal administration of magnesium do to prevent neonatal brain damage in very preterm infants? As reviewed previously, a number of pathways leading to neonatal neurologic damage have been proposed. In the first, hemorrhage occurs in the immature vasculature of the periventricular area of the brain during or soon after birth, presumably as a result of the poorly regulated cerebral blood flow of the preterm brain. In the second pathway, perinatal hypoxia combined with altered cerebral blood flow results in asphyxic damage to periventricular neurons, which appear as "PVL" at necropsy or as white matter echolucencies on neonatal cranial ultrasound. Also, *in utero* infection stimulates cytokine production that could affect periventricular neurons adversely, causing hemorrhage, PVL, or both.

First, magnesium may exert a beneficial effect by its known ability to stabilize vascular tone and thereby possibly prevent or diminish fluctuations in cerebral blood flow.

Second, magnesium may reduce reperfusion injury, possibly by blocking NMDA receptor activity and reducing calcium entry into neurons, thus protecting them from calcium-mediated damage or death (McDonald et al., 1990).

Third, magnesium may protect against infection-mediated damage because in pharmacologic doses, it appears to reduce cytokine and bacterial toxin synthesis (Kass et al., 1988; Weglicki et al., 1992).

Because of the ubiquitous nature of the magnesium ion and the still poorly understood pathophysiology of perinatal brain injury, other equally plausible pathways of injury and mechanisms of interruption by magnesium can be invoked.

Although to date, in several retrospective studies, magnesium in pharmacologic doses has been associated with an apparent reduction in cerebral palsy, proof of efficacy is lacking. A major concern in each of the published retrospective studies involves potential differences in the characteristics of the women selected for magnesium therapy and their controls. For example, most women treated with magnesium had preeclampsia, and many of the others were in relatively early preterm labor; the women in more advanced labor would not have received a tocolytic drug. It seems probable that women not treated with magnesium were more likely to have a uterine infection with elevated levels of inflammatory cytokines, more likely to undergo precipitous labor secondary to a placental separation, and more likely to be in hypoxic distress. Each of these characteristics could increase the risk of perinatal brain damage.

Because no prospective randomized trial has tested the hypothesis that predelivery magnesium sulfate reduces the risk of cerebral palsy, and because there are so many potential confounders that make the results of the retrospective studies nearly uninterpretable, only a well-designed prospective, randomized trial will provide entirely satisfactory evidence demonstrating the efficacy of magnesium in reducing the risk of cerebral palsy in very preterm infants (Goldenberg and Rouse, 1997).

A number of prospective randomized trials to test the efficacy of magnesium to prevent cerebral palsy are planned or underway both in the United States and abroad. If these studies are successful, the results will dictate whether to use magnesium to prevent cerebral palsy. In the interim, the use of magnesium sulfate outside of standard obstetric practice is not recommended. Mothers have been placed in serious jeopardy or even have died because of excessive magnesium administration, and many newborns are thought to be depressed for the same reason. Because several randomized trials are either under way or planned, awaiting their results seems an appropriate course of action.

■ S U M M A R Y

Cerebral palsy is an adverse outcome of pregnancy that occurs only rarely, is not a single entity, and has many known risk factors, but in only about half of cases is a plausible etiology discovered. Efforts to reduce its prevalence by various interventions, including widespread use of fetal monitoring and increasing use of cesarean section, have not been successful. Therefore, there is little reason to hope that the frequency of sporadic cases of cerebral palsy associated with asphyxia can be reduced substantially. Furthermore, it seems reasonably clear that even the universal availability of excellent medical care might eliminate only a small fraction of asphyxia-associated cerebral palsy cases.

Obviously, if one could reduce the rate of preterm birth, the risk of cerebral palsy would decrease substantially. The rate of spontaneous preterm birth, especially early spontaneous preterm birth, has not declined in recent decades, however, and in fact could be increasing. Unless the current studies showing attempts to reduce infection-related very early preterm births via antibiotics or other "anti-inflammatory" interventions demonstrate success of these strategies, there is little hope that the preterm delivery rate can be reduced substantially. Therefore, interventions aimed at reducing fetal or neonatal brain damage are the most likely to reduce cerebral palsy. These interventions, such as the use of corticosteroids and perhaps magnesium, and unstudied strategies, including the use of various antibiotics, anticytokines, or other anti-inflammatory agents, appear to be our best chances of reducing the neonatal brain damage that precedes cerebral palsy.

REFERENCES

Adinolfi M: Infectious diseases in pregnancy, cytokines and neurological impairment: A hypothesis. Dev Med Child Neurol 35:549, 1993.

Alberman E, Stanley F: Guidelines to the epidemiological approach. In Stanley F, Alberman E (eds): Clinics in Developmental Medicine No. 87: The Epidemiology of the Cerebral Palsies. Lavenham England, Lavenham Press, 1984, p. 27.

Allen MC: Developmental outcome and followup of the small for gestational age infant. Semin Perinatol 8:123, 1984.

Amato M, Donati F: Update on perinatal hypoxic insult: Mechanism, diagnosis and interventions. Eur J Paediatr Neurol 4(5):203, 2000.

American College of Obstetricians and Gynecologists (ACOG), Committee on Obstetric Practice: Antenatal corticosteroid therapy for fetal maturation. Committee opinion No. 147. Washington DC, ACOG, 1994.

American College of Obstetricians and Gynecologists, American Academy of Pediatrics: Neonatal Encephalopathy and Cerebral Palsy: Defining the pathogenesis and pathophysiology. A report by the Task Force on Neonatal Encephalopathy and Cerebral Palsy of the American College of Obstetricians and Gynecologists, Washington, DC, 2003.

Andrews WW, Goldenberg RL, Hauth JC: Preterm labor: Emerging role of genital tract infections. Infect Agents Dis 4:196, 1995.

Apgar V: A proposal for a new method of evaluation of the newborn infant. Curr Res Anesth Analg 32:260, 1953.

Aylward G, Pfieffer S, Wright A, et al: Outcome studies of low-birth-weight infants published in the last decade: A meta-analysis. J Pediatr 115:515, 1989.

Aziz K, Vickar DB, Sauve RS, et al: Province-based study of neurologic disability of children weighing 500 through 1249 grams at birth in relation to neonatal cerebral ultrasound findings. Pediatrics 95:837, 1995.

Baud O, Foix-L-Helias L, Kaminski M, et al. Antenatal glucocorticoid treatment and cystic periventricular leukomalacia in very premature infants. N Engl J Med 341:1190, 1999.

Bax M: Terminology and classification of cerebral palsy. Dev Med Child Neurol 6:295, 1964.

Bejar R, Vigliocco G, Gramajo H, et al: Antenatal origin of neurologic damage in newborn infants: II. Multiple gestations. Am J Obstet Gynecol 162:1230, 1990.

Bejar R, Wozniak P, Allard M, et al: Antenatal origin of neurologic damage in newborn infants: I. Preterm infants. Am J Obstet Gynecol 159:357, 1988.

Berg AT: Indices of fetal growth-retardation, perinatal hypoxia-related factors and childhood neurological morbidity. Early Hum Dev 19:271, 1989.

Blair E, Palmer L, Stanley F: Cerebral palsy in very low birthweight infants, pre-eclampsia and magnesium sulfate. Pediatrics 97:780, 1996.

Blair E, Stanley F: Intrapartum asphyxia: A rare cause of cerebral palsy. J Pediatr 112:515, 1988.

Blair E, Stanley F: Intrauterine growth and spastic cerebral palsy: I. Association with birth weight for gestational age. Am J Obstet Gynecol 162:229, 1990.

Blair E, Stanley F: Aetiological pathways to spastic cerebral palsy. Paediatr Perinat Epidemiol 7:302, 1993.

Bonacossa IA, Jocelyn LJ: Alloimmune thrombocytopenia of the newborn: Neurodevelopmental sequelae. Am J Perinatol 13:211, 1996.

Boyle CA, Yeargin-Allsopp M, Schendel DE, et al: Tocolytic magnesium sulfate exposure and risk of cerebral palsy among children with birth weights less than 1750 grams. Am J Epidemiol 152(2):120, 2000.

Brann AW: Factors during neonatal life that influence brain disorders. In Freeman JM (ed): Prenatal and Perinatal Factors Associated with Brain Disorders. Bethesda, Md, National Institutes of Health, 1985, p. 263.

Candy EJ, Joon AJ, Capute AJ, et al: MRI in motor delay: Important adjunct to classification of cerebral palsy. Pediatr Neurol 9:421, 1993.

Cans C: Surveillance of cerebral palsy in Europe: A collaboration of cerebral palsy surveys and registers. Dev Med Child Neurol 42:816, 2000.

Capute AJ, Accardo PJ: Cerebral palsy: The spectrum of motor dysfunction. In Capute AJ, Accardo PJ (eds): Developmental Disabilities in Infancy and Childhood, 2nd ed. Baltimore, Paul H. Brooks, 1996, p. 81.

Chalmers I: Randomized controlled trials of fetal monitoring 1973–1977. In Thalhammer O, Baumgarten K, Pollack A (eds): Perinatal Medicine. Stuttgart, Thieme, 1979, p. 260.

Chard T, Yoong A, MacIntosh M: The myth of fetal growth retardation at term. Br J Obstet Gynaecol 100:1076, 1993.

Cincotta RB, Gray PH, Ghythian G, et al: Long term outcome of twin-twin transfusion syndrome. Arch Dis Child Fetal Neonatal Ed 83:F171, 2000.

Colditz PB, Henderson-Smart DJ: Electronic fetal heart rate monitoring during labour: Does it prevent perinatal asphyxia and cerebral palsy? Med J Aust 153:88, 1990.

Colver AF, Givson M, Hey EN, et al: Increasing rates of cerebral palsy across the severity spectrum in north-east England 1964–1993. The North of England Collaborative Cerebral Palsy Survey. Arch Dis Child 83(1):F17, 2000.

Cooke RWI: Cerebral palsy in very low birthweight infants. Arch Dis Child 65:201, 1990.

Crowley P: Antenatal corticosteroid therapy: A meta-analysis of the randomized trials, 1972–1994. Am J Obstet Gynecol 173:322, 1995.

Cummins SK, Nelson KB, Grether JK, et al: Cerebral palsy in four northern California counties, births 1983 through 1985. J Pediatr 123:230, 1993.

Dammann O, Leviton A: Maternal intrauterine infection, cytokines, and brain damage in the preterm newborn. Pediatr Res 42:1, 1996.

Dammann O, Leviton A: The role of perinatal brain damage in developmental disabilities: An epidemiologic perspective. Ment Retard Dev Dis Res Rev 3:13, 1997.

Dammann O, Leviton A. Infection remote from the brain, neonatal white matter damage, and cerebral palsy in the preterm infant. Semin Pediatr Neurol 5(3):190, 1998.

Dammann O, Leviton A. The role of the fetus in perinatal infection and neonatal brain damage. Curr Opinion Pediatr 12(2):99, 2000.

Deguchi K, Mizuguchi M, Takashima S: Immunohistochemical expression of tumor necrosis factor-α in neonatal leukomalacia. Pediatr Neurol 14:13, 1996.

Doyle LW, Betheras FR, Ford GW, et al: Survival, cranial ultrasound and cerebral palsy in very low birthweight infants: 1980s versus 1990s. J Paediatr Child Health 36(1):7, 2000.

Duggan PJ, Maalouf EF, Watts TL, et al: Intrauterine T-cell activation and increased proinflammatory cytokine concentrations in preterm infants with cerebral lesions. Lancet 358:1600, 2001.

Ellenberg J, Nelson K: Birth weight and gestational age in children with cerebral palsy or seizure disorders. Am J Dis Child 133:1044, 1979.

Evans P, Elliott M, Alberman E, et al: Prevalence and disabilities in 4- to 8-year-olds with cerebral palsy. Arch Dis Child 60:940, 1985.

Fawer CL, Calame A, Perentes E, et al: Periventricular leukomalacia and neurodevelopmental outcome in preterm infants. Arch Dis Child 62:30, 1987.

Fee SC, Malee K, Deddish R, et al: Severe acidosis and subsequent neurologic status. Am J Obstet Gynecol 162:802, 1990.

Figueroa R, Martinez E, Sehgal P, et al: Elevated amniotic fluid interleukin-6 predicts neonatal periventricular leukomalacia and intraventricular hemorrhage. Am J Obstet Gynecol 174:330, 1996.

Finnstrom O, Otterblad-Olausson P, Sedin G, et al: Neurosensory outcome and growth at three years in extremely low birthweight infants: follow-up results from the Swedish national prospective study. Acta Paediatr 87:1055, 1998.

Fowler KB, Stagno S, Pass RG, et al: The outcome of congenital cytomegalovirus infection in relation to maternal antibody status. N Engl J Med 326:663, 1992.

Freeman JM (ed): Prenatal and Perinatal Factors Associated with Brain Disorders. Bethesda, Md, National Institutes of Health, 1985.

Freeman JM, Nelson KB: Intrapartum asphyxia and cerebral palsy. Pediatrics 82:240, 1988.

Freeman R: Intrapartum fetal monitoring—A disappointing story. N Engl J Med 322:624, 1990.

Freud S: Infantile cerebrallahumung. In Nothnagel's Specielle Pathologie and Therapie, Vol 12. Vienna, A. Holder, 1897.

Gaffney G, Flavell V, Johnson A, et al: Model to identify potentially preventable cerebral palsy of intrapartum origin. Arch Dis Child 73:F106, 1995.

Gaffney G, Squier MV, Johnson A, et al: Clinical associations of prenatal ischaemic white matter injury. Arch Dis Child 70:F101, 1994.

Garite TJ, Rumney PJ, Briggs GG, et al: A randomized placebo-controlled trial of betamethasone for the prevention of respiratory distress syndrome at 24 to 28 weeks' gestation. Am J Obstet Gynecol 166:646, 1992.

Gibbs RS, Romero MD, Hillier SL, et al: A review of premature birth and sub-clinical infection. Am J Obstet Gynecol 166:1515, 1992.

Gilbert SG, Grant-Webster KS: Neurobehavioral effects of developmental methylmercury exposure. Environ Health Perspect 103:135, 1995.

Gilles FH, Leviton A, Dooling EC: The Developing Human Brain: Growth and Epidemiologic Neuropathology. Boston, Wright, 1983.

Glinianaia SV, Pharoah POD, Wright C, et al: Fetal or infant death in twin pregnancy: Neurodevelopmental consequence for the survivor. Arch Dis Child 86:F9, 2002.

Goldenberg RL, Andrews WW: Intrauterine infection and why preterm prevention programs have failed (editorial). Am J Public Health 86:781, 1996.

Goldenberg RL, Andrews WW, Yuan AC, et al: Sexually transmitted diseases and adverse outcomes of pregnancy. Clin Perinatol 24:23, 1997.

Goldenberg RL, Hoffman HJ, Cliver SP: Neurodevelopmental outcome of small-for-gestational-age infants. Eur J Clin Nutr 52(Suppl 1):S54, 1998.

Goldenberg RL, Hoffman HJ, Foster JM, et al: Intrauterine growth retardation standards for diagnosis. Am J Obstet Gynecol 161:271, 1989.

Goldenberg RL, Huddleston JF, Nelson KG: Apgar scores and umbilical arterial pH in preterm newborns. Am J Obstet Gynecol 149:651, 1984.

Goldenberg RL, Rouse DJ: Preterm birth, cerebral palsy and magnesium: Where are we? Nature Med 3:146, 1997.

Goldenberg RL, Wright LL: Repeated courses of antenatal corticosteroids. Obstet Gynecol 97(2):316, 2001.

Grafe MR: The correlation of prenatal brain damage with placental pathology. J Neuropathol Exp Neurol 53:407, 1994.

Grant A: The relationship between obstetrically preventable intrapartum asphyxia, abnormal neonatal neurological signs and subsequent motor impairment in babies born at or after term. In Kubli F, Patel N, Schmidt W, et al (eds): Perinatal Events and Brain Damage in Surviving Children. Berlin, Springer-Verlag, 1988, p. 149.

Grant A, O'Brien N, Joy M-T, et al: Cerebral palsy among children born during the Dublin randomized trial of intrapartum monitoring. Lancet ii:1233, 1989.

Grether JK, Cummins SK, Nelson KB: The California cerebral palsy project. Paediatr Perinatol Epidemiol 6:339, 1992.

Grether JK, Hoogstrate J, Walsh-Greene E, et al: Magnesium sulfate for tocolysis and risk of spastic cerebral palsy in premature children born to women without preeclampsia. Am J Obstet Gynecol 183:717, 2000.

Grether JK, Nelson KB: Maternal infection and cerebral palsy in infants of normal birth weight. JAMA 278:207, 1997.

Grether JK, Nelson KB: Possible decrease in prevalence of cerebral palsy in premature infants. J Pediatr 136(1), 2000, p. 133.

Grether JK, Nelson KB, Emery ES III, et al: Prenatal and perinatal factors and cerebral palsy in very low birth weight infants. J Pediatr 128:407, 1996.

Groome LJ, Goldenberg RL, Cliver SP, et al: Neonatal periventricular-intraventricular hemorrhage after maternal beta-sympathomimetic tocolysis. Am J Obstet Gynecol 167:873, 1992.

Guzetta F, Shackelford GD, Volpe S, et al: Periventricular intraparenchymal echodensities in the premature newborn: Critical determinant of neurologic outcome. Pediatrics 78:995, 1986.

Hack M, Breslau N, Fanaroff A: Differential effects of intrauterine and post-natal brain growth failure in infants of very low birth weight. Am J Dis Child 143:63, 1989.

Hack M, Friedman H, Fanaroff AA: Outcomes of extremely low birth weight infants. Pediatrics 98:931, 1996.

Hagberg B, Hagberg G: Prenatal and perinatal risk factors in a survey of 681 Swedish cases. In Stanley F, Alberman E (eds): The Epidemiology of the Cerebral Palsies. Oxford, Blackwell Scientific Publications, 1984, p. 116.

Hagberg B, Hagberg G, Beckung E, et al: Changing panorama of cerebral palsy in Sweden. VIII. Prevalence and origin in the birth year period 1991-94. Acta Paediatr 90:271, 2001.

Hagberg B, Hagberg G, Olow I, et al: The changing panorama of cerebral palsy in Sweden: V. The birth year period 1979–82. Acta Paediatr Scand 78:283, 1989.

Halpern J-P, Boyages SC, Maberly GF, et al: The neurology of endemic cretinism: A study of two endemias. Brain 114:825, 1991.

Hansen AR, Collins MH, Genest D, et al: Very low birthweight infant's placenta and its relation to pregnancy and fetal characteristics. Pediatr Dev Path 3(5):519, 2000.

Hoon AH, Reinhardt EM, Kelley RI, et al: Brain magnetic resonance imaging in suspected extrapyramidal cerebral palsy: Observations in distinguishing genetic-metabolic from acquired cases. J Pediatr 131:240, 1997.

Ingram TTS: A historical review of the definition and classification of the cerebral palsies. In Stanley F, Alberman E (eds): The Epidemiology of the Cerebral Palsies. Oxford, Blackwell Scientific Publications, 1984, p. 1.

Jarvis S, Hey E: Measuring disability and handicap due to cerebral palsy. In Stanley F, Alberman E (eds): The Epidemiology of the Cerebral Palsies. Oxford, Blackwell Scientific Publications, 1984, p. 35.

Johnston MV, Trescher WH, Taylor GA: Hypoxic and ischemic central nervous system disorders in infants and children. Adv Pediatr 42:1, 1995.

Kari MA, Hallman M, Eronen M, et al: Prenatal dexamethasone treatment in conjunction with rescue therapy of human surfactant: A randomized placebo-controlled multicenter study. Pediatrics 93:730, 1994.

Kashlan F, Smulian J, Vintzileos A, et al: Umbilical vein interleukin-6 (IL-6) levels and intracranial events in very low birth weight infants. Pediatr Res 41:158a, 1997.

Kass EH, Schlievert PM, Parsonnet J, et al: Effect of magnesium on production of toxic-shock-syndrome toxin-1: A collaborative study. J Infect Dis 158:44, 1988.

Kitchen WA, Doyle LW, Fox GW, et al: Cerebral palsy in very low birthweight infants surviving to 2 years with modern perinatal intensive care. Am J Perinatol 4:29, 1987.

Kitchen WH, Ford GW, Doyle LW, et al: Cesarean section or vaginal delivery at 24 to 28 weeks' gestation. Comparison of survival and neonatal and two-year morbidity. Obstet Gynecol 66:149, 1985.

Koivisto M, Blanco-Sigueros M, Krause O: Neonatal symptomatic and asymptomatic hypoglycemia. A follow-up study. Dev Med Child Neurol 14:603, 1972.

Kraus FT: Cerebral palsy and thrombi in placental vessels of the fetus: Insights from litigation. Human Pathol 28(2):246, 1997.

Krebs L, Topp M, Langhoff-Roos J: The relation of breech presentation at term to cerebral palsy. Br J Obstet Gynaecol 106(9):943, 1999.

Kuban K, Sanocka U, Leviton A, et al: White matter disorders of prematurity: association with intraventricular hemorrhage and ventriculomegaly. The Developmental Epidemiology Network. J Pediatr 134(5):539, 1999.

Kuban KCK, Leviton A: Cerebral palsy. N Engl J Med 330:188, 1994.

Leviton A: Preterm birth and cerebral palsy: Is tumor necrosis factor the missing link? Dev Med Child Neurol 35:549, 1993.

Leviton A, Paneth N: White matter damage in preterm newborns—An epidemiologic perspective. Early Hum Dev 24:1, 1990.

Leviton A, Paneth N, Reuss ML, et al: Maternal infection, fetal inflammatory response, and brain damage in very low birth weight infants. Pediatric Res 46(5):566, 1999.

Liggins GC, Howie RN: A controlled trial of antepartum glucocorticoid treatment for prevention of the respiratory distress syndrome in premature infants. Pediatrics 50:515, 1972.

Lipton SA, Rosenberg PA: Excitatory amino acids as a final common pathway for neurologic disorders. N Engl J Med 330(9):613, 1994.

Little WJ: On the influence of abnormal parturition, difficult labors, premature birth, and asphyxia neonatorum, on the mental and physical condition of the child, especially in relation to deformities. Trans Obstet Soc London 3:293, 1861–1862.

Low J, Galbraith R, Muir D, et al: Intrauterine growth retardation: A study of long-term morbidity. Am J Obstet Gynecol 142:670, 1982.

MacDonald D: Cerebral palsy and intrapartum fetal monitoring. N Engl J Med 334:659, 1996.

MacDonald D, Grant A, Sheridan-Pereira M, et al: The Dublin randomized controlled trial of intrapartum fetal heart rate monitoring. Am J Obstet Gynecol 152:524, 1985.

MacLennan A, for the International Cerebral Palsy Task Force: A template for defining a causal relation between acute intrapartum events and cerebral palsy: International consensus statement. BMJ 319(16):1054, 1999.

Marcus JC: Neurological findings in the fetal alcohol syndrome. Neuropediatrics 18:158, 1987.

Matsuda Y, Kuono S, Hiroyama Y, et al: Intrauterine infection, magnesium sulfate exposure and cerebral palsy in infants born between 26 and 30 weeks of gestation. Eur J Obstet Gynecol Reprod Biol 91(2):159, 2000.

Mays J, Verma U, Klein S, et al: Acute appendicitis in pregnancy and the occurrence of major intraventricular hemorrhage and periventricular leukomalacia. Obstet Gynecol 86:650, 1995.

McCarrison R: Observations on endemic cretinism in the Chitral and Gilgit valleys. Lancet 2:1275, 1988.

McDonald JW, Silverstein FS, Johnston MV: Magnesium reduces N-methyl-D-aspartate (NMDA)-mediated brain injury in perinatal rats. Neurosci Lett 109:234, 1990.

Melnick M: Brain damage in survivor after in utero death in monozygous cotwin. Lancet ii:1287, 1977.

Murakami U: Organic mercury problems affecting intrauterine life. In Klingberg MA, Abromovic A, Clark J (eds): Drugs and Fetal Development: Proceedings of an International Symposium on the Effects of Prolonged Drug Usage on Fetal Development. New York, Plenum Press, 1972.

Murphy DJ, Sellers S, MacKenzie IZ, et al: Case-control study of antenatal and intrapartum risk factors for cerebral palsy in very preterm singleton babies. Lancet **346**:1449, 1995.

Nelson KB: Epidemiology of cerebral palsy. In Levene MI, Lilford RJ, Bennett MJ, Punt J (eds): Fetal and Neonatal Neurology and Neurosurgery. New York, Churchill Livingstone, 1995, p. 681.

Nelson KB: Magnesium sulfate and risk of cerebral palsy in very low-birth-weight infants. JAMA **278**(22):1843, 1996.

Nelson KB, Dambrosia JM, Ting TY, et al: Uncertain value of electronic fetal monitoring in predicting cerebral palsy. N Engl J Med **334**:613, 1996.

Nelson KB, Ellenberg JH: Epidemiology of cerebral palsy. Adv Neurol **19**:421, 1978.

Nelson KB, Ellenberg JH: Children who outgrow cerebral palsy. Pediatrics **69**:529, 1982.

Nelson KB, Ellenberg JH: Obstetric complications as risk factors for cerebral palsy or seizure disorders. JAMA **251**:1843, 1984.

Nelson KB, Ellenberg JH: Antecedents of cerebral palsy: Multivariate analysis of risk. N Engl J Med **315**:81, 1986.

Nelson KB, Ellenberg JH: Intrapartum events and cerebral palsy. In Kubli F, Patel N, Schmidt W, Linderkamp O (eds): Perinatal Events and Brain Damage in Surviving Children. Berlin, Springer-Verlag, 1988, p. 139.

Nelson KB, Grether JK: Can magnesium sulfate reduce the risk of cerebral palsy in very low birth weight infants? Pediatrics **95**:263, 1995.

Nelson KB, Grether JK: Potentially asphyxiating conditions and spastic cerebral palsy in infants of normal birth weight. Am J Obstet Gynecol **179**(2):507, 1998.

Nelson KB, Grether JK: Causes of cerebral palsy. Curr Opin Pediatr **11**(6):487, 1999.

NIH Consensus Development Panel. Antenatal corticosteroids revisited: Repeat courses—National Institutes of Health Consensus Development Conference Statement, August 17–18, 2000. Obstet Gynecol **98**(1):144, 2001.

NIH Consensus Development Panel on the Effect of Corticosteroids for Fetal Maturation on Perinatal Outcomes: Effect of corticosteroids for fetal maturation on perinatal outcomes. JAMA **273**:413, 1995.

Niswander K, Henson G, Elbourne D, et al: Adverse outcome of pregnancy and the quality of obstetric care. Lancet **2**:827, 1984.

O'Shea TM, Dammann O: Antecedents of cerebral palsy in very low birth-weight infants. Clin Perinatol **27**(2):285, 2000.

O'Shea TM, Kothadia JM, Klinepeter KL, et al: Randomized placebo-controlled trial of a 42-day tapering course of dexamethasone to reduce the duration of ventilator dependency in very low birth weight infants: Outcome of study participants at 1-year adjusted age. Pediatrics **104**:15–21, 1999.

Ozmen M, Caliskan M, Apak S, et al: 8-year clinical experience in cerebral palsy. J Trop Pediatr **39**:52, 1993.

Palmer L, Blair E, Petterson B, et al: Antenatal antecedent of moderate and severe cerebral palsy. Paediatr Perinat Epidemiol **9**:171, 1995.

Paneth N: Neonatal care and patterns of handicap in the community. Clin Dev Med **123/124**:232, 1992.

Paneth N: The causes of cerebral palsy: Recent evidence. Clin Invest Med **16**(2):95, 1993.

Paneth N, Kiely J: The frequency of cerebral palsy: A review of population studies in industrialised nations since 1950. In Stanley F, Alberman E (eds): The Epidemiology of the Cerebral Palsies. Oxford, Blackwell Scientific Publications, 1984, p. 46.

Paneth N, Rudelli R, Monte W, et al: White matter necrosis in very low birth weight infants: Neuropathologic and ultrasonic findings surviving six days or longer. J Pediatr **116**:975, 1990.

Papile L-A, Munsick-Bruno G, Schaefer A: Relationship of cerebral intraventricular hemorrhage and early childhood neurologic handicaps. J Pediatr **103**:273, 1983.

Perlman JM, Risser R, Broyles RS: Bilateral cystic periventricular leukomalacia in the premature infant: Associated risk factors. Pediatrics **97**(6):822, 1996.

Petterson B, Nelson KB, Watson L, et al: Twins, triplets, and cerebral palsy in births in Western Australia in the 1980s. BMJ **307**:1239, 1993.

Pharoah POD, Buttfield IH, Hetzel BS: Neurological damage to the fetus resulting from severe iodine deficiency during pregnancy. Lancet **i**:308, 1971.

Pharoah POD, Cooke T, Cooke RWI, et al: Birthweight specific trends in cerebral palsy. Arch Dis Child **65**:602, 1990.

Philip AGS, Allan WC, Tito AM, et al: Intraventricular hemorrhage in preterm infants: Declining incidence in the 1980s. Pediatrics **84**:797, 1989.

Pidcock FS, Graziani LJ, Stanley C, et al: Neurosonographic features of periventricular echodensities associated with cerebral palsy in preterm infants. J Pediatr **116**:417, 1990.

Pinto-Martin JA, Riolo S, Cnaan A, et al: Cranial ultrasound prediction of disabling and nondisabling cerebral palsy at age two in a low birth weight population. Pediatrics **95**:249, 1995.

Redline RW, O'Riordan MA: Placental lesions associated with cerebral palsy and neurologic impairment following term birth. Arch Pathol Lab Med **124**(12):1785, 2000.

Richmond S, Niswander K, Snodgrass CA, et al: The obstetric management of fetal distress and its association with cerebral palsy. Obstet Gynecol **83**:643, 1994.

Riikonen R, Raumavirta S, Sinivuori E, et al: Changing pattern of cerebral palsy in the southwest region of Finland. Acta Paediatr Scand **78**:581, 1989.

Robertson X, Etches P, Kyle J: Eight-year school performance and growth of preterm, small-for-gestational-age infants: A comparative study with subjects matched for birth weight or for gestational age. J Pediatr **116**:19, 1990.

Roth SC, Baudin J, McCormick DC, et al: Relation between ultrasound appearance of the brain of very preterm infants and neurodevelopmental impairment at eight years. Dev Med Child Neurol **35**:755, 1993.

Salafia CM, Minior VK, Rosenkrantz TS, et al: Maternal, placental, and neonatal associations with early germinal matrix/intraventricular hemorrhage in infants born before 23 weeks' gestation. Am J Perinatol **12**:429, 1995.

Scheller JM, Nelson KB: Twinning and neurologic morbidity. Am J Dis Child **146**:1110, 1992.

Schendel DE, Berg CJ, Yeargin-Allsopp M, et al: Prenatal magnesium sulfate exposure and the risk for cerebral palsy or mental retardation among very low-birth-weight children aged 3 to 5 years. JAMA **276**(22):1805, 1996.

Selmaj K, Raine CS, Path FRC, et al: Tumor necrosis factor mediates myelin and oligodendrocyte damage in vitro. Ann Neurol **23**:339, 1988.

Shankaran S, Bauer CR, Bain R, et al: Prenatal and perinatal risk and protective factors for neonatal intracranial hemorrhage. Arch Pediatr Adolesc Med **150**:491, 1996.

Shinwell ES, Karplus M, Reich D, et al: Early postnatal dexamethasone treatment and increased incidence of cerebral palsy. Arch Dis Child Fetal Neonat Ed **83**:F177, 2000.

Shy KK, Luthy DA, Bennett FC, et al: Effects of electronic fetal-heart-rate monitoring, as compared with periodic auscultation, on the neurologic development of premature infants. N Engl J Med **322**:588, 1990.

Sims ME: Brain injury and intrauterine death. Am J Obstet Gynecol **151**:721, 1985.

Stanley F: Social and biological determinants of the cerebral palsies. In Stanley F, Alberman E (eds): Clinics in Developmental Medicine No. 87: The Epidemiology of the Cerebral Palsies. Lavenham, England, Lavenham Press, 1984, p. 69.

Stanley FJ, Blair E, Hockey A, et al: Spastic quadriplegia in Western Australia: A genetic epidemiological study: I. Case population and perinatal risk factors. Dev Med Child Neurol **35**:191, 1993.

Stanley FJ, Watson L: Trends in perinatal mortality and cerebral palsy in Western Australia, 1967–1985. BMJ **304**:1658, 1992.

Stoll BJ, Gordon T, Korones SB, et al: Early-onset sepsis in very low birth weight neonates: A report from the National Institute of Child Health and Human Development Neonatal Research Network. J Pediatr **129**:72, 1995.

Stoll BJ, Gordon T, Korones SB, et al: Late-onset sepsis in very low birth weight neonates: A report from the National Institute of Child Health and Human Development Neonatal Research Network. J Pediatr **129**:63, 1996.

Strand C, Laptook AR, Dowling S, et al: Neonatal intracranial hemorrhage: I. Changing pattern in inborn low-birth-weight infants. Early Hum Dev **23**:117, 1990.

Susser M, Stein Z: Prenatal nutrition and subsequent development. In Reed DM, Stanley FJ (eds): The Epidemiology of Prematurity. Baltimore, Urban and Schwarzenberg, 1977, p. 177.

Susser M, Stein Z: Definitions, risks and indices. In Kubli F, Patel N, Schmidt W, et al (eds): Perinatal Events and Brain Damage in Surviving Children. Berlin, Springer-Verlag, 1988, p. 3.

Takeshita K, Anmdo Y, Ohtani K, et al: Cerebral palsy in Tottori, Japan. Neuroepidemiology **8**:184, 1989.

Torfs CP, van den Berg BJ, Oeschsli FW, et al: Prenatal and perinatal factors in the etiology of cerebral palsy. J Pediatr **116**:615, 1990.

Truwit CL, Barkovich AJ, Koch TK, et al: Cerebral palsy: MR findings in 40 patients. Am J Neuroradiol **13**:67, 1992.

Uvebrant P, Hagberg G: Intrauterine growth in children with cerebral palsy. Acta Paediatr **81**:407, 1992.

Veelken N, Stollhoff K, Claussen M: Development and perinatal risk factors of very low-birth-weight infants: Small versus appropriate for gestational age. Neuropediatrics **23**:102, 1992.

Weglicki WB, Phillips TM, Freedman AM, et al: Magnesium-deficiency elevates circulating levels of inflammatory cytokines and endothelin. Molec Cell Biochem **110**:169, 1992.

Wilson-Costello D, Borawski E, Friedman H, et al: Perinatal correlates of cerebral palsy and other neurologic impairment among very low birth weight children. Pediatrics **102**(2):315, 1998.

Winkler CL, Hauth JC, Tucker JM, et al: Neonatal complications at term as related to the degree of umbilical artery acidemia. Am J Obstet Gynecol **164**:637, 1991.

Wood NS, Marlow N, Costeloe K, et al: Neurologic and developmental disability after extremely preterm birth. EPICure Study Group. N Engl J Med **343**(6):378, 2000.

Wu YW, Colford JM Jr: Chorioamnionitis as a risk factor for cerebral palsy: A meta-analysis. JAMA **294**(11):1417, 2000.

Yeh TF, Lin YJ, Huang CC, et al: Early dexamethasone therapy in premature infants: A follow-up study. Pediatrics **101**:e7, 1998.

Yin R, Reddihough D, Ditchfield M, et al: Magnetic resonance imaging findings in cerebral palsy. J Paediatr Child Health **36**(2):139, 2000.

Yoon BH, Jun JK, Romero R, et al: Amniotic fluid inflammatory cytokines (interleukin-6, interleukin-1β, and tumor necrosis factor-alpha), neonatal brain white matter lesions, and cerebral palsy. Am J Obstet Gynecol **177**:19, 1997.

Yoon BH, Romero R, Kim CJ, et al: High expression of interleukin-6, interleukin-1β, and tumor necrosis factor-α in periventricular leukomalacia. Am J Obstet Gynecol **174**(319):399, 1996.

Yoon BH, Romero R, Park JS, et al: Fetal exposure to an intra-amniotic inflammation and the development of cerebral palsy at the age of three years. Am J Obstet Gynecol **182**(3):675, 2000.

Yoon BH, Romero R, Yang SH, et al: Interleukin-6 concentrations in umbilical cord plasma are elevated in neonates with periventricular white matter lesions associated with periventricular leukomalacia. Am J Obstet Gynecol **174**:1433, 1996.

Zupan V, Gonzalez P, Lacaze-Masmonteil T, et al: Periventricular leukomalacia: Risk factors revisited. Dev Med Child Neurol **38**:1061, 1996.

INDEX

Note: Page numbers followed by f refer to figures; page numbers followed by t refer to tables.

A

Abdomen, fetal
    maternal diabetes mellitus and, 1053
    measurement of, 325, 325f
Abdominal wall, defects of, 1297
Abortion
    septic, acute renal failure and, 918
    spontaneous. *See also* Recurrent pregnancy
        loss.
        after amniocentesis, 262–263, 270–271
        after chorionic villus sampling, 267–268,
            267t, 271, 271t
        alcohol use and, 293
        blocking antibodies and, 102
        caffeine and, 297
        chromosome abnormalities and, 22, 22t
        definition of, 623
        diabetes mellitus and, 1033
        hypothyroidism and, 1069
        in antiphospholipid syndrome, 584, 589,
            593, 1013, 1013t
        in Cushing syndrome, 1091
        in Sjögren syndrome, 1160
        in systemic lupus erythematosus, 1156
        mycoplasmal infection, 783
        nausea and vomiting and, 1114
        nicotine and, 296
        radioiodine therapy and, 1069
        reciprocal chromosomal translocations and,
            18
        thyroiditis after, 1078
    therapeutic
        cervical incompetence and, 608–609
        in breast cancer, 1234–1235
Abruptio placentae, 713–720
    abdominal pain in, 715
    cigarette smoking and, 714
    cocaine abuse and, 301, 715
    complications of, 717–720
    definition of, 713
    delivery in, 716–717
    diagnosis of, 715–716
    disseminated intravascular coagulation with,
        717–720, 718f, 719t
    etiology of, 713–715
    fetal complications of, 720
    hemorrhagic shock with, 717
    incidence of, 713
    intrauterine growth restriction and, 720
    management of, 716–717
    maternal age and, 714–715
    maternal hyperhomocystinemia and, 715
    maternal hypertension and, 714
    neonatal anemia and, 1288
    nicotine and, 296
    pathophysiology of, 713
    perinatal mortality and, 715
    premature rupture of membranes and, 715
    recurrence of, 715
    transfusion in, 717
    trauma and, 713–714, 714f

Abruptio placentae *(Continued)*
    ultrasonography in, 715–716
    umbilical cord anomaly and, 714
    uterine contractions in, 715, 716f
Abscess
    breast, 751, 751f
    pelvic, 697
    retropsoas, 697
Acarbose, in diabetes mellitus, 1052
Acardia, in twinning, 63–64, 64f, 65f, 527–528
Acetaminophen
    in migraine, 1170
    in rheumatoid arthritis, 1149–1150
    in systemic lupus erythematosus, 1158, 1159
Acetylcholinesterase, amniotic fluid, in neural
        tube defect screening, 246
Achondrogenesis, nonimmune hydrops with, 571
Achondroplasia, prenatal diagnosis of, 345
Achondroplastic dwarfism, anesthesia in,
        1257–1258
Acid indigestion, 162
Acid-base balance
    fetal, 429–438, 430f
        buffers in, 429–430
        carbonic acid in, 429
        continuous tissue measurement for, 437
        intrapartum monitoring of, 431–433, 431t,
            437
        metabolic factors in, 431
        monitoring of, 431–433, 431t, 432f
        noncarbonic acids in, 429
        pH determination in, 430
        physiology of, 429–431
        pulse oximetry for, 437
        respiratory factors in, 431
        scalp blood sampling for, 431t, 432–433, 432f
        terminology of, 430, 430t
        umbilical blood sampling for, 437. *See also*
            Cordocentesis.
    maternal, disturbances in, 207, 431
    newborn, umbilical cord blood analysis for,
        433–437, 434t, 435t, 436t. *See also*
        Umbilical cord, blood pH of.
Acidemia
    fetal, 405–406, 434–435, 435t
        delivery methods and, 436, 436t
        fetal heart rate and, 436, 436t
        infection and, 435, 436t
    newborn
        definition of, 430, 430f, 430t
        nuchal cord and, 435–436
        thickened meconium and, 436
Acidosis. *See also* Acid-base balance.
    definition of, 430, 430t
    fetal, meconium-stained fluid and, 444
    lactic
        in preeclampsia, 874
        in septic shock, 939
        with antiretroviral therapy, 810
    metabolic
        fetal, 431

Acidosis *(Continued)*
    maternal, 431
    neonatal, 1272
    respiratory
        fetal, 207, 431
        maternal, 431
        neonatal, 1272
Aciduria, amino, in pregnancy, 117
Acne vulgaris, 1208–1209
Acoustic neuroma, 1170
Acquired immunodeficiency syndrome (AIDS).
        See Human immunodeficiency virus (HIV).
Acrochordons, 1202
Acromegaly, 1089–1090
Actin, in uterine contraction, 72–73, 72f, 73f
Activin, 129
Acute leukemia, 989
Acute phase proteins, in innate immunity, 90
Acyclovir
    fetal effects of, 283
    in herpes simplex virus infection, 767
    in varicella pneumonia
Addison disease, 1095–1096, 1096t
Adenoma
    pituitary, 1170, 1171f. *See also* Prolactinoma.
    thyroid, 1073
Adenosine, in fetal arrhythmias, 477t
Adenovirus infection
    breast-feeding and, 149t
    nonimmune hydrops and, 571
Adolescent pregnancy, nutrition in, 161
Adrenal glands
    fetal, 176, 404, 1095
        congenital hyperplasia of, 1097–1098, 1098f
        heart rate and, 404
        in parturition, 81–82, 81f
    maternal, 1094–1099, 1094f
        disorders of, 1095–1099, 1096t. *See also*
            specific disorders.
        in preeclampsia, 870
        physiology of, 1094–1095, 1094f
Adrenal insufficiency
    maternal, 1095–1096, 1096t
    neonatal, 1091
β-Adrenergic agonists
    in maternal asthma, 965
    tocolytic, 649–651
        cardiovascular effects of, 649t, 650
        clinical efficacy of, 649
        dosage for, 650–651
        fetal effects of, 650
        hemodynamic monitoring in, 931, 931t
        maternal effects of, 649–650, 649t
        metabolic effects of, 649t, 650
        neonatal effects of, 650
        pharmacology of, 649
β-Adrenergic antagonists, 818, 819t
    adverse effects of, 819t
    in hypertension, 891, 891t
    in hyperthyroidism, 1071
Adrenergic receptors, fetal, 174, 175–176

1325